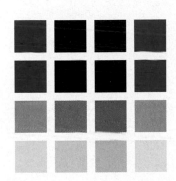

Creasy and Resnik's Maternal-Fetal Medicine

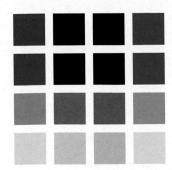

Creasy and Resnik's Maternal-Fetal Medicine: Principles and Practice

An Expert Consult Title: *Online + Print*

Sixth Edition

Editors

Robert K. Creasy, MD
Professor Emeritus
Department of Obstetrics, Gynecology, and Reproductive Sciences
University of Texas School of Medicine at Houston
Houston, Texas
Corte Madera, California

Robert Resnik, MD
Professor Emeritus
Department of Reproductive Medicine
University of California, San Diego, School of Medicine
San Diego, California

Jay D. Iams, MD
Frederick P. Zuspan Professor and Endowed Chair
Division of Maternal-Fetal Medicine
Vice Chair, Department of Obstetrics and Gynecology
The Ohio State University College of Medicine
Columbus, Ohio

Associate Editors

Charles J. Lockwood, MD
Anita O'Keefe Young Professor and Chair
Department of Obstetrics, Gynecology, and Reproductive Sciences
Yale University School of Medicine
New Haven, Connecticut

Thomas R. Moore, MD
Professor and Chairman
Department of Reproductive Medicine
University of California, San Diego, School of Medicine
San Diego, California

SAUNDERS
ELSEVIER

SAUNDERS
ELSEVIER

1600 John F. Kennedy Blvd.
Ste 1800
Philadelphia, PA 19103-2899

CREASY AND RESNIK'S MATERNAL-FETAL MEDICINE: PRINCIPLES AND PRACTICE, SIXTH EDITION ISBN: 978-1-4160-4224-2

Notice

Knowledge and best practice in this field are constantly changing. As new research and experience broaden our knowledge, changes in practice, treatment, and drug therapy may become necessary or appropriate. Readers are advised to check the most current information provided (i) on procedures featured or (ii) by the manufacturer of each product to be administered, to verify the recommended dose or formula, the method and duration of administration, and contraindications. It is the responsibility of the practitioner, relying on their own experience and knowledge of the patient, to make diagnoses, to determine dosages and the best treatment for each individual patient, and to take all appropriate safety precautions. To the fullest extent of the law, neither the Publisher nor the Editors assumes any liability for any injury and/or damage to persons or property arising out of or related to any use of the material contained in this book.

The Publisher

Library of Congress Cataloging-in-Publication Data

Creasy & Resnik's maternal-fetal medicine : principles and practice / editors, Robert K. Creasy, Robert Resnik, Jay D. Iams ; associate editors, Thomas R. Moore, Charles J. Lockwood.—6th ed.

p. ; cm.

Rev. ed. of: Maternal-fetal medicine. 5th ed. c2004.

Includes bibliographical references and index.

ISBN 978-1-4160-4224-2

1. Obstetrics. 2. Perinatology. I. Creasy, Robert K. II. Maternal-fetal medicine. III. Title: Creasy and Resnik's maternal-fetal medicine. IV. Title: Maternal-fetal medicine.

[DNLM: 1. Fetal Diseases. 2. Pregnancy—physiology. 3. Pregnancy Complications. 4. Prenatal Diagnosis. WQ 211 C912 2009]

RG526.M34 2009
618.2—dc22

2007051347

Acquisitions Editor: Rebecca Schmidt Gaertner
Developmental Editor: Kristina Oberle
Publishing Services Manager: Frank Polizzano
Project Manager: Rachel Miller
Design Direction: Lou Forgione

Printed in China

Last digit is the print number: 9 8 7 6 5 4 3 2 1

For

Judy, Lauren, Pat, Nancy, and Peggy

With love and gratitude—for everything

CONTRIBUTORS

Vikki M. Abrahams, PhD
Assistant Professor, Department of Obstetrics, Gynecology, and Reproductive Sciences, Yale University School of Medicine, New Haven, Connecticut
- The Immunology of Pregnancy

Michael J. Aminoff, MD, DSc, FRCP
Professor of Neurology, University of California, San Francisco, School of Medicine, Attending Physician, University of California Medical Center, San Francisco, California
- Neurologic Disorders

Marie H. Beall, MD
Professor of Obstetrics and Gynecology, Geffen School of Medicine at the University of California, Los Angeles; Vice Chair, Department of Obstetrics and Gynecology, Harbor–University of California, Los Angeles, Medical Center, Torrance, California
- Amniotic Fluid Dynamics

Kurt Benirschke, MD
Professor Emeritus, Reproductive Medicine and Pathology, University of California, San Diego, California
- Normal Early Development
- Multiple Gestation: The Biology of Twinning

Daniel G. Blanchard, MD, FACC
Professor of Medicine, Director, Cardiology Fellowship Program, University of California, San Diego, School of Medicine, La Jolla, California; Chief of Clinical Cardiology, Thornton Hospital, University of California, San Diego, Medical Center, San Diego, California
- Cardiac Diseases

Kristie Blum, MD
Assistant Professor of Medicine, Division of Hematology/Oncology, The Arthur G. James Cancer Hospital, The Ohio State University, Columbus, Ohio
- Malignancy and Pregnancy

Patrick Catalano, MD
Professor, Reproductive Biology, Case Western Reserve University; Chairman, Obstetrics and Gynecology, MetroHealth Medical Center, Cleveland, Ohio
- Diabetes in Pregnancy

Christina Chambers, PhD, MPH
Associate Professor, Departments of Pediatrics and Family and Preventive Medicine, University of California, San Diego, School of Medicine, La Jolla, California
- Teratogenesis and Environmental Exposure

Ronald Clyman, MD
Professor of Pediatrics, Investigator, Cardiovascular Research Institute, University of California, San Francisco
- Fetal Cardiovascular Physiology

David Cohn, MD
Donald and Patsy Jones Professor of Obstetrics and Gynecology, Division of Gynecologic Oncology, Arthur G. James Cancer Hospital and Richard J. Solove Research Institute, The Ohio State University College of Medicine, Columbus, Ohio
- Malignancy and Pregnancy

Robert K. Creasy, MD
Professor Emeritus, Department of Obstetrics, Gynecology, and Reproductive Sciences, University of Texas School of Medicine at Houston, Houston, Texas; Corte Madera, California
- Preterm Labor and Birth
- Intrauterine Growth Restriction

Mary E. D'Alton, MD, FACOG
Professor and Chair, Department of Obstetrics and Gynecology, Columbia University College of Physicians and Surgeons, New York, New York; Chair, Department of Obstetrics and Gynecology, Columbia University Medical Center, New York, New York
- Multiple Gestation: Clinical Characteristics and Management

John M. Davison, MD, FRCOG
Emeritus Professor of Obstetric Medicine, Institute of Cellular Medicine Medical School, Newcastle University; Consultant Obstetrician, Directorate of Women's Services, Royal Victoria Infirmary Newcastle upon Tyne, United Kingdom
- Renal Disorders

Jan A. Deprest, MD, PhD
Professor of Obstetrics and Gynecology, Division of Woman and Child, University Hospitals, Katholieke Universiteit Leuven, Leuven, Belgium
- Invasive Fetal Therapy

Mitchell P. Dombrowski, MD
Professor, Wayne State University, School of Medicine; Chief, Department of Obstetrics and Gynecology, St. John Hospital and Medical Center, Detroit, Michigan
- Respiratory Diseases in Pregnancy

Edward F. Donovan, MD
Emeritus, Professor of Pediatrics, University of Cincinnati College of Medicine; Medical Director, Child Policy Research Center, Cincinnati Children's Hospital Research Foundation, Cincinnati, Ohio
- Neonatal Morbidities of Prenatal and Perinatal Origin

Patrick Duff, MD
Professor and Residency Program Director, Associate Dean for Student Affairs, University of Florida College of Medicine, Gainesville, Florida
- Maternal and Fetal Infections

Rodney K. Edwards, MD, MS
Clinician, Phoenix Perinatal Associates, Scottsdale, Arizona
- Maternal and Fetal Infections

Doruk Erkan, MD
Assistant Professor of Medicine, Wall Medical College of Cornell University; Assistant Attending Physician, Hospital for Special Surgery, New York Presbyterian Hospital, New York, New York
- Pregnancy and Rheumatic Diseases

Jeffrey R. Fineman, MD
Professor of Pediatrics, Investigator, Cardiovascular Research Institute, University of California, San Francisco
- Fetal Cardiovascular Physiology

Michael Raymond Foley, MD
Clinical Professor, University of Arizona Medical School, Department of Obstetrics and Gynecology, Tucson, Arizona; Chief Academic Officer, Designated Institutional Officer, Scottsdale Healthcare System, Scottsdale, Arizona
- Intensive Care Monitoring of the Critically Ill Pregnant Patient

Edmund F. Funai, MD
Associate Professor of Obstetrics, Gynecology, and Reproductive Sciences, Yale University School of Medicine; Chief of Obstetrics, Yale–New Haven Hospital; Associate Chair for Clinical Affairs, Department of Obstetrics, Gynecology, and Reproductive Sciences, Yale University School of Medicine, New Haven, Connecticut
- Pregnancy-Related Hypertension

Robert Gagnon, MD, FRCSC
Professor, Departments of Obstetrics and Gynecology, and Physiology/Pharmacology and Pediatrics, University of Western Ontario, Schulich School of Medicine and Dentistry, London, Ontario, Canada
- Behavioral State Activity and Fetal Health and Development

Alessandro Ghidini, MD
Professor, Department of Obstetrics and Gynecology, Georgetown University Medical Center, Washington, D.C.; Executive Medical Director, Perinatal Diagnostic Center, Inova Alexandria Hospital, Alexandria, Virginia
- Benign Gynecologic Conditions in Pregnancy

Larry C. Gilstrap III, MD
Chair Emeritus, Department of Obstetrics and Gynecology and Reproductive Sciences, University of Texas at Houston Health Science Center, Houston, Texas; Clinical Professor, Obstetrics and Gynecology, University of Texas Southwestern Medical Center at Dallas, Dallas, Texas; Director of Evaluation, American Board of Obstetrics and Gynecology, Dallas, Texas
- Intrapartum Fetal Surveillance

Eduardo Gratacos, MD, PhD
Professor of Obstetrics; Chair, Department of Obstetrics, Hospital Clinic Barcelona, Barcelona, Spain
- Invasive Fetal Therapy

James M. Greenberg, MD
Associate Professor of Pediatrics, University of Cincinnati College of Medicine; Director, Division of Neonatology, Cincinnati Children's Hospital Research Foundation, Cincinnati, Ohio
- Neonatal Morbidities of Prenatal and Perinatal Origin

Beth Haberman, MD
Assistant Professor of Pediatrics, University of Cincinnati College of Medicine; Medical Director, Regional Center for Newborn Intensive Care, Cincinnati Children's Hospital Medical Center, Cincinnati, Ohio
- Neonatal Morbidities of Prenatal and Perinatal Origin

Bruce A. Hamilton, PhD
Associate Professor, Division of Genetics, Department of Medicine, University of California, San Diego, La Jolla, California
- Basic Genetics and Patterns of Inheritance

Mark Hanson, DPhil
Director, Developmental Origins of Health and Disease Division; British Heart Foundation Professor of Cardiovascular Science, University of Southampton, Southampton, United Kingdom
- Developmental Origins of Health and Disease

Christopher R. Harman, MD
Professor and Vice Chair, Department of Obstetrics, Gynecology, and Reproductive Sciences; Director, Center for Advanced Fetal Care, University of Maryland School of Medicine, Baltimore, Maryland
- Assessment of Fetal Health

Nazli Hossain, MBBS, FCPS
Associate Professor, Dow University of Health Sciences, Karachi, Pakistan
- Embryonic and Fetal Demise

Andrew D. Hull, MD, FRCOG, FACOG
Associate Professor of Clinical Reproductive Medicine; Director, Maternal-Fetal Medicine Fellowship, University of California, San Diego, La Jolla, California; Director, Fetal Care and Genetics Center, University of California, San Diego, Medical Center, San Diego, California
- Placenta Previa, Placenta Accreta, Abruptio Placentae, and Vasa Previa

Jay D. Iams, MD
Frederick P. Zuspan Endowed Chair, Division of Maternal-Fetal Medicine; Vice Chair, Department of Obstetrics and Gynecology, The Ohio State University College of Medicine, Columbus, Ohio
- Preterm Labor and Birth
- Cervical Insufficiency

Thomas M. Jenkins, MD
Director of Prenatal Diagnosis, Legacy Center for Maternal-Fetal Medicine, Legacy Health System, Portland, Oregon
- Prenatal Diagnosis of Congenital Disorders

Alan H. Jobe, MD, PhD
Professor of Pediatrics, University of Cincinnati School of Medicine; Director, Perinatal Biology, Cincinnati Children's Hospital, Cincinnati, Ohio
- **Fetal Lung Development and Surfactant**

Thomas F. Kelly, MD
Clinical Professor of Reproductive Medicine, Chief, Division of Perinatal Medicine, University of California, San Diego, School of Medicine, La Jolla, California; Director of Maternity Services, University of California, San Diego, Medical Center, San Diego, California
- **Gastrointestinal Disease in Pregnancy**

Nahla Khalek, MD
Assistant Clinical Professor, Department of Obstetrics and Gynecology, Divisions of Maternal-Fetal Medicine and Reproductive Genetics, Columbia University Medical Center; Assistant Clinical Professor, New York Presbyterian Hospital, Sloane Hospital for Women, New York, New York
- **Prenatal Diagnosis of Congenital Disorders**

Sarah J. Kilpatrick, MD, PhD
Professor, Head of the Department of Obstetrics and Gynecology, University of Illinois at Chicago; Vice Dean, University of Illinois College of Medicine, Chicago, Illinois
- **Anemia and Pregnancy**

Krzysztof M. Kuczkowski, MD
Associate Professor of Anesthesiology and Reproductive Medicine; Director of Obstetric Anesthesia, Departments of Anesthesiology and Reproductive Medicine, University of California, San Diego, California
- **Anesthetic Considerations for Complicated Pregnancies**

Robert M. Lawrence, MD
Clinical Associate Professor, Department of Pediatrics, University of Florida School of Medicine, Gainesville, Florida
- **The Breast and the Physiology of Lactation**

Ruth A. Lawrence, MD
Professor of Pediatrics, Obstetrics, and Gynecology, University of Rochester School of Medicine; Chief of Normal Newborn Services, Medical Director, Breastfeeding and Human Lactation Study Center, Golisano Children's Hospital at Strong Memorial Hospital, Rochester, New York
- **The Breast and the Physiology of Lactation**

Liesbeth Lewi, MD, PhD
Assistant Professor, Obstetrics and Gynecology, Division of Woman and Child, University Hospitals Katholieke Universiteit Leuven, Leuven, Belgium
- **Invasive Fetal Therapy**

James H. Liu, MD
Arthur H. Bill Professor and Chair, Department of Reproductive Biology, Case Western Reserve School of Medicine; Chair, University Hospitals, MacDonald Women's Hospital, Case Medical Center, Cleveland, Ohio
- **Endocrinology of Pregnancy**

Michael D. Lockshin, MD
Professor of Medicine and Obstetrics and Gynecology, Weill Medical College of Cornell University; Attending Physician, Hospital for Special Surgery, New York Presbyterian Hospital, New York, New York
- **Pregnancy and Rheumatic Diseases**

Charles J. Lockwood, MD
Anita O'Keefe Young Professor and Chair, Department of Obstetrics, Gynecology, and Reproductive Sciences, Yale University School of Medicine, New Haven, Connecticut
- **Pathogenesis of Spontaneous Preterm Labor**
- **Coagulation Disorders in Pregnancy**
- **Thromboembolic Disease in Pregnancy**

Stephen J. Lye, PhD
Vice President of Research, Mount Sinai Hospital; Associate Director, Samuel Lunenfeld Research Institute, Toronto, Canada
- **Biology of Parturition**

Lucy Mackillop, BM BCh, MA, MRCP
Senior Registrar in Obstetric Medicine, Queen Charlotte's and Chelsea Hospital, London, United Kingdom
- **Diseases of the Liver, Biliary System, and Pancreas**

George A. Macones, MD, MSCE
Professor and Head, Department of Obstetrics and Gynecology, Washington University School of Medicine in St. Louis; Chief of Obstetrics and Gynecology, Barnes-Jewish Hospital, St. Louis, Missouri
- **Evidence-Based Practice in Perinatal Medicine**

Fergal D. Malone, MD, FACOG, FRCPI, MRCOG
Professor and Chairman, Department of Obstetrics and Gynaecology, Royal College of Surgeons in Ireland; Chairman, Department of Obstetrics and Gynaecology, the Rotunda Hospital, Dublin, Ireland
- **Multiple Gestation: Clinical Characteristics and Management**

Frank A. Manning, MD, MSc FRCS
Professor, Department of Obstetrics and Gynecology, New York Medical College; Professor, Associate Director, Division of Maternal-Fetal Medicine, Department of Obstetrics and Gynecology, Westchester County Medical Center, Valhalla, New York
- **Imaging in the Diagnosis of Fetal Anomalies**

Stephanie Rae Martin, DO
Assistant Medical Director and Section Chief, Pikes Peak Maternal-Fetal Medicine, Memorial Health System, Colorado Springs, Colorado
- **Intensive Care Monitoring of the Critically Ill Pregnant Patient**

Brian M. Mercer, MD, FRCSC, FACOG
Professor of Reproductive Biology, Case Western Reserve University; Director of Obstetrics and Maternal-Fetal Medicine, Vice Chair of Hospitals, Obstetrics and Gynecology, MetroHealth Medical Center, Cleveland, Ohio
- **Assessment and Induction of Fetal Pulmonary Maturity**
- **Premature Rupture of the Membranes**

Giacomo Meschia, MD
Professor Emeritus of Physiology, University of Colorado School of Medicine, Denver, Colorado
- **Placental Respiratory Gas Exchange and Fetal Oxygenation**

Kenneth J. Moise, Jr., MD
Professor of Obstetrics and Gynecology, Baylor College of Medicine; Member, Texas Children's Fetal Center, Texas Children's Hospital, Houston, Texas
- **Hemolytic Disease of the Fetus and Newborn**

Manju Monga, MD
Berel Held Professor and Division Director, Maternal-Fetal Medicine; Director, Maternal-Fetal Medicine Fellowship, Department of Obstetrics, Gynecology, and Reproductive Sciences, University of Texas at Houston Health Science Center, Houston, Texas
- **Maternal Cardiovascular, Respiratory, and Renal Adaptation to Pregnancy**

Thomas R. Moore, MD
Professor and Chairman, Department of Reproductive Medicine, University of California, San Diego, School of Medicine, San Diego, California
- **Diabetes in Pregnancy**

Gil Mor, MD, PhD
Associate Professor, Yale University, School of Medicine, Department of Obstetrics, Gynecology, and Reproductive Sciences, New Haven, Connecticut
- **The Immunology of Pregnancy**

Shahla Nader, MD
Professor, Department of Obstetrics and Gynecology and Internal Medicine (Endocrine Division), University of Texas Medical School at Houston; Attending Physician, Memorial Hermann Hospital–Texas Medical Center, Houston, Texas
- **Thyroid Disease and Pregnancy**
- **Other Endocrine Disorders of Pregnancy**

Michael P. Nageotte, MD
Professor, Department of Obstetrics and Gynecology, University of California at Irvine, Orange, California; Associate Chief Medical Officer, Miller Children's, Long Beach Memorial Medical Center, Long Beach, California
- **Intrapartum Fetal Surveillance**

Vivek Narendran, MD
Associate Professor of Pediatrics, University of Cincinnati College of Medicine; Medical Director, University Hospital Neonatal Intensive Care Unit and Newborn Nurseries, Cincinnati Children's Hospital Research Foundation, University Hospital, Cincinnati, Ohio
- **Neonatal Morbidities of Prenatal and Perinatal Origin**

Errol R. Norwitz, MD, PhD
Professor; Co-director, Division of Maternal-Fetal Medicine; Director, Maternal-Fetal Medicine Fellowship Program; Director, Obstetrics and Gynecology Residency Program; Department of Obstetrics, Gynecology, and Reproductive Sciences, Yale University School of Medicine, New Haven, Connecticut
- **Biology of Parturition**

Michael J. Paidas, MD
Associate Professor, Co-director, Women and Children's Center for Blood Disorders, Department of Obstetrics, Gynecology, and Reproductive Sciences, Yale University School of Medicine, New Haven, Connecticut
- **Embryonic and Fetal Demise**

Lucilla Poston, PhD, FRCOG
Professor of Maternal and Fetal Health, King's College, London, United Kingdom
- **Developmental Origins of Health and Disease**

Bhuvaneswari Ramaswamy, MD, MRCP
Assistant Professor of Internal Medicine, Division of Hematology Oncology, Arthur G. James Cancer Hospital and Richard J. Solove Research Institute, The Ohio State University, Columbus, Ohio
- **Malignancy and Pregnancy**

Ronald P. Rapini, MD
Professor and Chairman, Department of Dermatology, University of Texas Medical School and MD Anderson Cancer Center, Houston, Texas
- **The Skin and Pregnancy**

Jamie L. Resnik, MD
Associate Clinical Professor of Reproductive Medicine, University of California, San Diego, School of Medicine; Physician, University of California Medical Center, San Diego, California
- **Post-term Pregnancy**

Robert Resnik, MD
Professor Emeritus, Department of Reproductive Medicine, University of California, San Diego, School of Medicine, San Diego, California
- **Post-term Pregnancy**
- **Intrauterine Growth Restriction**
- **Placenta Previa, Placenta Accreta, Abruptio Placentae, and Vasa Previa**

Bryan S. Richardson, MD, FRCSC
Professor and Chair, Department of Obstetrics and Gynecology, Professor, Departments of Physiology, Pharmacology, and Pediatrics, University of Western Ontario, Schulich School of Medicine and Dentistry, London, Ontario, Canada
- **Behavioral State Activity and Fetal Health and Development**

James M. Roberts, MD
Senior Scientist, Magee-Women's Research Institute, Professor of Obstetrics, Gynecology, and Reproductive Sciences and Epidemiology, University of Pittsburgh, Pittsburgh, Pennsylvania
- **Pregnancy-Related Hypertension**

Roberto Romero, MD
Professor of Molecular Obstetrics and Genetics, Wayne State University School of Medicine, Detroit, Michigan; Chief, Perinatology Research Branch, Program Director for Obstetrics and Perinatology, Intramural Division, Eunice Kennedy Shriver National Institute of Child Health and Human Development, National Institutes of Health, Bethesda, Maryland
- **Pathogenesis of Spontaneous Preterm Labor**
- **Preterm Labor and Birth**

Michael G. Ross, MD, MPH
Professor of Obstetrics and Gynecology and Public Health, Geffen School of Medicine, School of Public Health, University of California, Los Angeles, California; Chairman, Department of Obstetrics and Gynecology, Harbor-University of California, Los Angeles, Medical Center, Department of Obstetrics and Gynecology, Torrance, California
- **Amniotic Fluid Dynamics**

Jane E. Salmon, MD
Professor of Medicine and Obstetrics and Gynecology, Weill Medical College of Cornell University; Attending Physician, Hospital for Special Surgery New York Presbyterian Hospital, New York, New York
- **Pregnancy and Rheumatic Diseases**

Thomas J. Savides, MD
Professor of Clinical Medicine, Division of Gastroenterology, University of California, San Diego, La Jolla, California
- **Gastrointestinal Disease in Pregnancy**

Kurt R. Schibler, MD
Associate Professor of Pediatrics, University of Cincinnati College of Medicine; Director, Neonatology Clinical Research Program, Cincinnati Children's Hospital Research Foundation, Cincinnati, Ohio
- **Neonatal Morbidities of Prenatal and Perinatal Origin**

Ralph Shabetai, MD, FACC
Professor of Medicine, Emeritus, University of California, San Diego, School of Medicine; Chief, Emeritus, Cardiology Section, San Diego Veterans' Administration Medical Center, La Jolla, California
- **Cardiac Diseases**

Robert M. Silver, MD
Professor of Obstetrics and Gynecology; Chief, Maternal-Fetal Medicine, University of Utah Health Sciences Center, Salt Lake City, Utah
- **Coagulation Disorders in Pregnancy**

Mark Sklansky, MD
Associate Professor of Pediatrics and Obstetrics and Gynecology, University of Southern California, Keck School of Medicine; Director, Fetal Cardiology Program, Children's Hospital Los Angeles and CHLA-USC Institute for Maternal-Fetal Health, Los Angeles, California
- **Fetal Cardiac Malformations and Arrhythmias: Detection, Diagnosis, Management, and Prognosis**

Naomi E. Stotland, MD
Assistant Professor, Department of Obstetrics, Gynecology, and Reproductive Sciences, University of California, San Francisco, San Francisco, California
- **Maternal Nutrition**

Richard L. Sweet, MD
Professor of Obstetrics and Gynecology, University of California-Davis, Sacramento, California
- **Maternal and Fetal Infections**

John M. Thorp, Jr., MD
McAllister Distinguished Professor of Obstetrics and Gynecology, University of North Carolina School of Medicine; Professor of Maternal-Child Health, University of North Carolina School of Public Health, University of North Carolina, Chapel Hill, North Carolina
- **Clinical Aspects of Normal and Abnormal Labor**

Patrizia Vergani, MD
Associate Professor, University of Milano-Bicocco, School of Medicine; Director, Obstetrics, San Gerardo Hospital, Monza, Italy
- **Benign Gynecologic Conditions in Pregnancy**

Ronald J. Wapner, MD
Professor, Obstetrics and Gynecology, Columbia University; Director, Division of Maternal-Fetal Medicine, Columbia University Medical Center, New York, New York
- **Prenatal Diagnosis of Congenital Disorders**

Barbara B. Warner, MD
Associate Professor of Pediatrics, Washington University School of Medicine; Associate Professor of Pediatrics, Division of Newborn Medicine, St. Louis Children's Hospital, St. Louis, Missouri
- **Neonatal Morbidities of Prenatal and Perinatal Origin**

Carl P. Weiner, MD, MBA
K.E. Krantz Professor and Chair, Obstetrics and Gynecology, Professor, Molecular and Integrative Physiology, University of Kansas School of Medicine; Director of Women's Health, University of Kansas Hospital, Kansas City, Kansas
- **Teratogenesis and Environmental Exposure**

Janice E. Whitty, MD
Professor of Obstetrics and Gynecology, Director of Maternal and Fetal Medicine, Meharry Medical College; Chief of Obstetrics and Maternal Fetal Medicine, Nashville General Hospital, Nashville, Tennessee
- **Respiratory Diseases in Pregnancy**

Isabelle Wilkins, MD
Professor, Obstetrics and Gynecology, Director, Maternal-Fetal Medicine, University of Illinois at Chicago, Chicago, Illinois
- **Nonimmune Hydrops**

David J. Williams, PhD, FRCP
Consultant Obstetric Physician, Institute for Women's Health, University College London, London, United Kingdom
- **Renal Disorders**

Catherine Williamson, MD, FRCP
Professor of Obstetric Medicine, Institute of Reproductive and Developmental Biology, Imperial College London; Honorary Consultant in Obstetric Medicine, Queen Charlotte's and Chelsea Hospital, London, United Kingdom
- **Diseases of the Liver, Biliary System, and Pancreas**

Anthony Wynshaw-Boris, MD, PhD
Professor and Chief, Division of Genetics, Department of Pediatrics and Institute for Human Genetics, University of California, San Francisco, School of Medicine, San Francisco, California
- **Basic Genetics and Patterns of Inheritance**

Kimberly A. Yonkers, MD
Associate Professor of Psychiatry, Departments of Psychiatry and Obstetrics, Gynecology, and Reproductive Sciences and School of Epidemiology and Public Health, Yale University School of Medicine; Attending Physician, Yale–New Heaven Hospital, New Haven, Connecticut
- **Management of Depression and Psychoses in Pregnancy and the Puerperium**

PREFACE

With this new edition, we welcome Dr. Charles J. Lockwood and Dr. Thomas R. Moore as editors of this textbook. Their previous contributions have been of unique importance to the success of our efforts, and we look forward to a long and productive relationship.

The 6th edition brings many innovations, most prominent of which is that it will also be available as an Expert Consult title, www.expertconsult.com. The online version will be fully searchable, with all text, tables, and images included. Additional content that could not be included in print form will be presented in the Web edition. In recognition of how rapidly the field of maternal-fetal medicine is advancing, we will initiate quarterly updates with this edition as well. The text includes several new chapters: "Pathogenesis of Spontaneous Preterm Labor," "Benign Gynecologic Conditions in Pregnancy," "Developmental Origins of Health and Disease," and "Neonatal Morbidities of Prenatal and Perinatal Origin." All chapters have been extensively rewritten and updated, and we are, as always, deeply appreciative of the contributions of our many new and returning authors.

We also wish to express our appreciation and gratitude to our marvelous editors at Elsevier, particularly Kristina Oberle, our Developmental Editor, for her organizational skills and for always being available for counsel. We are also indebted to Rebecca Schmidt Gaertner for her overall supervision of the project and to Rachel Miller for moving the project through final production.

Finally, we are indebted to our families for their patience and support, because every hour spent producing this text was an hour spent away from them.

The Editors

CONTENTS

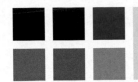

Part I
SCIENTIFIC BASIS OF PERINATAL BIOLOGY

CHAPTER 1
Basic Genetics and Patterns of Inheritance 3
Bruce A. Hamilton, PhD
Anthony Wynshaw-Boris, MD, PhD

CHAPTER 2
Normal Early Development 37
Kurt Benirschke, MD

CHAPTER 3
Amniotic Fluid Dynamics 47
Marie H. Beall, MD
Michael G. Ross, MD, MPH

CHAPTER 4
Multiple Gestation: The Biology of Twinning 55
Kurt Benirschke, MD

CHAPTER 5
Biology of Parturition 69
Errol R. Norwitz, MD, PhD
Stephen J. Lye, PhD

CHAPTER 6
The Immunology of Pregnancy 87
Gil Mor, MD, PhD
Vikki M. Abrahams, PhD

CHAPTER 7
Maternal Cardiovascular, Respiratory, and Renal Adaptation to Pregnancy 101
Manju Monga, MD

CHAPTER 8
Endocrinology of Pregnancy 111
James H. Liu, MD

CHAPTER 9
The Breast and the Physiology of Lactation 125
Robert M. Lawrence, MD
Ruth A. Lawrence, MD

CHAPTER 10
Maternal Nutrition 143
Naomi E. Stotland, MD

CHAPTER 11
Developmental Origins of Health and Disease 151
Lucilla Poston, PhD
Mark Hanson, DPhil

CHAPTER 12
Fetal Cardiovascular Physiology 159
Jeffrey R. Fineman, MD
Ronald Clyman, MD

CHAPTER 13
Behavioral State Activity and Fetal Health and Development 171
Bryan S. Richardson, MD
Robert Gagnon, MD

CHAPTER 14
Placental Respiratory Gas Exchange and Fetal Oxygenation 181
Giacomo Meschia, MD

CHAPTER 15
Fetal Lung Development and Surfactant 193
Alan H. Jobe, MD, PhD

CHAPTER 16
Evidence-Based Practice in Perinatal Medicine 207
George A. Macones, MD

Part II
FETAL DISORDERS: DIAGNOSIS AND THERAPY

CHAPTER 17
Prenatal Diagnosis of Congenital Disorders 221
Ronald J. Wapner, MD
Thomas M. Jenkins, MD
Nahla Khalek, MD

CHAPTER 18
Imaging in the Diagnosis of Fetal Anomalies 275
Frank A. Manning, MD, MSc

CHAPTER 19
Fetal Cardiac Malformations and Arrhythmias: Detection, Diagnosis, Management, and Prognosis 305
Mark Sklansky, MD

CHAPTER 20
Teratogenesis and Environmental Exposure 347
Christina Chambers, PhD, MPH
Carl P. Weiner, MD, MBA

CHAPTER 21
Assessment of Fetal Health 361
Christopher R. Harman, MD

CHAPTER 22
Intrapartum Fetal Surveillance 397
Michael P. Nageotte, MD
Larry C. Gilstrap III, MD

CHAPTER 23
Assessment and Induction of Fetal Pulmonary Maturity 419
Brian M. Mercer, MD

CHAPTER 24
Invasive Fetal Therapy 433
Jan A. Deprest, MD, PhD
Eduardo Gratacos, MD, PhD
Liesbeth Lewi, MD, PhD

CHAPTER 25
Multiple Gestation: Clinical Characteristics and Management 453
Fergal D. Malone, MD
Mary E. D'Alton, MD

CHAPTER 26
Hemolytic Disease of the Fetus and Newborn 477
Kenneth J. Moise, Jr., MD

CHAPTER 27
Nonimmune Hydrops 505
Isabelle Wilkins, MD

Part III
DISORDERS AT THE MATERNAL-FETAL INTERFACE

CHAPTER 28
Pathogenesis of Spontaneous Preterm Labor 521
Roberto Romero, MD
Charles J. Lockwood, MD

CHAPTER 29
Preterm Labor and Birth 545
Jay D. Iams, MD
Roberto Romero, MD
Robert K. Creasy, MD

CHAPTER 30
Cervical Insufficiency 583
Jay D. Iams, MD

CHAPTER 31
Premature Rupture of the Membranes 599
Brian M. Mercer, MD

CHAPTER 32
Post-term Pregnancy 613
Jamie L. Resnik, MD
Robert Resnik, MD

CHAPTER 33
Embryonic and Fetal Demise 619
Michael J. Paidas, MD
Nazli Hossain, MBBS

CHAPTER 34
Intrauterine Growth Restriction 635
Robert Resnik, MD
Robert K. Creasy, MD

CHAPTER 35
Pregnancy-Related Hypertension 651
James M. Roberts, MD
Edmund F. Funai, MD

Part IV
MATERNAL COMPLICATIONS

CHAPTER 36
Clinical Aspects of Normal and Abnormal Labor 691
John M. Thorp, Jr., MD

CHAPTER 37
Placenta Previa, Placenta Accreta, Abruptio Placentae, and Vasa Previa 725
Andrew D. Hull, MD
Robert Resnik, MD

CHAPTER 38
Maternal and Fetal Infections 739
Patrick Duff, MD
Richard L. Sweet, MD
Rodney K. Edwards, MD, MS

CHAPTER 39
Cardiac Diseases 797
Daniel G. Blanchard, MD
Ralph Shabetai, MD

CHAPTER 40
Coagulation Disorders in Pregnancy 825
Charles J. Lockwood, MD
Robert M. Silver, MD

CHAPTER 41
Thromboembolic Disease in Pregnancy 855
Charles J. Lockwood, MD

CHAPTER 42
Anemia and Pregnancy 869
Sarah J. Kilpatrick, MD, PhD

CHAPTER 43
Malignancy and Pregnancy 885
David Cohn, MD
Bhuvaneswari Ramaswamy, MD
Kristie Blum, MD

CHAPTER 44
Renal Disorders 905
David J. Williams, PhD
John M. Davison, MD

CHAPTER 45
Respiratory Diseases in Pregnancy 927
Janice E. Whitty, MD
Mitchell P. Dombrowski, MD

CHAPTER 46
Diabetes in Pregnancy 953
Thomas R. Moore, MD
Patrick Catalano, MD

CHAPTER 47
Thyroid Disease and Pregnancy 995
Shahla Nader, MD

CHAPTER 48
Other Endocrine Disorders of Pregnancy 1015
Shahla Nader, MD

CHAPTER 49
Gastrointestinal Disease in Pregnancy 1041
Thomas F. Kelly, MD
Thomas J. Savides, MD

CHAPTER 50
Diseases of the Liver, Biliary System, and Pancreas 1059
Catherine Williamson, MD
Lucy Mackillop, BM BCh, MA

CHAPTER 51
Pregnancy and Rheumatic Diseases 1079
Michael D. Lockshin, MD
Jane E. Salmon, MD
Doruk Erkan, MD

CHAPTER 52
Neurologic Disorders 1089
Michael J. Aminoff, MD, DSc

CHAPTER 53
Management of Depression and Psychoses in Pregnancy and the Puerperium 1113
Kimberly A. Yonkers, MD

CHAPTER 54
The Skin and Pregnancy 1123
Ronald P. Rapini, MD

CHAPTER 55
Benign Gynecologic Conditions in Pregnancy 1135
Alessandro Ghidini, MD
Patrizia Vergani, MD

CHAPTER 56
Anesthetic Considerations for Complicated Pregnancies 1147
Krzysztof M. Kuczkowski, MD

CHAPTER 57
Intensive Care Monitoring of the Critically Ill Pregnant Patient 1167
Stephanie Rae Martin, DO
Michael Raymond Foley, MD

Part V
THE NEONATE

CHAPTER 58
Neonatal Morbidities of Prenatal and Perinatal Origin 1197
James M. Greenberg, MD
Vivek Narendran, MD
Kurt R. Schibler, MD
Barbara B. Warner, MD
Beth Haberman, MD
Edward F. Donovan, MD

Index 1229

Part I

SCIENTIFIC BASIS OF PERINATAL BIOLOGY

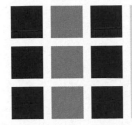

Chapter 1

Basic Genetics and Patterns of Inheritance

Bruce A. Hamilton, PhD, and Anthony Wynshaw-Boris, MD, PhD

Impact of Genetics and the Human Genome Project on Medicine in the 21st Century

For most of the 20th century, geneticists were considered to be outside the everyday clinical practice of medicine. The exceptions were those medical geneticists who studied rare chromosomal abnormalities and rare causes of birth defects and metabolic disorders. As recently as 20 years ago, genetics was generally not taught as part of the medical school curriculum, and most physicians' understanding of genetics was derived from undergraduate studies.[1] How things have changed in the 21st century! Genetics is now recognized as a contributing factor to virtually all human illnesses. In addition, the widespread reporting of genetic discoveries in the lay press and the plethora of genetic information available via the Internet has led to a great increase in the sophistication of patients and their families as medical consumers regarding genetics.

The importance of genetics in medical practice has grown as a consequence of the immense progress made in genetics and molecular biology during the 20th century. In the first year of that century, Mendel's laws were rediscovered and applied to many fields, including human disease. In 1953, Watson and Crick published the structure of DNA and ushered in the era of molecular biology. At nearly the same time, the era of cytogenetics began with the determination of the correct number of human chromosomes (46). In the 1970s, Sanger and Gilbert independently published techniques for determining the sequence of DNA. These findings, combined with automation of the Sanger method in the 1980s, led several prominent scientists to propose and initiate the Human Genome Project, with the goal of obtaining the complete human DNA sequence. At the time, it was hard to imagine that this goal could be achieved, but in the first year of the 21st century, a draft of the human genome was published simultaneously by the publicly funded Human Genome Project[2] and a private company, Celera.[3] Since then, additional public consortia and private companies have made systematic efforts to catalog DNA sequence variations that may predict or contribute to human disease. These include both single nucleotide polymorphisms (SNPs)[4] and copy number variations (CNVs)[5] of large blocks of sequence. Most of these data are available in public databases, and disease-related discoveries based on them are being reported at a rapid pace. The concepts, tools, and techniques of modern genetics and molecular biology have already had a profound impact on biomedical research and will continue to revolutionize our approach to human disease risk management, diagnosis, and treatment over the next decade and beyond.

Genetics plays an important role in the day-to-day practice of obstetrics and gynecology, perhaps more so than in any other specialty of medicine. In obstetric practice, genetic issues often arise before, during, and after pregnancy. Amniocentesis or chorionic villus sampling may detect potential chromosomal defects in the fetus. Fetuses examined during pregnancy by ultrasound may have possible birth defects. Specific prenatal diagnostic tests for genetic diseases may be requested by couples attempting to conceive who have a family history of that disorder. Infertile couples often require a workup for genetic causes of their infertility. In gynecology, genetics is particularly important in disorders of sexual development and gynecologic malignancies.

What Is a Gene?

Genes are the fundamental unit of heredity. As a concise description, a gene includes all the structural and regulatory information required to express a heritable quality, usually through production of an encoded protein or an RNA product. In addition to the more familiar genes encoding proteins (through messenger or mRNA) and RNAs that function in RNA processing (small nuclear or snRNA), ribosome assembly (small nucleolar or snoRNA), and protein translation (transfer or tRNA and ribosomal or rRNA), there are more recently appreciated classes of regulatory RNAs that function in control of gene expression, including microRNAs (miRNA), piwiRNAs (piRNAs), and other noncoding RNAs (ncRNA). Structural segments of the genome that do not encode an RNA or a protein may also be considered genes if their mutation produces observable effects. Humans are now thought to have 20,000 to 25,000 distinct protein-coding genes, although this number has fluctuated with improved methods for identifying genes. We shall now outline the chemical nature of genes, the biochemistry of gene function, and the classes and consequences of genetic mutations.

Chemical Nature of Genes

Human genes are composed of deoxyribonucleic acid (DNA) (Fig. 1-1). DNA is a negatively charged polymer of nucleotides. Each nucleotide is composed of a "base" attached to a 5-carbon deoxyribose sugar.

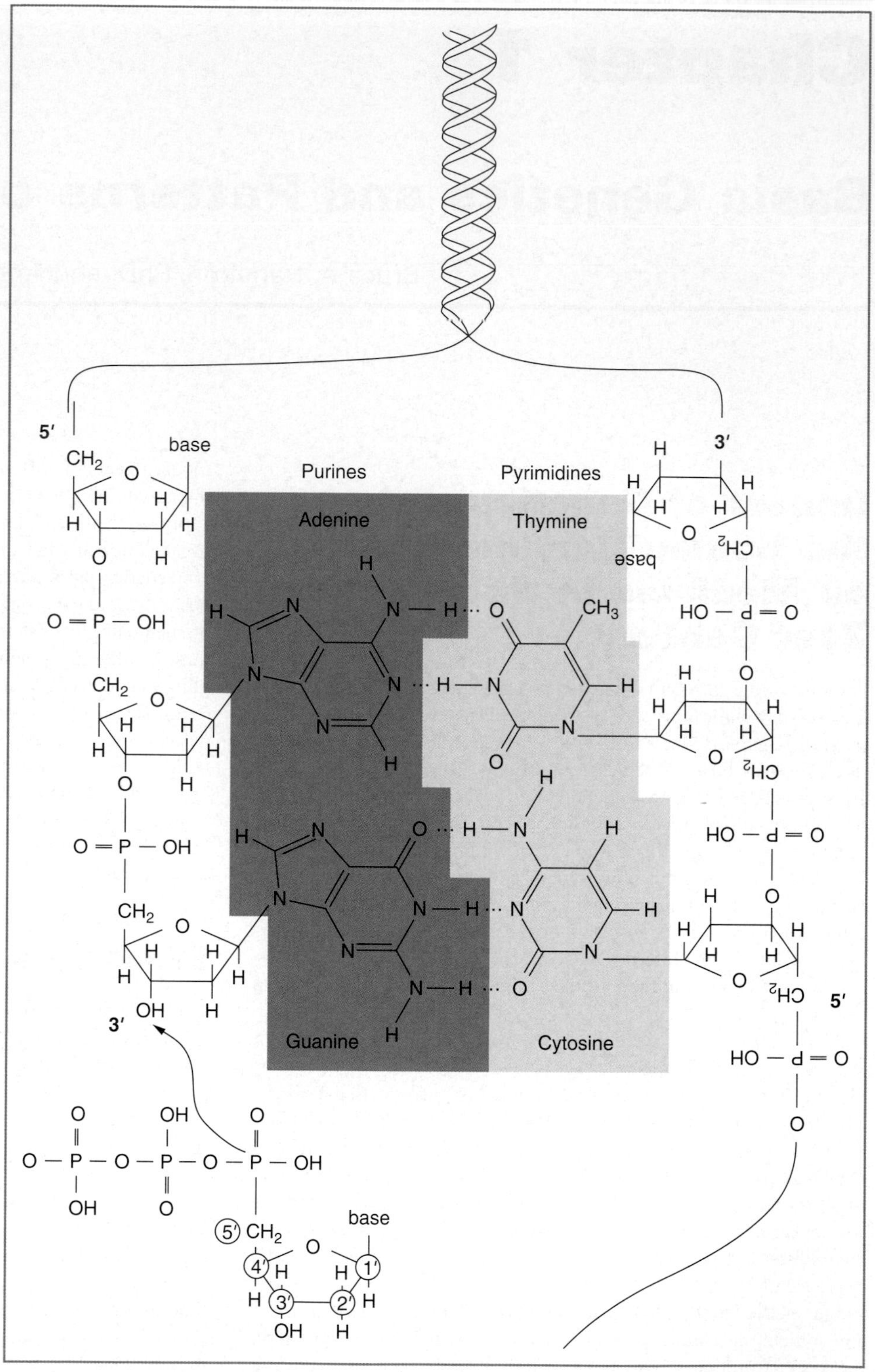

FIGURE 1-1 Schematic diagram of DNA structure. Each strand of the double helix is a polymer of deoxyribonucleotides. Hydrogen bonds (shown here as *dots* [···]) between base pairs hold the strands together. Each base pair includes one purine base (adenine or guanine) and its complementary pyrimidine base (thymine or cytosine). Two hydrogen bonds form between A:T pairs and three between G:C pairs. The two polymer strands run antiparallel to each other according to the polarity of their sugar backbone. As shown at the bottom, DNA synthesis proceeds in the 5′-to-3′ direction by addition of new nucleoside triphosphates. Energy stored in the triphosphate bond is used for the polymerization reaction. The numbering system for carbon atoms in the deoxyribose sugar is indicated.

Four bases are used in cellular DNA: two purines, adenine (A) and guanine (G), and two pyrimidines, cytosine (C) and thymine (T). The polymer is formed through phosphodiester bonds that connect the 5′ carbon atom of one sugar to the 3′ carbon of the next, which imparts directionality to the polymer.

Cellular DNA is a double-stranded helix. The two strands run antiparallel; that is, the 5′ to 3′ orientation of one strand runs in the opposite direction along the helix from its complementary strand. The bases in the two strands are paired: A with T, and G with C. Hydrogen bonds between the base pairs hold the strands together: two hydrogen bonds for A:T pairs and three for G:C pairs. Each base thus has a complementary base, and the sequence of bases on one strand implies the complementary sequence of the opposite strand. DNA is replicated in the 5′ to 3′ direction using the sequence of the complementary strand as a template. Nucleotide precursors used in DNA synthesis have 5′ triphosphate groups. Polymerase enzymes use the energy of this triphosphate to catalyze formation of a phosphoester bond with the hydroxyl group attached to the 3′ carbon of the extending strand.

Chemical attributes of DNA are the basis for clinical and forensic molecular diagnostic tests. Because nucleic acids form double-stranded duplexes, synthetic DNA and RNA molecules can be used to probe the integrity and composition of specific genes from patient samples. Noncomplementary base pairs formed by hybridization of DNA from a subject carrying a sequence variant relative to a reference sample are often detected by physicochemical properties such as reduced thermal stability of short (oligonucleotide) hybrids. In vitro DNA synthesis with recombinant polymerase enzymes are the basis for polymerase chain reaction (PCR) amplification of specific gene sequences. Increasingly, DNA sequencing methods are being used to detect small, nucleotide-level variations, and hybridization-based methods are used to discriminate between some known allelic differences and to assess structural variations such as variations in gene copy number.

First letter	Second letter: U		C		A		G		Third letter
U	UUU	phe	UCU	ser	UAU	tyr	UGU	cys	U
	UUC		UCC		UAC		UGC		C
	UUA	leu	UCA		UAA	ter*	UGA	ter*	A
	UUG		UCG		UAG		UGG	trp	G
C	CUU	leu	CCU	pro	CAU	his	CGU	arg	U
	CUC		CCC		CAC		CGC		C
	CUA		CCA		CAA	gln	CGA		A
	CUG		CCG		CAG		CGG		G
A	AUU	ile	ACU	thr	AAU	asn	AGU	ser	U
	AUC		ACC		AAC		AGC		C
	AUA		ACA		AAA	lys	AGA	arg	A
	AUG	met	ACG		AAG		AGG		G
G	GUU	val	GCU	ala	GAU	asp	GGU	gly	U
	GUC		GCC		GAC		GGC		C
	GUA		GCA		GAA	glu_	GGA		A
	GUG		GCG		GAG		GGG		G

FIGURE 1-2 The genetic code. The letters U, C, A, and G correspond to the nucleotide bases. In this diagram, U (uracil) is substituted for T (thymidine) to reflect the genetic code as it appears in messenger RNA. Three distinct triplets (codons)—UAA, UAG, and UGA—are "nonsense" codons and result in termination of messenger RNA translation into a polypeptide chain. All amino acids except methionine and tryptophan have more than one codon; thus the genetic code is degenerate. This is the primary reason that many single base–change mutations are "silent." For example, changing the terminal U in a UUU codon to a terminal C (UUC) still codes for phenylalanine. In contrast, an A to T (U) change (GAG to GUG) in the β-globin gene results in substitution of valine for glutamic acid at position 6 in the β-globin amino acid sequence, thus yielding "sickle cell" globin.

Biochemistry of Gene Function

Information Transfer

DNA is an information molecule. The central dogma of molecular biology is that information in DNA is *transcribed* to make RNA, and information in messenger RNA (mRNA) is *translated* to make protein. DNA is also the template for its own replication. In some instances, such as in retroviruses, RNA is reverse-transcribed into DNA. Although proteins are used to catalyze the synthesis of DNA, RNA, and proteins, proteins do not convey information back to genes. The sequence of RNA nucleotides (A, C, G, and uracil [U] bases coupled to ribose) is the same as the *coding* or *sense strand* of DNA (except that U replaces T), and the complementary antisense strand of DNA is the template for synthesis. The sequence of amino acids in a protein is determined by a three-letter code of nucleotides in its mRNA (Fig. 1-2). The phase of the reading frame for these three-letter codons is set from the first codon, usually an AUG, encoding the initial methionine.

Quality Control in Gene Expression

Several mechanisms protect the specificity and fidelity of gene expression in cells. *Promoter* and *enhancer* sequences are binding sites on DNA for proteins that direct transcription of RNA. Promoter sequences are typically adjacent and 5′ to the start of mRNA encoding sequences (although some promoter elements are also found downstream of the start site, particularly in introns), whereas enhancers may act at a considerable distance, from either the 5′ or 3′ direction. The combinations of binding sites present determine under what conditions the gene is transcribed.

Newly transcribed RNA is generally processed before it is used by a cell. Many processing steps occur cotranscriptionally, on the elongated RNA as it is synthesized. Pre-mRNAs generally receive a 5′ "cap" structure and a poly-adenylated 3′ tail. Protein-coding genes typically contain exons that remain in the processed RNA, and one or more introns that must be removed by *splicing* (Fig. 1-3). Nucleotide sequences in the RNA that are recognized by protein and RNA splicing factors determine where splicing occurs. Many RNAs can be spliced in more than one way to encode a related series of products, greatly increasing the complexity of products that can be encoded by a finite number of genes. For most genes, only spliced RNA is exported from the nucleus. Spliced RNAs that retain premature stop codons are rapidly degraded. Mutations in genes involved in these quality control steps appear in the clinic as early and severe genetic disorders, including spinal muscular atrophy (caused by mutations in *SMN1*, which encodes a splicing accessory factor) and fragile X syndrome (mutations in *FMR1*, which encodes an RNA-binding protein). Protein synthesis is also highly regulated. Translation, folding, modification, transport, and sometimes cleavage to create an active form of the protein are all regulated steps in the expression of protein-coding genes.

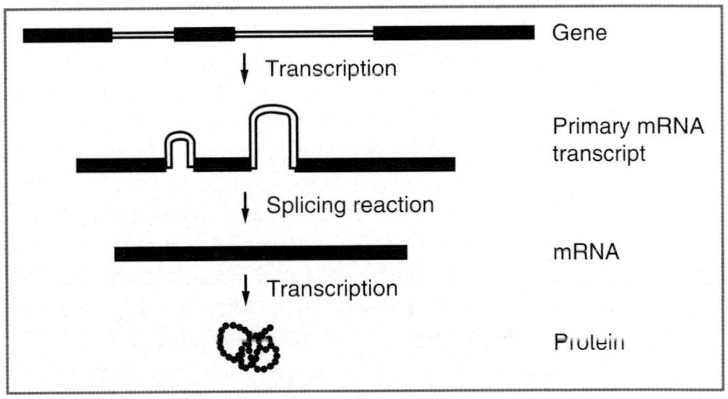

FIGURE 1-3 Transcription of DNA to RNA and translation of RNA to protein. Introns *(light sections)* are spliced out of the primary messenger RNA (mRNA) transcript and exons *(dark sections)* are joined together to form mature mRNA.

Mutations

Changes in the nucleotide sequence of a gene may occur through environmental damage to DNA, through errors in DNA replication, or

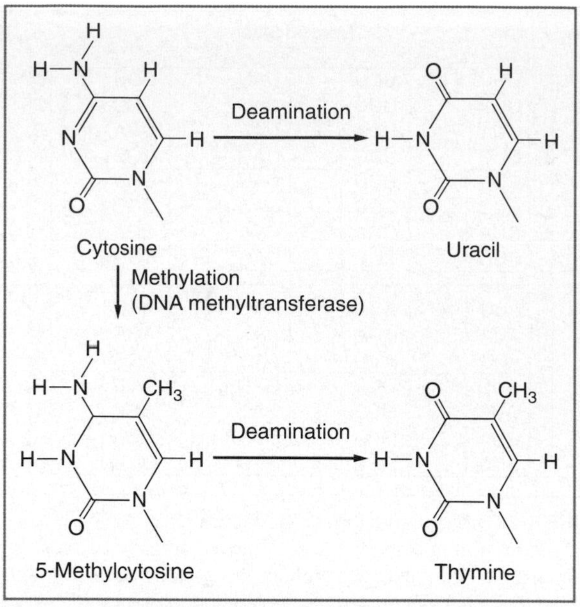

FIGURE 1-4 Deamination of cytosine. Deamination of cytosine or of its 5-methyl derivative produces a pyrimidine capable of pairing with adenine rather than guanine. Repair enzymes may remove the mispaired base before replication, but replication before repair (or repair of the wrong strand) results in the change becoming permanent. Spontaneous deamination of cytosine is a major mechanism of mutation in humans. Deamination of cytosine is also accelerated by some mutagenic chemicals, such as hydrazine.

TABLE 1-1	ONLINE RESOURCES FOR HUMAN GENETICS
Information on Individual Genes	
Online Mendelian Inheritance in Man (OMIM)	www.ncbi.nlm.nih.gov/entrez/query.fcgi?db=OMIM
GeneCards	http://bioinfo.weizmann.ac.il/cards/index.html
GenBank	www.ncbi.nlm.nih.gov/GenBank
Genome Browsers	
European Molecular Biology Organization/European Bioinformatics Institute	www.ensembl.org
National Center for Biotechnology Information (NCBI)	www.ncbi.nlm.nih.gov
University of California, Santa Cruz	http://genome.ucsc.edu
GeneLynx	www.genelynx.org

through unequal partitioning during meiosis. Ultraviolet light, ionizing radiation, and chemicals that intercalate, bind to, or covalently modify DNA are examples of mutation-causing agents. Replication errors often involve changes in the number of a repeated sequence; for example, changes in the number of $(CAG)_n$ repeats encoding polyglutamine in the *Huntintin* gene can result in alleles prone to Huntington disease. Replication also plays a crucial role in other mutations. Cells generally respond to high levels of DNA damage by blocking DNA replication and inducing a variety of DNA repair pathways. However, for any one site of DNA damage, replication may occur before repair. A frequent source of human mutation is spontaneous deamination of cytosine (Fig. 1-4). The modified base can be interpreted as a thymine if replication occurs before repair of the G:T mismatch pair. Ultraviolet light causes photochemical dimerization of adjacent thymine residues that may then be altered during repair or replication; in humans, this is more relevant to somatic mutations in exposed skin cells than to germline mutations. Ionizing radiation, by contrast, penetrates tissues and can cause both base changes and double-strand breaks in DNA. Errors in repair of double-strand breaks result in deletion, inversion, or translocation of large regions of DNA. Many chemicals, including alkylating agents and epoxides, can form chemical adducts with the bases of DNA. If the adduct is not recognized during the next round of DNA replication, the wrong base may be incorporated into the opposite strand. In addition, the human genome includes hundreds of thousands of endogenous retroviruses, retrotransposons, and other potentially mobile DNA elements. Movement of such elements or recombination between them is a source of spontaneous insertions and deletions, respectively.

Changes in the DNA sequence of a gene create distinct alleles of that gene. Alleles can be classified based on how they affect the function of that gene. An *amorphic* (or null) allele is a complete loss of function, *hypomorphic* is a partial loss of function, *hypermorphic* is a gain of normal function, *neomorphic* is a gain of novel function not encoded by the normal gene, and an *antimorphic* or dominant negative allele antagonizes normal function. A practical impact of allele classes is that distinct clinical syndromes may be caused by different alleles of the same gene. For example, different allelic mutations in the androgen receptor gene have been tied to partial or complete androgen insensitivity[6] (including hypospadias and Reifenstein syndrome), prostate cancer susceptibility, and spinal and bulbar muscular atrophy.[7] Similarly, mutations in the *CFTR* chloride channel cause cystic fibrosis, but some alleles are associated with pancreatitis or other less severe symptoms; mutations in the *DTDST* sulfate transporter cause diastrophic dysplasia, atelosteogenesis, or achondrogenesis, depending on the type of mutation present.

A small fraction of changes in genomic DNA affect gene function. Approximately 2% to 5% of the human genome encodes protein or confers regulatory specificity. Even within the protein coding sequences, many base changes do not alter the encoded amino acid, and these are called *silent substitutions*. Changes in DNA sequence that occurred long ago and do not alter gene function or whose impact is modest or uncertain are often referred to as *polymorphisms*, whereas *mutation* is reserved for newly created changes and changes that have significant impacts on gene function, such as in disease-causing alleles of disease-associated genes. Mutations that do affect gene function may occur in coding sequences or in sequences required for transcription, processing, or stability of the RNA. The rate of spontaneous mutation in humans can vary tremendously depending on the size and structural constraints of the gene involved, but estimates range from 10^{-4} per generation for large genes such as *NF1* down to 10^{-6} or 10^{-7} for smaller genes. Given current estimates of 20,000 to 25,000 human genes,[2,3] and given that more than 6 billion humans inhabit the earth, one may expect that each human is mutant for some gene and each gene is mutated in some humans. Several public databases that curate information about human genes and mutations are now available online (Table 1-1).

Chromosomes in Humans

Most genes reside in the nucleus and are packaged on the *chromosomes*. In the human, there are 46 chromosomes in a normal cell: 22 pairs of autosomes, and the X and Y sex chromosomes (see later). The autosomes are numbered from the largest (1) to the smallest (21 and 22). Each chromosome contains a *centromere,* a constricted region that forms the attachments to the mitotic spindle and governs chromosome movements during mitosis. The *chromosomal arms* radiate on each side of the centromere, terminating in the *telomere,* or end of each arm. Each chromosome contains a distinct set of genetic information. Each pair of autosomes is homologous and has an identical set of genes. Normal females have two X chromosomes, whereas normal males have one X and one Y chromosome. In addition to the nuclear chromosomes, the mitochondrial genome contains approximately 37 genes on a single chromosome that resides in this organelle.

Each chromosome is a continuous DNA double-helical strand, packaged into *chromatin,* which consists of protein and DNA. The protein moiety consists of basic *histone* and acidic *nonhistone* proteins. Five major groups of histones are important for proper packing of chromatin, whereas the heterogeneous nonhistone proteins are required for normal gene expression and higher-order chromosome packaging. Two each of the four core histones (H2A, H2B, H3, and H4) form a histone octamer nucleosome core that binds with DNA in a fashion that permits tight supercoiling and packaging of DNA in the chromosome-like thread on a spool. The fifth histone, H1, binds to DNA at the edge of each nucleosome in the spacer region. A single nucleosome core and spacer consists of about 200 base pairs of DNA. The nucleosome "beads" are further condensed into higher-order structures called solenoids, which can be packed into loops of chromatin that are attached to nonhistone matrix proteins. The orderly packaging of DNA into chromatin performs several functions, not the least of which is the packing of an enormous amount of DNA into the small volume of the nucleus. This orderly packing allows each chromosome to be faithfully wound and unwound during replication and cell division. Additionally, chromatin organization plays an important role in the control of gene expression.

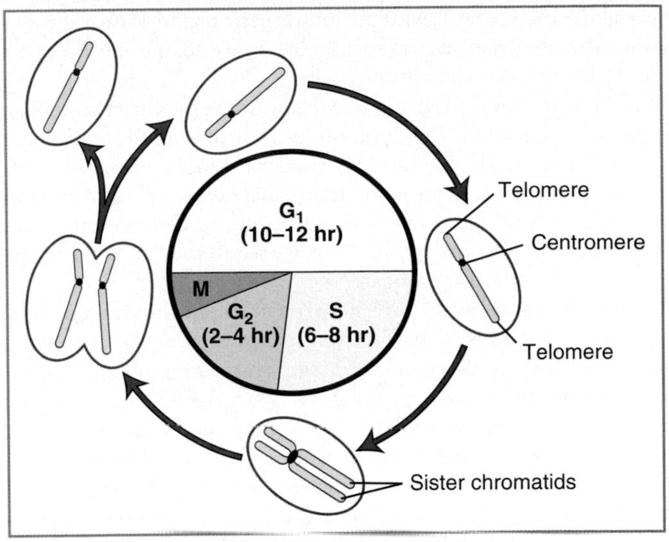

FIGURE 1-5 Cell cycle of a dividing mammalian cell, with approximate times in each phase of the cycle. In the G_1 phase, the diploid chromosome set (2n) is present once. After DNA synthesis (S phase), the diploid chromosome set is present in duplicate (4n). After mitosis (M), the DNA content returns to 2n. The telomeres, centromere, and sister chromatids are indicated. (From Nussbaum RL, McInnes RR, Willard HF: Thompson and Thompson's Genetics in Medicine, 6th ed. Philadelphia, WB Saunders, 2001.)

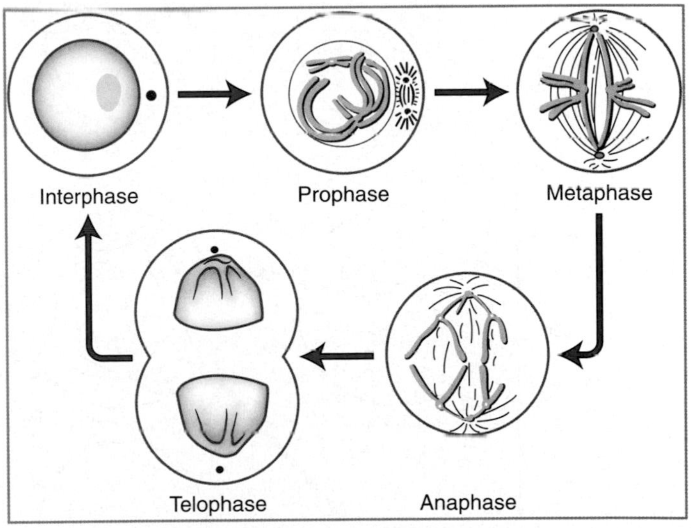

FIGURE 1-6 Schematic representation of mitosis. Only 2 of the 46 chromosomes are shown. (From Vogel F, Motulsky AG: Human Genetics: Problems and Approaches. New York, Springer-Verlag, 1979.)

Cell Cycle, Mitosis, and Meiosis

Cell Cycle

In replicating somatic cells, the complete diploid set of chromosomes is duplicated and the cell divides into two identical daughter cells, each with chromosomes and genes identical to those of the parent cell. The process of cell division is called *mitosis,* and the period between divisions is called *interphase.* Interphase can be divided into G_1, S, and G_2 *phases,* and a typical cell cycle is depicted in Figure 1-5. During the G_1 phase, synthesis of RNA and proteins occurs. In addition, the cell prepares for DNA replication. *S phase* ushers in the period of DNA replication. Not all chromosomes are replicated at the same time, and within a chromosome DNA is not synchronously replicated. Rather, DNA synthesis is initiated at thousands of origins of replication scattered along each chromosome. Between replication and division, called the G_2 phase, chromosome regions may be repaired and the cell is made ready for mitosis. In the G_1 phase, DNA of every chromosome of the diploid set (2n) is present once. Between the S and G_2 phases, every chromosome doubles to become two identical polynucleotides, referred to as *sister chromatids.* Thus, all DNA is now present twice ($2 \times 2n = 4n$).

Mitosis

The process of mitosis ensures that each daughter cell contains an identical and complete set of genetic information from the parent cell; this process is diagrammed in Figure 1-6. Mitosis is a continuous process that can be artificially divided into four stages based on the morphology of the chromosomes and the mitotic apparatus. The beginning of mitosis is characterized by swelling of chromatin, which becomes visible under the light microscope by the end of *prophase.* Only 2 of the 46 chromosomes are shown in Figure 1-6. In prophase, the two sister chromatids (chromosomes) lie closely adjacent. The nuclear membrane disappears, the nucleolus vanishes, and the spindle fibers begin to form from the microtubule-organizing centers, or *centrosomes,* that take positions perpendicular to the eventual plane of cleavage of the cell. A protein called *tubulin* forms the microtubules of the spindle and connects with the centromeric region of each chromosome. The chromosomes condense and move to the middle of the spindle at the eventual point of cleavage.

After prophase, the cell is in *metaphase,* when the chromosomes are maximally condensed. The chromosomes line up with the centromeres located on an equatorial plane between the spindle poles. This is the important phase for cytogenetic technology. When a cell is in metaphase, virtually all clinical methods of examining chromosomes cause arrest of further steps in mitosis. Thus, we see all sister chromatids (4n) in a standard clinical karyotype.

Anaphase begins as the two chromatids of each chromosome separate, connected at first only at the centromere region *(early anaphase).* Once the centromeres separate, the sister chromatids of each chromosome are drawn to the opposite poles by the spindle fibers. During telophase, chromosomes lose their visibility under the microscope, spindle fibers are degraded, tubulin is stored away for the next division, and a new nucleolus and nuclear membrane develop. The cytoplasm also divides along the same plane as the equatorial plate in a process called *cytokinesis.* Cytokinesis occurs once the segregating chromosomes approach the spindle poles. Thus, the elaborate process of mitosis and cytokinesis of a single cell results in the segregation of an equal complete set of chromosomes and genetic material in each of the resulting daughter cells.

Meiosis and the Meiotic Cell Cycle

In mitotic cell division, the number of chromosomes remains constant for each daughter cell. In contrast, a property of meiotic cell division is the reduction in the number of chromosomes from the diploid number in the germline to the haploid number in gametes (from 46 to 23 in humans). To accomplish this reduction, two successive rounds of meiotic division occur. The first division is a reduction division in which the chromosome number is reduced by one half, and it is accomplished by the pairing of homologous chromosomes. The second meiotic division is similar to most mitotic divisions, except the total number of chromosomes is haploid rather than diploid. The haploid number is found only in the germline; thus, after fertilization the diploid chromosome number is restored. The selection of chromosomes from each homologous pair in the haploid cell is completely random, thereby ensuring genetic variability in each germ cell. In addition, recombination occurs during the initial stages of chromosome pairing during the first phase of meiosis, providing an additional layer of genetic diversity in each of the gametes.

STAGES OF MEIOSIS

Figure 1-7 depicts the stages of meiosis. DNA synthesis has already occurred before the first meiotic division and does not occur again during the two stages of meiotic division. A major feature of *meiotic*

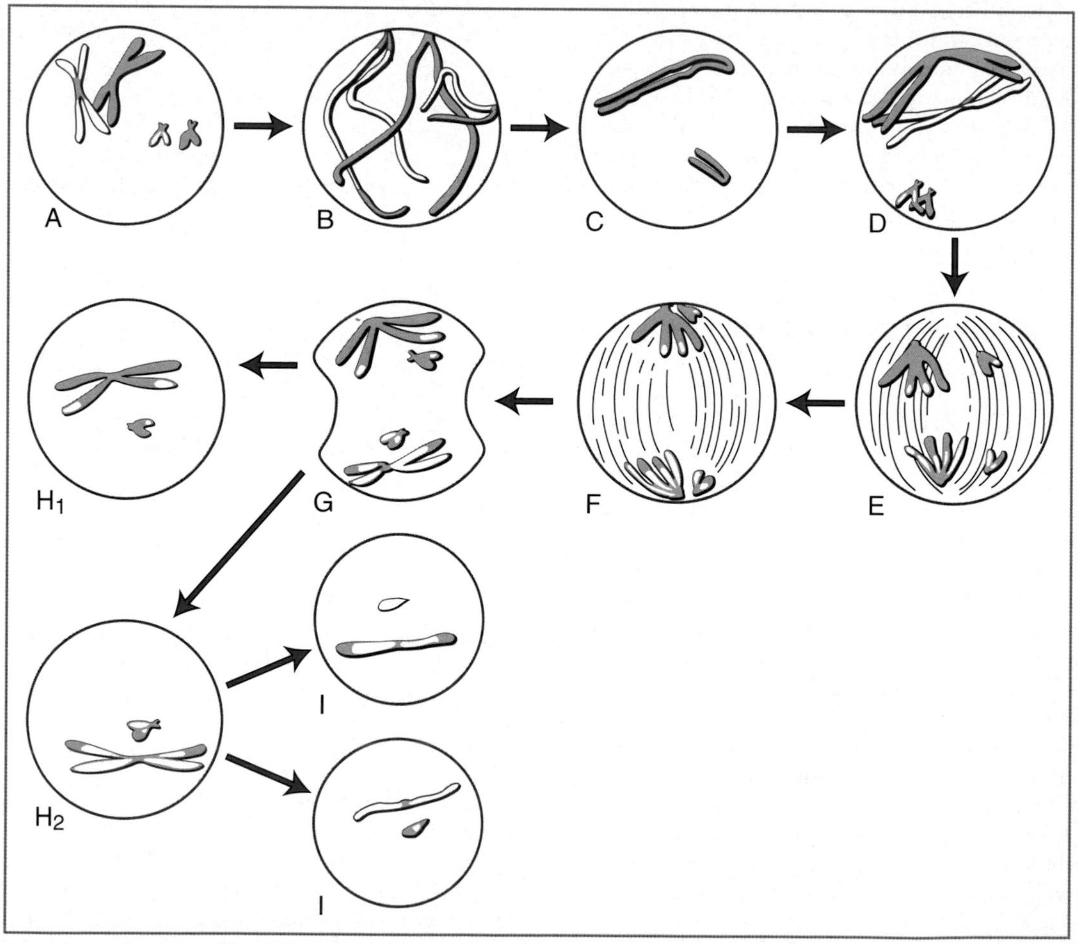

FIGURE 1-7 The stages of meiosis. Paternal chromosomes are *green;* maternal chromosomes are *white.* **A,** Condensed chromosomes in mitosis. **B,** Leptotene. **C,** Zygotene. **D,** Diplotene with crossing over. **E,** Diakinesis, anaphase I. **F,** Anaphase I. **G,** Telophase I. **H₁** and **H₂,** Metaphase II. **I,** Resolution of telophase II produces two haploid gametes. (From Vogel F, Motulsky AG: Human Genetics: Problems and Approaches. New York, Springer-Verlag, 1979.)

division I is the pairing of homologous chromosomes at homologous regions during prophase I; this is a complex stage in which many tasks are accomplished, and it can be subdivided into substages based on morphology of meiotic chromosomes. These stages are termed *leptonema, zygonema, pachynema, diplonema,* and *diakinesis.* Condensation and pairing occur during leptonema and zygonema (see Fig. 1-7C,D). The paired homologous chromosome regions are connected at a double-structured region, the *synaptonemal complex,* during pachynema. In diplonema, four chromatids of each kind are seen in close approximation side by side (see Fig. 1-7D). Nonsister chromatids become separated, whereas the sister chromatids remain paired; the chromatid crossings *(chiasmata)* between nonsister chromatids can be seen (see Fig. 1-7D). The chiasmata are believed to be sites of recombination. The chromosomes separate at diakinesis (see Fig. 1-7E). The chromosomes now enter meiotic metaphase I and telophase I (see Fig. 1-7F,G).

Meiotic division II is essentially a mitotic division of a fully copied set of haploid chromosomes. From each meiotic metaphase II, two daughter cells are formed (see Fig. 1-7H_1 and H_2), and a random assortment of DNA along the chromosome is accomplished at division (see Fig. 1-7I). After meiosis II, the genetic material is distributed to four cells as haploid chromosomes (23 in each cell). In addition to random crossing over, there is also random distribution of nonhomologous chromosomes to each of the final four haploid daughter cells. For these 23 chromosomes, the number of possible combinations in a single germ cell is 2^{23}, or 8,388,608. Thus $2^{23} \times 2^{23}$ equals the number of possible genotypes in the children of any particular combination of parents. This impressive number of variable genotypes is further enhanced by crossing over during prophase I of meiosis. Chiasma formation occurs during pairing and may be essential to this process, because there appears to be at least one chiasma per chromosome arm. A chiasma appears to be a point of crossover between two nonsister chromatids that occurs through breakage and reunion of nonsister chromatids at homologous points (Fig. 1-8).

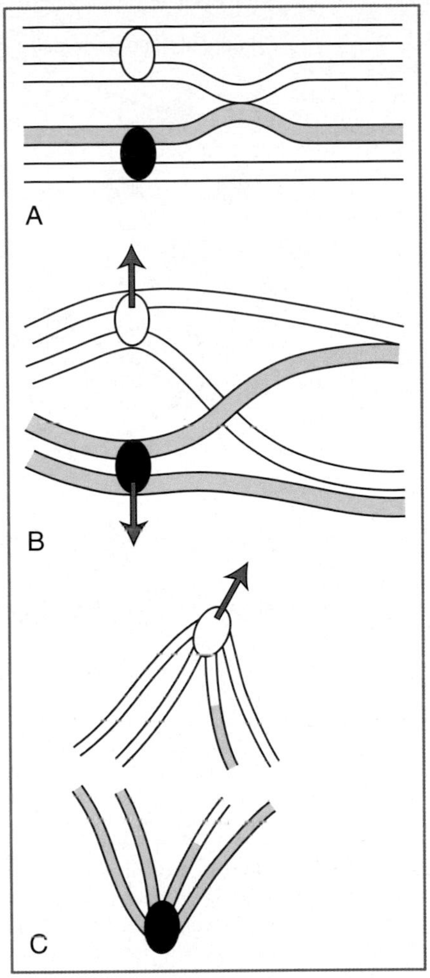

FIGURE 1-8 Crossing over and chiasma formation. **A,** Homologous chromatids are attached to each other. **B,** Crossing over with chiasma occurs. **C,** Chromatid separation occurs. (From Vogel F, Motulsky AG: Human Genetics: Problems and Approaches. New York, Springer-Verlag, 1979.)

SEX DIFFERENCES IN MEIOSIS

There are crucial distinctions between the two sexes in meiosis.

Males. In the male, meiosis is continuous in spermatocytes from puberty through adult life. After meiosis II, sperm cells acquire the ability to move effectively. The primordial fetal germ cells that produce oogonia in the female give rise to gonocytes at the same time in the male fetus. In these gonocytes, the tubules produce Ad (dark) spermatogonia (Fig. 1-9). During the middle of the second decade of life in males, spermatogenesis is fully established. At this point, the number of Ad spermatogonia is approximately 4.3 to 6.4×10^8 per testis. Ad spermatogonia undergo continuous divisions. During a given division, one cell may produce two Ad cells, whereas another produces two Ap (pale) cells. These Ap cells develop into B spermatogonia and hence into spermatocytes that undergo meiosis (see Fig. 1-9). Primary spermatocytes are in meiosis I, whereas secondary spermatocytes are in meiosis II. Vogel and Rathenberg[8] calculated approximations of the number of cell divisions according to age. On the basis of these approximations, it can be estimated further that from embryonic age to 28 years, the number of cell divisions of human sperm is approximately 15 times greater than the number of cell divisions in the life history of an oocyte.

Females. In the primitive gonad destined to become female, the number of ovarian stem cells increases rapidly by mitotic cell division. Between the 2nd and 3rd months of fetal life, oocytes begin to enter meiosis (Fig. 1-10). By the time of birth, mitosis in the female germ cells is finished and only the two meiotic divisions remain to be fulfilled. After birth, all oogonia are either transformed into oocytes or they degenerate. Fetal germ cells increase from 6×10^5 at 2 months' gestation to 6.8×10^6 during the 5th month. Decline begins at this time, to about 2×10^6 at birth. Meiosis remains arrested in the viable oocytes until puberty. At puberty, some oocytes start the division process again. An individual follicle matures at the time of ovulation. At the completion of meiosis I, one of the cells becomes the secondary oocyte, accumulating most of the cytoplasm and organelles, whereas the other cell becomes the first polar body. The maturing secondary oocyte completes meiotic metaphase II at the time of ovulation. If fertilization occurs, meiosis II in the oocyte is completed, with the formation of the second polar body. Only about 400 oocytes eventually mature during the reproductive lifetime of a woman, whereas the rest degenerate. In the female, only one of the four meiotic products develops into a mature oocyte; the other three become polar bodies that usually are not fertilized.

There are, then, three basic differences in meiosis between males and females:

1. In females, one division product becomes a mature germ cell and three become polar bodies. In the male, all four meiotic products become mature germ cells.

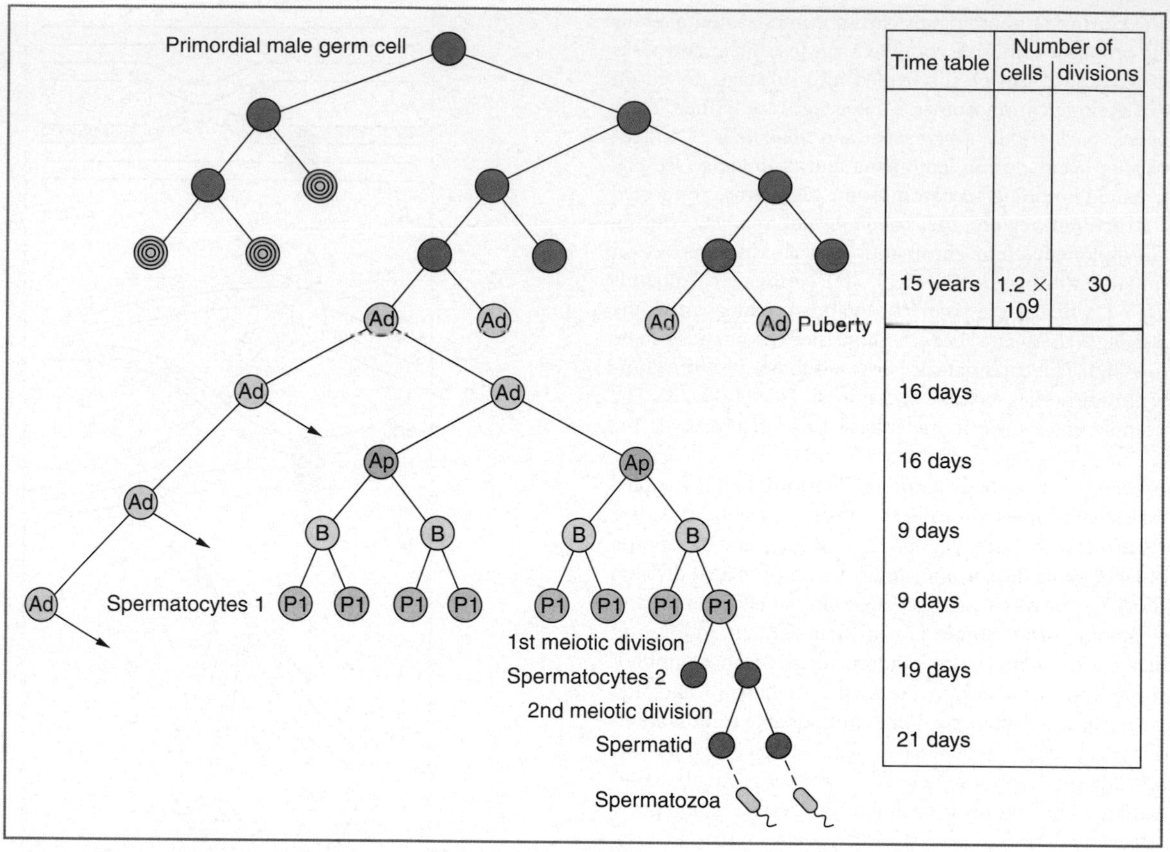

FIGURE 1-9 **Cell divisions during spermatogenesis.** The overall number of cell divisions is much higher than in oogenesis. It increases with advancing age. Ad, dark spermatogonia; Ap, pale spermatogonia; B, spermatogonia; P1, spermatocytes. *Concentric circles* indicate cell atrophy. (From Vogel F, Motulsky AG: Human Genetics: Problems and Approaches. New York, Springer-Verlag, 1979.)

2. In females, a low number of embryonic mitotic cell divisions occurs very early, followed by early embryonic meiotic cell division that continues to occur up to around the 9th month of gestation; division is then arrested for many years, commences again at puberty, and is completed only after fertilization. In the male, there is a much longer period of mitotic cell division, followed immediately by meiosis at puberty; meiosis is completed when spermatids develop into mature sperm.
3. In females, very few gametes are produced, and only one at a time, whereas in males, a large number of gametes are produced virtually continuously.

FERTILIZATION

The chromosomes of the egg and sperm are segregated after fertilization into the pronuclei, and each is surrounded by a nuclear membrane. The DNA of the diploid zygote replicates soon after fertilization, and after division two diploid daughter cells are formed, initiating embryonic development.

CLINICAL SIGNIFICANCE OF MITOSIS AND MEIOSIS

The proper segregation of chromosomes during meiosis and mitosis ensures that the progeny cells contain the appropriate genetic instructions. When errors occur in either process, the result is that an individual or cell lineage contains an abnormal number of chromosomes and an unbalanced genetic complement. Meiotic nondisjunction, occurring primarily during oogenesis, is responsible for chromosomally abnormal fetuses in several percent of recognized pregnancies. Mitotic nondisjunction can occur during tumor formation. In addition, if it occurs early after fertilization, it may result in chromosomally unbalanced embryos or mosaicism that may result in birth defects and mental retardation.

Analysis of Human Chromosomes

The era of clinical human cytogenetics began just about 50 years ago with the discovery that somatic cells in humans contain 46 chromosomes. The use of a simple procedure—hypotonic treatment for spreading the chromosomes of individual cells—enabled medical scientists and physicians to microscopically examine and study chromosomes in single cells rather than in tissue sections. Between 1956 and 1959, it was recognized that visible changes in the number or structure of chromosomes could result in a number of birth defects, such as Down syndrome (trisomy 21), Turner syndrome (45,XO), and Klinefelter syndrome (47,XXY). Chromosome disorders represent a large proportion of fetal loss, congenital defects, and mental retardation. In the practice of obstetrics and gynecology, clinical indications for chromosome analysis include abnormal phenotype in a newborn infant, unexplained first-trimester spontaneous abortion with no fetal karyotype, pregnancy resulting in stillborn or neonatal death, fertility problems, and pregnancy in women of advanced age.[9,10]

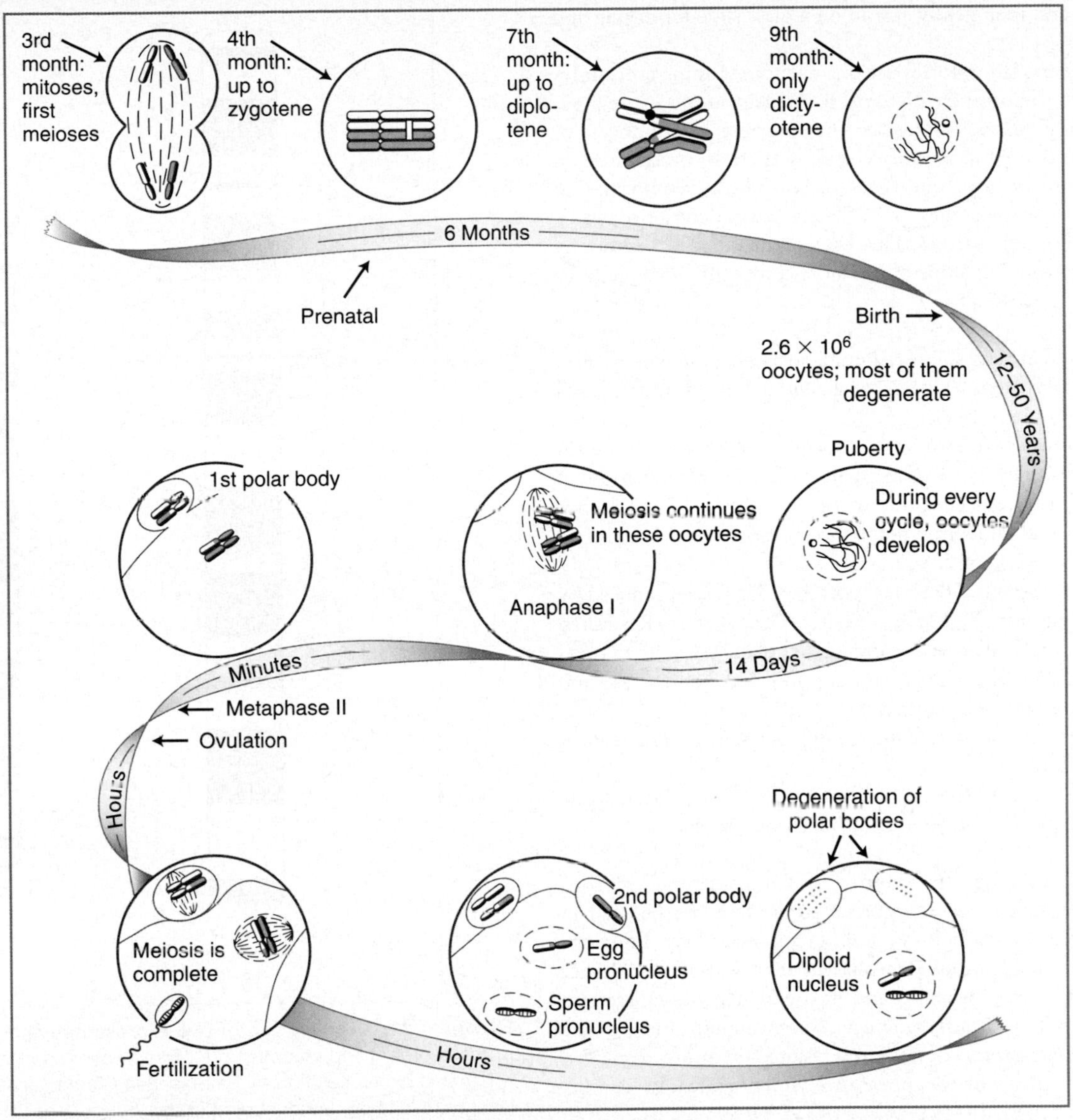

FIGURE 1-10 Meiosis in the human female. Meiosis starts after 3 months of development. During childhood, the cytoplasm of oocytes increases in volume, but the nucleus remains unchanged. About 90% of all oocytes degenerate at the onset of puberty. During the first half of every month, the luteinizing hormone of the pituitary stimulates meiosis, which is now almost completed (end of the prophase that began during embryonic stage; metaphase I, anaphase I, telophase I, and—within a few minutes—prophase II and metaphase II). Then meiosis stops again. A few hours after metaphase I is reached, ovulation is induced by luteinizing hormone. Fertilization occurs in the fallopian tube, and then the second meiotic division is complete. Nuclear membranes are formed around the maternal and paternal chromosomes. After some hours, the two "pronuclei" fuse and the first cleavage division begins. (From Bresch C, Haussmann R: Klassiche und Moleculare Genetik, 3rd ed. Berlin, Springer-Verlag, 1972.)

Preparation of Human Metaphase Chromosomes

Metaphase chromosomes can be prepared from any cell undergoing mitosis. Clinical and research cytogenetic laboratories routinely perform chromosome analysis on cells derived from peripheral blood, bone marrow, amniotic fluid, skin, or other tissues in situ and in tissue culture. For clinical cytogenetic diagnosis in living nonleukemic individuals, it is easiest to obtain metaphase cells from peripheral blood samples. To obtain adequate numbers of metaphase cells from peripheral blood, mitosis must be induced artificially, and in most procedures, *phytohemagglutinin,* a mitogen, is used for this purpose.

Specifically, T-cell lymphocytes are induced to undergo mitosis; thus, almost all chromosome analyses of human peripheral blood samples produce karyotypes of T lymphocytes. In general descriptive terms, a suspension of peripheral blood cells is incubated at 37°C in tissue culture media with mitogen for 72 hours to produce an actively dividing population of cells. The cells are then incubated for 1 to 3 hours in a dilute solution of a mitotic spindle poison such as colchicine to stop the cells in metaphase when chromosomes are condensed. Next, the nuclei containing the chromosomes are made fragile by swelling in a short treatment (10 to 30 minutes) in a hypotonic salt solution. The chromosomes are fixed in a mixture of alcohol and acetic acid and then gently spread on a glass slide for drying and staining.

Most cytogenetic laboratories use one or more staining procedures that stain each chromosome with variable intensity at specific regions, thereby providing "bands" along the chromosome; hence, the term *banding patterns* is used to identify chromosomes. All procedures are effective and provide different types of morphologic information about individual chromosomes. For convenience in descriptive terminology, various banding patterns have been named for the methods by which they were revealed. Some of the more commonly used methods are as follows:

1. *G bands* are revealed by Giemsa staining in association with various other secondary steps. This is probably the most widely used banding technique.
2. Quinacrine mustard and similar fluorochromes provide fluorescent staining for *Q bands*. The banding patterns are identical to those in G bands, but a fluorescence microscope is required. Q banding is particularly useful for identifying the Y chromosomes in both metaphase and interphase cells.
3. *R bands* are the result of "reverse" banding. They are produced by controlled denaturation, usually with heat. The pattern in R banding is opposite to that in G and Q banding; light bands produced on G and Q banding are dark on R banding, and dark bands on G and Q banding are light on R banding.
4. *T bands* are the result of specific staining of the telomeric regions of the chromosome.
5. *C bands* reflect constitutive heterochromatin and are located primarily on the pericentric regions of the chromosome.

Modifications and new procedures of band staining are constantly being developed. For example, a silver stain can be used to identify specifically the nucleolus organizer regions that were functionally active during the previous interphase. Other techniques enhance underlying chromosome instability and are useful in identifying certain aberrations associated with malignancies. Recent modifications of the basic culture-staining procedures have resulted in more elongated chromosomes, prophase-like in appearance, with more readily identifiable banding patterns.

Figure 1-11 depicts an ideogram of G banding in two normal chromosomes. Starting from the centromeric region, each chromosome is organized into two regions: the p region *(short arm)* and the q region *(long arm)*. Within each region, the area is further subdivided numerically. These numerical band designations greatly facilitate the descriptive identification of specific chromosomes. A complete male karyogram is depicted in Figure 1-12. A female karyogram would have two X chromosomes.

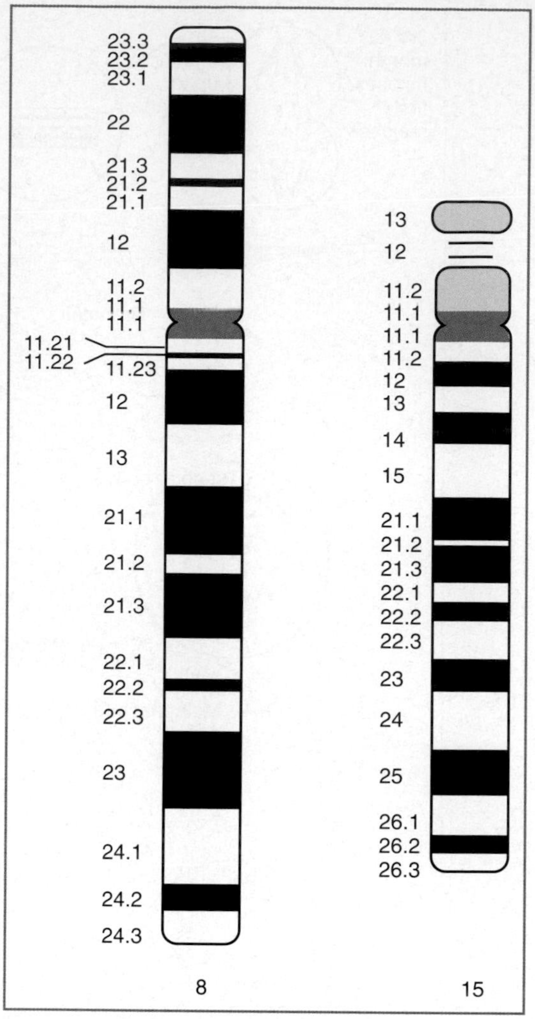

FIGURE 1-11 An ideogram of two representative chromosomes. Chromosome 8 and chromosome 15 represent arbitrary examples of schematic high-resolution mid-metaphase Giemsa banding. At the level of resolution demonstrated in this figure, a haploid set of 23 chromosomes has a combined total of approximately 550 bands. Light red areas represent the centromere, and the blue and white areas represent regions of variable size and staining intensity. The green area at the end of chromosome 15 is satellite DNA. A detailed ideogram of the entire human haploid set of chromosomes was published by the Standing Committee on Human Cytogenetic Nomenclature. (ISCN: Report of the Standing Committee on Human Cytogenetic Nomenclature. Basel, Karger, 1995.)

Molecular Cytogenetics: Fluorescence In Situ Hybridization and Multicolor Karyotyping

Besides routine karyotyping methods, more specific and sophisticated techniques have been developed that make use of fluorescence techniques and specific DNA sequences isolated by molecular biologic techniques. These techniques allow the evaluation of a chromosomal preparation for gain or loss of specific genes or chromosome regions and for the presence of translocations. In fluorescence in situ hybridization (FISH), DNA probes representing specific genes, chromosomal regions, and even whole chromosomes can be labeled with fluorescently tagged nucleotides. After hybridization to metaphase or interphase preparations of chromosomes (or both), these probes will specifically bind to the gene, region, or chromosome of interest (Fig. 1-13). This technique facilitates the detection of fine details of chromosome structure. For example, any single-copy gene is normally present in two copies in a diploid cell, one copy on each homologous chromosome. If one of the genes is missing in certain disease states, then only one copy will be detected by FISH with a probe specific for that gene. If the gene is present in numerous copies, as often occurs with certain oncogenes in tumors, multiple copies will be detected.

Similarly, entire chromosomes can be isolated by flow cytometry and probes prepared by labeling the entire chromosomal DNA complement (called a *chromosome paint probe*). When hybridized under appropriate conditions to metaphase or interphase preparations of chromosomes (or both), these probes will specifically detect the chromosome of interest. A translocation that occurs between two chromosomes can be easily detected with a chromosomal paint probe to one

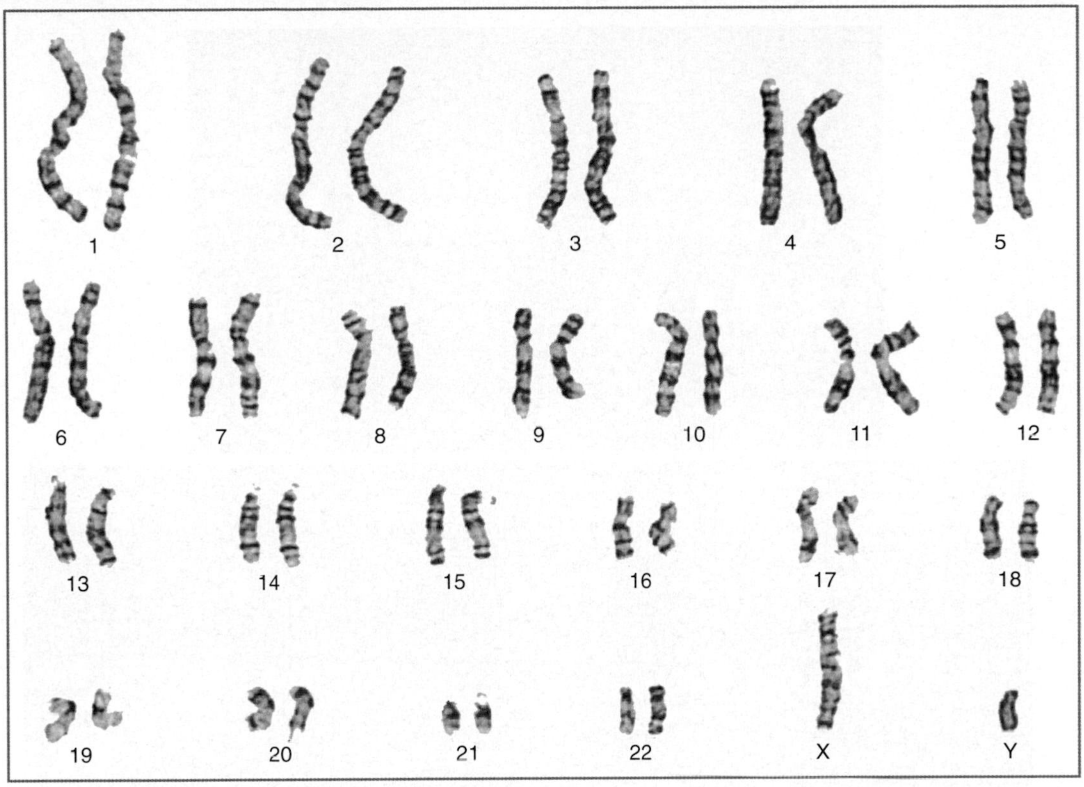

FIGURE 1-12 **A standard G-banded karyogram.** There is a total of approximately 550 bands in one haploid set of chromosomes in this karyogram. The sex karyotype is XY (male). A female karyogram would show two X chromosomes.

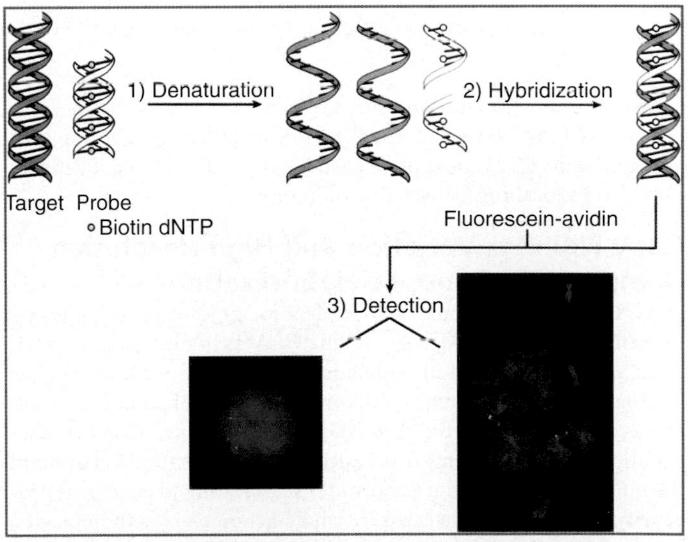

FIGURE 1-13 **A schematic representation of fluorescence in situ hybridization.** The DNA target (chromosome) and a short DNA fragment "probe" containing a nucleotide (e.g., deoxyribonucleotide triphosphate [dNTP]) labeled with biotin are denatured. The probe is specific for a chromosomal region containing the gene or genes of interest. During renaturation, some of the DNA molecules containing the region of interest hybridize with complementary nucleotide sequences in the probe, and with subsequent binding to a fluorochrome marker (fluorescein-avidin) a signal *(yellow-green)* is produced. The two lower panels demonstrate a metaphase cell and an interphase cell. The probe used is specific for chromosome 7. A control probe for band q36 on the long arm establishes the presence of two number 7 chromosomes. The second probe is specific for the Williams syndrome region at band 7q11.23. This signal is more intense and demonstrates no deletion at region 7q11.23 and essentially excludes the diagnosis of Williams syndrome. The signals are easily visible in both the metaphase and interphase cells.

of the translocation partners. Normally, this probe would identify two diploid chromosomes, and the entire length of each chromosome will be fluorescent. In contrast, the paint probe will identify a normal completely labeled chromosome and two new incompletely labeled chromosomes, representing the translocated fragments.

Recently, an extension of this methodology has been developed that is useful for the fluorescent detection and analysis of all chromosomes simultaneously. One such method is called *spectral karyotyping* (Fig. 1-14). A large number of fluorescent tags are available that can be used individually or in combination to prepare labeled chromosomes. It is possible to individually label each chromosome with unique combinations of these tags so that each one will emit a unique fluorescent signal when hybridized to chromosomal preparations. If all uniquely labeled chromosomal paint probes are mixed and hybridized to metaphase preparations simultaneously, each chromosome will emit a unique wavelength of light. These different wavelengths can be detected by a microscope-mounted spectrophotometer linked to a high-resolution camera. Sophisticated image analysis programs can then distinguish individual chromosomes, and a metaphase spread will appear as a multicolored array (see Fig. 1-14). With knowledge of the expected

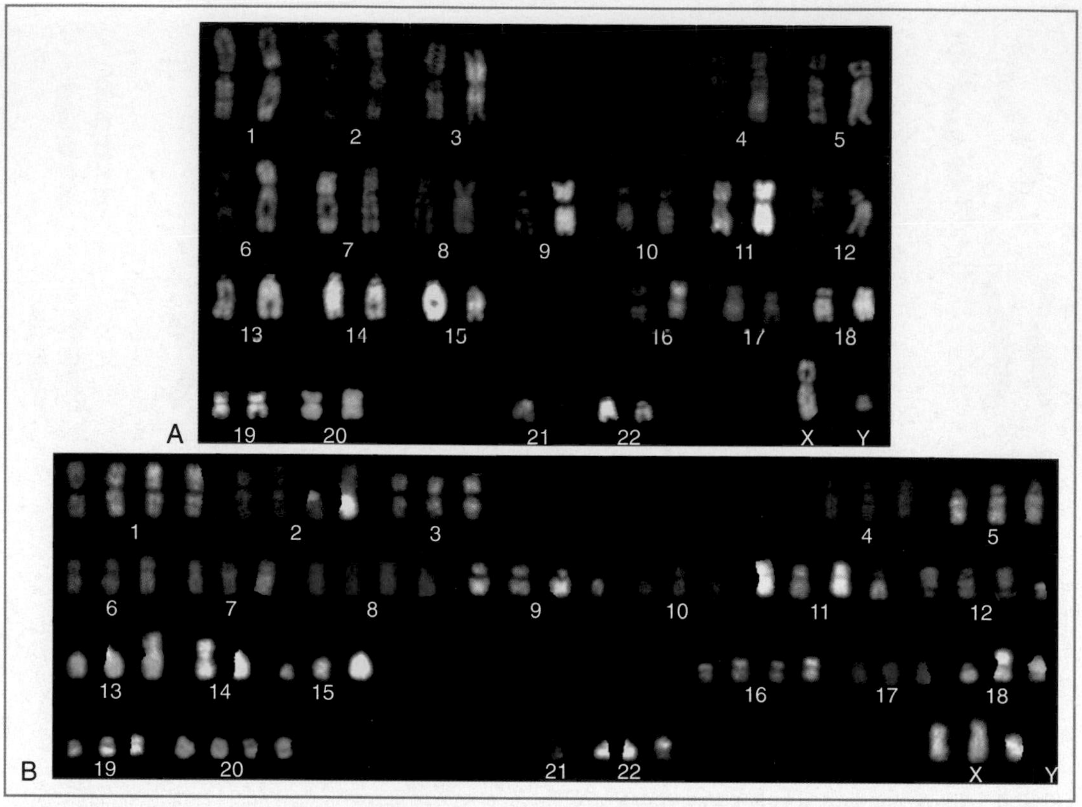

FIGURE 1-14 Spectral karyotyping (SKY). **A,** A normal human karyotype after SKY analysis, showing the presence of two copies of each chromosome, each pair with a different color. In addition, the X and Y chromosomes are different colors. **B,** SKY analysis of a tumor cell line, displaying extra copies of nearly all chromosomes, as well as translocations. These can be appreciated as chromosomes consisting of two colors. (Photos courtesy of Dr. Karen Arden, Ludwig Cancer Institute, UCSD School of Medicine.)

emission from each chromosome, the signal from each chromosome can be specifically identified, and the entire metaphase can be displayed as a karyogram. This method is particularly useful for the identification of translocations between chromosomes.

Copy Number Variation and High-Resolution Comparative Genomic Hybridization

Once the human genome was sequenced, producing an "average" human genome, the next phase of analysis was to find genome variations in individuals and in populations. One of the most remarkable findings was that individuals differ in the number of copies they have of pieces of DNA scattered throughout their genome.[5] Copy number variation (CNV) is the most prevalent type of structural variation in the human genome, and it contributes significantly to genetic heterogeneity. CNVs can be detected by whole-genome-array technologies, often referred to as *high-resolution comparative genomic hybridization* (hCGH), and careful measurement of intensities of hybridization to these arrays can provide a measure of regional duplication and deletion. Some of these CNVs are common in populations, but the extent of common CNVs has been difficult to estimate. Several array platforms were used in the early studies, making it difficult to compare one study with another. Also, more population studies and reference databases for control populations and populations with certain diseases are needed to determine the association between CNV frequency and disease. Some CNVs can contribute to human phenotype, including rare genomic disorders and mendelian diseases. Other CNVs are likely to be found to influence human phenotypic diversity and disease susceptibility. This is an active area of research that will very likely lead to findings with clinical importance in the near future.

Characteristics of the More Common Chromosome Aberrations in Humans

Abnormalities in Chromosome Number

Alteration of the number of chromosomes is called *heteroploidy*. A heteroploid individual is *euploid* if the number of chromosomes is a multiple of the haploid number of 23, and *aneuploid* if there is any other number of chromosomes. Abnormalities of single chromosomes are usually caused by nondisjunction or anaphase lag, whereas whole-genome abnormalities are referred to as *polyploidization.*

ANEUPLOIDY

Aneuploidy is the most frequently seen chromosome abnormality in clinical cytogenetics, occurring in 3% to 4% of clinically recognized pregnancies. Aneuploidy occurs during both meiosis and mitosis. The most significant cause of aneuploidy is *nondisjunction*, which may occur in both mitosis and meiosis but is observed more frequently in meiosis. One pair of chromosomes fails to separate (disjoin) and is transferred in anaphase to one pole. Meiotic nondisjunction can occur in meiosis I or II. The result is that one product will have both members of the pair and one will have neither of that pair (Fig. 1-15). After fertilization, the embryo will either contain an extra third chro-

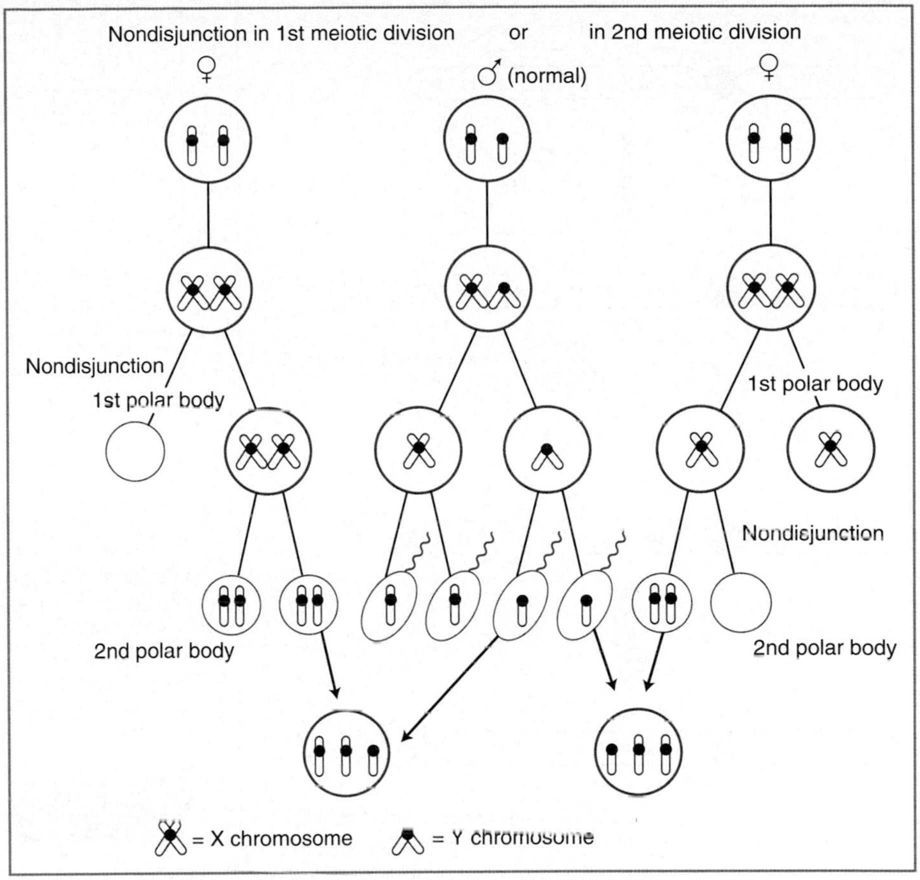

FIGURE 1-15 Nondisjunction of the X chromosome in the first and second meiotic divisions in a female. Fertilization is by a Y-bearing sperm. An XXY genotype and phenotype can result from both first and second meiotic division nondisjunction. (From Vogel F, Motulsky AG: Human Genetics: Problems and Approaches. New York, Springer-Verlag, 1979.)

mosome (trisomy) or have only one of the normal chromosome pair (monosomy).

Anaphase lag is another event that can lead to abnormalities in chromosome number. In this process, one chromosome of a pair does not move as rapidly during the anaphase process as its sister chromosome and is lost. Often this loss leads to a mosaic cell population, one euploid and one monosomic (e.g., 45,XO/46,XX mosaicism).

POLYPLOIDY

In affected fetuses that are polyploid, the whole genome is present more than once in every cell. When the increase is by a factor of one for each cell, the result is *triploidy,* with 69 chromosomes per cell. Triploidy is most often caused by fertilization of a single egg with two sperm, but rarely it results from the duplication of chromosomes during meiosis without division.

Alterations of Chromosome Structure

Structural alterations in chromosomes constitute the other major group of cytogenetic abnormalities. Such defects are seen less frequently in newborns than numerical defects and occur in about 0.0025% of newborns. However, chromosome rearrangements are a common occurrence in malignancies. Structural rearrangements are balanced if there is no net loss or gain of chromosomal material, or unbalanced if there is an abnormal genetic complement.

DELETIONS AND DUPLICATIONS

Deletions refer to the loss of a chromosome segment. Deletions may occur on the terminal segment of the short or long arm. Alternatively, an interstitial deletion may occur anywhere on the chromosome. Deletions can result from chromosomal breakage and when loss of the deleted fragment lacks a centromere (Fig. 1-16), or from unequal crossover between homologous chromosomes. One of the chromosomes carries a deletion, whereas the other reciprocal event is a duplication. A *ring chromosome* results from terminal deletions on both the short and long arms of the same chromosome (Fig. 1-17).

Autosomal Deletion and Duplication Syndromes

Autosomal deletions and duplications are often associated with clinically evident birth defects or milder dysmorphisms. Often the chromosomal defect is unique to that individual, and it is difficult to provide prognostic information to the family. In a few cases, a number of patients with similar phenotypic abnormalities were found to display similar cytogenetic defects. Some of these are cytogenetically detectable, whereas others are smaller and require molecular cytogenetic techniques. These are termed microdeletion and microduplication syndromes and merely reflect the size of the deletion or duplication. Table 1-2 summarizes some of the deletion and duplication syndromes that have been described and for which commercial FISH probes are available.

INSERTIONS

In the process of insertion, an interstitial deleted segment is inserted into a nonhomologous chromosome (Fig. 1-18).

INVERSIONS

Inversions more often involve the centromere *(pericentric)* rather than noncentromeric areas *(paracentric).* Figure 1-19 is a diagram-

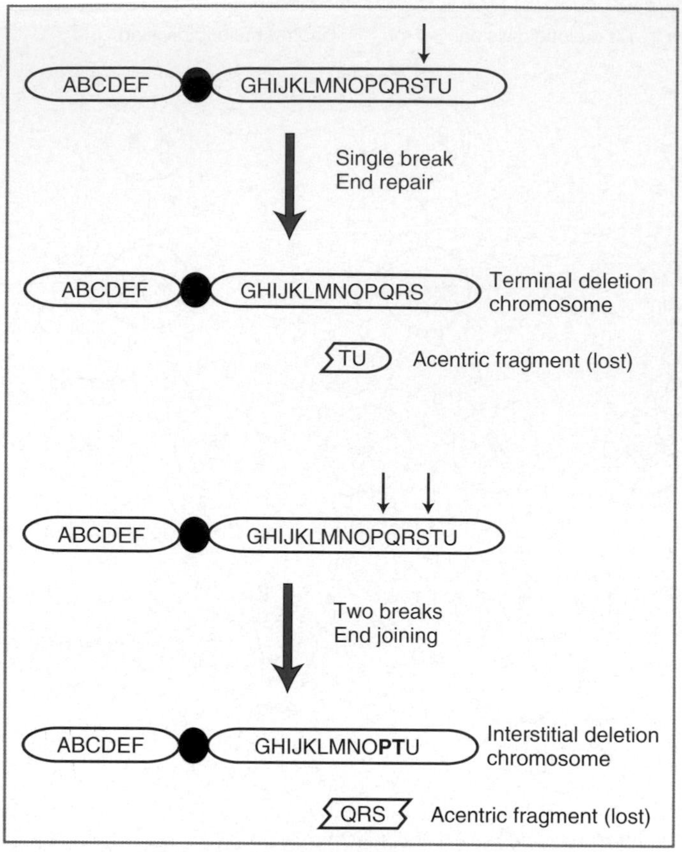

FIGURE 1-16 **Schematic representation of two kinds of deletion events.** A single double-strand break *(small black arrow)* may produce a terminal deletion if the end is repaired to retain telomere function. The telomeric fragment lacks a centromere (indicated by the *filled oval* in the intact chromosome) and will generally be lost in the next cell division. A chromosome with two double-strand breaks *(pair of black arrows)* may suffer an interstitial deletion if the break is repaired by end joining of the centromeric and telomeric fragments.

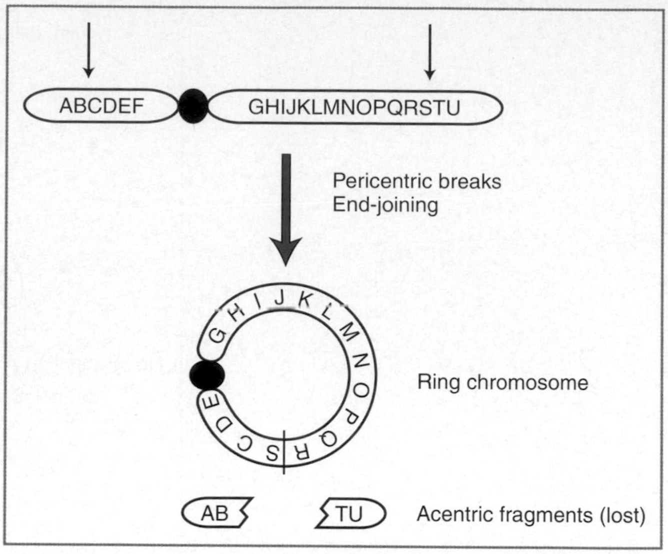

FIGURE 1-17 **Ring chromosome formation.** A chromosome with a double-strand break on each side of its centromere *(filled oval)* can result in terminal deletions (see Fig. 1-16), pericentric inversion, or formation of a ring chromosome by joining the two centromeric ends from the breaks. In the case of ring chromosome formation, the acentric fragments would be lost in the next cell division.

matic representation of a pericentric inversion. Inversions reduce pairing between homologous chromosomes, and crossing over may be suppressed within inverted heterozygote chromosomes. For homologous chromosomes to pair, one must form a loop in the region of the inversion (Fig. 1-20). If the inversion is pericentric, the centromere lies within the loop. When crossing over occurs, each of the two chromatids within the crossover has both a duplication and a deletion. If gametes are formed with the abnormal chromosomes, the fetus will be monosomic for one portion of the chromosome and trisomic for another portion. One result of abnormal chromosome recombinants might be increased fetal demise from duplication or deficiency of a chromosomal region.

When pericentric inversion occurs as a new mutation, usually the result is a phenotypically normal individual. However, when a carrier of a pericentric inversion reproduces, the pairing events just described may occur. If fertilization involves the abnormal gametes, there is a risk for abnormal progeny. When pericentric inversion is observed in a phenotypically abnormal child, parental karyotyping is indicated.

An exception to this rule involves a pericentric inversion in chromosome 9, the most common inversion noted in humans. The frequency of this inversion has been observed to be approximately 5% in 14,000 amniotic fluid cultures. In the 30 or so instances in which parental karyotyping was performed, invariably one or the other parent carried a pericentric inversion on one number 9 chromosome. One explanation for the apparently benign status of pericentric inversion in this chromosome is that the pericentric region on chromosome 9 contains many highly repetitive or genetically silent regions in the nucleotide sequence, so that inversion in this region is of no clinical consequence. Another explanation could be that inversions involving relatively short DNA sequences may not be involved in crossing over.

TABLE 1-2 DIAGNOSIS OF MICRODELETION SYNDROMES

Syndrome	Chromosome Band	Chromosome Defect
Alagille	20p12.1-p11.23	Deletion
Angelman	15q11-q13	Deletion (maternal genes)
Cri du chat	5p15.2-p15.3	Deletion
DiGeorge*	22q11.21-q11.23	Deletion
Miller-Dieker	17p13.3	Deletion
Prader-Willi	15q11-q13	Deletion (paternal genes)
Rubenstein-Taybi	16p13.3	Deletion
Smith-Magenis	17p11.2	Deletion
WAGR	11p13	Deletion
Williams	7q11.23	Deletion
Wolf-Hirschhorn	4p16.3	Deletion

***Patients with velocardiofacial (Shprintzen [catch 22] syndrome) also have deletions at 22q11.21-q11.23.**
WAGR, Wilms tumor, aniridia, genital anomalies, growth retardation.

TRANSLOCATIONS

A translocation is the most common form of chromosome structural rearrangement in humans. There are two types: *reciprocal* (Fig. 1-21) and *robertsonian* (Fig. 1-22).

Reciprocal Translocation. If a reciprocal translocation is balanced, phenotypic abnormalities are uncommon. Unbalanced translocations result in miscarriage, stillbirth, or live birth with multiple malformations, developmental delay, and mental retardation. Reciprocal translocations nearly always involve nonhomologous chromosomes among any of the 23 chromosome pairs, including chromosomes X and Y.

Gametogenesis in heterozygous carriers of translocations is especially significant because of the increased risk for chromosome segregation that produces gametes with unbalanced chromosomes in the diploid set (see Fig. 1-21). In a reciprocal translocation, there will be four chromosomes with segments in common (see Fig. 1-21). During meiosis, homologous segments must match for crossing over, so that in a translocation set of four, a *quadrivalent* is formed. During meiosis I, the four chromosomes may segregate randomly in two daughter cells with several results.

In 2:2 alternate segregation (see Fig. 1-21), one centromere segregates to one daughter cell and the next centromere segregates to the other daughter cell. This is the only mode that leads to a normal or balanced normal karyotype. Adjacent segregation and 3:1 nondisjunction segregation all produce unbalanced gametes.

If a gamete is chromosomally unbalanced, the odds are increased for spontaneous abortion. In familial translocations, the risk of unbalanced progeny seems to depend on the method of ascertainment. For example, if a familial reciprocal translocation is ascertained by a chromosomally unbalanced live birth or stillbirth, the risk for subsequent chromosomally unbalanced children is approximately 15% and the risk for spontaneous abortion or stillbirth is approximately 25%. In contrast, if the ascertainment is unbiased, risk for chromosomally unbalanced live birth is 1% to 2%, but the risk for miscarriage or stillbirth remains at 25%.

There appears to be a parental sex influence on the risk for chromosomally unbalanced progeny associated with certain types of segregants. In general, the risk for unbalanced progeny is higher if the female parent carries the translocation than it is with the paternal carrier. In addition, a viable conceptus is influenced by the type of configuration produced during meiosis by the translocated chromosomes. In general, larger translocated fragments and more asymmetrical pairing are associated with a greater likelihood for abnormal outcome of pregnancy.

Robertsonian Translocation. Robertsonian translocations involve only the *acrocentric* chromosome pairs 13, 14, 15, 21, and 22. They are joined end to end at the centromere and may be homologous (e.g., t21;21) or nonhomologous (e.g., t13;14). Robertsonian translocation is named for an insect cytogeneticist, W. R. B. Robertson, who in 1916 was the first to describe a translocation involving two acrocentric chromosomes. The robertsonian translocation is unique because the fusion of two acrocentric chromosomes usually involves the centromere (see Fig. 1-22) or regions close to the centromere. However, reciprocal translocations may also include acrocentric chromosomes.

Robertsonian translocations are nearly always nonhomologous. Most homologous robertsonian translocations produce nonviable conceptuses. For example, translocation 14;14 would result in either trisomy 14 or monosomy 14, and both are nonviable.

The most common nonhomologous robertsonian translocation in humans is 13;14. Approximately 80% of all nonhomologous robertsonian translocations involve chromosomes 13, 14, and 15. The next most common are translocations involving one chromosome from pairs 13, 14, and 15 and one chromosome from pairs 21 and 22.

Figure 1-23 illustrates gametogenesis in a nonhomologous 14;21 robertsonian translocation carrier and also represents the model for segregation during gametogenesis with any robertsonian translocation. Translocation carriers theoretically produce six types of gametes in equal proportions. Monosomic gametes are generally nonviable, as are many trisomies (e.g., trisomy 14 or 15). As illustrated, three gametes may result in viable conceptuses and one (B_1) may produce a liveborn abnormal infant.

Robertsonian translocation 14;21 is the most medically significant in terms of incidence and genetic risk. In contrast, the most

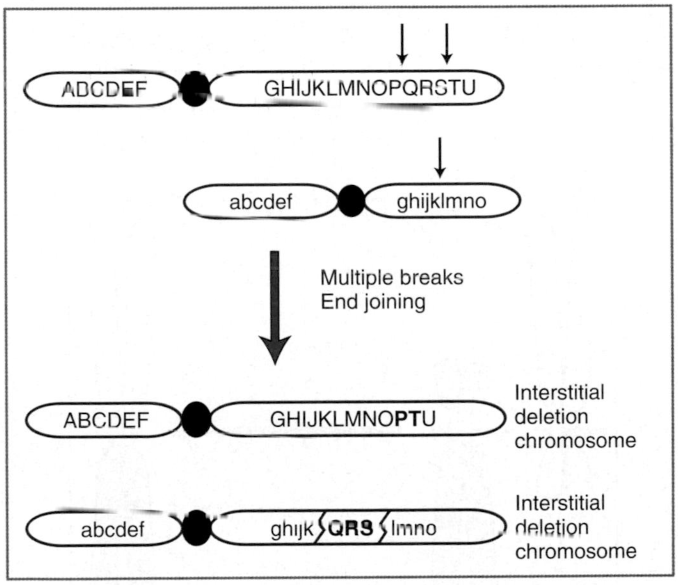

FIGURE 1-18 **Interstitial translocations.** Interstitial translocations can result from repair by end joining of fragments from nonhomologous chromosomes. In the example illustrated, a fragment QRS is liberated from one chromosome and inserted at a break between k and l in the recipient chromosome.

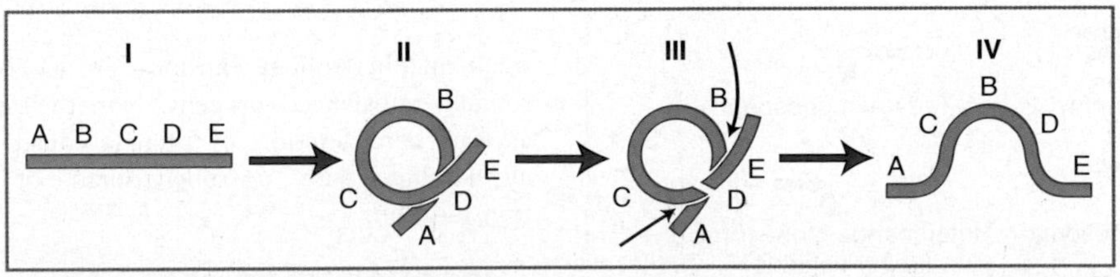

FIGURE 1-19 **An example of a possible mechanism for development of a pericentric inversion. I,** Normal sequence of coded information on the chromosome. **II,** Formation of a loop involving a chromosome region. **III,** Breakage and reunion at the *arrows,* where the chromosome loop intersects itself. **IV,** Formation of the inverted information sequence after reunion.

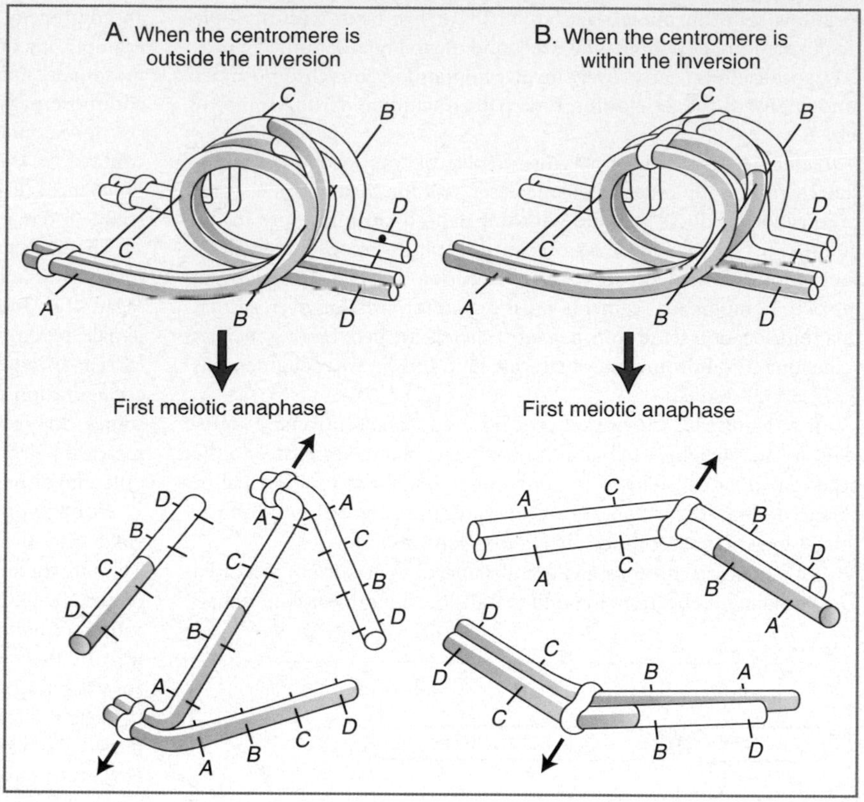

FIGURE 1-20 Inversions. Crossing over within the inversion loop of an inversion heterozygote results in aberrant chromatids with duplications or deficiencies. (From Srb AM, Owen RD, Edgar RS: General Genetics, 2nd ed. San Francisco, WH Freeman, 1965.)

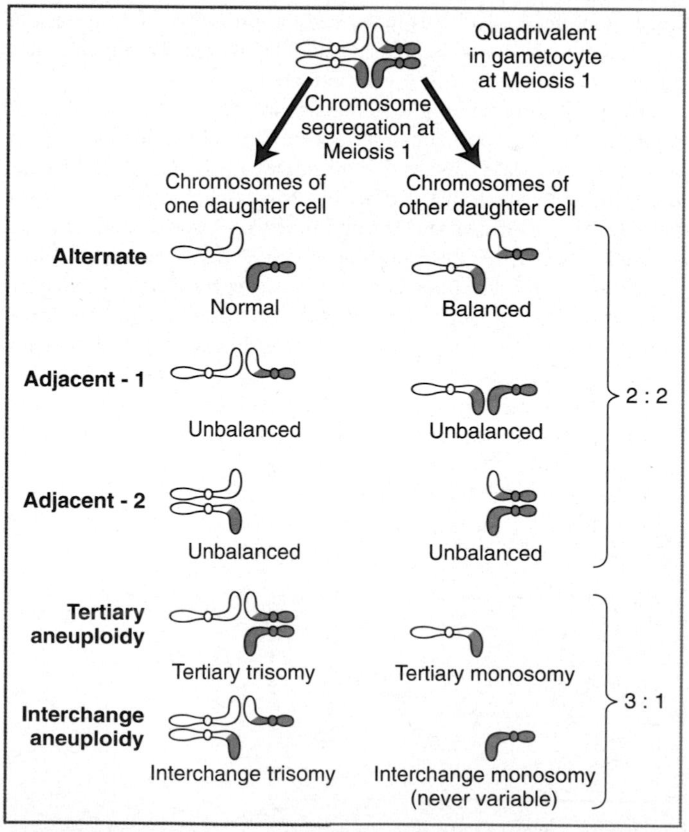

FIGURE 1-21 Chromosome segregation during meiosis in a reciprocal translocation heterozygote. (Modified from Gardner RJM, Sutherland GR: Chromosome Abnormalities and Genetic Counseling. New York, Oxford University Press, 1989.)

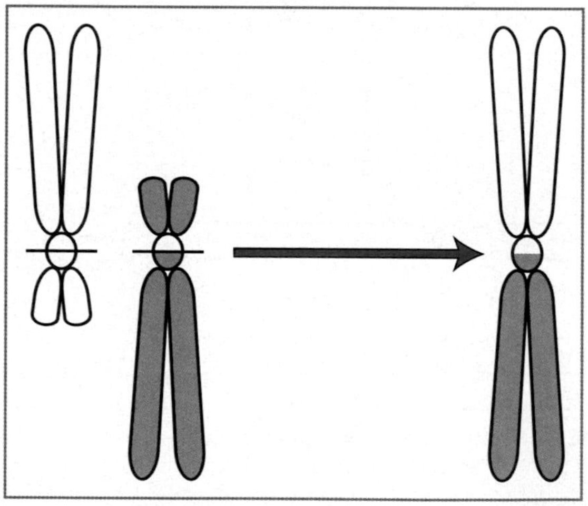

FIGURE 1-22 Formation of a centric fusion (monocentric) robertsonian translocation. Robertsonian translocations involve only the acrocentric chromosomes.

frequent robertsonian translocation, 13;14, rarely produces chromosomally unbalanced progeny. Nonetheless, genetic counseling and at least consideration of prenatal diagnosis is recommended for all families with a robertsonian or reciprocal chromosome translocation.

ISOCHROMOSOMES

An isochromosome is a structural rearrangement in which one arm of a chromosome is lost and the other arm is duplicated. The resulting chromosome is a mirror image of itself. Isochromosomes often involve the long arm of the X chromosome.

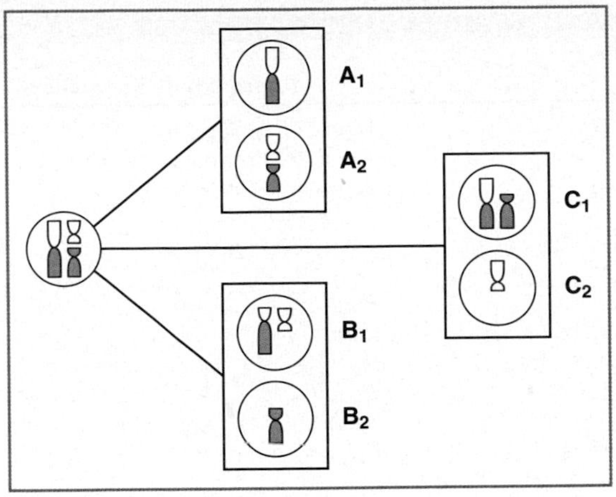

FIGURE 1-23 Gametogenesis for robertsonian translocation. A_1 is balanced with 22 chromosomes, including t(14q21q). A_2 is normal with 22 chromosomes. B_1 is abnormal with 23 chromosomes, including t(14q21q) and 21. This gamete would produce an infant with Down syndrome. B_2 is abnormal with 22 chromosomes and monosomy for chromosome 21. C_1 is abnormal with 23 chromosomes, including t(14q21q) and 14. C_2 is abnormal with 22 chromosomes and no chromosome 14.

Clinical and Biologic Considerations of the Sex Chromosomes

The X and Y chromosomes merit separate discussions. They have distinct patterns of inheritance and are structurally different. However, they pair in male meiosis because of the presence of the pseudoautosomal region at the ends of the short arms of the X and Y chromosomes. The pseudoautosomal region is the only region of homology between the X and Y chromosomes, and both pairing and recombination occur in this region.

The primitive gonad is undifferentiated, and phenotypic sex in humans is determined by the presence or absence of the Y chromosome. This is the case for two reasons. First, in the absence of the Y chromosome, the primitive gonad will differentiate into an ovary, and female genitalia will form. Thus, the female sex is the default sex. Second, the *SRY* gene, present on the Y chromosome, is necessary and sufficient for testis formation and for male external genitalia.

The X chromosome is present in two copies in females but only one copy in males. To equalize dosage (copy number) differences in critical genes on the X chromosomes between the two sexes, one of the X chromosomes is randomly inactivated in somatic cells of the female.[11] In addition, in cells with more than two X chromosomes, all but one of them are inactivated. This ensures that in any diploid cell, regardless of sex, only a single active X chromosome is present. X inactivation results in the complete inactivation of about 90% of the genes on the X chromosome. This is noteworthy because 10% of genes on the X chromosome escape *X inactivation.* Many of these are clustered on the short arm of X, so aneuploidies involving this region may have greater clinical significance than those on the long arm. X chromosome inactivation occurs because of the presence of an X inactivation center on Xq13 that contains a gene called *XIST* that is expressed on the allele of the inactive X chromosome. At the moment, the mechanism of action of *XIST* in X chromosome inactivation is unclear.

Although X inactivation is random in normal somatic cells, structural abnormalities of the X chromosome often result in nonrandom X inactivation. In general, when a structural abnormality involves only one X chromosome (i.e., deletion, isochromosome, ring chromosome), the abnormal X chromosome always appears to be the one inactivated.[10] If the structural abnormality is a translocation between part of one X chromosome and an autosome, the "normal" X seems to be the one genetically inactive. Although this pattern is not proven, it is assumed that if the X chromosome translocated to an autosome is genetically inactivated, part or all of that autosome might also become inactive, rendering that cell functionally monosomic for the autosome and thus nonviable. This phenomenon helps to explain why some females heterozygous for X-linked recessive biochemical disorders, such as Duchenne muscular dystrophy, have phenotypic expression of that disorder. In this instance, if the mutant X chromosome is the one involved in the X autosome translocation and the normal allele is inactive by virtue of being on the normal inactive X chromosome, it is likely that the female will express the disease.

Abnormalities of the sex chromosomes or genes on the sex chromosomes may affect any of the stages of sexual and reproductive development. Although an increased number of either the X or the Y chromosome enhances the likelihood of mental retardation and other anatomic anomalies, irrespective of the sex phenotype, aneuploidy of the sex chromosome does not alter prenatal fetal development nearly as much as aneuploidy of an autosome. Of note, many mutations or deletions in the X chromosome do result in X-linked mental retardation. Numeric and structural sex chromosome aneuploidies are summarized in Table 1-3, and we briefly describe only a few of the more common sex chromosome aberrations.

Turner Syndrome

Although Turner syndrome occurs in approximately 1 per 10,000 live born females, it is one of the chromosome abnormalities most commonly observed in studies of spontaneous abortuses. It is unknown why the same chromosomal defect usually results in spontaneous fetal loss but is also compatible with survival. It is often detected prenatally through ascertainment of a cystic hygroma by fetal ultrasound examination during the first or second trimester. Although there is wide variability in the phenotypic expression of Turner syndrome, it is one sex chromosome abnormality that should be identifiable by physical examination of the newborn.

Turner syndrome is associated with a 45,XO karyotype. Sex chromosome mosaics (such as 46,XX/45,XO) and structurally abnormal karyotypes (such as 46,X/delX and 46,X/isoX) are all phenotypic females like those with 45,XO Turner syndrome, but they have fewer of the typical manifestations associated with the 45,XO phenotype. The paternally derived X chromosome is more often missing in the 45,XO karyotype.

Some of the common features of the 45,XO phenotype and the frequencies with which they are seen are listed in Table 1-4. Mental retardation is not normally seen in this syndrome unless a small ring X chromosome is present. Although there is inadequate information at present to permit assessment of longevity and cause of death in adult life, the general health prognosis is good for childhood and young adult life with this phenotype. Renal anomalies, when present, rarely cause significant health problems, and when congenital heart disease is part of the phenotype, surgery is generally effective. The congenital lymphedema usually disappears during infancy, and when webbing of the neck poses a cosmetic problem, it can be corrected by plastic surgery. Short stature is a persistent problem. If a diagnosis is achieved early, height increase and external sexual development may be achieved with the collaboration of a knowledgeable endocrinologist. In particular, growth hormone therapy is standard and results in significant increases in adult height. Affected patients are nearly always sterile, and the

TABLE 1-3 NUMERIC AND STRUCTURAL X-CHROMOSOMAL ANEUPLOIDIES IN HUMANS

Karyotype	Phenotype	Approximate Frequency
XXY	Klinefelter syndrome	1 per 700 males
XXXY	Klinefelter variant	1 per 2500 males
XXXXY	Low-grade mental deficiency; severe sexual underdevelopment; radioulnar synostosis	Rare
XXX	Sometimes mild oligophrenia; occasionally disturbances of gonadal function	1 per 1000 females
XXXX	Growth retardation; severe mental retardation	Rare
XXXXX	Multiple physical defects; severe mental retardation	Rare
XXY/XY and XXY/XX mosaics	Klinefelter-like, sometimes milder in symptomatology	5% to 25% of all Klinefelter-like patients
XXX/XX mosaics	Like XXX	Rare
XO	Turner syndrome	1 per 2500 females at birth
XO/XX and XO/XXX mosaics	Like Turner syndrome, but very different degrees of manifestation	Not uncommon
Various structural anomalies of X chromosomes	—	Not uncommon
XYY	Increased stature; occasional behavioral abnormalities	1 per 800 males
XXYY	Increased stature; otherwise resembling Klinefelter syndrome	Rare

From Vogel F, Motulsky AG: Human Genetics: Problems and Approaches. New York, Springer-Verlag, 1979.

TABLE 1-4 45,XO PHENOTYPE: MAJOR FEATURES AND THEIR INCIDENCE

Feature	Incidence (%)
Small stature, often noted at birth	100
Ovarian dysgenesis with variable degree of hypoplasia of germinal elements	90+
Transient congenital lymphedema, especially notable over the dorsum of the hands and feet	80+
Shieldlike, broad chest with widely spaced, inverted, and/or hypoplastic nipples	80+
Prominent auricles	80+
Low posterior hairline, giving the appearance of a short neck	80+
Webbing of posterior neck	50
Anomalies of elbow, including cubitus valgus	70
Short metacarpal and/or metatarsal	50
Narrow, hyperconvex, and/or deepset nails	70
Renal anomalies	60+
Cardiac anomalies (coarctation of the aorta in 70% of cases)	20+
Perceptive hearing loss	50

emotional adjustment to this issue should be part of any medical management of gonadal dysgenesis.

When the diagnosis of 45,XO karyotype or a variant is missed during infancy or childhood, a complaint of persisting short stature or amenorrhea finally brings the patient to the physician. Often this delay precludes any specific therapy for the short stature. In rare variants of Turner syndrome, some cells may carry a Y chromosome, suggesting that such an individual was initially an X,Y male but the Y chromosome was lost. Occasionally, the Y chromosome line is found only in the germ cells, and the clinical manifestation in the individual may be virilization during adolescence or an unexplained growth spurt. In these cases, it is imperative to perform a gonadal biopsy for histologic and chromosome analysis. If a Y chromosome cell line is demonstrated in gonadal tissue, extirpation is indicated to prevent subsequent malignant transformation in gonadal cells.

Klinefelter Syndrome

Klinefelter syndrome, which occurs in approximately 1 per 700 to 1000 liveborn males, is associated with a 47,XXY karyotype. Major physical features of Klinefelter syndrome are as follows:

1. Relatively tall and slim body type, with relatively long limbs (especially the legs) is seen beginning in childhood.
2. Hypogonadism is seen at puberty, with small, soft testes and usually a small penis. Infertility is the rule. Gynecomastia is frequent, and cryptorchidism or hypospadias may be seen. Lack of virilization at puberty is common; indeed, it is often the reason for the patient to seek medical attention.
3. There is a tendency toward lower verbal comprehension and poorer performance on intelligence quotient tests, with learning disabilities a common feature. There is a higher incidence of behavioral and social problems, often requiring professional help.

There are several karyotypic variants of Klinefelter syndrome with more than two X chromosomes (such as the karyotype 48,XXXY). As the number of X chromosomes increases, there is a corresponding increase in the severity of the phenotype, with a greater incidence of mental retardation and with more physical abnormalities than in the typical syndrome. Approximately 15% of individuals with some of the Klinefelter phenotype have 47,XXY/46,XY mosaicism. Such mosaic individuals have more variable phenotypes and have a somewhat better prognosis for testicular function. In general, chromosome aneuploidies that include the Y chromosome are less likely to be diagnosed clinically during infancy or childhood. In fact, individuals are often first diagnosed during evaluation for infertility.

Prevalence of Chromosome Disorders in Humans

Identifiable abnormalities in the human karyotype occur more frequently than mutations, leading to mendelian hereditary disease. Table 1-5 summarizes studies on the incidence of sex chromosome and autosomal chromosomal abnormalities.[9]

TABLE 1-5 INCIDENCE OF CHROMOSOMAL ABNORMALITIES IN SURVEYS OF NEWBORNS

Type of Abnormality	Number	Approximate Incidence
Sex chromosome aneuploidy		
Males (43,612 newborns)		
47,XXY	45	1/1000
47,XYY	45	1/1000
Other X or Y aneuploidy	32	1/1350
Total	**122**	**1/360 male births**
Females (24,547 newborns)		
45,X	6	1/4000
47,XXX	27	1/900
Other X aneuploidy	9	1/2700
Total	**42**	**1/580 female births**
Autosomal aneuploidy (68,159 newborns)		
Trisomy 21	82	1/830
Trisomy 18	9	1/7500
Trisomy 13	3	1/22,700
Other aneuploidy	2	1/34,000
Total	**96**	**1/700 live births**
Structural abnormalities (68,159 newborns) (sex chromosomes and autosomes)		
Balanced rearrangements		
Robertsonian	62	1/1100
Other	77	1/885
Unbalanced rearrangements		
Robertsonian	5	1/13,600
Other	38	1/1800
Total	**182**	**1/375 live births**
All chromosome abnormalities	**442**	**1/154 live births**

From Hsu LYF: Prenatal diagnosis of chromosomal abnormalities through amniocentesis. In Milunsky A (ed): Genetic Disorders and the Fetus, 4th ed. Baltimore, Johns Hopkins University Press, 1998, p 179.

The most common autosomal numerical disorders in liveborn humans are trisomy 21, trisomy 18, and trisomy 13. Numerous studies have shown that trisomy 21 is the most common aneuploidy among liveborn humans. On the other hand, balanced reciprocal translocations occur almost as frequently. Trisomy 13 occurs at a much lower frequency than trisomy 18 or trisomy 21, possibly because of increased fetal demise with this mutation.[9] Among sex chromosomes, aneuploidies 45,X, 47,XYY, and 47,XXY are seen in liveborn infants.

It is noteworthy that the incidence of common chromosome abnormalities such as trisomy 21 is nearly 10 times greater than the incidence of genetic diseases such as achondroplasia, hemophilia A, and Duchenne muscular dystrophy. The cumulative data on chromosome abnormalities reveal an unanticipated finding. Chromosome analysis in newborns from several worldwide population samples shows the overall incidence of chromosome abnormalities to be 0.5% to 0.6%. In a large study series of nearly 55,000 infants, more than two thirds had no significant physical abnormality in association with these chromosomal defects, and of the one third with significant phenotype abnormalities, nearly 66% had trisomy 21.[9]

Chromosome Abnormalities in Abortuses and Stillbirths

About 15% of pregnancies terminate in spontaneous abortions, and at least 80% of those do so in the first trimester. The incidence of chromosome abnormalities in spontaneous abortuses during the first trimester has been reported to be as high as 61.5%.[12] Table 1-6 summarizes the karyotype incidence in chromosomally abnormal abortuses.[9] For comparison, note the incidence of chromosome abnormalities in liveborn infants (see Table 1-5). At an incidence of 19%, 45,XO is the most common chromosome abnormality found in first-trimester spontaneous abortions. Comparison with the relatively low incidence of 45,XO in liveborn infants suggests that most conceptuses with this karyotype are aborted spontaneously. Trisomic embryos are seen for all autosomes except chromosomes 1, 5, 11, 12, 17, and 19.

TABLE 1-6 FREQUENCY OF CHROMOSOME ABNORMALITIES IN SPONTANEOUS ABORTIONS WITH ABNORMAL KARYOTYPES

Type	Approximate Proportion of Abnormal Karyotypes
Aneuploidy	
Autosomal trisomy	0.52
Autosomal monosomy	<0.01
45,X	0.19
Triploidy	0.16
Tetraploidy	0.06
Other	0.07

Based on analysis of 8841 unselected spontaneous abortions, as summarized by Hsu LYF: Prenatal diagnosis of chromosomal abnormalities through amniocentesis. In Milunsky A (ed): Genetic Disorders and the Fetus, 4th ed. Baltimore, Johns Hopkins University Press, 1998, p 179.

The studies of Creasy and colleagues[13] and Hassold[14] offer a comparison between karyotypic abnormalities in live births and in spontaneous abortions (Table 1-7). Triploidy or tetraploidy, and trisomy 16 are the most common autosomal abnormalities in spontaneous abortuses but are never seen in live births. Comparison of the overall incidence of about 1 per 830 live births for trisomy 21 with the incidence in abortuses suggests that approximately 78% of trisomy 21 conceptuses are aborted spontaneously.

Summary of Maternal-Fetal Indications for Chromosome Analysis

Among all genetic aspects of maternal-fetal medicine, chromosome mutations and clinical syndromes associated with a dysmorphic phenotype constitute the category that most often requires the physician's attention. It is worthwhile, therefore, to review indications for the consideration, at least, of chromosome analysis as part of the evaluation of fetus, infant, or parents. The following situations would justify chromosome analysis.

Abnormal Phenotype in a Newborn Infant

Most abnormal phenotypes in the newborn resulting from chromosome abnormalities reflect abnormal autosomes. The important findings that should prompt karyotyping include (1) low birth weight or early evidence of failure to thrive; (2) any indication of developmental delay, in particular mental retardation; (3) abnormal (dysmorphic) features of the head and face, such as microcephaly, micrognathia, and abnormalities of eyes, ears, and mouth; (4) abnormalities of the hands and feet; and (5) congenital defects of various internal organs.

TABLE 1-7 OUTCOME OF 10,000 CONCEPTIONS

		Spontaneous Abortions		
Outcome	**Conceptions**	***n***	**%**	**Live Births**
Total	10,000	1,500	15	8,500
Normal chromosomes	9,200	750	8	8,450
Abnormal chromosomes				
Triploid/tetraploid	170	170	100	—
45,X	140	139	99	1
Trisomy 16	112	112	100	—
Trisomy 18	20	19	95	1
Trisomy 21	45	35	78	10
Trisomy, other	209	208	99.5	1
47,XXY, 47,XXX, 47,XYY	19	4	21	15
Unbalanced rearrangements	27	23	85	4
Balanced rearrangements	19	3	16	16
Other	39	37	95	2
Total abnormal	800	750	94	50

A single isolated malformation or a mental retardation without an associated physical malformation significantly reduces the likelihood of a chromosome abnormality. Disorders of the sex chromosomes are more likely to be associated with phenotypic ambiguity of the external genitalia and perhaps slight abnormality in growth pattern. Certainly, any newborn manifesting sexual ambiguity should undergo a chromosome analysis. In addition to helping to exclude the possibility of a life-threatening genetic disorder (e.g., adrenogenital syndrome), the identification of sex genotype by chromosome analysis will assist attending physicians in their decisions about therapy and counseling for the parents. For the infant suspected of having autosome abnormalities, in whom the chromosomal genotype is urgently needed for making decisions about the infant's care, rapid chromosome analysis can be obtained by culture of bone marrow aspirate. When a familial chromosome mutation, such as unbalanced translocation, is detected in the infant, karyotyping of other kindred is indicated.

Unexplained First-Trimester Spontaneous Abortion with No Fetal Karyotype

Usually, couples seek medical help because of recurrent first-trimester abortions, and there is no previous karyotype for aborted tissue. Many genetic centers now recommend parental karyotyping after several (usually two or three) spontaneous abortions have occurred. The likelihood of a parental genome mutation is probably greatest if the couple has already produced a child with birth defects. When a parental chromosome structural abnormality is identified, genetic counseling and prenatal fetal monitoring in all subsequent pregnancies are advised.

Stillbirth or Neonatal Death

Unless an explanation is obvious, any evaluation of a stillborn infant or a child dying in the neonatal period should include chromosome analysis. There is an approximately 10% incidence of chromosomal abnormalities in such individuals, compared with less than 1% for liveborn infants surviving the neonatal period. The likelihood of finding a chromosome mutation is increased significantly if intrauterine growth retardation or phenotypic birth defects are present.

Fertility Problems

In women presenting with amenorrhea and couples presenting with a history of infertility or spontaneous abortion, the incidence of chromosomal defects is between 3% and 6%.

In men presenting with infertility, deletions in the human Y chromosome have been found.[15] Among other disorders, these men can present with spermatogenic failure, or the absence of, or very low levels of, sperm production. It is known that the Y chromosome contains more than 100 testis-specific transcripts. Several deletions that remove some of these transcripts have been found that appear to cause spermatogenic failure. Screening for such deletions in infertile men is now a standard part of clinical evaluation. In addition, many other Y-chromosome structural variants have been described using techniques such as high-resolution comparative genomic hybridization (described earlier). Some of these structural variants affect gene copy number, although additional research is necessary to address the phenotypic effect of many of these structural variants.

Neoplasia

All patients with cancer present with some element of genomic instability, and specific chromosomal defects are often pathognomonic of certain specific cancers, especially hematologic malignancies.

Pregnancy in a Woman of Advanced Age

There is an increased risk of chromosomal abnormalities in fetuses conceived in women older than 30 to 35 years.[16] A karyotypic analysis of the fetus can be part of routine care in such pregnancies, or such women can be offered noninvasive screening.

Patterns of Inheritance

Single-gene traits are those inherited from a single locus. They segregate on the basis of two fundamental laws of genetics in diploid organisms established by Gregor Mendel using garden peas in 1857. These two laws are *segregation* (Fig. 1-24A) and *independent assortment* (see Fig. 1-24B). In medical genetics, the term *mendelian disorders* refers to single-gene phenotypes that segregate distinctly within families and generally occur in the proportions noted by Mendel in his experiments. Specific phenotypic or genotypic traits are inherited in distinct fashions, depending on whether the responsible gene is on the X chromosome or an autosome, and whether one or two copies of a gene are necessary for a phenotype. A phenotype is *dominant* if it is expressed when present on only one chromosome of a pair, whereas *recessive* traits are expressed only when present on both chromosomes. A purely dominant trait has the same phenotype when present on either one or

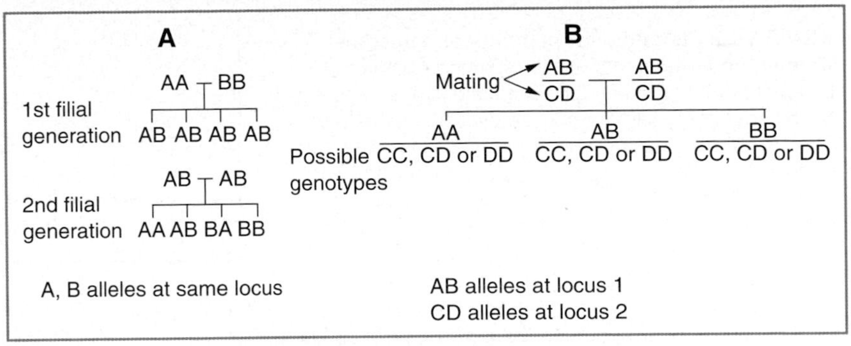

FIGURE 1-24 Mendel's first and second laws. **A,** With A and B representing alleles at the same locus, a mating of homozygous A and homozygous B individuals results in heterozygotes for A and B in each offspring. Mating of heterozygotes A,B results in the 1-2-1 segregation ratio in offspring. **B,** The segregation of genotypes for A and B at locus 1 is independent of the segregation of alleles C and D at locus 2. (From Kelly TE: Clinical Genetics and Genetic Counseling. Chicago, Year Book Medical, 1980.)

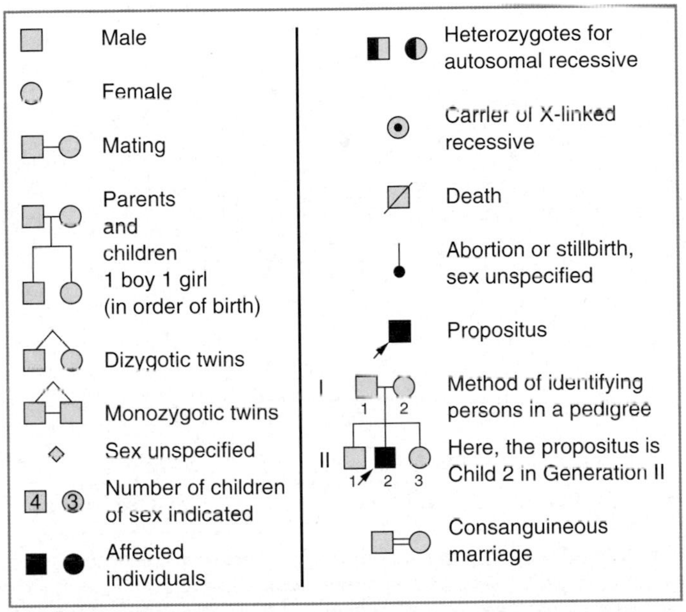

FIGURE 1-25 Symbols commonly used in pedigree charts. (From Nussbaum RL, McInnes RR, Willard HF: Thompson and Thompson's Genetics in Medicine, 6th ed. Philadelphia, WB Saunders, 2001.)

two chromosome pairs. However, if a phenotype is expressed when present as a single copy but is expressed more strongly when present on two chromosomes, the trait is *codominant.* Victor McKusick's catalog of single-gene phenotypes and mendelian disorders[17] is now available online[18] (see Table 1-1) and is an indispensable reference for human genetic traits and disorders.

Familial studies for genetic evaluation require development of a pedigree or a graphic representation of family history data. Figure 1-25 illustrates some of the symbols useful in this process. This aspect of data gathering serves several functions:

1. It assists the determination of transmission for the gene expression in question (recessive, dominant, sex-linked, or autosomal).
2. There is a greater likelihood that all possible genetic issues will be included in the data gathering when a formal pedigree chart is assembled.
3. When consanguinity is present, the pedigree chart helps to relate the consanguinity to individuals in subsequent generations who are expressing the phenotype of a particular inheritable disorder.

Autosomal Dominant Mode of Inheritance

In autosomal dominant inheritance, the disease is expressed in the heterozygote, and the probability of transmitting the gene to progeny is 50% with each pregnancy. The pedigree in Figure 1-26 demonstrates the features of inheritance of an autosomal dominant disease: gene expression in each generation, approximately half of the offspring affected (both males and females), and father-to-son transmission.

Criteria for Autosomal Dominant Inheritance

The criteria for autosomal dominant inheritance may be summarized as follows:

1. Expression of the gene rarely skips a generation.
2. Affected individuals, if reproductively fit, transmit the gene expression to progeny with a probability of 50%.
3. The sexes are affected equally, and there is father-to-son transmission.
4. A person in the kindred at risk who is not affected will not transmit the gene to progeny.

Other Characteristics

Other characteristics, although not exclusive properties of autosomal dominant disease, seem to be associated with this group of diseases more frequently.

VARIABLE EXPRESSIVITY

Variable expressivity refers to the degree of severity of expression of a trait and is commonly seen in kindreds with autosomal dominant traits. In neurofibromatosis, for example, a kindred may have a range of phenotypic expression in affected individuals, from some café au lait spots with a few tumors to extensive café au lait spots with massive neurofibromata.

PENETRANCE

Penetrance refers to whether there is any recognition of phenotypic expression of a particular mutant allele. If a gene is fully penetrant, it is always expressed as part of the genome of that individual. On the other hand, if a gene displays incomplete penetrance, not all individuals with that gene display any recognizable phenotype. For example, in the autosomal dominant form of retinoblastoma, the mutant gene is only 80% penetrant. This means that a person who receives the gene for retinoblastoma from a parent has a 20% chance that the disease phenotype will not be expressed.

Penetrance may also be influenced by the means available to detect expression of the gene. For example, in autosomal dominant hyper-

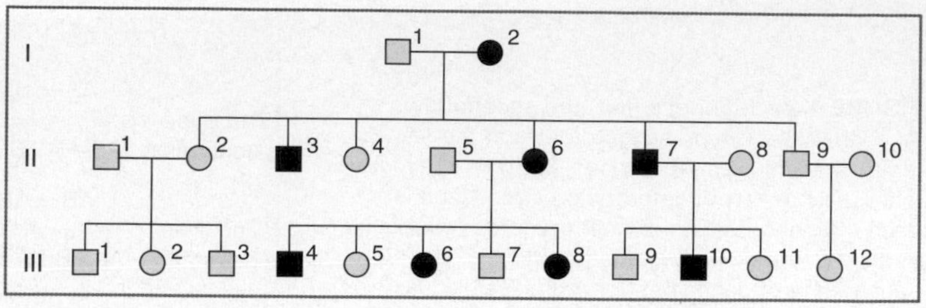

FIGURE 1-26 Stereotypical pedigree of autosomal dominant inheritance. Half the offspring of affected persons (7 of 14) are affected. The condition is transmitted only by affected family members, never by unaffected ones. Equal numbers of males and females are affected. Male-to-male transmission is seen. (From Nussbaum RL, McInnes RR, Willard HF: Thompson and Thompson's Genetics in Medicine, 6th ed. Philadelphia, WB Saunders, 2001.)

cholesterolemia, a myocardial infarction (a manifestation of gene expression and penetrance) may not appear until well into adult life. In this disorder, there is a laboratory test for expression, namely the serum cholesterol level, which becomes elevated quite early in life, well before the first chest pain of angina pectoris.

NEW MUTATIONS

It is not uncommon for an autosomal dominant disorder to manifest for the first time in a kindred as a new mutation. New mutations are also seen with sex-linked recessive disorders. For example, in a form of autosomal dominant dwarfism called achondroplasia, nearly 80% of individuals represent new mutations. When this phenomenon can be identified with certainty, parents may be reassured that the recurrence risk is probably no greater than that for the general population. The recurrence risk for offspring of the affected individual is 50%. New mutations for autosomal dominant diseases appear to be related to paternal age.

Autosomal Recessive Mode of Inheritance

For autosomal recessive diseases, mutant genes are expressed only in homozygous individuals. Consanguinity is often a clue for autosomal inheritance when the specific gene mutation has not been identified. A pedigree consistent with autosomal recessive inheritance is shown in Figure 1-27. Primary features consistent with autosomal recessive inheritance may be summarized as follows:

1. Both males and females are affected.
2. Unless consanguinity or random selection of heterozygous matings in each generation occurs, mutant gene expression may appear to skip generations, in contrast to autosomal dominant inheritance, which rarely skips generations.
3. Parents are usually unaffected, but unaffected sibs of affected homozygotes may be heterozygous carriers. Affected individuals rarely have affected children.
4. Subsequent to identification of a propositus, the recurrence risk for homozygous affected progeny in each subsequent pregnancy is one chance in four.
5. If the incidence of the disorder is rare, consanguineous parentage is often seen.

Sex-Linked Mode of Inheritance

In this discussion, sex-linked refers to inheritance from the X chromosome. For this group of genetic diseases, the male is considered to be hemizygous in relation to X-linked genes, whereas females are almost always heterozygous. However, because of patterns of X inactivation, females of some X-linked disorders may be more mildly affected than males with the same disorder.

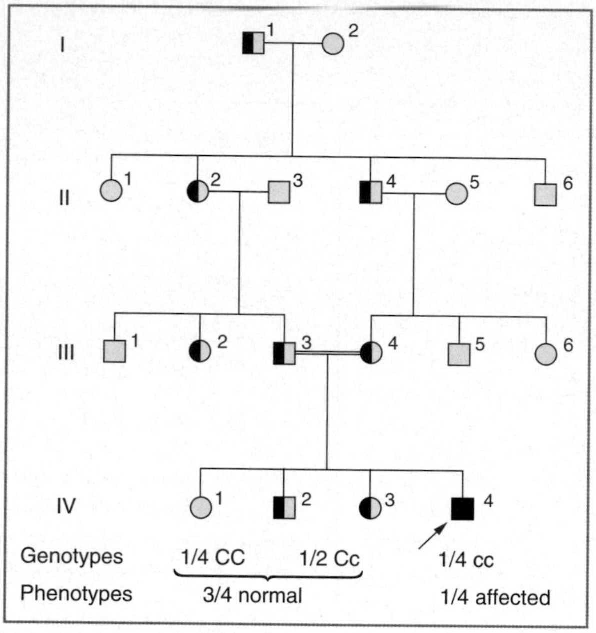

FIGURE 1-27 Stereotypical pedigree of autosomal recessive inheritance, including a cousin marriage. A gene from a common ancestor I-1 has been transmitted down two lines of descent to "meet itself" in IV-4 *(arrow)*. (From Nussbaum RL, McInnes RR, Willard HF: Thompson and Thompson's Genetics in Medicine, 6th ed. Philadelphia, WB Saunders, 2001.)

Hemophilia A is among the best-known X-linked recessive diseases. For illustrative purposes, we shall use the symbol X_h to represent the recessive allele for hemophilia A on the X chromosome and X_H to represent the normal or dominant allele. The diagrams in Figure 1-28 demonstrate progeny genotypes in matings between affected males and normal females as well as matings between normal males and heterozygous phenotypically normal females. When the father is affected, all sons will be normal and all daughters will be heterozygous carriers and phenotypically normal (see Fig. 1-28A). In the other mating cross, each daughter will have a 50% chance of being normal and a 50% chance of being a heterozygous carrier who is phenotypically normal (see Fig. 1-28B). Each son will have a 50% chance of being normal and a 50% chance of being affected.

Characteristics of X-linked recessive inheritance may be summarized as follows:

1. A higher incidence of the disorder is noted in males than in females.
2. The mutant gene expression is never transmitted directly from father to son.

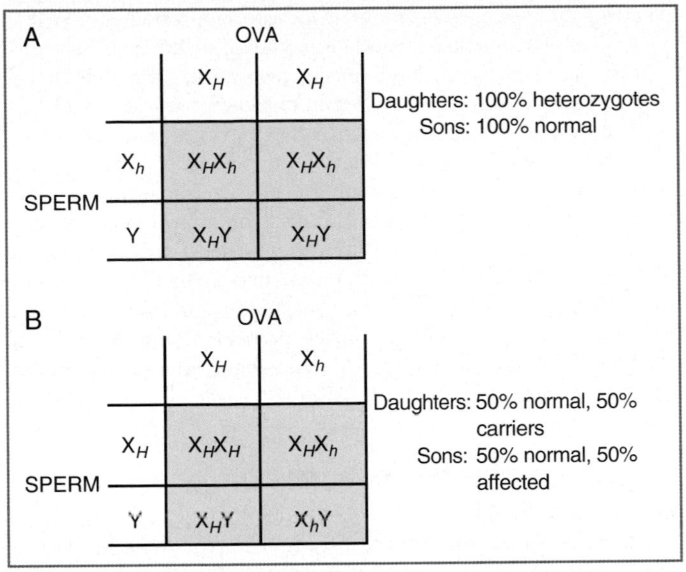

FIGURE 1-28 **Sex-linked recessive inheritance patterns.** See text. (From Nussbaum RL, McInnes RR, Willard HF: Thompson and Thompson's Genetics in Medicine, 6th ed. Philadelphia, WB Saunders, 2001.)

3. The mutant gene is transmitted from an affected male to all his daughters.
4. The trait is transmitted through a series of carrier females, and affected males in a kindred are related to one another through the females.
5. For sporadic cases, there may be an increase in the age of the maternal grandfather at which he fathered the mother of an affected child—similar to the increase in paternal age for certain new dominant mutations.

In contrast to X-linked recessive inheritance, X-linked dominant disorders are nearly twice as common in females as in males (Fig. 1-29). For example, none of the sons of a male affected with vitamin D–resistant rickets is affected, but all his daughters receive the mutant gene from him, and because the mutant is dominant, they all have the disease. A female with one X-linked mutant dominant allele will have the disease, and the transmission to her progeny, assuming a hemizygous normal mate, will be indistinguishable from that seen in autosomal dominant inheritance. As a group, the X-linked dominant disorders are relatively uncommon. Vitamin D–resistant rickets (hypophosphatemia) is one, and the X-linked blood group X is another.

The distinguishing features of X-linked dominant inheritance are summarized as follows:

1. All daughters of affected males have the disorder, but no sons are affected.
2. Heterozygous affected females transmit the mutant allele at a rate of 50% to progeny of both sexes. If the affected female is homozygous, all her children will be affected.
3. The incidence of X-linked dominant disease may be twice as common in females as in males.

Some rare disorders that are exclusively or nearly exclusively seen in females, such as Rett syndrome and incontinentia pigmenti type 2, appear to be X-linked dominant conditions in which affected males die before birth.

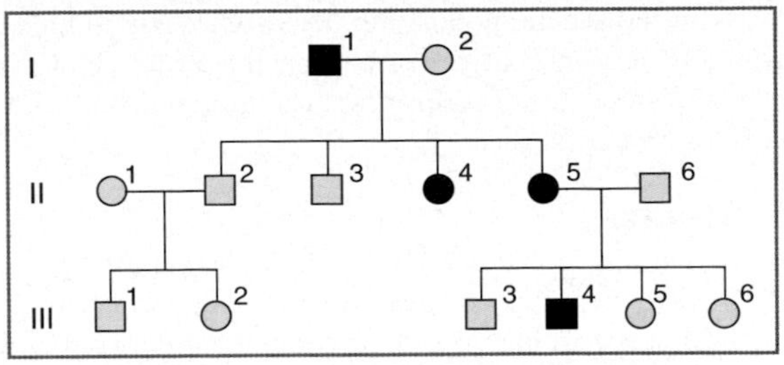

FIGURE 1-29 **Stereotypical pedigree of X-linked dominant inheritance.** Affected males have no affected sons and no normal daughters. (From Nussbaum RL, McInnes RR, Willard HF: Thompson and Thompson's Genetics in Medicine, 6th ed. Philadelphia, WB Saunders, 2001.)

Multifactorial Inheritance

In this age of genes and genomes, we should remember that not everything that runs in families is genetic and not everything that is genetic runs in families. Environmental and sociologic factors such as diet, age at first pregnancy, socioeconomic level, access to health care, and environmental conditions often segregate in families along with genes. An excellent example is the occurrence in families of cholera or tuberculosis. Although susceptibility to infectious diseases can be modulated by genetic inheritance, the susceptibility of a family to these diseases is most likely the result of unsanitary conditions (cholera) or chronic exposure (tuberculosis). On the other hand, some genetic disorders are sufficiently devastating that they are rarely if ever transmitted between generations, and most cases occur as de novo mutations. Examples of genetic disorders for which many patients have no family history include chromosomal abnormalities (e.g., Down syndrome), contiguous gene syndromes (e.g., Prader-Willi, Angelman, or Smith-Magenis syndrome), and single-gene disorders for which one copy of the gene is not enough (called *haploinsufficiency*) (e.g., neurofibromatosis type I). Clinicians should be aware that common disorders often have both genetic and nongenetic components to their etiology. A clinician who might encounter either familial clusters or rare genetic disorders should be familiar with the concepts used to distinguish genetic from nongenetic transmission.

Heritability

A measure of the genetic contribution to disease is heritability, which is the amount of phenotypic variation explained by genes relative to the total amount of variation. A more detailed treatment of statistical estimates of heritability can be found in texts devoted to genetic analysis.[19,20] High heritability does not imply the action of a single gene but rather a greater contribution of genes compared with environmental or stochastic factors for the characteristic being studied. Disorders (or susceptibility to them) may be inherited as monogenic, oligogenic, or polygenic in a given family. A disease with high heritability may also be inherited in different families through different genes. A disease caused by any of several mutations in the same gene is said to show *allelic heterogeneity.* A disease caused by changes in any of several different genes is said to show *locus heterogeneity.* A disease caused by environmental factors that mimics a genetic disorder is said to *phenocopy* that disorder.

Recurrence Risk

One common statistical measure used to estimate heritability is the recurrence risk to family members of an index case or proband. This is often expressed as the ratio of risk to a first-degree relative divided by the risk in the general population. Recurrence risk to full siblings is a common measure, but depending on the structure of available patient populations, first cousin, grandparent/grandchild, and other comparisons have been used.

Twin Studies

Twin studies are often extremely valuable in distinguishing effects of shared genes from effects of shared environment, particularly for diseases with complex etiology. A genetic component to a trait or disease can be seen as a difference in recurrence risk or concordance rate between monozygotic twins (derived from a single fertilization event and therefore genetically identical) and dizygotic twins (derived by independent fertilization of two eggs released in the same cycle and therefore sharing half of their genes). All twins generally share both prenatal and postnatal environments. Monozygotic twins also share all their genetic complement, but dizygotic twins share only half of theirs. Any substantial difference in concordance rate (or recurrence risk) between monozygotic and dizygotic twins as a group is taken as evidence of a genetic component.

Complex Inheritance

Many common disorders show complex inheritance. Allergy, asthma, autism, cancer, cleft lip and palate, diabetes, dizygotic twinning, handedness, hypertension, multiple sclerosis, neural tube defects, obesity, and schizophrenia are all examples of such complex traits with population frequencies greater than 1%. Such disorders may have rare single-gene (monogenic) forms, but most cases have more complex etiologies. Complex disorders include examples of polygenic inheritance, in which several genes contribute to the disease in the absence of environmental effects, and multifactorial inheritance, in which genes and environment interact to produce disease. In practice, a complex trait may have monogenic, polygenic, and multifactorial forms—and possibly more than one of each. Although such etiologic heterogeneity makes identification of the underlying genes (and environmental risk factors) more difficult, several characteristic features help to identify disorders with complex inheritance.

Complex inheritance may involve either *quantitative traits* or *qualitative traits*. In a quantitative trait, each causal gene or nongenetic factor contributes incrementally to a measurable outcome, such as height, body mass index, or age at onset of disease. A qualitative trait has alternative outcomes that either are nonquantitative or are very imprecisely quantified in practice; each causal gene contributes to meeting a threshold for expression of the trait or contributes to the probability of expressing the trait, such as susceptibility to disease. Note that these modes are not completely distinct: Susceptibility genes may act quantitatively on the probability of disease for each individual, but clinical outcome may be qualitative (e.g., the presence or absence of disease). Disease genes may also act additively to reach a qualitative threshold for disease and beyond the threshold contribute to increased severity of disease. Stratifying patients by intermediate phenotypes, disease severity, or known risk factors may simplify the inheritance patterns of some complex traits.

Recent technical advances have greatly increased our ability to identify individual genes in complex disorders. The public availability of the consensus human genome sequence, along with deep databases of single nucleotide polymorphisms, copy number variations, and high-throughput genotyping platforms, allows investigators to interrogate the entire genomes of clinical subjects for genetic linkage or statistical associations to clinical phenotypes. Maps defining common human haplotypes (arrangements of alleles at successive loci along an individual chromosome) have added further power to study designs for detecting disease genes in genome-wide association studies (GWAS—also called whole-genome association studies, or WGAS). Expanded repositories (and consortia of smaller repositories) for both clinical data and physical samples have begun to allow statistically highly significant genetic findings for disorders that previously had resisted less powerful analyses (e.g., see Wellcome Trust Case Control Consortium[21]). We should expect to see continued progress in identifying such genes over the next several years. This places additional importance on the ability of practicing doctors to identify clinical presentations and families that fit particular inheritance patterns. For the most up-to-date information on specific genes, loci, and disorders, the reader is encouraged to consult online sources, particularly the OMIM[18] and PubMed databases maintained by the National Center for Biotechnology Information in the National Library of Medicine (www.ncbi.nlm.nih.gov).

CHARACTERISTIC FEATURES OF COMPLEX TRAITS

Regression to the Mean. Because complex traits involve the inheritance (or environmental presence) of many factors, offspring from extreme individuals tend to be less extreme than the parents; that is, they regress to the mean of the population. Independent assortment in meiosis results in different combinations of genes being passed to offspring, and change of environment results in different factors being experienced by the offspring. Using a familiar example of a nondisease trait, very tall parents will have taller than average children, but in general children of the tallest parents will not inherit all of the "tall factors" that the parents have.

Heritability. Complex traits have heritability estimates over a wide range. They are by definition less heritable than fully penetrant monogenic traits but more heritable than would be expected by chance alone. The range of heritability reflects the varying degree to which genes determine the outcome of each trait. The higher the ratio of recurrence risk to a family member to risk in the general population (or the higher the ratio of monozygotic twin concordance to dizygotic twin concordance), the more genetically tractable the disease is likely to be.

Threshold Traits. The rate of development can determine outcome in a threshold trait. The idea of a threshold trait is that if an event does not happen by a specified time in development (a developmental threshold), then a consequent phenotype, such as a physical malformation or cognitive deficit, will ensue. Developmental rates are generally determined by a combination of genetic and environmental factors.

Penetrance, Probability, and Severity. The likelihood of having the disorder or trait, given the right genotype, is called the *penetrance*. For simple mendelian disorders, penetrance may be at or near 100%. For traits with environmental cofactors or developmental threshold effects, the penetrance can be much lower. For some disorders, the penetrance (in terms of either likelihood or severity of the disorder) is part of the pattern of inheritance within a family. Affected relatives of a severely affected proband are likely to be more severely affected than the average case. This is the other side of regression to the mean: Returning to our nondisease example, the children of very tall parents may not be as tall as their parents but will probably be taller than average. Taking a disease example, if a liveborn infant has unilateral cleft lip, the recurrence risk to future siblings is 2.5%, but for a liveborn infant with bilateral cleft lip and palate, the recurrence risk is 6% (see below).

Increased Risk across Diagnostic Categories. Another frequent feature of complex inheritance is that relatives of the proband may be at increased risk for related diagnostic categories. This has been suggested for categories of psychiatric illness, for some autoimmune disorders, and for some malformation syndromes. The implication of this is that overlapping sets of genes and environmental factors can lead to dysfunctions that present as related clinical entities.

Rarer Forms Show Increased Relative Risk. Forms of multifactorial disease that are less frequent in the general population tend to have higher recurrence risk ratios for families of an affected proband. For example, pyloric stenosis is five times more common in males than in females in the general population. As Table 1-8 shows, male relatives of any proband face a higher risk than their sisters, but relatives of female probands face much higher risk than relatives of male probands.

Common Disorders with Multifactorial Inheritance

CLEFT LIP AND CLEFT PALATE

The cleft lip malformation may occur with or without cleft palate (orofacial cleft) but is etiologically distinct from cleft palate alone.[22]

TABLE 1-8 RECURRENCE RISK OF PYLORIC STENOSIS FOR FIRST-DEGREE RELATIVES

	Risk (%)	Relative to General Population Risk
Male relatives of male patients	4.6	×10
Female relatives of male patients	2.6	×25
Male relatives of female patients	18.2	×35
Female relatives of female patients	8.1	×80

From Kelly TE: Clinical Genetics and Genetic Counseling. Copyright © 1980 by Year Book Medical, Chicago. Reproduced with permission.

These common malformations occur in more than 200 described human syndromes, including several single-gene disorders, chromosomal abnormalities, and syndromes of teratogen exposure (including thalidomide). Developmentally, cleft lip with or without cleft palate results from a failure in the fusion of the frontal prominence with the maxillary process at about 7 weeks of fetal development. Incidence is two- to fourfold higher in males than in females and varies among ethnogeographic groups: 0.4 per 1000 births in African Americans, 1 per 1000 births in whites, and 1.7 per 1000 births in Japanese. However, the recurrence risk to first-degree relatives is lower in Japan than in Europe, suggesting a higher environmental influence in Japan.[23] Within a population, the recurrence risk varies with the severity of defect in the proband, as noted previously. Examples are shown in Table 1-9. Several loci for syndromic and nonsyndromic orofacial cleft (OFC) have been implicated by genetic linkage and association studies, although for several loci the specific genes involved are not yet resolved.

CLEFT PALATE

In cleft palate without cleft lip, the secondary palate fails to fuse. The general incidence is approximately 1 in 2500 and it is more common in females than males. Little ethnic variation is noted, and the recurrence risk is approximately 2%. Isolated cleft palate appears genetically distinct from cleft lip with or without cleft palate. At least one gene for isolated cleft palate, *SATB2,* has been identified.[24,25]

NEURAL TUBE DEFECTS

This group of malformations is of special importance because they are prevalent, their risk can be significantly altered by diet, and there is a possibility of mid-trimester prenatal diagnosis and even perhaps prenatal screening of these disorders in all pregnancies. Expression of neural tube defects can be highly variable among individuals, ranging from anencephaly at one extreme to lumbar meningocele with little or no neurologic impairment at the other. The spectrum includes encephalocele, iniencephaly, meningomyelocele (usually involving the

TABLE 1-9 EXAMPLES OF RECURRENCE RISKS FOR CLEFT LIP, WITH OR WITHOUT CLEFT PALATE, AND FOR NEURAL TUBE MALFORMATIONS

Family History	Risk for Cleft Lip ± Cleft Palate (%)	Risk for Anencephaly and Spina Bifida (%)
No sibs affected		
Neither parent affected	0.1	0.3
One parent affected	3.0	4.5
Both parents affected	34.0	30.0
One sib affected		
Neither parent affected	3.0	4.0
One parent affected	11.0	12.0
Both parents affected	40.0	38.0
Two sibs affected		
Neither parent affected	9.0	10.0
One parent affected	19.0	20.0
Both parents affected	45.0	43.0
One sib and one second-degree relative affected		
Neither parent affected	6.0	7.0
One parent affected	16.0	18.0
Both parents affected	43.0	42.0
One sib and one third-degree relative affected		
Neither parent affected	4.0	5.5
One parent affected	14.0	16.0
Both parents affected	44.0	42.0

Adapted from Thompson MW: Thompson and Thompson's Genetics in Medicine, 4th ed. Philadelphia, WB Saunders, 1986; Based on data from Bonaiti-Pellié C: Risk tables for genetic counselling in some common congenital malformations. J Med Genet 11:374, 1974.

lower thoracic and lumbar spine and often called spina bifida cystica), and spina bifida. Defects arise through failure of the embryonic neural tube to close within 28 days from conception. The incidence in European-derived populations can vary substantially, from less than 1 per 1000 to nearly 1 per 100 births. One recent study of medical records showed an approximately 10-fold decrease in neural tube defects in England and Wales between 1964 and 2004, attributable both to a reduction in the occurrence of neural tube defects and to termination after early diagnosis.[26] The overall U.S. incidence is approximately 1 per 1000, but it is lower for individuals of African or Asian ancestry. Recurrence risks for anencephaly and spina bifida probands are shown in Table 1-9.

Epidemiologic and experimental animal studies have suggested that neural tube defects have characteristics of threshold traits as well as substantial environmental factors. For example, recent attention has been paid to the importance of dietary folate in preventing neural tube defects. Incidence of this defect in Canada decreased by 50% after folate supplementation of cereals in the United States and Canada in 1998.[27] Known genetic risk factors include genes for folate and homocysteine metabolism as well as loci thought to present folate-independent risk. Work in animal models has suggested inositol as another potential metabolic factor.[28-30]

PYLORIC STENOSIS

Pyloric stenosis is the most common disorder requiring corrective surgery in infants, with an incidence of 1 to 5 per 1000 live births. Heritability is inferred from the high recurrence risk to relatives. Carter and Evans first proposed sex-modified multifactorial inheritance in 1969.[31] Males are at higher risk than females, irrespective of family history, but the ratio of recurrence risk to general risk is higher in females (see Table 1-8). Mitchell and Risch[32] concluded that family studies were inconsistent with a single major locus causing pyloric stenosis and set model-based limits for the effect of any single locus at no more than a fivefold increase in recurrence risk across the general population. However, single-gene effects can be seen in some extended families. Evidence from patient material[33] and targeted mutations in mice[34,35] indicate that neuronal nitric oxide synthase gene, *NOS1*, is one locus for pyloric stenosis. An additional locus and further evidence for genetic heterogeneity have been identified by linkage analysis in a multigenerational family with 10 affected members.[36]

CELIAC DISEASE

Autoimmune reaction in celiac disease causes inflammatory injury to the mucosa of the small intestine, resulting in malabsorption. Once thought uncommon, celiac disease (or gluten-sensitive enteropathy) is now thought to affect as many as 1 in 120 to 1 in 300 people in Europe and North America. Several factors point to multifactorial inheritance. Recurrence risk to siblings is 10% or higher. Concordance rates for monozygotic twins is more than fourfold higher than for dizygotic twins.[37] Exposure to wheat gluten (or other grains, such as rye and barley) are environmental factors for genetically susceptible individuals. Genetic linkage to human leukocyte antigen has been reported, as well as linkage to several additional genetic loci.[38-40] Among regions showing significant linkage, variations in the *CTLA4* and *MYO9B* genes show strong association with disease.

INFLAMMATORY BOWEL DISEASE (CROHN DISEASE)

Genetic components of autoimmune disease directed against the gastrointestinal tract have also been mapped for findings of Crohn disease and ulcerative colitis. Together these somewhat overlapping diagnoses occur in 2 to 3 people per 1000 in the United States. Genetic effects of at least 11 distinct loci for inflammatory bowel disease have been identified in this complex trait, including linkage to the human leukocyte antigen region of chromosome 6p. As an interesting example of molecular analysis in a complex trait, Rioux and coworkers[41] mapped one locus on chromosome 5q, *IBD5*, to a cluster of inflammatory cytokine genes; several of the genes in this interval were polymorphic between patients and population control subjects, but causality for any one gene could not be determined because of strong linkage disequilibrium across the implicated region. An uncommon allele of IL-23R cytokine receptor was identified as a protective effect in a genome-wide association study.[42]

HIRSCHSPRUNG DISEASE

Congenital megacolon caused by lack of enteric ganglia along the intestine is a relatively well-studied complex genetic trait. Incidence is about 1 in 5000 births, including both short-segment and long-segment forms. Both dominant inheritance and recessive inheritance have been observed, and penetrance is variable. Single-gene mutations associated with varying penetrance for Hirschsprung disease have been identified that illuminate biochemical pathways with unique importance for the establishment of enteric ganglia. Aganglionic megacolon also occurs in more complicated disorders, including cartilage-hair hypoplasia, Smith-Lemli-Opitz syndrome type II, and primary central hypoventilation syndrome. Variations in the *RET* oncogene appear to be the major risk factor in Hirschsprung patients. Mutations in endothelin 3, endothelin receptor B, and endothelin converting enzyme, as well as neurturin, glial-derived neurotrophic factor, and the transcriptional regulator SOX10 have been identified as risk conferring in both human and animal studies. An exhaustive search for genetic linkage implicated two additional loci that act as oligogenic determinants of the expression of mild *RET* alleles.[43] Interestingly, mutation of a transcriptional enhancer of the autosomal *RET* gene confers sex-dependent risk for Hirschsprung disease.[44]

CONGENITAL HEART DEFECTS

The overall incidence of congenital heart disease is 5 to 7 live births per 1000 and is the leading cause of death from birth defects.[45] This heterogeneous group of defects can be caused by single-gene mutations, chromosomal abnormalities (trisomy 21), and teratogens such as rubella and maternal diabetes. Table 1-10, abstracted from the classic

TABLE 1-10 FREQUENCY OF SIX COMMON CONGENITAL HEART DEFECTS IN SIBS OF PROBANDS

Anomaly	Frequency in Sibs* (%)	Expected Frequency† (%)
Ventricular septal defect	4.3	4.2
Patent ductus arteriosus	3.2	2.9
Tetralogy of Fallot	2.2	2.6
Atrial septal defect	3.2	2.6
Pulmonary stenosis	2.9	2.6
Aortic stenosis	2.6	2.1

*Data from Nora JJ: Multifactorial inheritance hypothesis for the etiology of congenital heart disease: The genetic-environmental interaction. Circulation 38:604, 1968.
†$\sqrt{p}$, where p is the population frequency of the specific defect.
From Nussbaum RL, McInnes RR, Willard HF: Thompson and Thompson's Genetics in Medicine, 6th ed. Philadelphia, WB Saunders, 2001.

study of Nora,[46] summarizes the empiric recurrence risk for six common congenital heart defects. More recent familial recurrence data support heritability of additional congenital heart defects, including transposition of the great arteries and congenitally corrected transposition of the great arteries (reviewed by Calcagni and coworkers[47]). Patients with heart malformations associated with chromosomal abnormalities often present differently despite having the same cytologic findings. Allelic heterogeneity at some single-gene loci or modifying effects of either environmental factors or other genes may account for some diversity in clinical findings. For example, rare alleles of *NK2*, which encodes the transcription factor NKX2.5, have been separately implicated in atrial septal defects, hypoplastic left heart syndrome, and tetralogy of Fallot. Similarly, mutations in the *GATA4* transcription factor are reported for both atrioventricular canal defects and atrial septal defects. Mutations in the *Notch* signaling pathway are also seen in different forms of congenital heart defects.

Mitochondrial Inheritance

Mutations in mitochondria produce unique patterns of inheritance. All mitochondria inherited at conception come from the mother—termed *matrilineal* inheritance. Mitochondria are the only organelles in animal cells that carry their own DNA (mitochondrial DNA [mtDNA]). Human mitochondria contain a circular genome of 16,571 base pairs that encodes just 37 genes (GenBank reference sequence NC_001807). In contrast to nuclear genes, which are present in two copies per diploid cell, the mitochondrial genome is present once per mitochondrion and therefore in a variable number of copies per cell. Perhaps because of the generation of free radicals during energy production, mtDNA is subject to a relatively high rate of mutation. Mutations in mtDNA create a mixture of normal and mutant mitochondria, called *heteroplasmy*. At cell division, mitochondria segregate randomly to the two daughter cells. This *replicative segregation* can ultimately result in a cell lineage inheriting only mutant mtDNA *(homoplasmy)*. Segregation of either inherited or de novo mtDNA mutations among cell lineages can also result in a mosaic pattern across tissues of a single individual.

Phenotypic expression of mitochondrial mutations depends on the extent of heteroplasmy, the cell type involved, and the fraction of the cell type affected. Organ systems most frequently affected by mitochondrial mutations are those with high energy requirements, particularly muscle and brain. Mutations that reduce energy production by mitochondria may produce disease whenever energy production capacity falls below a threshold level. This may be episodic if the energy threshold is crossed only during exertion or other stressors. Leber optic atrophy is perhaps the best-known example of inherited disease caused by mutations in mtDNA. Mitochondrial myopathy (a complex including neurodegeneration, pigmentary retinopathy, and Leigh syndrome), MERRF disease (myoclonic epilepsy with ragged red fibers), MELAS (mitochondrial encephalomyopathy, lactic acidosis, and strokelike episodes), and hypertrophic cardiomyopathy are also attributable to mutations in mtDNA. Most of these are not identifiable at birth but become evident with age as later-onset, maternally inherited disorders.

Dynamic Mutations and Trinucleotide Repeats

Repetitive DNA sequences can give rise to mutations through a variety of mechanisms. Repeats of two, three, or four nucleotides are especially prone to changes in repeat length. The mutation rate depends on repeat length of the starting allele, the genomic context, and other factors. Small changes in allele repeat length have been attributed to "slippage" of the DNA polymerase (or more probably, the newly synthesized DNA fragment) during replication. Much larger changes in repeat length are more likely to be caused by unequal crossing over during meiosis.[48] Alleles that change within a pedigree are said to be *dynamic*. Dynamic mutations can show other unusual features of inheritance. *Premutation alleles* are those that are expanded sufficiently to be highly dynamic but are not yet disease causing. Further expansion of the repeat results in transmission of disease alleles to offspring at a high frequency. Disease alleles are themselves dynamic and if transmitted may give rise to alleles with more severe phenotypes and earlier onset. This is called *anticipation*. Most dynamic mutations seen in humans thus far are caused by instability of *trinucleotide repeats*—specifically, CAG repeats encoding polyglutamine in the protein and other trinucleotides in noncoding sequences that alter expression of the encoded products.

Expanded polyglutamine repeats cause neurodegenerative disorders that have several features in common. These disorders show dominant inheritance, mature onset, and neurologic symptoms that include motor signs. Examples include Huntington disease, several forms of spinocerebellar ataxia, dentatorubropallidoluysian atrophy, and spinobulbar muscular atrophy. Although these disorders typically have mature onset, age at onset varies inversely with the length of repeat, and extremely rare childhood Huntington disease patients have been reported as young as 2 years of age. Expanded polyglutamine-containing proteins have been shown to be cytotoxic in several experimental contexts. The interpretation of these disorders is that expanded polyglutamine destabilizes protein structure, and that the misfolded protein, often found in insoluble aggregates, impairs cell function and ultimately leads to cell death. For a given repeat length, toxicity increases with solubility,[49] which favors a surface area model for toxicity.[50]

Amplification of polyalanine homopolymers can also be associated with disease, including some evident at birth. An amplified GCG repeat encoding polyalanine in the poly(A)-binding protein gene *(PABPN1)* is associated with autosomal dominant oculopharyngeal muscular dystrophy, apparently through a toxic gain-of-function mechanism.[51] Nondynamic amplification of polyalanine (including each of the alanine codons) in the homeobox gene *HOXD13* causes synpolydactyly, and the severity of phenotypes correlates with the extent of amplification.[52,53] Expanded polyalanine in another homeobox gene, *ARX*, results in an X-linked infantile spasm syndrome equivalent to that seen by inactivating mutations of the same gene and recessive in female carriers, suggesting that, in at least one example, polyalanine expansions may act by inactivating the protein rather than through gain of toxicity. All 10 polyalanine expansions associated with human disease to date have been nucleic acid–binding proteins. In-frame loss of polyalanine repeats in at least some of these sites is also mutagenic, including premature ovarian failure for *FOXL2* polyalanine reductions and congenital central hypoventilation syndrome for *PHOX2B* and *ASCL1*.

Trinucleotide repeat expansions in noncoding sequences can also cause disease by altering gene expression. One example is Friedreich ataxia, an autosomal recessive neurologic disorder with juvenile onset. The most common form is caused by loss-of-function alleles of the *FRDA (frataxin)* gene. The most frequent class of *FRDA* allele in patients is expansion of a GAA repeat in an intron of the gene, accounting for 98% of mutant alleles.[54] Extremely long repeats induce an epigenetic loss of expression of that copy of the gene. GAA expansion alleles and rare protein-inactivating alleles have roughly the same effect on gene function. Another example of a mutation caused by a noncoding repeat expansion is fragile X syndrome (which includes mental retardation, macro-orchidism, and facial dysmorphology). The most frequent cause of fragile X syndrome is expansion of a CGG repeat in the 5′ untranslated region of the *FMR1* gene. CpG dinucleotides are targets for methylation,[55] and DNA of the expanded allele is hypermethylated compared with both normal and premutation (stable intermediate-length repeat) alleles. Hypermethylation in or near transcriptional control elements results in loss of *FMR1* expression of the expanded allele in affected males. Expanded CGG alleles are equivalent to isolated cases hemizygous for missense and splice site mutations, confirming that this repeat expansion acts as a loss-of-function allele. Autosomal dominant myotonic dystrophy (MD1) is a third example. Expansion of a CTG trinucleotide repeat in the 3′ untranslated region of the *DMPK* protein kinase gene is strongly correlated with the disease and shows anticipation in families; however, the pathogenic mechanism remains unclear.

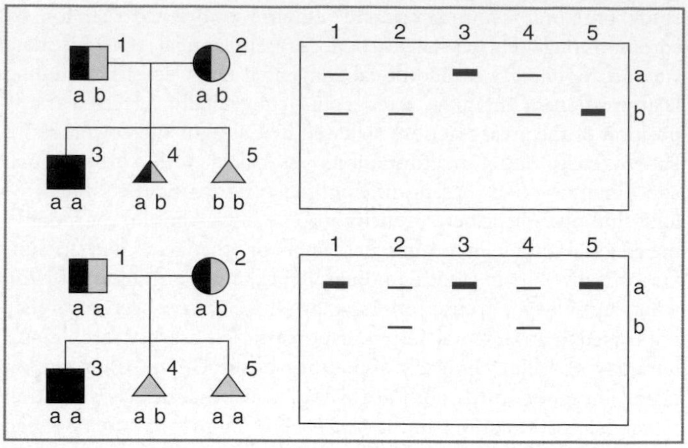

FIGURE 1-30 Schematic illustration of linkage by DNA probe analysis of restriction fragment length polymorphisms (RFLPs). **Left,** Pedigrees for two families. The *darker symbols* represent heterozygosity or homozygosity for the disease gene. Members tested are listed numerically. *Lighter triangles* represent fetuses in putative pregnancies. Letters *a* and *b* represent DNA restriction fragment lengths. **Right,** Gel electrophoresis patterns for the RFLPs. (Modified from Emery AEH: An Introduction to Recombinant DNA. New York, John Wiley & Sons, 1980.)

Imprinting

Besides the modes of inheritance already discussed, several atypical patterns of inheritance have been described. We discuss one of these patterns, called *imprinting*. Although most genes seem to have equivalent expression from alleles inherited from the father and the mother, it is now known that the expression of several genes differs between the parental alleles. This phenomenon has been termed genomic imprinting, because it appears that the two parental alleles are distinguished by some sort of mark. It appears that this mark is a reversible form of chromatin modification, perhaps methylation of one of the parental alleles, that occurs during gametogenesis and before fertilization. The mark then suppresses expression of this allele after conception. This mark is reversible in the germline, so that the parent-of-origin mark can be placed anew during gametogenesis.[56]

Prader-Willi and Angelman syndromes are good examples of the phenotypic effects of imprinting. Prader-Willi syndrome is characterized by neonatal hypotonia, childhood obesity with excessive eating, small hands and feet, hypogonadism, and mild mental retardation. Angelman syndrome is characterized by severe mental retardation, seizures, a characteristic spastic movement disorder, and an abnormal facial appearance. Although it is now known that these syndromes are caused by different genes, both syndromes can result from deletions of the same region of chromosome 15q11-q13. In about 70% of cases, Prader-Willi syndrome results from the deletion of this region inherited from the father, so they have only the maternal copy of this region. Strikingly, in about 70% of cases of Angelman syndrome, the same region is deleted and inherited from the mother, so they have only the paternal copy of this region.

Several rare disorders have now been attributed to imprinting effects. At this point, it is unclear if imprinting is an important factor in more common disorders, but it is likely that it is involved in several human genetic disorders.

Genetic Testing and DNA Diagnostics

The realization in the 1980s that DNA variations, or polymorphisms, between individuals occur fairly frequently led to the development of both DNA forensics and molecular diagnostics for genetic disorders and risk factors.[57] DNA diagnostics in medicine can use either direct assays for a specific mutation or linkage analysis with polymorphisms linked to a disease locus. Direct assays for specific mutations are most useful when relatively few distinct mutations account for most patients with a particular form of disease. As analysis methods become faster, cheaper, and more highly automated, performing direct tests on each nucleotide of a disease gene without knowing the precise mutation will become increasingly practical, particularly for genes in which a high proportion of patients have de novo mutations. Indirect assays using linkage analysis (Fig. 1-30) have traditionally been most useful for risk assessment when a disease gene has been mapped in pedigrees but not yet identified at the molecular level. Linkage analysis requires cooperation of other family members, including usually at least one affected member, to identify marker alleles on the disease-associated chromosome in that particular pedigree. Recombination between the marker and the disease gene is a potential caveat if a single marker is used; use of markers on each side of the disease gene at least makes this evident, and the likelihood of recombination can be built into the risk assessment. In practice, linkage assays for identified diseases become less necessary as a higher proportion of significant disease genes can be assayed directly. However, linkage analysis and family studies remain crucial to the successful identification of disease and disease susceptibility genes.

The initial molecular diagnostics to come out of the recombinant DNA revolution were based on restriction fragment length polymorphisms (RFLPs) (see Fig. 1-30). RFLPs are typically assayed by Southern blotting,[58] which requires substantial amounts of DNA and is relatively labor intensive and difficult to automate, making it relatively expensive. This approach is still used to identify large repeat expansions for genes known to be subject to dynamic mutations. The development of PCR by Mullis and coworkers in the mid-1980s allowed selective amplification of any desired sequence of DNA and radically changed the power of DNA diagnostics in terms of sample requirements and the types of assays one could perform.[59,60] Linkage markers in current use include simple sequence repeat length polymorphisms (SSLPs, or microsatellites) and, increasingly, biallelic SNPs. SNPs in particular have the advantage of being assayable in multiplex formats, such that many distinct polymorphic sites may be interrogated in a single biochemical reaction. Several different technologies for SNP detection have been and continue to be developed to allow simultaneous detection of larger numbers of loci at smaller marginal cost. Finally, as more is known about normal copy number variation and those associated with specific diseases, the detection of CNVs will become increasingly used in diagnostics.

Methods Used in Genetic Testing

Hybridization-Based Methods

Nucleic acid hybridization is a simple physical chemical process with well-described parameters,[61,62] and it forms the basis for a wide variety of molecular genetic tests. The rate and stability of nucleic acid duplexes depend on the concentration of each strand, temperature, ionic strength of the solution, and the presence of hydrogen bond competitors such as urea and formamide. Tests based on whole-genome Southern blots were among the first available for mutations with no cytologic correlate. As discussed earlier, hybridization of fluorescently labeled probes to fixed chromosomal spreads (FISH, spectral karyotyping) allows the identification of microdeletions, microduplications, translocations, and other cytologic abnormalities that would be difficult to detect without molecular probes. Other methods include hybridization of patient DNA to allele-specific oligonucleotides to discriminate single base changes. An example of detection by allele-specific oligonucleotides is given in the reverse dot-blot analysis shown in Figure 1-31. In a reverse dot-blot analysis, the probe sequence is bound to the support matrix while the amplified patient sample is labeled and hybridized to the oligonucleotides; using this approach, a patient sample can be tested for several mutations in a single assay.

Southern blotting is used to detect variations in size or amount of a defined DNA fragment (Fig. 1-32). To produce the defined fragments from whole genomic DNA, restriction endonuclease enzymes are used to cut intact DNA at specific sites. Restriction enzymes occur in bacteria, where they form part of the host defense against bacterial viruses. Different bacterial species produce enzymes that recognize and cleave

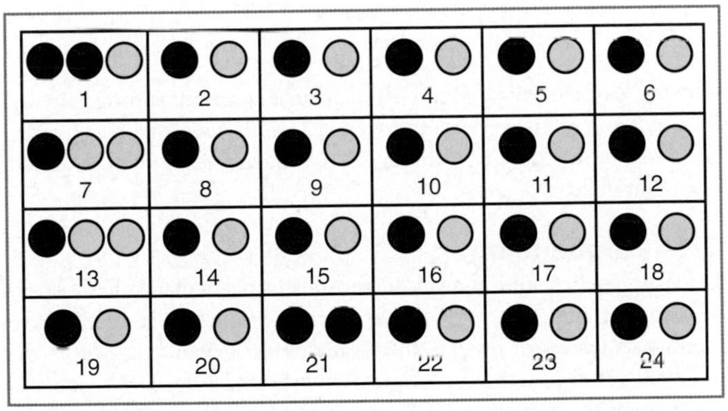

FIGURE 1-31 **Reverse dot-blot analysis for cystic fibrosis (CF) mutations.** Twenty-seven CF mutations were analyzed in this study. The complete panel in this figure represents a single filter, subdivided into 24 sections. Each section is numbered for specific mutation analysis. Sections 1, 7, and 13 analyze two separate mutations. Circles on the left in each numbered section contain normal oligonucleotide sequences from the CF gene region on chromosome 7. The sequences in each section represent different regions on the gene where a mutation has been identified. Thus, complementary normal sequences, amplified by polymerase chain reaction (PCR), hybridize as indicated by the *red circles.* The *blue circles* represent effort at hybridization between mutant sequences fixed to the filter and DNA sequences obtained from the patient and amplified by PCR. If the patient does not have a CF mutation among the group of 27 in this analysis, there is no hybridization and the circle remains open. In this analysis, sections 1 and 21 demonstrate that this patient has two CF mutations and would be designated a compound heterozygote. This individual would most likely have clinical manifestations of CF.

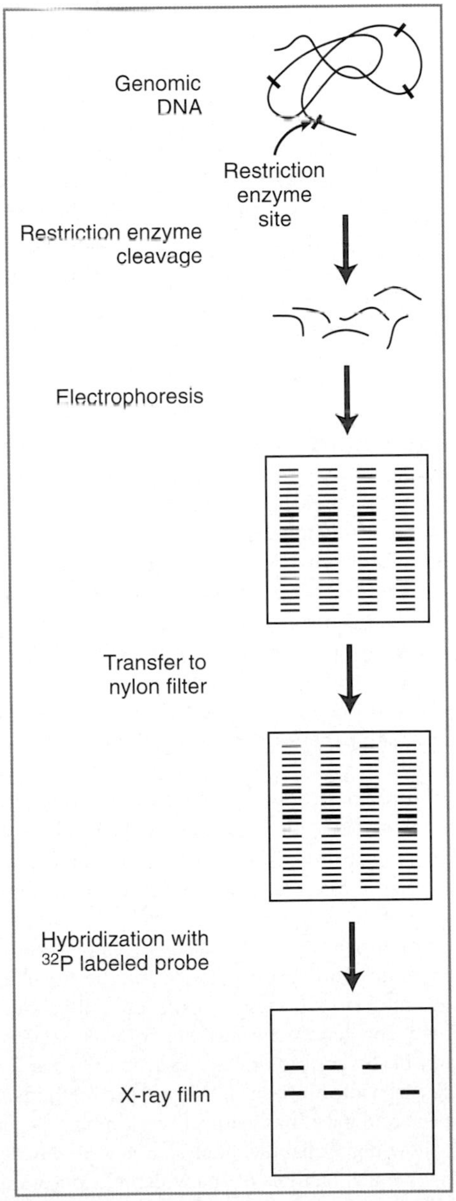

FIGURE 1-32 **Southern blotting.** DNA is cleaved by a restriction enzyme, separated according to size by agarose gel electrophoresis, and transferred to a filter. After hybridization of the DNA to a labeled probe and exposure of the filter to x-ray film, complementary sequences can be identified.

DNA at different sites. Each restriction enzyme cuts DNA at a defined sequence, usually a palindrome four to eight base pairs in length. For example, EcoRI cuts the palindromic site 5′-GAATTC-3′ between the G and the A:

$$\begin{matrix}5'\text{-GAATTC-}3' \\ 3'\text{-CTTAAG-}5'\end{matrix} \rightarrow \begin{matrix}5'\text{-G} + \text{AATTC-}3' \\ 3'\text{-CTTAA} + \text{G-}5'\end{matrix}$$

After digestion with restriction enzymes, DNA is size-fractionated by gel electrophoresis (moving through a gel matrix that retards larger fragments more than smaller fragments as they move in response to an electric field). DNA is then denatured into single strands by hydroxide and then transferred (blotted) from the gel to a membrane capable of binding the DNA, usually nitrocellulose or derivatized nylon. Single-stranded DNA on the membrane is then available for hybridization by base pairing with a "probe" sequence. The probe is labeled with either a radionuclide (usually phosphorus 32 [^{32}P]) or a chemical (biotin, digoxigenin, or fluorescein) tag for detection. After hybridization and removal of excess probe, the hybrid fragments are detected by film autoradiography for ^{32}P probes or antibody conjugate–based methods (chemiluminescence or chromatogenic reactions). By quantifying the radiologic signal from a Southern blot, it is also possible to assess the copy number of the DNA fragment in the genome relative to known standards. Southern blots have been used to detect insertions and deletions that change the length of the restriction fragment, sequence changes that affect a specific restriction site, and duplications and deficiencies that change the copy number of the fragment.

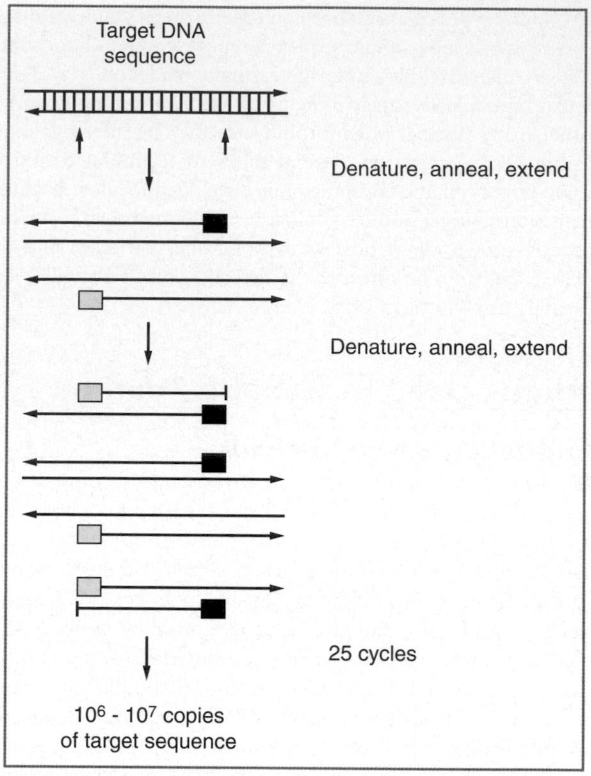

FIGURE 1-33 Polymerase chain reaction (PCR). Repeated synthesis of a specific target DNA sequence *(upward arrows)* results in exponential amplification. The reaction proceeds from the primers *(blue squares, red squares)* in the 3′ direction on each strand. The first two cycles of the PCR are shown.

Polymerase Chain Reaction

Amplification of DNA segments through PCR revolutionized DNA diagnostics for both medicine and forensics beginning in the mid-1980s.[59,63-65] Synthetic oligonucleotides are used to prime DNA synthesis so that synthesis directed from each primer includes the sequence complementary to the other primer (Fig. 1-33). Multiple cycles of DNA denaturation, primer annealing, and elongation of DNA synthesis create an exponential amplification of the DNA sequence between the two primers. The phases of this cycle are controlled by temperature. Using PCR to amplify specific DNA fragments, multiple diagnostic tests can be performed on minimal amounts of starting material.

Variations in length, such as in dynamic mutations, can be assayed directly by PCR amplification followed by gel electrophoresis to determine the size of the PCR product. For example, diagnostic tests for expanded alleles are available for dentatorubropallidoluysian atrophy, Huntington disease, and fragile X syndrome that are based on determining the size of the allele by amplification of patient DNA using oligonucleotide primers that flank the site of expansion.

Anonymous marker loci, such as SNPs and SSLPs, can be assayed in the same way for gene mapping and forensic studies. SNPs are amplified singly or in a multiplex combination of loci and detected by electrophoretic, hybridization, or spectroscopic methods. SNP-based assays are expected to have increasing clinical impact in coming years because they allow highly parallel analysis. Multiplex PCR amplifications can allow parallel analysis of many genetic loci simultaneously. Software modification can allow SNP-based assays to detect CNVs. As noted earlier, as more is known about normal CNVs and those associated with specific diseases, the detection of CNVs will become increasingly used in diagnostics.

Common mutations can also be assayed by PCR using primers specific for each allele or by allele-specific oligonucleotide hybridization. For genes in which no single mutation is common among patients, such as the hereditary hearing loss gene *JGB2,* novel sequence variations can be identified by direct DNA sequencing of PCR products from that gene.

DNA Sequencing

Modern genetics, and clinical diagnostics in particular, relies heavily on knowing the exact sequence of nucleotides in genes. Methods to identify sequences of small RNA molecules first began to appear in the late 1960s. However, the appearance of two methods for DNA sequencing of longer fragments in 1977 was a major breakthrough. The *chemical cleavage method*[66] uses base-specific chemistries to cleave a specified base from its sugar, followed by a second reaction to cleave the phosphodiester bond adjacent to the resulting abasic site. The *chain termination method*[67] uses enzymatic synthesis of DNA in the presence of dideoxynucleotides; dideoxynucleotides prevent further synthesis beyond their site of incorporation because they lack the 3′ hydroxyl group (see Fig. 1-1). The chain termination method is by far the most widely used today. It has been further developed to include fluorescent labels for automated detection and thermostable polymerase enzymes to allow multiple cycles of DNA synthesis for each template molecule. An important extension of this approach for diagnostics is the use of single nucleotide extension products (termed mini-sequencing) to determine alleles based on a single nucleotide change without the added labor and expense of gel or capillary electrophoresis. For example, tests for hereditary hemochromatosis use a version of mini-sequencing called Pyrosequencing to detect the *C282Y* mutation and the *H63D* and *S65C* alleles of the *HFE* gene.

Other Considerations

Current technology is quite powerful and still developing. Vanishingly small specimens can now be used to query ever-expanding numbers of known genes and anonymous DNA markers. Future developments seem likely to continue this trend toward making molecular genetic tests faster, less expensive, and more reliable. This technologic facility and the link between diagnostics and forensics raises numerous ethical, legal, and social issues (often referred to as ELSI). In current practice, one needs to pay particular attention to informed consent, restrictions on use of clinical material in research, and what has been termed genetic privacy. These issues are beyond the scope of this chapter but are as vital to the practitioner who requests genetic testing as they are to the practitioner in the diagnostic laboratory.

Linkage Analysis

Linkage analysis uses DNA polymorphisms as markers to follow the inheritance of a gene within a family. This approach is used to identify unknown genes that contribute to disease, and to follow disease-associated chromosomal segments in affected families before the causal mutation is pinpointed. Linkage analysis takes advantage of meiotic recombination by counting how frequently two loci are inherited together. By comparing the inheritance of a disease with inheritance of alleles at several known DNA polymorphisms (marker loci), it is possible to map the positions of disease genes. Theoretically, any single-gene disorder should be amenable to carrier identification and prenatal diagnosis by linkage analysis once the gene is mapped.

DNA polymorphisms are codominantly inherited, meaning each allele carried by an individual should be detected in a well-designed assay. Several kinds of DNA polymorphisms are frequent in the human genome and have been used in linkage studies.

RFLPs arise through insertions (often of mobile repetitive elements, such as Alu), deletions, and base changes at restriction sites (particularly through deamination of C residues in CG dinucleotides). Assays for RFLP markers by Southern blotting were described previously. RFLPs that have diagnostic importance are usually either converted to a PCR-based assay for the underlying sequence change or replaced for diagnostic use by a linked polymorphism that is more easily assayed.

Insertions and deletions occur frequently in the human genome. These range in size from a single base pair to multigene segments and arise by multiple mechanisms. Small insertion-deletion polymorphisms (also called indels) most likely occur through errors in DNA replication and repair. Larger insertions and deletions arise through several mechanisms, including retrotransposition (such as for Alu repeat sequences) and illegitimate recombination at sites of sequence homology (a frequent finding in microdeletion syndromes). Insertions and deletions were initially detected as RFLPs by Southern blotting. Now indel polymorphisms are usually detected using PCR-based methods designed to be compatible with detecting SNPs, CNVs, or both.

Variable number tandem repeats are more polymorphic than RFLPs and can occur in several alleles, varying by the number of repeat copies present at the locus. Variable number tandem repeats can be detected by Southern blot more sensitively than RFLPs because multiple copies are present. Some variable number tandem repeats are small enough to be assayed by PCR and can be used along with other PCR-based markers.

SSLPs (also called short tandem repeats, simple sequence repeats, or microsatellites) are simple repeats of two, three, or four nucleotides (such as CACACACACACA). Like variable number tandem repeats, SSLPs can have several possible alleles. The spontaneous mutation rate to a new allele size ranges from 10^{-3} to 10^{-6}. This high mutation rate makes microsatellites useful as markers for genetic mapping: They mutate frequently enough to be highly polymorphic in a population but are stable enough to be transmitted reliably in a pedigree. Simple sequence repeats (microsatellites) occur approximately every 30 kilobases in the human genome (depending on the repeat-length threshold one sets), and a high proportion are polymorphic to some extent across human populations. These markers are easily assayed on a moderate scale but still must be resolved by electrophoresis. Although this is practicable on a modest scale, such as diagnostics for linkage to a mapped but still unknown disease mutation segregating within a family, and has been used for genome-wide scans for genetic linkage, identifying the correct size of each allele is the most significant bottleneck for applications requiring very high throughput with many markers.

SNPs are by far the most frequent class of polymorphism in the human genome. On average, any two copies of the human genome have a polymorphism approximately every 1000 base pairs. Millions of SNPs have been cataloged across the human genome.[68] On a small scale, these polymorphisms can be detected using the direct analysis methods described for detecting specific mutations. However, for large linkage studies, the number of single genotypes that must be generated is quite large, and higher throughput methods have been and continue to be developed. Competing methods for large-scale genotyping include variations on allele-specific PCR that allow detection by hybridization, highly parallel allele specific oligonucleotide hybridization on high-density oligonucleotide arrays produced by photo lithography,[69] and mini-sequencing detected by fluorescence or mass spectroscopy.[70] These recently developed methods will impact DNA diagnostics in both the discovery of new genes involved in disease and in parallel testing for multiple disorders.

Identifying New Disease Genes

Linkage data to identify new disease genes are analyzed by computer algorithms that assess their statistical significance. Although many linkage analysis packages are available, a recurrent question arises with respect to the statistical threshold for declaring linkage. As pointed out by Lander and Kruglyak,[71] each genome scan is really a series of discrete hypotheses. Statistical thresholds must be set to account for the number of hypotheses tested. Lander and Kruglyak argue that in the current era, the number of hypotheses that must be accounted for in linkage studies is a function of genome size, as one could (and does) continue testing markers until the genome is covered. They suggested using statistical thresholds based on the likelihood of false-positive findings in a complete genome linkage scan (genome-wide significance) rather than in a discrete test of any one specific locus (pointwise significance). Computer simulations in the absence of linkage and permutation testing of real linkage data support the idea that genome-wide significance levels are needed to minimize reporting of false-positive findings.

Association and Linkage Disequilibrium

A concept related to linkage analysis is genetic association. Rather than explicitly following coinheritance of traits and markers through a family pedigree, association studies follow covariation of traits and markers in a population. Case and control samples are compared for alleles at each locus to ask whether one or more alleles are significantly overrepresented (disease-associated alleles) or underrepresented (protective alleles) in disease cases. One of the best-studied examples of genetic association is the increased risk of late-onset Alzheimer's disease for individuals with certain alleles of the apolipoprotein E gene (*APOE*).[72,73] The amino acid variants encoded by the E4 allele of *APOE* are thought to be directly responsible for the increased risk. However, a strong association of a polymorphism with disease does not necessarily mean that the polymorphism causes the disease, although it does provide immediate diagnostic value. Associations that are not causal occur by *linkage disequilibrium*. Linkage disequilibrium essentially means that specific alleles at two loci are inherited together throughout a population. This occurs when the genetic distance between the loci is small compared with the number of generations in which the two alleles could have separated by recombination in that population. Association studies that take best advantage of population-based linkage disequilibrium may provide the next opportunity to discover genes that act in multifactorial and genetically heterogeneous diseases. Current efforts in this area include both maps of human DNA polymorphisms[68] and maps of regions coinherited by linkage disequilibrium in the general population.[74]

The technical feasibility of simultaneously following very large numbers of DNA variations in large numbers of clinical subjects has allowed the development of very powerful genome-wide association studies, also called whole-genome association studies (as mentioned earlier). A substantial number of these studies first appeared in 2007, including a large study that combined analysis of several unrelated diseases and traits simultaneously.[21] By examining variations chosen to represent most if not all common variations (either directly or through linkage disequilibrium with the tested variations) and combining subjects ascertained by collaborating clinical groups, such studies have enormous statistical power for detecting previously unsuspected genetic susceptibilities for disease and will play a large role in the development of personalized medicine.

Impact of the Human Genome Project and Genomics

In 2001, a draft of the human genome was published simultaneously by the publicly funded Human Genome Project[2] and a private company, Celera.[3] Both groups had covered approximately 90% of the genome, and, as discussed previously, estimates of the number of genes had ranged from 30,000 to 40,000 human genes in these first published studies[2,3] to substantially higher estimates.[75,76] Then, in 2004 the complete human sequence became available from the Human Genome Project.[77] The International HapMap Consortium[4] determined a large fraction of the variations in DNA sequences over populations by cataloging SNPs, and more recently, efforts to catalog CNVs have begun.[5] As discussed in the introduction to this chapter, these tremendous advances have already had a profound impact on biomedical research. It is the consensus that this research will revolutionize our approach to diagnosis and treatment of human disease over the next decade and beyond, especially with respect to the identification of genetic risk factors for some of the most common disorders today, including cancer, hypertension, coronary artery disease, diabetes, susceptibility to infectious diseases, and obesity. Certainly, diagnostic testing by methods outlined in this chapter will be improved with this information. It is difficult to estimate when these advances will make their way into clinical practice, although some have ventured to gaze into the future.[1]

Conclusion

As noted in the beginning of this chapter, genetics plays an important role in the day-to-day practice of obstetrics. We have summarized the basic concepts of genetics as they apply to the understanding and treatment of human diseases and have emphasized those areas most pertinent to the practice of obstetrics. Clinical genetics will increasingly become a discipline that physicians will be expected to use for the care of their patients. Research in molecular biology and molecular genetics, along with the genetic information provided by the Human Genome Project and genomics, will provide the information necessary for physicians to formulate new clinical approaches to medical diagnostics and therapeutics.

Acknowledgments

We acknowledge the contributions of the authors of earlier editions of this book, O. W. Jones and T. C. Cahill, for the organization and many of the figures and tables used in the present chapter. We also thank Dr. Karen Arden for providing the spectral karyotyping image (see Fig. 1-14).

References

1. Collins FS, McKusick VA: Implications of the Human Genome Project for medical science. JAMA 285:540, 2001.
2. Lander ES, Linton LM, Birren B, et al: Initial sequencing and analysis of the human genome. Nature 409:860, 2001.
3. Venter JC, Adams MD, Myers EW, et al: The sequence of the human genome. Science 291:1304, 2001.
4. International HapMap Consortium. A haplotype map of the human genome. Nature 437:1299, 2005.
5. Redon R, Ishikawa S, Fitch KR, et al: Global variation in copy number in the human genome. Nature 444:444, 2006.
6. Brown TR, Lubahn DB, Wilson EM, et al: Deletion of the steroid-binding domain of the human androgen receptor gene in one family with complete androgen insensitivity syndrome: Evidence for further genetic heterogeneity in this syndrome. Proc Natl Acad Sci U S A 85:8151, 1988.
7. La Spada AR, Wilson EM, Lubahn DB, et al: Androgen receptor gene mutations in X-linked spinal and bulbar muscular atrophy. Nature 352:77, 1991.
8. Vogel F, Rathenberg R: Spontaneous mutation in man. Adv Hum Genet 5:223, 1975.
9. Hsu LYF: Prenatal diagnosis of chromosomal abnormalities through amniocentesis. In Milunsky A (ed): Genetic Disorders in the Fetus, 4th ed. Baltimore, Johns Hopkins University Press, 1998, p 179.
10. Nussbaum RL, McInnes RR, Willard HF: Thompson and Thompson's Genetics in Medicine, 6th ed. Philadelphia, WB Saunders, 2001.
11. Lyon MF: Gene action in the X-chromosome of the mouse (Mus musculus L). Nature 190:372, 1961.
12. Boueá J, Boueá A, Lazar P: Retrospective and prospective epidemiological studies of 1500 karyotyped spontaneous human abortions. Teratology 12:11, 1975.
13. Creasy MR, Crolla JA, Alberman ED: A cytogenetic study of human spontaneous abortions using banding techniques. Hum Genet 31:177, 1976.
14. Hassold TJ: A cytogenetic study of repeated spontaneous abortions. Am J Hum Genet 32:723, 1980.
15. Feng HL: Molecular biology of male infertility. Arch Androl 49:19, 2003.
16. Lamson SH, Hook EB: A simple function for maternal-age-specific rates of Down syndrome in the 20- to 49-year age range and its biological implications. Am J Hum Genet 32:743, 1980.

17. McKusick VA: Mendelian Inheritance in Man, 12th ed. Baltimore, Johns Hopkins University Press, 1998.
18. McKusick VA: Mendelian Inheritance in Man (National Center for Biotechnology Information). Available at www.ncbi.nlm.nih.gov/entrez/query.fcgi?db=OMIM (accessed January 24, 2008).
19. Hartl DL, Clark AG: Principles of Population Genetics. Sunderland, MA, Sinauer Associates, 2007.
20. Ott J: Analysis of Human Genetic Linkage, 3rd ed. Baltimore, Johns Hopkins University Press, 1999.
21. Wellcome Trust Case Control Consortium: Genome-wide association study of 14,000 cases of seven common diseases and 3,000 shared controls. Nature 447:661, 2007.
22. Fraser FC: The genetics of cleft lip and cleft palate. Am J Hum Genet 22:336, 1970.
23. Koguchi H: Recurrence rate in offspring and siblings of patients with cleft lip and/or cleft palate. Jinrui Idengaku Zasshi 20:207, 1975.
24. Brewer CM, Leek JP, Green AJ, et al: A locus for isolated cleft palate, located on human chromosome 2q32. Am J Hum Genet 65:387, 1999.
25. FitzPatrick DR, Carr IM, McLaren L, et al: Identification of *SATB2* as the cleft palate gene on 2q32-q33. Hum Mol Genet 12:2491, 2003.
26. Morris JK, Wald NJ: Prevalence of neural tube defect pregnancies in England and Wales from 1964 to 2004. J Med Screen 14:55, 2007.
27. DeWals P, Tairou F, Van Allen MI, et al: Reduction in neural-tube defects after folic acid fortification in Canada. N Engl J Med 357:135, 2007.
28. Copp AJ: Prevention of neural tube defects: Vitamins, enzymes and genes. Curr Opin Neurol 11:97, 1998.
29. Beemster P, Groenen P, Steegers-Theunissen R: Involvement of inositol in reproduction. Nutr Rev 60:80, 2002.
30. Cavalli P, Copp AJ: Inositol and folate resistant neural tube defects. J Med Genet 39:E5, 2002.
31. Carter CO, Evans KA: Inheritance of congenital pyloric stenosis. J Med Genet 6:233, 1969.
32. Mitchell LE, Risch N: The genetics of infantile hypertrophic pyloric stenosis: A reanalysis. Am J Dis Child 147:1203, 1993.
33. Subramaniam R, Doig CM, Moore L: Nitric oxide synthase is absent in only a subset of cases of pyloric stenosis. J Pediatr Surg 36:616, 2001.
34. Huang PL, Dawson TM, Bredt DS, et al: Targeted disruption of the neuronal nitric oxide synthase gene. Cell 75:1273, 1993.
35. Gyurko R, Leupen S, Huang PL: Deletion of exon 6 of the neuronal nitric oxide synthase gene in mice results in hypogonadism and infertility. Endocrinology 143:2767, 2002.
36. Capon F, Reece A, Ravindrarajah R, Chung E: Linkage of monogenic infantile hypertrophic pyloric stenosis to chromosome 16p12-p13 and evidence for genetic heterogeneity. Am J Hum Genet 79:378, 2006.
37. Greco L, Romino R, Coto I, et al: The first large population based twin study of coeliac disease. Gut 50:624, 2002.
38. Zhong F, McCombs CC, Olson JM, et al: An autosomal screen for genes that predispose to celiac disease in the western counties of Ireland. Nat Genet 14:329, 1996.
39. Greco L, Babron MC, Corazza GR, et al: Existence of a genetic risk factor on chromosome 5q in Italian coeliac disease families. Ann Hum Genet 65:35, 2001.
40. Liu J, Juo SH, Holopainen P, et al: Genomewide linkage analysis of celiac disease in Finnish families. Am J Hum Genet 70:51, 2002.
41. Rioux JD, Daly MJ, Silverberg MS, et al: Genetic variation in the 5q31 cytokine gene cluster confers susceptibility to Crohn disease. Nat Genet 29:223-228, 2001.
42. De Wals P, Tairou F, Van Allen MI, et al: A genome-wide association study identifies *IL23R* as an inflammatory bowel disease gene. Science 314:1461, 2006.
43. Gabriel SB, Salomon R, Pelet A, et al: Segregation at three loci explains familial and population risk in Hirschsprung disease. Nat Genet 31:89, 2002.
44. Emison ES, McCallion AS, Kashuk CS, et al: A common sex-dependent mutation in a *RET* enhancer underlies Hirschsprung disease risk. Nature 434:857, 2005.
45. Hoess K, Goldmuntz E, Pyeritz RE: Genetic counseling for congenital heart disease: New approaches for a new decade. Curr Cardiol Rep 4:68, 2002.
46. Nora JJ: Multifactorial inheritance hypothesis for the etiology of congenital heart diseases: The genetic-environmental interaction. Circulation 38:604, 1968.
47. Calcagni G, Digilio MC, Sarkozy A, et al: Familial recurrence of congenital heart disease: An overview and review of the literature. Eur J Pediatr 166:111, 2007.
48. Warren ST: Polyalanine expansion in synpolydactyly might result from unequal crossing-over of *HOXD13*. Science 275:408, 1997.
49. Watase K, Weeber EJ, Xu B, et al: A long CAG repeat in the mouse *Sca1* locus replicates SCA1 features and reveals the impact of protein solubility on selective neurodegeneration. Neuron 34:905, 2002.
50. Floyd JA, Hamilton BA: Intranuclear inclusions and the ubiquitin-proteasome pathway: Digestion of a red herring? Neuron 24:765, 1999.
51. Brais B, Bouchard JP, Xie YG, et al: Short GCG expansions in the *PABP2* gene cause oculopharyngeal muscular dystrophy. Nat Genet 18:164, 1998.
52. Muragaki Y, Mundlos S, Upton J, et al: Altered growth and branching patterns in synpolydactyly caused by mutations in *HOXD13*. Science 272:548, 1996.
53. Goodman FR, Mundlos S, Muragaki Y, et al: Synpolydactyly phenotypes correlate with size of expansions in *HOXD13* polyalanine tract. Proc Natl Acad Sci U S A 94:7458, 1997.
54. Delatycki MB, Knight M, Koenig M, et al: G130V, a common *FRDA* point mutation, appears to have arisen from a common founder. Hum Genet 105:343, 1999.
55. Bird A: The essentials of DNA methylation. Cell 70:5, 1992.
56. Tilghman SM: The sins of the fathers and mothers: Genomic imprinting in mammalian development. Cell 96:185, 1999.
57. Botstein D, White RL, Skolnick EM, et al: Construction of a genetic linkage map in man using restriction fragment length polymorphisms. Am J Hum Genet 32:314, 1980.
58. Southern EM: Detection of specific sequences among DNA fragments separated by gel electrophoresis. J Mol Biol 98:503, 1975.
59. Mullis K, Faloona F, Scharf S, et al: Specific enzymatic amplification of DNA in vitro: The polymerase chain reaction. Cold Spring Harb Symp Quant Biol 51:263, 1986.
60. Mullis KB, Faloona F: Specific synthesis of DNA in vitro via a polymerase-catalyzed chain reaction. Methods Enzymol 155:335, 1987.
61. Wetmur JG, Davidson N: Kinetics of renaturation of DNA. J Mol Biol 31:349, 1968.
62. Wetmur JG: Hybridization and renaturation kinetics of nucleic acids. Annu Rev Biophys Bioeng 5:337, 1976.
63. Saiki RK, Scharf S, Faloona F, et al: Enzymatic amplification of β-globin genomic sequences and restriction site analysis for diagnosis of sickle cell anemia. Science 230:1350, 1985.
64. Saiki RK, Bugawan TL, Horn GT, et al: Analysis of enzymatically amplified β-globin and HLA-DQα DNA with allele-specific oligonucleotide probes. Nature 324:163, 1986.
65. Saiki RK, Gelfand DH, Stoffel S, et al: Primer-directed enzymatic amplification of DNA with a thermostable DNA polymerase. Science 239:487, 1988.
66. Maxam AM, Gilbert W: A new method of sequencing DNA. Proc Natl Acad Sci U S A 74:560, 1977.
67. Sanger F, Nicklen S, Coulson AR: DNA sequencing with chain-terminating inhibitors. Proc Natl Acad Sci U S A 74:5463, 1977.
68. Sachidanandam R, Weissman D, Schmidt SC, et al: A map of human genome sequence variation containing 1.42 million single nucleotide polymorphisms. Nature 409:928, 2001.
69. Wang DG, Fan JB, Siao CJ, et al: Large-scale identification, mapping, and genotyping of single-nucleotide polymorphisms in the human genome. Science 280:1077, 1998.
70. Tang K, Fu DJ, Julien D, et al: Chip-based genotyping by mass spectrometry. Proc Natl Acad Sci U S A 96:10016, 1999.
71. Lander E, Kruglyak L: Genetic dissection of complex traits: guidelines for interpreting and reporting linkage results. Nat Genet 11:241, 1995.

72. Corder EH, Saunders AM, Strittmatter WJ, et al: Gene dose of apolipoprotein E type 4 allele and the risk of Alzheimer's disease in late onset families. Science 261:921, 1993.
73. Roses AD: Apolipoprotein E alleles as risk factors in Alzheimer's disease. Annu Rev Med 47:387, 1996.
74. Gabriel SB, Schaffner SF, Nguyen H, et al: The structure of haplotype blocks in the human genome. Science 23:23, 2002.
75. Liang F, Holt I, Pertea G, et al: Gene index analysis of the human genome estimates approximately 120,000 genes. Nat Genet 25:239, 2000.
76. Hogenesch JB, Ching KA, Batalov S, et al: A comparison of the Celera and Ensembl predicted gene sets reveals little overlap in novel genes. Cell 106:413, 2001.
77. International Human Genome Sequencing Consortium: Finishing the euchromatic sequence of the human genome. Nature 431:931, 2004.

Chapter 2

Normal Early Development

Kurt Benirschke, MD

The developing fertilized ovum enters the uterine cavity on about the 4th day after fertilization. During its journey through the fallopian tube, its cells proliferate within the zona pellucida (Fig. 2-1), and shortly before entering the uterus, a blastocyst cavity is formed. Differentiation of a human ovum into embryonic and future placental cells first occurs in a 58-cell morula, as described by Hertig.[1] His specimen was 6 days old and had five embryonic cells (the "inner cell mass," or "stem cells"), and 53 trophoblastic cells constituted the wall of this uterine blastocyst. The polar bodies and an apparently degenerating zona pellucida were still present in the specimen, features destined to be lost shortly before implantation. These landmarks are of importance now when embryonic stem cells are being harvested and when prenatal diagnosis, intracytoplasmic sperm injection (ICSI), and other aspects of assisted reproductive technology (ART) are actively being pursued.

Proliferation of the trophoblastic shell after this stage of development is rapid, and a segmentation cavity develops, with the more slowly reproducing embryonic cells assuming a marginal "polar" position. The adjacent trophoblastic cells enlarge and secure implantation, which is assumed to take place on about the 6th or 7th day after fertilization (Fig. 2-2). Attraction to certain regions of the endometrium is presumed to take place because of molecular signals expressed on the respective surfaces[2,3] and occurs only during the "window of receptivity" that is regulated by hormonal action on the endometrium.[4] With the very rapid enlargement occurring in the anchoring trophoblastic cells, the endometrial cells are dissociated by mechanisms to be discussed later (see Microscopic Development). The entire blastocyst thus comes to assume an "interstitial" position (i.e., it sinks entirely into the endometrium at the site of attachment). The process may well be aided by the collapse of the blastocyst cavity that occurs at this time (see Fig. 2-2). A deposition of fibrin or occasionally a coagulum at the site of penetration are common events thereafter, and then the implanted trophoblastic shell comes to be surrounded by endometrium (decidua) on all sides (Fig. 2-3). Perhaps some endometrial proliferation at the edges seals the defect.

The portion of decidua lying between blastocyst and myometrium is the decidua basalis; the portion covering the defect is the decidua capsularis. Eventually, the latter comes to lie on the outside of the placental membranes. The decidua of the opposite side of the uterus is the decidua vera. At the time of implantation, the 0.1-mm blastocyst can be detected only by a dissecting microscope. Within a few days, however, it will constitute a polypoid protrusion that can readily be seen by careful inspection of the endometrium. Thus, the approximately 14-day-old ovum (Fig. 2-4) looks like a polyp and already has a differentiated, elongated embryo with amnion and yolk sac cavities.

Occasionally, a small blood clot is attached to the implantation site, the *Schlusskoagulum*, whose presence may be detected clinically by spotting (Hartman sign) and may lead to misinterpretation of the length of gestation. Decidual hemorrhages and small areas of necrosis at the site of trophoblastic penetration are common at this time and later.

Macroscopic Development

In most recorded sites of early implantation, the ovum was found in the upper portion of the fundus and the development of the placenta has been followed by ultrasonography. Thus, Rizos and colleagues[5] found the 16-week placenta to be attached anteriorly in 37% of patients, posteriorly in 24%, in a fundal position in 34%, and both anteriorly and posteriorly in 4%. Others have used sonography to measure placental size and volume prenatally and have correlated their findings with fetal outcome.[6] Of interest in this context is the finding from sonographic study that low implantation of the placenta in the uterus occurs frequently, with the formation of an apparent placenta previa. Moreover, a low implantation may change through differential growth of the placenta and uterus and apparent marginal placental atrophy. Thus, even though low implantation is observed in early gestation, at term the situation often does not clinically resemble placenta previa.[7] In the report of Rizos and colleagues, only 5 of 47 patients in whom placenta previa was diagnosed with ultrasound between 16 and 18 weeks actually had this condition when delivery occurred at term. These findings are important in the interpretation of the shape of the placenta at term and necessitate revision of former impressions.

Most commonly, the placenta develops at the uterine fundus. Through rapid expansion of the extraembryonic cavity (the exocoelom) and proliferation of the trophoblastic shell, the ovum bulges into the endometrial cavity at the time of the first missed menstrual period. The surface is flecked by tiny hemorrhages and necrotic decidua. With continued expansion of the embryonic cavity, the surface becomes attenuated, the peripheral villi atrophy, and the future placental "membranes" form. They consist of decidua capsularis on the outside, hyalinized villi and trophoblast in the middle, and the membranous chorion laeve (and amnion) on the inside.

The relationship of these membranes to the remainder of the uterus was sequentially traced in numerous pregnant uteri in a series collected

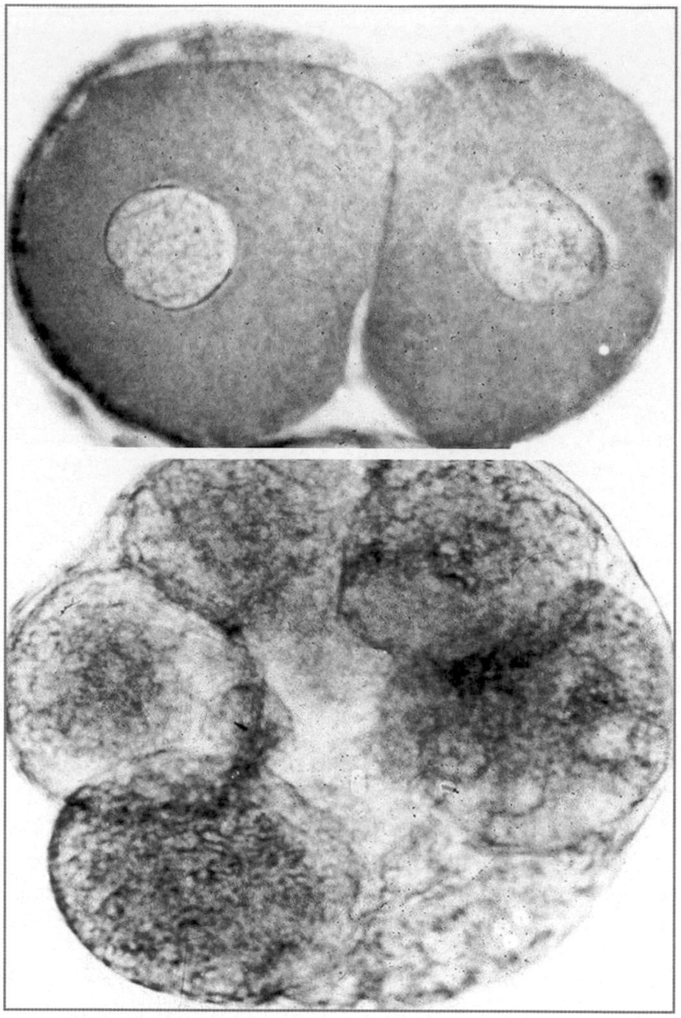

FIGURE 2-1 Two-cell stage (30 hours) and eight-cell morula.

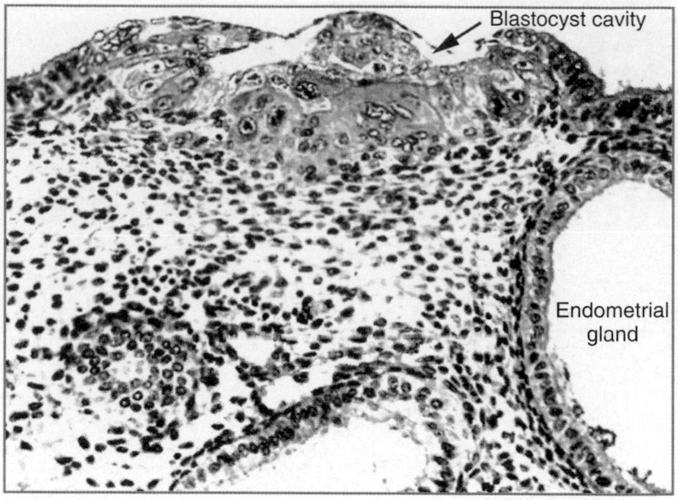

FIGURE 2-2 Implanted human embryo at a gestational age of approximately 7½ days. The blastocyst cavity has collapsed, and early invasion into the endometrial cavity has occurred with giant cells. The embryo is a small ball in the blastocyst cavity. (Courtesy of A. T. Hertig.)

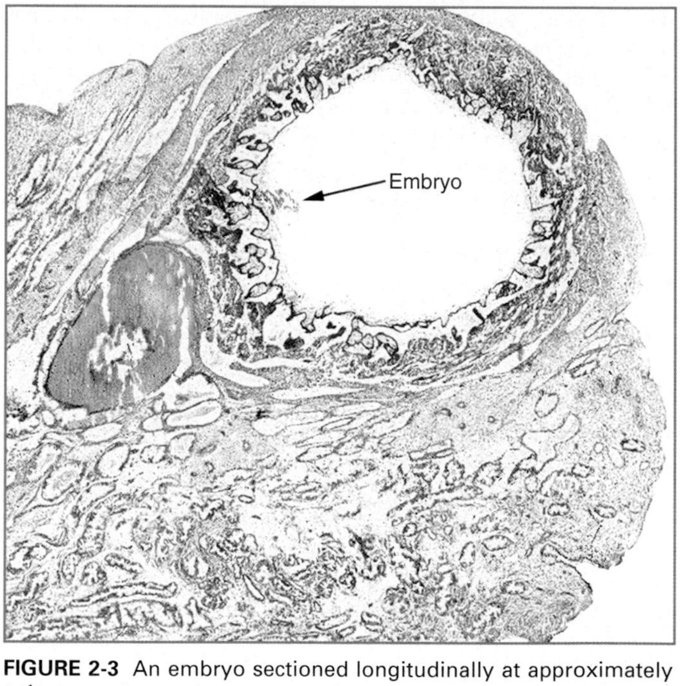

FIGURE 2-3 An embryo sectioned longitudinally at approximately 14½ days of gestation.

by Boyd and Hamilton.[8] Their observations suggested that the membranes truly fuse with the decidua vera of the side opposite to implantation in the 4th month of pregnancy, thereby obliterating the endometrial cavity. The decidua capsularis appeared to degenerate in their specimens before this time, and what is present on the outside of the term-delivered placenta was construed to be decidua vera attached to chorion. With the atrophy of peripheral villi and attachment of the membranes to the opposite side of the uterus, the macroscopic delineation of the placenta is essentially completed. Next, the formation of amnion, yolk sac, and body stalk is described.

Figures 2-3 through 2-7 demonstrate the developing placenta and finally an embryo at 7 weeks with an embryonic crown-rump length of 15 mm; the width of the entire specimen is approximately 25 mm. With the "herniation" of the chorion laeve into the endometrial cavity, its surface has been smoothed and stretched. At the edge, the decidua is thrown into a fold and minute coagula are present. When a tangential section is removed, the extension of the villous tissue for some distance onto the abembryonic pole of the cavity can be seen. The villi have already completely atrophied at the apex. The embryo is contained within the amniotic sac, which does not completely fill the chorionic cavity (see Fig. 2-8). It is suspended within the cavity by a gel (the magma reticulare) that liquefies on touching. When the sac is opened, the embryo and umbilical cord emerge (see Fig. 2-7).

An understanding of the morphogenesis of these structures is essential and can be gained from a study of Figure 2-4. In this histologic section, the embryo is sectioned longitudinally. The ectoderm appears as a dark streak and is contiguous with the amniotic sac epithelium that lies below. On the other side of the embryo lie the endoderm and yolk sac. The mesoderm is seen to "flow" from the left caudal pole of the embryo onto the inner surface of the trophoblastic shell. This streak of mesoderm ultimately becomes the substance of the umbilical cord. As the embryo grows and folds in such a manner as to enclose the endoderm, the amnion enlarges and the embryo may be thought of as herniating into this amniotic sac. A portion of the

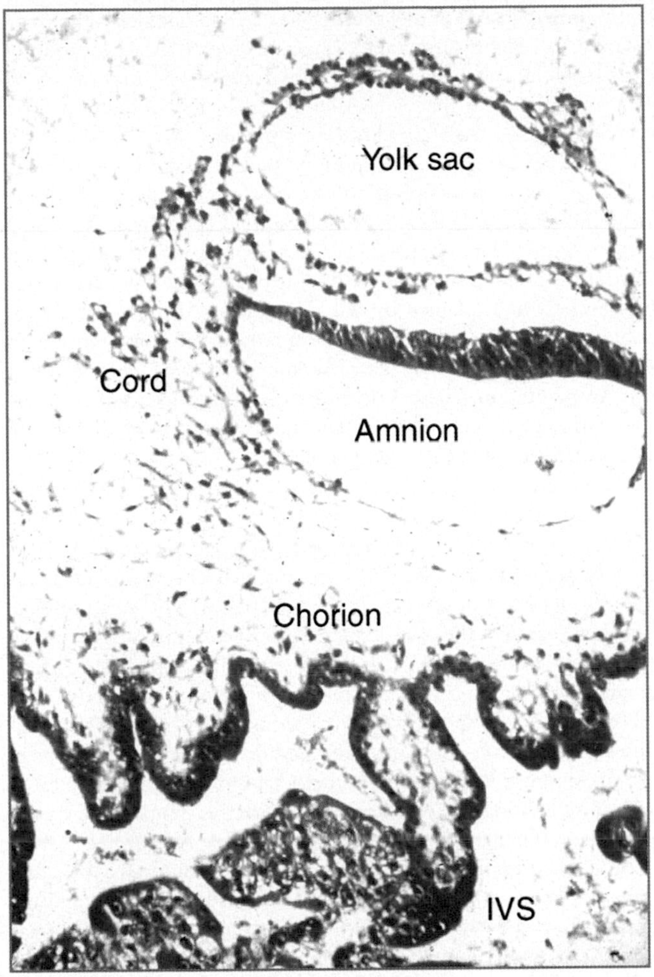

FIGURE 2-4 Human embryo at approximately 14 days' development. The chorion extends its connective tissue into the developing villi. The umbilical cord develops from the embryonic mesoderm. The amnion is contiguous with the embryonic ectoderm and will fill with fluid, and then the embryo will "herniate" into this amnionic cavity. IVS, intervillous space.

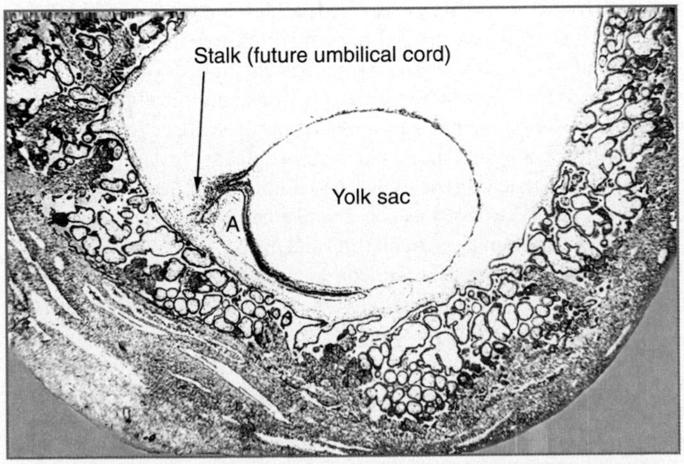

FIGURE 2-5 Implanted human embryo at 19 days' development, with villous development circumferentially. (Courtesy of A. T. Hertig.)

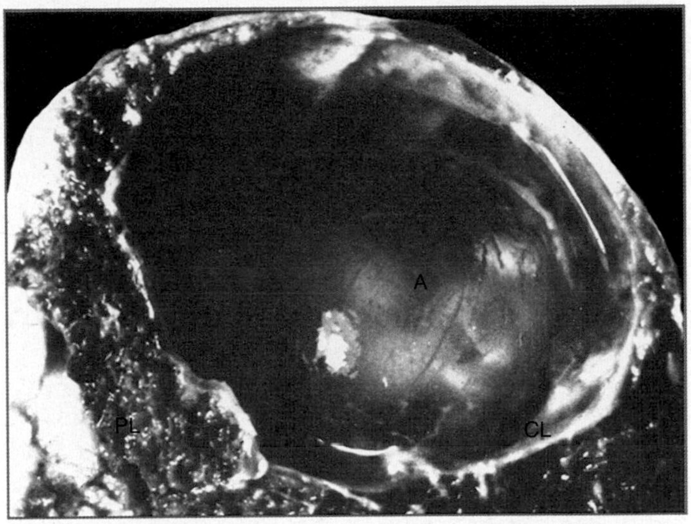

FIGURE 2-6 Seven-week gestation. A portion of the chorion laeve (CL) is removed to show partial atrophy of membranous villi, formation of definitive placenta (PL), and amniotic sac (A), which only partially fills the chorionic cavity at this age. (Courtesy of Dr. Jan E. Jirasek, Prague.)

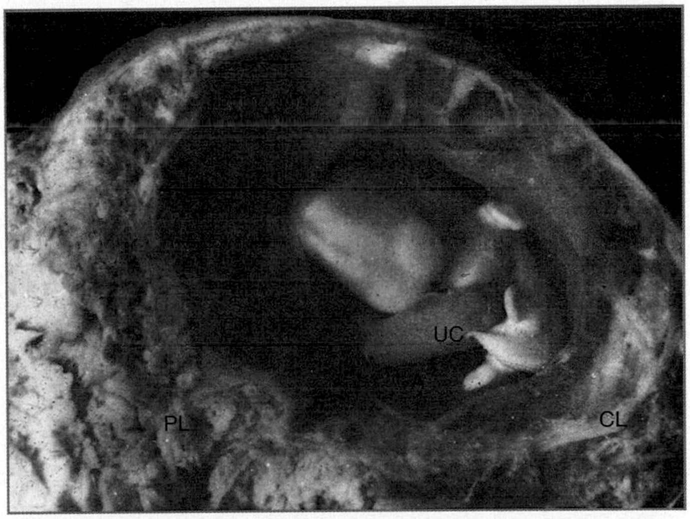

FIGURE 2-7 Seven-week gestation. Same specimen as in Figure 2-6, with the amnion (A) opened to disclose the 15-mm embryo and its umbilical cord (UC). CL, chorion laeve; PL, placenta. (Courtesy of Dr. Jan E. Jirasek, Prague.)

primitive yolk sac will be enclosed by the embryo to become its gut; another portion will be exteriorized (i.e., will lie outside the amniotic sac) and will be connected by the omphalomesenteric (vitelline) vessels and duct. Most often, these yolk structures disappear completely in later development; only in occasional term placentas can the calcified atrophic remnant of yolk sac be found at the periphery as a tiny (3-mm), yellow, extra-amniotic disk.

Once the amniotic sac has enclosed the entire embryo, it reflects on the umbilical cord, whose entire length it will eventually cover and to which it will be strongly adherent. At 8 weeks, the amnion is a thin translucent membrane (Fig. 2-8). It does not fully expand to cover the inside of the entire chorionic sac until about 12 weeks. It never completely grows together with the chorion, however, so that in most term

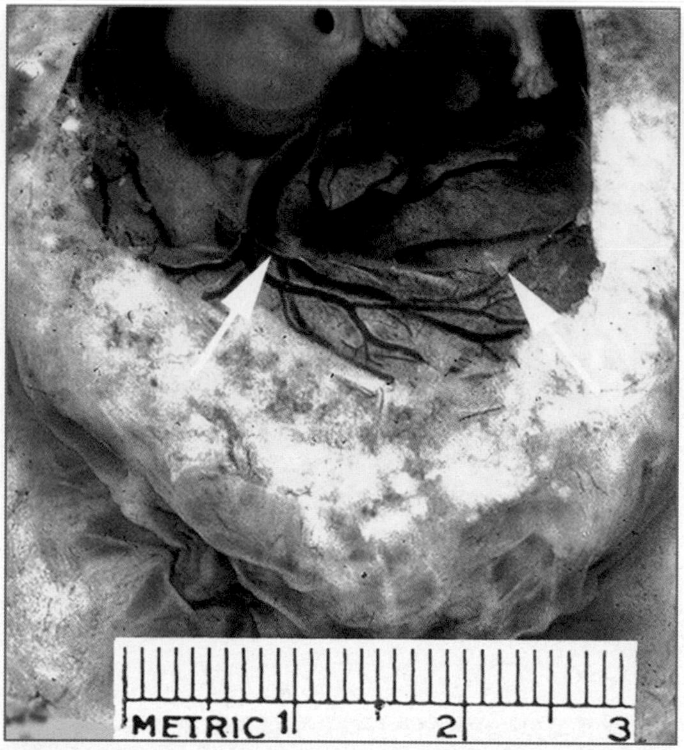

FIGURE 2-8 **Pregnancy at 8 weeks with 20-mm embryo.** The top portion of chorion laeve has been removed, thus disclosing amnion at *arrows*.

placentas the amnion may be dislodged from the chorion and the placental surface. This becomes particularly obvious in meconium discharge. The amnion does not have any blood vessels but is composed of a single layer of ectodermal epithelium, peripheral to which is a layer of delicate connective tissue with some macrophages.[9] Sophisticated studies have now shown that amnion and chorion also possess sheets of delicate elastic membranes.[10] It is presumed that these aid in the elasticity of the membranes and help prevent premature rupture. Betraying the ectodermal origin of the amnion are small plaques of squamous metaplasia near the insertion of the term placenta's umbilical cord that must not be mistaken for amnion nodosum.

When the embryonic cells differentiate into mesoderm, endoderm, and ectoderm, the mesoderm is first clearly seen at the caudal pole of the embryonic disk (see Fig. 2-4). The mesodermal cells rapidly proliferate and send a column of cells streaming toward the inner surface of the trophoblastic cavity, which they then come to line. This column is ultimately destined to become the umbilical cord, and blood vessels and a rudimentary allantoic sac grow into this body stalk from the primitive yolk sac—hence the term *chorioallantoic vessels*. It is commonly thought that the inner cell mass, the future embryo, lies centrally in the early stages of implantation and that for this reason the umbilical cord comes to be attached to the center of the placenta.

Aberrant attachment, such as at the margin or to the membranes (velamentous insertion), may be explained by one of two contradictory hypotheses. According to one hypothesis, the embryo had a less than perfect central position at the time of implantation and was perhaps even on the opposite side; thus, when the mesoderm proliferated, the location of the cord was established on the surface of the endometrium, the area destined to become membranes. The second hypothesis suggests that normal central implantation occurred but the area of implantation was less than optimal for placental development. Subsequently, the expansion of the placenta occurred to one side rather than in a uniform centrifugal manner. The already established location of the cord therefore changed from a central to a lateral position, a process called trophotropism that is also witnessed in the "migration" of a placenta that was earlier thought to be a previa.

This second hypothesis is supported by the much more common marginal or velamentous position of cords in multiple pregnancy, in which one can imagine there is competition for space by and collision of expanding placentas. In term placentas, moreover, marginal placental atrophy is often found, and the finding of succenturiate (accessory) lobes can best be explained by this mechanism. Also, the ultrasonographic finding of a "wandering" placenta favors this assumption, as does the fact that most of the few early embryos studied had a relatively central implantation. The first hypothesis is supported by the finding of a much higher frequency of velamentous insertion of the cord in aborted specimens than in term placentas.[11]

The umbilical cord measures approximately 55 cm in length at term, but extreme variations occur for largely unknown reasons. Because a normal cord weighs as much as 100 g and the segments of cord supplied with the placenta vary so much, the cord and membranes should be removed before the placental weight is ascertained. More often than not, the cord is spiraled, most commonly in a sinistral manner. Numerous theories have been presented to explain this helical arrangement, but the cause remains largely unknown. Because such twists do not exist in species with longitudinal orientation in bicornuate uteri and because of the observed mobility of the primate fetus in its uterus simplex, it is most likely that fetal movements are the cause of the cord twisting.[12,13] Further support for this explanation comes from the entwinement of cords in monoamniotic twins.

The cord contains two umbilical arteries and one vein. A second rudimentary vein, the omphalomesenteric (vitelline) vessels, and the allantoic duct of early embryonic stages atrophy, and only on rare occasions are often discontinuous remnants of these structures found in the term cord. The two umbilical arteries anastomose through a variably constructed vessel within 2 cm of the insertion of the cord in almost all normal placentas; this is the so-called Hyrtl anastomosis. There are no nerves in the cord. True knots occur in a few umbilical cords, particularly in very long ones, but much more common are so-called false knots. They represent redundancies (varicosities) of umbilical vessels that may protrude on the cord surface and have no clinical significance.

The surface vessels of the placenta represent ramifications of the umbilical vessels and pursue a predictable course on the chorionic surface. In general, one arterial branch is accompanied by one branch of the vein, and each terminal pair of vessels supplies one fetal cotyledon. The arteries may be recognized by their superficial location (i.e., they cross over the veins). Anastomoses between superficial vessels do not occur; for that matter, no such connections ever develop between villous vessels. Each district is isolated and distinct from the others.

Two types of surface vascular arrangements have been observed, a very coarse and sparse vasculature and finely dispersed vessels. No significantly different fetal outcomes correlate with these features, however, and mixtures of the two types exist in single placentas. The number of terminal perforating vessels determines the number of fetal-placental cotyledons or districts. In most placentas, this number is about 20, somewhat more than the number of lobules that can be seen from the maternal side of mature placentas. In general, there is correspondence of fetal lobules with maternal septal subdivisions when injection studies are performed of both circulations.[14]

Authors who have performed such dual injections envisage that the intervillous circulation is achieved by the injection of blood from a decidual artery into the center of a fetal cotyledon, which there disperses from a central cavity in the villous tissue to the periphery of the cotyledon and to the undersurface of the chorion, from where it is drained by veins in the septa and decidual base.[15] The loose central structure of cotyledons can easily be demonstrated when a placenta is horizontally sectioned. This more conventional model of cotyledonary arrangement of villous structure and intervillous circulation has been challenged by Gruenwald,[16] who envisaged a different lobular architecture, with arterial openings occurring at the periphery of cotyledons, a concept that has not yet been unequivocally refuted. The former notion that all intervillous blood flows laterally to the marginal sinus, however, is no longer acceptable.

The normal term placenta from which membranes and cord have been trimmed weighs between 400 and 500 g. There is enormous variability in placental size and shape, as there is in fetal weight. Some variations can be explained by racial differences, altitude, pathologic circumstances of implantation, diseases, or maternal habits such as smoking. In many cases, however, the deviations from "normal" are as difficult to explain as the factors that ultimately determine fetal and placental growth in general. Systematic studies of placental structure have given some insight into the complexities; they have been summarized in the careful analysis by Teasdale.[17] Absolute growth, as determined by DNA, RNA, and protein content, occurs in the placenta to the 36th week of gestation. Thereafter, proliferation of cells does not normally occur, and the placenta undergoes only further maturational changes. Previous studies have suggested an expansion of villous surface to between 11 and 13 m^2 at term, whereas Teasdale's careful measurements suggest that the maximum is reached with 10.6 m^2 at 36 weeks, decreasing to 9.4 m^2 at term. The fetal-to-placental ratio is estimated to change from 5:1 in the third trimester to 7:1 at term, most rapidly increasing during the last month of gestation. Reasons for discrepancies of these measurements reported in the literature are partly explained by inconsistent handling of the organ at delivery. Thus, a variable amount of blood may be trapped, depending on the time of cord clamping. It is widely accepted now that the delivered placenta has a smaller volume, in particular is less thick, than before delivery, as ascertained by sonography.[18] Therefore, for quantitative assessment, a histometric analysis must accompany such correlative study. Apparently, the slight increase in placental volume occurring in the last month of pregnancy results from an expansion of the "nonparenchymal" space (i.e., villous capillary size, decidua, septa, and fibrin). Thus, during the last month of gestation, fetal growth occurs without a commensurate increase in placental volume, indicating that changes must occur in perfusion or transport function of the placenta to ensure enhanced delivery of metabolic substrates to the fetus. Significant advances in technology are likely to discover new factors that regulate fetal and placental growth. Thus, the evolution of microarrays for the ascertainment of gene activity promises to become of major importance.[19]

Macroscopically, a delivered normal term placenta can be described as a disk-shaped, round, or ovoid structure measuring 18 × 20 cm in diameter and approximately 2 cm thick. The cord is normally inserted near the center of the disk (marginal in 7% and on the membranes in 1%); it measures 40 to 60 cm in length and 1.5 cm in thickness. It has two arteries, one vein, and a number of helical spirals. The membranes are attached at the periphery of the placental disk and have some degenerated yellow decidua on their outer surface and a smooth glistening inner amniotic surface. The amnion is only slightly adherent to the chorionic face of the placenta, from which it can be stripped by forceps, but it is firmly attached to the cord, upon which it reflects.

The fetal surface of the placenta is blue because of the fetal villous blood content seen through the membranes; most maternal blood has been expelled by the uterine contractions that expelled the placenta. Irregular whitish plaques of subchorionic fibrin project slightly between fetal vessels and produce what has been referred to as a bosselated surface; the plaques are indicative of a mature organ and result from eddying of the maternal blood in the intervillous space as it turns direction.

The maternal surface usually has a film of loosely attached blood clot, which when removed discloses the thin, grayish layer of decidua basalis and fibrin that comes away with delivery. In the fibrin, yellow granules and streaks of calcification characterize maturity. They are extremely variable in amount and have no clinical significance. The maternal surface is usually broken up into irregular lobules (cotyledons) by crevices that continue into partial or complete septa between fetal cotyledons. These septa are constructed of decidual cells and cellular trophoblast. On sectioning, the dark red villous tissue reflects the content of fetal blood. Loosely structured areas represent intervillous lakes, the presumed sites of first blood injections ("spurts") from decidual arteries.

Microscopic Development

It is likely that some adhesion molecules are essential for blastocyst attachment to the endometrium.[2,20] Once the trophoblastic shell has attached, marked changes occur on its surface and invasion is accomplished by dissociation and ingestion of endometrial cells. A completely interstitial implantation of the blastocyst is accomplished on the 9th day of gestation. The trophoblastic shell has proliferated appreciably, particularly at its basal portions, and most trophoblastic cells possess disproportionately large nuclei and form a syncytium. Within this mass of trophoblastic cells develop clefts (lacunae) that coalesce to form the most primitive type of the future intervillous space.

At about this time or on the next day, the somewhat congested decidual vessels are tapped into by the trophoblast. The first maternal leukocytes have been observed on day 11 in this primitive intervillous space, later to be followed by blood, thus establishing the primitive intervillous circulation.[1] At the same time, the trophoblastic cells can be seen to differentiate into a central cellular type (cytotrophoblast and extravillous trophoblast, and into the future Langhans layer) and peripheral syncytiotrophoblast (Fig. 2-9). The syncytial nuclei never undergo mitosis and grow only by the incorporation of cytotrophoblastic nuclei and cytoplasm; only the latter cells are capable of mitosis.[21,22] Recent studies indicate that the formation of the syncytium from cytotrophoblast is very complex. Thus, Debieve and Thomas[23] provided evidence that inhibin is involved; others have identified that it requires a protein ("syncytin") derived from a genetic contribution of a retroviral envelope gene.[24-26]

On day 13, the first connective tissue may be observed in the central portion of the future villi. It will rapidly expand peripherally into the cell columns of trophoblast. Evidence suggests that this connective tissue core derives from the mesoderm of the extraembryonic space and perhaps the body stalk (see Fig. 2-4) and not by central "delamination" from trophoblast. By the 30th day, a truly villous ovum is formed, and the basic future development of the villous structure is delineated. Villi are found around the entire circumference at first, only to atrophy over the pole later. Commencing almost simultaneously, on the 14th day and subsequently, is the development of villous capillaries. Moreover, fetal macrophages (the Hofbauer cells) infiltrate the villi. Although in 1968 Hertig[1] discussed in great detail how villous capillaries also derive from delaminated trophoblastic cells by the internal detachment of angioblastic cells, more likely their origin is from fetal mesoderm or endoderm. These are not idle problems of the embryologist but pertain directly to an understanding of the genesis of hydatidiform moles. If villous connective tissue and vessels are definitely derived from the embryo (rather than the trophoblast), hydatidiform moles must at one time have had an embryo. Occasionally, complete hydatidiform moles have been shown to contain degenerated embryos, but in most cases the embryo and its vessels have disappeared.[27,28] Villous vessels coalesce and connect to the omphalomesenteric and later allantoic vessels of the embryonic body stalk, and a true fetal circulation is active by 21 days.[29] The initial fetal blood cells come from yolk sac, and only after the 2nd month do they issue from fetal hematopoietic islands. With an established circulation, the villi are now called tertiary villi.[20]

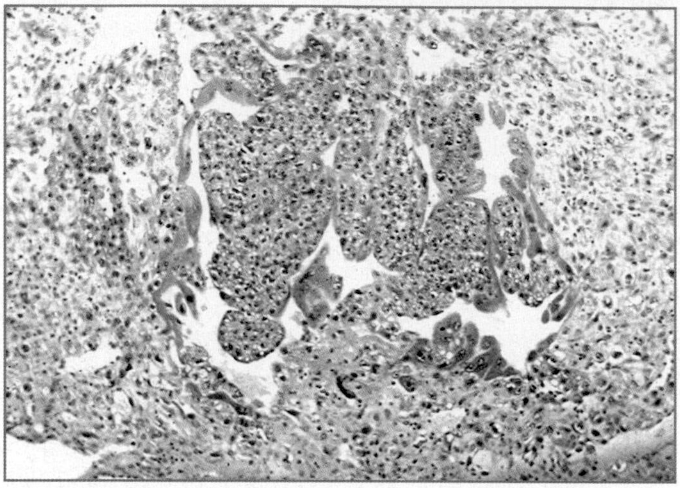

FIGURE 2-9 **Trophoblastic shell of a 13-day-old ovum.** Cell columns composed of solid cytotrophoblast are covered by syncytiotrophoblast lining the entire intervillous space, which is still devoid of maternal blood. H&E, ×300.

The villous structure changes appreciably during further development, and the gestational age can be crudely estimated from the histologic appearance of the villi. In young placentas, the mesenchymal core of villi is extremely loosely structured, appearing almost edematous (Fig. 2-10). Capillaries are filled with nucleated cells and lie very close to the villous surface. This surface is uniformly covered by an inner layer of cellular cytotrophoblast, which contains numerous mitoses and in turn is covered by a thick layer of syncytium that contains abundant organelles in its metabolically active cytoplasm. The syncytium is functionally the most important part of the placenta. With advancing age the villi elongate, lose their central edema, branch successively, and decrease in diameter. At term they contain little mesenchyma and are filled with distended capillaries. Cytotrophoblastic mitoses are rare after 36 weeks in normal placentas. The syncytium tends to form buds and "knots," many of which break loose and are swept into the intervillous circulation, by which they reach the maternal lung. They are destroyed in the lung as they have no mitotic capability, and they are presumably the source of the large quantities of "free DNA" in the maternal circulation that is now used for genotyping.[30] Fibrin and fibrinoid, also eosinophilic but composed of a variety of novel protein compounds, are normally accumulated in ever-increasing quantities on the surface of villi, in the subchorionic area,

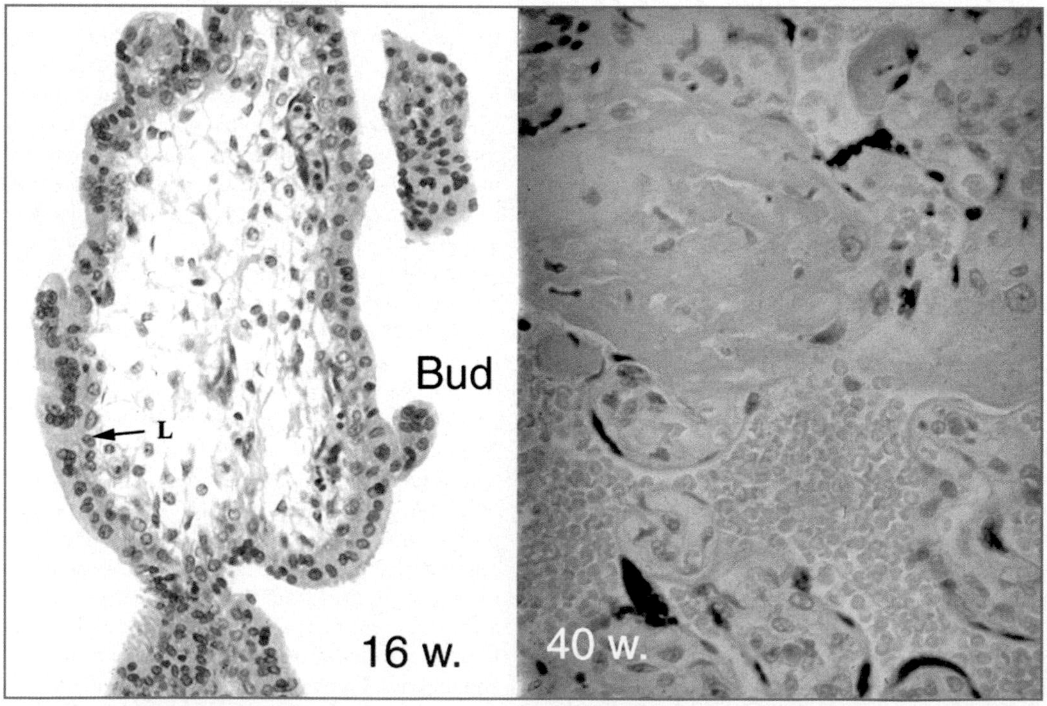

FIGURE 2-10 **Placental villi.** **Left:** Villi of 16-week-old placenta. Note the very loosely structured mesenchymal core containing isolated macrophages, the thin-walled fetal capillaries filled with nucleated red blood cells, and the double-layered trophoblastic surface. Langhans cells (L) at arrow (cytotrophoblast); syncytial "buds" begin to form. **Right:** A section of villi of a term placenta reveals dark syncytial buds and fibrinoid deposits. H&E, ×160.

and along the floor of the placenta, where the Rohr and Nitabuch fibrin layers mingle with the decidua basalis. Fibrinoid of the placenta is a complex admixture of true fibrin and a variety of proteins such as laminins and collagens.[31] Near term, some of these fibrin deposits become calcified in a normal process that may become excessive in the postmature placenta. The amount of calcium varies greatly but has no deleterious influence on placental function. The placental septa, composed of cellular extravillous trophoblast ("X cells" or intermediate trophoblast) and decidua, often undergo cystic change as a sign of maturity.

The X cell, now more commonly called the extravillous trophoblast, has recently been the focus of attention. It is a separate lineage of trophoblast that is intimately related to fibrinoid deposition, the production of the major basic protein and placental lactogen. Most so-called placental site giant cells are X cells and are often confused with decidual stromal elements.[27,32] From these basal trophoblastic elements come a variety of enzymes, especially stromelysin-3, to prepare for the invasion of the decidual floor and blood vessels.[33] These cells also infiltrate into the orifices of basal decidual spiral arterioles (Fig. 2-11). Hustin and colleagues[34,35] offered evidence that these extravillous trophoblastic cells completely occlude these vessels in early pregnancy, thus allowing only a filtrate of maternal blood to enter the intervillous space. This hypothesis was challenged with studies using Doppler flow in rhesus monkeys.[36] These investigations showed an early vascular connection of the maternal arterial circulation with the intervillous space, although flow was of low resistance and pulsatility from day 20 on. The population of Hofbauer cells derives from circulating fetal blood, increases in the first 36 weeks, and falls thereafter.[17] Although their precise function is not well understood, immunohistochemical studies show that this large population of cells represents fully differentiated phagocytes.[37] After hemolysis, they are seen to produce hemosiderin; in the chorionic surface, they actively transport meconium after its discharge, and it is speculated that they remove antifetal antibodies.

At the site of implantation, trophoblastic cells intermingle extensively with decidua basalis; indeed, they penetrate into the superficial portions of myometrium. These areas are often characterized by scattered lymphocyte infiltration and decidual necrosis.[38] Cytotrophoblastic cells enter the opened mouths of maternal arterioles and penetrate deeply along their endothelial linings; indeed, packets of villi "herniate" into open maternal vessels.[39] Some trophoblastic cells infiltrate the decidua and myometrium, often fusing to form placental giant cells (Fig. 2-12); others invade the spiral arterioles from the outside. They cause considerable local change, including fibrin deposition, and alter the normally contractile vessels to presumably rigid uteroplacental arteries. Thrombosis is not found normally but is a common finding when hypertensive changes are superimposed.

Electron microscopic study of placental villi in general supports the findings made by light microscopy, but it adds significant new details.

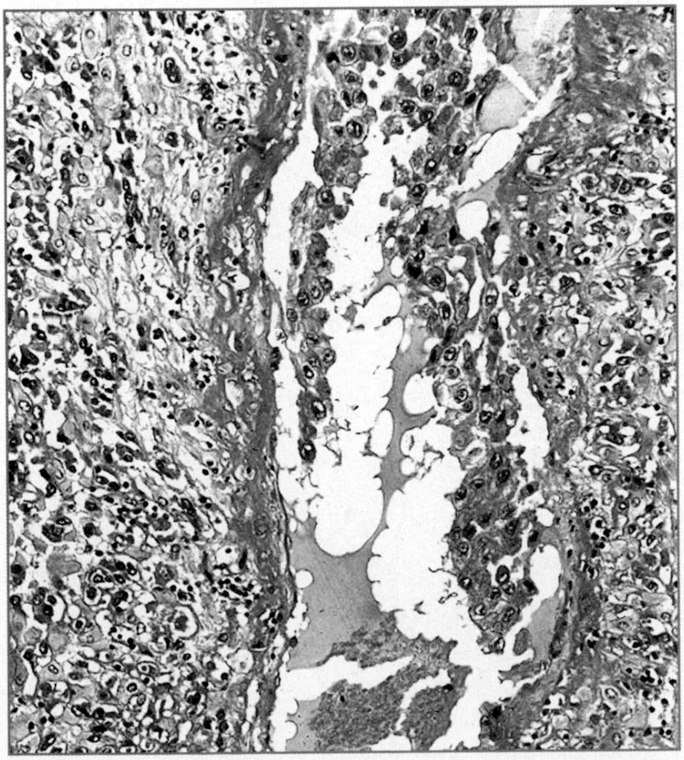

FIGURE 2-11 Term placental floor with infiltration of extravillous cytotrophoblast into a spiral arteriole. The walls of the arteriole have been transformed with fibrin deposits. The dark cells in the endometrial stroma are also extravillous trophoblast. H&E, ×128.

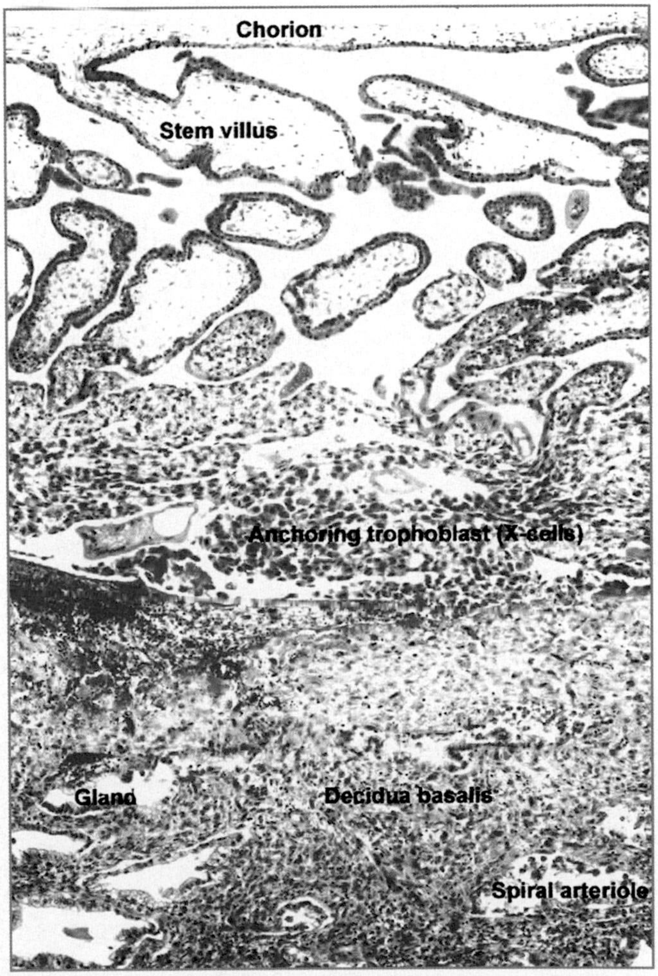

FIGURE 2-12 Implantation site of first-trimester placenta. The anchoring villi are composed of cytotrophoblast, and diffusely infiltrated placental giant cells can be seen. H&E, ×40. (From Benirschke K, Kaufmann P, Baergen RN: The Pathology of the Human Placenta, 5th ed. New York, Springer-Verlag, 2006.)

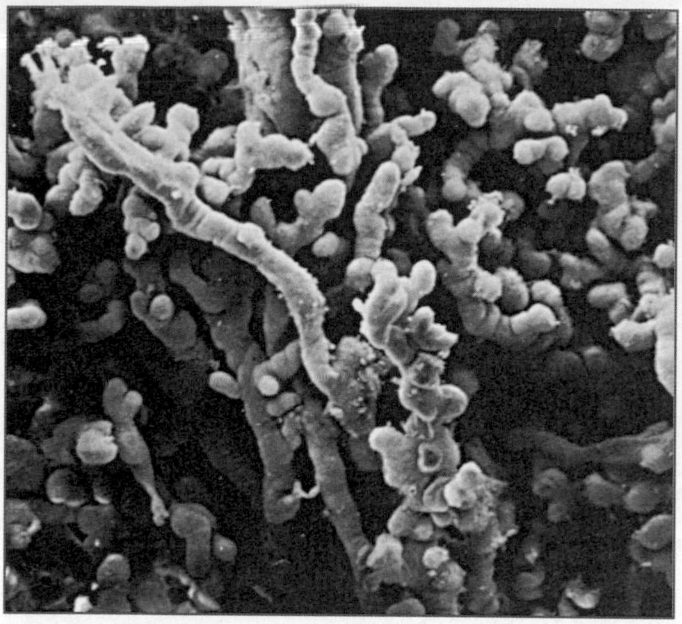

FIGURE 2-13 Scanning electron micrograph of mature villi at the periphery of the cotyledon. Note the fine uniform structure, rare adherence, and microvillous velvety surface of the terminal villi (×100). (From Sandstedt B: The placenta and low birth weight. Curr Top Pathol 66:1, 1979.)

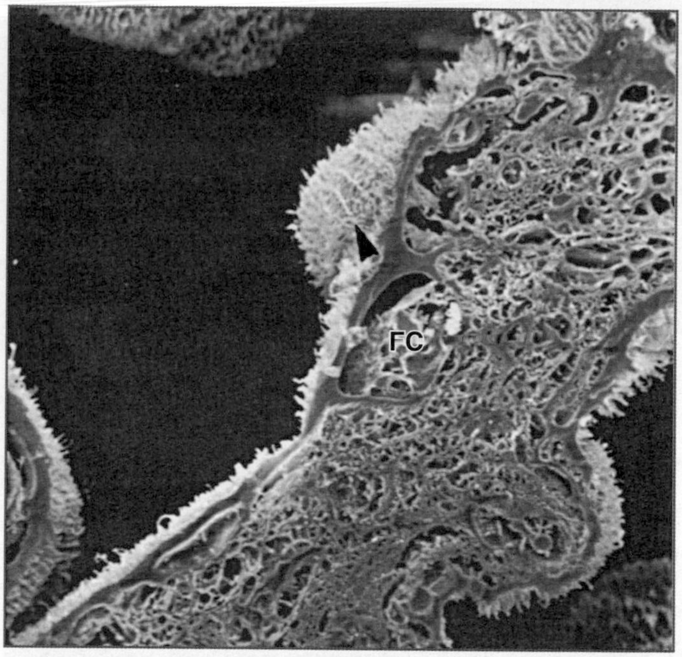

FIGURE 2-14 Term placental villus. The freeze-fracture scanning electron microphotograph (×250) shows the microvillous surface, often in rows *(arrowhead),* grayish trophoblast cytoplasm, and proximity of the fetal capillary (FC) to the black intervillous space. (From Sandstedt B: The placenta and low birth weight. Curr Top Pathol 66:1, 1979.)

The arborization of villi and their complexity are best appreciated in scanning electron micrographs (Fig. 2-13). In the more peripheral areas of cotyledons, the villi appear histologically more mature (i.e., they are smaller and have more branches and less stroma). The syncytial surface is covered by numerous minute microvilli, and syncytial bridges are occasionally seen. In the central portion of the cotyledon, the villi are plump and less branched. Freeze-fracture scanning electron microscopy discloses the proximity of fetal vessels to the basement membrane and the profusely microvillous surface of the syncytium (Fig. 2-14). With advancing maturity, the Langhans cytotrophoblastic layer not only becomes less prominent but also is interrupted in many more places. Here, then, the fetal capillaries abut a thin layer of syncytium, presumably the most efficient site of transfer.

These electron micrographic features of maturity are also found more frequently in the periphery of cotyledons than in their more immature-appearing centers, but qualitative differences do not exist.[40] The slightly different electron micrographic features of villi in part relate to the state of contraction of fetal capillaries (Fig. 2-15), and they may in part be the result of oxygen supply. Desmosomes have been identified by scanning and transmission electron microscopy in trophoblast.[41] They interlock syncytium with cytotrophoblast, and when found with free membranes in the cytoplasm of the syncytium, they presumably represent the remnants of the fusion-incorporation process of cytotrophoblast into syncytium. The structure of the syncytiotrophoblastic cytoplasm is extremely complex. It is filled with minute vacuoles, ribosomes, mitochondria, and the other usual cytoplasmic components. On the other hand, the cytotrophoblastic cytoplasm is relatively simple, reflecting its presumed primary function as precursor cells for syncytium.

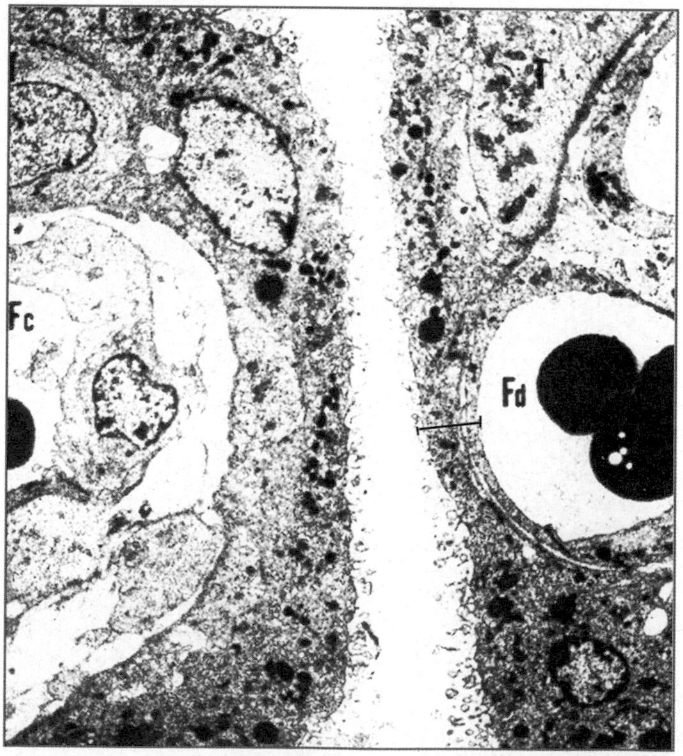

FIGURE 2-15 Transmission electron micrograph (×5000) of two placental villi at 30 weeks' gestation. The fetal capillary (Fc) at *left* is contracted. At *right,* several capillaries are dilated (Fd). Note microvilli and shortest maternal-fetal exchange distance (indicated by *bar*). (Courtesy of Dr. R. M. Wynn, Department of Obstetrics, Gynecology, and Pathology, SUNY Health Sciences Center, Brooklyn, NY.)

References

1. Hertig AT: Human Trophoblast. Springfield, IL, Charles C Thomas, 1968.
2. Bamberger A-M, Dudahl S, Löning T, et al: The adhesion molecule CEACAM1 (CD66a, C-CAM, BGP) is specifically expressed by the extravillous intermediate trophoblast. Am J Pathol 156:1165, 2000.
3. Genbacev OD, Prakobphol A, Foulk RA, et al: Trophoblast L-selectin-mediated adhesion at the maternal-fetal interface. Science 299:405, 2003.
4. Fazleabas AT, Strakova Z: Endometrial function: Cell specific changes in the uterine environment. Mol Cell Endocrinol 186:143, 2002.
5. Rizos N, Doran TA, Miskin M, et al: Natural history of placenta previa ascertained by diagnostic ultrasound. Obstet Gynecol 133:287, 1979.
6. Hoogland HJ, deHaan J, Martin CB: Placental size during early pregnancy and fetal outcome: A preliminary report of a sequential ultrasonographic study. Obstet Gynecol 138:441, 1980.
7. King DL: Placental migration demonstrated by ultrasonography. Radiology 109:167, 1973.
8. Boyd JD, Hamilton WJ: The Human Placenta. Cambridge, Heffer and Sons, 1970.
9. Bourne GL: The Human Amnion and Chorion. London, Lloyd-Luke, 1962.
10. Hieber AD, Corcino D, Motosue J, et al: Detection of elastin in the human fetal membranes: Proposed molecular basis for elasticity. Placenta 18:301, 1997.
11. Benirschke K: Anatomy. In Berger GS, Brenner WE, Keith LG (eds): Second Trimester Abortion. Boston, John Wright, 1981, p 39.
12. Monie IW: Velamentous insertion of the cord in early pregnancy. Am J Obstet Gynecol 93:276, 1965.
13. Lacro RV, Jones KL, Benirschke K: The umbilical cord twist: Origin, direction, and relevance. Am J Obstet Gynecol 157:833, 1987.
14. Wigglesworth JS: Vascular organization of the human placenta. Nature 216:1120, 1967.
15. Ramsey EM: New appraisal of an old organ: The placenta. Proc Am Philos Soc 113:296, 1969.
16. Gruenwald P: Lobular architecture of primate placentas. In Gruenwald P (ed): The Placenta and Its Maternal Supply Line. Baltimore, University Park Press, 1975.
17. Teasdale F: Gestational changes in the functional structure of the human placenta in relation to fetal growth: A morphometric study. Am J Obstet Gynecol 137:560, 1980.
18. Bleker OP, Kloosterman GJ, Breur W, et al: The volumetric growth of the human placenta: A longitudinal ultrasonic study. Am J Obstet Gynecol 127:657, 1977.
19. Ward K: Microarray technology in obstetrics and gynecology: A guide for clinicians. Am J Obstet Gynecol 195:364, 2006.
20. Enders AC: Perspectives on human implantation. Infertil Reprod Med Clin North Am 12:251, 2001.
21. Richart R: Studies of placental morphogenesis: I. Radioautographic studies of human placenta utilizing tritiated thymidine. Proc Soc Exp Biol 106:829, 1961.
22. Galton M: DNA content of placental nuclei. J Cell Biol 13:183, 1962.
23. Debieve F, Thomas K: Control of the human inhibin alpha chain promoter in cytotrophoblast cells differentiating into syncytium. Mol Hum Reprod 8:262, 2002.
24. Mi S, Lee X, Veldman GM, et al: Syncytin is a captive retroviral envelope protein involved in human placental morphogenesis. Nature 403:785, 2000.
25. Pötgens AJG, Schmitz U, Bose P, et al: Mechanism of syncytial fusion: A review. Placenta 23(Suppl A):S107, 2002.
26. Cáceres M, NISC Comp. Sequ. Progr., Thomas JW: The gene of retroviral origin syncytin 1 is specific to hominoids and is inactive in Old World monkeys. J Hered 97:100, 2006.
27. Benirschke K, Kaufmann P, Baergen RN: The Pathology of the Human Placenta, 5th ed. New York, Springer-Verlag, 2006.
28. Baergen RN, Kelly T, McGinnis MJ, et al: Complete hydatidiform mole with coexisting embryo. Hum Pathol 27:731, 1996.
29. Moore KL, Persaud TVN: The Developing Human: Clinically Oriented Embryology, 3rd ed. Philadelphia, WB Saunders, 1993.
30. Bianchi DW, Wataganara T, Lapaire O, et al: Fetal nucleic acids in maternal body fluids: An update. Ann N Y Acad Sci 1075:63, 2006.
31. Kaufmann P, Huppertz B, Frank H-G: The fibrinoids of the human placenta. Origin, composition and functional relevance. Ann Anat 178:485, 1996.
32. Wasmoen TL, Benirschke K, Gleich GJ: Demonstration of immunoreactive eosinophil granule major basic protein in the plasma and placentae of non-human primates. Placenta 8:283, 1987.
33. Maquoi E, Polette M, Nawrocki B, et al: Expression of stromelysin-3 in the human placenta and placental bed. Placenta 18:277, 1997.
34. Hustin J, Schaaps JP: Echocardiographic and anatomic studies of the maternotrophoblastic border during the first trimester of pregnancy. Am J Obstet Gynecol 157:162, 1987.
35. Hustin J, Schaaps JP, Lambotte R: Anatomical studies of the utero-placental vascularization in the first trimester of pregnancy. Trophoblast Res 3:49, 1988.
36. Simpson NAB, Nimrod C, De Vermette R, et al: Determination of intervillous flow in early pregnancy. Placenta 18:287, 1997.
37. Wetzka B, Clark DE, Charnock-Jones DS, et al: Isolation of macrophages (Hofbauer cells) from human term placenta and their prostaglandin E2 and thromboxane production. Hum Reprod 12:847, 1997.
38. Pijnenborg R, Dixon G, Robertson WB, et al: Trophoblastic invasion of human decidua from 8 to 18 weeks by pregnancy. Placenta 1:3, 1980.
39. Fujikura T: The openings of uteroplacental vessels with villous infiltration at different gestational ages. Arch Pathol Lab Med 129:382, 2005.
40. Schuhmann RA, Wynn RM: Regional ultrastructural differences in placental villi in cotyledons of a mature human placenta. Placenta 1:345-353, 1980.
41. Reale E, Wang T, Zaccheo D, et al: Junctions on the maternal blood surface of the human placental syncytium. Placenta 1:245-258, 1980.

Chapter 3

Amniotic Fluid Dynamics

Marie H. Beall, MD, and Michael G. Ross, MD, MPH

Amniotic fluid (AF) is necessary for normal human fetal growth and development. It protects the fetus from mechanical trauma, and its bacteriostatic properties may help to maintain a sterile intrauterine environment. The space created by the AF allows fetal movement and aids in the normal development of both lungs and limbs. Finally, AF offers convenient access to fetal cells and metabolic byproducts and therefore has been used for fetal diagnoses more often than any other gestational tissue.

The existence of AF has been appreciated since ancient times. Leonardo drew the fetus floating in the fluid, and William Harvey hypothesized that the fetus was nourished by it. Only in the late 19th century, however, did AF become available for study other than at delivery, and fluid sampling by amniocentesis was rarely performed until the second half of the 20th century. Genetic amniocentesis for fetal sex determination was first performed in 1956.[1] Research on the characteristics of AF is therefore a relatively recent development. This chapter reviews the current state of knowledge regarding the volume, composition, production, resorption, and volume regulation of AF.

Volume of Amniotic Fluid

In the first trimester of pregnancy, the amnion does not contact the placenta, and the amniotic cavity is surrounded by the fluid-filled exocoelomic cavity.[2] The exocoelomic fluid participates in the exchange of molecules between mother and fetus; at this stage, the function of the AF is uncertain.

By the end of the first trimester of human gestation, the exocoelomic cavity has been progressively obliterated, and the amniotic cavity becomes the only significant deposit of extrafetal fluid. AF volumes in the first half of pregnancy have been directly measured and are found to increase logarithmically.[3] AF volumes were first estimated in the latter two thirds of pregnancy using dilution techniques, and these original quantitative findings were supported by semiquantitative measurements performed with ultrasound (Fig. 3-1).[4] All methods demonstrate that AF volume increases progressively between 10 and 30 weeks of gestation. Typical volumes increase from less than 10 mL at 8 weeks[3] to 630 mL at 22 weeks, and to 770 mL at 28 weeks of gestation.[5] After 30 weeks, the increase slows, and AF volume may remain unchanged until 36 to 38 weeks, after which the volume tends to decrease. If the pregnancy proceeds after the term date, AF volume decreases sharply, averaging 515 mL at 41 weeks. Subsequently, there is a 33% decline in AF volume per week,[6-8] consistent with the increased incidence of oligohydramnios in post-term gestations.

The *rate* of change of AF volume depends on the gestational age. The rate of AF volume increase is 10 mL/wk at the beginning of the fetal period, and it increases to 50 to 60 mL/wk at 19 to 25 weeks' gestation before undergoing a gradual decrease until the rate of change equals zero (i.e., volume is at maximum) at 34 weeks. Thereafter, AF volume falls, with the decrease averaging 60 to 70 mL/wk at 40 weeks. Although the basic mechanisms that produce these alterations in AF volume throughout gestation are unclear, it is important to note that, when expressed as a percentage of total AF volume, the rate of change decreases consistently throughout the fetal period. Thus, the decrease in AF volume near term represents a natural progression rather than an aberration.

The volume of AF may be dramatically altered in pathologic states. Excessive AF (polyhydramnios) may total many liters, and the volume of AF in conditions of reduced fluid (oligohydramnios) may be near zero. Fetal anatomic abnormalities such as renal agenesis or esophageal atresia may impact on the normal processes for production and resorption of AF, leading to abnormal fluid volumes. In addition, transient changes, such as maternal dehydration or fetal anemia, may alter AF production or resorption and therefore AF volume. Abnormalities of AF volume may also occur without apparent cause and have been associated with poorer perinatal outcomes[9-12]; specifics are discussed elsewhere in the text.

Production of Amniotic Fluid

The AF in the first trimester of pregnancy has rarely been the subject of study. It appears that in the first trimester, human AF is isotonic with maternal or fetal plasma[13] but contains a minimal amount of protein. First-trimester AF also demonstrates an extremely low oxygen tension and exhibits an increased concentration of sugar alcohols, the product of anaerobic metabolism.[14] It is thought that early AF arises as a transudate of plasma, either from the fetus through non-keratinized fetal skin, or from the mother across the uterine decidua or placenta surface, or both, although the actual mechanism is unknown.[15]

In the second half of pregnancy, the human fetus produces dilute urine, which is a major component of AF and causes its composition to be different from that of serum. In particular, human AF osmolality decreases by 20 to 30 mOsm/kg with advancing gestation, to levels that are approximately 85% to 90% of maternal serum osmolality.[16] In the same period, amounts of AF urea, creatinine, and uric acid increase, resulting in AF concentrations of urinary byproducts two to three times higher than in fetal plasma.[16]

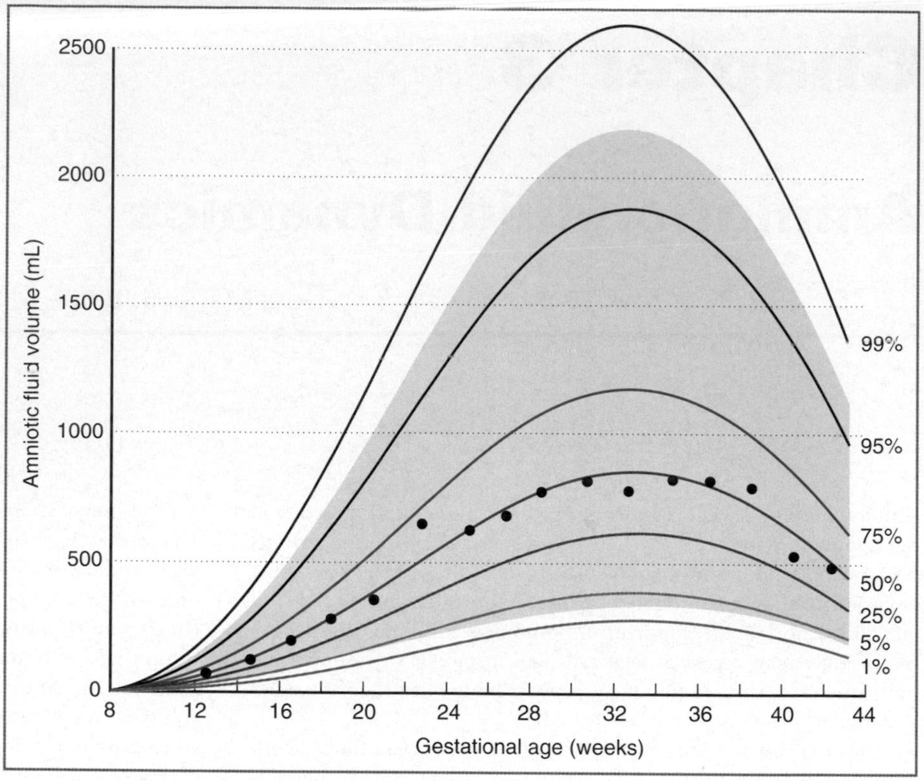

FIGURE 3-1 Amniotic fluid volumes from 8 to 44 weeks of human gestation. Dots represent mean measurement for each 2-week interval. Shaded area covers the 95% confidence interval (2.5 to 97.5 percentiles). (From Brace RA, Wolf EJ: Normal amniotic fluid volume changes throughout pregnancy. Am J Obstet Gynecol 161:382-388, 1989.)

AF production and resorption have been extensively studied in the latter half of pregnancy, most commonly in the sheep model. Evidence suggests that the entire volume of AF turns over on a daily basis,[17] making this a highly dynamic system. The volume of AF is influenced by a complex interplay of productive and absorptive mechanisms (Fig. 3-2).[18] These mechanisms act to maintain the AF volume, and there is some evidence that they may be regulated to normalize AF volume in pathologic conditions.

The major contributors to AF volume in the latter portion of pregnancy are fetal urine and fetal lung fluid. In addition, minor contributions occur from transudation across the umbilical cord and skin, and from water produced as a result of fetal metabolism. Although some data on these processes in the human fetus are available, the bulk of our information about fetal AF circulation is derived from animal models, primarily the sheep.

The largest contributor to late-gestation AF volume is the fetal urine. Although the mesonephros can produce urine by 5 weeks of gestation, the metanephros (the adult kidney) develops later, with nephrons formed at 9 to 11 weeks,[19] and at this point urine is excreted into the AF. The amount of urine produced increases progressively with advancing gestation, and it constitutes a significant proportion of the AF in the second half of pregnancy.[20] Human fetal urine production has been estimated by the use of ultrasound assessment of fetal bladder volume.[21] Although there continues to be uncertainty about the accuracy of noninvasive measurements, human fetal urine output appears to increase from 110 mL/kg/24 hr at 25 weeks to almost 200 mL/kg/24 hr at term,[21,22] in the range of 25% of bodyweight per day or nearly 1000 mL/day near term.[21,23] In near-term fetal sheep, with direct methods used for measuring urine production rates, similar high values have been found.[24-26] There may be a tendency for the urine flow rate to decrease after 40 weeks' gestation, particularly if oligohydramnios is present.[27]

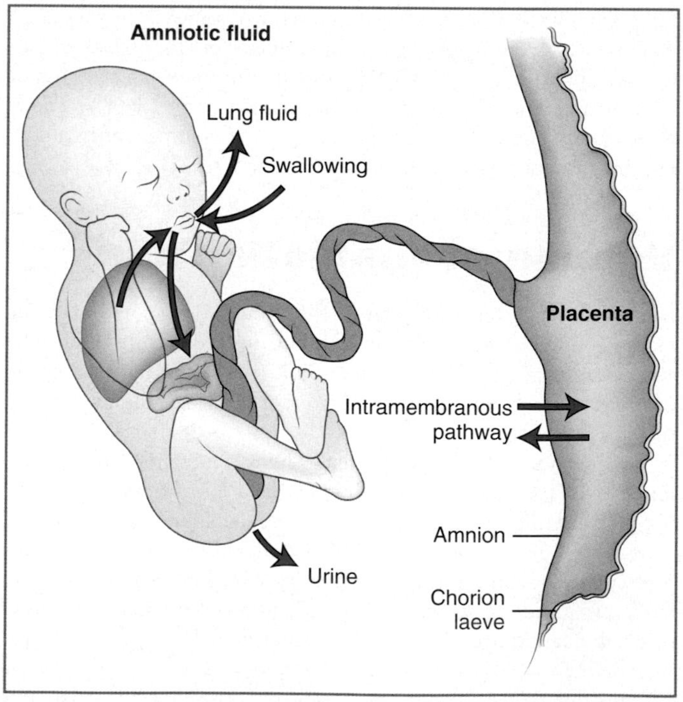

FIGURE 3-2 Circulation of amniotic fluid water to and from the fetus. (Modified from Seeds AE: Current concepts of amniotic fluid dynamics. Am J Obstet Gynecol 138:575, 1980.)

Reduction or absence of fetal urine flow is commonly associated with oligohydramnios, indicating that urine flow is very likely necessary to maintain normal AF volume. The mature fetus can also respond to changes in internal fluid status by modulating urine flow. In sheep, increased fetal blood pressure stimulates fetal secretion of atrial natriuretic factor[28] and an accompanying diuresis,[29] whereas increased plasma osmolality stimulates fetal arginine vasopressin (AVP) secretion and an antidiuretic response.[30,31] These findings indicate that AF volume could be regulated through the mechanism of altered fetal urine flow. Whereas human fetal hypoxia has been associated with oligohydramnios,[32,33] ovine fetal hypoxia is associated with increased urine flow,[34] during which AF volume is maintained. These data suggest that regulation of AF volume is mediated by other mechanisms in addition to changes in urine production.

The major secondary source of AF volume is fluid derived from the fetal lung. It appears that all mammalian fetuses secrete fluid from their lungs into the AF. The secretion of fetal alveolar phospholipids (lecithin, sphingomyelin, and phosphatidylglycerol) into the AF, used to predict human fetal lung maturity, is evidence that human fetuses are not exceptions to this statement. As the rate of fluid production by the human fetal lungs has not been directly measured, available data are derived from the ovine fetus. During the last third of gestation, the fetal lamb secretes an average of 100 mL/day/kg fetal weight from the lungs. Under physiologic conditions, half of the fluid exiting the lungs enters the AF and half is swallowed[35]; therefore, total lung fluid production approximates one-third that of urine production, whereas the net AF fluid contribution is only one-sixth that of urine. Fetal lung fluid flow is mediated by active transport of chloride ions across the lung epithelium,[36] and the lung fluid is isotonic to plasma, unlike the hypotonic urine. Lung fluid production is affected by a diversity of fetal physiologic and endocrine factors. Increased AVP,[37] catecholamines,[38] and cortisol[39] decrease lung fluid production, effects that may help explain enhanced clearance of lung fluid in fetuses delivered after labor, as compared with those delivered by elective cesarean section.[40,41] Nearly all active stimuli, including arginine vasopressin,[37] catecholamines,[38] and cortisol,[39] have been demonstrated to reduce fetal lung liquid secretion. Modulation of lung fluid production is therefore unlikely to be a significant regulator of AF volume. Current opinion is that fetal lung fluid secretion is probably most important in providing for pulmonary expansion, which promotes airway and alveolar development.

Other proposed sources for AF water include transudation across fetal skin before keratinization, transudation across the umbilical cord, saliva, and water produced as a byproduct of fetal metabolism. Fetal skin keratinizes at the beginning of the third trimester, making it an unlikely source for AF in the latter part of pregnancy.[42,43] Fetal oral and nasal secretions do not appear to be a significant source of AF water.[44] Little is known about the value of other sources of AF water, but they are not thought to be important contributors to AF volume.

Resorption of Amniotic Fluid

One major route of resorption of AF is fetal swallowing. Studies of near-term pregnancies suggest that the human fetus swallows 190 to 760 mL/day.[45,46] This is considerably less than the volume of urine produced each day, although these estimates may be unreliable, as fetal swallowing may be reduced beginning a few days before delivery.[47] In fetal sheep, the daily volume swallowed increases from approximately 130 mL/kg/day three-quarters of the way through gestation to over 400 mL/kg/day near term,[48] in contrast to a relatively constant urine production of 300 to 600 mL/kg/day,[49] again suggesting that the fluid produced exceeds the swallowed volume.

A series of studies have measured ovine fetal swallowing activity with esophageal electromyograms, and have measured swallowed volume using a flow probe placed around the fetal esophagus.[50] These studies demonstrate that near-term fetal swallowing increases in response to dipsogenic (e.g., central or systemic hypertonicity[51] or central angiotensin II[52]) or orexigenic (central neuropeptide Y[53]) stimulation, and decreases with acute arterial hypotension[54] or hypoxia.[35,55] Thus, near term, fetal swallowed volume is subject to periodic increases as mechanisms for "thirst" and "appetite" develop functionality. However, despite the fetal ability to modulate swallowing, this modulation is unlikely to be responsible for AF volume regulation. Fetal sheep subject to hypoxia maintain normal AF volume,[56] despite decreased swallowing and increased urine flow, suggesting that another mechanism is responsible for AF volume regulation.

The amount of fluid swallowed by the fetus does not equal the amount of fluid produced by the kidneys and lungs in either human or ovine gestation. As the volume of AF does not greatly increase during the last half of pregnancy, another route of fluid absorption is implied. The most likely route is the intramembranous (IM) pathway.

The IM pathway refers to the route of absorption from the amniotic cavity across the amnion into the fetal vessels. Injection of distilled water into the AF is followed by a lowering of fetal serum osmolality,[57] indicating absorption of free water. This occurs before any change in maternal osmolality, suggesting absorption directly to the fetus. In sheep, the permeability of the amnion to inert solutes such as technetium and inulin is greater from the AF to the fetal circulation than in the other direction. This asymmetry of membrane permeability is not seen in vitro. These findings suggest that a continuous flow of water and solutes from AF to the fetal circulation (IM flow) occurs in vivo,[58] and bidirectional (diffusional) flow is seen both in vivo and in vitro. Other experiments support the thesis that solutes can cross directly from the AF to the fetal circulation, as both vasopressin[59] and furosemide[60] are taken up into the fetal circulation and are biologically active when injected into the AF after fetal esophageal ligation. Experimental estimates of the net IM flow range from 200 to 400 mL/day in fetal sheep.[57,61,62] This, combined with fetal swallowing, approximately equals the flow of urine and lung liquid under homeostatic conditions. Although it has never been directly detected in humans, indirect evidence supports the presence of IM flow. For example, studies of intra-amniotic chromium-51 injection demonstrated appearance of the tracer in the circulation of fetuses with impaired swallowing.[63] In nonhuman primates, IM flow would explain the absorption of AF technetium[57] and vasopressin[59] in fetuses after esophageal ligation. Mathematical models of human AF dynamics also suggest significant IM water and electrolyte flows.[64,65] Other routes of absorption of AF have been investigated but were not found to be important in the movement of water out of the AF. In particular, transmembranous water flow (AF to maternal blood) is extremely small in comparison with IM flow.[66,67] In the following discussion, IM flow will be assumed to be the mechanism for fluid resorption from the AF by nonswallowing mechanisms, understanding that there is the potential for other pathways as yet undiscovered.

As just described, fetal urine and lung output and fetal swallowing can all be modulated, but there is little evidence that this modulation serves as a mechanism for the maintenance of normal AF volume. By contrast, some experimental observations suggest that IM flow rates may be regulated to normalize AF volume. In the following description of membrane water flow and fetal membrane anatomy, some proposals for the mechanism and regulation of IM flow are offered.

Membrane Water Flow

The AF serves as a fetal water compartment. Water ultimately derives from the mother via the placenta, making cell membrane water permeability of interest in the accumulation and in the circulation of AF. The water permeability of biologic membranes can be described mathematically, and values of membrane permeability thus defined can be used to compare one membrane with another. To discuss the possible mechanisms of water flux in pregnancy, a review of the basics of membrane water permeability is provided.

Five major routes of membrane transfer (of any moiety) can be distinguished as follows: (1) simple diffusion of lipophilic substances (e.g., oxygen), (2) diffusion of hydrophilic substances through transmembrane channels (the common mechanism for membrane water flow), (3) facilitated diffusion (as occurs with D-glucose), (4) active transport (as for certain electrolytes), and (5) receptor-mediated endocytosis (a mechanism of transfer of large molecules, such as IgG).[68] In addition to transcellular flow across the cell membrane, water and solutes may cross biologic membranes between cells (paracellular flow).

Except for the specific active transport systems, simple diffusion of any compound (moles per second) across the membrane along physical gradients can be described as follows:

$$J_s = PS(c_1 - c_2) + \frac{(c_1 - c_2)\cdot(1-\sigma)}{\ln(c_1/c_2)}\cdot J_v + \frac{t^+\cdot I}{F},$$

where it is assumed that c_1 and c_2 in mol/m^3 represent the unbound solute concentrations on opposite sides of the membrane, with c_1 greater than c_2. P represents the solute permeability of the membrane in m/sec, S stands for the surface area for diffusion in m^2, σ is the reflection coefficient (dimensionless, a measure of the exclusion of the solute by the membrane), J_v is the volume (water) flux in m^3/sec, t^+ is defined as the cationic transfer number, without dimension, with I as the electrical current in coulomb/sec and F as the Faraday constant in coulomb/equivalent.[69] J_s is influenced by the solubility of the compound under investigation, so lipid-insoluble compounds have low flow and, in turn, low permeability in the absence of membrane channels. Importantly, however, the mathematical description presented here makes no assumption about the route of passive membrane flow. The volume (water) flow can be simplified to become the well-known Starling equation, with R being the gas constant in Nm/kmol and T being the temperature in degrees Kelvin:

$$J_v = LpS[\Delta P - \sigma RT(c_1 - c_2)],$$

where the flow depends on the magnitude of the hydrostatic and osmotic pressure difference.[69-71]

Experimental studies on biologic membranes often report the membrane permeability *(P)* (usually in cm/sec) or the flux *(J)* (mL/sec/cm^2). At times, the filtration coefficient *(LpS)* (mL/min per unit of force [mm Hg or mOsm/L] per specimen [kilogram or organ]) is also reported. Flux is used when the reflection coefficient of the solute responsible for the osmotic force is unknown. The filtration coefficient is used when the surface area of the membrane being tested is unknown; this is often the case, for example, in whole-placenta preparations.[72] Membrane water permeabilities are reported as the permeability associated with flow of water in a given direction, and under a given type of force, or as the (bidirectional) diffusional permeability. As one membrane may have different osmotic, hydrostatic, and diffusional permeabilities,[73] an understanding of the forces driving membrane water flow is critical in understanding flow regulatory mechanisms (see later).

Understanding the forces driving membrane water flow may have real clinical relevance. There is evidence that maternal dehydration is associated with oligohydramnios, presumably on an osmotic basis,[74,75] and that rehydration can increase fetal urine flow and AF volume.[76,77] Hypoproteinemia, with decreased maternal plasma oncotic pressure, may be associated with an increase in AF.[78] In addition, water flow considerations have been used to describe the physiology of twin-twin transfusion syndrome, with an accurate prediction of the success of various treatment modalities.[79,80] Finally, knowledge of the natural mechanisms regulating AF volume may yield insights into possible therapies for abnormalities of AF volume.

The anatomy of the fetal membranes suggests mechanisms for IM flow. In sheep, an extensive network of microscopic blood vessels is located between the outer surface of the amnion and the chorion,[81] presumably providing the surface area for IM flow. In primates, including humans, IM flow most likely occurs across the fetal surface of the placenta, where fetal vessels course under the amnion. In vivo studies of ovine IM flow suggest that membrane water flow is proportionate to the AF volume, and that water flow can be independent of the clearance of other molecules.[82-84] In sheep, the filtration coefficient of the amnion has been estimated to be 0.00137 mL/min/mm Hg per kilogram fetal weight,[72] although IM flow rates under control conditions in vivo have not been directly measured. In the human, fetal membrane ultrastructural changes are noted with polyhydramnios or oligohydramnios,[85] suggesting that alterations in IM flow may contribute to idiopathic AF clinical abnormalities, or that marked changes in AF volume or pressure may have an impact on fetal membrane structure.

IM flow is presumably dependent on the water permeability of the fetal membranes and blood vessels. Despite the relative ease of measurement, chorioamnion permeability to water in vitro has rarely been assessed. In one experiment, human amnion overlying the chorionic plate was studied in a Ussing chamber at 38° C. The membrane diffusional permeability (P) to water was measured at 2.2×10^{-4} cm/sec.[86] Another experiment found an osmotic permeability of 1.5×10^{-2} cm/sec in human amnion.[73] These values are similar to values obtained in renal tubular epithelium[87-89] and would indicate that the amnion is a "leaky" epithelium with the potential for significant water flux, which would then be subject to modulation. When human amnion and chorion were both tested, the amnion appeared to be a more effective barrier to the diffusion of water.[90] Similarly, in the sheep, the permeability of amniochorion was $2.0 \pm 0.3 \times 10^{-4}$ cm/sec, not different from the permeability of amnion alone, which was $2.5 \pm 0.7 \times 10^{-4}$ cm/sec.[82] This, coupled with the fact that the fetal vessels occur between the amnion and chorion, would suggest that the amnion is the more likely to be involved in regulating IM water flow.

Studies in the ovine model suggest that flow through the IM pathway can be modulated to achieve AF volume homeostasis, specifically under conditions potentiating excess AF volume. Because fetal swallowing is a major route of AF fluid resorption, esophageal ligation would be expected to increase AF volume significantly. Although AF volume did increase significantly 3 days after ovine fetal esophageal occlusion,[91] longer periods (i.e., 9 days) of esophageal ligation reduced AF volume in preterm sheep despite continued production of urine.[56] Similarly, esophageal ligation of fetal sheep over a period of 1 month did not increase AF volume.[92] In the absence of swallowing, with continued fetal urine production, normalized AF volume suggests an increase in IM flow. In addition, AF resorption increased markedly after infusion of exogenous fluid to the AF cavity[93] or after increased fetal urine output stimulated by a fetal intravenous volume infusion.[84] Collectively, these studies suggest that IM flow may be under feedback regulation. That is, AF volume expansion increases IM resorption, ultimately resulting in a normalization of AF volume. Importantly, however, factors downregulating IM flow are less well characterized; there is no evidence of reduced IM resorption as an adaptive response to oligohydramnios. Downregulation of IM flow is possible, as prolactin reduces the upregulation of IM flow caused by osmotic challenge in the sheep model,[94] and it may reduce diffusional permeability to water in human[95] and guinea pig[96] amnion.

The specific mechanism and regulation of IM flow are probably the key to AF homeostasis. Bulk water flow across an epithelial membrane requires a motive force. IM flow may be driven by the significant osmotic gradient between the hypotonic AF and isotonic fetal plasma[57] in the human and sheep, although in rats and mice the osmotic gradient does not favor AF-to-plasma flow.[97-99] One explanation may be that solute concentration at the membrane surface may differ significantly from that in the plasma or AF as a whole, a phenomenon known as the "unstrirred layer" effect.[100] Gross hydrostatic forces are unlikely to drive AF-to-fetal flow, as the pressure in the fetal vessels exceeds that in the amniotic cavity. Hydrostatic forces could be developed between the AF and the interstitial space, with another force promoting water flow into the bloodstream. Local changes in hydrostatic or osmotic pressure have been proposed to drive IM flow, but none of these has been demonstrated in vivo.

A variety of mechanisms have been proposed for the regulation of IM flow. As esophageal ligation of fetal sheep resulted in upregulation of fetal chorioamnion vascular endothelial growth factor (VEGF) gene expression,[101] it was proposed that VEGF-induced neovascularization could potentiate AF water resorption. Those authors further speculated that fetal urine or lung fluid, or both, may contain factors that upregulate VEGF, although their recent work demonstrates no effect of lung liquid on the rate of IM flow (J. Jellyman, personal communication). The association of increased VEGF, and presumably vessel growth and permeability,[102] with increased IM flow, coupled with the difference noted between the asymmetrical flow in vivo and the symmetrical permeability of amnion in vitro, have also led to the suggestion that the rate of IM flow is regulated by the fetal vessel endothelium, rather than by the amnion.[58]

In animals in which the fetal urine output had been increased by an intravenous volume load, an increase in AF resorption occurred, despite a constant membrane diffusional permeability to technetium.[84] In addition, artificial alteration of the osmolality and oncotic pressure of the AF revealed that IM flow was highly correlated with osmotic differences; however, there was a component of IM flow that was not osmotic dependent. As this flow pathway was also permeable to protein, with a reflection coefficient of near zero, this residual flow was felt to be similar to fluid flow in the lymph system.[103] These findings, in aggregate, have been interpreted to indicate active transport of bulk fluid (i.e., water and solutes) from the AF to the fetal circulation, either in the amnion or in the fetal vessel wall. Daneshmand and colleagues[84] have proposed that this fluid transport occurs via membrane vesicles, and they point out the high prevalence of intracellular vesicles seen on electron microscopy of the amnion.[104] This theory has not been widely accepted, as vesicle water flow has not been demonstrated in any other tissue and would be highly energy dependent. Rather, most authors believe that IM flow occurs through conventional *para-* and *trans-*cellular channels, driven by osmotic and hydrostatic forces, perhaps modulated through an unstirred layer effect. Mathematical modeling indicates that relatively small IM sodium fluxes could be associated with significant changes in AF volume, suggesting that active transport of sodium may be a regulator of IM flow.[65] The observation that a portion of IM flow was independent of osmotic differences, however, suggests that other forces may also be significant.[103]

Importantly, upregulation of VEGF or sodium transfer alone cannot explain AF composition changes after fetal esophageal ligation, because AF electrolyte composition indicates that water flow increases disproportionately to solute (i.e., electrolyte) flow.[61] The passage of free water across a biologic membrane is a characteristic of transcellular flow, a process mediated by cell membrane water channels (aquaporins [AQPs]). AQPs are hydrophobic intramembranous proteins.[105,106] They organize in the cell membrane as tetramers, but each monomer forms a hydrophilic pore in its center and functions independently as a water channel.[106] Although the majority of AQP structural studies have been performed on AQP1, similarities in sequence suggest that the three-dimensional structure of all AQPs is similar, although in addition to water, some AQPs also allow passage of glycerol, urea, and larger molecules. Multiple AQPs have been identified (up to 13, depending on the species). Some are widely expressed throughout the body; others appear to be more tissue specific.

Regulation of water flux depends on the location and concentration of AQPs in the cell membrane. In the kidney, AQP3 and AQP4 are both present in the basolateral membrane of the collecting-duct principal cells, whereas AQP2 is present in the apical portion of the membrane of these cells.[107] The presence of different AQPs on different portions of the same cell is thought to regulate water transfer across the cell by differentially promoting water entry from the collecting duct lumen and from the interstitial fluid. AQP concentration in the membrane may be influenced by the insertion or removal of AQP into the membrane from the intracellular compartment, or by the promotion of AQP production. Both of these events may be the result of cellular stimulation by hormones or by the external environment. In the renal tubule, AQP2 is transferred from cytoplasm vesicles to the apical cell membrane in response to AVP[108] or forskolin (a stimulator of cAMP production).[109] AQP8 is similarly transferred from hepatocyte vesicles to the cell membrane in response to dibutyryl cAMP and glucagon.[110] In longer time frames, expression of various AQPs may be induced by external conditions. For example, AQP3 expression in cultured keratinocytes is increased in hypertonic medium.[111] In the intact organism, AQP3 expression in the kidney is upregulated by dehydration,[107] an effect mediated by AVP. Together with permeability data, these findings indicate that AQPs are important in the regulation of water flow across biologic membranes, and that their expression and activity are regulated according to the needs of the organism.

Studies have demonstrated AQP1, -3, -8, and -9 mRNA (gene) expression in fetal membrane and placenta in a variety of species. In addition, recent data suggest that membrane AQP1 may specifically regulate AF volume. Mice lacking the AQP1 gene have been reported to have significantly increased AF volume.[112] Furthermore, AQP1 expression was increased in human amnion derived from patients with increased AF volumes[113]; this upregulation was postulated to be a compensatory response to polyhydramnios. AQP1 protein increased in ovine chorioallantoic membranes when the fetus was made hypoxic, suggesting a mechanism for the increased IM flow associated with ovine fetal hypoxia.[114] AVP levels may be higher in the AF of fetuses with oligohydramnios,[115] and some work suggests that AVP and cAMP may upregulate AQP expression in cultured human amnion.[116-119] Upregulation of amnion AQP1 by AVP is a possible explanation for oligohydramnios resulting from increased IM flow. These results suggest that AQP1, and possibly -3, -8, and -9, could participate in the regulation of gestational water flow.

Summary

AF is an important component of successful gestation. When present in normal amounts, it provides an environment for normal development and an extrafetal water store. It also serves as a convenient source of diagnostic material. Normal AF volumes can vary widely between individuals, and a variety of pathologic conditions may be associated with frankly abnormal AF volume. Early in gestation, AF appears to be a transudate of fetal serum, although the specifics of AF production and resorption are little studied. In the second half of pregnancy, human AF is hypo-osmolar to serum and contains increased concentrations of urea and creatinine. Although the formation of AF is reasonably well described, the mechanisms for establishing and maintaining AF volume are poorly understood. Similarly, the cause of abnormal AF volumes in certain pathologic conditions is unknown. Although all of the major mechanisms for production and resorption of AF can be modulated by the near-term fetus, modulation of IM flow appears today to be the most likely to serve as a mechanism for normalizing AF volume. Regulation of AF volume remains an active area of investigation, as the ability to therapeutically alter the production or resorption of AF would represent an important advance in the management of pregnancy.

References

1. Fuchs F, RIIS P: Antenatal sex determination. Nature 177:330, 1956.
2. Calvo RM, Jauniaux E, Gulbis B, et al: Fetal tissues are exposed to biologically relevant free thyroxine concentrations during early phases of development. J Clin Endocrinol Metab 87:1768-1777, 2002.
3. Smith DL: Amniotic fluid volume: A measurement of the amniotic fluid present in 72 pregnancies during the first half of pregnancy. Am J Obstet Gynecol 110:166-172, 1971.
4. Geirsson RT, Patel NB, Christie AD: In-vivo accuracy of ultrasound measurements of intrauterine volume in pregnancy. BJOG 91:37-40, 1984.
5. Brace RA, Wolf EJ: Normal amniotic fluid volume changes throughout pregnancy. Am J Obstet Gynecol 161:382-388, 1989.
6. Gadd RL: The volume of the liquor amnii in normal and abnormal pregnancies. J Obstet Gynaecol Br Commonw 73:11-22, 1966.
7. Beischer NA, Brown JB, Townsend L: Studies in prolonged pregnancy: 3. Amniocentesis in prolonged pregnancy. Am J Obstet Gynecol 103:496-503, 1969.
8. Queenan JT, Von Gal HV, Kubarych SF: Amniography for clinical evaluation of erythroblastosis fetalis. Am J Obstet Gynecol 102:264-274, 1968.
9. Chamberlain PF, Manning FA, Morrison I, et al: Ultrasound evaluation of amniotic fluid volume: II. The relationship of increased amniotic fluid volume to perinatal outcome. Am J Obstet Gynecol 150:250-254, 1984.
10. Gumus II, Koktener A, Turhan NO: Perinatal outcomes of pregnancies with borderline amniotic fluid index. Arch Gynecol Obstet 276:17-19, 2007.
11. Volante E, Gramellini D, Moretti S, et al: Alteration of the amniotic fluid and neonatal outcome. Acta Biomed 75(Suppl 1):71-75, 2004.
12. Locatelli A, Vergani P, Toso L, et al: Perinatal outcome associated with oligohydramnios in uncomplicated term pregnancies. Arch Gynecol Obstet 269:130-133, 2004.
13. Campbell J, Wathen N, Macintosh M, et al: Biochemical composition of amniotic fluid and extraembryonic coelomic fluid in the first trimester of pregnancy. BJOG 99:563-565, 1992.
14. Jauniaux E, Hempstock J, Teng C, et al: Polyol concentrations in the fluid compartments of the human conceptus during the first trimester of pregnancy: Maintenance of redox potential in a low oxygen environment. J Clin Endocrinol Metab 90:1171-1175, 2005.
15. Gillibrand PN: Changes in the electrolytes, urea and osmolality of the amniotic fluid with advancing pregnancy. J Obstet Gynaecol Br Commonw 76:898-905, 1969.
16. Faber JJ, Gault CF, Green TJ, et al: Chloride and the generation of amniotic fluid in the early embryo. J Exp Zool 183:343-352, 1973.
17. Gitlin D, Kumate J, Morales C, et al: The turnover of amniotic fluid protein in the human conceptus. Am J Obstet Gynecol 113:632-645, 1972.
18. Seeds AE: Current concepts of amniotic fluid dynamics. Am J Obstet Gynecol 138:575-586, 1980.
19. Brophy BP, Robillard JE: Functional development of the kidney in utero. In Polin RA, Fox WW, Abman SH (eds): Fetal and Neonatal Physiology. Philadelphia, Saunders, 2004, p 1229.
20. Takeuchi H, Koyanagi T, Yoshizato T, et al: Fetal urine production at different gestational ages. Correlation to various compromised fetuses in utero. Early Hum Dev 40:1-11, 1994.
21. Rabinowitz R, Peters MT, Vyas S, et al: Measurement of fetal urine production in normal pregnancy by real-time ultrasonography. Am J Obstet Gynecol 161:1264-1266, 1989.
22. Lotgering FK, Wallenburg HC: Mechanisms of production and clearance of amniotic fluid. Semin Perinatol 10:94-102, 1986.
23. Fagerquist M, Fagerquist U, Oden A, Blomberg SG: Fetal urine production and accuracy when estimating fetal urinary bladder volume. Ultrasound Obstet Gynecol 17:132-139, 2001.
24. Gresham EL, Rankin JH, Makowski EL, et al: An evaluation of fetal renal function in a chronic sheep preparation. J Clin Invest 51:149-156, 1972.
25. Wlodek ME, Challis JR, Patrick J: Urethral and urachal urine output to the amniotic and allantoic sacs in fetal sheep. J Dev Physiol 10:309-319, 1988.
26. Brace RA, Moore TR: Diurnal rhythms in fetal urine flow, vascular pressures, and heart rate in sheep. Am J Physiol 261:R1015-1021, 1991.
27. Trimmer KJ, Leveno KJ, Peters MT, Kelly MA: Observations on the cause of oligohydramnios in prolonged pregnancy. Am J Obstet Gynecol 163:1900-1903, 1990.
28. Hargrave BY, Castle MC: Effects of phenylephrine induced increase in arterial pressure and closure of the ductus arteriosus on the secretion of atrial natriuretic peptide (ANP) and renin in the ovine fetus. Life Sci 57:31-43, 1995.
29. Silberbach M, Woods LL, Hohimer AR, et al: Role of endogenous atrial natriuretic peptide in chronic anemia in the ovine fetus: Effects of a non-peptide antagonist for atrial natriuretic peptide receptor. Pediatr Res 38:722-728, 1995.
30. Xu Z, Glenda C, Day L, et al: Osmotic threshold and sensitivity for vasopressin release and fos expression by hypertonic NaCl in ovine fetus. Am J Physiol Endocrinol Metab 279:E1207-1215, 2000.
31. Horne RS, MacIsaac RJ, Moritz KM, et al: Effect of arginine vasopressin and parathyroid hormone-related protein on renal function in the ovine foetus. Clin Exp Pharmacol Physiol 20:569-577, 1993.
32. Silva AM, Smith RN, Lehmann CU, et al: Neonatal nucleated red blood cells and the prediction of cerebral white matter injury in preterm infants. Obstet Gynecol 107:550-556, 2006.
33. Fignon A, Salihagic A, Akoka S, et al: Twenty-day cerebral and umbilical Doppler monitoring on a growth retarded and hypoxic fetus. Eur J Obstet Gynecol Reprod Biol 66:83-86, 1996.
34. Thurlow RW, Brace RA: Swallowing, urine flow, and amniotic fluid volume responses to prolonged hypoxia in the ovine fetus. Am J Obstet Gynecol 189:601-608, 2003.
35. Brace RA, Wlodek ME, Cock ML, Harding R: Swallowing of lung liquid and amniotic fluid by the ovine fetus under normoxic and hypoxic conditions. Am J Obstet Gynecol 171:764-770, 1994.
36. Carlton DP, Cummings JJ, Chapman DL, et al: Ion transport regulation of lung liquid secretion in foetal lambs. J Dev Physiol 17:99-107, 1992.
37. Ross MG, Ervin G, Leake RD, et al: Fetal lung liquid regulation by neuropeptides. Am J Obstet Gynecol 150:421-425, 1984.
38. Lawson EE, Brown ER, Torday JS, et al: The effect of epinephrine on tracheal fluid flow and surfactant efflux in fetal sheep. Am Rev Respir Dis 118:1023-1026, 1978.

39. Dodic M, Wintour EM: Effects of prolonged (48 h) infusion of cortisol on blood pressure, renal function and fetal fluids in the immature ovine foetus. Clin Exp Pharmacol Physiol 21:971-980, 1994.
40. Jain L, Eaton DC: Physiology of fetal lung fluid clearance and the effect of labor. Semin Perinatol 30:34-43, 2006.
41. Norlin A, Folkesson HG: Ca(2+)-dependent stimulation of alveolar fluid clearance in near-term fetal guinea pigs. Am J Physiol Lung Cell Mol Physiol 282:L642-649, 2002.
42. Stiles B, Power GG: Changes in permeability of fetal guinea pig skin during gestation. J Dev Physiol 5:405-411, 1983.
43. Parmley TH, Seeds AE: Fetal skin permeability to isotopic water (THO) in early pregnancy. Am J Obstet Gynecol 108:128-131, 1970.
44. Brace RA: Amniotic fluid volume and its relationship to fetal fluid balance: Review of experimental data. Semin Perinatol 10:103-112, 1986.
45. Pritchard JA: Fetal swallowing and amniotic fluid volume. Obstet Gynecol 28:606-610, 1966.
46. Abramovich DR, Garden A, Jandial L, Page KR: Fetal swallowing and voiding in relation to hydramnios. Obstet Gynecol 54:15-20, 1979.
47. Bradley RM, Mistretta CM: Swallowing in fetal sheep. Science 179:1016-1017, 1973.
48. Nijland MJ, Day L, Ross MG: Ovine fetal swallowing: expression of preterm neurobehavioral rhythms. J Matern Fetal Med 10:251-257, 2001.
49. Lumbers ER, Smith FG, Stevens AD: Measurement of net transplacental transfer of fluid to the fetal sheep. J Physiol 364:289-299, 1985.
50. Sherman DJ, Ross MG, Day L, Ervin MG: Fetal swallowing: Correlation of electromyography and esophageal fluid flow. Am J Physiol 258:R1386-1394, 1990.
51. Xu Z, Nijland MJ, Ross MG: Plasma osmolality dipsogenic thresholds and c-fos expression in the near-term ovine fetus. Pediatr Res 49:678-685, 2001.
52. El-Haddad MA, Ismail Y, Gayle D, Ross MG: Central angiotensin II AT1 receptors mediate fetal swallowing and pressor responses in the near term ovine fetus. Am J Physiol Regul Integr Comp Physiol 288:R1014-1020, 2004.
53. El-Haddad MA, Ismail Y, Guerra C, et al: Neuropeptide Y administered into cerebral ventricles stimulates sucrose ingestion in the near-term ovine fetus. Am J Obstet Gynecol 189:949-952, 2003.
54. El-Haddad MA, Ismail Y, Guerra C, et al: Effect of oral sucrose on ingestive behavior in the near-term ovine fetus. Am J Obstet Gynecol 187:898-901, 2002.
55. Sherman DJ, Ross MG, Day L, et al: Fetal swallowing: Response to graded maternal hypoxemia. J Appl Physiol 71:1856-1861, 1991.
56. Matsumoto LC, Cheung CY, Brace RA: Effect of esophageal ligation on amniotic fluid volume and urinary flow rate in fetal sheep. Am J Obstet Gynecol 182:699-705, 2000.
57. Gilbert WM, Brace RA: The missing link in amniotic fluid volume regulation: Intramembranous absorption. Obstet Gynecol 74:748-754, 1989.
58. Adams EA, Choi HM, Cheung CY, Brace RA: Comparison of amniotic and intramembranous unidirectional permeabilities in late-gestation sheep. Am J Obstet Gynecol 193:247-255, 2005.
59. Gilbert WM, Cheung CY, Brace RA: Rapid intramembranous absorption into the fetal circulation of arginine vasopressin injected intraamniotically. Am J Obstet Gynecol 164:1013-1018, 1991.
60. Gilbert WM, Newman PS, Brace RA: Potential route for fetal therapy: Intramembranous absorption of intraamniotically injected furosemide. Am J Obstet Gynecol 172:1471-1476, 1995.
61. Jang PR, Brace RA: Amniotic fluid composition changes during urine drainage and tracheoesophageal occlusion in fetal sheep. Am J Obstet Gynecol 167:1732-1741, 1992.
62. Brace RA: Physiology of amniotic fluid volume regulation. Clin Obstet Gynecol 40:280-289, 1997.
63. Queenan JT, Allen FH Jr, Fuchs F, et al: Studies on the method of intrauterine transfusion: I. Question of erythrocyte absorption from amniotic fluid. Am J Obstet Gynecol 92:1009-1013, 1965.
64. Mann SE, Nijland MJ, Ross MG: Mathematic modeling of human amniotic fluid dynamics. Am J Obstet Gynecol 175:937-944, 1996.
65. Curran MA, Nijland MJ, Mann SE, Ross MG: Human amniotic fluid mathematical model: Determination and effect of intramembranous sodium flux. Am J Obstet Gynecol 178:484-490, 1998.
66. Anderson DF, Faber JJ, Parks CM: Extraplacental transfer of water in the sheep. J Physiol 406:75-84, 1988.
67. Anderson DF, Borst NJ, Boyd RD, Faber JJ: Filtration of water from mother to conceptus via paths independent of fetal placental circulation in sheep. J Physiol 431:1-10, 1990.
68. Sibley CP, Boyd DH: Mechanisms of transfer across the human placenta. In Polin RA, Fox WW, Abman S (eds): Fetal and Neonatal Physiology. Philadelphia, WB Saunders, 2006, pp 111-122.
69. Schroder HJ: Basics of placental structures and transfer functions. In Brace RA, Ross MG, Robillard JE (eds): Reproductive and Perinatal Medicine, vol XI: Fetal and Neonatal Body Fluids. Ithaca, NY, Perinatology Press, 1989, pp 187-226.
70. Faber JJ, Binder ND, Thornburg KL: Electrophysiology of extrafetal membranes. Placenta 8:89-108, 1987.
71. Faber JJ, Thornburg KL: Placental Physiology: Structure and Function of Fetomaternal Exchange. New York, Raven Press, 1983.
72. Gilbert WM, Brace RA: Novel determination of filtration coefficient of ovine placenta and intramembranous pathway. Am J Physiol 259:R1281-1288, 1990.
73. Capurro C, Escobar E, Ibarra C, et al: Water permeability in different epithelial barriers. Biol Cell 66:145-148, 1989.
74. Sciscione AC, Costigan KA, Johnson TR: Increase in ambient temperature may explain decrease in amniotic fluid index. Am J Perinatol 14:249-251, 1997.
75. Hanson RS, Powrie RO, Larson L: Diabetes insipidus in pregnancy: A treatable cause of oligohydramnios. Obstet Gynecol 89:816-817, 1997.
76. Oosterhof H, Haak MC, Aarnoudse JG: Acute maternal rehydration increases the urine production rate in the near-term human fetus. Am J Obstet Gynecol 183:226-229, 2000.
77. Flack NJ, Sepulveda W, Bower S, Fisk NM: Acute maternal hydration in third-trimester oligohydramnios: Effects on amniotic fluid volume, utero-placental perfusion, and fetal blood flow and urine output. Am J Obstet Gynecol 173:1186-1191, 1995.
78. Okai T, Baba K, Kohzuma S, et al: [Nonimmunologic hydrops fetalis: A review of 30 cases.] Nippon Sanka Fujinka Gakkai Zasshi 36:1813-1821, 1984.
79. van den Wijngaard JP, Ross MG, van Gemert MJ: Twin-twin transfusion syndrome modeling. Ann N Y Acad Sci 1101:215-234, 2007.
80. van den Wijngaard JP, Ross MG, van der Sloot JA, et al: Simulation of therapy in a model of a nonhydropic and hydropic recipient in twin-twin transfusion syndrome. Am J Obstet Gynecol 193:1972-1980, 2005.
81. Brace RA, Gilbert WM, Thornburg KL: Vascularization of the ovine amnion and chorion: A morphometric characterization of the surface area of the intramembranous pathway. Am J Obstet Gynecol 167:1747-1755, 1992.
82. Lingwood BE, Wintour EM: Permeability of ovine amnion and amniochorion to urea and water. Obstet Gynecol 61:227-232, 1983.
83. Lingwood BE, Wintour EM: Amniotic fluid volume and in vivo permeability of ovine fetal membranes. Obstet Gynecol 64:368-372, 1984.
84. Daneshmand SS, Cheung CY, Brace RA: Regulation of amniotic fluid volume by intramembranous absorption in sheep: Role of passive permeability and vascular endothelial growth factor. Am J Obstet Gynecol 188:786-793, 2003.
85. Hebertson RM, Hammond ME, Bryson MJ: Amniotic epithelial ultrastructure in normal, polyhydramnic, and oligohydramnic pregnancies. Obstet Gynecol 68:74-79, 1986.
86. Leontic EA, Schruefer JJ, Andreassen B, et al: Further evidence for the role of prolactin on human fetoplacental osmoregulation. Am J Obstet Gynecol 133:435-438, 1979.
87. Kuwahara M, Verkman AS: Direct fluorescence measurement of diffusional water permeability in the vasopressin-sensitive kidney collecting tubule. Biophys J 54:587-593, 1988.

88. Chou CL, Ma T, Yang B, et al: Fourfold reduction of water permeability in inner medullary collecting duct of aquaporin-4 knockout mice. Am J Physiol 274:C549-554, 1998.
89. Berry CA, Verkman AS: Osmotic gradient dependence of osmotic water permeability in rabbit proximal convoluted tubule. J Membr Biol 105:33-43, 1988.
90. Hardy MA, Leonardi RT, Scheide JI: Cellular permeation pathways in a leaky epithelium: The human amniochorion. Biol Cell 66:149-153, 1989.
91. Fujino Y, Agnew CL, Schreyer P, et al: Amniotic fluid volume response to esophageal occlusion in fetal sheep. Am J Obstet Gynecol 165:1620-1626, 1991.
92. Wintour EM, Barnes A, Brown EH, et al: Regulation of amniotic fluid volume and composition in the ovine fetus. Obstet Gynecol 52:689-693, 1978.
93. Faber JJ, Anderson DF: Regulatory response of intramembranous absorption of amniotic fluid to infusion of exogenous fluid in sheep. Am J Physiol 277:R236-242, 1999.
94. Ross MG, Ervin MG, Leake RD, et al: Bulk flow of amniotic fluid water in response to maternal osmotic challenge. Am J Obstet Gynecol 147:697-701, 1983.
95. Leontic EA, Tyson JE: Prolactin and fetal osmoregulation: Water transport across isolated human amnion. Am J Physiol 232:R124-127, 1977.
96. Holt WF, Perks AM: The effect of prolactin on water movement through the isolated amniotic membrane of the guinea pig. Gen Comp Endocrinol 26:153-164, 1975.
97. Cheung CY, Brace RA: Amniotic fluid volume and composition in mouse pregnancy. J Soc Gynecol Investig 12:558-562, 2005.
98. Hedriana HL, Gilbert WM, Brace RA: Arginine vasopressin-induced changes in blood flow to the ovine chorion, amnion, and placenta across gestation. J Soc Gynecol Investig 4:203-208, 1997.
99. Desai M, Ladella S, Ross MG: Reversal of pregnancy-mediated plasma hypotonicity in the near-term rat. J Matern Fetal Neonatal Med 13:197-202, 2003.
100. Verkman AS, Dix JA: Effect of unstirred layers on binding and reaction kinetics at a membrane surface. Anal Biochem 142:109-116, 1984.
101. Matsumoto LC, Bogic L, Brace RA, Cheung CY: Fetal esophageal ligation induces expression of vascular endothelial growth factor messenger ribonucleic acid in fetal membranes. Am J Obstet Gynecol 184:175-184, 2001.
102. Bates DO, Hillman NJ, Williams B, et al: Regulation of microvascular permeability by vascular endothelial growth factors. J Anat 200:581-597, 2002.
103. Faber JJ, Anderson DF: Absorption of amniotic fluid by amniochorion in sheep. Am J Physiol Heart Circ Physiol 282:H850-854, 2002.
104. Wynn RM, French GL: Comparative ultrastructure of the mammalian amnion. Obstet Gynecol 31:759-774, 1968.
105. Verkman AS, Shi LB, Frigeri A, et al: Structure and function of kidney water channels. Kidney Int 48:1069-1081, 1995.
106. Knepper MA, Wade JB, Terris J, et al: Renal aquaporins. Kidney Int 49:1712-1717, 1996.
107. Nielsen S, Frokiaer J, Marples D, et al: Aquaporins in the kidney: From molecules to medicine. Physiol Rev 82:205-244, 2002.
108. Klussmann E, Maric K, Rosenthal W: The mechanisms of aquaporin control in the renal collecting duct. Rev Physiol Biochem Pharmacol 141:33-95, 2000.
109. Tajika Y, Matsuzaki T, Suzuki T, et al: Aquaporin-2 is retrieved to the apical storage compartment via early endosomes and phosphatidylinositol 3-kinase-dependent pathway. Endocrinology 145:4375-4383, 2004.
110. Gradilone SA, Garcia F, Huebert RC, et al: Glucagon induces the plasma membrane insertion of functional aquaporin-8 water channels in isolated rat hepatocytes. Hepatology 37:1435-1441, 2003.
111. Sugiyama Y, Ota Y, Hara M, Inoue S: Osmotic stress up-regulates aquaporin-3 gene expression in cultured human keratinocytes. Biochim Biophys Acta 1522:82-88, 2001.
112. Mann SE, Ricke EA, Torres EA, Taylor RN: A novel model of polyhydramnios: Amniotic fluid volume is increased in aquaporin 1 knockout mice. Am J Obstet Gynecol 192:2041-2044, 2005.
113. Mann SE, Dvorak N, Gilbert H, Taylor RN: Steady-state levels of aquaporin 1 mRNA expression are increased in idiopathic polyhydramnios. Am J Obstet Gynecol 194:884-887, 2006.
114. Bos HB, Nygard KL, Gratton RJ, Richardson BS: Expression of aquaporin 1 (AQP1) in chorioallantoic membranes of near term ovine fetuses with induced hypoxia. J Soc Gynecol Investig 12(2 Suppl):333A, 2005.
115. Bajoria R, Ward S, Sooranna SR: Influence of vasopressin in the pathogenesis of oligohydramnios-polyhydramnios in monochorionic twins. Eur J Obstet Gynecol Reprod Biol 113:49-55, 2004.
116. Wang S, Chen J, Au KT, Ross MG: Expression of aquaporin 8 and its up-regulation by cyclic adenosine monophosphate in human WISH cells. Am J Obstet Gynecol 188:997-1001, 2003.
117. Wang S, Amidi F, Beall MH, Ross MG: Differential regulation of aquaporin water channels in human amnion cell culture. J Soc Gynecol Investig 12(2 Suppl):344A, 2005.
118. Beall MH, Wang S, Amidi F, Ross MG: Mechanism of fetal hypoxia-induced oligohydramnios: Upregulation of amnion aquaporin 1 expression. J Soc Gynecol Investig 13(3 Suppl):299A, 2006.
119. Beall M, Wang S, Amidi F, Ross MG: Stimulation of aquaporin (AQP) gene expression in human fetal membrane explants. Am J Obstet Gynecol 193(6 Suppl):S168, 2005.

Chapter 4

Multiple Gestation

The Biology of Twinning

Kurt Benirschke, MD

Incidence of Twinning

The incidence of twinning is increasing as our population ages and a new technology—assisted reproductive technology (ART)—is becoming widely used. Not only have artificial reproductive techniques led to a marked increase in higher-order multiple births (triplets, quadruplets) but also they are followed by an increase in prematurity rates and congenital anomalies.[1-3] The statistics, which are usually derived from national or regional birth records and rely on reporting by physicians or other personnel attending births, do not accurately reflect the occurrence of twins at conception because the much higher prenatal mortality of twins (as abortion or fetus papyraceus) is not taken into account. Thoughtful reviews of the multiple gestation "epidemic" are available.[4-6] Some countries have chosen to deny transfer of more than one blastocyst.[7] An additional finding of interest is that there appears to be an increase in monozygotic twinning (identified as being monochorionic) when various ART procedures are used; also, placental abnormalities are more frequent.[8]

Guttmacher[9] suggested that 1.05% to 1.35% of pregnancies were twins, the reason for this wide variation being that the frequency of the twinning process varies widely among different populations. Data collated from various countries reveal that the variability relates largely to the ethnic stock of the population under consideration. Moreover, although the dizygotic (DZ) twinning rate varies widely under different circumstances, the monozygotic (MZ) twinning rate is considered to be "remarkably constant," usually between 3.5 and 4 per 1000,[10] although Murphy and Hey[11] found the rate to have slightly increased in recent years. In recent national statistics, of 4 million births in the United States, 3.3% were multiple, or 1 in 30 gestations.

When the twinning rate of a population is known, the frequencies of triplets, quadruplets, and so on can be roughly calculated by Hellin's hypothesis, which states that when the frequency of twinning is n, that of triplets is n^2, of quadruplets n^3, and so on. The highest number recorded so far is nine offspring.[12] Since 1973, there has been a steady rise in the incidence of twins and triplets, so that currently at least 1 in 43 births is a twin and 1 in 1341 pregnancies results in triplets.[2,13] In part, this increase was attributed to delayed childbearing, but the use of ovulation-enhancing drugs has also been implicated. Although acknowledging the increased DZ twinning frequency attributed to clomiphene, Tong and coworkers[14] found that the DZ-to-MZ ratio has significantly declined from 1.12 (1960) to 0.05 (1978) and suggested adverse environmental factors as a possible cause.

Types of Twins

Twins who possess characteristics that make them virtually indistinguishable are referred to as identical, whereas twins who are unlike are considered fraternal. Identical twins always have the same sex, but fraternal twins may be of different sexes. The terms *identical* and *fraternal,* although popular, are scientifically less useful and are best replaced by the terms *monozygotic* and *dizygotic*, respectively, to indicate the mechanism of origin of the two types of twins. An important reason for this preference is that MZ twins with discordant phenotypes (e.g., cleft lip) would be misclassified as fraternal.

To assess the frequency of MZ and DZ twins, investigators have commonly used the Weinberg differential method. This method suggests that the frequency of MZ twins can be deduced from a twin sample when the sex of the twin pairs is known. Thus, if the numbers of male and female conceptuses were approximately equal and all twins were fraternal (DZ), there would be 50 male-female pairs, 25 male-male pairs, and 25 female-female pairs in every 100 pairs of twins. Any excess of like-sex twins is therefore assumed to be the population of MZ twins. This number then can be calculated by using the following formula:

$$\text{MZ twins} = \text{like-sex pairs} - \text{unlike-sex pairs} \div \text{number of pregnancies}$$

When this formula is applied to national birth statistics, approximately one third of twins in the United States are MZ, although it must be said that the tautology of Weinberg, as Boklage[15] calls it, has often been criticized. Moreover, the very high twinning rate of the Yoruba tribe in Nigeria results from a higher frequency of double ovulation, whereas the low twinning rate in Japan is the result of a lower frequency of double ovulation. This formula also supports the notion that MZ twinning occurs with a relatively uniform incidence in different populations and rises only slightly with advancing maternal age.[10] In contrast, the rate of DZ twinning increases with maternal age to about 35 years and then falls abruptly. The rate also increases with parity, is higher in conceptions that occur in the first 3 months of marriage, and decreases in periods of malnutrition, such as during World War II. James[16] deduced that DZ twinning also increases with coital frequency, and numerous studies indicate that DZ twins occur in certain families, presumably because of the presence of genetic factors leading to double ovulation. These factors are expressed in the mother but may be transmitted through males. Only a few pedigrees suggest that MZ twinning is inherited, and most authorities have concluded that it is a random event. There is also some, occasionally disputed, evidence that assisted reproductive technology has increased the frequency of MZ twin births as well, perhaps because of damage to the blastocyst.[17-21]

Much has been written about the possible occurrence of "third twins," or the uncommon twins that may arise from possibly irregular ovulation events, such as polar body fertilization. Bulmer[10] concluded that such an event is unlikely to have been described. Bieber and colleagues,[22] however, suggested that the development of an acardiac triploid twin (a malformed MZ twin without a heart) represents such an example. As explained later, the topic is important only because the evidence that DZ twins come from two ovulations does not rest on very firm knowledge. Goldgar and Kimberling[23] developed a genetic model to discriminate between DZ and polar body twins. They found that only near-centromeric genetic loci can be confidently used to make such a crucial distinction.

Twins may also originate from fertilization by sperm of two fathers, and the suggestion by James[16] that DZ twinning is influenced by coital rates relates to this phenomenon of superfecundation. Few cases have been verified. In the ninth reported case, one white male twin and one African-American male twin were presumably conceived by two documented events 1 week apart.[24]

Causes of Twinning

The causes of both MZ and DZ twinning are incompletely understood. It is commonly assumed that DZ twinning occurs because of double ovulation, and occasional case descriptions support this assumption. Meyer and Meyer[25] described two 14-day implantation sites with two corpora lutea of similar age in contralateral ovaries. Moreover, multiple pregnancy can be induced by hormonal induction of ovulation, and the polyovulation can be followed via ultrasonography.[26,27] Serum gonadotropin levels in twin-prone Nigerian women are higher than in control subjects,[28] and lower levels are found in Japanese women, who are less likely to produce fraternal twins.[29] For these and other reasons, it is reasonable to assume that DZ twinning is the result of somewhat elevated serum gonadotropin levels, leading to double ovulation. Moreover, it is assumed that gonadotropin levels are influenced by maternal age, nutrition, parity, and, among other factors, maternal genotype. It has now also been found that DZ twinning correlates with a mutation on chromosome 3 that codes for a receptor gene,[30] whereas Healey and colleagues[31] questioned a relationship to the fragile X syndrome. More recently, a number of additional factors have been found to affect the ovulation rate. Thus, in sheep and cattle, specific mutations have been correlated with multiple ovulation,[32] and insulin-like growth factor-1 has been found to interact with ovulation and folliculogenesis.[33]

Although these assumptions may be correct, they are not proven, and the existence of two corpora lutea is rarely ascertained when twins are born. It is of interest to learn that the use of ovulation-enhancing agents has also led to an increase in MZ twins, but this is most easily identified in triplets.[34] We observed the same phenomenon in placental examination of triplets and quadruplets. This finding seems at first contradictory, but accidents in preservation of the zona pellucida have been witnessed in assisted reproduction of domestic animals, and these accidents are presumably also the basis for these unexpected events. In addition, the occurrence of two ova in one follicle is well documented, as are many abnormal fertilization events.

More important questions about the validity of this concept of DZ twinning are statistical, however, and they are as yet unanswered. Non–right handedness is found not only in MZ and DZ twins but also in their close relatives at a higher rate than would be expected in the general population.[35] The same observations have been made with respect to certain forms of schizophrenia, suggesting that the traditional MZ and DZ divisions may be incorrect, a full spectrum may exist between the two classes, and the MZ twinning process relates to a factor interfering with the brain symmetry development of the embryo. It has indeed been suggested that there is a continuum between the MZ and DZ twinning propensity.

The mechanism leading to MZ twinning is even more obscure. That such twins exist can be verified not only by their physical similarity but also by their identity in genetic characters. Exhaustive blood group analysis, finding no differences in the face of different parental markers, was formerly used to verify identity. Chromosomal markers had been used for the diagnosis of MZ twins with apparently greater assurance,[36,37] but most recently the direct comparison of DNA variations is being used for zygosity diagnosis. The determination of restriction fragment length polymorphism compares fragments of DNA and is decisive. Moreover, this technique can use a variety of tissues, including blood and placenta.[38,39] This methodology has now been greatly simplified and automated so that zygosity diagnosis can be achieved quickly, reliably, and inexpensively.[40] The facts that MZ twins occur slightly more frequently with advancing maternal age,[10] that discordant malformations often occur, that conjoined twins develop, and that MZ twinning can be induced by teratogens[41] have led to the hypothesis that MZ twins result from a teratologic event. Boklage[35] suggested a disturbance in the process of symmetry development in the embryo. It has been possible to produce MZ twins by the separation of early blastomeres in a few animal genera (e.g., *Triturus, Ovis, Bos, Mus*), but such physical events do not occur in early human embryonic stages. On the other hand, there is some evidence that MZ twinning may be more frequent after ART procedures although some have disputed this. Nevertheless, Steinman and Valderrama,[42,43] who have had an interest in the mechanism, have suggested that the possible reduction of calcium ions (needed for cell adhesion) may be causative because of the composition of the culture fluids and length of exposure in in vitro fertilization.

Because of these uncertainties, it has been convenient to speak of the "twinning impetus," an external and perhaps teratogenic agency, that is randomly distributed and that may lead to twins only up to a certain stage before the embryonic axis is established. Experiments in mice with vincristine support this hypothesis.[41] If teratogens had their effect later, twins would not be resulting; rather, anomalies in the singleton might develop. It is further assumed that this twinning impetus may lead to separation of only the embryonic cells but that it will not lead to the splitting of already formed cavities. Therefore, when the embryonic events are plotted against embryonic age, one may deduce from the placental configuration the approximate timing of the twinning process (Fig. 4-1).

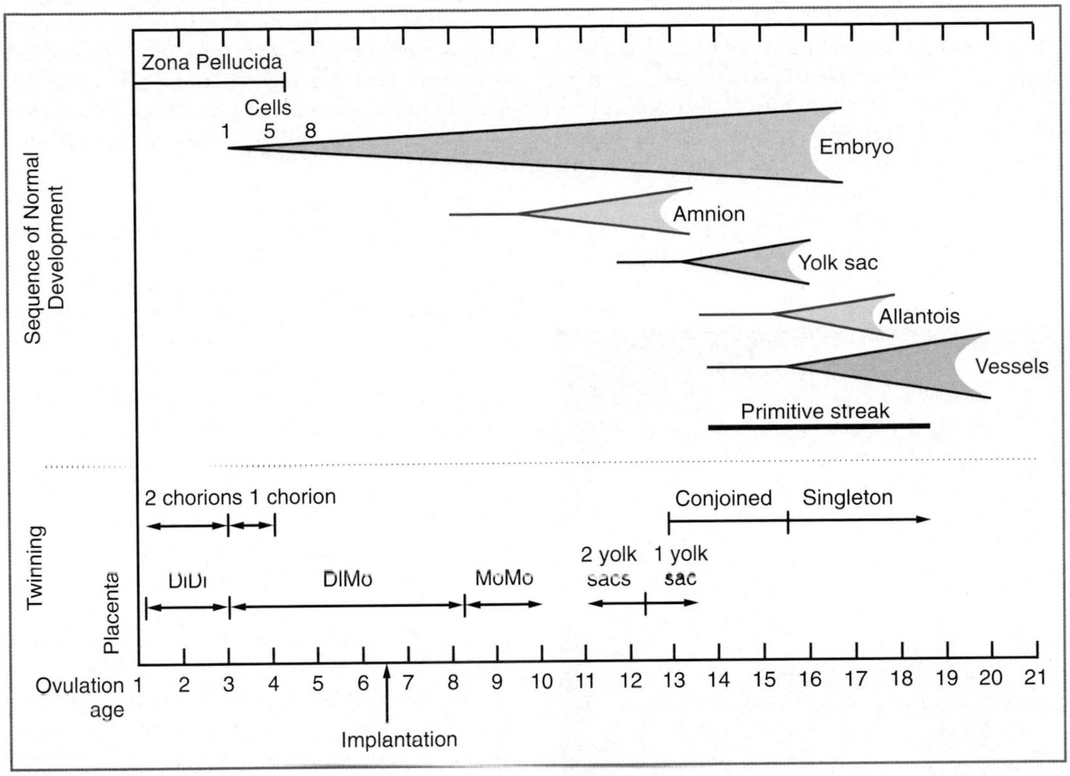

FIGURE 4-1 **Schematic representation of monozygotic twinning event superimposed on temporal events of embryogenesis.** The embryonic events in the upper portion are sketched according to the publications of early human embryos by Hertig (1968). The twinning event is depicted in the lower portion, with resulting placental types indicated. DiDi, diamniotic dichorionic; DIMo, diamniotic monochorionic; MoMo, monoamniotic monochorionic. (From Benirschke K, Kim CK: Multiple pregnancy. N Engl J Med 288:1276, 1973. Reprinted by permission from The New England Journal of Medicine.)

Placentation in Twinning

There are two principally different placental types, monochorionic and dichorionic placentas (Fig. 4-2), and it is essential that they be so identified at birth. Indeed, it is also desirable to differentiate these placentas prenatally by ascertaining the thickness of the "dividing membranes" sonographically. Winn and associates[44] established criteria for this measurement and suggested that, with an 82% accuracy, a maximal thickness of 2 mm is diagnostic of monochorionicity. More recent studies have shown the reliability of this methodology, especially in the mid-trimester. Oligohydramnios is its most serious limitation.[45,46] Numerous surveys of placental types of twins have shown that heterosexual (assuredly DZ) twins virtually always have a dichorionic placenta, and that monochorionic twins have always been of the same sex. These basic facts led us to assume that all monochorionic twins are MZ; however, exceptions have also been reported on very rare occasions.[47,48]

Some MZ twins may be endowed with dichorionic placentas (i.e., twins that separated in the first 2 days after fertilization) (see Fig. 4-1). Most MZ twins, however, have a placenta with diamniotic and monochorionic membranes (Fig. 4-3). Monoamniotic twins, which are by necessity also monochorionic, occur least commonly (approximate incidence, 1%). Conjoined twins are monoamniotic and are less common still, because it probably becomes increasingly difficult for a rapidly growing embryo to submit to the twinning impetus.

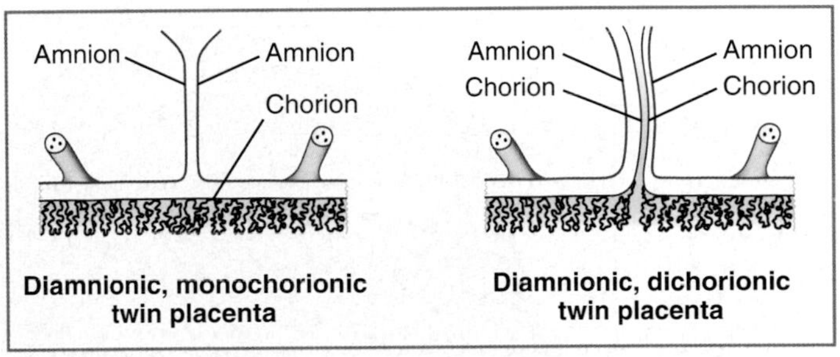

FIGURE 4-2 **The two principal types of twin placentation. Left,** Diamniotic monochorionic placenta, always monozygotic. **Right,** Diamniotic dichorionic placenta, which may or may not be fused.

DZ twins always have dichorionic placentation. Their placentas may be separated or intimately fused (Figs. 4-4 and 4-5). If the placentas are fused, a ridge develops in the central fusion plane that allows easy distinction from the monochorionic placenta. With rare exceptions,[49,50] blood vessels never cross from one side to the other in dichorionic twin placentas, and when the dividing membranes (that portion separating the two sacs) are carefully dissected, four separate layers can be identified: one amnion on either side and two chorions in the middle. Between the two chorions, one finds degenerated trophoblast and atrophied villi, features that render the dividing membranes of a diamniotic dichorionic twin pair opaque. Differential expansion of the fetal sacs often causes the membranes of one placenta to push away those of the other (Fig. 4-6), a feature that must not be confused with monochorionic placentation. It is referred to as *irregular chorionic fusion*. Very few verified DZ twins with monochorionic placenta have occurred, even with occasional anastomoses and with consequent blood chimerism. They are so rare that perhaps most have not been reported because they are not ascertained.

Although 20% to 30% of MZ twins have a dichorionic placentation, most often the placentas of monozygotic twins are monochorionic.

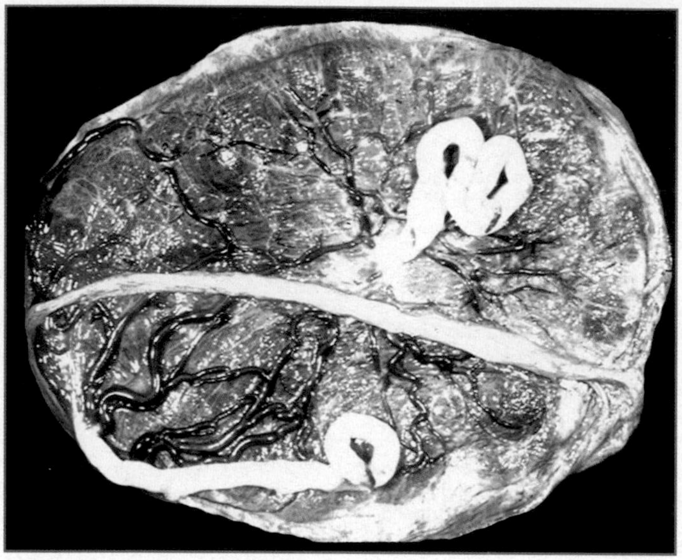

FIGURE 4-3 Diamniotic monochorionic twin placenta with numerous vascular anastomoses.

The latter type is invariably fused, and the dividing membranes consist of two translucent amnions only. When these amnions are separated from each other, the single chorion on the placental surface is evident. The chorion carries the fetal blood vessels and various types of interfetal vascular communications that occur regularly in monochorionic twins.

The two principal types of membrane relationships are shown in Figure 4-2. Monoamniotic twins are least common and carry a mortality rate of approximately 50% to 60% because of the frequent encircling of the cords, and knotting may lead to cessation of umbilical blood flow. Fetal demise usually occurs in the first part of pregnancy; after 32 weeks' gestation, no further mortality can be expected from entangling,[51,52] which can then be identified sonographically.[53] The chronic stasis induced by cord entanglement can lead to stillbirth and also to thrombosis with calcification of fetal vessels (Fig. 4-7). The possibility also exists that formerly diamniotic membranes become disrupted during gestation, with increased fetal mortality ensuing.[54] The perinatal mortality rate of diamniotic monochorionic twins is next highest (approximately 25%), because of the high frequency of the interfetal twin-to-twin-transfusion syndrome. The mortality rate is lowest for dichorionic twins (approximately 8.9%). This has been verified by a large study of twins in Belgium.[55]

The relationship of placentas among triplets, quadruplets, and higher-orders multiple births generally follows the same principles, except that monochorionic and dichorionic placentations may coexist (Fig. 4-8). With these higher numbers, there is more frequent association of placental anomalies, particularly marginal and velamentous insertions of the umbilical cord (see Figs. 4-8 and 4-9) and single umbilical artery (Fig. 4-9). The etiology of these anomalies may be related to the crowding of placentas and competition for space, or to primary disturbances of blastocyst nidation.

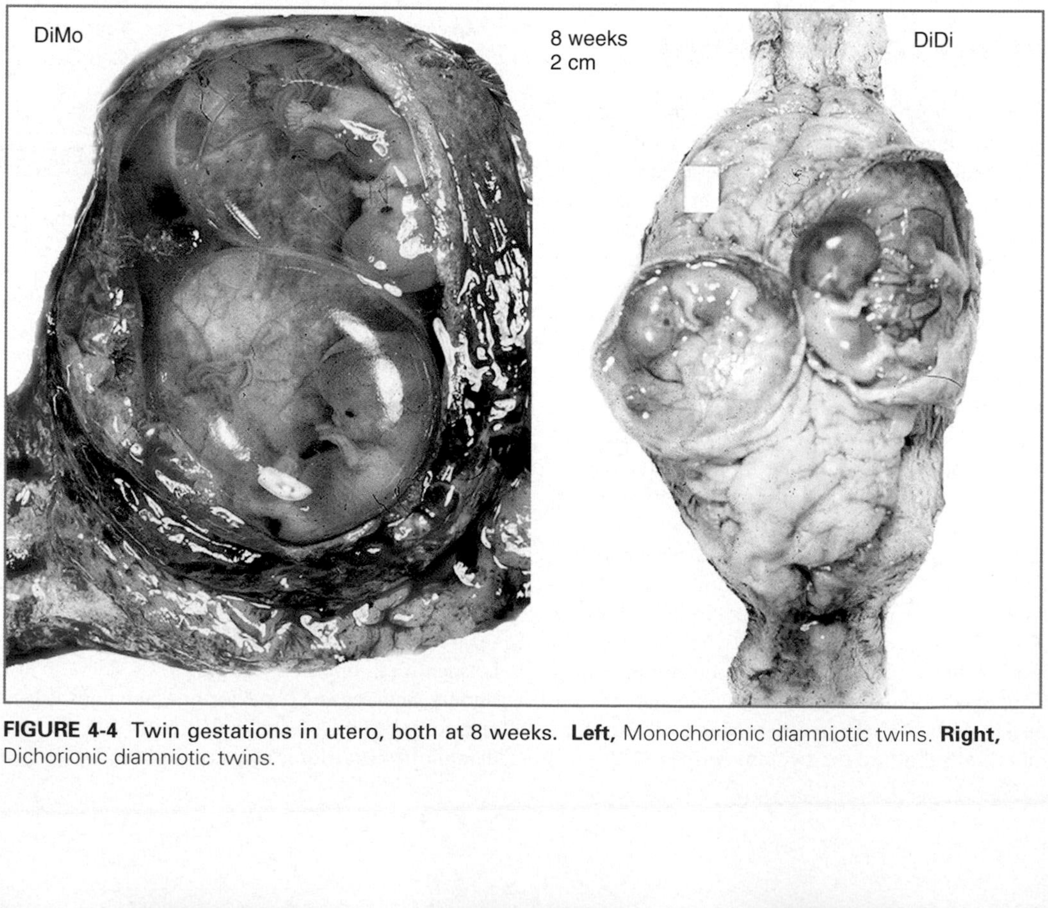

FIGURE 4-4 Twin gestations in utero, both at 8 weeks. **Left,** Monochorionic diamniotic twins. **Right,** Dichorionic diamniotic twins.

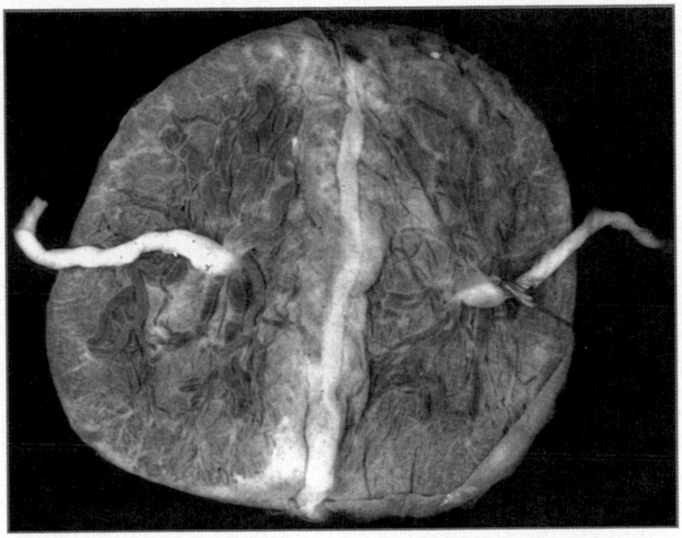

FIGURE 4-5 Diamniotic dichorionic twin placenta, fused. The umbilical cord on the left had a single umbilical artery. Note the close approximation of two placental disks with ridge formed by membranes in center.

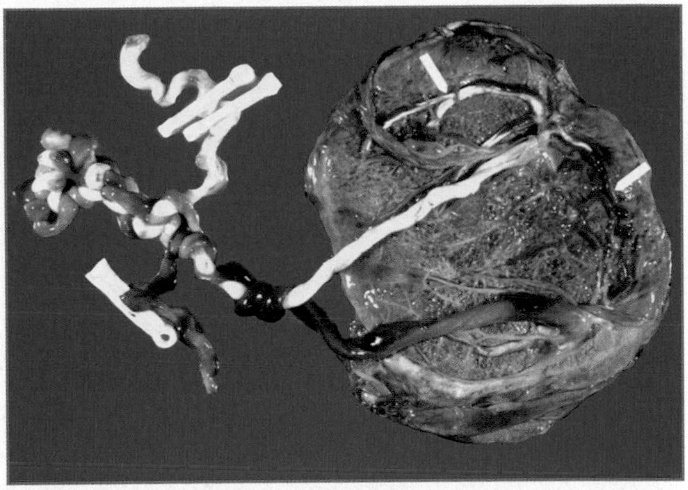

FIGURE 4-7 Monoamnionic twin placenta. There is marked encircling of the umbilical cords and fetal demise of dark cord's twin. The other twin died also and had massive CNS damage. Note the thrombosis of surface vessels and calcifications *(yellow)* of organized thrombi *(white arrows)*.

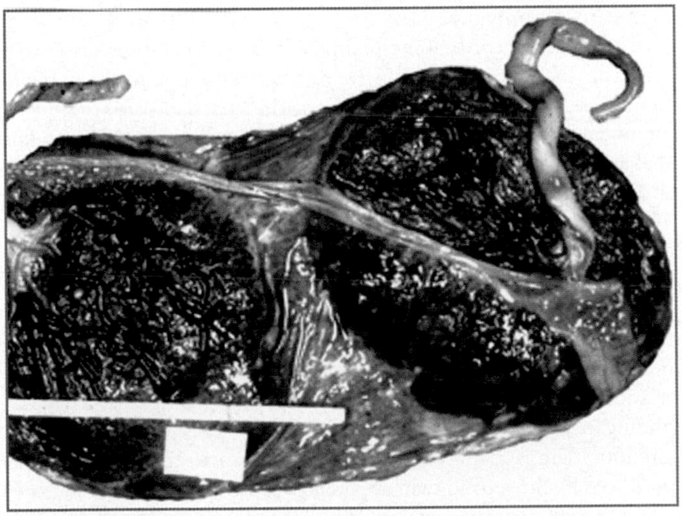

FIGURE 4-6 Diamniotic dichorionic (separate) twin placenta. The membranous sac of the left twin has pushed away the right membranes so that fusion of dividing membranes occurs over the right placenta ("irregular chorionic fusion").

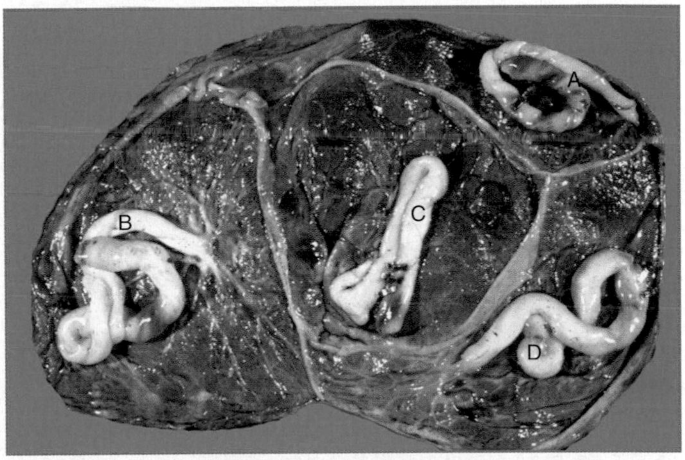

FIGURE 4-8 Placenta of quadruplets at 28.5 weeks. A, C, and D are female; B is male. Placenta is tetrachorionic and intimately fused. Birth order is indicated by letters. Cord A is marginally inserted. Despite intimate fusion, there are no anastomoses.

Velamentous Insertion of Umbilical Cord and Vasa Praevia

With the six- to nine-times-higher incidence of velamentous umbilical cord insertion in twin placentas and an even higher incidence in higher-order multiple births, the presence of vasa praevia in multiple pregnancy must be anticipated. It is a serious complication and often lethal because of exsanguination during delivery (see Fig. 4-10). Membranous vessels originating from a cord with velamentous insertion radiate toward the placental surface and are not protected by Wharton's jelly. Therefore, they may thrombose or may be compressed during labor. When the membranes are ruptured during delivery and these vessels accidentally have a transcervical position (vasa praevia), the rupture may lead to exsanguinating hemorrhage. Not only may the first twin exsanguinate but, as has been described, the second twin may exsanguinate through interfetal placental anastomoses if the placentation is monochorionic. Vasa praevia may exist not only over the cervical os but also over the dividing membrane when the second twin's cord has a velamentous insertion on the dividing membranes. Fetal hemorrhage leading to death within 3 minutes has been observed when the diamniotic dichorionic membranes of the second twin were ruptured.[56] In nine cases collected by Antoine and colleagues,[57] no first twin survived and 62.5% of the second twins eventually succumbed as the result of this hemorrhage. The clinical management of vasa praevia is discussed in detail in Chapter 37.

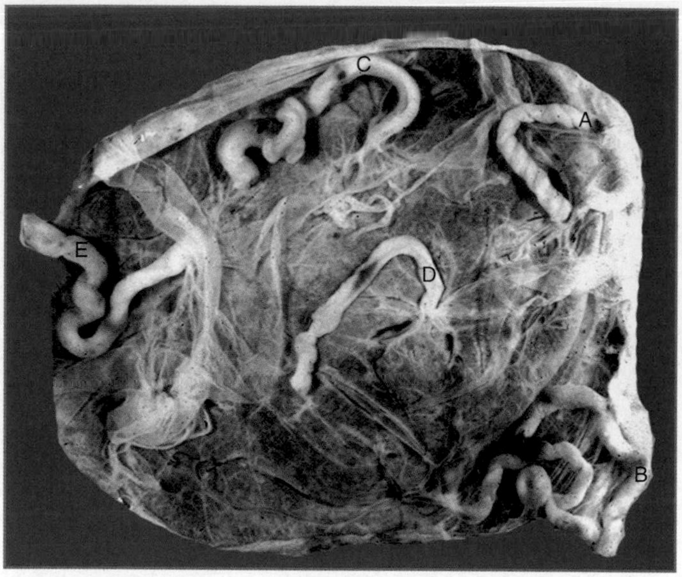

FIGURE 4-9 **Immature monochorionic quintuplet placenta.** All infants died from hyaline membrane disease and one had a single umbilical artery. There are numerous anastomoses. (From Benirschke K, Kaufmann P, Baergen RN: The Pathology of the Human Placenta. New York, Springer-Verlag, 2006.)

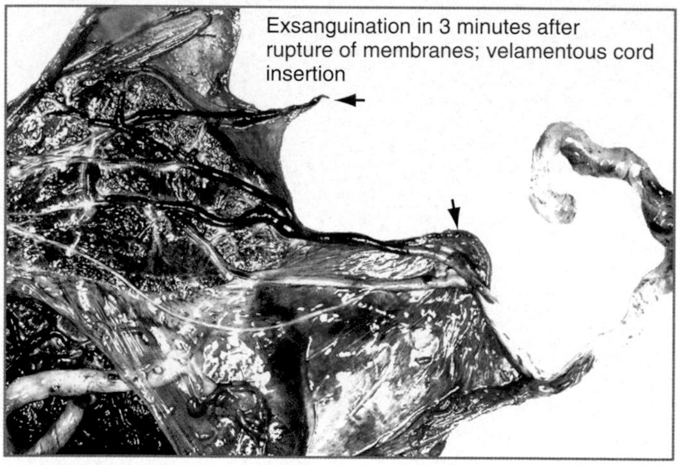

Exsanguination in 3 minutes after rupture of membranes; velamentous cord insertion

FIGURE 4-10 **Fatal vasa praevia in twin A of an intimately fused diamniotic dichorionic twin placenta.** The disrupted vessel is indicated by *arrows*. The mother was admitted 4 hours after rupture of membranes with no history of significant bleeding. Twin A had an Apgar score of 1 and could not be resuscitated. Twin B lived. The left half of the placenta had marked pallor (on maternal surface) because of fetal hemorrhage.

Monoamniotic Twins

Monoamniotic twins are all MZ, and all must also have a single chorion. Monoamniotic twins are the least common. Their occurrence is variably recorded as from 1 in 33 to 1 in 661 twin births. In the series reported by Benirschke and coworkers,[56] 3 of 250 pairs had this type of placenta, and three of the six fetuses died from various complications.

The most common complication is encircling and knotting of cords with cessation of umbilical blood flow (see Fig. 4-7). The extent of the knotting of cords is at times astonishing and testimony to the degree of fetal movements. In the past, double survival of monoamniotic twins was so uncommon that such cases were deemed worthy of report.[58] Preterm delivery, at 32 to 34 weeks' gestation, has led to increased survival of monoamniotic twins. Locking of the twins during delivery is rarely observed with monoamniotic twins, because almost all are delivered by cesarean section.

Most monochorionic twins have interfetal placental anastomoses, but such vessel communications are not invariably found. It was formerly believed that blood was exchanged between the twins through these anastomoses, and that if one twin succumbed before birth, thromboplastin, possibly originating in the macerating fetus, might lead to disseminated intravascular coagulation in the surviving twin. This phenomenon would be restricted to monochorionic placentation and was thought to occur in triplets as well. An alternative view for the demise of the second twin, and one that now has assumed greater likelihood, is that severe and acute hypotension develops through exsanguination into an already dead twin via large anastomoses,[58-60] very much like that which led to the demise of Eng when Chang of the notorious Siamese twins died.

Because of the high mortality rate, it is imperative to make an antepartum diagnosis. With such a diagnosis, a clear course of action awaited accumulation of adequate statistics that would delineate exactly when in the course of pregnancy one or both twins are likely to succumb from cord encircling. Rodis and colleagues[61] provided some of these data; they showed a 90% survival when adequate antenatal care was provided.

The umbilical cords of monoamniotic twins usually arise near each other on the placenta, and in rare circumstances they are partially fused. Less often, they are velamentous. The fusion of cords represents a gradual transition to the invariably monoamniotic conjoined twins that are thought to form only slightly later, at the end of the twinning spectrum shown in Figure 4-1. Conjoined twins may have two cords with three vessels each, forked cords, anomalous vessels, or, at the other end of the spectrum, one cord with only one artery and one vein. Congenital anomalies, although more common among twins in general, are particularly common in monoamniotic and conjoined twins. The more frequent occurrence of sirenomelia—100 to 150 times more common in twins than in singletons—has led to insights into the relationship of this anomaly with pulmonary hypoplasia, a regular finding in sirens because of a deficient urinary tract. When one monoamniotic twin is a siren and the other is normal, the amniotic fluid produced by the second twin apparently protects the siren from experiencing pulmonary hypoplasia. When the placenta is diamniotic, this protection does not occur.[62]

Diamniotic Monochorionic Twins

Diamniotic monochorionic twins are MZ, the placenta is fused, and the umbilical cords often have a marginal or velamentous insertion. The diagnosis is readily apparent from the absence of a ridge at the base of the dividing membranes (see Figs. 4-3 and 4-4) and the translucency of the dividing membranes. When the membranes are dissected, one amnion can be readily stripped from the other, leaving a single (placental) chorionic plate that carries the fetal blood vessels. The amnions do not necessarily meet at the vascular equator of the two placental beds but may shift irregularly from one side to the other, presumably because of fetal movements and the relative fluid contents of the two sacs. The diamniotic monochorionic placenta is the most common type seen in MZ twins; approximately 70% have this conformation (see Fig. 4-1), and a recent review details all its major complications.[63]

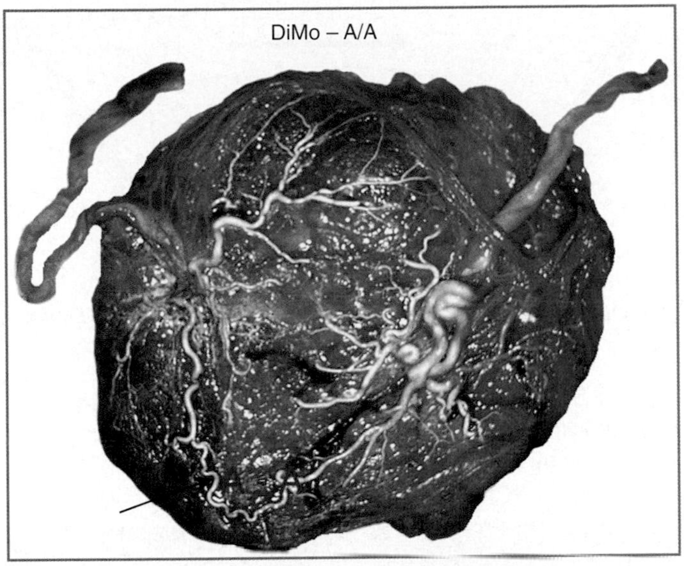

FIGURE 4-11 Diamniotic monochorionic (DiMo) twin placenta. One large direct A/A (artery-to-artery anastomosis) after injection with milk is shown.

The diamniotic monochorionic placenta and, less commonly, the monoamniotic twin placenta nearly always possess interfetal blood vessel communications (Fig. 4-11, and see Fig. 4-12). The anastomosis is more often an artery-to-artery (arterioarterial) (see Fig. 4-11) than a vein-to-vein communication, and sometimes both types are present and multiple. These vessels allow blood to shift readily from one side to the other, equalizing volumes and pressures. They are most readily demonstrated, after the amnion has been removed, by careful inspection, by stroking blood from one side to the other, or by injection. It is generally impractical to inject the entire placenta from the cord vessels, because rather large volumes are needed and the placental blood must not have been clotted. One can verify the existence of anastomoses more readily by first cutting off the cords and then injecting water or milk into those vessels that are thought to be anastomotic (see Fig. 4-12).

The large anastomoses have important practical clinical implications. Through these communications, the second twin may exsanguinate if vasa praevia of the first twin are ruptured or, of course, if the cord of the first twin is not clamped. In the rare event that the diagnosis of a twin gestation is not made until the time of delivery, the practice of permitting placental transfusion to occur, or removing umbilical cord blood, should be done only when it is confirmed that twins do not exist. Otherwise, the second twin may rapidly exsanguinate through these commonly large-caliber vessels (Fig. 4-13).

It must also be realized that the interfetal anastomoses of larger caliber may lead to significant shifts of blood between fetuses. This is particularly important when one fetus dies. The vascular bed of the dead twin relaxes, and a substantial amount of blood from the survivor may enter the dead twin, causing anemia in the survivor, possibly with destructive consequences. It now appears likely that the appreciable frequency of cerebral palsy of a surviving monochorionic twin results from acute hypotension after one twin dies, because of major blood shifts between the twins through placental anastomoses.[58,64] This feature is then grossly similar to the appearance of the twins shown in Figure 4-14, who died from the transfusion syndrome due to an arteriovenous anastomosis. One twin has much more blood than the other, and when this is the result of large blood vessel anastomoses rather than the arteriovenous shunt to be described next, such twins have been erroneously said to have the classic transfusion syndrome. Twins with such marked differences in blood content near term are never the result of the twin-to-twin transfusion syndrome (TTTS).

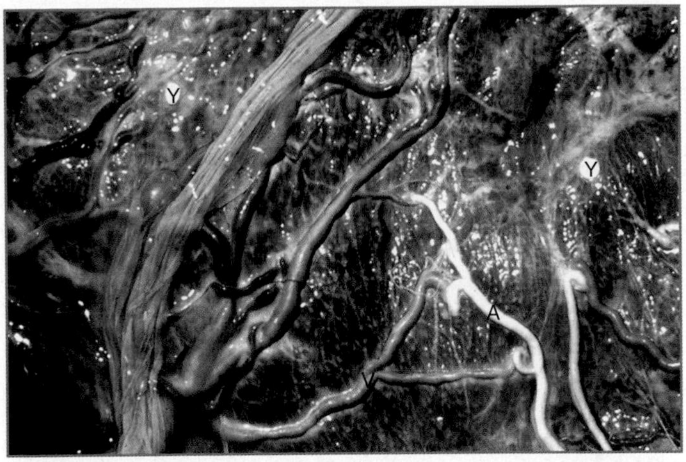

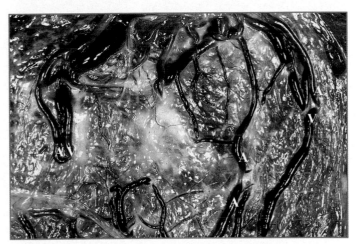

FIGURE 4-12 Placenta of twin-to-twin transfusion syndrome. Milk is being injected into the arteries of the donor twin. Several arteriovenous shared cotyledons can be seen. A, artery; V, vein; Y, remains of yolk sac.

FIGURE 4-13 Diamniotic monochorionic twin placenta showing a portion of the vascular equator. The amnions have been stripped off; only the chorionic surface is seen. Arteries lie on top of veins. Twin A *(top)* displays a normal cotyledonary supply at left, with an artery feeding the cotyledon and a vein returning it to the same fetus. Toward the right (*right* to the yellow patch of subchorionic fibrin) is an artery-to-artery (A/A) anastomosis. An arteriovenous shunt (A-V) is demonstrated at the right. These twins came to term because the A/A anastomosis immediately compensated for any irregularity of blood volume arising from the A-V shunt shown at the right.

The Twin-to-Twin Transfusion Syndrome

The most important anastomosis, the arteriovenous shunt, is also the most difficult to diagnose at inspection of the placenta after delivery. It is not a direct communication; instead, it occurs when one cotyledon

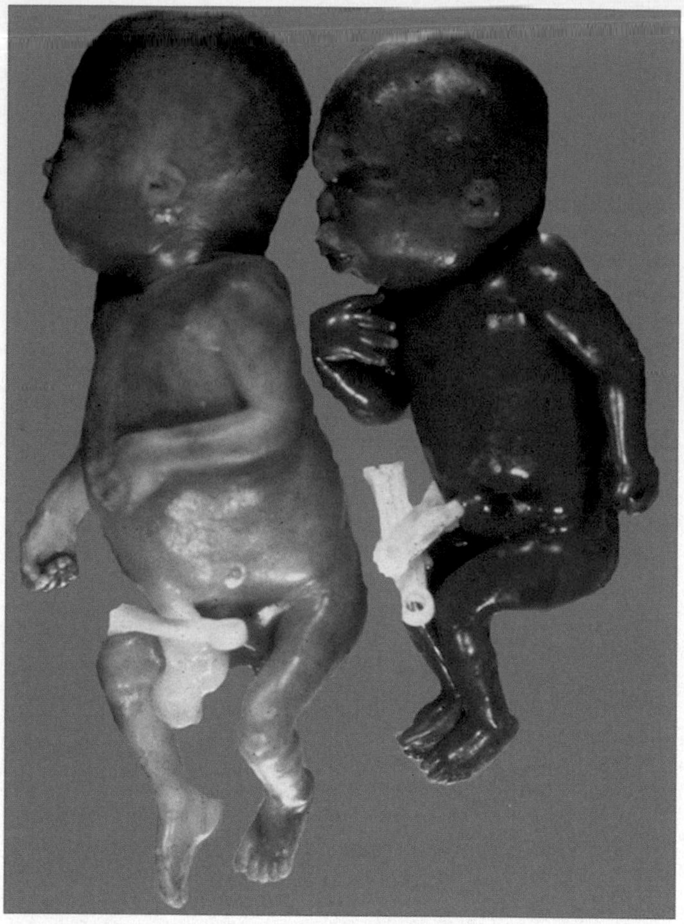

FIGURE 4-14 **Diamniotic monochorionic twins.** The plethoric twin *(right)* had died earlier and as a consequence, the larger fetus *(left)* bled back, through the shared vessels, into the now plethoric fetus. The smaller fetus had a velamentous cord insertion.

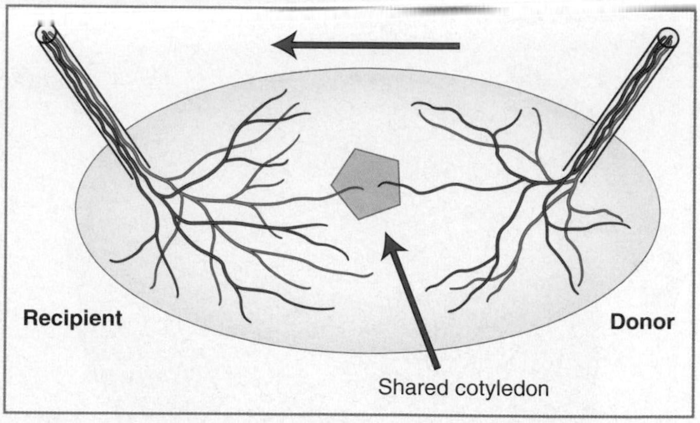

FIGURE 4-15 Diagram of the basis for the twin-to-twin transfusion syndrome.

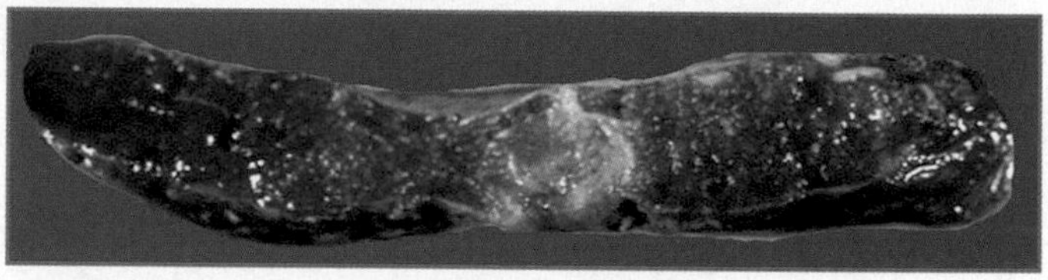

FIGURE 4-16 **Immature placenta.** In this cross section of an immature placenta, one cotyledon had been injected with water and, consequently, the villous tissue blanched. This "shared cotyledon" is the basis for the twin-to-twin transfusion syndrome.

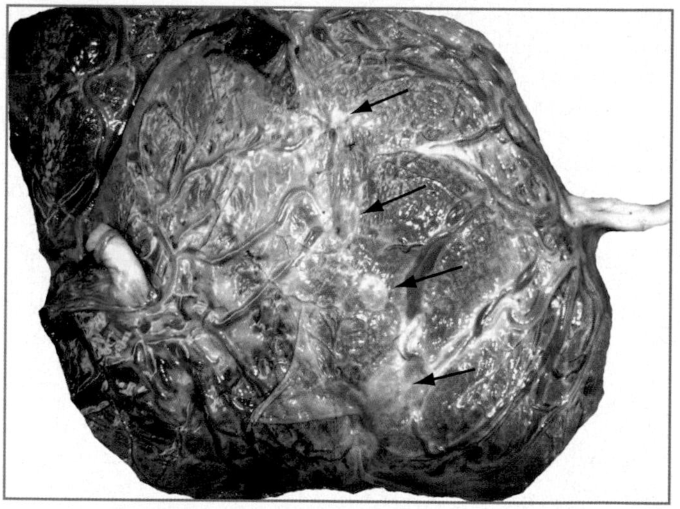

FIGURE 4-17 **Monochorionic twin placenta of a laser-treated, twin-to-twin transfusion syndrome pregnancy.** The laser-occluded districts are indicated by *arrows*. After laser therapy the pregnancy lasted another 2 months and the twins did well.

is fed by an artery from one twin and the blood is then drained by a vein into the other twin. The arteriovenous shunt is diagrammatically shown in Figure 4-15, and the common vascular relationships at a twin vascular equator are seen in Figure 4-13. To recognize such a shared cotyledon, one must follow all terminal arterial branches (arteries cross over veins) and ascertain whether a vein is returning to the same twin, as is normally the case (see Fig. 4-13, *left*) or whether the cotyledon is drained to the other twin (see Fig. 4-13, *right*). To verify the existence of a common or shared cotyledon, one may inject the artery with water; the shared cotyledon rises and blanches, and the water then drains from the vein of the other twin, thus blanching the common or shared cotyledon (Fig. 4-16). This arrangement has been referred to as the third circulation. It is incorrect, however, to assume that there are other "deep" anastomoses, as are often discussed. Villi are never connected only deep in the placenta, and they can exchange blood only through common shared cotyledons. The situation is different after laser surgery, as has recently been demonstrated (Fig. 4-17).[65]

Arteriovenous shunts may exist singly or may be multiple, and they may be in opposing directions. When they are not accompanied by artery-to-artery or vein-to-vein anastomoses, then one fetus continuously donates blood into the recipient (Figs. 4-18 through 4-20). This is the basis of the twin-to-twin transfusion syndrome, which leads to plethora and hypervolemia (hypertension) of the recipient and anemia (hypotension) of the donor. Cardiac compensation (hypertrophy in the recipient) ensues first and can be seen in abortuses afflicted by the TTTS; this is followed by a wide spectrum of bodily growth differences (Fig. 4-21, and see Fig. 4-18). A common symptom is rapid uterine expansion resulting from hydramnios of the recipient, presumed to be secondary to excessive fetal urination. The hydramnios usually manifests between 20 and 30 weeks of pregnancy, may reach enormous quantities, and is frequently the cause of preterm labor. The amniotic sac of the donor may be dry, and amnion nodosum may develop. The donor fetus is referred to as being "stuck." The severity and time of

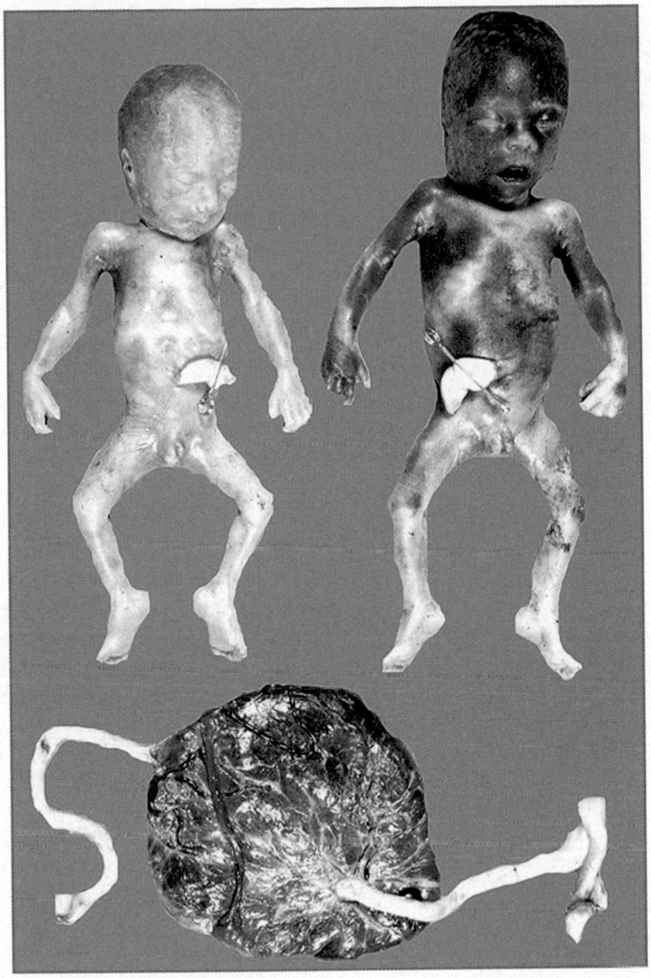

FIGURE 4-18 **Diamniotic monochorionic twin abortus resulting from twin-to-twin transfusion syndrome.** The recipient *(right)* is plethoric and larger, and the donor *(left)* is anemic and smaller. The monochorionic twin placenta is shown below, and its maternal side is seen in Figure 4-13.

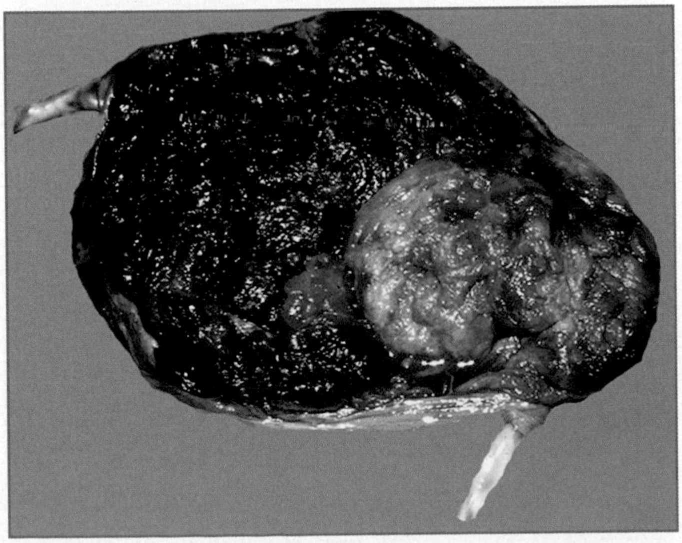

FIGURE 4-19 **Twin placenta of twins with twin-to-twin transfusion syndrome, maternal side.** This is the set of twins seen in Figure 4-18. Note the smaller quantity and anemia of the donor villous tissue.

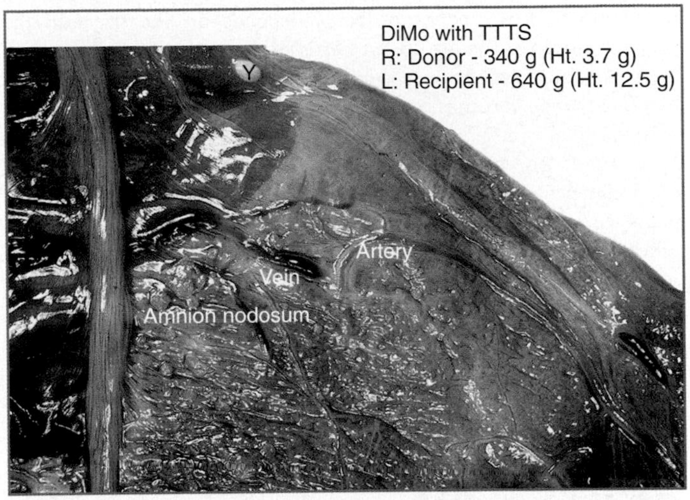

FIGURE 4-20 **Placenta of diamniotic monochorionic twins with twin-to-twin transfusion syndrome (TTTS).** A single arteriovenous anastomosis (A-V) with common district is present. The donor side had amnion nodosum; the diamnionic dividing membranes are seen at *left*. Y, remains of yolk sac.

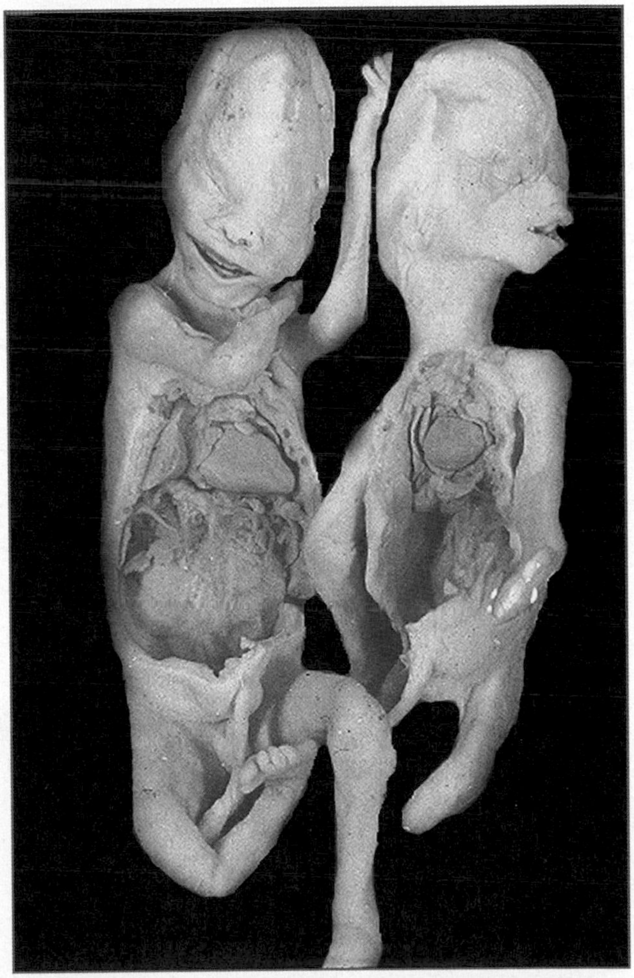

FIGURE 4-21 **Aborted monochorionic twins with twin-to-twin transfusion syndrome at 11 weeks' gestation.** The recipient *(left)* has a heart size of 440 mg; the donor's heart was 193 mg. Otherwise, the growth differential at this young gestational age is less significant (31 versus 20 g).

noted growth discrepancy probably depends on the size and the number as well as the direction of arteriovenous shunts. On occasion, the syndrome first becomes symptomatic when a formerly balanced blood exchange becomes unstable because of spontaneous thrombosis of a placental vein.[66]

At times, one twin dies in utero, the hydramnios disappears, and the pregnancy goes to term with one twin normal and the other a fetus papyraceus.[56] When the twins are born, usually prematurely, they may differ remarkably in size; indeed, they may be so discordant that they seem to be DZ twins. Catch-up growth occurs postnatally but often is incomplete, and the twins remain discordant even though they are MZ.

Clinical management of the various complications of twin gestation described here are outlined in detail in Chapter 25.

Abnormalities of Twin Gestation

Fetus Papyraceus

When one or more of the fetuses in a multiple gestation dies before birth and the pregnancy continues, the fluid of the dead twin's tissues is gradually absorbed, the amniotic fluid disappears, and the fetus is compressed and becomes incorporated into the membranes (Fig. 4-22). Hence, it is called a fetus compressus, fetus papyraceus, or membranous twin. The condition occurs in both DZ and MZ twins and is a regular finding when multiple gestations are surgically reduced. This has become much more common in recent years as many fetuses are conceived with ART.[67,68]

The existence of the fetus papyraceus has important practical and theoretical implications. First, a birth with such an association is not usually entered into statistics as a twin gestation; hence, the frequency of twinning is underestimated. Furthermore, the presence of a fetus papyraceus is often not recognized at birth. Figure 4-23 shows a twin placenta from what was thought to be an abruptio placentae of a singleton birth. One placenta was normal and the other was a shriveled, diminutive, and separate organ of a DZ fetus papyraceus. The small embryo presumably died early, but the preservation of the cord is remarkable. It is possible that this fetus papyraceus was a chromosomally abnormal conceptus that would ordinarily have been aborted had it not been for the normal twin. This would support one hypothesis for the rapid fall in the rate of twin gestations in women over age 35 years. Another less well understood hypothesis purports ovarian failure in older women to be the cause of the decline.[10] Such a fetus papyraceus in diamniotic monochorionic twins is also often overlooked. The example illustrated in Figure 4-23 was small and compressed. This fetus papyraceus is particularly interesting because it was associated with aplasia cutis of the surviving twin. The diffuse form of this unusual skin condition has always been associated with MZ twins, one a fetus papyraceus, in cases in which the placenta has been examined.[69] The inference is that diffuse patchy aplasia cutis (in contrast to that in the scalp midline) is the result of a prenatal insult associated with the death of one MZ twin.

Another insight into prenatal life afforded by the fetus papyraceus relates to the mechanism that leads to amnion nodosum. When one twin dies, so does the amnion of its sac. This occurs earliest on the diamniotic dividing membranes (Fig. 4-24). Because the amnion does not possess blood vessels, its growth and maintenance must be supported by nutrients and oxygen from adjacent tissues. The large area of dividing membranes, which are in contact only with amniotic fluid, must be maintained by this fluid. The amnion dies because of the disappearance of fluid or deficiency of its oxygen content. Amnion nodosum, or impaction of vernix, occurs secondarily after epithelial death.

Acardiac Twin

The most bizarre malformation recorded, acardiac twin, occurs only in one twin of a pair of MZ twins. The normal twin maintains the acardiac twin by perfusion through two anastomoses, one artery to artery and one vein to vein. The circulation of the acardiac twin is

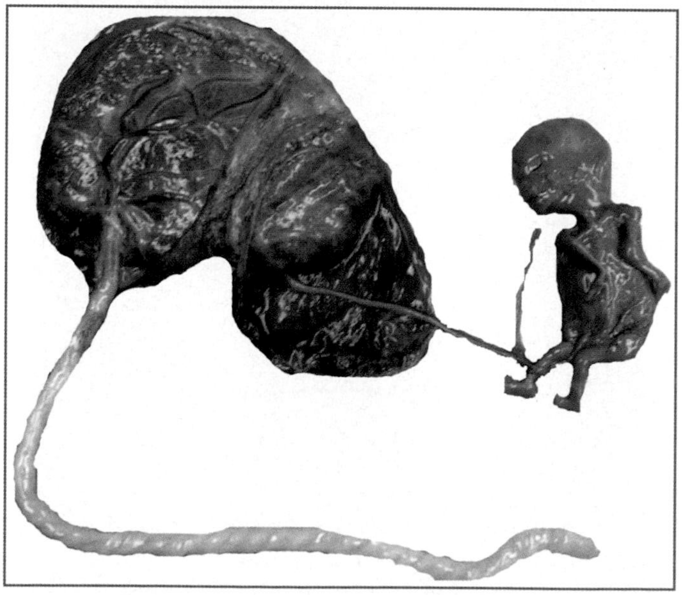

FIGURE 4-22 **Diamniotic dichorionic twin pregnancy with one fetus papyraceus.** This fetus had died because of cord entanglement around the leg.

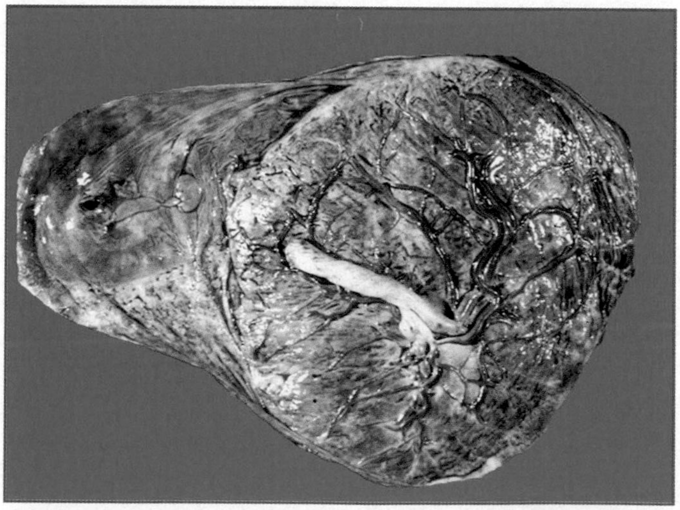

FIGURE 4-23 **Placenta of a 35-year-old woman thought to have abruptio placentae.** Diamniotic dichorionic separate twin placentas. Fetus papyraceus is attached to cord. Embryo was golden-yellow, about 1 cm. Surviving twin associated with this pregnancy had aplasia cutis.

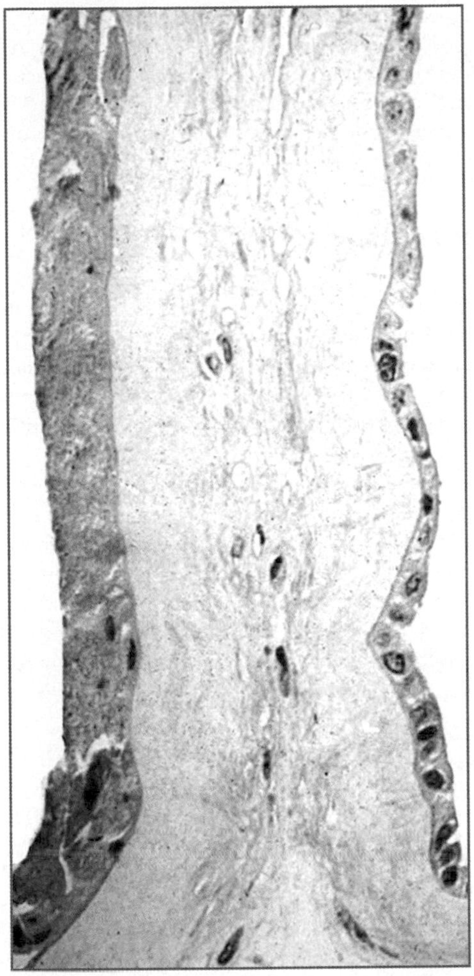

FIGURE 4-24 Cross section of diamnionic dividing membranes. The left twin had died and with it the entire amniotic epithelium.

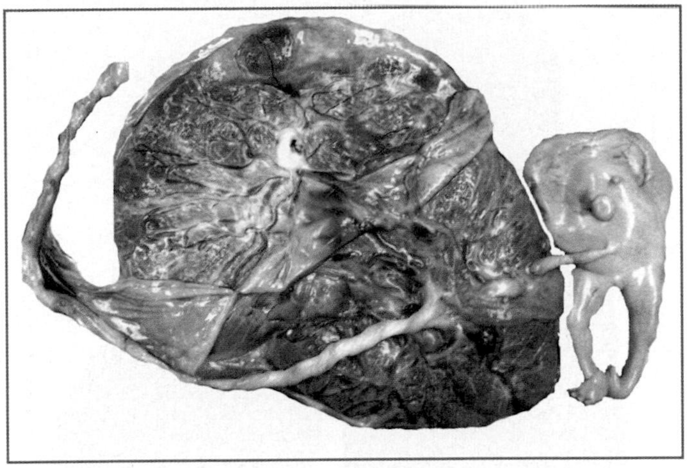

FIGURE 4-25 Triplet pregnancy with two survivors and one macerated acardiac fetus. This is a triamniotic dichorionic placenta, and the umbilical cord of the acardiac fetus had been interrupted by laser ablation 3 months earlier.

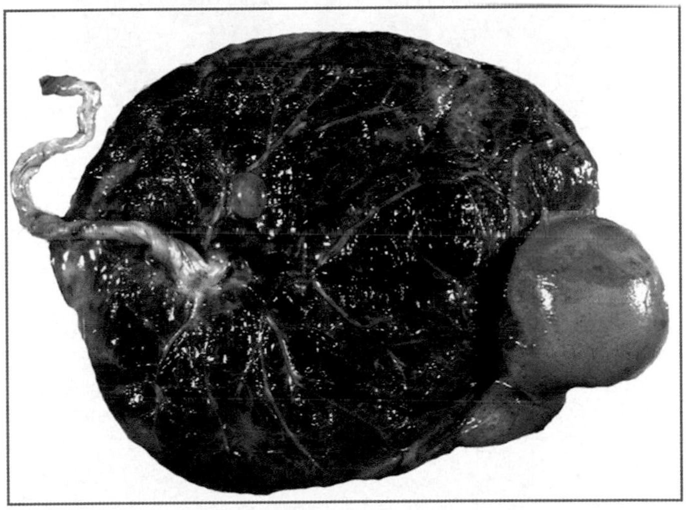

FIGURE 4-26 Diamniotic monochorionic term twin placenta. The (amorphus) acardiac twin is at right. It was a skin-covered ball of fat with few bones. The umbilical cord was very short. (Courtesy of the late N. Eastman, Johns Hopkins School of Medicine, Baltimore.)

therefore reversed, and most authors have assumed that this reversal of circulation may also be the cause of the malformation.[70] This concept is challenged by the occasional observation of an acardiac twin with different chromosomal constitution from that of the always diploid normal twin. Two trisomic acardiac fetuses and one triploid acardiac have been described, findings that suggest major errors in fertilization.[22,71] Genetic study in the case of Bieber and colleagues indicated the likelihood of origin by fertilization of a polar body for the triploid embryo. It is then remarkable that for every acardiac twin for which adequate placental examination has been made, a monochorionic (usually monoamniotic) placenta has been found, thought to be diagnostic of monozygosity.

Occasionally, an acardiac fetus is also a fetus papyraceus (Fig. 4-25), and only radiographs disclose its identity. Acardiac fetuses usually have no heart, as the name implies. Occasionally, however, a misshapen heart is found, commonly two chambered. The wide range of sizes and shapes among acardiac twins has led to a complex taxonomy. Most often, acardiac twins possess legs but lack arms and often have no head or have a head that is markedly abnormal. An acardiac fetus may look like an inside-out teratomatous mass (Fig. 4-26), although the fetus can be distinguished from a teratoma by the presence of an umbilical cord. The cord is almost invariably short, betraying the immobility of the acardiac fetus, and it usually possesses only one artery. Occasionally, however, acardiac fetuses have been witnessed to move, and then their cord may be quite long (Fig. 4-27).

Acardiac fetuses are often referred to as representing the twin reversed arterial perfusion syndrome; they can now be detected prenatally by the absence of cardiac activity and reversal of flow by Doppler sonography.[72] Because the normal twin perfuses this acardiac fetus in a reversed fashion, cardiac hypertrophy and failure may develop in the donor. Healey[73] identified a 35% mortality rate for the so-called pump twin, and prenatal removal, cord ligation, and other therapies have been advocated.

Other Anomalies

It has long been known that malformations occur more commonly in twins than in singletons; this increase results from the higher incidence of structural defects in MZ twins.[74] These anomalies may be concor-

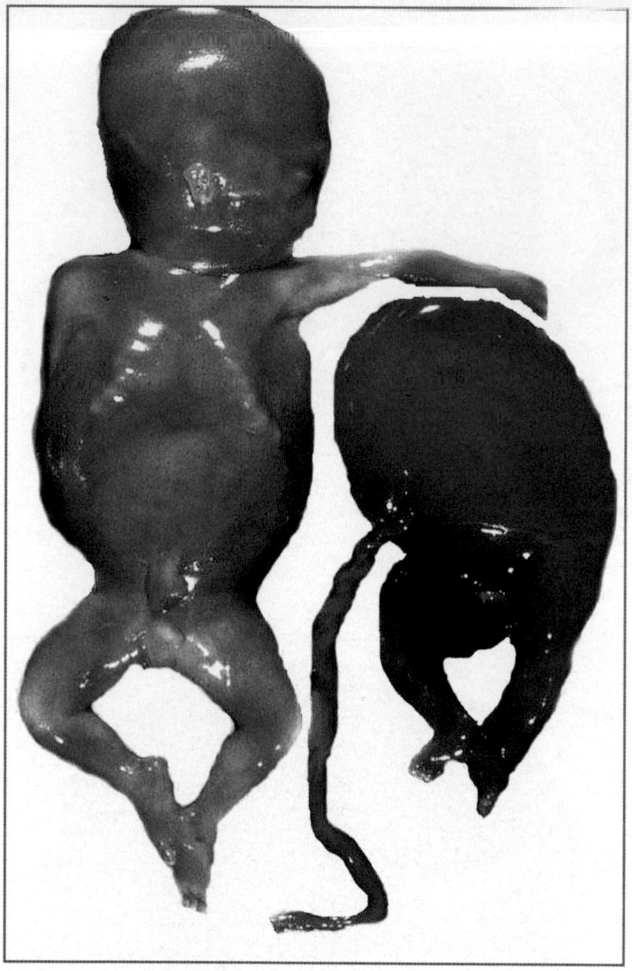

FIGURE 4-27 Monoamniotic twin pregnancy with plethoric acardiac fetus. The acardiac fetus has an unusually long umbilical cord. It had been seen to move sonographically; it had a spinal cord but no brain.

dant but more frequently are discordant, even in MZ twins. The reasons for the genesis of some anomalies are more readily comprehended than for others, such as the discordant development of conjoined twins and perhaps the acardiac anomaly and aplasia cutis that may be associated with sudden drops in blood pressure before birth. It is plausible that some other disruptions, such as porencephaly, occur as a result of interfetal vascular embolization or coagulation, and that other deformations are caused by crowding. In a large number of structural defects, however, the pathogenesis appears to be linked in some way to the twinning process itself. Thus, anencephaly and sirenomelia occur inexplicably commonly as discordant anomalies in MZ twins. These data suggest that further studies may provide significant insight into not only the poorly understood twinning process itself but also the pathogenesis of many congenital anomalies.[75]

Perhaps the most perplexing discordance occurs in the so-called heterokaryotic MZ twins (i.e., MZ twins with different karyotypes and phenotypes). On first impression, the idea of MZ twins with different karyotypes appears to be contradictory. If chromosomal nondisjunction of cells occurs just before or at the time of twinning, however, the process that causes mosaicism in a singleton may lead to MZ twins with different chromosome sets. Most often this has been described for the sex chromosomes, and XO/XXX, XO/XX, and even XO/XY twins have been reported with appropriate divergence of phenotypes. Sixteen such cases of divergence in gonadal dysgenesis were described by Pedersen and colleagues,[76] to which cases of discordance for trisomy 21 and some cases of acardiac twins must be added. These are the exceptional events, but they indicate the complexities of the twinning process.

"Disappearance" of a Twin

A word may be said about the apparent frequency of twins detected in early pregnancy by ultrasonography and their "disappearance" in later development. Figure 4-23 clearly indicates that even early embryonic death can be recognized in term placentas. A relevant inquiry resulted in the following findings—spontaneous reduction in twin pregnancies observed sonographically occurred in 36%, of triplets in 53%, and of quadruplets in 65%.[77]

Another reason for a vanishing twin, of course, is the selective fetal reduction of multifetal pregnancies. These multiple pregnancies are often hormonally induced, and selective reduction from triplets to twins improves the outcome of pregnancy.[78] The "reduced" twin may be detected in the placental membranes, but more often it is represented merely by a small amount of necrotic tissue. The many complications of selective reduction have been summarized by Berkovitz and associates.[79]

Chimeras

On rare occasions, blood grouping or lymphocyte karyotype examination of fraternal twins has shown the coexistence of two genetically dissimilar cell types. This state is referred to as blood chimerism because the solid tissues may not participate in the admixture of genotypes. Blood chimerism is best explained by the existence of transplacental anastomoses in fraternal twins that allowed migration of the bone marrow–like blood cell precursors, circulating in one embryo, to settle in the other twin. Because blood chimerism happens so early in embryonic life, this graft is tolerated as "self" and survives permanently without any ill effect. Although blood chimerism occurs with regularity in marmosets and frequently in twin cattle, where it may cause freemartinism, it must be very uncommon in humans, in whom such anastomoses between the presumably dichorionic twins have been identified only rarely.

Identification of Twin Zygosity

The zygosity of twins is of interest to the twins, their parents, physicians who may treat the children in the future, and to scientists. An attempt should be made to establish the zygosity at birth and to register the objective findings in the chart. Performing this task at the birth is particularly appropriate because of the availability of the placenta, examination of which can aid materially in the process. A good example for this need was provided by St. Clair and colleagues,[80] who treated presumed DZ twins for renal transplantation. DNA tests established "identity" only 15 years later when the transplant had been successful; immunosuppressive therapy was discontinued only then.

The most efficient way to identify zygosity is as follows: Gender examination allows the classification of male-female pairs as fraternal or DZ. The twins should also have a dichorionic placenta that may be separated or fused. Next, the placenta is studied in detail, and twins

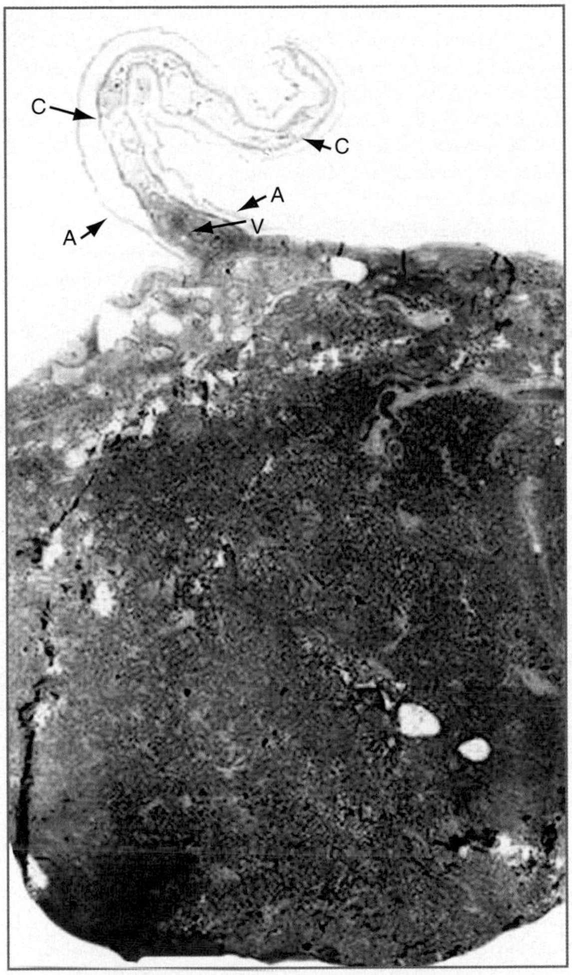

FIGURE 4-28 Fused twin placenta. Transverse-section at point of dividing membranes in diamniotic (A) dichorionic (C) fused twin placenta showing degenerated villi (V) and trophoblast *(dark area)* between the membranes. Inflammation of the chorial vessel is present *(left)*.

with a monochorionic placenta (monoamniotic or diamniotic) can be set aside as being of MZ ("identical") origin, whether or not they have dissimilar phenotypes. If doubt exists on gross examination of the dividing membranes, a transverse section (see Figs. 4-2 and 4-28) should be studied histologically. There then remain the like-sex twins with dichorionic placental membranes whose zygosity cannot instantly be known. They must be studied genetically, and the study of DNA polymorphism is currently the best way to approach these difficult problems.[38-40] Cameron[81] examined sex, placentas, and genotypes of 668 consecutive twin pairs in Birmingham, England, and found the following distribution:

- 35% DZ, because they were male and female
- 20% MZ, because they were monochorionic (and had the same sex)
- 45% of the same sex but with dichorionic membranes; when these last were genotyped, 36% were DZ because of genetic differences
- 8% MZ, because of genetic identity

References

1. Hansen M, Kurinczuk JJ, Bower C, Webb S: The risk of major birth defects after intracytoplasmic sperm injection and in vitro fertilization. N Engl J Med 346:725, 2002.
2. Martin JA, Hamilton BE, Sutton PD, et al: Births: final data for 2002. Natl Vital Stat Rep 52:1, 2003.
3. Gleicher N, Oleske DM, Tur-Kaspa I, et al: Reducing the risk of high order multiple pregnancy after ovarian stimulation with gonadotropins. N Engl J Med 343:57, 2000.
4. Templeton A: The multiple gestation epidemic: The role of the assisted reproductive technologies. Am J Obstet Gynecol 190:894, 2004.
5. Wilson EE: Assisted reproductive technologies and multiple gestations. Clin Perinatol 32:315, 2005.
6. Nunley WC Jr: The slippery slopes of advanced reproductive technologies. Presidential address. Am J Obstet Gynecol 191:588, 2004.
7. Thurin A, Hausken J, Hillensjö T, et al: Elective single-embryo transfer versus double-embryo transfer in in vitro fertilization. N Engl J Med 351:2392, 2004.
8. Daniel Y, Schreiber L, Geva E, et al: Morphologic and histopathologic characteristics of placentas from twin pregnancies spontaneously conceived and from reduced and nonreduced assisted reproductive technologies. J Reprod Med 46:735, 2001.
9. Guttmacher AF: The incidence of multiple births in man and some other uniparae. Obstet Gynecol 2:22, 1953.
10. Bulmer MG: The Biology of Twinning in Man. Oxford, Clarendon Press, 1970.
11. Murphy M, Hey K: Twinning rates. Lancet 349:1349, 1997.
12. Benirschke K, Kim CK: Multiple pregnancy. N Engl J Med 288:1276, 1973.
13. Luke B: The changing pattern of multiple births in the United States: Maternal and infant characteristics, 1973-1990. Obstet Gynecol 84:101, 1994.
14. Tong S, Caddy D, Short RV: Use of dizygotic to monozygotic twinning ratio as a measure of fertility. Lancet 349:843, 1997.
15. Boklage CE: The biology of human twinning: A needed change of perspective. In Blickstein I, Keith LG (eds): Multiple Pregnancy, 2nd ed. London, Taylor and Francis, 2005 (chapter 36).
16. James WH: Dizygotic twinning, marital stage and status and coital rates. Ann Hum Biol 8:371, 1981.
17. Sills ES, Tucker MJ, Palermo GD: Assisted reproductive technologies and monozygous twins: Implications for future study and clinical practice. Twin Res 3:217, 2000.
18. Platt MJ, Marshall A, Pharoah POD: The effects of assisted reproduction on the trends and zygosity of multiple births in England and Wales 1974-1999. Twin Res 4:417, 2001.
19. Schachter M, Raziel A, Friedler S, et al: Monozygotic twinning after assisted reproductive techniques: A phenomenon independent of micromanipulation. Hum Reprod 16:1264, 2001.
20. Alikani M, Cekleniak NA, Walters E, Cohen J: Monozygotic twinning following assisted conception: An analysis of 81 consecutive cases. Hum Reprod 18:1937, 2003.
21. Milki AA, Jun SH, Hinckley MD, et al: Incidence of monozygotic twinning with blastocyst transfer compared to cleavage-stage transfer. Fertil Steril 79:503, 2003.
22. Bieber FR, Nance WE, Morton CC, et al: Genetic studies of an acardiac monster: Evidence of polar body twinning in man. Science 213:775, 1981.
23. Goldgar DE, Kimberling WJ: Genetic expectations of polar body twinning. Acta Genet Med Gemellol (Roma) 30:257, 1981.
24. Harris DW: Letter to the editor. J Reprod Med 27:39, 1982.
25. Meyer WR, Meyer WW: Report on a very young dizygotic human twin pregnancy. Arch Gynecol 231:51, 1981.
26. Schenker JG, Yarkoni S, Granat M: Multiple pregnancies following induction of ovulation. Fertil Steril 35:105, 1981.
27. Martin NG, Shanley S, Butt K, et al: Excessive follicular recruitment and growth in mothers of spontaneous dizygotic twins. Acta Genet Med Gemellol (Roma) 40:291, 1991.

28. Nylander PPS: The factors that influence twinning rates. Acta Genet Med Gemellol (Roma) 30:189, 1981.
29. Soma H, Takayama M, Kiyokawa T, et al: Serum gonadotropin levels in Japanese women. Obstet Gynecol 46:311, 1975.
30. Busjahn A, Knoblauch H, Faulhaber H-D, et al: A region on chromosome 3 is linked to dizygotic twinning. Nat Genet 4:398, 2000.
31. Healey SC, Duffy DL, Martin NG, et al: Is fragile X syndrome a risk factor for dizygotic twinning? Am J Med Genet 72:245, 1997.
32. Galloway SM, McNatty KP, Cambridge LM, et al: Mutations in an oocyte-derived growth factor gene (BMP15) cause increased ovulation rate and infertility in a dosage-sensitive manner. Nat Genet 25:279, 2000.
33. Khamsi F, Roberge S, Yavas Y, et al: Recent discoveries in physiology of insulin-like growth factor-1 and its interaction with gonadotropins in folliculogenesis. Endocrine 16:151-165, 2001.
34. Derom C, Vlietinck R, Derom R, et al: Increased monozygotic twinning rate after ovulation induction. Lancet 1:1236, 1987.
35. Boklage CE: On the distribution of nonrighthandedness among twins and their families. Acta Genet Med Gemellol (Roma) 30:775, 1981.
36. McCracken AA, Daly PA, Zolnick MR, et al: Twins and Q-banded chromosome polymorphisms. Hum Genet 45:253, 1978.
37. Morton CC, Covey LA, Nance WE, et al: Quinacrine mustard and nucleolar organizer region heteromorphisms in twins. Acta Genet Med Gemellol (Roma) 30:39, 1981.
38. Derom C, Bakker E, Vlietinck R, et al: Zygosity determination in newborn twins using DNA variants. J Med Genet 22:279, 1985.
39. Hill AVS, Jeffreys AJ: Use of minisatellite DNA probes for determination of twin zygosity at birth. Lancet 2:1394, 1985.
40. Becker A, Busjahn A, Faulhaber HD, et al: Twin zygosity diagnosis: Automated determination with microsatellites. J Reprod Med 42:260, 1997.
41. Kaufman MH, O'Shea KS: Induction of monozygotic twinning in the mouse. Nature 276:707, 1978.
42. Steinman G, Valderrama E: Mechanisms of twinning: III. Placentation, calcium reduction and modified compaction. J Reprod Med 46:995, 2001.
43. Steinman G: Mechanisms of twinning: V. Conjoined twins, stem cells and the calcium model. J Reprod Med 47:313, 2002.
44. Winn HN, Gabrielli S, Reece EA, et al: Ultrasonographic criteria for the prenatal diagnosis of placental chorionicity in twin gestations. Am J Obstet Gynecol 161:1540, 1989.
45. Stagiannis KD, Sepulveda W, Southwell D, et al: Ultrasonographic measurement of the dividing membrane in twin pregnancy during the second and third trimesters: A reproducibility study. Am J Obstet Gynecol 173:1546, 1995.
46. Vayssiere CF, Heim N, Camus EP, et al: Determination of chorionicity in twin gestations by high-frequency abdominal ultrasonography: Counting the layers of the dividing membrane. Am J Obstet Gynecol 175:1529, 1996.
47. Nylander PPS, Osunloya BO: Unusual monochorionic placentation with heterosexual twins. Obstet Gynecol 36:621, 1970.
48. Souter VL, Kapur RP, Nyholt DR, et al: A report of dizygous monochorionic twins. N Engl J Med 349:154, 2003.
49. King AD, Soothill PW, Montemagno R, et al: Twin-to-twin blood transfusion in a dichorionic pregnancy without the oligohydramnious-polyhydramnious sequence. BJOG 102:334, 1995.
50. Molnar-Nadasdy G, Altshuler G: Perinatal pathology casebook. J Perinatol 16:507, 1996.
51. Carr SR, Aronson MP, Coustan DR: Survival rates of monoamniotic twins do not decrease after 30 weeks' gestation. Am J Obstet Gynecol 163:719, 1990.
52. Tessen JA, Zlatnik FJ: Monoamniotic twins: A retrospective controlled study. Obstet Gynecol 77:832, 1991.
53. Shahabi S, Donner C, Wallond J, et al: Monoamniotic twin cord entanglement: A case report with color flow Doppler ultrasonography for antenatal diagnosis. J Reprod Med 42:740, 1997.
54. Gilbert WM, Davis SE, Kaplan C, et al: Morbidity associated with prenatal disruption of the dividing membrane in twin gestations. Obstet Gynecol 78:623, 1991.
55. Loos R, Derom C, Vlietinck R, et al: The East Flanders prospective twin survey (Belgium): A population-based register. Twin Res 1:167, 1998.
56. Benirschke K, Kaufmann P, Baergen RN: The Pathology of the Human Placenta. New York, Springer-Verlag, 2006.
57. Antoine C, Young BK, Silverman F, et al: Sinusoidal fetal heart rate pattern with vasa previa in twin pregnancy. Obstet Gynecol 27:295-300, 1982.
58. Colburn DW, Pasquale SA: Monoamniotic twin pregnancy. J Reprod Med 27:165, 1982.
58. Yoshioka H, Kadomoto Y, Mino M, et al: Multicystic encephalomalacia in liveborn twin with a stillborn macerated co-twin. J Pediatr 95:798, 1979.
59. Yoshida K, Soma H: Outcome of the surviving cotwin of a fetus papyraceus or a dead fetus. Acta Genet Med Gemellol (Roma) 35:91, 1986.
60. Benirschke K: Intrauterine death of a twin: Mechanisms, implications for surviving twin, and placental pathology. Semin Diagn Pathol 10:222, 1993.
61. Rodis JF, McIlveen P, Egan JFX, et al: Monoamniotic twins: Improved perinatal survival with accurate prenatal diagnosis and antenatal fetal surveillance. Am J Obstet Gynecol 177:1046, 1997.
62. Wright JCY, Christopher CR: Sirenomelia, Potter's syndrome and their relationship to monozygotic twinning: A case report and discussion. J Reprod Med 27:291, 1982.
63. Trevett T, Johnson A: Monochorionic twin pregnancies. Clin Perinatol 32:475, 2005.
64. Liu S, Benirschke K, Scioscia AL, et al: Intrauterine death in multiple gestation. Acta Genet Med Gemellol (Roma) 41:5, 1992.
65. van den Wijngaard JP, Lopriore E, van der Salm SM, et al: Deep-hidden anastomoses in monochorionic twin placentae are harmless. Prenat Diagn 27:233-239, 2006.
66. Nikkels PJ, van Gemert MJC, Sollie-Szarynska KM, et al: Rapid onset of severe twin-twin transfusion syndrome caused by placental venous thrombosis. Pediatr Devel Pathol 5:310, 2002.
67. Stone J, Eddleman K, Lynch L, Berkowitz RL: A single center experience with 1000 consecutive cases of multifetal pregnancy reduction. Am J Obstet Gynecol 187:1163, 2002.
68. LaSala GB, Nucera G, Gallinelli A, et al: Spontaneous embryonic loss following in vitro fertilization: Incidence and effect on outcomes. Am J Obstet Gynecol 191:741, 2004.
69. Mannino FL, Jones KL, Benirschke K: Congenital skin defects and fetus papyraceus. J Pediatr 91:559, 1977.
70. Benirschke K, Harper V: The acardiac anomaly. Teratology 15:311, 1977.
71. Moore TR, Gale S, Benirschke K: Perinatal outcome of forty-nine pregnancies complicated by acardiac twinning. Am J Obstet Gynecol 163:907, 1990.
72. Zucchini S, Borghesani F, Soffriti G, et al: Transvaginal ultrasound diagnosis of twin reversed arterial perfusion syndrome at 9 weeks' gestation. Ultrasound Obstet Gynecol 3:209, 1993.
73. Healey MG: Acardia: Predictive risk factors for the co-twin survival. Teratology 50:205, 1994.
74. Schinzel AA, Smith DW, Miller JR: Monozygotic twinning and structural defects. J Pediatr 95:921-930, 1979.
75. Benirschke K, Masliah E: The placenta in multiple pregnancy: Outstanding issues. Reprod Fertil Dev 13:6, 2001.
76. Pedersen IK, Philip J, Sele V, et al: Monozygotic twins with dissimilar phenotypes and chromosome complements. Acta Obstet Gynecol Scand 59:459, 1980.
77. Dickey R, Taylor SN, Lu PY, et al: Spontaneous reduction of multiple pregnancy: Incidence and effect on outcome. Am J Obstet Gynecol 186:77, 2002.
78. Smith-Levitin M, Kowalik A, Birnholz J, et al: Selective reduction of multifetal pregnancies to twins improves outcome over nonreduced triplet gestations. Am J Obstet Gynecol 175:878, 1996.
79. Berkowitz RL, Lynch L, Stone J, et al: The current status of multifetal pregnancy reduction. Am J Obstet Gynecol 174:1265, 1996.
80. St. Clair DM, St. Clair JB, Swainson CP, et al: Twin zygosity testing for medical purposes. Am J Med Genet 77:412, 1998.
81. Cameron AH: The Birmingham twin survey. Proc Soc Med 61:229, 1968.

Chapter 5

Biology of Parturition

Errol R. Norwitz, MD, PhD, and Stephen J. Lye, PhD

Labor is the physiologic process by which the products of conception are passed from the uterus to the outside world, and it is common to all viviparous species. The timely onset of labor and birth is an important determinant of perinatal outcome. Considerable evidence suggests that the fetus is in control of the timing of labor, although maternal factors are also involved. Our progress in understanding of the molecular and cellular mechanisms responsible for the onset of labor is slow primarily because of the lack of an adequate animal model and because of the autocrine and paracrine nature of the parturition cascade in humans, which precludes direct investigation. This chapter summarizes the current state of knowledge on the biologic mechanisms responsible for the onset of labor at term in the human.

Morphologic Changes in the Reproductive Tract during Pregnancy

Pregnancy is associated with gestational age–dependent morphologic changes in all tissues of the reproductive tract. The most important changes occur in the uterus and cervix.

The Uterus

The uterus undergoes a dramatic increase in weight (from 4 to 70 g in the nonpregnant state to 1100 to 1200 g at term) and volume (from 10 mL to 5 L) during pregnancy. The number of myometrial cells increases in early pregnancy (referred to as myometrial hyperplasia), but thereafter it remains stable. Myometrial growth in the latter half of pregnancy results primarily from the increase in cell size (hypertrophy) that occurs under the influence of the sex steroids, especially estrogen.[1] This is accompanied by an increase in fibrous and connective tissue as well as blood vessels and lymphatics. In the latter half of pregnancy, distention leads to gradual thinning of the uterine wall. However, this thinning is not uniform throughout the uterus. For example, the lower portion of the uterus (the isthmus) does not undergo hypertrophy and becomes increasingly thin and distensible as pregnancy progresses, thereby forming the lower uterine segment.[2]

The increase in size of the uterus is accompanied by a 10-fold increase in uterine blood flow—from 2% of cardiac output in the nonpregnant state to 17% at term.[3,4] Moreover, pregnancy is associated with a redistribution of blood flow within the uterus. In the nonpregnant state, uterine blood flow is equally divided between myometrium and endometrium. As pregnancy progresses, 80% to 90% of uterine blood flow goes to the placenta, with the remainder distributed equally between the endometrium and myometrium.[5] Although the cellular mechanisms responsible for the increase in uteroplacental blood flow in pregnancy are not fully understood, the increase in flow parallels the increase in placental size and decrease in placental vascular resistance, most likely related to the sensitivity of the uterine vasculature to circulating levels of estrogen.[6] However, a number of other biologically active hormones may be involved at the level of the uterine arteries, including vascular endothelial growth factor,[7] angiotensin II,[8,9] nitric oxide,[9-11] and prostacyclin (also known as prostaglandin I_2 [PGI_2]).[11,12]

The Cervix

In contrast to the uterus, which is made up primarily of smooth muscle cells, the cervix is composed of fibrous connective tissue containing an extracellular matrix (collagen, elastin, and proteoglycans) and a number of different cell types (smooth muscle cells, fibroblasts, blood vessels, and epithelial cells). The cervix undergoes extensive remodeling during pregnancy. The amount of collagen decreases progressively, and the collagen fibrils become increasingly dispersed and disorganized, probably because of an increase in the amount of decorin, a low-molecular-weight dermatan sulfate proteoglycan, which coats and separates collagen fibrils.[13] Ongoing pregnancy is associated with enzymatic degradation of the cervical extracellular matrix caused by the increased activity of matrix metalloproteinases and elastases. Finally, the hormonal influence of estrogen, progesterone, and relaxin may result in increased collagenase activity as well as increased glycosaminoglycan content of the cervix.[14-16]

For several weeks before delivery, the connective tissues of the cervix undergo biochemical modifications in preparation for labor that result in changes to its elasticity and tensile strength. These include alterations in water, collagen, elastin, and proteoglycan composition. Advancing gestational age is associated with an increase in hyaluronic acid content within the cervix, which leads to increased water content and loosening and dispersal of collagen fibers.[16,17] These changes are mediated through the coordinated effort of a number of mechanical factors (such as cervical stretch and pressure of the fetal presenting part) and hormones, including oxytocin, relaxin, nitric oxide, and prostaglandins.[16] Thus, the factors responsible for cervical effacement (softening and shortening) and dilation during labor are most likely a combination of biochemical changes, the mechanical forces of traction caused by myometrial contractions, and pressure resulting from descent of the fetal head.[16]

Diagnosis of Labor

Labor is a clinical diagnosis. It is characterized clinically by regular, painful uterine contractions increasing in frequency and intensity and associated with progressive cervical effacement and dilation, leading, ultimately, to expulsion of the products of conception. In normal labor, there appears to be a time-dependent relationship between these factors. Biochemical connective tissue changes in the cervix usually precede uterine contractions and cervical dilation, which, in turn, occur before spontaneous rupture of the fetal membranes. Similarly, pro-contractile biochemical changes in the uterus precede active and effective uterine contractions. Cervical dilation in the absence of uterine contractions is seen most commonly in the second trimester and is suggestive of cervical insufficiency. Similarly, the presence of uterine contractions in the absence of cervical change does not meet criteria for the diagnosis of labor and should be referred to as preterm contractions.

Timing of Labor

The timely onset of labor and birth is an important determinant of perinatal outcome. The mean duration of a human singleton pregnancy is 280 days (40 weeks) from the first day of the last menstrual period. *Term* is defined as the period from 37 weeks of gestation to 42 weeks of gestation. Both preterm (defined as delivery before 37 weeks of gestation[18]) and post-term births (delivery after 42 weeks of gestation[19]) are associated with increased neonatal morbidity and mortality.

Considerable evidence suggests that, in most viviparous animals, the fetus is in control of the timing of labor.[20-27] During the time of Hippocrates, it was believed that the fetus presented head first so that it could kick its legs up against the fundus of the uterus and propel itself through the birth canal. We have moved away from this simple and mechanical view of labor, but the factors responsible for the initiation and maintenance of labor at term are still not well understood. The past few decades have seen a marked change in the nature of the hypotheses to explain the onset of labor. Initial investigations centered on changes in the profile of circulating hormone levels in the maternal and fetal circulations (endocrine events). More recent studies have focused on the biochemical dialog that occurs at the fetal-maternal interface (paracrine and autocrine events) in an attempt to understand in detail the molecular mechanisms that regulate parturition.

Genetic Influences on the Timing of Labor

Horse-donkey crossbreeding experiments performed in the 1950s resulted in a gestational length intermediate between that of horses (340 days) and that of donkeys (365 days), suggesting an important role for the *fetal* genotype in the initiation of labor.[22,23] Moreover, fetuses who fail to trigger labor at the appropriate gestational age, thereby allowing the pregnancy to continue after term, have an increased risk of both antepartum stillbirth and of unexplained death in the first year of life,[28-30] suggesting that such fetuses may have subtle abnormalities in their hypothalamic-pituitary-adrenal (HPA) axis.

Familial clustering,[31,32] racial disparities,[33-37] and the high incidence of recurrent preterm birth[38,39] all suggest an important role for *maternal* genetic factors in the timing of labor. For example, black (including African-American, African, and Afro-Caribbean) women in the United States have a preterm birth rate that is twofold higher than that observed in whites.[33-37] Even after adjusting for potential confounding demographic and behavioral variables, the rate of premature deliveries in black women remains higher than that in white women, and this is especially true of extremely premature deliveries before 28 weeks' gestation.[35,36] Interestingly, the risk of preterm birth in interracial (black-white) couples is significantly different and intermediate between that of white-white (8.6%) and black-black (14.8%) couples.[40]

Taken together, these data suggest that genetic influences of both the mother and the fetus may be involved in the timing of labor. More recent studies suggest that genetic factors—or more correctly, gene-environment factors—may account for up to 20% of preterm births.[41-43] For example, maternal carriage of the 308(G>A) polymorphism in the promoter region of the tumor necrosis factor α (TNF-α) gene is associated with an increased risk of spontaneous preterm birth (odds ratio [OR] = 2.7; 95% confidence interval [CI], 1.7 to 4.5),[44,45] which is further increased in the presence of bacterial vaginosis (OR = 6.1; 95% CI, 1.9 to 21.0).[44-46] Interestingly, the risk of spontaneous preterm birth is increased even further if the woman with the TNFα gene promoter polymorphism and bacterial vaginosis also happens to be black (OR = 17).[46]

The Hormonal Control of Labor

The hypothesis that the fetus is in control of the timing of labor has been elegantly demonstrated in domestic ruminants, such as sheep and cows, and involves activation at term of the fetal HPA axis.[47] In such animals, a sharp rise in the concentration of adrenocorticotropic hormone (ACTH) and cortisol in the fetal circulation 15 to 20 days before delivery[48] results in an increased expression in the ruminant placenta of the trophoblast cytochrome P450 enzyme 17α-hydroxylase/$C_{17,20}$-lyase, which catalyzes the conversion of pregnenolone to 17α-hydroxypregnenolone and dehydroepiandrostenedione. The resultant fall in progesterone and rise in estrone and 17β-estradiol levels in the maternal circulation stimulate the uterus to produce prostaglandin $F_{2\alpha}$ ($PGF_{2\alpha}$), which provides the impetus for labor.[25,48-50] Human placentas, however, lack the glucocorticoid-inducible 17α-hydroxylase/17,20-lyase enzyme,[23] and thus this mechanism does not apply. Despite these observations, recent data suggest that there may be more similarities than differences between these species. In both species, fetal adrenal C19 precursors are used to form estrogens. Androstenedione and dehydroepiandrosterone sulfate (DHEAS) are secreted by the fetal adrenal gland, and their secretion is stimulated by ACTH and hypoxia; DHEAS and androstenedione infused into the fetus can be metabolized into estrone and estradiol, respectively. The result is a progressive increase in conjugated estrogens in maternal plasma during the latter part of gestation, which precedes the sharp rise in estrogen that occurs just before delivery in response to cortisol-mediated induction of the cytochrome P450 enzyme in ruminants and other nonprimate species.

Recent studies in mice suggest that surfactant protein-A (SP-A) secreted from the lungs of near-term pups may provide an additional trigger for parturition in that species.[51] Whether SP-A has a comparable role in humans remains to be determined. As explained in the first paragraph of this chapter, we lack an adequate animal model for study of these events in humans.

It is likely that a parturition cascade (Fig. 5-1) exists in humans that is responsible for the removal of mechanisms maintaining uterine

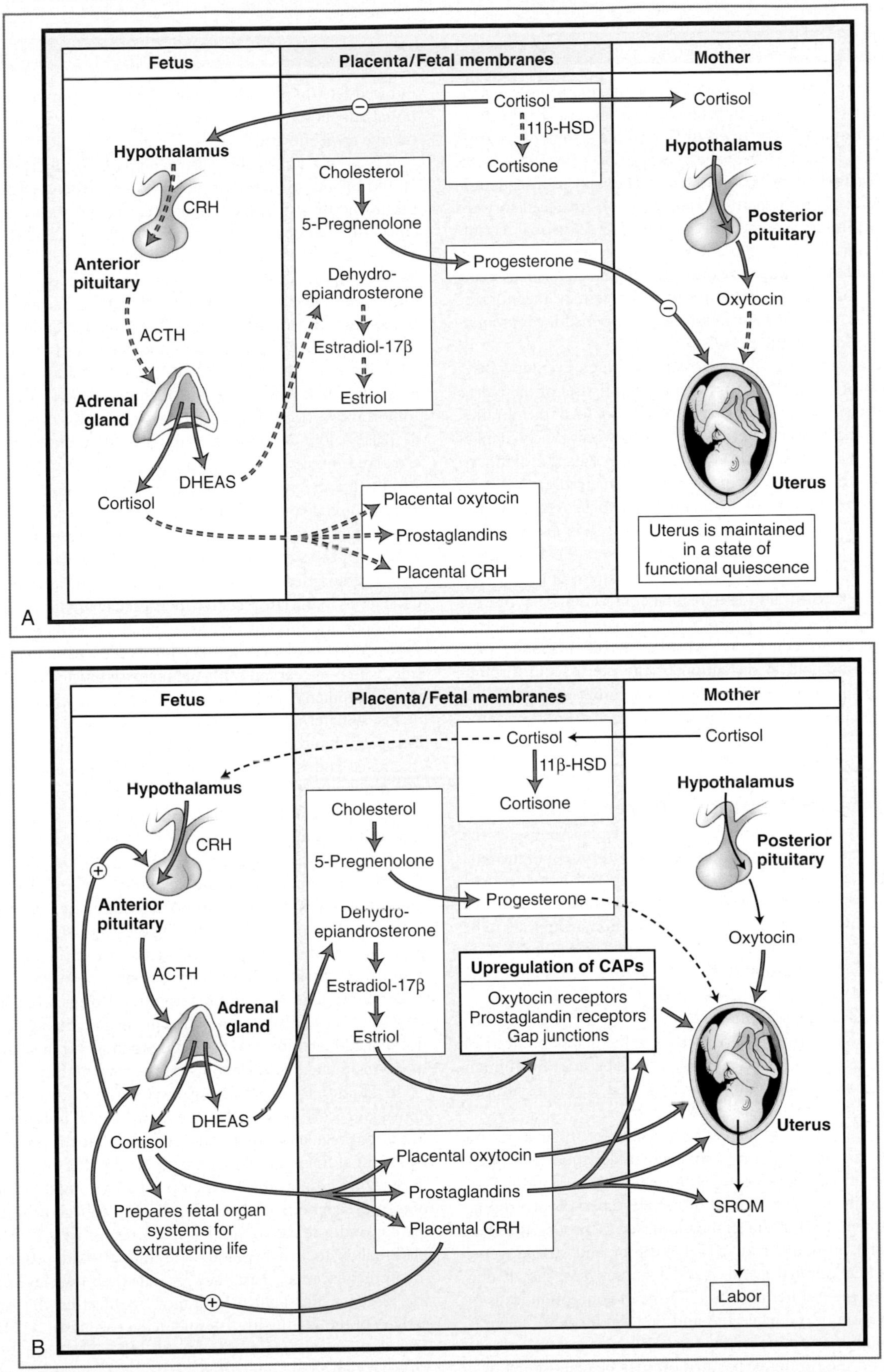

FIGURE 5-1 **Proposed parturition cascade for labor induction at term.** The spontaneous induction of labor at term in the human is regulated by a series of paracrine and autocrine hormones acting in an integrated parturition cascade. **A,** The factors responsible for maintaining uterine quiescence throughout gestation are shown. **B,** The factors responsible for the onset of labor are shown. They include the withdrawal of the inhibitory effects of progesterone on uterine contractility and the recruitment of cascades that promote estrogen (estriol) production and lead to upregulation of the contraction-associated proteins in the uterus. ACTH, adrenocorticotropic hormone (corticotropin); CAPs, contraction-associated proteins; CRH, corticotropin-releasing hormone; DHEAS, dehydroepiandrostenedione; 11β-HSD, 11β-hydroxysteroid dehydrogenase; SROM, spontaneous rupture of membranes.

quiescence and for the recruitment of factors acting to promote uterine activity.[26] Given its teleologic importance, such a cascade is likely to have multiple redundant loops to ensure a fail-safe system of securing pregnancy success and ultimately the preservation of the species. In such a model, each element is connected to the next in a sequential fashion, and many of the elements demonstrate positive feed-forward characteristics typical of a cascade mechanism. The sequential recruitment of signals that serve to augment the labor process suggest that it may not be possible to identify any one signaling mechanism as being uniquely responsible for the initiation of labor. It may therefore be prudent to describe such mechanisms as being responsible for *promoting*, rather than *initiating*, the process of labor.[52]

In brief, human labor is a multifactorial physiologic event involving an integrated set of changes within the maternal tissues of the uterus (myometrium, decidua, and uterine cervix) and fetal membranes, which occur gradually over a period of days to weeks. Such changes include, but are not limited to, an increase in prostaglandin synthesis and release within the uterus, an increase in myometrial gap junction formation, and upregulation of myometrial oxytocin receptors (i.e., uterine activation). Once the myometrium and cervix are prepared, endocrine and/or paracrine/autocrine factors from the fetal membranes and placenta bring about a switch in the pattern of myometrial activity from irregular contractures to regular contractions (i.e., uterine stimulation).[53] The fetus may coordinate this switch in myometrial activity through its influence on placental steroid hormone production, through mechanical distention of the uterus, and through secretion of neurohypophyseal hormones and other stimulators of prostaglandin synthesis. The roles of several specific hormones and pathways involved in the timing of labor will now be discussed further.

Fetal Hypothalamic-Pituitary-Adrenal Axis

In virtually every animal species studied, there is an increase in the concentration of the major adrenal glucocorticoid product in the fetal circulation in late gestation (cortisol in the sheep and human; corticosterone in the rat and mouse). As in other viviparous species, the final common pathway toward parturition in the human appears to be maturation and activation of the fetal HPA axis. The result is a dramatic increase in the production of the C19 steroid DHEAS from the intermediate (fetal) zone of the fetal adrenal. As noted, DHEAS is directly aromatized in the placenta to estrone, and it can also be 16-hydroxylated in the fetal liver and converted in the placenta to estriol (16-hydroxy-17β-estradiol) (see Fig. 5-1). This is because the human placenta is an incomplete steroidogenic organ, and estrogen synthesis by the placenta requires C19 as a steroid precursor.[25,54,55]

The cellular and molecular factors responsible for the maturation of the fetal HPA axis, although not completely understood, are associated with the gestational age–dependent upregulation of a number of critical genes within each component of the HPA axis: corticotropin-releasing hormone (CRH) in the fetal hypothalamus, proopiomelanocortin in the fetal pituitary, and ACTH receptor and steroidogenic enzymes in the fetal adrenal gland. Animal studies have shown that undernutrition of the mother around the time of conception leads to precocious activation of the fetal HPA and preterm birth,[56,57] suggesting that—although maturation of the fetal HPA axis is developmentally regulated and the timing of parturition may be determined by a "placental clock" set shortly after implantation—stress may accelerate this clock.[58] Thus, the length of gestation for any individual pregnancy appears to be established early in gestation, but some degree of flexibility may be possible. For example, rapid and profound activation of the fetal HPA axis has been demonstrated in the setting of experimentally induced fetal hypoxemia in the sheep, probably representing a functional adaptation and an effort by the fetus to escape a hostile intrauterine environment.[48]

Levels of CRH in the maternal circulation increase from between 10 and 100 pg/mL in nonpregnant women to between 500 and 3000 pg/mL in the third trimester of pregnancy, and then they decrease precipitously after delivery.[59] The source of this excess CRH is the placenta, and—in contrast to the situation in the hypothalamus, where corticosteroids suppress CRH expression in a classic endocrine feedback inhibition loop—the production of CRH by the placenta is upregulated by corticosteroids produced primarily by the fetal adrenal glands at the end of pregnancy.[60] Under the influence of estrogen, hepatic-derived CRH-binding protein (CRH-BP) concentrations also increase in pregnancy. CRH-BP binds and maintains CRH in an inactive form. Importantly, circulating CRH levels increase and CRH-BP levels decrease before the onset of both term and preterm labor, resulting in a marked increase in free (biologically active) CRH.[61] In addition to stimulating the production of ACTH by the fetal pituitary, CRH may also act directly on the fetal adrenal glands to promote the production of C19 steroid precursor (DHEAS).[62,63] For these reasons, some authorities have proposed that CRH may prime the placental clock that controls the duration of pregnancy, and that measurements of plasma CRH levels in the late second trimester may predict the onset of labor.[58] In support of this hypothesis, circulating levels of CRH have been shown to be increased in pregnant women with anxiety and depression, which may account for the increased incidence of preterm birth in such women.[64] However, recent studies have shown that measurements of maternal CRH are not clinically useful because of substantial intrapatient and interpatient variability,[65-67] which most likely reflects the mixed endocrine and paracrine role of placental, fetal membrane, and decidual CRH in the initiation of parturition.

At a molecular level, CRH acts by binding to specific nuclear receptors and affecting transcription of target genes. A number of CRH receptor isoforms have been described, and all have been identified in the myometrium, placenta, and fetal membranes.[68] During pregnancy, high-affinity CRH receptor isoforms dominate, and CRH promotes myometrial quiescence by inhibiting the production and increasing the degradation of prostaglandins, increasing intracellular cAMP, and stimulating nitric oxide synthase activity.[68,69] At term, CRH acts primarily through its low-affinity receptor isoforms, which promote myometrial contractility by stimulating prostaglandin production from the decidua and fetal membranes[70] and potentiating the contractile effects of oxytocin and prostaglandins on the myometrium.[71]

In addition to preparing organ systems for extrauterine life, endogenous glucocorticoids within the fetoplacental unit have a number of important regulatory functions. They regulate the production of prostaglandin at the maternal-fetal interface by affecting the expression of the enzymes responsible for their production and degradation—amnionic prostaglandin H synthase (PGHS) and chorionic 15-hydroxyprostaglandin dehydrogenase (PGDH), respectively.[72,73] They upregulate placental oxytocin expression[74] and interfere with progesterone signaling in the placenta.[27] Last, they regulate their own levels locally within the placenta and fetal membranes by affecting the expression and activity of the 11β-hydroxysteroid dehydrogenase (11β-HSD) enzyme. This enzyme exists in two isoforms: 11β-HSD-1 acts principally as a reductase enzyme, converting cortisone to cortisol, and is the predominant isoform found in the fetal membranes; 11β-HSD-2, which predominates in the placental syncytiotrophoblast, serves as a dehydrogenase that primarily oxidizes cortisol to inactive cortisone. It has been proposed that placental 11β-HSD-2 protects the fetus from high levels of maternal glucocorticoids.[75-77] Placental 11β-HSD-2

expression and activity is reduced in the setting of hypoxemia and in placentas from preeclamptic pregnancies, leading to increased passage of maternal cortisol into the fetal compartment, which may contribute to intrauterine growth restriction as well as fetal programming of subsequent adult disease.[78]

Progesterone

Progesterone is a steroid hormone that plays an integral role in each step of human pregnancy. It acts through its receptor, a member of the family of ligand-activated nuclear transcription regulators. Progesterone produced by the corpus luteum is critical to the maintenance of early pregnancy until the placenta takes over this function at 7 to 9 weeks of gestation—hence its name (progestational steroid hormone). Indeed, surgical removal of the corpus luteum[79] or the administration of a progesterone receptor (PR) antagonist such as mifepristone (RU-486)[80] readily induces abortion before 7 weeks (49 days) of gestation. The role of progesterone in later pregnancy, however, is less clear. It has been proposed that progesterone may be important in maintaining uterine quiescence in the latter half of pregnancy by limiting the production of stimulatory prostaglandins and inhibiting the expression of contraction-associated protein genes (ion channels, oxytocin and prostaglandin receptors, and gap junctions) within the myometrium.[26,27]

In most laboratory animals (with the noted exception of the guinea pig and armadillo), systemic withdrawal of progesterone is an essential component of parturition.[27] In humans, however, circulating progesterone levels during labor are similar to levels measured 1 week before labor, and levels remain elevated until after delivery of the placenta,[23,81] suggesting that systemic progesterone withdrawal is not a prerequisite for labor at term. However, circulating hormone levels do not necessarily reflect tissue levels. In the 1960s, Csapo and Pinto-Dantas put forth the idea of a "progesterone blockage," which suggested that the myometrial quiescence of human pregnancy was maintained by steady levels of progesterone, just as in pregnancies of other species.[82] The earliest studies looking at progesterone levels in labor were done separately in the 1970s by Csapo and colleagues[83] and Cousins and coworkers[84] and described a relative progesterone deficiency and an increase in the ratio of 17β-estradiol to progesterone in patients presenting in preterm labor, regardless of etiology. These and other findings have prompted extensive research into the potential mechanisms of progesterone action on the uterus and the possibility of progesterone therapy to prevent preterm birth.

Although systemic progesterone withdrawal may not correlate directly with the onset of labor in humans, there is increasing evidence to suggest that the onset of labor may be preceded by a physiologic (functional) withdrawal of progesterone activity at the level of the uterus.[26,27,85] The evidence in support of this hypothesis is mounting. For example, the administration of a PR antagonist (such as RU-486) at term leads to increased uterine activity and cervical ripening.[86] Moreover, antenatal supplementation with progesterone from 16 to 20 weeks through 34 to 36 weeks of gestation has been shown to reduce the rate of preterm birth in approximately one third of women judged to be at high risk by virtue of a prior spontaneous preterm birth.[87,88]

The molecular mechanisms by which progesterone is able to maintain uterine quiescence and prevent preterm birth in some high-risk women are not clear. However, six putative mechanisms have been proposed in the literature both by us and by other investigators. These are summarized briefly under the following headings:

Functional Progesterone Withdrawal before Labor May Be Mediated by Changes in PR-A and PR-B Expression with an Increase in the PR-A/PR-B Expression Ratio. The single-copy human PR gene uses separate promoters and translational start sites to produce two distinct isoforms, PR-A (94 kD) and PR-B (116 kD), which are identical except for an additional 165 amino acids that are present only in the amino terminus of PR-B.[89,90] Although PR-B shares many of its structural domains with PR-A, they are two functionally distinct transcripts that mediate their own response genes and physiologic effects, with little overlap. PR-B is an activator of progesterone-responsive genes, whereas PR-A acts, in general, as a repressor of PR-B function.[91] The onset of labor at term is associated with an increase in the myometrial PR-A/PR-B expression ratio, resulting in a functional withdrawal of progesterone action.[92-96] The factors responsible for this differential expression with the onset of labor are not known, but they may include prostaglandins (both PGE_2 and $PGF_{2\alpha}$), inflammatory cytokines (such as TNFα), and estrogen activation. The changes seen in the PR-A/PR-B ratio in the myometrium are also seen in the cervix[97] and fetal membranes.[98] Recent studies indicate that there may be an additional PR isoform (PR-C) that contributes to the onset of labor by inhibiting progesterone-PR signaling in the myometrium.[99]

Progesterone as an Anti-inflammatory Agent. Inflammation has a well-established role in the initiation and maintenance of parturition, both at term and preterm. Progesterone has been shown to inhibit the production and activity of key inflammatory mediators at the maternal-fetal interface, including cytokines (such as interleukin [IL]-1β and IL-8) and prostaglandins.[100-102] Recent data suggest that progesterone may also exert an anti-inflammatory effect at the level of the myometrium. For example, expression of the chemokine, monocyte chemoattractant protein-1 (MCP-1), increases in human myometrium during labor, both at term and preterm, and in association myometrial stretch.[103] In other model systems, MCP-1 has been shown to induce an influx of peripheral monocytes that differentiate into macrophages and secrete cytokines, matrix metalloproteinases, and prostaglandins, thereby contributing to an enhanced inflammatory state. Interestingly, myometrial MCP-1 expression can be inhibited by the administration of progesterone, both in vivo and in vitro.[103]

Progesterone Receptor Cofactors Mediate a Functional Withdrawal of Progesterone in the Myometrium at Term. The ability of progesterone to bind its receptor and affect transcription of target genes is reduced in uterine tissues obtained after, compared with before, the onset of labor.[104] Condon and colleagues[105] have shown that the PR coactivators cAMP-response element–binding protein (CREB)-binding protein and steroid receptor coactivators 2 and 3, as well as acetylated histone H3, are decreased in the myometrium of women in labor as compared with women not in labor. These data suggest that the decline in PR coactivator expression and histone acetylation in the uterus near term and during labor may impair progesterone-PR functioning. Progesterone-PR function may also be antagonized directly through the increased expression of PR co-repressors. Dong and coworkers[106] reported that *p*olypyrimidine tract binding protein–associated *s*plicing *f*actor (PSF) blocked PR binding to its DNA response element, thereby preventing the progesterone-PR complex from regulating the transcription of target genes. Interestingly, PSF appears to be expressed at higher levels in myometrium collected from the fundus than myometrium from the lower uterine segment,[107] and, at least in the rodent model, its expression is increased before the onset of labor.[106] Modulation of PR function by coactivators and co-repressors may therefore explain, at least in part, how it is possible to have a functional withdrawal of progesterone action at the level of the uterus without a significant change in circulating progesterone levels.

Progesterone May Interfere with Cortisol-Mediated Regulation of Placental Gene Expression. Cortisol and progesterone appear to have antagonistic actions within the fetoplacental unit. For example, cortisol increases, and progesterone decreases, prostaglandin[78] and CRH gene expression.[108] These data suggest that the cortisol-dominant environment of the fetoplacental unit just before the onset of labor may act locally through a series of autocrine and paracrine pathways to overcome the efforts of progesterone to maintain uterine quiescence and prevent myometrial contractions.

Progesterone May Act Also through Nongenomic Pathways. In addition to its well-described genomic effects, progesterone may also act through nongenomic (DNA-independent) pathways. For example, several investigators have shown that select progesterone metabolites (such as 5β-dihydroprogesterone)—but not progesterone itself—are capable of intercalating themselves into the lipid bilayer of the cell membrane, binding directly to and distorting the heptahelical oxytocin receptor, thereby inhibiting oxytocin binding and downstream signaling.[109-111] A functional withdrawal of this progesterone metabolite–mediated inhibition of oxytocin action on the myometrium at term would promote myometrial contractility and labor.

Possible Role for Cell Membrane–Bound PR in Myometrium. Recent studies have identified a specific membrane-bound PR in a number of human tissues, including uterine tissues, but the function of this receptor in pregnancy and labor has yet to be fully elucidated.

Estrogens

In the rhesus monkey, infusion of a C19 steroid precursor (androstenedione) leads to preterm delivery.[112] This effect is blocked by concurrent infusion of the aromatase inhibitor 4-hydroxyandrostenedione,[113] demonstrating that conversion of C19 steroid precursors to estrogen at the level of the fetoplacental unit is important. However, systemic infusion of estrogen failed to induce delivery, suggesting that the action of estrogen is most likely paracrine or autocrine, or both.[112,114] Levels of estrogen in the maternal circulation are significantly elevated throughout gestation and are derived primarily from the placenta. In contrast to the situation in many animal species (such as the sheep), the high circulating levels of estrogens in the human are already at the dissociation constant (K_d) for the estrogen receptor, which explains why there is no need for an additional increase in estrogen production at term.

At the cellular level, estrogens exert their effect by binding to specific nuclear receptors and effecting the transcription of target genes. Two distinct estrogen receptors are described: ERα and ERβ. Each is coded by its own gene (*ESR1* and *ESR2,* respectively), and requires dimerization before binding to its ligand. At the level of the uterus, ERα appears to be dominant. Expression of ERα increases in concert with an increase in the PR-A/PR-B expression ratio with increasing gestational age in nonlaboring myometrium.[115,116] These findings suggest that functional estrogen activation and functional progesterone withdrawal are linked. For most of pregnancy, progesterone decreases myometrial estrogen responsiveness by inhibiting ERα expression. Such an interaction would explain why the human myometrium is refractory to the high levels of circulating estrogens for most of pregnancy. At term, however, functional progesterone withdrawal removes the suppression of myometrial ERα expression, leading to an increase in myometrial estrogen responsiveness. Estrogen can then act to transform the myometrium into a contractile phenotype. This model may explain why disruption of progesterone action alone can trigger the parturition cascade. The link between functional progesterone withdrawal and functional estrogen activation may be a critical mechanism for the endocrine and paracrine control of human labor at term.

Prostaglandins

Endogenous levels of prostaglandins in the decidua are lower in pregnancy than in the endometrium at any stage of the menstrual cycle,[101,117] primarily because of a decrease in prostaglandin synthesis.[101] This is true also of prostaglandin production in other uterine tissues. These findings, along with the observation that the administration of exogenous prostaglandins, intravenously, intra-amniotically, or vaginally, in all species examined and at any stage of gestation, has the ability to induce abortion,[118-120] support the hypothesis that pregnancy is maintained by a mechanism that tonically suppresses prostaglandin synthesis, release, and activity throughout gestation.

Overwhelming evidence suggests a role for prostaglandins in the process of labor, both at term and preterm,[26,27] which is probably common to all viviparous species. For example, mice lacking a functional $PGF_{2\alpha}$ receptor, cytosolic phospholipase A_2 (PLA_2), or prostaglandin H_2 synthase type 1 (PGHS-1) protein all demonstrate a delay in the onset of labor.[121] In the human, exogenous prostaglandins stimulate uterine contractility both in vitro and in vivo,[122] and drugs that block prostaglandin synthesis can inhibit uterine contractility and prolong gestation.[123] All human uterine tissues contain receptors for the naturally occurring prostanoids and are capable of producing prostaglandins,[124] although their production is carefully regulated and compartmentalized within the uterus: the fetal membranes produce almost exclusively PGE_2, the decidua synthesizes mainly $PGF_{2\alpha}$ but also small amounts of PGE_2 and PGD_2, and the myometrium mainly produces prostacyclin (PGI_2). This is because, although these compounds are structurally similar, they can have different and often antagonistic actions. For example, $PGF_{2\alpha}$, thromboxane, PGE_1, and PGE_3 promote myometrial contractility by increasing calcium influx into myometrial cells and enhancing gap junction formation,[124-126] whereas PGE_2, PGD_2, and PGI_2 have the opposite effect and inhibit contractions.[124]

Prostaglandin levels increase in maternal plasma, urine, and amniotic fluid before the onset of uterine contractions,[124,127,128] suggesting that it is a cause and not a consequence of labor. Regulation of prostaglandin synthesis occurs at several different levels of the arachidonic acid cascade (Fig. 5-2). Prostaglandins are synthesized from unesterified (free) arachidonic acid released from membrane phospholipids through the action of a series of phospholipase enzymes, the most important of which appears to be phospholipase A_2 (PLA_2). Expression of PLA_2 increases gradually in the fetal membranes throughout gestation, but it does not appear to show further increase at the time of labor. Thereafter, arachidonic acid is metabolized to the intermediate metabolite (PGH_2) by PGHS enzymes, which have both cyclooxygenase and peroxidase activities. PGHS exists in two forms, each a product of a distinct gene: PGHS-1 (which is constitutively expressed) and PGHS-2 (also known as cyclooxygenase-2 [COX-2]), the inducible form that can be upregulated by growth factors and cytokines. Several studies have suggested that the transcription factor, nuclear factor kappa B (NF-κB), is an important regulator of PGHS-2 expression.[27]

PGH_2 is rapidly converted to one of the primary (biologically active) prostaglandins through different prostaglandin synthase enzymes (see Fig. 5-2). These hormones act locally in a paracrine or autocrine fashion (or both) by binding to specific prostaglandin receptors on adjacent cells. In addition, unesterified arachidonic acid can diffuse into the cell and interact directly with nuclear transcription factors to regulate the transcription of target genes, including cytokines and other hormones. The primary prostaglandins are then metabolized and excreted. The major pathway in the degradation of $PGE_{2\alpha}$ and $PGF_{2\alpha}$ involves the action of a nicotinamide adenine dinucleotide $(NAD)^+$-dependent PGDH that oxidizes 15-hydroxy groups, resulting in the formation of 15-keto and 13,14-dihydro-15-keto compounds

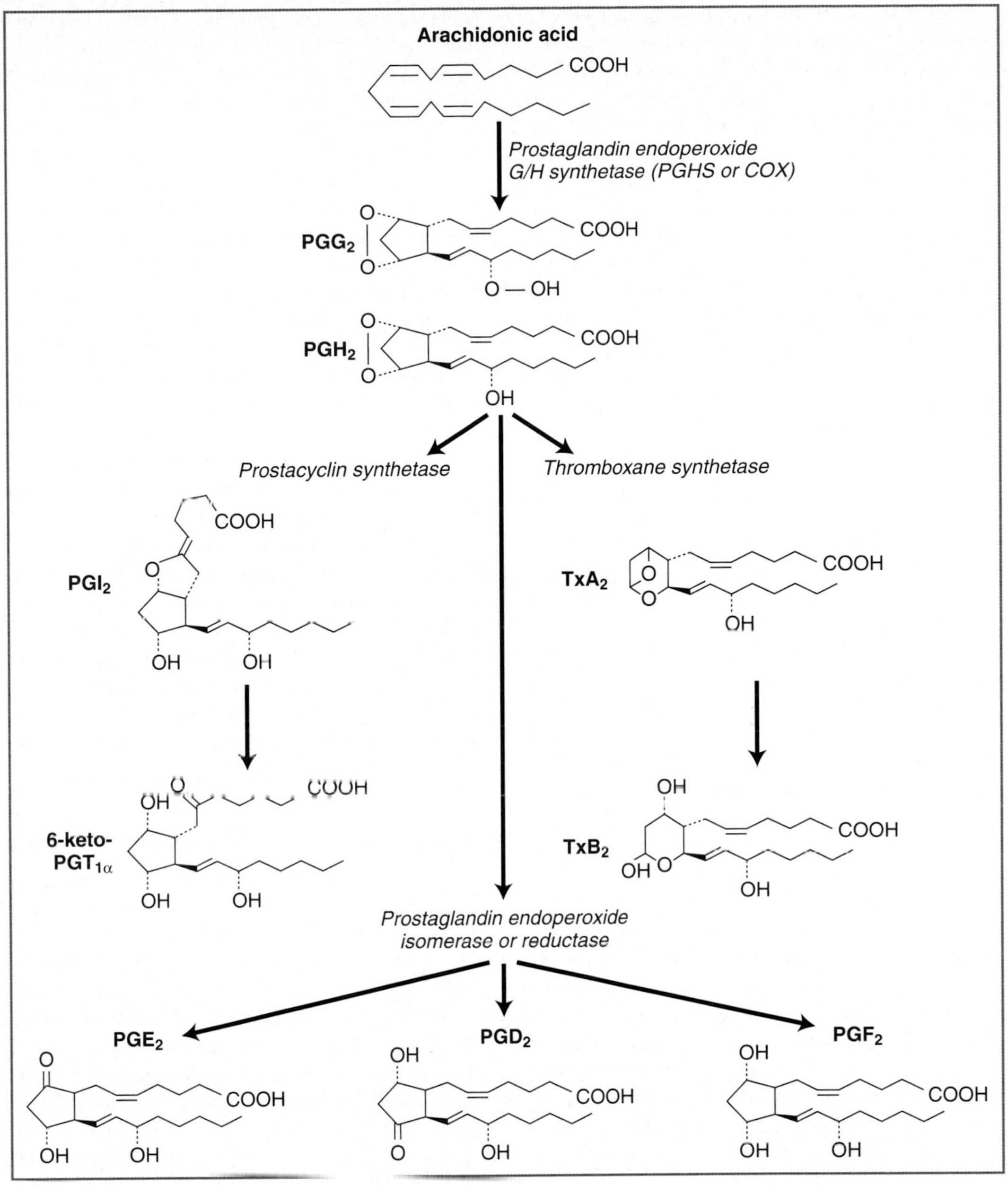

FIGURE 5-2 Schematic representation of the eicosanoid cascade. Dietary linoleic acid (18:3 ω-6) is lengthened and desaturated to form arachidonic acid, which is then esterified and incorporated into phospholipid within cell membranes. In response to a number of hormonal and inflammatory stimuli, phospholipase (PL) enzymes (primarily PLA_2) release free (unesterified) arachidonic acid from membrane phospholipid, which can then be enzymically converted to one of the eicosanoid metabolites. COX, cyclooxygenase; PG, prostaglandin; PGHS, prostaglandin H synthase.

with markedly reduced biologic activity. PGDH is abundantly expressed in the human chorion. In this way, the chorion serves as a protective barrier, preventing the transfer of the primary prostaglandins from the fetoplacental unit to the underlying decidua and myometrium.[129] Interestingly, the cells that express PDGH (chorionic trophoblasts) are decreased in preterm labor associated with chorioamnionitis resulting in a loss of this metabolic barrier.[130] The expression of PGDH is regulated by a variety of factors, including cytokines and steroid hormones. For example, progesterone tonically stimulates PGDH expression,[72] whereas cortisol increases prostaglandin production by the placenta and fetal membranes by upregulating PGHS-2 expression (in amnion and chorion) and downregulating PGDH expression (in chorionic trophoblast), thereby promoting cervical ripening and uterine contractions.[67,69,70] In the myometrium, the onset of labor, both at term and preterm, is associated with a significant decrease in PGDH but no change in PGHS-1 or -2 expression, suggesting that levels of prostaglandins in the myometrium may depend largely on catabolism rather than synthesis.[131]

Oxytocin

Maternally derived oxytocin is synthesized in the hypothalamus and released from the posterior pituitary in a pulsatile fashion. It is rapidly inactivated in the liver and kidney, resulting in a biologic half-life of 3 to 4 minutes in the maternal circulation. During pregnancy, oxytocin is degraded primarily by placental oxytocinase. Concentrations of oxytocin in the maternal circulation do not change significantly during pregnancy or before the onset of labor, but they do rise late in the second stage of labor.[132,133] Studies on fetal pituitary oxytocin production, the umbilical arteriovenous difference in oxytocin concentration, amniotic fluid oxytocin levels, and fetal urinary oxytocin output demonstrate conclusively that the fetus secretes oxytocin toward the maternal side.[134] Furthermore, the calculated rate of oxytocin secretion from the fetus increases from a baseline of 1 mU/min before labor to approximately 3 mU/min after spontaneous labor, which is similar to the amount normally administered to women to induce labor at term.

Specific receptors for oxytocin are present in the myometrium, and there appear to be regional differences in oxytocin receptor distribution, with large numbers of receptors in the fundal area and few receptors in the lower uterine segment and cervix.[135,136] Myometrial oxytocin receptor concentrations increase 50- to 100-fold in the first trimester of pregnancy compared with the nonpregnant state, and they increase an additional 200- to 300-fold during pregnancy, reaching a maximum during early labor.[124,130,131,135-137] This is mediated primarily by the sex steroid hormones, with estrogen promoting and progesterone inhibiting myometrial oxytocin receptor expression.[130] This rise in receptor concentration is paralleled by an increase in myometrial sensitivity to circulating levels of oxytocin.[124,130] Activation of myometrial oxytocin receptors results in interaction with the guanosine triphosphate binding proteins of the $G\alpha_{q/11}$ subfamily of G-proteins that stimulate phospholipase C activity resulting in increased production of inositol triphosphate[138] and calcium influx of calcium.[139]

Specific high-affinity oxytocin binding sites have also been isolated from amnion and decidua parietalis, but not from decidua vera.[133,140] However, neither amnion nor decidual cells are contractile, and the action of oxytocin on these tissues remains uncertain. It has been suggested that oxytocin plays a dual role in parturition. It may act directly through both oxytocin receptor-mediated and nonreceptor, voltage-mediated calcium channels to affect intracellular signal transduction pathways that promote uterine contractions. It may also act indirectly through stimulation of amniotic and decidual prostaglandin production.[133,137,140] Indeed, induction of labor at term is successful only when the oxytocin infusion is associated with an increase in $PGF_{2\alpha}$ production, in spite of seemingly adequate uterine contractions in both induction failures and successes.[133]

Myometrial Contractility

Regulation of Electrical Activity within the Uterus

During pregnancy, the pattern of electrical activity in the myometrium changes from irregular spikes to regular activity. As with other types of muscle, action potentials must be generated and propagated in the myometrium to effect contractions, in a process known as electromechanical coupling.[141,142] The generation of action potentials of +12 to +25 mV from a normal resting potential of −65 to −80 mV in pregnant myometrial cells relies on the rapid shifts of ions (especially calcium) through membrane ion channels,[143,144] the most important of which appear to be voltage-sensitive calcium channels and, at the end of pregnancy, fast sodium and potassium channels.[138,145-149] Autonomous pacemaker cells exist in the uterus. These cells have a higher resting transmembrane potential and spontaneously initiate action potentials.[150] Action potentials in the uterus occur in bursts, and the strength of contractions relies on their frequency and duration. This, in turn, determines the number of myometrial cells recruited for action. The action potential results in a rapid rise in intracellular calcium derived from both extracellular and intracellular sources, which trigger myometrial contractions by encouraging the relative movement of thick (myosin) and thin (actin) filaments within the contractile apparatus, resulting in shortening of the contractile unit. In this way, the electrical activity is translated into mechanical forces that are exerted on the intrauterine contents (Fig. 5-3).

The frequency of contractions correlates with the frequency of action potentials; the force of contractions correlates with the number of spikes in the action potential and the number of cells activated together; and the duration of contractions correlates with the duration of the action potentials. As labor progresses, electrical activity becomes more organized and increases in amplitude and duration. The strength of contractions, which is best measured as intrauterine pressure in millimeters of mercury (mm Hg), depends on the stage of labor. Early labor contractions have a peak intensity of +25 to +30 mm Hg, and this increases to +60 to +65 mm Hg during active labor.[151] A number of factors influence the strength of the uterine contractions, including parity, cervical status, exogenous oxytocin, and labor analgesia (especially epidural analgesia). For example, the more rapid labor observed in multiparous than in nulliparous women is caused not by increased intrauterine pressures during labor (indeed, multiparous women have lower intrauterine pressures than nulliparas)[152] but to a reduction in the resistance of the pelvic floor.

Mechanics of Myometrial Contractions

The structural basis for contractions is the relative movement of thick and thin filaments in the contractile apparatus, which allows them to slide over each other with resultant shortening of the myocyte. Although this movement is similar in all muscles, several structural and regulatory features are unique to smooth muscle including the myometrium.[153,154] In smooth muscle, the sarcomere arrangement of thick and thin filaments seen in striated muscle is present on a much smaller scale, and intermediate filaments of the cytoskeletal network maintain the structural integrity of these mini-sarcomeres. The thin filaments insert into dense bands linked by the cytoskeletal network, thereby allowing the generation of force in any direction within the cell. This allows smooth muscle cells to generate greater force (greater shortening) than striated muscle cells, and with relatively little energy expenditure.

Myosin makes up the thick filaments of the contractile apparatus. Smooth muscle myosin is a hexamer consisting of two heavy chain subunits (~200 kDa) and two pairs each of 20- and 17-kDa light chains (Fig. 5-4). Each heavy chain has a globular head that contains actin binding sites and sites with adenosine triphosphate (ATP) hydrolysis (ATPase) activity. A neck region connects the globular head to the α-helical tail, which interacts with the tail of the other heavy-chain subunits. In this way, multiple myosin molecules interact through their α-helical tails to make a coiled-coil rod, which forms the thick filament. Thin filaments are composed of actin, which polymerizes into a double-helical strand in association with a number of proteins. When the myosin head interacts with actin, the ATPase activity in the myosin head is activated. The energy generated from the hydrolysis of ATP allows the myosin head to move in the neck region, thereby changing the relative position of the thick and thin filaments with shortening of the contractile unit. The myosin head then detaches

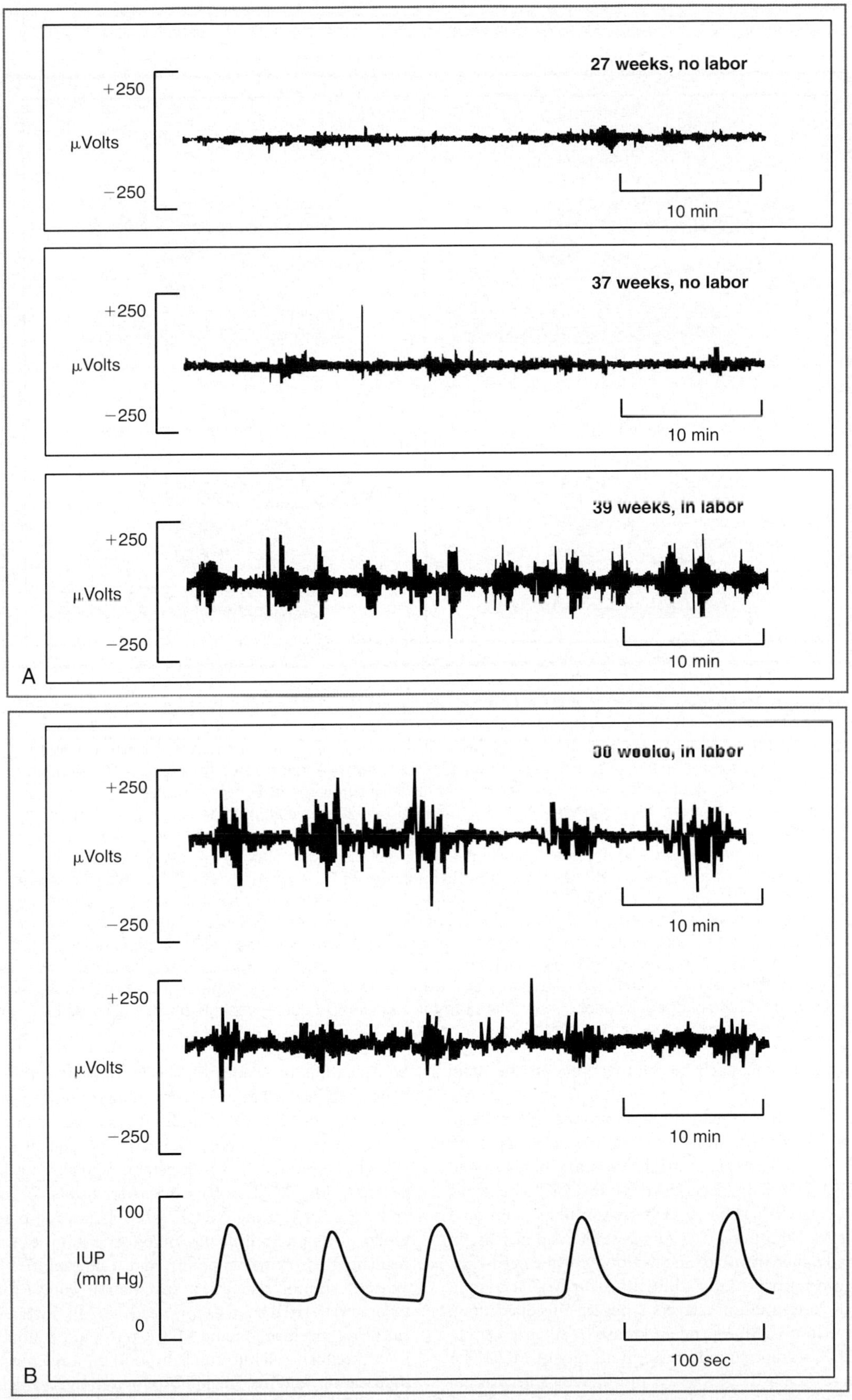

FIGURE 5-3 Uterine electrical activity during pregnancy and labor. A, During pregnancy, the pattern of electrical activity in the myometrium changes from irregular spikes to regular activity. Labor is associated with a further increase in the frequency, amplitude, and duration of action potential pulses. **B,** Electrical activity recorded noninvasively from two separate sites on the maternal abdomen is shown, which confirms electrical synchrony within the myometrium during labor. These electrical pulses correlate with uterine contractions as measured using an intrauterine pressure (IUP) catheter. (Modified from Buhimschi C, Buhimschi IA, Malinow AM, et al: The forces of labour. Fetal Matern Med Rev 14:273-307, 2003.)

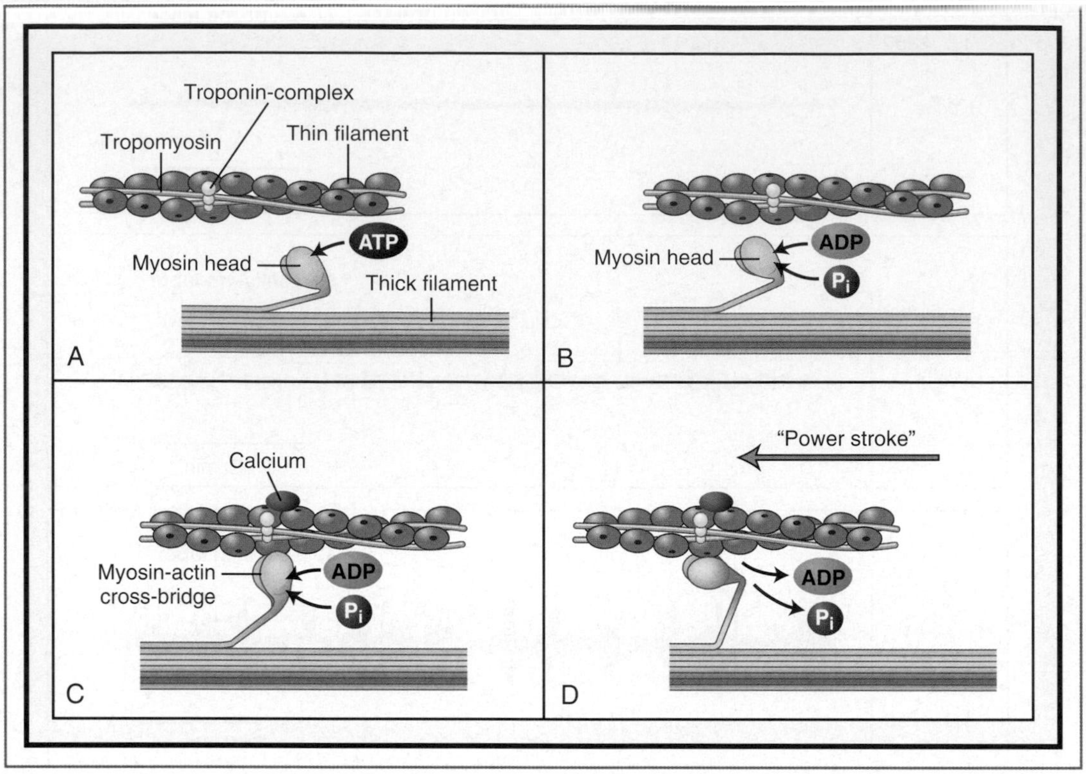

FIGURE 5-4 **Mechanics of muscle contraction. A,** The appearance of the contractile unit is illustrated. The thick filament refers to myosin; the thin filament is actin. Myosin-binding sites on the actin filaments are covered by a thin filament known as tropomyosin that obscures the myosin-binding sites, therefore preventing the myosin heads from attaching to actin and forming cross-bridges. Adenosine triphosphate (ATP) binds to the myosin head. The troponin complex is attached to the tropomyosin filament. **B,** The hydrolysis of ATP into adenosine diphosphate (ADP) and inorganic phosphate (Pi) allows the myosin head to assume its resting position. **C,** The binding of calcium to the troponin complex results in a conformational change that allows binding sites between actin and myosin to be exposed with the formation of actin-myosin cross-bridges. **D,** The formation of actin-myosin cross-bridges results in release of Pi and ADP, causing the myosin heads to bend and slide past the myosin fibers. This "power stroke" results in a shortening of the contractile unit and the generation of force within the muscle. At the end of the power stroke, the myosin head releases the actin-binding site, is cocked back to its furthest position, and binds to a new molecule of ATP in preparation for another contraction. The binding of myosin heads occurs asynchronously (i.e., some myosin heads are binding actin filaments while other heads are releasing them), which allows the muscle to generate a continuous smooth force. Cross-bridge formations must therefore form repeatedly during a single muscle contraction.

and, when reactivated, can reattach at another site on the actin filament.

Actin-myosin interaction is regulated by the intracellular calcium concentration, which is mediated through the calcium-binding protein calmodulin (CaM).[138,155,156] The calcium-CaM complex binds to and increases the activity of myosin light-chain kinase (MLCK), an enzyme responsible for phosphorylating the 20-kDa myosin light chain on a serine residue near the N-terminus.[156,157] This results in an increase in myosin ATPase activity, thereby increasing flexibility of the head-neck junction and increasing uterine contractility.[153] A further increase in intracellular calcium concentration triggers a negative-feedback loop with activation of calcium-CaM-dependent kinase II, an enzyme that phosphorylates MLCK, leading to a decrease in affinity of MLCK for calcium-CaM, a decrease in MLCK activity, and thereby a decrease in myometrial contractility.[156,158]

A number of intracellular proteins interact with actin and further regulate actin-myosin interactions. Tropomyosin does so by binding to calcium-CaM, making it less available for binding to MLCK; calponin directly inhibits myosin ATPase activity; and caldesmon acts through both of these mechanisms. The phosphatase group of enzymes also plays an important role in determining the sensitivity of the contractile apparatus to electrical stimuli and changes in intracellular calcium concentrations.[159-162] Phosphatases can be regulated by direct effects on catalytic subunits or by targeting regulatory proteins.[160,161,163] For example, MLCK phosphatase is responsible for dephosphorylating and thus inactivating MLCK; phosphatases also remove phosphate groups from and relieve the inhibitory actions of the actin-associated regulatory proteins calponin and caldesmon.[159,163] A number of external stimuli also affect myometrial contractility. For example, myometrial stretch (tension) leads to an increase in intracellular calcium concentration and MLCK phosphorylation.[155,159] The increase in intracellular calcium concentration typically precedes MLCK phosphorylation, and maximal phosphorylation is evident before maximal force is achieved. For the same amount of tension, less phosphorylation occurs in myometrium from late pregnant than from nonpregnant myometrium,[164] and this effect is seen without an increase in actin-myosin or phosphatase protein content with increasing gestational age.[155]

Multiple mechanisms are therefore responsible for the spontaneous contraction-relaxation cycles in human myometrium, including changes in intracellular calcium concentrations, alteration in membrane potential, phosphorylation and dephosphorylation (activation and inhibition) of MLCK, activation of phosphatases, and recruitment of a number of distinct intracellular signal transduction pathways.[138,149,154,155,158,162] This may explain why smooth muscle contractions can occur in response to external stimuli without a change in membrane potential or intracellular calcium concentration.[153,154]

Hormonal Regulation of Myometrial Contractility

As in other smooth muscles, myometrial contractions are mediated through the ATP-dependent binding of myosin to actin. In contrast to vascular smooth muscle cells, however, myometrial cells have a sparse innervation that is further reduced during pregnancy.[165] The regulation of the contractile mechanism of the uterus is therefore largely humoral or dependent on intrinsic factors within myometrial cells (or both). During pregnancy, the contractile activity of the uterus is maintained in a state of functional quiescence through the action of various putative inhibitors including, but not limited to, progesterone, prostacyclin (PGI_2), relaxin, parathyroid hormone–related peptide, nitric oxide, calcitonin gene–related peptide, adrenomedullin, and vasoactive intestinal peptide. The onset of uterine contractions at term is a consequence of release from the inhibitory effects of pregnancy on the myometrium as well as recruitment of uterine stimulants such as oxytocin and stimulatory prostaglandins (e.g., $PGF_{2\alpha}$, PGE_2).[166]

Not surprisingly, investigation of the control of myometrial contractility during pregnancy has focused on the physiologic, endocrine, and molecular events that occur a few days before the onset of labor, both at term and before term. Traditionally it was thought that, during the majority of pregnancy, the myometrium was a relatively inert organ whose role was limited to growing and protecting the products of conception. However, recent studies, primarily on rats, have challenged this notion and suggested that the myometrium undergoes a tightly regulated program of differentiation throughout pregnancy. In this model, labor can be viewed as the terminal differentiation state of the myometrium, with downregulation of inhibitory pathways and activation of contractile processes. This model explains why tocolysis in the setting of active preterm labor is largely ineffective.[26]

The program of myometrial differentiation includes four distinct states or phenotypes: proliferative, synthetic, contractile, and labor. In early pregnancy, uterine myocytes exhibit a high level of proliferation, as evidenced by increased expression of cell cycle markers and anti-apoptotic factors such as BCL2.[167] Myocyte proliferation during this phase is mediated in large part by estrogen-induced expression of insulin-like growth factor-1 (IGF-1).[168] In the rat, the proliferative phenotype ends abruptly on day 14 of 23 of gestation, and the myocytes differentiate to a synthetic phenotype. The switch from a proliferative to a synthetic phenotype most likely results from stretch-induced hypoxic injury to the myometrium that induces expression of stress-activated caspases.[167] The synthetic phase of myometrial differentiation is maintained by progesterone and tension on the uterine wall exerted by the expanding conception. During this phase, the myometrium expresses contractile protein isoforms typical of undifferentiated cells[169] and there is extensive tissue remodeling leading to loss of focal cell-matrix adhesion.[170] Growth of the myometrium during the synthetic period results not from cell proliferation but from myocyte hypertrophy and secretion of interstitial matrix proteins such as collagen I and fibronectin.[171]

At around day 19 of 23 in the rat, the myometrium switches to a contractile phenotype in preparation for labor. This change appears to be mediated by increased tension on the myometrium and a reduction in circulating progesterone levels, which together lead to an increased expression of more differentiated contractile protein isoforms in myocytes[169] and a switch from the synthesis of interstitial matrix proteins to basement membrane matrix proteins (such as laminin and collagen IV).[171] This serves to stabilize focal adhesions and allows myocytes to anchor more firmly into the underlying matrix,[170] which is critical to enable contraction and retraction (shortening) of the myometrium during labor. The slowdown in myocyte growth and continued growth of the fetus during this phase significantly increases myometrial tension which, in the setting of low circulating levels of progesterone (or an increase in the estrogen-to-progesterone ratio), is believed to provide the signal for terminal differentiation of the myometrium.[168] The resultant labor phenotype of the myometrium is associated with the upregulation of a series of "labor genes" or contraction-associated proteins (CAPs) associated with contractile activity, including ion channels that increase myocyte excitability, gap junctions (connexin 43) that increase the synchronization of contractions (Fig. 5-5), and receptors for uterotonic agonists (such as oxytocin and the stimulatory prostaglandins).

At a cellular and molecular level, the upregulation of the CAPs appears to be mediated at the level of gene transcription resulting from increased expression of cFos and other members of the activating protein (AP)-1 family of transcription factors (Fra-1, Fra-2) within myometrial cells caused by uterine stretch and hormonal factors, primarily estrogen.[167] There also appear to be regional differences in gene expression within the myometrium. For example, genes that promote contractile activity (such as connexin 43, oxytocin receptors, and the prostaglandin receptors EP1/4 and FP) are more highly expressed in the uterine fundus, whereas genes associated with contractile inhibition (EP2/4, CRH receptor subtype 1) are expressed more highly in the

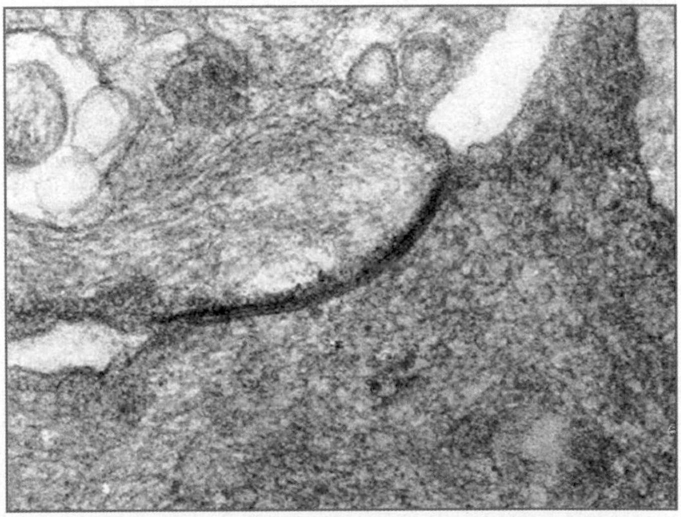

FIGURE 5-5 Electron micrograph of gap junction between adjacent myometrial cells. The transition of the uterus from a quiescent entity to a dynamic, contractile one comes through the recruitment of and communication between myometrial cells through gap junctions. An increase in gap junctions allows action potentials to be propagated between adjacent myometrial cells, thereby establishing electrical synchrony within the myometrium and allowing more effective coordination of contractions. (Reprinted from Buhimschi C, Buhimschi IA, Malinow AM, et al: The forces of labour. Fetal Matern Med Rev 14:273-307, 2003.)

lower uterine segment.[172,173] The molecular mechanisms responsible for the regionalization of gene expression within the uterus have yet to be determined, although recent reports of higher levels of the PR co-repressor, PSF, in the uterine fundus suggests the possibility of regionalized differences in functional withdrawal of progesterone.[107]

The role of a number of specific stimulants and relaxants involved in myometrial contractility during labor is discussed under the following headings:

Uterine Stimulants

Table 5-1 summarizes uterine stimulants implicated in uterine contractions during labor. *Oxytocin* is a potent endogenous uterotonic agent (discussed earlier) that is capable of stimulating uterine contractions if given exogenously at intravenous infusion rates of 1 to 2 mU/min at term. *Prostaglandins* (discussed earlier) cause uterine contractions and cervical effacement and dilation, and can be used clinically for induction of labor. A number of other less well recognized uterine factors have also been implicated in the generation of uterine contractions:

Endothelin. Endothelin is a 21–amino acid peptide with potent vasoconstrictor properties that binds to specific receptors on vascular endothelial cells to regulate vascular hemostasis. Endothelin receptors have been isolated in amnion, chorion, endometrium, and myometrium,[124,174] and they increase in the myometrium during labor.[174,175] Endothelin promotes uterine contractility directly by increasing intracellular calcium concentrations[124,176] and indirectly by stimulating prostaglandin production by the decidua and fetal membranes.[174]

Epidermal Growth Factor. Epidermal growth factor (EGF) is a ubiquitous growth factor that plays an important role in the regulation of cell growth, proliferation, and differentiation. It acts by binding to specific cell-surface tyrosine-kinase receptors that have been identified also in decidua and myometrium, and it appears to be upregulated by estrogen.[124] EGF appears to promote uterine contractility directly by increasing intracellular calcium concentrations[177] and indirectly by mobilizing arachidonic acid and increasing the synthesis and release of prostaglandins by the decidua and fetal membranes.[174]

TABLE 5-1 ENDOGENOUS AND EXOGENOUS FACTORS AFFECTING MYOMETRIAL CONTRACTILITY DURING LABOR

Uterine Stimulants	
Endogenous	Exogenous
Oxytocin	Oxytocin
Prostaglandins	Prostaglandins
Endothelin	
Epidermal growth factor	
Uterine Relaxants	
Endogenous	Exogenous
Relaxin	β-Adrenergic agonists (ritodrine hydrochloride, terbutaline sulfate, salbutamol, fenoterol)
Nitric oxide	Oxytocin receptor antagonist (atosiban)
L-Arginine	Magnesium sulfate
Magnesium	Calcium channel blockers (nifedipine, nitrendipine, diltiazem, verapamil)
Corticotropin-releasing hormone	Prostaglandin inhibitors (indomethacin)
Parathyroid hormone–related protein	Phosphodiesterase inhibitor (aminophylline)
Calcitonin gene–related peptide	Nitric oxide donor (nitroglycerin, sodium nitroprusside)
Adrenomedulin	
Progesterone	

Uterine Relaxants

A number of endogenous uterine relaxants have been described (see Table 5-1), although their role in labor and delivery are not well understood.

Relaxin. Relaxin is secreted by the corpus luteum, placenta, and myometrium, and relaxin binding sites have been identified on myometrial cells.[178] Relaxin acts in several ways to inhibit myometrial contractile activity: it decreases intracellular calcium concentrations by promoting calcium efflux and inhibiting agonist-mediated activation of calcium channels, and it directly inhibits MLCK phosphorylation.[138,149,178] Unfortunately, exogenous administration of relaxin has not been shown to consistently inhibit uterine contractile activity.[179]

Parathyroid Hormone–Related Protein. Parathyroid hormone–related protein (PTHrP) is produced by many tissues, and it has several functions both during development and in adult tissues, including regulation of vascular tone, bone remodeling, placental calcium transport, and myometrial relaxation. In rat myometrium, levels of PTHrP mRNA increase during late gestation and are higher in gravid than in nongravid myometrium.[180] In pregnant rats, administration of PTHrP-(1-34) inhibits spontaneous contractions in the longitudinal layer of the myometrium; in nonpregnant rats, PTHrP-(1-34) inhibits both oxytocin- and acetylcholine-stimulated uterine contractions[181,182] and delays but does not completely abrogate the increase in connexin 43 and oxytocin receptor gene expression.[183] PTHrP-(1-34) has been shown to exert a significant relaxant effect on human myometrium collected from late gestation tissues obtained before but not after the onset of labor.[184] Taken together, these data suggest that the onset of labor is associated with a removal of the ability of PTHrP to exert its myometrial relaxant effect.

Calcitonin Gene-Related Peptide and Adrenomedullin. Circulating levels of calcitonin gene–related peptide (CGRP) and adrenomedullin are increased during pregnancy, and both have been implicated in the maintenance of myometrial quiescence throughout gestation.[185-187] CGRP has been shown to inhibit myometrial contractility in rats,[185] humans,[188] and mice[189] during pregnancy. However, this effect disappears after the onset of labor, suggesting that progesterone may be required to mediate CGRP activity.[185] Adrenomedullin has been shown to inhibit spontaneous as well as bradykinin- and galanin-induced uterine contractions in rats,[186,190] but its role in human pregnancy is not well established.

Nitric Oxide. Nitric oxide and its substrate, L-arginine, as well as nitric oxide donors (such as sodium nitroprusside) have been shown to cause relaxation of myometrial contractile activity both in vitro and in vivo, and this effect is reversed by the nitric oxide synthase inhibitor, L-nitro-arginine methyl ester (L-NAME).[191] Nitric oxide activates the guanylate cyclase pathway leading to the production of cyclic guanosine monophosphate (cGMP), which decreases intracellular calcium concentrations and interferes with myosin light chain phosphorylation.[192,193]

Magnesium. Magnesium is present in the extracellular fluid of the myometrium in very high concentrations (10 nM), which results in increased intracellular magnesium levels, inhibition of calcium entry into myometrial cells via L- and T-type voltage-operated calcium channels, and enhanced sensitivity of potassium channels,[138,149] all of which lead to hyperpolarization and myometrial cell relaxation. Moreover, because they are both cations, magnesium competes with calcium within the cell for calmodulin binding, resulting in decreased affinity of calmodulin complexes for MLCK, which further favors myometrial relaxation.[194]

Non-naturally Occurring Uterine Relaxants. In addition to naturally occurring uterine relaxants, a number of such agents have been developed in an attempt to stop preterm labor (see Table 5-1). Unfortunately, the ability of these tocolytic agents to prevent preterm birth has been largely disappointing.[26]

β_2-Adrenergic receptor agonists act through specific receptors on myometrial cells to activate cAMP-dependent protein kinase A, which inhibits myosin light-chain phosphorylation[195] and decreases intracellular calcium concentrations,[138,149] thereby leading to myometrial relaxation.

Synthetic competitive *oxytocin receptor antagonists* such as atosiban (which has mixed vasopressin and oxytocin receptor specificity) inhibit uterine contractility both in vitro and in vivo.[196-198] The relative absence of oxytocin receptors in other organ systems suggests that such agents should have few side effects, and this has been borne out by a number of clinical trials.[199-201]

Calcium channel blockers function primarily by inhibiting the entry of calcium ions via voltage-dependent L-type calcium channels, which causes uterine relaxation but can also have adverse effects on the atrioventricular conduction pathway in the heart.

Prostaglandin synthesis inhibitors inactivate the cyclooxygenase enzyme responsible for the conversion of arachidonic acid to the intermediate metabolite (PGH_2), which is subsequently converted to PGE_2 and $PGF_{2\alpha}$. Aspirin causes irreversible acetylation of the cyclooxygenase enzyme, whereas indomethacin is a competitive (reversible) inhibitor. Although relatively effective, the adverse effects of these agents on the developing fetus (including premature closure of the ductus arteriosus and persistent pulmonary hypertension) have significantly limited their use. Moreover, these adverse effects can be seen with both nonselective cyclooxygenase inhibitors (such as indomethacin) and those that are selective for the inducible isoform, cyclooxygenase-2 (meloxicam, celecoxib).

Achieving a Successful Delivery

Labor is not a passive process in which uterine contractions push a rigid object through a fixed aperture. The ability of the fetus to successfully negotiate the pelvis during delivery depends on the complex interaction of three critical variables: the forces generated by the uterine musculature (the powers), the size and orientation of the fetus (the passenger), and the size, shape, and resistance of the bony pelvis and soft tissues of the pelvic floor (the passage). Because of the asymmetry in the shape of both the fetal head and the maternal pelvis, the fetus needs to undergo a series of orchestrated rotations (referred to as the cardinal movements) to allow it to negotiate the birth canal successfully. Further discussion of the mechanics of labor and delivery are beyond the scope of this chapter, but they have been reviewed in detail elsewhere.[166] Suffice it to say, the timely onset of labor does not guarantee an uneventful delivery and a healthy, undamaged child.

Conclusions

Labor is a physiologic and continuous process. The factors responsible for the onset and maintenance of normal labor at term are not completely understood and continue to be actively investigated. A better understanding of the mechanisms responsible for the onset of labor at term will further our knowledge about disorders of parturition, such as preterm and prolonged (post-term) labor, and will improve our ability to secure a successful pregnancy outcome.

References

1. Katzenellenbogen BS, Bhakoo HS, Ferguson ER, et al: Estrogen and antiestrogen action in reproductive tissues and tumors. Rec Prog Horm Res 35:259-300, 1979.
2. Danforth DN: The fibrous nature of the human cervix and its relation to the isthmic segment in the gravid and non-gravid uteri. Am J Obstet Gynecol 53:541, 1947.
3. Assali NS, Rauramo I, Peltonen T: Measurement of uterine blood low and uterine metabolism. Am J Obstet Gynecol 79:86-98, 1960.
4. Rekonen A, Luotola H, Pitkanen M, et al: Measurement of intervillous and myometrial blood flow by an intravenous 133Xe method. BJOG 83:723-728, 1976.
5. Makowski EL, Meschia G, Droegemueller W, Battaglia FC: Distribution of uterine blood flow in the pregnant sheep. Am J Obstet Gynecol 101:409-412, 1968.
6. Resnik R, Killam AP, Battaglia FC, et al: The stimulation of uterine blood flow by various estrogens. Endocrinology 94:1192-1196, 1974.
7. Cullinan-Bove K, Koos RD: Vascular endothelial growth factor/vascular permeability factor expression in the rat uterus: Rapid stimulation by estrogen correlates with estrogen induced increases in uterine capillary permeability and growth. Endocrinology 133:829-837, 1993.
8. Rosenfeld CR: Consideration of the uteroplacental circulation in intrauterine growth. Semin Perinatol 8:42-51, 1984.
9. Magness RR, Rosenfeld CR, Hassan A, Shaul PW. Endothelial vasodilator production by uterine and systemic arteries: I. Effects of ANG II on PGI2 and NO in pregnancy. Am J Physiol 270:1914-1923, 1996.
10. Magness RR, Shaw CE, Phernetton TM, et al: Endothelial vasodilator production by uterine and systemic arteries: II. Pregnancy effects on NO synthase expression. Am J Physiol 272:1730-1740, 1997.
11. Bird IM, Sullivan JA, Di T, et al: Pregnancy-dependent changes in cell signaling underlie changes in differential control of vasodilator production in uterine artery endothelial cells. Endocrinology 141:1107-1117, 2000.
12. Sladek SM, Magness RR, Conrad KP: Nitric oxide in pregnancy. Am J Physiol 272:441-463, 1997.
13. Rechberger T, Woessner JF Jr: Collagenase, its inhibitors and decorin in the lower uterine segment in pregnant women. Am J Obstet Gynecol 168:1598-1603, 1993.
14. Leppert PC: Anatomy and physiology of cervical ripening. Clin Obstet Gynecol 38:267-279, 1995.
15. Hwang JJ, Macinga D, Rorke EA: Relaxin modulates human cervical stromal activity. J Clin Endocrinol Metab 81:3379-3384, 1996.
16. Ludmir J, Sehdev HM: Anatomy and physiology of the uterine cervix. Clin Obstet Gynecol 43:433-439, 2000.
17. Winkler M, Rath W: Changes in the cervical extracellular matrix during pregnancy and parturition. J Perinat Med 27:45-60, 1999.
18. Wen SW, Smith G, Yang Q, Walker M: Epidemiology of preterm birth and neonatal outcome. Semin Fetal Neonatal Med 9:429-435, 2004.
19. American College of Obstetricians and Gynecologists: Management of postterm pregnancy. ACOG Practice Bulletin no. 55. Obstet Gynecol 104:639-466, 2004.
20. Thorburn GD, Challis JRG, Robinson JS: The endocrinology of parturition. In Wynn RM (ed): Cellular Biology of the Uterus. New York, Plenum Press, 1977, p 653.
21. Casey LM, MacDonald PC: The initiation of labor in women: Regulation of phospholipid and arachidonic acid metabolism and of prostaglandin production. Semin Perinatol 10:270, 1986.
22. Liggins GC: The onset of labour: An overview. In McNellis D, Challis JRG, MacDonald PC, et al (eds): The onset of labour: Cellular and integrative

mechanisms. A National Institute of Child Health and Human Development Research Planning Workshop (Nov 29-Dec 1, 1987). Ithaca, NY, Perinatology Press, 1988, pp 1-3.
23. Liggins GC: Initiation of labor. Biol Neonate 55:366-394, 1989.
24. Challis JRG, Gibb W: Control of parturition. Prenat Neonatal Med 1:283-291, 1996.
25. Nathanielsz PW: Comparative studies on the initiation of labor. Eur J Obstet Gynecol Reprod Biol 78:127-132, 1998.
26. Norwitz ER, Robinson JN, Challis JRG: The control of labor. N Engl J Med 341:660-667, 1999.
27. Challis JRG, Matthews SG, Gibb W, Lye SJ: Endocrine and paracrine regulation of birth at term and preterm. Endocr Rev 21:514-550, 2000.
28. Hilder L, Costeloe K, Thilaganathan B: Prolonged pregnancy: Evaluating gestation-specific risks of fetal and infant mortality. BJOG 105:169-173, 1998.
29. Cotzias CS, Paterson-Brown S, Fisk NM: Prospective risk of unexplained stillbirth in singleton pregnancies at term: Population based analysis. BMJ 1999 319:287-8.
30. Rand L, Robinson JN, Economy KE, Norwitz ER: Post-term induction of labor revisited. Obstet Gynecol 96:779-783, 2000.
31. Iams JD, Goldenberg RL, Mercer BM, et al: The Preterm Prediction Study: Recurrence risk of spontaneous preterm birth. The National Institute of Child Health and Human Development Maternal-Fetal Medicine Units Network. Am J Obstet Gynecol 178:1035-1040, 1998.
32. Winkvist A, Mogren I, Hogberg U: Familial patterns in birth characteristics: Impact on individual and population risks. Int J Epidemiol 27:248-254, 1998.
33. Carmichael SL, Iyasu S, Hatfield-Timajchy K: Cause-specific trends in neonatal mortality among black and white infants, United States, 1980-1995. Matern Child Health J 2:67-76, 1998.
34. Ventura SJ, Bachrach CA: Nonmarital childbearing in the United States, 1940-99. Natl Vital Stat Rep 48:1-10, 2000.
35. Blackmore CA, Ferre CD, Rowley DL, et al: Is race a risk factor or a risk marker for preterm delivery? Ethn Dis 3:372-377, 1993.
36. Blackmore-Prince C, Kieke B Jr, Kugaraj KA, et al: Racial differences in the patterns of singleton preterm delivery in the 1988 National Maternal and Infant Health Survey. Matern Child Health J 3:189-197, 1999.
37. Ekwo E, Moawad A: The risk for recurrence of premature births to African-American and white women. J Assoc Acad Minor Phys 9:16-21, 1998.
38. Mercer BM, Goldenberg RL, Moawad AH, et al: The preterm prediction study: Effect of gestational age and cause of preterm birth on subsequent obstetric outcome. The National Institute of Child Health and Human Development Maternal-Fetal Medicine Units Network. Am J Obstet Gynecol 181:1216-1221, 1999.
39. Ananth CV, Getahun D, Peltier MR, et al: Recurrence of spontaneous versus medically indicated preterm birth. Am J Obstet Gynecol 195:643-650, 2006.
40. Getahun D, Ananth CV, Selvam N, Demissie K: Adverse perinatal outcomes among interracial couples in the United States. Obstet Gynecol 106:81-88, 2005.
41. Esplin MS: Preterm birth: A review of genetic factors and future directions for genetic study. Obstet Gynecol Surv 61:800-806, 2006.
42. Gibson CS, MacLennan AH, Dekker GA, et al: Genetic polymorphisms and spontaneous preterm birth. Obstet Gynecol 109:384-391, 2007.
43. Menon R, Forunato SJ, Thorsen P, Williams S: Genetic associations in preterm birth: A primer of marker selection, study design, and data analysis. J Soc Gynecol Investig 13:531-541, 2006.
44. Genç MR, Vardhana S, Delaney ML, et al, MAP Study Group: TNF-308G>A polymorphism influences the TNF-alpha response to altered vaginal flora. Eur J Obstet Gynecol Reprod Biol 134:188-191, 2007.
45. Macones GA, Parry S, Elkousy M, et al: A polymorphism in the promoter region of TNF and bacterial vaginosis: Preliminary evidence of gene-environment interaction in the etiology of spontaneous preterm birth. Am J Obstet Gynecol 190:1504-1508, 2004.
46. Nguyen DP, Genç MR, Vardhana S, et al: Ethnic differences of polymorphisms in cytokine and innate immune system genes in pregnant women. Obstet Gynecol 104:293-300, 2004.
47. Liggins GC, Thorburn GD: Initiation of parturition. In Lamming GE (ed): Marshall's Physiology of Reproduction. London, Chapman & Hall, 1994, pp 863.
48. Matthews SG, Challis JRG: Regulation of the hypothalamo-pituitary-adrenocortical axis in fetal sheep. Trends Endocrinol Metab 7:239-246, 1996.
49. Liggins GC, Fairclough RJ, Grieves SA, et al: The mechanism of initiation of parturition in the ewe. Recent Prog Horm Res 1973 29:111-59.
50. Flint APF, Anderson ABM, Steele PA, Turnbull AC: The mechanism by which fetal cortisol controls the onset of parturition in the sheep. Biochem Soc Trans 3:1189-1194, 1975.
51. Condon JC, Jeyasuria P, Faust JM, Mendelson CR: Surfactant protein secreted by the maturing mouse fetal lung acts as a hormone that signals the initiation of parturition. Proc Natl Acad Sci U S A 101:4978-4983, 2004.
52. Myers DA, Nathanielsz PW: Biologic basis of term and preterm labor. Clin Perinatol 20:9-28, 1993.
53. Nathanielsz PW, Giussani DA, Wu WX: Stimulation of the switch in myometrial activity from contractures to contractions in the pregnant sheep and nonhuman primate. Equine Vet J 24:83-88, 1997.
54. Challis JRG: Characteristics of parturition. In Creasy RK, Resnick R (eds): Maternal-Fetal Medicine: Principles and Practice, 3rd ed. Philadelphia, WB Saunders, 1994, p 482.
55. Madden JD, Gant NF, MacDonald PC: Study of the kinetics of conversion of maternal plasma dehydroisoandrosterone sulfate to 16 alpha-hydroxydehydroisoandrosterone sulfate, estradiol, and estriol. Am J Obstet Gynecol 132:392-395, 1978.
56. Bloomfield FH, Oliver MH, Hawkins P, et al: A periconceptual nutritional origin for noninfectious preterm birth. Science 300:606, 2003.
57. Bloomfield FH, Oliver MH, Hawkins P, et al: Periconceptional undernutrition in sheep accelerates maturation of the fetal hypothalamic-pituitary-adrenal axis in late gestation. Endocrinology 145:4278-4285, 2004.
58. McLean M, Bisits A, Davies J, et al: A placental clock controlling the length of human pregnancy. Nat Med 1:460-463, 1995.
59. Goland RS, Wardlaw SL, Stark RI, et al: High levels of corticotropin releasing hormone immunoreactivity in maternal and fetal plasma during pregnancy. J Clin Endocrinol Metab 63:1199-203, 1986.
60. King BR, Smith R, Nicholson RC: The regulation of human corticotrophin-releasing hormone gene expression in the placenta. Peptides 22:1941-1947, 2001.
61. Hobel CJ, Arora CP, Korst LM: Corticotrophin-releasing hormone and CRH-binding protein: Differences between patients at risk for preterm birth and hypertension. Ann N Y Acad Sci 897:54-65, 1999.
62. Smith R, Mesiano S, Chan EC, et al: Corticotropin-releasing hormone directly and preferentially stimulates dehydroepiandrosterone sulfate secretion by human fetal adrenal cortical cells. J Clin Endocrinol Metab 83:2916-2920, 1998.
63. Chakravorty A, Mesiano S, Jaffe RB: Corticotropin-releasing hormone stimulates P450 17alpha-hydroxylase/17,20-lyase in human fetal adrenal cells via protein kinase C. J Clin Endocrinol Metab 84:3732-3738, 1999.
64. Hobel CJ, Dunkel-Schetter C, Roesch SC, et al: Maternal plasma corticotropin-releasing hormone associated with stress at 20 weeks' gestation in pregnancies ending in preterm delivery. Am J Obstet Gynecol 180:257-263, 1999.
65. Coleman MA, France JT, Schellenberg JC, et al: Corticotropin-releasing hormone, corticotropin-releasing hormone-binding protein, and activin A in maternal serum: Prediction of preterm delivery and response to glucocorticoids in women with symptoms of preterm labor. Am J Obstet Gynecol 183:643-648, 2000.
66. Inder WJ, Prickett TC, Ellis MJ, et al: The utility of plasma CRH as a predictor of preterm delivery. J Clin Endocrinol Metab 86:5706-5710, 2001.
67. McLean M, Smith R: Corticotropin-releasing hormone and human parturition. Reproduction 121:493-501, 2001.
68. Hillhouse EW, Grammatopoulos DK: Role of stress peptides during human pregnancy and labour. Reproduction 124:323-329, 2002.

69. McKeown KJ, Challis JRG: Regulation of expression of 15-hydroxyprostaglandin dehydrogenase by corticotrophin-releasing hormone through a calcium-dependent pathway in human chorion trophoblast cells. J Clin Endocrinol Metab 88:1737-1741, 2003.
70. Jones SA, Challis JRG: Local stimulation of prostaglandin production by corticotropin releasing hormone in human fetal membranes and placenta. Biochem Biophys Res Commun 159:192-199, 1989.
71. Benedetto C, Petraglia F, Marozio L, et al: Corticotropin-releasing hormone increases prostaglandin $F_{2\alpha}$ activity on human myometrium in vitro. Am J Obstet Gynecol 171:126-131, 1994.
72. Patel FA, Clifton VL, Chwalisz K, Challis JR: Steroid regulation of prostaglandin dehydrogenase activity and expression in human term placenta and chorio-decidua in relation to labor. J Clin Endocrinol Metab 84:291-299, 1999.
73. Patel FA, Challis JRG: Cortisol progesterone antagonism in the regulation of 15-hydroxy prostaglandin dehydrogenase activity and mRNA levels in human chorion and placental trophoblast cells at term. J Clin Endocrinol Metab 87:700-708, 2002.
74. Florio P, Lobardo M, Gallo R, et al: Activin A, corticotropin-releasing factor and prostaglandin F2 alpha increase immunoreactive oxytocin release from cultured human placental cells. Placenta 17:307-311, 1996.
75. Sun Y, Yang K, Challis JR: Regulation of 11beta-hydroxysteroid dehydrogenase type 2 by progesterone, estrogen, and the cyclic adenosine 5′-monophosphate pathway in cultured human placental and chorionic trophoblasts. Biol Reprod 58:1379-1384, 1998.
76. Alfaidy N, Xiong ZG, Myatt L, et al: Prostaglandin F2alpha potentiates cortisol production by stimulating 11beta-hydroxysteroid dehydrogenase 1: A novel feedback loop that may contribute to human labor. J Clin Endocrinol Metab 86:5585-5592, 2001.
77. Alfaidy N, Gupta S, DeMarco C, et al: Oxygen regulation of placental 11-beta-hydroxysteroid dehydrogenase-2: Physiological and pathological implications. J Clin Endocrinol Metab 87:4797-4805, 2002.
78. Challis JR, Sloboda DM, Alfaidy N, et al: Prostaglandins and mechanisms of preterm birth. Reproduction 124:1-17, 2002.
79. Csapo AI, Pulkkinen M: Indispensability of the human corpus luteum in the maintenance of early pregnancy: Luteectomy evidence. Obstet Gynecol Surv 33:69-81, 1978.
80. Peyron R, Aubeny E, Targosz V, et al: Early termination of pregnancy with mifepristone (RU 486) and the orally active prostaglandin misoprostol. N Engl J Med 328:1509-1513, 1993.
81. Hanssens MC, Selby C, Symonds EM: Sex steroid hormone concentrations in preterm labour and the outcome of treatment with ritodrine. BJOG 92:698-702, 1985.
82. Csapo AI, Pinto-Dantas CA: The effect of progesterone on the human uterus. Proc Natl Acad Sci U S A 54:1069-1076, 1965.
83. Csapo AI, Pohanka O, Kaihola HL: Progesterone deficiency and premature labour. BMJ 1:137-140, 1974.
84. Cousins LM, Hobel CJ, Chang RJ, et al: Serum progesterone and estradiol-17beta levels in premature and term labor. Am J Obstet Gynecol 127:612-615, 1977.
85. Romero R, Scoccia B, Mazor M, et al: Evidence for a local change in the progesterone/estrogen ratio in human parturition. Am J Obstet Gynecol 159:657-660, 1988.
86. Neilson JP: Mifepristone for induction of labour. Cochrane Database Syst Rev (4):CD002865, 2000.
87. Da Fonseca EB, Bittar RE, Carvalho MH, Zugaib M: Prophylactic administration of progesterone by vaginal suppository to reduce the incidence of spontaneous preterm birth in women at increased risk: A randomized placebo-controlled double-blind study. Am J Obstet Gynecol 188:419-424, 2003.
88. Meis PJ, Klebanoff M, Thom E, et al: Prevention of recurrent preterm delivery by 17 alpha-hydroxyprogesterone caproate. N Engl J Med 348:2379-2385, 2003.
89. Kastner P, Krust A, Turcotte B, et al: Two distinct estrogen-regulated promoters generate transcripts encoding the two functionally different human progesterone receptor forms A and B. EMBO J 9:1603-1614, 1990.
90. Sartorius CA, Melville MY, Hovland AR, et al: A third transactivation function (AF3) of human progesterone receptors located in the unique N-terminal segment of the B-isoform. Mol Endocrinol 8:1347-1360, 1994.
91. Pieber D, Allport VC, Hills F, et al: Interactions between progesterone receptor isoforms in myometrial cells in human labour. Mol Hum Reprod 7:875-879, 2001.
92. Haluska GJ, Wells TR, Hirst JJ, et al: Progesterone receptor localization and isoforms in myometrium, decidua, and fetal membranes from rhesus macaques: Evidence for functional progesterone withdrawal at parturition. J Soc Gynecol Investig 9:125-136, 2002.
93. Mesiano S, Chan EC, Fitter JT, et al: Progesterone withdrawal and estrogen activation in human parturition are coordinated by progesterone receptor A expression in the myometrium. J Clin Endocrinol Metab 87:2924-2930, 2002.
94. Mesiano S: Myometrial progesterone responsiveness and the control of human parturition. J Soc Gynecol Investig 11:193-202, 2004.
95. Madsen G, Zakar T, Ku CY, et al: Prostaglandins differentially modulate progesterone receptor-A and -B expression in human myometrial cells: Evidence for prostaglandin-induced functional progesterone withdrawal. J Clin Endocrinol Metab 89:1010-1013, 2004
96. Ni X, Hou Y, Yang R, et al: Progesterone receptors A and B differentially modulate corticotropin-releasing hormone gene expression through a cAMP regulatory element. Cell Mol Life Sci 61:1114-1122, 2004.
97. Stjernholm-Vladic Y, Wang H, Stygar D, et al: Differential regulation of the progesterone receptor A and B in the human uterine cervix at parturition. Gynecol Endocrinol 18:41-46, 2004.
98. Oh SY, Kim CJ, Park I, et al: Progesterone receptor isoform (A/B) ratio of human fetal membranes increases during term parturition. Am J Obstet Gynecol 193:1156-1160, 2005.
99. Condon JC, Hardy DB, Kovaric K, Mendelson CR: Up-regulation of the progesterone receptor (PR)-C isoform in laboring myometrium by activation of nuclear factor-kappaB may contribute to the onset of labor through inhibition of PR function. Mol Endocrinol 20:764-775, 2006.
100. Allport VC, Pieber D, Slater DM, et al: Human labour is associated with nuclear factor-kappaB activity which mediates cyclo-oxygenase-2 expression and is involved with the "functional progesterone withdrawal." Mol Hum Reprod 7:581-586, 2001.
101. Norwitz ER, Wilson T: Secretory component: A potential regulator of endometrial-decidual prostaglandin production in early human pregnancy. Am J Obstet Gynecol 183:108-117, 2000.
102. Shields AD, Wright J, Paonessa DJ, et al: Progesterone modulation of inflammatory cytokine production in a fetoplacental artery explant model. Am J Obstet Gynecol 193:1144-1148, 2005.
103. Shynlova O, Dorogin A, Lye S: Monocyte chemoattractant protein-1 integrates mechanical and endocrine signals that mediate term and preterm labor. Abstract 539, Society for Gynecologic Investigation, Reno, NV, 2007.
104. Henderson D, Wilson T: Reduced binding of progesterone receptor to its nuclear response element after human labor onset. Am J Obstet Gynecol 185:579-585, 2001.
105. Condon JC, Jeyasuria P, Faust JM, et al: A decline in the levels of progesterone receptor coactivators in the pregnant uterus at term may antagonize progesterone receptor function and contribute to the initiation of parturition. Proc Natl Acad Sci U S A 100:9518-9523, 2003.
106. Dong X, Shylnova O, Challis JR, Lye SJ: Identification and characterization of the protein-associated splicing factor as a negative co-regulator of the progesterone receptor. J Biol Chem 280:13329-13340, 2005.
107. Tyson-Capper AJ, Robson SC: PSF and the regulation of the progesterone receptor gene in the human myometrium during pregnancy. Abstract 541, Society for Gynecologic Investigation, Reno, NV, 2007.
108. Karalis K, Goodwin G, Majzoub JA: Cortisol blockade of progesterone: A possible molecular mechanism involved in the initiation of human labor. Nat Med 2:556-560, 1996.
109. Grazzini E, Guillon G, Mouillac B, Zingg HH: Inhibition of oxytocin receptor function by direct binding of progesterone. Nature 392:509-512, 1998.

110. Astle S, Slater DM, Thornton S: The involvement of progesterone in the onset of human labour. Eur J Obstet Gynecol Reprod Biol 108:177-181, 2003.
111. Astle S, Khan RN, Thornton S: The effects of a progesterone metabolite, 5 beta-dihydroprogesterone, on oxytocin receptor binding in human myometrial membranes. BJOG 110:589-592, 2003.
112. Mecenas CA, Giussani DA, Owiny JR, et al: Production of premature delivery in pregnant rhesus monkeys by androstenedione infusion. Nat Med 2:443-448, 1996.
113. Figueroa JP, Honnebier MBOM, Binienda Z, et al: Effect of 48 hour intravenous Δ 4-androstenedione infusion on pregnant rhesus monkeys in the last third of gestation: Changes in maternal plasma estradiol concentrations and myometrial contractility. Am J Obstet Gynecol 161:481-486, 1989.
114. Nathanielsz PW, Jenkins SL, Tame JD, et al: Local paracrine effects of estradiol are central to parturition in the rhesus monkey. Nat Med 4:456-459, 1998.
115. Leonhardt SA, Boonyaratanakornkit V, Edwards DP: Progesterone receptor transcription and non-transcription signaling mechanisms. Steroids 68:761-770, 2003.
116. Cermik D, Karaca M, Taylor HS: HOXA10 expression is repressed by progesterone in the myometrium: Differential tissue-specific regulation of HOX gene expression in the reproductive tract. J Clin Endocrinol Metab 86:3387-3392, 2001.
117. Abel MH, Kelley RW: Differential production of prostaglandins within the human uterus. Prostaglandins 18:821-828, 1979.
118. Gibb W: The role of prostaglandins in human parturition. Ann Med 30:235-241, 1998.
119. Embrey M: PGE compounds for induction of labour and abortion. Ann N Y Acad Sci 180:518-523, 1971.
120. Casey ML, MacDonald PC: Biomolecular processes in the initiation of parturition: Decidual activation. Clin Obstet Gynecol 31:533-552, 1988.
121. Muglia LJ: Genetic analysis of fetal development and parturition control in the mouse. Pediatr Res 47:437-443, 2000.
122. Olson DM, Mijovic JE, Sadowsky DW: Control of human parturition. Semin Perinatol 19:52-63, 1995.
123. Garrioch DB: The effect of indomethacin on spontaneous activity in the isolated human myometrium and on the response to oxytocin and prostaglandin. BJOG 85:47-52, 1978.
124. Fuchs AR: Plasma membrane receptors regulating myometrial contractility and their hormonal modulation. Semin Perinatol 19:15-30, 1995.
125. Phaneuf S, Europe-Finner GN, Varnev M, et al: Oxytocin-stimulated phosphoinositide hydrolysis in human myometrial cells: Involvement of pertussis toxin-sensitive and -insensitive G-proteins. J Endocrinol 136:497-509, 1993.
126. Molnar M, Hertelendy F: Regulation of intracellular free calcium in human myometrial cells by prostaglandin F2 alpha: Comparison with oxytocin. J Clin Endocrinol Metab 71:1243-1250, 1990.
127. Keirse MJNC, Turnbull AC: E prostaglandins in amniotic fluid during late pregnancy and labour. J Obstet Gynaecol Br Commonw 80:970-973, 1973.
128. Romero R, Munoz H, Gomez R, et al: Increase in prostaglandin bioavailability precedes the onset of human parturition. Prostaglandins Leukot Essent Fatty Acids 54:187-191, 1996.
129. Sangha RK, Walton JC, Ensor CM, et al: Immunohistochemical localization, messenger ribonucleic acid abundance, and activity of 15-hydroxyprostaglandin dehydrogenase in placenta and fetal membranes during term and preterm labor. J Clin Endocrinol Metab 78:982-989, 1994.
130. van Meir CA, Matthews SG, Keirse MJ, et al: 15-hydroxy-prostaglandin dehydrogenase: Implications in preterm labor with and without ascending infection. J Clin Endocrinol Metab 82:969-976, 1997.
131. Giannoulias D, Patel FA, Holloway ACL, et al: Differential changes in 15-hydroxyprostaglandin dehydrogenase and prostaglandin H synthase (types I and II) in human pregnant myometrium. J Clin Endocrinol Metab 87:1345-1352, 2002.
132. Zeeman GG, Khan-Dawood FS, Dawood MY: Oxytocin and its receptor in pregnancy and parturition: Current concepts and clinical implications. Obstet Gynecol 89:873-883, 1997.
133. Fuchs A-R, Fuchs F: Endocrinology of human parturition: A review. BJOG 91:948-967, 1984.
134. Dawood MY, Wang CF, Gupta R, Fuchs F: Fetal contribution to oxytocin in human labor. Obstet Gynecol 52:205-209, 1978.
135. Fuchs AR, Fuchs F, Husslein P, et al: Oxytocin receptors and human parturition: A dual role for oxytocin in the initiation of labor. Science 215:1396-1398, 1982.
136. Fuchs AR, Fuchs F, Husslein P, Soloff MS: Oxytocin receptors in the human uterus during pregnancy and parturition. Am J Obstet Gynecol 150:734-741, 1984.
137. Husslein P, Fuchs A-R, Fuchs F: Oxytocin and the initiation of human parturition: I. Prostaglandin release during induction of labor with oxytocin. Am J Obstet Gynecol 141:688-693, 1981.
138. Sanborn BM: Hormones and calcium: Mechanisms controlling uterine smooth muscle contractile activity. Exp Physiol 86:223-237, 2001.
139. Yang M, Gupta A, Shlykov SG, et al: Multiple Trp isoforms implicated in capacitative calcium entry are expressed in human pregnant myometrium and myometrial cells. Biol Reprod 67:988-994, 2002.
140. Fuchs A-R, Husslein P, Fuchs F: Oxytocin and the initiation of human parturition: II. Stimulation of prostaglandin production in human decidua by oxytocin. Am J Obstet Gynecol 141:694-697, 1981.
141. Garfield RE, Sims S, Daniel EE: Gap junctions: Their presence and necessity in myometrium during parturition. Science 198:958-960, 1977.
142. Wolfs GM, van Leeuwen M: Electromyographic observations on the human uterus during labour. Acta Obstet Gynecol Scand 90:1-61, 1979.
143. Kumar D, Barnes AC: Studies in human myometrium during pregnancy: II. Resting membrane potential and comparative electrolyte levels. Am J Obstet Gynecol 82:736-741, 1961.
144. Kuriyama H, Csapo A: A study of the parturient uterus with the microelectrode technique. Endocrinology 68:1010-1025, 1961.
145. Wray S, Jones K, Kupittayanant S, et al: Calcium signaling and uterine contractility. J Soc Gynecol Investig 10:252-264, 2003.
146. Carvajal JA, Thompson LP, Weiner CP: Chorion-induced myometrial relaxation is mediated by large-conductance Ca2+-activated K+ channel opening in the guinea pig. Am J Obstet Gynecol 188:84-91, 2003.
147. Woodcock NA, Taylor CW, Thornton S: Effect of an oxytocin receptor antagonist and rho kinase inhibitor on the $[Ca^{++}]_i$ sensitivity of human myometrium. Am J Obstet Gynecol 190:222-228, 2004.
148. Papandreou L, Chasiotis G, Seferiadis K, et al: Calcium levels during the initiation of labor. Eur J Obstet Gynecol Reprod Biol 115:17-22, 2004.
149. Sanborn BM: Ion channels and the control of myometrial electrical activity. Semin Perinatol 19:31-40, 1995.
150. Kao CY: Long-term observations of spontaneous electrical activity of the uterine smooth muscle. Am J Physiol 196:343-350, 1959.
151. Buhimschi C, Buhimschi IA, Malinow AM, et al: The forces of labour. Fetal Matern Med Rev 14:273-307, 2003.
152. Arulkumaran S, Gibb DM, Lun KC, et al: The effect of parity on uterine activity in labour. BJOG 91:843-848, 1984.
153. Jiang H, Stephens NL: Calcium and smooth muscle contraction. Mol Cell Biochem 135:1-9, 1994.
154. Somlyo AP, Somlyo AV: Signal transduction and regulation of smooth muscle. Nature 372:231-236, 1994.
155. Word RA: Myosin phosphorylation and the control of myometrial contraction/relaxation. Semin Perinatol 19:3-14, 1995.
156. Gallagher PJ, Herring BP, Stull JT: Myosin light chain kinases. J Muscle Res Cell Motil 18:1-16, 1997.
157. MacKenzie LW, Word RA, Casey ML, Stull JT: Myosin light chain phosphorylation in human myometrial smooth muscle cells. Am J Physiol 258:92-98, 1990.
158. Word RA, Tang DC, Kamm KE: Activation properties of myosin light chain kinase during contraction/relaxation cycles of tonic and phasic smooth muscles. J Biol Chem 269:21596-21602, 1994.
159. Savineau JP, Marthan R: Modulation of the calcium sensitivity of the smooth muscle contractile apparatus: Molecular mechanisms, pharmaco-

logical and pathophysiological implications. Fundam Clin Pharmacol 11:289-299, 1997.
160. Hartshorne DJ: Myosin phosphatase: Subunits and interactions. Acta Physiol Scand 164:483-493, 1998.
161. Hartshorne DJ, Ito M, Erdodi F: Myosin light chain phosphatase: Subunit composition, interactions and regulation. J Muscle Res Cell Motil 19:325-341, 1998.
162. Somlyo AP, Somlyo AV: Signal transduction by G-proteins, rho-kinase and protein phosphatase to smooth muscle and non-muscle myosin II. J Physiol 522:177-185, 2000.
163. Pato MD, Tulloch AG, Walsh MP, Kerc E: Smooth muscle phosphatases: Structure, regulation, and function. Can J Physiol Pharmacol 72:1427-1433, 1994.
164. Word RA, Stull JT, Casey ML, Kamm KE: Contractile elements and myosin light chain phosphorylation in myometrial tissue from nonpregnant and pregnant women. J Clin Invest 92:29-37, 1993.
165. Pauerstein CJ, Zauder HL: Autonomic innervation, sex steroids and uterine contractility. Obstet Gynecol Surv 25:617-630, 1970.
166. Norwitz ER, Robinson JN, Repke JT: Labor and delivery. In Gabbe SG, Niebyl JR, Simpson JL (eds): Obstetrics: Normal and Problem Pregnancies, 4th ed. Philadelphia, WB Saunders, 2001, pp 353-394.
167. Shynlova O, Oldenhof A, Dorogin A, et al: Myometrial apoptosis: Activation of the caspase cascade in the pregnant rat myometrium at midgestation. Biol Reprod 74:839-849, 2006.
168. Lye SJ, Mitchell J, Nashman NO, et al: Role of mechanical signals in the onset of term and preterm labor. Front Horm Res 27:165-178, 2001.
169. Shynlova O, Tsui P, Dorogin A, et al: Expression and localization of alpha-smooth muscle and gamma-actins in the pregnant rat myometrium. Biol Reprod 73:773-780, 2005.
170. Macphee DJ, Lye SJ: Focal adhesion signaling in the rat myometrium is abruptly terminated with the onset of labor. Endocrinology 141:274-283, 2000.
171. Shynlova O, Mitchell JA, Tsampalieros A, et al: Progesterone and gravidity differentially regulate expression of extracellular matrix components in the pregnant rat myometrium. Biol Reprod 70:986-992, 2004.
172. Stevens MY, Challis JR, Lye SJ: Corticotropin-releasing hormone receptor subtype 1 is significantly up-regulated at the time of labor in the human myometrium. J Clin Endocrinol Metab 83:4107-4115, 1998.
173. Myatt L, Lye SJ: Expression, localization and function of prostaglandin receptors in myometrium. Prostaglandins Leukot Essent Fatty Acids 70:137-148, 2004.
174. Yallampalli C: Role of growth factors and cytokines in the control of uterine contractility. In Garfield RE, Tabb TN (eds): Control of Uterine Contractility. Boca Raton, FL, CRC Press, 1994, pp 285-294.
175. Honore JC, Robert B, Vacher-Lavenu MC, et al: Expression of endothelin receptors in human myometrium during pregnancy and in uterine leiomyomas. J Cardiovasc Pharmacol 36:386-389, 2000.
176. Kaya T, Cetin A, Cetin M, Sarioglu Y: Effects of endothelin-1 and calcium channel blockers on contractions in human myometrium. J Reprod Med 44:115-121, 1999.
177. Anwer K, Monga M, Sanborn BM: Epidermal growth factor increases phosphoinositide turnover and intracellular free calcium in an immortalized human myometrial cell line independent of the arachidonic acid metabolic pathway. Am J Obstet Gynecol 174:676-681, 1996.
178. Hollingsworth M, Downing SJ, Cheuk JMS, et al: Pharmacological strategies for uterine relaxation. In Garfield RE, Tabb TN (eds): Control of Uterine Contractility. Boca Raton, FL, CRC Press, 1994, pp 401.
179. Kelly AJ, Kavanagh J, Thomas J: Relaxin for cervical ripening and induction of labour. Cochrane Database Syst Rev (2):CD03103, 2001.
180. Thiede MA, Daifotis AG, Weir EC, et al: Intrauterine occupancy controls expression of the parathyroid hormone-related peptide gene in preterm rat myometrium. Proc Natl Acad Sci U S A 87:6969-6973, 1990.
181. Williams ED, Leaver DD, Danks JA, et al: Effect of parathyroid hormone-related protein (PTHrP) on the contractility of the myometrium and localization of PTHrP in the uterus of pregnant rats. J Reprod Fertil 102:209-214, 1994.
182. Barri ME, Abbas SK, Care AD: The effects in the rat of two fragments of parathyroid hormone-related protein on uterine contractions in situ. Exp Physiol 77:481-490, 1992.
183. Mitchell JA, Ting TC, Wong S, et al: Parathyroid hormone-related protein treatment of pregnant rats delays the increase in connexin 43 and oxytocin receptor expression in the myometrium. Biol Reprod 69:556-562, 2003.
184. Slattery MM, O'Leary MJ, Morrison JJ: Effect of parathyroid hormone-related peptide on human and rat myometrial contractility in vitro. Am J Obstet Gynecol 184:625-629, 2001.
185. Dong YL, Gangula PRR, Fang L, et al: Uterine relaxation responses to calcitonin gene-related peptide and calcitonin gene-related peptide receptors decreased during labor in rats. Am J Obstet Gynecol 179:497-506, 1998.
186. Upton PD, Austin C, Taylor GM, et al: Expression of adrenomedullin (ADM) and its binding sites in the rat uterus: Increased number of binding sites and ADM messenger ribonucleic acid in 20-day pregnant rats compared with nonpregnant rats. Endocrinology 138:2508-2514, 1997.
187. Gangula PRR, Wimalawansa SJ, Yallampalli C: Pregnancy and sex steroid hormones enhance circulating calcitonin gene-related peptide levels in rats. Hum Reprod 15:949-953, 2000.
188. Dong YL, Fang L, Kondapaka S, et al: Involvement of calcitonin gene-related peptide in the modulation of human myometrial contractility during pregnancy. J Clin Invest 104:559-565, 1999.
189. Naghashpour M, Dahl G: Relaxation of myometrium by calcitonin gene-related peptide is independent of nitric oxide synthase activity in mouse uterus. Biol Reprod 63:1421-1427, 2000.
190. Yanagita T, Yamamoto R, Sugano T, et al: Adrenomedullin inhibits spontaneous and bradykinin-induced but not oxytocin- or prostaglandin F(2alpha)-induced periodic contraction of rat uterus. Br J Pharmacol 130:1727-1730, 2000.
191. Garfield RE, Ali M, Yallampalli C, Izumi H: Role of gap junctions and nitric oxide in control of myometrial contractility. Semin Perinatol 19:41-51, 1995.
192. Wu X, Somlyo AV, Somlyo AP: Cyclic GMP-dependent stimulation reverses G-protein–coupled inhibition of smooth muscle myosin-light chain phosphatase. Biochem Biophys Res Commun 220:658-663, 1996.
193. Van Riper DA, McDaniel NL, Rembold CM: Myosin light chain kinase phosphorylation in nitrovasodilator-induced swine carotid artery relaxation. Biochim Biophys Acta 1355:323-330, 1997.
194. Ohki S, Ikura M, Zhang M: Identification of magnesium binding sites and the role of magnesium on target recognition by calmodulin. Biochemistry 36:4309-4316,1997.
195. Wen Y, Anwer K, Singh SP, Sanborn BM: Protein kinase-A inhibits phospholipase-C activity and alters protein phosphorylation in rat myometrial plasma membranes. Endocrinology 131:1377-1382, 1992.
196. Goodwin TM, Valenzuela G, Silver H, Creasy G: Dose ranging study of the oxytocin antagonist atosiban in the treatment of preterm labor. Obstet Gynecol 88:331-336, 1996.
197. Buscher U, Chen FC, Riesenkampff E, et al: Effects of oxytocin receptor antagonist atosiban on pregnant myometrium in vitro. Obstet Gynecol 98:117-121, 2001.
198. Wilson RJ, Allen MJ, Nandi M, et al: Spontaneous contractions of myometrium from humans, non-human primate and rodents are sensitive to selective oxytocin receptor antagonism in vitro. BJOG 108:960-966, 2001.
199. European Atosiban Study Group: The oxytocin antagonist atosiban versus the beta-agonist terbutaline in the treatment of preterm labor. A randomized, double-blind, controlled study. Acta Obstet Gynaecol Scand 80:413-422, 2001.
200. French/Australian Atosiban Investigators Group: Treatment of preterm labor with the oxytocin antagonist atosiban: A double-blind, randomized, controlled comparison with salbutamol. J Obstet Gynecol Reprod Biol 98:177-185, 2001.
201. Worldwide Atosiban versus Beta-agonists Study Group: Effectiveness and safety of the oxytocin antagonist atosiban versus beta-adrenergic agonists in the treatment of preterm labour. The Worldwide Atosiban versus Beta-agonists Study Group. BJOG 108:133-142, 2001.

Chapter 6

The Immunology of Pregnancy

Gil Mor, MD, PhD, and Vikki M. Abrahams, PhD

Pregnancy as an Allograft

Cases of recurrent abortion, preeclampsia, or hemolytic disease of the newborn raise the rhetorical question, "Why did your mother reject you?" However, considering that maternal-fetal immune interactions are complex and the number of successful pregnancies is vast, perhaps the more salient question is "Why *didn't* your mother reject you?" More than 50 years ago, the renowned transplant immunologist Sir Peter Medawar proposed a theory as to why the fetus, a semi-allograft, is not rejected by the maternal immune system.[1] He recognized for the first time the unique immunology of the maternal-fetal interface and its potential relevance for transplantation. In his original work, he described the "fetal allograft analogy," in which the fetus is viewed as a semi-allogeneic conceptus (made of paternal antigens and therefore foreign to the maternal immune system) that, by unknown mechanisms, has evaded rejection by the maternal immune system. Subsequent studies demonstrated the presence of an active maternal immune system at the implantation site, and this provided evidence to support Medawar's original notion. As a result, investigators began to pursue the mechanisms by which the fetus might escape such maternal immune surveillance. Moreover, alterations in these pathways in pregnancy complications such as recurrent abortion and preeclampsia, where the immune system is thought to play a central role, have been used as further evidence for the Medawar hypothesis of the semi-allogeneic fetus. As a consequence, since Medawar's original observation, numerous studies have been performed to explain this paradox, many of which have centered on how the fetus and placenta suppress an active and aggressive maternal immune system. The objective of this chapter is to review some of the significant events involved in human implantation as they relate to the interaction between the maternal immune system and the fetus, to challenge some traditional concepts, and to propose a new perspective for the role of the immune system in pregnancy.

Defining the Immunology of Pregnancy

In 1991, Colbern and Main redefined the conceptual framework of reproductive immunology as maternal-placental tolerance rather than a maternal-fetal tolerance, focusing on the interaction between the maternal immune system and the placenta rather than the fetus.[2] The blastocyst in early development divides into two groups of cells: the internal, inner cell mass, which gives rise to the embryo, and the external embryonic trophectoderm, which ultimately produces the placenta and fetal membranes. Cells from the placenta directly interact with the mother's uterine cells and, therefore, the maternal immune system, and these placental cells are able to evade immune rejection. The fetus itself has no direct contact with maternal cells. Moreover, the fetus is known to express paternal major histocompatibility complex (MHC) antigens. Thus, as postulated by Medawar, the fetus would be rejected as a true allograft if removed from its external trophoblast-embedded placental and chorionic "cocoon" and transplanted into the thigh muscle or kidney capsule of the mother.

General Concepts of Immunology

Types of Immune Responses

The immune system eliminates foreign material in two ways: through natural or innate immunity and through adaptive immunity. Innate immunity produces a relatively unsophisticated response that prevents access to the body by potential pathogens. This is a primitive, evolutionarily preserved system that does not require prior exposure to similar pathogens. The primary cell types involved in these responses are phagocytic cells, such as macrophages and granulocytes. These cells express pattern recognition receptors (PRRs) that sense conserved sequences on the surface of microbes, triggering an immune response. As a result, phagocytic cells produce proinflammatory cytokines, release degradative enzymes, generate intense respiratory bursts of free radicals, and ultimately engulf and destroy the invading microorganisms. Thus, the innate immune system provides the first line of defense against invading microbes, and it is critical for priming the adaptive immune response.

Adaptive immunity is an additional, more sophisticated response found in higher forms of species, including humans. Cells of the innate immune system process phagocytosed foreign material and present derived antigens to cells of the adaptive immune system to initiate possible reactions. This immune response is highly specific and normally is potentiated by repeated antigenic encounters. Adaptive immunity consists of two types of immune responses: humoral immunity, in which antibodies are produced; and cellular immunity, which involves infected or foreign cells being lysed by specialized lymphocytes (cytolytic T cells). Adaptive immunity is characterized by an anamnestic response that enables the immune cells to remember the foreign antigenic encounter and react to further exposures to the same antigen faster and more vigorously.

Cytokines and the Immune Response

Immune cells mediate their effects by releasing cytokines, and through these secreted factors, they establish particular microenvironments. In other words, immune cells through their cytokine production may create either a proinflammatory or anti-inflammatory environment. Moreover, the cytokine profile created by immune cells can shape the characteristics of subsequent immune responses. For example, naive T helper lymphocytes (T_H0) originate in the thymus and play a major role in creating specific microenvironments within the periphery, depending on their differentiation status. If a T_H0 cell then differentiates into a T_H1 cell, it secretes interleukin-2 (IL-2) and interferon-γ (INF-γ), setting the scene for a cellular, cytotoxic immune response. On the other hand, T_H2 lymphocytes secrete cytokines, such as IL-4, IL-6, and IL-10, which are predominantly involved in antibody production. Furthermore, the actions of T_H1 and T_H2 cells are closely intertwined, both acting in concert and responding to counter-regulatory effects of their cytokines. Thus, T_H1 cytokines produce proinflammatory cytokines that, although they act to reinforce the cytolytic immune response, also downregulate the production of T_H2-type cytokines.

As will be discussed, the pregnant endometrium is populated by maternal immune cells, both during implantation and throughout gestation. Furthermore, the maternal immune system interacts, at different stages and under various circumstances, with the invading trophoblast. Our objective is to understand the types of interactions that occur and their role in the support of a normal pregnancy. We will summarize some of the main hypotheses proposed to explain the trophoblast-maternal immune interaction.

Maternal Immune Response to the Trophoblast: The Pregnant Uterus as an Immune Privileged Site

Implantation is the process by which the blastocyst becomes intimately connected with the maternal gestational endometrium (i.e., the decidua). During this period, the semi-allogeneic trophoblast comes in direct contact with the maternal uterine and blood-borne immune cells. However, as mentioned, in most cases, fetal rejection by the maternal immune system is prevented by a mechanism or mechanisms as yet undefined, but several have been proposed. We will discuss five of the main ones that endeavor to account for the immune privileged state of the decidua: (1) a mechanical barrier effect of the placenta, (2) systemic suppression of the maternal immune system during pregnancy, (3) a local and systemic cytokine shift from a T_H1 to a T_H2 cytokine profile, (4) the absence of MHC class I molecules on the trophoblast, and (5) (a more recent proposal) local immune suppression mediated by the Fas/FasL system.

The Placenta as a Mechanical Barrier

Until the late 1980s, the most popular of the five theories was that a mechanical barrier formed by the placenta prevented the movement of immune cells in both directions across the maternal-fetal interface. The barrier thus created a state of immunologic ignorance in which fetal antigens were never presented to, and thus never detected by, the maternal immune system. Scientists believed that the barrier, which is formed in the pregnant uterus by the trophoblast and the decidua, prevents the movement of activated, alloreactive, immune cells from the maternal circulation to the fetal side. Similarly, this barrier would isolate the fetus and prevent the escape of fetal cells into the maternal circulation.[3]

Challenging the mechanical barrier theory are studies showing that the trophoblast-decidual interface is less inert or impermeable than first envisioned. Evidence for bidirectional trafficking across the maternal-fetus interface includes the migration of maternal cells into the fetus[3] and the presence of fetal cells in the maternal circulation.[4] This is now known to be the case in most of the body's other immune privileged tissues, including the brain's blood-brain barrier.[4] Indeed, fetal cells are observed in the mother decades after the pregnancy.[5] These cells, like stem cells, have the potential to infiltrate maternal tissues and differentiate into liver cells, muscle, skin, and so on, transforming the mother into a chimera. Originally it was thought that these fetal cells were responsible for triggering autoimmune diseases that more often afflict women.[6] However, more recent studies have demonstrated that the fetal cells may play a role in repairing maternal tissues that are damaged by a pathologic process. In one case study, a woman suffering from hepatitis stopped treatment (against medical advice), yet, despite this, she did well clinically and her disease abated. Moreover, her liver specimen was found to contain male cells that had originated from her previous pregnancies, suggesting that these leftover fetal cells in the mother's circulation produced new liver cells and were, at least in part, responsible for her recovery.[5,7,8]

Systemic Immune Suppression

The second theory postulates that pregnancy is a state of systemic immune suppression, and therefore the maternal immune cells are unable to reject the fetus. This concept has been studied by numerous investigators and has become the conventional wisdom. Indeed, a wide array of factors in human serum have been found to have profound in vitro immunosuppressive activities.[9] However, if we carefully analyze this hypothesis, it is difficult to imagine how, from an evolutionary point of view, pregnancy involves a stage of profound immune suppression. Early humans were not able to wash their hands or clean their food, and were continually exposed to bacteria, parasites, and other microorganisms. If pregnant women were systemically immunosuppressed, they would not have survived, and the human species would have become extinct. Even today, in many parts of the world, pregnant women are continually exposed to harsh, unsanitary conditions, and a suppressed immune system would make it impossible for the mother and fetus to survive. Where human immunodeficiency virus (HIV) is pandemic, such as in Africa, HIV-positive women do not develop acquired immunodeficiency syndrome (AIDS) during pregnancy. In fact, recent studies clearly demonstrate that the maternal antiviral immunity is not affected by pregnancy.[10] Together, these observations argue against the existence of such nonspecific immune suppression.

Cytokine Shift

As the definition of pregnancy as a T_H2 or anti-inflammatory state was enthusiastically embraced, numerous studies attempted to prove and support this hypothesis, which postulates that pregnancy is an anti-inflammatory condition,[11] and that a shift in the type of cytokines produced would lead to abortion or pregnancy complications. Many studies supported this hypothesis, but a similar number argued against it.[12,13] The reason for these contradictory results may have been oversimplification of the disparate observations made during pregnancy. Pregnancy was viewed as a single continuous event. However, it appears to have three distinct immunologic phases characterized by distinct biologic processes that mirror how the pregnant woman feels.

Implantation and placentation in the first trimester and early second trimester of pregnancy resemble an open wound and require a strong inflammatory response. During this first stage, the embryo has to break through the epithelial lining of the uterus to implant; it must damage the underlying endometrial tissue to invade; and it must replace the endothelium and vascular smooth muscle of the maternal blood vessels to secure an adequate blood supply. These activities create a veritable battleground of invading cells, dying cells, and repairing cells. An inflammatory environment is required to secure the adequate repair of the uterine epithelium and the removal of cellular debris. During this period, the mother's well-being is affected: if she feels terrible, it is because her whole body is struggling to adapt to the presence of the fetus. The resultant immune response and attendant hormonal changes (e.g., human chorionic gonadotropin production) are responsible for morning sickness. Thus, the first trimester of pregnancy is a proinflammatory phase (Fig. 6-1).

The second immunologic phase of pregnancy, a period of rapid fetal growth and development, is in many ways the optimal time for the mother. The mother, placenta, and fetus are symbiotic, and the predominant immunologic feature is induction of an anti-inflammatory state. The woman no longer suffers the nausea, extreme fatigue, and inflammatory symptoms that she did in the first phase, in part because the immune response is no longer the predominant endocrine feature.

During the last immunologic phase of pregnancy, the fetus has completed its development; its organs are functional and ready to deal with the external world. Now the mother needs to deliver the infant and this can be achieved only through renewed inflammation. Parturition is characterized by an influx of immune cells into the myometrium to promote recrudescence of an inflammatory process. This proinflammatory environment promotes the contraction of the uterus, expulsion of the infant, and rejection of the placenta. In conclusion, pregnancy is a proinflammatory and anti-inflammatory condition, depending on the stage of gestation (see Fig. 6-1).[14]

Lack of Expression of HLA Antigens

A more recently postulated theory is based on the fact that polymorphic class I and II molecules have not been detected on the trophoblast.[15] MHC class I antigens are expressed on the surface of most nucleated cells and serve as important recognition molecules. In humans, these antigens are also known as human leukocyte antigens (HLA). HLA class I genes, located on chromosomal region 6p.21.3, have been subdivided into two groups—the HLA class Ia and the HLA class Ib genes, according to their polymorphism, tissue distribution, and function. HLA-A, -B, and -C class Ia genes exhibit a very high level of polymorphism, they are almost ubiquitously expressed in somatic tissue, and their immunologic functions are well established. They modulate antiviral and antitumoral immune responses through their interaction with T and natural killer (NK) cell receptors. In contrast, HLA E, F, and G class Ib genes are characterized by their limited polymorphism and their restricted tissue distribution, and their roles are poorly understood.

The statement that the human placenta does not express polymorphic MHC class I molecules is not entirely accurate. The human placenta does not express the polymorphic HLA-A and HLA-B class I antigens, but it does express HLA C molecules. In addition, HLA-G and HLA-E molecules are also expressed by the human placenta.[16,17] Using immunostaining with antibodies against the class I molecule, King and colleagues divided the human trophoblast into two distinct populations: the villous trophoblast in contact with maternal blood at the intervillous interface, which is class I negative, and the extravillous trophoblast invading the uterine decidua, which is class I positive.[18,19] On the basis of these findings, it was suggested that there are two fetal-maternal interfaces in human reproduction and that they

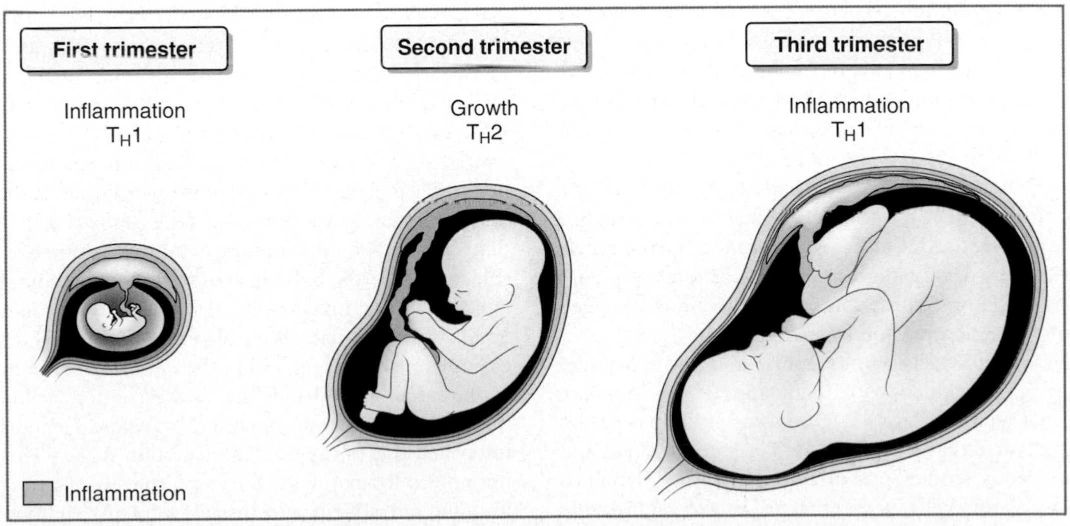

FIGURE 6-1 Inflammation and pregnancy. Each stage of pregnancy is characterized by a unique inflammatory environment. The first and third trimesters are proinflammatory (T_H1), whereas the second trimester represents an anti-inflammatory phase also known as T_H2 environment.

differ immunologically: a trophoblast population that is immunologically neutral in contact with the systemic maternal immune system, and a local immunologically active population of trophoblast cells migrating into the decidua, which can be stimulated by HLA class I.[20]

HLA-G was originally cloned in 1987, and it was demonstrated to be present in abundant amounts at the maternal-fetal interface.[21,22] On the basis of what was thought to be an almost exclusive expression of HLA-G at the maternal-fetal interface, it was suggested that this molecule maintains a very specialized role in this environment. Another unique feature of the HLA-G genes, which was postulated to be a prerequisite for maintenance of maternal immune tolerance, is the lack of polymorphism of the HLA-G nucleotide sequence.[23] However, new data have shown that this may not be the case. Thus, alternative splicing of the HLA-G mRNA yields different membrane-bound and soluble variants of the HLA-G protein and a limited number of variable sites in the DNA sequence of the HLA-G gene.[24-28] Therefore, the hypothesis that HLA-G is the mediator of fetal-maternal tolerance because of its monomorphism and immunologic neutrality needed to be revised.[23,29,30] In animal studies, it has been shown that murine trophoblast cells express MHC class I genes and alloantigens at high levels early in gestation. During those times, MHC class I is barely detectable on fetal tissues.[31,32] Therefore, it has been suggested by several investigators that it is highly unlikely that maternal T cells circulating through the murine maternal-fetal interface do not encounter cells of fetal origin. Thus, this pattern of MHC class I expression at the maternal-fetal interface is incompatible with the hypothesis that fetal tissues at the interface are antigenically immature and therefore do not provoke maternal T-cell responses.

In conclusion, although the apparent lack of classic MHC gene expression suggests that the preimplantation embryo is protected from direct immunologic attack by MHC-restricted T cells, the preimplantation embryo could still be vulnerable to a delayed-type hypersensitivity reaction, as well as to adverse effects of antibodies and cytokines by non-MHC-restricted effector cells.

Local Immune Suppression

The last main hypothesis is that there is a specific immune suppressor or regulatory mechanism during pregnancy. According to this hypothesis, immune cells that specifically recognize paternal alloantigens are deleted from the maternal immune system. This elimination process is thought to be achieved through either deletion of these alloreactive cells or through the suppression of their activity. One mechanism by which paternal antigen–recognizing T cells may be deleted is through the induction of cell death (apoptosis) by the Fas/Fas ligand (FasL) system (Fig. 6-2).[33-35] Our recent studies indicate that the proapoptotic protein FasL is not expressed at the cell surface membrane of trophoblast cells but instead is secreted via microvesicles and can then act on activated Fas receptor–expressing immune cells at locations away from the implantation site.[36] However, the role of this functional, secreted FasL is not fully understood and is under investigation.

Another way in which T cells may recognize and delete paternal antigens is through the production of indolamine 2,3-dioxygenase (IDO) at the maternal-fetal interface.[37] IDO is an enzyme that degrades tryptophan, an amino acid that is essential for T-cell proliferation and survival.[38-40] Most recently, studies have described a subset of lymphocytes known as T regulatory cells (Tregs) that are able to suppress the actions of alloreactive T cells to promote fetal-paternal immunotolerance.[41,42] Together, these are all potential mechanisms for the immunologic escape of the fetus.

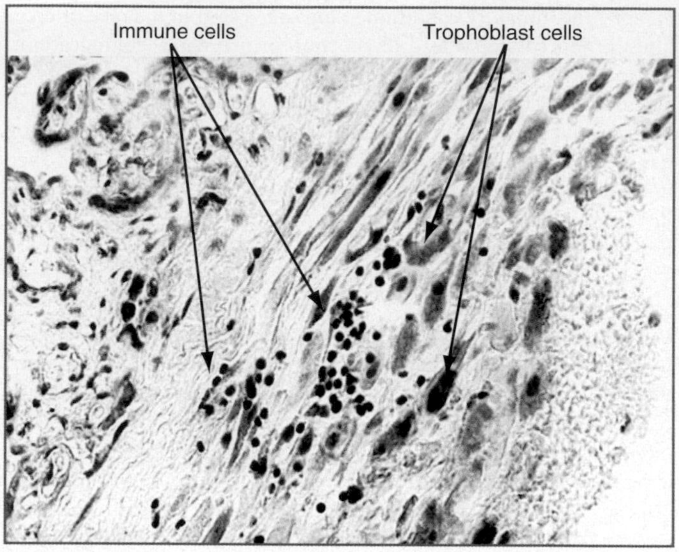

FIGURE 6-2 Expression of FasL in first-trimester trophoblast cells. The proapoptotic protein FasL is highly expressed in extravillous trophoblasts that are in close proximity to maternal immune cells present at the decidua.

The Role of the Innate Immune System in Pregnancy

During normal pregnancy, several of the cellular components of the innate immune system are found at the site of implantation. This has been taken as conclusive proof that the maternal immune system responds to the fetal allograft. During the first trimester, 70% of decidual leukocytes are NK cells, 20% to 25% are macrophages, and approximately 1.7% are dendritic cells.[43-45] These cells infiltrate the decidua and accumulate around the invading trophoblast cells. Furthermore, from the first trimester onward, circulating monocytes, granulocytes, and NK cells increase in number and acquire an activated phenotype. This evidence suggests that the maternal innate immune system is not indifferent to the fetus. However, where once these observations were thought to support the hypothesis of an immune response *against* the fetal allograft, animal studies using cell-deletion methods have proved quite the opposite. Indeed, depletion of NK cells during pregnancy, instead of being protective, has been shown to be detrimental for pregnancy outcome.[46] Much effort was focused on the susceptibility of the trophoblast to NK cell–mediated cytotoxicity,[20,47] until it was found that uterine NK cells are not cytotoxic.[48] Moreover, recently it was shown that uterine NK cells are important for promoting angiogenesis and trophoblast invasion, the two critical events in early pregnancy.[49] Similar findings have been observed with other immune cells. For example, macrophages within the decidua are important for clearing apoptotic and cellular debris, as well as for facilitating trophoblast migration throughout gestation,[50-52] whereas dendritic cells play an important role in the early implantation stage.[53] Therefore, the innate immune cells may have a critical role to play in the fetomaternal immune adjustment and in successful placentation. These findings challenge the conventional wisdom and the paradigm of pregnancy that has until now held that the maternal immune system was a threat to the developing fetus.

The field of reproductive immunology has always followed mainstream immunology, translating findings from transplantation to explain the immunology of the maternal-fetal relationship. However, these ideas have failed to conclusively prove the principle of semi-allograft acceptance by the mother and have also produced confusion over the role of the immune system during pregnancy. It is, therefore, time to reevaluate the basic underpinnings of the immunology of pregnancy: Does the fetal-placental unit truly act like an allograft that is in continual conflict with the maternal immune system?

Redefining Medawar's Hypothesis

Medawar's original observation was based on the assumption that the placenta was akin to a "piece of skin" with paternal antigens, which, under normal immunologic conditions, should be rejected. However, the placenta is more than just a transplanted organ. Our knowledge of placental biology has significantly increased over the past 50 years. We now know that the placenta is a complex organ; the original concept of it as an elaborate "egg cover" has evolved. Unlike transplanted grafts, pregnancy and implantation have been taking place for millions of years, and from an evolutionary point of view it is difficult to conceive that the placenta and the maternal immune system maintain an antagonistic status. Thus, although there should be an active mechanism preventing the potential recognition of paternal antigens by the maternal immune system, the trophoblast and the maternal immune system have evolved to a cooperative status, helping each other against common enemies—that is, against infectious microorganisms.

Today, research is focused on understanding how the trophoblast and the maternal immune system can work together to protect the fetus against infection. The results of our studies suggest that the trophoblast functions like the conductor of a symphony where the musicians are the cells of the maternal immune system. The success of the pregnancy depends on how well the trophoblast communicates with each immune cell type and then how all of them work together. At the molecular level, researchers are trying to understand how the trophoblast recognizes what is present, and, on the basis of that information, what types of signals are sent that would then coordinate the activities of the cellular components at the implantation site.

Current studies demonstrate that, like an innate immune cell, the trophoblast expresses PRRs that function as sensors of the surrounding environment.[54-58] Through these sensors, the trophoblast recognizes the presence of bacteria, viruses, dying cells, and damaged tissue. On recognition, the trophoblast often secretes a specific set of cytokines that, in turn, act on the immune cells within the decidua (e.g., macrophages, T regulatory cells, NK cells), "educating" them to work together in support of the growing fetus (Fig. 6-3).[59] Indeed, each immune cell type acquires specific properties related to implantation and placenta-

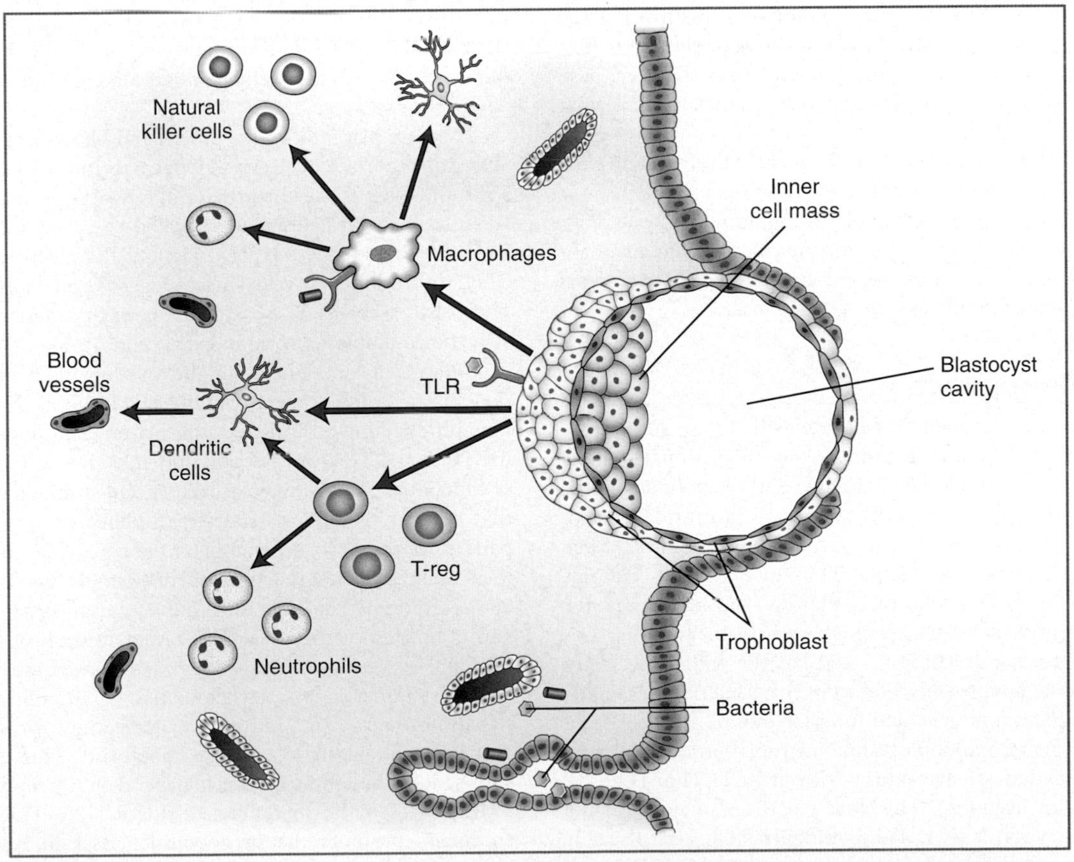

FIGURE 6-3 Trophoblast-immune interaction. The model summarizes a new perspective on trophoblast-immune interaction, in which the placenta and the maternal immune system positively interact for the success of pregnancy. The trophoblast recognizes, through Toll-like receptors (TLRs), microorganisms and the cellular components at the implantation site and responds to them with the production of cytokines and chemokines. These factors coordinate the migration, differentiation, and function of maternal immune cells.

tion, as already discussed. However, a viral or bacterial infection may perturb the harmony of these interactions.

Infection and Pregnancy

Bacterial and viral infections can pose a significant threat to a pregnancy, and to the well-being of the fetus, by gaining access to the placenta through one of three major routes: via the maternal circulation, by ascending into the uterus from the lower reproductive tract, or by descending into the uterus from the peritoneal cavity.[60] Clinical studies have established a strong association between pregnancy complications and intrauterine infections.[60-62] Indeed, infections have been reported as responsible for up to 60% of preterm delivery cases. Up to 80% of preterm deliveries occurring at less than 30 weeks of gestation have evidence of infection,[61-63] and other pregnancy complications, such as preeclampsia, may have an underlying infectious trigger.[64-66] How can a microorganism initiate a response that can induce preterm labor or abortion, or even preeclampsia? Interestingly, signals promoting such fetal rejection in the presence of an infection may be initiated by the same cells that promote fetal acceptance under normal conditions—that is, the trophoblast.[55]

Pattern Recognition Receptors

The innate immune system can distinguish between self and infectious nonself through a system of pattern recognition.[67-69] A series of innate immune receptors, the PRRs, recognize and bind to highly conserved sequences, known as pathogen-associated molecular patterns (PAMPs), that are expressed by microorganisms. Some of these PRRs can also recognize endogenous stress proteins or damage-associated molecular patterns (DAMPs).[70] The ligation of PRR by PAMPs or DAMPs often results in an inflammatory response.[71] PRRs include the large and well-defined family of Toll-like receptors (TLRs), which allow either the extracellular or lysosomal (or endosomal) recognition of a wide range of microbes,[72] whereas the newly identified nucleotide-binding oligomerization domain (NOD) proteins are cytoplasm-based receptors that facilitate responses to invasive intracellular bacteria.[73]

Toll-like Receptors

Toll-like receptors are transmembrane proteins that have an extracellular domain of leucine-rich repeat motifs, and the various receptors differ in specificity. So, although individually, TLRs respond to limited ligands, collectively the family of TLRs can respond to a wide range of PAMPs associated with bacteria, viruses, fungi, and parasites. Eleven mammalian TLRs have been identified (TLR1 to TLR11),[74,75] but only TLR1 to TLR10 have been found to be expressed in humans. TLR4, the first to be identified,[71] is the specific receptor for gram-negative bacterial lipopolysaccharide (LPS).[76] TLR2 has the widest specificity, recognizing bacterial lipoproteins, gram-positive bacterial peptidoglycan (PDG) and lipoteichoic acid, and fungal zymosan.[77-79] Also, TLR2 is unusual in that its recognition of some microbial products appears to require the formation of heterodimers with either TLR1 or TLR6.[80,81] Although the natural ligands for TLR7 and TLR10 are unknown, TLR3 is known to bind viral dsRNA, TLR5 recognizes bacterial flagellin, TLR8 recognizes viral ssRNA, and TLR9 binds microbial CpG DNA.[82-84] In addition, TLR4 and TLR2 can bind DAMPs, such as heat shock protein 60, heat shock protein 70, and fibrinogen.[85]

Ligation of TLRs by microbial products often results in the production of cytokines and antimicrobial factors. Such responses arise via a common intracellular signaling pathway. On ligand recognition, the TLRs recruit an intracellular signaling adapter protein, myeloid differentiation factor-88 (MyD88), and a subsequent kinase cascade triggers activation of the nuclear factor kappa B (NF-κB) pathway, which results in the generation of an inflammatory response.[85] However, TLR3 and TLR4 can also signal in a MyD88-independent manner.[86] Such MyD88-independent signaling occurs through another adapter protein, TRIF, which, although it can activate the NF-κB pathway, also results in the phosphorylation of interferon regulatory factor (IRF)-3. This alternative pathway generates an antiviral response associated with the production of type I interferons and interferon-inducible genes.[87]

Toll-like Receptors and Trophoblast Responses to Infection

The expression of all 10 TLRs has been described in the human placenta, and the dominant cell type expressing these TLRs is the trophoblast.[88-90] However, the expression of TLRs by trophoblasts differs with their differential stage and with gestational age. For example, first-trimester trophoblasts do not express TLR6, but this receptor *is* expressed by third-trimester trophoblasts.[88,91] Furthermore, in first-trimester placentas, the populations expressing TLR2 and TLR4 are the villous cytotrophoblast and the extravillous trophoblasts.[88,92,93] In contrast, syncytiotrophoblasts do not express these receptors. The lack of TLR expression by the outer trophoblast layer suggests that the first- and second-trimester placenta responds only to a microbe that has broken through this outer layer. Thus, a microorganism poses a threat to the fetus only if the TLR-negative syncytiotrophoblast layer is breached and the pathogen has entered the placental villous compartment.[57]

The term placenta, on the other hand, shows a different pattern of TLR expression, characterized by positive immunoreactivity for TLR2 and TLR4 on the cytoplasm of the syncytiotrophoblast.[89,93] More recently, Ma and colleagues evaluated the expression of TLR2 and TLR4 in third-trimester placentas and described the expression of TLR2 in endothelial cells, macrophages, syncytiotrophoblasts, and fibroblasts, whereas TLR4 expression was prominently expressed in syncytiotrophoblast and endothelial cells.[94]

In terms of function, Holmlund and coworkers first demonstrated that stimulation with zymosan and LPS induced IL-6 and IL-8 cytokine production by third-trimester placental cultures, without affecting TLR2 and TLR4 mRNA and protein expression levels,[89] suggestive of functional TLRs in the placenta. Recent studies have demonstrated that TLR-expressing first-trimester trophoblasts generate very distinct patterns of response, depending on the type of stimuli and, therefore, the specific TLR that is activated. For example, first-trimester trophoblasts respond in opposite directions to gram-negative bacterial LPS and gram-positive bacterial PDG. After ligation of TLR4 with LPS, trophoblasts generate a slow inflammatory response, characterized by a modest upregulation of chemokines.[56,88] In contrast, PDG, which signals through TLR2 rather than generating a cytokine response, induces trophoblasts to undergo apoptosis.[88] This unusual response after TLR2 stimulation appears to depend on the cooperative receptors TLR1 and TLR6. In trophoblasts that lack TLR6, TLR1 and TLR2 heterodimers promote the proapoptotic effect in response to PDG. However, in the presence of TLR6, cell death is prevented and a cytokine response ensues.[95] Other studies reporting the induction of trophoblast apoptosis through TLR2 include ultraviolet-inactivated human cytomegalovirus[96] and a recent report using recombinant chlamydial heat shock protein 60 through TLR4.[97]

In terms of their responses to viral infections, trophoblasts display some unique characteristics. TLR3 ligation by small amounts of viral dsRNA induces a rapid and highly potent inflammatory response characterized by a strong upregulation of chemokines and the production of type I interferons and interferon-inducible genes.[95] Moreover, the trophoblast has the ability to secrete antimicrobial factors that can act directly on the virus to inhibit its infectivity, suggesting that the placenta can actively prevent the transmission of certain viral infections to the fetus.

Together, these observations suggest that the trophoblast has the ability to discriminate between danger signals that jeopardize the pregnancy and microorganisms that may be necessary for the success of the pregnancy.[57,98] Viral infections, and possibly gram-positive bacterial infections, may be more likely to pose a threat to the fetus and to pregnancy outcome than an extracellular gram-negative bacterial infection. Indeed, the majority of lower-tract commensals are in this latter group.[60]

We believe that the expression of TLRs allows the trophoblast to recognize microorganisms as well as cellular debris and to coordinate a local immune response that, in principle, would not jeopardize the success of the pregnancy. Thus, the first step in our understanding of this interaction during the implantation process involves the attraction of monocytes by the invading trophoblast. Earlier work showed that trophoblasts constitutively secrete monocyte attractants, such as growth-related oncogene (GRO-α), monocyte chemoattractant protein (MCP-1), and IL-8, and that these trophoblasts are also able to recruit monocytes and macrophages.[54,57,59] A second step in this trophoblast-immune interaction involves a process of immune cell education, in which signals originating from the trophoblast could determine the subsequent cytokine profile generated by the local decidual immune cells. Thus, we found that first-trimester trophoblast cells induce the production of chemokines (GRO-α, MCP-1, IL-8, RANTES [regulated on activation, normal T cell expressed and secreted]) and TNF-α by monocytes.[59] We believe that this trophoblast-immune cell crosstalk is characteristic and essential for a normal early pregnancy.

However, a placental response to an infection, if intense enough or left unresolved, may subsequently alter the normal crosstalk between the trophoblast and decidual immune cells. Thus, TLR-mediated trophoblast inflammatory or apoptotic responses to an infection may affect the resident and recruited maternal immune cells by changing them from a supportive to an aggressive phenotype.[59] This may further promote a strong proinflammatory and proapoptotic microenvironment, and it may ultimately prove detrimental to pregnancy outcome by facilitating fetal rejection.[51] A number of animal models have supported this concept, as well as our in vitro observations. Gram-negative bacterial LPS cannot trigger prematurity in wild-type mice when delivered at low concentrations.[99,100] However, if bacterial LPS is administered at high doses, preterm labor is observed, and this has been shown to be mediated by TLR4.[101,102]

In vivo studies have also demonstrated that poly(I:C) promotes prematurity in a TLR3-dependent manner,[103,104] and this is associated with a type-I interferon response.[105] In addition, TLR2 stimulation triggers prematurity in vivo.[105-107] These studies, together with clinical data, make a strong case for TLRs as mediators of infection-associated prematurity. Possible therapeutic strategies are now being explored to determine whether the inhibition of TLR signaling might help prevent such pregnancy complications.

Chlamydial Infection and Pregnancy

Although no single infectious agent has been linked to poor pregnancy outcome, some bacteria (e.g., *Mycoplasma hominis*, *Ureaplasma urealyticum*, and *Gardnerella vaginalis*) are more often isolated from patients with preterm delivery than others.[61,108] One bacterium that has proved much harder to isolate and correlate with poor clinical outcome is *Chlamydia*.[109,110] *Chlamydia trachomatis* is the most common sexually transmitted infection in the United States[111] (Fig. 6-4). Chlamydial infection of the female genital tract can result in infertility, ectopic pregnancy, or pelvic inflammatory disease.[112] However, the link between chlamydial infection and pregnancy complications is more controver

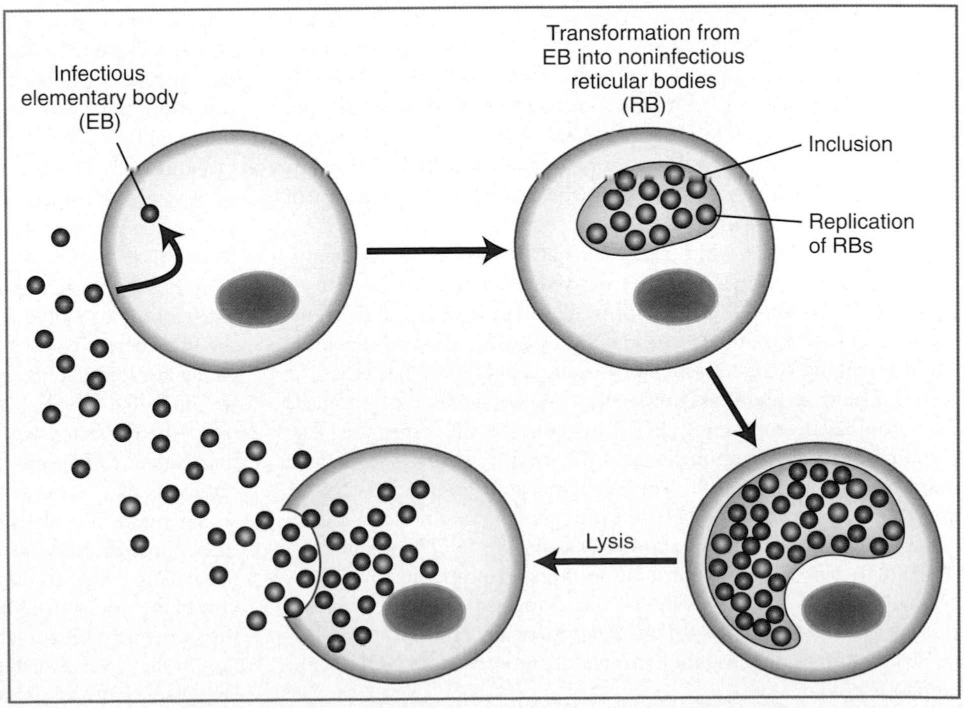

FIGURE 6-4 The life cycle of *Chlamydia*. *Chlamydia* is an obligate intracellular gram-negative bacterium. It invades the host cell as an infectious, nonreplicating extracellular elementary body (EB). Once in the cytoplasm, the EB differentiates into an intracellular reticulate body (RB), which then undergoes several rounds of binary fission. This occurs in a specialized compartment known as an inclusion. It is during this phase, if conditions are unfavorable, that a persistent infection can arise. During persistence, the RBs cease to replicate and the life cycle is arrested. However, under normal conditions, after replication, the RBs redifferentiate into infectious EBs, which are released from the host cell 2 to 3 days after infection, during a lytic process. The released EBs then infect neighboring cells.

sial. A recent study revealed that 17% of first-trimester placentas have evidence of chlamydial infection,[113] suggesting that the placenta is a target. Although the concept that chlamydial infection may adversely impact pregnancy has been supported by animal models,[114-116] clinical data are inconsistent. Studies have shown that a high proportion of spontaneous abortions are positive for *C. trachomatis,*[117] and that women positive for antibodies against *C. trachomatis* may be at greater risk for spontaneous abortion or preterm labor.[118-120] Moreover, a recent study reported that *Chlamydia*-infected women have an increased risk of preterm delivery compared with noninfected women.[121] However, other studies have reported no association between *Chlamydia* and prematurity.[122-125]

An alternative explanation for this discrepancy could be that it is not the *presence* of a chlamydial infection that defines whether a pregnancy will be negatively affected but instead the *status* of the infection, and this may be governed by the placental innate immune response. We propose that it is an *active* chlamydial infection that may adversely affect pregnancy outcome. Furthermore, it is the placenta that determines whether a chlamydial infection may lie dormant, in a state of persistence, or remain active and pose a threat to the pregnancy. A potential mechanism by which the trophoblast regulates such chlamydial infection is through the expression of a novel group of cytoplasmic receptors, the NOD proteins, which are capable of recognizing intracellular infections.

NOD Proteins and Trophoblast Responses to *Chlamydia*

The NOD proteins, NOD1 (*CARD4*) and NOD2 (*CARD15*), share some similarities with the TLRs, as both types of PRRs contain a leucine-rich repeat domain that is responsible for ligand recognition (Fig. 6-5).[126] However, unlike the TLRs, the NOD proteins lack a transmembrane domain and, therefore, their cellular localization is restricted to the cytoplasmic compartment, making them poised to respond to microbes that might otherwise escape external immune recognition by invading and replicating within a cell's cytosol. Indeed, NOD proteins have been shown to respond to intracellular pathogens, such as *Listeria, Shigella,* and *Chlamydia.*[127-130] In addition, NOD proteins also contain a central NOD domain that facilitates self-oligomerization, and CARD domains (one for NOD1 and two for NOD2), which interact with downstream adapter molecules, such as RIP-like interacting CLARP kinase (RICK), to mediate activation of the NF-κB and mitogen-activated protein kinase (MAPK) pathways.[131-134] Therefore, activation of NOD1 and NOD2 leads to a signaling cascade that generates an inflammatory response, characterized by the production of cytokines (see Fig. 6-5).[127,130,135]

Unlike other PRRs, which recognize native microbial components, NOD proteins recognize peptides derived from the degradation of bacterial PDG. Peptidoglycan from all gram-positive and gram-negative bacteria contain the NOD2 ligand, muramyldipeptide (MDP), making NOD2 a general cytosolic sensor of all bacteria.[136,137] NOD1 ligand recognition, however, is more selective, as it detects diaminopimelate-containing PDG, specifically the dipeptide γ-D-glutamyl-*meso*-diaminopimelic acid (iE-DAP), which is found in gram-negative bacteria.[127,128] The PDG motifs recognized by NOD1 and NOD2 are natural degradation products that are released during bacterial growth.[128] This is another reason why NOD proteins are thought to play a role in immune responses toward invasive intracellular bacteria that replicate in the cytoplasm of a host cell.[128] Indeed, studies have shown that *Chlamydia,* an obligate intracellular bacterium, contains the stimulatory motifs for NOD1 and NOD2.[138,139]

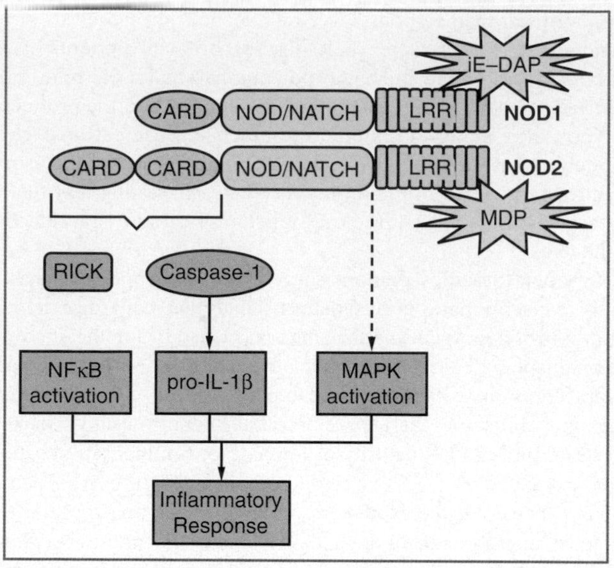

FIGURE 6-5 Structure of NOD1 and NOD2 and their signaling pathways. NOD1 and NOD2 contain a leucine-rich repeat (LRR) domain that is responsible for ligand recognition, and a central NOD/NATCH domain that facilitates self-oligomerization. NOD1 contains a single CARD domain, and NOD2 contains two CARD domains. After recognition of their specific ligands, NOD1 and NOD2 recruit RICK to their CARD domains, and RICK in turn activates the nuclear factor (NF)-κB pathway, resulting in the induction of an inflammatory response. NOD1 and NOD2 also have the capacity to bind and activate procaspase-1 through their CARD domains. Caspase-1 activation results in the processing of pro-interleukin-1 beta (IL-1β) into active IL-1β. NOD1 and NOD2 can also activate the mitogen-activated protein kinase (MAPK) pathway, although the upstream molecular mechanism of this is unknown at present. iE-DAP, γ-D-glutamyl-*meso*-diaminopimelic acid; MDP, muramyldipeptide.

NOD1 and NOD2 are expressed in first-trimester placenta and are localized to the villous cytotrophoblast and syncytiotrophoblast cells (Fig. 6-6).[58] In addition, isolated first-trimester trophoblast cells express NOD1 and NOD2 as well as the signaling effector protein RICK.[58] That the syncytiotrophoblast layer expresses these intracellular receptors is important because, as mentioned earlier, these cells lack the transmembrane TLRs.[88] This further supports the concept that the placenta responds only to a bacterium that has either breached this protective cell layer or gained access to the placenta via the decidua and/or intervillous space. Bacterial MDP through NOD2 triggers first-trimester trophoblasts to produce elevated levels of cytokines and chemokines,[58] as does NOD1 in response to iE-DAP (unpublished observations). Therefore, the trophoblast appears to be fully equipped to respond to the PDG derivatives that might be generated in the cytosol by a replicating intracellular bacterium such as *Chlamydia* (see Fig. 6-4). Indeed, we find that trophoblast cells mount an inflammatory response only when infected with an active chlamydial infection; ultraviolet-inactivated *Chlamydia* has no effect on these cells (unpublished observations).

Therefore, it is plausible that the response triggered by the trophoblast, through NOD proteins in response to a chlamydial infection, may change the infection from an active state into one of persistence. One of the mechanisms by which this process may be mediated involves the subsequent upregulation of IDO production.[37] A chlamydial infection in this persistent state would not be detrimental to the pregnancy (Fig. 6-7). However, should this infection remain active or become

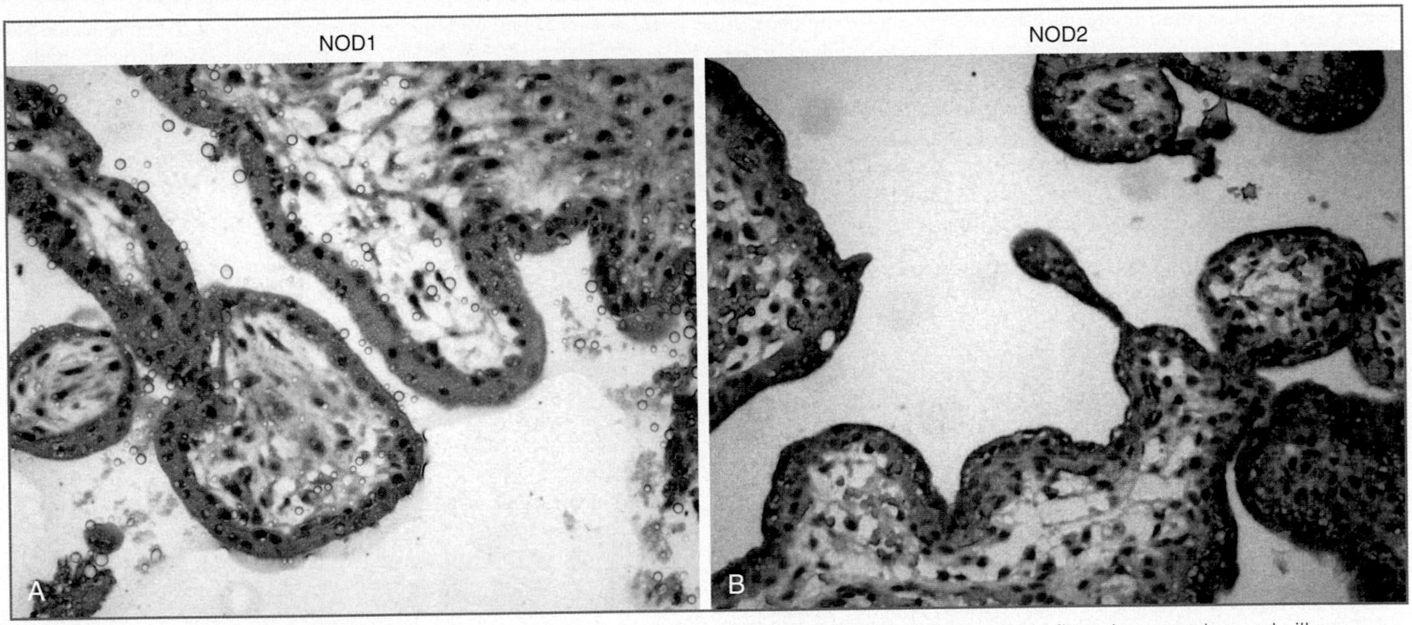

FIGURE 6-6 Expression of NOD1 and NOD2 by first-trimester placenta. NOD1 and NOD2 expression in first-trimester placental villous tissue was determined by immunohistochemistry. Tissue sections of first-trimester placental villi were stained for NOD1 and NOD2. **A,** Villous cytotrophoblast and syncytiotrophoblast cells both displayed strong positive staining for NOD1. **B,** Strong NOD2 expression is localized to the syncytiotrophoblast cells, with weaker NOD2 staining of the cytotrophoblast cells.

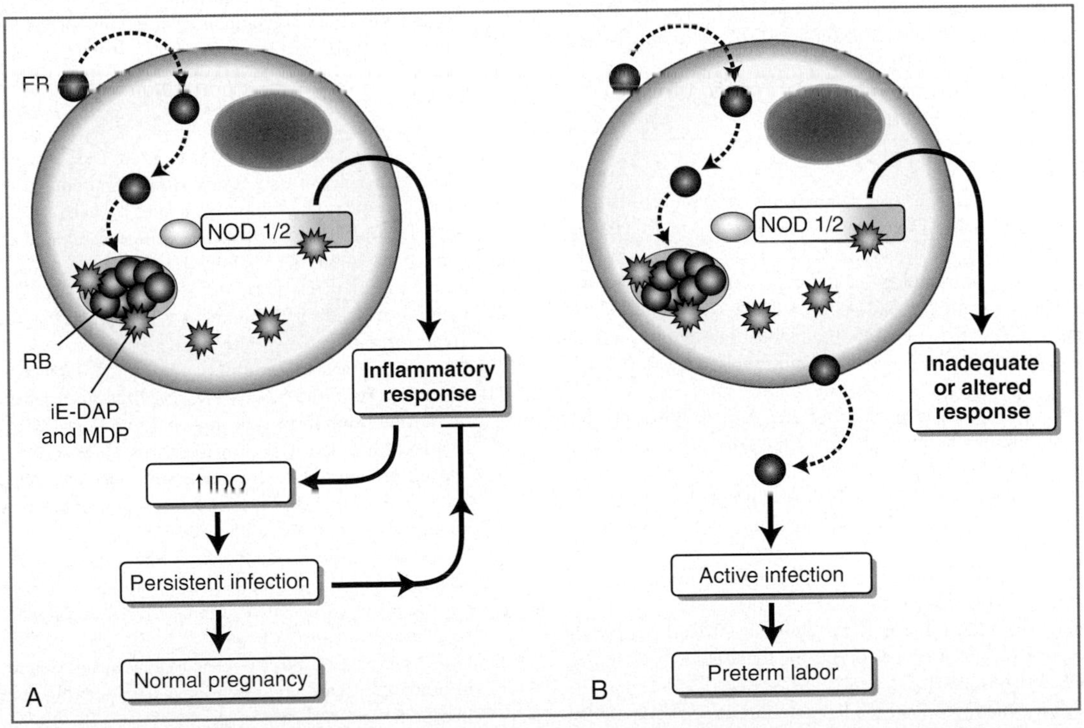

FIGURE 6-7 Trophoblast responses to *Chlamydia*. **A,** Infectious chlamydial elementary bodies (EBs) target the trophoblast. Once in the cell's cytosol, chlamydial EBs differentiate into replicating reticulate bodies (RBs), which undergo binary fission. During this replication stage, the dividing RBs generate the peptidoglycan-degradation products muramyldipeptide (MDP) and γ-D-glutamyl-*meso*-diaminopimelic acid (iE-DAP). MDP and iE-DAP produced by the invasive bacterium are then recognized by the cytoplasmic NOD proteins (NOD1 or NOD2), which, in turn, activate the trophoblast to produce cytokines and chemokines. This inflammatory response then upregulates indolamine 2,3-dioxygenase (IDO) production, which can promote a persistent infection. Once in a state of persistence, *Chlamydia* does not pose a threat to the pregnancy. **B,** Should the trophoblast response to the chlamydial infection be insufficient to upregulate IDO, or should it become altered in a way that results in a changed microenvironment, then the infection may remain active or become reactivated. An active *Chlamydia* infection may result in an adverse pregnancy outcome, such as preterm labor.

reactivated because of an inadequate response of the trophoblast, an adverse pregnancy outcome, such as preterm delivery, could occur (see Fig. 6-7).

Thus, although the prevalence of a chlamydial infection in placentas from normal and pathologic pregnancies may be the same, the *status* of the chlamydial infection may define whether a pregnancy is negatively affected, and the response by the trophoblast through NOD proteins may play an important role.

Summary

Together, our studies provide an alternative perspective on the role of the maternal innate immune system and its interactions with the trophoblast during pregnancy. The trophoblast and the maternal immune system act jointly to protect against infectious microorganisms. When the trophoblast identifies potentially dangerous molecular signatures, the maternal immune system responds with coordinate actions. Therefore, pregnancy might resemble an orchestra in which the trophoblast is the conductor and each immune cell type represents a different musical instrument. The success of the pregnancy depends on how well the trophoblast communicates and works together with each immune cell.

What was originally proposed to be only a graft-host interaction should now include a supportive regulatory interaction between the trophoblast and the maternal immune system. As we learn more about the regulation of the expression and function of TLRs and NOD proteins during pregnancy, we will better understand the cellular crosstalk existing at the maternal-fetal interface.

References

1. Medawar P: Some immunological and endocrinological problems raised by the evolution of viviparity in vertebrates. Symp Soc Exp Biol 7:320-338, 1952.
2. Colbern GT, Main EK: Immunology of the maternal-placental interface in normal pregnancy. Semin Perinatol 15:196-205, 1991.
3. Cserr H, Knopf P: Cervical lymphatics, the blood-brain barrier and the immunoreactivity of the brain: A new view. Immunol Today 13:507-512, 1992.
4. Bechmann I, Mor G, Nilsen J, et al: FasL (CD95L, Apo1L) is expressed in the normal rat and human brain: Evidence for the existence of an immunological brain barrier. Glia 27:62-74, 1999.
5. Bianchi DW, Zickwolf GK, Weil GJ, et al: Male fetal progenitor cells persist in maternal blood for as long as 27 years postpartum. Proc Natl Acad Sci U S A 93:705-708, 1996.
6. Adams KM, Nelson JL: Microchimerism: An investigative frontier in autoimmunity and transplantation. JAMA 291:1127-1131, 2004.
7. Khosrotehrani K, Reyes RR, Johnson KL, et al: Fetal cells participate over time in the response to specific types of murine maternal hepatic injury. Hum Reprod 22:654-661, 2007.
8. Lapaire O, Hosli I, Zanetti-Daellenbach R, et al: Impact of fetal-maternal microchimerism on women's health: A review. J Matern Fetal Neonatal Med 20:1-5, 2007.
9. Formby B: Immunologic response in pregnancy: Its role in endocrine disorders of pregnancy and influence on the course of maternal autoimmune diseases. Endocrinol Metab Clin North Am 24:187-205, 1995.
10. Read JS, Cahn P, Losso M, et al: Management of human immunodeficiency virus-infected pregnant women at Latin American and Caribbean sites. Obstet Gynecol 109:1358-1367, 2007.
11. Wegmann TG, Guilbert LJ: Immune signaling at the maternal-fetal interface and trophoblast differentiation. Dev Comp Immunol 16:425-430, 1992.
12. Saito S, Satomi M, Sasaki Y: Th1/Th2 Balance of the Implantation Site in Humans. Georgetown, TX, Landes Bioscience/Springer Science, 2006.
13. Chaouat G, Tranchot Diallo J, Volumenie JL, et al: Immune suppression and Th1/Th2 balance in pregnancy revisited: A (very) personal tribute to Tom Wegmann. Am J Reprod Immunol 37:427-434, 1997.
14. Mor G: Pregnancy reconceived. Natural History 116:36-41, 2007.
15. Kovats S, Main E, Librach C: HLA-G expressed in human trophoblast. Science 248:220-223, 1990.
16. Schmidt C, Orr H: Maternal/Fetal interactions: The roles of the MHC class I molecule HLA-G. Crit Rev Immunol 13:207-224, 1994.
17. Loke YW, Hiby S, King A: Human leucocyte antigen-G and reproduction. J Reprod Immunol 43:235-242, 1999.
18. King A, Burrows TD, Hiby SE, et al: Surface expression of HLA-C antigen by human extravillous trophoblast. Placenta 21:376-387, 2000.
19. King A, Hiby SE, Gardner L, et al: Recognition of trophoblast HLA class I molecules by decidual NK cell receptors. Placenta 21(Suppl A):S81-85, 2000.
20. Moffett-King A: Natural killer cells and pregnancy. Nat Rev Immunol 2:656-663, 2002.
21. Ellis SA, Sargent IL, Redman CW, McMichael AJ: Evidence for a novel HLA antigen on human extravillous trophoblast and a choriocarcinoma cell line. Immunology 59:595-601, 1986.
22. Ellis S, Palmer M, McMichael A: Human trophoblast and the choriocarcinoma cell line BeWo express a truncated HLA class molecule. J Immunol 144:731-735, 1990.
23. Hunt JS, Langat DK, McIntire RH, Morales PJ: The role of HLA-G in human pregnancy. Reprod Biol Endocrinol 4(Suppl 1):S10, 2006.
24. van der Ven K, Pfeiffer K, Skrablin S: HLA-G polymorphisms and molecule function: Questions and more questions—a review. Placenta 21(Suppl A):S86-92, 2000.
25. van der Ven K, Skrablin S, Ober C, Krebs D: HLA-G polymorphisms: Ethnic differences and implications for potential molecule function. Am J Reprod Immunol 40:145-157, 1998.
26. van der Ven K, Skrablin S, Engels G, Krebs D: HLA-G polymorphisms and allele frequencies in Caucasians. Hum Immunol 59:302-312, 1998.
27. Pace JL, Morales PJ, Phillips TA, Hunt JS: Analysis of the soluble isoforms of HLA-G mRNAs and proteins. Methods Mol Med 122:181-203, 2006.
28. Hunt JS, Geraghty DE: Soluble HLA-G isoforms: Technical deficiencies lead to misinterpretations. Mol Hum Reprod 11:715-717, 2005.
29. Bainbridge D, Ellis S, Le Bouteiller P, Sargent I: HLA-G remains a mystery. Trends Immunol 22:548-552, 2001.
30. Hunt JS: Stranger in a strange land. Immunol Rev 213:36-47, 2006.
31. Chatterjee-Hasrouni S, Lala PK: Localization of paternal H-2K antigens on murine trophoblast cells in vivo. J Exp Med 155:1679-1689, 1982.
32. Lala PK, Chatterjee-Hasrouni S, Kearns M, et al: Immunobiology of the feto-maternal interface. Immunol Rev 75:87-116, 1983.
33. Guller S: Role of Fas ligand in conferring immune privilege to non-lymphoid cells. Ann N Y Acad Sci 828:268-272, 1997.
34. Neale D, Demasio K, Illuzi J, et al: Maternal serum of women with pre-eclampsia reduces trophoblast cell viability: Evidence for an increased sensitivity to Fas-mediated apoptosis. J Matern Fetal Neonatal Med 13:39-44, 2003.
35. Mor G, Gutierrez L, Eliza M, et al: Fas-Fas ligand system induced apoptosis in human placenta and gestational trophoblastic disease. Am J Reprod Immunol 40:89-94, 1998.
36. Abrahams VM, Straszewski-Chavez SL, Guller S, Mor G: First trimester trophoblast cells secrete Fas ligand which induces immune cell apoptosis. Mol Hum Reprod 10:55-63, 2004.
37. Mellor AL, Chandler P, Lee GK, et al: Indoleamine 2,3-dioxygenase, immunosuppression and pregnancy. J Reprod Immunol 57:143-150, 2002.
38. Hogan RJ, Mathews SA, Mukhopadhyay S, et al: Chlamydial persistence: Beyond the biphasic paradigm. Infect Immun 72:1843-1855, 2004.
39. Paguirigan AM, Byrne GI, Becht S, Carlin JM: Cytokine-mediated indoleamine 2,3-dioxygenase induction in response to Chlamydia infection in human macrophage cultures. Infect Immun 62:1131-1136, 1994.

40. Pantoja LG, Miller RD, Ramirez JA, et al: Inhibition of Chlamydia pneumoniae replication in human aortic smooth muscle cells by gamma interferon-induced indoleamine 2,3-dioxygenase activity. Infect Immun 68:6478-6481, 2000.
41. Aluvihare VR, Kallikourdis M, Betz AG: Regulatory T cells mediate maternal tolerance to the fetus. Nat Immunol 5:266-271, 2004.
42. Zenclussen AC: CD4(+)CD25+ T regulatory cells in murine pregnancy. J Reprod Immunol 65:101-110, 2005.
43. Bulmer JN, Pace D, Ritson A: Immunoregulatory cells in human decidua: Morphology, immunohistochemistry and function. Reprod Nutr Dev 28:1599-1613, 1988.
44. King A, Wellings V, Gardner L, Loke YW: Immunocytochemical characterization of the unusual large granular lymphocytes in human endometrium throughout the menstrual cycle. Hum Immunol 24:195-205, 1989.
45. Gardner L, Moffett A: Dendritic cells in the human decidua. Biol Reprod 69:1438-1446, 2003.
46. Guimond MJ, Wang B, Croy BA: Engraftment of bone marrow from severe combined immunodeficient (SCID) mice reverses the reproductive deficits in natural killer cell-deficient tg epsilon 26 mice. J Exp Med 187:217-223, 1998.
47. Moffett-King A, Entrican G, Ellis S, et al: Natural killer cells and reproduction. Trends Immunol 23:332-333, 2002.
48. Kopcow HD, Allan DS, Chen X, et al: Human decidual NK cells form immature activating synapses and are not cytotoxic. Proc Natl Acad Sci U S A 102:15563-15568, 2005.
49. Hanna J, Goldman-Wohl D, Hamani Y, et al: Decidual NK cells regulate key developmental processes at the human fetal-maternal interface. Nat Med 12:1065-1074, 2006.
50. Mor G, Straszewski-Chavez SL, Abrahams VM: Macrophage-trophoblast interactions. Methods Mol Med 122:149-163, 2006.
51. Abrahams VM, Kim YM, Straszewski SL, et al: Macrophages and apoptotic cell clearance during pregnancy. Am J Reprod Immunol 51.275-282, 2004.
52. Aldo PB, Krikun G, Visintin I, et al: A novel three-dimensional in vitro system to study trophoblast-endothelium cell interactions. Am J Reprod Immunol 58:98-110, 2007.
53. Birnberg T, Plaks V, Berkutzki T, et al: Dendritic cells are crucial for decidual development during embryo implantation. Am J Reprod Immunol 57:342, 2007.
54. Abrahams VM, Visintin I, Aldo PB, et al: A role for TLRs in the regulation of immune cell migration by first trimester trophoblast cells. J Immunol 175:8096-8104, 2005.
55. Abrahams VM, Romero R, Mor G: TLR-3 and TLR-4 mediate differential chemokine production and immune cell recruitment by first trimester trophoblast cells. Am J Reprod Immunol 53:279-309, 2005 ASRI205-202 (Abstr).
56. Abrahams VM, Fahey JV, Schaefer TM, et al: Stimulation of first trimester trophoblast cells with Poly(I:C) induces SLPI secretion. Am J Reprod Immunol 53:280, 2005 ASRI205-204 (Abstr).
57. Mor G, Romero R, Aldo PB, Abrahams VM: Is the trophoblast an immune regulator? The role of toll-like receptors during pregnancy. Crit Rev Immunol 25:375-388, 2005.
58. Costello MJ, Joyce SK, Abrahams VM: NOD protein expression and function in first trimester trophoblast cells. Am J Reprod Immunol 57:67-80, 2007.
59. Fest S, Aldo PB, Abrahams VM, et al: Trophoblast-macrophage interactions: A regulatory network for the protection of pregnancy. Am J Reprod Immunol 57:55-66, 2007.
60. Espinoza J, Erez O, Romero R: Preconceptional antibiotic treatment to prevent preterm birth in women with a previous preterm delivery. Am J Obstet Gynecol 194:630-637, 2006.
61. Goldenberg RL, Hauth JC, Andrews WW: Intrauterine infection and preterm delivery. N Engl J Med 342:1500-1507, 2000.
62. Lamont RF: The role of infection in preterm labour and birth. Hosp Med 64:644-647, 2003.
63. Lamont RF: Infection in the prediction and antibiotics in the prevention of spontaneous preterm labour and preterm birth. BJOG 110(Suppl 20):71-75, 2003.
64. Hsu CD, Witter FR: Urogenital infection in preeclampsia. Int J Gynaecol Obstet 49:271-275, 1995.
65. Raynor BD, Bonney EA, Jang KT, et al: Preeclampsia and Chlamydia pneumoniae: Is there a link? Hypertens Pregnancy 23:129-134, 2004.
66. von Dadelszen P, Magee LA: Could an infectious trigger explain the differential maternal response to the shared placental pathology of preeclampsia and normotensive intrauterine growth restriction? Acta Obstet Gynecol Scand 81:642-648, 2002.
67. Janeway CA Jr: How the immune system protects the host from infection. Microbes Infect 3:1167-1171, 2001.
68. Janeway CA Jr, Medzhitov R: Innate immune recognition. Annu Rev Immunol 20:197-216, 2002.
69. Medzhitov R, Janeway CA Jr: Decoding the patterns of self and nonself by the innate immune system. Science 296:298-300, 2002.
70. Akira S: Toll-like receptor signaling. J Biol Chem 278:38105-38108, 2003.
71. Medzhitov R, Preston-Hurlburt P, Janeway CA Jr: A human homologue of the Drosophila Toll protein signals activation of adaptive immunity. Nature 388:394-397, 1997.
72. Uematsu S, Akira S: Toll-like receptors and innate immunity. J Mol Med 84:712-725, 2006.
73. Fritz JH, Ferrero RL, Philpott DJ, Girardin SE: Nod-like proteins in immunity, inflammation and disease. Nat Immunol 7:1250-1257, 2006.
74. Takeda K, Akira S: Roles of Toll-like receptors in innate immune responses. Genes Cells 6:733-742, 2001.
75. Zhang G, Ghosh S: Negative regulation of toll-like receptor mediated signaling by Tollip. J Biol Chem 277:7059-7065, 2002.
76. Poltorak A, He X, Smirnova I, et al: Defective LPS signaling in C3H/HeJ and C57BL/10ScCr mice: Mutations in Tlr4 gene. Science 282:2085-2088, 1998.
77. Aliprantis AO, Yang RB, Mark MR, et al: Cell activation and apoptosis by bacterial lipoproteins through toll-like receptor-2. Science 285:736-739, 1999.
78. Aliprantis AO, Yang RB, Weiss DS, et al: The apoptotic signaling pathway activated by Toll-like receptor-2. EMBO J 19:3325-3336, 2000.
79. Schwandner R, Dziarski R, Wesche H, et al: Peptidoglycan- and lipoteichoic acid-induced cell activation is mediated by toll-like receptor 2. J Biol Chem 274:17406-17409, 1999.
80. Krutzik SR, Ochoa MT, Sieling PA, et al: Activation and regulation of Toll-like receptors 2 and 1 in human leprosy. Nat Med 9:525-532, 2003.
81. Takahashi R, Deveraux Q, Tamm I, et al: A single BIR domain of XIAP sufficient for inhibiting caspases. J Biol Chem 273:7787-7790, 1998.
82. Heil F, Hemmi H, Hochrein H, et al: Species-specific recognition of single-stranded RNA via toll-like receptor 7 and 8. Science 303:1526-1529, 2004.
83. Takeda K, Kaisho T, Akira S: Toll-like receptors. Annu Rev Immunol 21:335-376, 2003.
84. Zhang D, Zhang G, Hayden MS, et al: A toll-like receptor that prevents infection by uropathogenic bacteria. Science 303:1522-1526, 2004.
85. Akira S, Hoshino K: Myeloid differentiation factor 88-dependent and -independent pathways in toll-like receptor signaling. J Infect Dis 187(Suppl 2):S356-363, 2003.
86. Yamamoto M, Sato S, Hemmi H, et al: Role of adaptor TRIF in the MyD88-independent toll-like receptor signaling pathway. Science 301:640-643, 2003.
87. Takeuchi O, Hoshino K, Akira S: Cutting edge: TLR2-deficient and MyD88-deficient mice are highly susceptible to Staphylococcus aureus infection. J Immunol 165:5392-5396, 2000.
88. Abrahams VM, Bole-Aldo P, Kim YM, et al: Divergent trophoblast responses to bacterial products mediated by TLRs. J Immunol 173:4286-4296, 2004.
89. Holmlund U, Cebers G, Dahlfors AR, et al: Expression and regulation of the pattern recognition receptors Toll-like receptor-2 and Toll-like receptor-4 in the human placenta. Immunology 107:145-151, 2002.
90. Kumazaki K, Nakayama M, Yanagihara I, et al: Immunohistochemical distribution of Toll-like receptor 4 in term and preterm human placentas

from normal and complicated pregnancy including chorioamnionitis. Hum Pathol 35:47-54, 2004.
91. Mitsunari M, Yoshida S, Shoji T, et al: Macrophage-activating lipopeptide-2 induces cyclooxygenase-2 and prostaglandin E(2) via toll-like receptor 2 in human placental trophoblast cells. J Reprod Immunol 72:46-59, 2006.
92. Rindsjo E, Holmlund U, Sverremark-Ekstrom E, et al: Toll-like receptor-2 expression in normal and pathologic human placenta. Hum Pathol 38:468-473, 2007.
93. Beijar EC, Mallard C, Powell TL: Expression and subcellular localization of TLR-4 in term and first trimester human placenta. Placenta 27:322-326, 2006.
94. Ma Y, Krikun G, Abrahams VM, et al: Cell type-specific expression and function of toll-like receptors 2 and 4 in human placenta: Implications in fetal infection. Placenta 28:1024-1031 2007.
95. Abrahams VM, Schaefer TM, Fahey JV, et al: Expression and secretion of antiviral factors by trophoblast cells following stimulation by the TLR-3 agonist, Poly(I: C). Hum Reprod 21:2432-2439, 2006.
96. Chan G, Guilbert LJ: Ultraviolet-inactivated human cytomegalovirus induces placental syncytiotrophoblast apoptosis in a Toll-like receptor-2 and tumour necrosis factor-alpha dependent manner. J Pathol 210:111-120, 2006.
97. Equils O, Lu D, Gatter M, et al: Chlamydia heat shock protein 60 induces trophoblast apoptosis through TLR4. J Immunol 177:1257-1263, 2006.
98. Kim YM, Romero R, Oh SY, et al: Toll-like receptor 4: A potential link between "danger signals," the innate immune system, and preeclampsia? Am J Obstet Gynecol 193:921-927, 2005.
99. Murphy SP, Fast LD, Hanna NN, Sharma S: Uterine NK cells mediate inflammation-induced fetal demise in IL-10-null mice. J Immunol 175:4084-4090, 2005.
100. Xu DX, Wang H, Zhao L, et al: Effects of low-dose lipopolysaccharide (LPS) pretreatment on LPS-induced intra-uterine fetal death and preterm labor. Toxicology 234:167-175, 2007.
101. Elovitz MA, Mrinalini C: Animal models of preterm birth. Trends Endocrinol Metab 15:479-487, 2004.
102. Elovitz MA, Wang Z, Chien EK, et al: A new model for inflammation-induced preterm birth: The role of platelet-activating factor and Toll-like receptor-4. Am J Pathol 163:2103-2111, 2003.
103. Lin Y, Zeng Y, Zeng S, Wang T: Potential role of toll-like receptor 3 in a murine model of polyinosinic-polycytidylic acid-induced embryo resorption. Fertil Steril 85(Suppl 1):1125-1129, 2006.
104. Lin Y, Liang Z, Chen Y, Zeng Y: TLR3-involved modulation of pregnancy tolerance in double-stranded RNA-stimulated NOD/SCID mice. J Immunol 176:4147-4154, 2006.
105. Ilievski V, Lu SJ, Hirsch E: Activation of toll-like receptors 2 or 3 and preterm delivery in the mouse. Reprod Sci 14:315-320, 2007.
106. Kakinuma C, Kuwayama C, Kaga N, et al: Trophoblastic apoptosis in mice with preterm delivery and its suppression by urinary trypsin inhibitor. Obstet Gynecol 90:117-124, 1997.
107. Kajikawa S, Kaga N, Futamura Y, et al: Lipoteichoic acid induces preterm delivery in mice. J Pharmacol Toxicol Methods 39:147-154, 1998.
108. Romero R, Maymon E, Pacora P, et al: Further observations on the fetal inflammatory response syndrome: A potential homeostatic role for the soluble receptors of tumor necrosis factor alpha. Am J Obstet Gynecol 183:1070-1077, 2000.
109. Romero R, Espinoza J, Chaiworapongsa T, Kalache K: Infection and prematurity and the role of preventive strategies. Semin Neonatol 7:259-274, 2002.
110. Romero R, Chaiworapongsa T, Espinoza J: Micronutrients and intrauterine infection, preterm birth and the fetal inflammatory response syndrome. J Nutr 133:1668S-1673, 2003.
111. Beagley KW, Timms P: Chlamydia trachomatis infection: Incidence, health costs and prospects for vaccine development. J Reprod Immunol 48:47-68, 2000.
112. Wiesenfeld HC, Hillier SL, Krohn MA, et al: Lower genital tract infection and endometritis: Insight into subclinical pelvic inflammatory disease. Obstet Gynecol 100:456-463, 2002.
113. McDonagh S, Maidji E, Ma W, et al: Viral and bacterial pathogens at the maternal-fetal interface. J Infect Dis 190:826-834, 2004.
114. Tuffrey M, Falder P, Gale J, Taylor-Robinson D: Failure of Chlamydia trachomatis to pass transplacentally to fetuses of TO mice infected during pregnancy. J Med Microbiol 25:1-5, 1988.
115. Buendia AJ, Sanchez J, Martinez MC, et al: Kinetics of infection and effects on placental cell populations in a murine model of Chlamydia psittaci-induced abortion. Infect Immun 66:2128-2134, 1998.
116. Pal S, Peterson EM, De La Maza LM: A murine model for the study of Chlamydia trachomatis genital infections during pregnancy. Infect Immun 67:2607-2610, 1999.
117. Magon T, Kluz S, Chrusciel A, et al: The PCR assessed prevalence of Chlamydia trachomatis in aborted tissues. Med Wieku Rozwoj 9:43-48, 2005.
118. Avasthi K, Garg T, Gupta S, et al: A study of prevalence of Chlamydia trachomatis infection in women with first trimester pregnancy losses. Indian J Pathol Microbiol 46:133-136, 2003.
119. Kishore J, Agarwal J, Agrawal S, Ayyagari A: Seroanalysis of Chlamydia trachomatis and S-TORCH agents in women with recurrent spontaneous abortions. Indian J Pathol Microbiol 46:684-687, 2003.
120. Witkin SS, Ledger WJ: Antibodies to Chlamydia trachomatis in sera of women with recurrent spontaneous abortions. Am J Obstet Gynecol 167:135-139, 1992.
121. Blas MM, Canchihuaman FA, Alva IE, Hawes SE: Pregnancy outcomes in women infected with Chlamydia trachomatis: A population-based cohort study in Washington State. Sex Transm Infect 83:314-318, 2007.
122. Alger LS, Lovchik JC, Hebel JR, et al: The association of Chlamydia trachomatis, Neisseria gonorrhoeae, and group B streptococci with preterm rupture of the membranes and pregnancy outcome. Am J Obstet Gynecol 159:397-404, 1988.
123. Cohen I, Tenenbaum E, Fejgin M, et al: Serum-specific antibodies for Chlamydia trachomatis in preterm premature rupture of the membranes. Gynecol Obstet Invest 30:155-158, 1990.
124. Rivlin ME, Morrison JC, Grossman JH 3rd: Comparison of pregnancy outcome between treated and untreated women with chlamydial cervicitis. J Miss State Med Assoc 38:404-407, 1997.
125. Andrews WW, Klebanoff MA, Thom EA, et al: Midpregnancy genitourinary tract infection with Chlamydia trachomatis: Association with subsequent preterm delivery in women with bacterial vaginosis and Trichomonas vaginalis. Am J Obstet Gynecol 194:493-500, 2006.
126. Murray PJ: NOD proteins: An intracellular pathogen-recognition system or signal transduction modifiers? Curr Opin Immunol 17:352-358, 2005.
127. Chamaillard M, Hashimoto M, Horie Y, et al: An essential role for NOD1 in host recognition of bacterial peptidoglycan containing diaminopimelic acid. Nat Immunol 4:702-707, 2003.
128. Girardin SE, Boneca IG, Carneiro LA, et al: Nod1 detects a unique muropeptide from gram-negative bacterial peptidoglycan. Science 300:1584-1587, 2003.
129. Girardin SE, Tournebize R, Mavris M, et al: CARD4/Nod1 mediates NF-kappaB and JNK activation by invasive Shigella flexneri. EMBO Rep 2:736-742, 2001.
130. Opitz B, Puschel A, Beermann W, et al: Listeria monocytogenes activated p38 MAPK and induced IL-8 secretion in a nucleotide-binding oligomerization domain 1-dependent manner in endothelial cells. J Immunol 176:484-490, 2006.
131. Chin AI, Dempsey PW, Bruhn K, et al: Involvement of receptor-interacting protein 2 in innate and adaptive immune responses. Nature 416:190-194, 2002.
132. Inohara N, Koseki T, Lin J, et al: An induced proximity model for NF-kappa B activation in the Nod1/RICK and RIP signaling pathways. J Biol Chem 275:27823-27831, 2000.
133. Kobayashi K, Inohara N, Hernandez LD, et al: RICK/Rip2/CARDIAK mediates signalling for receptors of the innate and adaptive immune systems. Nature 416:194-199, 2002.
134. Ogura Y, Inohara N, Benito A, et al: Nod2, a Nod1/Apaf-1 family member that is restricted to monocytes and activates NF-kappaB. J Biol Chem 276:4812-4818, 2001.

135. Uehara A, Yang S, Fujimoto Y, et al: Muramyldipeptide and diaminopimelic acid-containing desmuramylpeptides in combination with chemically synthesized Toll-like receptor agonists synergistically induced production of interleukin-8 in a NOD2- and NOD1-dependent manner, respectively, in human monocytic cells in culture. Cell Microbiol 7:53-61, 2005.
136. Girardin SE, Boneca IG, Viala J, et al: Nod2 is a general sensor of peptidoglycan through muramyl dipeptide (MDP) detection. J Biol Chem 278:8869-8872, 2003.
137. Inohara N, Ogura Y, Fontalba A, et al: Host recognition of bacterial muramyl dipeptide mediated through NOD2: Implications for Crohn's disease. J Biol Chem 278:5509-5512, 2003.
138. Opitz B, Forster S, Hocke AC, et al: Nod1-mediated endothelial cell activation by Chlamydophila pneumoniae. Circ Res 96:319-326, 2005.
139. Welter-Stahl L, Ojcius DM, Viala J, et al: Stimulation of the cytosolic receptor for peptidoglycan, Nod1, by infection with Chlamydia trachomatis or Chlamydia muridarum. Cell Microbiol 8:1047-1057, 2006.

Chapter 7

Maternal Cardiovascular, Respiratory, and Renal Adaptation to Pregnancy

Manju Monga, MD

Profound changes occur in the cardiovascular, respiratory, and renal systems during pregnancy. These remarkable adaptations begin early after conception and continue as gestation advances, yet most are almost totally reversible within weeks to months after delivery. These physiologic adaptations are usually well tolerated by the pregnant patient, but they must be understood so that normal can be distinguished from abnormal.

Cardiovascular System

Blood Volume

Plasma volume increases from 6 to 8 weeks of gestation, reaching a maximal volume of 4700 to 5200 mL at 32 weeks, an increase of 45% (1200 to 1600 mL) above nonpregnant values.[1,2] The mechanism of this plasma volume expansion is unclear, but it may be related to nitric oxide–mediated vasodilation, which induces the renin-angiotensin-aldosterone system and stimulates sodium and water retention, protecting the pregnant woman from hemodynamic instability after blood loss.[3] As maternal hypervolemia is present with hydatidiform mole, it is unlikely that the presence of a fetus is necessary for this volume expansion to occur.[4]

Red blood cell mass increases by 250 to 450 mL, an increase of 20% to 30% by term compared with prepregnancy values. This rise reflects increased production of red blood cells rather than prolongation of red blood cell life.[1] Placental chorionic somatomammotropin, progesterone, and perhaps prolactin are responsible for increased erythropoiesis,[5] which increases maternal demand for iron by 500 mg during pregnancy. In addition, 300 mg of iron is transferred from maternal stores to the fetus, and 200 mg of iron is required to compensate for normal daily losses during pregnancy. Erythrocyte 2,3-diphosphoglycerate concentration increases in pregnancy, lowering the affinity of maternal hemoglobin for oxygen. This facilitates dissociation of oxygen from hemoglobin, enhancing oxygen transfer to the fetus.[6]

Because plasma volume increases disproportionately to the increase in red blood cell mass, physiologic hemodilution occurs, resulting in a mild decrease in maternal hematocrit, which is maximal in the middle of the third trimester. This may have a protective function by decreasing blood viscosity to counter the predisposition to thromboembolic events in pregnancy and may be beneficial for intervillous perfusion.[7]

Anatomic Changes

Histologic and echocardiographic studies indicate that ventricular wall muscle mass and end-diastolic volume increase in pregnancy without an associated increase in end-systolic volume or end-diastolic pressure.[8,9] Ventricular mass increases in the first trimester, whereas end-diastolic volume increases in the second and early third trimesters.[8,10] This increases cardiac compliance (resulting in a physiologically dilated heart) without a concomitant reduction in ejection fraction, implying that myocardial contractility must also increase. This is supported by studies of systolic time intervals in pregnancy[11,12] and echocardiographic demonstration of a decreased ratio of the load-independent wall stress to the velocity of circumferential fiber shortening.[13] A recent echocardiographic study of left ventricular function during pregnancy suggests that changes in long-axis performance occur earlier than changes in transverse function and challenges the notion of dominance of circumferential fiber shortening.[14] Left atrial diameter increases in parallel with the rise in blood volume, starting early in pregnancy and plateauing by 30 weeks.[15]

A general softening of collagen occurs in the entire vascular system, associated with hypertrophy of the smooth muscle component. This results in increased compliance of capacitive (predominantly elastic wall) and conductive (predominantly muscular wall) arteries and veins that is evident as early as at 5 weeks of the beginning of amenorrhea.[16]

Cardiac Output

Cardiac output, the product of heart rate and stroke volume, is a measure of the functional capacity of the heart. Cardiac output may be calculated by invasive heart catheterization using dye dilution or thermodilution, or by noninvasive methods such as impedance cardiography and echocardiography. Limited data have been obtained from normal pregnant women by means of an invasive method.[17-19] M-mode echocardiography[20] and Doppler studies[21-23] have demonstrated good correlation with thermodilution methods. These validation studies have not been performed in healthy pregnant women, and reports are limited to critically ill patients. Yet to be determined is the most appropriate echocardiographic technique (pulsed-wave or continuous Doppler) and the most reproducible site through which to measure blood flow.[24] In contrast, thoracic electrical bioimpedance, which is influenced by intrathoracic fluid volume, hemoglobin, and chest configuration (all of which change in pregnancy), has had poor correlation with thermodilution techniques, with underestimation of cardiac output during pregnancy.[22,25,26]

Cardiac output increases by 30% to 50% during pregnancy,[13,17-19,23,27,28] and 50% of this increase occurs by 8 weeks of gestation.[28] A small decline in cardiac output at term results from a fall in stroke volume.[8,29-31]

Increased maternal cardiac output is caused by an increase in both stroke volume and heart rate. Stroke volume is primarily responsible for the early increase in cardiac output,[27,32] probably reflecting the increase in ventricular muscle mass and end-diastolic volume. Stroke volume declines toward term.[29] In contrast, maternal heart rate, which rises from 5 weeks' gestation to a maximal increment of 15 to 20 beats/min by 32 weeks' gestation, is maintained (Fig. 7-1).[27,29,33] Therefore, in the late third trimester, maternal tachycardia is primarily responsible for maintaining cardiac output.

Maternal posture significantly affects cardiac output. Turning from the left lateral recumbent to the supine position at term can result in a drop in cardiac output by as much as 25% to 30%.[29] This is the result of caval compression by the gravid uterus, which diminishes venous return from the lower extremities, decreasing stroke volume and cardiac output. Although most women do not become hypotensive with this maneuver, up to 8% of women do demonstrate the supine hypotensive syndrome, which is manifested by a sudden drop in blood pressure, bradycardia, and syncope.[34] This may result from inadequacy of the paravertebral collateral blood supply in these women, because symptomatic supine hypotensive syndrome does not appear to be associated with a decrease in baroreceptor response.[35]

This physiologic increase in cardiac output has a selective regional distribution. Uterine blood flow increases 10-fold to between 500 and 800 mL/min,[36] a shift from 2% of total cardiac output in the nonpregnant state to 17% at term. Renal blood flow increases significantly (by 50%) during pregnancy,[37] as does perfusion of the breasts and skin.[38,39] There does not appear to be any major alteration in blood flow to the brain or liver.

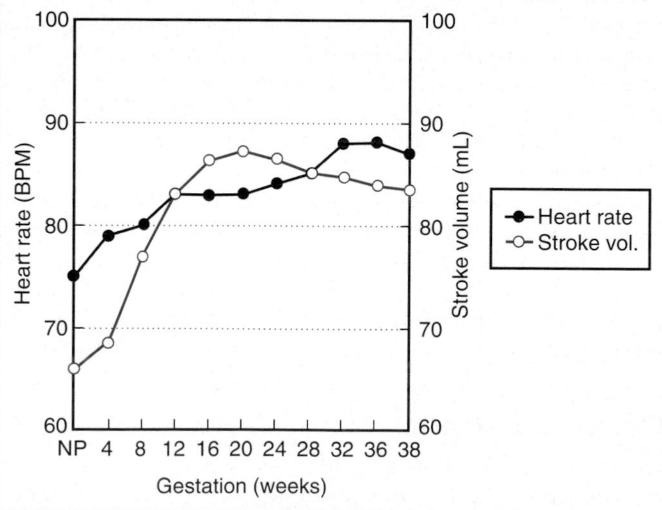

FIGURE 7-1 **Alteration in stroke volume and heart rate during pregnancy.** Stroke volume increases maximally during the first half of gestation. There is a slight decrease in stroke volume toward term. A mild increase in heart rate begins early in gestation and continues until term. (Adapted from Robson SC, Hunter S, Boys RJ, et al: Serial study of factors influencing changes in cardiac output during human pregnancy. Am J Physiol 256:H1060, 1989.)

Blood Pressure

Arterial blood pressure decreases in pregnancy beginning as early as the 7th week.[32] This early drop probably represents incomplete compensation for the decrease in peripheral vascular resistance by the increase in cardiac output. When measured in the sitting or standing positions, systolic blood pressure remains relatively stable throughout pregnancy, whereas diastolic blood pressure decreases by a maximum of 10 mm Hg at 28 weeks and then increases toward nonpregnant levels by term.[40] In contrast, when measured in the left lateral recumbent position, both systolic and diastolic blood pressures decrease to a level 5 to 10 mm Hg and 10 to 15 mm Hg, respectively, below nonpregnant values. This nadir occurs at 24 to 32 weeks' gestation and is followed by a rise toward nonpregnant values at term (Fig. 7-2).[40] Because diastolic pressures decrease to a greater extent than systolic pressures, there is a slight increase in pulse pressure in the early third trimester. Arterial blood pressures are approximately 10 mm Hg higher in the standing or sitting positions than in the lateral or supine positions; consistency in position during successive blood pressure measurements is essential for the accurate documentation of a trend during pregnancy.

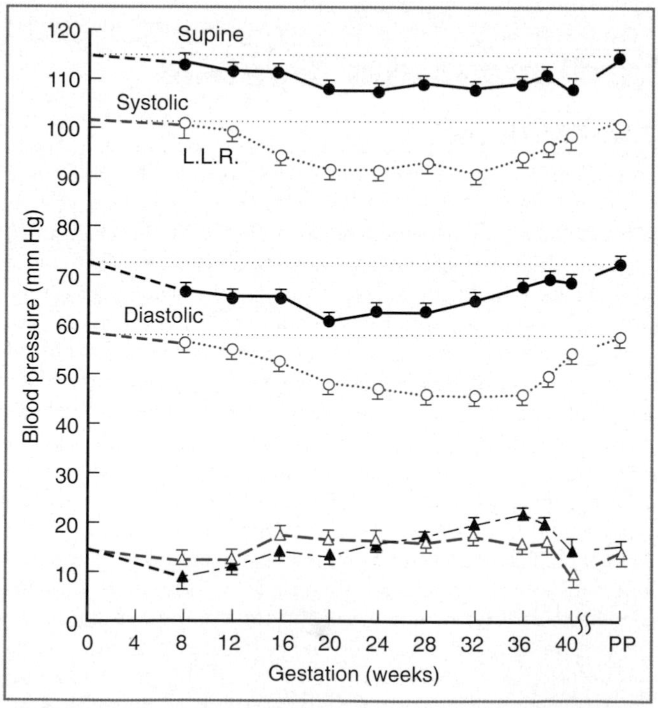

FIGURE 7-2 **Sequential changes in blood pressures throughout pregnancy.** The subjects were in supine *(closed circles)* or left lateral recumbent (L.L.R.) *(open circles)* positions. At the bottom of the graph, the changes in systolic *(open triangles)* and diastolic *(closed triangles)* blood pressures produced by movement from the left lateral recumbent to the supine position are shown. (From Wilson M, Morganti AA, Zervoudakis I, et al: Blood pressure, the renin-aldosterone system and sex steroids throughout normal pregnancy. Am J Med 68:97, 1980.)

Confusion has arisen with regard to the definition of diastolic blood pressure in pregnancy. Measurement of Korotkoff phase 4 (the point of muffling) results in mean diastolic pressures 13 mm Hg higher than measurement of Korotkoff phase 5 (the point of disappearance).[41] Use of Korotkoff phase 4 may be less reproducible.[42] Intra-arterial measurements of diastolic pressures may be 15 mm Hg lower than manual determinations,[43] whereas they may be significantly higher than automated cuff diastolic measurements.[44]

The use of ambulatory blood pressure monitoring has been validated in pregnancy.[45] Monitoring over a period of 24 hours has shown measurements that are either significantly lower[46] or higher[47] than office measurements. These differences cannot be explained by activity level, although work and job-related stress have been shown to increase blood pressure in late pregnancy.[47,48] Ambulatory blood pressure monitoring has shown marked circadian variation in blood pressure during pregnancy, with a nadir of systolic and diastolic blood pressures in the early morning hours and a peak in late afternoon and evening.[49]

Systemic Vascular Resistance

Systemic vascular resistance is calculated by the following equation:

$$(\text{Mean arterial pressure} - \text{central venous pressure}) \times 80 \text{ dyne-sec cm}^{-5}/\text{cardiac output}$$

Systemic vascular resistance decreases from as early as at 5 weeks of pregnancy as a result of the vasodilatory effect of progesterone and prostaglandins and perhaps the arteriovenous fistula–like function of the low-resistance uteroplacental circulation.[13,50-52] Alternatively, it has been proposed that increased production of endothelium-derived relaxant factors, such as nitric oxide, initiates vasodilation and a drop in systemic vascular resistance.[3,53] This decrease in systemic vascular tone may be the primary trigger for increasing heart rate, stroke volume, and cardiac output in the first few weeks of pregnancy.[3,52] The fall in systemic vascular resistance is paralleled by an increase in vascular compliance, which reaches a nadir at 14 to 24 weeks' gestation and then rises progressively toward term.[16,17]

Venous Vascular Bed

Venous compliance increases progressively during pregnancy as a result of the relaxant effect of progesterone or endothelium-derived relaxant factors on blood vessel smooth muscle, or as a result of altered elastic properties of the venous wall. This results in a decrease in flow velocity and leads to stasis.[54] Pregnant women are therefore more sensitive to autonomic blockade, which results in further venous pooling, decreased venous return, and a fall in cardiac output manifested as a sudden drop in arterial blood pressure. This may be seen in response to conduction anesthesia and ganglionic blockade.

Antepartum Hemodynamics

Clark and colleagues studied the effect of pregnancy on central hemodynamics by placing Swan-Ganz catheters and arterial lines in 10 normal primiparous women at 35 to 38 weeks' gestation and again at 11 to 13 postpartum weeks (Table 7-1).[19] Late pregnancy was characterized by significant elevations in heart rate, stroke volume, and cardiac output, in concert with significant decreases in systemic and pulmonary vascular resistance and serum colloid osmotic pressure. There was no significant alteration in pulmonary capillary wedge pressure, central venous pressure, or mean arterial blood pressure. The authors suggested that pulmonary capillary wedge pressure does not increase, despite significant increases in blood volume and stroke volume, because of ventricular dilation and the fall in pulmonary vascular resistance. They noted, however, that pregnant women were still at higher risk for pulmonary edema because of the significantly decreased gradient between colloid osmotic pressure and pulmonary capillary wedge pressure (gradient of 10.5 ± 2.7 mm Hg) compared with the nonpregnant state (gradient of 14.5 ± 2.5 mm Hg).

TABLE 7-1 HEMODYNAMIC PROFILES FOR NONPREGNANT AND PREGNANT PATIENTS IN THE THIRD TRIMESTER

	Nonpregnant	Pregnant	Change
Cardiac output (L/min)	4.3 ± 0.9	6.2 ± 1.0	+43%
Heart rate (beats/min)	71 ± 10	83 ± 10	+17%
SVR (dyne-sec cm^{-5})	1530 ± 520	1210 ± 266	−21%
PVR (dyne-sec cm^{-5})	119 ± 47	78 ± 22	−34%
CVP (mm Hg)	3.7 ± 2.6	3.6 ± 2.5	NS
COP (mm Hg)	20.8 ± 1.0	18.0 ± 1.5	−14%
PCWP (mm Hg)	6.3 ± 2.1	7.5 ± 1.8	NS
COP-PCWP (mm Hg)	14.5 ± 2.5	10.5 ± 2.7	−28%

COP, colloid osmotic pressure; COP-PCWP, gradient between COP and PCWP; CVP, central venous pressure; nonpregnant, at 11 to 13 weeks postpartum; NS, not significant; PCWP, pulmonary capillary wedge pressure; pregnant, at 36 to 38 weeks' gestation; PVR, pulmonary vascular resistance; SVR, systemic vascular resistance.
Adapted with permission from Clark SL, Cotton DB, Lee W, et al: Central hemodynamic assessment of normal term pregnancy. Am J Obstet Gynecol 161:1439, 1989.

Circulation time demonstrates a slight but progressive decline during pregnancy, reaching a minimal value of 10.2 seconds in the third trimester.[55] These findings have been interpreted to mean that blood flow velocity increases slightly in pregnancy.

Autonomic cardiovascular control in pregnancy has also been investigated. Although earlier studies indicated a blunted heart rate and blood pressure response to the Valsalva maneuver, possibly because of decreased vagal control of the heart,[33,56] a study of baroreceptor sensitivity using power spectral analysis of heart rate and blood pressure variability between 28 and 28 weeks' gestation indicated a significant negative correlation between baroreceptor sensitivity and cardiac output, and a positive correlation with total peripheral resistance. This suggests that baroreceptors respond to changes in cardiac output and peripheral vascular resistance to maintain blood pressure during pregnancy.[57]

Symptoms and Signs of Normal Pregnancy

Pregnant women report dyspnea with increased frequency as gestation advances (15% in the first trimester compared with 75% by the third).[58] The mechanism for this is unclear, but it may relate to the exaggerated ventilatory response (perhaps progesterone mediated) in response to increased metabolic demand. Easy fatigability and decreased exercise tolerance are also commonly reported, although mild to moderate exercise is well tolerated under normal circumstances.[59,60] Increased lower extremity venous pressure, caused by compression by the gravid uterus and lower colloid osmotic pressure, is commonly manifested as dependent edema—most often found in the distal lower extremities at term. Thigh-high support stockings significantly increase systemic vascular resistance by preventing venous pooling in the lower extremities and may be effective in decreasing peripheral edema in pregnancy.[61]

Cutforth and MacDonald documented clearly the alterations in heart sounds in pregnancy by a phonocardiographic study of 50 normal primigravid women.[62] Briefly, the first heart sound increased in loudness and was more widely split in approximately 90% of women (30 to 45 msec compared with 15 msec in the nonpregnant state). This results from early closure of the mitral valve, as demonstrated by the shortened interval between the Q wave of the electrocardiogram and the first heart sound. There was no significant change in the second heart sound until 30 weeks' gestation, when persistent splitting that does not vary with respiration may occur. A loud third heart sound was heard in up to 90% of pregnant women, whereas less than 5% had an audible fourth heart sound.

Systolic murmurs develop in more than 95% of pregnant women. These are heard best along the left sternal border and are most often either aortic or pulmonary in origin. Doppler echocardiography demonstrates an increased incidence of functional tricuspid regurgitation during pregnancy that may also lead to a systolic precordial murmur.[63] Although most of these changes in heart sounds are first audible between 12 and 20 weeks' gestation and regress by 1 week after the birth, nearly 20% have a persistent systolic murmur beyond the 4th week after delivery. Systolic murmurs louder than grade 2/4 and diastolic murmurs of any intensity are considered abnormal during pregnancy. However, 14% of women may have a continuous murmur of mammary vessel origin, which is heard maximally in the second intercostal space.[62]

Uterine growth results in upward displacement of the diaphragm, which is associated with superior, lateral, and anterior displacement of the heart within the thorax. This leads to lateral displacement of the point of maximal impulse and may suggest cardiomegaly on chest radiographs. This appearance is further enhanced by straightening of the left heart border and by prominence of the pulmonary outflow tracts; however, the cardiothoracic ratio is only slightly increased, if at all, in normal pregnancy.[64]

Intrapartum Hemodynamic Changes

Labor results in significant alteration in the cardiovascular measurements. The first stage of labor is associated with a 12% to 31% rise in cardiac output, primarily because of a 22% increase in stroke volume.[65,66] The second stage of labor is associated with an even greater increase in cardiac output (49%). Laboring in the left lateral decubitus position or analgesia decreases the magnitude of this increment. The increase in cardiac output is not completely abolished by relief of pain, because contractions result in the transfer of 300 to 500 mL of blood from the uterus to the general circulation.[67,68] Systolic and diastolic blood pressures transiently increase by 35 and 25 mm Hg, respectively, during labor.[66] For these reasons, women who have cardiovascular compromise may experience decompensation with labor, especially during the second stage.

Postpartum Hemodynamic Changes

Pregnant women with cardiac disease are perhaps at greatest risk for pulmonary edema in the immediate postpartum period. The immediate puerperium is associated with an 80% increase in cardiac output within 10 to 15 minutes after vaginal delivery with local anesthesia compared with 60% with caudal anesthesia.[69,70] Whole-body impedance cardiography was used to continuously study maternal hemodynamics and cardiovascular responses in 10 women having cesarean section under spinal analgesia.[71] Within 2 minutes of delivery, there was a 47% increase in cardiac index and a 39% decrease in systemic vascular index without appreciable change in mean arterial pressure. This immediate increase in cardiac output is caused by release of venacaval obstruction by the gravid uterus, autotransfusion of uteroplacental blood, and rapid mobilization of extravascular fluid. All these changes result in increased venous return to the heart and increased stroke volume. Cardiac output returns to prelabor values 1 hour after delivery.[70]

Vaginal delivery is associated with a blood loss of approximately 500 mL, whereas cesarean section may cause a loss of 1000 mL.[72] The pregnant woman is protected from postpartum blood loss in part by the expansion of blood volume associated with pregnancy.

M-mode echocardiographic studies have shown that left atrial dimensions increase 1 to 3 days after the birth, perhaps because of mobilization of excessive body fluids and increased venous return.[70] Atrial natriuretic levels also increase in the immediate postpartum period, which may stimulate diuresis and natriuresis in the early puerperium.[73]

Whereas left atrial dimensions and heart rate normalize within the first 10 postpartum days, left ventricular dimensions decrease gradually for 4 to 6 months. Cardiovascular measurements, such as stroke volume, cardiac output, and systemic vascular resistance, as measured by M-mode echocardiography, do not completely return to prepregnancy values by 12 postpartum weeks and may continue to decrease for 24 weeks before stabilizing.[28,70] Therefore, the early postpartum period may not accurately reflect the nonpregnant state in studies of pregnancy-related hemodynamic changes.

Respiratory System

There is a moderate decrease in functional residual capacity during pregnancy, attributed to a decrease in both expiratory reserve volume and residual volume (Table 7-2). This is primarily the result of upward displacement of the maternal diaphragm. Maternal tidal volume increases by 40% in pregnancy, and this increase results in maternal hyperventilation and hypocapnia.[74] Because maternal respiratory rate does not change during pregnancy, the 30% to 50% increase in minute ventilation that is noted as early as the first trimester is attributed to this increase in tidal volume alone.[75] Increased minute ventilation may be the result of increased progesterone and an increase in basal metabolic rate.

There is a decrease in the partial pressure of carbon dioxide from a pre-pregnancy level of 39 mm Hg to approximately 28 to 31 mm Hg at term. This hyperventilation facilitates the transfer of carbon dioxide from the fetus to the mother and is partially compensated for by an increased renal secretion of hydrogen ions, with a resultant serum bicarbonate level of 18 to 22 mEq/L. A mild respiratory alkalosis is therefore normal in pregnancy, with an arterial pH of 7.44, compared with 7.40 in the nonpregnant state. This mild respiratory alkalosis results in a shift to the left of the oxygen dissociation curve, increasing the affinity of maternal hemoglobin for oxygen (the Bohr effect) and reducing oxygen release to the fetus. This is compensated for by an alkalosis-stimulated increase in 2,3-diphosphoglycerate in maternal erythrocytes, which shifts the oxygen dissociation curve to the right, facilitating oxygen transfer to the fetus.[76]

TABLE 7-2 RESPIRATORY CHANGES DURING PREGNANCY

Lung Volume (mL)	Nonpregnant	Pregnant	Change
Total lung capacity (vital capacity + residual volume)	4200	4000	−4%
Vital capacity (total lung capacity − residual volume)	3200	3200	No change
Inspiratory capacity (vital capacity − expiratory reserve volume)	2500	2650	+6%
Tidal volume	450	600	+33%
Expiratory reserve volume (vital capacity − inspiratory capacity)	700	550	−20%
Inspiratory reserve volume (inspiratory capacity − tidal volume)	2050	2050	No change
Residual volume (result: decrease in total lung capacity)	1000	800	−20%
Functional residual capacity (residual volume + expiratory reserve volume)	1700	1350	−20%

Concomitant with the increase in maternal minute ventilation is a 20% to 40% increase in maternal oxygen consumption caused by increased oxygen requirements of the fetus, placenta, and maternal organs.[77] Because of the increase in maternal oxygen consumption and the decrease in functional residual capacity, pregnant women with asthma, pneumonia, or other respiratory pathology may be more susceptible to early decompensation.

Kidneys and Lower Urinary Tract

Dramatic changes in renal structure, dynamics, and function occur during pregnancy. These have recently been reviewed.[78]

Structure and Dynamics

Renal size and weight increase during pregnancy as a result of an increase in renal vascular and interstitial volume. Kidney length increases by approximately 1 cm,[79] and renal volume, as determined by computed nephrosonography, increases by approximately 30%.[80] More dramatic, however, is dilation of the urinary collecting system, which occurs in more than 80% of gravidas by mid-gestation.[81] Caliceal and ureteral dilation are more common on the right side than the left,[82,83] and the degree of caliceal dilation is more pronounced on the right than on the left (15 versus 5 mm).[84] The prominence of these changes on the right side may result from dextrorotation of the pregnant uterus, the location of the right ovarian vein that crosses the ureter, or the protective "cushion" effect of the sigmoid colon on the left side, or any combination of these. Ureteral dilation is rarely present below the level of the pelvic brim, and sonographic visualization demonstrates tapering of the ureters as they cross the common iliac artery.[85] Although obstruction plays a role in the physiologic pyelectasis of pregnancy, an associated increase in renal arterial resistance has not been consistently documented.[83] One reason for this may be the poor reproducibility of pulsed Doppler measurements in the maternal renal circulation as a result of high interobserver and intraobserver variability.[86] Progesterone, relaxin, and the nitric oxide pathway may play a concomitant role in ureteral smooth muscle relaxation, but there is no consensus on the influence of hormones on these anatomic alterations.[78,87]

The dilation of the urinary collecting system has several important clinical consequences, including an increase in ascending urinary tract infection, perhaps related to urinary stasis; difficulty in interpreting radiologic examinations of the urinary tract; and interference with evaluation of glomerular and tubular function, because these tests require high urine flow rates. Renal volume returns to normal within the first week of delivery,[80] but hydronephrosis and hydroureter may persist for 3 to 4 months after the birth.[84] This fact should be considered when radiologic or renal function studies on postpartum women are being interpreted. Ureteral peristalsis does not change in pregnancy; however, ureteral tone progressively increases, possibly as a result of mechanical obstruction, and then returns to normal shortly after delivery.[88] Controversy exists with regard to changes in urinary bladder pressures and capacity. In one study, urinary bladder pressure doubled between the first and third trimesters of pregnancy, implying a decrease in bladder capacity.[89] Previous studies demonstrated a relatively hypotonic bladder, with decreased pressure and increased capacity near term.[90] Urethral length and intraurethral closure pressure in pregnancy have also been determined by urodynamic studies and have been found to increase by 20%.[89] The latter may counter the increase in bladder pressure in an attempt to reduce stress incontinence, which is more common in pregnancy, occurring in 29% to 41% at term.[91]

Renal Function

Renal plasma flow, as estimated by para-aminohippurate clearance, increases by 60% to 80% over nonpregnant values by the middle of the second trimester and then falls to 50% above prepregnancy values in the third trimester.[92] Renal plasma flow, like cardiac output, is significantly higher when the patient is in the left lateral recumbent position than when she is sitting, standing, or supine. This reflects maximal venous return in the left lateral position.[93,94]

Glomerular filtration rate (GFR) is estimated by determination of inulin, iohexol, or creatinine clearance. Creatinine clearance, although most commonly used, is the least precise of the determinations because creatinine is secreted by the tubules in addition to being cleared by the glomeruli. Creatinine clearance can be calculated by dividing the total amount of urinary creatinine (in milligrams) by the duration of collection (in minutes). This value is then divided by the creatinine concentration in serum (in mg/mL). This yields a creatinine clearance in mL/min.

GFR begins to increase by as early as 6 weeks' gestation, with a peak of 50% over nonpregnant values by the end of the first trimester.[94] Although there are few data on the measurement of GFR after 36 weeks of gestation, GFR does not appear to decrease at term. Creatinine clearance is thus moderately increased in pregnancy (110 to 150 mL/min). This rate has a circadian variation of 80% to 125%, with maximal creatinine excretion between 2 PM and 10 PM and lowest excretion rates between 2 AM and 10 AM.[95]

The mechanisms behind the changes in renal hemodynamics are unclear, although study of pregnant rats suggests that GFR rises secondary to vasodilation of preglomerular and postglomerular resistance vessels without any alteration in glomerular capillary pressure.[96] This is further supported by the lack of continued increase in GFR after the first trimester of pregnancy despite decreasing serum albumin, implying independence from changes in oncotic pressure.[52]

Because the increase in renal plasma flow is initially greater than the rise in GFR, the filtration fraction (GFR divided by renal plasma flow) decreases until the third trimester of pregnancy, when a fall in renal plasma flow results in the return of the filtration fraction to a prepregnancy value of 1/5.[94] This alteration in filtration fraction parallels the change in mean arterial pressure described previously and may be related to circulating progesterone levels.[92,97]

Filtration capacity, which is estimated by the maximal GFR in response to a vasodilator stimulus, appears to be intact in pregnancy, as documented by studies of amino acid administration in rats[96] and protein loading in pregnant women.[98] As the resting GFR rises during pregnancy, the functional renal reserve (the difference between the filtration capacity and the resting GFR) decreases. One can therefore accurately assess renal function in pregnant patients with early renal disease by determining filtration capacity, but not by functional renal reserve.[98]

The pregnancy-associated rise in GFR (which normally occurs without any concomitant increase in production of urea or creatinine) results in decreased serum creatinine and urea concentrations in pregnancy.[97] Serum creatinine falls from prepregnancy values of 0.83 mg/dL to 0.7, 0.6, and 0.5 mg/dL in successive trimesters. Blood urea nitrogen decreases from 12 mg/dL in the nonpregnant state to 11, 9, and 10 mg/dL in the first, second, and third trimesters, respectively.

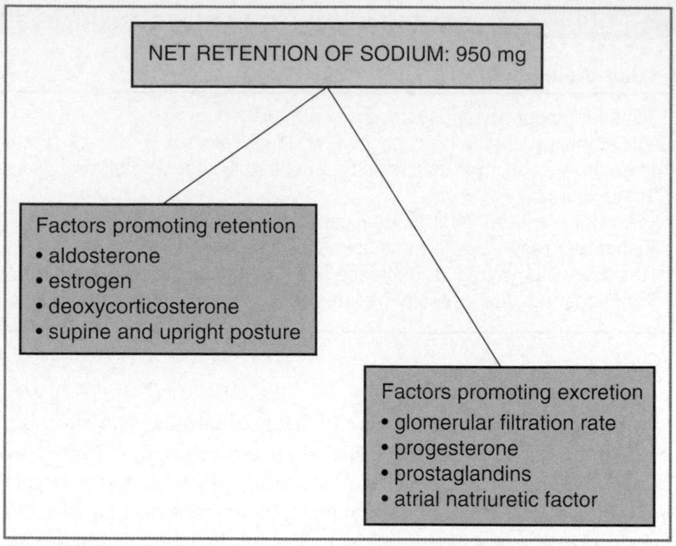

FIGURE 7-3 Factors influencing the regulation of sodium excretion in pregnancy.

Renal Tubular Function

Sodium

Several factors promote sodium excretion in pregnancy. There is an increase in the filtered load of sodium from approximately 20,000 to 30,000 mEq/day as a result of the 50% rise in GFR. Hormones that favor sodium excretion include the following:

Progesterone, a competitive inhibitor of aldosterone[99]
Vasodilatory prostaglandins[94]
Atrial natriuretic factor (although increased pregnancy-related production of atrial natriuretic factor has not been universally demonstrated)[100,101]

Despite these forces, there is a cumulative retention of approximately 950 mg of sodium during pregnancy. This is distributed between the maternal intravascular and interstitial compartments, the fetus, and the placenta.[102] The net reabsorption of sodium is one of the most remarkable adaptations of renal tubular function to pregnancy.

Factors that promote this sodium reabsorption include the increased production and secretion of aldosterone, deoxycorticosterone, and estrogen (Fig. 7-3).[99] These hormones may be regulated, in part, by the rise in plasma progesterone and vasodilatory prostaglandins, but they are also mediated by stimulation of the renin-angiotensin system. All components of the renin-angiotensin-aldosterone system increase in the first trimester of pregnancy and peak at 30 to 32 weeks' gestation.[3] Hepatic renin substrate is stimulated by estrogens and results in elevated renal production of renin. Renin stimulates increased conversion of angiotensinogen to angiotensins I and II. Sodium retention is also favored by postural changes in pregnancy; the supine and upright positions are associated with a marked decrease in sodium excretion.[37]

Potassium

Although the pregnancy-associated increase in plasma aldosterone would favor potassium excretion, a net retention of 300 to 350 mEq of potassium actually occurs. Increased kaliuresis may be prevented by the influence of progesterone on renal potassium excretion.[103] Because potassium reabsorption from the distal tubule and the loop of Henle decreases with pregnancy, it has been deduced that a significant increase in proximal tubular reabsorption occurs.[104]

Calcium

Urinary calcium excretion increases as a result of increased calcium clearance.[105] This is balanced by increased absorption of calcium from the small intestine, and therefore serum ionic (unbound) calcium levels remain stable. Total calcium levels fall in pregnancy from 4.75 mEq/L in the first trimester to 4.3 mEq/L at term because of a decrease in plasma albumin.[106] A rise in calcitriol in early pregnancy is paralleled by suppression of the parathyroid hormone and an increase in renal tubular phosphorus reabsorption.[107] This increase in calcitriol promotes reabsorption of calcium and phosphorus from the intestine and may facilitate bone mineralization in the fetus.

Glucose

Glucose excretion increases in pregnant women 10-fold to 100-fold over nonpregnant values of 100 mg/day.[108] This glycosuria, which occurs despite increased plasma insulin and decreased plasma glucose levels, is the result of impaired collecting tubule and loop of Henle reabsorption of the 5% of the filtered glucose that normally escapes proximal convoluted tubular reabsorption.[109] The clinical significance of this is that glycosuria cannot be accurately used to monitor pregnant women with diabetes mellitus.

Uric Acid

Plasma uric acid levels decrease by 25% at as early as 8 weeks' gestation, reaching a nadir of 2 to 3 mg/dL at 24 weeks' gestation, and then increase toward nonpregnant levels at term.[110] This may result from increased GFR and reduced proximal tubular reabsorption.[111] Conditions that lead to volume contraction, such as preeclampsia, may be associated with decreased uric acid clearance and increased plasma levels.

Amino Acids

The fractional excretion of alanine, glycine, histidine, serine, and threonine increases in pregnancy.[112] Cystine, leucine, lysine, phenylalanine, taurine, and tyrosine excretion increases early in pregnancy but then decreases in the second half of gestation. The excretion of arginine, asparagine, glutamic acid, isoleucine, methionine, and ornithine does not change. The mechanism of this selective amino aciduria is unknown. It is unclear whether renal excretion of albumin increases, decreases, or remains stable[113-115] in normal pregnancy. Urinary protein excretion does not normally exceed 300 mg per 24 hours.

Volume Homeostasis

Bodyweight increases by an average of 30 to 35 pounds in pregnancy.[116] Two thirds of this gain may be accounted for by an increase in total body water, with 6 to 7 L gained in the extracellular space and approximately 2 L gained in the intracellular space. Plasma volume expansion, as outlined previously, accounts for 25% of the increase in extracellular water, with the rest of the increment appearing as interstitial fluid.[102] As water is retained, plasma sodium and urea levels fall slightly, from 140.3 ± 1.7 to 136.6 ± 1.5 mM/L, and from 4.9 ± 0.9 to 2.9 ± 0.5 mM/L, respectively.[117] By 4 weeks after conception, plasma osmolality has decreased from 289 to 280.9. Because water deprivation in pregnant women leads to an appropriate increase in vasopressin and urine osmolality, and water loading results in a proportional decrease, it appears that the osmoregulation system is functioning normally but is "reset" at a lower threshold.[118] Further evidence to support this conclusion is that the osmotic threshold for thirst is decreased by 10 mOsm/kg in pregnancy.[103] The mechanism for this readjustment of the osmoregulatory system is unclear but may involve placental secretion of human chorionic gonadotropin.[119]

References

1. Pritchard JA: Changes in the blood volume during pregnancy and delivery. Anesthesiology 26:393, 1965.
2. Lund CJ, Donovan JC: Blood volume during pregnancy. Am J Obstet Gynecol 98:393, 1967.
3. Carbillon L, Uzan M, Uzan S: Pregnancy, vascular tone, and maternal hemodynamics: A crucial adaptation. Obstet Gynecol Surv 55:574, 2000.
4. Pritchard JA: Blood volume changes in pregnancy and the puerperiums: IV. Anemia associated with hydatidiform mole. Am J Obstet Gynecol 91:621, 1965.
5. Jepson JH: Endocrine control of maternal and fetal erythropoiesis. Can Med Assoc J 98:884, 1968.
6. Bille-Brahe NE, Rorth M: Red cell 2,3,-diphosphoglycerate in pregnancy. Acta Obstet Gynaecol Scand 58:19, 1979.
7. Pieters LLH, Verkeste CM, Saxena PR, et al: Relationship between maternal hemodynamics and hematocrit and hemodynamic effects of isovolemic hemodilution and hemoconcentration in the awake late-pregnant guinea pig. Pediatr Res 21:584, 1987.
8. Rubler S, Damani P, Pinto E: Cardiac size and performance during pregnancy estimated with echocardiography. Am J Cardiol 49:534, 1977.
9. Lard-Meeter K, van de Ley G, Bom T, et al: Cardiocirculatory adjustments during pregnancy: An echocardiographic study. Clin Cardiol 49:560, 1979.
10. Thompson JA, Hayes PM, Sagar KB, et al: Echocardiographic left ventricular mass to differentiate chronic hypertension from preeclampsia during pregnancy. Am J Obstet Gynecol 155:994, 1986.
11. Rubler S, Hammer N, Schneebaum R: Systolic time intervals in pregnancy and the postpartum period. Am Heart J 86:182, 1972.
12. Burg J, Dodek A, Kloster F, et al: Alterations of systolic time intervals during pregnancy. Circulation 49:560, 1974.
13. Gilson GJ, Samaan S, Crawford MH, et al: Changes in hemodynamics, ventricular remodeling, and ventricular contractility during normal pregnancy: A longitudinal study. Obstet Gynecol 89:957, 1997.
14. Kametas NA, McAuliffe F, Cook B, et al: Maternal left ventricular transverse and long axis systolic function during pregnancy. Ultrasound Obstet Gynecol 18:467-474, 2001.
15. Vered Z, Poler SM, Gibson P, et al: Noninvasive detection of the morphologic and hemodynamic changes during normal pregnancy. Clin Cardiol 14:327, 1991.
16. Spaanderman MEA, Willekes C, Hoeks APG, et al: The effect of pregnancy on the compliance of large arteries and veins in healthy parous control subjects and women with a history of preeclampsia. Am J Obstet Gynecol 183:1278, 2000.
17. Bader RA, Bader MG, Rose DJ, et al: Hemodynamics at rest and during exercise in normal pregnancy as studied by cardiac catheterization. J Clin Invest 34:1524, 1955.
18. Walters WAW, MacGregor WG, Hills M: Cardiac output at rest during pregnancy and the puerperium. Clin Sci (Colch) 30:1, 1966.
19. Clark SL, Cotton DB, Lee W, et al: Central hemodynamic assessment of normal term pregnancy. Am J Obstet Gynecol 161:1439, 1989.
20. Mashini IS, Albazzaz SJ, Fadel HE, et al: Serial noninvasive evaluation of cardiovascular hemodynamics during pregnancy. Am J Obstet Gynecol 156:1208, 1987.
21. Ihlen H, Amlie JP, Dale J, et al: Determination of cardiac output by Doppler echocardiography. Br Heart J 54:51, 1984.
22. Easterling TR, Watts H, Schmucker BC, et al: Measurement of cardiac output during pregnancy: Validation of Doppler technique and clinical observations in preeclampsia. Obstet Gynecol 69:845, 1987.
23. Easterling TR, Carlson KL, Schmucker BC, et al: Measurement of cardiac output in pregnancy by Doppler technique. Am J Perinatol 7:220, 1990.
24. Easterling TR, Benedetti TJ, Carlson KL, et al: Measurement of cardiac output in pregnancy by thermodilution and impedance techniques. BJOG 96:67, 1989.
25. Milsom I, Forssman L, Sivertsson R, et al: Measurement of cardiac stroke volume by impedance cardiography in the last trimester of pregnancy. Acta Obstet Gynaecol Scand 62:473, 1983.
26. Masaki DI, Greenspoon JS, Ouzounizn JG: Measurement of cardiac output by thoracic electrical bioimpedance and thermodilution. Am J Obstet Gynecol 161:680, 1989.
27. Robson SC, Hunter S, Boys RJ, et al: Serial study of factors influencing changes in cardiac output during human pregnancy. Am J Physiol 256: H1060, 1989.
28. Capeless EL, Clapp JF: When do cardiovascular parameters return to their preconception values? Am J Obstet Gynecol 165:883, 1991.
29. Ueland K, Novy M, Peterson E, et al: Maternal cardiovascular dynamics: IV. The influence of gestational age on the maternal cardiovascular response to posture and exercise. Am J Obstet Gynecol 104:856, 1969.
30. McLennan FM, Haites NE, Rawles JM: Stroke and minute distance in pregnancy: A longitudinal study using Doppler ultrasound. BJOG 94:499, 1987.
31. Easterling TR, Benedetti TJ, Schmucker BC, et al: Maternal hemodynamics in normal and preeclamptic pregnancies: A longitudinal study. Obstet Gynecol 76:1061, 1990.
32. Capeless EL, Clapp JF: Cardiovascular changes in early phase of pregnancy. Am J Obstet Gynecol 161:1449, 1989.
33. Stein PK, Hagley MT, Cole PL, et al: Changes in 24-hour heart rate variability during normal pregnancy. Am J Obstet Gynecol 180:978, 1999.
34. Holmes F: Incidence of the supine hypotensive syndrome in late pregnancy. J Obstet Gynaecol Br Emp 67:254, 1960.
35. Lanni SM, Tillinghast J, Silver HM: Hemodynamic changes and baroreflex gain in the supine hypotensive syndrome. Am J Obstet Gynecol 187:1636-1641, 2002.
36. Gant NF, Worley RJ: Measurement of uteroplacental blood flow in the human. In Rosenfeld CR (ed): The Uterine Circulation. Ithaca, Perinatology Press, 1989, p 53.

37. Chesley LC, Sloan DM: The effect of posture on renal function in late pregnancy. Am J Obstet Gynecol 89:754, 1964.
38. Katz M, Sokal MM: Skin perfusion in pregnancy. Am J Obstet Gynecol 137:30, 1980.
39. Frederiksen MC: Physiologic changes in pregnancy and their effect on drug disposition. Semin Perinatol 25:120, 2001.
40. Wilson M, Morganti AA, Zervoudakis I, et al: Blood pressure, the renin-aldosterone system and sex steroids throughout normal pregnancy. Am J Med 68:97, 1980.
41. Wickman K, Ryden G, Wickman G: The influence of different positions and Korotkoff sounds on the blood pressure measurements in pregnancy. Acta Obstet Gynaecol Scand 118(Suppl):25, 1984.
42. Johenning AR, Barron WM: Indirect blood pressure measurement in pregnancy: Korotkoff phase 4 versus phase 5. Am J Obstet Gynecol 167:577, 1992.
43. Koller O: The clinical significance of hemodilution during pregnancy. Obstet Gynecol Surv 37:649, 1982.
44. Kirshon B, Lee W, Cotton DB, et al: Indirect blood pressure monitoring in the obstetric patient. Obstet Gynecol 70:799, 1987.
45. Clark S, Hofmeyr GJ, Coats AJ, et al: Ambulatory blood pressure monitoring in pregnancy: Validation of the TM-420 monitor. Obstet Gynecol 77:152-155, 1991.
46. Halligan A, O'Brien E, O'Malley K, et al: Twenty four hour ambulatory blood pressure measurement in a primigravid population. J Hypertens 11:869, 1993.
47. Churchill D, Beevers DG: Differences between office and 24-hour ambulatory blood pressure measurement during pregnancy. Obstet Gynecol 88:455, 1996.
48. Walker SP, Permezel M, Brennecke SP, et al: Blood pressure in late pregnancy and work outside the home. Obstet Gynecol 97:361, 2001.
49. Hermida RC, Auala DE, Mojon A, et al: Blood pressure patterns in normal pregnancy, gestational hypertension, and preeclampsia. Hypertension 36:149, 2000.
50. Greiss FC, Anderson SG: Effect of ovarian hormones on the uterine vascular bed. Am J Obstet Gynecol 107:829, 1970.
51. Gerber JG, Payne HA, Murphy RC, et al: Prostacyclin produced by the pregnant uterus in the dog may act as a circulating vasodepressor substance. J Clin Invest 67:632, 1981.
52. Duvekot JJ, Cheriex EC, Pieters FAA, et al: Early pregnancy changes in hemodynamics and volume homeostasis are consecutive adjustments triggered by a primary fall in systemic vascular tone. Am J Obstet Gynecol 169:1382, 1993.
53. Duvekot JJ, Pieters LLH: Maternal cardiovascular hemodynamic adaptation to pregnancy. Obstet Gynecol Surv 49:S1, 1994.
54. Fawer R, Dettling A, Weihs D, et al: Effect of the menstrual cycle, oral contraception and pregnancy on forearm blood flow, venous distensibility and clotting factors. Eur J Clin Pharmacol 13:251, 1978.
55. Manchester B, Loube SD: The velocity of blood flow in normal pregnant women. Am Heart J 32:215, 1946.
56. Ekholm EMK, Erkkola RU: Autonomic cardiovascular control in pregnancy. Eur J Obstet Gynecol Reprod Biol 64:29, 1996.
57. Jayawardana MAJ: Baroreceptor sensitivity and hemodynamics in normal pregnancy. J Obstset Gynecol 21:559-562, 2001.
58. Milne JA, Howie AD, Pack AL: Dyspnoea during normal pregnancy. BJOG 85:260, 1978.
59. Kulpa PJ, White BM, Visscher R: Aerobic exercise in pregnancy. Am J Obstet Gynecol 156:1395, 1987.
60. Wolf LA, Hall P, Webb KA: Prescription of aerobic exercise during pregnancy. Sports Med. 8:273, 1989.
61. Hobel CJ, Castro L, Rosen D, et al: The effect of thigh-length support stockings on the hemodynamic response to ambulation in pregnancy. Am J Obstet Gynecol 174:1734, 1996.
62. Cutforth R, MacDonald CB: Heart sounds during normal pregnancy. Am Heart J 71:741, 1966.
63. Limacher MC, Ware JA, O'Meara ME, et al: Tricuspid regurgitation during pregnancy: Two-dimensional and pulsed Doppler echocardiographic observations. Am J Cardiol 55:1059, 1985.
64. Turner AF: The chest radiograph during pregnancy. Clin Obstet Gynecol 18:65, 1975.
65. Ueland K, Hansen JM: Maternal cardiovascular hemodynamics: III. Labor and delivery under local and caudal anesthesia. Am J Obstet Gynecol 103:8, 1969.
66. Robson SC, Dunlop W, Boys RJ, et al: Cardiac output during labor. Br Med J 295:1169, 1987.
67. Adams JQ, Alexander AM: Alterations in cardiovascular physiology during labor. Obstet Gynecol 12:542, 1958.
68. Hendricks CH, Quilligan EJ: Cardiac output during labor. Am J Obstet Gynecol 76:969, 1958.
69. Ueland K, Metcalfe J: Circulatory changes in pregnancy. Clin Obstet Gynecol 18:41, 1975.
70. Robson SC, Hunter S, Moore M, et al: Haemodynamic changes during the puerperium: A Doppler and M-mode echocardiographic study. BJOG 94:1028, 1987.
71. Tihtonen K, Koobi T, Yli-Hankala A, Uotila J: Maternal hemodynamics during caesarean delivery assessed by whole-body impedance cardiography. Acta Obstet Gynaecol Scand 84:355-361, 2005.
72. Ueland K: Maternal cardiovascular dynamics: VII. Intrapartum blood volume changes. Am J Obstet Gynecol 126:671, 1976.
73. Pouta AM, Raasanen JP, Airaksinen KEJ, et al: Changes in maternal heart dimensions and plasma atrial natriuretic peptide levels in the early puerperium of normal and pre-eclamptic pregnancies. BJOG 103:988, 1996.
74. Awe RJ, Nicotra MB, Newsom TD, et al: Arterial oxygenation and alveolar-arterial gradients in term pregnancy. Obstet Gynecol 53:182, 1979.
75. McAuliffe F. Kametas N, Costello J, et al: Respiratory function in singleton and twin pregnancy. BJOG 109:765-768, 2002.
76. Tsai CH, de Leeu NKM: Changes in 2,3-diphosphoglycerate during pregnancy and puerperium in normal women and in B-thalassemia heterozygous women. Am J Obstet Gynecol 142:520-526, 1982.
77. Crapo R: Normal cardiopulmonary physiology during pregnancy. Clin Obstet Gynecol 39:3-16, 1996.
78. Jeyabalan A, Lain KY: Anatomic and functional changes of the upper urinary tract during pregnancy. Urol Clin North Am 34:1-6, 2007.
79. Bailey RR, Rolleston GLI: Kidney length and ureteric dilatation in the puerperium. J Obstet Gynaecol Br Commonw 78:55, 1971.
80. Christensen T, Klebe JG, Bertelsen V, et al: Changes in renal volume during normal pregnancy. Acta Obstet Gynaecol Scand 68:541, 1989.
81. Rasmussen PE, Nielse FR: Hydronephrosis during pregnancy: A literature survey. Eur J Obstet Gynaecol Reprod Biol 27:249, 1988.
82. Schulman A, Herlinger H: Urinary tract dilatation in pregnancy. Br J Radiol 48:638, 1975.
83. Hertzberg BS, Carroll BA, Bowie JD, et al: Doppler USS assessment of maternal kidneys: Analysis of intrarenal resistivity indexes in normal pregnancy and physiologic pelvocaliectasis. Radiology 186:689, 1993.
84. Fried A, Woodring JH, Thompson TJ: Hydronephrosis of pregnancy. J Ultrasound Med 2:255, 1983.
85. MacNeily AE, Goldenberg SL, Allen GJJ, et al: Sonographic visualization of the ureter in pregnancy. J Urol 146:298, 1991.
86. Nakai A, Miyake H, Oya A, et al: Reproducibility of pulsed Doppler measurements of the maternal renal circulation in normal pregnancies and those with pregnancy-induced hypertension. Ultrasound Obstet Gynecol 19:598, 2002.
87. Marchant DJ: Effects of pregnancy and progestational agents on the urinary tract. Am J Obstet Gynecol 112:487, 1972.
88. Sala NL, Rubi RA: Ureteral function in pregnant women: II. Ureteral contractibility during normal pregnancy. Am J Obstet Gynecol 99:228, 1967.
89. Iosif S, Ingermarsson I, Ulmsten U: Urodynamics studies in normal pregnancy and in puerperium. Am J Obstet Gynecol 137:696, 1980.
90. Youssef AF: Cystometric studies in gynecology and obstetrics. Obstet Gynecol 8:181, 1956.
91. Kristiansson P, Samuelsson E, Von Schoultz B, et al: Reproductive hormones and stress urinary incontinence in pregnancy. Act Obstet Gynaecol Scand 80:1125, 2001.

92. Dunlop W: Serial changes in renal hemodynamics during normal human pregnancy. BJOG 88:1, 1981.
93. Equimokhai M, Davison JM, Philips PR, et al: Non-postural serial changes in renal function during the third trimester of normal human pregnancy. BJOG 88:465, 1981.
94. Davison JM, Dunlop W: Changes in renal hemodynamics and tubular function induced by normal human pregnancy. Semin Nephrol 4:198, 1984.
95. Kalousek G, Hlavecek C, Nedoss B, et al: Circadian rhythms of creatinine and electrolyte excretion in healthy pregnant women. Am J Obstet Gynecol 103:856, 1969.
96. Baylis C: The determinants of renal hemodynamics in pregnancy. Am J Kidney Dis 9:260, 1987.
97. Davison JM, Dunlop W: Renal hemodynamics and tubular function in normal human pregnancy. Kidney Int 18:152, 1980.
98. Ronco C, Brendolan A, Bragantini L, et al: Renal functional reserve in pregnancy. Nephrol Dial Transplant 2:157, 1988.
99. Barron WM, Lindheimer MD: Renal sodium and water handling in pregnancy. Obstet Gynecol Annu 13:35-69, 1984.
100. Bond AL, August P, Druzin ML, et al: Atrial natriuretic factor in normal and hypertensive pregnancy. Am J Obstet Gynecol 160:1112, 1989.
101. Marlettini MG, Cassani A, Boschi S, et al: Plasma concentrations of atrial natriuretic factor in normal pregnancy and early puerperium. Clin Exp Hypertens A 1989;11:531-552.
102. Hytten FE: Weight gain in pregnancy. In Hytten FE, Chamberlain G (eds): Clinical Physiology in Obstetrics. Oxford, Blackwell Scientific, 1991, pp 173-203.
103. Lindheimer MD, Barron WM, Davison JM: Osmoregulation of thirst and vasopressin release in pregnancy. Am J Physiol 257:F59, 1989.
104. Garland HO, Green R: Micropuncture study of changes in glomerular filtration and ion and water handling in the rat kidney during pregnancy. J Physiol (Lond) 329:389, 1982.
105. Roelofsen JMT, Berkel GM, Uttendorfsky OT, et al: Urinary excretion rates of calcium and magnesium in normal and complicated pregnancies. Eur J Obstet Gynaecol Reprod Biol 27:227, 1988.
106. Pitkin RM, Reynolds WA, Williams GA, et al: Calcium metabolism in pregnancy: A longitudinal study. Am J Obstet Gynecol 133:781, 1979.
107. Weiss M, Eisenstein Z, Ramot Y, et al: Renal reabsorption of inorganic phosphorus in pregnancy in relation to the calciotropic hormones. BJOG 105:195, 1998.
108. Davison JM, Hytten FE: The effect of pregnancy on the renal handling of glucose. J Obstet Gynaecol Br Commonw 82:374, 1975.
109. Bishop JHV, Green R: Effects of pregnancy on glucose reabsorption by the proximal convoluted tubule in the rat. J Physiol (Lond) 319:271, 1981.
110. Lind T, Godfrey KA, Otun H: Changes in serum uric acid concentration during normal pregnancy. BJOG 91:128, 1984.
111. Dunlop W, Davison JM: The effect of normal pregnancy upon the renal handling of uric acid. BJOG 84:13, 1977.
112. Hytten FE, Cheyne GA: The aminoaciduria of pregnancy. J Obstet Gynaecol Br Commonw 79:424, 1972.
113. Higby K, Suiter CR, Phelps JY, et al: Normal values of urinary albumin and total protein excretion during pregnancy. Am J Obstet Gynecol 171:984-989, 1994.
114. Misiani R, Marchesi D, Tiraboschi G, et al: Urinary albumin excretion in normal pregnancy and pregnancy-induced hypertension. Nephron 59:416, 1991.
115. Wright A, Steeke P, Bennet JR, et al: The urinary excretion of albumin in normal pregnancy. BJOG 94:408, 1987.
116. Abrams BF, Laros RK Jr: Prepregnancy weight, weight gain, and birth weight. Am J Obstet Gynecol 154:503, 1986.
117. Davison JM, Vallotton MB, Lindheimer MD: Plasma osmolality and urinary concentration and dilution during and after pregnancy. BJOG 88:472, 1981.
118. Davison JM, Gilmore EA, Durr J, et al: Altered osmotic thresholds for vasopressin secretion and thirst in human pregnancy. Am J Physiol 246: F105, 1984.
119. Davison JM, Shiells EA, Philips PR, et al: Serial evaluation of vasopressin and thirst in human pregnancy: Role of human chorionic gonadotropin on the osmoregulatory changes of gestation. J Clin Invest 81:798, 1988.

Chapter 8

Endocrinology of Pregnancy

James H. Liu, MD

The concept of the fetus, the placenta, and the mother as a functional unit originated in the 1950s. More recent is the recognition that the placenta itself is an endocrine organ capable of synthesizing virtually every hormone, growth factor, and cytokine thus far identified. The premise that the placenta, composed chiefly of two cell types (syncytiotrophoblast and cytotrophoblast), can synthesize and secrete a vast array of active substances could not even be contemplated until it was recognized in the 1970s that a single cell can, in fact, synthesize peptide and protein factors. This concept is even more remarkable because the placenta has no neural connections to either the mother or the fetus and is expelled after childbirth. Yet the placenta, an integral part of the fetal-placental-maternal unit, can be viewed as the most amazing endocrine organ of all. In this chapter, I review the hormonal interactions of the fetal-placental-maternal unit and the neuroendocrine and metabolic changes that occur in the mother and in the fetus during pregnancy and at parturition.

Implantation

Although early studies showed that the process of embryo implantation took place between 6 and 7 days after ovulation,[1,2] more contemporary results suggest that in most successful human pregnancies, the embryo implants approximately 8 to 10 days after ovulation.[3] This event involves a series of complex steps: (1) orientation of the blastocyst with respect to the endometrial surface, (2) initial adhesion of the blastocyst to the endometrium, (3) meeting of the microvilli on the surface of trophoblast with pinopodes (microprotrusions from the apical end of the uterine epithelium), (4) trophoblastic migration through the endometrial surface epithelium, (5) embryonic invasion with localized disruption of the endometrial capillary beds, and finally (6) remodeling of the capillary bed and formation of trophoblastic lacunae.[4,5] By day 10, the blastocyst is completely encased in the uterine stromal tissue. A diagrammatic representation of this process is shown in Figure 8-1.

Although recent work with in vitro fertilization (IVF)-related techniques such as embryo donation and frozen embryo transfer has contributed significantly to our understanding of this process, much of our present physiologic information is derived from other mammalian species, because human tissue experiments are limited by ethical constraints. The implantation process has been reviewed by Norwitz and colleagues.[5]

Results from assisted reproductive technologies suggest a window for implantation in which the endometrium is "receptive" to embryo implantation. In this concept, synchronization between embryonic and uterine receptivity is required for successful nidation. IVF-generated data suggest that implantation is successful usually after embryo transfer into the uterus, between 3 and 5 days after fertilization. The embryo is at the 6-8-cell to blastocyst stage of development. If the embryo is transferred outside this window or is in a different location, the likelihood of embryo demise or ectopic pregnancy increases. Although the process of embryo implantation requires a receptive endometrium, the process is not exclusive to the endometrium, because advanced ectopic (e.g., abdominal) pregnancies have been reported with a viable fetus.

During a typical IVF cycle, embryos are transferred to the uterus on day 3 or day 5 after fertilization. By day 3 of embryo culture, embryo development is at the six- to eight-cell stage. Embryos placed back into the uterus at this stage remain unattached to the endometrium and continue developing to the blastocyst stage, "hatch" or escape from the zona pellucida, and implant by day 6 or 7 of embryo life. In IVF programs that transfer on day 3, the chance of each embryo implanting is approximately 12% to 25%. Thus, to achieve a reasonable chance of overall pregnancy, most women undergoing IVF will have two to three good-quality embryos placed back into the uterus to achieve clinical pregnancy rates of 35% to 45% per IVF cycle. Because the implantation potential for each embryo is affected by the age of the mother, embryo morphology alone is imprecise in predicting likelihood of implantation. Transfer of multiple embryos can result in higher-order multiple pregnancies such as twins, triplets, or occasionally quadruplets. In 1997, the use of assisted reproductive technologies accounted for more than 40% of all triplets born in the United States.[6]

Many IVF programs have the capability to culture embryos for up to 5 days. Embryos at this stage are at the blastocyst or morula stage. The overall implantation rate for each good-quality embryo at this stage is between 30% and 50% per embryo. Thus, to achieve a reasonable chance of pregnancy, most women have only one or two good-quality blastocyst-staged embryos transferred to the uterus, reducing the chances of higher-order multiple pregnancies. A study from population-based control data indicates that the use of assisted reproductive technology accounts for a disproportionate number of low-birth-weight and very low birth weight infants partly because of multiple pregnancies and partly because even singleton infants conceived with this technology have lower birth weights.[7]

The cellular differentiation and remodeling of the endometrium induced by sequential exposure to estradiol and progesterone may play a major role in endometrial receptivity. The beginning of endometrial receptivity coincides with the downregulation of progesterone and estrogen receptors induced by the production of progesterone in the corpus luteum. It was thought that this process involved tight regulation, so that the morphologic development of microvilli (pinopodes)

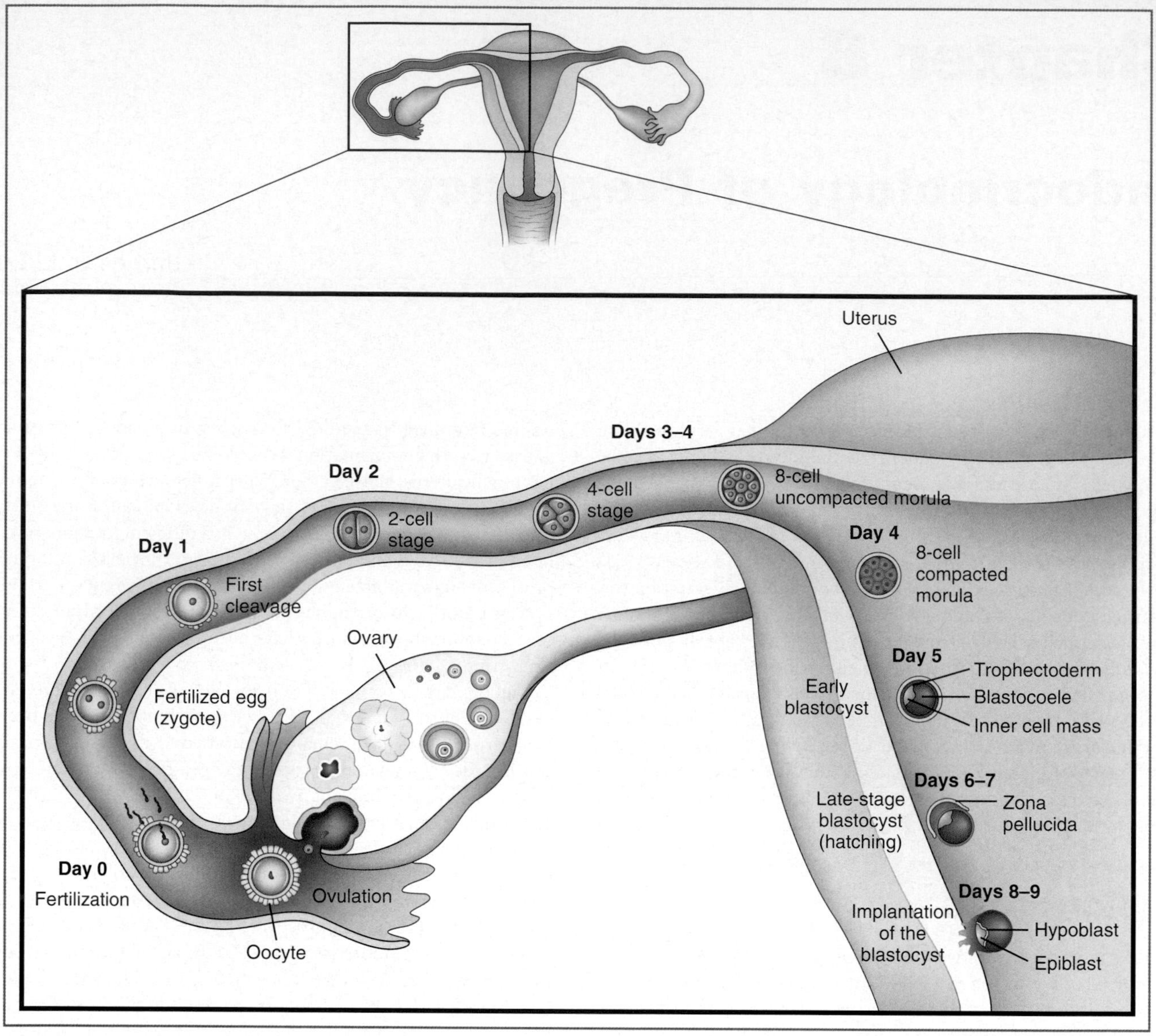

FIGURE 8-1 Diagrammatic sequence of embryo development from ovulation through the blastocyst stage of implantation in the human.

in glandular epithelium[8] and increased angiogenesis were required for successful embryo nidation. Experience with IVF techniques, however, suggests marked differences in endometrial morphology between different women at the same point in their cycle, as well as in the same woman from cycle to cycle.[9] Nevertheless, the current concept is that expression of factors produced by the blastocyst and the endometrium allows cell-to-cell communication so that successful nidation can take place.

Reviews of embryo implantation have identified an increasing number of factors, such as integrins, mucins, L-selectin, cytokines, proteinases, and glycoproteins, that are localized to either the embryo or the endometrium during the window of implantation.[10] Much information is derived from animal studies, and its application to human implantation is primarily circumstantial. Table 8-1 lists several of the factors believed to mediate embryo implantation.

Ultrasound studies of early human gestation show that most implantation sites are localized to the upper two thirds of the uterus and are closer to the side of the corpus luteum.[11] A growing body of literature suggests that the integrins, a class of adhesion molecules, are involved in implantation. Integrins are also essential components of the extracellular matrix and function as receptors that anchor extracellular adhesion proteins to cytoskeletal components.[12]

Integrins are a family of heterodimers composed of different α subunits and a common β subunit. At present, the integrin receptor family is composed of at least 14 distinct α subunits and more than nine β subunits,[13] making up to 20 integrin heterodimers.[14] Integrins are cell-surface receptors for fibrinogen, fibronectin, collagen, and laminin. These receptors recognize a common amino acid tripeptide, Arg-Gly-Asp (RGD), present in extracellular matrix proteins such as fibronectin. Integrins have been localized to sperm, oocyte, blastocyst, and endometrium.

One particular integrin, $\alpha_v\beta_3$, is expressed on endometrial cells after day 19 of the menstrual cycle. This integrin appears to be a marker for the implantation window. Integrin $\alpha_v\beta_3$ is also localized to trophoblast

TABLE 8-1 GROWTH FACTORS AND PROTEINS WITH A SIGNIFICANT ROLE IN EMBRYO IMPLANTATION

Factor	Putative Role	Reference
Leukemia inhibitory factor	Cytokine involved in implantation	Cullinan et al, 1996
Integrins	Cell-to-cell interactions	Sueoka et al, 1997
Transforming growth factor-β	Inhibits trophoblast invasion, stimulates syncytium formation	Graham et al, 1992
Epidermal growth factor	Mediates trophoblast invasion	Bass et al, 1994
Interleukin-1β	Mediates trophoblast invasion	Librach et al, 1994
Interleukin-10	Mediates implantation	Stewart et al, 1997
Matrix metalloproteinases	Mediates implantation	Stewart et al, 1997
Vascular endothelial growth factor	Mediates implantation	Stewart et al, 1997
L-selectin	Mediates implantation	Genbacev et al, 2003

cells, suggesting that it may participate in cell-to-cell interactions between the trophoblast and the endometrium, acting through a common bridging ligand. It is postulated that after hatching, the blastocyst, through its trophoblastic integrin receptors, attaches to the endometrial surface. Mouse primary trophoblast cells appear to interact with the fibronectin exclusively through the RGD recognition site.[15] The appearance of the β_3 integrin subunit depends on the downregulation of progesterone and estrogen receptors in the endometrial glands.[16] Subsequent changes in trophoblast adhesive and migratory behavior appear to stem from alterations in the expression of various integrin receptors. Antibodies to α_v or β-integrins inhibit the attachment activity of intact blastocysts.[17]

The role of integrins in trophoblast migration is not clear, but the expression of β_1-integrins appears to promote this phenomenon.[18] Work in the rhesus monkey suggests that the trophoblast migrates into the endometrium directly beneath the implantation site, invading small arterioles (but not veins).[19] L-selectins have recently been identified at the maternal-fetal interface, and they are postulated to function as an adhesion molecule necessary for successful implantation.[20]

Controlled invasion of the maternal vascular system by the trophoblast is necessary for the establishment of the hemochorial placenta. Studies with human placental villous explants suggest that chorionic villous cytotrophoblasts can differentiate along two distinct pathways: by fusing to form the syncytiotrophoblast layer and as extravillous trophoblasts that have the potential to invade the inner basalis layer of endometrium and the myometrium to reach the spiral arteries. Once trophoblasts have breached the endometrial blood vessels, decidualized stromal cells are believed to promote endometrial hemostasis by release of tissue factor and by thrombin generation.[21]

Three growth factors have been implicated in the regulation of this process. Epidermal growth factor (EGF)[22] and interleukin-1β[23] stimulate invasion by the extravillous trophoblast, whereas transforming growth factor β appears to inhibit the differentiation toward the invasive phenotype and serves to limit the invasiveness of extravillous trophoblast and to induce syncytium formation.[24] The process of invasion appears to peak by 12 weeks' gestation.[25] These trophoblasts proceed to form the chorionic villi, the functional units of the placenta, which consist of a central core of loose connective tissue and abundant capillaries connecting them with the fetal circulation. Around this core are the outer syncytiotrophoblast layer and the inner layer of cytotrophoblast. In general, both cytotrophoblast and syncytiotrophoblast produce peptide hormones, whereas the syncytiotrophoblast produces all of the steroid hormones.

Human Chorionic Gonadotropin Production

Human chorionic gonadotropin (hCG) is one of the earliest products of the cells forming the embryo, and it should be viewed as one of the first embryonic signals elaborated by the embryo, even before implantation.[26] This glycoprotein is a heterodimer (36 to 40 kDa). It is composed of a 92–amino acid α subunit that is homologous to thyroid-stimulating hormone, luteinizing hormone (LH), and follicle-stimulating hormone, and a 145–amino acid β subunit that is similar to LH. The α subunit gene for hCG has been localized to chromosome 6; the β subunit gene is located on chromosome 19, fairly close to the LH-β gene.

The presence of sialic acid residues on hCG-β accounts for its prolonged half-life in the circulation (longer than the half-life of LH). After implantation, hCG is produced principally by the syncytiotrophoblast layer of the chorionic villus and is secreted into the intervillous space. Cytotrophoblasts are also able to produce hCG.

Clinically, hCG can be detected in either the serum or the urine 7 to 8 days before expected menses, and it is the earliest biochemical marker for pregnancy (Fig. 8-2). In studies during IVF cycles in which embryos were transferred 2 days after fertilization, β-hCG was detected at as early as the eight-cell stage, whereas intact hCG was not detectable until 8 days after egg retrieval. The increase in hCG levels between days 5 and 9 after ovum collection is principally the result of free β hCG production, whereas by day 22 most of the circulating hCG is in the dimer form.

These observations correspond to in vitro studies that indicate a two-phase control of dimer hCG synthesis mediated principally through a supply of subunits. In contrast to LH secretion in the pituitary gland, hCG is secreted constitutively as the subunits become available, and it is not stored in secretory granules.[27] Initially, the immature syncytiotrophoblast produces free β-hCG subunits, and the cytotrophoblast's ability to produce the α subunit appears to lag by several days.[28] As the trophoblast matures, the ratio of α subunits to β subunits reaches 1:1, and the concentration of hCG reaches a peak of approximately 100,000 mU/mL by the 9th or 10th week of gestation (Fig. 8-3). By 22 weeks' gestation, the placenta produces more α subunit than β-hCG. At term gestation, the ratio of the release of α subunits to the release of hCG is approximately 10:1.[29]

The exponential rise of hCG after implantation is characterized by a doubling time of 30.9 ± 3.7 hours.[30] The hCG doubling time has been used as a marker by clinicians to differentiate normal from abnormal gestations (i.e., ectopic pregnancy). The inability to detect

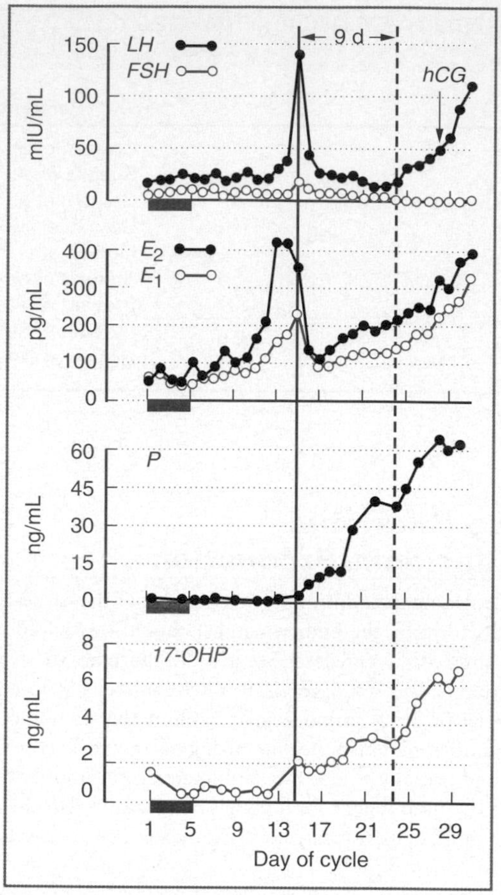

FIGURE 8-2 Hormone patterns during conception. Patterns of levels of luteinizing hormone (LH), follicle-stimulating hormone (FSH), estradiol (E_2), estrone (E_1), progesterone (P), and 17α-hydroxyprogesterone (17-OHP) during a conception cycle. Human chorionic gonadotropin (hCG) becomes detectable on cycle days 26 and 27.

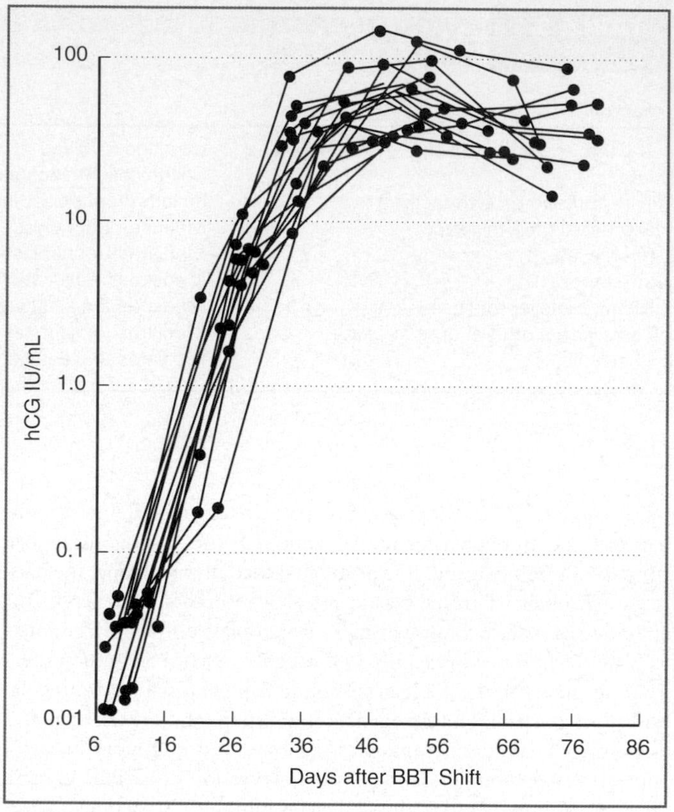

FIGURE 8-3 Chorionic gonadotropin levels after implantation. Exponential rise of circulating human chorionic gonadotropin (hCG) after implantation during the first trimester of pregnancy, with a subsequent plateau between the 11th and 12th weeks of gestation. BBT, basal body temperature. (From Braunstein GD, Kamdar V, Rasor J, et al: A chorionic gonadotropin-like substance in normal human tissues. J Clin Endocrinol Metab 49:917, 1979. Copyright © by the Endocrine Society.)

an intrauterine pregnancy (i.e., a gestational sac) by endovaginal ultrasound when serum hCG levels reach 1100 to 1500 mU/mL strongly suggests an abnormal gestation or ectopic pregnancy. Higher-than-normal hCG levels may indicate a molar pregnancy or multiple-gestational pregnancies. Levels of hCG in combination with maternal α-fetoprotein, unconjugated estriol, and inhibin have been used as a screening test for detection of fetal anomalies (see Chapter 17).

Maintenance of Early Pregnancy: Human Chorionic Gonadotropin and Corpus Luteum of Pregnancy

The major biologic role of hCG during early pregnancy is to "rescue" corpus luteum from its premature demise while maintaining progesterone production. Although the secretory pattern of hCG is not well characterized, hCG is required for rescue and maintenance of the corpus luteum until the luteal-placental shift in progesterone synthesis occurs. This concept is supported by observations that immunoneutralization of hCG results in early pregnancy loss.[31,32]

Studies in early pregnancy show that secretion of hCG and progesterone from the corpus luteum appears to be irregularly episodic with varying frequencies and peaks.[33,34] In first-trimester explant experiments, intermittent gonadotropin-releasing hormone administration enhances the pulse-like secretion of hCG from these explants, indirectly implicating placental gonadotropin-releasing hormone as a paracrine regulator of hCG secretion.[35] During nonconception cycles, the corpus luteum is preprogrammed to undergo luteolysis, a process that is not well understood. Acting through the LH receptor, hCG is also able to stimulate parallel production of estradiol, 17-hydroxyprogesterone, and other peptides such as relaxin and inhibin, from the corpus luteum.

Timing of the Luteal-Placental Shift

Ovarian progesterone production is essential for maintenance of early pregnancy. If progesterone action is blocked by a competitive progesterone antagonist, such as mifepristone, pregnancy termination results. During later gestation, placental production of progesterone is sufficient to maintain pregnancy. To uncover the timing of this luteal placental shift, Csapo and colleagues performed corpus luteum ablation

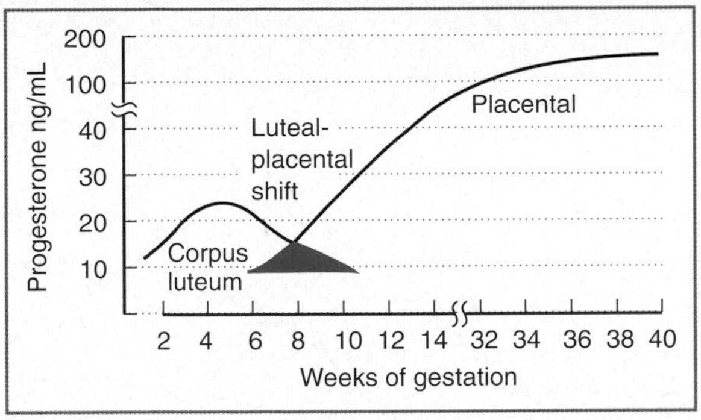

FIGURE 8-4 Shift in progesterone production. Diagrammatic representation of the shift in progesterone production from the corpus luteum to the placenta between the 7th and 9th weeks of gestation.

experiments. They demonstrated that removal of the corpus luteum before, but not after, the 7th week of gestation usually resulted in subsequent abortion.[32,36] Removal of the corpus luteum after the 9th week appears to have little or no influence on gestation (Fig. 8-4). Thus, progesterone supplementation is required if corpus luteum function is compromised before 9 to 10 weeks of gestation.

Fetoplacental Unit as an Endocrine Organ

The fetus and placenta must function together in an integrated fashion to control the growth and development of the unit and subsequent expulsion of the fetus from the uterus. Contributing to fetal and placental activity are the changes occurring in the maternal endocrine milieu. Estrogens, androgens, and progestins are involved in pregnancy from before implantation to parturition. They are synthesized and metabolized in complex pathways involving the fetus, the placenta, and the mother.

The fetal ovary is not active and does not secrete estrogens until puberty. In contrast, the Leydig cells of the fetal testes are capable of producing such large amounts of testosterone that the circulating testosterone concentration in the first-trimester male fetus is similar to that in the adult man.[37] Initial stimulus of the testes is by hCG. Fetal testosterone is required for promoting differentiation and masculinization of the male external and internal genitalia. In addition, local conversion of testosterone to dihydrotestosterone by 5α-reductase in the genital target tissues ensures final maturation of the external male genital structures. The maternal environment is protected from testosterone produced by the male fetus by the placental enzyme aromatase, which can convert testosterone to estradiol.

Progesterone

During most of pregnancy, the major source of progesterone is the placenta. For the first 6 to 10 weeks, however, the major source of progesterone is the corpus luteum. Exogenous progesterone must be administered during the first trimester to oocyte recipients who have no ovarian function.[38]

Progesterone is synthesized in the placenta mainly from circulating maternal cholesterol.[39] By the end of pregnancy, the placental production of progesterone approximates 250 mg/day, with circulating levels in the mother of about 130 to 150 ng/mL. In comparison, in the follicular phase, production of progesterone approximates 2.5 mg/day; in the luteal phase, it is about 25 mg/day. About 90% of the progesterone synthesized by the placenta enters the maternal compartment. Most of the progesterone in the maternal circulation is metabolized to pregnanediol and is excreted in the urine as a glucuronide.

During the first 6 weeks of pregnancy, 17α-hydroxyprogesterone is also elevated in the maternal circulation, to levels comparable to those of progesterone.[40] After 6 weeks of gestation, 17α-hydroxyprogesterone levels decrease progressively, becoming undetectable during the middle third of pregnancy, whereas progesterone levels fall transiently between 8 and 10 weeks of gestation and then increase thereafter. The decrease in 17α-hydroxyprogesterone and the dip in progesterone levels reflect the transition of progesterone secretion from the corpus luteum to the placenta. The 17α-hydroxyprogesterone secreted during the last third of pregnancy comes largely from the fetoplacental unit.

Estrogens

The major estrogen formed in pregnancy is estriol. Estriol is not secreted by the ovaries of nonpregnant women, but it comprises more than 90% of the known estrogen in the urine of pregnant women and is excreted as sulfate and glucuronide conjugates. Maternal serum levels of estriol increase to between 12 and 20 mg/mL by term (Fig. 8-5). Generally, circulating levels of estradiol are even higher than those of estriol. This is true because circulating estriol, in contrast to estrone and estradiol, has a very low affinity for sex hormone–binding globulin and is cleared much more rapidly from the circulation. During pregnancy, a woman produces more estrogen than a normal ovulatory woman could produce in more than 150 years.[40]

The biosynthesis of estrogens demonstrates the interdependence of the fetus, the placenta, and the maternal compartment. To form estrogens, the placenta, which has active aromatizing capacity, uses circulating androgens as the precursor substrate. The major androgenic precursor to placental estrogen formation is dehydroepiandrosterone sulfate (DHEAS), which is the major androgen produced by the fetal adrenal cortex. DHEAS is transported to the placenta and then is cleaved by sulfatase, which the placenta has in abundance, to form free unconjugated dehydroepiandrosterone, which is then aromatized by placental aromatase to estrone and estradiol. Very little estrone and estradiol is converted to estriol by the placenta. Near term, about 60% of the estradiol-17β and estrone is formed from fetal androgen precursors, and about 40% is formed from maternal DHEAS.[41]

The major portion of fetal DHEAS undergoes 16α-hydroxylation, primarily in the fetal liver but also in the fetal adrenal gland (Fig. 8-6). Fetal adrenal DHEAS in the circulation is taken up by syncytiotropho blast cells, where steroid sulfatase, a microsomal enzyme, converts it back to DHEA that is then aromatized to estriol.[42] Estriol is then secreted into the maternal circulation and conjugated in the maternal liver to form estriol sulfate, estriol glucosiduronate, and mixed conjugates and is excreted in the maternal urine.

Estetrol is an estrogen unique to pregnancy. It is the 15α-hydroxy derivative of estriol, and it is derived exclusively from fetal precursors. Although the measurement of estetrol in pregnancy was proposed as an aid in monitoring a fetus at risk for intrauterine death, it has not proved to be any better than measurement of urinary estriol.[43] Neither is currently used in the clinical setting.

Hydroxylation at the C_2 position of the phenolic A ring results in the formation of so-called catecholestrogens (2-hydroxyestrone, 2-hydroxyestradiol, and 2-hydroxyestriol) and is a major process in estrogen metabolism. 2-Hydroxyestrone is excreted in maternal urine in the

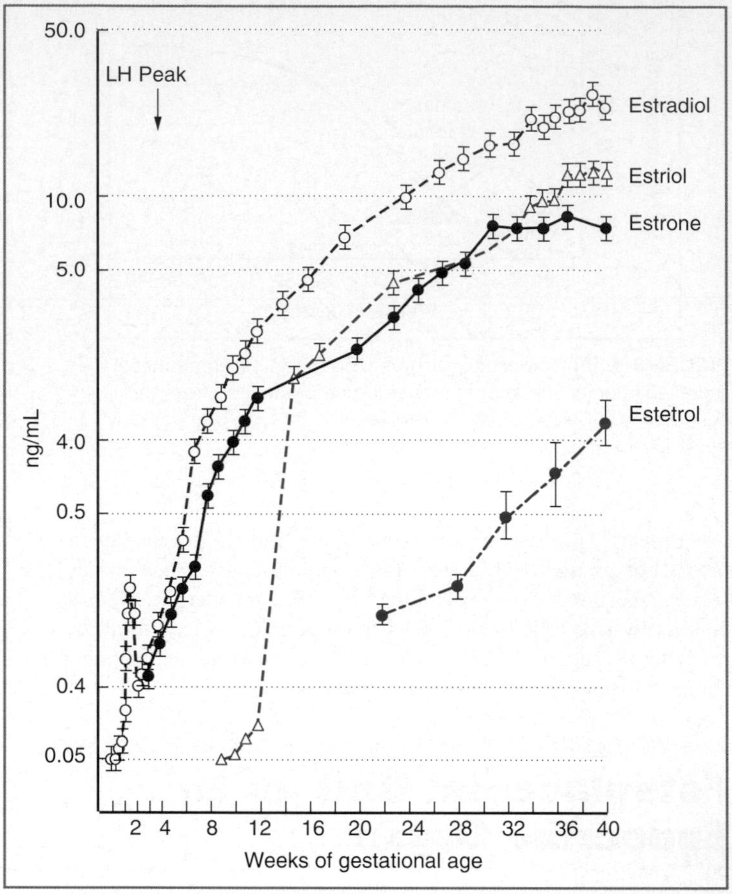

FIGURE 8-5 **Concentrations of estrogens in pregnancy.** The relative concentrations (mean ± standard error) of the four major estrogens during the course of pregnancy, plotted on log scale. LH, luteinizing hormone. (Courtesy of John Marshall, University of Virginia.)

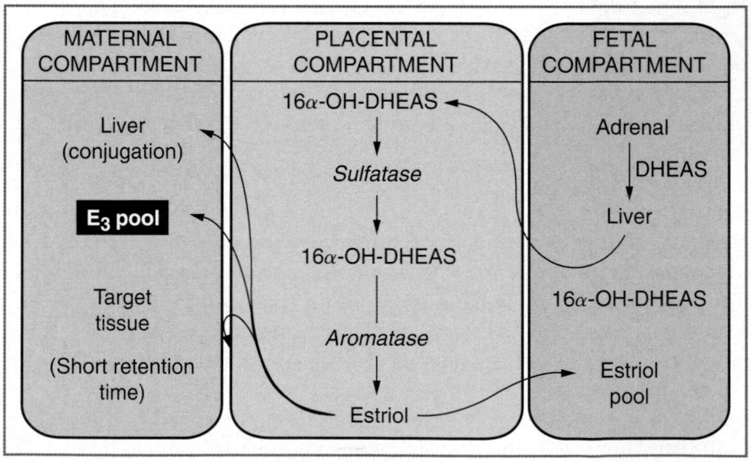

FIGURE 8-6 **Roles of the maternal-placental-fetal compartments in the formation of estriol.** Diagram of the roles of each compartment in the formation of estriol (E_3) from the fetal precursor 16α-hydroxydehydroepiandrosterone sulfate (16α-OH-DHEAS). DHEA, dehydroepiandrosterone.

largest amounts during pregnancy with marked individual variation (100 to 2500 mg/24 hr). Apparently, 2-hydroxyestrone levels increase during the first and second trimesters and decrease in the third trimester.[44] The physiologic significance of the catecholestrogens is unclear, particularly because they are rapidly cleared from the circulation; however, they do have the capacity to alter catecholamine synthesis and metabolism during pregnancy (inhibiting catecholamine inactivation via competition for carboxyl-*o*-methyl transferase, and reducing catecholamine synthesis via inhibition of tyrosine hydroxylase). Catecholestrogens also function as antiestrogens, competing with estrogens for receptors. Thus, catecholestrogens, when present in large quantities, may have significant effects in pregnancy. About 90% of the estradiol-17β and estriol secreted by the placenta enters the maternal compartment. Estrone is preferentially secreted into the fetal compartment.[44]

In the past, maternal estriol measurements were often used as an index of fetoplacental function. The numerous problems that have been documented in interpreting low estriol levels have limited the use of estriol. The normal range of urinary estriol concentrations at any given stage of gestation is quite large (typically, ±1 standard deviation). A single plasma measurement is meaningless because of moment-to-moment fluctuations. Body position (e.g., bed rest versus ambulation) affects blood flow to the uterus and kidney and therefore affects estriol levels. Moreover, numerous drugs, including glucocorticoids and ampicillin, affect estriol levels.

Two genetic diseases document that placental estrogen synthesis, at least at high levels, is apparently not required for maintenance of pregnancy. Human gestation proceeds to term when the fetus and placenta lack sulfatase.[45] In patients with this disorder, the gene has been localized to the distal short arm of the X chromosome, and the resulting male offspring manifest ichthyosis during the first few months of life. Pregnancies also reach term accompanied by severe fetal and placental aromatase deficiency.[46] Although pregnancy is maintained in both cases despite low placental estrogen synthesis, the changes in the reproductive tract that normally precede parturition, particularly ripening of the cervix, do not occur, revealing a significant role for placental estrogens in preparation for labor and birth. In addition, in the case of aromatase deficiency, both the fetus and the mother are virilized as a consequence of diminished aromatization of androgens.

Low levels of estrogens also occur after fetal demise and in most anencephalic pregnancies, in which fetal signals from the fetal hypothalamic-pituitary unit are diminished and do not stimulate synthesis of fetal adrenal androgens. In the absence of a fetus, as occurs in molar pregnancy and in pseudocyesis, estrogen levels are low as well.

Roles of Estrogens and Progestins during Pregnancy

Estrogens and progestins appear to play several important roles in pregnancy. They clearly induce the secretory endometrium, required for implantation. Progesterone appears to be important in maintaining uterine quiescence during pregnancy by actions on uterine smooth muscle.[47] Progesterone apparently suppresses uterine contraction by action through its two major progesterone receptor (PR) subtypes PR-A and PR-B.[48] PR-A appears to repress progesterone actions mediated by PR-B. At the time of labor, there is an increase in expression of PR-A.[49] Progesterone also inhibits uterine prostaglandin production,[50] presumably promoting uterine quiescence and delaying cervical ripening. Progesterone may also help to maintain pregnancy by inhibiting T lymphocyte–mediated processes that play a role in tissue rejection.[51] Thus, the high local concentrations of progesterone appear to contribute to the immunologically privileged status of the pregnant uterus. Progesterone is important in creating a barrier to penetration of pathogens into the uterus.

Estrogens are important for parturition at the appropriate time. The stimulatory effects of estrogen on phospholipid synthesis and turnover, prostaglandin production, and increased formation of lysosomes in the uterine endometrium, as well as estrogen modulation of adrenergic mechanisms in uterine myometrium, may be means by which estrogens act to time the onset of labor.[52] Estrogens also increase uterine blood flow,[53] which ensures an adequate supply of oxygen and nutrients to the fetus. It appears that estriol, an extremely weak estrogen, is just as effective as other estrogens in increasing uteroplacental blood flow.[53]

Estrogens are important in preparing the breast for lactation.[54] They also affect other endocrine systems during pregnancy, such as the renin-angiotensin system,[55] and stimulate production of hormone-binding globulins in the liver. Estrogens may play a role in fetal development and organ maturation, including increasing fetal lung surfactant production.[56]

The Placenta and Growth Factors

The functional roles for growth factors in the placenta can be divided into three areas:

1. Regulation of cell growth and differentiation
2. Local regulation of hormone release
3. Regulation of uterine contractility

Growth factors that are elaborated by the placenta are responsible for the following:

1. Regulation of amino acid transport
2. Increased glucose uptake
3. DNA synthesis and cell replication
4. RNA and protein synthesis

These processes may be regulated in an autocrine or paracrine manner within the placenta.

Although much of the research has been conducted in other mammalian systems and may not be directly applicable to humans, major similarities probably exist in the way growth factors operate to ensure continuing growth and development of the fetus. In the human, most of our knowledge has been limited to descriptive studies demonstrating localization of many growth factor systems. Unfortunately, our understanding of their functional roles has only begun. Table 8-2 is a partial listing of growth factors that have been identified in the

TABLE 8-2 GROWTH FACTORS, NEUROPEPTIDES, AND PROTEINS IDENTIFIED IN PLACENTAL TISSUES

Protein/Peptide Hormone	Neurohormone/Neuropeptide	Growth Factor	Binding Protein	Cytokine
Human chorionic gonadotropin	Gonadotropin-releasing hormone	Activin	Corticotropin-releasing hormone–binding protein (CRH-BP)	Interleukin-1 (IL-1)
Human placental lactogen	Thyrotropin-releasing hormone	Follistatin	Insulin-like growth factor–binding protein-1 (IGFBP-1)	IL-2
Growth hormone variant	Growth hormone–releasing hormone	Inhibin	IGFBP-2	IL-6
Adrenocorticotropic hormone	Somatostatin	Transforming growth factor-β and -α	IGFBP-3	IL-8
	Corticotropin-releasing hormone	Epidermal growth factor	IGFBP-4	Interferon-α
	Oxytocin	Insulin-like growth factor-I (IGF-I)	IGFBP-5	Interferon-β
	Neuropeptide Y	IGF-II	IGFBP-6	Interferon-γ
	β-Endorphin	Fibroblastic growth factor		Tumor necrosis factor-α
	Met-enkephalin	Platelet-derived growth factor		
	Dynorphin			

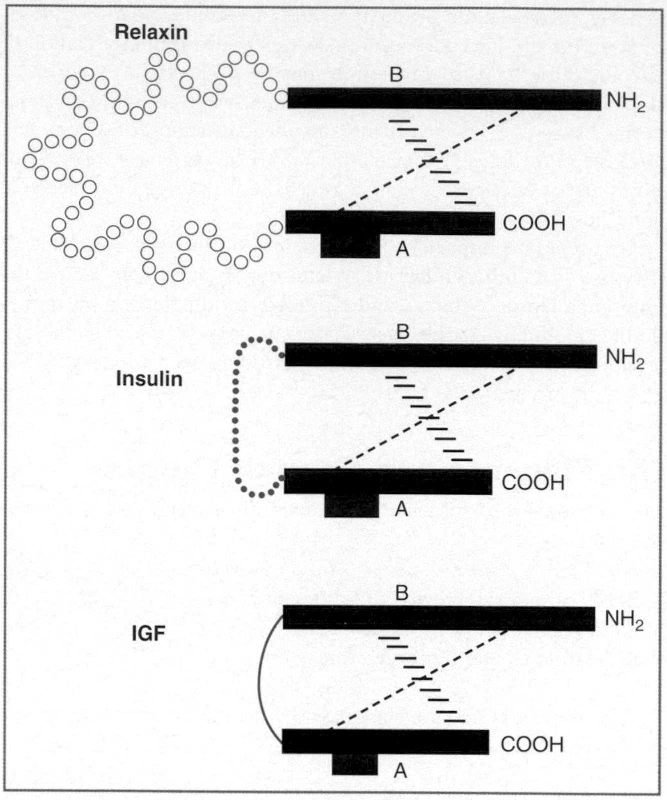

FIGURE 8-7 Structural similarities of relaxin, insulin, and insulin-like growth factor (IGF). A and B are chains linked by disulfide bonds.

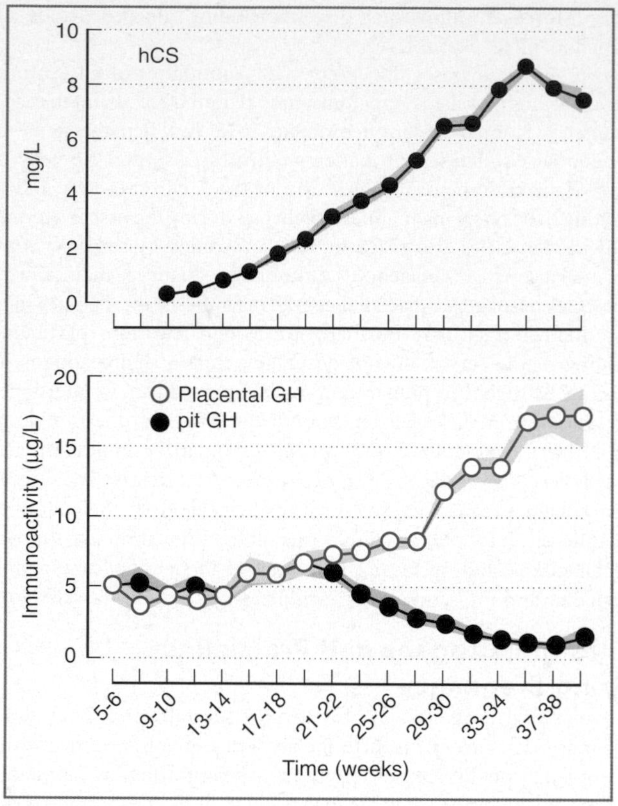

FIGURE 8-8 Comparison of serum levels of human chorionic somatomammotropin (hCS) with immunoactivity of placental growth hormone (GH) and pituitary growth hormone (pit GH) during human pregnancy. (Modified from Frankenne F, Closset J, Gomez F, et al: The physiology of growth hormones [GHs] in pregnant women and partial characterization of the placental GH variant. J Clin Endocrinol Metab 66:1171, 1988. Copyright © by the Endocrine Society.)

placenta. A detailed description of their respective roles is beyond the scope of this chapter. Only major growth factor systems are discussed.

Insulin-Like Growth Factor, Epidermal Growth Factor, and Transforming Growth Factor

In preimplantation embryos, the insulin-like growth factor (IGF), the transforming growth factor α, and the EGF systems have been studied extensively. In general, IGF-2/IGF-1 receptors are primarily responsible for regulation of cell proliferation, whereas cell differentiation is regulated by the transforming growth factor α and EGF-receptor systems.

IGF-1 appears to be an important modulator of fetal growth (Fig. 8-7). It is normally produced in response to pituitary growth hormone (GH) by the liver. In pregnancy, the levels of IGF-1 may be regulated in part by placental GH, a variant of pituitary GH. Fetal cord plasma IGF-1 levels are positively correlated to birth weight and length of the fetus.[57,58]

EGF and transforming growth factor α in the placenta both interact with the EGF receptor. Both growth factors are present in cytotrophoblast and syncytiotrophoblast. In these latter cells, EGF stimulates secretion of hCG and human placental lactogen.[59] The proliferative activities induced by a number of growth factors appear to overlap. These factors include IGF, platelet-derived growth factors, EGF, and fibroblastic growth factors.

Human Chorionic Somatomammotropin

Human chorionic somatomammotropin (hCS), initially named human placental lactogen when it was isolated from the human placenta in the 1960s,[60] has structural, biologic, and immunologic similarities to both pituitary human growth hormone (hGH) and prolactin. Now known to be a single-chain polypeptide (about 22 kDa) containing 191 amino acids and two disulfide bonds, hCS has up to 96% homology with GH and about 67% homology with prolactin.[61,62] The hCS/hGH gene cluster has been localized to the long arm of chromosome 17 and consists of five genes, two coding for hGH and three for hCS.[63] Two of the three hCS genes are expressed at approximately equivalent rates in the term placenta and synthesize identical proteins, and the third gene appears to be a pseudogene.[64]

Human chorionic somatomammotropin is produced only by syncytiotrophoblasts and appears to be transcribed at a constant rate throughout gestation.[65,66] As a consequence, serum levels of hCS correlate very well with placental mass as the placenta increases in size during pregnancy. At term, placental production of hCS approximates 1 to 4 g/day and maternal serum levels range from 5 to 15 µg/mL (Fig. 8-8), making it the most abundant secretory product of the placenta.

Despite the huge quantities produced during pregnancy, the function of hCS is poorly understood. It has been suggested that hCS must exert its major metabolic effects on the mother to ensure that the nutritional demands of the fetus are met, functioning as the "growth hormone" of pregnancy.[67] During pregnancy, maternal plasma glucose levels are decreased, plasma free fatty acids are increased, and insulin secretion is increased with resistance to endogenous insulin as a con-

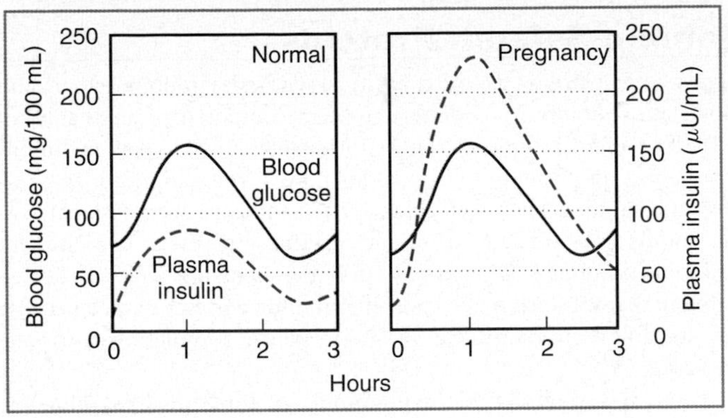

FIGURE 8-9 Insulin response to oral glucose. Comparison of the plasma insulin response to an oral glucose load (100 g) in women during late pregnancy and in nonpregnant ("normal") women.

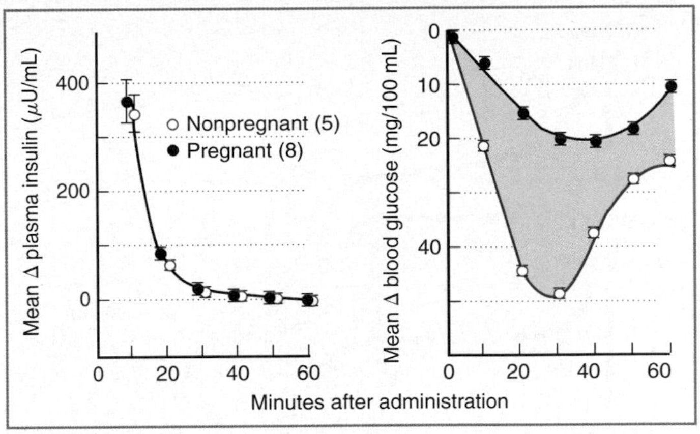

FIGURE 8-10 Disappearance of circulating insulin after injection of intravenous insulin. *Left,* Almost identical disappearance curves of circulating insulin after a bolus intravenous insulin injection (0.1 U/kg) in pregnant and nonpregnant women. *Right,* The marked decline in blood glucose in response to exogenous insulin in nonpregnant women as opposed to pregnant women suggests increased insulin resistance in the latter group. (From Burt RL, Davidson WF: Insulin half life and utilization in normal pregnancy. Obstet Gynecol 4:161, 1974. Reprinted with permission from the American College of Obstetricians and Gynecologists.)

sequence of the GH-like and contrainsulin effects of hCS (Fig. 8-9). Peripheral glucose uptake is inhibited in the mother but crosses the placenta freely. Amino acids are actively transported to the fetus against a concentration gradient, and transplacental passage of free fatty acids is slow. As a consequence, when the mother is in the fasting or starved state, glucose should be reserved largely for the fetus and free fatty acids would be used preferentially by the mother. The placenta is impermeable to insulin and other protein hormones.

Despite these presumptions, the regulation of hCS is also poorly understood. Factors that regulate pituitary GH secretion are largely ineffective in altering concentrations of hCS. In addition, despite its structural homology to GH and prolactin, hCS has very little (although definite) growth-promoting and lactogenic activity in humans.[67] Moreover, normal pregnancies resulting in delivery of healthy infants have been reported in individuals with very low to absent production of hCS.[68,69] Thus, it is possible that hCS is not essential for pregnancy but may serve as an evolutionary redundancy for pituitary GH and prolactin. Whether pregnancies with diminished hCS production would have good outcomes in the presence of nutritional deprivation, however, remains unknown.

Human Placental Growth Hormone

Only in the past several years has the existence of a placental GH been documented. The two forms of human placental GH present include a 22-kDa form and a glycosylated 25-kDa form. Both are encoded by the *hGH-V* gene in the hCS/hGH gene cluster on chromosome 17.[70,71] Pituitary hCG is encoded by the *hGH-N* gene in the same gene cluster.[72]

During the first trimester, pituitary GH is measurable in maternal serum and is secreted in a pulsatile fashion.[73] Human placental GH levels begin to rise thereafter as pituitary GH levels decrease; human placental GH is secreted in a relatively constant (in contrast to a pulsatile) manner.[73] It appears that human placental GH stimulates IGF-1 production, which in turn suppresses pituitary GH secretion in the second half of pregnancy.[74]

Endocrine and Metabolic Changes in Pregnancy

Pregnancy is accompanied by a series of metabolic changes, including hyperinsulinemia, insulin resistance, relative fasting hypoglycemia, increased circulating plasma lipids, and hypoaminoacidemia. All these changes seem intended to ensure an uninterrupted supply of metabolic fuels to the growing fetus. It is also now clear that these changes are directed by hormones elaborated by the fetoplacental unit.

The insulin resistance associated with pregnancy has been recognized for many years and is known to be accompanied by maternal islet cell hyperplasia (Fig. 8-10). The mechanism responsible for increasing insulin resistance throughout pregnancy is not entirely clear. It appears that hCS and human placental GH in particular reduce insulin receptor sites and glucose transport in insulin-sensitive tissues in the mother (Fig. 8-11).[75] There is no evidence that glucagon plays a significant role as a diabetogenic factor. The rapid return to normal glucose metabolism after delivery in women with gestational diabetes has been regarded as the best evidence that fetoplacental hormones are largely diabetogenic in the mother.[76]

Total plasma lipids increase significantly and progressively after 24 weeks of gestation, with the increases in triglycerides, cholesterol, and free fatty acids being most marked (Table 8-3).[77] Pre–β-lipoprotein, a very-low-density lipoprotein that normally represents a very small percentage of total lipoprotein, is increased in pregnancy. High-density-lipoprotein cholesterol levels increase in early pregnancy, whereas low-density-lipoprotein cholesterol levels increase later in pregnancy.[78]

Plasma triglyceride levels increase more in response to an oral glucose load in late pregnancy than in the nonpregnant state.[77] Because the placenta is poorly permeable to fat but readily permeable to glucose and amino acids, this mechanism helps ensure an adequate supply of glucose for the fetus.

Prolonged fasting in pregnancy is accompanied by exaggerated hypoglycemia, hypoinsulinism, and hyperketonemia.[79] Gluconeogenesis, however, is not increased, as would be expected. Thus, even though the demands of the fetus during maternal fasting are met in part by accelerated muscle breakdown, it is at the expense of the mother, in whom homeostatic mechanisms do not include sufficient gluconeogenesis to prevent maternal hypoglycemia. It is not clear whether

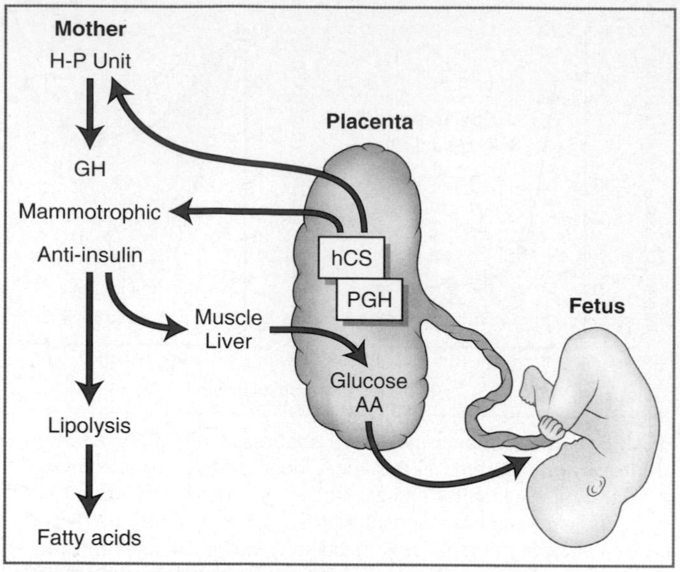

FIGURE 8-11 Maternal metabolic homeostasis. The proposed functional roles of human chorionic somatomammotropin (hCS) and placental growth hormone (PGH) in the readjustment of maternal metabolic homeostasis with preferential transfer of amino acid (AA) and glucose to the fetus. GH, pituitary growth hormone; H-P Unit, hypothalamic-pituitary unit.

TABLE 8-3 BASAL VALUES FOR INSULIN, GLUCAGON, AND PLASMA METABOLIC FUELS IN YOUNG WOMEN AFTER OVERNIGHT FAST

Plasma Metabolite	Units	Nongravid	Late Pregnancy
Glucose	(mg/dL)	79 ± 2.4	68 ± 1.5*
Insulin	(μU/mL)	9.8 ± 1.1	16.2 ± 2.0*
Glucagon	(pg/mL)	126 ± 6.1	130 ± 5.2 (NS)
Amino acids	(μmol/L)	3.82 ± 0.13	3.18 ± 0.11*
Alanine	(μmol/L)	286 ± 15	225 ± 9*
Free fatty acids	(μmol/L)	626 ± 42	725 ± 21*
	(mg/dL)	76.2 ± 7.0	181 ± 10*
Cholesterol	(mg/dL)	163 ± 8.7	205 ± 5.7*

***Significant difference between nongravid and late pregnancy values.**
NS, not significant.
Data from Freinkel N, Metzger BE, Nitzan M, et al: Facilitated anabolism in late pregnancy: Some novel maternal compensations for accelerated starvation. In Malaisse WJ, Pirart J (eds): Diabetes. International Series No. 312. Amsterdam, Excerpta Medica, 1973, p 474.

normal muscle catabolism simply cannot keep up with the loss of glucose and amino acids to the fetus during fasting or whether there are additional restraints on muscle breakdown during pregnancy.

Although cortisol is a potent diabetogenic hormone, inhibiting peripheral glucose uptake and promoting insulin secretion, and serum free cortisol levels clearly increase in late pregnancy,[80,81] it is unclear just how great a role cortisol plays in the diabetogenic nature of pregnancy. The increased circulating concentrations of estrogen and progesterone in pregnancy may also be important in the altered glucose-insulin homeostasis present during pregnancy.

Inhibin-Related Proteins

The human placenta has the capacity to synthesize inhibin, activin, and follistatin.[82] Inhibin is a dimeric protein composed of an α subunit (18 kDa) and a β subunit (14 kDa), originally shown to have an inhibitory effect on pituitary follicle-stimulating hormone release. Two different β subunits have been characterized and have been designated as β_A and β_B. Each different β subunit can thus give rise to two different inhibins (inhibin A, β_A, and inhibin B, β_B). Activin is a closely related protein that was discovered soon after inhibin and was named because of its ability to stimulate pituitary follicle-stimulating hormone release.

Activin is composed of two β subunits. All three possible configurations of activin have been identified—$\beta_A\beta_A$, $\beta_A\beta_B$, and $\beta_B\beta_B$. Follistatin is a single-chain glycoprotein that can functionally inhibit pituitary follicle-stimulating hormone release by binding of activin. Besides the human trophoblast, the maternal decidua, amnion, and chorion have been demonstrated to express messenger RNAs and immunoreactive proteins for inhibin, activin, and follistatin.

High levels of inhibin-like proteins have been reported in patients with fetal Down syndrome[83] and in patients with hydatidiform mole[84]; low levels have been observed in women with abnormal gestations, such as ectopic pregnancies[85] and pregnancies that end in abortion.[86] High levels of maternal activin A have been observed in pregnancies complicated by preeclampsia, diabetes, and preterm labor.[82]

At this point, there are no in vivo models to study the functional roles of inhibin-related proteins on placental hormone secretion, and thus the biologic roles of this system have been derived from in vitro cell cultures. In cultured placental cells, activin appears to increase the release of hCG and progesterone,[87] whereas inhibins decrease hCG and progesterone levels. Follistatin has been reported to reverse the activin-induced release of hCG and progesterone. These regulatory events appear to be parallel to that of the pituitary gland, where activin increases follicle-stimulating hormone release, whereas follistatin and inhibin oppose this effect.

Corticotropin-Releasing Hormone and Corticotropin-Releasing Hormone–Binding Protein System

The placenta, chorion, amnion, and decidua are all capable of synthesizing corticotropin-releasing hormone (CRH). This 41-amino acid peptide was first isolated from the hypothalamus and is responsible for stimulation of adrenocorticotropic hormone and proopiomelanocortin peptides from the pituitary. CRH is detectable by 7 to 8 weeks' gestation,[88] and maternal plasma levels of CRH rise progressively throughout gestation.[89] Maternal CRH levels increase significantly with labor, reaching a peak at delivery; levels remain stable in the absence of labor with cesarean section.[90] In the term placenta, CRH has been localized to both the cytotrophoblast and the syncytiotrophoblast.[91] The addition of CRH to human placental cells or amnion stimulates release of prostaglandin E and prostaglandin $F_{2\alpha}$, suggesting that locally elaborated CRH plays a major role in the initiation of myometrial contractility and labor.[92]

CRH-binding protein has also been identified in the placenta and appears to be produced by the syncytiotrophoblast,[93] the decidua, and fetal membranes.[94] This protein conceptually functions as a CRH receptor in the circulation, reduces the biologic activity of CRH, and thus may serve a modulatory role for localized CRH action.

Oxytocin

Oxytocin, a nonapeptide produced by the supraoptic and paraventricular nuclei of the hypothalamus, has now also been localized to the syncytiotrophoblast. In placental cell cultures, increased concentrations of estradiol are associated with increased levels of oxytocin mRNA. The levels of immunoreactive oxytocin increase throughout gestation and are parallel to levels in maternal blood. The placental oxytocin content is estimated to be fivefold greater than in the posterior pituitary lobe, suggesting that the placenta may be the main source of oxytocin during pregnancy.[95]

The role of maternal oxytocin in pregnancy and in parturition remains unclear. Circulating levels of oxytocin are low throughout pregnancy and increase markedly only during the second stage of labor.[96] Oxytocin receptors are present in myometrium and increase dramatically in number only shortly before the onset of labor.[97] The sensitivity of the myometrium, therefore, changes more dramatically in preparation for labor than do the circulating levels of the hormone. Oxytocin also can stimulate the production of prostaglandins by human decidua.[98] These data do not document any role for oxytocin in triggering the onset of parturition and imply that it is unlikely to be the initiator of human parturition.

Relaxin

Relaxin, a peptide hormone of approximately 6 kDa, belongs to the insulin family. It is composed of two disulfide-linked chains, A and B (see Fig. 8-7). Relaxin is produced in a number of sites, including the corpus luteum in pregnant and nonpregnant women, the decidua, the placenta, the prostate, and the atria of the heart.

Relaxin first appears in the serum of pregnant women at the same time hCG appears. Levels during pregnancy approximate 1 ng/mL. Relaxin concentrations are highest during the first trimester, peaking at about 1.2 ng/mL between the 8th and 12th weeks of pregnancy, and then gradually decrease to 1 ng/mL for the duration of pregnancy.[99] There is no evidence of any circadian rhythm, and no significant changes have been noted during labor.

The available evidence suggests that all relaxin circulating in the mother during pregnancy is of luteal origin. The relaxin concentration is highest in the blood draining the corpus luteum.[100] By immunohistochemistry profiles, relaxin can be detected only within the corpus luteum in the ovary. Luteectomy at term results in a prompt fall in circulating relaxin, with a half-life of less than 1 hour. In the absence of luteectomy, relaxin levels fall to undetectable levels over the first 3 days after delivery, consistent with the time frame for postpartum luteolysis. Perhaps most convincing is the observation that relaxin is undetectable in the serum of women pregnant by IVF and egg donation who have no corpora lutea.[101,102]

Relaxin appears to have a broad range of biologic activities. These include collagen remodeling and softening of the cervix and lower reproductive tract, and inhibition of uterine contractility.[103] However, circulating relaxin does not seem to be necessary for pregnancy maintenance or normal delivery in women. Women who become pregnant by egg donation go into labor at term and are capable of delivery vaginally.[104] It is possible, however, that the placenta and decidua provide sufficient relaxin for normal parturition under such circumstances.

Two conditions associated with an increase in circulating relaxin levels are multiple gestation and ovarian stimulation with the use of ovulation-inducing agents. Relaxin concentrations are higher in patients who become pregnant from IVF and exogenous gonadotropin treatment than in untreated pregnant control subjects. In both circumstances, there are multiple corpora lutea, and multiple gestations independently produce a significant increase in serum relaxin concentrations. Multiple gestations are associated with a higher risk of premature delivery, according to one group who suggested that first-trimester hyperrelaxinemia can predict the risk of preterm delivery.[104] This observation, potentially important, warrants further investigation.

Prolactin

During the first trimester of pregnancy, maternal serum prolactin levels rise progressively to achieve levels of approximately 125 to 180 ng/mL (Fig. 8-12).[105] The dramatic 10-fold increase in prolactin levels is believed to be a reflection of the estrogen-stimulated increase in size of the pituitary lactotropes, which contributes to a twofold to threefold enlargement of pituitary volume. Despite the increased magnitude of prolactin concentrations during pregnancy, the normal sleep-associated increase in prolactin remains preserved.[106] At delivery, the higher level of prolactin is responsible for priming the breast tissue in preparation for lactation.

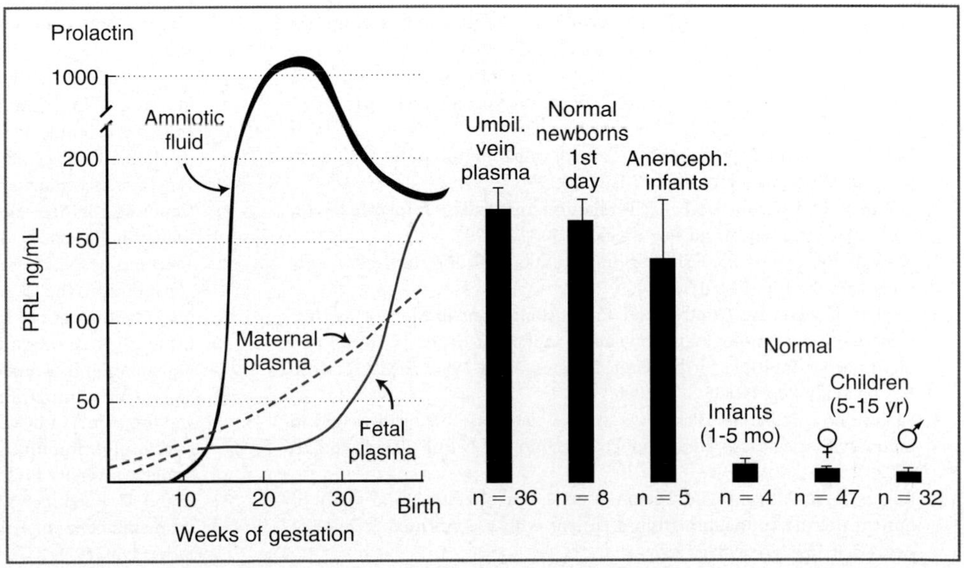

FIGURE 8-12 Prolactin levels in pregnancy. Approximate levels of prolactin (PRL) in amniotic fluid, maternal plasma, and fetal plasma during the course of pregnancy. Plasma levels in normal and anencephalic newborns are compared with levels in umbilical vein plasma and in normal infants and children. (Modified from Aubert ML, Grumbach MM, Kaplan SL: The ontogenesis of human fetal hormones: III. Prolactin. J Clin Endocrinol Metab 56:155, 1975. Copyright © by the Endocrine Society.)

After delivery, prolactin levels remain elevated at 200 to 250 ng/mL and fall gradually toward the normal range (<25 ng/mL) during a 3- to 4-week interval in nonbreastfeeding mothers.[107] In women who are breastfeeding, prolactin levels remain elevated and increase with each nursing episode. This constant hyperprolactinemic state may be partly responsible for the delay in return of ovulatory function in the breastfeeding woman.

The decidua is the major source of amniotic fluid prolactin. Decidual cells are capable of secretion of prolactin after day 23 of the menstrual cycle. Decidual prolactin is immunologically identical to the 23-kDa prolactin produced by the pituitary gland, and the complementary DNA from decidua appears virtually identical to pituitary prolactin.[108,109] Unlike that from the pituitary gland, decidual prolactin is not regulated by dopamine or thyrotropin-releasing hormone. The decidual prolactin synthesis is coupled to progesterone-induced decidualization. Once cells are stimulated to decidualize, prolactin production continues in culture even in the absence of progesterone. Because abnormal levels of amniotic fluid prolactin levels have been found in pregnancies complicated by polyhydramnios or oligohydramnios, it is believed that the biologic role of locally produced prolactin is to regulate solute and water transport in the amniotic compartment.[110]

Prostaglandins

Although concentrations of prostaglandin precursors are high in the endometrial compartment during pregnancy, there is a marked decrease in the production of prostaglandins by the endometrial decidua. Levels of cyclooxygenase-1, the constitutively expressed cyclooxygenase enzyme, fall precipitously during the mid-luteal phase of the menstrual cycle at the time of implantation. Under the influence of progesterone, the endometrial decidua produces secretory component, an endogenous inhibitor of prostaglandin synthesis.[111] The exogenous administration of prostaglandins is capable of inducing abortion or labor in all species, including humans. Taken together, these observations suggest multiple mechanisms that inhibit prostaglandin production during pregnancy. Progesterone may be one factor that suppresses synthesis of prostaglandins.

References

1. Hertig AT, Rock J, Adams EC: A description of 34 human ova within the first 17 days of development. Am J Anat 98:435, 1956.
2. O'Rahilly R: Developmental Stages in Human Embryos: Part A. Embryos of the First 3 Weeks (Stages 1 to 9). Publication No. 631. Washington, DC, Carnegie Institution, 1973.
3. Wilcox A, Baird DD, Weinberg C: Time of implantation of the conceptus and loss of pregnancy. N Engl J Med 340:1796, 1999.
4. Edelman GM, Crossin KL: Cell adhesion molecules: Implications for molecular histology. Annu Rev Biochem 60:155, 1991.
5. Norwitz ER, Schust DJ, Fisher SJ: Implantation and the survival of early pregnancy. N Engl J Med 345:1400, 2001.
6. Centers for Disease Control and Prevention: Contribution of assisted reproductive technology and ovulation-induction drugs to triplet and higher-order multiple births: United States, 1980-1997. MMWR Morb Mortal Wkly Rep 49:535-538, 2000.
7. Schieve LA, Meikle SF, Ferre C, et al: Low and very low birth weight in infants with use of assisted reproductive technology. N Engl J Med 346:731, 2002.
8. Rogers PAW, Murphy CR, Leeton J, et al: An ultrastructural study of human uterine epithelium from a patient with a confirmed pregnancy. Acta Anat 135:176, 1989.
9. Rogers PAW: Uterine receptivity. In Gardner D, Trounson AO (eds): Handbook of In Vitro Fertilization. Boca Raton, FL, CRC Press, 1993, p 263.
10. Lindhard A, Bentin-Ley U, Ravn V, et al: Biochemical evaluation of function at the time of implantation. Fertil Steril 78:221, 2002.
11. Kawakami Y, Andoh K, Mizunuma H, et al: Assessment of the implantation site by transvaginal ultrasound. Fertil Steril 59:1003, 1993.
12. Hynes RO: Integrins: Versatility, modulation, and signaling in cell adhesion. Cell 69:11, 1992.
13. Sueoka K, Shiokawa S, Miyazaki T, et al: Integrins and reproductive physiology: Expression and modulation in fertilization, embryogenesis, and implantation. Fertil Steril 67:799, 1997.
14. Lessey BA: Endometrial integrins and the establishment of uterine receptivity. Hum Reprod 13:347, 1998.
15. Armant DR, Kaplan HA, Mover H, et al: The effect of hexapeptides on attachment and outgrowth of mouse blastocysts cultured in vitro: Evidence for the involvement of the cell recognition tripeptide Arg-Gly-Asp. Proc Natl Acad Sci U S A 83:6751, 1986.
16. Lessey BA, Yeh I, Castelbaum AJ, et al: Endometrial progesterone receptors and markers of uterine receptivity in the window of implantation. Fertil Steril 65:477, 1996.
17. Schultz JF, Armant DR: Beta1- and beta3-class integrins mediate fibronectin binding activity at the surface of developing mouse peri-implantation blastocysts. J Biol Chem 270:11522, 1995.
18. Ruoslahti E, Pierschbacher MD: New perspective in cell adhesion: RGD and integrins. Science 238:491, 1987.
19. Enders AC, King BF: Early stages of trophoblastic invasion of the maternal vascular system during implantation in the macaque and baboon. Am J Anat 192:329, 1991.
20. Genbacev OD, Prakobphol A, Foulk RA, et al: Trophoblast L-selectin-mediated adhesion at the maternal fetal interface. Science 299:405-408, 2003.
21. Lockwood CJ, Krikun G, Hausknecht V, et al: Decidual cell regulation of hemostasis during implantation and menstruation. Ann N Y Acad Sci 828:188, 1997.
22. Bass KE, Morrish D, Roth I, et al: Human cytotrophoblast invasion is upregulated by epidermal growth factor: Evidence that paracrine factors modify this process. Dev Biol 164:550, 1994.
23. Librach CL, Feigenbaum SL, Bass KE, et al: Interleukin-1 beta regulates human cytotrophoblast metalloproteinase activity and invasion in vitro. J Biol Chem 269:17125-17131, 1994.
24. Graham CH, Lysiak JJ, McCrae KR, et al: Localization of transforming growth factor-beta at the human fetal-maternal interface: Role in trophoblast growth and differentiation. Biol Reprod 46:561, 1992.
25. Aplin JD: Implantation, trophoblast differentiation and haemochorial placentation: Mechanistic evidence in vivo and in vitro. J Cell Sci 99:681, 1991.
26. Hay DL, Lopata A: Chorionic gonadotropin secretion by human embryos in vitro. J Clin Endocrinol Metab 67:1322, 1988.
27. Muyan M, Boime I: Secretion of chorionic gonadotropin from human trophoblasts. Placenta 18:237, 1997.
28. Hay DL: Discordant and variable production of human chorionic gonadotropin and its free alpha- and beta-subunits in early pregnancy. J Clin Endocrinol Metab 61:1195, 1985.
29. Takemori M, Nishimura R, Ashitaka Y, et al: Release of human chorionic gonadotropin (hCG) and its alpha-subunit (hCGa) from perifused human placenta. Endocrinol Jpn 28:757-768, 1981.
30. Lenton EA, Woodward AJ: The endocrinology of conception cycles and implantation in women. J Reprod Fertil 36(Suppl):1, 1988.
31. Stevens VC: Antifertility effects from immunisation with intact subunits and fragments of hCG. In Edwards RG, Johnson MG (eds): Physiological Effects of Immunity against Reproductive Hormones. London, Cambridge University Press, 1975, p 249.
32. Csapo AI, Pulkkinen M: Indispensability of the human corpus luteum in the maintenance of early pregnancy: Luteectomy evidence. Obstet Gynecol Surv 33:69, 1978.

33. Owens OM, Ryan KJ, Tulchinsky D: Episodic secretion of human chorionic gonadotropin in early pregnancy. J Clin Endocrinol Metab 53:1307, 1981.
34. Nakajima ST, McAuliffe T, Gibson M: The 24-hour pattern of the levels of serum progesterone and immunoreactive human chorionic gonadotropin in normal early pregnancy. J Clin Endocrinol Metab 71:345, 1990.
35. Barnea ER, Kaplan M, Naor Z: Comparative stimulatory effect of gonadotropin releasing hormone (GnRH) and GnRH agonist upon pulsatile human chorionic gonadotropin secretion in superfused placental explants: Reversible inhibition by a GnRH antagonist. Hum Reprod 6:1063-1069, 1991.
36. Csapo AI, Pulkkinen MO, Wiest WG: Effect of luteectomy and progesterone replacement therapy in early pregnant patients. Am J Obstet Gynecol 115:756, 1973.
37. Tapanainen J, Kellokumpu-Lehtinen P, Pelliniem L, et al: Age-related changes in endogenous steroids of human testis during early and mid-pregnancy. J Clin Endocrinol Metab 52:98, 1981.
38. Rebar RW, Cedars MI: Hypergonadotropic forms of amenorrhea in young women. Pediatr Clin North Am 21:173, 1992.
39. Simpson ER, MacDonald PC: Endocrine physiology of the placenta. Annu Rev Physiol 43:163, 1981.
40. Tulchinsky D, Hobel CJ: Plasma human chorionic gonadotropin, estrone, estradiol, estriol, progesterone and 17α-hydroxyprogesterone in human pregnancy: III. Early normal pregnancy. Am J Obstet Gynecol 117:884, 1973.
41. Siiteri PK, MacDonald PC: The utilization of circulating dehydroisoandrosterone sulfate for estrogen synthesis during human pregnancy. Steroids 2:713, 1963.
42. Salido EC, Yen PH, Barajas L, et al: Steroid sulfatase expression in human placenta: Immunocytochemistry and in situ hybridization study. J Clin Endocrinol Metab 70:1564, 1990.
43. Tulchinsky D, Frigoletto F, Ryan KJ, et al: Plasma estetrol as an index of fetal well-being. J Clin Endocrinol Metab 40:560, 1975.
44. Gelbke HP, Bottger M, Knuppen R: Excretion of 2-hydroxyestrone in urine throughout human pregnancies. J Clin Endocrinol Metab 41:744, 1975.
45. Bradshaw KD, Carr BR: Placental sulfatase deficiency: Maternal and fetal expressions of steroid sulfatase deficiency and X-linked ichthyosis. Obstet Gynecol Surv 68:505, 1986.
46. Harada N: Genetic analysis of human aromatase deficiency. J Steroid Biochem Mol Biol 44:331, 1993.
47. Roberts JM, Lewis VL, Riemer RK: Hormonal control of uterine adrenergic response. In Bottari J, Thomas P, Vokser A, et al (eds): Uterine Contractility. New York, Masson, 1984, p 161.
48. Mesiano S: Myometrial progesterone responsiveness and the control of human parturition. J Soc Gynecol Invest 11:193-202, 2004.
49. Merlino AA, Welsh TN, Tan H, et al: Nuclear progesterone receptors in the human pregnancy myometrium: Evidence that parturition involves functional progesterone withdrawal mediated by increased expression of progesterone receptor-A. J Clin Endocrinol Metab 92:1927-1933, 2007.
50. Cane EM, Villee CA: The synthesis of prostaglandin F by human endometrium in organ culture. Prostaglandins 9:281, 1975.
51. Siiteri PK, Febres F, Clemens LE, et al: Progesterone and maintenance of pregnancy: Is progesterone nature's immunosuppressant? Ann N Y Acad Sci 286:384, 1977.
52. Casey ML, Winkel CA, Porter JC, et al: Endocrine regulation of the initiation and maintenance of parturition. Clin Perinatol 10:709, 1983.
53. Resnik R, Killam AP, Battaglia FC, et al: Stimulation of uterine blood flow by various estrogens. Endocrinology 94:1192, 1974.
54. Martin RH, Oakey RE: The role of antenatal oestrogen in postpartum human lactogenesis: Evidence from oestrogen-deficient pregnancies. Clin Endocrinol 17:403, 1982.
55. Carr BR, Gant NF: The endocrinology of pregnancy-induced hypertension. Clin Perinatol 10:737, 1983.
56. Parker CR Jr, Hankins GD, Guzick DS: Ontogeny of unconjugated estriol in fetal blood and the relation of estriol levels at birth to the development of respiratory distress syndrome. Pediatr Res 21:386, 1987.
57. Caufriez A, Frankenne F, Hennen G, et al: Regulation of maternal IGF-I by placental GH in normal and abnormal human pregnancies. Am J Physiol 265:E572, 1993.
58. Kniss DA, Shubert PJ, Zimmerman PD, et al: Insulin like growth factors: Their regulation of glucose and amino acid transport in placental trophoblasts isolated from first trimester chorionic villi. J Reprod Med 39:249, 1994.
59. Maruo T, Matsuo H, Murata K, et al: Gestational age-dependent dual action of epidermal growth factor on human placenta early in gestation. Endocrinology 75:1366, 1992.
60. Josimovich JB, MacLaren JA: Presence in the human placenta and term serum of a highly lactogenic substance immunologically related to pituitary growth hormone. Endocrinology 71:209, 1962.
61. Bewley TA, Dixon JS, Li CH: Sequence comparison of human pituitary growth hormone, human chorionic somatomammotropin, and ovine pituitary growth and lactogenic hormones. Int J Pept Protein Res 4:281, 1972.
62. Cooke NE, Coit D, Shine J: Human prolactin cDNA structural analysis and evolutionary comparisons. J Biol Chem 256:4007, 1981.
63. Owerbach D, Rutter WJ, Martial JA: Genes for growth hormone chorionic somatomammotropin and growth hormone–like gene on chromosomes 17 in humans. Science 209:289, 1980.
64. Barrera-Saldana HA, Seeburg PH, Saunders GF: Two structurally different genes produce the same secreted human placental lactogen hormone. Bio Chem 258:3787, 1983.
65. McWilliams D, Boime I: Cytological localization of placental lactogen messenger ribonucleic acid in syncytiotrophoblast layers of human placenta. Endocrinology 107:761, 1980.
66. Hoshina M, Boothby M, Boime I: Cytological localization of chorionic gonadotropin α and placental lactogen mRNAs during development of the human placenta. J Cell Biol 93:190, 1982.
67. Grumbach MM, Kaplan SL, Abrams CL, et al: Plasma free fatty acid response to the administration of chorionic "growth hormone-prolactin." J Clin Endocrinol Metab 26:478-482, 1966.
68. Nielsen PV, Pedersen H, Kampmann EM: Absence of human placental lactogen in an otherwise uneventful pregnancy. Am J Obstet Gynecol 135:322, 1979.
69. Parks JS, Nielsen PV, Sexton LA, et al: An effect of gene dosage on production of human chorionic somatomammotropin. J Clin Endocrinol Metab 60:994, 1985.
70. DeNoto FM, Moore DD, Goodman HM: Human growth hormone DNA sequence and mRNA structures: Possible alternative splicing. Nucleic Acids Res 9:719, 1981.
71. Seeburg PH: The human growth hormone gene family: Nucleotide sequences show recent divergence and predict a new polypeptide hormone. DNA 1:239-249, 1982.
72. Igout A, Scippo ML, Frankenne F, et al: Cloning and nucleotide sequence of placental hGH-V cDNA. Arch Int Physiol Biochim 96:63, 1988.
73. Eriksson L, Frankenne F, Eden S, et al: Growth hormone 24-hour serum profiles during pregnancy: Lack of pulsatility for the secretion of the placental variant. BJOG 96:949, 1989.
74. Frankenne F, Closset J, Gomez F, et al: The physiology of growth hormones (GHs) in pregnant women and partial characterization of the placental GH variant. J Clin Endocrinol Metab 66:1171, 1988.
75. Ciaraldi TP, Kettel LM, El-Roeiy A, et al: Mechanisms of cellular insulin resistance in human pregnancy. J Clin Endocrinol Metab 75:577, 1992.
76. Yen SSC, Tsai CC, Vela P: Gestational diabetogenesis: Quantitative analyses of glucose-insulin interrelationship between normal pregnancy and pregnancy with gestational diabetes. Am J Obstet Gynecol 11:792, 1971.
77. Freinkel N, Metzger BE, Nitzan M, et al: Facilitated anabolism in late pregnancy: Some novel maternal compensations for accelerated starvation. In Malaisse WJ, Pirart J (eds): Diabetes. International Series No. 312. Amsterdam, Excerpta Medica, 1973, p 47.
78. Potter JM, Nestel PJ: The hyperlipidemia of pregnancy in normal and complicated pregnancies. Am J Obstet Gynecol 133:165, 1979.

79. Felig P, Kim YJ, Lynch V, et al: Amino acid metabolism during starvation in human pregnancy. J Clin Invest 51:1195, 1972.
80. Cousins L, Rigg L, Hollinsworth D, et al: Qualitative and quantitative assessment of the circadian rhythm of cortisol in pregnancy. Am J Obstet Gynecol 145:411, 1983.
81. Abou-Samra AB, Pugeat M, Dechaud H, et al: Increased concentration of N-terminal lipotrophin and unbound cortisol during pregnancy. Clin Endocrinol (Oxf) 20:221-228, 1984.
82. Petraglia F, Florio P, Carmine N, et al: Peptide signaling in human placenta and membranes: Autocrine, paracrine, and endocrine mechanisms. Endocrinol Rev 17:156, 1996.
83. Van Lith JM, Pratt JJ, Beekhuis JR, et al: Second trimester maternal serum immunoreactive inhibin as a marker for fetal Down's syndrome. Prenat Diagn 12:801, 1992.
84. Yohkaichiya T, Fudaya T, Hoshiai H, et al: Inhibin, a new circulating marker in hydatidiform mole. BMJ 298:1684, 1989.
85. Yohkaichiya T, Polson DW, Hughes EG, et al: Serum immunoreactive inhibin levels in early pregnancy after in vitro fertilization and embryo transfer. Fertil Steril 59:1081, 1993.
86. Norman RJ, McLoughlin JW, Borthwick GM, et al: Inhibin and relaxin concentrations in early singleton, multiple, and failing pregnancy: Relationship to gonadotropin and steroid profiles. Fertil Steril 59:130, 1993.
87. Steele GL, Currie WD, Yuen BH, et al: Acute stimulation of human chorionic gonadotropin secretion by recombinant human activin-A in first trimester human trophoblast. Endocrinology 133:297, 1993.
88. Frim DM, Emanuel RL, Robinson BG, et al: Characterization and gestational regulation of corticotropin-releasing hormone messenger RNA in human placenta. J Clin Invest 82:287, 1988.
89. Goland RS, Wardlaw SL, Blum M, et al: Biologically active corticotropin-releasing hormone in maternal and fetal plasma during pregnancy. Am J Obstet Gynecol 159:884, 1988.
90. Petraglia F, Giardino L, Coukos G, et al: Corticotrophin-releasing factor at parturition: Plasma and amniotic fluid levels and placental binding. Obstet Gynecol 75:784, 1990.
91. Warren WB, Silverman AJ: Cellular localization of corticotrophin releasing hormone in the placenta, fetal membranes, and decidua. Placenta 9:16, 1995.
92. Jones SA, Challis JRG: Local stimulation of prostaglandin production by corticotropin-releasing hormone in human fetal membranes and placenta. Biochem Biophys Res Commun 159:192, 1989.
93. Berkowitz GS, Lapinski RH, Lockwood CJ, et al: Corticotropin-releasing factor and its binding protein: Maternal serum levels in term and preterm deliveries. Am J Obstet Gynecol 174:1477, 1996.
94. Challis JRG, Matthews SG, Van Meir C, et al: Current topic: The placental corticotropin-releasing hormone-adrenocorticotrophin axis. Placenta 16:481, 1995.
95. Nakazawa K, Makino T, Iizuka R, et al: Immunohistochemical study on oxytocin-like substance in the human placenta. Endocrinol Jpn 31:763, 1984.
96. Leake RD, Weitzman RE, Glatz TH, et al: Plasma oxytocin concentrations in man, nonpregnant women and pregnant women before and during spontaneous labor. J Clin Endocrinol Metab 53:730, 1981.
97. Fuchs A-R, Fuchs F, Husslein P, et al: Oxytocin receptors in the human uterus during pregnancy and parturition. Am J Obstet Gynecol 150:734, 1984.
98. Fuchs A-R, Fuchs R, Husslein P: Oxytocin receptors and human parturition: A dual role for oxytocin in the initiation of labor. Science 214:1396, 1982.
99. Bell RJ, Eddie LW, Lester AR: Relaxin in human pregnancy serum measured with an homologous radioimmunoassay. Obstet Gynecol 69:585, 1987.
100. Weiss G, O'Byrne EM, Steinetz BTG: Relaxin: A product of the human corpus luteum of pregnancy. Science 194:948, 1976.
101. Eddie LW, Cameron IT, Leeton JF: Ovarian relaxin is not essential for dilatation of cervix. Lancet 336:243, 1990.
102. Emmi AM, Skurnick J, Goldsmith LT: Ovarian control of pituitary hormone secretion in early human pregnancy. J Clin Endocrinol Metab 72:1359, 1991.
103. Bani D: Relaxin: A pleiotropic hormone. Gen Pharmacol 28:13-22, 1997.
104. Weiss G, Goldsmith LT, Sachdev R: Elevated first-trimester serum relaxin concentrations in pregnant women following ovarian stimulation predict prematurity risk and preterm delivery. Obstet Gynecol 82:821, 1993.
105. Riggs LA, Lein A, Yen SSC: The pattern of increase in circulating prolactin levels during human gestation. Am J Obstet Gynecol 129:454, 1977.
106. Boyar RM, Finkelstein JW, Kapen S, et al: Twenty-four hour prolactin (PRL) secretory patterns during pregnancy. J Clin Endocrinol Metab 40:1117, 1975.
107. Liu JH, Park KH: Gonadotropin and prolactin secretion increases during sleep during the puerperium in nonlactating women. J Clin Endocrinol Metab 66:839, 1988.
108. Bigazzi M: Specific endocrine function of human decidua. Semin Reprod Endocrinol 1:343, 1983.
109. Tyson JE, McCoshen JA: Decidual prolactin: An enigmatic cyber in human reproduction. Semin Reprod Endocrinol 1:197, 1983.
110. Handwerger S, Brar A: Placental lactogen, placental growth hormone, and decidual prolactin. Semin Reprod Endocrinol 10:106, 1992.
111. Norwitz ER, Wilson T: Secretory component: A potential regulator of endometrial-decidual prostaglandin production in early human pregnancy. Am J Obstet Gynecol 183:108, 2000.
112. Cullinan EB, Abbondanzo SJ, Anderson PS, et al: Leukemia inhibitory factor (LIF) and LIF receptor expression in human endometrium suggests a potential autocrine/paracrine function in regulating embryo implantation. Proc Natl Acad Sci 93:3115-3120, 1996.
113. Stewart CL, Cullinan EB: Preimplantation development of the mammalian embryo and its regulation by growth factors. Dev Genet 21:91-101, 1997.

Chapter 9

The Breast and the Physiology of Lactation

Robert M. Lawrence, MD, and Ruth A. Lawrence, MD

Universal breastfeeding is recommended by the American College of Obstetrics and Gynecology (ACOG), the World Health Organization (WHO), United Nations International Children's Emergency Fund, the American Academy of Pediatrics (AAP), and the Women, Infants and Children's Nutrition Program, but recommendations alone are not sufficient to promote breastfeeding. It is the responsibility of every physician to recommend and support breastfeeding enthusiastically. This is especially true in obstetrics, where a physician's advice can immediately influence a woman's informed decision concerning breastfeeding and create or diminish barriers to successful breastfeeding.

Benefits of Breastfeeding

Breastfeeding provides benefits for both the mother and the infant. Breast milk is species specific, made uniquely for the human infant.[1] Protein in breast milk is readily digested and is present in amounts that can be handled by the developing kidney. Various minerals (e.g., iron) and nutrients exist in a form and in conjunction with other components that make them easily absorbed to meet infants' needs during periods of rapid growth.[1,2] Cholesterol and docosahexaenoic acid have been shown to play a role in central nervous system development and may contribute to the enhanced intelligence quotient measurements reported in breastfed infants.[3-5]

Protection against infections, including otitis media, croup, pneumonia, and gastrointestinal infections, is mediated by the over 50 immunologically active components found in breast milk.[1,6] These immunologically active components include viable functioning cells (T and B lymphocytes, macrophages), T cell–secreted products, immunoglobulins (especially secretory IgA), carrier proteins such as lactoferrin and transferrin, enzymes (lysozyme and lipoprotein lipase), and nonspecific factors such as complement, bifidus factor, gangliosides, and nucleotides. Other immune factors in breast milk include hormones, hormone-like factors, and growth factors that contribute to the normal maturation of the mucosal barrier of the respiratory and gastrointestinal tracts as well as the developing infant's immune system. Breast milk is a very dynamic fluid, varying with the maternal-infant dyads' environment and needs, especially in the face of infection or stress (providing, for example, nucleotides, secretory IgA, interleukin, interferon, and cytokines).[7-10] There is also evidence that breastfeeding provides protection against some noninfectious illnesses such as asthmatic wheezing, eczema, childhood lymphoma, insulin-dependent childhood-onset diabetes, and obesity[6,10-15] in children who are exclusively breastfed for the first 4 to 6 months of life.

Cognitive and psychological benefits for breastfed infants have been suggested, including developmental performance,[16] visual acuity,[17-19] school performance,[20] and performance on standardized[20] and intelligence quotient[4] tests. More recent articles continue to support the impact of breastfeeding on intellectual development while fostering debate over the relative contributions of nutrition, genetics, and environment to the intellectual development of infants and the possible influence on the child's or adult's future cognitive abilities as measured by intelligence quotient testing.[21,22] The psychological benefits are more difficult to measure but are well described by Newton and Newton,[23] and indeed by most mothers who have successfully breastfed their infants. One of the most consistent findings of exclusive breastfeeding is its influence on later intelligence, with a few test point advantages to the breastfed infant.[5] Reports questioning this effect have been based on any breastfeeding, not exclusive breastfeeding.[24]

Potential benefits to the mother include improved postpartum recovery,[25] a lower incidence of subsequent obesity,[26] a decreased risk of osteoporosis, and reduced incidence of both breast and ovarian cancers.[27] Calcium and phosphorus concentrations are higher in lactating women, and the risk of osteoporosis is measurably less for women who have breastfed their infants.[28,29] Increasing number of pregnancies, longer oral contraceptive use, and increasing duration of lactation are all protective against ovarian cancer.[30-32] The incidence of breast cancer is lower among women who have nursed.[33,34]

It is essential that a discussion of the benefits of breastfeeding to infants, mothers, and families (fathers included) be presented alongside any potential risks or contraindications. The benefits of breastfeeding are tremendous, and the risks and contraindications are few. Summarized here are the conditions in which the risks of breastfeeding may outweigh its benefits.[35]

- Women who take street drugs or who do not control their alcohol intake.
- A woman who has an infant with galactosemia, because both human and cow's milk exacerbate the condition. A lactose-free formula is recommended for these infants.
- Women who are infected with the human immunodeficiency virus (HIV) (see Maternal Infections during Breastfeeding, later).
- Women who have active untreated tuberculosis. Because of the increased risk of airborne transmission associated with the close contact that is typical of breastfeeding, women with active tuberculosis should not feed their infant by *any* method until treatment is initiated. However, infected women can provide their pumped milk to their infants (see later).

- Women who are known or suspected to be infected with Ebola or Marburg virus or Lassa fever (see later).
- Women who take certain medications (see Medications while Breastfeeding, later).

Medical situations that indicate a potential risk from breastfeeding must be weighed against the benefits of breastfeeding in each maternal-infant dyad's unique situation.

Role of the Obstetrician in Promoting Breastfeeding

Obstetricians have many responsibilities for breastfeeding, including the following:

- Enthusiastic promotion and support for breastfeeding, based on the published literature of its benefits advocated by the major pediatric, obstetric, and women's health organizations[36]
- Imparting clinical information to the lactating mother about the physiology of lactogenesis[37] and lactation, before and after the birth
- Developing and supporting hospital policies that facilitate breastfeeding and actively remove any barriers to it
- Supporting community efforts to provide women with adequate information to make an informed decision about breastfeeding, including links to community breastfeeding resources
- Fostering a general acceptance of breastfeeding by promoting a normative portrayal of breastfeeding and supporting the provision of sufficient time and facilities in the workplace
- Performing breast examinations before and after the birth, and emphasizing lactation as the primary function of the breast
- Participating in breastfeeding education in medical and other health profession schools[38]

The mother's plan for infant feeding should be addressed early in prenatal care, with counseling, a medical history focused on breast health and breastfeeding, and a physical examination of the breast. Counseling can be modeled after "The Best Start Three-Step Breastfeeding Counseling Strategy" (available by e-mailing Beststart@mindspring.com),[39] a publication that advises beginning with open-ended questions about breastfeeding. An acknowledgment that feelings of doubt about the ability to breastfeed successfully are normal is a good place to begin. Education about breastfeeding then continues with discussion of how others have dealt with these concerns. This conversation will elucidate much about the woman's knowledge of breastfeeding, her previous experiences with breastfeeding, and her own attitudes and those of the infant's father, the extended family, and other potentially supportive persons in the mother's life.

To support breastfeeding adequately throughout the first 6 months of an infant's life, the concerns of family and friends must be addressed actively to foster support for breastfeeding on many levels. Misconceptions and potential barriers must be identified and reasonable solutions developed in partnership with the woman. These often include feelings of responsibility for every unexplained problem the infant displays; conflicts among a woman's several roles as mother, sexual partner, and worker outside the home; and, most commonly, a greater time commitment and fatigue than was expected. It is important to address these and other questions repeatedly throughout pregnancy and not just in the immediate postpartum period, working closely with the infant's pediatrician.[36]

Examination of the Breast

The medical history related to the breasts should include their development, previous experience with breastfeeding, systemic illnesses, infections, breast surgery or trauma, medications, allergies, self–breast examinations and findings, and any anatomic or physical concerns the mother has about her breasts.

The breast examination at prenatal and postpartum visits should include careful inspection and palpation. Inspection of the breasts is most effective in the sitting position, first with the arms overhead and then with hands on the hips. Skin changes, distortions in shape or contour, and the form and size of the areola and nipple should be noted. Palpation can begin in the sitting position, looking for axillary and supraclavicular adenopathy. Palpation in the supine position is easier for the complete examination of the breast and surrounding anterolateral chest wall. Size, shape, consistency, masses, scars, tenderness, and any abnormalities can be noted in both descriptive and picture form for future comparison. Serial examinations should document maturational changes of pregnancy (size, shape, fullness, enlargement of areola) and nipple position (inversion or eversion).

The changes in the breast during pregnancy provide important prognostic data regarding successful breastfeeding. With the increased frequency of cosmetic breast surgery, it is important to be aware of the nature of any surgery and to examine carefully for the location of the surgical scars. Many women successfully breastfeed after surgery for benign breast disease, breast augmentation, or breast reduction. However, a periareolar incision or "nipple translocation technique" for breast reduction can damage nerves and ducts, making this more difficult. Nipple piercing is another increasingly common procedure, after which breastfeeding can be successful with the jewelry removed. Such surgeries do not preclude successful breastfeeding but rather remind us that additional early support should be provided to these mothers from physicians, nurses, lactation consultants, and peer support groups.

Perinatal Period

The obstetrician can make important contributions to successful breastfeeding through the conduct of the labor, delivery, and puerperium. A stressful or exhausting labor and delivery has been shown to affect lactation adversely.[40] A safe delivery for both mother and infant is, of course, the most important outcome. During the delivery and afterward, any medications used should be compatible with breastfeeding and not interfere with the bonding and first feeding. Immediate skin-to-skin contact between mother and infant, and a first feeding within 1 hour of delivery are probably the most important intrapartum steps to increase the likelihood of successful breastfeeding. Having the infant in the mother's room, feeding on demand, and early breastfeeding support (including teaching appropriate techniques) within the first 24 to 36 hours can also help. Supplementation should be avoided unless medically indicated and ordered by the pediatrician.

For the breastfeeding woman, medication choices are very important (see Table 9-6). Most women and many health professionals assume that no medication can be safely administered to a lactating woman, but the number of contraindicated drugs is in fact quite small. Before assuming a medication is unsafe, expert advice should be consulted, available in texts, via a drug information telephone service (see Suggested Readings), or at carefully selected websites.

Early follow-up (2 to 4 days after discharge) with the infant's health provider should be arranged for all breastfeeding mothers. Continued support of breastfeeding for the mother should occur through the 6-week postpartum visit. Discussions about breastfeeding should cover techniques to ensure adequate emptying of the breast, nipple soreness or trauma, plugged duct (in the form of a small lump), mastitis, breast abscess, breast masses, and bloody nipple discharge, all of which can usually be treated without stopping breastfeeding.

The Breast

To fully understand the process of lactation, one needs to understand the anatomy and physiology of the breast as it applies to this function. The human mammary gland is the only organ that does not contain all the rudimentary tissues at birth. It experiences dramatic changes in size, shape, and function from birth through menarche, pregnancy, and lactation, and ultimately during involution. The three major phases of growth and development before pregnancy and lactation occur in utero, during the first 2 years of life, and at puberty (Fig. 9-1).

Embryonic Development

The milk streak appears in the 4th week of gestation when the embryo is approximately 2.5 mm long. It becomes the milk line, or milk ridge, during the 5th week of gestation (2.5 to 5.5 mm). The mammary gland itself begins to develop at 6 weeks of embryonic life, and proliferation of the milk ducts continues throughout embryonic growth. The process of forming the nipple in the human embryo begins with a thickened raised area of ectoderm in the region of the future gland by the 4th week of pregnancy. This thickened ectoderm becomes depressed into the underlying mesoderm, and thus the surface of the mammary area soon becomes flat and finally sinks below the level of the surrounding epidermis. The mesoderm that is in contact with the ingrowth of the ectoderm is compressed, and its elements become arranged in concentric layers that at a later stage give rise to the gland's stroma. By dividing and branching, the ingrowing mass of ectodermal cells gives rise to the future lobes and lobules, and much later to the alveoli.

By 16 weeks' gestation in the fetus, the branching stage has produced 15 to 25 epithelial strips that represent the future secretory alveoli. By 28 weeks' gestation, placental sex hormones enter the fetal circulation and induce canalization in the fetal mammary tissue. The lactiferous ducts and their branches are developed from outgrowth in the lumen. They open into a shallow epidermal depression known as the mammary pit. The pit becomes elevated as a result of mesenchymal proliferation, forming the nipple and areola. An inverted nipple is the failure of this pit to elevate.[41] At 32 weeks' gestation, the lumen has formed in the branching system, and by term there are four to 18 mammary ducts that form the fetal mammary gland.[42] Figure 9-2 shows the hormonal regulation of mammary development in the mouse.

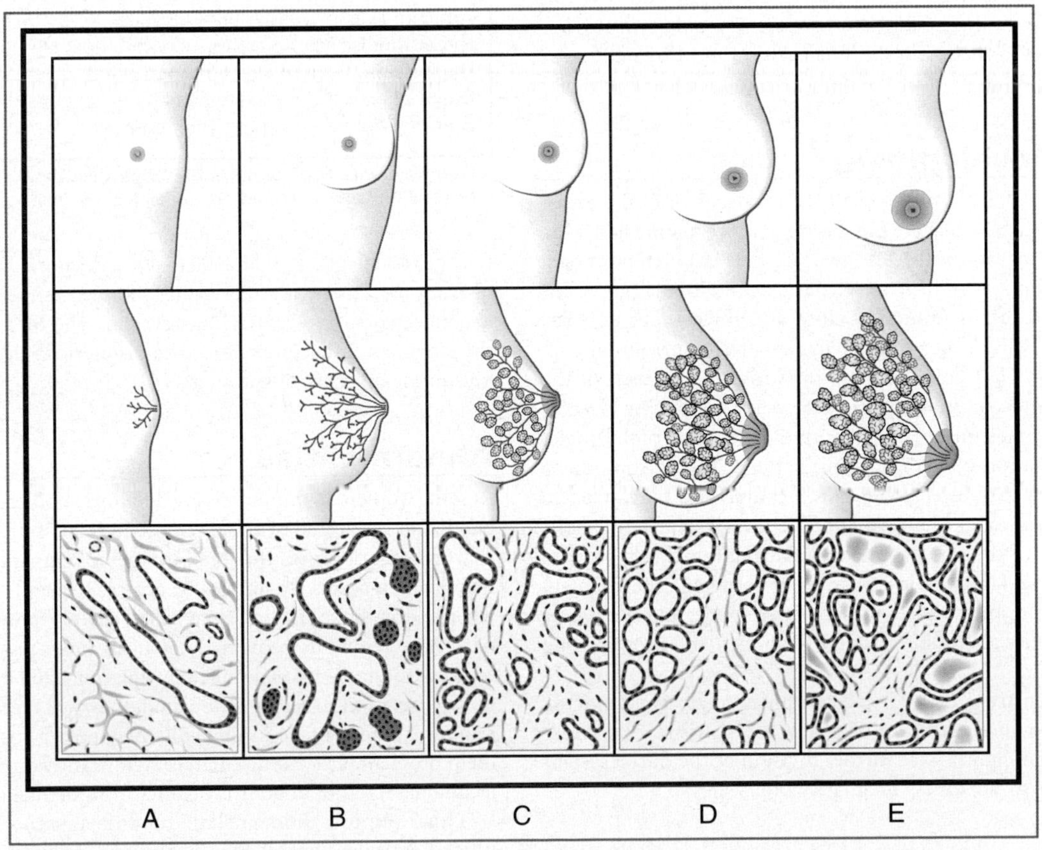

FIGURE 9-1 Female breast from infancy to lactation, with corresponding duct structure and tissue cross sections. **A, B,** and **C,** Gradual development of the well-differentiated ductular and peripheral lobular-alveolar system. **D,** Ductular sprouting and intensified peripheral lobular-alveolar development in pregnancy. Glandular luminal cells begin actively synthesizing milk fat and proteins near term; only small amounts are released into the lumen. **E,** With postpartum withdrawal of luteal and placental sex steroids and placental lactogen, prolactin is able to induce full secretory activity of alveolar cells and release of milk into alveoli and smaller ducts. (From Lawrence RA, Lawrence RM: Breastfeeding: A Guide for the Medical Profession, 6th ed. St. Louis, Mosby, 2005, p 43 [Fig. 2-3].)

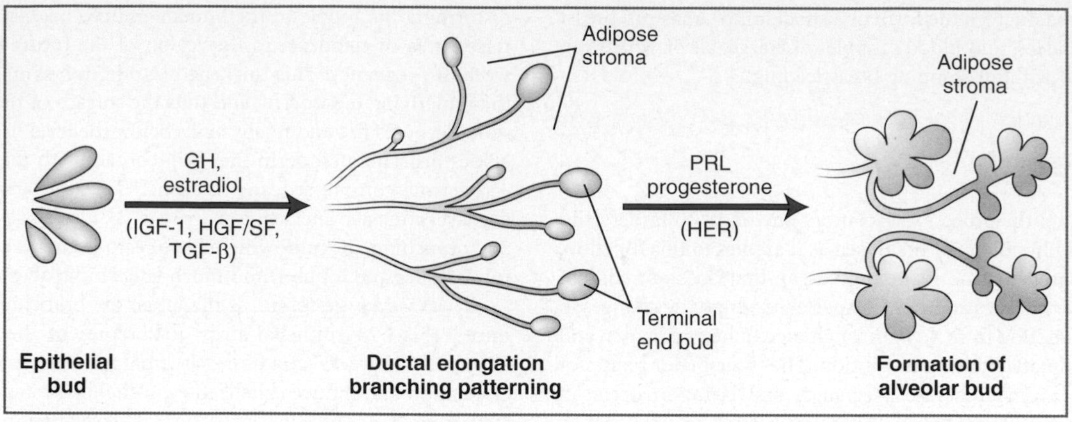

FIGURE 9-2 **Schema for hormonal regulation of mammary development in the mouse.** GH, growth hormone; HER, heregulin; HGF/SF, human growth factor/secretory factor; IGF-1, insulin-like growth factor 1; PRL, prolactin; TGF-β, transforming growth factor β. (From Neville MC: Mammary gland biology and lactation: A short course. Presented at the annual meeting of the International Society for Research on Human Milk and Lactation. Plymouth, Mass, October 1997.)

The nipple, areola, and breast bud are important landmarks for the determination of gestational age in the newborn. At 40 weeks, the nipple and areola are clearly seen and the breast bud is up to 1.0 cm in diameter. In the first weeks after delivery, the breast bud is visible and palpable; however, the gland then regresses to a quiescent stage as maternal hormones in the infant diminish. After this, the gland grows only in proportion to the rest of the body until puberty.

Pubertal Development

With the onset of puberty in the female, further growth of the breast occurs and the areolae enlarge and become more pigmented. The further development of the breast involves two distinct processes: organogenesis and milk production. The ductal and lobular growth is organogenesis, and this is initiated before and throughout puberty, resulting in the growth of breast parenchyma with its surrounding fat pad. The formation of alveolar buds begins within 1 to 2 years of the onset of menses and continues for several years, producing alveolar lobes. This menarchial stimulus begins with the extension of the ductal tree and the generation of its branching pattern. The existing ducts elongate. The ducts can develop bulbous terminal end buds that are the forerunners of alveoli. The formation of the alveolar bud begins within 1 to 2 years of the onset of menses. During this ductal growth, the alveoli enlarge and the nipple and areola become more pigmented. This growth involves an increase in connective tissue, adipose tissue, and vascular channels and is stimulated by estrogen and progesterone released by the ovary.[43]

During the menstrual cycle, there continues to be cyclic microscopic proliferation and regression of ductal breast tissue. The breast continues to enlarge slightly with further division of the ductal system until about the age of 28, unless pregnancy intervenes.

The Mature Breast

The mature breast is located in the superficial fascia between the second and sixth intercostal cartilages and is superficial to the pectoralis muscle. It measures 10 to 12 cm in diameter. It is located horizontally from the parasternal to the midaxillary line. The central thickness of the gland is 5 to 7 cm. In the nonpregnant state, the breast weighs about 200 g. During pregnancy, however, the size and weight increase to about 400 to 600 g and to 600 to 800 g during lactation. A projection of mammary tissue into the axilla is known as the tail of Spence and is connected to the central duct system. The breast is usually dome shaped or conic, becoming more hemispheric in the adult and pendulous in the older parous woman.

TABLE 9-1 BREAST ABNORMALITIES

Accessory breast: Any tissue outside the two major glands
Amastia: Congenital absence of breast or nipple
Amazia: Nipple without breast tissue
Hyperadenia: Mammary tissue without nipple
Hypoplasia: Underdevelopment of breast
Polythelia: Supernumerary nipple(s) (also hyperthelia)
Symmastia: Webbing between breasts

From Lawrence RA, Lawrence RM: Breastfeeding: A Guide for the Medical Profession, 6th ed. St. Louis, Mosby, 2005, p 45 (Box 2-1).

Abnormalities

In some women, mammary tissue develops at other sites in the galactic band. This is referred to as hypermastia, which is the presence of accessory mammary glands that are phylogenic remnants. These remnants may include accessory nipples or accessory gland tissue located anywhere along the milk line. From 2% to 6% of women have hypermastia. These remnants remain quiet until pregnancy, when they may respond to the hormonal milieu by enlarging and even secreting milk during lactation. If left unstimulated, they will regress after the birth. Major glandular tissue in the axilla may pose a cosmetic or management problem if the tissue enlarges significantly during pregnancy and lactation, secreting milk. It is distinct from the tail of Spence.

Other abnormalities include amastia (absence of the breast or nipple), amazia, hyperadenia, hypoplasia, polythelia, and symmastia (Table 9-1). Abnormalities of the kidneys have been associated with polythelia. Other variations include hyperplasia or hypoplasia in various combinations, as listed in Table 9-2. Gigantomastia is the excessive enlargement of the breasts in pregnancy and lactation, sometimes to life-threatening proportions. This enlargement may occur with the first or any pregnancy and may not recur. The enlargement recedes but rarely back to original size.[1] Breastfeeding has been suc-

TABLE 9-2	TYPES OF BREAST HYPOPLASIA, HYPERPLASIA, AND ACQUIRED ABNORMALITIES
Hypoplasia	
Unilateral hypoplasia, contralateral breast normal	
Unilateral hypoplasia, contralateral breast hyperplasia	
Unilateral hypoplasia of breast, thorax, and pectoral muscles (Poland syndrome)	
Bilateral hypoplasia with asymmetry	
Hyperplasia	
Unilateral hyperplasia, contralateral breast normal	
Bilateral hyperplasia with asymmetry	
Acquired Abnormalities	
Caused by trauma, burns, radiation treatment for hemangioma or intrathoracic disease, chest tube insertion in infancy, and preadolescent biopsy	

From Lawrence RA, Lawrence RM: Breastfeeding: A Guide for the Medical Profession, 6th ed. St. Louis, Mosby, 2005, p 46 (Box 2-2).

cessful in some cases of gigantomastia with appropriate professional support. In extreme cases, gigantomastia may require heroic measures, including emergency mastectomy.

Mothers with congenital abnormalities of the breast may wish to breastfeed. Not all abnormalities or variations preclude breastfeeding, and the decision is made on a case-by-case basis.

Nipple and Areola

The skin of the breast includes the nipple and areola and the thin, flexible, elastic skin that covers the body of the breast. The nipple is a conic elevation in the center of the areola at the level of about the fourth intercostal space, just below the midline of the breast. The nipple contains smooth muscle fibers and is richly innervated with sensory and pain fibers. It has a verrucous surface and has sebaceous and apocrine sweat glands, but not hair.

The areola surrounds the nipple and is also slightly pigmented and becomes deeply pigmented during pregnancy and lactation. The average diameter is 15 to 16 mm, but the range may exceed 5 cm during pregnancy. The sensory innervation is less than that of the nipple. The nipple and areola are very elastic and elongate into a teat when drawn into the mouth by the suckling infant.

The surface of the areola contains Montgomery glands, which hypertrophy during pregnancy and lactation and resemble vesicles. During lactation, they secrete a sebaceous material to lubricate the nipple and areola and protect the tissue while the infant suckles. These glands atrophy after weaning and are not visible to the naked eye except during pregnancy or lactation.

Each nipple contains four to 18 lactiferous ducts, of which five to eight are main ducts surrounded by fibromuscular tissue.[44] These ducts end as small orifices at the tip of the nipple from which the milk flows. The corpus mammae is an orderly conglomeration of a number of independent glands known as lobes. The morphology of the gland includes parenchyma that contains the ductular-lobular-alveolar structures. It also includes the stroma, which is composed of connective tissue, fat tissue, blood vessels, nerves, and lymphatics.

The mass of breast tissue consists of tubuloalveolar glands embedded in adipose tissue, which gives the gland its smooth, rounded contour. The mammary fat pad is essential for the proliferation and

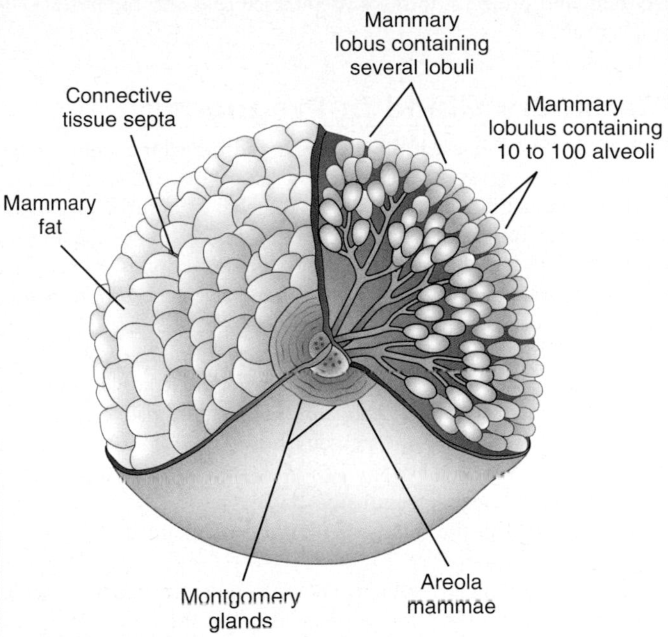

FIGURE 9-3 **Morphology of mature breast.** Diagrammatic dissection reveals mammary fat and duct system. (Modified from Lawrence RA, Lawrence RM: Breastfeeding: A Guide for the Medical Profession, 6th ed. St. Louis, Mosby, 2005, p 48 [Fig. 2-7].)

differentiation of the ductal arborization (Fig. 9-3). Each lobe is separated from the others by connective tissue, and opens into a duct that opens into the nipple. The extension of ducts is orderly and protected by an inhibitory zone into which other ducts cannot penetrate.[45]

Blood is supplied to the breast from branches of the intercostal arteries and perforating branches of the internal thoracic artery. The main blood supply comes from the internal mammary artery and the lateral thoracic artery. The venous supply parallels the arterial supply.

Lymphatic drainage has been thoroughly studied by researchers of breast cancer. The main drainage is to axillary nodes and the parasternal nodes along the thoracic artery within the thorax. The lymphatics of the breast originate in lymph capillaries of the mammary connective tissue and drain through the deep substance of the breast.

The breast is innervated from the branches of the fourth, fifth, and sixth intercostal nerves. The sensory innervation of the nipple and areola is extensive and includes both autonomic and sensory nerves. The innervation of the corpus mammae is meager by comparison and is predominantly autonomic. Neither parasympathetic nor cholinergic fibers supply any part of the breast. The efferent nerves are sympathetic adrenergic. Most of the mammary nerves follow the arteries. A few fibers course along the walls of the ducts. They may be sensory fibers that sense milk pressure. No innervation has been identified to supply the myoepithelial cells. Thus, the conclusion is that secretory activities of the acinar epithelium of the ducts depend on hormonal stimulation, such as oxytocin.

When sensory fibers are stimulated, the release of adenohypophyseal prolactin and neurohypophyseal oxytocin occurs. The areola is most sensitive to the stimulus of suckling, the nipple the least, and the skin of the breast is intermediate. The large number of dermal nerve endings results in high responsiveness to suckling. Pain fibers are more numerous in the nipple, with few in the areola. All cutaneous nerves run radially toward the nipple. Breast nerves can influence the mammary blood supply and therefore also influence the transport of oxytocin and prolactin to the myoepithelial cells and the lacteal cells, respectively.

Mammary Gland in Pregnancy

During the first trimester, rapid growth and branching from the terminal duct system into the adipose tissue is stimulated by the changing levels of circulating hormones. As epithelial structures proliferate, adipose tissue decreases. There is increased infiltration of the interstitial tissue with lymphatics, plasma cells, and eosinophils. By the third trimester, parenchymal cell growth slows and alveoli become distended with early colostrum. Alveolar proliferation is extensive.

The lactating mammary gland has a large number of alveoli that are made up of cuboidal, epithelial, and myoepithelial cells. Little connective tissue separates the alveoli. Lipid droplets are visible in the cells. By complex interplay of the nervous system and endocrine factors (progesterone, estrogen, thyroid, insulin, and growth factors), the mammary gland begins to function (lactogenesis stage I) and other hormones establish the milk secretion and maintain it (lactogenesis stage II).

Human prolactin has a significant role in both pregnancy and lactation. The levels are high during pregnancy, but the influence of prolactin on the breast itself is inhibited by a hormone produced by the placenta, originally referred to as prolactin-inhibiting hormone but believed to be progesterone.

Physiology of Lactation

Lactogenesis

Lactation is the physiologic completion of the reproductive cycle. The human infant is the most immature and dependent of all mammals except for marsupials, and thus the breast provides the most physiologically appropriate nutrients required by the human infant at birth. Throughout pregnancy, the breast develops and prepares to take over the role of fully nourishing the infant when the placenta is expelled. The breast is prepared for full lactation after 16 weeks' gestation. The physiologic adaptation of the mammary gland to its role in infant survival is a complex process, only the outline of which is discussed here. There are a number of complete reviews of the newer scientific studies on the physiology of lactation.[37,42,44,46] Hormonal control of lactation can be described in relationship to the five major changes in the development of the mammary gland: embryogenesis, mammogenesis or mammary growth, lactogenesis or initiation of milk secretion, lactation or full milk secretion, and involution (Table 9-3). Detailed explanation of mammary growth is beyond the scope of this discussion. The two most important hormones involved in lactation itself are prolactin and oxytocin, and these are described with respect to their impact on lactogenesis.

Lactogenesis is the initiation of milk secretion, beginning with the changes in the mammary epithelium in early pregnancy and progressing to full lactation. Stage I lactogenesis occurs during pregnancy and is achieved when the gland is sufficiently differentiated to secrete milk. It is prevented from doing so by high circulating plasma concentrations of progesterone.[47] Stage II is the onset of copious milk secretion associated with delivery of infant and the placenta. The progesterone level decreases sharply, by 10-fold in the first 4 days.[45] This is accompanied by the programmed transformation of the mammary epithelium.[48] By day 5, the infant has 500 to 750 mL of milk available (Fig. 9-4). The changes in milk composition that occur in the first 10 postpartum days should be viewed as part of a continuum in which the rapid changes of the first 4 days are followed by slower changes in various components of milk throughout lactation.[45] A change in permeability of the paracellular pathways results in a shift from high concentrations of sodium, chloride, and the protective immunoglobulins and lactoferrin, little lactose, and no casein in colostrum to increasing amounts of all milk components.[49]

TABLE 9-3 STAGES OF MAMMARY DEVELOPMENT

Developmental Stage	Hormonal Regulation	Local Factors	Description
Embryogenesis	?	Fat pad necessary for ductal extension	Epithelial bud develops in 18- to 19-week-old fetus, extending short distance into mammary fat pad with blind ducts that become canalized; some milk secretion may be present at birth
Mammogenesis			Anatomic development
Puberty			
Before onset of menses	Estrogen, GH	IGF-1, hGF, TGF-β; others?	Ductal extension into mammary fat pad; branching morphogenesis
After onset of menses	Estrogen, progesterone; PRL?		Lobular development with formation of terminal duct lobular unit
Pregnancy	Progesterone, PRL, hPL	HER; others?	Alveolus formation; partial cellular differentiation
Lactogenesis	Progesterone withdrawal, PRL, glucocorticoid	Not known	Onset of milk secretion Stage I: midpregnancy Stage II: parturition
Lactation	PRL, oxytocin	FIL	Ongoing milk secretion
Involution	PRL withdrawal	Milk stasis; FIL?	Alveolar epithelium undergoes apoptosis and remodeling; gland reverts to pre-pregnant state

FIL, feedback inhibition of lactation; GH, growth hormone; HER, heregulin; hGF, human growth factor; hPL, human placental lactogen; IGF-1, insulin-like growth factor 1; PRL, prolactin; TGF-β, transforming growth factor-beta.
Modified from Neville MC: Mammary gland biology and lactation: A short course. Presented at the biannual meeting of the International Society for Research on Human Milk and Lactation, Plymouth, Mass, October 1997.

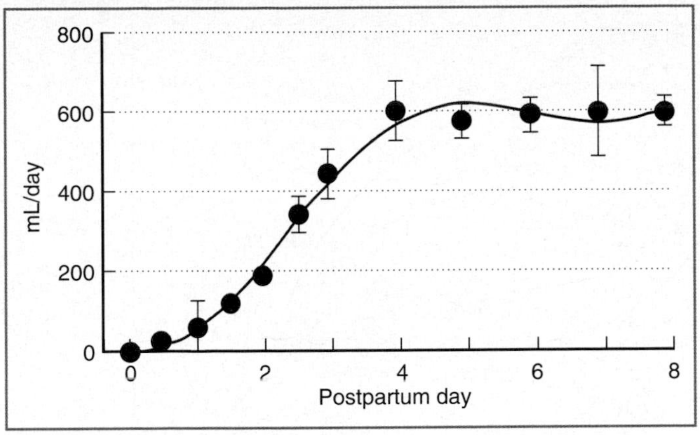

FIGURE 9-4 Milk volumes during 1st postpartum week. Mean values from 12 multiparous white women who test-weighed their infants before and after every feeding for the first 7 postpartum days. (Redrawn from Neville MC, Keller RP, Seacat J, et al: Studies in human lactation: Milk volumes in lactating women during the onset of lactation and full lactation. Am J Clin Nutr 48:1375-1386, 1988.)

Lactogenesis stage II results in an increase of milk from 100 mL in the first 24 hours to large volumes (500 to 750 mL/day) by day 4 or 5, gradually leveling off at 600 to 700 mL/day by day 8.[50] These volume changes are associated with a decrease in sodium and chloride concentration and an increase in lactose concentration. The production of lactose drives the production of milk. The early changes in sodium and chloride are a function of the closure of the tight junctions that block the paracellular pathway.[51,52] Secretory IgA and lactoferrin represent 10% by weight of the milk produced in the first 48 hours, and although their amounts remain the same, the increased volume of milk produced decreases their concentration. At 8 days, secretory IgA and lactoferrin are 1% by weight and 2 to 3 g/day.[53]

At 36 postpartum hours (in multiparas) and at up to 72 hours (in primiparas), milk production increases 10-fold (from 50 to 500 mL/day). Women refer to this as their milk "coming in". It reflects a massive increase in synthesis and secretion of the components of mature milk, including lactose, protein, and lipid.[54]

During pregnancy, hormones maintain the pregnancy and produce mammary tissue that is prepared to produce milk but does not do so. Progesterone, prolactin, and possibly placental lactogen are credited with the development of the alveoli. Progesterone has been identified as the major inhibitor of milk production during pregnancy.[55] Prolactin levels in pregnancy are greater than 200 ng/mL. Apparently, the continued high level of prolactin and a decrease in progesterone are necessary for stage II lactogenesis after parturition.[55] The placenta is the main source of progesterone in pregnancy. After the birth progesterone receptors are lost in the human breast and estrogen levels drop precipitously.

In addition to prolactin, insulin and corticoids are essential to milk synthesis.[56] Delayed lactogenesis is seen in women who had retained placenta, cesarean section, diabetes, and stress during delivery.[50,56-58] In the 1940s, Jackson[59] first noted that stressful labors influenced the early breastfeeding experience in the rooming-in unit. Stress may be the trigger for delayed lactogenesis in the conditions other than retained placenta. The significance of having a high sodium concentration in breast milk requires further study.[49] It has been observed that high sodium levels in early milk samples are seen in pregnancy, mastitis, involution (weaning), premature birth, and inhibition of prolactin secretion by bromocriptine. These observations suggest that junctional closure depends on adequate suckling or effective milk removal in the first 3 postpartum days.

If milk removal does not begin by 72 hours, the changes in milk composition associated with lactogenesis are reversed and the probability that lactation will be successful decreases. Thus, clinical efforts that facilitate early suckling by the newborn enhance the probability of lactation success. Early stimulation of the breast by pumping before 72 postpartum hours is essential when the infant is unable to nurse directly.

Let-Down (Ejection) Reflex

An effective let-down reflex is key to successful lactation. This reflex, also known as the ejection reflex, was first described in humans by Peterson and Ludwick in 1942,[60] and was later demonstrated clinically by Newton and Newton[23] to be caused by the release of oxytocin by the pituitary. Since that time, many refinements in the understanding of the process have been published, but the fundamental principles are unchanged (Fig. 9-5).

A mother may produce milk, but if it is not excreted, further production is eventually suppressed. The reflex is a complex function that depends on hormones, nerves, and glandular response and can be inhibited most easily by psychological influences.

Oxytocin is the hormone responsible for stimulating the myoepithelial cells to contract and eject the milk from the ductal system. The ducts begin at the alveoli, which are surrounded by a basket-like structure of myoepithelial cells that also surround the ducts all the way to the nipple. When the infant stimulates the breast by suckling, impulses sent to the central nervous system and to the posterior pituitary result in the release of oxytocin, which is then carried by the bloodstream to the myoepithelial cells. This is a neuroendocrine reflex. Oxytocin release can also be stimulated by other pathways of sight, sound, and smell that represent the infant. Oxytocin also stimulates the myoepithelial cells in the uterus, which are very sensitive to oxytocin during parturition and for a week or so after the birth. This causes the uterus to contract, decreases blood loss, and hastens postpartum involution. The uterus of a mother who breastfeeds returns to a pre-pregnant state more rapidly. The uterine cramping experienced while breastfeeding is a result of this stimulus (see Fig. 9-5).

Newton and Newton[23] demonstrated that pain and stress interfered with the let down reflex because it interfered with oxytocin release. In their experimental model, they stimulated stress with pain, loud noises, or pressure to solve mathematical problems. In other species, oxytocin release has been shown to stimulate mothering behaviors.[61] Levels of adrenocorticotropin and plasma cortisol are decreased in lactating women compared with nonlactating women in response to stress.

Prolactin is central to the production of milk and regulates the rate of synthesis. Its release depends on the suckling of the infant or the stimulation of the nipple by mechanical pumping or manual expression. Prolactin is also released through a neuroendocrine reflex. Its influence is modified, however, by the actual release of milk from the alveoli. Local factors in the ductal system or in the accumulated milk can inhibit milk release and thus inhibit further milk production. Prolactin is not released as a result of sound, sight, or smell of the infant, as is the case with oxytocin, but only by suckling (Fig. 9-6).

Initiation of Lactation

Although breastfeeding is a natural process in postpartum women, it is a learned skill, not a reflex. Because the incidence of breastfeeding in developed countries dropped to about 10% in the 1950s and 1960s,

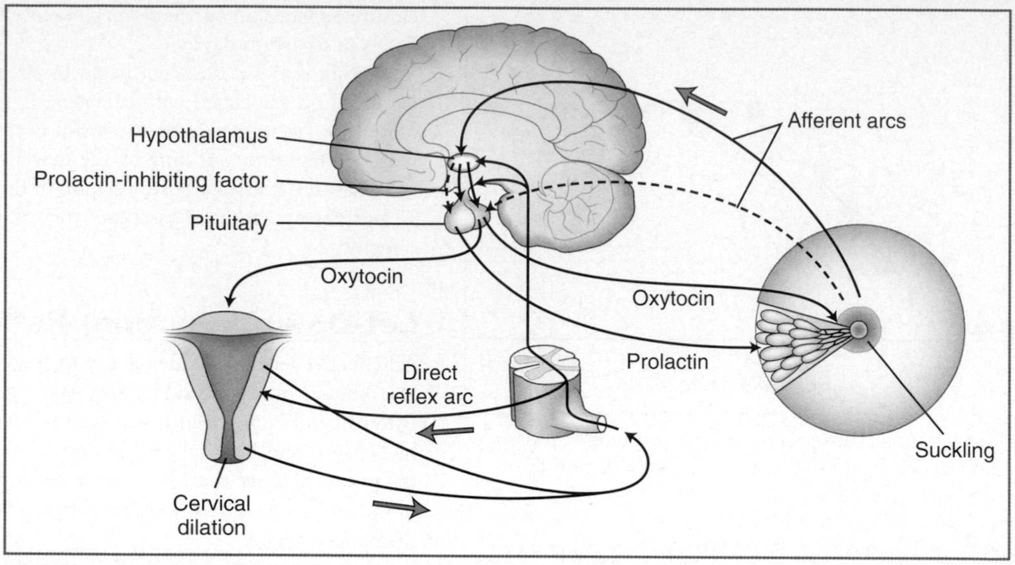

FIGURE 9-5 Neuroendocrine control of milk ejection. (Modified from Vorherr H: The Breast: Morphology, Physiology and Lactation. New York, Academic Press, 1974.)

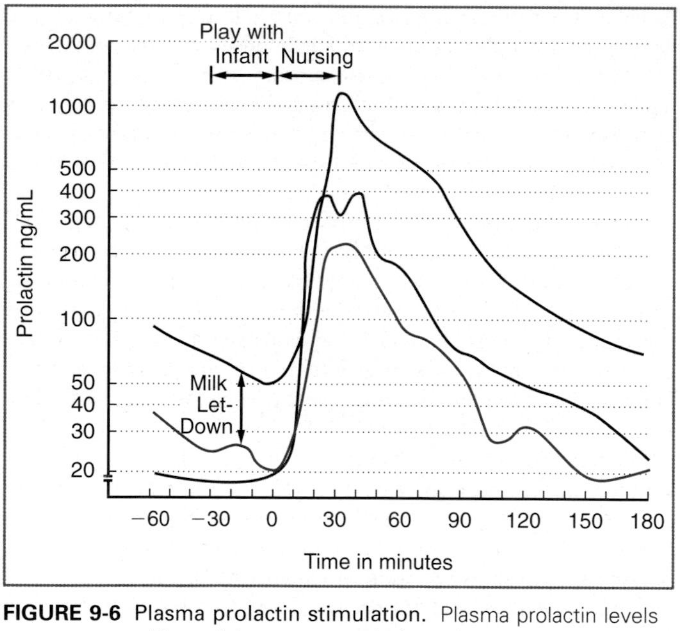

FIGURE 9-6 Plasma prolactin stimulation. Plasma prolactin levels were measured by radioimmunoassay before, during, and after a period of nursing in three mothers between 22 and 26 days after the birth. The levels rose with suckling but not with infant contact only. (Modified from Josimovich JB, Reynolds M, Cobo E: Lactogenic hormones, fetal nutrition, and lactation. In Josimovich JB, Reynolds M, Cobo E [eds]: Problems of Human Reproduction, vol 2. New York, John Wiley & Sons, 1974, p 1.)

there are few experienced role models available to support, encourage, and assist new mothers in feeding their infants at the breast. In the late 1940s, Edith Jackson at Yale, in cooperation with Herbert Thoms, established the first rooming-in unit in the United States, introduced "child birth without fear," and reestablished breastfeeding as the norm for mothers and infants at the Yale–New Haven Hospital.[62] Obstetric and pediatric residents were well schooled in the practical aspects of breastfeeding and human lactation. Jackson and her pediatric colleagues published the classic article on the management of breastfeeding,[63] on which decades of publications, both lay and professional, were based.

The obstetrician and pediatrician have become more involved in the decision to breastfeed and in the practical management of the mother-infant dyad. Medical schools are gradually adding breastfeeding and lactation to their curriculum. Although it is not the physician's role to put the infant to the breast, it is important to understand the process, to recognize problems, and to know how to solve them. Breastfeeding support is a team effort in which the physician works with many health care professionals, including nurses, midwives, doulas, and dietitians, to provide complete care to the perinatal patient. Lactation specialists may be nurses, dietitians, or nonmedical individuals with special training, or physicians with specialty designation. The physician should be sure that consultants are licensed and board certified by the International Board of Lactation Consultant Examiners, and that other physicians are recognized as a fellows of the Academy of Breastfeeding Medicine.

Except in extreme cases, breast size does not influence milk production. Augmentation mammoplasty does not interfere with lactation unless a periareolar incision was made and nerves were interrupted. If augmentation was done for cosmetic enhancement, the tissue should function well, but if there was little or no palpable breast tissue before surgery, lactation may be improbable.

Reduction mammoplasty is more invasive surgery, and results depend on the technique used. If many ducts were severed and the nipple and areolar transplanted, lactation is interfered with. If, however, the nipple and areolar remained intact on a pedicle of ducts, lactation could be successful. Other incisions (e.g., for lump removal) should be discussed but usually do not interfere with lactation.

During pregnancy, the obstetrician should document the changes in the breasts in response to pregnancy, when the nipple and areola should become more pigmented and enlarged and the breast should enlarge several cup sizes. Lack of breast changes should also be communicated to the pediatrician, as it represents a risk for early failure to thrive because of insufficient milk supply. A breast examination should be conducted late in the pregnancy to check for any new findings of masses, lumps, discharge, or pain. Berens[64] described the role of the obstetrician throughout pregnancy in detail.

Initiating Breastfeeding

The ideal time to initiate breastfeeding is immediately after birth (the Baby Friendly Initiative recommends within a half hour of birth). When left on the mother's abdomen to explore, the unmedicated newborn will move toward the breast, latch on, and begin suckling. This usually takes 20 to 30 minutes if unassisted.[65] The infant is ready to feed and has been sucking in utero since about 14 weeks' gestation, consuming amniotic fluid daily (about 1 g protein/kg of fetal weight is received daily from amniotic fluid). The infant at 28 weeks' gestation already has a rooting, sucking, and coordinated swallow while breastfeeding. The ability to coordinate suck and swallow while bottle feeding does not occur until 34 weeks.

Shortly after delivery, the mother should be offered the opportunity to breastfeed and should be assisted to assume a comfortable position, usually lying on her side. The infant can be placed beside her, tummy to tummy facing the breast. The mother should support her breast with her hand, keeping her fingers behind the areola so the infant can latch on. The mother should stroke the center of the lower lip with the breast. The infant should open the mouth wide, extend the tongue, and draw the nipple and areola into the mouth to form a teat. This teat is compressed against the palate by the tongue, and the gums and lips form a seal with the breast. It is the peristaltic motion of the tongue that stimulates the let-down reflex. The continued peristaltic motion travels to the posterior tongue, the pharynx, and down the esophagus as one coordinated motion so that swallowing is automatically coordinated with suckling during breastfeeding.

Ultrasound imaging of milk ejection in the breast of lactating women has provided a more detailed description of the process compared with the traditional serial sampling of plasma oxytocin levels and measurements of intraductal pressure. A significant increase in milk-duct diameter can be observed during milk ejection. Multiple milk ejections occur during the process and are correlated with milk flow and with the changes in milk-duct diameter, although they are not sensed by the mother.[66] The number of milk ejections influences the amount of milk available to the infant.

Sucking an artificial nipple is a very different tongue motion that is not coordinated with swallow. A newborn should not be given a bottle to test feeding ability before breastfeeding. It is wise to avoid all artificial nipples (bottles or pacifiers) in the early weeks of breastfeeding. If, for a medical necessity, the infant requires artificial formula, it can be given by medicine cup (cup feeding).[67,68]

The initial contact may be limited to exploration of the breast by the infant, with licking and nuzzling of the nipple, or the infant may latch on and suck for minutes. Timing is not necessary because the infant will interrupt him- or herself. The first hour after birth, the term unmedicated infant will be quietly alert. It is an opportunity for the mother, father, and infant to get acquainted.

Ideally, mother and infant recover in the same room together. The infant is fed on awakening, and the mother learns the early signs of hunger. Crying is a very late sign. She also learns about caring for her infant. There should be no schedules and no intervention unless an infant does not feed for over 6 hours. The nursing staff and lactation consultants ensure that the infant latches on well and the mother's questions are answered. Breastfeeding should not hurt; when it does, the process should be observed and adjusted. The pediatrician should observe a feeding as part of the infant's discharge examination. The

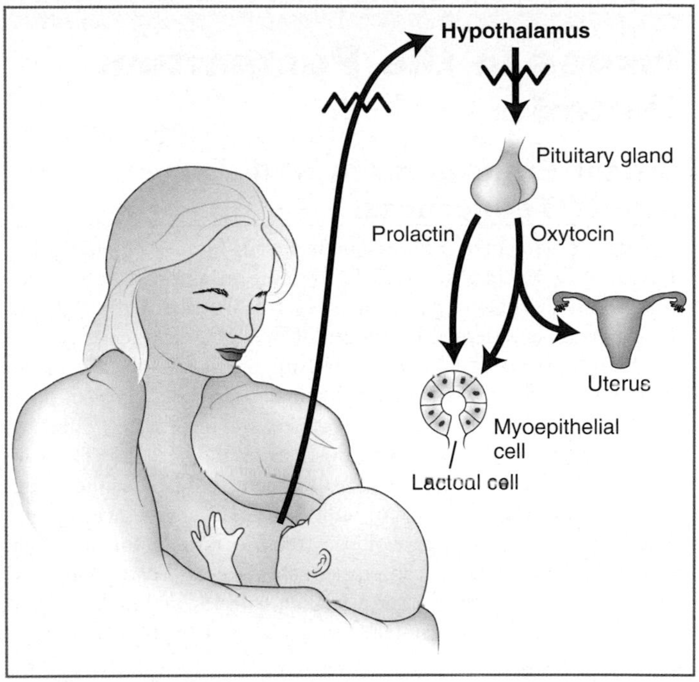

FIGURE 9-7 Diagram of ejection reflex arc. When the infant suckles the breast, mechanoreceptors in the nipple and areola are stimulated, which sends a stimulus along nerve pathways to the hypothalamus, which stimulates the posterior pituitary gland to release oxytocin. Oxytocin is carried via the bloodstream to the breast and uterus. Oxytocin stimulates myoepithelial cells in the breast to contract and eject milk from the alveolus. Prolactin is responsible for milk production in the lacteal cells lining the alveolus. Prolactin is secreted by the anterior pituitary gland in response to suckling. Stress (e.g., pain, anxiety) can inhibit the let-down reflex. Seeing or hearing the cry of the infant can stimulate the release of oxytocin but not prolactin. (From Lawrence RA, Lawrence RM: Breastfeeding: A Guide for the Medical Profession, 6th ed. St. Louis, Mosby, 2005, p 290 [Fig. 8-18].)

mother should be aware of the milk letting down by tingling in the breast or dripping from the opposite breast. The infant should be noted to swallow (Fig. 9-7).

The infant's weight is measured daily and again just before discharge. A weight loss of greater than 5% in the first 48 hours should be assessed by checking the feeding process and reviewing voidings and stoolings. Maximum weight loss should not exceed 7% in a breastfed infant by 72 hours. The weight should plateau after 72 hours. Birth weight should be regained by 7 days or, at the latest, 10 days. A healthy infant voids at least once and stools at least once in the first 24 hours, at least twice in the second 24 hours, and at least three times in the third 24 hours. From then on voidings should occur at least six times daily. An infant should stool at least once (and preferably three times) every day in the first month of life. After 3 to 4 months of age, a perfectly healthy breastfed infant may go a week without stooling and then pass a soft yellow stool, but this should not occur under 1 month of age.

Early discharge from the hospital has increased the need for newborn care visits within a few days after discharge and as required thereafter at 2- to 4-week intervals for assessment of weight and hydration. The AAP recommends a visit at 3 to 5 days of age for infants discharged at 48 hours or less.[38]

Issues in the Postpartum Period

Breast Engorgement and Nipple Tenderness

A little engorgement of the breast in the first 24 hours is physiologically normal as the vascular supply shifts from the once-gravid uterus to the breasts. Absence of any engorgement, such as absence of breast growth during pregnancy, is cause for concern. Not only is excess engorgement painful but the increased vascular pressure compresses the alveoli and ducts and interferes with milk production and release.[69] Prevention of excessive engorgement is the best treatment and involves the following: (1) wearing a well-fitting nursing brassiere even before the breasts are engorged, and around the clock, (2) frequent feedings for the infant, being sure to balance the use of both breasts, (3) gentle massage and softening of the areola before offering the breast to the infant, so that proper latch-on can be accomplished, (4) if necessary, applying cold packs or cold compresses after a feeding, and (5) taking acetaminophen or ibuprofen, which may be safely used by the mother for discomfort.

Peak engorgement usually occurs between 72 and 96 postpartum hours when the mother has arrived home and is on her own. At the peak of discomfort, standing in a warm shower to let milk drip or applying warm compresses before pumping to relieve the pressure and stimulate flow provides relief before the phenomenon subsides.

Sore nipples are a common complaint when early lactation has gone unassisted. It should not hurt to breastfeed. When it does hurt, the infant should be taken off the breast by breaking the suction with a finger and reattaching the infant carefully, following the steps previously described. The major cause of sore nipples is inadequate latch-on. It is not caused by breastfeeding too long or too frequently. A newborn usually feeds about every 2 hours in the first few weeks of life. Persistent sore nipples, cracks, or oozing may require the assistance of a licensed certified lactation consultant who can take the time and has the experience to work with the mother to identify the cause, determine effective treatment, and assist the dyad in maintaining pain-free breastfeeding.

Faltering Milk Supply

Many misconceptions lead to the impression that a failing milk supply is a common occurrence. Many women discontinue breastfeeding before 3 postpartum months, believing their milk is diminishing because their breasts are no longer engorged. Once supply and demand have been equilibrated and the breast makes what the infant needs, the breasts are soft and do not constantly drip. The emptying time of the stomach of the infant fed human milk is 90 minutes, fed formula it is 3 to 4 hours, and fed cow's milk it is 6 hours. Continuing to feed every 3 hours is a testimony to its digestibility, not its inadequacy. Weight gain in the infant is the better barometer of success. The ACOG supports the AAP statement that exclusive breastfeeding should continue for 6 months, with continued breastfeeding while adding weaning foods for the next 6 months, and then as long thereafter as mutually desired by mother and child.[38,70,71]

Genuine failure to produce enough milk may result from infant causes, such as increased need, increased fluid losses, or lack of adequate suckling, or to maternal causes, such as failure to let down or failure of production. Each case should be carefully reviewed because most situations are remediable. Ideally, the pediatrician is experienced in lactation management or has a staff member who is. Working together with a licensed certified lactation specialist, the issues can be resolved and breastfeeding can continue successfully.

Breastfeeding after Premature or Multiple Births

Human milk is beneficial in the management of the premature infant according to the Policy Statement of the AAP.[38] The benefits include infection protection; improvement in gastrointestinal function, digestion, and absorption of nutrients; and neurodevelopmental outcomes. The psychological well-being of the mother is enhanced when she provides her milk for her compromised infant.[72] Meeting the intrauterine rates of growth and nutrient accretion requires attention. Although human milk satisfies these needs for larger premature infants, it can be carefully supplemented for smaller infants and still preserve the benefits of human milk. Recently, a product created with 100% human milk has been developed to enhance mother's milk and replace supplementation made with cow's milk.[73]

Twins and triplets present problems of time management for the mother.[74] The mother will make enough milk, as supply will meet demand. Twins learn quickly to nurse simultaneously and will continue to do so for months or years. Breastfeeding ensures a mother's interaction with her infants. Helpful friends and relatives can perform the other household duties. The mother can also provide enough milk for triplets. Some mothers prefer to nurse two at a feeding, giving the third a bottle but rotating the three, feeding by feeding. Any breast milk is valuable in this situation. Mothers of multiples need help. It may be necessary for the physician to prescribe help and careful attention to proper rest. Mothers have also breastfed quadruplets and higher. Usually, they nurse several at each feeding and rotate bottle feeding. Exclusive breastfeeding of quadruplets for the first year has been reported by Berlin.[75]

Contraception

Lactation suppresses ovulation and thus helps prevent pregnancy for the first several months after delivery but should not be relied on as a sole method of contraception. Many couples resume coitus before the first postpartum visit and should be educated about the effects of breastfeeding on sexual function and fertility. Interest in sex may be reduced, not only by the endocrine environment of lactation but also by maternal fatigue, reduced vaginal lubrication during lactation, and the altered roles of wife and mother. Contraceptive choices are consequently affected by lactation.

Nonhormonal choices are preferred until ovulation resumes. ACOG recommends prelubricated condoms or other lubricated barrier methods such as a diaphragm. Intrauterine devices are appropriate once uterine involution has occurred. Supplemental lubrication may be required.

Use of hormonal contraceptives in breastfeeding women raises questions about maternal-fetal transfer of hormones, but the principal concerns relate to the effect on milk production and risk to the mother. Progestin-only contraceptives, such as the mini-pill tablet, injectable medroxyprogesterone acetate (Depo-Provera, Pharmacia), and levonorgestrel implants, are the hormonal methods of choice when nonhormonal methods are not acceptable. Unlike combined estrogen-progestin pills, the progestin-only methods have no effect on the quantity or quality of milk. The package inserts for progestin-only methods recommend initiation of use at 6 postpartum weeks for women who are breastfeeding exclusively, and at 3 weeks for those who supplement breast milk with formula. The injectable medroxyprogesterone acetate is recommended only at 6 weeks after delivery. The reasons for the delayed use of the progestin-only methods are primarily theoretical, related to concerns about an immediate effect on the onset of milk production if used within 3 days of birth and on the uncertain ability of the newborn to metabolize progesterone. However, concern about the impact of early initiation of progestin-only pills has been ameliorated by a recent report that found no adverse effects on continuation rates in exclusive breastfeeding or when supplements are used.[76] Medroxyprogesterone injections before 6 weeks have been observed to affect milk supply, but there are no controlled studies.[1]

Combined estrogen-progestin contraceptive tablets are not ideal during lactation because they reduce both the quantity and the quality of milk and may increase the risk of maternal thromboembolism in the already hypercoagulable postpartum period. If used at all, they should not be started until at least 6 postpartum weeks and after lactation is well established.

A thorough summary and suggested protocol, Contraception during Lactation, is available from the Academy of Breastfeeding Medicine.[77]

Maternal Infections during Breastfeeding

Although often a mother is concerned about the risk to a breastfeeding infant when she has an infectious illness, maternal infection is not a contraindication to breastfeeding in most cases (Table 9-4). Proscribing breastfeeding out of fear of infection deprives infants of significant immunologic, nutritional, and emotional benefits of breastfeeding when they are most needed.[1]

The decision-making process to breastfeed despite maternal infection should involve discussion of the usual route of infection transmission, reasonable infection control precautions, potential severity of infection in the infant or child, medications to treat the mother that are compatible with breastfeeding, the potential of prophylaxis for the infant, the protective effect of breast milk, and the acceptability of using expressed breast milk temporarily. The discussion should involve the mother (or both parents), weighing the known and potential risks of the infection against the known benefits of breastfeeding.[1]

For example, diphtheria and active pulmonary tuberculosis in the mother are commonly transmitted via the respiratory route, so contact between infant and mother should be proscribed regardless of how the infant is being fed. In the case of cutaneous diphtheria or tuberculosis mastitis, as long as there are no lesions on the breast, expressed breast milk can be given to the infant during the initial treatment of the mother (probable infectious periods are 5 days for diphtheria, and 14 days or until the sputum is negative for acid-fast tuberculous bacilli). Diphtheria and tuberculosis are not transmitted in the milk. Prophylactic antibiotics for the infant are appropriate in each case—penicillin or erythromycin for diphtheria and isoniazid for tuberculosis.[1,78,79]

In certain highly infectious and serious infections, such as the hemorrhagic fevers—specifically with Ebola or Marburg virus and Lassa fever—the risk of transmission from any contact with the infected mother is high, and the potential severity of the illness in mother or infant necessitates separation of the infant (breastfed or formula-fed) from the mother and proscription of breastfeeding as well as feeding expressed breast milk. For dengue virus or Hantavirus, standard precautions are appropriate, along with the temporary use of expressed breast milk and subsequent breastfeeding in the recovering mother.[1]

Possible West Nile virus (WNV) transmission to an infant through breastfeeding has been reported,[80] but the data on this infection in pregnant or breastfeeding women and their infants are limited. Hinckley and coworkers reported 10 instances of maternal or infant WNV-related illness while breastfeeding. In five cases, the transmission of WNV through breast milk could not be confirmed or ruled out, and in the other five cases, there was no evidence of vertical transmission. They concluded that the information they presented does not support a change in breastfeeding practices after infection with WNV, and that more information is needed.[81]

The hepatitis C virus (HCV) is a blood-borne infection. The rate of mother-to-infant transmission is about 6%. Several cohort studies suggest that most infants acquire HCV infection in utero or the peripartum period. HCV has been detected in colostrum and breast milk at low levels. Bhola and McGuire, in their analysis of three large cohort studies involving a total of 1854 mother-infant pairs, concluded that although the studies showed slightly higher percentages of HCV infection among the breastfed children, the proportions were not statistically significant.[82] Guidelines from the Centers for Disease Control and Prevention and from the AAP state that maternal HCV infection is not a contraindication to breastfeeding. HCV and HIV coinfection in the mother is a contraindication to breastfeeding in high-income countries. Because HCV is a blood-borne virus, some authorities recommend avoiding breastfeeding, at least temporarily, if a HCV-infected mother experiences nipples that are cracked or bleeding.

In the case of infections at specific sites, the management varies with the specific etiologic organism. For example, mastitis caused by *Staphylococcus* or group A *Streptococcus* requires contact precautions—delaying breastfeeding for 24 hours after beginning therapy in the mother and discarding the expressed breast milk for the first 24 hours. For endometritis caused by group B *Streptococcus*, standard precautions, breastfeeding after the initial 24 hours of therapy in the mother, and the use of expressed breast milk in the interim are appropriate. An example of the probable protective effect of breastfeeding is botulism.[83-85] *Candida* mastitis is a situation in which breastfeeding should continue while the mother and infant are treated simultaneously for at least 2 weeks to prevent reinfection of the breast from contact with the infant's oral candidiasis.

In mothers with hepatitis, identification of the etiologic agent is required before the appropriate management can be determined. Before the etiologic agent is identified, care must include precautions for all potential organisms. Suspension of breastfeeding (pumping and discarding breast milk) until the etiology is determined may be required. Consultation with an infectious disease specialist is often appropriate. For hepatitis A virus, infection in the newborn or young infant is uncommon and not associated with severe illness. Breastfeeding can continue, and if the diagnosis is made within 2 to 3 weeks of the infant's initial exposure to the infected mother, then immune serum globulin and hepatitis A virus vaccine simultaneously can decrease infection in the infant. With hepatitis B virus, the risk of chronic hepatitis B virus infection and its serious complications is high (up to 90%) when infection occurs perinatally or in early infancy. The hepatitis B immune globulin and the hepatitis B virus vaccine given simultaneously prevents hepatitis B virus transmission in over 95% of cases, regardless of whether the infant is fed by breast or bottle. Therefore, it is very appropriate to continue breastfeeding as soon as effective immune therapy is given.[79]

No clear data indicate hepatitis C virus transmission via breast milk in HIV-negative mothers (L. S. Barden, personal communication,

TABLE 9-4 BREASTFEEDING RECOMMENDATIONS FOR SELECTED MATERNAL INFECTIONS

Organism, Syndrome, or Condition*	Breastfeeding Acceptable[†]	Medications Compatible with Breastfeeding, Except as Noted[‡]
Candidiasis		
Candida albicans, Candida krusei: Mucocutaneous infection, vulvovaginitis	Yes (simultaneous therapy for infant and mother)[§]	Topical agents, fluconazole, ketoconazole, itraconazole, amphotericin B, flucytosine
Candida tropicalis invasive infections		
Chlamydia		
Chlamydia trachomatis: Urethritis, vaginitis, endometritis, salpingitis, lymphogranuloma venereum, conjunctivitis, pneumonia	Yes (consider treating the infant)	Erythromycin, azithromycin, clarithromycin, doxycycline, tetracycline, sulfisoxazole
Cytomegalovirus		
Asymptomatic infection	Yes (for term infants)	
Infectious mononucleosis	No (for premature or immunodeficient infants); do not give expressed breast milk	
Endometritis, Pelvic Inflammatory Disease		
Anaerobic organisms	Yes	Clindamycin, metronidazole, cefoxitin, cefmetazole
Chlamydia trachomatis	Yes	Erythromycin, azithromycin, tetracycline
Enterobacteriaceae	Yes	Ampicillin, aminoglycosides, cephalosporins
Group B streptococci	Yes (after 24 hr of therapy, breast milk is okay; observation	Penicillin, cephalosporins, macrolides
Mycoplasma hominis	Yes	Clindamycin, tetracycline
Neisseria gonorrhoeae	Yes[§]	Ceftriaxone, spectinomycin, doxycycline, azithromycin
Ureaplasma urealyticum	Yes	Erythromycin, azithromycin, clarithromycin, tetracycline
Gonorrhea		
Genital, pharyngeal, conjunctival, or disseminated infection; *Neisseria gonorrhoeae*	Yes[§]	Ceftriaxone, ciprofloxacin, spectinomycin, azithromycin, doxycycline
Hepatitis[§]		
A—Acute only	Yes (after immune serum globulin and vaccine)	
B—Chronic hepatitis, cirrhosis, hepatocellular carcinoma	Yes (after HBIG and vaccine)	
C—Chronic hepatitis, cirrhosis, hepatocellular carcinoma	Yes	
D—Associated with hepatitis B	Yes (after HBIG and vaccine)	
E—Severe disease in pregnant women	Yes	
G	Inadequate data	
Herpes Simplex Types 1, 2		
Mucocutaneous, neonatal, encephalitis	Yes (in the absence of breast lesions)	Acyclovir, valacyclovir, famciclovir
Human Immunodeficiency Viruses[§]		
Types 1 and 2	No/yes[‖]	Little or no information available on antiretrovirals in breast milk
Human T-Cell Leukemia Viruses[§]		
Type I (T-cell leukemia/lymphoma virus): myelopathy, dermatitis, adenitis, Sjögren syndrome	No[‖]	
Type II: Myelopathy, arthritis, glomerulonephritis	No[‖]	
Lyme Disease		
Borrelia burgdorferi: Multistaged illness of skin, joints, and peripheral or central nervous system	Yes, with informed discussion	Ceftriaxone, ampicillin, doxycycline

TABLE 9-4 BREASTFEEDING RECOMMENDATIONS FOR SELECTED MATERNAL INFECTIONS—cont'd

Organism, Syndrome, or Condition*	Breastfeeding Acceptable†	Medications Compatible with Breastfeeding, Except as Noted‡
Mastitis		
Candida albicans	Yes, with simultaneous treatment of the infant	Nystatin, ketoconazole
Enterobacteriaceae	Yes	Fluconazole
Staphylococcus aureus	Yes (after 24 hr of therapy, during which milk must be discarded)	Dicloxacillin, oxacillin, erythromycin, clindamycin, cotrimoxazole, azithromycin, linezolid, vancomycin
Group A streptococci		First-generation cephalosporins, penicillin, ampicillin, amoxicillin, erythromycin, azithromycin
Mycobacterium tuberculosis	No breast milk or breastfeeding for 2 weeks of maternal therapy; consider prophylactic isoniazid for the infant	Isoniazid, rifampin, ethambutol, pyrazinamide ethionamide
Pulmonary or extrapulmonary infection with *Mycobacterium tuberculosis*	Yes, expressed breast milk can be used during initial 2 weeks of maternal therapy, then breastfeeding can continue	Antituberculous medications are acceptable during breastfeeding
Trichomonas vaginalis		
Vaginitis, urethritis, or asymptomatic infections	Yes	Metronidazole
Adenoviruses		
Conjunctivitis, upper/lower respiratory infections, gastroenteritis	Yes¶	

***Patients with the syndromes or conditions listed may present with atypical signs and symptoms (e.g., neonates and adults with pertussis may not demonstrate paroxysmal or severe cough). The clinician's index of suspicion should be guided by the prevalence of specific conditions in the community and by clinical judgment. The organisms listed are not intended to represent the complete or even most likely diagnoses but rather possible etiologic agents.**

†*Yes* means that if the proposed precautions are followed for a hospitalized mother and infant, breastfeeding is acceptable and may be beneficial to the infant. Any infant breastfeeding during a maternal infection should be observed closely for signs or symptoms of illness.

‡Refer to Suggested Readings for a more complete discussion of medications and compatibility with breastfeeding.

§See text for more complete discussion.

‖*No,* in the United States and many other countries where safe alternatives to breast milk are available. *Yes,* in countries where there is no safe alternative to breast milk available.

¶Adenovirus types 4 and 7 have been known to cause severe respiratory disease in premature infants or individuals with immunodeficiency or underlying respiratory disease. In certain situations, feeding expressed breast milk to the infant may not be advisable.

HBIG, hepatitis B immunoglobulin.

Modified from Lawrence RA, Lawrence RM: Breastfeeding: A Guide for the Medical Profession, 6th ed. St. Louis, Mosby, 2005.

2000). However, given the multiple issues involved (e.g., low risk of hepatitis C virus transmission via breast milk, increased risk of transmission in association with HIV infection and high levels of hepatitis C virus RNA in maternal serum, lack of effective preventive treatments [vaccines or immune serum globulin] and the risk of chronic hepatitis C virus infection, and serious liver disease), it is essential to educate the parents about the possible risks of continued breastfeeding. If the mother is symptomatic, breastfeeding may not be indicated. If the mother is not symptomatic, breastfeeding is usually appropriate.

Maternal retroviral infection and breastfeeding is a highly controversial issue that continues to be evaluated and debated. HIV-1 is transmissible via breastfeeding and can significantly increase the risk of HIV infection in infants born to HIV-positive mothers. One meta-analysis of five studies of infants born to HIV-infected mothers reported the risk of HIV transmission to infants strictly from breastfeeding as 14% (95% confidence interval, 7% to 22%).[86] Among the many concerns about HIV and breastfeeding are the risk of transmission related to the duration of breastfeeding, the relative risks of exclusive versus nonexclusive breastfeeding, the risk of mortality and morbidity resulting from other infections and malnutrition associated with *not* breastfeeding, the significance of HIV viral loads and CD4 counts in the mother relative to transmission from breast milk, the potential protective effects of breast milk against HIV infection, and the degree to which antiretroviral therapy for the mother or infant will be protective against HIV infection. Social issues involved in this debate include the right of the mother to make choices for herself and her infant, the social stigma of not breastfeeding in certain cultures and communities, and the possibility that breastfeeding rates in HIV-negative mothers will be adversely affected by the advice given to HIV-positive mothers. In many countries, neither choice is optimal: Breastfeeding risks HIV infection in the infant, but not breastfeeding increases the risks of other infections and malnutrition. The lack of adequate data from controlled trials about the various factors contributing to infection adds to the difficulty of making straightforward recommendations applicable to diverse situations around the world. In the United States, it is appropriate to advise no breastfeeding for infants of HIV-infected mothers to decrease the risk of HIV transmission to the infant.[1,35]

There are limited reports that deal with the risk of HIV-2 transmission via breastfeeding. Studies suggest that HIV-2 transmission via breast milk is less common than HIV-1.[87] However, until adequate information is available, it is appropriate to use the same guidelines as for HIV-1. Until additional data are available from trials studying the administration of highly active antiretroviral therapy (HAART) to mothers during lactation, the optimal time and method for weaning, and the potential benefit of a perinatal vaccine, those concerned about breastfeeding and HIV in resource-limited countries should follow the current WHO recommendations for the prevention of mother-to-child transmission of HIV.[88]

Transmission of human T-cell leukemia virus type I (HTLV-I) infection is associated with breastfeeding, although short-term breastfeeding (<6 months) may pose no greater risk than the risk for formula-fed infants.[89-91] In Japan, where high rates of infection with this virus occur, proscription of breastfeeding is common. In the United States, when the mother has documented HTLV-I infection, it is appropriate to discuss the options, risks, and benefits of breastfeeding and to consider short-term breastfeeding. There are many uncertainties concerning HTLV-II, related to the diseases associated with infection and to whether transmission occurs via breast milk. Here again, it is appropriate to discuss the available data and to include an infectious disease consultant in the discussion.[1]

Numerous reviews[92-95] and studies[96,97] attempt to address the many issues of breastfeeding by HIV-positive mothers. The two most helpful resources related to breastfeeding and infection are the AAP's Report of the Committee on Infectious Diseases,[79] and Breastfeeding: A Guide for Medical Profession by Lawrence and Lawrence[1]; the latter contains a chapter and an appendix dedicated to the issue.

Complications of the Breast

Plugged Ducts

Tender lumps in the breast in a mother who is otherwise well are probably caused by plugging of a collecting duct. The best treatment is to continue nursing while manually massaging the area to initiate and ensure complete drainage. Holding the infant in a different position may encourage flow, as may application of hot packs before a feeding. If repeated plugging occurs, a check should be made for possible obstruction from a brassiere strap or other external forces. Some women can actually see small plugs ejected when they massage. For some, reducing polyunsaturated fats in the diet and adding lecithin[1] provides relief.

Galactocele

Milk-retention cysts are uncommon and are usually associated with lactation. The swelling is smooth and rounded and nontender. The cyst may be aspirated to confirm the diagnosis and to avoid surgery, but it will fill up again. The cyst can be removed with local anesthesia without interruption of the breastfeeding routine. The diagnosis can also be confirmed by ultrasound, by which the cyst and milk look similar but tumor is distinguishable.[1]

Mastitis

Mastitis is an infectious process in the breast producing localized tenderness, redness, and heat, together with systemic symptoms of a flulike illness with fever and malaise. It can be distinguished from engorgement and plugged duct (Table 9-5). Usually a red, tender, hot, swollen, wedge-shaped area of the breast is visible, and it corresponds to a lobe (Fig. 9-8). The common organisms are *Staphylococcus aureus, Escherichia coli,* and, rarely, *Streptococcus.*

The major points of management are as follows:

- Breastfeeding should continue on both breasts.
- Antibiotics appropriate to the probable cause and relevant sensitivities should be prescribed.
- Antibiotics should be given for no less than 10 days, and preferably 14. The antibiotic should be safe for the infant.
- Bed rest is necessary, and the mother should bring the infant to bed to nurse. She will need assistance for the rest of the household responsibilities.

The most common cause of recurrent mastitis is delayed or inadequate treatment of the initial disease. On recurrence, cultures of a midstream flow of milk should be sent and antibiotics chosen accordingly.

Candidiasis of Nipple and Breast

Candidiasis of the breast is frequently overdiagnosed because there are several causes for the breast pain that is described by mothers

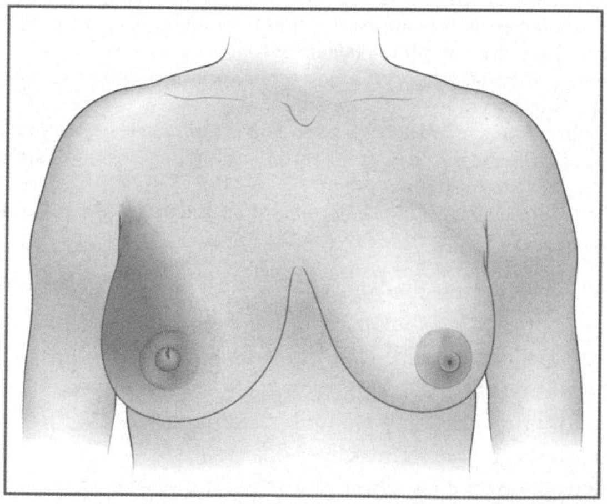

FIGURE 9-8 **Mastitis of right breast, upper outer quadrant.** (From Lawrence RA, Lawrence RM: Breastfeeding: A Guide for the Medical Profession, 6th ed. St. Louis, Mosby, 2005, p 563 [Fig. 16-1].)

TABLE 9-5 COMPARISON OF ENGORGEMENT, PLUGGED DUCT, AND MASTITIS

Symptom	Engorgement	Plugged Duct	Mastitis
Onset	Gradual, immediately after birth	Gradual, after feedings	Sudden, after 10 days
Site	Bilateral	Unilateral	Usually unilateral
Swelling and heat	Generalized	May shift; little or no heat	Localized, red, hot, swollen
Pain	Generalized	Mild but localized	Intense but localized
Body temperature	<38.4° C (101° F)	<38.4° C	>38.4° C
Systemic symptoms	Feels well	Feels well	Flulike symptoms

From Lawrence RA, Lawrence RM: Breastfeeding: A Guide for the Medical Profession, 6th ed. St. Louis, Mosby, 2005, p 279 (Table 8-5).

as feeling like "a stab with a hot poker." On examination, there may be little to see except a pinkish hue to the nipple and central areola. Rarely are white plaques seen on the nipple. If the mother has a history of vaginal candidiasis, the infant's mouth may have become colonized, and this could have resulted in inoculation of the nipples. The infant should also be examined for both thrush and diaper rash and treated simultaneously with the mother for a full 2 weeks. Nystatin ointment is applied after each feeding to nipples and areolae. The infant receives nystatin drops orally to the oral mucous membranes after each feeding. For a recurrent episode, the mother can be treated with 200 mg oral fluconazole systemically once daily for 3 days. The infant can be given 6 mg/kg on day 1 and then 3 mg/kg per dose every 24 hours orally. Pacifiers and bottle nipples that are put in the mouth should be discarded and new ones sterilized daily. Persistent thrush requires a complete evaluation of the mother and may require treatment for vaginal thrush, decreased sugar in diet, and colonization with lactobacillus by capsule or yogurt.

Medications while Breastfeeding

Questions about medication during breastfeeding are very commonly asked. The transfer of maternal drugs to the infant during lactation is different from transfer to the fetus during pregnancy. Although it is almost always better to breastfeed, the physician must weigh the benefit and risk of a medication against the substantial benefit of being breastfed for the infant. The risk-to-benefit ratio differs for each drug and clinical setting. Both scientific information and experienced clinical judgment are required to assess the risks and benefits and determine the therapeutic choice.

The AAP Committee on Drugs has published a list of commonly used drugs and chemicals that may transfer into human milk (Table 9-6).[98] The list is not all-inclusive and is revised intermittently.[97] Absence of a drug from the list merely indicates that the committee

TABLE 9-6 AAP DRUG GROUPS 1, 2, 3, AND 6

Group 1. Cytotoxic Drugs That May Interfere with Cellular Metabolism of the Nursing Infant

Possible immune suppression; unknown effect on growth or association with carcinogenesis; neutropenia

- Cyclophosphamide
- Cyclosporine
- Doxorubicin*
- Methotrexate

Group 2: Drugs of Abuse for Which Adverse Effects on the Infant during Breastfeeding Have Been Reported†

- Amphetamine*
- Cocaine
- Heroin
- Marijuana
- Phencyclidine

Group 3: Radioactive Compounds That Require Temporary Cessation of Breastfeeding

- Copper 64 (^{64}Cu)
- Gallium 67 (^{67}Ga)
- Indium 111 (^{111}In)
- Iodine 123 (^{123}I)
- Iodine 125 (^{125}I)
- Iodine 131 (^{131}I)
- Radioactive sodium
- Technetium 99m (^{99m}Tc)
- Macroaggregates, sodium pertechnetate ($^{99m}TcO_4$)

Group 6: Partial List of Selected Maternal Medications Usually Compatible with Breastfeeding

- Analgesics
  - Acetaminophen
  - Ibuprofen
  - Codeine
  - Antacids
- Antibiotics that can also be given to infants
  - Acyclovir
  - Amoxicillin
  - Cephalosporins
  - Erythromycin
  - Fluconazole
  - Gentamicin
  - Kanamycin
  - Miconazole
  - Penicillins
  - Spironolactone
  - Streptomycin
  - Vancomycin
- Cardiovascular or antihypertensive drugs
  - Captopril
  - Digoxin
  - Enalapril
  - Hydralazine
  - Labetalol
  - Metoprolol
  - Nifedipine
  - Nitrofurantoin
  - Quinidine
  - Quinine
  - Sotalol
  - Timolol
- Miscellaneous compounds
  - Lidocaine
  - Progesterone-only contraceptive pill
  - Magnesium sulfate
  - Prednisolone
  - Prednisone
  - Propylthiouracil
  - Scopolamine
  - Warfarin
  - Laxatives (bulk forming and stool softening)
  - Vaccines

***Drug is concentrated in human milk.**
†The AAP Committee on Drugs strongly believes that nursing mothers should not ingest drugs of abuse because they are hazardous to the nursing infant and to the health of the mother.
From American Academy of Pediatrics, Committee on Drugs: The transfer of drugs and other chemicals into human milk. Pediatrics 108:776, 2001.

did not study it in reference to lactation. The categories are as follows:

1. Cytotoxic drugs that may interfere with cellular metabolism of the nursing infant (see Table 9-6, group 1)
2. Drugs of abuse for which adverse effects on the infant during breastfeeding have been reported (see Table 9-6, group 2)
3. Radioactive compounds that require temporary cessation of breastfeeding (see Table 9-6, group 3)
4. Drugs for which the effect on nursing infants is unknown but that may be of concern—for example, bromocriptine, ergotamine compounds, and lithium
5. Drugs that have been associated with significant effects on some nursing infants and should be given to nursing mothers with caution
6. Maternal medication usually compatible with breastfeeding (see Table 9-6, group 6)
7. Food and environmental agents that might have an effect on the breastfeeding infant

A readily available and frequently updated handbook, *Medications and Mother's Milk,* is published by Hale.[99] This reference provides a scale that is roughly the reverse of the long-established classification system developed by the AAP. The Hale definitions are as follows:

- L1 safest
- L2 safer
- L3 moderately safe
- L4 possible hazardous
- L5 contraindicated

A lack of information about a drug does not necessarily require cessation of breastfeeding. Understanding the pharmacology of a drug, the dosing schedule, and the stage of growth and development of the infant inform the decision about whether it would affect the infant. Characteristics of the drug that influence its passage into milk include the size of the molecule, its solubility in lipid or water, whether it binds to protein, the pH, and the diffusion rates (Table 9-7). The route of administration influences the blood levels and therefore the milk levels. Passive diffusion is the principal transport mechanism. How the drug is metabolized influences whether it is present in the milk in its active form or as an inactive metabolite (Fig. 9-9).

The infant's ability to absorb, digest, metabolize, store, and excrete a drug must be considered when choosing a medication for a nursing mother. A drug that is not orally bioavailable will not be absorbed from the milk by the infant. The ability to absorb and metabolize a drug depends on the infant's developmental age and the chronologic age. An 18-month-old who nurses briefly about four times a day for comfort will get little medication, has a substantial diet other than mother's milk, and can metabolize and excrete more efficiently than a newborn. In the first weeks of life, the maturation or gestational age should be considered when determining the safety of a medication, because the less mature the infant is, the less mature are the liver and kidneys.

With the exception of radioactive compounds such as iodine 131, there is no drug whose possible presence in the milk would require immediate withholding of breastfeeding because the physician does not know the data. Therefore, the arbitrary interference with breastfeeding until information can be obtained is not justified. Ample references and information lines are available to resolve the issue. For medications used once or for a short time, the time required for the drug to clear the maternal system and her milk can be determined. The mother can pump and discard her milk for that period and return to breastfeeding (usually a few hours or days, not weeks).

TABLE 9-7 THE PASSAGE OF DRUGS INTO BREAST MILK

1. Mammary alveolar epithelium represents a lipid barrier with water-filled pores and is most permeable for drugs during the colostral phase of milk secretion (1st postpartum week).
2. Drug excretion into milk depends on the drug's degree of ionization, molecular weight, solubility in fat and water, and relationship of pH of plasma (7.4) to pH of milk (7.0).
3. Drugs enter mammary cells basally in the nonionized non–protein-bound form by diffusion or active transport.
4. Water-soluble drugs of molecular weight less than 200 pass through water-filled membranous pores.
5. Drugs leave mammary alveolar cells by diffusion or active transport.
6. Drugs may enter milk via spaces between mammary alveolar cells.
7. Most ingested drugs appear in milk; drug amounts in milk usually do not exceed 1% of ingested dosage, and levels in the milk are independent of milk volume.
8. Drugs are bound much less to milk proteins than to plasma proteins.
9. Drug-metabolizing capacity of mammary epithelium is not understood.

Modified from Lawrence RA, Lawrence RM: Breastfeeding: A Guide for the Medical Profession, 6th ed. St. Louis, Mosby, 2005.

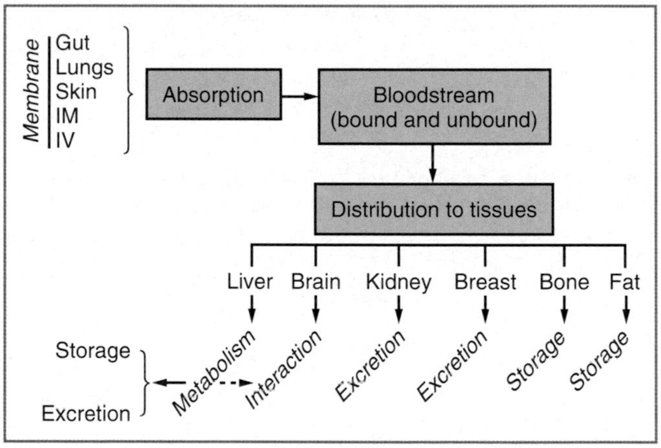

FIGURE 9-9 Distribution pathways for drugs. Distribution pathways vary with the drug and are relevant to advising the lactating mother about breastfeeding when drugs have been prescribed. IM, intramuscular; IV, intravenous. (Modified from Rivera-Calimlim L: Distribution pathways for drugs, once absorbed during lactation. Clin Perinatol 14:51, 1976.)

Milk-to-Plasma Ratio

The *milk-to-plasma ratio,* a term applied to drugs being used by a lactating mother, indicates the level of the drug in the milk compared with the level in the plasma at a given time. The dosage of the drug, including time and route of dosing, must be known to interpret the ratio. If there is a very low level in the plasma and the same very low level in the milk, the ratio is 1. A ratio of 1 means that the level is of concern, even though the actual level in milk is low. Most drugs have a milk-to-plasma ratio of less than 1. It is important to know peak plasma and peak milk levels, and peak plasma and peak milk times, to make appropriate recommendations to avoid feeding the infant when transfer of the drug would be greatest.

References

1. Lawrence RA, Lawrence RM: Breastfeeding: A Guide for the Medical Profession, 6th ed. St. Louis, Mosby, 2005.
2. Dewey KG: Nutrition, growth, and complementary feeding of the breastfed infant. Pediatr Clin North Am 48:87, 2001.
3. SanGiovanni JP, Berkey CS, Dwyer JT, et al: Dietary essential fatty acids, long-chain polyunsaturated fatty acids, and visual resolution acuity in healthy fullterm infants: A systematic review. Early Hum Dev 57:165, 2000.
4. Horwood LJ, Darlow BA, Mogridge N: Breast milk feeding and cognitive ability at 7-8 years. Arch Dis Child Fetal Neonatal Ed 84:F23, 2001.
5. Schack-Nielsen L, Michaelsen KF: Advances in our understanding of the biology of human milk and its effects on the offspring. J Nutr 137:503S, 2007.
6. American Academy of Pediatrics, Section on Breastfeeding: Breastfeeding and the use of human milk. Pediatrics 115:496, 2005.
7. Butte NF, Goldblum RM, Fehl LM, et al: Daily ingestion of immunologic components in human milk during the first four months of life. Acta Paediatr Scand 73:206, 1984.
8. Quan R, Barness LA, Uawy R: Do infants need nucleotide supplemented formula for optimal nutrition? J Pediatr Gastroenterol Nutr 11:429, 1990.
9. Srivastava MD, Srivastava A, Brouhard B, et al: Cytokines in human milk. Res Common Mol Pathol Pharmacol 93:263, 1996.
10. von Kries R, Koletzko B, Sauerwald, et al: Breastfeeding and obesity: Cross sectional study. BMJ 319:147, 1999.
11. Pickering LK, Granoff DM, Erickson JD, et al: Modulation of the immune system by human milk and infant formula containing nucleotides. Pediatrics 101:242, 1998.
12. Martin RM, Gunnell D, Owen CG, Smith GD: Breastfeeding and childhood cancer: A systematic review with metaanalysis. Int J Cancer 117:1020, 2005.
13. Mayer-Davis EJ, Rifas-Shiman SL, Zhou L, et al: Breastfeeding and risk for childhood obesity. Diabetes Care 29:2231-2237, 2006.
14. Owen CG, Martin RM, Whincup PH, et al: Does breastfeeding influence risk of type 2 diabetes in later life? A quantitative analysis of published evidence. Am J Clin Nutr 84:1043, 2006.
15. Scholtens S, Gehring U, Brunekreef B, et al: Breastfeeding, weight gain in infancy, and overweight at seven years of age: The prevention and incidence of asthma and mite allergy birth cohort study. Am J Epidemiol 165:919-926, 2007.
16. Lucas A, Morley R, Cole TJ, et al: Breast milk and subsequent intelligence quotient in children born preterm. Lancet 339:261, 1992.
17. Neuringer M: Infant vision and retinal function in studies of dietary long-chain polyunsaturated fatty acids: Methods, results, and implications. Am J Clin Nutr 71(Suppl):256, 2000.
18. Jorgensen MH, Hernell O, Lund P, et al: Visual acuity and erythrocyte docosahexaenoic acid-status in breastfed and formula-fed term infants during first four months of life. Lipids 31:99, 1996.
19. SanGiovanni JP, Parra-Cabrera S, Colditz GA, et al: Meta-analysis of dietary essential fatty acids and long-chain polyunsaturated fatty acids as they relate to visual resolution acuity in healthy preterm infants. Pediatrics 105:1292, 2000.
20. Horwood LJ, Fergusson DM: Breastfeeding and later cognitive and academic outcomes. Pediatrics 101:91, 1998.
21. Lucas A, Morley R, Cole TJ, et al: Randomized trial of early diet in preterm babies and later intelligence quotient. BMJ 317:1481, 1998.
22. Jacobson SW, Chiodo LM, Jacobson JL: Breastfeeding effects on intelligence in 4- and 11-year old children. Pediatrics 103:71, 1999.
23. Newton M, Newton NR: Psychologic aspects of lactation. N Engl J Med 277:1179, 1967.
24. Zhou SJ, Baghurst P, Gibson RA, Makrides M: Home environment, not duration of breast-feeding, predicts intelligence quotient of children at four years. Nutrition 23:236, 2007.
25. Groer MW, Davis MW: Cytokines, infections, stress, and dysphoric moods in breastfeeders and formula feeders. J Obstet Gynecol Neonatal Nurs 35:599-607, 2006.
26. Subcommittee on Nutrition during Lactation, Institute of Medicine: Nutrition during lactation. Washington, DC, National Academy of Sciences, National Academy Press, 1991.
27. Labbok MH: Effects of breastfeeding on the mother. Pediatr Clin North Am 48:143, 2001.
28. Kalkwarf HJ, Specker BL: Bone mineral loss during lactation and recovery after weaning. Obstet Gynecol 86:26, 1995.
29. Kalkwarf HJ, Specker BL, Heubi JE, et al: Intestinal calcium absorption of women during lactation and after weaning. Am J Clin Nutr 63:526, 1996.
30. Whitemore AS: Characteristics relating to ovarian cancer risk: Implications for prevention and detection. Gynecol Oncol 55(3 pt 2):515, 1994.
31. John EM, Whitemore AS, Harris R, et al: Characteristics relating to ovarian cancer risk: Collaborative analysis of seven US case-control studies—epithelial ovarian cancer in black women. Collaborative Ovarian Cancer Group. J Natl Cancer Inst 85:142, 1993.
32. Rosenblatt KA, Thomas DB: WHO collaborative study of neoplasia and steroid contraceptives: Lactation and the risk of epithelial ovarian cancer. Int J Epidemiol 22:192, 1993.
33. Newcomb PA, Storer BE, Longnecker MP, et al: Lactation and a reduced risk of premenopausal breast cancer. N Engl J Med 330:81, 1994.
34. Kim Y, Choi JY, Lee KM, et al: Dose-dependent protective effect of breast-feeding against breast cancer among ever-lactated women in Korea. Eur J Cancer Prev 16:124-129, 2007.
35. Lawrence RA: A Review of the Medical Benefits and Contraindications to Breastfeeding in the United States. Maternal and Child Health Technical Information Bulletin. Arlington, VA, National Center for Education in Maternal and Child Health, 1997.
36. Lockwood C, Riley L, Blackmon L, Lemons JA (eds): Guidelines for Perinatal Care, 6th ed. Washington, DC, American College of Obstetricians and Gynecologists, American Academy of Pediatrics, 2007.
37. Neville MC, Morton J, Umemura S: Lactogenesis: Transition from pregnancy to lactation. Pediatr Clin North Am 48:35, 2001.
38. Gartner LM, Morton J, Lawrence RA, et al: American Academy of Pediatrics Section on Breastfeeding: Breastfeeding and the use of human milk. Pediatrics 115:496-506, 2005.
39. Lazarov M, Evans A: Encouraging the best for low-income women. Zero to Three Aug/Sept:15, 2000. Available at www.zerotothree.org (site accessed January 31, 2008; registration required).
40. Dewey KG: Maternal and fetal stress are associated with impaired lactogenesis in humans. J Nutr 131:3012S, 2001.
41. Bland KJ, Romnell LJ: Congenital and acquired disturbances of breast development and growth. In Bland KI, Copeland EM III (eds): The Breast: Comprehensive Management of Benign and Malignant Diseases. Philadelphia, WB Saunders, 1991, p 69.
42. Neville MC: Mammary gland biology and lactation: A short course. Presented at biannual meeting of the International Society for Research on Human Milk and Lactation, Plymouth, MA, October 1997.
43. Osbourne MP: Breast development and anatomy. In Harris JR, Lippman ME, Morrow M, et al (eds): Diseases of the Breast. Philadelphia, Lippincott-Raven, 1996.
44. Ramsay DT, Kent JC, Hartmann RA, Hartmann PE: Anatomy of the lactating human breast redefined with ultrasound imaging. J Anat 206:525, 2005.
45. Neville MC: Anatomy and physiology of lactation. Pediatr Clin North Am 48:13, 2001.
46. Hartmann PE, Cregan MD, Ramsay DT: Physiology of lactation in preterm mothers: Initiation and maintenance. Pediatr Ann 32:351, 2003.
47. Kuhn NJ: Lactogenesis: The search for trigger mechanisms in different species. In Peaker M (ed): Comparative Aspects of Lactation. London, Academic Press, 1977, p 165.
48. Chen DC, Nommsen-Rivers L, Dewey KG, et al: Stress during labor and delivery and early lactation performance. Am J Clin Nutr 68:335, 1998.

49. Morton JA: The clinical usefulness of breast milk sodium in the assessment of lactogenesis. Pediatrics 93:802-806, 1994.
50. Neville MC, Keller RP, Seacat J, et al: Studies in human lactation: Milk volumes in lactating women during the onset of lactation and full lactation. Am J Clin Nutr 48:1375, 1988.
51. Kulski JK, Hartmann PE, Martin JD, Smith M: Effects of bromocriptine mesylate on the composition of the mammary section in non-breastfeeding women. Obstet Gynecol 52:38-42, 1978.
52. Aperia A, Broberger O, Herin P, Zetterström R: Salt content in human breast milk during the first three weeks after delivery. Acta Paediatr Scand 68:441-442, 1979.
53. Neville MC: Lactogenesis in women: A cascade of events revealed by milk composition. In Jensen RD (ed): The Composition of Milks. San Diego, Academic Press, 1995, p 87.
54. Neville MC, Allen JC, Archer P, et al: Studies in human lactation: Milk volume and nutrient composition during weaning and lactogenesis. Am J Clin Nutr 54:81, 1991.
55. Kuhn NJ: The biochemistry of lactogenesis. In Mepham TB (ed): Biochemistry of Lactation. Amsterdam, Elsevier, 1983, p 351.
56. Neubauer SH, Ferris AM, Chase CG, et al: Delayed lactogenesis in women with insulin-dependent diabetes mellitus. Am J Clin Nutr 58:54, 1993.
57. Neifert MR, McDonough SL, Neville MC: Failure of lactogenesis associated with placental retention. Am J Obstet Gynecol 140:477, 1981.
58. Sozmen M: Effects of early suckling of cesarean-born babies on lactation. Biol Neonate 62:67, 1992.
59. Jackson EB: Pediatric and psychiatric aspects of the Yale room-in project. Conn State Med J 14:616, 1950.
60. Peterson WE, Ludwick TM: Humoral nature of the factor causing let down of milk. Fed Proc 1:66-67, 1942.
61. Pedersen CA, Caldwell JD, Walker C: Oxytocin activates the postpartum onset of rat maternal behavior in the ventral tegmental and medial preoptic areas. Behav Neurosci 108:1163, 1994.
62. Jackson EB, Olmsted RW, Foord A, et al: A hospital rooming-in unit for four newborn infants and their mothers. Pediatrics 1:28, 1948.
63. Barnes GR, Lethin AN, Jackson EB, et al: Management of breastfeeding. JAMA 151:192, 1953.
64. Berens PD: Prenatal, intrapartum, and postpartum support of the lactating mother. Pediatr Clin North Am 48:365, 2001.
65. Righard L, Alade MO: Effect of delivery room routine on success of first breastfeed. Lancet 336:1105, 1990.
66. Ramsay DT, Mitoulas LR, Kent JC, et al: The use of ultrasound to characterize milk ejection in women using an electric breast pump. J Hum Lact 21:421, 2005.
67. Fredeen R: Cup feeding of newborn infants. Pediatrics 2:544, 1948.
68. Malhotra N, Vishwambaran L, Sundaram KR, et al: A controlled trial of alternative methods of oral feeding in neonates. Early Hum Dev 54:29, 1999.
69. Humerick SS, Hill PD, Anderson MA: Breast engorgement: Patterns and selected outcomes. J Hum Lact 10:87, 1994.
70. Lau C: Effect of stress on lactation. Pediatr Clin North Am 48:221, 2001.
71. Schanler RJ, Dooley S, Gartner LM, et al (eds): Breastfeeding Handbook for Physicians. Washington, DC, American College of Obstetricians and Gynecologists, American Academy of Pediatrics, 2006.
72. Schanler RJ: The use of human milk for premature infants. Pediatr Clin North Am 48:207, 2001.
73. Chan GM, Lee ML, Rechtman, DJ: Effects of a human milk-derived human milk fortifier on the antibacterial actions of human milk. Breastfeeding Medicine 2:205, 2007.
74. Gromada KK, Spangler AK: Breastfeeding twins and higher-order multiples. J Obstet Gynecol Neonatal Nurs 27:441, 1998.
75. Berlin CM Jr: Exclusive breastfeeding of quadruplets. Breastfeeding Medicine 2:125-126, 2007.
76. Halderman LD, Nelson AL: Impact of early postpartum administration of progestin-only hormonal contraceptives compared with nonhormonal contraceptives on short-term breastfeeding patterns. Am J Obstet Gynecol 186:1250, 2002.
77. Academy of Breastfeeding Medicine, Protocol Committee: Contraception during breastfeeding. Breastfeed Med 1:43-51, 2006.
78. Snider DE Jr, Powell KE: Should women taking antituberculous drugs breastfeed? Arch Intern Med 144:589, 1984.
79. American Academy of Pediatrics: Red Book 2000: Report of the Committee on Infectious Diseases, 25th ed. Elk Grove Village, IL, American Academy of Pediatrics, 2000.
80. Centers for Disease Control and Prevention: Possible West Nile virus transmission to an infant through breastfeeding. MMWR Morb Mortal Wkly Rep 51:877, 2002.
81. Hinckley AF, O'Leary DR, Hayes EB: Transmission of West Nile virus through human breast milk seems to be rare. Pediatrics 119:E666, 2007.
82. Bhola K, McGuire W: Does avoidance of breastfeeding reduce mother-to-infant transmission of hepatitis C virus infection? Arch Dis Child 92:365, 2007.
83. Arnon SS: Infant botulism. Annu Rev Med 31:541, 1980.
84. Arnon SS: Infant botulism: Anticipating the second decade. J Infect Dis 154:201, 1986.
85. Arnon SS, Damus K, Thompson B, et al: Protective role of human milk against sudden death from infant botulism. J Pediatr 100:568, 1982.
86. Dunn DT, Newell ML, Ades AE, et al: Risk of human immunodeficiency virus type 1 transmission through breastfeeding. Lancet 340:585, 1992.
87. Ekpini ER, Wiktor SZ, Satten GA, et al: Late postnatal mother-to-child transmission of HIV-1 in Abidjan, Côte D'Ivoire. Lancet 349:1054, 1997.
88. World Health Organization: Antiretroviral drugs for treating pregnant women and preventing HIV infection in infants: Guidelines on care, treatment and support of women living with HIV/AIDS and their children in resource-constrained settings. Available at www.who.int/hiv/pub/guidelines/pmtctguidelines2006.pdf (accessed January 31, 2008).
89. Hino S: Milk-borne transmission of HTLV-I as a major route in the endemic cycle. Acta Pediatr Jpn 31:428-435, 1989.
90. Hino S, Katamine S, Kawase K, et al: Intervention of maternal transmission of HTLV-I in Nagasaki, Japan. Leukemia 94:S68, 1993.
91. Takezaki T, Tajima K, Ito M, et al: Short-term breastfeeding may reduce the risk of vertical transmission of HTLV-I. Leukemia 11(Suppl 3):60, 1997.
92. Coutsoudis A: Breastfeeding and HIV. Best Pract Res Clin Obstet Gynaecol 19:185-196, 2005.
93. Wilfert CM, Fowler MG: Balancing maternal and infant benefits and the consequences of breastfeeding in the developing world during the era of HIV infection. J Infect Dis 195:165, 2007.
94. WHO Collaborative Study Team on the Role of Breastfeeding on the Prevention of Infant Mortality: Effect of breastfeeding on infant and child mortality due to infectious diseases in less developed countries: A pooled analysis. Lancet 355:451, 2000.
95. Andiman W: Transmission of HIV-1 from mother to infant. Curr Opin Pediatr 14:78, 2002.
96. Mbori-Ngacha D, Nduati R, John G, et al: Morbidity and mortality in breastfed and formula-fed infants of HIV-1 infected women: A randomized clinical trial. JAMA 286:2413, 2001.
97. Wolf LE, Lo B, Beckerman KP, et al: When parents reject interventions to reduce postnatal human immunodeficiency virus transmission. Arch Pediatr Adolesc Med 155:927, 2001.
98. American Academy of Pediatrics, Committee on Drugs: The transfer of drugs and other chemicals into human milk. Pediatrics 108:776, 2001.
99. Hale TW: Medications and Mothers' Milk, 12th ed. Amarillo, TX, Hale, 2006.

Suggested Readings

Briggs GG, Freeman RK, Yaffe SJ: Drugs in Pregnancy and Lactation, 7th ed. Philadelphia, Lippincott Williams & Wilkins, 2005.

Hale TW: Medications and Mothers' Milk, 12th ed. Amarillo, TX, Hale, 2006.

Lawrence RA, Lawrence RM: Breastfeeding: A Guide for the Medical Profession, 6th ed. St. Louis, Mosby, 2005.

Telephone Consultation Service for Physicians at the Breastfeeding and Human Lactation Study Center at the University of Rochester School of Medicine, 585-275-0088 (available weekdays).

Chapter 10

Maternal Nutrition

Naomi E. Stotland, MD

Despite ample evidence about the importance of nutrition on health in general as well as during pregnancy, the typical American diet is falling short of the mark. Surveys of pregnant women reveal that much of their caloric intake comes from high-calorie, nutrient-poor foods such as soft drinks and white bread. Intakes of calcium, iron, and folate are often below the recommended levels, and fat intake is generally high and in the form of harmful saturated fats rather than beneficial vegetable or marine sources.[1]

For much of the 20th century, the public health focus was on the prevention of undernutrition, as poor weight gain was considered a threat to optimal perinatal outcome. More recent studies reveal that excessive weight gain (above Institute of Medicine [IOM] guidelines) is increasingly common and is associated with multiple adverse outcomes. Overweight and obesity are now the norm, with 30.2% of reproductive-age women obese and 56.7% overweight.[2,3] Not only do pre-pregnancy overweight and excessive pregnancy weight gain adversely affect perinatal outcomes but women's long-term health is compromised, with higher rates of metabolic and cardiovascular illness later in life. Recent research has also emphasized the role of maternal nutritional and metabolic status on the long-term health of offspring. Although it has been recognized for some time that growth-restricted fetuses have higher rates of cardiovascular and metabolic problems as children and adults, it is now clear that excessive fetal growth, related to maternal obesity and hyperglycemia, also leads to higher rates of these adverse outcomes.[4,5] Despite this, approximately one third of prenatal patients report receiving no advice about weight gain during their pregnancy.[6,7] All clinicians caring for reproductive-age women should educate themselves and their patients about the importance of good nutritional health before, during, and after pregnancy.

Pre-conception Issues

Perinatal outcome may be influenced by the maternal nutritional and metabolic status at the time of conception as much as during pregnancy, or even more. Organogenesis occurs early in the first trimester before many women are aware of the pregnancy. Hence, women who may become pregnant or who are attempting to conceive should optimize their nutritional and metabolic status before pregnancy. Women with pregestational diabetes mellitus should strive to achieve euglycemia before conception, as higher levels of hemoglobin A_{1C} (a marker for hyperglycemia) are associated with progressively higher rates of congenital deformities.[8]

Folic Acid

Folic acid and folate are forms of vitamin B_9, which is essential for nucleic acid synthesis, red blood cell synthesis and maintenance, and fetal and placental growth. Maternal folic acid deficiency is associated with neural tube defects in the fetus and other congenital anomalies. The U.S. Centers for Disease Control and Prevention (CDC) recommends 0.4 mg/day of folic acid from diet or supplements for all women capable of becoming pregnant, to reduce the risk for neural tube defects.[9] Women with a previous pregnancy affected by a neural tube defect should take 4 mg of folic acid beginning 1 month before conception and throughout the first trimester. In 1998, the U.S. Food and Drug Administration (FDA) began requiring that most enriched breads, flours, corn meals, rice, noodles, macaroni, and other grain products be fortified with folic acid. After fortification, the incidence of pregnancies affected by neural tube defects decreased by 26%. The CDC had estimated a 50% reduction, and it is controversial whether intake of folic acid–fortified foods is adequate or whether additional supplementation is needed. Obese women have been found to have lower serum levels of folic acid, and they are also at increased risk for neural tube defects. However, a Canadian study found that the obesity-related risk for neural tube defects actually increased after the country instituted folic acid fortification of flour.[10] The mechanism underlying the association between obesity and neural tube defects is unclear, and some have suggested it may be related to a higher serum glucose rather than a folic acid deficit. The popularity of low-carbohydrate diets has led to some concern that decreased intake of fortified flours and other grain products would lead to an increase in neural tube defects, and data from the CDC show that serum folic acid levels in women of childbearing age actually decreased by 16% between 1999 and 2004.[11] It is unknown whether this decline was associated with an increase in neural tube defects.

There is also evidence of a small decrease in the rate of orofacial cleft anomalies after folic acid fortification.[12]

Body Mass Index and Obesity

Increasing epidemiologic evidence suggests that a woman's pre-pregnancy body mass index (BMI) and adiposity have a greater impact on some perinatal outcomes than her gestational weight gain. Women who begin pregnancy underweight are at increased risk for both preterm delivery and delivering a small-for-gestational-age (SGA) infant when compared with women of normal pre-pregnancy BMI. However, otherwise healthy but underweight women appear to be at *decreased* risk for multiple adverse outcomes, including macrosomia, cesarean delivery, and preeclampsia.[13,14] Women who begin pregnancy obese have increased rates of spontaneous abortion, congenital anomalies (e.g., neural tube defects, cardiac and gastrointestinal anomalies), gestational diabetes mellitus (GDM), intrauterine fetal death, hypertensive disorders of pregnancy, cesarean birth, failed vaginal birth after cesarean, thromboembolic disease, and postoperative complications. Higher BMI is associated with lower rates of births involving SGA infants or intrauterine growth restriction (IUGR); however, obese women with chronic hypertension or diabetic vasculopathy may be at increased risk for IUGR. Obese women have lower rates of spontaneous preterm birth; however, there is some evidence that morbidly obese women have increased rates of medically indicated preterm birth, probably related to the increased rates of preeclampsia and gestational diabetes.

Postconception Obesity-Related Risks

The risk for spontaneous abortion in the first trimester is greater for obese women than for lean women.[15] This increased risk is seen among both naturally conceived and in vitro fertilization pregnancies.[16] Obesity is associated with an increased risk for congenital anomalies, including neural tube defects and cardiac malformations, even in the absence of overt diabetes.[10,16] Although the mechanism linking obesity and congenital anomalies remains unclear, these same anomalies are associated with diabetes, and undiagnosed hyperglycemia early in gestation has been proposed as the mechanism. Such malformations are also more difficult to detect in obese women before the birth, because ultrasonography is less sensitive, and increased blood volume causes false-negative serum α-fetoprotein screening.[17]

Fetal Growth and Body Composition

Maternal pre-pregnancy weight and infant birth weight are highly correlated. Maternal obesity is a strong predictor of macrosomia or the birth of a large-for-gestational-age infant, even among women who are glucose tolerant.[18,19] Additionally, infants born to obese mothers have a higher percentage of body fat compared with infants born to normal-weight mothers. In a study of 220 infants born to glucose-tolerant mothers, infants born to women with a BMI of 25 or greater were heavier than those born to women with a BMI less than 25. Of note, the increase in birth weights between the two groups was explained by an excess of fat mass rather than lean body mass in the infants.[18] Although ultrasonographic detection of fetal anomalies may be impaired by maternal obesity,[17,20] studies have shown that ultrasonographic estimation of fetal weight is not significantly impaired by elevated maternal BMI.[21,22]

Intrauterine Growth Restriction

Underweight women are at increased risk of delivering an SGA infant, especially if gestational weight gain is inadequate,[19,23,24] and a low pre-pregnancy BMI is a strong predictor of IUGR or an SGA infant. There is evidence that overweight and obesity are protective against the birth of a SGA infant, but the data (cited earlier) showing decreased lean body mass and increased fat mass among infants born to obese women suggest that this protection may not lead to better health outcomes in children.

Obesity increases the risks for hypertension and type 2 diabetes, and if vascular sequelae are present, it increases the risk for IUGR in spite of significant obesity. In a Swedish cohort study, morbid obesity (BMI >40) was associated with an increased risk for the birth of a SGA infant, and this association lost statistical significance when subjects with preeclampsia were excluded, suggesting a possible mechanism.[25]

Hypertensive Disorders of Pregnancy

Obesity and higher pre-pregnancy BMI have been shown to increase the risk for gestational hypertension and preeclampsia in many epidemiologic studies.[26,27] A meta-analysis of BMI and preeclampsia showed a doubling of risk with each 5 to 7 kg/m^2 increase in maternal BMI.[28] This association persisted when accounting for confounders such as chronic hypertension, diabetes, and multiple gestations. The recent recognition of obesity as a chronic inflammatory state, characterized by elevated cytokine levels, has been hypothesized as playing a role in the association between obesity and preeclampsia. Subclinical hyperglycemia leading to decreased oxygen transfer to the uterus and abnormal placentation has also been proposed as a mechanism.[4]

Diabetes Mellitus

Obesity is a well-known risk factor for both pre-gestational and gestational diabetes mellitus. In a large U.S. cohort study, obese women (BMI, 30 to 34.9) had an adjusted odds ratio (OR) of 2.6 (range, 2.1 to 3.4), and morbidly obese women (BMI $\geq$ 35) had an adjusted OR of 4.0 (range, 3.1 to 5.2) for gestational diabetes, compared with women with a BMI of less than 30.[29]

Preterm Delivery

Most epidemiologic studies of pre-pregnancy BMI and preterm birth show an inverse relationship—that is, a lower BMI is associated with an increased risk for preterm birth.[30,31] There also appears to be an interaction between pre-pregnancy BMI and gestational weight gain, with underweight, low-gaining women at especially increased risk for preterm birth. Approximately 75% of preterm births are spontaneous, and 25% are medically indicated. Because obese women have higher rates of hypertensive and diabetic disorders of pregnancy, they may be at higher risk for medically indicated preterm birth. A large, population-based cohort study of births in Scotland found that parity altered the relationship between BMI and preterm birth.[32] For spontaneous preterm birth, lower BMI was associated with increased risk, and obesity was protective. BMI was a stronger predictor of spontaneous preterm birth among multiparous women. In contrast, risk for medically indicated preterm birth was increased with higher BMI, and this effect was stronger among nulliparous women.

Cesarean Birth

Higher BMI is associated with increased risk for cesarean birth.[13] Higher BMI is also associated with lower rates of successful vaginal birth after cesarean section among women undergoing a trial of labor.[33]

Intrauterine Fetal Demise

Overweight and obesity have been associated with increased rates of intrauterine fetal demise or stillbirth in large epidemiologic studies.[34,35] This association persisted even when analysis was restricted to women with early ultrasound dating, ruling out undiagnosed postdatism as the cause. Increased stillbirths are also seen among obese women even when women with overt hypertension and diabetes are excluded from the analyses. The mechanism remains unclear, but some investigators have suggested that subclinical hypertension and hyperglycemia may be the etiology. Fetal monitoring may be more difficult among morbidly obese women, and obesity has been associated with decreased maternal perception of fetal movement.[36] Overweight and obese women with hypertension or diabetes merit especially close antepartum monitoring, but the most beneficial and cost-effective regimen has not been established.

Postconception Nutritional Issues

Weight Gain During Pregnancy

The IOM established BMI-specific guidelines for gestational weight gain for women with singleton pregnancies in 1990 (Table 10-1).[37] Since that time, numerous epidemiologic studies have validated the IOM's recommended weight gain ranges, finding that gain within the guidelines is associated with the lowest rates of a number of adverse maternal and infant outcomes. However, controversy and uncertainty still exist over specific aspects of weight gain. In particular, the optimal weight gain range for obese women remains unclear, as is evidenced by the lack of an upper limit on the recommended range for this subgroup. In 2006, the IOM convened a workshop to review the current evidence on maternal weight and perinatal outcomes[38] (report available at www.iom.edu/CMS/12552/31379/41424.aspx [accessed February 2008]).

Conditions Associated with Inadequate Gestational Gain

Many studies have found an association between weight gain below the IOM guidelines and increased risk for spontaneous preterm birth.[30,39] These studies are usually limited by the fact that the rate of gestational weight gain is not constant throughout pregnancy, with the gain being less rapid in the first trimester, speeding up in the second and early third trimesters, and then slowing once again near term. Low gain is also associated with an increased risk for an SGA infant, and this association is strongest among women with a low pre-pregnancy BMI.[24] Among obese women, there is only a weak association between gestational gain and birth weight.[19] However, some studies have found an increased risk for an SGA infant even among obese women with inadequate gestational gain, so it is still unclear how much weight gain is necessary for optimal fetal growth and development among obese women.

In a hospital-based cohort, weight gain below IOM guidelines was not associated with increased neonatal morbidity in term infants, but extremely low weight gain (less than 7 kg) was associated with increased risk for seizures and prolonged hospital stay.[40]

TABLE 10-1 RECOMMENDED TOTAL WEIGHT GAIN RANGES FOR PREGNANT WOMEN BY PRE-PREGNANCY BMI*

	Recommended	Total	Gain
Weight for height	BMI	kg	lb
Underweight	<19.8	12.5-18	28-40
Normal weight	19.8-26.0	11.5-16	25-35
Overweight†	>26.0-29.0	7-11.5	15-25

*BMI (body mass index) is calculated using metric units.
†The recommended target weight gain for obese women (BMI >29.0) is at least 6.0 kg (15 lb).
Adapted from Institute of Medicine: Nutrition during Pregnancy, Weight Gain and Nutrient Supplements. Report of the Subcommittee on Nutritional Status and Weight Gain during Pregnancy, Subcommittee on Dietary Intake and Nutrient Supplements during Pregnancy, Committee on Nutritional Status during Pregnancy and Lactation, Food and Nutrition Board. Washington, DC, National Academy Press, 1990. Copyright 1990 by the National Academy of Sciences.

Conditions Associated with Excessive Gestational Gain

Preeclampsia and Gestational Hypertension

Cedergren found an increased risk for preeclampsia among women who gained more than 35 lb during pregnancy compared with those gaining between 18 and 35 lb.[41] This relationship held across all pre-pregnancy BMI categories.

Gestational Diabetes Mellitus

Although the relationship between high pre-pregnancy BMI and GDM is well established, it is difficult to study the role of gestational weight gain on GDM, as this diagnosis generally leads to dietary interventions and caloric restriction. Saldana and coworkers studied gestational weight gain up until the time the GDM diagnosis was made, and found that higher gain was associated with increased risk for GDM. Pre-pregnancy BMI was a much stronger predictor of GDM risk than weight gain, and there was an interaction between BMI and weight gain that indicated that excessive gain increased the risk for GDM only for those women who were overweight at the start of pregnancy.[42]

Cesarean Delivery

Many epidemiologic studies have linked excessive gestational weight gain to an increased risk for cesarean birth, independent of pre-pregnancy BMI and birth weight. Using U.S. population–based data, Dietz and colleagues found that women gaining 41 lb or more had an increased risk for cesarean birth.[13] Cedergren examined a cohort of Swedish women and found that regardless of pre-pregnancy BMI, a weight gain of greater than 35 lb was associated with cesarean birth.[41] Among overweight and obese women in the cohort, cesarean risk was reduced if weight gain was less than 18 lb.

Macrosomia

Although pre-pregnancy BMI appears to be a stronger predictor of birth weight than pregnancy weight gain, excessive gain is a predictor of macrosomia and the birth of a large-for-gestational-age infant. In a cohort of 45,245 births to nondiabetic women in a California HMO, women gaining more weight than set by IOM guidelines had an OR of 3.05 for macrosomia compared with women gaining within the guidelines.[43]

Neonatal Morbidity

In a hospital-based birth cohort, excessive gestational weight gain was associated with a low 5-minute Apgar score, neonatal seizures, hypoglycemia, polycythemia, meconium aspiration syndrome, and assisted ventilation.[40] In another study in a California HMO, weight gain greater than IOM guidelines was associated with neonatal hypoglycemia and hyperbilirubinemia.[43]

Postpartum Weight Retention

Many studies have shown an association between excessive gestational weight gain, higher postpartum weight retention, and a greater risk for postpartum overweight and obesity. Women who are overweight or obese at the start of pregnancy are at the highest risk of retaining pregnancy weight in the long term.[44,45]

Interventions to Optimize Gestational Weight Gain

Although the amount of weight gained during pregnancy is related to many factors beyond simple energy balance (calories consumed versus calories expended), epidemiologic evidence indicates that a high caloric intake or low physical activity level (or both) are risk factors for excessive gestational weight gain.[46,47] Olson and Strawderman examined the relative contributions of various biologic and psychosocial factors and gestational weight gain, and found that modifiable factors such as increased food intake and decreased physical activity explained 27% of the variance in gestational weight gain.[47]

Few clinical trials have assessed the efficacy of specific prenatal interventions and programs to optimize weight gain during pregnancy. Polley and coworkers randomized pregnant women to a control arm or to an intervention that included diet and exercise counseling, weekly newsletters, and personalized goal-setting and weight gain graphs.[48] Among subjects with a normal pre-pregnancy BMI, there was a lower rate of excessive weight gain in the intervention group (33% versus 58%, $P < .05$). However, among overweight and obese women, the intervention group showed a trend toward a higher rate of excessive gain (59% versus 32%, $P < .09$). Interestingly, the overweight and obese women in the control arm had a much lower rate of excessive gain than is reported in observational studies. Olson and coworkers tested a weight gain intervention in pregnancy and compared outcomes to historical controls.[49] Gestational weight gains in the intervention group were monitored by health care providers, and this group received by-mail patient education. Among the low-income subgroup, the intervention reduced excessive weight gain more than in controls (OR = 0.41, 95% confidence interval [CI], 0.20 to 0.81), but no effect was seem among higher-income subjects.

Supplementation

Recommendations for vitamin and mineral intakes during pregnancy and lactation are shown in Table 10-2.

TABLE 10-2 RECOMMENDED VITAMIN AND MINERAL SUPPLEMENTATION

All Women Who May Become Pregnant and in the First Trimester of Pregnancy			
Folic acid	0.4 mg		
Multivitamin-Mineral Preparation for Women with Poor Diets or in High-Risk Categories			
Iron	30 mg	Vitamin B_6	2 mg
Zinc	15 mg	Folic acid	0.4 mg
Copper	2 mg	Vitamin C	50 mg
Calcium	250 mg	Vitamin D	5 µg
Supplementation for Women in Special Circumstances			
Complete vegetarians, who consume no animal products whatsoever			
10 µg (400 IU) vitamin D			
2 µg vitamin B_{12}			
Women under age 25 whose daily intake of calcium is less than 600 mg			
600 mg calcium			
Women with low intake of vitamin D–fortified milk, especially those who have minimal exposure to sunlight			
10 µg (400 IU) vitamin D			

Adapted and reprinted with permission from Institute of Medicine: Nutrition during Pregnancy, Weight Gain and Nutrient Supplements. Report of the Subcommittee on Nutritional Status and Weight Gain during Pregnancy, Subcommittee on Dietary Intake and Nutrient Supplements during Pregnancy, Committee on Nutritional Status during Pregnancy and Lactation, Food and Nutrition Board. Washington, DC, National Academy Press, 1990. Copyright 1990 by the National Academy of Sciences.

Multivitamin Supplementation

As noted earlier, surveys have shown that a large percentage of pregnant women in the United States consume diets inadequate in several vitamins and minerals. Prescription of "prenatal" multivitamin supplements during pregnancy is common practice in the United States. Although data exist supporting the benefits of folic acid and iron supplementation, the risks and benefits of routine prenatal multivitamin use in the U.S. population have not been clearly documented. One concern is that interactions between nutrients may inhibit or enhance the absorption or bioavailability of individual vitamins and minerals when consumed together in a multivitamin.[50] For example, magnesium and calcium inhibit iron absorption. An observational study of a cohort of low-income pregnant women in New Jersey found an association between first and second trimester multivitamin use and reduced risk for preterm delivery.[51] In a multivariable analysis, risk for delivery before 33 weeks was reduced fourfold among first-trimester vitamin users. There are no randomized, controlled trials of prenatal multivitamin use in the U.S. population.

Iron Supplementation

Epidemiologic data show an association between lower hemoglobin levels and adverse perinatal outcomes, including low birth weight, prematurity, and maternal and infant mortality. The IOM recommends an iron intake of 27 mg/day during pregnancy.[37] Most pregnant women need a supplement to achieve this intake. A Cochrane Collaboration review of routine iron supplementation during pregnancy concluded that antenatal supplementation with iron or iron plus folic acid reduces the risk for anemia (hemoglobin levels below 10 to 10.5 g/L) at or near term.[52] The review concluded that there was insufficient evidence that iron supplementation had any other benefits or any adverse effects on pregnancy outcome. However, a randomized trial in low-income pregnant women in North Carolina showed reductions in preterm birth and higher birth weights among women taking iron supplements.[53] Iron supplements are best absorbed when taken with citrus juices, as the vitamin C enhances absorption. Coffee, tea, milk, and calcium supplements inhibit iron absorption and thus should be consumed separately from iron supplements.

Calcium

Less than half of U.S. women meet the recommendation for dietary intake of calcium. The recommended daily intake of calcium for women 19 to 39 years old (whether pregnant or not) is 1000 mg/day. For women under age 18, 1300 mg/day is recommended.[9] For optimal benefit, calcium should be taken with adequate doses of vitamin D and magnesium. Women with inadequate baseline calcium intake may also benefit from supplementation, which may reduce their risk for preeclampsia and the risk for bone loss.[54] Adequate calcium intake may also be protective against lead toxicity to the fetus, as lead is stored in bone, and increased bone turnover during pregnancy may release lead into the bloodstream.[55]

Dietary Guidelines

Macronutrient Intake

The following is a general guide for otherwise healthy pregnant women with singleton gestations. Pregnant women with normal pre-pregnancy BMI should consume an additional 300 kcal/day above a normal nonpregnant intake.

Fruits and Vegetables. Pregnant women should eat seven or more servings of fruits and vegetables (in any combination) per day. This is necessary for adequate fiber intake, as well as for folic acid, vitamin C, vitamin A, and other nutrients. Consumption of higher-fiber diets is associated with lower risk for excessive gestational weight gain among obese women.[16] One serving of fruit means, for example, one medium apple or one medium banana. One serving of vegetables means 1 cup raw leafy vegetables or one-half cup of other vegetables (raw or cooked).

Carbohydrates. Carbohydrates should make up between 45% and 65% of calories. Pregnant women should consume six to nine servings of whole grains a day, such as whole wheat bread and whole grain cereals. Whole grains provide fiber as well as B vitamins and minerals. One serving of bread or cereal means one slice of bread, and one-half cup of cooked cereal, rice, or pasta.

Dairy Products. Pregnant women should eat at least four servings of low-fat or non-fat dairy products per day. Dairy products are good sources of calcium, vitamins A and D, protein, and B vitamins. Women who are lactose intolerant can get these nutrients from other food sources: cheese and yogurt are low in lactose, and reduced-lactose milk is commercially available. Women who avoid dairy products can choose other calcium-rich foods such as calcium-fortified citrus juice or soy milk, tofu made with calcium sulfate, canned salmon or sardines (with bones), ground sesame seeds, and leafy green vegetables.

Protein. Pregnant women need about 60 g of protein daily, 10 g above the requirement for nonpregnant women. However, most Americans consume more protein than necessary, and much of it is from animal sources high in saturated fat. Beneficial sources of protein include lean meats such as chicken without skin, fish, beans, tofu, nuts, and eggs. One serving of protein means 2 to 3 oz of cooked lean meat, poultry, or fish; one half cup tofu or cooked dried beans; one egg; one-third cup of nuts; or two tablespoons of peanut butter.

Fats. Total fat intake should be between 20% and 35% of calories. Beneficial fats include polyunsaturated fatty acids found in fish, nuts, and vegetable oils. Women should limit the intake of saturated fats and avoid *trans* fats.

Food-Borne Infections

Because pregnant women and fetuses are especially vulnerable to food-borne illnesses such as toxoplasmosis and listeriosis, pregnant women should avoid uncooked and undercooked meats and fish. More information on how to avoid infection with listeriosis can be found on the CDC website, www.cdc.gov/ncidod/dbmd/diseaseinfo/listeriosis_g.htm (accessed February 2008). General information on food safety in pregnancy can be found on the FDA website, www.cfsan.fda.gov/~pregnant/pregnant.html (accessed February 2008).

Fish Consumption: Mercury and Omega-3 Fatty Acids

In 2004, the U.S. government issued health advisories recommending that pregnant women limit their fish consumption to avoid exposure to methyl mercury, a heavy metal and industrial pollutant or contaminant that accumulates in some seafood. Mercury is neurotoxic, and the developing fetus is especially vulnerable. These recommendations were based primarily on data from studies conducted in the Faroe Islands and New Zealand,[56,57] which demonstrated worse performance on neurobehavioral tests among children exposed to higher levels of mercury-contaminated fish. However, a similar study from the Seychelles Islands showed no adverse effect of higher maternal fish consumption.[58] Subsequent to the governmental fish advisories, studies demonstrated that fish consumption dropped among women of reproductive age in the United States.[59]

TABLE 10-3 MERCURY IN COMMONLY EATEN FISH AND SEAFOOD

Fish high in mercury (avoid)	Shark Tilefish Swordfish King mackerel
Fish low in mercury	Salmon Shrimp Canned light tuna Pollock Catfish

However, fish is a primary source of omega-3 fatty acids, which are important in fetal neurologic development. Higher consumption of dietary fish oils has also been associated in epidemiologic studies with lower rates of preterm birth, low birth weight, and preeclampsia.[60-62] In a large population-based study published in 2007 from the United Kingdom, lower maternal fish consumption was associated with lower verbal intelligence quotient scores and other neurobehavioral measures in children 6 months to 8 years of age.[63] Thus, controversy persists over the optimal fish intake during pregnancy. It remains unclear whether the benefits of higher seafood consumption outweigh the risks of mercury exposure. Avoidance of fish known to contain higher levels of mercury is prudent (Table 10-3), and more research is needed about the risks related to typical seafood consumption among U.S. women of reproductive age. The U.S. Environmental Protection Agency advisory related to mercury and fish can be found on their website, www.epa.gov/waterscience/fishadvice/advice.html (accessed February 2008).

Fish Oil Supplements in Pregnancy

Because of the observed epidemiologic associations between higher fish consumption and reduced rates of preterm birth, low birth weight, and preeclampsia, large multicenter trials were initiated to study whether fish oil supplements would prevent such adverse outcomes in pregnancy. Unlike dietary fish, supplements can be prepared to minimize mercury and other toxin contamination. A 2005 Cochrane review of existing trials of fish oil supplementation during pregnancy concluded that there was insufficient evidence to support routine use, although small beneficial effects were seen on birth weight and length of gestation.[64]

Special Diets in Pregnancy

Vegetarian

Although the current prevalence of strict vegetarianism in the United States is not reported, data from the 1990s suggest that approximately

2.5% of U.S. adults consider themselves vegetarian.[65] Interestingly, only 0.9% of those surveyed reported eating no animal flesh, with over half of self-described vegetarians consuming some meat or fish. There is also a lack of data on the relationship of vegetarian and vegan diets during pregnancy to perinatal outcomes. The primary concern about vegetarian diets is vitamin B_{12} deficiency, as this vitamin is found primarily in animal food sources. Women who are ovolactovegetarians (who consume eggs or dairy products, or both) may have adequate B_{12} intake from dairy products. However, a German cohort study found that 39% of ovolactovegetarians had low serum levels of B_{12} during at least one trimester of pregnancy (versus 3% of controls, $P < .001$), although clinical outcomes were not reported.[66] Vegans (those who consume no animal products) generally require a B_{12} supplement for adequate intake. Vegans can also increase their B_{12} intake with B_{12}-fortified vegetarian foods such as soy milk and meat substitutes. The vegan diet may also be so high in fiber and low in fat that caloric intake may be insufficient for pregnancy, and adherents to vegan diets are more likely to have a BMI in the underweight range. Intakes of calcium, vitamin D, riboflavin, and iron may also be inadequate. With dietary assessment and counseling, such women can maintain their diet and have an adequate nutritional intake during pregnancy.

Clinical Issues

Multiple Gestation

Women carrying more than one fetus should increase their caloric intake by 300 kcal/day per fetus. As is true for women carrying singleton gestations, optimal weight gain for twin pregnancies varies by pre-pregnancy BMI. In a large, multicenter cohort of liveborn twins, optimal gestational age and birth weight outcomes were associated with the following patterns of maternal gain[67]:

- Underweight women: 1.25 to 1.75 lb/wk until 20 weeks, 1.50 to 1.75 lb/wk between 20 and 28 weeks, and 1.25 lb/wk from 28 weeks to delivery
- Normal-weight women: 1.0 to 1.5 lb/wk until 20 weeks, 1.25 to 1.75 lb/wk between 20 and 28 weeks, and 1.0 lb/wk from 28 weeks to delivery
- Overweight women: 1.0 to 1.25 lb/wk until 20 weeks, 1.0 to 1.5 lb/wk between 20 and 28 weeks, and 1.0 lb/wk from 28 weeks to delivery
- Obese women: 0.75 to 1.0 lb/wk until 20 weeks, 0.75 to 1.25 lb/wk between 20 and 28 weeks, and 0.75 lb/wk from 28 weeks to delivery

Women with triplets should aim for a total gain of at least 50 to 60 lb. Eating at least five times a day may help women achieve this large caloric intake. Vitamin supplementation is especially helpful in multiple gestations, and additional calcium, magnesium, and zinc may improve outcomes.[68]

Nausea and Vomiting

A majority of pregnant women report some nausea and vomiting during pregnancy. Symptoms virtually always appear before 9 weeks of gestation, so a new onset of nausea or vomiting after 9 weeks should prompt a medical workup for other etiologies. Hyperemesis gravidarum is found in only 0.5% to 2% of pregnancies; this is usually defined as severe persistent vomiting with no other clear etiology accompanied by large ketonuria or weight loss of at least 5% of pre-pregnancy body weight. Excluding cases of hyperemesis gravidarum, women who experience nausea and vomiting of pregnancy actually have better pregnancy outcomes than women who do not experience these symptoms. First-line therapy should be vitamin B_6, 10 to 25 mg, three or four times per day. Ginger has also been effective in clinical trials. Doxylamine, 12.5 mg three or four times per day, added to the vitamin B_6 regimen, may be of additional benefit.[69]

References

1. Siega-Riz AM, Bodnar LM, Savitz DA: What are pregnant women eating? Nutrient and food group differences by race. Am J Obstet Gynecol 186:480-486, 2002.
2. Flegal KM, Carroll MD, Ogden CL, Johnson CL: Prevalence and trends in obesity among US adults, 1999-2000. JAMA 288:1723-1727, 2002.
3. Hedley AA, Ogden CL, Johnson CL, et al: Prevalence of overweight and obesity among US children, adolescents, and adults, 1999-2002. JAMA 291:2847-2850, 2004.
4. King JC: Maternal obesity, metabolism, and pregnancy outcomes. Annu Rev Nutr 26:271-291, 2006.
5. Catalano PM: Management of obesity in pregnancy. Obstet Gynecol 109:419-433, 2007.
6. Stotland NE, Haas JS, Brawarsky P, et al: Body mass index, provider advice, and target gestational weight gain. Obstet Gynecol 105:633-638, 2005.
7. Cogswell ME, Scanlon KS, Fein SB, Schieve LA: Medically advised, mother's personal target, and actual weight gain during pregnancy. Obstet Gynecol 94:616-622, 1999.
8. Rosenn B, Miodovnik M, Combs CA, et al: Glycemic thresholds for spontaneous abortion and congenital malformations in insulin-dependent diabetes mellitus. Obstet Gynecol 84:515-520, 1994.
9. Otten JJ, Hellwig JP, Meyers LD (eds): Dietary Reference Intakes: The Essential Guide to Nutrient Requirements. Institute of Medicine of the National Academies. Washington, DC, National Academies Press, 2006.
10. Ray JG, Wyatt PR, Vermeulen MJ, et al: Greater maternal weight and the ongoing risk of neural tube defects after folic acid flour fortification. Obstet Gynecol 105:261-265, 2005.
11. Boulet SL, Yang Q, Mai C, et al: Folate status in women of childbearing age, by race/ethnicity—United States, 1999-2000, 2001-2002, and 2003-2004. MMWR Morb Mortal Wklt Rep 55:1377-1380, 2007.
12. Yazdy MM, Honein MA, Xing J: Reduction in orofacial clefts following folic acid fortification of the U.S. grain supply. Birth Defects Res A Clin Mol Teratol 79:16-23, 2007.
13. Dietz PM, Callaghan WM, Morrow B, Cogswell ME: Population-based assessment of the risk of primary cesarean delivery due to excess prepregnancy weight among nulliparous women delivering term infants. Matern Child Health J 9:237-244, 2005.
14. Abenhaim HA, Kinch RA, Morin L, et al: Effect of prepregnancy body mass index categories on obstetrical and neonatal outcomes. Arch Gynecol Obstet 275:39-43, 2007.
15. Lashen H, Fear K, Sturdee DW: Obesity is associated with increased risk of first trimester and recurrent miscarriage: matched case-control study. Hum Reprod 19:1644-1646, 2004.
16. Fedorcsak P, Storeng R, Dale PO, et al: Obesity is a risk factor for early pregnancy loss after IVF or ICSI. Acta Obstet Gynecol Scand 79:43-48, 2000.
17. Hendler I, Blackwell SC, Bujold E, et al: The impact of maternal obesity on midtrimester sonographic visualization of fetal cardiac and craniospinal structures. Int J Obes Relat Metab Disord 28:1607-1611, 2004.
18. Sewell MF, Huston-Presley L, Super DM, Catalano P: Increased neonatal fat mass, not lean body mass, is associated with maternal obesity. Am J Obstet Gynecol 195:1100-1103, 2006.
19. Abrams BF, Laros RK Jr: Prepregnancy weight, weight gain, and birth weight. Am J Obstet Gynecol 154:503-509, 1986.

20. Wolfe HM, Sokol RJ, Martier SM, Zador IE: Maternal obesity: A potential source of error in sonographic prenatal diagnosis. Obstet Gynecol 76:339-342, 1990.
21. Field NT, Piper JM, Langer O: The effect of maternal obesity on the accuracy of fetal weight estimation. Obstet Gynecol 86:102-107, 1995.
22. Farrell T, Holmes R, Stone P: The effect of body mass index on three methods of fetal weight estimation. BJOG 109:651-657, 2002.
23. Cheng CJ, Bommarito K, Noguchi A, et al: Body mass index change between pregnancies and small for gestational age births. Obstet Gynecol 104:286-292, 2004.
24. Cnattingius S, Bergstrom R, Lipworth L, Kramer MS: Prepregnancy weight and the risk of adverse pregnancy outcomes. N Engl J Med 338:147-152, 1998.
25. Cedergren MI: Maternal morbid obesity and the risk of adverse pregnancy outcome. Obstet Gynecol 103:219-224, 2004.
26. Morris CD, Jacobson SL, Anand R, et al: Nutrient intake and hypertensive disorders of pregnancy: Evidence from a large prospective cohort. Am J Obstet Gynecol 184:643-651, 2001.
27. Sibai BM, Gordon T, Thom E, et al: Risk factors for preeclampsia in healthy nulliparous women: A prospective multicenter study. The National Institute of Child Health and Human Development Network of Maternal-Fetal Medicine Units. Am J Obstet Gynecol 172:642-648, 1995.
28. O'Brien TE, Ray JG, Chan WS: Maternal body mass index and the risk of preeclampsia: A systematic overview. Epidemiology 14:368-374, 2003.
29. Weiss JL, Malone FD, Emig D, et al: Obesity, obstetric complications and çesarean delivery rate: A population-based screening study. Am J Obstet Gynecol 190:1091-1097, 2004.
30. Dietz PM, Callaghan WM, Cogswell ME, et al: Combined effects of pre-pregnancy body mass index and weight gain during pregnancy on the risk of preterm delivery. Epidemiology 17:170-177, 2006.
31. Schieve LA, Cogswell ME, Scanlon KS: Maternal weight gain and preterm delivery: Differential effects by body mass index. Epidemiology 10:141-147, 1999.
32. Smith GC, Shah I, Pell JP, et al: Maternal obesity in early pregnancy and risk of spontaneous and elective preterm deliveries: A retrospective cohort study. Am J Public Health 97:157-162, 2007.
33. Bujold E, Hammoud A, Schild C, et al: The role of maternal body mass index in outcomes of vaginal births after cesarean. Am J Obstet Gynecol 193:1517-1521, 2005.
34. Nohr EA, Bech BH, Davies MJ, et al: Prepregnancy obesity and fetal death: A study within the Danish National Birth Cohort. Obstet Gynecol 106:250-259, 2005.
35. Huang DY, Usher RH, Kramer MS, et al: Determinants of unexplained antepartum fetal deaths. Obstet Gynecol 95:215-221, 2000.
36. Tuffnell DJ, Cartmill RS, Lilford RJ: Fetal movements factors affecting their perception. Eur J Obstet Gynecol Reprod Biol 39:165-167, 1991.
37. Institute of Medicine (U.S.) Subcommittee on Nutritional Status and Weight Gain during Pregnancy, Subcommittee on Dietary Intake and Nutrient Supplements during Pregnancy: Nutrition during pregnancy: I. Weight gain; II. Nutrient supplements. Washington, DC, National Academy Press, 1990.
38. National Research Council, Institute of Medicine: Influence of pregnancy weight on maternal and child health: Workshop report. Washington, DC, 2007.
39. Carmichael SL, Abrams B: A critical review of the relationship between gestational weight gain and preterm delivery. Obstet Gynecol 89:865-873, 1997.
40. Stotland NE, Cheng YW, Hopkins LM, Caughey AB: Gestational weight gain and adverse neonatal outcome among term infants. Obstet Gynecol 108:635-643, 2006.
41. Cedergren M: Effects of gestational weight gain and body mass index on obstetric outcome in Sweden. Int J Gynaecol Obstet 93:269-274, 2006.
42. Saldana TM, Siega-Riz AM, Adair LS, Suchindran C: The relationship between pregnancy weight gain and glucose tolerance status among black and white women in central North Carolina. Am J Obstet Gynecol 195:1629-1635, 2006.
43. Hedderson MM, Weiss NS, Sacks DA, et al: Pregnancy weight gain and risk of neonatal complications: Macrosomia, hypoglycemia, and hyperbilirubinemia. Obstet Gynecol 108:1153-1161, 2006.
44. Gunderson EP, Abrams B, Selvin S: Does the pattern of postpartum weight change differ according to pregravid body size? Int J Obes Relat Metab Disord 25:853-862, 2001.
45. Gunderson EP, Abrams B, Selvin S: The relative importance of gestational gain and maternal characteristics associated with the risk of becoming overweight after pregnancy. Int J Obes Relat Metab Disord 24:1660-1668, 2000.
46. Olafsdottir AS, Skuladottir GV, Thorsdottir I, et al: Maternal diet in early and late pregnancy in relation to weight gain. Int J Obes (Lond) 30:492-499, 2006.
47. Olson CM, Strawderman MS: Modifiable behavioral factors in a biopsychosocial model predict inadequate and excessive gestational weight gain. J Am Diet Assoc 103:48-54, 2003.
48. Polley BA, Wing RR, Sims CJ: Randomized controlled trial to prevent excessive weight gain in pregnant women. Int J Obes Relat Metab Disord 26:1494-1502, 2002.
49. Olson CM, Strawderman MS, Reed RG: Efficacy of an intervention to prevent excessive gestational weight gain. Am J Obstet Gynecol 191:530-536, 2004.
50. Yetley EA: Multivitamin and multimineral dietary supplements: Definitions, characterization, bioavailability, and drug interactions. Am J Clin Nutr 85:269S-276, 2007.
51. Scholl TO, Hediger ML, Bendich A, et al: Use of multivitamin/mineral prenatal supplements: Influence on the outcome of pregnancy. Am J Epidemiol 146:134-141, 1997.
52. Pena-Rosas JP, Viteri FE: Effects of routine oral iron supplementation with or without folic acid for women during pregnancy. Cochrane Database Syst Rev (3):CD004736, 2006.
53. Siega-Riz AM, Hartzema AG, Turnbull C, et al: The effects of prophylactic iron given in prenatal supplements on iron status and birth outcomes: A randomized controlled trial. Am J Obstet Gynecol 194:512-519, 2006.
54. Hofmeyr GJ, Atallah AN, Duley L: Calcium supplementation during pregnancy for preventing hypertensive disorders and related problems. Cochrane Database Syst Rev (3):CD001059, 2006.
55. Ettinger AS, Hu H, Hernandez-Avila M: Dietary calcium supplementation to lower blood lead levels in pregnancy and lactation. J Nutr Biochem 18:172-178, 2007.
56. Grandjean P, White RF, Weihe P, Jorgensen PJ: Neurotoxic risk caused by stable and variable exposure to methylmercury from seafood. Ambul Pediatr 3:18-23, 2003.
57. Crump KS, Kjellstrom T, Shipp AM, et al: Influence of prenatal mercury exposure upon scholastic and psychological test performance: Benchmark analysis of a New Zealand cohort. Risk Anal 18:701-713, 1998.
58. Myers GJ, Davidson PW, Cox C, et al: Prenatal methylmercury exposure from ocean fish consumption in the Seychelles child development study. Lancet 361:1686-1692, 2003.
59. Oken E, Kleinman KP, Berland WE, et al: Decline in fish consumption among pregnant women after a national mercury advisory. Obstet Gynecol 102:346-351, 2003.
60. Olsen SF, Osterdal ML, Salvig JD, et al: Duration of pregnancy in relation to seafood intake during early and mid pregnancy: Prospective cohort. Eur J Epidemiol 21:749-758, 2006.
61. Olsen SF, Secher NJ: Low consumption of seafood in early pregnancy as a risk factor for preterm delivery: Prospective cohort study. BMJ 324:447, 2002.
62. Olafsdottir AS, Skuladottir GV, Thorsdottir I, et al: Relationship between high consumption of marine fatty acids in early pregnancy and hypertensive disorders in pregnancy. BJOG 113:301-309, 2006.
63. Hibbeln JR, Davis JM, Steer C, et al: Maternal seafood consumption in pregnancy and neurodevelopmental outcomes in childhood (ALSPAC study): An observational cohort study. Lancet 369:578-585, 2007.
64. Makrides M, Duley L, Olsen SF: Marine oil, and other prostaglandin precursor, supplementation for pregnancy uncomplicated by pre-eclampsia or

intrauterine growth restriction. Cochrane Database Syst Rev (3):CD003402, 2006.

65. Haddad EH, Tanzman JS: What do vegetarians in the United States eat? Am J Clin Nutr 78:626S-632, 2003.
66. Koebnick C, Hoffmann I, Dagnelie PC, et al: Long-term ovo-lacto vegetarian diet impairs vitamin B-12 status in pregnant women. J Nutr 134:3319-3326, 2004.
67. Luke B, Hediger ML, Nugent C, et al: Body mass index: Specific weight gains associated with optimal birth weights in twin pregnancies. J Reprod Med 48:217-224, 2003.
68. Luke B: Nutrition and multiple gestation. Semin Perinatol 29:349-354, 2005.
69. ACOG (American College of Obstetrics and Gynecology) Practice Bulletin: Nausea and vomiting of pregnancy. Obstet Gynecol 103:803-814, 2004.

Chapter 11

Developmental Origins of Health and Disease

Lucilla Poston, PhD, and Mark Hanson, DPhil

Environmental agents that are active at a sensitive or critical period of development are well recognized to cause teratogenic effects in the embryo or fetus. Obstetricians are also very familiar with the infant mortality and morbidity associated with compromised fetal growth (e.g., the growth restriction of preeclampsia or the macrosomia of maternal diabetes). The more subtle and persistent consequences of perturbations of in utero growth and nutrition are less widely appreciated, but even modest changes in growth and development may have unforeseen consequences that extend into adulthood. Although not immediately evident in the newborn period, these can alter an individual's response to the subsequent challenges of life, leading, ultimately, to a greater risk for adult disease.

The suggestion that compromised growth in utero may enhance risk for adult disease came from early studies implying that small size at birth conferred greater risk for chronic noncommunicable diseases such as cardiovascular disease (coronary heart disease, hypertension, stroke), type 2 diabetes, and osteoporosis.[1,2] Indeed, the majority of work in this area has concentrated on perturbations in the nutritional environment during prenatal and early postnatal life. Other environmental influences have been implicated in animal models, including temperature, oxygen tension, fluid balance, and stress,[3,4] but in this review we will concentrate largely on the human situation and early nutritional influences, discussing the evidence, the proposed underlying mechanisms, and possible interventions.

Associations between Low Birth Weight and Adult Disease

How the Concept Arose—The Early Studies

The concept of developmental programming was largely inspired by the reports from Barker and his colleagues in the 1980s, indicating an association between risk for cardiovascular disease and low birth weight in cohorts of middle-aged men and women in the United Kingdom for whom detailed birth records were available.[1] These followed Forsdahl's early study of Norwegian populations suggesting that chronic adult disease was linked to deficiencies in the early childhood environment. Forsdahl stressed that these effects persisted even if circumstances improved in later years.[5] Similarly, Lucas had proposed that detrimental influences in early life may increase risk for later disease.[6] The early papers from Barker and colleagues were followed by others showing that low birth weight was associated not only with increased risk for death from cardiovascular disease but also with insulin resistance and obesity—in fact, with each of the criteria that define the metabolic syndrome. It was proposed that in utero nutritional status could influence risk for both cardiovascular and metabolic disease in later life.

Contemporary Viewpoints

Now, almost 20 years since the "fetal programming" concept was first proposed, we have come to recognize that birth weight is a weak index of in utero nutrition and growth. Smallness at birth can arise either from poor growth beginning in early gestation or from early rapid growth followed by slow growth in late gestation—each likely to arise from different causes. However as growth trajectory data are usually not available for historical cohorts, most studies continue to investigate relationships between birth weight and incidence of later disease.

The validity of the concept has been questioned because of the wide variability reported among associations between birth weight and proxy markers of disease (e.g., adult blood pressure),[7] but associations are much stronger, and criticism therefore less warranted, when the outcome measure is clinical disease.[8] It must be kept in mind that pregnancies in the historical cohorts occurred when nutrition and health care were very different from those of contemporary developed societies. The lower-birth-weight individuals in these cohorts, for example, would be unlikely to include fetuses born long before term or with intrauterine growth restriction, and the higher-birth-weight group would be unlikely to include fetuses of diabetic mothers, as these would not have survived in those days.

Testing the Concept in Different Populations

The strength of the idea, however, lies in the reproducibility of the many geographically dispersed cohort studies that have now accumulated. Most, including those from countries other than the United Kingdom, have replicated the original association between lower birth weight and not only adult death from ischemic heart disease[9] but also nonfatal coronary artery disease and stroke.[10] Indeed, a recent study of

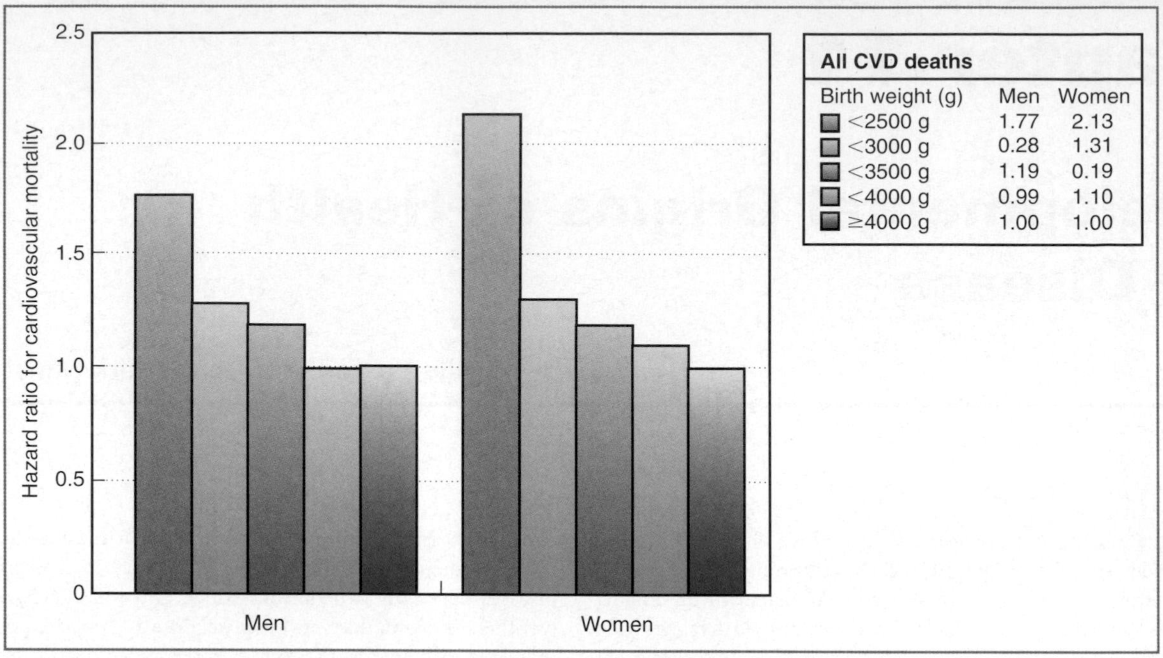

FIGURE 11-1 **Risk for cardiovascular disease (CVD) mortality stratified by birth weight.** The difference between the sexes is also shown. (Adapted from Kajantie E, Osmond C, Barker D, et al: Size at birth as a predictor of mortality in adulthood: A follow-up study of 350,000 person-years. Int J Epidemiol 34:655-663, 2005.)

13,830 men and women for whom records were available from the Finnish National Death Registry showed an association between low birth weight and *all cause* mortality among women.[11] The relationship between birth weight and cardiovascular mortality risk for men and women is shown in Figure 11-1.

A recent follow-up study of 10,803 children born in Aberdeen, Scotland, in the 1950s, at a time when environmental influences were more favorable for infants than in earlier studies, has confirmed an inverse association between birth weight and later coronary artery disease and stroke.[12] Other large cohort studies, such as that of almost 90,000 Swedish army recruits born between 1973 and 1981, have also continued to show that lower birth weight is linked to higher adulthood blood pressure and, although small in magnitude, the increment in blood pressure was independent of socioeconomic factors or familial effects.[13]

Even a small rise in blood pressure is important when viewed from the perspective of risk for later disease.[14] A recent meta-analysis of data from 198,000 individuals in 20 Nordic studies (1910 to 1987 cohorts) shows unequivocally an inverse and linear association between birth weight in males, but a U-shaped relationship for females, those with birth weight higher than 4 kg having a higher systolic blood pressure in adult life.[15] Similar confirmation of the association with low birth weight and raised systolic blood pressure has been derived from a British birth cohort study of 3157 men and women born in 1946.[16] Some but not all studies correct adulthood outcomes for current body mass index (BMI), an adjustment that has led to a continuing controversy, as has the failure to account for the influence of growth trajectories at different stages of life and inclusion of subjects taking antihypertensive medication.[17,18] These criticisms have themselves proved controversial.

A recent review of the literature investigating associations between low birth weight and insulin resistance shows that people with lower weight at birth generally have an adverse profile of later glucose and insulin metabolism, which is related to insulin resistance rather than altered insulin secretion.[19] Associations of low birth weight and adulthood obesity have also generally stood the test of time,[20] and criticisms that the use of BMI, an inaccurate assessment of central obesity, confounded interpretation have been countered by descriptions of inverse associations between birth weight and raised adulthood fat mass, and with reduced lean mass.[21,22]

Associations between Maternal Weight, Birth Weight, and Adulthood Disease

Diabetes

The rising birth weight in developed countries (with the possible exception of Japan[23]), associated with the prevalence of obesity in pregnancy and related gestational diabetes, may also have the potential for detrimental influences on the developing child.[24,25] After the original suggestion by a few studies showing a U- or J-shaped relationship between birth weight and later insulin resistance and obesity, there is now good evidence that children of women who are diabetic in pregnancy are themselves more likely to develop insulin resistance in later life and to become overweight.[26] Although this may represent in part a genetically inherited disorder, studies of sib pairs discordant for maternal diabetes show that this relationship holds only in the offspring prenatally exposed to diabetes, strongly suggesting an acquired diabetic trait.[27,28] Also, independent of birth weight, infants of mothers with gestational diabetes have a greater neonatal fat mass,[29] and a rather alarming report documents a higher rate of childhood metabolic syndrome (central adiposity, insulin resistance, and hypertension) in large-for-gestational-age (LGA) infants born to mothers with gestational diabetes[30] than in appropriate-(weight)-for-gestational-age (AGA) infants. Importantly, the risk for metabolic syndrome was also present, but to a lesser extent, in LGA infants from normoglycemic mothers. Higher birth weight in normoglycemic pregnancies is generally associated with raised adulthood BMI, and larger infants tend to become heavier adults. However, detailed investigation of the relative contributions of lean and fat mass have sometimes suggested that this association reflects increased lean body mass rather that fat mass,[31] although a recent study of infants from obese normoglycemic mothers shows clear evidence of increased adiposity.[32]

There have been few attempts to define accurately the relationship between maternal, childhood, and adulthood body composition over any range of maternal BMIs. Ongoing prospective longitudinal studies in contemporary cohorts such as the Avon Longitudinal Study of Parents and Children (ALSPAC) cohort in Avon[33] and the Southampton Women's Survey[34] (both in the United Kingdom) will be very informative in this regard. In the latter, it is already clear that a woman's body composition and dietary balance before pregnancy can affect fetal cardiovascular development in late gestation.[35]

Disorders Associated with Lower Birth Weight

The primary focus in this field has been on developmental origins of cardiovascular disease and disorders of glucose homeostasis, but associations have also been reported between low birth weight and adulthood reduced bone density,[36] schizophrenia,[37] breast cancer,[38] and asthma.[39] These have been reviewed recently.[40]

Breastfeeding

Longitudinal studies that have tracked height and weight of the participants have suggested that children who demonstrate rapid growth, either in early infancy or in early childhood, are at risk for adulthood cardiovascular and metabolic disease—children who are small at birth being the most vulnerable.

Investigations among cohorts of very premature children have shown that rapid growth in the first weeks or even days of neonatal life associated with formula feeding may lead to increased risk for cardiovascular disease in adolescents.[41] Rapid weight gain in infancy has, in many studies, been linked to childhood obesity,[25,42,43] and formula feeding promotes rapid growth in early infancy[44] and thus may confer an increased risk for obesity in childhood and adolescence.[45] A study from a U.S. cohort has suggested that obesity in adults (20 to 32 years of age) may be linked to rapid growth in only the first 8 days of life in normal-birth-weight infants fed formula milk.[46] A meta-analysis of 61 studies has shown that breastfed infants have a reduced incidence of childhood or adulthood obesity compared with those whose mothers opted to feed their infants with formula milk.[47] These observations fit into the broader framework of greater risk associated with greater "mismatch" between the environment during development and that in later life.[48]

Childhood Growth

One of the largest cohort studies published has linked coronary events to birth weight and early life growth trajectories.[49] Among 8760 Finnish men and women born between 1934 and 1944, those who suffered coronary events were more likely to have been small at birth and thin at 2 years, and to have subsequently experienced a greater increase in BMI by 11 years of age. Lower BMI at 2 years of age and increased BMI from age 2 to 11 were also associated with a highly significant elevation of fasting insulin concentrations. Although this study noted a lower risk for coronary events with weight gain at 3 months, no analysis was presented of weight gain in the earliest weeks of life (see previous paragraph), although graphic representation did suggest a rapid growth trajectory in the first few weeks of life for those who had coronary events. Nonetheless, the overall growth trajectory closely resembled that found in India among men and women who developed insulin resistance or diabetes in adulthood.[50]

Importantly, the influences of birth weight and growth during some critical period of childhood remain to be fully established in contemporary cohorts. The different conclusions drawn by Singhal and Lucas[6] and Barker and colleagues[49] on the relative importance of postnatal growth may relate to the different historical periods studied, but it may also relate to differences in the subjects (e.g., preterm versus term). Preterm birth itself is also associated with increased risks of type 2 diabetes, independent of size for gestational age.[51] Studies such as those from Finland and the United Kingdom investigated adults who were born in times when nutrition was not abundant and may have been unbalanced, particularly for those born in Finland around the Second World War. The rapid postnatal growth hypothesis has nonetheless been shown to hold in two contemporary studies. One is a study from the ALSPAC cohort of children born in the 1990s, which reported that increased insulin resistance and raised abdominal girth are evident in 8-year-olds born small and those who demonstrated greater weight gain between birth and 3 years.[52] The other is a report on a young U.K. cohort (22 years of age) that showed that systolic blood pressure is highest in those who were born small but demonstrated rapid weight gain between the ages of 1 and 5.[53] Of course, growth from conception onward lies on a continuum, so it is difficult in all these studies to determine the time at which environmental influences induce effects, some of which are manifest later.

Developmental Effects of Antenatal Glucocorticoids

Antenatal steroids are widely used to hasten fetal lung maturation when premature delivery is threatened. However, antenatal administration of steroids in experimental animals evokes persistent and deleterious effects in the developing offspring, which become manifest only in adulthood. The administration of an exogenous glucocorticoid such as dexamethasone during a critical window of early development is detrimental to cardiovascular and renal function and to glucose homeostasis in several species.[54-57] Whether this reflects exaggeration of naturally occurring prenatal processes inducing a change in the offspring phenotype or a disruption of *normal* development is not known, but understandable concern has arisen over the prolonged effects of antenatal glucocorticoids given to pregnant women at risk for preterm delivery, despite the uncontested improvement in neonatal respiratory outcome. A recent report has shown elevation of neonatal blood pressure 2 standard deviations above the normal range in 67% of children exposed to multiple courses and 24% exposed to a single course.[58] However, 31-year-olds who had been exposed to a single course of betamethasone in utero showed no difference in psychological functioning and health-related quality of life compared with those antenatally randomized to placebo.[59] A report from the same cohort at age 30 years showed a higher plasma insulin concentration at 30 minutes after a 75-g oral glucose tolerance test, possibly indicative of insulin resistance, although cardiovascular indices were unaffected.[60]

The authors suggested that this modest influence on adulthood risk factors does not contraindicate the use of a single course of betamethasone. We must conclude that the gain from administration of antenatal corticosteroids significantly outweighs the potential disadvantage.

The pronounced consequences of maternal glucocorticoid administration described in the animal studies has logically led to concern over the potential effects of maternal stress on the fetus. Several studies in rodents have shown that stress in pregnancy can lead to altered behavior of the offspring and also to altered biochemical responses to stress.[61] Cardiovascular function in adult offspring may also be compromised.[62] Studies in humans are also strongly indicative of a deleterious and persistent effect of maternal stress on the offspring, with 14 independent prospective studies showing a link between antenatal maternal anxiety (or stress) and cognitive, behavioral, and emotional problems in the child.[63]

Animal Models

The concept of developmental origins of health and disease has stimulated wide-ranging investigations in animal models.[64-66] Studies in rats, mice, sheep, guinea pigs, and nonhuman primates lend strong support to the hypothesis. Most notably, several characteristics of the offspring phenotypes arising from a range of nutritional interventions are shared across species. Indeed, it has proved remarkably easy to demonstrate characteristics equivalent to human disease, particularly features of the metabolic syndrome, through experimental manipulation of the diet of the pregnant animal or her offspring. The effects include aspects of cardiovascular function and glucose homeostasis in the offspring. Adulthood adiposity has also been induced by maternal nutritional intervention, both by undernutrition and overnutrition. In addition, the behavioral effects on the offspring include reduced exploratory behavior and activity levels, and even impaired learning behavior.[67] These animal models offer the potential for investigation of mechanisms, and thereby suggestions for intervention. The most effective interventions reported have been supplementation of a low-protein diet during pregnancy in the rat with glycine[68,69] or folate,[70] and neonatal treatment of the pups with leptin.[71]

Mechanistic Insights

Some clear leads regarding mechanisms of developmental programming are beginning to emerge. That sustained effects on the offspring can be produced in very early pregnancy, or even in the preimplantation environment, focuses attention on the early embryo[72] and raises potential concern about the possible long-term effects of in vitro fertilization procedures. Even embryo transfer, with or without culture to blastocyst stage in vitro, produces elevated blood pressure in offspring.[73] Perhaps changes in the "test tube" milieu explain the increased rate of abnormalities associated with defects of genomic imprinting reported in vitro fertilization infants.[74]

Permanent epigenetic changes are proposed to occur in fetal or neonatal nuclear DNA, either by changes in methylation or in histone packaging, that alter gene expression permanently. Moreover, these changes can be reversed by dietary supplements that promote the provision of methyl groups.[75] More recently, epigenetic changes have been demonstrated for the first time in nonimprinted genes in the liver of rat offspring, effects that were inversely related to gene expression and that were reversed by maternal dietary folate supplementation.[76] The effects are associated with changes in DNA methyltransferase activity[77] and can be passed to grand-offspring.[78]

Permanent alteration to mitochondrial DNA (mtDNA) offers another plausible hypothesis for developmental programming[79,80] that may be additive to the effects on nuclear DNA. Persistent alteration to mtDNA has been proposed to explain the transgenerational transmission of disorders observed in several animal models[81,82] and to development of metabolic disorders.

Induction of a phenotype with greater risk for later disease does not have to involve an overall reduction in somatic growth, as suggested by some of the epidemiologic studies and many of the animal models. It appears, therefore, that reduced body growth may not lie directly on the causal pathway to such disease. This does not of course preclude changes in the growth or structure of individual organs, especially if the environmental challenge occurs during sensitive developmental windows. A prime candidate is the kidney. Smaller-birth-weight children have a reduced nephron complement, and deficiency in nephron number has also been linked to the development of hypertension in humans.[83] Animal studies using unbalanced nutrition during pregnancy or glucocorticoid treatment have reported reduced nephron number in the offspring.[84] Moreover, reduction in fetal growth produced by uterine artery ligation in the rat produces epigenetic effects on expression of genes associated with apoptosis in the kidney.[85] Nearly all nutritional models and a model of reduced uterine blood flow have shown persistent alteration in the pancreatic structure, including a reduction in pancreatic beta cell density.[86] This may contribute to early pancreatic failure in the presence of peripheral insulin resistance and to the development of overt diabetes later in life. Intriguingly, many studies have suggested that persistent alteration in the appetite centers of the hypothalamus could play a role in inducing later hyperphagia and contribute to obesity.[87,88]

Time for Intervention?

Nutrient Supplementation

In light of clinical and cohort studies, and indeed of all that is already accepted in relationship to infant morbidity and mortality in children who were small for their gestational age, low birth weight should clearly be prevented whenever possible. Balanced energy and protein supplementation may reduce the risk of delivering a small-for-gestational-age infant in an undernourished woman,[89] but prevention of low birth weight has proved to be an intractable problem in developed countries.[90,91] Nutritional interventions with micronutrients may have small effects but have largely failed to show a significant impact,[92] although it has been argued that the majority of studies have been of inadequate design, and that well-conducted randomized control trials of adequate sample size and appropriate outcome measures are still required.[93] Such a study is now under way in Mumbai, India. The Pune nutritional trial[94] has shown that birth weight is strongly related to maternal folate status and green vegetable intake at 28 weeks' gestation.

Maternal Body Composition

Optimization of maternal pre-pregnancy body composition and nutrition are likely to minimize the "developmental origins" problem, as may improved antenatal and maternal health care in developing countries. Animal models are likely to provide specific direction for effective intervention. For example, maternal administration of the amino acids taurine and glycine has already been shown to have potential for reversal of disorders of cardiovascular function and glucose metabolism induced by unbalanced maternal nutrition. Importantly, prospective cohort studies are moving away from birth weight as a primary outcome, toward more accurate indices of body composition such as dual-energy x-ray absorptiometry (DEXA). Longitudinal studies of fetal growth trajectories, not just of the fetal body but also of organs such as the liver, kidneys, and placenta, are underway and will be linked to maternal pre-pregnancy characteristics as well as to measures of pregnancy outcome. These studies will have to be continued into childhood with measures of body composition, metabolism and physical activity, cardiovascular function, and glucose and lipid homeostasis. This will be expensive, but it will be an investment that will pay great dividends when translated into public health policy to identify in early life individuals who will be susceptible to later chronic disease, and to give them more individually based advice and interventions.

Maternal Obesity: An Important Public Health Problem

The numerous studies that implicate maternal obesity and associated gestational diabetes in impaired later health of the offspring provide a clear and immediate public health agenda, strongly supporting the benefits of pre-conceptual weight loss in obese women intending to conceive. A recent large cohort study from Scandinavia showing that weight gain between first and second pregnancies is a risk for adverse outcome in the second pregnancy reemphasizes the need to avoid excessive weight gain in pregnancy.[95] Although it is unwise to recommend calorie restriction in pregnant women, there is a need to identify ideal weight gain in pregnancy, and this will require careful consideration of pre-pregnancy weight, parity, and ethnicity. The Southampton Women's Survey has already made clear that maternal thinness, as judged from skinfold thicknesses, and imprudent diet produce adverse effects on the circulatory adaptations of the late-gestation fetus.[35] A range of maternal characteristics, including body composition, smoking, and strenuous exercise in pregnancy, are also associated with lower neonatal bone mineral density,[96] and most recently a marked correlation between maternal and neonatal adiposity has been observed.[97] Dietary and exercise interventions that aim to improve insulin sensitivity rather than reduce calorie intake may prove efficacious in improving pregnancy outcome.

Neonatal Feeding Regimens

Optimal neonatal feeding strategies need to be better defined in regard to subsequent risk for obesity and cardiovascular disease, and large randomized controlled trials are underway to define the optimal constituents of formula milk for infants of mothers unable or unwilling to breastfeed. These will also evaluate relationships between neonatal growth rates and risk for later disease.

Developmental Effects on the Human Phenotype: Pathology or Survival?

The acquisition of disease risk in utero as a result of imbalances in the nutritional environment is likely to confer advantage in terms of Darwinian fitness (i.e., survival to reproduce), or the underlying mechanisms would not have been selected during human evolution. The "thrifty phenotype hypothesis" of David Barker and the late Nicholas Hales[98] concerns a rather special case of this broader phenomenon, in which fetal phenotypic adaptations are induced in response to nutritional imbalance in utero. These adaptations confer an immediate fetal and neonatal survival advantage, but the individual has to trade this advantage for later detrimental effects in terms of increased risk for adult disease. If disease were to occur only in the post-reproductive phase of life, then it would have no impact on fitness. Fetal blood flow for example, is directed to areas of the body where nutrient delivery is prioritized (e.g., brain, thus depriving the skeletal muscle, which grows less). In later life, the lack of skeletal muscle would confer the advantage of reducing glucose consumption when food was in poor supply—often thought to have been a valuable adaptive response in our hunter-gatherer ancestors. However, should nutritional status be surprisingly good or even excessive, as it is today in many developed nations, the poor capacity of the muscle to take up glucose could eventually contribute to the development of the insulin resistance of type 2 diabetes. In the case of placental insufficiency, the fetus would be tricked into the need to prepare for a life of nutritional inadequacy, when in reality the postpartum life today in developed nations is frequently one of nutritional plenty.

Thrifty Phenotype and Predictive Adaptive Models

The thrifty phenotype hypothesis seems valid in the case of the small-for-gestational-age infant, but it becomes problematic when we consider the graded relationship between, for example, size at birth and risk for later disease, which is manifest across the entire normal range of size at birth. The predictive adaptive response hypothesis proposed by Gluckman and Hanson[99] suggests that aspects of the prenatal environment are able to induce phenotypic changes in the embryo and fetus that confer advantage in terms of Darwinian fitness because they predict aspects of the postnatal environment. According to this view, the phenotype of the offspring has not been set to cope with a prenatal challenge, but to be best able to respond to predicted postnatal challenges. An accurate prediction would confer greater likelihood of health in the predicted environment, but an inaccurate or inappropriate prediction, such as might occur with a change in the environment caused by socioeconomic change or migration, would be associated with greater risk for disease. Thus it is the mismatch between the predicted and the actual environment that raises risk for disease.[48] Several lines of experimental evidence in animals now support this concept,[82,100-102] and evidence is emerging in humans in terms of reproductive functions.[102]

Conclusions

Epidemiologic studies from contemporary and historical cohorts implicate a role for prenatal influences on the risk for later development of adult disease. The influences considered to date have focused largely on maternal diet and body composition, but there is increasing evidence for important effects from maternal smoking, strenuous exercise, stress, drugs such as steroids, pathogens, and environmental pollutants that can act as endocrine disruptors. Many studies have linked lower birth weight with greater risk for adulthood cardiovascular morbidity, obesity, and insulin resistance. Also, considerable data support an association between maternal obesity, or gestational diabetes, and acquisition of risk for type 2 diabetes in the offspring.

Given this foundation of information, there is now a need to conduct more robust, prospective cohort studies to define the prenatal and postnatal phenotypic characteristics that are associated with later risk for disease, and then to develop prognostic intermediate outcome markers and pilot potential interventions. A few are now underway. It is as yet too early to suggest any specific intervention in pregnancy or in the neonate, except to recommend that obese women lose weight before becoming pregnant and that regular exercise and a balanced diet be adapted. The concepts discussed support a focus for public health measures that aim to optimize nutrition for the mother and child as strategies to prevent obesity and insulin resistance in the population. A new focus on development as part of a life-course perspective is likely to have a very substantial effect in reducing the burden of chronic noncommunicable disease in both developed and developing societies.

Acknowledgment

The authors thank the British Heart Foundation for support, and Professor Poston is grateful to Tommy's, the Baby Charity.

References

1. Barker DJ, Osmond C: Infant mortality, childhood nutrition and ischaemic heart disease in England and Wales. Lancet 1:1077-1081, 1986.
2. Barker DJP: Mothers, Babies and Health in Later Life. Edinburgh, Churchill Livingstone, 1998.
3. Gluckman PD, Hanson MA, Spencer HG, Bateson P: Environmental influences during development and their later consequences for health and disease: Implications for the interpretation of empirical studies. Proc Biol Soc 272:671-677, 2005.
4. Gluckman P, Hanson M: The Fetal Matrix: Evolution, Development and Disease. Cambridge, Cambridge University Press, 2005.
5. Forsdahl A: Living conditions in childhood and subsequent development of risk factors for arteriosclerotic heart disease: The cardiovascular survey in Finnmark 1974-75. J Epidemiol Community Health 32:34-37, 1978.
6. Singhal A, Lucas A: Early origins of cardiovascular disease: Is there a unifying hypothesis? Lancet 363:1642-1645, 2004.
7. Huxley R, Neil A, Collins R: Unravelling the fetal origins hypothesis: Is there really an inverse association between birthweight and subsequent blood pressure? Lancet 360:659-665, 2002.
8. Curhan GC, Chertow GM, Willett WC, et al: Birth weight and adult hypertension and obesity in women. Circulation 94:1310-1315, 1996.
9. Koupilova I, Leon DA, NcKeigue PM, Lithell HO: Is the effect of birth weight on cardiovascular mortality mediated through high blood pressure? J Hypertens 17:19-25, 1999.
10. Rich Edwards J, Stampfer MJ, Manson JE, et al: Birth weight and risk of cardiovascular disease in a cohort of women followed up since 1976. BMJ 315:396-400, 1997.
11. Kajantie E, Osmond C, Barker D, et al: Size at birth as a predictor of mortality in adulthood: A follow-up study of 350,000 person-years. Int J Epidemiol 34:655-663, 2005.
12. Lawlor DA, Ronalds G, Clark H, et al: Birth weight is inversely associated with incident coronary heart disease and stroke among individuals born in the 1950s: Findings from the Aberdeen Children of the 1950s prospective cohort study. Circulation 112:1414-1418, 2005.
13. Bergvall N, Iliadou A, Tuvemo T, Cnattingius S: Birth characteristics and risk of high systolic blood pressure in early adulthood: Socio-economic factors and familial effects. Epidemiology 16:635-640, 2005.
14. Vasan RS, Pencine MJ, Cobain M, et al: Estimated risks for developing obesity in the Framingham Study. Ann Intern Med 143:473-480, 2005.
15. Gamborg M, Byberg L, Rasmussen F, et al: Birth weight and systolic blood pressure in adolescence and adulthood: Meta-regression analysis of sex- and age-specific results from 20 Nordic studies. Am J Epidemiol 166:634-645, 2007.
16. Hardy R, Wadsworth ME, Langenberg C, Kuh D: Birthweight, childhood growth and blood pressure at 43 years in a British birth cohort. Int J Epidemiol 33:121-129, 2004.
17. Schluchter MD: Publication bias and heterogeneity in the relationship between systolic blood pressure, birth weight, and catch-up growth: A meta analysis. J Hypertens 21:273-279, 2003.
18. Tu YK, West R, Ellison GTH, Gilthorpe MS: Why evidence for the fetal origins of adult disease might be a statistical artifact: The "reversal paradox" for the relation between birth weight and blood pressure in later life. Am J Epidemiol 161:27-32, 2005.
19. Newsome CA, Shiell AW, Fall CHD, et al: Is birth weight related to later glucose and insulin metabolism? A systematic review. Diabet Med 20:339-348, 2003.
20. Rogers I: Birth weight and obesity and fat distribution in later life. Birth Defects Res A Clin Mol Teratol 73:485-486, 2005.
21. Singhal A, Wells J, Cole TJ, et al: Programming of lean body mass: A link between birth weight, obesity and cardiovascular disease. Am J Clin Nutr 77:726-730, 2003.
22. Kensara OA, Wootton SA, Phillips DI, et al: Hertfordshire Study Group: Fetal programming of body composition: Relation between birthweight and body composition measured with dual-energy X-ray absorptiometry and anthropometric methods in older Englishmen. Am J Clin Nutr 82:980-987, 2005.
23. Gluckman PD, Yap Seng C, Fukuoka H, et al: Low birthweight and subsequent obesity in Japan. Lancet 369:1081-1082, 2007.
24. Catalano P: Obesity and pregnancy: The propagation of a viscous cycle? J Clin Endocrinol Metab 88:3505-3506, 2003.
25. Oken E, Gillman MW: Fetal origins of obesity. Obes Res 11:496-506, 2003.
26. Dörner G, Plagemann A: Perinatal hyperinsulinism as possible predisposing factor for diabetes mellitus, obesity and enhanced cardiovascular risk in later life. Horm Metab Res 26:213-221, 1994.
27. Dabelea D, Hanson RL, Lindsay RS, et al: Intrauterine exposure to diabetes conveys risks for type 2 diabetes and obesity: A study of discordant sibships. Diabetes 49:2208-2211, 2000.
28. Dabelea D, Pettitt DJ: Intrauterine diabetic environment confers risks for type 2 diabetes mellitus and obesity in the offspring, in addition to genetic susceptibility. J Pediatr Endocrinol Metab 14:1085-1091, 2001.
29. Catalano PM, Thomas A, Huston-Presley L, Amini SB: Increased fetal adiposity: A very sensitive marker of abnormal in utero development. Am J Obstet Gynecol 189:1698-1704, 2003.
30. Boney CM, Verma A, Tucker R, Vohr BR: Metabolic syndrome in childhood: Association with birth weight, maternal obesity, and gestational diabetes mellitus. Pediatrics 115:290-296, 2005.
31. Sayer AA, Syddall HE, Dennison EM, et al: Birth weight, weight at 1 y of age, and body composition in older men: Findings from the Hertfordshire Cohort Study. Am J Clin Nutr 80:199-203, 2004.
32. Sewell MF, Huston-Presley L, Super DM, Catalano P: Increased neonatal fat mass, not lean body mass, is associated with maternal obesity. Am J Obstet Gynecol 195:1100-1103, 2006.
33. Ness AR: The Avon Longitudinal Study of Parents and Children (ALSPAC): A resource for the study of the environmental determinants of childhood obesity. Eur J Endocrinol 151:U141-1419, 2004.
34. Inskip H, Godfrey KM, Robinson SM, et al: SWS Study Group: Cohort profile: The Southampton Women's Survey. Int J Epidemiol 35:42-48, 2006.
35. Haugen G, Hanson M, Kieerud T, et al: Fetal liver-sparing cardiovascular adaptations linked to mother's slimness and diet. Circ Res 96:12-14, 2005.
36. Harvey N, Cooper C: The developmental origins of osteoporotic fracture. J Br Menopause Soc 10:14-15, 29, 2004.
37. Nilsson E, Stalberg G, Lichtenstein P, et al: Fetal growth restriction and schizophrenia: A Swedish twin study. Twin Res Hum Genet 8:402-408, 2005.
38. Michels KB, Trichopoulos D, Robins JM, et al: Birthweight as a risk factor for breast cancer. Lancet 348:1542-1546, 1996.
39. Steffensen FH, Sorensen HT, Gillman MW, et al: Low birth weight and preterm delivery as risk factors for asthma and atopic dermatitis in young adult males. Epidemiology 2:185-188, 2000.

40. Gluckman PD, Hanson MA (eds): Developmental Origins of Health and Disease. Cambridge, Cambridge University Press, 2007.
41. Singhal A, Lucas A: Early origins of cardiovascular disease: Is there a unifying hypothesis? Lancet 363:1642-1645, 2004.
42. Ong KKL, Ahmed ML, Emmett PM, et al: Association between postnatal catch-up growth and obesity in childhood: Prospective cohort study. BMJ 320:967-971, 2000.
43. Stettler N, Zemal BS, Kumanyika S, Stallings VA: Infant weight gain and childhood overweight status in a multicentre, cohort study. Pediatrics 109:194-199, 2002.
44. Baker JL, Michaelson KF, Rasmussen KM, Sorensen TI: Maternal prepregnant body mass index, duration of breastfeeding, and timing of complementary food introduction are associated with infant weight gain. Am J Clin Nutr 80:1579-1588, 2004.
45. Gillman MW, Rifas-Shiman SL, Camargo CA Jr, et al: Risk of overweight among adolescents who were breastfed as infants. JAMA 285:2461-2467, 2001.
46. Stettler N, Stallings VA, Troxel AB, et al: Weight gain in the first week of life and overweight in adulthood: A cohort study of European American subjects fed infant formula. Circulation 111:1897-1903, 2005.
47. Owen C, Martin RM, Whincup PH, et al: Effect of infant feeding on the risk of obesity across the life course: A quantitative review of published evidence. Pediatrics 115:1367-1377, 2005.
48. Gluckman PD, Hanson MA: Mismatch: Why Our World No Longer Fits Our Bodies. Oxford, UK, Oxford University Press, 2006.
49. Barker DJP, Osmond C, Forsen TJ, et al: Trajectories of growth among children who have coronary events as adults. N Engl J Med 353:1802-1809, 2005.
50. Bhargava SK, Sachdev HS, Fall CH, et al: Relation of serial changes in childhood body-mass index to impaired glucose tolerance in young adulthood. N Engl J Med 350:865-875, 2004.
51. Hovi P, Andersson S, Eriksson JG, et al: Glucose regulation in young adults with very low birth weight. N Engl J Med 356:2053-2063, 2007.
52. Ong KK, Petry CJ, Emmett PM, et al: ALSPAC Study Team: Insulin sensitivity and secretion in normal children related to size at birth, postnatal growth, and plasma insulin-like growth factor-I levels. Diabetologia 47:1064-1070, 2004.
53. Law CM, Shiell AW, Newsome CA, et al: Fetal, infant, and childhood growth and adult blood pressure: A longitudinal study from birth to 22 years. Circulation 105:1088-1092, 2002.
54. Langley-Evans SC: Fetal programming of cardiovascular function through exposure to maternal undernutrition. Proc Nutr Soc 60:505-513, 2001.
55. Dodic M, Abouantoun T, O'Conor A, et al: Programming effects of short prenatal exposure to dexamethasone in sheep. Hypertension 40:729-734, 2002.
56. Seckl JR: Prenatal glucocorticoids and long-term programming. Eur J Endocrinol 151:U49-62, 2004.
57. Matthews SG: Early programming of the hypothalamo-pituitary axis. Trends Endocrinol Metab 13:373-380, 2002.
58. Mildenhall LFJ, Battin MR, Morton SMB, et al: Exposure to repeat doses of antenatal glucocorticoids is associated with altered cardiovascular status after birth. Arch Dis Child Fetal Neonatal Ed 91:F56-60, 2006.
59. Dalziel SR, Lim VK, Lambert A, et al: Antenatal exposure to betamethasone: Psychological functioning and health related quality of life 31 years after inclusion in randomised controlled trial. BMJ 331:665, 2005.
60. Dalziel SR, Walker NK, Parag V, et al: Cardiovascular risk factors after antenatal exposure to betamethasone: 30-year follow-up of a randomised controlled trial. Lancet 365:1856-1862, 2005.
61. de Kloet ER, Sibug RM, Helmerhorst FM, Schmidt M: Stress, genes and the mechanism of programming the brain for later life. Neurosci Biobehav Rev 29:271-281, 2005.
62. Igosheva N, Klimova O, Anishchenko T, Glover V: Prenatal stress alters cardiovascular responses in adult rats. J Physiol 2004:557:273-285.
63. Van den Bergh BR, Mulder EJ, Mennes M, Glover V: Antenatal maternal anxiety and stress and the neurobehavioural development of the fetus and child: Links and possible mechanisms—A review. Neurosci Biobehav Rev 29:237-258, 2005.
64. Bertram CE, Hanson MA: Animal models and programming of the metabolic syndrome. Br Med Bull 60:103-121, 2001.
65. McMillen IC, Robinson JS: Developmental origins of the metabolic syndrome: Prediction, plasticity, and programming. Physiol Rev 85:571-633, 2005.
66. Armitage J, Taylor P, Poston L: Experimental models of developmental programming: Consequences of exposure to an energy rich diet during development. J Physiol 565:3-8, 2005.
67. Vickers MH, Breier BH, Cutfield WS, et al: Fetal origins of hyperphagia, obesity, and hypertension and postnatal amplification by hypercaloric nutrition. Am J Physiol Endocrinol Metab 279:E83-87, 2000.
68. Jackson AA, Dunn RL, Marchand MC, et al: Increased systolic blood pressure in rat induced by a maternal low-protein diet is reversed by dietary supplementation with glycine. Clin Sci 103:633-639, 2002.
69. Brawley L, Torrens C, Anthony FW, et al: Glycine rectifies vascular dysfunction induced by dietary protein imbalance during pregnancy. J Physiol 554:497-504, 2004.
70. Torrens C, Brawley L, Anthony FW, et al: Folate supplementation during pregnancy improves offspring cardiovascular dysfunction induced by protein restriction. Hypertension 47:982-987, 2006.
71. Vickers MH, Gluckman PD, Coveny AH, et al: Neonatal leptin treatment reverses developmental programming. Endocrinology 146:4211-4216, 2005.
72. Kwong WY, Wild AE, Roberts P, et al: Maternal undernutrition during the pre-implantation period of rat development causes blastocyst abnormalities and programming of postnatal hypertension. Development 127:4195-4202, 2000.
73. Watkins AJ, Platt D, Papenbrock T, et al: Mouse embryo culture induces changes in postnatal phenotype including raised systolic blood pressure. Proc Natl Acad Sci U S A 104:5449-5454, 2007.
74. Allen C, Reardon W: Assisted reproduction technology and defects of genomic imprinting. BJOG 112:1589-1594, 2005.
75. Waterland RA, Jirtle RL: Early nutrition, epigenetic changes at transposons and imprinted genes, and enhanced susceptibility to adult chronic diseases. Nutrition 20:63-68, 2004.
76. Lillycrop KA, Phillips ES, Jackson AA, et al: Dietary protein restriction of pregnant rats induces and folic acid supplementation prevents epigenetic modification of hepatic gene expression in the offspring. J Nutr 135:1382-1386, 2005.
77. Lillycrop KA, Slater-Jefferies JL, Hanson MA, et al: Induction of altered epigenetic regulation of the hepatic glucocorticoid receptor in the offspring of rats fed a protein-restricted diet during pregnancy suggests that reduced DNA methyltransferase-1 expression is involved in impaired DNA methylation and changes in histone modifications. Br J Nutr 97:1064-1073, 2007.
78. Burdge GC, Torren C, Phillips E, et al: Dietary protein restriction of pregnant rats in the F_0 generation induces altered methylation of hepatic gene promoters in the adult male offspring in the F_1 and F_2 generations. Br J Nutr 97:435-439, 2007.
79. Taylor PD, McConnell J, Khan IY, et al: Impaired glucose homeostasis and mitochondrial abnormalities in offspring of rats fed a fat-rich diet in pregnancy. Am J Physiol 288:R134-139, 2005.
80. Simmons RA, Suponitsky-Kroyter I, Selak MA: Progressive accumulation of mitochondrial DNA mutations and decline in mitochondrial function lead to beta-cell failure. J Biol Chem 280:28785-28791, 2005.
81. Aerts L, Holemans K, Van Assche FA: Maternal diabetes during pregnancy; consequences for the offspring. Diabetes Metab Rev 6:147-167, 1990.
82. Zambrano E, Martinez-Samayoa PM, Bautista CJ, et al: Sex differences in transgenerational alterations of growth and metabolism in progeny (F2) of female offspring (F1) of rats fed a low protein diet during pregnancy and lactation. J Physiol 566:225-236, 2005.
83. Luyckx VA, Brenner BM: Low birth weight, nephron number, and kidney disease. Kidney Int Suppl 97:S68-S77, 2005.
84. Moritz KM, Dodic M, Wintour EM: Kidney development and the fetal programming of adult disease. Bioessays 25:212-220, 2003.

85. Pham TD, MacLennan NK, Chiu CT, et al: Uteroplacental insufficiency increases apoptosis and alters p53 gene expression in the full-term IUGR rat kidney. Am J Physiol 285:R933-934, 2003.
86. Holness MJ, Langdown ML, Sugden MC: Early-life programming of susceptibility to dysregulation of glucose metabolism and the development of type 2 diabetes mellitus. Biochem J 349:657-665, 2000.
87. McMillen C, Adam CL, Muhlhausler BS: Early origins of obesity: Programming the appetite regulatory system. J Physiol 565:9-17, 2005.
88. Terroni PL, Anthony FW, Hanson MA, Campanang FR: Expression of agouti-related peptide, neuropeptide Y, pro-opiomelanocortin and the leptin receptor isoforms in fetal mouse brain from pregnant dams on a protein restricted diet. Brain Res Mol Brain Res 140:111-115, 2005.
89. Kramer MS, Kakuma R: Energy and protein intake in pregnancy. Cochrane Database Syst Rev (4):CD000032, 2003.
90. Hodnett ED, Fredericks S: Support during pregnancy for women at increased risk of low birthweight babies. Cochrane Database Syst Rev (3): CD000198, 2003.
91. Lu MC, Tache V, Alexander GR, et al: Preventing low birth weight: Is prenatal care the answer? J Matern Fetal Neonatal Med 13:362-380, 2003.
92. Fall CH, Yajnik CS, Rao S, et al: Micronutrients and fetal growth. Nutrition 133:1747S-1756, 2003.
93. Merialdi M, Carroli G, Villar J, et al: Nutritional interventions during pregnancy for the prevention or treatment of impaired fetal growth: An overview of randomised controlled trials. J Nutr 133:1626S-1631, 2003.
94. Rao S, Yajnik CS, Kanade A, et al: Intake of micronutrient-rich foods in rural Indian mothers is associated with the size of their babies at birth: The Pune Maternal Nutrition Study. J Nutr 131:1217-1224, 2001.
95. Villamor E, Cnattingius S: Interpregnancy weight change and risk of adverse pregnancy outcomes: A population-based study. Lancet 368:1164-1170, 2006.
96. Cooper C, Westlake S, Harvey N, et al: Review: Developmental origins of osteoporotic fracture. Osteoporosis Int 17:337-347, 2006.
97. Harvey NC, Poole JR, Javaid MK, et al: SWS Study Group: Parental determinants of neonatal body composition. J Clin Endocrinol Metab 92:523-526, 2007.
98. Hales CN, Barker DJ: Type 2 (non-insulin-dependent) diabetes mellitus: The thrifty phenotype hypothesis. Diabetologia 35:595-601, 1992.
99. Gluckman PD, Hanson MA: Living with the past: Evolution, development and patterns of disease. Science 305:1733-1736, 2004.
100. Norman JF, LeVeen RE: Maternal atherogenic diet in swine is protective against early atherosclerotic development in offspring consuming an atherogenic diet post-natally. Atherosclerosis 157:41-47, 2001.
101. Khan I, Dekou V, Hanson M, et al: Predictive adaptive responses to maternal high-fat diet prevent endothelial dysfunction but not hypertension in adult rat offspring. Circulation 110:1097-1102, 2004.
102. Jasienska G, Thune I, Ellison PT: Fatness at birth predicts adult susceptibility to ovarian suppression: An empirical test of the Predictive Adaptive Response hypothesis. Proc Natl Acad Sci U S A 103:12759-12762, 2006.

Chapter 12

Fetal Cardiovascular Physiology

Jeffrey R. Fineman, MD, and Ronald Clyman, MD

Blood Flow Patterns and Oxygen Delivery

In the mammalian adult, oxygenation occurs in the lungs, and oxygenated blood returns via the pulmonary veins to the left side of the heart to be ejected by the left ventricle into the systemic circulation. In the fetus, gas exchange occurs in the placenta, and the fetal lungs are nonfunctional as far as the transfer of oxygen and carbon dioxide is concerned. For oxygenated blood derived from the placenta to reach the systemic circulation, the fetal circulation is so arranged that several sites of intercommunication (shunts) are present. In addition, preferential flow and streaming occur to limit the disadvantages of intermixing the oxygenated and deoxygenated blood that returns to the heart. The patterns of blood flow to and from the fetal heart are shown diagrammatically in Figure 12-1. With fetal stress, these preferential streaming patterns may be modified even more to mitigate the adverse effects of disorders such as reduced umbilical blood flow and fetal hypoxemia. Little quantitative information regarding primate fetal circulation is available; the data presented here were obtained mainly from fetal lambs.

Venous Return to the Heart

About 40% of total fetal cardiac output (thus about 200 mL/kg of fetal bodyweight per minute) is distributed to the placental circulation; a similar amount returns to the heart via the umbilical venous system. Because umbilical venous blood is the most highly oxygen-saturated blood in the fetal circulation, distribution of umbilical venous return is most important in determining oxygen delivery to fetal tissues. After entering the intra-abdominal portion of the umbilical vein, a portion of umbilical venous blood flow supplies the liver; the remainder passes through the ductus venosus, which directly connects the umbilical vein–portal sinus confluence to the inferior vena cava (see Fig. 12-1). Unlike the umbilical and portal veins, the ductus venosus has no direct branches to the liver. Umbilical venous blood can enter the ductus venosus directly. Portal venous return, however, can reach the ductus venosus only through the portal sinus.[1] Approximately 50% of umbilical blood flow passes through the ductus venosus; the remainder enters the hepatic-portal venous system and passes through the hepatic vasculature.[2]

The fetal liver receives its blood supply not only from the umbilical vein but also from the portal vein and hepatic artery. In normal fetal lambs in utero, umbilical venous blood flow contributes approximately 75% to 80% of total blood supply of the liver.[2-4] Portal venous blood flow accounts for about 15%, and hepatic arterial blood flow from the aorta represents only 4% to 5%. The blood from these sources is distributed differently to the various parts of the liver. Hepatic arterial blood flow to the liver is equally distributed to the right and left lobes, but the left lobe is supplied almost exclusively (>95%) by umbilical venous blood. In contrast, the right lobe receives both umbilical venous blood (approximately 60%) and portal venous blood (approximately 30%). Because umbilical venous blood supplies a major portion of flow to the right liver lobe by traversing the portal sinus, little if any portal venous blood reaches the ductus venosus. The blood in the ductus venosus, therefore, has pH, blood gas values, and hemoglobin oxygen saturation values similar to those of umbilical venous blood. The portion of umbilical venous blood flow that passes via the ductus venosus directly into the inferior vena cava meets the systemic venous drainage from the lower body.

Blood flow through the thoracic inferior vena cava represents approximately 65% to 70% of venous return to the heart; flow from the ductus venosus accounts for about one third of this.[2,5] The two streams (one from the abdominal inferior vena cava and one from the ductus venosus) do not mix, and they demonstrate definite streaming in the thoracic inferior vena cava; the well-oxygenated blood derived from the ductus venosus occupies the dorsal and leftward portion of the inferior vena cava.[6] This separation of the more highly saturated umbilical venous stream and the desaturated inferior vena caval stream returning from the lower body produces preferential flow of umbilical venous return into the left atrium and then into the left ventricle and ascending aorta.[6-8] Of particular importance is preferential streaming of umbilical venous blood to the brain and myocardium.

The preferential streaming of umbilical venous return to the left lobe of the liver and portal venous return to the right lobe also affects the distribution of oxygenated blood to the fetal body. The left hepatic lobe is perfused with umbilical venous blood, which has an oxygen saturation of 80% to 85%; the right lobe is perfused by a mixture of umbilical and portal venous blood, which has a much lower oxygen saturation (approximately 35%). The oxygen saturation of blood in the hepatic veins reflects this difference in perfusion saturation.[1,4] The oxygen saturation in left hepatic venous blood is about 10% lower than that in umbilical venous blood but about 10% higher than that in right hepatic venous blood, in which the saturation more closely approximates that in the descending aorta.

In fetal lambs, the ductus venosus and left hepatic vein drain into the inferior vena cava, essentially at a common point; partial valves are seen over the entrance of the hepatic vein and ductus venosus into the

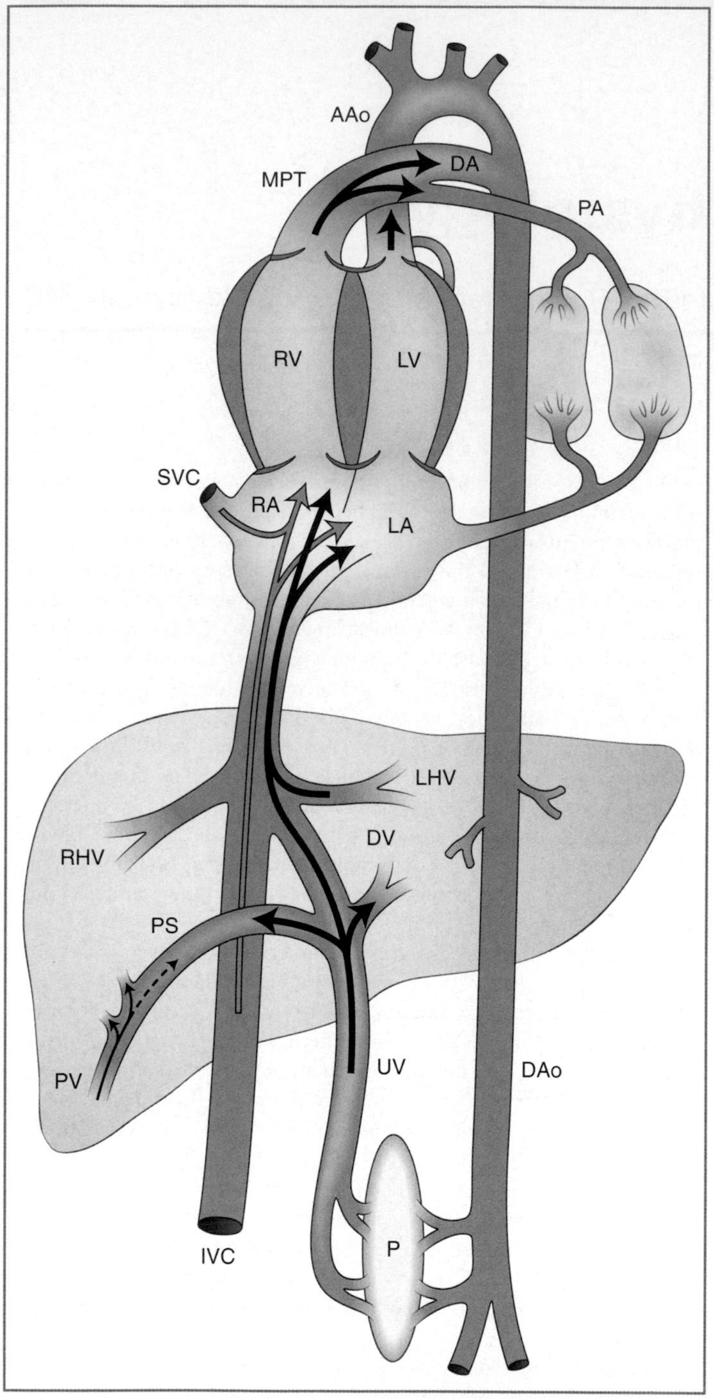

FIGURE 12-1 Diagrammatic representation of the normal fetal circulation and major fetal blood flow patterns. AAo, ascending aorta; DA, ductus arteriosus; DAo, descending aorta; DV, ductus venosus; IVC, inferior vena cava; LA, left atrium; LHV, left hepatic vein; LV, left ventricle; MPT, main pulmonary trunk; P, placenta; PA, main branch pulmonary arteries; PS, portal sinus; PV, portal vein; RA, right atrium; RHV, right hepatic vein; RV, right ventricle; SVC, superior vena cava; UV, umbilical vein.

inferior vena cava.[1] Similarly, the entrance of the right hepatic vein into the inferior vena cava has a valvelike membrane overlying the ostium. This arrangement probably allows left hepatic venous blood to be distributed in a manner similar to that of ductus venosus blood, whereas right hepatic venous blood is distributed similarly to the abdominal inferior vena caval stream. This is particularly important because about half of umbilical venous return passes through the liver, thereby accounting for about 20% of total venous return to the heart. In fetal lambs, left hepatic venous blood flow follows the same pattern as ductus venosus flow, with preferential streaming to the brain and heart.[4] Similarly, right hepatic blood flow follows the distribution pattern of abdominal inferior vena caval blood flow.

The inferior vena caval blood then enters the right atrium, and because of the position of the foramen ovale, more preferential streaming occurs. The foramen ovale is situated low in the interatrial septum, close to the inferior vena cava. The cephalad margin of the foramen, formed by the lower margin of the septum secundum, lies on the right side of the atrial septum; it is called the crista dividens and is positioned so that it overrides the orifice of the inferior vena cava. The crista dividens therefore splits the inferior vena caval bloodstream into an anterior and rightward stream that enters the right atrium, and a posterior and leftward stream that passes through the foramen ovale into the left atrium. It is this latter stream that has the more highly saturated blood returning from the umbilical circulation through the ductus venosus and left hepatic lobe. Despite this anatomic arrangement and the preferential streaming in the inferior vena cava, some mixing of blood does occur; a portion of the more highly saturated umbilical venous blood passes directly into the right atrium, and some desaturated abdominal inferior vena caval blood passes into the left atrium. The net result, however, is still a significantly higher saturation in the left atrium than in the right (Fig. 12-2).

Blood returning to the heart via the superior vena cava also streams preferentially once it reaches the right atrium. The crista interveniens, situated in the posterolateral aspect of the right atrial wall, effectively directs superior vena caval blood toward the tricuspid valve. The coronary sinus, which drains blood from the left ventricular myocardium, enters the right atrium between the crista dividens and the tricuspid valve; the very desaturated coronary venous return (saturation approximately 20%) is therefore also preferentially directed toward the tricuspid valve. This preferential streaming of superior vena caval and coronary sinus venous return to the right ventricle is also advantageous in the fetal circulation, because this very desaturated blood is preferentially directed toward the placenta for reoxygenation. Pulmonary venous return to the heart enters the left atrium, where it mixes with the portion of inferior vena caval blood that has crossed the foramen ovale to enter the left atrium.

Approximately 65% of total cardiac output reaches the lower body and placenta and returns via the thoracic inferior vena cava to the heart. Of this inferior vena caval return, approximately 40% crosses the foramen ovale to the left atrium; the remaining 60% enters the right ventricle across the tricuspid valve. The amount of inferior vena caval return crossing the foramen ovale therefore represents about 27% of total fetal cardiac output. This blood then combines with pulmonary venous return (approximately 8% of total fetal cardiac output) and represents the output of the left ventricle, or approximately 35% of total fetal cardiac output. The venous return from the superior vena cava, the coronary sinus, and the remainder of the inferior vena caval return (approximately 40% of total fetal cardiac output) enters the right ventricle and represents the portion of total fetal cardiac output ejected by the right ventricle (approximately 65% of total fetal cardiac output).

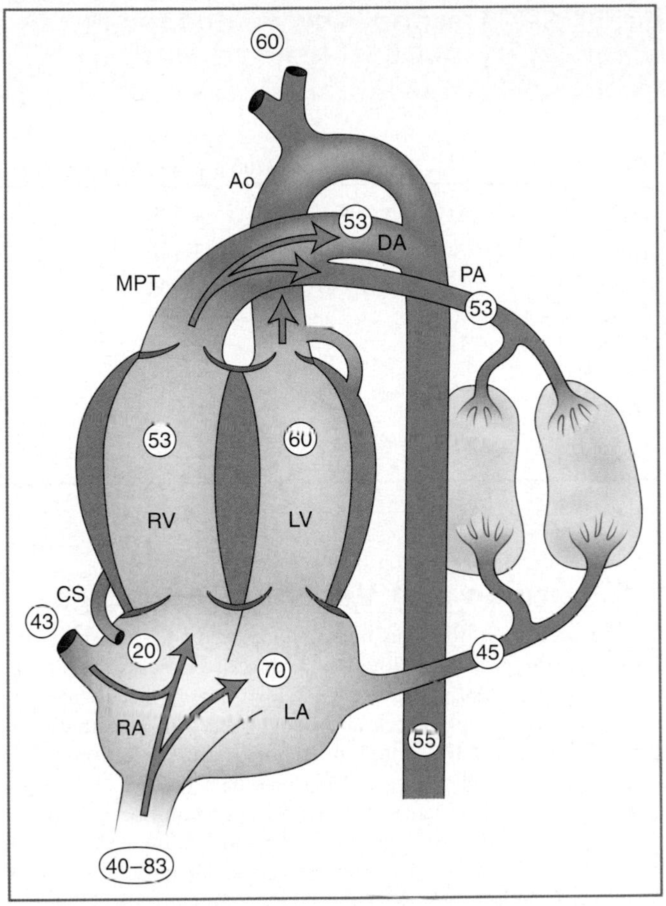

FIGURE 12-2 Hemoglobin oxygen saturation. Representative normal hemoglobin oxygen saturation data (*circled numbers* indicate percent saturation) in the heart and major vascular channels in fetal lambs. Ao, aorta; CS, coronary sinus; DA, ductus arteriosus; LA, left atrium; LV, left ventricle; MPT, main pulmonary trunk; PA, main branch pulmonary arteries; RA, right atrium; RV, right ventricle.

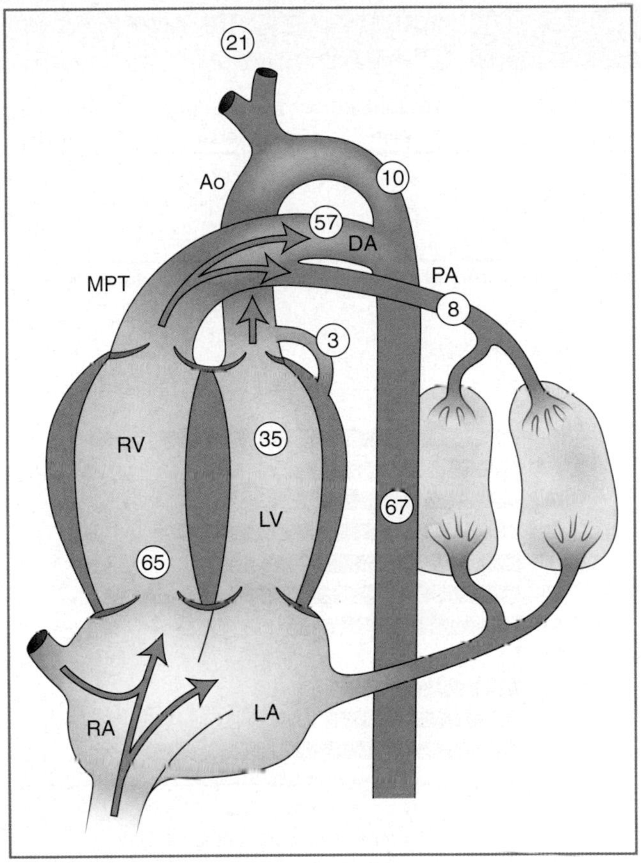

FIGURE 12-3 Cardiac output leaving the heart. Representative normal values for percentages (*circled numbers*) of total cardiac output (combined ventricular output) ejected by the heart and passing through the major arteries leaving the heart in fetal lambs. Ao, aorta; DA, ductus arteriosus; LA, left atrium; LV, left ventricle; MPT, main pulmonary trunk; PA, main branch pulmonary arteries; RA, right atrium; RV, right ventricle.

Cardiac Output and Its Distribution

In the fetus, because of the blood flow across the ductus arteriosus into the descending aorta, lower body organs are perfused by both the right and left ventricles (across the aortic isthmus). For this reason and because of intracardiac shunting, it is customary to consider fetal cardiac output as being the total output of the heart, or the combined ventricular output. In fetal lambs, this is about 450 mL/kg/min. Unlike in the adult, and because of the various sites of intracardiac and extracardiac shunting, the left and right ventricles in the fetus do not eject in series and therefore do not need to have the same stroke volume. In fact, as shown in Figure 12-3, the right ventricle ejects approximately two thirds of total fetal cardiac output (approximately 300 mL/kg/min), whereas the left ventricle ejects only a little more than one third (approximately 150 mL/kg/min).[9]

Echocardiographic studies in human pregnancy have suggested that in humans also, the right ventricle dominates the left.[10-14] Of the 65% of cardiac output ejected by the right ventricle, only a small amount (8%) flows through the pulmonary arteries to the lungs. The remainder (57%) crosses the ductus arteriosus and enters the descending aorta. Because right ventricular output contains all superior vena caval and coronary sinus return, it allows this unoxygenated venous blood to be preferentially returned to the placenta. Left ventricular output (approximately 35% of cardiac output) enters the ascending aorta; in the fetal lamb, approximately 21% reaches the brain, head, upper limbs, and upper thorax. About 10% of cardiac output traverses the aortic isthmus and joins the blood flowing across the ductus arteriosus to perfuse the descending aorta.

The level of hemoglobin oxygen saturation in the ventricles and great arteries is determined by the streaming patterns into, through, and out of the fetal heart. The highly saturated umbilical venous return streams preferentially across the foramen ovale into the left atrium, where it mixes with the relatively small amount of desaturated blood returning from the pulmonary veins. The net result is that blood ejected by the left ventricle to the ascending aorta is relatively well oxygenated (saturation about 60%). On the other hand, the extremely desaturated coronary sinus venous return and the desaturated blood returning from the brain and upper body flow almost exclusively across the tricuspid valve into the right ventricle. This blood mixes with the inferior vena caval stream, which is primarily composed of desaturated blood returning from the lower body but also contains some umbilical venous return. The net result is that the oxygen saturation of blood in the right ventricle is lower than that in the left. This blood perfuses the fetal lungs and traverses the ductus arteriosus to the descending aorta, from which it perfuses lower body organs and reaches the placenta for reoxygenation.

TABLE 12-1 NORMAL FETAL pH AND BLOOD GAS DATA

	Umbilical Vein	Descending Aorta	Ascending Aorta
pH	7.40-7.43	7.36-7.39	7.37-7.40
Po_2 (mm Hg)	28-32	20-23	21-25
Pco_2 (mm Hg)	38-42	43-48	41-45

Pco_2, partial pressure of carbon dioxide; Po_2, partial pressure of oxygen.

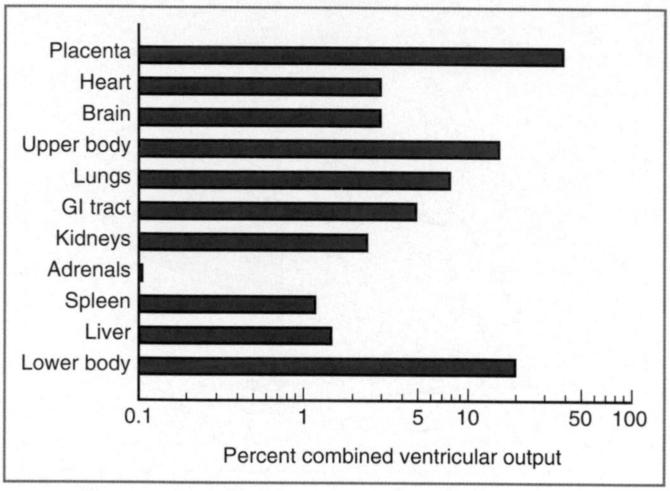

FIGURE 12-4 Cardiac output to organs. Representative normal values for the percentages of total cardiac output (combined ventricular output) distributed to different organs or parts in fetal lambs. GI, gastrointestinal.

Blood gas and pH values in the fetus also reflect the preferential streaming patterns. The data shown in Table 12-1 represent values usually found in healthy catheterized fetal animals. Both daily variability and variability between animals are seen. During a normal uterine contraction, arterial blood has a lower partial pressure of oxygen than under truly resting conditions. In addition, during the last 7 to 10 days of gestation, partial pressure of oxygen declines slightly and partial pressure of carbon dioxide increases commensurately.

The distribution of blood flow to individual organs is shown in Figure 12-4. Because arterial blood supply to lower body organs is derived from both the left and right ventricles, it is customary to express organ flow as a percentage of the combined output of both ventricles (i.e., the combined ventricular output), and the values shown in Figure 12-4 are typical.[5,15] These values remain fairly constant throughout the last third of gestation, the period in which such measurements have been made. There is, however, a slight increase in the percentage of combined ventricular output distributed to the heart, brain, and gastrointestinal tract in the 10 days before parturition. The flow distributed to the lungs increases from approximately 4% to 8% of combined ventricular output between 125 and 130 days (0.85) of gestation. Organ blood flows are shown in Table 12-2. Umbilical placental blood flow, like combined ventricular output, is usually not considered in relationship to placental weight, which is quite variable, but rather is expressed in relationship to fetal weight. Placental blood flow is approximately 200 mL/kg/min.

TABLE 12-2 BLOOD FLOW TO ORGANS IN NORMAL, NEAR-TERM FETAL LAMBS

Organ	Blood Flow (mL/100 g organ weight/min)
Heart	180
Brain	125
Upper body	25
Lungs	100
Gastrointestinal tract	70
Kidneys	150
Adrenals	200
Spleen	200
Liver (hepatic arterial)	20
Lower body	25

Intracardiac and Vascular Pressures

Vascular pressure in the fetus reflects the preferential streaming patterns described previously. Although the ductus venosus is a fairly large and widely dilated structure, there is a high flow returning from the placenta through the umbilical veins, and therefore this structure offers some resistance to flow. Umbilical venous pressure is generally 3 to 5 mm Hg higher than that in the inferior vena cava (Fig. 12-5). Right atrial pressure is also higher than left atrial pressure because of the greater volume of flow through the right atrium. Although the ductus arteriosus is widely patent, it too offers a small resistance to flow. Therefore, systolic pressures in the main pulmonary trunk and the right ventricle are slightly higher (1 to 2 mm Hg) than those in the aorta and left ventricle.

The representative pressure data shown in Figure 12-5 would be expected in a fetus close to term. Arterial pressures increase slowly and progressively over the last third of gestation, reaching these values shortly before parturition. Measurement of intravascular pressures in the fetus reflects the additional amniotic pressure not found after birth. Because intra-amniotic pressure is used as the zero reference point, the values presented exclude this additional pressure and are therefore true vascular pressures.

Myocardial Function

Cardiac output is determined by the interrelationships of preload, afterload, myocardial contractility, and heart rate. Preload (ventricular filling pressure) reflects the initial muscle length, which by the Frank-Starling principle influences the development of myocardial force. Afterload (the impedance to ejection from the ventricles) is reflected basically by arterial pressure. Contractility reflects the intrinsic inotropic capability of the myocardium.

Studies of fetal myocardium show immaturity of structure, function, and sympathetic innervation relative to the adult.[16-20] At all muscle lengths along the curve of length versus tension, the active tension generated by fetal myocardium is lower than that generated by adult myocardium.[16] In addition, resting, or passive, tension is higher in fetuses than in adults, suggesting lower compliance of fetal myocardium.

Studies in chronically instrumented intact fetal lambs showed that after volume loading by the infusion of blood or saline, the right

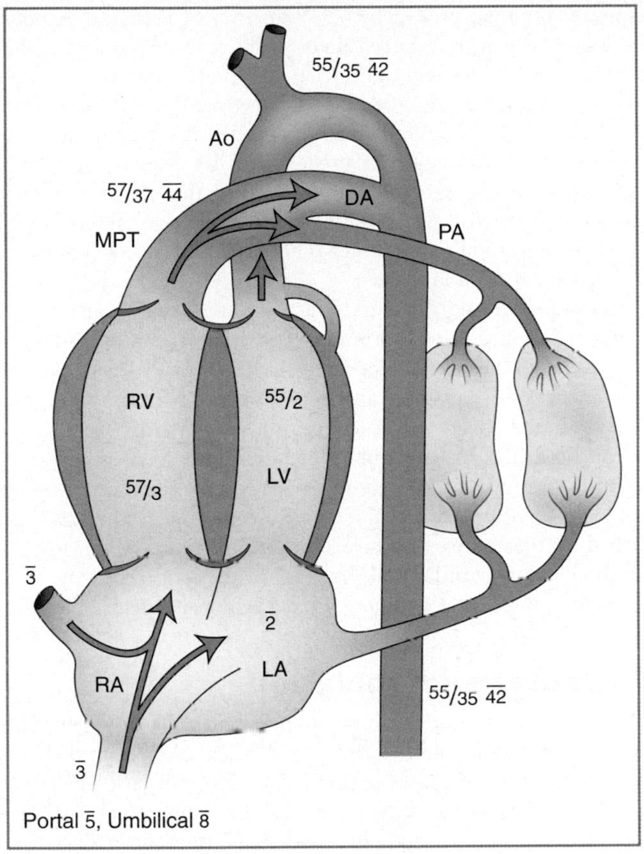

FIGURE 12-5 Normal vessel and chamber pressures. Representative normal pressures in millimeters of mercury (mm Hg) in various vessels and cardiac chambers in fetal lambs. (Measurements given as systolic pressure/diastolic pressure; ¯ indicates mean pressure.) Ao, aorta; DA, ductus arteriosus; LA, left atrium; LV, left ventricle; MPT, main pulmonary trunk; PA, main branch pulmonary arteries; RA, right atrium; RV, right ventricle.

ventricle is unable to increase stroke work or output to the same extent as in the adult.[17] This is particularly true in less-mature fetuses, in whom right ventricular end-diastolic pressure is markedly elevated without any obvious change in right ventricular stroke work. Similar results are found for both the left and right ventricles but with some ability to increase output or work at lower pressures, between 2 and 5 mm Hg.[18-20] Limitations in stroke work increase with increasing filling pressure have been shown to be afterload dependent and, for the left ventricle, are probably affected by right ventricular mechanical constraint.[21,22]

Fetal and adult sarcomeres have equivalent lengths,[23] but there are major ultrastructural differences between fetal myocardium and adult myocardium. The diameter of the fetal cells is smaller and, perhaps more importantly, the proportion of noncontractile mass (i.e., of nuclei, mitochondria, and surface membranes) to the number of myofibrils is significantly greater than in the adult. In the fetal myocardium, only about 30% of the muscle mass consists of contractile elements; in the adult, the proportion is about 60%. These ultrastructural differences are probably responsible for the age-dependent differences in performance.[16]

In newborn lambs, stroke volume is decreased at afterload levels considered low for adult animals.[24] Gilbert[20] showed that in fetal animals, an increase in arterial pressure of about 15 mm Hg, produced by methoxamine infusion, depresses the cardiac function curve so that cardiac output averages 25% to 30% less than normal. The extent of shortening is less in the fetus at any level of tension than in the adult—a potential explanation for the effects of afterload on stroke volume.[16]

In chronically instrumented fetal lambs, there is a close relationship between cardiac output and heart rate. Spontaneous and induced changes in heart rate are associated with corresponding changes in left or right ventricular output. Increasing heart rate from the resting level of about 180 up to 250 to 300 beats/min increases cardiac output 15% to 20%. Likewise, decreasing heart rate below the resting level significantly decreases ventricular output.

The fetal heart normally appears to operate near the top of its cardiac function curve. An increase in heart rate results in only a modest increase in output; however, bradycardia can reduce output significantly. At an atrial filling pressure of greater than approximately 8 mm Hg, there is little or no increase in output because the length-to-tension relationship has reached a plateau. In addition, the fetal heart is sensitive to changes in afterload.

Sympathetic and Parasympathetic Innervation

Isolated fetal cardiac tissue has a lower threshold of response to the inotropic effects of norepinephrine than does adult cardiac tissue and is more sensitive to norepinephrine throughout dose-response curves.[16] Because isoproterenol, a direct β-adrenergic agonist that is not taken up and stored in sympathetic nerves, has similar effects on fetal and adult myocardium, the supersensitivity of fetal myocardium to norepinephrine is probably the result of incomplete development of sympathetic innervation in fetal myocardium. Myocardial concentrations of norepinephrine in the fetus within several weeks of term are significantly lower than in newborn animals, and activity of tyrosine hydroxylase, the intraneuronal enzyme responsible for the first transformation in catecholamine biosynthesis, is also reduced.[16] In contrast, adrenal gland tyrosine hydroxylase activity at the same gestational age is not suppressed, possibly because the decrease in myocardial activity is related to delayed sympathetic innervation rather than to a generalized immaturity.

Monoamine oxidase, the enzyme responsible for oxidative deamination of norepinephrine, is also present in lower concentrations in the fetal heart than in the adult. Histochemical evaluation of the development of sympathetic innervation using the monoamine fluorescence technique has further substantiated the delayed development of sympathetic innervation of the fetal myocardium. At term, sympathetic innervation is incomplete. Patterns of staining indicate a progression of innervation, starting at the area of the sinoatrial node and progressing toward the left ventricular apex.[25,26]

Although sympathetic nervous innervation appears to begin developing in the fetal heart by about 0.55 of gestation, β-adrenergic receptors seem to be present much earlier and can be stimulated by appropriate agonists before 0.4 of gestation.[27] Before about 0.55 of gestation (80 days of gestation in the lamb), fetal myocardium may be affected by circulating catecholamines, but local reflex activity through the sympathetic nervous system is not likely to play a major role in circulatory regulation.

Vagal stimulation at about 0.85 of gestation produces bradycardia. Administering atropine at 0.55 of gestation produces a modest increase in fetal heart rate,[28] indicating that vagal innervation is present by this stage of development. Histochemical staining for acetylcholinesterase in close-to-term fetuses has shown that the concentrations of this enzyme, which is responsible for metabolism of acetylcholine, are similar to those found in adults.

Energy Metabolism

In the normal unstressed fetus, myocardial blood flow is about 180 mL/min/100 g tissue, approximately 80% more than in the adult. Fetal myocardial oxygen consumption, as measured in the left ventricular free wall, is about 400 mM/100 g/min, similar to that in the adult. In adult sheep, free fatty acids provide the major source of energy for the myocardium, and carbohydrate accounts for only about 40% of myocardial oxygen consumption.[29] In fetal sheep under normal conditions, however, free fatty acid concentrations are extremely low, and almost all the oxygen consumed can be accounted for by carbohydrate metabolism—glucose for 33%, pyruvate for 6%, and lactate for 58% of the oxygen consumed by the left ventricular free wall.

ATPase activity in fetal myocardium is equal to that in adult myocardium, suggesting that energy utilization by the contractile apparatus is similar in fetal and adult myocardium.[16] Mitochondria from fetal myocardium demonstrate higher oxidative phosphorylation than those from adult myocardium. The higher oxygen consumption in fetal mitochondria uncoupled by deoxyribonucleoprotein suggests that the augmented respiratory rate in mitochondria is a reflection of increased electron transport.[16] This is consistent with the greater cytochrome oxidase activity in fetal mitochondria.

Control of the Cardiovascular System

Maintenance of normal cardiovascular function, blood pressure, heart rate, and distribution of blood flow represents a complex interrelationship between local vascular and reflex effects. These effects are initiated by the stimulation of various receptors, and they are mediated through the autonomic nervous system as well as through hormonal influences. Although some information is available about how these mechanisms affect the circulation after stress, little is known about their role in normal fetal cardiovascular homeostasis. To complicate the situation, other factors, such as sleep state, electrocortical activity, and uterine activity, transiently affect the circulation. As a result, this area of fetal physiology is difficult to study and the data are difficult to interpret.

Local Regulation

As the oxygen content of blood perfusing the fetus falls, blood flow to the brain, myocardium, and adrenal gland increases; on the other hand, pulmonary blood flow falls as oxygen content decreases. Local effects of changes in oxygen environment are less clearly established for other organs.

Many adult organs exhibit autoregulation, the ability to maintain constant blood flow over a fairly wide range of perfusion pressures. In the fetus, the umbilical-placental circulation does not exhibit autoregulation, and blood flow changes in relation to changes in arterial perfusion pressure.[30] On the other hand, the cerebral circulation in fetal lambs does show autoregulatory capability.[31]

Baroreflex Regulation

In chronically instrumented fetal lambs, the fetal heart rate slows after an acute increase in systemic arterial pressure.[32,33] This baroreflex response, although present by 0.55 (80 days) of gestation, is poorly developed early on, but the sensitivity of the reflex to induced changes in pressure increases with advancing gestation. Carotid denervation partially inhibits the response, and combined carotid and aortic denervation abolishes it. Parasympathetic blockade with atropine also abolishes the reflex. Although the existence of the arterial baroreflex is established, Dawes and associates[34] suggested that the threshold for fetal baroreflex activity is above the range of the normal fetal arterial blood pressure and that this reflex is not important in controlling cardiovascular function in utero.

Carotid sinus and vagus nerve activity are synchronous with the arterial pulse, suggesting continuous baroreceptor activity.[35,36] Marked fluctuations in the arterial blood pressure and heart rate are observed after sinoaortic denervation, although the average arterial blood pressure and heart rate are not different from those in controls.[37]

The baroreflex in fetal animals requires fairly marked changes in pressures to produce relatively minor responses. Sinoaortic denervation increases heart rate and blood pressure variability, however. Under normal circumstances, therefore, baroreceptor function acts to stabilize the heart rate and blood pressure. In the fetus, as in the adult, baroreflex control is also influenced by hormonal systems.[38]

Chemoreflex Regulation

In general, chemoreceptor stimulation by sodium cyanide injection induces hypertension and bradycardia.[39,40] Central or carotid chemoreceptor stimulation causes hypertension and mild tachycardia with increased respiratory activity, whereas aortic chemoreceptor stimulation produces bradycardia with modest increases in arterial blood pressure. Because the carotid chemoreceptors are less sensitive than the aortic chemoreceptors, hypertension and bradycardia usually result. In chronically instrumented fetal lambs, sodium cyanide produces bradycardia with variable blood pressure changes, responses abolished by sinoaortic denervation.[41] Fetal hypoxia produces bradycardia and hypertension, which are abolished by carotid sinus denervation.[42]

Autonomic Nervous System and Adrenal Medulla

As described earlier, sympathetic innervation of the heart is not complete until term or, in some species, until after delivery. In contrast, cholinergic innervation, as measured by the presence of acetylcholinesterase, appears to be fully developed during fetal life. The innervation of other vascular beds also appears to proceed at different rates during gestation.[43]

Adrenergic receptors are present in the fetus and have been demonstrated in myocardium.[44-46] Receptor populations that have been studied in the fetus exhibit characteristics similar to those in adults.[47,48] The fetus possesses mature adrenergic receptors fairly early in gestation, but the concentration of receptors is different from that in adult organs.[44] The fetal concentration of receptors can be altered by administering thyroid hormone or isoxsuprine to the mother.

Injecting cholinergic or adrenergic agonists into fetal sheep produces responses at as early as 0.4 (60 days) of gestation.[27,49] α-Adrenergic stimulation with methoxamine produces an increase in arterial blood pressure, a small decrease in cardiac output, an increase in blood flow to the lungs, and a marked decrease in kidney and peripheral blood flow at as early as 0.5 of gestation. β-Adrenergic stimulation by isoproterenol causes a response earlier in gestation and an increase in heart rate with little or no change in arterial blood pressure and cardiac output. Blood flow to both the myocardium and the lungs is increased. Administration of acetylcholine decreases blood pressure and heart rate and increases pulmonary blood flow markedly, particularly in fetuses close to term.

Although receptor affinity is well developed during fetal life, the response to a specific agonist is blunted relative to the adult. The maximal constrictor response to norepinephrine or nerve stimulation increases throughout the latter part of gestation, and even more after birth.[50] The increase might result from gestational differences in neurotransmitter release in the fetus. During the last trimester of gestation, there is a progressive increase in maximal pressor response to ephedrine, which exerts its effect indirectly through neurotransmitter release; phenylephrine has a direct pressor effect.[51] In addition, neurotransmitter reuptake in sympathetic nerve terminals is not fully mature in the fetus.[48] Similarly, the differences between fetal and adult myocardium with respect to threshold and sensitivity to norepinephrine indicate an immature reuptake mechanism for norepinephrine in the fetus.[16]

As gestation progresses, these variable rates of maturation of different components of the autonomic nervous system modify control mechanisms relating to the autonomic nervous system. The role of β-adrenergic stimulation in resting circulatory regulation has been evaluated by pharmacologic blockade of β-adrenergic receptors with propranolol. This component of the sympathetic nervous system exerts a positive influence over fetal heart rate that first appears at about 0.6 (80 to 90 days) of gestation,[28] but this influence is relatively small.[52] During stress such as hypoxia or hemorrhage, however, β-adrenergic activity appears to be increased because propranolol produces much greater changes in heart rate.

α-Adrenergic control of the circulation has a somewhat clearer developmental pattern. α-Adrenergic blockade with phentolamine or phenoxybenzamine reduces arterial blood pressure very little, if at all, before 0.75 (100 to 110 days) of gestation; thereafter, there is a progressive increase in response, indicating a progressive increase in resting vascular tone attributed to α-adrenergic nervous activity. The parasympathetic nervous system exerts an inhibitory influence over fetal heart rate that is present by 0.55 (80 days) of gestation.[28,52] Parasympathetic blockade with atropine produces small changes at this age, with a progressive increase in parasympathetic control as gestation advances. After approximately 0.85 (120 to 130 days) of gestation, no further increase is evident.

Hypoxemia or asphyxia increases circulating plasma catecholamine concentrations in fetal sheep.[53-55] In fetuses younger than about 120 days' gestation, when the adrenal gland becomes innervated, extremely low fetal blood oxygen concentrations are required to stimulate the adrenal gland; thereafter, catecholamine secretion can be induced by more moderate hypoxemia.[53] Infusing catecholamines to reach plasma concentrations that mimic those observed during hypoxemia produces circulatory changes similar to those seen during hypoxemia.[56] Adrenal medullary responses to stress appear to play a role in circulatory adjustments; whether catecholamine secretion exerts a continuous regulatory function is not clear.

Hormonal Regulation of the Circulation Renin-Angiotensin System

The renin-angiotensin system is important in regulating the normal fetal circulation and its response to hemorrhage. The juxtaglomerular apparatus in the kidneys is well developed in fetuses and is present by 0.6 (90 days) of gestation.[57] Plasma renin activity, as well as circulating angiotensin II, is present in fetal plasma as early as about 0.6 (90 days) of gestation.[58-60] The effects of fetal stress such as hemorrhage and hypoxia on the renin-angiotensin system are not absolutely clear. In some studies, small amounts of hemorrhage increase plasma renin activity[57,58]; other studies, however, have shown little effect.[61] Similarly, the effects of hypoxemia on the renin-angiotensin system in the fetus are controversial, but most likely hypoxemia is of little consequence.

When angiotensin II is infused to achieve plasma concentrations similar to those that occur after a moderate (15% to 20%) hemorrhage, there are broad cardiovascular effects.[62] Arterial blood pressure increases markedly, and after an initial abrupt bradycardia, heart rate increases. Combined ventricular output increases, as does blood flow to the lungs and myocardium. Renal blood flow decreases, but umbilical placental flow is unchanged; this latter phenomenon indicates vascular constriction in the umbilical-placental circulation because arterial blood pressure increases but flow does not. The increase in myocardial blood flow is probably caused by an increase in stroke work, and the large increase in pulmonary blood flow probably reflects the release of some other local pulmonary vasodilating substance, such as one of the prostaglandins.[63]

Inhibiting the action of angiotensin II by specific inhibitors, such as saralasin, has somewhat variable effects. In unstressed fetal animals, however, generally a fall in mean arterial pressure and a slight decrease in heart rate occur.[59] Combined ventricular output is unaltered, but umbilical-placental blood flow falls, probably in association with the fall in systemic arterial pressure. Blood flow to the peripheral tissues, adrenal glands, and myocardium increases. During hemorrhage, the effects of saralasin are markedly accentuated and result in profound hypotension and bradycardia.

Under normal resting conditions, endogenous angiotensin II appears to exert a tonic vasoconstriction on the peripheral vascular bed, thereby maintaining systemic arterial blood pressure and umbilical-placental blood flow. In response to hemorrhage, angiotensin II is released and produces more vasoconstriction in the periphery, as well as other cardiovascular effects, thereby maintaining systemic arterial blood pressure and umbilical blood flow.

Vasopressin

Arginine vasopressin (antidiuretic hormone) has been detected at as early as 0.4 (60 days) of gestation in fetal lambs.[64] Although hypoxia and hemorrhage, as well as many other stimuli such as hypotension and hypernatremia, induced a marked increase in plasma vasopressin concentrations,[64,65] it is unlikely that vasopressin plays a major role in normal circulatory regulation. Maximal antidiuresis in adults occurs with vasopressin concentrations that have no discernible effects on systemic blood pressure. Fetal vasopressin concentrations are below this level.

Infusing vasopressin into fetal sheep to produce concentrations similar to those observed during fetal hypoxemia produces hypertension and bradycardia.[60] Combined ventricular output decreases slightly, but the proportion distributed to the gastrointestinal tract and peripheral circulations falls, whereas that to the umbilical-placental, myocardial, and cerebral circulations increases. These findings indicate that vasopressin probably participates in fetal circulatory responses to stress not only directly but also by enhancing pressor responses to other vasoactive substances. Under resting conditions, however, vasopressin apparently has little regulatory function.

Natriuretic Peptides

Atrial natriuretic peptide (ANP) and B-type natriuretic peptide (BNP), belong to a potent volume-regulating family of cardiac hormones released from the atria and ventricles in response to myocyte stretch, and other stimuli such as α-agonist stimulation, endothelin 1 (ET-1), and cytokines.[66] These peptides have potent vasodilatory, diuretic, natriuretic, and growth inhibitory actions via the secondary messenger cGMP. The natriuretic system appears to be functional by mid gestation, and it is able to regulate systemic and pulmonary blood pressures as well as salt and water balance in the fetus. In addition, these peptides are regulated during heart development, suggesting an important role for the natriuretic peptides in the developing cardiovascular system. Finally, both ANP and BNP have potent vasodilating properties in the placenta and thus may be important regulators of placental blood flow.[67,68]

Arachidonic Acid Metabolites

Although prostaglandins generally are locally active substances that do not normally circulate in adult blood, relatively high concentrations do normally circulate in the fetus.[69,70] It is likely that these prostaglandins are derived from the placenta. The fetal vasculature is also capable of producing prostaglandins, and the umbilical vessels, ductus arteriosus, and aorta produce significant amounts of prostaglandin E and prostacyclin (also known as prostaglandin I_2 [PGI_2]).

Prostaglandins administered to the fetus have diverse and extensive cardiovascular effects. Prostaglandin E_1 (PGE_1) and prostaglandin E_2 (PGE_2) constrict the umbilical-placental circulation.[71,72] Prostaglandin $F_{2\alpha}$ and thromboxane also cause constriction, whereas PGI_2 dilates the umbilical-placental circulation. PGE_1, PGE_2, PGI_2, and prostaglandin D_2 produce pulmonary vasodilatation in the fetus, whereas prostaglandin $F_{2\alpha}$ produces constriction.[73] Infusing PGE_1 into fetal sheep has no effect on cardiac output or systemic pressure, but in addition to a reduction in umbilical-placental blood flow, there are increases in flow to the myocardium, adrenals, gastrointestinal tract, and peripheral tissues.[74]

Of great interest is the role of prostaglandins in maintaining patency of the ductus arteriosus in the fetus. Circulating prostaglandins, as well as PGE_2 and PGI_2 produced locally in the ductus arteriosus, play a major role in maintaining the ductus arteriosus in a dilated state in utero.[75-77] For details of the overall physiologic regulation of the ductus arteriosus (see Ductus Arteriosus, later).

The role of endogenous prostaglandin production in regulating other fetal vascular beds has been elucidated by administering inhibitors of prostaglandin synthesis to the fetus. Although PGE_2 produces umbilical-placental vasoconstriction, inhibition of prostaglandin synthesis has little effect on umbilical-placental vascular resistance, suggesting that prostaglandins do not normally regulate the umbilical-placental circulation. When prostaglandin synthesis is inhibited, the proportion of blood flow to the gastrointestinal tract, kidneys, and peripheral circulation decreases, indicating an increase in vascular resistance in these tissues. Vascular resistances to other tissues are essentially unchanged.

Although prostaglandins do not appear to be central to regulation of the resting fetal pulmonary circulation, PGI_2 may act to modulate tone and thereby maintain pulmonary vascular resistance relatively constant. However, leukotrienes, also metabolites of arachidonic acid and potent smooth muscle constrictors, may play an active role in maintenance of the normally high fetal pulmonary vascular resistance. In newborns,[78] leukotriene inhibition attenuates hypoxic pulmonary vasoconstriction. In fetal lambs, leukotriene receptor blockade[79] or synthesis inhibition[80] increases pulmonary blood flow about eightfold, suggesting a role for leukotrienes in the maintenance of the normally high fetal pulmonary vascular resistance; the presence of leukotrienes in fetal tracheal fluid further supports this.[81]

Endothelial-Derived Factors and Endothelin

In addition to PGI_2, vascular endothelial cells can be stimulated to produce other important vasoactive factors, including potent vasoconstrictors, such as endothelin, and potent vasodilators, such as endothelium-derived nitric oxide (EDNO).[82] EDNO is produced by most endothelial cells in response to various stimuli, generally involving specific receptors or changes in shear stress; smooth muscle relaxation is produced through several messenger systems, such as guanylyl cyclase/cyclic guanosine monophosphate, K channels, or PGI_2/cyclic adenosine monophosphate. In the fetus, EDNO is produced by umbilical vascular endothelium[83,84]; nitroso compounds reduce umbilical vascular resistance in vitro,[85] and EDNO modulates resting umbilical vascular tone in fetal sheep in utero.[86] Disturbances in normal EDNO production may also be involved in the genesis of preeclampsia.[87]

EDNO clearly is involved in regulation of vascular tone in the fetal pulmonary circulation, although it plays a far more important role in postnatal transition to air breathing.[88] Superfused fetal sheep pulmonary arteries release endothelium-derived relaxing factor when stimulated with bradykinin.[89] In fetal lambs, the vasodilating effects of bradykinin are attenuated by methylene blue and resting tone increases with Nω-nitro-L-arginine, an inhibitor of NO synthesis by NO synthase from precursor L-arginine,[90] suggesting that a cyclic guanosine monophosphate–dependent mechanism, such as EDNO production, continuously modulates or offsets the increased tone of the resting fetal pulmonary circulation. Inhibition of EDNO synthesis also blocks the pulmonary vasodilatation with oxygenation of fetal lungs in utero and markedly attenuates the increase in pulmonary blood flow with ventilation at birth.[90,91]

Endothelin 1, a 21-amino acid polypeptide, also produced by vascular endothelial cells, has potent vasoactive properties.[92] The hemodynamic effects of ET-1 are mediated by at least two distinct receptor populations, ET_A and ET_B, the densities of which are different depending on the vascular bed studied. The ET_A receptors are located on vascular smooth muscle cells and mediate vasoconstriction, whereas the predominant subpopulation of ET_B receptors is located on endothelial cells and mediates vasodilation.[93-95] However, a second subpopulation of ET_B receptors is located on smooth muscle cells and mediates vasoconstriction.[96] The vasodilating effects of ET-1 are associated with the release of NO and potassium channel activation.[97-101] The vasoconstricting effects of ET-1 are associated with phospholipase activation, the hydrolysis of phosphoinositol to inositol-1,4,5-triphosphate and diacylglycerol, and the subsequent release of Ca^{2+}.[102] In addition to its vasoactive properties, ET-1 has mitogenic activity on vascular smooth muscle cells and may participate in vascular remodeling.[103]

The predominant effect of exogenous ET-1 in the fetal and newborn sheep pulmonary circulation is vasodilation, mediated via ET_B receptor activation and NO release. However, the predominant effect in the juvenile and adult pulmonary circulations is vasoconstriction, mediated via ET_A receptor activation. In fetal lambs, selective ET_A receptor blockade produces small decreases in resting fetal pulmonary vascular resistance. This suggests a potential minor role for basal ET-1–induced vasoconstriction in maintaining the high fetal pulmonary vascular resistance.[98,100] Although plasma and urinary concentrations of ET-1 are increased at birth,[104,105] in vivo studies suggest that basal ET-1 activity does not play an important role in mediating the transitional pulmonary circulation.[106] ET-1 causes fetal renal vasodilation[107] and thus may be involved in the regulation of fetal renal blood flow.

Other factors, such as calcitonin gene–related peptide and a related substance, adrenomedullin, have vasodilatory effects on the fetal pulmonary circulation and too may play a role in the regulation of pulmonary vascular tone in the fetus.[108,109] The effects of these substances probably also are mediated by NO release.[110]

Ductus Arteriosus

Patency of the fetal ductus arteriosus is regulated by both dilating and contracting factors. The factors that promote ductus arteriosus constriction in the fetus have yet to be fully identified. The ductus arteriosus maintains a tonic degree of constriction in utero that appears to be both dependent and independent of extracellular calcium.[111] ET-1 also appears to play a role in producing the basal tone of the ductus arteriosus.[112]

The factors that oppose ductus arteriosus constriction in utero are better understood. The vascular pressure within the ductus arteriosus lumen opposes ductus arteriosus constriction.[113] Vasodilator prostaglandins appear to be the most important factors opposing ductus arteriosus constriction in the latter part of gestation.[111,114] Inhibitors of prostaglandin synthesis (e.g., indomethacin) constrict the fetal ductus arteriosus both in vitro and in vivo.[76,115,116] Their vasoconstrictive effects appear to be most pronounced beyond 30 weeks' gestation in humans. Both the cyclooxygenase-1 and cyclooxygenase-2 isoforms of cyclooxygenase are present within the fetal ductus arteriosus and are responsible for synthesizing the prostaglandins that maintain ductus arteriosus patency.[117] Inhibitors of both cyclooxygenase-1 and cyclooxygenase-2 will individually produce fetal ductus arteriosus constriction in vivo.[117] On the other hand, PGE_2 will dilate the constricted ductus arteriosus both in vitro and in vivo. PGE_2 produces ductus arteriosus relaxation by interacting with several of the PGE receptors (EP_2, EP_3, and EP_4).[118] The EP_4 receptor appears to play a prominent role in ductus arteriosus vasodilation.[119,120] NO also is made by the fetal ductus arteriosus and appears to play an important role in maintaining ductus arteriosus patency in rodent fetuses.[114] Although NO is also made in the ductus arteriosus of larger species, its importance in maintaining ductus arteriosus patency under normal conditions has not been conclusively demonstrated[121] (see next paragraph for the role in fetuses exposed to indomethacin tocolysis).

Although pharmacologic inhibition of prostaglandin synthesis produces ductus arteriosus constriction in utero, genetic interruptions of either prostaglandin synthesis (i.e., homozygous combined cyclooxygenase-1 and cyclooxygenase-2 knockout mice)[122] or signaling (i.e., homozygous EP_4 receptor knockout mice)[120] do not lead to ductus arteriosus constriction in utero. Contrary to expectations, both genetic interruptions produce newborn mice in which the ductus arteriosus fails to close after birth. The mechanisms through which the absence of prostaglandins early in gestation alter the normal balance of other vasoactive factors in the ductus arteriosus have yet to be elucidated. It is interesting to note that pharmacologic inhibition of prostaglandin synthesis in human pregnancy also is associated with an increased incidence of patent ductus arteriosus after birth.[123] When the fetus is exposed to indomethacin in utero, the ductus arteriosus constricts. Ductus arteriosus constriction in utero produces ischemic hypoxia, increased NO production, and smooth muscle cell death in the ductus arteriosus wall. These factors prevent the ductus arteriosus from constricting normally after birth and make it resistant to the constrictive effects of indomethacin administered postnatally.[124,125]

References

1. Bristow J, Rudolph AM, Itskovitz J: A preparation for studying liver blood flow, oxygen consumption, and metabolism in the fetal lamb in utero. J Dev Physiol 3:255, 1981.
2. Edelstone DI, Rudolph AM, Heymann MA: Liver and ductus venosus blood flows in fetal lambs in utero. Circ Res 42:426, 1978.
3. Edelstone DI, Rudolph AM, Heymann MA: Effects of hypoxemia and decreasing umbilical flow on liver and ductus venosus blood flows in fetal lambs. Am J Physiol 238:H656, 1980.
4. Bristow J, Rudolph AM, Itskovitz J, et al: Hepatic oxygen and glucose metabolism in the fetal lamb. J Clin Invest 71:1, 1983.
5. Rudolph AM, Heymann MA: Circulatory changes during growth in the fetal lamb. Circ Res 26:289, 1970.
6. Edelstone DI, Rudolph AM: Preferential streaming of ductus venosus blood to the brain and heart in fetal lambs. Am J Physiol 237:H724, 1979.
7. Behrman RE, Lees MH, Peterson EN, et al: Distribution of the circulation in the normal and asphyxiated fetal primate. Am J Obstet Gynecol 108:956, 1970.
8. Reuss ML, Rudolph AM, Heymann MA: Selective distribution of microspheres injected into the umbilical veins and inferior venae cavae of fetal sheep. Am J Obstet Gynecol 141:427, 1981.
9. Heymann MA, Creasy RK, Rudolph AM: Quantitation of blood flow patterns in the foetal lamb in utero. In Comline RS, Cross KW, Dawes GS, et al (eds): Proceedings of the Sir Joseph Barcroft Centenary Symposium: Foetal and Neonatal Physiology. Cambridge, Cambridge University Press, 1973.
10. Sahn DJ, Lange LW, Allen HD, et al: Quantitative real-time cross-sectional echocardiography in the developing normal human fetus and newborn. Circulation 62:588, 1980.
11. Reed KL, Meijboom EJ, Sahn DJ, et al: Cardiac Doppler flow velocities in human fetuses. Circulation 73:41, 1986.
12. DeSmedt MCH, Visser GHA, Meijboom EJ: Fetal cardiac output estimated by Doppler echocardiography during mid and late gestation. Am J Cardiol 60:338, 1987.
13. Rasanen J, Wood DC, Weiner S, et al: Role of the pulmonary circulation in the distribution of human fetal cardiac output during the second half of pregnancy. Circulation 94:1068, 1996.
14. Harada K, Rice MJ, Shiota T, et al: Gestational age- and growth-related alterations in fetal right and left ventricular diastolic filling patterns. Am J Cardiol 79:173, 1997.
15. Peeters LLH, Sheldon RE, Jones MD Jr, et al: Blood flow to fetal organs as a function of arterial oxygen content. Am J Obstet Gynecol 135:637, 1979.
16. Friedman WF: The intrinsic physiologic properties of the developing heart. In Friedman WF, Lesch M, Sonnenblick EH (eds): Neonatal Heart Disease. New York, Grune & Stratton, 1973.
17. Heymann MA, Rudolph AM: Effects of increasing preload on right ventricular output in fetal lambs in utero [abstract]. Circulation 48:IV-37, 1973.
18. Kirkpatrick SE, Pitlick PT, Naliboff JB, et al: Frank-Starling relationship as an important determinant of fetal cardiac output. Am J Physiol 231:495, 1976.
19. Gilbert RD: Control of fetal cardiac output during changes in blood volume. Am J Physiol 238:H80, 1980.
20. Gilbert RD: Effects of afterload and baroreceptors on cardiac function in fetal sheep. J Dev Physiol 4:299, 1982.
21. Hawkins J, Van Hare GF, Schmidt KG, et al: Effects of increasing afterload on left ventricular output in fetal lambs. Circ Res 65:127, 1989.
22. Teitel DF, Dalinghaus M, Cassidy SC, et al: In utero ventilation augments the left ventricular response to isoproterenol and volume loading in fetal sheep. Pediatr Res 29:466, 1991.
23. Sheldon CA, Friedman WF, Sybers HD: Scanning electron microscopy of fetal and neonatal lamb cardiac cells. J Mol Cell Cardiol 8:853, 1976.
24. Downing SE, Talner NS, Gardner TM: Ventricular function in the newborn lamb. Am J Physiol 208:931, 1965.
25. Friedman WF, Pool PE, Jacobowitz D, et al: Sympathetic innervation of the developing rabbit heart. Circ Res 23:25, 1968.
26. Lebowitz EA, Novick JS, Rudolph AM: Development of myocardial sympathetic innervation in the fetal lamb. Pediatr Res 6:887, 1972.

27. Barrett CT, Heymann MA, Rudolph AM: Alpha and beta adrenergic function in fetal sheep. Am J Obstet Gynecol 112:1114, 1972.
28. Vapaavouri EK, Shinebourne EA, Williams RL, et al: Development of cardiovascular responses to autonomic blockade in intact fetal and neonatal lambs. Biol Neonate 22:177, 1973.
29. Fisher DJ, Heymann MA, Rudolph AM: Myocardial oxygen and carbohydrate consumption in fetal lambs in utero and in adult sheep. Am J Physiol 238:H399, 1980.
30. Berman W Jr, Goodlin RC, Heymann MA, et al: Pressure-flow relationships in the umbilical and uterine circulations of the sheep. Circ Res 38:262, 1976.
31. Papile L, Rudolph AM, Heymann MA: Autoregulation of cerebral blood flow in the preterm fetal lamb. Pediatr Res 19:159, 1985.
32. Shinebourne EA, Vapaavouri EK, Williams RL, et al: Development of baroreflex activity in unanesthetized fetal and neonatal lambs. Circ Res 31:710, 1972.
33. Maloney JE, Cannata JP, Dowling MH, et al: Baroreflex activity in conscious fetal and newborn lambs. Biol Neonate 31:340, 1977.
34. Dawes GS, Johnston BM, Walker DW: Relationship of arterial pressure and heart rate in fetal, newborn, and adult sheep. J Physiol (Lond) 309:405, 1980.
35. Biscoe TJ, Purves MJ, Sampson SR: Types of nervous activity which may be recorded from the carotid sinus nerve in the sheep foetus. J Physiol (Lond) 202:1, 1969.
36. Ponte J, Purves MJ: Types of afferent nervous activity which may be measured in the vagus nerve of the sheep foetus. J Physiol (Lond) 229:51, 1973.
37. Itskovitz J, LaGamma EF, Rudolph AM: Baroreflex control of the circulation of chronically instrumented fetal lambs. Circ Res 52:589, 1983.
38. Segar JL: Ontogeny of the arterial and cardiopulmonary baroreflex during fetal and postnatal life. Am J Physiol 273:R457, 1997.
39. Dawes GS, Duncan LB, Lewis BV, et al: Cyanide stimulation of the systemic arterial chemoreceptors in foetal lambs. J Physiol (Lond) 201:117, 1969.
40. Goodlin RC, Rudolph AM: Factors associated with initiation of breathing. In Hodari AA, Mariona FG (eds): Proceedings of the International Symposium on Physiological Biochemistry of the Fetus. Springfield, IL, Charles C Thomas, 1972.
41. Itskovitz J, Rudolph AM: Denervation of arterial chemoreceptors and baroreceptors in fetal lambs in utero. Am J Physiol 242:H916, 1982.
42. Bartelds B, van Bel F, Teitel DF, et al: Carotid, not aortic, chemoreceptors mediate the fetal cardiovascular response to acute hypoxemia in lambs. Pediatr Res 34:51, 1993.
43. Zink J, Van Petten GR: Noradrenergic control of blood vessels in the premature lamb fetus. Biol Neonate 39:61, 1981.
44. Cheng JB, Cornett LE, Goldfien A, et al: Decreased concentration of myocardial alpha-adrenoceptors with increasing age in foetal lambs. Br J Pharmacol 70:515, 1980.
45. Cheng JB, Goldfien A, Cornett LE, et al: Identification of beta-adrenergic receptors using (3H)dihydroalprenolol in fetal sheep heart: Direct evidence of qualitative similarity to the receptors in adult sheep heart. Pediatr Res 15:1083, 1981.
46. Whitsett JA, Pollinger J, Matz S: β-Adrenergic receptors and catecholamine-sensitive adenylate cyclase in developing rat ventricular myocardium: Effect of thyroid status. Pediatr Res 16:463, 1982.
47. Nuwayhid B, Brinkman CR III, Su C, et al: Systemic and pulmonary hemodynamic responses to adrenergic and cholinergic agonists during fetal development. Biol Neonate 26:301, 1975.
48. Harris WH, Van Petten GR: Development of cardiovascular responses to noradrenaline, normetanephrine and metanephrine in the unanesthetised fetus. Can J Physiol Pharmacol 57:242, 1979.
49. Assali NS, Brinkman CR III, Woods JR Jr, et al: Development of neurohumoral control of fetal, neonatal, and adult cardiovascular functions. Am J Obstet Gynecol 129:748, 1977.
50. Wyse DG, Van Petten GR, Harris WH: Responses to electrical stimulation, noradrenaline, serotonin, and vasopressin in the isolated ear artery of the developing lamb and ewe. Can J Physiol Pharmacol 55:1001, 1977.
51. Harris WH, Van Petten GR: Development of cardiovascular responses to sympathomimetic amines and autonomic blockade in the unanesthetised fetus. Can J Physiol Pharmacol 56:400, 1978.
52. Walker AM, Cannata J, Dowling MH, et al: Sympathetic and parasympathetic control of heart rate in unanesthetised fetal and newborn lambs. Biol Neonate 33:135, 1978.
53. Comline RS, Silver IA, Silver M: Factors responsible for the stimulation of the adrenal medulla during asphyxia in the foetal lamb. J Physiol (Lond) 178:211, 1965.
54. Jones CT, Robinson RD: Plasma catecholamines in fetal and adult sheep. J Physiol (Lond) 248:15, 1975.
55. Lewis AB, Evans WN, Sischo W: Plasma catecholamine responses to hypoxemia in fetal lambs. Biol Neonate 41:115, 1982.
56. Lorijn RWH, Longo LD: Norepinephrine elevation in the fetal lamb: Oxygen consumption and cardiac output. Am J Physiol 239:R115, 1980.
57. Smith FG Jr, Lupu AN, Barajas L, et al: The renin-angiotensin system in the fetal lamb. Pediatr Res 8:611, 1974.
58. Broughton-Pipkin F, Lumbers ER, Mott JC: Factors influencing plasma renin and angiotensin II in the conscious pregnant ewe and its foetus. J Physiol (Lond) 243:619, 1974.
59. Iwamoto HS, Rudolph AM: Effects of endogenous angiotensin II on the fetal circulation. J Dev Physiol 1:283, 1979.
60. Iwamoto HS, Rudolph AM, Keil LC, et al: Hemodynamic responses of the sheep fetus to vasopressin infusion. Circ Res 44:430, 1979.
61. Robillard JE, Weitzman RE: Developmental aspects of the fetal renal response to exogenous arginine vasopressin. Am J Physiol 238:F407, 1980.
62. Iwamoto HS, Rudolph AM: Effects of angiotensin II on the blood flow and its distribution in fetal lambs. Circ Res 48:183, 1982.
63. Gryglewski RJ: The lung as a generator of prostacyclin. CIBA Found Symp 78:147, 1980.
64. Drummond WH, Rudolph AM, Keil LC, et al: Arginine vasopressin and prolactin after hemorrhage in the fetal lamb. Am J Physiol 238:E214, 1980.
65. Rurak DW: Plasma vasopressin levels during hypoxaemia and the cardiovascular effects of exogenous vasopressin in foetal and adult sheep. J Physiol (Lond) 277:341, 1978.
66. Levin ER, Gardner DG, Samson WK: Natriuretic peptides. N Engl J Med 339:321-328, 1998.
67. Cameron VA, Ellmers LJ: Minireview: Natriuretic peptides during development of the fetal heart and circulation. Endocrinology 144:2191-2194, 2003.
68. Walther T, Schultheiss HP, Tschope C, Stepan H: Natriuretic peptide system in fetal heart and circulation. J Hypertens 20:785-791, 2002.
69. Mitchell MD, Flint AP, Bibby J, et al: Plasma concentrations of prostaglandins during late human pregnancy: Influence of normal and preterm labor. J Clin Endocrinol Metab 46:947, 1978.
70. Challis JRG, Patrick JE: The production of prostaglandins and thromboxanes in the feto-placental unit and their effects on the developing fetus. Semin Perinatol 4:23, 1980.
71. Novy MJ, Piasecki G, Jackson BT: Effect of prostaglandins E2 and F2-alpha on umbilical blood flow and fetal hemodynamics. Prostaglandins 5:543, 1974.
72. Berman W Jr, Goodlin RC, Heymann MA, et al: Effects of pharmacologic agents on umbilical blood flow in fetal lambs in utero. Biol Neonate 33:225, 1978.
73. Cassin S: Role of prostaglandins, thromboxanes, and leukotrienes in the control of the pulmonary circulation in the fetus and newborn. Semin Perinatol 11:53, 1987.
74. Tripp ME, Heymann MA, Rudolph AM: Hemodynamic effects of prostaglandin E1 on lambs in utero. In Coceani F, Olley PM (eds): Prostaglandins and Perinatal Medicine. Advances in Prostaglandin and Thromboxane Research, vol 4. New York, Raven Press, 1978.

75. Olley PM, Bodach E, Heaton J, et al: Further evidence implicating E-type prostaglandins in the patency of the lamb ductus arteriosus. Eur J Pharmacol 34:247, 1975.
76. Clyman RI: Ontogeny of the ductus arteriosus response to prostaglandins and inhibitors of their synthesis. Semin Perinatol 4:115, 1980.
77. Clyman RI: Ductus arteriosus: Current theories of prenatal and postnatal regulation. Semin Perinatol 11:64, 1987.
78. Schreiber MD, Heymann MA, Soifer SJ: Leukotriene inhibition prevents and reverses hypoxic pulmonary vasoconstriction in newborn lambs. Pediatr Res 19:437, 1985.
79. Soifer SJ, Loitz RD, Roman C, et al: Leukotriene end-organ antagonists increase pulmonary blood flow in fetal lambs. Am J Physiol 249:H570, 1985.
80. LeBidois J, Soifer SJ, Clyman RI, et al: Piriprost: A putative leukotriene synthesis inhibitor increases pulmonary blood flow in fetal lambs. Pediatr Res 22:350, 1987.
81. Velvis H, Krusell J, Roman C, et al: Leukotrienes C4, D4, and E4 in fetal lamb tracheal fluid. J Dev Physiol 14:13, 1990.
82. Ignarro LJ: Biological actions and properties of endothelium-derived nitric oxide formed and released from artery and vein. Circ Res 65:1, 1989.
83. Van de Voorde J, Vanderstichele H, Leusen I: Release of endothelium-derived relaxing factor from human umbilical vessels. Circ Res 60:517, 1987.
84. Chaudhuri G, Buga GM, Gold ME, et al: Characterization and actions of human umbilical endothelium derived relaxing factor. Br J Pharmacol 102:331, 1991.
85. Myatt L, Brewer A, Brockman D: The action of nitric oxide in the perfused human fetal-placental circulation. Am J Obstet Gynecol 164:687, 1991.
86. Chang J-K, Roman C, Heymann MA: Effect of endothelium-derived relaxing factor inhibition on the umbilical-placental circulation in fetal lambs in utero. Am J Obstet Gynecol 166:727, 1992.
87. Pinto A, Sorrentino R, Sorrentino P, et al: Endothelial-derived relaxing factor released by endothelial cells of human umbilical vessels and its impairment in pregnancy-induced hypertension. Am J Obstet Gynecol 164:507, 1991.
88. Fineman JR, Soifer SJ, Heymann MA: Regulation of pulmonary vascular tone in the perinatal period. Annu Rev Physiol 57:115, 1995.
89. Glasgow RE, Heymann MA: Endothelium-derived relaxing factor as a mediator of bradykinin-induced perinatal pulmonary vasodilatation. Clin Res 38:211A, 1990.
90. Moore P, Velvis H, Fineman JR, et al: Endothelium derived relaxing factor inhibition attenuates the increase in pulmonary blood flow due to oxygen ventilation in fetal lambs. J Appl Physiol 73:2151, 1992.
91. Fineman JR, Wong J, Morin FC, et al: Chronic nitric oxide inhibition in utero produces persistent pulmonary hypertension in newborn lambs. J Clin Invest 93:2675, 1994.
92. Yanagisawa M, Kurihara H, Kimura S, et al: A novel potent vasoconstrictor peptide produced by vascular endothelial cells. Nature 332:411, 1988.
93. Arai H, Hori S, Aramori I, et al: Cloning and expression of a cDNA encoding an endothelin receptor. Nature 348:730, 1990.
94. Sakurai T, Yanagisawa M, Takuwa Y, et al: Cloning of a cDNA encoding a non-isopeptide-selective subtype of the endothelin receptor. Nature 348:732, 1990.
95. Wong J, Vanderford PA, Winters J, et al: Endothelin b receptor agonists produce pulmonary vasodilation in the intact newborn lamb with pulmonary hypertension. J Cardiovasc Pharm 25:207, 1995.
96. Shetty SS, Toshikazu O, Webb RL, et al: Functionally distinct endothelin B receptors in vascular endothelium and smooth muscle. Biochem Biophys Res Commun 191:459, 1993.
97. Cassin S, Kristova V, Davis T, et al: Tone-dependent responses to endothelin in isolated perfused fetal sheep pulmonary circulation in situ. J Appl Physiol 70:1228, 1991.
98. Ivy DD, Kinsella JP, Abman SH: Physiologic characterization of endothelin A and B receptor activity in the ovine fetal pulmonary circulation. J Clin Invest 93:2141, 1994.
99. Wong J, Vanderford PA, Fineman JR, et al: Endothelin-1 produces pulmonary vasodilation in the intact newborn lamb. Am J Physiol 265:H1318, 1993.
100. Wong J, Fineman JR, Heymann MA: The role of endothelin and endothelin receptor subtypes in regulation of fetal pulmonary vascular tone. Pediatr Res 35:664, 1994.
101. Wong J, Vanderford PA, Fineman JR, et al: Developmental effects of endothelin-1 on the pulmonary circulation in sheep. Pediatr Res 36:394, 1994.
102. La M, Reid JJ: Endothelin-1 and the regulation of vascular tone. Clin Exp Pharmacol Physiol 22:315, 1995.
103. Hassoun PM, Thappa V, Landman MJ, et al: Endothelin 1: Mitogenic activity on pulmonary artery smooth muscle cells and release from hypoxic endothelial cells. Proc Exp Bio Med 199:165, 1992.
104. Malamitsi-Puchner A, Economou E, Efstathopoulos T, et al: Endothelin 1-21 plasma concentrations on days 1 and 4 of life in healthy and ill preterm neonates. Biol Neonate 67:317, 1995.
105. Sulyok E, Ertl T, Adamovits K, et al: Urinary endothelin excretion in the neonate: Influence of maturity and perinatal pathology. Pediatr Nephrol 7:881, 1993.
106. Winters J, Wong J, Van Dyke D, et al: Endothelin receptor blockade does not alter the increase in pulmonary blood flow due to oxygen ventilation in fetal lambs. Pediatr Res 40:152, 1996.
107. Bogaert GA, Kogan BA, Mevorach RA, et al: Exogenous endothelin-1 causes renal vasodilation in the fetal lamb. J Urol 156:847, 1996.
108. DeVroomen M, Takahashi Y, Gournay V, et al: Adrenomedullin increases pulmonary blood flow in fetal sheep. Pediatr Res 41:493, 1997.
109. DeVroomen M, Takahashi Y, Roman C, et al: Calcitonin gene-related peptide increases pulmonary blood flow in fetal sheep. Am J Physiol 274:H277, 1998.
110. Takahashi Y, de Vrooman M, Roman C, et al: Mechanisms of calcitonin gene related peptide (CGRP)-induced increases of pulmonary blood flow in fetal sheep. Am J Physiol 279:H1654, 2000.
111. Kajino H, Chen YQ, Seidner SR, et al: Factors that increase the contractile tone of the ductus arteriosus also regulate its anatomic remodeling. Am J Physiol 281:R291, 2001.
112. Coceani F, Liu Y, Seidlitz E, et al: Endothelin A receptor is necessary for O_2 constriction but not closure of ductus arteriosus. Am J Physiol 277:H1521, 1999.
113. Clyman RI, Mauray F, Heymann MA, et al: Influence of increased pulmonary vascular pressures on the closure of the ductus arteriosus in newborn lambs. Pediatr Res 25:136, 1989.
114. Momma K, Toyono M: The role of nitric oxide in dilating the fetal ductus arteriosus in rats. Pediatr Res 46:311, 1999.
115. Sharpe GL, Larsson KS, Thalme B: Studies on closure of the ductus arteriosus: XII. In utero effects of indomethacin and sodium salicylate in rats and rabbits. Prostaglandins 9:585, 1975.
116. Heymann MA, Rudolph AM: Effects of acetylsalicylic acid on the ductus arteriosus and circulation in fetal lambs in utero. Circ Res 38:418, 1976.
117. Takahashi Y, Roman C, Chemtob S, et al: Cyclooxygenase-2 inhibitors constrict the fetal lamb ductus arteriosus both in vitro and in vivo. Am J Physiol 278:R1496, 2000.
118. Bouayad A, Kajino H, Waleh N, et al: Characterization of PGE_2 receptors in fetal and newborn lamb ductus arteriosus. Am J Physiol 280:H2342, 2001.
119. Smith GCS, Coleman RA, McGrath JC: Characterization of dilator prostanoid receptors in the fetal rabbit ductus arteriosus. J Pharmacol Exp Ther 271:390, 1994.
120. Nguyen M, Camenisch T, Snouwaert JN, et al: The prostaglandin receptor EP4 triggers remodelling of the cardiovascular system at birth. Nature 390:78, 1997.
121. Fox JJ, Ziegler JW, Dunbar DI, et al: Role of nitric oxide and cGMP system in regulation of ductus arteriosus tone in ovine fetus. Am J Physiol 271:H2638, 1996.

122. Loftin CD, Trivedi DB, Tiano HF, et al: Failure of ductus arteriosus closure and remodeling in neonatal mice deficient in cyclooxygenase-1 and cyclooxygenase-2. Proc Natl Acad Sci U S A 98:1059, 2001.
123. Norton ME, Merrill J, Cooper BAB, et al: Neonatal complications after the administration of indomethacin for preterm labor. N Engl J Med 329:1602, 1993.
124. Clyman RI, Chen YQ, Chemtob S, et al: In utero remodeling of the fetal lamb ductus arteriosus: The role of antenatal indomethacin and avascular zone thickness on vasa vasorum proliferation, neointima formation, and cell death. Circulation 103:1806, 2001.
125. Goldbarg SH, Takahashi Y, Cruz C, et al: In utero indomethacin alters O_2 delivery to the fetal ductus arteriosus: Implications for postnatal patency. Am J Physiol 282:R184, 2002.

Chapter 13

Behavioral State Activity and Fetal Health and Development

Bryan S. Richardson, MD, and Robert Gagnon, MD

Studies in human adults more than 50 years ago first demonstrated that sleep occurs in two distinct phases—rapid eye movements (REM) sleep and slow-wave sleep (SWS), or non-REM sleep—which are recognized by temporal patterns in various electrophysiologic and behavioral parameters. Since that time, much study has been directed at the nature of these so-called sleep states, including their physiologic correlates, control mechanisms, and possible function, and their use as an expression of neurodysfunction with apparent maldevelopment. Sleep states have been shown to exist in apparently healthy newborn infants, although they are not evident in preterm infants born much before 36 weeks of gestation.

Over the past 3 decades, the use of chronic catheterization techniques in fetal animals, primarily sheep, and the use of high-resolution ultrasound equipment for the study of the human fetus have firmly established the existence of activity or behavioral states in utero that have similarities to postnatal sleep states. From such study, it has become evident that fetal behavioral activities are important and necessary for normal growth and development of the lungs and musculoskeletal system. These activities also serve to characterize the healthy fetus, and they become altered when oxygenation is compromised, providing a basis for the use of activity parameters in the biophysical assessment of fetal health. Moreover, a developmental process is evident whereby the REM behavioral state predominates in early life, which may have functional importance for the growth and development of the brain.

Fetal Behavioral State Activity

Animal Studies

Studies involving chronic placement of electrodes and pressor sensors in unanesthetized fetal animals near term have identified the equivalents of behavioral or sleep states with similarities to those described after birth in neonates and adults. Most of these studies have involved the use of the chronic fetal sheep preparation, which has been the primary animal model for the study of fetal behavioral activity. Behavioral state classification is based for the most part on electrophysiologic recordings (electrocortical activity with an electrocorticogram [ECoG], electro-ocular activity with an electro-oculogram [EOG], and nuchal muscle activity with an electromyogram [EMG]) (Fig. 13-1), with the following states recognized[1-3]:

- High-voltage (HV) ECoG/NREM—high-voltage, low-frequency ECoG activity, eye movements absent, nuchal muscle tone mainly present
- Low-voltage (LV) ECoG/REM—low-voltage, high-frequency ECoG activity, rapid eye movements, nuchal muscle atonia
- Awake—low-voltage, high-frequency ECoG activity, eye movements present or absent, nuchal muscle tone present

The HV/NREM and LV/REM behavioral states described for the ovine fetus are directly comparable to these same states seen after birth and thus are seen to represent in utero sleep state activity.[1-3] The third behavioral state (wakefulness) can also be characterized using criteria used to identify postnatal wakefulness. Direct observations of exteriorized sheep fetuses, behavioral responses to external stimuli, and the different effects of evoked potentials in skeletal muscles provide further support for the existence of a fetal awake-like state.[1-4]

As seen with sleep state activity after birth, additional physiologic parameters are recorded as consistent concomitants to fetal behavioral state activity, although species differences may be evident. In the ovine fetus, rapid irregular breathing movements, as identified in recordings of tracheal pressure, occur only during the LV/REM state.[4] They are not continuous, however, as approximately one third of LV/REM time is not associated with breathing movements, and thus this parameter cannot be used as a criterion for defining the presence or absence of this state. Similarly, in the ovine fetus, wakefulness or arousal is generally associated with higher blood pressure and heart rate, whereas heart rate is lower during HV/NREM and further decreased during LV/REM, which is thought to be mediated by a decrease in sympathetic activity.[4-6] On the other hand, fetal heart rate variability is generally increased during LV/REM in association with the presence of breathing movements, and this can be attributed in part to a respiratory sinus arrhythmia.[4] In fetal sheep, episodes of repeated swallowing (resembling postnatal feeding episodes) and bladder contractions (indicative of bladder emptying) are also influenced by behavioral state. Near term, both of these activities mainly occur during LV ECoG activity in association with eye movements and increased nuchal muscle activity, suggesting a state of heightened arousal resembling wakefulness (Fig. 13-2).[7,8]

Detection of temporal patterns in individual state criteria as well as concomitant physiologic parameters, as noted, that are relatively

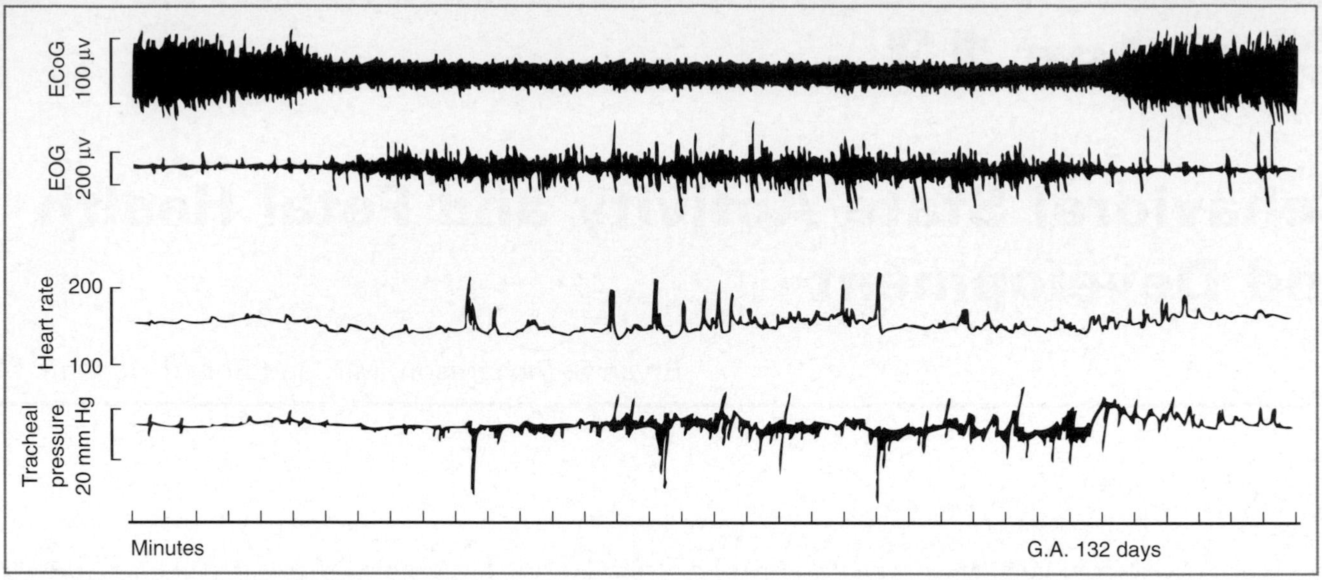

FIGURE 13-1 Electro-ocular activity and fetal breathing movements. Chart recording demonstrating that electro-ocular activity (EOG) and fetal breathing movements normally occur during times of low-voltage electrocortical activity (ECoG). G.A., gestational age.

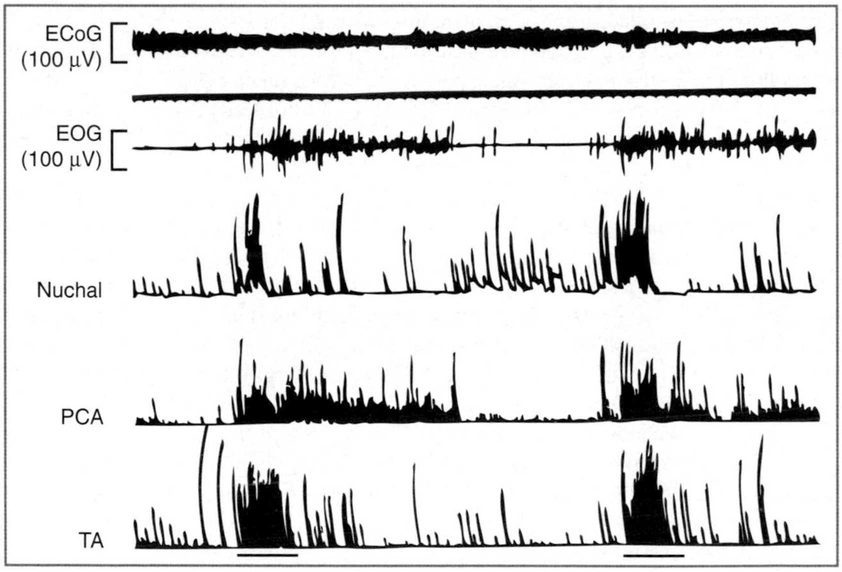

FIGURE 13-2 Phasic activity in the thyroarytenoid muscle. Chart recording demonstrating two bouts of swallowing *(underlined)* noted by the phasic activity in the thyroarytenoid (TA) muscle. Each bout occurs during low-voltage rapid eye movements (LV/REM) with phasic activity in the nuchal and posterior cricoarytenoid (PCA) muscles (the latter as a measure of breathing activity). Electromyographs of PCA, TA, and nuchal muscles are shown in an integrated form. ECoG, electrocorticogram; EOG, electro-oculogram. (From Harding R, Sigger JH, Poore ER, Johnson P: Ingestion in fetal sheep and its relation to sleep states and breathing movements. Q J Exp Physiol 69:477-486, 1984.)

stable and repeat over time provide evidence for the existence of fetal behavioral states in other animal species, including the rhesus monkey,[9] baboon,[10] and guinea pig.[11]

Human Studies

Body movement and heart rate patterns in the human fetus near term reveal a cyclicity which, by reference to postnatal patterns, appear to also have a state-related basis (Fig. 13-3). Initial studies used fetal body movements and heart rate patterns as scoring criteria for behavioral state assessment.[12,13] With improvement in real-time ultrasound imaging the scoring of fetal eye movements also became possible. One set of state definitions widely used is that introduced by Nijhuis et al.[14] based on parameters observed with ultrasound and the simultaneous recording of fetal heart rate patterns. Following the strategy used for the newborn infant by Prechtl et al.,[15] four distinct behavioral states were recognized from the stability of the temporal association of parameters over prolonged periods, and by the simultaneous changes in these parameters at state transition.

State 1F (fetal)—quiescence (occasional brief gross body movements), eye movements absent, fetal heart rate stable with a narrow oscillation bandwidth;

State 2F—frequent gross body movements, eye movements continually present, fetal heart rate with a wider oscillation bandwidth and frequent accelerations during body movements;

State 3F—no gross body movements, eye movements continually present, fetal heart rate stable but with a wider oscillation bandwidth than for state 1F;

State 4F—frequent and vigorous gross body movements, eye movements continually present, fetal heart rate unstable with large and long-lasting accelerations.

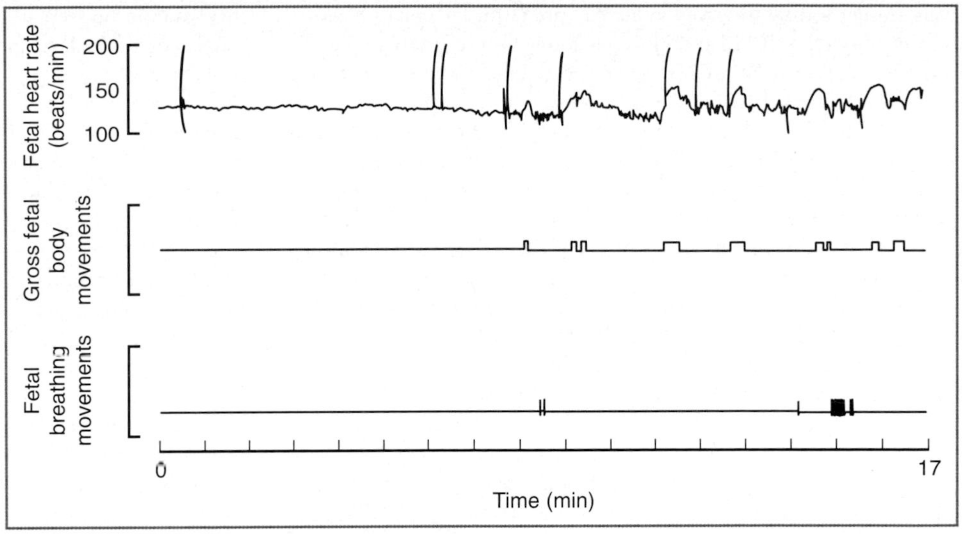

FIGURE 13-3 A chart recording of behavioral parameters from a healthy human fetus near term. For the first 8 minutes, there are no gross body movements and the heart rate pattern demonstrates no accelerations. From 8 to 17 minutes, a normal episode of gross body movements accompanied by accelerations in the heart rate occurs. (From Richardson BS, Campbell K, Carmichael L, Patrick J: Effects of external physical stimulation on fetuses near term. Am J Obstet Gynecol 139:344-352, 1981.)

When eye movements, body movements, and heart rate patterns are compared, states 1F and 2F are directly comparable to NREM or quiet sleep, and REM or active sleep, respectively, in the newborn. However, comparisons between fetal states 3 and 4 and postnatal states are less clear, as state 3F is seldom seen and the frequency of body movements for state 4F is somewhat less than that seen in active wakefulness after birth. Nonetheless, the behavioral response of the human fetus to external stimuli including vibroacoustic stimulation supports the existence of a fetal awake state near term[16,17] in keeping with comparable findings in the ovine fetus.

Additional behavioral parameters are evident as state-related concomitants, but are not continuously present and thus again are unsuitable for use as state-defining criteria. Fetal breathing movements are more regular during state 1F than 2F, while their incidence is increased during 2F.[18,19] Fetal micturition detected by ultrasound recognition of bladder emptying, while inhibited during episodes of low heart rate variation suggestive of state 1F, appears facilitated by a change to an episode of high heart rate variation with rapid eye movements and fetal breathing movements suggesting state 2F or possibly 4F.[20] Conversely, regular mouthing movements, as in the neonate, only occur during periods of quiescence and can be considered a concomitant for state 1F.[21]

Developmental Changes

The study of the temporal relationship between behavioral and physiologic parameters has firmly established not only the existence of behavioral states in the fetus, which are analogous to postnatal sleep states, but also developmental changes whose timing is species dependent and intricately linked to brain maturation.

For the ovine fetus (term, approximately 145 days), well-differentiated ECoG patterns are evident from approximately 120 days of gestation onward, with a temporal relationship to episodic muscle and breathing activity that is indicative of behavioral states.[3] Initially, there is a high proportion (>50%) of time in the LV/REM state, with approximately 40% of the time in the HV/NREM state and only brief periods of apparent wakefulness. Thereafter, there is a progressive decrease in the incidence of LV/REM, to approximately 40% by term, mainly because of an increase in periods of wakefulness, although HV/NREM is also increased.[3] Postnatally, there is a marked falloff in the incidence of LV/REM sleep, to less than 10%, again primarily because of an increase in time spent awake.[1,3] The durations of both HV/NREM and LV/REM also show a developmental increase with advancing gestation until a stable level is attained at 130 days.[3] At this time, the average duration of a sleep cycle is 20 minutes, with approximately 11 minutes in LV/REM and 8 minutes in HV/NREM, interspersed with brief periods of wakefulness lasting no more than 2 to 4 minutes.[3] The ovine fetus also has a cycling of behavioral parameters before the appearance of a differentiated ECoG, but these are not well synchronized, and episodic breathing and ocular movements are initially associated with increased, rather than decreased, activity in the neck muscles.[22]

The human fetus first demonstrates clearly defined behavioral states at approximately 36 weeks of gestation with stable alignment of behavioral parameters and synchrony of change at state transitions.[14] At this time, state 2F (or REM sleep) predominates, occurring approximately 40% of the time (Table 13-1). State 1F (or NREM sleep) occurs approximately 25% of the time, and state 4F (or wakefulness) occurs but briefly. Behavioral states cannot be identified approximately 20% of the time. With advancing gestation, the incidence of NREM sleep and wakefulness increases, that of the REM state remains little changed, whereas the percentage of time with no identifiable states decreases. This time course of behavioral state development in utero is qualita-

TABLE 13-1 COINCIDENCE* OF HUMAN FETAL STATES 1F AND 2F

	Gestational Age (wk)			
	25-30†	32‡	36‡	40‡
1F (%)	6	15	20	36
2F (%)	17	46	38	42
No coincidence (%)	77	29	22	9

*Shown as percentage of total recording time.
†Data (mean values) from Drogtrop AP, Ubels R, Nijhuis JG: The association between fetal body movements, eye movements and heart rate patterns in pregnancies between 25 and 30 weeks of gestation. Early Hum Dev 23:67-73, 1990.
‡Data (median values) from Nijhuis JG, Prechtl HFR, Martin CB Jr, Bots RS: Are there behavioural states in the human fetus? Early Hum Dev 6:177-195, 1982.

tively similar to that observed in healthy premature neonates.[15] Moreover, although the NREM and REM states are observed more frequently in the fetus at term (approximately 80%) than in the neonate during early infancy (approximately 70%), the ratio of these two states remains similar.[14,15] Before 36 weeks of gestation, periods of activity and quiescence are again evident, but although the coinciding behavioral parameters may mimic states, they lack stability in temporal relationship and synchrony of change at transition of states (see Table 13-1).[14,23] Of note, the duration of this activity-quiescence cycle also shows a maturational change, with a progressive increase from about 20 minutes at 28 weeks' gestation to about 60 minutes by term, and this length is similar to that of the REM-NREM cycle of the newborn infant.[14,15]

Observations on the maturation of ECoG patterns in utero or of behavioral state activity after birth provide insights into the development of sleep-wake states in other species. The organization of ECoG activity in the guinea pig fetus is similar to that in the ovine fetus, with the onset of cyclic differentiation occurring prenatally and with progressive maturation in ECoG waveforms thereafter.[11] Likewise, fetal baboons show well-differentiated ECoG patterns near term with maturational changes thereafter.[10] Newborn guinea pigs, monkeys, baboons, and sheep clearly demonstrate the behavioral state aspects of NREM sleep, REM sleep, and wakefulness at the time of birth.[1,10,11,24] On the other hand, the adult-like ECoG aspects of sleep and wakefulness are not fully developed until several postnatal days in the rat, rabbit, and cat, with an associated delay in the appearance of delineated sleep states.[25,26] Although comparison between the immature of several species of animals thus indicates considerable difference in the rate of development of sleep-wake patterns, all demonstrate a similarly high proportion of the REM state with the establishment of well-defined behavioral states.

Hypoxia and Intrauterine Growth Restriction

In the near-term ovine fetus, moderate hypoxemia of short-term duration[27] and prolonged and graded reductions in fetal oxygenation over several days[28] result in little change in ECoG activity until hypoxemia is severe enough to result in associated metabolic acidosis with a decrease in the incidence of the LV ECoG state, whereas forelimb, eye, and breathing movements are variably decreased with lesser degrees of hypoxemia (Fig. 13-4). This hierarchical response of fetal activities to hypoxia can be seen as protective, as ECoG activity that may have an impact on brain development (see later) is initially minimally changed, whereas movement activities that result in increased energy expenditure[29,30] are variably decreased. However, it should be noted that a marked decrease in fetal movement activity with chronic hypoxemia is also seen only at the level at which acidemia becomes apparent.[28] Thus, clinical assessment of fetal movement should be used as a marker for moderate to severe hypoxemic change.

Growth is known to account for a consequential fraction of the substrate consumption of fetal sheep near term.[31] With both prolonged reduction in fetal O_2 delivery over several days[32] and induced intrauterine growth restriction (IUGR),[33] total O_2 consumption by the fetus is reduced approximately 20%. This decrease in oxidative metabolism represents the energy savings from decreased tissue growth, but it also reflects, in part, changes in behavioral activity and associated energy requirements. Worthington and colleagues[34] studied the effects of reducing placental size in sheep with resultant asymmetrical IUGR and chronic hypoxemia without acidemia. The incidence of fetal breathing movements was marginally decreased to approximately 20% of the time, thereby providing a decrease in oxidative needs. However, there has been no similar study of the effects on ECoG activity, although these are likely to be minimal given the findings with induced hypoxemia of shorter duration.[27,28]

In human pregnancies with IUGR and presumed chronic fetal hypoxemia, the incidence of fetal breathing movements and gross body movements is generally decreased but appears to depend on the severity of the IUGR and the conditions of study.[35-40] Although the related decrease in energy expenditure is probably biologically important, there is considerable overlap with population norms, which limits the clinical usefulness of these movement parameters as markers for IUGR. When behavioral state organization was assessed in growth-restricted fetuses during the latter part of human pregnancy, little difference was noted in the incidence of the coincidence of states 1F and 2F when compared with that of appropriately grown fetuses.[41] This finding is similar to the ECoG findings in the ovine fetus with prolonged hypoxemia in the absence of any acidemia.[28] However, subtle differences are noted: IUGR fetuses show a delay in the appearance of well-delineated behavioral states with a lack of synchrony in parameter change at state transition and the interruption of stable associations by periods of no coincidence. This indicates that some aspects of central nervous system function are disturbed.[41,42]

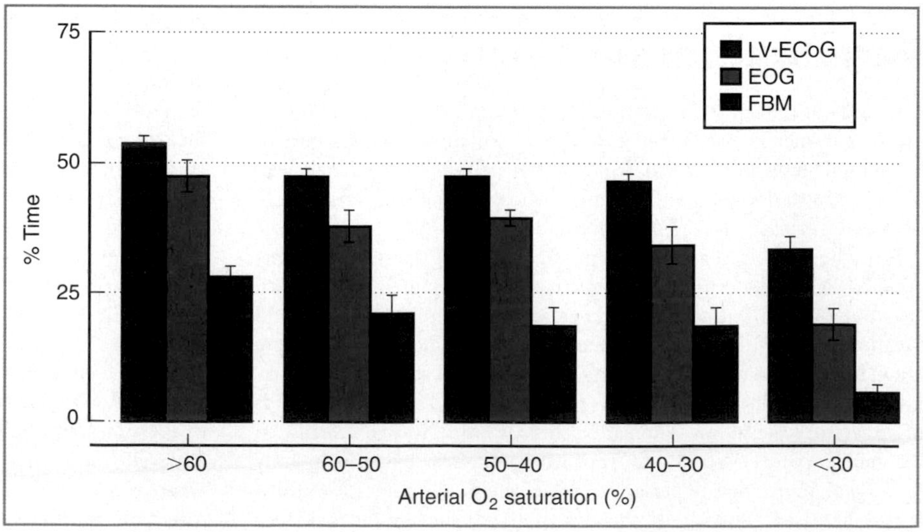

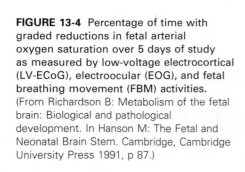

FIGURE 13-4 Percentage of time with graded reductions in fetal arterial oxygen saturation over 5 days of study as measured by low-voltage electrocortical (LV-ECoG), electroocular (EOG), and fetal breathing movement (FBM) activities. (From Richardson B: Metabolism of the fetal brain: Biological and pathological development. In Hanson M: The Fetal and Neonatal Brain Stem. Cambridge, Cambridge University Press 1991, p 87.)

Assessment of Fetal Health

Breathing Activity and Body Movements

The recognition of the presence of episodic fetal breathing movements (FBM) and gross fetal body movements (GFBM) in animal studies[4] and their subsequent inhibition by acute hypoxia[43] has formed the basis for using these biophysical parameters as part of an ultrasound-based assessment of fetal health (see Chapter 21). The resultant composite biophysical profile score includes markers of both acute and chronic fetal compromise. The markers for acute fetal compromise and fetal oxygenation include FBM, GFBM, fetal tone, and fetal heart rate (FHR) reactivity. Amniotic fluid volume is usually considered a marker of chronic fetal or placental compromise, although acute deterioration in amniotic fluid volume preceding fetal death has been reported.[44] According to Manning and colleagues,[45] both fetal breathing and body movements are assessed using a semiquantitative scoring method and are given a score of 2 if present or a score of 0 if absent by predefined criteria. Assessment of fetal tone, FHR reactivity, and amniotic fluid volume are combined with that score for a maximum score of 10 out of 10 if all five criteria are met (see Table 21-1 in Chapter 21). The negative predictive value for a normal perinatal outcome is high (>95%) among the four dynamic biophysical variables (FBM, GFBM, fetal tone, and reactive nonstress test).[46,47] However, it is only when test results are combined into a composite score that the positive predictive value for abnormal outcome is improved.[46,47] A score of either 10 of 10 or 8 of 10 with normal amniotic fluid volume, or 8 of 8 without nonstress testing, is interpreted as indicative of fetal health, and interventions for fetal indications are not recommended.[45] Repeat testing is recommended at specific intervals depending on the risk situation[48,49] (see Chapter 21). However, antepartum fetal health assessment reflects the metabolic fetal status *at the time of the test*, and furthermore, the frequency at which it should be repeated in high-risk pregnancies is still uncertain.

Acute biophysical markers of fetal assessment are also affected by rest-activity cycles reflecting fetal behavioral activity,[14] gestational age,[50,51] and IUGR,[17] which may lead to false-positive results and unnecessary early premature deliveries. Fetal breathing and body movements are more likely to be falsely abnormal at 26 to 33 weeks' gestation when compared with results at 34 to 41 weeks,[50] reflecting the maturational changes in these biophysical dynamic variables. Similarly, nonstress testing is more likely to be falsely nonreactive before 30 weeks' gestation,[51] because of both the maturational changes in fetal biophysical parameters and the autonomic control of the fetal heart with advancing gestation.[17] Growth-restricted fetuses experience lower incidences of FBM and GFBM in addition to lower FHR reactivity than fetuses growing normally in the absence of metabolic acidosis.[39,40] Therefore, different strategies have been used to decrease the false-positive rate of an abnormal biophysical profile, such as an immediate extension of the biophysical profile if a score of 4 or less is found after 30 minutes.[45] Assessment of FHR reactivity has included the use of objective computerized FHR analysis to take into account gestational age and to identify the lower-amplitude FHR accelerations expected in healthy, normally growing premature (<30 weeks) fetuses and in growth-restricted fetuses,[51,52] in addition to providing a more accurate assessment of FHR variability.[53] Although Devoe and coworkers[54] have tried to adjust FBM and GFBM scoring criteria for gestational age to reduce the false-positive rate and improve positive predictive value, this approach has not been tested in large population–based studies. Also, because of the inherent periodicity in FBM and GFBM, it is unlikely that such an approach would be sufficient to improve the positive predictive value of the current biophysical profile scoring system for growth-restricted fetuses.

Each of the four acute markers of fetal metabolic status has a different time course during which it becomes abnormal in relationship to the metabolic status of the fetus. A nonreactive nonstress test and absent FBM are early and therefore sensitive markers of fetal hypoxemia or metabolic acidosis, but they can be expected to have higher false-positive rate.[55,56] Furthermore, GFBM and fetal tone are late markers and therefore can be expected to have a better positive predictive value.[55,56] Current protocols for responding to abnormal scores (i.e., less than 8) are detailed in Chapter 21. The risk for fetal metabolic acidosis and perinatal mortality rises exponentially with progressive decrease in biophysical profile score.[57]

In the presence of preterm premature rupture of membranes, there may be a reduction in amniotic fluid volume. In addition, there is a significant risk of intrauterine infection, which may compromise neonatal outcome. An early retrospective report from Vintzileos and colleagues[58] suggested that with the onset of intrauterine infection, an abnormal biophysical profile may occur, and it could correlate with the subsequent development of neonatal sepsis. However, subsequent reports[59,60] in prospective cohorts could not confirm these observations, indicating that changes in biophysical profile scoring cannot be used as a reliable marker for intrauterine infection but still can be used to assess fetal metabolic status.

Fetal Movements versus Other Means of Fetal Surveillance

Currently, the biophysical profile is the primary method to indirectly estimate fetal oxygenation and the onset of metabolic acidosis. Umbilical artery Doppler ultrasound is a placental function test that provides important diagnostic and prognostic information in growth-restricted fetuses and is a useful addition to the assessment of fetal health by the dynamic biophysical profile score[61] (see Chapter 21). Umbilical artery Doppler velocimetry has shown a significant correlation with the umbilical artery pH and is also a sensitive indicator of fetal acidosis, comparable to the biophysical profile score.[61] In the presence of abnormal umbilical artery Doppler, fetal growth rate is reduced likely associated with a reduction in fetal oxygen consumption as a survival mechanism. Under clinical conditions where prematurity is a concern within the context of IUGR, the addition of assessment of the fetal circulation, and particularly the ductus venosus Doppler, appears to be a useful adjunct to identify IUGR fetuses at high risk for adverse outcome (particularly stillbirth), and thus requiring delivery, independent of the umbilical artery Doppler waveform and biophysical profile testing.[62,63] It is against these complex interactions between causative factors of fetal hypoxemia and reactive or adaptive responses that the different means of fetal health surveillance can be compared and the clinical decision made to deliver the compromised fetus.

Fetal Growth and Development

Brain

Brain growth and development are characterized by a series of events that include the proliferation and migration of nerve cells, gliogenesis, the growth of axons and dendrites, the formation of functional synapses, cell death, myelination of axons, and the fine tuning of neuronal specificity. These events proceed in a temporally and regionally dependent manner that is well coordinated, and for the most part the events are similar across mammalian species, albeit with considerable variance in their degree of advancement at the time of birth. For the ovine species, the increase in brain weight occurs in two phases: one up to 90 days after conception and the second a more rapid and longer increase after 90 days that continues to birth,[64] leading to the classification of sheep as prenatal brain developers. These two phases appear to reflect an increase in neuroblast multiplication followed by neuroglial multiplication and myelination.[64,65] For monkeys, neurogenesis is also largely complete well before birth, although the most rapid phase of synaptogenesis occurs thereafter within a time-window of approximately 40 days, centered on birth.[66] Although early neuronal connectivity with synaptogenesis and dendritic arborization is largely mediated by an intrinsic growth program, specific refinement occurs later on to generate class-specific dendritic morphologies regulated in part by patterns of synaptic activity.[67] Sensory-driven activity contributes to this during postnatal brain development, and recent study has pointed to a similar requirement for endogenous neural activity generated by the nervous system itself before sensory input is widely available, and presumably more so for those species whose development is extensively prenatal.[68] From a comparative standpoint using the timing for peaks in growth velocity of brain development, guinea pigs as well as monkeys can also be classified as prenatal brain developers, humans as perinatal brain developers, and cats and rats as postnatal brain developers.[64]

The anatomic development of the brain as studied across species thus appears to correlate with its electrophysiologic development as indicated by behavioral state maturation. Thus, whereas sheep and guinea pigs as prenatal brain developers from a neuroanatomic standpoint have relatively mature electrocortical patterns at birth, rats as postnatal brain developers have a poorly differentiated ECoG. This neurodevelopmental correlation, along with the high proportion of REM sleep or behavioral like activity during early life, indicate that the immature being has a high requirement for such activity and that the REM state itself might play a role in the brain's growth and development. The concept of a functional role for the REM state mechanism in brain development is further supported by the finding in the ovine fetus of an increase in cerebral metabolic rate at this time, which is most pronounced in mid brain and pontine structures[69-71] (Table 13-2), presumably reflecting increased neuronal activity associated with the generation of the REM state. Doppler flow velocity studies in the human fetus suggest a similar REM state effect, given the tight flow-metabolism coupling reported for the brain.[72] There is also a maturational increase in the cerebral metabolic rate of the ovine fetal LV/REM state[70] (see Table 13-2) which, along with the reported maturational change in the power spectrum of the ECoG waveform,[73] may thus reflect increasing endogenous stimulation of and by the brain as proposed by Roffwarg and coworkers[74] for the REM state over 40 years ago. For the ovine fetus, the cerebral metabolic rate of the prenatal LV/REM state at term is also similar to that of the awake state at 24 hours after birth, a time of increasing exogenous stimulation for the brain's functional activity (see Table 13-2).[70] Thus, it is not surprising that drug-induced REM sleep deprivation in rat pups during the period of rapid brain maturation and when there is normally a high amount of REM sleep, results in disturbed sleep-wake patterns during later life and a significant reduction in the size of the cerebral cortex.[75] Although these findings are not conclusive, collectively they support a role for REM state activity during early brain development, most likely with the provision of endogenous stimulation that might then promote synapse refinement and the formation of orderly connections during the critical period of synaptic plasticity.[68,76]

TABLE 13-2 CEREBRAL OXYGEN CONSUMPTION (μmol/100 g/min) IN THE OVINE FETUS

	Near Term* (~130 days GA)	Term† (~140 days GA)	Newborn† (At 24 hr)
HV/NREM	126 ± 7	133 ± 14	128 ± 8
LV/REM	152 ± 7	203 ± 13	—
Awake	—	—	170 ± 8

*Data (mean values ± SEM) from Richardson BS, Patrick JE, Abduljabbar H: Cerebral oxidative metabolism in the fetal lamb: Relationship to electrocortical state. Am J Obstet Gynecol 153:426-431, 1985.
†Data (mean values ± SEM) from Richardson BS, Carmichael L, Homan J, Gagnon R: Cerebral oxidative metabolism in lambs during perinatal period: Relationship to electrocortical state. Am J Physiol 257:R1251-1257, 1989.
GA, gestational age; HV/NREM, high-voltage, nonrapid eye movement state; LV/REM, low-voltage, rapid eye movement state.

Although most study and speculation has been directed at the REM state, there is reason to believe that the NREM state may also be important for the brain's development. The developmental change in NREM sleep coincides with the formation of thalamocortical and intracortical patterns of innervation and thereby with periods of heightened synaptogenesis, and it may also be associated with important processes in synaptic remodeling.[77,78] Furthermore, study in the near-term ovine fetus with infusion of an amino acid tracer has shown that leucine uptake by the brain is increased during the HV/NREM state rather than during the LV/REM state, indicating that protein synthesis and degradation must also be increased at this time.[79] This finding is consistent with that in adult animals, where higher rates of cerebral protein synthesis have been shown to be positively correlated with the occurrence of NREM sleep.[80,81] These studies also indicate that the decrease in the brain's metabolic demand during NREM sleep as seen in the ovine fetus[69,70] and in other species postnatally, including humans,[82] does not result from a decrease in biosynthetic activity and may, in fact, favor the synthesis of new proteins. This would support the restorative theory of sleep[83] whereby energy conservation during NREM sleep favors the anabolic restoration of tissues. Thus, REM and NREM sleep state activity may both have an impact on the brain's development, with the former providing a degree of endogenous stimulation through neuronal activity and leading to synaptic remodeling with increased protein synthesis or degradation,[84] which subsequently occurs during the following NREM period when energy needs for neuronal activity are lower. An interaction between sleep state and the brain's development is also supported by the finding in the near-term ovine fetus that HV/NREM episode duration is positively correlated with the duration of the previous LV/REM episode,[85] in keeping with a homeostatic model of REM/NREM sleep control as proposed for the adult rat.[86]

Lungs

Evidence from animal experimentation and from observations of human fetuses has indicated that fetal breathing movements are important for the normal development of the fetal lungs. Studies in fetal rabbits[87] and sheep[88] have shown that, after section of the upper cervical spinal cord and elimination of phasic respiratory movements of the diaphragm, the DNA content of the lungs was reduced. Circumstantial evidence from anomalous development of human fetuses also supports the conclusion that loss of fetal breathing movements plays a role in abnormal lung growth with pulmonary hypoplasia, although loss of thoracic volume may be just as important if not more so.[89] Although the mechanisms whereby fetal breathing movements affect lung growth are not well understood, phasic distortion of the lungs leading to pulmonary cell division and the maintenance of lung liquid volume or distention appear to be important.[90] Of interest, the experimental induction of growth restriction in fetal sheep does lead to a reduction in lung growth that affects the airways and alveoli.[91,92] However, the extent to which these growth effects are the result of an associated decrease in fetal breathing activity, or the related chronic hypoxemia, and the longer-term consequences for pulmonary function remain to be determined.

Because fetal breathing movements are important for lung growth, they have been studied in patients with oligohydramnios in relation to the subsequent development of pulmonary hypoplasia.[93-96] Although fetal breathing movements appear to be variably decreased or absent in fetuses who are subsequently shown to have pulmonary hypoplasia,[95,96] this may depend on the gestational age studied. Fetuses with preterm rupture of the membranes and oligohydramnios, as studied during the latter half of pregnancy, are certainly capable of making breathing movements.[58,97] Moreover, fetuses with renal agenesis and oligohydramnios and subsequently shown to have pulmonary hypoplasia, but studied after 29 weeks of gestation, are also seen to make breathing movements.[93] Thus, fetal breathing movements may be seen as decreased or absent in the younger fetus with oligohydramnios as a result of developing pulmonary hypoplasia and increased "lung stiffness." With advancing gestation and an increase in the stimuli for respiratory movements and chest wall excursion, breathing movement activity may now be evident despite underlying pulmonary hypoplasia. However, it is also possible that oligohydramnios of a marked degree mechanically restricts chest wall movement in the younger fetus, in turn contributing to the development of pulmonary hypoplasia.

Musculoskeletal

The loss of muscle mass and strength in later life is called sarcopenia, and it influences the proportion of lean mass. In vivo studies show that lean body mass represents 98% of total weight of term growth-restricted infants. In contrast, lean body mass is 87% in normally grown newborn infants, which suggests a reduction in fat deposition with fetal growth restriction.[98] Padoan and colleagues[99] recently used ultrasound estimation of fetal body fat and lean mass to demonstrate that growth-restricted fetuses have reduced subcutaneous fat and lean mass compared with control fetuses, particularly in the presence of adverse perinatal outcome. However, it is unknown if this relative sarcopenia persists into adulthood. A number of studies have demonstrated a significant, positive association between birthweight and muscle mass at different stages of life. Furthermore, there is evidence that small size at birth is associated not only with reduced muscle mass and strength but also with changes in metabolic function, with a small study showing that impaired fetal growth was associated with reduced muscle glycolysis in adult life as revealed by phosphorus 31 magnetic resonance spectroscopy.[100] However, the link between the mechanical and metabolic functions of muscle remains unclear, and there was no evidence in this study for differences in skeletal morphology according to size at birth. Although evidence from animal models suggests that early influences on the growth and development of muscle fibers may underlie the relationship between size at birth and adult muscle mass and function, the concept that there is a fixed number of muscle fibers determined at birth appears outdated. Recent evidence suggests that postmitotic myonuclei lying within mature myofibers might be able to reform myoblasts or stem cells, and there is increasing recognition of the role that satellite cells play in postnatal muscle growth and regeneration.[101]

De Vries and Fong[102] recently described the changes in the pattern of fetal body movements and motility associated with several genetic fetal anomalies. Hypokinetic fetal movement patterns were associated with several autosomal recessive disorders, whereas other chromosomal anomalies were associated with hyperkinetic gross fetal body movements but restriction in distal joint mobility resulting in clenched wrists. Therefore, abnormal fetal body movement patterns or the quality of movement activity may be associated with major fetal anomalies and contribute to abnormal neuromuscular development. However, although the neural activity of fetal motility and its motor effects may contribute to the development of muscles, joints, and even the fine structure of the central nervous system itself,[103] there has been little study, either experimental or clinical, in this area to date.

References

1. Ruckebusch Y, Gaujoux M, Eghbali R: Sleep cycles and kinesis in the foetal lamb. Electroencephalogr Clin Neurophysiol 42:226-237, 1977.
2. Ioffe S, Jansen AH, Russell BJ, et al: Sleep, wakefulness and the monosynaptic reflex in fetal and newborn lambs. Pflugers Arch 388:149-157, 1980.
3. Szeto HH, Hinman DJ: Prenatal development of sleep-wake patterns in sheep. Sleep 8:347-355, 1985.
4. Dawes GS, Fox HE, Leduc BM, et al: Respiratory movements and rapid eye movement sleep in the foetal lamb. J Physiol (London) 220:119-143, 1972.
5. Clapp JF, Szeto HH, Abrams RM, et al: Physiologic variability and fetal electrocortical activity. Am J Obstet Gynecol 136:1045-1050, 1980.
6. Zhu YS, Szeto HH: Cyclic variation in fetal heart rate and sympathetic activity. Am J Obstet Gynecol 156:1001-1005, 1987.
7. Harding R, Sigger JN, Poore ER, Johnson P: Ingestion in fetal sheep and its relation to sleep states and breathing movements. Q J Exp Physiol 69:477-486, 1984.
8. Wlodek ME, Thorburn GD, Harding R: Bladder contractions and micturition in fetal sheep: Their relation to behavioural states. Am J Physiol Regul Integr Comp Physiol 357:R1526-R1532, 1989.
9. Martin CB, Murata Y, Petrie RH, Parer JT: Respiratory movements in fetal rhesus monkeys. Am J Obstet Gynecol 119:939-948, 1974.
10. Grieve PG, Myers MM, Stark RI: Behavioral states in the fetal baboon. Early Hum Dev 39:159-175, 1994.
11. Umans JG, Cox MJ, Hinman DJ, et al: The development of electrocortical activity in the fetal and neonatal guinea pig. Am J Obstet Gynecol 153:467-471, 1985.
12. Junge HD: Behavioral states and state related heart rate and motor activity patterns in the newborn infant and the fetus antepartum—A comparative study: I. Technique, illustration of recordings, and general results. J Perinat Med 7:85-103, 1979.
13. Timor-Tritsch IE, Dierker LJ, Hertz RH, et al: Studies of antepartum behavioral states in the human fetus at term. Am J Obstet Gynecol 132:524-528, 1978.
14. Nijhuis JG, Prechtl HFR, Martin CB, et al: Are there behavioural states in the human fetus? Early Hum Dev 6:177-195, 1982.
15. Prechtl HFR: The behavioural states of the newborn infant (a review). Brain Res 76:185-212, 1974.
16. Gagnon R, Hunse C, Carmichael L, et al: Effects of vibratory acoustic stimulation on human fetal breathing and gross fetal body movements near term. Am J Obstet Gynecol 155:1227-1230, 1986.

17. Gagnon R, Hunse C, Carmichael L, et al: Human fetal responses to vibratory acoustic stimulation from twenty-six weeks to term. Am J Obstet Gynecol 157:1375-1381, 1987.
18. Junge HD, Walter H: Behavioral states and breathing activity in the fetus near term. J Perinat Med 8:150-157, 1980.
19. Nijhuis JG, Martin CB, Gommers S, et al: The rhythmicity of fetal breathing varies with behavioural state in the human fetus. Early Hum Dev 9:1-7, 1983.
20. Visser GHA, Goodman JDS, Levine DH, Dawes GS: Micturition and the heart period cycle in the human fetus. BJOG 88:803-805, 1981.
21. Nijhuis JG: Behavioural states: Concomitants, clinical implications and the assessment of the condition of the nervous system. Eur J Obstet Gynaecol Reprod Biol 21:301-308, 1986.
22. Clewlow F, Dawes GS, Johnston BM, et al: Changes in breathing electrocortical and muscle activity in unanaesthetized fetal lambs with age. J Physiol 341:463-476, 1983.
23. Drogtrop AP, Ubels R, Nijhuis JG: The association between fetal body movements, eye movements, and heart rate patterns in pregnancies between 25 and 30 weeks of gestation. Early Hum Dev 23:67-73, 1990.
24. Meier GW, Berger RJ: Development of sleep and wakefulness patterns in the infant rhesus monkey. Exp Neurol 12:257-277, 1965.
25. Jouvet-Mounier D, Astic L, Lacote D: Ontogenesis of the states of sleep in rat, cat and guinea pig during the fist postnatal month. Dev Psychobiol 2:216-239, 1970.
26. Shimizu A, Himwich HE: The ontogeny of sleep in kittens and young rabbits. Electroencephlogr Clin Neurophysiol 24:307-318, 1968.
27. Bocking AD: Fetal behavioural states: Pathological alteration with hypoxia. Semin Perinatol 16:252-257, 1992.
28. Richardson BS, Carmichael L, Homan J, Patrick JE: Electrocortical activity, electroocular activity, and breathing movements in fetal sheep with prolonged and graded hypoxemia. Am J Obstet Gynecol 167:553-558, 1992.
29. Rurak DW, Gruber NC: Increased oxygen consumption associated with breathing activity in fetal lambs. J Appl Physiol 54:702-707, 1983.
30. Rurak DW, Gruber NC: The effect of neuromuscular blockade on oxygen consumption and blood gases in the fetal lamb. Am J Obstet Gynecol 145:258-262, 1983.
31. Battaglia FC, Meschia G: Principal substrates of fetal metabolism. Physiol Rev 58:499-527, 1978.
32. Anderson DF, Parks CM, Faber JJ: Fetal O_2 consumption in sheep during controlled long-term reductions in umbilical blood flow. Am J Physiol 250:H1037-1042, 1986.
33. Clapp JF, Szeto HH, Larrow R, et al: Fetal metabolic response to experimental placental vascular damage. Am J Obstet Gynecol 140:446-451, 1981
34. Worthington D, Piercy WN, Smith BT: Effects of reduction of placental size in sheep. Obstet Gynecol 58:215-221, 1981.
35. van Vliet MAT, Martin CB, Nijhuis JG, et al: The relationship between fetal activity and behavioral states and fetal breathing movements in normal and growth-retarded fetuses. Am J Obstet Gynecol 153:582-588, 1985.
36. Ruedrich DA, Devoe LD, Searle N: Effects of maternal hyperoxia on the biophysical assessment of fetuses with suspected intrauterine growth retardation. Am J Obstet Gynecol 161:188-192, 1989.
37. Gagnon R, Hunse C, Vijan S: The effect of maternal hyperoxia on behavioral activity in growth-retarded human fetuses. Am J Obstet Gynecol 163:1894-1899, 1990.
38. Bekedam DJ, Mulder EJH, Snijders RJM, et al: The effects of maternal hyperoxia on fetal breathing movements, body movements and heart rate variation in growth retarded fetuses. Early Hum Dev 27:223-232, 1991.
39. Bekedam DJ, Visser GHA, de Vries JJ, et al: Motor behavior in the growth retarded fetus. Early Hum Dev 12:155-165, 1985.
40. Gagnon R, Hunse C, Fellows F, et al: Fetal heart rate and activity patterns in growth-retarded fetuses: Changes after vibratory acoustic stimulation. Am J Obstet Gynecol 158:265-271, 1988.
41. van Vliet MAT, Martin CB Jr, Nijhuis JG, Prechtl HFR: Behavioural states in growth-retarded human fetuses. Early Hum Dev 12:183-197, 1985.
42. Arduini D, Rizzo G, Caforio L, et al: Behavioural state transitions in healthy and growth retarded fetuses. Early Hum Dev 19:155-165, 1989.
43. Natale R, Clewlow F, Dawes GS: Measurement of fetal forelimb movements in the lamb in utero. Am J Obstet Gynecol 140:545-551, 1981.
44. Sherer DM, Dayal AK, Schwartz BM, et al: Acute oligohydramnios and deteriorating fetal biophysical profile associated with severe preeclampsia. J Matern Fetal Med 8:193-195, 1999.
45. Manning FA, Morrison I, Lange IR, et al: Fetal assessment based on fetal biophysical profile scoring: experience in 12,620 referred high-risk pregnancies: I. Perinatal mortality by frequency and etiology. Am J Obstet Gynecol 151:343-350, 1985.
46. Manning FA: Assessment of fetal condition and risk: Analysis of single and combined biophysical variable monitoring. Semin Perinatol 9:168-183, 1985.
47. Manning FA, Morrison I, Harman CR, et al: Fetal assessment based on fetal biophysical profile scoring: Experience in 19,221 referred high-risk pregnancies: II. An analysis of false-negative fetal deaths. Am J Obstet Gynecol 157:880-884, 1987.
48. Johnson JM, Harman CR, Lange IR, Manning FA: Biophysical profile scoring in the management of the postterm pregnancy: An analysis of 307 patients. Am J Obstet Gynecol 154:269-273, 1986.
49. Johnson JM, Lange IR, Harman CR, et al: Biophysical profile scoring in the management of the diabetic pregnancy. Obstet Gynecol 72:841-846, 1988.
50. Natale R, Nasello-Paterson C, Connors G: Patterns of fetal breathing activity in the human fetus at 24 to 28 weeks of gestation. Am J Obstet Gynecol 158:317-321, 1988.
51. Gagnon R, Campbell K, Hunse C, Patrick J: Patterns of human fetal heart rate accelerations from 26 weeks to term. Am J Obstet Gynecol 157:743-748, 1987.
52. Gagnon R, Hunse C, Bocking AD: Fetal heart rate patterns in the small-for-gestational-age human fetus. Am J Obstet Gynecol 161:779-784, 1989.
53. Gagnon R, Campbell MK, Hunse C: A comparison between visual and computer analysis of antepartum fetal heart rate tracings. Am J Obstet Gynecol 168:842-847, 1993.
54. Devoe LD, Searle N, Searle J, et al: Computer-assisted assessment of the fetal biophysical profile. Am J Obstet Gynecol 153:317-321, 1985.
55. Bekedam DJ, Visser GH: Effects of hypoxemic events on breathing, body movements, and heart rate variation: A study in growth-retarded human fetuses. Am J Obstet Gynecol 153:52-56, 1985.
56. Manning FA, Morrison I, Harman CR, Menticoglou SM: The abnormal fetal biophysical profile score: V. Predictive accuracy according to score composition. Am J Obstet Gynecol 162:918-924; discussion, 924-927, 1990.
57. Manning FA, Snijders R, Harman CR, et al: Fetal biophysical profile score: VI. Correlation with antepartum umbilical venous fetal pH. Am J Obstet Gynecol 169:755-763, 1993.
58. Vintzileos AM, Campbell WA, Nochimson DJ, et al: The fetal biophysical profile in patients with premature rupture of the membranes: An early predictor of fetal infection. Am J Obstet Gynecol 152:510-516, 1985.
59. Miller JM Jr, Kho MS, Brown HL, Gabert HA: Clinical chorioamnionitis is not predicted by an ultrasonic biophysical profile in patients with premature rupture of membranes. Obstet Gynecol 76:1051-1054, 1990.
60. Lewis DF, Adair CD, Weeks JW, et al: A randomized clinical trial of daily nonstress testing versus biophysical profile in the management of preterm premature rupture of membranes. Am J Obstet Gynecol 181:1495-1499, 1999.
61. Alfirevic Z, Neilson JP: Doppler ultrasonography in high-risk pregnancies: Systematic review with meta-analysis. Am J Obstet Gynecol 172:1379-1387, 1995.
62. Baschat AA, Harman CR: Venous Doppler in the assessment of fetal cardiovascular status. Curr Opin Obstet Gynecol 18:156-163, 2006.
63. Gagnon R, Van den Hof M, Diagnostic Imaging Committee, Executive and Council of the Society of Obstetricians and Gynaecologists of Canada:

The use of fetal Doppler in obstetrics. J Obstet Gynaecol Can 25:601-614, 2003.

64. McIntosh GH, Baghurst KI, Potter BJ, Hetzel B: Foetal brain development in the sheep. Neuropathol Appl Neurobiol 5:103-114, 1979.
65. Mallard EC, Rees S, Stringer M, et al: Effects of chronic placental insufficiency on brain development in fetal sheep. Pediatr Res 43:262-270, 1998.
66. Bourgeois JP: Synaptogenesis, heterochrony and epigenesis in the mammalian neocortex. Acta Paediatr Suppl 422:27-33, 1997.
67. Whitford KL, Dijkhuizen P, Polleux F, Ghosh A: Molecular control of cortical dendrite development. Annu Rev Neurosci 25:127-149, 2002.
68. Penn AA, Shatz CJ: Brain waves and brain wiring: The role of endogenous and sensory-driven neural activity in development. Pediatr Res 45:447-458, 1999.
69. Richardson BS, Patrick JE, Abduljabbar H: Cerebral oxidative metabolism in the fetal lamb: Relationship to electrocortical state. Am J Obstet Gynecol 153:426-431, 1985.
70. Richardson BS, Carmichael L, Homan J, Gagnon R: Cerebral oxidative metabolism in lambs during perinatal period: Relationship to electrocortical state. Am J Physiol 257:R1251-1257, 1989.
71. Richardson BS, Caetano H, Homan J, Carmichael L: Regional brain blood flow in the ovine fetus during transition to the low-voltage electrocortical state. Dev Brain Res 81:10-16, 1994.
72. Connors G, Gillis S, Hunse C, et al: The interaction of behavioural state, heart rate and resistance index in the human fetus. J Dev Physiol 15:331-336, 1991.
73. Szeto HH: Spectral edge frequency as a simple quantitative measure of the maturation of electrocortical activity. Pediatr Res 27:289-292, 1990.
74. Roffwarg HP, Muzio JN, Dement WC: Ontogenetic development of the human sleep-dream cycle. Science 152:604-619, 1966.
75. Mirmiran M, Mass YGH, Ariagno RL: Development of fetal and neonatal sleep and circadian rhythms. Sleep Med Rev 7:321-334, 2003.
76. Blumberg MS, Lucas DE: A developmental and component analysis of active sleep. Dev Psychobiol 29:1-22, 1996.
77. Bear MF, Malenka RC: Synaptic plasticity: LTP and LTD. Curr Opin Neurobiol 4:389-399, 1994.
78. Cramer KS, Sur M: Activity dependent remodeling of connections in the mammalian visual system. Curr Opin Neurobiol 5:106-111, 1995.
79. Czikk MJ, Sweeley JC, Homan JH, et al: Cerebral leucine uptake and protein synthesis in the near-term ovine fetus: relationship to fetal behavioural state. Am J Physiol Regul Integr Comp Physiol 284:R200-207, 2003.
80. Nakanishi H, Sun Y, Nakamura RK, et al: Positive correlations between cerebral protein synthesis rates and deep sleep in *Macaca mulatta*. Eur J Neurosci 9:271-279, 1997.
81. Ramm P, Smith CT: Rates of cerebral protein synthesis are linked to slow wave sleep in the rat. Physiol Behav 48:749-753, 1990.
82. Madsen PL, Vorstrup S: Cerebral blood flow and metabolism during sleep. Cerebrovasc Brain Metab Rev 3:281-296, 1991.
83. Adam K: Sleep as a restorative process and theory to explain why. Prog Brain Res 53:289-305, 1980.
84. Jiang C, Schuman EM: Regulation and function of local protein synthesis in neuronal dendrites. Trends Biochem Sci 27:506-513, 2002.
85. Rao N, Czikk M, Totten S, Richardson B: Behavioural state linkage in the ovine fetus near term support a homeostatic model of REM/nREM sleep control. J Soc Gynecol Investig II:(Suppl), 2004.
86. Benington JH, Heller HC: REM-sleep timing is controlled homeostatically by accumulation of REM-sleep propensity in non-REM sleep. Am J Physiol 266:R1992-2000, 1994.
87. Wigglesworth JS, Desai R: Effects on lung growth of cervical cord section in the rabbit fetus. Early Human Dev 3:51-65, 1979.
88. Harding R, Hooper SB, Han VKM: Abolition of fetal breathing movements by spinal cord transaction leads to reductions in fetal lung liquid volume, lung growth and IGF-II gene expression. Pediatr Res 34:148-153, 1993.
89. Liggins GC: Growth of the fetal lung. J Dev Physiol 6:237-248, 1984.
90. Harding R: Development of the respiratory system. In Thorburn GD, Harding R (eds): Texbook of Fetal Physiology. Oxford, Oxford University Press, 1994, pp 140-167.
91. Cock ML, Joyce BJ, Hooper SB, et al: Pulmonary elastin synthesis and deposition in developing and mature sheep: Effects of intrauterine growth restriction. Exp Lung Res 30:405-418, 2004.
92. Maritz GS, Cock ML, Louey S, et al: Fetal growth restriction has long-term effects of postnatal lung structure in sheep. Pediatr Res 55:287-295, 2004.
93. Fox HE, Moessinger AC: Fetal breathing movements and lung hypoplasia: Preliminary human observations. Am J Obstet Gynecol 151:531-533, 1985.
94. Moessinger AC, Fox HE, Higgins A, Rey HR: Fetal breathing movements are not a reliable predictor of continued lung development in pregnancies complicated by oligohydramnios. Lancet 2:1297-1300, 1987.
95. Blott M, Greenough A, Nicolaides KH, Campbell S: The ultrasonographic assessment of the fetal thorax and fetal breathing movements in the prediction of pulmonary hypoplasia. Early Hum Dev 21:143-151, 1990.
96. Blott M, Greenough A, Nicolaides KH: Fetal breathing movements in pregnancies complicated by premature membrane rupture in the second trimester. Early Hum Dev 21:41-48, 1990.
97. Richardson B, Natale R, Patrick J: Human fetal breathing activity during electively induced labor at term. Am J Obstet Gynecol 133:247-255, 1979.
98. Peterson S, Gotfredsen A, Knudsen FU: Lean body mass in small for gestational age and appropriate for gestational age infants. J Pediatr 113:886-889, 1998.
99. Padoan A, Rigano S, Ferrazzi E, et al: Differences in fat and lean mass proportions in normal and growth-restricted fetuses. Am J Obstet Gynecol 191:1459-1464, 2004.
100. Taylor DJ, Thompson CH, Kemp GJ, et al: A relationship between impaired fetal growth and reduced muscle glycolysis revealed by ^{31}P magnetic resonance spectroscopy. Diabetologia 38:1205-1212, 1995.
101. Maltin CA, Delday MI, Sinclair KD, et al: Impact of manipulations of myogenesis in utero on the performance of adult skeletal muscle. Reproduction 122:359-374, 2001.
102. de Vries JI, Fong BF: Changes in fetal motility as a result of congenital disorders: An overview. Ultrasound Obstet Gynecol 29:590-599, 2007.
103. Prechtl HFR: Perinatal development of postnatal behaviour. In Rauh H, Steinhausen H (eds): Psychobiology and Early Development, pp 231-238. North-Holland, Elsevier Science, 1987.

Chapter 14

Placental Respiratory Gas Exchange and Fetal Oxygenation

Giacomo Meschia, MD

Knowledge of respiratory gas exchange across the human placenta depends on the integrating of observations in pregnant patients with experimental findings in laboratory animals. This integration is necessary because data on the physiology of the human fetus are scant and cannot be interpreted correctly in the absence of experimental evidence. The evidence in laboratory animals consists of a fairly comprehensive set of data in sheep with chronically implanted vascular catheters in the maternal and fetal circulation, and a more limited but important set of data in nonhuman primates and other mammals.

Transport of Atmospheric Oxygen to the Gravid Uterus

The transport of oxygen (O_2) from the atmosphere to fetal tissues can be visualized as a sequence of six steps that alternate bulk transport with transport by diffusion (Fig. 14-1).[1] The first three steps of this process are part of general physiologic knowledge and therefore are presented here briefly.

In step 1, transport from the atmosphere to the alveoli is by action of the respiratory muscles, which move air in and out of the maternal lungs. This action maintains the partial pressure of oxygen (P_{O_2}) in the alveoli at a level that is regulated by several physiologic mechanisms, some of which are driven by sensors of the P_{O_2}, of partial pressure of carbon dioxide (P_{CO_2}), and of maternal blood pH. During pregnancy, the maternal organism is set to regulate arterial P_{CO_2} at a lower level than in the nonpregnant state.

In step 2, oxygen diffuses from the alveoli into the maternal red blood cells that circulate through the lungs. In the normal organism at sea level, the diffusion rate is so rapid that the P_{O_2} at the venous end of the pulmonary capillaries becomes virtually equal to the P_{O_2} in the adjacent alveoli. Nevertheless, the P_{O_2} of maternal arterial blood is somewhat less than the P_{O_2} in a sample of alveolar air, in part because some deoxygenated blood bypasses the lungs and in part because ventilation and perfusion of the alveoli are not matched evenly throughout the lungs. Under pathologic conditions that prevent the equilibration of P_{O_2} between alveoli and blood, increase the degree of uneven ventilation-perfusion, or shunt more deoxygenated blood directly into the arterial system, the P_{O_2} difference between alveolar air and arterial blood becomes larger.

In step 3, maternal blood, propelled by action of the maternal heart, transports oxygen from the lungs to the gravid uterus via the pulmonary veins, left atrium, left ventricle, aorta, uterine arteries, and branches of the ovarian and vaginal arteries. Oxygen is transported by blood in two forms, free and bound to hemoglobin. In any blood samples, these two forms are in reversible equilibrium. The special nomenclature for the components of this equilibrium is summarized in Table 14-1.

Oxygen Uptake by the Uterus and Fetus

The oxygen uptake by the uterus and the fetus can be calculated by measuring simultaneously uterine and umbilical blood flows and the oxygen content of blood samples drawn from four blood vessels: maternal artery, uterine vein, umbilical vein, and umbilical artery. A numerical example of these calculations is presented in Figure 14-2.

The rationale, commonly known as the Fick principle, is as follows. Each milliliter of maternal blood in passing through the pregnant uterus gives up a certain amount of oxygen, which can be calculated by measuring the difference in oxygen content between maternal arterial blood and uterine venous blood. The quantity of oxygen lost by each milliliter of blood is then multiplied by the milliliters of blood flowing through the pregnant uterus to obtain the uterine oxygen uptake.

To calculate the rate at which the fetus takes up oxygen from the placenta, exactly the same reasoning can be applied to the umbilical blood data. Note that the oxygen uptake by the gravid uterus is greater than the oxygen uptake by the fetus. This is so because the placenta is metabolically active and consumes a relatively large fraction of the oxygen that the uterine circulation delivers to the gravid uterus.

Fetal growth is accompanied by an increase in fetal oxygen uptake. However, oxygen uptake and fetal weight do not increase proportionally. A 200-g mid-gestation fetal lamb has an average oxygen uptake of 0.460 μmol/min/g, whereas a 3000-g near-term fetus has an average uptake of 0.340 μmol/min/g.[2] The differences in uptake are much larger if the uptake is related to fetal dry weight because fetal growth is accompanied by a decrease in fetal water content. Oxygen uptake expressed per unit fetal dry weight is about 2.5 times higher at mid-gestation.

Given this complexity and the lack of comparable information for the human fetus, it is important to ask whether fetal oxygen uptake measurements in experimental animals can be used to estimate human fetal oxygen uptake. If the aim is an accurate estimate, the answer must

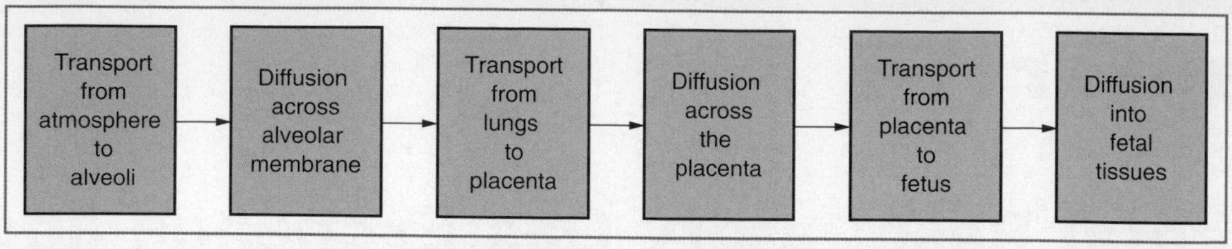

FIGURE 14-1 Transport of oxygen to fetal tissues. Transport of oxygen from the atmosphere to the fetal tissues in a sequence of steps that alternate bulk and diffusional transport. (From Meschia G: Supply of oxygen to the fetus. J Reprod Med 23:160, 1979.)

TABLE 14-1 BLOOD OXYGEN TRANSPORT: TERMINOLOGY, MEASUREMENT, AND RELATIONSHIPS

Nomenclature	Symbol	Units	Methods of Measurement
Free O_2	$[O_2]$	mM*	—
O_2 bound to hemoglobin	$[HbO_2]$	mM*	—
O_2 content	$[O_2$ Tot$]$	mM*	e.g., Van Slyke apparatus
O_2 pressure	Po_2	mm Hg	Po_2 electrode
Hemoglobin	[Hb]	mM*	Spectrophotometer
O_2 capacity	$[O_2$ CAP$]$	mM*	—
O_2 saturation	S	—	Spectrophotometer
O_2 saturation x 100	% S	—	—

$[O_2 \text{ Tot}] = [HbO_2] + [O_2]$
$[O_2 \text{ CAP}] = 4\,[Hb]^{\dagger}$
$S = [HbO_2] \div [O_2 \text{ CAP}]$
$[O_2] = \alpha O_2\, Po_2$ (where αO_2 = O_2 solubility coefficient).

***Another unit used often in reporting quantities of O_2 is mL_{STP} (1 millimole = 22.4 mL_{STP}).**
†Each hemoglobin molecule can combine with four molecules of oxygen.

Measured Quantities

Maternal arterial O_2 content (A): 0.143 mL_{STP}/mL of blood
Uterine venous O_2 content (V): 0.109 mL_{STP}/mL of blood
Umbilical arterial O_2 content (a): 0.078 mL_{STP}/mL of blood
Umbilical venous O_2 content (v): 0.115 mL_{STP}/mL of blood
Uterine blood flow (F): 1412 mL/min
Umbilical blood flow (f): 716 mL/min
Fetal body weight (BW): 4.0 kg
Uteroplacental unit weight (UPW): 1.0 kg

Calculations

O_2 uptake by the gravid uterus:	$(A - V) \times F = 48.0\ mL_{STP}$/min
O_2 uptake by the fetus:	$(v - a) \times f = 26.5\ mL_{STP}$/min
O_2 uptake per kg by fetus:	$(v - a) \times f \div BW = 6.6\ mL_{STP}$/min/kg
O_2 uptake per kg by fetus and uteroplacental unit:	$(A - V) \times F \div (BW + UPW) = 9.6\ mL_{STP}$/min/kg

FIGURE 14-2 The Fick principle. Application of the Fick principle to a calculation of oxygen uptake by the pregnant uterus and the fetus using representative data from experiments in chronic sheep preparations during the last 2 weeks of pregnancy. STP, standard temperature and pressure.

be No, because several interspecies differences are likely to affect oxygen demand. For example, in comparing near-term ovine and human fetuses of equal bodyweight, one must note that the human fetus has a much larger brain mass, has more adipose tissue, lives at a lower body temperature, and grows more slowly. It would be surprising if all these differences did not add up to a significant difference in oxygen uptake. However, attempts to measure near-term fetal oxygen consumption rates in different species (horse, cattle, rhesus monkey, guinea pig) have yielded values of oxygen uptake per gram wet weight that are within ±20% of the fetal lamb value despite very large differences in body size, rate of growth, and body composition.[3] Therefore, it may be assumed that data in experimental animals provide an approximate estimate of human fetal oxygen demand.

Oxygen Pressures in Uterine and Umbilical Circulations

The Po_2 of umbilical venous blood (i.e., the blood that transports O_2 from placenta to fetus) is quite low in comparison with maternal arterial and uterine venous Po_2, even under normal physiologic conditions. Table 14-2 presents representative data for sheep.[4] A large Po_2 difference is also present across the human and rhesus monkey placentas, suggesting that what has been learned about the transplacental Po_2 difference in sheep is relevant to human fetal physiology.

TABLE 14-2 REPRESENTATIVE Po_2 VALUES IN UTERINE AND UMBILICAL CIRCULATIONS OF SHEEP HOMOZYGOUS FOR OVINE B HEMOGLOBIN

Location	Po_2 (mm Hg)
Uterine artery	72
Uterine vein	48
Umbilical vein	27
Umbilical artery	19

In any given near-term, normal ovine pregnancy, umbilical venous Po_2 varies as a function of uterine venous Po_2, and the uterine-umbilical venous Po_2 difference remains virtually constant in response to wide Po_2 changes. Figure 14-3 shows the umbilical venous Po_2 response to variations of uterine venous Po_2 that were induced by changing the percentage of O_2 in maternal inspired air, or by shifting to the right the oxyhemoglobin dissociation curve of maternal blood via a decrease in the pH of maternal blood.[5] Figure 14-4 shows the results of experiments in five animals in which the uterine venous Po_2

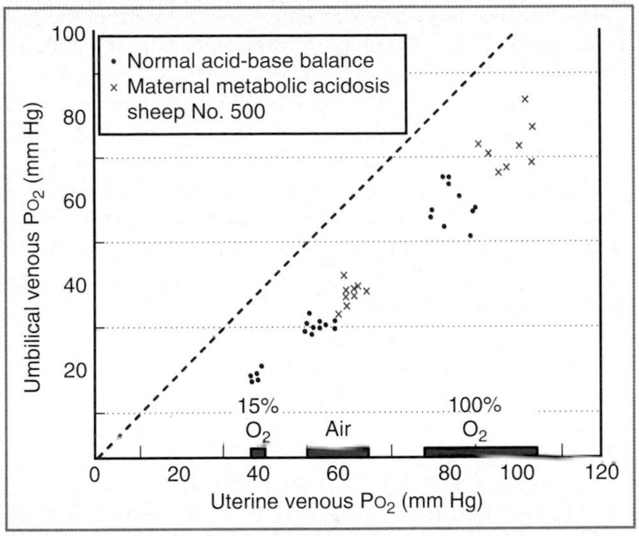

FIGURE 14-3 Relationship of umbilical venous Po_2 to uterine venous Po_2 in a near-term pregnant sheep. Uterine venous Po_2 was varied by administration of different gas mixtures to the mother and by displacing the maternal hemoglobin dissociation curve to the right via a decrease of maternal blood pH. The *dashed line* is the identity line. (From Rankin JHG, Meschia G, Makowski EL, et al: Relationship between uterine and umbilical venous Po_2 in sheep. Am J Physiol 220:1688, 1971.)

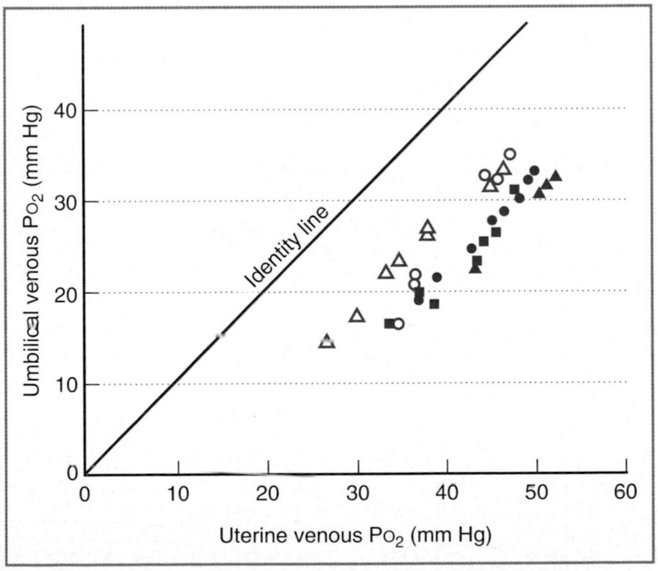

FIGURE 14-4 Relationship of umbilical to uterine venous Po_2 in five near-term sheep. The uterine venous Po_2 was decreased by decreasing uterine blood flow. Each animal is represented by a different symbol. (From Wilkening RB, Meschia G: Fetal oxygen uptake, oxygenation, and acid-base balance as a function of uterine blood flow. Am J Physiol 244:H749, 1983.)

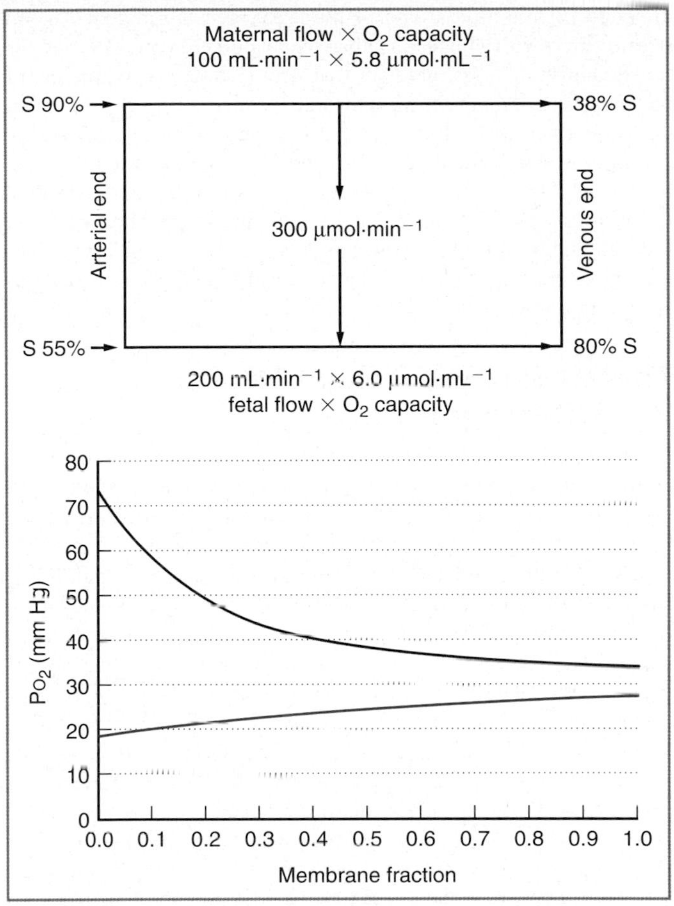

FIGURE 14-5 Concurrent blood flow model of O_2 transport across a structurally homogeneous membrane that does not consume any oxygen. In this model, the fetal O_2 saturations (S), blood flow, and O_2 capacity are representative of normal values at two-thirds gestation. The membrane is assumed to have an O_2-diffusing capacity that provides almost complete Po_2 equilibration at the venous end of the exchanger. The graph of Po_2 versus membrane fraction shows the Po_2 changes from the arterial to the venous end within the maternal (*red line*) and the fetal (*blue line*) vascular channels.

was decreased by decreasing uterine blood flow.[6] It is apparent that the two figures demonstrate a similar umbilical-versus-uterine venous Po_2 relationship, despite the different means that were used to vary uterine venous Po_2. Changes in the percentage of O_2 in maternal inspired air cause changes of Po_2 and O_2 content in maternal arterial blood, but they have virtually no effect on uterine blood flow.[7] In contrast, a decrease of uterine blood flow does not change the oxygenation of maternal arterial blood.

In an attempt to explain this basic information, it is useful to address two questions: (1) why does umbilical venous Po_2 vary as a function of uterine venous Po_2? and (2) why is umbilical venous Po_2 so much less than uterine venous Po_2?

The Venous Equilibration Model of Transplacental Exchange

Studies on the transplacental diffusion of molecules that rapidly cross the placental barrier (e.g., tritiated water, ethanol) have established that, in sheep, the maternal and fetal placental circulations form an exchange system that tends to equilibrate the venous concentrations of any molecule that diffuses across the barrier.[8]

The physiologic concept of venous equilibration is easy to grasp by considering the hypothetical model shown in Figure 14-5. This model assumes that the basic unit of transplacental exchange consists of a membrane that separates two bloodstreams flowing in the same direction. At the arterial end of the exchanger, the maternal bloodstream enters with a higher Po_2 than fetal blood (72 versus 19 mm Hg), thus establishing a Po_2 gradient that drives O_2 across the membrane into fetal blood. As the two streams flow concurrently past the membrane, transfer of O_2 into the fetal circulation causes a progressive decrease of Po_2 in the maternal stream and a progressive increase of Po_2 in the fetal stream, so that the transmembrane Po_2 difference at the venous end tends toward zero. This model explains why, in a venous equilibration system, umbilical venous Po_2 depends directly on uterine venous Po_2, whereas it has no direct relationship to maternal arterial Po_2.

The Uterine-Umbilical Venous Po_2 Difference

Several theories have been proposed to explain why the placenta maintains umbilical venous Po_2 to a much lower level than uterine venous Po_2 even under normal conditions. The following explanation is what I consider the one that best fits our current knowledge.

The placental epithelial barrier that separates maternal and fetal blood consumes O_2. Because O_2 transport into and across the barrier is by diffusion, the placenta has no intrinsic mechanisms that would make it utilize O_2 drawn from the maternal rather than the fetal circulation. The mother-to-fetus polarity of placental O_2 transport depends on extrinsic mechanisms that maintain a positive Po_2 difference between the maternal and the fetal circulation. This transplacental Po_2 difference is the sum of two terms—the Po_2 difference that is generated by the O_2 consumption of the placental barrier and the Po_2 difference that draws O_2 all across the barrier from the maternal to the fetal circulation. If we try to imagine how the transplacental Po_2 difference changes from the arterial to the venous end of the barrier, it becomes apparent that its two components do not behave the same. The Po_2 difference that draws O_2 into fetal blood decreases toward zero as O_2 is transferred from one circulation to the other. In contrast, the Po_2 difference that is generated by the O_2-consuming barrier does not change systematically from the arterial to the venous end. Placental mitochondria, like those in other organs, do not appreciably change their O_2 utilization rate in response to changes in Po_2, as long as the Po_2 is kept above a critical level, which is generally quite low. As a consequence, the Po_2 difference generated by placental O_2 consumption can be a larger fraction of the transplacental Po_2 difference at the venous, than at the arterial, end of the placental barrier. Furthermore, it contributes to the remarkable stability of the uterine-umbilical venous Po_2 difference in response to changes in uterine venous Po_2.

For any given value of umbilical O_2 uptake and placental O_2 consumption, the magnitude of the transplacental Po_2 difference depends on the surface and thickness of the placental barrier. It can be understood intuitively, for example, that a large difference would be necessary to maintain a high rate of O_2 transport into and across a thick barrier with a small surface. Respiratory physiologists would say that such a barrier has a low "O_2-diffusing capacity." Placental O_2-diffusing capacity has been estimated indirectly, via measurements of CO-diffusing capacity.[9] These measurements have led to the conjecture that the O_2-diffusing capacity of a normal placenta is sufficient to allow a virtually complete vein-to-vein Po_2 equilibration in the placental microcirculation, and that the uterine-umbilical vein Po_2 difference results entirely from shunting of uterine and umbilical blood flows across the placenta and from uneven maternal-to-fetal blood perfusion ratios within the placenta itself.[9] However, the conjecture that placental O_2 transport is not diffusion-limited is based on the assumption that umbilical O_2 uptake is the only O_2 flux that generates the transplacental Po_2 gradient. The more realistic assumption—that some of this gradient is caused by O_2 consumption by the placental barrier—leads to an alternative interpretation of experimental evidence. The importance of placental oxidative metabolism in determining the uterine-umbilical venous Po_2 difference and the uterine-to-umbilical blood flow ratio is best illustrated by contrasting two models of fetal oxygenation.

In the model that was used to explain the concept of venous equilibration (see Fig. 14-5), two bloodstreams flowing concurrently at the same rate are separated by a structurally homogeneous membrane that does not consume O_2. The two streams have virtually the same hemoglobin content per milliliter of blood but are assumed to have the highly different oxyhemoglobin dissociation curves of fetal sheep and pregnant sheep homozygous for ovine hemoglobin B. The numerical example of this model assumes the O_2-diffusing capacity to be high enough to produce almost complete venous Po_2 equilibration and a normal level of arterial and venous O_2 saturation of the fetal bloodstream.

In the second model (Fig. 14-6), the membrane is assumed to have an O_2-diffusing capacity identical to that in the first model. In contrast to the first model, however, the membrane is assumed to consume O_2 at constant rate per unit of surface and to have a total O_2 consumption

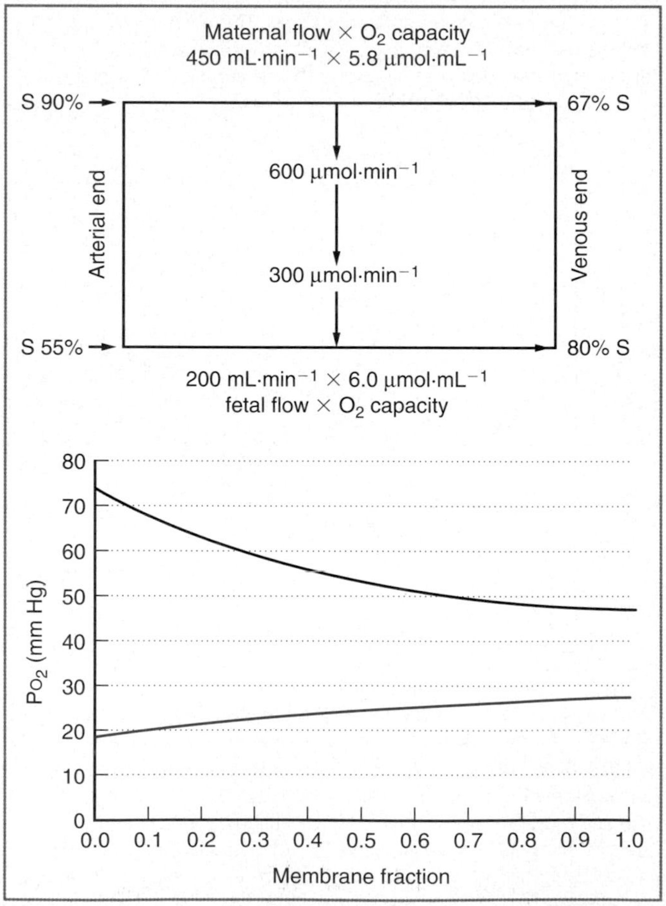

FIGURE 14-6 O_2 transport across a homogeneous membrane that consumes oxygen. Model of O_2 transport across a structurally and metabolically homogeneous membrane that is assumed to have the same O_2-diffusing capacity as in the Figure 14-5 model, and to consume O_2 at a rate that is equal to fetal O_2 uptake. Oxygen consumption by the membrane requires a greater transmembrane Po_2 gradient and a greater maternal blood flow to provide the same level of fetal oxygenation as in the Figure 14-5 model. *Red line,* maternal; *blue line,* fetal.

that is equal to fetal O_2 uptake. Because it takes a smaller PO_2 difference to draw O_2 into the membrane than across the whole membrane, the PO_2 difference generated by membrane O_2 consumption is assumed to be only 75% of the PO_2 difference that is required to transport the same amount of O_2 from maternal to fetal blood. Fetal placental blood flow and oxygenation are as in the first model. It is apparent that O_2 consumption by the membrane requires a much larger vein-to-vein PO_2 difference (approximately 20 versus 6 mm Hg) and a markedly higher maternal-to-fetal flow ratio (2.25 versus 0.5).

The doubling of O_2 flux through the maternal surface of the membrane requires a disproportionally greater increase of maternal blood flow, because a proportional increase would have left the maternal PO_2 unchanged. The increase in the ratio of maternal flow to O_2 flux decelerates the decrease of maternal PO_2 from arterial to venous end and maintains the greater transplacental PO_2 difference that is required to maintain a normal level of fetal oxygenation.

Developmental Changes in Placental Oxygen Transport

Under normal physiologic conditions, the O_2 saturations and PO_2 of umbilical blood decline in the time interval between mid-gestation and two-thirds gestation and then show no further systematic change. In the fetal lamb, O_2 saturations decline, approximately, from 90% to 80% in the umbilical vein, and from 65% to 55% in the umbilical artery. These are remarkably small variations in view of the enormous and complex changes in O_2 uptake, placental blood flow, and placental structure that take place throughout pregnancy.

At mid-gestation, the placenta consumes, approximately, four times more O_2 than the fetus,[10] and the placental villi show a smaller degree of branching than at later stages.[11] The hindrance to transplacental O_2 diffusion that is produced by these conditions is compensated for by a very high uterine blood flow. At this stage of development, the ratio of uterine blood flow to fetal O_2 uptake is about 6 mL/µmol of O_2 (500 mL · min^{-1}/80 µmol · min^{-1}). From mid-gestation to two-thirds gestation, this ratio declines to about 1.7 (500/300). The two major factors that produce this change are (1) an elongation and branching of the placental villi without any increase in placental O_2 consumption, and (2) an increase in umbilical blood flow (approximately from 70 to 200 mL · min^{-1}). The increase in placental villous surface without a commensurate increase in placental O_2 consumption suggests a radical change in placental energy metabolism. Unfortunately, there is no clue as to the nature of this change. The mathematical model presented in Figure 14-6 is meant to be a schematic representation of placental O_2 transport at two-thirds gestation when umbilical O_2 uptake has become about equal to placental O_2 consumption.

From two-thirds to near-term gestation, there is a further, large increase in umbilical O_2 uptake (approximately from 300 to 1000 µmol · min^{-1}). There is also an increase in placental O_2 consumption, which is, however, smaller than the increase in umbilical uptake (approximately from 300 to 600 µmol · min^{-1}). The increase in O_2 transport across the placenta is determined by synchronous increases in placental O_2-diffusing capacity and in uterine and umbilical blood flows. Under normal physiologic conditions, these changes in diffusing capacity and flows maintain virtually constant the transplacental PO_2 difference.[17] In this final stage of development, the increase in O_2-diffusing capacity results primarily from a process of placental differentiation that produces extremely thin regions of the placental epithelium. Presumably, the thinning of the epithelium involves also a local reduction in mitochondrial density per unit surface. In essence, the placental epithelial barrier progressively evolves into a structurally and metabolically uneven barrier that tends to separate the respiratory gas exchange function from other functions that require a high rate of oxidative metabolism. A likely, concomitant process is that the regions of the barrier that acquire specialized functions become perfused at different rates by maternal and fetal blood, thus creating a more complex condition of placental O_2 transport than the one depicted in Figure 14-6.

It is important to note that the maternal and the fetal blood flow to the placental cotyledons are only a fraction of the uterine and the umbilical flows, respectively. In sheep, the fraction of uterine flow perfusing the cotyledons is approximately 80% from mid-gestation[10] to term.[13] The fraction of umbilical flow to the cotyledons is about 93%.[14] For this reason alone, any model that represents the placenta as a structurally and metabolically homogeneous membrane that is perfused evenly at rates equal to the uterine and the umbilical flow is no more than an approximate representation of the real system at any developmental stage. It is not clear, however, whether conditions of physiologically significant uneven O_2 exchange are present in the placental cotyledons in early development or become a distinctive feature of placental function in the last third of gestation only.

The uterine-umbilical venous PO_2 difference varies widely among pregnancies. According to our present understanding of placental O_2 transport, this is the expression of variability in the ratio of the placental O_2-diffusing capacity to the placental and fetal O_2 consumption. At comparable values of placental and fetal oxidative metabolism, the greater the O_2-diffusing capacity of the placental membrane is, the smaller the vein-to-vein transplacental PO_2 difference is. Under conditions of normal placental development, variations in placental O_2-diffusing capacity have the function of adapting placental O_2 transport to the PO_2 in the maternal circulation. For example, ewes who are homozygous for high-O_2-affinity hemoglobin maintain a smaller PO_2 in the uterine circulation than ewes that carry the low-O_2-affinity hemoglobin type.[4] The placental membrane adapts to the low maternal PO_2 by developing a greater O_2-diffusing capacity. This developmental change requires a smaller transmembrane PO_2 gradient to draw O_2 at a normal rate into and across the barrier. The result of this adaptation is a smaller uterine-umbilical venous PO_2 difference and a normal level of fetal oxygenation. There are conditions, however, that inhibit placental development to various degrees, widen the transplacental PO_2 gradient, and generate a state of chronic fetal hypoxia. An extreme example of this type of fetal hypoxia has been produced experimentally by exposing pregnant ewes to high environmental temperatures for most of gestation.[15] Near term, these ewes carry severely hypoxic, growth-restricted fetuses. This form of fetal hypoxia is characterized by the presence of a uterine-umbilical venous PO_2 difference that is about twice the normal value. The umbilical venous PO_2 and O_2 saturation are about 20 mm Hg and 50%, respectively. This is a level of oxygenation that alters the distribution of fetal cardiac output, decreases O_2 consumption by some fetal tissues (e.g., skeletal muscle), and is close to the limit of fetal viability.

There is evidence that human fetal growth restriction is also associated with a uterine-umbilical venous PO_2 difference that is greater than normal (Fig. 14-7).[16] Furthermore, the terminal villi in the placentas of severely hypoxic, growth-restricted human fetuses occupy a significantly smaller fraction of placental volume than normal[17] and show signs of trophoblastic degeneration.[18] Because in the differentiation of the placental barrier, the areas with the smallest interhemal distance are located preferentially in the terminal villi, these data support the hypothesis that the hypoxia of growth-restricted fetuses is the result of a disproportionate reduction of those regions of the placental barrier that facilitate the transplacental diffusion of oxygen.

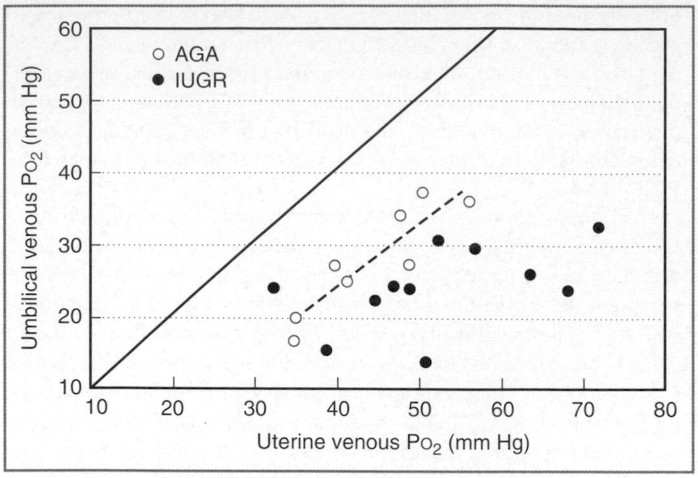

FIGURE 14-7 Uterine venous and umbilical venous partial pressures of oxygen. Relationship between uterine venous and umbilical venous partial pressure of oxygen (Po_2) in normal human pregnancies *(open circles)* and pregnancies with intrauterine growth restriction (IUGR) *(closed circles)*. AGA, appropriate for gestational age. (From Pardi G, Cetin I, Marconi AM, et al: Venous drainage of the human uterus: Respiratory gas studies in normal and fetal growth retarded pregnancies. Am J Obstet Gynecol 166:699, 1992.)

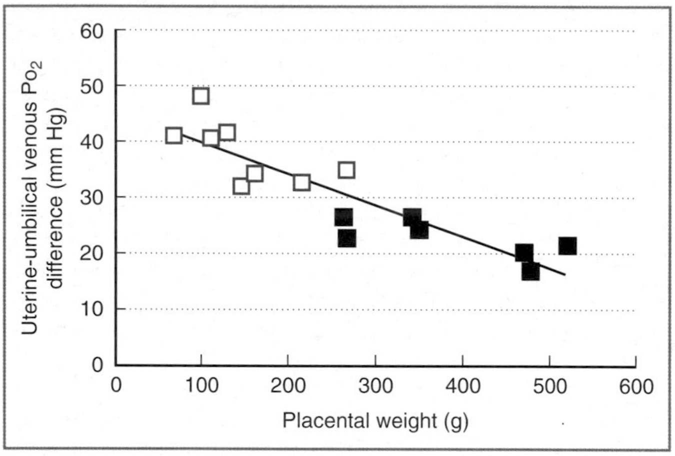

FIGURE 14-8 Uterine-umbilical venous Po_2 difference versus placental weight. Correlation of the uterine-umbilical venous Po_2 difference with placental weight in normal *(closed squares)* and growth-restricted *(open squares)* fetal sheep (R^2 = 0.79). (From Regnault TR, de Vrijer B, Galan HL, et al: Development and mechanisms of fetal hypoxia in severe fetal growth restriction. Placenta 28:714-723, 2007.)

Studies on placental respiratory gas exchange under normal physiologic conditions have shown that the uterine-umbilical venous Po_2 difference is inversely correlated to placental weight. This negative correlation becomes highly significant if the placentas of growth-restricted fetuses are included in the analysis (Fig. 14-8).[15] A likely explanation for this finding is that the growth of placental mass and the differentiation of the placental epithelium are controlled, at least in part, by common factors. This explanation is supported by the results of a study on the effects of deleting, in mice, the placental-specific insulin-like growth factor 2 gene (*IGF2*).[19] This deletion causes both a decrease in placental mass and an increase in the mean thickness of the trophoblast.

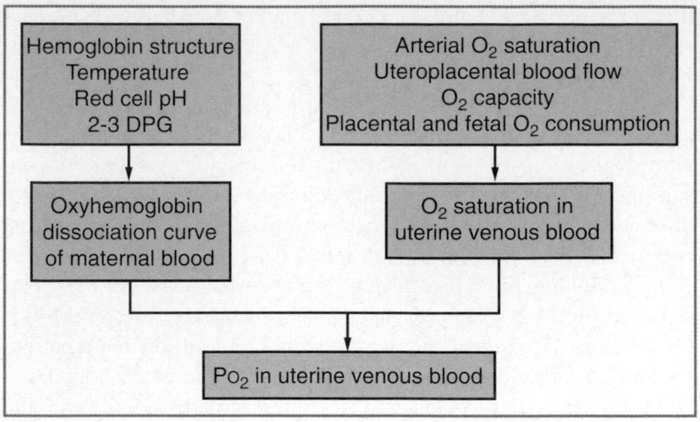

FIGURE 14-9 Factors that determine uterine venous partial pressure of oxygen (Po_2). 2-3 DPG, 2,3-diphosphoglycerate.

Factors That Determine Uterine Venous Po_2

The evidence in sheep, rhesus monkeys, and humans points to uterine venous Po_2 as being the primary determinant of umbilical venous blood Po_2 in these species. The factors that determine uterine venous Po_2 are shown in Figure 14-9, and of these, the immediate causative factors are the oxygen saturation and oxyhemoglobin dissociation curve of venous blood. The position of the oxyhemoglobin dissociation curve is shifted by pH, so that at any given saturation, the Po_2 is inversely related to pH (the Bohr effect). Because of the Bohr effect, maternal alkalosis can be detrimental to fetal oxygenation via its effect on uterine venous Po_2 (Fig. 14-10).

The oxygen saturation of uterine venous blood, S_V, is a function of four variables and can be calculated with the following equation:

$$S_V = S_A - \dot{V}O_2/F\ [O_2\ CAP],$$

where S_A is the oxygen saturation of maternal arterial blood, O_2 CAP is the oxygen capacity of maternal blood, F is the uterine blood flow, and $\dot{V}O_2$ is the oxygen consumption rate of the gravid uterus. This equation, an application of the Fick principle,* is an approximation that neglects the small contribution of free oxygen to the oxygen content of blood. Implicit in the equation are the three main types of hypoxia listed in textbooks of physiology:

---

*Derivation of the equation for oxygen saturation of venous blood. Let $\dot{V}O_2$ = uterine O_2 consumption (mmol/min), F = uterine blood flow (mL/min), A = arterial oxygen content (mmol/mL), V = uterine venous oxygen content (mmol/mL), [O_2 CAP] = oxygen capacity (mmol/mL), S_A = oxygen saturation of arterial blood, and S_V = oxygen saturation of uterine venous blood. According to the Fick principle,

$$\dot{V}O_2 = F(A - V).$$

Divide both sides of the equation by oxygen capacity: $\dot{V}O_2/[O_2\ CAP] = F\{A/[O_2\ CAP] - V/[O_2\ CAP]\}$. If we neglect the contribution of free oxygen to A and V, $A/[O_2\ CAP] = S_A$, and $V/[O_2\ CAP] = S_V$.

$$\text{Therefore, } \dot{V}O_2/[O_2\ CAP] = F(S_A - S_V)$$
$$\text{and } S_V = S_A - \dot{V}O_2/F[O_2\ CAP].$$

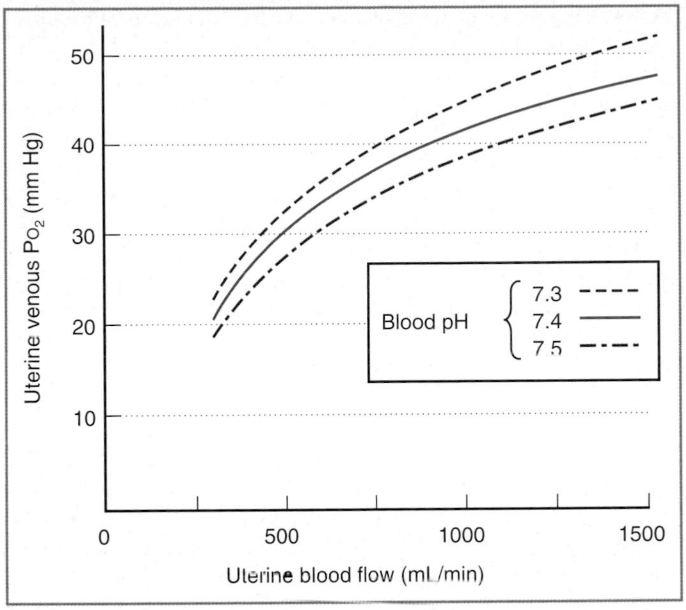

FIGURE 14-10 Uterine venous partial pressure of oxygen (Po_2) as a function of uterine blood flow in a pregnant patient close to term. The figure was constructed with the assumption that the following values were constant: maternal arterial Po_2, 80 mm Hg; maternal oxygen capacity, 17.4 volumes percent; oxygen consumption rate of the gravid uterus, 30 mL_{STP}/min. STP, standard temperature and pressure.

- Low saturation of arterial blood (hypoxic hypoxia)
- Reduced oxygen capacity (anemic hypoxia)
- Reduction in blood flow (circulatory hypoxia)

These types of hypoxia, alone or in combination, decrease uterine venous saturation. A decrease in uterine venous oxygen saturation implies a decrease of uterine venous Po_2 and impairment of fetal oxygenation.

An important consequence of the inefficiency of a placenta—which is a venous equilibrator, consumes O_2 at a rapid rate, and has a low oxygen-diffusing capacity—is that it requires a relatively high uterine blood flow to provide a normal level of fetal oxygenation. For example, if we consider as valid the evidence that under normal physiologic conditions the umbilical venous Po_2 of a 35-week-old human fetus is about 30 mm Hg[20] and that uterine venous Po_2 must be at least 10 mm Hg higher than umbilical venous Po_2,[16] according to Figure 14-10 the uterine blood flow in late human pregnancy should normally be about 1 L. Early estimates based on Doppler technology were considerably lower.[21] However, using improved Doppler imaging, Konje and colleagues[22] reported the mean blood flow carried by the two uterine arteries to be 942 mL/min at 36 weeks. Knowing the normal value of uterine blood flow is necessary to construct a correct model of fetal oxygenation.

Transport of Oxygen to Fetal Tissue

In recent years, improved techniques for blood flow measurement and umbilical blood sampling in utero have led to considerable progress in the exploration of human fetal physiology. The results of this effort, together with comparative data in sheep, allow us to construct a tentative picture of normal human fetal oxygenation and blood oxygen transport (Table 14-3).

TABLE 14-3 REPRESENTATIVE DATA FOR BLOOD OXYGEN TRANSPORT IN A 35-WEEK HUMAN FETUS AND A SHEEP FETUS AT A COMPARABLE DEVELOPMENTAL STAGE

	Human Fetus (35 wk)	Sheep Fetus (19 wk)
Blood O_2 capacity (mM)	9.4	6.7
Umbilical venous O_2 saturation (%)	70.0	81.0
Umbilical venous O_2 content (mM)	6.6	5.4
Umbilical venous Po_2 (mm Hg)	28.0	28.0
Umbilical arterial O_2 saturation (%)	40.0	56.0
Umbilical arterial O_2 content (mM)	3.8	3.8
Umbilical arterial Po_2 (mm Hg)	19.0	19.0
Cardiac output (mL/min/kg)	500.0	500.0
Umbilical blood flow (mL/min/kg)	120.0	216.0
Umbilical flow/cardiac output	0.24	0.43

In both the human and ovine fetuses, arterial Po_2 is about one-fourth the maternal arterial Po_2 at sea level. This is a consequence partly of the structural and functional characteristics of the placenta, which require that the oxygenation of fetal blood take place at a low Po_2, and partly of the anatomy of the fetal circulation, which forms arterial blood by mixing the blood that returns from the placenta with deoxygenated blood returning from the fetal tissues.

Despite the very low Po_2 of its blood, the fetus is capable of transporting large amounts of oxygen from the placenta to the sites of oxygen consumption in the fetal body. Three major adaptations make this possible:

- The hemoglobin of fetal red blood cells has a high affinity for oxygen (i.e., it binds oxygen at low Po_2 values). This property enables the fetal red blood cells that circulate through the placenta to become highly saturated with oxygen.
- The fetus has a very high cardiac output relative to its body size and metabolic rate.
- The distribution of cardiac output between placenta and fetus and within the fetus creates a well-balanced oxygen uptake and delivery system.

Available data for the human fetus indicate that this adaptive strategy has some intriguing quantitative differences from the ovine model. At mid-gestation, the oxygen capacity of human fetal blood is approximately 6.5 mM; umbilical venous oxygen saturation and Po_2 are about 90% and 50 mm Hg, respectively.[23] In comparison, the mid-gestation ovine fetus has a somewhat lower oxygen capacity (5.7 ± 0.3 mM) and an equally high umbilical venous oxygen saturation (89% ± 1%). Note that a 90% oxygen saturation is close to the highest value that can reasonably be expected for the oxygenation of blood by any respiratory organ.

As gestation progresses past mid-term, umbilical venous oxygen saturation and Po_2 decline concomitantly with an increase in oxygen capacity. These changes occur in both species, but those described in humans are larger,[20,23] so that in late gestation the human fetus has blood with substantially greater oxygen capacity and about 10% lower umbilical venous oxygen saturation than the ovine fetus.

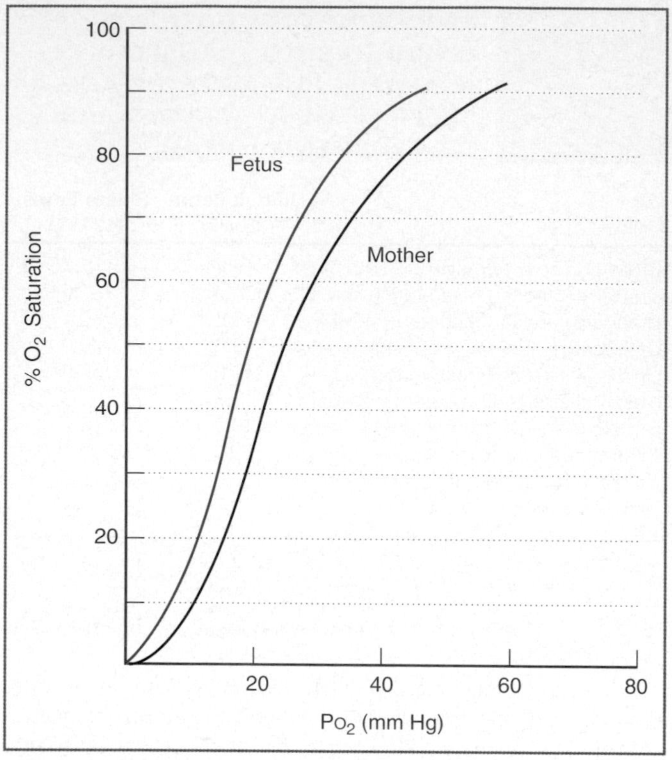

FIGURE 14-11 The oxyhemoglobin dissociation curves of maternal (*red line*) and fetal (*blue line*) human blood at pH 7.4 and 37° C. Po_2, partial pressure of oxygen. (From Hellegers AE, Schruefer JJ: Nomograms and empirical equations relating oxygen tension, percentage saturation and pH in maternal and fetal blood. Am J Obstet Gynecol 81:377, 1961.)

Despite the difference in oxygen saturation, the two species have comparable umbilical venous Po_2 values because human fetal blood has slightly lower oxygen affinity than ovine fetal blood. Although the oxygen affinity of human fetal blood is not as high as in sheep, it still represents an important adaptation to the low Po_2 at which the human placenta oxygenates the fetus. Figure 14-11 compares the oxyhemoglobin dissociation curves of human adult and fetal blood.[24] At a Po_2 of 30 mm Hg and blood pH 7.4, fetal blood is 73% saturated with oxygen; adult blood is only 60% saturated.

In addition to umbilical venous Po_2 and oxygen saturation, we must consider oxygen content, which is the product of oxygen saturation and capacity. The umbilical venous blood of the late-gestation human fetus has a higher oxygen content than that of the sheep fetus because the higher oxygen capacity more than compensates for the lower saturation.

The next two important factors to be considered are umbilical blood flow and fetal cardiac output. The human umbilical blood flow is approximately 120 mL/min/kg fetal bodyweight,[25] which is about 40% lower than umbilical blood flow measured in sheep.[3] Initial attempts to measure human fetal cardiac output suggested that it is also relatively small, but further investigations indicate that cardiac output is as high in the human as in the sheep fetus and approximately equal to 500 mL/min/kg fetal bodyweight.[26-28] Therefore, there seems to be a major difference between the two species in the distribution of fetal cardiac output. In fetal sheep, umbilical blood flow represents approximately 40% of cardiac output; in the late-gestation human fetus, umbilical blood flow is less than 30% of cardiac output (see Table 14-3). This large difference may result, in part, from errors of measurement. It seems clear, however, that in comparison with the ovine fetus, a high blood oxygen capacity (i.e., high hemoglobin content and hematocrit) and a low ratio of umbilical blood flow to cardiac output are distinctive normal characteristics of the human fetus. Umbilical blood flow and oxygen capacity are interrelated. In anemic human fetuses, umbilical blood flow becomes greater than 120 mL/min/kg fetal bodyweight and can be as high as in the sheep fetus.[29]

The function of the fetal circulation as an oxygen delivery system depends on an appropriate balance between umbilical blood flow and fetal somatic blood flow. It can be understood intuitively that directing too much cardiac output into the somatic circulation would impair the umbilical uptake of oxygen, and that directing too much cardiac output into the umbilical circulation would impair the supply of oxygen to fetal organs. It may seem that, theoretically, the optimal balance is to split the distribution of cardiac output evenly between the umbilical and somatic circulations. However, the experimental evidence shows a balance tilted toward the somatic circulation. The enormous growth of the human fetal brain is probably the major factor that creates the demand for a smaller umbilical flow in the human than in the ovine fetus. At term, the human fetus and the ovine fetus weigh about the same, but the mass of the fetal human brain is about eight times greater. A larger cerebral mass implies a greater oxygen demand and requires a greater percentage of cardiac output directed to the fetal upper body at the expense of the fetal lower body and the umbilical circulation. The high O_2 capacity of human fetal blood can be viewed as a compensatory mechanism that allows the human fetus to maintain a relatively low umbilical blood flow without compromising umbilical O_2 uptake.

Because of its low blood Po_2, the fetus is more hypoxic than the neonate. Normally, however, the fetus has access to all the oxygen it needs and does not use anaerobic glycolysis as a terminal source of energy.[30] Furthermore, the low level of Po_2 in fetal arterial blood is physiologically useful because it is an essential component of the mechanisms that keep the ductus arteriosus open and the pulmonary vascular bed constricted. To counteract the pathologic connotation of the word *hypoxia,* it is advisable to use the expression *physiologic hypoxia* to refer to the normal state of fetal oxygenation.

In the ordinary usage of the term, fetal hypoxia means any decrease below normal in the level of fetal oxygenation. Such a decrease can come about in different ways, most commonly as a reduction in the Po_2 of umbilical venous blood, which in turn determines a decrease of fetal arterial Po_2, in the oxygen capacity of fetal blood (anemic hypoxia, elevated levels of carbon monoxide), or in the perfusion rate of the umbilical circulation.

The circulation of an unanesthetized, otherwise healthy fetus reacts to an acute decrease in umbilical venous and arterial Po_2 in a predictable manner.[31,32] As the Po_2 falls, blood flow is increased to the central nervous system (CNS) and the heart, although cardiac output and placental blood flow tend to remain constant. As a consequence, acute fetal hypoxia is characterized by a redistribution of cardiac output favoring the CNS and heart at the expense of other parts of the fetal body.

The fraction of cardiac output directed to the CNS and heart increases hyperbolically as the arterial oxygen content decreases (Fig. 14-12). The functional meaning of this relationship is that to mount a successful defense against hypoxia, the fetus must keep constant (or nearly so) the flow of oxygen to the CNS and heart (i.e., the product of blood flow times the oxygen content per milliliter of arterial blood). The limit of a successful circulatory defense against acute hypoxia is reached when the perfusion rate of the CNS and the heart has reached

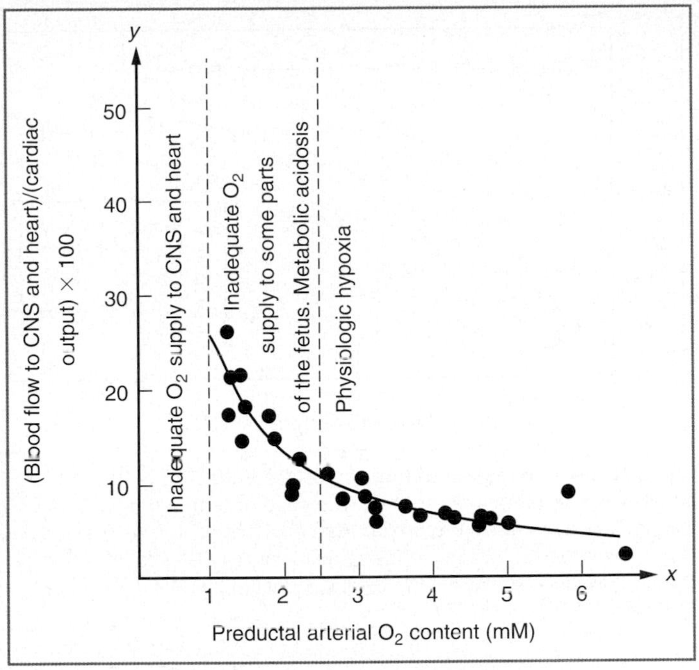

FIGURE 14-12 **Hyperbolic relationship between the oxygen content in the preductal arteries of a fetal lamb and the percentage of cardiac output directed to the heart and the central nervous system (CNS).** The curve was drawn according to the equation $y \times x = 0.26$. (From Sheldon RE, Peeters LLH, Jones MD Jr, et al: Redistribution of cardiac output and oxygen delivery in the hypoxemic fetal lamb. Am J Obstet Gynecol 135:1071, 1979.)

TABLE 14-4 PO_2 OF MATERNAL AND UMBILICAL BLOOD AT DIFFERENT LEVELS OF MATERNAL OXYGENATION

	PO_2 (mm Hg)			
Location	**Rhesus Monkey***		**Human†**	
Maternal artery	108	257	91	583
Uterine vein	37	44	—	—
Umbilical vein	22	30	32	40
Umbilical artery	15	21	11	16

*From Behrman RE, Peterson EN, Delannoy CW: The supply of O_2 to the primate fetus with two different O_2 tensions and anesthetics. Respir Physiol 6:271, 1969.
†From Wulf KH, Künzel W, Lehmann V: Clinical aspects of placental gas exchange. In Longo LD, Bartels H (eds): Respiratory Gas Exchange and Blood Flow in the Placenta. Washington, DC, DHEW Publications (National Institutes of Health), 1972.

its maximum. In the fetal lamb, this limit is attained when the oxygen content in the supraductal arteries is approximately 1 mM. At this level, the flow of blood per gram of tissue is extremely high in the brain (approximately 4 mL/min/g) and in the heart (approximately 7 mL/min/g). Furthermore, the combined CNS and heart flow has become 26% of fetal cardiac output (see Fig. 14-12).[31] The circulations of the human and ovine fetus react similarly to acute hypoxia. Under normal physiologic conditions, however, the large oxygen demand of the human fetal brain requires a larger contribution of cardiac output to cerebral perfusion than that of the fetal lamb. As a consequence, in response to acute hypoxia the human fetus may not be able to produce a percentage increase in cerebral blood flow as dramatic as in a species with a small brain.

Between the region of oxygenation that defines physiologic hypoxia and the limit below which there is an insufficient oxygen supply to the CNS and heart, there is a broad range (approximately between 2.5 and 1 mM arterial oxygen content in the fetal lamb) in which the supply of oxygen to some parts of the fetal body other than the CNS and heart (e.g., skeletal muscle) cannot sustain a normal level of O_2 consumption.[33]

Oxygen Therapy

The inhalation of oxygen by a pregnant patient can dramatically increase the PO_2 of maternal arterial blood but causes only a small increase in fetal arterial PO_2 (Table 14-4).[34,35] This observation seems to contradict the empirical knowledge that oxygen therapy can be an effective measure for the improvement of fetal oxygenation. Indeed, some investigators have claimed that maternal oxygen inhalation cannot ameliorate fetal hypoxia because its effect on fetal PO_2 is "negligible." Others have claimed that the discrepancy of PO_2 changes in mother and fetus is the consequence of severe placental vasoconstriction in response to the high PO_2 of maternal blood. To dispel these misconceptions, it is necessary first to understand why fetal arterial PO_2 increases much less than maternal arterial PO_2 and then to focus attention on the effect that oxygen therapy has on the oxygen content of fetal blood.

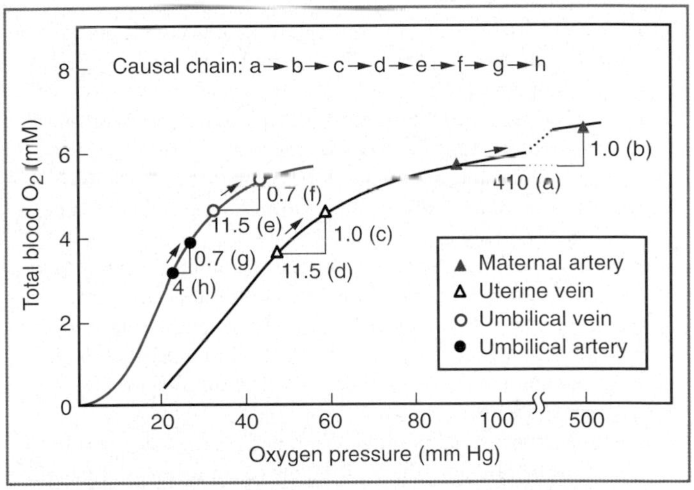

FIGURE 14-13 **Oxygen therapy.** Example of the relationship between oxygen content and partial pressure of oxygen in maternal (*red line*) and fetal (*blue line*) blood before and after maternal inhalation of 100% oxygen. (From Meschia G: Transfer of oxygen across the placenta. In Gluck L [ed]: Intrauterine Asphyxia and the Developing Fetal Brain. Chicago, Year Book Medical, 1977.)

The venous equilibration model of placental exchange and the characteristics of the maternal and fetal oxyhemoglobin dissociation curves readily explain the "small" effect of oxygen therapy on fetal PO_2. In the example shown in Figure 14-13,[36] the oxygen contents of maternal and fetal blood are plotted against PO_2:

- The inhalation of 100% oxygen by the mother causes the PO_2 of maternal arterial blood to increase from 90 to 500 mm Hg (step a).

- This increase in Po_2 causes an increase of maternal arterial oxygen content equal to 1 mM (step b). These changes in arterial Po_2 and oxygen content do not cause any appreciable change in the uterine blood flow.
- If we assume they do not increase the uterine oxygen consumption rate—a correct assumption if fetal oxygen supply was already adequate before oxygen therapy—the law of conservation of matter requires that uterine venous oxygen content also increase 1 mM (step c).
- The increase in uterine venous oxygen content causes the uterine venous Po_2 to increase 11.5 mm Hg (step d). Note that the "S" shape of the maternal oxyhemoglobin dissociation curve and the different positions of the arterial and venous points on this curve determine that an equal change of oxygen content is associated with a markedly smaller change of Po_2 in the uterine vein than in the maternal arteries. Note also that the assumption of a constant oxygen consumption rate maximizes the increase in venous Po_2. If the oxygen consumption of the gravid uterus were to increase in response to oxygen therapy, the increase of venous Po_2 would be less than indicated.
- Given an increase of 11.5 mm Hg in the uterine venous Po_2, the umbilical venous Po_2 will increase by an approximately equal value (step e).
- The increase in umbilical venous Po_2 is associated with an increase in umbilical venous oxygen content (step f), whose magnitude is dictated by the slope of the oxyhemoglobin dissociation curve and by the position of the umbilical venous point on that curve.
- In this example, the oxygen content of umbilical venous blood increases 0.7 mM. If we assume no appreciable change in umbilical blood flow or oxygen uptake, it follows (again by application of the law of conservation of matter) that the oxygen content in the umbilical artery must also increase 0.7 mM (step g).
- Because the arterial point is positioned on the steep part of the fetal oxyhemoglobin dissociation curve, an increase of 0.7 mM in oxygen content is associated with a Po_2 increase of only 4 mm Hg (step h).

The conclusion of this chain of events is that a Po_2 change of 410 mm Hg in maternal arterial blood results in a Po_2 change of 4 mm Hg in umbilical arterial blood.

If we focus our attention on fetal Po_2 changes by excluding other considerations, we might be tempted to conclude that maternal oxygen therapy has no appreciable effect on fetal oxygenation. However, oxygen therapy can cause similar increments in the oxygen content of maternal and fetal blood. In the example, an increase of 1 mM in maternal blood was associated with an increase of 0.7 mM in fetal blood. Under somewhat different circumstances, the oxygen content of fetal blood can actually increase more than the oxygen content of maternal blood (Fig. 14-14).[36]

Oxygen therapy is commonly used in the treatment of acute fetal hypoxia. It may be valuable also in the treatment of chronic fetal hypoxia. In two studies, 55% oxygen was administered for several days to pregnant patients with intrauterine growth restriction.[37,38] There were significant increases in umbilical venous Po_2 and oxygen saturation and a significant improvement in Doppler flow patterns.

Finally, it is important to consider the issue of oxygen toxicity. Breathing oxygen at high concentrations can be harmful to the lungs of the mother. Because of this concern, breathing 100% oxygen at atmospheric pressure must be limited to a few hours only. Breathing 50% oxygen at atmospheric pressure is considered safe. However, the question of whether pregnancy alters the tolerance of the mother to hyperoxia has not been addressed. In general, there is no concern that maternal hyperoxia would increase fetal Po_2 to toxic levels, as long as the oxygen is administered at atmospheric pressure and for the purpose of treating fetal hypoxia.

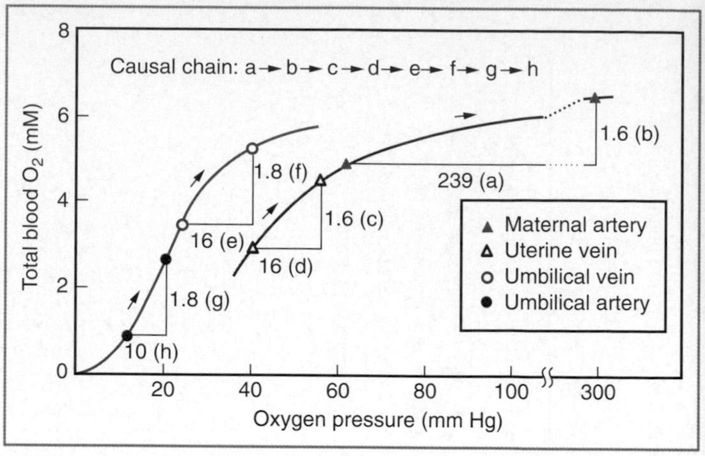

FIGURE 14-14 Example of the pronounced effect of oxygen therapy on fetal oxygen content in a case of fetal hypoxia secondary to maternal hypoxia. *Red line,* maternal; *blue line,* fetal. (From Meschia G: Transfer of oxygen across the placenta. In Gluck L [ed]: Intrauterine Asphyxia and the Developing Fetal Brain. Chicago, Year Book Medical, 1977.)

Placental Carbon Dioxide Transfer

Carbon dioxide is an end product of fetal metabolism. In the fetal lamb, the respiratory quotient (i.e., the moles of CO_2 produced per mole of oxygen consumed) is approximately 0.94. The CO_2 produced by the fetus diffuses from the umbilical circulation into the placenta and from the placenta into the maternal blood, which brings it to the lungs for excretion. The diffusional transfer of CO_2 from fetus to mother requires the Pco_2 of fetal blood to be higher than the Pco_2 of maternal blood. In chronic sheep preparations, umbilical venous Pco_2 is approximately 5 mm Hg higher than uterine venous Pco_2. The factors responsible for determining the magnitude of the Pco_2 gradient between fetal and maternal blood have not been analyzed in detail. A consequence of the high diffusibility of CO_2 across the placenta is that respiratory disturbances of acid-base balance in the mother cause—with a delay of a few minutes only—analogous disturbances in the fetus, as long as the two organisms are in communication via a well-perfused placenta. An abnormally low fetal Pco_2 (fetal respiratory alkalosis) is always secondary to a low maternal Pco_2. However, an abnormally high fetal Pco_2 (fetal respiratory acidosis) can be caused by a high maternal arterial Pco_2, inadequate gas exchange across the placenta, or a combination of these two conditions.

There are probably substantial differences among mammals in the permeability of the placental barrier to bicarbonate ions. The epitheliochorial placenta of sheep has a very low permeability to bicarbonate and to other small anions, such as chloride ions and ketoacids. If maternal metabolic acidosis or alkalosis develops, the bicarbonate concentration of fetal blood remains normal for several days; however, the hemochorial placenta of the rabbit or rhesus monkey is much more permeable to chloride ions than an epitheliochorial placenta. This suggests that the hemochorial placenta is permeable to bicarbonate and other ions, in which case metabolic disturbances of acid-base balance in the mother would cause analogous disturbances in the fetus. Unfortunately, there is no exact information, in the human or any other species with a hemochorial placenta, about the rate at which a metabolic disturbance of acid-base balance in the maternal compartment is transmitted to the fetal compartment.

References

1. Meschia G: Supply of oxygen to the fetus. J Reprod Med 23:160, 1979.
2. Bell AW, Kennaugh JM, Battaglia FC, et al: Metabolic and circulatory studies of fetal lamb at midgestation. Am J Physiol 250:E538, 1986.
3. Battaglia FC, Meschia G: An Introduction to Fetal Physiology. New York, Academic Press, 1986.
4. Wilkening RB, Molina RD, Meschia G: Placental oxygen transport in sheep with different haemoglobin types. Am J Physiol 254:R585-589, 1988.
5. Rankin JHG, Meschia G, Makowski EL, et al: Relationship between uterine and umbilical venous Po_2 in sheep. Am J Physiol 220:1688, 1971.
6. Wilkening RB, Meschia G: Fetal oxygen uptake, oxygenation, and acid-base balance as a function of uterine blood flow. Am J Physiol 244:H749-755, 1983.
7. Makowski EL, Hertz RH, Meschia G: Effects of acute maternal hypoxia and hyperoxia on the blood flow to the pregnant uterus. Am J Obstet Gynecol 115:624, 1973.
8. Wilkening RB, Anderson S, Martensson L, Meschia G: Placental transfer as a function of uterine blood flow. Am J Physiol 242:H429, 1982.
9. Longo LD, Ching KS: Placental diffusing capacity for carbon monoxide and oxygen in unanesthetized sheep. J Appl Physiol 43:885-893, 1977.
10. Molina RD, Meschia G, Wilkening RB: Uterine blood flow, oxygen and glucose uptakes at mid-gestation in the sheep. Proc Soc Exp Biol Med 195:379-385, 1990.
11. Stegeman JHJ: Placental development in the sheep and its relation to fetal development. Bijdragen tot de Dierkunde 44:4, 1974.
12. Meschia G, Makowski EL, Battaglia FC: The use of indwelling catheters in the uterine and umbilical veins of sheep for a description of fetal acid-base balance and oxygenation. Yale J Biol Med 42:154, 1969.
13. Makowski EL, Meschia G, Droegemueller W, Battaglia FC: Distribution of uterine blood flow in the pregnant sheep. Am J Obstet Gynecol 101:409, 1968.
14. Makowski EL, Meschia G, Droegemueller W, Battaglia FC: Measurement of umbilical arterial blood flow to the sheep placenta and fetus in utero Circulation Res 23:623, 1968.
15. Regnault TRH, de Vrijer B, Galan HL, et al: Development and mechanisms of fetal hypoxia in severe fetal growth restriction. Placenta 28:714, 2007.
16. Pardi G, Cetin I, Marconi AM, et al: Venous drainage of the human uterus: Respiratory gas studies in normal and fetal growth retarded pregnancies. Am J Obstet Gynecol 166:699, 1992.
17. Jackson MR, Walsh AJ, Morrow RJ, et al: Reduced placental villous tree elaboration in small-for-gestational-age pregnancies: Relationship with umbilical artery Doppler waveforms. Am J Obstet Gynecol 172(2 Pt 1):518, 1995.
18. Macara L, Kingdom JCP, Kaufmann P, et al: Structural analysis of placental terminal villi from growth-restricted pregnancies with abnormal umbilical artery Doppler waveforms. Placenta 17:37, 1996.
19. Constancia M, Hemberger M, Hughes J, et al: Placental-specific IGF-II is a major modulator of placental and fetal growth. Nature 417:945-948, 2002.
20. Soothill P, Nicolaides KH, Rodeck CH, et al: Effect of gestational age on fetal and intervillous blood gas and acid base values in human pregnancy. Fetal Ther 1:168, 1986.
21. Thaler I, Manor D, Itskovitz G, et al: Changes in uterine blood flow during human pregnancy. Am J Obstet Gynecol 162:121, 1990.
22. Konje J, Kaufmann P, Bell SC, et al: A longitudinal study of quantitative uterine blood flow with the use of color power angiography in appropriate for gestational age pregnancies. Am J Obstet Gynecol 185:608, 2001.
23. Bozzetti P, Buscaglia M, Cetin I, et al: Respiratory gases, acid-base balance and lactate concentrations of the midterm human fetus. Biol Neonate 51:188, 1987.
24. Hellegers AE, Schruefer JJ: Nomograms and empirical equations relating oxygen tension, percentage saturation and pH in maternal and fetal blood. Am J Obstet Gynecol 81:377, 1961.
25. Gill RW, Kossoff G, Warren PS, et al: Umbilical venous flow in normal and complicated pregnancy. Ultrasound Med Biol 10:349, 1984.
26. Kenny JF, Plappert T, Doubilet P, et al: Changes in intracardiac blood flow velocities and right and left ventricular stroke volumes in the gestational age in the normal human fetus: A prospective Doppler echocardiographic study. Circulation 74:1208, 1986.
27. DeSmedt MCH, Visser GHA, Meijboom EJ: Fetal cardiac output estimated by Doppler echocardiography during mid and late gestation. Am J Cardiol 60:338, 1987.
28. Rizzo G, Arduini D: Fetal cardiac function in intrauterine growth retardation. Am J Obstet Gynecol 165:876, 1991.
29. Jouppila P, Kirkinen P: Umbilical vein blood flow in the human fetus in cases of maternal and fetal anemia and uterine bleeding. Ultrasound Med Biol 10:365, 1984.
30. Battaglia FC, Meschia G: Principal substrates of fetal metabolism. Physiol Rev 58:499, 1978.
31. Sheldon RE, Peeters LLH, Jones MD Jr, et al: Redistribution of cardiac output and oxygen delivery in the hypoxemic fetal lamb. Am J Obstet Gynecol 135:1071, 1979.
32. Peeters LLH, Sheldon RE, Jones MD Jr, et al: Blood flow to fetal organs as a function of arterial oxygen content. Am J Obstet Gynecol 135:637, 1979.
33. Boyle DW, Meschia G, Wilkening RB: Metabolic adaptation of fetal hindlimb to severe, nonlethal hypoxia. Am J Physiol. 263:R1130, 1992.
34. Wulf KH, Künzel W, Lehmann V: Clinical aspects of placental gas exchange. In Longo LD, Bartels H (eds): Respiratory Gas Exchange and Blood Flow in the Placenta. Washington, DC, DHEW Publications (National Institutes of Health), 1972.
35. Behrman RE, Peterson EN, Delannoy CW: The supply of O_2 to the primate fetus with two different O_2 tensions and anesthetics. Respir Physiol 6:271, 1969.
36. Meschia G: Transfer of oxygen across the placenta. In Gluck L (ed): Intrauterine Asphyxia and the Developing Fetal Brain. Chicago, Year Book Medical, 1977, pp 109-115.
37. Nicolaides KH, Econimides DL, Soothill PW: Blood gases, pH and lactate in appropriate-and-small-for-gestational-age fetuses. Am J Obstet Gynecol 161:996, 1989.
38. Battaglia FC, Artini PG, B'Ambrogio G, et al: Maternal hyperoxygenation in the treatment of intrauterine growth retardation. Am J Obstet Gynecol 167:430, 1992.

Chapter 15

Fetal Lung Development and Surfactant

Alan H. Jobe, MD, PhD

In the recent past, lung immaturity in the preterm newborn often resulted in death. With intensive clinical management, lung function no longer limits the survival of most preterm newborns. That management includes the use of antenatal corticosteroids to mature the fetal lung, improvements in neonatal ventilatory techniques, and surfactant treatments. Understanding the process of lung maturation involves anatomy, physiology, and cell and molecular biology. Although the anatomy and physiology of lung development in the human and in experimental animals have been characterized, the cell biology and genetics are now revealing the mechanisms underlying the developmental program.

Hyaline membranes were described in association with respiratory deaths early in the twentieth century. However, there was no substantial increase in the understanding of lung immaturity until Avery and Mead correlated respiratory failure with decreased surfactant levels in saline extracts of the lungs of infants who died of respiratory distress syndrome (RDS) in 1959.[1] Once the association between atelectasis with hyaline membranes and surfactant levels was appreciated, a large research effort was focused on the surfactant system. The first direct clinical benefit was the development by Gluck and colleagues in 1971 of the lecithin-to-sphingomyelin ratio using amniotic fluid to predict the risk of RDS in preterm infants.[2] The usefulness of phosphatidylglycerol measurements for lung maturity testing then was recognized.[3] The maturational effects of corticosteroids on developing systems were apparent by the late 1960s, and in 1972 Liggins and Howie demonstrated a decreased incidence in RDS with maternal corticosteroid treatments.[4] The subsequent development of surfactant treatment for RDS and other neonatal lung diseases has had a major beneficial impact on outcomes.[5] Further progress in the pulmonary outcomes of infants will result from new information about how antenatal and postnatal abnormalities contribute to lung development, injury, and repair.

Lung Structural Development

Embryonic Stage

The lung first appears in the embryo at about 26 days as a ventral bud off the esophagus just caudal to the laryngotracheal sulcus.[6] The grooves between the lung bud and the esophagus deepen, and the bud elongates within the surrounding mesenchyme and divides to form the future mainstem bronchi (Fig. 15-1).[7] Several factors that determine lung bud formation have been identified using transgenic mouse models. Deletion of fibroblast growth factor 10 (FGF-10) or a compound deletion of the zinc finger DNA-binding proteins Gli2 and Gli3 prevent lung development by disrupting tracheal development (Table 15-1).[8,9] Subsequent dichotomous branching of the trachea gives rise to the conducting airways and lobar structures of the lungs. Branching is controlled by the underlying mesoderm because removal of the mesenchyme stops branching, and transplantation of the mesenchyme from a branching airway to a more proximal airway or the trachea induces budding in the new location. Lobar airways are formed by about 37 days with progression to segmental airways by 42 days and subsegmental bronchi by 48 days in the human.[6]

Some of the diffusible factors responsible for airway branching have been identified.[8,9] Several members of the large family of fibroblast growth factors acting through specific fibroblast growth factor receptors modulate airway branching and parenchymal development. For example, overexpression of FGF-7 (also known as keratinocyte growth factor) results in lung tumors similar to cystic adenomatoid malformations. Several factors are associated with the development of tracheoesophageal fistula in transgenic mice. These and other genes have very precise spatial and temporal expression patterns that choreograph lung structural development. Newly developed techniques to turn on or turn off specific genes in mouse models will result in a more complete understanding of early lung development.

Pseudoglandular Stage

The pseudoglandular period, from about the 6th to 17th week of human gestation, is characterized by progressive division to generate 15 to 20 generations of airways depending on airway segment length and lobar position.[10] The developing airways are lined with simple cuboidal cells that contain large amounts of glycogen. Epithelial differentiation is centrifugal in that the most distal tubules are lined with undifferentiated cells, with progressive differentiation in the more proximal airways. Pulmonary arteries grow in conjunction with the airways, and the principal arteries are present by 14 weeks. The pulmonary microvasculature develops in the mesenchyme around the developing airways by the processes of angiogenesis by the sprouting of new vessels from preexisting vessels, and of vasculogenesis, in which primitive vascular plexuses fuse and then connect with vessels under control of factors such as vascular endothelial growth factor[8] (VEGF). Pulmonary venous development occurs in parallel by both angiogeneses and vasculogeneses, but with a different pattern that demarcates lung segments and subsegments. By the end of the pseudoglandular stage, airways, arteries, and veins have developed in a pattern corresponding to that found in the adult. The diaphragm separates the chest from the abdomen during this stage of lung development, and failure to close results in diaphragmatic hernia and lung hypoplasia.

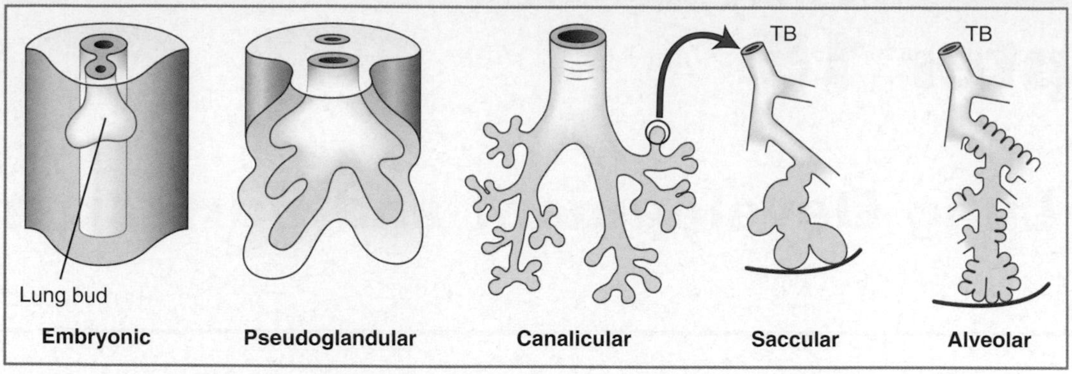

FIGURE 15-1 **Morphologic development of the human lung.** Schematic representations of stages of development. TB, terminal bronchiole. (Courtesy of Jeffrey Whitsett, Cincinnati Children's Hospital.)

TABLE 15-1 LUNG DEVELOPMENT IN THE HUMAN FETUS

Stage of Development	Fetal Age (wk)	Structural Events	Regulators of Lung Growth and Differentiation	Associated Abnormalities
Embryonic	3-6	Lung bud formation, trachea, lobar and segmental bronchi	TTF-1, FGF-10, Shh, Gli	TE fistula, pulmonary agenesis, hypoplasia, asymmetries
Pseudoglandular	6-16	Subsegmental bronchi, terminal bronchi, mucous glands, cartilage, smooth muscle, early vasculature and epithelial differentiation	TTF-1, FGFs, FOXa1/a2	Sequestration, abnormal lobation, cystic adenomatoid malformation, lymphangiectasias, congenital diaphragmatic hernia
Canalicular	16-26	Respiratory bronchioles, acinar saccules, thinning of capillary-epithelial space, type I and type II epithelial cells	Glucocorticoid receptors, VEGF	Pulmonary hypoplasia, alveolar-capillary dysplasia
Saccular	26-36	Division of acinar saccules, microvascular expansion, increase in gas-exchange surface area	Glucocorticoid receptors, VEGF	Pulmonary hypoplasia, pulmonary hypertension
Alveolar	32 wk to 2 yr	Septation of saccules and alveoli, maturation of type II cells, surfactant	Glucocorticoid receptors, retinoic acid receptors, inflammatory mediators	SP-B, SP-C, and ABCA3 transporter deficiencies, pulmonary hypertension

FGF-10, fibroblast growth factor 10; FOXa1/a2, forkhead box a1/a2; Shh, sonic hedgehog homolog; TTF-1, thyroid-specific transcription factor 1; VEGF, vascular endothelial growth factor.

Canalicular Stage

The canalicular stage, between about 16 and 26 weeks' gestation, represents the transformation of the previable lung to the potentially viable lung that can exchange gases. The three major events during this stage are the "birth" of the acinus, epithelial differentiation with the development of the potential air-blood barrier, and the start of surfactant synthesis within recognizable type II cells.[11] The acinus is the tuft of distal airways originating from a terminal bronchiole. Its initial development is the critical first step for the development of the future gas exchange surface of the lung. The initially poorly vascularized mesenchyme surrounding the airways becomes more vascular and more closely aligned with the airway epithelial cells. The capillaries initially form a double capillary network between future airspaces. These capillaries subsequently fuse to form a single capillary bed between the future gas exchange surfaces, with close apposition to the saccular walls to form a structure by about 19 weeks similar to the thin air-blood barrier in the adult lung. If the double capillary network does not fuse, the infant will have severe hypoxemia and the histopathologic findings of alveolar-capillary dysplasia. The total surface area occupied by the air-blood barrier increases exponentially through the canalicular stage, with a resultant fall in the mean wall thickness and with an increased potential for gas exchange. Epithelial differentiation is characterized by proximal-to-distal thinning of the epithelium by transformation of cuboidal cells into thin cells that line wide tubes. The tubes grow both in length and in width with attenuation of the mesenchyme, which is simultaneously vascularized. After about 20 weeks' gestation in the human fetus, these cuboidal cells rich in glycogen begin to have lamellar bodies in their cytoplasm, indicating the initiation of surfactant production.

Saccular Stage

The saccular stage is the period of lung development that is present in most potentially viable preterm fetuses from about 26 weeks to 36 weeks of gestation. The saccule is the terminal structural element of the fetal lung, which divides or septates through perhaps three generations with formation of respiratory bronchioles, and a further three generations to form alveolar ducts before the initiation of "secondary" septation of these saccules to form alveoli.[6] During this saccular stage of lung development, airspace number increases from about 65,000 at 18 weeks to 4 million by 32 to 36 weeks of gestation (Fig. 15-2). Micro-

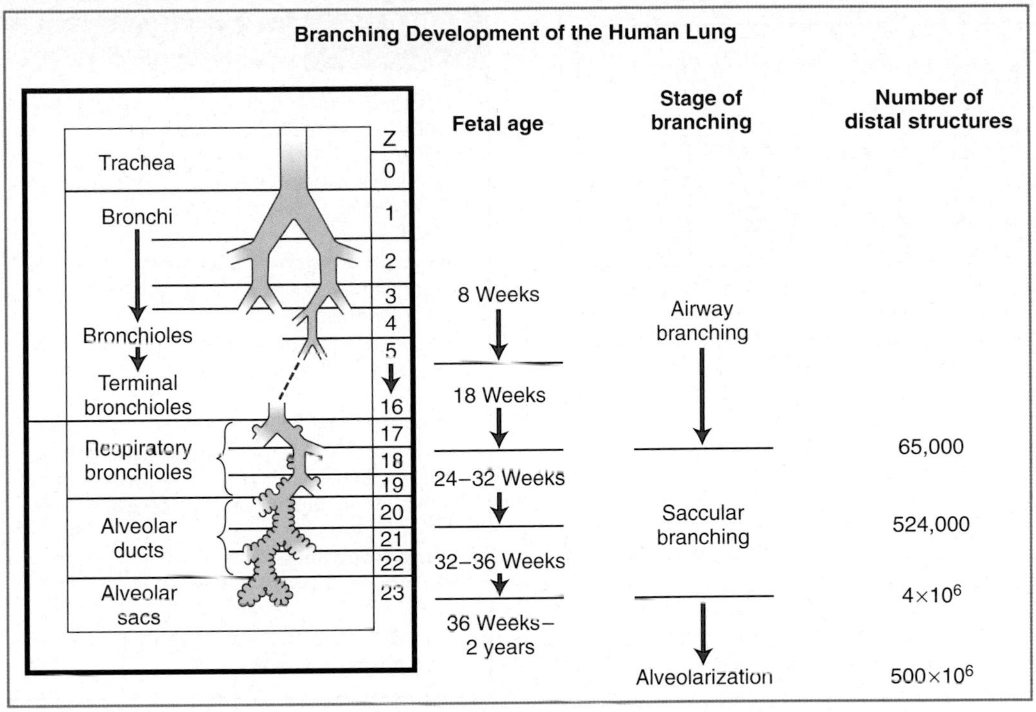

FIGURE 15-2 Airway branching, fetal age, and number of branches during lung development. Airway branching results in about 16 generations of airways by about 18 weeks' gestation. Branching of distal saccular structures yields respiratory bronchioles and alveolar ducts in the saccular lung by about 32 weeks' gestation. Alveolarization continues from 32 to 36 weeks until 2 years of age. (Modified from Burri PW: Development and growth of the human lung. In Fishman AP, Fisher AB [eds]: Handbook of Physiology: The Respiratory System. Bethesda, MD, American Physiology Society, 1986, p 1.)

vascularity continues to increase, as does the gas-exchange surface area of the lung. The fetal lung is sensitive to glucocorticoid stimulation of surfactant and lung structural changes and to the development of pulmonary hypoplasia. Very little is known about the modulators of saccular septation. Saccular septation and the associated vascularization are the critical stages of lung development that may be influenced by common obstetric interventions.

Alveolar Stage

Alveolarization is initiated at 32 to 36 weeks from the terminal saccules by the appearance of septa composed of capillaries, elastin fibers, and collagen fibers (see Fig. 15-1). The saccules and new alveoli rapidly septate to generate about 100 million alveoli at term and about 500 million alveoli in the adult human.[12,13] The rate of alveolar formation is maximal between about 36 weeks' gestation and several months after birth and may be complete by about 2 years of age. The important concept is that alveolar development is a late fetal event that is at its maximal rate during the stages of fetal development after early preterm labor and delivery. Once alveoli are formed, the lung subsequently loses alveoli with age, although under some circumstances the adult lung may be able to develop new alveoli.[14] However, if alveolarization is disrupted during the period of rapid accumulation between about 32 weeks' gestation and term, then there may be adverse short-term and long-term effects on lung function in the newborn.

A number of clinical interventions and agents are known to disrupt normal alveolarization in developing animals (Table 15-2). Hyperoxia, hypoxia, and mechanical ventilation all can interfere with alveolarization.[15] The preterm infant that is mechanically ventilated will be exposed to these factors as well as to nutritional deficits.[16] Recent pathology from infants with very low birth weight who have died of bronchopulmonary dysplasia (BPD) demonstrates an arrest of alveolar development with lungs that contain fewer and larger alveoli.[17] These lungs also demonstrate less airway injury, inflammation, and fibrosis than the lungs of infants who died from bronchopulmonary dysplasia in earlier eras.

New concepts about inflammatory mediators are being developed that link the clinical observations that chorioamnionitis can be associated with altered lung development.[18] In transgenic mouse models, the overexpression of proinflammatory cytokines during the period of postnatal alveolarization disrupts alveolar formation. These same cyto-

TABLE 15-2 MODULATORS OF ALVEOLARIZATION

Factors That Delay or Interfere with Alveolarization
Mechanical ventilation of the preterm infant
Glucocorticoids
Proinflammatory cytokines (TNF-α, TGF-α, IL-11, IL-6)
Chorioamnionitis
Hyperoxia or hypoxia
Poor nutrition
Nicotine
Factors That Stimulate Alveolarization
Vitamin A (retinoic acid)
Thyroxine

IL, interleukin; TGF-α, transforming growth factor-α; TNF-α, tumor necrosis factor-α.

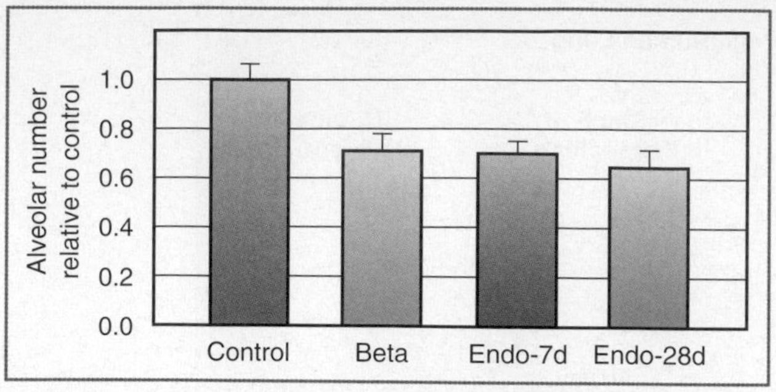

FIGURE 15-3 Effect of maternal betamethasone (Beta) or intra-amniotic endotoxin (Endo) on alveolar number in preterm lambs. The betamethasone treatment (0.5 mg/kg) was given 7 days before preterm delivery at 125 days' gestation. Endotoxin (*Escherichia coli* 055:B5) (20 mg) was given by intra-amniotic injection 6 days before preterm delivery at 125 days, or continuously from day 80 to day 108 at a rate of 0.6 mg/day into the amniotic fluid using an Alzet pump. The interventions decreased alveolarization of the fetal lung. (Data from Willet KE, Jobe AH, Ikegami M, et al: Antenatal endotoxin and glucocorticoid effects on lung morphometry in preterm lambs. Pediatr Res 48:782, 2000; and Moss TJM, Newnham JP, Willet KE, et al: Early gestational intra-amniotic endotoxin: Lung function, surfactant and morphometry. Am J Respir Crit Care Med 165:805, 2002.)

TABLE 15-3 CLINICAL ASSOCIATIONS WITH PULMONARY HYPOPLASIA

Thoracic Compression
Renal agenesis (Potter syndrome)
Urinary tract outflow obstruction
Oligohydramnios before 28 weeks' gestational age
Extra-amniotic fetal development
Decreased Intrathoracic Space
Diaphragmatic hernia
Pleural effusions
Abdominal distention sufficient to limit chest volume
Thoracic dystrophies
Decreased Fetal Breathing
Intrauterine central nervous system damage
Fetal Werdnig-Hoffmann syndrome
Other neuropathies and myopathies
Other Associations
Primary pulmonary hypoplasia
Trisomy 21
Multiple congenital anomalies
Erythroblastosis fetalis

kines are elevated in amniotic fluid, cord blood, and tracheal aspirate samples of infants exposed to chorioamnionitis before preterm delivery. In an experimental model of chorioamnionitis caused by the intra-amniotic injection of endotoxin, alveolar numbers were decreased after preterm delivery in sheep (Fig. 15-3).[19,20]

Another clinically relevant observation is that glucocorticoids can cause an arrest in alveolarization. Glucocorticoids cause permanent abnormalities in alveolar and vascular development in mice and rats.[14] Maternal glucocorticoids given to the monkey at the saccular stage of lung development decrease the mesenchyme and make the lung appear more mature, but at term the lung has a lower gas volume and fewer alveoli.[21] In sheep, single or repetitive weekly maternal glucocorticoid treatments cause a decrease in alveolar number and an increase in alveolar size after preterm birth (see Fig. 15-3).[22] However, the alveolar numbers were normal at term, demonstrating that recovery from an inhibition of alveolar development is possible. A concern is that many infants with very low birth weight who are exposed to chorioamnionitis also are exposed to antenatal and postnatal glucocorticoid therapy.

Pulmonary Hypoplasia

Although embryonic developmental anomalies occasionally result in unilateral pulmonary atresias and abnormal lung segmentation syndromes, pulmonary hypoplasia syndromes are much more common. Pulmonary hypoplasia diagnosed by low lung weight was found in 15% to 20% of an unselected autopsy series.[23] The diagnosis of pulmonary hypoplasia by the anatomic criteria of decreased airway numbers and decreased radial alveolar counts is time consuming and not routine. Measurements of lung DNA content relative to body weight also can identify infants with pulmonary hypoplasia. However, generally the diagnosis is made clinically on the basis of the severity of respiratory failure and the clinical associations. The fetus must maintain the appropriate volume of fetal lung fluid in the airways and have the normal frequency and amplitude of fetal breathing movements for the lung to grow normally.[24] Fetal lung fluid volume can be decreased either by external chest compression (e.g., oligohydramnios) or by space occupation in the chest cavity (e.g., diaphragmatic hernia). Conditions associated with pulmonary hypoplasia are listed in Table 15-3. Thoracic compression syndromes are most destructive to lung growth during the canalicular period of human lung development from 16 to 24 weeks' gestation. Oligohydramnios not associated with renal anomalies does not invariably result in pulmonary hypoplasia; however, the earlier it is in gestation, the more severe and the longer the oligohydramnios lasts, the more likely it is that severe pulmonary hypoplasia will occur.[25] Some infants delivered because of premature preterm rupture of membranes after many weeks of oligohydramnios can have good lung function.[26] Pulmonary hypoplasia, despite maintenance of apparently normal fetal lung fluid and amniotic fluid volumes, can occur in infants with severe central nervous system damage from infectious or developmental neuropathies and myopathies.

Diaphragmatic hernia is the most common cause of pulmonary hypoplasia resulting from lung compression. The lung on the side of the diaphragmatic hernia is often severely hypoplastic, but the contralateral lung also is hypoplastic, although less so. Studies in animal models indicate that maturation of the surfactant system is delayed in the hypoplastic lungs, and surfactant components are decreased in amniotic fluid from infants with diaphragmatic hernia.[27] Attempts to surgically correct the diaphragmatic hernia in utero have seldom succeeded. Obstruction of the trachea will distend the fetal lung with fetal lung fluid and stimulate lung growth. Although the lung grows larger, the constant stretch can result in decreased numbers of type II cells and decreased surfactant.[28] As a general rule, the fetal lung develops abnormally if it is compressed, collapsed because of loss of fetal lung fluid, or overstretched.

Infants with diaphragmatic hernia and with less severe degrees of pulmonary hypoplasia can be supported with mechanical ventilation. Attempting to achieve normal gas exchange and oxygenation with excessive mechanical ventilation results in severe lung injury. Gentle approaches to mechanical ventilation together with the selective use of extracorporeal membrane oxygenation and delayed surgical correction of diaphragmatic hernias is resulting in survivals of 80% or better. Infants with trisomy 21 or other syndromes may have anomalous lung development or may have abnormal fetal breathing patterns that may result in pulmonary hypoplasia.

Fetal Lung Fluid

The fetal airways are filled with fluid until delivery and the initiation of ventilation. Quantitative information about fetal lung fluid is from the fetal lamb, with sonographic and pathologic correlates available for the human. The fetal lung close to term contains enough fluid to maintain the airway volume approximately at the same volume as the functional residual capacity once air breathing is established. This volume is about 25 mL/kg body weight in the fetal lamb. The composition of fetal lung fluid is unique relative to other fetal fluids.[29] The chloride content is high, and the bicarbonate and protein contents are low. The fetal epithelium is essentially impermeable to protein. The fetal lung fluid is in equilibrium with fetal partial pressure of carbon dioxide values of about 45 mm Hg, which results in a low pH in fetal lung fluid. This electrolyte composition is maintained by transepithelial chloride secretion with bicarbonate reabsorption. However, there are species differences in fetal lung fluid, and bicarbonate and pH are higher in the primate. Active chloride transport by epithelial cells results in passive water movement into the fetal airspaces, with a net production rate for fetal lung fluid of 4 to 5 mL/kg/hr.[30] The production of fetal lung fluid is about 400 mL/day for a 4-kg fetus. In humans, about half of this fluid is swallowed and about half mixes with the amniotic fluid. The pressure in the fetal trachea exceeds that in the amniotic fluid by about 2 mm Hg, generating an outflow resistance that maintains the fetal lung fluid volume. The secretion of fetal lung fluid is primarily an intrinsic metabolic function of the developing alveolar and airway epithelium, because changes in vascular hydrostatic pressures, tracheal pressures, and fetal breathing movements do not greatly affect fetal lung fluid production.

Although the presence of fetal lung fluid is essential for normal lung development, its clearance is equally essential for normal neonatal respiratory adaptation. Fetal lung fluid production can be completely stopped and fluid adsorption initiated in near-term fetal sheep by infusions of epinephrine at concentrations that approximate the levels of epinephrine present during labor.[31] The epinephrine-responsive change in the airspace epithelium from fluid secretion to absorption is absent in preterm fetal sheep and can be induced by short-term cortisol and triiodothyronine infusions.[32] In term guinea pigs, the Na^+ channel blocker amiloride delays fluid clearance and causes respiratory distress, demonstrating that Na^+,K^+ adenosine triphosphatase function is essential for the clearance of airway fluid after birth.[29]

Fetal lung fluid production may decrease in the days just before labor. Fetal lung fluid volume decreases in fetal sheep to about 65% of the maximal volumes present during fetal life.[30] During active labor and delivery, another 30% of the fluid is cleared from the airways and alveoli, leaving only about 35% of the fetal lung fluid to be adsorbed and cleared from the lungs with breathing. Most of the fluid moves rapidly into the interstitial spaces and then directly into the pulmonary vasculature, with less than 20% of the fluid being cleared by pulmonary lymphatics. Clearance of the fluid from the interstitial spaces occurs over many hours. Alveolar fluid volume in the normal lung is only about 0.3 mL/kg. The sequence of prelabor, labor, and delivery is an important regulator of the fetal lung fluid volume present at the initiation of air breathing.

Cesarean delivery of fetuses who have not experienced labor can result in decreased lung compliance, early respiratory distress, and transient tachypnea of the newborn.[33,34] The magnitude of the potential problem can be appreciated by the following estimates. Assume the apneic term newborn born without labor has a fetal lung fluid volume of 25 mL/kg, a normal blood volume of 80 mL/kg, and a hematocrit of 50%. The fetal lung fluid, which contains essentially no protein, would be equivalent to 62% of the plasma volume. Cesarean delivery, intubation, and ventilation could result in a crystalloid volume challenge of 25 mL/kg, which could destabilize cardiopulmonary function. Although this scenario is the extreme, many subtle abnormalities and a few severe difficulties of neonatal adaptation result from the presence of large amounts of alveolar and interstitial fluid in the lungs of infants.

Surfactant

Lipids

Surfactant from lungs of all mammalian species contains 70% to 80% phospholipids, about 8% protein, and about 8% neutral lipids, primarily cholesterol (Fig. 15-4). The phosphatidylcholine species of the phospholipids contribute about 70% by weight to surfactant and are about 80% of the phospholipids.[35] The composition of the phospholipids in surfactant is unique relative to the lipid composition of the lung or other organs. About 50% of the phosphatidylcholine species are saturated, in that most of the fatty acid esterified to the glycerolphosphorylcholine backbone is the 16-carbon saturated fatty acid palmitic acid. The other major phosphatidylcholine species of surfactant has a fatty acid with one double bond in the 2-acyl position of the molecule.

Saturated phosphatidylcholine is the principal surface-active component of surfactant. The acidic phospholipid, phosphatidylglycerol, is 4% to 15% of the phospholipids in surfactant from different species. The composition of the phospholipids in the surfactant lipoprotein complex changes during late gestation. Surfactant phospholipids from the immature fetus or newborn contain relatively large amounts of phosphatidylinositol, and these amounts decrease as phosphatidylglycerol appears with lung maturity.[36] Although phosphatidylglycerol is a convenient marker for lung maturity, its presence is not necessary for normal surfactant function.

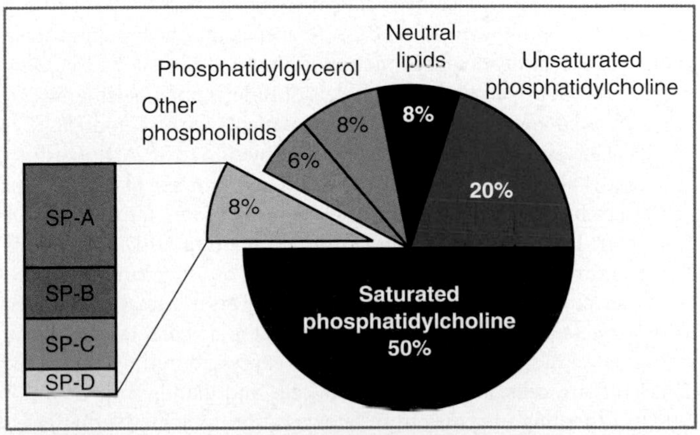

FIGURE 15-4 Composition of surfactant. The major component is saturated phosphatidylcholine. The surfactant proteins (SP) contribute about 8% to the mass of surfactant.

Proteins

Much of the protein isolated with surfactant from alveolar lavages is serum protein that is not specific to surfactant. However, four surfactant proteins have been characterized and their functions in part elucidated.[37] Two of the proteins (SP-A and SP-D) have related structures and are classified as collectins because they bind carbohydrate lectins in a calcium-dependent manner.

The 26-kDa monomer of SP-A is heavily glycosylated and assembled as a six-tetramer complex of about 650 kDa.[38] The protein has a collagen-like domain that facilitates tetramer formation, and a carbohydrate recognition domain. SP-A is expressed predominantly in type II cells and Clara cells in the late-gestation and mature lung. SP-A appears in fetal lung fluid and amniotic fluid in parallel with the surfactant phospholipids during late gestation. It is secreted constitutively and separately from the surfactant complex contained in the lamellar bodies. Once in the airspace, SP-A associates with surfactant and is required for tubular myelin formation. SP-A may contribute to the biophysical function of surfactant primarily by making surfactant less sensitive to inactivation by edema fluid and inflammatory products in the injured lung. Mice that lack SP-A have essentially normal surfactant function and metabolism unless the lung is injured.

SP-A functions primarily as an innate host defense protein in the alveolus and airways.[38] The ability of SP-A to bind carbohydrates and to interact with immune cells in the lungs contributes to host defense. It binds endotoxin avidly, and it also binds a wide range of gram-positive and gram-negative organisms, fungi (such as *Aspergillus fumigatus*), and other organisms such as mycobacteria and *Pneumocystis carinii*. Macrophages have receptors for SP-A, and SP-A promotes phagocytosis and killing of microorganisms by alveolar macrophages. SP-A also acts as an opsonin for the phagocytosis of viruses, such as herpes simplex, influenza A, and respiratory syncytial virus. Mice that lack SP-A have less effective clearance and killing of bacteria and viruses, and infections are more likely to become systemic.[39] The defect in host defenses can be corrected by treating SP-A–deficient mice with SP-A.

Another component of the host defense role of SP-A is modulation of the inflammatory response to infection. Nitric oxide production by macrophages is increased by SP-A to promote pathogen killing. SP-A also downregulates the general inflammatory response of the lung that generates tumor necrosis factor-α and other proinflammatory cytokines.

Two closely related genes express SP-A in humans, and no genetically based deficiency state has been identified. However, genetic polymorphisms in SP-A have been linked to an increased risk of RDS.[40] Infants born with low ratios of SP-A to surfactant phospholipid are at increased risk of death and bronchopulmonary dysplasia.[41] SP-A levels are also low in preterm baboon models of BPD, in infants with respiratory syncytial virus pneumonia, and in patients with acute RDS.

SP-D has similarities in structure and function to SP-A, but distinct differences also are apparent.[38] The 43-kDa monomer of SP-D forms tetramers by collagen domains and then associates into a 560-kDa multimer. The carbohydrate recognition domain of SP-D binds endotoxin, gram-negative organisms, and a variety of other lung pathogens with a specificity that overlaps with SP-A. SP-D is minimally associated with surfactant lipids. The protein is present in alveolar lavage fluid at 10% to 30% of the level of SP-A. SP-D is expressed in the lung in type II cells, Clara cells, and other airway cells and glands. Expression of SP-D in the lung increases from late gestation to achieve adult levels after term, and glucocorticoids increase SP-D expression.

SP-D has the characteristics of an innate host defense protein. It binds bacteria and fungi, aggregates viruses, and promotes opsonization and phagocytosis by macrophages. It also may modulate the proinflammatory responses of leukocytes in the lung. In contrast to SP-A, SP-D increases with acute lung injury. Mice that lack SP-D have increased tissue and alveolar pools of surfactant lipids and develop emphysema.[42] Mice that are SP-D deficient have a greater inflammatory response when given respiratory syncytial virus. No SP-D deficiency has been identified in humans, and its contribution to the pathogenesis of BPD and lung infections in newborns has not been defined.

SP-B is a small, 79-amino-acid homodimer of about 18 kDa that comprises about 2% of surfactant by weight.[38] The essential function of SP-B is its absolute requirement for normal packaging of the surfactant phospholipids into lamellar bodies for secretion. In the absence of SP-B, type II cells have no lamellar bodies and SP-C is incompletely processed. Therefore, functionally, SP-B deficiency also results in SP-C deficiency. Mice and humans that lack SP-B die soon after birth with a severe RDS-like syndrome.[43] Surfactant treatment is not effective, presumably because there are no pathways for reprocessing of the surfactant components.

Deficiency of SP-B most frequently occurs because of a frame-shift mutation, although multiple compound mutations have been described. The gene frequency of this frame-shift maturation is 1 per 1000 to 3000 individuals.[44] Deficiency of SP-B from all mutations accounts for about 30% of term infants who die of severe RDS at birth as a result of possible genetic causes for the respiratory failure. An antenatal diagnosis of SP-B deficiency can be made using amniotic fluid. Some mutations result in low expression that may increase with glucocorticoid treatment. Infants with low expression may have a chronic progressive lung disease indistinguishable from bronchopulmonary dysplasia. Acute lung injury and inflammation resulting in release of tumor necrosis factor in the lungs depresses SP-B levels.

SP-C is a 35-amino-acid, 4.5-kDa monomer that is about 2% of surfactant by weight.[37] This extremely hydrophobic protein promotes surfactant film adsorption. The SP-C sequence is highly conserved across species, and messenger RNA is expressed in the developing tips of the branching airways during early lung development. During late gestation, SP-C is expressed, processed, and secreted with SP-B and the surfactant lipids in lamellar bodies only by type II cells. A deficiency of SP-C in mice results in no lung developmental abnormalities or striking abnormalities in surfactant function.[45] However, the mice get a progressive interstitial lung disease as they age. SP-C deficiency in humans can also cause a progressive interstitial lung disease that can present in infancy and may make the individual susceptible to developing acute RDS.[46] The clinical spectrum of genetically based SP-C abnormalities in humans has not been well defined yet. Acute lung injury will decrease the expression of SP-C, but how this may affect lung function is not known.

Deficiency of the ABCA3 transporter has recently been described as a cause of severe lethal RDS in term infants resulting from surfactant deficiency.[47] This transporter is a member of a family of ATP-binding cassette transporters that localize to the limiting membranes of lamellar bodies in type II cells. Its deficiency seems to disrupt lipid transport and lamellar body formation, resulting in severe surfactant deficiency. This genetically based deficiency disease in term infants is more common than are SP-B or SP-C deficiencies.

Surfactant Metabolism

Type II cells and macrophages are the cells responsible for the major pathways involved in surfactant metabolism (Fig. 15-5). The synthesis and secretion pathways in type II cells are complex sequences of bio-

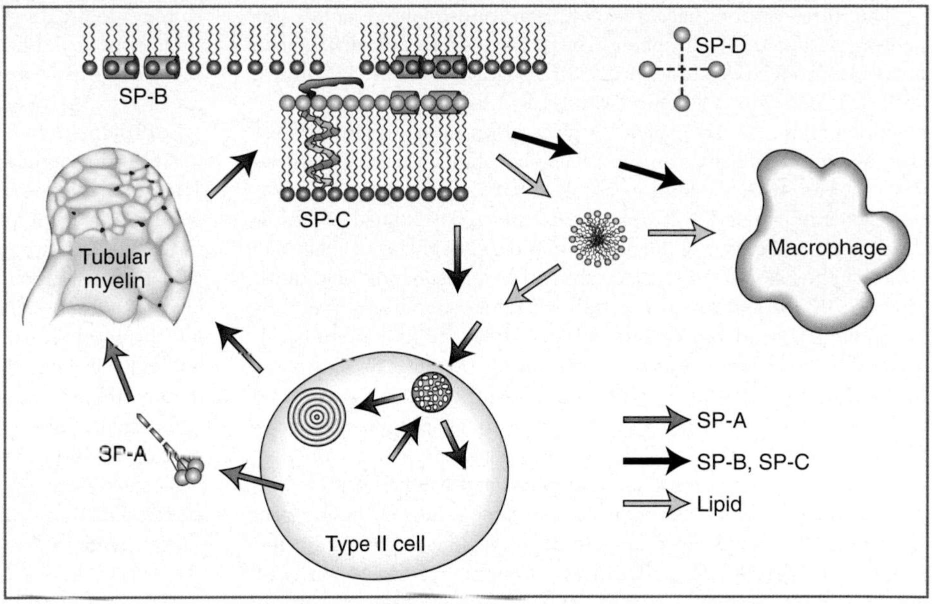

FIGURE 15-5 Diagram of surfactant metabolism. The lipid-associated surfactant proteins B (SP-B) and SP-C *(solid red arrows)* track with the lipid from synthesis to secretion of lamellar bodies. SP-A is secreted and combines to form tubular myelin with SP-B, SP-C, and the lipids. The surface film is shown as a monolayer of lipids with SP-B. The hypophase of bilayer lipids is a reservoir of surfactant that can add to the monolayer. SP-B and SP-C leave the monolayer without lipids and are catabolized by macrophages. Lipids leave the monolayer as vesicles and are either catabolized or recycled back to type II cells.

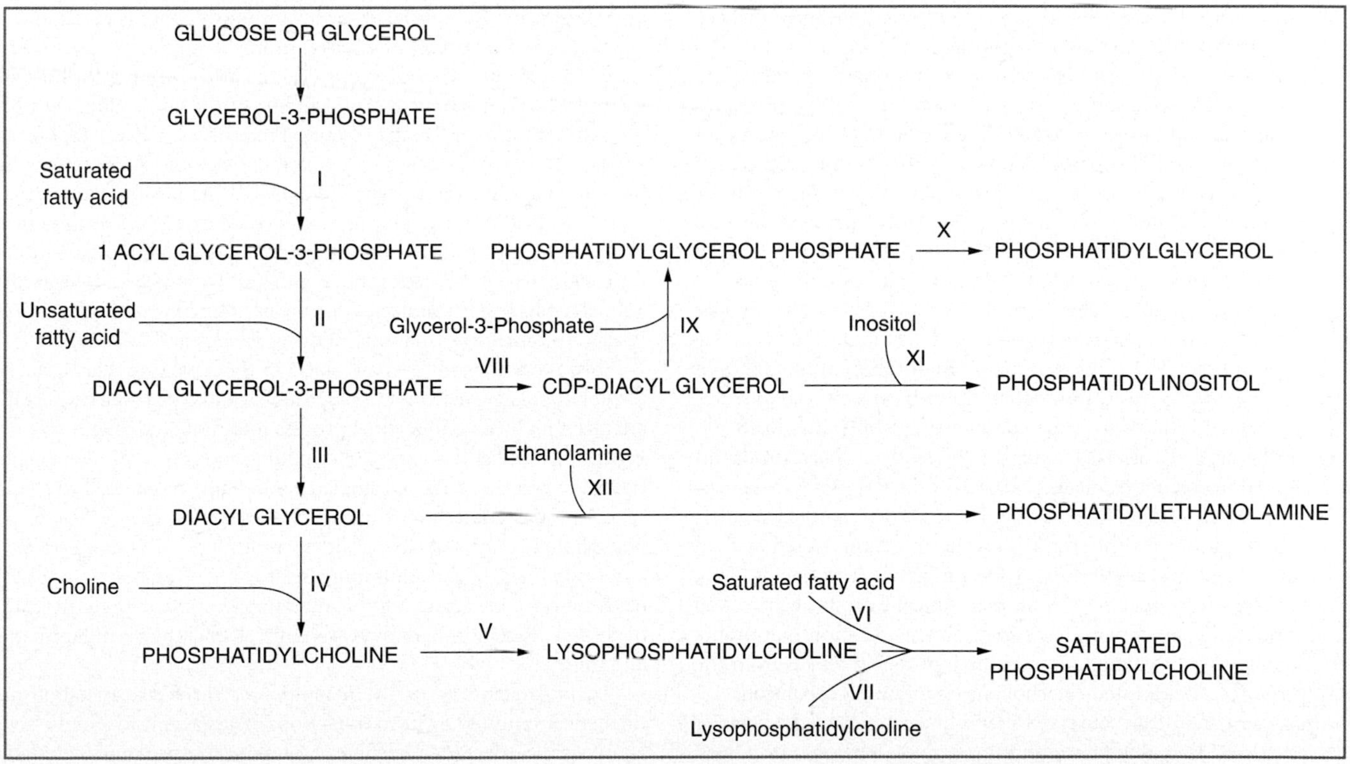

FIGURE 15-6 Biosynthesis of lung phospholipids. The major pathways and precursors for the synthesis of saturated phosphatidylcholine, phosphatidylethanolamine, phosphatidylinositol, and phosphatidylglycerol are outlined. The enzymes specific for each step are indicated by roman numerals: I, glycerophosphate acyltransferase; II, 1-acyl-glycerolphosphate phosphotransferase; III, phosphatidic acid phosphatase; IV, cytidine-5′-diphospho (CDP)-choline diacylglycerol phosphotransferase; V, phospholipase A_2; VI, lysophosphatidylcholine acyl transferase; VII, lysophosphatidylcholine-lysophosphatidylcholine acyl transferase; VIII, phosphatidate cytidyltransferase; IX, glycerophosphate phosphatidyltransferase; X, phosphatidylglycerol phosphatase; XI, CDP-inositol diacylglycerol phosphotransferase; XII, ethanolamine diacylglycerol phosphotransferase.

chemical events that result in lipid, SP-B, and SP-C release in lamellar bodies to the alveolus by exocytosis. Specific enzymes within the endoplasmic reticulum use glucose, phosphate, and fatty acids as substrates for phospholipid synthesis. The uniqueness of a phospholipid is determined by the fatty acid side chains esterified to the glycerol carbon backbone and by the head group (e.g., choline, glycerol, inositol) linked to the phosphate. The interrelated pathways for the synthesis of lung phospholipids are outlined in Figure 15-6, and the enzymes discussed in the next paragraph are identified by roman numerals on that figure.

The three-carbon backbone of each phospholipid enters the pathway as glycerol-3-phosphate. The de novo synthetic pathway then proceeds through two sequential acyltransferase reactions. A saturated fatty acyl-coenzyme A (usually palmitic acid) is esterified to the 1-acyl position of glycerol-3-phosphate by glycerol-phosphate acyltransferase (I). Then the 1-acyl-glycerol-phosphate phosphotransferase (II) esterifies either an unsaturated or a saturated fatty acid to the 2-acyl position, generating diacylglycerophosphate (phosphatidic acid), which is the common precursor of the phospholipids. Phosphatidic acid is then either dephosphorylated to diacylglycerol by phosphatidic acid phosphatase (III) or converted to cytidine-5′-diphosphodiacylglycerol by phosphatidate cytidyltransferase (VIII). Cytidine-5′-diphosphodiacylglycerol is the common precursor of phosphatidylglycerol and phosphatidylinositol. Phosphatidylglycerol is synthesized by a two-step pathway involving the enzymes glycerol-phosphate phosphatidyltransferase (IX) and phosphatidylglycerol phosphatase (X). The diacylglycerol is the direct precursor of both phosphatidylethanolamine and phosphatidylcholine after the transfer of ethanolamine or choline from the cytidine-5′-diphosphoethanolamine or cytidine-5′-diphosphocholine to the diacylglycerol by the appropriate phosphotransferase (IV, XII). However, the resulting phosphatidylcholines are largely 1-acyl saturated, 2-acyl unsaturated.

A remodeling of some of the 2-acyl-unsaturated phosphatidylcholines from the de novo synthetic pathway occurs in the type II cell before packaging of the resulting saturated phosphatidylcholine into lamellar bodies for secretion. The direct re-acylation of lysophosphatidylcholine with palmitoyl-coenzyme A (enzyme VI) is the important pathway for saturated phosphatidylcholine synthesis in type II cells.[48]

Although the overall synthetic pathways are known, the details of how the components of surfactant condense to form the surfactant lipoprotein complex containing the phospholipids SP-B and SP-C in lamellar bodies remain obscure. Lipids and the hydrophobic surfactant proteins are essential to lamellar body formation, because the lamellar bodies are absent or abnormal from type II cells that lack SP-B or the ABCA3 transporter. The development and maturation of the ability of the immature lung to process surfactant lipids from synthesis to secretion are essential if the fetus is to ventilate successfully after birth.

Once the type II cell has matured sufficiently to have surfactant stores, secretion can be stimulated.[49] Type II cells respond to beta agonists by increased surfactant secretion. Purines such as adenosine tri phosphate are more potent stimulators of surfactant secretion than beta agonists and may be important for surfactant secretion at birth. Surfactant secretion also occurs with mechanical stimuli, such as lung distention and hyperventilation. The surfactant secretion that occurs with the initiation of ventilation after birth probably results from the combined effects of elevated catecholamines and lung expansion.

After Avery and Mead[1] observed that saline extracts of the lungs of infants with RDS had high minimum surface tensions, decreased alveolar and tissue surfactant pools were documented in developing animals. In general, surfactant pool sizes correlate with lung compliance during development, although other factors, such as structural maturation of the lung, also influence compliance measurements. Infants with RDS have surfactant pool sizes on the order of 2 to 10 mg/kg of bodyweight.[50] The quantity is similar to the amount of surfactant found in the alveoli of healthy adult animals and humans, but much less than the amount of surfactant recovered from healthy term animals, which have surfactant pool sizes of 100 mg/kg of bodyweight.

The rate of increase in the pool size of alveolar surfactant after preterm birth has been measured in ventilated preterm monkeys recovering from RDS.[51] The surfactant pool size increases from about 5 mg/kg toward the 100 mg/kg value measured in term monkeys within 3 to 4 days. Although there are no comparable pool size measurements for humans, the concentration of saturated phosphatidylcholine in airway samples from infants recovering from RDS increased over a 4- to 5-day period to become comparable with values for normal or surfactant-treated infants.[41] This slow increase in pool size explains why the uncomplicated clinical course of RDS lasts from 3 to 5 days. The explanation for why surfactant pool sizes increase slowly after preterm birth is apparent from measurements of the kinetics of surfactant secretion and clearance in the newborn.[52] Incorporation of precursors into lung phosphatidylcholine is rapid. However, there are long delays between synthesis and the movement of surfactant components from the endoplasmic reticulum through the Golgi to lamellar bodies for eventual secretion. The time lag from surfactant phospholipid synthesis to peak secretion of labeled surfactant is about 40 hours in term newborn lambs. Ventilated preterm baboons with RDS that are developing BPD have small alveolar pool sizes of surfactant, a low percentage secretion of de novo synthesized lipids, and decreased surfactant function.[53] The peak time for secretion of surfactant lipids labeled with ^{13}C-glucose was about 70 hours in infants with RDS (Fig. 15-7).[54]

The slow increase in the alveolar surfactant pool from de novo synthesis is balanced in the term and preterm lung by slow catabolism and clearance.[55] Radiolabeled surfactant phospholipids given into the airspaces of term lambs are cleared from the lung with a half-life on the order of 6 days. This slow lung clearance is in striking contrast with the more rapid catabolism characteristic of the adult lung, with half-life values on the order of 12 hours. Preterm ventilated baboons that are developing BPD degrade a treatment dose of surfactant with a half-life of about 2 days.[53] The biologic half-life of surfactant lipids in infants with RDS was about 35 hours (see Fig. 15-7).[56] Although the measurements of surfactant metabolism in preterm infants are limited, the consistency of the values between infants with RDS and the preterm animal models clearly indicates that the preterm lung requires a number of days to achieve normal surfactant pool sizes and metabolism.

Surfactant does not remain static in the airspaces. The surfactant phospholipids move from the airspaces back to type II cells, where they are taken up by an endocytotic process into multivesicular bodies (see Fig. 15-5).[55] In the term and preterm lung, about 90% of the phospholipids are recycled back to lamellar bodies and re-secreted to the airspace. In the adult lung, this process is about 25% efficient. The phospholipids are recycled as intact molecules without degradation and resynthesis. In the adult lung, macrophages catabolize about 50% of the surfactant. There are few macrophages in the preterm lung at birth, but their numbers increase with postnatal age, inflammation, and injury.

An understanding of the dynamics of surfactant metabolism is further complicated by form transitions of surfactant within the alveolar space.[55] Surfactant phosphatidylcholine moves from secretion as lamellar bodies to a tubular myelin pool that is the reservoir in the hypo-phase from which the surface film is maintained. SP-A is essential for this transition. Area compression of the surface film is then thought to concentrate saturated phosphatidylcholine by squeezing out other lipids and surfactant proteins. New surfactant adsorbs into the surface film and "used" surfactant leaves in the form of small vesicles, which then are cleared from the airspaces.

Physiologic Effects of Surfactant on the Preterm Lung

The effects of surfactant on the preterm surfactant-deficient lung can be demonstrated by the pressure-volume relationships during quasi-

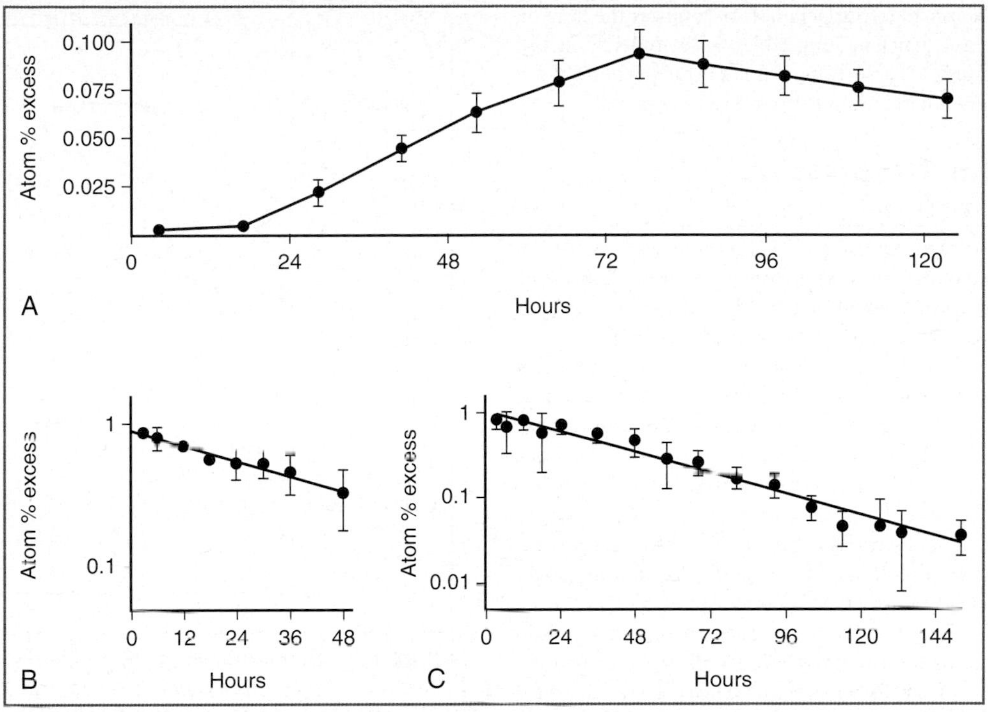

FIGURE 15-7 Measurements of surfactant metabolism in preterm infants with respiratory distress syndrome using stable isotopes. A, Curve for the ^{13}C labeling of palmitate in phosphatidylcholine recovered from airway aspirates of 11 preterm infants who received ^{13}C-glucose infusion for the first 24 hours of life. The time to maximal enrichment expressed as atom % excess ^{13}C was 77 ± 8 hours. The half-life after peak enrichment was about 100 hours. **B** and **C,** Loss of ^{13}C dipalmitoyl phosphatidylcholine from treatment doses of surfactant given to eight preterm infants at a mean age of 4.6 hours (**B**), and for a second dose of surfactant given at a mean age of 37 hours (**C**). The half-life of the label in the airway aspirates was about 34 hours. (Data in **A** from Bunt JE, Carnielli VP, Darcos Wattimena JL, et al: The effect in premature infants of prenatal corticosteroids on endogenous surfactant synthesis as measured with stable isotopes. Am J Respir Crit Care Med 162:844, 2000; data in **C** from Torresin M, Zimmermann LJ, Cogo PE, et al: Exogenous surfactant kinetics in infant respiratory distress syndrome: A novel method with stable isotopes. Am J Respir Crit Care Med 161:1584, 2000.)

static inflation and deflation.[5] The pressure needed to open a lung unit is related to the radius of curvature and surface tension of the meniscus of fluid in the airway to that unit. With surfactant deficiency, surface tensions are high and variable. The uninflated lung contains fluid-filled airways with different radii. The units served by airways with larger radii and with lower surface tensions "pop" open first, making lung inflation nonuniform with surfactant deficiency. Preterm surfactant-deficient rabbit lungs do not inflate until pressures exceed 25 cm H_2O (Fig. 15-8).

Surfactant treatment results in a striking decrease in the opening pressure to about 15 cm H_2O. Because the treatment does not alter the radii of the airways, the decreased opening pressure results from adsorption of the surfactant to the menisci. Inflation is more uniform because low surface tensions make aeration of airways less dependent on airway size. More units are opening at lower pressures, and there is less overdistention of the units that do open. Inflation is less uniform in the surfactant-deficient lung.

A striking effect of surfactant on the surfactant-deficient lung is the 2.5 times increase in maximal volume at 35 cm H_2O airway pressure (see Fig. 15-8). Pressures higher than 35 cm H_2O rupture the surfactant-deficient control lungs and result in little further volume accumulation. This difference in the lung gas volume caused by surfactant treatment is lung volume that will increase the surface area of the lung

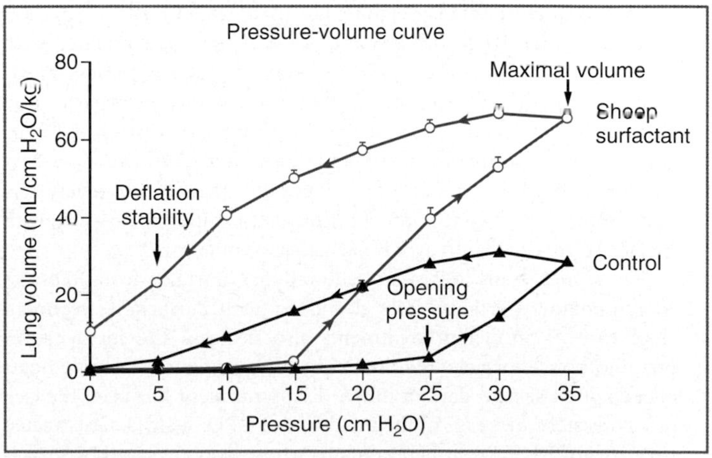

FIGURE 15-8 Pressure-volume relationships for the inflation and deflation of surfactant-deficient and surfactant-treated preterm rabbit lungs. The *arrowheads* on the curves indicate the direction of the inflation-deflation sequence. The control lungs are from 27-day preterm rabbits. Surfactant deficiency is indicated by the high opening pressure, the low maximal volume at a distending pressure of 35 cm H_2O, and the lack of deflation stability at low pressures on deflation. In contrast, treatment of 27-day preterm rabbits with a natural surfactant strikingly alters the pressure-volume relationships.

and provide better gas exchange. Surfactant also stabilizes the lung on deflation. The surfactant-deficient lung collapses completely at low transpulmonary pressures. The surfactant-treated lung retains about 36% of the lung volume on deflation to 5 cm H_2O pressure.

Surfactant for Respiratory Distress Syndrome

Fujiwara and associates first reported in 1980 that airway instillation of surfactant improved oxygenation in infants with severe RDS.[57] Surfactant for RDS became available for general clinical use in 1990 after extensive clinical trials.[58] Three surfactants prepared from pig or cow lungs are currently in use in the United States. They are not equivalent to natural surfactant in composition or function because they have altered surfactant protein and phospholipid compositions and somewhat different biophysical characteristics. However, the metabolic characteristics of surfactant in the preterm are favorable for surfactant treatment.[5] In the infant with RDS, alveolar and tissue pool sizes are small, and the alveolar pool increases slowly after birth. Treatment acutely increases both the alveolar and tissue pools because the exogenously administered surfactant is taken up into type II cells and processed for re-secretion. The surfactant given as treatment becomes substrate for the preterm lung to metabolize and can improve the function of the surfactant used for treatment.[59] The surfactant used for treatment remains in the lungs and is not rapidly degraded (see Fig. 15-7). Treatment doses of surfactant do not feedback inhibit the endogenous synthesis of saturated phosphatidylcholine or the surfactant proteins. No adverse metabolic consequences of surfactant treatment on the endogenous metabolism of surfactant or other lung functions have been identified. There are no clinically important differences between the surfactants used clinically to treat RDS.

Surfactants have been evaluated as treatment in two situations: for preterm infants at risk for RDS immediately after birth, and for infants with established RDS.[60] Either treatment strategy effectively decreases the severity of respiratory symptoms and infant mortality. The choice of treatment strategy probably does not influence complications or outcomes for larger infants with RDS, but early treatment may benefit the very immature infant weighing less than 1 kg at birth.

In the initial trials, delivery room treatment was compared with treatment many hours after birth. In clinical practice, the two treatment strategies now are less distinct because treatment is given as soon after birth as is practical and when some respiratory distress is apparent.[61] A surfactant treatment should not interfere with neonatal resuscitation and initial stabilization. Clinical treatment strategies also include the use of continuous positive end-expiratory pressure with surfactant treatments to avoid mechanical ventilation.[62]

The clinical trials consistently showed that mortality from RDS and overall infant mortality rates decreased with surfactant treatment (Fig. 15-9).[60] Surfactant treatments also decrease the incidence of pneumothorax, oxygen requirements, and ventilatory requirements over the first several days of life. A disappointment has been the lack of a consistent decrease in the incidence of BPD in surfactant-treated survivors of RDS. Presumably, infants whose lives are saved by surfactant treatment are those most likely to develop BPD, thus in part explaining the lack of decrease of this chronic lung disease. Fortunately, the severity of BPD has decreased despite the survival of more immature infants. Although isolated trials report either increases or decreases in the occurrences of common neonatal problems, such as patent ductus arteriosus and intraventricular hemorrhage, surfactant treatments do not seem to affect the nonpulmonary complications of prematurity.

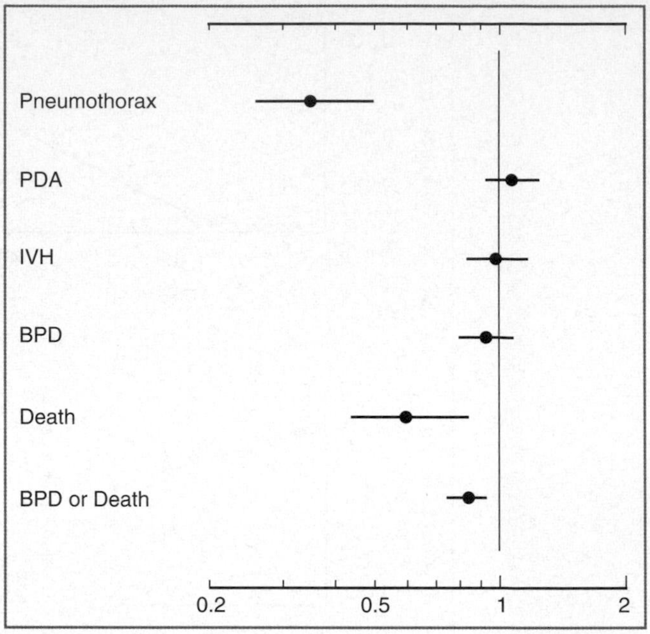

FIGURE 15-9 **Meta-analysis of eight randomized controlled trials of surfactant for the treatment of respiratory distress syndrome.** Results are given as odds ratios and 95% confidence intervals for 988 randomized patients. BPD, bronchopulmonary dysplasia; IVH, intraventricular hemorrhage; PDA, patent ductus arteriosus. (Data from Soll RF, Morley C: Prophylactic versus selective use of surfactant for preventing morbidity and mortality in preterm infants. Cochrane Database Syst Rev [2]:CD000510, 2001.)

Infants with primarily surfactant deficiency should respond well to surfactant. Reasons for poor responses are injury to the preterm lung by inflammation or ventilatory injury before surfactant treatment, unrecognized pulmonary hypoplasia, or very immature lung structure. Antenatal corticosteroid treatments before preterm birth seem to act synergistically with surfactant to improve outcomes for infants by improving respiratory function and decreasing pneumothorax and intraventricular hemorrhage.[63] Multiple beneficial interactions between antenatal corticosteroids and postnatal surfactant treatments can be demonstrated in experimental models.[64] The corticosteroid exposure makes the endogenous surfactant less resistant to inhibition by proteins and inflammatory mediators. The corticosteroid-induced increases in airspace volume and decreased permeability of the airway epithelium decreases the dosage of exogenous surfactant needed to improve lung function and decreases surfactant inactivation. Other effects of corticosteroids on fluid clearance and inflammation also probably contribute to improved clinical responses. The availability of surfactant treatments is not a reason to withhold antenatal corticosteroid treatment to women at risk of preterm delivery.

Induced Lung Maturation

Normally, lung maturation does not occur until after 36 or 37 weeks' gestation in an infant destined to deliver at term. However, the incidence of RDS is only about 30% at 30 weeks' gestation, and infants as early as 25 weeks' gestation often do not have severe RDS.[62] Therefore, spontaneous "early maturation" is frequent and is thought to result from fetal stress inducing endogenous fetal cortisol and other hormones that result in early lung maturation responses. Clinical experience and recent results in transgenic mouse models suggest that endogenous cortisol is not as absolutely required for normal lung development as previously thought.[65] Explants of mid-gestation fetal human lung differentiate and develop mature type II cells and surfactant in the absence of glucocorticoids. Infants born at term without hypothalamic-pituitary function generally have normal lungs. The simplest interpretation of these observations is that the fetal human lung can develop without cortisol. However, some maternal cortisol crosses the placenta to the fetus, as demonstrated by experiments with transgenic mice. Disruption of the corticotropin-releasing hormone (CRH) gene *(Crh$^{-/-}$)* results in adult mice with very low plasma corticosterone levels that require corticosterone supplementation to reproduce.[66] CRH$^{-/-}$ fetuses from CRH$^{-/-}$ mice die after birth with lungs that have an arrest in thinning of the saccules, although the surfactant system matures relatively normally. Corticosterone supplementation in the water of the CRH$^{-/-}$ dam prevents the delayed lung development in CRH$^{-/-}$ fetuses, because the glucocorticoid leaks from dam to fetus. The lungs of CRH$^{-/-}$ fetuses develop normally in CRH^{+} dams because corticosterone is transferred to the fetus during the circadian peak in maternal glucocorticoid secretion.[67] Low levels of fetal glucocorticoid exposure are sufficient to support normal lung maturation.

The clinical issues regarding diagnosis and induction of fetal lung maturation are developed in Chapter 23. However, a few points pertaining to basic mechanisms are pertinent at this juncture. Pharmacologic induction of early lung maturation is the rationale for the clinical use of antenatal glucocorticoids in women at risk for preterm delivery. Numerous animal models and the clinical trials demonstrate that glucocorticoids can induce maturation of lung and other organs. However, the fetal stress presumed to accompany fetal growth restriction, preeclampsia, or premature rupture of membranes is not consistently associated with a decrease in the incidence of RDS in the clinical literature.[68] Thus, the link between presumed fetal stress and early lung maturation is not apparent.

A provocative clinical observation is that histologic chorioamnionitis is associated with a decreased incidence of RDS in preterm infants.[69] This observation has been explored in fetal sheep using intra-amniotic injections of endotoxin, the proinflammatory cytokine interleukin (IL)-1α, and live *Ureaplasma* organisms as inflammatory stimuli.[70-73] Endotoxin induces chorioamnionitis and lung inflammation followed by a change in lung structure comparable to the maternal betamethasone effect. The surfactant system is stimulated more by inflammatory mediators than by maternal betamethasone (Fig. 15-10).[71-73] Fetal plasma cortisol is not increased by the inflammatory stimuli, demonstrating that the lung maturational effect is not mediated by cortisol. In fetal sheep, maternal betamethasone causes fetal growth restriction and thymic involution, and both adverse effects are prevented if the fetus also is exposed to intra-amniotic endotoxin.[74] These results with inflammatory mediators and the clinical observations indicate that inflammatory pathways are contributing to the early lung maturation that frequently accompanies preterm birth.

Although many hormones influence lung maturation in experimental systems (Table 15-4), the only lung maturational agent other than corticosteroid that has been systematically evaluated in the human is thyrotropin-releasing hormone (TRH). The rationale for the use of TRH is that thyroid hormone induces lung maturation when given to the fetus, and the combined use of thyroid hormone and corticosteroid stimulates surfactant synthesis in vitro in human lung explants and lung tissues from other animals more rapidly and to a greater extent than either agent alone. Thyroid hormones are not a good choice for maternal treatment, because high and toxic maternal doses would be required to achieve placental transfer. TRH does cross

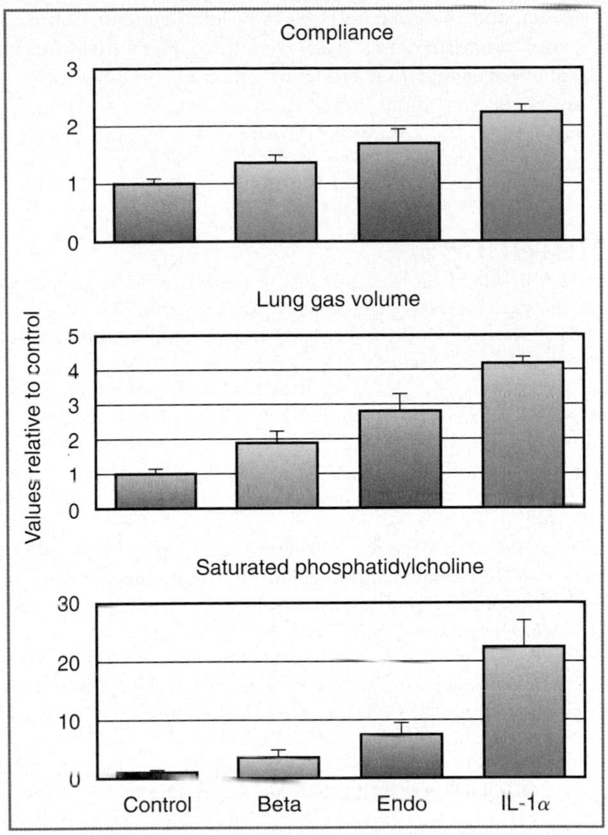

FIGURE 15-10 **Induction of lung maturation.** Relative effects on lung compliance, lung gas volume measured at 40 cm H_2O pressure, and the amount of saturated phosphatidylcholine in alveolar washes 7 days after fetal exposure to 0.5 mg/kg maternal betamethasone (Beta), 10 mg intra-amniotic endotoxin (Endo), or 150 mg recombinant ovine interleukin 1α (IL-1α). The endotoxin or IL-1α stimulus improved lung function and increased surfactant. (Data from Jobe AH, Newnham JP, Willet KE, et al: Endotoxin-induced lung maturation in preterm lambs is not mediated by cortisol. Am J Respir Crit Care Med 162:1656, 2000; and Willet K, Kramer BW, Kallapur SG, et al: Intra-amniotic injection of IL-1 induces inflammation and maturation in fetal sheep lung. Am J Physiol 282:L411, 2001.)

TABLE 15-4 EXPERIMENTAL EFFECTORS THAT ALTER LUNG MATURATION

Accelerate Maturation
Corticosteroids
Thyrotropin-releasing hormone
Triiodothyronine
β-Agonists
Prolactin
Epidermal growth factor
Transforming growth factor-α
Estrogen
Bombesin
Delay Maturation
Insulin
Androgens

the placenta, and maternal TRH elevates fetal triiodothyronine, thyroxine, and prolactin levels. However, three large trials found no beneficial effect of maternal TRH, and one trial suggested some acute risks and concerns about longer-term outcomes for infants who received TRH.[75] TRH cannot be recommended to induce early lung maturation.

References

1. Avery ME, Mead J: Surface properties in relation to atelectasis and hyaline membrane disease. Am J Dis Child 97:517-523, 1959.
2. Gluck L, Kulovich M, Borer RC, et al: Diagnosis of the respiratory distress syndrome by amniocentesis. Am J Obstet Gynecol 109:440-445, 1971.
3. Hallman M, Kulovich M, Kirkpatrick E, et al: Phosphatidylinositol and phosphatidylglycerol in amniotic fluid: Indices of lung maturity. Am J Obstet Gynecol 125:613-617, 1976.
4. Liggins GC, Howie RN: A controlled trial of antepartum glucocorticoid treatment for prevention of RDS in premature infants. Pediatrics 50:515-525, 1972.
5. Jobe AH: Pulmonary surfactant therapy. N Engl J Med 328:861-868, 1993.
6. Burri PW: Development and growth of the human lung. In Fishman AP, Fisher AB (eds): Handbook of Physiology: The Respiratory System. Bethesda, MD, American Physiologic Society, 1985, pp 1-46.
7. Whitsett JA, Wert S: Molecular determinants of lung morphogenesis. In Chernick V, Boat TF, Wilmott RW, Bush A (eds): Kendig's Disorders of the Respiratory Tract in Children. Philadelphia, Saunders/Elsevier, 2006, pp 1-16.
8. Whitsett JA, Wert SE, Trapnell BC: Genetic disorders influencing lung formation and function at birth. Hum Mol Genet 13(Spec No 2):R207-215, 2004.
9. Whitsett JA, Matsuzaki Y: Transcriptional regulation of perinatal lung maturation. Pediatr Clin North Am 53:873-887, viii, 2006.
10. Zeltner TB, Burri PH: The postnatal development and growth of the human lung: II. Morphology. Respir Physiol 67:269-282, 1987.
11. Burri PH: Structural aspects of prenatal and postnatal development and growth of the lung. In McDonald JA (ed): Lung Growth and Development. New York, Marcel Dekker, 1997, pp 1-35.
12. Hislop AA, Wigglesworth JS, Desai R: Alveolar development in the human fetus and infant. Early Hum Dev 13:1-11, 1986.
13. Langston C, Kida D, Reed M, et al: Human lung growth in late gestation and in the neonate. Am Rev Respir Dis 129:607-613, 1984.
14. Massaro GD, Radaeva S, Clerch LB, et al: Lung alveoli: Endogenous programmed destruction and regeneration. Am J Physiol Lung Cell Mol Physiol 283:L305-309, 2002.
15. Jobe AH: The new BPD: An arrest of lung development. Pediatr Res 46:641-643, 1999.
16. Massaro D, Massaro GD, Baras A, et al: Calorie-related rapid onset of alveolar loss, regeneration, and changes in mouse lung gene expression. Am J Physiol Lung Cell Mol Physiol 286:L896-906, 2004.
17. Thibeault DW, Mabry SM, Ekekezie I, et al: Lung elastic tissue maturation and perturbations during the evolution of chronic lung disease. Pediatrics 106:1452-1459, 2000.
18. Kramer BW, Jobe AH: The clever fetus: Responding to inflammation to minimize lung injury. Biol Neonate 88:202-207, 2005.
19. Moss TM, Newnham J, Willet K, et al: Early gestational intra-amniotic endotoxin: Lung function, surfactant and morphometry. Am J Respir Crit Care Med 165:805-811, 2002.
20. Willet K, Jobe A, Ikegami M, et al: Antenatal endotoxin and glucocorticoid effects on lung morphometry in preterm lambs. Pediatr Res 48:782-788, 2000.
21. Johnson JWC, Mitzner W, Beck JC, et al: Long-term effects of betamethasone on fetal development. Am J Obstet Gynecol 141:1053-1061, 1981.
22. Willet KE, Jobe AH, Ikegami M, et al: Lung morphometry after repetitive antenatal glucocorticoid treatment in preterm sheep. Am J Respir Crit Care Med 163:1437-1443, 2001.
23. Wigglesworth JS, Desai R: Is fetal respiratory function a major determinant of perinatal survival? Lancet 1:264-267, 1982.
24. Liggins GC: Growth of the fetal lung. J Dev Physiol 6:237-248, 1984.
25. Thibeault DW, Beatty EC Jr, Hall RT, et al: Neonatal pulmonary hypoplasia with premature rupture of fetal membranes and oligohydramnios. J Pediatr 107:273-277, 1985.
26. Lindner W, Pohlandt F, Grab D, et al: Acute respiratory failure and short-term outcome after premature rupture of the membranes and oligohydramnios before 20 weeks of gestation. J Pediatr 140:177-182, 2002.
27. Wilcox DT, Glick PL, Karamanoukian HL, et al: Contributions by individual lungs to the surfactant status in congenital diaphragmatic hernia. Pediatr Res 41:686-691, 1997.
28. Kay S, Laberge JM, Flageole H, et al: Use of antenatal steroids to counteract the negative effects of tracheal occlusion in the fetal lamb model. Pediatr Res 50:495-501, 2001.
29. O'Brodovich H: Fetal lung liquid secretion: Insights using the tools of inhibitors and genetic knock-out experiments. Am J Respir Cell Mol Biol 25:8-10, 2001.
30. Bland RD: Lung epithelial ion transport and fluid movement during the perinatal period. Am J Physiol 259:L30-37, 1990.
31. Brown MJ, Oliver RE, Ramoden CA, et al: Effects of adrenaline and of spontaneous labor on the secretion and adsorption of lung liquid in the fetal lamb. J Physiol (Lond) 344:137, 1983.
32. Barker PM, Markiewicz M, Parker KA, et al: Synergistic action of triiodothyronine and hydrocortisone on epinephrine induced readsorption of fetal lung fluid. Pediatr Res 27:588-591, 1990.
33. Gerten KA, Coonrod DV, Bay RC, et al: Cesarean delivery and respiratory distress syndrome: Does labor make a difference? Am J Obstet Gynecol 193:1061-1064, 2005.
34. Kolas T, Saugstad OD, Daltveit AK, et al: Planned cesarean versus planned vaginal delivery at term: Comparison of newborn infant outcomes. Am J Obstet Gynecol 195:1538-1543, 2006.
35. Veldhuizen R, Nag K, Orgeig S, et al: The role of lipids in pulmonary surfactant. Biochim Biophys Acta 1408:90-108, 1998.
36. Kulovich MV, Hallman M, Gluck L: The lung profile: Normal pregnancy. Am J Obstet Gynecol 135:57-63, 1979.
37. Weaver TE, Conkright JJ: Function of surfactant proteins B and C. Annu Rev Physiol 63:555-578, 2001.
38. Crouch E, Wright JR: Surfactant proteins a and d and pulmonary host defense. Annu Rev Physiol 63:521-554, 2001.
39. LeVine AM, Whitsett J: Pulmonary collectins and innate host defense of the lung. Microbes Infect 3:161-166, 2001.
40. Ramet M, Haataja R, Marttila R, et al: Association between the surfactant protein A (SP-A) gene locus and respiratory-distress syndrome in the Finnish population. Am J Hum Genet 66:1569-1579, 2000.
41. Hallman M, Merritt TA, Akino T, et al: Surfactant protein-A, phosphatidylcholine, and surfactant inhibitors in epithelial lining fluid: Correlation with surface activity, severity of respiratory distress syndrome, and outcome in small premature infants. Am Rev Respir Dis 144:1376-1384, 1991.
42. Wert SE, Yoshida M, LeVine AM, et al: Increased metalloproteinase activity, oxidant production, and emphysema in surfactant protein D gene-inactivated mice. Proc Natl Acad Sci U S A 97:5972-5977, 2000.
43. Cole FS, Hamvas A, Nogee LM: Genetic disorders of neonatal respiratory function. Pediatr Res 50:157-162, 2001.
44. Cole FS, Hamvas A, Rubinstein P, et al: Population-based estimates of surfactant protein B deficiency. Pediatrics 105:538-541, 2000.
45. Glasser SW, Detmer EA, Ikegami M, et al: Interstitial pneumonitis in SP-C gene targeted mice. J Biol Chem 278:14291-14298, 2003.
46. Nogee LM, Dunbar AE 3rd, Wert S, et al: Mutations in the surfactant protein C gene associated with interstitial lung disease. Chest 121:20S-21, 2002.
47. Shulenin S, Nogee LM, Annilo T, et al: ABCA3 gene mutations in newborns with fatal surfactant deficiency. N Engl J Med 350:1296-1303, 2004.
48. Van Golde LM, Batenburg JJ, Robertson B: The pulmonary surfactant system: Biochemical aspects and functional significance. Physiol Rev 68:374-455, 1988.

49. Mason RJ, Voelker DR: Regulatory mechanisms of surfactant secretion. Biochim Biophys Acta 1408:226-240, 1998.
50. Hallman M, Merritt TA, Pohjavuori M, et al: Effect of surfactant substitution on lung effluent phospholipids in respiratory distress syndrome: Evaluation of surfactant phospholipid turnover, pool size, and the relationship to severity of respiratory failure. Pediatr Res 20:1228-1235, 1986.
51. Jackson JC, Palmer S, Truog WE, et al: Surfactant quantity and composition during recovery from hyaline membrane disease. Pediatr Res 20:1243:1247, 1986.
52. Ikegami M, Jobe A, Yamada T, et al: Surfactant metabolism in surfactant-treated preterm ventilated lambs. J Appl Physiol 67:429-437, 1989.
53. Seidner SR, Jobe AH, Coalson JJ, et al: Abnormal surfactant metabolism and function in preterm ventilated baboons. Am J Respir Crit Care Med 158:1982-1989, 1998.
54. Bunt JE, Carnielli VP, Darcos Wattimena JL, et al: The effect in premature infants of prenatal corticosteroids on endogenous surfactant synthesis as measured with stable isotopes. Am J Respir Crit Care Med 162:844-849, 2000.
55. Jobe AH, Ikegami M: Surfactant metabolism. Clin Perinatol 20:683-696, 1993.
56. Torresin M, Zimmermann LJ, Cogo PE, et al: Exogenous surfactant kinetics in infant respiratory distress syndrome: A novel method with stable isotopes. Am J Respir Crit Care Med 161:1584-1589, 2000.
57. Fujiwara T, Chida S, Watabe Y, et al: Artificial surfactant therapy in hyaline-membrane disease. Lancet 1:55-59, 1980.
58. Soll RF, Morley C: Prophylactic versus selective use of surfactant for preventing morbidity and mortality in preterm infants. Cochrane Database Syst Rev (2):CD000510, 2001.
59. Ikegami M, Ueda T, Absolom D, et al: Changes in exogenous surfactant in ventilated preterm lamb lungs. Am Rev Respir Dis 148:837-844, 1993.
60. Horbar JD, Carpenter JH, Buzas J, et al: Timing of initial surfactant treatment for infants 23 to 29 weeks' gestation: Is routine practice evidence based? Pediatrics 113:1593-1602, 2004.
61. Horbar JD, Carpenter JH, Buzas J, et al: Collaborative quality improvement to promote evidence based surfactant for preterm infants: A cluster randomised trial. BMJ 329:1004, 2004.
62. Ammari A, Suri MS, Milisavljevic V, et al: Variables associated with the early failure of nasal CPAP in very low birth weight infants. J Pediatr 147:341-347, 2005.
63. Jobe AH, Mitchell BR, Gunkel JH: Beneficial effects of the combined use of prenatal corticosteroids and postnatal surfactant on preterm infants. Am J Obstet Gynecol 168:508-513, 1993.
64. Jobe AH: Animal models of antenatal corticosteroids: Clinical implications. Clin Obstet Gynecol 46:174-189, 2003.
65. Jobe AH, Ikegami M: Fetal responses to glucocorticoids. In Mendelson CR (ed): Endocrinology of the Lung. Totowa, NJ, Humana Press, 2000, pp 45-57.
66. Muglia LJ, Bae DS, Brown TT, et al: Proliferation and differentiation defects during lung development in corticotropin-releasing hormone-deficient mice. Am J Respir Cell Mol Biol 20:181-188, 1999.
67. Venihaki M, Carrigan A, Dikkes P, et al: Circadian rise in maternal glucocorticoid prevents pulmonary dysplasia in fetal mice with adrenal insufficiency. Proc Natl Acad Sci U S A 97:7336-7341, 2000.
68. Chang EY, Menard MK, Vermillion ST, et al: The association between hyaline membrane disease and preeclampsia. Am J Obstet Gynecol 191:1414-1417, 2004.
69. Andrews WW, Goldenberg RL, Faye-Petersen O, et al: The Alabama Preterm Birth study: Polymorphonuclear and mononuclear cell placental infiltrations, other markers of inflammation, and outcomes in 23- to 32-week preterm newborn infants. Am J Obstet Gynecol 195:803-808, 2006.
70. Willet K, Kramer BW, Kallapur SG, et al: Intra-amniotic injection of IL-1 induces inflammation and maturation in fetal sheep lung. Am J Physiol 282:L411-420, 2002.
71. Sosenko IR, Kallapur SG, Nitsos I, et al: IL-1α causes lung inflammation and maturation by direct effects on preterm fetal lamb lungs. Pediatr Res 60:294-298, 2006.
72. Moss TJM, Nitsos I, Ikegami M, et al: Experimental intra-uterine *Ureaplasma* infection in sheep. Am J Obstet Gynecol 192:1179-1186, 2005.
73. Jobe AH, Newnham JP, Willet KE, et al: Endotoxin induced lung maturation in preterm lambs is not mediated by cortisol. Am J Respirt Crit Care Med 162:1656-1661, 2000.
74. Newnham JP, Moss TJ, Padbury JF, et al: The interactive effects of endotoxin with prenatal glucocorticoids on short-term lung function in sheep. Am J Obstet Gynecol 185:190-197, 2001.
75. Australian Collaborative Trial of Antenatal Thyrotropin-Releasing Hormone (ACTOBAT) for prevention of neonatal respiratory disease. Lancet 345:877-882, 1995.

Chapter 16

Evidence-Based Practice in Perinatal Medicine

George A. Macones, MD

All those who drink of this remedy recover in a short time, except those whom it does not help, who die. Therefore, it is obvious that it fails only in incurable cases.

—Galen (circa 100 AD)

Evidence-Based Medicine in Perspective

Many of the improvements in medical care for women in the past 30 years have come about as a result of carefully designed studies of interventions aimed at improving health. Before this time, physicians relied on anecdote and personal experience to guide patient care.

Evidence-based medicine is a style of practice best described as "integrating individual clinical expertise with the best-available external clinical evidence from systematic research."[1] Thus, contrary to what many believe, evidence-based medicine combines understanding of the literature with individual expertise. It is this blend of evidence and clinical intuition that makes evidence-based medicine so attractive and essential to the practice of modern medicine.

Why is evidence-based medicine important in maternal-fetal medicine? First, the practice of evidence-based medicine allows us to provide the best care to our patients. Instances in obstetrics are easily found where an incomplete or improper assessment of the evidence has led to problems with care. The classic example is the emergence of electronic fetal heart rate monitoring (see Chapter 22). This device, novel when it was introduced, generated new information that was widely expected to lead to improved perinatal outcomes. Unfortunately, electronic fetal monitoring was widely implemented before evidence of benefit existed, and it became firmly rooted in obstetrics in the United States and many other countries. As has been well documented, it is uncertain whether continuous electronic fetal monitoring confers any benefit beyond that of intermittent auscultation in low-risk patients, and it has been a major contributing factor in the rise in the rate of cesarean delivery.

Second, clinical research is growing exponentially, as evidenced by the number of medical journals, research publications, and scientific societies. Some have estimated that 1000 articles are added to MEDLINE per day. In addition, clinical research has gained in importance, with programs at the National Institutes of Health and other funding agencies focused on clinical research. With the volume and rapid access to such information (for both physicians and patients), it is essential for practicing clinicians to be able to assess the medical literature to determine a best course of action for an individual patient.

Finally, in perinatal medicine we are today faced with several important yet unanswered questions:

- What (if any) treatment should we recommend for women with a short cervix seen on an ultrasound scan?
- Can preeclampsia be prevented or reduced through prenatal screening and treatment programs?
- Should we screen women for inherited thrombophilias if they have a history of poor pregnancy outcome? If so, how should we treat those who are positive?

How do we, as physicians and researchers, reach sound decisions for such questions? We start by learning to assess the quality of available medical evidence. In this chapter, we review the principles that serve as a basis for learning to interpret clinical research, including clinical research study designs, measures of effect, sources of error in clinical research (systematic and random), and screening and diagnosis. This will provide the reader with the information that will advance the journey toward becoming an evidence-based medicine practitioner.

Types of Clinical Research Studies

Several study designs are reported in the medical literature.

Descriptive Studies

Case reports and case series are simply descriptions of either a single case or a number of cases, and these are termed descriptive studies.[2] Often they focus on an unusual disease, an unusual presentation of a disease, or an unusual treatment for a disease. In case reports and case series, there is no control group. Because of this, drawing any inference on causality is impossible. Such studies are useful mainly for hypothesis *generation*, rather than hypothesis *testing*. However, case reports and case series can be very valuable in the scientific process, because many important observations were initially made by a single case or series of cases. For example, in the early 1980s, physicians in California noted an unusual respiratory illness in homosexual men. The astute observation of these physicians led to the discovery of the acquired immunodeficiency syndrome epidemic in the United States.

Observational Studies

The two main types of observational studies are case-control studies and cohort studies.[2,3,4] These study designs attempt to assess the relationship between an exposure and an outcome (Table 16-1).

In case-control studies, subjects are identified on the basis of disease rather than on exposure. Groups of subjects with and without disease are identified, and then exposures of interest are retrospectively sought. Comparisons of the distribution of exposures are then made between cases and controls. Case-control studies are useful for the study of rare conditions. Advantages of case-control studies include efficient use of time, low cost, and the ability to assess the impact of multiple exposures. However, case-control studies cannot be used to calculate an incidence of disease given a particular exposure, and they carry substantial potential for confounding and bias.

Cohort studies identify subjects on the basis of exposure and then assess the relationship between the exposure and the clinical outcome of interest. Cohort studies can be either retrospective or prospective. In a retrospective cohort study, the exposed population is identified after the event of interest has occurred. In a prospective cohort study, exposed and unexposed subjects are followed over time to see if the outcome of interest occurs. Cohort studies are useful in the study of rare exposures. The advantages of cohort studies are that the incidence of disease in exposed and unexposed individuals can be assessed, and there is less potential for bias (especially if prospective). The main disadvantage of prospective cohort studies is that they can be time-consuming, sometimes requiring years to complete (if prospective), and are thus often expensive.

A clinical example may help to contrast these study designs. The relationship between anticonvulsant use in pregnancy and the occurrence of neural tube defects could be assessed with either a case-control or a cohort study. In a case-control study, one would identify a group of cases of fetuses or neonates with neural tube defects and a group of controls (i.e., children without a neural tube defect). The maternal record could be reviewed to determine whether exposure to anticonvulsants has occurred. To study this question with a cohort study, one would first identify a population of women taking anticonvulsants in pregnancy and a group not taking anticonvulsants, and then follow both groups through pregnancy and delivery to determine the frequency of neural tube defects in each group.

TABLE 16-1 COMPARISON OF CASE-CONTROL STUDIES AND COHORT STUDIES

Case-Control Studies	Cohort Studies
Good for rare disease	Good for common disease
Study multiple exposures	Study multiple outcomes
Done quickly	Long follow-up
Inexpensive	Expensive (prospective)
No incidence data	Can directly calculate incidence
Prone to bias	Less prone to bias

Cohort studies can be either prospective or retrospective, whereas case-control studies are almost always retrospective. The advantage of a prospective cohort study is that the type and amount of data being collected can be determined by the investigator, based on the research question. In a retrospective cohort study, one almost always relies on inpatient or outpatient records for data collection, so the study is limited by the type and quality of the data included in these sources. For example, suppose an investigator is interested in the relationship between maternal cocaine use and fetal growth restriction. In a prospective cohort study, one would have the opportunity for a very accurate assessment of this exposure, perhaps by obtaining a hair sample. A retrospective study would have to rely on what was recorded in the medical record, which is most likely based on patient self-report.

There is a common misconception that an analysis performed using data prospectively collected and contained in a database is equivalent to a prospective cohort study. In fact, unless the research question was defined a priori (i.e., before the start of data collection), this is best termed a *retrospective secondary analysis of prospectively collected data.* In many cases, such analyses are more similar to a retrospective cohort study, because important clinical information may not have been collected as completely or systematically as it could have been had the research question been specified in advance.

Interventional Studies

The randomized clinical trial is the gold standard of clinical research design.[5] In a clinical trial, eligible consenting participants are randomly allocated to receive different therapies. Differences in clinical outcomes are then compared on the basis of the treatment assignment. Clinical trials are powerful because the likelihood of confounding and bias influencing the results is minimized. However, clinical trials are logistically difficult and expensive, and they can take years to complete. There are also concerns about whether the results of clinical trials can be generalized—that is, applied to clinical practice with the expectation that the same results will occur. Specifically, people who consent to be part of a trial may differ from those who do not consent in that they may be more likely to comply with an intervention or have a generally more healthy lifestyle than persons who decline to enter the study. In addition, well-performed clinical trials often have strict inclusion and exclusion criteria, with strict follow-up procedures. In real-life clinical situations, such rigor in follow-up rarely occurs. Standards for reporting prospective randomized trials have been developed to ensure that results from all trial participants are reported. These have been published as the CONSORT statement.[6]

Despite these concerns, clinical trials provide the best evidence to guide practice. An excellent example of a practice-guiding clinical trial was the screening and treatment study of bacterial vaginosis (BV) in pregnancy performed by the Maternal-Fetal Medicine Units (MFMU) Network.[7] A variety of studies from around the world suggested that symptomatic and asymptomatic BV was associated with spontaneous preterm birth.[8-10] In addition, secondary analyses of data from clinical trials with high-risk women suggested that screening and treating BV in pregnancy might reduce the occurrence of spontaneous preterm delivery.[11,12] Many assumed that screening and treating all pregnant women might reduce the incidence of preterm birth if applied to all pregnant women. To answer this question, the MFMU Network performed a placebo-controlled clinical trial comparing treatment with metronidazole to placebo for women who screened positive for BV in pregnancy.[7] This study demonstrated that treating asymptomatic BV in pregnancy did not affect the occurrence of preterm birth.

Another benefit of randomized clinical trials is that subgroup analyses from such data can be used to generate hypotheses for future research. One example is the study cited earlier by Hauth and colleagues.[11] After the primary analysis of their randomized clinical trial of metronidazole and erythromycin to reduce the risk for preterm birth in women with a prior preterm birth or other historical risk factors demonstrated a reduction of preterm birth, a secondary analysis found that the benefit was limited to women with BV. This secondary analysis (and a similar secondary analysis of another randomized clinical trial[12]) should have prompted a new randomized trial of antibiotic treatment, for which women would be enrolled if they had both BV and a historical risk for preterm birth.

Other Study Designs

Two other study designs deserve mention: meta-analysis and decision analysis. Both are valuable tools for the evidence-based medicine practitioner.

Meta-Analysis

In a meta-analysis, the results of a series of randomized clinical trials (or observational studies) can be statistically combined to obtain a *summary estimate* for the effect of a given treatment.[13] Meta-analyses are also termed systematic reviews, and they should be differentiated from other, less data-driven review articles in which authors present their own interpretation of data. The strength of a meta-analysis comes from its being an analysis of combined results from multiple clinical trials, thereby increasing the "power" to detect differences in treatment. This is an especially important methodology in obstetrics, as we have few large randomized clinical trials to guide our treatments. Numerous meta-analyses have been performed for topics in obstetrics,[14,15] many in the Cochrane Database of Systemic Reviews.[16] Two such analyses (Figs. 16-1 and 16-2) are taken from the Cochrane Library meta-analysis of the effect on neonatal outcome of antibiotics given antenatally to women with preterm prematurely ruptured amniotic membranes.[17] In Figure 16-1, a comparison of neonatal infectious complications between those who received antibiotics and those who did not is made, and the data are pooled for all available studies. Each of 11 randomized trials that met inclusion criteria for this analysis is listed, with the number of subjects and the frequency of the outcome in the treatment and control groups noted. The relative risk and 95% confidence interval (see Assessing Random Error, later) for each study, weighted for their sample size, are shown. The total number of subjects with the outcome of interest is summed and the combined relative risk and 95% confidence interval calculated. In this example, a number of small trials show a nonsignificant trend in favor of antibiotic treatment. The pooled (i.e., statistically combined) relative risk was 0.67, with a 95% confidence interval from 0.52 to 0.85. The point estimate (i.e., the relative risk) suggests that the "best guess" is that antibiotics reduce the risk for neonatal infection by 33%. The confidence interval suggests that the data are consistent with as much as a 48% reduction in risk (1 − 0.52) or as little as a 15% (1 − 0.85) reduction in risk. Even the upper bound of the confidence interval suggests a protective effect of antibiotics on neonatal infection.

Compare this summary graph with that for the effect of antibiotics on perinatal death in women with preterm premature rupture of membranes (see Fig. 16-2). Here, the pooled estimate yields a point estimate relative risk of 0.89, with a 95% confidence interval from 0.67 to 1.18. The point estimate suggests that the best estimate is that antibiotics reduce the occurrence of perinatal death by 11%. The confidence interval suggests that the data are consistent with as much as a 33% reduction in perinatal death or an 18% increase in perinatal death with antibiotics. Because the confidence interval crosses a relative risk of 1.0, the data are consistent with "no difference" between the groups.

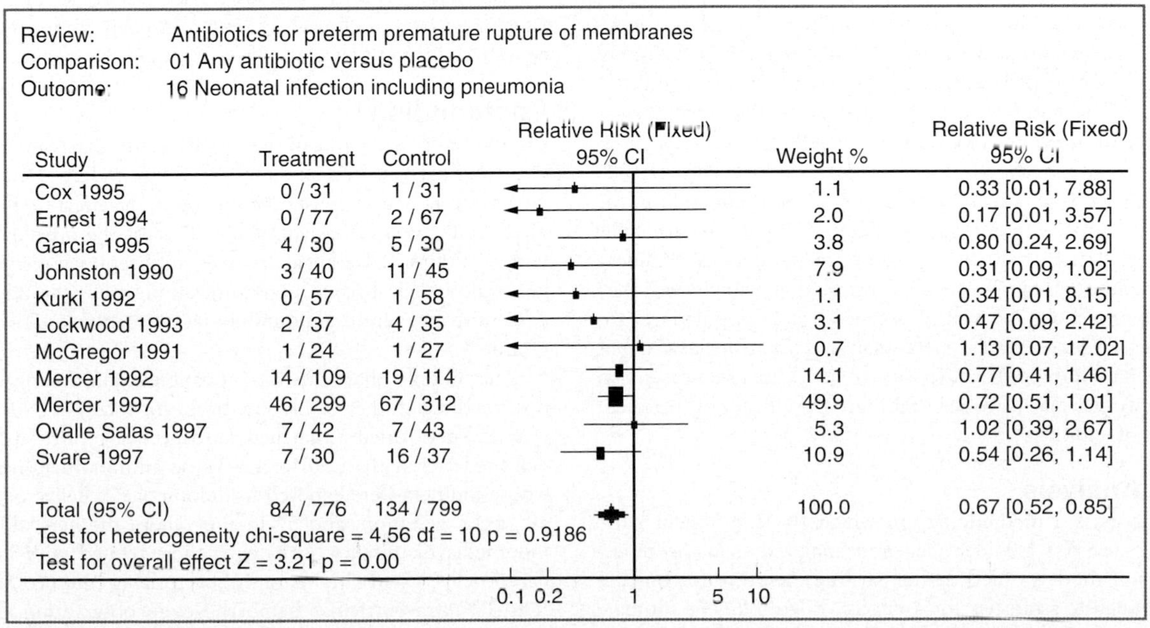
Review: Antibiotics for preterm premature rupture of membranes
Comparison: 01 Any antibiotic versus placebo
Outcome: 16 Neonatal infection including pneumonia
Study | Treatment | Control | Relative Risk (Fixed) 95% CI | Weight % | Relative Risk (Fixed) 95% CI
Cox 1995 | 0 / 31 | 1 / 31 | 1.1 | 0.33 [0.01, 7.88]
Ernest 1994 | 0 / 77 | 2 / 67 | 2.0 | 0.17 [0.01, 3.57]
Garcia 1995 | 4 / 30 | 5 / 30 | 3.8 | 0.80 [0.24, 2.69]
Johnston 1990 | 3 / 40 | 11 / 45 | 7.9 | 0.31 [0.09, 1.02]
Kurki 1992 | 0 / 57 | 1 / 58 | 1.1 | 0.34 [0.01, 8.15]
Lockwood 1993 | 2 / 37 | 4 / 35 | 3.1 | 0.47 [0.09, 2.42]
McGregor 1991 | 1 / 24 | 1 / 27 | 0.7 | 1.13 [0.07, 17.02]
Mercer 1992 | 14 / 109 | 19 / 114 | 14.1 | 0.77 [0.41, 1.46]
Mercer 1997 | 46 / 299 | 67 / 312 | 49.9 | 0.72 [0.51, 1.01]
Ovalle Salas 1997 | 7 / 42 | 7 / 43 | 5.3 | 1.02 [0.39, 2.67]
Svare 1997 | 7 / 30 | 16 / 37 | 10.9 | 0.54 [0.26, 1.14]
Total (95% CI) | 84 / 776 | 134 / 799 | 100.0 | 0.67 [0.52, 0.85]
Test for heterogeneity chi-square = 4.56 df = 10 p = 0.9186
Test for overall effect Z = 3.21 p = 0.00
0.1 0.2 1 5 10

FIGURE 16-1 Meta-analysis summary graph for neonatal infection. The effect of maternal antibiotic administration on the occurrence of neonatal infection in women with preterm premature rupture of membranes. 95% CI, 95% confidence interval. (From Kenyon S, Boulvain M, Neilson J: Antibiotics for preterm premature rupture of membranes. Cochrane Database Syst Rev [4]:CD001058, 2001.)

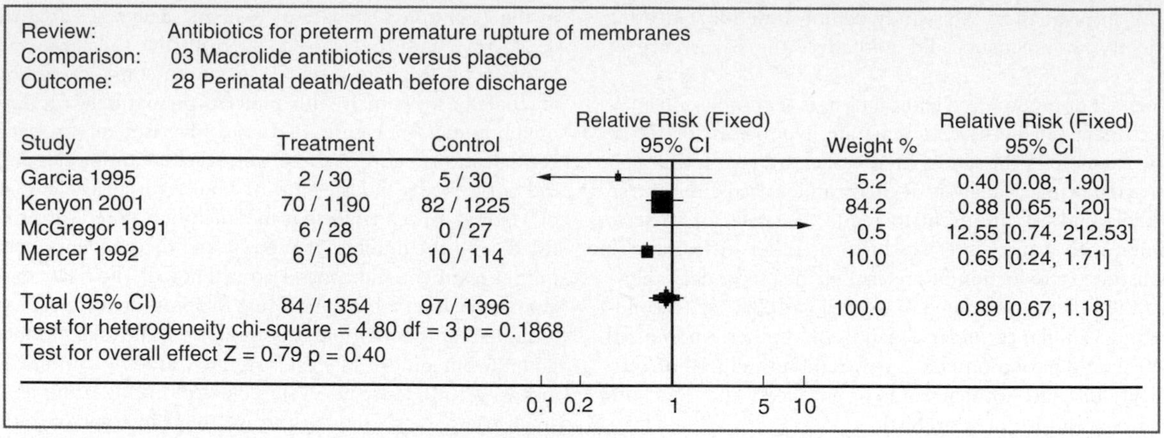

Study	Treatment	Control	Weight %	Relative Risk (Fixed) 95% CI
Garcia 1995	2 / 30	5 / 30	5.2	0.40 [0.08, 1.90]
Kenyon 2001	70 / 1190	82 / 1225	84.2	0.88 [0.65, 1.20]
McGregor 1991	6 / 28	0 / 27	0.5	12.55 [0.74, 212.53]
Mercer 1992	6 / 106	10 / 114	10.0	0.65 [0.24, 1.71]
Total (95% CI)	84 / 1354	97 / 1396	100.0	0.89 [0.67, 1.18]

Test for heterogeneity chi-square = 4.80 df = 3 p = 0.1868
Test for overall effect Z = 0.79 p = 0.40

FIGURE 16-2 Meta-analysis summary graph for perinatal death. The effect of maternal antibiotic administration on the occurrence of perinatal death or death before discharge in women with preterm premature rupture of membranes. 95% CI, 95% confidence interval. (From Kenyon S, Boulvain M, Neilson J: Antibiotics for preterm premature rupture of membranes. Cochrane Database Syst Rev [4]:CD001058, 2001.)

A notable limitation of meta-analysis is that clinical trials on the same general topic seldom enroll populations or employ treatments that are the same. Thus, at times, meta-analysis can seem like mixing apples with oranges.[13,18-20] It is incumbent on the reader to make such a determination. Guidelines for publication of quality meta-analyses have been promulgated by the QUOROM statement, proposed by a consortium of journal editors[21] and, like the CONSORT statement, they are subscribed to by the *American Journal of Obstetrics and Gynecology, Obstetrics and Gynecology*, and general medical journals such as *The Lancet*, the *New England Journal of Medicine*, and the *Journal of the American Medical Association*.

Two other issues are pertinent to the subject of meta-analyses. First, performing a meta-analysis requires significant methodological skill, so not all meta-analyses are of the same quality. The Cochrane Library, for example, includes very high quality meta-analyses on a number of obstetric topics. Second, there is debate about the role of meta-analyses when large clinical trials are available. This issue was raised in a recent meta-analysis of antiplatelet agents for the secondary prevention of preeclampsia.[22] The authors suggested that antiplatelet agents may reduce the risk for preeclampsia and for birth before 34 weeks of gestation. In this meta-analysis, out of five studies that enrolled over 1000 women in each treatment arm, four did not show a reduction in the risk for preeclampsia with antiplatelet therapy. How do we reconcile the role of large clinical trials with the role of meta-analyses in guiding our practice? Although opinions vary, I believe that a single, well-performed randomized clinical trial in a generalizable population provides stronger evidence than a meta-analysis (where heterogeneous studies must be combined). On the other hand, meta-analyses that include large studies may provide insight into the efficacy of treatment in subgroups of subjects.

Decision Analysis

Decision analysis is a methodology in which the component parts of a complex decision are identified and analyzed in a theoretical model. Decision models often use the existing literature to compare different therapeutic strategies for a clinical dilemma. The ultimate goal of any decision analysis is to reach a clinical decision. Importantly, decision models are often the foundation for formal economic analysis, such as cost-effectiveness analysis.[23] Decision and economic analyses are fairly common in the obstetric literature. Such analyses have been published on group B streptococci screening,[24] indomethacin use for preterm labor,[25] tocolysis at advanced gestational ages,[26] and thromboprophylaxis at cesarean delivery.[27] Interested readers should consider reading review articles on this subject.[23,28]

Sources of Error in Clinical Research

Broadly speaking, two types of error can occur in clinical research studies: *systematic* error and *random* error.[3,4] Systematic error is generally introduced by the investigator in the study design. Sources of systematic error include confounding and bias.[29-31] Random error is assessed using various methods for hypothesis testing, as described later. As readers of clinical research, our goals are to understand and to try to interpret the role of these errors in the studies we read.

Confounding

Confounding is a type of systematic error that can be present in observational research studies.[29,31,32] Confounding occurs when two factors are associated with each other and the effect of one factor on a given outcome is distorted by the effect of the other factor. Importantly, randomized clinical trials of sufficient size generally cannot be confounded, because randomization itself should lead to an equal distribution of confounding factors between various treatment groups.[5]

An example that illustrates possible confounding comes from observational studies of indomethacin for tocolysis. Norton and colleagues[33] performed a matched retrospective cohort study of infants delivered at less than 30 weeks. These authors identified 57 infants whose mothers were exposed to indomethacin delivered at or before 30 weeks' gestation, and 57 infants whose mothers did not receive indomethacin. Infants born to mothers treated with indomethacin before delivery had a higher rate of necrotizing enterocolitis and grades II to IV intraventricular hemorrhage, an observation also noted in other observational studies.[34-36] However, the proper interpretation of observational studies requires that potential sources of systematic error such as confounding and bias be considered. In this example, it is possible that confounding may explain the association between indomethacin and the neonatal morbidity observed in this observational study.[37] Specifically, because indomethacin is generally not a first-line tocolytic in practice, it is likely that this drug was used mainly in subjects who failed first-line tocolysis. If failing first-line tocolysis is itself a risk factor for adverse neonatal outcome, then the association between indomethacin and adverse neonatal outcome can be confounded. Thus, a principal question in the interpretation of these studies is whether patients who are failing first-line tocolysis are themselves at higher risk for adverse neonatal outcomes (whether exposed to indomethacin or not) than those who respond to first-line tocolysis. Existing data suggest that women whose labor does not stop after first-line tocolysis have an increased risk for adverse neonatal consequences because of the well-established relationship between tocolytic failure and subclinical and intra-amniotic infection, both of which are associated with adverse neonatal outcome.

Because of the relationships between refractory preterm labor and subclinical infection, and between subclinical infection and major neonatal morbidity,[38-40] it is uncertain whether the association between indomethacin and adverse neonatal outcome in these retrospective observational studies is a "true" association or a spurious association resulting from confounding. We hypothesize that in the observational studies, exposure to indomethacin may be nothing more than a sign of inflammation-driven preterm labor, which itself is associated with major neonatal complications.[37]

Bias

Bias is defined as a "process at any stage of inference tending to produce results that depart systematically from true results."[41] Bias usually occurs at the study design stage.[30,31] There are two main types of bias to consider. *Selection* bias occurs when an error is made in the selection of a study population. For example, a recent study by Nicholson and colleagues[42] sought to determine the association between "preventive" induction and a reduced rate of cesarean birth. The authors designed a retrospective cohort study, comparing outcomes of women managed by physicians who use preventive induction, to outcomes of women managed by physicians who do not use preventive induction. The results suggest that those cared for by physicians who use preventive induction have, surprisingly, lower cesarean rates. However, the physicians who practiced preventive induction in this study were trained in family medicine, whereas those who practiced without preventive induction were trained as obstetric/gynecologic specialists. Because it is likely that these two groups of physicians cared for different types of patients and probably had differences in clinical management, the possibility of selection bias exists. Such bias cannot be controlled for analytically. In this example, the authors correctly acknowledged the possibility of selection bias as an explanation for their findings.

Information bias occurs when a systematic error is made in the measurement of exposure or outcome information. A *recall* bias is a type of information bias that occurs when subjects recall past events differently, and the difference is related to the exposure status or the disease outcome. Recall bias occurs commonly in observational studies of teratogenesis. In a case-control study to assess whether exposure to medications is associated with cleft lip,[43] cases of cleft lip were ascertained after delivery occurred. Controls were women who delivered children without a birth defect. Mothers of cases and controls were asked about medication use during the pregnancy. The question that should be asked when reading such a study is whether women who have delivered a child with a birth defect are more likely to recall medication use than a woman who has delivered a normal child. To the extent that there is differential recall, there may be significant recall bias that would lead to an inflated estimate of the relationship between medications and cleft lip.

Assessing the Role of Systematic Error in Clinical Research

Clinicians must be able to assess the role of systematic error in clinical research. Although a detailed discussion is beyond the scope of this chapter, there are several useful maxims for reading clinical research:

1. Systematic error is of greater concern for observational studies than for clinical trials. Because of randomization, confounding seldom occurs in clinical trials.[44]
2. Retrospective observational studies are often more likely to be biased than prospective studies (although bias can still occur in prospective observational studies).
3. In any observational study, one should always carefully read the methods section and consider whether there is the potential for bias.
4. Even if one believes a study to have a serious bias, the study should not automatically be discarded. It is important to consider not just the *presence* of bias but also the *direction* of the bias.[31] Consider again the example of the case-control study of medications and cleft palate just described. Now assume that the results of the study suggested no association between medications and cleft palate. Given the study design, concern about recall bias is appropriate, but in this case the recall bias would have led to an overestimate of the association between medications and cleft lip. Because the study showed *no* association, it is unlikely that the recall bias would lead to a change in the overall interpretation of the results of the study.
5. Likewise, confounding should always be considered as an explanation of observed results. Readers should consider whether relevant confounding factors were measured and, if they were unmeasured, the direction of the possible confounding. There are statistical techniques to adjust for measured confounding factors, such as multivariate analysis and logistic regression.[45] In modern observational clinical research, it is unacceptable to report only unadjusted associations when measured confounders can be adjusted for, using appropriate statistical techniques.

Assessing Random Error: Hypothesis Testing and Measures of Effect in Clinical Research

In clinical research, one is often interested in whether an exposure is significantly associated with an outcome, or whether an intervention can improve a given outcome. Commonly, interpretation of the results of clinical research is focused on the assessment of a significance test, such as a probability value. This type of testing provides information on the role of chance (i.e., random error) to explain the observed results in a given study. Although assessing the role of random error is important when reading medical literature, it is equally important to assess the role of systematic error (i.e., bias and confounding) in clinical research.

Let us consider a recent randomized trial that was designed to assess whether vitamin C and E supplementation in pregnancy would reduce the incidence of preeclampsia and perinatal complications.[46] To answer this question, the authors randomly allocated 935 women to active treatment with vitamins, and 942 to placebo (Table 16-2). The association between treatment with vitamins C and E and preeclampsia can be expressed in several ways: by probability value, by relative risk with

TABLE 16-2 VITAMINS C AND E TO PREVENT PREECLAMPSIA

	Preeclampsia		
	Yes	No	Total
Vitamins C and E	56	879	935
Placebo	47	895	942
Total	103	1774	1877

Data from Rumbold AR, Crowther CA, Haslam RR, et al: Vitamins C and E and the risks of preeclampsia and perinatal complications. N Engl J Med 354:1796-1806, 2006.

95% confidence intervals, and by several other measures of effect, including odds ratio and risk difference.

Probability Value

A probability value is defined as the likelihood of obtaining the observed differences in the sample if there is no true difference in the population. For example, a probability value of 0.05 means that there is a 5% probability of achieving the observed difference if in fact the null hypothesis of no true difference is true. Thus, the smaller the probability value, the smaller the possibility of chance as the explanation for an observed difference. In the MFMU Network example[7] (in which treatment with metronidazole was compared to placebo for women who screened positive for BV in pregnancy), the probability value was 0.95, indicating a high likelihood that chance explained the small difference in the rate of preterm birth between the groups.

Traditionally, a probability value of less than 0.05 has indicated "significance," whereas a probability value of more than 0.05 has indicated "no significance." In fact, many journals still allow probability values to be reported in this way. However, with the definition of a probability value in mind (see preceding paragraph), readers should wonder whether a probability value of 0.049 is different from a probability value of 0.051. Clearly, there is more to the interpretation of a probability value than the absolute number.

Relative Risk with 95% Confidence Intervals

A relative risk is defined as the incidence of the outcome in the exposed group divided by the incidence of disease in the unexposed (untreated) group. Thus, in the vitamin study (see Table 16-2), the relative risk was as follows:

$$\text{Relative risk} = \frac{56/935}{47/942} = \frac{0.06}{0.05} = 1.20$$

A relative risk of 1.0 means that the incidence of the outcome is identical in the exposed and unexposed subjects. A relative risk of less than 1.0 means that the incidence of the outcome is less in the exposed group, whereas a relative risk of more than 1.0 means that the incidence is greater in the exposed group.

The point estimate is the best estimate of the association between an exposure and an outcome, but it does not give information about the stability or statistical precision of the estimate. Clearly, the precision of such an estimate is related to the power of the study. The precision of a relative risk or other measure of effect is often described as a 95% confidence interval.[47] A 95% confidence interval is interpreted as follows: If a study is without bias, there is a 95% chance that the true point estimate lies within the bounds of the confidence interval. The narrower the confidence interval is, the greater is precision in the estimate. The wider the confidence interval is, the less certainty there is in the estimate.

Confidence intervals also provide information about statistical significance. In general, if a relative risk of 1.0 falls within the bounds of the 95% confidence interval for a given association, then the corresponding probability value will be more than 0.05. Likewise, if a relative risk of 1.0 is *not* included in the bounds of a 95% confidence interval, then the corresponding probability value will most likely be less than 0.05.

Other Measures of Effect

An odds ratio is another popular measure of effect that can be calculated from either observational studies or clinical trials.[48] Odds ratios are good approximations of relative risks in cases where the disease of interest is rare. They are most commonly calculated in case-control studies when the calculation of a relative risk is impossible because the denominator is not known. Odds ratios are also the output for most statistical packages when multivariable logistic regressions are performed. In general, relative risks are preferred over odds ratios when data are available to calculate a relative risk, such as in cohort studies or clinical trials.

Using the example from Table 16-2, the odds ratio for the association between vitamin treatment and preeclampsia is as follows:

$$\text{Odds ratio} = \frac{56 \times 895}{879 \times 47} = 1.21$$

An odds ratio is interpreted in exactly the same manner as a relative risk. Thus, an odds ratio of 2.0 would be interpreted as a twofold increase in risk, whereas an odds ratio of 0.5 would mean a 50% reduction in risk. The 95% confidence intervals are also interpreted in the same fashion as those for relative risks. Remember that the preferred measure of effect to calculate in clinical trials and cohort studies is a relative risk (or risk difference). Odds ratios can be used as surrogates for relative risks when the disease in question is rare.

The risk difference is the simple arithmetic difference in incidence between groups and can be calculated from clinical trial data or from cohort studies (but not from case-control studies). In the case of the vitamin study data (see Table 16-2), the risk difference is 0.06 – 0.05 = 0.01.

A risk difference is interpreted differently from a relative risk or an odds ratio. A risk difference of zero means that there is no difference in the incidence of disease between groups. A positive risk difference means that the incidence of the outcome is greater in the experimental group, whereas a negative risk difference means that the incidence of the outcome is greater in the control group. In the example of vitamin C and E treatment to prevent preeclampsia, the risk difference means that there is a 1.0% increase in the risk for preeclampsia in those exposed to vitamins C and E. The 95% confidence interval includes zero, which signifies that the data are consistent with there being no difference in the incidence between groups (and corresponds to a probability value of more than 0.05).

The measure of effect that is appropriate is largely determined by the aims of the study and the study design.[48]

Approach to Assessing Random Error

Approaching the analysis of research data can seem a daunting task. However, apprehension can be minimized by forming a clear plan at the start or in the planning phase of a research study. The following are some key steps to consider in the analysis of clinical research data.

STEP 1. GRAPH AND SUMMARIZE

Graph and summarize (e.g., means, range, standard deviation) all outcomes and exposures. This simple process allows the researcher to see a snapshot of the data to appreciate the distribution of a variable (e.g., is it a normal distribution?) and to identify implausible data elements.

STEP 2. PERFORM UNIVARIATE DATA ANALYSES

This critical step provides the foundation for the next steps: stratified and multivariable analysis. Univariate analysis allows assessment of associations between any given single exposure and outcome. The choice of the statistical test (or tests) in univariate analysis will vary with the design of the study and the type of outcome and exposure. An important design criterion that influences the univariate statistical test employed is whether or not the study is matched. *Matching* refers to the process of making a study group and comparison group comparable with respect to extraneous factors. A matched study design must be followed by a matched analysis.

There are several commonly used univariate statistical tests:

- Chi-square and Fisher's exact tests: These tests are used when both the outcome and exposure of interest are binary (yes/no). These tests compare the observed distribution of numbers in the cells of a 2 × 2 table, and they compare them to the expected distribution. Chi-square and Fisher's exact tests are used when data are unmatched. If the study is matched, then the appropriate test is the McNemar test.
- Student *t* test: A *t* test is used to compare means between two groups. For example, if one wished to compare the mean maternal age of women who develop preeclampsia with the age of those who do not, a *t* test would be appropriate. A *t* test can be either paired (for matched data) or unpaired (for unmatched data).

STEP 3. PERFORM STRATIFIED ANALYSIS

Stratified analysis is a way to assess confounding factors and effect modification. This can help to identify the variables to be included in multivariable analysis. The following is an example of a stratified analysis for a hypothetical case-control study to assess the association between alcohol use and preeclampsia. Table 16-3 is a 2 × 2 table generated from this case-control study.

The unadjusted odds ratio is 2.26; 95% confidence interval (CI), 1.2 to 4.2. This unadjusted analysis suggests that alcohol use increases the risk for preeclampsia, but in an observational study, confounding factors that may distort the relationship between alcohol and preeclampsia must be considered. One possible confounding factor is parity, because it may be associated with both alcohol use and preeclampsia. To assess whether parity confounds the association between alcohol use and preeclampsia, a stratified analysis can be performed to assess the alcohol-preeclampsia association separately in multiparous and in nulliparous women. This stratified analysis of this hypothetical dataset generates Tables 16-4 and 16-5.

In addition to these stratum-specific odds ratios, a stratified analysis also generates a Mantel-Haenszel summary odds ratio, which in this case is 1.0; 95% CI, 0.42 to 2.34. The proper interpretation of this summary odds ratio is that it represents the association between alcohol use and preeclampsia, after adjusting for the effect of parity. Thus, in this hypothetical example, although the unadjusted odds ratio suggested an association, the adjusted results did not. Stated differently, parity confounds the association between alcohol and preeclampsia.

A stratified analysis is thus a key step in assessing potential confounders, but it is limited because one can stratify only one or two factors simultaneously. Therefore, stratified analysis is more useful to assess potential confounders that should be included in multivariable models.

STEP 4. PERFORM MULTIVARIABLE ANALYSIS

A multivariable analysis is essential for observational studies, and it can be used occasionally in interventional studies. It allows assessment of the independent effects of many exposures on an outcome, while controlling for confounding factors. The performance of a multivariable analysis is complex and beyond the scope of this chapter. It is generally useful to consult with a biostatistician or with someone who has significant expertise in this area.

Sample Size and Power

So far, we have focused mainly on the assessment of type I (or alpha) error in clinical research, defined as the probability of rejecting the null hypothesis when in fact the null is correct. Type II (or beta) error is

TABLE 16-3 2 × 2 TABLE FROM CASE-CONTROL STUDY TO ASSESS ALCOHOL USE AND PREECLAMPSIA

	Preeclampsia +	Preeclampsia –	Total
Alcohol +	71	52	—
Alcohol –	29	48	—
Total	100	100	200

TABLE 16-4 ALCOHOL-PREECLAMPSIA ASSOCIATION IN NULLIPAROUS SUBJECTS

	Preeclampsia +	Preeclampsia –	Total
Alcohol +	8	16	—
Alcohol –	22	44	—
Total	30	60	90

Odds ratio = 1.0 (95% confidence interval, 0.33 to 2.9).

TABLE 16-5 ALCOHOL-PREECLAMPSIA ASSOCIATION IN MULTIPAROUS SUBJECTS

	Preeclampsia +	Preeclampsia –	Total
Alcohol +	63	36	—
Alcohol –	7	4	—
Total	70	40	110

Odds ratio = 1.0 (95% confidence interval, 0.23 to 4.2).

defined as the probability of accepting the null hypothesis when in fact it is false. In a study with type II error, the results are falsely reported as negative, and thus a true difference is missed. This typically occurs when the sample size is insufficient.

This concept of a false-negative study emphasizes the importance of sample size estimation and statistical power (*power* is defined as 1 minus the beta error). Sample size estimates should be performed prior to any observational or interventional study. The following are the key components of a sample size estimate for cohort studies or clinical trials, and for case-control studies (that have a binary outcome).

Sample size estimate for cohort study or clinical trial
Alpha error
Beta error
Incidence of outcome in unexposed subjects
Ratio of exposed to unexposed subjects
Minimum detectable relative risk

Sample size estimate for case-control study
Alpha error
Beta error
Prevalence of exposure in controls
Ratio of controls to cases
Minimum detectable odds ratio

Some of these components deserve discussion. First, alpha error, by tradition, is set at 0.05, reflecting the intent to perform a study whose results will be falsely declared to be positive less than 5% of the time. Second, beta error is usually set somewhere between 0.05 and 0.20, reflecting the intent to identify a true relationship at least 80% of the time when a relationship truly exists, and, simultaneously, a willingness to miss finding a true relationship 20% of the time. This means that such a study is described as having 80% to 95% power. Third, the incidence of exposure or the prevalence of exposure can generally be estimated from the literature or from pilot data. Last, the minimum detectable odds ratio or relative risk is that meant to be clinically relevant. In practice, there is a tradeoff between wanting to detect as small a difference as possible and wanting to maintain a reasonable sample size (from a logistical and cost perspective).

Sample size estimates should be performed before beginning a research study and should be reported as part of the study's design. As readers of the literature, we should be especially cognizant of sample size and statistical power in cases of a negative study.

Assessing Research on Screening and Diagnosis

Screening and diagnostic tests are an integral part of clinical medicine. For example, measurement of fundal height, a screening test for fetal growth disturbances and amniotic fluid abnormalities, is a routine part of prenatal care. If the fundal height measures significantly less than anticipated, a diagnostic test, in this case an ultrasound examination, is performed. The same sequence of screening followed by diagnostic testing occurs commonly in obstetric practice—for example, a family history (screening test) that leads to a "targeted" ultrasound (which may be diagnostic for some disorders or a screening test for others) and eventually to amniocentesis (diagnostic test). Because such testing dominates our clinical lives, it is essential that physicians understand the principles of screening and diagnostic tests.[49] Only by understanding the difference between screening and diagnostic testing can physicians make rational decisions about the proper interpretation of test results, and about whether a new test should be incorporated into clinical practice.

Screening versus Diagnosis

Screening has been defined as "the presumptive identification of an unrecognized disease or defect by the application of tests, examination or other procedures which can be applied rapidly. . . . A screening test is not meant to be diagnostic. Persons with positive or suspicious findings must be referred to their physicians for diagnosis and treatment."[41] Thus, screening tests are those that are widely applied to a population and require follow-up with a diagnostic test (if an individual screens positive). In general, a successful screening program must meet the following criteria:

- The condition screened for must have a significant burden on health.
- There must be effective early treatment for those who screen positive.
- The test must be sufficiently sensitive and specific (see later).
- The screening test must be inexpensive and easy to perform.
- The screening test must be safe and acceptable to patients.

Cervical cytology screening for premalignant lesions of the cervix is an example of a successful screening program that fulfills all of these criteria. In contrast, although cytomegalovirus infection of the fetus and neonate creates a significant burden of disease, a screening program for this virus has no value because there is no successful intervention. Similarly, although cervicovaginal fetal fibronectin screening can identify as many as 60% of women destined for preterm birth before 28 weeks,[50] there is currently no effective intervention that could be applied to screen-positive women to reduce the risk for preterm delivery.[51]

Sensitivity, Specificity, and Predictive Values

It is critical to understand the characteristics of both screening and diagnostic tests. Sensitivity and specificity are characteristics inherent in the test and are independent of the prevalence of the disease.[49,52] Sensitivity is the probability, expressed as a percentage, that if the disease is present, the test is positive. The numerator is the number of subjects with the disease who have a positive test, and the denominator is the total number of diseased subjects.

Specificity is the probability, expressed as a percentage, that if the disease is absent, the test is negative. The numerator is the number of subjects without disease who have a negative test, and the denominator is the total number of nondiseased subjects. Although the sensitivity and specificity of a test are important considerations when deciding whether or not to order a test, we become more interested in the predictive values when the test results have returned. Predictive values, unlike sensitivity and specificity, depend on the prevalence of the outcome in the population tested.

A positive predictive value (PPV) is the probability that if the test is positive, the subject has the disease. The numerator is the number of subjects with the disease who have a positive test, and the denominator is the total number of those with a positive test. A negative predictive value (NPV) is the probability that if the test is negative, the subject does not have the disease. The numerator is the number of subjects

TABLE 16-6 FETAL FIBRONECTIN (FFN) TO PREDICT DELIVERY WITHIN 7 DAYS OF TESTING

	Delivery, <7 Days		
	Yes	No	Total
FFN +	20	130	150
FFN −	3	610	613
Total	23	740	763

Prevalence = 23/763 = 3%.
Sensitivity = 20/23 = 87%; specificity = 610/740 = 82%
PPV = 20/150 = 13%; NPV = 610/613 = 99.5%.
NPV, negative predictive value; PPV, positive predictive value.
Data from Peaceman AM, Andrews WW, Thorp JM, et al: Fetal fibronectin as a predictor of preterm birth in patients with symptoms: A multicenter trial. Am J Obstet Gynecol 177:13, 1997.

TABLE 16-7 FETAL FIBRONECTIN (FFN) TEST TO PREDICT DELIVERY WITHIN 7 DAYS OF TESTING: HYPOTHETICAL ANALYSIS OF A HIGH-PREVALENCE GROUP

	Delivery < 7 Days		
	Yes	No	Total
FFN +	99	117	216
FFN −	15	532	547
Total	114	649	763

Prevalence = 114/763 = 15%.
Sensitivity = 99/114 = 87%; specificity = 532/649 = 82%.
PPV = 99/216 = 45%; NPV = 532/547 = 97%.
NPV, negative predictive value; PPV, positive predictive value.

without disease who have a negative test, and the denominator is the total number of those with negative tests. Given the same sensitivity and specificity, the PPV will increase and the NPV will decrease as the prevalence rises. Likewise, as the prevalence decreases, the PPV decreases and the NPV increases.

These abstract concepts are best demonstrated with a clinical example. Peaceman and colleagues[53] performed a prospective cohort study at multiple centers to assess whether cervicovaginal fetal fibronectin could be used as a diagnostic test in women with symptoms of preterm labor; fetal fibronectin has also been assessed in other studies as a screening test.[50] In the Peaceman study, women with symptoms of early preterm labor were enrolled, and cervicovaginal swabs for fibronectin testing were obtained. Treating physicians and patients were blinded to the results of the fibronectin test, a strength of the study. The outcomes assessed were the occurrence of delivery within 7 days, within 2 weeks, and before 37 weeks' gestation. The results of the analysis of delivery within 7 days (Table 16-6) may be used as an example to illustrate sensitivity, specificity, and PPV and NPV.

Some would look at these results and the high NPV and suggest that fetal fibronectin is a useful tool in this setting to rule out an imminent delivery. Another way of looking at these same data would be to look closely at the low prevalence of delivery within 7 days (3%). After reading this article, the following questions emerge: Is it appropriate to use a diagnostic test in such a low prevalence group? And, more importantly, what would be the impact of testing a higher-prevalence population (i.e., a population with a greater chance of preterm birth within 7 days)?

Physicians may look at these results differently. Some may argue that the treatment for preterm labor has risk, is of questionable efficacy, and is overused. Thus, a test that could avoid overtreatment with tocolytics might be helpful. Others could argue that the very high NPV with fetal fibronectin was obtained only when testing patients with a very low prevalence of preterm delivery and that no diagnostic test is needed in such a low-prevalence population. Furthermore, when this test is used in a higher-prevalence group, the NPV will decrease, making it much less useful. The value of a test with these characteristics is thus population dependent, according to the prevalence of preterm birth and the prevailing pattern of clinical care regarding tocolytic drugs for women with minimal symptoms.

For example, let us assume the population tested could be selected by adding clinical data to define a group with a higher prevalence of delivery within 7 days. Table 16-7 illustrates the effect of the increased prevalence on PPV and NPV. Remember that the sensitivity and specificity stay constant regardless of the disease prevalence. As expected, the PPV increases somewhat, and the NPV is decreased to 97%. Another way of looking at the NPV is that 3% of those with a negative test will go on to deliver within 7 days. Is this rate of false-negative testing acceptable for a patient who presents at 24 weeks with symptoms of preterm labor? Once again, the answer is determined by patient- and physician-related factors that are unique to the clinical setting.

Likelihood Ratios

Likelihood ratios, another method to describe test performance, can be used to calculate post-test probabilities, just like predictive values. In literature from the United States, predictive values are commonly reported, whereas likelihood ratios are preferred in many European and South American journals. A likelihood ratio is defined as the probability of the test result in the presence of outcome, divided by the probability of the result in those without the outcome. Separate likelihood ratios are calculated for positive tests and negative tests. Likelihood ratios express how many times more (or less) likely a test result is to be found in those with the outcome compared with those without the outcome.

As an example, the positive likelihood ratios from the data on delivery within 7 days in the previously cited Peaceman study[53] can be calculated as shown here, by dividing the proportion of women with a positive test who did deliver within 7 days, by the proportion of women with a positive test who did not deliver within 7 days:

$$\text{Positive likelihood ratio} = \frac{20/23}{130/740} = \frac{0.87}{0.18} = 4.8$$

Likelihood ratios can also be used to calculate a post-test probability (PPV), which is what we use in clinical practice. To do this, however, the pretest probability (prevalence) must be converted to pretest odds using the following formula:

$$\text{Odds} = \text{probability of event}/(1 - \text{probability of event})$$
$$\text{Probability} = \text{odds}/(1 + \text{odds})$$

Using the Peaceman data for a positive test, the prevalence of delivery within 7 days is 3%. In odds, this translates to 0.031. Then, we can calculate the post-test odds using the formula

$$\text{Pretest odds} \times \text{likelihood ratio} = \text{post-test odds}$$

In this case, the post-test odds are $0.031 \times 4.8 = 0.1488$. When the post-test odds are converted to a post-test probability (i.e., a PPV), the result is $0.1488/1.1488 = 13.0\%$, the same as the PPV calculation we saw in Table 16-6.

Thus, looking at the positive and negative likelihood ratios is another way to assess the utility of a test, and these ratios can be used to convert pretest probabilities to post-test probabilities. For the latter issue, this can be somewhat cumbersome, and many individuals prefer to simply use a 2 × 2 table to calculate predictive values.

Receiver Operating Characteristic Curves

Although test results may be categorical (i.e., positive or negative), they are more often expressed in clinical medicine as a point on a continuum. As clinicians, we evaluate test results and try to discriminate "normal" from "abnormal." Although it would be ideal to have tests that are simultaneously very sensitive and specific, this is seldom the case. Thus, we are faced with selecting thresholds that trade between degrees of sensitivity and specificity. A graphic method that makes these tradeoffs explicit and aids in the selection of cut points is the *receiver operating characteristic (ROC) curve*. The sensitivity is placed on the y axis versus 1 minus the specificity (the false-positive rate) on the x axis for the entire range of cut points. Tests that discriminate well tend to generate a curve that occupies the upper left corner of the graph. Poorly discriminating tests generate a curve that falls along the diagonal that follows from the lower left corner to the upper right corner. A 45-degree line along this diagonal describes a nondiscriminating test, which is one that has no threshold value.

ROC curves have three primary uses: to select a cut point for an individual test, to assess the overall accuracy of the individual test, and to compare the overall accuracy of two tests for the same condition. The last is most often done by calculating and comparing the area under the ROC curve.

A recent example of the clinical use of ROC curves in selecting an appropriate cut point was published by Owen and colleagues[54] and focused on mid-trimester transvaginal cervical length measurements to predict preterm birth before 35 weeks' gestation in high-risk women. To assess this question, the authors performed a multicenter prospective study of transvaginal ultrasound cervical measurements every 2 weeks in 183 women with a prior birth at less than 32 weeks. Figure 16-3 shows a comparison of ROC curves for shortest observed cervical length to the cervical length at the first examination, for the prediction of spontaneous preterm birth before 35 weeks' gestation. Figure 16-3 suggests the following:

1. The shortest observed cervical length is a better discriminator than the initial cervical length for the prediction of spontaneous preterm birth at less than 35 weeks.
2. Although the shortest observed cervical length is better than the initial examination, neither test is particularly discriminating (as evidenced by the fact that neither curve is very close to the left upper corner of the graph).
3. The optimal cut point for the shortest observed cervical length is 25 mm. At this level, however, the sensitivity is only about 70%, with a false-positive rate of about 20%.

Iams and colleagues[55] reported a study of several tests to predict preterm birth in pregnant women. Cervical examinations by digital examination (expressed as a Bishop score) and by ultrasound (expressed as the length of the cervical canal) were compared with monitored

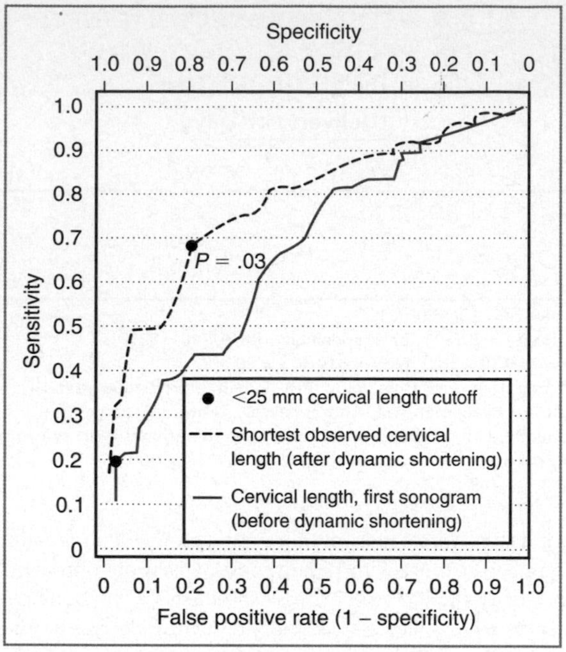

FIGURE 16-3 Comparison of ROC curves for cervical length. Receiver operating characteristic (ROC) curves of cervical length cutoffs for the prediction of spontaneous preterm birth before 35 weeks' gestation. (From Owen J, Yost N, Berghella V, et al: Mid-trimester endovaginal sonography in women at high risk for spontaneous preterm birth. JAMA 286:1340, 2000.)

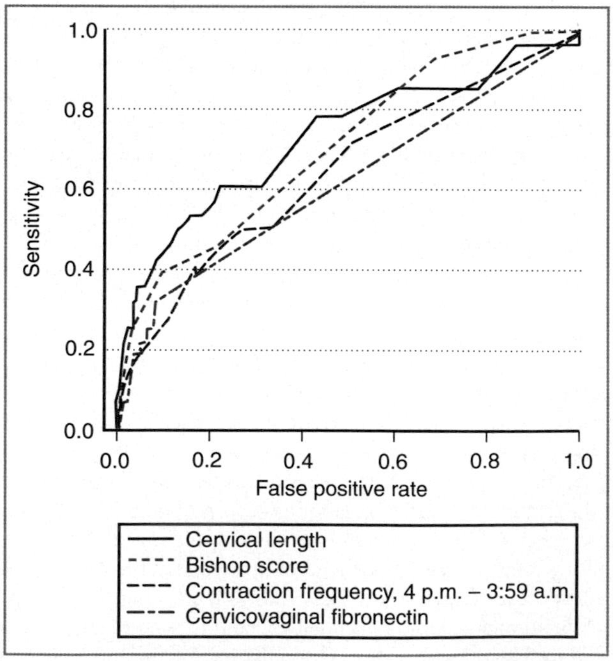

FIGURE 16-4 Comparison of tests to predict preterm birth. Receiver operating characteristic curves for cervical length, Bishop score, frequency of contractions, and presence or absence of fetal fibronectin in cervicovaginal secretions at 27 to 28 weeks in the prediction of spontaneous preterm delivery (less than 35 weeks). (From Iams JD, Newman RB, Thom EA, et al, for the National Institute of Child Health and Human Development Network of Maternal-Fetal Medicine Units: Frequency of uterine contractions and the risk of spontaneous preterm delivery. N Engl J Med 346:250, 2002.)

uterine contraction frequency and fetal fibronectin in cervicovaginal secretions using ROC curves. The performance of each test was displayed on a common graph of their ROC curves (Fig. 16-4). Cervical length by ultrasound, though far from an ideal test, had the "best" performance, as the uppermost line of the curves displayed.

Summary

This overview of study design and methods to analyze and report data in perinatal medicine can serve as a starting point to integrate research data appropriately into clinical care. As with any skill, it is mastered by frequent repetition and especially by analyzing and presenting one's own data with one of the methods described.

References

1. Centre for Evidence-Based Medicine, Oxford University, available at www.cebm.net (accessed February 28, 2008).
2. Peipert JF, Phipps MG: Observational studies. Clin Obstet Gynecol 41:235, 1998.
3. Hennekens CH, Buring JE: Epidemiology in Medicine. Boston, Little, Brown, 1987.
4. Kelsey JL, Whittemore AS, Evans AE, et al: Methods in Observational Epidemiology. New York, Oxford University Press, 1996.
5. Meinert CL: Clinical Trials: Design, Conduct, and Analysis. New York, Oxford University Press, 1986.
6. Moher D, Schulz KF, Altman D: The CONSORT statement: Revised recommendations for improving the quality of reports of parallel-group randomized trials. JAMA 285:1987, 2001.
7. Carey JC, Klebanoff MA, Hauth JC, et al, for the National Institute of Child Health and Human Development Network of Maternal-Fetal Medicine Units: Metronidazole to prevent preterm delivery in pregnant women with asymptomatic bacterial vaginosis. N Engl J Med 342:534, 2000.
8. Kurki T, Sivonen A, Renkonen O, et al: Bacterial vaginosis in early pregnancy and pregnancy outcome. Obstet Gynecol 80:173, 1992.
9. Riduan JM, Hillier SL, Utomo B, et al: Bacterial vaginosis and prematurity in Indonesia: Association in early and late pregnancy. Am J Obstet Gynecol 169:175, 1993.
10. Hillier SL, Nugent RP, Eschenbach DA, et al: Association between bacterial vaginosis and preterm delivery of a low-birth-weight infant. The Vaginal Infections and Prematurity Study Group. N Engl J Med 333:1737, 1995.
11. Hauth JC, Goldenberg RL, Andrews WW, et al: Reduced incidence of preterm delivery with metronidazole and erythromycin in women with bacterial vaginosis. N Engl J Med 333:1732, 1995.
12. McGregor JA, French JI, Parker R, et al: Prevention of premature birth by screening and treatment for common genital tract infections: Results of a prospective controlled evaluation. Am J Obstet Gynecol 173:157-167, 1995.
13. Peipert JF, Bracken MB: Systematic reviews of medical evidence: The use of meta-analysis in obstetrics and gynecology. Obstet Gynecol 89:628, 1997.
14. Sanchez-Ramos L, Kaunitz AM, Gaudier FL, et al: Efficacy of maintenance therapy after acute tocolysis: A meta-analysis. Am J Obstet Gynecol 181:484, 1999.
15. Tsatsaris V, Papatsonis D, Goffinet F, et al: Tocolysis with nifedipine or beta-adrenergic agonists: A meta-analysis. Obstet Gynecol 97:840, 2001.
16. Cochrane Database of Systematic Reviews: The Cochrane Library, issue 4. Oxford, 2002. Update software; available online at www.cochrane.org. Look for the Cochrane Pregnancy and Childbirth Group. Abstracts of Cochrane Reviews.
17. Kenyon S, Boulvain M, Neilson J: Antibiotics for preterm premature rupture of membranes. Cochrane Database Syst Rev (4):CD001058, 2001.
18. Cook D, Guyatt G: The professional meta-analyst: An evolutionary advantage. J Clin Epidemiol 47:1327, 1994.
19. LeLorier J, Gregoire G, Benhaddad A, et al: Discrepancies between meta-analyses and subsequent large randomized, controlled trials. N Engl J Med 337:536, 1997.
20. Villar J, Paggio G, Carroli G, et al: Factors affecting the comparability of meta-analyses and largest trials results in perinatology. J Clin Epidemiol 50:997, 1997.
21. Moher D, Cook DJ, Eastwood S, et al: Improving the quality of reports of meta-analyses of randomised controlled trials: The QUOROM statement. Quality of Reporting of Meta-Analyses. Lancet 354:1896, 1999.
22. Askie LM, Duley L, Henderson-Smart DJ, Stewart LA: Antiplatelet agents for prevention of preeclampsia: A meta-analysis of individual patient data. Lancet 369:1791-1798, 2007.
23. Macones G, Goldie S, Peipert J: Economic analyses in obstetrics and gynecology: A guide for clinicians and researchers. Obstet Gynecol Surv 54:663, 1999.
24. Rouse D, Goldenberg R, Cliver S, et al: Strategies for the prevention of early-onset neonatal group B streptococcal sepsis: A decision analysis. Obstet Gynecol 83:483, 1994.
25. Macones G, Robinson C: Is there justification for using indomethacin in preterm labor? An analysis of risks and benefits. Am J Obstet Gynecol 177:819, 1997.
26. Macones GM, Bader TJ, Asch DA: Optimising maternal-fetal outcomes in preterm labour: A decision analysis. BJOG 105:541, 1998.
27. Casele H, Grobman W: Cost-effectiveness of thromboprophylaxis with intermittent pneumatic compression at cesarean delivery. Obstet Gynecol 108:535-540, 2006.
28. Grobman WA: Decision analysis in obstetrics and gynecology. Obstet Gynecol Surv 61:602-607, 2006.
29. Datta M. You cannot exclude the explanation you have not considered. Lancet 342:345, 1993.
30. Sitthi-amorn C, Poshyachinda V: Bias. Lancet 342:286-288, 1993.
31. Grimes DA, Schulz KF: Bias and causal associations in observational research. Lancet 359:248, 2002.
32. Leon D: Failed or misleading adjustment for confounding. Lancet 342:479, 1993.
33. Norton ME, Merrill J, Cooper BA, et al: Neonatal complications after the administration of indomethacin for preterm labor. N Engl J Med 329:1602, 1993.
34. Itskovitz J, Abramovici H, Brandes J: Oligohydramnion, meconium and perinatal death concurrent with indomethacin treatment in human pregnancy. J Reprod Med 24:137-140, 1980.
35. Major C, Lewis D, Harding J, et al: Tocolysis with indomethacin increases the incidence of necrotizing enterocolitis in the low birth weight neonate. Am J Obstet Gynecol 170:102, 1994.
36. Iannucci T, Besinger R, Fisher S, et al: Effect of dual tocolysis on the incidence of severe intraventricular hemorrhage among extremely low-birth-weight infants. Am J Obstet Gynecol 175:1043, 1996.
37. Macones G, Marder S, Clothier B, et al: The controversy surrounding indomethacin for tocolysis. Am J Obstet Gynecol 184:264, 2001.
38. Romero R, Sirtori M, Oyarzun E: Infection and labor: V. Prevalence, microbiology, and clinical significance of intraamniotic infection in women with preterm labor and intact membranes. Am J Obstet Gynecol 161:817, 1989.
39. Romero R, Gomez R, Ghezzi F, et al: A fetal systemic inflammatory response is followed by the spontaneous onset of preterm parturition. Am J Obstet Gynecol 179:186, 1998.
40. Yoon B, Kim C, Romero R, et al: Experimentally induced intrauterine infection causes fetal brain white matter lesions in rabbits. Am J Obstet Gynecol 177:797, 1997.
41. Last JL: A Dictionary of Epidemiology. New York, Oxford University Press, 1995.
42. Nicholson JM, Kellar LC, Cronholm PF, Macones GA: Active management of risk in pregnancy at term is an urban population: An association between a higher induction of labor rate and a lower caesarean delivery rate. Am J Obstet Gynecol 191:1516-1528, 2004.
43. Czeizel AE, Rockenbauer M: A population based case-control teratologic study of oral metronidazole treatment during pregnancy. BJOG 105:322, 1998.

44. Schulz KF, Grimes DA: Generation of allocation sequences in randomised trials: Chance not choice. Lancet 359:515, 2002.
45. Hosmer D, Lemeshow D: Applied Logistic Regression. New York, Wiley, 1989.
46. Rumbold AR, Crowther CA, Haslam RR, et al: Vitamins C and E and the risks of preeclampsia and perinatal complications. N Engl J Med 354:1796-1806, 2006.
47. Shakespeare TP, Gebski VJ, Veness MJ, et al: Improving interpretation of clinical studies by use of confidence levels, clinical significance curves, and risk-benefit contours. Lancet 357:1349, 2001.
48. Victora C: What's the denominator? Lancet 342:97, 1993.
49. Boardman LA, Peipert JF: Screening and diagnostic testing. Clin Obstet Gynecol 41:267, 1998.
50. Goldenberg RL, Mercer BM, Meis PJ, et al: The preterm prediction study: Fetal fibronectin testing and spontaneous preterm birth. NICHD Maternal Fetal Medicine Units Network. Obstet Gynecol 87:643, 1996.
51. Andrews WW, Sibai BM, Thom EA, et al, for the National Institute of Child Health and Human Development: Maternal-Fetal Medicine Units Network: Randomized clinical trial of metronidazole plus erythromycin to prevent spontaneous preterm delivery in fetal fibronectin positive women. Obstet Gynecol 101(5 Pt 1):847-855, 2003.
52. Clarke J: A scientific approach to surgical reasoning: I. Diagnostic accuracy. Theoret Surg 5:206, 1990.
53. Peaceman AM, Andrews WW, Thorp JM, et al: Fetal fibronectin as a predictor of preterm birth in patients with symptoms: A multicenter trial. Am J Obstet Gynecol 177:13, 1997.
54. Owen J, Yost N, Berghella V, et al: Mid-trimester endovaginal sonography in women at high risk for spontaneous preterm birth. JAMA 286:1340, 2000.
55. Iams JD, Newman RB, Thom EA, et al, for The National Institute of Child Health and Human Development Network of Maternal-Fetal Medicine Units: Frequency of uterine contractions and the risk of spontaneous preterm delivery. N Engl J Med 346:250, 2002.

Part II

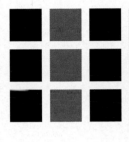

FETAL DISORDERS: DIAGNOSIS AND THERAPY

Chapter 17

Prenatal Diagnosis of Congenital Disorders

Ronald J. Wapner, MD, Thomas M. Jenkins, MD, and Nahla Khalek, MD

Prenatal diagnosis, a term once considered synonymous with invasive fetal testing and karyotype evaluation, now encompasses pedigree analysis, population screening, fetal risk assessment, genetic counseling, and fetal diagnostic testing. Although prenatal evaluation of the fetus for genetic disorders can have a huge impact on individual families, most screening and testing is done for events that occur in less than 1% of pregnancies. In this chapter, we describe different modalities available for in utero fetal diagnosis of congenital disorders, the approach to screening ongoing pregnancies for genetic disease, and the counseling requirement for each.

Screening for Fetal Genetic Disorders

Detecting or defining risk for disease in an asymptomatic low-risk population is the goal of screening. As opposed to diagnostic testing, intended to identify or confirm an affected individual, screening is intended to identify populations who have an increased risk for a specific disorder, and for whom diagnostic testing may be warranted. An ideal perinatal genetic screening test should fulfill the following criteria:

- Identify common or important fetal disorders
- Be cost-effective and easy to perform
- Have a high detection rate and a low false-positive rate
- Be reliable and reproducible
- Test for disorders for which a diagnostic test exists
- Be positive early enough in gestation to permit safe and legal options for pregnancy termination if desired

Sensitivity and specificity are two key concepts in screening test performance (see Chapter 16). Sensitivity is the percentage of affected pregnancies that are screen positive. Specificity is the percentage of individuals with unaffected pregnancies who screen negative. The reciprocal of specificity is the false-positive rate. Sensitivity and specificity are independent of disease frequency, and they describe the anticipated performance of a screening test in the population. Alternatively, positive and negative predictive values are dependent on disease prevalence and are vital in the interpretation of the test result for an individual patient. These latter two values represent, respectively, the likelihood that a person with a positive or negative test does or does not have an affected pregnancy. The impact of the prevalence of the disease on the positive and negative predictive values is described in Chapter 16 and is shown in Tables 16-6 and 16-7.

Use of screening tests requires that cutoff values for "positive" tests be set. Performance of the test depends on this cutoff; for example, increased detection rate can be obtained by lowering the cutoff threshold, but the concomitant lowered specificity would result in more false-positive results. Table 17-1 shows the performance of second-trimester maternal serum screening for Down syndrome based on various cutoffs.[1] A receiver operating curve can be used as a statistical method to find the "best" balance between sensitivity and specificity. A line diagram is plotted with sensitivity on the vertical axis and the false-positive rate plotted horizontally (Fig. 17-1). The greater the area under the curve (toward the upper left corner), the better the test's performance is, with increasing sensitivity and a reduced false-positive rate.

When screening for Down syndrome, cutoff values are important for laboratories that provide the testing and for clinicians who interpret the results. When viewed from the patient's perspective, reporting tests as positive or negative can be confusing. Receipt of a "positive" result of 1 in 250 may lead to a choice of a diagnostic test that carries a risk of complications, whereas a "negative" result of 1 in 290 may provide greater reassurance than intended, when in fact the actual risk of Down syndrome is similar for both patients. Often, explaining the significance of a positive or negative result before the screening test is performed will assist patients in understanding their results. Many centers report the absolute risk to the patient to further help in interpretation. Regardless of the counseling approach, understanding the concept of screening is difficult for many patients. From the perspective of the laboratory or clinician, selection of a cutoff that is too high or too low will lead to overutilization or underutilization of diagnostic tests and the consequent risk of procedure-related pregnancy loss or false reassurance, respectively.

Likelihood Ratios

The impact of a positive screening test depends on the pretest (a priori) risk of an affected pregnancy. Likelihood ratios are statistical means to modify an individual's risk based on known data for a population. For binary risk factors that are either present or absent, likelihood ratios are determined by comparing the frequency of positive tests in affected pregnancies to the frequency in normal pregnancies. This is calculated as the sensitivity of the test divided by its false-positive rate (likelihood ratio = sensitivity/false-positive rate). For tests that use continuous variables (such as serum marker measurements), likeli-

TABLE 17-1 DOWN SYNDROME DETECTION: FALSE-POSITIVE RATES (FPR) AT DIFFERENT CUTOFF VALUES

Triple Screen Cutoff	Detection Rate	FPR	Quadruple Screen Cutoff	Detection Rate	FPR
1:200	57	4.3	1:200	60	3.5
1:250	61	5.6	1:250	64	4.5
1:300	64	6.8	1:300	67	5.5
1:350	67	8.1	1:350	69	6.5
1:400	69	9.3	1:400	72	7.6

Data from Huang T, Watt H, Wald N: The effect of differences in the distribution of maternal age in England and Wales on the performance of prenatal screening for Down's syndrome. Prenat Diagn 17:615, 1997.

TABLE 17-2 ADJUSTING THE RISK FOR DOWN SYNDROME USING LIKELIHOOD RATIOS FOR BINARY ULTRASOUND MARKERS

A priori risk of Down syndrome (age or serum screen)	1:1000
Positive ultrasound marker for Down syndrome	
Rate in Down syndrome population (sensitivity of marker)	10%
Rate in general population (FPR of marker)	1.0%
Likelihood ratio (sens/FPR)	10.0
Adjusted risk for Down syndrome	
(A priori risk × likelihood ratio) = $^1/_{1000} \times 10$	1:100

FPR, false-positive rate; sens, sensitivity.

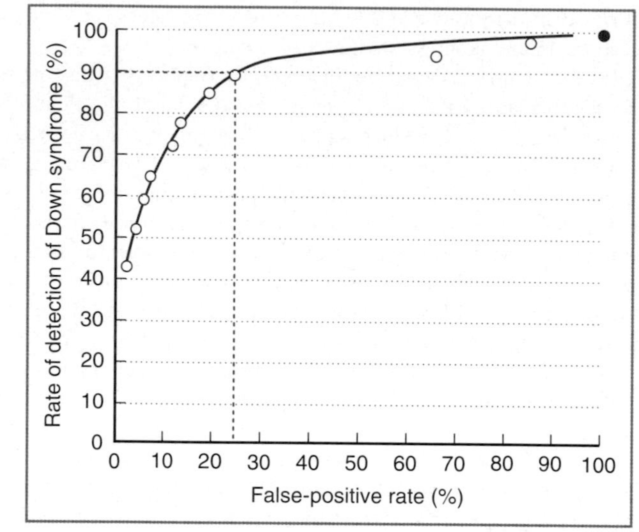

FIGURE 17-1 Receiver operating curve demonstrating sensitivity for Down syndrome detection versus false-positive rate. Cutoff points for sensitivity versus false-positive rate are determined by these curves. (From Haddow JE, Palomaki GE, Knight GJ, et al: Reducing the need for amniocentesis in women 35 years of age or older with serum markers for screening. N Engl J Med 330:1114, 1994.)

hood ratios are calculated from the log gaussian distributions of normal and affected pregnancies. Once a likelihood ratio is determined, it can be used to modify the a priori risk (Table 17-2). If more than one likelihood ratio is available and is independent of other parameters, it also can be used to modify risk. In this way, multiple factors (such as maternal age, serum analytes, and ultrasound findings) can be simultaneously used to modify risk.

Antenatal Screening for Down Syndrome

There has been a general consensus in the United States that invasive testing for Down syndrome should be offered to women with a second-trimester risk of 1:270 or higher (liveborn risk of 1:380). The cutoff level and subsequent public policy was determined more than 25 years ago and was based on a maternal age risk of 35 years at delivery. The factors considered in determining this value included the prevalence of disease, a perceived significant increase in the trisomy 21 risk after this age, the risk of invasive testing, the availability of resources, and a cost-to-benefit analysis. Since that time, a number of additional screening tests for Down syndrome have become available that challenge the validity of maternal age as a single indication for invasive testing.

Maternal Age as a Screening Test

The association of Down syndrome with advancing maternal age was first reported in 1909.[2] Fifty years later, karyotype analysis was developed and correlated the Down syndrome phenotype with an extra G chromosome.[3] This led to the development of genetic amniocentesis, through which the prenatal diagnosis of Down syndrome became feasible. To standardize the use of this emerging technology, a consensus report from the National Institutes of Health in 1979 suggested that amniocentesis be routinely offered to women aged 35 years or older at delivery. At that time, maternal age risks of Down syndrome were available only in 5-year groupings. Using these data, the age of 35 seemed a natural cutoff, because women in the 30- to 34-year grouping had a risk of 1:880, and the risk for women aged 35 to 40 was almost fourfold higher. This cutoff was based on a number of factors, including the availability of experienced operators and cytogenetics laboratories, the cost-to-benefit ratio, and the balance between procedure-related losses and the possibility of a positive finding. This cutoff continues to be used, and the second-trimester risk of 1:270 or liveborn risk of 1:380 remains the standard value for offering women invasive testing.

The risk for Down syndrome is now recognized to be continuous, which emphasizes the arbitrary nature of an absolute age threshold of 35. In addition to maternal age, the risk of trisomy 21 depends on the gestational age at which testing is performed, because only 69% of first-trimester and 76% of second-trimester Down syndrome pregnancies are viable (Table 17-3).[4] Currently, more than 80% of diagnostic procedures to determine fetal karyotype performed in the United States are performed solely for "advanced maternal age," yet 70% of affected pregnancies are born to women outside this group. With many women delaying childbirth until later in life, more than 14% of pregnant women in the United States are being offered testing based on age alone. In Switzerland and the United Kingdom, almost 15% of births now occur in women older than 35.

TABLE 17-3 RISK FOR DOWN SYNDROME BASED ON MATERNAL AND GESTATIONAL AGES

Maternal Age (yr)	Gestational Age 12 Wk	16 Wk	20 Wk	Liveborn
20	1/1068	1/1200	1/1295	1/1527
25	1/946	1/1062	1/1147	1/1352
30	1/626	1/703	1/759	1/895
31	1/543	1/610	1/658	1/776
32	1/461	1/518	1/559	1/659
33	1/383	1/430	1/464	1/547
34	1/312	1/350	1/378	1/446
35	1/249	1/280	1/302	1/356
36	1/196	1/220	1/238	1/280
37	1/152	1/171	1/185	1/218
38	1/117	1/131	1/142	1/167
39	1/89	1/100	1/108	1/128
40	1/68	1/76	1/82	1/97
42	1/38	1/43	1/46	1/55
44	1/21	1/24	1/26	1/30
45	1/16	1/18	1/19	1/23

Data from Hook EB: Rates of chromosome abnormalities at different maternal ages. Obstet Gynecol 58:282, 1981.

Second-Trimester Maternal Serum Screening

Serum screening may be used to identify the 70% of Down syndrome pregnancies in women less than 35 years of age. This approach is derived from a 1984 report of lower maternal serum α-fetoprotein (MSAFP) levels in women carrying a Down syndrome fetus. Women with Down syndrome pregnancies had a median MSAFP value of 0.75 multiples of the unaffected median (MoM).[5,6] Using this deviation to calculate a likelihood ratio, the age-related risk for Down syndrome could be modified. When the standard 1:270 cutoff was used, approximately 25% of Down syndrome pregnancies among women less than 35 years of age were screen-positive.[7-9]

Elevated human chorionic gonadotropin (hCG) (mean, 2.3 MoM) and reduced levels of unconjugated estriol (mean, 0.7 MoM) were subsequently linked to an increased risk of trisomy 21.[6,10,11] hCG or reduced levels of unconjugated estriol used alone to modify the maternal age risk has a Down syndrome detection rate of only 20% to 30%. However, because they are independent variables, they can be analyzed simultaneously with maternal age and AFP to form a composite risk calculation (frequently called a triple screen).

The sensitivity of the triple screen for Down syndrome detection in women younger than 35 years ranges between 57% and 67% if the false-positive rate is held constant at 5%.[12-15] Overall, the odds of having an affected pregnancy with a positive screen are approximately 1 in 33 to 1 in 62, depending on the age range of the population studied,[16,17] an improvement over the 1:100 odds when maternal age is the sole screening parameter. Because of the impact of maternal age on the risk analysis, screening women who will be 35 years of age or more increases the sensitivity using the same cutoffs to approximately 87% but with a false-positive rate of nearly 25%.[13,18]

Inhibin A, a protein produced initially by the corpus luteum and later by the placenta, is now routinely included in second-trimester Down syndrome screening resulting in a "quad screen." Inhibin A levels are elevated in Down syndrome pregnancies (1.3 to 2.5 MoM) and do not vary with gestational age in the second trimester. There is, however, a small correlation with hCG levels, making the added sensitivity for Down syndrome detection less robust.[19] Detection rates when a quad screen of α-fetoprotein (AFP), hCG, unconjugated estriol, and inhibin A are used are about 75% (screen positive rate, 5%) in the population under age 35 years.[20] For women older than 35, the detection rate is approximately 92% with a screen-positive rate of 13%.

Other analytes or combinations of analytes have been tested to further increase sensitivity. Hyperglycosylated hCG excreted in maternal urine has been tested as a marker for Down syndrome. One study of nearly 1500 women (1448 control subjects and 39 Down syndrome pregnancies) reported a sensitivity of 96% of affected pregnancies with a 5% false-positive rate and 71% detection with a 1% false-positive rate when a combination of hyperglycosylated hCG, urine β-core hCG fragment, MSAFP, and maternal age was used.[21] This detection rate, however, has not been duplicated by others.

With the addition of extra markers, the potential benefit must be balanced against the cost. With each additional marker, costs to society can balloon into the millions because of the number of pregnancies tested each year with only a minimal improvement in detection. The relative cost and value of raising the sensitivity or lowering the false-positive rate a few percentage points is an ongoing debate.

Abnormal Second Trimester Maternal Serum Markers in Pregnancies with a Normal Karyotype

Unexplained Elevated Maternal Serum α-Fetoprotein

When an elevated MSAFP is reported in pregnancies in which the gestational age is correctly assigned and the fetus is structurally normal, and the amniotic fluid AFP (AFAFP) is normal, the biologic explanation is almost always a breach in the maternal-fetal interface. This leads to higher AFP levels in the maternal circulation. Not surprisingly, women with unexplained elevation in AFP levels have been found to have increased risk of obstetric complications, including fetal growth restriction, fetal death, prematurity, oligohydramnios, abruptio placentae, and preeclampsia. Table 17-4 summarizes the numerous reports; the higher the MSAFP level is, the greater the risk. Crandall and colleagues[22] studied 1002 women with MSAFP values greater than 2.5 MoM and stratified them by the degree of elevation. In those with a normal ultrasound and amniocentesis, the risk of adverse outcome was 27% overall but varied with the degree of elevation. Adverse outcome occurred in 16% when the MSAFP was 2.5 to 2.9 MoM, 29% when it was 3.0 to 5.0 MoM, and 70% when it was greater than 5.0 MoM. Waller and coworkers[23-25] investigated 51,008 women screened with MSAFP in California to evaluate the predictive value of high MSAFP compared with low levels. The risk of delivery before 28 weeks was 0.4% with low values (<0.81 MoM) and 3.2% for those with high values (>2.5 MoM), an eightfold difference. The rates for delivery before 37 weeks were 2.6% for the low MSAFP group and 24.3% for the high MSAFP group. Notably, women with MSAFP values greater than 2.5 MoM had a 10.5-fold increase in preeclampsia and a 10-fold increased risk of placental complications, suggesting that an elevated value in the absence of an anomaly may derive from a fetal-maternal hemorrhage of sufficient volume to have clinical significance. This observation may explain the elevation in MSAFP, but to date no management protocol has been demonstrated to improve outcome in these cases.

TABLE 17-4 STUDIES EVALUATING THE RELATION OF UNEXPLAINED ELEVATIONS OF MSAFP AND POOR PREGNANCY OUTCOME

Source	Location (Year)	Pregnancies Screened	MoM Cutoff	LBW Risk	IUGR Risk	Premature Delivery Risk	Abruption Risk	IUFD Risk	Perinatal Death
Brock et al (505, 506)	Scotland (1977, 1979)	15,481	2.3	2.5×				+	+
Wald et al (507, 508)	England (1977, 1980)	3,194	3.0	4.7×		5.8×			3.5×
		4,198							
Macri et al (509)	New York (1978)	6,031	2.0	2.0×					
Gordon et al (510)	England (1978)	1,055	2.0			3.5×			4.5×
Smith (511)	England (1980)	1,500	2.0	+	+	+			+
Evans and Stokes (512)	Wales (1984)	2,913	2.0	3.0×			+		8.0×
Burton et al (513, 514)	North Carolina (1983, 1988)	42,037	2.5	2.0×				8.0×	10.0×
Persson et al (515)	Sweden (1983)	10,147	2.3	2.8×		2.0×	10.0×		3.0×
Haddow et al (516)	Maine (1983)	3,636	2.0	3.6×		2.0×			
Purdie et al (517)	Scotland (1983)	7,223	2.5	2.5×			20.0×		
Fuhrmann and Weitzel (518)	West Germany (1985)	50,000	2.5	3.5×				8.6×	
Williamson et al (519)	Iowa (1986)	1,161		Poor outcomes					
Robinson et al (520)	California (1989)	35,787	2.0	3.5×					
Ghosh et al (521)	Hong Kong (1986)	9,838	2.0	+					
Schnittger and Kjessler (522)	Sweden (1984)	18,037	2.0	+			+		
Hamilton et al (523)	Scotland (1985)	10,885	2.5	10.0×	2×	>10.0×	3.0×		8.0×
Doran et al (524)	Ontario (1987)	8,140	2.0	6.0×				+	
Milunsky et al (525)	Massachusetts (1989)	13,486	2.0	4.0×			3.0×	8.0×	+

IUFD, intrauterine fetal demise; IUGR, intrauterine growth retardation; LBW, low birth weight; MoM, multiple of the median; MSAFP; maternal serum α-fetoprotein; +, increased risk but unquantified.

Data from Milunsky A (ed): Genetic Disorders and the Fetus: Diagnosis, Prevention, and Treatment, 3rd ed. Baltimore, Johns Hopkins University Press, 1992, p 656.

Unexplained Elevated Human Chorionic Gonadotropin Levels

The risk for adverse pregnancy outcome with elevated hCG levels appears to be independent of those associated with elevated AFP. Studies have shown that unexplained elevated hCG (greater than 2.0 MoM) is associated with an increased risk of preeclampsia, preterm birth, low birth weight, fetal demise, and possibly hypertension.[26] It appears that the higher the hCG is, the greater the risk.

Elevated Human Chorionic Gonadotropin and Maternal Serum α-Fetoprotein

The combination of elevated MSAFP and hCG levels occurs rarely but may have an overall pregnancy complication rate exceeding 50%. A study of 66 singleton and 33 multiple pregnancies with an MSAFP of more than 2 MoM and an hCG of more than 3.0 MoM found that 60% of singletons and 81% of twins had at least one of several obstetric complications, including preeclampsia, preterm birth, growth restriction, placental abnormalities, and fetal death.[27] Confined placental mosaicism for chromosome 16 has been reported to be associated with extremely high levels of both analytes, as well as with similarly poor outcomes.[28,29]

Low Second-Trimester Maternal Serum Estriol

Low maternal serum unconjugated estriol levels have been linked to adverse pregnancy outcomes.[30,31] Very low or absent estriol levels of 0.0 to 0.15 MoM suggest biochemical abnormalities of the fetus or placenta, including placental steroid sulfatase deficiency, Smith-Lemli-Opitz syndrome, congenital adrenal hypoplasia, adrenocorticotropin deficiency, hypothalamic corticotropin deficiency, and anencephaly.

Smith-Lemli-Opitz syndrome is an autosomal recessive disorder resulting from a defect in 3αβ-hydroxysteroid-α7-reductase, altering cholesterol synthesis and resulting in low cholesterol levels and the accumulation of the cholesterol precursor 7-dehydrocholesterol in blood and amniotic fluid. Because cholesterol is a precursor of estriol, the defect results in reduced or undetectable levels of estriol in maternal serum and amniotic fluid. Smith-Lemli-Opitz syndrome is characterized by low birth weight, failure to thrive, and moderate to severe mental retardation. It is associated with multiple structural anomalies, including syndactyly of the second and third toes, microcephaly, ptosis, and a typical-appearing facies.[32-34] Undermasculinization of the genetalia including complete sex reversal can be seen in male fetuses.

Bradley and colleagues[35] summarized findings in 33 women who delivered infants with Smith-Lemli-Opitz syndrome. Twenty-four of 26 women who had second-trimester estriol values obtained had levels less than the 5th percentile (<0.5 MoM). The median level in this group was 0.23 MoM (below the first percentile). A risk assessment based on low maternal serum unconjugated estriol levels has been suggested but is not presently available.[36] Reliable and inexpensive prenatal testing for Smith-Lemli-Opitz syndrome based on amniotic fluid cholesterol or 7-dehydrocholesterol levels is available.[37]

Placental steroid sulfatase deficiency is an X-linked recessive disorder resulting from deletion of Xp22.3. This enzyme deficiency prevents removal of the sulfate molecule from fetal estrogen precursors, preventing conversion to estriol. The fetal phenotype depends on the extent of the deletion, with greater than 90% of cases presenting as X-linked ichthyosis that can be treated with topical keratolytic agents. However, in about 5% of cases, there can be a deletion of contiguous genes causing mental retardation. The deletion can, on occasion, extend to cause Kallman syndrome or chondrodysplasia punctata. The lack of estrogen biosynthesis may result in delayed onset of labor, prolonged labor, or stillbirth.

Prenatal diagnosis for the deletion leading to placental sulfatase deficiency and congenital ichthyosis can be performed by identifying the gene deletion by karyotype or fluorescence in situ hybridization.[38-40] Although very low estriol levels, usually below the level of detection, can identify males at risk for this disorder, testing in these cases is not routinely offered because the phenotype is usually mild. However, the rarer, more serious cases of extensive deletions will be missed.[41]

Second-Trimester Ultrasound Markers of Down Syndrome

The clinical suspicion of Down syndrome is suspected when an infant is found to have specific physical findings that occur frequently in Down syndrome infants but can also occur in normal individuals. These include a simian crease in the fetal hand, a short femur or humerus, clinodactyly, and excessive nuchal skin. Similarly, the in utero diagnosis of Down syndrome can be suspected when anomalies or physical features that occur more frequently in Down syndrome than in the general population are noted on an ultrasound examination. Certain of these congenital anomalies, such as atrioventricular canal or duodenal atresia, strongly suggest the possibility of Down syndrome and are independent indications to offer invasive testing. Although when these anomalies are present there is a high risk of trisomy 21, these anomalies have low sensitivity and thus are not useful in screening. For example, when duodenal atresia is identified, there is an approximate 40% risk of Down syndrome, yet it is seen in only 8% of affected fetuses. Physical characteristics that are not themselves anomalies but that occur more commonly in fetuses with Down syndrome are called *markers*. By comparing the prevalence of markers in Down syndrome fetuses to their prevalence in the normal population, a likelihood ratio can be calculated that can be used to modify the a priori age or serum screening risk. This is the basis for ultrasound screening for Down syndrome.

For a marker to be useful for Down syndrome screening, it should be sensitive (i.e., present in a high proportion of Down syndrome pregnancies), specific (i.e., rarely seen in normal fetuses), easily imaged in standard sonographic examination, and present early enough in the second trimester that subsequent diagnostic testing by amniocentesis can be performed so that results are available when pregnancy termination remains an option. A list of available markers and their likelihood ratios are seen in Tables 17-5 and 17-6, respectively.

Before considering each marker individually, it is important to remember that the predictive value of any test (e.g., a marker) depends on the prevalence in the population of the condition being tested for. In the case of sonographic markers for trisomy 21, the clinical importance of a marker, therefore, varies according to the a priori risk as determined by maternal age, the results of multiple serum markers, and the presence of any other sonographic markers detected at the same examination. It is wise, therefore, to defer discussion of the impact of markers until the ultrasound examination has been completed and the results of serum screening have been reported. Markers commonly sought to assess the risk of Down syndrome include the following:

TABLE 17-5 SECOND-TRIMESTER ULTRASOUND MARKERS ASSOCIATED WITH DOWN SYNDROME
Brachycephaly
Increased nuchal thickness
Congenital heart defects
Hyperechoic bowel
Shortened femur
Shortened humerus
Renal pyelectasis
Duodenal atresia
Hypoplasia of the midphalanx of the fifth digit
Echogenic intracardiac focus
"Sandal gap" of the foot
Widened ischial spine angle
Foot length
Short or absent nasal bone

1. An increased nuchal fold (>6 mm) in the second trimester is the most distinctive marker. The fetal head is imaged in a transverse plane similar to that for measuring the biparietal diameter. The thalami and the upper portion of the cerebellum should be in the plane of the image. The distance between the external surface of the occipital bone and the external surface of the skin is then measured. About 35% of Down syndrome fetuses but only 0.7% of normal fetuses have a nuchal skin fold measurement greater than 5 mm. This ratio yields a likelihood ratio of 50 but includes fetuses with more than one marker. When an increased nuchal fold is an isolated finding, the likelihood ratio is still strong at 20-fold. This high likelihood ratio is obtained because of the rarity of an increased nuchal fold in an unaffected population (i.e., high specificity). For women with an a priori risk of less than 1:1600 (age-related risk for a 20-year-old), a 20-fold increase results in a risk estimate of at least 1:270. Thus, the presence of an increased nuchal fold alone is an indication to offer invasive testing.[42-47]
2. The fetal nasal bone has been demonstrated to be hypoplastic or absent in up to 60% of Down syndrome pregnancies imaged in the second trimester and only about 1% to 2% of unaffected pregnancies. Complete absence will occur in about 37% of affected cases with hypoplasia occuring in about half. In normal pregnancies, absence is seen in 0.9% of cases and hypoplasia in 2.4%. Nasal bone length can be converted to a likelihood ratio and used for Down syndrome risk assessment. When performed by experienced operators, nasal bone evaluation may be the best single ultrasound marker for second trimester risk assessment.[48]
3. Down syndrome fetuses in the second trimester may have short proximal extremities (humerus and femur) relative to the expected length for their biparietal diameter. This can be used to identify at-risk pregnancies by calculating a ratio of observed to expected femur length based on the fetus's biparietal diameter. An observed-to-expected ratio of less than 0.91 or a biparietal diameter-to-femur ratio of more than 1.5 has a reported likelihood ratio of 1.5 to 2.7 when present as an isolated finding. A short humerus is more strongly related to Down syndrome, with reported likelihood ratios

TABLE 17-6 LIKELIHOOD RATIOS (LR) FOR ISOLATED MARKERS IN THREE STUDIES

Sonographic Marker	AAURA LR* (N = 1042)	Nyberg et al. LR (95% CI)† (N = 8830)	Smith-Bindman et al. LR (95% CI)‡ (N = meta-analysis of >131,000)
Nuchal thickening	18.6	11.0 (5.2-22)	17.0 (8.0-38)
Hyperechoic bowel	5.5	6.7 (2.7-16.8)	6.1 (3.0-12.6)
Short humerus	2.5	5.1 (1.6-16.5)	7.5 (4.7-12)
Short femur	2.2	1.5 (0.8-2.8)	2.7 (1.2-6)
Echogenic intracardiac focus	2.0	1.8 (1.0-3)	2.8 (1.5-5.5)
Pyelectasis	1.5	1.5 (0.6-3.6)	1.9 (0.7-5.1)

*LR assumed by the original age-adjusted ultrasound risk adjustment (AAURA) model by Nyberg DA, Luthy DA, Resta RG, et al: Age-adjusted ultrasound risk assessment for fetal Down's syndrome during the second trimester: Description of the method and analysis of 142 cases. Ultrasound Obstet Gynecol 12:8, 1998.
†Nyberg DA, Souter VL, El-Bastawissi A, et al: Isolated sonographic markers for detection of fetal Down syndrome in the second trimester of pregnancy. J Ultrasound Med 20:1053, 2001.
‡LR of meta-analysis by Smith-Bindman R, Hosmer W, Feldstein VA, et al: Second-trimester ultrasound to detect fetuses with Down syndrome: A meta-analysis. JAMA 285:1044, 2001.
CI, confidence interval.

ranging from 2.5 to 7.5. Bahado-Singh and coworkers[49] combined humerus length with nuchal skin fold to estimate Down syndrome risk and calculated the likelihood ratios for various measurements to adjust estimated Down syndrome risk for each patient.

4. Echogenic intracardiac foci occur in up to 5% of normal pregnancies and in approximately 13% to 18% of Down syndrome gestations.[50] The likelihood ratio for Down syndrome when an echogenic focus is present as an isolated marker has ranged from 1.8 to 2.8. The risk does not seem to vary if the focus is in the right or left ventricle or if it is unilateral or bilateral.
5. Increased echogenicity of the fetal bowel, when brighter than the surrounding bone, has a Down syndrome likelihood ratio of 5.5 to 6.7.[51-53] This finding can also be seen with fetal cystic fibrosis (CF), congenital cytomegalovirus infection, swallowed bloody amniotic fluid, and severe intrauterine growth restriction. Therefore, if amniocentesis is performed for this finding, testing for the other potential etiologies should be considered.
6. Mild fetal pyelectasis (a renal pelvis anterior-posterior diameter greater than 4 mm) has been suggested as a potential marker for Down syndrome. As an isolated marker, the likelihood ratio ranges from 1.5 to 1.9 (see Table 17-6). This has been found by Snijders and coworkers[54] not to be significantly more frequent in Down syndrome pregnancies than in normal pregnancies (i.e., low specificity).
7. Other markers described include a hypoplastic fifth middle phalanx of the hand,[55] short ears, a sandal gap between the first and second toes,[56,57] an abnormal iliac wing angle,[58] and an altered foot-to-femur ratio.[59] These markers are inconsistently used because of the time and expertise required to obtain them.

Use of Second-Trimester Ultrasound to Estimate the Risk of Down Syndrome

As with other screening modalities, second-trimester ultrasound can be used to alter the a priori risk in either direction. A benign second-trimester scan having none of the known markers and no anomalies has been suggested to have a likelihood ratio of 0.4, assuming the image quality is satisfactory. Nyberg and coworkers[60] used this approach to calculate an age-adjusted ultrasound risk assessment for Down syndrome in 8914 pregnancies (186 fetuses with Down syndrome, 8728 control subjects). Some type of sonographic finding (major abnormality, minor marker, or both) was observed in 68.8% of fetuses with trisomy 21 compared with 13.6% of control fetuses ($P < .001$). The observation that about one third of fetuses with Down syndrome have neither a marker nor an anomaly has been used to adjust the estimated risk of Down syndrome downward by approximately 60% to 65% (likelihood ratio, 0.4) when the "genetic ultrasound" is normal. This sensitivity was observed in a single experienced center. It is doubtful that the same sensitivity can be achieved in every center.[61]

A positive likelihood ratio can be used to estimate an increase in risk. The magnitude of the increase depends on the marker(s) or anomalies seen. Nyberg and colleagues reviewed their own data[60,62] and the data of others[63] to estimate a likelihood ratio for each marker as an isolated finding (see Table 17-6). An isolated minor or "soft" marker was the only sonographic finding in 42 (22.6%) of 186 fetuses with trisomy 21, compared with 987 (11.3%) of 8728 control fetuses ($P < .001$). Nuchal thickening, nasal bone hypoplasia, and hyperechoic bowel showed the strongest association with trisomy 21 as isolated markers, followed by shortened humerus, echogenic intracardiac focus, shortened femur, and pyelectasis. Echogenic intracardiac focus was the single most common isolated marker in both affected fetuses (7.1%) and control fetuses (3.9%) but carried a low risk.

Combined Ultrasound and Second-Trimester Maternal Serum Marker Risk Assessment

Ultrasound markers can also be combined with serum markers if they are independent. Souter and coworkers[64] demonstrated a relatively small correlation that needs to be taken into consideration if a quantitative approach is used. Bahado-Singh and colleagues[65] combined ultrasound markers with maternal analytes, including urinary hyperglycosylated hCG and urinary α-core fragment of hCG. In a sample of 585 pregnancies, the sensitivity was 93.7%, with a false-positive rate of 5%.

TABLE 17-7 ASSOCIATION OF ULTRASOUND MARKERS WITH ANEUPLOIDY

Ultrasound Finding	Isolated (%)	Multiple (%)	Trisomy 13	Trisomy 18	Trisomy 21	Other	45X
Holoprosencephaly *n* = 132	4	39	30	7	—	7	—
Choroid plexus cysts *n* = 1806	1	46	11	121	18	11	—
Facial cleft *n* = 118	0	51	25	16	—	6	—
Cystic hygroma *n* = 276	52	71	—	13	26	11	163
Nuchal skin fold	19	45	—	9	85	19	10
Diaphragmatic hernia *n* = 173	2	34	—	18	—	14	—
Ventriculomegaly *n* = 690	2	17	10	23	13	14	—
Posterior fossa cyst *n* = 101	0	52	10	22	—	8	—
Major heart defects *n* = 829	16	66	30	82	68	31	30
Duodenal atresia *n* = 44	38	64	—	—	21	2	—
Hyperechoic bowel *n* = 196	7	42	—	—	22	17	—
Omphalocele *n* = 475	13	46	28	108	—	31	—
Renal anomalies *n* = 1825	3	24	40	52	48	62	—
Mild hydronephrosis *n* = 631	2	33	8	6	27	9	—
Intrauterine growth restriction (early) *n* = 621	4	38	11	47	—	18	36 (triploidy)
Talipes *n* = 127	0	33	—	—	—	—	—

Isolated, isolated finding; multiple, multiple findings on ultrasound.
Adapted from Snijders RJM, Nicolaides KH: Ultrasound Markers for Fetal Chromosomal Defects. New York, Parthenon, 1996.

Second-Trimester Ultrasound Screening for Other Chromosomal Abnormalities

Fetal aneuploidy other than Down syndrome can be suspected based on ultrasound findings (Table 17-7). Choroid plexus cysts occur in 1% of fetuses between 16 and 24 weeks' gestation and have been associated with trisomy 18. Thirty percent to 35% of fetuses with trisomy 18 have choroid plexus cysts. Among fetuses with a choroid plexus cyst, about 3% have trisomy 18, most (65% to 90%) of whom have other ultrasound findings (Table 17-8). Although an isolated choroid plexus cyst was estimated to yield a probability of trisomy 18 of 1 of 150 in one review, many of the series reviewed contained a high proportion of older women, which would overstate the risk. Snijders and coworkers[66] calculated that an isolated choroid plexus cyst has a likelihood ratio for trisomy 18 of 1.5 and can be used to calculate an individual's risk for trisomy 18. The size, location, or persistence of the cyst does not alter this risk.[67-71]

Table 17-7 displays the magnitude of the associations between various ultrasound findings and aneuploid conditions as estimated from a referral population. The rates noted may overestimate the strength of the association when such findings are noted on a screening examination.

First-Trimester Ultrasound Screening for Aneuploidy

In his initial description of the syndrome that bears his name, Langdon Down described skin so deficient in elasticity that it appeared to be too large for the body. This was particularly noticeable in the neck area. The skin in the fetal neck can now be seen with ultrasound at as early as 10 to 12 weeks of gestation and is known as a nuchal translucency (NT). The quantification of this additional "skin behind the neck" can be used for first-trimester Down syndrome screening.[72]

The NT is a fluid-filled space in the posterior fetal nuchal area. NT is defined as a collection of fluid under the skin behind the neck in fetuses between 11 and 14 weeks' gestation. This can be successfully measured by transabdominal ultrasound examination in approximately 95% of cases.

Studies conducted in women with increased risk of aneuploidy demonstrated an association between increased NT and chromosomal defects.[73-90] Subsequent studies demonstrated that an NT thickness above the 95th percentile was present in approximately 80% of trisomy 21 fetuses.[89] As with other serum and ultrasound markers, the significance of the NT thickness depends on the a priori risk for a chromosomal abnormality. NT thickness increases with gestational age or crown-rump length. Figure 17-2 illustrates the NT between 11 and 14

TABLE 17-8 ULTRASOUND FINDINGS ASSOCIATED WITH TRISOMY 18

Finding	Frequency (%)
Growth restriction	46
Hand or foot abnormalities*	39
Cardiac abnormality	31
CNS abnormality	29
Diaphragmatic hernia	13
Ventral wall defect	10
Facial abnormality	7
At least one abnormality	90

*Including rocker bottom feet, overlapping fingers.
CNS, central nervous system.
From Gupta JK, Cave M, Lilford RJ, et al: Clinical significance of fetal choroid plexus cysts. Lancet 346:724, 1995.

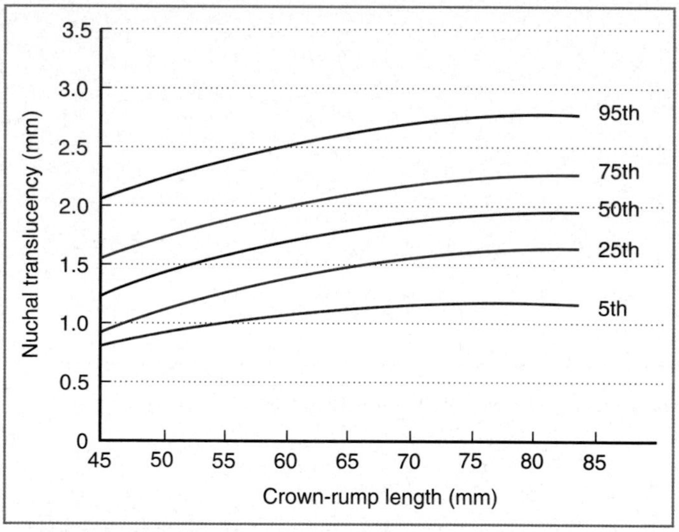

FIGURE 17-2 Normative curves for nuchal translucency measurement between 11 and 14 weeks' gestation. (From Nicolaides KH, Sebire NJ, Snijders RJM: The 11-14 Week Scan. New York, Parthenon, 1999.)

weeks' gestation. These observations suggested that NT could be used as a screening test for Down syndrome by converting the deviation from the expected mean to a likelihood ratio.

NT combined with the maternal and gestational age to assess the risk for Down syndrome was studied in more than 100,000 pregnancies.[91] NT was greater than the 95th percentile in more than 70% of fetuses with trisomy 21. The risk of Down syndrome was calculated by the maternal age and gestational age prevalence multiplied by the likelihood ratio. A cutoff of 1:300 was used. The studied sample included 326 fetuses with trisomy 21. Eighty-two percent of trisomy 21 fetuses were identified, with a false-positive rate of 8.3%.[91] When a screen-positive rate of 5% was selected, the sensitivity was 77% (95% confidence interval [CI], 72% to 82%). Subsequent studies have demonstrated similar Down syndrome detection rates, between 70% and 75% (Table 17-9).

The screening paradigm using an ultrasound measurement to determine a likelihood ratio is reliable only if NT is measured in a standard fashion. Standards for NT measurements include the following:

1. The minimal crown length should be 45 mm and the maximal, 84 mm. The success rate for accomplishing a measurement for these gestational ages is between 98% and 100%. The success rate falls to 90% at 14 weeks and onward.[92]
2. Either transabdominal or transvaginal scanning can be used, with about 95% of cases able to be imaged by the transabdominal route.[93]
3. A true sagittal section of the fetus as for measuring the fetal crown-rump length must be obtained.
4. The magnification must be such that the fetus occupies at least three fourths of the image. The magnification should be increased so that each increment in the distance between calipers should only be 0.1 mm. Studies have demonstrated that ultrasound measurements can be accurate to the nearest 0.1 to 0.2 mm.[94]
5. Care must be taken to clearly distinguish between the fetal skin and the amnion. At this gestational age, both structures appear as thin membranes. This can be accomplished by either waiting for spontaneous fetal movement away from the amniotic membrane or by bouncing the fetus off the amnion by asking the mother to cough or tap on her abdomen (Fig. 17-3).
6. The maximal thickness of this subcutaneous translucency between the skin and the soft tissue overlying the cervical spine should be measured by placing the calipers on the lines as illustrated in Figure 17-4.

TABLE 17-9 STUDIES OF IMPLEMENTATION OF FETAL NUCHAL TRANSLUCENCY (NT) SCREENING

Source (ref)	Gestation (wk)	*N*	Successful Measurement	NT Cutoff (mm)	False-Positive Rate (%)	Detection Rate of Trisomy 21
Pandya (89), 1995	10-14	1,763	100%	>2.5	3.6	3 of 4 (75%)
Szabo (90), 1995	9-12	3,380	100%	>3.0	1.6	28 of 31 (90%)
Bewley (97), 1995	8-13	1,704	66%	>3.0	6.0	1 of 3 (33%)
Bower et al (526), 1995	8-14	1,481	97%	>3.0	6.3	4 of 8 (50%)
Kornman et al (527), 1996	8-13	923	58%	>3.0	6.3	2 of 4 (50%)
Zimmerman et al (528), 1996	10-13	1,131	100%	>3.0	1.9	2 of 3 (67%)
Taipale et al (529), 1997	10-16	10,010	99%	>3.0	0.8	7 of 13 (54%)
Hafner (179), 1998	10-14	4,371	100%	>2.5	1.7	4 of 7 (57%)
Pajkrt (181), 1998	10-14	1,547	96%	>3.0	2.2	6 of 9 (67%)

Adapted from Nicolaides KH, Sebire NJ, Snijders RJM: The 11-14 Week Scan. New York, Parthenon, 1999.

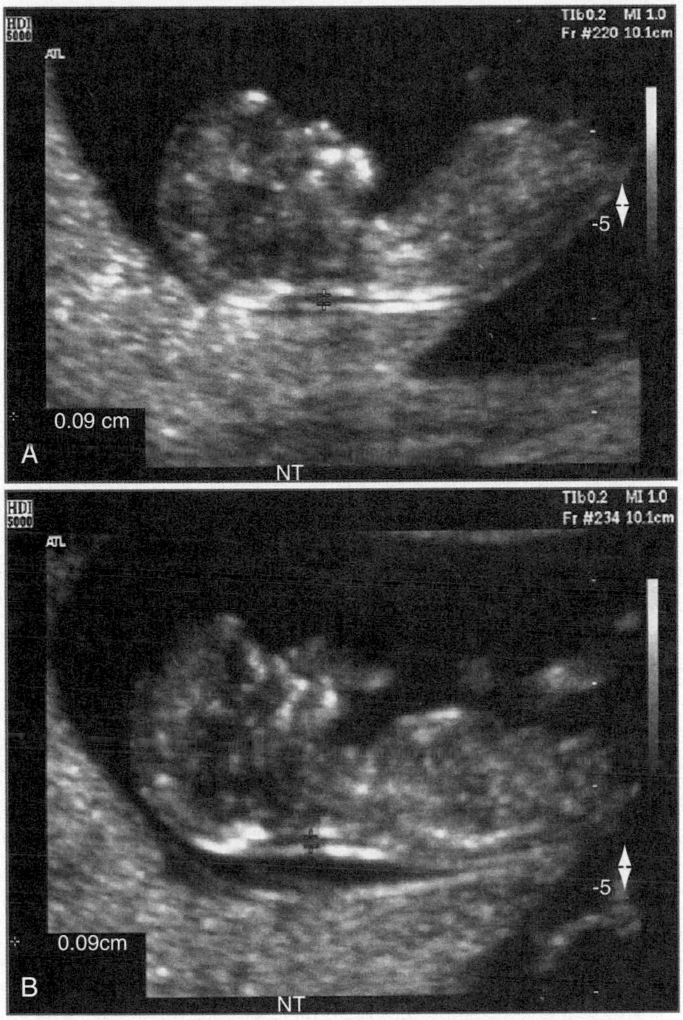

FIGURE 17-3 **First-trimester nuchal translucency (NT) measurement.** Clear distinction of the amnion as opposed to the skin edge is made by waiting for fetal movement. Measurement before the fetus moves (**A**) is less accurate than after fetal movement (**B**).

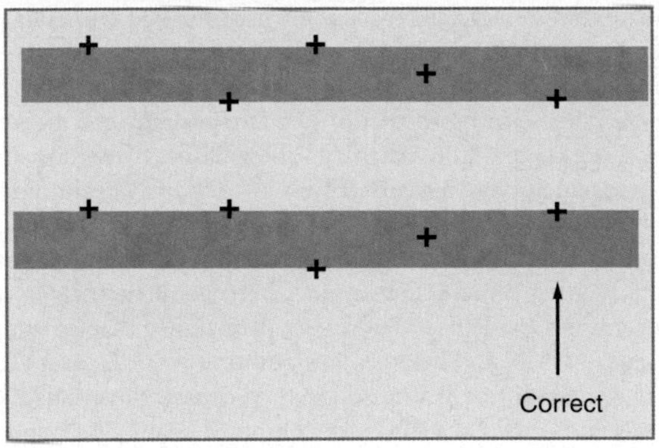

FIGURE 17-4 **Proper placement of the calipers for measuring the nuchal translucency.** (From Nicolaides KH, Sebire NJ, Snijders RJM: The 11-14 Week Scan. New York, Parthenon, 1999.)

7. During the scan, these measurements should be taken and the maximum one recorded and used for Down syndrome risk calculation.
8. The NT should be measured with the fetal head in the neutral position. When the fetal neck is hyperextended, the measurement can be increased by 0.6 mm, and when the neck is flexed, the measurement can be decreased by 0.4 mm.[95]
9. The umbilical cord may be found around the fetal neck in approximately 5% to 10% of cases, which may produce a falsely increased NT, adding about 0.8 mm to the measurement.[96] In such cases, the measurements of NT above and below the cord differ, and the smaller measurement is the most appropriate.

Even with these criteria, standardization of NT measurements remains difficult. Certification courses are available with continuous quality assessment to maintain proper technique. The ability to achieve a reliable measurement has been linked to the motivation of the sonographer. A study comparing the results obtained from hospitals where NT was clinically used compared with those where they were merely measured but were not acted on, reported that, in the interventional groups, successful measurement was achieved in 100% of cases, whereas the noninterventional centers were successful in only 85%.[97] In a recent prospective study,[98] the NT was measured by two to four operators in 200 pregnant women, demonstrating that after an initial measurement, a second one made by the same operator or another operator varied from the initial measurement by less than 0.5 and 0.6 mm, respectively, in 95% of cases. It is suggested that a large part of the variation between operators can be accounted for by placement of the calipers rather than generation of the appropriate image. Subsequent studies[99-101] have continued to report small interoperator differences.

Because NT values are incorporated into a standardized algorithm along with biochemical analytes, it is critical that these ultrasound measurements be performed and monitored appropriately. To accomplish this, certification and quality review programs have been developed to ensure that accurate and precise NT measurements are obtained. The Fetal Medicine Foundation of London was the first to offer formalized NT training and quality review. In the United States, the Nuchal Translucency Quality Review (NTQR) program was initiated in 2005. Both programs teach the mechanics of obtaining an NT measurement, have an image review process to ensure that the standard technique is used correctly, and perform ongoing epidemiologic monitoring of sonographer and sonologist performance. Two studies have evaluated the techniques used to ensure consistent NT results. Both confirmed that ongoing expert review of images is an inefficient and impractical approach. Epidemiologic monitoring in which individual operator's performance is compared with expected standards is preferable.[101,102]

First-Trimester Biochemical Screening

Two serum analytes are useful for first-trimester screening. Pregnancy-associated plasma protein A has been demonstrated to have a mean value of 0.4 MoM in trisomy 21 pregnancies. The free β subunit of hCG is elevated in Down syndrome pregnancies, with a mean value of 1.8 MoM. Screening using pregnancy-associated plasma protein A (PAPP-A) alone identifies about 40% to 45% of trisomy 21 pregnancies, and free β-hCG identifies about 23%, both with a false-positive rate of 5%.[103-105] Combining both free β-hCG and PAPP-A can identify 60% to 65% of trisomy 21 pregnancies, for a similar 5% false-positive rate.[106] This is a serum analyte detection rate similar to that seen with triple screening in the second trimester.

The total hCG molecule can also be used for first-trimester screening but has slightly less discrimination power than does the free β subunit,[107] especially at less than 11 weeks' gestation. Free β-hCG begins to increase in performance as a Down syndrome marker at as early as 9 weeks' gestation, reaching values almost twice those in unaffected pregnancies by 13 weeks. Levels of total hCG begin to increase above those in unaffected gestations at 11 weeks.[108,109] The impact of substituting total hCG for the free β subunit on overall Down syndrome screening remains uncertain. A recent meta-analysis showed that in younger patients (<35 years), detection of Down syndrome increased by 4, 5, 6, and 7 percentage points at 9, 10, 11, and 12 weeks, respectively, when free β was added to pregnancy-associated plasma protein A and nuchal translucency compared with 0, 0, 2, and 4 percentage points when intact human chorionic gonadotropin was added.[110] In patients with advanced maternal age (>35), inclusion of free β-hCG reduced the false-positive rate by 2.5, 3.1, 3.8, and 4.4 percentage points compared with 0.1, 0.3, 1.0, and 2.2 percentage points for intact hCG at 9, 10, 11, and 12 weeks, respectively. Other authors have found less impact. Using samples from the FASTER study, Canick and coworkers[111] showed that at 12 weeks' gestation, the addition of free β-hCG to NT and PAPP-A added only 0.9% (−3.3 to 6.3) detection. However, at earlier gestational ages the impact of free β-hCG would be greater.

Combined First-Trimester Nuchal Translucency and Biochemistry Screening

Combining NT with serum analytes improves first-trimester Down syndrome detection rates. Table 17-10 summarizes the large international experience with first-trimester Down syndrome screening using free β-hCG, PAPP-A, and NT measurements. Overall, for a 5% false-positive rate, combined first-trimester risk assessment provides a Down syndrome detection rate of approximately 88% (95% CI, 84.0% to 89.4%). In women older than 35, 90% to 92% of trisomy 21 pregnancies can be identified with a 16% to 22% false-positive rate.[20,112] First-trimester screening can also identify trisomy 18 pregnancies. Over 90% of such pregnancies are screen positive when combined biochemical and NT screening is used.[112]

When combining analytes, differences in gestational age–specific performance should be considered.[113-115] At all gestational ages between 9 and 12 weeks, NT and PAPP-A are the most efficient markers. In combination, they are most efficient at 11 weeks, when free and total hCG are least efficient. In practice, screening is performed between 11 and 13 weeks of gestation.

Additional First-Trimester Markers of Down Syndrome

Biochemical Markers

ADAM 12 is the secreted form of a disintegrin and metalloprotease 12, a glycoprotein of the Meltrin family synthesized by the placenta and secreted throughout pregnancy. ADAM 12 has proteolytic function against insulin-like growth factor (IGF) binding proteins IGFBP-3 and IGFBP-5 and regulates the bioavailability and action of IGF-1 and -2.[116] Studies have shown that first-trimester ADAM 12 levels are reduced in women carrying a Down syndrome pregnancy, and that the reduction is more pronounced in earlier gestation.[117-119] Discrimination appears best at around 8 to 10 weeks, with an overall median MoM of 0.79 in Down syndrome pregnancies.[119] Population modeling shows that a combination of ADAM 12 and PAPP-A measured at 8 to 9 weeks, combined with NT and free β-hCG measured at 12 weeks, could achieve a detection rate of 97% with a 5% false-positive rate, or 89% with a 1% false-positive rate.[119]

Ultrasound Markers

Nasal Bone. Similar to findings in the second trimester, investigators have suggested that assessment of the fetal nasal bone (NB) can be used in the first trimester to predict trisomy 21. This is based on the flat nasal bridge area, which is a well-described component of the Down syndrome phenotype, as well as on several histopathologic and radiographic studies demonstrating differences in the nasal bones of Down syndrome fetuses. Stempfle and colleagues[120] found that NB ossification was absent in one quarter of Down syndrome fetuses investigated between 15 and 40 weeks' gestation, compared with none of the controls. Similarly, Tuxen and colleagues[121] evaluated Down syndrome fetuses between 14 and 25 weeks' gestational age by radiograph and pathologic study and found that the NB was absent in one third.

Sonek and colleagues[48] published the first large prospective trial of aneuploid risk evaluation using first-trimester ultrasound assessment of the fetal nasal bone. They determined that the fetal nasal bone could routinely be imaged and that its absence was associated with trisomy 21 (Fig. 17-5). The NB was absent in 73% of trisomy 21 fetuses compared with only 0.5% of euploid fetuses. They estimated that if NB assessment were combined with maternal age and NT measurement, 93% of Down syndrome cases would be detected at a false-positive rate of 5%, and 85% with a false-positive rate of 1%.

A recent review of the literature by Rosen and D'Alton[122] evaluated 35,312 women having first-trimester ultrasound assessment for NB. In 33,314 cases (94.3%), the NB was successfully imaged. The sensitivity

TABLE 17-10 STUDIES OF DOWN SYNDROME DETECTION RATES IN FIRST-TRIMESTER SCREENING

Study (ref)	Pregnancies Screened	Down Syndrome Cases (Screen-Positive/Total)	Detection Rate
BUN (Wapner [112], 2003)	8,216	48/61	79%
FASTER (Malone [20], 2005)	38,033	100/117	86%
SURUSS (Wald [138], 2003)	47,053	84/101	83%
Nicolaides ([143], 2005)	75,821	321/325	93%
TOTAL	167,210	533/604	88.2%

Screening tests were for free β-subunit of human chorionic gonadotropin, pregnancy-associated plasma protein A, and nuchal translucency (with a 5% false-positive rate).

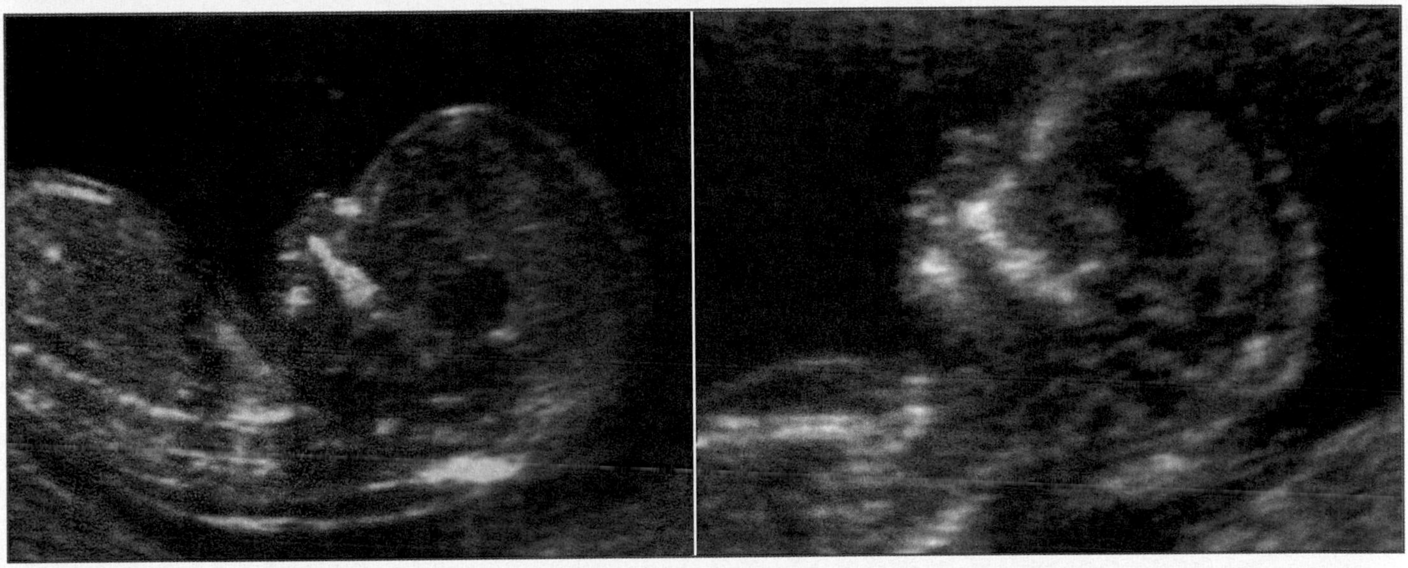

FIGURE 17-5 Ultrasound images of the fetal nasal bone (NB) in the first trimester. First-trimester ultrasound images of euploid *(left)* and trisomy 21 *(right)* fetuses demonstrate the presence of the nasal bone in the normal gestation and its absence in trisomy 21. Scanning techniques are those suggested by the Fetal-Medicine Foundation for assessing NB and include the following: (1) The image is magnified so that each movement of the calipers causes a 0.1-mm incremental change. (2) A midsagittal view of the fetal profile is obtained. (3) The angle between the ultrasound transducer and a line passing from the fetal forehead to the chin is 45 degrees. (4) When the NB is present, three echogenic lines should be visible. The NB and overlying skin look like an equal sign. In the same view, the skin over the nasal tip should be visible. If both the nasal tip and skin are present, and the NB echo cannot be visualized or is less echogenic than the skin, the NB is considered absent. (Fetal-Medicine Foundation, available at http://www.fetalmedicinefoundation.com/nasal.htm.)

of NB alone for detecting trisomy 21 was 65% with a false-positive rate of 0.8%. The positive predictive value of the screen was 54%, meaning that approximately 1 in 2 fetuses with an absent NB had trisomy 21. If the NB was absent, the likelihood that a fetus had trisomy 21 was increased 87-fold. The negative likelihood ratio with a normal NB was 0.35 (95% CI, 0.32 to 0.39).

As experience with NB has increased, relationships between absent NB, fetal crown-rump length (i.e., gestational age), NT, and ethnicity have been established. The current data demonstrate that in euploid pregnancies, NB absence occurs more frequently with increasing NT. In a series of 5851 high-risk patients containing 333 trisomy 21 fetuses, absence of the NB had a likelihood ratio of 37.1 when the NT was less than the 95th percentile, and this was reduced to 13.4 when the NT was 4 or greater.[123] The same study showed that the NB was more likely to be absent at earlier gestational ages. For example, in euploid fetuses with a crown-rump length between 45 and 54 mm, the NB was absent in 4.7% of cases. At a crown-rump length between 75 and 84 mm, the NB was absent in only 1.0% of cases. Prefumo and colleagues[124] found that NB hypoplasia was more common in the euploid fetuses of women of African descent when compared with either Asian or white populations (odds ratio, 2.3). Cicero and colleagues[125] also found an increased incidence of absent fetal NB in the first trimester in women of Afro-Caribbean and southern Asian descent. The NB was absent in 2.5%, 9.0%, and 5.0% of white, Afro-Caribbean, and southern Asian populations, respectively. Likelihood ratios for trisomy 21 with absent NB were 31.3, 8.8, and 14.2, respectively, in these three populations.

NB status is independent of serum biochemistry, allowing NB assessment to be combined with measurements of NT and maternal serum markers to increase first-trimester screening performance.[126] In a retrospective case-control study of a high-risk population with a median maternal age of more than 38 years assessed by NT, NB, and biochemistry, it was estimated that 97% of Down syndrome cases would be detected at a false-positive rate of 5%.[127] For a false-positive rate of 0.5%, the detection rate would be 90.5%. Although these data are promising, detection rates using this combined screen would be expected to be significantly lower in an unselected population using a similar 5% false-positive rate. In addition, appropriate imaging of the NB appears to be technologically more difficult than measurement of the NT, making its use in a primary screening program less attractive.[128]

Tricuspid Regurgitation. Another potential ultrasound marker is tricuspid regurgitation determined by pulsed wave Doppler ultrasonography.[129,130] This finding is present in around 8% of normal fetuses and 65% of those with trisomy 21. Combining tricuspid regurgitation with NT and PAPP-A would be expected to achieve a detection rate of 95% with a 5% false-positive rate, or 90% with a 2% false-positive rate.[131]

Ductus Venosus Wave Form. A third potential marker is abnormal blood flow through the ductus venosus. Studies have shown that pulsation of the ductus venosus gives detection rates of 65% to 75% with a 4% to 5% false-positive rate,[132] and the rate increased to 75% to 80% when NT was added. When serum biochemical markers measured at 10 weeks were also added, the modeled detection rate increased to 92% at a 5% false-positive rate, or 84% at a 1% false-positive rate.[133]

Impact of Spontaneous Miscarriages on First-Trimester Screening

A potential disadvantage of earlier screening is that chromosomally abnormal pregnancies that are destined to miscarry will be identified. The impact of this can be evaluated because 69% of trisomy 21 fetuses living in the first trimester and 76% of those alive in the second trimester will be born alive.[4] Using this information, Dunstan and Nix[134] calculated that a detection rate of 80% in the first trimester is approximately equivalent to a second-trimester sensitivity of 75%, suggesting that when early spontaneous losses of trisomy 21 pregnancies are considered, first-trimester screening is superior to that presently available in the second trimester.

First-trimester screening would be less desirable if screen-positive pregnancies or those with enlarged NTs were preferentially lost. In a study of 108 fetuses with trisomy 21 diagnosed in the first trimester because of increased NT, Hyett and colleagues found that six patients elected to continue the pregnancy.[135] In five of the six fetuses the translucency resolved, and at the second-trimester scan the nuchal fold thickness was normal. All six of these trisomy 21 fetuses were born alive. Wapner and colleagues[112] calculated that greater than 80% of screen-positive trisomy 21 pregnancies would be born alive.

Other Approaches to Down Syndrome Screening: Combining First- and Second-Trimester Screening Tests

Screening performance may be improved by combining analytes performed at different gestational ages.[136,137] These approaches include the following.

Integrated Aneuploidy Screening (Noninformative Sequential). Wald and colleagues[137] described a protocol for screening based on tests performed during both the first (NT and PAPP-A) and second trimesters (quad screen). A single risk estimate is calculated in the second trimester using all six of the measured analytes. Integrated screening has a detection rate of approximately 95% with a 5% false-positive rate.[20,137] Approximately 85% of affected pregnancies would be detected with a false-positive rate of only 0.9%.[137,138] Although this screening approach is quite sensitive and specific, withholding the risk estimate until the second trimester precludes earlier prenatal diagnosis by chorionic villus sampling (CVS) and is not an acceptable approach for many women.[139]

If NT scanning is not available, an integrated serum screen may be performed (PAPP-A in the first trimester and a quad screen in the second trimester). This approach has a detection rate of 86% to 90% at a 5% false-positive rate.[20,137]

Sequential Testing. In an attempt to maximize screening performance by combining first- and second-trimester analytes yet retain the benefit of first-trimester diagnosis, various methods of sequential screening have been proposed. In these approaches, first-trimester risk results are calculated and used for clinical management, with second-trimester testing performed in selected cases.

Three approaches to sequential risk assessment are presently available. In independent sequential testing, a first-trimester combined risk is calculated with a 1:270 screen-positive cutoff. Decisions on invasive testing are made on the basis of these results. In the second trimester, a quad screen is performed and calculated independent of the first-trimester results. This approach provides detection rates greater than 95%,[20,136] but it has an unacceptably high false-positive rate of greater than 10% because independent calculation of the quad screen risk does not take into consideration the reduced second-trimester prevalence of Down syndrome pregnancies after first-trimester prenatal diagnosis.

Stepwise sequential testing reduces the high false-positive rate of independent sequential testing and offers the highest risk patients the option of first trimester invasive testing by using a high first-trimester risk cutoff and calculating the second-trimester risk by integrating information from both trimesters.[140] For example, using a 1:65 cutoff in the first trimester identifies 70% of affected pregnancies with only a 1% false-positive rate. If all screen-negative patients proceed to second-trimester screening, an overall detection rate of 95% can be obtained with a 5% false-positive rate. Although this approach has excellent performance, with a high proportion of affected pregnancies identified in the first trimester, it is logistically demanding.

Contingent sequential screening is similar to stepwise sequential screening, but patients with a very low first-trimester combined risk do not have second-trimester analysis performed. Using an approach in which patients with a first-trimester risk of 1:1300 or less complete screening in the first trimester, only 15% to 20% of patients have to return for second-trimester analysis.[141,142] Contingent sequential screening has a detection rate of 92% to 94% for a 5% screen positive rate.[140]

Nasal Bone Contingency Screening. Nasal bone assessment is technically more difficult to perform than NT, which may limit availability. To address this Nicolaides and colleagues[143] proposed a two-stage screen, reserving NB assessment for patients at intermediate risk after the combined first-trimester screen is complete. In this model, patients evaluated by NT and serum markers with a risk of 1 in 100 or greater would be offered CVS, and those with a risk of less than 1:1000 would be deemed to have such a low risk that no further testing is offered. Those with a risk between 1:101 and 1:1000 would have NB evaluation. In initial studies, performance of this two-stage approach was similar to using NB assessment as part of the initial screen. The two-stage approach would have a significant advantage because only about 15% of pregnancies would require NB evaluation, which could be performed in centers that have developed special expertise in this technique.

Can Maternal Age Be Eliminated as an Indication for Invasive Prenatal Diagnosis?

Maternal age of 35 or older has been a standard indication for invasive testing for more than 35 years. When it was initially suggested, approximately 5% of births were to women older than 35 years, as were 30% of trisomy 21 gestations. Presently, almost three times as many women giving birth are older than 35, and this group contains about 50% of trisomy 21 conceptions. For every invasive procedure done with maternal age as the only indication, the odds of being affected are approximately 1:100.[20] As screening has improved, the importance of maternal age as a single indication for testing has been reevaluated.

In women aged 35 years and older, 87% of Down syndrome pregnancies and 25% of unaffected pregnancies will be triple-screen positive at a cutoff of 1:250.[18] The incidence of Down syndrome in this age group is approximately 1:100. Table 17-11 demonstrates that performing an amniocentesis on screen-negative women (risk <1:270) aged 35 years or older would lead to the loss of three normal pregnancies from procedure-induced complications for every Down syndrome pregnancy identified. First-trimester screening has greater than a 90% sensitivity with a 15% false-positive rate in women aged 35 years or older.[112] Using the approach illustrated in Table 17-1, it can be calculated that almost four normal pregnancies will be lost for each Down syndrome pregnancy identified.

Screening the entire population of pregnant women regardless of age provides the most effective use of resources. Presently, 14.2% of women older than 35 are offered invasive testing, as are about 5% of women under age 35 who are screen positive, making greater than 18% of pregnant women eligible for testing. If second-trimester screening were used for all patients regardless of age and only screen-positive patients were offered invasive testing, the number of procedures would

TABLE 17-11 COMPARISON OF SCREENING APPROACHES FOR WOMEN AGED 35 YEARS AND OLDER*

	Invasive Procedures for All Women ≥35 Years (*N* = 10,000)	First-Trimester Screening for All Women ≥35 Years (*N* = 10,000)	Second-Trimester Screening for All Women ≥35 Years (*N* = 10,000)
Down syndrome pregnancies	100	100.0	100
Down syndrome detected	100	90.0	87
Down syndrome missed	0	10.0	13
Invasive procedures performed	10,000	1500.0	2500
Pregnancies lost due to procedure	50	7.5	13
Pregnancies lost to diagnose one trisomy 21 pregnancy in screen-negative women	N/A	4.3	3

Based on population of 10,000 pregnant women ≥35 years old
***Assumes one procedure-related loss for every 200 invasive procedures performed. First-trimester screening: sensitivity, 90%; false-positive rate, 16%. Second-trimester screening: sensitivity, 87%; false-positive rate, 25%.**

be reduced to only 6.4% of the pregnant population. If first-trimester screening is used, the number of eligible patients is only 3.8%.

Age-related autosomal and sex chromosome trisomies other than trisomy 21 would potentially be missed if invasive testing for age were abandoned. Presently, both second- and first-trimester screening for trisomy 18 are available and efficient. Wapner[112] showed a 100% detection rate using first-trimester combined screening in women aged 35 years and older. About 50% of the sex chromosome abnormalities will be screen positive in the second trimester in women aged 35 years and older.[144]

The American College of Obstetricians and Gynecologists has recommended that maternal age of 35 years should no longer be used as a cutoff to determine who is offered screening and who is offered invasive testing.[145] This approach has to be preceded by explicit patient counseling to explain the risks and advantages of both options.

Maternal Serum α-Fetoprotein Screening for Neural Tube and Other Structural Defects

Physiology

Maternal serum screening for neural tube defects was the initial foray into pregnancy screening for congenital anomalies. Because 95% of neural tube defects occurred in families without a history of a previously affected offspring, prenatal detection of these defects was largely fortuitous before 1980. Screening is based on elevated levels of MSAFP, which occurs in anencephaly and spina bifida.

AFP is a fetal-specific globin similar to albumin in molecular weight and charge but with a different primary structure and distinct antigenic properties. The gene for AFP is located on chromosome 4q. AFP is synthesized early in gestation by the yolk sac and subsequently by the fetal gastrointestinal tract and liver. The level of fetal plasma AFP peaks between 10 and 13 weeks of gestation and declines exponentially from 14 to 32 weeks and then more sharply until term. The exponential fall in fetal plasma AFP is most likely the result of the dilution effect of increasing fetal blood volume, as well as of a decline in the amounts synthesized by the fetus, as fetal albumin is increasingly produced as the primary oncotic protein in fetal blood.

AFP enters the fetal urine and is excreted into the amniotic fluid. Peak levels of amniotic fluid AFP are reached between 12 and 14 weeks' gestation, declining between 10% and 15% per week during the second trimester, and levels are almost undetectable at term.

Maternal serum AFP levels rise above nonpregnant levels as early as the 7th week of gestation. MSAFP levels are significantly lower than AFAFP levels but progressively increase during gestation until 28 and 32 weeks, when they peak. This paradoxical rise in MSAFP when amniotic fluid and serum levels are decreasing is believed to be accounted for by increasing placental mass and progressive permeability to fetal plasma proteins. Thus the amount of AFP detected in maternal serum is increased in the presence of multiple placentas (i.e., in multifetal gestation).

In normal pregnancies, transport of AFAFP into maternal serum contributes little to the MSAFP compartment. The significant difference in fetal serum AFP compared with that in the amniotic fluid and maternal serum serves as the basis for using this fetal protein to screen for fetal lesions such as neural tube defects, which potentially leak high levels of AFP into the amniotic fluid and, hence, the maternal serum. The concentration gradient between fetal plasma and AFAFP is about 150 to 200 : 1. The concentration differential between fetal and maternal serum is about 50,000 : 1. Thus, the presence of a small volume of fetal blood or serum in the amniotic fluid can raise the AFP level significantly.

Screening

MSAFP screening for neural tube defects is ideally performed between 16 and 18 weeks of pregnancy. Cutoffs between 2.0 and 2.5 MoM yield detection rates of almost 100% for anencephaly and 85% to 92% for open spina bifida, with a false-positive rate between 2% and 5%. As with all screening modalities, the positive predictive value for an individual patient depends on the population risk. Table 17-12 demonstrates the odds of an individual woman having a child with a neural tube defect, based on the degree of elevation of her serum AFP and on her a priori risk of having a child with a neural tube defect. Because MSAFP values rise between 16% and 18% per week during the second trimester, use of gestational age-corrected MSAFP MoM for comparison between laboratories is recommended. The median is preferred to the mean because it is less influenced by occasional outliers.

MSAFP is performed using an enzyme immunoassay. All laboratories performing this test should have their own normal ranges and a mechanism for continuous quality control assessment. The College of American Pathologists operates a nationwide external proficiency test

TABLE 17-12 ODDS OF HAVING A FETUS WITH OPEN SPINA BIFIDA BASED ON SERUM α-FETOPROTEIN (AFP) LEVEL AT 16 TO 18 WEEKS' GESTATION

Serum AFP (MoM)	A Priori Birth Incidence*: 1 per 1000	2 per 1000
2.0	1:800	1:400
2.5	1:290	1:140
3.0	1:120	1:59
3.5	1:53	1:27
4.0	1:26	1:13
4.5	1:14	1:7
5.0	1:7	1:4

*In the absence of antenatal diagnosis. Multiple pregnancies excluded by ultrasonography.
MoM, multiple of the median.
From Milunsky A (ed): Genetic Disorders and the Fetus: Diagnosis, Prevention, and Treatment, 3rd ed. Baltimore, Johns Hopkins University Press, 1992, p 656.

TABLE 17-13 FETAL ANOMALIES IDENTIFIED BY AN ELEVATED AMNIOTIC FLUID α-FETOPROTEIN, ENHANCED BY ACETYLCHOLINESTERASE (AChE)

Positive AChE	Negative AChE
Anencephaly	Aneuploidy
Open spina bifida	Intrauterine fetal demise
Encephalocele	Obstructive uropathy
Omphalocele	Cleft lip/palate
Gastroschisis	Omphalocele
Esophageal atresia	Gastroschisis
Teratoma	Fetal hydrops
Intrauterine fetal demise	Intrauterine growth restriction
Cystic hygroma	Congenital nephrosis
Acardiac twin	Normal gestation
Cloacal extrophy	
Epidermolysis bullosa	
Aplasia cutis congenita	
Normal gestation	

that is an essential element in population-based screening programs. Most laboratories presently use an upper-limit cutoff of 2.0 MoM. Some laboratories use a somewhat higher cutoff, up to 2.5 MoM. The choice of a specific cutoff is a balance between the anticipated detection rate and the false-positive rate. Because ultrasound screening for the evaluation of elevated numbers of neural tube defects has replaced the need for amniocentesis in many cases, a trend toward choosing a lower AFP threshold to gain a higher detection rate with slightly more false-positives has occurred.

Because of interlaboratory variation and interassay variation, many clinics repeat an MSAFP that initially falls between 2 and 3 MoM. If the repeat value is normal, no further evaluation is required. However, the variance of MSAFP by gestational week related to assay precision or individual fluctuation yields no practical value in performing a repeat MSAFP on either the same or a second sample taken up to 1 month later. Most centers thus choose to obtain an ultrasound after any elevated MSAFP level.

A number of factors influence the interpretation of an MSAFP value. The most important factor for efficient MSAFP screening is the accuracy of the gestational age determination. Because there is an exponential rise in MSAFP over the recommended screening period of 15 to 20 weeks, a variation of 2 weeks between the actual gestational age and that used for MSAFP interpretation can be misleading. A potential confounding factor is that fetuses with spina bifida may have biparietal diameters that are reduced by approximately 2 weeks. Consequently, femur length and biparietal diameter should be measured to confirm gestational age for AFP screening. A first-trimester ultrasound is the preferable means of documenting gestational age; results of this ultrasound can be submitted to the laboratory in place of the last menstrual period.

Maternal weight affects the MSAFP concentration. The heavier the woman, the lower the MSAFP value as a result of dilution in the larger blood volume. Adjusting MSAFP values for maternal weight increases the detection rate for open spina bifida. Dividing the observed MoM by the expected MoM for a given weight enables adjustment for differences in weight. Correction for weights greater than 250 pounds significantly increases the rate of elevated MSAFP results, suggesting overcorrection. Therefore, some laboratories recommend linear correction of MSAFP only up to a weight of 200 pounds. Presently, weight correction of MSAFP reports is routinely performed.

Maternal ethnicity may also alter the interpretation of an MSAFP level, because black women have a 10% to 15% higher MSAFP than nonblacks.[146] This is important because the incidence of neural tube defects in blacks is lower. Other ethnic groups also have slightly different MSAFP levels, but they do not vary sufficiently to warrant corrections. Pregnant women with insulin-dependent diabetes mellitus have MSAFP values that are significantly lower than nondiabetic women in the second trimester,[147,148] which requires adjustments in the interpretation. This is critical because there is up to a 10-fold higher frequency of neural tube defects in the offspring of these patients. MSAFP also must be altered in multiple gestations, and this adjustment is discussed later.

There may be a genetic component to raised MSAFP. Women with an elevated MSAFP in one pregnancy appear to have an increased risk of elevated values in subsequent gestations. A false-positive AFP has been seen in multiple members of some families.[149,150]

Evaluation

Once an elevated MSAFP has been detected, the next step is ultrasound evaluation to confirm the gestational age, rule out twin gestation, identify other causes of elevated MSAFP such as fetal demise and oligohydramnios, and identify other structural defects that can cause elevated MSAFP, such as omphalocele, gastroschisis, and duodenal atresia (Table 17-13). The most important aspect of this ultrasound is confirmation of gestational age. In up to 50% of cases, incorrect dating is identified, and adjustment of the initial value resolves the issue. If the elevated MSAFP remains unexplained, further testing by either amniocentesis or targeted ultrasound is required.

Until recently, the standard diagnostic test for an elevated MSAFP was amniocentesis with evaluation of AFAFP and acetylcholinesterase (AChE) levels. AFAFP determination has nearly a 100% detection rate for anencephaly and a 96% to 99% detection rate for open spina bifida, with a false-positive rate of 0.7% to 1.0%.[149] The accuracy of amniotic fluid determination is enhanced by the addition of AChE. As opposed to AFP, which is a fetal serum protein, AChE is predominantly neuronally derived, giving it additional specificity for nervous system lesions.

The most common assay for AChE is a polyacrylamide gel electrophoresis, in which AChE can be distinguished from nonspecific cholinesterases on the basis of mobility. A combined use of AFP and AChE together appears to be the most sensitive and specific in determining neural tube defects.

As with AFP, there are a number of potential confounders with AChE. When fetal blood is present in the amniotic fluid, interpretation of AChE might be complicated and inaccurate. In addition, false-positive AChE results have been clearly documented in normal pregnancies before 15 weeks' gestation and may be seen in up to one third of cases under 12 weeks' gestation.

In experienced hands, targeted ultrasound for elevated MSAFP has been found to be as sensitive and specific as amniotic fluid AFP and AChE levels.[151,152] Although ultrasound as a primary screening tool for spina bifida may identify only 60% to 80% of neural tube defects, targeted sonographic evaluation in high-risk cases is remarkably accurate. Sensitivities have been reported between 97% and 100%, with 100% specificity.

Ultrasound diagnosis of meningomyelocele is frequently based on the finding of a cystic mass protruding from the dorsal vertebral bodies without skin covering. This is ideally seen in the transverse plane as a wide separation of the lateral processes of the lamina. In the coronal plane, widening of the parallel lines of the normal spine can be seen. It should be cautioned that occasionally coronal and sagittal views can be misleading, and the present standard for spina bifida screening by ultrasound is an image of transverse planes of individual vertebrae. Some cases of meningomyelocele do not have a cystic structure and are identified only by a subtle widening of the posterior processes.

Indirect sonographic signs of meningomyelocele have been found to be as important as visualization of the spinal lesion and are somewhat easier to image. These include ventriculomegaly, microcephaly, frontal bone scalloping (lemon sign), and obliteration of the cisterna magna with either an "absent" cerebellum or abnormal anterior curvature of the cerebellar hemispheres (banana sign) (Fig. 17-6).[153] These findings are seen in more than 95% of cases of neural tube defects imaged in the middle of the second trimester. The banana sign and lemon sign may not be present after 22 to 24 weeks' gestation. Anencephaly should routinely be identified by ultrasound as early as 11 or 12 weeks' gestation but should be reconfirmed by a scan at around 13 weeks because ossification of the skull in some cases may not be completed until that time (see Chapter 18).

Presently, the best approach to evaluate an elevated MSAFP is a combination of ultrasound imaging and amniocentesis. When ultrasound expertise is available and optimal images can be obtained of both the spine and the central nervous system, amniocentesis can be avoided. If ultrasound expertise or high-resolution equipment is not available or fetal position or maternal body habitus prevents optimal fetal visualization, further evaluation by amniocentesis should be offered.

Other Fetal Causes of Elevated Maternal Serum α-Fetoprotein and Amniotic Fluid α-Fetoprotein

The greater the elevation in both MSAFP and AFAFP is, the greater the risk of fetal abnormalities. Crandall and Chua[154] analyzed 1086 amniotic fluid samples with elevated AFP levels and found abnormalities associated with AFAFP elevations of 2.0 to 4.9, 5.0 to 9.9, and more than 10.0 MoM in 25%, 88.1%, and 97.7% of pregnancies, respectively.

In addition to neural tube defects, other lesions leaking fetal serum into the amniotic fluid can cause elevations of both MSAFP and AFAFP. These include fetal abdominal wall defects such as omphalocele, gastroschisis, or extrophy of the bladder; weeping skin lesions such as epidermolysis bullosa or aplasia cutis; and some cases of sacrococcygeal teratoma and fetal urinary tract obstruction. Table 17-13 lists other fetal conditions associated with elevated MSAFP with and without elevations of AChE.

Because AFP is produced in the fetal gastrointestinal tract and liver, reduced intestinal AFP clearance with regurgitation of intestinal contents has been associated with elevated MSAFP and AFAFP. Reflux of lung fluid can also cause elevated levels. This occurs with duodenal atresia, annular pancreas, intestinal atresia, pharyngeal teratoma, and congenital cystic adenomatoid malformation of the lung.

Exceedingly high MSAFP and AFAFP levels are associated with the rare condition of congenital fetal nephrosis.[155-157] The elevated AFP is a result of altered filtering capabilities of the fetal glomeruli. Congenital nephrosis is an autosomal recessive disorder, with the most common mutations mapping to chromosome 19q, the nephrin gene *(NPHS1)*. In the Finnish population, 36 mutations have been located within the gene, with two, Finmajor and Finminor, accounting for 94% of cases.[158] Lenkkeri and colleagues[159] reported that 20% (7 of 35) of non-Finnish cases have no detectable mutation along the nephrin gene sequence. Therefore, non-Finnish cases may have mutations in other sequences or on other chromosomes.[158,159]

The condition is lethal in infancy if untreated, with an average lifespan of 7 months.[160] More aggressive treatments have been attempted, including dialysis and bilateral nephrectomy with subsequent renal transplant, resulting in some survivors. Unfortunately, a transplant cannot be performed until 2 years of age, on average.[161]

In Finland, where the disorder occurs in 1 of 2600 to 8000 pregnancies, screening programs using mid-trimester MSAFP have been used successfully to identify this condition.[150-162] In other areas of the world, when markedly elevated AFP levels are found without ultrasound-detected anomalies, congenital nephrosis must be considered.

The diagnosis is strongly suggested with the finding of an elevated MSAFP (usually greater than 5 to 6 MoM) followed by an extremely elevated (frequently more than 10 MoM) level in the amniotic fluid. Although one case of congenital nephrosis with a low AFP level (<2.5) has been described,[150] this is extremely unusual and probably was related to too early testing because the degree of elevation of AFAFP increases with gestational age, proportionate to the contribution that fetal urine makes to the amniotic fluid. Consistent with this is a case report in which serial amniocenteses showed a rapid increase in AFP levels between 14 and 18 weeks.[163] Other amniotic fluid markers of congenital proteinuria such as transferrin and albumin have been examined to help make a more definitive diagnosis, but the sensitivity of these substances is not sufficient.[164,165]

Confirming congenital nephrosis in utero is confounded by the lack of ultrasound findings. Although echogenic and slightly enlarged kidneys have been described, in most cases the kidneys appear normal, the amount of amniotic fluid is normal, and placentomegaly, which may occur, does not appear until late in gestation. If no ultrasound anomalies are seen, the karyotype is normal, and elevated AFAFP is confirmed, congenital nephrosis must be suspected, but a normal gestation (false-positive) is possible.[150] In these cases, in utero fetal kidney biopsy provides a means to examine the renal cortex, glomerular basement membrane structure, and podocyte morphology,[166] because the pathologic characteristics are present in the second trimester.[167] Electron microscopic evaluation of the biopsy sample is required to visualize altered podocyte morphology diagnostic of this condition.

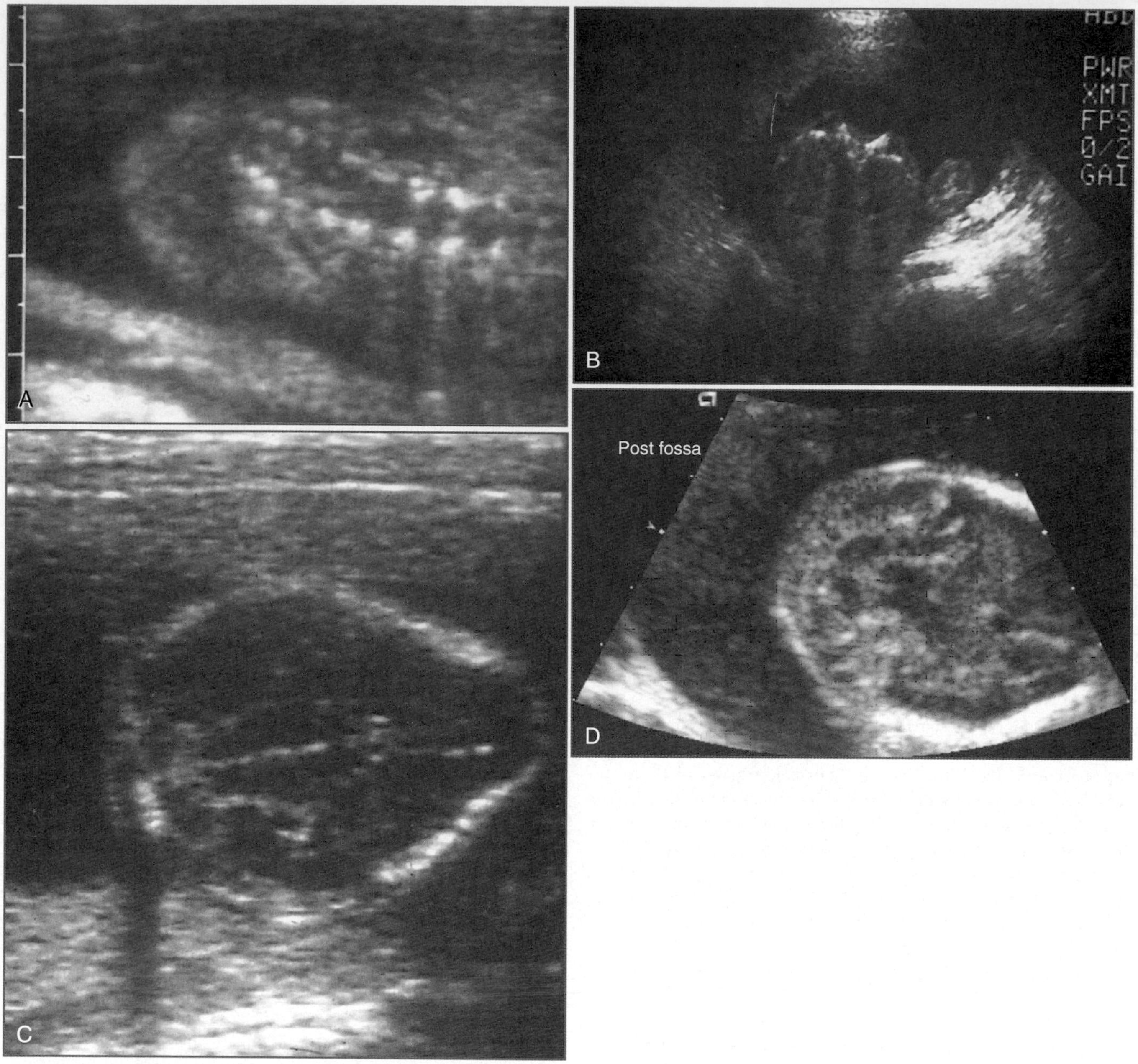

FIGURE 17-6 Ultrasound of a fetus with a neural tube defect. Sagittal (**A**) and transverse (**B**) views of the spine. Transverse view of the skull, with scalloping of the frontal bones, the lemon sign (**C**), and herniation of the cerebellum, the banana sign (**D**).

Ultrasound Screening for Fetal Congenital Anomalies

The value of routine second-trimester ultrasound as a screening test is unknown. The Routine Antenatal Diagnostic Imaging Ultrasound Study[61] was a randomized controlled trial to test whether routine ultrasound during pregnancy would reduce perinatal morbidity and mortality. This study concluded that routine ultrasound did not alter perinatal outcomes and therefore should not be routinely performed on all women. Limitations to this study are numerous; for example, nearly 70% of the control group received an ultrasound examination at some point in their pregnancy, more congenital anomalies were detected in the screened group, but the overall rate of detected anomalies was only 35%, and experienced referral centers demonstrated a 23% higher detection rate (35% versus 13%) than nontertiary centers.

At present, the American College of Obstetricians and Gynecologists does not recommend ultrasound as a routine part of prenatal care,[168] but other authors argue that denial of access to universal ultrasound with its current abilities may be unethical.[169] Whether routine or targeted, anatomic screening should be done by experienced centers to increase detection of anomalies and limit false-positive results.[170]

Increased Nuchal Translucency and Normal Karyotype

An increased NT has been described with certain nonchromosomal fetal disorders.[79,80,82-84,86,171-183] In some cases, this may be coincidental. However, in others, such as cardiac defects, diaphragmatic hernias, and fetal skeletal and neurologic abnormalities, a true relationship appears likely. Additionally, an association between increased NT and poor perinatal outcomes, including miscarriage and perinatal death, exists.[184] This information is important in counseling patients who have an elevated NT and a normal karyotype.

In approximately 90% of explored cases in which the NT is greater than the 99th percentile but below 4.5 mm, a healthy infant can be expected. With NTs between 4.5 and 6.4 mm, about 80% of births will result in a healthy newborn. Measurements greater than 6.5 mm have only a 45% incidence of normal results.[184]

The association of increased NT with fetal cardiac and great vessel defects is significant (Table 17-14).[185-194] A large series from the Fetal Medicine Foundation Project showed that the prevalence of major cardiovascular abnormalities increases with increasing NT.[184] With an NT measurement between the 95th percentile and 3.4 mm, the frequency of heart and great vessel anomalies was 4 per 1000. When the NT was between 3.5 and 4.5 mm, the incidence increased to 27 per 1000, and when the NT was greater than 6.5 mm, the frequency was 170 per 1000. In a similar, but retrospective, study of approximately 30,000 chromosomally normal singleton pregnancies, the prevalence of cardiac defects increased from 0.8 per 1000 in individuals with an NT below the 95th percentile, to almost 64 per 1000 when the NT was above the 99th percentile.[195] Alternatively, approximately 40% of all fetuses with cardiac defects will have an NT above the 99th percentile, and 66% will be above the 95th percentile.[195]

This information strongly suggests that the presence of an NT above the 99th percentile, and perhaps above the 95th, should be followed with a fetal echocardiogram. In this group of individuals, the frequency of major cardiac defects would be anticipated to be about 2%, which is higher than the threshold risk for pregnancies presently receiving echocardiograms, such as those with a mother affected with diabetes mellitus or a family history of an affected offspring. If a cutoff at the 95th percentile is used and 5% of all pregnancies would be offered testing, resources to accomplish this may be insufficient. However, if a 99th percentile NT measurement is used, only about 1% of patients would require echocardiograms, with an incidence of positive findings of approximately 6%. Recent improvements in the resolution of ultrasound and increasing experience with first-trimester cardiac scanning suggest that major cardiac defects could be identified by the end of the first trimester.[186,196-199] This means that patients identified with an enlarged NT who presently have their echocardiograms performed at 20 weeks may not need to delay testing.

Fetal anomalies occur frequently enough after an elevated NT that follow-up scans in the second trimester are recommended. These anomalies include diaphragmatic hernias, severe skeletal defects, and omphaloceles.[184] Table 17-15 lists the anomalies with a possible relationship with an increased NT.

The most difficult counseling issue involves patients with an elevated NT, a normal karyotype, and a normal second trimester ultrasound. In a certain percentage of these cases, genetic syndromes not identifiable by ultrasound may be present, including Noonan syndrome, as well as others listed in Table 17-15. Recently, there has also been some speculation of an increased frequency of unexplained developmental delay in some of these infants (E. Pergament, personal communication, 2002). Presently, there is insufficient information to counsel patients specifically; however, in most cases, patients can be reassured that this frequency appears to be less than 10%.[200]

TABLE 17-14 PREVALENCE OF MAJOR DEFECTS OF THE HEART AND GREAT ARTERIES IN CHROMOSOMALLY NORMAL FETUSES BY NUCHAL TRANSLUCENCY THICKNESS

Nuchal Translucency (mm)	*n*	Major Cardiac Defects	Prevalence (per 1000)
<95th percentile	27,332	22	0.8
≥95th percentile to 3.4	1,507	8	5.3
3.5 to 4.4	208	6	28.9
4.5 to 5.4	66	6	90.0
≥5.5	41	8	195.1
Total	29,154	50	1.7

From Hyett J, Perdu M, Sharland G, et al: Using fetal nuchal translucency to screen for major congenital cardiac defects at 10-14 weeks of gestation: Population based cohort study. BMJ 318:81, 1999.

TABLE 17-15 FETAL ABNORMALITIES AND GENETIC SYNDROMES ASSOCIATED WITH INCREASED NUCHAL TRANSLUCENCY

Diaphragmatic hernia
Cardiac defects
Exomphalos
Achondrogenesis type II
Achondroplasia
Asphyxiating thoracic dystrophy
Beckwith-Wiedemann syndrome
Blomstrand osteochondrodysplasia
Body stalk anomaly
Campomelic dysplasia
EEC syndrome
Fetal akinesia deformation sequence
Fryn syndrome
GM_1 gangliosidosis
Hydrolethalus syndrome
Joubert syndrome
Jarcho-Levin syndrome
Meckel-Gruber syndrome
Nance-Sweeny syndrome
Noonan syndrome
Osteogenesis imperfecta type II
Perlman syndrome
Roberts syndrome
Short-rib polydactyly syndrome
Smith-Lemli-Opitz syndrome
Spinal muscular atrophy type 1
Thanatophoric dysplasia
Trigonocephaly "C" syndrome
VACTERL association
Zellweger syndrome

EEC syndrome, ectrodactyly-ectodermal dysplasia-cleft palate syndrome; VACTERL association, *v*ertebral abnormality, *a*nal atresia, *c*ardiac defect, *t*racheo*e*sophageal fistula, *r*enal and radial *l*imb abnormality.

TABLE 17-16 COMMON AUTOSOMAL RECESSIVE DISORDERS IN ETHNIC GROUPS: CARRIER SCREENING RECOMMENDED

Ethnic Group	Genetic Disorder	Carrier Frequency in Ethnic Group	Frequency of Carrier Couples	Screening Test Available?	Detection Rate (%)
African ancestry	Sickle cell disease (HbS and C)	1:10-HbS 1:20-HbC	1:130	Hb electrophoresis	100
	Sickle cell S–β-thalassemia			MCV, Hb electrophoresis	
	α-Thalassemia			MCV, DNA	
Ashkenazi Jews (and Jews of unknown descent)	Tay-Sachs disease	1:30	1:150	Hexosaminidase A level	98
	Canavan disease	1:40	1:1600	DNA mutation	
Chinese	α-Thalassemia		1:625	MCV	
French Canadian, Cajun	Tay-Sachs disease			Hexosaminidase A level	
Mediterranean (Italian/Greek/Turks/Spaniards)	β-Thalassemia		1:900	MCV	
All patients seeking pre-conception counseling (especially whites of European origin)	Cystic fibrosis	1:25-29	1:625	DNA mutation	80*

***Depends on ethnic group: 70% for southern European descent, 90% for northern European descent.**
Hb, hemoglobin; MCV, mean corpuscular volume.

Screening for Gene Mutations That Lead to Fetal Disease

Certain populations have an increased frequency of specific, identifiable, disease-causing gene mutations. This may occur because the population has remained relatively isolated, because many individuals in the population are descended from a few common relatives having a specific mutation (founder effect), or because the carrier state has a beneficial effect on survival in a particular environment (sickle cell carrier state protection from malaria). It has become a part of routine obstetric care to identify these at-risk individuals. Presently, candidates for screening are identified because of their race or heritage. Table 17-16 lists the standard screening tests that should be offered to pregnant patients based on their ethnicity.

The goal of testing is to provide individuals with information that will permit them to make informed reproductive decisions. Such testing is of maximal benefit when it is part of a comprehensive screening program. Components of this program should include patient education, counseling, and a relationship with medical facilities capable of performing invasive diagnostic testing when needed. To be responsive to patient needs, information related to genetics, in general and specific to their individual risks, should be given. This should include basic inheritance patterns, the variable nature of disease expression, the risk of occurrence, and the diagnostic and therapeutic options available. Educating a couple can be accomplished by using direct counseling, printed materials, or interactive online systems.

Before carrier testing is performed, informed consent should be obtained. This should demonstrate that the individual has fully understood the multiple options that ensue from testing. It is equally important to ensure that those who decline testing do so knowledgeably, and this should be documented. Any testing performed must be voluntary, and patients must be assured that every effort will be made to ensure confidentiality. As molecular diagnostics has become more available, the complexity of gene-based diagnosis and screening has become clear. The vast number of mutations with their varying phenotypic consequences frequently require sophisticated laboratory capabilities and subsequent counseling by individuals explicitly trained in this area.

Cystic Fibrosis Screening

Cystic fibrosis (CF) is a multisystem genetic disorder in which defective chloride transport across membranes causes dehydrated secretions, leading to tenacious mucus in the lungs, mucous plugs in the pancreas, and high sweat chloride levels. CF is an autosomal recessive disorder with the responsible gene on chromosome 7 coding for the CF transmembrane conductance regulator (CFTR). CF can have a highly variable presentation and course, which ranges from severe pulmonary and gastrointestinal disease in infancy to relatively mild disease when initial presentation is during young adulthood. Mutations of the CF gene can lead to otherwise normal men with congenital absence of the vas deferens or women with chronic sinusitis or bronchitis as their only morbidity.

CF is one of the most common genetic diseases in the white population, with an incidence of about 1 in 3300 individuals. The gene is also relatively common in Ashkenazi Jews and has a fairly high incidence among Hispanics (1 in 9550). The disease is rare in native Africans and Asians (<1 in 50,000) but somewhat higher in American populations of these ethnic groups (1 in 15,300 and 1 in 32,100, respectively). Table 17-17 demonstrates the incidence of CF and the carrier frequency in various ethnic groups.

The gene causing CF was first cloned in 1989 and provided the initial ability to screen individuals with no family history. More than 600 mutations and DNA sequence variations have since been identified. The ΔF508 mutation, the most common, is a frame-shift mutation caused by a three-base pair deletion in exon 10 of the CF transmembrane conductance regulator that codes for phenylalanine at the 508th amino acid. Although present in almost all populations, its relative frequency varies among different geographies and ethnic groups. The highest frequency is observed in the white population, where it accounts for approximately 70% of CF mutations. Some 15 to 20 other "common" mutations account for 2% to 15% of CF alleles, depending on the ethnic composition of the patient group.

TABLE 17-17 CARRIER FREQUENCY DISTRIBUTION OF COMMON CYSTIC FIBROSIS ALLELES IN VARIOUS ETHNIC GROUPS

Group	Incidence	Carrier Frequency	Delta F508 (%)	Common White Alleles (%)	Group-Specific Alleles (%)	Approximate Mutation Detection Rate (%)
Whites in North America	1/3,300	1/29	70	14	—	80-85
Hispanics	1/8,900	1/46	46	11	—	57
Ashkenazi Jews	1/3,970	1/29	30	67	—	97
Native Americans	1/1,500		0	25	69	94
African Americans	1/15,300	1/60-65	48	4	23	75
Asian Americans	1/32,100	1/90	30			30

From Cutting GR: Genetic epidemiology and genotype/phenotype correlations. Presented at the NIH Consensus Development Conference on Genetic Testing for Cystic Fibrosis, Washington, DC, April 14-16, 1997.

TABLE 17-18 RECOMMENDED CORE MUTATION PANEL FOR CYSTIC FIBROSIS CARRIER SCREENING IN GENERAL POPULATION

Standard Mutation Panel					
ΔF508	ΔI507	G542X	G551D	W1282X	N1
R553X →	621+1G T	R117H	1717-G1 A	A455E	Rb
R1162X →	G85E	R334W	R347P	711+1G T	189
2184delA → →	1078delT	3849+10kbC T	2789+5G A	3659delC	114
3120+1G → A					
Reflex Tests					
1506V,* 1507V,* F508C*					
5T/7T/9T†					

***Benign variants. This test distinguishes between a cystic fibrosis mutation and these benign variants. 1506V, 1507V, and F508C are tests performed for unexpected homozygosity for ΔF508 and/or Δ1507.**
†5T in *cis* can modify R117H phenotype or alone can contribute to congenital bilateral absence of vas deferens (CBA VD); 5T analysis.

The sensitivity of CF screening using DNA mutation analysis depends on the frequency of common identifiable mutations in the screened population. Although greater than 90% carrier detection is presently possible in a number of ethnic groups, a standard panel of mutations has been developed to maximize overall screening efficiency that provides the greatest pan-ethnic detection and can be practically performed (Table 17-18). This panel was initially composed of 25 mutations but in 2004 the number was reduced to 23.[201] The panel contains all CF-causing mutations with an allele frequency of at least 0.1% in the general U.S. population. An understanding of the distribution of mutations in the CF transmembrane conductance regulator is continually advancing, and it is likely that this panel will continue to evolve. Panels with more mutations are available, as is complete gene sequencing, and may be useful in certain specific clinical situations.

There has been much discussion and debate over which ethnic and racial groups should be offered CF carrier testing. Some maintain that screening should be limited to the highest-risk populations, such as non-Jewish whites of European ancestry and Ashkenazi Jews, in which both the carrier frequency (1:25 to 1:30) and the mutation detection rate (25 mutations detect more than 80% of CF alleles) are sufficiently high to make screening cost-effective. This would exclude African Americans, with a detection rate of only about 75%. Hispanics would also be excluded, despite their relatively high incidence of the disease, because detectable alleles account for only 57% of their CF mutations. Screening would be even less effective in Asian Americans, who would have only 30% sensitivity. Others argue that the admixture of populations in the United States makes it difficult to exclude patients on the basis of specific ethnic group and that even attempting to make such a determination in a busy clinical setting may place an undue burden on primary care physicians.

To resolve this debate, the National Institutes of Health issued a consensus statement in 1997 indicating that CF testing should be offered to adults with a positive family history of CF, to partners of people with CF, to all couples planning a pregnancy, and to couples seeking prenatal testing, particularly those in high-risk populations. It was believed that genetic testing should be offered in the prenatal setting to enhance the ability to make reproductive choices and to engage individuals when their interest and use of the information was maximal.

A second National Institutes of Health–sponsored conference focusing on implementation of the consensus recommendations was held in 1998. Shortly thereafter, the American Colleges of Medical Genetics and Obstetrics and Gynecology, in conjunction with the National Human Genome Research Institute, issued a joint opinion entitled "Preconception and Prenatal Carrier Screening for Cystic Fibrosis." This document recommended narrowing the population screened to non-Jewish whites and Ashkenazi Jews. Information about screening should be made available to other ethnic and racial groups through educational brochures or other efficient methods. These lower-risk groups should be informed of the availability of testing but should also be advised of the limitations encountered for their particular situation. For example, Asian Americans, African Americans, and Native Americans without significant white mixture should be informed of the rarity of the disease and the low yield of the test in their respective populations.[202,203] Pre-conception testing should be encouraged, but for practical purposes, most testing should continue to occur in the prenatal setting.

In appropriate populations, there are two possible approaches to screening. In sequential screening, one member of the couple (usually the woman) is tested first, and only if a positive result is obtained is the partner tested. Alternatively, couple-based screening analyzes specimens from both partners, with each informed of his or her specific results. Present recommendations are that either is appropriate, with the method depending on the target population, the nature of the clinical setting, and the judgment of the practitioner. Couple-based testing is recommended for white couples of northern European and Ashkenazi Jewish descent, particularly when concurrently testing for other common genetic disorders. Sequential screening is believed to be more useful for groups in which the carrier frequency is lower and when obtaining a simultaneous sample from the partner is impractical. In general, the individual provider or center should choose the method they believe is most practical in their setting.

All patients with negative screen results should be reminded that carrier screening is not 100% sensitive. This is particularly pertinent in couples when one partner is found to carry a mutation. The residual risk after a negative CF carrier test depends on the ethnic and racial group of the patient (Table 17-19). In northern and eastern European populations in which CF mutation screening detects up to 90% of mutant alleles and in which the carrier frequency is 1 in 25, a negative screen reduces the risk of being a carrier to 1 in 241. Screen-negative couples will then reduce their risk of having an affected child from 1 in 2500 ($^1/_4 \times ^1/_{25} \times ^1/_{25}$) to 1 in 232,324 ($^1/_4 \times ^1/_{241} \times ^1/_{241}$). If one parent has a mutation and the other is negative, the risk of an affected child is 1 in 964 ($^1/_4 \times 1 \times ^1/_{241}$). When both parents are found to have identifiable mutations, the risk of an affected child is 1 in 4. Prenatal diagnosis by either chorionic villus sampling or amniocentesis, along with genetic counseling, would be recommended.

For individuals with a family history of CF, medical records identifying the mutation should be obtained. If the mutation has not been identified, screening with an expanded panel of mutations, or in some cases complete sequencing, may be necessary. Individuals with a reproductive partner with either CF or congenital bilateral absence of the vas deferens may also benefit from either an expanded panel or gene sequencing.

In most cases, interpretation of the screening results is straightforward, but complicated situations may occur and frequently involve the 5T variant polymorphism. This is one of three poly(T) (thymidine) alleles (5T, 7T, and 9T) in intron 8 of the CF transmembrane conductance regulator gene. It occurs in about 5% of the population and decreases production of the CFTR protein. The 5T mutation can cause congenital bilateral absence of the vas deferens or atypical CF when present in a male in *trans* with a common CF allele. This arrangement has no clinical significance in females. Accordingly, identification of the 5T variant will produce complicated counseling issues, because it expands the risk ascertainment beyond classic CF. Because of this, most laboratories do not offer 5T analysis as part of routine screening. Testing for this variant is only appropriate as a reflex test when the R117H mutation is detected on the primary screen. This is required because classic CF occurs when 5T is in *cis* with R117H on one chromosome and a CFTR mutation is present on the other chromosome. Accordingly, patients positive for both R117H and 5T require further analysis to determine if the 5T is in *cis* or *trans* with the R117H allele. To accomplish this, the laboratory requests specimens from appropriate family members. Using this approach, the initial screening is for classic CF rather than fertility of the fetus.

Jewish Disease Testing

A number of recessive disorders occur more frequently in the Ashkenazi Jewish population. Carrier testing for two of these, Tay-Sachs disease and Canavan disease, is now considered standard of care.[204]

Tay-Sachs Disease. Tay-Sachs disease is an autosomal recessive lysosomal storage disorder caused by deficiency of the enzyme hexosaminidase A. This results in a group of neurodegenerative disorders caused by intralysosomal storage of the specific glycosphingolipid GM2 ganglioside. Classic Tay-Sachs disease is characterized by loss of motor skills beginning between 3 and 6 months of age, with progressive neurodegeneration, including seizures, blindness, and eventual total incapacitation and death usually before the age of 4. The juvenile (subacute), chronic, and adult-onset variants of the hexosaminidase A deficiencies have later onsets, slower progression, and more variable neurologic findings, including progressive dystonia, spinocerebellar degeneration, motor neuron disease, and, in some individuals with adult-onset disease, a bipolar form of psychosis.

TABLE 17-19 IMPACT OF A NEGATIVE CYSTIC FIBROSIS (CF) SCREENING PANEL (25 MUTATIONS) ON THE CARRIER RISK*

Ethnic Group	Detection Rate (%)	Estimated Carrier Risk: Before Test	Estimated Carrier Risk: After Negative Test
Ashkenazi Jews	97	1/29	Approx. 1 in 930
European white	80	1/29	Approx. 1 in 140
African American	69	1/65	Approx. 1 in 207
Hispanic American†	57	1/46	Approx. 1 in 105
European white with positive family history	80		
Sibling with CF		2/3	Approx. 1 in 3.5
Carrier parent		1/2	Approx. 1 in 6
Carrier grandparent		1/4	Approx. 1 in 14

*Residual carrier risk after a negative test is modified by the presence of a positive family history.
†This is a pooled set of data and requires additional information to accurately predict risk for specific Hispanic populations.

The incidence of the Tay-Sachs carrier state is between 1:27 and 1:30 in the Ashkenazi Jewish population (i.e., from Central and Eastern Europe), resulting in a birth prevalence of 1 in 3600 infants. Among Sephardic Jews and all non-Jews, the disease frequency is approximately 100 times less, corresponding to a 10-fold lower carrier frequency (1 in 250 to 1 in 300). As the result of extensive genetic counseling of carriers and prenatal diagnosis, the incidence of Tay-Sachs disease in Ashkenazi Jews in North America has already been reduced by greater than 90%.[205,206]

In addition to occurring in Ashkenazi Jews, Tay-Sachs disease can occur in children of any ethnic, racial, or religious group, but certain populations that are relatively isolated genetically, such as French Canadians of the eastern St. Lawrence River valley area of Quebec, Cajuns from Louisiana, and the Amish in Pennsylvania, have been found to carry hexosaminidase A mutations with frequencies comparable with, or even greater than, those observed in Ashkenazi Jews.

Population screening for the carrier state of Tay-Sachs disease uses serum or leukocyte determination of hexosaminidase A enzyme activity using synthetic substrate. Carriers have significantly reduced levels compared with noncarriers. Serum samples are used for testing all males and for nonpregnant women not on oral contraceptives. Pregnant women, those on oral contraceptives, and women who have a tissue destructive disorder such as diabetes mellitus, hepatitis, or rheumatoid arthritis should have a white blood cell determination of enzyme activity, because these conditions artificially lower the serum hexosaminidase A level, leading to a false diagnosis of the carrier state. When the enzymatic testing is abnormal or inconclusive, DNA analysis of the hexosaminidase A gene is performed to confirm the diagnosis, identify the specific mutation, and rule out the presence of a pseudodeficiency allele that is present in approximately 2% of the Ashkenazi Jewish population and approximately 35% of the non-Jewish population.[207]

Two pseudodeficiency alleles exist and can be tested for. Individuals heterozygous for the pseudodeficiency allele have an apparent deficiency of hexosaminidase A enzymatic activity with the synthetic substrate but not with the natural substrate, GM2 ganglioside. Their levels are similar to those of Tay-Sachs carriers, leading to a potential incorrect determination of a carrier. Homozygous pseudodeficient individuals have extremely low or absent hexosaminidase A levels similar to individuals affected with Tay-Sachs disease. Neither compound heterozygotes having one Tay-Sachs allele and one pseudodeficient allele nor homozygotes for the pseudodeficient allele have any neurologic abnormality.

There are more than 90 disease-causing mutations in the hexosaminidase A gene, but routine mutation analysis tests for only the six most common mutations.[208] Molecular analysis of the six-mutation hexosaminidase panel will identify between 92% and 98% of Jewish carriers but only between 23% and 46% of non-Jewish carriers (Table 17-20). Some laboratories use mutation analysis as their primary screening approach in the Ashkenazi population. However, this will identify only 92% to 94% of carriers, so some will be missed. Laboratories seeing a high proportion of French-Canadian patients may offer extended panels or test for selected mutations that are specific to that population. In Quebec, a 7.6-kb deletion is the most common allele associated with Tay-Sachs disease. Accordingly, when testing individuals from the French-Canadian population or other populations with founder mutations, care should be taken to identify a laboratory performing analysis for the appropriate mutations. It is not uncommon for a couple in which one partner is Jewish and the other is not to inquire about testing. It is presently recommended that such couples be offered carrier analysis by enzymatic testing, because DNA analysis with the routine six-mutation panel would fail to detect a significant proportion of the non-Jewish carriers. Also, individuals who have French-Canadian, Cajun, and Amish ancestry should be offered carrier testing. Individuals who are pursuing reproductive technologies that involve gamete donation and who are at increased risk of being heterozygous for hexosaminidase A because of their ethnic background should also be screened.

Prenatal diagnosis for Tay-Sachs disease is possible by enzymatic analysis of either amniocytes or chorionic villi. Hexosaminidase A deficiency can be identified by CVS within 30 minutes of retrieval or from uncultured amniotic fluid.[209-211] However, very few laboratories use this approach, preferring to use mutation analysis if the disease-causing mutation has been identified in both parents. Prenatal testing may also be recommended when one parent is a known heterozygote and the other has inconclusive enzymatic activity without a disease-causing mutation found on DNA analysis. It also may be recommended when the mother is a known heterozygote and the father is either unknown or unavailable for testing. Both of these latter scenarios require intensive genetic counseling.

TABLE 17-20 MOLECULAR GENETIC TESTING USED IN HEXOSAMINIDASE A DEFICIENCY

		% of Heterozygotes			
		Obligate*		Screening†	
Allele	Allele Status	Jewish	Non-Jewish	Jewish	Non-Jewish
+TAC1278	Null	81	32	80	8.0
+1 IVS 12	Null	15	0	9	0.0
+1 IVS 9	Null	0	14	0	10.3‡
G269S	Adult onset	2	0	3	5.0
R247W	Pseudodeficiency	0	0	2	32.0
R249W	Pseudodeficiency	0	0	0	4.0
Disease-causing alleles detected using the six-mutation HEX A panel (%)	98	46	92	23.0	

*Obligate heterozygotes (i.e., parents of a child with hexosaminidase A deficiency).
†Individuals identified in screening programs as having levels of hexosaminidase A enzymatic activity in the heterozygous range.
‡Primarily persons of Celtic, French, Cajun, or Pennsylvania Dutch background.
From Kaback M, Lim-Steele J, Dabholkar D, et al: Tay-Sachs disease-carrier screening, prenatal diagnosis, and the molecular era: An international perspective, 1970 to 1993. The International TSD Data Collection Network. JAMA 270:2307, 1993.

Canavan Disease. Screening of Ashkenazi Jewish patients or couples for Canavan disease is now part of routine obstetric care.[212] This disorder is caused by a deficiency in aspartoacylase and is characterized by developmental delay by the age of 3 to 5 months, with severe hypotonia and failure to achieve independent sitting, ambulation, or speech.[213] Hypotonia eventually changes to spasticity, requiring assistance with feeding. Life expectancy is usually into the teens.[214] Because about 99% of disease-causing mutations in persons of Ashkenazi Jewish heritage is identified by only three alleles, carrier testing is done by DNA mutation analysis.[215,216] Testing by biochemical analysis is not routinely available because it relies on a complex enzyme assay and cultured skin fibroblasts.[217] Fifty-five percent of disease-causing alleles in non-Jewish individuals are identified by analysis of these three alleles as well.[218] Prenatal testing for pregnancies that are at 25% risk can be performed by either amniocentesis or CVS using mutation analysis. For the unusual couple where one partner is known to be a carrier and a mutation or the carrier status of the other is uncertain or unknown, prenatal testing can be performed by measuring the level of *N*-acetyl aspartic acid in amniotic fluid at 16 to 18 weeks.[219,220]

Other Diseases Increased in the Jewish Population. A number of other disorders have been found to occur more frequently among the Ashkenazi Jewish population (Table 17-21).[221] The gene frequency for these disorders varies compared with those for Tay-Sachs or Canavan disease.[222] In some of these disorders, such as Gaucher disease type I, the phenotype in some individuals is relatively benign or treatable. Although this autosomal recessive lysosomal storage disease has a carrier frequency of 1 in 18 in Ashkenazi Jewish individuals, the clinical course is heterogeneous, ranging from early onset of severe disease, with major disability or death in childhood, to a mild disease compatible with a normal productive life. The phenotype in this disorder is well correlated with the genotype. Of the more than 200 mutations in the affected acid α-glucosidase gene, four mutations (N370S, 84GG, L444P, and IVS2) account for 95% of those in Ashkenazi Jews. Although an affected individual who carries two copies of any combination of the 84GG, L444P, and IVS2 mutations will have severe neurodegenerative disease, individuals homozygous for the most common N370S mutation have a non-neurologic disorder with an average age at onset of 30. Some individuals may never come to medical attention. Individuals having the N370S mutation with one of the other three common mutations will also have non-neurologic disease but of a somewhat more severe phenotype than in N370S homozygotes. This predominance of relatively mild non-neurologic disease in the Ashkenazi Jewish population has led some to question whether screening in this population is appropriate. In addition, effective treatment of type I Gaucher disease with enzyme replacement exists.

Presently, in some centers, the availability of these carrier tests is discussed with Jewish couples so they can make individualized decisions about whether to have them performed. Overall, if these nine

TABLE 17-21 POTENTIAL SCREENING AVAILABLE FOR AUTOSOMAL RECESSIVE DISORDERS IN THE ASHKENAZI JEWISH POPULATION

Disease	Status	Genetic Defect	Carrier Frequency in Ashkenazi Jews	Comments
Cystic fibrosis	S	Transmembrane conductance regulator (CFTR) mutation	1:26	97% detection rate with 97 mutation panel
Tay-Sachs	S	Hexosaminidase A deficiency	1:30	Screening done by enzyme analysis. Carrier screening during pregnancy, while on oral contraceptives, or with debilitating illness requires leukocyte analysis. Pseudodeficient allele exists. 97% to 98% detection with enzyme analysis and 92% to 94% with mutation analysis.
Canavan	S	Aspartoacylase (ASPA) deficiency	1:40	Three common mutations account for 99% of disease-causing alleles.
Niemann-Pick type A	A	Acid sphingomyelinase deficiency	1:90	Three mutations with 95% detection.
Gaucher disease type 1	A	Glucocerebrosidase deficiency	1:14	The type 1 Gaucher disease seen in this population is the mild variant with no CNS involvement. Some affected individuals with mild disease may be identified through screening. Five mutations with 95% detection
Fanconi anemia	A	Chromosome breakage	1:89	One mutation with 99% detection
Bloom syndrome	A	Chromosome breakage	1:100	One mutation with 97% detection
Congenital deafness	A	Connexin 26 mutation	1:21	Wide variability in severity of disease
Glycogen storage disease type IA	A	Glucose 6 phosphatase	1:71	Two mutations with 99% detection
Maple syrup urine disease	A	Branched-chain alpha-ketoacid dehydrogenase (BCKAD) complex	1:81	Four mutations with 99% detection
Mucolipidosis type IV	A	*MCOLN1*	1:122	Two mutations with 96% detection
Familial dysautonomia	A	*IKBKAP* gene mutation	1:30	Two mutations with 99% detection

A, available for screening at-risk families (could be used for population screening); CNS, central nervous system; S, standard of care.

diseases are screened for, one in six Ashkenazi Jews will be determined to be a carrier for at least one disorder. To avoid the anxiety that such a high carrier rate may engender, it is recommended that both members of a couple be screened simultaneously, so that genetic counseling need be provided only to carrier couples.[223]

Hemoglobinopathies

Sickle Cell Syndromes

Sickle cell diseases are a common group of inherited hemoglobin disorders characterized by chronic hemolytic anemia, heightened susceptibility to infection, end-organ damage, and intermittent attacks of vascular occlusion causing both acute and chronic pain. Approximately 70,000 Americans of different ethnic backgrounds have sickle cell disease. In the United States, sickle cell syndromes are most frequently present in African Americans and occur at a frequency of 1:400. The disease is also found in high frequency in individuals from certain areas of the Mediterranean basin, the Middle East, and India.[224]

Sickle cell syndromes include sickle cell anemia, variant hemoglobin sickle cell disease, and hemoglobin S–β-thalassemia. Normal hemoglobin consists of hemoglobin A (α, β), hemoglobin F (α, γ), and hemoglobin A_2 (α, δ). The protein sequences are coded on chromosome 11 for the β, δ, and γ chains, and the β variants such as hemoglobin S, hemoglobin C, and hemoglobin D all occur from a mutation of this gene. Sickle cell anemia is the most common variant and results when an individual inherits a substitution of valine for the normal glutamic acid in the sixth amino acid position of the β globin chain. This substitution alters the hemoglobin molecule so that it crystallizes and alters the red cell into a sickle shape when the hemoglobin loses oxygen. Hemoglobin C is caused by a substitution of lysine in the same location.

Screening for sickle cell disease should be offered to individuals of African and African-American descent and to those from the Mediterranean basin, the Middle East, and India. Approximately 1 in 12 African Americans has sickle cell trait. The definitive test to determine the carrier state of sickle cell disease is hemoglobin electrophoresis, which is based on the altered electrical charge of abnormal hemoglobins caused by the amino acid substitutions. A simple sickle cell preparation fails to identify individuals carrying β-thalassemia or certain sickle cell variants (hemoglobins C, D, and E) and is no longer acceptable for screening. In addition, routine cellulose acetate gel hemoglobin electrophoresis cannot delineate all hemoglobin variants. If routine electrophoresis is abnormal, further testing by high-performance liquid chromatography may be necessary.

HEMOGLOBIN VARIANTS

Hemoglobin C occurs in higher frequency in individuals with heritage from West Africa, Italy, Greece, Turkey, and the Middle East. Individuals who are hemoglobin C homozygotes have a mild hemolytic anemia, microcytosis, and target cell formation. They may very occasionally have episodes of joint and abdominal pain. Splenomegaly is common, and aplastic crisis and gallstones may occur. Compound-heterozygous patients with hemoglobin S and C have a sickle syndrome that is very similar to sickle cell anemia. Hemoglobin C carriers have no anemia but usually have target cells on blood smear and may have a slightly low mean corpuscular volume (MCV) with no other clinical problems. Individuals who are compound heterozygotes for hemoglobin C and β-thalassemia who inherit a β^0 mutation have a moderately severe anemia, splenomegaly, and may have bone changes. Individuals who inherit a β^+ mutation with hemoglobin C have only a mild anemia, low MCV, and target cells on blood smear.

On occasion, hemoglobin E is seen by electrophoresis. This is a structurally abnormal hemoglobin caused by a substitution of lysine for glutamic acid at the 26th position of the β globin chain, which causes abnormal processing of pre–messenger RNA to functional messenger RNA, resulting in decreased synthesis of hemoglobin E. The hemoglobin E gene is very common in areas of Southeast Asia, India, and China. Heterozygotes for hemoglobin E and hemoglobin A have no anemia, a low MCV, and target cells on blood smear. Hemoglobin electrophoresis shows approximately 75% hemoglobin A and 25% hemoglobin E. Homozygotes for hemoglobin E may have normal hemoglobin levels or only a slight anemia. The MCV is low, and many target cells are present. There is a single band in the hemoglobin C or A position on cellulose acetate electrophoresis and increased hemoglobin F (10% to 15%). There are no clinically significant problems. Individuals who are compound heterozygotes for hemoglobin E and β^0-thalassemia can have a severe disease with profound anemia, microcytosis, splenomegaly, jaundice, and expansion of marrow space. Hemoglobin electrophoresis in these individuals shows hemoglobin E and a significant increase in hemoglobin F (30% to 60%). Individuals who are compound heterozygote for hemoglobin E and β^+-thalassemia have a moderate disease with anemia, microcytosis, splenomegaly, and jaundice. Hemoglobin electrophoresis shows hemoglobin E at approximately 40%, hemoglobin A at 1% to 30%, and a significant increase in hemoglobin F (at approximately 30% to 50%).

SICKLE THALASSEMIAS

Beta-thalassemias are caused by mutations that reduce or abolish the production of the β globin subunits of hemoglobin. Compound heterozygotes of β-thalassemia and hemoglobin S have very significant clinical problems. In hemoglobin S–β^0-thalassemia, no normal hemoglobin A is made, so electrophoresis of hemoglobin shows only hemoglobin S, increased hemoglobin A_2, and increased hemoglobin F. In hemoglobin S–β^+-thalassemia, hemoglobin A is reduced, so hemoglobin electrophoresis shows hemoglobin A (5% to 25%), hemoglobin F, hemoglobin S, and increased hemoglobin A_2. The severity of the clinical manifestations of sickle cell thalassemia can vary greatly between patients. Most individuals with the hemoglobin S–β^+-thalassemia have preservation of spleen function and fewer problems with infections, fewer pain episodes, and less organ damage than those with sickle cell disease. Individuals with hemoglobin S–β^0-thalassemia may have very severe disease identical to disease in those homozygous for sickle cell anemia.

Sickle cell anemias are inherited as autosomal recessive disorders. Therefore, when both parents carry the hemoglobin S gene, the couple has a 1:4 risk of having an affected child. Prenatal diagnosis using molecular DNA detection of the mutation is routine. When one parent has a hemoglobin S mutation and the other is a carrier of β-thalassemia, the couple has a 25% risk of having a child with sickle thalassemia. If the specific parental mutation responsible for thalassemia is known, the gene can be detected by molecular analysis of villi or amniocytes and an affected child identified. If the thalassemia mutation is not identifiable, fetal blood sampling for globin chain synthesis may be required.

Beta-Thalassemia

Beta-thalassemia is characterized by reduced hemoglobin β-chain production and results in microcytic, hypochromic anemia, and an abnormal peripheral blood smear with nucleated red cells. There are reduced (β^+) to absent (β^0) amounts of hemoglobin A on hemoglobin electrophoresis.[225] Patients homozygous for a β-thalassemia mutation have thalassemia major with severe anemia and hepatosplenomegaly. They usually come to medical attention within the first 2 years of life, and without treatment affected children have severe failure to thrive and a shortened life expectancy. Treatment requires a program of regular transfusions and chelation therapy, which can result in normal growth and development.

β-Thalassemia is inherited in an autosomal recessive manner, with two carrier parents having a 25% chance of an affected child. Heterozygotes are clinically asymptomatic and may have only slight anemia. Carriers are referred to as having thalassemia minor.[226] The β-thalassemias result from more than 200 different hemoglobin β chain mutations.[227] Despite this marked molecular heterogeneity, the prevalent molecular defects are limited in each at-risk population—that is, each racial or ethnic population has only four to 10 mutations that account for the large majority of the disease-causing alleles in that population (Table 17-22). For example, in individuals of Mediterranean, Middle Eastern, Indian, Thai, or Chinese extraction, a limited number of population-specific mutations account for between 90% and 95% of the disease genes. In Africans and African Americans, common mutations account for approximately 75% to 80%. This phenomenon has significantly facilitated molecular genetic testing.

Screening for thalassemia should be offered to all individuals of Mediterranean, Middle Eastern, Transcaucasian, Central Asian, Indian, and Far Eastern groups. Because thalassemia is also common in individuals of African heritage, carrier testing should be offered to all African Americans. As with sickle cell disease, the distribution is probably related to selective pressure from malaria, because the disease distribution is similar to that of endemic *Plasmodium falciparum* malaria.[226] However, because of population migration and, in limited part, the slave trade, β-thalassemia is now also commonly seen in northern Europe, North and South America, the Caribbean, and Australia.

Carriers are identified by evaluation of the red blood cell indices, quantitative hemoglobin analysis, and hemoglobin β chain mutation studies. Carriers are initially identified by their red blood cell indices that show microcytosis (low MCV, <80) and a reduced content of hemoglobin per cell (low mean corpuscular hemoglobin). Next, a hemoglobin electrophoresis displays a hemoglobin A_2 of more than 3.5% (Table 17-23). On rare occasions, carrier identification using MCV can be misleading. For example, coinheritance of an α-thalassemia gene may normalize red blood cell indices. Also, coinheritance of the δ-thalassemia gene can reduce the normal increased hemoglobin A_2 levels typical of β-thalassemia. Likewise, screening using only a routine hemoglobin electrophoresis as the primary test is insufficient, because thalassemia carriers can easily be missed when hemoglobin levels are normal, and the subtle increases in hemoglobin A_2 and F on electrophoresis may be overlooked. Therefore, a complete blood count with MCV and red cell count should be obtained and a quantitative hemoglobin electrophoresis should be performed, because the MCV is almost always low in β-thalassemia and the red cell count is elevated. Quantitative hemoglobin electrophoresis for hemoglobin A_2 and F is diagnostic.[225]

When the initial hematologic analysis is abnormal and the couple is at risk for having a child with either homozygous β-thalassemia or thalassemia–sickle cell disease syndrome, DNA analysis of the hemoglobin β chain is indicated to identify the disease-causing mutation. This helps identify carriers of mild and silent mutations of β-thalassemia that result in attenuated forms of the disease. Knowledge of the specific mutations will also be required if subsequent prenatal diagnosis is performed. However, the sensitivity of molecular testing remains less than 100%, so for some individuals a specific mutation cannot be identified.

Prenatal diagnosis is offered to couples when both members are carriers of β-thalassemia and their gene mutations have been identified. In these cases, mutation analysis can be performed by DNA extracted from either CVS or amniocentesis. Prenatal testing is occasionally offered to families in which one parent is a definitive heterozygote and the other parent has a β-thalassemia–like hematologic picture but no mutation can be identified by sequence analysis. If the father of a pregnancy with a known heterozygote mother is unavailable for testing and belongs to a population at risk, prenatal diagnosis can be offered. In either of the latter two situations, if the known mutation

TABLE 17-22 MOLECULAR GENETIC TESTING USED FOR β-THALASSEMIA

Population	Patients with Positive Results (%)	Most Common Hemoglobin Mutations in At-Risk Populations
Mediterranean	91-95	−87 C→G, IVS1-1 G→A, IVS1-6 T→C, IVS1-110 G→A, cd 39 C–
Middle East	91-95	cd 8 -AA, cd 8/9 + G, IVS1-5 G→C, cd 39 C→T, cd 44-C, IVS2-1 G→A
Indian	91-95	−619 bp deletion, cd 8/9 + G, IVS1-1 G→T, IVS1-5 G→C, 41/42-TTCT
Thai	91-95	−28 A→G, 17 A→T, 19 A→G, IVS1-5 G→C, 41/42-TTCT, IVS2-654 C→T
Chinese	91-95	−28 A→G, 17 A→T, 41/42-TTCT, IVS2-654 C→T
African and African-American	75-80	−88 C→T, −29 A→AG, IVS1-5 G→T, cd 24 T→A, IVS11-949 A→G, A→C

TABLE 17-23 RED BLOOD CELL INDICES IN β-THALASSEMIA

Red Blood Cell Index	Normal Male	Normal Female	Affected β-Thalassemia Major	Carrier β-Thalassemia Minor
Mean corpuscular volume, fL	80.0-100.0	80.0-100.0	50-70	<80
Mean corpuscular hemoglobin, pg	27.5-33.2	27.5-33.2	12-20	18-22
Hemoglobin, g/dL	14-18	12-16	<7	11-14

From Hann IM, Gibson BES, Letsky EA: Fetal and Neonatal Haematology. Philadelphia, WB Saunders, 1991.

is identified by CVS or amniocentesis, globin chain synthesis analysis is available for definitive diagnosis.

Alpha-Thalassemia

Alpha-thalassemia is a hemoglobinopathy caused by the deficiency or absence of α globin chain synthesis. The α globin gene cluster is located on chromosome 16 and includes two adult genes ($\alpha 1$ and $\alpha 2$) so that normal individuals have four α globin genes ($\alpha 1\alpha 2/\alpha 1\alpha 2$). α-Thalassemia can be divided into two forms based on the number of functioning genes. A severe form called α^0-thalassemia results in a typical thalassemic blood picture in heterozygotes and a severe, perinatally lethal form in homozygotes. α^0-Thalassemia results from 1 of 17 gene deletions, all of which delete both α globin genes on each chromosome. Alternatively, α^+-thalassemia is milder and is almost completely silent in heterozygotes. This form is commonly caused by one of six deletions that remove one of the two α globin genes on chromosome 16.

The homozygous state of α^0-thalassemia resulting from deletions of all four α globin genes (—/—) causes severe hydrops fetalis and the predominance of hemoglobin Barts ($\gamma 4$) and a small amount of hemoglobin Portland ($\zeta 2\gamma 2$) in the fetus. This is routinely lethal in utero or in the early neonatal period if untreated. Although cases of fetal survival after in utero transfusion have been described, this must be followed by repetitive transfusions of the infant and subsequent bone marrow transplant. This approach is not routinely recommended. Maternal risks of hemoglobin Barts hydrops fetalis syndrome include preeclampsia and postpartum hemorrhage.

Hemoglobin H disease results from the compound heterozygous state for α^0 and α^+ (—/–α)-thalassemia, leading to the deletion of three of the four α chain genes. These individuals have a moderately severe hypochromic microcytic anemia and produce large amounts of hemoglobin H (β^4) because of the excessive quantities of β chains in their reticulocytes. In the most common form, these individuals lead a relatively normal life but may have fatigue, general discomfort, and splenomegaly. They rarely require hospitalization. There is a rare, more severe form of hemoglobin H disease arising from a compound heterozygous state of α^0-thalassemia and nondeletion α^+-thalassemia involving the more dominant α^2 gene.

α^0-Thalassemia gene deletions are found in high frequency in individuals from Southeast Asia, South China, the Philippine Islands, Thailand, and a few Mediterranean countries, such as Greece and Cyprus. Because these populations are at risk for the homozygous state leading to hemoglobin Barts disease, they should be screened for the presence of the gene. The α^+-thalassemia genes are frequent in Africa, the Mediterranean area, the Middle East, the Indian subcontinent, Melanesia, Southeast Asia, and the Pacific area. Because this leads to a mild form of thalassemia, routine screening for α-thalassemia in these populations is not recommended.

The carrier state for α^0-thalassemia is identified by performing a complete blood count with indices. Carriers (—/$\alpha\alpha$) have a decreased MCV (<80 fL) and a mean corpuscular hemoglobin level (<27 pg), as seen with α-thalassemia, but the carriers are differentiated by having a normal hemoglobin A_2 level (<3.5%). The diagnosis is confirmed by DNA testing, which can identify the specific deletion. Prenatal diagnosis is available by CVS or amniocentesis and is based on the molecular determination of the gene status.

Fragile X Syndrome

Fragile X syndrome is characterized by relatively typical phenotypic characteristics and moderate mental retardation in affected males. Affected females have somewhat milder mental retardation.[228] Classic features become more prevalent with age, including long face, large ears, prominent jaw, and macrotestes. There is delayed attainment of motor milestones and speech. Abnormal temperament is frequently associated with hyperactivity, hand flapping, hand biting, and autism spectrum disorder. Behaviors in postpubertal males include tactile defensiveness, poor eye contact, and perseverative speech. Physical and behavioral features can be seen in female heterozygotes, but with a lower frequency and milder involvement. Adult manifestations of the fragile X premutation carrier state occur. The fragile X–associated tremor/ataxia syndrome (FXTAS) is characterized by late-onset, progressive cerebellar ataxia and intention tremor in males who have a premutation.[229] Other neurologic findings include short-term memory loss, executive function deficits, cognitive decline, parkinsonism, peripheral neuropathy, lower-limb proximal muscle weakness, and autonomic dysfunction. Penetrance is age related; symptoms in men are seen in 17% aged 50 to 59 years, in 38% aged 60 to 69 years, in 47% aged 70 to 79 years, and in 75% aged 80 years and older. Some female premutation carriers may also develop tremor and ataxia. In girls and women, premature ovarian failure (POF), defined as cessation of menses before age 40 years, has been observed in carriers of premutation alleles.[230] A review by Sherman[231] concluded that the risk for POF was 21% (estimates ranged from 15% to 27% in various studies) in premutation carriers compared with a 1% background risk. In this review, an odds ratio of 2.5 was estimated for intermediate repeat sizes of 41 to 58. Ovarian failure occurred at as early as 11 years of age. In contrast, carriers of full mutation alleles are not at increased risk for POF.

Prevalence estimates of the fragile X syndrome have been revised downward since the isolation of the gene in 1991. Despite this, the original estimates are still occasionally quoted in the fragile X literature. Most recent studies using molecular genetic testing have estimated a prevalence of 1 in 4000 males. The prevalence of affected females is presumed to be approximately one half of the male prevalence.

Fragile X syndrome is inherited in X-linked dominant fashion. The molecular mutations leading to this syndrome result from expansion of a trinucleotide repeat (CGG) causing aberrant methylation of the gene. This results in decreased or complete absence of the protein gene product termed *fragile X mental retardation 1 protein* (FMR-1 protein). This protein is found in the cytoplasm of many cells but is most abundant in neurons.[232] The function of the protein remains unknown, but its absence leads to developmental abnormalities.

FMR-1 alleles are categorized according to the repeat number, which is correlated with the likelihood of expansion during maternal meiosis and the clinical manifestations. However, the distinction between allele categories is not absolute and must be made by considering both family history and repeat instability. Normal alleles are approximately 5 to 40 repeats. Alleles of this size are stably transmitted without any increase or decrease in repeat number. In these stable normal alleles, the CGG region is interrupted by an AGG triplet after every nine or 10 CGG repeats. These AGG triplets are believed to maintain repeat integrity by preventing DNA strand slippage during replication. Mutable normal alleles or intermediate alleles (also termed gray zone) may be broadly defined as 41 to 58 repeats. The risk for instability of alleles with 41 to 49 repeats when transmitted from parent to child is minimal. Any changes in repeat number are typically very small (plus or minus one or two repeats). Historically, the largest repeat included in the intermediate range has been 54. In fact, the intermediate range may extend slightly higher, as no transmission of alleles with 58 or fewer repeats is known to have resulted in an affected individual. Because most clinical testing laboratories state that repeat measurements are plus or minus two to three repeats, it may be wise to consider reported test results with 55 to 58 repeats as potential premutations.

Premutation alleles of approximately 59 to 200 repeats have an increased risk of expansion to a full mutation and of causing the clinical phenotype. Alleles of this size are not associated with mental retardation but do convey increased risk for FXTAS and POF. Because of potential repeat instability with transmission of premutation alleles through maternal meiosis, women with alleles in this range are considered to be at risk for having children affected with fragile X syndrome and should consider prenatal diagnosis. Full mutation alleles are those with more than 200 repeats, with several hundred to several thousand repeats being typical. Aberrant hypermethylation of the deoxycytidylate residues contained in the CGG repeats usually occurs once repeat expansion exceeds approximately 200, leading to complete absence of FMR-1. This results in the complete fragile X phenotype in males. The phenotype of full mutation females, although also dependent on the size of the mutation, can be modified by random inactivation of either the normal or mutated X chromosome in the brain.[233] Approximately 50% of females who have a full fragile X mutation are mentally retarded but are usually less severely affected than males with the full mutation.[234] Importantly, about 50% of females who are heterozygotes for the full mutation are intellectually normal.[235]

The probability of a carrier of a premutation having a child with a full mutation depends on both the size of the premutation and the sex of the carrier. When premutations are transmitted by the father, only small increases in the trinucleotide repeat number may occur, and they do not result in full mutations. All daughters of "transmitting males" are unaffected premutation carriers, with the potential of subsequent expansion in their offspring. Women who are premutation carriers have a 50% risk of transmitting the abnormal chromosome in each pregnancy.[236] Their risk of having an offspring with a full mutation is based on their premutation size. Table 17-24 demonstrates the likelihood of expansion to a full mutation based on the maternal premutation size. In these cases, prenatal diagnosis should be offered.

The presence of normal transmitting males and the variable likelihood of full expansion by females carrying a premutation will lead to pedigrees with skipped generations or the seemingly spontaneous occurrence of the fragile X syndrome.[237] Therefore, carrier testing should be offered to all individuals seeking reproductive counseling who have either a family history of fragile X syndrome or undiagnosed mental retardation in individuals of either sex.[227]

Some centers offer all women seeking prenatal diagnosis the opportunity to have fragile X testing performed as part of routine screening. This approach is based on evidence that the frequency of the premutation is relatively high in the general population. One study of a French-Canadian population found that 1 in 259 women had a premutation in the FMR-1 gene.[238] A more recent study of 14,334 Israeli women of child-bearing age identified 127 carriers with greater than 54 repeats, including three asymptomatic women with full mutations, representing a prevalence of 1 in 113 (885 in 100,000).[237] The benefits of such a screening strategy have not been demonstrated.

Methodologies for molecular testing vary from laboratory to laboratory. Most laboratories screen patient DNA samples by the polymerase chain reaction (PCR) specific for the trinucleotide repeat region of the FMR-1 gene.[239] This technique has high sensitivity for FMR-1 repeats in the normal and lower premutation range but may rarely fail to detect FMR-1 alleles in the upper premutation range. It also can fail to detect full mutations with a high repeat number (especially when used for prenatal testing). Because of these limitations, many laboratories also perform Southern blot analysis, which will detect the presence of full mutations and large premutations. When PCR reveals a normal or premutation allele size in male patients or two alleles within the normal or premutation range in female patients, further testing by Southern blot is not necessary.[240,241]

Prenatal testing for fetuses at increased risk for FMR-1 full mutations is performed using DNA extracted from either amniocytes or chorionic villi. The Southern blot patterns for DNA expansions derived from amniocytes are identical to those found in adult tissues. However, unreliable methylation patterns can occur in DNA from cells obtained by CVS because methylation of villus tissue may occur at varying gestational ages.[242] Because the methylation pattern is predictive of gene function, it is occasionally used to make the distinction between a large premutation and a small full mutation. As a result, on occasion, follow-up amniocentesis or testing using PCR to determine the size of the FMR-1 alleles may be required. Chromosome analysis for fragile X status using modified culture techniques to induce the fragile sites seen in the affected X chromosomes is no longer used for diagnosis because of low sensitivity and increased cost when compared with DNA testing. Because of the complexity of FMR-1 trinucleotide repeat expansion detection and the accompanying methylation issues, a laboratory with known competence for FMR-1 prenatal molecular testing is strongly suggested.[239,241,243]

TABLE 17-24 RISKS FOR EXPANSION FROM A MATERNAL PREMUTATION TO A FULL MUTATION WHEN TRANSMITTED TO OFFSPRING

Number of Maternal Premutation CGG Repeats	Total Maternal Transmissions	Expansions to Full Mutations (%)*
55-59	27	1 (3.7%)
60-69	113	6 (5.3%)
70-79	90	28 (31.1%)
80-89	140	81 (57.8%)
90-99	111	89 (80.1%)
100-109	70	70 (100%)
110-119	54	53 (98.1%)
120-129	36	35 (97.2%)
130-139	18	17 (94.4%)
140-200	19	19 (100%)

***Unlike in classic X-linked dominant disorders, in which all females with a mutation are affected, only about 50% of females with a full mutation are mentally retarded. This variability in phenotype is likely to be related to X-chromosome inactivation, a phenomenon independent of *FMR1* mutations.**

Adapted from Nolin SL, Brown WT, Glicksman A, et al: Expansion of the fragile X CGG repeat in females with premutation or intermediate alleles. Am J Hum Genet 72:454-464, 2003.

Diagnostic Tests

Indications for Invasive Testing

Indications for diagnostic testing are dominated by advanced maternal age (>35 years) and positive screening tests and have been discussed. A prior history of a fetus with a chromosomal abnormality is the next most frequent indication for cytogenetic testing. The recurrence risk after the birth of one child with trisomy 21 varies in the literature, with most studies quoting an empiric risk of approximately 1% to 1.5% for any trisomy.[244] Closer scrutiny suggests that the risk depends on the age of the mother at the birth of the initial trisomic child. Warburton and colleagues[245] demonstrated that if the initial trisomic child is born when a mother is less than 30 years old, a future pregnancy born while the mother is still under 30 years old has an eightfold increased risk over maternal age risk. This usually results in a risk of just under 1%. If the initial trisomy 21 birth occurred when the mother was older than 30, the risk of another trisomic child is not statistically greater than her age-related risk at the time of the next pregnancy.

The risk of a liveborn trisomic child after a trisomy 21 conception that was either spontaneously or electively terminated is uncertain. The work of Warburton and colleagues[246] suggests that the karyotype of a miscarried pregnancy may predict the karyotype of subsequent miscarriages, but the relevance of this to live births is uncertain. Presently, most authorities recommend the conservative approach of offering the same risks as for a liveborn conception, so prenatal diagnosis in subsequent pregnancies is recommended.

After the birth of two or more trisomy 21 pregnancies, the possibility that one of the parents is either a somatic or germ cell mosaic for Down syndrome must be considered, and peripheral blood chromosome studies of the parents should be offered. Uchida and Freeman[247] reported parental mosaicism in 2.7% to 4.3% of peripheral karyotypes in such parents. Mothers appeared to have a higher risk than fathers. The risk of recurrence in these families may be as high as 10% to 20%, and prenatal testing is indicated.

About 3% to 5% of Down syndrome cases are secondary to either a de novo or an inherited Robertsonian translocation. If the translocation is de novo, risk of another affected child is minimal, although gonadal mosaicism leading to a recurrence has been suspected in some families. Prenatal diagnosis may be offered in these cases. If the balanced translocation is present in the mother, the overall risk of an unbalanced liveborn Down syndrome child is 10% to 15% but varies according to the specific translocation (Table 17-25). If the translocation is paternal, the risk of an unbalanced offspring is approximately 0.5%, but this also depends on the nature of the translocation. In all cases of parental translocation, prenatal diagnosis is indicated.

Some offspring with inherited balanced Robertsonian translocations have been found to have uniparental disomy (UPD). This can have phenotypic consequences if chromosome 14 or 15 is involved. When a balanced Robertsonian translocation involving one of these acrocentric chromosomes is present in a pregnancy, additional testing for UPD is indicated.[248]

TABLE 17-25 PARENTAL CARRIER OF ROBERTSONIAN TRANSLOCATION: EMPIRIC RISK FOR DOWN SYNDROME LIVE BIRTH

Carrier	Risk for Down Syndrome Live Births
Mother: 13/21, 14/21, 15/21 translocation	10.0%-15%
Mother: 21/22 translocation	4.0%-15%
Father: 13/21, 14/21, 15/21 translocation	0.5%-5%
Father: 21/22 translocation	0.5%-2%
Either parent: 21/21	100%

The recurrence risk after the birth of a child with a trisomy other than 21 is poorly quantified. In a recent collaborative study of 1076 Japanese women with a history of a previous trisomy in whom second-trimester amniocentesis was performed, none of the 170 women with previous trisomy 18 offspring and none of the 46 women with a previous trisomy 13 offspring had another such fetus.[249] In general, an empiric risk of about 1% is appropriate, and prenatal diagnosis should be offered.

A previous 45X pregnancy does not significantly increase the risk of a recurrence, but cases of maternal 45X/46XX mosaicism leading to a second affected child have been described.[250] The recurrence after a triploid pregnancy is exceedingly low but has been reported to occur.[200]

Other cytogenetic indications for invasive testing include a parental reciprocal translocation or inversion, a parent or previous child with a mosaic karyotype or marker chromosome, or a sex chromosome/autosome translocation. The risk of an unbalanced offspring in these cases depends on the mode of ascertainment and the specific rearrangement, and genetic counseling is recommended.

Prenatal invasive testing is also indicated to obtain material for biochemical or DNA studies. The molecular abnormalities responsible for many disorders are being identified at a rapid rate, and any listing of these is soon outdated. A list of the more common genetic conditions for which DNA-based prenatal diagnosis is available is given in Table 17-26. A more detailed list, and a list of the centers performing each test, can be found at www.genetests.org. Many of these conditions are rare and their diagnosis is complex, so consultation with a genetics unit is encouraged before performing an invasive test.

Ultrasound identification of fetal structural anomalies is increasing in frequency as an indication for invasive testing. In addition to major structural defects that have long been known to be associated with fetal aneuploidy, more subtle markers have been demonstrated to increase the risk.[251,252] In addition, ultrasound markers for fetal infection, anemia, or other disorders frequently requires evaluation by amniocentesis.

Amniocentesis

Historical Perspective

Amniocentesis was first performed in the 1880s for decompression of polyhydramnios.[253,254] It was during the 1950s that it became a significant diagnostic tool, when measurement of amniotic fluid bilirubin concentration began to be used in the monitoring of Rh isoimmunization.[255,256] In that same decade, amniotic fluid investigation for fetal chromosome analysis was initiated, as laboratory techniques for cell culture and karyotyping were developed. The first reported applications were limited to fetal sex determination by Barr body analysis.[257] The feasibility of culturing and karyotyping amniotic fluid cells was demonstrated in 1966,[258] and the first prenatal diagnosis of an abnormal karyotype, a balanced translocation, was reported in 1967.[259]

Technique of Amniocentesis

Mid-trimester amniocentesis for genetic evaluation is most commonly performed between 15 and 18 weeks' gestation. At this age, the amount of fluid is adequate (approximately 150 mL), and the ratio of viable to nonviable cells is greatest. Before the procedure, an ultrasound scan is performed to determine the number of fetuses, confirm gestational age, ensure fetal viability, document anatomy, and locate the placenta

TABLE 17-26 COMMON CONDITIONS FOR WHICH MOLECULAR PRENATAL DIAGNOSIS IS AVAILABLE

Disorder	Mode of Inheritance	Prenatal Diagnosis
α_1-Antitrypsin deficiency	AR	Determine PiZZ allele. Not all homozygotes have liver involvement; pre-procedure genetic counseling critical.
α-Thalassemia	AR	α-Hemoglobin gene mutation (see text)
Adult polycystic kidney	AD	PKD1 and PKD2 gene mutations. In large families, linkage is possible in >90%. Gene mutation identifiable in ~50% of PKD1 and 75% of PKD2.
β-Thalassemia	AR	β-Hemoglobin gene mutation (see text)
Congenital adrenal hyperplasia	AR	*CYP21A2* gene mutations/deletions. Nine common mutations/deletions detect 90% to 95% of carriers. Sequencing available.
Cystic fibrosis	AR	CFTR gene mutation (see text)
Duchenne/Becker muscular dystrophy	XLR	Dystrophin gene mutation
Fragile X syndrome	XLR	CGG repeat number (see text)
Hemoglobinopathy (SS, SC)	AR	β-Chain gene mutation (see text)
Hemophilia A	XLR	Factor VIII gene inversion 45%, other gene mutations 45% (not available in all labs), linkage analysis in appropriate families.
Huntington disease	AD	CAG repeat length (PGD and non-informing PND possible to avoid disclosing presymptomatic parents' disease status).
Marfan syndrome	AD	Fibrillin (FBN-1) gene mutation. Linkage in large families. Approximately 70% have mutation identified (not always clinically available).
Myotonic dystrophy	AD	CTG expansion in the *DMPK* gene
Neurofibromatosis type 1	AD	NF1 gene mutation identifiable in >95% of cases but requires sequencing. Linkage in appropriate families.
Phenylketonuria	AR	4 to 15 common mutations, 40% to 50% detection. Further mutation analysis > 99%.
Spinal muscular atrophy	AR/AD	
Tay-Sachs disease	AR	Enzyme absence; gene mutation (see text)

AD, autosomal dominant; AR, autosomal recessive; PGD, preimplantation genetic diagnosis; PND, prenatal diagnosis; XLR, X-linked recessive.

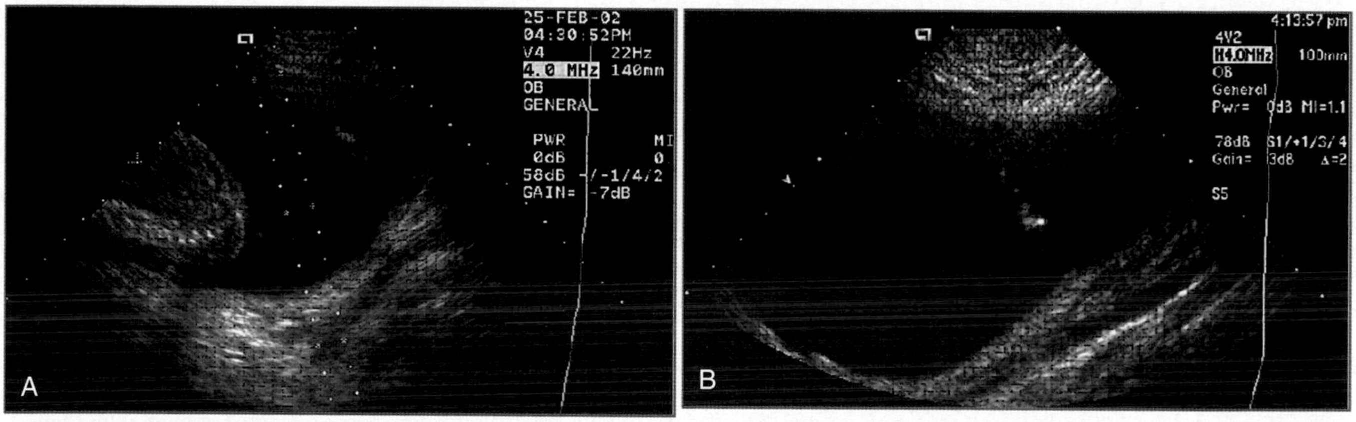

FIGURE 17-7 Ultrasound for amniocentesis procedure. Amniocentesis can be performed with a needle guide (**A**) or by free-hand technique (**B**). Either technique can be used, and the choice is usually by practitioner preference. Needle guides can be helpful when one member of the team (operator or sonographer) is less experienced or when dealing with oligohydramnios or morbid obesity.

and cord insertion. After an appropriate sampling path has been chosen, the maternal abdomen is washed with antiseptic solution. Continuously guided by ultrasound, a 20- to 22-gauge needle is introduced into a pocket of amniotic fluid free of fetal parts and umbilical cord (Fig. 17-7). The pocket should be large enough to allow advancement of the needle tip through the free-floating amniotic membrane that may occasionally obstruct the flow of fluid. The first 1 to 2 mL of aspirated amniotic fluid is discarded to prevent maternal cell contamination of the tissue culture, and then 20 to 30 mL of amniotic fluid is withdrawn. Fetal heart rate and activity are documented immediately after the procedure.

Transplacental passage of the needle should be avoided when possible, but if it is unavoidable, attempts should be made to traverse the thinnest portion, away from the placental edge and the umbilical cord insertion.[260] If the placenta must be traversed, color Doppler is helpful to avoid any large fetal vessels at the sampling site. The area close to the placental cord insertion should be avoided, because it contains the largest vessels. Using this approach, transplacental amniocentesis does not increase fetal loss rates in the hands of experienced operators.[261,262]

Amniocentesis should be performed using continuous ultrasound guidance. Guidance should be maintained throughout the procedure to avoid inadvertent puncture of the fetus and to identify uterine contractions that occasionally retract the needle tip back into the myometrium. Romero and colleagues[263] showed that continuous guidance decreases the number of insertions as well as of dry and bloody taps.

The procedure may be performed either freehand or with a needle guide.[260,264] The freehand technique allows easier manipulation of the needle if the position of the target is abruptly altered by a uterine contraction or fetal movement. On the other hand, a needle guide allows more certain ascertainment of the needle entry point and a more precise pre-entry determination of the sampling path. The guide may allow easier sampling in certain situations, such as when oligohydramnios is present or for patients who are morbidly obese. A needle guide is especially helpful for relatively inexperienced operators or sonographers. Most guides now allow easy intraoperative removal of the needle from the guide and quick adaptation to freehand guidance once the uterus has been entered.[265]

If the initial attempt to obtain fluid is unsuccessful, a second attempt in another location should be performed after reevaluation of the fetal and placental positions. Amniotic membrane tenting and the development of needle-induced uterine wall contractions are most frequently the cause of initial failure. No more than two attempts should be made at any single session. If two attempts have been unsuccessful, the patient may be rescheduled in several days. Studies have demonstrated that fetal loss rate increases with the number of insertions. Marthin and coworkers[262] reported a postamniocentesis loss rate of 3.8% after three insertions, compared with 1.2% after a single pass. Loss rates do not increase with the number of separate procedures. In experienced centers, return visits are rarely required, occurring in less than 1% of cases.[266]

Laboratory Considerations for Amniocentesis

The cells within the amniotic fluid arise from the fetal skin, respiratory tract, urinary tract, gastrointestinal tract, and placenta. After retrieval, the cells are put into tissue culture, either in flasks or more often on coverslips. After 3 to 7 days of growth, sufficient mitoses are present for staining and karyotype analysis. Cells grown in flasks are harvested and analyzed together, whereas those grown on coverslips are analyzed in situ as individual colonies. Amniocyte culture is quite reliable, with failure occurring in less than 1% of cases.

MOSAIC RESULTS

Chromosomal mosaicism—the presence of two or more cell lines with different karyotypes in a single sample—occurs in approximately 0.1% to 0.3% of amniocentesis cases. This most frequently results from postzygotic nondisjunction,[267] but it can also occur from meiotic errors with trisomic rescue (see Laboratory Aspects of Chorionic Villus Sampling, later). The most common etiology is pseudomosaicism,[267] where the abnormality is evident in only one of several flasks or confined to a single colony on a coverslip. In this case, the abnormal cells have arisen in vitro, are not present in the fetus, and are not clinically important. Even the observation of multiple cell lines on more than one coverslip or in more than one flask in a sample does not necessarily mean that the fetus is mosaic, because the results are confirmed in only 70% of cases.[268] Some mosaic results (e.g., trisomy 20) occur in the amniotic fluid relatively frequently but are rarely confirmed in the fetus.[269]

True fetal mosaicism is rare, occurring in 0.25% of amniocenteses, but can be clinically important, leading to phenotypic or developmental abnormalities.[267] In many cases, the question of whether amniotic fluid mosaicism involves the fetus can be resolved by karyotyping fetal lymphocytes obtained by percutaneous umbilical blood sampling (PUBS).[270] However, this approach may not be valid in all cases, because the mosaic cell line may involve fetal tissues but be excluded from the fetal hematopoietic compartment and therefore not present in a fetal blood sample.[269] Certain chromosomes, such as 22, are notorious for exclusion from fetal blood and may require testing of additional fetal tissues such as the skin.[271]

Evaluation of mosaic results should include detailed ultrasound assessment to assess fetal growth and exclude structural anomalies. If both ultrasound and fetal sampling are normal, the parents can be reassured that, in most cases, the fetus is unaffected.[270] However, a small chance of fetal involvement still exists because the presence of an undetectable but clinically significant abnormal cell line can never be absolutely excluded. Because of the complexity of interpreting mosaic amniotic fluid results, consultation with a cytogenetics laboratory and a clinical geneticist is recommended.

USE OF FLUORESCENCE IN SITU HYBRIDIZATION

Fluorescence in situ hybridization (FISH) probes are relatively short, fluorescence-labeled DNA sequences that are hybridized to a known location on a specific chromosome and allow the number and location of specific DNA sequences to be determined. Interphase cells are evaluated by counting the number of discrete fluorescent signals from each probe. A normal diploid cell queried with a probe for the centromere of chromosome 18 would have two signals, whereas a trisomy 18 cell would have three.

Prenatal interphase evaluation of uncultured amniotic fluid can detect aneuploidies caused by monosomies, free trisomies, trisomies associated with robertsonian translocations, triploidy, and other numerical chromosomal abnormalities. In standard practice, probes involving chromosomes 13, 18, 21, X, and Y are used. This technology does not routinely detect cytogenetic abnormalities such as mosaics, translocations, and rare aneuploidies.[272,273]

Since 1993, the position of the American College of Medical Genetics has been that prenatal FISH is investigational. In 1997, the U.S. Food and Drug Administration cleared the specific FISH probes to enumerate chromosomes 13, 18, 21, X, and Y for prenatal diagnosis. Subsequent studies demonstrate an extremely high concordance rate between FISH and standard cytogenetics (99.8%) for the specific abnormalities that the assay is designed to detect.[274-277] These performance characteristics support the use of FISH for prenatal testing when a diagnosis of aneuploidy of chromosome 13, 18, 21, X, or Y is highly suspected by virtue of maternal age, positive maternal serum biochemical screening, or abnormal ultrasound findings.[278]

Presently, it is suggested that FISH analysis not be used as a primary screening test on all genetic amniocenteses because of its inability to detect structural rearrangements, mosaicism, markers, and uncommon trisomies. Evans and coworkers[279] surveyed the results of almost 73,000 prenatal cases from seven centers and reported that only 67% of abnormalities would have been detected by routine FISH. This interpretation may be misleading in that some of the missed abnormalities would not have had an impact on fetal development. Because all abnormalities would be detectable by tissue culture, FISH analysis is not cost-effective. Most laboratories use FISH to offer quick reassurance to patients with an unusually high degree of anxiety, or to test fetuses at the highest risk, such as those with ultrasound anomalies. It is also beneficial when rapid results are crucial to subsequent management, such as with advanced gestational age. FISH on metaphase chromosomes using probes for unique sequences has greatly expanded the resolution of conventional chromosome analysis. This has been demonstrated in countless case reports by the diagnosis of structural changes at the submicroscopic level (e.g., microdeletion syndromes) or by the determination of the origin of marker chromosomes and complex structural changes.[200]

Complications of Amniocentesis

A common finding after amniocentesis is cramping that lasts for 1 to 2 hours. Lower abdominal discomfort may occur for up to 48 hours after the procedure but is usually not severe. Fortunately, serious maternal complications such as septic shock are rare. Amnionitis occurs in 0.1% of cases[280] and can occur from contamination of the amniotic fluid with skin flora or from inadvertent puncture of the maternal bowel. It may also follow procedure-induced amnion rupture. Postamniocentesis chorioamnionitis can have an insidious onset and frequently appears with flulike symptoms and with few early localizing signs. This can evolve into a systemic infection with marked maternal morbidity unless early aggressive treatment is undertaken. Therefore, a high index of suspicion is necessary.

The development of rhesus isoimmunization occurs in approximately 1% of Rh-negative women undergoing amniocentesis,[281-283] but it can be avoided by prophylactic administration of anti-D immunoglobulin after the procedure.

Amniotic fluid leakage or vaginal bleeding is noted by 2% to 3% of patients after amniocentesis. Unlike spontaneous second-trimester amnion rupture, which has a dismal prognosis, fluid leakage after amniocentesis usually resolves after a few days of bed rest. Successful pregnancy outcome after such an event is common.[284] Occasionally, leakage of amniotic fluid persists throughout pregnancy,[285,286] but if the amniotic fluid volume remains adequate, a good outcome can be anticipated.

Pregnancy Loss after Mid-Trimester Amniocentesis

The safety of mid-trimester amniocentesis was documented in the mid 1970s by three collaborative studies performed in the United Kingdom, the United States, and Canada.[285,287,288] These studies, performed prior to the clinical use of ultrasound, were not randomized but rather included unsampled matched control groups. The U.S. and Canadian studies showed similar loss rates (spontaneous abortions, stillbirths, and neonatal deaths) between the two groups. A greater risk of loss occurred with needles of 19 gauge or larger and with more than two needle insertions per procedure. Both studies reported total postprocedure loss rates of 3% to 4%.

In contrast to these studies, the British Collaborative Study found an excess of fetal loss (1% to 1.5%) in the amniocentesis group compared with control subjects. This study has been criticized for a number of concerns, including a significant proportion of sampled patients with elevated MSAFP levels, an unusually low complication rate in the control group, and a change in the matching criteria during the study.

Seeds[289] performed a contemporary review of more than 68,000 amniocenteses from centers reporting 1000 or more procedures and analyzed results from both controlled and noncontrolled studies (Table 17-27). From this analysis he concluded the following:

TABLE 17-27 STUDIES* DESCRIBING ULTRASOUND GUIDANCE TO VISUALIZE NEEDLE PLACEMENT

Study (ref)	Amniocentesis cases (N)	Losses at ≤28 Weeks' Gestation (n)	Control Type, No. of Losses (No. of Control Subjects)	Comment
Farahani et al (530), 1984	2100	19 (0.9%)	Unmatched, 11 (2200)	No fetal trauma detected
Leschot et al (531), 1985	2920	64 (2.19%)		First 1500 cases were in Verjaal and Leschot
Dacus et al (293), 1985	1981	32 (1.6%)		Risk increased with the number of passes, bloody fluid, or no ultrasound scan
Tabor et al (294), 1986	2242	29 (1.3%)	Randomized, 8 (2270)	18-gauge needle; more risk with transplacental; losses through 24 wk of gestation
Andreason and Kristoffersen (532), 1989	1289	28 (2.2%)	Unmatched, 2 (258)	More risk with transplacental
Bombard et al (261), 1995	1000	12 (1.3%)		More risk, but not significant with transplacental
Marthin et al (262), 1997	2083	28 (1.3%)		No increase with transplacental
Canadian Early and Mid Trimester Amniocentesis Trial (266), 1999	2090	40 (1.9%)		
Eiben et al (533), 1997	1802	12 (0.8%)		
Tongsong et al (534), 1998	2045	36 (1.8%)	Matched, 29 (2045)	
Roper et al (535), 1999	2924	35 (1.2%)		
Reid et al (536), 1999	3774	29 (0.8%)		More risk, but not significant with transplacental
Antsaklis et al (291), 2000	3696	79 (2.1%)	Unmatched, 80 (5324)	
Horger et al (537), 2001	4198	35 (0.83%)		Losses only to 60 days after procedure
Totals	34,144	478 (1.4%)	130/12097 (1.08%)	

*Studies include those with at least 1000 cases, with or without control subjects.
From Seeds JW: Diagnostic mid trimester amniocentesis: How safe? Am J Obstet Gynecol 191:607-615, 2004.

1. Amniocentesis with concurrent ultrasound guidance is associated with a procedure-related rate of excess pregnancy loss of 0.33% (95% CI, 0.09 to 0.56) in a comparison of all studies. . Among only controlled studies, the procedure-related rate of loss is 0.6% (95% CI, 0.31 to 0.90). When calculating the total postprocedure rate of loss (to 28 weeks' gestation), the procedure-induced losses should be added to the 1.08% rate of natural losses occurring in women not undergoing amniocentesis.
2. The use of concurrent ultrasound guidance appears to reduce the number of punctures and the incidence of bloody fluid. In a comparison of all studies, pregnancy loss is diminished with the use of concurrent ultrasound guidance; however, when only controlled studies are compared, this trend remains, but the advantage is not significant.
3. The reported experience does not support an increased rate of pregnancy loss after placental puncture. Transplacental amniocentesis is associated with an aggregate rate of reported loss of 1.4%, which is identical to the overall rate of loss among all amniocentesis patients and lower than that reported from controlled studies.

Certain clinical factors influence the risk of pregnancy loss, independent of the amniocentesis procedure. For example, spontaneous abortion is more common in older patients and may be more common among patients of any age with an abnormal serum screen result. A prior pregnancy loss is reported to increase the risk, as is previous vaginal bleeding. The number of needle placements, the observation of bloody fluid, and especially the observation of green or murky fluid are seen to be associated with a significantly increased risk of pregnancy loss after amniocentesis.[290-295]

The only prospective randomized controlled trial evaluating the safety of second-trimester amniocentesis is a Danish study, which reported on 4606 low-risk healthy women, 25 to 34 years old, who were randomly allocated to either amniocentesis or ultrasound examination.[294] The total fetal loss rate in the amniocentesis group was 1.7% and in the control subjects, 0.7% ($P < .01$). The observed difference of 1% (95% CI, 0.3 to 1.5) gave a relative risk of 2.3. The conclusions of this study were initially criticized because the original report stated that a 17-gauge needle (which is associated with higher risks than smaller needles) was used. Tabor and colleagues[295] subsequently reported that they had in fact used a 20-gauge needle for most of the procedures.

Both the U.K. and Danish studies[290,294] found an increase in respiratory distress syndrome and pneumonia in neonates from the amniocentesis groups. Other studies have not found this association. The U.K. study also showed an increased incidence of talipes and dislocation of the hip in the amniocentesis group.[288] This finding has not been confirmed.

In early experience with amniocentesis, needle puncture of the fetus was reported in 0.1% to 3.0% of cases[285,296] and was associated with fetal exsanguination,[297] intestinal atresia,[298,299] ileocutaneous fistula,[300] gangrene of a fetal limb,[301] uniocular blindness,[302] porencephalic cysts,[303] patellar tendon disruption,[304] skin dimples,[305] and peripheral nerve damage.[296] Continuous use of ultrasound to guide the needle minimizes needle puncture of the fetus, which, in experienced centers, is an exceedingly rare but still seen complication.[289]

No long-term adverse effects have been demonstrated in children undergoing amniocentesis. Baird and colleagues[306] compared 1296 liveborn children whose mothers had a mid-trimester amniocentesis to unsampled control subjects. With the exception of hemolytic disease resulting from isoimmunization, the offspring of women who had amniocentesis were no more likely than control subjects to have a disability during childhood and adolescence. Finegan and colleagues[307] reported an increased incidence of middle-ear abnormalities in children whose mothers had amniocentesis.

Amniocentesis Performed before 15 Weeks' Gestation (Early Amniocentesis)

The desire for a first-trimester diagnosis stimulated interest in the feasibility of performing amniocentesis at less than 15 weeks' gestation. The technique at this gestational age varies from conventional amniocentesis in that less fluid is available and incomplete fusion of the amnion and chorion frequently cause tenting of the membranes, resulting in failed procedures in 2% to 3% of cases.[266,308]

Although initial experience with early amniocentesis was reassuring,[309-312] subsequent studies have raised serious concerns about its safety. In 1994, Nicolaides and coworkers[313] reported on more than 1300 women undergoing first-trimester diagnoses. In this study, significantly higher rates of fetal loss (5.3% versus 2.3%) were seen in the early amniocentesis group. This finding was echoed by Vandenbussche and coworkers,[314] who reported a 6.7% higher occurrence of pregnancy loss for early amniocentesis compared with CVS. Sundberg and colleagues,[315] in a prospective randomized comparison of CVS to early amniocentesis, also found a higher loss rate with early amniocentesis but had to terminate the study early because of an unanticipated increase in talipes equinovarus (clubfoot) in the early amniocentesis group. Higher loss rates have also been found when comparing early amniocentesis to second-trimester amniocentesis. The Canadian Early and Mid-Trimester Amniocentesis trial reported a 1.7% higher incidence of fetal loss in the early amniocentesis group compared with second-trimester sampling when taking all fetal losses into account (7.6% versus 5.9%).[308] There is also an increased frequency of culture failure and ruptured membranes compared with later procedures.[308,313,315]

Of most concern is that fetal talipes equinovarus occurs in 1% to 2% of cases sampled by early amniocentesis.[308,313,315,316] This rate is 10-fold higher than the 1 per 1000 births seen in the U.S. population. The clubfoot deformities are believed to occur secondary to procedure-induced fluid leakage, because they occurred in 1% of cases in which no leakage occurred and in 15% of cases when leakage occurred.[308] For these reasons, amniocentesis should rarely, if ever, be performed before the 13th week of gestation. The safety of amniocentesis in weeks 13 and 14 is uncertain. Until its safety can be ensured, it is best to delay routine sampling until week 15 or 16 of pregnancy.

Chorionic Villus Sampling

The major drawbacks of conventional second-trimester genetic amniocentesis are the delayed availability of the karyotype and the increased medical risks of a pregnancy termination late in pregnancy. Furthermore, delaying the procedure until after fetal movement is appreciated by the mother is believed to inflict a severe emotional burden on the patient. As a result of these concerns, attempts have been made to move prenatal diagnosis into the first trimester. CVS, which samples the developing placenta rather than penetrating the amniotic membrane, has been the most successful approach to date at accomplishing this.

History of Chorionic Villus Sampling

The ability to sample and analyze villus tissue was demonstrated more than 25 years ago by the Chinese, who, in an attempt to develop a technique for fetal sex determination, inserted a thin catheter into the uterus guided only by tactile sensation.[317] When resistance from the gestational sac was felt, suction was applied and small pieces of villi were aspirated. Although this approach seems crude by today's standards of ultrasonically guided invasive procedures, their diagnostic accuracy and low miscarriage rate demonstrated the feasibility of first-trimester sampling.

Initial experiences in other parts of the world were not as promising. In 1968, Hahnemann and Mohr[318] attempted blind transcervical trophoblast biopsy in 12 patients using a 6-mm diameter instrument. Although successful tissue culture was possible, half of these subjects subsequently aborted. In 1973, Kullander and Sandahl[319] used a 5-mm-diameter fiberoptic endocervicoscope with biopsy forceps to perform transcervical CVS in patients requesting pregnancy termination. Although tissue culture was successful in approximately half of the cases, two subjects subsequently became septic.

In 1974, Hahnemann[320] described further experience with first-trimester prenatal diagnosis using a 2.5-mm hysteroscope and a cylindrical biopsy knife. Once again, significant complications, including inadvertent rupture of the amniotic sac, were encountered. By this time, the safety of mid-trimester genetic amniocentesis had become well established, and further attempts at first-trimester prenatal diagnosis were temporarily abandoned in the Western Hemisphere.

Two technologic advances occurred in the early 1980s that allowed reintroduction of CVS. The first of these was the development of real-time sonography, making continuous guidance possible. At the same time, sampling instruments were miniaturized and refined. In 1982, Kazy and associates[321] reported the first transcervical CVS performed with real-time sonographic guidance. That same year, Old and colleagues[322] reported the first-trimester diagnosis of β-thalassemia major using DNA from chorionic villi obtained by sonographically guided transcervical aspiration with a 1.5-mm-diameter polyethylene catheter. Using a similar sampling technique, Brambati and Simoni[323] diagnosed trisomy 21 at 11 weeks' gestation.

After these preliminary reports, several CVS programs were established both in Europe and the United States, with the outcomes informally reported to a World Health Organization (WHO)-sponsored registry maintained at Jefferson Medical College in Philadelphia. This registry, along with single-center reports, was used to estimate the safety of CVS until 1989, when two prospective multicenter studies, one from Canada[324] and one from the United States,[325] were published and confirmed the safety of the procedure.

Technique of Transcervical Chorionic Villus Sampling

Ultrasound examination immediately before the procedure confirms fetal heart activity, appropriate size, and placental location. The position of the uterus and cervix is determined, and a catheter path is mapped. If the uterus is anteverted, additional filling of the bladder can be used to straighten the uterine position. Although most procedures require a moderately filled bladder, an overfilled bladder is discouraged, because it lifts the uterus out of the pelvis, lengthening the sampling path, which can diminish the flexibility required for catheter manipulation. Occasionally, a uterine contraction interferes with passage of the catheter. Delaying the procedure until the contraction dissipates is suggested (Fig. 17-8).

When the uterine condition and location are favorable, the patient is placed in the lithotomy position, and the vulva and vagina are aseptically prepared with povidone-iodine solution. A speculum is inserted, and the cervix is similarly prepared. The distal 3 to 5 cm of the sampling catheter is molded into a slightly curved shape and the catheter gently passed under ultrasound guidance through the cervix until a loss of resistance is felt at the endocervix. The operator then waits until the sonographer visualizes the catheter tip. The catheter is then advanced parallel to the chorionic membranes to the distal edge of the placenta. The stylet is then removed and a 20-mL syringe containing nutrient medium is attached. Negative pressure is applied by means of the syringe and the catheter removed slowly.

The syringe is then visually inspected for villi. These can frequently be seen with the naked eye as white branching structures floating in the medium. On occasion, however, viewing the samples under a low-power dissecting microscope is necessary to confirm the presence of sufficient villi. Maternal decidua is frequently retrieved with the sample but is usually easily recognized by its amorphous appearance. If sufficient villi are not retrieved with the initial pass, a second insertion can be made with minimal impact on pregnancy loss rate.

Technique of Transabdominal Chorionic Villus Sampling

Continuous ultrasound is used to direct a 19- or 20-gauge spinal needle into the long axis of the placenta (Fig. 17-9). After removal of the stylet, villi are aspirated into a 20-mL syringe containing tissue culture media. Because the needle is somewhat smaller than

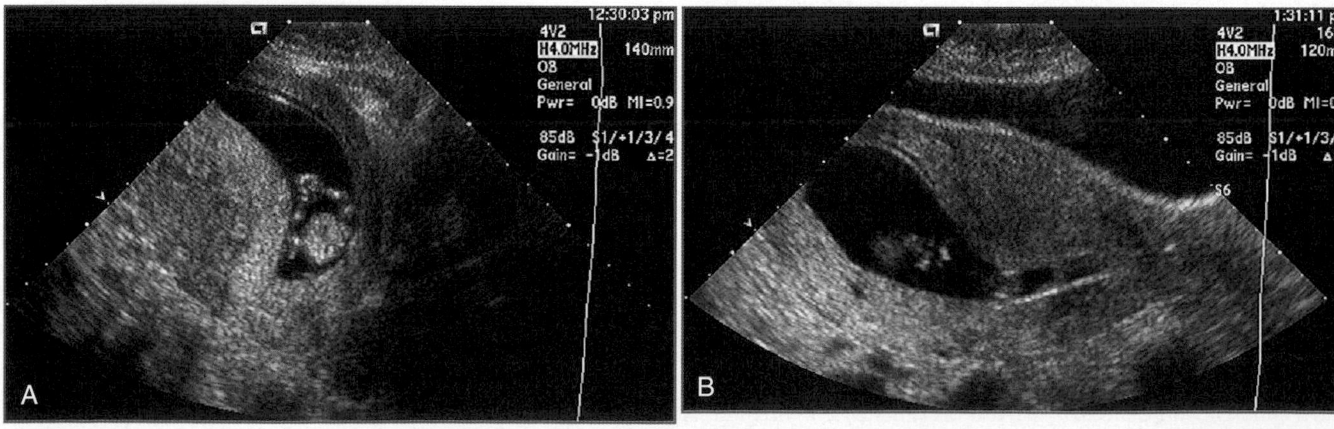

FIGURE 17-8 Ultrasound photos of a transcervical chorionic villus sampling. **A,** Typical uterine focal contraction characteristic of this gestational age involves the posterior wall of the uterus. **B,** The same patient 60 minutes later. The contraction has dissipated, the bladder has filled, and the operator is now able to pass the catheter into the posterior chorionic frondosum.

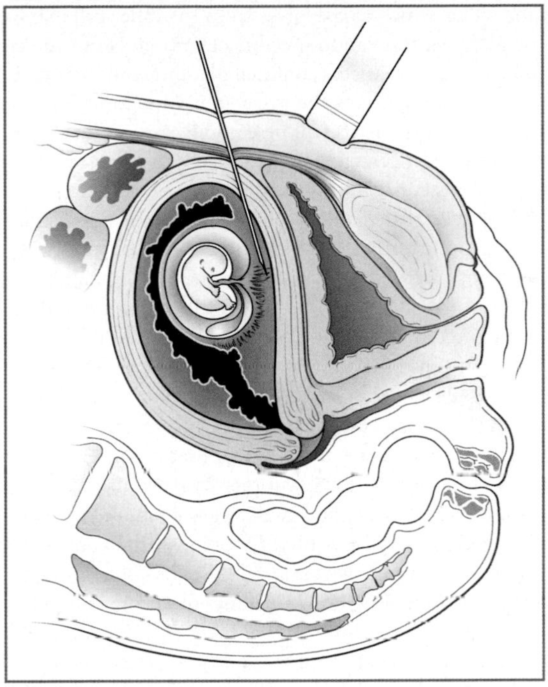

FIGURE 17-9 Transabdominal chorionic villus sampling. Continuous ultrasound guidance is used to help guide the needle into the chorionic frondosum, remaining parallel to the plate. The sample is then obtained by back-and-forth movement of the needle while maintaining negative pressure. The needle tip is continuously kept in sight via ultrasound. (From Scioscia AL: Reproductive genetics. In Moore TR, Reiter RC, Rebar RW, et al [eds]: Obstetrics and Gynecology: A Longitudinal Approach. New York, Churchill Livingstone, 1993, p 72.)

the cervical sampling catheter, three or four to-and-fro passes of the needle tip through the body of the placenta are required to retrieve the villi. Unlike transcervical CVS, which is best performed before 14 weeks' gestation, the transabdominal procedure can be performed throughout pregnancy and therefore constitutes an alternative to amniocentesis or PUBS when a karyotype is needed. If oligohydramnios is present, transabdominal CVS may be the only approach available.

Comparison of Transcervical and Transabdominal Chorionic Villus Sampling

The transabdominal and transcervical approaches to villus sampling have been shown to be equally safe.[326,327] In most cases, operator or patient choice determines the sampling route; however, in about 3% to 5% of cases, one approach is clearly preferred, so operators must be skilled in both. For example, a posterior placenta is sampled most easily by the transcervical route, whereas a fundal placenta is more simply approached transabdominally. Bowel in the sampling path may preclude transabdominal CVS in some cases, whereas necrotic cervical polyps or an active herpetic lesion should lead to transabdominal sampling.

More chorionic tissue is obtained by the transcervical method, but the proportion of cases in which less than 10 mg is obtained is similar in both groups. There are no differences in birth weight, gestational age at delivery, or congenital malformations with either method.

Laboratory Aspects of Chorionic Villus Sampling

Chorionic villi have three major components: an outer layer of hormonally active and invasive syncytiotrophoblast, a middle layer of cytotrophoblast from which syncytiotrophoblast cells are derived, and an inner mesodermal core containing blood capillaries.

The average sample from a transcervical aspiration contains 15 to 30 mg of villous material. The villi identified in the syringe are carefully and aseptically transferred for inspection and dissection under a microscope. The villi are cleaned of adherent decidua and then exposed to trypsin to digest and separate the cytotrophoblast from the underlying mesodermal core. The cytotrophoblast has a high mitotic index, with many spontaneous mitoses available for immediate chromosome analysis. The liquid suspension containing the cytotrophoblast is either dropped immediately onto a slide for analysis or may undergo a short incubation.[320,329] This "direct" chromosome preparation can give preliminary results within 2 to 3 hours. However, most laboratories now use an overnight incubation to improve karyotype quality and thus report results within 2 to 4 days. The remaining villus core is placed in tissue culture and is typically ready for harvest and chromosome analysis within 1 week.[330]

The direct method has the advantage of providing a rapid result and minimizing the decidual contamination, whereas tissue culture is better for interpreting discrepancies between the cytotrophoblast and the actual fetal state. Ideally, both the direct and culture methods should be used, because they each evaluate slightly different tissue sources. Although the direct preparation is less likely to be representative of the fetus, its use minimizes the likelihood of maternal cell contamination, and, if culture fails, a nonmosaic normal direct preparation result can be considered conclusive, although rare cases of false-negative rates for trisomy 21 and 18 have been reported.[331,332] Abnormalities in either may have clinical implications.

Most biochemical diagnoses that can be made from amniotic fluid or cultured amniocytes can usually be made from chorionic villi.[333] In many cases, the results are available more rapidly and efficiently when villi are used, because sufficient enzyme is present to allow direct analysis rather than the products of tissue culture being required. However, for certain rare biochemical diagnoses, villi are not an appropriate or reliable diagnostic source.[334] To ensure that appropriate testing is possible, the laboratory should be consulted before sampling.

Accuracy of Chorionic Villus Sampling: Cytogenetic Results

CVS is now considered a reliable method of prenatal diagnosis, but early in its development incorrect results were reported.[329,335,336] The major sources of these errors included maternal cell contamination and misinterpretation of mosaicism confined to the placenta. Today, genetic evaluation of chorionic villi provides a high degree of success and accuracy, particularly in regard to the diagnosis of common trisomies.[337,338] The U.S. collaborative study revealed a 99.7% rate of successful cytogenetic diagnosis, with only 1.1% of the patients requiring a second diagnostic test such as amniocentesis or fetal blood analysis to further interpret the results.[338] In most cases, the additional testing was required to delineate the clinical significance of mosaic or other ambiguous results (76%), whereas laboratory failure (21%) and maternal cell contamination (3%) also required follow-up testing.

MATERNAL CELL CONTAMINATION

Chorionic villus samples typically contain a mixture of placental villi and maternally derived decidua. Although specimens are thoroughly washed and inspected under a microscope after collection, some maternal cells may remain and grow in the culture. As a result, two cell lines, one fetal and the other maternal, may be identified. In other cases, the maternal cell line may completely overgrow the culture, thereby leading to diagnostic errors, including incorrect sex determination,[339-341] and potentially to false-negative diagnoses, although there are no published reports of the latter. Direct preparations of chorionic villi are generally thought to prevent maternal cell contamination,[328,339] whereas long-term culture has a rate varying from 1.8% to 4%.[340] Because, in contrast to cytotrophoblast, maternal decidua has a low mitotic index, it is highly desirable for laboratories to offer a direct chromosome preparation as well as a long-term culture on all samples of chorionic villus. Even in culture, the contaminating cells are easily identified as maternal and should not lead to clinical errors. Interestingly, for reasons still uncertain, maternal cell contamination occurs more frequently in specimens retrieved by the transcervical route.[340]

Contamination of samples with significant amounts of maternal decidual tissue is almost always the result of small sample size, making selection of appropriate tissue difficult. In experienced centers in which adequate quantities of villi are available, this problem has disappeared. Choosing only whole, clearly typical villus material and discarding any atypical fragments, small pieces, or fragments with adherent decidua avoids confusion.[342] Therefore, if the initial aspiration is small, a second pass should be performed rather than risk inaccurate results. When proper care is taken and good cooperation and communication exist between the sampler and the laboratory, absence of even small amounts of contaminating maternal tissue can be accomplished.

CONFINED PLACENTAL MOSAICISM

The second major source of potential diagnostic error associated with CVS is mosaicism confined to the placenta. Although the fetus and placenta have a common ancestry, chorionic villus tissue does not always reflect fetal genotype.[338,343] Although initially there was concern that this might invalidate CVS as a prenatal diagnostic tool, subsequent investigations have led to a clearer understanding of villus biology, so that accurate clinical interpretation is now possible. This understanding has also revealed new information about the etiology of pregnancy loss, discovered a new cause of intrauterine growth retardation, and clarified the basic mechanism of UPD.

Discrepancies between the cytogenetics of the placenta and the fetus occur because the cells contributing to the chorionic villi become separate and distinct from those forming the embryo in early development. Specifically, at approximately the 32- to 64-cell stage, only three to four cells become compartmentalized into the inner cell mass to form the embryo, whereas the remainder become precursors of the extraembryonic tissues.[344] Mosaicism can then occur through two possible mechanisms.[344] An initial meiotic error in one of the gametes can lead to a trisomic conceptus that would normally spontaneously abort. However, if during subsequent mitotic divisions one or more of the early aneuploid cells loses one of the trisomic chromosomes through anaphase lag, the embryo can be "rescued" by reduction of a portion of its cells to disomy. This results in a mosaic morula with the percentage of normal cells dependent on the cell division at which rescue occurred. More abnormal cells are present when correction is delayed to the second or a subsequent cell division. Because most cells in the morula proceed to the trophoblast cell lineage (processed by the direct preparation), it is highly probable that that lineage will continue to contain a significant number of trisomic cells. On the other hand, because only a small proportion of cells are incorporated into the inner cell mass, involvement of the fetus depends on the random distribution of the aneuploid progenitor cells. Involvement of the mesenchymal core of the villus, which also evolves from the inner cell mass, is similarly dependent on this random cell distribution. Noninvolvement of the fetal cell lineage produces "confined placental mosaicism," in which the trophoblast and perhaps the extraembryonic mesoderm will have aneuploid cells but the fetus will be euploid.

In the second mechanism, mitotic postzygotic errors produce mosaicism with the distribution and percent of aneuploid cells in the morula or blastocyst dependent on the timing of nondisjunction. If mitotic errors occur early in the development of the morula, they may segregate to the inner cell mass and have the same potential to produce an affected fetus as do meiotic errors. Mitotic errors occurring after primary cell differentiation and compartmentalization have been completed lead to cytogenetic abnormalities in only one lineage.

Meiotic rescue can lead to UPD. This occurs because the original trisomic cell contained two chromosomes from one parent and one from the other. After rescue, there is a theoretical one-in-three chance that the resulting pair of chromosomes came from the same parent, which is called UPD. UPD may have clinical consequences if the chromosomes involved carry imprinted genes in which expression is based on the parent of origin. For example, Prader-Willi syndrome may result from uniparental maternal disomy for chromosome 15. Therefore, a CVS diagnosis of confined placental mosaicism for trisomy 15 may be the initial clue that UPD could be present and lead to an affected child.[345,346] Because of this, all cases in which trisomy 15 (either complete or mosaic) is confined to the placenta should be evaluated for UPD by amniotic fluid analysis. In addition to chromosome 15, chromosomes 7, 11, 14, and 22 are believed to be imprinted and require similar follow-up.[347]

Confined placental mosaicism (unassociated with UPD) can alter placental function and lead to fetal growth failure or perinatal death.[344,348-353] The exact mechanism by which abnormal cells within the placenta alter function is unknown, but the effect is limited to specific chromosomes. For example, confined placental mosaicism for chromosome 16 leads to severe intrauterine growth restriction, prematurity, or perinatal death, with less than 30% of pregnancies resulting in normal, appropriate-for-gestational-age, full-term infants.[15,29,349,354,355]

Mosaicism occurs in about 1% of all CVS samples[337,340,354,356] but is confirmed in the fetus in only 10% to 40% of these cases. In most cases, if the mosaic results are confined to the placenta, fetal development will be normal. If the mosaic cell line involves the fetus, significant phenotypic consequences are possible. The probability of fetal involvement appears to be related to the tissue source in which the aneuploid cells were detected, with culture results more likely than direct preparation to reflect a true fetal mosaicism.

The specific chromosome involved also predicts the likelihood of fetal involvement.[347] Phillips and coworkers[15] demonstrated that autosomal mosaicism involving common trisomies (i.e., 21, 18, and 13) was confirmed in the fetus in 19% of cases, whereas uncommon trisomies involved the fetus in only 3%. When sex chromosome mosaicism was found in the placenta, the abnormal cell line was confirmed in the fetus in 16% of cases.

When placental mosaicism is discovered, amniocentesis can be performed to elucidate the extent of fetal involvement. When mosaicism is limited to the direct preparation, amniocentesis correlates perfectly with fetal genotype.[15] When a mosaicism is observed in tissue culture, amniocentesis predicts the true fetal karyotype in approximately 94% of cases, with both false-positive and false-negative results seen.[15] Three cases were reported of mosaic trisomy 21 on villus culture, and despite a normal amniotic fluid analysis, a fetus or newborn was born with mosaic aneuploidy.[338]

If mosaicism is found, follow-up amniocentesis should be offered in most cases. Under no circumstances should a decision to terminate a pregnancy be based entirely on a CVS mosaic result. For CVS mosaicism involving sex chromosome abnormalities, polyploidy, marker chromosomes, structural rearrangements, and most uncommon trisomies, the patient can be reassured if amniocentesis results are euploid and detailed ultrasonographic examination is normal. However, no guarantees should be made. As described previously, in certain cases testing for UPD is indicated. If common trisomies (21, 18, 13) are involved, amniocentesis should be offered, but the patient must be advised of the possibilities of a false-negative result. Follow-up may include detailed ultrasonography, fetal blood sampling, or fetal skin biopsy. At present, the predictive accuracy of these additional tests is uncertain.

Pregnancy Loss after Chorionic Villus Sampling

Although loss rates after CVS (calculated from the time of the procedure until 28 weeks' gestation) are approximately 1% greater than those after amniocentesis (2.5% versus 1.5%), this comparison fails to take into consideration that the background miscarriage rate at 11 to 13 weeks is about 1% greater than at 15 to 16 weeks. To appropriately compare the two procedures, studies must enroll all patients in the first trimester, assign them to either approach, and then calculate the frequency of all subsequent losses, including spontaneous and induced abortions. In 1989, the Canadian Collaborative CVS/Amniocentesis Clinical Trial Group[324] reported such a prospective randomized trial and demonstrated equivalent safety of CVS and second-trimester amniocentesis. In more than 2650 patients assigned to either procedure, there was a 7.6% loss rate in the CVS group and a 7.0% loss rate in the amniocentesis group (relative risk [RR] = 1.10; 95% CI, 0.92 to 1.30). No significant differences were noted in the incidence of preterm birth, low birth weight, or rate of maternal complication.

A U.S. multicenter prospective nonrandomized study enrolled 2235 women in the first trimester who chose either transcervical CVS or second-trimester amniocentesis.[325] An excess pregnancy loss rate of 0.8% in the CVS group over the amniocentesis group was calculated, which was not statistically significant. Repeated catheter insertions were significantly associated with pregnancy loss, with cases requiring three or more passes having a 10.8% spontaneous abortion rate, compared with 2.9% in cases that required only one pass.

Further information comes from a Danish randomized trial, which assigned 1068 patients to transcervical CVS, 1078 to transabdominal CVS, and 1158 to second-trimester amniocentesis. There was no difference in loss rates between transabdominal CVS and amniocentesis (RR = 0.9; 95% CI, 0.66 to 1.23). Overall, there was a slightly increased risk of pregnancy loss after CVS (RR = 1.30; 95% CI, 1.01 to 1.67) compared with amniocentesis, which was completely accounted for by an excess of losses in the group sampled transcervically (RR = 1.70; 95% CI, 1.30 to 2.22)—the technique with which this group of investigators had the least experience. Excess loss after transcervical CVS has not been replicated in four other direct comparisons.[326,327,357,358]

A prospective, randomized, collaborative comparison of more than 3200 pregnancies, sponsored by the European Medical Research Council,[359] reported that CVS had a 4.6% greater pregnancy loss rate than amniocentesis (RR = 1.51; 95% CI, 1.24 to 1.84). The present consensus is that operator inexperience with CVS accounts for the discrepancy between this trial and the other major studies. The U.S. trial consisted of seven experienced centers and the Canadian trial 11, whereas the Medical Research Council trial used 31. There were, on average, 325 cases per center in the U.S. study, 106 in the Canadian study, and 52 in the European trial.

In conclusion, when appropriately compared, CVS and amniocentesis are equally safe, but the impact of operator experience cannot be underestimated. CVS, particularly the transcervical approach, has a relatively prolonged learning curve. Saura and colleagues[360] suggested that more than 400 cases may be required before safety is maximized. The role of experience is further demonstrated by three sequential trials sponsored by the National Institute of Child Health and Human Development in which the majority of operators remained relatively constant. The postprocedure loss rate after CVS fell from 3.2% in the initial trial performed from 1985 to 1987,[325] to 2.4% for the trial performed from 1987 to 1989,[327] to only 1.3% in their most recent experience of 1997 to 2001.[316] Most recently, Caughey and coworkers[361] confirmed the continuing improvement seen with experience. When outcomes from their center were analyzed in 5-year time intervals, the overall postprocedure loss rate decreased from 4.4% in the interval from 1983 to 1987, to 1.9% from 1998 to 2003. When compared with their amniocentesis loss rates, no statistical or clinical difference between the two procedures was seen in the most recent interval.

Other Complications of Chorionic Villus Sampling

Postprocedure bleeding is the most common complaint after CVS. Most centers report postprocedure bleeding in 7% to 10% of patients sampled transcervically, whereas bleeding or spotting is relatively uncommon after transabdominal sampling, occurring in 1% or less of cases.[325] Minimal spotting may occur in up to one third of women sampled by the transcervical route.[325] On occasion, a small subchorionic hematoma may be seen after sampling.[362] This usually resolves spontaneously within a few weeks and is rarely associated with adverse outcome. Hematomas occur when the catheter is passed too deeply into the underlying vascular decidua basalis. Because passage into the decidua gives a "gritty" sensation, careful attention to the feel of the catheter can minimize this complication. Operators should also avoid sampling near or within large placental "lakes," which also leads to bleeding.[363]

Since the initial development of transcervical CVS, there has been concern that transvaginal passage of an instrument would introduce vaginal flora into the uterus. Although cultures of catheter tips have isolated bacteria in 30% of transcervical CVS cases,[364-367] the incidence of chorioamnionitis is extremely low and occurs equally infrequently after either the transcervical or transabdominal procedure. In the U.S. collaborative trial, infection was suspected as a possible etiology of pregnancy loss in only 0.3% of cases.[325]

Early in the development of transcervical CVS, two life-threatening pelvic infections were reported.[368,369] The practice of using a new sterile catheter for each insertion was subsequently universally adopted, and there have been no additional reports of serious infections. Infection after transabdominal CVS has been demonstrated and may result from inadvertent bowel puncture by the sampling needle.[326]

Acute rupture of membranes is exceedingly rare in experienced centers.[325] Fluid leakage with oligohydramnios has been reported days to weeks after the procedure.[370,371] In most cases, this is unrelated to the procedure but occasionally may be secondary to a procedure-induced hematoma.

An acute rise in MSAFP after CVS has consistently been reported, implying a detectable degree of fetomaternal bleeding.[371-374] The MSAFP elevation is not related to the technique used to retrieve villi but seems to depend on the quantity of tissue aspirated.[374] Levels return to normal ranges by 16 to 18 weeks of gestation, thus allowing

MSAFP serum screening to proceed according to usual prenatal protocols. All Rh-negative nonsensitized women undergoing CVS should receive Rh-D immune globulin after the procedure. Exacerbation of preexisting Rh immunization after CVS has been described. Existing Rh sensitization, therefore, represents a contraindication to the procedure.[375]

Risk of Fetal Abnormality after Chorionic Villus Sampling

Firth and colleagues[376] reported five occurrences of severe limb abnormalities out of 289 pregnancies sampled by CVS between 56 and 66 days. Four of these cases had the unusual but severe oromandibular-limb hypogenesis syndrome, which occurs in the general population at a rate of 1 per 175,000 births.[376] Burton and coworkers[377] then reported on 14 more post-CVS cases of limb reduction defects (LRD), ranging from mild to severe, only two of which occurred when sampling was performed beyond 9.5 weeks. After these two early reports, the WHO gathered additional data from its CVS registry, published reports,[376,377] and case-controlled studies[378,379] and concluded that "far greater data supporting CVS not being associated with LRD were available in various collaborative studies, in individual centers having the greatest experience, and in the WHO-initiated registry comprising 138,996 procedures."[380] They further concluded that CVS was not associated with LRD when performed after 8 completed weeks of pregnancy.[381] This infrequent occurrence of LRD after CVS was echoed by the American College of Obstetricians and Gynecologists, who stated that a risk for LRD of 1 in 3000 would be a prudent upper limit for counseling patients. Data on 216,381 procedures are now in the WHO CVS registry and have been reported.[380] This report analyzed the frequency of limb anomalies, their pattern, and their associated gestational age at sampling and found no overall increased risk of LRD or any difference in the pattern of defects compared with the general population. To analyze a possible temporal relationship between CVS and LRD, a subset of 106,383 cases was stratified by the week at which the procedure was performed. The incidence of LRD was 11.7, 4.9, 3.8, 3.4, and 2.3 per 10,000 CVS procedures in weeks 8, 9, 10, 11, and more than 12, respectively. Only the rate at week 8 exceeded the background risk of 6.0 per 10,000 births. If cases from the cluster seen in the original report of Firth and coworkers[376] are removed, the rate for week 8 procedures also falls below baseline. Brambati and colleagues,[382] in a small series of early CVS cases, had an LRD incidence of 1.6% for procedures performed in weeks 6 and 7, 0.1% in week 8, and (population frequency) 0.059% in week 9.

Present data confirm that performing CVS in the standard gestational window of 10 to 13 weeks does not increase the risk of LRD. Sampling before 10 weeks is not recommended, except in very unusual circumstances, such as when a patient's religious beliefs may preclude a pregnancy termination beyond a specific gestational age.[112] These patients, however, must be informed that the incidence of severe LRD could be as high as 1% to 2%.

Prenatal Diagnosis and Multiple Gestation

Risk of Fetal Aneuploidy in Multiple Gestations

The overall probability that a given multiple gestation contains an aneuploid fetus depends on its zygosity. Because monozygotic twins originate from the same gamete, both fetuses possess the same karyotype, and the overall risk of aneuploidy is that of a singleton. Although this construct ignores the very small possibility of mitotic nondisjunction, such a possibility is such a rare occurrence that it should not change the overall risk calculation. In dizygotic twins, on the other hand, either one or both fetuses may be affected, with the chance for aneuploidy in either fetus being independent.

The risk of both dizygotic twin fetuses being affected is low (the singleton risk squared), whereas the risk of at least one affected fetus is approximately twice the singleton risk.[383] These risks can be used to counsel patients if the zygosity is known.

If zygosity is unknown, the ratio of the risk of at least one fetus (in a twin pregnancy) being aneuploid to the risk of a singleton gestation being aneuploid can be approximated as 5:3. This approximation is based on the assumption that one third of all twin gestations are monozygotic twins. Despite the slight inaccuracy of this approach caused by the varying rates of monozygotic twins and dizygotic twins twinning with maternal age and ethnicity, this approximation is quite satisfactory for patient counseling. A more accurate determination taking these variations into account has been published by Meyers and colleagues.[384] Based on these calculations, a 32-year-old woman with twins has nearly the same risk of having at least one aneuploid fetus as a 35-year-old woman with a singleton. Present recommendations are that invasive prenatal diagnosis be offered at this cutoff. Table 17-28 demonstrates the risk of fetal aneuploidy at different maternal ages in twin gestations using these calculations.

Higher-order multiple gestations resulting from assisted reproductive technology (ART) have a greater predilection for polyzygosity than naturally occurring multiples. The risk of at least one aneuploid fetus can be approximated as the singleton risk multiplied by the number of fetuses. Despite the fact that recent studies have shown that monozygotic twin pregnancies occur more frequently than anticipated after the use of ART,[385,386] their frequency still remains low enough that this estimate is appropriate.

An even steeper increase in the risk of gene transmission for pregnancies at risk for mendelian disorders occurs with multiple gestations. For example, for a twin gestation at risk for an autosomal recessive disorder, there is a three-in-eight chance of at least one fetus being affected, and a one-in-eight chance that both will inherit the affected genes.

Screening Tests in Twins

SECOND TRIMESTER

For singleton pregnancies, second-trimester biochemical screening is a routine practice. For twins, however, the value and accuracy of serum screening is much less certain because the contribution of an abnormal fetus will, on average, be brought closer to the normal mean

TABLE 17-28 CALCULATED RISK, AT TERM, OF DOWN SYNDROME IN AT LEAST ONE FETUS IN TWIN GESTATIONS

Maternal Age (yr)	Singleton Risk	Equivalent Twin Risk	Equivalent Maternal Age Risk
25	1/1,250	1/679	32.5
30	1/952	1/508	33.8
32	1/769	1/409	34.7
35	1/378	1/199	37.5
40	1/106	1/56	42.5

From Meyers C, Adam R, Dungan J, et al: Aneuploidy in twin gestations: When is maternal age advanced? Obstet Gynecol 89:248, 1997.

TABLE 17-29 SERUM ANALYTE VALUES IN TWIN GESTATIONS (MoMs)

Second Trimester					First Trimester			
Source (ref)	*N*	AFP	hCG	Unconjugated Estriol	Source (ref)	*N*	PAPP-A	Free β-hCG
Wald et al (538), 1991	200	2.13	1.84	1.67	Spencer et al (541), 2008	1914	2.12	2.02
Canick et al (13), 1990	35	2.30	1.90	1.70				
Räty et al (539), 2000	145	2.18	1.83	—				
Muller et al (540), 2003	3043	2.10	2.11	—				
All	3423	2.11	2.08	1.60				

AFP, α-fetoprotein; hCG, human chorionic gonadotropin; PAPP-A, pregnancy-associated plasma protein A.

by an unaffected co-twin. This tends to decrease the overall screening sensitivity. Screening, however, can be useful nonetheless.

The mean and median values of MSAFP, unconjugated estriol, and hCG in twins have been studied and are presented in Table 17-29. Dividing the measured result by the twin median can be used to estimate a twin MoM for each analyte. These MoM values can then be used in singleton algorithms to estimate a risk of aneuploidy. Neveux and coworkers[387] evaluated this approach and, based on a calculated model, predicted that 73% of monozygotic twin and 43% of dizygotic twin cases with a Down syndrome fetus would be detected with a 5% false-positive rate. In their clinical sample of 274 twin pregnancies, 5.5% screened positive. They had no cases of Down syndrome, making evaluation of the sensitivity difficult. Presently, the use of biochemical markers for aneuploidy screening in multiple gestations is extremely limited and is not recommended for general practice.

For the detection of neural tube defects, the levels of maternal AFP are again affected by the presence of a co-fetus. The mean MSAFP level in twin pregnancies ranges from 2.0 to 2.5 MoM. This is not surprising, considering double production. In singleton gestations, an MSAFP upper cutoff of 2.5 MoM will identify 75% of fetuses with a neural tube defect and has a false-positive rate between 2% and 3.3%. A similar cutoff in twin gestations would identify 99% of anencephalic fetuses and 89% of open neural tube defects,[388] but this would be associated with an unacceptably high false-positive rate of 30%. A twin false-positive rate similar to that for singletons can be calculated by doubling the singleton cutoff level; for example, choosing an MSAFP cutoff value of 5.0 MoM for twins would have the same false positive rate as a 2.5 MoM cutoff in singletons. The detection rate will be lower, however, because, when only one fetus has a neural tube defect, the normal coexisting fetus will contribute an AFP level near the singleton median. Maintaining the 75% sensitivity accomplished with singleton screening would require an MSAFP elevation of approximately 3.5 MoM, which would have a false-positive rate of 15%.

Presently, there is no standard agreement on the MSAFP elevation that warrants further evaluation in twins. Some centers use a cutoff of 4.0 MoM, which would identify approximately 60% of fetuses with open spina bifida but has approximately an 8% incidence of false-positive results. Other centers use a cutoff of 4.5 MoM, which has a sensitivity of approximately 50%.

FIRST TRIMESTER

First-trimester combined screening (NT, PAPP-A, hCG) for Down syndrome can be performed in twin gestations and may be preferable to second-trimester screening, as a fetus-specific risk rather than a pregnancy-specific risk can be obtained.[115,389] The analyte levels are adjusted for twins as done for second-trimester screening (see Table 17-29). In dichorionic gestations, the NT of individual fetuses is measured, and then a fetus-specific risk is obtained using maternal age and analyte levels. In monochorionic gestations in which the fetal karyotypes are identical, the NT measurements are averaged and a single likelihood ratio is calculated. This is combined with maternal age and serum analyte levels, resulting in a pregnancy-specific risk.

Overall, first-trimester combined Down syndrome screening in twins has a 72% detection rate with a 5% false-positive rate.[389] Using NT alone is less efficient, with a 69% detection rate. The performance of this approach is better for monochorionic gestations, as both fetuses will be affected and the analyte values from each will trend in the same direction. In dichorionic pregnancies, which are more likely to be dizygotic and have discordant karyotypes, the abnormal biochemical analytes from an affected gestation may be diluted by those from the normal fetus. Theoretical modeling suggests that combined screening has an 84% detection rate with a 5% false-positive rate in monochorionic gestations, compared with 70% in dichorionic twins. Performance in these subgroups is better when biochemical analytes are added to NT measurements.

Amniocentesis in Multifetal Gestations

Amniocentesis in multifetal pregnancy involves puncture of the first sac, withdrawal of amniotic fluid, injection of dye to mark the sampled sac, and then a new needle insertion to puncture the second sac.[390] If the fluid aspirated after the second puncture is clear, this is confirmation that the first sac was not resampled. If color-tinged fluid is retrieved, the needle should be removed and another attempt at sampling the second sac should be made.

History has shown the possible toxic effects of dye instillation. Methylene blue is associated with small bowel atresia[391,392] and an increased risk of fetal death.[393] Its use is now contraindicated. Use of indigo carmine (the dye of choice) has been reviewed in large series by both Cragan and coworkers[394] and Pruggmayer and coworkers,[395] and no increased risk for small bowel atresia or any other congenital anomaly has been found. However, because of the theoretical risk of intra-amniotic dye, instillation-free techniques have evolved.[264,396]

A single-puncture method has been described in which the site of needle insertion is determined by the position of the dividing membrane.[264] After entry into the first sac and aspiration of amniotic fluid, the same needle is advanced through the dividing membrane into the second sac. To avoid contamination of the second sample with fluid from the first, the first 1 mL of fluid from the second sample is discarded. This method may cause iatrogenic rupture of the dividing membrane, with creation of a monoamniotic sac and its attendant risk of cord entanglement.[397] This appears to occur almost exclusively in monochorionic gestations.

Bahado-Singh and colleagues[398] described a technique of twin amniocentesis that entails identifying the separating membranes with a curvilinear or linear transducer. The first needle is inserted, fluid retrieved, and the needle left in place while a second needle is inserted

TABLE 17-30 PREGNANCY OUTCOMES AFTER TWIN AMNIOCENTESIS

Source (ref)	Years of Procedures	Continuous Guidance	*N*	Success Rate	Loss to 20 Wk	Loss to 28 Wk
Pijpers et al (542), 1989	1980-1985	No	83	93%	1.2%	4.8%
Anderson et al (543), 1991	1969-1990	No	330	99%	—	3.6%
Pruggmayer et al (544), 1991	1982-1989	Yes	98	100%	6.1%	8.1%
Pruggmayer et al (395), 1992	1981-1990	Yes	529	100%	2.3%	3.7%
Wapner et al (407), 1993	1984-1990	Yes	73	100%	1.4%	2.9%
Ghidini et al (402), 1993	1987-1992	Yes	101	100%	0.0%	3.0%
Ko et al (545), 1998	1986-1997	Yes	128	100%	4.5%	—
Yukobowich et al (403), 2001	1990-1997	Yes	476	100%	2.7%*	—

*Loss within 4 weeks of procedure.

into the coexisting sac. Visualization of the two needle tips on alternate sides of the membrane confirms sampling of both fetuses. Patient tolerance of this technique may be a problem, as well as the potential requirement of two operators when sampling.

Complications of Amniocentesis in Multiple Gestation. A comparison of the relative safety of any invasive procedure in multiple gestations must take into consideration that, at any gestational age, loss rates for multiples are significantly higher than for singletons. Evaluation of the safety of invasive procedures, therefore, needs to be kept in context. Most series report postprocedure loss rates between 2% and 5% (Table 17-30). Literature evaluating the risk of pregnancy loss before 28 weeks in unsampled twins with a normal second-trimester ultrasound demonstrates rates of 4.5%,[399] 5.8%,[400] and 7.2%,[401] which helps to put the increase in postprocedure rates into perspective. However, the ideal way to evaluate procedure-induced loss rates is to compare similar cohorts of sampled and unsampled twins. Ghidini and colleagues[402] evaluated the risk of amniocentesis in twins by comparing 101 sampled pregnancies with an unsampled control group scanned at a matching gestational age. No significant difference in total loss rate was detected. A recent report attributed a 2% higher loss rate with amniocentesis (2.7% versus 0.6%) as compared with singletons or nonsampled twin gestations, with 13 losses in 476 pregnancies (95% CI, 1.5 to 4.6).[403] The makeup of the sampled group was 47% with maternal age of at least 35 years, 21% with abnormal MSAFP, and 11% with abnormal ultrasound, which could have affected loss rates. No study in the current literature has the power to definitively quantify the procedure-induced loss rate in twins. Empirically, the procedure-related loss rate is 1% to 1.5%.

Patients with twins must also be counseled about the risk of finding a karyotypically abnormal child, which, because of the presence of two fetuses, is approximately twice that after a singleton procedure.[383] Amniocentesis in twins does raise some very painful questions. Families need to consider the possibility of a test showing that one of the twins is normal and the other has an abnormality. Selective termination of the affected fetus is now a routine procedure and can be accomplished in 100% of cases with a postprocedure loss rate of 5% to 10% in experienced centers.[279] However, this approach is also associated with an increased risk of preterm birth, especially when performed after 20 weeks' gestation or if the presenting fetus is terminated.[404]

Chorionic Villus Sampling in Multiple Gestations

Twin, as well as higher-order multiple, gestations have been sampled successfully using CVS.[405-408] Each distinct placental site must be identified and sampled individually. Because no dye marker is available to ensure retrieval from a gestation, if there is any suspicion that two separate samples have not been obtained, a backup amniocentesis should be offered if the fetal sexes are concordant.[405] However, this is rarely required if meticulous intraoperative ultrasound placement of the needle or catheter is performed. Another difficulty is the possible cross-contamination of samples when both placentas are on the same uterine wall (i.e., both anterior or both posterior). In these cases, sampling the lower sac transcervically and the upper transabdominally minimizes the chance of contamination. When a biochemical diagnosis is required, the potential for misinterpretation is even greater because a small amount of normal tissue could significantly alter the test result. These cases should only be sampled in experienced centers.

TABLE 17-31 SAFETY OF CHORIONIC VILLUS SAMPLING WITH TWINS

Source (ref)	*n*	Success Rate	Pregnancy Loss Rate (to 28 wk)
Wapner et al (407), 1993	161	100.0%	2.8%
Pergament et al (406), 1992	128	99.2%	2.4%
Brambati et al (87), 1991	66	100.0%	1.6%
De Catte et al (408), 2000	262	99.0%	3.1%*

*Loss before 22 weeks.

Complications of Chorionic Villus Sampling in Multiple Gestations. Studies assessing procedure-related loss rates after CVS sampling of twins are shown in Table 17-31. In experienced centers, no increased procedure-related loss risks are seen compared with second-trimester amniocentesis.

Which Procedure to Perform?

Whether to perform a first- or second-trimester procedure depends on a number of factors, including local availability of the procedures described. If both CVS and amniocentesis are available, the relative risks and the advantages of an earlier diagnosis need to be considered. Second-trimester amniocentesis is more readily available and technically easier to perform, but CVS provides the information more than 1 month sooner, thus giving earlier reassurance. When discordant results are encountered, if selective termination is chosen, its complications and loss rates are markedly decreased if performed at less than 16 weeks' gestation.[279]

Only one study to date has analyzed outcomes for twins after CVS compared with after second-trimester amniocentesis.[407] In this work,

81 women had amniocentesis and 161 had CVS. Loss of the entire pregnancy before the 28th week followed amniocentesis in 2.9% of the cases and CVS in 3.2%. The fetal loss rate, which included loss of one fetus, was 9.3% for amniocentesis and 4.9% for CVS.

Percutaneous Umbilical Blood Sampling

In 1983, Daffos and coworkers[409] described a method of obtaining fetal blood using ultrasound guidance of a 20- to 22-gauge spinal needle through the maternal abdomen into the umbilical cord. This technique (variously called PUBS, fetal blood sampling, cordocentesis, or funipuncture) offered considerable advantage in both efficacy and safety over the fetoscopic methods previously used to obtain fetal blood.

Until recently, a common reason for PUBS was the need for rapid karyotype. With the advent of rapid and safer cytogenetic diagnosis by either FISH of amniocytes or the rapid analysis of chorionic villi obtained by placental biopsy, the diagnostic indications for PUBS have changed. Currently, the primary genetic indication is evaluation of mosaic results found on amniocentesis or CVS. Most mendelian disorders that previously required fetal blood for diagnosis are now made using molecular DNA analysis of amniocytes or chorionic villi. PUBS is necessary only for the rare cases in which the specific mutation is not known. The most frequent nongenetic indications are assessment for fetal anemia, infection, and thrombocytopenia. These indications are described in detail in Chapters 24, 26, 27, and 38.

The main complication of PUBS is fetal loss, which is estimated to be approximately 2% higher than background risk.[374,410] This exact risk is difficult to quantify because many of the fetuses studied had severe congenital malformations.

Best estimates for procedure-related risk are from the North American PUBS registry, which collected data from 16 centers in the United States and Canada. Information on 7462 diagnostic procedures performed on 6023 patients is available.[411] Fetal loss is defined as intrauterine fetal death within 14 days of the procedure. The fetal loss rate in these cases is calculated to be 1.1% per procedure and 1.3% per patient.

The major causes for fetal loss were chorioamnionitis, rupture of membranes, puncture site bleeding, severe bradycardia, and thrombosis. The range of losses for participating centers varied from 1% to 6.7%, which reflects operator experience and differences in patient selection. These figures are subjective, relying on the operator's impression that a pregnancy loss was directly related to the procedure and not to the underlying fetal condition.

Technique of Percutaneous Umbilical Blood Sampling

Fetal vessels can be accessed within either the cord or the fetus itself. The cord is most reliably entered at the placental insertion site where it is anchored. Color Doppler imaging enhances visualization of the insertion site and is especially useful when oligohydramnios is present. Entering the cord near the umbilical insertion site or into a free loop is possible but can be more difficult. The hepatic vein is the most accessible and safe intrafetal location.[412]

It is essential to verify that the blood sample is fetal in origin. The most definitive way to establish this is to compare the MCV of the retrieved red cells with a sample of maternal blood. This comparison is easily performed on small aliquots of blood by a standard channeling instrument. Fetal red blood cells are considerably larger than those of an adult, but the value is gestational-age dependent. The mean MCV decreases from 145 fL at 16 weeks to 113 fL at 36 weeks of gestation.[413] Alternatively, one can visually confirm appropriate location of the needle by injecting a small amount of sterile saline. If the needle is in the umbilical vein, microbubbles can be seen moving toward the fetus.

Forestier and colleagues[414] recommended performing biochemical studies on the aspirated blood that include a complete blood count with differential analysis and determination of anti-I and anti-i cold agglutinin, β-hCG, factors IX and VIIIC, and AFP levels. It is not general practice to perform all these studies.

Other Invasive Diagnostic Procedures

On infrequent occasions, analysis of other fetal tissues may be required. Fetal skin biopsy is performed to diagnose fetal genetic skin disorders when molecular testing is not available, and it can also be helpful in the workup of fetal mosaicism for chromosomes (such as 22) known not to be manifested in fetal blood.[271] Fetal muscle biopsy for dystrophin analysis is used to diagnose muscular dystrophy in a male fetus if DNA testing is not informative.[415] Fetal kidney biopsy has diagnosed congenital nephrosis in utero,[164] and aspiration and analysis of fetal urine is imperative in the pre-shunt evaluation of fetal renal function.[416] Each of these procedures is performed under ultrasound guidance. Because they are only rarely required, their use is usually confined to only a few regional referral centers in hopes of limiting procedural risk.

Preimplantation Genetic Screening

Over the past two decades, methods of in vitro fertilization and embryo culture and transfer have developed into routine clinical practice. Simultaneously, the introduction of increasingly sophisticated genetic diagnostic procedures now allows prenatal diagnoses to be performed by testing one or two cells of a developing preimplantation embryo. This technique was developed initially to benefit patients at high risk for a fetal genetic disorder and for whom termination of an affected fetus was not an option. Most of these diagnoses were for relatively rare mendelian disorders. However, as the technology has progressed and the ability to perform cytogenetic analysis by FISH on single cells has improved, preimplantation genetic screening (PGS) has been used to improve outcomes for in vitro fertilization (IVF), patients with repetitive miscarriages, and women of advanced maternal age. As characterized by the European Society of Human Reproduction and Embryology, PGS is now divided into two general categories. High-risk PGS refers to analysis carried out for patients at risk of transmitting a genetic or chromosomal abnormality to their offspring. This includes single-gene defects as well as translocations and structural aberrations. Low-risk PGS (also referred to as PGS aneuploidy screening [PGD-AS]) is reserved for infertility patients undergoing in vitro fertilization, with the goal of increasing pregnancy rates by screening for aneuploidy.[417]

The techniques available to retrieve preimplantation cells include polar body biopsy of prefertilized oocytes, biopsy of one or two cells (called blastomeres) from the six- to eight-cell early cleavage stage embryo on day 3, or removal of five to 12 cells from the trophectoderm of the 5- to 7-day blastocyst.[418] In all cases, removal of the cells is well tolerated, with continued development of the embryo and no increased risk of congenital anomalies.[419]

PGS for Karyotype Analysis

In 2003, more than 100,000 IVF cycles with PGS were reported in the United States, resulting in the birth of 48,000 babies.[420] The most common indication was chromosomal evaluation for aneuploidy, including evaluation for both structural rearrangements and numerical abnormalities. Reciprocal translocation is the most common structural anomaly for which PGS is used. Analysis of chromosome number using FISH for chromosomes 21, 13, 18, X, and Y is performed for the indications of maternal age, a previous child with aneuploidy, repeated IVF failures, recurrent spontaneous abortions, or a combination of these.

As techniques have improved, cytogenetic results can be obtained in almost 90% of cases.[421,422] However, clinical interpretive errors have occurred, probably because early-stage embryos are frequently mosaic, with mosaicism rates of 42% to 50%.[421,423] Abnormal-appearing zygotes have the highest rates of mosaicism,[421,424] but those appearing normal still carry a risk of approximately 20%.[421] Rates of mosaicism within the inner cell mass are similar to those in trophoblast precursors,[425] showing that there is not a selection bias against aneuploid cells from integrating into the fetal precursor cells. Accordingly, the rate of misdiagnosis with one biopsied blastomere is at least 5.4%. Because of this potential for error, invasive prenatal diagnosis by CVS or amniocentesis is recommended for appropriate indications even when PGS has been performed. In contrast to blastomere biopsy, no misdiagnosis of aneuploidy has been reported with polar body biopsy to date.

Aneuploid screening and preselection of normal embryos is now used to improve in vitro fertilization implantation and pregnancy rates even if no genetic indication for testing is present. When this is performed, about 40% of embryos are suitable for transfer. The success of this approach has led to its being extended to other indications, such as repetitive aborters with normal parental karyotypes and multiple in vitro fertilization failures.

PGS for Monogenetic Disorders

PGS for monogenetic disorders requires the ability to evaluate the DNA of a single cell. To accomplish this, the DNA content of a single blastomere is amplified by PCR and then analyzed. The most common monogenetic disorders evaluated by PGS are CF, thalassemia, and spinal muscular atrophy among the autosomal recessive disorders; myotonic dystrophy, Huntington disease, and Charcot-Marie-Tooth disease among the dominant disorders; and fragile X, Duchenne/Becker muscular dystrophy, and hemophilia among the X-linked disorders. PGS is especially valuable for adult-onset autosomal disorders such as Huntington disease, when the parents want to avoid the birth of an affected child but do not wish to have their own diagnosis confirmed. Using PGS, only unaffected zygotes can be implanted without informing the parents of whether the gene was present. However, to maintain parental nondisclosure, this approach must be performed on all subsequent pregnancies, even if no evidence of the gene is seen in prior cycles.

Although the molecular diagnosis is considered to be quite accurate, errors have occurred. For example, an error may occur as a result of the failure of a primer to anneal to a relevant sequence, a phenomenon called allele dropout (ADO). This may lead to an incorrect diagnosis, especially when there is a compound heterozygote. Real-time PCR has become the optimal choice for high-risk PGS because of the limited quantity of DNA in a sample, and because of the need to provide a genotype result within a specified and limited amount of time. The sensitivity of real-time PCR maximizes the detection of amplified DNA copies even when present in low amounts, which in turn reduces rates of amplification failure and ADO.[426] Recent improvements in this technology have made errors exceedingly uncommon, with some centers now reporting 100% accuracy. Despite this, invasive prenatal diagnosis should still be performed to confirm the PGS result.

Perinatal Risks of IVF and PGS

Assisted reproductive technologies, including IVF, are a significant contributor to preterm delivery, predominantly through an increased rate of multiple gestations. Over 30% of ART pregnancies are twins or higher-order multiple gestations (triplets or greater), and more than half of all ART neonates are the products of multiple gestations.[427,428] Furthermore, the frequency of monozygotic gestations and their additional perinatal risks is increased; especially with blastocyst transfers.[428-432]

Only recently have sufficiently sized and appropriately performed studies and meta-analyses been available to explore the perinatal effects of IVF in singleton gestations.[427,433-438] Although the majority of pregnancies are uncomplicated, there are higher rates of adverse pregnancy outcomes. These include an increased frequency of preterm and term low birth weight, preterm deliveries, and perinatal mortality. Two well-performed meta-analyses have recently been reported. One meta-analysis of 15 studies comprising 12,283 IVF singleton offspring and 1.9 million spontaneously conceived infants demonstrated approximately a 1.6- to 2.7-fold increased risk for these outcomes.[438] The second meta-analysis of 25 studies showed similar results, with a 1.7- to 3.0-fold increased risk in these same outcomes.[434] Although evidence of the effect is convincing, questions remain about whether this is secondary to a treatment effect or to the underlying infertility.

Women with IVF-conceived singletons are at increased risk of preeclampsia, gestational diabetes, placenta previa, and stillbirth.[439] They are also at a significantly higher risk of having induction of labor and both emergent and elective cesarean deliveries. Thus, some of the adverse outcomes, including low birth weight, very low birth weight, and preterm delivery, may be attributable, in part, to iatrogenic intervention. An increased incidence of abnormal placentation, including a 2.4-fold increased risk of placental abruption and a 6.0-fold increased risk of placenta previa, have been noted in IVF pregnancies compared with controls.

One of the most frequently evaluated effects of IVF is the occurrence of birth defects.[436,437-446] Despite numerous studies, the results remain uncertain because of concerns including small sample size for specific anomalies, incomplete ascertainment of birth defects, confounding effects such as the cause of the infertility, and the potential of a parental genetic contribution. Two recent population-based studies with sufficient data to evaluate potential confounders demonstrate an increased risk for birth defects among ART infants.[440,441] One registry-based study[442] stands out because of its large sample size, including 4555 IVF children, 4467 other ART children, and 27,078 controls from the Finnish Registry of Congenital Malformations. The adjusted odds ratio for major malformations was 1.3 (95% CI, 1.1 to 1.6). The major malformation increased was hypospadias (rate of 76/10,000 births compared with 29/10,000 in controls). Other strongly associated malformations include other genitourinary anomalies, neural tube defects, gastrointestinal defects, musculoskeletal defects, and cardiovascular defects. A meta-analysis of the prevalence of birth defects in infants after IVF or intracytoplasmic sperm injection (ICSI) compared with spontaneously conceived infants revealed a pooled odds ratio of 1.29

for 19 studies (95% CI, 1.01 to 1.67). Thus, the effect of IVF and other ART modifications on birth defects appears real but small.

Chromosomal abnormalities also appear to be slightly increased, especially after ICSI for male factor disorders.[447] In one study of 8319 liveborn ICSI children, there was a slight but significant increase in sex chromosomal aneuploidy (0.6% versus 0.2%) and de novo chromosomal abnormalities (0.4% versus 0.07%). For all of these anomalies, it is not presently possible to distinguish the treatment effect from the effect of the etiology of the infertility because infertile males have a higher frequency of chromosomal abnormalities including microdeletions and translocations. Similarly, female partners of couples undergoing ART have an increased risk of chromosomal abnormalities.[448] Although this risk is not high enough to routinely offer invasive testing to all women undergoing IVF, those having invasive testing to confirm PGS results should have a full karyotype analysis.

Noninvasive Prenatal Diagnosis

Many studies have demonstrated that both intact fetal cells and cell-free nucleic acids circulate freely in maternal blood. Because invasive prenatal diagnosis techniques such as CVS and amniocentesis can be expensive and associated with small risks to the mother and fetus, alternative noninvasive methods, such as searching for fetal cells and nucleic acids from maternal blood samples, are being explored. This is particularly relevant because as of January 2007, the American College of Obstetricians and Gynecologists recommended that all women who present for prenatal care before 20 weeks of gestation be offered screening and invasive testing for aneuploidy, irrespective of age, and be counseled about the differences between screening and invasive diagnostic testing.[145] Screening tests such as nuchal translucency and the quadruple maternal serum screen are noninvasive, but invasive procedures are required for diagnosis. Isolating fetal DNA from the maternal circulation in a reliable and reproducible manner has the potential to eradicate the small, albeit present, risks of invasive testing.

Prenatal Diagnosis Using Fetal Cells in the Maternal Circulation

Cytogenetic evaluation of fetal cells retrieved from the maternal peripheral circulation for analysis has demonstrated potential to become a noninvasive diagnostic test.[449] The most promising results have been with the retrieval of fetal nucleated red blood cells. This cell line appears to be the most appropriate target, because they have specific antigens that can be used to enhance isolation[450] and contaminating maternal nucleated red cells are rare. The staggeringly small number of fetal cells (0 to 20 cells in 20 mL of maternal blood) and their low concentration (one fetal cell per 100,000 to 10 million maternal cells) have hampered consistent retrieval. Over the years, laboratory techniques such as diffusion gradients, fluorescent cell sorting, and magnetic cell separation have been used to improve the yield and concentration of the fetal cells.[451] These approaches can increase the concentration of fetal nucleated red cells to approximately 1 in 3000 or greater. Once enriched, the cells can be analyzed using FISH probes for specific aneuploidies.

There have been a number of reports of successful retrieval of aneuploid cells from the maternal circulation of women carrying affected pregnancies.[452-455] Most studies have shown sufficient enrichment for clinical analysis in approximately 50% of cases. The National Institute of Child Health and Human Development Fetal Cell Isolation Study (NIFTY) concluded that the fetal sex detection rate was 41.4%.[456] However, aneuploid pregnancies may have higher rates of fetal-maternal cell trafficking than euploid gestations, facilitating the diagnosis of abnormal pregnancies.[453]

Although fetal cell retrieval remains an intriguing option for noninvasive prenatal diagnosis, it is likely that routine feasibility will require the development of newer technologies. Work is underway on a number of possibilities. Many of these are using microfluidics to better separate the cells, and improved approaches to antibody-based isolation. In another approach, computer scanning technology is being used to rapidly survey the large number of cells on a slide and selectively identify those that are fetal. This technique requires the development of markers that are uniquely fetal, such as stains for early embryonic fetal hemoglobin. Once these rare cells are identified, there still remains the task of analyzing their genetic content. Although FISH for specific chromosomes has been used, fetal cell isolation and detection techniques cause cell injury, making FISH interpretation difficult and at times unreliable. The development of techniques to remove single cells from a slide and individually evaluate them using molecular technology is underway. Single-cell PCR may also allow the diagnosis of single-gene disorders.[457]

Free fetal DNA has also been detected in maternal plasma and has been explored as a potential approach to fetal diagnosis. This has certain technical advantages. It is less labor intensive because the amount of free fetal DNA is greater than the number of fetal cells and may account for greater than 3% of the total DNA in a maternal sample.[458]

Noninvasive Prenatal Diagnosis using Free Fetal DNA in the Maternal Circulation

Following the discovery of large amounts of cell-free tumor DNA in the plasma of patients with cancer, it was extrapolated that a rapidly growing fetus and placenta also possess tumor-like qualities. The presence of male fetal DNA sequences was demonstrated in maternal serum using standard PCR amplification of Y-specific DNA sequences to detect fetal DNA in the plasma of women carrying male fetuses.[459] This prompted a new area of research as it was established that perhaps 25 times more fetal DNA is present in a pregnant woman's serum than can be extracted from the cellular fraction of maternal blood.[460] There is an increase in fetal DNA concentration as gestation advances; in early pregnancy, the mean fractional concentration in maternal plasma is 3.4%, whereas in later pregnancy that value is 6.2%.[458] Maternal plasma or serum analysis of fetal DNA has the advantage of being reliable, rapid, and reproducible, and it can be performed for a large number of samples. The main limitation is the availability of uniquely fetal gene sequences that identify the presence of fetal DNA in both male and female fetuses.[461]

Identifying fetal DNA in the maternal circulation also prompted insights into physiology. Turnover of circulating fetal DNA in the maternal circulation was studied and it was determined that levels were undetectable by about 2 postpartum hours.[462] The mean half-life was estimated to be 16 minutes. This led to speculation that fetal DNA is continuously liberated into the maternal circulation. There is also indirect evidence to support that circulating fetal DNA fragments are small (less than 450 base pairs) and that it is protected within apoptotic bodies or within nucleosomes.[463]

Circulating fetal DNA has been hypothesized to arise from three sources: fetal hematopoietic cells, the placenta, and direct transfer of

DNA molecules. Data from studies on fetal cellular and nucleic acid trafficking in specific complications of pregnancy and preterm labor have demonstrated that fetal erythroblasts are not the exclusive source of fetal DNA.[464-466] Because of its size and abundant cellular activity, the placenta is probably the primary source for circulating fetal DNA. This conclusion is based primarily on the direct relationship between the amount of cell-free fetal DNA and advancing gestation.[458,467,468] Furthermore, Guibert and associates[469] demonstrated fetal SRY gene sequences as early as 18 days after embryo transfer, whereas the definitive fetoplacental circulation is not established until 28 days after conception. These data advocate the theory that the source of fetal DNA is the trophoblast and not fetal hematopoietic cells.

Prenatal diagnostic techniques using free fetal DNA are limited because of the presence of contaminating maternal DNA, requiring that the fetal sequence of interest be distinguished from that of the mother. For example, in attempting to diagnose a fetal autosomal recessive disorder, mutations in the DNA of a carrier mother could not be differentiated from those of the fetus. However, if the father carries a mutation different from that of the mother, lack of the paternal allele in the maternal circulation would preclude the need for invasive testing. To diagnose an autosomal dominant disorder, the mutation would have to be de novo or of paternal origin. This approach is still investigational, and false-positive and false-negative results occur.

Clinical Implications of Fetal DNA in the Maternal Circulation

GENDER DETECTION

One clinically valuable application of fetal DNA analysis is the determination of fetal sex. Positive signals for Y chromosome DNA sequences indicate a male fetus, whereas absence indicates a female fetus.[459,470] With the advent of real-time PCR, cell-free fetal DNA in the maternal plasma can be analyzed to determine fetal sex at as early as 5 to 7 weeks of gestation with a documented 100% sensitivity and specificity.[456,467,471]

Early, noninvasive fetal sex determination has a number of valid clinical indications. For pregnancies at risk for an X-linked disorder, determination of the fetal sex helps determine whether invasive testing should be performed for diagnostic purposes. Another use is in the management of congenital adrenal hyperplasia, in which prenatal treatment of a female fetus with maternal dexamethasone to prevent masculinization of the genitalia must be initiated before 9 weeks' gestation. Using fetal DNA analysis, fetal sex can be determined earlier and unnecessary treatment of male fetuses can be avoided.[472]

FETAL RED BLOOD CELL GENOTYPE DETERMINATION

Antigens of the Rh blood group system are encoded by two genes, RhD and RhCE. These genes, which are 93.8% homologous, are organized into 10 exons in a tail-to-tail configuration (5′-RhD-3′-3′-RhCE-5′).[473] RhD-negative individuals are lacking the RhD gene locus located on chromosome 1p36.2-p34. Exceptions to this rule occur when the gene is present but not translated or not expressed, or when the epitopes of the antigen are composed of weak D (epitopes weakly expressed) or partial D (epitopes are absent) phenotypes.[474] In whites, the majority of RhD-negative individuals are the result of a gene deletion. In Africans, however, the Rh-negative phenotype is most frequently the result of genes that contain RhD sequences but do not produce D antigen; these are the RhD-pseudogene and RhD-CE-Ds. The distribution of these genes differs between black Africans, African Americans, and black South Africans. False-negative results occur because of undetected or absent fetal DNA in the maternal sample, early gestational age, or insensitive methods. To address this, techniques that separate fetal DNA from maternal DNA are being actively sought.[475]

Detection of the RhD sequence in plasma or serum from an RhD-negative pregnant woman would indicate an Rh-positive fetus, and its absence an Rh-negative pregnancy. In 1998, it was demonstrated that this could be accomplished with high sensitivity and specificity.[476,477] Accuracy of fetal Rh genotyping has been reported to be approximately 95%, and many centers report 100% accurate results.[478,479] False-positive and false-negative results occur because of gene variation, presence of atypical mutations, or gene deletions. For example, false positives can occur because of the presence of RhD variants.[479] In the presence of a pseudogene, prenatal determination of fetal Rh type from maternal blood will reveal an RhD-positive type in a mother tested as Rh-negative by serology because of the abundant maternal D gene sequences that are not expressed but are amplified. Accordingly, primers for multiplex PCR amplification of RhD have to be selected carefully and designed around the RhD gene variants that are common in the studied population.

Prenatal determination of fetal red blood cell phenotype has two important clinical uses. First, in Rh-negative sensitized pregnancies for which the father is known to be heterozygous for the D allele, identification of an Rh-negative fetus prevents unnecessary surveillance or intervention. Secondly, a Rh-negative unsensitized woman carrying Rh-negative fetuses will not require antenatal RhoGAM administration.

Fetal blood typing has become a routine prenatal practice in Europe, specifically in the United Kingdom, France, and The Netherlands.[480,481] Despite the wide availability of similar technology in the United States, it has not yet been widely adapted. Major obstacles include lack of standardized protocols, cost, reproducibility, and quality control.

Noninvasive Diagnosis of Fetal Aneuploidy

Aneuploid pregnancies appear to have altered levels of free and cellular fetal DNA compared with euploid gestations. Bianchi and coworkers[453] have demonstrated elevations in DNA from intact fetal cells in trisomy 21 pregnancies. This has also been observed for free fetal DNA in maternal plasma. The median concentration of circulating fetal DNA in the second trimester has been found to be twice as high in women carrying fetuses with trisomy 21.[482] Fetal DNA levels have been found to be significantly elevated in trisomy 13 pregnancies but not in trisomy 18.[483] Although the differences between normal and aneuploid pregnancies are not diagnostic, some authors have suggested that they may be useful as part of a screening algorithm.

Single Gene Disorders

Specific single-gene disorders identified using analysis of fetal DNA in the maternal circulation include myotonic dystrophy, achondroplasia, cystic fibrosis, β-thalassemia, and congenital adrenal hyperplasia.[484-486] As discussed earlier, this is possible only if the mutation of interest is not present in the mother.

Nucleic Acids in Other Body Fluids

Fetal nucleic acids have been reported in other maternal fluid compartments, including cerebrospinal fluid,[487] peritoneal cavity fluid,[488] and maternal urine.[489] However, these alternative sources have proved to be unreliable in terms of yield, sensitivity, and specificity. Advancements in reverse transcription PCR will enable more specific and sensitive detection of nucleic acids, particularly in maternal urine, which could allow for the truest form of noninvasive prenatal diagnosis.

Cell-free fetal DNA has been amplified and analyzed from amniotic fluid samples using quantitative PCR and used for the rapid identification of specific fetal chromosome abnormalities, including aneuploidies of chromosomes 21, 18, 13, X, and Y.[490] Using comparative genomic hybridization, on commercially available microarrays that encompass genetic sequences from all 24 human chromosomes, whole-chromosome and segmental aneuploidies can be determined. This suggests that cell-free fetal DNA in amniotic fluid samples may enhance the clinical application of the traditional metaphase karyotype (molecular karyotype), which could provide information not only about the presence or absence of whole-chromosome aneuploidy but also about subtle deletions or unbalanced rearrangements.[491]

Fetal Cell-Free RNA in the Maternal Circulation

The mother and fetus share approximately half of their genomic DNA sequences, which can be viewed as being a major limitation to using DNA in maternal blood for prenatal testing. RNA analysis has therefore become a candidate for an independent fetal marker. Fetal mRNA sequences can be detected in the maternal plasma of women in early and in late pregnancy.[492] This mRNA is stable in peripheral blood, probably protected in the circulation by its association with particles.[493]

Genetic Evaluation of Stillbirth

A considerable proportion of stillbirths may occur from genetic causes. Six percent to 12% result from karyotype abnormalities,[494,495] but in many cases, tissue cultures are unsuccessful, which contributes to a significant underestimation.[496] The use of molecular-cytogenetic approaches that do not require culturing should be considered in these cases. Even in the presence of a normal karyotype, genetic abnormalities are present in 25% to 35% of perinatal autopsies.[497] The American College of Obstetrics and Gynecology issued a committee opinion in 2001 suggesting that autopsy findings supplemented by genetic studies are invaluable in determining the potential etiology of fetal death.[498] Evaluation should include a perinatal and family history, as well as physical examination of the fetus, photographs, autopsy, and placental examination. Cytogenetic, molecular, biochemical, and infectious disease studies should be considered when appropriate.

The most useful examination is the gross autopsy, which will reveal a change in diagnosis or additional findings in 22% to 76% of cases.[499-502] Alternatives to autopsy have been explored (e.g., magnetic resonance imaging [MRI]), as there may be cultural or social restrictions limiting autopsy evaluation. However, a review of 100 fetal autopsies in which MRI was also used concluded that postmortem examination was better.[503] Fetal skeletal radiographs have not been found to be useful in fetuses without an abnormality on ultrasound.[504]

References

1. Huang T, Watt H, Wald N: The effect of differences in the distribution of maternal age in England and Wales on the performance of prenatal screening for Down's syndrome. Prenat Diagn 17:615, 1997.
2. Shuttleworth G: Mongolian imbecility. BMJ 2:661, 1909.
3. Lejeune J: Les chromosomes humains en culture de tissues. C R Acad Sci 248:602, 1959.
4. Morris JK, Wald NJ, Watt HC: Fetal loss in Down syndrome pregnancies. Prenat Diagn 19:142, 1999.
5. Merkatz IR, Nitowsky HM, Macri JN, et al: An association between low maternal serum alpha-fetoprotein and fetal chromosomal abnormalities. Am J Obstet Gynecol 148:886, 1984.
6. Haddow J, Palomaki G: Prenatal screening for Down syndrome. In Simpson J, Elias S (eds): Essentials of Prenatal Diagnosis. New York, Churchill Livingstone, 1993, p 185.
7. Cuckle HS, Wald NJ, Lindenbaum RH: Maternal serum alpha-fetoprotein measurement: A screening test for Down syndrome. Lancet 1:926, 1984.
8. DiMaio MS, Baumgarten A, Greenstein RM, et al: Screening for fetal Down's syndrome in pregnancy by measuring maternal serum alpha-fetoprotein levels. N Engl J Med 317:342, 1987.
9. New England Regional Genetics Group Prenatal Collaborative Study of Down Syndrome Screening: Combining maternal serum alpha-fetoprotein, human chorionic gonadotropin, and unconjugated estriol. Am J Obstet Gynecol 169:526, 1989.
10. Bogart MH, Pandian MR, Jones OW: Abnormal maternal serum chorionic gonadotropin levels in pregnancies with fetal chromosome abnormalities. Prenat Diagn 7:623, 1987.
11. Canick JA, Knight GJ, Palomaki GE, et al: Low second trimester maternal serum unconjugated oestriol in pregnancies with Down's syndrome. BJOG 95:330, 1988.
12. Wald NJ, Cuckle HS, Densem JW, et al: Maternal serum screening for Down's syndrome in early pregnancy. BMJ 297:883, 1988.
13. Heyl PS, Miller W, Canick JA: Maternal serum screening for aneuploid pregnancy by alpha fetoprotein, hCG, and unconjugated estriol. Obstet Gynecol 76:1025, 1990.
14. MacDonald ML, Wagner RM, Slotnick RN: Sensitivity and specificity of screening for Down syndrome with alpha-fetoprotein, hCG, unconjugated estriol, and maternal age. Obstet Gynecol 77:63, 1991.
15. Phillips O, Tharapel A, Lerner J, et al: Risk of fetal mosaicism when placental mosaicism is diagnosed by chorionic villus sampling. Am J Obstet Gynecol 174:850, 1996.
16. Burton BK, Prins GS, Verp MS: A prospective trial of prenatal screening for Down syndrome by means of maternal serum alpha-fetoprotein, human chorionic gonadotropin, and unconjugated estriol. Am J Obstet Gynecol 169:526, 1993.
17. Haddow JE, Palomaki GE, Knight GJ, et al: Prenatal screening for Down's syndrome with use of maternal serum markers. N Engl J Med 327:588, 1992.
18. Haddow JE, Palomaki GE, Knight GJ, et al: Reducing the need for amniocentesis in women 35 years of age or older with serum markers for screening. N Engl J Med 330:1114, 1994.
19. Renier MA, Vereecken A, Van Herck E, et al: Second trimester maternal dimeric inhibin-A in the multiple-marker screening test for Down's syndrome. Hum Reprod 13:744, 1998.
20. Malone FD, Canick JA, Ball RH, et al: First- and Second-Trimester Evaluation of Risk (FASTER) Research Consortium. First-trimester or second-trimester screening, or both, for Down's syndrome. N Engl J Med 353:2001-2011, 2005.
21. Cole LA, Shahabi S, Oz UA, et al: Hyperglycosylated human chorionic gonadotropin (invasive trophoblast antigen) immunoassay: A new basis for gestational Down syndrome screening. Clin Chem 45:2109, 1999.
22. Crandall BF, Robinson L, Grau P: Risks associated with an elevated maternal serum alpha-fetoprotein level. Am J Obstet Gynecol 165:581, 1991.
23. Waller DK, Lustig LS, Cunningham GC, et al: Second-trimester maternal serum alpha-fetoprotein levels and the risk of subsequent fetal death. N Engl J Med 325:6, 1991.
24. Waller DK, Lustig LS, Cunningham GC, et al: The association between maternal serum alpha-fetoprotein and preterm birth, small for gestational age infants, preeclampsia, and placental complications. Obstet Gynecol 88:816, 1996.
25. Waller DK, Lustig LS, Smith AH, et al: Alpha-fetoprotein: A biomarker for pregnancy outcome. Epidemiology 4:471, 1993.

26. Yaron Y, Cherry M, Kramer RL, et al: Second-trimester maternal serum marker screening: Maternal serum alpha-fetoprotein, beta-human chorionic gonadotropin, estriol, and their various combination as predictors of pregnancy outcome. Am J Obstet Gynecol 181:968, 1999.
27. Kuller JA, Sellati LE, Chescheir NC, et al: Outcome of pregnancies with elevation of both maternal serum alpha-fetoprotein and human chorionic gonadotropin. Am J Perinatol 12:93, 1995.
28. Morssink LP, Kornman LH, Beekhuis JR, et al: Abnormal levels of maternal serum human chorionic gonadotropin and alpha-fetoprotein in the second trimester: Relation to fetal weight and preterm delivery. Prenat Diagn 15:1041, 1995.
29. Benn P: Trisomy 16 and trisomy 16 mosaicism: A review. Am J Med Genet 79:121-133, 1998.
30. Santolaya-Forgas J, Jessup J, Burd LI, et al: Pregnancy outcome in women with low midtrimester maternal serum unconjugated estriol. J Reprod Med 41:87, 1996.
31. Kowalczyk TD, Cabaniss ML, Cusmano L: Association of low unconjugated estriol in the second trimester and adverse pregnancy outcome. Obstet Gynecol 91:396, 1998.
32. Bitzer MG, Kelley RI, Schwartz MF: Abnormal maternal serum marker pattern associated with Smith-Lemli-Opitz (SLO) syndrome. Am J Hum Genet 55:A277, 1994.
33. Canick JA, Abuelo DN, Bradley LA, et al: Maternal serum marker levels in two pregnancies affected with Smith-Lemli-Opitz syndrome. Prenat Diagn 17:187, 1997.
34. Tint GS, Abuelo D, Till M, et al: Fetal Smith-Lemli-Opitz syndrome can be detected accurately and reliably by measuring amniotic fluid dehydrocholesterols. Prenat Diagn 18:651, 1998.
35. Bradley LA, Palomaki GE, Knight GJ, et al: Levels of unconjugated estriol and other maternal serum markers in pregnancies with Smith-Lemli-Opitz (RSH) syndrome fetuses. Am J Med Genet 82:355, 1999.
36. Palomaki GE, Bradley LA, Knight GJ, et al: Assigning risk for Smith-Lemli-Opitz syndrome as part of 2nd trimester screening for Down's syndrome. J Med Screen 9:43, 2002.
37. Kratz LE, Kelley RI: Prenatal diagnosis of the RSH/Smith-Lemli-Opitz syndrome. Am J Med Genet 82:376, 1999.
38. Zalel Y, Kedar I, Tepper R, et al: Differential diagnosis and management of very low second trimester maternal serum unconjugated estriol levels, with special emphasis on the diagnosis of X-linked ichthyosis. Obstet Gynecol Surv 51:200, 1996.
39. Bradley LA, Canick JA, Palomaki GE, et al: Undetectable maternal serum unconjugated estriol levels in the second trimester: Risk of perinatal complications associated with placental sulfatase deficiency. Am J Obstet Gynecol 176:531, 1997.
40. Santolaya-Forgas J, Cohen L, Vengalil S, et al: Prenatal diagnosis of X-linked ichthyosis using molecular cytogenetics. Fetal Diagn Ther 12:36, 1997.
41. Schleifer RA, Bradley LA, Richards DS, et al: Pregnancy outcome for women with very low levels of maternal serum unconjugated estriol on second-trimester screening. Am J Obstet Gynecol 173:1152, 1995.
42. Benacerraf BR, Gelman R, Frigoletto FD Jr: Sonographic identification of second-trimester fetuses with Down's syndrome. N Engl J Med 317:1371, 1987.
43. Perella R, Duerinckx AJ, Grant EG, et al: Second-trimester sonographic diagnosis of Down syndrome: Role of femur-length shortening and nuchal-fold thickening. AJR Am J Roentgenol 151:981, 1988.
44. Nyberg DA, Resta RG, Hickok DE, et al: Femur length shortening in the detection of Down syndrome: Is prenatal screening feasible? Am J Obstet Gynecol 162:1247, 1990.
45. Crane JP, Gray DL: Sonographically measured nuchal skinfold thickness as a screening tool for Down syndrome: Results of a prospective clinical trial. Obstet Gynecol 77:533, 1991.
46. Donnenfeld AE: Sonographic screening for Down syndrome. Genet Teratol 1:1, 1992.
47. Borrell A, Costa D, Martinez JM, et al: Early midtrimester fetal nuchal thickness: Effectiveness as a marker of Down syndrome. Am J Obstet Gynecol 175:45, 1996.
48. Sonek JD, Cicero S, Neifer R, et al: Nasal bone assessment in prenatal screening for trisomy 21. Am J Obstet Gynecol 195:1219-1230, 2000.
49. Bahado-Singh R, Deren O, Oz U, et al: An alternative for women initially declining genetic amniocentesis: Individual Down syndrome odds on the basis of maternal age and multiple ultrasonographic markers. Am J Obstet Gynecol 179:514, 1998.
50. Bromley B, Lieberman E, Shipp TD, et al: Significance of an echogenic intracardiac focus in fetuses at high and low risk for aneuploidy. J Ultrasound Med 17:127, 1998.
51. Nyberg DA, Resta RG, Mahony T, et al: Fetal hyperechogenic bowel and Down's syndrome. Ultrasound Obstet Gynecol 3:330, 1993.
52. MacGregor SN, Tamura R, Sabbagha R, et al: Isolated hyperechoic fetal bowel: Significance and implications for management. Am J Obstet Gynecol 173:1254, 1995.
53. Corteville JE, Gray DL, Langer JC: Bowel abnormalities in the fetus: Correlation of prenatal ultrasonographic findings with outcome. Am J Obstet Gynecol 175:724, 1996.
54. Snijders RJ, Sebire NJ, Faria M, et al: Fetal mild hydronephrosis and chromosomal defects: Relation to maternal age and gestation. Fetal Diagn Ther 10:349, 1995.
55. Benacerraf BR, Osathanondh R, Frigoletto FD: Sonographic demonstration of hypoplasia of the middle phalanx of the fifth digit: A finding associated with Down syndrome. Am J Obstet Gynecol 159:181, 1988.
56. Drugan A, Johnson MP, Evans MI: Ultrasound screening for fetal chromosome anomalies. Am J Med Genet 90:98, 2000.
57. Shipp TD, Benacerraf BR: Second trimester ultrasound screening for chromosomal abnormalities. Prenat Diagn 22:296, 2002.
58. Paladini D, Tartaglione A, Agangi A, et al: The association between congenital heart disease and Down syndrome in prenatal life. Ultrasound Obstet Gynecol 15:104, 2000.
59. Johnson MP, Barr M Jr, Treadwell MC, et al: Fetal leg and femur/foot length ratio: A marker for trisomy 21. Am J Obstet Gynecol 169:557, 1993.
60. Nyberg DA, Luthy DA, Resta RG, et al: Age-adjusted ultrasound risk assessment for fetal Down's syndrome during the second trimester: Description of the method and analysis of 142 cases. Ultrasound Obstet Gynecol 12:8, 1998.
61. Crane JP, LeFevre ML, Winborn RC, et al: A randomized trial of prenatal ultrasonographic screening: Impact on the detection, management, and outcome of anomalous fetuses. The RADIUS Study Group. Am J Obstet Gynecol 171:392, 1994.
62. Nyberg DA, Souter VL, El-Bastawissi A, et al: Isolated sonographic markers for detection of fetal Down syndrome in the second trimester of pregnancy. J Ultrasound Med 20:1053, 2001.
63. Smith-Bindman R, Hosmer W, Feldstein VA, et al: Second-trimester ultrasound to detect fetuses with Down syndrome: A meta-analysis. JAMA 285:1044, 2001.
64. Souter VL, Nyberg DA, El-Bastawissi A, et al: Correlation of ultrasound findings and biochemical markers in the second trimester of pregnancy in fetuses with trisomy 21. Prenat Diagn 22:175, 2002.
65. Bahado-Singh R, Shahabi S, Karaca M, et al: The comprehensive midtrimester test: High-sensitivity Down syndrome test. Am J Obstet Gynecol 186:803, 2002.
66. Snijders RJ, Shawa L, Nicolaides KH: Fetal choroid plexus cysts and trisomy 18: Assessment of risk based on ultrasound findings and maternal age. Prenat Diagn 14:1119, 1994.
67. Shunagshoti S, Netsky MG: Neuroepithelial (colloid) cysts of the nervous system: Further observation of pathogenesis, location, incidence and histochemistry. Neurology 16:887, 1966.
68. Nadel AS, Bromley BS, Frigoletto FD Jr, et al: Isolated choroid plexus cysts in the second-trimester fetus: Is amniocentesis really indicated? Radiology 185:545, 1992.
69. Riebel T, Nasir R, Weber K: Choroid plexus cysts: A normal finding on ultrasound. Pediatr Radiol 22:410, 1992.
70. Porto M, Murata Y, Warneke LA, et al: Fetal choroid plexus cysts: An independent risk factor for chromosomal anomalies. J Clin Ultrasound 21:103, 1993.

71. Nava S, Godmillow L, Reeser S, et al: Significance of sonographically detected second-trimester choroid plexus cysts: A series of 211 cases and a review of the literature. Ultrasound Obstet Gynecol 4:448, 1994.
72. Nicolaides KH, Sebire NJ, Snijders RJM: The 11-14 Week Scan. New York, Parthenon, 1999.
73. Cullen MT, Gabrielli S, Green JJ, et al: Diagnosis and significance of cystic hygroma in the first trimester. Prenat Diagn 10:643, 1990.
74. Szabo J, Gellen J: Nuchal fluid accumulation in trisomy-21 detected by vaginosonography in first trimester. Lancet 336:1133, 1990.
75. Nicolaides KH, Azar G, Byrne D, et al: Fetal nuchal translucency: Ultrasound screening for chromosomal defects in first trimester of pregnancy. BMJ 304:867, 1992.
76. Schulte-Vallentin M, Schindler H: Non-echogenic nuchal oedema as a marker in trisomy 21 screening. Lancet 339:1053, 1992.
77. Shulman LP, Emerson DS, Felker RE, et al: High frequency of cytogenetic abnormalities in fetuses with cystic hygroma diagnosed in the first trimester. Obstet Gynecol 80:80, 1992.
78. Suchet IB, van der Westhuizen NG, Labatte MF: Fetal cystic hygromas: Further insights into their natural history. Can Assoc Radiol J 43:420, 1992.
79. van Zalen-Sprock MM, van Vugt JMG, van Geijn HP: First-trimester diagnosis of cystic hygroma: Course and outcome. Am J Obstet Gynecol 167:94, 1992.
80. Ville Y, Lalondrelle C, Doumerc S, et al: First-trimester diagnosis of nuchal anomalies: Significance and fetal outcomes. Ultrasound Obstet Gynecol 2:314, 1992.
81. Wilson RD, Venir N, Farquharson DF: Fetal nuchal fluid: Physiological or pathological? In pregnancies less than 17 menstrual weeks. Prenat Diagn 12:755, 1992.
82. Hewitt B: Nuchal translucency in the first trimester. Aust N Z J Obstet Gynaecol 33:389, 1993.
83. Johnson MP, Johnson A, Holzgreve W, et al: First-trimester simple hygroma: Cause and outcome. Am J Obstet Gynecol 168:156, 1993.
84. Nadel A, Bromley B, Benacerraf BR: Nuchal thickening or cystic hygromas in first- and early second-trimester fetuses: Prognosis and outcome. Obstet Gynecol 82:43, 1993.
85. Savoldelli G, Binkert F, Achermann J, et al: Ultrasound screening for chromosomal anomalies in the first trimester of pregnancy. Prenat Diagn 13:513, 1993.
86. Trauffer PM, Anderson CE, Johnson A, et al: The natural history of euploid pregnancies with first-trimester cystic hygromas. Am J Obstet Gynecol 170:1279, 1994.
87. Brambati B, Cislaghi C, Tului L, et al: First-trimester Down's syndrome screening using nuchal translucency: A prospective study in patients undergoing chorionic villus sampling. Ultrasound Obstet Gynecol 5:9, 1995.
88. Comas C, Martinez JM, Ojuel J, et al: First-trimester nuchal edema as a marker of aneuploidy. Ultrasound Obstet Gynecol 5:26, 1995.
89. Pandya PP, Kondylios A, Hilbert L, et al: Chromosomal defects and outcome in 1015 fetuses with increased nuchal translucency. Ultrasound Obstet Gynecol 5:15, 1995.
90. Szabo J, Gellen J, Szemere G: First-trimester ultrasound screening for fetal aneuploidies in women over 35 and under 35 years of age. Ultrasound Obstet Gynecol 5:161, 1995.
91. Snijders RJ, Noble P, Sebire N, et al: UK multicentre project on assessment of risk of trisomy 21 by maternal age and fetal nuchal-translucency thickness at 10-14 weeks of gestation: Fetal Medicine Foundation First Trimester Screening Group. Lancet 352:343, 1998.
92. Whitlow BJ, Economides DL: The optimal gestational age to examine fetal anatomy and measure nuchal translucency in the first trimester. Ultrasound Obstet Gynecol 11:258, 1998.
93. Braithwaite JM, Economides DL: The measurement of nuchal translucency with transabdominal and transvaginal sonography: Success rates, repeatability and levels of agreement. Br J Radiol 68:720, 1995.
94. Braithwaite JM, Morris RW, Economides DL: Nuchal translucency measurements: Frequency distribution and changes with gestation in a general population. BJOG 103:1201, 1996.
95. Whitlow BJ, Chatzipapas IK, Economides DL: The effect of fetal neck position on nuchal translucency measurement. BJOG 105:872, 1998.
96. Schaefer M, Laurichesse-Delmas H, Ville Y: The effect of nuchal cord on nuchal translucency measurement at 10-14 weeks. Ultrasound Obstet Gynecol 11:271, 1998.
97. Roberts LJ, Bewley S, Mackinson AM, et al: First trimester fetal nuchal translucency: Problems with screening the general population. BJOG 102:381, 1995.
98. Pandya PP, Altman DG, Brizot ML, et al: Repeatability of measurement of fetal nuchal translucency thickness. Ultrasound Obstet Gynecol 5:334, 1995.
99. Herman A, Maymon R, Dreazen E, et al: Utilization of the nuchal translucency image-scoring method during training of new examiners. Fetal Diagn Ther 14:234, 1999.
100. Pajkrt E, Mol BW, Boer K, et al: Intra- and interoperator repeatability of the nuchal translucency measurement. Ultrasound Obstet Gynecol 15:297, 2000.
101. Snijders RJ, Thom EA, Zachary JM, et al: First-trimester trisomy screening: Nuchal translucency measurement training and quality assurance to correct and unify technique. Ultrasound Obstet Gynecol 19:353-359, 2002.
102. D'Alton ME, Cleary-Goldman J: Education and quality review for nuchal translucency ultrasound. Semin Perinatol 29:380-385, 2005.
103. Macri JN, Spencer K, Garver K, et al: Maternal serum free beta hCG screening: Results of studies including 480 cases of Down syndrome. Prenat Diagn 14:97, 1994.
104. Berry E, Aitken DA, Crossley JA, et al: Analysis of maternal serum alpha-fetoprotein and free beta human chorionic gonadotrophin in the first trimester: Implications for Down's syndrome screening. Prenat Diagn 15:555, 1995.
105. Cuckle HS, van Lith JM: Appropriate biochemical parameters in first-trimester screening for Down syndrome. Prenat Diagn 19:505, 1999.
106. Krantz DA, Larsen JW, Buchanan PD, et al: First-trimester Down syndrome screening: Free beta-human chorionic gonadotropin and pregnancy-associated plasma protein A. Am J Obstet Gynecol 174:612, 1996.
107. Hallahan T, Krantz D, Orlandi F, et al: First trimester biochemical screening for Down syndrome: Free Beta hCG versus intact hCG. Prenat Diagn 20:785-789, 2000.
108. Spencer K, Crossley JA, Aitken DA, et al: Temporal changes in maternal serum biochemical markers of trisomy 21 across the first and second trimester of pregnancy. Ann Clin Biochem 39:567-576, 2002.
109. Palomaki GE, Neveux LM, Haddow JE, et al: Hyperglycosylated-hCG (h-hCG) and Down syndrome screening in the first and second trimesters of pregnancy. Prenat Diagn 27:808-813, 2007.
110. Evans MI, Krantz DA, Hallahan TW, Galen RS: Meta-analysis of first trimester Down syndrome screening studies: Free beta-human chorionic gonadotropin significantly outperforms intact human chorionic gonadotropin in a multimarker protocol. Am J Obstet Gynecol 196:198-205, 2007.
111. Canick JA, Lambert-Messerlian GM, Palomaki GE, et al: First and Second Trimester Evaluation of Risk (FASTER) Trial Research Consortium. Comparison of serum markers in first-trimester down syndrome screening. Obstet Gynecol 108:1192-1199, 2006.
112. Wapner RJ, Thom E, Simpson JL, et al: First Trimester Maternal Serum Biochemistry and Fetal Nuchal Translucency Screening (BUN) Study Group. First-trimester screening for trisomies 21 and 18. N Engl J Med 349:1405-1413, 2003.
113. Wald NJ, Rodeck C, Hackshaw AK, Rudnicka A: SURUSS in perspective. BJOG 111:521-531, 2004.
114. Spencer K, Bindra R, Nix AB, et al: Delta-NT or NT MoM: Which is the most appropriate method for calculating accurate patient-specific risks for trisomy 21 in the first trimester? Ultrasound Obstet Gynecol 22:142-148, 2003.
115. Spencer K: Screening for trisomy 21 in twin pregnancies in the first trimester using free β-hCG and PAPP-A, combined with fetal nuchal translucency thickness. Prenat Diagn 20:91-95, 2000.

116. Wewer UM, Engvall E, Albrechtsen R: Adam 12: The long and the short of it. In Hooper NM, Lendeckel U (eds): The ADAM Family of Proteases, vol 4. The Netherlands, Springer, pp 123-146, 2005.
117. Laigaard J, Christiansen M, Frohlich C, et al: The level of ADAM12 in maternal serum is an early first-trimester marker of fetal trisomy 18. Prenat Diagn 25:45-46, 2005.
118. Laigaard J, Cuckle H, Wewer UM, Christiansen M: Maternal serum ADAM12 levels in Down's and Edwards' syndrome pregnancies at 9-12 weeks gestation. Prenat Diagn 26:689-691, 2006.
119. Laigaard J, Spencer K, Christiansen M, et al: ADAM12 as a first trimester maternal serum marker in screening for Down's syndrome. Prenat Diagn 26:973-979, 2006.
120. Stempfle N, Huten Y, Fredouille C, et al: Skeletal abnormalities in fetuses with Down's syndrome: A radiographic post-mortem study. Pediatr Radiol 29:682-688, 1999.
121. Tuxen A, Keeling JW, Reintoft I, et al: A histological and radiological investigation of the nasal bone in fetuses with Down syndrome. Ultrasound Obstet Gynecol 22:22-26, 2003.
122. Rosen T, D'Alton ME: Down syndrome screening in the first and second trimesters: What do the data show? Semin Perinatol 29:367-375, 2005.
123. Cicero S, Rembouskos G, Vandecruys H, et al: Likelihood ratio for trisomy 21 in fetuses with absent nasal bone at the 11-14-week scan. Ultrasound Obstet Gynecol 23:218-223, 2004.
124. Prefumo F, Sairam S, Bhide A, et al: Maternal ethnic origin and fetal nasal bones at 11-14 weeks of gestation. BJOG 111:109-112, 2004.
125. Cicero S, Rembouskos G, Vandecruys H, et al: Likelihood ratio for trisomy 21 in fetuses with absent nasal bone at the 11-14-week scan. Ultrasound Obstet Gynecol 23:218-223, 2004.
126. Cicero S, Spencer K, Avgidou K, et al: Maternal serum biochemistry at 11-13(+6) weeks in relation to the presence or absence of the fetal nasal bone on ultrasonography in chromosomally abnormal fetuses: An updated analysis of integrated ultrasound and biochemical screening. Prenat Diagn 25:977-983, 2005.
127. Cicero S, Bindra R, Rembouskos G, et al: Integrated ultrasound and biochemical screening for trisomy 21 using fetal nuchal translucency, absent fetal nasal bone, free beta-hCG and PAPP-A at 11 to 14 weeks. Prenat Diagn 23:306-310, 2003.
128. Cicero S, Dezerega V, Andrade E, et al: Learning curve for sonographic examination of the fetal nasal bone at 11-14 weeks. Ultrasound Obstet Gynecol 22:135-137, 2003.
129. Huggon IC, DeFigueiredo DB, Allan LD: Tricuspid regurgitation in the diagnosis of chromosomal anomalies in the fetus at 11-14 weeks. Heart 89:1071-1073, 2003.
130. Faiola S, Tsoi E, Huggon IC, et al: Likelihood ratio for trisomy 21 in fetuses with tricuspid regurgitation at the 11 to 13+6-week scan. Ultrasound Obstet Gynecol 26:22-27, 2005.
131. Falcon O, Auer M, Gerovassili A, et al: Screening for trisomy 21 by fetal tricuspid regurgitation, nuchal translucency and maternal serum free bhCG and PAPP-A at 11+0 to 13+6 weeks. Ultrasound Obstet Gynecol 27:151-155, 2006.
132. Borrell A: The ductus venosus in early pregnancy and congenital anomalies. Prenat Diagn 24:688-692, 2004.
133. Borrell A, Gonce A, Martinez JM, et al: First trimester screening for Down syndrome with ductus venosus Doppler studies in addition to nuchal translucency and serum markers. Prenat Diagn 25:901-905, 2005.
134. Dunstan FDJ, Nix ABJ: Screening for Down's syndrome: The effect of test date on the detection rate. Ann Clin Biochem 35:57, 1998.
135. Hyett JA, Sebire NJ, Snijders RJ, Nicolaides KH: Intrauterine lethality of trisomy 21 fetuses with increased nuchal translucency thickness. Ultrasound Obstet Gynecol 7:101-103, 1996.
136. Platt LD, Greene N, Johnson A, et al: First Trimester Maternal Serum Biochemistry and Fetal Nuchal Translucency Screening (BUN) Study Group. Sequential pathways of testing after first-trimester screening for trisomy 21. Obstet Gynecol 104:661-666, 2004.
137. Wald NJ, Watt HC, Hackshaw AK: Integrated screening for Down's syndrome on the basis of tests performed during the first and second trimesters. N Engl J Med 341:461, 1999.
138. Wald NJ, Rodeck C, Hackshaw AK, et al: First and second trimester antenatal screening for Down's syndrome: The results of the Serum, Urine and Ultrasound Screening Study (SURUSS). Health Technol Assess 7:1-77, 2003.
139. Jenkins TM, Wapner RJ: Integrated screening for Down's syndrome. N Engl J Med 341:1935, 1999.
140. Cuckle H, Benn P, Wright D: Down syndrome screening in the first and/or second trimester: model predicted performance using meta-analysis parameters. Semin Perinatol 29:252-257, 2005.
141. Benn P, Wright D, Cuckle H: Practical strategies in contingent sequential screening for Down syndrome. Prenat Diagn 25:645-652, 2005.
142. Reddy UM, Wapner RJ: Comparison of first and second trimester aneuploidy risk assessment. Clin Obstet Gynecol 50:442-453, 2007.
143. Nicolaides KH, Spencer K, Avgidou K, et al: Multicenter study of first-trimester screening for trisomy 21 in 75,821 pregnancies: Results and estimation of the potential impact of individual risk orientated two-stage first-trimester screening. Ultrasound Obstet Gynecol 25:221-226, 2005.
144. Rose NC, Palomaki GE, Haddow JE, et al: Maternal serum alpha-fetoprotein screening for chromosomal abnormalities: A prospective study in women aged 35 and older. Am J Obstet Gynecol 170:1073, 1994.
145. American College of Obstetricians and Gynecologists: ACOG Pract Bull No 77: Screening for fetal chromosome abnormalities. Obstet Gynecol 109:217-227, 2007.
146. O'Brien JE, Dvorin E, Drugan A, et al: Race-ethnicity-specific variation in multiple-marker biochemical screening: Alpha-fetoprotein, hCG, and estriol. Obstet Gynecol 89:355 1997.
147. Wald NJ, Cuckle H, Boreham J, et al: Maternal serum alpha-fetoprotein and diabetes mellitus. BJOG 86:101, 1979.
148. Crossley JA, Berry E, Aitken DA, et al: Insulin-dependent diabetes mellitus and prenatal screening results: Current experience from a regional screening programme. Prenat Diagn 16:1039, 1996.
149. Crandall BF, Matsumoto M: Routine amniotic fluid alphafetoprotein assay: Experience with 40,000 pregnancies. Am J Med Genet 24:143, 1986.
150. Heinonen S, Ryynanen M, Kirkinen P, et al: Prenatal screening for congenital nephrosis in east Finland: Results and impact on the birth prevalence of the disease. Prenat Diagn 16:207, 1996.
151. Lennon CA, Gray DL: Sensitivity and specificity of ultrasound for the detection of neural tube and ventral wall defects in a high-risk population. Obstet Gynecol 94:562, 1999.
152. Boyd PA, Wellesley DG, De Walle HE, et al: Evaluation of the prenatal diagnosis of neural tube defects by fetal ultrasonographic examination in different centres across Europe. J Med Screen 7:169, 2000.
153. Nicolaides KH, Campbell S, Gabbe SG, et al: Ultrasound screening for spina bifida: Cranial and cerebellar signs. Lancet 2:72, 1986.
154. Crandall BF, Chua C: Risks for fetal abnormalities after very and moderately elevated AF-AFPs. Prenat Diagn 17:837, 1997.
155. Seppala M, Ruoslahti E: Alpha fetoprotein in amniotic fluid: An index of gestational age. Am J Obstet Gynecol 114:595, 1972.
156. Seppala M, Rapola J, Huttunen NP, et al: Congenital nephrotic syndrome: Prenatal diagnosis and genetic counselling by estimation of amniotic-fluid and maternal serum alpha-fetoprotein. Lancet 2:123, 1976.
157. Kjessler B, Johansson SG, Sherman M, et al: Alpha-fetoprotein in antenatal diagnosis of congenital nephrosis. Lancet 1:432, 1975.
158. Kestila M, Lenkkeri U, Mannikko M, et al: Positionally cloned gene for a novel glomerular protein: Nephrin is mutated in congenital nephrotic syndrome. Mol Cell 1:575, 1998.
159. Lenkkeri U, Mannikko M, McCready P, et al: Structure of the gene for congenital nephrotic syndrome of the Finnish type *(NPHS1)* and characterization of mutations. Am J Hum Genet 64:51, 1999.
160. Hallman N, Hjelt L: Congenital nephrotic syndrome. J Pediatr 55:152, 1959.
161. Holmberg C, Jalanko H, Koskimies O, et al: Renal transplantation in small children with congenital nephrotic syndrome of the Finnish type. Transplant Proc 23:1378, 1991.

162. Ryynanen M, Seppala M, Kuusela P, et al: Antenatal screening for congenital nephrosis in Finland by maternal serum alpha-fetoprotein. BJOG 90:437, 1983.
163. Crow YJ, Tolmie JL, Crossley JA, et al: Maternal serum alpha-fetoprotein levels in congenital nephrosis. Prenat Diagn 17:1089, 1997.
164. Suren A, Grone HJ, Kallerhoff M, et al: Prenatal diagnosis of congenital nephrosis of the Finnish type (CNF) in the second trimester. Int J Gynaecol Obstet 41:165, 1993.
165. Ghidini A, Alvarez M, Silverberg G, et al: Congenital nephrosis in low-risk pregnancies. Prenat Diagn 14:599, 1994.
166. Wapner RJ, Jenkins TM, Silverman N, et al: Prenatal diagnosis of congenital nephrosis by in utero kidney biopsy. Prenat Diagn 21:256, 2001.
167. Rapola J: Renal pathology of fetal congenital nephrosis. Acta Pathol Microbiol Scand [A] 89:63, 1981.
168. American College of Obstetricians and Gynecologists: Committee on Technical Bulletins: Ultrasonography in pregnancy. Tech Bull No 187. Washington, DC, ACOG, 1993.
169. Chasen ST, Chervenak FA: What is the relationship between the universal use of ultrasound, the rate of detection of twins, and outcome differences? Clin Obstet Gynecol 41:66, 1998.
170. Filly RA, Crane JP: Routine obstetric sonography. J Ultrasound Med 21:713, 2002.
171. Shulman LP, Emerson DS, Grevengood C, et al: Clinical course and outcome of fetuses with isolated cystic nuchal lesions and normal karyotypes detected in the first trimester. Am J Obstet Gynecol 171:1278, 1994.
172. Salvesen DR, Goble O: Early amniocentesis and fetal nuchal translucency in women requesting karyotyping for advanced maternal age. Prenat Diagn 15:971, 1995.
173. Hewitt BG, de Crespigny L, Sampson AJ, et al: Correlation between nuchal thickness and abnormal karyotype in first trimester fetuses. Med J Aust 165:365, 1996.
174. Moselhi M, Thilaganathan B: Nuchal translucency: A marker for the antenatal diagnosis of aortic coarctation. BJOG 103:1044, 1996.
175. Fukada Y, Yasumizu T, Takizawa M, et al: The prognosis of fetuses with transient nuchal translucency in the first and early second trimester. Acta Obstet Gynaecol Scand 76:913, 1997.
176. Hernadi L, Torocsik M: Screening for fetal anomalies in the 12th week of pregnancy by transvaginal sonography in an unselected population. Prenat Diagn 17:753, 1997.
177. Reynders CS, Pauker SP, Benacerraf BR: First trimester isolated fetal nuchal lucency: Significance and outcome. J Ultrasound Med 16:101, 1997.
178. Thilaganathan B, Slack A, Wathen NC: Effect of first-trimester nuchal translucency on second-trimester maternal serum biochemical screening for Down's syndrome. Ultrasound Obstet Gynecol 10:261, 1997.
179. Hafner E, Schuchter K, Liebhart E, et al: Results of routine fetal nuchal translucency measurement at weeks 10-13 in 4233 unselected pregnant women. Prenat Diagn 18:29, 1998.
180. Bilardo CM, Pajkrt E, de Graaf I, et al: Outcome of fetuses with enlarged nuchal translucency and normal karyotype. Ultrasound Obstet Gynecol 11:401, 1998.
181. Pajkrt E, van Lith JM, Mol BW, et al: Screening for Down's syndrome by fetal nuchal translucency measurement in a general obstetric population. Ultrasound Obstet Gynecol 12:163, 1998.
182. Van Vugt JM, Tinnemans BW, Van Zalen-Sprock RM: Outcome and early childhood follow-up of chromosomally normal fetuses with increased nuchal translucency at 10-14 weeks' gestation. Ultrasound Obstet Gynecol 11:407, 1998.
183. Adekunle O, Gopee A, el-Sayed M, et al: Increased first trimester nuchal translucency: Pregnancy and infant outcomes after routine screening for Down's syndrome in an unselected antenatal population. Br J Radiol 72:457, 1999.
184. Souka AP, Snijders RJ, Novakov A, et al: Defects and syndromes in chromosomally normal fetuses with increased nuchal translucency thickness at 10-14 weeks of gestation. Ultrasound Obstet Gynecol 11:391, 1998.
185. Bronshtein M, Siegler E, Yoffe N, et al: Prenatal diagnosis of ventricular septal defect and overriding aorta at 14 weeks' gestation, using transvaginal sonography. Prenat Diagn 10:697, 1990.
186. Gembruch U, Knopfle G, Bald R, et al: Early diagnosis of fetal congenital heart disease by transvaginal echocardiography. Ultrasound Obstet Gynecol 3:310, 1993.
187. Gembruch U, Knopfle G, Chatterjee M, et al: First-trimester diagnosis of fetal congenital heart disease by transvaginal two-dimensional and Doppler echocardiography. Obstet Gynecol 75:496, 1990.
188. Achiron R, Rotstein Z, Lipitz S, et al: First-trimester diagnosis of fetal congenital heart disease by transvaginal ultrasonography. Obstet Gynecol 84:69, 1994.
189. Hyett J, Moscoso G, Nicolaides K: Increased nuchal translucency in trisomy 21 fetuses: Relationship to narrowing of the aortic isthmus. Hum Reprod 10:3049, 1995.
190. Hyett J, Moscoso G, Nicolaides K: Morphometric analysis of the great vessels in early fetal life. Hum Reprod 10:3045, 1995.
191. Hyett J, Moscoso G, Nicolaides KH: Cardiac defects in 1st-trimester fetuses with trisomy 18. Fetal Diagn Ther 10:381, 1995.
192. Hyett J, Moscoso G, Nicolaides KH: First-trimester nuchal translucency and cardiac septal defects in fetuses with trisomy 21. Am J Obstet Gynecol 172:1411, 1995.
193. Hyett J, Moscoso G, Nicolaides K: Abnormalities of the heart and great arteries in first trimester chromosomally abnormal fetuses. Am J Med Genet 69:207, 1997.
194. Hyett J, Perdu M, Sharland GK, et al: Increased nuchal translucency at 10-14 weeks of gestation as a marker for major cardiac defects. Ultrasound Obstet Gynecol 10:242, 1997.
195. Hyett J, Perdu M, Sharland G, et al: Using fetal nuchal translucency to screen for major congenital cardiac defects at 10-14 weeks of gestation: Population based cohort study. BMJ 318:81, 1999.
196. Dolkart LA, Reimers FT: Transvaginal fetal echocardiography in early pregnancy: Normative data. Am J Obstet Gynecol 165:688, 1991.
197. Carvalho JS, Moscoso G, Ville Y: First-trimester transabdominal fetal echocardiography. Lancet 351:1023, 1998.
198. Sharland G: First-trimester transabdominal fetal echocardiography. Lancet 351:1662, 1998.
199. Zosmer N, Souter VL, Chan CS, et al: Early diagnosis of major cardiac defects in chromosomally normal fetuses with increased nuchal translucency. BJOG 106:829, 1999.
200. Pergament E: The application of fluorescence in-situ hybridization to prenatal diagnosis. Curr Opin Obstet Gynecol 12:73, 2000.
201. Watson MS, Cutting GR, Desnick RJ, et al: Cystic fibrosis population carrier screening: 2004 revision of American College of Medical Genetics mutation panel. Genet Med 6:387-391, 2004.
202. Mennuti MT, Thomson E, Press N: Screening for cystic fibrosis carrier state. Obstet Gynecol 93:456, 1999.
203. Grody WW, Cutting GR, Klinger KW, et al: Laboratory standards and guidelines for population-based cystic fibrosis carrier screening. Genet Med 3:149, 2001.
204. American College of Obstetricians and Gynecologists: Committee on Obstetricians: Screening for Tay-Sachs Disease. No 162. Washington, DC, ACOG, 1995.
205. Kaback M, Lim-Steele J, Dabholkar D, et al: Tay-Sachs disease:Carrier screening, prenatal diagnosis, and the molecular era. An international perspective, 1970 to 1993. The International TSD Data Collection Network. JAMA 270:2307, 1993.
206. Kaback MM: Population-based genetic screening for reproductive counseling: The Tay-Sachs disease model. Eur J Pediatr 159(Suppl 3):S192, 2000.
207. Akerman BR, Natowicz MR, Kaback MM, et al: Novel mutations and DNA-based screening in non-Jewish carriers of Tay-Sachs disease. Am J Hum Genet 60:1099, 1997.
208. Gravel RA, Kaback MM, Proia RL, et al: The GM2 gangliosidoses. In Scriver CR, Beaudet AL, Sly WS, et al (eds): The Metabolic and Molecular Bases of Inherited Diseases, vol 3, 8th ed. New York, McGraw-Hill, 2001, p 3827.

209. Grebner EE, Jackson LG: Prenatal diagnosis of Tay-Sachs disease: Studies on the reliability of hexosaminidase levels in amniotic fluid. Am J Obstet Gynecol 134:547, 1979.
210. Grebner EE, Jackson LG: Prenatal diagnosis of neurolipidoses. Ann Clin Lab Sci 12:381, 1982.
211. Grebner EE, Jackson LG: Prenatal diagnosis for Tay-Sachs disease using chorionic villus sampling. Prenat Diagn 5:313, 1985.
212. American College of Medical Genetics position statement on carrier testing for Canavan disease. 1998.
213. Elpeleg ON, Shaag A, Anikster Y, et al: Prenatal detection of Canavan disease (aspartoacylase deficiency) by DNA analysis. J Inherit Metab Dis 17:664, 1994.
214. Matalon R, Michals K, Kaul R: Canavan disease: From spongy degeneration to molecular analysis. J Pediatr 127:511, 1995.
215. Kaul R, Gao GP, Aloya M, et al: Canavan disease: Mutations among Jewish and non-Jewish patients. Am J Hum Genet 55:34, 1994.
216. Kaul R, Gao GP, Balamurugan K, et al: Spectrum of Canavan mutations among Jewish and non-Jewish patients. Am J Hum Genet 55:A212, 1994.
217. Matalon R, Michals-Matalon K: Molecular basis of Canavan disease. Eur J Paediatr Neurol 2:69, 1998.
218. Kaul R, Gao GP, Matalon R, et al: Identification and expression of eight novel mutations among non-Jewish patients with Canavan disease. Am J Hum Genet 59:95, 1996.
219. Bennett MJ, Gibson KM, Sherwood WG, et al: Reliable prenatal diagnosis of Canavan disease (aspartoacylase deficiency): Comparison of enzymatic and metabolite analysis. J Inherit Metab Dis 16:831, 1993.
220. Kelley RI: Prenatal detection of Canavan disease by measurement of *N*-acetyl-l-aspartate in amniotic fluid. J Inherit Metab Dis 16:918, 1993.
221. Sugarman EA, Allitto BA: Carrier testing for seven diseases common in the Ashkenazi Jewish population: Implications for counseling and testing. Obstet Gynecol 97:S38, 2001.
222. Kronn D, Oddoux C, Phillips J, et al: Prevalence of Canavan disease heterozygotes in the New York metropolitan Ashkenazi Jewish population. Am J Hum Genet 57:1250, 1995.
223. Eng CM, Desnick RJ: Experiences in molecular-based prenatal screening for Ashkenazi Jewish genetic diseases. Adv Genet 44:275, 2001.
224. Stein J, Berg C, Jones JA, et al: A screening protocol for a prenatal population at risk for inherited hemoglobin disorders: Results of its application to a group of Southeast Asians and blacks. Am J Obstet Gynecol 150:333, 1984.
225. Cao A, Saba L, Galanello R, et al: Molecular diagnosis and carrier screening for beta thalassemia. JAMA 278:1273, 1997.
226. Flint J, Harding RM, Boyce AJ, et al: The population genetics of the haemoglobinopathies. Baillieres Clin Haematol 11:1, 1998.
227. Huisman THJ, Carver MFH, Baysal E: A Syllabus of Thalassemia Mutations. Augusta, GA, Sickle Cell Anemia Foundation, 1997.
228. Curry CJ, Stevenson RE, Aughton D, et al: Evaluation of mental retardation: Recommendations of a Consensus Conference: American College of Medical Genetics. Am J Med Genet 72:468, 1997.
229. Jacquemont S, Hagerman RJ, Leehey MA, et al: Penetrance of the fragile X-associated tremor/ataxia syndrome in a premutation carrier population. JAMA 291:460-469, 2004.
230. Schwartz CE, Dean J, Howard-Peebles PN, et al: Obstetrical and gynecological complications in fragile X carriers: A multicenter study. Am J Med Genet 51:400-402, 1994.
231. Sherman S: Clinical implications of gray-zone FMR1 alleles. Abstract #308. Presented at American College of Medical Genetics meeting, Dallas, TX, 2005.
232. Devys D, Lutz Y, Rouyer N, et al: The FMR-1 protein is cytoplasmic, most abundant in neurons and appears normal in carriers of a fragile X premutation. Nat Genet 4:335, 1993.
233. Franke P, Maier W, Hautzinger M, et al: Fragile-X carrier females: Evidence for a distinct psychopathological phenotype? Am J Med Genet 64:334, 1996.
234. Riddle JE, Cheema A, Sobesky WE, et al: Phenotypic involvement in females with the FMR1 gene mutation. Am J Ment Retard 102:590, 1998.
235. Turner G, Webb T, Wake S, et al: Prevalence of fragile X syndrome. Am J Med Genet 64:196, 1996.
236. Nolin SL, Lewis FA 3rd, Ye LL, et al: Familial transmission of the FMR1 CGG repeat. Am J Hum Genet 59:1252, 1996.
237. Toledano-Alhadef H, Basel-Vanagaite L, Magal N, et al: Fragile-X carrier screening and the prevalence of premutation and full-mutation carriers in Israel. Am J Hum Genet 69:351, 2001.
238. Rousseau F, Rouillard P, Morel ML, et al: Prevalence of carriers of premutation-size alleles of the FMRI gene, and implications for the population genetics of the fragile X syndrome. Am J Hum Genet 57:1006, 1995.
239. Oostra BA, Willemsen R: Diagnostic tests for fragile X syndrome. Expert Rev Mol Diagn 1:226-232, 2001.
240. Tarleton JC, Saul RA: Molecular genetic advances in fragile X syndrome. J Pediatr 122:169, 1993.
241. Maddalena A, Richards CS, McGinniss MJ, et al: Technical standards and guidelines for fragile X: The first of a series of disease-specific supplements to the Standards and Guidelines for Clinical Genetics Laboratories of the American College of Medical Genetics. Quality Assurance Subcommittee of the Laboratory Practice Committee. Genet Med 3:200, 2001.
242. Sutcliffe JS, Nelson DL, Zhang F, et al: DNA methylation represses FMR-1 transcription in fragile X syndrome. Hum Mol Genet 1:397, 1992.
243. Hagerman RJ: Medical follow-up and pharmacotherapy. In Hagerman RJ, Cronister A (eds): Fragile X Syndrome: Diagnosis, Treatment and Research, 2nd ed. Baltimore, The Johns Hopkins University Press, 1996, p 283.
244. Gardner RJM, Sutherland GR: Chromosome Abnormalities and Genetic Counseling. New York, Oxford University Press, 1996, p 243.
245. Warburton D, Byrne J, Canki N: Chromosome Anomalies and Prenatal Development: An Atlas. Oxford Monographs on Medical Genetics No. 20. New York, Oxford University Press, 1991.
246. Warburton D, Kline J, Stein Z, et al: Does the karyotype of a spontaneous abortion predict the karyotype of a subsequent abortion? Evidence from 273 women with two karyotyped spontaneous abortions. Am J Hum Genet 41:465, 1987.
247. Uchida IA, Freeman VCP: Trisomy 21 Down syndrome: II. Structural chromosome rearrangements in the parents. Hum Genet 72:118, 1986.
248. Berend SA, Horwitz J, McCaskill C, et al: Identification of uniparental disomy following prenatal detection of Robertsonian translocations and isochromosomes. Am J Hum Genet 66:1787, 2000.
249. Uehara S, Yaegashi N, MaedaT, et al: Risk of recurrence of fetal chromosomal aberrations: Analysis of trisomy 21, trisomy 18, trisomy 13, and 45,X in 1,076 Japanese mothers. J Obstet Gynaecol Res 25:373, 1999.
250. Khur AS, Chattopadhyay A, Datta S, et al: Familial mosaic Turner syndrome. Clin Genet 46:382, 1994.
251. Nyberg DA, Resta RG, Luthy DA, et al: Humerus and femur length shortening in the detection of Down's syndrome. Am J Obstet Gynecol 168:534, 1993.
252. Rotmensch S, Liberati M, Bronshtein M, et al: Prenatal sonographic findings in 187 fetuses with Down syndrome. Prenat Diagn 17:1001, 1997.
253. Lambl D: Ein seltener Fall von Hydramnios. Zentrabl Gynaskol 5:329, 1881.
254. Schatz F: Eine besondere Art von ein seitiger Oligohydramnie bei Zwillingen. Arch Gynecol 65:329, 1992.
255. Bevis D: Composition of liquor amnii in haemolytic disease of the newborn. Lancet 2:443, 1950.
256. Walker A: Liquor amnii studies in the prediction of haemolytic disease of the newborn. BMJ 2:376, 1957.
257. Fuchs F, Riis P: Antenatal sex determination. Nature 177:330, 1956.
258. Steele M, Breg W Jr: Chromosome analysis of human amniotic-fluid cells. Lancet 1:383, 1966.
259. Jacobson C, Barter R: Intrauterine diagnosis and management of genetic defects. Am J Obstet Gynecol 99:795, 1967.
260. Lenke RR, Ashwood ER, Cyr DR, et al: Genetic amniocentesis: Significance of intraamniotic bleeding and placental location. Obstet Gynecol 65:798, 1985.

261. Bombard AT, Powers JF, Carter S, et al: Procedure-related fetal losses in transplacental versus nontransplacental genetic amniocentesis. Am J Obstet Gynecol 172:868, 1995.
262. Marthin T, Liedgren S, Hammar M: Transplacental needle passage and other risk-factors associated with second trimester amniocentesis. Acta Obstet Gynaecol Scand 76:728, 1997.
263. Romero R, Jeanty P, Reece EA, et al: Sonographically monitored amniocentesis to decrease intraoperative complications. Obstet Gynecol 65:426, 1985.
264. Jeanty P, Shah D, Roussis P: Single-needle insertion in twin amniocentesis. J Ultrasound Med 9:511, 1990.
265. Sonek J, Nicolaides K, Sadowsky G, et al: Articulated needle guide: Report on the first 30 cases. Obstet Gynecol 74:821, 1989.
266. Johnson JM, Wilson RD, Singer J, et al: Technical factors in early amniocentesis predict adverse outcome: Results of the Canadian Early (EA) versus Mid-trimester (MA) Amniocentesis Trial. Prenat Diagn 19:732, 1999.
267. Hsu LY, Perlis TE: United States survey on chromosome mosaicism and pseudomosaicism in prenatal diagnosis. Prenat Diagn 4:97, 1984.
268. Bui TH, Iselius L, Lindsten J: European collaborative study on prenatal diagnosis: Mosaicism, pseudomosaicism and single abnormal cells in amniotic fluid cell cultures. Prenat Diagn 4:145, 1984.
269. Johnson A, Wapner RJ: Mosaicism: Implications for postnatal outcome. Curr Opin Obstet Gynecol 9:126, 1997.
270. Gosden C, Nicolaides KH, Rodeck CH: Fetal blood sampling in investigation of chromosome mosaicism in amniotic fluid cell culture. Lancet 1:613, 1988.
271. Berghella V, Wapner RJ, Yang-Feng T, et al: Prenatal confirmation of true fetal trisomy 22 mosaicism by fetal skin biopsy following normal fetal blood sampling. Prenat Diagn 18:384, 1998.
272. Klinger K, Landes G, Shook D, et al: Rapid detection of chromosome aneuploidies in uncultured amniocytes by using fluorescence in situ hybridization (FISH). Am J Hum Genet 51:55, 1992.
273. Ward BE, Gersen SL, Carelli MP, et al: Rapid prenatal diagnosis of chromosomal aneuploidies by fluorescence in situ hybridization: Clinical experience with 4,500 specimens. Am J Hum Genet 52:854, 1993.
274. Cheong Leung W, Chitayat D, Seaward G, et al: Role of amniotic fluid interphase fluorescence in situ hybridization (FISH) analysis in patient management. Prenat Diagn 21:327, 2001.
275. Sawa R, Hayashi Z, Tanaka T, et al: Rapid detection of chromosome aneuploidies by prenatal interphase FISH (fluorescence in situ hybridization) and its clinical utility in Japan. J Obstet Gynaecol Res 27:41, 2001.
276. Tepperberg J, Pettenati MJ, Rao PN, et al: Prenatal diagnosis using interphase fluorescence in situ hybridization (FISH): 2 year multi center retrospective study and review of the literature. Prenat Diagn 21:293, 2001.
277. Weremowicz S, Sandstrom DJ, Morton CC, et al: Fluorescence in situ hybridization (FISH) for rapid detection of aneuploidy: Experience in 911 prenatal cases. Prenat Diagn 21:262, 2001.
278. Technical and clinical assessment of fluorescence in situ hybridization: An ACMG/ASHG position statement: I. Technical considerations. Test and Technology. Transfer Committee. Genet Med 2:356, 2000.
279. Evans MI, Goldberg JD, Horenstein J, et al: Selective termination for structural, chromosomal, and mendelian anomalies: International experience. Am J Obstet Gynecol 181:893, 1999.
280. Turnbull AC, MacKenzie IZ: Second-trimester amniocentesis and termination of pregnancy. Br Med Bull 39:315, 1983.
281. Golbus MS, Loughman WD, Epstein CJ, et al: Prenatal genetic diagnosis in 3000 amniocenteses. N Engl J Med 300:157, 1979.
282. Hill LM, Platt LD, Kellogg B: Rh sensitization after genetic amniocentesis. Obstet Gynecol 56:459, 1980.
283. Tabor A, Jerne D, Bock JE: Incidence of rhesus immunisation after genetic amniocentesis. BMJ (Clin Res Ed) 293:533, 1986.
284. Kishida T, Yamada H, Sagawa T, et al: Spontaneous reseal of high-leak PROM following genetic amniocentesis. Int J Gynaecol Obstet 47:55, 1994.
285. NICHD Amniocentesis Registry: Midtrimester amniocentesis for prenatal diagnosis: Safety and accuracy. JAMA 236:1471, 1976.
286. Simpson JL, Socol ML, Aladjem S, et al: Normal fetal growth despite persistent amniotic fluid leakage after genetic amniocentesis. Prenat Diagn 1:277, 1981.
287. Medical Research Council: Diagnosis of Genetic Disease by Amniocentesis during the Second Trimester of Pregnancy. Ottawa, Canada, MRC, 1977.
288. Working Party on Amniocentesis: An assessment of hazards of amniocentesis. BJOG 85:1, 1978.
289. Seeds JW: Diagnostic mid trimester amniocentesis: How safe? Am J Obstet Gynecol 191:607-615, 2004.
290. Andreasen E, Kristoffersen K: Incidence of spontaneous abortion after amniocentesis: Influence of placental localization and past obstetric and gynecologic history. Am J Perinatol 6:268-273, 1989.
291. Antsaklis A, Papantoniou N, Xygakis A, et al: Genetic amniocentesis in women 20-34 years old: Associated risks, Prenat Diagn 20:247-250, 2000.
292. Hanson FW, Tennant FR, Zorn E, Samuels S: Analysis of 2136 genetic amniocenteses: Experience of a single physician. Am J Obstet Gynecol 152:436-443, 1985.
293. Dacus JV, Wilroy RS, Summitt R, et al: Genetic amniocentesis: A twelve years' experience, Am J Med Genet 20:443-452, 1985.
294. Tabor A, Philip J, Madsen M, et al: Randomised controlled trial of genetic amniocentesis in 4606 low-risk women. Lancet 1:1287, 1986.
295. Tabor A, Philip J, Bang J, et al: Needle size and risk of miscarriage after amniocentesis. Lancet 1:183, 1988.
296. Karp LE, Hayden PW: Fetal puncture during midtrimester amniocentesis. Obstet Gynecol 49:115, 1977.
297. Young PE, Matson MR, Jones OW: Fetal exsanguination and other vascular injuries from midtrimester genetic amniocentesis. Am J Obstet Gynecol 129:21, 1977.
298. Swift PG, Driscoll IB, Vowles KD: Neonatal small-bowel obstruction associated with amniocentesis. BMJ 1:720, 1979.
299. Therkelsen AJ, Rehder H: Intestinal atresia caused by second trimester amniocentesis: Case report. BJOG 88:559, 1981.
300. Rickwood AM: A case of ileal atresia and ileocutaneous fistula caused by amniocentesis. J Pediatr 91:312, 1977.
301. Lamb MP: Gangrene of a fetal limb due to amniocentesis. BJOG 82:829, 1975.
302. Merin M, Beyth Y: Uniocular congenital blindness as a complication of midtrimester amniocentesis. Am J Ophthalmol 89:299, 1980.
303. Youroukos S, Papadelis F, Matsaniotis N: Porencephalic cysts after amniocentesis. Arch Dis Child 55:814, 1980.
304. Epley SL, Hanson JW, Cruikshank DP: Fetal injury with midtrimester diagnostic amniocentesis. Obstet Gynecol 53:77, 1979.
305. Broome DL, Wilson MG, Weiss B, et al: Needle puncture of fetus: A complication of second-trimester amniocentesis. Am J Obstet Gynecol 126:247, 1976.
306. Baird PA, Yee IM, Sadovnick AD: Population-based study of long-term outcomes after amniocentesis. Lancet 344:1134, 1994.
307. Finegan JA, Quarrington BJ, Hughes HE, et al: Child outcome following mid-trimester amniocentesis: Development, behaviour, and physical status at age 4 years. BJOG 97:32, 1990.
308. Anonymous: Randomized trial to assess safety and fetal outcome of early and midtrimester amniocentesis. The Canadian Early and Mid-Trimester Amniocentesis Trial (CEMAT) Group. Lancet 351:242, 1998.
309. Penso CA, Sandstrom MM, Garber MF, et al: Early amniocentesis: Report of 407 cases with neonatal follow-up. Obstet Gynecol 76:1032, 1990.
310. Assel BG, Lewis SM, Dickerman LH, et al: Single-operator comparison of early and mid-second-trimester amniocentesis. Obstet Gynecol 79:940, 1992.
311. Hanson F, Tennant F, Hune S, et al: Early amniocentesis: Outcome, risks, and technical problems at less than or equal to 12.8 weeks. Am J Obstet Gynecol 166:1707, 1992.
312. Henry GP, Miller WA: Early amniocentesis. J Reprod Med 37:396, 1992.

313. Nicolaides K, Brizot Mde L, Patel F, et al: Comparison of chorionic villus sampling and amniocentesis for fetal karyotyping at 10-13 weeks' gestation. Lancet 344:435, 1994.
314. Vandenbussche FP, Kanhai HH, Keirse MJ: Safety of early amniocentesis. Lancet 344:1032, 1994.
315. Sundberg K, Bang J, Smidt-Jensen S, et al: Randomised study of risk of fetal loss related to early amniocentesis versus chorionic villus sampling. Lancet 350:697, 1997.
316. Philip J, Silver RK, Wilson RD, et al; NICHD EATA Trial Group: Late first-trimester invasive prenatal diagnosis: Results of an international randomized trial. Obstet Gynecol 103:1164-1173, 2004.
317. Department of Obstetrics and Gynecology, Tietung Hospital of Anshan Iron and Steel Co., Anshan, China: Fetal sex prediction by sex chromatin of chorionic villi cells during early pregnancy. Chin Med J (Engl) 1:117, 1975.
318. Hahnemann N, Mohr J: Genetic diagnosis in the embryo by means of biopsy from extraembryonic membranes. Bull Eur Soc Hum Genet 2:23, 1968.
319. Kullander S, Sandahl B: Fetal chromosome analysis after transcervical placental biopsies during early pregnancy. Acta Obstet Gynecol Scand 52:355, 1973.
320. Hahnemann N: Early prenatal diagnosis: A study of biopsy techniques and cell culturing from extraembryonic membranes. Clin Genet 6:294, 1974.
321. Kazy Z, Rozovdky I, Bakhaev V: Chorion biopsy in early pregnancy: A method of early prenatal diagnosis for inherited disorders. Prenat Diagn 2:39, 1982.
322. Old JM, Ward RH, Petrou M, et al: First-trimester fetal diagnosis for haemoglobinopathies: Three cases. Lancet 2:1413, 1982.
323. Brambati B, Simoni G: Diagnosis of fetal trisomy 21 in first trimester. Lancet 1:586, 1983.
324. Canadian Collaborative CVS/Amniocentesis Clinical Trial Group: Multicentre randomized clinical trial of chorionic villus sampling and amniocentesis. Lancet 1:1, 1989.
325. Rhoads GG, Jackson LG, Schlesselman SE, et al: The safety and efficacy of chorionic villus sampling for early prenatal diagnosis of cytogenetic abnormalities. N Engl J Med 320:609, 1989.
326. Brambati B, Terzian E, Tognoni G: Randomized clinical trial of transabdominal versus transcervical chorionic villus sampling methods. Prenat Diagn 11:285, 1991.
327. Jackson LG, Zachary JM, Fowler SE, et al: A randomized comparison of transcervical and transabdominal chorionic-villus sampling. The U.S. National Institute of Child Health and Human Development Chorionic-Villus Sampling and Amniocentesis Study Group. N Engl J Med 327:594, 1992.
328. Gregson N, Seabright N: Handling of chorionic villi for direct chromosome studies. Lancet 2:1491, 1983.
329. Simoni G, Brambati B, Danesino C, et al: Efficient direct chromosome analyses and enzyme determinations from chorionic villi samples in the first trimester of pregnancy. Hum Genet 63:349, 1983.
330. Chang HC, Jones OW, Masui H: Human amniotic fluid cells grown in a hormone-supplemented medium: Suitability for prenatal diagnosis. Proc Natl Acad Sci U S A 79:4795, 1982.
331. Martin AO, Simpson JL, Rosinsky BJ, et al: Chorionic villus sampling in continuing pregnancies: II. Cytogenetic reliability. Am J Obstet Gynecol 154:1353, 1986.
332. Bartels I, Hansmann I, Holland U, et al: Down syndrome at birth not detected by first-trimester chorionic villus sampling. Am J Med Genet 34:606, 1989.
333. Poenaru L: First trimester prenatal diagnosis of metabolic diseases: A survey in countries from the European community. Prenat Diagn 7:333, 1987.
334. Gray RG, Green A, Cole T, et al: A misdiagnosis of X-linked adrenoleukodystrophy in cultured chorionic villus cells by the measurement of very long chain fatty acids. Prenat Diagn 15:486, 1995.
335. Martin A, Elias S, Rosinsky B, et al: False-negative findings on chorionic villus sampling. Lancet 2:391, 1986.
336. Cheung SW, Crane JP, Beaver HA, et al: Chromosome mosaicism and maternal cell contamination in chorionic villi. Prenat Diagn 7:535, 1987.
337. Mikkelsen M, Ayme S: Chromosomal findings in chorionic villi. In Vogel F, Sperling K (eds): Human Genetics. Heidelberg, Springer-Verlag, 1987.
338. Ledbetter DH, Martin AO, Verlinsky Y, et al: Cytogenetic results of chorionic villus sampling: High success rate and diagnostic accuracy in the United States collaborative study. Am J Obstet Gynecol 162:495, 1990.
339. Williams J, Madearis A, Chun W, et al: Maternal cell contamination in cultured chorionic villi: Comparison of chromosome Q-polymorphisms derived from villi, fetal skin, and maternal lymphocytes. Prenat Diagn 7:315, 1987.
340. Ledbetter DH, Zachary JM, Simpson JL, et al: Cytogenetic results from the U.S. Collaborative Study on CVS. Prenat Diagn 12:317, 1992.
341. Boehm FH, Salyer SL, Dev VG, et al: Chorionic villus sampling: Quality control—A continuous improvement model. Am J Obstet Gynecol 168:1766, 1993.
342. Elles RG, Williamson R, Niazi M, et al: Absence of maternal contamination of chorionic villi used for fetal-gene analysis. N Engl J Med 308:1433, 1983.
343. Karkut I, Zakrzewski S, Sperling K: Mixed karyotypes obtained by chorionic villi analysis: Mosaicism and maternal contamination. In Fraccaro M, Brambati B, Simoni G (eds): First Trimester Fetal Diagnosis. Heidelberg, Springer-Verlag, 1985.
344. Wolstenholme J: Confined placental mosaicism for trisomies 2, 3, 7, 8, 9, 16, and 22: Their incidence, likely origins, and mechanisms for cell lineage compartmentalization. Prenat Diagn 16:511, 1996.
345. Cassidy SB, Lai LW, Erickson RP, et al: Trisomy 15 with loss of the paternal 15 as a cause of Prader-Willi syndrome due to maternal disomy. Am J Hum Genet 51:701, 1992.
346. Purvis-Smith SG, Saville T, Manass S, et al: Uniparental disomy 15 resulting from "correction" of an initial trisomy 15. Am J Hum Genet 50:1348, 1992.
347. Ledbetter DH, Engel E: Uniparental disomy in humans: Development of an imprinting map and its implications for prenatal diagnosis. Hum Mol Genet 4:1757, 1995.
348. Worton RG, Stern R: A Canadian collaborative study of mosaicism in amniotic fluid cell cultures. Prenat Diagn 4:131, 1984.
349. Kalousek DK, Dill FJ, Pantzar T, et al: Confined chorionic mosaicism in prenatal diagnosis. Hum Genet 77:163, 1987.
350. Kalousek DK, Howard-Peebles PN, Olson SB, et al: Confirmation of CVS mosaicism in term placentae and high frequency of intrauterine growth retardation association with confined placental mosaicism. Prenat Diagn 11:743, 1991.
351. Goldberg JD, Porter AE, Golbus MS: Current assessment of fetal losses as a direct consequence of chorionic villus sampling. Am J Med Genet 35:174, 1990.
352. Johnson A, Wapner RJ, Davis GH, et al: Mosaicism in chorionic villus sampling: An association with poor perinatal outcome. Obstet Gynecol 75:573, 1990.
353. Wapner RJ, Simpson JL, Golbus MS, et al: Chorionic mosaicism: Association with fetal loss but not with adverse perinatal outcome. Prenat Diagn 12:347, 1992.
354. Breed AS, Mantingh A, Vosters R, et al: Follow-up and pregnancy outcome after a diagnosis of mosaicism in CVS. Prenat Diagn 11:577, 1991.
355. Post JG, Nijhuis JG: Trisomy 16 confined to the placenta. Prenat Diagn 12:1001, 1992.
356. Vejerslev LO, Mikkelsen M: The European collaborative study on mosaicism in chorionic villus sampling: Data from 1986 to 1987. Prenat Diagn 9:575, 1989.
357. Bovicelli L, Rizzo N, Montacuti V, et al: Transabdominal vs. transcervical routes for chorionic villus sampling. Lancet 2:290, 1986.
358. Tomassini A, Campagna G, Paolucci M, et al: Transvaginal CVS vs. transabdominal CVS (our randomized cases). XI European Congress of Prenatal Medicine, 1104, 1988.
359. MRC Working Party on the Evaluation of Chorion Villus Sampling: Medical Research Council European trial of chorion villus sampling. Lancet 337:1491, 1991.

360. Saura R, Gauthier B, Taine L, et al: Operator experience and fetal loss rate in transabdominal CVS. Prenat Diagn 14:70, 1994.
361. Caughey AB, Hopkins LM, Norton ME: Chorionic villus sampling compared with amniocentesis and the difference in the rate of pregnancy loss. Obstet Gynecol 108(3 Pt 1):612-616, 2006.
362. Brambati B, Oldrini A, Ferrazzi E, et al: Chorionic villus sampling: An analysis of the obstetric experience of 1,000 cases. Prenat Diagn 7:157, 1987.
363. Liu D, Agbaje R, Preston C, et al: Intraplacental sonolucent spaces: Incidences and relevance to chorionic villus sampling. Prenat Diagn 11:805, 1991.
364. Brambati B, Varotto F: Infection and chorionic villus sampling. Lancet 2:609, 1985.
365. McFadyen I, Taylor-Robinson D, Furr P, et al: Infections and chorionic villus sampling. Lancet 2:610, 1985.
366. Wass D, Bennett M: Infection and chorionic villus sampling. Lancet 2:338, 1985.
367. Brambati B, Matarrelli M, Varotto F: Septic complications after chorionic villus sampling. Lancet 1:1212, 1987.
368. Blakemore K, Mahoney J, Hobbins J: Infection and chorionic villus sampling. Lancet 2:339, 1985.
369. Barela AI, Kleinman GE, Golditch IM, et al: Septic shock with renal failure after chorionic villus sampling. Am J Obstet Gynecol 154:1100, 1986.
370. Hogge WA, Schonberg SA, Golbus MS: Chorionic villus sampling: Experience of the first 1000 cases. Am J Obstet Gynecol 154:1249, 1986.
371. Cheng EY, Luthy DA, Hickok DE, et al: Transcervical chorionic villus sampling and midtrimester oligohydramnios. Am J Obstet Gynecol 165:1063, 1991.
372. Blakemore KJ, Baumgarten A, Schoenfeld-Dimaio M, et al: Rise in maternal serum alpha-fetoprotein concentration after chorionic villus sampling and the possibility of isoimmunization. Am J Obstet Gynecol 155:988, 1986.
373. Brambati B, Guercilena S, Bonacchi I, et al: Feto-maternal transfusion after chorionic villus sampling: Clinical implications. Hum Reprod 1:37, 1986.
374. Shulman LP, Elias S: Percutaneous umbilical blood sampling, fetal skin sampling, and fetal liver biopsy. Semin Perinatol 14:456, 1990.
375. Moise KJ Jr, Carpenter RJ Jr: Increased severity of fetal hemolytic disease with known rhesus alloimmunization after first-trimester transcervical chorionic villus biopsy. Fetal Diagn Ther 5:76, 1990.
376. Firth HV, Boyd PA, Chamberlain P, et al: Severe limb abnormalities after chorion villus sampling at 56-66 days' gestation. Lancet 337:762, 1991.
377. Burton BK, Schulz CJ, Burd LI: Spectrum of limb disruption defects associated with chorionic villus sampling. Pediatrics 91:989, 1993.
378. Mastroiacovo P, Botto LD, Cavalcanti DP, et al: Limb anomalies following chorionic villus sampling: A registry based case-control study. Am J Med Genet 44:856, 1992.
379. Olney RS, Khoury MJ, Botto LD, et al: Limb defects and gestational age at chorionic villus sampling. Lancet 344:476, 1994.
380. WHO/PAHO: Consultation on CVS: Evaluation of chorionic villus sampling safety. Prenat Diagn 19:97, 1999.
381. Froster UG, Jackson L: Limb defects and chorionic villus sampling: Results from an international registry, 1992-94. Lancet 347:489, 1996.
382. Brambati B, Simoni G, Travi M, et al: Genetic diagnosis by chorionic villus sampling before 8 gestational weeks: Efficiency, reliability, and risks on 317 completed pregnancies. Prenat Diagn 12:789, 1992.
383. Rodis JF, Egan JF, Craffey A, et al: Calculated risk of chromosomal abnormalities in twin gestations. Obstet Gynecol 76:1037, 1990.
384. Meyers C, Adam R, Dungan J, et al: Aneuploidy in twin gestations: When is maternal age advanced? Obstet Gynecol 89:248, 1997.
385. Hook EB: Rates of chromosome abnormalities at different maternal ages. Obstet Gynecol 58:282, 1981.
386. Wenstrom KD, Syrop CH, Hammitt DG, et al: Increased risk of monochorionic twinning associated with assisted reproduction. Fertil Steril 60:510, 1993.
387. Neveux LM, Palomaki GE, Knight GJ, et al: Multiple marker screening for Down syndrome in twin pregnancies. Prenat Diagn 16:29, 1996.
388. Cuckle H, Wald N, Stevenson JD, et al: Maternal serum alpha-fetoprotein screening for open neural tube defects in twin pregnancies. Prenat Diagn 10:71, 1990.
389. Wald NJ, Rish S: Prenatal screening for Down syndrome and neural tube defects in twin pregnancies. Prenat Diagn 25:740-745, 2005.
390. Elias S, Gerbie A, Simpson J, et al: Genetic amniocentesis in twin gestations. Am J Obstet Gynecol 138:169, 1980.
391. Nicolini U, Monni G: Intestinal obstruction in babies exposed in utero to methylene blue. Lancet 336:1258, 1990.
392. Van der Pol J, Volf H, Boer K, et al: Jejunal atresia related to the use of methylene blue in genetic amniocentesis in twins. BJOG 99:141, 1992.
393. Kidd S, Lancaster P, Anderson J, et al: Fetal death after exposure to methylene blue dye during mid-trimester amniocentesis in twin pregnancy. Prenat Diagn 16:39, 1996.
394. Cragan JD, Martin ML, Khoury MJ, et al: Dye use during amniocentesis and birth defects. Lancet 341:1352, 1993.
395. Pruggmayer M, Johoda M, Van der Pol J: Genetic amniocentesis in twin pregnancies: Results of a multicenter study of 529 cases. Ultrasound Obstet Gynecol 2:6, 1992.
396. Sebire NJ, Noble PL, Odibo A, et al: Single uterine entry for genetic amniocentesis in twin pregnancies. Ultrasound Obstet Gynecol 7:26, 1996.
397. Megory E, Weiner E, Shalev E, et al: Pseudomonoamniotic twins with cord entanglement following genetic funipuncture. Obstet Gynecol 78:915, 1991.
398. Bahado-Singh R, Schmitt R, Hobbins J: New technique for genetic amniocentesis in twins. Obstet Gynecol 70:304, 1992.
399. Prompelan H, Madiam H, Schillinger H: Prognose von sonographisch fruh diagnostizierter awillingsschwangerschafter. Geburtsh Frauv 49:715, 1989.
400. Coleman B, Grumback K, Arger P, et al: Twin gestations: Monitoring of complications and anomalies with ultrasound. Radiology 165:449, 1987.
401. Pretorious D, Budorick N, Scioscia A, et al: Twin pregnancies in the second trimester in an α-fetoprotein screening program: Sonographic evaluation and outcome. AJR Am J Roentgenol 161:1001, 1993.
402. Ghidini A, Lynch L, Hicks C, et al: The risk of second-trimester amniocentesis in twin gestations: A case-control study. Am J Obstet Gynecol 169:1013, 1993.
403. Yukobowich E, Anteby EY, Cohen SM, et al: Risk of fetal loss in twin pregnancies undergoing second trimester amniocentesis (1). Obstet Gynecol 98:231, 2001.
404. Lynch L, Berkowitz RL, Stone J, et al: Preterm delivery after selective termination in twin pregnancies. Obstet Gynecol 87:366, 1996.
405. Brambati B, Tului L, Lanzani A, et al: First-trimester genetic diagnosis in multiple pregnancy: Principles and potential pitfalls. Prenat Diagn 11:767, 1991.
406. Pergament E, Schulman JD, Copeland K, et al: The risk and efficacy of chorionic villus sampling in multiple gestations. Prenat Diagn 12:377, 1992.
407. Wapner RJ, Johnson A, Davis G, et al: Prenatal diagnosis in twin gestations: A comparison between second-trimester amniocentesis and first-trimester chorionic villus sampling. Obstet Gynecol 82:49, 1993.
408. De Catte L, Liebaers I, Foulon W: Outcome of twin gestations after first trimester chorionic villus sampling. Obstet Gynecol 96:714, 2000.
409. Daffos F, Capella-Pavlovsky M, Forestier F: Fetal blood sampling via the umbilical cord using a needle guided by ultrasound: Report of 66 cases. Prenat Diagn 3:271, 1983.
410. Daffos F, Capella-Pavlovsky M, Forestier F: Fetal blood sampling during pregnancy with use of a needle guided by ultrasound: A study of 606 consecutive cases. Am J Obstet Gynecol 153:655, 1985.
411. Ludomirsky A: Intrauterine fetal blood sampling: A multicenter registry: Evaluation of 7462 procedures between 1987-1991. Am J Obstet Gynecol 168:318, 1993.

412. Nicolini U, Nicolaidis P, Fisk NM, et al: Fetal blood sampling from the intrahepatic vein: Analysis of safety and clinical experience with 214 procedures. Obstet Gynecol 76:47, 1990.
413. Nicolaides KH, Snijders RJ, Thorpe-Beeston JG, et al: Mean red cell volume in normal, anemic, small, trisomic, and triploid fetuses. Fetal Ther 4:1-13, 1989.
414. Forestier F, Cox WL, Daffos F, et al: The assessment of fetal blood samples. Am J Obstet Gynecol 158:1184, 1988.
415. Evans MI, Krivchenia EL, Johnson MP, et al: In utero fetal muscle biopsy alters diagnosis and carrier risks in Duchenne and Becker muscular dystrophy. Fetal Diagn Ther 10:71, 1995.
416. Johnson M, Bukowdki T, Reitleman C, et al: In utero surgical treatment of fetal obstructive uropathy: A new comprehensive approach to identify appropriate candidates for vesicoamniotic shunt therapy. Am J Obstet Gynecol 170:1770, 1994.
417. Thornhill AR, deDie-Smulders CE, Geraedts JP, et al: ESHRE PGD Consortium 'Best practice guidelines for clinical preimplantation genetic diagnosis (PGD) and preimplantation genetic screening (PGS)'. Hum Reprod 20:35, 2005.
418. Harper JC, Delhanty JD: Preimplantation genetic diagnosis. Curr Opin Obstet Gynecol 12:67, 2000.
419. Hardy K, Martin KL, Leese HJ, et al: Human preimplantation development in vitro is not adversely affected by biopsy at the 8-cell stage. Hum Reprod 5:708, 1990.
420. Van Voorhis BJ: In vitro fertilization. N Engl J Med 356:379, 2007.
421. Munne S, Sultan KM, Weier HU, et al: Assessment of numeric abnormalities of X, Y, 18, and 16 chromosomes in preimplantation human embryos before transfer. Am J Obstet Gynecol 172:1191, 1995.
422. Geraedts J, Handyside A, Harper J, et al: ESHRE Preimplantation Genetic Diagnosis (PGD) Consortium: Preliminary assessment of data from January 1997 to September 1998. ESHRE PGD Consortium Steering Committee. Hum Reprod 14:3138, 1999.
423. Laverge H, Van der Elst J, De Sutter P, et al: Fluorescent in-situ hybridization on human embryos showing cleavage arrest after freezing and thawing. Hum Reprod 13:425, 1998.
424. Kligman I, Benadiva C, Alikani M, et al: The presence of multinucleated blastomeres in human embryos is correlated with chromosomal abnormalities. Hum Reprod 11:1492, 1996.
425. Evsikov S, Verlinsky Y: Mosaicism in the inner cell mass of human blastocysts. Hum Reprod 13:3151, 1998.
426. Traeger-Synodinos J: Real-time PCR for prenatal and preimplantation genetic diagnosis of monogenic diseases. Mol Aspects Med 27:176, 2006.
427. Pinborg A: IVF/ICSI twin pregnancies: Risks and prevention. Hum Reprod 11:575-593, 2005.
428. Dare M, Crowther C, Dodd J, Norman R: Single or multiple embryo transfer following in vitro fertilisation for improved neonatal outcome: A systematic review of the literature. Aust N Z J Obstet Gynecol 44:283-291, 2004.
429. Derom C, Derom R, Vlietnck R, et al: Increased monozygotic twinning rate after ovulation induction. Lancet 1:1236-1238, 1987.
430. Blickstein I, Verhoeven HC, Keith LG: Zygotic splitting after assisted reproduction. N Engl J Med 340:738-739, 1999.
431. Alikani M, Cekleniak NA, Walters E, Cohen J: Monozygotic twining following assisted conception: Analysis of 81 consecutive cases. Hum Reprod 18:1937-1943, 2003.
432. Schachter M, Raziel A, Friedler S, et al: Monozygotic twinning after assisted reproductive techniques: A phenomenon independent of micromanipulation. Hum Reprod 16:1264-1269, 2001.
433. Pinborg A, Loft A, Rasmussen S, Nyboe Andersen A: Neonatal outcome in a Danish national cohort of 8602 children born after in vitro fertilization or intracytoplasmic sperm injection: The role of twin pregnancy. Acta Obstet Gynecol Scand 83:1071, 2004.
434. Helmerhorst FM, Perquin DA, Donker D, Keirse MJ: Perinatal outcome of singletons and twins after assisted conception: A systematic review of controlled studies. BMJ 328:261-265, 2004.
435. McGovern PG, Llorens AJ, Skurnick JH, et al: Increased risk of preterm birth in singleton pregnancies resulting from in vitro fertilization-embryo transfer or gamete intrafallopian transfer: A meta-analysis. Fertil Steril 82:1514-1520, 2004.
436. Rimm AA, Katayama AC, Diaz M, Katayama KP: A meta-analysis of controlled studies comparing major malformation rates in IVF and ICSI infants with naturally conceived children. J Assist Reprod Genet 21:437-443, 2004.
437. Olson C, Keppler-Noreuil KM, Romitti PA, et al: In vitro-fertilization is associated with an increase in major birth defects. Fertility and Sterility 84:1308-1315, 2005.
438. Jackson RA, Gibson KA, Wu YW, et al: Perinatal outcomes in singletons following in vitro fertilization: A meta-analysis. Obstet Gynecol 103:551-563, 2004.
439. Shevell T, Malone FD, Vidaver J, et al: Assisted reproductive technology and pregnancy outcome. Obstet Gynecol 106(5 Pt 1):1039-1045, 2005.
440. Schieve L, Rasmussen S, Buck G, et al: Are children born after assisted reproduction technology at increased risk for adverse health outcomes. Obstet Gynecol 103:1154-1162, 2004.
441. Hansen M, Kurinczuk JJ, Bower C, Webb S: The risk of major birth defects after intracytoplasmic sperm injection and in vitro fertilization. N Engl J Med 346:725-730, 2002.
442. Ericson A, Kallen B: Congenital malformations in infants born after IVF: A population-based study. Hum Reprod. 16:504-509, 2001.
443. Wennerholm U, Bergh C, Hamberger L, et al, Incidence of congenital malformations in children born after ICSI. Hum Reprod 15:944-948, 2000.
444. Wood H, Trock BP, Gearhart JP: In vitro fertilization and the cloacal-bladder exstrophy-epispadias complex: Is there an association? Human Urol 169:1512-1515, 2003.
445. MRC Working Party on Children Conceived by In Vitro Fertilisation: Births in Great Britain resulting from assisted conception, 1978-1987. BMJ 300:1229-1233, 1990.
446. Anthony S, Buitendijk SE, Dorrepall CA, et al: Congenital malformations in 4224 children conceived after IVF. Hum Reprod 17:2089-2095, 2002.
447. Bonduelle M, Liebaers I, Deketelaere V, et al: Neonatal data on a cohort of 2889 infants born after ICSI (1991-1999) and of 2995 infants born after IVF (1983-1999). Hum Reprod 17:671-694, 2002.
448. Schreurs A, Legius E, Meuleman C, et al: Increased frequency of chromosomal abnormalities in female partners of couples undergoing in vitro fertilization or intracytoplasmic sperm injection. Fertil Steril 74:94-96, 2000.
449. Bianchi DW: Fetal cells in the mother: From genetic diagnosis to diseases associated with fetal cell microchimerism. Eur J Obstet Gynaecol Reprod Biol 92:103, 2000.
450. Adinolfi M: Non- or minimally invasive prenatal diagnostic tests on maternal blood samples or transcervical cells. Prenat Diagn 15:889, 1995.
451. Jackson L: Fetal cells and DNA in maternal blood. Prenat Diagn 23:837, 2003.
452. Bianchi DW, Shuber AP, DeMaria MA, et al: Fetal cells in maternal blood: Determination of purity and yield by quantitative polymerase chain reaction. Am J Obstet Gynecol 171:922, 1994.
453. Bianchi DW, Williams JM, Sullivan LM, et al: PCR quantitation of fetal cells in maternal blood in normal and aneuploid pregnancies. Am J Hum Genet 61:822, 1997.
454. Bianchi DW, Simpson JL, Jackson LG, et al: Fetal cells in maternal blood: NIFTY clinical trial interim analysis. DM-STAT. NICHD fetal cell study (NIFTY) group. Prenat Diagn 19:994, 1999.
455. de la Cruz F, Shifrin H, Elias S, et al: Low false-positive rate of aneuploidy detection using fetal cells isolated from maternal blood. Fetal Diagn Ther 13:380, 1998.
456. Bianchi DW, Simpson JL, Jackson GL, et al: Fetal gender and aneuploidy detection using fetal cells in maternal blood: Analysis if NIFTY I data. Prenat Diagn 22:609, 2002.
457. Hahn S, Zhong XY, Troeger C, et al: Current applications of single-cell PCR. Cell Mol Life Sci 57:96, 2000.

458. Lo YM, Tein MS, Lau TK, et al: Quantitative analysis of fetal DNA in maternal plasma and serum: Implications for noninvasive prenatal diagnosis. Am J Hum Genet 62:768, 1998.
459. Lo YM, Corbetta N, Chamberlain PF, et al: Presence of fetal DNA in maternal plasma and serum. Lancet 350:485, 1997.
460. Lo YM: Fetal DNA in maternal plasma: Biology and diagnostic applications. Clin Chem 46:1903, 2000.
461. Bianchi DW. Circulating fetal DNA: Its origin and diagnostic potential-a review. Placenta 25(Suppl A):S93, 2004.
462. Lo YM, Zhang J, Leung TN, et al: Rapid clearance of fetal DNA from maternal plasma. Am J Hum Genet 64:218, 1999.
463. Halicka HD, Bedner E, Darzynkiewicz Z: Segregation of RNA and separate packaging of DNA in apoptotic bodies during apoptosis. Exp Cell Res 260:248, 2000.
464. Bianchi DW, Lo YM: Fetomaternal cellular and plasma DNA trafficking: The Yin and the Yang. Ann N Y Acad Sci 945:119, 2001.
465. Zhong XY, Holzgreve W, Hahn S: Cell-free fetal DNA in the maternal circulation does not stem from the transplacental passage of fetal erythroblasts. Mol Hum Reprod 8:864, 2002.
466. Angert RM, Le Shane ES, Lo YM, et al: Fetal cell-free plasma DNA concentrations in maternal blood are stable 24 hours after collection: Analysis of first- and third-trimester samples. Clin Chem 49:195, 2003.
467. Honda H, Miharu N, Ohashi Y, et al: Fetal gender determination in early pregnancy through qualitative and quantitative analysis of fetal DNA in maternal serum. Hum Genet 110:75, 2002.
468. Chan LY, Leung TN, Chan KC, et al: Serial analysis of fetal DNA concentrations in maternal plasma in late pregnancy. Clin Chem 49:678, 2003.
469. Guibert J, Benachi A, Grebille AG, et al: Kinetics of SRY gene appearance in maternal serum: Detection by real time PCR in early pregnancy after assisted reproductive techniques. Hum Reprod 18:1733, 2003.
470. Guetta E: Noninvasive detection of fetal sex: The laboratory diagnostician's view. Prenat Diagn 26:635, 2006.
471. Rijnders RJ, van der Schoot CE, Bossers B, et al: Fetal sex determination from maternal plasma in pregnancies at risk for congenital adrenal hyperplasia. Obstet Gynecol 98:374, 2001.
472. Avent ND, Chitty LS: Non-invasive diagnosis of fetal sex: Utilisation of free fetal DNA in maternal plasma and ultrasound. Prenat Diagn 26:598-603, 2006.
473. Avent ND, Reid ME: The Rh blood group system: A review. Blood 95:375-387, 2000.
474. Wagner FF, Gassner C, Muller TH, et al: Molecular basis of weak D phenotypes. Blood 93:385-393, 1999.
475. Lo YM, Lun FM, Chan KC, et al: Digital PCR for the molecular detection of fetal chromosomal aneuploidy. Proc Natl Acad Sci U S A 104:13116-13121, 2007.
476. Faas BH, Beuling EA, Christiaens GC, et al: Specific sequences in maternal plasma. Lancet 352:1196, 1998.
477. Lo YM, Hjelm NM, Fidler C, et al: Prenatal diagnosis of fetal RhD status by molecular analysis of maternal plasma. N Engl J Med 339:1734, 1998.
478. Geifman-Holtzman O, Grotegut C, Gaughan J: Diagnostic accuracy of non-invasive fetal Rh genotyping from maternal blood: A meta analysis. Am J Obstet Gynecol 195:1163-1173, 2006.
479. Roulliac-Le Sciellour C, Puillandre P, Gillot R, et al: Large scale prenatal diagnosis study of fetal RHD genotyping by PCR on plasma DNA from RhD-negative pregnant women. Mol Diagn 8:23, 2004.
480. Finning KM, Martin PG, Soothill PW, Avent ND: Prediction of fetal D status from maternal plasma: Introduction of a new noninvasive fetal RHD genotyping service. Transfusion 42:1079, 2002.
481. Bianchi DW, Avent ND, Costa JM: Noninvasive prenatal diagnosis of fetal Rhesus D: Ready for prime(r) time. Obstet Gynecol 106:841, 2005.
482. Lo YM, Lau TK, Zhang J, et al: Increased fetal DNA concentrations in the plasma of pregnant women carrying fetuses with trisomy 21. Clin Chem 45:1747, 1999.
483. Wataganara T, LeShane ES, Farina A, et al: Maternal serum cell-free fetal DNA levels are increased in cases of trisomy 13 but not trisomy 18. Hum Genet 112:204, 2003.
484. Gonzalez-Gonzalez MC, Garcia-Hoyos M, Trujillo MJ, et al: Prenatal detection of a cystic fibrosis mutation in fetal DNA from maternal plasma. Prenat Diagn 22:946, 2002.
485. Chiu RW, Lau TK, Cheung PT, et al: Noninvasive prenatal exclusion of congenital adrenal hyperplasia by maternal plasma analysis: A maternal feasibility study. Clin Chem 48:778, 2002.
486. Chiu RW, Lau TK, Leung TN, et al: Prenatal exclusion of beta thalassemia major by examination of maternal plasma. Lancet 360:998, 2002.
487. Angert RM, LeShane ES, Yarnell RW, et al: Cell-free fetal DNA in the cerebrospinal fluid of peripartum women. Am J Obstet Gynecol 190:1087, 2004.
488. Cioni R, Bussani C, Scarselli B, et al: Detection of fetal DNA in the peritoneal cavity during pregnancy. Eur J Obstet Gynecol Reprod Biol 107:210, 2003.
489. Al-Yatama MK, Mustafa AS, Ali S, et al: Detection of Y chromosome-specific DNA in the plasma and urine of pregnant women using nested polymerase chain reaction. Prenat Diagn 21:399, 2001.
490. Shaffer LG, Bui T-H: Molecular cytogenetic and rapid aneuploidy detection methods in prenatal diagnosis. Am J Med Genet C Semin Med Genet 145:87-98, 2007.
491. Larrabee PB, LeShane ES, Pestova E, et al: The prenatal molecular karyotype: DNA microarray analysis of cell free fetal DNA (cffDNA) in amniotic fluid. Am J Hum Genet 73(Suppl):599, 2003.
492. Poon LL, Leung TN, Lau TK, Lo YM: Presence of fetal RNA in maternal plasma. Clin Chem 46:1832, 2000.
493. Ng EK, Tsui NB, Lau TK, et al: mRNA of placental origin is readily detectable in maternal plasma. Proc Natl Acad Sci U S A 100:4360, 2003.
494. Wapner RJ, Lewis D: Genetics and metabolic causes of stillbirth. Semin Perinatol 26:70, 2002.
495. Christiaens GC, Vissers J, Poddighe PJ, de Pater JM: Comparative genomic hybridization for cytogenetic evaluation of stillbirth. Obstet Gynecol 96:281, 2000.
496. Saal HM, Rodis J, Weinbaum PJ, et al: Cytogenetic evaluation of fetal death: The role of amniocentesis. Obstet Gynecol 70:601, 1987.
497. Faye-Petersen OM, Guinn DA, Wenstrom KD: Value of perinatal autopsy. Obstet Gynecol 94:915, 1999.
498. American College of Obstetricians and Gynecologists (ACOG) Committee Opinion: Committee on Genetics. Genetic evaluation of stillbirths and neonatal deaths. Obstet Gynecol 97(5 Pt 1):suppl 1-3, 2001.
499. Mueller RF, Sybert VP, Johnson J, et al: Evaluation of a protocol for post-mortem examination of stillbirths. N Engl J Med 309:586, 1983.
500. Meier PR, Manchester DK, Shikes RH, et al: Perinatal autopsy: Its clinical value. Obstet Gynecol 67:349, 1986.
501. Gordijn SJ, Erwich JJ, Khong TY: Value of the perinatal autopsy: Critique. Pedatr Dev Pathol 5:480, 2002.
502. Bohra U, Regan C, O'Connell MP, et al: The role of investigations for term stillbirths. J Obstet Gynaecol 24:133, 2004.
503. Cohen M, Paley M, Griffiths P, Whitby E: Less invasive autopsy: Benefits and limitations of the use of magnetic resonance imaging in the perinatal post-mortem. Pediatr Dev Pathol 22:1, 2007.
504. Bourliere-Najean B, Russel AS, Paneul M, et al: Value of fetal skeletal radiographs in the diagnosis of fetal death. Eur Radiol 13:1046, 2003.
505. Brock DJ, Barron L, Duncan P, et al: Significance of elevated mid-trimester maternal plasma-alpha-fetoprotein values. Lancet 1:1281-1282, 1979.
506. Brock DJ, Barron L, Jelen P, et al: Maternal serum-alpha-fetoprotein measurements as an early indicator of low birth-weight. Lancet 2:267-268, 1977.
507. Wald N, Cuckle H, Stirrat GM, et al: Maternal serum-alpha-fetoprotein and low birth-weight. Lancet 2:268-270, 1977.
508. Wald NJ, Cuckle H: Maternal serum alpha-fetoprotein and birth weight in twin pregnancies. BJOG 85:582-584, 1978.
509. Macri JN, Haddow JE, Weiss RR: Screening for neural tube defects in the United States. A summary of the Scarborough Conference. Am J Obstet Gynecol 133:119-125, 1979.
510. Gordon YB, Grudzinskas JG, Kitau MJ, et al: Fetal wastage as a result of an alpha-fetoprotein screening programme. Lancet 1:677-678, 1978.

511. Smith ML: Raised maternal serum alpha-fetoprotein levels and low birth weight babies. BJOG 87:1099-1102, 1980.
512. Evans J, Stokes IM: Outcome of pregnancies associated with raised serum and normal amniotic fluid alpha fetoprotein concentrations. BMJ 288:1494, 1984.
513. Burton BK, Sowers SG, Nelson LH: Maternal serum alpha-fetoprotein screening in North Carolina: Experience with more than twelve thousand pregnancies. Am J Obstet Gynecol 146:439-444, 1983.
514. Burton BK: Outcome of pregnancy in patients with unexplained elevated or low levels of maternal serum alpha-fetoprotein. Obstet Gynecol 72:709-713, 1988.
515. Persson PH, Kullander S, Gennser G, et al: Screening for fetal malformations using ultrasound and measurements of alpha-fetoprotein in maternal serum. BMJ 286:747-749, 1983.
516. Haddow JE, Kloza EM, Smith DE, et al: Data from an alpha-fetoprotein pilot screening program in Maine. Obstet Gynecol 62:556-560, 1983.
517. Purdie DW, Young JL, Guthrie KA, et al: Fetal growth achievement and elevated maternal serum alpha-fetoprotein. BJOG 90:433-436, 1983.
518. Fuhrmann W, Weitzel HK: Maternal serum alpha-fetoprotein screening for neural tube defects. Report of a combined study in Germany and short overview on screening in populations with low birth prevalence of neural tube defects. Hum Genet 69:47-61, 1985.
519. Williamson RA, Hanson JW, Grant SS: Maternal serum alpha-fetoprotein screening: Report of a pilot project in Iowa. Iowa Med 76:61-64, 1986.
520. Robinson L, Grau P, Crandall BF: Pregnancy outcomes after increasing maternal serum alpha-fetoprotein levels. Obstet Gynecol 74:17-20, 1989.
521. Ghosh A, Tang MH, Tai D, et al: Justification of maternal serum alpha-fetoprotein screening in a population with low incidence of neural tube defects. Prenat Diagn 6:83-87, 1986.
522. Schnittger A, Kjessler B: Alpha-fetoprotein screening in obstetric practice. Acta Obstet Gynecol Scand Suppl 119:1-47, 1984.
523. Hamilton MP, Abdalla HI, Whitfield CR: Significance of raised maternal serum alpha-fetoprotein in singleton pregnancies with normally formed fetuses. Obstet Gynecol 65:465-470, 1985.
524. Doran TA, Valentine GH, Wong PY, et al: Maternal serum alpha-fetoprotein screening: Report of a Canadian pilot project. CMAJ 137:285-293, 1987.
525. Milunsky A, Jick SS, Bruell CL, et al: Predictive values, relative risks, and overall benefits of high and low maternal serum alpha-fetoprotein screening in singleton pregnancies: New epidemiologic data. Am J Obstet Gynecol 161:291-297, 1989.
526. Bower S, Chitty L, Bewley S, et al: First trimester nuchal translucency screening of the general population: Data from three centres [abstract]. Presented at the 27th British Congress of Obstetrics and Gynaecology. Dublin, Royal College Obstetrics and Gynaecology, 1995.
527. Kornman LH, Morssink LP, Beekhuis JR, et al: Nuchal translucency cannot be used as a screening test for chromosomal abnormalities in the first trimester of pregnancy in a routine ultrasound practice. Prenat Diagn 16:797-805, 1996.
528. Zimmerman R, Hucha A, Salvoldelli G, et al: Serum parameters and nuchal translucency in first trimester screening for fetal chromosomal abnormalities. BJOG 103:1009-1014, 1996.
529. Taipale P, Hiilesmaa V, Salonen R, et al: Increased nuchal translucency as a marker for fetal chromosomal defects. N Engl J Med 337:1654-1658, 1997.
530. Farahani G, Goldman MA, Davis JG, et al: Use of the ultrasound aspiration transducer in midtrimester amniocentesis. J Reprod Med 29:227-231, 1984.
531. Leschot NJ, Verjaal M, Treffers PE: Risks of midtrimester amniocentesis: Assessment in 3000 pregnancies. BJOG 92:804-807, 1985.
532. Andreasen E, Kristoffersen K: Incidence of spontaneous abortion after amniocentesis: Influence of placental localization and past obstetric and gynecologic history. Am J Perinatol 6:268-273, 1989.
533. Eiben B, Hammans W, Hansen S, et al: On the complication risk of early amniocentesis versus standard amniocentesis. Fetal Diagn Ther 12:140-144, 1997.
534. Tongsong T, Wanapirak C, Sirivatanapa P, et al: Amniocentesis-related fetal loss: A cohort study. Obstet Gynecol 92:64-67, 1998.
535. Roper EC, Konje JC, De Chazal RC, et al: Genetic amniocentesis: Gestation specific pregnancy outcome and comparison of outcome following early and traditional amniocentesis. Prenat Diagn 19:803-807, 1999.
536. Reid KP, Gurrin LC, Dickinson JE, et al: Pregnancy loss rates following second trimester genetic amniocentesis. Aust N Z J Obstet Gynaecol 39:281-285, 1999.
537. Horger EO, Finch H, Vincent VA: A single physician's experience with four thousand six hundred genetic amniocenteses. Am J Obstet Gynecol 185:279-288, 2001.
538. Wald N, Cuckle H, Wu TS, et al: Maternal serum unconjugated oestriol and human chorionic gonadotrophin levels in twin pregnancies: Implications for screening for Down's syndrome. BJOG 98:905-908, 1991.
539. Räty R, Virtanen A, Koskinen P, et al: Maternal midtrimester serum AFP and free beta-hCG levels in in vitro fertilization twin pregnancies. Prenat Diagn 20:221-223, 2000.
540. Muller F, Dreux S, Dupoizat H, et al: Second-trimester Down syndrome maternal serum screening in twin pregnancies: Impact of chorionicity. Prenat Diagn 23:331-335, 2003.
541. Spencer K, Kagan KO, Nicolaides KH: Screening for trisomy 21 in twin pregnancies in the first trimester: An update of the impact of chorionicity on maternal serum markers. Prenat Diagn 28:49-52, 2008.
542. Pijpers L, Jahoda MG, Reuss A, et al: Selective birth in a dyzygotic twin pregnancy with discordancy for Down's syndrome. Fetal Ther 4:58-60, 1989.
543. Anderson RL, Goldberg JD, Golbus MS: Prenatal diagnosis in multiple gestation: 20 years' experience with amniocentesis. Prenat Diagn 11:263-270, 1991.
544. Pruggmayer M, Baumann P, Schütte H, et al: Incidence of abortion after genetic amniocentesis in twin pregnancies. Prenat Diagn 11:637-640, 1991.
545. Ko TM, Tseng LH, Hwa HL: Second-trimester genetic amniocentesis in twin pregnancy. Int J Gynaecol Obstet 61:285-287, 1998.

Chapter 18

Imaging in the Diagnosis of Fetal Anomalies

Frank A. Manning, MD, MSc

Congenital Anomalies: Definition and Population Frequency

Human development is a complex process by which the fusion of two haploid cells progresses by genetically signaled repeated cell division and exquisitely timed biochemical and biophysical differentiation so as to evolve through embryonic, fetal, and postnatal life expressing the unique characteristics of the individual's genome but sharing a commonality of structure and function with all humans. Phenotypic structural and functional variation occurs across the life span including the prenatal period. In embryonic/fetal life, most of these macroscopic phenotypic variations are insignificant, and they are not recognized nor do they have any impact on survival or the quality of postnatal life.

In contrast, some phenotypic variations result in either death or serious disability, and these phenotypic variations are termed *major congenital anomalies*. There are approximately 275 discrete macroscopic anomalies that have been described and hundreds of combinations of anomalies compiled as syndromes. In about 50% of cases, no cause for the anomaly is recognized, and in about 40% of cases there is either a chromosomal abnormality or a proven or suspect gene alteration. Teratogens (3%), uterine factors (2.5%), and multiple gestation (0.5%) are the remaining causes.[1]

The measurement of the incidence of major congenital anomalies remains imprecise. Determination of the incidence of major anomalies at birth underestimates the true rate, because fetal deaths of anomalous fetuses are excluded and some anomalies are inapparent in the neonate. Estimates of the frequency of major anomalies derived from antepartum ultrasound assessment are inaccurate because of the limitations of the imaging methods. Nevertheless, the overall incidence of major anomalies is considered to be in the range of 2% to 3% of all pregnancies.[2-5] The incidence of major anomalies can be expected to vary according to specifics of the study population, including ethnic heterogeneity, environmental conditions and exposures, maternal (but not paternal) age at conception,[6,7] and the presence of comorbidities such as diabetes[8] and obesity.[9]

Antenatal Recognition of Congenital Anomalies: Methods and Limitations

Whereas antenatal maternal serum *screening* for structural and chromosomal congenital anomalies is based on analysis of specific marker analytes in the maternal circulation (e.g., elevated serum α-fetoprotein in fetuses with neural tube defects,[10] abnormal serum analyte pattern in aneuploid pregnancies[11]) or on recognition of a marker (e.g., nuchal lucency) discrete from the specific anomaly,[12,13] the *diagnosis* of an anomaly depends on direct visualization of the malformed or absent organ or organ systems, often coupled with evidence of dysfunctional sequelae. Over the years, a variety of methods have been introduced to visualize the fetus, including radiography, direct visualization through either the transparent membranes (transvaginal embryoscopy) or the amniotic fluid (fetoscopy), ultrasound, and magnetic resonance imaging. Each modality has advantages and limitations. In contemporary fetal medicine *dynamic ultrasound* is the primary method for detection of fetal structural defects, and the other modalities are reserved specific for confirmatory circumstances.

Currently, two-dimensional dynamic ultrasound imaging is the most commonly used method although three- and four-dimensional ultrasound techniques are becoming increasingly available and appear to offer improved recognition of some anomalies (e.g., facial clefts[14]) (Fig. 18-1). The sensitivity of ultrasound for detection of major anomalies is variable but in general surprisingly low. One important study[2] compared the major anomaly detection rate in a general population with scheduled ultrasound evaluations at 15 to 20 weeks and at 31 to 35 weeks to the anomaly detection rate in a population in whom ultrasound was done only for clinical indications. The incidence of fetal anomaly in this combined population of 15,281 women was 2.3%, but the anomaly *detection* rate in the scheduled ultrasound population was 35% as compared to 11% in the control group. These differences, although statistically significant, created controversy, because the prevailing belief was that the ultrasound detection rate was actually much higher. Subsequent reports for the most part have confirmed these data, with reported detection rates ranging from 22% to 55%.[3,5,15,16] A secondary analysis of these data revealed no evident improvement in

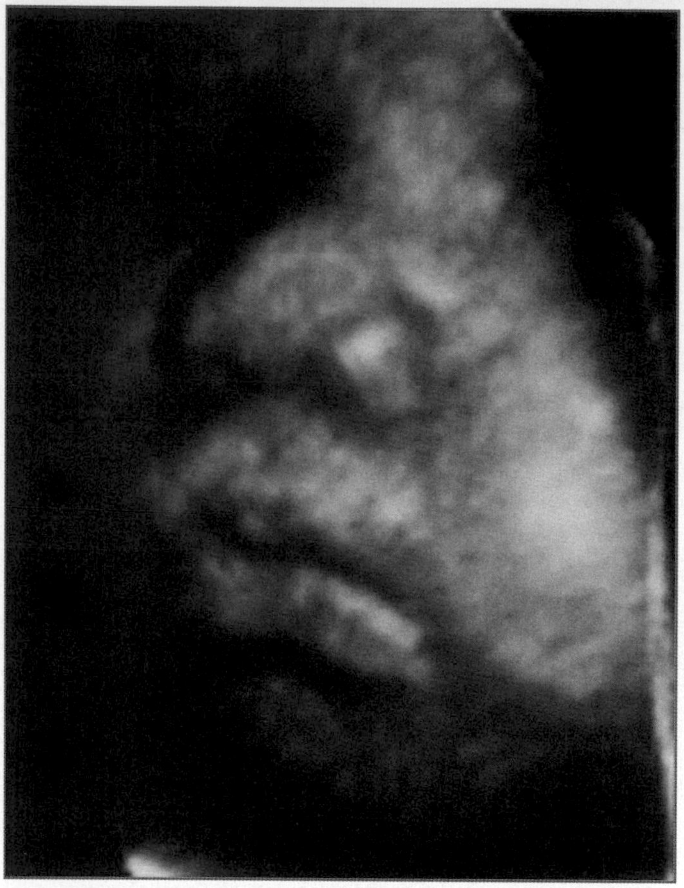

FIGURE 18-1 The frontal view of the face of a near-term fetus produced by three-dimensional ultrasound imaging. Note the striking clarity of detail of the lips, philtrum, and nose. (Courtesy of Professor Delores Pretorius, Department of Radiology, University of California, San Diego.)

maternal and perinatal outcome between the screened and control population.[17]

The following factors influence the ultrasound detection rate of fetal anomalies:

- *Fetal anomaly type.* The detection rate by ultrasound varies widely according to the specific anomaly. The best detection rates are seen for major central nervous system (CNS) anomalies such as anencephaly (94% to 100%[18,19]), with major fetal cardiac defects in the mid range (25% to 60%[20]) and facial clefts tending to be lowest.[21,22] The ultrasound detection rate is significantly increased when multiple anomalies are present,[18] which underscores a clinical axiom: If you find one anomaly, look for more. The detection rate further increases as more scans are done: when patients are subjected to sequenced serial ultrasound anatomic surveys in the first and second trimesters, the detection rate nearly doubles.[23]
- *Gestational age.* Although the genesis of most fetal structural anomalies occurs during the embryonic period, detection by ultrasound is possible for most lesions in later gestational ages. Large anomalies such as anencephaly or limb–body wall defects can be recognized almost as soon as failure of normal development occurs. Other anomalies of embryonic origin are too small to be seen with early ultrasound and do not become manifest until functional abnormality occurs (e.g., aqueductal stenosis is not recognized until the mid to late second trimester and then only because of progressive obstructive fetal ventriculomegaly). Anomalies such as renal agenesis may not be suspected until there is severe oligohydramnios. Some anomalies are the result of failure of completion of a normal developmental process and are identified only at the conclusion of an adjacent normal event. For example, although omphalocele appears to be a result of failure of fusion of the lateral ecto-mesodermic folds to fuse in the midline, an event normally completed by about 28 days of embryonic life,[24] this anomaly cannot be recognized before the normal retraction of the midgut into the abdominal cavity from the umbilical cord at approximately 10 to 11 weeks.
- *Risk factors.* The detection rate for a specific anomaly improves substantially when risk factors are present. For example, a history of a previous anomalous fetus raises the risk by about 50% in autosomal dominant conditions, by about 25% in autosomal recessive conditions, and by about 5% to 10% in multifactorial inheritance conditions. Risk is also increased three- to six-fold with a family history of anomaly, exposure to environmental toxins, or concurrent maternal disease such as pregestational diabetes[25] and obesity.[26,27] Risk is increased in the presence of abnormal maternal serum analytes[28] or of nonspecific fetal markers such as nuchal lucency, oligohydramnios, and polyhydramios.[3] Thus when risk factors are present, targeting ultrasound imaging to specific areas of concern improves anomaly detection.
- *Imaging method and image quality.* The advances in ultrasound imaging methods over the past 2 decades have been remarkable. They have evolved from single-line, to static B-mode, to gray-scale, to real-time (dynamic) B-mode, and now to real-time three-dimensional B-mode (four-dimensional) ultrasound. Concurrently, the introduction of new multifrequency transducers, a wider ultrasound frequency range, higher-speed computing, and real-time duplex and color Doppler have improved image quality and diagnostic precision. As a result, the detection rate for some anomalies (e.g., neural tube defects) has risen to almost 100% in skilled hands.

Nevertheless, limitations remain in the ability of ultrasound to produce fetal images of adequate resolution to ensure that every possible anomaly can be detected. Ultrasound resolution is a function of sound frequency, target density, and distance and variation from adjacent tissues. Resolution is best at the interface between high- and low-density tissues (e.g., skin and amniotic fluid) and worst between tissues of similar tissue density (e.g., liver and gut, kidney and adrenal). Resolution also depends on the incidence angle of the ultrasound beam. Because bone attenuates the ultrasound signal, fetal position can have a profound impact on image quality; for example, fetal cardiac imaging is virtually impossible when the fetal spine lies between the ultrasound beam and the fetal heart. Similarly, maternal body fat attenuates the ultrasound signal, leading to poor image quality in up to 36% of obese patients,[29] and this limitation persists despite repeated examinations.[30] In obese patients, transvaginal scanning can produce improved image quality, as can application of a high-frequency vaginal transducer to the maternal umbilicus, but this is limited to early pregnancy and target distances of less than 10 cm.[31] Thus it is important for medicolegal reasons to ensure that maternal weight is recorded in patients referred for ultrasound and to note in the report whether image quality was compromised by maternal body habitus.

TABLE 18-1 INTRAUTERINE FETAL INVASIVE TREATMENT: METHODS AND RELATIVE SURVIVALS

Fetal Anomaly (ref)	Treatment Method and Survival	Survival of Concurrently Untreated Fetus	Comment
Hydrocephalus (187)	Ventriculoamniotic shunt 83% (34/44) survival	—	10% operative mortality 33% intact survival
Myelomeningocele (68, 69)	Open or fetoscopic repair 90% (56/60) survival	—	44% (87/175) shunt dependent No obvious improvement in limb paresis Randomized trial underway
Congenital diaphragmatic hernia	Open repair[123] 61% (32/53) survival	55% (11/20) survival	No advantage to open in utero repair
	Fetoscopic tracheal occlusion[124] 73% (8/11) survival	77% (10/13) survival	Randomized trial stopped because of no benefit
Pleural effusion or congenital cystic adenomatoid malformation (188)	Thoracoamniotic shunt 67% (13/19) survival	—	
Aortic/pulmonary valve stenosis (189)	Balloon valvuloplasty 15% (3/20) clinical success	—	20% operative mortality Only 70% of attempts successful
Lower urinary tract obstruction (190)	Vesicoamniotic shunt 68% (74/109) survival	40% (23/58) survival	Significant survival improvement only in severe cases Postnatal renal failure, 33%

The Management of Fetal Structural Anomalies

The clinical management of the pregnancy complicated by a fetal anomaly depends on integration of fetal, obstetric, and maternal factors. The ultimate decision regarding management rests with the parents, but the health care team has the responsibility to acquire all available information to assist parents with their decision (Table 18-1). The following four factors affect fetal management.

Prognosis

Some anomalies (e.g., thanatophoric dwarfism, renal agenesis, anencephaly) are always *lethal*, with death occurring either in utero or in the early neonatal period. When the fetal prognosis is hopeless, clinical management is directed to preventing maternal morbidity. In early gestation, pregnancy termination is the usual management. In late pregnancy, management is generally to induce labor when the cervix is favorable and to avoid cesarean section for fetal distress.

Some fetuses have anomalies that are compatible with limited survival but associated with certain and very severe neurologic disabilities (e.g., hydrencephaly, trisomy 18). Management of these fetuses generally follows that for fetuses with lethal anomalies.

At the opposite extreme are fetal anomalies with recognizable anatomic manifestations but with lesions that in postnatal life can be repaired, limiting or eliminating debilitating functional sequelae (e.g., cleft lip). In such circumstances, educating the parents about the anomaly can be beneficial, allowing time for adjustment, acceptance, and arranging postnatal care.

Unfortunately, most anomalies fall into a category in which the prognosis is generally good but cannot be assigned with any degree of certainty (e.g., mild cerebral ventriculomegaly), with a spectrum of outcomes ranging from severe physical limitation but usually intact mental faculties (e.g., spinal bifida) to intact physical faculties but uncertain mental faculties (e.g., agenesis of the corpus callosum).

Gestational Age at Diagnosis

Gestational age at the time of diagnosis of an anomaly has a powerful impact on management decisions. As a general rule, the earlier the gestational age is at the time of diagnosis, the more severe the defect and the worse the prognosis. This association exists in part because the younger the fetus is, the larger the defect must be to be recognized, and the larger the defect is, the greater the likelihood of damaging or disrupting both adjacent and remote tissues. In the mature fetus, delivery and postnatal evaluation may be the most appropriate management. In the immature fetus, termination of pregnancy is often selected, especially when the anomaly is associated with either a hopeless or very poor prognosis.

Progression

The management of an anomaly varies according to whether the lesion is stable and lacking downstream consequences, or whether it is progressive and apt to cause damage to other organs. Many anomalies, such as some cardiac lesions, are nonprogressive, have few functional effects in fetal life, and become manifest as causes of morbidity or mortality only in the neonate (e.g., a small VSD), whereas some anomalies cause a progressive deterioration in function and structure of the local and remote tissues (e.g., renal agenesis). For example, myelomeningocele is usually nonprogressive at the spine, but the tethering of the spinal cord can produce herniation of the cerebellar tonsils into the foramen magnum, resulting in progressive obstructive hydrocephalus. Management of the fetus with anomalies of a progressive, deteriorating character depends on balancing the risks associated with progression with the risks of preterm delivery.

Rarely, anomalous conditions spontaneously resolve in utero. Spontaneous resolution of obstructive hydrocephalus, obstructive uropathy, nonimmune hydrops, and some cardiac arrhythmias is

TABLE 18-2 RELATIVE AND ABSOLUTE INCIDENCE OF MAJOR CONGENITAL HEART LESIONS AND THEIR RECURRENCE RATES

Lesion*	Percentage of All CHD 25% to 75% (Median)	Per Million Live-Born Children 25% to 75% (Median)	% Recurrence	
			Siblings	Offspring
Ventricular septal defect	27.1-42.0 (32.4)	1667-3142 (2267)	4-6	2-22
Atrial septal defect	6.8-11.7 (7.5)	403-910 (563)	3	2-14
Patent ductus arteriosus†	5.3-11.0 (7.1)	350-774 (471)	2.5-3	2-11
Pulmonic stenosis	5.0-8.6 (7.0)	280-641 (404)	3	3-18
Coarctation of the aorta	3.8-5.8 (5.0)	289-419 (332)	2-7	2-8
Transposition of the great arteries	3.5-5.3 (4.5)	275-380 (327)	2	0¶-5
Tetralogy of Fallot	3.9-6.8 (5.2)	261-500 (311)	2-3	1-4
Atrioventricular septal defect‡	2.6-5.1 (3.8)	213-346 (284)	2-3	5-15
Aortic stenosis	3.3-5.9 (4.0)	155-339 (283)	3	3-18
Hypoplastic left heart§	1.6-3.4 (2.9)	151-255 (230)	1-4	—
Hypoplastic right heart‖	1.4-3.2 (2.3)	105-197 (171)	1	5
Double-inlet left ventricle	0.7-1.7 (1.4)	54-126 (87)	3	5
Persistent truncus arteriosus	0.7-1.7 (1.4)	61-145 (86)	1-14	8
Double-outlet right ventricle	1.0-3.9 (1.2)	69-238 (79)	2	4
Total anomalous pulmonary venous connection	0.6-1.7 (1.0)	47-93 (53)	3	5
Miscellaneous	8.0-14.8 (11.4)	536-1058 (804)		

*Lesions are arranged in order of absolute incidence rates.
†Excluding preterm infants.
‡Excluding trisomy 21.
§Mainly aortic and mitral atresia.
‖Mainly tricuspid atresia and pulmonary atresia with an intact ventricular septum.
¶Close to xero for simple transposition of the great arteries.
From Hoffman JI, Christianson R: Congenital heart disease in a cohort of 19,502 births with long-term follow-up. Am J Cardiol 42:641-647, 1978.

known to occur. Management of the fetus with a resolved anomaly is usually conservative with the expectation of a good outcome.

Availability of Fetal or Neonatal Treatment

The availability of methods to correct or ameliorate fetal structural defects has a significant impact on management. Most truly effective treatments are applied in the neonatal period. The usual goal of managing a fetus with a nonlethal anomaly for which there is a reasonable prospect of minimal postnatal disability is to delay delivery until the fetus is mature (Table 18-2). Prenatal consultation with the neonatal team greatly facilitates care coordination and reduces mortality and morbidity.

In a few, very select cases, in utero intervention may be the treatment of choice. However, the initial optimism that accompanied the introduction of in utero treatment of the anomalous fetus has waned significantly as better-constructed studies have demonstrated that the treatment is often ineffective and associated with increased fetal and maternal morbidity.

Cardiovascular Anomalies: Incidence, Causes, Embryologic Development

Approximately 1% of all liveborn children have a structural cardiac anomaly. This rate is even higher when abortuses and stillbirths are included. The distribution of congenital heart anomalies is not equal among the various structural defects, and ventriculoseptal defects (VSDs) are by far the most common lesion (Table 18-3). In most instances, the precise cause of the maldevelopment of the fetal heart is unknown. Approximately 8% of cardiac anomalies are associated with recognizable genetic disease, including 5% that are associated with major aneuploidies (trisomy 21, monosomy X, trisomy 18, trisomy 13) and 3% that are associated with a single gene mutation, including Noonan syndrome (pulmonary stenosis and hypertrophic cardiomyopathy as the most common cardiac structural abnormalities), Apert syndrome (VSD, coarctation of aorta), Holt-Oram syndrome (atrioseptal defect [ASD]/VSD), and Ellis–van Creveld syndrome (single atrium).

TABLE 18-3 CONGENITAL HEART DISEASE: RISK OF RECURRENCE

Defect	Recurrence Risks (%)		
	One Sibling Affected	Father Affected	Mother Affected
Aortic stenosis	2	3	13-18
Atrial septal defect	2.5	1.5	4-4.5
Atrioventricular canal	2	1	14
Coarctation	2	2	4
Patent ductus arteriosus	3	2.5	3.5-4
Pulmonary stenosis	2	2	4-6.5
Tetralogy of Fallot	2.5	1.5	2.5
Ventricular septal defect	3	2	6-10

Modified from Nora JJ, Nora AH: The evolution of specific genetic and environmental counseling in congenital heart diseases. Circulation 57:205-213, 1978.

Most cardiac malformations are inherited in multifactorial fashion, giving a 1% to 2% risk with no family history. However, the risk is increased when there is a *family history:* 4% to 6% with a single affected sibling, 8% to 12% with two first-degree relatives, and 5% to 10% if the mother has congenital heart disease. Fetal structural cardiac defects may also occur after *teratogen* exposure in utero. Lithium ingestion is associated with valvular defects (Ebstein anomaly). Retinoic acid can cause a variety of severe cardiac defects. *Fetal viral infections* are a recognized cause of fetal cardiac defects, rubella virus can cause pulmonary stenosis, mumps virus may cause endocardial fibroelastosis, and Cocksackie B virus is suspected to cause a variety of cardiac defects.

The fetal heart begins development as a simple contractile tube with four segments: from cranial to caudad they are the sinoatrial segment (the origin of the atria), the primitive ventricle (the origin of the left ventricle), the bulbus cordis (the origin of the right ventricle), and the conotruncus (the origin of the pulmonary artery and aorta). By about the 26th day, the contracting of the evolving heart can be visualized by ultrasound. The cardiac tube divides into two parallel tracts, each with an atrium, a ventricle, and an outflow tract, and concurrently the primitive tube moves ventrally and to the right so that the bulbus cordis (the origin of the right ventricle) moves to the right and anterior and the primitive ventricle (the origin of the left ventricle) moves to the left. The completion of this movement (termed cardiac looping) results in the normal configuration of the right ventricle anterior and to the right, and the left ventricle posterior and to the left.

The atria develop by division of the sinoatrial segment by the septum primum and secundum and the migration of mesenchyme to form the four discrete atrioventricular cushions and subsequently the tricuspid and mitral valves and the proximal portion of the ventricular septum. The atrioventricular canal rotates to the right and the ventricular septum posterior to the left, bringing the right atrium over the right ventricle and the left atrium over the left ventricle. The bulboarteriosus divides into two tracts and undergoes spiral rotation, bringing the pulmonary artery over the right ventricle and the aorta over the left ventricle. This complex process of division, differential growth, and rotation is completed by about the 7th week of fetal life. Thereafter, the heart grows in size but the structure remains essentially the same. Errors in migration result in univentricle, double-outlet right ventricle, and ventricle inversus. Failed cardiac looping results in transposition of the great vessels. Failure of division of the conoarteriosus results in truncus arteriosus.

For detailed information about specific cardiac malformations, diagnosis, and management, see Chapter 19.

Central Nervous System Anomalies

Embryologic Development

Developmentally, the CNS begins as a midline fold in the ectodermal neural plate that progresses to form an open-ended tube. As a result of differential growth, the tube folds cranially, initially to form the midbrain and then the hindbrain and forebrain; the caudal end remains unfolded and forms the spinal cord. These events occur very early in embryonic life, and by 4 weeks the CNS is fully differentiated into these four regions. By week 5, the forebrain (prosencephalon) divides into the cerebral primordial and the diencephalons, the midbrain (mesencephalon) remains unchanged and the hindbrain (rhombencephalon) divides into the cerebellum and pons and the medulla oblongata.

The initial ectodermic tube remains hollow, and the epencephalon cavity forms the lateral ventricles and third ventricle and the rhombencephalon forms the fourth ventricle. The choroid plexus develops from pia mater and blood vessels invaginated into the inner walls of the developing ventricles, and by the 6th week they are producing cerebral spinal fluid (CSF). The caudal end of the ectodermic tube (neuropore) closes first, followed later by closure of the rostral (distal) neuropore. Closure of the neuropore depends on normal folate in the fetus. The vessels of the brain arise from mesenchyme migration. Anomalies of the CNS generally occur very early in embryogenesis, arising from abnormally programmed proliferation of the ectodermal segmental folds. Most CNS anomalies are contained within a particular ectodermal developmental region, and CNS anomalies in adjacent regions are usually the result of pressure distortions.

Hydrocephalus (Ventriculomegaly)

Diagnosis. Hydrocephalus, or more precisely ventriculomegaly, is a condition characterized by abnormal enlargement of the lateral ventricles with or without dilation of the third and fourth ventricle. Isolated third or fourth ventriculomegaly does not occur. Because the lateral ventricles are filled with CSF, visualization by ultrasound is easy and reliable. In contrast, because the third and fourth ventricles function more as CSF conduits, these structures are not normally visualized by prenatal ultrasound. The lateral ventricles are shaped like curved elongated ovals, and planar measurement is difficult. By convention, the size of the lateral ventricle is determined by the span measured at the midportion of the ventricle (Fig. 18-2), and nomograms for normal ventricle size and growth either as absolute values or as a ratio of hemisphere widths are available.[32]

Obstruction to CSF flow is the most common cause of ventriculomegaly. Given the relatively large amount of CSF produced in the lateral ventricle by the choroid plexus and the lack of rigidity of the ventricular wall and surrounding cerebrum, in the presence of obstruction the ventricle dilates quickly and dramatically and thus ultrasound recognition is usually easy and reliable (Figs. 18-3 and 18-4). Typically, as the ventricle enlarges, the space between the choroid plexus on the

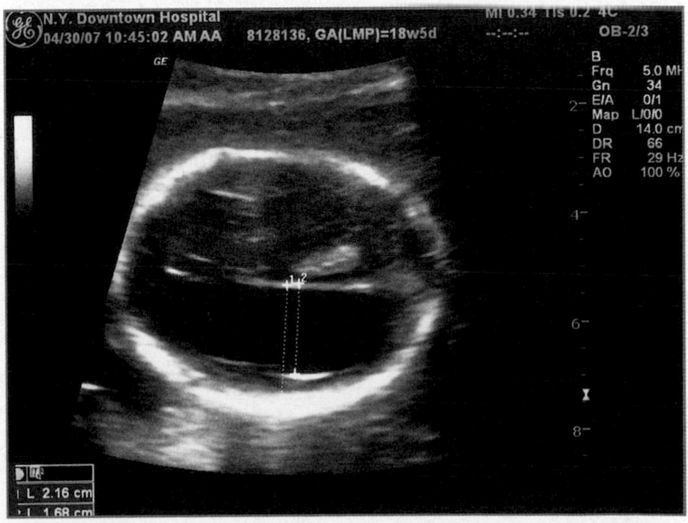

FIGURE 18-2 **Fetus with mild ventriculomegaly.** In this 20-week fetus, the ratio of lateral ventricular width to hemisphere width (LVW:HW ratio) was 1.23 (>95th percentile).

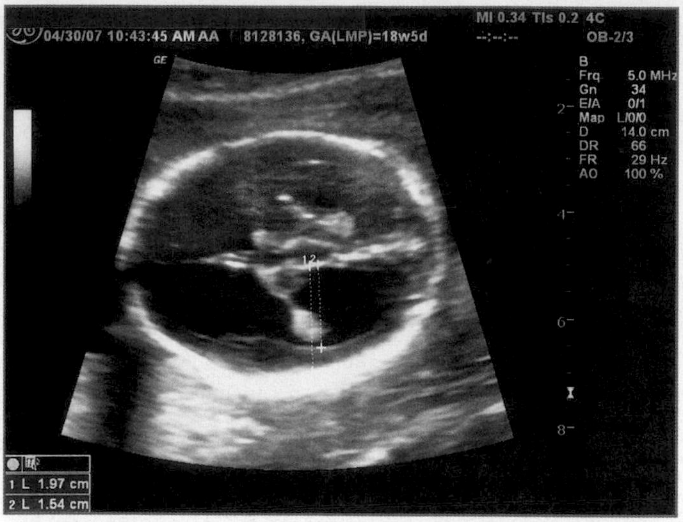

FIGURE 18-3 **Mild to moderate ventriculomegaly.** Note the choroid plexus, which seems to "dangle" into the lateral ventricle.

inner ventricle wall and the lateral wall widens, giving the impression of a "dangling" choroid.

Ventriculomegaly can arise from stenosis of either the third or fourth ventricle or of both. Third-ventricle stenosis occurs most commonly at the connection between the third and fourth ventricles (the aqueduct of Sylvius). *Aqueduct stenosis* results in pressure ventriculomegaly of the third and lateral ventricles and is usually a result of either restrictive gliotic reaction to infectious inflammation (50% of cases), genetic-origin developmental narrowing (25% of cases), sporadic idiopathic stenosis (20% of cases), or obstruction secondary to tumors (5% of cases). Inflammatory obstructive gliosis can be related to infection caused by *Toxoplasma*,[33] cytomegalic inclusion virus,[34] herpes simplex,[35] varicella, herpes zoster,[36] enterovirus,[37] lymphocytic choriomeningitis virus,[38] or parvovirus B19.[39]

Genetic-origin aqueductal stenosis is most commonly related to X-linked recessive inheritance,[40] and in about half of these cases there are abduction anomalies of the thumbs. Autosomal recessive inheritance has also been observed in some cases,[41] as well as uncertain inheritance.[42] Tumors that obstruct the aqueduct include papilla, teratoma,[43] hamartoma,[44] cavum velum cyst,[45] primary neoplasms, and metastatic neoplasia, including that from the mother.[46] Associated anomalies generally occur only with aqueductal stenosis of genetic origin. These anomalies include other CNS anomalies such as agenesis of the corpus callosum, vascular abnormalities, and arachnoid cysts.[47]

Prognosis. The prognosis of ventriculomegaly from aqueductal stenosis varies according to the cause, degree, and permanence of the obstruction. X-linked and autosomal recessive aqueductal stenosis have a very poor prognosis with high mortality (90%) and serious neurodevelopmental anomalies among the few survivors. For inflammatory aqueduct stenosis, the prognosis generally depends on the degree of ventriculomegaly, defined by the transverse diameter of the atrium.[48] Severe ventriculomegaly (i.e., transverse diameter >15 mm) is associated with severe neurodevelopmental delay in 90% of cases.[48] In contrast, isolated mild ventriculomegaly (transverse diameter of the atrium between 10 and 15 mm) has a very high postnatal survival, and normal development is observed in 80% of cases, mild disability in about 10%, and severe disability in about 10%.[49]

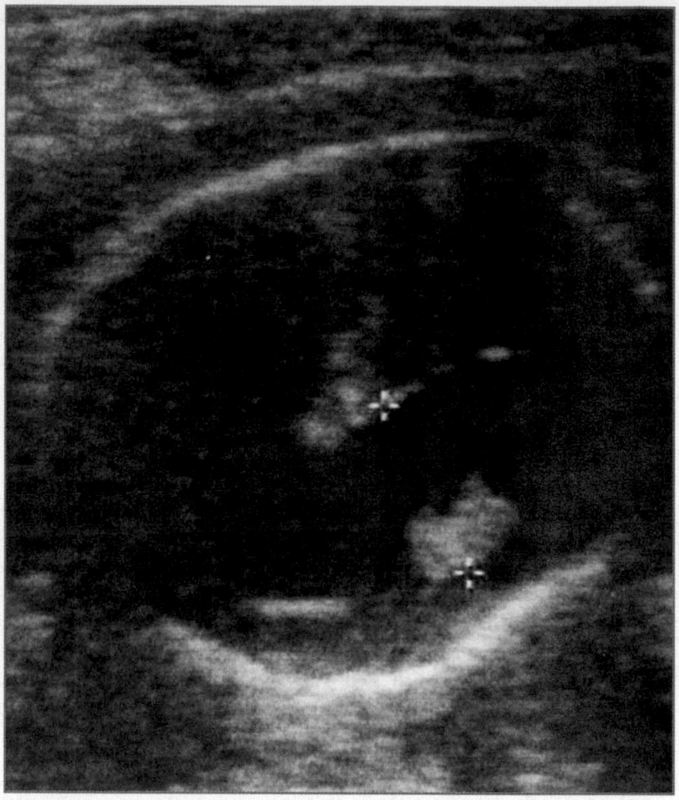

FIGURE 18-4 **Cerebral ventriculomegaly.** Fetal ventriculomegaly at 21 weeks' gestation secondary to aqueductal stenosis. The fetal head is normal in shape and size. The calipers measure the maximal width of the lateral ventricle. The key diagnostic features are the increase in ventricle size, as evidenced by an abnormal ventricle-to-hemisphere ratio (0.8125 in this case) and a prominent lateral shift of the choroid plexus. The midline structures were stable, and the cortical mantle was seen. Disease was rapidly progressive; the fetus was delivered at 24 weeks and died.

In utero fetal decompression of ventriculomegaly has been proposed as a means to halt or reverse progression of disease, relieve cortical compression, and prevent neurodevelopmental damage. Percutaneous ventriculoamniotic shunt placement, although technically feasible, did not benefit postnatal outcome, as 50% of treated survivors had severe disability.[50] Based on these poor results, the Fetal Medicine and Surgery Society recommended this therapy be abandoned. More recently, Bruner and colleagues[51] used an open surgical approach (hysterotomy) to place ventriculoamniotic shunts in four fetuses with severe ventriculomegaly due to isolated aqueduct stenosis. The results were dismal, with one perinatal death related to chorioamnionitis and the three survivors having serious neurologic handicap. Clearly, at present, there is no role for in utero treatment of ventriculomegaly.

Dandy-Walker Malformation

Diagnosis. Dandy-Walker complex is characterized by a posterior fossa cyst that allows communication of the cyst with the fourth ventricle, resulting in obstructive ventriculomegaly of the third and lateral ventricles, often of a major degree. The ultrasound diagnosis of Dandy-Walker syndrome is relatively straightforward. In the transcerebellar axial plane, enlargement of the posterior fossa, overt splaying of the cerebellar hemispheres, a connection between the foramen magnum

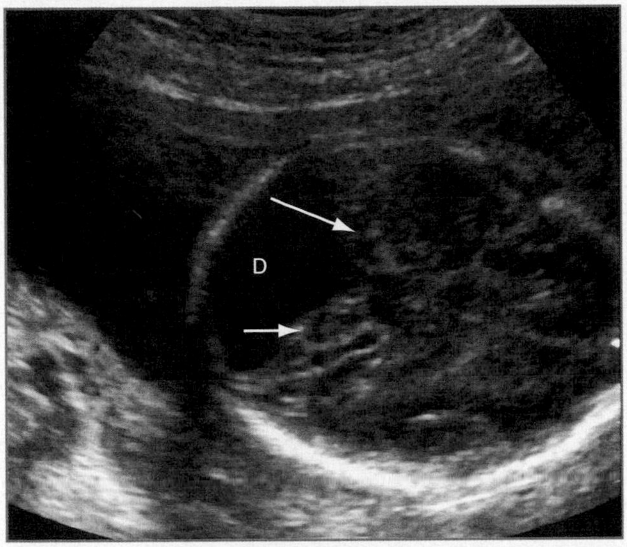

FIGURE 18-5 Dandy-Walker cyst. A small dysplastic cerebellar configuration (*arrows*) adjacent to the Dandy-Walker cyst (D). (From Sanders R, Blackmon L, Hogge W, et al: Structural Fetal Abnormalities, 2nd ed. Philadelphia, Mosby, 2002.

and the fourth ventricle (Fig. 18-5), and lateral ventriculomegaly are evident. The anomaly can be diagnosed by ultrasound in the first trimester.[52]

A variant of the Dandy-Walker malformation with partial agenesis of the vermis and mild expansion of the foramen magnum can occur. It is critical to confirm the vermis abnormality, as simple enlargement of the foramen magnum (>10 mm) is a minor anomaly and associated with an excellent outcome. Dandy-Walker variant malformation is commonly (50% to 70%) associated with other anomalies, including other CNS anomalies (agenesis of the corpus callosum, holoprosencephaly), other organ system anomalies (polycystic kidney, facial clefting), and chromosomal anomalies including a 5p deletion[53] and a 13q deletion.[54]

Prognosis. The prognosis for Dandy-Walker syndrome is very poor. In a recent study of 47 fetuses diagnosed with Dandy-Walker malformation or Dandy-Walker variant, 41 (82%) had associated anomalies, 44 died (mortality rate 94%), and all three survivors had serious neurodevelopmental handicap.[55]

Neural Tube Defects

Failure of closure of the cranial end of the ectodermal neurotube results in anencephaly, and failure of closure of the caudal end results in defects in the dorsum of the vertebrae that may result in herniation of either the meninges (meningocele) or the meninges and spinal cord (meningomyelocele). In the United States, neural tube defects occur at a frequency of about 2 per 1000 live births. However, the frequency of this condition is decreasing because prevention by prenatal administration of folate,[56] implementation of universal maternal serum α-fetoprotein screening,[10] and highly reliable ultrasound diagnosis.[57]

Diagnosis. The ultrasound diagnosis of anencephaly is usually obvious: the calvarium and neocortex are absent (Fig. 18-6). Anencephaly is one of the few CNS anomalies that can be routinely diagnosed in the first trimester,[58] and in the second trimester a diagnostic rate of 100% is expected. The perinatal prognosis is hopeless.

Encephalocele

Diagnosis. Encephaloceles (posterior or anterior) are variants of neural tube defects. These conditions can also be diagnosed in early pregnancy and by the second trimester should be recognizable in most instances. The salient ultrasound feature is an echolucent bulge, most commonly in the posterior occipital region (Fig. 18-7).

Prognosis. The prognosis of encephalocele is completely dependent on whether there is associated herniation of brain tissue into the meningeal sac. When brain tissue herniation occurs, the mortality is high and intact survival rate very poor.[59] In contrast, when there is meningeal herniation only, rates of both survival and intact postnatal development are excellent.[60]

Spina Bifida

Diagnosis. The ultrasound diagnosis of spina bifida in the second trimester is highly reliable with a skilled operator and in many studies superior to maternal serum alpha-protein screening.[57,61] The most reliable ultrasound markers are intracranial and occur as a tethering of the spinal cord such that continued fetal growth results in herniation of the cerebellar tonsils into the foramen magnum (the Arnold-Chiari malformation). As a result of the downward migration of the brainstem, the frontal lobes retract and the anterior calvarium collapses to form a "lemon sign" (Fig. 18-8), which is present to varying degrees in almost every case.[62,63] Normal cranial shape (i.e., a negative lemon sign) is an extremely accurate indication of the *absence* of spinal bifida. The hindbrain herniation with spina bifida causes flattening of the cerebellar hemispheres against the posterior calvarium, producing a characteristic "banana sign." This sign is slightly less reliable than the lemon sign, and it never occurs as a sole finding with spina bifida. Ventriculomegaly to varying degrees is always present with spina bifida and characteristically worsens as pregnancy advances.

The defect in the spine occurs in the low lumbar area in 60% of cases, in the high lumbar, low thoracic area in 35%, and in the sacral area in 5%. The key ultrasound features of the spine are the absence of the dorsal aspect of the vertebrae and a protuberant cystic mass, which usually contains elements of spinal cord (meningomyelocele) (Fig. 18-9) but may be composed of meninges only (meningocele). Abnormal angulation of the spine may also be present (kyphosis or gibbus).

Recognized causal associations with neural tube defects are multifactorial inheritance patterns (the recurrence rate in subsequent pregnancies is 5% or higher), single gene defects (e.g., Meckel syndrome, Robert syndrome, Jarcho-Levin syndrome), chromosome abnormalities (especially trisomy 13 and 18), poorly controlled maternal diabetes, and teratogenic drugs such as valproic acid and retinoid A. Neural tube defects do not have a major impact on the fetus in utero, although occasionally anencephaly may result in swallowing disorders, causing hydramnios. With spina bifida, limb movements are usually normal and bladder filling and emptying may be observed.

Prognosis. The postnatal prognosis of spina bifida depends on the size and location of the lesion: in general, the lower and smaller the lesion, the better the outcome.[64] Pregnancy termination is common. Postnatal mortality is reported to be at least 15% in the first year of life, usually related to respiratory compromise caused by hindbrain herniation.[65] Lower limb paresis is very common. Bladder denervation is common, and renal failure is a significant cause of late infant death. Progressive obstructive hydrocephaly is very common, and at least 85% of infants born with spina bifida will require ventricular shunts.[66] In utero repair of myelomeningocele is possible.[67] Despite the lack of a randomized trial, more than 250 fetuses from four major academic centers have undergone prenatal surgical repair of

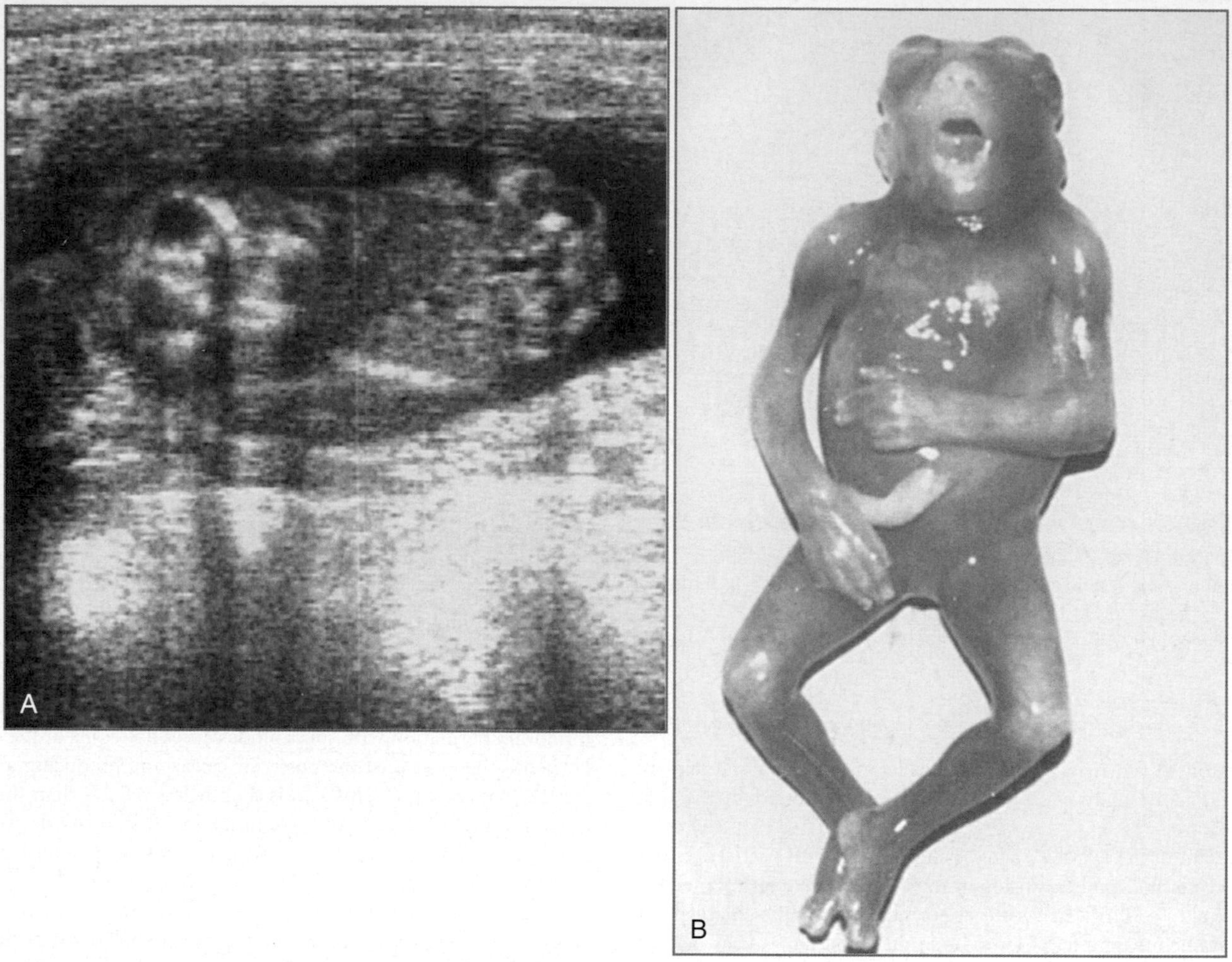

FIGURE 18-6 Anencephaly. **A,** An ultrasound view in the longitudinal coronal plane of an anencephalic fetus. The fetal calvarium is totally absent, and the fetal orbits appear relatively large and prominent. **B,** Same anencephalic fetus as in **A**. Note the prominence of the eyes and the complete absence of the calvarium.

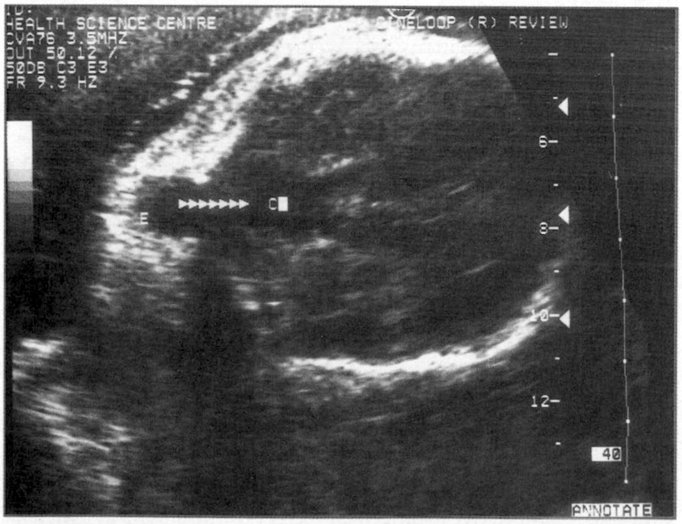

FIGURE 18-7 Posterior encephalocele. The echolucent mass (E) is the meningeal sac protruding through a defect in the posterior occiput. No elements of brain tissue were identified in this mass.

myelomeningocele.[66,68-70] In utero repair probably reduces the need for postnatal shunting of ventriculomegaly (to 50% in treated patients versus 85% in untreated patients). In utero treatment does reverse hindbrain herniation but does not prevent or halt ventriculomegaly,[70] and it does not prevent cortical mantle thinning.[71] There is no evidence that in utero repair prevents or moderates lower limb paresis. Postnatal bladder function is not improved,[72] and in one study it was worse.[73] There is no evidence that neurodevelopmental outcome at age 2 years is improved with in utero treatment.[74] Serious complications have been reported with in utero open surgery for myelomeningocele, including fetal and neonatal death[69] and abruption.[75] The results of an ongoing multicenter prospective randomized trial should make it clear whether the surgery is warranted.

Fetal Intracranial Cystic Lesions

Holoprosencephaly

Diagnosis. Holoprosencephaly occurs as a result of failure of normal development of the prosencephalon. The anomaly has three

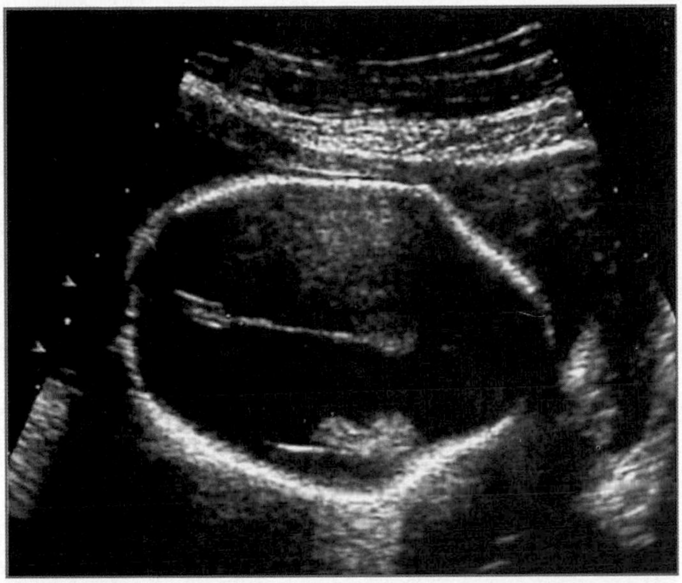

FIGURE 18-8 The "lemon sign" in spina bifida. This transverse scan of the fetal head in the plane of the biparietal diameter demonstrates collapse of the anterior calvarium, which results in the lemon sign. The collapse of the frontal bone plates of the skull occurs because of downward movement of the frontal lobes, in turn a result of tethering of the spinal cord. The lemon sign is pathognomonic for neural tube defect and is present to varying degrees in virtually every case.

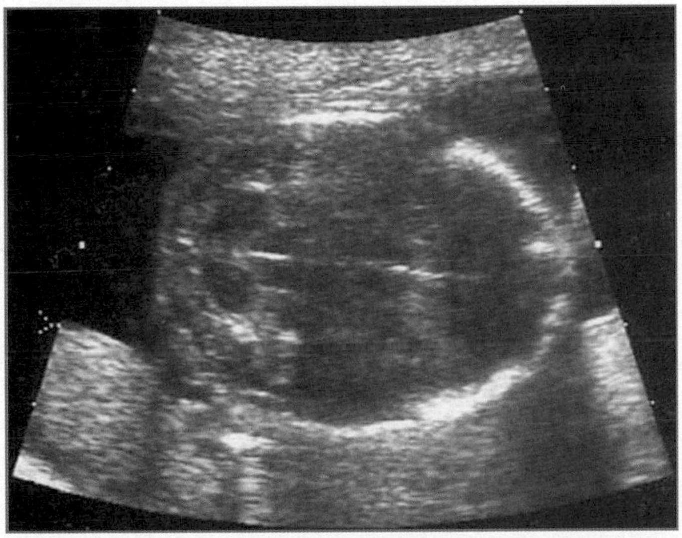

FIGURE 18-9 The "banana sign" in neural tube defect. This transverse scan of the fetal head demonstrates the flattening of the cerebellar hemispheres and the relative loss of the space of the foramen magnum. This banana sign is a result of herniation of the brainstem. The banana sign is very commonly but not universally observed in the fetus with a neural tube defect.

variants: alobar, semi-lobar, and lobar. Both alobar and semi-lobar holoprosencephaly have complete absence of normal cerebral cortex but vary only by degrees of disruption. Both feature a common fused lateral ventricle and both are associated with major mid-facial defects including fused eyes (cyclopia), proboscis defect, and facial clefts. The diagnosis can usually be made from as early as 10 weeks.

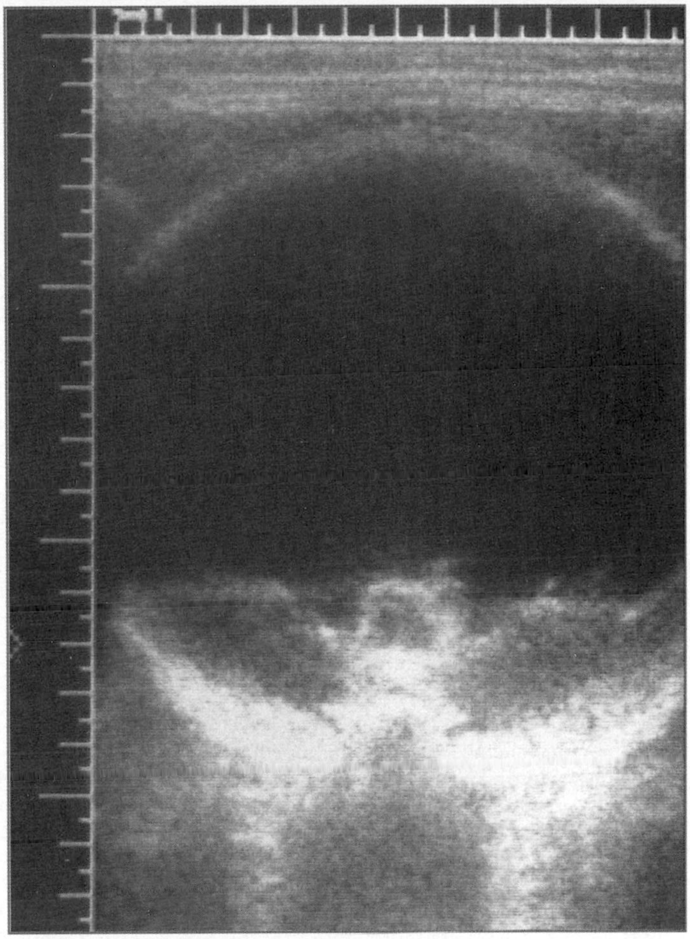

FIGURE 18-10 Holoprosencephaly. In this coronal view of the fetal head, there is complete absence of any cortical structures, including the intercerebral fissure. The brainstem structures are visible. The prognosis for a fetus with this condition is hopeless.

Prognosis. The prognosis is always hopeless. Liveborn infants with alobar holoprosencephaly usually die within the first year of life, and those with the semi-lobar form may survive for longer but always have major neurodevelopmental deficit. Lobar holoprosencephaly is characterized by fusion of the frontal horns of the lateral ventricles and is rarely diagnosed in utero. Holoprosencephaly is associated with trisomy 13 and trisomy 13/15 and less commonly with trisomy 18.

Hydrencephaly and Porencephaly

Diagnosis. Occlusion of cerebral vessels in early fetal life can result in cavitating necrosis of brain tissue. Occlusion of the internal carotid arteries results in loss of both cerebral hemispheres, which are replaced by a fluid-filled cyst (hydrencephaly), whereas occlusion of intracerebral vessels or intracerebral hemorrhage can result in localized cysts distributed in any area of the cerebrum (porencephaly). These lesions are easily recognized on ultrasound as echolucencies without any internal structure. Hydrencephaly can superficially resemble severe hydrocephaly, but with detailed scanning the absence of any midline cerebral structures aids in differentiation (Fig. 18-10).

Porencephaly is recognized with the characteristic isolated round echolucent "holes" in the brain tissue. In contrast, arachnoid cyst and aneurysm of the great vein of Galen, lesions that can also present as cystic structures, are easily differentiated by Doppler ultrasound and by confirmation of an extracerebral location. Occasionally, a porencephalic cyst may communicate with a lateral ventricle. In most instances, the cause of the vascular occlusion is unknown, but it may result from embolic showers during intrauterine transfusion (my unpublished observations), from infection,[76] as a consequence of severe acute ischemia in twin-to-twin transfusion syndrome,[77] from the trauma of fetal invasive procedures such as amniocentesis and possibly chorionic villus sampling,[78] and from fetal thrombocytopenia.[79]

Prognosis. The prognosis for fetuses with hydrencephaly is uniformly hopeless, and there is no prospect of intact survival. In contrast, the prognosis for fetuses with porencephalic cysts, although generally poor, is much more variable and depends on the location, size, number, and progression.[80] Differentiation of a porencephalic cyst from an arachnoid cyst is clinically important, because the prognosis of an arachnoid cyst may be excellent.[81,82] Aneurysm of the great vein of Galen is a very rare fetal anomaly characterized on gray-scale ultrasound as an echolucent cystic mass that lights up with color Doppler. This lesion is usually associated with other vascular malformations and can cause high output failure in the fetus, with resulting hydrops. The long-term prognosis, although not hopeless, is generally poor.[83]

Intracranial Tumors and Cystic Malformations

Intracranial neoplasms can occur in the fetus and can appear as either cystic or solid lesions or as both, and by mass effect they may distort adjacent normal tissue and cause obstructive hydrocephalus. Intracranial tumors include glioblastoma multiforme,[84] astrocytoma,[85] primitive neuroectodermal tumor,[86] craniopharyngioma, teratoma, and hemangioma.[87] The prognosis of fetal tumors varies with the cause and size, but it is generally very poor. Specific tissue diagnosis of fetal brain tumor is possible by ultrasound-guided biopsy, but this is rarely if ever indicated.

Choroid Plexus Cysts

Diagnosis. Choroid plexus cysts result from obstruction of the microtubules connecting the fluid-producing cells with the lateral ventricle (Fig. 18-11). These cysts may be unilateral or bilateral, single or multiple, and they are relatively common, occurring in at least 1% of all fetuses.

Prognosis. By themselves the cysts are innocuous and almost always resolve spontaneously. The cyst per se does not cause brain injury, nor is there any direct association between these cysts and postnatal brain dysfunction. The major clinical issue associated with choroid plexus cysts is their association with aneuploidy, especially trisomy 18 and to a much lesser degree trisomy 21.[88] It is estimated that somewhere between 50% and 66% of fetuses with trisomy 18 have choroid plexus cysts (or a single cyst) as an associated ultrasound finding.[89] However, choroids plexus cysts are almost never the only anomaly identified in the fetus with trisomy 18. Further, a significant proportion of trisomy 18 can now be accurately recognized in early gestation by nuchal lucency and maternal serum analytes and in the second trimester by detailed survey of fetal hands and the fetal heart. The role of amniocentesis for a fetus with isolated choroid plexus cysts is highly controversial.[90]

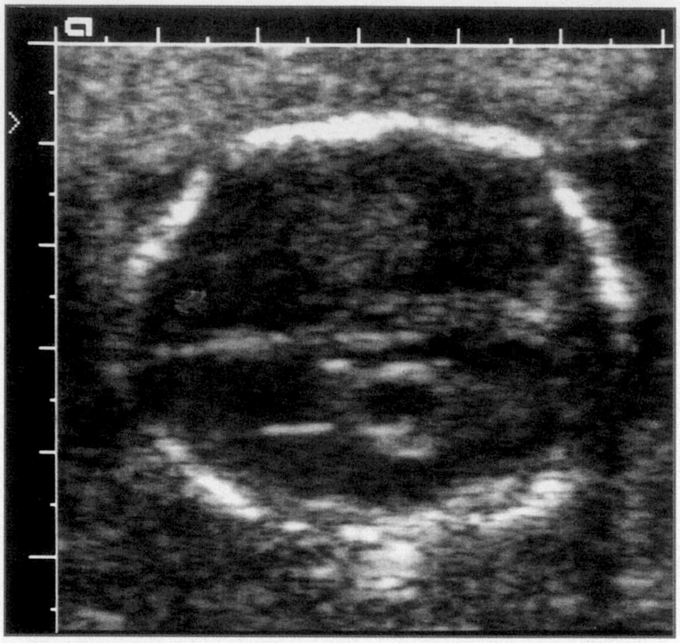

FIGURE 18-11 Choroid plexus cyst. In this transverse view of the fetal head made in the plane of the biparietal diameter, the proximal choroid is normal, and in the distal choroid a solitary cyst is identified.

Fetal Craniofacial Abnormalities

Microcephaly

Diagnosis. Microcephaly is identified when the fetal head is pathologically small (as opposed to small as a result of normal distribution). True microcephaly is diagnosed when fetal head size, as measured in utero by head circumference, is more than 4 standard deviations below the mean. A sloping forehead is a common finding.

Prognosis. Great care must be taken in assigning a prognosis to fetal microcephaly, because 50% of fetuses with a head circumference less than 2 standard deviations below the mean have normal intelligence, and 18% of fetuses with a head circumference less than 3 standard deviations below the mean have normal intelligence.[91,92]

Craniosynostosis

Diagnosis. Craniosynostosis is the result of early and abnormal fusion of the cranial plates, and it can cause a wide range of abnormal head shapes. Wide separation of the cranial plates can occur with *thanatophoric dysplasia*, and frontal bossing and relative macrocephaly may be observed with *achondroplastic dwarfism*. The intraocular diameter can be measured in utero and standard nomograms[32] are available to determine the presence of increased intraocular width (*hypertelorism*) or an abnormally narrow width (*hypotelorism*). Hypertelorism is associated with numerous malformations and syndromes, including facial defects, skull dysplasias, skeletal malformations, and chromosomal abnormalities. Similarly, hypotelorism is associated with conditions such as holoprosencephaly, microcephaly, aneuploidies (including trisomy 13, 18, and 21), and with maternal metabolic disorders such as phenylketonuria.

Prognosis. The prognosis varies with the underlying cause and associated abnormalities.

Fetal Facial Anomalies: Facial Clefts

Diagnosis. Facial clefts are among the most common of all fetal anomalies, occurring with a frequency of approximately 1.2 per 1000 births[93] and accounting for about 13% of all reported anomalies, second in incidence only to fetal cardiovascular defects.[94] The recurrence of cleft lip or cleft palate conforms to a polygenic multifactorial inheritance pattern. With normal parents and one affected infant, or when one parent has the abnormality, the recurrence risk in the sub-

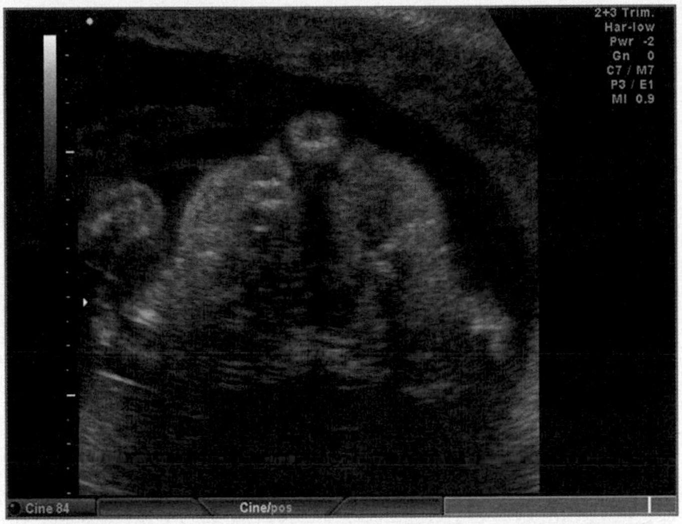

FIGURE 18-12 Two-dimensional ultrasound image of the fetal face in the transverse plane. Note the bilateral facial cleft. (Courtesy of Dr. Christopher Harman.)

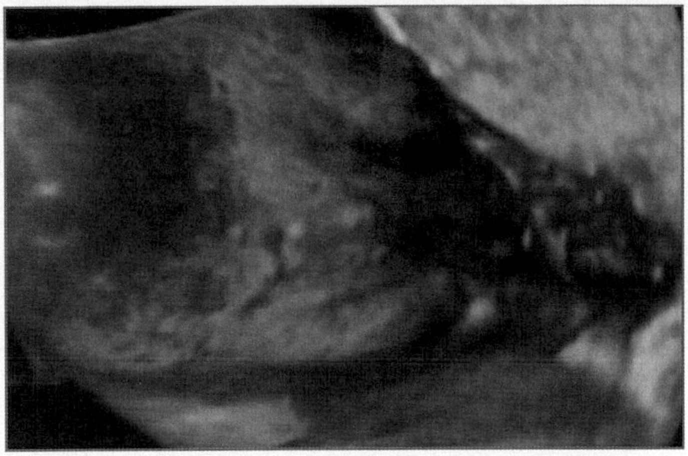

FIGURE 18-13 Three-dimensional ultrasound of the fetal face. In the frontal view, the bilateral facial clefts are clearly visible. (Courtesy of Dr. Christopher Harman.)

sequent fetus is about 4%. When both parents are affected, the risk is about 35%. The risk in subsequent fetuses rises as more siblings have the anomaly. Abnormal findings in the parents may be subtle and expressed as a bifid uvula, a submucous cleft of the soft palate, or linear lip indentations. In about 50% of affected fetuses, the facial cleft involves the lip and palate, and the remaining cases are roughly equally divided between isolated cleft lip (25%) and cleft palate (25%). Cleft lip usually cannot be identified before about the midpoint of the second trimester, and isolated cleft palate is infrequently diagnosed in utero.[22]

The two-dimensional ultrasound diagnosis of cleft lip requires a frontal view of the lower face at its outmost projection (Fig. 18-12). Because the fetal head is usually flexed, with the chin resting on the anterior thorax, the best imaging of the fetal lips and nose often occurs while the fetal heart is being evaluated. The diagnosis of facial clefts is enhanced with three-dimensional ultrasound[95] (Fig. 18-13), and specialized views may improve the recognition of cleft palate.[96,97] However, overall routine ultrasound screening is relatively poor in detecting cleft lip or palate. In prospective studies in the general population, the detection of cleft lip ranged from 44% to 60%.[94,98]

Prognosis. About one third of fetuses with a cleft lip or palate have an associated major anomaly, such as Goldenhar syndrome (oculoauriculovertebral dysplasia), Pierre Robin syndrome (micrognathia), and Treacher Collins syndrome (mandibulofacial dysostosis), and aneuploidies, especially trisomy 13 and less frequently trisomy 18. In the absence of associated anomalies, the prognosis for cleft lip or palate is good, and remarkable postnatal cosmetic repair is achievable.

Anomalies of the midface such as fused orbits (cyclopia) and nose anomalies (in the extreme form, proboscis lateralis) are typically associated with trisomy 13 or more rarely are a manifestation of hemifacial microsomia and otocephaly. The diagnosis of micrognathia is usually made by visual assessment, but nomograms for mandibular length per gestational age are published.[99] The Pierre Robin syndrome is characterized by a short mandible (micrognathia), a posterior displacement of the tongue (glossoptosis), and a U-shaped cleft palate. These facial abnormalities can lead to feeding problems in the newborn. Other conditions associated with micrognathia include Treacher Collins syndrome and various aneuploidies including triploidy.

Anomalies of the Neck and Chest

Fetal Lung Anomalies

By about day 26 of fetal life, the endodermal primordia of the fetal lung derive from the respiratory diverticulum arising from the floor of the pharynx, and by about day 28 the two lung buds grow out from the caudal end of the diverticulum and draw along the splanchnic mesenchyme. These two components ultimately form the functional lung, with the endoderm complement giving rise to the bronchial tree and alveoli and the mesenchyme giving rise to the vascular component. Abnormal development of the lung buds can lead to three major lung anomalies: bronchogenic cyst, bronchopulmonary sequestration (BPS), and congenital cystic adenomatoid malformation (CCAM).

Bronchogenic Cyst

Diagnosis. A bronchogenic cyst is a rare anomaly (incidence, approximately 1 in 15,000 live births) that develops when a component of the growing lung bud becomes isolated from the main bifurcation process. These cysts are thin walled and usually located in the mediastinum near the membranous portion of the posterior trachea, but they can occur anywhere throughout the lung and can be attached to the pericardium, the mediastinum, below the diaphragm, and in the upper airway including the mouth. The interior of the cyst often contains cartilaginous nests, mucous glands, and primitive respiratory epithelium. Typically there is a single cyst, but multiple cysts can occur. The ultrasound diagnosis of bronchogenic cyst is quite straightforward. It is usually seen as a simple round empty cystic structure prominent in the fetal lung. The cyst can be multilobular and is often large (Fig. 18-14).

Prognosis. The cyst per se is benign but the compressing effect on contiguous tissue can cause fetal compromise. Compression of the esophagus can occur, with subsequent hydramnios and preterm labor. Compression of a mainstem bronchus, evident as increased echogenicity in the distal lung, can result in airway compromise at birth. Fetal hydrops appears not to be a complication of bronchogenic cyst, and accordingly the fetal prognosis is excellent. In most instances postnatal resection of the cyst is required.

Bronchopulmonary Sequestration

Diagnosis. A pulmonary sequestration is a rare sporadic lung anomaly arising as a echogenic mass of lung tissue that has no connection to the trachea and receives blood supply from one or more anomalous vessels. The sequestrated mass is thought to derive from an aberrant secondary lung bud developing in the embryonic fetal foregut distal to the tracheobronchial bud. As the aberrant lung bud develops, it brings its own splanchnic blood supply and can develop a separate pleural membrane. BPS can occur anywhere in the distribution of the primitive foregut, but in most cases (75%) the semisolid mass is confined to a lobe of the lung, and in about 25% of cases it is extralobar, either within the mediastinum or below the diaphragm. The key diagnostic points are the recognition of an echogenic mass (often extremely dense) and a separate feeding vessel demonstrated with Doppler ultrasound (Fig. 18-15). Pleural effusion, displacement of the mediastinum, hydrops, and hydramnios are frequently associated ultrasound findings.[100]

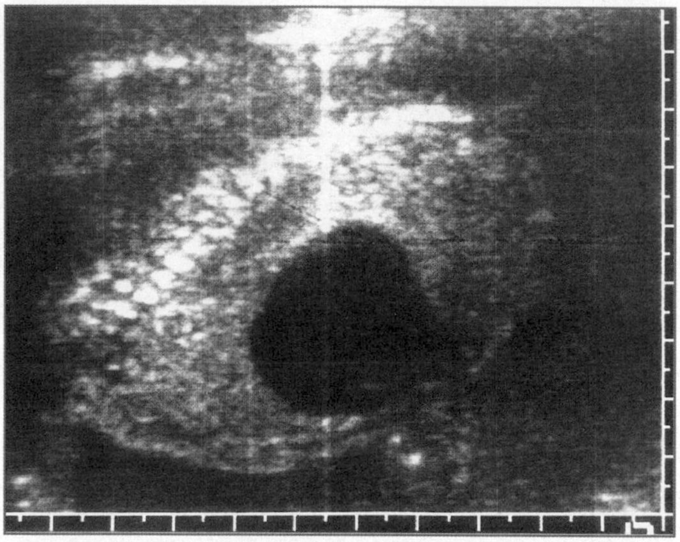

FIGURE 18-14 Bronchogenic cyst. This large simple cyst is in the left hemithorax.

Prognosis. Initially, it was reported that BPS was lethal in the majority (66%) of cases overall and in all cases when hydrops was present.[101] It is now understood that BPS may evolve along three pathways. First, in some cases, BPS may resolve spontaneously in utero.[102,103] The mechanism for resolution appears to be occlusion of the feeding aberrant vessel and subsequent involution, although reestablishing a connection with the main tracheobronchial tree is a remote possibility. In utero resolution is not associated with any postnatal consequences. Second, in some cases, the lesion remains relatively stable in utero and causes no fetal consequences. Postnatal resection is required in most cases but usually can be delayed until the infant is at least 6 months old.[104,105] Postnatal survival in these infants is at least 95%.[106]

Third, in about 20% of cases, generalized hydrops develops in association with BPS. The mechanism for hydrops is unknown but may be related to compression of veins and lymphatics. The development of hydrops with BPS gravely affects the prognosis. In the absence of intervention, most if not all of these fetuses die. Treatment options vary according to gestational age. In the fetus at or beyond 26 weeks, the treatment of choice includes steroids, delivery, and postnatal care. In the grossly immature fetus, open in utero resection of the mass is an option: Grethel and colleagues[106] reported a 50% survival (15 of 30 cases) with open surgery, compared with a 3% survival (1 of 33) in those managed conservatively. Ultrasound-guided laser fulguration of the feeding vessels of the sequestrated mass has been reported to be an effective and less invasive method of treatment.[107] Extralobar sequestration can undergo torsion, causing pleural effusion, which when progressive and severe may require pleuroamniotic shunting.

Congenital Cystic Adenomatoid Malformation

Diagnosis. Congenital cystic adenomatoid malformation is an uncommon lung lesion that appears to arise with an arrest in development of a lobule of the lung. The mass is almost always singular, unilobular (in 90% of cases), and unilateral (in 99% of cases), and it always communicates with the parent tracheobronchial tree, although the connections are minute and tortuous. The arterial and venous blood supply arises from the normal pulmonary circulation (as

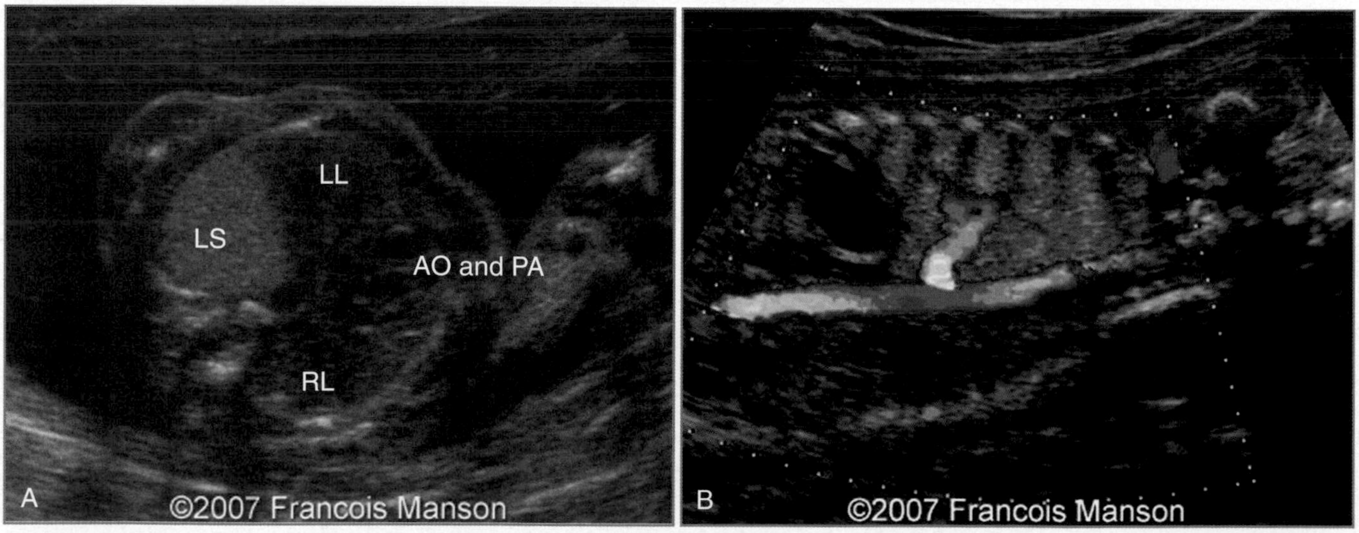

FIGURE 18-15 Bronchopulmonary sequestration. **A,** The echodense mass occupies a significant portion of the lower hemithorax. **B,** Color Doppler image of a single large feeding vessel arising from below the diaphragm. AO, aorta; LL, left lung; LS, lung sequestration; PA, pulmonary artery; RL, right lung. (Courtesy of Dr. Phillipe Jeanty.)

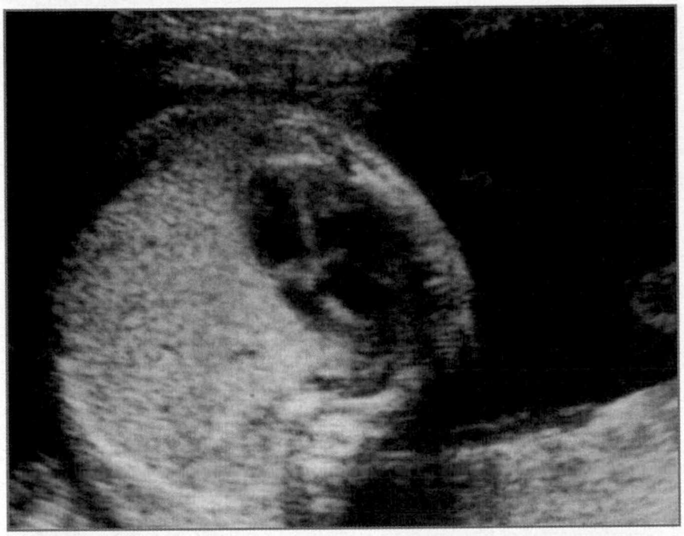

FIGURE 18-16 Congenital cystic adenomatoid malformation of the lung, type 1. This echodense mass occupies almost the entire hemithorax. Note the mass effect resulting in a slight mediastinal shift. (Courtesy of Dr. Phillipe Jeanty.)

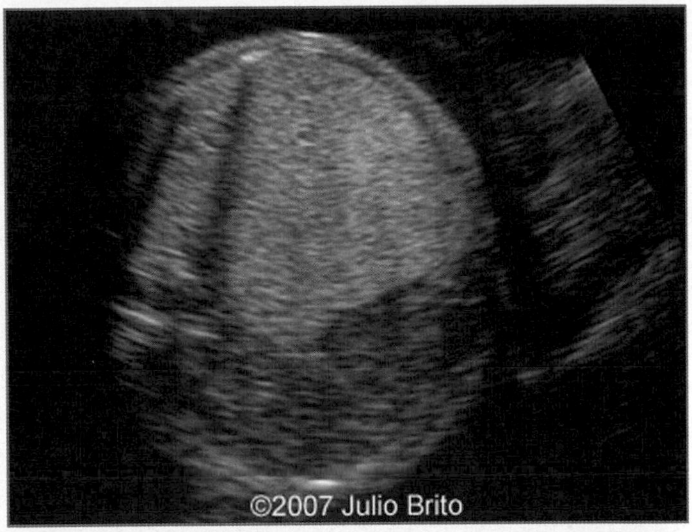

FIGURE 18-17 Congenital cystic adenomatoid malformation, type III. Note the extreme displacement and compression of the fetal heart. (Courtesy of Dr. Phillipe Jeanty.)

opposed to the aberrant blood supply seen in BPS). The macroscopic, histologic, and ultrasound appearances of CCAM vary according to the time that development was arrested.[108] Type I CCAM (Fig. 18-16) mimics late lung development and has the characteristic features of large (up to 10 cm), single or multiple simple cysts. Type I is the most commonly observed variant of CCAM (50% of postnatal cases) and has an excellent prognosis. Type II CCAM resembles the pseudoglandular phase of lung development and is characterized by the presence of multiple small (typically between 3 and 10 mm in diameter) cysts within the mass. About 40% of all CCAMs are classified as type II lesions. Type III CCAM resembles the very early developing lung and is composed of regularly spaced bronchiole-like structures and primitive alveolar sacs. Type III lesions are characterized by the absence of visible cysts and the appearance of a large echodense mass usually involving the entire lobe of the lung (Fig. 18-17). Microcysts can be identified by histologic examination. Type III CCAM is the least common type (approximately 10%), and it is the most lethal.

Associated anomalies are rare with type I lesions. In contrast, associated anomalies such as truncus arteriosus, tetralogy of Fallot, and jejunal atresia occur in about 15% of fetuses with type II lesions and an even higher proportion of fetuses with type III lesions.[108]

Prognosis. The natural outcome varies according to CCAM type and ranges from excellent (near 100% survival) with type I, to good survival in type II (the outcome depends mostly on the presence or absence of associated anomalies), to poor with type III, to hopeless with type III with hydrops. At least 15% of cases of CCAM resolve spontaneously in utero.[109] The prognosis can be improved with in utero therapy, including open resection of the lesion and reduction of lung compression by placing a pleuroamniotic shunt. Adzick and coworkers[102] reported outcomes in 120 fetuses with CCAM (of all types). The 101 fetuses who did not develop hydrops were managed conservatively (observation/intervention at fetal maturity) and all survived (100% survival). Of the 120 fetuses, 38 (31.5%) developed hydrops (most with type III lesions). In this group, 25 fetuses were managed conservatively and all died (100% mortality), and 13 were treated in utero by open resection and eight survived (61%). An additional six with a very large solitary cyst and without hydrops received a percutaneous procedure to place a shunt between the cyst and the amniotic cavity, and five of these six fetuses survived.

In a reported British experience of 67 fetuses,[104] 35 cases were microcystic (CCAM types II and III), 27 cases (40%) were macrocystic (predominantly CCAM type 1), and five cases (8%) were mixed (type II). Fetal hydrops was uncommon, occurring in only five fetuses (7%). None of these fetuses had open surgery. Survival was 96% (64 of 67 fetuses). Most (63%) required postnatal surgery.

Diaphragmatic Hernia

In the developing fetus, the mesenchymal muscular diaphragm closes before 9 weeks' gestation and before the midgut retreats into the abdomen from its temporary umbilical cord herniation. If the midgut returns to the abdomen before the diaphragm closes, there is the potential for herniation of the viscera, including the liver, typically through a posterior lateral defect into the thoracic cavity, resulting in a congenital diaphragmatic hernia (CHD).

Diagnosis. Congenital diaphragmatic hernia is a relatively uncommon anomaly occurring at a frequency of about 1 per 7000 live births, and more frequently in stillborn infants.[110] In at least 40% of cases, CDH is associated with other major anomalies including aneuploidy (18% of cases) and cardiac defects.[111,112] Only about half of all cases of CDH are diagnosed prenatally. The classic ultrasound diagnostic features of CDH are the presence of a cystic mass in the hemithorax (usually the left) and often with evident peristaltic movements, the absence of the normal fluid-filled stomach "bubble" sited in the fetal abdomen, the presence of a scaphoid abdominal wall, a shift of the mediastinum, lateral deviation or kinking of the umbilical portion of the portal sinus, and varying degrees of hydramnios (Fig. 18-18). The actual diaphragmatic defect is almost never identified by ultrasound.

Prognosis. The prognosis for fetuses with CDH is determined almost exclusively by the presence and degree of pulmonary hypoplasia, which in turn appears to be a direct result of compression of the lung by the herniated viscera. The degree of pulmonary hypoplasia depends on the timing of the herniation (the earlier the hernia, the greater the degree of hypoplasia), the volume of the herniated viscera (pulmonary hypoplasia is greatest when the left lobe of the liver is

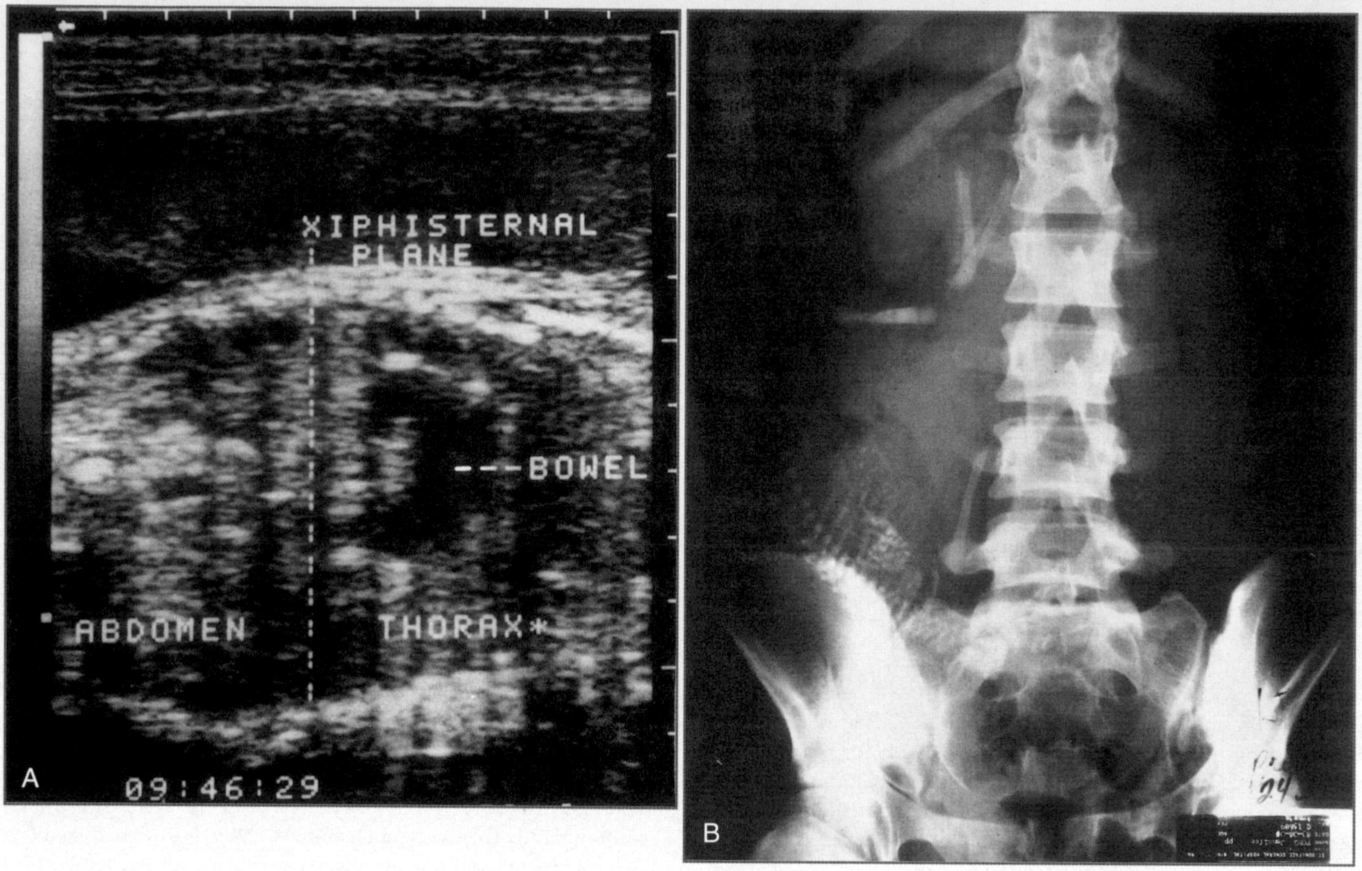

FIGURE 18-18 Diaphragmatic hernia. **A,** Longitudinal view of the fetal chest and abdomen demonstrates an echolucent mass in the fetal chest (stomach and small bowel). Note the absence of stomach in the abdomen and the relative scaphoid anterior abdominal wall. **B,** This maternal abdominal radiograph demonstrates a fetus in cephalic presentation with the fetal spine to the maternal right. In this case, Renographin had been introduced into the amniotic fluid, was swallowed by the fetus, and is concentrated in the small bowel. The radiopaque Renographin outlines the fetal small bowel and clearly confirms its presence within the fetal thorax.

herniated into the chest and least when the hernia is only stomach and small bowel), and on the persistence of the hernia. Paradoxically, in some instances, the diaphragmatic defect may allow a sliding type of hernia, in which case the risk of pulmonary hypoplasia is very low. When CDH is present but not recognized despite prenatal ultrasound screening (in about 50% of cases), the implication is either that the hernia is of the sliding variety or it is relatively small and does not contain liver. The perinatal survival when CDH is diagnosed after birth is reported to be in the range of 66%, compared with 33% in those cases of CDH diagnosed prenatally.[111] Polyhydramnios is an important prognostic feature: 11% of fetuses survive when hydramnios is present, whereas 55% survive when amniotic fluid volume is normal.[113]

Open fetal surgery to reduce the hernia and close the diaphragm defect was advanced as a novel and potentially effective therapy. In a series of elegant experiments in sheep and primate fetuses, Harrison and colleagues[114] were able to demonstrate that creating a diaphragmatic hernia could cause lethal pulmonary hypoplasia, and that subsequent repair of the iatrogenic hernia would restore lung growth and allow for survival of some of the experimental animals. Unfortunately, these observations have not translated into effective treatment in the affected human fetus. In an initial human clinical trial involving 14 fetuses treated by open surgery before 24 weeks' gestation, five died intraoperatively (often when a herniated left lobe of liver could not be reduced), three died in utero despite apparent successful repair of the defect, and two delivered prematurely and died. The overall survival was 28.5%.[115] The survival rate for patients referred to the same center but electing to defer surgery was 41%. In a subsequent randomized trial, survival was not improved by in utero repair of CDH and accordingly the procedure is now no longer accepted or practiced.[116]

It remains clear, however, that fetuses with CDH containing the left lobe of the liver are at greatest risk for death from pulmonary hypoplasia. Furthermore, it has been reported that the ratio of the right lung to the head circumference (LHR) might be useful as a sonographic predictor of the degree of pulmonary hypoplasia and survival in the fetus with CDH.[117] In 55 affected fetuses, there were no survivors when the LHR was less than 0.6, all fetuses survived when the LHR was greater than 1.35, and 61% of fetuses survived when the values were intermediate. In a more recent study, Jani and coworkers[118] noted that the LHR was a good predictor: survival with an LHR of 0.4 to 0.5 was 17%, between 0.6 and 0.7 it was 62%, and between 0.8 and 0.9 it was 78%. The prognostic value of LHR is disputed. Heling and colleagues[119] reported no prognostic value of this ratio among 22 fetuses with isolated CDH, and Arkovitz and coworkers,[120] in a study of 28 fetuses, could find no correlation of the LHR to outcome.

As it has been known for some time that occlusion of the trachea can result in exaggerated lung growth,[121] in utero tracheal occlusion has been advocated to treat this most severe form of CDH. Initial attempts at open tracheal occlusion have been unsuccessful, with only five of 15 fetuses (33%) surviving.[122] An initial clinical experience with fetal tracheal occlusion using a fetoscopic approach to place an occluding clip appeared more successful, with six of eight fetuses (75%) surviving, compared with 15% survival in those treated by open surgery to occlude the trachea and 38% survival in affected fetuses managed conservatively.[123] However, in a subsequent prospective trial of fetoscopic tracheal occlusion for severe congenital diaphragmatic hernia conducted in 24 randomized patients (11 to fetoscopic tracheal occlusion and 13 to observation only), there were no observed differences in outcome (73% survival treated versus 77% survival not treated). The trial was stopped and it was concluded that tracheal occlusion did not improve survival or morbidity rates among a cohort of fetuses with the most severe form of congenital diaphragmatic hernia.[124] Subsequently, in a nonrandomized trial, Deprest and colleagues[125] reported that survival rate to discharge was 50% for 20 fetuses with severe CDH treated by fetoscopically placed balloon occlusion of the trachea (fetoscopic endoluminal tracheal occlusion [FETO]). The consensus of the published data to 2007 suggests that tracheal occlusion remains experimental, and any conclusions as to its value await more extensive randomized trials.

Chylothorax and Other Fetal Pleural Effusions

Diagnosis. Accumulation of fluid in the pleural cavity of the fetus can occur either because of abnormal lymphatic drainage of the pleural space (chylothorax), as a result of local pathology in or adjacent to the pleural space (diaphragmatic hernia, extralobar sequestration), or as a result of a generalized disease process associated with hypoproteinemia, anemia, or increased venous compression (immune and nonimmune hydrops). Chylothorax is usually bilateral, is usually not associated with any mediastinal shift, and has a good prognosis (Fig. 18-19).

The pathognomonic diagnostic feature in the newborn—chyle-stained (milky white) pleural drainage—does not occur in the fetus. Fluid aspirated from the fetus with chylothorax is clear, and when it is examined microscopically, it exhibits a high proportion of lymphocytes, nearly always more than 80% and often almost 100%. Chylothorax is usually a late-onset disease in the fetus and is seldom seen before 30 weeks' gestation.

Prognosis. The condition is relatively benign for the fetus but life threatening for the newborn. Treatment can include either thoracocentesis immediately before delivery or continuous drainage by ultrasound-guided percutaneous placement of a pleuroamniotic shunt. Because lymphatic fluid accumulates quickly, there is no benefit to serial fetal thoracocentesis.

The prognosis for fetuses with chylothorax is very good, with at least 85% surviving without long-term morbidity. Pleural effusions from causes other that chylothorax have a very different outcome. These effusions are associated with an abnormal karyotype in at least 5% of cases and with severe congenital heart disease in about 5% of cases. Secondary pleural effusions associated with or resulting from hydrops carry a very poor prognosis, mostly as a result of the underlying cause of the hydrops. The reported mortality of secondary pleural effusions is 53%,[126] although more recent reports indicate improved survival, which is now in the range of 75%.[127] Despite in utero treatment by chronic pleuroamniotic shunting, the outcome of fetuses with pleural effusion and hydrops still remains guarded. In a study of 16 fetuses with pleural effusions associated with hydrops treated in utero, seven survived (44%) and two procedure-related deaths occurred.[128]

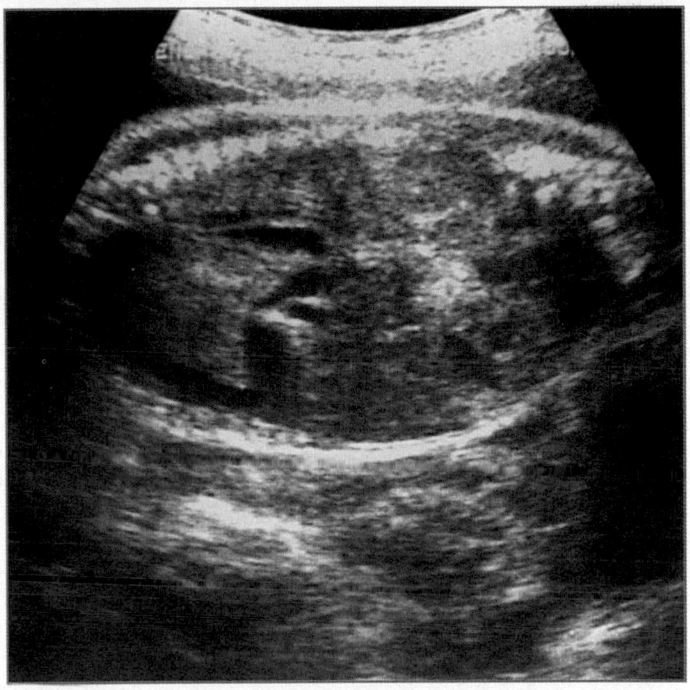

FIGURE 18-19 **Pleural effusion.** Sagittal scan of the thorax in a 31-week fetus with bilateral pleural effusions. The effusion is greater in the right hemithorax, and there is no associated ascites or skin edema. In this fetus, the discovery of pleural effusion was incidental, and it was the result of chylothorax. It is likely that this observation was critical to the survival of this perinate.

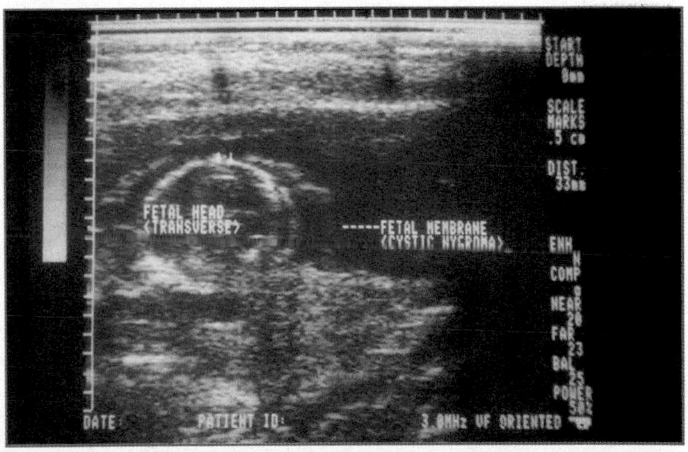

FIGURE 18-20 **Cystic hygroma.** In this transverse view of the fetal head in the plane of the biparietal diameter, bilateral large echolucent cysts are evident. This fetus had a normal karyotype but developed hydrops and died in utero.

Cystic Hygroma

Diagnosis. Cystic hygroma (also termed lymphatic hamartoma or cystic lymphangioma) consists of loculated tissue sacs distended with lymphatic fluid (Fig. 18-20). These lesions are most commonly in the region of the posterior neck, but they can also occur in the mediastinum and the axilla. The lesions may be huge and extend from the neck to the entire dorsum of the fetus, or extend around the fetus to engulf the head. The cause of cystic hygroma is not certain, but in most instances it is thought to be the result of abnormal communication between the primitive jugular lymphatic and the internal jugular vein. There is no communication between the hygroma and the normal lymphatic drainage.

Prognosis. The mortality rate associated with cystic hygroma diagnosed before 30 weeks' gestation is high (93%) and most of the fetal deaths (84%) are associated with progressive nonimmne hydrops.[129] There is a high rate of association between cystic hygroma and aneuploidies, especially trisomy 21, Turner syndrome, and Noonan syndrome. Occasionally, a cystic hygroma resolves spontaneously in utero and is associated with survival and normal outcome. Pregnancy termination is a common management option, however. In the patient electing pregnancy continuation, amniocentesis is strongly indicated. If the amniocentesis result is normal and nonimmune hydrops does not develop, expectant management is reasonable. It is important to determine the relationship between the edges of the hygroma and the trachea and upper airway, as obstruction can occur at birth. Ex utero intrapartum treatment (EXIT) may be indicated in such cases and may enhance survival.[130]

Anomalies of the Gastrointestinal Tract and Abdominal Wall

Esophageal Atresia and Tracheoesophageal Fistula

Esophageal atresia, although among the most commonly observed anomalies of the gastrointestinal tract, is a relatively rare defect occurring at an estimated frequency of 1 per 4000 live births.[131] The esophagus and trachea both develop as a common diverticulum from primitive foregut and then separate into the two separate structures as a result of proliferation of the endodermal components. This process is completed early in gestational life, and by about 26 days the esophagus and trachea appear as separate structures.

Disruption of the normal separation of the esophagus and the trachea results in a spectrum of anomalous variations (Fig. 18-21), of

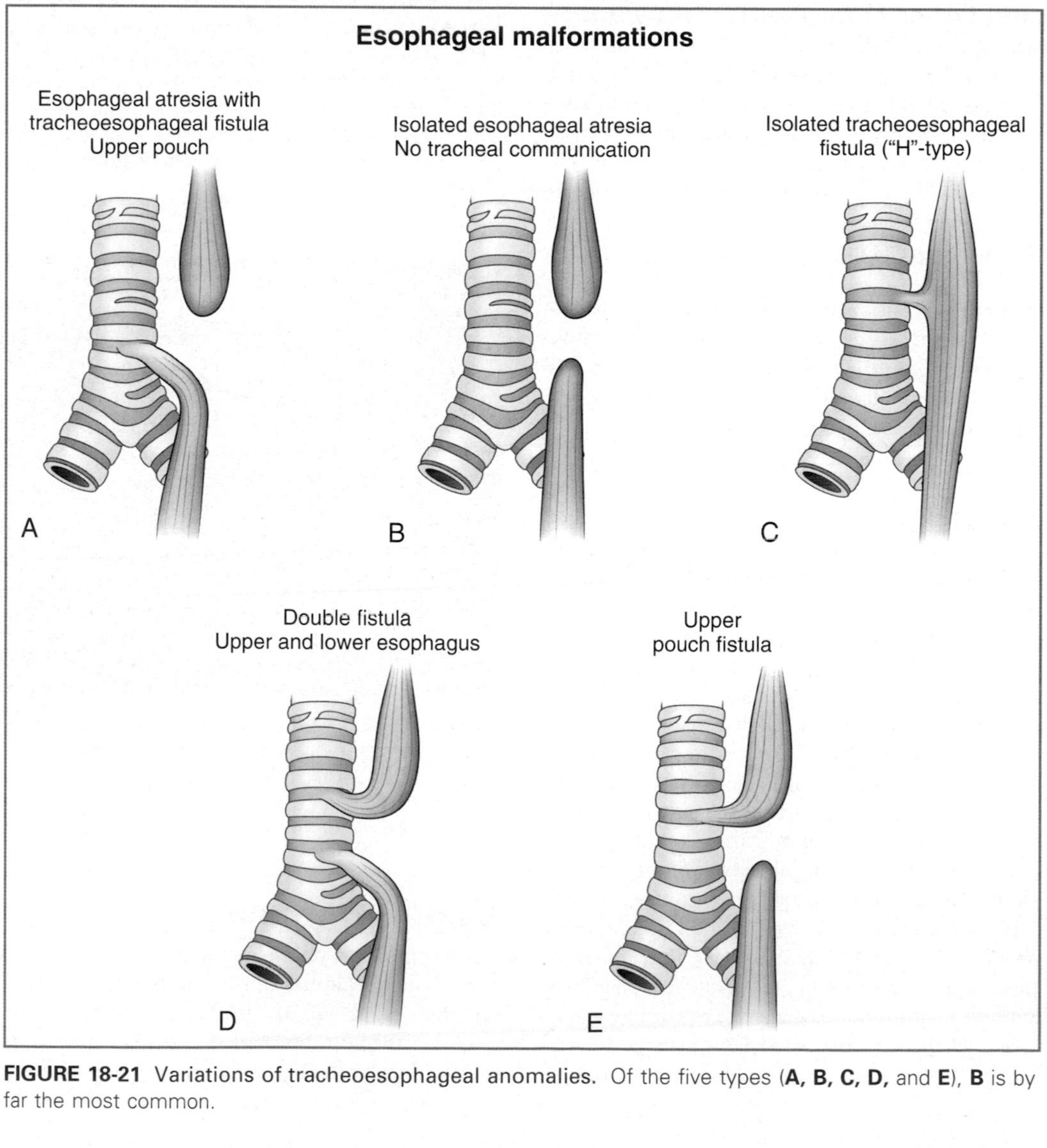

FIGURE 18-21 Variations of tracheoesophageal anomalies. Of the five types (**A, B, C, D,** and **E**), **B** is by far the most common.

which the most common (90% of cases) is a blind upper esophageal pouch, with the separated lower esophagus communicating with the trachea via a short fistulous connection. The esophageal atresia–tracheoesophageal (TE) fistula complex has no direct fetal effects, and growth and development are normal. However, there is a strong association between this anomaly and anomalies of other organ systems. Major cardiac anomalies are present in at least 25% of fetuses with esophageal atresia–TE fistula, and about 5% of affected fetuses have aneuploidies, most commonly trisomy 13, trisomy 18, and less commonly trisomy 21.[132] Esophageal atresia–TE fistula complex is also found in association with other anomalies of the gastrointestinal tract, heart, vertebrae, kidneys, and limbs, and these anomalies often occur together with a specific spectrum of anomalies known as the VACTERL association: *v*ertebral abnormality, *a*nal atresia, *c*ardiac defect, *t*racheo-*e*sophageal fistula, *r*enal and radial *l*imb abnormality.

Diagnosis. The diagnosis of esophageal atresia–TE fistula is usually made by inference from the ultrasound findings of hydramnios and absence of a visible stomach bubble *made over serial observations.* A normal fluid-filled stomach is routinely seen by 15 weeks' gestation, and although physiologic emptying of the stomach does occur, complete emptying is unusual and refilling is rapid.[133] Neither of these findings is specific to the condition, but persistence increases the probability of the diagnosis. Occasionally, the blind dilated proximal esophageal pouch can be visualized,[134] and it is pathognomonic for esophageal atresia. Furthermore, in affected fetuses observed with real-time ultrasound, it is not uncommon to see repetitive swallowing efforts and intermittent episodes of rapid egress of fluid from the mouth (my personal observations, 2007). As imaging methods have improved, the diagnosis of the condition is more common.

Prognosis. Khorshid and coworkers[135] reported on an experience of 78 cases diagnosed antenatally. Fetal prognosis varies according to associated anomalies. Usually, the hydramnios is moderate and preterm delivery is not a common problem. The newborn is at risk for reflux and aspiration. Long-term sequelae include a high incidence of metaplasia of the esophageal mucosa, and esophageal cancer in young adulthood has been reported.[136]

Duodenal and Small Bowel Atresia

Anomalous luminal occlusion can occur as an isolated or a repeated defect anywhere in the small bowel, but it most commonly affects the proximal duodenum. Small bowel atresias appear to be the result of failure of recanalization of the invading epithelial core. Swallowed and secreted fluid accumulates proximal to the obstruction and distends the bowel. Furthermore, the more proximal the obstruction is, the less swallowed amniotic fluid is absorbed and accordingly the greater is the degree of hydramnios.

Duodenal Atresia

Diagnosis. Duodenal atresia is by far the most common small bowel obstruction. The classic ultrasound findings are echolucent distended proximal duodenum coupled with a normal or moderately distended stomach, producing the "double-bubble" sign (Fig. 18-22). The signs of duodenal atresia are relatively slow to develop, but rarely

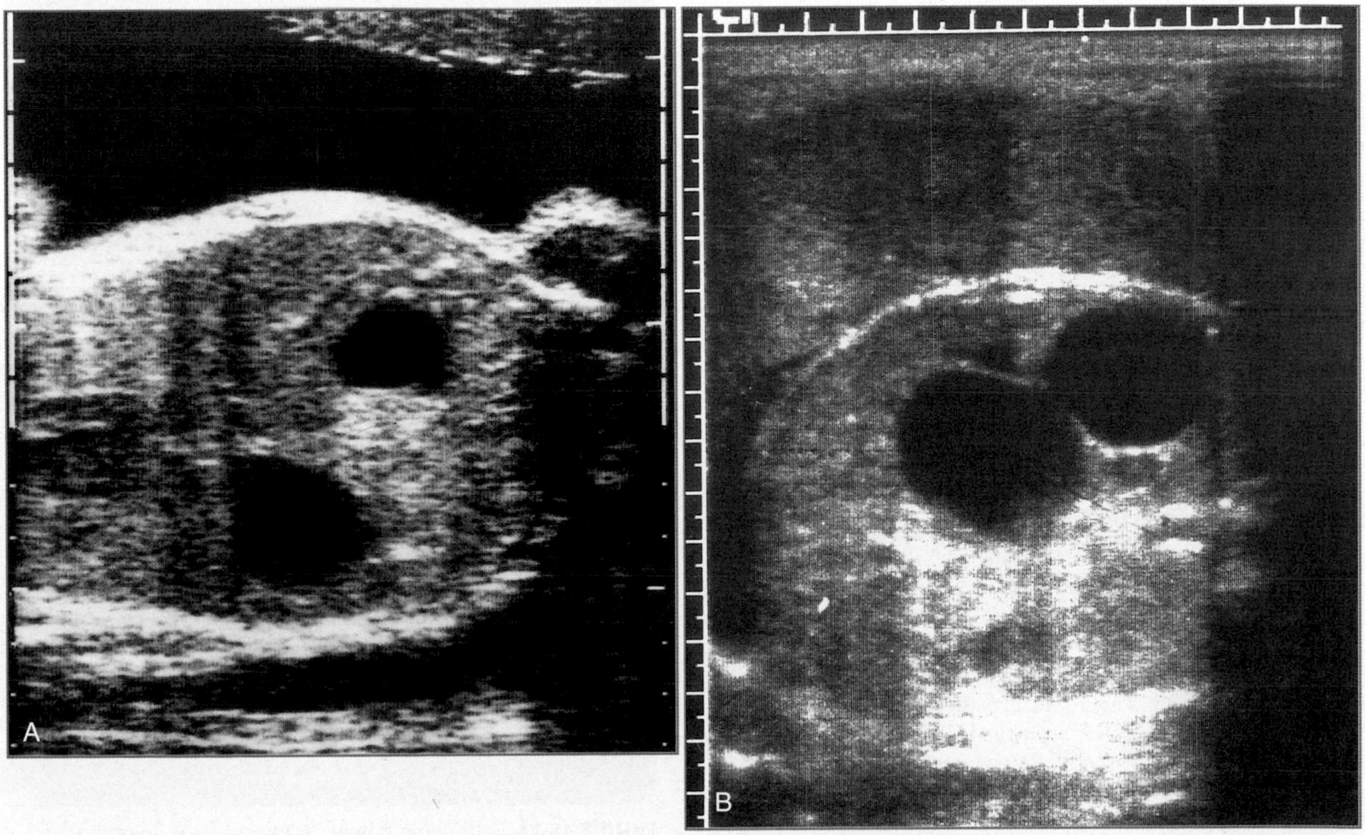

FIGURE 18-22 Duodenal atresia. **A,** Longitudinal view of the abdomen of a fetus with duodenal atresia. Note the two discrete cystic structures. The inferior structure is the dilated stomach, and the cystic mass to the upper right is the distended proximal duodenum. **B,** Transverse view of the fetal abdomen in a fetus with duodenal atresia.

they may be present as early as 15 weeks.[137] It is much more typical for them to appear in the late second trimester. The associated hydramnios usually has an insidious course, although occasionally it may appear as massive acute distention of the uterus. Other anomalies are present in at least 50% of fetuses with duodenal atresia, and cardiac anomalies are the most commonly associated structural defects. At least 25% of fetuses with duodenal atresia have trisomy 21.[138] A detailed anatomic survey and an amniocentesis are required aspects in the management of the fetus with duodenal atresia.

Duodenal obstruction can occur for causes other than atresia, and the ultrasound findings may be identical to those observed with luminal atresia. Other causes of duodenal obstruction in the fetus include annular pancreas,[139] duodenal web, occlusion by an anomalous portal vein crossing over the duodenum,[140] and an abnormal location of the common bile duct.[141] Rarely, the proximity of other intra-abdominal cysts, such as a choledochal cyst, renal cyst, or mesenteric cyst to the duodenum, can lead to the wrong diagnosis of duodenal obstruction.

Prognosis. When the duodenal atresia is an isolated finding and the karyotype is normal, the long-term prognosis is excellent. The hydramnios associated with duodenal atresia is usually slowly progressive and rarely causes maternal distress or compromise. Symptomatic hydramnios can be treated either with serial-reduction amniocentesis or with maternal indomethacin therapy, or with both. Preterm delivery related to hydramnios is a common complication and occurs in at least 46% of cases.[142] Postnatal surgical repair is usually very successful, with survival rates in the range of 90%, although intraoperative mortality of up to 4% is reported[143] and late mortality occurs in up to 6% of affected infants.[143]

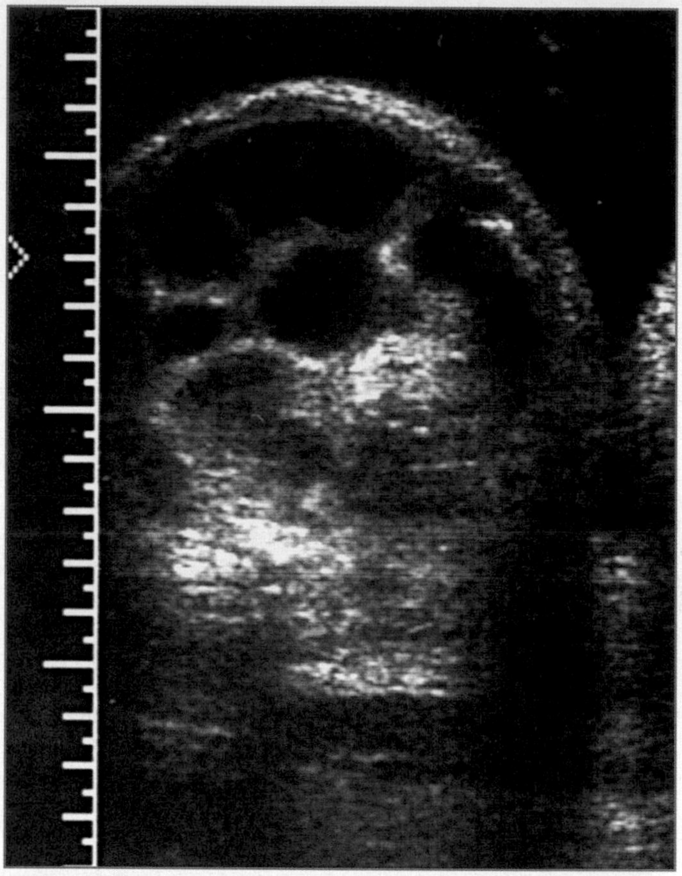

FIGURE 18-23 Small bowel obstruction. Transverse view of the fetal abdomen in a fetus with distal ileal atresia. Note the multiple loops of dilated small bowel. During real-time ultrasound scanning, hyperperistaltic activity in most of the dilated bowel loops was observed.

Small Bowel Obstruction (Intestinal Atresia)

Diagnosis. Intestinal atresia can occur at any level below the duodenum but is most commonly seen in the jejunum and less commonly in the ileum. Obstruction of the small bowel is characterized by multiple echolucent loops of small bowel proximal to the areas of obstruction (Fig. 18-23). Unlike duodenal atresia, jejunal and ileal atresias are usually isolated findings and are rarely associated with aneuploidies and other organ anomalies. The cause of small bowel atresia is usually not known, although in some cases segmental arterial occlusion is observed. The lumen of terminal ileum can be obstructed with viscous meconium, especially in infants with cystic fibrosis.[144]

Prognosis. Hydramnios is usually absent or mild with intestinal atresia, and the pregnancies usually continue to term. Surgical repair is necessary in the early neonatal period, and postnatal survival is excellent.[142]

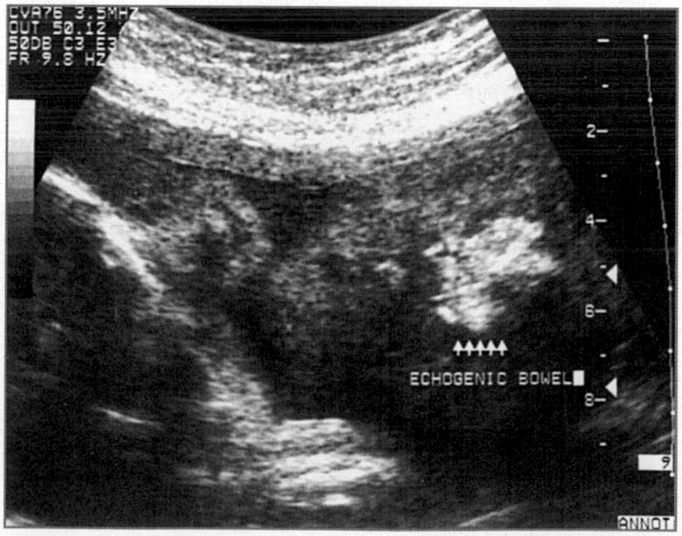

FIGURE 18-24 Echogenic bowel. A transverse scan of the abdomen in a 19-week fetus demonstrating intense echogenicity of the small bowel. The bowel echogenicity is comparable to that of bone.

Echogenic Bowel

Diagnosis. The finding of speckled or echogenic bowel is a common ultrasound observation (Fig. 18-24). The condition is characterized by increased echodensity of the small bowel. The diagnosis is subjective, and as the quality of ultrasound imaging has improved, an accurate diagnosis has become more difficult and overdiagnosis has become very common. The essential pathologic ultrasound sign is *echogenicity of the small bowel approximating the echodensity of long bones and the sacrum.*

Prognosis. True echogenic bowel is associated with cystic fibrosis, fetal infection (e.g., by cytomegalic inclusion virus),[145] and splanchnic ischemia associated with dysmature intrauterine growth restriction.[146] Echogenic bowel may be associated with swallowing of fetal blood from the amniotic cavity and thus may be a transient finding.[147] The association of echogenic bowel with aneuploidies, especially trisomy 13, 18, or 21, is very tenuous, and the occurrence of echogenic bowel as the *only marker of trisomy 21 probably never occurs.*[148]

Large Bowel Obstruction

Diagnosis. Obstruction of the fetal colon is uncommon and is notoriously difficult to diagnose by ultrasound. In the normal fetus, meconium normally accumulates in the colon with advancing gestational age, and it can produce an ultrasound image not dissimilar to obstruction. True large bowel obstruction can occur as a result of a mechanical plug produced by meconium, as a result of abnormal innervation of the large bowel (e.g., with Hirschsprung disease[149]), and in association with other anorectal anomalies (e.g., isolated defects such as anal and rectal atresia), or in association with multiple organ anomaly syndromes (e.g., VACTERL association).

Prognosis. Large bowel obstruction rarely if ever results in fetal compromise in utero, and the problems associated with this anomaly are usually confined to the immediate neonatal period. Occasionally, meconium obstruction of the large bowel results in rupture and leakage of meconium into adjacent tissues. The fetal inflammatory response is intense and walls off these areas, which ultimately calcify. Accordingly, multiple calcified echogenic foci scattered throughout the abdomen are a sign of meconium ileus.

Hepatic Masses

Diagnosis. The fetal liver is easily visualized in utero, and the size, shape, and echogenic texture can be assessed. Hepatomegaly in the fetus is almost always secondary to acquired fetal disease such as alloimmune anemia and infections. Liver tumors including teratoma, hamartoma, adenoma, and angiomas can be recognized in utero. Occasionally, these fetal liver tumors become very large and cause vascular compression and fetal death (Fig. 18-25). Fetal infection with cytomegalic virus or *Toxoplasma* can cause focal hepatitis with necrotic calcifications seen as multiple small very bright echoes distributed randomly throughout the liver parenchyma. The fetal gallbladder is usually easily visualized. Fetal gallstones do occur.[150] Significant anomalies of the fetal biliary tree are uncommon and rarely recognized in utero, with the exception of the *choledochal cyst.* A choledochal cyst appears as an echolucent mass in the right upper quadrant adjacent to but separate from the liver.

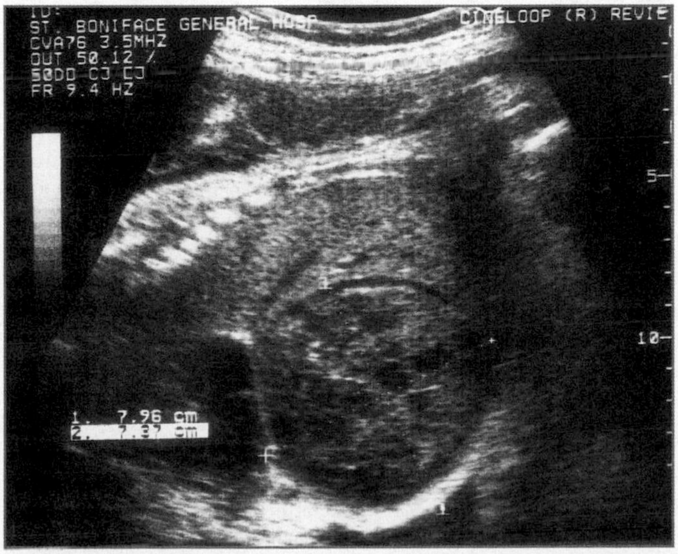

FIGURE 18-25 Cystic mass in the fetal liver. The cause of this large (approximately 8 × 8 cm) semisolid or cystic mass was never determined.

Prognosis. Choledochal cysts left undetected can cause progressive and irreversible cirrhosis and liver failure. Neoplastic degeneration can occur in later life. Choledochal cysts may be associated with communicating cavernous ectasia of the biliary tree (Caroli disease) and may ultimately require liver transplantation.

Abnormalities of the Anterior Abdominal Wall

The anterior abdominal wall develops as a thin layer of ectodermal endothelium and mesoderm overlying the abdominal organs. The abdominal wall muscles develop from invading mesenchymal myoblasts, which by the end of about 8 weeks have met and fused at the midline (linea alba) The umbilical vessels pass through the body stalk formed by fusion of the cephalic, caudal, and lateral embryonic body folds.

Omphalocele

Diagnosis. Omphalocele is a *midline* anomalous herniation of abdominal contents through the body stalk at the base of the umbilicus (Fig. 18-26). The herniation may be central or epigastric. Omphalocele has several defining characteristic features. First, the hernia sac is always contained within a peritoneal membrane and, accordingly, contents such as small bowel remain contiguous and contained. Second, the hernia sac can always be traced to a midline origin. Third, liver herniation is almost unique to omphalocele and only rarely is present with other abdominal wall defects. In at least 50% of cases, omphalocele is associated with chromosomal abnormalities, notably trisomy 13 and trisomy 18,[151] and more than 80% of affected fetuses have other major structural anomalies.[152] Omphalocele is a component of the pentalogy of Cantrell (midline omphalocele, defect of lower sternum, absent diaphragmatic pericardium, diaphragmatic hernia, and cardiac anomaly) and is a component of Beckwith-Weidemann syndrome (macroglossia, exomphalos, visceromegaly, omphalocele).

Prognosis. The prognosis of omphalocele is extremely poor, with less than 20% of affected perinates surviving. Amniocentesis and detailed repeated ultrasound anatomic surveys are always indicated if the pregnancy is planned to continue. Pregnancy termination is a frequently chosen management option.[152]

Gastroschisis

Diagnosis. Herniation of small bowel and other abdominal contents through a *lateral* abdominal wall defect is termed gastroschisis. This appears to be the result of an ischemic interruption of the closure of the abdominal wall at or near the right umbilical vein (which normally involutes by about 4 weeks' gestation) or the omphalomesenteric artery. As a consequence, the abdominal wall defect of gastroschisis is always a full-thickness defect and is usually located to the *right* side of the midline. The orifice of the defect is usually small and as a result only loops of small bowel herniate. The herniated bowel is not contained in a membrane and thus appears to be free-floating in the amniotic cavity (Fig. 18-27).

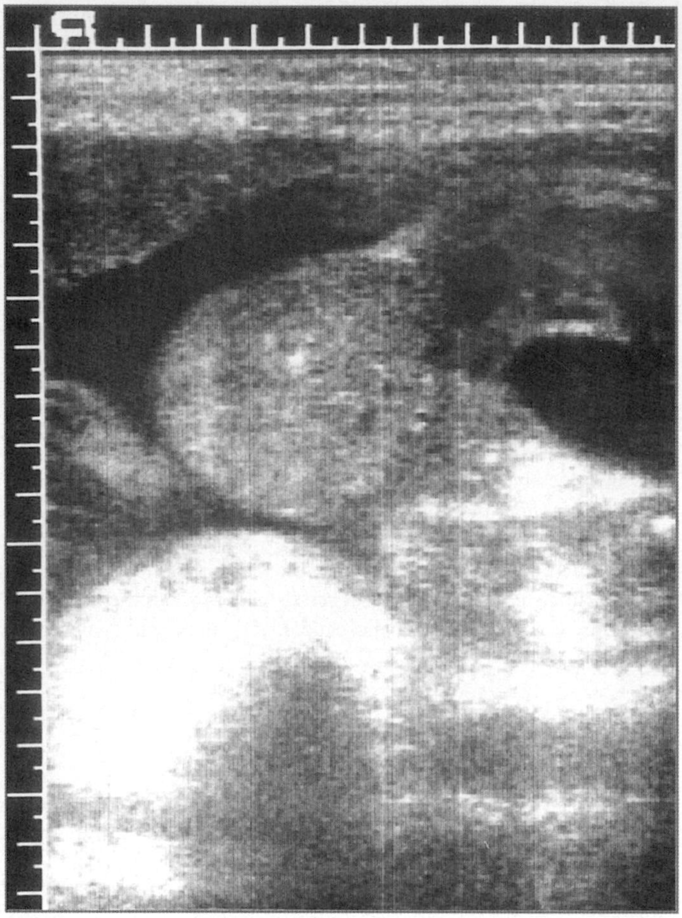

FIGURE 18-26 Omphalocele. Transverse view of the fetal abdomen. The mass protruding from the midline of the anterior abdominal wall is an omphalocele. This fetus had trisomy 21.

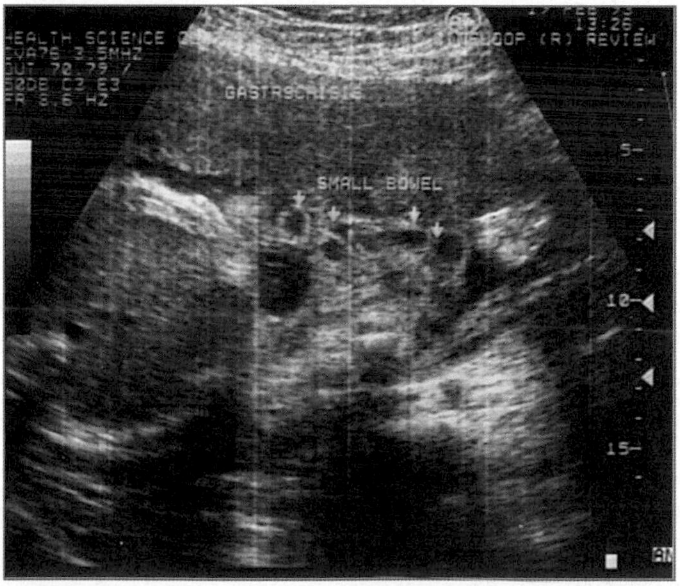

FIGURE 18-27 Gastroschisis. Gastroschisis in a third-trimester fetus. Multiple loops of dilated small bowel float freely in the amniotic fluid. The fetal liver is in the fetal abdomen. By real-time imaging, bowel peristalsis appeared diminished in this fetus.

Prognosis. The free loops of bowel often acquire a fibrinous covering thought to be the result of inflammation induced by amniotic fluid. As a result, the bowel evolves to a matted complex with altered motility. The incidence of aneuploidy is not increased with gastroschisis, nor is there an increase in anomalies of other organ systems. The incidence of jejunal atresia is increased in fetuses with gastroschisis, possibly resulting from a common vascular ischemic mechanism.

Gastroschisis is associated with a 25% or greater rate of intrauterine growth restriction.[153] There is no reported advantage to delivery by cesarean section.[154] Infants born with gastroschisis require surgical repair, often sequenced, and they are at risk of long-term gastrointestinal complications such as stricture, adhesions, and volvulus. However, long-term intact survival is usually excellent, exceeding 97%.[155]

Body stalk anomaly occurs as a result of complete failure of closure of body folds and is characterized by absence of the umbilicus and umbilical cord. Survival is extremely rare with this condition.[156]

Bladder Exstrophy

Diagnosis. Bladder exstrophy is an anterior abdominal wall anomaly that occurs as a result of failure of fusion of the caudal components of the ecto-mesodermal body folds. As a result, there is protrusion of the urinary bladder with communication to the amniotic cavity and with separation of the symphysis pubis. Obstruction of the upper urinary tract is commonly associated. The occurrence of normal amniotic fluid, dilated ureter (one or both), and inability to visualize the urinary bladder despite repeated observations at intervals strongly suggests the diagnosis. Bladder exstrophy is associated with abnormalities of the phallus and may occur in conjunction with cloacal exstrophy.

Prognosis. Isolated bladder exstrophy can be corrected after the birth and has a generally good long-term prognosis.[157] In contrast, the prognosis of cloacal exstrophy, either alone or in association with bladder exstrophy, is very poor in terms of both survival and quality of life.[158]

Abnormalities of the Fetal Genitourinary Tract

The fetal kidney has three embryonic components, the pronephros, the mesonephros, and the metanephros. The functional fetal kidney arises from the fusion of the ureteral bud, which grows cranially to fuse with the metanephros. The ureteral bud gives origin to the ureter, renal pelvis, papillae, and collecting system, whereas the mesonephros gives rise to the functional nephrons. Fusion of the ureteral bud and the metanephros is completed early in gestational life (by 7 weeks) and the production of urine with drainage to the amniotic cavity begins shortly thereafter.

The kidney continues to grow and differentiate throughout fetal life, and nomograms can be used to differentiate normal from abnormal kidney dimensions for given gestational ages.[159] Because fetal urine is the major source of amniotic fluid from the early second trimester onward, the presence of normal amniotic fluid volume implies normal urine production, whereas oligohydramnios is the hallmark sign of renal dysfunction or obstruction. Fetal urine production can be estimated from measurement of fetal bladder filling and emptying.[160] Because the fetal kidneys are easily visualized by ultrasound, obstruction of urine outflow always results in proximal echolucent dilation, and because oligohydramnios complicates obstruction or decreased

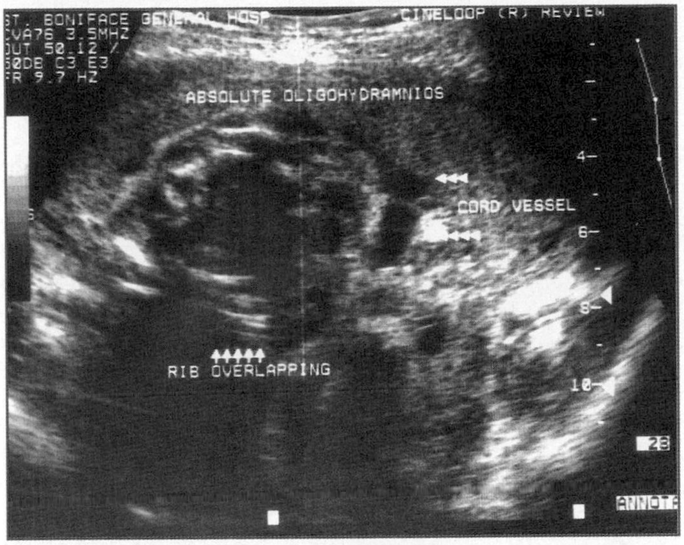

FIGURE 18-28 **Absolute oligohydramnios associated with renal agenesis.** The only echolucency in the amniotic cavity is produced by bunching of the fetal cord and layering of echolucent segments of the umbilical vein. The renal fossae contain no visible structures.

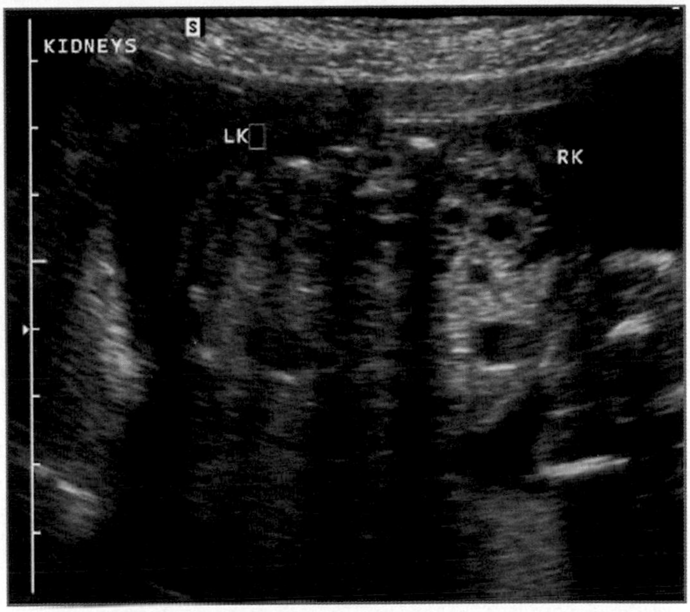

FIGURE 18-29 **Multicystic dysplastic kidney.** In this axial view through the lower fetal abdomen, the right kidney (RK) has multiple cysts with echogenic renal parenchyma surrounding them. The left kidney (LK) is normal.

production of urine, genitourinary anomalies are among the most easily and consistently recognized in utero. Therefore, the detection rate of genitourinary anomalies by ultrasound in the second and third trimesters is at least 80%.[161]

Anomalies of the Fetal Kidney

Renal Agenesis

Diagnosis. Failure of the fetal kidneys to develop is thought to arise from the failure of development of the ureteric bud and may affect one (unilateral) or both kidneys (bilateral). Unilateral renal agenesis is rarely diagnosed in utero (because of the lack of positive signs) and is associated with a normal prognosis. In contrast, bilateral renal agenesis is easily diagnosed by the constellation of absolute oligohydramnios (Fig. 18-28), failure to identify a urinary bladder on serial observations or in response to administration of furosemide to the mother or directly to the fetus, and the failure to identify normal fetal kidneys. Absence of normal fetal kidneys is difficult to confirm because in the absence of renal tissue, the fetal adrenal expands into the renal fossa and may have an echotexture similar to the kidney.

Prognosis. The oligohydramnios resulting from bilateral renal agenesis causes pulmonary hypoplasia, which is the cause of death in the immediate postpartum or early neonatal period. Oligohydramnios also leads to facial compression, producing Potter facies. Renal agenesis may occur as an isolated anomaly or as part of a syndrome such as TAR syndrome (thrombocytopenia, renal agenesis, hypoplasia of the radius), Fraser syndrome (cryptophthalmos, cleft palate, laryngeal abnormalities), cerebro-oculo-facioskeletal syndrome, and acrorenal-mandibular syndrome. Pregnancy interruption or nonintervention for fetal indications is always indicated for bilateral renal agenesis.

Multicystic Dysplastic Kidney

Diagnosis. Multicystic dysplastic kidney (MDK) results from incomplete union of the ureteric bud to the metanephros, resulting in dilation of all or some of the collecting tubules in the renal pelvis (Fig. 18-29). On ultrasound, the affected kidney appears enlarged, with multiple cystic and abnormally echogenic foci, some of which may be calcified, distributed throughout the kidney. The dysplastic areas are always dysfunctional. Unilateral disease is associated with abnormalities in the contralateral kidney, most commonly dilation of the renal pelvis (ureteropelvic junction [UPJ] anomaly).

Prognosis. The prognosis for bilateral multicystic dysplastic kidney is hopeless. However, with unilateral disease, the functioning contralateral kidney maintains normal amniotic fluid volume, so pulmonary hypoplasia is not a complication. The unilateral multicystic kidney usually atrophies in childhood and surgical resection is rarely required.[162]

Infantile Polycystic Kidney (Autosomal Recessive Polycystic Kidney Disease)

Diagnosis. Autosomal recessive polycystic kidney disease is characterized by massive bilateral enlargement of the kidneys, with cystic dilation of the renal tubules, often associated with degrees of hepatic fibrosis (Fig. 18-30).

Prognosis. When diagnosed in utero, the prognosis is very poor. Postnatal survival has been reported but only when the cystic degeneration involves only a segment of the kidney. Infantile polycystic kidneys are usually associated with severe oligohydramnios and pulmonary hypoplasia, resulting in fetal or neonatal death. Infantile polycystic kidney anomaly can be diagnosed in utero from as early as the end of the first trimester.[163]

Autosomal Dominant Polycystic Kidney Disease (Adult Polycystic Disease)

Diagnosis. Autosomal dominant polycystic kidney disease rarely manifests first in utero. Renal masses secondary to neoplasia (mesoblastic nephroma, hamartoma, Wilms tumor, neuroblastoma) occur rarely and are evidenced by the unilateral location, size (often massive),

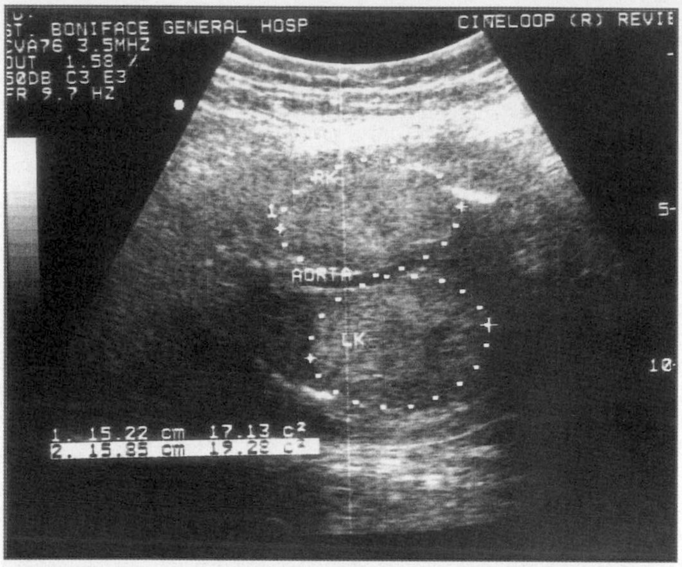

FIGURE 18-30 **Infantile polycystic kidney (autosomal recessive polycystic kidney disease).** In this coronal view of the fetal abdomen, the fetal kidneys are huge (15 × 19 cm) and have a homogeneous echotexture with recognizable internal structure. Note the associated oligohydramnios. These are the typical findings in the infantile polycystic kidney anomaly. LK, left kidney; RK, right kidney.

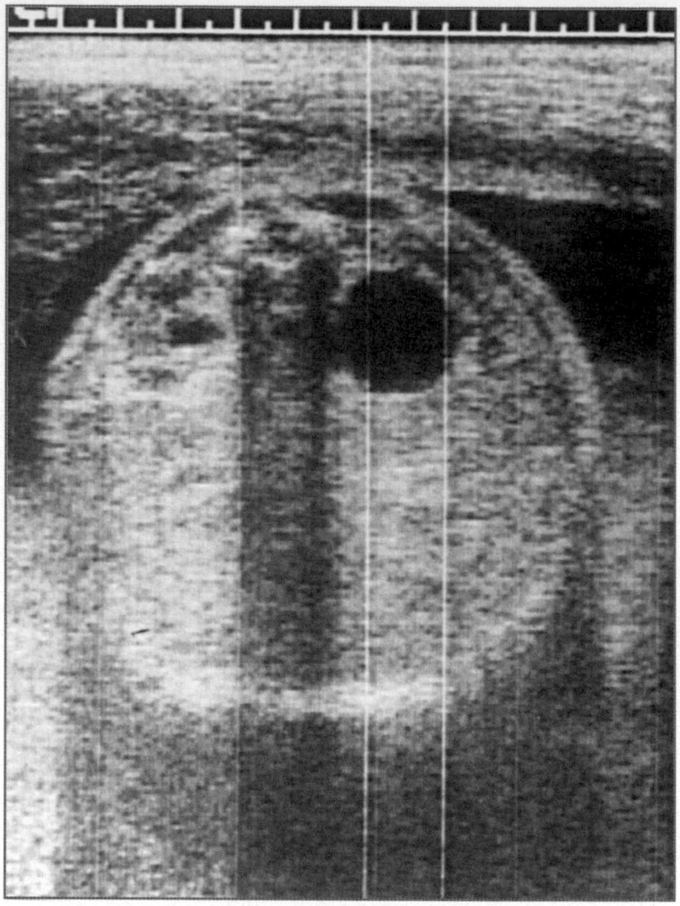

FIGURE 18-31 **Ureteropelvic obstruction.** Severe bilateral ureteropelvic obstruction at 31 weeks of gestation. Note the asymmetrical dilation of the renal pelves (greater on the left) and the less pronounced dilation of the calyces. Amniotic fluid volume is normal.

and distortion of the renal architecture. Isolated renal cysts can occur and usually have no impact on the kidney unless they are massive.

Ureteropelvic Junction Obstruction

Diagnosis. Ureteropelvic junction obstruction is among the most commonly identified renal anomalies. In the normal fetal kidney, the major renal calyces contain a small amount of urine visible by ultrasound. UPJ obstruction is diagnosed when the anteroposterior diameter of the renal pelvis exceeds 7 to 10 mm at or beyond 28 weeks' gestation (Fig. 18-31). The obstruction is usually unilateral but is occasionally bilateral, and it may progress, regress, or disappear.

Prognosis. In general, the larger the dilation of the renal pelvis is, the more likely the need for postnatal medical or surgical treatment. Postnatal intervention is required in about 50% of fetuses with third-trimester calyceal enlargement of 1.5 cm, and in almost all fetuses when the renal pelvis exceeds 2 cm.[164] Management of the fetus with UPJ is usually conservative, as early intervention has not been shown to reduce morbidity.[165] In utero treatment (needle decompression, shunting) has not been shown to be beneficial and has been associated with fetal complications.[166]

Megaureter

Diagnosis. When megaureter occurs as an isolated finding, it is thought to be the result of abnormal enervation of ureteral smooth muscle, resulting in reverse peristalsis. Most commonly, megaureter occurs as a result of obstruction of the ureter as it enters the bladder, as a result of vesicoureteric reflux, or as a result of distal bladder obstruction. The dilated ureter appears as multiple fluid-filled loops in the abdomen. In the absence of bladder obstruction, differentiating megaureter from small bowel obstruction can be difficult.

Prognosis. The prognosis for primary megaureter is excellent, whereas the prognosis for secondary megaureter depends on the underlying cause. Megaureter secondary to vesicoureteric reflux has a good prognosis, but megaureter in association with bladder outlet obstruction has a much more guarded prognosis.

Megacystis

Diagnosis. Primary megacystis is a subjective ultrasound observation, usually very apparent, and the diagnosis is easily made. Megacystis is the result of absent or abnormal enervation of the bladder associated with conditions such as megacystis-microcolon-intestinal hypoperistalsis syndrome (MMIHS)[167] or a neurogenic bladder associated with meningomyelocele.[168]

Prognosis. The prognosis of neurogenic megacystis is generally very poor.[169] Analysis of amniotic fluid digestive enzymes and fetal urinalysis has been proposed as a method for identifying MMIHS. However, although an elevated amniotic fluid digestive enzyme profile, presumed secondary to fetal vomiting, is prevalent in fetuses with MMIHS, it is not a universal finding, and elevated enzymes may also occasionally be present in the fetus without MMIHS.[170]

Obstructive megacystis is caused by an obstruction of the outflow tract, secondary to either posterior urethral valves or urethral atresia (Fig. 18-32), and it is almost exclusively an anomaly of male fetuses.

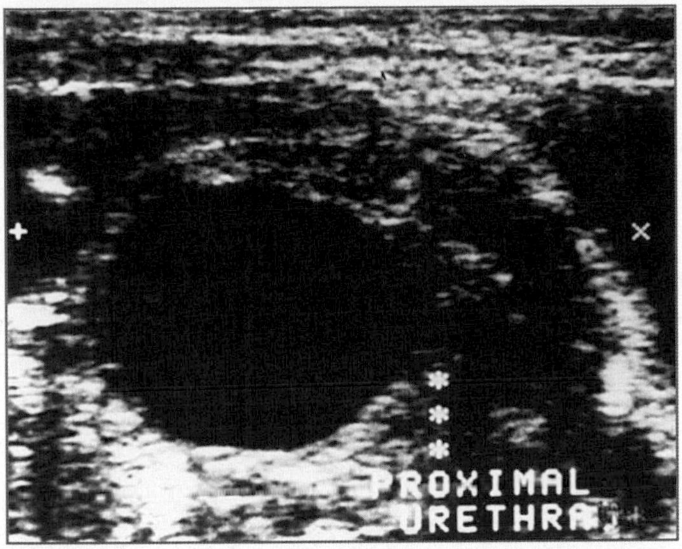

FIGURE 18-32 Magnified view of the bladder and proximal urethra in a fetus with posterior urethral valves. Note the dilation of the proximal urethra and the absence of visualization of the distal urethra. The bladder wall is thickened and relatively echogenic.

The bladder outlet obstruction results in progressive enlargement of the bladder, often to massive proportions, dilation of the ureters and renal pelves, and oligohydramnios.

Posterior Urethral Valves

Diagnosis. Tissue folds at the junction of the urethra and bladder resulting in a "valve" are the most common cause of bladder outlet obstruction. Posterior urethral valves typically occur in male fetuses. The obstructing valves are created by folding of the urethral mucosa distal to the vesicoureteric junction. The dilated proximal urethra creates the classic "key-hole" abnormality. Bladder outlet obstruction can also occur as a result of ureteral stenosis. This anomaly is much rarer than posterior urethral valves and can affect both male and female fetuses.

Prognosis. In utero therapy is a consideration, because left untreated, the bladder outflow obstruction will cause progressive hydronephrosis with loss of renal parenchyma and abnormal fetal urine chemistry, and it can cause severe oligohydramnios, leading to lethal pulmonary hypoplasia. Although this condition is easily recognized in utero, and because it is possible to divert the obstruction by placing a tube between the bladder and the amniotic cavity, effectively bypassing the obstruction,[171] or by using a fetoscope to fulgurate the obstructing valves,[172] fetal surgery for bladder outlet obstruction has been attempted; however, its role is uncertain. Sequential analyses of fetal urine chemistry are useful in selecting fetuses most likely to benefit from in utero treatment[173] and in predicting postnatal renal function.[174]

Comparative analyses of outcomes among 35 treated and 46 untreated perinates indicate that survival is worse in treated cases (43% mortality), and that the incidence of postnatal renal disease, stratified by severity, is about 50% and is similar for perinates treated prenatally and those treated postnatally.[175,176] As of May 2008 there are no randomized clinical trials confirming any significant reduction in mortality and morbidity by any form of fetal surgery for bladder outlet obstruction.

Skeletal Anomalies

The skeleton develops from three components of mesenchymal origin: bone, cartilage, and fibrous tissue. Congenital skeletal anomalies arise as a result of abnormalities of growth, shape, and intrinsic integrity of each of these components, either in isolation or in combination. With advances in molecular medicine, it has become possible to unravel some of the genetic mechanisms that regulate skeletal development and growth, and to identify gene abnormalities underlying some skeletal anomalies. The idea of a genetic basis for skeletal anomalies is important in the field of prenatal diagnosis because it opens the possibility of diagnosis based on DNA analysis rather than the conventional (and confusing) ultrasound-based morphologic classification.

Several DNA sites regulate skeletal growth. The homeobox *(HOX) genes* are active in the growth and shape of bones.[177] The growth of each limb is regulated by a specific sequence of HOX genes. For example, upper arm growth is regulated by genes in the 9 to 10 group, the lower arm by the 10, 11, and 12 groups, and the digits by the 11, 12, and 13 groups.[178] In addition to gene sequences, skeletal growth is also regulated by pairing of HOX genes, referred to as Pax (paired-like, homeobox-containing) sequences. A second gene sequence, the HMG box, contains gene combinations (SOX and TBX) that are active in regulation skeletal growth. The *fibroblastic growth factor receptors* (e.g., FGFR3) are a group of polypeptide gene products that regulate maturation and function of chondrocytes.[179] Bone mineralization and development is regulated in part by *parathyroid hormone–related protein receptor* (PTHrPR). Collagen, the essential component of the extracellular matrix, is regulated by *collagen gene loci* (genes *COL1A1* and *COL2A1*). The noncollagen component of the extracellular matrix, the *cartilage oligomeric matrix protein* (COMP), is regulated by a gene sequence located on chromosome 19. Cartilage maturation is controlled by transfer of sulfate groups to the proteoglycans in the extracellular matrix. This process of sulfonation of proteoglycans is regulated by a sulfate transport protein, in turn controlled by a gene combination termed the *diastrophic dysplasia sulfate transporter* (DTDST).

Abnormalities in these regulatory genes have been found in a number of skeletal dysplasias (Table 18-4). Abnormalities in these regulatory genes and gene products can be combined with biochemical and radiologic abnormalities to produce a logical classification of the skeletal dysplasias. This molecular, biochemical, radiologic morphology classification contains 372 specific diagnoses arranged in 37 different categories.[180]

Diagnosis. The diagnosis of fetal skeletal dysplasia depends on ultrasound findings of abnormalities in bone length, shape, and echodensity (abnormal mineralization), the complete absence of a bone or presence of additional bones, abnormalities of cartilage evident at the epiphyseal ends of bone, and abnormal shapes of complex structures such as the thorax, skull, and face caused by abnormal growth of the bone and cartilage components. Accordingly, ultrasound screening for anomalies should always include assessment of all long bones to determine presence, shape, density, and proportion; of the thorax to determine shape and to assess relative size; and of the skull and face to evaluate shape and proportions.

In almost all cases, the presence of a fetal skeletal anomaly is obvious and it can be identified by gross characteristics. However, recognition of a skeletal anomaly is only a first step, and the final diagnosis and assignment of prognosis depends on detailed measurements of all the long bones and expert assessment of all shape and structural charac-

TABLE 18-4 GENE ABNORMALITIES ASSOCIATED WITH SKELETAL DYSPLASIAS

Gene	Syndrome
Disorders of Mesenchymal Condensation and Differentiation	
SOX9	Camptomelic dysplasia
HOX13	Synpolydactyly
PAX3	Waardenburg's syndrome
CDMP1	Hunter-Thompson type acromesomelic dysplasia
	Brachydactyly type C
TBX5	Holt-Oram syndrome
Disorders of Maturation of Cartilage	
FGFR1	Pfeiffer's syndrome
	Apert's syndrome
	Jackson-Weiss syndrome
FGFR2	Crouzon's syndrome
	Thanatophoric dysplasia
	Achondroplasia
FGFR3	Hypochondroplasia
	Jansen's metaphyseal chondrodysplasia
PTHrPR	Blomstrand osteochondrodysplasia
Disorders in Collagenous and Noncollagenous Extracellular Matrix	
COL1A1, COL1A2	Osteogenesis imperfecta types I-IV
COL2A1	Achondrogenesis
	Hypochondrogenesis
	Kniest's dysplasia
	Stickler's dysplasia
COL9A2	Multiple epiphyseal dysplasia
COL10A1	Schmid's metaphyseal chondrodysplasia
COMP	Pseudoachondroplasia
DTDST	Achondrogenesis type IB
	Atelosteogenesis type II
	Diastrophic dysplasia

From Maymon E, Romero R, Ghezzi F, et al: Fetal skeletal anomalies. In Fleischer A, Manning FA, Jeanty P, Romero R (eds): Sonography in Obstetrics and Gynecology: Principles and Practice, 6th ed. New York, McGraw-Hill, 2001.

teristics and associations between abnormalities of long bones, digits, skull, face, chest, and vertebrae. Nomograms are available for all long bones and long bone length ratios, the foot, the mandible, and thoracic dimensions.[181] In the individual case, classification of a sporadic or first-affected fetus is challenging. The diagnosis when a sibling is affected is considerably easier and more accurate. Skeletal anomalies are rare, occurring a frequency of about 2 per 10,000 live births, but they are present about 18 times more frequently in surveys of perinatal deaths.[182] The incidence of skeletal anomalies varies by population and may be 10-fold higher when consanguinity is common.[183]

The most commonly encountered skeletal anomalies, in order of decreasing frequency, are thanatophoric dysplasia, osteogenesis imperfecta, chondrodysplasia punctata, camptomelic syndrome (achondroplasia), and osteogenesis imperfecta type I. It is critical to arrive at a correct diagnosis to assign appropriate prognoses. The problem is compounded because the expression (penetrance) of the underlying genetic disorder is variable, and because the fetal age at initial expression varies widely within and between conditions.

Prognosis. Several skeletal dysplasias can be associated with postnatal survival. Heterozygous achondroplasia is a short-limb dystrophy characterized by proximal long-bone shortening (rhizomelic dwarfism), bowing of the limbs (especially the lower limbs), a large skull, and depression of the nasal bridge. The condition is transmitted in an autosomal dominant manner with variable penetrance, so the incidence of an affected fetus is 50% if one parent is affected. If both parents are affected, the incidence of homozygous achondroplasia (uniformly lethal) is 25%, the incidence of heterozygous achondroplasia is 50%, and in 25% of cases the perinate is not affected. Interestingly, achondroplasia is one of the few conditions associated with advanced paternal age.[184] The ultrasound diagnosis depends on identification of bilateral short femurs, modest shortening of the humerus, normal length of radius, ulna, tibia, and fibula, normal mineralization, mild cephalomegaly, and normal thoracic dimensions. Postnatal survival is usual and morbidity is minimal.

Osteogenesis Imperfecta

The multiple syndromes of osteogenesis imperfecta are conditions characterized by inadequate mineralization of bones, making them fragile and subject to fracture, and by generalized diminished long bone growth. The penetrance varies. In two forms of osteogenesis imperfecta (type I and type III), the long bones may be fragile and subject to easy fracture but generally are near normal length, and they (especially the femur) may exhibit slight bowing. Type I and type III osteogenesis imperfecta are not associated with increased perinatal mortality. Type III disease is very minimal and may be evident only postnatally by mild deafness and a bluish sclera. Type I disease is somewhat more severe, with a higher propensity for fracture and again an association with deafness and a blue sclera. The features that distinguish types I and III osteogenesis from the lethal forms (types II and IV) are the presence in the former of normal thoracic architecture, normal or near-normal long bone length, and the absence of in utero fractures.

Other Skeletal Dysplasias

Diastrophic dystrophy is an autosomal recessive disorder characterized by predominantly rhizomelic long bone dysplasia, multiple joint flexures and the classic hand abnormality in which fingers are short and widely spaced and the thumb is abducted (the "hitchhiker thumb"). Frequently associated abnormalities of the face include micrognathia and cleft palate. Postnatal survival is generally not affected, and intellect appears intact. *Mesomelic dysplasia* is an autosomal dominant condition typically characterized by shortening and bowing of the distal limb bones. Prenatal diagnosis is rare. The long-term prognosis is generally good. *Camptomelic dysplasia* is characterized by extreme bowing of the long bones, and the diagnosis is usually obvious. Facial abnormalities including micrognathia, cleft palate, and macrocephaly are almost always present. Prenatal diagnosis is reported and survival is possible but rare: in most instances, early infant death occurs.[185,186] *Chondroectodermal dysplasia* (Ellis–van Creveld syndrome) is an autosomal recessive condition characterized by acromelia and polydactyly. The condition is frequently associated with major cardiac anomalies, and early infant death is common. Long-term survival with intact intellectual function can occur.

The common lethal skeletal dysplasias typically have a combination of thoracic deformities (thanatophoric dwarfism, short rib–polydactyly syndrome, asphyxiating thoracic dystrophy), extreme limb shortening (osteogenesis imperfecta types II and IV, achondrogenesis), demineralization (hypophosphatasia, fibrochondrogenesis, achondrogenesis), macrocrania (achondrogenesis), and facial abnormalities.

Bone abnormalities may also occur because of absence of bone development (dysostoses) or abnormal fusions of bones. *Craniosynostosis* occurs when there is premature fusion of the calvarial sutures, resulting in a wide spectrum of abnormal skull shapes. Craniosynostosis is frequently associated with other anomalies, which typically determine the prognosis. *Radial aplasia*, or severe dysplasia as an isolated skeletal anomaly, can be associated with cardiac anomalies (Holt-Oram syndrome) or with thrombocytopenia, often severe (the TAR syndrome mentioned earlier). Congenital contractures with varus or valgus malrotation of the foot (clubfoot) can be an isolated finding or can be associated with numerous syndromes and trisomies. Unilateral absence of digits, foot and hand, or lower limb can occur as a result of in utero amputation secondary to amniotic band syndrome. Abnormal fixation of limbs and joints is a characteristic of arthrogryposis multiplex congenita.

Summary

Congenital abnormalities are among the most common causes of perinatal mortality and of infant and adult morbidity and mortality. As prenatal care improves and mortality of structurally normal perinates declines, the relative importance of identifying congenital anomalies before birth increases. The tremendous advances occurring in fetal imaging and in molecular biology have made the diagnosis of anomalies in utero more accurate and have pushed back the gestational age at which the diagnosis can be made. Advances in postnatal care have improved survival and functional prognosis for many of the structural anomalies, especially the cardiac anomalies. The initial hope that prenatal intervention and surgical repair or reconstruction of anomalies has been more recently tempered with reality, but antenatal intervention remains an important area of future investigation and still holds promise as a means to further reduce the mortality and morbidity of fetal anomalies. The promise for continued advances in the spectrum and quality of care is virtually certain.

References

1. Nelson K, Holmes LB: Malformations due to spontaneous mutations of newborn infants. N Engl J Med 320:19-26, 1989.
2. Crane JP, LeFevre ML, Winborn RC, et al: A randomized trial of prenatal ultrasound screening: Impact on detection, management and outcome of anomalous fetuses. The RADIUS Study Group. Am J Obstet Gynecol 171:392-399, 1994.
3. Boyd PA, Chamberlain PFC, Hicks NR: 6-year experience of prenatal diagnosis in an unselected population in Oxford, UK. Lancet 352:1577-1581, 1998.
4. Garne E, Loane M, Dolk H, et al: Prenatal diagnosis of severe structural congenital malformations in Europe. Ultrasound Obstet Gynecol 25:6-11, 2005.
5. Nikkila A, Rydhstroem H, Kallen B, Jorgensen C: Ultrasound screening for fetal anomalies in southern Sweden: A population based study. Acta Obstet Gynecol Scand 85:688-693, 2006.
6. Reefhuis J, Honein MA: Maternal age and non-chromosomal birth defects, Atlanta 1968-2000: Teenager or thirty-something, who is at risk. Birth Defects Res A Clin Mol Teratol 70:572-579, 2004.
7. Zhu JL, Madsen KM, Vestergaard M, et al: Paternal age and congenital malformations. Hum Reprod 20:3173-3177, 2005.
8. Wong SF, Chan FY, Cincotta RB, et al: directly in the amniotic fluid (fetoscopy): Routine ultrasound screening in diabetic pregnancies. Ultrasound Obstet Gynecol 19:171-176, 2002.
9. Watkins ML, Rasmussen SA, Honein MA, et al: Maternal obesity and risk for birth defects. Pediatrics 111(5 Pt 2):1152-1158, 2003.
10. Canick JA, Kellner LH, Bombard AT: Prenatal screening for open neural tube defects. Clin Lab Med 23:385-394, 2003.
11. Haddow JE, Palomaki GE, Knight GJ, et al: Prenatal screening for Down's syndrome with use of maternal serum markers.N Engl J Med 327:588-593, 1992.
12. Bahado-Singh RO, Wapner R, Thom E, et al: Elevated first-trimester nuchal translucency increases the risk of congenital heart defects. Am J Obstet Gynecol 192:1357-1361, 2005.
13. Simpson LL, Malone FD, Bianchi DW, et al: Nuchal translucency and the risk of congenital heart disease. Obstet Gynecol 109:376-383, 2007.
14. Kurjak A, Azumendi G, Andonotopo W, Salihagic-Kadic A: Three-and four dimensional ultrasonography for the structural and functional evaluation of the fetal face. Am J Obstet Gynecol 196:16-28, 2007.
15. Eugenics K, Axelsson O, Cnattingius S, et al: Second trimester ultrasound screening performed by midwives: Sensitivity for detection of fetal anomalies. Acta Obstet Gynecol Scand 78:98-104, 1999.
16. Saltvedt S, Almstrom H, Kublickas H, et al: Detection of malformations in chromosomally normal fetuses by routine ultrasound at 12 or 18 weeks of gestation: A randomized controlled trial in 39572 pregnancies. BJOG 113:664-674, 2006.
17. LeFevre ML, Bain RP, Ewigman BG, et al: A randomized trial of prenatal ultrasonographic screening: Impact on maternal management and outcome. RADIUS Study Group. Am J Obstet Gynecol 169:483-489, 1993.
18. Garne E, Loane M, Dolk H, et al: Prenatal diagnosis of severe structural congenital malformations in Europe. Ultrasound Obstet Gynecol 25:6-11, 2005.
19. Stoll C, Dott B, Alembik Y, Roth MP: Evaluation of routine prenatal diagnosis by a registry of congenital anomalies. Prenat Diag 15:791-800, 1995.
20. Gascard-Battisti C, Dubois-Lebbe C, Chatelet-Cheront C, et al: Antenatal screening for congenital heart disease: A retrospective analysis of 20 years experience. J Obstet Biol Reprod 35:472-476, 2006.
21. Clementi M, Tendon R, Bianchi F, Stoll C: Evaluation of prenatal diagnosis of cleft lip with or without cleft palate by ultrasound: Experience from 20 European registries. Prenat Diag 20:870-875, 2000.
22. Hanikeri M, Savundra J, Gillett D, et al: Transabdominal ultrasound detection of cleft lip and palate in Western Australia from 1996-2003. Cleft Palate Craniofac J 43:61-66, 2006.
23. Souka AP, Pilalis A, Kavalakis I, et al: Screening for major structural anomalies at the 11-14 week ultrasound scan. Am J Obstet Gynecol 194:393-396, 2006.
24. Dimmick JE, Kalouset DE (eds): Developmental Pathology of the Embryo and Fetus. Philadelphia, Lippincott, 1992, p 527.
25. Yang J, Cummings EA, O'Connell C, Jangaard K: Fetal and neonatal outcomes in diabetic pregnancies. Obstet Gynecol 108(3 Pt 1):644-650, 2006.
26. Waller DK, Mills JL, Simpson JL, et al: Are obese women at higher risk for producing malformed offspring? Am J Obstet Gynecol 170:541-548, 1994.
27. Watkins ML, Rasmussen SA, Honeru MA, et al: Maternal obesity and the risk for birth defects. Pediatrics 111:1152-1158, 2003.
28. Malone FD, Canick J, Ball RH, et al: First-trimester and second-trimester screening, or both, for Down's syndrome N Engl J Med 353:2001-2011, 2005.
29. Hendler I, Blackwell SC, Bujold E, et al: The impact of maternal obesity on mid-trimester sonographic visualization of fetal cardiac and craniospinal structures. Int J Obes Gynecol Rel Metab Disord 28:1607-1615, 2004.
30. Hendler I, Blackwell SC, Bujold E, et al: Suboptimal second-trimester ultrasonographic visualization of the fetal heart in obese woman: Should we repeat the examination? J Ultrasound Med 24:1205-1209, 2005.
31. Rosenberg JC, Guzman ER, Vintzileos AM, Knuppel RA: Transumbilical placement of the vaginal probe in obese pregnant women. Obstet Gynecol 85:132-134, 1995.

32. Romero R, Pilu J, Jeanty P, et al: The central nervous system: Normal sonographic anatomy of the central nervous system. In: Prenatal Diagnosis of Congenital Anomalies. Norwalk, CT, Appleton Lange, 1988, p 4.
33. Gay-Andrieu F, Marty P, Pialat J, Sournes G, et al: Fetal toxoplasmosis and negative amniocentesis: Necessity of ultrasound follow-up. Prenat Diag 23:558-560, 2003.
34. Ornoy A, Diav-Citrin O: Fetal effects of primary and secondary cytomegalovirus infection in pregnancy. Reprod Toxicol 21:399-409, 2006.
35. Hoppen T, Eis-Hubinger AM, Schild RL, et al: Intrauterine herpes simplex infection. Klin Padiatr 213:63-68, 2001.
36. Mazzella M, Arioni C, Bellini C, et al: Severe hydrocephalus associated with congenital varicella syndrome. CMAJ 168:561-563, 2003.
37. Chow KC, Lee CC, Shen WC, et al: Congenital enterovirus 71 infection: A case study with virology and immunohistochemistry. Clin Infect Dis 31:509-512, 2000.
38. Barton LL, Mets MB, Beauchamp CL: Lymphocytic choriomeningitis virus: Emerging fetal teratogen. Am J Obstet Gynecol 187:1715-1716, 2002.
39. Katz VL, McCoy MC, Kuller JA, Hansen WF: An association between fetal parvovirus B19 and fetal anomalies: Report of two cases. Am J Perinatol 13:43-45, 1996.
40. Halliday J, Chow CW, Wallace D, Danks DM: X-linked hydrocephalus: A survey of a 20 year period in Victoria Australia. J Med Genet 23:23-31, 1986.
41. Hamada H, Watanabe H, Sigimoto M, et al: Autosomal recessive hydrocephalus due to congenital stenosis of the aqueduct of Sylvius. Prenat Diag 19:1067-1069, 1999.
42. Zlotogoro J, Sagi M, Cohen T: Familial hydrocephalus of prenatal onset. Am J Med Genet 49:202-204, 1994.
43. Racket CH, Probes-Cousin S, Louwen F, et al: Congenital immature teratoma of the fetal brain. Childs Nerv Syst 13:556-559, 1997.
44. Marcorelle P, Fallet-Bianco C, Oury JF, et al: Fetal aqueduct glioneuronal hamartoma: Clinicopathological and pathophysiological study of three cases. Clin Neuropathol 24:155-162, 2005.
45. Eisenberg VH, Hoffmann C, Feldman Z, Achiron R: Prenatal diagnosis of cavum velum interpositum cysts: Significance and outcome Prenat Diag 23:779-783, 2003.
46. Trumble ER, Smith RM, Pearl G, Wall J: Transplacental transmission of metastatic melanoma to the posterior fossa: Case report. J Neurosurg 103(2 Suppl):191-193, 2005.
47. Greco P, Vimercati A, DeCosmo L, et al: Mild ventriculomegaly as counseling challenge. Fetal Diag Ther 16:398-401, 2001.
48. Graham E, Duhl A, Ural S, et al: The degree of antenatal ventriculomegaly is related to pediatric neurological morbidity. J Matern Fetal Med 10:258-263, 2001.
49. Laskin MD, Kingdom J, Toi A, et al: Perinatal and neurodevelopmental outcome with isolated ventriculomegaly : A systemic review. J Matern Fetal Neonatal Med 18:289-298, 2005.
50. Manning FA: Ultrasound guided invasive fetal therapy: Current status. In Fleischer A, Manning FA, Jeanty P, Romero R (eds): Sonography in Obstetrics and Gynecology: Principles and Practice, 6th ed. New York, McGraw-Hill, 2001, p 813.
51. Bruner JP, Davis G, Talipan N: Intrauterine shunt for obstructive hydrocephalus: Still not ready. Fetal Diag Ther 21:532-539, 2006.
52. Nizard J, Bernard JP, Ville Y: Fetal cystic malformations of the posterior fossa in the first trimester of pregnancy. Fetal Diag Ther 20:146-151, 2005.
53. Vialard F, Robyr R, Hillion Y, et al: Dandy Walker syndrome and corpus callosum agenesis in 5p deletion. Prenat Diag 25:311-313, 2005.
54. Guia A, Cebeci A, Erol O, et al: Prenatal diagnosis of 13q-syndrome in a fetus with Dandy-Walker malformation. Obstet Gynecol 105:1227-1229, 2005.
55. Long A, Moran P, Robson S: Outcome of fetal cerebral posterior fossa anomalies. Prenat Diag 26:707-710, 2006.
56. Pitkin RM: Folate and neural tube defects. Am J Clin Nutr 85:285-288, 2007.
57. Norem CT, Schoen EJ, Walton DL, et al: Routine ultrasonography compared with maternal serum alpha-fetoprotein for neural tube defect screening. Obstet Gynecol 106:747-752, 2005.
58. Cedergren M, Selbing A: Detection of fetal structural abnormalities by an 11-14 week ultrasound scan in an unselected Swedish population. Acta Obstet Gynecol Scand 85:912-915, 2006.
59. Lorber J: The prognosis of occipital encephalocoele. Dev Child Neurol (Suppl) 13:75, 1966.
60. Bannister CM, Russell SA, Rimmer S, et al: Can prognostic indicators be identified in a fetus with an encephalocoele? Eur J Pediatr Surg Suppl 1:20-23, 2000.
61. Kyle PM, Harman CR, Evans JA, et al: Life without amniocentesis: Elevated maternal serum alpha feto-protein in the Manitoba program 1986-1991. Ultrasound Obstet Gynecol 4:199-204, 1994.
62. Nicolaides KH, Campbell S, Gabbe SG, Guidetti R: Ultrasound screening for spina bifida: Cranial and cerebellar signs. Lancet 2:72-74, 1986.
63. Campbell J, Gilbert WM, Nicolaides KH, Campbell S: Ultrasound screening for spinal bifida: Cranial and cerebellar signs in a high-risk population. Obstet Gynecol 70:247-250, 1987.
64. Budorick NE, Pretorius DH, Nelson TR: Sonography of the fetal spine: Technique, imaging findings, and clinical implications. AJR Am J Roentgenol 164:421-428, 1995.
65. Rauzzino M, Oakes WJ: Chiari malformation II and syringomyelia. Neurosurg Clin North Am 6:293-307, 1995.
66. Johnson MP, Sutton LN, Rintoul N, et al: Fetal myelomenigocoele repair: Short-term clinical outcomes. Am J Obstet Gynecol 189:482-487, 2003.
67. Tulipan N, Bruner JP: Menigomyelocoele repair in utero: A report of three cases. Pediatr Neurosurg 28:177-180, 1999.
68. Bruner JP, Tulipan N, Reed G, et al: Intrauterine repair of spina bifida: Preoperative predictors of shunt-dependent hydrocephalus. Am J Obstet Gynecol 190:1305-1312, 2004.
69. Farmer DL, von Koch CS, Peacock WJ, et al: In utero repair of myelomeningocoele: Experimental, pathophysiology, initial clinical experience and outcomes. Arch Surg 138:872-878, 2003.
70. Adelberg A, Blotzer A, Koch G, et al: Impact of maternal-fetal surgery for myelomeningocoele on the progression of ventriculomegaly in utero. Am J Obstet Gynecol 193:727-731, 2005.
71. Danzer E, Johnson MP, Bebbington M, et al: Fetal head biometry assessed by fetal magnetic resonance imaging following in utero myelomeningocoele repair. Fetal Diag Ther 22:1-6, 2007.
72. Holmes NM, Nguyen HT, Harrison MR, et al: Fetal intervention for myelomeningocoele: Effect on postnatal bladder function. J Urol 166:2383-1286, 2001.
73. Koh CJ, DeFilippo RE, Borer JG, et al: Bladder and external urethral sphincter function after prenatal closure of myelomeningocele. J Urol 176:2232-2236, 2006.
74. Johnson MP, Gerdes M, Rintoul N, et al: Maternal-fetal surgery for myelomeingocoele: Neurodevelopment outcomes at 2 years of age. 194:1145-1150, 2006.
75. Barini R, Barreto MW, Cursino K, et al: Abruptio placentae during fetal myelomeningocoele repair. Fetal Diag Ther 21:115-117, 2006.
76. Moinuddin A, McKinstry RC, Martin KA, Neil JJ: Intracranial hemorrhage progressing to porencephaly as a result of congenitally acquired cytomegalovirus infection. Prenat Diag 23:797-800, 2003.
77. Simonazzi G, Segata M, Ghi T, et al: Accurate neurosonographic prediction of brain injury in the surviving fetus after the death of a monochorionic cotwin. Ultrasound Obstet Gynecol 27:517-521, 2006.
78. Eller KM, Kuller JA: Porencephaly secondary to fetal trauma during amniocentesis. Obstet Gynecol 85:865-867, 1995.
79. Sharif U, Kuban K: Prenatal intracranial hemorrhage and neurological complications in alloimmune thrombocytopenia. J Child Neurol 16:838-842, 2001.
80. Eller KM, Kuller JA: Fetal porencephaly: A review of etiology, diagnosis and prognosis. Obstet Gynecol Survey 50:684-687, 1995.
81. Pilu G, Falco P, Perolo A, et al: Differential diagnosis and outcome of intracranial hypoechoic lesions: A report of 21 cases. Ultrasound Obstet Gynecol 9:229-236, 1997.

82. Bannister CM, Russell SA, Rimmer S, Mowle DH: Fetal arachnoid cysts: Their site, prognosis and differential diagnosis. Eur J Pediatr Surg 9(Suppl 1):27-28, 1999.
83. Sasidharan CK, Anoop P, Vijayakumar M, Jayakrishnan MP: Spectrum of clinical presentation of vein of Galen aneurysm. Indian J Pediatr 71:459-463, 2004.
84. Seker A, Ozek MM: Congenital glioblastoma multiforme: Case report and review of the literature. J Neurosurg 105:473-479, 2006.
85. Heckel S, Favre R, Gasser B, Christmann D: Prenatal diagnosis of a congenital astrocytoma: A case report and literature review. Ultrasound Obstet Gynecol 5:63-66, 1995.
86. Kosal Y, Varan A, Akalan N, et al: Congenital cerebellar primitive neuroectodermal tumor in a newborn. Am J Perinatol 23:173-176, 2006.
87. Ortega-Aznar A, Romero-Vidal FJ, de la Torre J, et al: Neonatal tumors of the CNS: A report of 9 cases and a review of the literature. Clin Neuropathol 20:181-189, 2001.
88. Yoder PR, Sabbagha RE, Gross SJ, Zelop CM: The second trimester fetus with isolated choroid plexus cysts: A meta-analysis of risk of trisomy 18 and trisomy 21. Obstet Gynecol 93:869-872, 1999.
89. Achiron R, Barkal G, Katznelson B, et al: Fetal lateral ventricle choroid plexus cysts: The dilemma of amniocentesis. Obstet Gynecol 78:815-818, 1991.
90. Silva SR, Jeanty J: Fetal syndromes. In Fleischer A, Manning FA, Jeanty P, Romero R (eds): Sonography in Obstetrics and Gynecology: Principles and Practice, 6th ed. New York, McGraw-Hill, 2001, p 591.
91. Avery GB, Menses L, Lodge A: The clinical significance of measured microcephaly. Am J Dis Child 123:214-220, 1972.
92. Martin HP: Microcephaly and mental retardation Am J Dis Child 119:128-132, 1972.
93. Shaw GM, Carmichael SL, Yang W, et al: Congenital malformations with orofacial clefts among 3.6 million California births, 1983-1997. Am J Med Genet A 125:250-256, 2004.
94. Gorlin RJ, Cervenka J, Pruzansky S: Facial clefting and its syndromes. Birth Defects 7:3-11, 1971.
95. Mittermayer C, Blaicher W, Brugger PC, et al: Foetal facial clefts: Prenatal evaluation of lip and palate by 2D and 3D ultrasound. Ultraschall Med 25:120-125, 2004.
96. Campbell S, Lees C, Moscoso G, Hall P: Ultrasound antenatal diagnosis of cleft palate by a new technique: The 3D "reverse face" view. Ultrasound Obstet Gynecol 25:12-18, 2005.
97. Platt LD, Devore GR, Pretorius DH: Improving cleft palate/cleft lip antenatal diagnosis by 3-dimensional sonography: The "flipped face" view. J Ultrasound Med 25:1423-1430, 2006.
98. Cash C, Set P, Coleman N: The accuracy of antenatal ultrasound in the detection of facial clefts in a low-risk screening population. Ultrasound Obstet Gynecol 18:432-436, 2001.
99. Chitty LS, Campbell S, Altman DG: Measurement of the fetal mandible: Feasibility and construction of a centile chart. Prenat Diagn 13:749-756, 1993.
100. Winters WD, Efland EL: Congenital masses of the lung: Prenatal and postnatal imaging evaluation. J Thorac Imaging 16:196-206, 2001.
101. Adzick NS: Fetal thoracic lesions. Semin Pediat Surg 2:103-108, 1993.
102. Adzick NS, Harrison MR, Crombleholme TM, et al: Fetal lung lesions: Management and outcome. Am J Obstet Gynecol 179:884-889, 1998.
103. Illanes S, Hunter A, Evans M, et al: Prenatal diagnosis of echogenic lung: Evolution and outcome. Ultrasound Obstet Gynecol 26:145-149, 2005.
104. Davenport M, Warnes SA, Cacciaguerra S, et al: Current outcome of antenatally diagnosed cystic lung disease, J Pediatr Surg 39:549-556, 2004.
105. Shanmugam G, MacArthur K, Pollock JC: Congenital lung malformations: Antenatal and postnatal evaluation and management. Eur J Cardiothorac Surg 27:45-52, 2005.
106. Grethel EJ, Wagner AJ, Clifton MS, et al: Fetal intervention for mass lesions and hydrops improves outcome: A 15-year experience. J Pediatr Surg 42:117-123, 2007.
107. Oepkes D, Devlieger R, Lopriore E, Klumper FJ: Successful ultrasound-guided laser treatment of fetal hydrops caused buy pulmonary sequestration. Ultrasound Obstet Gynecol 29:457-459, 2007.
108. Stocker JT, Madewell JE, Drake RM: Congenital cystic adenoid malformation of the lung. Hum Pathol 82:155-161, 1977.
109. Wilson RD, Hedrick HL, Liechty KW, et al: Cystic adenoid malformation of the lung: Review of genetics, prenatal diagnosis and in utero treatment. Am J Med Gen A 140:151-155, 2006.
110. Yang W, Carmichael SL, Harris JA, Shaw GM: Epidemiological characteristics of congenital diaphragmatic hernia among 2.5 million California births, 1989-1997. Birth Defects Res A Clin Mol Teratol 76:170-174, 2006.
111. Colvin J, Bower C, Dickenson JE, Sokol J: Outcomes of congenital diaphragmatic hernia: A population based study in Western Australia. Pediatrics 116:356-363, 2006.
112. Crane JP: Familial diaphragmatic hernia: Prenatal diagnostic approach and analysis of twelve families. Clin Genet 16:244-248, 1979.
113. Adzick NS, Harrison MR, Glick PL, et al: Diaphragmatic hernia in the fetus: Prenatal diagnosis and outcome in 94 cases. J Pediatr Surg 20:357-362, 1985.
114. Harrison MR, Bressack MA, Churg AM: Correction of congenital diaphragmatic hernia in utero: II. Simulated correction permits fetal lung growth with survival at birth. Surgery 88:260-268, 1980.
115. Harrison MR, Adzick NS, Estes JM, et al: A prospective study of the outcome of fetuses with diaphragmatic hernia. JAMA 271:382-384, 1994.
116. Harrison MR, Adzick NS, Bullard K, et al: Correction of congenital diaphragmatic hernia in utero: VII. A prospective trial. J Pediatr Surg 31:1637-1642, 1997.
117. Metkus AP, Filly RA, Stringer MD, et al: Sonographic predictors of survival in fetal diaphragmatic hernia. J Pediatr Surg 31:148-151, 1996.
118. Jani JC, Nicolaides KH, Gratacos E, et al: Fetal head-to-lung ratio in the prediction of survival in severe left-sided diaphragmatic hernia treated by fetal endoscopic tracheal occlusion (FETO). Am J Obstet Gynecol 195:1646-1650, 2006.
119. Heling KS, Wauer RR, Hammer H, et al: Reliability of the lung-to-head ratio in predicting outcome and neonatal ventilation parameters in fetuses with congenital diaphragmatic hernia. Ultrasound Obstet Gynecol 25:112-118, 2005.
120. Arkovitz MS, Russo M, Devine P, et al: Fetal lung-head ratio is not related to outcome for antenatal diagnosed congenital diaphragmatic hernia. J Pediatr Surg 42:107-110, 2007.
121. Alcorn D, Adamson T, Lambert T: Morphological effects of chronic tracheal ligation and drainage in the fetal lamb lung. J Anat 22:649-657, 1976.
122. Flake AW, Crombleholme TM, Johnson MP, et al: Treatment of severe congenital diaphragmatic hernia by fetal tracheal occlusion: Clinical experience with fifteen cases. Am J Obstet Gynecol 183:1059-1066, 2000.
123. Harrison MR, Mychaliska GB, Albanese CT, et al: Correction of congenital diaphragmatic hernia in utero: IX. Fetuses with poor prognosis—Liver herniation and low lung-to-head ratio can be saved by fetoscopic temporary tracheal occlusion. J Pediatr Surg 33:1017-1022, 1998.
124. Harrison MR, Keller RL, Hawgood SB, et al: A randomized trial of fetal endoscopic tracheal occlusion for severe fetal congenital diaphragmatic hernia. N Engl J Med 349:1916-1924, 2003.
125. Deprest J, Jani J, Gratacos E, et al: Fetal intervention for congenital diaphragmatic hernia: The European experience. Semin Perinatol 29:94-103, 2005.
126. Longaker MT, Laberge JM, Dansereau J, et al: Primary fetal hydrothorax: Natural history and management J Pediatr Surg 24:573-576, 1989.
127. Klam S, Bigras JL, Hudon L: Predicting outcome in primary fetal hydrothorax. Fetal Diagn Ther 20:366-370, 2005.
128. Smith RP, Illanes S, Denbow ML, Soothill PW: Outcome of pleural effusions treated by thoracoamniotic shunting. Ultrasound Obstet Gynecol 26:63-66, 2005.
129. Langer JC, Fitzgerald PG, Desa D, et al: Cervical cystic hygroma in the fetus: Clinical spectrum and outcome. J Pediatr Surg 25:58-62, 1990.

130. Bouchard S, Johnson MP, Flake AW, Howell LJ, et al: The EXIT procedure: Experience and outcome in 31 cases. J Pediatr Surg 37:418-426, 2002.
131. Canfield MA, Honein MA, Yuskiv N, et al: National estimates and race/ethnic-specific variation of birth defects in the United States, 1999-2001. Birth Defects Res A Clin Mol Teratol 76:747-756, 2006.
132. Beasley SW, Allen M, Myers N: The effects of Down syndrome and other chromosomal abnormalities on survival and management in esophageal atresia. Pediatr Surg Int 12:550-551, 1997.
133. Nagata S, Koyanagi T, Horimoto N, et al: Chronological development of the fetal stomach assessed using real time ultrasound. Early Human Dev 22:15-22, 1990.
134. Centini G, Rosignoli L, Kenanidis A, Petraglia F: Prenatal diagnosis of esophageal atresia with the pouch sign. Ultrasound Obstet Gynecol 21:494-497, 2003.
135. Khorshid EA, Dokhan AL, Turkistani AF, et al: Five year experience in prenatal ultrasound diagnosis of esophageal atresia in Saudi Arabia. Ann Saudi Med 23:132-134, 2003.
136. Deurloo JA, Aronson DC: Possibility of esophageal atresia (EA) carries an increased risk for esophageal carcinoma. J Pediatr Surg 41:876-877, 2006.
137. Zimmer EZ, Bronshtein M: Early diagnosis of duodenal atresia and possible monographic pitfalls. Prenatal Diagn 16:564-566, 1996.
138. Miro J, Bard H: Congenital atresia and stenosis of the duodenum: The impact of a prenatal diagnosis. Am J Obstet Gynecol 158:555-559, 1988.
139. Weiss H, Sherer DM, Manning FA: Ultrasonography of fetal annular pancreas. Obstet Gynecol 94:853, 1999.
140. Choi SO, Park WH: Preduodenal portal vein: A cause for prenatally diagnosed duodenal obstruction. J Pediatr Surg 30:1521-1522, 1995.
141. Muraoka I, Ohno Y, Kobayashi K, et al: Preduodenal position of the common bile duct associated with annular pancreas: Case report and literature review. Pancreas 3:283-385, 2005.
142. Dalla Vecchia LK, Grosfeld JL, West KW, et al: Intestinal atresia and stenosis: A 25 year experience with 277 cases. Arch Surg 113:490-496, 1998.
143. Escobar MA, Ladd AP, Grosfeld JL, et al: Duodenal atresia and stenosis: long term follow-up over 30 years. J Pediatr Surg 39:867-871, 2004.
144. Sigalas I, Dafopoulos K, Galazios G, et al: Fetal small bowel obstruction: A report of two cases. Clin Exp Obstet Gynecol 30:161-163, 2003.
145. Al-Kouatly HB, Chasen ST, Streltzoff J, Chervenak FA: The clinical significance of fetal echogenic bowel. Am J Obstet Gynecol 185:1035-1038, 2001.
146. Achiron R, Mazkereth R, Orvieto R, et al: Echogenic bowel in intrauterine growth restricted fetuses: Does this jeopardize the gut? Obstet Gynecol 100:120-125, 2002.
147. Sepulveda W, Reid R, Nicolaides P, et al: Second trimester echogenic bowel and intraamniotic bleeding: Association between fetal bowel echogenicity and amniotic fluid spectrophotometry at 410 nm. Am J Obstet Gynecol 174:839-842, 1996.
148. Smith-Bindman R, Chu P, Goldberg JD: Second trimester prenatal ultrasound for the detection of pregnancies at increased risk of Down syndrome. Prenat Diagn 27:535-544, 2007.
149. Eliyahu S, Yanai N, Blondheim O, et al: Sonographic presentation of Hirschsprung's disease: A case of an entirely ganglion colon and ileum. Prenat Diagn 14:1170-1172, 1004.
150. Beretsky I, Lankin DH: Diagnosis of fetal cholelithiasis using real-time high-resolution imaging employing digital detection. J Ultrasound Med 2:381-383, 1983.
151. Chen CP: Chromosomal abnormalities associated with omphalocoele. Taiwan J Obstet Gynecol 46:1-8, 2007.
152. Lakasing L, Cicero S, Davenport M, et al: Current outcome of antenatally diagnosed exomphalos: An 11 year review. J Pediatr Surg 41:1403-1406, 2006.
153. Raynor BD, Richards D: Growth retardation in fetuses with gastroschisis. J Ultrasound Med 16:13-16, 1997.
154. Puligandla PS, Janvier A, Flageole H, et al: Routine cesarean delivery does not improve outcome of infants with gastroschisis. J Pediatr Surg 39:742-745, 2004.
155. Saxena AK, Hulskamp G, Schleef J, et al: Gastroschisis: A 15 year, single-center experience. Pediatr Surg Int 18:420-424, 2002.
156. Kanamori Y, Hashizume K, Sugiyama M, et al: Long term survival of a baby with body stalk anomaly: Report of a case. Surg Today 37:30-33, 2007.
157. van Leeuwen MA, Dik P, Klijn AJ, et al: Primary repair of bladder exstrophy followed by clean intermittent catherization: Outcome of 15 years' experience. Urology 67:394-398, 2006.
158. Hyun J: Cloacal exstrophy. Neonatal Netw 25:101-115, 2006.
159. Grannum P, Bracken M, Silverman R, et al: Assessment of fetal kidney size in normal gestation by comparison of kidney circumference to abdominal circumference. Am J Obstet Gynecol 136:249-253, 1980.
160. Campbell S, Wladimiroff JW, Dewhurst CJ: The antenatal measurement of fetal urine production. J Obstet Gyneacol Br Commonw 80:680-682, 1980.
161. Wiesel A, Queisser-luft A, Clementi M, et al: Prenatal detection of congenital renal malformations by fetal ultrasonographic examination: An analysis of 709,030 births in 12 European countries. Eur J Med Genet 48:131-144, 2005.
162. Kuwertz-Broeking E, Brinkmann OA, Von Lengerke HJ, et al: Unilateral multicystic dysplastic kidney: Experience in children. Br J Urol Int 93:388-392, 2004.
163. Bronshtein M, Yoffe N, Brandes JM, Blumenfeld Z: First and second trimester diagnosis of fetal urinary tract anomalies using transvaginal ultrasound. Prenat Diagn 10:653-656, 1990.
164. Nguyen HT, Kogan BA: Upper urinary tract obstruction: Experimental and clinical aspects. Br J Urol 81:13-21, 1998.
165. Thorup J, MortensenT, Diemer H, et al: The prognosis of surgically treated congenital hydronephrosis after diagnosis in utero. J Urol 134:914-923, 1985.
166. Lunacek A, Oswald J, Schwentner C, et al: Prenatal puncture of a unilateral hydronephrosis leading to fetal urinoma and postnatal nephrectomy. Urology 63:982-984, 2004.
167. Young ID, McKeever PA, Brown LA: Prenatal diagnosis of the megacystis-microcolon-intestinal peristalsis syndrome. J Med Genet 26:403-406, 1989.
168. Louie A, Arger PH: Fetal genitourinary tract. Semin Roentgen 4:342-352, 1990.
169. Verbruggen SC, Wijnen RM, van den Berg P: Megacystis-microcolon-intestinal hypoperistalsis syndrome: A case report. J Matern Fetal Neonatal Med 16:140-141, 2004.
170. Muller F, Dreux S, Vaast P, et al: Prenatal diagnosis of megacystis-microcolon-intestinal hypoperistalsis syndrome: Contribution of amniotic fluid digestive enzyme assay and fetal urinalysis. Prenat Diagn 25:203-209, 2005.
171. Manning FA, Harman CR, Lange I, et al: Antepartum chronic vesicoamniotic shunts for obstructive uropathy: A report of two cases. Am J Obstet Gynecol 145:819-823, 1983.
172. Quintero RA, Hume R, Smith C, et al: Percutaneous fetal cystoscopy and endoscopic fulguration of posterior urethral valves. Am J Obstet Gynecol 172:206-209, 1995.
173. Nicolaides KK, Cheng HH, Snijders RJ, Moniz CF: Fetal urine biochemistry in the assessment of obstructive uropathy. Am J Obstet Gynecol 166:932-937, 1992.
174. Miguelez J, Blunduki V, Yoshizaki CT, et al: Fetal obstructive uropathy: Is urine sampling useful for prenatal counseling. Prenat Diagn 26:81-84, 2006.
175. McLorie G, Farhat W, Khoury A, et al: Outcome analysis of vesicoamniotic shunting in a comprehensive population. J Urol 166:1036-1040, 2001.
176. Holmes N, Harrison MR, Baskin LS: Fetal surgery for posterior urethral valves: Long-term postnatal outcomes. Pediatrics 108:E7, 2001.
177. Morgan BA, Tabin C: The role of Hox genes in limb development. Curr Opin Genetic Dev 4:668-674, 1993.
178. Zanaky J, Duboule D: Hox genes in digit development and evolution. Cell Tissue Res 296:19-25, 1999.
179. Johnson DE, Williams LT: Structural and functional diversity of the FGF receptor multigene family. Adv Cancer Res 60:1-41, 1993.

180. Superti-Furga A, Unger S: Nosology and classification of genetic skeletal disorders: 2006 revision. Am J Med Genet A 143:1-18, 2007.
181. Maymon E, Romero R, Ghezzi F, et al: Fetal skeletal anomalies. In Fleischer A, Manning FA, Jeanty P, Romero R (eds): Sonography in Obstetrics and Gynecology: Principles and Practice, 6th ed. New York, McGraw-Hill, 2001, p 459.
182. Connor JM, Connor RAC, Sweet EM, et al: Lethal neonatal chondrodysplasias in the west of Scotland 1970-1983, with a description of thanatophoric, dysplasialike, autosomal recessive disorder, Glasgow variant. Am J Med Genet 22:43-46, 1985.
183. Al-Gazali LI, Bakir M, Hamid Z, et al: Birth prevalence and pattern of osteochondrodysplasias in an inbred high-risk population. Birth Defects Res A Clin Mol Tetatol 67:125-132, 2003.
184. Murdoch JL, Walker BA, Hall JG: Achondroplasia: A genetic and statistical survey. Ann Hum Genet 33:227-231, 1970.
185. Nagar AM, Sangle PM, Morani AC, Rajpal ND: Antenatal diagnosis of camptomelic dysplasia. J Postgrad Med 52:69-70, 2006.
186. Beluffi G, Fraccaro M: Genetic and clinical aspects of campomelic dysplasia. Prog Clin Biol Res 104:53-58, 1982.
187. Manning FA, Harrison MR, Rodeck C: Catheter shunts for fetal hydronephrosis and hydrocephalus: Reprint of the International Fetal Surgery Registry. N Engl J Med 315:336-340, 1986.
188. Wilson RD, Baxter JK, Johnson MP, et al: Thoraco-amniotic shunts: Fetal treatment for pleural effusions and congenital cystic adenomatoid malformations. Fetal Diagn Ther 19:413-420, 2004.
189. Tworetzky W, Wilkins-Haug L, Jennings RW, et al: Balloon dilation of severe aortic stenosis in the fetus: Potential for prevention of hypoplastic left heart syndrome–Candidate selection, technique, and results of successful intervention. Circulation 110:2125-2131, 2004.
190. Clark TJ, Martin WL, Divakaran TC, et al: Prenatal bladder drainage in the management of fetal lower urinary tract obstruction: A systematic review and meta-analysis. Obstet Gynecol 102:367-82, 2003.

Chapter 19

Fetal Cardiac Malformations and Arrhythmias

Detection, Diagnosis, Management, and Prognosis

Mark Sklansky, MD

Over the years, as the practice of fetal ultrasonography has evolved, a consensus has formed among sonographers, radiologists, obstetricians, and maternal-fetal medicine subspecialists: screening for fetal heart disease deserves the dubious distinction of being one of the most challenging and least successful aspects of fetal ultrasonography.[1-3] Because of the challenges inherent with screening the fetus for congenital heart disease (CHD), the rate of prenatal detection of even severe forms of CHD remains disappointingly low.[1,3-7] Furthermore, when a fetal heart defect or arrhythmia is suspected, many professionals feel uncomfortable with much more than referring the patient to someone else for further evaluation.

This chapter aims neither to make everyone involved with fetal ultrasonography into an expert fetal echocardiographer, nor to provide an exhaustive, encyclopedic review of the field of fetal cardiology; such detailed reviews may be found elsewhere.[8,9] Instead, the chapter takes a distinctive clinical bent, aiming to help those involved with fetal cardiac imaging (1) to become better at screening the fetal heart for CHD, (2) to become better at diagnosing and evaluating common forms of fetal cardiac malformations and arrhythmias, (3) to understand the basic approach to fetal and neonatal management of the most common forms of fetal cardiac malformations and arrhythmias, and (4) to understand the general prognosis associated with the most common forms of fetal heart disease.

After a brief discussion of the epidemiology of fetal heart disease, this chapter reviews the basic approach to screening in low-risk pregnancies for fetal heart disease. The next section reviews the more detailed technique of formal fetal echocardiography in pregnancies at high risk for fetal CHD, including a description of the fetal presentation of fetal congestive heart failure (CHF) and a discussion of the potential role of three-dimensional (3D) fetal echocardiography. The last two sections discuss the diagnosis, management, and prognosis of the most common and clinically important forms of fetal cardiac malformations and arrhythmias.

Incidence of Congenital Heart Disease in the Fetus

CHD represents by far the most common major congenital malformation.[10,11] Although most studies suggest an incidence of approximately 8 of 1000 live births,[11-13] this figure includes many forms of disease (e.g., secundum atrial septal defect [ASD], mild valvar pulmonary stenosis, and small muscular or membranous ventricular septal defects [VSDs]) that never will require either medical or surgical attention. In fact, 3 or 4 of every 1000 live newborn infants have some form of CHD that is likely to require medical if not surgical intervention.[1] Because cases of fetal heart disease, particularly those associated with aneuploidy or extracardiac malformations, may end in fetal demise, and because many VSDs may close spontaneously before birth,[14] the incidence of CHD during the first and second trimesters should be considerably higher than the incidence at term.

At the same time, some forms of CHD probably have a higher incidence at term than during the first or early second trimesters. Many forms of CHD evolve dramatically from first trimester to term.[15,16] Mild aortic or pulmonary valve stenosis, for instance, may evolve prenatally into severe forms of critical pulmonary or aortic stenosis or may even adversely affect ventricular development to the point of manifesting as hypoplastic left or right heart syndrome at term. Similarly, cardiac tumors such as cardiac rhabdomyomas or intrapericardial teratomas may not develop significantly until the second trimester,[17] and they may continue to enlarge dramatically from mid-gestation to term. Ductal constriction or closure of the foramen ovale may not develop until late in gestation,[18] and the same may be said for fetal arrhythmias, valvar regurgitation, myocardial dysfunction, and CHF.[16]

Risk Factors for Congenital Heart Disease in the Fetus

Inasmuch as most cases of CHD occur in pregnancies not identified as being at high risk,[19,20] effective screening for CHD in low-risk pregnancies remains tremendously important. Nevertheless, many risk factors (fetal, maternal, and familial) for fetal heart disease have been identified (Tables 19-1, 19-2, and 19-3).[21-36] Some anomalies, such as omphalocele with diaphragmatic hernia and tracheoesophageal fistula,[26] cleft lip/palate,[25] aneuploidies such as trisomy,[21,23,30] or maternal CHD,[24,27,28,31,32] carry significantly increased risks for fetal heart disease. Other associations, such as a family history of CHD,[24,34] many cases of maternal diabetes,[23,36] fetal exposure to many of the known

TABLE 19-1 RISK FACTORS FOR FETAL HEART DISEASE

Fetal
Abnormal visceral/cardiac situs
Abnormal four-chamber view or outflow tracts
Arrhythmia
Aneuploidy
Two-vessel umbilical cord
Extracardiac structural malformation
Intrauterine growth restriction
Polyhydramnios
Pericardial effusion/pleural effusion/ascites
Twins
Increased nuchal translucency thickness
Maternal
Systemic erythematosus
Diabetes mellitus
Phenylketonuria
Viral syndrome (mumps, Coxsackie virus, influenza, rubella, cytomegalovirus)
Congenital heart disease
Teratogen exposure
In-vitro fertilization?
Familial
First-degree relative with congenital heart disease
First-degree relative with cardiac syndrome
DiGeorge syndrome
Long QT syndrome
Noonan syndrome
Marfan syndrome
Tuberous sclerosis
Williams syndrome

TABLE 19-2 EXTRACARDIAC STRUCTURAL MALFORMATIONS ASSOCIATED WITH FETAL HEART DISEASE

Central Nervous System
Neural tube defect
Hydrocephalus
Absent corpus callosum
Arnold-Chiari malformation
Dandy-Walker malformation
Thoracic
Tracheoesophageal fistula
Cystic adenomatoid malformation of the lung
Diaphragmatic hernia
Skeletal
Holt-Oram syndrome
Apert syndrome
Thrombocytopenia/absent radii
Ellis–van Creveld syndrome
Fanconi syndrome
Gastrointestinal
Omphalocele
Duodenal atresia
Imperforate anus
Gastroschisis
Urogenital
Dysplastic/absent kidney
Horseshoe kidney
Ureteral obstruction

teratogens,[23,29,35] and fetal ureteral obstruction or gastroschisis,[26] carry only moderately increased risks for CHD. Many syndromes (familial, sporadic, or related to known teratogens) convey variable risks for CHD.[23] Finally, additional risk factors for CHD will undoubtedly be recognized in the future. For instance, increased nuchal translucency thickness in the first trimester (10 to 14 weeks) represents an important newly discovered risk factor for fetal heart disease, even in the presence of normal fetal chromosomes.[22,33] This subject is addressed in detail in Chapter 17.

A distinction should be recognized between "fetal risk factor for CHD" and "indication for fetal echocardiography." Because not all risk factors for fetal heart disease are equal, the primary obstetrician or perinatologist should weigh the likelihood of fetal heart disease when considering whether further evaluation is indicated. However, the expertise of primary obstetricians, perinatologists, and radiologists, as well as pediatric cardiologists, in evaluating the fetal heart varies tremendously. Therefore, the determination of which pregnancies to refer for formal echocardiography should depend on the degree of added expertise in fetal cardiac imaging, management of fetal heart disease, and counseling for fetal heart disease offered by the consultant. Ultimately, the decision of whom to refer for formal fetal echocardiography should reflect both the perceived likelihood of fetal heart disease and the additional expertise anticipated from referral.

TABLE 19-3 SUBSTANCES BELIEVED TO CAUSE FETAL HEART DISEASE

Anticonvulsants
Valproic acid
Carbamazepine
Phenytoin
Phenobarbital
Warfarin
Aspirin/ibuprofen
Tricyclic antidepressants
Lithium
Alcohol
Recreational drugs (including cocaine)
Isotretinoin

Screening for Congenital Heart Disease in the Fetus

Background

The prenatal detection of CHD in the low-risk pregnancy has long represented the fetal sonographer's Achilles' heel.[37] Although CHD occurs more frequently than any other major congenital anomaly, the rate of detection has remained disappointingly low.[1,3-7] This weakness in fetal screening sonography represents a real problem. Not only is CHD responsible for most neonatal mortality from congenital malformations,[10] but prenatal detection and diagnosis also can improve the outcome of fetuses and neonates with CHD.[38-43] For these reasons, more improvement needs to be made in prenatal detection of the patient at low risk than in the detailed fetal diagnosis of CHD.[5,19,44]

For years, those involved with fetal imaging have attempted to improve the prenatal detection of CHD. Soon after the development of two-dimensional (2D) fetal cardiac imaging, investigators proposed the four-chamber view (4CV) as an effective approach to screening the fetus for CHD.[45-47] To this day, the 4CV has remained the standard of care for the screening fetal ultrasound evaluation of low-risk pregnancies, although probably not for much longer.[2,48,49] In practice, the 4CV has not resulted in the high rates of detection initially anticipated.[1,4,6,50-52]

To improve detection further, others have suggested that color flow imaging, performed along with the 4CV, could improve detection rates,[53] but this technique requires specialized expertise and equipment and probably adds little to the detection of major forms of CHD. On the other hand, there has been an important push toward attempting to include visualization of the outflow tracts along with the 4CV,[54-59] because many defects (e.g., double-outlet right ventricle [DORV], tetralogy of Fallot [TOF], transposition of the great arteries [TGA], truncus arteriosus) can have normal-appearing 4CVs. Routine inclusion of the outflow tracts has been somewhat problematic, however, in part because the outflow tracts, unlike the 4CV, do not reside in a single plane. Nevertheless, inclusion of outflow tracts along with the 4CV for the low-risk standard fetal ultrasound evaluation makes sense and is swiftly becoming the standard of care.[2,48,49]

More recently, multiple investigators have suggested that 3D imaging, wherein volumes may be acquired within seconds and subsequently interactively reviewed, allowing the display of virtually any plane, may facilitate and improve the evaluation of both the 4CV and the outflow tracts.[60-62] However, image resolution with 3D imaging remains low, and considerable expertise currently is required to evaluate volume data sets, despite a wealth of evolving algorithms and display techniques aimed at facilitating and improving analysis.[60-64]

Despite these developments, prenatal fetal cardiac anatomy screening remains flawed, for several reasons. First, the practice of prenatal screening for CHD remains heavily dependent on both the expertise of the sonographer[3,65] and the quality of the equipment. Second, and equally important, effective screening requires an experienced reviewer to evaluate the fetal heart.[55] And third, although it makes sense to evaluate static fetal structures as still-frame images, it does not make sense—and does not work—to evaluate the heart as a single still-frame image of the 4CV, or even as a series of still-frame images of the 4CV and outflow tracts.[37]

For these reasons, the beating 4CV (plus outflow tracts) should supplant the 4CV as the centerpiece of screening the fetus for CHD.[37] Visualization of valve and myocardial motion facilitates and enhances the evaluation of cardiac structure[4,66] and makes reviewers less likely to miss a major structural defect. Ideally, screening should also include evaluation of both outflow tracts; however, the addition of just the left ventricular outflow tract (LVOT) would probably effectively detect most major anomalies typically missed with 4CV imaging alone.[56] The following paragraphs describe the routine (second-trimester) evaluation of low-risk pregnancies for fetal heart disease; descriptions of first-trimester evaluation of the fetal heart may be found elsewhere.[15,67-70]

Technique

Extracardiac Evaluation

Prenatal screening for CHD should begin with an evaluation for extracardiac abnormalities associated with CHD. The umbilical cord should have three vessels; the heart and stomach should both be on the fetal left (above and below the diaphragm, respectively); and there should be no ascites (Fig. 19-1) or pericardial or pleural effusions. A trivial amount of pericardial fluid may normally be seen adjacent to the right and left ventricular free walls.[71] Abnormalities of any of these findings should raise the suspicion for CHD and prompt more than just a routine evaluation.

Beating Four-Chamber View

The 4CV (Figs. 19-2 and 19-3) always deserves a close, detailed evaluation, even as part of a general screening fetal ultrasound study. In fact, given the current low rates of prenatal detection of CHD,[1,3-7] the 4CV probably deserves more attention than it has been receiving. Evaluation of the beating 4CV should assess situs, size, symmetry, structure, and squeeze.

SITUS

The heart should be located within the left thorax, with the apex directed approximately 45 degrees to the left. Hearts on the right (dextrocardia), in the middle (mesocardia), or with the apex directed toward the left (left axis deviation)[72] have all been associated with CHD. Moreover, should the space around the heart be filled with fluid, either circumferentially or with a depth of greater than 2 mm, further evaluation may be indicated.[71]

SIZE

The heart should occupy no more than approximately one third of the cross-sectional area of the thorax.[73] Alternatively, the circumference of the fetal heart should be no more than approximately half the transverse circumference of the thorax. However, no quantitative threshold outperforms an experienced eye. An enlarged fetal heart, by

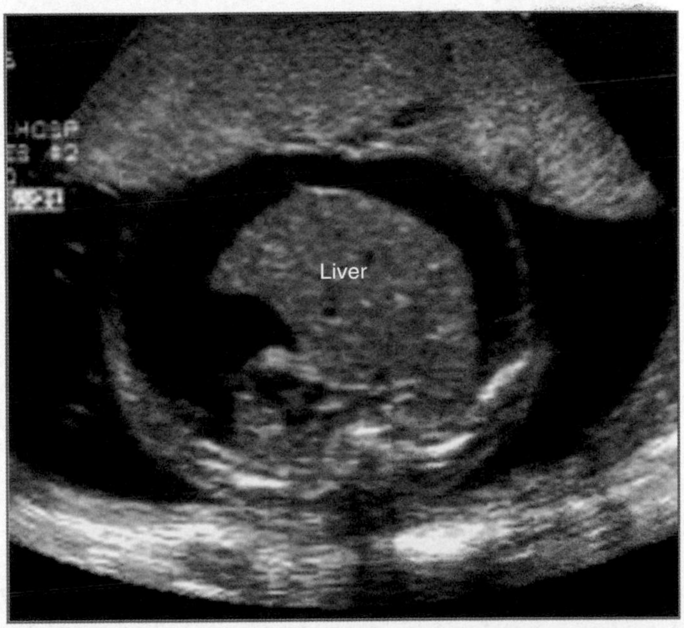

FIGURE 19-1 Fetal ultrasonographic image of severe ascites.

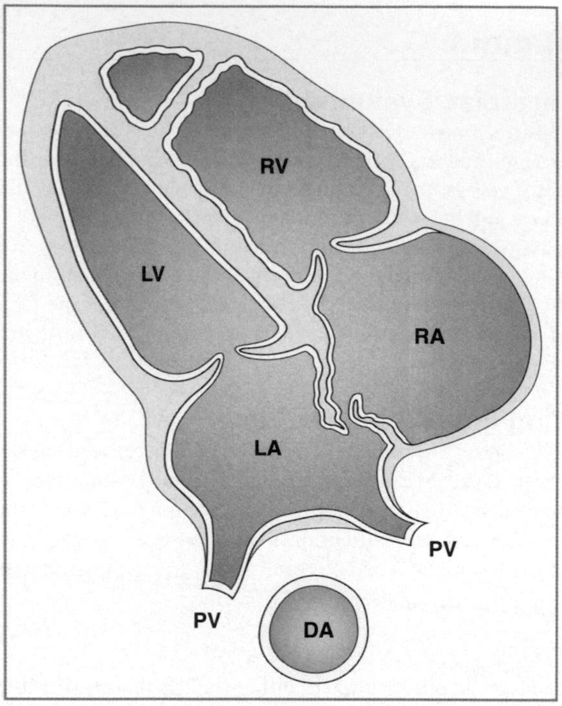

FIGURE 19-2 Schematic diagram of fetal four-chamber view. The right side of the heart appears slightly larger than the left side. The pulmonary veins (PV) enter the left atrium. The flap of the foramen ovale resides within the left atrium. The tricuspid valve inserts onto the ventricular septum slightly apical to the mitral valve insertion. The moderator band characterizes the right ventricular apex. Both ventricles contribute to the cardiac apex. DA, descending aorta; LA, left atrium; LV, left ventricle; RA, right atrium; RV, right ventricle. (Diagram courtesy of Irving R. Tessler, M.D.)

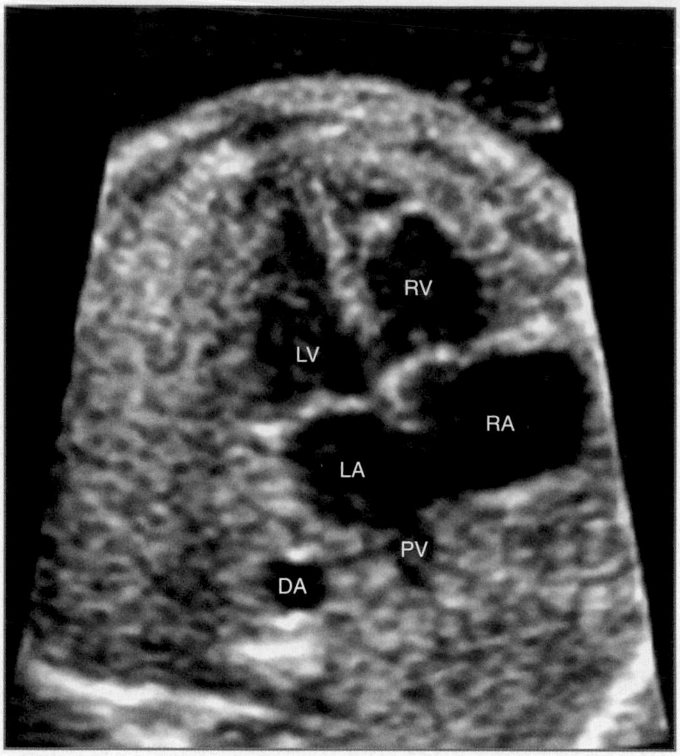

FIGURE 19-3 Fetal echocardiographic image of four-chamber view. Compare with Figure 19-2. The right side of the heart appears slightly larger than the left. A right-sided pulmonary vein (PV) drains into the left atrium (LA). The tricuspid valve inserts onto the ventricular septum slightly more apically than does the mitral valve. The moderator band characterizes the right ventricular apex. Both ventricles contribute to the cardiac apex. DA, descending aorta; LV, left ventricle; RA, right atrium; RV, right ventricle.

any means of measurement, should be considered a strong indicator of CHD and should prompt a more detailed evaluation.

SYMMETRY

The right and left sides of the fetal heart should appear generally symmetrical, with the right side slightly larger. During the third trimester, this right-sided predominance may become more pronounced.[74] If the left side of the heart appears larger than the right, or if the right side appears substantially larger than the left, further evaluation may be prudent.

Frequently, there is a question as to whether the right side is enlarged or the left side is small. Commonly, it may be a little of both, with fetal cardiac output simply redistributing. In other cases, however, the pathology is truly one-sided. The more important questions to consider may be (1) why is there an abnormal ratio between the right and left sides of the heart, and (2) what is the primary lesion?

STRUCTURE

Even for the purposes of screening for CHD, several aspects of the structure of the 4CV should be evaluated. First, the flap of the foramen ovale should be visualized deviated into the left atrium. This flap may not be well visualized, but certainly a flap that is deviated toward the right atrium should raise the concern for right-sided volume or pressure overload and prompt further evaluation. Second, the lowest portion of the atrial septum, just above the insertion point of the mitral valve, should always be visualized. Third, the septal leaflet of the tricuspid valve should attach to the ventricular septum slightly more toward the apex than the septal leaflet of the mitral valve does. In practice, this normal offset may be subtle, difficult to appreciate, and honestly not critical to note for the purposes of screening for CHD.

Fourth, the mitral and tricuspid valves should be thin and delicate, with the tricuspid valve slightly larger than the mitral valve, and the valves should open symmetrically during diastole. Fifth, the left ventricle (aligned with the left atrium) should be smooth walled and should extend to the apex. The right ventricle should appear more heavily trabeculated and should extend toward the cardiac apex along with the left ventricle. Finally, the ventricular septum should appear intact with 2D imaging.

SQUEEZE

The 4CV, even for the purposes of screening for CHD, should be evaluated with the heart beating. The heart rate should range roughly between 120 and 160 beats/min, with no pauses and no skipped or extra beats, other than transient bradycardia during deep transducer pressure. The mitral and tricuspid valves should open and close symmetrically, and both ventricles should squeeze well. Abnormalities of rhythm, valvar function, or myocardial motion may reflect important forms of fetal heart disease and may be overlooked with evaluation of only still-frame images.[37]

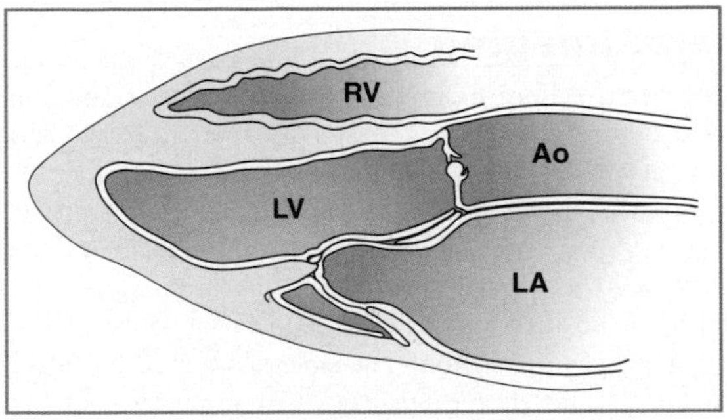

FIGURE 19-4 **Schematic diagram of fetal left ventricular long-axis view.** Note that it is preferable to obtain the image perpendicular to left ventricular outflow tract. Ao, aorta; LA, left atrium; LV, left ventricle; RV, right ventricle. (Diagram courtesy of Irving R. Tessler, M.D.)

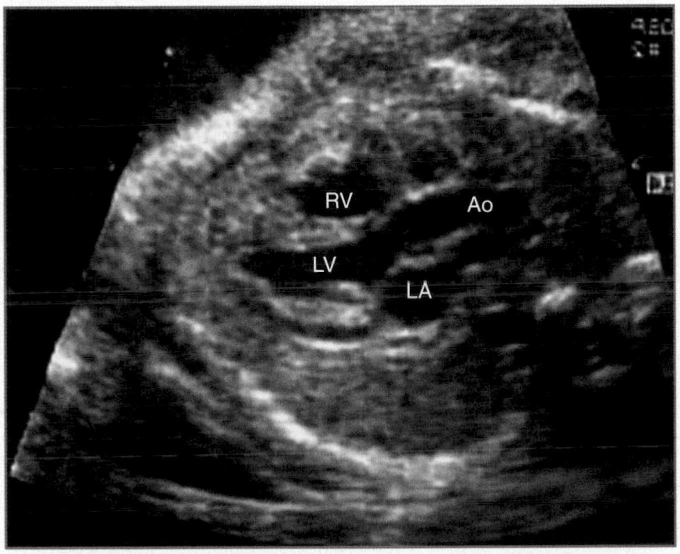

FIGURE 19-5 **Fetal echocardiographic image of left ventricular long-axis view.** Compare with Figure 19-4. Ao, aorta; LA, left atrium; LV, left ventricle; RV, right ventricle.

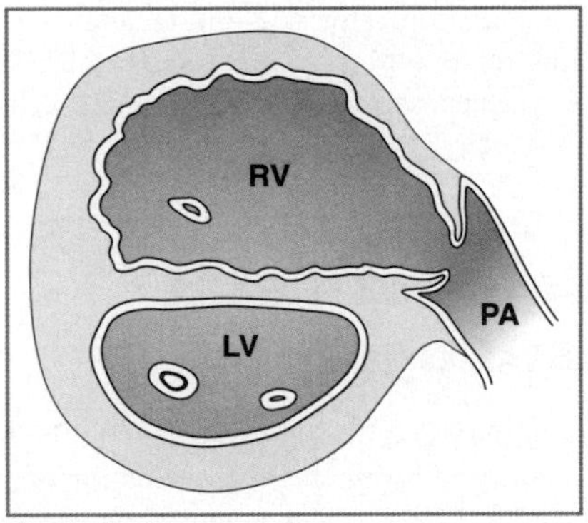

FIGURE 19-6 **Schematic diagram of right ventricular outflow tract crossing view.** LV, left ventricle; PA, main pulmonary artery; RV, right ventricle. (Diagram courtesy of Irving R. Tessler, M.D.)

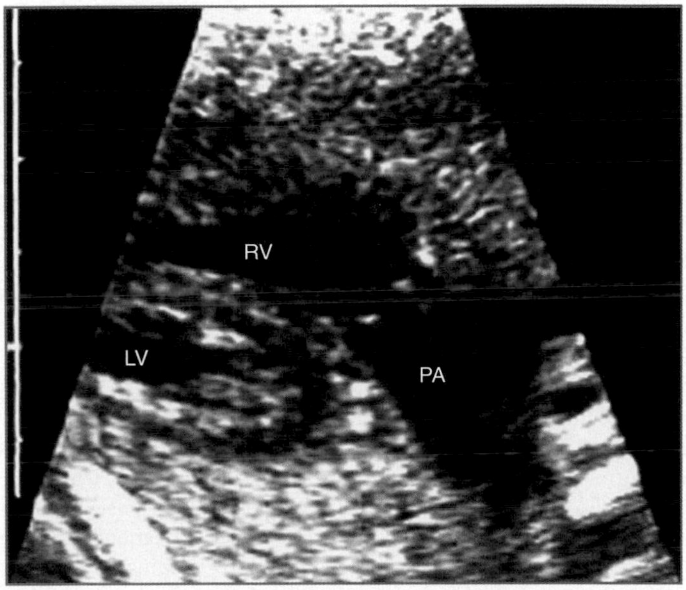

FIGURE 19-7 **Fetal echocardiographic image of right ventricular outflow tract crossing view.** Note that the pulmonary artery aims to the left of the spine. Compare with Figure 19-6. LV, left ventricle; PA, main pulmonary artery; RV, right ventricle.

Outflow Tracts

Ideally, prenatal screening for CHD should include visualization of both outflow tracts. In practice, appropriate evaluation of the outflow tracts may be more challenging than visualization of the 4CV. Nevertheless, because of the ability of the outflow tract views to detect major forms of CHD not visualized with the 4CV, a serious attempt should be made to evaluate the LVOT at the very least, and evaluation of both outflow tracts is becoming the standard of care.[2,48,49]

Slight angulation of the transducer cephalad from the 4CV should demonstrate the aortic valve and ascending aorta arising from the left ventricle (Figs. 19-4 and 19-5). The aortic valve should appear thin and delicate. The ventricular septum should be noted to extend, uninterrupted, from the cardiac apex all the way to the lateral aspect of the ascending aorta. The ascending aorta, or aortic root, should point toward the right of the spine. The left ventricular long-axis view should be able to detect most forms of CHD involving the outflow tracts.[56] However, with just slight further cephalic angulation of the transducer, the right ventricular outflow tract, or RVOT (pulmonary valve and pulmonary artery), can be visualized arising from the right ventricle and crossing the aortic root (Figs. 19-6 and 19-7). The pulmonary valve should be thin and delicate, and the pulmonary valve and main pulmonary artery should be slightly larger than the aortic valve and aortic root. The main pulmonary artery should point to the left of the spine.

Prenatal Screening Using Three-Dimensional Imaging

Although the current standard for screening the low-risk pregnancy for CHD uses 2D imaging, 3D imaging may ultimately facilitate the prenatal detection of CHD by allowing virtual[60] or automated[63,75] evaluation of the entire fetal heart after a simple, short acquisition. When desired, volume data sets may be transmitted electronically to experts at remote locations, who can perform a virtual examination as if actually scanning the patient themselves.[76] Ultimately, 3D fetal cardiac imaging may make acquisition of fetal cardiac data sets less dependent on time and operator skill and facilitate evaluation of the 4CV and outflow tracts offline.[60,77] 3D fetal cardiac imaging is discussed further in the next section, which covers fetal echocardiography in high-risk pregnancies.

Technique of Fetal Echocardiography

Detailed fetal echocardiography in the pregnancy at high risk for CHD provides an in-depth and comprehensive evaluation of fetal cardiovascular structure and function.[78] In experienced hands, and particularly when performed beyond 18 weeks' gestation, fetal echocardiography has been shown to have high degree sensitivity for almost all forms of fetal heart disease.[19,79,80] First-trimester fetal echocardiography, performed between 10 and 14 weeks' gestation either transvaginally or transabdominally, does not have the same degree of sensitivity for CHD as second-trimester imaging, in part because many forms of CHD evolve significantly between the late first trimester and term (e.g., aortic and pulmonary valvar stenosis, ventricular hypoplasia, valvar regurgitation, arrhythmias, cardiac tumors, restriction of the ductus arteriosus or foramen ovale).[16,81,82] Although first-trimester fetal echocardiography undoubtedly will have an increasing clinical role as the technique's resolution improves,[15,67-70,83] it is not discussed here in any further detail. Instead, this section reviews the technique of fetal echocardiography as performed transabdominally beyond 16 to 18 weeks' gestation. Solely to optimize image quality, fetal echocardiography optimally should be performed between 22 and 28 weeks' gestation. However, because earlier diagnosis may be desired for various management and emerging therapeutic options, fetal echocardiography should be performed generally between 18 and 22 weeks' gestation.

Formal fetal echocardiography involves evaluation of the fetal heart and cardiovascular system using several modalities: 2D imaging, color flow imaging, spectral/continuous wave Doppler evaluation, quantitative assessment of ventricular function, and 3D imaging. In practice, the fetal heart and cardiovascular system is probably best evaluated in an anatomically systematic fashion, using various modalities in combination for each anatomic component of the evaluation. However, the order in which individual components of the evaluation are performed may vary with case-specific clinical and imaging considerations.

Various quantitative measurements[8,9,84-94] may be performed if an abnormality is suspected, if doubt remains regarding normalcy, or if measurements for a database are desired. Spectral Doppler echocardiography should routinely be used to assess flow across vessels or valves with suspected pathology.[84,86,91-94] Any structure that appears small or large should be measured several times, with the best-guess measurement plotted on nomograms according to gestational age.[95-100] Color flow imaging, which is exquisitely sensitive to valvar regurgitation, flow through small VSDs, and pulmonary/systemic venous returns, should be used routinely to demonstrate normalcy and to assess pathology. More sophisticated tissue Doppler studies[89,101,102] or other quantitative means of evaluation of ventricular diastolic[91-94] or combined diastolic/systolic[87,88] function may be used in special circumstances. This section describes a clinical approach to the formal fetal echocardiographic evaluation, with an emphasis on the importance of routine 2D and color flow imaging. Readers should note that this approach might be somewhat less rigorous and comprehensive than that described in previously published guidelines,[78] but it may also be more clinically practical in many settings.

General Imaging

The formal fetal echocardiogram begins with a determination of the number of fetuses, their levels of activity, their respective positions, and their gestational ages. The number of fetuses and their respective positions matter because the lie, late in the third trimester, may affect delivery plans. With multiple-gestation pregnancies, each fetus should undergo its own detailed fetal echocardiogram, and noting the fetal lie or position helps to distinguish one fetus from another. Gestational age determination (1) enables assessment of fetal growth, (2) may affect counseling or management strategies, and (3) allows assessment of cardiac structures that vary in appearance with gestational age.

Umbilical Cord

Next comes evaluation of the umbilical cord (Fig. 19-8). Spectral Doppler evaluation of the umbilical artery provides information on placental resistance, which may affect fetal cardiovascular function and reflect overall fetal well-being. In cases of suspected placental pathology, calculation of a pulsatility index enables a quantitative assessment of placental resistance. Doppler evaluation of the umbilical vein in free-floating cord is most useful in cases of suspected fetal heart failure.[86] Normally, the umbilical venous waveform pulsates in response to fetal breathing, but it should not vary with the fetal cardiac cycle. Pulsatile flow in the free-floating umbilical cord, reflecting fetal cardiac contractions, suggests markedly elevated fetal right atrial pressure and represents a manifestation of significant CHF.[103]

Hydrops

Initial evaluation of the fetus itself should assess for the presence of fluid accumulation suggestive of CHF. Normally, no more than a trivial (loculated and <2 mm) pericardial effusion should be present.[71] Greater accumulation of pericardial fluid (circumferential or >2 mm) or the presence of any pleural fluid or ascites (see Fig. 19-1) should be considered abnormal, with a differential diagnosis including CHF, myopericarditis, viral infection, anemia, and aneuploidy.

Visceroatrial Situs

Following the determination of fetal number, position, gestational age, umbilical waveforms, and presence or absence of hydrops, attention should be directed toward the structure and function of the fetal cardiovascular system itself. This assessment should begin with an

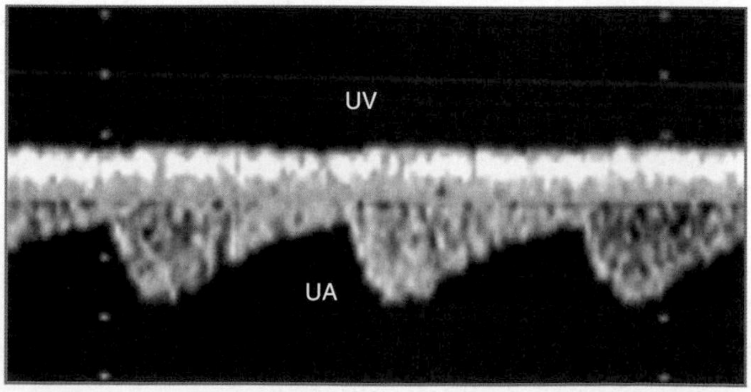

FIGURE 19-8 Spectral Doppler display of flow within free-floating umbilical cord. UA, umbilical artery; UV, umbilical vein.

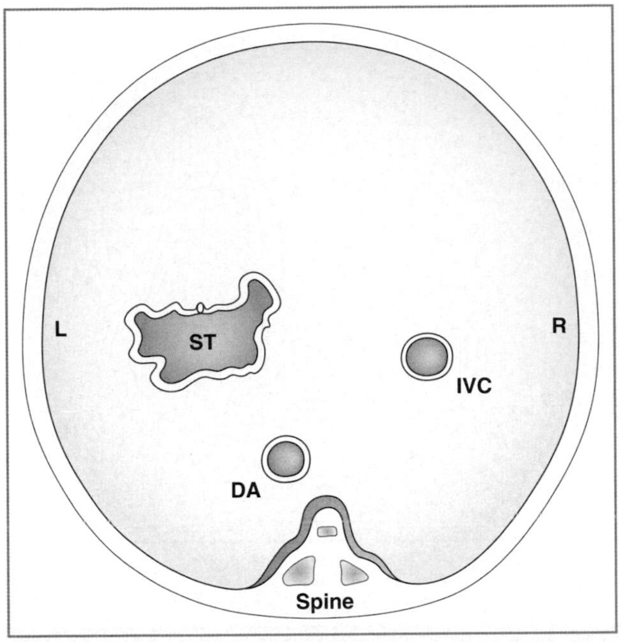

FIGURE 19-9 Schematic diagram of abdominal situs view. DA, descending aorta; IVC, inferior vena cava; L, fetal left; R, fetal right; ST, stomach. (Diagram courtesy of Irving R. Tessler, M.D.)

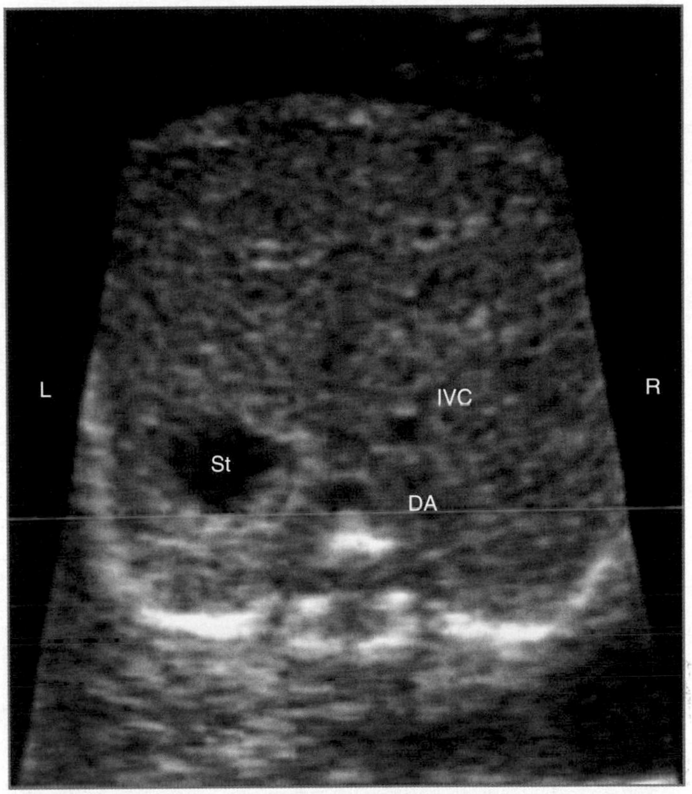

FIGURE 19-10 Fetal echocardiographic image of abdominal situs view. Compare with Figure 19-9. DA, descending aorta; IVC, inferior vena cava; L, fetal left; R, fetal right; ST, stomach.

abdominal assessment of visceral situs (Figs. 19-9 and 19-10). Transverse imaging of the abdomen should demonstrate the descending aorta, in cross section, just anterior and slightly leftward of the spine. The stomach should be anterior and leftward, and the inferior vena cava (IVC) and liver should both be anterior and rightward. A prominent vein (usually the azygos) should not be visualized posterior to the descending aorta. Angulation of the probe from transverse to sagittal imaging should demonstrate the IVC draining into the right atrium. Finally, transverse imaging of the thorax should demonstrate the heart on the left, with the apex directed anteriorly and leftward. Abnormalities of any of these features should prompt further evaluation for situs abnormalities (asplenia or polysplenia) or associated CHD or both.

Beating Four-Chamber View

Central to screening for CHD, the 4CV also represents a critically important aspect of the formal fetal echocardiogram.[8,9,104] As with screening, detailed fetal echocardiography begins by demonstrating the fetal heart to be in the left thorax with the apex directed approximately 45 degrees to the left (see Figs. 19-2 and 19-3). The heart should fill less than one third of the area of the thorax,[73] and the heart's circumference should be less than half the thoracic circumference. These quantitative measurements, like most such measurements in fetal echocardiography, should be considered optional unless an abnormality is suspected, normalcy is in doubt, or measurements are desired for incorporation into a database.

The fetal heart's right-sided structures should be equal to or, more commonly, slightly larger than their respective left-sided structures.[74] Mild right heart disproportion appears to occur in some cases of trisomy 21, even in the absence of structural disease.[105] With advancing gestation, the right side of the heart becomes progressively more dominant, making the diagnosis of right heart disproportion much more common during the third trimester than during the second.[74] For this reason, false-positive diagnoses of coarctation of the aorta occur most frequently late in gestation.

Venous Drainage

Although evaluation of systemic and pulmonary venous drainage may be accomplished with 2D imaging alone, color flow imaging helps to confirm the anatomy and to demonstrate areas of obstruction,[106] and spectral Doppler may help to assess cardiovascular status still further.[86,90,91,103] With slight inferior angulation or tilting of the transducer from the 4CV, the coronary sinus should be seen coursing from left to right just above the mitral groove (Fig. 19-11). At the level of the 4CV, the coronary sinus sometimes may be seen in cross section laterally, adjacent to the left atrial free wall just above the mitral annulus. However, enlargement of the coronary sinus should prompt evaluation for either a left-sided superior vena cava (LSVC)[107,108] or drainage of some or all pulmonary veins directly into the coronary sinus. All four pulmonary veins may be seen, but such visualization can be time-consuming and challenging; therefore, visualization by color flow Doppler of even one or two pulmonary veins (Figs. 19-12 and 19-13; see Fig. 19-3) draining normally to the left atrium is generally sufficient[1,85] in the absence of suspected disease. The presence of a ridge of tissue (normal pericardial reflection, or infolding of tissue between the left atrial appendage and left pulmonary vein) extending a short distance medially from the posterior/lateral aspect of the left atrium helps to rule out total anomalous pulmonary venous return. Color flow imaging should be performed to confirm normal, unobstructed pulmonary venous return to the left atrium. Spectral Doppler analysis may be performed if color Doppler suggests pathol-

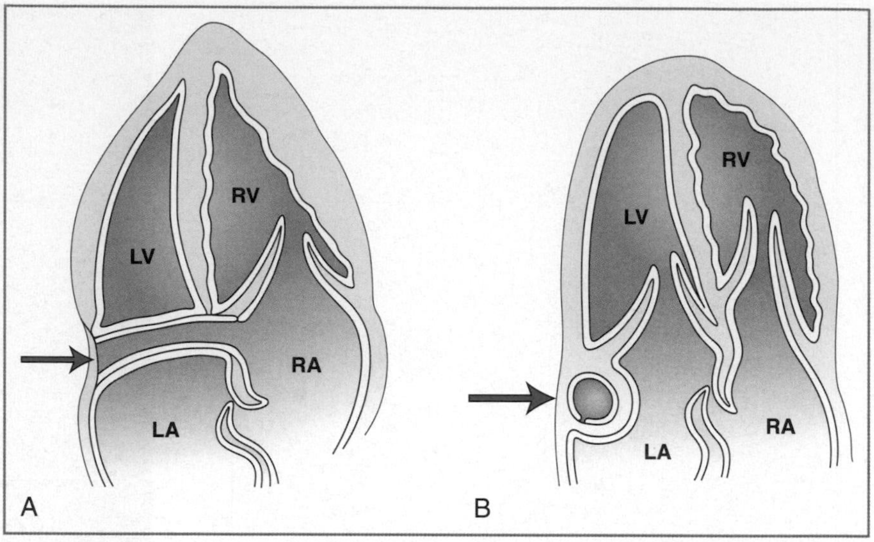

FIGURE 19-11 Schematic diagrams of coronary sinus views. **A,** Longitudinal coronary sinus view obtained with slight inferior angulation from the four-chamber view. The coronary sinus *(arrow)* drains along the mitral annulus before opening into the right atrium and can be seen in normal fetuses. **B,** Four-chamber view demonstrating dilated coronary sinus in cross section *(arrow)* at the lateral aspect of the mitral annulus. A normal coronary sinus is usually small or not seen at all with this perspective. LA, left atrium; LV, left ventricle; RA, right atrium; RV, right ventricle. (Diagrams courtesy of Irving R. Tessler, M.D.)

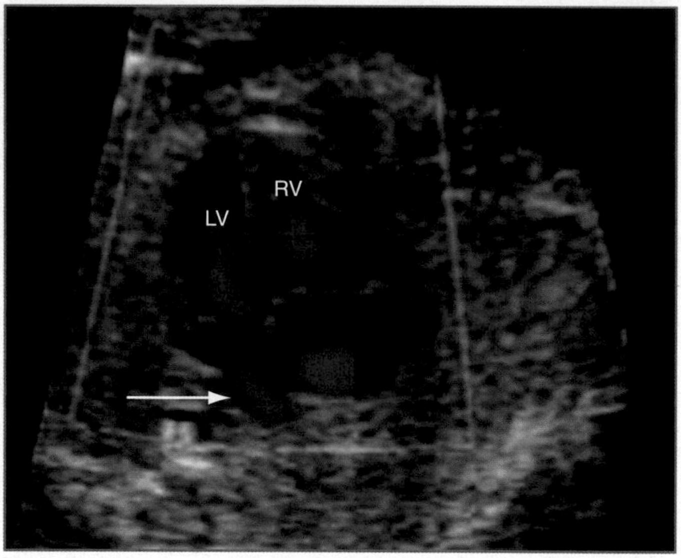

FIGURE 19-12 Fetal echocardiographic image of four-chamber view. Color flow imaging demonstrates a right-sided pulmonary vein *(arrow)* draining into the left atrium. LV, left ventricle; RV, right ventricle.

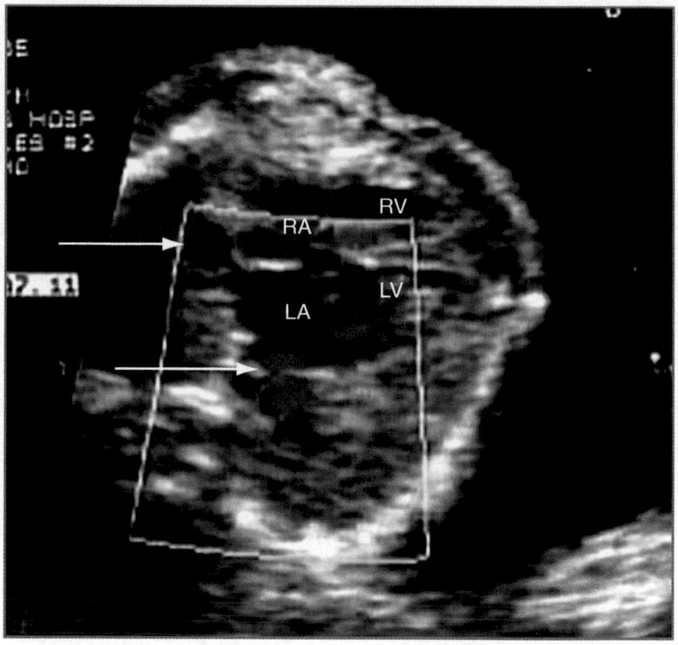

FIGURE 19-13 Fetal echocardiographic image of four-chamber view. Color flow imaging demonstrates right and left pulmonary veins *(arrows)* draining into the left atrium. LA, left atrium; LV, left ventricle; RA, right atrium; RV, right ventricle.

ogy.[91] Structural abnormalities of venous return raise the possibility of heterotaxy.[106,109,110]

Atrial Septum

Because the foramen ovale normally shunts oxygenated blood from the right atrium to the left atrium, the flap of the foramen ovale should be deviated toward the left atrium. Although this flap typically moves back and forth during the cardiac cycle, the dominant position should be leftward (see Fig. 19-2). The flap itself should occupy a central position within the atrial septum, and it should extend increasingly further into the left atrium with advancing gestational age. Both the superior and inferior aspects of the atrial septum should appear intact, although the superior rim may not always be seen with routine screening. Occasionally, particularly when dilated, the coronary sinus (seen longitudinally) may generate the appearance of an absent inferior portion of the atrial septum (Fig. 19-14).[107] For this reason, if this portion of the atrial septum appears deficient, care must be taken to confirm that the image plane has not simply been directed too far posteriorly/inferiorly from the 4CV.

Atrioventricular Valves

The atrioventricular valve morphology and function should be evaluated, along with the rest of the heart, during real-time motion. Both valves may be evaluated in their entirety from the 4CV (see Figs. 19-2 and 19-3), although visualization from other views may be useful, particularly if abnormalities are present or suspected. The tricuspid valve annulus should be the same size or slightly larger than the mitral

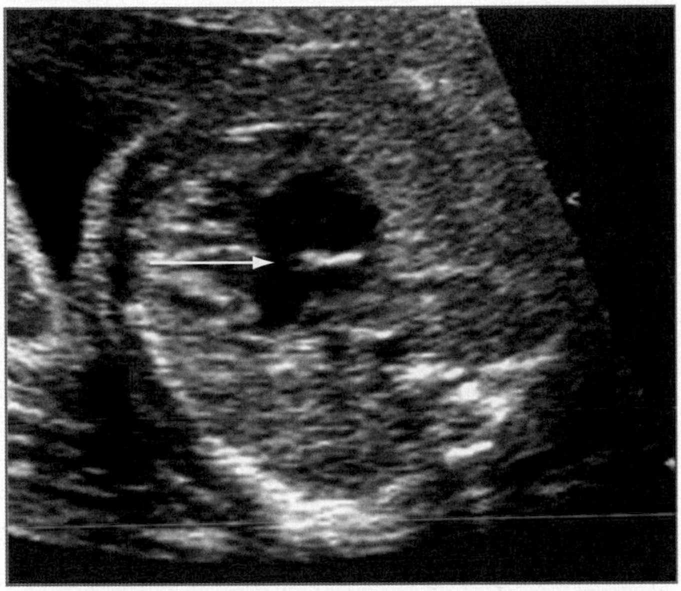

FIGURE 19-14 Fetal echocardiographic image of dilated coronary sinus, obtained with slight inferior angulation from the four chamber view. The dilated coronary sinus orifice *(arrow)* mimics ostium primum atrial septal defect.

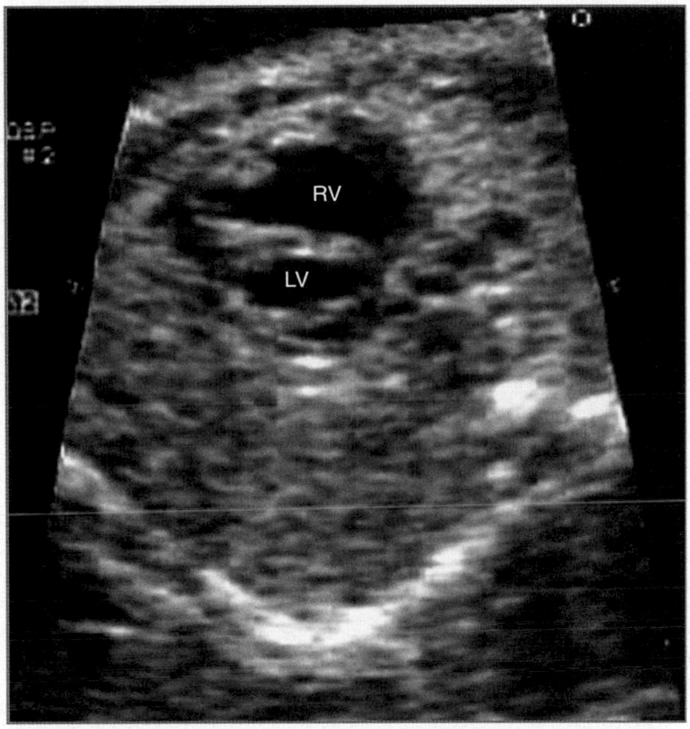

FIGURE 19-15 Fetal echocardiographic image of apical short-axis view. Right ventricular disproportion is demonstrated. LV, left ventricle; RV, right ventricle.

annulus. The leaflets should appear thin and delicate, with unrestricted diastolic excursion into their respective ventricles. A subtle abnormality of either valve early in the second trimester may progress to a severe abnormality, or even to hypoplastic right or left heart syndrome, at term. The septal leaflet of the tricuspid valve should insert slightly more apically onto the ventricular septum than the septal leaflet of the mitral valve does. The papillary muscles of the tricuspid valve should have attachments to the ventricular septum and right ventricular free wall. In contrast, the papillary muscles of the mitral valve should have no attachments to the ventricular septum. Evaluation of the atrioventricular valves should always include color flow imaging to assess for diastolic turbulence or valvar regurgitation. A trace amount of early systolic tricuspid regurgitation probably is normal,[111] although many investigators consider any tricuspid regurgitation prenatally to be abnormal.[112] Prenatal valvar regurgitation of any other valve is generally considered abnormal. Fetuses with trisomy appear to have an increased incidence of tricuspid regurgitation, even in the presence of a structurally normal heart.[105] Measurement of tricuspid and mitral valve annulus size,[95-97,99,100] as well as spectral Doppler evaluation of inflow patterns,[92-94] should be performed if an abnormality is suspected, if normalcy cannot be confirmed, or if additions to a database are desired.

Ventricles

The structure and function of both ventricles should be evaluated in detail. The 4CV provides the single best perspective to evaluate ventricular structure (see Figs. 19-2 and 19-3). Both ventricles should extend to the cardiac apex, and both should squeeze symmetrically during systole. The left ventricle should be smooth walled, aligned with the mitral valve, and located leftward and posterior to the right ventricle. The right ventricle should be more heavily trabeculated, should have a moderator band of tissue crossing the ventricle near the apex, should be aligned with the tricuspid valve, and should be located rightward and anterior to the left ventricle. The right ventricle should be equal in size or, more commonly, slightly larger than the left ventricle, with right heart predominance increasing normally with advancing gestational age. Mild right heart disproportion (Fig. 19-15) has been associated with trisomy 21.[105] Quantitative assessment of ventricular systolic and diastolic function[86-89,92-94,102,113] may be performed if an abnormality is suspected, if normalcy cannot be confirmed, or if additions to a database are desired. However, close attention to ventricular systolic function should always be made qualitatively and from multiple views, including the 4CV and basal short-axis view (obtained from a sagittal fetal orientation). Ventricular dysfunction may be isolated and primary,[114] or it may be associated with structural heart disease.

The presence of small, circumscribed echogenic densities, foci, or reflectors within the chordal apparatus of the mitral valve (or, less commonly, tricuspid valve) should probably be considered, from a cardiovascular standpoint, as benign variants of normal.[115-117] If doubt exists regarding the diagnosis, further evaluation should be performed to rule out CHD. Although the data remain somewhat controversial, such echogenic foci do appear to be more prevalent among fetuses with aneuploidy than among those with normal chromosomes.[116-119]

Ventricular Septum

The ventricular septum should be evaluated for thickness, motion, and the presence of a VSD. The ventricular septum should be roughly the same thickness as the left ventricular posterior free wall, and it should contract symmetrically with the left ventricular free wall. Ventricular septal thickness may be evaluated from the 4CV and the basal short-axis view. In cases of suspected septal hypertrophy, the septal thickness should be measured, typically during both diastole and systole. The entirety of the ventricular septum then needs to be evaluated for VSDs. 2D imaging should be performed from multiple views and with multiple sweeps, seeking to identify any defect in any portion of the ven-

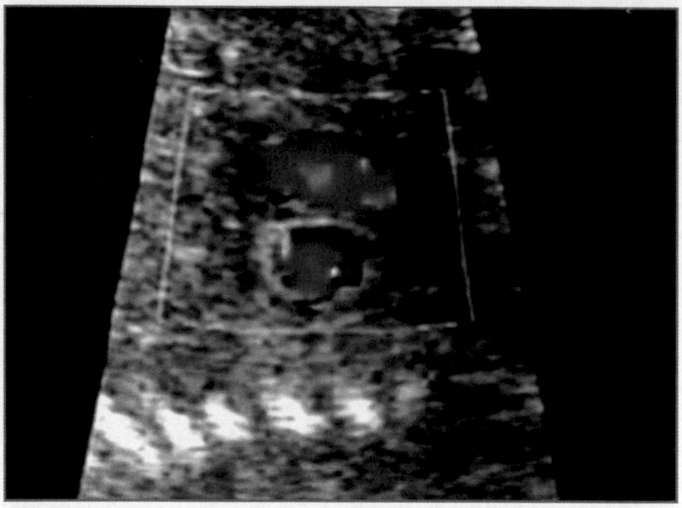

FIGURE 19-16 Fetal echocardiographic image of apical short-axis view. Color flow imaging demonstrates intact muscular ventricular septum.

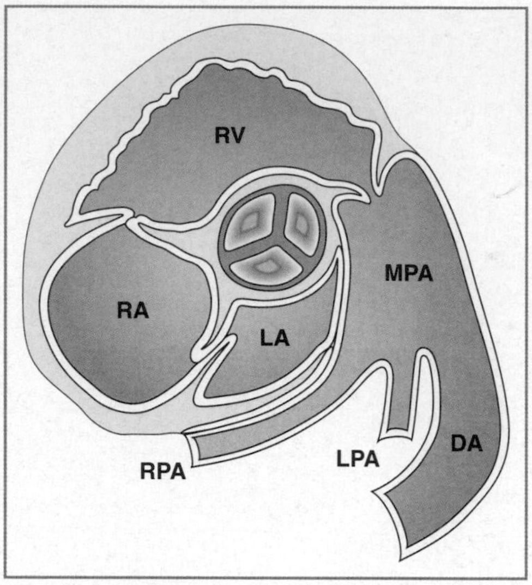

FIGURE 19-17 Schematic diagram of fetal basal short-axis/ductal arch view. The left pulmonary artery and ductus arteriosus commonly appear superimposed in this view. DA, ductus arteriosus; LA, left atrium; LPA, left pulmonary artery; MPA, main pulmonary artery; RA, right atrium; RPA, right pulmonary artery; RV, right ventricle. (Diagram courtesy of Irving R. Tessler, M.D.)

tricular septum. To avoid false-positive "drop out" in the inlet and membranous portions of the ventricular septum, 2D imaging should be performed as perpendicular as possible to the ventricular septum and with the transducer angled slowly from the 4CV into the left ventricular long-axis view (see Figs. 19-4 and 19-5). Color flow imaging should also always be performed in search of VSDs (Fig. 19-16), using the same perpendicular orientations and sweeps; some defects may not be visualized with 2D imaging alone.

Outflow Tracts in Motion

Semilunar Valves

The semilunar (aortic and pulmonary) valves should be evaluated with the same attention to anatomy and function that is given to the evaluation of the atrioventricular valves. Consistent with the right-sided predominance seen at the levels of the atrium, atrioventricular valve, and ventricle, the pulmonary valve annulus should be equal in size or, more commonly, slightly larger than the aortic valve annulus. The aortic valve may be best visualized with a left ventricular long-axis view (see Fig. 19-5), which is obtained with slight anterior/superior angulation from the 4CV. In addition, ideally, the probe may be rotated slightly from a transverse cut toward a partially sagittal plane. The aortic valve may be evaluated further with a basal short-axis view, which is obtained from a sagittal fetal orientation. The pulmonary valve (RVOT crossing view) (see Fig. 19-7) may be evaluated with slight anterior/superior angulation from the left ventricular long-axis view. In addition, the pulmonary valve may be evaluated further with a basal short-axis view. The aortic valve should arise from the anterior aspect of the left ventricle, and the pulmonary valve from the anterior aspect of the right ventricle. Both aortic and pulmonary valves should be thin and delicate, with unrestricted excursion during systole, resulting in the valve's practically disappearing from view when fully open (see Fig. 19-5). During diastole, the aortic and pulmonary valves should appear as central points or symmetrical, thin plates. The aortic valve, during diastole, should appear on the left ventricular long-axis view as a thin, central plate, parallel to the axis of the aortic root. The pulmonary valve during diastole, in contrast, should appear on the basal short-axis view also as a thin plate but perpendicular to the axis of the main pulmonary artery. A subtle abnormality of either valve during the early second trimester may progress to a severe valve abnormality, or even to hypoplastic left or right heart syndrome, at term. Measurement of aortic or pulmonary valve annulus size, or evaluation of the systolic Doppler flow profile, or both, should be performed if an abnormality is suspected, if normalcy cannot be confirmed, or if additions to a database are desired. However, evaluation of aortic and pulmonary valves should always include color flow imaging to assess for aortic or pulmonary regurgitation (always abnormal) or systolic turbulence suggestive of increased flow volume or anatomic obstruction.

Great Arteries and Ductal and Aortic Arches

The ascending aorta (aortic root) and main pulmonary artery should arise from the left and right ventricles, respectively, and then cross at an angle of roughly 45 to 90 degrees. Demonstration of great artery crossing represents an important finding on the normal fetal echocardiogram. This crossing can be seen either with transverse imaging (slight anterior/superior angulation from the 4CV to left ventricular long-axis view to RVOT crossing view) or with sagittal imaging (slight leftward angulation from sagittal aortic arch view to ductal arch view). In general, the aortic root should point to the right of the spine (see Fig. 19-5), and the main pulmonary artery should point to the left of the spine (see Fig. 19-7). As with other right-left ratios in the fetal heart, the main pulmonary artery should be equal in size or, more commonly, slightly larger than the aortic root. The ductal arch and basal short-axis views (Figs. 19-17, 19-18, and 19-19) should demonstrate the trifurcation of the main pulmonary artery into the right pulmonary artery (which wraps around the aorta in the basal short-axis view), the left pulmonary artery, and the ductus arteriosus (the largest of the three branches).

In cases of suspected pathology, the branch pulmonary arteries should be measured and their Doppler flow profiles obtained. For instance, fetal pulmonary artery diameter may correlate with outcome in cases of congenital diaphragmatic hernia.[120] In cases of suspected ductal constriction (i.e., tricuspid and pulmonary regurgitation across

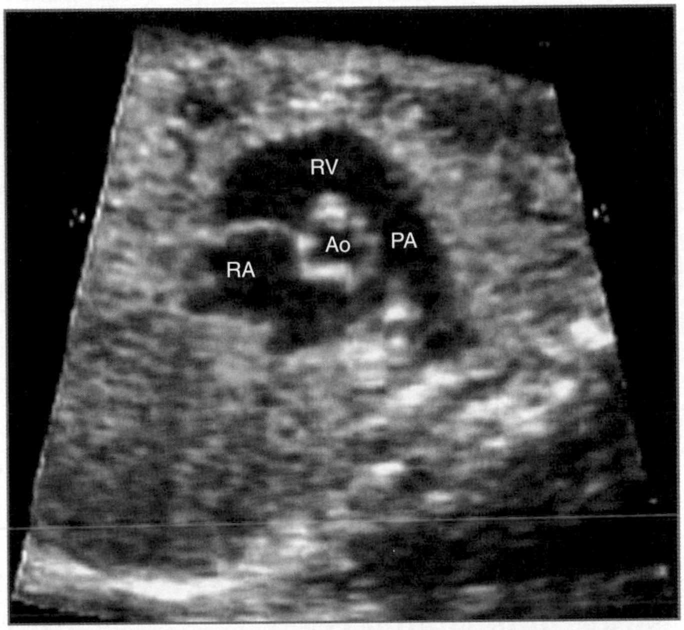

FIGURE 19-18 Fetal echocardiographic image of basal short-axis view during systole. The pulmonary artery bifurcates into the right and left pulmonary arteries. The ductus arteriosus appears superimposed over the left pulmonary artery. The pulmonary valve is open and is closely opposed to the main pulmonary artery. Ao, aorta; PA, main pulmonary artery; RA, right atrium; RV, right ventricle.

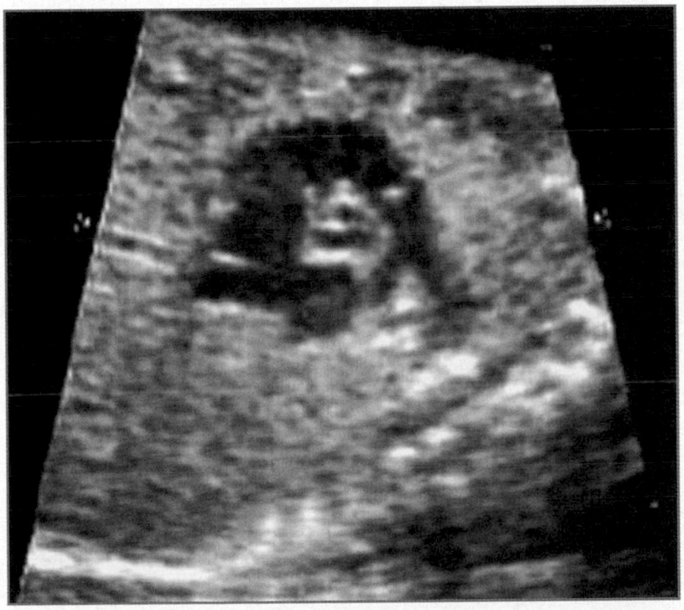

FIGURE 19-19 Fetal echocardiographic image of basal short-axis view during diastole. The aortic and pulmonary valves appear in their closed positions, and the tricuspid valve is open.

normal-appearing valves, or simply fetal exposure to indomethacin[121]), the flow profile of the ductus arteriosus should be obtained parallel to flow on the sagittal ductal arch view. A pulsatility index of less than 1.9 suggests ductal constriction,[121] whereas a pulsatility index greater than 3 suggests increased right ventricular output and left heart obstruction.[122] The sagittal aortic arch view (Figs. 19-20 and 19-21), obtained with rightward angulation from the ductal arch view, dem-

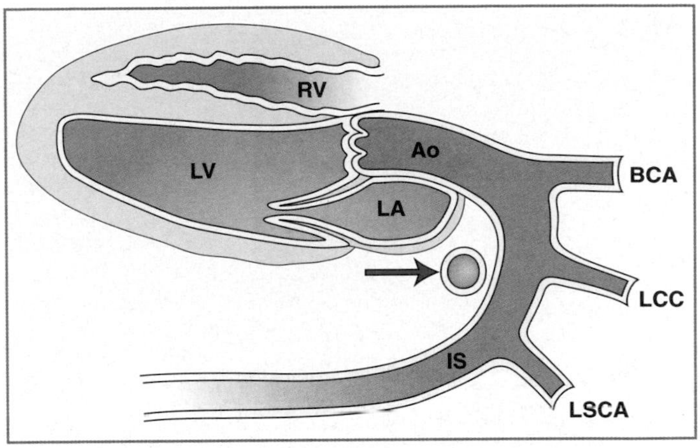

FIGURE 19-20 Schematic diagram of fetal sagittal aortic arch view. The aortic arch crosses over the right pulmonary artery *(arrow).* Ao, aortic arch; BCA, brachiocephalic artery; IS, aortic isthmus; LA, left atrium; LCC, left common carotid artery; LSCA, left subclavian artery; LV, left ventricle; RV, right ventricle. (Diagram courtesy of Irving R. Tessler, M.D.)

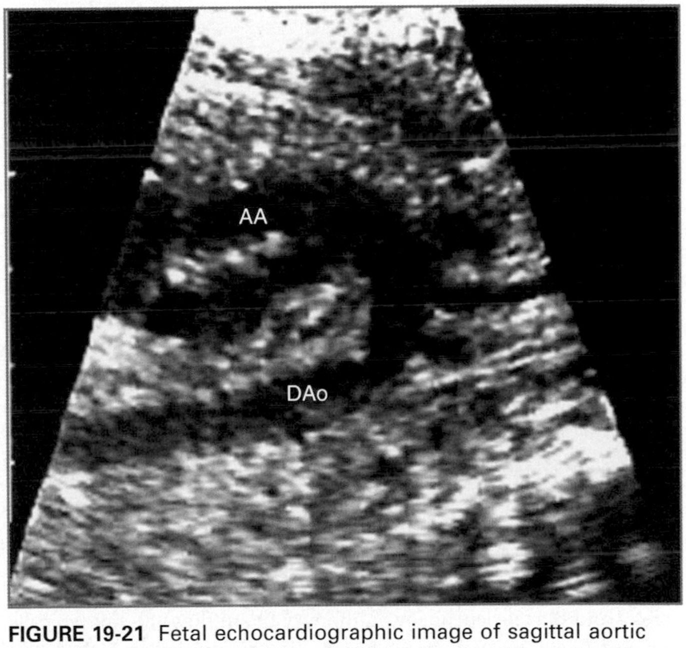

FIGURE 19-21 Fetal echocardiographic image of sagittal aortic arch view. Compare with Figure 19-20. AA, ascending aorta; DAo, descending aorta.

onstrates the aortic arch in its entirety, including aortic root, transverse aortic arch, aortic isthmus, and descending aorta. Color flow imaging should always be performed of the entire aortic (Fig. 19-22) and ductal arches. Measurements of aortic dimensions[95,96,98] should be obtained if an abnormality is suspected, if normalcy cannot be confirmed, or if additions to a database are desired.

Evaluation for Fetal Congestive Heart Failure

Fetal CHF may be related to extracardiac disease (e.g., anemia, cerebral arteriovenous fistula, twin-twin transfusion syndrome) or to fetal

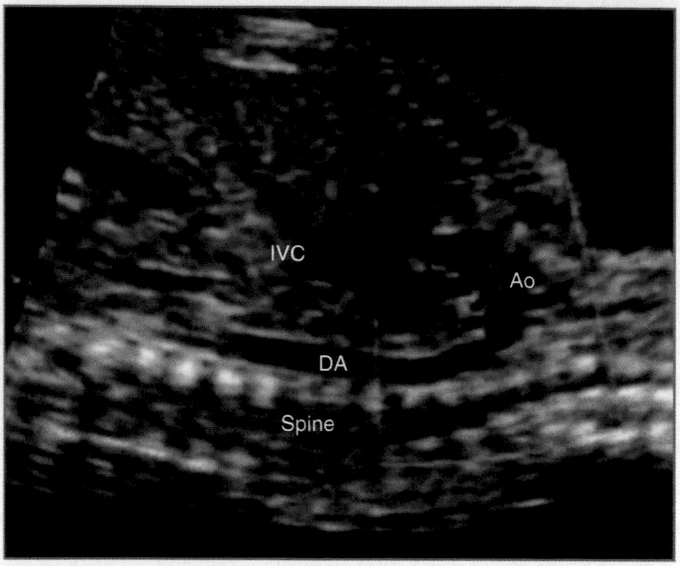

FIGURE 19-22 Fetal echocardiographic image of sagittal aortic arch view. Color flow imaging demonstrates prograde flow into aortic arch (Ao) and descending aorta (DA). IVC, inferior vena cava.

TABLE 19-4 CAUSES OF FETAL CONGESTIVE HEART FAILURE
Anemia
Twin-twin transfusion syndrome
Arteriovenous malformation
Diaphragmatic hernia
Pericardial effusion
Cardiac Causes
Hypertrophic cardiomyopathy
Dilated cardiomyopathy
Sustained bradycardia/tachycardia
Valvar regurgitation
Restrictive foramen ovale
Ductal constriction

heart disease (Table 19-4). Some of the most severe forms of CHD (e.g., hypoplastic left heart syndrome [HLHS], TOF with pulmonary atresia and ductal-dependent pulmonary blood flow) do not typically generate fetal CHF. Rather, fetal heart disease that causes CHF almost invariably includes one or more of the following[103,123,124]: sustained tachycardia or bradycardia (i.e., supraventricular tachycardia [SVT] or complete heart block), myocardial dysfunction (i.e., dilated cardiomyopathy), valvar regurgitation (i.e., Ebstein anomaly of the tricuspid valve or TOF with absent pulmonary valve), or restrictive flow across the foramen ovale or ductus arteriosus.[122] The fetus with absence of a valve (e.g., tricuspid atresia) or absence of a ventricle (e.g., HLHS) generally does better prenatally than one with a poorly functioning valve or ventricle.

Unlike the postnatal diagnosis of CHF, which relies more on clinical signs (tachycardia, tachypnea, hepatomegaly, rales, and peripheral edema) than on radiographic or echocardiographic findings, the prenatal diagnosis of CHF relies exclusively on sonographic findings.[86,103,123,124] The sonographic findings associated with fetal CHF from any cause include (1) dilated, poorly squeezing ventricle with systolic and diastolic dysfunction; (2) cardiomegaly; (3) pericardial

TABLE 19-5 SONOGRAPHIC FINDINGS IN FETAL CONGESTIVE HEART FAILURE
Cardiomegaly
Tricuspid regurgitation
Pericardial effusion
Diminished ventricular systolic function
Increased atrial flow reversal in systemic veins

effusion; (4) tricuspid regurgitation; and (5) increased atrial flow reversal in the systemic veins (Table 19-5). More detailed cardiac and peripheral Doppler evaluation also may be performed.[86,103,124,125] Severe forms of CHF lead to hydrops and cardiac pulsations within the free-floating umbilical vein. The diagnosis of fetal CHF or hydrops should prompt further evaluation for clues to the etiology, as well as serial follow-up studies, given the potential for progression of disease and even fetal demise.

Three-dimensional Fetal Cardiac Imaging

Background

At the current time, 3D fetal cardiac imaging[60-62,64,77,126-149] remains predominantly an investigational tool for academic centers seeking to improve and enhance the prenatal detection and diagnosis of CHD. Because of persistent challenges related to image resolution, substantial learning curves, and expensive equipment, 3D fetal cardiac imaging has not yet become an acceptable alternative to conventional 2D imaging.

That said, compared with 2D fetal cardiac imaging, 3D imaging carries important advantages that promise to revolutionize the clinical approach to fetal cardiac imaging.[60,63,131,140] First, 3D imaging, by acquiring a comprehensive volume dataset within a matter of a few seconds, makes fetal cardiac imaging less operator dependent and less time-consuming to perform. Second, 3D volume datasets may be evaluated interactively offline, enabling virtual examinations of the entire fetal heart, with reconstruction of any plane or sweep, after the initial, short acquisition. Such interactive evaluations may be performed at the bedside, remotely by centers with expertise,[76] or even, potentially, automatically using evolving algorithms designed to automate the process of screening for CHD.[63,75] Third, volume-rendering algorithms display data as "surgeon's-eye views," enabling visualization of the internal architecture and anatomy of the fetal heart (Figs. 19-23 and 19-24) or great arteries from any perspective. Such displays improve comprehension of complex forms of CHD, leading to improved patient counseling and patient selection for fetal interventions. Moreover, evolving technology allows the 3D visualization of color-flow jets within volume-rendered displays or as stand-alone "angiograms."[135,138] Finally, 3D volume datasets enable more accurate quantitative measurements of ventricular size and function,[139,141] which can translate into improved ability to predict the prenatal and postnatal courses of CHD from early in the second trimester (or even earlier).

Technique

Three-dimensional fetal cardiac imaging may be performed with either a reconstructive[61,62,126-130,142-144] or a real-time[60,132,133,136,137,139,145,146] approach. Reconstructive approaches use specialized probes to image

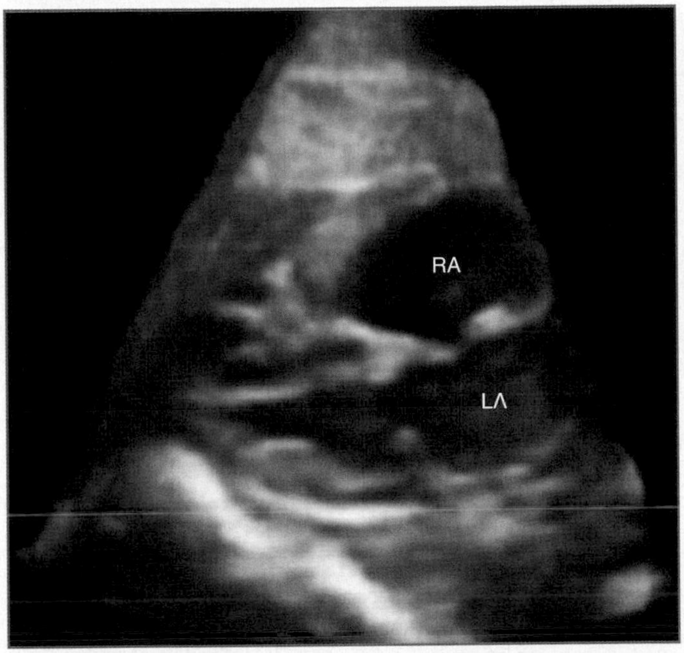

FIGURE 19-23 **Fetal echocardiographic real-time three-dimensional rendered image of normal four-chamber view.** LA, left atrium. RA, right atrium.

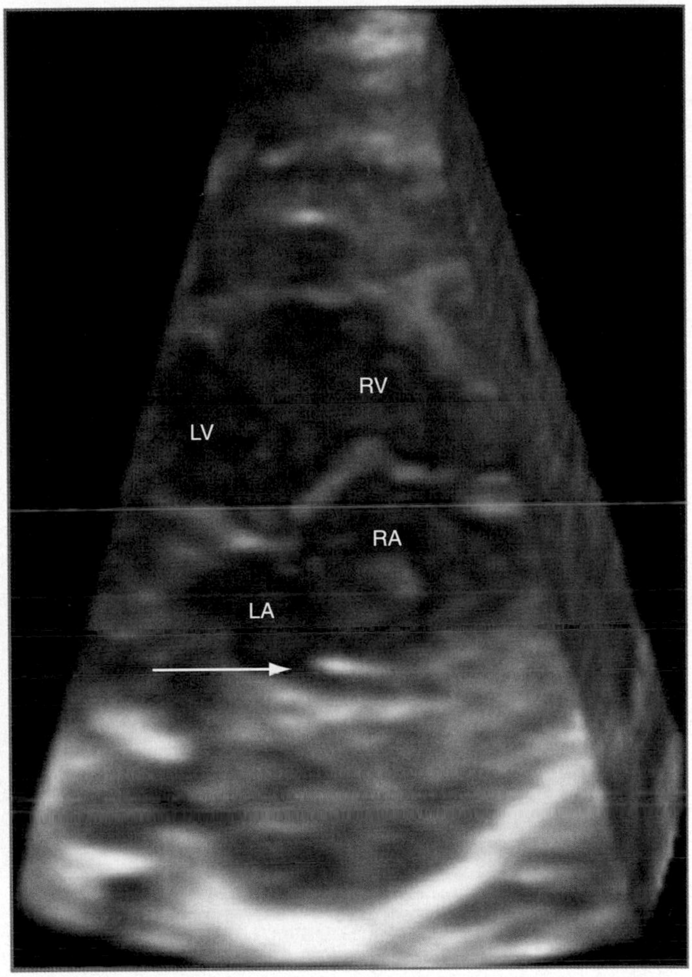

FIGURE 19-24 **Fetal echocardiographic real-time three-dimensional rendered image of mitral atresia with hypoplastic left ventricle.** Arrow points to right-sided pulmonary vein draining to left atrium. LA, left atrium; LV, left ventricle; RA, right atrium; RV, right ventricle.

the fetal heart as an automated sweep, acquiring a series of parallel planar images over 7 to 15 seconds. The images and their spatial coordinates are subsequently reconstructed into a volume dataset or, using gating algorithms to view cardiac motion,[126,129,142,147] into a series of volume datasets for subsequent display and review. Reconstructive approaches have a disadvantage in that they require the fetus and mother to be relatively motionless throughout the acquisition; any fetal or maternal motion distorts the reconstructed volume dataset.

In contrast, real-time approaches use specialized probes to image the fetal heart as a volume, acquiring the entire fetal heart (or portion thereof) virtually instantaneously. The volume data do not require reconstruction, and they do not require gating algorithms (as do reconstructive techniques) to view cardiac motion. Real-time approaches make the most sense for imaging the fetal heart, given their quick acquisition time (2 seconds), relative resistance to artifact derived from random fetal motion, and lack of a need for cardiac gating.[60,132,136,137,145,146] However, real-time approaches are unable to acquire large volumes in real time, and they have relatively poor image resolution compared with reconstructive approaches.

After volume data have been acquired, via either reconstructive or real-time techniques, volume datasets may be reviewed interactively, displaying any plane,[62,128] rendered volume,[60,62,143,144] or sweep of interest and allowing precise quantitative measurements of ventricular size and function.[147-149] Investigators continue to develop new ways to display volume data,[77,138,144] in an effort maximally to exploit the potential clinical utility of 3D sonographic data (Figs. 19-25 and 19-26).

The Future

Within the next 10 years, 3D imaging (most likely real-time rather than reconstructive imaging) may become the standard of care, both for prenatal screening for CHD and for detailed evaluation of complex CHD using rendered displays, color flow imaging, and quantitative measurements. Ultimately, 3D imaging may automate the display of important planes and sweeps, representing a novel form of computer-aided prenatal detection and diagnosis of CHD.[63,75]

Fetal Cardiac Malformations: Diagnosis, Management, and Prognosis

This section aims to help the obstetrician, perinatologist, radiologist, cardiologist, and sonographer to recognize and diagnose the most common and important forms of fetal cardiac malformations (Table 19-6) and to understand their management and prognosis. The embryology of certain defects is described briefly; more detailed descriptions may be found elsewhere.[8,9,150-153] Likewise, more thorough descriptions of individual defects, as well as lesion-specific management and prognosis, may be found elsewhere in standard texts.[8,9,152,153]

Readers should keep in mind that any single heart defect may occur in conjunction with other cardiac defects; often, the most difficult fetal cardiac defect to detect is the second one. Because of the

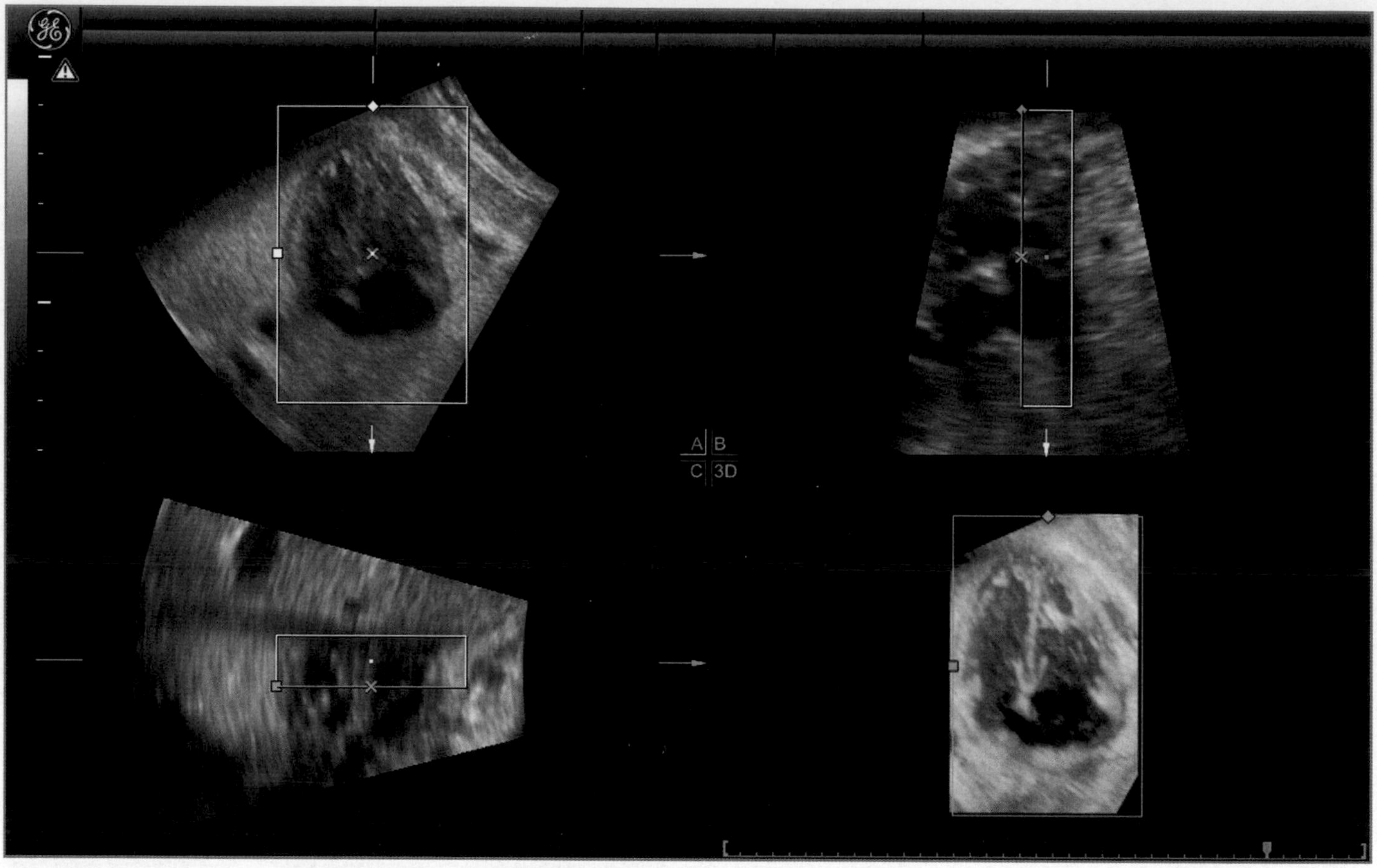

FIGURE 19-25 **Fetal echocardiographic reconstructive three-dimensional multiplanar display.** Normal fetal cardiac anatomy is demonstrated from three orthogonal planes and in a rendered image at lower right. (Image courtesy of Greggory R. DeVore, M.D.)

complexity of various forms of fetal structural heart defects, as well as their common association with maternal or extracardiac fetal disease, a multidisciplinary team (potentially including an obstetrician, perinatologist, radiologist, pediatric cardiologist, neonatologist, social worker, genetics counselor, nurse, and cardiothoracic surgeon) should jointly manage pregnancies complicated by complex fetal heart disease.

Systemic Venous Anomalies

Persistent Umbilical Vein

Normally, during embryonic development, bilateral umbilical veins course along each side of the fetal liver, carrying oxygenated blood from the placenta to the fetal heart. The right umbilical vein involutes, along with the left umbilical vein's connection to the heart. The persistent portion of the left umbilical vein becomes the fetal umbilical vein, which carries oxygenated blood to the IVC via the ductus venosus. Rarely, the right umbilical vein fails to involute. In such cases, the fetus may be found to have a large, unobstructed vein connecting from the cordal insertion site directly to the right atrium (Fig. 19-27). A persistent right umbilical vein may be associated with structural cardiac defects, right heart disproportion, extracardiac defects, or aneuploidy, or it may simply be an isolated anomaly, usually well tolerated but occasionally associated with CHF.[154-156] Commonly, a persistent right umbilical vein is associated with absence of the ductus venosus.

The finding of a persistent right umbilical vein should prompt a detailed evaluation for other structural defects, cardiac and extracardiac, as well as cardiac function.[154-156] Patients also should be advised of the potential for aneuploidy. All cases deserve neonatal clinical and echocardiographic follow-up, although, if the anomaly is isolated, the infant typically does well as the persistent umbilical vein involutes after occlusion of the cord at delivery.

Persistent Left-sided Superior Vena Cava

Normally, during embryogenesis, the right-sided superior vena cava forms from the right anterior cardinal vein and the right common cardinal vein. Abnormal persistence of the left anterior cardinal vein, which normally involutes during embryogenesis, leads to the presence of a persistent LSVC in the fetus and newborn. A persistent LSVC typically drains through the coronary sinus and into the right atrium (Fig. 19-28; see Figs. 19-11 and 19-14). In such cases, a right-sided superior vena cava (normal) may or may not be present (Fig. 19-29).

Cases of persistent LSVC may be detected in the fetus by visualization of an enlarged coronary sinus (see Fig. 19-11) in the 4CV[106,107] or by direct visualization of the LSVC (see Fig. 19-28). The finding of a persistent LSVC may be isolated, resulting in physiological return of deoxygenated blood to the right atrium, albeit via an abnormal pathway. Such cases represent variations of normal and do not require any intervention, either prenatally or after birth. However, persistent LSVC may be associated with left-sided obstructive lesions (e.g., coarctation of the aorta, valvar aortic stenosis, HLHS),[108] so the finding should prompt a detailed fetal echocardiographic evaluation and, probably, neonatal echocardiographic follow-up. In some cases,

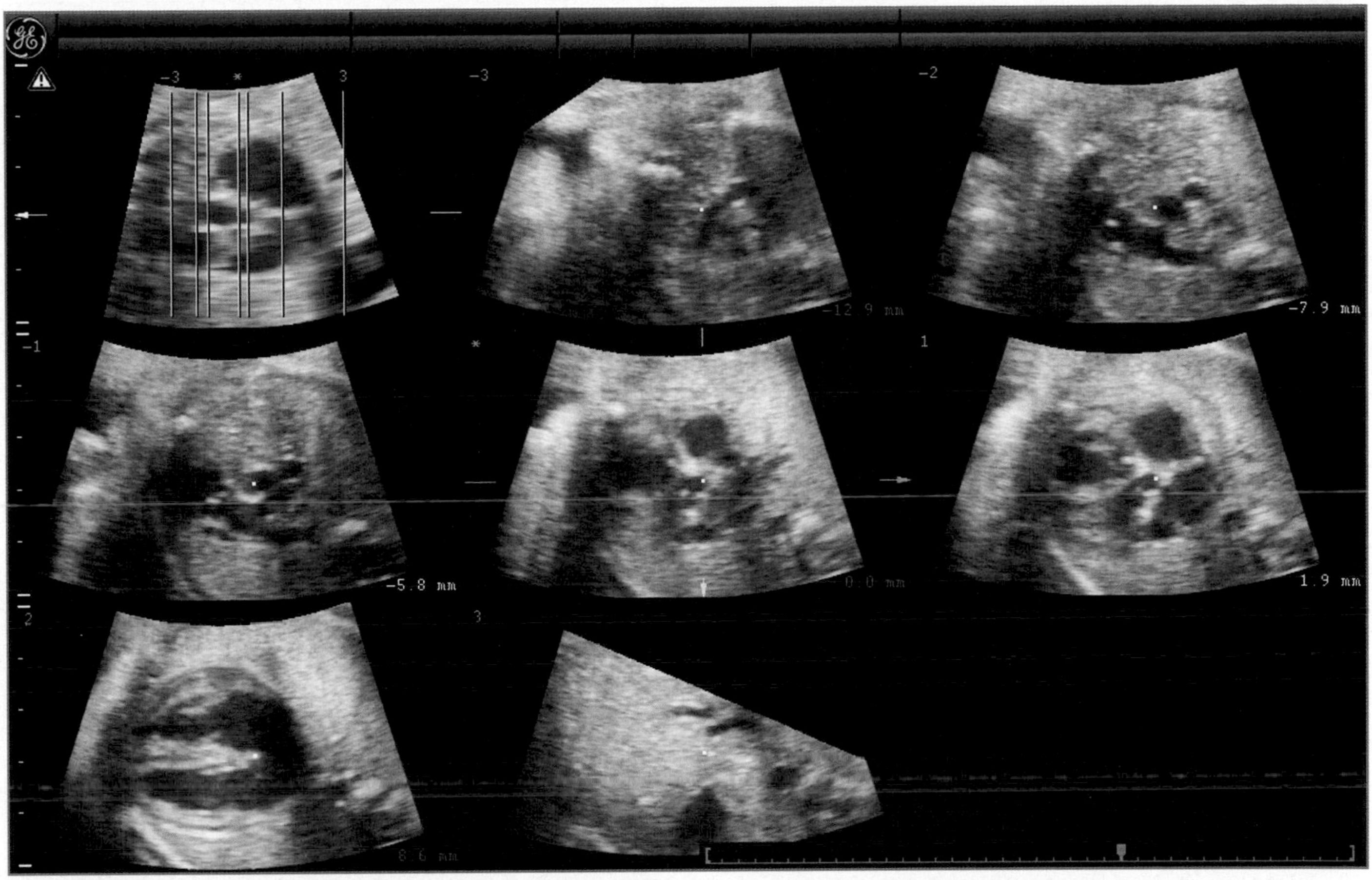

FIGURE 19-26 Fetal echocardiographic reconstructive three-dimensional tomographic ultrasonic image display. Normal fetal cardiac anatomy is demonstrated from multiple parallel planes. (Image courtesy of Greggory R. DeVore, M.D.)

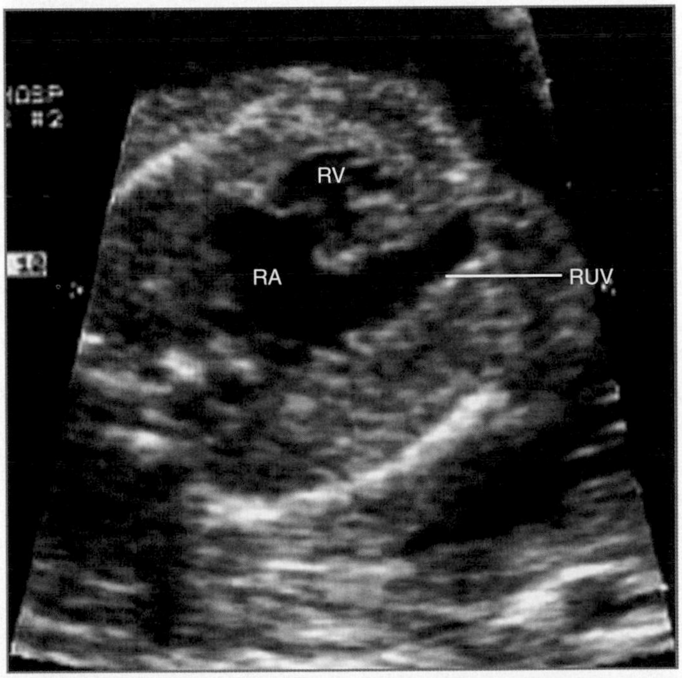

FIGURE 19-27 Fetal echocardiographic image of persistent right umbilical vein. The persistent right umbilical vein (RUV) is shown draining to the right atrium (RA). RV, right ventricle.

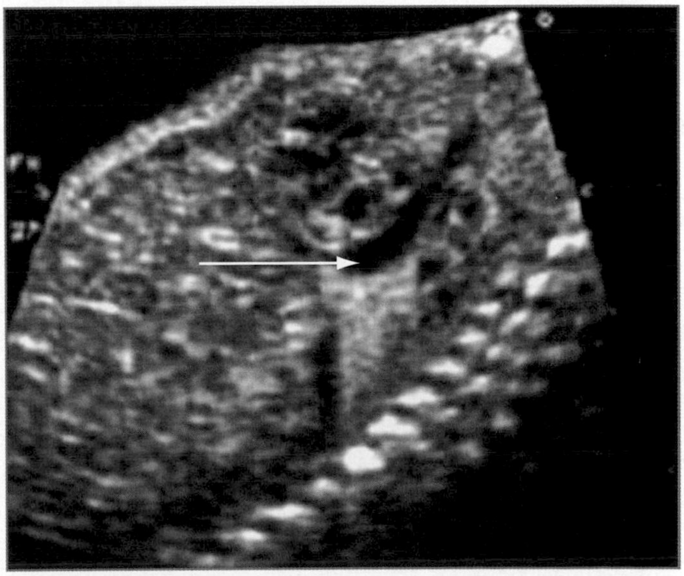

FIGURE 19-28 Fetal echocardiographic sagittal image of left-sided superior vena cava. The persistent left-sided superior vena cava *(arrow)* is shown draining into the coronary sinus.

TABLE 19-6 FETAL CARDIAC MALFORMATIONS

Systemic Venous Abnormalities
Persistent umbilical vein
Interrupted inferior vena cava
Persistent left-sided superior vena cava
Pulmonary Venous Abnormalities
Partial anomalous pulmonary venous return
Total anomalous pulmonary venous return
Shunt Lesions
Atrial septal defect
Ventricular septal defect
Atrioventricular Canal Defect
Complete
Partial
Transitional
Tricuspid Valve Dysplasia and Ebstein Anomaly
Right Heart Obstructive Lesions
Tricuspid atresia
Pulmonary atresia with intact ventricular septum
Left Heart Obstructive Lesions
Mitral stenosis/atresia (hypoplastic left heart syndrome)
Valvar aortic stenosis/atresia
Coarctation of the aorta
Outflow Tract Abnormalities
Tetralogy of Fallot
Double-outlet right ventricle
Transposition of the great arteries
Truncus arteriosus
Tumors
Rhabdomyoma
Intrapericardial teratoma

persistent LSVC is associated with extracardiac abnormalities or heterotaxy.[109,110,157]

Interrupted Inferior Vena Cava

Normally, during embryogenesis, the IVC forms from the right supracardinal vein, subcardinal-supracardinal anastomosis, right subcardinal vein, hepatic vein, and hepatic sinusoids. Occasionally, the hepatic portion of the IVC fails to form, resulting in an interruption of the IVC.[154] In such cases, venous return from the lower half of the fetus drains via a so-called "azygos continuation" of the IVC. The azygous vein returns deoxygenated blood to the right atrium via the superior vena cava.

Interrupted IVC with azygos continuation may be diagnosed prenatally from a transverse view of the abdomen (Fig. 19-30). The cross-sectional image will show, in place of the IVC (within the liver), a cross-sectional image of an azygos vein located posterior to the descending aorta. Sagittal imaging confirms the absence of a direct connection from the IVC to the right atrium; only the hepatic veins are seen to connect directly. Using both 2D and low-velocity color flow sagittal imaging, the azygos vein can be seen longitudinally, located posterior to the aorta and coursing superiorly and anteriorly (Fig. 19-31) to its termination in the superior vena cava.[106]

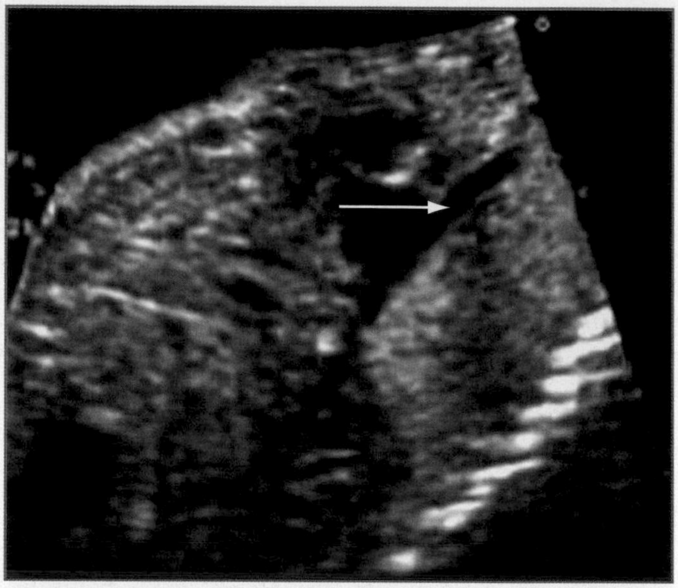

FIGURE 19-29 **Fetal echocardiographic sagittal image of right-sided superior vena cava.** The normal right-sided superior vena cava *(arrow)* is shown draining into the right atrium. Note inferior vena cava draining into right atrium from below.

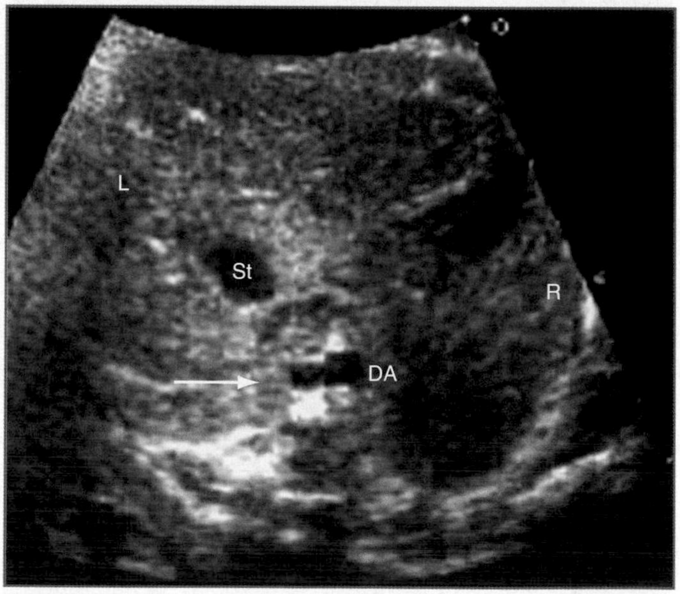

FIGURE 19-30 **Ultrasonographic transverse image of fetal abdomen demonstrating an interrupted inferior vena cava with azygos continuation.** The azygos vein *(arrow)* appears posterior to the descending aorta (DA), and the intrahepatic inferior vena cava is not visualized. L, fetal left; R, fetal right; St, fetal stomach.

The presence of an IVC with azygos continuation does not, in itself, require any treatment, either prenatally or postnatally. However, this finding should prompt detailed fetal and neonatal echocardiographic evaluations because of the association of interrupted IVC with polysplenia[110,154,157] with or without structural heart disease. The diagnosis of polysplenia may be further suggested by the presence of a midline liver or fetal bradycardia (absent sinus node). All cases deserve neonatal echocardiographic follow-up.

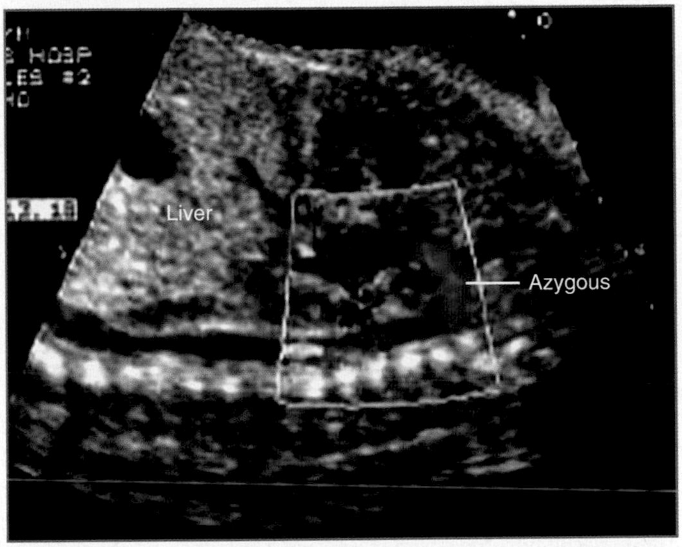

FIGURE 19-31 **Fetal echocardiographic sagittal image of azygos vein draining into the superior vena cava.** In contrast to retrograde flow into either the aorta or the pulmonary artery (pulsatile), venous flow appears continuous during real-time imaging.

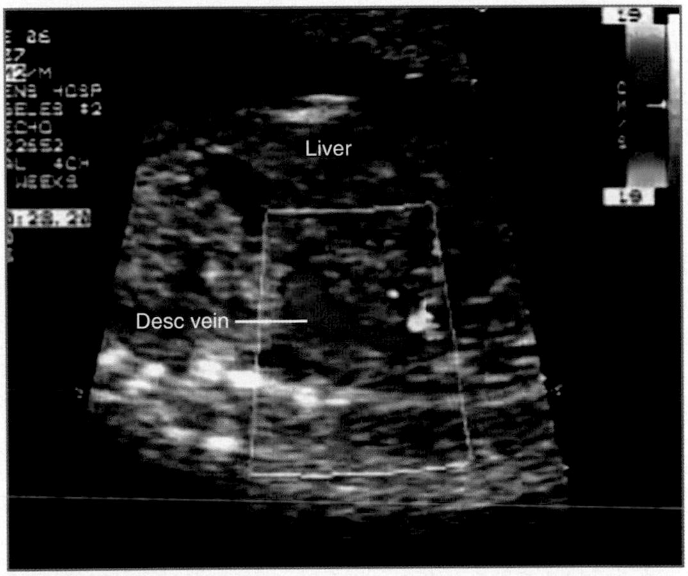

FIGURE 19-32 **Fetal echocardiographic sagittal image of infradiaphragmatic total anomalous pulmonary venous return.** Color flow imaging demonstrates the descending vein as continuous flow directed inferiorly toward the liver. Desc vein, descending vein.

Pulmonary Venous Abnormalities

Normally, during embryonic development, the common pulmonary vein evolves to form not only four separate pulmonary veins but also much of the left atrium itself. Cases of partial anomalous pulmonary venous return (PAPVR), involving one to three veins, or total anomalous pulmonary venous return (TAPVR), involving all four veins, result from abnormalities of this portion of embryogenesis.[150-154] As with abnormalities of systemic venous return, both 2D and color flow imaging play important roles in the diagnosis of anomalous pulmonary venous return. Color flow imaging can facilitate visualization of normal (see Figs. 19-12 and 19-13) or anomalous (Figs. 19-32 and 19-33) pulmonary venous return when the scale has been adjusted for low-velocity flows. Anomalous pulmonary venous return frequently occurs in association with heterotaxy.[106,110,157]

Partial Anomalous Pulmonary Venous Return

Because even detailed fetal echocardiography may not routinely demonstrate all four pulmonary veins, many cases of PAPVR may be overlooked prenatally, unless they are associated with other cardiac abnormalities. This section discusses two types of PAPVR that may be detectable before birth because of associated findings. In general, however, PAPVR usually does not require neonatal intervention and carries an excellent long-term prognosis.

Scimitar syndrome represents an unusual form of PAPVR in which the right-sided pulmonary vein (or veins) returns to a vein that descends through the diaphragm before joining the IVC just proximal to the right atrium. Postnatally, this vein may appear radiographically like a sword, or scimitar; hence, the name of the syndrome. In addition, typically, a collateral vessel arising from the descending aorta supplies a separate part of the right lung. Color flow imaging may demonstrate anomalously draining right-sided pulmonary venous return. Further evaluation may demonstrate a collateral vessel arising from the descending aorta and supplying a portion of the right lung. The fetus with scimitar syndrome may have minimal or no right heart disproportion but frequently presents with dextrocardia or mesocardia.[158] Commonly, the syndrome occurs in association with a secundum ASD, which similarly presents a diagnostic challenge prenatally. Fortunately, most infants with scimitar syndrome do quite well, and neonatal intervention is rarely required.

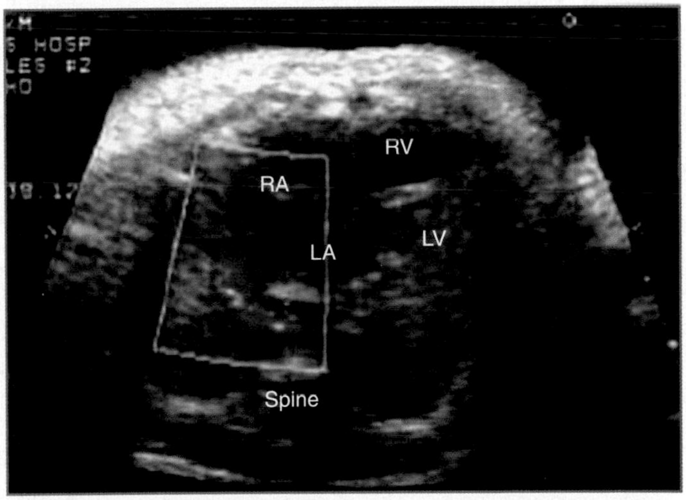

FIGURE 19-33 **Fetal echocardiographic transverse image of supracardiac total anomalous pulmonary venous return.** Color flow imaging demonstrates the pulmonary confluence draining continuously toward the right atrium. LA, left atrium; LV, left ventricle; RA, right atrium; RV, right ventricle.

Sinus venosus ASDs (discussed in more detail later) typically occur in association with anomalous pulmonary venous return of one or both right-sided pulmonary veins to the superior vena cava. Although affected fetuses may not present with right heart disproportion, the ASD high in the atrial septum may be detectable prenatally, with an absent superior rim of the atrial septum. Color flow imaging may demonstrate anomalously draining right-sided pulmonary veins. Sinus venosus defects do not generally require intervention during infancy;

ultimately, however, closure of the defect is required, with baffling of the right-sided pulmonary venous drainage to the left atrium.

Total Anomalous Pulmonary Venous Return

TAPVR can usually be diagnosed prenatally.[159-161] Although right heart disproportion is present in many cases, in others it is minimal or absent.[161] However, affected fetuses do not have the normal infolding of tissue between the left atrial appendage and left pulmonary vein, and color flow imaging will demonstrate absence of pulmonary venous return to the left atrium. Other prenatal sonographic findings in TAPVR depend on the specific type of TAPVR and associated cardiac or extracardiac abnormalities.[110,157] With intracardiac TAPVR, the pulmonary veins drain to the coronary sinus, causing the coronary sinus to be markedly dilated. Infradiaphragmatic TAPVR may manifest as a dilated IVC, because the pulmonary veins turn below the diaphragm and form a common vein before draining into the IVC. The descending vein, which typically partially obstructs within the liver, should be evaluated with color flow imaging (see Fig. 19-32). Finally, in cases of supracardiac TAPVR, 2D and color flow imaging may demonstrate a large common vein draining cephalad toward a left-sided vertical vein or toward a right-sided superior vena cava[160] (see Fig. 19-33).

Obstructed forms of TAPVR (infradiaphragmatic and some cases of supracardiac TAPVR) usually manifest in the immediate neonatal period with respiratory distress and cyanosis. In such instances, prostaglandin is contraindicated, despite the presence of cyanotic CHD, because the result would be exacerbation of pulmonary venous obstruction and edema. Infants with obstructed forms of TAPVR (usually infradiaphragmatic) are at risk for pulmonary hypertension and usually require surgical repair relatively emergently as newborns. For this reason, delivery should be performed at facilities prepared to manage such high-risk cases. Obstructed TAPVR carries a guarded prognosis, but infants who do well with the initial surgical intervention may have a good long-term prognosis in the absence of significant pulmonary hypertension. Nonobstructed forms of TAPVR usually require repair during infancy, although typically not emergently; occasionally, repair may be postponed for several months.

Septal Defects

This section discusses ASD and VSD, two of the most common forms of CHD. Prenatally, the aortic isthmus normally shunts flow between the right and left heart distributions. The foramen ovale allows oxygenated blood flow to stream from right atrium to left atrium, and the ductus arteriosus directs the majority of right ventricular output toward the fetal body, away from the high-resistance pulmonary circuit. Postnatally, the ductus arteriosus closes via constriction, and the foramen ovale closes via pressure-related closure of a one-way valve or flap-door. Thus, the normal fetus has a right-to-left atrial shunt, as well as a patent ductus arteriosus, but never a communication between right and left ventricles.

Atrial Septal Defect

A secundum ASD represents a deficiency of the middle portion of the atrial septum, in the same general location as the normal foramen ovale. Prenatally differentiating a normal foramen ovale from a secundum ASD can be challenging, if not impossible. Even postnatally, this distinction can be difficult to make. A secundum ASD results, embryologically, from either inadequate development of the septum secundum or excessive resorption of the septum primum. Unlike most forms of CHD, the secundum ASD occurs far more commonly in females than in males. During the second and third trimesters, the flap of the foramen ovale (septum primum) becomes progressively more aneurysmal and more deviated into the left atrium. In some cases, the flap appears more aneurysmal than normal for gestational age, or the foramen itself appears to occupy a greater proportion of the atrial septum than normal. In such cases, a detailed evaluation for associated cardiac abnormalities, such as right heart obstruction in the case of excessive deviation, should be performed. However, no convincing association has yet been demonstrated between an abnormal prenatal appearance of the foramen ovale and the postnatal diagnosis of a true secundum ASD. Fortunately, isolated ASDs, which are probably more common than currently suspected, usually close spontaneously and rarely require intervention during infancy. If the foramen ovale does appear abnormal prenatally, particularly in association with other cardiac abnormalities or other risk factors for fetal heart disease, elective postnatal echocardiography would be prudent.

Sinus venosus ASDs occur far less commonly than secundum ASDs, and they typically occur in conjunction with anomalous return of the right-sided pulmonary veins to the superior vena cava or right atrium. Unlike secundum ASDs, sinus venosus defects may be readily diagnosed prenatally by demonstrating absence of the superior rim of the atrial septum. Moreover, the right-sided pulmonary veins occasionally may be demonstrated to drain anomalously to the superior vena cava on 2D and color flow imaging. Like secundum ASDs, these defects rarely require any neonatal intervention. Unlike secundum ASDs, however, sinus venosus defects never close spontaneously, and they typically require surgical repair electively during the first 5 years of life. Long-term prognosis is excellent.

The most important ASDs to detect prenatally are the ostium primum ASDs, which are common, always require surgery, and frequently are associated with trisomy 21. These defects can and should be readily detected, even on a standard fetal ultrasound study. Ostium primum defects result from failure of fusion of the septum primum with the endocardial cushions. These defects, also known as partial atrioventricular canal (AVC) defects, commonly occur in conjunction with a cleft mitral valve. However, the most reliable and consistent prenatal sonographic finding is absence of the lower, inferior portion of the atrial septum. Care should be taken to avoid false-positive diagnoses, because posterior/inferior angulation of the probe from the 4CV opens up a longitudinal view of the coronary sinus (see Figs. 19-11 and 19-14), which may appear similar to an ostium primum ASD. The distinction may be made simply with anterior/superior angulation of the probe: A true ostium primum ASD is evident on a true 4CV, whereas the coronary sinus should mimic this defect only with posterior/inferior angulation.

The diagnosis of an ostium primum ASD carries prenatal and postnatal implications. First, these defects carry an increased risk for trisomy 21,[23,30] so karyotype analysis may be indicated. Second, ostium primum ASDs commonly occur in conjunction with other cardiac and extracardiac abnormalities, so detailed prenatal evaluation should be performed. Finally, isolated defects generally do not require neonatal intervention, but they uniformly require surgical repair, usually during the first 5 years of life. Long-term prognosis is usually excellent, although abnormalities of the mitral valve rarely can persist and may require additional medical or surgical attention.

Ventricular Septal Defect

VSDs probably represent the most common form of CHD, excluding patent ductus arteriosus and bicommissural aortic valve. The size and type (location) of a VSD and its associated cardiac abnormalities, if any, dictate both the prenatal and postnatal clinical implications and the approach to, and feasibility of, prenatal detection.

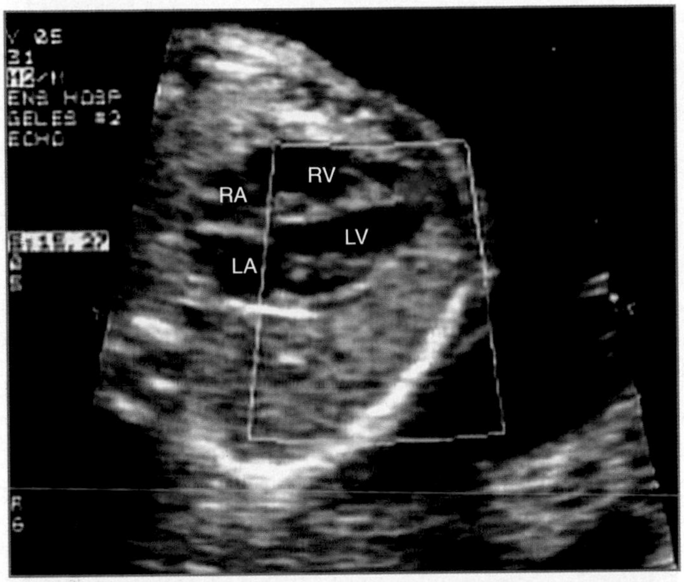

FIGURE 19-34 **Fetal echocardiographic image of the four-chamber view.** Color flow imaging demonstrates a small apical ventricular septal defect with left-to-right shunting. LA, left atrium; LV, left ventricle; RA, right atrium; RV, right ventricle.

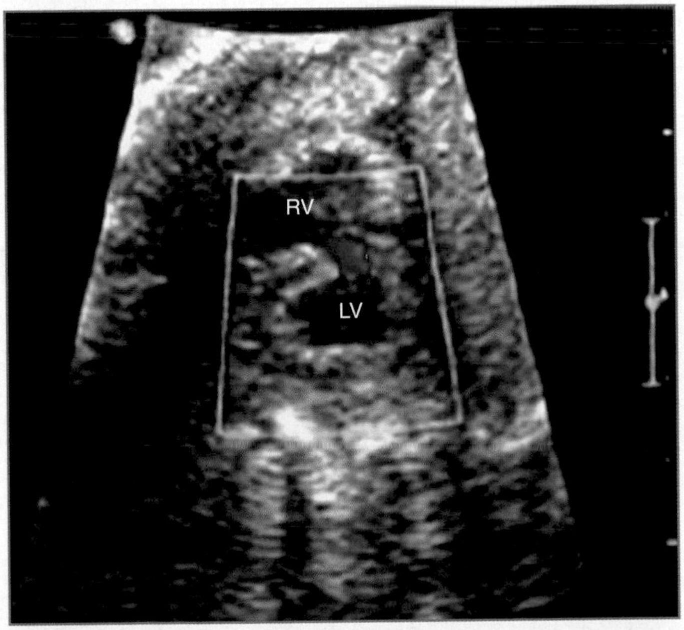

FIGURE 19-35 **Fetal echocardiographic image of apical short-axis view.** Color flow imaging demonstrates a moderate-sized mid-muscular ventricular septal defect with left-to-right shunting. LV, left ventricle; RV, right ventricle.

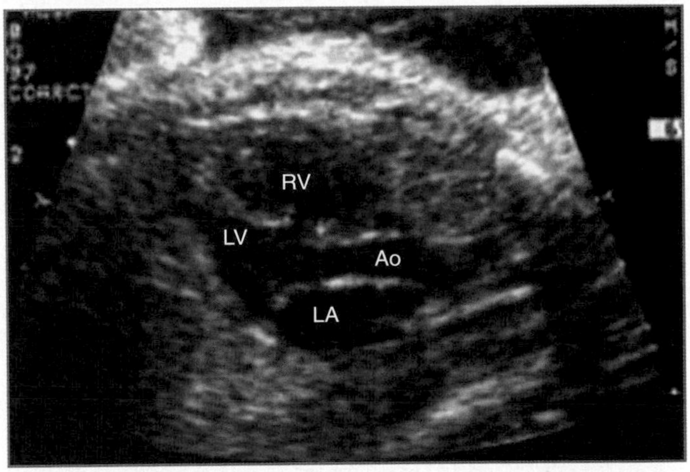

FIGURE 19-36 **Fetal echocardiographic image of membranous ventricular septal defect seen in left ventricular long-axis view.** Ao, aorta; LA, left atrium; LV, left ventricle; RV, right ventricle.

The most common forms of VSD (muscular and membranous) represent, fortuitously, the only types known to close spontaneously, either prenatally or postnatally.[14] Muscular VSDs may be visualized on the 4CV (Fig. 19-34) or short-axis view (Fig. 19-35). By definition, muscular VSDs do not reside immediately beneath the mitral and tricuspid valves; such inlet VSDs occur in conjunction with abnormalities of the mitral and tricuspid valves and represent an AVC type of VSD. Inlet defects, although detectable on the 4CV, do not close spontaneously and usually require surgery. Such inlet defects are discussed in detail in the next section.

Muscular VSDs may be demonstrated with 2D imaging if they are moderate or large, but small ones may be difficult to detect without color flow imaging. Color flow imaging helps confirm the diagnosis, but spectral Doppler evaluation should also be performed. Muscular VSDs, like membranous VSDs, usually shunt predominantly left-to-right prenatally (see Figs. 19-34 and 19-35); predominant right-to-left shunting should prompt further evaluation for right-sided obstructive lesions. Small or moderate muscular defects may close prenatally or within the first few years after delivery.

Large, muscular defects manifest in infancy with tachypnea and failure to thrive and may require surgical closure during the first year of life. Because muscular defects occur within a heavily trabeculated portion of the ventricular septum, effective surgical closure can be difficult to achieve. Alternative approaches include pulmonary artery banding, followed by removal of the band once the defect has decreased in size; or, rarely, such VSDs may be closed percutaneously with a device. The long-term prognosis is usually excellent unless delayed surgery has allowed the development of pulmonary vascular disease.

Membranous VSDs, like muscular VSDs, may close spontaneously. However, unlike muscular VSDs, they cannot be visualized on the 4CV. The membranous septum resides anteriorly, a small distance beneath the aortic valve. A left ventricular long-axis view of the LVOT represents the ideal approach for visualizing a membranous VSD (Fig. 19-36). Moreover, because false-positive dropout through the thin (i.e., membranous) septum occurs commonly when the ultrasound beam is oriented parallel with the septum, the diagnosis can best be confirmed with the ultrasound beam perpendicular to the ventricular septum. Small defects may be missed, although color flow imaging and spectral Doppler evaluation are helpful for both prenatal detection and confirmation. Because of the proximity of the membranous septum to the aortic valve, membranous VSDs may cause the gradual development of aortic regurgitation, with or without prolapse of one or more aortic cusps into the defect. Although most membranous VSDs close spontaneously, larger defects may require surgical closure within the first year in infants with failure to thrive or progressive aortic regurgitation. Long-term prognosis is usually excellent unless irreversible

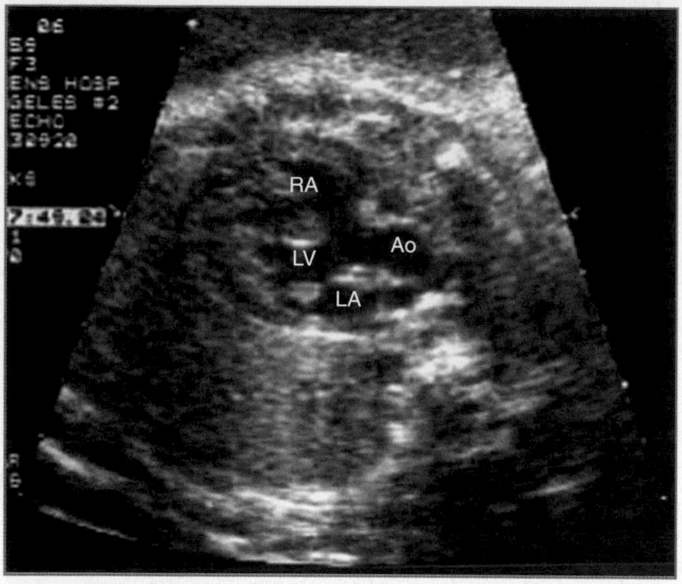

FIGURE 19-37 Fetal echocardiographic image of tetralogy of Fallot seen in left ventricular long-axis view. The aorta overrides the crest of the ventricular septum. Ao, aorta; LA, left atrium; LV, left ventricle; RV, right ventricle.

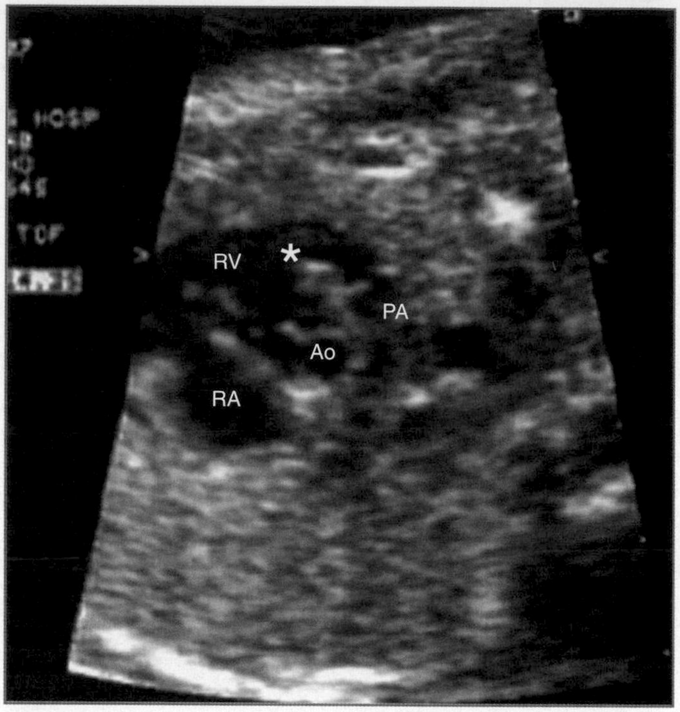

FIGURE 19-38 Fetal echocardiographic image of tetralogy of Fallot seen in apical short-axis view. The conal septum *(asterisk)* deviates anteriorly into the right ventricular outflow tract, causing subvalvar pulmonary stenosis, aortic override, and an anterior malalignment ventricular septal defect. Note that the pulmonary valve appears smaller than the aortic valve. Ao, aorta; PA, pulmonary artery; RA, right atrium; RV, right ventricle.

damage to the aortic valve has occurred. In such cases, aortic valve repair or even replacement may be necessary.

Subarterial VSDs commonly occur in conjunction with other cardiac abnormalities. These defects never close spontaneously and cannot be seen on the 4CV; prenatal detection requires evaluation of the outflow tracts. Subarterial defects may be predominantly under the aortic valve (subaortic) or the pulmonary valve (subpulmonary). Unlike membranous VSDs, which occur close to, but not immediately beneath, the aortic valve, subarterial defects occur immediately beneath one or both semilunar valves. These defects almost invariably require surgical correction within the first year of life. The prognosis, although generally good, relates in part to associated cardiac abnormalities and to any residual aortic or pulmonary pathology.

Malalignment VSDs occur when the upper (conal/infundibular) portion of the ventricular septum separates from the rest of the septum and deviates either anteriorly into the RVOT or posteriorly into the LVOT. Malalignment VSDs secondary to anterior deviation of the conal septum generate RVOT obstruction (subvalvar and valvar pulmonary stenosis and pulmonary artery hypoplasia); TOF is the most common manifestation of such a defect (Figs. 19-37 and 19-38). In contrast, posterior malalignment of the conal septum generates a malalignment VSD in association with LVOT obstruction (e.g., aortic stenosis, bicommissural aortic valve, aortic arch hypoplasia, coarctation of the aorta) (Fig. 19-39). Like subarterial VSDs, malalignment VSDs may appear normal on 4CV, but both the VSD and its associated outflow tract abnormalities should be seen with outflow tract imaging. Management and prognosis depend on the type and severity of outflow tract obstruction. Severe malalignment in either direction may generate severe enough outflow tract obstruction to require maintenance of ductal patency (with prostaglandin) after delivery.

Atrioventricular Canal Defect

Normally, during embryonic development, the septum primum and the endocardial cushions fuse together. Abnormal development of

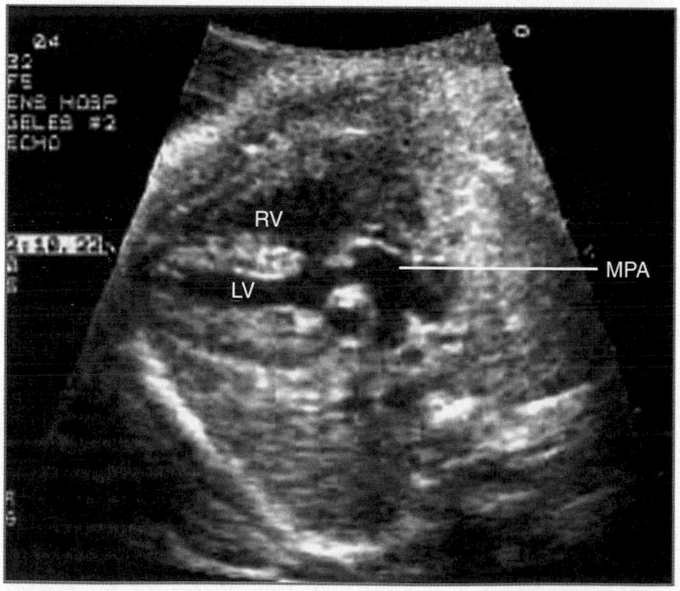

FIGURE 19-39 Fetal echocardiographic image of transposition with subvalvar and valvar pulmonary stenosis seen in left ventricular long-axis view. The conal septum deviates posteriorly into the left ventricular outflow tract, causing subvalvar pulmonary stenosis and a posterior malalignment ventricular septal defect. With normally related great arteries, posterior malalignment of the conal septum would cause aortic rather than pulmonary obstruction. LV, left ventricle; MPA, main pulmonary artery; RV, right ventricle.

these structures results in several forms of AVC defect, all of which should be detected with standard fetal screening ultrasound evaluations as well as with detailed fetal echocardiography. Moreover, all forms of AVC defects ultimately require surgical intervention, and most have relatively high associations with trisomy 21[23,30] or other cardiac abnormalities.[162] The prognosis is generally good but depends on the associated cardiac and extracardiac abnormalities,[163] as well as postoperative mitral, tricuspid, and ventricular function.

Partial Atrioventricular Canal Defect

In partial AVC defects, the septum primum fails to fuse with the endocardial cushions. As a result, the fetal heart develops an ostium primum ASD and, typically, a cleft in the mitral valve (with some degree of mitral regurgitation). In part because of this defect's close association with trisomy 21 or heterotaxy,[23,30,162] great care should be taken not to miss a partial AVC defect on routine screening ultrasonography. Partial AVC defects may be readily detected in the 4CV by the conspicuous absence of the septum primum (the lowest, most inferior portion of the atrial septum). Moreover, the absence of an atrioventricular septum results in absence of the normal apical displacement of the septal leaflet of the tricuspid valve; instead, the septal leaflets of the mitral and tricuspid valves insert onto the ventricular septum at the same level. Care should be taken not to confuse this defect with a dilated coronary sinus (usually secondary to a persistent LSVC), which would be seen in a plane immediately posterior/inferior to the 4CV (see Figs. 19-11 and 19-14).[107] True AVC defects will be noted with anterior/superior angulation of the probe from the level of the coronary sinus into a true 4CV.

Partial AVC defects manifest clinically similar to secundum ASDs, usually with a heart murmur in an asymptomatic child between 2 months and 2 years of age. Many patients have trisomy 21[30] or other cardiac disease (heterotaxy).[162] The cleft in the mitral valve typically does not generate signs or symptoms unless it is associated with more severe degrees of mitral regurgitation. The long-term prognosis after surgical closure during the first several years of life is usually excellent, unless significant mitral valve pathology persists.

Complete Atrioventricular Canal Defect

In complete AVC defects, the endocardial cushions fail to fuse, and the septum primum fails to fuse with the endocardial cushions. As a result, the fetal heart has not only an ostium primum ASD and cleft mitral valve but also a large inlet VSD (contiguous with the ostium primum ASD) and a single, common atrioventricular valve. This type of AVC defect should be readily detected with a routine 4CV (Figs. 19-40 and 19-41). Although isolated forms of complete AVC defects carry an exceptionally high association with trisomy 21,[23,30] complete AVC defects in association with other cardiac abnormalities carry a high association with heterotaxy syndrome.[162,163] Beyond the diagnosis of complete AVC defect, detailed fetal echocardiographic evaluation should include assessment of atrioventricular valvar regurgitation using color flow imaging and close attention to the relative development of both ventricles and possible outflow tract obstruction.

When complete AVC defects occur with well-balanced right and left ventricles (so-called balanced complete AVC), corrective surgery may be offered at 3 to 6 months of age. Such patients usually have an excellent long-term prognosis in the absence of severe residual atrioventricular valve regurgitation. On the other hand, the fetus with a hypoplastic right ventricle (left ventricle–dominant AVC) (Fig. 19-42) or a hypoplastic left ventricle (right ventricle–dominant AVC) is likely to require single-ventricle palliation, meaning three palliative surgical procedures within the first 2 to 3 years of life. Some of these patients may undergo early pulmonary artery banding (during the first month after delivery), to provide a controlled source of pulmonary blood flow for the first 6 months and to avoid the development of pulmonary vascular disease. Because single-ventricle palliation involves rerouting of the systemic venous return through the lungs without the benefit of a subpulmonary ventricle, elevated pulmonary vascular resistance may be considered a relative contraindication (or at least a risk factor) for subsequent palliative procedures (i.e., Glenn and Fontan proce-

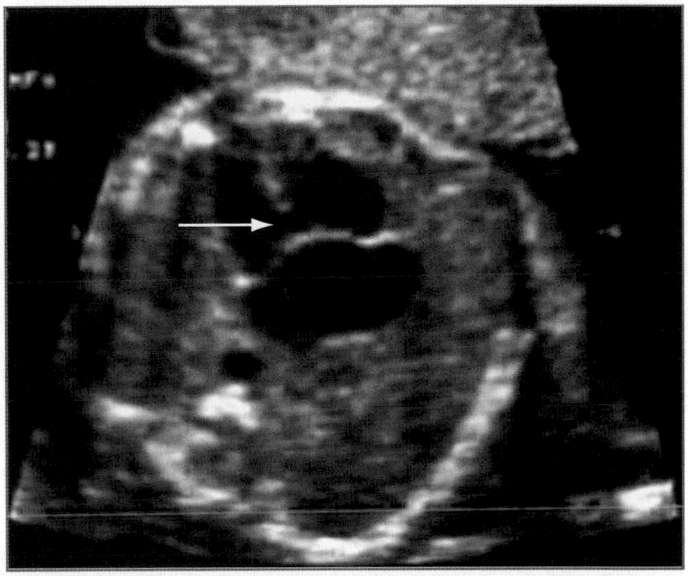

FIGURE 19-40 **Fetal echocardiographic image of four-chamber view demonstrating a balanced complete atrioventricular canal defect.** During systole, the common atrioventricular valve is closed, and the large atrial and ventricular *(arrow)* defects are readily apparent. Note the absence of the septum primum.

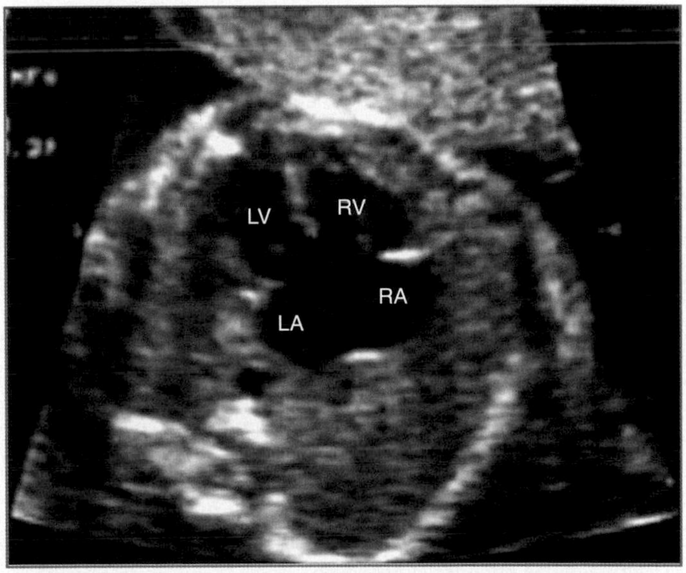

FIGURE 19-41 **Fetal echocardiographic image of four-chamber view demonstrating a balanced complete atrioventricular canal defect.** During diastole, the common atrioventricular valve is open, and the large atrial and ventricular defects (in continuity) are readily apparent. LA, left atrium; LV, left ventricle; RA, right atrium; RV, right ventricle.

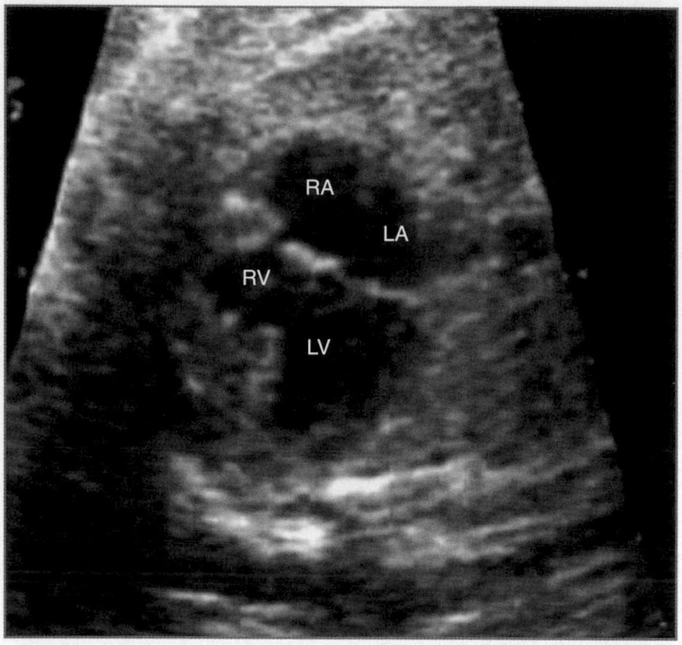

FIGURE 19-42 Fetal echocardiographic image of four-chamber view demonstrating an unbalanced, left ventricle–dominant atrioventricular canal. Note the large primum atrial septal defect and large inlet ventricular septal defect, as well as the hypoplastic right ventricle (RV). LA, left atrium; LV, left ventricle; RA, right atrium.

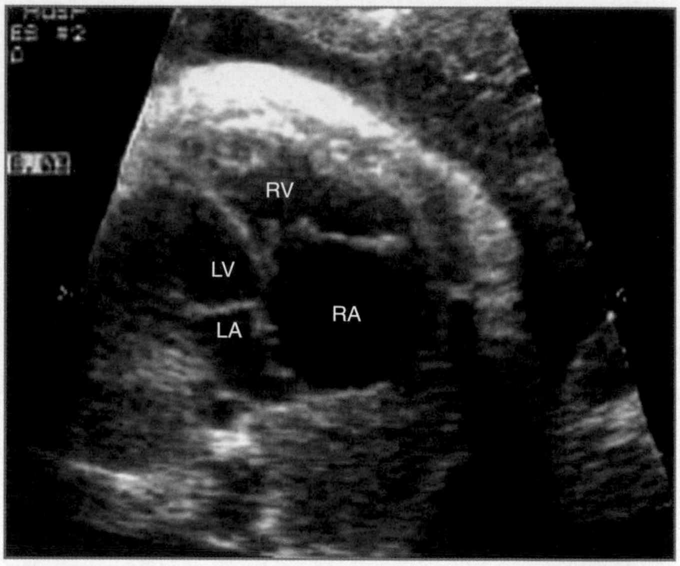

FIGURE 19-43 Fetal echocardiographic image of four-chamber view demonstrating tricuspid valve dysplasia. Note absence of apical displacement of the septal insertion site of the tricuspid valve. LA, left atrium; LV, left ventricle; RA, right atrium; RV, right ventricle.

dures, which redirect, respectively, the superior vena cava or the IVC directly to the right pulmonary artery). In the best of cases, the patient with an unbalanced complete AVC defect faces a much more guarded, palliated long-term prognosis than the patient with a balanced complete AVC defect. Therefore, making such a distinction in a fetus is of great importance.

Transitional Atrioventricular Canal Defect

A transitional AVC defect should be recognized readily from the 4CV. Affected fetuses have an ostium primum defect and, with absence of the atrioventricular septum, the mitral and tricuspid valves insert onto the crest of the ventricular septum at the same level. The mitral valve is frequently cleft, with some degree of mitral regurgitation visualized with color flow imaging. In contrast to a complete AVC defect, transitional AVC defects may have two relatively well-formed mitral and tricuspid valves, and the inlet VSD is only small to moderate in size, largely occluded by mitral and tricuspid valve tissue. Transitional AVC defects, when balanced and not associated with other cardiac defects, typically require a single surgical procedure between 6 months and 5 years of age, and generally carry a good long-term prognosis.

Ebstein Anomaly of the Tricuspid Valve and Tricuspid Valve Dysplasia

Both fetal Ebstein anomaly of the tricuspid valve and tricuspid valve dysplasia carry a wide spectrum of potential outcomes, depending on severity.[164,165] Fortuitously, the more severe cases are those that should be most readily detected on a standard 4CV.

Tricuspid valve dysplasia refers to thickening and distortion of the tricuspid valve leaflets and supportive apparatus, with the primary pathophysiologic manifestation being tricuspid regurgitation. The more severe the tricuspid regurgitation, the more dilated the right atrium and right ventricle, the more likely the development of pulmonary valve stenosis/atresia (related to diminished antegrade flow), and the more likely the development of hydrops or pulmonary hypoplasia or both (related to elevated right atrial pressure and right-sided heart enlargement).

Sharing similar pathophysiology, Ebstein anomaly of the tricuspid valve may be considered a subset of tricuspid valve dysplasia. In Ebstein anomaly, the dysplastic tricuspid valve is partially fused against the ventricular septum, causing the coaptation point to be apically displaced within the right ventricle. Both disorders carry an association with episodic SVT and Wolff-Parkinson-White (WPW) syndrome.

Both Ebstein anomaly and tricuspid valve dysplasia may be visualized on the 4CV, with enlargement of the right side of the heart (particularly the right atrium), dysplasia of the tricuspid valve (Fig. 19-43), and apical displacement of the tricuspid valve coaptation point in the case of Ebstein anomaly (Fig. 19-44). Color flow imaging is useful to demonstrate the degree of tricuspid regurgitation (Fig. 19-45), although such information should be suspected from the degree of right atrial enlargement. In cases of severe tricuspid regurgitation, Ebstein anomaly and tricuspid valve dysplasia commonly have some degree of pulmonary valve stenosis, or even atresia, along with hypoplasia of the main and branch pulmonary arteries; such findings should be evident on evaluation of the outflow tracts.

Although Ebstein anomaly and tricuspid valve dysplasia are occasionally associated with fetal exposure to maternal lithium, most cases occur in pregnancies not identified as high risk. The risk for associated aneuploidy is probably mildly increased over that in the general fetal population. Ebstein anomaly represents a common finding in the rare setting of congenitally corrected transposition (discussed later). However, most of the time, the overriding determinants of short- and long-term survival are the degree of fetal heart failure or hydrops, the degree of pulmonary hypoplasia, and the degree of left ventricular dysfunction. Progressive fetal CHF (related to tricuspid regurgitation, SVT, and/or ventricular dysfunction) puts the fetus at risk for hydrops and fetal demise. Newborns with a history of hydrops prenatally may present with diffuse edema or anasarca, and they face significant

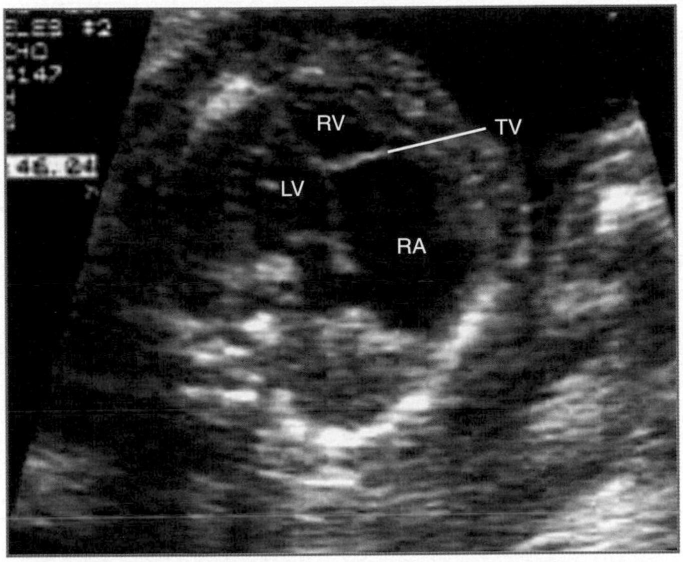

FIGURE 19-44 **Fetal echocardiographic image of four-chamber view demonstrating Ebstein anomaly of the tricuspid valve.** Note apical displacement of the septal insertion site of the tricuspid valve. Compare with Figure 19-43. LV, left ventricle; RA, right atrium; RV, right ventricle; TV, tricuspid valve.

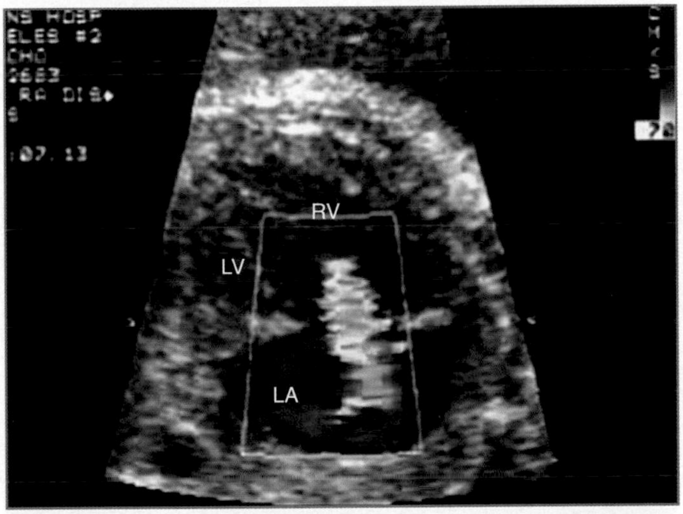

FIGURE 19-45 **Fetal echocardiographic image of four-chamber view demonstrating Ebstein anomaly of the tricuspid valve.** Color flow imaging demonstrates tricuspid regurgitation jet arising from within the right ventricle. LA, left atrium; LV, left ventricle; RV, right ventricle.

neonatal morbidity and mortality. Pulmonary hypoplasia, related to marked cardiomegaly, particularly early in gestation, represents the other primary determinant of neonatal survival and may not always be accurately predicted with prenatal assessments. Fetuses with moderate or severe forms of Ebstein anomaly or tricuspid valve dysplasia should be delivered at centers that can provide optimal medical and surgical care for high-risk neonates.

Tricuspid Atresia

Tricuspid atresia represents the most basic form of single ventricle and generally carries the best long-term prognosis among single-ventricle

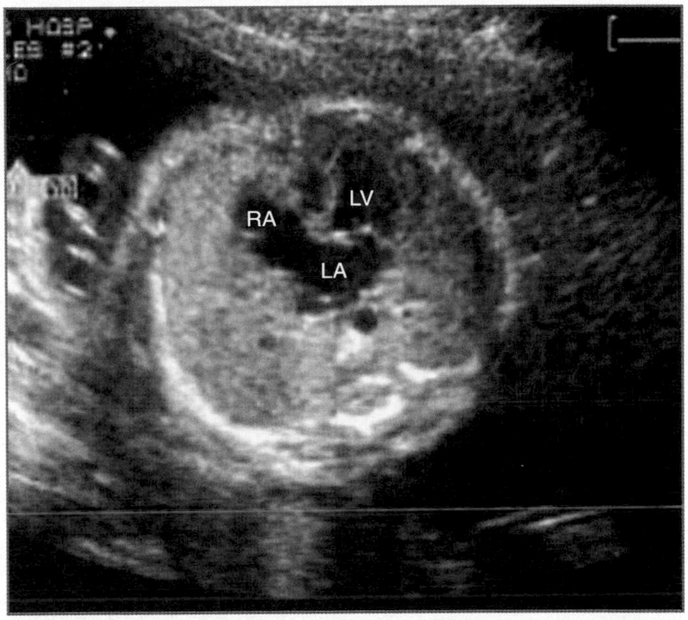

FIGURE 19-46 **Fetal echocardiographic image of four-chamber view demonstrating tricuspid atresia.** Note hypoplastic right ventricle, atretic and membranous tricuspid valve, and bowing of the atrial septum laterally into the left atrium. LA, left atrium; LV, left ventricle; RA, right atrium.

disorders. In tricuspid atresia, the tricuspid valve either is not formed or otherwise simply does not open. As a result, all flow entering the right atrium must cross the foramen ovale into the left atrium and, from there, into the left ventricle. From the left ventricle, some portion of the blood exits via the aortic valve, and some passes through a VSD (usually present with tricuspid atresia) and into the pulmonary artery. Because flow into the right ventricle and pulmonary artery must come via the VSD, the right ventricle and pulmonary artery generally appear hypoplastic, and the pulmonary valve is usually stenotic, if not atretic. However, when tricuspid atresia occurs in conjunction with transposition of the great arteries (TGA), the pulmonary valve and pulmonary artery (in this case arising from the left ventricle) are usually well formed, whereas the aortic valve may be stenotic, with a hypoplastic aortic arch and possible coarctation.

In the fetus, tricuspid atresia manifests with an abnormal 4CV (Fig. 19-46), including an abnormal (or absent) tricuspid valve and hypoplastic right ventricle.[166] Rarely, color flow imaging demonstrates the foramen ovale to be restrictive to flow. The outflow tracts also demand close attention, given the close association of tricuspid atresia with TGA or with underdevelopment of the great artery arising from the right ventricle, or both.

After delivery, most affected babies appear cyanotic, but ductal dependency is determined by the amount of pulmonary blood flow (in normally related great arteries) or by the presence of aortic stenosis, coarctation, or inadequate mixing (in TGA). Infants with tricuspid atresia ultimately require palliation with a Glenn procedure (anastomosis of the cephalic end of the superior vena cava to the right pulmonary artery, usually at about 6 months of age) followed by a Fontan procedure (anastomosis of the IVC directly to the right pulmonary artery with interposition graft, usually at 2 to 3 years of age). Whether a neonatal shunt or arch repair is needed depends on the details of the anatomy and pathophysiology. Long-term prognosis for tricuspid atresia tends to be better than for other forms of single ventricle, but the child will still have increasing risks for heart failure and arrhythmias and possible need for cardiac transplantation in later decades.

Pulmonary Atresia with Intact Ventricular Septum

In pulmonary atresia with intact ventricular septum, the RVOT ends blindly (pulmonary atresia). As a result, during fetal life, the right side of the heart must direct its share of cardiac output entirely through the foramen ovale. In the presence of a competent tricuspid valve (which is typical), the right ventricle hypertrophies in response to the high pressure generated by absence of egress. This lesion may result, in some cases, from prenatal progression of pulmonary stenosis to pulmonary atresia.[16] The right ventricle, along with its tricuspid valve, typically develops some degree of hypoplasia. Those fetuses with markedly elevated right ventricular pressure may develop sinusoidal connections between the right ventricular cavity and the coronary arteries. Such sinusoids may occur in association with significant coronary artery stenoses, placing these patients at risk for acute myocardial infarction.

Pulmonary atresia with intact ventricular septum usually manifests in fetal life with an abnormal 4CV (Figs. 19-47 and 19-48), including an abnormal-appearing tricuspid valve and a hypoplastic, hypertrophied, poorly functioning right ventricle. Occasionally, the degree of tricuspid valve and right ventricular hypoplasia is mild enough to be missed on a cursory 4CV; other cases may mimic tricuspid atresia (compare Figs. 19-46 and 19-47). Color flow imaging should be used to evaluate the tricuspid valve for evidence of tricuspid regurgitation. Color flow imaging may also detect significant sinusoids within the ventricular septum or right ventricular free wall or both. Careful evaluation of the 4CV in real time should almost always detect some abnormality in size, structure, or function of the tricuspid valve or right ventricle. Imaging of the outflow tracts should invariably demonstrate the pulmonary valve to be atretic, with no prograde flow from right ventricle to pulmonary artery. Detailed cardiac imaging should include evaluation of the continuity and size of the main and branch pulmonary arteries, supplied retrograde through the ductus arteriosus.

After delivery, babies with this lesion require prostaglandin to maintain patency of the ductus arteriosus for pulmonary blood flow. Neonatal surgery is always necessary; it usually includes placement of a shunt, and sometimes reconstruction of the RVOT. Long-term prognosis varies from an excellent two-ventricle repair to single-ventricle palliation, and those patients with coronary artery abnormalities face additional short- and long-term risks of myocardial infarction. Some fetal echocardiographic parameters, including tricuspid valve size and the presence of tricuspid regurgitation, can help predict outcome.[167,168]

Hypoplastic Left Heart Syndrome

One of the most common and most feared cardiac diagnoses, HLHS represents a heterogeneous constellation of various forms of CHD, the result of which in the newborn infant is a left heart with a surgically resistant inability to sustain systemic cardiac output. Most cases of HLHS carry an increased risk for congenital or acquired central nervous system abnormalities,[41,169] as well as some increased risk for

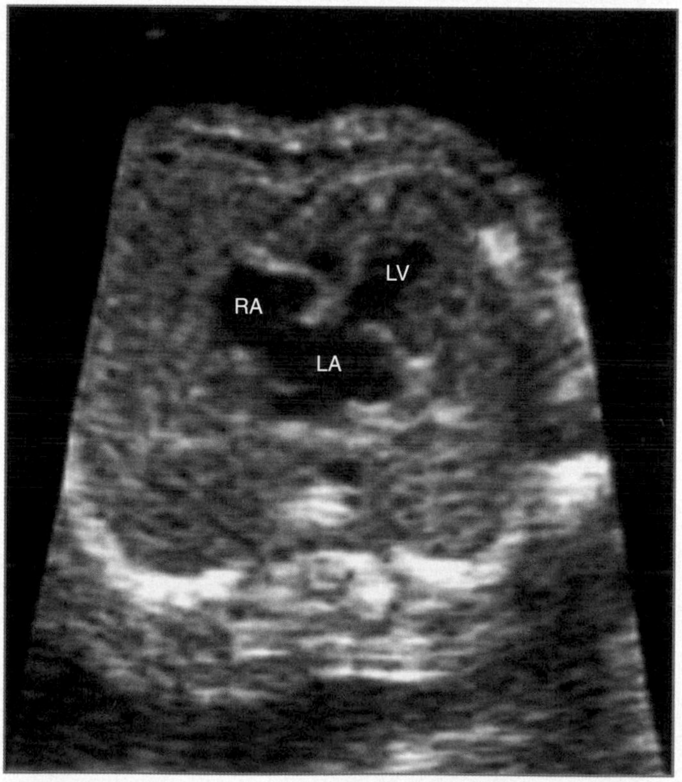

FIGURE 19-47 Fetal echocardiographic image of four-chamber view demonstrating pulmonary atresia with intact ventricular septum. Note similarity to tricuspid atresia (Figure 19-46), but with a more normal appearance to the tricuspid valve. LA, left atrium; LV, left ventricle; RA, right atrium.

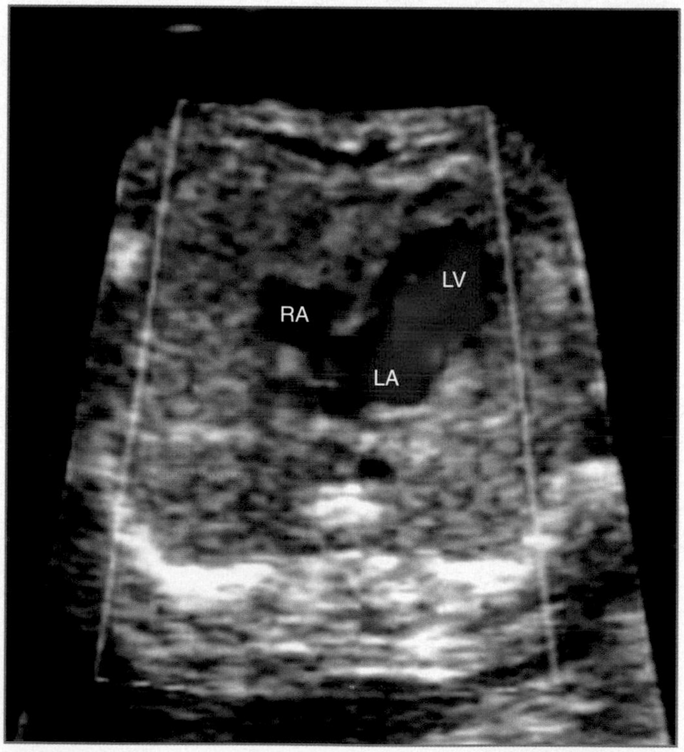

FIGURE 19-48 Fetal echocardiographic image of four-chamber view of fetus with pulmonary atresia with intact ventricular septum. Color flow imaging demonstrates absence of prograde flow across the tricuspid valve during diastole and right-to-left flow across the atrial septum. LA, left atrium; LV, left ventricle; RA, right atrium.

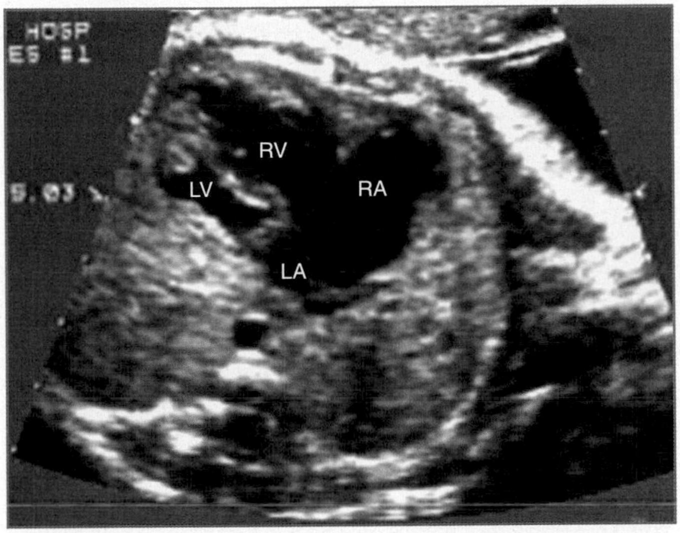

FIGURE 19-49 Fetal echocardiographic image of four-chamber view demonstrating hypoplastic left heart syndrome with mitral atresia and ventricular septal defect. The ventricular septal defect, although not visualized, may be inferred from the presence of a moderately well-formed left ventricle with mitral atresia. LA, left atrium; LV, left ventricle; RA, right atrium; RV, right ventricle.

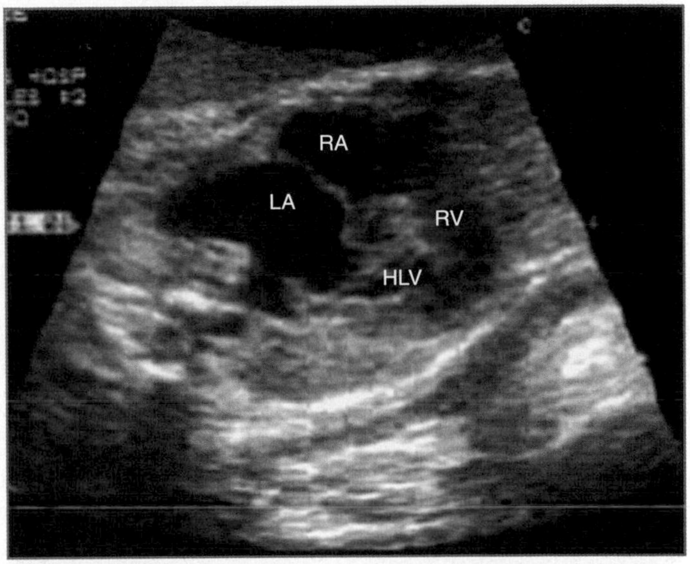

FIGURE 19-50 Fetal echocardiographic image of four-chamber view demonstrating hypoplastic left heart syndrome with restrictive foramen ovale. The left atrium and pulmonary veins appear dilated in response to left atrial hypertension (lack of egress of pulmonary venous return from left atrium). HLV, hypoplastic left ventricle; LA, left atrium; RA, right atrium; RV, right ventricle.

aneuploidy. Some forms of multiple left-sided obstructive lesions (e.g., Shone syndrome) may be corrected with surgical procedures addressing the left ventricular inflow tract, outflow tract, and aortic arch; these cases do not qualify as HLHS. Although this distinction is of tremendous clinical importance, it sometimes is subtle, even postnatally.

This section discusses the most common and classic form of HLHS, mitral and aortic atresia, with the caution that other forms of HLHS may differ in their prenatal appearance and postnatal course. Mitral or aortic stenosis, for example, may manifest with a relatively well-formed left ventricle at mid-gestation but with HLHS at term.[16,82,170] In fetuses with mitral and aortic atresia, there is a markedly abnormal 4CV at mid-gestation, with no inflow into the left ventricle (effectively no mitral valve) and a severely hypoplastic left ventricle (Fig. 19-49; see Fig. 19-24). The foramen ovale needs close prenatal evaluation with 2D and color flow imaging, because restriction to flow (left-to-right) may lead to pulmonary venous congestion (Fig. 19-50) and irreversible pulmonary vascular disease.[171] Such restriction to flow occasionally may not develop until late in the third trimester. Some fetuses with HLHS and a restrictive foramen ovale may be candidates for percutaneous enlargement of the foramen ovale during the second trimester, with the hope of avoiding the development of pulmonary vascular disease and improving long-term survival.[171] The aortic arch fills retrograde from the ductus arteriosus (Fig. 19-51), and may be visualized with both 2D and color flow imaging. Tricuspid valve and right ventricular structure and function also require close evaluation, using both 2D and color flow imaging to assess for tricuspid regurgitation and right ventricular dysfunction.

The fetus with HLHS should be delivered at a tertiary care center experienced with complex CHD in newborns. All newborns with HLHS, by definition, are ductal dependent for systemic blood flow, so prostaglandin infusion should be initiated. Supplemental oxygen generally should be avoided, because in these patients it usually worsens pulmonary overcirculation and systemic hypoperfusion. The newborn with HLHS and a restrictive foramen ovale may require emergent atrial

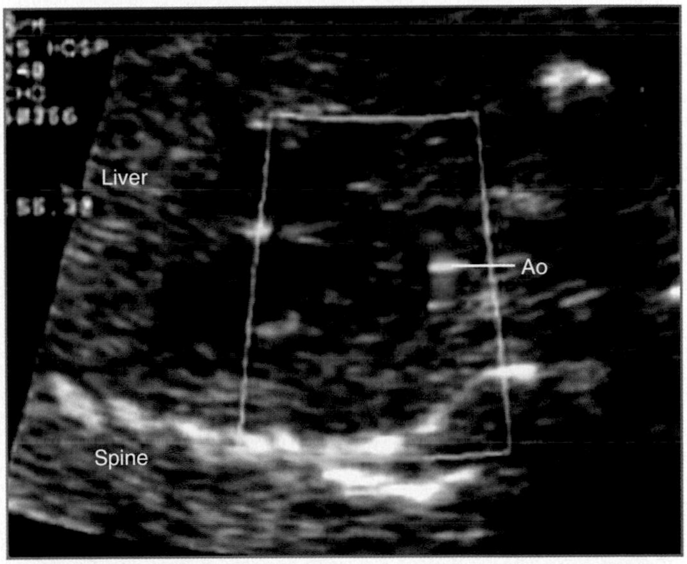

FIGURE 19-51 Fetal echocardiographic sagittal image of aortic arch in fetus with hypoplastic left heart syndrome. Color flow imaging demonstrates pulsatile, retrograde flow into the transverse aortic arch. Ao, aortic arch.

septostomy/septectomy within the first several hours after delivery. In general, infants with HLHS require the first of three palliative surgical procedures (the Norwood operation) within the first week after delivery, followed by a Glenn procedure at approximately 6 months and a Fontan procedure at 2 to 3 years. Some patients undergo cardiac transplantation,[172] and others receive comfort care only.[172,173] With surgery, the current long-term prognosis begins with a 5-year survival rate of 75% to 80% at the best and largest centers. Although many patients do extremely well early on, long-term data are lacking because the surgical approach is so new.[172-174] Many survivors have some degree of

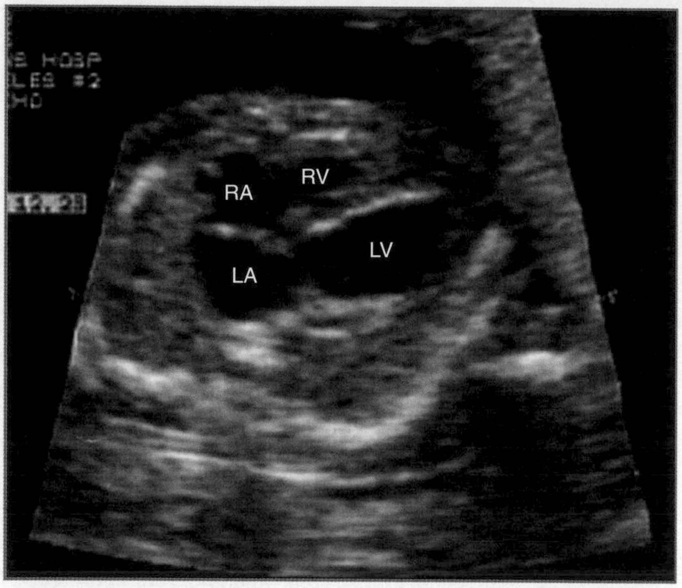

FIGURE 19-52 **Fetal echocardiographic image of four-chamber view demonstrating a dilated left ventricle with endocardial fibroelastosis in a fetus with severe aortic stenosis.** Note the presence of left-sided heart disproportion. LA, left atrium; LV, left ventricle; RA, right atrium; RV, right ventricle.

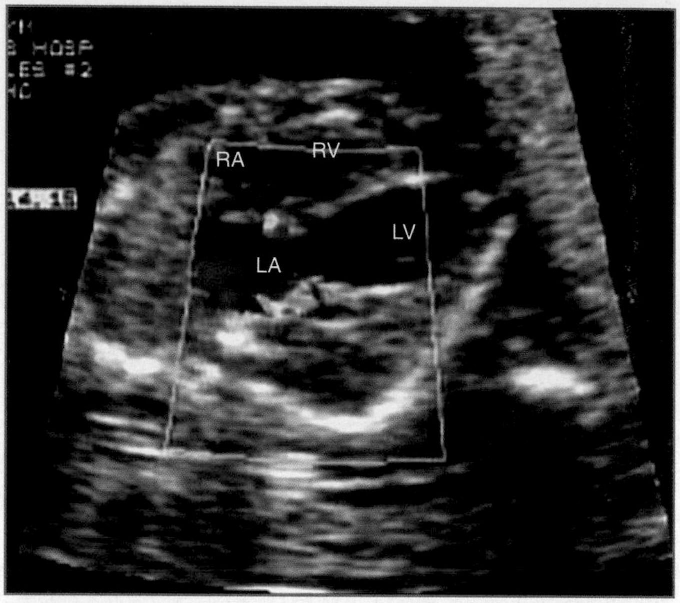

FIGURE 19-53 **Fetal echocardiographic image of four-chamber view demonstrating a dilated left ventricle with endocardial fibroelastosis in a fetus with severe aortic stenosis.** Color flow imaging demonstrates mitral regurgitation and left-to-right flow across the foramen ovale. LA, left atrium; LV, left ventricle; RA, right atrium; RV, right ventricle.

neurodevelopmental delay.[41,169] Long-term survivors with progressive right-sided heart failure may require cardiac transplantation during adulthood.

Valvar Aortic Stenosis

Valvar aortic stenosis, usually secondary to a thickened, bicommissural aortic valve, represents one of the most common lesions known to have the potential to evolve dramatically during the second and third trimesters.[16] Severe cases of valvar aortic stenosis, particularly if present by 18 to 20 weeks' gestation, may adversely affect the prenatal development of the left ventricle, potentially generating a form of dilated cardiomyopathy that then evolves into HLHS.[170,175] All degrees of valvar aortic stenosis may occur in conjunction with coarctation of the aorta. From a flow-related explanation of CHD, either lesion may actually cause the other.

Mild to moderate valvar aortic stenosis may be detected prenatally by visualization of a thickened, usually small aortic valve on imaging of the LVOT. The 4CV view typically appears normal. Spectral and color flow Doppler imaging may demonstrate flow acceleration with an increased velocity in the ascending aorta; rarely, this lesion may also have some degree of aortic regurgitation.

Severe forms of valvar aortic stenosis may manifest during the second trimester with abnormalities of both the 4CV and the outflow tracts. The 4CV may include a dilated, poorly functioning left ventricle (Fig. 19-52); in some cases, diminished diastolic excursion of the mitral valve, mitral valve regurgitation, and, often, endocardial fibroelastosis (brightened left ventricular endocardium) are present. The foramen ovale may shunt predominantly left-to-right (Fig. 19-53). The outflow tract views may demonstrate a small, thickened aortic valve with diminished excursion, and color flow imaging of the aortic arch may demonstrate retrograde (see Fig. 19-51) or bidirectional flow in the transverse arch. Some cases of severe valvar aortic stenosis may evolve into HLHS by term, whereas others manifest in the newborn period with valvar aortic stenosis and a well-formed but poorly functioning left ventricle.[170,175]

In a subset of those cases judged most likely to evolve into HLHS, the fetus may be a candidate for second-trimester dilation of the aortic valve.[170,175] Such fetal intracardiac interventions may prevent the development of some cases of HLHS and allow a neonatal two-ventricle repair rather than single-ventricle palliation. Some fetuses may also benefit from the procedure's ability to establish prograde, pulsatile flow to the brain. However, the procedure carries risks for both mother and fetus. Although the safety of the procedure and the ability to predict which cases will evolve into HLHS both improve with advancing gestation, the likelihood of procedural efficacy decreases with advancing gestational age. The procedure, and the data to support it, both remain inadequately developed.

After delivery, mild to moderate valvar aortic stenosis usually requires observation over months to years; transcatheter or surgical intervention is postponed until the disease has significantly progressed. In contrast, severe valvar aortic stenosis typically manifests immediately after delivery with poor left ventricular systolic and diastolic function. These newborns require prostaglandin to maintain ductal patency for systemic blood flow. Affected infants undergo, soon after birth, either transcatheter balloon dilation of the aortic valve, surgical aortic valvuloplasty, or the Ross procedure (replacement of the patient's own aortic valve with the patient's own pulmonary valve and placement of a pulmonary homograft into the patient's RVOT). Most cases of severe valvar aortic stenosis ultimately require valve replacement, but the prognosis remains quite good as long as left ventricular function recovers after the initial intervention.

Coarctation of the Aorta

Coarctation of the aorta represents not only one of the most common forms of ductal-dependent CHD but also one of the most difficult

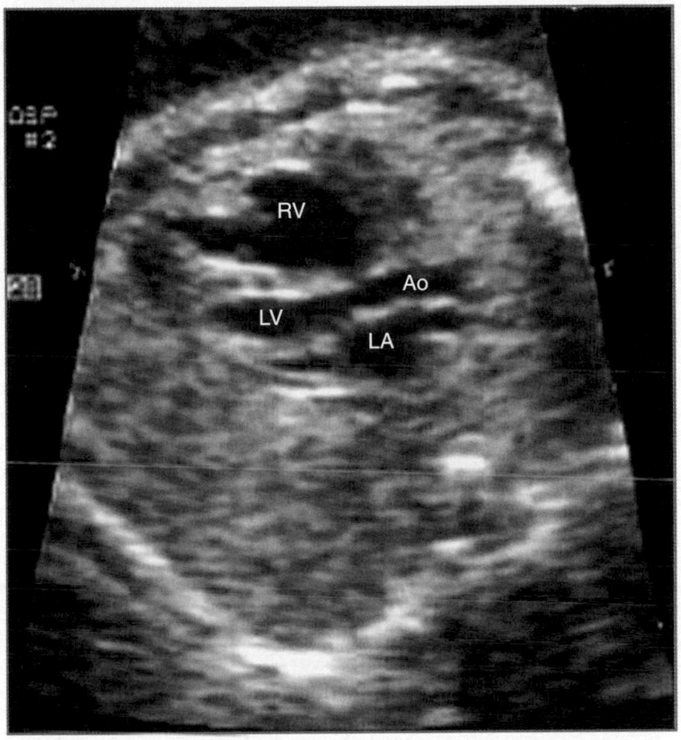

FIGURE 19-54 Fetal echocardiographic image of left ventricular long-axis view demonstrating right heart disproportion suggestive of coarctation. The presence of a bicommissural aortic valve, possibly thickened, would help to support the diagnosis of coarctation. Ao, aorta; LA, left atrium; LV, left ventricle; RV, right ventricle.

cardiac lesions to detect prenatally.[176,177] Normally, the fetal left ventricle supplies the coronary and cerebral circulations, with only a relatively small component of left ventricular cardiac output crossing the aortic isthmus to supply the lower body. The fetal right ventricle, in contrast, normally supplies most of the lower body of the fetus, with most of the right ventricular output passing right-to-left through the ductus arteriosus and joining the descending aorta just distal to the aortic isthmus. Coarctation of the aorta represents a narrowing of the aortic isthmus, but it frequently may also involve hypoplasia of the transverse and distal aortic arches. Prenatally, coarctation may be difficult to detect as long as the ductus arteriosus remains widely patent. With closure of the ductus arteriosus postnatally, ductal tissue extending circumferentially around the descending aorta and isthmus constricts, allowing a previously unrecognized coarctation to become manifest.

As a result, the prenatal detection and diagnosis of coarctation remains challenging, particularly with relatively discrete forms of the disease.[176-178] Mild and moderate forms of coarctation may appear normal prenatally. More severe forms of coarctation, however, commonly result in abnormalities of the 4CV and outflow tracts (Fig. 19-54). The right atrium and ventricle commonly appear larger than expected (right heart disproportion), probably related to redistribution of flow to the right side of the heart, and color flow imaging may detect some degree of tricuspid regurgitation. A persistent LSVC draining to the coronary sinus represents a commonly associated finding[108] and should increase the suspicion for coarctation of the aorta. Evaluation of the outflow tracts should again demonstrate right heart disproportion. Because a bicommissural aortic valve is another commonly associated finding, the aortic valve may appear mildly thickened or eccentric. The aortic valve annulus, aortic root, transverse aortic arch, and aortic isthmus may all appear small. Quantitative measurements of the aortic annulus and arch may be useful.[82,98,178] Finally, in the presence of coarctation, the third main branch of the aortic arch, the left subclavian artery, may have its origin somewhat distally displaced, closer to the isthmus than normal.

More severe forms of coarctation of the aorta represent ductal-dependent lesions requiring initiation of prostaglandin after delivery to maintain systemic cardiac output. These patients require neonatal repair, via either transcatheter dilation or surgical correction. Prenatal detection may prevent the inadvertent discharge to home of a newborn with severe coarctation whose ductus arteriosus has not yet closed.[39] Unless end-organ damage occurs at home before the diagnosis is made, the prognosis is generally excellent for isolated coarctation of the aorta. However, up to 50% of cases with neonatal repair require reintervention for recoarctation, and many patients, even with successful repair, have lifelong systemic hypertension.

Tetralogy of Fallot

TOF represents both the most common form of cyanotic CHD and the most common major CHD associated with a normal 4CV. Although most cases of TOF occur in isolation, TOF is also one of the most common forms of CHD associated with maternal diabetes, trisomy 21, DiGeorge syndrome,[179] omphalocele, and pentalogy of Cantrell, among other conditions.[23] TOF comprises a series of four cardiac findings, all believed to be related to anterior, superior, and rightward deviation of the conal septum into the RVOT. As a result of this deviation of the conal septum, TOF manifests with pulmonary stenosis, malalignment VSD, overriding aorta, and, postnatally, right ventricular hypertrophy secondary to persistent exposure of the right ventricle to systemic pressure. The detection, management, and prognosis of TOF depend on details of the anatomy and physiology. The following categories of TOF are discussed in this section: TOF with pulmonary stenosis, TOF with pulmonary atresia (TOF/PA), and TOF with absent pulmonary valve (TOF/APV).

Tetralogy of Fallot with Pulmonary Stenosis

In TOF with pulmonary stenosis, the degree of RVOT obstruction and the degree of hypoplasia of the main and branch pulmonary arteries determine the extent of cyanosis after delivery, the timing for initial surgical intervention, and, to some degree, the prognosis. The pulmonary stenosis in a fetus with TOF usually progresses prenatally, although at a variable rate.[16,81]

In a fetus with TOF with pulmonary stenosis, the 4CV is usually normal. Occasionally, the right ventricle appears slightly dilated or hypertrophied. Evaluation of the outflow tracts demonstrates a large malalignment VSD beneath the aortic valve and an overriding aorta (Fig. 19-55; see Figs. 19-37 and 19-38).[180,181] The pulmonary valve appears small and thickened (see Fig. 19-38) in all but the mildest cases, and the main and branch pulmonary arteries typically appear somewhat hypoplastic.

Patients with TOF with pulmonary stenosis may or may not require any neonatal intervention. After postnatal confirmation of the diagnosis, those with mild pulmonary stenosis may be discharged home without neonatal surgery or medical treatment, with definitive repair planned for sometime during the first year of life. Those with more severe pulmonary stenosis will require earlier surgical intervention, either primary intracardiac repair (reconstruction of the RVOT and closure of the VSD) or early placement of an aortopulmonary shunt

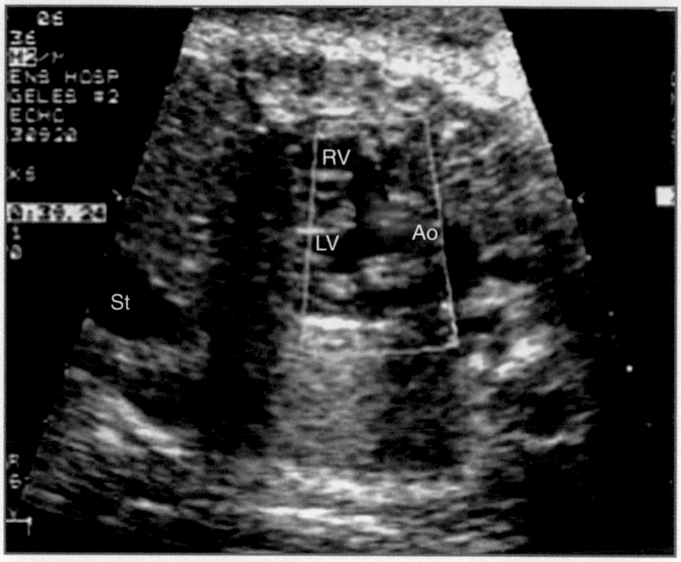

FIGURE 19-55 Fetal echocardiographic image of tetralogy of Fallot demonstrated in left ventricular long-axis view. Compare with Figure 19-37. Color flow demonstrates right-to-left shunting across the malalignment ventricular septal defect. Ao, aorta; LV, left ventricle; RV, right ventricle; St, fetal stomach.

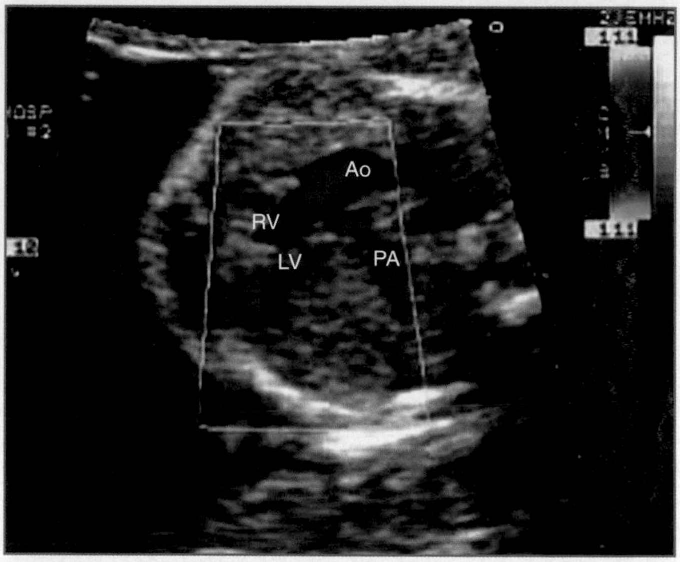

FIGURE 19-56 Fetal echocardiographic image of tetralogy of Fallot with pulmonary atresia. Color flow imaging demonstrates retrograde flow into the pulmonary artery, helping to distinguish this lesion from truncus arteriosus. Ao, aorta; LV, left ventricle; PA, pulmonary artery; RV, right ventricle.

(to augment pulmonary blood flow) followed by intracardiac repair later during the first year. The outlook for these patients is generally excellent,[180] although those with more severely affected pulmonary valves may require multiple pulmonary valve replacements over a lifetime.

Tetralogy of Fallot with Pulmonary Atresia

In TOF/PA the lungs receive their blood supply either from retrograde flow through the ductus arteriosus or through multiple aortopulmonary collaterals arising from various points along the aortic arch. Patients with ductal-dependent pulmonary blood flow usually have well-formed pulmonary arteries; their long-term prognosis is excellent and is comparable to that of patients with TOF and severe pulmonary stenosis. In contrast, patients with pulmonary blood flow dependent on aortopulmonary collaterals usually have severely hypoplastic or absent true pulmonary arteries and face a much more guarded long-term prognosis.

TOF/PA, like TOF with pulmonary stenosis, typically exhibits a normal 4CV prenatally. Evaluation of the outflow tracts demonstrates an atretic pulmonary valve and, often, absence of the main pulmonary artery.[181] Patients with ductal-dependent pulmonary blood flow have a large, tortuous ductus arteriosus flowing into hypoplastic but relatively well-formed branch pulmonary arteries (Fig. 19-56). In contrast, patients with collateral-dependent pulmonary blood flow have severely hypoplastic or absent pulmonary arteries, an absent ductus arteriosus, and multiple aortopulmonary collaterals visible with color flow imaging of the aortic arch.[144]

After delivery, some patients with TOF/PA may require cardiac catheterization to visualize the source of pulmonary blood flow. Patients with ductal-dependent pulmonary blood flow may undergo neonatal placement of an aortopulmonary shunt. Those patients with collateral-dependent pulmonary blood flow face a far more complicated course, requiring case-specific medical and surgical management, and a much more guarded prognosis.

Tetralogy of Fallot with Absent Pulmonary Valve

TOF/APV represents an unusual lesion with risks for both cardiac and pulmonary complications. In TOF/APV, primitive, donut-shaped pulmonary valve tissue causes both pulmonary stenosis and pulmonary regurgitation. As a result, the right ventricle and tricuspid valve annulus dilate, frequently causing tricuspid regurgitation and the potential for CHF, or even hydrops, prenatally. Typically, the ductus arteriosus is absent, even during fetal life. The combination of an augmented right ventricular stroke volume and absent ductus arteriosus causes the branch pulmonary arteries to dilate aneurysmally. As a result, patients with TOF/APV may be born with pulmonary hypoplasia or severe airway disease, or both, related to chronic extrinsic compression by markedly dilated pulmonary arteries during fetal life.

Unlike simple forms of TOF, TOF/APV manifests typically during fetal life with both an abnormal 4CV and abnormal outflow tracts.[182-184] Because of the pulmonary regurgitation, the right ventricle typically appears dilated. With significant stretch of the tricuspid valve annulus, tricuspid regurgitation may cause right atrial enlargement. In addition, elevated right ventricular diastolic pressure contributes to right atrial enlargement. Scanning into the LVOT demonstrates the malalignment VSD and overriding aorta. Angulation toward the RVOT demonstrates a small, donut-like pulmonary valve annulus, with pulmonary stenosis and regurgitation seen with color flow imaging. Probably the most recognizable features of TOF/APV are its aneurysmally dilated branch pulmonary arteries (Fig. 19-57), which may resemble "Mickey Mouse" ears and may appear to pulsate.

After delivery, many newborns with TOF/APV suffer from pulmonary hypoplasia or severe airway disease. This type of presentation carries a poor prognosis. Many infants without respiratory compromise have a good long-term prognosis,[182-184] albeit with multiple pulmonary valve replacements during a lifetime. Because patients with TOF/APV typically do not have a ductus arteriosus, prostaglandin

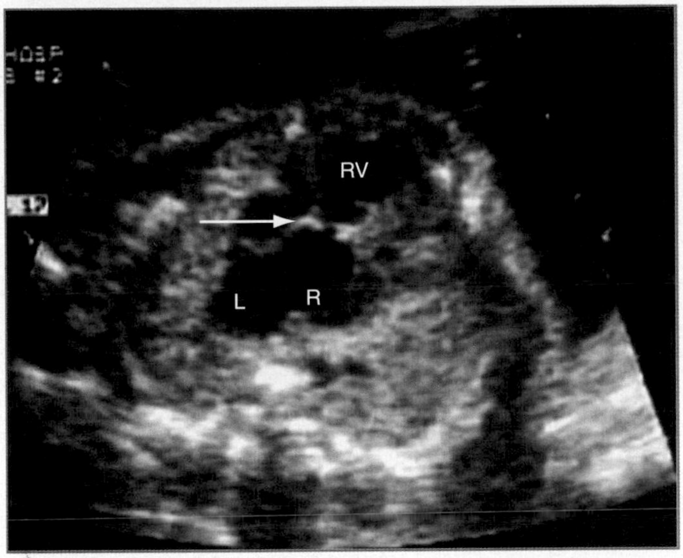

FIGURE 19-57 Fetal echocardiographic image of tetralogy of Fallot with absent pulmonary valve. Primitive tissue at the level of the pulmonary annulus *(arrow)* allows for both pulmonary stenosis and pulmonary regurgitation, which in turn leads to aneurysmal dilation of the branch pulmonary arteries and dilation of the right ventricle. L, left pulmonary artery; R, right pulmonary artery; RV, right ventricle.

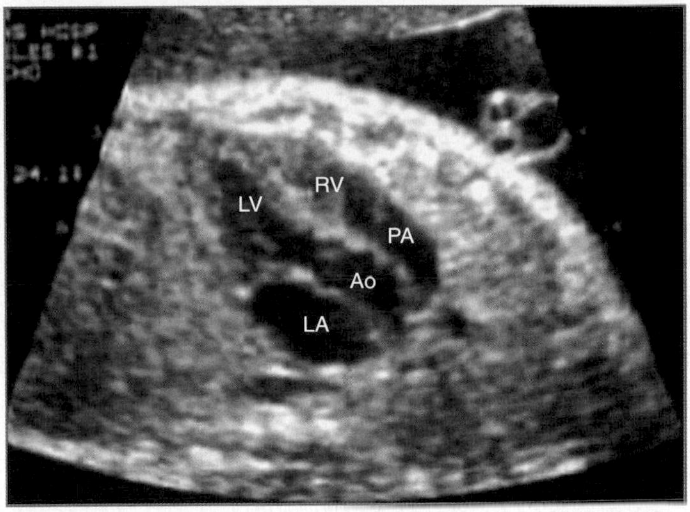

FIGURE 19-58 Fetal echocardiographic image of transposition of the great arteries. Note the absence of crossing of the great arteries. Ao, aorta; LA, left atrium; LV, left ventricle; PA, pulmonary artery; RV, right ventricle.

generally has little benefit during the neonatal period. Those infants without respiratory compromise need detailed echocardiographic and clinical evaluation to determine the appropriate timing for surgical intervention.

Double-outlet Right Ventricle

DORV represents a heterogeneous group of congenital heart defects that have in common the origin of both great arteries from the right ventricle. Technically, DORV also implies mitral-aortic discontinuity, with conal tissue beneath both great arteries. Because of varying size and location of the VSD, as well as variable degrees of pulmonary stenosis, infants with DORV may present with the pathophysiology of TOF, TGA, VSD, or single ventricle. DORV also commonly occurs in conjunction with other structural defects.[185] Neonatal management and prognosis vary accordingly.

Although some cases of DORV exhibit a large VSD or ventricular asymmetry on the 4CV, virtually all fetuses with DORV have abnormalities of the outflow tracts.[180] The left ventricular long-axis view does not demonstrate the aorta arising from the left ventricle. Instead, the aorta is seen to arise entirely or in part from the right ventricle. The pulmonary artery similarly arises entirely or in part from the right ventricle. If either great artery arises partially from the left and partially from the right ventricle, a VSD will be seen immediately beneath the straddling great artery. In addition, in DORV, the relative spatial relationship between the aortic and pulmonary valves may vary considerably. The great arteries in DORV commonly, but not always, lack the normal crossing seen in hearts with normally related great arteries. Finally, DORV typically manifests with pulmonary stenosis, and rarely with aortic stenosis. As with other cardiac lesions, pulmonary stenosis commonly coexists with pulmonary artery hypoplasia, and aortic stenosis commonly coexists with aortic arch hypoplasia and coarctation of the aorta.

The approach to management of DORV in the neonate requires detailed clinical and echocardiographic evaluation after delivery, because details of the anatomy and pathophysiology dictate the medical and surgical approach. Prognosis varies from that of mild TOF (excellent) to that of HLHS with hypoplastic pulmonary arteries (very poor).[180]

Transposition of the Great Arteries

In TGA, the aorta arises from the right ventricle, and the pulmonary artery arises from the left ventricle. Management and prognosis vary widely, depending on details of the anatomy and pathophysiology. Two major types of TGA have been described: dextro- or D-TGA and levo- or L-TGA. These are discussed separately.

D-TGA

Generally, D-TGA refers to TGA in which the visceral situs is normal (stomach on the left and liver on the right) and the ventricular looping is normal (D-looped). In D-TGA, the aortic valve is typically anterior and rightward of the pulmonary valve. As a result, systemic venous return passes from right atrium to right ventricle to aorta, and pulmonary venous return passes from left atrium to left ventricle to pulmonary artery. The patient with D-TGA may or may not have a VSD, other cardiac abnormalities, or heterotaxy.[110,157]

The fetus with isolated D-TGA usually has an entirely normal 4CV but markedly abnormal views of the outflow tracts.[180] Any restriction to flow at the level of the foramen ovale should be noted with spectral and color flow Doppler evaluations,[18,186] because newborns with restricted interatrial communications may require emergent balloon atrial septostomies, something not available at most hospitals. Unlike normally related great arteries, the great arteries in D-TGA do not cross each other (Fig. 19-58; see Fig. 19-39). Instead, the pulmonary artery arises from the left ventricle and heads posteriorly, and the aorta arises from the right ventricle and heads superiorly to give off the head and neck vessels before joining the descending aorta at the isthmus. In addition, in D-TGA, the pulmonary valve and main pulmonary artery (both arising from the left ventricle) should appear slightly larger than the aortic valve and aortic root (both arising from the right ventricle). The ductus arteriosus should be evaluated with 2D imaging and color/spectral Doppler for evidence of ductal constriction.[18,186]

The newborn with D-TGA usually is dependent on the ductus arteriosus for adequate oxygenation. In addition, unless a large VSD is present, oxygenation relies on a large atrial communication. As a result, patients with D-TGA usually require prostaglandin infusion and may require balloon atrial septostomy relatively emergently after delivery. Subsequently, patients with straightforward D-TGA usually undergo the arterial switch operation within the first 1 to 2 weeks after delivery. The prognosis can be excellent but depends largely on associated cardiac (see Fig. 19-39) and extracardiac abnormalities.[180]

L-TGA

The term L-TGA describes the heart with normal visceral situs, L-looped ventricles, and TGA. Usually, in L-TGA, the aortic valve sits anterior and leftward of the pulmonary valve. In L-TGA, the systemic venous return passes from right atrium to left ventricle to pulmonary artery, and the pulmonary venous return passes from left atrium to right ventricle to aorta. For this reason, L-TGA has been described as "congenitally corrected transposition." In many cases, however, L-TGA occurs in conjunction with a VSD, Ebstein anomaly of the left-sided tricuspid valve, heart block, pulmonary stenosis/atresia, or some combination of these. Such associated abnormalities affect the prenatal and postnatal presentation, management, and prognosis.

Typically, L-TGA manifests in the fetus with both an abnormal 4CV and abnormal outflow tracts.[187,188] L-looped ventricles are present on the 4CV, with a left ventricle anterior and rightward of a posterior and leftward right ventricle (Fig. 19-59). The right ventricle can be distinguished from the left ventricle by the presence of coarse trabeculations and moderator band, and by a tricuspid valve that inserts onto the ventricular septum slightly more apically than the left ventricle's mitral valve. In addition, those fetuses with associated Ebstein anomaly of the tricuspid valve, which is always associated with the right ventricle, have that lesion's characteristic findings (but with left atrial rather than right atrial dilation). Imaging of the outflow tracts demonstrates absence of crossing of one outflow over the other. The aortic valve, arising anterior and leftward of the pulmonary valve, gives rise to the aorta, which heads superiorly. In contrast, the pulmonary valve, arising posterior and rightward of the aortic valve, gives rise to the pulmonary artery, which heads posteriorly. Pulmonary stenosis or atresia is detectable with 2D and color flow imaging and may affect the development of the main and branch pulmonary arteries. The presence of a VSD may be seen on either the 4CV or outflow tract views, depending on the size and location of the VSD: The more anterior the VSD, the more likely it is to be seen with imaging of the outflow tracts, and the less likely to be seen on the 4CV. Finally, heart block may develop at any time prenatally or after birth and may be documented with 2D imaging, spectral Doppler, or M-mode evaluation (see later discussion).

After delivery, patients with straightforward L-TGA may not require any intervention, even for many years. However, the presence of any associated abnormalities may require neonatal or subsequent medical or surgical intervention. All patients require close clinical, echocardiographic, and electrocardiographic evaluation postnatally. Long-term prognosis varies widely, but, without surgery, all patients remain at risk for heart failure and arrhythmias because of their systemic right ventricle.[187,188]

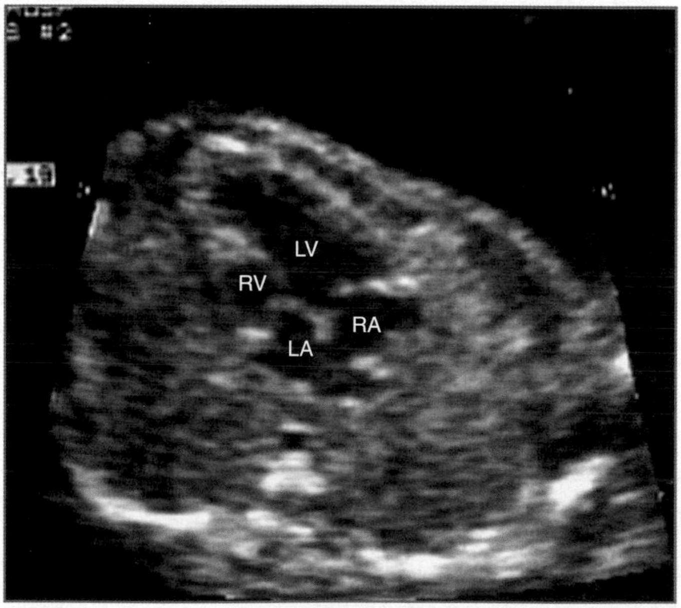

FIGURE 19-59 Fetal echocardiographic image of the four-chamber view demonstrating congenitally corrected transposition of the great arteries. Note the presence of a smooth-walled left ventricle anteriorly and rightward and a more trabeculated right ventricle posteriorly and leftward. The tricuspid valve, associated with the right ventricle, inserts more apically onto the ventricular septum than does the right-sided mitral valve. LA, left atrium; LV, left ventricle; RA, right atrium; RV, right ventricle.

Truncus Arteriosus

Truncus arteriosus represents a complex conotruncal malformation wherein a single arterial trunk arises from the heart and gives rise to the systemic, pulmonary, and coronary circulations. Truncus arteriosus arises from abnormal development of the truncal ridges and aortopulmonary septum and carries a strong association with DiGeorge syndrome.[23] Most cases have no ductus arteriosus during fetal life, except in the rare form associated with interrupted aortic arch.

Prenatally, truncus arteriosus exhibits a normal 4CV but markedly abnormal outflow tract views.[180,189,190] The truncal valve commonly appears mildly thickened, overrides a large VSD, and may have some degree of regurgitation on color flow imaging. The pulmonary arteries arise from the truncal root either as a common main pulmonary artery (Fig. 19-60) or as separate origins of right and left branch pulmonary arteries. It can be difficult to differentiate truncus arteriosus from TOF/PA prenatally. Both lesions show a single semilunar valve overriding a VSD. Both lesions have a normal 4CV, and both have strong associations with DiGeorge syndrome.[23] The distinction may be made, however, by assessing the direction of blood flow within the pulmonary arteries. In the case of TOF/PA, blood flow in the pulmonary arteries is retrograde from the ductus arteriosus (see Fig. 19-56), or it may not be seen at all in the case of collateral-dependent pulmonary blood flow. In truncus arteriosus, blood from the pulmonary arteries is prograde from the truncal root. In addition, whereas the aortic valve in TOF/PA usually appears large but thin and delicate, the truncal valve in truncus arteriosus typically appears somewhat thickened, eccentric, and, occasionally, regurgitant.

After delivery, all patients require close clinical and echocardiographic evaluation, as well as evaluation for DiGeorge syndrome. Commonly, patients with truncus arteriosus undergo surgical repair within the first few weeks after delivery, with VSD closure and placement of a pulmonary homograft into the RVOT. As with TOF/PA, the

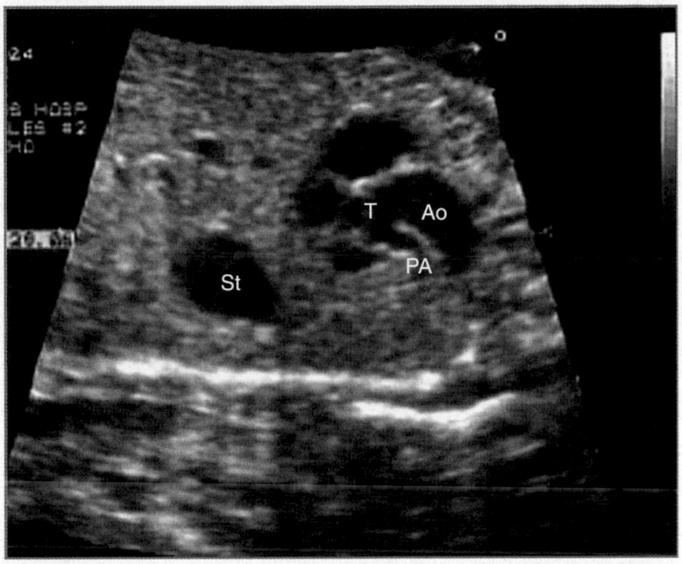

FIGURE 19-60 Fetal echocardiographic sagittal image of truncus arteriosus. The pulmonary artery arises from the proximal truncal root. Ao, aorta; PA, pulmonary artery; St, stomach; T, truncal root.

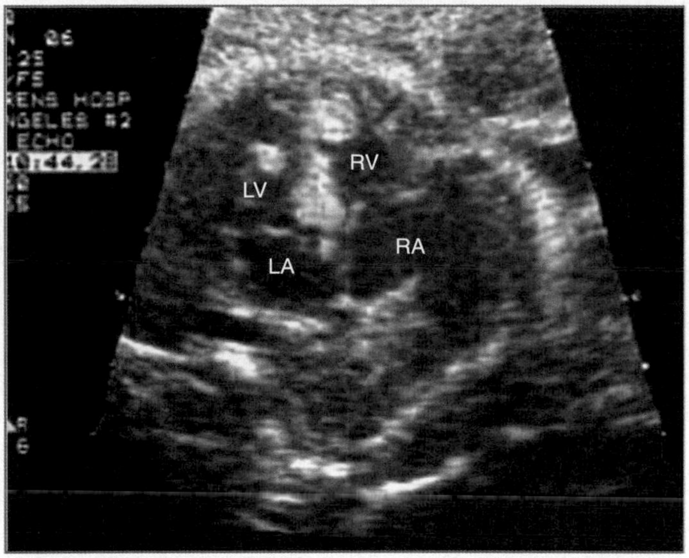

FIGURE 19-61 Fetal echocardiographic image of four-chamber view demonstrating multiple ventricular rhabdomyomas. LA, left atrium; LV, left ventricle; RA, right atrium; RV, right ventricle.

pulmonary homograft will require multiple replacements during a lifetime. Long term prognosis depends on the associated abnormalities and truncal valve function but can be quite good if all goes well.[189,190]

Cardiac Tumors

Fetal cardiac tumors, although rarely malignant in the oncologic sense, may be life-threatening in their own right or may be associated with systemic syndromes. This section reviews two of the most common cardiac tumors seen in the fetus: rhabdomyoma and intrapericardial teratoma. Both appear to have their greatest period of growth from mid-gestation to term. Readers may consult other sources for more detailed discussions of fetal cardiac tumors.[8,9,152,153,191,192]

Cardiac Rhabdomyoma

By far the most common fetal cardiac tumor,[191,192] cardiac rhabdomyoma may occur as an isolated, single cardiac mass or, more commonly, as a collection of well-circumscribed tumors. In a substantial percentage of cases, cardiac rhabdomyomas occur as one manifestation of tuberous sclerosis.[193,194] Although tuberous sclerosis may be associated with significant neurologic disease, including seizures, developmental delay, and cognitive impairment,[23] cardiac rhabdomyomas often do not cause cardiovascular pathology, either prenatally or after delivery. Occasionally, however, cardiac rhabdomyomas may become obstructive to flow in or out of one or both ventricles, may adversely affect myocardial function, may generate atrial or ventricular arrhythmias, and may be associated with WPW syndrome. In the absence of fetal arrhythmias, diminished ventricular function, obstruction to flow, or CHF, the fetus with cardiac rhabdomyomas rarely will develop cardiovascular pathology postnatally, short of SVT in the presence of WPW. In fact, cardiac rhabdomyomas typically regress or remain stable in size postnatally,[193,194] in contrast to other tumors, which may grow substantially after delivery.

The diagnosis of cardiac rhabdomyomas can generally be made from a 4CV. Most cardiac rhabdomyomas manifest as echogenic, homogeneous, well-circumscribed masses within or extending partially into the ventricular free wall or ventricular septum or both (Fig. 19-61). Rarely, cardiac rhabdomyomas reside predominantly within the walls of the right or left atrium. In contrast, benign echogenic reflectors or foci reside exclusively within the chordal apparatus of the mitral or tricuspid valves and do not extend into the ventricular myocardium.

The fetus with suspected cardiac rhabdomyomas should be evaluated thoroughly for tuberous sclerosis, possibly including sonography, magnetic resonance imaging, and/or genetic means of analysis. After delivery, affected infants should again undergo comprehensive evaluation for tuberous sclerosis, a repeat echocardiographic evaluation, and an electrocardiogram to assess for WPW. Long-term prognosis, from a cardiovascular standpoint, is excellent if no significant rhythm, ventricular dysfunction, or hemodynamic obstruction manifests during the late fetal or neonatal periods.

Intrapericardial Teratoma

The intrapericardial teratoma is probably the second most common primary fetal cardiac tumor. Like the cardiac rhabdomyoma, it may be considered benign in the oncologic sense,[8,152,191,192] but affected fetuses may develop CHF or hydrops secondary to progressive enlargement of the pericardial effusion. Histologically, the intrapericardial teratoma represents a combination of cystic areas, lined by various forms of epithelium, surrounded by solid areas composed of muscle, nerve, pancreas, cartilage, thyroid, or bone tissues. Intrapericardial teratomas typically arise from the ascending aorta and secrete fluid into the pericardial space. Over time, the expanding pericardial effusion can impede cardiac output, and the resultant tamponade physiology can result in fetal demise. After delivery, mass effect of the tumor may impede cardiac output or cause respiratory compromise by compressing the trachea or mainstem bronchi.[195]

The diagnosis of intrapericardial teratoma may be suspected in the fetus with a pericardial effusion in conjunction with a heterogeneous, cystic mass with areas of calcification that arises from the ascending aorta (Fig. 19-62). After the diagnosis is made, affected fetuses require close observation and may benefit from pericardiocentesis for progres-

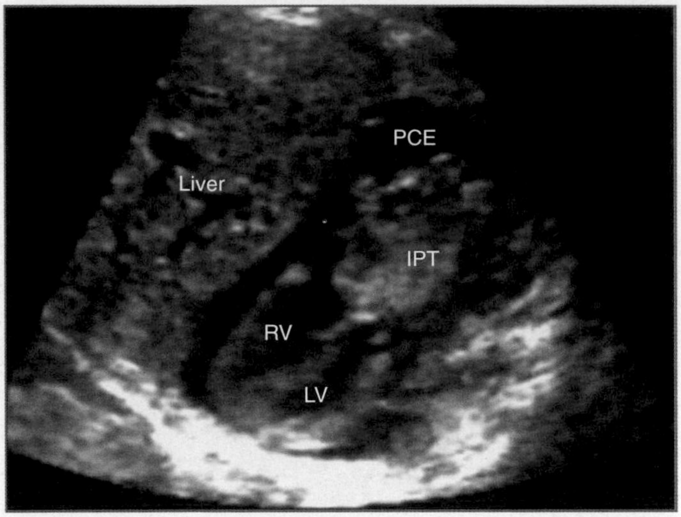

FIGURE 19-62 Fetal echocardiographic image of intrapericardial teratoma arising from the ascending aorta. Note the heterogeneous appearance of the tumor. IPT, intrapericardial teratoma; LV, left ventricle; PCE, pericardial effusion; RV, right ventricle.

TABLE 19-7 FETAL ARRHYTHMIAS

Irregular Rhythm
Premature atrial contractions/couplets
Second-degree heart block
Sustained Bradycardia
Sinus bradycardia
Atrial bradycardia
Blocked atrial bigeminy
Atrial flutter with high-degree block
Complete heart block
Sustained Tachycardia
Sinus tachycardia
Supraventricular tachycardia
Atrial flutter
Ventricular tachycardia

sive enlargement of the pericardial effusion and worsening tamponade.[195] Delivery should be arranged to allow for rapid intubation, if necessary, and subsequent early surgical resection of the tumor. Long-term prognosis after expeditious, early resection is excellent, with little chance for recurrence.

Fetal Arrhythmias: Diagnosis, Management, and Prognosis

This section reviews the diagnosis, management, and prognosis of the most common and important fetal arrhythmias (Table 19-7), with a distinctively clinical approach. For more detailed discussions of fetal arrhythmias, readers may refer to other, more comprehensive reviews.[8,9,152,196-198]

Beyond demonstrating a normal transverse abdominal view, 4CV, and standard views of the outflow tracts, the normal fetal screening

TABLE 19-8 ANTIARRHYTHMIC MEDICATIONS FOR FETAL ARRHYTHMIAS

Fetal Arrhythmia	Potential Treatments*
Premature atrial/ventricular contractions	None
Atrial bigeminy (blocked or conducted)	None
Nonsustained SVT	Usually none (see text)
Sustained SVT	Digoxin
	Flecainide
	Amiodarone
	Propranolol
Atrial flutter	Digoxin
	Sotalol
	Propranolol
	Amiodarone
Ventricular tachycardia	Propranolol
	Sotalol
	Mexiletine
	Amiodarone
First/second/third-degree heart block (positive antibodies)	Dexamethasone?

***Note that all antiarrhythmic medications have the potential for serious, possibly fatal maternal and/or fetal proarrhythmia. Treatment of a specific fetus for an arrhythmia should be done only after careful consideration of anticipated benefits and potential risks and after full disclosure has been made to the mother.**
SVT, supraventricular tachycardia.

ultrasound evaluation should demonstrate physiologic rate and variability of the fetal heartbeat. The fetal heart rate should be physiologic (120 to 160 beats/min) and should have physiologic variability (small but real changes in heart rate during scanning, with prolonged or severe bradycardia only during periods of deep transducer pressure). Abnormal variability (irregular beats or extrasystoles) and abnormalities in rate (sustained bradycardia or tachycardia) should be noted, evaluated, and, if appropriate, treated. Most fetal arrhythmias are benign, are self-resolving, and do not require treatment.[196-198] Treatment of a fetus for arrhythmia should be undertaken only after careful weighing of desired benefits against potential maternal and fetal complications and after full disclosure to the mother. Table 19-8 lists some of the most common antiarrhythmic medications used to treat fetal arrhythmias.

Premature Atrial Contractions

Premature atrial contractions (PACs), the most common fetal arrhythmia,[196-199] manifest as an irregularly irregular variability in fetal heart rate, usually beginning between 18 and 24 weeks' gestation, but occasionally appearing initially during the third trimester. The diagnosis of PACs typically is made empirically by observing the rhythm with 2D imaging. However, to confirm the diagnosis, spectral Doppler inflow and outflow evaluation of the left ventricle or M-mode analysis should be performed.

Normally, by orienting the ultrasound beam in parallel with both left ventricular inflow and outflow (Fig. 19-63), spectral Doppler evaluation of sinus rhythm will demonstrate a biphasic inflow pattern for every atrial contraction (i.e., early passive filling followed by atrial contraction) and a single, uniphasic outflow pattern after each ventricular contraction (Fig. 19-64).[200,201] PACs, by definition, come early, and they typically lack the early passive filling component (E wave) of the Doppler waveform (Fig. 19-65). Alternatively, M-mode

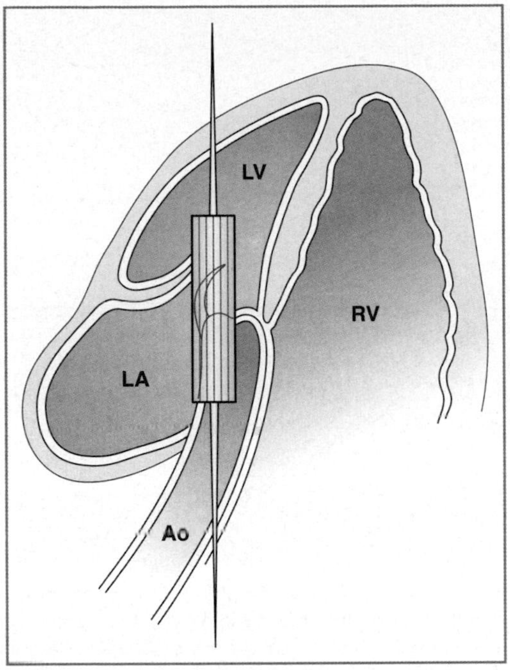

FIGURE 19-63 **Schematic diagram of left ventricular inflow and outflow.** The Doppler cursor is positioned in parallel with mitral and aortic flows to assist with the diagnosis of fetal arrhythmias. Ao, aorta; LA, left atrium; LV, left ventricle; RV, right ventricle. (Diagram courtesy of Irving R. Tessler, M.D.)

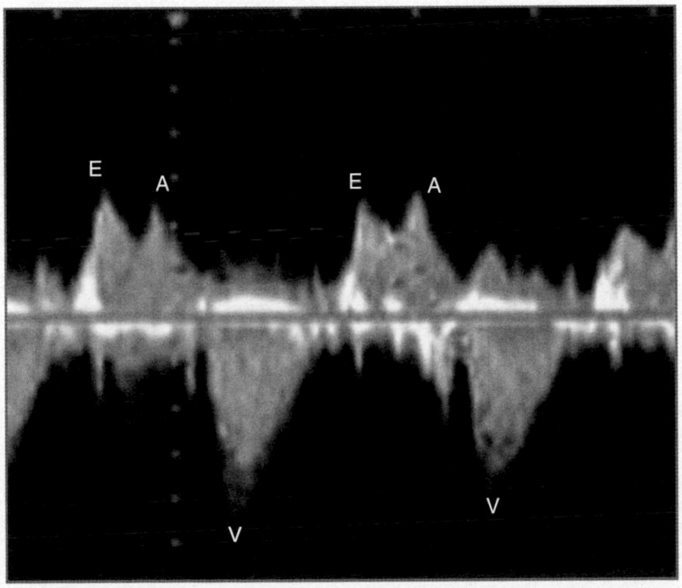

FIGURE 19-64 **Fetal Doppler waveform obtained from left ventricular inflow and outflow demonstrating sinus rhythm.** The Doppler cursor is positioned as in Figure 19-63. Note the biphasic mitral inflow, with passive early inflow (E wave) followed by atrial contraction (A wave). Each mitral inflow pattern is followed by single outflow. A, atrial contraction; E, early passive filling; V, ventricular contraction.

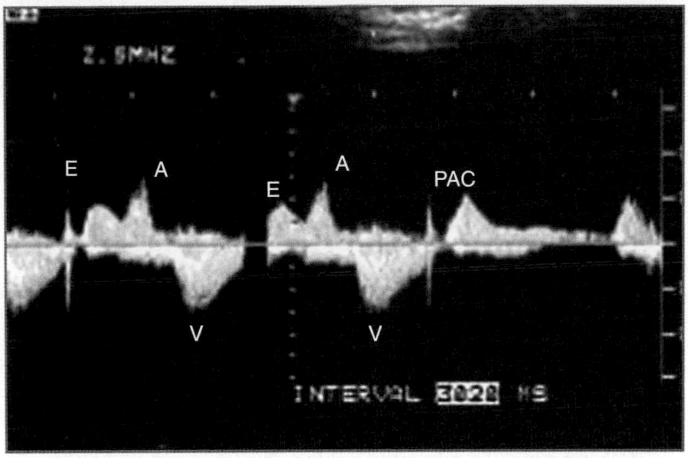

FIGURE 19-65 **Fetal Doppler waveform obtained from left ventricular inflow and outflow demonstrating sinus rhythm with premature atrial contraction.** The Doppler cursor is positioned as in Figure 19-63. The premature atrial contraction (PAC) comes early and is monophasic; it is blocked (i.e., not followed by ventricular contraction). A, atrial contraction; E, early passive filling; V, ventricular contraction.

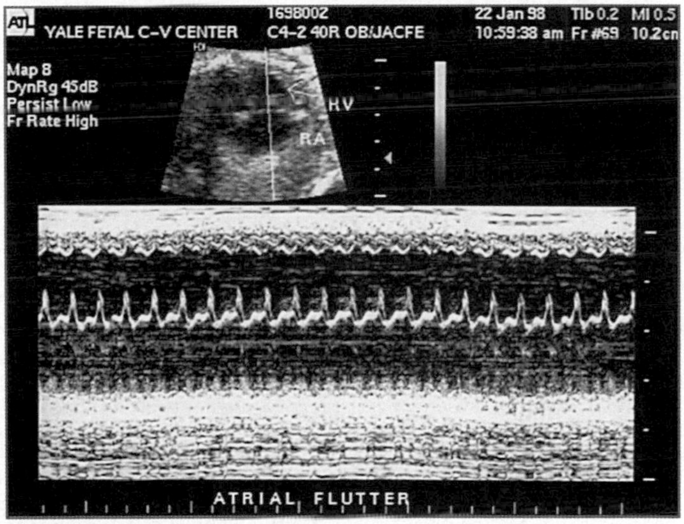

FIGURE 19-66 **Fetal echocardiographic image of M-mode analysis of fetal arrhythmia.** The M-mode cursor is placed across the right atrium and right ventricle *(inset).* This M-mode image demonstrates atrial flutter. (Image courtesy of Charles Kleinman, MD, Joshua Copel, MD, and Rodrigo Nehgme, MD.)

echocardiography allows visualization of atrial and ventricular contractions simultaneously when, guided by a 2D image, the M-mode sampling line is directed through the fetal atrium and ventricle (Fig. 19-66).[202] Other. more sophisticated approaches to evaluating fetal arrhythmias have also been developed.[101]

Rarely, PACs are associated with intermittent SVT. PACs may be exacerbated by ingestion of caffeine, decongestant medications (stimulants), or tobacco. Typically, PACs resolve spontaneously within 2 to 3 weeks after diagnosis. PACs do not represent any real risk to the fetus, and they do not require treatment. However, a small percentage of fetuses with isolated PACs develop SVT. Referral for further evaluation should be considered if concerns persist regarding the diagnosis or the possibility of additional arrhythmias or structural CHD.

Sustained Bradycardia

A sustained fetal heart rate of less than 120 beats/min represents fetal bradycardia and merits further evaluation. In contrast, fetal bradycardia related to deep transducer pressure or a particular maternal lie might represent a normal fetal response to stress. In such cases, if the fetal heart rate normalizes after relief of transducer pressure or change in maternal or fetal position, no further cardiac evaluation may be necessary.

The differential diagnosis of fetal bradycardia includes sinus bradycardia, atrial bradycardia, blocked atrial bigeminy, atrial flutter with high-degree block, and complete heart block. Treatment approaches and prognosis depend on the precise diagnosis. Sinus bradycardia, manifesting with a slow rate but with physiologic variability and with 1:1 conduction between the atria and ventricles, may represent fetal distress and therefore should prompt a thorough evaluation of fetal well-being and placental function. Particularly if it is associated with some degree of heart block, fetal sinus bradycardia may, rarely, be the first sign of long QT syndrome.[203] Affected fetuses and newborns are at risk for ventricular tachycardia. For this reason, fetuses in good health that demonstrate unexplained sinus bradycardia without fetal distress should undergo electrocardiographic evaluation after delivery. In addition, because long QT syndrome may run in families, a family history for long QT syndrome, recurrent syncope, or sudden infant death syndrome should be sought. In contrast, atrial bradycardia may appear identical to sinus bradycardia, but it actually represents the normal rate of an accessory atrial pacemaker in the absence of an effective sinus node. Such an atrial bradycardia commonly occurs in conjunction with polysplenia, so the suspicion of this rhythm should prompt evaluation for the cardiac and abdominal abnormalities seen with polysplenia.[106,110,157]

Occasionally, fetal sinus bradycardia represents blocked atrial bigeminy, in which normal sinus beats alternate with blocked PACs. In atrial bigeminy, the premature beats may be blocked if they occur very early, when the atrioventricular node is still refractory. In such cases, only sinus beats conduct, generating a uniform ventricular rate exactly half of the atrial rate. No specific therapy is warranted other than close observation and avoidance of caffeine, decongestant medications, and tobacco. Prognosis is excellent.

In some cases, atrial flutter may conduct consistently 3:1 or 4:1, and such fetuses may present with bradycardia. Close inspection of the heart with 2D imaging, M-mode, or spectral Doppler can diagnose the arrhythmia and assess the degree of conduction. Although atrial flutter usually has an atrial rate of 300 to 500 beats/min, high degrees of atrioventricular block may lead to fetal bradycardia; for example, atrial flutter with a flutter rate of 300 beats/min and a 3:1 conduction would present with a fetal ventricular rate of 100 beats/min. Unlike SVT, atrial flutter rarely manifests as intermittent tachycardia; flutter typically is incessant, although the ventricular response rate may vary. Like other fetal arrhythmias, fetal atrial flutter may be associated with structural heart disease. Treatment of atrial flutter, typically with maternal orally administered pharmacologic therapy (e.g., digoxin, sotalol, amiodarone) can slow the ventricular response rate and decrease the likelihood of development of fetal CHF or hydrops. Some investigators believe that sotalol has emerged as a potential first-line agent for the treatment of atrial flutter.[204]

Complete heart block (CHB) in the fetus typically manifests with a sustained fetal heart rate in the range of 40 to 70 beats/min (Fig. 19-67). In the fetus with complete heart block, the atrial rate remains normal but atrial contractions do not conduct to the ventricles. As a result, the ventricles depolarize with their own intrinsic rate. Approximately 50% of cases of fetal complete heart block occur in the presence of structural heart disease (L-looped ventricles, atrioventricular septal defects, or complex forms of heart disease associated with polysplenia).[157,196,205] These cases have a relatively poor prognosis, with a high rate of fetal demise related to progressive heart failure and hydrops. Therapy with maternal oral agents such as terbutaline or other sympathomimetics has not been shown to improve the outcome.

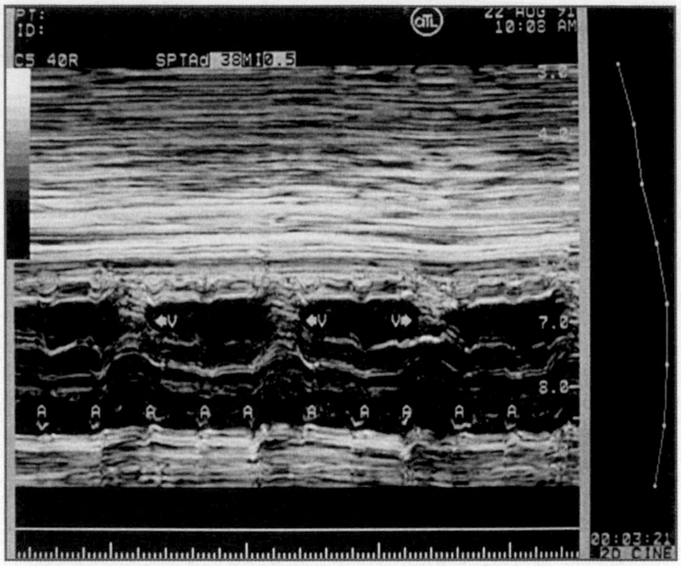

FIGURE 19-67 Fetal echocardiographic image of M-mode demonstration of complete heart block. A, atrial contraction; V, ventricular contraction. (Image courtesy of Charles Kleinman, MD, Joshua Copel, MD, and Rodrigo Nehgme, MD.)

The other 50% of cases of fetal heart block occur secondary to damage to the fetal atrioventricular node by maternal anti-Ro and/or anti-La antibodies,[205-207] usually in the context of maternal systemic lupus erythematosus, Sjögren's syndrome, or related connective tissue disorders. In some of these cases, maternal treatment with dexamethasone has improved fetal outcome, probably by improving myocardial function in the face of presumptive immune-mediated myocarditis.[208-210] Some investigators have used sympathomimetics agents to increase ventricular rates in this setting, particularly for rates that remain slower than 55 beats/min,[211] but sustained increases in fetal heart rate have rarely been achieved. Pregnancies complicated by anti-Ro or anti-La antibodies carry a risk of approximately 1% for the development of fetal heart block,[212] and the recurrence rate for a second fetus with heart block in antibody-positive pregnancies may be as high as 15%.[207] Spectral Doppler evaluation of the fetal PR interval has been shown to be a useful way to identify fetuses in anti-Ro or anti-La antibody–positive pregnancies with evidence of atrioventricular node disease.[213,214] Treatment of fetuses at risk (first-, second-, or third-degree heart block in antibody-positive pregnancies) with dexamethasone may prevent the progression to CHB or otherwise improve outcome by enhancing myocardial function, but such management remains controversial.[208-210,215,216]

Sustained Tachycardia

SVT represents the great majority of instances of sustained fetal tachycardia. Sinus tachycardia represents an unusual response to fetal heart failure or distress. Fetal ventricular tachycardia occurs still far less commonly.

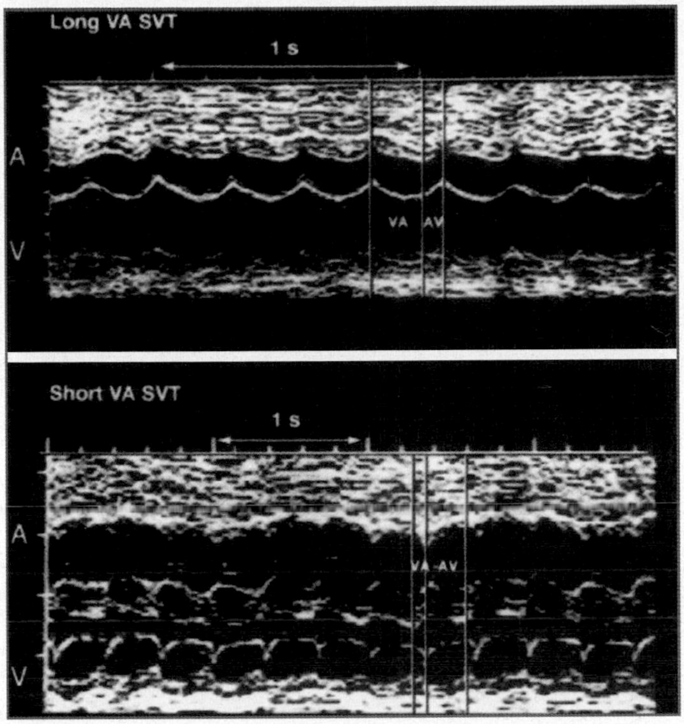

FIGURE 19-68 Fetal echocardiographic image of M-mode demonstration of two types of supraventricular tachycardia. In contrast to ventricular tachycardia, both types (i.e., long and short VA SVT) have 1 : 1 atrioventricular association. A, atrial contraction; AV, interval between atrial and ventricular contraction; SVT, supraventricular tachycardia; V, ventricular contraction; VA, interval between ventricular and atrial contraction. (Reproduced with permission from Jaeggi E, Fouron JC, Fournier A, et al: Ventriculo-atrial time interval measured on M-mode echocardiography: A determining element in diagnosis, treatment, and prognosis of fetal supraventricular tachycardia. Heart 79:582, 1998. Image courtesy of Charles Kleinman, MD, Joshua Copel, MD, and Rodrigo Nehgme, MD.)

Supraventricular Tachycardia

Fetal SVT typically occurs via an accessory pathway, although autonomic forms of fetal SVT also occur relatively commonly. Fetal SVT, usually in the range of 240 to 280 beats/min, occurs most frequently in fetuses with structurally normal hearts and rarely occurs in the setting of structural CHD. However, fetal SVT may be associated with WPW syndrome. The diagnosis of SVT may be suggested by 2D imaging, by spectral Doppler assessment of the left ventricular inflow and outflow tracts (see Fig. 19-63), or by M-mode analysis (Fig. 19-68). Ventricular tachycardia, which is typically slower but less well tolerated than SVT, may be associated with ventricular structural abnormalities or tumors or may occur in the context of long QT interval. Ventricular tachycardia can be difficult to discriminate from fetal SVT, even with M-mode or spectral Doppler analysis,[196,197,217] although ventricular tachycardia is typically far less well tolerated. Because fetal SVT typically manifests as an intermittent, nonsustained arrhythmia, the presence of PACs or atrial couplets can help strengthen the certainty of the diagnosis. Moreover, unlike ventricular tachycardia, SVT usually conducts 1 : 1 from atria to ventricles.

Although few would dispute treatment of fetal SVT in the face of hydrops and in the absence of lung maturity, no consensus exists on the approach to the second-trimester (or early third-trimester) fetus with SVT in the absence of hydrops.[196,197,217-219] As would be expected, SVT in a fetus with structural heart disease is far less well tolerated than SVT in one with a structurally normal heart. However, therapeutic strategies advocated for the nonhydropic, immature fetus with SVT remain largely divergent, ranging from treatment of any documented SVT to treatment only with the development of hydrops.[217] No consensus has been reached on the exact relationship between heart rate, type of SVT, and development of hydrops in the context of fetal SVT. Antiarrhythmic agents, dosing schedules, and routes of administration represent separate areas of controversy and disagreement, similarly without consensus.

Although each case may be handled somewhat differently, depending on patient characteristics and physician biases, the following represents our institution's approach. The presence of structural heart disease in the context of SVT lowers the tolerance for shortened diastolic filling times and elevated central venous pressure, so such fetuses typically receive treatment earlier than do fetuses with structurally normal hearts. When fetal SVT becomes complicated by hydrops, the threshold for treatment falls much further. In the absence of fetal structural heart disease or hydrops, fetal SVT usually receives treatment if the tachycardia occurs more than 33% of the time. However, beyond 32 to 34 weeks' gestation, many cases of fetal tachycardia may be better approached with delivery than with maternally administered medications, all of which have variable efficacy and carry the potential for both maternal and fetal toxicity. Before treatment, all potential precipitating factors (tobacco, decongestant medications, and caffeine) are withdrawn, and the fetal rhythm is monitored in-house for 8 to 24 hours to assess the percentage of time during which the fetus is in tachycardia. The mother is informed of all possible fetal and maternal risks to therapy, as well as the anticipated benefit to treatment. All antiarrhythmic agents have the potential for maternal and/or fetal proarrhythmia. Because maternal serum factors rarely may react with assays for digoxin,[220] a maternal serum digoxin level is determined, along with a set of electrolytes and creatinine. A maternal electrocardiogram and, ideally, consultation with an adult cardiologist is performed before therapy is initiated. The presence of WPW or other abnormality on the maternal electrocardiogram may contraindicate the use of certain forms of antiarrhythmic therapy (e.g., digoxin).

When indicated, and only in the absence of any contraindication, treatment may begin with a digoxin load, using 0.5 mg intravenously every 6 to 8 hours, with a maternal serum digoxin measurement and electrocardiogram performed before each dose. Loading continues until effect (<25% tachycardia or decreased hydrops or both), therapeutic level (2.0 μg/mL), maternal toxicity (maternal symptoms or electrocardiographic abnormalities beyond first-degree heart block), or fetal toxicity (worsening of arrhythmia) is reached, whichever comes first. After a desired effect has been safely achieved, digoxin is administered orally two to four times daily, usually at 0.25 to 0.5 mg per dose. Often, consultation with the hospital pharmacologist is useful. Patients are discharged after a steady state has been achieved with acceptable control of the fetal arrhythmia, acceptable maternal serum digoxin levels, and absence of maternal or fetal toxicity. However, close outpatient follow-up is essential to confirm continued effect and lack of toxicity, and occasionally to increase dosing as maternal volumes of distribution continue to increase during the second and third trimesters. If digoxin fails to achieve adequate control, second-line agents such as propranolol,[196,197] flecainide,[221] or amiodarone[222] may be substituted or added, but the potential for toxicity increases and the likelihood for efficacy decreases.[196,197]

Atrial Flutter

In contrast to fetal SVT, fetal atrial flutter ranges between 300 and 500 atrial contractions per minute, with a ventricular rate that may vary from less than 100 to more than 300 beats/min.[196,197,223] In atrial flutter, the atrioventricular node refractory periods may vary, occasionally producing 1:1 conduction but more typically allowing only every second or third atrial contraction to conduct to the ventricles (2:1 or 3:1 conduction, respectively) (see Fig. 19-66). Flutter usually manifests in a much more sustained fashion than does SVT, which commonly produces intermittent runs of tachycardia interspersed with periods of sinus rhythm. Compared with SVT, atrial flutter has a higher association with structural heart disease, although structural heart disease is still rare in the neonate with atrial flutter.[224] Finally, although flutter may be successfully treated with maternally administered digoxin, recent reports suggest that sotalol is an excellent second-line agent, and some centers have chosen sotalol as their first-line therapy for fetal atrial flutter.[204] Propranolol has also been used successfully to control the ventricular response rate in the fetus with atrial flutter.[197]

Ventricular Tachycardia

Ventricular tachycardia in the fetus, as in newborns and children, represents a commonly fatal arrhythmia when sustained. In part for this reason, fetal ventricular tachycardia is diagnosed far less often than fetal SVT, although fetal ventricular tachycardia is also far less common than fetal SVT. Fetal ventricular tachycardia usually manifests with fetal rates between 180 and 300 beats/min and, often, poor ventricular function. Discrimination of ventricular tachycardia from SVT can be challenging but is important, because digoxin is contraindicated for ventricular tachycardia. Unlike SVT, ventricular tachycardia has dissociation between atrial and ventricular contractions (Fig. 19-69). Ventricular tachycardia that is associated with structural heart disease carries a particularly poor prognosis. Fetal ventricular tachycardia has been associated with tumors (usually rhabdomyomas), structural heart disease (cardiomyopathy, severe right or left ventricular hypertrophy or coronary abnormalities), prolonged QT interval,[203] and fetal distress or acidosis. Lower ventricular rates (180 to 220 beats/min) may be better tolerated, with improved outcomes compared with higher ventricular rates. In some cases, treatment may be attempted with lidocaine (administered directly into the fetal umbilical vein) or with oral maternal administration of propranolol, mexiletine, sotalol, or amiodarone, but the prognosis remains guarded.[196,197,222]

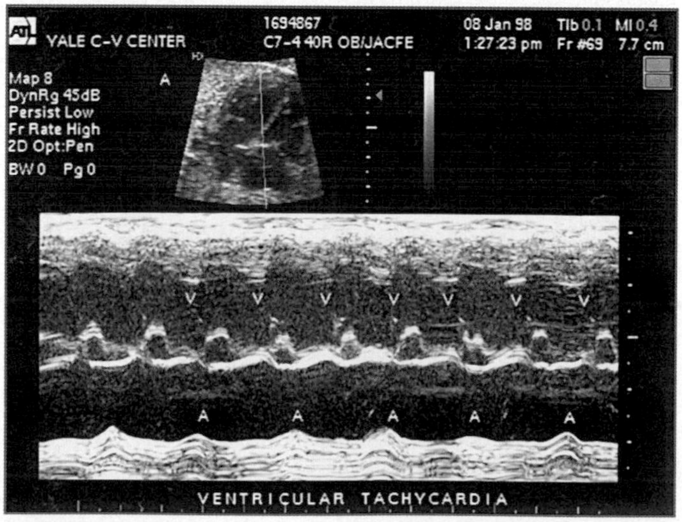

FIGURE 19-69 Fetal echocardiographic image of M-mode demonstration of ventricular tachycardia. Note atrioventricular dissociation, with ventricular rate faster than atrial rate. A, atrial contraction; V, ventricular contraction. (Image courtesy of Charles Kleinman, MD, Joshua Copel, MD, and Rodrigo Nehgme, MD.)

Conclusions

The detection, diagnosis, and management of fetal structural heart defects and arrhythmias remain important challenges for those involved in fetal screening ultrasonography or detailed evaluation of the fetal heart. The assessment and management of the fetal heart, in both low-risk and high-risk pregnancies, requires attention to detail, experience, and a collaborative effort among multiple specialists caring for the fetal patient.

References

1. Allan L, Benacerraf B, Copel J, et al: Isolated major congenital heart disease. Ultrasound Obstet Gynecol 17:370, 2001.
2. International Society of Ultrasound in Obstetrics and Gynecology: Cardiac screening examination of the fetus: Guidelines for performing the "basic" and "extended basic" cardiac scan. Ultrasound Obstet Gynecol 27:107, 2006.
3. Tegnander E, Eik-Nes S: The examiner's ultrasound experience has a significant impact on the detection rate of congenital heart defects at the second-trimester fetal examination. Ultrasound Obstet Gynecol 28:8, 2006.
4. Chaoui R: The four-chamber view: Four reasons why it seems to fail in screening for cardiac abnormalities and suggestions to improve detection rates. Ultrasound Obstet Gynecol 22:3, 2003.
5. Jaeggi E, Sholler G, Jones O, et al: Comparative analysis of pattern, management and outcome or pre- versus postnatally diagnosed major congenital heart disease: A population-based study. Ultrasound Obstet Gynecol 17:380, 2001.
6. Garne E, Stoll C, Clementi M; Euroscan Group: Evaluation of prenatal diagnosis of congenital heart diseases by ultrasound: Experience from 20 European registries. Ultrasound Obstet Gynecol 17:386, 2001.
7. Heide H, Thomson J, Wharton G, et al: Poor sensitivity of routine fetal anomaly ultrasound screening for antenatal detection of atrioventricular septal defect. Heart 90:916, 2004.
8. Allan L, Hornberger L, Sharland G (eds): Textbook of Fetal Cardiology. London, Greenwich Medical Media, 2000.
9. Yagel S, Silverman N, Gembruch U (eds): Fetal Cardiology. London, Martin Dunitz, 2003.
10. Centers for Disease Control and Prevention: Trends in infant mortality attributable to birth defects—United States, 1980-1995. MMWR Morb Mortal Wkly Rep 47:773, 1998.
11. Ferencz C, Rubin JD, Mc Carter RJ, et al: Congenital heart disease: Prevalence at live birth. The Baltimore-Washington Infant Study. Am J Epidemiol 121:31, 1985.
12. Hoffman J: Incidence of congenital heart disease: I. Postnatal incidence. Pediatr Cardiol 16:103, 1995.
13. Hoffman J, Christianson R: Congenital heart disease in a cohort of 19,502 births with long-term follow-up. Am J Cardiol 42:641, 1978.
14. Axt-Fliedner R, Schwarze A, Smrcek J, et al: Isolated ventricular septal defects detected by color Doppler imaging: Evolution during fetal and first year of postnatal life. Ultrasound Obstet Gynecol 27:266, 2006.
15. Smrcek J, Berg C, Geipel A, et al: Detection rate of early fetal echocardiography and in utero development of congenital heart defects. J Ultrasound Med 25:187, 2006.
16. Trines J, Hornberger LK: Evolution of heart disease in utero. Pediatr Cardiol 25:287, 2004.

17. Weber H, Kleinman C, Hellenbrand W, et al: Development of a benign intrapericardial tumor between 20 and 40 weeks of gestation. Pediatr Cardiol 9:153, 1988.
18. Maeno Y, Kamenir S, Sinclair B, et al: Prenatal features of ductus arteriosus constriction and restrictive foramen ovale in d-transposition of the great arteries. Circulation 99:1209, 1999.
19. Stumfplen I, Stumfplen A, Wimmer M, et al: Effect of detailed fetal echocardiography as part of routine prenatal ultrasonographic screening on detection of congenital heart disease. Lancet 348:854, 1996.
20. Cooper M, Enderlein M, Dyson D, et al: Fetal echocardiography: Retrospective review of clinical experience and an evaluation of indications. Obstet Gynecol 86:577, 1995.
21. Small M, Copel JA: Indications for fetal echocardiography. Pediatr Cardiol 25:210, 2004.
22. Carvalho J: The fetal heart or the lymphatic system or . . . ? The quest for the etiology of increased nuchal translucency. Ultrasound Obstet Gynecol 25:215, 2005.
23. Jones K. Smith's Recognizable Patterns of Human Malformation, 6th ed. Philadelphia, Elsevier Saunders, 2006.
24. Gill HK, Splitt M, Sharland GK, et al: Patterns of recurrence of congenital heart disease: An analysis of 6,640 consecutive pregnancies evaluated by detailed fetal echocardiography. J Am Coll Cardiol 42:923, 2003.
25. Milerad J, Larson O, Hagberg C, et al: Associated malformations in infants with cleft lip and palate: A prospective, population-based study. Pediatrics 100:180, 1997.
26. Copel JA, Pilu G, Kleinman CS: Congenital heart disease and extracardiac anomalies: Associations and indications for fetal echocardiography. Am J Obstet Gynecol 154:1121, 1986.
27. Nora JJ, Nora AH: Maternal transmission of congenital heart diseases. New recurrence risk figures and the questions of cytoplasmic inheritance and vulnerability to teratogens. Am J Cardiol 59:459, 1987.
28. Allan L, Crawford D, Chita S, et al: Familial recurrence of congenital heart disease in a prospective series of mothers referred for fetal echocardiography. Am J Cardiol 58:334, 1986.
29. Zierler S: Maternal drugs and congenital heart disease. Obstet Gynecol 65:155, 1985.
30. Cooley WC, Graham JM Jr: Down syndrome: An update and review for the primary pediatrician. Clin Pediatr 30:233, 1991.
31. Boughman JA, Berg KA, Astemborski JA, et al: Familial risks of congenital heart defect in a population-based epidemiological study. Am J Med Genet 26:839, 1987.
32. Whittemore R, Wells J, Castellsague X: A second-generation study of 427 probands with congenital heart defects and their 837 children. J Am Coll Cardiol 23:1459, 1994.
33. Hyett J, Perdu M, Sharland G, et al: Using fetal nuchal translucency to screen for major congenital cardiac defects at 10-14 weeks of gestation: Population based cohort study. BMJ 318:81, 1999.
34. Burn J, Brennan P, Little J, et al: Recurrence risks in offspring of adults with major heart defects: Results from first cohort of British collaborative study. Lancet 351:311, 1998.
35. Van Marter L, Leviton A, Allred E, et al: Persistent pulmonary hypertension of the newborn and smoking and aspirin and nonsteroidal anti-inflammatory drug consumption during pregnancy. Pediatrics 97:658, 1996.
36. Becerra JE, Khoury MJ, Cordero JF, et al: Diabetes mellitus during pregnancy and the risks for specific birth defects: A population-based case control study. Pediatrics 85:1, 1990.
37. Sklansky M: Prenatal screening for congenital heart disease: A moving proposal. J Ultrasound Med 26:1, 2007.
38. Khoshnood B, Vigan C, Vodovar V, et al: Trends in prenatal diagnosis, pregnancy termination, and perinatal mortality of newborns with congenital heart disease in France, 1983-2000: A population-based evaluation. Pediatrics 115:95, 2005.
39. Franklin O, Burch M, Manning N, et al: Prenatal diagnosis of coarctation of the aorta improves survival and reduces morbidity. Heart 87:67, 2002.
40. Verheijen PM, Lisowski LA, Stoutenbeek P, et al: Prenatal diagnosis of congenital heart disease affects preoperative acidosis in the newborn infant. J Thorac Cardiovasc Surg 121:798, 2001.
41. Mahle W, Clancy R, McGaurn S, et al: Impact of prenatal diagnosis on survival and early neurologic morbidity in neonates with the hypoplastic left heart syndrome. Pediatrics 107:1277, 2001.
42. Kovalchin JP, Silverman NH: The impact of fetal echocardiography. Pediatr Cardiol 25:299, 2004.
43. Bonnet D, Coltri A, Butera G, et al: Detection of transposition of the great arteries in fetuses reduces neonatal morbidity and mortality. Circulation 99:916, 1999.
44. Meyer-Wittkopf M, Cooper S, Sholler G: Correlation between fetal cardiac diagnosis by obstetric and pediatric cardiologist sonographers and comparison with postnatal findings. Ultrasound Obstet Gynecol 17:392, 2001.
45. Copel JA, Pilu G, Green J, et al: Fetal echocardiographic screening for congenital heart disease: The importance of the four-chamber view. Am J Obstet Gynecol 157:648, 1987.
46. Allan LD, Crawford DC, Chita SK, et al: Prenatal screening for congenital heart disease. BMJ 292:1717, 1986.
47. DeVore GR: The prenatal diagnosis of congenital heart disease: A practical approach for the fetal sonographer. J Clin Ultrasound 13:229, 1985.
48. American Institute of Ultrasound in Medicine: AIUM Practice Guideline for the Performance of an Antepartum Obstetric Ultrasound Examination. Laurel, MD, AIUM, 2003.
49. American College of Obstetrics and Gynecology: ACOG Practice Bulletin No. 58: Ultrasonography in Pregnancy. Obstet Gynecol 104:1449, 2004.
50. Tegnander E, Eik-Nes SH, Johansen OJ, et al: Prenatal detection of heart defects at the routine fetal examination at 18 weeks in a non-selected population. Ultrasound Obstet Gynecol 5:373, 1995.
51. Crane JP, Lefevre ML, Winborn RC, et al: A randomized trial of prenatal ultrasonographic screening: Impact on the detection, management and outcome of anomalous fetuses. The RADIUS Study Group. Am J Obstet Gynecol 171:393, 1994.
52. Todros T, Faggiano F, Chiappa E, et al: Accuracy of routine ultrasonography in screening heart disease prenatally. Prenat Diagn 17:901, 1997.
53. DeVore GR, Horenstein J, Siassi B, et al: Fetal echocardiography: VII. Doppler color flow mapping: A new technique for the diagnosis of congenital heart disease. Am J Obstet Gynecol 156:1054, 1987.
54. Carvalho J, Mavrides E, Shinebourne E, et al: Improving the effectiveness of routine prenatal screening for major congenital heart defects. Heart 88:387, 2002.
55. Ogge G, Gaglioti P, Maccanti S, et al: Prenatal screening for congenital heart disease with four-chamber and outflow-tract views: A multicenter study. Ultrasound Obstet Gynecol 28:779, 2006.
56. Kirk JS, Riggs TW, Comstock CH, et al: Prenatal screening for cardiac anomalies: The value of routine addition of the aortic root to the four-chamber view. Obstet Gynecol 84:427, 1994.
57. Kirk JS, Comstock CH, Lee W, et al: Sonographic screening to detect fetal cardiac anomalies: A 5-year experience with 111 abnormal cases. Obstet Gynecol 89:227, 1997.
58. DeVore GR: The aortic and pulmonary outflow tract screening in the human fetus. J Ultrasound Med 11:345, 1992.
59. Bromley B, Estroff JA, Sanders SP, et al: Fetal echocardiography: Accuracy and limitations in a population at high and low risk for heart defects. Am J Obstet Gynecol 166:1473, 1992.
60. Sklansky M, Miller D, DeVore G, et al: Prenatal screening for congenital heart disease using real-time three-dimensional echocardiography and a novel "sweep volume" acquisition technique. Ultrasound Obstet Gynecol 25:435, 2005.
61. DeVore GR, Polanco B, Sklansky MS, et al: The "spin" technique: A new method for examination of the fetal outflow tracts using three-dimensional ultrasound. Ultrasound Obstet Gynecol 24:72, 2004.
62. Goncalves L, Lee W, Espinoza J, et al: Examination of the fetal heart by four-dimensional (4D) ultrasound with spatio-temporal image correlation (STIC). Ultrasound Obstet Gynecol 27:336, 2006.

63. Abuhamad A: Automated multiplanar imaging: A novel approach to ultrasonography. J Ultrasound Med 23:573, 2004.
64. Espinoza J, Kusanovic JP, Gonçalves LF, et al: A novel algorithm for comprehensive fetal echocardiography using 4-dimensional ultrasonography and tomographic imaging. J Ultrasound Med 25:947, 2006.
65. Wong S, Chan F, Cincotta B, et al: Factors influencing the prenatal detection of structural congenital heart diseases. Ultrasound Obstet Gynecol 21:19, 2003.
66. Sklansky MS, Nelson TR, Pretorius DH: Three-dimensional echocardiography: Gated versus nongated techniques. J Ultrasound Med 17:451, 1998.
67. Carvalho JS, Moscoso G, Tekay A, et al: Clinical impact of first and early second trimester fetal echocardiography on high risk pregnancies. Heart 90:921, 2004.
68. Haak MC, Twisk JW, Van Vugt JM: How successful is fetal echocardiographic examination in the first trimester of pregnancy? Ultrasound Obstet Gynecol 20:9, 2002.
69. Haak M, Van Vugt JMG: Echocardiography in early pregnancy: Review of literature. J Ultrasound Med 22:271, 2003.
70. Huggon IC, Ghi T, Cook AC, et al: Fetal cardiac abnormalities identified prior to 14 weeks gestation. Ultrasound Obstet Gynecol 20:22, 2002.
71. Dizon-Townson D, Dildy G, Clark S: A prospective evaluation of fetal pericardial fluid in 506 second-trimester low-risk pregnancies. Obstet Gynecol 90:958, 1997.
72. Smith R, Comstock C, Kirk J, et al: Ultrasonographic left cardiac axis deviation: A marker for fetal anomalies. Obstet Gynecol 85:187, 1995.
73. Respondek M, Respondek A, Huhta J, et al: 2D echocardiographic assessment of the fetal heart size in the 2nd and 3rd trimester of uncomplicated pregnancy. Eur J Obstet Gynecol Reprod Biol 44:185, 1992.
74. Kirk J, Comstock C, Lee W, et al: Fetal cardiac asymmetry: A marker for congenital heart disease. Obstet Gynecol 93:189, 1999.
75. Abuhamad A, Falkensammer P, Zhao Y: Automated sonography: Defining the spatial relationship of standard diagnostic fetal cardiac planes in the second trimester of pregnancy. J Ultrasound Med 26:501, 2007.
76. Michailidis GC, Simpson JM, Karidas C, et al: Detailed three-dimensional fetal echocardiography facilitated by an internet link. Ultrasound Obstet Gynecol 18:325, 2001.
77. DeVore GR, Polanko B: Tomographic ultrasound imaging of the fetal heart: A new technique for identifying normal and abnormal cardiac anatomy. J Ultrasound Med 24:1685, 2005.
78. Rychik J, Ayres N, Cuneo B, et al: American Society of Echocardiography Guidelines and Standards for Performance of the Fetal Echocardiogram. J Am Soc Echocardiogr 17:803, 2004.
79. Allan LD, Chita SK, Sharland GK, et al: The accuracy of fetal echocardiography in the diagnosis of congenital heart disease. Int J Cardiol 25:279, 1989.
80. Allan L, Sharland G, Milburn A, et al: Prospective diagnosis of 1,006 consecutive cases of congenital heart disease in the fetus. J Am Coll Cardiol 23:1452, 1994.
81. Hornberger LK, Sanders SP, Sahn DJ, et al: In utero pulmonary artery and aortic growth and potential for progression of pulmonary outflow tract obstruction in tetralogy of Fallot. J Am Coll Cardiol 25:739, 1995.
82. Hornberger LK, Sanders SP, Rein AJ, et al: Left heart obstructive lesions and left ventricular growth in the midtrimester fetus: A longitudinal study. Circulation 92:1531, 1995.
83. Lombardi C, Bellotti M, Fesslova V, et al: Fetal echocardiography at the time of the nuchal translucency scan. Ultrasound Obstet Gynecol 29:249, 2007.
84. Del Rio M, Martinez J, Figueras F, et al: Reference ranges for Doppler parameters of the fetal aortic isthmus during the second half of pregnancy. Ultrasound Obstet Gynecol 28:71, 2006.
85. Allan L, Dangel J, Fesslova V, et al: Recommendations for the practice of fetal cardiology in Europe. Cardiol Young 14:109, 2004.
86. Michelfelder E: Doppler echocardiographic characterization of the fetus in distress. Prog Pediatr Cardiol 22:31, 2006.
87. Eidem B, Edwards J, Cetta F: Quantitative assessment of fetal ventricular function: Establishing normal values of the myocardial performance index in the fetus. Echocardiography 18:9, 2001.
88. Mori Y, Rice M, McDonald R, et al: Evaluation of systolic and diastolic ventricular performance of the right ventricle in fetuses with ductal constriction using the Doppler Tei index. Am J Cardiol 88:1173, 2001.
89. Larsen L, Peterson O, Norrild K, et al: Strain rate derived from color Doppler myocardial imaging for assessment of fetal cardiac function. Ultrasound Obstet Gynecol 27:210, 2006.
90. Mari G, Uerpairojkit B, Copel J: Abdominal venous system in the normal fetus. Obstet Gynecol 86:729, 1995.
91. Better D, Kaufman S, Allan L: The normal pattern of pulmonary venous flow on pulsed Doppler examination of the human fetus. J Am Soc Echocardiogr 9:281, 1996.
92. Harada K, Rice M, Shiota T, et al: Gestational age- and growth-related alterations in fetal right and left ventricular diastolic filling patterns. Am J Cardiol 79:173, 1997.
93. Weiner Z, Efrat Z, Zimmer E, et al: Fetal atrioventricular blood flow throughout gestation. Am J Cardiol 80:658, 1997.
94. Splunder P, Stijnen T, Wladimiroff J: Fetal atrioventricular flow-velocity waveforms and their relation to arterial and venous flow-velocity waveforms at 8 to 20 weeks of gestation. Circulation 94:1372, 1996.
95. Schneider C, McCrindle B, Carvalho S, et al: Development of Z-scores for fetal cardiac dimensions from echocardiography. Ultrasound Obstet Gynecol 26:599,2005.
96. DeVore G: The use of Z-scores in the analysis of fetal cardiac dimensions. Ultrasound Obstet Gynecol 26:596, 2005.
97. Firpo C, Hoffman J, Silverman N: Evaluation of fetal heart dimensions from 12 weeks to term. Am J Cardiol 87:594, 2001.
98. Hornberger LK, Weintraub RG, Pesonen E, et al: Echocardiographic study of the morphology and growth of the aortic arch in the human fetus. Circulation 86:741, 1992.
99. Sharland GK, Allan LD: Normal fetal cardiac measurements derived by cross-sectional echocardiography. Ultrasound Obstet Gynecol 2:175, 1992.
100. Tan J, Silverman NH, Hoffman JI, et al: Cardiac dimensions determined by cross-sectional echocardiography in the normal human fetus from 18 weeks to term. Am J Cardiol 70:1459, 1992.
101. Rein A, O'Donnell C, Geva T, et al: Use of tissue velocity imaging in the diagnosis of fetal cardiac arrhythmias. Circulation 106:1827, 2002.
102. Paladini D, Lamberti A, Teodoro A, et al: Tissue Doppler imaging of the fetal heart. Ultrasound Obstet Gynecol 16:530, 2000.
103. Huhta JC: Guidelines for the evaluation of heart failure in the fetus with or without hydrops. Pediatr Cardiol 25:274, 2004.
104. Allan L: Technique of fetal echocardiography. Pediatr Cardiol 25:223, 2004.
105. DeVore G: Trisomy 21: 91% Detection rate using second-trimester ultrasound markers. Ultrasound Obstet Gynecol 16:133, 2000.
106. Yeager S, Parness I, Spevak P, et al: Prenatal echocardiographic diagnosis of pulmonary and systemic venous anomalies. Am Heart J 128:397, 1994.
107. Chaoui R, Heling K, Kalache K: Caliber of the coronary sinus in fetuses with cardiac defects with and without left persistent superior vena cava and in growth-restricted fetuses with heart-sparing effect. Prenat Diagn 23:552, 2003.
108. Agnoletti G, Annecchino F, Preda L, et al: Persistence of the left superior caval vein: Can it potentiate obstructive lesions of the left ventricle? Cardiol Young 9:285, 1999.
109. Berg C, Knuppel M, Geipel A, et al: Prenatal diagnosis of persistent left superior vena cava and its associated congenital anomalies. Ultrasound Obstet Gynecol 27:274, 2006.
110. Atkinson D, Drant S: Diagnosis of heterotaxy syndrome by fetal echocardiography. Am J Cardiol 82:1147, 1998.
111. Messing B, Porat S, Imbar T, et al: Mild tricuspid regurgitation: A benign fetal finding at various stages of pregnancy. Ultrasound Obstet Gynecol 26:60, 2005.

112. Respondek M, Kammermeier M, Ludomirsky A, et al: The prevalence and clinical significance of fetal tricuspid valve regurgitation with normal heart anatomy. Am J Obstet Gynecol 171:1265, 1994.
113. Nii M, Roman K, Kingdom J, et al: Assessment of the evolution of normal fetal diastolic function during mid and late gestation by spectral Doppler tissue echocardiography. J Am Soc Echocardiogr 19:1431, 2006.
114. Pedra S, Smallhorn J, Ryan G, et al: Fetal cardiomyopathies: Pathogenic mechanisms, hemodynamic findings, and clinical outcome. Circulation 106:585, 2002.
115. Barsoom M, Feldman D, Borgida A, et al: Is an isolated fetal cardiac echogenic focus an indication for fetal echocardiography? J Ultrasound Med 20:1043, 2001.
116. Doubilet P, Copel J, Benson C, et al: Choroid plexus cyst and echogenic intracardiac focus in women at low risk for chromosomal anomalies: The obligation to inform the mother. J Ultrasound Med 23:88, 2004.
117. Filly R, Benacerraf B, Nyberg D, et al: Choroid plexus cyst and echogenic intracardiac focus in women at low risk for chromosomal anomalies. J Ultrasound Med 23:447, 2004.
118. Sotiriadis A, Makrydimas G, Ioannides J: Diagnostic performance of intracardiac echogenic foci for Down syndrome: A meta-analysis. Obstet Gynecol 101:1009, 2003.
119. Vibhakar N, Budorick N, Scioscia A, et al: Prevalence of aneuploidy with a cardiac intraventricular echogenic focus in an at-risk patient population. J Ultrasound Med 18:265, 1999.
120. Sokol J, Shimizu N, Bohn D, et al: Fetal pulmonary artery diameter measurements as a predictor of morbidity in antenatally diagnosed congenital diaphragmatic hernia: A prospective study. Am J Obstet Gynecol 195:470, 2006.
121. Tulzer G, Gudmundsson S, Tews G, et al: Incidence of indomethacin-induced human fetal ductal constriction. J Matern Fetal Invest 1:267, 1992.
122. Tulzer G, Gudmundsson S, Sharkey AM, et al: Doppler echocardiography of fetal ductus arteriosus constriction versus increased right ventricular output. J Am Coll Cardiol 18:532, 1991.
123. Kleinman C, Donnerstein R, DeVore G, et al: Fetal echocardiography for evaluation of in utero congestive heart failure. N Engl J Med 306:568, 1982.
124. Hecher K, Campbell S, Doyle P, et al: Assessment of fetal compromise by Doppler ultrasound investigation of the fetal circulation. Circulation 91:129, 1995.
125. Rychik J: Fetal cardiovascular physiology. Pediatr Cardiol 25:201, 2004.
126. Nelson T, Pretorius D, Sklansky M, et al: Three-dimensional echocardiographic evaluation of fetal heart anatomy and function: Acquisition, analysis and display. J Ultrasound Med 15:1, 1996.
127. Deng J, Gardener JE, Rodeck CH, et al: Fetal echocardiography in three and four dimensions. Ultrasound Med Biol 22:979, 1996.
128. Sklansky MS, Nelson TR, Pretorius DH: Usefulness of gated three-dimensional fetal echocardiography to reconstruct and display structures not visualized with two-dimensional imaging. Am J Cardiol 80:665, 1997.
129. DeVore GR, Falkensammer P, Sklansky MS, et al: Spatio-temporal image correlation (STIC): A new technology for evaluation of the fetal heart. Ultrasound Obstet Gynecol 22:380, 2003.
130. Gonçalves LF, Lee W, Chaiworapongsa T, et al: Four-dimensional ultrasonography of the fetal heart with spatiotemporal image correlation. Am J Obstet Gynecol 189:1792, 2003.
131. Deng J, Rodeck C: Current applications of fetal cardiac imaging technology. Curr Opin Obstet Gynecol 18:177, 2006.
132. Maulik D, Nanda NC, Singh V, et al: Live three-dimensional echocardiography of the human fetus. Echocardiography 20:715, 2003.
133. Deng J, Sullivan ID, Yates R, et al: Real-time three-dimensional fetal echocardiography: optimal imaging windows. Ultrasound Med Biol 28:1099, 2002.
134. Viñals F, Poblete P, Giuliano A: Spatio-temporal image correlation (STIC): A new tool for the prenatal screening of congenital heart defects. Ultrasound Obstet Gynecol 22:388, 2003.
135. Chaoui R, Hoffmann J, Heling KS: Three-dimensional (3D) and 4D color Doppler fetal echocardiography using spatiotemporal image correlation (STIC). Ultrasound Obstet Gynecol 23:535, 2004.
136. Sklansky MS, Nelson T, Strachan M, et al: Real-time three-dimensional fetal echocardiography: Initial feasibility study. J Ultrasound Med 18:745, 1999.
137. Sklansky MS, DeVore GR, Wong PC: Real-time 3-dimensional fetal echocardiography with an instantaneous volume-rendered display: Early description and pictorial essay. J Ultrasound Med 23:283, 2004.
138. Goncalves LF, Romero R, Espinoza J, et al: Four-dimensional ultrasonography of the fetal heart using color Doppler spatiotemporal image correlation. J Ultrasound Med 23:473, 2004.
139. Schindera ST, Mehwald PS, Sahn DJ, et al: Accuracy of real-time three-dimensional echocardiography for quantifying right ventricular volume. J Ultrasound Med 21:1069, 2002.
140. DeVore G, Sklansky M: Three-dimensional imaging of the fetal heart: Current applications and future directions. Progr Pediatr Cardiol 22:9, 2006.
141. Meyer-Wittkopf M, Cole A, Cooper SG, et al: Three-dimensional quantitative echocardiographic assessment of ventricular volume in healthy human fetuses and in fetuses with congenital heart disease. J Ultrasound Med 20:317, 2001.
142. Deng J, Ruff C, Linney A, et al: Simultaneous use of two ultrasound scanners for motion-gated three-dimensional fetal echocardiography. Ultrasound Med Biol 26:1021, 2000.
143. Yagel S, Benachi A, Bonnet D, et al: Rendering in fetal cardiac scanning: The intracardiac septa and the coronal atrioventricular valve planes. Ultrasound Obstet Gynecol 28:266, 2006.
144. Volpe P, Campobasso G, Stanziano A, et al: Novel application of 4D sonography with B-flow imaging and spatio-temporal image correlation (STIC) in the assessment of the anatomy of pulmonary arteries in fetuses with pulmonary atresia and ventricular septal defect. Ultrasound Obstet Gynecol 28:40, 2006.
145. Acar P, Dulac Y, Taktak A, et al: Real-time three-dimensional fetal echocardiography using matrix probe. Prenat Diagn 25:370, 2005.
146. Scharf A, Geka F, Steinborn A, et al: 3D real-time imaging of the fetal heart. Fetal Diagn Ther 15:267, 2000.
147. Meyer-Wittkopf M, Rappe N, Sierra R, et al: Three-dimensional (3-D) ultrasonography for obtaining the four and five-chamber view: Comparison with cross-sectional (2-D) fetal sonographic screening. Ultrasound Obstet Gynecol 15:397, 2000.
148. Hejmadi A, Corbett V, Carpenter N, et al: Fetal ventricular mass determination on three-dimensional echocardiography: Studies in normal fetuses and validation experiments. Circulation 110:1054, 2004.
149. Chang F, Hsu K, Ko H, et al: Fetal heart volume assessment by three-dimensional ultrasound. Ultrasound Obstet Gynecol 9:42, 1997.
150. Moore K, Persaud T: The Developing Human: Clinically Oriented Embryology, 6th ed. Philadelphia, Saunders, 1998.
151. Abdulla R, Blew G, Holterman M: Cardiovascular embryology. Pediatr Cardiol 25:191, 2004.
152. Allen H, Gutgesell H, Clark E, et al (eds): Moss and Adams' Heart Disease in Infants, Children and Adolescents Including the Fetus and Young Adult, 6th ed. Philadelphia, Lippincott Williams & Wilkins, 2001.
153. Keane J, Lock J, Fyler D, et al (eds): Nadas' Pediatric Cardiology, 2nd ed. Philadelphia, Saunders, 2006.
154. Fasouliotis S, Achiron R, Kivilevitch Z, et al: The human fetal venous system: Normal embryologic, anatomic, and physiologic characteristics and developmental abnormalities. J Ultrasound Med 21:1145, 2002.
155. Lai W: Prenatal diagnosis of abnormal persistence of the right or left umbilical vein: Report of 4 cases and literature review. J Am Soc Echocardiogr 11:905, 1998.
156. Kirsch C, Feldstein V, Goldstein R, et al: Persistent intrahepatic right umbilical vein: A prenatal sonographic series without significant anomalies. J Ultrasound Med 15:371, 1996.
157. Lim J, McCrindle B, Smallhorn J, et al: Clinical features, management, and outcome of children with fetal and postnatal diagnoses of isomerism syndromes. Circulation 112:2454, 2005.

158. Michailidis G, Simpson J, Tulloh R, Economides D: Retrospective prenatal diagnosis of scimitar syndrome aided by three-dimensional power Doppler imaging. Ultrasound Obstet Gynecol 17:449, 2001.
159. Patel C, Lane J, Spector M, et al: Totally anomalous pulmonary venous connection and complex congenital heart disease. J Ultrasound Med 24:1191, 2005.
160. Patel C, Lane J, Sallee D: In utero diagnosis of isolated obstructed supracardiac total anomalous pulmonary venous connection. J Ultrasound Med 573, 2002.
161. Allan L, Sharland G: The echocardiographic diagnosis of totally anomalous pulmonary venous connection in the fetus. Heart 85:434, 2001.
162. Friedberg M, Kim N, Silverman N: Atrioventricular septal defect recently diagnosed by fetal echocardiography: Echocardiographic features, associated anomalies, and outcomes. Congenit Heart Dis 2:110, 2007.
163. Huggon I, Cook A, Smeeton N, et al: Atrioventricular septal defects diagnosed in fetal life: Associated cardiac and extra-cardiac abnormalities and outcome. J Am Coll Cardiol 36:593, 2000.
164. Hornberger L, Sahn D, Kleinman C, et al: Tricuspid valve disease with significant tricuspid insufficiency in the fetus: Diagnosis and outcome. J Am Coll Cardiol 17:167, 1991.
165. Sharland G, Chita S, Allan L: Tricuspid valve dysplasia or displacement in intrauterine life. J Am Coll Cardiol 17:944, 1991.
166. Tongsong T, Sittiwangkul R, Wanapirak C, et al: Prenatal diagnosis of isolated tricuspid valve atresia. J Ultrasound Med 23:945, 2004.
167. Peterson R, Levi D, Williams R, et al: Echocardiographic predictors of outcome in fetuses with pulmonary atresia with intact ventricular septum. J Am Soc Echocardiogr 19:1393, 2006.
168. Salvin J, McElhinney D, Colan S, et al: Fetal tricuspid valve size and growth as predictors of outcome in pulmonary atresia with intact ventricular septum. Pediatrics 118:e415, 2006.
169. Mahle W, Clancy R, Moss E, et al: Neurodevelopmental outcome and lifestyle assessment in school-aged and adolescent children with hypoplastic left heart syndrome. Pediatrics 105:1082, 2000.
170. Tworetzky W, Wilkins-Haug L, Jennings RW, et al: Balloon dilation of severe aortic stenosis in the fetus. Circulation 11;2125, 2004.
171. Marshall A, van der Velde M, Tworetsky W, et al: Creation of an atrial septal defect in utero for fetuses with hypoplastic left heart syndrome and intact or highly restrictive atrial septum. Circulation 110:25, 2004.
172. Chang R-K, Chen A, Klitzner T: Clinical management of infants with hypoplastic left heart syndrome in the United States, 1988-1997. Pediatrics 110:292, 2002.
173. Byrne P, Murphy A: Informed consent and hypoplastic left heart syndrome. Acta Paediactrica 94:1171, 2005.
174. Cohen M, Marino B, McElhinney D, et al: Neo-aortic root dilation and valve regurgitation up to 21 years after staged reconstruction for hypoplastic left heart syndrome. J Am Coll Cardiol 42:533, 2003.
175. Makikallio K, McElhinney D, Levine J, et al: Fetal aortic valve stenosis and the evolution of hypoplastic left heart syndrome: Patient selection for fetal intervention. Circulation 113:1401, 2006.
176. Head C, Jowett V, Sharland G, et al: Timing of presentation and postnatal outcome of infants suspected of having coarctation of the aorta during fetal life. Heart 91:1070, 2005.
177. Sharland G, Chan K-Y, Allan L: Coarctation of the aorta: Difficulties in prenatal diagnosis. Br Heart J 71:70, 1994.
178. Hornberger L, Sahn D, Kleinman C, et al: Antenatal diagnosis of coarctation of the aorta: A multicenter experience. J Am Coll Cardiol 23:417, 1994.
179. Botto LD, May K, Fernhoff PM, et al: A population-based study of the 22q11.2 deletion: Phenotype, incidence, and contribution to major birth defects in the population. Pediatrics 112:101, 2003.
180. Tometzki A, Suda K, Kohl T, et al: Accuracy of prenatal echocardiographic diagnosis and prognosis of fetuses with conotruncal anomalies. J Am Coll Cardiol 33:1696, 1999.
181. Lee W, Smith R, Comstock C, et al: Tetralogy of Fallot: Prenatal diagnosis and postnatal survival. Obstet Gynecol 86:583, 1995.
182. Moon-Grady A, Tacy T, Brook M, et al: Value of clinical and echocardiographic features in predicting outcome in the fetus, infant, and child with tetralogy of Fallot with absent pulmonary valve complex. Am J Cardiol 89:1280, 2002.
183. Razavi R, Sharland G, Simpson J: Prenatal diagnosis by echocardiogram and outcome of absent pulmonary valve syndrome. Am J Cardiol 91:429, 2003.
184. Galindo A, Gutierrez-Larraya F, Martinez J, et al: Prenatal diagnosis and outcome for fetuses with congenital absence of the pulmonary valve. Ultrasound Obstet Gynecol 28:32, 2006.
185. Gelehrter S, Owens S, Russell M, et al: Accuracy of the fetal echocardiogram in double-outlet right ventricle. Congenit Heart Dis 2:32, 2007.
186. Donofrio M: Premature closure of the foramen ovale and ductus arteriosus in a fetus with transposition of the great arteries. Circulation 105:e65, 2002.
187. Paladini D, Volpe P, Marasini M, et al: Diagnosis, characterization and outcome of congenitally corrected transposition of the great arteries in the fetus: A multicenter series of 30 cases. Ultrasound Obstet Gynecol 27:281, 2006.
188. Sharland G, Tingay R, Jones A, et al: Atrioventricular and ventriculoarterial discordance (congenitally corrected transposition of the great arteries): Echocardiographic features, associations, and outcome in 34 fetuses. Heart 91:1453, 2005.
189. Volpe P, Paladini D, Marasini M, et al: Common arterial trunk in the fetus: Characteristics, associations, and outcome in a multicenter series of 23. Heart 89:1437, 2003.
190. Duke C, Sharland G, Jones A, et al: Echocardiographic features and outcome of truncus arteriosus diagnosed during fetal life. Am J Cardiol 88:1379, 2001.
191. Isaacs H Jr: Fetal and neonatal tumors. Pediatr Cardiol 25:252, 2004.
192. Holley D, Martin G, Brenner J, et al: Diagnosis and management of fetal cardiac tumors: A multicenter experience and review of published papers. J Am Coll Cardiol 26:516, 1995.
193. Tworetsky W, McElhinney D, Margossian R, et al: Association between cardiac tumors and tuberous sclerosis in the fetus and neonate. Am J Cardiol 92:487, 2003.
194. Bader R, Chitayat D, Kelly E, et al: Fetal rhabdomyoma: Prenatal diagnosis, clinical outcome, and incidence of associated tuberous sclerosis complex. J Pediatr 143:620, 2003.
195. Sklansky M, Greenberg M, Lucas V, et al: Intrapericardial teratoma in a twin fetus: Diagnosis and management. Obstet Gynecol 89:807, 1997.
196. Kleinman CS, Nehgme RA: Cardiac arrhythmias in the human fetus. Pediatr Cardiol 25:234, 2004.
197. Kleinman C, Nehgme R, Copel J: Fetal cardiac arrhythmias: Diagnosis and therapy. In Creasy R, Resnik R, Iams J (eds): Maternal-Fetal Medicine, 5th ed. Philadelphia, Saunders, 2003.
198. Simpson J: Fetal arrhythmias. Ultrasound Obstet Gynecol 27:599, 2006.
199. Respondek M, Wloch A, Kaczmarek P, et al: Diagnostic and perinatal management of fetal extrasystole. Pediatr Cardiol 18:361, 1997.
200. Strasburger J, Huhta J, Carpenter R, et al: Doppler echocardiography in the diagnosis and management of persistent fetal arrhythmias. J Am Coll Cardiol 7:1386,1986.
201. Kleinman C, Copel J, Hobbins J: Combined echocardiographic and Doppler assessment of fetal congenital atrioventricular block. BJOG 94:967, 1987.
202. Jeaggi E, Fouron J, Fournier A, et al: Ventriculo-atrial time interval measured on M-mode echocardiography: A determining element in diagnosis, treatment, and prognosis of fetal supraventricular tachycardia. Heart 79:582, 1998.
203. Hofbeck M, Ulmer H, Beinder E, et al: Prenatal findings in patients with prolonged QT interval in the neonatal period. Heart 77:198, 1997.
204. Oudijk MA, Michon MM, Kleinman CS, et al: Sotalol in the treatment of fetal dysrhythmias. Circulation 101:2721, 2000.
205. Schmidt LG, Ulmer HE, Silverman NH, et al: Perinatal outcome of fetal complete atrioventricular block: A multicenter experience. J Am Coll Cardiol 91:1360, 1991.
206. Buyon JP, Clancey R, Di Donato F, et al: Cardiac 5-HT serotoninergic receptors, 52KD SSA/Ro and autoimmune-associated congenital heart block. J Autoimmun 19:79, 2002.

207. Buyon JP, Hiebert R, Copel JA, et al: Autoimmune-associated congenital heart block: Mortality, morbidity and recurrence rates obtained from a national neonatal lupus registry. J Am Coll Cardiol 31:165, 1998.
208. Nield LE, Silverman ED, Smallhorn JF, et al: Endocardial fibroelastosis associated with maternal anti-Ro and anti-La antibodies in the absence of atrioventricular block. J Am Coll Cardiol 40:796, 2002.
209. Jaeggi ET, Fouron JC, Silverman ED, et al: Transplacental fetal treatment improves the outcome of prenatally diagnosed complete atrioventricular block without structural heart disease. Circulation 110:1542, 2004.
210. Copel J, Buyon J, Kleinman C: Successful in utero therapy of fetal heart block. Am J Obstet Gynecol 173:1384, 1995.
211. Groves AM, Allan LD, Rosenthal E: Therapeutic trial of sympathomimetics in three cases of complete heart block in the fetus. Circulation 92:3394, 1995.
212. Brucato A, Frassi M, Franceschini F, et al: Risk of congenital complete heart block in newborns of mothers with anti-Ro/SSA antibodies detected by counterimmunoelectrophoresis: A prospective study of 100 women. Arthritis Rheum 44:1832, 2001.
213. Glickstein J, Buyon J, Friedman D: Pulsed Doppler echocardiographic assessment of the fetal PR interval. Am J Cardiol 86:236, 2000.
214. Bergman G, Jacobsson L, Wahren-Herlenius M, et al: Doppler echocardiographic and electrocardiographic atrioventricular time intervals in newborn infants: Evaluation of techniques for surveillance of fetuses at risk for congenital heart block. Ultrasound Obstet Gynecol 28:57, 2006.
215. Jaeggi E, Hamilton R, Silverman E, et al: Outcome of children with fetal, neonatal or childhood diagnosis of isolated congenital atrioventricular block. J Am Coll Cardiol 39:130, 2002.
216. Saleeb S, Copel J, Friedman D, et al: Comparison of treatment with fluorinated glucocorticoids to the natural history of autoantibody-associated congenital heart block: Retrospective review of the Research Registry for Neonatal Lupus. Arthritis Rheum 42:2335, 1999.
217. Simpson LL, Marx GR, D'Alton ME: Supraventricular tachycardia in the fetus: Conservative management in the absence of hemodynamic compromise. J Ultrasound Med 16:459, 1997.
218. Cuneo BF, Strasburger JF: Management strategy for fetal tachycardia. Obstet Gynecol 96:575, 2000.
219. Van Engelen A, Weijtens O, Brenner J, et al: Management outcome and follow-up of fetal tachycardia. J Am Coll Cardiol 24:1371, 1994.
220. Lupoglazoff J, Jacoz-Aigrain E, Guyot B, et al: Endogenous digoxin-like immunoreactivity during pregnancy and at birth. Br J Clin Pharmac 35:251, 1993.
221. Allan L, Chita S, Sharland G, et al. Flecainide in the treatment of fetal tachycardia. Br Heart J 65:46, 1991.
222. Strasburger J, Cuneo B, Michon M, et al. Amiodarone therapy for drug-refractory fetal tachycardia. Circulation 109:375, 2004.
223. Lisowski L, Verheijen P, Benatar A, et al: Atrial flutter in the perinatal age group: Diagnosis, management and outcome. J Am Coll Cardiol 35:771, 2000.
224. Texter KM, Kertesz N, Friedman R, et al: Atrial flutter in infants. J Am Coll Cardiol 48:1040, 2006.

Chapter 20

Teratogenesis and Environmental Exposure

Christina Chambers, PhD, MPH, and Carl P. Weiner, MD, MBA

A teratogenic agent is defined as one that has the potential to interfere with the normal functional or structural development of an embryo or fetus. A teratogenic exposure occurs when a pregnant woman is exposed to an agent that increases risk. Although teratogenic exposures are generally thought of as those that increase the risk for major congenital anomalies, in the broader sense, teratogenic exposures also increase the risk for a spectrum of adverse pregnancy outcomes, including spontaneous abortion, stillbirth, minor structural anomalies, shortened gestational age, growth restriction, and behavioral or cognitive deficits. However, excess risks for these latter events are much more difficult to recognize.

The currently known teratogenic exposures comprise a wide range of agents, including some prescription and over-the-counter medications, recreational drugs and alcohol, chemicals, physical agents, and maternal diseases. Although studies specifically evaluating human teratogenicity are lacking for most environmental agents, including prescription medications, it is generally estimated that at least 10% of major birth defects are attributable to environmental exposures and therefore are, to some extent, preventable.[1] As a result, the possible teratogenicity of agents to which a woman may be exposed during pregnancy is of great concern to the general public and requires that clinicians develop expertise in evaluating these risks on behalf of their patients.

Historical Perspective

Before the 1940s, it was somewhat naively thought that the placenta provided a protective barrier for the developing embryo and fetus, so that agents to which the mother was exposed could not interfere with normal prenatal development. The revolutionary concept that a maternal exposure could pose a risk to the developing embryo or fetus was first raised, not by a scientist or an obstetrician, but rather by an Australian ophthalmologist, Norman Gregg, who observed in his own clinical practice an unusual number of children diagnosed with congenital cataracts shortly after a rubella epidemic. Gregg's work led to investigations that identified additional features of a variable but characteristic pattern of developmental abnormalities associated with fetal rubella infection, including congenital heart defects, hearing deficits, and endocrine abnormalities, all of which came to be known as the congenital rubella syndrome.[2]

In the early 1960s, an Australian obstetrician and a German geneticist independently recognized that first-trimester maternal use of thalidomide, a sedative-hypnotic drug, was associated with a dramatic increase in risk for a characteristic pattern of limb reduction anomalies and other defects.[3,4] Although the drug had undergone premarket testing in rodents, it had not shown any evidence of adverse outcomes in these species. The subsequent recognition that therapeutic agents could induce malformations was a major stimulus for the implementation of the Kefauver-Harris Amendment to the Food, Drug and Cosmetic Act in the United States, which expanded the role of the Food and Drug Administration (FDA) as a regulatory agency charged with ensuring both the efficacy and the safety of products.[5]

Although the thalidomide experience raised public awareness of the potential risks of prenatal exposures, it was accompanied by misunderstandings about how to differentiate exposures that actually cause birth defects from coincidental exposures occurring in women whose pregnancy outcome is abnormal for other, unrelated reasons. A classic example is doxylamine succinate and pyridoxine hydrochloride with or without dicyclomine hydrochloride (Bendectin®), a once popular antiemetic medication used by as many as 30% of American women for the treatment of nausea and vomiting of pregnancy. In 1983, this agent was voluntarily withdrawn from the market after anecdotal concerns for teratogenicity triggered on onslaught of litigation, despite voluminous scientific evidence to the contrary.[6]

Within the last 40 years, research in the field of teratology has advanced, and several new human teratogens have been identified, including several anticonvulsants, selected antineoplastic agents, inhibitors of enzymes in the angiotensinogen-angiotensin pathway, methylmercury, cocaine, alcohol, hyperthermia, tetracycline, warfarin, and isotretinoin.[7] Work continues to better define the range of adverse outcomes associated with these exposures, the magnitude of the risk for a given dose at a specific gestational age, and the subpopulations of mothers and infants who may be at particularly increased risk because of their genotype. However, major knowledge gaps exist for most agents—few of which have been adequately evaluated in human pregnancy.[8]

Concerns regarding the inadequacy of accurate information for the developmental effects of a majority of therapeutic and over-the-counter agents are critical. Studies indicate that drug exposure during pregnancy is extremely common: in one U.S. health care system sample of 98,182 deliveries, 64% of women were prescribed at least one medication during their pregnancy other than a vitamin or mineral supplement.[9] In another U.S. population–based sample of women, more than 70% reported the use of one or more over-the-counter medications during pregnancy.[10] Therefore, a theoretical and practical framework is necessary to aid clinicians in advising patients, who are likely to have experienced several exposures by the time their pregnancy is recognized, and to help support evidence-based clinical decision making in the common situations in which pregnancy exposures can be anticipated.

Principles of Teratology

Wilson and Fraser[11] outlined the basic principles of teratology in the early 1970s to aid in identifying those agents with teratogenic potential and to provide a basis for establishing causality. Appreciation of these principles can help clinicians place into context research findings from the literature as well as individual patient histories. The principles discussed here are species specificity, genetic susceptibility, gestational timing, dose response, route of administration, spectrum of outcomes, and specific mechanisms leading to pathogenesis.

The principle of *species specificity,* in combination with the concept of *genetic susceptibility,* holds that agents that are teratogenic in one species may not be so in another. Similarly, the manifestations of a teratogenic exposure may differ across susceptible species, and, even within species, certain strains or individuals may be at higher risk than others.

These two principles have implications for the predictive value of preclinical animal reproductive toxicity studies; for example, thalidomide was not teratogenic in the species initially tested, and only after its recognition as a human teratogen was the most sensitive animal species identified.[12] Variability in susceptibility is also evident within species, including humans, where no teratogenic agent at typical doses has been demonstrated to produce adverse effects in 100% of conceptuses. Even potent, known human teratogens such as thalidomide and isotretinoin affect fewer than 50% of exposed infants. In some cases, this variability in susceptibility has been linked to specific genetic polymorphisms that interact with the agent to create a particularly susceptible subgroup of mothers or fetuses.

For example, women with infants who have cleft lip with or without cleft palate or isolated cleft palate are approximately twice as likely to report heavy first-trimester tobacco use than are mothers of normal newborns; however, women who have a certain transforming growth factor-α (TGF-α) polymorphism and who smoke heavily have a 3 to 11 times higher risk of having a child with an oral cleft, suggesting a gene-environment interaction. Furthermore, this risk appears to be lessened by maternal multivitamin use.[13,14] Similarly, a low level of epoxide hydrolase enzyme activity influenced by epoxide hydrolase polymorphisms has been implicated as a risk factor for fetal hydantoin syndrome in children whose mothers have taken phenytoin for the treatment of a seizure disorder during pregnancy.[15]

The principle of *gestational timing,* or critical developmental windows of exposure, requires that the exposure occur during the stage in development when the maturational process is most susceptible. For example, the critical window for an agent that interferes with closure of the neural tube in the human embryo is approximately the first 3 weeks after conception. Carbamazepine, an anticonvulsant linked to a 10-fold increased risk for neural tube defects, does not produce the defect if maternal exposure occurs after the second month of pregnancy.[16,17]

A corollary to this principle is that, depending on the precise gestational timing of teratogenic exposure, a range of adverse outcomes may be induced. For example, coumarin-derived anticoagulants are associated with a pattern of nasal hypoplasia and skeletal abnormalities when prenatal exposure occurs during a critical window in the latter portion of the first trimester, whereas later gestational exposure is associated with central nervous system (CNS) effects.[18] The former abnormality likely reflects a vitamin K deficiency, the latter a complication of fetal bleeding.

Consistent with these concepts, very early gestational exposure, limited in general to the first 2 weeks after conception, is thought to pose little potential for teratogenicity. This is true in part because of the limited biologic availability to the embryo of an agent that is taken and eliminated by the mother before the completion of placentation. Further, pluripotent cells of the early embryo may be resilient in recovering from a teratogenic insult, or, alternatively, they may be particularly vulnerable to a teratogenic exposure, resulting in spontaneous abortion before the clinical recognition of pregnancy.[11]

The principle of *dose response* suggests that, for those agents that are teratogenic, there is a threshold dose below which no effect is detected, and higher doses produce stronger effects relative to lower doses, with the highest doses being lethal. For example, when the anticonvulsant valproic acid is ingested by a pregnant woman during the critical window for neural tube closure, the risk for that defect increases by approximately 10- to 20-fold, from a baseline risk of 0.1% to a risk of 1% to 2% . However, there is evidence that the risk is dose-related, because valproate-treated mothers who deliver infants with spina bifida on average have taken significantly higher doses than valproate-treated mothers of normal newborns.[19]

The principle of *route of administration* is closely linked to the principle of dose response from the standpoint of influencing the effective dose that is biologically available to the embryo or fetus. This is a critical element in the design of animal reproductive and developmental toxicity studies in terms of their comparability to human pregnancy exposures. This principle can be applied to studies regarding the relative toxicity of human exposures resulting from oral dosing versus topical application. For example, retinoids as a class have been identified as human teratogens with effects that depend on the dose and timing of exposure in gestation. Isotretinoin taken as an oral medication is one of the most potent known human teratogens. Exposure to isotretinoin limited to as little as a few days in early pregnancy results in an approximate 20% risk of a pattern of brain, heart, ear, and thymus abnormalities and mental deficiency in liveborn children.[20] In contrast, topical retinoids, when used sparingly in the first trimester for blemishes or to reduce signs of skin aging, have not been associated with a measurably increased risk for the same pattern of adverse effects.[21,22] These findings do not rule out the teratogenic potential of topical retinoids but simply suggest that the maternal blood levels of retinoids delivered via skin absorption may represent a teratogenic risk that is so low as to be undetectable without very large sample sizes.

The principle of *spectrum of outcomes* indicates that, depending on dose and timing in gestation, adverse outcomes associated with a given teratogen may encompass effects ranging from spontaneous abortion or stillbirth to major and minor structural defects, prenatal or postnatal growth deficiency, preterm delivery, and functional deficits or learning disabilities. For example, moderate to heavy maternal alcohol intake, particularly if consumed in a "binge" pattern, has been demonstrated to increase the risks for spontaneous abortion, stillbirth, a characteristic pattern of minor craniofacial abnormalities, selected specific major structural defects including heart defects and oral clefts, prenatal and postnatal growth deficiency, deficits in global IQ, and specific behavioral and learning abnormalities.[23] Animal and human studies consistently support the notion that the entire spectrum of outcomes associated with alcohol may not be manifested in any single affected pregnancy; rather, the results vary by dose and pattern of drinking, differ with gestational timing of exposure, and are influenced by genetic susceptibility and other modifying factors such as maternal nutrition.

Finally, the principle of *specific mechanisms leading to pathogenesis* specifies that teratogenic agents do not increase the risk of all adverse outcomes; rather, they act on specific targets to produce a characteristic pattern of effects. This principle underlies the methods by which many human teratogens have been recognized; that is, a pattern of abnormalities associated with a particular teratogenic exposure helps to identify that exposure as a cause of the outcome. For example, the characteristic pattern of abnormalities comprising the fetal alcohol syndrome includes minor craniofacial features (short palpebral fissures, smooth philtrum, and thin vermilion of the upper lip) accompanied by microcephaly, growth deficiency, and cognitive and behavioral deficits. The prenatal effects of alcohol, although pervasive, nevertheless represent a constellation or pattern of features that is unlikely to randomly occur without exposure to alcohol in substantial doses and during certain gestational weeks.

It therefore appears likely that there are a few general mechanisms that lead to abnormal development. For example, a teratogenic agent can interact with a receptor, bind to DNA or protein, degrade cell membranes or proteins, inhibit an enzyme, or modify proteins. These mechanisms ultimately manifest as one or more types of abnormal embryogenesis, including excessive or reduced cell death, failed cell interactions, reduced biosynthesis, impeded morphogenetic movement, or mechanical disruption of tissues. For this reason, several specific teratogens may have the same end result on development by acting through a common pathway. For example, some anticonvulsants, trimethoprim, and triamterine may increase the risk for neural tube defects via folate antagonism.[24] Angiotensin I–converting enzyme (ACE) inhibitors such as enalapril and lisinopril may induce the risk for ACE-inhibitor fetopathy, which consists of renal tubular dysplasia and hypocalvarium, possibly through the mechanism of drug-induced fetal hypotension leading to hypoperfusion and oligohydramnios.[25]

Sources of Safety Data on Exposures in Pregnancy

In the ideal world, clinicians would have access to complete information about the human teratogenic potential of all environmental exposures, including medications, recreational drugs, nutrients and nutrient supplements, occupational exposures, toxic exposures or poisonings, household chemicals and cosmetics, environmental contaminants or pollutants, and physical agents such as heat and radiation. Unfortunately, for many if not most exposures, reliable information is limited. Sufficient human data are commonly lacking for even prescription medications whose safety is monitored by the FDA. In one study reviewing the human safety data for prescription medications marketed in the United States over the previous 20 years, Lo and Friedman[8] concluded there were insufficient data to confirm or rule out teratogenicity for more than 80% of these agents.

There are many reasons for this situation, some inherent to the difficulty of conducting pregnancy outcome research and some related to the lack of a standard surveillance system for studying agents to which women of reproductive age are likely to be exposed. Clinical trials for prescription medications are not typically conducted in human pregnancy, and the pharmaceutical industry has no incentive to do so even when there is an apparent clinical need. Animal reproductive and developmental toxicity studies are used to estimate the potential for human teratogenicity. For almost all known human teratogens, there is an animal model; however, animal studies are not completely predictive of human pregnancy outcomes due to species sensitivity and differences in dosing and exposure timing.

Adverse Case Reports

When new medications are marketed in the United States, initial reports of pregnancy exposures with adverse outcomes may appear as case reports in the literature, or through safety data provided to the FDA by manufacturers, or in voluntary reports by clinicians or patients. Although individual adverse outcome reports have the potential to generate a hypothesis regarding teratogenicity—especially if the outcome reported is an unusual pattern of malformation—these data sources lack critical information about the number of exposed pregnancies with normal outcomes and therefore can confuse the process of determining whether the adverse event reports represent an excess risk over the baseline for that event.

Pregnancy Registries

Additional sources of pregnancy safety information on new drugs sometimes include pregnancy registries. Registries typically collect data regarding exposures to a specific drug or class of drugs, both retrospectively and prospectively. The outcome of primary interest in traditional pregnancy registries is major birth defects. Registry data are periodically summarized and reviewed for possible "signals" that might lead to recommendations for initiation of a hypothesis-testing study. Strengths of registries include their potential for gathering early information about a new drug and the possibility of identifying a unique pattern of malformation that is associated with exposure to the drug of interest. However, traditional registries lack formal comparison groups and typically have outcome data on relatively small numbers of pregnancies. As a result, they usually have insufficient sample size to detect increased frequencies of specific and relatively rare birth defects.[26] Nevertheless, collaborative registry designs such as the Antiepileptic Drugs in Pregnancy Registry have demonstrated success in identifying signals or establishing higher than expected rates for major birth defects after selected exposures.[27]

Observational Cohort Studies

Another source of pregnancy safety data originates from observational cohort studies that are initiated with the goal of testing a specific hypothesis. These include prospectively designed exposure cohort studies in which women with and without the exposure of interest are enrolled during pregnancy and followed to outcome. Such studies have the ability to evaluate a spectrum of outcomes, including major and minor malformations, and to collect early information on a new drug. They also have the advantage of including a comparison group or groups, allowing for the control of key factors that may be confounders, such as maternal age, socioeconomic status, and alcohol or tobacco use. Such a study design was successful identifying carbamazepine as a human teratogen.[28] One disadvantage of this approach is that the sample sizes are typically too small to rule out anything but the most dramatically increased prevalence of specific major birth defects.

Database Cohorts

A variation of the observational cohort involves construction of an historical cohort using archived information in existing databases. For example, health maintenance organization claims data and records from government-supported healthcare agencies are increasingly being analyzed for information on pregnancies with or without specific medication exposures. The strengths of this approach include the potential cost savings for collecting data for a given number of pregnancies, but the limitations include sample sizes that are too small to detect increased risks for many, if not most, specific birth defects. In addition, because database studies rely on information not collected primarily for research purposes, validation of exposure and outcome, as well as data on some key potential confounders, may be difficult or impossible to obtain. Nevertheless, database cohorts have been used, for example, to identify a possible link between paroxetine and congenital heart defects.[29]

Case-Control Studies

In case-control study designs, pregnancies are retrospectively selected for having a specific outcome, such as a particular birth defect. The frequency of exposure to an agent of interest among mothers of affected infants is compared with the frequency among mothers whose pregnancies did not result in that birth defect. A major strength of case-control studies is that, with proper numbers of cases and controls, they can provide sufficient power to detect increased risks for rare outcomes. In addition, because they include a comparison group, they can collect information on important potential confounding variables such as age, socioeconomic status, and alcohol and tobacco use. The case-control approach was used successfully to identify the association of misoprostol (used to induce abortion) with a very high risk for a rare congenital facial nerve paralysis, Möbius syndrome.[30] Limitations to case-control studies include the lag time inherent in collecting information on a new drug, especially if it is infrequently used by pregnant women. Another limitation is the inability to evaluate an agent for a spectrum of outcomes that are as yet unidentified as part of the anomaly pattern. Finally, it is possible that women who are already aware of a negative outcome of their pregnancy may recall exposures more carefully (or incorrectly) than those who had a normal outcome.

Summary of Data Sources

In summary, the strengths and weaknesses of the methodologies that are available to evaluate for potential teratogenicity reveal that no single approach is sufficient. From the clinical perspective, this means that conclusions drawn from one type of study must be interpreted with caution until they are either confirmed or refuted by other types of studies. This is especially important in recognizing high-risk exposures (and perhaps even more so for identifying agents that are not teratogenic), so that appropriate treatment decisions can be made. From a public health perspective, a combination of complementary study designs is required, one that ideally is initiated in a coordinated, systematic fashion so as to provide clinicians and patients with the best and earliest possible information.[31]

Risk Assessments and Resources

The U.S. FDA established a widely used pregnancy safety category system that is incorporated into the product label with the intent of informing clinicians and pregnant women of the teratogenic risks associated with prescription drugs. However, this category system is frequently misunderstood by health care providers and patients alike. The categories are summarized in Table 20-1.

TABLE 20-1 FDA PREGNANCY CATEGORIES

Category	Definition
A	Adequate and well-controlled studies have failed to demonstrate a risk to the fetus in the first trimester of pregnancy (and there is no evidence of risk in later trimesters).
B	Animal reproduction studies have failed to demonstrate a risk to the fetus and there are no adequate and well-controlled studies in pregnant women.
C	Animal reproduction studies have shown an adverse effect on the fetus and there are no adequate and well-controlled studies in humans, but potential benefits may warrant use of the drug in pregnant women despite potential risks.
D	There is positive evidence of human fetal risk based on adverse reaction data from investigational or marketing experience or studies in humans, but potential benefits may warrant use of the drug in pregnant women despite potential risks.
X	Studies in animals or humans have demonstrated fetal abnormalities and/or there is positive evidence of human fetal risk based on adverse reaction data from investigational or marketing experience, and the risk involved in use of the drug in pregnant women clearly outweighs potential benefits.

In practice, the FDA category assigned to a medication often misrepresents or oversimplifies the actual evidence. For example, the category assignments do not take into consideration factors such as exposure timing in gestation or dose and route of administration. Although several drugs assigned to category X (i.e., contraindicated in pregnancy) are indeed known human teratogens (e.g., isotretinoin), others, such as ribavirin and the "statins," were assigned to that category based on theoretical concerns or animal data without conclusive human data to establish a teratogenic risk.[32] Further, incorporation of new data into the label and classification updates is often slow.

Communication of potential risk to a woman regarding a category X exposure that has already taken place varies substantially from that for an exposure that is anticipated. An example is the communication of information regarding risk from an exposure to ribavirin (to treat hepatitis C) that occurred during an unplanned pregnancy compared with the communication of concern if the clinician and patient are prospectively determining whether ribavirin is an appropriate medication to use. Such nuances are not reflected in the category statements. In recognition of these limitations and weaknesses, the FDA has worked with an advisory committee to develop recommended revisions to the category system and the label format.[33]

Other sources of information readily available to the clinician include a number of print resources, each with different approaches to providing summary information. Some of these references are available in hard copy, compact disk (CD-ROM), and personal digital assistant (PDA) versions.[34,35] Online databases that provide summary statements prepared by experts in the field of teratology and updated on a frequent basis include TERIS and REPROTOX (available at http://www.micromedex.com/reprorisk [accessed January 14, 2008]). In addition, the Organization of Teratology Information Specialists

(OTIS) provides individualized information to clinicians as well as the public via toll-free telephone access (see http://otispregnancy.org [accessed January 14, 2008]). Clinicians or patients who are interested in pregnancy registries that are open for enrollment can locate a current list at the FDA's Office of Women's Health Web site (available at http://www.fda.gov/womens/registries [accessed January 14, 2008]).

Selected Human Teratogens

Table 20-2 presents the potential effects of selected human teratogens, some of which are discussed further in the following sections.

Vitamin K Antagonists

A specific pattern of congenital anomalies referred to as the *fetal warfarin syndrome* has been identified in some children born to mothers who use medications such as phenprocoumon, acenocoumarol, fluindione, warfarin, and phenindione, which are vitamin K antagonists. The features include nasal hypoplasia, stippled epiphyses visible on radiographs, and growth restriction. Central nervous system (CNS) and eye abnormalities including microcephaly, hydrocephalus, Dandy-Walker malformation, agenesis of the corpus callosum, optic atrophy, cataracts, and mental retardation occur occasionally.[36,37] The critical period for the warfarin embryopathy appears to be between 6 and 9 weeks' gestation. A systematic review of 17 studies involving a total of 979 exposed pregnancies estimated a 6% incidence of warfarin embryopathy. In addition, 22% of exposed pregnancies ended in spontaneous abortion, 4% in stillbirth, and 13% in preterm delivery.[38] A large multicenter study of 666 pregnancies with exposure to vitamin K antagonists reported a significant increase in the rate of major birth defects overall, relative to unexposed healthy comparison women (odds ratio [OR], 3.86; 95% confidence interval [CI], 1.76 to 8.00). In that study, only 2 infants (0.6%) were thought to have warfarin embryopathy. In addition, the rate of preterm delivery was increased (16.0% versus 7.6%; OR, 2.61; CI, 1.76 to 3.86); the mean birth weight of term infants was significantly lower (3166 versus 3411 g); and the rate of spontaneous abortion was significantly higher (42% versus 14%; OR, 3.36; CI, 2.28 to 4.93) with exposure.[18]

In one study of 71 pregnancies occurring in 52 women with prosthetic heart valves who were being treated with warfarin, the risk for

TABLE 20-2 EFFECTS OF SELECTED TERATOGENS

Drug	Potential Effects	Comments
ACE inhibitors	Calvarial hypoplasia, renal dysgenesis, oligohydramnios, IUGR, and neonatal renal failure	Risk seen with use in second and third trimester
Alcohol	Syndrome: prenatal and postnatal growth restriction, microcephaly, craniofacial dysmorphology (1-4/1000 live births); renal, cardiac, and other major malformations increased	Risk not limited to first trimester; late pregnancy use is associated with IUGR and developmental delay; incidence is 4-44% among "heavy drinkers"
Antidepressants (SSRIs)	Possible cardiac defects, NTDs, omphalocele; neonatal pulmonary hypertension and withdrawal syndrome	—
Aminopterin and methotrexate	Syndrome: calvarial hypoplasia, craniofacial abnormalities, limb defects; possible developmental delay	Syndrome associated with methotrexate >10 mg/wk
Androgens and norprogesterones	Masculinization of external female genitalia	Labioscrotal fusion can occur with exposure; as many as 50% of those exposed are affected
Carbamazepine	NTDs (1%); possible facial hypoplasia and developmental delay	—
Corticosteroids	Cleft lip/palate increased threefold to sixfold; IUGR increased with high doses	—
Diethylstilbestrol	Clear cell adenocarcinoma of the vagina, vaginal adenosis, abnormalities of the cervix and uterus, testicular abnormalities, male/female infertility	—
Isotretinoin	Syndrome: CNS malformations, microtia/anotia, micrognathia, thymus abnormalities, cleft palate, cardiac abnormalities, eye anomalies, limb reduction defects (28%); miscarriage (22%), developmental delay (47%)	—
Lithium	Small increase in Ebstein cardiac anomaly	—
Penicillamine	Cutis laxa with chronic use	—
Phenytoin	Syndrome: IUGR, microcephaly, facial hypoplasia, hypertelorism, prominent upper lip (10%); possible developmental delay	Full syndrome in 10%; up to 30% exhibit some features
Streptomycin	Hearing loss, eighth nerve damage	—
Tetracycline	Discoloration of deciduous teeth and enamel hypoplasia	Risk only in second and third trimester
Tobacco	Oral clefts: relative risk, 1.22-1.34; IUGR, IUFD, abruption	—
Trimethadione	Syndrome: oral clefts, craniofacial abnormalities, developmental delay (80%)	—
Valproic acid	NTDs (1-2%); facial hypoplasia, possible developmental delay	—
Warfarin	Syndrome: nasal hypoplasia, stippled epiphyses, growth restriction (6%); also increased microcephaly, Dandy-Walker syndrome, IUGR, preterm birth, mental retardation	Greatest risk is at 6-9 wk

ACE, angiotensin-converting enzyme; CNS, central nervous system; IUGR, intrauterine growth restriction; NTD, neural tube defect.

adverse outcome was found to be significantly greater with doses greater than 5 mg/day.[39] A review of 85 pregnancies involving exposure to a coumarin drug only after the first trimester reported that 1 pregnancy ended in stillbirth, 3 in spontaneous abortion, and 19 in preterm births; 1 infant had a CNS anomaly, and none had the warfarin embryopathy.[38] In addition, in one large study that evaluated the cognitive performance of 307 children prenatally exposed to warfarin, compared with that of nonexposed children, mean IQ scores did not differ significantly, but low intelligence scores (IQ < 80) occurred more frequently in those children whose exposure was limited to the second and third trimester.[40]

Antiepileptic Drugs

As a group, most older drugs used to treat seizure disorders are associated with an increase in the risk of congenital malformations.[41,42] This has been suggested to indicate that the underlying disease is the teratogenic cause. Newer studies have challenged this concept[42-44]; however, it is difficult to separate the effects of the disease from those of treatment, especially for more severe epilepsy, which is unlikely to be untreated during pregnancy. The use of multiple anticonvulsant medications (polytherapy) as opposed to a single drug (monotherapy) is associated with greater risk of structural defects.[43,45,46] It is unclear whether this is a result of drug-drug interactions, more severe disease in women requiring treatment with polytherapy, or a combination of the two.

Diphenylhydantoin

Phenytoin as a treatment for seizure disorders has been associated with an increased risk for oral clefts and for a pattern of anomalies known as the *fetal hydantoin syndrome.* This pattern is estimated to occur in 10% of infants with prenatal exposure and includes prenatal or postnatal growth restriction, microcephaly, hypoplasia of the digits and nails, and craniofacial abnormalities (i.e., short nose with low nasal bridge, ocular hypertelorism, abnormal ears, and a wide mouth with a prominent upper lip).[47-49] Initial reports suggested that mental deficiency was also a common feature of fetal hydantoin syndrome.[50] However, the limited subsequently published data suggest that neurobehavioral effects may be more mild.[51] For example, Scolnik and colleagues[52] reported that average IQ scores were 10 points lower in children exposed to phenytoin monotherapy, compared with unexposed children born to mothers who were matched on age and socioeconomic status.

Valproic Acid

Studies over the last 2 decades have associated early first-trimester exposure to valproic acid with an increased risk for neural tube defects, specifically spina bifida. The estimated risk is about 1% to 2%, with higher doses thought to be associated with higher risk.[19,53] It has been estimated that the overall risk for major birth defects is increased by fourfold to sevenfold after valproate monotherapy, with increased risks for specific cardiovascular, limb, and genital anomalies noted in some reports.[27] As with other anticonvulsants, a pattern of minor malformations and growth deficiency has also been identified for valproic acid; it includes midface hypoplasia, epicanthal folds, short nose, broad nasal bridge, thin upper lip, thick lower lip, micrognathia, and subtle limb defects (primarily hyperconvex fingernails).[54] In addition, there is some evidence that valproic acid monotherapy is associated with reduced cognitive ability and additional educational needs in children prenatally exposed.[55,56]

Carbamazepine

Similar to valproic acid, carbamazepine has been associated with an increased risk for spina bifida (approximately 1%) with exposure in the early first trimester.[16] It has also been linked to a pattern of minor craniofacial abnormalities, including upslanting palpebral fissures, a long philtrum, and nail hypoplasia, as well as growth deficiency and microcephaly.[28] Although some small studies have suggested developmental delay after prenatal exposure to carbamazapine,[57] others have not.[58,59]

Other Antiepileptic Drugs

A number of newer antiepileptic medications have been introduced into practice over the past several years, including lamotrigine, gabapentin, and topiramate. Although these agents are currently being studied, insufficient information has been collected to rule out or identify risks similar to those seen with older anticonvulsants. Furthermore, specific risks associated with the use of older- and newer-generation anticonvulsants for other indications, such as treatment of mood disorders, has not been well studied.

Chemotherapeutic and Immunosuppressive Agents

Cyclophosphamide

Eight case reports documenting a unique pattern of malformation in infants prenatally exposed to cyclophosphamide have been published.[60] Features include growth deficiency, craniofacial anomalies, and absent fingers and toes. In three of these cases, the infant survived and developmental information was available; significant delays were noted in all three. The magnitude of the risk is unknown.

Methotrexate

Both aminopterin and its methyl derivative, methotrexate, have been associated with a specific pattern of malformation that includes prenatal-onset growth deficiency, severe lack of calvarial ossification, hypoplastic supraorbital ridges, small low-set ears, micrognathia, limb abnormalities, and, in some cases, developmental delay.[61,62] The majority of affected infants have been born to women treated with high-dose methotrexate for psoriasis or neoplastic disease or as an abortifacient. Although the magnitude of the risk is unknown, it has been suggested that the dose necessary to produce the aminopterin/methotrexate syndrome is greater than 10 mg/wk.[63,64]

Adrenal Corticosteroids

Among four recent case-control studies, three concluded that systemic corticosteroid use in the first trimester appears to be associated with a threefold to sixfold increased risk for cleft lip with or without cleft palate and possibly cleft palate alone.[65-68] It is unclear to what extent this association was caused by the various underlying maternal diseases involved in these studies. If only the positive studies are considered, this relative risk translates to a risk of approximately 3 to 6 cases per 1000 pregnancies exposed in the critical period for lip and palate closure. Furthermore, an association has long been recognized between prenatal exposure to corticosteroids and intrauterine growth restriction in humans. The risk appears to be dose-related, suggesting that this concern can be minimized with lower doses.[69,70]

Antihypertensive Medications

Angiotensin I Converting Enzyme (ACE) Inhibitors and Angiotensin II Receptor Antagonists

Based on case reports and case series, prenatal exposure to an ACE inhibitor (benazepril, captopril, enalapril, enalaprilat, fosinopril, lisinopril, moexipril, quinapril, ramipril) or to an angiotensin II receptor antagonist (losartan, candesartan, valsartan, tasosartan, telmisartan) during the second or third trimester of pregnancy is associated with an increased risk for fetal hypotension, renal failure, and oligohydramnios leading to fetal growth restriction, joint contractures, pulmonary hypoplasia, and stillbirth or neonatal death. Calvarial hypoplasia has also been reported as part of the fetopathy. In children who survive the neonatal period, renal insufficiency often occurs. The magnitude of the risk after second- or third-trimester exposure is not known.[25,71]

First-trimester exposure to ACE inhibitors or to angiotensin II receptor antagonists has not been well studied. One recent database linkage study suggested an increased risk for cardiovascular defects (risk ratio [RR], 3.72; CI, 1.89 to 7.30) and CNS defects (RR, 4.39; CI, 1.37 to 14.02) in infants born to mothers who had received a prescription for an ACE inhibitor in the first trimester of pregnancy, compared with infants born to women with no exposure to antihypertensive medications during pregnancy. However, these findings have not yet been replicated, and it is possible that they were confounded by inability to completely control for maternal diabetes.[72]

Psychotherapeutic Medications

Lithium

Early reports from a lithium exposure registry[73] included information on 143 infants exposed to lithium in utero; 13 of these were reported to have malformations, 4 of which were Ebstein anomaly (downward displacement of the tricuspid valves within the right ventricle). This finding represented an excess over expected numbers, because the baseline incidence of Ebstein anomaly is approximately 1 in 20,000 births. A subsequent prospective cohort study involving follow-up of 148 women with first-trimester exposure to lithium noted one case of Ebstein anomaly, with no other cardiac malformations identified in the sample.[74] In contrast, a case-control study published by Zalzstein and associates[75] found no prenatal exposure to lithium among 59 patients with Ebstein anomaly. In summary, the available data suggest that, if there is a risk at all, the use of lithium in the first trimester of pregnancy is associated with a very small increased risk for Ebstein anomaly.

Selective Serotonin Reuptake Inhibitors

Although medications within the selective serotonin reuptake inhibitor (SSRI) class of antidepressants (fluoxetine, paroxetine, sertraline, citalopram, escitalopram, fluvoxamine) have been studied extensively in pregnancy, most investigations have had insufficient sample sizes to rule out increased risks for specific malformations associated with individual medications. Several recent studies have suggested a small increased risk for cardiac defects (approximately twofold) specifically with first-trimester exposure to paroxetine.[76,77] One recent large, multisite, case-control study did not find an overall increase in cardiac defects but found increased risks for other selected malformations in association with first-trimester use of all SSRIs combined. These specific defects included anencephaly (adjusted OR, 2.4; CI 1.1 to 5.1), craniosynostosis (adjusted OR, 2.5; CI, 1.5 to 4.0), and omphalocele (adjusted OR, 2.8; CI, 1.3 to 5.7).[78] A second large, multisite, case-control study did not confirm these findings with respect to craniosynostosis, omphalocele, neural tube defects, or cardiac defects when all SSRIs were evaluated as a group but did find significantly increased risks with specific drugs. With first-trimester sertraline use, the odds were increased for omphalocele (adjusted OR, 5.7; CI, 1.6 to 20.7) and septal defects (adjusted OR, 2.0; CI, 1.2 to 4.0).[79] With first-trimester paroxetine use, the odds were increased for right ventricular outflow tract obstruction defects (adjusted OR, 3.3; CI, 1.3 to 8.8).

In addition to these findings with respect to structural defects, several other adverse outcomes have been associated with late pregnancy exposure to SSRIs. These include a possible small increased risk for persistent pulmonary hypertension of the newborn[80] and a well-established increased risk for a neonatal withdrawal or toxicity syndrome consisting primarily of CNS, motor, respiratory, and gastrointestinal signs that are generally mild and resolve by 2 weeks of age.[81]

Retinoids

Vitamin A (Retinol)

The teratogenic potential of excessive doses of preformed vitamin A is well described in animal models[82,83]; however, the threshold dose at which naturally occurring vitamin A might be teratogenic in humans remains controversial. Two studies suggested that preformed vitamin A supplementation at amounts greater than 10,000 IU per day in the first trimester of pregnancy is associated with a small increased risk of selected defects that are consistent with those known to be induced by synthetic retinoids.[84,85] However, other studies did not confirm these findings or suggested that the elevated risk is concentrated at doses greater than 40,000 IU per day.[86-88] The current recommended daily allowance (RDA) for pregnant women carrying a single fetus is 2560 IU of vitamin A. To avoid any of these potential concerns, many prenatal vitamin formulations have replaced retinol with β-carotene.

Isotretinoin and Other Oral Synthetic Retinoids

Consistent with animal data, an increased risk of pregnancy loss and a characteristic pattern of malformations and mental deficiency have been identified after prenatal exposure to isotretinoin. This pattern includes CNS malformations, microtia/anotia, micrognathia, cleft palate, cardiac and great vessel defects, thymic abnormalities, eye anomalies, and, occasionally, limb reduction defects.[20,89] The estimated risks are at least as high as 22% for spontaneous abortion, 28% for structural defects, and 47% for mild to moderate mental deficiency, even if no structural abnormalities are present.[20,90,91] Affected children have been reported with exposures to usual therapeutic doses and with treatment for durations shorter than 1 week in the first trimester. There does not appear to be a risk of malformations when the drug is discontinued before conception, which is consistent with the half-life of isotretinoin.[92,93] Pregnancy prevention among women who are prescribed isotretinoin continues to be a challenge. A third-generation restricted distribution program, iPledge, was implemented in March 2006; it mandates close monitoring of birth control practices and negative pregnancy testing before dispensing of prescriptions for isotretinoin.

Risks for the retinoid embryopathy are also found with other oral synthetic retinoids such as etretinate and its metabolite, acitretin, which are used for the treatment of psoriasis.[94] The extremely long half-life of etretinate led to its removal from the U.S. market in 1998. The half-life of acitretin is considerably longer than that of isotretinoin (50 to 60 hours), and it can be converted to etretinate with maternal ingestion of alcohol. Therefore, the drug must be discontinued before pregnancy, and alcohol must be avoided during the entire period of treatment and for at least 2 months after discontinuation of therapy.[95,96]

Ionizing Radiation

Prenatal exposure to high-dose radiation is associated with an increased risk of microcephaly, mental deficiency, and growth deficiency based on data derived from a small number of pregnant survivors of the atomic bombs in Nagasaki and Hiroshima.[97] It is estimated that doses of 50 rad (50 cGy) or greater to the uterus are required to produce these effects. The highest risk appears to be associated with exposures between 8 and 15 weeks' gestation, with a higher threshold dose at more advanced gestational ages.[98] The available data do not support an increase in the risk of mental retardation associated with high-dose radiation exposure beyond 25 weeks or before 8 weeks of gestation.[97] Based on dose-response calculations, it is not thought that diagnostic procedures involving radiation have the potential to pose a risk to the fetus unless the cumulative dose to the uterus is greater than 10 cGy; conservative guidelines suggest that doses should be kept below 5 cGy to the uterus during pregnancy if radiation exposure is required.[99]

Environmental Agents

Methylmercury

Prenatal exposure to methylmercury has been recognized as a neurodevelopmental teratogen since the experience of environmental contaminations in Japan (Minamata Bay) and Iraq in the mid-20th century.[100,101] The reported effects, termed *fetal methylmercury syndrome* or *congenital Minamata disease,* include cerebral palsy and a variety of neurologic and functional problems as well as mental deficiency.[102] Although the lower limit of exposure that may pose a risk in prenatal development remains controversial, an independent U.S. National Research Council expert committee concluded that limiting maternal intake to no more than 0.1 μg/kg/day was sufficient to protect the fetus.[103] Currently, consumption of contaminated fish or marine mammals is the major source of methylmercury exposure in most populations. The U.S. Environmental Protection Agency and FDA have advised pregnant women and women of childbearing age who may become pregnant to avoid eating shark, swordfish, king mackerel, and tilefish and to limit their average consumption of other cooked fish to 12 ounces (340 g) per week in order to prevent fetal exposure to excessive amounts of methylmercury.[104] Similarly, limiting tuna consumption to no more than three servings per week is recommended because of methylmercury concerns.

Lead

In utero exposure to very high levels of lead (maternal blood concentrations >30 μg/dL) has been associated with an increase in spontaneous abortion, preterm birth, and mental deficiency.[105,106] Prenatal exposure to lower levels (>10 μg/dL) may be associated with subtle neurobehavioral effects; however, these effects may not persist into older childhood.[107-109] Occupational and environmental exposures to lead that precede pregnancy may result in fetal exposure due to mobilization of lead stored in maternal bone. These effects may be modified by maternal intake of calcium.[110]

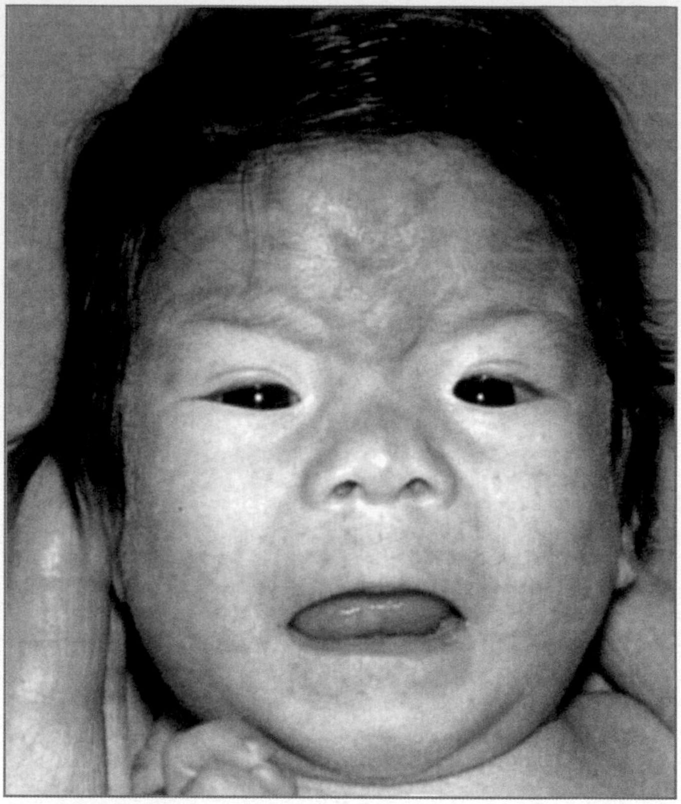

FIGURE 20-1 Nine-month-old infant with fetal alcohol syndrome. (From Streissguth AP, Aase JM, Clarren SK, et al: Fetal alcohol syndrome in adolescents and adults. JAMA 265:1961, 1991. Copyright 1991, American Medical Association.)

Social and Illicit Drugs

Alcohol

A pattern of anomalies, known as the *fetal alcohol syndrome (FAS),* was first described more than 35 years ago in a case series of infants born to alcoholic women.[111] The characteristic features of this disorder are prenatal and/or postnatal growth retardation, microcephaly or other CNS dysfunction including neurobehavioral deficits and neurologic impairment, and characteristic facial anomalies consisting of short palpebral fissures and a smooth philtrum, with a smooth, thin vermilion border of the upper lip (Fig. 20-1).[112,113] Although FAS is difficult to diagnose, particularly in the newborn period, estimates of its incidence in selected U.S. and Western European populations are approximately 1 to 4 per 1000 live births.[114]

Many more children are thought to have alcohol-related neurobehavioral or neurologic impairment with or without some structural features. In addition, congenital heart defects, oral clefts, and abnormalities of the eyes, brain, and kidneys are more common than expected among the children of women who drink moderately to heavily during pregnancy.[115-118] These children, variably described as having partial FAS, alcohol-related neurodevelopmental abnormalities (ARND), or alcohol-related birth defects (ARBD), are now thought of as representing a continuum known as fetal alcohol spectrum disorders (FASD). Accurate estimates of the prevalence of FASD are lacking; however, one population-based study in the Seattle, Washington, area suggested that the rates may be as high as 1 per 100 children.[114] Increased risks for spontaneous abortion, stillbirth, and sudden infant death syndrome have also been linked to prenatal alcohol exposure, particularly exposure from alcohol consumed in a heavy episodic or binge pattern.[119-122]

Both animal and human data support a dose-response relation in terms of risk for FAS/FASD. However, because of variabilities in diagnosis and difficulties in obtaining and validating exposure information reported by pregnant women, estimates vary widely regarding the magnitude of the risk. For example, estimates for the full-blown syndrome range from about 4% to 44% of children born to women who drink heavily during pregnancy.[123,124] The women at highest risk appear to be those who have already had an affected child and who continue to consume alcohol in subsequent pregnancies. Lower levels of maternal alcohol consumption have been associated with less severe neurobehavioral outcomes and persistent growth effects.[125-127] However, the exact threshold doses and patterns of consumption for these effects are not well understood. For example, full-blown FAS is typically seen among the children of women who report consuming an average of six or more standard drinks (beer, wine, or spirits) per day during pregnancy. However, some studies have suggested that women who consume more than two standard drinks per day during pregnancy are at increased risk. These risks may be mediated or ameliorated by the pattern of drinking (i.e., binge drinking versus more frequent and lesser quantities), maternal age, nutrition, and genetic susceptibility.[118,128-130] Furthermore, the duration of exposure is likely to be important, in that CNS development continues throughout gestation.[131]

At present, the data are insufficient to assign a risk to certain common patterns of prenatal alcohol exposure, such as alcohol consumption limited to occasional binge episodes before recognition of pregnancy. However, the data do support the notion that reduction or discontinuation of alcohol consumption at any point in pregnancy may be beneficial. A lower threshold of exposure, below which no effects will be seen, has not been defined. Therefore, for those women who are planning pregnancy or who have the potential to become pregnant, the U.S. Surgeon General has recommended that the safest course is to avoid alcohol entirely during pregnancy.[132]

Tobacco

Maternal cigarette smoking is associated with a variety of harmful effects on the embryo and fetus, including increased risks for specific congenital malformations, spontaneous abortion, placental complications, preterm delivery, reduced birth weight, and sudden infant death syndrome. The structural malformations that have been significantly associated with first-trimester smoking include oral clefts and gastroschisis. A recent meta-analysis of 24 studies estimated the risk for oral clefts to be low: the relative risk for cleft lip with or without cleft palate was 1.34 (CI, 1.25 to 1.44), and for cleft palate alone it was 1.22 (CI, 1.10 to 1.35).[133] Some studies have suggested gene-environment interactions in susceptibility for oral clefts when mothers smoke during early pregnancy. Infants who have a null deletion of the detoxifying gene *GSTT1*, or infant genotype at the Taq1 site for transforming growth factor-α and whose mothers smoke are at higher risk for certain oral clefts than infants with either risk factor alone.[134,135] The elevated risks for gastroschisis after maternal smoking are also estimated to be low.[136] However, as with oral clefts, there is some evidence for gene-environment interaction between maternal smoking and polymorphisms of fetal genes involved in vascular response.[137] Other defects reported to occur with increased frequency after pregnancy exposure to tobacco smoke include craniosynostosis and club foot.[138-140] Most studies with dose information available have suggested a dose-response relation for each of these defects, with the heaviest smokers being at highest risk.

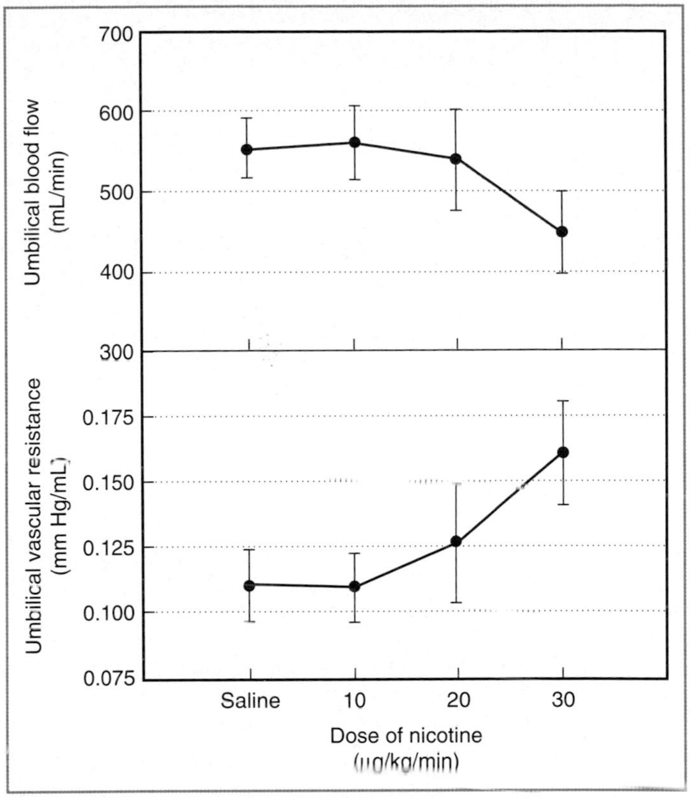

FIGURE 20-2 Umbilical blood flow and umbilical vascular resistance response to maternally administered nicotine. Maternal administration produced a decrease in umbilical blood flow from a baseline of 554 ± 37 to 449 ± 52 mL/min, which was significant only at the 30 μg/kg/min dose ($P < .05$). Umbilical vascular resistance increased from a baseline of 0.110 ± 0.013 to 0.161 ± 0.020 mm Hg/mL, which was significant only at the 30 μg/kg/min dose ($P < .05$). For the 20 μg/kg/min dose, $n = 6$. For saline solution and all other doses, $n = 8$. (From Clark KE, Irion GL: Fetal hemodynamic response to maternal intravenous nicotine administration. Am J Obstet Gynecol 167:1624, 1992.)

The deleterious effects of cigarette smoking on other pregnancy outcomes are well documented. Intrauterine growth restriction is the most consistently reported adverse outcome. On average, babies born to women who smoke during pregnancy are 200 g lighter than those born to comparable women who do not smoke, with a clear dose-response gradient.[141] This may be a result, in part, of the reduction in uterine blood flow associated with rising levels of plasma nicotine in women who smoke (Fig. 20-2).[142] Lesser reductions in birth weight have also been noted when exposure is limited to environmental or passive smoke.[143] A strong gene-environment and gene-gene–environment interaction has been demonstrated between the cytochrome P450 isozyme *CYP1A1* and *GSTT1* maternal metabolic genes and infant birth weight in mothers who smoke.[144]

Perinatal mortality is also increased with maternal smoking, in part because of the increased risks of placental complications and preterm delivery. In one large study, the combined risk for fetal or infant death for primiparous women who smoked less than one pack per day was estimated to be 25% higher than that for nonsmoking women, and the risk was 56% higher for those who smoked one pack per day or more.[145] However, if smoking is discontinued in the first half of gestation, evidence indicates that the effects on birth weight can be eliminated.[146-148]

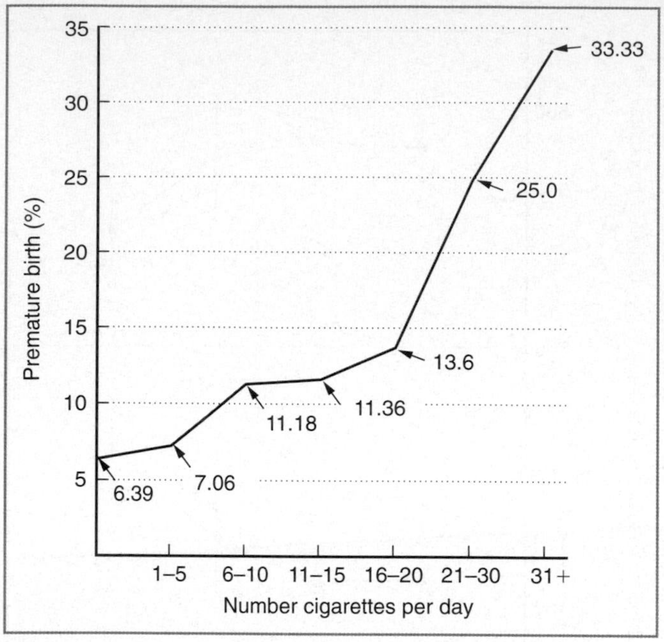

FIGURE 20-3 **Dose-response relationship of cigarette smoking and prematurity.** (From Simpson WJ: A preliminary report on cigarette smoking and the incidence of prematurity. Am J Obstet Gynecol 73:808, 1957.)

Furthermore, based on dose-response data, any reduction in the number of cigarettes smoked may reduce risk for low birth weight, preterm birth, and placental complications (Fig. 20-3).[149-153]

Cocaine

Various structural defects have been reported in newborns prenatally exposed to cocaine and are thought to be the result of intrauterine vascular accidents; they include cavitary CNS lesions, genitourinary anomalies, terminal transverse limb reduction defects, and intestinal atresia/infarction.[154-157] In addition to these structural defects, an increased risk for placental abruption and premature rupture of membranes was documented in a systematic review.[158] However, assessment of the absolute risk for these outcomes after cocaine exposure is complicated by the fact that affected pregnancies often involve use of other drugs, tobacco, and alcohol as well as cocaine; the purity and dose of the drug is often not known, and multiple potential other confounding factors could be involved.

The most consistently reported effects of prenatal cocaine exposure are a small but statistically significant increase in intrauterine growth restriction[159,160] and abnormalities in neonatal state regulation and motor performance.[161] However, based on a synthesis of 36 published studies of children 6 years of age or younger, Frank and colleagues[162] concluded that no consistent negative association existed between prenatal cocaine exposure and postnatal physical growth, developmental test scores, receptive language, or standardized parent and teacher reports of child behavior. An association between prenatal cocaine exposure and decreased emotional expressiveness has been suggested.[163]

References

1. Moore KL, Persaud TVN: The Developing Human: Clinically Oriented Embryology, 7th ed. Philadelphia: Saunders, 2002.
2. Forrest JM, Turnbull FM, Sholler GF, et al: Gregg's congenital rubella patients 60 years later. Med J Aust 177:664, 2002.
3. McBride WG: Thalidomide and congenital abnormalities. Lancet 2:1358, 1961.
4. Lenz W: Diskussionbemerkung zu dem Vortrag von RA Pfeiffer and K Kosenow: Zur Frage der exogenen Entstehung schwere Extremitatens-missbil-dungen. Tagung Rheinischwestful Kinderarztevere Dusseldorf 19:11, 1961.
5. Krantz JC: New drugs and the Kefauver-Harris amendment. J New Drugs 6:77, 1966.
6. Kutcher JS, Engle A, Firth J, et al: Bendectin and birth defects II: Ecological analyses. Birth Defects Res A Clin Molec Teratol 67:88, 2003.
7. Koren G, Pastuszak A, Ito S: Drugs in pregnancy. N Engl J Med 338:1128, 1998.
8. Lo WY, Friedman JM: Teratogenicity of recently introduced medications in human pregnancy. Obstet Gynecol 100:465, 2002.
9. Andrade SE, Gurwitz JH, Davis RL, et al: Prescription drug use in pregnancy. Am J Obstet Gynecol 191:398, 2004.
10. Werler MM, Mitchell AA, Hernandez-Diaz S, et al: Use of over-the-counter medications during pregnancy. Am J Obstet Gynecol 193:771, 2005.
11. Wilson JG, Fraser FC (eds): Handbook of Teratology. Vol. 1: General Principles and Etiology. New York, Plenum Press, 1977, pp 49-62.
12. Fratta ID, Sigg EB, Maiorana K: Teratogenic effects of thalidomide in rabbits, rats, hamsters, and mice. Toxicol Appl Pharmacol 7:268, 1965.
13. Shaw GM, Wasserman CR, Lammer EJ, et al: Orofacial clefts, parental cigarette smoking, and transforming growth factor-alpha gene variants. Am J Hum Genet 58:551, 1996.
14. Shaw GM, Wasserman CR, Murray JC, et al: Infant TGF-alpha genotype, orofacial clefts, and maternal periconceptional multivitamin use. Cleft Palate-Craniofac J 35:366, 1997.
15. Buehler BA, Delimont D, van Waes M, et al: Prenatal prediction of risk of the fetal hydantoin syndrome. N Engl J Med 322:1567, 1990.
16. Rosa FW: Spina bifida in infants of women treated with carbamazepine during pregnancy. N Engl J Med 321:674, 1991.
17. Matalon S, Schechtman S, Goldzweig G, et al: The teratogenic effect of carbamazepine: A meta-analysis of 1255 exposures. Reprod Toxicol 16:9, 2002.
18. Schaeffer C, Hanneman D, Meister R, et al: Vitamin K antagonists and pregnancy outcome: A multi-centre prospective study. Thromb Haemost 95:949, 2006.
19. Omtzigt JG, Los FJ, Grobbee DE, et al: The risk of spina bifida aperta after first-trimester exposure to valproate in a prenatal cohort. Neurology 42:119, 1992.
20. Lammer EJ, Chen DT, Hoar RM, et al: Retinoic acid embryopathy. N Engl J Med 313:837, 1985.
21. Shapiro L, Pastuszak A, Curto G, et al: Safety of first-trimester exposure to topical tretinoin: Prospective cohort study. Lancet 250:1143, 1997.
22. Loureiro KD, Kao KK, Jones KL, et al: Minor malformations characteristic of the retinoic acid embryopathy and other birth outcomes in children of women exposed to topical tretinoin during early pregnancy. Am J Med Genet A 136:117, 2005.
23. Floyd RL, O'Connor MJ, Sokol RJ, et al: Recognition and prevention of fetal alcohol syndrome. Obstet Gynecol 106:1059, 2005.
24. Hernandez-Diaz S, Werler MM, Walker AM, et al: Neural tube defects in relation to use of folic acid antagonists during pregnancy. Am J Epidemiol 153:961, 2001.
25. Barr M: Teratogen update: angiotensin-converting enzyme inhibitors. Teratology 50:399, 1994.
26. Honein MA, Paulozzi LJ, Cragan JD, et al: Evaluation of selected characteristics of pregnancy drug registries. Teratology 60:356, 1999.
27. Wyszynski DF, Nambisan M, Surve T, et al: Antiepileptic Drug Pregnancy Registry: Increased rate of major malformations in offspring exposed to valproate during pregnancy. Neurology 64:961, 2005.
28. Jones KL, Lacro RV, Johnson KA, et al: Pattern of malformations in the children of women treated with carbamazepine during pregnancy. N Engl J Med 320:1661, 1989.

29. Glaxo Smith Kline: Paroxetine Studies: EPIP083. Available at http://ctr.gsk.co.uk/summary/paroxetine/studylist.asp (accessed January 14, 2008).
30. Pastuszak AL, Schuler L, Speck-Martins CE, et al: Use of misoprostol during pregnancy and Mobius' syndrome in infants. N Engl J Med 339:1553, 1998.
31. Mitchell AA: Systematic identification of drugs that cause birth defects: A new opportunity. N Engl J Med 349:2556, 2003.
32. Polifka J, Friedman JM: Developmental toxicity of Ribavirin/IFalpha combination therapy: Is the label more dangerous than the drugs? Birth Defects Res A Clin Molec Teratol 67:8, 2003.
33. Scialli A, Buelke-Sam JL, Chambers CD, et al: Communicating risk during pregnancy: A workshop on the use of data from animal developmental toxicity studies in pregnancy labels for drugs. Birth Defects Res A Clin Molec Teratol 70:7, 2004.
34. Weiner CP, Buhimschi C: Drugs for Pregnant and Lactating Women, 2nd ed. New York: Churchill Livingstone, 2007.
35. Schaeffer C, Peters PWJ, Miller RK (eds): Drugs During Pregnancy and Lactation: Treatment Options and Risk Assessment. New York: Academic Press, 2007.
36. Holzgreve W, Carey JC, Hall BD: Warfarin-induced fetal abnormalities. Lancet 2:914, 1976.
37. Hall JG, Pauli RM, Wilson KM: Maternal and fetal sequelae of anticoagulation during pregnancy. Am J Med 68:122, 1980.
38. van Driel D, Wesseling J, Sauer PJ, et al: Teratogen update: Fetal effects after in utero exposure to coumarins overview of cases, follow-up findings, and pathogenesis. Teratology 66:127, 2002.
39. Cotrufo M, DeFeo M, DeSanto LS, et al: Risk of warfarin during pregnancy with mechanical valve prostheses. Obstet Gynecol 99:35, 2002.
40. van Driel D, Wesseling J, Sauer PJ, et al: In utero exposure to coumarins and cognition at 8-14 years. Pediatrics 107:123, 2001.
41. Gilmore J, Pennell PB, Stern BJ: Medication use during pregnancy for neurologic conditions. Neurol Clin 16:189, 1998.
42. Canger R, Battino D, Canevini MP, et al: Malformations in offspring of women with epilepsy: A prospective study. Epilepsia 40:1231, 1999.
43. Holmes LB, Harvey EA, Coull BA, et al: The teratogenicity of anticonvulsant drugs. N Engl J Med 344:1132, 2001.
44. Yerby MS: Epilepsy and pregnancy: New issues for an old disorder. Neurol Clin 11:777, 1993.
45. Kaneko S, Otani K, Fukushima Y, et al: Teratogenicity of antiepileptic drugs: An analysis of possible risk factors. Epilepsia 29:459, 1988.
46. Koch S, Losche G, Jager-Roman E, et al: Major and minor birth malformations and antiepileptic drugs. Neurology 42:83, 1992.
47. Hanson JW, Smith DW: The fetal hydantoin syndrome. J Pediatr 87:285, 1975.
48. Hanson JW, Myrianthopoulos NC, Harvey MA, et al: Risks to offspring of women treated with hydantoin anticonvulsants with emphasis on the fetal hydantoin syndrome. J Pediatr 89:662, 1976.
49. Kelly TE, Rein M, Edwards P: Teratogenicity of anticonvulsant drugs I: Review of the literature. Am J Med Genet 19:413, 1984.
50. Hanson JW: Teratogen update: Fetal hydantoin effects. Teratology 33:349, 1986.
51. Adams J, Voorhees CV, Middaugh LD: Developmental neurotoxicity of anticonvulsants: Human and animal evidence on phenytoin. Neurotoxicol Teratol 12:203, 1990.
52. Scolnik D, Nulman I, Rovet J, et al: Neurodevelopment of children exposed in utero to phenytoin and carbamazepine monotherapy. JAMA 271:767, 1994.
53. Robert E, Guibaud P: Maternal valproic acid and congenital neural tube defects. Lancet 2:937, 1982.
54. DiLiberti JH, Farndon PA, Dennis NR, et al: The fetal valproate syndrome. Am J Med Genet 19:473, 1984.
55. Adab N, Jacoby A, Smith D, et al: Additional educational needs in children born to mother with epilepsy. J Neurol Neurosurg Psychiatry 70:15, 2001.
56. Adab N, Kini V, Vinten J, et al: The longer-term outcome of children born to mothers with epilepsy. J Neurol Neurosurg Psychiatry 75:1575, 2004.
57. Ornoy A, Cohen E: Outcome of children born to epileptic mothers treated with carbamazepine during pregnancy. Arch Dis Child 75:517, 1996.
58. Nulman I, Scolnik D, Chitayat D, et al: Findings in children exposed in utero to phenytoin and carbamazepine monotherapy: Independent effects of epilepsy and medications. Am J Med Genet 68:18-24, 1997.
59. Wide K, Henning E, Tomson T, Winbladh B: Psychomotor development in preschool children exposed to antiepileptic drugs in utero. Acta Paediatr 91:409, 2002.
60. Vaux KK, Kahole NCO, Jones KL: Cyclophosphamide, methotrexate and cytarabine embryopathy: Is apoptosis the common pathway? Birth Defects Res A Clin Mol Teratol 67:403, 2003.
61. Milunsky A, Graef JW, Gaynor MF Jr: Methotrexate-induced congenital malformations. J Pediatr 72:790, 1968.
62. Del Campo M, Kosaki K, Bennett FC, et al: Developmental delay in fetal aminopterin/methotrexate syndrome. Teratology 60:10, 1999.
63. Feldkamp M, Carey JC: Clinical teratology counseling and consultation case report: Low dose methotrexate exposure in the early weeks of pregnancy. Teratology 47:553, 1993.
64. Lewden B, Vial T, Elefant E, et al: Low dose methotrexate in the first trimester of pregnancy: Results of a French collaborative study. J Rheumatol 31:2360, 2004.
65. Rodriguez-Pinilla E, Martinez-Frias ML: Corticosteroids during pregnancy and oral clefts: A case-control study. Teratology 58:2, 1988.
66. Czeizel AE, Rockenbauer M: Population-based case-controls study of teratogenic potential of corticosteroids. Teratology 56:335, 1997.
67. Carmichael SL, Shaw GM: Maternal corticosteroid use and risk of selected congenital anomalies. Am J Med Genet 86:242, 1999.
68. Pradat P, Robert-Gnasia E, Di Tanna GL, et al: First trimester exposure to corticosteroids and oral clefts. Birth Defects Res A Clin Mol Teratol 67:968, 2003.
69. Reinisch JM, Simon NG, Karow WG, et al: Prenatal exposure to prednisone in humans and animals retards intrauterine growth. Science 202:436, 1978.
70. Rayburn WF. Glucocorticord therapy for rheumatic diseases: Maternal, fetal, and breast-feeding considerations. Am J Reprod Immunol 28:138, 1992.
71. Alwan S, Polifka JE, Friedman JM: Angiotensin II receptor antagonists treatment during pregnancy. Birth Defects Res A Clin Mol Teratol 73:123, 2005.
72. Cooper WO, Hernandez-Diaz S, Arbogast PG et al: Angiotensin converting enzyme inhibitors and the risk of major congenital malformations. N Engl J Med 354:2443, 2006.
73. Weinstein MR, Goldfield M: Cardiovascular malformations with lithium use during pregnancy. Am J Psychiatry 132:529-531, 1975.
74. Jacobson SJ, Jones K, Johnson K, et al: Prospective multicentre study of pregnancy outcome after lithium exposure during first trimester. Lancet 339:869, 1992.
75. Zalzstein E, Koren G, Einarson T, Freedom RM: A case-control study on the association between first trimester exposure to lithium and Ebstein's anomaly. Am J Cardiol 65:817-818, 1990.
76. Kallen BAJ, Olausson PO: Maternal use of selective serotonin re-uptake inhibitors in early pregnancy and infant congenital malformations. Birth Defects Res A Clin Mol Teratol 79:301, 2007.
77. Berard A, Ramos E, Rey E, et al: First trimester exposure to paroxetine and risk of cardiac malformations in infants: The importance of dosage. Birth Defects Res B Reprod Toxicol 80:18, 2007.
78. Alwan S, Reefhuis J, Rasmussen SA, et al: Use of selective serotonin-reuptake inhibitors in pregnancy and the risk of birth defects. N Engl J Med 354:2684, 2007.
79. Louik C, Lin AE, Werler MM, et al: First-trimester use of selective serotonin-reuptake inhibitors and the risk of birth defects. N Engl J Med 356:2675, 2007.
80. Chambers CD, Hernandez-Diaz S, Van Marter LJ, et al: Selective serotonin-reuptake inhibitors and risk fo persistent pulmonary hypertension of the newborn. N Engl J Med 354:579, 2006.
81. Moses-Kolko EL, Bogen D, Perel J, et al: Neonatal signs after late in utero exposure to serotonin reuptake inhibitors JAMA 293:2372, 2005.

82. Geelen JA, Langman J, Lowdon JD: The influence of excess vitamin A on neural tube closure in the mouse embryo. Anat Embryol (Berl) 159:223, 1980.
83. Rosa FW, Wilk AL, Kelsey FP: Teratogen update: Vitamin A congeners. Teratology 33:355, 1986.
84. Rothman KJ, Moore LL, Singer MR, et al: Teratogenicity of high vitamin A intake. N Engl J Med 333:1369, 1995.
85. Botto LD, Loffredo C, Scanlon KS, et al: Vitamin A and cardiac outflow tract defects. Epidemiology 12:491, 2000.
86. Werler MM, Lammer EJ, Rosenberg L, et al: Maternal vitamin A supplementation in relation to selected birth defects. Teratology 42:497, 1990.
87. Mills JL, Simpson JL, Cunningham GC, et al: Vitamin A and birth defects. Am J Obstet Gynecol 177:31, 1997.
88. Martinez-Frias ML, Salvador J: Epidemiological aspects of prenatal exposure to high doses of vitamin A in Spain. Eur J Epidemiol 6:118, 1990.
89. Rizzo R, Lammer EJ, Parano E, et al: Limb reduction defects in humans associated with prenatal isotretinoin exposure. Teratology 44:599, 1991.
90. Dai WS, LaBraico JM, Stern RS: Epidemiology of isotretinoin exposure during pregnancy. J Am Acad Dermatol 26:599, 1992.
91. Adams J, Lammer EJ: Neurobehavioral teratology of isotretinoin. Reprod Toxicol 7:175, 1993.
92. Dai WS, Hsu M-A, Itri LM: Safety of pregnancy after discontinuation of isotretinoin. Arch Dermatol 125:362, 1989.
93. Kallen B: Restriction of the use of drugs with teratogenic properties: Swedish experiences with isotretinoin. Teratology 60:53, 1999.
94. Geiger J-M, Baudin M, Saurat J-H: Teratogenic risk with etretinate and acitretin treatment. Dermatology 189:109, 1994.
95. Maradit H, Geiger J-M: Potential risk of birth defects after acitretin discontinuation. Dermatology 198:3, 1999.
96. Grønhøj Larsen F, Steinkjer B, Jakobsen P, et al: Acitretin is converted to etretinate only during concomitant alcohol intake. Br J Dermatol 143:116, 2000.
97. Otake M, Schull WJ: In utero exposure to A-bomb radiation and mental retardation: A reassessment. Br J Radiol 57:409, 1984.
98. Yamazaki JN, Schull WJ: Perinatal loss and neurological abnormalities among children of the atomic bomb: Nagasaki and Hiroshima revisited, 1949 to 1989. JAMA 265:605-609, 1990.
99. Brent RJ: The effect of embryonic and fetal exposure to x-ray, microwaves, and ultrasound: Counseling the pregnant and nonpregnant patient about these risks. Semin Oncol 16:347, 1989.
100. Matsumoto H, Koya G, Takeuchi T: Fetal Minimata disease: A neuropathological study of two cases of intrauterine intoxication by a methylmercury compound. J Neuropath Exp Neurol 24:563, 1965.
101. Bakir F, Damluji SF, Amin-Zaki L, et al: Methylmercury poisoning in Iraq: An interuniversity report. Science 181:230, 1973.
102. Kondo K: Congenital Minamata disease: Warnings from Japan's experience. J Child Neurol 15:458, 2000.
103. Mahaffey KR: Recent advances in recognition of low-level methylmercury poisoning. Curr Opin Neurol 13:699, 2000.
104. U.S. Environmental Protection Agency and U.S. Food and Drug Administration: What You Need to Know about Mercury in Fish and Shellfish. Available at http://www.epa.gov/waterscience/fishadvice/advice.html (accessed January 14, 2008).
105. Rom WN: Effects of lead on the female and reproduction: A review. Mt Sinai J Med 43:542-53, 1976.
106. Hertz-Picciotto I: The evidence that lead increases the risk for spontaneous abortion. Am J Ind Med 38:300, 2000.
107. Bellinger D, Leviton A, Waternaux C, et al: Longitudinal analyses of prenatal and postnatal lead exposure and early cognitive development. N Engl J Med 316:1037, 1987.
108. Dietrich KN, Krafft KM, Bornschein RL, et al: Low-level fetal lead exposure effect on neurobehavioral development in early infancy. Pediatrics 80:721, 1987.
109. Tong SL, Baghurst P, McMichael A, et al: Lifetime exposure to environmental lead and children's intelligence at 11-13 years: The Port Pirie cohort study. BMJ 312:1569, 1996.
110. Hertz-Picciotto I, Schramm M, Watt-Morse M, et al: Patterns and determinants of blood lead during pregnancy. Am J Epidemiol 152:829, 2000.
111. Jones KL, Smith DW, Ulleland CN, et al: Pattern of malformation in offspring of chronic alcoholic mothers. Lancet 1:1267, 1973.
112. Streissguth AP, Aase JM, Clarren SK, et al: Fetal alcohol syndrome in adolescents and adults. JAMA 265:1961, 1991.
113. Hoyme HE, May PA, Kalberg WO, et al: A practical clinical approach to diagnosis of fetal alcohol spectrum disorders: Clarification of the 1996 institute of medicine criteria. Pediatrics 115:39, 2005.
114. Sampson PD, Streissguth AP, Bookstein FL, et al: Incidence of fetal alcohol syndrome and prevalence of alcohol-related neurodevelopmental disorder. Teratology 56:317, 1997.
115. Moore CA, Khoury MJ, Liu Y: Does light-to-moderate alcohol consumption during pregnancy increase the risk for renal anomalies among offspring? Pediatrics 99:E11, 1997.
116. Shaw GM, Lammer EJ: Maternal periconceptional alcohol consumption and risk for orofacial clefts. J Pediatr 134:298, 1999.
117. Williams LJ, Correa A, Rasmussen S: Maternal lifestyle factors and risk for ventricular septal defects. Birth Defects Res A Clin Mol Teratol 70:59, 2004.
118. Martínez-Frías ML, Bermejo E, Rodríguez-Pinilla E, et al: Risk for congenital anomalies associated with different sporadic and daily doses of alcohol consumption during pregnancy: A case-control study. Birth Defects Res A Clin Mol Teratol 70:194, 2004.
119. Kesmodel U, Wisborg K, Olsen SF, et al: Moderate alcohol intake in pregnancy and the risk of spontaneous abortion. Alcohol Alcohol 37:87, 2002.
120. Kesmodel U, Wisborg K, Olsen SF, et al: Moderate alcohol intake during pregnancy and the risk of stillbirth and death in the first year of life. Am J Epidemiol 155:305, 2002.
121. Iyasu S, Randall LL, Welty TK, et al: Risk factors for sudden infant death syndrome among northern plains Indians. JAMA 288:2717, 2002.
122. Carpenter RG, Irgens LM, Blair PS, et al: Sudden unexplained infant death in 20 regions in Europe: Case control study. Lancet 363:185, 2004.
123. Abel EL: An update on the incidence of FAS: FAS is not an equal opportunity birth defect. Neurotoxicol Teratol 17:437, 1995.
124. Jones KL, Smith DW: The fetal alcohol syndrome. Teratology 12:1, 1975.
125. Streissguth AP, Barr HM, Sampson PD: Moderate prenatal alcohol exposure: Effects on child IQ and learning problems at age 7 1/2 years. Alcohol Clin Exp Res 14:662, 1990.
126. Day NL, Leech SL, Richardson GA, et al: Prenatal alcohol exposure predicts continued deficits in offspring size at 14 years of age. Alcohol Clin Exp Res 26:1584, 2002.
127. Jacobson SW: Specificity of neurobehavioral outcomes associated with prenatal alcohol exposure. Alcohol Clin Exp Res 22:313-320, 1998.
128. Jacobson SW, Jacobson JL, Sokol RJ, et al: Maternal age, alcohol abuse history, and quality of parenting as moderators of the effects of prenatal alcohol exposure on 7.5-year intellectual function. Alcohol Clin Exp Res 28:1732, 2004.
129. Khaole NC, Ramchandani VA, Viljoen DL, et al: A pilot study of alcohol exposure and pharmacokinetics in women with or without children with fetal alcohol syndrome. Alcohol Alcohol 39:503, 2004.
130. Warren KR, Li T-K: Genetic polymorphisms: Impact on the risk of fetal alcohol spectrum disorders. Birth Defects Res A Clin Mol Teratol 73:195, 2005.
131. Goodlett CR, West JR: Fetal alcohol effects: Rat model of alcohol exposure during the brain growth spurt. In Zagon IS, Slotkin TA (eds). Maternal Substance Abuse and the Developing Nervous System. San Diego, Academic Press, 1992, pp 45-75.
132. U.S. Department of Health and Human Services, Office of the Surgeon General: News Release: U.S. Surgeon General Releases Advisory on Alcohol Use in Pregnancy, February 21, 2005. Available at http://www.surgeongeneral.gov/pressreleases/sg02222005.html (accessed January 14, 2008).

133. Little J, Cardy A, Munger RG: Tobacco smoking and oral clefts: A meta-analysis. Bull World Health Organ 82:213, 2004.
134. Shi M, Christensen K, Weinberg CR, et al: Orofacial cleft risk is increased with maternal smoking and specific detoxification-gene variants. Am J Hum Genet 80:76, 2006.
135. Zeiger JS, Beaty TH, Liang KY: Oral clefts, maternal smoking, and TGFA: A meta-analysis of gene-environment interaction. Cleft Palate Craniofac J 42:58, 2005.
136. Haddow JE, Palomaki GE, Holman MS: Young maternal age and smoking during pregnancy as risk factors for gastroschisis. Teratology 47:225, 1993.
137. Torfs CP, Christianson RE, Iovannisci DM, et al: Selected gene polymorphisms and their interaction with maternal smoking, as risk factors for gastroschisis. Birth Defects Res A Clin Mol Teratol 76:723, 2006.
138. Honein MA, Rasmussen SA: Further evidence for an association between maternal smoking and craniosynostosis. Teratology 62:145, 2000.
139. Honein MA, Paulozzi LJ, Watkins ML: Maternal smoking and birth defects: Validity of birth certificate data for effect estimation. Public Health Rep 116:327, 2001.
140. Skelly AC, Holt VL, Mosca VS, et al: Talipes equinovarus and maternal smoking: A population-based case-control study in Washington state. Teratology 66:91, 2002.
141. Eskenazi B, Prehn AW, Christianson RE: Passive and active maternal smoking as measured by serum cotinine: The effect on birthweight. Am J Public Health 85:395-398, 1995.
142. Clark KE, Irion GL: Fetal hemodynamic response to maternal intravenous nicotine administration. Am J Obstet Gynecol 167:1624, 1992.
143. Windham GC, Eaton A, Hopkins B. Evidence for an association between environmental tobacco smoke exposure and birthweight: A meta-analysis and new data. Paediatr Perinat Epidemiol 13:35-57, 1999.
144. Wang X, Zuckerman B, Pearson C, et al: Maternal cigarette smoking, metabolic gene polymorphism, and infant birth weight. JAMA 287:195, 2002.
145. Kleinman JC, Pierre MB Jr, Madans JH, et al: The effects of maternal smoking on fetal and infant mortality. Am J Epidemiol 127:274, 1988.
146. MacArthur C, Knox EG: Smoking in pregnancy: Effects of stopping at different stages. BJOG 95:551, 1988.
147. McDonald AD, Armstrong BG, Sloan M: Cigarette, alcohol, and coffee consumption and prematurity. Am J Public Health 82:87, 1992.
148. Lindley AA, Becker S, Gray RH, et al: Effect of continuing or stopping smoking during pregnancy on infant birth weight, crown-heel length, head circumference, ponderal index, and brain:body weight ratio. Am J Epidemiol 152:219, 2000.
149. Naeye RL: Abruptio placentae and placenta previa: Frequency, perinatal mortality, and cigarette smoking. Obstet Gynecol 55:701, 1980.
150. Sexton M, Hebel JR: A clinical trial of change in maternal smoking and its effect on birth weight. JAMA 251:911, 1984.
151. Dolan-Mullen P, Ramírez G, Groff JY: A meta-analysis of randomized trials of prenatal smoking cessation interventions. Am J Obstet Gynecol 171:1328, 1994.
152. Mainous AG 3rd, Hueston WJ: The effect of smoking cessation during pregnancy on preterm delivery and low birthweight. J Fam Pract 38:262, 1994.
153. Simpson WJ: A preliminary report on cigarette smoking and the incidence of prematurity. Am J Obstet Gynecol 73:808, 1957.
154. Hoyme HE, Jones KL, Dixon SD, et al: Prenatal cocaine exposure and fetal vascular disruption. Pediatrics 85:743, 1991.
155. Dixon SD, Bejar R: Echoencephalographic findings in neonates associated with with maternal cocaine and methamphetamine use: Incidence and clinical correlates. J Pediatr 115:770, 1989.
156. Bingol N, Fuchs M, Diaz V, et al: Teratogenicity of cocaine in humans. J Pediatr 110:93, 1987.
157. Chavez GF, Mulinare J, Cordero JF: Maternal cocaine use during early pregnancy as a risk factor for congenital urogenital anomalies. JAMA 262:795, 1989.
158. Addis A, Moretti ME, Syed FA, et al: Fetal effects of cocaine: An updated meta-analysis. Reprod Toxicol 15: 341, 2001.
159. Lutiger B, Grahm K, Einarson TR, et al: Relationship between gestational cocaine use and pregnancy outcome. Teratology 44:405, 1991.
160. Holzman C, Paneth N: Maternal cocaine use during pregnancy and perinatal outcome. Epidemiol Rev 16:315, 1994.
161. Held JR, Riggs ML, Dorman C: The effect of prenatal cocaine exposure on neurobehavioral outcome. Neurotoxicol Teratol 21:619, 1999.
162. Frank DA, Augustyn M, Knight WG, et al: Growth, development and behavior in early childhood following prenatal cocaine exposure JAMA 285:1613, 2001.
163. Allesandri S, Sullivan MW, Imaizumi S, et al: Learning and emotional responsivity in cocaine-exposed infants. Dev Psychol 29:989, 1993.

Chapter 21

Assessment of Fetal Health

Christopher R. Harman, MD

Defining fetal status clarifies many perinatal decisions. If fetal condition is reassuring and the situation is stable, management is confidently conservative, seeking further intrauterine time for maturation. If fetal status is uncertain, management will depend on gestational age: near term, delivery may be the best option; before then, enhanced surveillance and preparation for delivery is indicated; remote from term, intrauterine therapy might be in order. When fetal compromise is certain, our primary responses are delivery and neonatal management—down to the frontiers of viability. So, what we do is determined by what we think of fetal status.

Just as fetal status indicates management, fetal and maternal conditions modify our approach to surveillance. Risk assignment, and the corresponding acuity of our monitoring, is a process of constant revision. Historical factors are important, but they give way as more specific information becomes available from first- and second-trimester screening and the performance of the individual fetus. Maternal conditions change as well, with advancing gestation, worsening disease, and interaction of maternal treatment all superimposed on changes in placental function and fetal demands. Monitoring must cope with these many complexities.

As the interlocutor between maternal-fetal status and clinical action, assessment of fetal well-being must meet many demands. These requirements, and the complex situations in which they must apply, dictate the prime directive of all fetal assessment: No single parameter can suffice. The aim of this chapter is to describe the integration of multiple components in a comprehensive approach to fetal assessment.

Normal Fetal Behavior

If we can reliably equate normal behavior with normal healthy status, many types of fetal activity provide avenues for evaluation of fetal status. Beginning with pioneering work focused on fetal breathing,[1,2] it became clear that the absence of specific fetal behaviors could mean serious hypoxemia or acidosis.[3-5] The number of parameters has multiplied, and their application has extended to progressively lower gestational ages, but the general pattern has endured for most variables: present equals normal, and absent equals abnormal.

Basic Functions

Even the most primary functions are subject to marked variability that conditions monitoring techniques and interpretation. Fetal heart rate (FHR) comes under increasing parasympathetic dominance as pregnancy progresses, resulting in a gradual decrease in heart rate, increase in variability, increasing responsiveness (both accelerations and decelerations), and the emergence of complex relationships with other behaviors.[6] Variability in basic functions is not restricted to neurologic interactions; as placental and fetal vascular systems mature, so do Doppler resistance characteristics, regionalization of blood flow, and cardiovascular reflexes.[7] Even at term, changes in cerebral circulation may reflect maturation patterns.[8] In short, the interpretation of fetal vital functions requires detailed understanding of the fetal environment.

Individual Behaviors

Coordinated activities such as thumbsucking, respiratory movements, and apparently deliberate changes in position begin very early. A large repertoire of fetal activities is already established by 10 to 12 weeks. These individual behaviors change throughout pregnancy, and their distribution may alter dramatically. For example, fetal hiccups are the most dominant form of early diaphragmatic activity, giving way later to rhythmic fetal breathing movement.[9] Fetal breathing movements, in turn, become much more responsive to maternal glucose levels, the emergence of behavioral states, and circadian rhythms, and they may even show patterns of carbon dioxide responsiveness identical to those of newborn infants as pregnancy progresses.[10,11] Fetal body movement also demonstrates increasing sophistication with advancing gestation. The wriggling activity seen at 8 to 10 weeks gives way to the total body jumping activity that gradually diminishes as the second trimester begins. By that time, defined kicking, delicate hand movements, fetal breathing, and virtually all the individual behaviors of the term fetus can be demonstrated. The distribution of individual behaviors changes markedly over the remainder of pregnancy, including the often dramatic reduction in fetal kicking at 34 to 38 weeks with the onset of small-amplitude highly coordinated movements typical of infants. Chapter 13 addresses fetal breathing and body movements in greater detail.

Patterned Behavior

As individual behaviors change, so do their relationships with one another. In the first trimester, individual behaviors are present, often to the virtual exclusion of others (e.g., the fetus almost never hiccups while moving). By 18 to 20 weeks, there are periods of high and low activity, during which many behaviors may appear simultaneously.

Beginning at this time, diurnal patterns are evident in fetal urine production, adrenal steroid production, heart rate, Doppler arterial velocities, and virtually all complex behaviors.[12-14]

Fetal Behavioral States

By the beginning of the third trimester, behavioral states 1F to 4F can be defined,[4,9,15] and they are directly analogous to the neonatal behavioral states originally described by Prechtl.[16] Two patterns dominate—quiet sleep and active sleep. In quiet sleep, state 1F, rapid eye movements and repetitive mouthing movements are present, but almost all other movements are absent. As term approaches, this level of inactivity extends, from a mean of about 220 seconds in mid-trimester, to as long as 110 minutes by 40 weeks.[9,17] During state 2F, active sleep, movements are grouped, providing efficient monitoring, because multiple activities overlap. In state 4F (active awake), the "jogging fetus" illustrates a high level of voluntary activity and also a sustained high heart rate where return to baseline may be interpreted as decelerations. As with its neonatal equivalent, state 3F (quiet awake) is unusual and short and is seldom present before term. Clearly, fetal assessment using any or all of these variables must account for their complex presentation and for their influence on basic functions, such as Doppler characteristics.[18,19]

Coupled Behaviors

Several behavioral characteristics provide advantages for monitoring because they are coupled. The classic association of FHR accelerations with fetal movement, the basis of the nonstress test (NST), is so reliable that an acceleration of significant amplitude can be inferred to prove fetal activity.[20] Fetal breathing movements and maternal glucose levels are reliably connected, so that fetal assessment units operate most efficiently in the 2 to 3 hours after each mealtime.[21] Of course, fetal breathing movements produce effects in many other individual parameters (Fig. 21-1). Over the longer term, the pairing of sleep and wake cycles may be the most reliable evidence available of normal fetal oxygen status.[22]

Fetal-to-Neonatal Transition

True "infant" behavior in term fetuses is seen in many systems. Sometimes this responsiveness is problematic; even earlier than term, the fetal ductus arteriosus may begin to close with indomethacin exposure.[23] During behavioral state 4F, in addition to unusually vigorous activity, the "jogging fetus" coordinates combined facial and chest movements that can be seen clearly as "crying." During these short periods at term, it appears the fetus is actually awake. Finally, the fetus exposed to high concentrations of oxygen will initiate carbon dioxide–dependent breathing activity that includes deep inhalation and expiration movements, moving much more pulmonary fluid than in normal fetal breathing movement activity.[11] This "true breathing" includes a series of cardiovascular changes similar to those of infancy, all of which may be reversed by allowing fetal oxygen levels to decline back to normal. These levels of responsiveness, including Doppler evaluation of flow changes, may provide detailed information about fetal maturity.[23]

Fetal Responses to Hypoxemia

Fetal evaluation relies on inference: alterations in fetal behavior imply alteration in fetal status. For many reasons, such inference must be cautious. First, oxygen in the fetal environment is not easily measured: with oxygen partial pressure seldom exceeding 60 mm Hg throughout pregnancy, simply measuring PO_2 is imprecise; exacting methodology measuring oxygen content is more accurate. Second, PO_2 normally declines throughout gestation, provoking many normal adaptations. Next, responses to abnormal drops in oxygen may be only temporary responses to a variety of acute, chronic, or acute-superimposed-on-chronic insults,[24] so the mechanisms of compensation are highly individualized.[25,26] For discussion, fetal compensatory responses can be grouped into three phases:

1. *Increase oxygen supply.* Several temporary responses will increase oxygen availability. Although these produce the marginal increments necessary to respond to most incidental issues, they are unlikely to suffice in the case of placental insufficiency or marginal fetal status subject to the onset of labor. These include increase in baseline heart rate, increase in hemoglobin concentration, improved cardiac contractility or efficiency, and increased oxygen extraction.[24,27] These steps are limited in capacity. Whereas mild intrauterine growth restriction (IUGR) features increased nucleated red cell liberation and a tendency toward polycythemia, more severe IUGR features even higher libera-

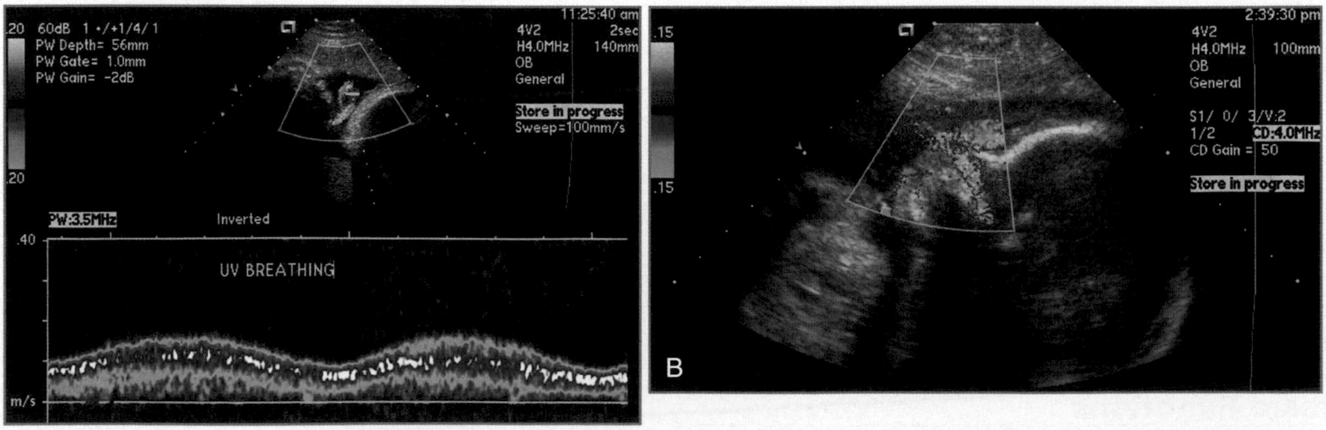

FIGURE 21-1 Fetal breathing movement. **A,** Umbilical venous fluctuations accompanying diaphragmatic excursion during fetal breathing movements. **B,** Nasal flaring of expelled lung fluid during fetal breathing movement.

tion of premature red cell forms but worsening anemia.[28] On the other hand, during "normal" situations of decreased oxygen (e.g., during contractions in term labor), increased oxygen extraction may contribute up to 14% additional oxygen on a virtually instantaneous basis.[29] Even these initial responses may be complex—rising placental resistance may be met by increased fetal blood pressure, with the result that changes in cardiac function and cerebral perfusion, once thought to be caused by hypoxemia, may in fact be part of the fetal hypertensive state.[30]

2. Control oxygen distribution. The distribution of blood flow results in preservation of oxygenation in vital centers of the brain, heart, adrenals, and placenta, with corresponding reduction to mesenteric, renal, and distal aortic outflow tracts (see Chapter 14).[31,32] The resulting differences in perfusion will lead to differential growth rates and asymmetrical IUGR and will have long-term implications far beyond fetal and neonatal health. Many of these hemodynamic adaptations can be depicted on serial Doppler evaluation of placental and fetal systemic circulations (see later), which occur before acute changes in other fetal behaviors. Initial steps may be subtle—changes in the proportion of resistance in the cerebral and placental circulations may be the first signs of beneficial diversion of flow toward the brain.[33] Later, overt increases in brain blood flow depicted in the middle cerebral artery with Doppler, most likely represent interaction of increases in perfusion resulting from systemic hypertension, and decreases in regional resistance resulting from hypoxemic vasodilation. Such changes occur in many organs, including the brain, liver, and adrenal glands, with corresponding shunting away from organs less critical to fetal survival. Thus, "brain-sparing" depiction of increased brain flow in the face of rising placental vascular resistance may signal shunting of blood away from somatic arterial beds.[34] "Heart-sparing" dilation of the fetal coronary arteries appears to be a much later hemodynamic change, associated with marked placental insufficiency.[35] The onset of these hemodynamic responses may be very subtle, including minor shifts in the cortical proportion of renal blood flow or slight reductions in gut perfusion. Progressive redistribution, up until cardiac decompensation, is an effective means of rationing the limited or declining oxygen supply.[4] Most fetuses experiencing chronic limitations in oxygen can maintain normal pH, neurologic function, and cardiac efficiency through a range of very low umbilical venous PO_2.[26,36]

3. Reduce oxygen consumption. This sophisticated mechanism of fetal adaptation to oxygen limits should not be confused with the obtundation induced by severe absolute cerebral hypoxemia. Most fetal responses that decrease oxygen consumption are voluntary and can be rapidly turned on and off.[37] These are initiated with minor increases in time between activity cycles and may extend all the way to complete abolition of fetal activity, rapidly reversible mere minutes after delivery. Fetal oxygen consumption may fall more than 15% during inactivity, and when this is coupled with redistribution and extraction, there may even be significant increases in oxygen supply to critical organs.[38] Different elements of fetal behavior may illustrate different sensitivities to declining oxygen levels. Heart rate reactivity tends to disappear before fetal breathing movements, which are almost always absent before fetal movements disappear (Fig. 21-2).[39]

These pathways of response are sequential, overlapping, and potentially reversible.[40] The IUGR fetus, for example, may deal effectively with increasing placental insufficiency with a combination of increasing oxygen extraction, increased hemoglobin concentration, and diversion of flow, such that temporary reduction in fetal activity may be restored and amniotic fluid volume maintained.[41] The extent to which these changes are reversible in utero will vary, but they include increased fetal activity with maternal supplemental oxygen and improved Doppler resistance patterns when oligohydramnios is restored by amnioinfusion.

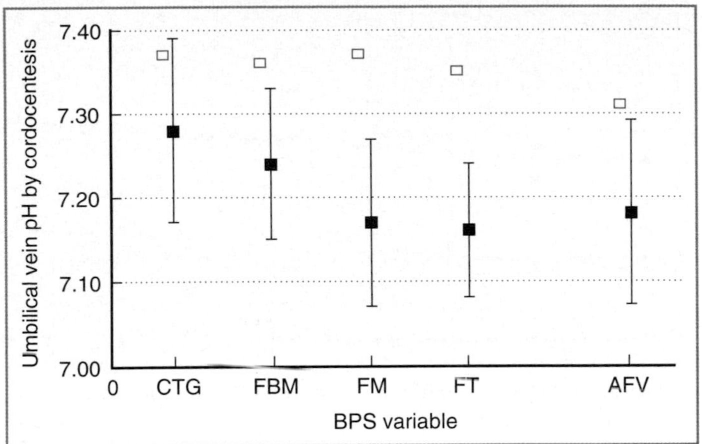

FIGURE 21-2 **Changes in fetal behavior with declining pH.** As umbilical venous pH falls, various behaviors become less frequent and eventually disappear. The graph summarizes cordocentesis data relating antepartum pH to individual biophysical profile score (BPS) variables. *Open squares,* mean pH when the variable was present (normal); *Filled squares,* mean pH ± 1 standard deviation when the variable was absent (abnormal). Data suggest that loss of individual variables is sequential. AFV, amniotic fluid volume; CTG, cardiotocogram; FBM, fetal breathing movement; FM, fetal movement; FT, fetal tone.

Fetal Compromise

As compensatory mechanisms reach their limits, metabolic consequences of hypoxemia arise—lactic acidemia, cardiac dysfunction, and progressive acidosis. Identification of these end points has become a critical role of fetal monitoring in the markedly premature. Even when venous Doppler indices have deteriorated, suggesting cardiac decompensation, acute fetal monitoring may still be used to coax a few more days of gestation, as well as to allow administration of antenatal steroids, with resulting improvement in long term outcome.[42] Understanding the interaction between arterial and venous Doppler tracings and biophysical fetal behavior becomes critical in this situation.

Absent Fetal Behavior: How Long Is too Long?

Fetal behavioral state 1F is known as quiet sleep. The fetal electroencephalogram features low-frequency, high-voltage patterns, occasional twitches but few voluntary movements, individual breathing movements without sustained episodes, marked diminution in heart rate variability, odd mouthing movements, and absence of acceleration-movement coupling.[43]

Near term, such profound inactivity, illustrated by the nonreactive NST (Fig. 21-3), is readily confused with fetal compromise. This confusion led to many inappropriate interventions during the initial development of FHR monitoring. Although state 1F and the nonreactive NST seldom persist longer than 40 minutes, intervals approaching 2 hours are still most likely normal.[44] The definition of these abnormal periods depends very much on the modality of testing. Multitransducer real-time observation of fetal activity often discloses frequent

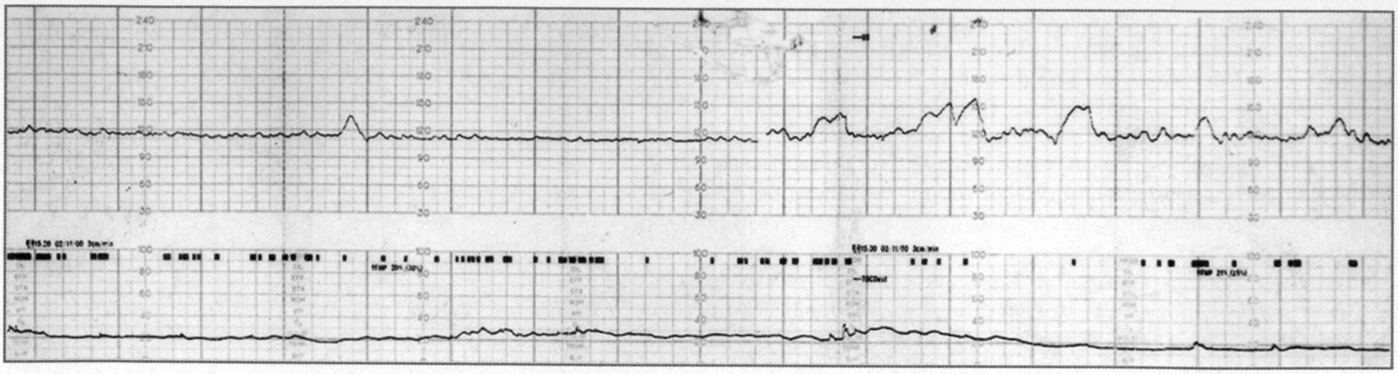

FIGURE 21-3 Eighteen-minute sleep-wake cycle in the term fetus. Virtually no activity (one kick, one acceleration) in the first 9 minutes, with low-variability fetal heart rate, behavioral state 1F. In the next 9 minutes, 60 discrete fetal movements on real-time ultrasound, multiple accelerations, increased variation between accelerations (2F).

small movements of hands, mouth, and trunk when less rigorous assessment describes complete inactivity. Clearly, any fetal testing modality must address this critical distinction: nearly dead or just napping.

Principles of Monitoring

To account for all these potential variables, the ideal monitoring system would gather a wide range of information, with versatility for all maternal and fetal conditions and flexibility for all gestational ages, allowing for varying degrees of onset, severity, and duration of intrauterine challenges.[39] In meeting these objectives, an ideal antenatal monitoring system would do the following:

1. Detect fetal peril with specificity, sensitivity, and timeliness to allow preventive intervention. Achieving these qualities entails the following:
   - Correlation with measurable standards of fetal compromise (antepartum pH; postdelivery outcome such as blood gases, Apgar scores, and neonatal performance)
   - Proportionality between test results and outcome (the worst score equals the highest risk of permanent handicap or perinatal mortality)
   - A low false-alarm rate, especially as prematurity deepens
   - Application to all ranges of perinatal morbidity as well as basic perinatal mortality
   - A reliable relationship to compromise that yields intervention early enough to prevent permanent damage but late enough to be certain of the need for intervention and to minimize the risks of prematurity
2. Reliably exclude stillbirth or permanent injury over a significant period of time. However, allowing for the possibility of acute change such as placental abruption, a normal test must exclude abnormal outcomes for a clinically important length of time, most commonly 7 days.
3. Exclude lethal congenital anomalies. This mandates at least one high-resolution comprehensive fetal examination but does not dictate that this must be repeated at every testing opportunity.
4. Incorporate multiple variables. This principle reflects the only way in which a monitoring system can address both the complexity of normal fetal behavior and the individual nature of fetal compensation.
5. Apply to fetal compromise from a variety of basic sources, including asphyxia, poisoning, metabolic abnormalities, anemia, and chance obstetric factors such as cord accident, to address the many origins of adverse outcome. These should be applicable in outpatient settings, with readily available equipment, accessible technicality, and high reproducibility.
6. Have measurable benefits to high-risk populations, in reduction of perinatal mortality and perinatal morbidity, at least in part by safely extending intrauterine time. Meeting these objectives simultaneously will, by definition, be cost effective.

In the context of the great variability in normal behavior and the complex cascades of responses to abnormal conditions, no single parameter could satisfy all these objectives. In balancing the risks of stillbirth from intrauterine decompensation against the likelihood of neonatal death from prematurity, single-modality tests have an impressive record of failure. The recent perinatal literature is full of such examples, including the use of the biparietal diameter as the unequivocal measurement for definition of IUGR,[45] nonstress testing as the single parameter to determine obstetric management,[46] or a series of Doppler parameters (absent diastolic velocities, cerebralization of blood flow, umbilical-venous pulsations, in that historical order) where knee-jerk responses, in the form of delivery as soon as the observation was made, have resulted in a litany of iatrogenic problems.[47]

Tests of Fetal Health: Monitoring Methods

Biophysical Profile Scoring

The biophysical profile score (BPS) presumes that multiple parameters of well-being are better predictors of outcome than single parameters.[48] Figure 21-4 shows one example of the detailed evaluation of outcome variables performed during development.[49,50] The traditional BPS study includes five variables (Table 21-1), with a total possible score of 10, but several variations have been proposed. Vintzileos and colleagues[51] added placental grading, for a total possible score of 12. Several authors proposed a modified biophysical profile that usually includes heart rate monitoring and amniotic fluid evaluation.[52,53] There may be modest differences in these approaches, but all emphasize the principle of multivariable fetal assessment.

Biophysical Profile Score Variables

AMNIOTIC FLUID MEASUREMENT

With the transducer vertical to the maternal abdomen, the maximum vertical depth of a clear amniotic fluid pocket is recorded. The transducer is then rotated 90 degrees in the same vertical axis, confirming that the measured pocket has true biplanar dimensions. The phrase *2 × 2 pocket* does not mean the pocket is 2 cm deep and 2 cm wide; it refers to the documentation that the pocket is 2 cm deep in at least two intersecting ultrasound planes, avoiding the possibility that a "sliver" of amniotic fluid is misconstrued as a true three-dimensional pocket. Amniotic fluid is measured in real time, and when there is doubt about a true clear pocket, it is confirmed by pulsed Doppler. Continuous color imaging may lead to the false impression of oligohydramnios (Fig. 21-5).[54] This method reflects the relative amount of amniotic fluid and was not meant as an absolute physiologic parameter.[55]

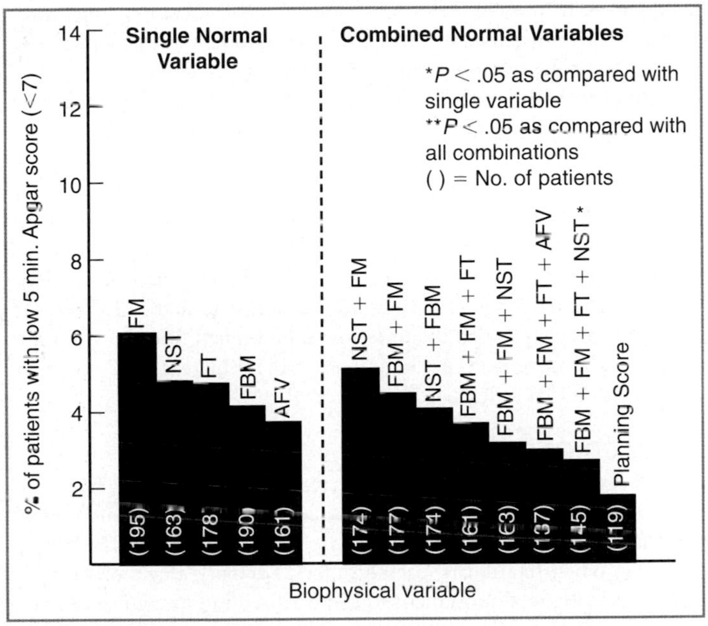

FIGURE 21-4 Prediction of outcome by individual biophysical profile score variables *(left)* or combinations of variables *(right)*. In this example, a 5-minute Apgar score less than 7 was best predicted by a combination of all five variables. (The Planning Score, named for Platt and Manning, was the first full biophysical profile score.) AFV, amniotic fluid volume; FBM, fetal breathing movement; FM, fetal movement; FT, fetal tone; NST, nonstress test.

Amniotic Fluid Volume. Maximum amniotic fluid pocket depth less than 2 cm or more than 8 cm mandates a detailed fetal evaluation to exclude anatomic and anomalous explanations.[56,57] For moderately increased fluid (maximum vertical pocket depth, 8 to 12 cm), the most common explanations are structural abnormalities, fetal macrosomia resulting from maternal diabetes, and idiopathic polyhydramnios, and fetal testing is likely to reflect fetal neurologic status accurately.[58] For pockets deeper than 12 cm in singleton pregnancies, neurologic issues and structural defects associated with aneuploidy are more likely and the BPS may not be valid.[59] Through the normal range (maximum vertical pocket depth, 3 to 8 cm), the maximum vertical depth assigns "normal" status accurately, although it may not correlate precisely with absolute volumes. As amniotic fluid volume decreases, the statistical value of the maximum vertical pocket method improves.

Subjectively Reduced Amniotic Fluid. In this situation, the minimum criterion of a 2-cm pocket depth is met, but there is no cord-free pocket greater than 3 cm. This suggests that fluid is significantly less than average, and subjective findings often include restricted extension of fetal movement, the uterus or the placenta molding to the contours of the fetus (or both), FHR decelerations with transducer pressure, spontaneous decelerations associated with fetal movement, and maternal reports of decreased fetal movement.[39]

Oligohydramnios. The original criterion for this diagnosis was a maximum vertical pocket of only 1 cm. Although this finding is highly

TABLE 21-1 INTERPRETATION OF BIOPHYSICAL PROFILE SCORE (BPS) VARIABLES

Fetal Variable	Normal Behavior (score = 2)	Abnormal Behavior (score = 0)
Fetal breathing movements (FBM)	Intermittent, multiple episodes of more than 30-sec duration, within 30-min BPS time frame. Hiccups count. Continuous FBM for 30 min, rule out fetal acidosis.	Continuous breathing without cessation. Completely absent breathing or no sustained episodes.
Body or limb movements	At least four discrete body movements in 30 min. Continuous active movement episodes = single movement. Includes fine motor movements, rolling movements, and so on, but not rapid eye movements or mouthing movements.	Three or fewer body or limb movements in a 30-min observation period.
Fetal tone/posture	Demonstration of active extension with rapid return to flexion of fetal limbs and brisk repositioning or trunk rotation. Opening and closing of hand or mouth, kicking, and so on.	Low-velocity movement only. Incomplete flexion, flaccid extremity positions, abnormal fetal posture. Must score 0 when fetal movement (FM) is completely absent.
Cardiotocogram (CTG)	Normal mean variation (computerized fetal heart rate interpretation), accelerations associated with maternal palpation FM (accelerations graded for gestation), 20-min CTG.	FM and accelerations not coupled. Insufficient accelerations, absent accelerations, or decelerative trace. Mean variation <20 or short-term variation <4.5 msec on numerical analysis of CTG.
Amniotic fluid evaluation	At least one pocket >2 cm with no umbilical cord. See text regarding subjectively decreased fluid.	No cord-free pocket >2 cm, or multiple definite elements of subjectively reduced amniotic fluid volume.

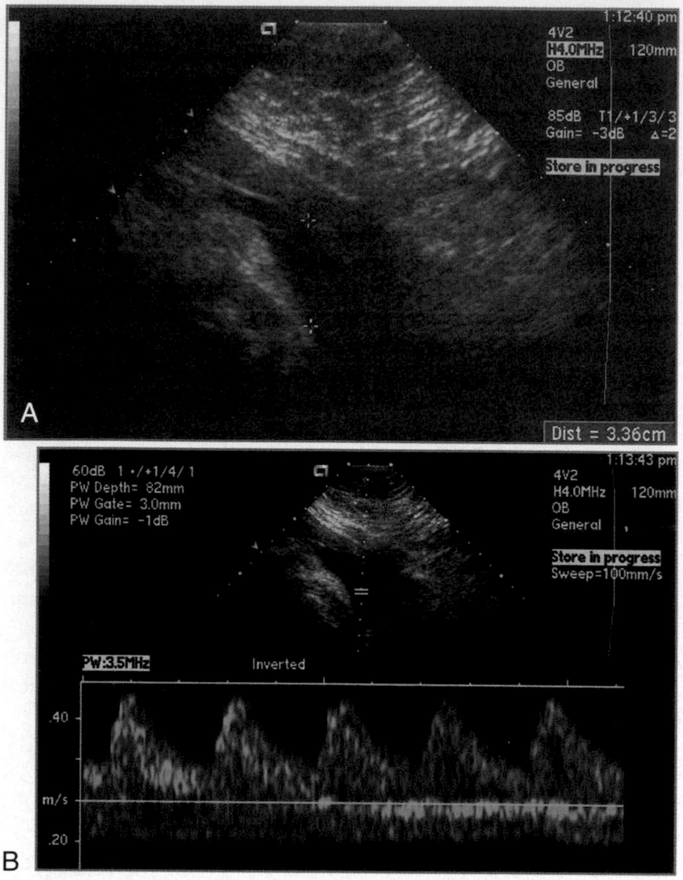

FIGURE 21-5 Fluid pocket verification. **A,** Amniotic fluid apparently meets vertical pocket criteria of the biophysical profile score. **B,** Pulsed Doppler demonstrates that this is a vertical pocket of umbilical cord, with no measurable amniotic fluid.

correlated with IUGR, it is so rare as to be clinically insignificant. The 2-cm standard for oligohydramnios has good reliability as a test for potential fetal compromise, as a correlate of IUGR and as a correlate of repetitive decelerations in labor, leading to a decision for cesarean delivery. Because of its reduced likelihood of false-alarm diagnosis, reduced intervention, and the corresponding reduced maternal morbidity despite identical outcome predictions, the maximum vertical pocket method is superior to the four-quadrant amniotic fluid index (AFI).[60,61] The use of maximum vertical pocket depth, and not the four-quadrant AFI, in traditional BPS is validated by current research.[62] The underlying principle, fetal oliguria, is a component of redistribution of fetal blood flow and segmental renal hemodynamics,[63] reflected in abnormal placental Doppler indices. For predicting adverse fetal outcome, there is an excellent complementary association between oligohydramnios and worsening placental function.[64]

FETAL BREATHING MOVEMENTS

Either rhythmic fetal diaphragm contractions or hiccups lasting more than 30 seconds meet normal criteria. This fetal behavior is the one most easily suppressed by hypoxemia, but it is also the most episodic in normal fetuses. Because the amplitude of fetal breathing depends on gestational age, maternal glucose, exposure to increased oxygen concentrations, and many medications (e.g., xanthenes), careful evaluation of all parameters is necessary before intervention is precipitated.[65] The unusual presence of continuous monotonous fetal breathing, or fetal gasping, with complete absence of all other behavior for an extended period, may indicate acidosis, especially in the fetus of a diabetic mother.[66-68]

FETAL MOVEMENT AND TONE

One of the interpretive pitfalls of BPS is that at least some movement must be present to evaluate tone.[39] Tone is not simply the flexed posture of a normal fetus. The evaluation of tone is indeed subjective, but absent tone is strongly correlated with fetal acidosis.

Fine motor movement of the face and hands, purposeful movement such as swallowing, facial expressions, sucking, yawning, large kicks, small kicks, rolling motions, and so on may all be included as movements. When a fetus does not move for a period of 30 minutes, extended testing is required,[69] and completion of heart rate testing is also performed to extend the time of continuous observation. In practice, fetal movement is referenced to previous BPS experience with this fetus, maternal reports, and gestational age. The markedly preterm fetus moves virtually all the time, and a movement frequency of only five to eight movements per hour would call for increased testing, even though minimal criteria are met.

CARDIOTOCOGRAM

An experienced observer can derive much information from the systematic recording of the FHR with simultaneous documentation of uterine activity, which comprises the cardiotocogram (CTG) (Fig. 21-6).[70] When fetal heart rate and uterine activity are recorded passively, relating fetal movement to standardized interpretation of FHR accelerations, a nonstress test is defined as reactive (a score of 2 meets criteria for accelerations associated with fetal movement) or nonreactive (a score of 0 means acceleration criteria are not met).[71] These data can be acquired digitally by a computerized system that not only interprets accelerations and decelerations but also numerically analyzes FHR variability within gestational-age-normalized paradigms.[72,73] This significantly reduces the impact of gestational age on FHR testing, making it more interpretable at gestational ages progressively less than 32 weeks.

A valuable component of the CTG is elicited uterine activity. Contraction patterns may suggest uterine irritability, such as in preterm labor, with uterine infection, or with impending abruptio placentae. The minimal deceleration pattern illustrated in Figure 21-7 suggests oligohydramnios. Fetal breathing often produces characteristic deflections of the tocodynamometer, as well as irregularities in FHR (Fig. 21-8).[74] Normal variability with a monotonous repetitive (sawtooth) pattern for more than 40 minutes may indicate fetal anemia, whereas overt sinusoidal heart rate is indicative of more severe fetal compromise, including hydropic anemia, drug intoxication (e.g., narcotics), or abnormalities of the central nervous system with decorticate behavior.[75,76]

CTG is never used alone in biophysical profile scoring.[77,78] Any of the patterns just mentioned would immediately call for performance of all ultrasound parameters in the BPS. The CTG must be interpreted within the context of gestational age.[79] Modification of the interpretation of the NST is shown in Table 21-1 and reflects the potential benefits of computerized CTG in the preterm fetus.[80,81]

Biophysical Profile Score Technique

Table 21-2 shows how the BPS is systematically interpreted and applied to management. More detailed instructions on the application of BPS are available elsewhere,[39,82] but some technical points deserve emphasis.

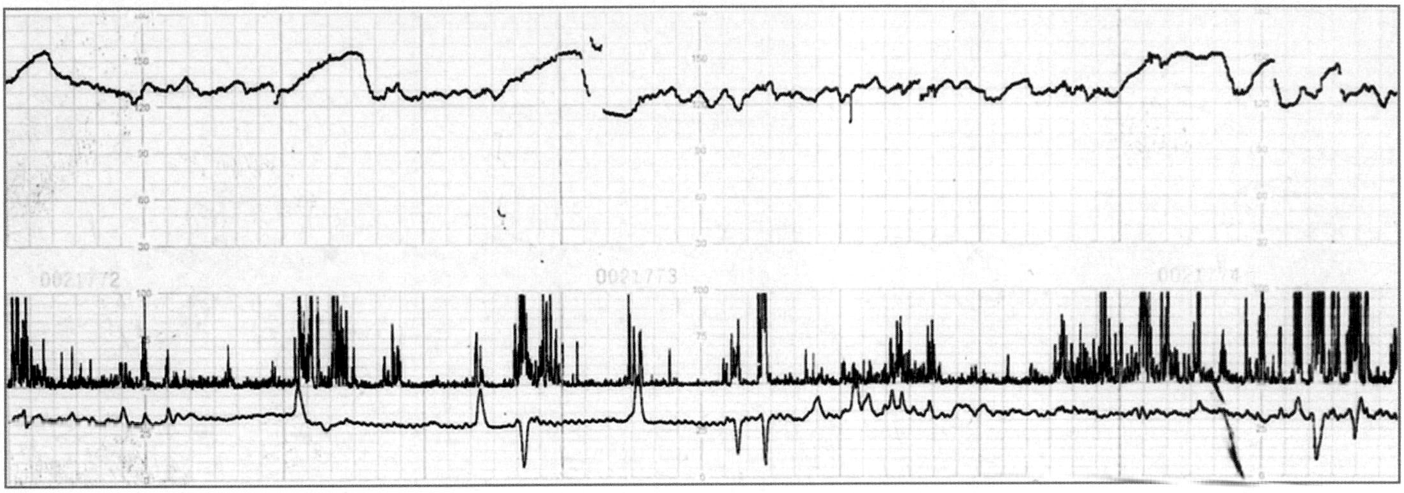

FIGURE 21-6 Reactive nonstress test. Prominent fetal heart rate accelerations associated with palpated fetal movements (also documented by this type of monitor, *second tracing from bottom*). Between large accelerations, normal variability, classified as moderate by the National Institute of Child Health and Human Development criteria. No detectable uterine contractions *(bottom tracing)*.

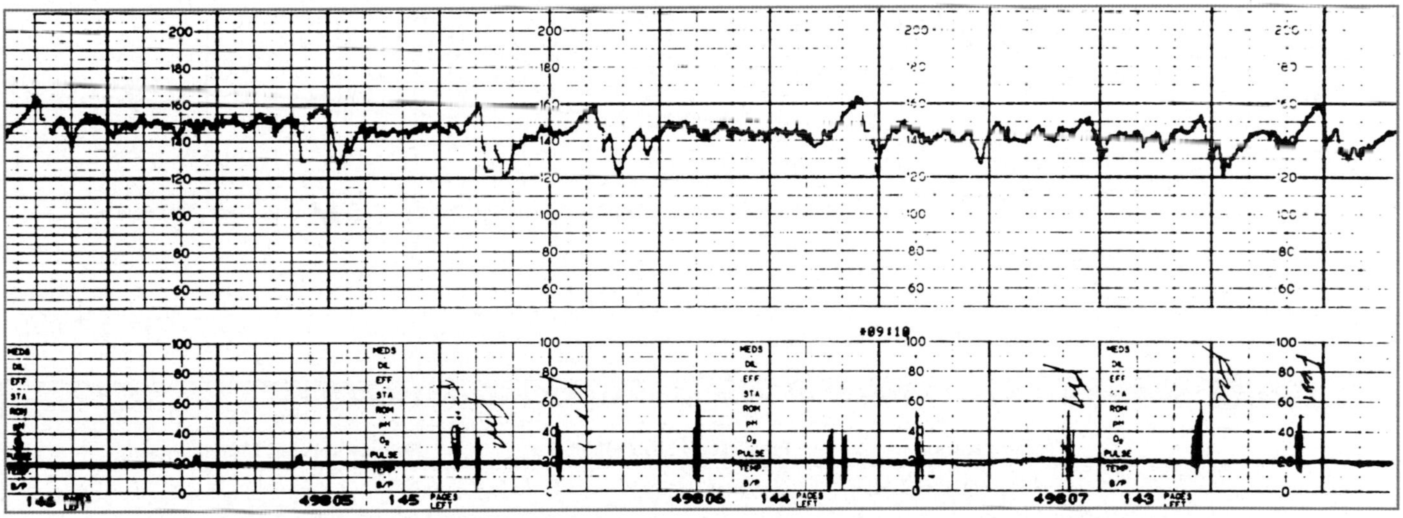

FIGURE 21-7 "Minimal variable" FHR pattern. Numerous fetal movements (marked FM on *lower tracing*), were associated with small decelerations caused by cord compression. Biophysical profile score was 6/10, with equivocal nonstress test and no amniotic fluid pocket more than 2.0 cm. Fetus failed induction because of repetitive decelerations despite amnioinfusion in labor.

Score of 10. A score of "6/8" is not a BPS. When the four ultrasound variables are performed first, but at least one of them is absent, the CTG must be performed before the BPS is complete, and the score will then be reported as 6 or 8/10. The only score that is allowed to stand after only the ultrasound variables have been evaluated is 8/8. In that case, the CTG is not required. Based on randomized controlled trial data, the NST is used selectively after ultrasound variables have been performed. When this protocol is followed, the NST is required in only about 10% of cases.[39,78] Exceptions to this design include high-risk fetuses with hemodynamic abnormalities; the presence of multiple medical disorders (especially active lupus, thrombophilia, and the combination of hypertension and diabetes); volatile situations such as chronic abruption, fetal infection and arrhythmias; and in recognition of prior adverse outcome. Fetuses who always require a five-variable BPS (a score "out of 10") are those with Doppler-defined placental insufficiency, including absent or reversed end-diastolic velocities (REDV) or venous Doppler abnormalities (see later).

8/10-Oligohydramnios. The recommendation to proceed with delivery when there is no pocket of 2 cm or greater is based on the close association with adverse outcome[83]—that is, on a high perinatal mortality (up to 560 per 1000 in fetuses with no amniotic fluid pocket greater than 1 cm). At term, the recommendation is to proceed with a trial of labor, noting that up to 45% of the time, cesarean delivery is required for repetitive FHR decelerations. For preterm gestations, if the remainder of fetal behavior is within normal limits, additional time may be taken to administer antenatal steroids, transfer to a tertiary center, and prepare the maternal cervix, provided close monitoring continues. Extending this rationale to less severe oligohydramnios (e.g., when using an AFI of 5 cm) has caused confusion on this point. Using maximum vertical pocket depth will avoid undue interference in most cases. Remote from term, diagnostic amnioinfusion reveals occult rupture of membranes in up to 19%.[84] The role of chronic amnioinfusion to preserve fluid volume has not been substantiated in randomized control trials.

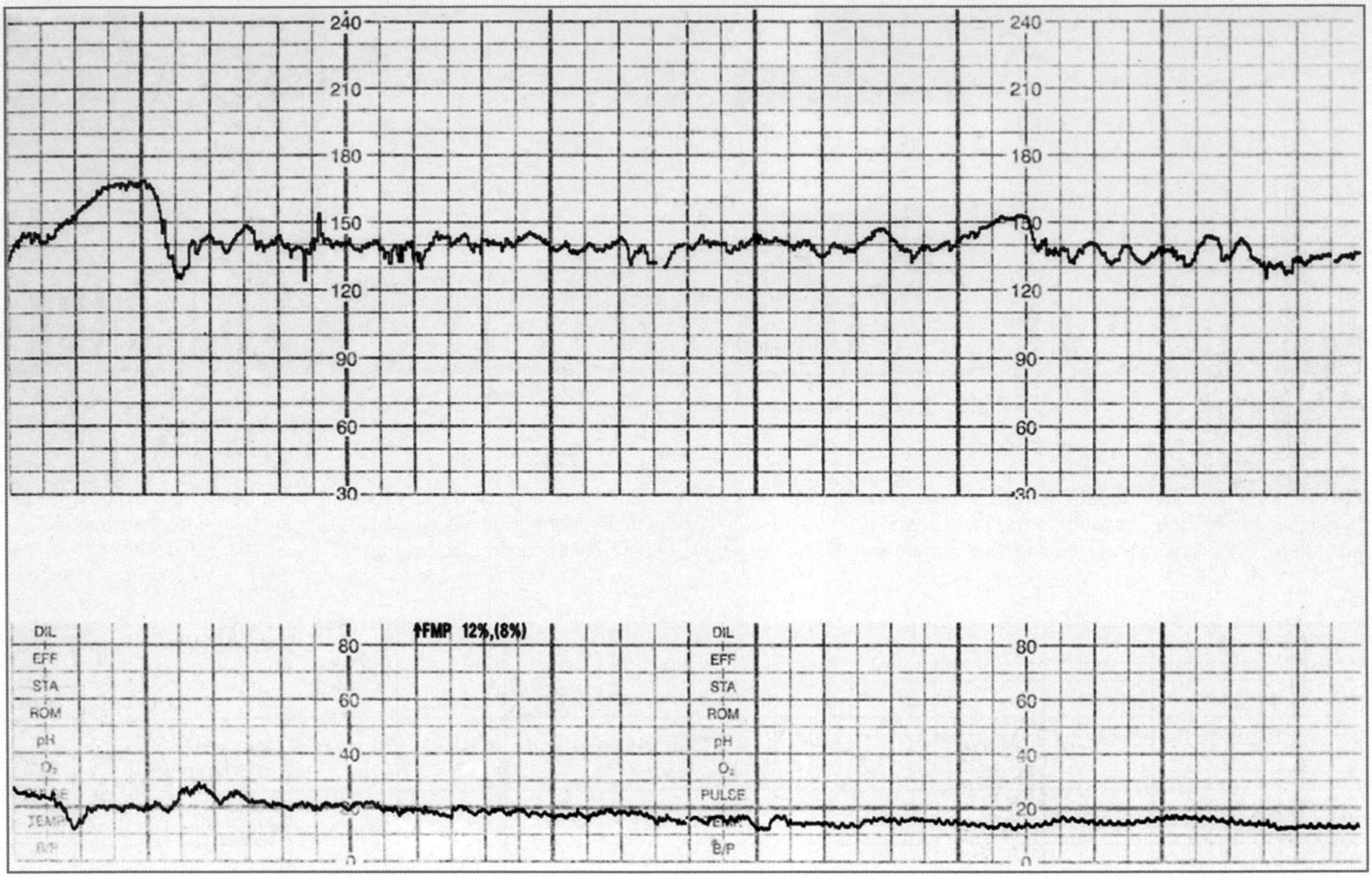

FIGURE 21-8 Active fetus with "respiratory arrhythmia." Simultaneous real-time ultrasound showed episodic fetal breathing for most of this tracing after the first large acceleration. *Upper tracing* shows increased short-term variability; *lower tracing* shows maternal abdomen moving in small-amplitude waves (20 to 30/min) caused by fetal chest movement.

TABLE 21-2 SYSTEMATIC APPLICATION OF BIOPHYSICAL PROFILE SCORING (BPS)

BPS	Interpretation	Predicted PNM/1000*	Recommended Management
10/10 8/8 8/10 (AFV normal)	No evidence of fetal asphyxia present.	Less than 1/1000	No acute intervention on fetal basis. Serial testing indicated by disorder-specific protocols.
8/10-oligohydramnios	Chronic fetal compromise likely (unless ROM is proven)	89/1000	For absolute oligohydramnios, prove normal urinary tract, disprove undiagnosed ROM, consider antenatal steroids, then deliver.
6/10 (AFV normal)	Equivocal test, fetal asphyxia is not excluded	Depends on progression (61/1000 on average)	Repeat testing immediately, before assigning final value. If score is 6/10, then 10/10, in two continuous 30-min periods, manage as 10/10. For persistent 6/10, deliver the mature fetus, repeat within 24 hours in the immature fetus, then deliver if less than 6/10.
4/10	Acute fetal asphyxia likely. If AFV-oligo, acute on chronic asphyxia very likely.	91/1000	Deliver by obstetrically appropriate method, with continuous monitoring.
2/10	Acute fetal asphyxia, most likely with chronic decompensation.	125/1000	Deliver for fetal indications (usually cesarean section).
0/10	Severe, acute asphyxia virtually certain.	600/1000	If fetal status is viable, deliver immediately by cesarean section.

***Per test, within 1 week of the result shown, if no intervention. For scores of 0, 2, or 4, intervention should begin virtually immediately, provided the fetus is viable. For all interventions, lethal anomaly should be excluded as a potential cause of the abnormal behavior.**
AFV, amniotic fluid volume; PNM, perinatal mortality; ROM, rupture of membranes.

Equivocal or Abnormal Scores. The correlation between abnormal scores and high risk of poor outcome has been demonstrated in large population studies and produces a characteristically shaped outcome curve (Fig. 21-9).[85] Statistically, the most likely correlate of an equivocal score is coincidental absence of behavior in a normal fetus. Even an abnormal score carries a differential diagnosis, including many obstetrical factors (Table 21-3). Extending the testing period, retesting after a brief interval, or adding ancillary tests can be done before moving to delivery for equivocal scores. When a score of 0 to 4/10 is found for a fetus whose screening in the first and second trimesters was normal, and especially when biophysical parameters and anatomic review were normal in the recent past, undue delay in delivery is usually not advisable.

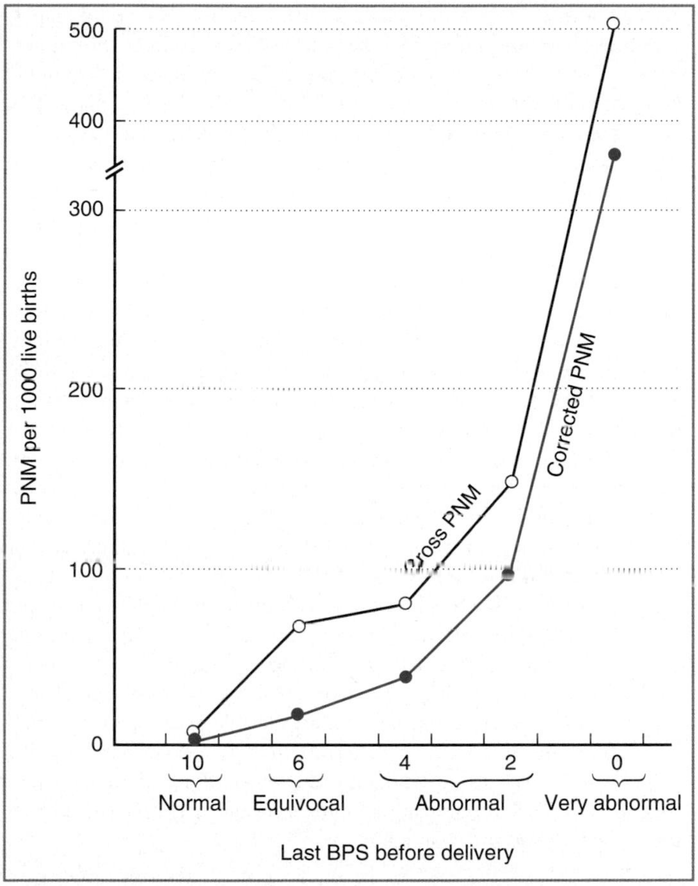

FIGURE 21-9 Perinatal mortality and BPS. Perinatal mortality (PNM) varies exponentially with declining biophysical profile score (BPS). The important contribution of lethal fetal anomalies accounts for the difference between the two curves.

The Monitoring Context. The *process* of obtaining the BPS can provide important information. Further investigation may be stimulated by, for example, the mother's observations, the uterine response to stimulation by the transducer, or observation of individual abnormal behavior. This interactive style of monitoring is preferable to the rigid application of a simple BPS.[86] Performance of BPS; routine ultrasound observation of the uterus, placenta, and membranes; measurement of fetal growth parameters; and comprehensive Doppler survey, as well as identification of subjective changes such as echogenic bowel or behavioral ones such as reduced tone, all constitute information gathering.

Fetal Heart Rate Monitoring

Isolated use of FHR testing, whether by classic NST or by the introduction of contraction challenges (oxytocin challenge test or contraction stress test), is not considered standard of care for high-risk fetuses. There may be economic or logistic reasons why ultrasound is not available to women with no identifiable risks who are receiving routine prenatal care, but even in that population, it may not be appropriate to use the NST as the sole surveillance tool (Table 21-4). A valuable component of virtually all multivariable systems, the NST recognizes the unique coupling of fetal neurologic status to cardiovascular reflex responses.[87] It is one of the factors that tends to disappear earliest during progressive fetal compromise,[39,88] and many studies have shown it to be the most sensitive of the four shorter-term variables that indicate worsening hypoxemia or acidosis.[89,90] In modified BPS systems, a fully reactive NST may be used to infer fetal movement. Any abnormality in such test results, including the nonreactive NST, occasional decelerations, decreased variability, and persistent minor decelerations, calls for complete ultrasound evaluation.

TABLE 21-3 FACTORS THAT INFLUENCE BIOPHYSICAL PROFILE SCORING PERFORMANCE

Agent	Fetal Effect
Drugs	
Sedatives/sedative side effects (e.g., Aldomet)	Diminished activity of all varieties; abolition of none
Excitatory (e.g., theophylline)	Continuous, "picket fence" FBM
Street drugs (e.g., crack cocaine)	Rachitic, rigid, furious, bizarre FM
Indomethacin	Oligohydramnios
Maternal cigarette smoking	Various observations: FBM abolished or attenuated but some report no change; FM reduced
Maternal hyperglycemia (iatrogenic or unregulated)	Sustained FBM or acidosis, diminution or abolition of FM or FT or CTG-reactivity
Maternal hypoglycemia (e.g., poor nutrition, insulin excess)	Abnormal paucity of all behaviors, normal AFV
Single Parameter Removed by Perinatal Condition	
Persistent fetal arrhythmia	Uninterpretable CTG
Spontaneous premature rupture of membranes	Obligatory oligohydramnios
Periodic decelerations (e.g., in proteinuric preeclampsia)	CTG defined as non-reactive
Acute Disasters (eclampsia, abruptio placentae, ketoacidosis)	May invalidate predictive accuracy

AFV, amniotic fluid volume; CTG, cardiotocogram; FBM, fetal breathing movements; FM, fetal movement; FT, fetal tone.

TABLE 21-4 PROBLEMS WITH USING NONSTRESS TESTING ALONE

Detection Failure	
	Oligohydramnios
	Lethal anomalies
	Cord presentation, abnormalities
	Placental abnormalities
	Growth disorders
	Twin demise
	Anomalies requiring intervention
	Overall sensitivity, 50% (all outcomes)
Nonreactive Test	
	Poor specificity for compromise
	Poor specificity for fetal death
Reactive Test	
	Falsely reassuring rate,* 6/1000
	Unreliable as backup test*

***Falsely reassuring rate for post-term pregnancy, 20/1000. Falsely reassuring rate for decreased fetal movement, 24/1000.**

The Nonstress Test

The coupled presence of palpable fetal movements and FHR acceleration is the essence of the NST. The classic criteria for a reactive NST are at least two FHR accelerations lasting at least 15 seconds and rising at least 15 beats/min above the established baseline heart rate.[91] Most term fetuses have many of these accelerations in each 20- to 30-minute period of active sleep (behavioral state 2F), and the term fetus seldom goes more than 60 minutes, and certainly not more than 100 minutes, without meeting these criteria.[44] On the other hand, preterm fetuses, IUGR fetuses at similar gestations, or fetuses with maternal medication such as sedatives or magnesium sulfate frequently have paired accelerations—movements that do not meet these criteria.[79] Modification of these criteria in BPS (e.g., including accelerations of 10 beats/min lasting 10 seconds on a background of normal FHR variability, for fetuses less than 32 weeks) accepts the principle that earlier fetuses have smaller accelerations but that they should always demonstrate some degree of FHR acceleration with palpated fetal movements.

NST reactivity may be inferred. Experienced nurses listening to a heart rate monitor can detect accelerations and properly classify a reactive NST without looking at the paper record.[92] Real-time ultrasound observation of concurrent FHR accelerations and movements also correlates perfectly with reactive NST.

Falsely reassuring NSTs do occur, at a rate of four to five per 1000 in the largest studies.[46,93,94] These are most problematic in fetuses with asymmetrical IUGR, oligohydramnios, or metabolic problems associated with severe macrosomia, for whom false-reassuring rates may reach 15%. Thus, NST has significant liabilities in the groups at highest risk. Strong evidence, including data from randomized trials, shows that NST should not be used in isolation in determining the antenatal status of such fetuses.

The nonreactive NST is defined by an FHR monitoring interval that does not meet the criteria just described. However, there is a large variation in the total duration allowed, and it ranges from a minimum of 10 minutes of monitoring to 40 minutes or even 60 minutes according to some authors.[95,96] In the context of BPS, 30 minutes is allowed for the NST to reach reactivity. About 10% to 12% of fetuses in the third trimester do not meet these criteria at 30 minutes. This number falls below 6% by 40 minutes.[44] Clearly, the choice of time end point is critical in determining the false-alarm rate, its major clinical drawback. In fact, because most normal fetuses demonstrate normal ultrasound BPS (i.e., a score of 8/8) within 15 minutes, spending the additional time to perform NST is optional. By far the most common explanation for the nonreactive NST is the presence of a longer-than-average sleep cycle in a normal fetus.[6] A nonreactive NST, especially if variability remains present and there are no decelerations, should not be assumed to indicate fetal compromise. The standard of care indicates that ultrasound evaluation (a full BPS) should be available as the backup test. Although fetal nonstress testing in isolation has frequently been the reference test for post-term pregnancies, decreased fetal movement on maternal movement counting programs, and other published protocols for first-line monitoring, the standard of care now indicates a much more comprehensive evaluation.[97]

Ultrasound may resolve apparently abnormal NST as well. For example, repetitive nonreactive NST in a fetus with normal serial ultrasound variables may lead to a diagnosis of central nervous system abnormalities, drug ingestion, or prior fetal central nervous system injury. As well, late deceleration or variable decelerations may occur in the context of NST monitoring, with no deflection of the uterine pressure monitor. Uterine activity is probably responsible, but the situation (placental insufficiency in the case of late decelerations, umbilical cord compression in the case of variable decelerations) is so precarious that even minor changes in uterine tone may provoke them. Either pattern should call for immediate evaluation by real-time and Doppler ultrasound to exclude IUGR, direct fetal compromise, oligohydramnios, chronic placental insufficiency, or more acute events such as abruption. This should be done immediately, as the explanation may be imminent cord prolapse or evolving placental separation without significant maternal findings. Or it may be simpler: variable decelerations lasting up to 2 minutes may occur as the term fetus squeezes the cord with its hand.[98] In the context of modern fetal evaluation, all these issues suggest that FHR monitoring should be done in a unit capable of immediate ultrasound evaluation.

Computerized Cardiotocography

The binary reactive or nonreactive interpretation of FHR has been evaluated in many ways, but more detailed visual analysis has not proved superior.[46] Computerized storage and interpretation of FHR records obtained with conventional monitors has a clear advantage. Objective interpretation using digitized analysis of heart rate patterns can clarify the information available from the CTG.[99,100] This is essentially a computerized extension of the National Institutes of Health workshop on electronic heart rate monitoring,[101] which categorized heart rate variability as undetectable, minimal, moderate, marked, or sinusoidal. Computerized analysis can depict variability as a continuous output variable, analyzing beat-to-beat variability (short-term variation, which has a mean of 3 to 8 msec), or as overall variation, depicted as mean minute variability from the established baseline.[102] Normal mean minute variation is correlated with gestational age. An example is shown in Figure 21-10. The interpretation algorithm is very complex and includes correlation of gestational age for the definitions of accelerations, variability, baseline heart rate, movement frequency, and the depiction of fetal state.[72] Although the subtleties of states 3F and 4F are not depicted, states 1F (low variability, fetal movements) and 2F (high variability and significantly increased movement frequency) are correctly classified.[103] Finally, variations within periods of high episodes and low episodes are also analyzed and compared with gestational age–corrected means. Data stored on a hard disk are used to examine serial changes.

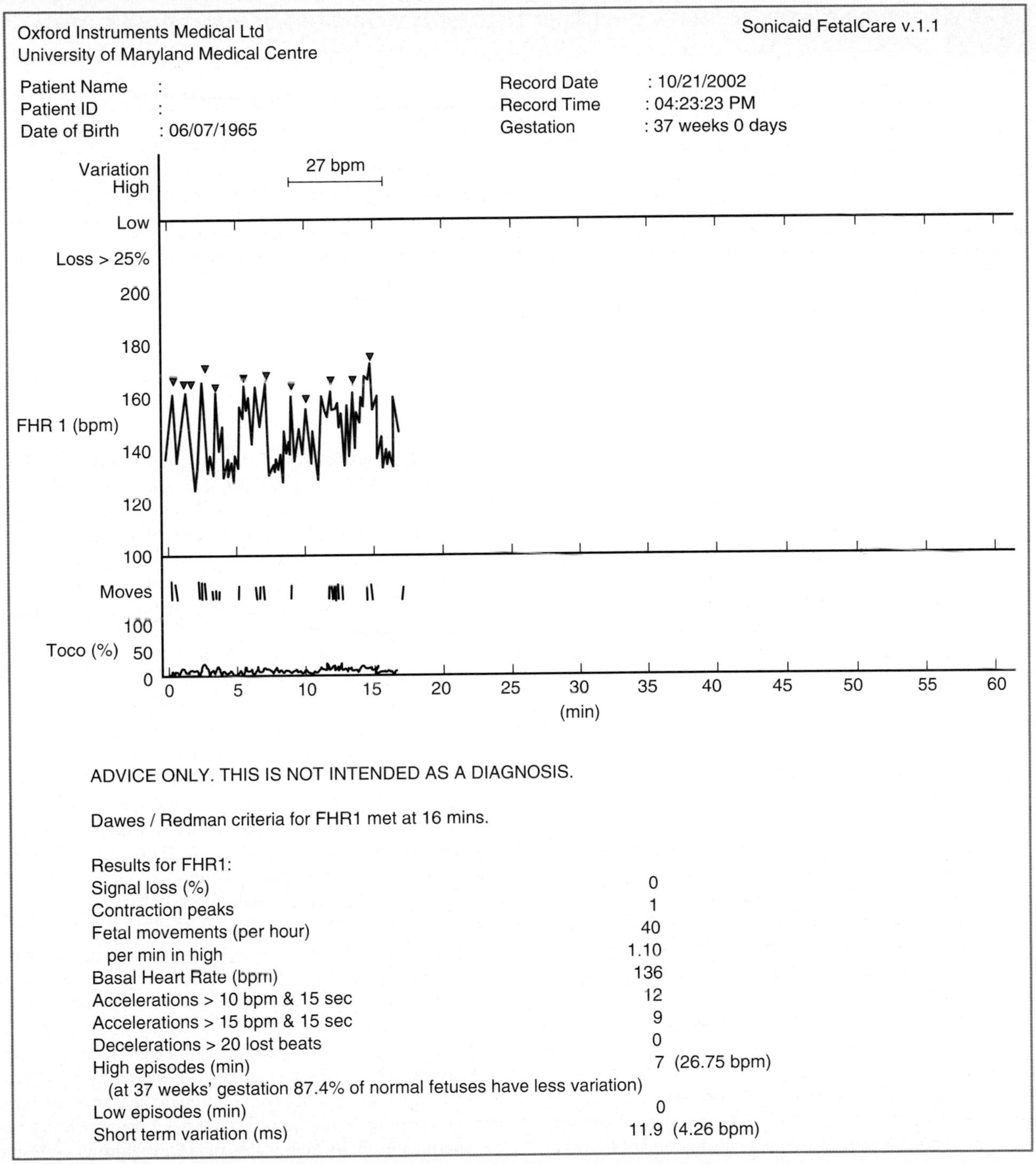

FIGURE 21-10 Output from Oxford Sonicaid System 8002 computerized cardiotocogram (CTG) interpretation algorithm. bpm, beats per minute; FHR, fetal heart rate.

Computerized cardiotocography (CCTG) outperforms NST by expanding the applicable gestational age and making objective interpretations. Statistically, this means better positive and negative predictive accuracy, fewer equivocal test results, and superior performance at less than 32 weeks' gestation. Although good evidence suggests CCTG, like the NST, should not be used as a solitary method of fetal surveillance, increasing evidence supports a central role in multivariable testing when maintaining fetal safety to gain critical time is the goal (e.g., with severe placenta-based IUGR at the lower limits of viability).[104] In more common populations undergoing fetal surveillance, however, this degree of precision is generally not required, and the binary format of the NST suffices.

Doppler Ultrasound

In the overall context of fetal evaluation, Doppler velocimetry defines placental status and, therefore, the relative risk of sudden deterioration.[34,105] For example, Doppler categories of risk mandate the frequency of biophysical profile scoring (Table 21-5).[39] Extreme Doppler abnormalities may indicate intervention, but Doppler is not used in

TABLE 21-5 DOPPLER ABNORMALITY DICTATES FREQUENCY OF BIOPHYSICAL PROFILE SCORING (BPS)*

Abnormality†	BPS Frequency‡	Decision to Deliver (Fetal)§
Elevated indices only	Weekly	Abnormal BPS‖ or Term or >36 weeks with no fetal growth
AEDV	Twice weekly	Abnormal BPS‖ or >34 weeks proven maturity of Conversion to REDV
REDV	Daily	Any BPS < 10/10¶ or >32 weeks dexamethasone given
REDV-UVP	Three times daily	Any BPS < 10/10¶ or >28 weeks dexamethasone given

***BPS determines management. Must be viable to enter: >25 weeks gestation, >500 g, normal anatomy, normal karyotype.**
†Umbilical artery and complete venous-tree Doppler; cerebralization of blood flow confirms umbilical artery abnormality as serious, does not directly alter management.
‡*Minimum* testing frequency, increased on basis of severity: maternal condition(s), degree of IUGR, gestation.
§Neonatal consultation, maternal condition/instability, direct fetal parameter by cordocentesis, all will impact this decision.
‖Any BPS ≤ 4/10, or 8/10—Oligo, or repeated 6/10.
¶BPS 8/10 cyclic absence of FBM is the only exception, in which case, repeat BPS < 6 hr.
AEDV, absent end-diastolic velocity; FBM, fetal breathing movement; IUGR, intrauterine growth retardation; REDV, reversed end-diastolic velocity; UVP, umbilical venous pulsations.

isolation, and evaluation of fetal status using all available tools is imperative.

Fetal Doppler Velocimetry

Fetal Doppler studies have evolved from simple evaluation of the umbilical outflow to assess the placenta[106] to comprehensive multivessel evaluation of fetal circulatory status.[105] Although most literature is focused on umbilical artery velocimetry by itself, current standards of practice require both placental and fetal systemic Doppler studies to adequately assess the compromised fetus.[107-110]

Umbilical Artery

Hemodynamics. The umbilical arteries arise from the common iliac arteries and represent the dominant outflow of the distal aortic circulation. Because there are no somatic branches after their origin, the umbilical arteries purely reflect the downstream resistance of the placental circulation. Normal umbilical artery resistance falls progressively through pregnancy, reflecting increased numbers of tertiary stem villous vessels (Fig. 21-11).[111] In a number of pathologic conditions, increased resistance in the umbilical arteries represents placental injury with loss of cross-sectional arterial outflow.[112] In the sheep model, infarction of multiple small vessels by infusing microspheres can be titrated to induce precise rises in umbilical artery resistance.[113,114] As umbilical artery resistance rises (Fig. 21-12), diastolic velocities fall, and ultimately these are absent (absent end-diastolic velocities [AEDV]).[113] As resistance rises even further, an elastic component is added, which will induce REDV, as the insufficient, rigid placental circulation recoils after being distended by pulse pressure.[115] This latter condition is terminal and can exist for only a short period of time; our longest recorded healthy survivor had 13 days of REDV, whereas our longest survivor with AEDV had more than 14 weeks.[39]

Measurement. As with all Doppler evaluations, the sample gate is enlarged to encompass the entire vessel, and transducer position is adjusted to eliminate aliasing, to minimize the Doppler angle, and to sample a single umbilical artery.[116] In the initial Doppler evaluation of any compromised fetus, both umbilical arteries should be sampled, and information from the best umbilical artery should be used in clinical decisions.[117] There is no established standard as to where along the course of the umbilical artery the definitive evaluation should be made. Especially for the compromised IUGR fetus, the length of the cord may represent substantial resistance in itself (Fig. 21-13). Although all these waveforms are abnormal, the mid-cord waveform may be most representative.

Clinical Significance. In isolation, elevated umbilical artery indices suggest placental liability but correlate with IUGR in less than 60% of cases.[118] Monitoring of fetal growth, proportions, amniotic fluid volume, and well-being are indicated, but intervention is seldom justified by elevated umbilical artery resistance by itself. Markedly elevated umbilical artery resistance suggests placental injury, mandating increased fetal surveillance, including multivessel systemic Doppler assessment and BPS.[119,120]

AEDV may exist in equilibrium, but in many fetuses, AEDV is not stable and will progress to REDV over time. Many fetuses with AEDV also have altered brain blood flow, with increased diastolic velocities—the brain-sparing phenomenon.[32] Not all fetuses with this degree of placental resistance have functional evidence of placental insufficiency in the form of acidosis or hypoxemia, but AEDV is not usually compatible with term pregnancy. It is not surprising that the majority (80% to 100%) of such fetuses are delivered by cesarean section, often electively, or provoked by fetal distress in labor. Clearly, the combination of prematurity, IUGR, and potential placental respiratory insufficiency suggests that tertiary delivery is indicated for most of these fetuses.

AEDV is an indication to prepare for delivery, including appropriate referral, administration of antenatal steroids, and detailed maternal evaluation to exclude undiagnosed hypertension, renal disorders, connective tissue disorders, or thrombophilias. Furthermore, because up to 20% of such fetuses have malformations or overt aneuploidy, a diligent review of fetal anatomy, and in some cases invasive fetal testing for fetal karyotype, is indicated.[121] Although the latter may seem unduly invasive considering the short intrauterine time remaining, avoidance of maternal morbidity (about 35% of those requiring cesarean delivery undergo classic cesarean sections) and exclusion of fetal karyotypic abnormality are important. Even in fetuses with no visible anomalies, the combination of IUGR, including fetal disproportion, and abnormal placental Doppler parameters may be associated with 5% to 8% aneuploidy.[122]

Monitoring the fetus with AEDV requires multivariable assessment. Fetal heart rate monitoring alone is insufficient, as most of these fetuses have reduced heart rate variability and small accelerations. Relying on composite scoring of the BPS means a lower rate of false-positive tests but does require the observer to become attuned to the movement pattern of the individual fetus. In this precarious situation, subjectively reduced amniotic fluid volume, overall reductions in total fetal activity, long intervals between periods of fetal breathing, and spontaneous FHR decelerations observed on real-time ultrasound may

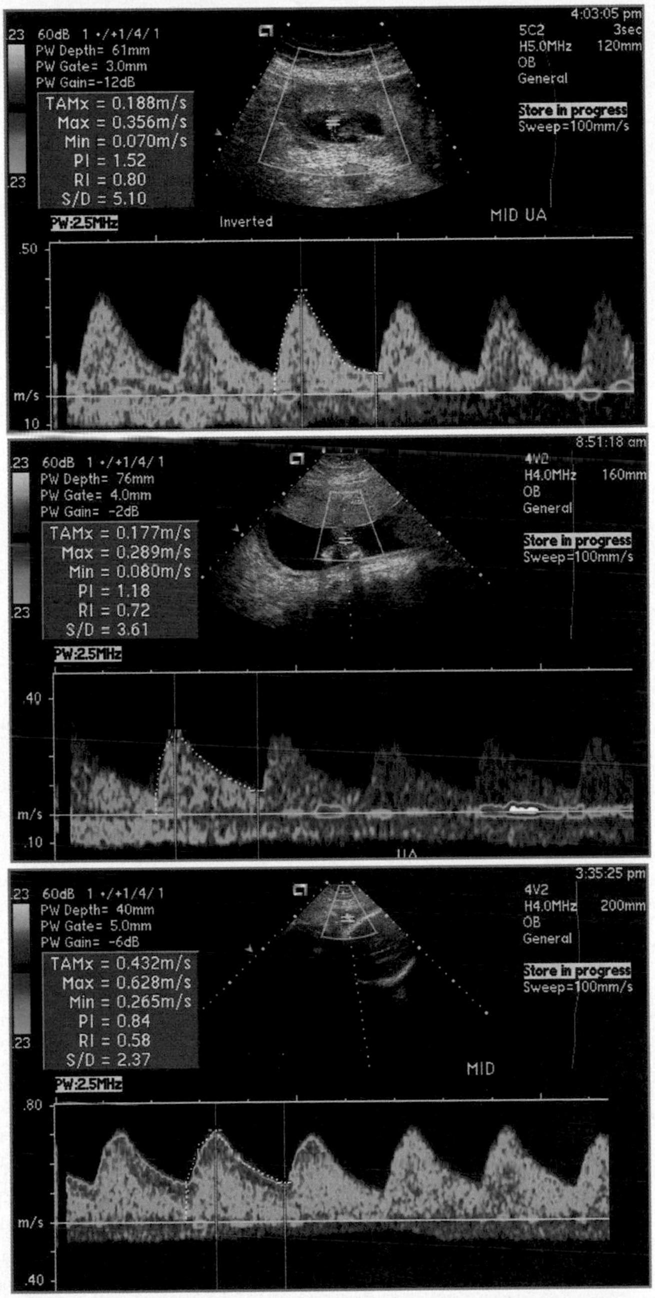

FIGURE 21-11 Evolution of normal umbilical artery resistance, measured in mid cord. Although there is an increase in diastolic velocities and a corresponding gradual decline in systolic-to-diastolic ratio from first trimester to third (**A** to **C**), there is already well-developed diastolic flow in the earlier waveform.

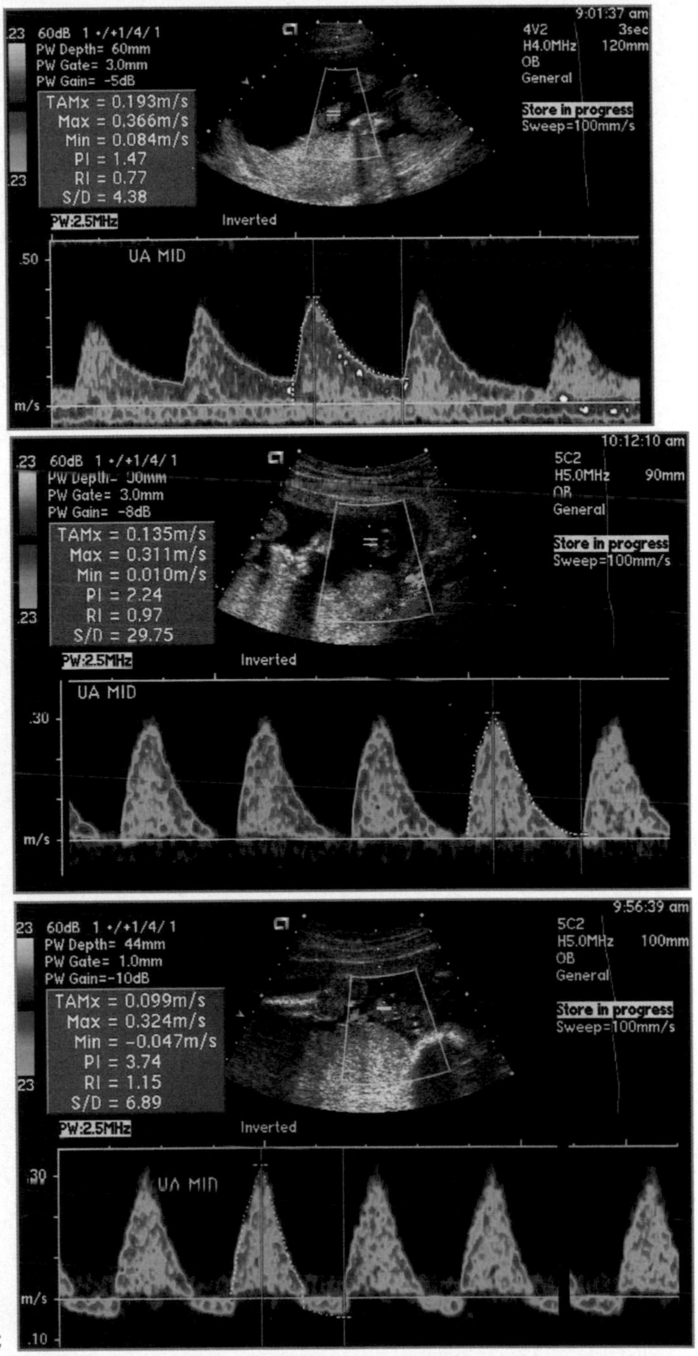

FIGURE 21-12 Progressive abnormality of umbilical artery resistance. Initially nearly normal at 18 weeks (pulsatility index, 1.47) (**A**), by 24 weeks (**B**) the umbilical artery shows absent end-diastolic velocities, which progressed to reversal of flow for 25% of the cardiac cycle (**C**). The infant had an umbilical venous pH of 7.18 after nonlabored cesarean section. All measurements in the mid cord.

lie above the baseline threshold for BPS variables and yet indicate progressive deterioration in fetal status. This level of awareness required of the ultrasound observer may explain some authors' dissatisfaction with withholding delivery of these fetuses.[123,124] Infants who had AEDV as fetuses are at risk for many neonatal complications because of placental insufficiency, asphyxial events surrounding delivery, and the significant impacts of prematurity (Table 21-6).[125-127] Progression to AEDV, or from AEDV to REDV, calls for enhanced fetal assessment, with shorter intervals, BPS scored out of 10, and arterial and venous Doppler studies together. Monitoring such fetuses by simple NST and repeated single umbilical artery Doppler does not satisfactorily ascertain fetal status.[128,129]

REDV magnifies these dangers and risks. In almost every fetal situation, this is a very unstable, often rapidly changing fetal-placental process. Acute vascular accidents (abruption, intraplacental bleeding, or fetal maternal hemorrhage) are frequent end points. Thus, many authors have recommended delivery as soon as possible.[130-132] Because

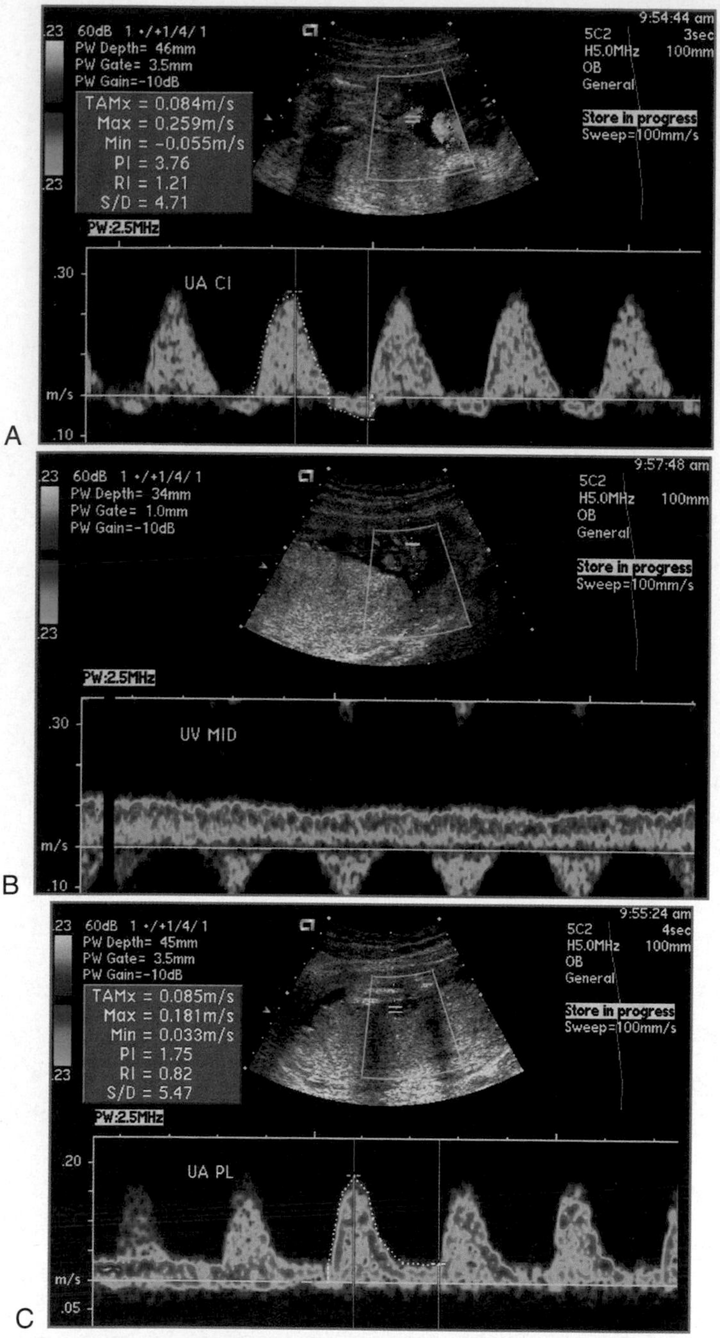

FIGURE 21-13 Umbilical artery resistance may vary extremely from one point on the umbilical cord to another. **A,** Abdominal cord insertion shows reverse end-diastolic velocities. **B,** At mid cord, end-diastolic velocities are absent (waveforms inverted in this image). **C,** At placental cord insertion, there is elevated resistance, but positive diastolic flow is demonstrated.

many cases of REDV are discovered on the first evaluation (e.g., on referral for evaluation of clinical IUGR), the progression for an individual fetus is difficult to determine. If the BPS is normal and amniotic fluid is adequate, there are no decelerations on the CTG, mean minute variation is greater than 3 msec, and most importantly if venous Doppler parameters are normal, time can be taken to administer antenatal steroids and to evaluate maternal condition before delivery. Because REDV is often associated with very significant abnormality of cerebral and venous circulations, it is linked to the highest frequency of fetal compromise, neonatal complications, perinatal mortality, and perinatal morbidity. Reducing the superimposed impacts of prematurity on such infants is effective in achieving the highest rate of intact survival.[105,119]

TABLE 21-6 ABNORMAL UMBILICAL ARTERY DOPPLER PREDICTS ADVERSE OUTCOMES*

Cesarean section for fetal distress
Acidosis
Hypoxemia
Low Apgar—5
Ventilator required
Long-term oxygen
Bronchopulmonary dysplasia
Anemia
Increased nucleated red blood cells (NRBC)
Thrombocytopenia
Prolonged NRBC release
Neutropenia
Transfusions required
Intraventricular hemorrhage
Necrotizing enterocolitis
Perinatal mortality

***The frequency of all of these outcomes rises exponentially from abnormal indices to absent end-diastolic velocities to reversed end-diastolic velocities.**

Middle Cerebral Artery

Hemodynamics. The middle cerebral artery (MCA) is short, straight, and uniformly positioned relative to the fetal skull and other intracranial landmarks. Doppler measurements taken from this vessel are more reproducible than those taken from other vascular beds and have few collateral circulatory influences, while representing a critical component of the fetal circulation, and the MCA is usually readily accessible throughout gestation.[133] Because the Doppler angle can be minimized, direct interpretation of the peak systolic velocity can be used to evaluate the absolute speed of blood flow, which has direct application in fetal anemia.[134,135] As the blood becomes thinner, cardiac ejection fraction increases and transaortic velocities increase, and the MCA offers an ideal location for direct interpretation of this increase in velocity as a decline in fetal hematocrit (Fig. 21-14).[136]

Placental insufficiency may alter peak systolic velocity, in some fetuses by anemia, transmitted hypertension, or both, but the key MCA abnormality expressed by the compromised fetus is centralization.[137,138] This is an increase in diastolic velocities and represents increased brain blood flow (Fig. 21-15). A significant question is whether such changes are compensatory (parenchymal vasodilation by active mechanisms) or involuntary (increased shunting of blood away from somatic circulations, under the force of hypertension dictated by accelerating placental vascular resistance).[139] As fetal compromise progresses, it is likely that both mechanisms are operant. Cerebral blood flow as depicted by the MCA may be responsive to a number of stimuli, including maternal administration of oxygen (increased resistance),[140] carbon dioxide (decreased resistance),[141] or nicotine (increased resistance, and lack of responsiveness).[142] These changes may occur gradually, indicated by subtle changes in the cerebroplacental ratio,[143] which reflects the calculated ratio of resistance indices in the MCA and umbilical artery. This ratio changes in response to redistribution of blood flow, the first stage of brain sparing.[144] The cerebroplacental ratio may therefore provide an early warning system to initiate more detailed fetal surveillance.

Measurement. The ideal location for Doppler assessment of the MCA is 2 mm after its origin from the internal carotid.[145] As demonstrated in Figures 21-14 and 2-15, the gate is opened to encompass the vessel, and short periods of insonation are used to minimize the amount of direct multiformat ultrasound delivered to the fetal brain. Most authorities recommend fetal MCA velocimetry should not be studied in the first trimester.

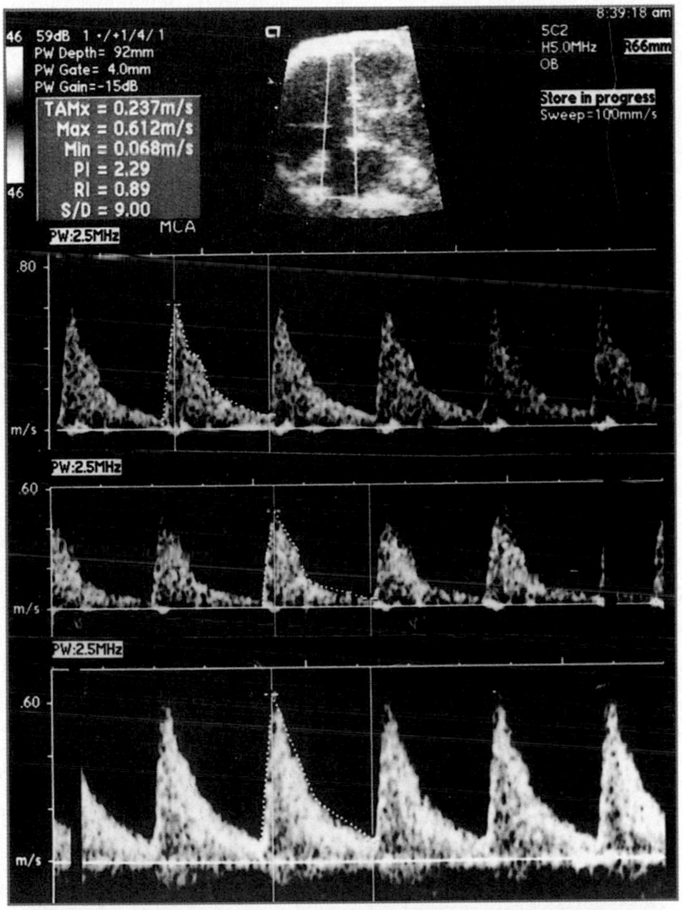

FIGURE 21-14 **The peak systolic velocity (PSV) in the middle cerebral artery (MCA) reflects fetal hematocrit accurately.** This fetus had serious anti-D isoimmune anemia. *Top,* Pretransfusion, MCA PSV of 60 cm/sec accurately predicted anemia (hematocrit, 19.0). After intrauterine transfusion, the MCA peak fell to 41 cm/sec as hematocrit rose to 44.0. Before the next transfusion *(bottom),* the MCA rose to 62 cm/sec and hematocrit had fallen to 20.0.

Clinical Significance. As IUGR worsens and compensatory mechanisms take place, MCA diastolic velocities rise. This centralization continues to increase in most fetuses with AEDV, and in many with REDV.[146] At the point when REDV and fetal hypoxemia result in cardiac decompensation, MCA diastolic velocities may fall, returning to an apparently high-resistance pattern because cardiac output is no longer sufficient to force blood into the fetal circulation (fetal cerebrovascular tone and fetal brain edema are thought to contribute here). This reversion resulting from heart failure has been called normalization, and it is an ominous sign meriting consideration for delivery.[147] Separate information may come from individual parameters of the waveform. In some fetuses, the MCA peak systolic velocity may be a better indicator of poor outcome than the Doppler index itself.[148] This relationship is independent of fetal anemia, for which MCA peak systolic velocity is not a reliable tool in growth-restricted fetuses.[149] Other than these infrequent findings, the MCA indicates the need for further testing rather than dictating clinical management by itself.[150] Critical examination suggests that the value of MCA Doppler information is minor when umbilical artery, precordial veins, and BPS are combined. Shifts in the cerebroplacental ratio or overt centralization of the MCA indicates a need for comprehensive fetal examination, testing using multivessel Doppler, and BPS (scored out of 10), on a frequent basis.[105] An exception to this rule occurs close to term, where MCA centralization without abnormal umbilical arteries or precordial veins may be associated with acidosis and hypoxemia and poor perinatal outcome.[151] The frequency of this finding in completely normal fetuses is unknown.

Fetal Venous Doppler Studies

Clinical Significance. There is evidence that venous Doppler studies are crucial in predicting severe compromise in fetal growth restriction (FGR) and other fetal-placental vascular abnormalities.[152-154] Without the use of venous Doppler, prediction of outcome (including perinatal mortality, acid-base status, birth asphyxia, and requirement for intensive neonatal support) is incomplete. Ductus venosus deterioration precedes, but strongly predicts, changes in BPS that require delivery. Although MCA Doppler changes are not statistically predictive of increased adverse outcome, ductus venosus resistance elevation and depression of the a-wave correlate with a threefold

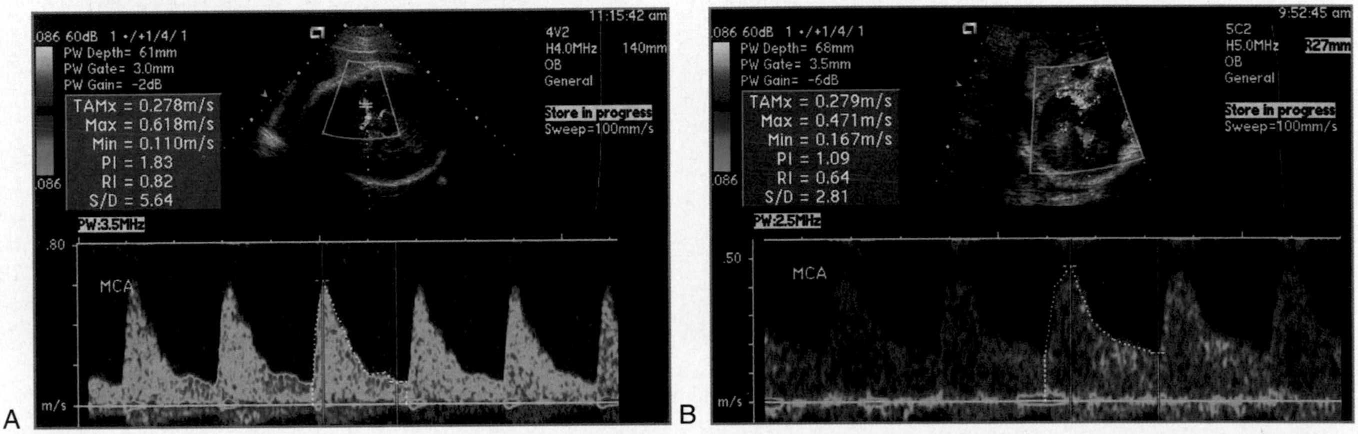

FIGURE 21-15 **Centralization of blood flow. A,** Normal middle cerebral artery (MCA) shows high resistance, low diastolic velocities. **B,** As placental resistance rises, brain blood flow increases, with falling resistance and increased diastolic velocities in the MCA.

rise in major neonatal complications. When both phases of the ductus venosus are abnormal and are also associated with umbilical venous pulsations, this relative risk exceeds 11.[155] Perhaps more important than the correlations of poor ductus venosus waveform with poor outcome is the reassurance of normal ductus venosus flow. Even in the presence of significant arterial abnormalities, the preservation of normal ductus venosus flow and normal biophysical variables is strongly correlated with normal fetal status, allowing successful extension of the pregnancy. There is strong agreement between abnormal venous Doppler parameters and an abnormal BPS in predicting fetuses who need delivery. However, venous Doppler studies and BPS are not strictly concordant: some fetuses who show deterioration manifest this primarily in umbilical and ductus venosus waveforms, with late decline in fetal behavior. Others demonstrate declining biophysical performance and yet maintain reasonably normal venous waveforms. These two systems are complementary—only with dual application is outcome optimized.[156]

Ductus Venosus. The ductus venosus is a sharply tapered conduit from the proximal umbilical vein into the inferior vena cava, directly at its connection to the right atrium. Its hourglass shape regulates inflow to the central circulation through a narrow aperture that is constricted in the healthy near-term fetus, allowing only 20% of umbilical venous return into the right atrium. Because of the Venturi effect, this narrow jet delivers highly oxygenated blood at high velocity directly to the foramen ovale, keeping it open and promoting right-to-left shunting of this nutrient-rich stream. In healthy fetuses, the ductus venosus regulates the distribution of oxygen and placental nutrients by restricting the centralization of flow. The high-velocity flow through the ductus venosus makes it easy to identify with color flow Doppler. When this short vessel is identified, Doppler insonation and depiction of the characteristic waveform (Fig. 21-16A) is relatively straightforward. The reflected wave seen in the ductus venosus waveform represents the impact of cardiac actions (directly analogous to the adult jugular venous waveform). The phases of the ductus venosus correspond to cardiac events as depicted in Figure 21-16B. During atrial systole, reduction in forward flow always occurs, producing the most notable characteristic of this waveform, the a-wave. The a-wave becomes progressively deeper as high afterload develops as a result of adverse placentation. It is further magnified as poor cardiac function superimposes (e.g., with hydrops, viral infection, endstage anemia) or as severe placental resistance results in respiratory dysfunction and direct hypoxemia. A retrograde a-wave (see Fig. 21-16C) signifies the onset of significant cardiac impairment. When cardiac function deteriorates toward preterminal pump failure, dramatic changes occur in both the atrial and ventricular phases of the ductus venosus (see Fig. 21-16D).

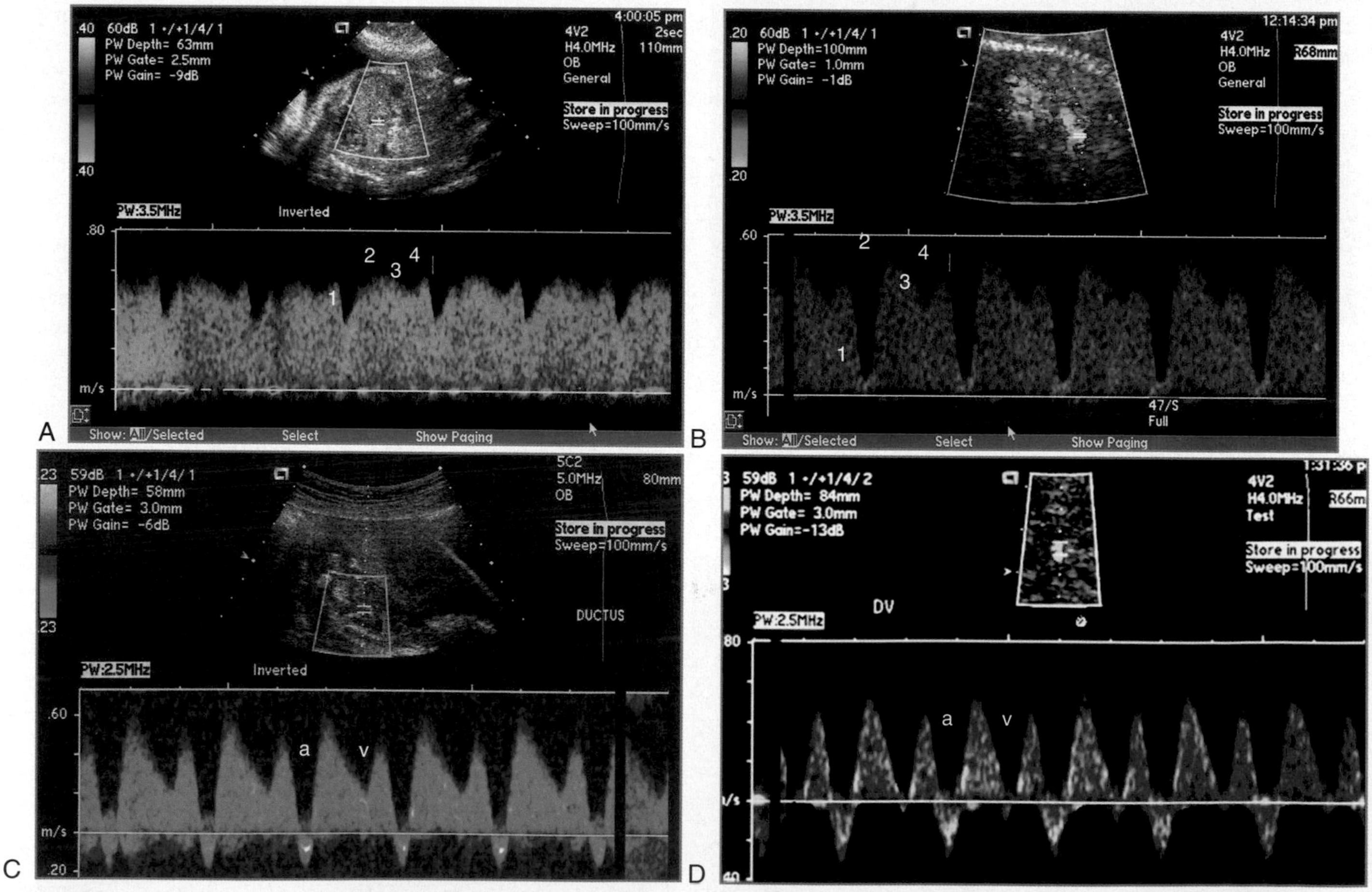

FIGURE 21-16 **Ductus venosus waveforms.** **A,** Normal four-phase waveform (1, atrial contraction, called an a-wave; 2, ventricular systole; 3, ascent of annulus; 4, diastole) with a-wave showing only modest normal reduction in forward flow. **B,** In fetuses with growth restriction, increased afterload (from placental resistance) is reflected through the heart as markedly abnormal forward cardiac function, with a nearly retrograde a-wave. **C,** Cardiac effects are also reflected distally. Note retrograde a-wave as well as cardiac function producing distortion of v-descent (compare to 3 in normal wave form). **D,** Severe cardiac decompensation results in both phases being negative.

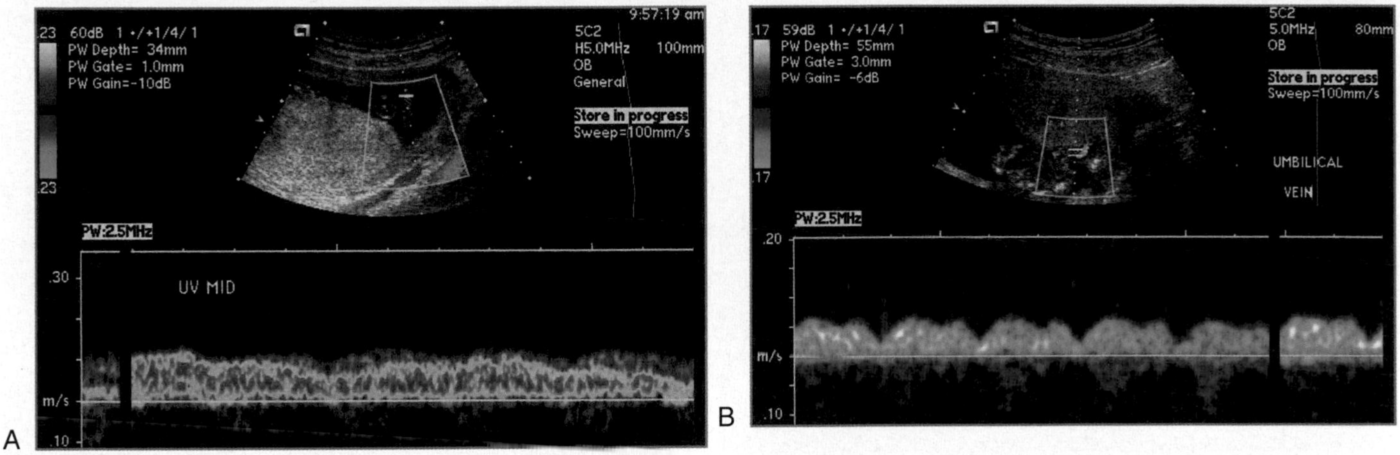

FIGURE 21-17 Umbilical venous pulsations. **A,** Moderate pulsatility, increased placental resistance in intrauterine growth restriction. **B,** Cardiac failure with tricuspid regurgitation reflected as retrograde flow all the way back to mid cord. Note timing relationship to arterial pulsations *(below line)*.

The ductus venosus offers dual insights into oxygen-regulated flow and cardiovascular function. These factors, as well as the ease of identification throughout gestation, suggest that the ductus venosus is the precordial vein of choice. Multiple venous systems have been studied, and there is no statistical basis for choosing the inferior vena cava, umbilical vein within the free abdomen, or other venous index over the ductus venosus for accuracy in predicting fetal compromise. Furthermore, only the ductus venosus can actively dilate with hypoxemia, an added benefit that supports its superior application.

Functionally, the retrograde a-wave is frequently associated with umbilical venous pulsations (see Fig. 21-17). These pulsations reflect retrograde conduction of the a-wave impulse (facilitated by the dilated ductus venosus) and a distended column of blood extending directly back from the heart into the free portion of the umbilical vein. Umbilical venous pulsations are infrequent, so they are not a practical marker with a high rate of detection of the compromised fetus. When seen in association with ductus venosus abnormality, umbilical venous pulsations call for prompt referral to a tertiary center and preparation for delivery.

Umbilical Vein. Pulsations in the umbilical vein occur for a number of reasons.[157] During fetal heart rate accelerations, temporary pulsation may reflect increased cardiac dynamic action. If the cord is tightly coiled around the body or limb, or temporarily constricted by fetal position, umbilical venous pulsations may be documented. It is important to retain the context of these observations, because a series of umbilical vein pulsations in isolation, or umbilical venous pulsations with normal ductus venosus waveform, are of uncertain significance. There is also the possibility of specific vascular anomalies, including a partially occluded or even absent ductus venosus. Although the pulsation pattern has been suggested as a discriminator,[158] other investigators have not been able to duplicate these correlations (Fig. 21-17). Many groups have demonstrated that umbilical venous pulsations are an ominous finding and frequently lead to intrauterine demise or serious neonatal compromise.[159] The lack of standard definitions means that there are many false positives, and action based solely on umbilical venous pulsations appears unwarranted. Thus, umbilical venous pulsations are the best example of the warning that Doppler investigations are not to be taken in isolation, out of context with other fetal observations.[160]

Other Veins. The inferior vena cava (IVC) shares some characteristics with the ductus venosus but is not easily interpreted. It is normal to have a retrograde a-wave in the IVC, so meticulous measurement of the venous resistance index is required. Second, the IVC does not vary with hypoxemia, so reflection distally cannot be inferred as a marker for sequential fetal compromise. Similar observations can be obtained from cerebral veins, hepatic veins, or regional venous vessels. All the precordial veins are involved in the fetal responses to hypoxemia.[161] The apparent ease of ductus venosus recognition seems to be the reason it is suggested as the standard for this information.

Maternal Doppler Studies

Uterine Artery

The uterine arteries normally demonstrate progressive reduction in resistance and increased diastolic velocities throughout gestation (Fig. 21-18).[162] This depends on absence of maternal hypertension and presence of normal placental invasion.[163] Pre-pregnancy, high-impedance characteristics of uterine artery circulation, including high resistance, persistence of diastolic notching, and even absent end-systolic forward flow, can persist throughout pregnancy if placentation is inadequate.[164] Different components of uterine artery abnormality have different sensitivities and specificities for placental malfunction and for maternal hypertensive disorders, or both. These findings may be of diagnostic benefit in a hypertensive mother (to evaluate the possibility of preeclampsia) or for a small fetus (to assess the possibility of FGR based on placental insufficiency). Failure of complete development of a uterine artery pattern (Fig. 21-19), especially in patients with a history of prior severe preeclampsia or eclampsia, may be indicative of recurrent maternal disease or FGR. Prophylactic trials using first-trimester uterine artery Doppler screening to allocate low-dose aspirin offer promise.[165,166] However, a monitoring role for uterine artery Doppler in the third trimester has not been established, because as many as two thirds of preeclamptic mothers have normal uterine artery Doppler tracings.

Maternal Cerebral Doppler Studies

Initial interest in maternal MCA Doppler in the monitoring and pharmacologic management of serious preeclampsia has not become standard of practice.[167,168] The maternal MCA can be visualized through the thin temporal window just anterior to the temporal artery. Characteristics in normal and hypertensive pregnancies are shown in

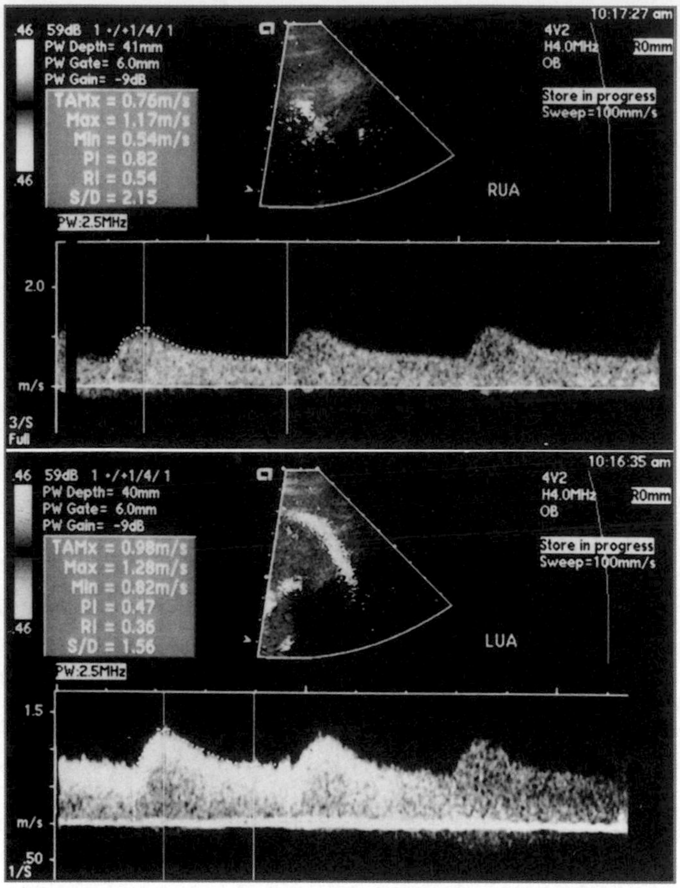

FIGURE 21-18 Normal maternal Doppler studies from right (RUA) and left (LUA) uterine arteries. Low resistance, high diastolic flow, and little difference from one side to the other characterize normal placentation.

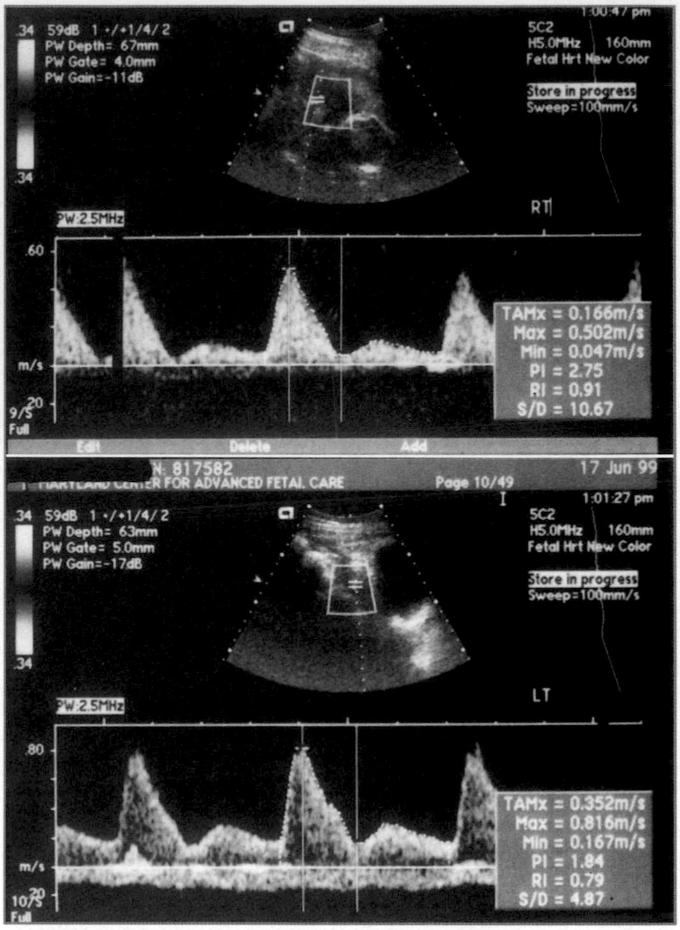

FIGURE 21-19 Uterine arteries. Markedly abnormal uterine arteries in mother with lupus, hypertension, superimposed preeclampsia, and intrauterine growth restriction (at same gestational age as woman in Fig. 21-18). Note the increased resistance, the persistent diastolic notching, and the significant difference between right (RT) and left (LT).

Figure 21-20. Monitoring of maternal cerebral circulation, especially in women who were eclamptic and are being treated with multiple antihypertensive drugs including acute vasodilators such as nitroprusside, may offer a role for serial monitoring of these vessels.[169] In general, however, the research demonstrating the powerful and almost immediate effect of magnesium sulfate in producing dilation of the cerebrovasculature, thus releasing arterial spasm, means that clinical application of maternal MCA Doppler is seldom mandatory.[170] More recent studies, with a better understanding of maternal MCA characteristics specific to pregnancy, have focused on monitoring changes.[171,172]

Doppler Application

Important applications of Doppler technology exist from the first trimester to near term. Evaluation of placentation through uterine arteries can predict the frequency and severity of preeclampsia and placenta-based FGR. Umbilical artery Doppler provides insight into the fetal aspects of placentation, directly reflecting placental vascular resistance. These findings are strongly correlated with FGR and multiple critical fetal and neonatal outcome characteristics, progressively worsening as reduction, loss, and reversal of diastolic flow follow in deteriorating sequence. As umbilical artery abnormalities advance, direct assessment of the fetal circulation, using a combination of systemic arterial and venous Doppler waveforms (MCA and precordial veins, respectively), becomes of increasing importance in accurately depicting fetal status. Combining these Doppler techniques can be done efficiently in the context of a regular fetal assessment examination. Doppler information from all these sources (placental, systemic arterial, and systemic venous), coupled with biophysical variables, provides the ideal depiction of fetal status. Although these techniques have evolved separately, the reasons to use this multivessel approach are compelling.

Patterns of Deterioration

In general, placental abnormalities may persist for months before other Doppler parameters deteriorate. As placental resistance increases (e.g., as more and more placental infarcts occur), the cerebroplacental ratio shifts, reflecting a change in balance between placental and systemic perfusion—that is, there is redistribution. Then, brain sparing is invoked, with progressive abnormalities in umbilical artery circulation (AEDV, progressing to REDV) being associated with increasingly higher diastolic velocities in the MCA. By this time, subjective elements of behavior, such as increasing intervals of quiet sleep (state 1F), decreased velocity of fetal movements (often perceived by the mother as "weaker" movements), and elements of subjectively decreased

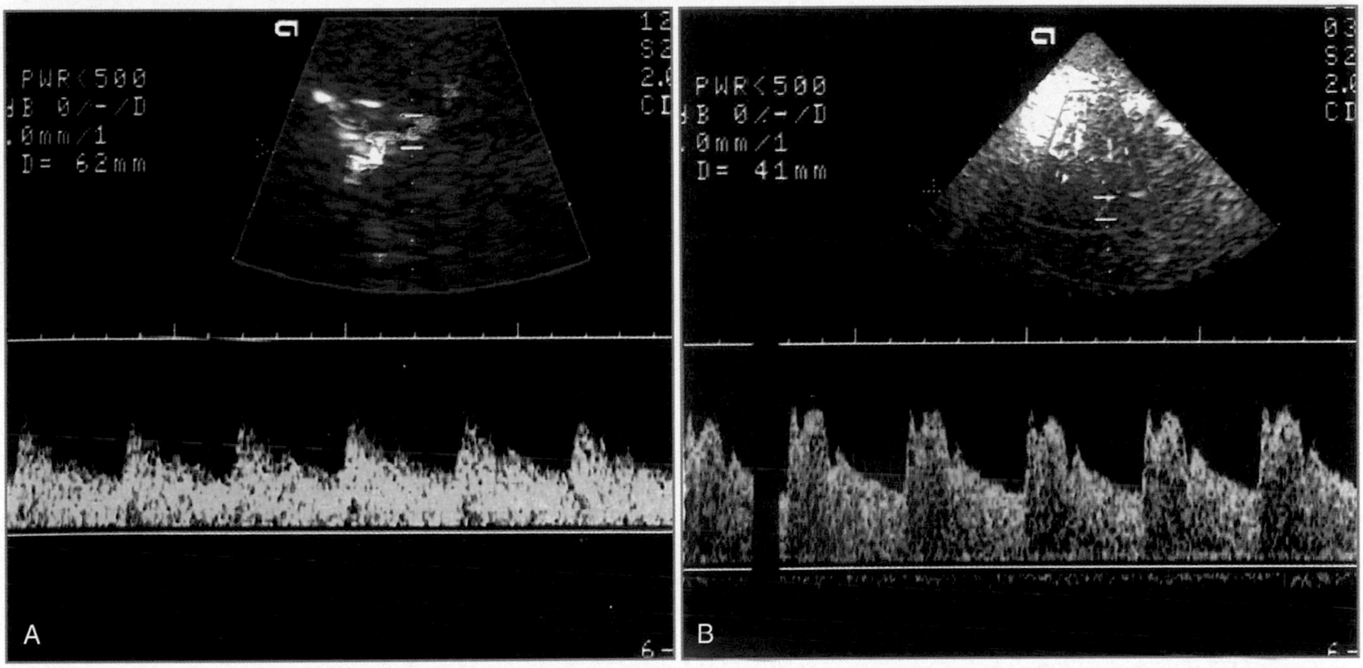

FIGURE 21-20 **Maternal intracranial Doppler examination.** **A,** Normal middle cerebral artery (MCA) Doppler waveform has a modest systolic peak less than 60 cm/sec, a diastolic peak less than 30 cm/sec, and slight notching. **B,** Abnormal maternal MCA in preeclamptic woman at 26 weeks has higher velocities (102 and 50 cm/sec, respectively), with systolic and diastolic notching.

amniotic fluid, may begin to appear.[107] With onset of AEDV, progressive redistribution yields overt centralization, and oligohydramnios becomes more common. The NST often becomes flatter, with overt nonreactivity at or just before deterioration of precordial veins, including retrograde ductus venosus a-wave. At about this time, reversal of end-diastolic velocities in the umbilical artery may occur (although this progression is completed in only 20% of fetuses with severe IUGR), with progressive loss of fetal breathing movements, followed by loss of fetal tone, and then abolition of all movements, as the BPS becomes overtly abnormal (Fig. 21-21).[34]

Integrated Fetal Testing

This stereotypical path of deterioration is not always followed, and it does not always progress at a predictable rate. Thus, management strategies cannot be based on the anticipation that one specific finding inevitably means that delivery must occur within a specified short period of time. The Growth Restriction Intervention Trial (GRIT) (see later) demonstrated that reacting to Doppler findings in such an automatic fashion led to unnecessary prematurity, with long-term neurologic consequences.[173] Responding to absent end-diastolic umbilical artery velocities simply by delivery is not only unnecessary but has substantial consequences. When IUGR is studied using multiformat testing (multiple Doppler indices plus biophysical parameters), the overriding principle is that gestational age determines outcome over a wide range.[42] Only as severely compromised fetuses reach the third trimester does umbilical venous Doppler become a statistically important correlate of outcome, and its performance in indicating delivery is inferior to ductus venosus Doppler plus biophysical parameters. Studies to date constitute complex observations in severely compromised FGR fetuses. These are difficult studies, requiring intensive detail of both multivessel Doppler and BPS, but the resulting data produce many valuable insights into monitoring. They are not, however, randomized controlled trials. So, the system of combined Doppler and biophysical parameters displayed in Table 21-7, although it follows the principles clarified in those studies, remains to be validated as a superior method by randomized controlled trials.

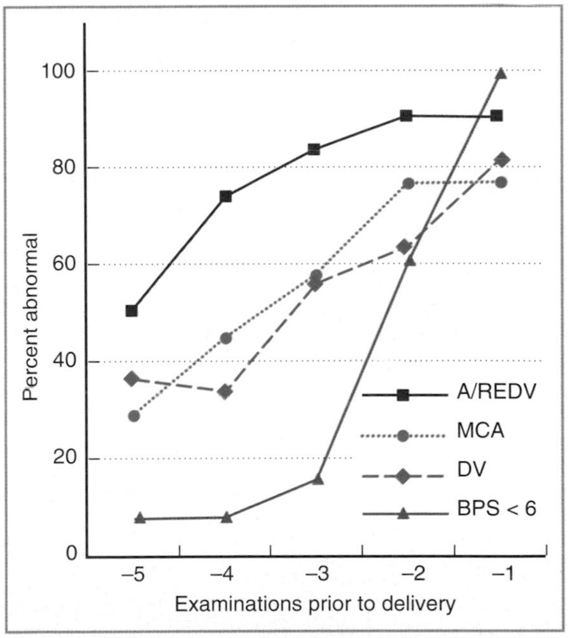

FIGURE 21-21 **Deterioration in Doppler waveforms before delivery for abnormal biophysical profile score (BPS).** All fetuses had prospective Doppler studies, and management decisions were made according to BPS. A/REDV, Absent or reversed end-diastolic velocity; DV, ductus venosus; MCA, middle cerebral artery.

In our clinical application of this protocol, the rigorous monitoring of all systems inevitably generates data that can further refine its

TABLE 21-7 PROTOCOL FOR MANAGEMENT OF SUSPECTED INTRAUTERINE GROWTH RESTRICTION (IUGR) BY INTEGRATED FETAL TESTING

IUGR Unlikely
Normal AC, AC growth rate, and HC/AC ratio.
UA and MCA Doppler normal, BPS and AFV normal.
Asphyxia very rare, low risk for intrapartum distress.
Monitor growth monthly. Deliver for obstetric or maternal factors.

IUGR Uncomplicated
AC < 5th percentile, slow AC growth rate, high HC/AC ratio.
UA elevated, MCA and DV normal. BPS and AFV normal.
Asphyxia very rare, at risk for intrapartum distress.
Monitor with weekly BPS, multivessel Doppler biweekly. Deliver for obstetric or maternal factors.

IUGR with Blood Flow Redistribution
IUGR is diagnosed based on above criteria. MCA centralized, DV normal.
BPS and AFV normal.
Hypoxemia possible, asphyxia rare. Increased risk for intrapartum distress.
Monitor with BPS twice per week, weekly Doppler. Deliver for obstetric or maternal factors, or at term.

IUGR with Marked Blood Flow Redistribution
Umbilical artery progresses to A/REDV, MCA continues centralized, DV normal. BPS ≥ 6/10, oligohydramnios frequent.
These Doppler changes mark the onset of fetal compromise. Hypoxemia common, acidemia or overt asphyxia are possible.
>34 weeks: deliver. Majority will not tolerate labor with oligohydramnios. (Cesarean section rate 85% for this group.) Before 34 weeks, monitor daily with integrated fetal testing, give antenatal steroids, consider transfer to tertiary center.

IUGR with Proven Fetal Compromise
Significant redistribution is present, evident by markedly abnormal UA resistance, MCA centralization, increased DV pulsatility, without a-wave reversal or UV pulsations. BPS ≥ 6/10, oligohydramnios is frequent.
More serious fetal compromise, delivery decision is imminent. Acidemia or asphyxia increasingly possible.
Integrated fetal testing daily, up to three times daily, depending on individual characteristics. Beyond 32 weeks, steroids given, deliver at tertiary center. Before 32 weeks, admit for monitoring, give steroids, transfer to tertiary center.

IUGR with Fetal Decompensation
All the above criteria are met. DV abnormalities progress to absent or reversed a-wave, with or without pulsatile UV.
BPS must be 6/10 or greater to delay delivery.
This is the preterminal stage of fetal compensation, featuring cardiovascular instability, metabolic compromise, imminent stillbirth, high perinatal mortality irrespective of intervention.
Beyond 28 weeks or if steroids given, deliver by cesarean section at a tertiary care center with highest level NICU. Before 28 weeks, monitor continuously and administer at least one dose of antenatal steroids.

AC, abdominal circumference; AFV, amniotic fluid volume; A/REDV, absent/reversed end diastolic velocity; BPS, biophysical profile scoring; DV, ductus venosus; HC, head circumference; NRFHR, nonreassuring fetal heart rate; MCA, middle cerebral artery; NICU, neonatal intensive care unit; UA, umbilical artery; UV, umbilical vein.

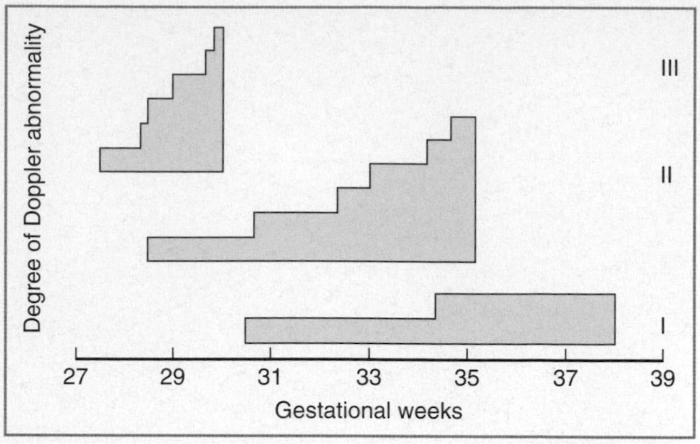

FIGURE 21-22 Patterns of Doppler deterioration in severe placental disease. In pattern I *(lower box)*, diagnosis is at average of 29 to 30 weeks. Progression from abnormal umbilical artery alone to umbilical artery abnormalities plus brain sparing occurs in some, but deterioration to severe placental insufficiency generally does not occur and delivery is close to term. In pattern II *(middle box)*, gradual escalation with changes in stages occurring about every 10-14 days causes gradual progression to severe Doppler parameter changes in a minority. Onset is at 28 to 30 weeks and delivery somewhat before term, but outcome is generally favorable. In pattern III *(upper box)*, progression is rapid, with deterioration from the relatively early onset of multiple vessel disease to full involvement of all vascular targets requiring urgent premature delivery of potentially compromised fetuses over only 2 to 3 weeks. A primary advantage of identification of these patterns is that differentiation is enabled in the first few weeks of careful monitoring using integrated fetal testing, allowing timely planning, individualized monitoring, and optimal delivery conditions.

application. These findings emphasize the need for flexibility, even when integrated fetal testing is applied. There are generally three patterns of change after a diagnosis of placenta-based FGR by umbilical artery Doppler criteria; these three patterns follow different time courses, and they require different levels of monitoring and different degrees of intervention (Fig. 21-22). Clearly, although the acute group requires intensive monitoring over a short period of time, that degree of resource allocation would be redundant in the other groups. That these patterns can be discriminated from one another during as few as 2 weeks of careful assessment means valuable resources can be properly allocated.

In many situations, a maternal disorder has a prominent vascular component (e.g., lupus, chronic renal disease, chronic hypertension, diabetes with vascular involvement, monochorionic twins, and dichorionic twins with marked discordance). When the vascular abnormalities of such conditions affect the fetus and placenta, integrated fetal testing may be ideal for fetal monitoring. The management of the fetus with IUGR is also addressed in detail in Chapter 34.

Ancillary Tests

As with any patient, the history and physical come first. Maternal risk factors, such as cigarette smoking, hypertension, antiphospholipid antibody syndrome, thrombophilia, vascular effects of diabetes, cocaine and other toxic substance abuse, and other sources of placental impairment, have a primary role in indicating surveillance for fetuses. Nuchal translucency and first-trimester maternal serum analytes, detailed review of fetal anatomy, serial evaluation of growth, amniotic fluid volume, and Doppler patterns all set the stage for the monitoring protocols described here. Overlapping risk factors mean modifying surveillance protocols to focus on vascular issues, reduce testing intervals based on severity, and apply ancillary testing. The provision of adequate prenatal care is itself a monitoring tool, capable of direct impact on perinatal and long-term outcome.[174-176] Such information is not static, and sonographers should interact freely with patients at every visit. Receptiveness to all channels of information about maternal and fetal well-being is a statistically important supplement to any monitoring technique.

Contraction Stress Test and Oxytocin Challenge Test

The contraction stress test (CST) and the oxytocin challenge test (OCT) are active tests using FHR responses to uterine activity to evaluate fetal health. The CST uses spontaneously occurring contractions or contractions induced by maternal nipple stimulation.[177] The OCT uses intravenous oxytocin to cause repetitive uterine activity[178] (Fig. 21-23). Interpretation includes standard NST parameters (accelerations, FHR baseline, and variability) and the FHR response once a contraction pattern has been established.

The technique is similar to that of the NST, except that the mother may not be monitored sitting or supine. (Postural artifact and restriction of fetal movement in response to contractions may generate falsely alarming tests.) Once a contraction pattern is established, with at least three contractions in 10 minutes, evaluation is possible. A negative OCT has no decelerations or other unclassifiable changes from baseline with contractions.[178] There may be isolated decelerations or times when the FHR is not adequately monitored, so normal criteria suggested by Schifrin[179] include any monitored segment in which three consecutive contractions are not associated with FHR decelerations.

Interpretation of a positive (abnormal) CST or OCT is also disputed. The classic standard is that FHR decelerations must accompany at least three consecutive contractions.[179] Another interpretation categorizes the CST as positive if at least 50% of the contractions cause late decelerations (when there are at least three contractions in 10 minutes), or when all the contractions are associated with late decelerations but there are fewer than three in 10 minutes.[180] An equivocal CST or OCT demonstrates repetitive decelerations not late in timing and pattern, usually classified as variable decelerations. Because this is a marker for oligohydramnios or cord entrapment, further assessment is required for this category of tests as well.[181,182]

For the OCT, intravenous oxytocin by continuous infusion pump is started at 0.5 mU/min, titrating upward in 1-mU increments until three contractions occur in each 10-minute window. This is done in a hospital setting to enable emergency response to hyperstimulation, unrelenting contractions despite discontinuing the oxytocin, tetanic

A

B

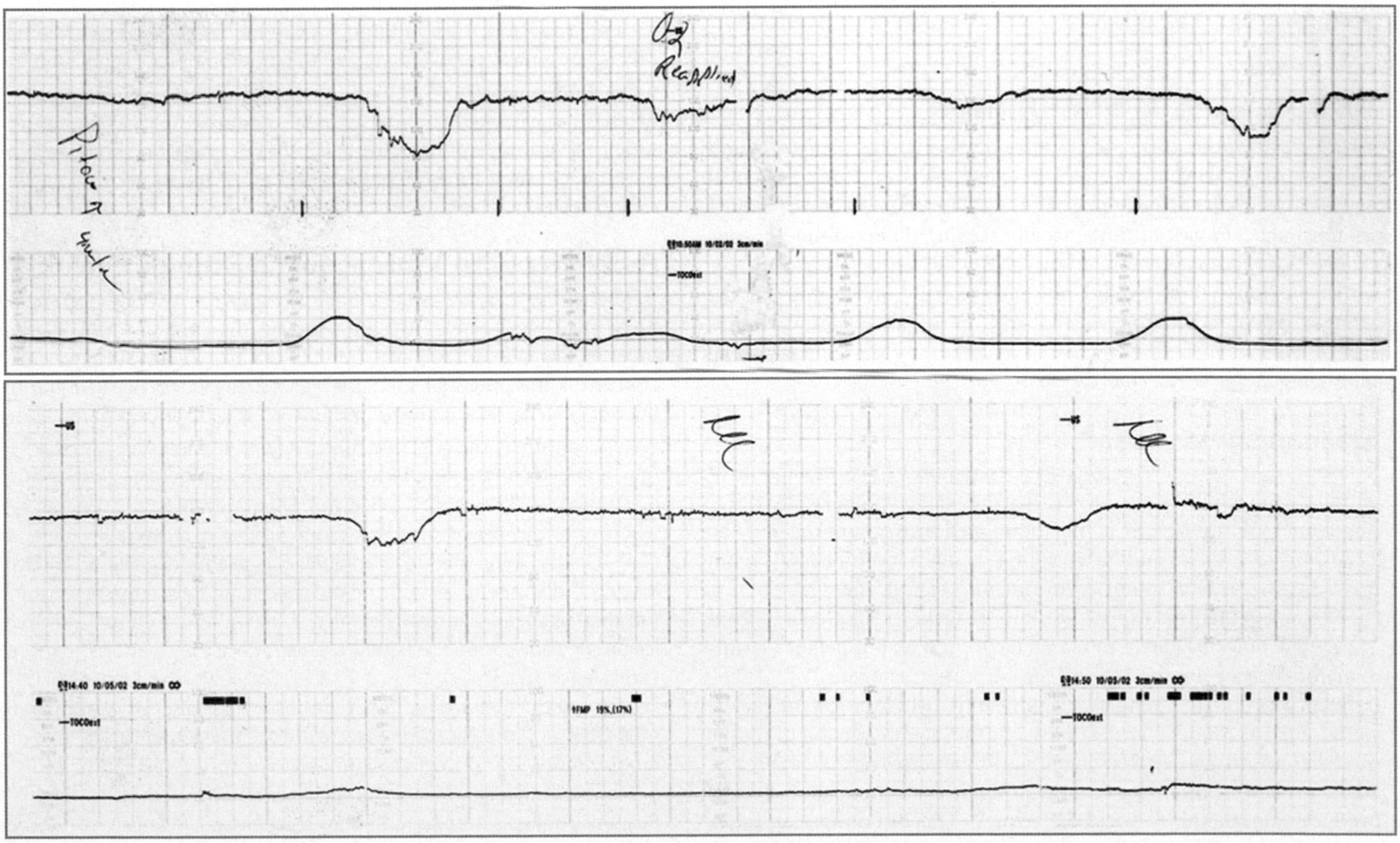

FIGURE 21-23 **Oxytocin challenge test and contraction stress test.** **A,** Oxytocin challenge test. Once contractions were established, repetitive late decelerations occurred with each contraction (a positive oxytocin challenge test). Delivery was by cesarean section because of fetal distress as induction of labor was attempted. Note that different strengths of contractions produced different depths of deceleration, all late in timing. **B,** Contraction stress test. Even trivial uterine activity caused late decelerations (a positive contraction stress test) in this fetus with severe intrauterine growth restriction and with abnormal Doppler parameters. Biophysical profile score was 4/10 at 25 weeks.

contractions, and fixed fetal bradycardia. Although the more dangerous consequences of these events are rare, hyperstimulation occurs in more than 10% of tests.[183]

Clinical application of these tests has become marginalized for several reasons. First, the method may have significant complications. Second, even for normal testing, the method is time consuming and expensive, usually taking up to 40 minutes to provoke contractions and ensure normality, and much longer if the test is equivocal or abnormal. Third, although these tests are good indicators of fetal well-being when negative (negative predictive values exceeding 99.8%), a positive test is not accurate enough to form the basis for clinical action. Positive predictive values for perinatal mortality of 8.7% to 14.9%, and for morbidity up to 70% for low 5-minute Apgar scores, fetal distress, and cesarean delivery for abnormal FHR in labor, show correlations but do not justify emergency delivery. When BPS is the backup test for a positive CST or OCT, at least 50% of pregnancies may be safely allowed to continue 1 week or more.[52] Furthermore, when multivariable testing is evaluated, outcomes correlate better with BPS variables than with elements of the CST or OCT, and the stress portions of the testing are irrelevant.[184,185] Few centers use either of these tests as a first-line method for high-risk pregnancy fetal monitoring. A residual role for OCT may be in allowing a trial of labor in patients with third-trimester FGR and oligohydramnios (if OCT is negative) and in monitoring some fetuses with unique presentations. For the preterm fetus with FGR who has normal amniotic fluid and normal BPS but who also has markedly abnormal Doppler velocimetry in multiple vessels, highly suggestive of placental insufficiency, the combination of stressed testing and fetal blood sampling for pH and cord blood gases may allow continuation of the pregnancy.

Vibroacoustic Stimulation

Where NST or other forms of FHR monitoring are the primary means of evaluating fetal health, the nonreactive test resulting from fetal quiet sleep (state 1F) is a major source of falsely alarming tests and consumes an inordinate amount of time (usually nursing time) waiting for state change. Vibroacoustic stimulation (VAS) (i.e., stimulating the fetus with a noxious vibration and noise) is effective in producing state change, fetal startle movements, and increased FHR variability, and thus in shortening the time it takes to demonstrate fetal well-being.[186,187]

Mechanism of Action

It is not clear whether these responses require the combination of vibration and audible noise or whether they can be provoked by vibration alone. Vibration sense is fully developed throughout the body by 22 to 24 weeks,[188] and auditory response about a month later.[189] From this time on, the fetal sound environment is significant.

The normal fetus is exposed to low-frequency sound energy from a variety of sources. Direct human data are scarce, but detailed evaluation of hearing in the fetal sheep appears analogous.[190,191] High-frequency sound is attenuated significantly, whereas low-frequency sound, such as thunder, airport noise, or the rhythm section of music, produces measurable evoked potentials in the cerebrum and appropriate deformation within the fetal ear.[192] High-decibel impact may even produce damage in low-frequency areas.[193] This discrimination probably extends to differentiation of vowels (low frequency, easily heard) from consonants (higher frequency, probably heard poorly) and produces apparent learning behavior.[194] The latter includes recognition of or favoring the maternal voice over other voices, apparent recognition of music played in fetal life (whether it is the actual music and its multiple tones or simply the rhythm is unclear), and perceived responsiveness to intrauterine music.[195] Again, it is unclear whether it is the actual music or merely its vibratory pattern that the fetus favors; apparently low-amplitude music with a slow rhythm is soothing, whereas high-amplitude, high-frequency, high-rate rhythmic music produces significant accelerations[196] and perhaps even a state change to hyperactive 4F.[197]

Given these observations about fetal hearing and the exquisite sense of vibration that is developed even earlier, it is not surprising the fetus can be "stimulated" by electromechanical devices that induce a very broad band of atonal white noise from 0.1 to 10 kHz.[198] Depending on the instrument used, this may deliver sound pressure exceeding 130 decibels (enough to produce permanent damage) and at almost all points in the entire range in excess of 70 decibels (comfortable hearing).[199] A number of different instruments, including ordinary alarm clocks, tin cans, electric toothbrushes, clapping hands, and electric door buzzers, have been used to provoke the classic fetal response.

VAS induces reproducible state changes in fetuses.[197] When the fetus is in quiet sleep (1F), even short bursts of VAS provoke the movement patterns, type of movement, fetal posture, FHR, and FHR variability typical of state 2F. If the fetus is already in state 2F (moving actively), the VAS may generate conversion to 4F (hyperactive "jogging" fetus) and almost always results in increased frequency of movements, amplitude of movements, rise in heart rate, and exaggerated FHR variability. On occasion, fetal bradycardia has been incited.[200] That VAS is useful in persuading a breech-presenting fetus to turn spontaneously into the transverse position with one or two applications[201] is seen by some as a useful or even essential adjunct to external cephalic version[202] but by others as undue punishment for malpresentation.[203] The high frequency of state change in the human fetus, especially close to term, means that VAS achieves its purpose of shortening the monitoring time, converting a nonreactive NST to a reactive one, and avoiding prolonged testing times,[204] but even the most recent review expresses safety concerns.[205]

Problems with Vibroacoustic Stimulation

A large number of studies demonstrated false-positive rates as high as 67%.[206,207] This characteristic means that the backup test (full BPS) must be available on site for the majority of patients. Of even more concern is the potential for falsely reassuring rates. Because the frequency of true fetal compromise, manifest as asphyxia before labor, intrapartum fetal distress, low Apgar scores, and abnormal pH, is very low in most of these populations, very large numbers of patients must be studied to evaluate the liability of failed detection. In trials of VAS where the prevalence of adverse outcome was reasonably high, the false-negative rate was unacceptable. For example, Serafini and colleagues[208] documented a 55% falsely reassuring rate in the detection of intrapartum fetal distress (prevalence 20%), and Kuhlman and colleagues[209] showed a 53% falsely reassuring rate for pH less than 7.20 (prevalence 16%).

Among the higher-risk target groups, where cases of oligohydramnios, FGR, and preterm fetuses were not excluded, preterm infants may require more sound to elicit significant responses, raising the odds of hearing injury when VAS is applied before 33 weeks' gestation.[210,211] Responsiveness is decreased in abnormal fetuses,[212] fetuses of mothers with hypertension,[213] fetuses exposed to cocaine in fetal life,[197] fetuses whose mothers have depression,[214] and fetuses with severe IUGR[215] treated with magnesium, antenatal steroids, or β-mimetics for preterm labor.[216,217] Thus, the greatest liability for inaccuracies with VAS is compounded in those fetuses at greatest need for monitoring.

Is There a Role for Vibroacoustic Stimulation?

When the BPS ultrasound variables are normal (score, 8/8), there is no need for additional reassurance by NST in the majority of cases, and testing time averages 11 minutes in routine antenatal surveillance. When specifically studied in a trial of multiformat testing in FGR, VAS offered no additional information beyond the combination of biophysical and Doppler assessments. The proven convenience of VAS in shortening NST times is simply outweighed by the combination of safety concerns, an annoying false-negative rate, and a dangerous falsely reassuring rate. VAS should not be part of routine testing in high-risk pregnancies.

Fetal Movement Counting

Maternal awareness of fetal activity in the unprovoked setting has been documented for many generations. Multiple factors may influence the systematic application of movement counting as a method of fetal surveillance (Table 21-8). Sudden absolute cessation of fetal movement is alarming, but this may be a premortem event, rather than one with any realistic warning period. Second, NST alone is ineffective in monitoring the fetus with decreased movement, as shown in a large randomized trial.[218] That trial used the count-to-10 method and produced several interesting effects. First, the control group experienced a very significant drop in perinatal mortality compared with patients not enrolled in the study at all—a clear example of the Hawthorne effect, where the presence of a trial in the community produces responses even in those not undergoing the experimental maneuver. Second, the compliance for immediate reporting of decreased fetal movement was low compared with other studies. It is critical, of course, that women report the decrease on the day it happens and not at their next prenatal visit. Finally, the rescue methodology was simple FHR monitoring, with the result that a large proportion of the fetuses who ultimately died were monitored and discharged without ultrasound evaluation. The authors concluded that "routine daily counting . . . seems to offer no advantage over informal inquiry about movements during standard antenatal care." Recent reviews of 24 available studies including two trials,[218,219] however, conclude that positive benefits may be found, but that properly constructed trials are needed before clinical implementation is merited.[220,221] It may well be that the information about fetal activity, especially focusing on significant changes in routine rather than absolute loss of movement, may be effective, especially in the context of multisystem monitoring.

Invasive Fetal Testing

Fetal Blood Sampling

Fetal blood sampling as early as 17 to 18 weeks, reliably in almost every fetus by 22 weeks, has led to a wealth of experience in determining fetal metabolic, respiratory, hematologic, and genetic correlates in normal and abnormal situations. These studies offered tremendous insight into the mechanisms of disease and the application of normative values. At the same time, a catalog of noninvasive observations was also assembled—ultrasound, heart rate testing, and Doppler—which all provide key correlations to values obtained invasively. As experience was gained, it became clear that virtually any test possible in the newborn or infant could be obtained and evaluated with reliability in the fetus. Although the risks of these techniques were measurable, experienced teams were able to perform ultrasound-guided fetal blood sampling in normal-appearing fetuses (e.g., for rapid karyotype of women who attended genetic counseling late) with fetal loss rates much less than 1%, and in several series only modestly more than amniocentesis.[222-224]

Fetal blood sampling has specific applications:

- For fetal abnormalities, especially hydrops (red cell alloimmunization, viral infection, asphyxial injury)
- When history, maternal alloimmune titers, or MCA Doppler studies indicate a risk of anemia
- For rare metabolic, hematologic, or gene disorders testable only by fetal blood sampling
- For infrequent confirmation of ambiguous test results from amniocentesis or chorionic villus sampling
- Even more rarely, for documentation of fetal respiratory status

Ultimately, the noninvasive correlates, proven through the experience of fetal blood sampling, have rendered the actual blood test less important. Key examples include MCA Doppler peak velocity to assess the degree of fetal anemia, which has markedly reduced the need for initial fetal blood sampling.[135] The correlation between BPS and fetal

TABLE 21-8 PROBLEMS WITH FETAL MOVEMENT COUNTING (FMC)

Factors	Effect
Highly variable methodology	Confusion and inconsistent instructions
Efficacy	Physician noncompliance
Fetal/maternal variation:	
Different activity between fetuses	These factors require flexible, individualized FMC methodology.
Changing activity in the same fetus	
Different perceptions between mothers	
Different perceptions by same mother	
Public misinformation (e.g., it's OK for the baby to stop moving before labor)	Failure to follow protocol directions in unusual circumstances
Poor maternal compliance	Up to 20% of women do not count, and may falsify records
Faulty clinical response	Despite proper maternal performance, no definitive testing or intervention is undertaken, or too much reliance placed on the cardiotocogram alone. Biophysical profile scoring is the only acceptable response to bona fide decreased fetal movement.
Lack of public awareness	Insufficient family participation

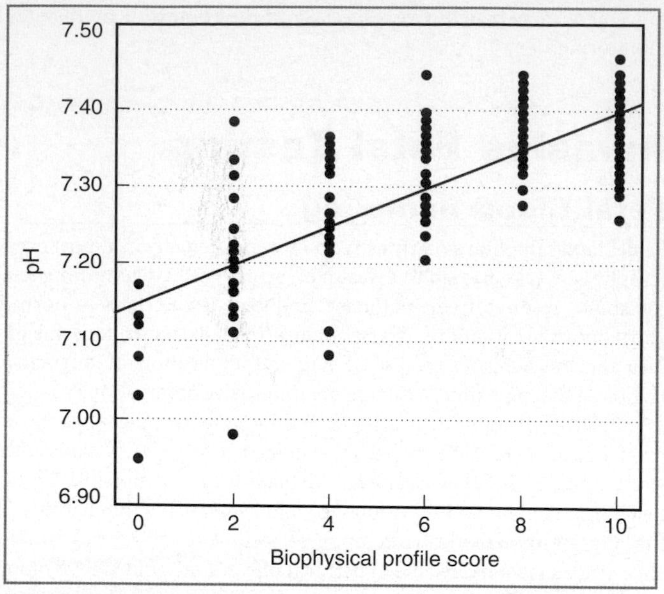

FIGURE 21-24 Correlation between biophysical profile score (BPS) and fetal pH on cordocentesis. Cordocentesis in 493 fetuses with concomitant BPS shows correlation of score with unlabored fetal umbilical venous pH. (BPS 10/10, pH > 7.20 in 100%. BPS 0/10, pH always < 7.20.) Note wide variation in pH for scores of 2 to 4/10.

pH on cordocentesis (Fig. 21-24 and see Fig. 21-2) means that BPS can be safely relied on to indicate fetal pH without the blood test.[89] Furthermore, the application of sensitive polymerase chain reaction techniques for gene amplification (together with the emergence of many new genetic markers) has replaced essential blood tests with tests of improved accuracy from fetal cells obtained by simple amniocentesis. Table 21-9 lists changes in indications for cordocentesis, noting that the modern distribution of the procedure reflects a 90% reduction in application of cordocentesis.

Cordocentesis Procedure

The umbilical vein is the target of choice, and it may be approached at virtually any point in its course. At the placental insertion, it is stable and usually easily entered, but this is also true of free loops of cord that may be pinned against the posterior wall of the uterus, the umbilical vein at the abdominal skin insertion, or in the intrahepatic portion of the vessel. The procedure itself has been greatly simplified and can usually be accomplished in a few minutes. Several previous adjuncts have been discarded, including maternal sedation, narcotic analgesia, prophylactic antibiotics, tocolysis, and admission to the hospital. Except in unusual circumstances, the mother is not prepared for emergency surgery and does not have an intravenous catheter, standby services such as obstetric anesthesia, or a reserved operating room.

A 22-gauge spinal needle of appropriate length usually suffices. Echotip needles and larger-bore introducers are seldom needed. Figure 21-25 demonstrates use of a needle guide, fixed to the ultrasound transducer. This limits excursion and angulation of the needle shaft, and the path of the needle is illustrated by software additions to standard ultrasound machines. Whereas debate has been vigorous in the last decade about measurable differences in outcome related to the use of the needle guide,[225] it now appears to be truly a matter of personal preference. Most senior authors reporting large series do not use needle guides.

TABLE 21-9 CHANGE IN INDICATIONS FOR CORDOCENTESIS FROM 1991 TO 2007

Indication	1991	2007
Rapid karyotype	28%	0%
Investigate other abnormal tests	10%	15%
Red blood cell alloimmunization	23%	20%
Infection	10%	15%
Nonimmune hydrops	7%	23%
Blood gases and pH	5%	3%
Twin-twin transfusion	5%	0%
Neonatal alloimmune thrombocytopenia	5%	13%
Immune thrombocytopenia	2%	—
Immune deficiency	2%	3%
Coagulopathy	1%	—
Hemoglobinopathy	1%	2%
Paralysis for fetal magnetic resonance imaging	—	2%
Late feticide (anomalies)	—	4%

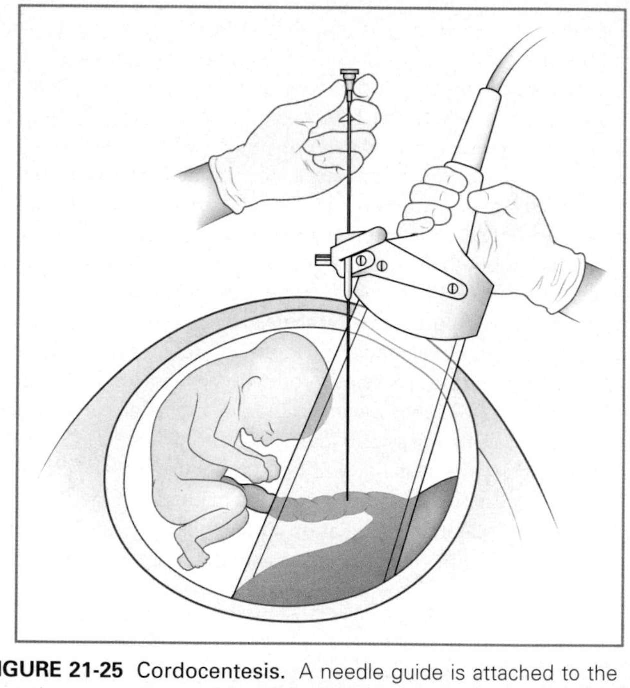

FIGURE 21-25 Cordocentesis. A needle guide is attached to the transducer, and the shaft of the needle is visualized in the ultrasound plane for this style of cordocentesis.

The maternal skin is marked for the approximate point of needle insertion, taking as much time as necessary to define the ideal approach to the clearest target vessel. Under sterile technique, the needle is inserted into the skin and imaged continuously. As the needle approaches the target vessel, the magnified field feature of the ultrasound machine is used, and the last few millimeters are completed to allow the needle tip to rest against the vessel wall. This is followed by a sharp 3- to 5-mm "pop" to overcome tissue resistance. Once the needle is seen in the lumen of the vessel, the stylette is removed and backflow is observed, which will usually gently fill the needle hub. The sample is obtained by directed flow rather than vigorous suction, as the latter tends to pull the vessel wall up against the needle and stop

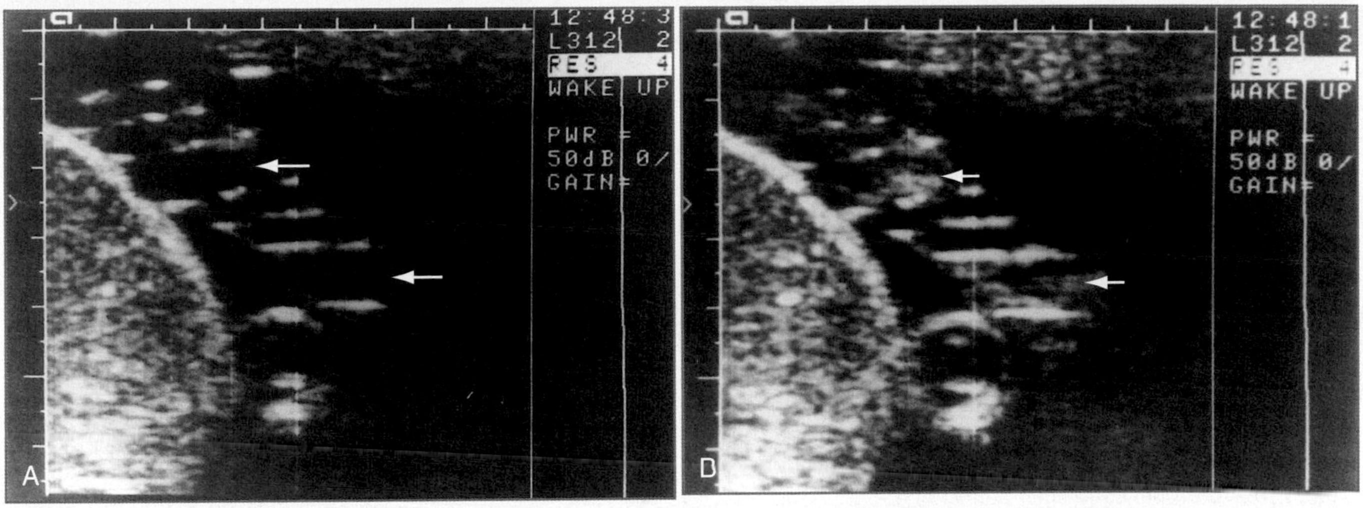

FIGURE 21-26 Turbulence during cordocentesis procedure. **A,** The umbilical cord in longitudinal section, adjacent to the fetal abdomen. The needle produced excellent return of fetal blood. No infusion. **B,** Infusion of 250 μL of normal saline demonstrates bright turbulence, identifying the umbilical vein *(arrows)*.

flow altogether. If free blood flow is not obtained, the needle is withdrawn in very small increments, with continuous gentle suction and rotation of the needle through a few degrees. The stylette is not replaced unnecessarily, because each stylette insertion introduces an echogenic microbubble into the ultrasound field directly above the target.

Vessel identity is confirmed by infusion of a small bolus (0.2 to 0.3 mL) of normal saline, which usually produces unmistakable turbulence (Fig. 21-26). Samples that may have been contaminated by amniotic fluid should not be discarded, because they are as reliable as pure fetal blood for polymerase chain reaction techniques or other genetic testing. On the other hand, metabolic measurements, fetal blood gases and pH, and especially hematologic measurements require absolutely pure fetal blood obtained under free-flowing conditions (without heparin in the syringe) and delivered immediately into the appropriate tubes for testing.[226-229] For routine blood sampling, the needle is in the fetal vessel for a very short time (usually less than 2 minutes) and fetal movement is not perilous—paralysis with intravenous pancuronium (0.4 to 0.6 mg) is now rarely used.[230]

The needle is withdrawn gently but firmly, without changing the angle used to insert it. Bleeding from the needle puncture site is visible for all transamniotic punctures, but because this is variable, it is always monitored to cessation. Later in gestation, when a free loop is used, Wharton jelly in the cord is usually completely hemostatic, and only one or two drops escape. If vessel puncture through an anterior placenta has been completely extra-amniotic, bleeding may exist but will be invisible, so postprocedure monitoring would be hemodynamic rather than visible. Ten minutes of direct Doppler-assisted ultrasound monitoring will account for that small possibility. In the Rh-negative woman, anti-D immunoglobulin is given at the end of the procedure.

Typical turbulence and a free-flowing blood sample provide assurance that the needle was properly placed. Laboratory confirmation should be obtained that the sample is pure fetal blood without maternal contamination, which can be ensured by a variety of tests. At term, there may be a broad distribution of fetal cell sizes, so the final confirmation of pure fetal origin is not morphologic but by the Kleihauer-Betke test.[231] This test takes 45 to 70 minutes to complete and is thus not suitable for bedside use; only after it is reported to show 100% fetal cells should a final interpretation of results be made.

TABLE 21-10 FETAL CONDITION AND CORDOCENTESIS LOSS

Condition	Average (%)	Range (%)
Nonimmune hydrops	35	3-80
Hydramnios	20	5-33
IUGR/oligohydramnios	9.3	1-14
Single anomaly*	5.8	1-13
Multiple anomalies*	4.8	1-12
Rh, platelets	3.4	0-17
Risk of infection	0.6	1-1.3
Normal, DS risk only	0.48	0-1.3

*Statistically not different.
DS, Down syndrome; IUGR, intrauterine growth restriction.

Postprocedural Monitoring

When the immediate procedural monitoring is completed, the fetus should be moving and should have a stable heart beat with no active bleeding. The uterus should relax completely between any contractions that may have been provoked by the procedure, and the absence of a prelabor contraction pattern is confirmed by a brief period (30 minutes or less) of cardiotocography. Sample validation and verification of normal maternal and fetal status after the procedure allow discharge from the hospital, usually within 1 hour.

Complications

Overall pregnancy loss rate depends largely on the fetal condition for which the cordocentesis was done (Table 21-10).[232,233] The rate of pregnancy loss is worse in cases of fetal hydrops, multiple anomalies, and abnormal karyotype.[234]

Immediate Complications

Fetal bradycardia has been reported in as many as 52% of procedures and is the most common complication of cordocentesis. It is almost always of short duration, self-limited, and usually with no long-term consequences. More serious bradycardia may occur as often as 3% of

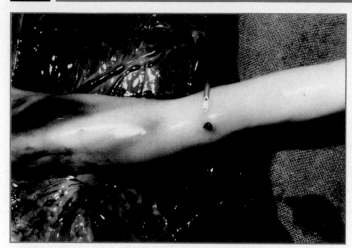

FIGURE 21-27 Cord puncture site. Normal small bruise when transamniotic needle insertion is through Wharton's jelly. Cordocentesis produced no visible bleeding when needle was withdrawn.

TABLE 21-11 FETAL BLOOD GAS AND pH WITH ADVANCING GESTATION

Parameter	Mean Values 22 Wk	28 Wk	34 Wk	40 Wk
UV (pH)	7.416	7.407	3.398	7.388
UV (Po_2)	47.600	42.000	36.300	30.600
UV (Pco_2)	33.600	34.900	36.200	37.500
UV (Hco_3)	22.300	23.000	23.700	24.300
UA (pH)	7.390	7.379	7.368	7.357
UA (Po_2)	28.300	26.300	24.300	22.300
UV pressure (mm Hg)	3.800	5.200	6.500	—

UA, umbilical artery; UV, umbilical vein.
Data from Soothill PW, Nicolaides KH, Rodeck CH, et al: Effect of gestational age on fetal and intervillous blood gas and acid-base values in human pregnancy. Fetal Ther 1:168, 1986; Nicolaides KH, Economides DL, Soothill PW: Blood gases, pH, and lactate in inappropriate- and small-for-gestational-age fetuses. Am J Obstet Gynecol 161:996, 1989; and Weiner CP, Sipes SL, Wenstrom K: The effect of fetal age upon normal fetal laboratory values and venous pressure. Obstet Gynecol 79:713, 1992.

the time and may indicate umbilical artery spasm. Maternal oxygen administration may relieve this spasm, and frequently it relents after a few minutes without untoward fetal effect.[11]

In about 1 in 300 cordocentesis procedures, profound or prolonged bradycardia occurs. Undetected cord hematoma, transplacental hemorrhage, uterine activity, or combinations of these may lead to fetal death on these rare occasions.[230,235] Reinsertion of the needle to try to aspirate a hematoma is usually unsuccessful and may cause further intrafundic bleeding.

Fetal bleeding is common, and 50% to 60% of simple vein punctures bleed for 15 to 60 seconds. Bleeding over 300 seconds or massive hemorrhage requiring resuscitation occurs less than once per 200 cordocentesis procedures.[230] When this does occur, frequently the result of severe fetal thrombocytopenia, the time to act is short.[236]

Most often, cord hematoma is not specifically detected but is noted incidentally after delivery or as a result of emergency intervention for intractable bradycardia (Fig. 21-27). The incidence of symptomatic cord hematoma causing significant fetal bradycardia is very low.[237] This is more commonly the result of difficult procedures with multiple attempts, including infusion of saline to try to identify the needle tip, infusion of pancuronium to paralyze a very active fetus,[238] or deliberate infusion of platelets or blood,[239] with malposition of the needle tip.

Acute maternal complications are rarely seen. Cordocentesis takes longer than amniocentesis, and the mother is likely to have more discomfort. The test is less uncomfortable than transabdominal chorion villus sampling, so for most women pain, contractions, and anxiety are not dominant complaints. Acute rupture of membranes is rare and usually associated with gross hydramnios or prolonged difficult procedures. Preterm labor is very rare.

Delayed Complications

Evidence for transmission of viral infection to the fetus from contaminated amniotic fluid or transplacentally from mothers with active diseases is not convincing. Amniocentesis does not increase hepatitis B transmission,[240] so it has been argued that cordocentesis for human immunodeficiency virus (HIV) testing may also be safe.[241] However, the possibility of vertical transmission exists.[242] Therefore, the application of fetal blood sampling in mothers infected with HIV may be of very limited value. Chorioamnionitis after cordocentesis in previously uninfected women is unusual but may be severe on rare occasions.[243] Infectious agents are skin staphylococcal species and enteric organisms.

In the case of maternal alloimmunization, fetal transfusion with donor blood may cause new red cell antibody development in up to 20% of women. For simple cordocentesis, however, serologic data are much less pronounced. Between 15% and 26% of women do show significant volumes of transplacental bleeding, as judged by maternal Kleihauer-Betke test, or up to 40% as judged by elevation of maternal serum α-fetoprotein after the test.[244] This is associated with transplacental insertion, and infrequently (in 7 of 90 women) it results in elevation of already present red cell antibody levels.[245] No cases of clinically significant new alloimmunization developed as a consequence of cordocentesis within a 17-year surveillance window.[230] This experience includes the following:

- Knowing maternal Rh before all procedures
- Administration of Rh immune globulin at the end of the procedure
- Maternal Kleihauer test after all procedures
- Follow-up additional Rh immune globulin for any case of transplacental hemorrhage of more than 10 mL of fetal red blood cells
- Avoiding the placenta if at all possible in women with known fetal-maternal incompatibility

Fetal Respiratory Status by Cordocentesis

Table 21-11 presents normative data for fetal blood gases and pH and demonstrates the progression of changes in these values with advancing gestation.[246-248] Of course, on the rare occasions when fetal blood sampling is performed to evaluate indices of infection, acidosis in the macrosomic diabetic fetus, hematologic indices in cases of hydrops, intracranial hemorrhage, or other presentation with abnormal fetal testing, specific knowledge of the individual variables, within the gestational age limitations, is essential.

TABLE 21-12 INDICATIONS FOR ANTENATAL SURVEILLANCE*

Maternal Conditions	Placental Conditions	Fetal Conditions	Miscellaneous
Severe hyperthyroidism Symptomatic hemoglobinopathy Cyanotic heart disease Chronic renal disease Type I diabetes Marked uterine anomalies	Antiphospholipid antibody syndrome Systemic lupus erythematosus Hypertensive disorders, including pregnancy-induced hypertension of all severities Thrombophilia Marked placental anomalies	Decreased fetal movement Oligohydramnios Polyhydramnios Intrauterine growth restriction Post-term pregnancy Alloimmunization Macrosomia Fetal anomalies or aneuploidy Multiple gestation (all)	In vitro fertilization pregnancy Teratogen exposure Previous stillbirth Prior neurologic injury Previous recurrent abruption

***Monitoring of pregnancies with abnormal Doppler parameters and no apparent underlying disorder remains controversial.**
Modified from American College of Obstetricians and Gynecologists Practice Bulletin #9, October 1999.

TABLE 21-13 SUGGESTED ANTENATAL FETAL SURVEILLANCE

Condition	Begin Surveillance*	Timing
Pregnancy-induced hypertension	At diagnosis	Weekly UA Doppler
Preeclampsia	At diagnosis	Twice weekly UA Doppler + BPS
Chronic hypertension	28-32 weeks	Weekly BPS or MBPS
Fetal growth restriction (FGR)	At diagnosis	Integrated fetal testing
Gestational diabetes		
A1	At 40 weeks	Weekly BPS or MBPS
A2	At 36 weeks	Weekly BPS or MBPS
Pregestational diabetes	At 28-32 weeks	Twice weekly BPS/MBPS
Diabetes w/macrosomia	At diagnosis	Twice weekly BPS/MBPS
Vascular disease	At 24-28 weeks	Integrated fetal testing
Postterm	At 41 weeks	Twice weekly BPS/MBPS
Multiple gestation, concordant fetus FGR	At 32-34 weeks	Weekly BPS/MBPS
Multiple gestation, discordant fetus FGR	At diagnosis	Integrated fetal testing

***Start earlier for severe disease, complicated disease, prior pregnancy losses. Patient care should be individualized. Some patients may require biophysical profile scoring, amniotic fluid index, Doppler flow studies, or other testing in addition.**
BPS, modified biophysical profile score; MBPS, modified BPS, consisting of fetal nonstress test and ultrasound measurement of amniotic fluid maximum vertical pocket depth; UA, uterine artery.

Practical Fetal Testing

Who, When, How to Test

The monitoring methods discussed to this point lack the certainty of multiple randomized controlled trials. At the same time, an inference is clear—outcome improves in monitored populations. Table 21-12 shows factors that should prompt scheduled fetal surveillance. This table is not exclusive, as many historical factors and combinations of influences dictate fetal surveillance. There is not yet general agreement on whether isolated Doppler findings indicate a full program of surveillance, or simply repeating the Doppler studies after an appropriate interval (e.g., 4 to 6 weeks when uterine artery Doppler parameters are abnormal in the mid trimester). For a number of pregnancy complications of vascular origin, Doppler surveillance has been proven effective in randomized controlled fashion. Thus, in many circumstances, abnormal umbilical artery Doppler studies might indicate placental conditions, and abnormal fetal systemic Doppler studies might indicate fetal conditions.

When to initiate monitoring has not been established by randomized trial, nor is it likely to be. General guidelines, such as those established by the American College of Obstetricians and Gynecologists, suggest starting monitoring at 32 to 34 weeks. If the threshold of viability at a tertiary institution is 24 weeks and the presentation is one of severe fetal growth restriction, monitoring is likely to be started early and repeated often, customized to the maternal and fetal status. Testing frequency is also determined by the severity of the disorder and varies from 6 weeks for general review of fetal growth, to three times a day for severe FGR with abnormal venous Doppler. Some examples of onset and testing frequency are displayed in Table 21-13. This table emphasizes the individualization of fetal testing and the important principle of disorder-specific surveillance. Understanding the mechanism by which the high-risk disorder affects the fetus is the key for selecting the monitoring method and adding other variables, such as modifying recommended intervals and prioritizing specific observations. For example, in chronic placental insufficiency with asymmetric IUGR, a combination of multivessel Doppler, measuring fetal growth, and modifying heart rate interpretation (FGR fetuses have delayed maturation of heart rate variability) is added to the base BPS framework.[104]

Why? Impacts of Monitoring on Perinatal Mortality

Two examples are useful here. First, using BPS in the context of a multidisciplinary perinatal team is associated with significant changes in perinatal mortality (Table 21-14).[53,249-251] These data reflect changes not only in monitoring but also in referral patterns, awareness of complications, and a comprehensive management scheme, not just statistical associations with outcome. Although the strength of this evidence is not ideal, it becomes difficult to evaluate further such a relationship, because this level of monitoring is now considered standard of practice. It seems clear from these results, however, that an ultrasound-based system of fetal assessment can produce important benefits. The power of these studies is in the large number of subjects, giving these data effective strength similar to a smaller randomized trial.

Similar analysis has demonstrated the impact of Doppler velocimetry on perinatal mortality. This assessment is more complicated because of the number of Doppler techniques, the various thresholds for intervention, and the degree of integration of biophysical variables. In general, perinatal mortality frequency rises exponentially—from isolated umbilical artery Doppler index elevation, to complex Doppler abnormalities, including REDV in the umbilical artery and reversal of the a-wave in the ductus venosus. The data[252-255] displayed in Table 21-15 are not sufficiently uniform to form a cohesive meta-analysis. Several studies that examined umbilical artery Doppler alone are more than a decade old. More modern studies looked at umbilical artery Doppler in the context of multivessel Doppler, with or without FHR testing, full BPS or integrated fetal testing. On the other hand, the conclusion seems clear that when pregnancy is complicated by vascular disorders (including placenta-based IUGR), Doppler should form part of the monitoring scheme. This principle will be further clarified with publication of the TRUFFLE (Trial of Umbilical and Fetal Flow in Europe) study and others examining randomized clinical application.

Testing the Tests

Even more important than short-term measures are the impacts on long-term development. Randomized trials are not yet available that prove the impact of antenatal monitoring on long-term neurologic and intellectual health. Long-term outcome studies are expensive, are difficult to construct, and suffer from progress: by the time most such studies are completed, their premises have been overcome by further advances. Two examples, however, are illustrative.

Growth Restriction Intervention Trial

The Growth Restriction Intervention Trial (GRIT)[256] studied 573 high-risk pregnancies in a multicenter randomized intervention trial. When physicians enrolled patients with clinical IUGR, the patients were randomly allocated to be delivered immediately or to have delivery delayed until the clinician was certain that delivery was required. No set criteria were mandated by the trial about when that certainty was reached. As such, the results of GRIT, displayed in Table 21-16, represent a management approach with an extremely variable intervention arm. Perinatal mortality was the same with either approach. Those who were delivered immediately had a lower stillbirth rate (0.67%) but a much higher neonatal death rate from prematurity (9%). In contrast, those who waited until diagnostic certainty before delivery had a stillbirth rate of 2.4% and neonatal death rate of 6%. Cesarean delivery was almost three times as likely in those who were delivered immediately. Critical information about GRIT, which became available when follow-up data were presented, included differences in cerebral palsy and total disability rate among survivors and clearly favored retention of the pregnancy, optimizing intrauterine time.

TABLE 21-14 PERINATAL MORTALITY (PNM) CHANGES WITH BIOPHYSICAL PROFILE SCORE (BPS) APPLICATION

		PNM per 1000	
Program (ref)	***N***	**Tested**	**Not Tested**
Ireland (250)	3,200	4.1	10.7
Nova Scotia (249)	5,000	3.1	6.6
Manitoba (251)	56,000	1.9	7.7
California (53)	15,000	1.3	8.8

TABLE 21-15 UMBILICAL ARTERY DOPPLER ALTERS PERINATAL MORTALITY

Review (ref)	Studies	Patients	RR	CI
Giles, 1993 (252)	6	2102	0.54*	0.50-1.01
Divon, 1995 (253)	8	6838	0.66	0.46-0.94
Neilson, 2000 (255)	11	7000	0.71	0.32-0.89
Westergaard, 2001 (254)	13	8465	0.67	0.47-0.97

*Stillbirth rate only.
CI, 95% confidence interval; RR, relative risk.

TABLE 21-16 RESULTS FROM THE GROWTH RESTRICTION INTERVENTION TRIAL (GRIT)

Outcome	Immediate Delivery	Delayed Delivery	Odds Ratio
Cesarean section rate	91%	79%	2.7 (CI, 1.6-4.5)
Early PNM	10%	9%	1.1 (CI, 0.61-1.8)
Late PNM	2%	2%	1.0
Cerebral palsy	5%	1%	Not calculated
All disabilities	8%	4%	Not calculated
Death or disability at 2 years	55/290 (19%)	44/283 (15.5%)	1.1 (CI, 0.7-1.8)

CI, 95% confidence interval; PNM, perinatal mortality.

TABLE 21-17 CHILDHOOD NEUROLOGIC SEQUELAE IN POPULATIONS TESTED AND NOT TESTED WITH BIOPHYSICAL PROFILE SCORE (BPS)

Outcome	BPS Tested	Not Tested	Odds Ratio
Cerebral palsy	1.33*	4.74	3.6, $P < .001$
Cortical blindness	0.66	1.04	1.6, $P < .01$
Cortical deafness	0.90	2.2	2.4, $P < .005$
Mental retardation	0.80	3.1	3.9, $P < .001$
Attention deficit hyperactivity disorder	4.7	28.1	6.0, $P < .001$
Emotional disorders of childhood (control variable)	1.2	1.0	1.2, NS

*Rates are per 1000 live births.

Neurologic Outcome in Biophysical Profile Score Management

Manning and colleagues did use the fixed criteria of BPS to indicate delivery timing.[257-260] However, this study (Table 21-17) includes high-risk pregnancies of many kinds, including pregnancies with maternal complications such as diabetes and hypertension, which did not necessarily include IUGR or Doppler abnormalities. They used health records of children who were live-born after BPS was used to manage the complicated pregnancy, compared with all other children born during the same years in a regional health district in Canada. Patients were not randomized. In fact, the preferential selection of high-risk cases for monitoring means that differences in pregnancy parameters favored the untested group, whose outcomes could have been expected to improve. Differences in mean birth weight (2090 g versus 2280 g), frequency of babies less than 1 kg (14% versus 6.7%), mean gestational age (32.4 weeks versus 34.4 weeks), and deliveries before 28 weeks (13.5% versus 10.9%) meant that the tested population had higher frequencies of factors expected to have adverse neurologic outcomes. The diagnostic grouping "emotional disorders of childhood" did not differ between groups, excluding the role of ascertainment bias. As discussed (see Biophysical Profile Scoring earlier), there is a direct correlation between worsening scores and increased cerebral palsy rate.[261] The data displayed in Figure 21-28 suggest that intervention on the basis of BPS may lower that rate. Review of the origins of cerebral palsy demonstrates meaningful reduction in intrapartum causes (6% in the tested group, 9% in the untested group) and neonatal time period (28% versus 33%, respectively).[257]

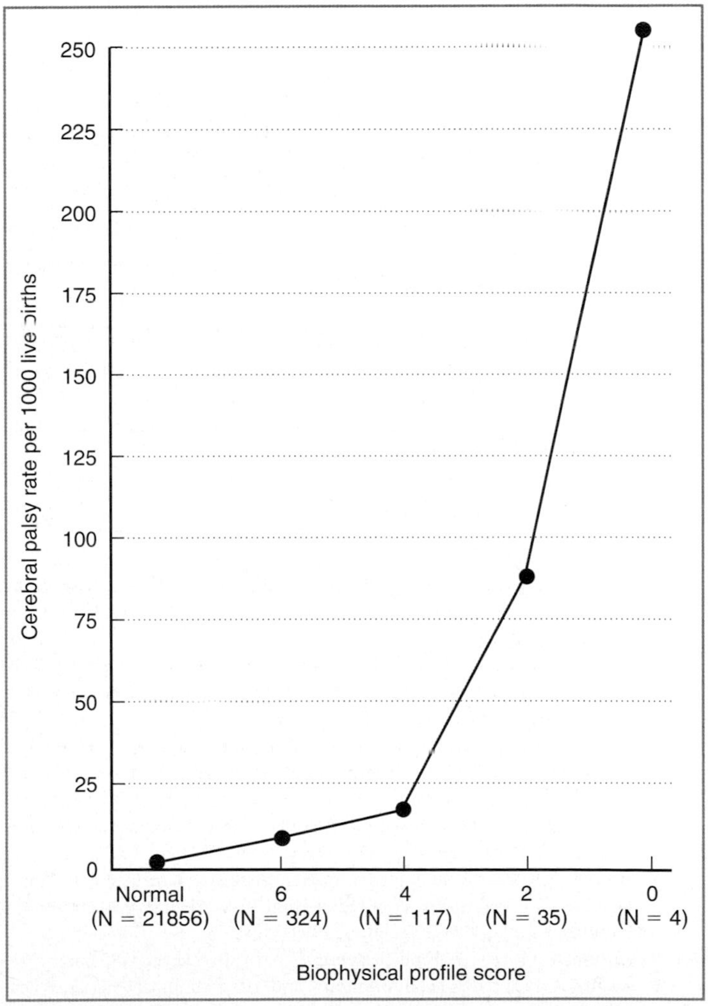

FIGURE 21-28 Abnormal biophysical profile score (BPS) reflects cerebral palsy rate. Cerebral palsy rate is related exponentially to worsening BPS.

Summary

The first prenatal visit initiates a process of monitoring. Identification of family, historical, and maternal risk factors begin to customize fetal monitoring at the onset. Specific fetal data, including first- and second-trimester screening, biochemical testing, and growth evaluation, further refine that assessment. As indicated by the presence of risk factors, multivariable fetal assessment, biophysical profile scoring as a central element, and the liberal addition of multivessel Doppler assessment of placental and fetal circulations can achieve the optimal balance between maturity and safety. The process continually renews the balance between the risks of neonatal injury resulting from prematurity and the risks of stillbirth and permanent injury from waiting too long. The details of fetal testing continue to evolve as further data become available, but these principles endure: multivariable testing, individualized testing reflecting maternal and fetal condition, continuous validation by reliable outcome measures.

References

1. Dawes GS, Fox HE, Leduc BM, et al: Respiratory movements and paradoxical sleep in the foetal lamb. J Physiol (Lond) 210:47, 1970.

2. Dawes GS, Fox HE, Leduc BM, et al: Respiratory movements and rapid eye movement sleep in the foetal lamb. J Physiol (Lond) 220:119, 1972.
3. Boddy K, Dawes GS, Fisher R, et al: Foetal respiratory movements, electrocortical and cardiovascular responses to hypoxemia and hypercapnia in sheep. J Physiol (Lond) 243:599, 1974.
4. Nijhuis JG, Prechtl HFR, Martin CB Jr, et al: Are there behavioral states in the human fetus? Early Hum Dev 6:177, 1982.
5. Bocking AD, Gagnon R, White SE, et al: Circulatory responses to prolonged hypoxemia in fetal sheep. Am J Obstet Gynecol 159:1418, 1988.
6. Pillai M, James D: The development of fetal heart rate patterns during normal pregnancy. Obstet Gynecol 76:812, 1990b.
7. Van Eyck J, Wladimiroff JW, Noordam MJ, et al: The blood flow velocity waveform in the fetal descending aorta: Its relationship to fetal behavior state in normal pregnancy at 37-38 weeks. Early Hum Dev 12:137, 1985.
8. Simanaviciute D, Gudmundsson S: Fetal middle cerebral to uterine artery pulsatility index ratios in normal and pre-eclamptic pregnancies. Ultrasound Obstet Gynecol 28:794-801, 2006.
9. Pillai M, James D: Development of human fetal behavior: A review. Fetal Diagn Ther 5:15, 1990a.
10. Baier RJ, Hasan SU, Cates DB, et al: Effects of various concentrations of O_2 and umbilical cord occlusion on fetal breathing and behavior. J Appl Physiol 68:1597, 1990.
11. Baier RJ, Hasan SU, Cates DB, et al: Hyperoxemia profoundly alters breathing pattern and arouses the fetal sheep. J Dev Physiol 18:143, 1992.
12. Patrick J, Campbell K, Carmichael L, et al: Patterns of human fetal breathing movements during the last 10 weeks of pregnancy. Obstet Gynecol 56:24, 1980.
13. Chamberlain PF, Manning FA, Morrison I, et al: Circadian rhythm in bladder volumes in the term human fetus. Obstet Gynecol 64:657, 1984.
14. Arduini D, Rizzo G, Parlati E, et al: Modifications of ultradian and circadian rhythms of fetal heart rate after fetal-maternal adrenal gland suppression: A double blind study. Prenat Diagn 6:409, 1986.
15. Martin CB Jr: Behavioral states in the human fetus. J Reprod Med 26:425, 1981.
16. Prechtl HFR: The behavioral states of the newborn infant [review]. Brain Res 76:185, 1974.
17. de Vries JIP, Visser GHA, Mulder EJH, et al: Diurnal and other variations in fetal movement and heart rate patterns at 20 to 22 weeks. Early Hum Dev 15:333, 1987.
18. Sallout BI, Fung KF, Wen SW, et al: The effect of fetal behavioral states on middle cerebral artery peak systolic velocity. Am J Obstet Gynecol 191:1283-1287, 2004.
19. Boito SM, Ursem NT, Struijk PC, et al: Umbilical venous volume flow and fetal behavioral states in the normally developing fetus. Ultrasound Obstet Gynecol 23:138-142, 2004.
20. Lee CY, DiLoreto PC, O'Lane JM: A study of fetal heart rate acceleration patterns. Obstet Gynecol 45:142, 1975.
21. Harman CR, Menticoglou S, Manning FA: Assessing fetal health. In James DK, Steer PJ, Weiner CP, et al (eds): High Risk Pregnancy Management Options. New York, WB Saunders, 1999, p 249.
22. Arduini D, Rizzo G: Fetal behavioral states. In Dawes GS, Burruto F, Zacutti A, et al (eds): Fetal Autonomy and Adaptation. Chichester, Wiley, 1990, p 55.
23. de Vries JIP, Visser GHA, Prechtl HFR: The emergence of fetal behavior: III. Individual differences and consistencies. Early Hum Dev 16:85, 1988.
24. Richardson BS: Fetal adaptive responses to asphyxia. Clin Perinat 16:595, 1989.
25. Rudolph AM: The fetal circulation and its response to stress. J Dev Physiol 16:595, 1984.
26. Bocking AD, Gagnon R, Milne KM, et al: Behavioral activity during prolonged hypoxemia in fetal sheep. J Appl Physiol 65:2420, 1988.
27. Rurak DW, Richardson BS, Patrick JE, et al: Oxygen consumption in the fetal lamb during sustained hypoxemia with progressive acidemia. Am J Physiol 258:1108, 1990.
28. Baschat AA, Gembruch U, Reiss I, et al: Neonatal nucleated red blood cell counts in growth-restricted fetuses: Relationship to arterial and venous Doppler studies. Am J Obstet Gynecol 181:190, 1999.
29. Rurak DW, Selke P, Fisher M, et al: Fetal oxygen extraction: comparison of the human and sheep. Am J Obstet Gynecol 156:360, 1987.
30. Galan HL, Anthony RV, Rigano S, et al: Fetal hypertension and abnormal Doppler velocimetry in an ovine model of intrauterine growth restriction. Am J Obstet Gynecol 192:272-279, 2005.
31. Sheldon RE, Peeters LLH, Jones MD, et al: Redistribution of cardiac output and oxygen delivery in the hypoxemic fetal lamb. Am J Obstet Gynecol 135:1071, 1979.
32. Baschat AA, Gembruch U, Reiss I, et al: Relationship between arterial and venous Doppler and perinatal outcome in fetal growth restriction. Ultrasound Obstet Gynecol 16:407, 2000.
33. Wladimiroff JW, vd Wijngaard JA, Degani S, et al: Cerebral and umbilical arterial blood flow velocity waveforms in normal and growth-retarded pregnancies. Obstet Gynecol 69:705, 1987.
34. Baschat AA, Gembruch U, Harman CR: The sequence of changes in Doppler and biophysical parameters as severe fetal growth restriction worsens. Ultrasound Obstet Gynecol 18:571, 2001.
35. Baschat AA, Gembruch U, Gortner L, et al: Coronary artery blood flow visualization signifies hemodynamic deterioration in growth-restricted fetuses. Ultrasound Obstet Gynecol 16:425, 2000.
36. Pillai M, James D: Continuation of normal neurobehavioral development in fetuses with absent umbilical arterial end diastolic velocities. BJOG 98:277, 1991.
37. Anderson DF, Parks CM, Faber JJ: Fetal O_2 consumption in sheep during controlled long-term reductions in umbilical blood flow. Am J Physiol 250:H1037, 1986.
38. Rurak DW, Gruber NC: Effect of neuromuscular blockade on oxygen consumption and blood gases. Am J Obstet Gynecol 145:258, 1983.
39. Harman CR: Fetal biophysical variables and fetal status. In Maulik D (ed): Asphyxia and Brain Damage. New York, Wiley-Liss, 1999, p 279.
40. Koos B, Kitanaka T, Matsuda K, et al: Fetal breathing adaptation to prolonged hypoxaemia in sheep. J Dev Physiol 10:161, 1988.
41. Kitanaka T, Alonso JG, Gilbert RD, et al: Fetal responses to long-term hypoxaemia in sheep. Am J Physiol 256:R1340, 1989.
42. Baschat AA, Cosmi E, Bilardo CM, et al: Predictors of neonatal outcome in early onset placental dysfunction. Obstet Gynecol 109:253-261, 2007.
43. Pillai M, James D: Human fetal mouthing movements: A potential biophysical variable for distinguishing state 1F from abnormal fetal behavior—Report of four cases. Eur J Obstet Gynaecol Reprod Biol 38:151, 1991.
44. Brown R, Patrick J: The nonstress test: How long is enough. Am J Obstet Gynecol 151:646, 1981.
45. Duff GB, Evans LJ: Measurement of the fetal biparietal diameter by ultrasound is not an accurate method of detecting fetal growth retardation. N Z Med J 94:312-314, 1981.
46. Devoe LD: The non-stress test. In Eden RD, Boehm FH (eds): Assessment and Care of the Fetus: Physiological, Clinical and Medicolegal Principles. Norwalk, CT, Appleton & Lange, 1990, p 265.
47. Woo JSK, Liang ST, Lo RLS: Significance of an absent or reversed end diastolic flow in Doppler umbilical artery waveforms. J Ultrasound Med 6:291, 1987.
48. Manning FA, Platt LD, Sipos L: Antepartum fetal evaluation: Development of a fetal biophysical profile score. Am J Obstet Gynecol 136:787, 1980.
49. Platt LD, Manning FA, LeMay M, et al: Human fetal breathing: Relationships to fetal condition. Am J Obstet Gynecol 132:514, 1978.
50. Manning FA, Platt LD, Sipos L, et al: Fetal breathing movements and the nonstress test in high-risk pregnancies. Am J Obstet Gynecol 135:511, 1979.
51. Vintzileos AM, Campbell WA, Ingardia CJ, et al: The fetal biophysical profile and its predictive value. Obstet Gynecol 62:271, 1983.
52. Nageotte MP, Towers CV, Asrat T, et al: The value of a negative antepartum test: Contraction stress test and modified biophysical profile. Obstet Gynecol 84:231, 1994.

53. Miller DA, Rabello YA, Paul RH: The modified biophysical profile: Antepartum testing in the 1990s. Am J Obstet Gynecol 174:812, 1996.
54. Magann EF, Chauhan SP, Barrilleaux PS, et al: Ultrasound estimate of amniotic fluid volume: Color Doppler overdiagnosis of oligohydramnios. Obstet Gynecol 98:71, 2001.
55. Manning FA, Hill LM, Platt LD: Qualitative amniotic fluid volume determination by ultrasound: Antepartum detection of intrauterine growth retardation. Am J Obstet Gynecol 139:254, 1981.
56. Chamberlain PF, Manning FA, Morrison I, et al: Ultrasound evaluation of amniotic fluid volume: I. The relationship of marginal and decreased amniotic fluid volumes to perinatal outcome. Am J Obstet Gynecol 150:245, 1984.
57. Harman CR: Comprehensive examination of the human fetus. Fetal Med 1:125, 1989.
58. Chamberlain PF, Manning FA, Morrison I, et al: Ultrasound evaluation of amniotic fluid volume: II. The relationship of increased amniotic fluid volume to perinatal outcome. Am J Obstet Gynecol 150:250, 1984.
59. Manning FA, Baskett TF, Morrison I, et al: Fetal biophysical profile scoring: A prospective study in 1184 high-risk patients. Am J Obstet Gynecol 140:289, 1981.
60. Phelan JP, Ahn MO, Smith CV, et al: Amniotic fluid index measurements during pregnancy. J Reprod Med 32:601, 1987.
61. Moore TR, Cayle JE: The amniotic fluid index in normal pregnancy. Am J Obstet Gynecol 162:1168, 1990.
62. Magann EF, Chauhan SP, Doherty DA, et al: The evidence for abandoning the amniotic fluid index in favor of the single deepest pocket. Am J Perinatol 24:549-555, 2007.
63. Groome LJ, Owen J, Neely CL: Oligohydramnios: Antepartum fetal urine production and intrapartum fetal distress. Am J Obstet Gynecol 165:1077, 1991.
64. Harman CR, Baschat AA, Gembruch U, Weiner C: Oligohydramnios and hemodynamic deterioration are related, in compromised fetuses with intrauterine growth restriction (IUGR). Annual Meeting of the Society for Maternal-Fetal Medicine. Am J Obstet Gynecol 184:S104, 2001.
65. Manning FA, Martin CB Jr, Murata Y, et al: Breathing movements before death in the primate fetus. Am J Obstet Gynecol 135:71, 1979.
66. Molteni RA, Melmed MH, Sheldon RE, et al: Induction of fetal breathing by metabolic acidemia and its effect on blood flow to the respiratory muscles. Am J Obstet Gynecol 36:609, 1980.
67. Hohimer AR, Bissonnette JM: Effect of metabolic acidosis on fetal breathing movements in utero. Respir Physiol 43:99, 1981.
68. Manning FA, Heaman M, Boyce D, et al: Intrauterine fetal tachypnea. Obstet Gynecol 58:398, 1981.
69. Manning FA, Harman CR, Morrison I, et al: Fetal assessment based on fetal biophysical profile scoring: III. Positive predictive accuracy of the very abnormal test (biophysical profile score = 0). Am J Obstet Gynecol 162:398, 1990.
70. Martin CB Jr: Regulation of the fetal heart rate and genesis of FHR patterns. Semin Perinatol 2:131, 1978.
71. Lavery JP: Nonstress fetal heart rate testing. Clin Obstet Gynecol 25:689, 1982.
72. Dawes GS, Moulden M, Redman CWG: System 8000: Computerized antenatal FHR analysis. J Perinat Med 19:47, 1991.
73. Guzman ER, Vintzileos AM, Martins M, et al: The efficacy of individual computer heart rate indices in detecting acidemia at birth in growth-restricted fetuses. Obstet Gynecol 87:969, 1996.
74. Fouron J-C, Korcaz Y, Leduc B: Cardiovascular changes associated with fetal breathing. Am J Obstet Gynecol 123:868, 1975.
75. Nijhuis JG, Crevels AJ, van Dongen PWJ: Fetal brain death: The definition of a fetal heart rate pattern and its clinical consequences. Obstet Gynecol Surv 45:229, 1990.
76. Yaffe H, Kreisberg GA, Gale R: Sinusoidal heart rate pattern and normal biophysical profile in a severely compromised fetus. Acta Obstet Gynaecol Scand 68:561, 1989.
77. Manning FA, Lange IR, Morrison I, et al: Fetal biophysical profile score and the nonstress test: A comparative trial. Obstet Gynecol 64:326, 1984.
78. Manning FA, Morrison I, Lange IR, et al: Fetal biophysical profile scoring: Selective use of the nonstress test. Am J Obstet Gynecol 156:709, 1987.
79. Castillo RA, Devoe LD, Arthur M, et al: The preterm nonstress test: Effects of gestational age and length of study. Am J Obstet Gynecol 160:172, 1989.
80. Baskett TF: Gestational age and fetal biophysical assessment. Am J Obstet Gynecol 158:332, 1988.
81. Ribbert LSM, Fidler V, Visser GHA: Computer-assisted analysis of normal second trimester fetal heart rate patterns. J Perinat Med 19:53, 1991.
82. Manning FA: Fetal biophysical profile scoring: Theoretical considerations and clinical application. In Fetal Medicine Principles and Practice, vol 6. Norwalk, CT, Appleton & Lange, 1995, p 221.
83. Bastide A, Manning F, Harman CR, et al: Ultrasound evaluation of amniotic fluid: Outcome of pregnancies with severe oligohydramnios. Am J Obstet Gynecol 154:895, 1986.
84. Harman CR: Amniotic fluid abnormalities. Semin Perinatol 2008 (in press).
85. Manning FA, Morrison I, Lange IR, et al: Fetal assessment based on fetal biophysical profile scoring: Experience in 12,620 referred high-risk pregnancies—I. Perinatal mortality by frequency and etiology. Am J Obstet Gynecol 151:343, 1985.
86. Yoon BH, Romero R, Roh CR, et al: Relationship between the fetal biophysical profile score, umbilical artery Doppler velocimetry, and fetal blood acid-base status determined by cordocentesis. Am J Obstet Gynecol 169:1586, 1993.
87. Baser I, Johnson TRB, Paine LL: Coupling of fetal movement and fetal heart rate accelerations as an indicator of fetal health. Obstet Gynecol 80:62, 1992.
88. Vintzileos AM, Flemming AD, Scorza WE, et al: Relationship between fetal biophysical activities and umbilical cord blood gas values. Am J Obstet Gynecol 165:707, 1991.
89. Manning FA, Snijders R, Harman CR, et al: Fetal biophysical profile scoring: VI. Correlations with antepartum umbilical venous pH. Am J Obstet Gynecol 169:755, 1993.
90. Morrison I, Menticoglou S, Manning FA, et al: Comparison of antepartum test results to perinatal outcome. J Matern Fetal Med 3:75, 1994.
91. Druzin ML: Antepartum fetal heart rate monitoring: State of the art. Clin Perinatol 16:627, 1989.
92. Baskett TF, Boyce CD, Lohre MA, et al: Simplified antepartum fetal heart assessment. BJOG 88:395, 1981.
93. Druzin ML, Gratacos J, Paul RH: Antepartum fetal heart rate testing: VI. Predictive reliability of "normal" tests in the prevention of antepartum deaths. Am J Obstet Gynecol 137:745, 1980.
94. Freeman RK, Anderson G, Dorchester W: A prospective multi-institutional study of antepartum fetal heart rate monitoring: I. Risk of perinatal mortality and morbidity according to antepartum fetal heart rate results. Am J Obstet Gynecol 143:771, 1982.
95. Nochimson DJ, Turbeville JS, Terry JE, et al: The non-stress test. Obstet Gynecol 51:419, 1978.
96. Schifrin BS, Foye G, Amato J, et al: Routine fetal heart rate monitoring in the antepartum period. Obstet Gynecol 54:21, 1979.
97. American College of Obstetricians and Gynecologists: ACOG Practice Bulletin. Antepartum Fetal Surveillance. In Compendium 2001. Washington, DC, ACOG, 2001, p 119.
98. Petrikovsky BM, Kaplan GP: Fetal grasping of the umbilical cord causing variable fetal heart rate decelerations. J Clin Ultrasound 21:642, 1993.
99. Borgatta A, Shrout L, Divon MY: Reliability and reproducibility of nonstress test readings. Am J Obstet Gynecol 159:554, 1988.
100. Dawes GS, Moulden M, Redman CWG: The advantages of computerized fetal heart rate analysis. J Perinat Med 19:39, 1991.
101. National Institute of Child Health & Human Development Research Planning Workshop: Electronic fetal heart rate monitoring: Research guidelines for interpretation. J Obstet Gynecol Neonat Nurs 26:635, 1997.
102. Dawes GS, Redman CWG: Numerical analysis of the normal human antenatal fetal heart rate. BJOG 88:792, 1981.
103. Pillai M, James D: The importance of the behavioral state in biophysical assessment of the term human fetus. BJOG 97:1130, 1990.

104. Turan S, Turan OM, Berg C, et al: Computerized fetal heart rate analysis, Doppler ultrasound and biophysical profile score in the prediction of acid-base status of growth-restricted fetuses. Ultrasound Obstet Gynecol 30:750-756, 2007.
105. Baschat AA, Harman CR: Antenatal assessment of the growth restricted fetus. Curr Opin Obstet Gynecol 13:161, 2001.
106. Snijders R, Hyett J: Fetal testing in intra-uterine growth retardation. Curr Opin Obstet Gynecol 9:91, 1997.
107. Hecher K, Bilardo CM, Stigter RH, et al: Monitoring of fetuses with intrauterine growth restriction: A longitudinal study. Ultrasound Obstet Gynecol 18:564, 2001.
108. Muller T, Nanan R, Rehn M, et al: Arterial and ductus venosus Doppler in fetuses with absent or reverse end-diastolic flow in the umbilical artery: Correlation with short-term perinatal outcome. Acta Obstet Gynecol Scand 81:860-866, 2002.
109. Harman CR, Baschat AA: Comprehensive assessment of fetal wellbeing: Which Doppler tests should be performed? Curr Opin Obstet Gynecol 15:147, 2003.
110. Baschat AA: Arterial and venous Doppler in the diagnosis and management of early onset fetal growth restriction. Early Hum Devel 81:877-887, 2005.
111. Stuart B, Drumm J, Fitzgerald DE, et al: Fetal blood velocity waveforms in normal pregnancy. BJOG 87:780, 1980.
112. Giles WB, Trudinger BJ, Baird PJ: Fetal umbilical artery flow velocity waveforms and placental resistance: Pathological correlations. BJOG 92:31, 1985.
113. Trudinger BJ, Stevens D, Connelly A, et al: Umbilical artery flow velocity waveforms and placental resistance: The effects of embolization of the umbilical circulation. Am J Obstet Gynecol 157:1443, 1987.
114. Morrow RJ, Adamson SL, Bull SB, et al: Effect of placental embolization on the umbilical arterial waveform in fetal sheep. Am J Obstet Gynecol 161:1055, 1989.
115. Arabin B, Siebert M, Jimenez R, et al: Obstetrical characteristics of a loss of end diastolic velocities in the fetal aorta and/or umbilical artery using Doppler ultrasound. Gynecol Obstet Invest 25:173, 1988.
116. Eik-Nes SH, Marshal K, Kristoffersen K: Methodology and basic problems related to blood flow studies in the human fetus. Ultrasound Med Biol 10:329, 1984.
117. Maulik D, Saini VD, Nanda NC, et al: Doppler evaluation of fetal hemodynamics. Ultrasound Med Biol 8:705, 1982.
118. Pollack RN, Divon MY: Intrauterine growth retardation: Diagnosis. In Copel JA, Reed KL (eds): Doppler Ultrasound in Obstetrics and Gynecology. New York, Raven Press, 1995, p 171.
119. Divon MY, Girz BA, Lieblish R, et al: Clinical management of the fetus with markedly diminished umbilical artery end-diastolic flow. Am J Obstet Gynecol 161:1523, 1989.
120. Hecher K, Campbell S, Doyle P, et al: Assessment of fetal compromise by Doppler ultrasound investigation of the fetal circulation. Circulation 91:129, 1995.
121. Hsieh FJ, Chang FM, Ko TM, et al: Umbilical artery flow velocity waveforms in fetuses dying with congenital abnormalities. BJOG 95:478, 1988.
122. Farine D, Kelly EN, Ryan G, et al: Absent and reversed umbilical artery end-diastolic velocity. In Copel JA, Reed KL (eds): Doppler Ultrasound in Obstetrics and Gynecology. New York, Raven Press, 1995, p 187.
123. Yoon BH, Syn HC, Kim SW: The efficacy of Doppler umbilical artery velocimetry in identifying fetal acidosis: A comparison with fetal biophysical profile. J Ultrasound Med 11:1, 1992.
124. Battaglia C, Artini PG, Galli PA, et al: Absent or reversed end-diastolic flow in umbilical artery and severe intrauterine growth retardation: An ominous association. Acta Obstet Gynecol Scand 72:167, 1993.
125. Trudinger BJ, Cook CM, Giles WB, et al: Fetal umbilical artery velocity waveforms and subsequent neonatal outcome. BJOG 98:378, 1991.
126. Kelly E, Ryan G, Farine D, et al: Absent end diastolic umbilical artery velocity (AEVD): Short and long-term outcome. J Matern Fetal Investig 3:203, 1993.
127. Zelop CM, Richardson DK, Heffner LJ: Outcomes of severely abnormal umbilical artery Doppler velocimetry in structurally normal singleton fetuses. Obstet Gynecol 87:434, 1996.
128. Gramellini D, Piantelli G, Verrotti C, et al: Doppler velocimetry and non-stress test in severe fetal growth restriction. Clin Exp Obstet Gynecol 28:33-39, 2001.
129. Hartung J, Kalache KD, Heyna C, et al: Outcome of 60 neonates who had ARED flow prenatally compared with a matched control group of appropriate-for-gestational age preterm neonates. Ultrsound Obstet Gynecol 25:566-572, 2005.
130. Pattinson RC, Norman K, Kirsten G, et al: Relationship between the fetal heart rate pattern and perinatal mortality in fetuses with absent end-diastolic velocities of the umbilical artery: A case-controlled study. Am J Perinatol 12:286, 1995.
131. Madazli R, Uludag S, Ocak V: Doppler assessment of umbilical artery, thoracic aorta and middle cerebral artery in the management of pregnancies with growth restriction. Acta Obstet Gynecol Scand 80:702-707, 2001.
132. Malhotra N, Chanana C, Kumar S, et al: Comparison of perinatal outcome of growth-restricted fetuses with normal and abnormal umbilical artery Doppler waveforms. Indian J Med Sci 60:311-317, 2006.
133. Van den Wijngaard JAGW, Groenenberg IAL, Wladimiroff JW, et al: Cerebral Doppler ultrasound of the human fetus. BJOG 96:845, 1989.
134. Harman CR: Ultrasound in the management of the alloimmunized pregnancy. In Fleisher AC, Manning FA, Jeanty P, et al (eds): Sonography in Obstetrics and Gynecology, 5th ed. Norwalk, CT, Appleton & Lange, 1996, p 683.
135. Mari G, Detti L, Oz U, et al: Accurate prediction of fetal hemoglobin by Doppler ultrasonography. Obstet Gynecol 99:589-593, 2002.
136. Copel JA, Grannum PA, Belanger K, et al: Pulsed Doppler flow-velocity waveforms before and after intrauterine intravascular transfusion for severe erythroblastosis fetalis. Am J Obstet Gynecol 158:768, 1988.
137. Chandran R, Serra-Serra V, Sellers SM, et al: Fetal cerebral Doppler in the recognition of fetal compromise. BJOG 100:139, 1993.
138. Hecher K, Ville Y, Snijders R, et al: Doppler studies of the fetal circulation in twin-twin transfusion syndrome. Ultrasound Obstet Gynecol 5:318, 1995.
139. Picklesimer AH, Oepkes D, Moise KJ Jr, et al: Determinants of the middle cerebral artery peak systolic velocity in the human fetus. Am J Obstet Gynecol 197:526, 2007.
140. Arduini D, Rizzo G, Romanini C, et al: Hemodynamic changes in growth retarded fetuses during maternal oxygen administration as predictors of fetal outcome. J Ultrasound Med 8:193, 1989.
141. Potts P, Connors G, Gillis S, et al: The effect of carbon dioxide on Doppler flow velocity waveforms in the human fetus. J Dev Physiol 17:119, 1992.
142. Arbeille P, Bosc M, Vaillant MC, et al: Nicotine-induced changes in the cerebral circulation in ovine fetuses. Am J Perinatol 9:270, 1992.
143. Arbeille P, Roncin A, Berson M, et al: Exploration of the fetal cerebral blood flow by duplex Doppler–linear array system in normal and pathological pregnancies. Ultrasound Med Biol 13:329, 1987.
144. Arbeille P, Body G, Saliba E, et al: Fetal cerebral circulation assessment by Doppler ultrasound in normal and pathological pregnancies. Eur J Obstet Gynecol Reprod Biol 29:261, 1988.
145. Mari G, Abuhamad AZ, Cosmi E, et al: Middle cerebral artery peak systolic velocity: Technique and variability. J Ultrasound Med 24:425-430, 2005.
146. Karsdorp VH, van Vugt JM, van Geijn HP, et al: Clinical significance of absent or reversed end diastolic velocity waveforms in umbilical artery. Lancet 344:1664, 1994.
147. Jensen A, Garnier Y, Berger R: Dynamics of fetal circulatory responses to hypoxia and asphyxia. Eur J Obstet Gynaecol Reprod Biol 84:155, 1999.
148. Mari G, Hanif F, Kruger M, et al: Middle cerebral artery peak systolic velocity: A new Doppler parameter in the assessment of growth-restricted fetuses. Ultrasound Obstet Gynecol 29:310-316, 2007.
149. Makh DS, Harman CR, Baschat AA: Is Doppler prediction of anemia effective in the growth-restricted fetus? Ultrasound Obstet Gynecol 22:489-492, 2003.

150. Turan OM, Turan S, Makh DS, et al: Middle cerebral artery peak systolic velocity (MCA PSV): Its role as an outcome predictor in fetal growth restriction (FGR). Ultrasound Obstet Gynecol 2008 (in press).
151. Hershkovitz R, Kingdom JC, Geary M, et al: Fetal cerebral blood flow redistribution in late gestation: Identification of compromise in small fetuses with normal umbilical artery Doppler. Ultrasound Obstet Gynecol 15:209, 2000.
152. Baschat AA, Cuclu S, Kush ML, et al: Venous Doppler in the prediction of acid-base status of growth-restricted fetuses with elevated placental blood flow resistance. Am J Obstet Gynecol 191:277-284, 2004.
153. Schwarze A, Gembruch U, Krapp M, et al: Qualitative venous Doppler flow waveform analysis in preterm intrauterine growth-restricted fetuses with ARED flow in the umbilical artery: Correlation with short-term outcome. Ultrasound Obstet Gynecol 25:573-579, 2005.
154. Baschat AA, Harman CR: Venous Doppler in the assessment of fetal cardiovascular status. Curr Opin Obstet Gynecol 18:156-163, 2006.
155. Bilardo CM, Wolf H, Stigter RH, et al: Relationship between monitoring parameters and perinatal outcome in severe, early intrauterine growth restriction. Ultrasound Obstet Gynecol 23:119-125, 2004.
156. Baschat AA, Galan HL, Bhide A, et al: Doppler and biophysical assessment in growth-restricted fetuses: Distribution of test results. Ultrasound Obstet Gynecol 27:41-47, 2006.
157. Rizzo G, Arduini D, Romanini C: Umbilical vein pulsations: A physiologic finding in early gestation. Am J Obstet Gynecol 167:676-677, 1992.
158. Hofstaetter C, Gudmundsson S, Hansmann M: Venous Doppler velocimetry in the surveillance of severely compromised fetuses. Ultrasound Obstet Gynecol 20:233-239, 2002.
159. Hofstaetter C, Hansmann M, Eik-Nes SH, et al: A cardiovascular profile score in the surveillance of fetal hydrops. J Matern Fetal Neonatal Med 19:407-413, 2006.
160. Kiserud T: The ductus venosus. Semin Perinatol 25:11, 2001.
161. Bellotti M, Pennati G, De Gasperi C, et al: Simultaneous measurements of umbilical venous, fetal hepatic and ductus venosus blood flow in growth-restricted fetuses. Am J Obstet Gynecol 190:1347-1358, 2004.
162. Trudinger BJ, Giles WB, Cook CM: Uteroplacental blood flow velocity-time waveforms in normal and complicated pregnancy. BJOG 92:39, 1985.
163. Rotmensch S, Liberati M, Santolaya-Forgas J, et al: Uteroplacental and intraplacental circulation. In Copel JA, Reed KL (eds): Doppler Ultrasound in Obstetrics and Gynecology, vol 11. New York, Raven, 1995, p 115.
164. Schulman H, Fleischer A, Fannakides G, et al: Development of uterine artery compliance in pregnancy as detected by Doppler ultrasound. Am J Obstet Gynecol 155:1031, 1986.
165. Vainio M, Kujansuu E, Iso-Mustajarvi M, Maenpaa J: Low dose acetylsalicylic acid in prevention of pregnancy-induced hypertension and intrauterine growth retardation in women with bilateral uterine artery notches. BJOG 109:161-167, 2002.
166. Li H, Gudnason H, Olofsson P, et al: Increased uterine artery vascular impedence is related to adverse outcome of pregnancy, but is present in only one-third of late third-trimester pre-eclamptic women. Ultrasound Obstet Gynecol 25:459-463, 2005.
167. Williams K, McLean C: Maternal cerebral vasospasm in eclampsia assessed by transcranial Doppler. Am J Perinatol 10:243, 1993.
168. Williams K, Wilson S: Maternal middle cerebral artery blood flow velocity variation with gestational age. Obstet Gynecol 84:445, 1994.
169. Kyle PM, Buckley D, Redman CWG: Noninvasive assessment of the maternal cerebral circulation by transcranial Doppler ultrasound during angiotensin II infusion. BJOG 100:85, 1993.
170. Belfort MA, Moise KJ: Effect of magnesium sulfate on maternal brain blood flow in preeclampsia: A randomized, placebo-controlled study. Am J Obstet Gynecol 167:661, 1992.
171. Riskin-Mashia S, Belfort MA, Saade GR, Herd JA: Transcranial Doppler measurement of cerebral velocity indices as a predictor of pre-eclampsia. Am J Obstet Gynecol 187:1667-1672, 2002.
172. Lindqvist PG, Marsal K, Pirhonen JP: Maternal cerebral Doppler velocimetry before, during, and after a normal pregnancy: A longitudinal study. Acta Obstet Gynecol Scand 85:1299-1303, 2006.
173. Thornton JG, Hornbuckle J, Vail A, et al: GRIT Study Group. Infant well being at 2 years of age in the Growth Restriction Intervention Trial (GRIT): Multicentered randomized controlled trial. Lancet 364:513-520, 2004.
174. Vintzileos AM, Ananth CV, Smulian JC, et al: The impact of prenatal care on postnatal deaths in the presence and absence of antenatal high-risk conditions. Am J Obstet Gynecol 187:1258-1262, 2002.
175. Ickovics JR, Kershaw TS, Westdahl C, et al: Group prenatal care and perinatal outcomes: A randomized controlled trial. Obstet Gynecol 110:330-339, 2007.
176. Panaretto KS, Mitchell MR, Anderson L, et al: Sustainable antenatal care services in an urban indigenous community: The Townsville experience. Med J Aust 187:18-22, 2007.
177. Lenke RR, Nemes JML: Use of nipple stimulation to obtain contraction stress test. Obstet Gynecol 63:345, 1984.
178. Ray M, Freeman RK, Pine S: Clinical experience with the oxytocin challenge test. Am J Obstet Gynecol 114:1, 1972.
179. Schifrin BS: The rationale for antepartum fetal heart rate monitoring. J Reprod Med 23:213, 1979.
180. Huddlestone JF, Sutliff G, Robinson D: Contraction stress test by intermittent nipple stimulation. Obstet Gynecol 63:660, 1984.
181. Collea JV, Holls WM: The contraction stress test. Clin Obstet Gynecol 4:707, 1982.
182. Merrill PA, Porto M, Lovett SM, et al: Evaluation of the nonreactive positive contraction stress test prior to 32 weeks: The role of the biophysical profile. Am J Perinatol 12:229, 1995.
183. Freeman RK, Lagnew DC Jr: The contraction stress test. In Eden RD, Boehm FM (eds): Assessment and Care of the Fetus: Physiological, Clinical and Medicolegal Principles. Norwalk, CT, Appleton & Lange, 1990, 351.
184. Arabin B, Becker R, Mohnhaupt A, et al: Prediction of fetal distress and poor outcome in intrauterine growth retardation: A comparison of fetal heart rate monitoring combined with stress tests and Doppler ultrasound. Fetal Diagn Ther 8:234-240, 1993.
185. Arabin B, Becker R, Mohnhaupt A, et al: Prediction of fetal distress and poor outcome in prolonged pregnancy using Doppler ultrasound and fetal heart rate monitoring combined with stress tests. Fetal Diagn Ther 9:1-6, 1994.
186. Ohel G, Birkenfield A, Rabinowitz R, et al: Fetal response to vibratory acoustic stimulation in periods of low heart rate reactivity and low activity. Am J Obstet Gynecol 154:619, 1986.
187. Gagnon R, Hunse C, Carmichael L, et al: Effects of vibratory acoustic stimulation on human fetal breathing and gross body movements near term. Am J Obstet Gynecol 155:1227, 1986.
188. Patrick JE, Gagnon R: Adaptation to vibroacoustic stimulation. In Dawes GS, Zacutti A, Borruto F, et al (eds): Fetal Autonomy and Adaptation. Chichester, England, Wiley, 1990, p 39.
189. Woods JR, Plessinger M, Mack C: The fetal auditory brainstem response. Pediatr Res 18:83, 1984.
190. Vince MA, Armitage SE: Sound stimulation available to the sheep fetus. Reprod Nutr Dev 20:801, 1980.
191. Lecanuet JP, Gautheron B, Locatelli A, et al: What sounds reach fetuses: Biological and nonbiological modeling of the transmission of pure tones. Dev Psychobiol 33:203, 1998.
192. Bauer R, Schwab M, Abrams RM, et al: Electrocortical and heart rate response during vibroacoustic stimulation in fetal sheep. Am J Obstet Gynecol 177:66, 1997.
193. Abrams RM, Peters AJ, Gerhardt KJ: Effect of abdominal vibroacoustic stimulation on sound and acceleration levels at the head of the fetal sheep. Obstet Gynecol 90:216, 1997.
194. Gerhardt KJ, Abrams RM: Fetal exposures to sound and vibroacoustic stimulation. J Perinatol 30:S21, 2000.
195. Poreba A, Dudkieqicz D, Drygalski M: The influence of the sounds of music on chosen cardiotocographic parameters in mature pregnancies. Ginekol Pol 71:915, 2000.

196. Groome LJ, Mooney DM, Holland SB, et al: Behavioral state affects heart rate response to low-intensity sound in human fetuses. Early Hum Dev 54:39, 1999.
197. Gingras JL, O'Donnell KJ: State control in the substance-exposed fetus: I. The fetal neurobehavioral profile—An assessment of fetal state, arousal, and regulation competency. Ann N Y Acad Sci 846:262, 1998.
198. Abrams RM, Gerhardt KJ, Rosa C, et al: Fetal acoustic stimulation test: Stimulus features of three artificial larynges recorded in sheep. Am J Obstet Gynecol 173:1372, 1995.
199. Gerhardt KJ, Abrams RM, Kovatz BM, et al: Intrauterine noise levels produced in pregnant ewes by sound applied to the abdomen. Am J Obstet Gynecol 159:228, 1988.
200. Sherer DM, Menashe M, Sadovsky E: Severe fetal bradycardia caused by external vibratory acoustic stimulation. Am J Obstet Gynecol 159:334, 1988.
201. Johnson RL, Elliott JP: Fetal acoustic stimulation, an adjunct to external cephalic version: A blinded, randomized crossover study. Am J Obstet Gynecol 173:1369, 1995.
202. Hofmeyr GJ: Interventions to help external cephalic version for breech presentation at term. Cochrane Database Syst Rev (2):CD000184, 2002.
203. Kiuchi M, Nagata N, Ikeno S, et al: The relationship between the response to external light stimulation and behavioral states in the human fetus: How it differs from vibroacoustic stimulation. Early Hum Dev 58:153, 2000.
204. Newnham JP, Burns SE, Roberman BD: Effect of vibratory acoustic stimulation on the duration of fetal heart rate monitoring tests. Am J Perinatol 7:232, 1990.
205. Tan KH, Smyth R: Fetal vibroacoustic stimulation for facilitation of tests of fetal well being. Cochrane Database Syst Rev (1):CD002963, 2001.
206. Kamel HS, Makhlouf AM, Youssef AA: Simplified biophysical profile: An antepartum fetal screening test. Gynecol Obstet Invest 47:223, 1999.
207. Gagnon R: Acoustic stimulation: Effect on heart rate and other biophysical variables. Clin Perinatol 16:643, 1989.
208. Serafini P, Lindsay MBJ, Nagy DA, et al: Antepartum fetal heart rate response to sound stimulation: The acoustic stimulation test. Am J Obstet Gynecol 148:41, 1984.
209. Kuhlman KA, Kayreen AB, Depp R, et al: Ultrasonic imaging of normal fetal response to external vibratory acoustic stimulation. Am J Obstet Gynecol 158:47, 1988.
210. Bartnicki J, Dimer JA, Hertqig K, et al: Computerized cardiotocography following vibroacoustic stimulation of premature fetuses. Gynecol Obstet Invest 45:73, 1998.
211. Kisilevsky BS, Pang L, Hains SM: Maturation of human fetal responses to airborne sound in low- and high-risk fetuses. Early Hum Dev 58:179, 2000.
212. Vindla S, James D, Sahota D: Comparison of unstimulated and stimulated behavior in human fetuses with congenital abnormalities. Fetal Diagn Ther 14:156, 1999.
213. Warner J, Hains SM, Kisilevsky BS: An exploratory study of fetal behavior at 33 and 36 weeks gestational age in hypertensive women. Dev Psychobiol 41:156, 2002.
214. Allister L, Lester BP, Carr S, et al: The effects of maternal depression on fetal heart rate response to vibroacoustic stimulation. Dev Neuropsychol 20:639, 2001.
215. Gagnon R, Hunse C, Carmichael L, et al: Vibratory acoustic stimulation in 26- to 32-week, small-for-gestational-age fetus. Am J Obstet Gynecol 160:160, 1989.
216. Rotmensch S, Celentano C, Liberati M, et al: The effect of antenatal steroid administration on the fetal response to vibroacoustic stimulation. Acta Obstet Gynaecol Scand 78:847, 1999.
217. Sherer DM: Blunted fetal response to vibroacoustic stimulation associated with maternal intravenous magnesium sulfate therapy. Am J Perinatol 11:401, 1994.
218. Grant A, Elbourne D, Valentin L, et al: Routine formal fetal movement counting and risk of antepartum late death in normally formed singletons. Lancet 2:345, 1982.
219. Neldam S: Fetal movements as an indicator of fetal well being. Dan Med Bull 33:213, 1986.
220. Froen JF: A kick from within: Fetal movement counting and the cancelled progress in antenatal care. J Perinat Med 32:13-24, 2004.
221. Mangesi L, Hofmeyr GJ: Fetal movement counting for assessment of fetal well being. Cochrane Database Syst Rev (1):CD004909, 2007.
222. Daffos F, Capella-Pavlovsky M, Forestier F: Fetal blood sampling via the umbilical cord using a needle guided by ultrasound: Report of 66 cases. Prenat Diagn 3:271, 1983.
223. Weiner CP: The role of cordocentesis in fetal diagnosis. Clin Obstet Gynecol 31:285, 1988.
224. Nicolini U, Nicolaidis P, Fisk NM, et al: Fetal blood sampling from the intrahepatic vein: Analysis of safety and clinical experience with 214 procedures. Obstet Gynecol 76:47, 1990.
225. Weiner CP, Okamura K: Diagnostic fetal blood sampling technique-related losses. Fetal Diagn Ther 11:169, 1996.
226. Moniz CF, Nicolaides KH, Bamforth FJ, et al: Normal reference ranges for biochemical substances relating to renal, hepatic, and bone function in fetal and maternal plasma throughout pregnancy. J Clin Pathol 38:468, 1985.
227. Forestier F, Daffos F, Galacteros F, et al: Hematological values of 163 normal fetuses between 18 and 30 weeks of gestation. Pediatr Res 20:342, 1986.
228. Weiner CP: The biochemical assessment of the human fetus: Norms and applications. In Harman CR (ed): Invasive Fetal Testing and Treatment. Cambridge, Blackwell, 1995, p 93.
229. Nava S, Bocconi L, Zuliani G, et al: Aspects of fetal physiology from 18 to 37 weeks' gestation as assessed by blood sampling. Obstet Gynecol 87:975, 1996.
230. Harman CR: Invasive techniques in the management of alloimmune anemia. In Harman CR (ed): Invasive Fetal Testing and Treatment. Cambridge, Blackwell, 1995, p 109.
231. Kleihauer E, Stein G, Schmidt G: Demonstration of fetal hemoglobin in blood stains dependent upon their age. Z Gesamte Exp Med 144:105, 1967.
232. Duchatel F, Oury JF, Mennesson B, et al: Complications of diagnostic ultrasound-guided percutaneous umbilical blood sampling: Analysis of a series of 341 cases and review of the literature. Eur J Obstet Gynaecol Reprod Biol 52:95, 1993.
233. Manning FA: Amniotic fluid volume. In Fetal Medicine Principles and Practice. Norwalk, CT, Appleton & Lange, 1995, p 173.
234. Wilson RD, Farquharson DF, Wittmann BK, et al: Cordocentesis: Overall pregnancy loss rate as important as procedure loss rate. Fetal Diagn Ther 9:142, 1994.
235. Paidas MI, Berkowitz RL, Lynch L, et al: Alloimmune thrombocytopenia: Fetal and neonatal losses related to cordocentesis. Am J Obstet Gynecol 172:475, 1995.
236. Harman CR, Bowman JM, Menticoglou SM, et al: Profound fetal thrombocytopenia in Rhesus disease: Serious hazard at intravascular transfusion. Lancet 2:741, 1988.
237. Jauniaux E, Nicolaides KH, Campbell S, et al: Hematoma of the umbilical cord secondary to cordocentesis for intrauterine fetal transfusion. Prenat Diagn 10:477, 1990.
238. Seeds JW, Chescheir NC, Bowes WA Jr, et al: Fetal death as a complication of intrauterine intravascular transfusion. Obstet Gynecol 74:461, 1989.
239. Doyle LW, de Crespigny L, Kelly EA: Haematoma complicating fetal intravascular transfusions. Aust N Z J Obstet Gynaecol 33:208, 1993.
240. Ko TM, Tseng LH, Chang MH, et al: Amniocentesis in mothers who are hepatitis B virus carriers does not expose the infant to an increased risk of hepatitis B virus infection. Arch Gynecol Obstet 255:25, 1994.
241. Viscarello RR, Cullen MT, DeGennaro NJ, et al: Fetal blood sampling in human immunodeficiency virus-seropositive women before elective midtrimester termination of pregnancy. Am J Obstet Gynecol 167:1075, 1992.
242. Mandelbrot L, Schlienger I, Bongain A, et al: Thrombocytopenia in pregnant women infected with human immunodeficiency virus: Maternal and neonatal outcome. Am J Obstet Gynecol 171:252, 1994.

243. Wilkins I, Mezrow G, Lynch L, et al: Amnionitis and life-threatening respiratory distress after percutaneous umbilical blood sampling. Am J Obstet Gynecol 160:427, 1989.
244. Nicolini U, Santolaya I, Ojo OE, et al: The fetal intrahepatic umbilical vein as an alternative to cord needling for prenatal diagnosis and therapy. Prenat Diagn 8:665, 1988.
245. Bowman JM, Pollock JM, Peterson LE, et al: Fetomaternal hemorrhage following funipuncture: Increase in severity of maternal red cell alloimmunization. Obstet Gynecol 84:839, 1994.
246. Soothill PW, Nicolaides KH, Rodeck CH, et al: Effect of gestational age on fetal and intervillous blood gas and acid-base values in human pregnancy. Fetal Ther 1:168, 1986.
247. Nicolaides KH, Economides DL, Soothill PW: Blood gases, Ph, and lactate in appropriate- and small-for-gestational-age fetuses. Am J Obstet Gynecol 161:996, 1989.
248. Weiner CP, Sipes SL, Wenstrom K: The effect of fetal age upon normal fetal laboratory values and venous pressure. Obstet Gynecol 79:713, 1992.
249. Baskett TF, Allen AC, Gray JH, et al: Fetal biophysical profile and perinatal death. Obstet Gynecol 70:357, 1987.
250. Chamberlain PF: Later fetal death: Has ultrasound a role to play in its prevention? Irish J Med Sci 160:251, 1991.
251. Manning FA: Cordocentesis: Clinical considerations. In Harman CR (ed): Invasive Fetal Testing and Treatment. Cambridge, Blackwell, 1995, p 49.
252. Giles W, Bisits A: Clinical use of Doppler ultrasound in pregnancy: information from six randomized trials. Fetal Diagn Ther 8:247-255, 1993.
253. Divon MY: Randomized controlled trials of umbilical artery Doppler velocimetry: How many are too many? Ultrasound Obstet Gynecol 6:377-379, 1995.
254. Westergaard HB, Langhoff-Roos J, Lingman G, et al: A critical appraisal of the use of umbilical artery Doppler ultrasound in high-risk pregnancies: Use of meta-analysis in evidence-based obstetrics. Ultrasound Obstet Gynecol 17:464-465, 2001.
255. Neilson JP, Alfirevic Z: Doppler ultrasound for fetal assessment in high risk pregnancies. Cochrane Database Syst Rev (2)CD000073, 2000.
256. GRIT Study Group: A randomized trial of timed delivery for the compromised pre-term fetus: Short-term outcomes and Bayesian interpretation. BJOG 110:27, 2003.
257. Manning FA, Bondagji N, Harman CR, et al: Fetal assessment based on biophysical profile scoring: VIII. The incidence of cerebral palsy in tested and non-tested perinates. Am J Obstet Gynecol 178:696, 1998.
258. Manning FA, Harman CR, Menticoglou S, et al: Attention deficit disorder: Relationship to fetal biophysical profile. Am J Obstet Gynecol 182:S72, 2000.
259. Manning FA, Harman CR, Menticoglou S, et al: Mental retardation: Prevalence and etiologic factors in a large obstetric population. Am J Obstet Gynecol 182:S110, 2000.
260. Manning FA, Harman CR, Menticoglou S, et al: The prevalence of non-specific emotional disorder of childhood is unrelated to adverse perinatal factors. Am J Obstet Gynecol 182:S110, 2000.
261. Manning FA, Bondagji N, Harman CR, et al: Fetal assessment based on the fetal biophysical profile score: VII. Relationship of last BPS result to subsequent cerebral palsy. J Gynecol Obstet Biol Reprod 26:720, 1997.

Chapter 22

Intrapartum Fetal Surveillance

Michael P. Nageotte, MD, and Larry C. Gilstrap III, MD

Factors Controlling Fetal Heart Rate

Fetal heart rate (FHR) analysis is the most common means by which a fetus is evaluated for adequacy of oxygenation. Knowledge of the rate and regulation of the fetal heart is therefore of great importance to the obstetrician. At 20 weeks of gestation, the average FHR is 155 beats/min; at 30 weeks, it is 144 beats/min; and at term, it is 140 beats/min. This progression is thought to be related to maturation of vagal tone, with consequent slowing of the baseline FHR. Variations of 20 beats/min faster or slower than these baseline values are present in normal fetuses.

The fetal heart is similar to the adult heart in that it has its own intrinsic pacemaker activity which results in rhythmic myocardial contractions. The sinoatrial node, found in one wall of the right atrium, has the fastest rate of conduction and sets the rate in the normal heart. The next fastest pacemaker rate is found in the atrium. Finally, the ventricle has a slower rate than either the sinoatrial node or the atrium. In cases of complete or partial heart block in the fetus, variations in rate markedly slower than normal can be seen. The rate in a fetus with a complete heart block is often 60 to 80 beats/min.

Variability of the FHR is important clinically and is of prognostic value with respect to its specific amplitude as part of the FHR pattern. The heart rate is the result of many physiologic factors that modulate the intrinsic rate of the fetal heart, the most common being signals from the autonomic nervous system.

Parasympathetic Nervous System

The parasympathetic nervous system consists primarily of the vagus nerve (10th cranial nerve), which originates in the medulla oblongata. The vagus nerve innervates both the sinoatrial and the atrioventricular nodes. Stimulation of the vagus nerve results in a decrease in FHR in the normal fetus, because vagal influence on the sinoatrial node decreases its rate of firing. In a similar fashion, blockade of this nerve in a normal fetus causes an increase in the FHR of approximately 20 beats/min at term.[1] This finding demonstrates a normally constant vagal influence on the FHR, which tends to decrease it from its intrinsic rate.

The vagus nerve has another very important function: It is responsible for transmission of impulses causing beat-to-beat variability of FHR. Blockade of the vagus nerve results in disappearance of this variability. Hence, there are two possible vagal influences on the heart: a tonic influence tending to decrease FHR and an oscillatory influence that results in FHR variability.[2] Further, vagal tone is not necessarily constant. Its influence increases with gestational age.[3] In fetal sheep, vagal activity increases as much as fourfold during acute hypoxia[4] or experimentally produced fetal growth restriction.[5]

Sympathetic Nervous System

Sympathetic nerves are widely distributed in the muscle of the heart at term. Stimulation of the sympathetic nerves releases norepinephrine and causes increases in both the rate and the strength of fetal cardiac contractions, resulting in higher cardiac output. The sympathetic nerves are a reserve mechanism to improve the pumping activity of the heart during intermittent stressful situations. There is normally a tonic sympathetic influence on the heart. Blocking the action of these sympathetic nerves causes a decrease in FHR of approximately 10 beats/min. As with the vagal tone, tonic sympathetic influence increases as much as twofold during fetal hypoxia.

Chemoreceptors

Chemoreceptors are found in both the peripheral and the central nervous system. They have their most dramatic effects on the regulation of respiration but are also important in control of the circulation. The peripheral chemoreceptors are in the aortic and carotid bodies, which are located in the arch of the aorta and the area of the carotid sinus, respectively. The central chemoreceptors in the medulla oblongata respond to changes in oxygen and carbon dioxide tension in the blood or in the cerebrospinal fluid perfusing this area.

In the adult, when oxygen is decreased or the carbon dioxide content is increased in the arterial blood perfusing the central chemoreceptors, a reflex tachycardia occurs. There is also a substantial increase in arterial blood pressure, particularly when the carbon dioxide concentration is increased. Both effects are thought to be protective, representing an attempt to circulate more blood through the affected areas and thereby bring about a decrease in carbon dioxide tension (PCO_2) or an increase in oxygen tension (PO_2). Selective hypoxia or hypercapnia of the peripheral chemoreceptors alone in the adult produces a bradycardia, in contrast to the tachycardia and hypertension that results from central hypoxia or hypercapnia.

The interaction of the central and peripheral chemoreceptors in the fetus is poorly understood. It is known that the net result of hypoxia or hypercapnia in the unanesthetized fetus is bradycardia with hypertension. During basal conditions, the chemoreceptors contribute to stabilization of FHR and blood pressure.[6]

Baroreceptors

In the arch of the aorta, and in the carotid sinus at the junction of the internal and external carotid arteries, are small stretch receptors in the vessel walls that are sensitive to increases in blood pressure. When pressure rises, impulses are sent from these receptors via the vagus or glossopharyngeal nerve to the midbrain; this results in further impulses' being sent via the vagus nerve to the heart, tending to slow it. This is an extremely rapid response, occurring almost with the first systolic rise of blood pressure. It is a protective, stabilizing attempt by the body to lower blood pressure by decreasing the heart rate and cardiac output when blood pressure is increasing.

Central Nervous System

In the adult, the higher centers of the brain influence the heart rate. Heart rate is increased by emotional stimuli such as fear and sexual arousal. In fetal lambs and monkeys, the electroencephalogram or electro-oculogram shows increased activity, at times in association with increased variability of the FHR and body movements. At other times, apparently when the fetus is sleeping, body movement slows and FHR variability decreases, suggesting an association between these two factors and central nervous system activity.[7]

The medulla oblongata contains the vasomotor centers, integrative centers in which the net result of all the inputs is either acceleration or deceleration of the FHR. It is probably in these centers that the net result of numerous central and peripheral inputs is processed to generate irregular oscillatory vagal impulses, giving rise to FHR variability.

Hormonal Regulation

Adrenal Medulla

The fetal adrenal medulla produces epinephrine and norepinephrine in response to stress. Both substances act on the heart and cardiovascular system in a way similar to sympathetic stimulation to produce a faster FHR, greater force of contraction of the heart, and higher arterial blood pressure.

Renin-Angiotensin System

Angiotensin II may play a role in fetal circulatory regulation at rest, but its main activity is observed during hemorrhagic stress on a fetus.

Prostaglandins

Various prostaglandins and arachidonic acid metabolites are found in the fetal circulation and in many fetal tissues. Their main roles with respect to cardiovascular function seem to be regulating umbilical blood flow and maintaining the patency of the ductus arteriosus during fetal life.

Other Hormones

Other hormones, such as nitric oxide, α-melanocyte–stimulating hormone, atrial natriuretic hormone, neuropeptide Y, thyrotropin-releasing hormone, cortisol, and metabolites such as adenosine, are also present in the fetus and participate in the regulation of circulatory function.

Blood Volume Control

Capillary Fluid Shift

In the adult, when the blood pressure is elevated by excessive blood volume, fluid moves out of the capillaries into interstitial spaces, thereby decreasing the blood volume toward normal. Conversely, if the adult loses blood through hemorrhage, some fluid shifts out of the interstitial spaces into the circulation, increasing the blood volume toward normal. There is normally a delicate balance between the pressures inside and outside the capillaries. This mechanism of regulating blood pressure is slower than the almost instantaneous regulation observed with the reflex mechanisms discussed previously. Its role in the fetus is imperfectly understood, although imbalances may be responsible for the hydrops seen in some cases of red cell alloimmunization and the high-output failure sometimes seen with supraventricular tachycardia.

Intraplacental Pressures

Fluid moves along hydrostatic pressure gradients and in response to osmotic pressure gradients. The specific role of these factors within the human placenta, where fetal and maternal blood closely approximate, is unclear. It seems likely, however, that some delicate balancing mechanisms within the placenta prevent rapid fluid shifts between mother and fetus. The mean arterial blood pressure of the mother (approximately 100 mm Hg) is much higher than that of the fetus (approximately 55 mm Hg), but the osmotic pressures are not substantially different. Therefore, some compensatory mechanism must be present to equalize the effective pressures at the exchange points so as to prevent dramatic fluid shifts.

Frank-Starling Mechanism

The amount of blood pumped by the heart is determined by the amount of blood returning to the heart; that is, the heart normally pumps the blood that flows into it without excessive damming of blood in the venous circulation. When the cardiac muscle is stretched before contraction by an increased inflow of blood, it contracts with a greater force and is able to pump out more blood. This mechanism of response to preload is apparently not the same in the fetal heart as in the adult heart. In the fetus, increases in preload produce minor, if any, changes in combined ventricular output, suggesting that the fetal heart normally operates near the peak of its function curve.

The output of the fetal heart is essentially related to the FHR. Some researchers have shown that spontaneous variations of FHR relate directly to cardiac output (i.e., as the rate increases, output also increases). However, different responses have been observed during right or left atrial pacing studies.[8] Clearly, additional factors are required to explain such differences. In addition to FHR and preload, cardiac output depends on afterload and intrinsic contractility.[8,9]

The fetal heart appears to be highly sensitive to changes in afterload, represented by the fetal arterial blood pressure. Increases in afterload dramatically reduce the stroke volume or cardiac output. As already stated, the fetal heart is incompletely developed. Many ultrastructural differences between the fetal and adult heart account for a lower intrinsic capacity of the fetal heart to alter its contraction efficiency. The determinants of cardiac output do not work separately; each interacts dynamically to modulate the fetal cardiac output during changing physiologic conditions. In clinical practice, it is reasonable to assume that modest variations of FHR from the normal range produce relatively small effects on the cardiac output. However, at the extremes (e.g., tachycardia >240 beats/min, bradycardia <60 beats/min), cardiac output and umbilical blood flow are likely to be substantially decreased.

Umbilical Blood Flow

The umbilical blood flow is approximately 40% of the combined fetal ventricular output, and not all of this blood flow to the placenta exchanges with maternal blood. Umbilical blood flow is unaffected by acute moderate hypoxia but is decreased by severe hypoxia affecting the myocardial function. There is no innervation of the umbilical cord, and there are no known means of increasing umbilical flow. However, variable decelerations in the FHR commonly occur with transient umbilical cord compression, and flow is certainly diminished or stopped for a time, depending on the degree and duration of cord compression or occlusion.

Fetal Heart Rate Monitor

The electronic FHR monitor is a device with two components: One establishes the FHR, and the other measures uterine contractions.[10] To recognize FHR, the device uses either the R wave of the fetal electrocardiogram (ECG) complex (fetal scalp electrode) or the modulation of an ultrasound signal generated by movement of a cardiovascular structure (Doppler ultrasound transducer or cardiotachometer). Uterine contractions are detected either directly, by a pressure transducer attached to a catheter within the amniotic cavity (intrauterine pressure catheter), or by an belt-like external device (tocodynamometer) that recognizes the tightening of the uterus during a contraction. Monitoring with devices attached directly to the fetus or placed within the uterine cavity is called "internal," and monitoring with devices that are on the maternal abdomen is called "external."

Fetal Heart Rate Detection

Fetal Electrode

The fetal electrode consists of a small, stainless steel, spiral wire that is typically attached to the fetal scalp. A second contact is bathed by the vaginal fluids. The wires traverse the vaginal canal and are connected to a maternal leg plate, which in turn is attached to the fetal monitor. The internal mode gives the most accurate FHR tracing, because this technique directly measures the fetal cardiac electrical signal and true beat-to-beat variability.

Doppler Ultrasound Transducer

The FHR monitoring device most commonly employed is the cardiotachometer or Doppler ultrasound transducer. This device emits a high-frequency ultrasound signal (approximately 2.5 MHz) that is reflected from any moving structure (e.g., ventricle wall, valvular leaflets), with the reflected signal being altered in frequency. The change in frequency with each systole is recognized as a cardiac contraction and is processed by the transducer. The interval between cardiac events is measured (in seconds) and then divided into 60 to yield a rate for each interval between beats. These calculated rates are transcribed onto a paper strip that is moving at a specific speed (usually 3 cm/min). The resulting tracing appears as a jiggly line and is a very close representation of true FHR variability. If the intervals between heartbeats are persistently identical, the resultant FHR line is straight, suggesting minimal or absent variability.

Although this device is simple to apply, it is often inconsistent in obtaining a signal because of interference caused by maternal and fetal movements. Improvements in the logic and technology of the monitors have made the external devices more accurate and easier to use. In particular, the technique of "autocorrelation" is now used to define the timing of the cardiac contraction more accurately. A very large number of points on the "curve" depicting the Doppler frequency shift are analyzed, and this produces a signal that much more accurately represents the FHR variability.

Uterine Activity Detection

Intra-amniotic Catheter

The internal means of detecting uterine activity typically uses a soft plastic, transducer-tipped catheter placed transcervically into the amniotic cavity. The pressure of the baseline uterine tone and that of any uterine contraction is translated into an electrical signal, which is calibrated and displayed directly (in millimeters of mercury of pressure).

Tocodynamometer

The tocodynamometer is an external device that is placed on the maternal abdominal wall, over the uterine fundus. The tightening of the fundus with each contraction is detected by pressure on a small button in the center of the transducer, and uterine activity is displayed on the recorder. It acts just like a hand placed on the uterine fundus through the abdominal wall to detect uterine activity. This device detects the frequency and duration of uterine contractions but not true contraction intensity. One disadvantage of the tocodynamometer is that it works best with the mother in the supine position. This limitation may not always be compatible with maternal comfort, fetal well-being, or progression of labor. With repositioning of the patient, it is important to reestablish accurate monitoring of both the fetal heart and uterine activity.

Fetal Responses to Hypoxia/Acidemia

Studies of chronically prepared animals have shown that a number of responses occur during acute hypoxia or acidemia in the previously normoxemic fetus. Little or no change in combined cardiac output and umbilical (placental) blood flow occurs, but there is a redistribution of blood flow favoring certain vital organs—namely, heart, brain, and adrenal gland—and a decrease in blood flow to the gut, spleen, kidneys, and carcass.[11] This initial response is presumed to be advantageous to a fetus in the same way as the diving reflex is advantageous to an adult seal, in that the blood containing the available oxygen and other nutrients is supplied preferentially to vital organs. This series of responses may be thought of as temporary compensatory mechanisms that enable a fetus to survive for moderately long periods (e.g., up to 30 minutes) of limited oxygen supply without decompensation of vital organs, particularly the brain and heart.

The close matching of blood flow to oxygen availability to achieve a constancy of oxygen consumption has been demonstrated in the fetal cerebral circulation[12] and in the fetal myocardium.[13] In studies on hypoxic lamb fetuses, cerebral oxygen consumption was constant over a wide range of arterial oxygen concentrations, because the decrease in arteriovenous oxygen content accompanying hypoxia was offset by an increase in cerebral blood flow. However, during more severe acidemia or sustained hypoxemia, these responses were no longer maintained, and decreases in cardiac output, arterial blood pressure, and blood flow to the brain and heart resulted.[14] These changes may be considered to be a stage of decompensation after which tissue damage and even fetal death may follow.[15] The implications of such a scenario are of obvious importance to the fetus in utero.

Fetal Acid-Base Balance

Physiology

Normal metabolism in the fetus results in the production of both carbonic and organic acids. These acids are buffered by various mechanisms which regulate the fetal pH within a very narrow range. Although the concentration of hydrogen ions is extremely low, changes in fetal pH as small as 0.1 unit can have profound effects on metabolic activity and on the cardiovascular and central nervous systems. Extreme changes in pH can be fatal.

The maternal acid-base status can adversely affect fetal acid-base status. In normal pregnancies, the difference between maternal and fetal pH is usually 0.05 to 0.10 units.[16]

Carbonic Acid

Carbonic acid (H_2CO_3) is a volatile acid that is produced from the metabolism of glucose and fatty acids. During fetal oxidative metabolism (i.e., aerobic glycolysis or cellular respiration), the oxidation of glucose uses oxygen (O_2) and produces carbon dioxide (CO_2).

From a practical standpoint, carbonic acid formation is equivalent to carbon dioxide generation, and most of the free hydrogen ion formed is buffered intracellularly. As blood passes through the placenta (or through the lung in the adult), bicarbonate ion (HCO_3^-) reenters erythrocytes and combines with hydrogen ions to form carbonic acid, which then dissociates to carbon dioxide and water. The carbon dioxide thus formed in the fetus diffuses across the placenta and is excreted by the maternal lung. Carbon dioxide diffuses rapidly across the human placenta, so that even large quantities produced by the fetus can be eliminated rapidly if maternal respiration, uteroplacental blood flow, and umbilical blood flow are normal.

The rate of fetal carbon dioxide production is roughly equivalent to the fetal oxygen consumption rate.[17] In order for carbon dioxide to diffuse from fetus to mother, a gradient must be maintained between $P\text{CO}_2$ in fetal umbilical blood and that in maternal uteroplacental blood; in addition, adequate perfusion of both sides of the placenta must be preserved. Secondary to progesterone-stimulated maternal hyperventilation, the maternal arterial $P\text{CO}_2$ is reduced from a mean of 39 mm Hg during nonpregnancy to a mean of 31 mm Hg during pregnancy. Renal compensation, in turn, results in an increase in bicarbonate excretion, resulting in plasma levels of 18 to 22 mEq/L during pregnancy.[18]

Noncarbonic Acids

Anaerobic metabolism in the fetus results in the production of nonvolatile or noncarbonic acids via two mechanisms: (1) use of non–sulfur-containing amino acids, which results in uric acid formation, and (2) incomplete combustion of carbohydrates and fatty acids, which results in the production of lactic acid and the ketoacids (e.g., β-hydroxybutyric acid).

Because of relatively immature renal function, the fetus is unable to effectively excrete these acids; instead, they are transported to the placenta, where they diffuse slowly (in contradistinction to carbon dioxide) into the maternal circulation. The maternal kidney excretes noncarbonic acids produced by both maternal and fetal metabolism and thus helps regenerate bicarbonate. Because the maternal glomerular filtration rate increases significantly during normal pregnancy, the maternal kidney filters and reabsorbs large quantities of bicarbonate daily.

The fetus does have the ability to metabolize accumulated lactate in the presence of sufficient oxygen; however, this is a slow process, and for practical purposes it is not thought to account for a large proportion of lactic acid elimination from the fetal compartment.

Buffers

Dramatic changes in pH are minimized by the action of buffers. The two major buffers are plasma bicarbonate and hemoglobin. Other, quantitatively less important buffers include erythrocyte bicarbonate and inorganic phosphates.[19]

Terms that are used for the expression of buffering capacity include the following:

1. *Delta base*—a measure of "change" in the buffering capacity of bicarbonate
2. *Base deficit*—bicarbonate values lower than normal
3. *Base excess*—bicarbonate values higher than normal

Although the fetus has a limited ability to buffer an increase in acid production with bicarbonate and hemoglobin, the placental bicarbonate pool could also play a role in buffering the fetus against changes in maternal pH or blood gas status. Aarnoudse and colleagues[20] studied bicarbonate permeability in the perfused human placental cotyledon model and found that acidification of the maternal circulation to pH 7.06 for 30 minutes did not significantly alter fetal pH. Instead, there was an efflux of total carbon dioxide from the placenta into the maternal circulation in the form of bicarbonate, which was not matched by an influx of total carbon dioxide from the fetal circulation. By this mechanism, bicarbonate transfer could take place between the placental tissue pool and the maternal circulation, while the transmission of maternal pH and blood gas changes to the fetal circulation would be minimized.

pH Determination

The pH is a measure of the acid-base status of various body fluids. Specifically, pH is the negative logarithm of the hydrogen ion concentration. It is directly related to the concentration of bicarbonate (base) and inversely related to the concentration of carbonic acid (acid). The H_2CO_3 equals $0.03 \times P\text{CO}_2$ and the pK equals 6.11 for normal plasma at 37°C. This relation is best illustrated by the Henderson-Hasselbalch equation for determining the pH of a buffered system, in which pK is the negative logarithm of the acid dissociation constant:

$$\text{pH} = \text{pK} + \log\frac{[\text{base}]}{[\text{acid}]}$$

In the case of fetal acid-base balance determinations,

$$\text{pH} = \text{pK} + \log\frac{[\text{HCO}_3^-]}{[\text{H}_2\text{CO}_3]}$$

$$\text{pH} = \text{pK} + \log\frac{[\text{HCO}_3^-](\text{mEq/L})}{0.03[P\text{CO}_2](\text{mm Hg})}$$

In simplest terms, the HCO_3^- represents the "metabolic" component, whereas the H_2CO_3 (or PCO_2) represents the "respiratory" component.[21]

Terminology

Acidemia refers to an increase in hydrogen ions in the blood; *acidosis* refers to an increase in hydrogen ions in tissue. Similarly, *hypoxemia* is a decrease in oxygen content in blood, whereas *hypoxia* is a decrease in oxygen content in tissue (Table 22-1).

Although an umbilical artery pH of less than 7.20 has traditionally been used to define newborn acidemia, most clinicians define acidemia as two standard deviations below the mean umbilical artery pH (7.10 to 7.18). The concept of clinically significant or "pathologic" acidemia is discussed later in this chapter.

Acidemia in the newborn can be classified into three basic types: metabolic, respiratory, and mixed. The type is based primarily on the levels of HCO_3^- and PCO_2 (Table 22-2). With marked elevations of the PCO_2, there is a compensatory increase in HCO_3^- of 1 mEq/L for each 10 mm Hg increase in PCO_2.[22]

Factors Affecting Acid-Base Balance

With regard to acid-base balance in the fetus, the placenta acts as both "lungs" and "kidneys" by supplying oxygen and removing carbon dioxide and various metabolites. The pH in the fetus is thus controlled within a very tight range. Umbilical blood oxygen content and saturation and fetal arterial delta base depend primarily on uterine blood flow. Oxygen supply, in turn, depends on the following:

- Adequate maternal oxygenation
- Blood flow to the placenta
- Transfer across the placenta
- Fetal oxygenation
- Delivery to fetal tissues

TABLE 22-1 TERMINOLOGY

Acidemia	Increased concentration of hydrogen ions in blood
Acidosis	Increased concentration of hydrogen ions in tissue
Asphyxia	Hypoxia with metabolic acidosis
Base deficit	HCO_3^- concentration lower than normal
Base excess	HCO_3^- concentration higher than normal
Delta base	Measure of change in buffering capacity of bicarbonate
Hypoxemia	Decreased oxygen content in blood
Hypoxia	Decreased level of oxygen in tissue
pH	Negative logarithm of hydrogen ion concentration

Adapted from American College of Obstetricians and Gynecologists: Umbilical Artery Blood Acid-Base Analysis. Technical Bulletin No. 216. Washington, DC, ACOG, November 1995.

TABLE 22-2 TYPES OF ACIDEMIA*

Metabolic	Normal PCO_2 and decreased HCO_3^-
Respiratory	Increased PCO_2 and normal HCO_3^- (after correction of PCO_2)
Mixed	Increased PCO_2 and decreased HCO_3^-

***Umbilical artery pH <7.10.**

Removal of carbon dioxide depends on fetal blood flow to the placenta and transport across the placenta. Fixed-acid equilibrium depends on a continued state of balance between production and removal.

Respiratory Factors

Respiratory acidosis results from increased PCO_2 and subsequently decreased pH. In the fetus, this picture is usually associated with a decrease in PO_2 as well. The most common cause of acute respiratory acidosis in the fetus is a sudden decrease in placental or umbilical perfusion. Umbilical cord compression, uterine hyperstimulation, and abruptio placentae are good examples, with transient cord compression being the most common factor.

Conditions associated with maternal hypoventilation or hypoxia can also result in respiratory acidosis in the fetus (and in metabolic acidosis, if severe enough). Coleman and Rund[23] reviewed the association of maternal hypoxia with nonobstetric conditions (e.g., asthma, epilepsy) during pregnancy, noting that the normal physiologic changes that occur during pregnancy may make early recognition of maternal hypoxia difficult. For example, in a mother with asthma, a pH of less than 7.35 and a PCO_2 higher than 38 mm Hg could indicate respiratory compromise.[24] To minimize the risk of concurrent hypoxemia in the fetus, early intubation in mothers who have borderline or poor blood gas values or evidence of respiratory compromise is recommended.

Other conditions can result in maternal hypoventilation (acute or chronic) during pregnancy. Induction of anesthesia or narcotic overdose can depress the medullary respiratory center. Hypokalemia, neuromuscular disorders (e.g., myasthenia gravis), and drugs that impair neuromuscular transmission (e.g., magnesium sulfate) can, in toxic doses, result in hypoventilation or even paralysis of the respiratory muscles. Finally, airway obstruction from foreign bodies can also result in maternal respiratory acidosis. Restoration of normal fetal acid-base balance depends on the reversibility of maternal etiologic factors.

Maternal respiratory alkalosis may occur when hyperventilation reduces the PCO_2 and subsequently increases pH. Severe anxiety, acute salicylate toxicity, fever, sepsis, pneumonia, pulmonary emboli, and acclimation to high altitudes are etiologic factors. As in respiratory acidosis, restoration of the maternal acid-base balance by appropriate treatment of causative factors results in normalization of fetal blood gases.

Metabolic Factors

Fetal metabolic acidosis is characterized by loss of bicarbonate, high base deficit, and a subsequent fall in pH. This type of acidosis results from protracted periods of oxygen deficiency to a degree that results in anaerobic metabolism. The etiology can be fetal or maternal and usually implies the existence of a chronic metabolic derangement. Conditions such as growth restriction resulting from chronic uteroplacental hypoperfusion can be associated with fetal metabolic acidosis secondary to decreased oxygen delivery.

Maternal metabolic acidosis can also cause fetal metabolic acidosis and is classified according to the status of the anion gap. In addition to bicarbonate and chloride, the remaining anions required to balance the plasma sodium concentration are referred to as "unmeasured anions" or the *anion gap*. Reduced excretion of inorganic acids (as in renal failure) or accumulation of organic acids (as in alcoholic, diabetic, or starvation ketoacidosis and lactic acidosis) results in an increased anion gap metabolic acidosis. Bicarbonate loss (as in renal tubular acidosis, hyperparathyroidism, and diarrheal states) or failure of bicarbonate regeneration results in metabolic acidosis characterized

TABLE 22-3 FETAL SCALP BLOOD VALUES IN LABOR*

Measurement	Early First Stage	Late First Stage	Second Stage
pH	7.33 ± 0.03	7.32 ± 0.02	7.29 ± 0.04
PCO_2 (mm Hg)	44.00 ± 4.05	42.00 ± 5.1	46.30 ± 4.2
PO_2 (mm Hg)	21.8 ± 2.6	21.3 ± 2.1	16.5 ± 1.4
Bicarbonate (mMol/L)	20.1 ± 1.2	19.1 ± 2.1	17 ± 2
Base excess (mMol/L)	3.9 ± 1.9	4.1 ± 2.5	6.4 ± 1.8

*Mean ± standard deviation.
From Huch R, Huch A: Maternal-fetal acid-base balance and blood gas measurement. In Beard RW, Nathanielsz PW (eds): Fetal Physiology and Medicine. New York, Marcel Dekker, 1984, p 713.

by a normal anion gap. Fetal responses to these maternal conditions are manifested by a pure metabolic acidosis with normal respiratory gas exchange as long as placental perfusion remains normal.

Prolonged fetal respiratory acidosis (as in cord compression and abruptio placentae) can also result in accumulation of noncarbonic acids produced by anaerobic metabolism; this condition is characterized by blood gas measurements that reflect a mixed respiratory and metabolic acidosis.

Effects of Labor

Each uterine contraction transiently diminishes uterine blood flow, reduces placental perfusion, and impairs transplacental gaseous exchange. A sample of blood may be obtained from the fetal presenting part to help evaluate fetal status during labor. Typical fetal scalp blood values during labor are shown in Table 22-3.

Umbilical Cord Blood Acid-Base Analysis

Umbilical cord blood acid-base analysis provides an objective method of evaluating a newborn's condition, especially with regard to hypoxia and acidemia.[16] Assessing umbilical cord blood pH has become an important adjunct in defining perinatal hypoxia that is severe enough to result in acute neurologic injury.[25] Moreover, the technique is simple and relatively inexpensive.

Technique

A segment of cord (approximately 10 to 20 cm) should be doubly clamped immediately after delivery in all women, in the event that cord blood analysis is desired or deemed necessary. The cord is clamped immediately because a delay as short as 20 seconds can significantly alter the arterial pH and PCO_2.[26] Specimens should be obtained ideally from the umbilical artery and the umbilical vein, but the umbilical artery sample provides a more direct assessment of fetal condition, whereas the umbilical vein reflects placental acid-base status. In cases such as cord prolapse, the umbilical artery pH may be extremely low, even in the presence of a normal umbilical vein pH.[27] Nevertheless, some clinicians still prefer to use the umbilical vein, which is easier to access for drawing blood, especially in the very premature infant. In one study of 453 term infants, D'Souza and colleagues[28] determined that umbilical venous and arterial blood pH are significantly related to each other and that umbilical venous pH measurements do provide useful information regarding newborn acidemia at birth.

Samples should be drawn in plastic or glass syringes that have been flushed with heparin (1000 U/mL). Commercial syringes (1 to 2 mL) containing lyophilized heparin are also available for obtaining specimens. Kirshon and Moise[29] reported that the addition of 0.2 mL of 10,000 U/mL of heparin to 0.2 mL of blood significantly decreased the pH, PCO_2, and bicarbonate. Therefore, any residual heparin (as well as air) should be ejected, and the needle should be capped.

A few practical points merit mention. First, it is not necessary to draw the sample from the umbilical artery immediately, provided that the cord is clamped. Adequate specimens have been obtained from a clamped segment of cord as long as 60 minutes after delivery without significant changes in pH or PCO_2.[30] Moreover, once the specimens have been drawn into the syringe, they are relatively stable at room temperature for up to 60 minutes[31] and do not need to be transported to the laboratory on ice.[32] The same may not be true for specimens obtained from placental vessels.[33]

Chauhan and colleagues[34] prepared a mathematical model that allows for the calculation of umbilical artery pH for up to 60 hours after delivery. This model permits the estimation of fetal pH at birth.

Normal Values

Although there is no consensus as to what the most appropriate umbilical artery pH cutoff should be to define acidemia, the mean pH values from four studies are shown in Table 22-4. The mean value for umbilical artery pH appears to be very close to 7.28. The subjects in the study reported by Riley and Johnson[27] were from 3522 unselected women undergoing vaginal delivery.

The mean pH for umbilical venous blood has been reported to be 7.32 to 7.35. In a study of umbilical venous blood pH, D'Souza and associates[28] reported a mean venous pH of 7.34 (± 0.07). Huisjes and Aarnoudse[35] also reported good correlation between umbilical venous and arterial pH.

Although the Apgar scores of premature infants may be low because of immaturity, mean values for both arterial and venous pH and blood gas values are similar to those of the term infant. Mean values for almost 2000 premature infants are summarized in Table 22-5.

Pathologic Fetal Acidemia

What level of umbilical artery pH should be considered abnormal, "pathologic," or clinically significant? It is now well established that the former pH cutoff of 7.20 is not appropriate.[16,36] Most newborns with an umbilical artery pH lower than 7.20 are vigorous and without systemic evidence of hypoxia. Recent evidence suggests that significant neonatal morbidity is more likely to occur in neonates with umbilical artery pH values lower than 7.00, especially if associated with a low Apgar score (i.e., ≤3). For example, in a study of 2738 term newborns, hypotonia, seizures, and need for intubation were significantly correlated with an umbilical artery pH of less than 7.00 and an Apgar score of 3 or less at 1 minute.[37] The authors concluded that a newborn must be severely depressed at birth for birth hypoxia to be implicated as the cause of seizures.

TABLE 22-4 NORMAL UMBILICAL CORD BLOOD pH AND BLOOD GAS VALUES IN TERM NEWBORNS (MEAN ± SD)

Measurement	Yeomans et al., 1985 (*n* = 146)	Ramin et al., 1989 (*n* = 1292)	Riley and Johnson, 1993 (*n* = 3520)	Thorp et al., 1989 (*n* = 1924)
Arterial Blood (*n* = 1694)				
pH	7.28 ± 0.05	7.28 ± 0.07	7.27 ± 0.07	7.24 ± 0.07
P_{CO_2} (mm Hg)	49.20 ± 8.4	49.90 ± 14.2	50.30 ± 11.1	56.30 ± 8.6
HCO_3^- (mEq/L)	22.30 ± 2.5	23.10 ± 2.8	22.00 ± 3.6	24.10 ± 2.2
Base excess (mEq/L)	—	−3.60 ± 2.8	−2.70 ± 2.8	−3.60 ± 2.7
Venous Blood (*n* = 1820)				
pH	7.35 ± 0.05	—	7.34 ± 0.06	7.32 ± 0.06
P_{CO_2} (mm Hg)	38.20 ± 5.6	—	40.70 ± 7.9	43.80 ± 6.7
HCO_3^- (mEq/L)	20.40 ± 4.1	—	21.40 ± 2.5	22.60 ± 2.1
Base excess (mEq/L)	—	—	−2.40 ± 2.0	2.90 ± 2.4

Data from Yeomans ER, Hauth JC, Gilstrap LC, et al: Umbilical cord pH, P_{CO_2} and bicarbonate following uncomplicated term vaginal deliveries. Am J Obstet Gynecol 151:798, 1985; Ramin SM, Gilstrap LC, Leveno KJ, et al: Umbilical artery acid-base status in the preterm infant. Obstet Gynecol 74:256, 1989; Riley RJ, Johnson JWC: Collecting and analyzing cord blood gases. Clin Obstet Gynecol 36:13, 1993; Thorp JA, Boylan PC, Parisi VM, et al: Effects of high-dose oxytocin augmentation on umbilical cord blood gas values in primigravid women. Am J Obstet Gynecol 159:670, 1988.

TABLE 22-5 NORMAL ARTERY BLOOD GAS VALUES FOR PREMATURE INFANTS (MEAN ± SD)

Measurement	Dickenson et al., 1992 (*n* = 949)	Riley and Johnson, 1993 (*n* = 1015)
pH	7.27 ± 0.07	7.28 ± 0.089
P_{CO_2} (mm Hg)	51.60 ± 9.4	50.20 ± 12.3
HCO_3^- (mEq/L)	23.90 ± 2.1	22.40 ± 3.5
Base excess (mEq/L)	−3.00 ± 2.5	−2.50 ± 3.0

From Dickenson JE, Eriksen NL, Meyer BA, et al: The effect of preterm birth on umbilical cord blood gases. Obstet Gynecol 79:575, 1992; Riley RJ, Johnson JWC: Collecting and analyzing cord blood gases. Clin Obstet Gynecol 36:13, 1993.

TABLE 22-6 NEONATAL MORBIDITY AND MORTALITY ACCORDING TO pH CUTOFF

pH	*N*	Neonatal Deaths	Seizures	Both
7.15-7.19	2236	3 (0.1%)	2 (0.1%)	1 (0.05%)
7.10-7.14	798	3 (0.4%)	1 (0.1%)	0 (0.00%)
7.05-7.09	290	0 (0.0%)	0 (0.0%)	1 (1.1%)
7.00-7.04	95	1 (1.1%)	1 (1.1%)	1 (1.1%)
<7.00	87	7 (8.0%)*	8 (9.2%)*	2 (2.3%)

*$P < .05$.
From Goldaber KG, Gilstrap LC, Leveno KJ, et al: Pathologic fetal acidemia. Obstet Gynecol 78:1103, 1991.

Goldaber and coworkers,[22] in an attempt to better define the critical cutoff for pathologic fetal acidemia, studied the neonatal outcome of 3506 term newborns. They determined the critical pH cutoff point to be 7.00 (Table 22-6). Many of these babies, however, had no complications and went to the newborn nursery. In a follow-up study from the same institution, King and associates[38] reported on 35 term newborns with an umbilical artery pH greater than 7.00 who were triaged to the newborn nursery. These authors concluded that term newborns who had this degree of acidemia at birth but had a stable appearance in the delivery room (and were without other complications) did not have evidence of hypoxia or ischemia during the 48 hours after birth. It has been reported that fewer than half of neonates with an umbilical artery pH lower than 7.00 actually have neonatal complications.[39]

The critical pH cutoff for neonatal morbidity may actually be even lower than 7.00. Data presented by Andres and colleagues[40] suggest a value closer to 6.90. In a review of 93 neonates (>34 weeks' gestational age) with an umbilical artery pH greater than 7.00, the median pH for the group was 6.92 (range, 6.62 to 6.99); however, the median pH was 6.75 for neonates with seizures (25th to 75th percentile, 6.72 to 6.88), compared with 6.93 for those without seizures ($P = .02$). The median pH for newborns with hypoxic-ischemic encephalopathy was also significantly lower (6.69; 25th to 75th percentile, 6.62 to 6.75) than for those without this diagnosis (6.93; 25th to 75th percentile, 6.85 to 6.97; $P = .03$). The median pH was also less than 6.90 in newborns who required intubation (6.83) or cardiopulmonary resuscitation (6.83) and was significantly lower ($P < .05$) than in newborns without these complications It should also be noted that the median P_{CO_2} and base deficit were significantly higher in neonates with these morbidities.[40]

Acute Neurologic Injury

There is poor correlation between neurologic outcome and the 1-minute and 5-minute Apgar scores. The correlation does improve if the scores remain between 0 and 3 at 10, 15, and 20 minutes; however, many such babies will still be "normal" if they survive. Similarly, a low umbilical artery pH in and of itself also has poor correlation with adverse outcome. The American College of Obstetricians and Gynecologists (ACOG)[41] has established the following essential criteria (all four must be met) to indicate hypoxia proximate to delivery severe enough to be associated with acute neurologic injury:

1. Evidence of a metabolic acidosis in fetal umbilical cord arterial blood obtained at delivery (pH <7 and base deficit ≥12 mmol/L)
2. Early onset of severe or moderate neonatal encephalopathy in infants born at 34 or more weeks of gestation

3. Cerebral palsy of the spastic quadriplegic or dyskinetic type
4. Exclusion of other identifiable etiologies, such as trauma, coagulation disorders, infectious conditions, or genetic disorders

In two publications, Low and associates[42,43] reported on the association of severe or significant metabolic acidosis (as determined by the umbilical artery blood gas profile) and newborn complications. Low[43] proposed a classification of intrapartum fetal asphyxia, the severity of which is based on newborn encephalopathy and other organ system dysfunction.

Other Clinical Events and Umbilical Blood Acid-Base Analysis

Beyond its use in assessing prematurity and neurologic injury, umbilical blood gas analysis has been reported in a variety of clinical situations, such as acute chorioamnionitis, nuchal cords, meconium, prolonged pregnancy, FHR anomalies, operative vaginal delivery, breech delivery, and use of oxytocin.[36] Such analysis may also prove useful in assessing the interval to delivery in shoulder dystocia cases.

ACUTE CHORIOAMNIONITIS

In one study of 123 women with acute chorioamnionitis, compared with more than 6000 noninfected women, Maberry and coauthors[44] found no significant association between infection and fetal acidemia (Table 22-7). Hankins and colleagues[45] found no association between acute chorioamnionitis and newborn acidemia. Meyer and colleagues,[46] however, reported an association of fetal sepsis with a decrease in umbilical artery pH compared with controls (7.21 versus 7.26).

NUCHAL CORDS

In a study of 110 newborns with nuchal cords, Hankins and colleagues[47] reported that significantly more newborns with nuchal cords were acidemic (umbilical artery pH <7.20), compared with controls (20% versus 12%; $P < .05$); however, there were no significant differences in mean pH (7.25 versus 7.27); P_{CO_2} (49 versus 48 mm Hg), or HCO_3^- (20.5 versus 21.0 mEq/L).

MECONIUM

In one study of 53 term pregnancies with moderate to thick meconium, Mitchell and colleagues[48] reported that approximately half of the newborns were acidemic, and that significantly more acidemic newborns had meconium below the cords, compared with controls (32% versus 0%; $P < .05$). These authors, however, used an umbilical artery pH cutoff of 7.25 to define acidemia.

In another report of 323 newborns with meconium by Yeomans and associates,[49] there was a significantly increased frequency of meconium below the cords in acidemic fetuses than in nonacidemic fetuses (31% versus 18%; $P < .05$). Meconium aspiration syndrome, however, was an uncommon event, occurring in only 3% of newborns. Ramin and colleagues,[50] in a study of meconium, reported that 55% of meconium aspiration syndrome cases occurred in newborns with an umbilical artery pH greater than 7.20.

In a review of 4985 term neonates born to mothers with meconium-stained amniotic fluid, Blackwell and colleagues[51] identified 48 cases of severe meconium aspiration syndrome in which umbilical artery pH measurements were obtained; the pH was 7.20 or higher in 29 of these patients and less than 7.20 in 19. There was no difference in frequency of seizures between the two pH groups. The authors concluded that severe meconium aspiration syndrome occurred in the presence of normal acid-base status at delivery in many of the cases, suggesting that a "preexisting injury or a nonhypoxic mechanism is often involved."[51]

PROLONGED PREGNANCY

In a study of 108 women with a prolonged pregnancy, Silver and colleagues[52] reported a mean umbilical artery pH of 7.25. Moreover, significantly more newborns who were delivered for FHR indications had acidemia than newborns who were not (45% versus 13%; $P < .05$).

FETAL HEART RATE ABNORMALITIES

Gilstrap and colleagues,[53] in a study of 403 term newborns with FHR abnormalities in the second stage of labor compared with 430 control newborns, reported an association of abnormalities and acidemia (Table 22-8). This was confirmed in a follow-up study.[54] Honjo and Yamaguchi[55] also reported a correlation between second-stage baseline FHR abnormalities and fetal acidemia at birth. Although there may be an association between FHR abnormalities and acidemia, the association with adverse long-term neurologic outcome is uncommon. For example, Nelson and colleagues,[56] in a population-based study of children with cerebral palsy and a birth weight of 2500 g or more, reported that specific FHR abnormalities (i.e., late deceleration and decreased beat-to-beat variability) were associated with an increased risk of cerebral palsy. However, of all the children with these abnormal FHR findings only 0.19% had cerebral palsy. Therefore, the false-positive rate was 99.8%.

TABLE 22-7 COMPARISON OF UMBILICAL ARTERY pH IN PATIENTS WITH AND WITHOUT ACUTE CHORIOAMNIONITIS

Umbilical Artery pH	Patients with Chorioamnionitis (*n* = 123)	Controls (*n* = 6769)
<7.20	18 (15.0%)	701 (10.0%)
<7.15	4 (3.0%)	242 (4.0%)
<7.00	0	6 (0.1%)
Metabolic acidemia	1 (0.8%)	9 (0.1%)

From Maberry MC, Ramin SM, Gilstrap LC, et al: Intrapartum asphyxia in pregnancies complicated by intraamniotic infection. Obstet Gynecol 76:351, 1990. Reprinted with permission from the American College of Obstetricians and Gynecologists.

TABLE 22-8 ASSOCIATION OF UMBILICAL ARTERY ACIDEMIA AND SECOND-STAGE FETAL HEART RATE (FHR) ABNORMALITIES IN NEWBORNS

FHR Pattern	*N*	Umbilical Artery pH <7.20
Tachycardia*	117	15%
Mild bradycardia*	165	18%
Moderate/marked bradycardia*	121	27%
Normal	430	4%

*P < .0001 compared with normals.
Modified from Gilstrap LC, Hauth JC, Toussaint S: Second stage fetal heart rate abnormalities and neonatal acidosis. Obstet Gynecol 63:209, 1984. Reprinted with permission from the American College of Obstetricians and Gynecologists.

TABLE 22-9 METHOD OF DELIVERY AND FETAL ACIDEMIA

Method of Delivery	*N*	% with Acidemia*
Spontaneous	303	7
Elective outlet/low forceps	177	9
Indicated outlet/low forceps	293	18
Indicated midforceps	234	21
Cesarean delivery	111	18

*Umbilical artery pH <7.20.
From Gilstrap LC, Hauth JC, Shiano S, et al: Neonatal acidosis and method of delivery. Obstet Gynecol 63:681, 1984. Reprinted with permission from the American College of Obstetricians and Gynecologists.

OPERATIVE VAGINAL DELIVERY

Gilstrap and coworkers[57] found no significant difference in the frequency of newborn acidemia according to method of delivery (Table 22-9). This was true even when the indication for delivery was fetal distress.

BREECH DELIVERY

Although the mean umbilical artery pH was lower for infants delivered vaginally in breech presentations compared with cephalic presentations in two studies,[58,59] pH levels were not significantly low from a clinical standpoint (7.23 and 7.16, respectively). It seems unlikely that delivery of breech presentations by the vaginal route is related to significant newborn acidemia.

SHOULDER DYSTOCIA

Most adverse outcomes associated with shoulder dystocia are due to actual physical injury to the brachial plexus[60] and not to acidemia or asphyxia (unless an extremely protracted period is needed to extract the fetus). In a review of 134 infants born after shoulder dystocia, Stallings and colleagues[61] reported that this complication was associated with a "statistically significant but clinically insignificant" reduction in mean umbilical artery pH levels, compared to their obstetric population (7.23 versus 7.27).

OXYTOCIN

In a study of 556 women who received oxytocin compared with 704 who did not, Thorp and colleagues[62] found no significant difference in mean umbilical artery pH measurements (7.23 versus 7.24, respectively).

Summary

The fetus maintains its pH within a very limited range and is dependent on the placenta and the maternal circulation to maintain acid-base balance. Several methods for assessing fetal-newborn acid-base status have been described. Of these methods, umbilical blood gas analysis is probably the most useful and the easiest (and relatively the least expensive) to perform.

There are few data to justify a policy of umbilical blood gas analysis for all newborns. In a survey of 133 universities in the United States, Johnson and Riley[63] reported that approximately 27% of centers used cord blood for assessing newborn acid-base status in all deliveries. Two thirds of the programs used them for tracing abnormal FHRs or for low Apgar scores. The Royal College of Obstetricians and Gynecologists and the Royal College of Midwives[64] recommend routine cord blood measurements for all cesarean deliveries and instrumental deliveries for fetal distress. The ACOG[41] recommends umbilical cord blood acid-base analysis in the following situations:

- Cesarean delivery for fetal compromise
- Low 5-minute Apgar score
- Severe growth restriction
- Abnormal FHR tracing
- Maternal thyroid disease
- Intrapartum fever
- Multifetal gestations

Characteristics of Fetal Heart Rate Patterns

Basic Patterns

The characteristics of the FHR pattern are classified as baseline or periodic/episodic.[65,66] The *baseline* features—rate and variability—are those recorded between uterine contractions. *Periodic* changes occur in association with uterine contractions, and *episodic* changes are those not obviously associated with uterine contractions.

Baseline Features

The baseline features of the FHR are those predominant characteristics that can be recognized between uterine contractions. They are the baseline rate and variability of the FHR.

BASELINE RATE

The definition of baseline rate is the FHR recorded between contractions. More rigidly described, it is the approximate mean FHR rounded to 5 beats/min during a 10-minute segment, excluding the following: (1) periodic or episodic changes, (2) periods of marked FHR variability, and (3) segments of the baseline that differ by at least 25 beats/min. In any 10-minute window, the minimum baseline duration must be at least 2 minutes; otherwise, the baseline for that period is indeterminate.

The normal baseline FHR is between 110 and 160 beats/min. Rates slower than 110 beats/min are termed *bradycardia,* and rates faster than 160 beats/min are termed *tachycardia.* Baseline bradycardia and tachycardia are quantified by the actual rate observed in keeping with the definition of baseline rate.

FETAL HEART RATE VARIABILITY

Electronic fetal heart rate monitoring (EFM) in most cases produces a tracing with an irregular line, demonstrating the FHR variability. The irregularities represent the slight differences in time interval, and therefore in calculated FHR, that occur from beat to beat. If all intervals between heartbeats were identical, the line would be straight. Fluctuations in the baseline FHR are irregular in amplitude and frequency. (A pattern called "sinusoidal," discussed later, differs from variability in that it has a smooth sine wave of regular frequency and amplitude and therefore is excluded from the definition of FHR variability.)

Baseline variability is defined as fluctuations in the FHR of 2 or more cycles per minute and is quantitated as the peak-to-trough amplitude of the FHR in beats per minute. Variability is *absent* when the amplitude range is undetectable. It is *minimal* when there is an amplitude range but it is less than 5 beats/min. Variability is *normal* or *moderate* when the amplitude is between 6 and 25 beats/min. Variability is *marked* when the amplitude ranges greater than 25 beats/min[67] (see Classification and Significance of Baseline Variability).

Periodic Heart Rate Patterns

Periodic patterns are the alterations in FHR that are associated with uterine contractions or changes in blood flow within the umbilical cord vessels. These patterns are termed late decelerations, early decelerations, variable decelerations, and accelerations. In each case, the decrease or increase in FHR is calculated from the most recently determined portion of the baseline.

LATE DECELERATIONS

In late deceleration of the FHR, there is a visually apparent decrease and subsequent return to baseline FHR that is associated with a uterine contraction. The decrease is gradual, with the time from onset of deceleration to nadir being at least 30 seconds, and is delayed in timing, with the nadir of the deceleration occurring late in relation to the peak of the uterine contraction. In most cases, the onset, nadir, and recovery are all late in relation to the beginning, peak, and ending of the contraction, respectively.

EARLY DECELERATIONS

Early deceleration of the FHR is similar to late deceleration except that the decrease is coincident in timing, with the nadir of the deceleration occurring at the same time as the peak of the uterine contraction. In most cases, the onset, nadir, and recovery are all coincident with the beginning, peak, and ending of the contraction, respectively.

VARIABLE DECELERATIONS

Variable deceleration is defined as a visually apparent *abrupt* decrease (less than 30 seconds from onset of deceleration to beginning of nadir) in FHR from the baseline. The decrease in FHR is at least 15 beats/min, and its duration (from baseline to baseline) is at least 15 seconds but not more than 2 minutes. When variable decelerations are associated with uterine contractions, their onset, depth, and duration commonly vary with successive contractions.

Prolonged deceleration is a visually apparent abrupt decrease in FHR below the baseline of at least 15 beats/min that has a duration between 2 and 10 minutes from onset to return to baseline.

ACCELERATIONS

Acceleration is defined as a visually apparent abrupt increase (<30 seconds from onset of acceleration to peak) in FHR above the baseline. The acme is at least 15 beats/min above the baseline, and the acceleration lasts between 15 seconds and 2 minutes from onset to return to baseline. Before 32 weeks of gestation, accelerations are defined as having an acme of at least 10 beats/min above the baseline and a duration of at least 10 seconds. *Prolonged* acceleration is an acceleration that lasts at least 2 minutes but less than 10 minutes.

There is a close association between the presence of accelerations and normal FHR variability. At times it may be difficult to decide whether a recorded pattern represents "acceleration" or a normal long-term variability complex. The final decision is not important, because both accelerations and normal variability have the same positive prognostic significance, indicating normal fetal oxygenation.

QUANTIFICATION

Any deceleration is quantified by the depth of the nadir in beats per minute below the baseline. The duration is quantified in minutes and seconds from the beginning to the end of the deceleration. Acceleration is quantified similarly. Decelerations are defined as recurrent or persistent if they occur with more than 50% of uterine contractions in any 20-minute period. Bradycardia and tachycardia are quantified by the actual FHR in beats per minute.

Normal and Abnormal Heart Rate Patterns

The normal or reassuring FHR pattern (Fig. 22-1) is accepted as that with a baseline FHR of between 110 and 160 beats/min; an FHR variability amplitude between 6 and 25 beats/min; and no decelerative periodic changes (although there may be periodic or episodic accelerations). It is widely accepted in clinical practice that a fetus born with this FHR pattern is normally oxygenated if delivery occurs when the normal FHR pattern is traced.[4,68,69]

In contrast to the high predictability of fetal normoxia and vigor in the presence of the normal pattern, variant patterns are not as accurately predictive of fetal compromise. However, when these nonreassuring patterns are placed in the context of the clinical case (e.g., the progressive change in the patterns, the duration of the variant patterns), one can make reasonable judgments about the likelihood of fetal decompensation. With this screening approach, impending intolerable fetal acidosis can be presumed or, in certain cases, ruled out by the use of ancillary techniques (e.g., fetal scalp stimulation, vibroacoustic stimulation, fetal scalp blood sampling).

As a predictor for significant neurologic morbidity such as cerebral palsy, EFM has a very poor specificity and positive predictive value. The positive predictive value of a nonreassuring FHR is stated to be 0.14%. This means that for every 1000 fetuses born with a nonreassuring FHR tracing, 1 or 2 of them develop cerebral palsy.[70] Thus, the false-positive rate is greater than 99%.

Baseline Rate

BRADYCARDIA

Bradycardia is defined as a baseline FHR slower than 110 beats/min. Certain fetuses have a baseline FHR of less than 110 beats/min and are cardiovascularly normal. Their baseline FHR simply represents a variation outside the limits of normal. Others with an FHR slower than 110 beats/min may have congenital heart block and a well-compensated status despite a low FHR.

Bradycardia is a term that relates to baseline FHR and is distinguished from a deceleration. However, a prolonged deceleration resulting in a new baseline bradycardia may result from vagal activity in response to fetal hypoxia (Fig. 22-2). Reasons for such decreases in FHR include the following:

1. A sudden drop in oxygenation, such as occurs with placental abruption, maternal apnea, or amniotic fluid embolus
2. A decrease or cessation in umbilical blood flow, such as occurs with a prolapsed cord or uterine rupture
3. A decrease in uterine blood flow, such as occurs with severe maternal hypotension

TACHYCARDIA

Tachycardia is defined as a baseline FHR of more than 160 beats/min; it is distinguished from an acceleration in that its duration is at least 10 minutes. With tachycardia, there is commonly a loss of variability of the FHR. Although fetal tachycardia is potentially associated with fetal hypoxia, particularly when it is accompanied by decelerations of the FHR, the more common association is with maternal or

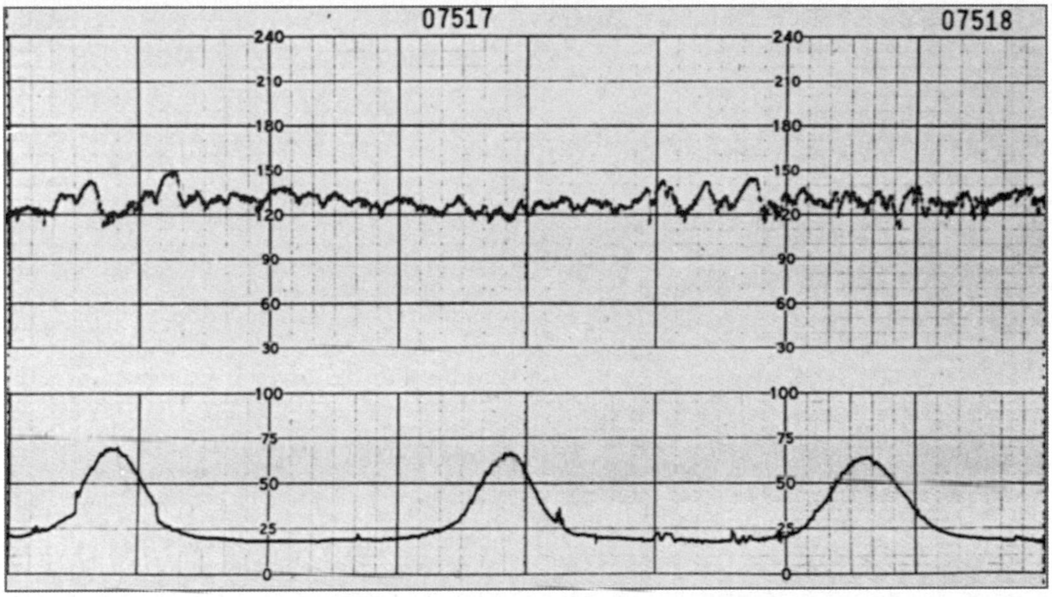

FIGURE 22-1 **Normal fetal heart rate pattern.** The tracing exhibits normal rate (approximately 130 beats/min), normal variability (amplitude range about 15 beats/min), and absence of periodic changes. This pattern represents a nonacidemic fetus without evidence of hypoxic stress. Uterine contractions are 2 to 3 minutes apart and about 60 to 70 mm Hg in intensity.

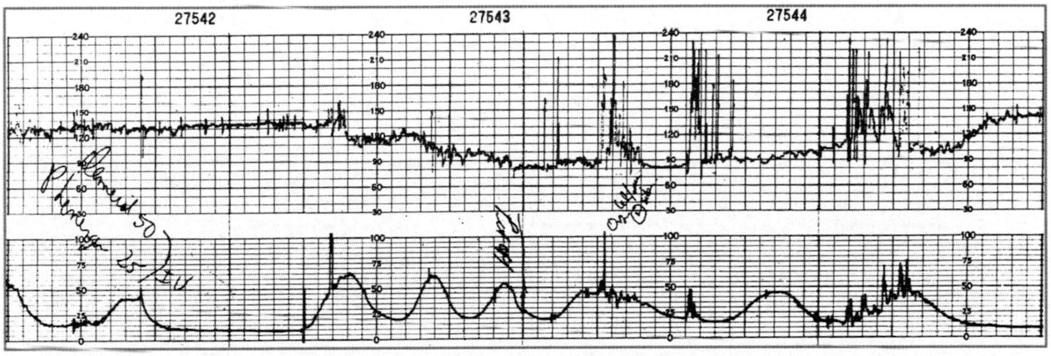

FIGURE 22-2 **Prolonged fetal bradycardia resulting from excessive oxytocin-induced hyperstimulation of the uterus after intravenous infusion of meperidine (Demerol) and promethazine (Phenergan) into the same tubing.** The heart rate is returning to normal at the end of the tracing, after appropriate treatment (signified by the notes "Pit off," "O_2 6 L/min," and "side"). Note that fetal heart rate variability was maintained throughout this asphyxial stress, signifying adequate central oxygenation.

fetal infection (e.g., chorioamnionitis). In most of these instances, the fetus is not hypoxic but has an elevated baseline FHR.

It is not uncommon for the FHR baseline to rise in the second stage of labor. Certain drugs also cause tachycardia, such as β-mimetic agents used for attempted tocolysis or illicit drugs such as methamphetamine and cocaine.

Tachycardia should not be confused with the rarer finding of a fetal cardiac tachyarrhythmia, in which the FHR is faster than 240 beats/min. These arrhythmias may be intermittent or persistent and are the result of abnormalities of the intrinsic determinants of cardiac rhythm. Such findings of supraventricular tachyarrhythmias need to be monitored closely and possibly treated with medical therapy or delivery, because they may be associated with deterioration of the fetal status.

Classification and Significance of Baseline Variability

As described earlier, FHR variability may be absent, minimal, moderate, or marked, based on the amplitude range. The moderate (normal) amplitude range is between 6 and 25 beats/min. If the FHR variability is normal, regardless of what other FHR patterns may be present, the fetus is not experiencing cerebral tissue acidemia. This is because the fetus is able to centralize the available oxygen and is thus physiologically compensated. If excessive hypoxic stress persists, however, this compensation may break down, and the fetus may have progressive hypoxia in cerebral and myocardial tissues. In such cases, the FHR variability decreases and eventually is lost.

There are several possible nonhypoxic causes of decreased or absent FHR variability:

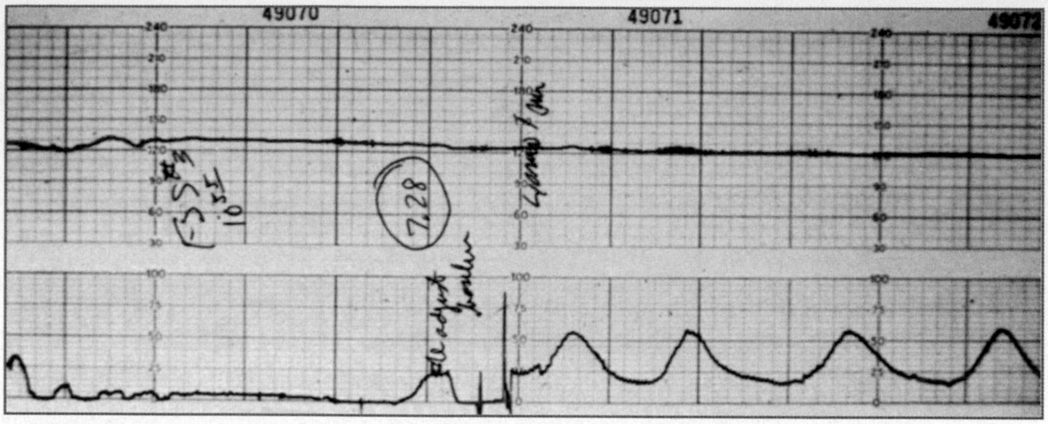

FIGURE 22-3 **No variability of fetal heart rate.** The mother had severe preeclampsia and was receiving magnesium sulfate and narcotics. The normal scalp blood pH (7.28) ensures that the absence of variability is nonasphyxic in origin and that the fetus is not chronically asphyxiated and decompensating. The uterine activity channel has an inaccurate trace in the first half.

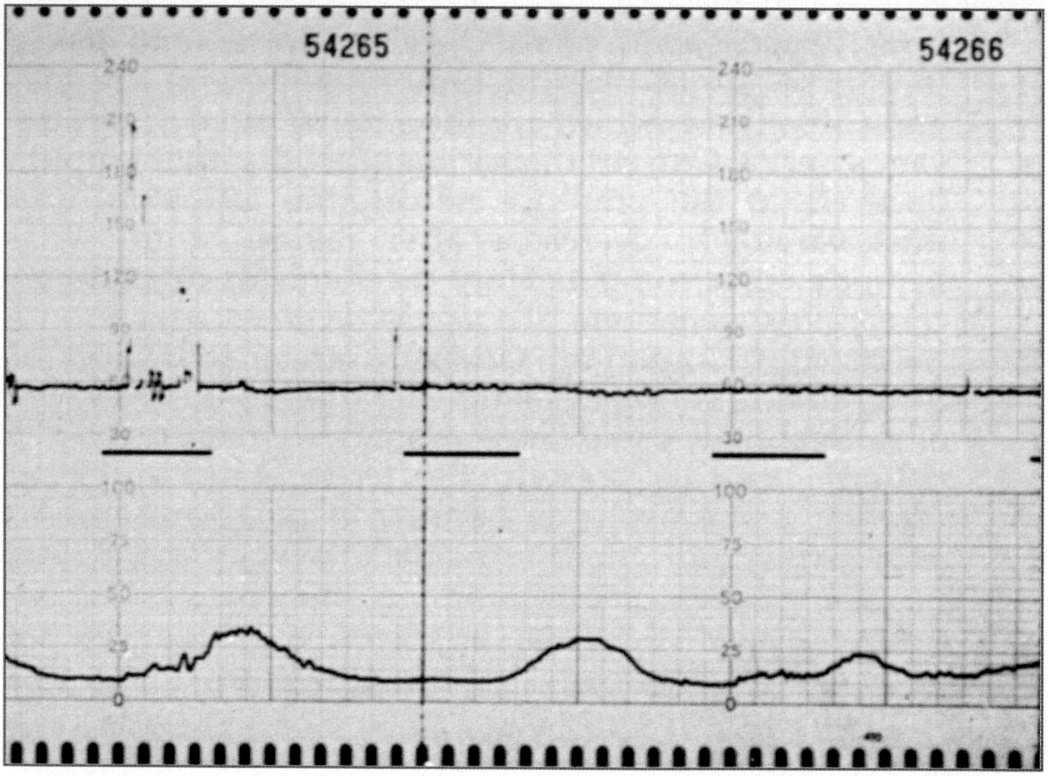

FIGURE 22-4 **Unremitting fetal bradycardia.** This tracing does not signify asphyxia, because this fetus had complete heart block, with a ventricular rate of about 55 beats/min. Note the absence of fetal heart rate variability. There were serious cardiac structural defects, and the fetus died shortly after birth.

1. Absence of the cortex (anencephaly)
2. Narcotized or drugged higher centers (e.g., by morphine, meperidine, diazepam) (Fig. 22-3)
3. Vagal blockade (e.g., by atropine or scopolamine)
4. Defective cardiac conduction system (e.g., complete heart block) (Fig. 22-4)

Periodic Changes in Fetal Heart Rate

LATE DECELERATIONS

Late decelerations (Fig. 22-5) are of two varieties: reflex and nonreflex.[4,71-73]

Reflex late deceleration is sometimes seen when an acute insult (e.g., reduced uterine blood flow resulting from maternal hypotension) is superimposed on a previously normally oxygenated fetus in the presence of contractions. These late decelerations are caused by a decrease in uterine blood flow (with the uterine contraction) beyond the capacity of the fetus to extract sufficient oxygen. The relatively deoxygenated blood is carried from the fetal placenta through the umbilical vein to the heart and is distributed to the aorta, neck vessels, and head. Here, the low PO_2 is sensed by chemoreceptors, and neuronal activity results in a vagal discharge, which causes the transient deceleration. The deceleration is presumed to be "late" because of the circulation time from

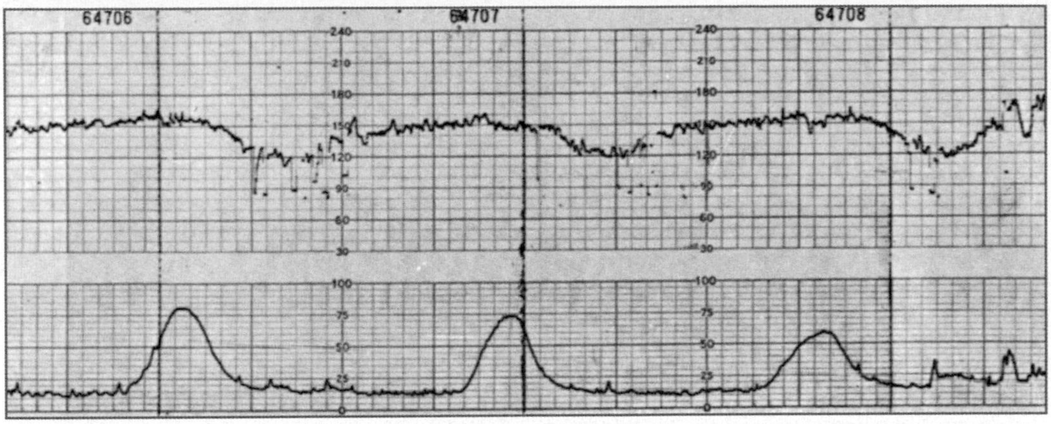

FIGURE 22-5 **Late decelerations.** These were recorded via Doppler ultrasound in the antepartum period in a severely growth-restricted (1700-g) term infant born to a 32-year old preeclamptic primipara. Delivery was by cesarean section because neither a direct fetal electrocardiogram nor a fetal blood sample could be obtained due to a firm closed posterior cervix. The infant subsequently did well.

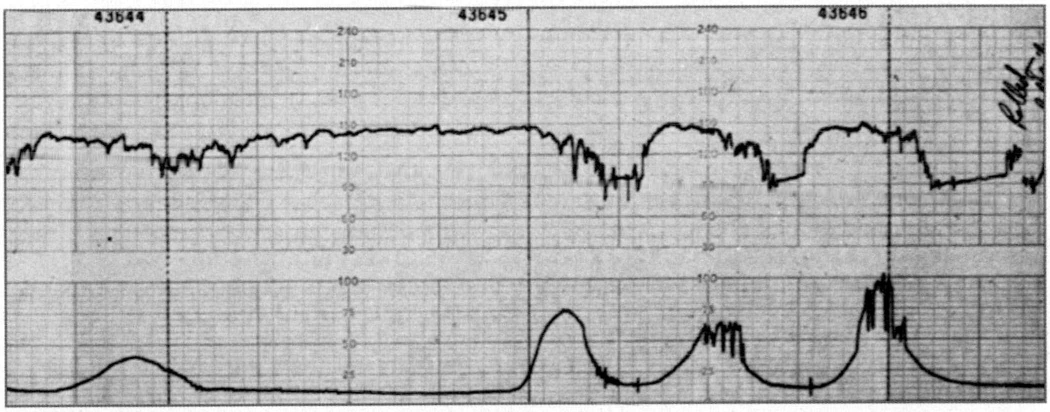

FIGURE 22-6 **Reflex late decelerations.** The fetal heart rate pattern was previously normal, but late decelerations appeared after severe maternal hypotension (70/30 mm Hg), which was a result of sympathetic blockade caused by a caudal anesthetic agent.

the fetal placental site to the chemoreceptors and because the progressively decreasing P_{O_2} must reach a certain threshold before vagal activity occurs. There may also be baroreceptor activity causing the vagal discharge.[71] Between contractions, oxygen delivery is adequate and there is no additional vagal activity, so the baseline FHR is normal. These reflex late decelerations are accompanied by normal FHR variability and thus signify normal central nervous system integrity (i.e., the fetus is physiologically "compensated" in the vital organs) (Fig. 22-6).

The second type of late deceleration results from the same initial mechanism, except that the deoxygenated bolus of blood from the placenta is presumed to be insufficient to support myocardial action. Thus, for the period of the contraction, there is direct myocardial hypoxic depression (or failure) and vagal activity.[71,73] These *nonreflex late decelerations* are seen without variability (Fig. 22-7), signifying fetal "decompensation" (i.e., inadequate fetal cerebral and myocardial oxygenation). They are seen most commonly in states of decreased placental reserve (e.g., preeclampsia, intrauterine growth restriction) or after prolonged hypoxic stress (e.g., a long period of severe reflex late decelerations).

Further support for the two etiologic mechanisms of late decelerations comes from observations on chronically catheterized fetal monkeys in spontaneous labor during the course of intrauterine death.[74] The animals were initially observed with normal blood gases, normal FHR variability, presence of accelerations, and no persistent periodic changes. After a variable period of time, they first demonstrated late decelerations and retained accelerations. This period was associated with a small decline in ascending aortic P_{O_2}, from 28 to 24 mm Hg, and a normal acid-base state. These late decelerations were probably of the vagal reflex type caused by chemoreceptor activity. At an average of more than 3 days after the onset of these reflex decelerations, accelerations were lost in the presence of worsening hypoxia (P_{O_2}, 19 mm Hg) and acidemia (pH, 7.22). Fetal death followed an average of 36 hours of persistent late decelerations, and these latter decelerations without accelerations were presumed to be of the nonreflex myocardial depression type.

When late decelerations are present, one should make efforts to optimize placental blood flow and maternal oxygenation and ensure that maternal blood pressure is normal.

VARIABLE DECELERATIONS

Variable decelerations (Fig. 22-8), have the following characteristics:

1. They are variable in duration, depth, and shape.
2. They are usually abrupt in onset and cessation.

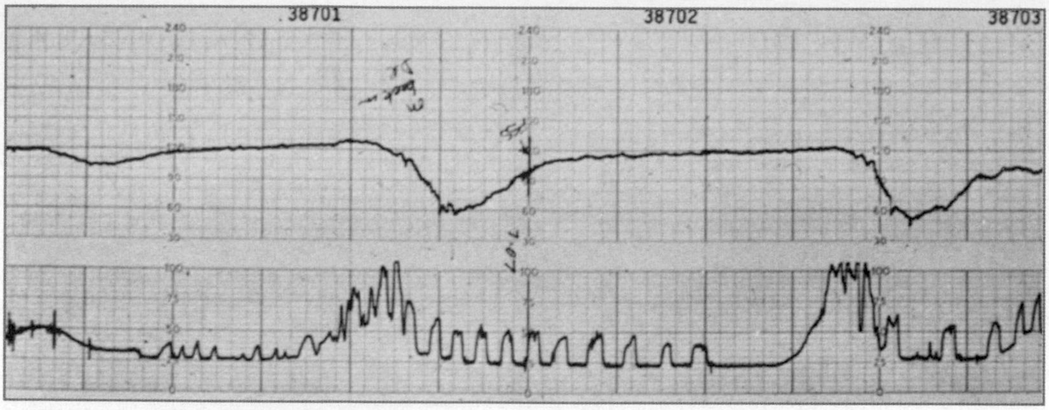

FIGURE 22-7 **Nonreflex late decelerations with virtual absence of fetal heart rate (FHR) variability.** The decelerations represent transient asphyxic myocardial failure as well as intermittent vagal decreases in heart rate. The lack of FHR variability also signifies decreased cerebral oxygenation. Note the acidemia in fetal scalp blood (7.07). The infant, a 3340-g girl with Apgar scores of 3 (1 minute) and 4 (5 minutes) was delivered soon after this tracing. Cesarean section was considered to be contraindicated because of a severe preeclamptic coagulopathy.

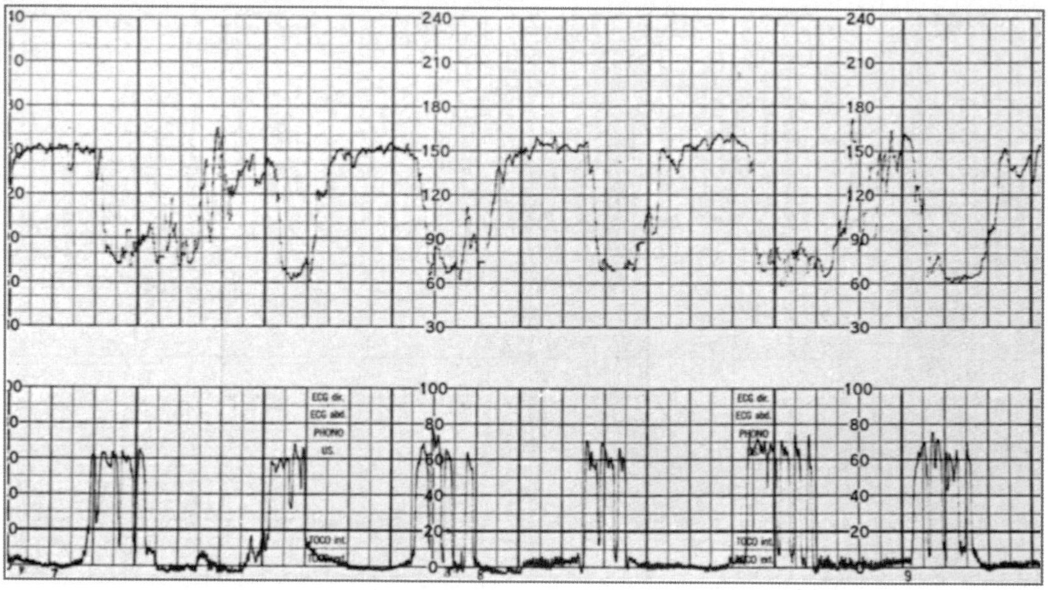

FIGURE 22-8 **Variable decelerations.** Intrapartum recording using fetal scalp electrode and tocodynamometer. The spikes in the uterine activity channel represent maternal pushing efforts in the second stage of labor. The normal baseline variability between contractions signifies normal central oxygenation despite the intermittent hypoxic stress represented by the moderate variable decelerations.

3. They are not reassuring when there is either a slow return to baseline, a rise in baseline, or an absence of variability in the baseline between decelerations.

EFFECT OF IN UTERO TREATMENT

Fetal oxygenation can be improved, acidemia relieved, and variant FHR patterns abolished by certain modes of treatment. The events that result in fetal stress (recognized by FHR patterns) are presented in Table 22-10 together with the recommended treatment maneuvers and presumed mechanisms for improving fetal oxygenation. These should be the primary maneuvers carried out; if the hypoxic event is acute and the fetus was previously normoxic, there is an excellent chance that the undesired FHR pattern will be abolished.

If the FHR pattern cannot be improved (i.e., if the stress patterns indicative of peripheral tissue or central tissue hypoxia persist for a significant period), further diagnostic steps or delivery may be indicated. Certain patterns are of such a severe character that immediate delivery is warranted if they cannot rapidly be relieved (Figs. 22-9 and 22-10).

Other Patterns

SINUSOIDAL PATTERN

The sinusoidal pattern is a regular, smooth, sine wave–like baseline, with a frequency of approximately 3 to 6 cycles per minute and an amplitude range of up to 30 beats/min. The regularity of the waves distinguishes this pattern from long-term variability complexes, which are crudely shaped and irregular. Another distinguishing feature is the absence of beat-to-beat or short-term variability (Fig. 22-11).

The sinusoidal pattern was first described in a group of severely affected Rh-alloimmunized fetuses but was subsequently noted in

TABLE 22-10 INTRAUTERINE TREATMENT FOR VARIANT FETAL HEART RATE (FHR) PATTERNS

Causes	Possible Resulting FHR Patterns	Corrective Maneuver	Mechanism
Hypotension (e.g., supine hypotension, conduction anesthesia)	Bradycardia, late decelerations	Intravenous fluids, position change, ephedrine	Return of uterine blood flow toward normal
Excessive uterine activity	Bradycardia, late decelerations	Decrease in oxytocin, lateral position	Same as above
Transient umbilical cord compression	Variable decelerations	Change in maternal position (e.g., left or right lateral, Trendelenburg) Amnioinfusion	Presumably removes fetal part from cord Relieves compression of cord
Head compression	Early or variable decelerations	Push only with alternate contractions	Allows fetal recovery
Decreased uterine blood flow associated with uterine contraction	Late decelerations	Change in maternal position (e.g., left lateral or Trendelenburg) Tocolytic agents (e.g., terbutaline)	Enhancement of uterine blood flow toward optimum Decrease in contractions or tone
Prolonged asphyxia	Decreasing FHR variability*	Change in maternal position (e.g., left lateral or Trendelenburg), establishment of maternal hyperoxia	Enhancement of uterine blood flow to optimum, increase in maternal-fetal oxygen gradient

***During labor, this is virtually always preceded by a heart rate pattern signifying asphyxial stress (e.g., late decelerations, usually severe), severe variable decelerations, or a prolonged bradycardia. This is not necessarily so in the antepartum period, before the onset of uterine contractions.**

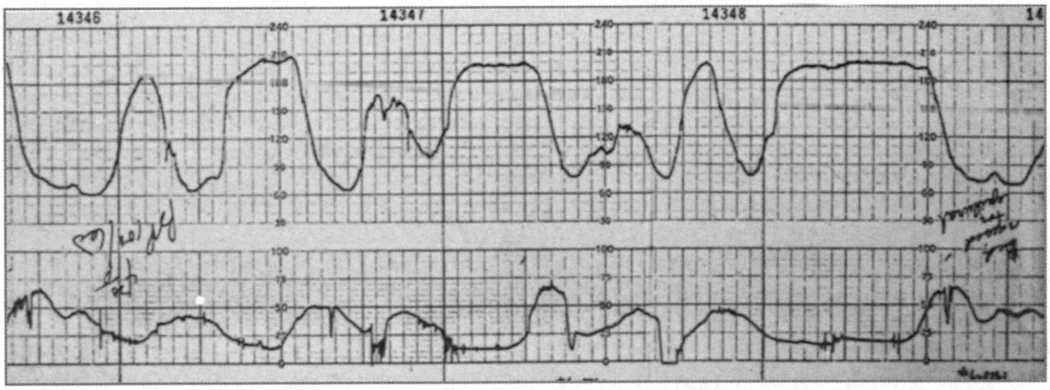

FIGURE 22-9 **Sinister heart rate pattern in a 28-week fetus (gestational age determined after delivery) with baseline tachycardia, absence of heart rate variability, and severe periodic changes.** The scalp blood pH was 7.0, and the fetus died shortly after this tracing was made. Cesarean section was not performed because the fetus was believed to be previable, although in fact it weighed 1100 g. There is much artifact in the uterine activity channel.

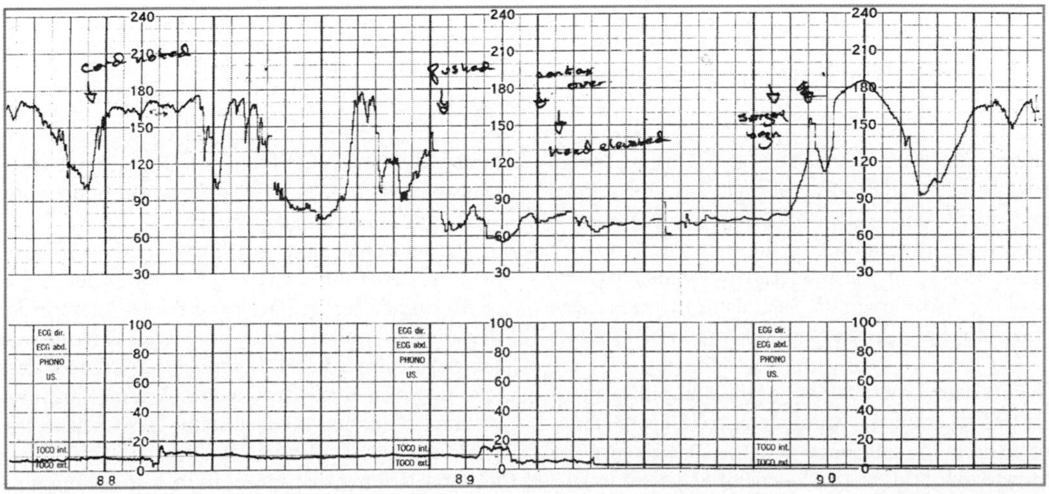

FIGURE 22-10 **Bradycardia resulting from cord prolapse.** The infant was delivered by cesarean section and did well.

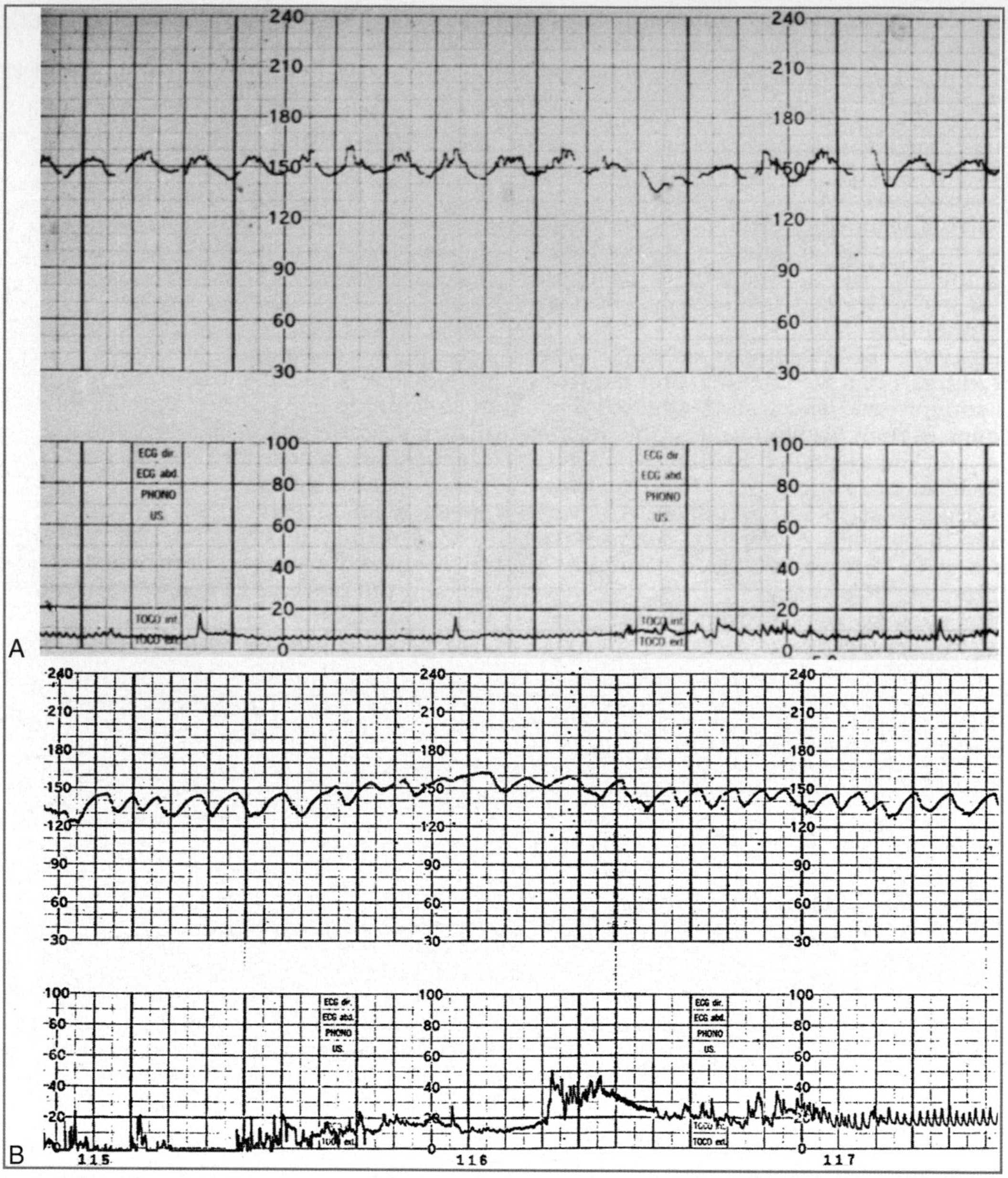

FIGURE 22-11 Sinusoidal pattern. **A** and **B,** Sinusoidal pattern in a term fetus with severe hemolysis caused by Rh disease. Cord hematocrit was 20%, and the infant, delivered by cesarean section, was subsequently normal. Recording by direct fetal electrode.

association with fetuses that were anemic for other reasons and in severely depressed infants. It was also described in cases of normal infants born without depression or acid-base abnormalities, but in these cases there is dispute about whether the patterns were truly sinusoidal or whether, because of the moderately irregular pattern, they were variants of long-term variability. Such patterns, often called pseudosinusoidal, may also be seen after administration of narcotics to the mother.

It is believed that an essential characteristic of the sinusoidal pattern is extreme regularity and smoothness. Murata and colleagues[75] implicated arginine vasopressin in the sinusoidal pattern. The presence of a sinusoidal pattern or variant of this in an Rh-sensitized patient usually suggests anemia with a fetal hematocrit value of less than 30%. The presence of hydrops in such a fetus suggests a fetal hematocrit of 15% or lower. Many severely anemic Rh-affected fetuses do not have a sinusoidal pattern but rather have a rounded, blunted pattern, and accelerations are usually absent.

If a sinusoidal pattern is seen in an Rh-sensitized patient and severe hemolysis is confirmed (by peak systolic velocity measurement of flow in the middle cerebral artery of the fetus, by cordocentesis, or by the deviation in optical density at 450 nm determination by spectrophotometry of amniotic fluid), rapid intervention is needed. This step may take the form of delivery or intrauterine transfusion, depending on gestational age and the fetal status (see Chapter 26).

Management of a sinusoidal pattern in the absence of alloimmunization is somewhat more difficult to recommend. If the pattern is persistent, monotonously regular, and unaccompanied by short-term variability and cannot be abolished by the maneuvers just described,

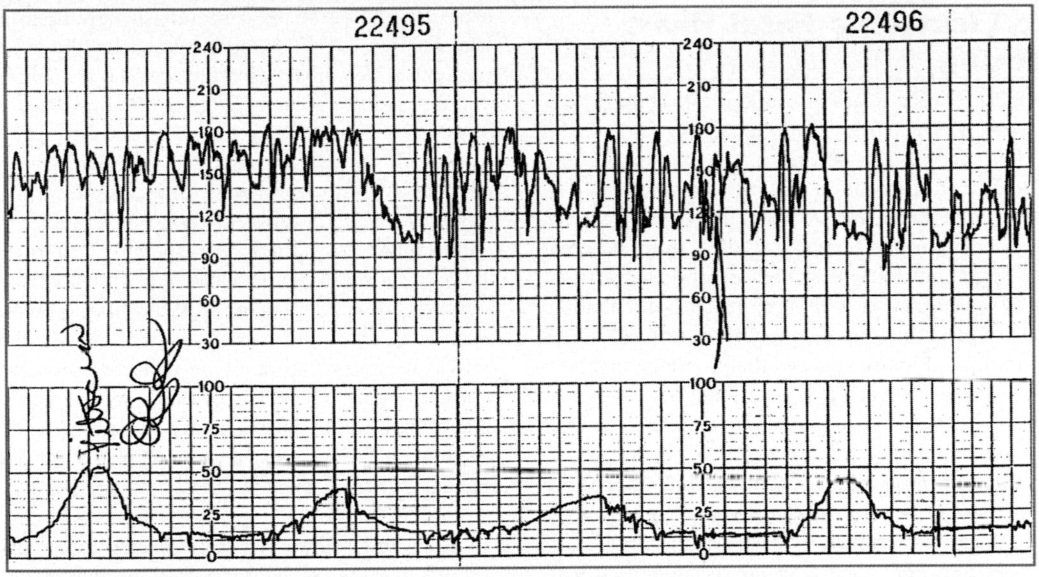

FIGURE 22-12 Saltatory pattern. Saltatory pattern showing excessive fetal heart rate variability of up to 60 beats/min in brief intervals, probably representing mild hypoxic stress.

further workup and evaluation of the adequacy of fetal oxygenation (e.g., contraction stress test, fetal stimulation test, biophysical profile, fetal blood sampling) are indicated. Nonalloimmune sinusoidal patterns have been associated with severe fetal acidemia and with fetal anemia resulting from fetal-maternal bleeding. The latter diagnosis is supported by the identification of fetal red blood cells in maternal blood, detected by the Kleihauer-Betke test. If the pattern is irregularly sinusoidal or pseudosinusoidal, intermittently present, and not associated with intervening periodic decelerations, fetal compromise is unlikely, and immediate delivery is not warranted.

SALTATORY PATTERN

The saltatory pattern consists of rapid variations in FHR with a frequency of 3 to 6 cycles per minute and an amplitude range greater than 25 beats/min (Fig. 22-12). It is qualitatively described as a marked variability, and the variations have a strikingly bizarre appearance. The saltatory pattern is seen during labor rather than in the antepartum period. The etiology is uncertain, but it may be similar to that of the increased FHR variability seen in animal experiments with brief and acute hypoxia in a previously normoxic fetus. Therefore, efforts should be made to optimize placental blood flow and fetal oxygenation if such a pattern appears during labor.

Congenital Anomalies

Except as described for the dysrhythmias, most fetuses with congenital anomalies have essentially normal FHR patterns and respond to hypoxia in a manner similar to the normal fetus. There are several exceptions, including complete heart block and anencephaly. Aneuploid fetuses and fetuses with aplastic lungs, meningomyelocele, and/or hydrocephalus may give no FHR warning of such underlying defects, because they are not necessarily experiencing hypoxia or acidosis. However, even though there was no pathognomonic pattern in such fetuses, the rate of cesarean section for fetal intolerance to labor was reported to be significantly increased, presumably because of nonreassuring patterns during or preceding labor.[76]

Efficacy, Risks, and Recommendations for Usage

Electronic Monitoring versus Auscultation

Because there are no prospective randomized clinical trials comparing EFM with no fetal heart monitoring during labor, most efforts to suggest its efficacy have relied on research reports comparing EFM with intermittent auscultation. Efficacy is generally held to be an expected decrease in complications, which, for FHR monitoring, could include fetal death in labor or severe neonatal and pediatric morbidity (e.g., neonatal seizures, cerebral palsy). Ideally, the improved outcomes would be accompanied by appropriate interventions and appropriate noninterventions.

In a meta-analysis of the nine published clinical studies comparing EFM with intermittent auscultation of the FHR, several conclusions were reached.[77] (It should be noted that in several of these trials, patients with conditions considered to be high risk were not randomized for study inclusion.) The use of EFM was associated with significant increases in the rate of cesarean delivery for fetal intolerance to labor, the overall cesarean delivery rate, and the use of instrumentation for vaginal delivery (both vacuum and forceps). However, there was no reduced overall perinatal mortality in these patients. As a result of such reports, either option of monitoring the fetus during labor is acceptable for patients not considered to be at high risk.[67] However, it should be noted that the optimal frequency for intermittent auscultation in such low-risk patients has not been established. At a minimum, the FHR should be assessed at least every 30 minutes in the first stage of labor and every 15 minutes in the second stage.[67] Another method is to auscultate and record FHR every 15 minutes in the active first stage of labor and every 5 minutes in the second stage, without limiting such a modality to low-risk patients.[78]

Adjuncts to Electronic Fetal Heart Rate Monitoring

The initial belief with EFM when it was introduced into clinical practice more than 35 years ago was that it would identify fetuses with impending stillbirth or damaging asphyxia in an appropriate and timely manner to allow for the prevention of untoward outcomes. The result would be improved perinatal and neonatal outcomes. However, several well-designed, randomized clinical studies from different clinical centers involving almost 40,000 women in labor suggest that intrapartum EFM, when compared with intermittent auscultation, does not result in any measurable improvement in outcome.[79,80] This is certainly disappointing, and it also suggests that the thinking about the risks associated with intrapartum events and adverse long-term neurologic outcomes needs to be re-evaluated. Of note, these studies did reveal a strong correlation between certain EFM patterns and fetal acidosis as measured by both the base deficit and the umbilical artery pH. In addition, with respect to the specific end point of neonatal seizures, several of these trials reported that there were significantly fewer such cases after intrapartum EFM than after labors monitored with intermittent auscultation. This end point, however, does not serve as a true surrogate for long-term neurologic brain damage, because, in many of these cases, damage was no longer evident with repeat examination as the child grew older.

Nevertheless, the clinical reality is that, because of the labor intensity demanded of the nursing staff when intermittent auscultation is employed as in these prospective studies, along with the diminishing number of nurses available to most hospital labor and delivery units, it is not practical to offer most laboring patients the option of intermittent auscultation. This is particularly true for "high-risk" patients, and, as a result, EFM has become the default option for most modern obstetric units. At least for the foreseeable future, despite its limitations and disappointments, EFM will continue to be utilized frequently in the management of labor in this country.

With full knowledge of these issues, as well as the significant lack of concordance in the interpretation of monitor data showing anything but a reassuring pattern, efforts continue to be made to provide appropriate adjuncts to EFM. There continues to be an unacceptably high-false positive rate with EFM, as well as an occasional false-negative result. Historically, fetal scalp blood sampling was used in an effort to accurately identify the fetus with an acidotic pH. Unfortunately, this is a cumbersome and challenging procedure that is associated with complications and is currently not an option in most hospitals providing obstetric care. Efforts to obtain a continuous measure of the fetal pH have also been unsuccessful for a number of reasons.

More recently, efforts to directly assess fetal oxygenation (fetal pulse oximetry) or to more closely interpret the fetal ECG (ST-waveform analysis) have been studied as complementary technologies to improve both sensitivity and specificity for prediction of fetal intrapartum hypoxia and/or acidosis.

Fetal Pulse Oximetry

EFM is intended to assess fetal oxygenation indirectly, as reflected in specific changes in FHR. FHR monitoring is not a direct measure of fetal oxygenation, and it has insufficient specificity and sensitivity to correctly identify the fetus who is in oxygen debt. Continuous direct assessment of fetal oxygenation has been proposed as a technique to overcome the suboptimal specificity and sensitivity of continuous FHR monitoring. Ideally, a monitor that measures fetal oxygenation or pH directly would be preferable to accurately identify the physiologically compromised fetus. Efforts to develop instrumentation to measure fetal oxygenation or pH continuously have been limited by difficulty with fetal access, safety, and accuracy of the information generated (e.g., stasis of capillary blood in the fetal scalp during active labor).

Pulse oximetry has been a significant advance in the assessment of oxygenation status for adult and pediatric patients. Essentially all patients in surgery, recovery, and intensive care units are monitored continuously with a noninvasive, transcutaneously applied pulse oximeter. Pulse oximetry provides a continuous source of reliable information about oxygen status in intraoperative and critically ill patients that has been shown to dramatically reduce the number of hypoxia-related anesthetic deaths.[81] Several obstacles have prevented the use of this technology for intrapartum fetal assessment, including access to the fetus (ruptured membranes are required), an appropriate surface on which to apply the sensor (a stable surface is needed that will not change significantly during labor), and differences in fetal versus adult physiology (the fetal blood pressure is lower, whereas the pulse and hemoglobin are higher, and the oxyhemoglobin dissociation is different than in the adult).

Adult and pediatric pulse oximetry uses transmission oximetry technology, in which light is passed through tissue to a sensor on the opposite side of the patient's finger or earlobe. The noninvasive determination of oxygen saturation is founded on the differential absorption of red and infrared light by oxyhemoglobin and deoxyhemoglobin: Less red light and more infrared light are absorbed by oxyhemoglobin than by deoxyhemoglobin. The ratio of these differences is used to measure the oxygen saturation during each arterial pulse.

Detection of oxygen saturation in the fetus has been difficult because the fetus has no body part that can be used for transmission oximetry. This technical problem has been addressed by the development of a sensor that remains stable when applied to the fetal cheek or back and that uses reflectance oximetry, in which light is emitted and then reflected to a photosensor located on the same probe by the underlying fetal tissue (OxiFirst Fetal Oxygen Saturation Monitoring System, Mallinckrodt/Nellcor, Pleasanton, CA).

Studies have related the oxygen saturation as measured by reflectance pulse oximetry to fetal arterial oxygen saturation measured directly in fetal lambs[82] and to fetal scalp pH in humans.[83] Dildy and coworkers[84] suggested that an arterial oxygen saturation of 30% is a reasonable threshold to detect acidemia. This conclusion was based on their analysis of 1101 paired umbilical artery and vein gases, in which significant umbilical acidemia (arterial pH <7.13) occurred rarely (1.6%) when arterial oxygen saturation exceeded 30%; acidemia was more common (10.4%) when the arterial oxygen saturation was lower than 30%. Other studies[85,86] investigated the time required to produce metabolic acidosis in the human fetus in labor. They found that fetal acidemia did not occur unless the fetal pulse oximeter revealed a saturation lower than a critical threshold of 30% for longer than 2 minutes.

Garite and colleagues[87] applied fetal pulse oximetry to a population of more than 1000 laboring women who had FHR tracings that were worrisome but not sufficiently ominous to require immediate delivery, including (1) mild or moderate decelerations for longer than 30 minutes, (2) a baseline FHR of 100 to 110 beats/min without accelerations, (3) a baseline FHR of less than 100 or more than 160 beats/min, (4) variability less than 5 or greater than 25 beats/min, (5) late decelerations, or (6) prolonged decelerations. Patients were randomly assigned to receive FHR monitoring alone or FHR plus fetal pulse oximetry. In those assigned to the latter group, if the FHR tracing was reassuring, labor was allowed to continue regardless of the fetal pulse oximetry level. If the FHR tracing was ominous, delivery was accomplished, again regardless of the fetal pulse oximetry data. However, the pulse oximetry data were used if the FHR tracing was nonreassuring which was not uncommon in these patients. In such cases, labor was allowed to continue if the fetal oxygen saturation was greater than 30%, and delivery was recommended if the fetal oxygen saturation was lower than 30% for the entire interval between two contractions. The primary end point was the rate of cesarean section performed for fetal intolerance to labor. This rate was significantly decreased with fetal pulse oximetry, but the rate of cesarean delivery for dystocia was correspondingly increased, and the overall rate of cesarean section was not different in the FHR versus FHR plus pulse oximetry groups.

In response to the various reports of the potential use of fetal pulse oximetry, the ACOG Committee on Obstetric Practice did not endorse the adoption of this device "because of concerns that its introduction could further escalate the cost of medical care without necessarily improving clinical outcome."[88] As with other technologic developments, obstetricians have been anxious to adopt new techniques despite the lack of adequate trials demonstrating clinical efficacy. In a recent large study, use of fetal pulse oximetry was not associated with a reduction in cesarean delivery rate or improved neonatal outcome in patients monitored continuously with EFM.[89] Although other investigators have reported clinical efficacy with this modality and the argument can be made that this added information regarding fetal status during labor is helpful in selected patients, the discussion regarding the clinical value of fetal pulse oximetry is now moot, because the device is no longer being produced and marketed for use in this country.

ST Analysis of Fetal Electrocardiography

Adult humans experiencing metabolic acidosis, anaerobic metabolism, and hypoxia of the myocardium demonstrate changes in their ECG. Specifically, there may be depression or elevation of the ST segment, as well as T wave changes. An increase in the ST segment and in the T wave of the fetal ECG in response to hypoxia has been demonstrated in fetal animal studies.[90] T-wave height compared with QRS height (T/QRS ratio) can be used as a means to express such changes.[91]

ST analysis, or STAN (Neoventa Medical, Moelndal, Sweden), is a fetal monitoring technology that has evolved to address these basic physiologic changes associated with hypoxia. STAN combines the routine visual assessment of the intrapartum EFM tracing with an automated analysis of the fetal ECG. A modified gold-plated fetal scalp electrode is used.. STAN performs a computer analysis of the fetal ECG specific to the detection of ST-segment changes that may be predictive of fetal hypoxia during labor. In a randomized control trial, Swedish investigators reported that fetal ECG analysis using STAN, when combined with the standard EFM techniques, lowered the rates of operative delivery for fetal intolerance to labor, severe fetal metabolic acidosis (pH <7.05 and base deficit >12 mmol/L), and neonatal encephalopathy, compared with EFM alone, in term laboring patients who were deemed to be candidates for continuous EFM.[92,93] In a report from the United States, the appropriate use of STAN technology was measured and confirmed.[94] In this nonrandomized feasibility study, trained clinicians demonstrated the ability to appropriately apply STAN in cases requiring delivery interventions or noninterventions, compared with experienced STAN users. A negative predictive value of 95.2% was reported for nonintervention in cases with nonreassuring EFM patterns, with normal STAN readings and normal neonatal outcomes with umbilical arterial pH greater than 7.12. Further, there was an 84% agreement for intervention and a 90% agreement for nonintervention between investigators and three STAN experts when the cases were retrospectively reviewed.

It is important to note that these reports are essentially limited to singleton pregnancies in labor at or beyond 36 weeks' gestation. In addition, the STAN system requires a period of time, usually 20 minutes, to assess the fetal ECG and establish the normal and abnormal parameters before it is able to identify significant changes suggestive of fetal hypoxia. Other concerns include a frequency of 2% to 3% for missing ST data due to poor signal quality or continuous absence of data for unclear reasons. With correct scalp electrode placement and further improvements in the processing of the ECG signal, it is hoped that these errors will become less frequent.

References

1. Mendez-Bauer C, Poseirio JJ, Arellano-Hernandez G, et al: Effects of atropine on the heart rate of the human fetus during labor. Am J Obstet Gynecol 85:1033, 1963.
2. DeHaan J, Stolte LAM, Veth AFL, et al: The significance of short-term irregularity in the fetal heart rate pattern. In Dudenhausen JW, Saling E (eds): Perinatale Medezin, vol 4. Stuttgart, Thieme Verlag, 1973, p 398.
3. Schifferli PY, Caldeyro-Barcia R: Effect of atropine and beta adrenergic drugs on the heart rate of the human fetus. In Boreus L (ed): Fetal Pharmacology. New York, Raven Press, 1973.
4. Parer JT: Handbook of Fetal Heart Rate Monitoring, 2nd ed. Philadelphia, Saunders, 1997.
5. Llanos AJ, Green JR, Creasy RK, et al: Increased heart rate response to parasympathetic and beta-adrenergic blockade in growth-retarded fetal lambs. Am J Obstet Gynecol 136:808, 1980.
6. Hanson MA: The importance of baro- and chemo-reflexes in the control of the fetal cardiovascular system. J Dev Physiol 10:491, 1988.
7. Nijhuis JG, Prechtl HFR, Martin CB Jr, et al: Are there behavioural states in the human fetus? Early Hum Dev 6:177, 1982.
8. Anderson PAW, Glick KL, Killam AP, et al: The effect of heart rate on in utero left ventricular output in the fetal sheep. J Physiol 372:557, 1986.
9. Anderson PAW, Killam AP, Mainwaring RD, et al: In utero right ventricular output in the fetal lamb: The effect of heart rate. J Physiol 387:297, 1987.
10. Hon EH: An Atlas of Fetal Heart Rate Patterns. New Haven, Harty Press, 1968.
11. Cohn HE, Sacks EJ, Heymann MA, et al: Cardiovascular responses to hypoxemia and acidemia in fetal lambs. Am J Obstet Gynecol 120:817, 1974.
12. Jones MD, Sheldon RE, Peeters LL, et al: Fetal cerebral oxygen consumption at different levels of oxygenation. J Appl Physiol 43:1080, 1977.
13. Fisher DS, Heymann MA, Rudolph AM: Fetal myocardial oxygen and carbohydrate consumption during acutely induced hypoxemia. Am J Physiol 242:H657, 1982.
14. Yaffe H, Parer JT, Block BS, et al: Cardiorespiratory responses to graded reductions of uterine blood flow in the sheep fetus. J Dev Physiol 9:325, 1987.
15. Myers RE: Two patterns of brain damage and their conditions of occurrence. Am J Obstet Gynecol 112:246, 1972.
16. American College of Obstetricians and Gynecologists (ACOG): Obstetricians and Gynecologists: Umbilical Artery Blood Acid-Base Analysis. Technical Bulletin No. 216. Washington, DC, ACOG, November 1995.
17. James EJ, Raye JR, Gresham EL, et al: Fetal oxygen consumption, carbon dioxide production and glucose uptake in a chronic sheep preparation. Pediatrics 50:361, 1972.
18. Landon MB: Acid-base disorders during pregnancy. Clin Obstet Gynecol 37:16, 1994.
19. Blechner JN: Maternal-fetal acid-base physiology. Clin Obstet Gynecol 36:3, 1993.
20. Aarnoudse JG, Deesley NP, Penfold P, et al: Permeability of the human placenta to bicarbonate: In vitro perfusion studies. BJOG 91:1096, 1984.
21. Cunningham FGC, Gant NF, Leveno KJ, et al: The newborn infant. In Cunningham FGC, Gant NF, Leveno KJ, et al (eds): Williams Obstetrics, 21st ed. New York, McGraw-Hill, 2001, p 385.
22. Goldaber KG, Gilstrap LC, Leveno KJ, et al: Pathologic fetal acidemia. Obstet Gynecol 78:1103, 1991.

23. Coleman MT, Rund DA: Nonobstetric conditions causing hypoxia during pregnancy: Asthma and epilepsy. Am J Obstet Gynecol 177:1, 1997.
24. Huff RW: Asthma in pregnancy. Med Clin North Am 73:653, 1989.
25. American College of Obstetricians and Gynecologists Committee on Obstetric Practice: Use and Abuse of the Apgar Score. Committee Opinion No. 174. Washington, DC, ACOG, July 1996.
26. Lievaart M, de Jong PA: Acid-base equilibrium in umbilical cord blood and time of cord clamping. Obstet Gynecol 63:44, 1984.
27. Riley RJ, Johnson JWC: Collecting and analyzing cord blood gases. Clin Obstet Gynecol 36:13, 1993.
28. D'Souza SW, Black P, Cadman J, et al: Umbilical venous blood pH: A useful aid in the diagnosis of asphyxia at birth. Arch Dis Child 58:15, 1983.
29. Kirshon B, Moise KJ: Effect of heparin on umbilical arterial blood gases. J Reprod Med 34:955-959, 1989.
30. Duerbeck NB, Chaffin DG, Seeds JW: A practical approach to umbilical artery pH and blood gas determinations. Obstet Gynecol 79:959, 1992.
31. Valenzuela P, Guijarro R: The effects of time on pH and gas values in the blood contained in the umbilical cord. Acta Obstet Gynecol Scand 85:1307-1309, 2006.
32. Strickland DM, Gilstrap LC III, Hauth JC, et al: Umbilical cord pH and PCO2: Effect of interval from delivery to determination. Am J Obstet Gynecol 148:191, 1984.
33. Meyer BA, Thorp JA, Cohen GR, et al: Umbilical cord blood gases: The effect of smoking on delayed sampling from the placenta (abstract no. 158). Am J Obstet Gynecol 170:320, 1994.
34. Chauhan SP, Cowan BD, Meydrech EF, et al: Determination of fetal acidemia at birth from a remote umbilical arterial blood gas analysis. Am J Obstet Gynecol 170:1705, 1994.
35. Huisjes HJ, Aarnoudse JG: Arterial or venous umbilical pH as a measure of neonatal morbidity? Early Hum Dev 3:155, 1979.
36. Goldaber KG, Gilstrap LC III: Correlations between obstetric clinical events and umbilical cord acid-base and blood gas values. Clin Obstet Gynecol 36:47, 1993.
37. Gilstrap LC, Leveno KJ, Burris JB, et al: Diagnoses of birth asphyxia based on fetal pH, Apgar score and newborn cerebral dysfunction. Am J Obstet Gynecol 161:825, 1989.
38. King TA, Jackson GL, Josey AS, et al: The effect of profound umbilical artery acidemia in term neonates admitted to a newborn nursery. J Pediatr 132:624, 1998.
39. Sehdev HM, Stamilio DM, Macones GA, et al: Predictive factors for neonatal morbidity in neonates with an umbilical arterial pH less than 7.00. Am J Obstet Gynecol 177:1030, 1997.
40. Andres RL, Saade MD, Gilstrap LC, et al: Association between umbilical blood gas parameters and neonatal morbidity and death in neonates with pathologic fetal acidemia. Am J Obstet Gynecol 181:867, 1999.
41. American College of Obstetricians and Gynecologists: ACOG Committee Opinion No. 348, November 2006: Umbilical cord blood gas and acid-base analysis. Obstet Gynecol 108:1319, 2006.
42. Low JA, Panagiotopoulos C, Derrick EJ, et al: Newborn complications after intrapartum asphyxia with metabolic acidosis in the term fetus. Am J Obstet Gynecol 170:1081, 1994.
43. Low JA: Intrapartum fetal asphyxia: Definition, diagnosis, and classification. Am J Obstet Gynecol 176:957, 1997.
44. Maberry MC, Ramin SM, Gilstrap LC, et al: Intrapartum asphyxia in pregnancies complicated by intraamniotic infection. Obstet Gynecol 76:351, 1990.
45. Hankins GDV, Snyder RR, Yeomans ER: Umbilical arterial and venous acid-base and blood gas values and the effect of chorioamnionitis on those values in a cohort of preterm infants. Am J Obstet Gynecol 164:1261, 1991.
46. Meyer BA, Dickinson JE, Chamber C, et al: The effect of fetal sepsis on umbilical cord blood gases. Am J Obstet Gynecol 166:612, 1992.
47. Hankins GDV, Snyder RR, Hauth JC, et al: Nuchal cords and neonatal outcome. Obstet Gynecol 70:687, 1987.
48. Mitchell J, Schulman H, Fleischer A, et al: Meconium aspiration and fetal acidosis. Obstet Gynecol 65:352, 1985.
49. Yeomans ER, Gilstrap LC, Leveno KL, et al: Meconium in the amniotic fluid and fetal acid-base status. Obstet Gynecol 73:175, 1989.
50. Ramin KD, Leveno KJ, Kelly MA, et al: Amniotic fluid meconium: A fetal environmental hazard. Obstet Gynecol 87:181, 1996.
51. Blackwell SC, Moldenhauer J, Hassan SS, et al: Meconium aspiration syndrome in term neonates with normal acid-base status at delivery: Is it different? Am J Obstet Gynecol 184:1422, 2001.
52. Silver RK, Dooley SL, MacGregor SN, et al: Fetal acidosis in prolonged pregnancy cannot be attributed to cord compression alone. Am J Obstet Gynecol 159:666, 1988.
53. Gilstrap LC, Hauth JC, Toussaint S: Second stage fetal heart rate abnormalities and neonatal acidosis. Obstet Gynecol 63:209, 1984.
54. Gilstrap LC, Hauth JC, Hankins GD, et al: Second-stage fetal heart rate abnormalities and type of neonatal acidemia. Obstet Gynecol 70:191, 1987.
55. Honjo S, Yamaguchi M: Umbilical artery blood acid-base analysis and fetal heart rate baseline in the second stage of labor. J Obstet Gynaecol Res 27:249, 2001.
56. Nelson KB, Dambrosia JM, Ting TY, et al: Uncertain value of electronic fetal monitoring in predicting cerebral palsy. N Engl J Med 334:613, 1996.
57. Gilstrap LC, Hauth JC, Schiano S, et al: Neonatal acidosis and method of delivery. Obstet Gynecol 63:681, 1984.
58. Luterkort M, Marsaál K: Umbilical cord acid-base state and Apgar score in term breech neonates. Acta Obstet Gynecol Scand 66:57, 1987.
59. Christian SS, Brady K: Cord blood acid-base values in breech-presenting infants born vaginally. Obstet Gynecol 78:778, 1991.
60. Gherman RB, Ouzounian JG, Goodwin TM: Obstetric maneuvers for shoulder dystocia and associated fetal morbidity. Am J Obstet Gynecol 178:1126, 1998.
61. Stallings SP, Edwards RK, Johnson JW: Correlation of head-to-body delivery intervals in shoulder dystocia and umbilical artery acidosis. Am J Obstet Gynecol 185:268, 2001.
62. Thorp JA, Boylan PC, Parisi VM, et al: Effects of high-dose oxytocin augmentation on umbilical cord blood gas values in primigravid women. Am J Obstet Gynecol 159:670, 1988.
63. Johnson JWC, Riley W: Cord blood gas studies: A survey. Clin Obstet Gynecol 36:99, 1993.
64. Royal College of Obstetricians and Gynaecologists, Royal College of Midwives: Toward safer childbirth: Minimum standards for the organization of labour wards. Report of a joint working party. London, RCOG Press, 1999, p 22.
65. Hon EH, Quilligan EJ: The classification of fetal heart rate. Conn Med 31:779, 1967.
66. National Institute of Child Health and Human Development Research Planning Workshop: Electronic fetal heart rate monitoring: Research guidelines for interpretation. Am J Obstet Gynecol 177:1385, 1997.
67. American College of Obstetricians and Gynecologists: Intrapartum Fetal Heart Rate Monitoring. Practice Bulletin No. 70. Washington, DC, ACOG, Decenber 2005.
68. Paul RH, Suidan AK, Yeh SY, et al: Clinical fetal monitoring: VII. The evaluation and significance of intrapartum baseline fetal heart rate variability. Am J Obstet Gynecol 123:206, 1975.
69. Krebs HB, Petres RE, Dunn LJ, et al: Intrapartum fetal heart rate monitoring: I. Classification and prognosis of fetal heart rate patterns. Am J Obstet Gynecol 133:762, 1979.
70. Nelson KB, Dambrosia JM, Ting TY, Grether JK: Uncertain value of electronic fetal monitoring in predicting cerbral palsy. N Engl J Med 324:613-618, 1996.
71. Martin CB Jr, DeHann J, van der Wildt B, et al: Mechanisms of late decelerations in the fetal heart rate: A study with autonomic blocking agents in fetal lambs. Eur J Obstet Gynaecol Reprod Biol 9:361, 1979.
72. Parer JT, Krueger TR, Harris JL: Fetal oxygen consumption and mechanisms of heart rate response during artificially produced late decelerations of fetal heart rate in sheep. Am J Obstet Gynecol 136:478, 1980.
73. Harris JL, Krueger TR, Parer JT: Mechanisms of late decelerations of the fetal heart rate during hypoxia. Am J Obstet Gynecol 144:491, 1982.

74. Murata Y, Martin CB, Ikenoue T, et al: Fetal heart rate accelerations and late decelerations during the course of intrauterine death in chronically catheterized rhesus monkeys. Am J Obstet Gynecol 144:218, 1982.
75. Murata Y, Miyake Y, Yamamoto T, et al: Experimentally produced sinusoidal fetal heart rate patterns in the chronically instrumented fetal lamb. Am J Obstet Gynecol 153:693, 1985.
76. Garite TJ, Linzey EM, Freeman RK, et al: Fetal heart rate patterns and fetal distress in fetuses with congenital anomalies. Obstet Gynecol 53:716, 1979.
77. Vintzileos AM, Nochimson DJ, Guzman EF, et al: Intrapartum fetal heart rate monitoring versus intermittent auscultation: A meta-analysis. Obstet Gynecol 85:149-155, 1995.
78. Vintzileos AM, Nochimson DJ, Antsaklis A, et al: Comparison of intrapartum electronic fetal heart rate monitoring versus intermittent auscultation in detecting fetal acidemia at birth. Am J Obste Gynecol 173:1021-1024, 1995.
79. Alfirevic Z, Devane D, Gyte GM: Continuous cariotocography (CTG) as a form of electronic fetal monitoring (EFM) for fetal assessment during labour. Cochrane Database Syst Rev. 2006;(3):CD006066.
80. Graham EM, Petersen SM, Christo DK, et al: Intrapartum electronic fetal heart rate monitoring and the prevention of perinatal brain injury. Obstet Gynecol 108:656-666, 2006.
81. Johnson N: Development and potential of pulse oximetry. Contemp Rev Obstet Gynecol 3:193, 1991.
82. Nijiland R, Jongsma HW, Nijhuis JG: Arterial oxygen saturation in relation to metabolic acidosis in fetal lambs. Am J Obstet Gynecol 172:810, 1995.
83. Kuhnert M, Seelback-Gobel B, Butterwegge M: Predictive agreement between the fetal arterial oxygen saturation and fetal scalp pH: Results of the German multicenter study. Am J Obstet Gynecol 178:330, 1998.
84. Dildy GA, Thorp JA, Yeast JD: The relationship between oxygen saturation and pH in umbilical blood: Implications for intrapartum fetal oxygen saturation monitoring. Am J Obstet Gynecol 175:682, 1996.
85. Dildy GA, van den Berg PP, Katz M, et al: Intrapartum fetal pulse oximetry: Fetal oxygen saturation trends during labor and relation to delivery outcome. Am J Obstet Gynecol 171:679, 1994.
86. Bloom SL, Swindle RG, McIntire DD, et al: Fetal pulse oximetry: Duration of desaturation and intrapartum outcome. Obstet Gynecol 93:1036, 1999.
87. Garite TJ, Dildy GA, McNamara H, et al: A multicenter controlled trial of fetal pulse oximetry in the intrapartum management of nonreassuring fetal heart rate patterns. Am J Obstet Gynecol 183:1049, 2000.
88. American College of Obstetricians and Gynecologists: Fetal pulse oximetry. Committee Opinion No. 258. Obstet Gynecol 98:523, 2001.
89. Bloom SL, Spong CY, Thom E, et al: and the Maternal-Fetal Medicine Units Network. Fetal pulse oximetry and cesarean delivery. N Engl J Med 355:2195-2202, 2006.
90. Greene KR: The ECG waveform. In Whittle M (ed): Bailliere's Clinical Obstetrics and Gynecology, 1:131-155, 1987.
91. Rosen KG, Lindcrantz K: STAN: The Gothenburg model for fetal surveillance during labour by ST analysis of the fetal ECG: Clin Phys Physiol Meas 10(Suppl B):51-56, 1989.
92. Amer-Wahlin I, Hellsten C, Noren H, et al: Intrapartum fetal monitoring: Cardiotocography versus cardiotocography plus ST analysis of the fetal ECG. A Swedish randomized controlled trial. Lancet 358:534-538, 2001.
93. Noren H, Amer-Wahlin I, Hagberg H, et al: Fetal electrocardiography in labor and neonatal outcome: Data from the Swedish randomized controlled trila on intrapartum fetal monitoring. Am J Obstet Gynecol 188:183-192, 2003.
94. Devoe LD, Ross M, Wilde C, et al: United States multicenter clinical usage study of the STAN 21 electronic fetal monitoring system. Am J Obstet Gynecol 195:729-734, 2006.

Chapter 23

Assessment and Induction of Fetal Pulmonary Maturity

Brian M. Mercer, MD

Respiratory distress syndrome (RDS) results when immature lungs fail to produce adequate surface-acting proteins and phospholipids to reduce alveolar surface tension and prevent alveolar collapse during expiration. Because the work necessary to open a collapsed alveolus is much more than that needed to expand an already open alveolus, the increased work of breathing leads to muscular exhaustion and mechanical respiratory failure. Alveolar collapse, fluid buildup in the immature alveolus, and diminished respiratory gas exchange lead to hypoxia, hypercarbia, and, consequently, acidosis. RDS is the most common major acute morbidity at any gestational age between viability and 36 weeks. Neonatal RDS and complications of its treatment are associated with an increased risk of serious acute and long-term morbidities, including intraventricular hemorrhage (IVH), patent ductus arteriosus, retinopathy of prematurity, and chronic lung diseases, including bronchopulmonary dysplasia. Although the frequency and severity of RDS tend to be worse when delivery occurs remote from term, RDS occurring near term can also lead to serious complications or even death.

When preterm delivery is inevitable, treatment is directed to optimizing the timing of delivery, newborn condition, and resources for neonatal care. If continuation of pregnancy is an option, the relative fetal and maternal risks of conservative management versus delivery must be considered. Because cardiopulmonary function is a principal requirement for neonatal survival, identification of fetuses at risk for RDS and methods to induce fetal maturity before preterm birth are important.

Assessment of Fetal Pulmonary Maturity

Direct Evaluation of Amniotic Fluid

Both invasive and noninvasive tests for prediction of fetal pulmonary maturity have been evaluated. An optimal test of maturity would provide clear discrimination between the mature fetus and the fetus likely to suffer RDS. Because central respiratory drive, muscular strength, infection, hypoxia, and hypotension can also alter the clinical course, antenatal pulmonary maturity testing cannot completely differentiate between the mature and the immature fetus. Currently, biochemical and biophysical analyses of the amniotic fluid offer the most accurate means to predict fetal pulmonary maturity. In general, the predictive value of a test indicating maturity is 97% to 100%. The risk of RDS after a test indicating immaturity varies from 5% to almost 100%, depending on gestational age and the degree of immaturity predicted by the test.

Clinical tests to determine fetal pulmonary maturity from amniotic fluid specimens have been available since the early 1970s, when Gluck and coworkers first introduced the lecithin/sphingomyelin ratio (L/S ratio).[1,2] The relative proportions of lecithin (disaturated phosphatidylcholine) and sphingomyelin are stable until the middle of the third trimester, at which time the pulmonary active phospholipid, lecithin, increases relative to the nonpulmonary sphingomyelin. An L/S ratio of at least 2:1 is considered indicative of fetal maturity.

The L/S ratio has in the past been considered the gold standard for assessment of fetal pulmonary maturity, but it is neither 100% sensitive nor specific. Phosphatidylglycerol (PG) is one of the last pulmonary phospholipids to become evident in the amniotic fluid, and its detection is highly predictive of fetal pulmonary maturity.[3,4] An advantage of PG determination is reliability in the presence of blood, meconium, or vaginal secretions. However, when the test is performed before 36 weeks' gestation, it carries a high false immaturity rate. The slide agglutination test for PG can provide more rapid results and requires less technical expertise than traditional thin-layer chromatography.[5-8]

Recognizing that the relative proportions of the fetal pulmonary phospholipids change with increasing gestational age, Kulovich and associates introduced the fetal "lung profile" in 1979.[9] The lung profile includes information obtained by two-dimensional thin-layer chromatography regarding the L/S ratio, the presence of PG, and the relative fractions of lecithin, PG, and phosphatidylinositol (PI); the PI fraction typically rises to 35 weeks and then declines with the appearance of PG in the amniotic fluid. The lung profile was proposed to improve prediction of pulmonary maturity and to help determine the optimal timing of subsequent testing if immaturity was recognized.

Each of these traditional tests requires considerable time, technical expertise, and cost to perform. Therefore, the L/S ratio determination and the PG assay are used as secondary tests, should simpler and less expensive automated testing indicate immaturity, or as primary tests in special clinical circumstances. Amniotic fluid prolactin, cholesterol palmitate, desmosine, surfactant apoproteins, fluorescent polarization microviscosity, and drop volume have also been related to fetal pulmonary maturity but are not commonly assessed in clinical practice.

Several functional tests of fetal pulmonary maturity were developed in the 1970s and 1980s, including the shake test, the Foam Stability Index (FSI), the automated Lumadex-FSI (Beckman Instruments, Carlsbad, CA), and the tap test. Each assessed the ability of the fetal pulmonary surfactants to maintain a stable ring of foam bubbles when amniotic fluid was diluted and mixed with various reagents.[10-13] Each test was highly predictive of the presence of fetal pulmonary maturity, but false immature results were common, and these tests are not often used in clinical practice in North America today. Indirect amniotic fluid markers of fetal pulmonary maturity include amniotic fluid density based on spectrophotometric absorbance at 650 nm, amniotic fluid turbidity, and evaluation for the presence of vernix caseosum in the amniotic fluid. Although each of these measurements is correlated to fetal pulmonary maturity, they are not adequately accurate to supplant biochemical testing. Like the PG and L/S ratio, functional tests and assessment of indirect amniotic fluid markers have largely been replaced by simpler automated tests. Currently, the surfactant/albumin ratio (S/A ratio) and the lamellar body count (LBC) are commonly used primary tests for assessment of fetal pulmonary maturity in clinical practice.

Developed in the late 1980s, the S/A ratio is performed by evaluating competitive binding to surfactant and albumin by a ligand that exhibits fluorescence polarization (TDx FLM, Abbott Laboratories, Abbott Park, IL).[14,15] The TDx FLM assay is simple to perform, accurate, and reproducible. Results are independent of amniotic fluid volume. Because the test can be performed with equipment already found in clinical laboratories, no additional equipment or special expertise is needed. The TDx FLM assay and its subsequent modification, the TDx FLM II assay, have compared favorably with the L/S ratio, shake test, FSI, and PG test.[16-19] In a multicenter study, Russell and colleagues found the sensitivity and specificity of the TDx FLM to be 96% and 58%, respectively, using a cutoff of 50 mg/g; in addition, the results of the TDx FLM test in predicting pulmonary maturity were similar to those of the PG test and the L/S ratio.[14] In a subsequent study of 218 pregnancies, Winn-MacMillan and Karon found a TDx FLM result of 45 mg/g or greater to be 100% predictive of the absence of newborn RDS.[20]

Lamellar bodies are surfactant-containing particles secreted by type II pneumocytes; they are 1 to 5 μm in diameter (1.28 to 6.4 fL).[21,22] The number of lamellar bodies found in the amniotic fluid increases with the onset of functional fetal pulmonary maturity. Because lamellar bodies are similar in size to platelets (2 to 20 fL), they can be estimated using an automated particle counter calibrated for platelet quantitation. Centrifugation of the specimen leads to underestimation of the total lamellar body number. In a study of 833 women who delivered within 72 hours of testing, the LBC compared favorably with the L/S ratio and the PG test in predicting fetal pulmonary maturity, with predictive values of 97.7%, 96.8%, and 94.7%, respectively.[23] In an attempt to introduce standardization in LBC testing, Neerhof and associates formed a consensus group that reached agreement on the following points:[24]

1. Centrifugation is not required to remove cellular debris in the amniotic fluid and should be abandoned.
2. In the absence of centrifugation, a count greater than or equal to 50,000/μL should be considered to indicate maturity, and a count less than or equal to 15,000/μL should be considered to indicate immaturity. A transitional count of 15,000-50,000/μL should lead to consideration of an additional test to clarify the result.
3. Because meconium can interfere with the cell counter and can reduce the count, either the LBC should not be performed in the presence of meconium, or clinical judgment should be exercised in interpretation of the results.
4. If there is blood contamination, a hematocrit (Hct) should be performed, and the clinician should be notified if the value is greater than 1%.
5. Although vaginal pool specimens may be acceptable, such specimens should not be analyzed if there is evident mucus, because it can obstruct the counter channels.
6. Severe oligohydramnios can increase the LBC, and polyhydramnios can lead to a false determination of immaturity.

Should centrifugation be performed, a cutoff of 30,000/μL has been suggested for prediction of fetal pulmonary maturity.[25,26]

Noninvasive Assessment of Fetal Pulmonary Maturity

Amniocentesis is not without risk, even when it is performed near term. Before ultrasound was used routinely to guide amniocentesis, invasive testing was associated with high rates of complications (19%), including tachycardia and bradycardia (1%), spontaneous membrane rupture (3%), bloody specimens (15%), and failure to obtain fluid (11%).[27] Although ultrasound guidance is associated with a much lower failure rate (1.6%), there remains a low but significant risk of complications in experienced hands, including a 0.7% risk of emergent delivery and a 6.6% risk of bloody fluid.[28] Because of these concerns, noninvasive markers, including direct and ultrasonographic amniotic fluid visualization, placental grading, fetal biometry, and fetal lung imaging, have been studied for their predictive value regarding fetal pulmonary maturity.

At term, free-floating particles visualized on ultrasound correlate to the presence of fetal vernix,[29] but such particles may be seen at any gestational age[30] and do not correlate well with biochemical fetal pulmonary maturity test results.[31] Although a grade III placenta at term has been correlated to a mature L/S ratio, placental grade before preterm birth correlates less well with the L/S ratio (7% immature) and the PG test (25% absent), limiting the utility of this finding.[32] When assessed at term, a biparietal diameter of at least 92 mm or the presence of a grade III placenta has been found to correlate to the absence of neonatal pulmonary complications,[33,34] but the correlation with biochemical testing at term and the relationship with pulmonary complications for those delivering preterm are not consistent.[35,36] These restrictions severely limit the potential utility of biometric and placental grade evaluations for assessment of fetal pulmonary maturity, particularly for women with unsure dating and those who are anticipating preterm delivery.

Noninvasive imaging of the fetal lung has been proposed to predict fetal pulmonary maturity. In evaluations of lung echogenicity, texture, and through-transmission, Cayea and colleagues[37] and Fried and associates[38] found a poor correlation between ultrasound findings and mature amniotic fluid indices. Lecithin has a characteristic magnetic resonance signal that may be amenable to assessment by magnetic resonance spectroscopy or by echoplanar magnetic resonance imaging.[39,40] Although the preliminary data are interesting, technical difficulties in these modalities remain to be resolved, and the cost related to such testing is likely to be prohibitive.

Impact of Gestational Age on Fetal Pulmonary Maturity Testing

Because fetal pulmonary maturity is highly correlated with gestational age, the predictive value of the test result varies significantly with the gestational age at which the test is performed (Fig. 23-1).[41] At term, the

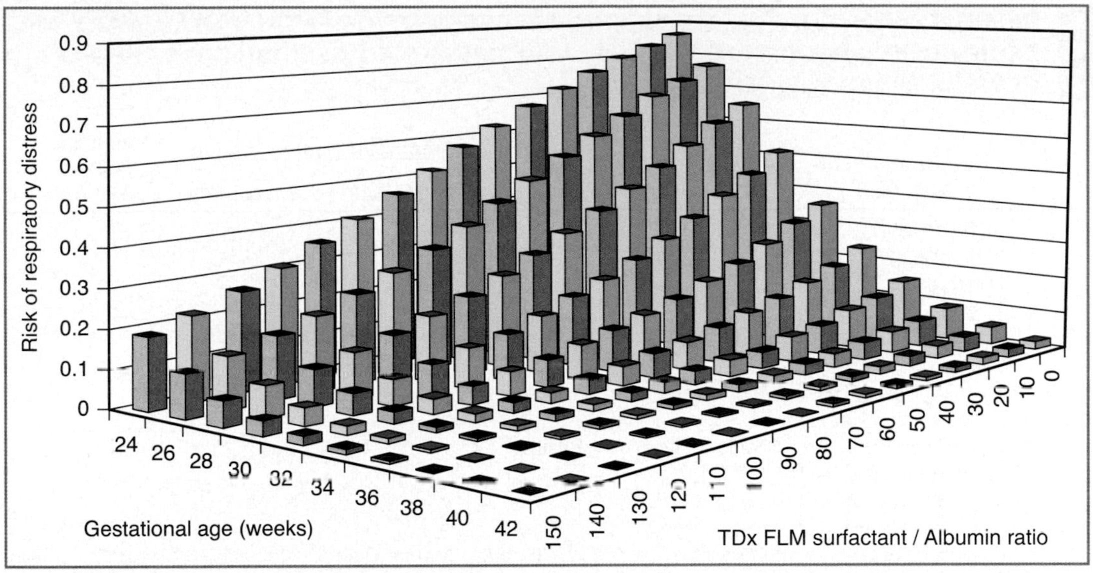

FIGURE 23-1 Risk of neonatal respiratory distress based on gestational age and TDx FLM surfactant/albumin assay result (mg/g). (Adapted from Tanasijevic MJJ, Wybenga DR, Richardson D, et al: A predictive model for fetal lung maturity employing gestational age and test results. Am J Clin Pathol 102:788, 1994.)

risk of RDS resulting from pulmonary immaturity is 1% or less. Although a test result indicating immaturity at term is associated with RDS, the risk is low, and severe disease is unlikely. However, in a preterm infant delivered remote from term, an amniotic fluid test suggesting fetal pulmonary immaturity carries a high risk of RDS.

Both at and near term, the likelihood of RDS is low after a test result indicating pulmonary maturity. On the other hand, significant risks of RDS (19.2%), severe IVH (8.1%), and necrotizing enterocolitis (4.8%) were found to exist despite a mature L/S ratio or a positive PG test when preterm birth occurred before 34 weeks.[42] Lauria and associates found a similar progressive increase in infant morbidity, despite a mature L/S ratio or a positive PG test, with decreasing gestational age at delivery; they also found a low risk of RDS (8.3%) after an immature result at term.[43]

Assessment of Fetal Pulmonary Maturity in Special Groups

Several investigators have found a lower incidence of RDS among African-American infants and a lower risk of RDS among African-American infants at any cutoff value for the TDx FLM assay.[44,45] Similarly, female fetuses appear to have higher L/S ratios at any given gestational age and earlier appearance of PG than males.[46] When matched for gestational age at delivery, twin neonates and singletons have similar morbidity rates,[47,48] but twin fetuses may have accelerated TDx FLM results after 31 weeks.[49] It remains controversial whether there is an altered risk for RDS in pregnancies affected by Rh isoimmunization, growth restriction, or preeclampsia, compared with gestational age–matched controls.[50-55] Regardless of potential differences in the rate of fetal pulmonary maturation or the predictive value of testing in any of these settings, the differences that are observed do not adequately allow differentiation between those who will and will not suffer pulmonary complications, and recommendations for testing and cutoff values for fetal maturity are not altered.

Diabetes complicating pregnancy can alter the rate of fetal lung development and has been proposed to alter the validity of diagnostic tests for fetal pulmonary maturity. Delayed pulmonary maturity in fetuses of women with class A, B, and C diabetes mellitus (White classification; see Chapter 46), despite a mature L/S ratio of 2:1, has been reported,[56-58] and some have suggested that an L/S ratio cutoff value of 3:1 should be used in the setting of diabetes. The apparently false maturity associated with a "mature" L/S ratio in such cases was elucidated by a case-control study of 295 subjects in which the L/S ratio was found to be comparable between diabetic and nondiabetic women with increasing gestational age whereas PI levels were significantly higher in women with pregestational diabetes at 33 to 35 weeks' gestation, and the onset of PG production was delayed by 1 to 1½ weeks in the diabetic pregnancies.[59] The increased risk of RDS despite a mature L/S ratio and the delayed appearance of PG could result in part from increased levels of myoinositol with hyperglycemia,[60] because myoinositol enhances PI production to the detriment of PG synthesis.[61]

The major factor that influences pulmonary maturation in diabetic progeny appears to be blood glucose control, because those with good control do not have delayed maturation.[62,63] PG appears later in poorly controlled diabetic pregnancies.[64,65] The presence of PG, however, is reliable in prediction of fetal pulmonary maturity.[66] Women with more advanced diabetes (White class D, R, or F) may demonstrate accelerated fetal maturation,[56] possibly related to uteroplacental dysfunction leading to fetal growth restriction. The S/A ratio, with a cutoff of 70 mg/g, is a reliable predictor of pulmonary maturity in women with diabetes, as is a mature LBC.[23,67] In a comparison of LBC with PG and L/S ratio in 90 diabetic pregnancies at term,[68] a centrifuged LBC count greater than 37,000/μL was consistent with fetal pulmonary maturity based on PG and L/S ratio testing. Because the potential impact of delayed fetal pulmonary maturation with diabetes is resolved by 38 weeks' gestation, well-dated pregnancies with good blood glucose control generally do not require assessment of fetal pulmonary maturity after 38 completed weeks.[69] When a term infant of a diabetic mother suffers RDS, other possible causes, such as hypertrophic cardiomyopathy, cardiac malformations, and isolated ventricular septal hypertrophy, should be considered.

TABLE 23-1 SELECTED ANTENATAL TESTS FOR ASSESSMENT OF FETAL PULMONARY MATURITY: TECHNIQUE, PREDICTIVE VALUES, AND PREDICTED RELIABILITY BASED ON CONTAMINATION AND SOURCE

Test	Author and Year (Ref. No.)	Technique	Cutoff	Impact of Contamination: Blood	Impact of Contamination: Meconium	Vaginal Pool Collection	Comments
L/S ratio	Gluck 1973 (56) Buhi 1975 (70) Cotton 1984 (71)	Thin-layer chromatography	2.0:1	Mature result valid	Not valid	Valid*	Blood decreases mature and increases immature result.
PG	Hallman 1976 (3) Hallman 1977 (4) Schumacher 1985 (5)	Thin-layer chromatography	Present	Valid	Valid	Valid†	—
Amniostat-FLM PG	Garite 1983 (6) Halvorson 1985 (7) Pastorek 1988 (8)	Slide agglutination	Positive (>2%)	Valid	Valid	Valid†	Rapid test kit. Little technical expertise required.
TDx-FLM S/A ratio	Russell 1989 (14) Steinfeld 1992 (17) Tanasijevic 1994 (41)	Fluorescent polarization	50-70 mg/g	Mature result valid	Not valid?	Valid*	Blood decreases test result.
TDx-FLM II S/A ratio	Carlan 1997 (73)	Fluorescent polarization	55 mg/g	Mature result valid	Not valid?	Valid*	Blood decreases test result.
LBC, uncentrifuged	Neerhof 2001 (23)	Cell counter	50,000/μL	Mature result valid	Reduces count	Valid‡	Reliable if Hct <1%. Platelets initially increase count. Coagulation subsequently decreases count.
LBC, centrifuged	Fakhoury 1994 (25) Dalence 1995 (26)	Cell counter	30,000/μL	Mature result valid	Reduces count	Valid‡	Reliable if Hct <1%. Platelets initially increase count. Coagulation subsequently decreases count.

*Free-flowing vaginal fluid may be valid if no blood or meconium is present.
†Heavy genital bacterial contamination may yield false mature result due to bacterial phospholipid production.
‡Vaginal fluid may be valid if no blood, meconium, or mucus is present.
FLM, fetal lung maturity; Hct, hematocrit; LBC, lamellar body count; L/S ratio, lecithin/sphingomyelin ratio; PG, phosphatidyl glycerol; S/A ratio, surfactant/albumin ratio.

Impact of Contaminants on Fetal Pulmonary Testing Results

Because of the presence of nonpulmonary phospholipids, contamination of amniotic fluid with blood can alter the results of nonspecific fetal pulmonary maturity tests for pulmonary phospholipids (Table 23-1). Maternal serum has been shown to have an intrinsic L/S ratio of between 1.3:1 and 1.9:1, raising the possibility that blood contamination could falsely lower a mature result.[70,71] On the other hand, a mature result can be considered reassuring, because blood contamination could not be expected to increase an immature value to the level of a mature result. In one study, meconium contamination increased the L/S ratio by 0.1 to 0.2 in preterm infants and by as much as 0.5 after 35 weeks' gestation,[72] leading the authors to recommend cutoffs of 2.2:1 and 2.5:1 for preterm and term pregnancies, respectively, when meconium staining is present.

The PG test is not affected by blood contamination. Blood contamination can falsely lower the TDx FLM II assay result, but a mature result reliably predicts fetal pulmonary maturity.[73] Because red blood cell phospholipids may interfere with the TDx FLM result, some elect not to perform aTDx FLM II assay if there is blood in the specimen.[74] Dubin suggested that the LBC is not affected by osmotically lysed blood.[21] Others, however, have suggested that blood contamination may alter the LBC in a biphasic manner, initially increasing the count as a result of the presence of platelets and subsequently decreasing the count as a result of sequestration of lamellar bodies with coagulation.[75] As such, the LBC should be treated with caution if there is greater than 1% contamination with blood.

Assessment of Fetal Pulmonary Maturity from Vaginal Fluid Specimens

Clinical studies support a role for vaginally collected amniotic fluid specimens after preterm premature rupture of the membranes (pPROM). Shaver and coworkers obtained amniotic fluid by amniocentesis and from the vaginal pool of women admitted with pPROM.[76] There was a close correlation between L/S ratios obtained from vaginal pool specimens and those obtained from amniocentesis ($r = .88$), and there was an 89% concordance regarding fetal pulmonary maturity. The mean L/S ratio from vaginal pool specimens was not significantly higher than from amniocentesis (2.6 versus 2.3 : 1; $P = .06$). Similarly, the correlation coefficient for PG was 0.94, and all patients with a positive amniocentesis result also had PG present in the vaginal pool. In addition, PI, phosphatidylethanolamine, and phosphatidylserine levels were similar between amniocentesis and vaginal pool specimens. Other studies have found no evident lecithin or sphingomyelin in lavage fluid from the vagina[77] and no differences in the L/S ratio or in the amounts of lecithin between vaginal and amniocentesis specimens.[78]

Although prolonged exposure to vaginal fluids has been suggested to yield inaccurate results because of bacterial degradation or phospholipid production, the L/S ratio, PG, and PI levels were similar when fluid was collected directly from the vagina or collected over a period of hours from perineal pads,[79] and RDS did not occur among infants delivered after a mature PG result from vaginal pool fluid.[80] In 447 women with PROM, PG determinations from vaginal fluid collected via perineal pads were highly predictive of fetal pulmonary maturity (97.8%), and they were similarly predictive of pulmonary immaturity when compared with specimens collected by amniocentesis (33.7%).[81] In a study of 60 vaginally collected samples, no cases of RDS occurred after a mature L/S ratio, PG, or TDx FLM result greater than 50 mg/g was found.[14] Regarding the vaginally collected fluid for TDx FLM II analysis, a mature S/A ratio (≥55 mg/g) had a predictive value of 97.6% in a study of 153 women with pPROM at 30 to 36 weeks, and 24.4% of infants with an immature result (<40 mg/g) suffered RDS.[82] The LBC can be falsely elevated by vaginal mucus, which also can block Coulter analyzer channels.[75]

Because vaginally collected amniotic fluid samples yield results similar to those of amniocentesis specimens, it is reasonable to evaluate free-flowing vaginal fluid samples by L/S ratio, S/A ratio, PG determination, and the LBC, provided there is no evident blood, meconium, or mucus in the sample. Perineal collection appears appropriate for L/S ratio and PG determinations, but it is not known whether perineal pad collection is appropriate for TDx FLM II analysis or LBC. Blood and meconium have the potential to alter testing results, as delineated in the foregoing discussion. Practically, if significant blood or meconium is present in a vaginal pool specimen, consideration should be given to expeditious delivery for fetal indication rather than conservative management.

Induction of Fetal Pulmonary Maturity

The mainstay of efforts directed toward acceleration of fetal maturation is maternal administration of antenatal corticosteroids before preterm birth. Glucocorticoids act through reversible binding to the promoter region of genes that code for functional and structural proteins in various organs.[83,84] In the lung, glucocorticoids induce lipogenic enzymes necessary for surfactant phospholipid synthesis and conversion of unsaturated to disaturated phosphatidylcholine, stimulate production of antioxidants and surfactant proteins (SP-A through SP-D), and induce enzymes responsible for sodium and potassium channel ion and fluid flux.[85] The physiologic effects of glucocorticoids on the lung include increased compliance and maximal lung volume, decreased vascular permeability, enhanced lung water clearance, parenchymal structural maturation, and improved respiratory function, in addition to an enhanced response to postnatal surfactant treatment. In addition, glucocorticoids have demonstrated maturational effects in the brain, heart, skin, digestive system, and kidney through cytodifferentiation, enzyme induction, and protein synthesis.

Betamethasone and dexamethasone are long-acting synthetic corticosteroids with similar glucocorticoid potency and negligible mineralocorticoid effects (Table 23-2).[84] Because of differences in albumin binding, placental transfer, and glucocorticoid receptor affinity, substantially higher doses of cortisol, cortisone, hydrocortisone, prednisone, and prednisolone are required to reach dose equivalency to betamethasone and dexamethasone in the fetus. Women receiving corticosteroids other than betamethasone or dexamethasone should not be considered to have received an adequate dose to stimulate fetal pulmonary maturation.

Prolactin, ambroxol, aminophylline, Intralipid, and β-adrenergic agents, among others, have also been evaluated as potential treatments to enhance fetal pulmonary maturation but have not been consistently effective. Thyroxine has been shown to act directly on the type II pneumocyte to induce surfactant synthesis in animal and human models, but, because thyroxine crosses the placenta poorly, intra-

TABLE 23-2 RELATIVE GLUCOCORTICOID AND MINERALOCORTICOID ACTIVITIES AND EQUIVALENT DOSES OF NATURAL AND SYNTHETIC ADRENAL STEROIDS

Glucocorticoid	Approximate Equivalent Dose (mg)	Relative Anti-inflammatory (Glucocorticoid) Potency	Relative Mineralocorticoid Potency
Cortisone	25	0.8	2
Hydrocortisone	20	1	2
Prednisone	5	4	1
Prednisolone	5	4	1
Triamcinolone	4	5	0
Methylprednisolone	4	5	0
Dexamethasone	0.75	20-30	0
Betamethasone	0.65-0.75	20-30	0

From Drug Facts and Comparisons. St. Louis, Facts and Comparisons, 1995, p 504.

amniotic thyroxine instillation with fetal ingestion would be necessary to achieve therapeutic fetal levels. Alternatively, thyrotropin-releasing hormone administered to the mother can cross the placenta to induce fetal thyroxine synthesis via production of thyroid-stimulating hormone. Despite early encouraging results, a meta-analysis of this approach failed to demonstrate benefit of concurrent antenatal maternal thyrotropin-releasing hormone and corticosteroid administration.[85] In one study, adverse neurologic outcomes—including delayed motor and sensory development as well as social delay—were seen with thyrotropin-releasing hormone exposure.[86]

Antenatal Corticosteroids

Neonatal Outcomes

First demonstrated to reduce RDS and neonatal death by Liggins and Howie in 1972, antenatal corticosteroid administration is one of the most effective and cost-efficient prenatal interventions for preventing perinatal morbidity and mortality related to preterm birth.[87] Meta-analysis of 21 randomized clinical trials, including 4269 infants, confirmed that antenatal corticosteroids administered to women at risk for preterm birth significantly reduced the incidences of RDS (relative risk [RR], 0.66), IVH (RR, 0.54), necrotizing enterocolitis (RR, 0.46) and neonatal death (RR, 0.69), without increasing maternal or neonatal infection (Fig. 23-2).[88] Antenatal corticosteroid administration is effective regardless of infant gender or race.[89] The beneficial impact of antenatal corticosteroids on perinatal outcomes is similar when pPROM occurs before the onset of treatment (Fig. 23-3).[88] Although Liggins' original trial suggested that corticosteroids might increase the risk of fetal death in the setting of maternal hypertension, this was not confirmed in subsequent studies.[90-92] It is generally believed that optimal corticosteroid effects are achieved when delivery occurs 24 hours or longer after initiation of therapy, but significant reductions in the rates of IVH (odds ratio [OR], 0.42), neonatal death (OR, 0.31), and need for vasopressors (OR, 0.35) have been observed when delivery occurs before the second dose of betamethasone is administered.[93]

It has been suggested that the immunosuppressive effects of corticosteroids could predispose to maternal or neonatal infection. In a retrospective evaluation of 1260 infants weighing less than 1750 g at birth, administration of antenatal corticosteroids was found to reduce the incidence of RDS, IVH, periventricular leukomalacia, and neonatal death without increasing neonatal sepsis when delivery occurred in the presence of histologic chorioamnionitis.[94] A retrospective evaluation of 457 pregnancies delivering at 23 to 32 weeks' gestation found no increases in neonatal morbidities after corticosteroid exposure when intrauterine infection or inflammation was evident, and fetal systemic inflammatory response syndrome was less common in this setting if the fetus was exposed to corticosteroid treatment before birth.[95]

Although several studies have suggested that betamethasone is more protective against periventricular leukomalacia than dexamethasone, review of published trials reveals no apparent difference in efficacy with either agent regarding prevention of RDS, IVH, or neonatal

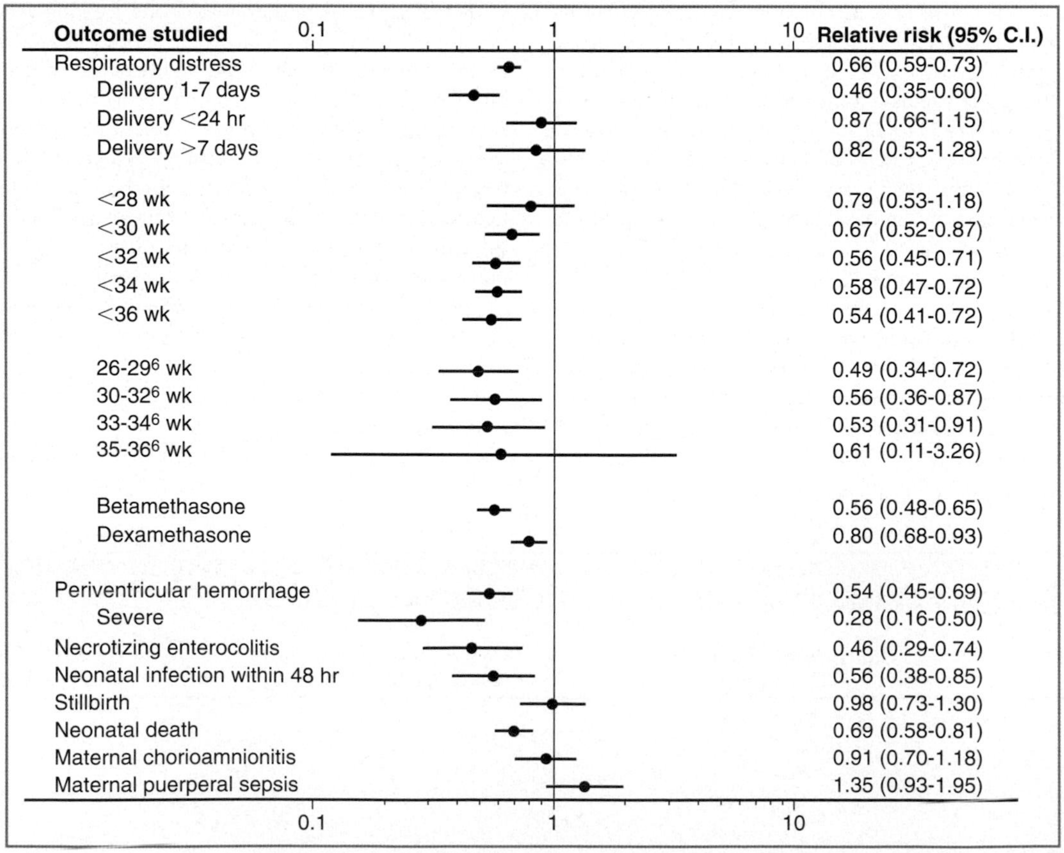

FIGURE 23-2 **Impact of antenatal corticosteroids before anticipated preterm birth on perinatal outcomes. C.I., confidence interval.** (Data from Roberts D, Dalziel S: Antenatal corticosteroids for accelerating fetal lung maturation for women at risk of preterm birth. Cochrane Database Syst Rev (3): CD004454, 2006.)

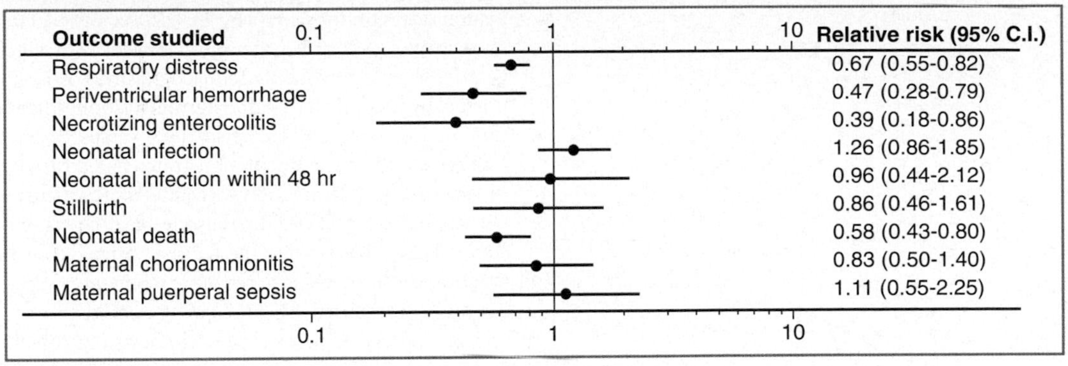

FIGURE 23-3 Impact of antenatal corticosteroids before anticipated preterm birth on perinatal outcomes when premature rupture of the membranes occurred before initiation of treatment. C.I., confidence interval. (Data from Roberts D, Dalziel S: Antenatal corticosteroids for accelerating fetal lung maturation for women at risk of preterm birth. Cochrane Database Syst Rev (3):CD004454, 2006.)

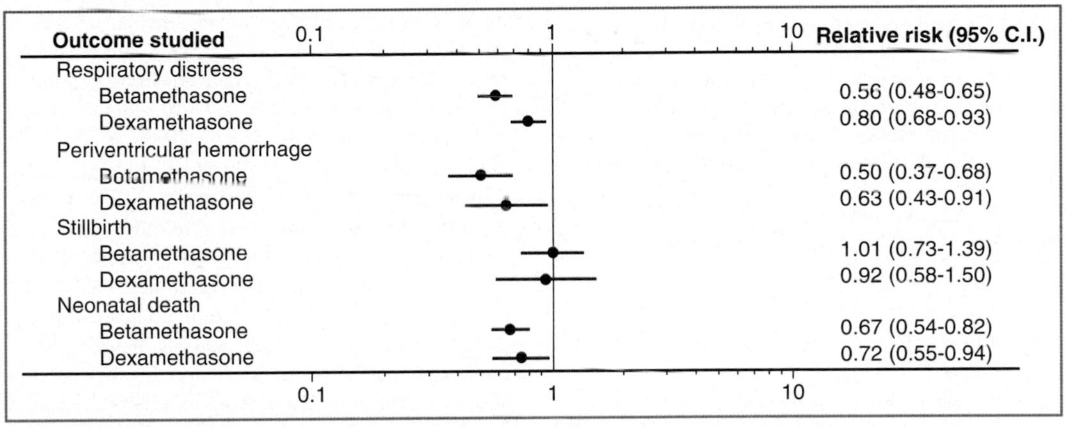

FIGURE 23-4 Impact of antenatal betamethasone and dexamethasone before anticipated preterm birth on perinatal outcomes. C.I., confidence interval. (Data from Roberts D, Dalziel S: Antenatal corticosteroids for accelerating fetal lung maturation for women at risk of preterm birth. Cochrane Database Syst Rev (3): CD004454, 2006.)

death (Fig. 23-4).[88,96-98] In 2007, a randomized, controlled trial that directly compared betamethasone and dexamethasone in 299 pregnancies found similar neonatal outcomes between the two treatments, with the exception of IVH, which was more common after betamethasone (17.0 versus 5.7%; $P = .02$). Further study to clarify the relative benefits and risks of these two agents is needed.[99] Despite a pharmacokinetic profile similar to that of intramuscular injection, oral administration of dexamethasone is not recommended because it has been associated with an increased risk of neonatal IVH and sepsis when compared with intramuscular injection.[100,101] Because placental transfer of betamethasone and dexamethasone is rapid, there is no rationale for direct fetal administration.

The potential benefit of antenatal corticosteroids varies according to the a priori risk of fetal morbidity due to prematurity (Fig. 23-5).[102] The most recent meta-analysis evaluated the benefits of antenatal corticosteroids across the spectrum of gestational age and found evident benefit with corticosteroid administration up to 34 weeks and 6 days of gestation (see Fig. 23-2).[88] Although significant benefit was not demonstrated at 35 to 36 weeks' gestation, the relative risk of RDS after antenatal corticosteroid exposure (0.66) was similar to that at earlier gestations. The Collaborative Group on Antenatal Steroid Therapy permitted enrollment of women beyond 34 weeks if an L/S ratio yielded an immature result and excluded those with a mature result at any gestational age.[91] Infants born after an immature L/S ratio had a significant reduction in RDS with antenatal dexamethasone exposure (8.7% versus 17.3%; $P = .03$). Amniotic fluid testing for fetal pulmonary maturity identifies women with fetuses at higher risk for RDS and also those who will not benefit from antenatal corticosteroids. Antenatal corticosteroid administration may therefore be considered when an immature fetal pulmonary maturity result is identified between 34 and 36 completed weeks of gestation.

Other Fetal and Neonatal Effects

A number of investigators have evaluated the impact of antenatal corticosteroid exposure on fetal biophysical and heart rate activity. These studies have found that betamethasone and dexamethasone reduce fetal breathing and body movements, with inconsistent findings regarding elevation of the baseline fetal heart rate.[103-109] Although it is unclear whether antenatal corticosteroids reduce the frequency of nonreactive fetal heart rate patterns, a decrease in the frequency of accelerations after corticosteroid administration has been reported.[107-109] Overall, the fetal biophysical effects of betamethasone appear to be

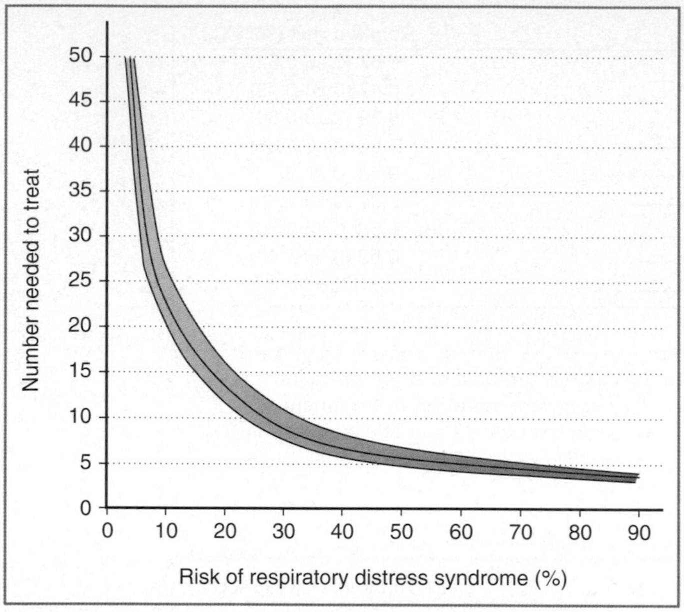

FIGURE 23-5 Number of women who must be treated with antenatal corticosteroids to prevent one case of neonatal respiratory distress syndrome based on the a priori risk of respiratory distress. Shaded zone shows 95% confidence limits. (From Sinclair JC: Meta-analysis of randomized controlled trials of antenatal corticosteroid for the prevention of respiratory distress syndrome: Discussion. Am J Obstet Gynecol 173:335, 1995.)

more pronounced than those of dexamethasone and resolve within 3 to 7 days after administration.[104,106-109]

Neonatal white blood cell counts are generally not affected by maternal glucocorticoid administration.[110] Sporadic case reports of neonatal Cushing syndrome and adrenal dysfunction have been reported with prolonged antenatal exposure to steroids.[111,112] However, Terrone and coworkers found no significant decrease in cortisol levels with increasing antenatal corticosteroid exposure after controlling for other variables,[113] and several studies have found normal neonatal responsiveness to adrenocorticotropic hormone (ACTH) stimulation after exposure to antenatal corticosteroids.[114-117] Isolated cases of neonatal hypertrophic cardiomyopathy, a known complication in infants of diabetic mothers and with postnatal corticosteroid exposure, have also been reported after antenatal corticosteroid exposure in the absence of significant maternal glucose intolerance.[117] A direct cause-effect relationship and the biologic mechanism of this finding remain to be elucidated.

Maternal Consequences

Antenatal corticosteroid administration has been associated with a transient increase in maternal white blood cell count that becomes evident within 24 hours.[118] The maternal leukocyte count increases by 4.4×10^3 cells/mL on average but is not expected to rise above 20,000 $\times 10^3$ cells/mL. Glucose intolerance can occur, with transient maternal hyperglycemia in nondiabetic women and increasing insulin requirements in diabetic women.[119,120] Assessment for gestational diabetes is best delayed at least 1 week after corticosteroid administration. Mathiesen and colleagues found that daily insulin requirements increased by 6%, 38%, 36%, 27%, and 17%, respectively, on days 1 through 5 after corticosteroid administration and suggested an algorithm of increasing insulin doses on those days by 25%, 40%, 40%, 20%, and 10% to 20%, respectively, to compensate for this need.[121] In Liggins' original trial, betamethasone transiently reduced plasma cortisol; levels returned to normal by the fourth day after administration.[87] In addition to a reduction in basal maternal cortisol (1.9 versus 26.5 μg/mL; $P < .001$), McKenna and colleagues demonstrated a decreased maternal response to corticotropin stimulation with antenatal corticosteroids.[122] Although betamethasone and dexamethasone have virtually no mineralocorticoid effects, it has been suggested that antenatal corticosteroid administration could predispose pregnant women to pulmonary edema. This issue is confounded by concurrent administration of fluid boluses, administration of tocolytics, and coexisting infection as a cause of preterm labor, all of which can lead to pulmonary edema. Current data do not support an independent role for antenatal treatment with either betamethasone or dexamethasone in the pathogenesis of maternal pulmonary edema.

Repeated Courses

Review of published research in animals reveals a consistent improvement in lung function at the expense of decreased fetal growth and adverse effects on brain development with repeated courses of antenatal corticosteroids.[123] Jobe and coworkers found that both a single course and three weekly courses of antenatal betamethasone caused a dose-dependent reduction in birth weight in preterm and term lambs, as well as decreased head size in term lambs.[124] Reduced brain growth, nerve growth, and myelination have been demonstrated after exposure to antenatal corticosteroids, particularly with repeated courses.[125-128] A review of eight trials demonstrated a consistent pattern of neurologic abnormalities, including altered optic nerve myelination, decreased eye diameter and retinal thickening, altered sciatic nerve development, reduced brain volume, neuronal degeneration in sheep and monkeys.[123] Growth restriction, low body weight, low blood pressure at 3 months, and a persistent decrease in brain weight at 3.5 years were noted in a randomized, controlled trial of repeated corticosteroids in sheep.[129] Postnatal cortisol exposure in rats was associated with reduced total body weight (50%) and brain weight (30%), with a proportional reduction in cerebral (30%) and cerebellar (20%) cell number, suggesting a reduction in cell division during the first 2 weeks of life.[130]

Retrospective and observational studies in humans have revealed similar effects on fetal pulmonary function and brain growth with multiple courses of antenatal corticosteroids. Infants exposed to more than one course of antenatal steroids had smaller head circumferences (28.1 versus 28.4 cm; $P = .01$) and a lower incidence of RDS (34.9% versus 45.2%; $P = .005$).[131] In an observational study of 447 infants born before 33 weeks' gestation, a dose-dependent reduction in birth weight (122 g; $P = .01$) and head circumference (1.02 cm; $P = .002$) occurred after three or more courses of antenatal corticosteroids.[132] In a post hoc analysis of 710 fetuses exposed to various doses of antenatal corticosteroids in a trial of antenatal thyrotropin-releasing hormone, exposure to more than one course of antenatal corticosteroids was associated with a 32-g decrease in birth weight for infants born before 32 weeks' gestation and an 80-g reduction for infants born after 32 weeks' gestation.[133] A review of retrospective and nonrandomized observational studies of antenatal corticosteroids in humans found that multiple courses were associated with significantly reduced RDS (OR, 0.79) and patent ductus arteriosus (OR, 0.56) but no differences in mortality, IVH, bronchopulmonary dysplasia, or necrotizing enterocolitis when compared with a single course.[134] Overall, these studies revealed no consistent increase in the risk of neonatal sepsis or amnionitis with multiple courses despite an increased rate of endometritis (OR, 3.22).

No significant differences in functional residual capacity, respiratory compliance, head circumference, or birth weight were found in a recent study between infants delivered within 7 days after at least two courses of antenatal betamethasone, infants delivered more than 7 days after a single course, and untreated controls.[135] Although postnatal systemic corticosteroid administration has been shown to reduce chronic lung disease and ventilatory requirements, short-term peripartum treatment of preterm infants is also associated with hyperglycemia, hypertension, hypertrophic cardiomyopathy, and growth failure.[136]

Long-term data regarding the effects of antenatal corticosteroid exposure in humans are limited. The Collaborative Group on Antenatal Steroid Therapy monitored infants exposed antenatally to dexamethasone for 3 years.[91] Steroid-exposed infants were slightly heavier and taller (3%; $P = .05$); the placebo group had more respiratory complications (3.5% versus 0.5%; $P = .02$) and heart murmurs (11.2% versus 5.6%; $P = .04$). Head circumferences and neurologic outcomes were similar in the placebo and steroid groups. Infants evaluated 10 to 12 years after participating in a randomized, placebo-controlled trial of antenatal betamethasone demonstrated more admissions for infections during the first years of life but no differences in weight, height, head circumference, neurologic development, pulmonary function, or visual acuity.[137] Long-term evaluation of the preterm infants revealed catch-up growth after exposure to multiple courses of antenatal corticosteroids, with no differences in infant weight, length, or head circumference at 3 years.[132]

Data are available from several prospective, randomized clinical trials of repeated antenatal corticosteroids in humans. In a study of 502 women randomized to receive either weekly betamethasone to 34 weeks or no further treatment after an initial course of antenatal corticosteroids, repeated antenatal corticosteroids did not significantly reduce composite morbidity (severe RDS, bronchopulmonary dysplasia, severe IVH, periventricular leukomalacia, sepsis, necrotizing enterocolitis, or death; 22.5% versus 28.0%, $P = .16$).[138] However, severe RDS (15.3% versus 24.1%; $P = .01$) and composite morbidity were decreased if delivery occurred between 24 and 27 weeks (77.4% versus 96.4%; $P = .03$) after repeated doses. The relative risk of composite morbidity after repeated corticosteroids declined with increasing gestational age at birth. There was no significant relationship between birth weight and repeated steroids (2009 versus 2139 g; $P = .10$), but the effect size was similar to that previously described.[132,133] The National Institute of Child Health and Human Development Maternal-Fetal Medicine Units (NICHD-MFMU) Network study randomly assigned 495 women at 23 to 32 weeks' gestation to receive either weekly betamethasone or placebo 7 to 10 days after an initial course and found no significant reduction in the composite primary morbidity outcome (8.0% versus 9.1%; $P = .67$) with repeated corticosteroid treatments.[139] However, repeated treatment was associated with less frequent neonatal surfactant administration ($P = .02$), mechanical ventilation ($P = .004$), continuous positive airway pressure ($P = .05$), and pneumothoraces ($P = .03$). The group receiving repeated corticosteroids had more neonates weighing less than the 10th percentile (23.7% versus 15.3%; $P = .02$), and those receiving four or more courses were significantly smaller.

Crowther and colleagues randomly assigned 982 women at risk for preterm birth at less than 32 weeks' gestation after a single course of antenatal corticosteroids to receive repeated weekly betamethasone or placebo weekly.[140] Repeated corticosteroid treatment led to less frequent RDS (33% versus 41%; $P = .01$) and severe lung disease (12% versus 20%; $P = .0003$), as well as less frequent oxygen therapy and shorter duration of mechanical ventilation. In the only reported trial to evaluate rescue corticosteroid treatments, Mercer and associates randomly allocated women at risk for preterm birth to weekly betamethasone through 34 weeks or rescue therapy if needed.[141] Those assigned to repeated weekly corticosteroids were twice as likely to receive corticosteroids within 1 week of birth before 35 weeks; only 37% of those assigned to rescue therapy receiving corticosteroids in a timely fashion before early preterm birth ($P = .001$). As in the NICHD-

TABLE 23-3 SUMMARY OF THE 1994 AND 2000 NATIONAL INSTITUTES OF HEALTH CONSENSUS PANEL GUIDELINES REGARDING ANTENATAL CORTICOSTEROIDS FOR FETAL MATURATION

The benefits of antenatal administration of corticosteroids to fetuses at risk of preterm delivery vastly outweigh the potential risks. These benefits include not only a reduction in the risk of RDS but also a substantial reduction in mortality and IVH. Optimal benefit begins 24 hours after initiation of therapy and lasts at least 7 to 14 days.
All pregnant women between 24 and 34 weeks' gestation who are at risk of preterm delivery within 7 days should be considered candidates for antenatal treatment with a single course of corticosteroids.
Treatment consists of two doses of betamethasone, 12 mg given IM 24 hours apart, or four doses of dexamethasone, 6 mg given IM 12 hours apart. There is no proof of efficacy for any other regimen.
Because treatment with corticosteroids for less than 24 hours is still associated with significant reductions in neonatal mortality, RDS, and IVH, antenatal corticosteroids should be given unless immediate delivery is anticipated.
The decision to use antenatal corticosteroids should not be altered by fetal race or gender or by the availability of surfactant replacement therapy. Patients who are eligible for therapy with tocolytics should also be eligible for treatment with antenatal corticosteroids.
In complicated pregnancies where delivery before 34 weeks' gestation is likely, antenatal corticosteroid use is recommended unless there is evidence that corticosteroids will have an adverse effect on the mother or delivery is imminent.
In preterm premature rupture of the membranes at less than 30 to 32 weeks' gestation in the absence of clinical chorioamnionitis, antenatal corticosteroid use is recommended because of the high risk of IVH at these early gestational ages.
Because of insufficient scientific data from randomized clinical trials regarding efficacy and safety, repeated courses of corticosteroids should not be used routinely. In general, repeated courses should be reserved for patients enrolled in randomized, controlled trials.

IVH, intraventricular hemorrhage; RDS, respiratory distress syndrome.
Adapted from the Effect of corticosteroids for fetal maturation on perinatal outcomes. National Institutes of Health Consensus Development Conference Statement, February 28–March 24, 1994. Am J Obstet Gynecol 173:246, 1995; and Antenatal corticosteroids revisited: Repeat courses. National Institutes of Health Consensus Development Conference Statement, August 17-18, 2000. Obstet Gynecol 98:144-150, 2001.

MFMU trial, multivariate analysis revealed a dose-dependent reduction in birth weight ($P < .02$) with increasing exposure to antenatal corticosteroids.[142] Further study is needed to determine the optimal approach to achieve timely antenatal corticosteroid treatment while minimizing fetal exposure.

National Institutes of Health Consensus Panel on Antenatal Steroids

In 1994, a National Institutes of Health (NIH) consensus panel reviewed the available literature and published guidelines regarding antenatal corticosteroid administration.[143] In response to the rapid adoption into clinical practice of repeated antenatal corticosteroid administration to women at high risk for preterm birth and the accumulating data suggesting potential risks associated with this approach, the consensus panel was reconvened to review the available literature regarding repeated corticosteroid administration in August, 2000.[144] This review reaffirmed the benefits of antenatal corticosteroid administration and recommended against routine administration of repeated courses of corticosteroids. The recommendations of these two conferences are summarized in Table 23-3.

Summary

The induction of fetal maturation through timely antenatal administration of betamethasone or dexamethasone is one of the most effective prenatal interventions available for reduction of perinatal morbidity and mortality related to preterm birth. Like many medications with strong effects, antenatal corticosteroids have the potential for significant side effects. The optimal timing and dosage of antenatal steroids before anticipated preterm birth is the subject of important ongoing research. In the meantime, unless delivery is imminent, a single course of antenatal corticosteroids should be considered when preterm birth before 34 completed weeks is anticipated, and repeated courses should not be administered routinely outside the setting of randomized clinical trials. Alternative techniques to promote fetal pulmonary maturation are not recommended. Fetal pulmonary maturity testing through amniotic fluid analysis can be helpful in determining the relative risks of neonatal complications. If amniotic fluid testing indicates fetal pulmonary maturity, aggressive attempts at pregnancy prolongation for infant benefit may not be worthwhile, but an immature result can identify those who may benefit from pregnancy prolongation for antenatal corticosteroid administration. In any case, delivery should not be delayed for the purpose of fetal maturation in the setting of nonreassuring fetal testing, suspected intrauterine infection, or worsening maternal or fetal condition that places the mother or fetus in imminent jeopardy.

References

1. Gluck L: Biochemical development of the lung: Clinical aspects of surfactant development, RDS and the intrauterine assessment of lung maturity. Clin Obstet Gynecol 14:710, 1971.
2. Gluck L, Kulovich MV, Borer RC Jr, et al: Diagnosis of the respiratory distress syndrome by amniocentesis. Am J Obstet Gynecol 109:440, 1971.
3. Hallman M, Kulovich M, Kirkpatrick E, et al: Phosphatidylinositol and phosphatidylglycerol in amniotic fluid: Indices of lung maturity. Am J Obstet Gynecol 125:613, 1976.
4. Hallman M, Feldman BH, Kirkpatrick E, et al: Absence of phosphatidylglycerol (PG) in respiratory distress syndrome in the newborn: Study of the minor surfactant phospholipids in newborns. Pediatr Res 11:714, 1977.
5. Schumacher RE, Parisi VM, Steady HM, et al: Bacteria causing false positive test for phosphatidylglycerol in amniotic fluid. Am J Obstet Gynecol 151:1067, 1985.
6. Garite TJ, Yabusaki KK, Moberg LJ, et al: A new rapid slide agglutination test for amniotic fluid phosphatidylglycerol: Laboratory and clinical correlation. Am J Obstet Gynecol 147:681, 1983.
7. Halvorsen PR, Gross TL: Laboratory and clinical evaluation of a rapid slide agglutination test for phosphatidylglycerol. Am J Obstet Gynecol 151:1061, 1985.
8. Pastorek JG II, Letellier RL, Gebbia K: Production of a phosphatidylglycerol-like substance by genital flora bacteria. Am J Obstet Gynecol 159:199, 1988.
9. Kulovich MV, Hallman MB, Gluck L: The lung profile: I. Normal pregnancy. Am J Obstet Gynecol 135:57, 1979.
10. Clements JA, Platzker ACG, Tierney DF, et al: Assessment of the risk of respiratory distress syndrome by a rapid test for surfactant in amniotic fluid. N Engl J Med 286:1077, 1972.
11. Sher G, Statland BE, Freer DE, et al: Assessing fetal lung maturation by the foam index stability test. Obstet Gynecol 52:673, 1978.
12. Sher G, Statland BE: Assessment of fetal pulmonary maturity by the Lumadex Foam Stability Index Test. Obstet Gynecol 61:444, 1983.
13. Socol ML, Sing E, Depp OR: The tap test: A rapid indicator of fetal pulmonary maturity. Am J Obstet Gynecol 148:445, 1984.
14. Russell JC, Cooper CM, Ketchum CH, et al: Multicenter evaluation of TDx test for assessing fetal lung maturity. Clin Chem 35:1005, 1989.
15. Herbert WN, Chapman JF, Schnoor MM: Role of the TDx FLM assay in fetal lung maturity. Am J Obstet Gynecol 168:808, 1993.
16. Ashwood ER, Tait JF, Foerder CA, et al: Improved fluorescence polarization assay for use in evaluating fetal lung maturity: III. Retrospective clinical evaluation and comparison with the lecithin/sphingomyelin ratio. Clin Chem 32:260, 1986.
17. Steinfeld JD, Samuels P, Bulley MA, et al: The utility of the TDx test in the assessment of fetal lung maturity. Obstet Gynecol 79:460, 1992.
18. Bender TM, Stone LR, Amenta JS: Diagnostic power of lecithin/sphingomyelin ratio and fluorescence polarization assays for RDS compared by relative operating characteristic curves. Clin Chem 40:541, 1994.
19. Bonebrake RG, Towers CV, Rumney PJ, et al: Is fluorescence polarization reliable and cost efficient in a fetal lung maturity cascade? Am J Obstet Gynecol 177:835, 1997.
20. Winn-McMillan T, Karon BS: Comparison of the TDx-FLM II and lecithin to sphingomyelin ratio assays in predicting fetal lung maturity. Am J Obstet Gynecol 193:778-82, 2005.
21. Dubin SB: Characterization of amniotic fluid lamellar bodies by resistive-pulse counting: Relationship to measures of fetal lung maturity. Clin Chem 35:612, 1989.
22. Ashwood ER, Oldroyd RG, Palmer SE: Measuring the number of lamellar body particles in amniotic fluid. Obstet Gynecol 75:289, 1990.
23. Neerhof MG, Haney EI, Silver RK, et al: Lamellar body counts compared with traditional phospholipid analysis as an assay for evaluating fetal lung maturity. Obstet Gynecol 97:305, 2001.
24. Neerhof MG, Dohnal JC, Ashwood ER, et al: Lamellar body counts: A consensus on protocol. Obstet Gynecol 97:318, 2001.
25. Fakhoury G, Daikoku NH, Benser J, et al: Lamellar body concentrations and the prediction of fetal pulmonary maturity. Am J Obstet Gynecol 170:72, 1994.
26. Dalence CR, Bowie LJ, Dohnal JC, et al: Amniotic fluid lamellar body count: A rapid and reliable fetal lung maturity test. Obstet Gynecol 86:235, 1995.
27. Sabbagha R, Salvino C: Report on third trimester amniocentesis at Prentice Women's Hospital of Northwestern University Medical School, Chicago, Illinois. Antenatal Diagnosis. NIH Consensus Statement. National

Institutes of Health. Bethesda, Md. 2:61, 1979. In Stark CM, Smith RS, Lagrandeur RM, et al: Need for urgent delivery after third-trimester amniocentesis. Obstet Gynecol 95:48, 2000.
28. Stark CM, Smith RS, Lagrandeur RM, et al: Need for urgent delivery after third-trimester amniocentesis. Obstet Gynecol 95:48, 2000.
29. Brown DL, Polger M, Clark PK, et al: Very echogenic amniotic fluid: Ultrasonography-amniocentesis correlation. J Ultrasound Med 13:95, 1994.
30. Parulekar SG: Ultrasonographic demonstration of floating particles in amniotic fluid. J Ultrasound Med 2:107, 1983.
31. Helewa M, Manning F, Harman C: Amniotic fluid particles: Are they related to a mature amniotic fluid phospholipid profile? Obstet Gynecol 74:893, 1989.
32. Harman CR, Manning FA, Stearns E, et al: The correlation of ultrasonic placental grading and fetal pulmonary maturation in five hundred sixty-three pregnancies. Am J Obstet Gynecol 143:941, 1982.
33. Petrucha RA, Golde SH, Platt LD: The use of ultrasound in the prediction of fetal pulmonary maturity. Am J Obstet Gynecol 144:931, 1982.
34. Golde SH, Tahilramaney MP, Platt LD: Use of ultrasound to predict fetal lung maturity in 247 consecutive elective cesarean deliveries. J Reprod Med 29:9, 1984.
35. Spellacy WN, Gelman SR, Wood SD, et al: Comparison of fetal maturity evaluation with ultrasonic biparietal diameter and amniotic fluid lecithin-sphingomyelin ratio. Obstet Gynecol 51:109, 1978.
36. Newton ER, Cetrulo CL, Kosa DJ: Biparietal diameter as a predictor of fetal lung maturity. J Reprod Med 7:480, 1983.
37. Cayea PD, Grant DC, Doubilet PM, et al: Prediction of fetal lung maturity inaccuracy of study using conventional ultrasound instruments. Radiology 155:473, 1985.
38. Fried AM, Loh FK, Umer MA, et al: Echogenicity of fetal lung relation to fetal age and maturity. AJR Am J Roentgenol 145:591, 1985.
39. Fenton BW, Lin CS, Ascher S, et al: Magnetic resonance spectroscopy to detect lecithin in amniotic fluid and fetal lung. Obstet Gynecol 95:457, 2000.
40. Moore RJ, Strachan B, Tyler DJ, et al: In vivo diffusion measurements as an indication of fetal lung maturation using echo planar imaging at 0.5T. Magn Reson Med 45:247, 2001.
41. Tanasijevic MJ, Wybenga DR, Richardson D, et al: A predictive model for fetal lung maturity employing gestational age and test results. Am J Clin Pathol 102:788, 1994.
42. Wigton TR, Tamura RK, Wickstrom E, et al: Neonatal morbidity after preterm delivery in the presence of documented lung maturity. Am J Obstet Gynecol 169:951, 1993.
43. Lauria MR, Dombrowski MP, Delaney-Black V, et al: Lung maturity tests: Relation to source, clarity, gestational age and neonatal outcome. J Reprod Med 41:685, 1996.
44. Richardson DK, Torday JS: Racial differences in predictive value of the lecithin/sphingomyelin ratio. Am J Obstet Gynecol 170:1273, 1994.
45. Berman S, Tanasijevic MJ, Alvarez JG, et al: Racial differences in the predictive value of the TDx fetal lung maturity assay. Am J Obstet Gynecol 175:73, 1996.
46. Fleisher B, Kulovich MV, Hallman M, et al: Lung profile sex differences in normal pregnancy. Obstet Gynecol 66:327, 1985.
47. Nielson HC, Harvey-Wilkes K, MacKinnon B, et al. Neonatal outcome of very premature infants from multiple and singleton gestations. Am J Obstet Gynecol 177:563, 1997.
48. Donovan EF, Ehrenkranz RA, Shankaran S, et al: Outcomes of very low birth weight twins cared for in the National Institute of Child Health and Human Development Neonatal Research Network's intensive care units. Am J Obstet Gynecol 179:742, 1998.
49. McElrath TF, Norwitz ER, Robinson JN, et al: Differences in TDx fetal lung maturity assay values between twin and singleton gestations. Am J Obstet Gynecol 182:1110, 2000.
50. Quinlan RW, Buhi WC, Cruz AC: Fetal pulmonary maturity in isoimmunized pregnancies. Am J Obstet Gynecol 148:787, 1984.
51. Horenstein J, Golde SH, Platt LD: Lung profiles in the isoimmunized pregnancy. Am J Obstet Gynecol 153:443, 1985.
52. Winn HN, Romero R, Roberts A, et al: Comparison of fetal lung maturation in preterm singleton and twin pregnancies. Am J Perinatol 9:326, 1992.
53. Schiff E, Friedman SA, Mercer BM, et al: Fetal lung maturity is not accelerated in preeclamptic pregnancies. Am J Obstet Gynecol 169:1096, 1993.
54. Piazze JJ, Maranghi L, Nigro G, et al: The effect of glucocorticoid therapy on fetal lung maturity indices in hypertensive pregnancies. Obstet Gynecol 92:220, 1998.
55. Winn HN, Klosterman A, Amon E, et al: Does preeclampsia influence fetal lung maturity? J Perinat Med 28:210, 2000.
56. Gluck L, Kulovich MV: Lecithin-sphingomyelin ratios in amniotic fluid in normal and abnormal pregnancy. Am J Obstet Gynecol 115:539, 1973.
57. Cruz AC, Buhi WC, Birk SA, et al: Respiratory distress syndrome with mature lecithin/sphingomyelin ratios: Diabetes mellitus and low Apgar scores. Am J Obstet Gynecol 126:78, 1976.
58. Tabsh KM, Brinkman CR III, Bashore RA: Lecithin:sphingomyelin ratio in pregnancies complicated by insulin-dependent diabetes mellitus. Obstet Gynecol 59:353, 1982.
59. Moore TR: A comparison of amniotic fluid fetal pulmonary phospholipids in normal and diabetic pregnancy. Am J Obstet Gynecol 186:641-650, 2002.
60. Hallman M, Wermer D, Epstein BL, et al: Effects of maternal insulin or glucose infusion on the fetus: Study on lung surfactant phospholipids, plasma myoinositol, and fetal growth in the rabbit. Am J Obstet Gynecol 142:877, 1982.
61. Bourbon JR, Doucet E, Rieutort M, et al: Role of myo-inositol in impairment of fetal lung phosphatidylglycerol biosynthesis in the diabetic pregnancy: Physiological consequences of a phosphatidylglycerol-deficient surfactant in the newborn rat. Exp Lung Res 11:195, 1986
62. Curet LB, Olson RW, Schneider JM, et al: Effect of diabetes mellitus on amniotic fluid lecithin/sphingomyelin ratio and respiratory distress syndrome. Am J Obstet Gynecol 135:10, 1979.
63. Dudley DK, Black DM: Reliability of lecithin/sphingomyelin ratios in diabetic pregnancy. Obstet Gynecol 66:521, 1985.
64. Piper JM, Langer O: Does maternal diabetes delay fetal pulmonary maturity? Am J Obstet Gynecol 168:783, 1993.
65. Piper JM, Xenakis EM, Langer O: Delayed appearance of pulmonary maturation markers is associated with poor glucose control in diabetic pregnancies. J Matern Fetal Med 7:148, 1998.
66. Kulovich MV, Gluck L: The lung profile: II. Complicated pregnancy. Am J Obstet Gynecol 135:64, 1979.
67. Tanasijevic MJ, Winkelman JW, Wybenga DR, et al: Prediction of fetal lung maturity in infants of diabetic mothers using the FLM S/A and disaturated phosphatidylcholine tests. Am J Clin Pathol 105:17, 1996.
68. DeRoche ME, Ingardia CJ, Guerette PJ, et al: The use of lamellar body counts to predict fetal lung maturity in pregnancies complicated by diabetes mellitus. Am J Obstet Gynecol 187:908-912, 2002.
69. Berkowitz K, Reyes C, Saadat P, et al: Fetal lung maturation: Comparison of biochemical indices in gestational diabetic and nondiabetic pregnancies. J Reprod Med 42:793, 1997.
70. Buhi WC, Spellacy WN: Effects of blood or meconium on the determination of the amniotic fluid lecithin/sphingomyelin ratio. Am J Obstet Gynecol 121:321, 1975.
71. Cotton DB, Spillman T, Bretaudiere JP: Effect of blood contamination on lecithin to sphingomyelin ratio in amniotic fluid by different detection methods. Clin Chim Acta 137:299, 1984.
72. Tabsh KM, Brinkman CR III, Bashore R: Effect of meconium contamination on amniotic fluid lecithin:sphingomyelin ratio. Obstet Gynecol 58:605, 1981.
73. Carlan SJ, Gearity D, O'Brien WF: The effect of maternal blood contamination on the TDx-FLM II assay. Am J Perinatol 14:491, 1997.
74. Apple FS, Bilodeau L, Preese LM, et al: Clinical implementation of a rapid, automated assay for assessing fetal lung maturity. J Reprod Med 39:883, 1994.
75. Ashwood ER, Palmer SE, Taylor JS, et al: Lamellar body counts for rapid fetal lung maturity testing. Obstet Gynecol 81:619, 1993.

76. Shaver DC, Spinnato JA, Whybrew D, et al: Comparison of phospholipids in vaginal and amniocentesis specimens of patients with premature rupture of membranes. Am J Obstet Gynecol 156:454, 1987.
77. Sbarra AJ, Blake G, Cetrulo CL, et al: The effect of cervical/vaginal secretions on measurements of lecithin/sphingomyelin ratio and optical density at 650 nm. Am J Obstet Gynecol 139:214, 1981.
78. Phillippe M, Acker D, Torday J, et al: The effects of vaginal contamination on two pulmonary phospholipid assays. J Reprod Med 27:283, 1982.
79. Golde SH: Use of obstetric perineal pads in collection of amniotic fluid in patients with rupture of the membranes. Am J Obstet Gynecol 146:710, 1983.
80. Lewis DF, Towers CV, Major CA, et al: Use of Amniostat-FLM in detecting the presence of phosphatidylglycerol in vaginal pool samples in preterm premature rupture of membranes. Am J Obstet Gynecol 169:573, 1993.
81. Estol PC, Poseiro JJ, Schwarcz R: Phosphatidylglycerol determination in the amniotic fluid from a PAD placed over the vulva: A method for diagnosis of fetal lung maturity in cases of premature ruptured membranes. J Perinat Med 20:65, 1992.
82. Edwards RK, Duff P, Ross KC: Amniotic fluid indices of fetal pulmonary maturity with preterm premature rupture of membranes. Obstet Gynecol 96:102, 2000.
83. Ballard PL, Ballard RA: Scientific basis and therapeutic regimens for use of antenatal glucocorticoids. Am J Obstet Gynecol 173:254, 1995.
84. Drug Facts and Comparisons. St Louis, Facts and Comparisons, 1995, p 504.
85. Crowther CA, Alfirevic Z, Haslam RR: Prenatal thyrotropin-releasing hormone for preterm birth. Cochrane Database Syst Rev (2):CD000019, 2000.
86. ACTOBAT Study Group. Australian Collaborative Trial of Antenatal Thyrotropin-releasing hormone (ACTOBAT) for the prevention of neonatal respiratory disease. Lancet 345:877, 1995.
87. Liggins GC, Howie RN: A controlled trial of antepartum glucocorticoid treatment for prevention of the respiratory distress syndrome in premature infants. Pediatrics 50:515, 1972.
88. Roberts D, Dalziel S: Antenatal corticosteroids for accelerating fetal lung maturation for women at risk of preterm birth. Cochrane Database Syst Rev (3):CD004454, 2006.
89. Crowley PA: Antenatal corticosteroid therapy: A meta-analysis of the randomized trials, 1972 to 1994. Am J Obstet Gynecol 173:322, 1995.
90. Gamsu HR, Mullinger BM, Donnai P, et al: Antenatal administration of betamethasone to prevent respiratory distress syndrome in preterm infants: Report of a UK multicentre trial. BJOG 96:401, 1989.
91. Collaborative Group on Antenatal Steroid Therapy: Effect of antenatal dexamethasone administration on the prevention of respiratory distress syndrome. Am J Obstet Gynecol 141:276, 1981.
92. Kari MA, Hallman M, Eronen M, et al: Prenatal dexamethasone treatment in conjunction with rescue therapy of human surfactant: A randomized placebo-controlled multicenter study. Pediatrics 93:730, 1994.
93. Elimian A, Figueroa R, Spitzer AR, et al: Antenatal corticosteroids: Are incomplete courses beneficial? Obstet Gynecol 102:352-355, 2003.
94. Elimian A, Verma U, Beneck D, et al: Histologic chorioamnionitis, antenatal steroids, and perinatal outcomes. Obstet Gynecol 96:333-336, 2000.
95. Goldenberg RL, Andrews WW, Faye-Petersen OM, et al: The Alabama preterm birth study: Corticosteroids and neonatal outcomes in 23- to 32-week newborns with various markers of intrauterine infection. Am J Obstet Gynecol 195:1020-1024, 2006.
96. Baud O, Foix-L'Helias L, Kaminski M, et al: Antenatal glucocorticoid treatment and cystic periventricular leukomalacia in very premature infants. N Engl J Med 341:1190, 1999.
97. Spinillo A, Viazzo F, Colleoni R, et al: Two-year infant neurodevelopmental outcome after single or multiple antenatal courses of corticosteroids to prevent complications of prematurity. Am J Obstet Gynecol 191:217-224, 2004.
98. Lee BH, Stoll BJ, McDonald SA, Higgins RD; National Institute of Child Health and Human Development Neonatal Research Network: Adverse neonatal outcomes associated with antenatal dexamethasone versus antenatal betamethasone. Pediatrics 117:1503-1510, 2006.
99. Elimian A, Garry D, Figueroa R, et al: Antenatal betamethasone compared with dexamethasone (Betacode trial). Obstet Gynecol 110:26-30, 2007.
100. Egerman RS, Mercer BM, Doss JL, et al: A randomized, controlled trial of oral and intramuscular dexamethasone in the prevention of neonatal respiratory distress syndrome. Am J Obstet Gynecol 179:1120, 1998.
101. Egerman RS, Pierce WF IV, Andersen RN, et al: A comparison of the bioavailability of oral and intramuscular dexamethasone in women in late pregnancy. Obstet Gynecol 89:276, 1997.
102. Sinclair JC: Meta-analysis of randomized controlled trials of antenatal corticosteroid for the prevention of respiratory distress syndrome: Discussion. Am J Obstet Gynecol 173:335, 1995.
103. Magee LA, Dawes GS, Moulden M, et al: A randomised controlled comparison of betamethasone with dexamethasone: Effects on the antenatal fetal heart rate. BJOG 104:1233, 1997.
104. Mulder EJ, Derks JB, Visser GH: Antenatal corticosteroid therapy and fetal behaviour: A randomised study of the effects of betamethasone and dexamethasone. BJOG 104:1239, 1997.
105. Mushkat Y, Ascher-Landsberg J, Keidar R, et al: The effect of betamethasone versus dexamethasone on fetal biophysical parameters. Eur J Obstet Gynecol Reprod Biol 97:50-52, 2001.
106. Senat MV, Minoui S, Multon O, et al: Effect of dexamethasone and betamethasone on fetal heart rate variability in preterm labour: A randomised study. BJOG 105:749, 1998.
107. Rotmensch S, Liberati M, Vishne TH, et al: The effect of betamethasone and dexamethasone on fetal heart rate patterns and biophysical activities: A prospective randomized trial. Acta Obstet Gynecol Scand 78:493, 1999.
108. Subtil D, Tiberghien P, Devos P, et al: Immediate and delayed effects of antenatal corticosteroids on fetal heart rate: A randomized trial that compares betamethasone acetate and phosphate, betamethasone phosphate, and dexamethasone. Am J Obstet Gynecol 188:524-531, 2003.
109. Rotmensch S, Lev S, Kovo M, et al: Effect of betamethasone administration on fetal heart rate tracing: A blinded longitudinal study. Fetal Diagn Ther 20:371-376, 2005.
110. Zachman RD, Bauer CR, Boehm J, et al: Effect of antenatal dexamethasone on neonatal leukocyte count. J Perinatol 8:111, 1988.
111. Grajwer LA, Lilien LD, Pildes RS: Neonatal subclinical adrenal insufficiency: Result of maternal steroid therapy. JAMA 238:1279, 1977.
112. Bradley BS, Kumar SP, Mehta PN, et al: Neonatal cushingoid syndrome resulting from serial courses of antenatal betamethasone. Obstet Gynecol 83:869, 1994.
113. Terrone DA, Smith LG Jr, Wolf EJ, et al: Neonatal effects and serum cortisol levels after multiple courses of maternal corticosteroids. Obstet Gynecol 90:819, 1997.
114. Ohrlander S, Gennser G, Nilsson KO, et al: ACTH test to neonates after administration of corticosteroids during gestation. Obstet Gynecol 49:691, 1977.
115. Teramo K, Hallman M, Raivio KO: Maternal glucocorticoid in unplanned premature labor: Controlled study on the effects of betamethasone phosphate on the phospholipids of the gastric aspirate and on the adrenal cortical function of the newborn infant. Pediatr Res 14:326, 1980.
116. Terrone DA, Rinehart BK, Rhodes PG, et al: Multiple courses of betamethasone to enhance fetal lung maturation do not suppress neonatal adrenal response. Am J Obstet Gynecol 180:1349, 1999.
117. Yunis KA, Bitar FF, Hayek P, et al: Transient hypertrophic cardiomyopathy in the newborn following multiple doses of antenatal corticosteroids. Am J Perinatol 16:17, 1999.
118. Diebel ND, Parsons MT, Spellacy WN: The effects of betamethasone on white blood cells during pregnancy with pPROM. J Perinat Med 26:204, 1998.
119. Fisher JE, Smith RS, Lagrandeur R, et al: Gestational diabetes mellitus in women receiving beta-adrenergics and corticosteroids for threatened preterm delivery. Obstet Gynecol 90:880, 1997.

120. Bedalov A, Balasubramanyam A: Glucocorticoid-induced ketoacidosis in gestational diabetes: Sequela of the acute treatment of preterm labor. A case report. Diabetes Care 20:922, 1997.
121. Mathiesen ER, Christensen AB, Hellmuth E, et al: Insulin dose during glucocorticoid treatment for fetal lung maturation in diabetic pregnancy: Test of an algorithm. Acta Obstet Gynaecol Scand 81:835-839, 2002.
122. McKenna DS, Wittber GM, Nagaraja HN, et al: The effects of repeat doses of antenatal corticosteroids on maternal adrenal function. Am J Obstet Gynecol 183:669, 2000.
123. Aghajafari F, Murphy K, Matthews S, et al: Repeated doses of antenatal corticosteroids in animals: A systematic review. Am J Obstet Gynecol 186:843, 2002.
124. Jobe AH, Wada N, Berry LM, et al: Single and repetitive maternal glucocorticoid exposures reduce fetal growth in sheep. Am J Obstet Gynecol 178:880, 1998.
125. Dunlop SA, Archer MA, Quinlivan JA, et al: Repeated prenatal corticosteroids delay myelination in the ovine central nervous system. J Matern Fetal Med 6:309, 1997
126. Huang WL, Beazley LD, Quinlivan JA, et al: Effect of corticosteroids on brain growth in fetal sheep. Obstet Gynecol 94:213, 1999.
127. Quinlivan JA, Archer MA, Evans SF, et al: Fetal sciatic nerve growth is delayed following repeated maternal injections of corticosteroid in sheep. J Perinat Med 28:26, 2000.
128. Huang WL, Harper CG, Evans SF, et al: Repeated prenatal corticosteroid administration delays myelination of the corpus callosum in fetal sheep. Int J Dev Neurosci 19:415, 2001.
129. Moss TJ, Doherty DA, Nitsos I, et al: Effects into adulthood of single or repeated antenatal corticosteroids in sheep. Am J Obstet Gynecol 192:146-152, 2005.
130. Cotterrell M, Balazs R, Johnson AL: Effects of corticosteroids on the biochemical maturation of rat brain: Postnatal cell formation. J Neurochem 19:2151, 1972.
131. Abbasi S, Hirsch D, Davis J, et al: Effect of single versus multiple courses of antenatal corticosteroids on maternal and neonatal outcome. Am J Obstet Gynecol 182:1243, 2000.
132. French NP, Hagan R, Evans SF, et al: Repeated antenatal corticosteroids: Size at birth and subsequent development. Am J Obstet Gynecol 180:114, 1999.
133. Banks BA, Cnaan A, Morgan MA, et al: Multiple courses of antenatal corticosteroids and outcome of premature neonates. North American Thyrotropin-Releasing Hormone Study Group. Am J Obstet Gynecol 181:709, 1999.
134. Aghajafari F, Murphy K, Willan A, et al: Multiple courses of antenatal corticosteroids: A systematic review and meta-analysis. Am J Obstet Gynecol 185:1073, 2001.
135. McEvoy C, Bowling S, Williamson K, et al: The effect of a single remote course versus weekly courses of antenatal corticosteroids on functional residual capacity in preterm infants: A randomized trial. Pediatrics 110:280-284, 2002.
136. Halliday HL, Ehrenkranz RA: Early postnatal (<96 hours) corticosteroids for preventing chronic lung disease in preterm infants. Cochrane Database Syst Rev (1):CD001146, 2003.
137. Smolders-de Haas H, Neuvel J, Schmand B, et al: Physical development and medical history of children who were treated antenatally with corticosteroids to prevent respiratory distress syndrome: A 10- to 12-year follow-up. Pediatrics 86:65, 1990.
138. Guinn DA, Atkinson MW, Sullivan L, et al: Single vs weekly courses of antenatal corticosteroids for women at risk of preterm delivery: A randomized controlled trial. JAMA 286:1581, 2001.
139. Wapner RJ, Sorokin Y, Thom EA, et al; National Institute of Child Health and Human Development Maternal Fetal Medicine Units Network. Single versus weekly courses of antenatal corticosteroids: Evaluation of safety and efficacy. Am J Obstet Gynecol 195:633-642, 2006.
140. Crowther CA, Haslam RR, Hiller JE, et al; Australasian Collaborative Trial of Repeat Doses of Steroids (ACTORDS) Study Group. Neonatal respiratory distress syndrome after repeat exposure to antenatal corticosteroids: A randomised controlled trial. Lancet 367:1913-1919, 2006.
141. Mercer B, Egerman R, Beazley D, et al: Antenatal corticosteroids in women at risk for preterm birth: A randomized trial. Am J Obstet Gynecol 184: S6, 2001.
142. Mercer B, Egerman R, Beazley D, et al: Steroids reduce fetal growth: Analysis of a prospective trial. Am J Obstet Gynecol 184:S6, 2001.
143. National Institutes of Health Consensus Development Conference Statement: Effect of corticosteroids for fetal maturation on perinatal outcomes, February 28-March 24, 1994. Am J Obstet Gynecol 173:246, 1995.
144. National Institutes of Health Consensus Development Conference Statement, August 17-18, 2000: Antenatal corticosteroids revisited: Repeat courses. Obstet Gynecol 98:144-150, 2001.

Chapter 24

Invasive Fetal Therapy

Jan A. Deprest, MD, PhD, Eduardo Gratacos, MD, PhD, and Liesbeth Lewi, MD, PhD

The availability of high-resolution ultrasound imaging and screening programs has made the unborn child a true patient. When fetal malformations, genetic diseases, or in utero acquired conditions are suspected, patients are referred to tertiary care units with more specialized skills, technical equipment, experience, and multidisciplinary counselors to define potential options. In some cases, intervention before birth may be desirable, which often does not require direct access to the fetus—for example, transplacental administration of pharmacologic agents for cardiac arrhythmias or antibiotics in case of fetal infection. Other conditions can be treated only by invasive access to fetus. In utero transfusion of a hydropic fetus to treat the anemia of Rh isoimmunization, first described in 1961, was probably the first successful invasive therapeutic procedure. Today, blood transfusion through the umbilical cord, intrahepatic vein, or (exceptionally) directly into the fetal heart is widely offered, with good fetal and long-term outcome when procedures are done by experienced operators.

Some conditions are amenable to surgical correction, and in the majority of cases this is best done after birth. Occasionally, prenatal surgery is required to save the life of the fetus, or to prevent permanent organ damage. This can be achieved by correcting the malformation, by arresting the progression of the disease, or by treating some of the immediately life-threatening effects of the condition, delaying more definitive repair until after birth. Because of the potential complications, risks and benefits of the intervention must be weighed against each other. Table 24-1 summarizes the indications and rationale for in utero surgery on the fetus, placenta, cord, or membranes.

A consensus, endorsed by the International Fetal Medicine and Surgery Society (IFMSS), has been reached on the criteria and indications for fetal surgery (Table 24-2).[1] In the 1980s to 1990s, only a few conditions met these criteria, and surgical intervention required maternal laparotomy, partial exteriorization of the fetus through a stapled hysterotomy. These "open" procedures were initially associated with high fetal-maternal morbidity, raising the question for some of the value of claimed benefits.

The growing availability of videoendoscopic surgery in the 1990s, combined with earlier experience with fetoscopy, paved the way for the concept of *endoscopic fetal surgery*. The rationale was that minimally invasive access to the amniotic cavity would reduce the frequency of preterm labor and diminish maternal morbidity. Investigators at the Centre for Surgical Technologies (CST) in Leuven, Belgium, have helped advance the application of these techniques by first establishing an ovine model for endoscopic fetal surgery.[2] That experience laid the basis for the first successful umbilical cord ligation in Europe,[3] almost simultaneously with, but independently from, a successful procedure done by Quintero a few months earlier. The Leuven group subsequently set up the Eurofoetus consortium supported by the European Commission (E.C.), acting as liaison between selected European fetal medicine units and an endoscopic instrument maker to design new endoscopes and instruments to improve management of specific conditions.[4,5] The later execution of a successful randomized trial on laser coagulation of twin-twin transfusion syndrome (TTTS) prompted in Europe wide clinical acceptance of fetoscopy.

Progress in the practice of fetal surgery has been slowed by the paucity of randomized trials, by patient and practitioner reluctance, by availability of local operator expertise, and even by the lack of regulatory approval of novel surgical instrumentation. For example, open fetal surgery can now be performed with significantly improved outcomes and fewer side effects compared with a decade ago. Despite that, such procedures are rarely done in Europe, with the exception of operations on placental support.[6] In the United States, slow regulatory acceptance of new fetoscopic instruments has contributed to the controversy regarding the place of fetoscopic treatment of TTTS,[7,8] together with a historically stronger preference for open procedures, including even for nonethical conditions. Indeed, in utero repair of myelomeningocele (MMC) is currently being performed in the MOMS trial (see Outcome of Antenatal Neural Tube Defect Repair, later), sponsored by the National Institutes of Health, which tests the hypothesis that antenatal repair will reduce morbidity in survivors compared with postnatal repair. Should the results of the MOMS trial be positive, undoubtedly European centers will have to reconsider the issue of open surgery, just as increasing experience and more encouraging long-term results of fetoscopic procedures from Europe have spurred the spread of minimally invasive procedures throughout the United States.

Open Fetal Surgery

Open fetal surgery is a complex enterprise that should be undertaken only in centers staffed with skilled personnel. Because of the high incidence of preterm labor, prophylactic tocolysis is essential, using for instance indomethacin or nifedipine. Large-bore venous access is established, but fluid administration is conservative and meticulously managed to reduce the risk for pulmonary edema that frequently occurs with certain tocolytics. Open surgical procedures are typically performed using general endotracheal anesthesia, taking advantage of the myorelaxant and uterine contraction suppression qualities of halogenated anesthetic gases. The uterus is exposed by a large laparotomy and opened with specially designed, resorbable lactomer surgical staples

TABLE 24-1 INDICATIONS AND RATIONALE FOR IN UTERO SURGERY ON THE FETUS, PLACENTA, CORD, OR MEMBRANES

	Pathophysiology	Rationale for In Utero Intervention
Surgery on the Fetus		
1. Congenital diaphragmatic hernia	Pulmonary hypoplasia and anatomic substrate for pulmonary hypertension	Reverse pulmonary hypoplasia and reduce degree of pulmonary hypertension; repair of actual defect delayed until after birth
2. Lower urinary tract obstruction	Progressive renal damage by obstructive uropathy Pulmonary hypoplasia by oligohydramnios	Prevention of renal failure and pulmonary hypoplasia by anatomic correction or urinary deviation
3. Sacrococcygeal teratoma	High-output cardiac failure by arteriovenous shunting and/or bleeding	Reduction of functional impact of the tumor by its ablation or (part of) its vasculature
	Direct anatomic effects of the tumoral mass	Reduction of anatomic effects by draining cysts or bladder
	Polyhydramnios-related preterm labor	Amnioreduction preventing obstetric complications
4. Thoracic space-occupying lesions	Pulmonary hypoplasia (space-occupying mass)	Creating space for lung development
	Hydrops by impaired venous return (mediastinal compression)	Reverse process of cardiac failure
5. Neural tube defects	Damage to exposed neural tube Chronic cerebrospinal fluid leak, leading to Arnold-Chiari malformation and hydrocephalus	Prevention of exposure of the spinal cord to amniotic fluid; restoration of CSF pressure, correcting Arnold-Chiari malformation
6. Cardiac malformations	Critical lesions causing irreversible hypoplasia or damage to developing heart	Reverse process by anatomic correction of restrictive pathology
Surgery on the Placenta, Cord, or Membranes		
7. Chorioangioma	High-output cardiac failure by arteriovenous shunting Effects of polyhydramnios	Reverse process of cardiac failure and hydrops fetoplacentalis by ablation or reduction of flow
8. Amniotic bands	Progressive constrictions causing irreversible neurologic or vascular damage	Prevention of amniotic band syndrome leading to deformities and function loss
9. Abnormal monochorionic twinning: twin-to-twin transfusion	Intertwin transfusion leads to oligopolyhydramnios sequence, hemodynamic changes; preterm labor and rupture of the membranes; in utero damage to brain, heart, or other organs In utero fetal death may cause damage to co-twin	Arrest intertwin transfusion, prevent or reverse cardiac failure and/or neurologic damage, including at the time of in utero death Prolongation of gestation
Fetus acardiacus and discordant anomalies	Cardiac failure of pump twin and consequences of polyhydramnios	Selective feticide: to arrest parasitic relationship, to prevent consequences of in utero fetal death
	Serious anomaly raises question for termination of pregnancy or selective feticide	To avoid termination of the entire pregnancy

Historically, in utero treatment of hydrocephalus was attempted but abandoned. In the late 1990s, indications 5 and 6 were added; 7 to 9 were typical results of the introduction of obstetric endoscopy in fetal surgery programs.

TABLE 24-2 CRITERIA FOR FETAL SURGERY

1. Accurate diagnosis and staging is possible, with exclusion of associated anomalies
2. Natural history of the disease is documented, and prognosis established.
3. Currently no effective postnatal therapy.
4. In utero surgery proven feasible in animal models, reversing deleterious effects of the condition.
5. Interventions performed in specialized multidisciplinary fetal treatment centers with strict protocols and approval of the local ethics committee, and with informed consent of the mother or parents.

Adapted from Harrison MR, Adzick NS: The fetus as a patient: Surgical considerations. Ann Surg 213:279-291; discussion, 277-278, 1991.

(Premium Poly CS 57, US Surgical, Norwalk, CT) to prevent intraoperative maternal hemorrhage. Location of the uterine incision largely depends on placental position, as determined by sterile ultrasound.

The fetus is partially exposed, and sometimes exteriorized, and monitored while the procedure is performed, using ultrasound, pulse-oximetry, or direct fetal electrocardiography.[9] Additional analgesics, atropine, and pancuronium or vecuronium are given to the fetus to suppress the fetal stress response, bradycardia, as well as to immobilize it. The fetus is kept warm through the use of intrauterine infusion of Ringer's lactate at body temperature, and intrauterine volume and pressure are maintained as close as possible to physiologic levels. After completion of the fetal portion of the procedure, the uterus is closed in two layers with resorbable sutures, amniotic fluid volume is restored, and intra-amniotic antibiotics are administered. The hysterotomy is covered with an omental flap. Postoperatively, the patient is managed in intensive care while receiving aggressive tocolysis with magnesium sulfate and, when required, additional agents.

Complications of open fetal surgery include preterm contractions, maternal morbidity from tocolysis, rupture of membranes, and fetal distress. Postoperative uterine contractions are the Achilles' heel of open fetal surgery, but new tocolytic regimes have improved tocolytic efficacy while limiting maternal side effects. Amniotic fluid leakage through the hysterotomy site (or, more commonly, vaginally because of membrane rupture) can occur. With significant postoperative oligohydramnios, delivery may be necessary because of fetal distress. In recent case series on myelomeningocele repair, patients left the hospital within a few days, a much shorter interval than previously.[10,11] Delivery by cesarean section is mandatory to prevent uterine rupture.

The EXIT Procedure

The EXIT (ex utero intrapartum treatment) procedure is increasingly used for selected fetal conditions and is an example of open fetal surgery—in this instance, to establish functional and reliable fetal airway control while keeping the fetus attached to the uteroplacental circulation by delivering only a portion of the fetus through a hysterotomy incision. EXIT is done under maximal uterine relaxation, so the maternal risks of this procedure are mainly hemorrhagic. Because of the complex interactions necessary between the anesthesia, obstetric, and pediatric personnel, EXIT procedures require significant advance preparation and preassignment of the roles for the many physicians and nurses involved. The indications for EXIT include congenital airway obstruction from laryngeal atresia, large head and neck tumors, and malformations of the face and jaw. For more information on EXIT, please refer to the Online Edition of this chapter.

Fetoscopy

Instrumentation

Fetoscopic procedures are minimally invasive interventions that can be considered a cross between ultrasound-guided and formal surgical procedures. Fetoscopy must be organized so that the surgical team can see simultaneously both the ultrasound and the fetoscopic image. Specifically designed fetoscopes typically have deported eyepieces to reduce weight and facilitate precise movements. Nearly all are flexible fiber-endoscopes rather than conventional rod lens scopes, and as the number of pixels has increased, image quality has improved markedly. Working length must be sufficient to reach all regions of the intrauterine space. Amniotic access is facilitated by thin-walled, semiflexible disposable, or larger-diameter reusable metal cannulas, so that instrument changes are possible. Once inside the amniotic cavity, the obturator is replaced by the fetoscope. Technical handbooks provide details of use of these instruments and a discussion of distention media.[3,4] Instrument insertion is facilitated with local or locoregional anesthesia, which is injected along the anticipated track of the cannula down to the myometrium.

Despite the minimally invasive nature of fetoscopy, it continues to be associated with iatrogenic preterm premature rupture of membranes (pPROM) (Table 24-3). Initiatives that have been evaluated to treat or prevent this condition[12] include attempts to repair defects with various tissue sealants applied either intracervically or intra-amniotically. These efforts have met with limited success, because fetal membranes have limited ability to heal.[13] The use of amniopatch as a treatment modality for symptomatic iatrogenic pPROM was first described by Quintero in 1996,[14] and since then a number of case series have been published[15] for iatrogenic membrane rupture after amniocentesis, fetoscopy, or chorionic villus sampling.[16] Chorionic membrane separation, without obvious amniorrhexis, is another complication that may be treated with amniopatch.[17]

Fetal Pain Relief during Procedures

Pain is a subjective experience occurring in response to impending or actual tissue damage. The subjective experience of pain requires nociception and an emotional reaction. Nociception requires an intact sensory system, whereas an emotional reaction requires some form of consciousness. It is difficult to know the extent to which the fetus experiences pain. However, several indirect methods have suggested that the fetus at least *can* feel pain. Anand and colleagues and Fisk and coworkers demonstrated that premature infants and fetuses display several stress responses during invasive procedures.[18-20] These data indicate that the mid-gestational fetus responds to noxious stimuli by mounting a distinct stress response as evidenced by an outpouring of catecholamines and other stress hormones as well as hemodynamic changes. Consequently, management of fetal pain and associated stress response in utero during invasive fetal interventions is important.[20]

TABLE 24-3 RISK FOR PRETERM PREMATURE RUPTURE OF MEMBRANES (pPROM) AFTER FETOSCOPIC PROCEDURES

Procedure	Risk for pPROM (At Assessment)	Diameter Instrument	Reference
Amniocentesis	1%-1.7%	22 ga (0.7 mm)	Tabor et al, 1986; Eddleman et al, 2006
Amniodrainage	1% per tap	18 ga (1.2 mm)	Umur et al, 2001
			Mari et al, 2000
Cordocentesis	3.7% (<37 wks)	20 ga (0.9 mm)	Tsongsong et al, 2001
Shunt	15% (thorax)	7 Fr (2.3 mm)	Picone et al, 2004 (thorax)
	32% (bladder)		Freedman, 1996 (bladder)
Fetoscopic laser	7% (<1 wk)	10 Fr (3.3 mm)	Yamamoto and Ville, 2005
(twins: 6%)	45% (<37 wks)		Lewi et al, 2006
Cord occlusion	10% (<4 wks)	10 Fr (3.3 mm)	Robyr et al, 2005
FETO	20% (<32 wks)	10 Fr (3.3 mm)	Jani et al, 2006

FETO, fetal endoscopic tracheal occlusion.

Fetal Therapy for Complicated Monochorionic Twin Pregnancies

Monochorionic twins constitute about 30% of all twin pregnancies[21] and by definition share a single placenta and nearly always have vascular anastomoses interconnecting their circulations.[22] Because of often unequal placental circulatory districts as well as cross-connecting placental vessels, monochorionic twins have substantially greater morbidity and mortality than their dichorionic counterparts.[23] These result from complications such as TTTS, twin reversed arterial perfusion (TRAP) sequence, and, in the event of single intrauterine fetal demise (IUFD), acute exsanguination of the surviving twin into the vascular space of the demised twin.[24]

Twin-Twin Transfusion Syndrome

TTTS occurs in 8% to 9% of monochorionic twin pregnancies and represents the most important cause of mortality. The complication typically becomes clinically evident between 16 and 26 weeks of gestation.[25,26] The pathology is usually explained by unbalanced circulatory sharing between the twins across placental vascular anastomoses. These anastomoses are denoted as arterioarterial (AA), venovenous (VV) or arteriovenous (AV).[27] AA and VV anastomoses are bidirectional anastomoses, whereas AV anastomoses are unidirectional and hence may create imbalance in interfetal circulation, leading to TTTS. The artery and vein of an AV anastomosis can be visualized on the placental surface as an unpaired artery and vein that pierce the chorionic plate at close proximity. Bidirectional AA anastomoses are believed to protect against the development of TTTS, as most non-TTTS monochorionic placentas (84%) have AA anastomoses in contrast to TTTS placentas (24%). Although vascular anastomoses are an anatomic prerequisite for the development of TTTS, the pathogenesis of TTTS is probably more complex,[28] involving vasoactive mediators produced by both donor and recipient.[29]

Diagnosis

The diagnosis of TTTS is based on stringent sonographic criteria of amniotic fluid and bladder filling discordance. In the donor, there is oliguric oligohydramnios, with the deepest vertical pocket (DVP) being 2 cm, while the recipient twin presents with polyuric polyhydramnios (DVP cutoff of 8 cm before 20 weeks' gestation and 10 cm after 20 weeks).[7] Although growth restriction is often present in the donor twin, it is not essential for the diagnosis of TTTS. In severe cases of TTTS, ultrasound signs of congestive cardiac failure resulting from fluid overload in the recipient include a negative or reverse a-wave in the ductus venosus, pulsatile flow in the umbilical vein, tricuspid regurgitation, and signs of hypovolemia or increased vascular resistance in the donor, with absent or reversed flow in the umbilical artery.

The differential diagnosis includes monoamnionicity, discordant growth, isolated polyhydramnios or oligohydramnios, and severe intertwin hemoglobin differences at the time of birth. TTTS does occur in monoamniotic pregnancies and is characterized by polyhydramnios of the common amniotic cavity with discordant bladder sizes. However, monoamniotic twins can move freely and usually their umbilical cords are entangled, whereas in diamniotic twins with TTTS, the donor is usually stuck against the uterine wall. Severe discordant growth is also often confused with TTTS, as the growth restricted twin may appear stuck because of oligohydramnios, but the appropriately grown twin invariably has normal amniotic fluid or only a mild degree of polyhydramnios that does not fulfill the criteria of TTTS.

Staging

TTTS is currently staged according to the Quintero staging system,[30] which is based on relative amniotic fluid volume, Doppler waveforms, and the bladder status in the donor (Table 24-4). Although the Quintero staging system predicts outcome, it better reflects manifestations of disease rather than a time sequence, as it is clear that cases can progress directly from stage I to stage V, and TTTS can appear as stage III. Attempts are now being made to improve the current staging system by incorporating a cardiac function score with echocardiographic features.[31,32] However, its additional value for predicting outcome or the choice of treatment remains to be demonstrated.[33]

Treatment

The mortality of untreated mid-trimester TTTS is more than 80% because of extreme prematurity with labor or pPROM with polyhydramnios, or as a result of fetal demise of one or both twins from cardiac failure in the recipient or poor perfusion in the donor. In view of the poor outcome, the general consensus is that treatment should

TABLE 24-4 QUINTERO STAGING SYSTEM

Time in Pregnancy	DVP Recipient	DVP of Donor
<20 weeks*	≥8 cm	<2 cm
≥20 weeks*	≥10 cm*	<2 cm

With Either

Stage I	Stage II	Stage III	Stage IV	Stage V
Bladder filling in donor	Absent bladder filling in donor	Abnormal Doppler findings: Absent/reversed EDF umbilical artery (donor); Reversed a-wave ductus venosus (recipient)	Hydrops fetalis	Intra-uterine fetal death

DVP, deepest vertical amniotic fluid pocket; EDF, end-diastolic flow.
Twin-twin transfusion syndrome cases should have a deepest pool of 8 cm on the recipient side and a deepest pool of less than 2 cm on the donor side. Classification is further made by the filling status of the bladder in the donor (Stages I and II). Additional (Doppler) ultrasound features upgrade stage.
*In European centers, most use a cutoff of 10 cm for gestation over 20 weeks. For earlier presentations than 18 weeks, cutoffs have not been agreed upon.

be offered. Unfortunately, even with the latest treatment modalities, the risk for adverse outcome remains significant and the pregnancy must be followed carefully regardless. The option of pregnancy termination should be part of patient counseling.

AMNIOREDUCTION

Serial amnioreduction was the first procedure offered to reduce polyhydramnios and intrauterine pressure in the hopes of alleviating contractions and prolonging the pregnancy. Theoretically, amnioreduction might also improve fetal hemodynamics by reducing the amniotic fluid pressure on the placental vessels. Amnioreduction is a relatively simple procedure involving aspiration of amniotic fluid via an 18-gauge needle under local anesthesia until restoration of normal amniotic fluid volume can be measured sonographically. The main shortcoming of amnioreduction is its failure to address the cause of the disease, because the vascular anastomoses remain patent. Furthermore, even if amnioreduction can resolve or stabilize stage I or II disease, it fails in one third of cases,[33] and, after failed amnioreduction, subsequent laser coagulation may be hampered by intra-amniotic bleeding, membrane separation, or unintentional septostomy.

SEPTOSTOMY

Intentional puncturing of the intertwin septum (i.e., septostomy), with or without amnioreduction, has been suggested to have beneficial effects largely based on the rarity of TTTS in monoamniotic twins. It is proposed that the donor may be able to restore blood volume and improve perfusion by swallowing amniotic fluid. A randomized trial comparing septostomy with amnioreduction found similar rates of survival of at least one twin. However, patients undergoing septostomy were more likely to require only a single procedure.[34] Nevertheless, septostomy brings with it the potential risks of cord entanglement resulting from an iatrogenic monoamnionic state, and it makes laser coagulation of the vascular anastomoses for progressive disease technically much more challenging.

SELECTIVE FETICIDE

This procedure is usually performed by umbilical cord coagulation with laser or bipolar energy and is associated with an overall survival rate of the remaining twin of about 70% to 80%.[8,9] The most important drawback of this approach is its maximum survival rate of 50%. Also, it may be unacceptable for many parents to sacrifice one twin without obvious structural pathology, and it may not be easy to determine which twin has the highest risk for adverse outcome. Therefore, this technique should be reserved for cases with severe discordant anomalies, with an inaccessible vascular equator, with pPROM of one sac, or with imminent IUFD.

FETOSCOPIC LASER COAGULATION

Laser coagulation of the vascular anastomoses was first reported in 1990 by De Lia and colleagues,[35] who described nonselective coagulation of all vessels crossing the intertwin membrane, thus arresting the transfusion of blood and vascular mediators from donor to recipient and functionally making the placenta dichorionic. However, nonselective coagulation of all vessels along the intertwin membrane causes significant parenchymal placental damage and probably increases the procedure-related fetal loss. Most fetoscopic laser centers therefore avoid coagulation of nonanastomosing vessels and instead perform selective coagulation of all visible anastomosing vessels along the vascular equator.

Fetoscopic laser coagulation is usually performed between 16 and 26 weeks of gestation. Before 16 weeks, the amniotic membrane may still be separated from the chorion, hampering amniotic access and making the degree of oligohydramnios or polyhydramnios difficult to measure. After 26 weeks, fetoscopic laser coagulation remains a valid treatment option and appears to be associated with less major neonatal morbidity than repeated amnioreduction.[36] From 32 weeks onward, elective preterm delivery should be considered if lung maturation can be documented.

Preoperatively, a detailed ultrasound scan is performed for disease staging and to exclude discordant anomalies. Prophylactic antibiotics and prophylactic tocolytics are used. Fetoscopy is performed percutaneously through a 3- to 4-mm incision under local or regional anesthesia. High-quality videoendoscopic hardware with an excellent light source, video camera, and monitor, and with specifically designed 20- to 30-cm fiberoptic or rod lens fetoscopes with a diameter of 1 to 3 mm, is used. For laser coagulation, a neodymium-yttrium aluminum garnet (Nd-YAG) laser (minimal power requirements, 60 to 100 W) or a diode laser (30 to 60 W) with fibers of 400 to 600 μm provide optimal efficacy.

Next, the positions of the fetuses, umbilical cord insertions, and placenta are mapped by ultrasound. Under ultrasound guidance, the cannula or fetoscopic sheath is inserted into the recipient's sac. Preferentially, the site of the trocar insertion is remote from the donor's sac to avoid the risk of unintentional septostomy, and the trocar is aimed to achieve a 90-degree angle with the vascular equator, as this provides the best opportunity for optimal coagulation. The vascular equator can usually not be visualized on ultrasound unless there is a marked difference in echogenicity between the two placental districts.[37] The trocar is therefore optimally inserted halfway along the imaginary line between the two cord insertions. Occasionally, vision is hampered by blood or debris, in which case amnioexchange with warmed Hartmann's solution (heated by a blood warmer or a special amnio-irrigator) can improve visibility.

A systematic inspection of the entire vascular equator is performed. The placental insertion of the intertwin septum is easily identified as a thin white line on the chorionic surface, and anastomosing vessels leaving the donor usually cross under the septum in the direction of the recipient. Anastomosing vessels can also be identified starting from the recipient's or donor's cord insertion. Arteries are distinguishable from veins, as they cross over the veins and have a darker color because of their lower oxygen saturation.[38] Not uncommonly, it may be impossible, because of the position of the intertwin septum, placenta, fetus, or other physical limitations, to determine whether vessels anastomose. In these instances, these vessels are coagulated as well, as the aim is to separate the two fetal circulations completely.

Coagulation is performed at a distance of approximately 1 cm and ideally at a 90-degree angle, using a nontouch technique (Fig. 24-1), starting at one placental border and finishing at the other end. Recently the sequential approach selecting A-V anastomoses first has been advocated.[39] Sections of 1 to 2 cm are coagulated with shots of about 3 to 4 seconds, according to the tissue response. The use of excessive laser power levels should be avoided, as this may cause vessel perforation and fetal hemorrhage. Once all vessels are coagulated, the vascular equator is inspected once more to ascertain that all anastomoses have been fully coagulated and that flow has not resumed. The procedure is completed by amnioreduction until normal amniotic fluid volume (DVP, 5 to 6 μm) is measured by ultrasound.

With an anterior placenta, the recipient's sac as well as the anastomosing vessels may be much more difficult to access. Instruments for anterior placentas have been developed, but it is still unclear whether these improve performance. Nonflexible rod lens telescopes have been fabricated with angles of inclination up to 30 degrees, or with an associ-

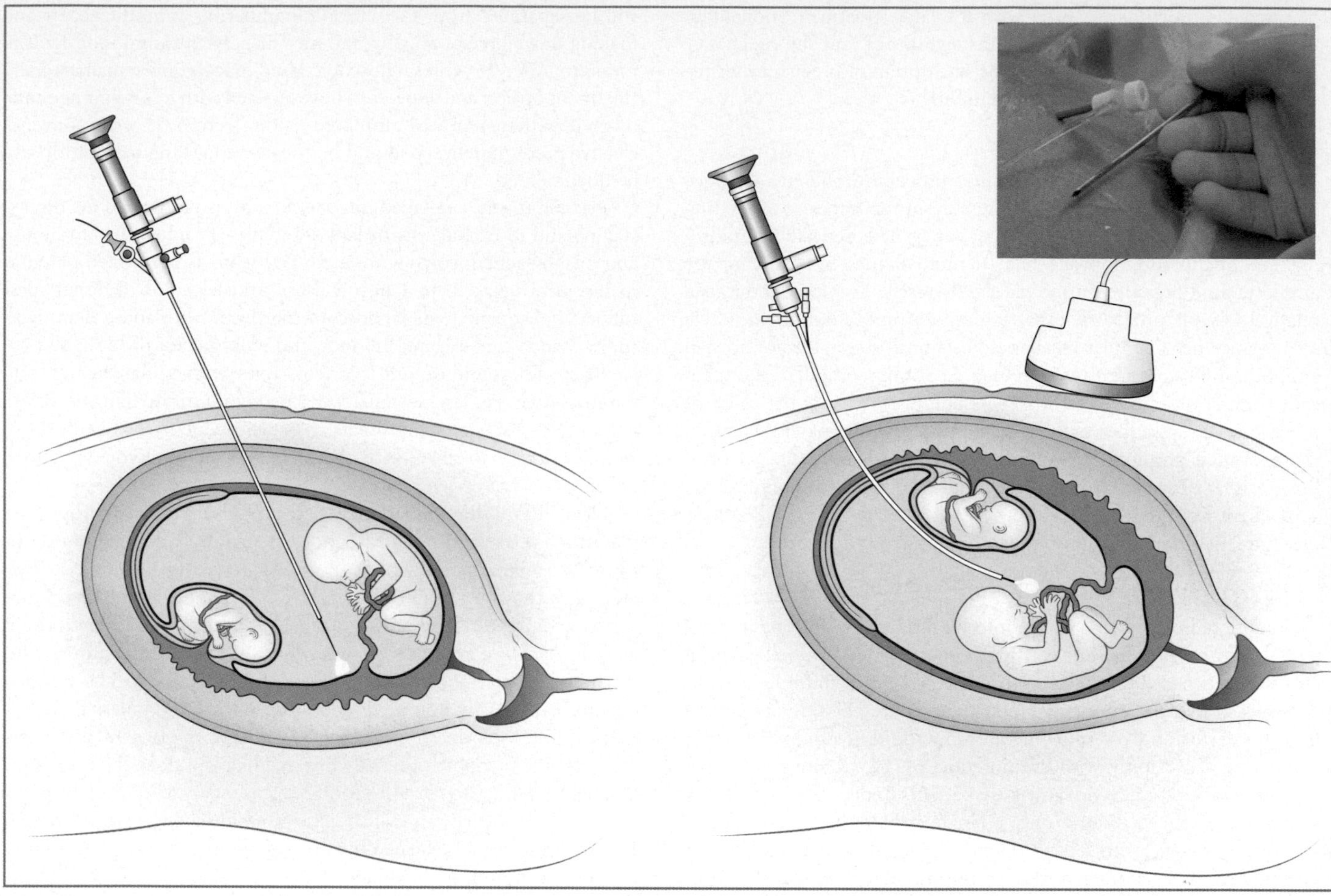

FIGURE 24-1 Schematic drawing of fetoscopic laser coagulation. When the placenta is posterior, the scope can be directly inserted through the sheath without using a cannula *(left)*. When the placenta is anterior *(right)*, a curved sheath and a flexible cannula *(inset)* can be used. This allows a change of instruments. (Drawing by K. Dalkowski, and modified with permission of Endopress Karl Storz.)

ated deflecting mechanism for the laser fiber.[40] Thus far, similar outcomes have been reported for anterior and posterior placentas.[7]

Postoperatively, the patient should remain in the hospital for 1 to 2 days while daily ultrasound scans are performed to document fetal viability, amniotic fluid volume, and changes in the phenotypic features of TTTS, particularly bladder filling and Doppler parameters. Postoperative transient hydropic changes and absent or reversed a-wave in the ductus venosus may occur in the donor twin.[41,42] For fetuses with absent end-diastolic flow preoperatively, reappearance of end-diastolic flow is observed in 53%.[43] Laser coagulation may equalize previously discordant umbilical venous blood flow between donor and recipient.[44,45] Catch-up fetal growth has also been described.

Fetal complications after laser treatment include fetal demise, isolated severe intertwin hemoglobin discordance, and persistent TTTS. Postoperative single IUFD occurs in about 33% and double IUFD in 4% of pregnancies. Single IUFD seems to affect donor and recipient equally,[46] and approximately 60% are diagnosed within 24 hours and 75% within 1 week. Persistent TTTS complicates up to 14% of pregnancies with two surviving fetuses 1 week after laser treatment[47] and appears to be related to missed, large, unidirectional anastomoses.[48] Possible treatment options include repeat laser with backup cord coagulation, amnioreduction, and elective delivery. A number of other, rarer complications have been described, most of them occurring after amnioreduction as well. Please also refer to the Online Edition of this chapter.

AMNIOREDUCTION VERSUS LASER COAGULATION

The Eurofoetus trial,[7] with 142 enrolled patients with stage I to IV disease diagnosed between 15 and 26 weeks of gestation, demonstrated that fetoscopic laser coagulation is currently the best available treatment option for TTTS (Table 24-5). Compared with amnioreduction, use of the laser was associated with a significantly higher likelihood of the survival of at least one twin to 28 days of life (76% versus 56%). Also, the median gestational age at delivery was higher in the laser than in the amnioreduction group (33.3 weeks versus 29.0 weeks' gestation), with 42% and 69% women, respectively, delivering at less than 32 weeks. Also, infants in the laser group had a lower incidence of cystic periventricular leukomalacia (laser 6% versus amnioreduction 14%). Importantly, the Eurofoetus trial demonstrated that more than half of severe cerebral lesions identified postnatally appear to have had an antenatal origin.[24,49] A recent systematic review of the Eurofoetus randomized controlled trial and two other observational studies confirmed that laser coagulation appears to be more effective in the treatment of TTTS, with less perinatal neurologic morbidity and mortality.[50]

Huber and coworkers[51] similarly demonstrated, in a consecutive series of 200 pregnancies, a significant trend toward reduced survival after fetoscopic laser treatment with increasing stage. Survival of both twins was 75.9% for stage I, 60.5% for stage II, 53.8% for stage III, and 50% for stage IV. At least one twin survived in 93.1% of pairs at stage

TABLE 24-5 LASER COAGULATION VERSUS AMNIOREDUCTION

	Laser (*N* = 72)	Amnioreduction (*N* = 70)	*P* Value
Gestational age at randomization (wks)	20.6 (2.4)	20.9 (2.5)	ns
Quintero stage at randomization			
Stage I	6 (8.3%)	5 (7.1%)	ns
Stage II	31 (43.1%)	31 (44.3%)	ns
Stage III	34 (47.2%)	33 (47.1%)	ns
Stage IV	1 (1.4%)	1 (1.4%)	ns
Number of procedures	1*	2.6 (1.9)	—
AFV drained per procedure (mL) or in total overall amniodrainages: median (range)	1725 (500-5500)	2000 (243-4000)	ns
		3800 (600-18,000)	<.001
Pregnancy loss at or within 7 days of the initial procedure	8 (11.6%)	2 (2.9%)	.10
Premature rupture of membranes at or within 7 days of the first procedure	4 (5.8%)	1 (1.5%)	.37
Premature rupture of membranes at or within 28 days of the first procedure	6 (8.7%)	6 (8.8%)	.98
Intrauterine death ≤7 days of the first procedure†	16/138 (11.6%)	9/136 (6.6%)	.23
At least one survivor at 6 months of life	55 (76.4%)	36 (51.4%)	.002
No survivors	17 (23.6%)	34 (48.6%)	
One survivor	29 (40.3%)	18 (25.7%)	
Two survivors	26 (36.1%)	18 (25.7%)	
At least one survivor at 6 months stratified by stage			
Quintero stages I and II	32/37 (86.5%)	21/36 (58.3%)	.007
Quintero stages III and IV	23/35 (65.7%)	15/34 (44.1%)	.07
Gestational age at delivery—median (interquartile range)	33.3 (26.1-35.6)	29.0 (25.6-33.3)	.004
Neonatal and infant death	12 (8.3%)	41 (29.3%)	
≤24 hours after delivery	6 (4.2%)	26 (18.6%)	
1 to 7 days after delivery	4 (2.8%)	6 (4.3%)	
7 to 28 days after delivery	1 (0.7%)	5 (0.0%)	
28 days or more after delivery	1 (0.7%)	4 (2.9%)	
Intraventricular hemorrhage (grades III and IV)‡	2 (1.4%)	8 (5.7%)	.10*
Donor	2 (2.8%)	2 (2.9%)	1.0
Recipient	0 (0.0%)	6 (8.6%)	.02
Cystic periventricular leukomalacia§	8 (5.6%)	20 (14.3%)	.02*
Donor	2/72 (2.8%)	5/70 (7.1%)	.27
Recipient	6/72 (8.3%)	15/70 (21.4%)	.03

Baseline characteristics according to group. Results reported as number of pregnancies [n (%)]. AFV, amniotic fluid valve.
***Two patients had two laser procedures.**
†With number of fetuses as denominator (P value adjusted for clustering).
‡Severe intraventricular hemorrhage was defined as ventricular bleeding with dilation of the cerebral ventricles (grade III) or parenchymal hemorrhage (grade IV).
§Cystic periventricular leukomalacia was defined as periventricular densities evolving into extensive cystic lesions (grade III) or extending into the deep white matter evolving into cystic lesions (grade IV).

I, 82.7% at stage II, 82.5% at stage III, and 70% at stage IV. The survival rate of donors (70.5%) was similar to that of recipients (72.5%). Hecher and associates demonstrated the importance of the learning curve in laser photocoagulation, with increased experience leading to improved survival,[52] later gestational age at delivery, and a decrease in neurodevelopmental impairment.[53]

With regard to long-term follow-up, a study of surviving infants (aged 14 to 44 months) from a laser photocoagulation series laser demonstrated neurologic problems in 22% of survivors,[54] of which 11% were mild and 11% were severe. In a later series by the same group, 7% of infants showed minor and 6% showed major neurologic abnormalities.[53] The reduced neurologic impairment in the second report may be explained by increased operator experience. These results are significantly better than the 16% minor and 26% major abnormalities in a cohort treated with amnioreduction.[55]

Selective feticide may be indicated for cases with a severe discordant structural or chromosomal anomaly, with severe discordant growth and a high risk for IUFD, or with TRAP sequence, and it may be indicated for selected cases with TTTS. However, because monochorionic multiple fetuses share a single placenta with multiple vascular anastomoses, selective feticide by intravascular injection of potassium chloride may embolize the healthy fetus. Fetoscopic umbilical cord ligation has been largely abandoned because it is a cumbersome and lengthy procedure, although it achieved an immediate and complete cord occlusion.[56]

Selective Feticide for Other Complications

For fetuses with TRAP sequence, needle-based coagulation techniques using laser, monopolar, and radiofrequency energy[57-59] have been adopted, involving the insertion of a 14- to 17-gauge needle into the acardiac twin's abdomen under ultrasound guidance, and aiming for the intra-abdominal rather than umbilical vessels. The largest series, of 29 monochorionic multiple pregnancies treated with radiofrequency energy between 18 and 24 weeks, reported a survival rate of 86%.[59] Median gestational age at delivery was 38 weeks (range, 24 to 40 weeks). In another recent smaller series[60] of 13 cases treated with radiofrequency energy between 17 and 24 weeks, the survival rate was 94%. All patients delivered after 32 weeks, except for one patient complicated by pPROM at 26 weeks.

Umbilical Cord Occlusion

At present, laser or bipolar coagulation of the umbilical cord is our preferred approach and can be used for all indications from 16 weeks onward.[48,61] Early on, a double-needle loaded with a 1-mm fetoscope and a 400-μm laser fiber is used.[62] Lasering of the cord allows optimal visual control but may fail beyond 20 weeks because of the increasing size of the umbilical cord vessels.[63,64] Ultrasound-guided bipolar cord coagulation was therefore introduced for later gestational ages.

Bipolar coagulation is performed with a 2.4- or 3-mm reusable or disposable forceps. Under ultrasound guidance, a portion of the umbilical cord is grasped at a convenient location and coagulation current is applied in progressive increments until the appearance of turbulence and steam bubbles indicates tissue coagulation. Confirmation of arrest of flow distal to the occlusion is performed by color Doppler. Even if there is no longer any visible flow, two additional cord segments (preferably at a site more proximal to the target fetus) are coagulated. After completion of the coagulation procedure, amnioreduction of excessive fluid is carried out before removal of the cannula. The survival rates of umbilical cord coagulation in monochorionic twins is approximately 80%. In dichorionic and monochorionic triplets, the technique resulted in similar survival rates of 79%. About half of the losses are attributable to intrauterine demise of the healthy co-twin and about half to postnatal losses related to the very preterm birth, mostly related to pPROM.[47,48]

Twin Reversed Arterial Perfusion Sequence

An extreme manifestation of TTTS is the TRAP sequence, which complicates about 1% of monochorionic twin pregnancies. In the TRAP sequence, blood flows from an umbilical artery of the pump twin in a reversed direction into the umbilical artery of the perfused twin, via an AA anastomosis. The perfused twin's blood supply is by definition deoxygenated and results in variable degrees of deficient development of the head, heart, and upper limb structures. Two criteria are necessary for the development of a TRAP sequence: an AA anastomosis and a discordant development[65] or intrauterine death of one twin,[66] allowing reversal of blood flow.

The increased burden to perfuse the parasitic twin puts the pump twin at risk for congestive heart failure and hydrops.[67] Because of the rarity of the disorder, the natural history of antenatally diagnosed cases is still poorly documented, with reported survival rates for the pump twin varying between 14%[68] and 90%.[69] Data on long-term outcome are not available, although the risk for cardiac and neurodevelopmental sequelae may be high as a result of vascular imbalances in utero.[70,71] Several factors have been suggested to indicate a poor prognosis, such as a high ratio of the weight of the acardiac twin to that of the pump twin,[72] a rapid increase in the acardiac mass,[73] and small differences in the umbilical artery Doppler values.[74,75] These parameters were, however, mostly studied in the late second and third trimesters and do not necessary apply in the early second trimester, where spontaneous resolution as well as sudden death of the pump twin remain unpredictable. Early intervention is an option, as the diagnosis is now usually made at an early stage in pregnancy, although the pump twin may survive without any intervention in at least half of cases. For later procedures, umbilical cord coagulation as well as needle-based intrafetal coagulation techniques are both suitable treatment options. The largest experience with fetoscopic laser coagulation for this indication was reported by Hecher and coworkers ($N = 60$) with an 80% survival rate.[76]

More discussion of the techniques of management of TTTS, together with figures, tables, and references, can be found in the Online Edition of this chapter.

Isolated Congenital Diaphragmatic Hernia

Congenital diaphragmatic hernia (CDH) occurs sporadically, with an incidence of 1 in 2500 to 1 in 5000 newborns. The term *congenital diaphragmatic hernia* designates a range of lesions, and outcomes are accordingly diverse.[77] Ultimately, all the phenotypes of CDH arise from genetic mutations in one or several developmental pathways common for tissues of the fetal diaphragm and adjacent organs.

Eighty-four percent of lesions are left-sided, 13% are right-sided, and 2% are bilateral. Complete diaphragmatic agenesis, with herniation of the central tendineus portion and eventration, are other rare manifestations. Associated anomalies are present in 40% of cases, which confers an increased risk for neonatal death, and less than 15% of infants in this group survive.[78,79] In the majority, however, CDH is an isolated defect. Although CDH is in essence a defect in the diaphragm, the abnormal lung development that ensues confers its clinical impact. CDH lungs have a reduced number of alveoli, thickened alveolar walls, increased interstitial tissue, and markedly diminished alveolar air space and gas-exchange surface area. The conducting airways and associated blood vessels are diminished as well. Both lungs are typically affected, the ipsilateral more than the contralateral. There may be other anatomic aberrations present in the diaphragm and in the upper gastrointestinal tract, such as the position of the liver, lower esophagus, and stomach.

Prenatal Diagnosis of Congenital Diaphragmatic Hernia

The diagnosis of CDH is usually made in the prenatal period when cystic masses are visualized in the chest or when cardiac deviation is noted in the axial view of the thorax (Fig. 24-2). Left-sided CDH typically appears with rightward shift of the heart and the echolucent stomach and intestines in the left chest. Right-sided CDH is more difficult to diagnose because the echogenicity of liver is similar to that of the mid-trimester fetal lung. The diagnosis is suggested when the fetal heart is shifted farther into the left chest, or when color Doppler interrogation of the umbilical vein and hepatic vessels are shown to cross the diaphragmatic boundary. The differential diagnosis includes cystic or mixed masses (cystic adenomatoid malformation, bronchogenic, enteric and neuroenteric cysts, mediastinal teratoma, and thymic cysts), bronchopulmonary sequestration, and bronchial atresia. In these conditions, abdominal organs are not displaced into the chest.

When CDH is suspected, the patient should be examined for associated cardiac, renal, central nervous system, and gastrointestinal anomalies.[80] Chromosomal anomalies are increased in CDH, so amniocentesis and genetic consultation are mandatory. For management, patients should be referred to tertiary centers accustomed to managing complex congenital anomalies, in prenatal and in postnatal periods, to optimize the necessary comprehensive diagnostic and prognostic assessments, provide counseling on which parents can base further decisions, and eventually offer timed delivery followed by optimal postnatal care.

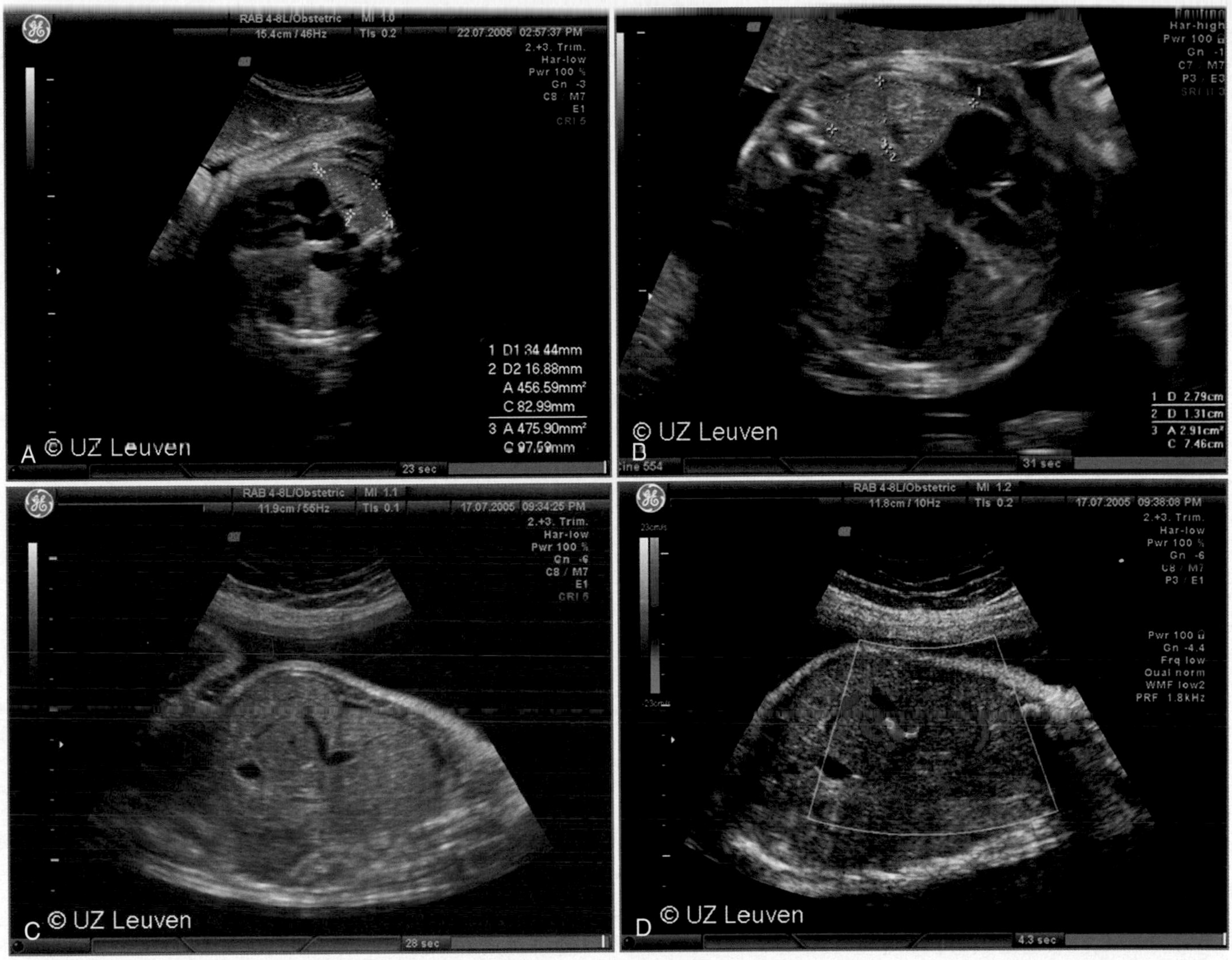

FIGURE 24-2 Ultrasound of a fetus with congenital diaphragmatic hernia. **A,** Measurement of the lung-to-head ratio (LHR) in a section through the four-chamber view, with the longest-axis method and the tracing method. **B,** Measurement of LHR, 1 day after balloon insertion. Echogenicity has changed. **C,** Herniation of the liver. **D,** Visualization of the major vessels helps identify the liver position.

Prognostic Indicators for Congenital Diaphragmatic Hernia

Multiple prognostic measures have been proposed, including proportions of the cardiac ventricles, amniotic fluid volume, degree of mediastinal shift, and position of the stomach. However, most have not been shown to reliably provide clinically useful correlations. Because the most critical problems of the neonate with CDH are lung hypoplasia and pulmonary hypertension, quantitation of relative pulmonary mass using a variety of imaging techniques has been most successful.[81]

The best validated measurement is the ratio of lung area (assessed by two-dimensional ultrasound through the contralateral lung) to head circumference (LHR).[82] Although different methods for measuring the LHR have been proposed, the most reproducible and accurate involves tracing the lung contours (see Fig. 24-2).[83] The predictive value of LHR was validated in 184 consecutive cases of isolated left-sided CDH; the fetuses were examined at 22 to 28 weeks of gestation and were born live beyond 30 weeks at 10 centers (Table 24-6).[83-85] Liver herniation has also been shown to be an independent predictor of outcome.[86] Because the echogenicity of liver is comparable to that of the lung, Doppler interrogation of the umbilical vein and hepatic vessels helps in determining its position above or below the diaphragm.

From 12 to 32 weeks, lung area in the fetus increases four times faster than head circumference, so the LHR must be referenced to gestational age.[35] The gestational effect on LHR can be accommodated by expressing the observed LHR as a ratio of the expected mean for gestation. A study from the CDH antenatal registry (354 fetuses) with unilateral isolated CDH evaluated these measures between 18 and 38 weeks.[85] Observed-to-expected (O/E) LHR predicted outcome well, regardless of the gestational age at measurement, and also correlates with short-term morbidity indicators (Fig. 24-3).[87]

Prediction of Pulmonary Arterial Hypertension

In utero assessment of lung vasculature can be obtained by measuring the number of branches and vessel diameters, and by performing mea-

TABLE 24-6 NEONATAL OUTCOME AS A FUNCTION OF LHR IN FETUSES WITH LEFT-SIDED ISOLATED CDH AND LIVER HERNIATION, EXPECTANTLY MANAGED VERSUS AFTER FETO

Degree of Pulmonary Hypoplasia	LHR	N	Expectant Management*	LHR	N	FETO†
Extreme	0.4-0.5	2	0 (0%)	0.4-0.5	6	1 (16.7%)
Severe	0.6-0.7	6	0 (0%)	0.6-0.7	13	8 (61.5%)
	0.8-0.9	19	3 (15.8%)	0.8-0.9	9	7 (77.8%)
	LHR < 1.0	*27*	*3 (11.1%)*	*LHR < 1.0*	*28*	*16 (57.1%)*
Moderate	1.0-1.1	23	14 (60.9%)	1.0-1.1		na
	1.2-1.3	19	13 (68.4%)	1.2-1.3		na
Mild	1.4-1.5	11	8 (72.7%)	1.4-1.5		na
	≥1.6	6	5 (83.3%)	≥1.6		na
	total	*86*	*43 (50%)*			

*Data from Kinsella J, Parker T, Dunbar I, et al: Noninvasive delivery of inhaled nitric oxide therapy for late pulmonary hypertension in newborn infants with congenital diaphragmatic hernia. J Pediatr 142:397-401, 2003.

†Data from Jani J, Nicolaides KH, Gratacos E, et al, and the FETO task group: Fetal lung-to-head ratio in the prediction of survival in severe left-sided diaphragmatic hernia treated by fetal endoscopic tracheal occlusion (FETO). Am J Obstet Gynecol 195:1646-1650, 2006.

CDH, congenital diaphragmatic hernia; FETO, fetal endoscopic tracheal occlusion; LHR, fetal lung-to-head circumference ratio; na, not applicable because these fetuses were not eligible for FETO.

surements of flow and resistance with two- or three-dimensional techniques. The Toronto group demonstrated that the diameter of the ipsilateral branch of the main pulmonary artery is related to the severity of hypoplasia in the prenatal as well as in the postnatal period, where it is also a significant predictor of morbidity.[88-90] Recently, Ruano and colleagues established nomograms for main pulmonary artery branch diameters, which will allow proper validation of this concept.[91] They also proposed three-dimensional power Doppler to assess the entire lung vasculature, and to predict neonatal survival and the occurrence of pulmonary hypoplasia.[92]

Postnatal Management of Congenital Diaphragmatic Hernia

The ill development of the fetal lung leads to variable degrees of respiratory insufficiency and pulmonary hypertension after birth. The aberrant vasculature is also more sensitive to hypoxic vasoconstriction, leading to pulmonary hypertension and further increasing right-to-left shunt. This creates a vicious cycle that prevents gas exchange of the shunted blood and increases acidosis and hypoxia. Pulmonary hypertension is increasingly being treated by inhaled nitric oxide.[93] Administration of prostaglandin E_1 has been advocated to keep the ductus arteriosus patent in cases with severe secondary left ventricular cardiac dysfunction.[94,95] Survival statistics for postnatally managed CDH are optimized in specialized centers: in France, referral centers have higher survival rates (41% to 66%; $P = .03$)[96]; in Canada, high-volume centers (>12 CDH admissions over the 22-month period) with centralized management report a 13% higher survival rate than low-volume centers.[97]

Antenatal Management for Congenital Diaphragmatic Hernia

Meticulous preparation for a possible antenatal surgical procedure for CDH is critical. Informed consent requires counseling that includes describing the typical postnatal course of a newborn with CDH, together with the range of expected morbidities that might be encountered. Counseling should also include individualized information derived from the imaging assessments (O/E LHR < 25%). In mild or moderate cases, the predicted survival rate is more than 60%, so planned delivery at a referral center is appropriate. In more severe cases, especially with associated anomalies, other options should be discussed, including termination of pregnancy.

The patients with a poorer prognosis are also candidates for an antenatal intervention that could reduce the likelihood of lethal pulmonary hypoplasia. Previously, antenatal therapy consisting of in utero anatomic repair using hysterotomy and direct fetal surgery was advocated, but this has been abandoned because of poor results. Subsequently, Di Fiore and colleagues revived the concept of triggering lung growth by tracheal occlusion,[98] based on the observation that fetuses with congenital high airway obstruction syndrome (CHAOS) display impressive lung growth, probably because of the lung-distending pressure of the trapped pulmonary secretions. However, lung growth alone is not adequate for postnatal pulmonary function, as lung epithelial maturation is also necessary. Under normal circumstances, fetal breathing movements promote fluid flow out of the airways, creating cycles of tissue stretch and relaxation. It is now clear that breathing movements are important for an appropriate balance between growth and differentiation.[99]

Temporary tracheal occlusion takes advantage of this principle, its beneficial effects being a function of the timing and duration of the occlusion. When sustained until birth, lung growth is vigorous but airway epithelial maturation is compromised. Experimental models, now confirmed with clinical experience, demonstrate that in utero placement, then reversal of occlusion (plug-unplug sequence) achieves improved lung volume and maturation.[100] Antenatal tracheal occlusion is clinically applied at 26 to 28 weeks under locoregional anesthesia using fetoscopy to insert a balloon into the fetal trachea. The occlusion is reversed by removing the balloon fetoscopically at 34 weeks to allow fetal breathing and epithelial maturation.[101,102] If preterm labor precludes fetoscopic removal, emergency peripartum removal by laryngotracheoscopy or an EXIT procedure may be required.[103]

A recent report of a randomized controlled trial by Harrison and coworkers showed that prenatal tracheal occlusion did not increase survival.[104] In that study, however, fetuses with O/E LHR up to 36% (LHR = 1.4) were offered fetal therapy. It is therefore not surprising that postnatal management yielded results equivalent to those of antenatal surgery. There were not enough cases with extreme or severe

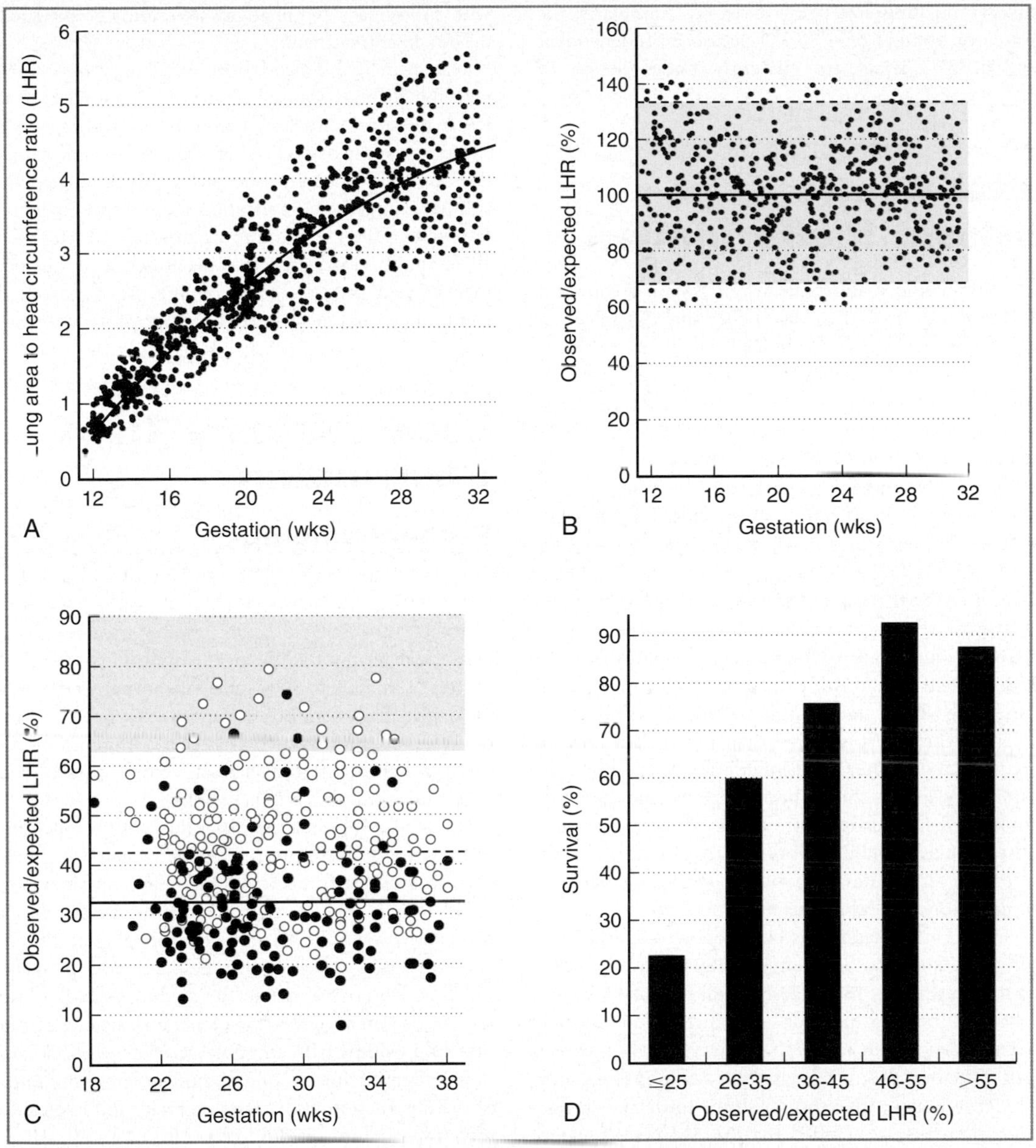

FIGURE 24-3 Ratio of lung area to head circumference (LHR). **A,** Measurements of right LHR in normal fetuses throughout pregnancy. The curve shows LHR as a function of gestational age. **B,** Plot of the observed-to-expected (O/E) LHR with the mean and the 95th and 5th percentiles in normal fetuses. **C,** Right O/E LHR in fetuses with isolated left-sided diaphragmatic hernia. The shaded area depicts the lower part of the normal range. *Closed circles* (observations), *solid line* (mean), nonsurvivors; *open circles* (observations), *dotted line* (mean), survivors. **D,** Survival rates according to the O/E LHR in fetuses with isolated left-sided diaphragmatic hernia and liver herniation ($N = 161$). (**A** and **B** from Peralta CF, Cavoretto P, Csapo B, et al: Assessment of lung area in normal fetuses at 12-32 weeks. Ultrasound Obstet Gynecol 26:718-724, 2005; **C** and **D** modified from Jani J, Nicolaides KH, Keller RL, et al: Observed to expected lung area to head circumference ratio in the prediction of survival in fetuses with isolated diaphragmatic hernia. Ultrasound Obstet Gynecol 30:67-71, 2007.)

hypoplasia. These are the subjects who are offered fetal endoscopic tracheal occlusion (FETO) in the current European programs, where the presence of liver herniation and O/E LHR < 27% to 28% (corresponding to LHR < 1.0 in the early third trimester) are strict criteria today.

The European FETO task force has reported a survival rate of 50% to 57% in this group of fetuses with otherwise poor predicted survival.[105] Iatrogenic pPROM remains a major complication. In such cases, patients are managed expectantly in the hospital so that the tracheal balloon can be promptly removed once labor or chorioamnionitis occurs. Thus far, more than 75% of patients have delivered beyond 34 weeks (mean gestational age at birth, 36 weeks), significantly later than the 31 weeks observed by Harrison and colleagues.[104] Neonatal survival rate is higher with prenatal than with perinatal balloon retrieval (83.3% versus 33.3%; $P = .013$), a trend persisting until discharge (67% versus 33%; NS). Major predictors of survival are gestational age at delivery and lung size prior to FETO.[74] Similarly, the increase in lung area or volume after FETO is also an independent predictor of survival.[106,107] Trials are currently under design in Europe.

Congenital Cystic Adenomatoid Malformation

Congenital cystic adenomatoid malformation (CCAM) is a common pulmonary malformation estimated to occur in approximately 1 in 3000 to 5000 pregnancies. CCAM is a dysplastic or hamartomatous tumor with overgrowth of terminal bronchioles and reduction in number of alveoli. Patients usually present with a thoracic mass involving only one pulmonary lobe. In approximately 40%, the CCAM may have a systemic vascular supply, similar to bronchopulmonary sequestration (BPS), and these forms are defined as hybrid CCAM-BPS. The classic pathologic classification as proposed by Stocker established three types.[108] Chapter 18 gives details of diagnosis and prognosis.

When the CCAM is larger, there is an increased risk for pulmonary compression and hydrops. Use of the ratio of the mass area to head circumference (CCAM volume ratio [CVR]) has been proposed as a gestational-age-independent prognostic measure.[109] CCAM volume (in milliliters) is measured using the formula for an ellipse (length × height × width × 0.52). When CVR is higher than 1.6, an 80% risk for fetal hydrops is predicted. When the CVR is high but fetal age is greater than 34 weeks, respiratory distress should be anticipated, and the EXIT procedure with lobectomy in a tertiary care center should be considered.[110] Hydrops after viability should prompt delivery. In the previable period, fetal intervention can be lifesaving, but no large series is available to judge among options. Percutaneous puncture and thoracoamniotic shunting of macrocystic masses has been reported and has the advantage of minimal invasiveness.[111] Wilson recently reviewed experience with 23 shunted cases at a mean gestational age of 21 to 22 weeks.[112] The mean CVR in this group was 2.4, which fell to 0.7 after shunting. The mean interval from shunt to delivery was 11.8 weeks (36.3 weeks at birth). The overall survival was 74%, with one fetal and five neonatal deaths, correlating with a shorter shunt-to-delivery interval. A recent systematic review concluded that CCAM cyst drainage improves perinatal survival among hydropic fetuses.[113]

For solid lesions, lobectomy via open fetal surgery can be considered. In a series of 22 cases receiving surgery between 21 and 31 weeks, there were 11 long-term survivors who were developmentally normal (up to 12 years of age).[114] Hydrops resolved in 1 to 2 weeks, followed by normalization of the mediastinum, and the remaining lung underwent impressive catch-up growth. Causes of fetal death despite fetal surgery were termination of pregnancy for Ballentyne syndrome (one patient), preterm labor and/or chorioamnionitis (two patients), and fetal hemodynamic compromise leading to intraoperative death in six fetuses and postoperative death in another two.

Other Thoracic Lesions

Pleural effusion or fetal hydrothorax is a typical symptom of other pathology. Pleural effusions have the potential to cause mediastinal shift, abnormal venous return and secondary lung compression, hydrops, and intrauterine demise. Most primary effusions are lymphatic in origin, but they may be associated with other anomalies (25%), including aneuploidy (7%).[115] Bilateral effusions are associated with pulmonary lymphangiectasia, and the prognosis remains poor despite fetal treatment.

The principal indication for fetal intervention for pleural effusions is fetal hydrops, because the survival rate is 30%, compared with 80% when there are effusions without fetal hydrops.[113] Thoracoamniotic shunting is performed using a double-pigtail catheter or via serial thoracentesis.[116] There is no proof that serial puncture is better than shunting, and the complication rate of this procedure is about 15%. Iatrogenic pPROM[117] and procedure-related fetal loss occurs in 5% to 10%. Shunt dislodgment has been described, but posterior insertion may prevent the fetus from pulling the shunt out. Preterm birth is common, with a mean gestational age of 34 to 35 weeks.

Lower Urinary Tract Obstruction

Pathophysiology

Congenital anomalies of the genitourinary tract are the most commonly identified during prenatal ultrasound screening, with an incidence of up to 0.4%. *Lower urinary tract obstruction* (LUTO) is a descriptive term for a heterogeneous group of relatively common conditions (1 in 5000 to 8000 male newborns). Posterior urethral valves is by far the most common cause (at least one third in autopsy series), but other conditions such as stenosis of the urethral meatus, anterior urethral valves, urethral atresia, ectopic insertion of a ureter, and (peri)vesical tumors are included.

LUTO leads to bladder distention with compensatory hypertrophy of the smooth muscle of the bladder wall. Over time, bladder compliance and elasticity decrease and may contribute to poor postnatal bladder function. Elevated bladder pressure inhibits urinary inflow from above, resulting in reflux hydronephrosis. Progressive pyelectasis and calyectasis compress the delicate renal parenchyma, leading to functional abnormalities in the medullary and eventually the cortical regions, leading eventually to renal insufficiency. Concurrently, amniotic fluid volume falls, and pulmonary hypoplasia evolves. This condition is reproducible in animal models, and more importantly, reversal of the obstruction both experimentally and clinically leads to reaccumulation of amniotic fluid.[118]

Case Selection

Because LUTO can result in neonatal lethal pulmonary hypoplasia and renal failure, careful selection of candidates for antenatal intervention is paramount, ensuring that procedures to relieve LUTO are offered only to fetuses with sufficient renal function.[119] Because fetal renal function cannot be determined on a single urine sample, the best prediction is obtained by two or more sequential vesicocenteses several days apart.[120] The commonly recognized prognostic thresholds are shown in Table 24-7.

The prenatal evaluation of fetuses with the sonographic findings of LUTO must be comprehensive, and coexisting structural and chromosomal anomalies must be excluded before intervention can be considered.[121] Female fetuses very often have more complex syndromes of cloacal malformations that may not benefit from in utero shunt therapy. Because of the presence of oligohydramnios or anhydramnios, it may be necessary to obtain karyotype by transabdominal chorionic villus or fetal blood sampling and thorough structural assessment of the fetus after amnioinfusion.

TABLE 24-7 FETAL URINE ANALYSIS PROGNOSTIC THRESHOLDS

Electrolytes	Good Prognosis	Poor Prognosis
Sodium	<90 mmol/L	>100 mmol/L
Chloride	<90 mmol/L	>100 mmol/L
Osmolality	<180 mOsm/L	>200 mOsm/L
Total protein	<20 mg/dL	>40 mg/dL
β_2-microglobulin	<6 mg/L	>10 mg/L

Outcomes for Antenatal Therapy of Lower Urinary Tract Obstruction

Vesicoamniotic shunts bypass the urethral obstruction, diverting the urine into the amniotic space and allowing drainage of the upper urinary tract and prevention of pulmonary hypoplasia by restoration of amniotic fluid volume. Initial experience showed good outcomes.[122] In the largest and longest-term documented experience from Biard and coworkers,[123] postnatal diagnosis of the type of urinary obstruction was highly predictive of long-term renal outcome. Fetuses with posterior urethral valves had better outcomes than those with urethral atresia or the prune belly syndrome. Most children were developmentally normal, but pulmonary problems may persist. Among 18 survivors, six had acceptable renal function, four had mild insufficiency, and six required dialysis and transplantation.

Other case series have had similar results, suggesting that even with favorable pre-procedure urine profiles, up to half of survivors have chronic renal insufficiency in childhood.[124,125] The systematic review by Clark and coworkers[124] indicated that there was a lack of high-quality evidence to reliably support the clinical practice of vesicoamniotic shunting despite an improvement in perinatal survival (odds ratio [OR], 2.5; 95% confidence interval [CI], 1.0 to 5.9; $P < .03$). Subgroup analysis indicated that improved survival was most likely in fetuses with a defined poor prognosis (based on a combination of ultrasound appearance and fetal urinary analytes) (OR, 8.0; CI, 1.2 to 52.9; $P < .03$). It has now been proposed to evaluated this therapy in a multicenter randomized trial, referred to as a PLUTO trial.[122]

Congenital Heart Defects

The first fetal cardiac intervention was an attempt by Carpenter and colleagues[126] at fetal pacing for complete heart block because of circulating anti-Ro/La antibodies. In 1991, Maxwell and coworkers[127] performed two percutaneous valvuloplasties, and since then, there has been an increase in experience with minimally invasive treatment for congenital heart defects. Still, most centers only have sporadic experience, and only a few, such as Children's Hospital in Boston, have achieved a wider experience.[128]

Most congenital heart defects can be operated on postnatally with low (<5%) mortality and good quality of life in survivors. However, when this is not the case, and when the abnormal cardiac anatomy would lead to progressive myocardial and pulmonary damage during the pregnancy and would ultimately preclude effective postnatal treatment, timely fetal intervention can be lifesaving. Antenatal intervention theoretically reduces intraventricular pressure, improves coronary perfusion, reduces ischemic damage, allows ventricular growth, and avoids induction of myocardial fibroelastosis, thus enabling improved functional postnatal repair. However, the exact timing and selection of patients for performing such interventions remains unclear. Furthermore, in utero fetal cardiac intervention is still frequently bound by technical limitations, the often late timing of diagnosis, and our current insufficient understanding of these diseases.

Antenatal Intervention for Congenital Heart Defects

Fetal valvuloplasty is the most frequent intrauterine intervention, with indications including management of critical aortic and pulmonary stenosis or atresia, atrial septostomy for highly restrictive foramen ovale with aortic stenosis, and hypoplastic left heart syndrome (HLHS). Table 24-8 summarizes experiences with conditions that are currently claimed to be candidates for prenatal intervention, as recently summarized by Matsui and Gardiner.[128]

In utero valvuloplasty is typically done by a team of fetal medicine specialists familiar with intrauterine invasive procedures, and interventional pediatric cardiologists. Levine and Tworetzky recently reviewed their experience with this procedure.[129] External version is performed as required, and the fetus is positioned with the left chest facing anteriorly and the insertion track free of limbs or cord. Achieving these optimal but essential conditions sometimes requires a laparotomy. Fetal analgesia and immobilization are required; the mother can be sedated or more rarely is given general anesthesia. Bradycardia during the procedure occurs in 9% and hemopericardium in less than 1%, and the fetal loss rate has been reported as 3.8%.[130] Under ultrasound guidance, the valve is dilated with a balloon up to 1.2 to 1.5 times the size of the annulus.

HLHS is a particularly severe valvular abnormality amenable to prenatal intervention. The range of HLHS structural malformations includes critical aortic stenosis, unbalanced atrioventricular septal defects with hypoplasia of the left heart and aorta, severe aortal coarctation, and the association of atresia or hypoplasia of both the aortic and mitral valve. Currently, the only available neonatal treatment is staged palliative surgery (Norwood operation, followed by a Fontan procedure), with an overall 5-year survival of 70%. However, more than half will require further surgery before the age of 5 years.[131]

Balloon valvuloplasty for HLHS was first technically successful in 1991, and by 2000, 12 cases had been performed world-wide and compiled. However, technical problems were frequent, with a 50% balloon rupture rate and a 75% incidence of bradycardia. Only two patients survived, and one of them had a two-ventricle circulation after birth.[132] However, the more extensive experience of the Boston group learns what can be achieved after the learning curve. From the initial 20 cases,[133] there were 13 successful procedures between 21 and 29 weeks. In their most recent series, 28 of 38 treated fetuses survived. Nevertheless, three died in utero after the procedure, one was born prematurely, and two patients opted for termination. Postprocedure assessments of the left heart showed growth of the ventricle, of the mitral and aortic valves, and of ascending aorta. Of the seven born live, three were surviving with biventricular circulation, and another had palliative surgery.

There are also other indications for in utero valvuloplasty and disruption of the atrial septum. More information on these indications and procedures for fetal cardiac diseases is available in the Online Edition of this chapter.

Myelomeningocele

Neural tube defects (NTD) are a major source of mortality and morbidity. The pathophysiology and details of diagnosis are discussed in

TABLE 24-8 REPORTED EXPERIENCES WITH FETAL VALVULOPLASTY

Procedure/References	Number of Fetuses	Technical Success	Prenatal Loss, Including TOP	Neonatal or Infant Death	Alive
Atrial Septostomy					
Marshall et al, 2004	14	13/14	1/14	8/14	5/14
Quintero et al, 2005	2	2/2	0	1/2	1/2
Aortic Valvuloplasty					
Kohl et al, 2000	12	8/12*	4/12	6/12	2
Tulzer et al, 2002	8	5/8			
Tworetzky et al, 2004	38	29/38	6/38	2/38	28
Gardiner and Kumar, 2005	4	4/4	2/4	1/4	1/4
Suh et al, 2006; Huhta et al, 2004	2	2/2	0	1/2	1/2
Pulmonary Valvuloplasty					
Tulzer et al, 2002; Galindo et al, 2006	3	3/3*	0	1/3	3
Tworetzky et al, 2004	8	4/8	NA	NA	NA
Tulzer et al, 2002; Gardiner and Kumar, 2005	2	1/2	0/2	1/2	1/2

***Two procedures required on one fetus.**
NA, not available; TOP, termination of pregnancy.
Reported experience with fetal valvuloplasty as summarized in Matsui H, Gardiner H: Fetal intervention for cardiac disease: The cutting edge of perinatal care. Semin Fetal Neonatal Med 12:482-489, 2007.

Chapter 18. The 5-year mortality of patients with neonatally repaired spina bifida is 79 in 1000 births. Mortality can be as high as 35% among patients with symptoms of brainstem dysfunction, and 81% of children have hydrocephalus requiring treatment. More than 70% of NTD survivors have an IQ above 80 but only 37% can live independently as adults. The vast majority have anal sphincteric dysfunction and lower extremity paralysis.[134]

The technique of closure of the NTD in the fetus is identical to that of the postnatal surgical procedure. The fringe of full-thickness skin is incised circumferentially down to the fascia and the sac is mobilized medially. It is then excised from the placode, removing all epithelial tissue to avoid inclusion cysts later on. Because the spinal cord in the fetus is extremely frail, no attempt is made to re-neurulate the placode. The defect is then closed with dura or undermined fascia, or both. The skin is closed primarily, at times requiring lateral relaxing incisions or even dermal graft material.

Outcome of Antenatal Neural Tube Defect Repair

Preliminary experience at Vanderbilt[135] and Children's Hospital of Philadelphia[136] did demonstrate improvement in outcome with intrauterine microsurgical closure of myelomeningocele compared with postnatal repair. These centers noted a decreased requirement for ventriculoperitoneal (V-P) shunting, attributed in part to reversal of cerebellar herniation. The other potential outcomes such as thinning of the corpus callosum and polymicrogyria were not affected by in utero surgery. Fetal head size, typically lower after postnatal repair, has also been shown to increase, which is believed to be the result of restoration of cerebrospinal volume.

Although the relatively decreased need for shunting among babies repaired in utero diminishes with passing time, a number of them never require shunts. The combined experience suggests an overall incidence of approximately 30% (hence a lower incidence) of V-P shunting. This is clinically important, because the placing of a shunt increases the possibility of surgical complications and infection, thus affecting cognitive functioning in later life. Another important codeterminant of long-term outcome is the upper level of the lesion.[135] For each increase in vertebral level, the risk of receiving a shunt increases accordingly. A final determinant of outcome quality is the gestational age at repair: shunt rate drops significantly (from 71% to 39%) when fetal surgery is done before or after 25 weeks, respectively.

Improvement in lower extremity function or urinary continence with in utero NTD repair has been more difficult to demonstrate. However, although postnatally repaired patients have neurologic function that corresponds with the bony level of the defect, prenatally repaired patients, who have maintained leg function in the prenatal period and had an early repair, have in the majority (57%) of cases a "better than predicted" leg function when evaluated over the short term.[11] However, a major cognitive improvement in prenatally repaired fetuses is not expected.[137] An interesting observation is that in utero repairs showed a surprisingly impressive cosmetic result, confirming that fetal epithelial wound healing is more favorable.

These data were taken into account when planning the Management of Myelomeningocele study (MOMS) on in utero closure of fetal MMC (available at www.spinabifidamoms.com, accessed March 9, 2008). Selection criteria for this trial were gestation less than 26 weeks, normal karyotype, structural examination confirming normal leg movement and absence of talipes, a maximum lateral ventricle diameter of less than 17 mm, and grade III (severe) Chiari type II malformation. The MOMS trial is a nonblinded randomized study requiring 200 patients offered either in utero repair at 28 to 25 weeks or postnatal repair at one of the three participating institutions. In the United States, no fetal MMC repair is offered outside the trial. By the beginning of 2007, recruitment efforts had enrolled just over half of the required subjects. The primary outcome measure is placement of a V-P shunt at the age of 1 year, with predefined shunting criteria. Secondary

TABLE 24-9 OBSTETRIC AND SHORT-TERM OUTCOMES ON MYELOMENINGOCELE REPAIR

	Children's Hospital of Philadelphia (*N* = 51)	Vanderbilt (*N* = 178)
Gestation at surgery (wks and days)	23 + 0 (20 + 0 to 25 + 4)	(19-30); later <26 wks
Gestation at delivery (wks and days)	34 + 4 (25 + 4 to 37)*	33 + 5 (25-38)
Chiari malformation	14%/86%	7%/0%
Before (moderate/severe)	100%/0%	
After		
Postnatal shunt (postnatal age)	46% (21 wks)	46% (12 wks)
Perinatal losses	3/51 (prematurity)	5/178 (2.8%) (not specified)
Length of hospital stay	4 days	3.3 days (3-7)
Oligohydramnios		25% early on with 30% readmission rate
Delivery <30 wks	5/47(10.6%)[†]	11.8%
Delivery >32 wks	40/47 (85%)[†]	(not specified)
Maternal complications	None reported, including dehiscence or rupture; one amniotic fluid leak through hysterotomy	9 (5.1%) mild pulmonary edema 1 bowel obstruction 4 (2.2%) dehiscence, asymptomatic in 3

***Includes all patients.**
[†]Denominator is survivors only.
Children's Hospital of Philadelphia data from Johnson MP, Sutton LN, Rintoul N, et al: Fetal myelomeningocele repair: Short-term clinical outcomes. Am J Obstet Gynecol 189:482-487, 2003.
Vanderbilt data from Bruner J, Tulipan N: Intra-uterine repair of spina bifida. Clin Obstet Gynecol 48:942-955, 2005.

end points include neurologic function, cognitive outcome, and maternal morbidity.

Table 24-9 summarizes important outcome variables from the earlier published experience on MMC repair. From these data, it appears that open fetal surgery has a significant but possibly acceptable maternal risk given the debilitating nature of MMC for the fetus. Maternal pulmonary edema after aggressive tocolytic therapy has been initially frequent, but this is potentially reducible by improved tocolytic regimens. Transfusions are uncommon (2.2% in the Vanderbilt experience), and maternal bowel obstruction happened in a single case. Preterm birth before 30 weeks occurs in approximately 10% to 15% despite aggressive tocolysis. Postoperative oligohydramnios is not uncommon but is usually without significant clinical consequences, although occasional lethal fetal pulmonary hypoplasia has been observed. The risk for perinatal death at the time of surgery or associated with preterm delivery in the available studies was 3% to 6%.

Summary

In utero fetal therapy is an evolving science significantly hampered by the lack of adequately studied animal models and practice in a wide variety of perinatal centers with a generally uncontrolled range of interventions. Nevertheless, laser photocoagulation for TTTS has been shown via randomized trials to be beneficial. The judgment regarding efficacy for antenatal treatment of congenital diaphragmatic hernia, urinary tract obstruction, and congenital cardiac lesions is yet incomplete.

Acknowledgment

We thank the European Commission for supporting EuroTwin2Twin (5th Framework Programme, QLG1-CT-2002-01632) and EuroSTEC (6th Framework Programme, EuroSTEC; LSHC-CT-2006-037409).

References

1. Harrison MR, Adzick NS: The fetus as a patient: Surgical considerations. Ann Surg 213:279-291; discussion, 277-278, 1991.
2. Deprest J, Luks F, Peers K, et al: Intra-uterine endoscopic creation of urinary tract obstruction in the fetal lamb: A model for fetal surgery. Am J Obstet Gynecol 172:1422-1426, 1995.
3. Deprest J, Evrard V, Van Schoubroeck D, Vandenberghe K: Fetoscopic cord ligation [letter]. Lancet 348:890-891, 1996.
4. Deprest J, Ville Y, Barki G, et al: The Eurofoetus Group, Jan Deprest (ed). Endoscopy in Fetal Medicine. Germany, Endopress Tuttlingen, 2004, pp 1-58.
5. Deprest J, Barki G, Lewi L, et al: Fetoscopic instrumentation and techniques. In Van Vught J, Schulman L (eds): Fetal Medicine. New York, M Dekker, 2006, pp 473-491.
6. Bouchard S, Johnson P, Flake A, et al: The EXIT procedure: Experience and outcome in 31 cases. J Pediatr Surg 37:418-426, 2002.
7. Crombleholme TM, Shera D, Lee H, et al: A prospective, randomized, multicenter trial of amnioreduction vs selective fetoscopic laser photocoagulation for the treatment of severe twin-twin transfusion syndrome. Am J Obstet Gynecol 197:396.e1-9, 2007.
8. Rossi AC, D'Addario V: Laser therapy and serial amnioreduction as treatment for twin-twin transfusion syndrome: A metaanalysis and review of literature. Am J Obstet Gynecol 198:147-152, 2008.
9. Keswani SG, Crombleholme TM, Rychik J, et al: Impact of continuous intraoperative monitoring on outcomes in open fetal surgery. Fetal Diagn Ther 20:316-320, 2005.
10. Bruner JP: Intrauterine surgery in myelomeningocele. Semin Fetal Neonat Med 12:471-476, 2007.
11. Johnson MP, Sutton LN, Rintoul N, et al: Fetal myelomeningocele repair: Short-term clinical outcomes. Am J Obstet Gynecol 189:482-487, 2003.
12. Devlieger R, Millar LK, Bryant-Greenwood G, et al: Fetal membrane healing after spontaneous and iatrogenic membrane rupture: A review of current evidence. Am J Obstet Gynecol 195:1512-1520, 2006.
13. Gratacos E, Sanin-Blair J, Lewi L, et al: A histological study of fetoscopic membrane defects to document membrane healing. Placenta 27:452-456, 2006.
14. Quintero RA, Romero R, Dzieczkowski J, et al: Sealing of ruptured amniotic membranes with intra-amniotic platelet-cryoprecipitate plug [letter]. Lancet 347:1117, 1996.
15. Lewi L, Van Schoubroeck D, Van Ranst M, et al: Successful patching of iatrogenic rupture of fetal membranes. Placenta 25:352-356, 2004.
16. Cobo T, Borrell A, Fortuny A, et al: Treatment with amniopatch of premature rupture of membranes after first-trimester chorionic villus sampling. Prenat Diagn 27:1024-1027, 2007.

17. Chang YL, Chao AS, Hsieh PCC, et al: Transient chorioamniotic membrane separation after fetoscope guide laser therapy for twin-twin transfusion syndrome: A case report. Fetal Diagn Ther 22:180-182, 2007.
18. Anand KJ, Hickey PR: Pain and its effects in the human neonate and fetus. N Engl J Med 317:1321-1329, 1987.
19. Giannakoulopoulos X, Sepulveda W, Kourtis P, et al: Fetal plasma cortisol and beta-endorphin response to intrauterine needling. Lancet 344:77-81, 1994.
20. Fisk NM, Gitau R, Teixeira JM, et al: Effect of direct fetal opioid analgesia on fetal hormonal and hemodynamic stress response to intrauterine needling. Anesthesiology 95:828-835, 2001.
21. Dubé J, Dodds L, Armson BA: Does chorionicity or zygosity predict adverse perinatal outcomes in twins? Am J Obstet Gynecol 186:579-583, 2002.
22. Denbow ML, Cox P, Taylor M, et al: Placental angioarchitecture in monochorionic twin pregnancies: Relationship to fetal growth, fetofetal transfusion syndrome, and pregnancy outcome. Am J Obstet Gynecol 182:417-426, 2000.
23. Sebire NJ, Snijders RJ, Hughes K, et al: The hidden mortality of monochorionic twin pregnancies. Br J Obstet Gynaecol 104:1203-1207, 1997.
24. Lewi L, Van Schoubroeck D, Gratacos E, et al: Monochorionic diamniotic twins: Complications and management options. Curr Opin Obstet Gynecol 15:177-194, 2003.
25. Acosta-Rojas R, Becker J, Munoz-Abellana B, et al: Catalunya and Balears Monochorionic Network: Twin chorionicity and the risk of adverse perinatal outcome. Int J Gynaecol Obstet 96:98-102, 2007.
26. Lewi L, Jani J, Boes AS, et al: The natural history of monochorionic twins and the role of prenatal ultrasound scan. Ultrasound Obstet Gynecol 30:401-402, 2007.
27. De Lia J, Fisk N, Hecher K, et al: Twin-to-twin transfusion syndrome: Debates on the etiology, natural history and management. Ultrasound Obstet Gynecol 16:210-213, 2000.
28. Denbow M, Fogliani R, Kyle P, et al: Haematological indices at fetal blood sampling in monochorionic pregnancies complicated by feto-fetal transfusion syndrome. Prenat Diagn 18:941-946, 1998.
29. Mahieu-Caputo D, Meulemans A, Martinovic J, et al: Paradoxic activation of the renin-angiotensin system in twin-twin transfusion syndrome: An explanation for cardiovascular disturbances in the recipient. Pediatr Res 58:685-688, 2005.
30. Quintero RA, Morales WJ, Allen MH, et al: Staging of twin-twin transfusion syndrome. J Perinatol 19:550-555, 1999.
31. Rychik J, Tian Z, Bebbington M, et al: The twin-twin transfusion syndrome: Spectrum of cardiovascular abnormality and development of a cardiovascular score to assess severity of disease. Am J Obstet Gynecol 197:392.e1-8, 2007.
32. Muñoz-Abellana B, Hernandez-Andrade E, Figueroa-Diesel H, et al: Hypertrophic cardiomyopathy-like changes in monochorionic twin pregnancies with selective intrauterine growth restriction and intermittent absent/reversed end-diastolic flow in the umbilical artery. Ultrasound Obstet Gynecol 30:977-982, 2007.
33. Wee LY, Fisk NM: The twin-twin transfusion syndrome. Semin Neonatol 7:187-202, 2002.
34. Moise KJ Jr, Dorman K, Lamvu G, et al: A randomized trial of amnioreduction versus septostomy in the treatment of twin-twin transfusion syndrome. Am J Obstet Gynecol 193:701-707, 2005.
35. De Lia JE, Cruikshank DP, Keye WR Jr: Fetoscopic neodymium:YAG laser occlusion of placental vessels in severe twin-twin transfusion syndrome. Obstet Gynecol 75:1046-1053, 1990.
36. Middeldorp JM, Lopriore E, Sueters M, et al: Twin-to-twin transfusion syndrome after 26 weeks of gestation: Is there a role for fetoscopic laser surgery? BJOG 114:694-698, 2007.
37. Keunen J, Berger H, Bereskova O, et al: Placental discordance before selective laser ablation as a predictor of perinatal outcome and birth weight discordance in twin-twin transfusion syndrome (TTTS). Ultrasound Obstet Gynecol 30:489-490, 2007.
38. Benirschke K, Driscoll S: The Pathology of the Human Placenta. New York, Springer-Verlag, 1967.
39. Quintero RA, Ishii K, Chmait RH, et al: Sequential selective laser photocoagulation of communicating vessels in twin-twin transfusion syndrome. J Matern Fetal Neonatal Med 20:763-768, 2007.
40. Huber A, Baschat AA, Bregenzer T, et al: Laser coagulation of placental anastomoses in severe mid-trimester twin-twin transfusion syndrome and anterior placenta with a 30 degrees fetoscope. Ultrasound Obstet Gynecol 30:403, 2007.
41. Gratacós E, Van Schoubroeck D, Carreras E, et al: Impact of laser coagulation in severe twin-twin transfusion syndrome on fetal Doppler indices and venous blood flow volume. Ultrasound Obstet Gynecol 20:125-130, 2002.
42. Gratacós E, Van Schoubroeck D, Carreras E, et al: Transient hydropic signs in the donor fetus after fetoscopic laser coagulation in severe twin-twin transfusion syndrome: Incidence and clinical relevance. Ultrasound Obstet Gynecol 19:449-453, 2002.
43. Zikulnig L, Hecher K, Bregenzer T, et al: Prognostic factors in severe twin-twin transfusion syndrome treated by endoscopic laser surgery. Ultrasound Obstet Gynecol 14:380-387, 1999.
44. Ishii K, Chmait RH, Martinez JM, et al: Ultrasound assessment of venous blood flow before and after laser therapy: Approach to understanding the pathophysiology of twin-twin transfusion syndrome. Ultrasound Obstet Gynecol 24:164-168, 2004.
45. Yamamoto M, Nasr B, Ortqvist L, et al: Intertwin discordance in umbilical venous volume flow: A reflection of blood volume imbalance in twin-to-twin transfusion syndrome. Ultrasound Obstet Gynecol 29:317-320, 2007.
46. Cavicchioni O, Yamamoto M, Robyr R, et al: Intrauterine fetal demise following laser treatment in twin-to-twin transfusion syndrome. BJOG 113:590-594, 2006.
47. Robyr R, Lewi L, Salomon LJ, et al: Prevalence and management of late fetal complications following successful selective laser coagulation of chorionic plate anastomoses in twin-to-twin transfusion syndrome. Am J Obstet Gynecol 194:796-803, 2006.
48. Lewi L, Gratacos E, Ortibus E, et al: Pregnancy and infant outcome of 80 consecutive cord coagulations in complicated monochorionic multiple pregnancies. Am J Obstet Gynecol 194:782-789, 2006.
49. Lopriore E, van Wezel-Meijler G, Middeldorp JM, et al: Incidence, origin, and character of cerebral injury in twin-to-twin transfusion syndrome treated with fetoscopic laser surgery. Am J Obstet Gynecol 194:1215-1220, 2006.
50. Fox C, Kilby MD, Khan KS: Contemporary treatments for twin-twin transfusion syndrome. Obstet Gynecol 105:1469-1477, 2005.
51. Huber A, Diehl W, Bregenzer T, et al: Stage-related outcome in twin-twin transfusion syndrome treated by fetoscopic laser coagulation. Obstet Gynecol 108:333-337, 2006.
52. Hecher K, Diehl W, Zikulnig L, et al: Endoscopic laser coagulation of placental anastomoses in 200 pregnancies with severe mid-trimester twin-to-twin transfusion syndrome. Eur J Obstet Gynecol Reprod Biol 92:135-139, 2000.
53. Graef C, Ellenrieder B, Hecher K, et al: Long-term neurodevelopmental outcome of 167 children after intrauterine laser treatment for severe twin-twin transfusion syndrome. Am J Obstet Gynecol 194:303-308, 2006.
54. Banek CS, Hecher K, Hackeloer BJ, Bartmann P: Long-term neurodevelopmental outcome after intrauterine laser treatment for severe twin-twin transfusion syndrome. Am J Obstet Gynecol 188:876-880, 2003.
55. Frusca T, Soregaroli M, Fichera A, et al: Pregnancies complicated by twin-twin transfusion syndrome: Outcome and long-term neurological follow-up. Eur J Obstet Gynecol Reprod Biol 25:145-150, 2003.
56. Deprest JA, Van Ballaer PP, Evrard VA, et al: Experience with fetoscopic cord ligation. Eur J Obstet Gynecol Reprod Biol 81:157-164, 1998.
57. Jolly M, Taylor M, Rose G, et al: Interstitial laser: A new surgical technique for twin reversed arterial perfusion sequence in early pregnancy. BJOG 108:1098-1102, 2001.

58. Rodeck C, Deans A, Jauniaux E: Thermocoagulation for the early treatment of pregnancy with an acardiac twin. New Engl J Med 339:1293-1294, 1998.
59. Lee H, Wagner AJ, Sy E, et al: Efficacy of radiofrequency ablation for twin-reversed arterial perfusion sequence. Am J Obstet Gynecol 196:459.e1-e4, 2007.
60. Livingston JC, Lim FY, Polzin W, et al: Intrafetal radiofrequency ablation for twin reversed arterial perfusion (TRAP): A single-center experience. Am J Obstet Gynecol 197:399.e1-e3, 2007.
61. Robyr R, Yamamoto M, Ville Y: Selective feticide in complicated monochorionic twin pregnancies using ultrasound-guided bipolar cord coagulation. BJOG 112:1344-1348, 2005.
62. Hecher K, Hackeloer BJ, Ville Y: Umbilical cord coagulation by operative microendoscopy at 16 weeks' gestation in an acardiac twin. Ultrasound Obstet Gynecol 10:130-132, 1997.
63. Ville Y, Hyett JA, Vandenbussche FP, et al: Endoscopic laser coagulation of umbilical cord vessels in twin reversed arterial perfusion sequence. Ultrasound Obstet Gynecol 4:396-398, 1994.
64. Ville Y: Selective feticide in monochorionic pregnancies: Toys for the boys or standard of care? Ultrasound Obstet Gynecol 22:448-450, 2003.
65. Van Allen MI, Smith DW, Shephard TH: Twin reversed arterial perfusion (TRAP) sequence: A study of 14 twin pregnancies with acardiacus. Semin Perinatol 7:285-293, 1983.
66. Gembruch U, Viski S, Bagamery K, et al: Twin reversed arterial perfusion sequence in twin-to-twin transfusion syndrome after the death of the donor co-twin in the second trimester. Ultrasound Obstet Gynecol 17:153-156, 2001.
67. Gillham DL, Hendricks CH. Holoacardius: Review of literature and case report. Obstet Gynecol 2:647-653, 1953.
68. Sogaard K, Skibsted L, Brocks V: Acardiac twins: Pathophysiology, diagnosis, outcome and treatment—Six cases and review of the literature. Fetal Diagn Ther 14:53-59, 1999.
69. Sullivan AE, Varner MW, Ball RH, et al: The management of acardiac twins: A conservative approach. Am J Obstet Gynecol 189:1310-1313, 2003.
70. Chandra S, Crane JM, Young DC, Shah S: Acardiac twin pregnancy with neonatal resolution of donor twin cardiomyopathy. Obstet Gynecol 96(5 Pt 2):820-821, 2000.
71. Kosno-Kruszewska E, Deregowski K, Schmidt-Sidor B, et al: Neuropathological and anatomopathological analyses of acardiac and "normal" siblings in an acardiac-twin pregnancy. Folia Neuropathol 41:103-109, 2003.
72. Moore TR, Gale S, Benirschke K: Perinatal outcome of forty-nine pregnancies complicated by acardiac twinning. Am J Obstet Gynecol 163:907-912, 1990.
73. Brassard M, Fouron JC, Leduc L, et al: Prognostic markers in twin pregnancies with an acardiac fetus. Obstet Gynecol 94:409-414, 1999.
74. Sherer DM, Armstrong B, Shah YG, et al: Prenatal sonographic diagnosis, Doppler velocimetric umbilical cord studies, and subsequent management of an acardiac twin pregnancy. Obstet Gynecol 74:472-475, 1989.
75. Dashe JS, Fernandez CO, Twickler DM: Utility of Doppler velocimetry in predicting outcome in twin reversed-arterial perfusion sequence. Am J Obstet Gynecol 185:135-139, 2001.
76. Hecher K, Lewi L, Gratacos E, et al: Twin reversed arterial perfusion: Fetoscopic laser coagulation of placental anastomoses or the umbilical cord. Ultrasound Obstet Gynecol 28:688-691, 2006.
77. Ackerman KG, Pober BR: Congenital diaphragmatic hernia and pulmonary hypoplasia: New insights from developmental biology and genetics. Am J Med Genet C Semin Med Genet 145C:105-108, 2007.
78. Rottier R, Tibboel D: Fetal lung and diaphragm development in congenital diaphragmatic hernia. Semin Perinatol 29:86-93, 2005.
79. Skari H, Bjornland K, Haugen G, et al: Congenital diaphragmatic hernia: A meta-analysis of mortality factors. J Pediatr Surg 35:1187-1197, 2000.
80. Graham G, Devine PC: Antenatal diagnosis of congenital diaphragmatic hernia. Semin Perinatol 29:69-76, 2005.
81. Deprest J, Jani J, Cannie M, et al: Progress in intrauterine assessment of the fetal lung and prediction of neonatal function. Ultrasound Obstet Gynecol 25:108-111, 2005.
82. Metkus AP, Filly RA, Stringer MD, et al: Sonographic predictors of survival in fetal diaphragmatic hernia. J Pediatr Surg 31:148-152, 1996.
83. Peralta CF, Cavoretto P, Csapo B, et al: Assessment of lung area in normal fetuses at 12-32 weeks. Ultrasound Obstet Gynecol 26:718-724, 2005.
84. Jani J, Keller RL, Benachi A, et al: Prenatal prediction of survival in isolated left-sided diaphragmatic hernia. Ultrasound Obstet Gynecol 27:18-22, 2006.
85. Jani J, Nicolaides KH, Keller RL, et al, on behalf of the antenatal-CDH-Registry Group: Observed to expected lung area to head circumference ratio in the prediction of survival in fetuses with isolated diaphragmatic hernia. Ultrasound Obstet Gynecol 30:67-71, 2007.
86. Hedrick HL, Danzer E, Merchant A, et al: Liver position and lung-to-head ratio for prediction of extracorporeal membrane oxygenation and survival in isolated left congenital diaphragmatic hernia. Am J Obstet Gynecol 197:422.e1-4, 2007.
87. Jani J, Benachi A, Mitanchez D, et al: Lung-to-head ratio and liver position to predict neonatal morbidity in fetuses with isolated congenital diaphragmatic hernia: A multicenter study. Am J Obstet Gynecol 195:S60, 2006.
88. Suda K, Bigras JL, Bohn D, et al: Echocardiographic predictors of outcome in newborns with CDH. Pediatrics 105:1106-1109, 2000.
89. Sokol J, Bohn D, Lacro RV, et al: Fetal pulmonary artery diameters and their association with lung hypoplasia and postnatal outcome in congenital diaphragmatic hernia. Am J Obstet Gynecol 186:1085-1090, 2002.
90. Sokol J, Shimizu, Bohn D, et al. Fetal pulmonary artery diameter measurements as a predictor of morbidity in antenatally diagnosed congenital diaphragmatic hernia: A prospective study. Am J Obstet Gynecol 195:470-477, 2006.
91. Ruano R, de Fatima Yukie Maeda M, Niigaki JI, et al: Pulmonary artery diameters in healthy fetuses from 19-40 weeks gestation. J Ultrasound Med 26:309-316, 2007.
92. Ruano R, Aubry MC, Barthe B, et al: Quantitative analysis of pulmonary vasculature by 3D- power Doppler ultrasonography in isolated congenital diaphragmatic hernia. Am J Obstet Gynecol 195:1720-1728, 2006.
93. Kinsella J, Parker T, Dunbar I, Abman S: Noninvasive delivery of inhaled nitric oxide therapy for late pulmonary hypertension in newborn infants with congenital diaphragmatic hernia. J Pediatr 142:397-401, 2003.
94. Kinsella J, Dunbar I, Abman S: Pulmonary vasodilator therapy in congenital diaphragmatic hernia: Acute, late, and chronic pulmonary hypertension. Semin Perinatol 29:123-128, 2005.
95. Inamura N, Kubota A, Nakajima T, et al: A proposal of new therapeutic strategy for antenatally diagnosed congenital diaphragmatic hernia. J Pediatr Surg 40:1315-1319, 2005.
96. Gallot D, Boda C, Ughetto S, et al: Prenatal detection and outcomes of congenital diaphragmatic hernia: A French registry-based study. Ultrasound Obstet Gynecol 29:276-283, 2007.
97. Javid P, Jaksic T, Skarsgard E, Lee S: Canadian Neonatal Network. Survival rate in congenital diaphragmatic hernia: The experience of the Canadian Neonatal Network. J Pediatr Surg 39:657-660, 2004.
98. Di Fiore JW, Fauza DO, Slavin R, et al: Experimental fetal tracheal ligation reverses the structural and physiological effects of pulmonary hypoplasia in CDH. J Pediatr Surg 29:248-256, 1997.
99. Nelson SM, Hajivassiliou CA, Haddock G, et al: Rescue of the hypoplastic lung by prenatal cyclical strain. Am J Respir Crit Care Med 171:1395-1402, 2005.
100. Flageole H, Evrard V, Piedboeuf B, et al, The plug-unplug sequence: An important step to achieve type II pneumocyte maturation in the fetal lamb model. J Pediatr Surg 33:299-303, 1998.
101. Kohl T, Gembruch U, Tchatcheva K, Schaible T: Deliberately delayed and shortened fetoscopic tracheal occlusion: A different strategy after prenatal diagnosis of life-threatening congenital diaphragmatic hernias [letter]. J Pediatr Surg 41:1344-1345, 2006.

102. Jani J, Gratacos E, Greenough A, et al, and the FETO task group: Percutaneous fetal endoscopic tracheal occlusion (FETO) for severe left sided congenital diaphragmatic hernia. Clin Obstet Gynecol 48:910-922, 2005.
103. Deprest J, Gratacos E, Nicolaides KH: Fetoscopic tracheal occlusion (FETO) for severe congenital diaphragmatic hernia: Evolution of a technique and preliminary results. Ultrasound Obstet Gynecol 24:121-126, 2004.
104. Harrison MR, Keller RL, Hawgood SB, et al: A randomized trial of fetal endoscopic tracheal occlusion for severe fetal congential diaphragmatic hernia. N Engl J Med 349:1916-1924, 2003.
105. Jani J, Nicolaides KH, Gratacos E, et al: and the FETO task group: Fetal lung-to-head ratio in the prediction of survival in severe left-sided diaphragmatic hernia treated by fetal endoscopic tracheal occlusion (FETO). Am J Obstet Gynecol 195:1646-1650, 2006.
106. Peralta CFA, Jani J, Van Schoubroeck D, et al: Fetal lung volume after endoscopic tracheal occlusion in the prediction of postnatal outcome. Am J Obstet Gynecol 198:60.e1-e5, 2008.
107. Cannie M, Jani J, de Keyzer F, et al: Lung response to fetal tracheal occlusion is better prior to 29 weeks than after. Am J Obstet Gynecol 197:554, 2007.
108. Stocker JT, Madewell JE, Drake RM: Congenital cystic adenomatoid malformation of the lung. Classification and morphologic spectrum. Hum Pathol 8:155-171, 1977.
109. Crombleholme TM, Coleman B, Hedrick H, et al: Cystic adenomatoid malformation volume ratio predicts outcome in prenatally diagnosed cystic adenomatoid malformation of the lung. J Pediatr Surg 37:331-338, 2002.
110. Hedrick HL, Flake AW, Crombleholme TM, et al: The ex utero intrapartum therapy procedure for high-risk fetal lung lesions. J Pediatr Surg 40:1038-1043; discussion, 1044, 2005.
111. Wilson RD, Baxter JK, Johnson MP, et al: Thoracoamniotic shunts: Fetal treatment of pleural effusions and congenital cystic adenomatoid malformations. Fetal Diagn Ther 19:413-420, 2004.
112. Wilson RD, Hedrick HL, Liechty KW, et al: Cystic adenomatoid malformation of the lung: review of genetics, prenatal diagnosis, and in utero treatment. Am J Med Genet A 140:151-155, 2006.
113. Knox EM, Kilby MD, Martin WL, Khan KS: In utero pulmonary drainage in the management of primary hydrothorax and congenital cysti lung lesion: A systematic review. Ultrasound Obstet Gynecol 28:726-734, 2006.
114. Adzick NS: Management of fetal lung lesions. Clin Perinatol 30:481-492, 2003.
115. Deurlo K, Devlieger R, Lopriore E, et al: Isolated fetal hydrothorax with hydrops: A systematic review of prenatal treatment options. Prenat Diagn 27:893-899, 2007.
116. Tanemura M, Nishikawa N, Kojima K, et al: A case of successful fetal therapy for congenital chylothorax by intrapleural injection of OK-432. Ultrasound Obstet Gynecol 4:371-375, 2001.
117. Picone O, Benachi A, Mandelbrot L, et al: Thoracoamniotic shunting for fetal pleural effusions with hydrops. Am J Obstet Gynecol 6:2047-2050, 2004.
118. Manning FA, Harman CR, Lange IR, et al: Antepartum chronic fetal vesicoamniotic shunts for obstructive uropathy: A report of two cases. Am J Obstet Gynecol 145:819, 1983.
119. Johnson MP, Bukowski TP, Reitleman C, et al: In utero surgical treatment of fetal obstructive uropathy: A new comprehensive approach to identify appropriate candidates for vesicoamniotic shunt therapy. Am J Obstet Gynecol 170:1770-1776; discussion, 1776-1779, 1994.
120. Johnson MP, Corsi P, Bradfield W, et al: Sequential fetal urine analysis provides greater precision in the evaluation of fetal obstructive uropathy. Am J Obstet Gynecol 173:59-65, 1995.
121. Morris RK, Kilby MD: Congenital urinary tract obstruction. Best Pract Res Clin Obstet Gynaecol 22:97-122, 2008.
122. Freedman AL, Bukowski TP, Smith CA, et al: Fetal therapy for obstructive uropathy: Specific outcomes diagnosis. J Urol 156:720-724, 1996.
123. Biard JM, Johnson MP, Carr MC, et al: Long-term outcomes in children treated by prenatal vesicoamniotic shunting for lower urinary tract obstruction. Obstet Gynecol 106:503-508, 2005.
124. Clark TJ, Martin WL, Divakaran TG, et al: Prenatal bladder drainage in the management of fetal lower urinary tract obstruction: A systematic review and meta-analysis. Obstet Gynecol 102:367-382, 2003.
125. Holmes N, Harrison MR, Baskin LS: Fetal surgery for posterior urethral valves: long-term postnatal outcomes. Pediatrics 108:E7, 2001.
126. Carpenter RJ, Strasburger JF, Garson A, et al: Fetal ventricular pacing for hydrops secondary to complete atrioventricular block. J Am Coll Cardiol 8:1434-1436, 1986.
127. Maxwell D, Allan L, Tynan MJ: Balloon dilatation of the aortic valve in the fetus: A report of two cases. Br Heart J 65:256-258, 1991.
128. Matsui H, Gardiner H: Fetal intervention for cardiac disease: The cutting edge of perinatal care. Semin Fetal Neonatal Med 12:482-489, 2007.
129. Levine J, Tworetzky W: Intervention for severe aortic stenosis in the fetus: Altering the progression of left sided heart disease. Prog Pediatr Cardiol 22:71-78, 2006.
130. Antsaklis AI, Papantinoiou NE, Mesogitis SA, et al: Cardiocentesis: An alternative method for fetal blood sampling for the prenatal diagnosis of hemoglobinopathies. Obstet Gynecol 79:630-633, 1992.
131. McCrindle BW, Blackstone EH, Williams WG, et al: Are outcomes of surgical versus transcatheter balloon valvotomy equivalent in neonatal critical aortic stenosis? Circulation 104(Suppl 1):I152-158, 2001.
132. Kohl T, Sharland G, Allan LD, et al: World experience of percutaneous ultrasound-guided balloon valvuloplasty in human fetuses with severe aortic valve obstruction. Am J Cardiol 85:1230-1233, 2000.
133. Tworetzky W, Wilkins-Haug L, Jennings RW, et al: Balloon dilatation of severe aortic stenosis in the fetus: Candidate selection, technique, and results of successful intervention. Circulation 110:2125-2131, 2004.
134. Rintoul N, Sutton L, Hubbard A, et al: A new look at myelomeningoceles: Functional level, vertebral level, shunting and the implications for fetal intervention. Pediatrics 109:409-413, 2002.
135. Bruner J, Tulipan N: Intra-uterine repair of spina bifida. Clin Obstet Gynecol 48:942-955, 2005.
136. Johnson MP, Gerdes M, Rintoul N, et al: Maternal-fetal surgery for myelomeningocele: Neurodevelopmental outcomes at 2 years of age. Am J Obstet Gynecol 194:1145-1150, 2006.
137. Nejat F, Kazmi SS, Habibi Z, et al: Intelligence quotient in children with meningomyeloceles: A case control study. J Neurosurg 106:106-110, 2007.
138. Tabor A, Philip J, Madsen M, et al: Randomised controlled trial of genetic amniocentesis in 4606 low-risk women. Lancet 1:1287-1293, 1986.
139. Eddleman KA, Malone FD, Sullivan L, et al: Pregnancy loss rates after midtrimester amniocentesis. Obstet Gynecol 108:1067-1072, 2006.
140. Umur A, van Gemert MJ, Ross MG: Fetal urine and amniotic fluid in monochorionic twins with twin-twin transfusion syndrome: Simulations of therapy. Am J Obstet Gynecol 185:996-1003, 2001.
141. Mari G, Detti L, Oz U, et al: Long-term outcome in twin-twin transfusion syndrome treated with serial aggressive amnioreduction. Am J Obstet Gynecol 183:211-217, 2000.
142. Tongsong T, Wanapirak C, Kunavikatikul C, et al: Fetal loss rate associated with cordocentesis at midgestation. Am J Obstet Gynecol 184:719-723, 2001.
143. Yamamoto M, Ville Y: Recent findings on laser treatment of twin-to-twin transfusion syndrome. Curr Opin Obstet Gynecol 18:87-92, 2006.
144. Lewi L, Gratacos E, Ortibus E, et al: Pregnancy and infant outcome of 80 consecutive cord coagulations in complicated monochorionic multiple pregnancies. Am J Obstet Gynecol 194:782-789, 2006.
145. Robyr R, Yamamoto M, Ville Y: Selective feticide in complicated monochorionic twin pregnancies using ultrasound-guided bipolar cord coagulation. BJOG 112:1344-1348, 2005.
146. Vida VL, Bacha EA, Larrazabal A, et al: Hypoplastic left heart syndrome with intact or highly restrictive atrial septum: Surgical experience from a single center. Ann Thorac Surg 84:581-585, 2007.

147. Quintero RA, Huhta J, Suh E, et al: In utero cardiac fetal surgery: Laser atrial septotomy in the treatment of hypoplastic left heart syndrome with intact atrial septum. Am J Obstet Gynecol 193:1424-1428, 2005.
148. Marshall AC, van der Velde ME, Tworetzky W, et al: Creation of an atrial septal defect in utero for fetuses with hypoplastic left heart syndrome and intact or highly restrictive atrial septum. Circulation 110:253-258, 2004.
149. Tulzer G, Arzt W, Franklin RC, et al: Fetal pulmonary valvuloplasty for critical pulmonary stenosis or atresia with intact septum. Lancet 360:1567-1568, 2002.
150. Tworetzky W, Wilkins-Haug L, Jennings RW, et al: Balloon dilation of severe aortic stenosis in the fetus: Potential for prevention of hypoplastic left heart syndrome: Candidate selection, technique, and results of successful intervention. Circulation 110:2125-2131, 2004.
151. Gardiner HM, Kumar S: Fetal cardiac interventions. Clin Obstet Gynecol 48:956e6, 2005.
152. Suh E, Quintessenza J, Huhta J, et al: How to grow a heart: Fiberoptic guided fetal aortic valvotomy. Cardiol Young 16(suppl. 1):43e6, 2006.
153. Huhta J, Quintero RA, Suh E, et al: Advances in fetal cardiac intervention. Curr Opin Pediatr 16:487e93, 2004.
154. Galindo A, Gutierrez-Larraya F, Velasco JM, et al: Pulmonary balloon valvuloplasty in a fetus with critical pulmonary stenosis/atresia with intact ventricular septum and heart failure. Fetal Diagn Ther 21:100e4, 2006.

Chapter 25

Multiple Gestation

Clinical Characteristics and Management

Fergal D. Malone, MD, and Mary E. D'Alton, MD

The incidence of multiple gestation continues to increase, and multiple gestations now account for more than 3% of all live births in the United States.[1] Over the last several decades, the rate of twin births in the United States has increased every year, to a current rate of 32.2 per 1000 total births. In the decade from 1995 to 2004, the number of twin births increased by 37% (Table 25-1). The two major factors accounting for these increases are the widespread availability of assisted reproductive technologies and increasing maternal age at childbirth. The number of triplet, quadruplet, and higher-order multiple births has peaked or dropped slightly, most likely due to voluntary limits imposed by many assisted reproduction centers in the number of embryos transferred and to the availability and acceptance of multifetal pregnancy reduction (MFPR) procedures.[2] Because perinatal and maternal morbidity and mortality are increased in multiple gestation, contemporary data about pregnancy outcome and management options are essential. Congenital abnormalities are also increased in multiple gestation, making management decisions more complex, because the fates of sibling fetuses are necessarily linked. For these reasons, women with complicated multiple gestation are increasingly cared for under the supervision of an appropriately trained specialist.[3,4]

Perinatal Mortality and Morbidity

Prematurity, monochorionicity, and growth restriction pose the main risks to fetuses and neonates in multiple gestations. Perinatal deaths have decreased, but the risk of prematurity has not changed significantly. The mean duration of pregnancy is 35 weeks for twin gestations, 32 weeks for triplets, and 29 weeks for quadruplets.[1] The mean gestational age at delivery in multiple pregnancies can be misleading because it does not reveal the true incidence of extreme prematurity, which has greater clinical significance. Although the incidence of very premature delivery (before 32 weeks) for singletons in the United States is 1.6%, that incidence increases to 12% for twin and 36% for triplet gestations.[1] The perinatal mortality rate for twins is at least threefold higher than for singletons. In a Swedish population database of more than 2.2 million births, the fetal and infant mortality rates for singletons were 4.1 and 5.0 per 1000 births, respectively; the rates for twins were 12.0 and 16.0 per 1000 births.[5] Mortality rates are significantly higher among same-gender twins compared with discordant-gender twins. It therefore appears that the two most important factors explaining increased mortality in twin gestations are increased rates of prematurity and complications of monochorionicity. The risk that twins will weigh less than 1500 g at birth is 10 times the risk for singletons. These increased risks are more pronounced in male-male pairs, in black infants, and in infants of younger mothers.[6]

Most published data on perinatal outcome for higher-order multiple gestations (triplets or greater) are limited by (1) noncontemporary study periods, (2) small sample size, (3) long duration of sample collection, (4) lack of control groups for comparison, and (5) accumulation of data from multiple centers with differing management practices. These limitations are even more pronounced for pregnancies with four or more fetuses. In one recent population study, stillbirth rates were noted to increase from 6.8 per 1000 for singletons to 16.1 for twins and 21.5 for triplets, and infant mortality rates increased from 5 to 23.4 and 51.2 per 1000 births, respectively[7] (Figs. 25-1 and 25-2). Two recent, large studies summarized perinatal outcome of triplet pregnancies. One suggested an incidence of preterm delivery before 28 weeks of 14%, with a perinatal mortality rate of 103 per 1000, and the second showed an incidence of preterm delivery before 30 weeks of 24%, with a perinatal mortality rate of 150 per 1000.[8,9] Perinatal mortality in triplet gestations is significantly worse in dichorionic compared with trichorionic pregnancies.[9] In addition, the rate of spontaneous loss before 24 weeks for triplet pregnancies with confirmed cardiac activity may be as high as 20%.[10] Once cardiac activity is confirmed at 10 to 14 weeks in a triplet pregnancy, the risk of miscarriage before 24 weeks is 4.4%.[11] Some quadruplet pregnancy series have suggested perinatal mortality rates ranging from 0 to 67 per 1000 quadruplet births.[12,13] However, caution is needed when interpreting studies of higher-order multiple gestations, because often only pregnancies reaching "viability" are included, producing an overly positive view of perinatal outcome.

Perinatal morbidity is also more likely in multiple gestations. Although multiple gestation accounts for only 3% of all births in the United States, infants of multiple gestations comprise almost one quarter of very-low-birth-weight infants.[14] The incidence of severe handicap among neonatal survivors of multiple gestation is also increased: 34.0 and 57.5 per 1000 twin and triplet survivors, respec-

TABLE 25-1 INCIDENCE OF MULTIPLE BIRTHS IN THE UNITED STATES

Year	Twins	Triplets	Quadruplets	Quintuplets and Higher Order
2004	132,219	6,750	439	86
2003	128,665	7,110	468	85
2002	125,134	6,898	434	69
2001	121,246	6,885	501	85
2000	118,916	6,742	506	77
1999	114,307	6,742	512	67
1998	110,670	6,919	627	79
1997	104,137	6,148	510	79
1996	100,750	5,298	560	81
1995	96,736	4,551	365	57

From Martin JA, Hamilton BE, Sutton PD, et al: Births: Final Data for 2004. Natl Vital Stat Rep 55(1):80-81, 2006.

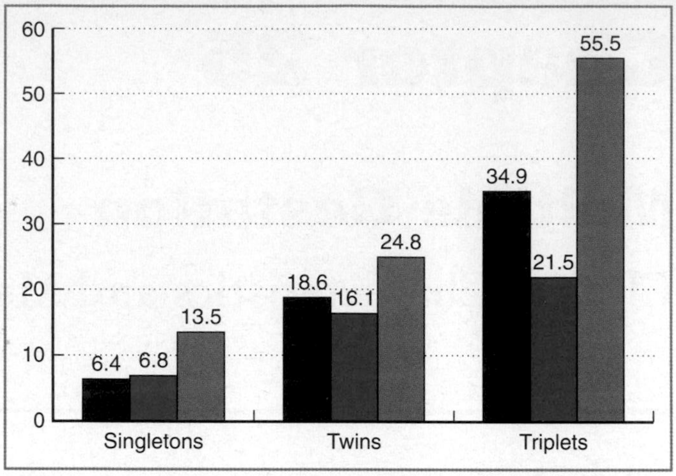

FIGURE 25-1 Rates of stillbirth in the United States. Crude stillbirth rates for singletons, twins, and triplets by race/ethnicity. Purple bars, blacks; blue bars, whites; red bars, Hispanics. (Modified from Salihu HM, Garces IC, Sharma PP, et al: Stillbirth and infant mortality among Hispanic singletons, twins, and triplets in the United States. Obstet Gynecol 106:789-796, 2005.)

tively, compared with 19.7 per 1000 singleton survivors.[15] Twins account for 5% to 10% of all cases of cerebral palsy in the United States.[16] The risk of producing at least one infant with cerebral palsy from one pregnancy has been reported to be 1.5% for twin, 8.0% for triplet, and 42.9% for quadruplet gestations.[17]

In the United States, mean birth weight is significantly lower for twin neonates (2333 g) and triplet neonates (1700 g), compared with singletons (3316 g).[1] However, there is no evidence that twin or triplet neonates have outcomes different from those of gestational age–matched singletons. When matched by gestational age at delivery, singleton, twin, and triplet neonates have similar birth weights and similar rates of morbidity and mortality.[18]

Maternal Mortality and Morbidity

Given the low rate of maternal mortality in developed countries and the small sample sizes in published series, it is difficult to determine the incidence of maternal death in contemporarily managed multiple gestations. However, maternal morbidity is significantly increased in mothers with multiple gestations and is apparently related to the number of fetuses. Twin pregnancies are associated with significantly higher risks of hypertension (2.5-fold), abruption (3-fold), anemia (2.5-fold), and urinary tract infections (1.5-fold) than singleton pregnancies.[19]

The risk of significant maternal morbidity is also increased in triplet pregnancies. In a comparison of maternal morbidity among twin, triplet, and quadruplet pregnancies, the risks of gestational hypertension, eclampsia, diabetes, placental abruption, and preterm premature rupture of membranes (pPROM) were all significantly increased.[20] In a study of 100 triplet pregnancies, almost all women had at least one antenatal complication and almost half developed postpartum complications.[8] These risks include preterm labor (78%); preeclampsia (26%); hemolysis, elevated liver enzymes, or low platelets (HELLP) syndrome (9%); anemia (24%); pPROM (24%); gestational diabetes (14%); acute fatty liver (4%); chorioendometritis (16%); and postpartum hemorrhage (9%). No differences in the frequency of complications were noted between spontaneous triplets and those arising from ovulation induction or in vitro fertilization. Preterm labor occurs in nearly all quadruplet pregnancies, and the risk of gestational hypertension ranges from 32% to 90%.[12,13] In addition, preeclampsia in higher-order multiple gestations occurs at an earlier gestational age, is more severe, and more likely to have an atypical clinical presentation than preeclampsia in singleton gestations.[8,21]

Maternal Adaptations

The normal maternal physiologic adaptations seen in singleton pregnancy are exaggerated in multiple gestation. These physiologic responses consist of both observed changes and expected changes extrapolated from singleton pregnancy physiology.[22,23] Serum levels of progesterone, estradiol, estriol, human placental lactogen, human chorionic gonadotropin (hCG), and α-fetoprotein (AFP) are all significantly higher in multiple than in singleton gestations.

Heart rate and stroke volume are significantly increased in gravidas with twins during the third trimester, leading to a significant increase in cardiac output and cardiac index compared with singleton pregnanciess.[24] In one study of 119 twin pregnancies, stroke volume was increased by 15%, heart rate by 4%, and cardiac output by 20%, compared with singletons.[25] These increases most likely occur secondary to increased myocardial contractility and blood volume in the setting of multiple gestation. Systolic and diastolic blood pressures mirror the changes seen during singleton pregnancy, with an even greater drop in pressures noted during the second trimester in twin pregnancy. However, by the time of delivery, mean maternal blood pressures are significantly higher in multiple compared with singleton pregnancies.[26] Depending on the number of fetuses, plasma volume increases by 50% to 100%, which may lead to dilutional anemia.

Uterine volume increases rapidly in multiple gestation. A 25-week twin-gestation uterus is equal in size to a term singleton uterus.[27] Uterine blood flow increases significantly in a twin pregnancy and is related to both increased cardiac output and decreased uterine artery resistance.[28] In multiple gestations, the normal increase in tidal volume and oxygen consumption is probably increased further, which may lead to an even more alkalotic arterial pH than that seen with singleton pregnancy. Similarly, the normal increase in glomerular filtration rate and size of the renal collecting system is probably more marked in women with multiple gestations.

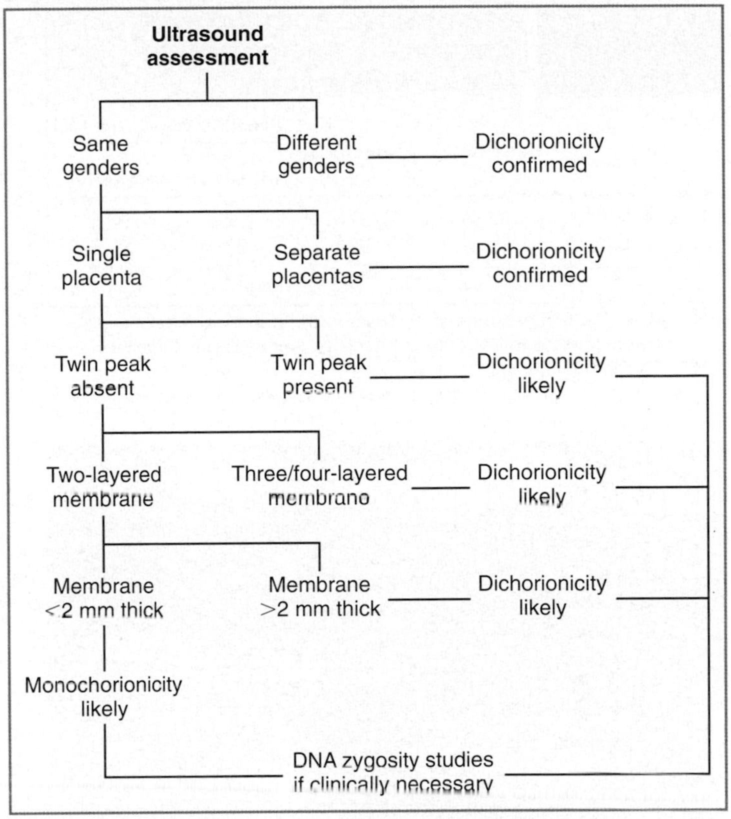

FIGURE 25-2 Determining chorionicity. Flow chart for determining chorionicity in multiple gestation.

It is recommended that daily caloric intake increase to 3000 to 4000 kcal (depending on whether the pregravid body mass index suggests underweight or overweight) in multiple gestations, compared with 2400 kcal/day in singleton gestations.[29] The recommended maternal weight gain for twin pregnancies is 1 to 1.5 pounds per week, for a total pregnancy weight gain of 35 to 45 pounds. An easy-to-remember recommendation of 24 pounds by 24 weeks' gestation has been suggested to achieve this goal.[29] Although specific recommendations have not been issued, ideal weight gain in higher-order multiple gestations is likely to be significantly greater than in twin gestations. Some have suggested that optimal fetal growth in higher order multiple gestations can be achieved with maternal weight gain of at least 1.5 pounds per week during the first 24 weeks of pregnancy.[30]

Ultrasonography

Routine prenatal ultrasonography has proved valuable for early detection of multiple gestation.[31] It is only after diagnosis of a multiple gestation that steps can be taken to reduce the perinatal and maternal morbidity associated with the condition. Prenatal ultrasonography in multiple gestation is useful for the following:

- Confirming a diagnosis of multiple gestation
- Determining chorionicity
- Detecting fetal anomalies
- Guiding invasive procedures
- Evaluating fetal growth
- Measuring cervical length
- Confirming fetal well-being
- Assisting in delivery

Diagnosis of Multiple Gestation

Positive sonographic diagnosis of multiple gestation can be made by visualizing multiple gestational sacs with yolk sacs by 5 weeks of gestation and multiple embryos with cardiac activity by 6 weeks. If two gestational sacs are seen on early ultrasound studies, the chance of delivering twins is 57%, but this increases to 87% if two embryonic poles with cardiac activity are visualized.[32] If three gestational sacs are seen on early ultrasound, the chance of delivering triplets is 20%, increasing to 68% if three embryonic poles with cardiac activity are visualized. In addition to twins, the early sonographic visualization of two intrauterine fluid collections may represent a singleton in a bicornuate uterus, a singleton with a subchorionic hemorrhage, or a vanishing twin, which can occur in 20% to 50% of cases of early multiple gestation diagnoses.[33]

Chorionicity

Because 20% of twins are monochorionic and such pregnancies are associated with a perinatal mortality risk of up to 26%, accurate determination of chorionicity is essential for clinical management.[34,35] In most women, sonographic assessment can determine chorionicity (see Fig. 25-2). Sonographic determination of chorionicity should be attempted in all multiple gestations and is best performed in the first trimester. Before 8 weeks' gestation, obvious separate gestational sacs, each surrounded by a thick echogenic ring, is suggestive of dichorionicity.[36] If separate echogenic rings are not visible, monochorionicity is likely. In such situations, counting the number of yolk sacs may assist in establishing amnionicity. Two fetal poles with two yolk sacs in a monochorionic gestation suggests diamnionicity, whereas the presence of two fetal poles with only one yolk sac suggests a monoamniotic

TABLE 25-2 STATISTICAL ACCURACY OF ANTENATAL PREDICTION OF MONOCHORIONICITY

	Sensitivity (%)	Specificity (%)	Predictive Value (%)	
			Positive	Negative
Overall	88.9	97.7	92.6	96.5
1st trimester	89.8	99.5	97.8	97.5
2nd trimester	88	94.7	88	94.7

From Lee YM, Cleary-Goldman J, Thaker HM, et al: Antenatal sonographic prediction of twin chorionicity. Am J Obstet Gynecol 195:863, 2006 (Table 1).

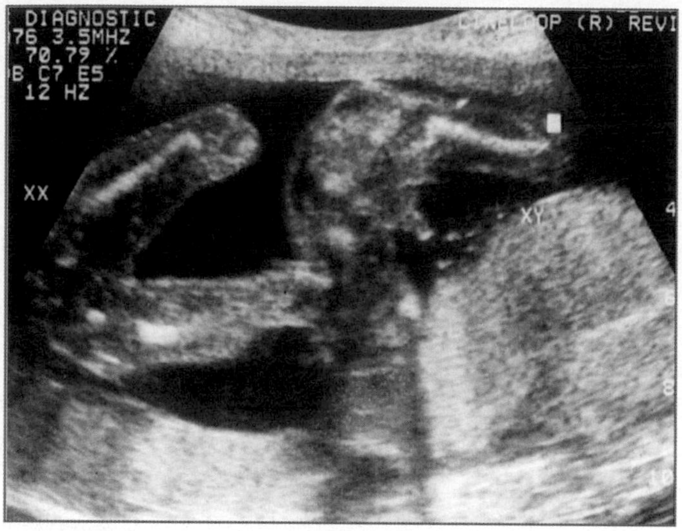

FIGURE 25-3 Dichorionic gestation. A single ultrasound view demonstrates female external genitalia on the left and male external genitalia on the right, confirming dichorionic twin gestation with certainty. (Courtesy of Sabrina Craigo, MD, New England Medical Center, Boston.)

gestation.[37] However, the specificity of this finding for monoamnionicity is uncertain.[38,39] The sensitivity of first- and second-trimester ultrasound for predicting monochorionicity is approximately 90%; the specificity falls from 99% for first-trimester sonography to 95% in the second trimester (Table 25-2).[40] Later in gestation, if the fetuses are discordant for gender or two distinct placentas are seen, a dichorionic gestation can be confirmed with confidence (Fig. 25-3). In the absence of these findings, monochorionicity is possible, and other sonographic features should be assessed.

The visualization of only one placental mass has a positive predictive value for monochorionicity of only 42%, because many dichorionic gestations develop apparent fusion of separate placentas as pregnancy progresses.[41] Counting the number of layers in the dividing membrane, near its insertion into the placenta, is 100% predictive of dichorionicity but is not as reliable in predicting monochorionicity.[42,43] When this method is used, it is assumed that the placentation is monochorionic if only two layers are present; the presence of three or four layers suggests dichorionicity. The use of a membrane thickness cutoff value of 2 mm has also been reported to correctly assign chorionicity in more than 90% of cases, but the reproducibility of this measurement has been questioned.[44] Visualization of a triangular projection of placenta between the layers of the dividing membrane (known as the *twin-peak* or *lambda* sign) is also useful in diagnosis of dichorionicity, but its absence is not as reliable to predict monochorionicity. Although each of these sonographic features individually has a poor positive predictive value for monochorionicity, use of a composite sonographic approach (i.e., one placenta, gender concordance, thin dividing membrane, and absence of the twin-peak sign) may yield a positive predictive value for monochorionicity of 92%.[41]

The use of transvaginal sonography in the first trimester, together with this composite approach, produces correct assignment of chorionicity and amnionicity in almost 100% of cases.[38] If the initial ultrasound examination is not performed until the second trimester, its precision in assigning chorionicity declines.[45] Although the sensitivity is not perfect, the specificity for monochorionicity is almost 100% when this approach is used in the first trimester, falling to 95% in the second trimester.[40] In certain clinical situations, such as the presence of fetal anomalies or of twins discordant for growth, management requires the reliable exclusion of monochorionicity. If monochorionicity cannot be reliably excluded, invasive testing to assign chorionicity by DNA zygosity studies on amniocytes can be performed if clinically indicated.[46]

Detection of Fetal Anomalies

Careful sonographic surveys of fetal anatomy are indicated in multifetal pregnancies, because the risk of congenital anomalies is increased. The accuracy of ultrasonography to detect congenital fetal anomalies in multiple gestations has not been adequately studied in large series. Smaller, single-center series have tried to establish the predictive value of prenatal ultrasound for the detection of anomalies in multiple gestations. In a series of 24 anomalous fetuses in twin gestations, serial ultrasonography at a specialist center achieved an 88% detection rate, with 100% specificity, for the prenatal diagnosis of anomalies.[47] An 83% rate of detecting fetuses with Down syndrome in twin pregnancies was achieved by combining risks derived from maternal age and nuchal translucency thickness measurement at 10 to 14 weeks' gestation, with a 5% false-positive rate.[48] The finding of increased nuchal translucency in one fetus of a monochorionic pair may also presage the development of twin-twin transfusion syndrome (TTTS).

Evaluation of Fetal Growth

Serial ultrasonography is the most accurate method to assess fetal growth in multiple gestation. Intrauterine growth of twins is similar to that of singletons until 30 to 32 weeks' gestation, when the abdominal circumference measurements of twins begin to lag behind those of singletons.[49] Composite assessments of fetal weight appear to be superior to individual biometric parameters (e.g., abdominal circumference, femur length) for predicting growth discordance.[50] Although the predictive value of all biometric assessments to identify growth discordance has been questioned, no other sonographic markers for discordance have yet been validated.[51]

Although individual growth curves for twin and triplet gestations have been described, singleton fetal weight standards are still commonly used to assess growth in multiple gestation. A prospective study of serial biometric measurements in twins found no significant differences in fetal growth between twin and singleton gestations.[52] Because growth restriction is a dynamic process and sibling fetuses are immediately available for comparison, we consider it reasonable to assess growth in multiple gestation with serial evaluations, based on singleton growth curves, using as many biometric parameters as possible and comparing sibling estimated fetal weights for discordance. Typically, a 20% to 25% difference in estimated fetal weight between sibling fetuses, expressed as a percentage of the larger fetal weight, suggests clinically significant growth discordance.[38,53] In a study of 460 twin pregnancies, weight discordance of 25% or more was associated with a 6.5-fold increase in the rate of stillbirth, compared with nondiscordant twins, and an overall perinatal death rate of 9.7%.[54] In another study of 1370 twin pregnancies in which weight discordance was stratified in 5% increments, a statistically significant increase in fetal death occurred only with weight discordance greater than 30%.[55] Growth discordance greater than 20% has also been shown to be an important predictor for adverse perinatal outcomes, even in situations where individual fetal size is appropriate for gestational age.[56]

Much of the increased mortality associated with growth discordance is likely related to monochorionicity. In one study, birth weight discordance of at least 15% was associated with highest risk of perinatal mortality among same-gender twins, but discordance of at least 30% was required for significant perinatal mortality among gender-discordant twins.[57] It is unclear whether adverse outcomes seen with significant weight discordance are related to continuation of pregnancy within a hostile intrauterine environment or to iatrogenic prematurity. In general, we use the finding of significant weight discordance as an indication for close fetal surveillance rather than an indication for immediate delivery. Decisions regarding delivery are then made based on the results of tests of fetal well-being, together with gestational age, rather than solely on the basis of significant weight discordance.

Measurement of Cervical Length

Ultrasound surveillance of cervical length in multiple gestation can identify those at increased risk of preterm delivery. The Maternal-Fetal Medicine Units Network of the National Institute of Child Health and Human Development (NICHD) performed a Preterm Prediction Study of risk factors for preterm birth in twins. A transvaginal sonographic measurement of cervical length of 2.5 cm or less at 24 weeks' gestation was associated with a 6.9-fold increased risk of delivery before 32 weeks' gestation,[58] but a short cervix at 28 weeks' gestation was no longer predictive of preterm birth. A study of cervical length in 215 twin gestations reported that the sensitivity of a cervical length of 2.5 cm or less at 23 weeks' gestation was 100% for preterm delivery at or before 28 weeks, 80% for delivery at or before 30 weeks, and 47% for delivery at or before 32 weeks.[59] Approximately 11% to 17% of all twin gestations can be expected to have cervical lengths less than or equal to 2.5 cm.[58,59] In a study of 66 triplet gestations, a cervical length cutoff of 2 cm at 24 weeks' gestation was significantly associated with preterm delivery.[60]

When evaluating cervical length with ultrasound, the maternal bladder should first be emptied. Transvaginal sonography is the preferred approach. Care must be taken to avoid pressure on the cervix from the ultrasound probe. A sagittal view should be obtained, with an echogenic endocervical mucosa visible along the length of the cervical canal. Measurements should be taken between the V-shaped notch at the internal os and the triangular echolucent area at the external os. The optimal interval at which to perform sonographic assessments of cervical length during gestation is unclear. Our practice has been to measure cervical length every 2 weeks from 16 to 24 weeks in selected cases of multiple gestation deemed to be at highest risk for preterm delivery (e.g., higher-order multiple gestations, history of preterm deliveries). For all other multiple gestations, we perform sonographic assessment of cervical length at the time of sonography for fetal anatomy or growth. Two studies found that cervical length measurement of 3.5 cm or greater at 24 weeks can identify twin pregnancies with a very low (3% to 4%) risk of preterm birth before 34 weeks.[61,62] The major limitation of routine cervical length assessment for multiple gestations is the lack of a proven effective intervention when a short cervix is noted[4] (see later discussion on prophylaxis of preterm birth).

Confirmation of Fetal Well-Being

Ultrasonography is useful to confirm fetal well-being in multiple pregnancies. Nonstress testing (NST) in multiple gestation is discussed later (see Fetal Surveillance). The biophysical profile may also be of benefit in multiple gestation if an NST is not reassuring or in cases of higher-order multiple gestation, in which an NST can be impractical to perform. There is no evidence that routine biophysical profile testing in the absence of specific additional high-risk factors has any benefit in multiple gestations.[4]

Doppler velocimetry may also be used to evaluate fetal well-being in multiple gestations. Umbilical artery systolic-to-diastolic ratios are similar in singleton and twin gestations. A deterioration in this ratio may occur before the sonographic detection of growth restriction. Normal Doppler velocimetry indices of other fetal vessels, such as the middle cerebral artery and the descending aorta, are similar between singleton, twin, and triplet fetuses.[63] An absolute difference of 0.4 (or 15%) or greater in umbilical artery systolic-to-diastolic ratios between sibling fetuses identifies growth discordance as accurately as a difference in estimated fetal weight, presumably because such differences represent unequal fetoplacental perfusion.[31] We employ Doppler velocimetry whenever multiple gestation is complicated by significant growth restriction or discordance.

Sonographic measurement of amniotic fluid volume is an important tool to evaluate fetal well-being. In a dye-dilution study of diamniotic twin pregnancies, the amniotic fluid volume in each amniotic sac was noted to be independent of the volume in the neighboring sac and was similar to singleton fluid volumes.[64] There is no agreement on the optimal sonographic method to assess amniotic fluid volume in multiple gestations. Methods in use include the following[65,66]:

- A single overall amniotic fluid index without reference to the dividing membrane
- Individual amniotic fluid indices for each sac
- Largest two-diameter pocket in each sac
- Subjective assessment of the relative distribution of fluid between sacs

No one method, however, has been shown to be optimal to predict perinatal outcome in multiple gestation.

Prenatal Diagnosis

Prenatal diagnosis and genetic counseling are important in the management of multiple gestation, inasmuch as such patients are at higher risk of fetal anomalies because of (1) the presence of a multiple gestation and (2) the positive association between twinning and maternal age.

In dizygotic twin pregnancies, each fetus has its own independent risk of aneuploidy; thus, the chance of at least one abnormal fetus is increased. In addition, both monozygotic and dizygotic pregnancies are at increased risk for many structural anomalies. Monozygotic twins may not necessarily be concordant for chromosomal abnormalities, because the phenomenon of postzygotic nondisjunction can result in heterokaryotypic twins. Because of this phenomenon, and because the diagnosis of monochorionicity is rarely made with certainty, consideration should be given to sampling each gestation separately whenever prenatal diagnosis is indicated.

The role of ultrasonography to detect fetal anomalies in multiple gestations has been discussed previously.

Risks of Chromosomal Abnormalities

Risks for Down syndrome and other chromosomal aneuploidies have been calculated for twin gestations at various maternal ages.[67] In the population studied by Rodis and coworkers, the risk that one fetus in a twin pregnancy would have Down syndrome for a 33-year-old woman was similar to that for a 35-year-old woman with a singleton gestation. These specific risks do change, depending on the incidence of dizygotic twinning, which is dependent on the maternal age and race profiles of the study population. After correction for different rates of dizygosity based on maternal age and race, it was suggested that invasive prenatal diagnosis should be offered to women in the United States with twin gestations who are 31 years of age or older (Table 25-3).[68] In a triplet gestation, the chance that a 28-year-old woman will have at least one fetus with Down syndrome may be similar to that of a 35-year-old woman with a single fetus. These alterations in risk assessment for chromosomal abnormalities are important, because invasive prenatal diagnosis may be considered at an even earlier maternal age for gravidas with higher-order multiple gestations. However, recent advances in multiple-marker screening have led to decreased use of maternal age alone as a threshold for offering invasive testing of fetal karyotype. For this reason, a policy of offering chorionic villus sampling (CVS) or amniocentesis to all patients with twin pregnancy who are 31 or 33 years of age or older is difficult to justify.[69] All women, regardless of age, should be made aware of the relative advantages and disadvantages of screening versus diagnostic tests for fetal aneuploidy. Women with multiple gestations who are concerned about aneuploidy risk should be counseled and supported to make their own personal decision whether to choose a screening test, a diagnostic test, or no testing at all.[69]

Serum Screening for Down Syndrome

Screening for Down syndrome using maternal serum levels of AFP, hCG, unconjugated estriol, and inhibin-A, together with maternal age, is commonly performed in the United States during the second trimester for singleton pregnancies. In twin pregnancies, experience with such screening is limited. Average levels of AFP, hCG, and unconjugated estriol are increased 2.04-fold, 1.93-fold, and 1.64-fold, respectively, in twin compared with singleton pregnancies.[70] In one prospective evaluation of screening with multiple serum markers in twins, the screen-positive rate remained at 5%, but no cases of Down syndrome were detected in the study population.[71] Using statistical modeling and maintaining a 5% false-positive rate, the authors estimated that 73% of monozygotic twins and 43% of dizygotic twins with Down syndrome would be detected. In another series of 420 twin pregnancies, AFP and hCG levels were twice the levels seen in singletons.[72] The authors postulated that risk prediction from singletons could be extrapolated to twin gestations using a twin correction method in which the multiple of the median (MoM) value is divided by the mean MoM of the twin population. This process with AFP and hCG screening was predicted to yield a 51% detection rate for Down syndrome, with a 5% rate of false-positive results.[72] Although second trimester serum screening for Down syndrome represents an improvement over the use of maternal age alone, it is also clear that the accuracy of such

TABLE 25-3 RISK OF AT LEAST ONE CHROMOSOMAL ABNORMALITY IN WHITE SINGLETON AND TWIN GESTATIONS BASED ON MATERNAL AGE AT THE TIME OF AMNIOCENTESIS

	Singleton Gestation		Twin Gestation	
Maternal Age (yr)	Down Syndrome	All Chromosomal Abnormalities	Down Syndrome	All Chromosomal Abnormalities
25	1/885	1/1533	1/481	1/833
26	1/826	1/1202	1/447	1/650
27	1/769	1/943	1/415	1/509
28	1/719	1/740	1/387	1/398
29	1/680	1/580	1/364	1/310
30	1/641	1/455	1/342	1/243
31	1/610	1/357	1/324	1/190
32	1/481	1/280	1/256	1/149
33	1/389	1/219	1/206	1/116
34	1/303	1/172	1/160	1/91
35	1/237	1/135	1/125	1/71
36	1/185	1/106	1/98	1/56
37	1/145	1/83	1/77	1/44
38	1/113	1/65	1/60	1/35
39	1/89	1/51	1/47	1/27
40	1/69	1/40	1/37	1/21
41	1/55	1/31	1/29	1/17
42	1/43	1/25	1/23	1/13
43	1/33	1/19	1/18	1/10
44	1/26	1/15	1/14	1/8
45	1/21	1/12	1/11	1/6

From Meyers C, Adam R, Dungan J, et al: Aneuploidy in twin gestations: When is maternal age advanced? Obstet Gynecol 89:248; 1997. Reprinted with permission from the American College of Obstetricians and Gynecologists.

an approach is considerably less than that of serum screening in singleton pregnancies.[73] Given the effective alternative of nuchal translucency sonography, we do not routinely offer serum marker evaluation for aneuploidy screening with multiple gestation.

First-Trimester Screening

With the availability of late first-trimester MFPR procedures in higher-order multiple gestations, there is now increasing interest in screening tests for fetal abnormalities in the first trimester. Although combined screening for Down syndrome with nuchal translucency, free β-hCG, and pregnancy-associated plasma protein A (PAPP-A) has been reported in singletons, less is known about the performance of first-trimester screening in multiples.[69] Similar to second-trimester serum markers, first-trimester free β-hCG and PAPP-A levels are about twice as high in twin compared with singleton pregnancies.[73] In studies of normal twin pregnancies, average first-trimester free β-hCG levels were 1.86 MoM and PAPP-A levels were 2.10 MoM.[73,74]

At present, we use only increased nuchal translucency thickness to screen for aneuploidies in multiple gestations in the first trimester, given the limitations of interpreting serum marker results in the setting of multiple gestation. In one study of 448 twin gestations, this form of screening delivered an 88% detection rate for Down syndrome, with a 7.3% screen-positive rate.[75] In another series of 24 multiple gestations and 79 singleton control subjects, the distribution of nuchal translucency measurements, including 95th percentile values, was similar in all cases, implying that this form of screening could be implemented using established normative data from singleton populations.[76] If MFPR is being planned, we incorporate the nuchal translucency measurement into consideration in deciding which fetus or fetuses to target for reduction.

Screening for Neural Tube Defects

A second-trimester maternal serum AFP level greater than 2.0 or 2.5 MoM has been used to screen for neural tube defects in singleton gestations. Because the maternal serum AFP level is approximately doubled in normal twin pregnancy, different cutoff values are needed to interpret this test if it is used in multiple gestations. If a 2.5 MoM cutoff in twin pregnancy is used, 99% of cases of anencephaly and 89% of open neural tube defects are detected but at the expense of generating a 30% false-positive rate.[77] Raising the twin cutoff value to 5.0 MoM decreases the false-positive rate to 3% but also decreases the detection of anencephaly to 83% and that of open neural tube defects to 39%.

The most commonly used cutoff for neural tube defect screening is 4.5 MoM, which has a detection rate of 50% to 85%, based on a 5% false-positive rate.[70] Amniotic fluid AFP and acetylcholinesterase levels in different amniotic sacs are independent of each other in dichorionic twins but are interdependent in monochorionic twins.[78] Because serum screening for fetal abnormalities in multiple gestation will always be limited by the inability to confirm which fetus is affected, many centers do not offer serum screening in multiple gestation, even for neural tube defects. Sonographic evaluation alone may be more efficient to screen for fetal neural tube defects in multiple gestations. Use of this approach relies on identifying either the neural tube defect along the fetal spine or the secondary intracranial effects (e.g., Chiari malformation). These sonographic features include the "lemon" sign, representing scalloping of the frontal bones, and the "banana" sign, representing downward displacement of the cerebellum toward the foramen magnum.

Genetic Amniocentesis

Genetic amniocentesis in twins is most commonly performed with an ultrasound-guided double-needle approach.[70] After the first sac has been entered and amniotic fluid aspirated, several milliliters of the blue dye indigo carmine are instilled and the needle is removed. A new needle is then placed into the second sac, and aspiration of clear fluid confirms successful sampling of two separate sacs. Methylene blue dye should not be used because of the risks of fetal hemolytic anemia, small-intestine atresia, and fetal demise. This procedure can be extended sequentially to perform triplet and quadruplet genetic amniocenteses.[79]

Careful sonographic mapping of placentas and sacs is mandatory to assist in future management plans when karyotype results return, which may be as long as 2 weeks later if rapid diagnostic techniques such as polymerase chain reaction (PCR) or fluorescence in situ hybridization (FISH) are not utilized. The rate of pregnancy loss after genetic amniocentesis in twins has been considered similar to that observed with singletons,[80] but a comparison of pregnancy outcomes after amniocentesis in 476 twin pregnancies with a similar number of control twins and singleton pregnancies suggested a 2% increased risk of loss in women with twins.[81] A higher loss rate after amniocentesis in twins may reflect the higher spontaneous loss rate seen in twins.[70] No data exist on loss rates for amniocentesis with higher-order multiple gestation or on loss rates for early amniocentesis (<14 weeks) with multiple gestations. However, early amniocentesis is no longer recommended in singleton or multiple gestations, because its safety compares unfavorably with that of CVS.[79]

Chorionic Villus Sampling

CVS is usually performed in twin gestations at 10 to 13 weeks. It is considered to be an equally safe alternative to amniocentesis in twins.[82] The needle tip must be kept under constant sonographic visualization to ensure that both chorion frondosum sites have been separately sampled. If monochorionicity has been confirmed, then a single-placenta sampling procedure is reasonable. A combination of transabdominal and transcervical approaches to the two placentas of a dichorionic pregnancy may ensure that separate placental sites have indeed been sampled.[79] Because as many as 2% to 4% of samples show evidence of twin-twin contamination, the cytogenetic laboratory should be made aware that a twin CVS has been performed.[70,79] As with twin amniocentesis, careful sonographic mapping of placentas and sacs is mandatory to assist in future management plans after karyotype results become available. Although data on the safety of twin or triplet CVS are limited, at least one series of 208 procedures at a single center demonstrated very low pregnancy loss rates.[83]

Antepartum Management

The incidence and range of maternal and fetal complications in multiple gestation suggest that these pregnancies should be managed under the supervision of an appropriately trained specialist.[3,4,84] In a nonrandomized study comparing the outcome of 67 triplet gestations managed by maternal-fetal medicine specialists with 24 triplet gestations managed by generalist physicians, significant increases in gestational age at delivery and birth weight were observed for cases managed by specialists,[84] as well as significant reductions in neonatal intensive care unit length of stay and cost.

Interventions to improve outcome cannot reasonably be expected to work unless an early diagnosis of multiple gestation has been made. This supports our practice of offering routine ultrasonography to all pregnant patients. If ultrasound diagnosis is not offered, vigilance should be maintained for early clinical signs of multiple gestation, such as size greater than dates, excessive maternal weight gain, auscultation of more than one fetal heart rate, elevated maternal serum AFP levels, or unexplained severe anemia.

Preterm Labor and Delivery

Preterm birth occurs in more than 40% of twin and 75% of triplet gestations.[8,85] Although patient education regarding the early signs of preterm labor in multiple gestations is important, surveillance for cervical change may also be helpful in predicting premature delivery. Other parameters used to predict preterm delivery in multiple gestations include sonographic assessment of cervical length and cervicovaginal assays for fetal fibronectin. As described previously, these factors were evaluated in large prospective studies of twin gestations.[58,59] In women with twins who are screened at 24 weeks, a cervical length of less than 25 mm is significantly associated with preterm delivery before 32 weeks (odds ratio, 6.9), as well as a 27% rate of spontaneous preterm birth before 32 weeks, compared with 5% in twin gestations with a longer cervical length. A positive cervicovaginal fetal fibronectin assay at 28 weeks is also significantly associated with preterm delivery before 32 weeks, with an odds ratio of 9.4 and a spontaneous preterm birth rate (<32 weeks) of 29%, compared with 4% for a twin gestation with negative fetal fibronectin. The main value of a single negative fetal fibronectin test for twin pregnancy is in its very high negative predictive value for subsequent preterm delivery.[4,58] No other risk factors were significantly associated with preterm delivery of twins in the NICHD study.[58]

Interventions to prevent preterm labor and prolong pregnancy in multiple gestations have been disappointing. There is no evidence that prophylactic cervical cerclage or prophylactic tocolytic agents are beneficial.[86,87] An observational study of 128 twin pregnancies with cervical length less than 2.5 mm at 18 to 26 weeks' gestation revealed no benefit for any outcome measure after cerclage placement.[88] There are no randomized trials indicating a benefit to cerclage for a shortened cervix in multiple gestations. In a comparison of 16 triplet gestations treated by prophylactic cervical cerclage and 52 triplet gestations without cerclage, the mean gestational age at delivery was 34 weeks in both groups, and the perinatal mortality rates were 104 per 1000 births with cerclage versus 71 per 1000 with no cerclage.[89] In another observational study of 59 triplet gestations, 20 received prophylactic cervical cerclage, and the remaining 39 were expectantly managed.[90] Although the authors reported fewer infants with extremely low birth weight in the cerclage group, there were no significant differences in mean gestational age at delivery or any other measure of neonatal outcome. We reserve cervical cerclage in multiple gestation for women who also meet historical criteria for cervical insufficiency (see Chapter 30).

Cerclage placement has been considered in women with multiple gestation when sonographic surveillance of cervical length demonstrates progressive cervical shortening, but a meta-analysis of data from four prospective trials found a twofold *increase* in preterm birth in women with twins and short cervix who received a cerclage.[87] Current data are insufficient to exclude or confirm a benefit of cerclage in multiple gestation.[4,87,91]

Based on studies showing reduced rates of preterm birth after treatment with progesterone compounds in singleton gestations at risk of preterm birth,[92,93] prophylactic progesterone was investigated in a randomized, placebo-controlled trial of 661 twin pregnancies. Weekly intramuscular injections of 17α-hydroxyprogesterone caproate (17P) had no effect on outcome. Forty-two percent of treated women delivered before 35 weeks, compared with 37% in those who received placebo injections.[94]

Long-term maintenance administration of tocolytic drugs (e.g., oral terbutaline or nifedipine, rectal indomethacin, subcutaneous infusion of terbutaline) does not prolong pregnancy or prevent prematurity in multiple gestation. Caution is advised when tocolytic agents are given to women with multiple gestation because of the significant potential for maternal cardiovascular and pulmonary morbidity. The combination of one or more tocolytic agents, corticosteroids, and intravenous fluid replacement in the setting of the increased blood volume of multiple gestation leads to a significant risk of pulmonary edema. We suggest that acute tocolysis be reserved for women with documented preterm labor, to delay delivery and allow transport to an appropriate medical center and antenatal treatment with betamethasone. Betamethasone (12 mg IM, two doses, 24 hours apart) is given whenever there is a high risk of delivery between 24 and 34 weeks of gestation. Use of repeated courses of antenatal corticosteroids is discussed in Chapter 23.

Bed rest, at home or in hospital, is not effective in prolonging pregnancy or preventing preterm labor or delivery.[4,95] Retrospective studies suggested that hospitalization and bed rest might improve outcome in multiple gestation, but subsequent prospective trials and meta-analyses have not supported this intervention. A review of six randomized trials involving more than 600 multiple gestations noted a trend toward a decrease in low-birth-weight infants with inpatient bed rest.[96] However, there was no decrease in very-low-birth-weight infants, and inpatient bed rest was actually associated with an increased risk of delivery before 34 weeks' gestation in women with uncomplicated twin pregnancies. There have been no recent prospective trials evaluating the role of bed rest at home for patients with multiple gestation. Because it is extremely difficult to standardize home bed rest and, consequently, difficult to refute the possibility of potential benefit, we advise modified rest at home for women with higher-order multiple gestations, starting at approximately 20 weeks of gestation.[3] For example, one suggested care algorithm for triplet gestation recommends lateral recumbent rest for 4 to 6 hr/day beginning at 16 weeks' gestation, increasing to 6 to 8 hr/day by 20 weeks and extending to rest for most of the day by 24 weeks.[97] Others omit a recommendation for bed rest in women with multiple gestation if cervical sonography indicates a length greater than 35 mm at 24 weeks' gestation.[61,62]

Outpatient uterine activity monitoring does not prolong pregnancy or prevent preterm labor and delivery in either singleton or multiple gestations.[98,99] A meta-analysis of six randomized trials showed no significant benefit of home uterine activity monitoring to reduce the risk of preterm birth in twin gestations.[100] A randomized trial of weekly nurse contact, daily nurse contact, or daily nurse contact plus home uterine activity monitoring conducted in 2422 women at risk of preterm birth found no differences in frequency of birth before 35 weeks' gestation overall and, specifically, no benefit in the 844 women with twin gestations.[98] Outpatient uterine activity monitoring has not been studied in women who have undergone fetal reduction procedures in higher-order multiple gestation or in utero fetal surgery.

Preeclampsia

Pregnancy-related hypertension, including gestational hypertension and preeclampsia, is increased in multifetal gestations, ranging from 10% to 20% in twin, 25% to 60% in triplet, and up to 90% in quadruplet pregnancies.[8,13,19,21,85] The incidence of preeclampsia may be further increased in multiple pregnancies that follow assisted reproductive technologies, but it does not appear to be related to zygosity.[101,102] When preeclampsia occurs in higher-order multiple gestations, it more often occurs earlier, is more severe, and is atypical.[4,8,21] A multicenter study of 87 twin and 143 singleton gestations with preeclampsia demonstrated lower gestational age at delivery, lower birth weight, and a higher rate of cesarean delivery among the twin gestations.[103] These data emphasize the importance of specialist supervision of multiple gestations and regular monitoring for early signs and symptoms of preeclampsia. To date, however, no prophylactic interventions (e.g., low-dose aspirin, calcium supplementation) have been found to prevent or reduce the incidence of preeclampsia in these high-risk pregnancies. In one study in which 688 women with multiple gestation were randomized to receive low-dose aspirin or placebo between 13 and 26 weeks' gestation, the incidence of preeclampsia was 12% with aspirin and 16% with placebo, a difference that was not significant (relative risk, 0.7; 95% confidence interval, 0.5 to 1.1).[104]

Other Maternal Complications

Daily supplementation with at least 60 mg of elemental iron and 1 mg of folic acid is recommended because of the increased risk of iron- and folate-deficiency anemia in multiple gestation. Surveillance for other potential maternal complications of higher-order multiple gestations, including acute fatty liver of pregnancy, gestational diabetes, urinary tract infections, and intervertebral disk disease, is important as well.[4,8] Although there are no data to guide timing or frequency of screening for gestational diabetes in multiple gestations, it may be reasonable to perform glucose challenge testing at 20 to 24 weeks' gestation, followed by a repeat screen at 28 to 32 weeks' gestation. In particular, multiple gestation is a risk factor for the development of acute fatty liver of pregnancy, perhaps because of the increase in placental mass.[105] Acute fatty liver should be carefully considered in the differential diagnosis if hepatic dysfunction is found in a woman with multiple gestation.

Fetal Surveillance

As described earlier, serial sonographic assessment of fetal growth is recommended for multiple gestations. We evaluate fetal weight and growth discordance every 3 to 4 weeks from approximately 18 weeks' gestation, or every 2 weeks if growth restriction or growth discordance (>20%) is discovered. Although some obstetricians routinely monitor all multiple gestations using weekly NST or biophysical profiles beginning at 34 weeks, this practice has not been validated by prospective studies.[4] Surveillance with NST or biophysical profile is reserved for multiple pregnancies with the following indications:

- Significant growth restriction in either fetus
- Growth discordance
- Oligohydramnios
- Decreased fetal movement
- Maternal medical complications

Fetal testing for monoamniotic twins, TTTS, demise of one fetus, and anomalous twins is discussed later (see Special Considerations in Management).

As soon as the diagnosis of significant growth discordance is confirmed, fetal testing should begin intensively. In our practice, this consists of twice-weekly NST supplemented by biophysical profiles and umbilical artery Doppler velocimetry. If absent or reversed end-diastolic flow is discovered, delivery should be considered if gestational age is sufficiently advanced that the healthy twin would not be significantly compromised by delivery. Selecting the appropriate time for delivery is extremely difficult in such cases, because an effort that is intended to save a twin that may already be significantly compromised may lead to iatrogenic morbidity in the healthy twin. Daily, or twice-daily, fetal testing should be performed in cases of absent or reversed end-diastolic flow until delivery is accomplished.

Determination of fetal lung maturity is sometimes helpful if multiple gestation is complicated by preterm labor, ruptured membranes, diabetes mellitus, growth restriction, or growth discordance. In most instances, only one sac is sampled, because lung maturity studies are usually similar.[106] In the case of discordant twins, it is difficult to predict which fetus will have higher lung maturity indices. In one series, 9 of 15 discordant twin pairs showed higher lung maturity indices in the larger twin, whereas theoretically the growth-restricted fetus would be predicted to have more advanced lung maturity owing to stress responses.[107] Therefore, we believe each amniotic sac should be sampled in selected cases if the results of lung maturity testing will affect management.[4]

Intrapartum Management

Preparations

The nadir of perinatal mortality for dichorionic twin pregnancies occurs at approximately 38 weeks, and for triplets at about 35 weeks.[4,108] All twin fetuses should therefore be delivered by 39 weeks of gestation because of the rising perinatal morbidity and mortality beyond that date. The rate of stillbirth in multiple gestations at 39 weeks surpassed the risk for singleton gestations at greater than 42 weeks' gestation in one study.[109] A retrospective review of 5594 twin pregnancies demonstrated an increase in the rate of stillbirth beyond 36 weeks' gestation.[110] The lowest rate of perinatal morbidity and mortality occurred at 37 weeks' gestation. Whether elective delivery at this gestational age for all twins will optimize outcomes is unclear and is the subject of ongoing study.[110] Until more data are available, it is reasonable to consider delivery of uncomplicated dichorionic twins by 37 or 38 weeks' gestation.[111] For uncomplicated monochorionic twins, even in the setting of intensive fetal surveillance, the risk of sudden death after 32 weeks' gestation is significant, reaching 5%.[112] For this reason, and given the unique challenges of monochorionicity together with the relatively low risk of serious neonatal morbidity, we believe that it is reasonable to consider elective delivery of uncomplicated monochorionic twins by 34 to 35 weeks' gestation.

The use of prostaglandins for induction and oxytocin for induction or augmentation of labor is acceptable in twin gestation. An attempt at vaginal birth after a previous low transverse cesarean delivery is considered by some to be an acceptable alternative to elective repeated cesarean section in twin gestation.[113] However, it should be noted that no randomized studies are available to confirm the safety of vaginal birth after cesarean (VBAC) in the setting of multiple gestation. A multicenter registry of 186 attempts at VBAC in twin pregnancies demonstrated a 65% success rate.[114] In 30 of the 66 patients in whom a trial of labor failed, the first twin was successfully delivered vaginally, and a cesarean delivery was required for the second twin. Maternal and perinatal morbidity and mortality rates were similar in women with twins who attempted VBAC and those who delivered by repeat cesarean delivery[114] in this observational study. However, such studies to date have lacked power to address the safety of this approach.

Intrapartum management of the parturient with a multiple gestation requires multidisciplinary cooperation. Adequate obstetric and nursing staff, together with an anesthesiologist and at least one neonatologist or pediatrician, should be present for delivery. Intravenous access and prompt availability of blood products should be ensured.[111]

As soon as possible after admission to the delivery unit, ultrasonography should be performed to determine fetal presentations and size before choosing the mode of delivery. Electronic fetal heart monitoring should be available; this is usually best achieved by placing a fetal scalp electrode for the first twin and using an external monitor for the second twin. If a trial of labor is elected, continuous lumbar epidural anesthesia should be strongly recommended, because it allows a full range of obstetric interventions to be performed rapidly if needed. Vaginal deliveries should be performed in an operating room, because emergent cesarean section may be required for the second twin in a significant number of cases.[115] Before vaginal delivery of a second twin, prompt availability of ultrasonography in the operating room may be very helpful in confirming presentation and fetal well-being.

Vertex-Vertex Twins

The vertex-vertex presentation occurs in 40% to 45% of all twin pregnancies. In the absence of obstetric indications for cesarean delivery, vaginal birth should be planned regardless of gestational age.[111,115] Routine cesarean delivery for all vertex-vertex twins is not supported by the literature; no improvement in perinatal outcome has been found.[116]

After delivery of the first twin, the cord should be clamped. No blood samples should be obtained until after delivery of the second twin. Unless the presentation is obviously vertex by clinical examination, ultrasonography should be performed to confirm presentation of the second twin and to exclude a funis presentation. With the availability of continuous electronic fetal heart monitoring, there is no absolute indication to deliver the second twin within a specified time limit. However, active intervention to complete the delivery (amniotomy, if safe, and oxytocin augmentation) is encouraged by studies that link length of delivery interval to fetal acid-base status. In one series of 118 cases of twin deliveries, significant negative correlations were noted between the length of the delivery interval and umbilical cord pH and base excess.[117] The rate of umbilical arterial pH of 7.00 or less was zero when the delivery interval was less than 15 minutes, increasing to 6% for an interval of 16 to 30 minutes, and to 27% for intervals longer than 30 minutes. Undue delay may also allow time for the fully dilated cervix to contract, thereby limiting the range of options for urgent delivery of the second twin should a problem develop. The cesarean section rate for the second twin also increases with increasing delivery interval.[115]

Vertex-Nonvertex Twins

Vertex-breech or vertex-transverse presentation occurs in 35% to 40% of all twin pregnancies. Selection of mode of delivery depends on (1) the size of the second twin; (2) the presence of growth discordance (estimated weight of second twin at least 25% greater than first twin); and (3) the availability of obstetric staff skilled in assisted breech delivery, internal podalic version, and total breech extraction. In the absence of an appropriately skilled obstetrician, or if the second twin is significantly larger than the first, cesarean delivery is recommended.

Another option is external cephalic version of the second twin immediately after delivery of the first. This method is successful in up to 70% of cases of vertex-nonvertex twins.[118] Vaginal delivery is not always possible after successful external version of the second twin and may be associated with complications, such as cord prolapse and placental abruption, that require emergent cesarean delivery of the second twin. For these reasons, breech extraction may be a better alternative, with success rates of more than 95%.[119] It has also been suggested that external cephalic version should no longer be attempted for a second twin because of the very high rate of emergency cesarean delivery required for the second twin.[111,119,120]

Vaginal breech delivery of the second twin appears to be reasonable in appropriately selected cases. The adverse perinatal outcome associated with breech second twins is more often related to prematurity or growth restriction rather than mode of delivery.[115] A liberal cesarean delivery policy for the nonvertex second twin has not significantly improved perinatal outcome. For fetuses with birth weights of 1500 g or more, there is no apparent benefit to cesarean delivery over vaginal breech delivery for the nonvertex second twin.[15] Data for fetuses with estimated birth weights less than 1500 g are insufficient to make such a firm conclusion, but vaginal breech delivery of such fetuses is not absolutely contraindicated. In a series of 141 twin deliveries in which the second twin was nonvertex, including 35 cases of vaginal delivery, there was no evidence of benefit from cesarean delivery when gestational age was greater than 24 weeks and the birth weight exceeded 1500 g.[121] It seems reasonable to offer vaginal breech delivery for the nonvertex second twin with an estimated birth weight between 1500 and 3500 g, provided it is not significantly larger than the first twin and the head is not hyperextended. An estimated fetal weight of 2000 g as a lower threshold of fetal size allows for the imprecision of fetal ultrasound in accurately predicting birth weight.

If a vaginal breech delivery is planned for the second twin, the delivery of the presenting vertex twin is performed as previously described. If the second twin is in a frank or complete breech presentation and the fetal heart tracing is reassuring, membranes may be left intact until engagement of the presenting part, and an assisted breech delivery can be performed.

If the second twin is in a transverse lie or a footling breech presentation, or if fetal testing is not reassuring, membranes should be left intact until the feet can be secured in the pelvis, after which immediate amniotomy and total breech extraction should be performed.[115] Whenever total breech extraction is indicated, it should be performed as soon as possible after delivery of the first twin, while the cervix is still fully dilated.[111]

Nonvertex First Twin

Breech-vertex or breech-breech presentation occurs in 15% to 20% of all twin pregnancies. Such cases are almost always managed by cesarean delivery. Historically, this was practiced because of concern about interlocking fetal heads in breech-vertex twins. However, this complication is so rare that some centers offer vaginal delivery when the breech twin of a breech-vertex pair meets the selection criteria for singleton vaginal breech deliveries. Among 239 vaginal deliveries in which the first twin was breech, there was no evidence of depressed Apgar scores or increased neonatal deaths when the first twin's weight was greater than 1500 g.[122] However, Apgar scores and neonatal deaths were significantly increased for first twins weighing less than 1500 g who were delivered vaginally from breech presentation. External cephalic version of a breech-presenting twin has also been described.[123] In the absence of prospective studies validating these approaches, cesarean section for the nonvertex first twin is likely to be the optimal mode of delivery.

Higher-Order Multiple Gestations

Although case series of successful vaginal delivery of triplets exist, there are no prospective series large enough to establish the safety of vaginal delivery over cesarean delivery.[124-126] One center described a protocol for vaginal delivery in selected cases of triplet gestation and reported that 8 of 11 women who were eligible successfully underwent vaginal delivery.[127] No increase in maternal or neonatal morbidity was noted in this small series. Another review suggested that there was a sixfold increased risk of stillbirth and a threefold increased risk of neonatal death when vaginal delivery of viable triplets was attempted.[128] Because of practical difficulties in adequately monitoring three or more fetuses in labor and through delivery, we recommend cesarean delivery under regional anesthesia for all patients with three or more live fetuses that are of a viable gestational age. There is no conclusive evidence to recommend one type of uterine incision over another in higher-order multiple gestation.

Asynchronous Delivery

Asynchronous delivery, or delayed interval delivery, refers to delivery of one fetus in a multiple gestation that is not followed promptly by delivery of the remaining fetus or fetuses. This extremely rare scenario is acceptable only in the management of extreme prematurity, when the remaining fetus is either previable or would be at very high risk for severe complications of prematurity if delivered. Clinical conditions that typically contraindicate asynchronous delivery include monochorionicity, intra-amniotic infection, placental abruption, and the coexistence of preeclampsia. Successful outcomes have been reported in carefully selected cases.[129] In a report of 24 twins and triplets managed with delayed interval delivery, a protocol of amniocentesis of the remaining sac to exclude infection, ligation of the cord of the delivered fetus with absorbable suture near the placenta, aggressive tocolysis, placement of a cerclage, broad-spectrum antibiotics for up to 7 days, bed rest, and close surveillance were instituted.[130] The mean latency interval was 36 days; the range was 3 to 123 days. In 16 of the 24 cases, the gestational age was 24 weeks or less at the time of presentation; 10 (63%) of these reached 24 weeks, and 8 (44%) of the 18 remaining infants survived. Given the limitations of these data, it is essential that careful counseling be provided and informed consent be obtained from the mother regarding risks to her health before such management is attempted. Eligible women should be monitored closely for the development of chorioamnionitis or maternal sepsis. Cervical cerclage and tocolytic agents should be used with extreme caution and only after excluding chorioamnionitis. Data are insufficient to comment on the role of prophylactic antibiotics or amniocentesis in this setting.

Special Considerations in Management

Twin-Twin Transfusion Syndrome

Background and Pathogenesis

TTTS occurs because of an imbalance in blood flow through vascular communications in the placenta which leads to overperfusion of one twin and underperfusion of its co-twin (Fig. 25-4). It occurs exclusively

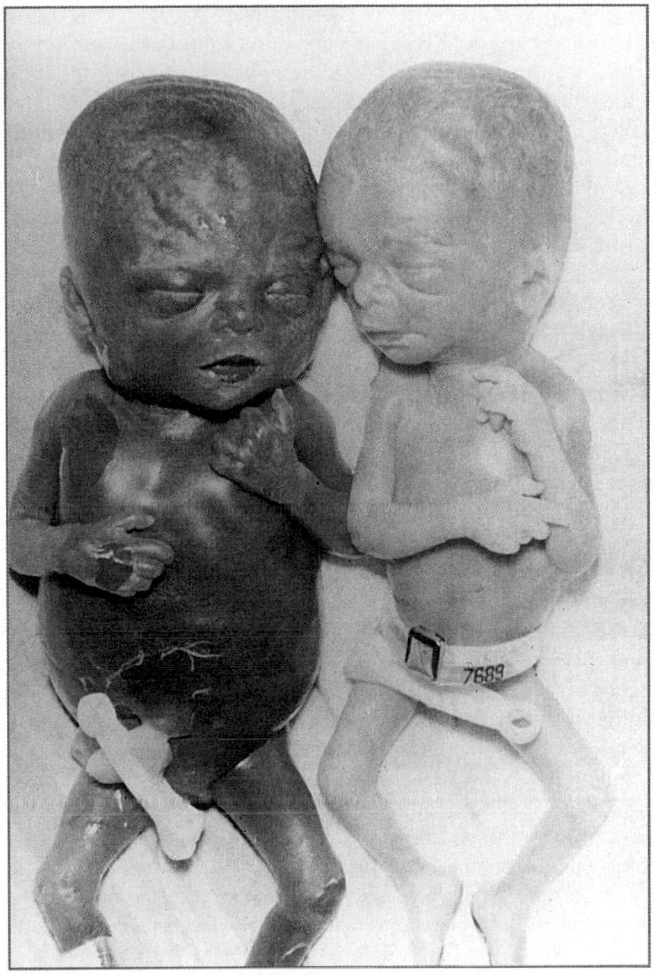

FIGURE 25-4 **Twin-twin transfusion syndrome.** Twin-twin transfusion syndrome resulted in pregnancy loss at 22 weeks' gestation; the plethoric recipient twin is on the left and the anemic donor twin on the right. (Courtesy of Steven Ralston, MD, New England Medical Center, Boston, MA.)

in monochorionic twin pregnancies and is estimated to occur in at least 15% of such pregnancies.[131,132] Theoretically, TTTS should not occur in dichorionic twin pregnancies, but it has been demonstrated at least once in a fused dichorionic twin gestation.[133] The precise incidence of TTTS is extremely difficult to define, because the syndrome is associated with a wide spectrum of clinical presentations, ranging from the vanishing-twin phenomenon in the first trimester to unexplained fetal demise in the third trimester. There is even disagreement on terminology defining the syndrome. Some authors suggest that "twin oligohydramnios-polyhydramnios sequence" is a more precise term.[134,135]

The precise cause of TTTS is unknown. Initial theories suggested that pregnancies affected by TTTS demonstrate significantly fewer placental anastomoses, and the few anastomoses present are more likely to be deep than superficial.[136] This theory implies that TTTS is likely to be the result of a paucity of placental anastomoses, which interferes with the placenta's ability to regulate blood flow equally between the twins. More recent work has demonstrated that it is the anatomic type of placental anastomoses, rather than simply their number, that underlies the pathophysiology of TTTS. Arteriovenous (AV) anastomoses have been described on the placental surface as a single unpaired artery carrying blood from the donor twin to a placental cotyledon, together with a single unpaired vein carrying blood from that cotyledon back to the recipient twin.[137] Although these vessels run along the surface of the placenta separately, they enter the same placental cotyledon. It is theorized that these AV anastomoses result in net transfusion of blood from the donor to the recipient fetus. However, such AV anastomoses are present in up to 70% of monochorionic placentas, whereas the clinical syndrome of TTTS is far less common (15%).[138] Therefore, a protective mechanism must be in place that prevents TTTS from developing in the majority of monochorionic pregnancies. It has been suggested that arterioarterial anastomoses are bidirectional and that the presence of a large number of such anastomoses in a monochorionic placenta may compensate for unidirectional AV anastomotic flow, thereby preventing the appearance of TTTS.[138,139] This theory is consistent with earlier studies suggesting that a lack of superficial placental anastomoses (presumably arterioarterial), together with the existence of a number of deep placental anastomoses (presumably AV), explains the pathophysiology of TTTS.[136,139,140]

Clinical and Sonographic Features

The clinical features of TTTS can be explained by the placental architecture findings just described. The donor fetus is relatively hypoperfused, demonstrating signs of intrauterine growth restriction and oligohydramnios. Eventually, anhydramnios develops, and this fetus attains the typical "stuck twin" appearance because of inability to visualize the dividing membrane separate from the fetal body. Fetal blood sampling studies have demonstrated that this donor fetus has a significantly lower hematocrit than the recipient fetus (36% versus 47%).[141] Echocardiographic studies have not shown any specific pattern of abnormal findings among donor fetuses.[142,143] By contrast, the recipient fetus is relatively hyperperfused, becomes hypertensive, and produces increasing amounts of atrial and brain natriuretic peptides in an effort to handle its larger blood volume.[144] Recipient fetuses demonstrate biventricular hypertrophy and diastolic dysfunction, which tends to be progressive without definitive therapy.[145] This results in significant polyhydramnios and increasing intrauterine pressure. Uterine overdistention and raised intrauterine pressure may then contribute to increased rates of preterm labor or pPROM, as well as exacerbating hypoperfusion of the donor fetus through compression effects. Echocardiographic features in the recipient twin include ventricular hypertrophy and dilation, tricuspid regurgitation, and cardiac failure.[142,143] Additionally, acquired progressive right ventricular outflow tract obstruction, possibly leading to right ventricular outflow atresia, has been described in up to 9% of recipient fetuses.[146]

Prenatal diagnosis of TTTS depends on a high degree of clinical suspicion in monochorionic pregnancies, together with the visualization of certain ultrasonographic criteria. These include the following[34]

- Presence of a single placenta
- Gender concordance
- Significant growth discordance (usually >20%)
- Discrepancy in amniotic fluid volume between the two amniotic sacs (usually oligohydramnios and polyhydramnios)
- Discrepancy in size of the umbilical cords
- Presence of fetal hydrops or cardiac dysfunction
- Abnormal umbilical artery Doppler findings, such as absent end-diastolic flow in the donor fetus

Not all sonographic criteria need to be met to make the diagnosis of TTTS, and none of the criteria is specific for TTTS. For example, a significant growth discrepancy between monochorionic fetuses is not required to make a diagnosis of TTTS, because acute TTTS is known to occur; it leads to marked inequality in amniotic fluid volume in each sac but with insufficient time for significant fetal size discordance to become apparent. The most important criterion appears to be discrepancy in amniotic fluid volume, with a maximum vertical pocket of less than 2 cm expected around the donor fetus and a maximum vertical pocket greater than 8 cm around the recipient fetus. An early sonographic marker of TTTS may be significant discrepancy in nuchal translucency measurements at 10 to 14 weeks' gestation in a monochorionic twin.[147] The differential diagnosis of significant growth discordance or stuck twin phenomenon includes uteroplacental insufficiency, structural or chromosomal fetal abnormalities, abnormal cord insertion, and intrauterine infection (e.g., cytomegalovirus infection). Although abnormal cord insertions can coexist with TTTS, it does not appear that this contributes to the incidence of TTTS. In one study of monochorionic twins with and without TTTS, the incidence of velamentous cord insertion was approximately 15% in both groups.[148]

Other methods of prenatal diagnosis of TTTS have included (1) fetal blood sampling to detect a difference in hemoglobin concentration between twins and (2) transfusion of adult rhesus-negative red blood cells into the donor twin, followed by Kleihauer detection in the recipient twin. Although fetal blood sampling studies have demonstrated significantly lower hematocrit values in donor compared with recipient fetuses, only some cases of TTTS have sufficient hematocrit differences to be of diagnostic value.[141] Neonatal diagnosis of TTTS also relies on significant birth-weight discordance and on the demonstration of a difference of at least 5 g/dL in initial neonatal hemoglobin levels. However, because weight and hemoglobin differences are common in most monochorionic gestations, with or without TTTS, it is difficult to use these criteria alone for diagnosis.[149] Because great clinical variability exists in the appearance of TTTS, sonographic criteria have been proposed to classify severity. The clinical value of scoring systems to improve fetal outcome has not yet been determined, but they may foster comparison of published treatment strategies. One system uses the following markers, with the stage being assigned based on the worst sonographic features documented[150]:

Stage I: Donor twin bladder still visible, fetal Doppler values normal
Stage II: Donor twin bladder no longer visible, fetal Doppler values normal
Stage III: Donor twin bladder no longer visible, fetal Doppler values critically abnormal
Stage IV: Presence of hydrops
Stage V: Intrauterine death of one or both fetuses

It should be noted that fetuses with TTTS may not show an orderly progression through these stages and that ultimate prognosis is likely determined by the final stage at the time of definitive therapy rather than the stage at initial diagnosis.

Management

Because the diagnosis of TTTS is essentially one of exclusion, management first involves excluding other causes of significant growth discordance or stuck twin phenomenon. This requires careful sonographic assessment of fetal anatomy (in particular, the presence of normal fetal kidneys), cardiac function, and placental cord insertions for both fetuses. Although consideration should be given to the performance of amniocentesis to exclude chromosomal anomaly or infection, this procedure may interfere with subsequent management if fetoscopic laser therapy is a possibility.[151] It is preferable, therefore, to defer amniocentesis until the time of definitive fetal therapy. Expectant management is associated with high rates of perinatal mortality, as high as 80% to 100% if the diagnosis is made before 24 weeks' gestation.[152,153] If only one twin dies, there is a significant risk (as high as 20%) of profound neurologic handicap in the surviving twin.[154] Medical management with maternal administration of digoxin has not been widely used, and administration of indomethacin is no longer practiced because of a high likelihood of intrauterine demise, presumably due to interference with fetal renal perfusion.[155]

Three possible management approaches have been described for the treatment of TTTS: serial reduction amniocenteses, amniotic septostomy, and selective fetoscopic laser photocoagulation of placental anastomoses. Serial reduction amniocenteses have been suggested in an effort to equilibrate amniotic fluid volume across the dividing membrane and to reduce overall intrauterine pressure, although the precise mechanism of action is unclear. The main advantage of this approach is that it is simple to perform and is widely accessible to the vast majority of patients and obstetricians, with up to 20% of patients showing resolution of TTTS.[156] With this technique, aggressive decompression amniocentesis is performed under ultrasound guidance. An 18-gauge needle is used to drain off as much fluid as possible from around the recipient twin. The procedure is repeated as often as necessary to maintain near-normal amniotic fluid volume; in particular, it is repeated when the maximum pocket of fluid in the recipient sac increases again toward 10 cm. The rationale for amnioreduction is that a decrease in uterine distention leads to reduced risk of preterm labor and pPROM, thereby prolonging gestation and improving perinatal outcome. However, an improvement in fetal condition has also been noted after reduction amniocentesis, which suggests that this therapy may also provide direct benefit for the fetus. Because amnioreduction does not affect the placental anastomoses that are the basis of TTTS, the mechanism by which reduction amniocentesis improves the fetal condition is uncertain. A reduction in polyhydramnios and intrauterine pressure may improve circulation in superficial arterioarterial anastomotic placental vessels at the donor side, leading to increased fetal renal perfusion and formation of urine, and to increased amniotic fluid volume in the donor sac.

Perinatal survival rates when serial reduction amniocentesis is chosen as primary therapy for TTTS range from 37% to 83%.[157] The variability in reported performance of reduction amniocenteses may be the result of reporting bias, small study sizes, and variations in the timing and volume of fluid removed. An international registry of 223 twin pregnancies with TTTS detected before 28 weeks' gestation and managed with reduction amniocenteses reported an overall survival rate of 78%.[152] The median number of amnioreduction procedures performed was two, with a median of 1400 mL of amniotic fluid removed per procedure. Predictors of poor outcome included earlier gestational age at diagnosis, absent end-diastolic umbilical arterial blood flow in the donor fetus, and the presence of hydrops. Survival at 4 weeks of age was 60%, and approximately 25% of survivors had abnormal intracranial ultrasound findings.[152] However, the prevalence of long-term neurologic abnormality may be lower than is suggested by these sonographic data. In a series of 33 TTTS pregnancies in which surviving infants were monitored until 2 years of age, there were only two cases (4.9%) of cerebral palsy, one of which was an infant who survived after an intrauterine demise of its co-twin, and the other an infant who also had cardiac malformations.[158]

Amniotic septostomy involves deliberate perforation of the dividing membrane.[159,160] The mechanism of action for this approach is unclear, but it may involve equalization of fluid across the dividing membrane that results in ingestion of a fluid bolus by the donor twin and resultant expansion in its intravascular volume. However, such a theory has not been proven and does not explain the finding of TTTS in up to 10% of monoamniotic twin pregnancies.[161] In 12 twin pregnancies managed with amniotic septostomy, a survival rate of 83% was achieved.[162] In another observational report of 14 cases, 7 managed with serial reduction amniocentesis and 7 with amniotic septostomy, there was no difference in overall survival, but there was significantly greater pregnancy prolongation with septostomy.[163] In another report of three cases of amniotic septostomy, all fetuses were lost within 5 days of the procedure.[164] A randomized trial of 73 patients comparing amniotic septostomy and reduction amniocentesis failed to demonstrate any difference in outcome between the two therapeutic approaches.[160] Septostomy has been criticized because it may result in an iatrogenic monoamniotic twin pregnancy, with all the negative implications of this condition. Additionally, creation of an undulating dividing membrane may limit the success of a subsequent fetoscopic laser procedure if one is required.[153] Some have advocated microseptostomy, in which a single needle perforation is made in the dividing membrane to reduce the likelihood of iatrogenic monoamnionicity. Comparison of amnioreduction and septostomy is difficult, because septostomy may inadvertently occur during amnioreduction and because many cases of septostomy are treated with amnioreduction as well.

Probably the most effective management option for TTTS is selective fetoscopic photocoagulation of the anastomotic vessels on the surface of the placenta, using a fetoscopically placed neodymium-yttrium aluminum garnet (neo-YAG) laser or diode laser. A 2- to 3-mm fetoscope is placed into the polyhydramniotic recipient twin's sac under ultrasound guidance, and the vessels on the surface of the placenta are inspected. AV anastomoses are easily identifiable as a single unpaired artery coming from the donor side and entering a foramen on the placental surface, together with a single unpaired vein exiting the same area on the placental surface with blood flowing toward the recipient twin. Selective photocoagulation involves placement of a 0.4-mm neo-YAG laser fiber through the fetoscope and ablating all visible anastomoses that communicate between the fetuses. Debate continues as to the benefit of ablating all anastomoses or just the AV anastomoses.[138,165] It would appear to be preferable to ablate all vascular communications that connect the two fetal circulations, because this would prevent reverse fetal transfusion and neurologic injury if one fetus dies. Whereas the selective approach to laser ablation involves ablating all anastomoses that connect the two fetal circulations, it also involves leaving intact those vessels that drain an area of placenta both to and from one particular fetus. Amnioreduction is also performed as part of the same procedure. An apparent advantage of selective photocoagulation is that it is the only therapy that directly addresses the underlying pathophysiology of TTTS. By ablation of the AV anastomoses, the net transfusion of blood from donor to recipient can be reduced. Ablation of all placental anastomoses that connect the fetuses essentially makes the pregnancy dichorionic.

Overall survival rates of 55%, 69%, 65%, and 57% have been reported from series of 144, 93, 200, and 72 TTTS pregnancies, respectively.[166-169] The mean survival rate for the 471 TTTS cases in these series was 62%, with a 5% incidence of neurologic injury among survivors. Comparing the outcome of survivors of TTTS cases managed by laser or reduction amniocentesis has been difficult. In one single-center study, of 137 survivors of TTTS therapy, death or severe cerebral injury was significantly more common after reduction amniocentesis than after laser therapy.[170] Additionally, the incidence of adverse outcome was similar between survivors of laser therapy and gestational age–matched dichorionic twin controls.

A major advance in the debate on the comparative performance of reduction amniocenteses versus laser ablation for TTTS occurred in 2004 with the publication of the Eurofoetus Consortium randomized trial of these two approaches.[171] This multicenter trial, based at centers of excellence for fetoscopy in Europe, randomized 142 patients with severe TTTS before 26 weeks' gestation to either serial reduction amniocenteses or fetoscopic laser ablation of placental vessels. The trial was stopped early because of the significance of the results in favor of laser therapy. Compared with the group undergoing amniocenteses, the laser ablation group had significantly prolonged median gestational age at delivery (33 versus 29 weeks), significantly more cases with at least one survivor at 6 months of age (76% versus 51%), and significantly fewer instances of major neurologic damage among surviving infants at 6 months of age (5% versus 10%). Overall, patients can be counseled based on such data that in about one third of cases both fetuses will die, in about one third one fetus will die, and in only one third of cases will both fetuses survive.[156,171] The fact that two out of three patients with this condition will deliver a dead or neurologically impaired infant, despite optimal therapy, is sobering.

In another recent randomized trial of fetoscopic laser ablation and reduction amniocenteses for TTTS, no difference was found between the two approaches.[172] However, the success rate of reduction amniocentesis appeared to be better than that found by the Eurofoetus investigators, whereas the efficacy of laser ablation appeared considerably worse than that seen by the Eurofoetus authors and other investigators. However, this trial, which was sponsored by the U.S. National Institutes of Health (NIH), differed significantly from the Eurofoetus trial and was significantly underpowered to make any conclusions regarding the relative efficacy of the two therapies. The NIH study randomized patients to either fetoscopic laser ablation of placental vessels or reduction amniocenteses only after patients first failed a trial of initial reduction amniocentesis. Power analysis suggested that 146 patients would need to be randomized, but the trial was stopped early, after only 42 patients had been enrolled over a study period of more than 5 years. The main reason for early cessation of the trial was difficulty encountered in recruiting patients. Therefore, it is hard to draw any meaningful conclusions regarding optimal therapy for TTTS from this trial.

Although these randomized trial data are of great utility in counseling patients with TTTS, there are still areas of uncertainty related to management. It is unclear whether fetoscopic laser surgery should be considered first-line therapy in all cases of TTTS, or whether it should be reserved for early and severe cases. Given that laser ablation is a significantly more invasive procedure and is available only at a limited number of centers, there will likely remain a role for reduction amniocentesis in certain situations. In any case, frequent sonographic follow-up is required after the initial therapy. Intensive fetal surveillance should be performed when viability is reached. Betamethasone administration is recommended because of the high likelihood of early delivery. Delivery should be based on usual obstetric indications, although cesarean section is likely. If complete laser separation of shared vessels within the placenta has been confidently achieved, and if TTTS features resolve, some experts believe that it is reasonable to maintain the pregnancy until 37 weeks. However, given the difficulty in confirming with certainty that all placental anastomoses have been ablated, it may also be reasonable to electively deliver TTTS cases at 34 weeks after successful earlier therapy. Two neonatal resuscitation teams should be present at delivery. Surviving infants are at increased risk for long-term morbidity, including cardiomyopathy and periventricular leukomalacia.[171,173] There have been no reports of recurrent TTTS in subsequent pregnancies.

Studies of long-term outcome after laser treatment for TTTS have also confirmed that a significant number of survivors have neurologic impairment. In one series reporting on 2 years' follow-up of 115 survivors after laser treatment for TTTS, 17% had neurodevelopmental impairment, mostly cerebral palsy or developmental delay.[174] In another study of 89 survivors of laser treatment for TTTS at a median age of 21 months, 11% had major neurologic deficits, and a further 11% had minor deficits.[175] However, it is likely that much of the neurologic injury seen in survivors of laser therapy for TTTS occurs antenatally. In a comparison of neurologic injury in survivors of laser-treated TTTS pregnancies versus survivors of monochorionic pregnancies without TTTS, severe cerebral lesions were diagnosed in 14% of the TTTS group and in only 6% of the control group, with two-thirds of these lesions being diagnosed antenatally.[176]

Monoamniotic Twins

Monoamniotic twinning results in a single amniotic sac containing both twins and occurs in approximately 1% of monozygotic gestations.[34] Prenatal diagnosis is established when a dividing membrane cannot be identified by an experienced sonographer in a twin gestation. The diagnosis is also confirmed after sonographic identification of entangled umbilical cords (Fig. 25-5); this feature has been reported in 70% to 100% of cases.[177,178] Cord entanglement has been diagnosed by color Doppler ultrasonography as early as 10 weeks' gestation.[179] It can be difficult to visualize the dividing membrane sonographically in certain situations, especially in the early first trimester. Other techniques used to diagnose monoamnionicity include sonographic visualization of only one yolk sac in a twin gestation at less than 10 weeks' gestation and amniography with iopamidol or indigo carmine–air mixture.[37,180,181] However, the specificity of the visualization of only one yolk sac for the diagnosis of monoamnionicity is unclear.[39]

Monoamniotic twins historically carried a higher risk of perinatal morbidity and mortality than diamniotic twins, with a perinatal mor-

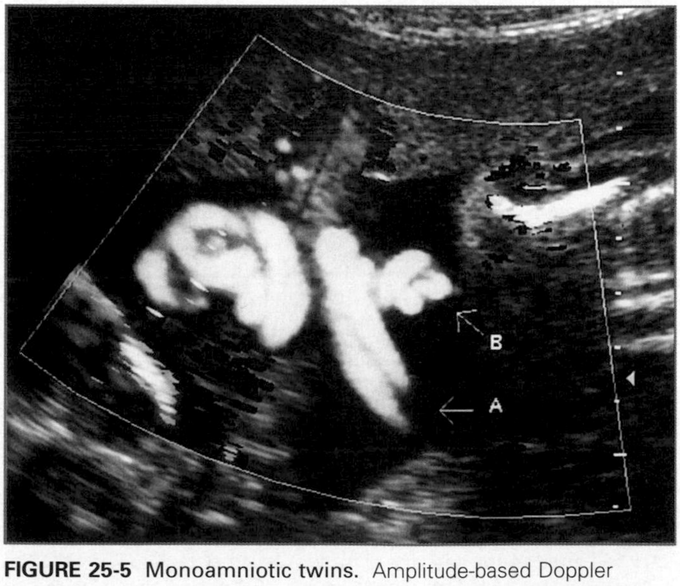

FIGURE 25-5 Monoamniotic twins. Amplitude-based Doppler image of monoamniotic twins at 29 weeks' gestation demonstrates entangled umbilical cords of twins A and B. (Courtesy of Achilles Athanassiou, MD, New England Medical Center, Boston.)

tality rate greater than 50%.[182] However, more recent series and reviews of prenatally diagnosed cases of monoamniotic twins suggest mortality rates ranging from 10% to 21%.[178,183] This risk may be secondary to premature delivery, growth restriction, congenital anomalies, vascular anastomoses between twins, and umbilical cord entanglement or cord accidents. Because umbilical cord accidents (e.g., cord prolapse, cord compression between fetuses) seem to be the primary cause of fetal death, most management protocols for monoamniotic twins emphasize intensive fetal surveillance.[184] Such surveillance should occur from the time of fetal viability, because intrauterine fetal demise has been documented in monoamniotic twins throughout gestation.[178,179,185,186] Additionally, surveillance must be repeated frequently, because fetal compromise and death have been documented despite twice-weekly fetal testing.[178] The only intervention proposed to reduce the likelihood of cord accidents in monoamniotic twins is maternal administration of sulindac, a prostaglandin inhibitor that results in decreased amniotic fluid volume, which may, in turn, stabilize fetal lie and theoretically reduce the risk of cord entanglement.[187] However, because of a lack of evidence to support its safety and efficacy, this approach must be considered to be experimental.

Because umbilical cord accidents are not predictable by current methods of fetal surveillance and continuous fetal heart monitoring throughout pregnancy is not feasible, we have managed monoamniotic twin gestations with daily NSTs beginning at 24 to 26 weeks' gestation to determine the frequency of variable decelerations.[184] If variable decelerations increase in frequency, we perform continuous fetal heart monitoring and intervene with cesarean delivery if fetal heart testing becomes nonreassuring.

In the absence of nonreassuring fetal heart testing, the timing and mode of delivery of monoamniotic twins are controversial. In two series of 44 sets of monoamniotic twins, Carr and colleagues[182] and Tessen and Zlatnik[188] reported no fetal deaths after 32 weeks, suggesting that prophylactic early delivery was not indicated.[182,188] In an addendum to the latter series, however, it was noted that a double fetal death occurred at 35 weeks' gestation in one monoamniotic twin set, calling into question the safety of expectant management of monoamniotic twins beyond a gestational age at which neonatal morbidity is likely to be low. In these two series, vaginal delivery was achieved in more than 70% of cases, although in the series by Carr and coauthors the diagnosis of monoamniotic twins was not known prenatally in 80% of cases. Although vaginal delivery of monoamniotic twins is clearly possible, the incidence of cesarean delivery is high when fetal testing is nonreassuring. In addition, case reports have described cutting of the nuchal cord of the second twin after delivery of the first twin's head.[189,190]

Because of these concerns, we and others electively perform cesarean delivery at 32 to 34 weeks' gestation after maternal administration of betamethasone.[111,184,191] It is difficult to recommend continuation of pregnancy beyond 34 weeks' gestation, given the ongoing risk of stillbirth and the high rates of infant survival beyond this gestational age.[185] Whereas the majority of recent studies have suggested elective cesarean section, vaginal delivery may be acceptable if the fetal heart rates are continuously monitored and the mother has been informed that an emergent cesarean delivery may be necessary.

Twin Reversed Arterial Perfusion Sequence

Twin reversed arterial perfusion (TRAP) sequence, or acardiac twinning, is a unique abnormality of monochorionic multiple gestations in which one twin has an absent, rudimentary, or nonfunctioning heart. The incidence is estimated to occur in 1% of monozygotic twin pregnancies, with birth estimates ranging from 1 in 35,000 to 1 in 150,000 births.[34] The condition occurs because of early development of arterial-to-arterial anastomoses between the umbilical arteries of twin fetuses that share a fused placenta.[192]

The donor, or "pump twin," provides circulation for itself and for the recipient, or "perfused twin," through a direct umbilical arterial–to–umbilical arterial anastomosis at the placental surface. There is reversal of blood flow in the umbilical artery of the acardiac twin, with the artery bringing deoxygenated blood from the co-twin to the acardiac twin. This perfusion is usually asymmetric in the recipient twin, with relative hypoperfusion of the upper part of the body, leading to significant structural anomalies. A bizarre range of anomalies can be seen in the acardiac twin, including anencephaly, holoprosencephaly, absent limbs, absent lungs or heart, intestinal atresias, abdominal wall defects, and absent liver, spleen, or kidneys.[192] Up to one third of the fetuses also have an abnormal karyotype.[193]

Prenatal diagnosis of TRAP is based on the recognition of one normal-appearing fetus and an additional, profoundly abnormal-appearing fetus or amorphous mass of tissue. The pregnancy should be clearly monochorionic, and two thirds of cases demonstrate a single umbilical artery. The acardiac fetus may be unrecognizable as a fetus or may have an abnormally appearing head or trunk with no obvious heart. Sonographic signs of cardiac failure may be visible in the pump twin, including polyhydramnios, cardiomegaly, and tricuspid regurgitation. The differential diagnosis of TRAP includes intrauterine fetal demise of one fetus and anencephaly. Doppler velocimetry of the umbilical cords demonstrating reversed direction of flow in the umbilical artery and vein may be helpful in confirming the diagnosis.[194]

The goal of antepartum management of TRAP pregnancies is to maximize outcome for the structurally normal pump twin. The pump twin is at risk for development of hydrops or congestive cardiac failure. In one series of 49 cases of TRAP, the overall perinatal mortality rate for the pump twin was 55%, with polyhydramnios leading to prematurity being a major factor in prognosis.[195] Prediction of prognosis for the pump twin depends on the ratio of the weight of the perfused twin to the weight of the pump twin, with a 30% chance of congestive cardiac failure when the ratio is greater than 0.70, compared with 10% when the ratio is less than 0.70.[195] Other criteria that may suggest the need for intervention include an abdominal circumference measurement in the acardiac twin greater than or equal to that of the pump twin, polyhydramnios with maximum vertical fluid pocket greater than 8 cm, abnormal Doppler indices, hydrops in the pump twin, or TRAP in the setting of monoamnionicity.[196]

In the absence of such poor prognostic features, expectant management with serial sonographic evaluation may be reasonable.[157,197,198] Serial weekly echocardiographic surveillance of the pump twin is recommended for early signs of cardiac failure, such as atrial or ventricular enlargement, tricuspid regurgitation, or decreased ventricular fractional shortening capacity. Rapid growth of the acardiac fetus may also be a sign of poor outcome.[199] Antenatal corticosteroid administration should be given if delivery is expected to occur between 24 and 34 weeks' gestation. Signs of cardiac decompensation after 32 to 34 weeks' gestation should prompt consideration for delivery. Antenatal intervention on behalf of the pump twin should be considered if poor prognostic criteria, as summarized earlier, are noted before 32 to 34 weeks' gestation.

Invasive management has included selective delivery by hysterotomy of the acardiac recipient fetus, as well as percutaneous injection of various sclerosants into the umbilical cord of the acardiac twin.[200,201]

These options are now of only historical interest because of the availability of a range of less invasive and more effective percutaneous approaches to selective termination of the acardiac fetus. Currently, percutaneous approaches for interrupting blood flow to the acardiac twin include fetoscopic cord ligation or laser ablation and radiofrequency thermablation of the acardiac twin's cord using a special needle device.[196,202] In 45 cases managed by fetoscopic cord ligation or laser ablation, 30 pump twins (67%) survived,[196] Twenty-five (86%) of 29 pump twins managed exclusively with percutaneous radiofrequency thermablation survived, with a mean gestational age at delivery of 35 weeks.[202] No direct comparative studies have been performed. The advantage of the radiofrequency ablation technique is use of a single 14- or 17-gauge needle, compared with a typical 2- to 3-mm fetoscope for cord ligation approaches. The recurrence risk for TRAP is estimated at 1 in 10,000.[192]

Conjoined Twins

Conjoined twins are a subset of monozygotic twin gestations in which incomplete embryonic division occurs 13 to 15 days after conception, resulting in varying degrees of fusion of the two fetuses. The estimated frequency of conjoined twinning is 1 in 50,000 births.[34] The prenatal diagnosis should be straightforward and is confirmed by failure to visualize two fetuses separately in what appears to be a single amniotic sac. Other sonographic features that assist in making the diagnosis include bifid appearance of the first-trimester fetal pole, more than three umbilical cord vessels, heads persistently at the same level and body plane, and failure of the fetuses to change position relative to each other over time.[203] Prenatal diagnosis of conjoined twins has been made in the first trimester with the aid of three-dimensional sonography.[204] However, caution should be exercised in making a definite diagnosis of conjoined twins at less than 10 weeks' gestation, because false-positive diagnoses have been documented.[205]

By careful sonographic survey of the shared anatomy, it should be possible to classify conjoined twins into one of the following five types:

1. Thoracopagus, in which the two fetuses face each other, accounts for 75% of conjoined twins (Fig. 25-6). The fetuses usually have common sternum, diaphragm, upper abdominal wall, liver, pericardium, and gastrointestinal tract. Because 75% of thoracopagus twins have joined hearts, prognosis for surgical division is extremely poor.
2. Omphalopagus (or xiphopagus) is a rare subgroup of thoracopagus in which there is an abdominal wall connection, often also with common liver. Because joined hearts are rare in omphalopagus, twins in this subgroup have a much better surgical prognosis than twins with other forms of thoracopagus.
3. Pygopagus accounts for 20% of cases; the twins share a common sacrum and face away from each other. There is a single rectum and bladder, and prognosis for surgical separation is usually good.
4. Ischiopagus, in which the twins share a single common bony pelvis, accounts for 5% of conjoined twins. Surgical prognosis is good, although the remaining lower spines are often abnormal.
5. Craniopagus accounts for 1% of cases and is marked by partial or complete fusion of skull, meninges, and vascular structures. Surgical prognosis depends on the degree of fusion of vascular structures, in particular the presence of an adequate superior sagittal sinus to allow venous drainage.[203]

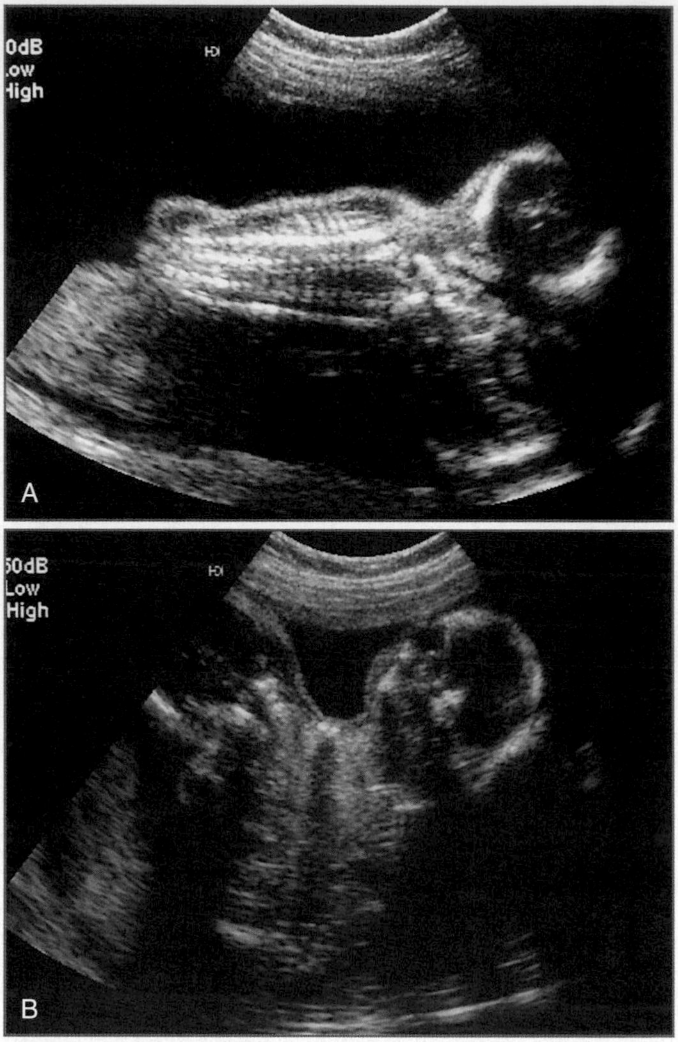

FIGURE 25-6 Conjoined twins. Thoracopagus conjoined twins at 20 weeks' gestation, demonstrating a single trunk containing two parallel spines (**A**) and leading to two separate heads (**B**).

Termination of pregnancy is commonly requested by parents of conjoined twins, especially in cases of thoracopagus with joined hearts. If expectant management is selected by the parents, fetal echocardiography and possibly magnetic resonance imaging should be used to delineate the exact extent of union and assist in neonatal surgical planning.[206] In addition, a careful search must be made to exclude other anomalies that commonly coexist with conjoined twins. In one series of 14 sets of prenatally diagnosed conjoined twin pregnancies from a single center, the combination of prenatal ultrasonography, echocardiography, and magnetic resonance imaging accurately defined the anatomy in all cases.[207] In this series, 3 pregnancies were terminated, 1 resulted in intrauterine death; of the remaining 10 pregnancies delivered after viability, 5 individual fetuses survived. When expectant management is selected, cesarean section (usually through a classical incision) is the delivery method of choice to minimize maternal and fetal trauma.[34,111] Vaginal delivery is reasonable only in cases of extreme prematurity in which fetal survival is not an issue and maternal trauma should be less likely than with a cesarean section.

The surgical separation of conjoined twins, although beyond the scope of this chapter, has been summarized in the surgical literature.[208,209] One of the largest series of conjoined twins managed at a single center was reported from South Africa, where 46 pairs of conjoined twins were seen over 40 years. In total, 17 sets underwent surgical separation, with 22 children (65%) surviving.[210] A survival rate of 85% was reported from another series of 10 sets of conjoined twins treated by surgical separation.[206] Tremendously complex moral and ethical issues occur in the neonatal period regarding appropriate surgical options in conjoined twins when only one twin has the potential of survival.[211] We are unaware of any reported cases of recurrence after the diagnosis of conjoined twins.

Intrauterine Demise of One Fetus

Intrauterine demise of one fetus in a multiple gestation during the first trimester is common and was originally thought to have no effect on the prognosis for the surviving fetus or fetuses. Such a "vanishing twin" has been reported to occur in 21% of twin pregnancies, with no obvious detrimental effect on the remaining fetus.[212] However, it now appears that intrauterine demise of one fetus in a monochorionic twin pregnancy as early as 12 weeks' gestation can result in profound neurologic injury to the surviving fetus.[213] In a series of 55 spontaneous first-trimester twin deaths in dichorionic pregnancies, there was an increased rate of preeclampsia and lower birth weight among surviving co-twins, compared with singleton pregnancies.[214] A further series of 642 surviving fetuses from vanishing twin pregnancies also confirmed an increased risk of small for gestational age, with risk being proportional to the gestational age at time of co-twin demise.[215] Intrauterine demise of one fetus in the second or third trimester is rarer (2% to 5% of twin pregnancies; 14% to 17% of triplet pregnancies) and probably has far greater potential for significant morbidity to the surviving fetus or fetuses.[34] After the death of one twin in a monochorionic gestation, approximately 12% of remaining fetuses also die, compared with approximately 4% of remaining fetuses in a dichorionic gestation.[216] The outcome of multiple gestations complicated by a single intrauterine demise is worse for monochorionic than for dichorionic gestations, with mean gestational ages at delivery of 30.6 and 32.9 weeks, respectively.[217]

The risk of significant neurologic morbidity is increased after intrauterine death of one fetus in a monochorionic, but not in a dichorionic, gestation. Serious neurologic abnormality, such as multicystic encephalomalacia leading to profound neurologic handicap, occurs in 18% of surviving fetuses after the death of a co-twin in a monochorionic gestation.[154] Neurologic morbidity has been reported after the death of a co-twin as early as 12 weeks of gestation.[213] In a review of birth certificate data from the United Kingdom, 434 gender-concordant twin pregnancies were found in which intrauterine demise of one fetus had occurred.[218] The prevalence of cerebral palsy among surviving fetuses was 10.6%, and the prevalence of other neurologic injury was 11.4%. The main limitation of such birth certificate data is the inability to be sure of the prevalence of monochorionicity among the gender-concordant pairs. In a literature review of 119 monochorionic twin pregnancies complicated by single intrauterine fetal death, 9% of surviving fetuses subsequently died in utero, a further 10% subsequently died in the neonatal period, and 24% had serious neonatal morbidity, including porencephaly, multicystic encephalomalacia, renal cortical necrosis, and small-bowel atresia.[219]

Neurologic injury in the surviving fetus probably occurs because of significant hypotension at the time of death of the co-twin. Fetal disseminated intravascular coagulopathy resulting from fetal-to-fetal transfer of thromboplastic material from the dead fetus was once advanced as a cause of neurologic injury but is unlikely.[220] In a series of fetal blood sampling studies performed immediately before and after intrauterine death of one twin, primarily in the setting of evaluation of TTTS, no evidence of fetal anemia was noted before fetal death, but all surviving fetuses were found to be anemic after death of the co-twin.[220] This study suggested that acute blood loss from the surviving fetus into the dead fetus occurs proximate to fetal demise and that subsequent obstetric intervention may be too late to influence outcome for the surviving twin.

Because the risk of neurologic morbidity is present from the moment one twin dies, expectant management may not be appropriate for monochorionic gestations in which one fetus appears to be in a premorbid condition.[221] This 18% risk of profound neurologic injury after demise of a co-twin must be weighed against the risk of complications of prematurity with a premorbid fetus in a monochorionic multiple gestation. If fetal demise has already occurred, close surveillance of the surviving fetuses is recommended, although this may not prevent neurologic injury, which may already have occurred. Antenatal neurologic injury (e.g., multicystic encephalomalacia) may not be predictable by ultrasound or cardiotocographic monitoring. Delivery at 37 weeks, or after lung indices suggest maturity, is reasonable in such situations.

The maternal risks after intrauterine death of one fetus have probably been overestimated. The risk of maternal disseminated intravascular coagulopathy was once estimated at 25%, but in recent reviews of spontaneous fetal deaths and selective terminations in multiple gestations, no clinical cases of disseminated intravascular coagulopathy were noted. Our practice has been to obtain a baseline set of coagulation indices after diagnosis of the death of one fetus; subsequent laboratory surveillance with coagulopathy studies is probably unnecessary.[221]

Selective Termination of an Anomalous Fetus

When a multiple gestation is complicated by the discovery of a significant anomaly in one fetus, counseling of the parents and management decisions are difficult. Factors to incorporate into the decision-making analysis include the following:

- Severity of the anomaly
- Chorionicity of the pregnancy
- Effect of the anomalous fetus on the normal co-twin or co-triplets
- Ethical beliefs of the parents

Three main choices are available[221]: expectant management, termination of the entire pregnancy, and selective termination of the anomalous fetus.

The phrase "selective termination" refers specifically to deliberate termination of an anomalous fetus in a multiple gestation, typically in the second trimester. Selective termination is performed to optimize outcome for the normal fetus and to prevent delivery of an abnormal fetus. This differs from "multifetal reduction," which refers to a nonspecific reduction in the number of fetuses present in a higher-order multiple gestation, almost always in the first trimester, to lower the risk of prematurity for the remaining fetuses.[222]

Expectant management of a multiple gestation complicated by a single anomalous fetus leads to a 20% increase in the risk of preterm delivery attributable to the presence of an anomalous fetus, a correspondingly lower birth weight, and a higher cesarean delivery rate than is reported in normal twin gestations.[223] In addition, expectant management of twins discordant for anencephaly is associated with an increased rate of intrauterine death of the normal co-twin in monochorionic gestations, as well as an increased rate of premature delivery, probably secondary to polyhydramnios, in both monochorionic and dichorionic gestations.[224] Amnioreduction to reduce the incidence of prematurity may be considered if significant polyhydramnios develops in twins discordant for anencephaly.

The method of selective termination depends on the chorionicity.[221] In dichorionic gestations, ultrasound-guided intracardiac injection of potassium chloride is the most common technique; in monochorionic gestations, complete ablation of the umbilical cord of the anomalous fetus is required to avoid death or neurologic injury in the normal fetus. When selective termination in a monochorionic gestation is considered in contemporary obstetric practice, ultrasound-guided cord occlusion, fetoscopic cord occlusion, or laser ablation is most commonly used.[225,226] Techniques such as hysterotomy and injection of cord sclerosants are no longer used.[200,227]

These selective termination procedures for monochorionic gestations are significantly more complicated than the potassium chloride injection procedure used for dichorionic gestations. Few data are available to counsel patients about the safety and efficacy of these monochorionic techniques. Fetoscopic cord ligation may be associated with a 10% procedure failure rate and up to a 30% risk of pPROM.[225] In one series of 80 consecutive monochorionic cord coagulation procedures, the overall perinatal survival rate was 83%, and there was a 10% rate of unexpected intrauterine fetal death, most of which was related to pPROM before viability.[228] Reports of mistaken fetoscopic ligation of the cord of the normal fetus have also been described.[229] Bipolar cautery and aortic thermocoagulation using single fetoscopic ports or single spinal needle access with sonographic guidance may be safer, but there are insufficient data to recommend an optimal choice for selective termination in monochorionic gestations.

Before performing the procedure, the physician must confirm that the targeted fetus has the anomaly in question. If the abnormal fetus has a structural anomaly, correct fetal identification is straightforward. If a chromosomal abnormality exists without structural markers and there is doubt about the position of the target fetus, repeated chromosomal analysis using rapid techniques (PCR or FISH) is required immediately before termination. The physician must be certain of the chorionicity of the pregnancy. Potassium chloride injection is contraindicated if dichorionicity cannot be confirmed with certainty. If such sonographic confirmation cannot be obtained, DNA zygosity studies on amniocytes may be required to exclude monochorionicity.[46]

Results of selective termination from a large multicenter study of 402 cases of twins, triplets, quadruplets, and quintuplets demonstrated a 100% technical success rate, with an 8% rate of pregnancy loss before 24 weeks (5% if the procedure was performed before 12 weeks, 9% if performed between 13 and 18 weeks, and 7% if performed between 19 and 24 weeks).[230] All procedures used intracardiac potassium chloride injection. In addition, another 6% of patients delivered between 25 and 28 weeks, 8% between 29 and 32 weeks, and 17% between 33 and 36 weeks. There were no cases of laboratory or clinical coagulopathies or other complications in the mothers.[230]

A series of 200 cases of twins, triplets, and quadruplets at one center demonstrated increased risks of preterm delivery if the presenting twin was terminated and an increased risk of pregnancy loss among triplet pregnancies.[231] The overall rate of unintended pregnancy loss before 24 weeks' gestation at this center was 4%, but the rate increased to 11% for selective termination in triplet gestations. The pregnancy loss rate may increase to as high as 43% with the termination of more than one anomalous fetus in a pregnancy. There does not appear to be a significant difference in pregnancy loss rates at various gestational ages.[79,231]

Selective termination of a single anomalous fetus in a multiple gestation therefore seems to be a reasonable management option. These data should be used to counsel patients according to the unique circumstances of each case.

Multifetal Pregnancy Reduction

The goal of first-trimester MFPR is to reduce the number of fetuses in a higher-order multiple gestation so as to decrease the chance of premature delivery and thereby to improve the outcome for the remaining fetuses. Higher-order multiple gestations are associated with a significant risk of delivery before viability. Fetuses that reach viability have a significant risk of birth before 28 weeks, when serious long-term neonatal morbidity is likely.

The natural history of triplet gestation suggests a 7% to 8% risk of delivery between 24 and 28 weeks' gestation.[8,79,232] The natural history of quadruplet gestation suggests a 14% risk of delivery before 28 weeks' gestation.[79,232] The risk of spontaneous loss of a triplet pregnancy before 24 weeks' gestation is approximately 11%.[232] The risk of losing the entire pregnancy before 20 or 24 weeks in quadruplet or higher gestations is unknown, because, in general, only pregnancies that successfully reach 20 weeks' gestation are reported in the literature. In addition, the risks to maternal health of expectantly managed higher-order multiple gestations are significant. The risks just described should be carefully discussed with each couple during counseling before a management plan is selected in all cases of higher-order multiple gestations.

The technique of transabdominal MFPR, as typically performed between 10 and 13 weeks' gestation, is straightforward.[233] The patient is given a single oral antibiotic dose (dicloxacillin, 500 mg) immediately before the procedure. Ultrasonography is used to map the location of all gestations precisely within the uterus, and measurements are taken of crown-rump length and nuchal translucency thickness. If an abnormality is found or these measurements are abnormal in a particular fetus, that fetus is selected for reduction. Otherwise, the fetus or fetuses that are technically easiest to access are chosen, with the exception of the fetus overlying the internal os, which is rarely selected. If a monochorionic pair of fetuses exists within a higher-order multiple gestation, that pair is usually selected for reduction.[79] Under continuous ultrasound guidance with sterile technique, a 22-gauge needle is placed into the thorax of the targeted fetus, 2 to 3 mEq of potassium chloride is injected, and asystole is observed for at least 3 minutes. The procedure is then repeated for additional fetuses as required, with a different needle. Another ultrasound study is performed 1 hour after the procedure and again 1 week later to confirm demise of the targeted fetuses and viability of the remaining fetuses. Transvaginal MFPR is less commonly performed because it is associated with significantly higher loss rates when compared with the transabdominal approach (12% versus 5%).[234]

A current area of debate with MFPR is the role of prenatal diagnosis before or after the procedure. Options include amniocentesis for surviving fetuses 4 weeks after MFPR and CVS for some or all fetuses before MFPR. Amniocentesis after MFPR does not appear to further increase the risk of pregnancy loss.[235] The main drawback of amniocentesis is that, if an abnormality is discovered, patients may have to consider yet another reduction procedure. CVS has also been shown to be safe when it is performed before MFPR, with success rates greater than 99% and with no obvious increase in the risk of pregnancy loss.[236] Decisions of which placentas to sample are made based on starting fetal number, finishing fetal number, likely target fetuses, and ease of access to particular placentas. Fetuses that are chromosomally abnormal or untested are preferentially selected for reduction.[79] For example, in a quadruplet pregnancy to be reduced to twins, it is reasonable to perform CVS only for the two fetuses being retained; if these fetuses are confirmed to be chromosomally normal, the remaining two fetuses can then be reduced.

The overall pregnancy loss rate before 24 weeks for transabdominal MFPR procedures has fallen from 8% to 5%, reflecting a procedure-related learning curve.[234] The relative contribution to the overall loss rate of procedure-related loss, as opposed to the spontaneous loss typical of multiple gestations, is uncertain. International collaborative MFPR data from more than 3500 pregnancies documented a loss rate before 24 weeks that was directly related to both the starting and the finishing number of fetuses.[234] This loss rate decreased, respectively, from 22% to 15%, 12%, 6%, and 6% with six, five, four, three, and two fetuses present at the start of the procedure. In addition, the risk of very premature delivery at 25 to 28 weeks decreased from 6% to 6%, 4%, 3%, and 1%, respectively. The optimal finishing number of fetuses appeared to be twins, with a loss rate before 24 weeks of 9%, compared with 20% for triplets. Reflecting the importance of the learning curve, these authors reported that the pregnancy loss rates for MFPR procedures performed most recently (1995 to 1998) were 4% for triplets reduced to twins and 7% for quadruplets reduced to twins.[234] A single-center series of MFPR described 1000 cases, with a pregnancy loss rate of 5% before 24 weeks' gestation.[237] This group subsequently updated their experience from 2000 consecutive MFPR cases and noted an increase in the number of patients choosing to reduce to a singleton.[238] These authors also noted a significant increase in the number of patients undergoing CVS before the MFPR procedure (1.5% in the first 1000 cases, and 44% in the second 1000 cases). The documented safety of CVS, as well as the increasing desire of patients to be more selective about which fetuses to reduce and to be confident of not leaving viable fetuses with chromosomal abnormalities, appear to underlie these changing trends.[238]

For fetuses that reach viability after MFPR, 85% to 90% can be expected to be born at 32 weeks' gestation or later, with only 3% to 5% born between 25 and 28 weeks.[233,239] It is now clear that MFPR is associated with better outcomes for patients with quadruplet and higher gestations. When counseling such patients, the option of MFPR should be presented, and patients should be informed that their best chance of delivering healthy, surviving infants is by undergoing MFPR. Much debate still exists, however, on the role of MFPR for triplet gestation. Over the last 15 years, there have been 17 studies published in which the outcome of expectantly managed triplet gestations was compared with the outcome after reduction of triplets to twins, with some also comparing outcome to nonreduced twin pregnancies.[11] The results from a meta-analysis of these data are summarized in Table 25-4. Reduction of triplets to twins yields a significant prolongation of gestation, but at the expense of an increased rate of earlier miscarriage. From a total of 893 triplet pregnancies reviewed, 411 were expectantly managed and 482 underwent MFPR to twins. The rate of miscarriage before 24 weeks was 4% in the expectantly managed group but 8% in the MFPR group. This worse outcome with MFPR was offset by a reduction in the rate of preterm delivery between 24 and 32 weeks, from 27% in the expectantly managed group to 10% in the MFPR group.[11] Additionally, some data suggest that maternal complications can also be decreased when triplets are reduced to twins, with one study indicating a 22% incidence of gestational diabetes among nonreduced triplet pregnancies, compared with 6% among triplets reduced to twins.[240]

The data in Table 25-4 may be a little misleading, however, particularly with reference to perinatal mortality. MFPR involves the obligate death of one fetus in a triplet gestation, so the overall fetal mortality rate for triplets reduced to twins must be at least 333 per 1000. This may not be clear to patients if only perinatal mortality rates focusing on survivors of the MFPR procedure are presented. Additionally, no long-term outcome data for the survivors of reduced triplet pregnancies are available. We believe the available information does make a convincing argument to include MFPR in the counseling of all patients with triplet gestations. For an individual patient to select MFPR with triplets, she must decide whether the obligate death of one fetus, together with an increased risk of procedure-related pregnancy loss, justifies a 50% reduction in the risk of delivery before 32 weeks' gestation. This decision should be individualized in all cases.

After the MFPR procedure, patients should be observed closely for the usual complications of multiple gestation. Surveillance for appropriate fetal growth is recommended, because there may be an increased risk of intrauterine growth restriction after MFPR.[241] In addition, the psychological implications for mothers who have undergone MFPR can be significant. Seventy percent of these women demonstrate grief reactions, and 84% describe the procedure as very stressful.[242]

In view of the complex issues involved, MFPR should not be considered a simple solution to the problems of higher-order multiple gestations in this era of assisted reproductive technologies.[233] Instead, attention should be focused on prevention of the problem, which may be alleviated at least in part through careful supervision of assisted reproductive practices. The American College of Obstetricians and Gynecologists recommends that it is preferable to terminate an ovulation induction cycle if a higher-order multiple gestation appears to be likely, and to limit the number of embryos transferred in an in vitro fertilization, rather than allow a situation to develop in which patients have to consider the option of MFPR.[243] The ethical challenges associated with MFPR decision making are complex and are different from those concerning elective abortion. In the latter situation, the patient's intent is to avoid the birth of a child, whereas in the former, the opposite scenario exists: the patient is considering MFPR precisely because she wants to maximize her chance of having a healthy child.[243]

TABLE 25-4 META-ANALYSIS OF STUDIES COMPARING OUTCOME OF EXPECTANTLY MANAGED TRIPLET GESTATIONS WITH THAT OF TRIPLETS REDUCED TO TWINS

Management	Number of Pregnancies	Pregnancy Loss (<24 Wk)	Preterm Delivery (24-31 wk)
Expectant management	411	18/411 (4%)	105/393 (27%)
Reduction to twins	482	39/482 (8%)	46/443 (10%)

From Papageorghiou AT, Avgidou K, Bakoulas V, et al: Risk of miscarriage and early preterm birth in trichorionic triplet pregnancies with embryo reduction versus expectant management: New data and systematic review. Hum Reprod 21:1912, 2006.

References

1. Martin JA, Hamilton BE, Sutton PD, et al: Births: Final Data for 2004. Natl Vital Stat Rep 55(1):80-81, 2006.
2. Blickstein I, Keith LG: The decreased rates of triplet births: Temporal trends and biologic speculations. Am J Obstet Gynecol 193:327, 2005.
3. Newman RB, Ellings JM: Antepartum management of the multiple gestation: The case for specialized care. Semin Perinatol 19:387, 1995.
4. American College of Obstetricians and Gynecologists: Multiple Gestation: Complicated Twin, Triplet, and High-Order Multifetal Pregnancy. (Practice Bulletin No. 56). Washington, DC: ACOG, 2004.
5. Rydhstroem H, Heraib F: Gestational duration, and fetal and infant mortality for twins vs singletons. Twin Res 4:227, 2001.
6. Powers WF, Wampler NS: Further defining the risks confronting twins. Am J Obstet Gynecol 175:1522, 1996.
7. Salihu HM, Garces IC, Sharma PP, et al: Stillbirth and infant mortality among hispanic singletons, twins, and triplets in the United States. Obstet Gynecol 106:789, 2005.
8. Devine PC, Malone FD, Athanassiou A, et al: Maternal and neonatal outcome of 100 consecutive triplet pregnancies. Am J Perinatol 18:225, 2001.
9. Bajoria R, Ward SB, Adegbite AL: Comparative study of perinatal outcome of dichorionic and trichorionic iatrogenic triplets. Am J Obstet Gynecol 194:415, 2006.
10. Lipitz S, Reichman B, Uval J, et al: A prospective comparison of the outcome of triplet pregnancies managed expectantly or by multifetal reduction to twins. Am J Obstet Gynecol 170:874, 1994.
11. Papageorghiou AT, Avgidou K, Bakoulas V, et al: Risk of miscarriage and early preterm birth in trichorionic triplet pregnancies with embryo reduction versus expectant management: New data and systematic review. Hum Reprod 21:1912, 2006.
12. Collins MS, Bleyl JA: Seventy-one quadruplet pregnancies: Management and outcome. Am J Obstet Gynecol 162:1384, 1990.
13. Elliott JP, Radin TG: Quadruplet pregnancy: Contemporary management and outcome. Obstet Gynecol 80:421, 1992.
14. Martin JA, Hamilton BE, Sutton PD, et al: Births: Final Data for 2003. Natl Vital Stat Rep 54(2):1-116, 2005.
15. Luke B, Keith LG: The contribution of singletons, twins and triplets to low birth weight, infant mortality and handicap in the United States. J Reprod Med 37:661, 1992.
16. Scheller JM, Nelson KB: Twinning and neurologic morbidity. Am J Dis Child 146:1110, 1992.
17. Yokoyama Y, Shimizu T, Hayakawa K: Prevalence of cerebral palsy in twins, triplets and quadruplets. Int J Epidemiol 24:943, 1995.
18. Kaufman GE, Malone FD, Harvey-Wilkes KB, et al: Neonatal morbidity and mortality associated with triplet pregnancy. Obstet Gynecol 91:342, 1998.
19. Spellacy WN, Handler A, Ferre CD: A case-control study of 1253 twin pregnancies from a 1982-1987 perinatal data base. Obstet Gynecol 75:168, 1990.
20. Wen SW, Demissie K, Yang Q, et al: Maternal morbidity and obstetric complications in triplet pregnancies and quadruplet and higher-order multiple pregnancies. Am J Obstet Gynecol 191:254, 2004.
21. Hardardottir H, Kelly K, Bork MD, et al: Atypical presentation of preeclampsia in high-order multifetal gestations. Obstet Gynecol 87:370, 1996.
22. Yeast JD: Maternal physiologic adaptation to twin gestation. Clin Obstet Gynecol 33:10, 1990.
23. Gardner MO, Wenstrom KD: Maternal adaptation. In Gall SA (ed): Multiple Pregnancy and Delivery. St. Louis: Mosby, 1996, p 99.
24. Veille JC, Morton MJ, Burry KJ: Maternal cardiovascular adaptations to twin pregnancy. Am J Obstet Gynecol 153:261, 1985.
25. Kametas NA, McAuliffe F, Krampl E, et al: Maternal cardiac function in twin pregnancy. Obstet Gynecol 102:806, 2003.
26. Campbell DM: Maternal adaptation in twin pregnancy. Semin Perinatol 10:14, 1986.
27. Redford DHA: Uterine growth in twin pregnancy by measurement of total intrauterine volume. Acta Genet Med Gemmell 32:145, 1982.
28. Rizzo G, Arduini D, Romanini C: Uterine artery Doppler velocity waveforms in twin pregnancies. Obstet Gynecol 82:978, 1993.
29. Luke B: Nutrition in multiple gestations. Clin Perinatol 32:403, 2005.
30. Luke B, Bryan E, Sweetland C, et al: Prenatal weight gain and the birthweight of triplets. Acta Genet Med Gemell 44:93, 1995.
31. LeFevre ML, Bain RP, Ewigman BG, the RADIUS Study Group: A randomized trial of prenatal ultrasonographic screening: Impact on maternal management and outcome. Am J Obstet Gynecol 169:483, 1993.
32. Dickey RP, Olar TT, Curole DN, et al: The probability of multiple births when multiple gestational sacs or viable embryos are diagnosed at first trimester ultrasound. Hum Reprod 5:880, 1990.
33. Divon MY, Weiner Z: Ultrasound in twin pregnancy. Semin Perinatol 19:404, 1995.
34. D'Alton ME, Simpson LL: Syndromes in twins. Semin Perinatol 19:375, 1995.
35. Pasquini L, Wimalasundera RC, Fisk NM: Management of other complications specific to monochorionic twin pregnancies. Best Pract Res Clin Obstet Gynaecol 18:577, 2004.
36. Barss VA, Benacerraf BR, Frigoletto FD: Ultrasonographic determination of chorion type in twin gestation. Obstet Gynecol 66:779, 1985.
37. Bromley B, Benacerraf B: Using the number of yolk sacs to determine amnionicity in early first trimester monochorionic twins. J Ultrasound Med 14:415, 1995.
38. Monteagudo A, Roman AS: Ultrasound in multiple gestations: Twins and other multifetal pregnancies. Clin Perinatol 32:329, 2005.
39. Shen O, Samueloff A, Beller U, et al: Number of yolk sacs does not predict amnionicity in early first-trimester monochorionic multiple gestations. Ultrasound Obstet Gynecol 27:53, 2006.
40. Lee YM, Cleary-Goldman J, Thaker HM, et al: Antenatal sonographic prediction of twin chorionicity. Am J Obstet Gynecol 195:863, 2006.
41. Scardo JA, Ellings JM, Newman RB: Prospective determination of chorionicity, amnionicity, and zygosity in twin gestations. Am J Obstet Gynecol 173:1376, 1995.
42. D'Alton ME, Dudley DK: The ultrasonographic prediction of chorionicity in twin gestation. Am J Obstet Gynecol 160:557, 1989.
43. Vayssiere CF, Heim N, Camus EP, et al: Determination of chorionicity in twin gestations by high-frequency abdominal ultrasonography: Counting the layers of the dividing membrane. Am J Obstet Gynecol 175:1529, 1996.
44. Stagiannis KD, Sepulveda W, Southwell D, et al: Ultrasonographic measurement of the dividing membrane in twin pregnancy during the second and third trimesters: A reproducibility study. Am J Obstet Gynecol 173:1546, 1995.
45. Stenhouse E, Hardwick C, Maharaj S, et al: Chorionicity determination in twin pregnancies: How accurate are we? Ultrasound Obstet Gynecol 19:350, 2002.
46. Norton ME, D'Alton ME, Bianchi DW: Molecular zygosity studies aid in the management of discordant multiple gestations. J Perinatol 17:202, 1997.
47. Edwards MS, Ellings JM, Newman RB, et al: Predictive value of antepartum ultrasound examination for anomalies in twin gestations. Ultrasound Obstet Gynecol 6:43, 1995.
48. Chasen ST, Perni SC, Kalish RB, et al: First trimester risk assessment for trisomies 21 and 18 in twin pregnancy. Am J Obstet Gynecol 197:374, 2007.
49. Grumbach K, Coleman BG, Arger PH, et al: Twin and singleton growth patterns compared using ultrasound. Radiology 158:237, 1986.
50. Hill LM, Guzick D, Chenevey P, et al: The sonographic assessment of twin growth discordancy. Obstet Gynecol 84:501, 1994.
51. Caravello JW, Chauhan SP, Morrison JC, et al: Sonographic examination does not predict twin growth discordance accurately. Obstet Gynecol 89:529, 1997.
52. Reece EA, Yarkoni S, Abdalla M, et al: A prospective study of growth in twin gestations compared with growth in singleton pregnancies. I: The fetal head. J Ultrasound Med 10:439, 1991.

53. D'Alton ME, Mercer BM: Antepartum management of twin gestation: Ultrasound. Clin Obstet Gynecol 33:42, 1990.
54. Erkkola R, Ala-Mello S, Piiroinen O, et al: Growth discordancy in twin pregnancies: A risk factor not detected by measurements of biparietal diameter. Obstet Gynecol 66:203, 1985.
55. Hollier LM, McIntire DD, Leveno KJ: Outcome of twin pregnancies according to intrapair birth weight differences. Obstet Gynecol 94:1006, 1999.
56. Amaru RC, Bush MC, Berkowitz RL, et al: Is discordant growth in twins an independent risk factor for adverse neonatal outcome? Obstet Gynecol 103:71, 2004.
57. Ananth CV, Demissie K, Hanley ML: Birth weight discordancy and adverse perinatal outcomes among twin gestations in the United States: The effect of placental abruption. Am J Obstet Gynecol 188:954, 2003.
58. Goldenberg RL, Iams JD, Miodovnik M; National Institute of Child Health and Human Development Maternal-Fetal Medicine Units Network: The preterm prediction study: Risk factors in twin gestations. Am J Obstet Gynecol 175:1047, 1996.
59. Souka AP, Heath V, Flint S, et al: Cervical length at 23 weeks in twins in predicting spontaneous preterm delivery. Obstet Gynecol 94:450, 1999.
60. McElrath T, Kaimal A, Benson C, et al: Gestational age at delivery of triplet pregnancies as a function of cervical length throughout gestation. Am J Obstet Gynecol 185:S250, 2001.
61. Imseis HM, Albert TA, Iams JD: Identifying twin gestations at low risk for preterm birth with a transvaginal ultrasonographic cervical measurement at 24-26 weeks' gestation. Am J Obstet Gynecol 177:1149, 1997.
62. Yang JH, Kuhlman K, Daly S, et al: Prediction of preterm birth by second trimester cervical sonography in twin gestations. Ultrasound Obstet Gynecol 15:288, 2000.
63. Akiyama M, Kuno A, Tanake Y, et al: Comparison of alterations in fetal regional arterial vascular resistance in appropriate-for-gestational-age singleton, twin and triplet pregnancies. Hum Reprod 14:2635, 1999.
64. Magann EF, Whitworth NS, Bass JD, et al: Amniotic fluid volume of third-trimester diamniotic twin pregnancies. Obstet Gynecol 85:957, 1995.
65. Chau AC, Kjos SL, Kovacs BW: Ultrasonographic measurement of amniotic fluid volume in normal diamniotic twin pregnancies. Am J Obstet Gynecol 174:1003, 1996.
66. Porter TF, Dildy GA, Blanchard JR, et al: Normal values for amniotic fluid index during uncomplicated twin pregnancy. Obstet Gynecol 87:699, 1996.
67. Rodis JF, Egan JFX, Craffey A, et al: Calculated risks of chromosomal abnormalities in twin gestations. Obstet Gynecol 76:1037, 1990.
68. Meyers C, Adam R, Dungan J, et al: Aneuploidy in twin gestations: When is maternal age advanced? Obstet Gynecol 89:248, 1997.
69. American College of Obstetricians and Gynecologists: Screening for Fetal Chromosomal Abnormalities. (Practice Bulletin No. 77). Washington, DC: ACOG, 2007.
70. Wapner RJ: Genetic diagnosis in multiple pregnancies. Semin Perinatol 19:351, 1995.
71. Neveux LM, Palomaki GE, Knight GJ, et al: Multiple marker screening for Down syndrome in twin pregnancies. Prenat Diagn 16:29, 1996.
72. Spencer K, Salonen R, Muller F: Down's syndrome screening in multiple pregnancies using alpha-fetoprotein and free beta hCG. Prenat Diagn 15:94, 1995.
73. Bush MC, Malone FD: Down syndrome screening in twins. Clin Perinatol 32:373, 2005.
74. Niemimaa M, Suonapaa M, Heinonen S, et al: Maternal serum human chorionic gonadotrophin and pregnancy-associated plasma protein A in twin pregnancies in the first trimester. Prenat Diagn 22:183, 2002.
75. Sebire NJ, Snijders RJM, Hughes K, et al: Screening for trisomy 21 in twin pregnancies by maternal age and fetal nuchal translucency thickness at 10-14 weeks of gestation. BJOG 103:999, 1996.
76. Maymon R, Dreazen E, Tovbin Y, et al: The feasibility of nuchal translucency measurement in higher order multiple gestations achieved by assisted reproduction. Hum Reprod 14:2102, 1999.
77. Cuckle H, Wald N, Stevenson JD, et al: Maternal serum alpha-fetoprotein screening for open neural tube defects in twin pregnancies. Prenat Diagn 10:71, 1990.
78. Stiller RJ, Lockwood CJ, Belanger K, et al: Amniotic fluid alpha-fetoprotein concentrations in twin gestations: Dependence on placental membrane anatomy. Am J Obstet Gynecol 158:1088, 1988.
79. Rochon M, Eddleman KA, Stone J: Invasive procedures in multifetal pregnancies. Clin Perinatol 32:355, 2005.
80. Ghidini A, Lynch L, Hicks C, et al: The risk of second-trimester amniocentesis in twin gestations: A case-control study. Am J Obstet Gynecol 169:1013, 1993.
81. Yukobowich E, Anteby EY, Cohen SM, et al: Risk of fetal loss in twin pregnancies undergoing second trimester amniocentesis. Obstet Gynecol 98:231, 2001.
82. Wapner RJ, Johnson A, Davis G: Prenatal diagnosis in twin gestations: A comparison between second trimester amniocentesis and first trimester chorionic villus sampling. Obstet Gynecol 82:49, 1993.
83. Brambati B, Tului L, Guercilena S, et al: Outcome of first-trimester chorionic villus sampling for genetic investigation in multiple pregnancy. Ultrasound Obstet Gynecol 17:209, 2001.
84. Meyer B, Elimian A, Royek A: Comparison of clinical and financial outcomes of triplet gestations managed by maternal-fetal medicine versus community physicians. Am J Obstet Gynecol 185:S102, 2001.
85. Kovacs BW, Kirschbaum TH, Paul RH: Twin gestations. I: Antenatal care and complications. Obstet Gynecol 74:313, 1989.
86. Keirse MJNC, Grant A, King JF: Preterm labour. In Chalmers I, Enkin M, Keirse MJNC (eds): Effective Care in Pregnancy and Childbirth. New York: Oxford University Press, 1989, p 644.
87. Berghella V, Odibo AO, To MS, et al: Cerclage for short cervix on ultrasonography: Meta-analysis of trials using individual patient-level data. Obstet Gynecol 106:181, 2005.
88. Newman RB, Krombach RS, Myers MC, et al: Effect of cerclage on obstetric outcome in twin gestations with a shortened cervical length. Am J Obstet Gynecol 186:634, 2002.
89. Lipitz S, Reichman B, Paret G, et al: The improving outcome of triplet pregnancies. Am J Obstet Gynecol 161:1279, 1989.
90. Elimian A, Figueroa R, Nigam S, et al: Perinatal outcome of triplet gestation: Does prophylactic cerclage make a difference? J Maternal Fetal Med 8:119, 1999.
91. Rebarber A, Roman AS, Istwan N, et al: Prophylactic cerclage in the management of triplet pregnancies. Am J Obstet Gynecol 193:1193, 2005.
92. da Fonseca EB, Bittar RE, Carvalho MH, et al: Prophylactic administration of progesterone by vaginal suppository to reduce the incidence of spontaneous preterm birth in women at increased risk: A randomized placebo-controlled double-blind study. Am J Obstet Gynecol 188:419, 2003.
93. Meis PJ, Klebanoff M, Thom E, et al: Prevention of recurrent preterm delivery by 17 alpha-hydroxyprogesterone caproate. N Engl J Med 348:2379, 2003.
94. Rouse DJ, Caritis SN, Peaceman AM, et al: A trial of 17 alpha-hydroxyprogesterone caproate to prevent prematurity in twins. N Engl J Med 357:499, 2007.
95. MacLennan AH, Green RC, O'Shea R, et al: Routine hospital admission in twin pregnancy between 26 and 30 weeks' gestation. Lancet 335:267, 1990.
96. Crowther CA: Hospitalisation and bed rest for multiple pregnancy. Cochrane Database Syst Rev (1):CD000110, 2001.
97. Adams DM, Sholl JS, Haney EI, et al: Perinatal outcome associated with outpatient management of triplet pregnancy. Am J Obstet Gynecol 178:843, 1998.
98. Dyson DC, Danbe KH, Bamber JA, et al: Monitoring women at risk for preterm labor. N Engl J Med 338:15, 1998.
99. American College of Obstetricians and Gynecologists: Special Problems of Multiple Gestation (Educational Bulletin No. 253). Washington, DC, American College of Obstetricians and Gynecologists, 1998.
100. Colton T, Kayne HL, Zhang Y, et al: A meta-analysis of home uterine activity monitoring. Am J Obstet Gynecol 173:1499, 1995.

101. Maxwell CV, Lieberman E, Norton M, et al: Relationship of twin zygosity and risk of preeclampsia. Am J Obstet Gynecol 185:819, 2001.
102. Lynch A, McDuffie R, Murphy J, et al: Preeclampsia in multiple gestations: The role of assisted reproductive technologies. Obstet Gynecol 99:445, 2002.
103. Sibai BM, Hauth J, Caritis S, et al: Hypertensive disorders in twin versus singleton gestations. Am J Obstet Gynecol 182:938, 2000.
104. Caritis S, Sibai B, Hauth J, et al: Low-dose aspirin to prevent preeclampsia in women at high risk. N Engl J Med 338:701, 1998.
105. Davidson KM, Simpson LL, Knox TA, et al: Acute fatty liver of pregnancy in triplet gestation. Obstet Gynceol 91:806, 1998.
106. Norman RJ, Joubert SM, Marivate M: Amniotic fluid phospholipids and glucocorticoids in multiple pregnancy. BJOG 90:51, 1983.
107. Leveno KJ, Quirk JG, Whalley PJ, et al: Fetal lung maturity in twin gestation. Am J Obstet Gynecol 148:405, 1984.
108. Luke B: Reducing fetal deaths in multiple births: Optimal birthweights and gestational ages for infants of twin and triplet births. Acta Genet Med Gemell 45:333, 1996.
109. Sairam S, Costeloe K, Thilaganathan B: Prospective risk of stillbirth in multiple-gestation pregnancies: A population-based analysis. Obstet Gynecol 100:638, 2002.
110. Dodd JM, Crowther CA: Should we deliver twins electively at 37 weeks' gestation? Curr Opin Obstet Gynecol 17:579, 2005.
111. Cruikshank DP: Intrapartum management of twin gestations. Obstet Gynecol 109:1167, 2007.
112. Barigve O, Pasquini L, Galea P, et al: High risk of unexpected late fetal death in monochorionic twins despite intensive ultrasound surveillance: a cohort study. PLoS Med 2:e172, 2005.
113. Miller DA, Mullin P, Hou D, et al: Vaginal birth after cesarean section in twin gestations. Am J Obstet Gynecol 175:194, 1996.
114. Varner MW, Leindecker S, Spong CY, et al: The Maternal-Fetal Medicine Unit cesarean registry: Trial of labor with a twin gestation. Am J Obstet Gynecol 193:135, 2005.
115. Simpson LL, D'Alton ME: Multiple pregnancy. In Creasy RK (ed): Management of Labor and Delivery. Malden, MA: Blackwell, 1997, p 395.
116. Hogle KL, Hutton EK, McBrien KA, et al: Cesarean delivery for twins: A systematic review and meta-analysis. Am J Obstet Gynecol 188:220, 2003.
117. Leung TY, Tam WH, Leung TN, et al: Effect of twin-to-twin delivery interval on umbilical cord blood gas in the second twins. BJOG 109:63, 2002.
118. Chervenak FA, Johnson RE, Berkowitz RL, et al: Intrapartum external version of the second twin. Obstet Gynecol 62:160, 1983.
119. Gocke SE, Nageotte MP, Garite T, et al: Management of the nonvertex second twin: Primary cesarean section, external version, or primary breech extraction. Am J Obstet Gynecol 161:111, 1989.
120. Persad VL, Baskett TF, O'Connell CM, et al: Combined vaginal-cesarean delivery of twin pregnancies. Obstet Gynecol 98:1032, 2001.
121. Winn HN, Cimino J, Powers J, et al: Intrapartum management of nonvertex second-born twins: A critical analysis. Am J Obstet Gynecol 185:1204, 2001.
122. Blickstein I, Goldman RD, Kupferminc M: Delivery of breech first twins: A multicenter retrospective study. Obstet Gynecol 95:37, 2000.
123. Bloomfield MM, Philipson EH: External cephalic version of twin A. Obstet Gynecol 89:814, 1997.
124. Thiery M, Kermans G, Derom R: Triplet and higher-order births: What is the optimal delivery route? Acta Genet Med Gemell 37:89, 1988.
125. Clarke JP, Roman JD: A review of 19 sets of triplets: The positive results of vaginal delivery. Aust N Z J Obstet Gynaecol 34:50, 1994.
126. Dommergues M, Mahieu-Caputo D, Mandelbrot L, et al: Delivery of uncomplicated triplet pregnancies: Is the vaginal route safer? Am J Obstet Gynecol 172:513, 1995.
127. Alamia V, Royek AB, Jaekle RK, et al: Preliminary experience with a prospective protocol for planned vaginal delivery of triplet gestations. Am J Obstet Gynecol 179:1133, 1998.
128. Vintzelios AM, Ananth CV, Kontopoulos E, et al: Mode of delivery and risk of stillbirth and infant mortality in triplet gestations: United States, 1995 through 1998. Am J Obstet Gynecol 192:464, 2005.
129. Lavery JP, Austin RF, Schaefer DS, et al: Asynchronous multiple birth: A report of five cases. J Reprod Med 39:55, 1994.
130. Farkouh LJ, Sabin ED, Heyborne KD, et al: Delayed-interval delivery: Extended series from a single maternal-fetal medicine practice. Am J Obstet Gynecol 183:1499, 2000.
131. Benirschke K, Kim CK: Multiple pregnancy. N Engl J Med 288:1276, 1973.
132. Huber A, Hecher K: How can we diagnose and manage twin-twin transfusion syndrome? Best Pract Res Clin Obstet Gynaecol 18:543, 2004.
133. Lage JM, Vanmarter LJ, Mikhail E: Vascular anastomoses in fused, dichorionic twin placentas resulting in twin transfusion syndrome. Placenta 10:55, 1989.
134. Bruner JP, Rosemond RL: Twin-to-twin transfusion syndrome: A subset of the twin oligohydramnios-polyhydramnios sequence. Am J Obstet Gynecol 169:925, 1993.
135. King AD, Soothill PW, Montemagno R, et al: Twin-to-twin blood transfusion in a dichorionic pregnancy without the oligohydramnios-polyhydramnios sequence. BJOG 102:334, 1995.
136. Bajoria R, Wigglesworth J, Fisk NM: Angioarchitecture of monochorionic placentas in relation to the twin-twin transfusion syndrome. Am J Obstet Gynecol 172:856, 1995.
137. Machin GA, Feldstein VA, Van Gemert MJ, et al: Doppler sonographic demonstration of arterio-venous anastomoses in monochorionic twin gestation. Ultrasound Obstet Gynecol 16:214, 2000.
138. De Lia J, Fisk N, Hecher K, et al: Twin-to-twin transfusion syndrome: Debates on the etiology, natural history and management. Ultrasound Obstet Gynecol 16:210, 2000.
139. Denbow ML, Cox P, Taylor M, et al: Placental angioarchitecture in monochorionic twin pregnancies: Relationship to fetal growth, fetofetal transfusion syndrome, and pregnancy outcome. Am J Obstet Gynecol 182:417, 2000.
140. Diehl W, Hecher K, Zikulnig L, et al: Placental vascular anastomoses visualized during fetoscopic laser surgery in severe mid-trimester twin-twin transfusion syndrome. Placenta 22:876, 2001.
141. Denbow M, Fogliani R, Kyle P, et al: Hematological indices at fetal blood sampling in monochorionic pregnancies complicated by feto-fetal transfusion syndrome. Prenat Diagn 18:941, 1998.
142. Fesslova V, Villa L, Nava S, et al: Fetal and neonatal echocardiographic findings in twin-twin transfusion syndrome. Am J Obstet Gynecol 179:1056, 1998.
143. Simpson LL, Marx GR, Elkadry EA, et al: Cardiac dysfunction in twin-twin transfusion syndrome: A prospective, longitudinal study. Obstet Gynecol 92:557, 1998.
144. Bajoria R, Ward S, Chatterjee R: Natriuretic peptides in the pathogenesis of cardiac dysfunction in the recipient fetus of twin-twin transfusion syndrome. Am J Obstet Gynecol 186:121, 2002.
145. Barrea C, Alkazaleh F, Ryan G, et al: Prenatal cardiovascular manifestations in the twin-to-twin transfusion syndrome recipients and the impact of therapeutic amnioreduction. Am J Obstet Gynecol 192, 892, 2005.
146. Lougheed J, Sinclair BG, Fung Kee Fung K, et al: Acquired right ventricular outflow tract obstruction in the recipient twin in twin-twin transfusion syndrome. J Am Coll Cardiol 38:1533, 2001.
147. Sebire NJ, Souka A, Skentou H, et al: Early prediction of severe twin-to-twin transfusion syndrome. Hum Reprod 15:2008, 2000.
148. Lopriore E, Sueters M, Middeldorp JM, et al: Velamentous cord insertion and unequal placental territories in monochorionic twins with and without twin-to-twin transfusion syndrome. Am J Obstet Gynecol 196:159, 2007.
149. Wenstrom KD, Tessen JA, Zlatnik FJ, et al: Frequency, distribution, and theoretical mechanisms of hematologic and weight discordance in monochorionic twins. Obstet Gynecol 80:257, 1992.
150. Quintero RA, Morales WJ, Allen MH, et al: Staging of twin-twin transfusion syndrome. J Perinatol 19:550, 1999.

151. Quintero RA, Kontopoulos EV, Chmait R, et al: Management of twin-twin transfusion syndrome in pregnancies with iatrogenic detachment of membranes following therapeutic amniocentesis and the role of interim amniopatch. Ultrasound Obstet Gynecol 26:628-633, 2005.
152. Mari G, Roberts A, Detti L, et al: Perinatal morbidity and mortality rates in severe twin-twin transfusion syndrome: Results of the International Amnioreduction Registry. Am J Obstet Gynecol 185:708, 2001.
153. Trevett T, Johnson A: Monochorionic twin pregnancies. Clin Perinatol 32:475, 2005.
154. Ong SS, Zamora J, Khan KS, et al: Prognosis for the co-twin following single-twin death: A systematic review. BJOG 113:992, 2006.
155. Jones JM, Sbarra AJ, Delillo L, et al: Indomethacin in severe twin-to-twin transfusion syndrome. Am J Perinatol 10:24, 1993.
156. Fisk NM, Galea P: Twin-twin transfusion: As good as it gets? N Engl J Med 351:182, 2004.
157. Malone FD, D'Alton ME: Anomalies peculiar to multiple gestations. Clin Perinatol 27:1033, 2000.
158. Mari G, Dett L, Oz U, et al: Long-term outcome in twin-twin transfusion syndrome treated with serial aggressive amnioreduction. Am J Obstet Gynecol 183:211, 2000.
159. Saade GR, Olson G, Belfort MA, et al: Amniotomy: A new approach to the "stuck twin" syndrome. Am J Obstet Gynecol 172:429, 1995.
160. Moise KJ, Dorman K, Lamvu G, et al: A randomized trial of amnioreduction versus septostomy in the treatment of twin-twin transfusion syndrome. Am J Obstet Gynecol 701:193, 2005.
161. Suzuki S, Kaneko K, Shin S, et al: Incidence of intrauterine complications in monoamniotic twin gestation. Arch Gynecol Obstet 265:57, 2001.
162. Saade GR, Belfort MA, Berry DL, et al: Amniotic septostomy for the treatment of twin oligohydramnios-polyhydramnios sequence. Fetal Diagn Ther 13:86, 1998.
163. Johnson JR, Rossi KQ, O'Shaughnessy RW: Amnioreduction versus septostomy in twin-twin transfusion syndrome. Am J Obstet Gynecol 185:1044, 2001.
164. Pistorius LR, Howarth GR: Failure of amniotic septostomy in the management of 3 subsequent cases of severe previable twin-twin transfusion syndrome. Fetal Diagn Ther 14:337, 1999.
165. Quintero RA, Morales WJ, Mendoza G, et al: Selective photocoagulation of placental vessels in twin-twin transfusion syndrome: Evolution of a surgical technique. Obstst Gynecol Survey 53:597-603, 1998.
166. Ville Y, Hecher K, Gagnon A, et al: Endoscopic laser coagulation in the management of severe twin-to-twin transfusion syndrome. BJOG 105:446, 1998.
167. De Lia JE, Kuhlmann RS, Lopez KP: Treating previable twin-twin transfusion syndrome with fetoscopic laser surgery: Outcomes following the learning curve. J Perinat Med 27:61, 1999.
168. Hecher K, Diehl W, Zikulnig L, et al: Endoscopic laser coagulation of placental anastomoses in 200 pregnancies with severe mid-trimester twin-to-twin transfusion syndrome. Eur J Obstet Gynaecol Reprod Biol 92:135, 2000.
169. Quintero RA, Bornick PW, Allen MH, et al: Selective laser photocoagulation of communicating vessels in severe twin-twin transfusion syndrome in women with an anterior placenta. Obstet Gynecol 97:477, 2001.
170. Lenclen R, Paupe A, Ciarlo G, et al: Neonatal outcome in preterm monochorionic twins with twin-to-twin transfusion syndrome after intrauterine treatment with amnioreduction or fetoscopic laser surgery: Comparison with dichorionic twins. Am J Obstet Gynecol 196:450.e1-450.e7, 2007.
171. Senat MW, Deprest J, Boulvain M, et al: Endoscopic laser surgery versus serial amnioreduction for severe twin-to-twin transfusion syndrome. N Engl J Med 351:136, 2004.
172. Crombleholme TM, Shera D, Lee H, et al: A prospective, randomized, multicenter trial of amnioreduction vs selective fetoscopic laser photocoagulation for the treatment of severe twin-twin transfusion syndrome. Am J Obstet Gynecol 197:396, 2007.
173. Cincotta R, Oldham J, Sampson A: Antepartum and postpartum complications of twin-twin transfusion. Aust N Z J Obstet Gynaecol 36:303, 1996.
174. Lopriore E, Middeldorp JM, Sueters M, et al: Long-term neurodevelopmental outcome in twin-to-twin transfusion syndrome treated with fetoscopic laser surgery. Am J Obstet Gynecol 196:231, 2007.
175. Banek CS, Hecher K, Hackeloer BJ, et al: Long-term neurodevelopmental outcome after intrauterine laser treatment for severe twin-twin transfusion syndrome. Am J Obstet Gynecol 188:876, 2003.
176. Lopriore E, van Wezel-Meijler G, Middeldorp JM, et al: Incidence, origin, and character of cerebral injury in twin-to-twin transfusion syndrome treated with fetoscopic laser surgery. Am J Obstet Gynecol 194:1215, 2006.
177. Lee CY: Management of monoamniotic twins diagnosed antenatally by ultrasound. Am J Gynecol Health 6:25, 1992.
178. Rodis JF, McIlveen PF, Egan JF, et al: Monoamniotic twins: Improved perinatal survival with accurate prenatal diagnosis and antenatal surveillance. Am J Obstet Gynecol 177:1046, 1997.
179. Arabin B, Laurini RN, van Eyck J: Early prenatal diagnosis of cord entanglement in monoamniotic multiple pregnancies. Ultrasound Obstet Gynecol 13:181, 1999.
180. Lavery J, Gadwood KA: Amniography for confirming the diagnosis of monoamniotic twinning: A case report. J Reprod Med 35:911, 1990.
181. Tabsh K: Genetic amniocentesis in multiple gestation: A new technique to diagnose monoamniotic twins. Obstet Gynecol 75:296, 1990.
182. Carr SR, Aronson MP, Coustan DR: Survival rates of monoamniotic twins do not decrease after 30 weeks' gestation. Am J Obstet Gynecol 163:719, 1990.
183. Allen VM, Windrim R, Barrett J, et al: Management of monoamniotic twin pregnancies: A case series and systematic review of the literature. BJOG 108:931, 2001.
184. Heyborne KD, Porreco RP, Garite TJ, et al: Improved perinatal survival of monoamniotic twins with intensive inpatient monitoring. Am J Obstet Gynecol 192:96, 2005.
185. Roque H, Gillen-Goldstein J, Funai E, et al: Perinatal outcomes in monoamniotic gestations. J Mat Fet Neonat Med 13:414, 2003.
186. Demaria F, Goffinet F, Kayem G, et al: Monoamniotic twin pregnancies: Antenatal management and perinatal results of 19 consecutive cases. BJOG 111:22, 2004.
187. Peek MJ, McCarthy A, Kyle P, et al: Medical amnioreduction with sulindac to reduce cord complications in monoamniotic twins. Am J Obstet Gynecol 176:334, 1997.
188. Tessen JA, Zlatnik FJ: Monoamniotic twins: A retrospective controlled study. Obstet Gynecol 77:832, 1991.
189. McLeod FN, McCoy DR: Monoamniotic twins with an unusual cord complication. BJOG 88:774, 1981.
190. Katanka KS, Buchmann EJ: Vaginal delivery of monoamniotic twins with umbilical cord entanglement: A case report. J Reprod Med 46:275, 2001.
191. Dickinson JE: Monoamniotic twin pregnancy: A review of contemporary practice. Aust N Z J Obstet Gynaecol 45:474, 2005.
192. Van Allen MI, Smith SW, Shepard TH: Twin reversed arterial perfusion (TRAP) sequence: A study of 14 twin pregnancies with acardius. Semin Perinatol 7:285, 1983.
193. Healey MG: Acardia: Predictive risk factors for the co-twin's survival. Teratology 50:205, 1994.
194. Langlotz H, Sauerbrei E, Murray S: Transvaginal Doppler sonographic diagnosis of an acardiac twin at 12 weeks' gestation. J Ultrasound Med 10:175, 1991.
195. Moore TR, Gale S, Benirschke K: Perinatal outcome of forty-nine pregnancies complicated by acardiac twinning. Am J Obstet Gynecol 163:907, 1990.
196. Quintero RA, Chmait RH, Murakoshi T, et al: Surgical management of twin reversed arterial perfusion sequence. Am J Obstet Gynecol 194:982, 2006.
197. Sullivan AE, Varner MW, Ball RH, et al: The management of acardiac twins: A conservative approach. Am J Obstet Gynecol 189:1310, 2003.
198. Wong AE, Sepulveda W: Acardiac anomaly: Current issues in prenatal assessment and treatment. Prenat Diagn 25:796, 2005.
199. Brassard M, Fouron JC, Leduc L, et al: Prognostic markers in twin pregnancies with an acardiac fetus. Obstet Gynecol 94:409, 1999.

200. Fries MH, Goldberg JD, Golbus MA: Treatment of acardiac-acephalus twin gestations by hysterotomy and selective delivery. Obstet Gynecol 79:601, 1992.
201. Holzgreve W, Tercanli S, Krings W, et al: A simpler technique for umbilical-cord blockade of an acardiac twin. N Engl J Med 331:56, 1994.
202. Lee H, Wagner AJ, Sy E, et al: Efficacy of radiofrequency ablation for twin-reversed arterial perfusion sequence. Am J Obstet Gynecol 196:459, 2007.
203. Van Den Brand SFJJ, Nijhuis JG, Van Dongen PWJ: Prenatal ultrasound diagnosis of conjoined twins. Obstet Gynecol Surv 49:656, 1994.
204. Maymon R, Halperin R, Weinraub Z, et al: Three-dimensional transvaginal sonography of conjoined twins at 10 weeks: A case report. Ultrasound Obstet Gynecol 11:292, 1998.
205. Usta IM, Awwad JT: A false positive diagnosis of conjoined twins in a triplet pregnancy: Pitfalls of first trimester ultrasonographic prenatal diagnosis. Prenat Diagn 20:169, 2000.
206. Spitz L: Conjoined twins. Prenat Diagn 25:814, 2005.
207. Mackenzie TC, Crombleholme TM, Johnson MP, et al: The natural history of prenatally diagnosed conjoined twins. J Pediatr Surg 37:303, 2002.
208. Kiesewetter WB: Surgery on conjoined (Siamese) twins. Surgery 59:860, 1996.
209. Al Rabeeah A: Conjoined twins: Past, present and future. J Pediatr Surg 41:1000, 2006.
210. Rode H, Fleggen AG, Brown RA, et al: Four decades of conjoined twins at Red Cross Children's Hospital: Lessons learned. S African Med J 96:931, 2006.
211. Annas GJ: Conjoined twins: The limits of law at the limits of life. N Engl J Med 344:1104, 2001.
212. Landy HJ, Weiner S, Corson SL, et al: The "vanishing twin": Ultrasonographic assessment of fetal disappearance in the first trimester. Am J Obstet Gynecol 155:14, 1986.
213. Weiss JL, Cleary-Goldman J, Tanji K, et al: Multicystic encephalomalacia after first-trimester intrauterine fetal death in monochorionic twins. Am J Obstet Gynecol 190:563, 2004.
214. Chasen ST, Luo G, Perni SC, et al: Are in vitro fertilization pregnancies with early spontaneous reduction high risk? Am J Obstet Gynecol 195, 814, 2006.
215. Pinborg A, Lidegaard O, Freiesleben NC, et al: Vanishing twins: A predictor of small-for-gestational age in IVF singletons. Hum Reprod 22:2707, 2007.
216. Ong SS, Zamora J, Khan KS, et al: Prognosis for the co-twin following single-twin death: A systematic review. BJOG 113:992, 2006.
217. Eglowstein MS, D'Alton ME: Single intra-uterine demise in twin gestation. J Maternal Fetal Med 2:272, 1993.
218. Pharoah PO, Adi Y: Consequences of in-utero death in a twin pregnancy. Lancet 355:1597, 2000.
219. Nicolini U, Poblete A: Single intrauterine death in monochorionic twin pregnancies. Ultrasound Obstet Gynecol 14:297, 1999.
220. Nicolini U, Pisoni MP, Cela E, et al: Fetal blood sampling immediately before and within 24 hours of death in monochorionic twin pregnancies complicated by single intrauterine death. Am J Obstet Gynecol 179:800, 1998.
221. Malone FD, D'Alton ME: Management of multiple gestations complicated by a single anomalous fetus. Curr Opin Obstet Gynecol 9:213, 1997.
222. Berkowitz RL, Lynch L: Selective reduction: An unfortunate misnomer. Obstet Gynecol 75:873, 1990.
223. Malone FD, Craigo SD, Chelmow D, et al: Outcome of twin gestations complicated by a single anomalous fetus. Obstet Gynecol 88:1, 1996.
224. Sebire NJ, Sepulveda W, Hughes KS, et al: Management of twin pregnancies discordant for anencephaly. BJOG 107:216, 1997.
225. Challis D, Gratacos E, Deprest JA: Cord occlusion techniques for selective termination in monochorionic twins. J Perinat Med 27:327, 1999.
226. Robyr R, Yamamoto M, Ville Y: Selective feticide in complicated monochorionic twin pregnancies using ultrasound-guided bipolar cord coagulation. BJOG 112:1344, 2005.
227. Sepulveda W, Bower S, Hassan J, et al: Ablation of acardiac twin by alcohol injection into the intra-abdominal umbilical artery. Obstet Gynecol 86:680, 1995.
228. Lewi L, Gratacos E, Ortibus E, et al: Pregnancy and infant outcome of 80 consecutive cord coagulations in complicated monochorionic multiple pregnancies. Am J Obstet Gynecol 194:782, 2006.
229. Young BK, Roque H, Abdelhak Y, et al: Endoscopic ligation of the umbilical cord at 19 weeks' gestation in monoamniotic monochorionic twins discordant for hypoplastic left heart syndrome. Fetal Diagn Ther 16:61, 2001.
230. Evans MI, Goldberg JD, Horenstein J, et al: Selective termination for structural, chromosomal and mendelian anomalies: International experience. Am J Obstet Gynecol 181:893, 1999.
231. Eddleman K, Stone J, Lynch L, et al: Selective termination of anomalous fetuses in multifetal pregnancies: Two hundred cases at a single center. Am J Obstet Gynecol 187:1168, 2002.
232. Stone J, Eddleman K: Multifetal pregnancy reduction. Curr Opin Obstet Gynecol 12:491, 2000.
233. Berkowitz RL, Lynch L, Stone J, Alvarez M: The current status of multifetal pregnancy reduction. Am J Obstet Gynecol 174:1265, 1996.
234. Evans MI, Berkowitz RL, Wapner RJ, et al: Improvement in outcomes of multifetal pregnancy reduction with increased experience. Am J Obstet Gynecol 184:97, 2001.
235. McLean LK, Evans MI, Carpenter RJ, et al: Genetic amniocentesis following multifetal pregnancy reduction does not increase the risk of pregnancy loss. Prenat Diagn 18:186, 1998.
236. Eddleman KA, Stone JL, Lynch L, et al: Chorionic villus sampling before multifetal pregnancy reduction. Am J Obstet Gynecol 183:1078, 2000.
237. Stone J, Eddleman K, Lynch L, et al: A single center experience with 1000 consecutive cases of multifetal pregnancy reduction. Am J Obstet Gynecol 187:1163, 2002.
238. Stone J, Belogolovkin V, Matho A, et al: Evolving trends in 2000 cases of multifetal pregnancy reduction: A single-center experience. Am J Obstet Gynecol 197:394, 2007.
239. Evans MI, Britt D: Fetal reduction. Semin Perinatol 29:321, 2005.
240. Sivan E, Maman E, Homko CJ, et al: Impact of fetal reduction on the incidence of gestational diabetes. Obstet Gynecol 99:91, 2002.
241. Depp R, Macone GA, Rosenn MF, et al: Multifetal pregnancy reduction: Evaluation of fetal growth in the remaining twins. Am J Obstet Gynecol 174:1233, 1996.
242. Schreiner-Engel P, Walther VN, Mindes J, et al: First-trimester multifetal pregnancy reduction: Acute and persistent psychologic reactions. Am J Obstet Gynecol 172:541, 1995.
243. American College of Obstetricians and Gynecologists: Multifetal Pregnancy Reduction. (Committee Opinion No. 369). Washington, DC: ACOG, 2007.

Chapter 26

Hemolytic Disease of the Fetus and Newborn

Kenneth J. Moise, Jr., MD

Red Cell Alloimmunization in Pregnancy

Terminology

Maternal antibodies to red blood cell antigens can pass across the placenta, attach to fetal red cells, and lead to their destruction. Historically, the perinatal effects of these antibodies could not be assessed until after delivery, and the descriptive term *hemolytic disease of the newborn* (HDN) was used. The advent of such diagnostic tools as ultrasound and fetal blood sampling (FBS) has allowed for the diagnosis of fetal anemia and hydrops fetalis before delivery. For this reason, the term *hemolytic disease of the fetus and newborn* (HDFN) is more appropriate to describe this disorder. Another historical term, *erythroblastosis fetalis,* was first used when neonatal studies revealed a large percentage of circulating erythroblasts in patients with severe HDFN. This represents a profound state of fetal anemia that probably occurs in only a small percentage of cases of HDFN. Therefore, the term *erythroblastosis fetalis* should be replaced by *HDFN.* Finally, the maternal etiology of HDFN, namely the formation of antibodies to red cell antigens, should be called *red cell alloimmunization* instead of the older term of *red cell isoimmunization.*

Historical Perspectives

The first case of HDFN was probably described in 1609 in the French literature by a midwife.[1] The case was a twin gestation in which the first fetus was stillborn and the second twin developed jaundice and died soon after birth. There is some suggestion that HDFN caused by the rhesus D (RhD) antibody may have played a role in the ultimate formation of the Anglican Church.[2] Henry VIII's first wife, Katherine of Aragon, conceived six children; five died in the perinatal period from presumed HDFN. Only one daughter, Mary Tudor, survived the union. The ultimate inability of Katherine to bear a viable male heir to the English throne resulted in a divorce that the Roman Pope would not grant. This led to Henry's declaration of the formation of the Church of England. The modern era of Rhesus disease probably began in 1939 when Levine and Stetson[3] described an antibody in a woman who gave birth to a stillborn fetus. The patient experienced a severe hemolytic transfusion reaction after later receiving her husband's blood. In 1940, Landsteiner and Weiner[4] injected red cells from rhesus monkeys into guinea pigs. The antibody that was isolated from the guinea pigs was used to test human blood samples from Caucasian individuals, and agglutination was noted in 85% of them. One year later, Levine and associates[5] were able to demonstrate a causal relationship between RhD antibodies in RhD-negative women and HDFN in their offspring.

The advent of therapy for HDFN began in 1945 with the description by Wallerstein[6] of the technique of neonatal exchange transfusion. Later, Bevis[7] and then Liley[8] proposed the use of amniotic fluid bilirubin assessment as an indirect measure of the degree of fetal hemolysis. Sir William Liley's[9] major contribution to the story of rhesus disease was the introduction of the intraperitoneal fetal transfusion (IPT). He learned from a visiting geneticist who had returned from Africa that the infusion of red cells into the peritoneal cavity of neonates with sickle cell disease produced normal-appearing red blood cells on peripheral blood smear. Liley realized that he had previously inadvertently entered the peritoneal cavity of fetuses at the time of amniocentesis, as indicated by the marked contrast in the yellow hue of the ascitic fluid compared with amniotic fluid. He postulated that purposeful entry into the fetal peritoneal cavity could be accomplished. After three unsuccessful attempts that resulted in fetal deaths, the fourth fetus was delivered at 34 weeks and 4 days of gestation after undergoing two IPTs at 32 weeks 1 day and 33 weeks 4 days.[9] Several investigators made futile attempts to transfuse the fetus by direct access via hysterotomy using the fetal femoral artery, saphenous vein, and internal jugular vein.[10-12]

Early attempts at IPT used fluoroscopy for needle guidance. With the introduction of real-time ultrasound in the early 1980s, IPTs became a safer procedure as fluoroscopy was abandoned. Rodeck and coworkers[13] are credited with the first intravascular fetal transfusion (IVT); they used a fetoscope to guide the transfusion needle into a placental plate vessel. Bang and coworkers[14] performed the first ultrasound-guided IVT using the intrahepatic portion of the umbilical vein.

The 1990s saw the introduction of genetic techniques using amniocentesis to perform fetal red cell typing. With the dawn of the new millennium, the noninvasive detection of fetal anemia through Doppler ultrasound became a reality. The noninvasive determination of fetal antigen status using free DNA in the maternal circulation has also now entered clinical practice.

Incidence

The advent of the routine administration of antenatal and postpartum rhesus immune globulin (RhIG) resulted in a marked reduction in cases of red cell alloimmunization secondary to the RhD antigen. A report from surveillance hospitals of the Centers for Disease Control and Prevention noted in 1991 that 1 in every 1000 liveborn infants exhibited some effect from rhesus hemolytic disease.[15] Data from a 2003 review of the national registry of U.S. birth certificates indicated an incidence of 6.8 cases per 1000 live births.[16] Although this would appear to indicate an increasing incidence, reporting bias in the latter study probably explains this difference. Clearly, a shift to other red cell antibodies associated with HDFN has occurred as a result of the decreasing incidence of RhD alloimmunization.

Geifman-Holtzman and coworkers[17] evaluated 37,506 serum samples from female patients at two New York blood centers between the years of 1993 and 1995. Sixty percent of the women were of childbearing age. A positive screen for an antibody previously reported to be associated with HDFN was identified in 424 (1.1%) of the samples. Rhesus antibodies were the most common, accounting for more than half of significant antibodies, with the RhD antibody accounting for almost one fourth of all antibodies. Kell antibodies were next most frequent (29%), followed by Duffy (7%), MNS (6%), Kidd, and anti-U. These authors compared their findings with previous investigations of antibody prevalence. As expected, secondary to the widespread adoption of RhIG prophylaxis, the incidence of RhD alloimmunization decreased from 43.3 per 1000 samples in 1967 to 2.6 per 1000 in 1996 (Fig. 26-1).[18] Kell alloimmunization was higher in the 1996 series (3.2 per 1000), compared with studies of the U.S. population in 1967 (1.6 per 1000); this increase was thought to be related to enhanced detection of antibodies through improvement of blood banking techniques. Alternatively, increasing maternal age could result in a higher likelihood of exposure to blood transfusions that have the potential to result in Kell sensitization. Finally, these investigators noted important differences in the incidence of such antibodies as Kell when comparing the U.S. population with similar populations in Australia[19] or Sweden[20] (Kell incidence, 3.2, 0.5, and 0.4 per 1000, respectively). These differences are most likely explained by geographic variations in gene frequency, although specific national transfusion practices could also have an influence.

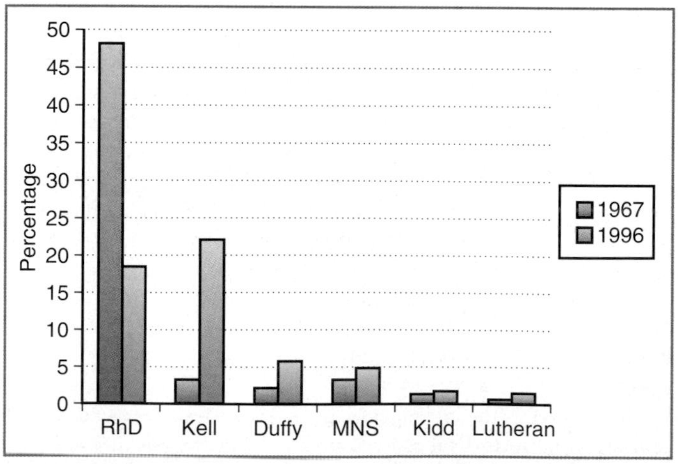

FIGURE 26-1 Incidence of maternal anti–red cell antibodies associated with hemolytic disease of the fetus and newborn in women of reproductive age. Graph shows changes in incidence from 1967 to 1996 in the United States.

Pathophysiology

It is well established that the fetal-maternal interface is not an absolute barrier, because there is evidence that considerable trafficking of many types of cells occurs between the fetus and the mother throughout gestation. In most cases, the antigenic load of a putative antigen on the fetal erythrocytes and erythrocytic precursors is insufficient to stimulate the maternal immune system. However, in the case of a large antenatal fetomaternal hemorrhage (FMH) or an FMH at delivery, B lymphocyte clones that recognize the foreign red cell antigen are established. The initial maternal production of immunoglobulin M (IgM) is short-lived and is followed by a rapid change to an IgG response. A human antiglobulin titer can usually be detected by 5 to 16 weeks after the sensitizing event.

The anti-D immune response is the best characterized of the anti–red cell antibodies associated with HDFN. In one third of cases, only subclass IgG1 is produced; in the remainder of cases, a combination of IgG1 and IgG3 subclasses are found.[21] IgG3 anti-D is thought to promote monocyte–red cell interaction more efficiently than IgG1. A longer hinge region in its structure enables the IgG3 molecule to more easily bridge the gap between sensitized red cells and reticuloendothelial cells.[22] Anti-D IgG is a nonagglutinating antibody that does not bind complement.

After the initial antigenic exposure, memory B lymphocytes await the appearance of red cells containing the putative antigen in a subsequent pregnancy. If stimulated by fetal erythrocytes, these B lymphocytes differentiate into plasma cells that can rapidly proliferate and produce IgG antibodies and an increase in the maternal titer. Maternal IgG crosses the placenta and attaches to fetal erythrocytes that have expressed the paternal antigen. These cells are then sequestered by macrophages in the fetal spleen, where they undergo extravascular hemolysis, producing fetal anemia. Fetal sex may play a significant role in the fetal response to maternal antibodies. Ulm and associates[23] reported that the chance for hydrops fetalis was increased by 13-fold in RhD-positive male fetuses compared with their female counterparts; the adjusted odds ratio for perinatal mortality was 3.38 in male fetuses.

Several important physiologic responses occur in fetuses as a result of this anemia. An enhanced bone marrow production of reticulocytes is noted when the fetal hemoglobin deficit exceeds 2 g/dL, compared with norms for gestational age, and erythroblasts from the fetal liver occur at a hemoglobin deficit of 7 g/dL or greater.[24] Cardiac output increases, and 2,3-diphosphoglycerate levels are enhanced. Tissue hypoxia appears as anemia progresses. An increased umbilical artery lactate level occurs when the fetal hemoglobin falls below 8 g/dL, and increased venous lactate is noted with a hemoglobin below 4 g/dL.[25]

Hydrops fetalis, a collection of fluid in serous compartments, heralds end-stage disease, with hemoglobin deficits of 7 g/dL or greater.[24] It first manifests as fetal ascites; later, there are findings of pleural effusion and scalp edema. The exact pathophysiology of this condition is unknown. Lower serum albumin levels have been reported, presumably owing to depressed synthesis by the fetal liver, which shifts to an erythropoietic function.[26] Colloid osmotic pressure also appears to decrease.[27] However, congenital analbuminemia is not associated with hydrops fetalis, and experimental removal of fetal plasma proteins does not produce hydrops.[28,29] Recently, Pasman and colleagues[30] studied albumin levels of 224 fetuses in Rh-alloimmunized pregnancies. A serum albumin concentration of less than 2 standard deviations below the mean was noted in only 14% of fetuses with mild hydrops and in 63% of fetuses with severe hydrops. An alternative hypothesis suggests that tissue hypoxia resulting from anemia enhances capillary permeability. Iron overload resulting from ongoing hemolysis may contribute to free radical formation and endothelial cell dysfunction.[31] Central venous pressures do appear to be elevated in the hydropic fetus with HDFN.[27] This may cause a functional blockage of the lymphatic system at the level of the thoracic duct as it empties into the left brachiocephalic vein. This theory is supported by reports of poor absorption of donor red blood cells infused into the intraperitoneal cavity in cases of hydrops.[32]

Several specific antibody situations probably affect the pathophysiology of HDFN. Spong and coworkers[33] reported an increased degree of fetal anemia when multiple maternal antibodies associated with HDFN were present, compared with anti-D alone. Red cell sensitization to multiple antibodies was associated with a 1.8 fold increased need for intrauterine transfusions (IUTs), compared with patients who had only anti-D. The body of in vitro and in vivo evidence suggests that fetal anemia in cases of Kell (anti-K1) sensitization is secondary to two mechanisms: hemolysis and erythropoietic suppression. Vaughan and coworkers[34] studied 11 anemic fetuses from pregnancies with Kell alloimmunization who were matched for gestational age and hematocrit (Hct) with 11 anemic fetuses from pregnancies complicated by RhD alloimmunization. The anti-Kell group was noted to have a lower level of both reticulocytosis and erythroblastosis. Weiner and Widness[35] compared 11 fetuses from Kell-sensitized pregnancies with 54 from RhD-sensitized pregnancies. Like the previous investigators, they noted an inverse correlation between fetal hemoglobin concentration and reticulocyte count in the RhD fetuses; such a correlation could not be demonstrated in the Kell fetuses. Finally, Vaughan and colleagues[36] undertook an in vitro analysis of erythroid progenitors to assess the impact of anti-K1 antibodies compared with anti-D antibodies. Kell– and Kell+ erythroid cell lines were established from umbilical cord blood. Serum from 22 women sensitized to Kell suppressed the growth of Kell+ erythroid burst-forming and colony-forming units; no suppression occurred in Kell– cultures. Monoclonal anti-K1 antibody caused a dose-dependent suppression of growth in Kell+ cell lines but not in Kell– cell lines. Monoclonal anti-RhD antibody exhibited no suppression in either cell line. The role of the Kell antigen in red cell physiology is unknown; however, the Kell protein has structural similarities to endopeptidases and therefore may be involved in protein regulation and cell growth in the erythroid cells. At this time, little is known as to whether other anti–red cell antibodies are associated with suppression of fetal erythropoiesis.

Rhesus Alloimmunization and Hemolytic Disease of the Fetus and Newborn

Genetics

Fischer and Race[37] first proposed the concept of three genes that encode for the three major Rh antigen groups—D, C/c, and E/e. Some 45 years later, the Rh locus was localized to the short arm of chromosome 1.[38] Only two genes were identified—an RhD gene and an RhCE gene. Each gene is 10 exons in length, and there is 96% homology between the genes. This led some to conclude that these genes represent a duplication of a common ancestral gene. Production of two distinct proteins from the *RHCE* gene probably occurs as a result of alternative splicing of messenger RNA.[39] One nucleotide difference, a change from cytosine to thymine in exon 2 of the *RHCE* gene, results in a single amino

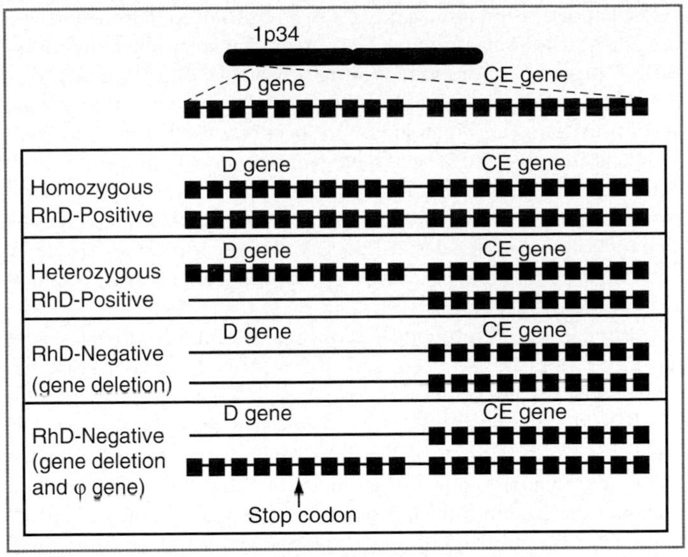

FIGURE 26-2 Schematic diagram of Rh gene locus on chromosome 1. Four genotypes are demonstrated: homozygous RhD-positive, heterozygous RhD-positive, typical RhD-negative, and RhD-negative with pseudogene (ψ).

acid change of a serine to proline. This causes the expression of the C antigen as opposed to the c antigen.[40] A single cytosine-to-guanine change in exon 5 of the *RHCE* gene produces a single amino acid change of a proline to alanine, resulting in formation of the e antigen instead of the E antigen.[41]

The gene frequency found in various ethnic groups can be traced to the Spanish colonization in the 15th and 16th centuries. Native populations of certain land masses (Eskimos, Native Americans, Japanese, and Chinese individuals) have less than a 1% incidence of RhD negativity. The Basque tribe in Spain is noted to have a 30% incidence of Rh negativity. This may well be the origin of the RhD gene deletion that is the most common genetic basis of the RhD– state in whites (Fig. 26-2). Whites of European descent exhibit a 15% incidence of RhD negativity, whereas an 8% incidence occurs in African Americans and Hispanics of Mexico and Central America. This latter incidence probably reflects ethnic diversity secondary to Spanish colonization of the New World.

An RhD pseudogene has been described in 69% of South African blacks and 24% of African Americans (see Fig. 26-2).[42] In this situation, all 10 exons of the RhD gene are present; however, translation of the gene into a messenger RNA product does not occur because of the presence of a stop codon in the intron between exons 3 and 4. Therefore, no RhD protein is synthesized, and the patient is serologically RhD–. The presence of this gene in an RhD– pregnant patient has important implications for the prenatal diagnosis of the fetal blood type using amniocentesis, chorion villus biopsy, or free fetal DNA (see later discussion).

Prevention of RhD Hemolytic Disease of the Fetus and Newborn

Four RhIG preparations are currently available in the United States for the prevention of RhD alloimmunization. Two of the products (RhoGAM, Ortho-Clinical Diagnostics, Raritan, NJ, and HyperRHO S/D, Talecris Biotherapeutics-USA, Research Triangle Park, NC) are limited to intramuscular use because they are manufactured by Cohn cold ethanol fractionation, a process that results in contamination with IgA and other plasma proteins. The remaining two products (WinRho-SDF, Cangene Corporation, Winnipeg, Canada, and Rhophlac, CSL Behring, Marburg, Germany) are prepared through sepharose column and ion-exchange chromatography, respectively. Currently, all available products are subject to solvent detergent treatment to inactivate enveloped viruses; many manufacturers also employ an additional micropore filtration step to further reduce the chance of viral contamination. Thimerosal, a mercury-derived preservative used to prevent bacterial and fungal contamination, has been removed from all RhIG products used in the United States.

Although Rh(D) antibody was once produced from the plasma of sensitized women, the decreasing prevalence of rhesus disease has necessitated the use of male donors who undergo repeated injections of RhD+ red blood cells. Because of concerns regarding Creutzfeldt-Jakob disease in the United Kingdom, only plasma from the United States is used as the source of antibody for RhIG preparation in that region at the current time. Occasional outbreaks of hepatitis C related to the administration of RhIG were reported in Ireland[43] and Germany[44] in the late 1970s, although none has occurred in the United States. Because RhIG is a blood derivative, patients who choose not to accept blood products secondary to religious beliefs should be informed of its source and asked for informed consent. Although most RhIG is issued from hospital blood banks, various manufacturers' products can be purchased by private physicians for use in their offices. A past recall by one manufacturer warrants that careful records of lot numbers be documented in the patient's medical chart and in a general clinic logbook.

The exact mechanism by which RhIG prevents alloimmunization to the RhD antigen is unknown. Studies using intramuscular human monoclonal anti-D antibodies revealed that only about 8% of RhD antigenic sites are bound by anti-D antibody after injection.[45] This negates the theory that masking of antigenic sites is the explanation for the effectiveness of RhIG. Passive anti-K has been shown to prevent the formation of anti-D in K− RhD− patients exposed to K+ RhD+ red cells.[46] Exogenous anti-D bound to RhD sites on the red cell is thought to bind to the IgG Fc receptors FcγRI, FcγRIIA, and FcγRIIIA on effector cells (macrophages and natural killer cells), thereby resulting in clearance of RhD+ red cells from circulation.[47] Inhibition of the activation of B lymphocytes through binding with FcγRIIB1 receptors also has been proposed as part of the mechanism for prevention of alloimmunization.[47]

The limited resource of donors and issues with the safety of injection of exogenous red cells led several investigators to develop monoclonal anti-D preparations to replace the current polyclonal products that are on the market.[48] Polyclonal anti-D is composed of approximately 85% IgG1 and 15% IgG3. Trials have been reported with mixtures of monoclonal antibodies such as BRAD-5/BRAD-3.[49] Although most clinical trials have revealed enhanced clearance of RhD+ red cells from the circulation of RhD− subjects, most of the monoclones tested have not achieved rates of clearance that equal those of polyclonal anti-D. One of the larger trials using a BRAD-5/BRAD-3 combination monoclonal antibody revealed a failure rate of 2% for the prevention of alloimmunization.[49] Only the monoclonal antibody T125 has shown promise for red blood cell clearance equal to polyclonal anti-D in a mouse model of severe combined immunodeficiency disease (SCID).[47]

All pregnant patients should undergo an antibody screen at the first prenatal visit. If there is no evidence of anti-D alloimmunization in the RhD− woman, recommendations in North America include the intramuscular administration of 300 μg of RhIG at 28 weeks of gestation.[50] This practice has been reported to reduce the incidence of antenatal alloimmunization from 2% to 0.1%.[51] In the United Kingdom, an antenatal protocol of administering 100 μg (500 IU) of RhIG at 28 and 34 weeks is used.[52] Limited resources have not allowed for extension of this protocol to all subsequent pregnancies. The American Association of Blood Banks recommends that a repeat antibody screen be obtained before administration of antenatal RhIG, although the incidence of alloimmunization before 28 weeks is very low.[53] The cost-effectiveness of this practice has been questioned by the American College of Obstetricians and Gynecologists.[50] If a repeat antibody screen is to be undertaken, a maternal blood sample can be drawn at the same office visit as the RhIG injection. Although the administration of the exogenous anti-D will eventually result in a weakly positive titer, this will not occur in the short interval of several hours because of the slow absorption from the intramuscular site. Some experts recommend that a second dose of RhIG be given if the patient has not delivered by 40 weeks' gestation.

Although they have not been well studied, additional indications for the antepartum administration of RhIG include spontaneous abortion, elective abortion, ectopic pregnancy, genetic amniocentesis, chorion villous sampling, and FBS. A dose of 50 μg of RhIG is effective until 12 weeks' gestation because of the small volume of red cells in the fetoplacental circulation.[50] From a practical sense, most hospitals and offices do not stock this dose of RhIG; therefore, a standard dose of 300 μg is often given. Data supporting use of RhIG in other scenarios in which the fetoplacental barrier is breached are lacking. However, most experts agree that such events as hydatidiform mole, threatened abortion, fetal death in the second or third trimester, blunt trauma to the abdomen, and external cephalic version warrant strong consideration for the use of RhIG. The administration of RhIG after a postpartum tubal ligation is controversial. The possibility of a new partner in conjunction with the availability of in vitro fertilization would seem to make the use of RhIG in these situations prudent. RhIG is not effective once alloimmunization to the RhD antigen has occurred. Currently, prophylactic immune globulin preparations to prevent other forms of red cell alloimmunization, such as anti-K1 (Kell), do not exist.

Because the half-life of RhIG is approximately 16 days, 15% to 20% of patients receiving it at 28 weeks will have a very low anti-D titer (usually 2 or 4) detected at the time of admission for labor at term.[54] In North America, the recommendation is to administer 300 μg of RhIG within 72 hours after delivery if umbilical cord blood typing reveals an RhD+ infant.[50] This is sufficient to protect from sensitization secondary to an FMH of 30 mL of fetal whole blood. In the United Kingdom, 100 μg of RhIG is given at delivery.[53]

Approximately 1 in 1000 deliveries is associated with an excessive FMH; risk factors identify only 50% of these.[55,56] Routine screening of all women at the time of delivery for excessive FMH should therefore be undertaken. A qualitative yet sensitive test for FMH, the rosette test, is first performed. Results return as positive or negative. A negative result warrants administration of a standard dose of RhIG. If the rosette is positive, a Kleihauer-Betke stain or fetal cell stain using flow cytometry is undertaken. The percentage of fetal blood cells is multiplied by a factor of 50 to estimate the volume of the FMH. Because this calculation includes an inaccurate estimation of the maternal blood volume, the blood bank typically indicates that an additional dose of RhIG should be administered beyond the calculated amount. No more than five standard doses (1500 μg, 2.5 mL) of RhIG should be administered by the intramuscular route in one 24-hour period. Should a large dose of RhIG be necessary, an alternative method would be to give the entire calculated dose using the intravenous preparations of RhIG that are now available. The total dose should be calculated and administered in increments of 600 µg (3000 U) every 8 hours. Should RhIG be inadvertently omitted after delivery, it has been shown that some protection is provided by administration within 13 days; recommendations have been made to administer it as late as 28 days after delivery.[55] If delivery occurs less than 3 weeks from the administration of RhIG used for antenatal indications such as amniocentesis for fetal lung maturity or external cephalic version, a repeat dose is unnecessary unless a large FMH is detected at the time of delivery.[50] Despite the widespread acceptance of similar guidelines, studies from Scotland revealed that two thirds of rhesus-alloimmunized cases were secondary to antepartum sensitization, whereas an additional 13% were caused by failure to administer RhIG for the usual obstetric indications.[57]

Diagnostic Methods

Maternal Antibody Determination

The maternal titer is the first step in the evaluation of the RhD-sensitized patient. Previous methodologies using albumin or saline should no longer be practiced because they detect varying levels of IgM antibody. Because the pentamer structure of this class of antibody does not allow for transplacental passage, the contribution of IgM to the titer quantitation has no clinical relevance. The human antiglobulin titer (indirect Coombs) is used to determine the degree of alloimmunization, because it measures the maternal IgG response.

By convention, titer values are reported as the reciprocal of the last tube dilution that led to a positive agglutination reaction; that is, a titer of 16 is the equivalent of a dilution of 1:16. Variation in results between laboratories is not uncommon, because many commercial laboratories use enzymatic treatment of red cells to prevent failure of detection of low-titer samples. However, in a single laboratory, the titer should not vary by more than one dilution if the two samples are run in tandem. This means that an initial titer of 8 that returns at 16 may not represent a true increase in the amount of antibody in the maternal circulation. A critical titer is defined as the titer associated with a significant risk for fetal hydrops. If a critical titer is present, further fetal surveillance is required. This titer varies with the institution and the methodologies used; however, most centers use a critical value for anti-D between 8 and 32.

In the United Kingdom, quantitation of anti-D is undertaken through the use of an automated device known as an autoanalyzer. Red cell samples are mixed with agents that enhance agglutination by the anti-D antibodies. Agglutinated cells are separated from nonagglutinated cells and then lysed. The amount of released hemoglobin is then compared with an international standard; results are reported as international units (IU) per milliliter. Levels of less than 4 IU/mL are rarely associated with HDFN. In one series of 42 fetuses undergoing serial FBS, a maternal anti-D level of less than 15 IU/mL was associated with only mild fetal anemia.[58] An increase in the maternal anti-D level of more than 15 IU/mL over a 2- to 3-week interval was associated with the development of moderate to severe fetal anemia in approximately 50% of cases.

In Vitro Tests

Because measurements of maternal anti-D have been poor predictors of HDFN, there has been considerable interest in in vitro assays that might better predict fetal disease by mimicking the red cell destruction that occurs in the fetus.[59] Typically, maternal serum containing anti–red cell antibodies is mixed with adult red cells heterozygous for the specific antigen. These sensitized red cells are then combined with various types of reticuloendothelial cells, such as macrophages, monocytes, or lymphocytes. The degree of red cells hemolysis or activation of the reticuloendothelial cells is then quantitated. The three tests most commonly used are the antibody-dependent cell-mediated cytotoxicity (ADCC) assay, the monocyte monolayer assay, and the monocyte chemiluminescence test. In the ADCC assay, the release of chromium 51 from sensitized red cells previously incubated with this isotope is used as a measure of the in vitro destruction caused by the monocytes. The percentage of total monocytes involved in adherence or phagocytosis of red cells is assessed by microscopic examination in the monocyte monolayer assay. The chemiluminescence assay uses the photoactivity of luminol, a compound that generates light as it reacts with oxygen free radicals released from the activated monocytes.

Many of the original studies using these assays sought to predict the neonatal outcome of HDFN. In a multicenter trial using FBS to assess fetal disease, the percentage of phagocytosis in the monocyte monolayer assay was similar in antigen-negative fetuses; nonanemic, antigen-positive fetuses; and anemic, antigen-positive fetuses,[60] indicating that the monocyte monolayer assay was not useful to forecast the need for IUT. Zupanska and coworkers[61] studied the ability of the chemiluminescence and ADCC assays to predict a fetal hemoglobin deficit of more than 3 g/dL, their threshold for IUT, in 37 pregnancies with anti-D sensitization. The chemiluminescence test was 89% predictive, whereas the ADCC was 78% predictive; the former was associated with fewer false positive findings. Negative tests for the assays always predicted that FBS was not necessary.

These assays do not enjoy widespread use in the United States, although countries such as the Netherlands routinely use the ADCC performed at one central location (Central Laboratory of the Netherlands Red Cross) to decide when to proceed with invasive testing in the fetus.

Fetal Blood Typing through Genetics

Paternal zygosity plays an important role in the management of the red cell–alloimmunized pregnancy. In cases of a heterozygous paternal genotype, 50% of the fetuses will not express the involved red cell antigen and therefore will escape the hemolytic effects of the maternal anti–red cell antibody. In these cases, further maternal and fetal testing can be eliminated. Because the RhC/c and RhE/e antigens are inherited in a closely linked fashion to RhD, antisera for these antigens can be used with gene frequency tables based on ethnicity to determine the paternal zygosity at the RhD locus. Mathematic modeling should be employed to modify the incidence of heterozygosity based on the paternal history of previous RhD+ offspring.[62] As an example, a white partner whose serologic testing results indicate a *Dce* phenotype and who has no history of an RhD+ progeny, has a 94% chance of being heterozygous. A history of repeated RhD+ offspring, however, would markedly decrease the chance of a heterozygous state (Table 26-1). Ethnicity must be taken into account when calculating the likelihood of heterozygosity, because disparate results can be noted with similar serologic findings.

Direct paternal zygosity testing is now available through quantitative polymerase chain reaction (PCR) techniques.[63] The PCR signal intensities of *RHD* exons 5 and 7 are compared with internal control genes (exon 7 of the *RHCE* genes) to determine the heterozygous or homozygous paternal state for the *RHD* gene (Fig. 26-3). The assay has also proved effective in detecting the RhD pseudogene.

First described in 1993, amniocytes have become the primary source used to test the fetal blood type in cases of a heterozygous

TABLE 26-1 INCIDENCE OF PATERNAL HETEROZYGOSITY (%) BASED ON SEROLOGY, ETHNIC BACKGROUND, AND NUMBER OF PREVIOUS RhD-POSITIVE OFFSPRING

	White No. of RhD+ Infants						Black No. of RhD+ Infants						Hispanic No. of RhD+ Infants					
Serologic Type	**0**	**1**	**2**	**3**	**4**	**5**	**0**	**1**	**2**	**3**	**4**	**5**	**0**	**1**	**2**	**3**	**4**	**5**
DCce	90	82	69	53	36.0	22.0	41	26.0	15.0	8.0	4.0	2.0	85	74.0	59.0	42.0	26.0	15.0
DCe	9	5	2	1	0.6	0.3	19	11.0	6.0	3.0	1.0	0.7	5	2.0	1.0	0.6	0.3	0.1
DCEe	90	82	69	53	36.0	22.0	37	23.0	13.0	7.0	4.0	2.0	85	74.0	59.0	42.0	26.0	15.0
DcE	13	7	4	2	0.9	0.5	1	0.5	0.3	0.1	0.1	0.0	2	0.9	0.5	0.2	0.1	0.1
DCcEe	11	6	3	2	0.8	0.4	10	5.0	3.0	1.0	0.7	0.3	12	6.0	3.0	2.0	0.8	0.4
Dce	94	89	80	66	50.0	33.0	54	37.0	23.0	13.0	7.0	4.0	92	85.0	74.0	59.0	42.0	26.0

Reproduced with permission from Moise KJ: Modern management of rhesus alloimmunization in pregnancy. Obstet Gynecol 100:600, 2002. Elsevier Science Company, copyright 2002.

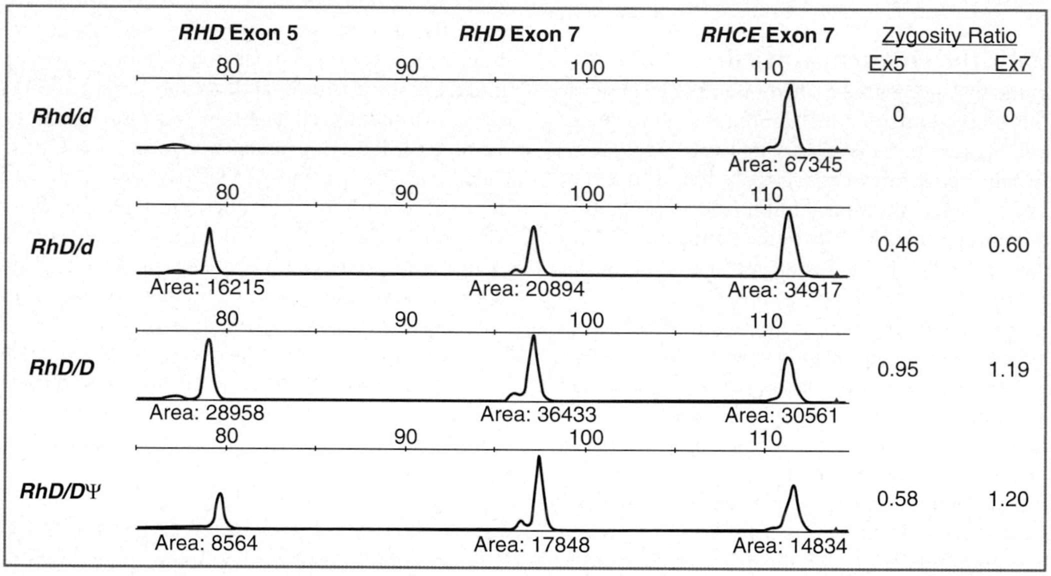

FIGURE 26-3 Paternal zygosity testing. Quantitative fluorescent polymerase chain reaction (PCR) was used to amplify exons 5 and 7 of the *RHD* gene as well as an internal control gene, exon 7 of the two *RHCE* genes. PCR products were analyzed on an automated sequencer. The ratio of *RHD* exon 5 or 7 peak areas was compared to the peak area derived from the two copies of exon 7 of the *RHCE* genes. *Upper panel: RHD* negative genotype (Rhd/d); no peak is seen for *RHD* exon 5 or *RHD* exon 7. *Upper middle panel: RHD* positive, heterozygous state (RhD/d); peaks for *RHD* exons 5 and 7 are approximately half of the peak area seen for the *RHCE* genes (ratios of 0.46 and 0.60). *Lower middle panel: RHD* positive, homozygous state (RhD/D); peaks for the RHD exons 5 and 7 are approximately equal to the peak area for the RHCE genes (ratios of 0.95 and 1.19). *Lower panel: RHD* positive, one copy of *RHD* gene and one copy of the RhD pseudogene (*RHDψ*) noted. The RHD exon 5 primers detect only *RHD* and not *RHDψ*, whereas the RHD exon 7 primers detect both *RHD* and *RHDψ*, explaining the copy number discrepancy in the *RHD*/D*ψ* sample (peak ratios of 0.58 and 1.20 versus the *RHCE* genes). (Courtesy of Daniel Bellissimo, PhD, Molecular Diagnostics Laboratory, The Blood Center of Wisconsin, with permission.)

paternal genotype.[64] Amniocentesis to detect fetal blood type actually assesses the fetal genotype instead of the fetal phenotype, which is the expression of the RhD antigen on the fetal red cells as determined by serology. Serologic fetal red cell typing can be performed on blood obtained by ultrasound-directed FBS, but this technique is associated with a rate of perinatal loss at least fourfold greater than with amniocentesis. Extensive experience with the use of amniocentesis for determining fetal blood type has revealed rare discrepancies. In the event of a DNA result that reveals an RhD– fetus when the fetus is RhD+ by serology, usual surveillance techniques would not be used and fetal loss can occur. In one series of 500 amniocenteses, this occurred in 1.5% of cases.[65] Aside from erroneous paternity, the most likely etiology for this inconsistency is a rearrangement at the paternal RhD gene locus. Such rearrangements have been documented in approximately 2% of individuals.[66] Checking of the paternal blood, the source of the fetal RhD gene, with the same PCR primers used on the amniotic fluid verifies that a gene rearrangement is not a potential source of error. For this reason, most laboratories that offer fetal red cell typing on amniotic fluid require an accompanying paternal blood sample. Multiplex PCR, which targets at least two different exons of the RhD gene, is used by many centers to decrease the chance of nondetection of a gene rearrangement (Fig. 26-4).

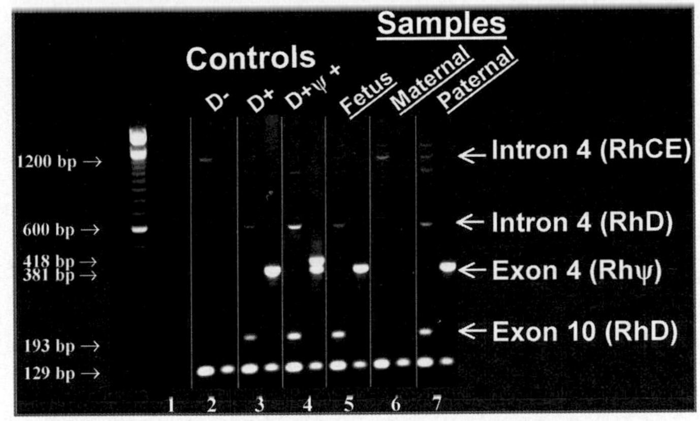

FIGURE 26-4 **Electrophoresis gel of maternal, paternal, and amniotic fluid analysis for fetal RhD testing using multiplex polymerase chain reaction.** Intron 4 of the *RHCE* gene (internal control), intron 4 and exon 10 of the *RHD* gene, and exon 4 of the RhD pseudogene (*RHDψ*) are used in the analysis. Lane numbers are indicated at bottom of figure. Lane 1, molecular weight ladder. Lane 2, RhD-negative control; a 1200-base pair (bp) band is noted, indicating *RHCE* amplification as internal control. Lane 3, RhD-positive control; the 1200-bp band for the *RHCE* gene is present, and additional bands of 600 bp (intron 4) and 193 bp (exon 10) are also noted, indicating the presence of the *RHD* gene. Lane 4, RhD/Dψ heterozygous control; 1200-bp (*RHCE*) as well as 600-bp and 193-bp (*RHD*) bands are noted. Additional bands are noted at 418 and 381 bp, indicating the presence of the Rh pseudogene. Lane 5, fetal sample, RhD positive: 1200-bp (*RHCE*) as well as 600-bp and 193-bp (*RHD*) bands are present, but the 381-bp band is noted only from exon 4, indicating absence of the Rh pseudogene. Lane 6, maternal sample, RhD-negative: only the 1200-bp band is noted (RHCE). No *RHD* or *RhDψ* bands are present. Lane 7, paternal sample, RhD-positive: bands are present at 1200 bp (*RHCE*), as well as 600 pb and 193 bp (*RHD*), but only 381 bp of exon 4 is present, indicating absence of the Rh pseudogene. (Courtesy of Daniel Bellissimo, PhD, Molecular Diagnostics Laboratory, The Blood Center of Wisconsin, with permission.)

In situations where paternity is not assured or there is no partner available to send a blood sample for confirmation of PCR primers, the result of an RhD– fetal blood type performed by amniocentesis should be considered suspect. Hopkins[67] assessed serial titers in patients with RhD alloimmunization who subsequently delivered RhD– offspring and noted that serial maternal titers rose by fourfold in less than 2% of cases. In situations of questionable paternity, a repeat maternal antiglobulin titer should be obtained 4 to 6 weeks after the results of the amniocentesis as a confirmatory strategy (Fig. 26-5). If a fourfold rise in antibody titer is noted, then an RhD– PCR result on amniotic fluid should be questioned. Repeat amniocentesis to evaluate the spectral analysis of amniotic fluid at 450 nm (ΔOD_{450}) or FBS to determine the fetal RhD status using serologic techniques should be considered.

If the maternal ethnicity is black, then the presence of a maternal pseudogene must be excluded. In this situation, the pregnant patient is RhD– on serologic testing, but the entire RhD gene is present. Because the fetus inherits one of its RhD genes from the mother, amniotic PCR testing would yield a false-positive result—that is, the fetus would be RhD+ by genotype testing but RhD– by serology. This could lead to unnecessary intervention with its inherent risks. For this reason, a maternal blood sample should also accompany the amniotic fluid sent for fetal RhD testing, in an effort to rule out the presence of a maternal RhD pseudogene. If the maternal sample is positive for this variant, then fetal testing for the pseudogene should also be performed (see Fig. 26-5).

Chorionic villus biopsy has been used for fetal red cell typing, but this technique should be discouraged in patients who wish to continue their pregnancy in the event that the fetus is found to be RhD+. Disruption of the chorionic villi during the procedure can result in FMH and a rise in maternal titer, thereby worsening the fetal disease.[68]

Noninvasive fetal testing for the RhD gene now enjoys widespread clinical use in Europe and only recently has become available in North America.[69] Cell-free fetal DNA is now known to be present in the maternal circulation as early as 38 days of gestation; by term, it comprises 6% of the total DNA pool.[70,71] The source of this DNA is thought to be apoptosis of placental trophoblasts; this would account for its relatively short half-life, measured in minutes after delivery. It is an attractive source for prenatal diagnosis, because there should not be any residual fetal DNA from previous gestations.[72] The use of free DNA to determine fetal RhD status was first reported by Lo and associates in 1998.[73] Since that time, numerous reports have appeared in the literature. Geifman-Holtzman and colleagues[74] compiled reports of more than 2000 patients for whom fetal RhD status was determined from free DNA in maternal plasma, with an accuracy of 97%. A single center in the Netherlands has reported a 99.4% accuracy in more than 1200 cases.[75] Noninvasive fetal RhCc, RhE, and Kell typing are now available at some European centers using free fetal DNA as well.[76]

Amniocentesis to Monitor the Severity of Hemolytic Disease of the Fetus and Newborn

Since it was first introduced to clinical practice by Bevis,[7] the ΔOD_{450} has been used to measure the level of bilirubin, an indirect indicator of the degree of fetal hemolysis. Liley[8] proposed a management scheme involving three zones based on gestational ages between 27 and 42 weeks. The Liley curve is useful for monitoring alloimmunized pregnancies, but extrapolation of Liley curves to gestational ages before 27 weeks has proved erroneous. Nicolaides and coworkers[77] correlated fetal hematologic values in 59 RhD-sensitized pregnancies between 18 and 25 weeks' gestation with ΔOD_{450} values on a Liley curve extrapolated to 18 weeks' gestation. They found that, if intervention were reserved for fetuses with ΔOD_{450} values in zone 3, 70% of cases of fetal anemia would not be detected. Even if all cases of fetal hydrops were excluded, 56% of cases of fetal anemia would still have been misdiagnosed. For a brief period after this report, many centers used FBS exclusively in cases of severe red cell alloimmunization if fetal assessment was indicated before 27 weeks' gestation. A modified ΔOD_{450} curve for such situations was proposed by Queenan and coworkers[78] from a series of 789 amniotic fluid samples obtained between 14 and 40 weeks' gestation (Fig. 26-6). Oepkes and associates[79] monitored 165 fetuses at risk for fetal anemia secondary to maternal red cell alloimmunization; 74 were subsequently found to exhibit severe anemia at the time of FBS. Serial ΔOD_{450} analysis using the Queenan curve was found to be superior to the Liley curve for the prediction of severe anemia (sensitivity, 81% versus 76%; specificity, 81% versus 77%). When limited to gestations of less than 27 weeks, the Queenan curve also proved to be more predictive than the modified Liley curve (sensitivity, 90% versus 84%).

If amniocentesis is used to monitor fetal disease, serial procedures are undertaken at intervals of 10 days to 2 weeks and continued until delivery to follow trends in the ΔOD_{450} values. Transplacental passage of the needle should be diligently avoided, because it can lead to FMH and a rise in maternal antibody titer. A rising or plateauing ΔOD_{450} value that approaches the IUT zone of the Queenan curve

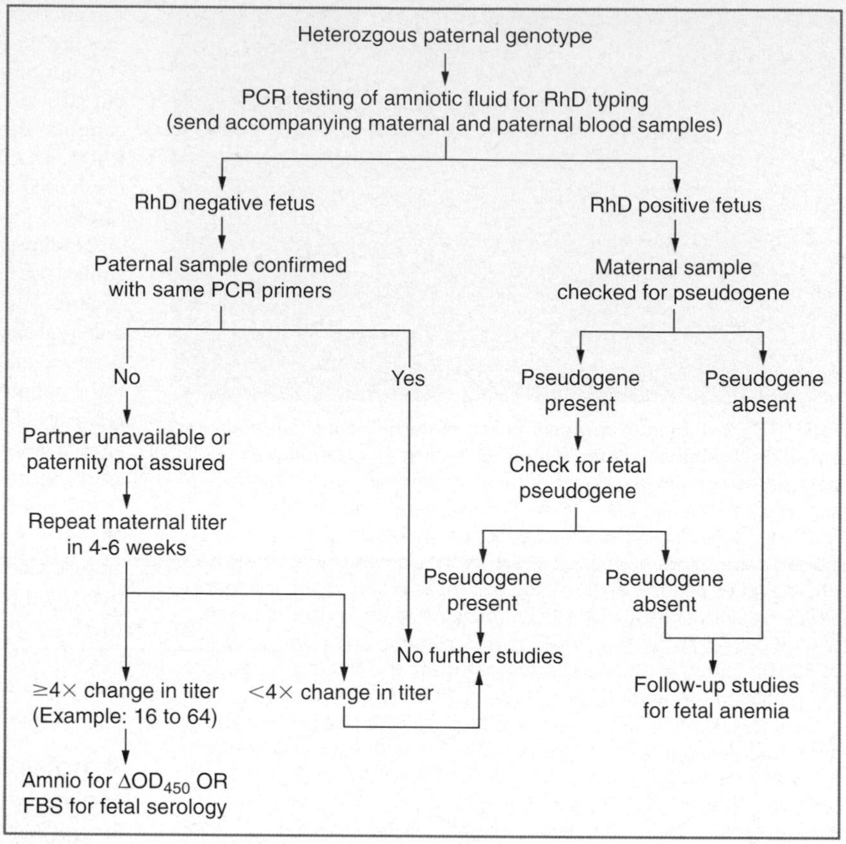

FIGURE 26-5 Algorithm for fetal RhD testing in the case of a heterozygous paternal phenotype. ΔOD_{450}, deviation in optical density at 450 nm wavelength; Amnio, amniocentesis; FBS, fetal blood sampling; PCR, polymerase chain reaction.

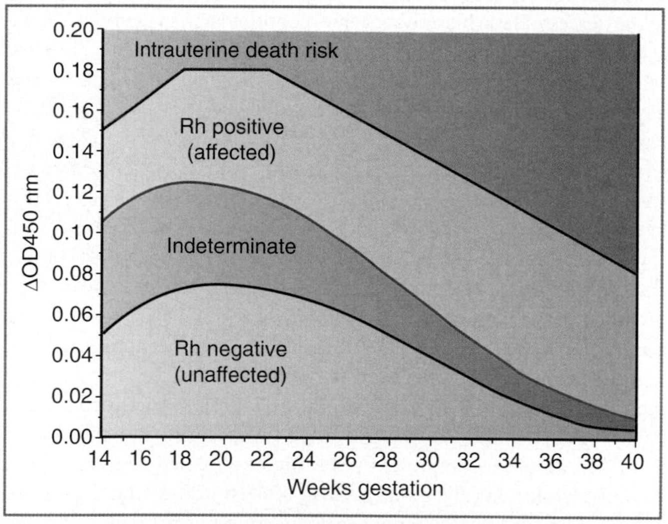

FIGURE 26-6 Queenan curve for monitoring of Rh-immunized pregnancies. ΔOD_{450}, deviation in amniotic fluid optical density at 450 nm wavelength. (With permission from Queenan JT, Tomai TP, Ural SH, et al: Deviation in amniotic fluid optical density at a wavelength of 450 nm in Rh-immunized pregnancies from 14 to 40 weeks' gestation: A proposal for clinical management. Am J Obstet Gynecol 168:1370, 1993. Mosby, Inc., copyright 2001.)

or reaches the 80th percentile of zone 2 of the Liley curve requires further investigation by FBS. After 37 weeks' gestation, fetal lung maturity testing may be assessed, because induction of labor can be considered with a determination of maturity, instead of further amniocenteses.

Fetal Blood Sampling

Ultrasound-directed FBS (also called percutaneous umbilical blood sampling, cordocentesis, or funipuncture) allows direct access to the fetal circulation to obtain important laboratory values such as Hct, direct Coombs, fetal blood type, reticulocyte count, and total bilirubin. Serial FBS has been proposed as a primary method of fetal surveillance after a maternal critical titer is reached. Weiner and coworkers[80] studied 128 red cell–alloimmunized pregnancies and described four patterns that could be used to predict fetal anemia based on fetal values for hematocrit (Hct), direct Coombs assay, and reticulocyte count. FBS is associated with a 1% to 2% rate of fetal loss and up to a 50% risk for FMH with subsequent worsening of the alloimmunization.[81] For these reasons, it is usually reserved for patients with elevated peak middle cerebral artery (MCA) Doppler velocities or elevated ΔOD_{450} values. However, if the fetal Hct is normal at the time of sampling, use of the direct Coombs and reticulocyte count may be of value to time subsequent procedures. Weiner[82] also noted that a fetal umbilical venous total serum bilirubin concentration greater than 3 mg/dL was associated with the development of severe fetal anemia or postnatal hyperbilirubinemia in 94% of cases. If a transplacental approach has been used for FBS, a maternal antibody titer should be repeated in 1 week. If a large increase is noted as a result of an anamnestic response, the interval to the next FBS should be reduced, because the onset of fetal anemia can be rapid in these circumstances. When FBS is indicated by other first-line diagnostic modalities, blood should be immediately available for IVT if fetal anemia is detected (Hct <30% or <2 standard deviations for gestational age).

Ultrasound

Ultrasound plays a key role in the management of the alloimmunized pregnancy. It should be used early in the pregnancy to establish the correct gestational age, because this parameter becomes important in determining such normative laboratory values as ΔOD_{450} levels and fetal hematologic values. Although hydrops fetalis can be easily detected with ultrasound, its presence represents the end-stage state of fetal anemia. Therefore, many investigators have sought alternative ultrasound parameters that could predict the early onset of anemia. In one large series, fetal abdominal circumference, head-to-abdomen circumference ratio, intraperitoneal volume, intrahepatic and extrahepatic umbilical vein diameter, and placental thickness were assessed to predict severe fetal anemia, defined as a fetal hemoglobin concentration of less than 5 g/dL.[83] Placental thickness and intraperitoneal volume detected only one fourth of cases, and the other parameters detected no more than 10% of severe cases.

Because the fetal liver is a site of extramedullary hematopoiesis in cases of severe fetal anemia, ultrasound has been used to measure the length of the right lobe as a marker of hepatomegaly.[84,85] In one series, a liver length greater than the 95th percentile correctly predicted fetal anemia in 64 (93%) of 69 cases. The spleen is also a site of extramedullary hematopoiesis and destruction and sequestration of sensitized red cells in cases of severe HDFN. Determination of a splenic perimeter ([length + width] × 1.57) greater than 2 standard deviations above the mean was predictive of severe fetal anemia in 94% and 100% of cases in two studies.[86,87] Despite these data, hepatic length and splenic perimeter have not enjoyed widespread use for noninvasive surveillance in cases of red cell alloimmunization.

Many investigations have attempted to use Doppler ultrasound to correlate blood velocities in various fetal vessels to the level of fetal hemoglobin. Sites of study have included the descending aorta,[88] umbilical vein,[89] splenic artery,[90] and common carotid artery.[91] The rationale for this approach is that decreasing fetal hemoglobin is associated with a lower blood viscosity, which produces less shearing in blood vessels, resulting in higher blood velocities. Alternatively, the increased cardiac output associated with fetal anemia may contribute to the higher blood velocities. Vyas and coworkers[92] first described Doppler velocity in the MCA to detect fetal anemia. Using the intensity-weighted, time-averaged mean velocity of the MCA, these authors found one of the best correlations with fetal hemoglobin reported to date ($R = -0.77$). However, only 50% of the cases of fetal anemia were detected. Measurement of the peak systolic velocity in the fetal MCA has subsequently been shown to be the most accurate Doppler method for determination of fetal anemia. In the initial report by Mari and coworkers,[93] normative data for gestational age was established. Using receiver operating characteristic curve (ROC) analysis, a threshold value of 1.5 multiples of the median (MoM) was used to predict moderate to severe anemia (<0.65 MoM for fetal hemoglobin) (Fig. 26-7). These authors calculated that more than 70% of invasive tests could be avoided if this modality were used to monitor alloimmunized pregnancies.

A meta-analysis of noninvasive monitoring of alloimmunized pregnancies reported that the diagnostic test with the highest methodologic quality was the peak MCA velocity (positive likelihood ratio, 8.45; 95% confidence interval [CI], 4.7 to 15.6); negative likelihood ratio, 0.02 (CI, 0.001 to 0.25).[94] In the first multicenter intent-to-treat prospective study, the peak MCA velocity proved accurate to detect moderate to severe anemia in 98% of fetuses from whom longitudinal measurements were obtained.[95] In the two cases of anemia that were not detected (neonatal hemoglobin concentrations, 5 and 8.2 g/dL), intervals of 17 and 21 days, respectively, had elapsed between the last Doppler study and delivery. In a prospective series, Oepkes and coworkers[79] found that the peak MCA Doppler value was superior to ΔOD_{450} measurements using both the Queenan and Liley curves in the detection of severe fetal anemia. The accuracy of MCA Doppler assessment was 85%, compared with 76% for the Liley curve and 81% for the Queenan curve.

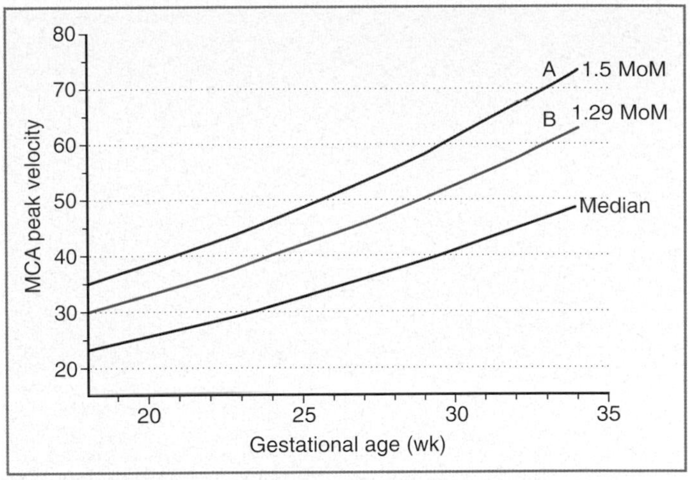

FIGURE 26-7 Middle cerebral artery (MCA) Doppler peak velocities based on gestational age. Zone A indicates moderate to severe anemia; zone B, mild anemia. MoM, multiples of the median. (Reproduced with permission from Moise KJ: Modern management of Rhesus alloimmunization in pregnancy. Obstet Gynecol 100:600, 2002. Elsevier Science Company, copyright 2002.)

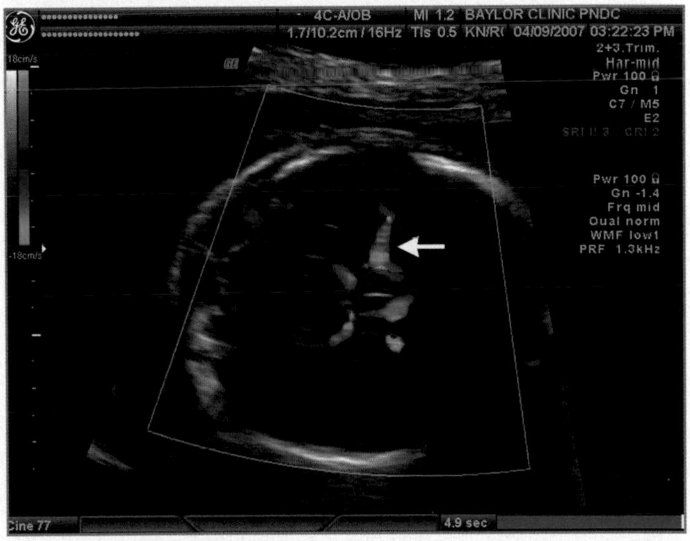

FIGURE 26-8 Middle cerebral artery showing location of Doppler gate. Arrow indicates location for correctly measuring the peak velocity.

The fetal MCA closest to the maternal skin should be evaluated using a minimal angle of insonation; angle correction can be used if necessary (Fig. 26-8). If the MCA vessel on the opposite side of the fetal head appears to provide a better angle for insonation, studies have shown that the results are comparable.[96] The Doppler gate is placed over the vessel just where it bifurcates from the carotid siphon. Placement of the gate on the more peripheral aspects of the MCA vessel will result in a false depression of the true peak systolic velocity. Color Doppler aids in determining the correct location. During the measurement, the Doppler baseline should be adjusted close to zero; the pulse

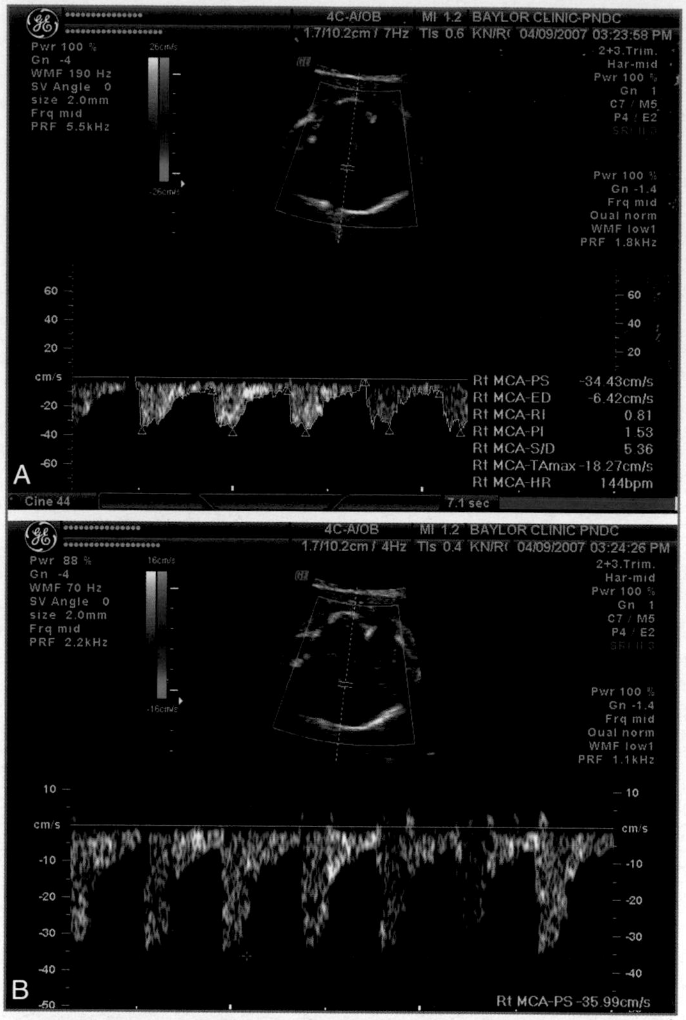

FIGURE 26-9 Optimization of Doppler parameters. **A,** Baseline and pulse repetition frequency (PRF) not optimized; automated software is used to measure a peak velocity of 34 cm/sec. **B,** Doppler baseline changed to 10 cm/sec, PRF optimized; manual caliper is used to measure a peak velocity of 36 cm/sec.

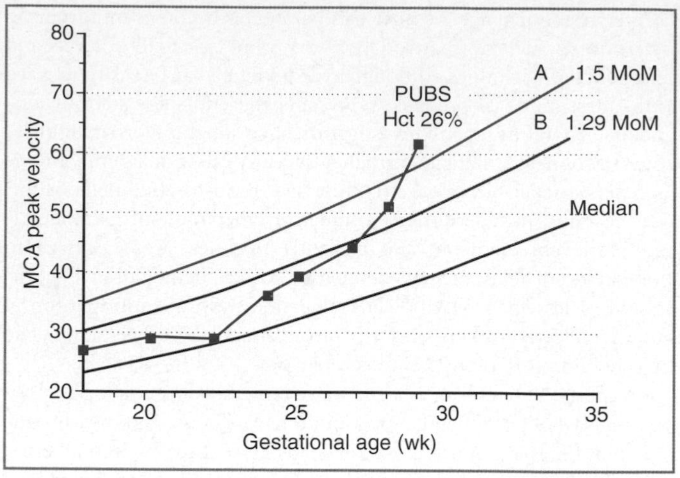

FIGURE 26-10 Serial middle cerebral artery (MCA) Doppler ultrasound studies. Zone A indicates moderate to severe anemia; zone B, mild anemia. Hct, hematocrit; MoM, multiples of the median; PUBS, percutaneous umbilical blood sampling.

repetition frequency (PRF) should then be optimized to the approximate peak velocity (Fig. 26-9). These adjustments optimize the appearance of the waveform and make the true peak velocity more discernible. Peak systolic measurements should be made with the use of electronic calipers; automated software to trace the waveform typically underestimates the true peak velocity. Measurements can be initiated as early as 16 to 18 weeks' gestation and should be performed weekly (Fig. 26-10). Values should be reported in MoM to account for changes in gestational age. Internet-based calculators are available (see http://www.perinatology.com/calculators2.htm). After 35 weeks' gestation, the false-positive rate for the prediction of anemia increases, presumably secondary to fetal heart rate accelerations as a result of changes in the fetal behavioral state.[95,97] In cases of a normal MCA peak velocity after 35 weeks, serial weekly measurements may be continued until induction of labor is scheduled.

Because a learning curve is associated with performing MCA Doppler measurements, Mari[98] suggested that a center having minimal experience with this technique should perform it in conjunction with serial amniocenteses for ΔOD_{450}. MCA Doppler assessment has revolutionized the care of the RhD-sensitized pregnancy by minimizing invasive diagnostic testing.[99]

Summary of Clinical Management

The approach using the available diagnostic tools is based on the patient's past history of fetal or neonatal manifestations of HDFN. As a general rule, the patient's first RhD-sensitized pregnancy involves minimal fetal or neonatal disease, and subsequent gestations are associated with a worsening degree of anemia.

First Affected Pregnancy

Once sensitization to the RhD antigen is detected (Fig. 26-11), maternal titers are repeated every month until approximately 24 weeks; titers are repeated every 2 weeks thereafter. Paternal blood is drawn to determine RhD status and zygosity. In the case of an RhD− paternal blood type, further maternal and fetal monitoring is unwarranted as long as paternity is assured (see Fig. 26-5).

Once a critical titer is reached (usually 32), the MCA peak systolic velocity is measured every week starting at about 24 weeks' gestation. MCA Doppler assessments may be started as early as 18 weeks' gestation if the maternal titer is significantly elevated (≥128). If a perinatal center skilled in the MCA Doppler technique is not geographically nearby, serial amniocenteses for ΔOD_{450} may be initiated and repeated at intervals of 10 days to 2 weeks. The Queenan curve should be used to analyze the results. In cases of a heterozygous paternal phenotype, an amniotic fluid sample along with maternal and paternal blood samples should be sent to a DNA reference laboratory at the time of the first amniocentesis to determine the fetal RhD status (this can be done at 24 weeks if one is following the Doppler protocol). If an RhD− result returns, further maternal and fetal testing can be eliminated.

If there is evidence of an RhD+ fetus (homozygous paternal phenotype or RhD+ fetus by PCR testing on amniotic fluid), serial MCA Doppler measurements are continued weekly. If the peak MCA exceeds 1.5 MoM (or if the ΔOD_{450} value on serial amniocenteses enters the upper aspect of the Rh+ affected zone of the Queenan curve), one should perform cordocentesis, with blood readied for IUT if the fetal Hct is found to be less than 30%.

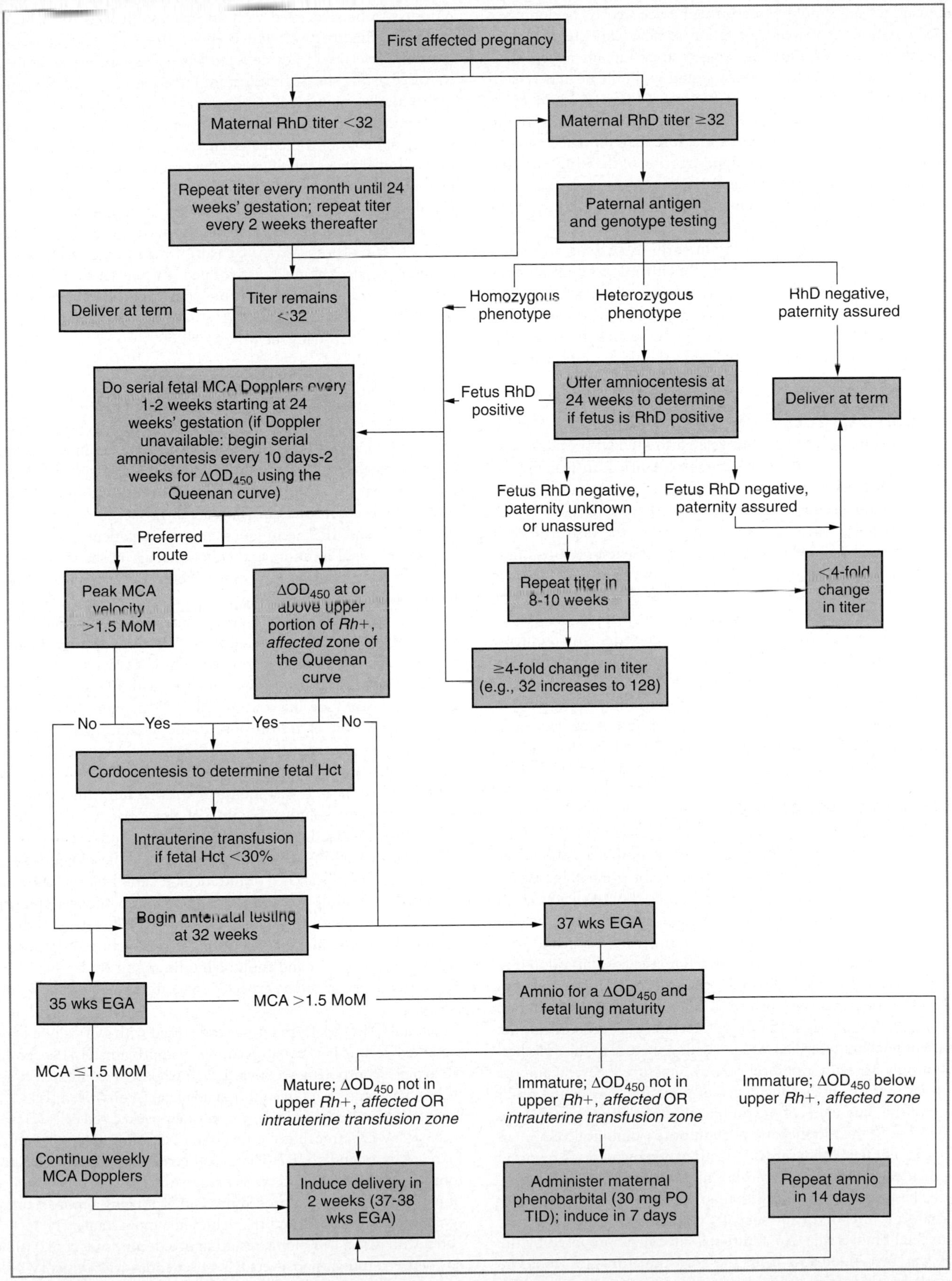

FIGURE 26-11 **Algorithm for overall clinical management of the first red cell–sensitized gestation.** ΔOD_{450}, deviation in optical density at 450 nm wavelength; amnio, amniocentesis; EGA, estimated gestational age; Hct, hematocrit; MCA, middle cerebral artery; MOM, multiples of the median. (Modified from Moise KJ: Diagnosis, management, and prevention of rhesus (Rh) alloimmunization. In UpToDate, Rose BD (ed): UpToDate, Wellesley, MA, 2008. Copyright 2008 UpToDate, Inc. For more information visit www.uptodate.com.)

Antenatal testing should be performed twice weekly, beginning at 32 weeks' gestation. At 35 weeks' gestation, serial weekly MCA Doppler assessments can be continued as long as they remain at less than 1.5 MoM. Induction at 37 to 38 weeks' gestation should be undertaken. If the MCA Doppler measurement is greater than 1.5 MoM at 35 weeks, amniocentesis for ΔOD_{450} should be considered because of the high false-positive rate of the Doppler measurement for detecting fetal anemia. If the ΔOD_{450} is below the upper portion of the RhD+ affected zone of the Queenan curve and fetal lung maturity is noted, labor should be induced in 2 weeks to allow time for hepatic maturity. If the ΔOD_{450} is at or above the upper portion of the RhD+ affected zone of the Queenan curve and fetal lung immaturity is present, treatment with 7 days of maternal phenobarbital (see Other Treatment Modalities) to enhance fetal hepatic maturity should be considered, with induction in 1 week. Finally, if the ΔOD_{450} is below the upper portion of the RhD+ affected zone of the Queenan curve and the fetal lungs are found to be immature, amniocentesis should be repeated in 2 weeks.

Previously Affected Fetus or Infant

If there is a history of perinatal loss related to HDFN, previous need for IUT, or previous need for neonatal exchange transfusions, the patient should be referred to a tertiary care center with experience in management of the severely alloimmunized pregnancy (Fig. 26-12). In these cases, maternal titers are not predictive of the degree of fetal anemia. In the case of a heterozygous paternal phenotype, an amniocentesis at 15 weeks' gestation to determine the fetal RhD status is indicated. The preferred method of surveillance is serial MCA Doppler measurements initiated at 18 weeks' gestation. If Doppler studies are not available at an otherwise experienced center, serial amniocenteses for measurement of ΔOD_{450} may be used, with the Queenan curve for reference values. If a rising value for peak MCA Doppler velocity greater than 1.5 MoM or a rising ΔOD_{450} value into the upper portion of the Rh+ affected zone of the Queenan curve is found, cordocentesis is recommended with blood readied for IUT if the fetal Hct is found to be less than 30%.

Intrauterine Transfusion

ACCESS SITE

The cord insertion proximate to the fetal umbilicus should be avoided because vagal innervation is thought to be present, increasing the likelihood of fetal bradycardia. Weiner and coworkers[81] also noted that puncture of the midsegment of the umbilical cord was associated with a 2.5-fold higher incidence of fetal bradycardia, compared with puncture at the placental insertion. Therefore, the cord insertion into the placenta is the preferred site for access. The vessel of interrogation should be the umbilical vein instead of one of the umbilical arteries. In one series of 750 diagnostic or therapeutic FBS procedures, the incidence of fetal bradycardia was 21% with puncture of the umbilical artery but only 3% with umbilical venous puncture.[81] Several authors conjectured that this higher incidence of puncture may be the result of spasm of the muscularis of the umbilical artery. Other centers have advocated use of the intrahepatic portion of the umbilical vein in an effort to prevent fetal bradycardia. Nicolini and coworkers[100] reported a 2.3% incidence of fetal bradycardia using this approach in 214 procedures. These authors proposed that absence of the umbilical artery at the anatomic level of the intrahepatic vein explained their low incidence of fetal bradycardia. An additional advantage proposed by the authors was that blood loss from the cord puncture site would be minimized by absorption from the peritoneal cavity. Despite these theoretical advantages, IUTs using the intrahepatic vein have been reported to be associated with an increase in fetal stress hormones (noradrenaline, cortisol, and β-endorphin).[101,102] Similar changes in hormone levels were not detected when the cord placental insertion was used as the site of transfusion. Puncture of the intrahepatic vein is technically more challenging than use of the placental insertion, predominantly because of fetal movement. The fetus must present with its spine toward the maternal back to allow access. Most centers in the United States therefore use the umbilical cord insertion into the placenta as the primary site of access for IUT. However, in cases of poor visualization, use of the intrahepatic vein is an option.

Direct cardiac puncture has been reported as a method of access for IUT. It has been associated with a high rate of fetal death, and therefore its use cannot be advocated. In one series of 158 cases of diagnostic cardiocentesis for the prenatal diagnosis of hemoglobinopathies, the corrected fetal loss rate was 5.6%, significantly higher than the 1% loss rate usually identified for FBS.[103]

METHOD OF TRANSFUSION

Until the direct IVT was introduced in the mid-1980s, the IPT was the method of IUT for almost 20 years. With the advent of ultrasound-directed FBS, direct transfusion of cells into the umbilical circulation became the preferred method for IUT. Experience in hydropic fetuses indicated that the absorption of transfused red cells from the peritoneal cavity is compromised. Harman and colleagues[104] compared the direct IVT and IPT techniques, matching patients for severity of disease, placental location, and gestational age at the start of transfusions. Several important outcome differences were noted. When the fetuses were divided into nonhydropic and hydropic groups at the time of the first transfusion, a 13% greater survival was observed in nonhydropic fetuses for IVT compared with IPT; in the hydropic fetuses, the rate of survival was almost doubled with IVT. IVT resulted in fewer neonatal exchange transfusions compared with IPT and a shorter stay in the intensive care nursery. Direct IVT therefore has become the preferred method of transfusion of the anemic fetus (Fig. 26-13). Initial interest in performing the IVT by an exchange technique, much like neonatal exchange transfusions, waned after further experience with the direct IVT. It was soon realized that the fetus could tolerate large transfusion volumes because of the capacity of the placental vasculature to vasodilate. The IPT remains a practical method for delivery of red cells to the nonhydropic fetus if there is difficulty with access to the umbilical cord or intrahepatic umbilical vein. Bowman[105] proposed a formula for calculating the intraperitoneal transfusion volume that has withstood the test of time. The volume of red cells to be infused (in milliliters) is calculated by subtracting 20 from the gestational age in weeks and multiplying the result by 10. Blood in the peritoneal reservoir can be expected to be absorbed over a 7- to 10-day period.

Serial Hct values from fetuses transfused with IVTs alone revealed a marked decline between procedures of approximately 1% per day.[106] To avoid this problem, we investigated whether a combined IPT/IVT technique would result in a more stable fetal Hct between IUTs.[107] The technique involved administering enough packed red cells (Hct, 75% to 85%) by IVT to achieve a final fetal Hct of 35% to 40%; this was followed by a standard IPT. The hypothesis was that the intraperitoneal infusion of blood would serve as a reservoir, allowing the slow absorption of red cells between procedures and producing a more stable Hct. A combined direct IVT and IPT achieved a more stable fetal Hct compared with direct IVT alone, resulting in a decline in Hct of 0.01% per day between transfusions, versus 1.14% per day with direct IVT alone. Although these data suggest several theoretical advantages of a combined transfusion technique, most centers exclusively use the direct

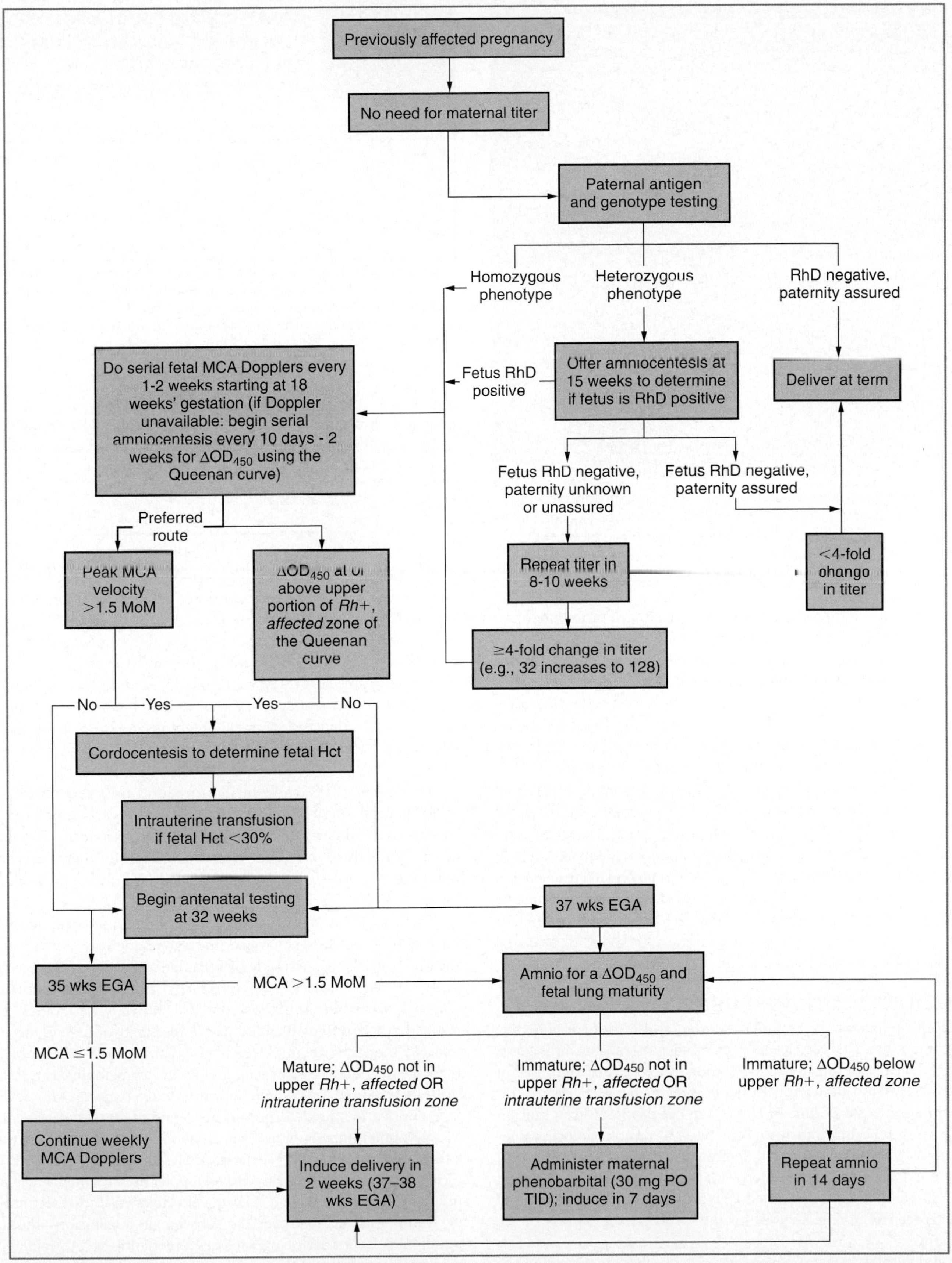

FIGURE 26-12 **Algorithm for overall clinical management of a subsequent red cell–sensitized gestation.** ΔOD_{450}, deviation in optical density at 450 nm wavelength; amnio, amniocentesis; EGA, estimated gestational age; Hct, hematocrit; MCA, middle cerebral artery; MOM, multiples of the median. (Modified from Moise KJ: Diagnosis, management, and prevention of rhesus (Rh) alloimmunization. In UpToDate, Rose BD (ed): UpToDate, Wellesley, MA, 2008. Copyright 2008 UpToDate, Inc. For more information visit www.uptodate.com.)

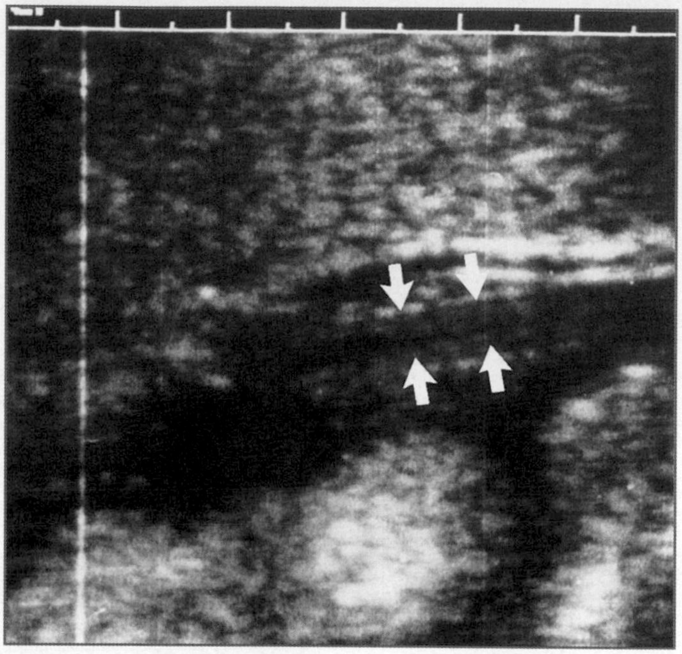

FIGURE 26-13 Direct intravascular transfusion through the umbilical vein. Arrows indicate outer walls of the vein. Echoes in the vein are the result of the streaming of infused red blood cells. Placental cord insertion is seen to the left of the arrows.

IVT, citing the need for two punctures and prolonged procedure times as the disadvantages of a combined approach.

Data on IUTs in twin gestations are limited to case reports. In one series of nine pregnancies complicated by RhD alloimmunization, five required IUT.[108] In four of the five cases, the twins were dizygotic based on first-trimester ultrasound. In one case, only one fetus was RhD+, illustrating the need to sample each fetus for antigen testing. In one case of monozygotic gestation, the IUT of one fetus was quickly followed by movement of donor red blood cells through intraplacental anastomoses, as illustrated by a positive Kleihauer-Betke stain at the time of FBS of the second twin. In subsequent IUTs, the transfusion of only one member of the twin pair resulted in adequate levels of hemoglobin in both twins. Therefore, caution against overtransfusion should be observed in the monozygotic gestation. The intrahepatic portion of the umbilical vein may be the preferred target for vascular access when transfusing a twin gestation if the corresponding placental cord insertions are difficult to identify.

AMOUNT TO TRANSFUSE

The end point for the completion of an IUT varies considerably. Most centers use a target Hct to decide when a transfusion is completed. Advocates of direct IVT often transfuse to a final Hct value of 50% to 65%. This allows a reasonable interval between procedures based on a projected decline in Hct of 1% per day. However, caution should be exercised in transfusing the fetus to nonphysiologic values for Hct. Welch and coworkers[109] demonstrated that a marked rise in whole blood viscosity is associated with fetal Hct values greater than 50%. Centers that use a combined IVT/IPT technique usually choose a final target Hct of 35% to 40% for the intravascular portion of the procedure.

Several authors have proposed formulas to calculate the volume of red blood cells to be transfused. The method of Mandelbrot and coworkers[110] requires calculation of the fetoplacental volume (mL) from the ultrasound estimate of the fetal weight by multiplying the weight in grams by a factor of 0.14. The volume of red cells in milliliters to be transfused is then calculated by the following formula:

$$V_{\text{transfused}} = \frac{V_{\text{fetoplacental}}\,(\text{Hct}_{\text{final}} - \text{Hct}_{\text{initial}})}{\text{Hct}_{\text{transfused blood}}}$$

Giannina and coworkers[111] proposed a simpler method of calculating the volume of packed red cells needed for IUT. Assuming an Hct of approximately 75% for the donor unit, a series of transfusion coefficients were determined for raising the initial fetal Hct to a desired final value (Table 26-2). The operator simply multiplies the coefficient by the ultrasound estimation of fetal weight in grams to calculate the volume of the transfusion in milliliters needed to achieve the final desired fetal Hct. This practical approach is used exclusively at our center.

TABLE 26-2 COEFFICIENT FOR CALCULATING VOLUME OF PACKED RED BLOOD CELLS NEEDED FOR INTRAUTERINE TRANSFUSION

Target Increase in Fetal Hematocrit (%)	Transfusion Coefficient
10	0.02
15	0.03
20	0.04
25	0.05
30	0.06

Reproduced with permission from Moise KJ, Whitecar PW: Antenatal therapy for haemolytic disease. In Hadley A, Soothill P (eds): Alloimmune Disorders of Pregnancy: Anaemia, Thrombocytopenia and Neutropenia in the Fetus and Newborn. Cambridge, UK, Cambridge University Press, 2002, p 182. Copyright 2002.

After the first IUT, subsequent procedures are scheduled at 14-day intervals until suppression of fetal erythropoiesis is noted on Kleihauer-Betke stain or fetal cell stain using flow cytometry. This usually occurs by the third IUT. Thereafter, the interval for repeat procedures (usually 3 to 4 weeks) can be determined based on the decline in Hct for the individual fetus.

The peak MCA velocity can be used to determine the transfusion interval.[112] In 64 fetuses that had undergone one IUT, a threshold for the MCA of 1.69 MoM yielded a sensitivity of 100% and a specificity of 94% for the prediction of severe fetal anemia (fetal hemoglobin <0.55 MoM) at the time of the second IUT. An MCA value of 1.32 MoM resulted in a sensitivity of 100% with a specificity of 63% in the ability to detect moderate anemia (fetal hemoglobin, 0.65 to 0.55 MoM). The rheology of the mixture of fetal and adult hemoglobins as a result of the transfused red cells would appear to make the peak MCA velocity less sensitive for the detection of moderate to severe fetal anemia. If MCA Doppler ultrasonography is used to time the second transfusion, a threshold of 1.32 MoM for the peak MCA should be used. Although serial monitoring with weekly MCA Doppler measurements may prove useful in timing the second IUT, the effectiveness of this technique in determining when to undertake subsequent transfusions should be questioned. In one series of 39 fetuses undergoing MCA peak Doppler measurements before a third IUT, a threshold value of 1.5 MoM failed to detect 5 cases of severe anemia and 4 of the 7 cases of moderate anemia.[113]

The Severely Anemic Early-Second-Trimester Fetus

The severely anemic fetus at 18 to 24 weeks' gestation presents a special challenge to the perinatologist. Often, technical limitations do not allow ready access to the fetal circulation through cordocentesis. Kilby and colleagues[114] reported on six pregnancies with a history of severe fetal anemia and hydrops before 20 weeks' gestation; perinatal mortality was 60% with attempted IUTs. In the subsequent pregnancies, IPTs were initiated at 16 weeks' gestation until IVTs could be undertaken at 22 weeks; this approach resulted in perinatal survival in five of six cases. The severely anemic second-trimester fetus is less able to adapt to the acute correction of its anemia by IVT, resulting in a higher perinatal mortality rate. An increase of greater than 10 mm Hg in umbilical venous pressure at the conclusion of an IVT correctly predicted fetal death within 24 hours with a sensitivity of 80%.[115] This finding may be the result of cardiac failure in these fetuses secondary to an acute change in viscosity associated with correction of the fetal Hct into the normal range. Radunovic and coworkers[116] reported 37% mortality within 72 hours after IVT in fetuses presenting with severe anemia and hydrops. These authors recommended that, in the severely anemic fetus, the final post-transfusion Hct after IVT should not exceed a value of 25% or a fourfold increase from the pretransfusion value.

If severe anemia occurs in the fetus at less than 24 weeks' gestation, a stepwise progression in correction of the fetal Hct should be undertaken, using the fourfold rule for increase in Hct at the time of the first procedure. A repeat IVT is performed within 48 hours to correct the fetal Hct into the normal range; the third procedure is scheduled in 7 to 10 days. Thereafter, repeat transfusions are undertaken based on the results of fetal Hct and Kleihauer-Betke stain. If a combined procedure is used, an IPT should not be undertaken until there is resolution of fetal hydrops, owing to impaired absorption associated with this condition. A stepwise correction of the Hct in cases of severe fetal anemia after 24 weeks' gestation is rarely necessary, because these fetuses can compensate for an acute change in Hct into the normal range.

Adjunctive Measures

The safety of fetal transfusion is enhanced by the use of fetal paralysis during the procedure. Before this modification, fetal movement often resulted in injury to fetal viscera during IPT or umbilical cord damage during IVT. Fetal paralysis was first introduced by de Crespigny and colleagues[117] in Australia. Initial use in the United States involved the intramuscular injection of D-tubocurarine into the fetal thigh under ultrasound guidance.[118] Later, pancuronium bromide was used intravascularly.[119] More recently, short-acting agents such as atracurium besylate and vecuronium bromide have been used.[120,121] The latter agents do not appear to cause the fetal tachycardia and loss of short-term heart rate variability associated with pancuronium.[122] A vecuronium dose of 0.1 mg/kg of the ultrasound-estimated fetal weight produces almost immediate cessation of fetal movement after intravascular injection at the start of the IUT. Fetal paralysis can be expected to last 1 to 2 hours. No untoward effects have been observed in neonates treated in this manner. In cases of anterior placentation, some centers do not routinely use fetal paralysis. Anecdotally, we have noted cord trauma resulting from fetal movement even in this scenario; therefore, we use vecuronium in all cases of IUT.

Prophylactic antibiotics have not been studied in association with IUT but are used by many centers. A broad-spectrum cephalosporin with coverage that includes gram-positive skin flora would appear to be appropriate.

Source of Red Blood Cells

Red cells used for IUT must undergo the same rigorous testing that occurs for any allogeneic donation. In the United States, this includes a written questionnaire that inquires about illicit substance abuse, high-risk sexual behavior, and travel outside of the continental United States. Serum testing for antibodies to syphilis, hepatitis B core antigen, human immunodeficiency viruses (HIV) types 1 and 2, hepatitis C virus, and human lymphotropic viruses types I and II, as well as testing for the p24 antigen of the HIV, the hepatitis B surface antigen, and alanine aspartate transferase, is undertaken. Additional testing by nucleic acid amplification for the HIV, hepatitis C virus, and West Nile virus is also done. In the United Kingdom, all donors are screened for the hepatitis B surface antigen and antibodies against HIV types 1 and 2, hepatitis C virus, and syphilis. In both countries, red cells to be used for IUT are often cytomegalovirus (CMV) seronegative or leukocyte reduced to decrease the risk of transmitting CMV. A fresh unit is preferred to stored blood, to enhance the level of 2,3-diphosphoglycerate. Standards in the United Kingdom require that red cells used for IUT have a shelf life of less than 5 days. A 1997 review reported that six cases of graft-versus-host reaction have been reported in infants who underwent IUT.[123] Bohm and colleagues[124] proposed that this was due to the induction of immune tolerance to engrafting lymphocytes that gained entry into the fetal circulation through large volumes of blood infused during IUTs. The standards of the British Blood Transfusion Task Force[125] and the American Association of Blood Banks[126] require that red cell units for IUT undergo γ-irradiation using 25 Gy to prevent graft-versus-host reaction. Leukodepletion is required in the United Kingdom. It is not routinely practiced in the United States but is often used to reduce CMV risk and will probably be universally accepted soon.

Maternal blood donation is an excellent source of red cells for IUT. In a series of 21 patients, up to six units of blood per patient were harvested for IUT.[127] No serious maternal or fetal effects were noted. Theoretical advantages to the use of maternal blood include a decreased risk for sensitization to new red cell antigens, a longer circulating half-life in the fetus because of the fresh source of cells, and a decreased risk for transmission of viral agents. Vietor and coworkers[128] investigated the source of new red cell antibodies in 91 patients undergoing 280 IUTs. Twenty-six percent of the women developed new antibodies. In 14 cases, the source of the sensitizing antigen could be determined; in one fifth of these cases, donor red cells carried the involved antigen. Therefore, it appears that the use of maternal blood as the source of red cells for IUT would theoretically prevent the development of new anti–red cell antibodies in 5% of cases.

In a study of the fetal effects of maternal red cells ($n = 76$) versus unrelated donor red cells ($n = 213$) for IUT,[129] the fetal Hct did not decline as rapidly when maternal red cells were used; however, this difference did not manifest until after 33 weeks' gestation. Infants who received maternal blood required fewer neonatal transfusions than those who received unrelated donor cells. The authors conjectured that this finding could be related to an increased maternal reticulocytosis that probably occurs secondary to repeated blood donation. Such reticulocytosis would result in a younger population of red cells with a longer half-life in the fetus. They concluded that maternal red cells were preferred over unrelated donor red cells because they offered the potential advantage of decreasing the total number of IUTs necessary for the treatment of a particular fetus. To date, no study has compared maternal versus unrelated donor red cells in regard to the risk of fetal viral infection.

In a maternal blood donation program, if IUTs are likely, the patient can donate a unit of red cells after the first trimester. The unit can be separated into two smaller aliquots and refrigerated for up to 42 days. If not used by this time interval, the unit can then be frozen for use for up to 10 years. Patients should be supplemented with iron therapy (324 mg ferrous sulfate twice daily) and folate (1 mg daily) in addition to prenatal vitamins. The left lateral recumbent position should be used during the donation, and the donated volume should be replaced with isotonic intravenous fluids. Fetal monitoring during the procedure is unnecessary.[130] A standard volume of 450 ± 45 mL is taken, because subsequent processing will markedly reduce the final volume available for IUT. The blood is washed several times to remove the offending antibody present in any contaminating plasma. The use of maternal blood in the CMV-seropositive patient is controversial. Dormant CMV virus is noted to reside in the polymorphonuclear leukocytes. Both leukoreduction and washing have been demonstrated to be effective mechanisms to reduce transmission of CMV.[131] For this reason, use of maternal CMV-seropositive blood, after careful counseling of the patient, can be considered. Finally, the use of ABO-incompatible maternal red cells for IUT has raised concern. With fetal typing now available at the first FBS, situations may arise in which the patient is found to be type A or B and the fetus is typed as O. We have used maternal blood in two such cases with no deleterious effects noted in the fetus. Follow-up at 3 years of age in one of these infants revealed anti-A and anti-B titers that were appropriate for age.

Timing of Delivery

Until the introduction of the direct IVT, fetuses were routinely delivered by 32 weeks' gestation. Hyaline membrane disease and the need for neonatal exchange transfusions for the treatment of hyperbilirubinemia were common. As experience with IVT became widespread, several centers began to question this policy of premature delivery. Klumper and colleagues[132] compared perinatal mortality for IUTs undertaken before and after 32 weeks' gestation. Perinatal loss occurred in 3.4% of 409 early IUTs and in 1% of 200 procedures performed after 32 weeks' gestation. Most experienced centers now perform the final IUT at up to 35 weeks' gestation, with delivery anticipated at 37 to 38 weeks. This practice allows maturation of the hepatic enzyme systems, which virtually eliminates the need for neonatal exchange transfusions. After a viable gestational age is attained, performing the transfusion in immediate proximity to the labor and delivery suite and allowing the patient nothing by mouth in the preoperative period appear to be prudent measures, so that cesarean section can be undertaken if fetal distress should occur.

Outcome

Survival after IUT varies with the center, with experience, and with the presence of hydrops fetalis. Overall survival in one review was 84%; up to one fourth fewer hydropic fetuses survived with IUT (70%), compared with fetuses who underwent their first IUT when they were not hydropic (92%).[133] The experience of a single treatment center with 213 fetuses receiving 599 IUTs was very similar. Survival with any degree of hydrops was 78%, compared with 92% for nonhydropic fetuses.[134] The authors further classified hydrops as mild (only mild ascites) or severe (significant ascites with scalp edema and pericardial effusion or pleural effusion). Mild hydrops reversed in 88% of cases, whereas severe hydrops reversed in 39%, a finding clearly linked to overall perinatal survival: 98% of fetuses survived after reversal of hydrops. With persistent hydrops, 39% of fetuses survived; if the hydrops was severe and persisted, only one fourth survived.

Immediate follow-up studies of infants treated with IVTs in utero revealed a need for top-up transfusions in the early months of life. Typically, these infants are born with a virtual absence of reticulocytes and a red cell population consisting mainly of transfused red cells containing adult hemoglobin. Exchange transfusions for hyperbilirubinemia are rarely necessary. However, at 1 month of age, these infants often require a simple transfusion because of symptoms associated with anemia. In our series of 36 infants who had undergone IUTs, 50% required top-up transfusions at a mean age of 38 days, with a range of 20 to 68 days.[135] Studies of these infants indicated erythroid hypoplasia of the bone marrow accompanied by low levels of circulating erythropoietin and reticulocytes.[136] This finding led Ovali and coworkers[137] to study the use of exogenous erythropoietin in neonates after IUTs. Twenty infants were randomized to receive 200 U/kg of recombinant human erythropoietin or saline placebo administered subcutaneously three times a week between the second and eighth week of life. Infants in the treatment group required a mean of 1.8 red cell transfusions, compared with a mean of 4.2 transfusions in the placebo group. Recovery of the neonate's bone marrow occurred earlier in the treatment group in control subjects.

Because of this phenomenon, neonatal Hct and reticulocyte determinations should be checked weekly until hematopoiesis recovers in infants who have undergone IUTs. Proposed criteria for transfusion of the infant vary and are usually described for premature infants. A more conservative approach was advocated by Maier and coworkers.[138] A threshold for transfusion is an Hct of less than 27% if the infant is asymptomatic, or less than 32% with symptoms. Shannon and colleagues[139] proposed a threshold value for Hct of less than 20% without symptoms or less than 30% in conjunction with symptoms. If erythropoietin is to be used, initiation in the first week of life in the infant with a persistent low circulating reticulocyte count may prove beneficial. Supplemental iron therapy is unnecessary because of the high levels of circulating iron in these infants secondary to ongoing hemolysis in utero. Supplemental folate therapy (0.5 mg/day) should be considered.

Investigations regarding the long-term neurologic evaluation of infants who have been treated with IUTs are limited. Hardyment and colleagues[140] reported a series of fetuses transfused with IPT between 1966 and 1975, when the survival rate was only 48%. Twenty-one of the 27 fetuses underwent evaluation, and evidence of cerebral palsy was found in 10%. Advancements in treatment techniques suggest that more moribund and severely anemic fetuses now survive. Doyle and coworkers[141] evaluated 38 surviving infants at 2 years of age. They noted one case of cerebral palsy, one case of mild disability with a mental developmental index of 72, and one case of severe developmental delay associated with seizures. Comparison with a group of 51 randomly selected infants of normal birth weight who underwent a similar assessment at 2 years of age yielded no significant differences in the incidence of sensorineural outcomes. Janssens and coworkers[142] studied 69 infants for 6 months to 6 years of age. Seven percent of the children exhibited some evidence of neurologic handicap; 4% were diagnosed with cerebral palsy. Sixteen percent of the children were noted to have developmental delay: six cases showed mild delay, and five others exhibited severe delay. The overall 10% rate of disability in their group was comparable with that in a cohort of normal Dutch children with 6% disability and a cohort of high-risk children with 12% disability. We observed 40 surviving infants for up to 62 months of age; only one case of spastic hemiplegia was detected. Gesell and McCarthy developmental scores were similar to norms for the general population.[143] Grab and colleagues[144] monitored 30 infants and noted mild sensorineural disabilities in 2. One infant exhibited delayed speech development at 24 months; the second had mild psychomotor developmental delay at 1 year that had resolved by 6 years of age.

Hearing loss in the neonate has been reported in association with high bilirubin levels. Because red cell destruction can lead to high levels of in utero bilirubin and elevated levels in neonatal life, HDFN could be associated with sensorineural hearing loss. Janssens and colleagues[142] found that 14% of 58 children screened at 9 months had evidence of hearing loss. However, five of these cases were thought to be conductive in nature because of their association with middle ear or respiratory infection and the transient nature of the findings. Hudon and coworkers[143] tested 21 infants just before discharge. Two infants had mild peripheral sensitivity loss, with recovery noted in one at 5 months of age; the other child was lost to follow-up. A third child exhibited severe bilateral deafness. Based on these studies, it would appear that the prevalence of hearing loss is increased 5- to 10-fold over the general population in infants requiring in utero therapy for HDFN. Therefore, careful follow-up of these infants is warranted.

The issue of enhanced survival of the hydropic fetus and its relationship to long-term outcome was addressed in two investigations. Using a two-sample analysis, Janssens and coworkers[142] found no correlation between either the presence of hydrops or the number of IUTs and poor neonatal neurologic outcome. Using a multivariate analysis, our group[143] could find no relationship between global developmental scores and the number of IUTs, the lowest fetal Hct, or the presence of hydrops. These data are reassuring in counseling couples with a severely anemic fetus. A normal neurologic outcome can be expected in more than 90% of surviving infants, even if hydrops fetalis is noted at the time of the first IUT.

Other Treatment Modalities

Plasmapheresis

Plasmapheresis has been relegated to an historical treatment modality for HDFN since the advent of modern IUT techniques. Most literature reports include single cases or relatively small case series. Reported protocols vary considerably, but all involve repeated procedures because of a rebound increase in antibody titer. In animal studies, Bystryn and coworkers[145] experimentally lowered antibody levels by exchange transfusion. Antibody levels were noted to rebound to more than 200% of the initial levels, with the greatest increase (50% to 80%) seen in the first 48 hours. Most reports suggested starting plasmapheresis after 12 weeks of gestation. This approach seems reasonable in view of the documented transplacental passage of up to 60% of maternal IgG1 and 30% of IgG3 antibodies by this period of gestation.[146] The plasma that is removed requires replacement; saline, plasma protein fraction, Rh− plasma, and albumin have all been used. With modern concerns regarding viral transmission through blood products, 5% albumin would seem to be the preferred fluid. Automated cell separators are now routinely used for the procedure, with citrate being used in the machine's extracorporeal circuit to prevent coagulation. Angela and coworkers[147] reported a 15% incidence of complications among 261 procedures in pregnant women. These included delayed vertigo, headache, allergic reaction to plasma, peripheral edema, and syncope; 10 cases involved mild citrate toxicity. The latter is usually heralded by circumoral paresthesia and can be treated with oral calcium. In some cases, intravenous calcium gluconate is required at the conclusion of the procedure.

Intravenous Immune Globulin

Intravenous immune globulin (IVIG) has been used effectively as the sole antenatal treatment for HDFN. In the largest series reported to date, Margulies and coworkers[148] described the use of IVIG without IUTs in 24 patients with severe rhesus disease. The study population represented a high-risk group, with more than half the patients having experienced a fetal or neonatal death in a previous pregnancy and 12% having had two or more perinatal losses. All patients in the series were noted to have an RhD+ fetus, three having undergone FBS because of a heterozygous paternal genotype. Patients received a total dose of 2 g/kg IVIG administered over 4 consecutive days (400 mg/kg/day); the dose was repeated at 2- to 3-week intervals throughout the pregnancy. The patients were divided into three groups based on gestational age at the initiation of IVIG therapy: less than 20 weeks' gestation, 20 to 28 weeks' gestation, and more than 28 weeks' gestation. There was a total of three fetal losses in groups 1 and 2; all three fetuses were noted to be hydropic at the start of therapy. There were no neonatal deaths, yielding a perinatal survival rate for the series of 88%. Half the neonates in group 1, one third of those in group 2, and 88% of those in group 3 required exchange transfusions, leading the authors to conclude that IVIG is not effective if initiated after 28 weeks' gestation. Interestingly, the maternal anti-D titers declined in all three groups, although this difference was not statistically significant in group 2.

In a follow-up case-control study of 69 patients, this same group of investigators compared the outcomes of pregnancies treated with IVIG before 20 weeks' gestation followed by IUT versus the use of only IUTs after 20 weeks.[149] Again, the study group represented cases of severe rhesus alloimmunization, in that 73% of the IVIG group and 56% of the IUT group had experienced previous perinatal losses. Significant differences were noted between the groups. Hydrops at the first IUT occurred in one fourth of the IVIG/IUT group, compared with three fourths of the IUT-alone group. The first IUT was performed a median of 1.5 weeks later in those patients who had received IVIG. Fetal death was 2.5-fold more likely in the IUT-only group (51% versus 20%). Neonatal death occurred in 8% of the IVIG–IUT group and in 21% of the IUT-only group, although this difference did not achieve statistical significance.

The mechanism of action of IVIG in cases of severe HDFN is not well understood. At least three different theories for its effect have been postulated: decreased production of maternal anti–red cell antibodies, decreased placental transport of antibodies, and fetal reticuloendothelial blockade. Dooren and coworkers[150] randomized 20 patients to receive either IVT alone or IVT in conjunction with direct fetal infusion of IVIG. No significant differences in transfusion requirement or clinical outcome could be demonstrated between the two groups. However, the average fetal IVIG dose of 85 mg/kg was fairly low compared with the 500-mg/kg dose usually used to treat neonatal HDFN.[151] In a case report, Alonso and coworkers[152] used between 406 and 481 mg/kg of IVIG and administered this directly to the fetus on four occasions at the time of FBS. Fetal Hct increased and ΔOD_{450} values decreased with advancing gestation. To further elucidate the protective mechanism of IVIG, one investigation compared six pregnancies treated with maternal IVIG with seven control sensitized pregnancies that were monitored only with serial FBS.[153] No obvious inhibitory effect on transplacental passage of anti-D or on maternal anti-D production was noted. Finally, Besalduch and colleagues[154] reported a case in which IVIG was used in a patient with early hydrops fetalis secondary to anti-E alloimmunization. These authors used a pepsin-treated preparation resulting in a purified IgG product with loss of Fc receptors. Fetal hydrops and hepatosplenomegaly were noted to resolve with repeated IVIG administration. The authors postulated that the effectiveness of the IVIG in their case was related to suppression of maternal antibody levels, because their product could not have crossed the placenta owing to the lack of Fc receptors.

Yu and Lennon[155] proposed a mechanism to explain the potential ability of IVIG to cause the accelerated catabolism of circulating anti–red cell antibodies. An intracellular Fc receptor abundant in endothelial cells normally binds the IgG that has entered the cell through pinocytosis and presents it to the surface of the cell for release back into the microcirculation. In cases of excess circulating IgG secondary to IVIG, the protective intracellular Fc receptors become saturated, allowing accelerated catabolism of free IgG molecules that enter the endothelial cells. These data would lead one to conclude that multiple mechanisms may contribute to the effectiveness of IVIG. Although the primary effect may be suppression of the level of maternal antibody, a fetal reticuloendothelial blockade may also be involved.

Combined Plasmapheresis and Intravenous Immune Globulin

Berlin and coworkers[156] used a combined plasmaphereses/IVIG approach when problems with continued venous access precluded continued plasmaphereses in a patient with severe anti-D alloimmunization. A total of 10 L of plasma was exchanged over 4 days at 25 weeks' gestation. This was followed by an IVIG dose of 0.4 g/kg/day over 5 consecutive days. Ruma and associates[157] reported on a series of nine patients treated with a combined plasmapheresis/IVIG protocol. Among the seven women with a previous history of a perinatal loss, a live birth was achieved in all treated cases. Their protocol included a single-volume plasmapheresis every other day for three procedures in the 12th week of gestation, with 5% albumin used for volume replacement. The IgG pool was replaced after the third procedure by administering a 1 g/kg loading dose of IVIG diluted in normal saline. The 10% IVIG infusion was started at a rate of 60 mL/hr and increased by 30 mL/hr every 30 minutes to a maximum rate of 240 mL/hr. A second dose of 1 g/kg IVIG was given the following day. The patients were then treated with a weekly dose of 1 g/kg IVIG until 20 weeks' gestation. All patients eventually required IUT therapy.

Typical side effects encountered during IVIG administration include urticaria and severe headache.[158] Premedication with 1000 mg of oral acetaminophen several hours before the scheduled infusion and administration of 25 mg of intravenous diphenhydramine HCl just before treatment aids in preventing these symptoms. In some situations, a change to a different manufacturer results in fewer headaches in some patients. On occasion, patients complain of a mild desquamation of the palmar surface of the hands; the cause of this phenomenon is unknown.

In the case of a heterozygous paternal genotype, an amniocentesis is undertaken at 15 weeks' gestation using DNA techniques to determine the fetal red cell antigen status. If the fetus is found to be antigen negative, the IVIG is discontinued. Standard noninvasive or invasive fetal testing is used to determine the timing of the first IUT in the case of a homozygous paternal phenotype or an RhD+ fetus by amniocentesis. In our experience, this approach is successful in deferring the need for the first IUT until approximately 24 to 26 weeks' gestation.

Oral Tolerance

Studies to date attempting oral desensitization to red cell antigens have revealed conflicting results. In 1979, Bierme and associates[159] investigated the use of oral RhD antigen in seven severely alloimmunized women. All previous pregnancies had resulted in intrauterine death, even though IUTs were used in four cases. RhD titers were noted to remain stable in all cases. In some cases, a new anti-Rh class of antibody appeared, of the IgM or IgA variety. In six of the seven treated cases, an RhD+ infant was born at 35 weeks' gestation in good condition. In an attempt to duplicate these results, American investigators treated four patients with RhD alloimmunization who had a history of severe HDN with oral erythrocytes using the method of Bierme and associates.[160] All four cases resulted in either fetal or neonatal death; hydrops fetalis was noted in all cases. In a rebuttal letter to the editor, Bierme's group reported on a larger series of 16 pregnancies that resulted in 12 live births using oral erythrocyte therapy in conjunction with oral promethazine.[161] The authors proposed that a therapeutic trial should be undertaken.

Three years later, Barnes and coworkers[162] conducted a scientific investigation to study the effects of oral erythrocyte membrane therapy in the nonpregnant patient. Six previously sensitized women were administered a 2-g/day dose of a lyophilized preparation of erythrocyte membranes for 4 weeks. Half of the patients received an erythrocyte preparation made from RhD– red cells, and half received RhD+ red cell preparations. In three subjects, there was no change in antibody levels; in the remaining three, there was a clear elevation in antibody titers. Two of these three had received RhD+ oral antigen. These findings led the authors to conclude that their oral preparation was not tolerogenic but in fact immunogenic. No further reports can be found in peer-reviewed literature regarding this therapy, because it appears to have been abandoned as a potential treatment with the advent of more effective methods of IUT.

Chemotherapeutic Agents

In vitro, promethazine interferes with the ability of human fetal macrophages to phagocytize red cells coated with anti-RhD antibodies.[163] This finding led several investigators to use this agent in an effort to ameliorate the effects of maternal anti–red cell antibodies in HDFN. Gusdon and associates[164] treated 72 patients with RhD alloimmunization with promethazine, 3.7 to 5.0 mg/kg/day divided in four doses beginning as early as 14 weeks' gestation. The lower dose was used in patients with their first affected pregnancy, whereas the highest dose was used in patients with a history of previous IUTs or fetal death. When compared with previous pregnancy, there was a marked improvement in outcome. Three perinatal deaths occurred in the pregnancies treated with promethazine, compared with eight deaths in previous pregnancies. The infants in 28% of the treated pregnancies required neonatal exchange transfusion, whereas 44% needed neonatal exchange transfusion in the previous pregnancies in these patients. A similar investigation in 21 pregnancies was undertaken,[165] giving a general impression that promethazine was not beneficial in view of the continued need for IUTs. However, a therapeutic effect was possibly seen in some gestations in women with previous neonatal death.

Steroids have been proposed as a treatment for HDFN, but no case series have been published.[166] Agents such as betamethasone and dexamethasone cross the placenta and have been associated with decreases in ΔOD_{450}.[167] However, these changes have not been associated with a decrease in the severity of HDFN but instead are probably related to alterations in fetal bilirubin metabolism.[166]

Antenatal treatment with maternal phenobarbital has been proposed as a method to decrease the need for neonatal exchange transfusions for hyperbilirubinemia. This agent has been shown to enhance the neonatal hepatic capacity to conjugate and eliminate bilirubin through stimulation of gluronyl transferase. Trevett and colleagues[168] retrospectively evaluated 71 pregnancies that had been treated with serial IUTs; 31 of these were treated with 30 mg of oral phenobarbital three times daily for the last 7 to 10 days before anticipated delivery. The need for any neonatal exchange transfusion was 9% in those cases treated with phenobarbital, compared with 52% in those not receiving the drug. After controlling for confounding variables, maternal phenobarbital treatment was associated with a 75% reduction in the need for neonatal exchange transfusions.

Sensitization to Paternal Leukocyte Antigens

In vitro data and clinical case reports suggest that maternal alloantibodies to paternal leukocytes may result in an Fc blockade, thereby protecting the fetal red cells from hemolysis in cases of RhD alloimmunization. Neppert and coworkers[169] reported that human sera with human leukocyte antigen (HLA)-A, -B, -C, and -DR antibodies inhibited the binding activity and phagocytosis of monocytes. The authors proposed that this inhibitory effect of maternal anti-HLA antibodies on the fetal reticuloendothelial system may explain the lack of clinical disease in cases of HDFN with a strongly positive direct Coombs finding at birth.[170] Dooren and coworkers[171] studied 12 cases of RhD alloimmunization in which the ADCC assay predicted severe fetal disease but the neonatal clinical course was instead benign. When donor monocytes were replaced in the assay by paternal cells (monocytes that should share HLA antigens with the neonate), seven of the repeat assays revealed lack of lysis of the sensitized red cells. Six of these seven cases involved maternal monocyte-reactive antibodies of the paternal HLA-DR specificity. Three reports of clinical cases have appeared in the literature in which maternal HLA antibodies were thought to be the explanation for the mild clinical course in HDN.[172,173] In two cases, the specificity of the maternal antibody was HLA-DR, whereas in the remaining case the antibody was directed against the HLA-A10 and -DR13 antigens. Data suggest that these alloantibodies prevent the binding of anti-D–sensitized fetal red cells to FcγR-bearing splenic phagocytes, thus reducing the severity of HDN.[174,175]

We showed in a rabbit model for HDFN that alloimmunization to paternal leukocytes produces fetal hemoglobin levels that approach normal in does previously sensitized to red cells.[176] Limitations of this method of treatment for severe red cell alloimmunization are substantial. In human trials, any contamination of the paternal leukocytes with red cells could produce a substantial anamnestic effect in the maternal antibody titer. Maternal sensitization to paternal HLA antigens could produce alloimmune thrombocytopenic purpura in the fetus or neonate.

Nasal Tolerance to the RhD Antigen

Hall and associates[177] developed transgenic mice for the human HLA-DR15 gene and then immunized them to purified human RhD protein. Four candidate peptides were developed that represented significant epitopes for helper T cells; these were then administered intranasally to the immunized mice. A blunted antibody response was noted when the mice were rechallenged with the purified RhD protein. If confirmed in subsequent human clinical trials, such therapy may prove useful in the treatment of the severely alloimmunized pregnant patient.

Hemolytic Disease of the Fetus and Newborn Caused by Non-RhD Antibodies

More than 50 different red cell antigens have been reported to be associated with HDFN (Table 26-3). However, the antibodies frequently associated with severe HDFN appear to include those against RhD, Rhc, and Kell (K1). In a series from Manitoba, Canada, encompassing the years 1962 to 1988, 1022 cases of non-RhD

TABLE 26-3 NON-RhD ANTIBODIES AND ASSOCIATED HEMOLYTIC DISEASE OF THE FETUS AND NEWBORN

Antigen System	Specific Antigens
Frequently Associated with Severe Disease	
Kell	-K (K1)
Rhesus	-c
Infrequently Associated with Severe Disease	
Colton	-Co^a -Co3
Diego	-ELO -Di^a -Di^b -Wr^a -Wr^b
Duffy	-Fy^a
Kell	-Js^a -Js^b -k (K2) -Kp^a -Kp^b -K11 -K22 -Ku -Ul^a
Kidd	-Jk^a
MNS	-En^a Far -Hil -Hut -M -Mi^a -Mit -Mt^a -MUT -Mur -M^v -s -s^D -S -U -Vw
Rhesus	-Be^a -C -Ce -C^w -C^x -ce -D^w -E -E^w -Evans -e -G -Go^a -Hr -Hr$_o$ -JAL -HOFM -LOCR -Riv -Rh29 -Rh32 -Rh42 -Rh46 -STEM -Tar
Other antigens	-HJK -JFV -JONES -Kg -MAM -REIT -Rd
Associated with Mild Disease	
Dombrock	-Do^a -Gy^a -Hy -Jo^a
Duffy	-Fy^b -Fy^3
Gerbich	-Ge^2 -Ge^3 -Ge^4 -Ls^a
Kidd	-Jk^b -Jk^3
Scianna	-Sc2
Other	-Vel -Lan -At^a -Jr^a

From Issitt PD, Anstee DJ: Hemolytic disease of the newborn. In Issitt PD, Anstee DJ (eds): Applied Blood Group Serology. Durham, NC, Montgomery Scientific Publications, 1998, p 1045; Daniels G: Blood group antibodies in haemolytic disease of the fetus and newborn. In Hadley A, Soothill P (eds): Alloimmune Disorders in Pregnancy: Anaemia, Thrombocytopenia, and Neutropenia in the Fetus and Newborn. Cambridge, UK, Cambridge University Press, 2002, p 21.

alloimmunization were accumulated.[178] Only anti-c was associated with severe HDFN that ended in a hydropic stillbirth or necessitated IUT. Anti-c resulted in twofold and sevenfold greater incidence of hemolytic disease compared with anti-K1 and anti-E antibodies, respectively. Anti-c and anti-K1 antibodies were equally likely to be associated with the need for neonatal exchange transfusion or phototherapy; anti-E was half as likely to require neonatal treatment. A selected population of 22 patients was referred from outside Manitoba during the same time period.[178] Antibodies against the following antigens were associated with the need for IUTs: K1 ($n = 9$), k (1), c (7), cE (1), Fy^a (1), Jk^a (1), CC^w (1), and E (1). In a series of 258 pregnancies managed with IUTs at a single national referral center in the Netherlands from 1988 to 2001, 85% of cases involved RhD alloimmunization.[134] Ten percent of cases involved anti-K1, and 3.5% involved anti-c; anti-RhE, anti-Rhe, and anti-Fy^a were each associated with a single case.

Antibodies to the red cell antigens Lewis, I, and P are often encountered through antibody screening during prenatal care. Because these antibodies are typically of the IgM class, they are not associated with HDFN.[179]

Rhesus

Anti-Rhc

Anti-c antibody has been associated with severe HDFN of a similar magnitude to that caused by anti-D. In one series, more than half of pregnant patients had a history of a previous blood transfusion.[180] These authors reported a series of 177 pregnancies with 1 neonatal death secondary to hydrops and 11 other infants requiring exchange transfusions. Wenk and associates[181] reported 70 cases of maternal alloimmunization to Rhc with a known c-antigen–positive infant. Eight cases resulted in hydropic stillborns or perinatal deaths, 26% of cases had mild HDFN and did not require transfusions after birth, and an additional 29% had moderate HDFN requiring transfusion therapy. Kozlowski and coworkers[182] reported that, among 100 c-antigen–positive neonates born to alloimmunized parturients, only one pregnancy required IUTs, whereas 14% of the infants required neonatal exchange transfusions. Finally, Hackney and colleagues[183] found that 25% of c-antigen–positive fetuses exhibited severe HDFN; 7% of the total group were hydropic, and 17% required IUTs.

Anti-RhC, -RhE, and -Rhe

Antibodies against the rhesus antigens C, E, and e are usually found as a low titer in conjunction with anti-RhD antibody (for example, anti-D, 128, with anti-C, 2). Their presence may be additive to the hemolytic effect of the anti-D on the fetus.[33] IUTs are only rarely reported when these antibodies occur as the sole finding.[134,184] Joy and coworkers[185] reported 32 pregnancies alloimmunized exclusively to RhE. Fifteen percent of offspring were noted to have evidence of fetal or neonatal anemia; one fetus presented with hydrops fetalis.

Anti-RhG

In some patients, the anti-D and anti-C titers are observed to be equal; alternatively, the value of the anti-C titer may actually exceed that of the anti-D (for example, anti-D, 128, with anti-C, 256). In these cases, one should suspect the presence of anti-RhG. Consultation with a blood bank pathologist should be undertaken to clarify whether anti-RhG is present. Previous case reports have indicated that anti-G is associated with mild HDFN; however, a high titer can be associated with significant fetal disease necessitating IUT.[186] Importantly, if invasive fetal procedures are indicated, RhIG should be administered to prevent the formation of anti-D.

Kell

The Kell red cell antigen system includes 23 different members. Individual antigens in the system are designated by name, letter abbreviation, or number. Antibodies to at least nine of the antigens have been associated with HDFN. The most common of these are Kell (K, or K1) and Cellano (k, or K2). Additional antibodies that have been reported to be causative for HDFN include anti-Penny (Kp^a, or K3), -Rautenberg (Kp^b, or K4), -Peltz (Ku, or K5), -Sutter (Js^a, or K6), -Matthews (Js^b, or K7), -Karhula (Ul^a, or K10), and -K22.[187]

Anti-K (K1)

The K1 antigen is found on the red cells of 9% of whites and 2% of blacks, with virtually all antigen-positive individuals being heterozygous (Table 26-4). Kell antibody was detected in 127 of 127,076 pregnancies in one series, yet, because of the low gene frequency, only 13 cases resulted in Kell+ fetuses.[188] Hydrops fetalis was noted in four cases; three of these infants suffered in utero or neonatal death. Bowman and colleagues[189] reported a 46-year experience of 459 Kell–alloimmunized pregnancies in 311 women. Fourteen percent of these pregnancies ended in spontaneous or induced abortion, 82% resulted in Kell– infants or infants with no recorded clinical disease, and the remaining 4% were affected. Among these last 20 infants, there was 1 neonatal death, and 3 fetuses with hydrops died in utero. In a referral series of 16 pregnancies that occurred between 1970 and 1985, the authors reported a perinatal mortality rate of 67% before the advent of IVT, compared with a rate of 10% after this technique began to be used.

Berkowitz and colleagues[190] described a case of Kell alloimmunization with a maternal titer of 2048. Amniocenteses at 20 and 21 weeks revealed a declining trend in the ΔOD_{450} values; however, a hydropic fetal death was noted at 24 weeks' gestation. Amniocentesis at that time revealed a ΔOD_{450} value lower than the previous ones. These findings led the authors to conclude that ultrasound detection of fetal hydrops could be a better predictor of fetal deterioration than amniotic fluid bilirubin. Four years later, Caine and Mueller-Heubach[188] reported on three cases of poor perinatal outcome, with fetal hydrops in two cases and one neonatal death. ΔOD_{450} values 1 week before delivery were noted to be in upper zone 2 of the Liley curve. In a matched comparison, Vaughan and coworkers[34] noted lower amniotic fluid bilirubin levels in Kell-alloimmunized pregnancies compared with pregnancies complicated by RhD alloimmunization. They suggested that, for this reason, serial amniocenteses were not a reliable method of management of the Kell-alloimmunized pregnancy. In a similar matched comparison, Weiner and Widness[35] noted that Kell-affected fetuses exhibited a lower total serum bilirubin concentration than their RhD counterparts. These authors suggested that serial FBS, rather than ΔOD_{450} analysis, would appear to be the preferred method for monitoring the pregnancy complicated by Kell alloimmunization.

Bowman's group[189] suggested that ΔOD_{450} values are still useful in the management of the Kell-alloimmunized pregnancy. Twelve Kell+ fetuses were monitored with amniocenteses. Two cases involved hydropic losses at 21 and 24 weeks after a previous low or mid–zone 2 reading. Combining these results with the ΔOD_{450} values in the Kell– fetuses, the authors suggested an 83% to 89% accuracy for serial amniocenteses, compared with an accuracy of 95% cited for rhesus disease. They recommended use of a ΔOD_{450} value greater than 0.15 before 20 weeks' gestation and a subsequent value in excess of the 65th

TABLE 26-4 GENE FREQUENCIES AND ZYGOSITY FOR NON-RhD RED CELL ANTIGENS ASSOCIATED WITH HEMOLYTIC DISEASE OF THE NEWBORN

	White		Black		Hispanic	
Antigen	Antigen+(%)	Heterozygous(%)	Antigen+(%)	Heterozygous(%)	Antigen+(%)	Heterozygous(%)
C	70.0	50.0	30.0	32.0	81.0	51.0
c	80.0	50.0	96.0	32.0	76.0	51.0
E	32.0	29.0	23.0	21.0	41.0	36.0
e	97.0	29.0	98.0	21.0	95.0	36.0
K (K1)	9.0	97.8	2	100		
k (K2)	99.8	8.8	100	2		
M	78.0	64.0	70	63		
N	77.0	65.0	74	60		
S	55.0	80.0	31	90		
s	89.0	50.0	97	29		
U	100.0	—	99	—		
Fy^a	66.0	26.0	10	90		
Fy^b	83.0	41.0	23	96		
Jk^a	77.0	36.0	91	63		
Jk^b	72.0	32.0	43	21		

Reproduced with permission from Moise KJ: Red cell alloimmunization. In Gabbe SG, Simpson JL, Niebyl JR, et al. (eds): Obstetrics: Normal and Abnormal Pregnancies, 5th ed. New York, Churchill Livingstone, 2007.

percentile of zone 2 of the Liley curve as the threshold to initiate FBS and suggested that a critical maternal titer of 8 be used, instead of 16 or 32, as the threshold for initiating serial amniocenteses.

Use of the peak MCA systolic velocity has proved successful for the detection of fetal anemia in cases of K1 alloimmunization. Van Dongen and colleagues[191] reported on 27 pregnancies complicated by Kell alloimmunization; 17 fetuses were noted to have severe anemia at the time of cordocentesis. A peak MCA of greater than 1.5 MoM yielded an 89% sensitivity and specificity (false-positive rate, 1%) for detecting the subgroup with anemia. When those fetuses with ultrasound evidence of hydrops were excluded, the sensitivity and specificity for the detection of severe anemia was unchanged. Similarly, Rimon and coworkers[192] observed eight fetuses that were documented to be K1+ by amniocentesis and at risk for severe HDFN. They were successful in detecting all cases of severe anemia with weekly MCA Doppler assessments.

Management of the K1-sensitized pregnancy should entail paternal red cell typing and genotype testing. If the paternal typing returns a K1− genotype (*kk*) and paternity is assured, no further maternal testing is undertaken. If paternal testing reveals a positive result, maternal titers of less than 4 should be reassessed monthly until a critical value of 8 is attained. At that time, if the paternal genotype is heterozygous, amniocentesis for DNA typing of the fetus should be offered after 15 weeks' gestation, because 50% of fetuses will be unaffected. Paternal blood should be studied simultaneously with amniotic fluid, using the same PCR primers, to assess for the accuracy of the technique. However, cases of gene rearrangements in the Kell gene have not been reported to date. If the fetus is found to be K1−, no further fetal or maternal testing is warranted. In the case of a homozygous paternal genotype or a K1+ fetus, serial MCA Doppler measurements are repeated every 1 to 2 weeks starting at 18 weeks' gestation. An elevated value of more than 1.50 MoM is followed by FBS with blood readied for IUT.

Anti-k (K2)

Bowman and colleagues[193] reviewed 20 years of antibody screening of approximately 350,000 pregnancies in a Manitoba population and detected only 1 case of anti-k alloimmunization. Levine and colleagues[194] reported the first case of HDN secondary to anti-k, which resulted in a mildly affected infant; this was followed by the report of a second mild case by Bryant.[195] Additional individual cases of HDFN have required treatment with a single neonatal exchange transfusion, a single simple neonatal transfusion, and a simple neonatal transfusion followed by a top-up transfusion for delayed neonatal anemia.[193,196,197] A sixth case referred to Bowman's group[193] required three IUTs beginning at 30 weeks' gestation The maternal titer was noted to be 16. In the second case reported from their institution, the maternal antiglobulin titer was 8. These findings led these investigators to surmise that anti-k antibody, analogous to anti-K1 antibody, may produce fetal erythropoietic suppression at lower maternal titers than are typically used for a critical value in cases of anti-RhD.

MNS

The MNS system consists of 40 red cell antigens, with antibodies to the M, N, S, s, and U antigens representing the members of this group that have been more commonly associated with HDFN. The M and N antigens can be expressed simultaneously on the glycophorin A molecule, or they can be expressed alone. The S, s, and U antigens are expressed on the glycophorin B molecule in various combinations. In most cases, the paternal genotype is positive for antigen, with most genotypes being heterozygous (see Table 26-4).

Anti-M

Anti-M is a naturally occurring IgM antibody that typically presents as a cold agglutinin. An IgG type can occur rarely and can be associated with HDFN. A total of six patients with severe HDFN have been reported in the English literature. The first case involved a maternal anti-M albumin titer of 1000 in association with a hydropic fetal death in one twin and the need for exchange transfusions in the sibling.[198] A second patient with a titer of 2048 was noted to have a history of four fetal deaths.[199] Matsumoto and colleagues[200] reported a patient who had experienced three fetal losses in conjunction with a maternal anti-M titer of 1024. Furukawa and coworkers[201] reported a patient with a history of three perinatal losses. A successful outcome was achieved in a fourth pregnancy after intensive plasmapheresis to treat a titer of 4096; the infant required only phototherapy. Duguid and coworkers[202] described a patient with a titer of 16 who gave birth to a child requiring phototherapy and exchange transfusion. Kanra and colleagues[203] investigated a patient who had experienced seven pregnancies with losses occurring between 10 and 33 weeks' gestation secondary to in utero or neonatal death; five of these pregnancies were associated with hydrops fetalis. A maternal anti-M titer of 512 was detected, although little information is available regarding the evaluation of the neonates.

De Young-Owens and colleagues[204] reviewed a 26-year experience at their institution and noted an anti-M antibody in 115 pregnancies in 90 women. They reported a threefold to sevenfold increased incidence of detection over the course of the study period; anti-M comprised 10% of all pregnant patients with a positive antibody screen. Explanations offered for the increasing frequency included a change in antibody screening technique from albumin to ethylene glycol and the addition of indicator red cells homozygous for the M antigen to their red cell screening panel. The antiglobulin titer was less than 4 in 90% of cases. In five cases, there was more than a two-tube increase in titer. However, the fetuses were noted to be negative for the M antigen in four of these five cases; in the fifth case, the M antigen status of the fetus was unknown. In 42 cases of antigen-positive fetuses, there was no increase in maternal titer. Clinical outcome for the fetuses revealed minimal disease. Of the 70 infants who tested positive for the M antigen, only 17% had a positive direct Coombs test at birth. Only one of these infants required phototherapy. In that case, the maternal anti-M antibody titer was 1, and the finding of a neonatal 3+ direct Coombs result was believed to be related to an ABO incompatibility. Four additional infants required phototherapy; all had negative direct Coombs testing and were associated with a maternal titer of less than 2. The authors proposed that prematurity accounted for the need for phototherapy, because all four infants were born at less than 36 weeks' gestation.

These data led De Young-Owens and coworkers[204] to conclude that, if there is no previous history of an affected pregnancy, an initial titer of 4 or less requires no further evaluation. If the titer is greater than 4 or there is a history of a previously affected fetus or infant, serial titers should be obtained. Bowman[178] recommended amniocentesis for ΔOD_{450} assessment if the indirect Coombs titer is 64 or higher. At our center, we elected to use serial maternal titers until a value of 32 is reached. Consultation with the transfusion service is then obtained to determine whether the antibody class is predominantly IgM or a combination of IgM and IgG.[205] This can be accomplished by treating the serum with dithiothreitol or 2-mercaptoethanol. These agents disrupt the disulfide bonds between the components of the pentamer structure of the IgM molecule, thereby abolishing its agglutinating and complement-binding properties. Serum treated with dithiothreitol containing only an IgM antibody exhibits a loss of reactivity and a subsequent negative titer. Serum containing a mixture of IgM and IgG antibody exhibits a decrease in the original titer. Once the IgG component of the titer reaches 32, we proceed with serial MCA Doppler assessments. If the paternal genotype is heterozygous, fetal typing using PCR techniques on amniotic fluid is available for the M antigen (M. J. Hessner, personal communication, The Blood Center of Wisconsin), using a technique previously described by Corfield and colleagues.[206]

Anti-S

In one series of 175,000 pregnancies during a 5-year period in the Oxford region of England, anti-S antibody was detected in 22 pregnancies in 19 women.[207] Previous transfusions were believed to be the likely source of sensitization in 13 patients. A positive direct Coombs assay was noted in only four cases; one infant required exchange transfusions. Most cases of HDFN described in the literature involve mild neonatal disease.[208] Only three cases of severe disease have been described. The first case was reported in 1952; the infant died of kernicterus at 60 hours of life.[209] Griffith[210] described a case of stillbirth at 41 weeks' gestation complicated by the finding of a maternal anti-S antibody and autopsy findings consistent with erythroblastosis fetalis. Finally, Mayne and coworkers[207] reported a case of maternal anti-S alloimmunization that resulted in the birth of a neonate requiring three exchange transfusions and 5 days of phototherapy.

Anti-s

Three cases of severe HDFN and one case of mild HDN associated with anti-s have been reported.[211]

Anti-N

One case of mild HDFN associated with anti-N, which required only phototherapy, has been reported.[212] PCR typing of the fetus in amniotic fluid has proved problematic, particularly in the black race, where there is up to 15% discordance between paternal serology and genotype (M. J. Hessner, personal communication, The Blood Center of Wisconsin).

Anti-U

The U antigen is a high-frequency antigen: It is universally found in the white population and only rarely absent in patients of African heritage. Smith and colleagues[213] reviewed six of their own cases of HDFN secondary to anti-U alloimmunization and an additional nine cases from peer-reviewed literature. The neonates in four cases managed at their institution required only phototherapy for treatment despite maternal antibody titers of as high as 4000 in conjunction with a strongly positive direct Coombs assay on cord blood. One patient delivered an infant who required six simple transfusions after birth. A subsequent pregnancy in this same patient was complicated by the need for four IUTs. After delivery, two additional exchange transfusions and three simple transfusions were necessary during the neonatal course. Their review of the nine cases reported in the literature described one stillbirth at 35 weeks,[214] three neonates requiring exchange transfusions,[215-217] one infant with late-onset of anemia at 3 weeks of age,[218] and four additional cases with minimal evidence of HDFN.[219-221] Based on the clinical course noted in these 15 cases, the authors recommended a threshold for a critical titer of 128 if there was no HDFN in a previous pregnancy. Experience in several of their cases indicated that amniocentesis for ΔOD_{450} was an accurate method of assessing the severity of fetal anemia.

In cases of anti-U alloimmunization requiring treatment with IUT, maternal blood should be strongly considered as the primary source of red cells, because fresh U− blood is often not readily available due to the high frequency of this antigen in the white population, the primary source of the donor pool.[127] Alternatively, maternal siblings or parents may be tested to determine whether they can serve as donors.

Duffy

The Duffy antigen system consists of two antigens, Fy^a and Fy^b. Inheritance is by codominant alleles that result in four possible phenotypes. Only anti-Fy^b antibodies have been associated with mild HDFN. A review of 19 cases of HDFN secondary to anti-Fy^a antibody between 1956 and 1975 revealed a neonatal mortality rate of 18%, with almost one third of the infants requiring neonatal exchange transfusion.[222] Maternal titers as low as 8 were associated with moderate HDFN necessitating exchange transfusion. PCR typing of the fetus through amniocentesis is available in cases of a heterozygous paternal genotype.[223]

Kidd

The Kidd antigen system consists of two antigens, Jk^a and Jk^b. Inheritance is by codominant alleles that produce four possible phenotypes, although the Jk^a–/Jk^b– genotype is extremely rare. Rare cases of mild hemolytic disease have been reported. PCR typing of the fetus through amniocentesis is available in cases of a heterozygous paternal genotype.[224]

Summary

Irregular anti–red cell antibodies associated with HDFN will continue to challenge the practitioner, because the development of these antibodies is often related to transfusion therapy necessitated by complications in pregnancy. Prophylactic immune globulins are unlikely to be developed because of the rarity of these situations. In Australia, only K1– red cells are used for transfusion in female children and women of reproductive age, in an effort to markedly decrease the incidence of Kell alloimmunization. Such policies should receive further consideration in other countries.

Guidelines for intervention in cases of irregular antibodies are limited by the bias of anecdotal reports in the literature in favor of severe cases of HDFN. Large published series of patients with anti-K1 or anti-M in which most fetuses and neonates were minimally affected or unaffected substantiate this bias. In general, principles used in the management of the RhD alloimmunized patient should be followed in most cases of irregular anti–red cell antibodies as well. A notable exception is K1 or K2 alloimmunization. A lower maternal critical titer of 8 and serial MCA Doppler studies should be used to decide when to proceed to cordocentesis.

References

1. Bowman JM: RhD hemolytic disease of the newborn. N Engl J Med 339:1775-1777, 1998.
2. Rosse WF: Clinical Immunohematology: Basic Concepts in Clinical Applications, vol. 1. Boston, Blackwell Scientific, 1990.
3. Levine P, Stetson R: An usual case of intragroup agglutination. JAMA 113:126-127, 1939.
4. Landsteiner K, Weiner AS: An agglutinable factor in human blood recognized by immune sera for rhesus blood. Proc Soc Exp Biol Med 43:223, 1940.
5. Levine P, Katzin EM, Burham L: Isoimmunzation in pregnancy: Its possible bearing on etiology of erythroblastosis foetalis. JAMA 116:825-827, 1941.
6. Wallerstein H: Treatment of severe erythroblastosis by simultaneous removal and replacement of blood of the newborn infant. Science 103:583-584, 1946.
7. Bevis DC: Blood pigments in haemolytic disease of newborn. J Obstet Gynaecol Br Emp 63:68-75, 1956.
8. Liley AW: Liquor amnii analysis in the management of pregnancy complicated by rhesus sensitization. Am J Obstet Gynecol 82:1359-1370, 1961.
9. Liley AW: Intrauterine transfusion of foetus in haemolytic disease. BMJ 2:1107-1109, 1963.
10. Freda VJ, Adamsons K: Exchange transfusion in utero: Report of a case. Obstet Gynecol 89:817-821, 1964.
11. Asensio SH, Figueroa-Longo JG, Pelegrina IA: Intrauterine exchange transfusion. Am J Obstet Gynecol 95:1129-1133, 1966.
12. Asensio SH, Figueroa-Longo JG, Pelegrina IA: Intrauterine exchange transfusion: A new technic. Obstet Gynecol 32:350-355, 1968.
13. Rodeck CH, Kemp JR, Holman CA, et al: Direct intravascular fetal blood transfusion by fetoscopy in severe rhesus isoimmunisation. Lancet 1:625-627, 1981.
14. Bang J, Bock JE, Trolle D: Ultrasound-guided fetal intravenous transfusion for severe rhesus haemolytic disease. BMJ 284:373-374, 1982.
15. Chavez GF, Mulinare J, Edmonds LD: Epidemiology of Rh hemolytic disease of the newborn in the United States. JAMA 265:3270-3274, 1991.
16. Martin JA, Hamilton BE, Sutton PD, et al: Births: Final data for 2003. Natl Vital Stat Rep 54:1-116, 2005.
17. Geifman-Holtzman O, Wojtowycz M, Kosmas E, et al: Female alloimmunization with antibodies known to cause hemolytic disease. Obstet Gynecol 89:272-275, 1997.
18. Queenan JT, Smith BD, Haber JM, et al: Irregular antibodies in the obstetric patient. Obstet Gynecol 34:767-771, 1969.
19. Pepperell RJ, Barrie JU, Fliegner JR: Significance of red-cell irregular antibodies in the obstetric patient. Med J Aust 2:453-456, 1977.
20. Filbey D, Hanson U, Wesstrom G: The prevalence of red cell antibodies in pregnancy correlated to the outcome of the newborn: A 12 year study in central Sweden. Acta Obstet Gynecol Scand 74:687-692, 1995.
21. Pollock JM, Bowman JM: Anti-Rh(D) IgG subclasses and severity of Rh hemolytic disease of the newborn. Vox Sang 59:176-179, 1990.
22. Hadley AG, Kumpel BM: Synergistic effect of blending IgG1 and IgG3 monoclonal anti-D in promoting the metabolic response of monocytes to sensitized red cells. Immunology 67:550-552, 1989.
23. Ulm B, Svolba G, Ulm MR, et al: Male fetuses are particularly affected by maternal alloimmunization to D antigen. Transfusion 39:169-173, 1999.
24. Nicolaides KH, Thilaganathan B, Rodeck CH, et al: Erythroblastosis and reticulocytosis in anemic fetuses. Am J Obstet Gynecol 159:1063-1065, 1988.
25. Soothill PW, Nicolaides KH, Rodeck CH, et al: Relationship of fetal hemoglobin and oxygen content to lactate concentration in Rh isoimmunized pregnancies. Obstet Gynecol 69:268-271, 1987.
26. Nicolaides KH, Warenski JC, Rodeck CH: The relationship of fetal plasma protein concentration and hemoglobin level to the development of hydrops in rhesus isoimmunization. Am J Obstet Gynecol 152:341-344, 1985.
27. Moise KJ Jr, Carpenter RJ Jr, Hesketh DE: Do abnormal Starling forces cause fetal hydrops in red blood cell alloimmunization? Am J Obstet Gynecol 167:907-912, 1992.
28. Cormode EJ, Lyster DM, Israels S: Analbuminemia in a neonate. J Pediatr 86:862-867, 1975.
29. Moise AA, Gest AL, Weickmann PH, et al: Reduction in plasma protein does not affect body water content in fetal sheep. Pediatr Res 29:623-626, 1991.
30. Pasman SA, Meerman RH, Vandenbussche FP, et al: Hypoalbuminemia: A cause of fetal hydrops? Am J Obstet Gynecol 194:972-975, 2006.
31. Berger HM, Lindeman JH, van Zoeren-Grobben D, et al: Iron overload, free radical damage, and rhesus haemolytic disease. Lancet 335:933-936, 1990.
32. Lewis M, Bowman JM, Pollock J, et al: Absorption of red cells from the peritoneal cavity of an hydropic twin. Transfusion 13:37-40, 1973.
33. Spong CY, Porter AE, Queenan JT: Management of isoimmunization in the presence of multiple maternal antibodies. Am J Obstet Gynecol 185:481-484, 2001.
34. Vaughan JI, Warwick R, Letsky E, et al: Erythropoietic suppression in fetal anemia because of Kell alloimmunization. Am J Obstet Gynecol 171:247-252, 1994.
35. Weiner CP, Widness JA: Decreased fetal erythropoiesis and hemolysis in Kell hemolytic anemia. Am J Obstet Gynecol 174:547-551, 1996.
36. Vaughan JI, Manning M, Warwick RM, et al: Inhibition of erythroid progenitor cells by anti-Kell antibodies in fetal alloimmune anemia. N Engl J Med 338:798-803, 1998.

37. Fischer RA, Race RR: Rh gene frequencies in Britain. Nature 157:48-49, 1946.
38. Cherif-Zahar B, Mattei MG, Le Van Kim C, et al: Localization of the human Rh blood group gene structure to chromosome region 1p34.3-1p36.1 by in situ hybridization. Hum Genet 86:398-400, 1991.
39. Le Van Kim C, Cherif-Zahar B, Raynal V, et al: Multiple Rh messenger RNA isoforms are produced by alternative splicing. Blood 80:1074-1078, 1992.
40. Carritt B, Kemp TJ, Poulter M: Evolution of the human Rh (rhesus) blood group genes: A 50 year old prediction (partially) fulfilled. Hum Mol Genet 6:843-850, 1997.
41. Avent ND: Fetal genotyping. In Hadley A, Soothill P (eds): Alloimmune Disorders in Pregnancy: Anaemia, Thrombocytopenia, and Neutropenia in the Fetus and Newborn, vol. 1. Cambridge, UK: Cambridge University Press, 2002.
42. Singleton BK, Green CA, Avent ND, et al: The presence of an RHD pseudogene containing a 37 base pair duplication and a nonsense mutation in africans with the Rh D-negative blood group phenotype. Blood 95:12-18, 2000.
43. Yap PL: Viral transmission by blood products: A perspective of events covered by the recent tribunal of enquiry into the Irish Blood Transfusion Board. Ir Med J 90:84-88, 1997.
44. Wiese M, Berr F, Lafrenz M, et al: Low frequency of cirrhosis in a hepatitis C (genotype 1b) single-source outbreak in Germany: A 20-year multicenter study. Hepatology 32:91-96, 2000.
45. Kumpel BM, Elson CJ: Mechanism of anti-D-mediated immune suppression: A paradox awaiting resolution? Trends Immunol 22:26-31, 2001.
46. Woodrow JC, Clarke CA, Donohow WT, et al: Mechanism of Rh prophylaxis: An experimental study on specificity of immunosuppression. BMJ 2:57-59, 1975.
47. Siberil S, de Romeuf C, Bihoreau N, et al: Selection of a human anti-RhD monoclonal antibody for therapeutic use: Impact of IgG glycosylation on activating and inhibitory Fc gamma R functions. Clin Immunol 118:170-179, 2006.
48. Beliard R: Monoclonal anti-D antibodies to prevent alloimmunization: Lessons from clinical trials. Transfus Clin Biol 13:58-64, 2006.
49. Smith NA, Ala FA, Lee D, et al: A multi-centre trial of monoclonal anti-D in the prevention of RhD immunization of RhD– male volunteers by RhD+ cells. Transfus Med 10:8, 2000.
50. American College of Obstetricians and Gynecologists: Prevention of RhD Alloimmunization. ACOG Practice Bulletin No. 4. Washington, DC, ACOG, 1999.
51. Bowman JM: The prevention of Rh immunization. Transfus Med Rev 2:129-150, 1988.
52. National Institute for Clinical Excellence: Guidance on the Use of Routine Antenatal Anti-D Prophylaxis for RhD-Negative Women. Technology Appraised Guidance No. 41. London, National Institute for Clinical Excellence, 2002.
53. American Association of Blood Banks: Prevention of hemolytic disease of the newborn due to anti-D: Prenatal/perinatal testing and Rh immune globulin administration. Association Bulletin Number 98, 1998. Bethesda, MD, American Association of Blood Banks.
54. Goodrick J, Kumpel B, Pamphilon D, et al: Plasma half-lives and bioavailability of human monoclonal Rh D antibodies BRAD-3 and BRAD-5 following intramuscular injection into Rh D-negative volunteers. Clin Exp Immunol 98:17-20, 1994.
55. Bowman JM: Controversies in Rh prophylaxis: Who needs Rh immune globulin and when should it be given? Am J Obstet Gynecol 151:289-294, 1985.
56. Ness PM, Baldwin ML, Niebyl JR: Clinical high-risk designation does not predict excess fetal-maternal hemorrhage. Am J Obstet Gynecol 156:154-158, 1987.
57. Hughes RG, Craig JI, Murphy WG, et al: Causes and clinical consequences of rhesus (D) haemolytic disease of the newborn: A study of a Scottish population, 1985-1990. BJOG 101:297-300, 1994.
58. Nicolaides KH, Rodeck CH: Maternal serum anti-D antibody concentration and assessment of rhesus isoimmunisation. BMJ 304:1155-1156, 1992.
59. Hadley AG: In vitro assays to predict the severity of hemolytic disease of the newborn. Transfus Med Rev 9:302-313, 1995.
60. Moise KJ Jr, Perkins JT, Sosler SD, et al: The predictive value of maternal serum testing for detection of fetal anemia in red blood cell alloimmunization. Am J Obstet Gynecol 172:1003-1009, 1995.
61. Zupanska B, Lenkiewicz B, Michalewska B, et al: The ability of cellular assays to predict the necessity for cordocenteses in pregnancies at risk of haemolytic disease of the newborn. Vox Sang 80:234, 2001.
62. Kanter MH: Derivation of new mathematic formulas for determining whether a D-positive father is heterozygous or homozygous for the D antigen. Am J Obstet Gynecol 166:61-63, 1992.
63. Pirelli K, Pietz B, Johnson S, et al: Molecular determination of RhD zygosity. Am J Obstet Gynecol 195:S172, 2006.
64. Bennett PR, Le Van Kim C, Colin Y, et al: Prenatal determination of fetal RhD type by DNA amplification. N Engl J Med 329:607-610, 1993.
65. Van den Veyver IB, Moise KJ Jr: Fetal RhD typing by polymerase chain reaction in pregnancies complicated by rhesus alloimmunization. Obstet Gynecol 88:1061-1067, 1996.
66. Simsek S, Faas BH, Bleeker PM, et al. Rapid Rh D genotyping by polymerase chain reaction–based amplification of DNA. Blood 85:2975-2980, 1995.
67. Hopkins DF: Maternal anti-Rh(D) and the D-negative fetus. Am J Obstet Gynecol 108:268-271, 1970.
68. Moise KJ Jr, Carpenter RJ Jr: Chorionic villus sampling for Rh typing: Clinical implications. Am J Obstet Gynecol 168:1002-1003, 1993.
69. Brown S, Kellner LH, Munson M, et al: Noninvasive prenatal testing: Strategies to achieve testing of cell free fetal DNA (CFFDNA) RhD genotype in a clinical lab. Am J Obstet Gynecol 197:5173, 2007.
70. Lo YM, Tein MS, Lau TK, et al: Quantitative analysis of fetal DNA in maternal plasma and serum: Implications for noninvasive prenatal diagnosis. Am J Hum Genet 62:768-775, 1998.
71. Wataganara T, Chen AY, LeShane ES, et al: Cell-free fetal DNA levels in maternal plasma after elective first-trimester termination of pregnancy. Fertil Steril 81:638-644, 2004.
72. Moise KJ: Fetal RhD typing with free DNA in maternal plasma. Am J Obstet Gynecol 192:663-665, 2005.
73. Lo YM, Hjelm NM, Fidler C, et al: Prenatal diagnosis of fetal RhD status by molecular analysis of maternal plasma. N Engl J Med 339:1734-1738, 1998.
74. Geifman-Holtzman O, Grotegut CA, Gaughan JP: Diagnostic accuracy of noninvasive fetal Rh genotyping from maternal blood: A meta-analysis. Am J Obstet Gynecol 195:1163-1173, 2006.
75. van der Schoot CE, Hahn S, Chitty LS: Noninvasive prenatal diagnosis and determination of fetal Rh status. Semin Fetal and Neonatal Med 13:63-68, 2008.
76. Finning K, Martin P, Summers J, Daniels G: Fetal genotyping for the K (kell) and RhC, c, and E blood groups on cell-free fetal DNA in maternal plasma. Transfusion 47:2126-2133, 2007.
77. Nicolaides KH, Rodeck CH, Mibashan RS, et al: Have Liley charts outlived their usefulness? Am J Obstet Gynecol 155:90-94, 1986.
78. Queenan JT, Tomai TP, Ural SH, et al: Deviation in amniotic fluid optical density at a wavelength of 450 nm in Rh-immunized pregnancies from 14 to 40 weeks' gestation: A proposal for clinical management. Am J Obstet Gynecol 168:1370-1376, 1993.
79. Oepkes D, Seaward PG, Vandenbussche FP, et al: Doppler ultrasonography versus amniocentesis to predict fetal anemia. N Engl J Med 355:156-164, 2006.
80. Weiner CP, Williamson RA, Wenstrom KD, et al: Management of fetal hemolytic disease by cordocentesis: I. Prediction of fetal anemia. Am J Obstet Gynecol 165:546-553, 1991.
81. Weiner CP, Wenstrom KD, Sipes SL, et al: Risk factors for cordocentesis and fetal intravascular transfusion. Am J Obstet Gynecol 165:1020-1025, 1991.

82. Weiner CP: Human fetal bilirubin levels and fetal hemolytic disease. Am J Obstet Gynecol 166:1449-1454, 1992.
83. Nicolaides KH, Fontanarosa M, Gabbe SG, et al: Failure of ultrasonographic parameters to predict the severity of fetal anemia in rhesus isoimmunization. Am J Obstet Gynecol 158:920-926, 1988.
84. Vintzileos AM, Campbell WA, Storlazzi E, et al: Fetal liver ultrasound measurements in isoimmunized pregnancies. Obstet Gynecol 68:162-167, 1986.
85. Roberts AB, Mitchell JM, Lake Y, et al: Ultrasonographic surveillance in red blood cell alloimmunization. Am J Obstet Gynecol 184:1251-1255, 2001.
86. Oepkes D, Meerman RH, Vandenbussche FP, et al: Ultrasonographic fetal spleen measurements in red blood cell-alloimmunized pregnancies. Am J Obstet Gynecol 169:121-128, 1993.
87. Bahado-Singh R, Oz U, Mari G, et al: Fetal splenic size in anemia due to Rh-alloimmunization. Obstet Gynecol 92:828-832, 1998.
88. Rightmire DA, Nicolaides KH, Rodeck CH, et al: Fetal blood velocities in Rh isoimmunization: Relationship to gestational age and to fetal hematocrit. Obstet Gynecol 68:233-236, 1986.
89. Kirkinen P, Jouppila P, Eik-Nes S: Umbilical vein blood flow in rhesus-isoimmunization. BJOG 90:640-643, 1983.
90. Bahado-Singh R, Oz U, Deren O, et al: Splenic artery Doppler peak systolic velocity predicts severe fetal anemia in rhesus disease. Am J Obstet Gynecol 182:1222-1226, 2000.
91. Bilardo CM, Nicolaides KH, Campbell S: Doppler studies in red cell isoimmunization. Clin Obstet Gynecol 32:719-727, 1989.
92. Vyas S, Nicolaides KH, Campbell S: Doppler examination of the middle cerebral artery in anemic fetuses. Am J Obstet Gynecol 162:1066-1068, 1990.
93. Mari G; for the Collaborative Group for Doppler Assessment of the Blood Velocity in Anemic Fetuses: Noninvasive diagnosis by Doppler ultrasonography of fetal anemia due to maternal red-cell alloimmunization. N Engl J Med 342:9-14, 2000.
94. Divakaran TG, Waugh J, Clark TJ, et al: Noninvasive techniques to detect fetal anemia due to red blood cell alloimmunization: A systematic review. Obstet Gynecol 98:509-517, 2001.
95. Zimmerman R, Carpenter RJ Jr, Durig P, et al: Longitudinal measurement of peak systolic velocity in the fetal middle cerebral artery for monitoring pregnancies complicated by red cell alloimmunisation: A prospective multicentre trial with intention-to-treat. BJOG 109:746-752, 2002.
96. Abel DE, Grambow SC, Brancazio LR, et al: Ultrasound assessment of the fetal middle cerebral artery peak systolic velocity: A comparison of the near-field versus far-field vessel. Am J Obstet Gynecol 189:986-989, 2003.
97. Sallout BI, Fung KF, Wen SW, et al: The effect of fetal behavioral states on middle cerebral artery peak systolic velocity. Am J Obstet Gynecol 191:1283-1287, 2004.
98. Mari G: Middle cerebral artery peak systolic velocity: Is it the standard of care for the diagnosis of fetal anemia? J Ultrasound Med 24:697-702, 2005.
99. Moise KJ Jr: Diagnosing hemolytic disease of the fetus: Time to put the needles away? N Engl J Med 355:192-194, 2006.
100. Nicolini U, Santolaya J, Ojo OE, et al: The fetal intrahepatic umbilical vein as an alternative to cord needling for prenatal diagnosis and therapy. Prenat Diagn 8:665-671, 1988.
101. Giannakoulopoulos X, Sepulveda W, Kourtis P, et al: Fetal plasma cortisol and beta-endorphin response to intrauterine needling. Lancet 344:77-81, 1994.
102. Giannakoulopoulos X, Teixeira J, Fisk N, et al: Human fetal and maternal noradrenaline responses to invasive procedures. Pediatr Res 45:494-499, 1999.
103. Antsaklis AI, Papantoniou NE, Mesogitis SA, et al: Cardiocentesis: An alternative method of fetal blood sampling for the prenatal diagnosis of hemoglobinopathies. Obstet Gynecol 79:630-633, 1992.
104. Harman CR, Bowman JM, Manning FA, et al: Intrauterine transfusion: Intraperitoneal versus intravascular approach. A case-control comparison. Am J Obstet Gynecol 162:1053-1059, 1990.
105. Bowman JM: The management of Rh-isoimmunization. Obstet Gynecol 52:1-16, 1978.
106. Berkowitz RL, Chitkara U, Goldberg JD, et al: Intrauterine intravascular transfusions for severe red blood cell isoimmunization: Ultrasound-guided percutaneous approach. Am J Obstet Gynecol 155:574-581, 1986.
107. Moise KJ Jr, Carpenter RJ Jr, Kirshon B, et al: Comparison of four types of intrauterine transfusion: Effect on fetal hematocrit. Fetal Ther 4:126-137, 1989.
108. Lepercq J, Poissonnier MH, Coutanceau MJ, et al: Management and outcome of fetomaternal Rh alloimmunization in twin pregnancies. Fetal Diagn Ther 14:26-30, 1999.
109. Welch R, Rampling MW, Anwar A, et al: Changes in hemorheology with fetal intravascular transfusion. Am J Obstet Gynecol 170:726-732, 1994.
110. Mandelbrot L, Daffos F, Forestier F, et al: Assessment of fetal blood volume for computer-assisted management of in utero transfusion. Fetal Ther 3:60-66, 1988.
111. Giannina G, Moise KJ Jr, Dorman K: A simple method to estimate the volume for fetal intravascular transfusion. Fetal Diagn Ther 13:94-97, 1998.
112. Detti L, Oz U, Guney I, et al: Doppler ultrasound velocimetry for timing the second intrauterine transfusion in fetuses with anemia from red cell alloimmunization. Am J Obstet Gynecol 185:1048-1051, 2001.
113. Mari G, Zimmermann R, Moise KJ Jr, et al: Correlation between middle cerebral artery peak systolic velocity and fetal hemoglobin after 2 previous intrauterine transfusions. Am J Obstet Gynecol 193:1117-1120, 2005.
114. Kilby M, Martin W, Whittle M: Early intraperitoneal transfusion and adjuvant maternal immunoglobulin in severe alloimmunisation, prior to fetal intravascular transfusion. Am J Obstet Gynecol 195:S191, 2006.
115. Hallak M, Moise KJ Jr, Hesketh DE, et al: Intravascular transfusion of fetuses with rhesus incompatibility: Prediction of fetal outcome by changes in umbilical venous pressure. Obstet Gynecol 80:286-290, 1992.
116. Radunovic N, Lockwood CJ, Alvarez M, et al: The severely anemic and hydropic isoimmune fetus: Changes in fetal hematocrit associated with intrauterine death. Obstet Gynecol 79:390-393, 1992.
117. de Crespigny LC, Robinson HP, Quinn M, et al: Ultrasound-guided fetal blood transfusion for severe rhesus isoimmunization. Obstet Gynecol 66:529-532, 1985.
118. Moise KJ Jr, Carpenter RJ Jr, Deter RL, et al: The use of fetal neuromuscular blockade during intrauterine procedures. Am J Obstet Gynecol 157:874-879, 1987.
119. Moise KJ Jr, Deter RL, Kirshon B, et al: Intravenous pancuronium bromide for fetal neuromuscular blockade during intrauterine transfusion for red-cell alloimmunization. Obstet Gynecol 74:905-908, 1989.
120. Bernstein HH, Chitkara U, Plosker H, et al: Use of atracurium besylate to arrest fetal activity during intrauterine intravascular transfusions. Obstet Gynecol 72:813-816, 1988.
121. Daffos F, Forestier F, Mac Aleese J, et al: Fetal curarization for prenatal magnetic resonance imaging. Prenat Diagn 8:312-314, 1988.
122. Pielet BW, Socol ML, MacGregor SN, et al: Fetal heart rate changes after fetal intravascular treatment with pancuronium bromide. Am J Obstet Gynecol 159:640-643, 1988.
123. Harte G, Payton D, Carmody F, et al: Graft versus host disease following intrauterine and exchange transfusions for rhesus haemolytic disease. Aust N Z J Obstet Gynaecol 37:319-322, 1997.
124. Bohm N, Kleine W, Enzel U: [Graft-versus-host disease in two newborns after repeated blood transfusions because of rhesus incompatibility.] Beitr Pathol 160:381-400, 1977.
125. Guidelines on gamma irradiation of blood components for the prevention of transfusion-associated graft-versus-host disease. Transfus Med 6:261-271, 1996.
126. Brecher ME: Technical Manual of the American Association of Blood Banks. Bethesda, MD, American Association of Blood Banks, 2005.
127. Gonsoulin WJ, Moise KJ Jr, Milam JD, et al: Serial maternal blood donations for intrauterine transfusion. Obstet Gynecol 75:158-162, 1990.
128. Vietor HE, Kanhai HH, Brand A: Induction of additional red cell alloantibodies after intrauterine transfusions. Transfusion 34:970-974, 1994.

129. el-Azeem SA, Samuels P, Rose RL, et al: The effect of the source of transfused blood on the rate of consumption of transfused red blood cells in pregnancies affected by red blood cell alloimmunization. Am J Obstet Gynecol 177:753-757, 1997.
130. Herbert WN, Owen HG, Collins ML: Autologous blood storage in obstetrics. Obstet Gynecol 72:166-170, 1988.
131. Pamphilon DH, Rider JR, Barbara JA, et al: Prevention of transfusion-transmitted cytomegalovirus infection. Transfus Med 9:115-123, 1999.
132. Klumper FJ, van Kamp IL, Vandenbussche FP, et al: Benefits and risks of fetal red-cell transfusion after 32 weeks gestation. Eur J Obstet Gynecol Reprod Biol 92:91-96, 2000.
133. Schumacher B, Moise KJ Jr: Fetal transfusion for red blood cell alloimmunization in pregnancy. Obstet Gynecol 88:137-150, 1996.
134. van Kamp IL, Klumper FJ, Bakkum RS, et al: The severity of immune fetal hydrops is predictive of fetal outcome after intrauterine treatment. Am J Obstet Gynecol 185:668-673, 2001.
135. Saade GR, Moise KJ, Belfort MA, et al: Fetal and neonatal hematologic parameters in red cell alloimmunization: Predicting the need for late neonatal transfusions. Fetal Diagn Ther 8:161-164, 1993.
136. Koenig JM, Ashton RD, De Vore GR, et al: Late hyporegenerative anemia in Rh hemolytic disease. J Pediatr 115:315-318, 1989.
137. Ovali F, Samanci N, Dagoglu T: Management of late anemia in rhesus hemolytic disease: Use of recombinant human erythropoietin (a pilot study). Pediatr Res 39:831-834, 1996.
138. Maier RF, Obladen M, Scigalla P, et al: The effect of epoetin beta (recombinant human erythropoietin) on the need for transfusion in very-low-birth-weight infants. European Multicentre Erythropoietin Study Group. N Engl J Med 330:1173-1178, 1994.
139. Shannon KM, Mentzer WC, Abels RI, et al: Recombinant human erythropoietin in the anemia of prematurity: Results of a placebo-controlled pilot study. J Pediatr 118:949-955, 1991.
140. Hardyment AF, Salvador HS, Towell ME, et al: Follow-up of intrauterine transfused surviving children. Am J Obstet Gynecol 133:235-241, 1979.
141. Doyle LW, Kelly EA, Rickards AL, et al: Sensorineural outcome at 2 years for survivors of erythroblastosis treated with fetal intravascular transfusions. Obstet Gynecol 81:931-935, 1993.
142. Janssens HM, de Haan MJ, van Kamp IL, et al: Outcome for children treated with fetal intravascular transfusions because of severe blood group antagonism. J Pediatr 131:373-380, 1997.
143. Hudon L, Moise KJ Jr, Hegemier SE, et al: Long-term neurodevelopmental outcome after intrauterine transfusion for the treatment of fetal hemolytic disease. Am J Obstet Gynecol 179:858-863, 1998.
144. Grab D, Paulus WE, Bommer A, et al: Treatment of fetal erythroblastosis by intravascular transfusions: Outcome at 6 years. Obstet Gynecol 93:165-168, 1999.
145. Bystryn JC, Graf MW, Uhr JW: Regulation of antibody formation by serum antibody: II. Removal of specific antibody by means of exchange transfusion. J Exp Med 132:1279-1287, 1970.
146. Schur PH, Alpert E, Alper C: Gamma G subgroups in human fetal, cord, and maternal sera. Clin Immunol Immunopathol 2:62-66, 1973.
147. Angela E, Robinson E, Tovey LA: Intensive plasma exchange in the management of severe Rh disease. Br J Haematol 45:621-631, 1980.
148. Margulies M, Voto LS, Mathet E: High-dose intravenous IgG for the treatment of severe rhesus alloimmunization. Vox Sang 61:181-189, 1991.
149. Voto LS, Mathet ER, Zapaterio JL, et al: High-dose gammaglobulin (IVIG) followed by intrauterine transfusions (IUTs): A new alternative for the treatment of severe fetal hemolytic disease. J Perinat Med 25:85-88, 1997.
150. Dooren MC, van Kamp IL, Scherpenisse JW, et al. No beneficial effect of low-dose fetal intravenous gammaglobulin administration in combination with intravascular transfusions in severe Rh D haemolytic disease. Vox Sang 66:253-257, 1994.
151. Rubo J, Albrecht K, Lasch P, et al: High-dose intravenous immune globulin therapy for hyperbilirubinemia caused by Rh hemolytic disease. J Pediatr 121:93-97, 1992.
152. Alonso JG, Decaro J, Marrero A, et al: Repeated direct fetal intravascular high-dose immunoglobulin therapy for the treatment of Rh hemolytic disease. J Perinat Med 22:415-419, 1994.
153. Gottvall T, Selbing A: Alloimmunization during pregnancy treated with high dose intravenous immunoglobulin: Effects on fetal hemoglobin concentration and anti-D concentrations in the mother and fetus. Acta Obstet Gynecol Scand 74:777-783, 1995.
154. Besalduch J, Forteza A, Duran MA, et al: Rh hemolytic disease of the newborn treated with high-dose intravenous immunoglobulin and plasmapheresis. Transfusion 31:380-381, 1991.
155. Yu Z, Lennon VA: Mechanism of intravenous immune globulin therapy in antibody-mediated autoimmune diseases. N Engl J Med 340:227-228, 1999.
156. Berlin G, Selbing A, Ryden G: Rhesus haemolytic disease treated with high-dose intravenous immunoglobulin. Lancet 1:1153, 1985.
157. Ruma MS, Moise KJ, Kim E, et al: Combined plasmapheresis and intravenous immune globulin for the treatment of maternal red cell alloimmunization. Am J Obstet Gynecol 196:138.e1-e6, 2006.
158. Hamrock DJ: Adverse events associated with intravenous immunoglobulin therapy. Int Immunopharmacol 6:535-542, 2006.
159. Bierme SJ, Blanc M, Abbal M, et al: Oral Rh treatment for severely immunised mothers. Lancet 1:604-605, 1979.
160. Gold WR Jr, Queenan JT, Woody J, et al: Oral desensitization in Rh disease. Am J Obstet Gynecol 146:980-981, 1983.
161. Parinaud J, Bierme S, Fournie A, et al: Oral Rh treatment for severely immunized mother. Am J Obstet Gynecol 150:902, 1984.
162. Barnes RM, Duguid JK, Roberts FM, et al: Oral administration of erythrocyte membrane antigen does not suppress anti-Rh(D) antibody responses in humans. Clin Exp Immunol 67:220-226, 1987.
163. Gusdon JP Jr, Caudle MR, Herbst GA, et al: Phagocytosis and erythroblastosis: I. Modification of the neonatal response by promethazine hydrochloride. Am J Obstet Gynecol 125:224-226, 1976.
164. Gusdon JP Jr: The treatment of erythroblastosis with promethazine hydrochloride. J Reprod Med 26:454-458, 1981.
165. Stenchever MA: Promethazine hydrochloride: Use in patients with Rh isoimmunizationlyophilized preparation of erythrocyte membranes. Am J Obstet Gynecol 130:665-668, 1978.
166. Caudle MR, Scott JR: The potential role of immunosuppression, plasmapheresis, and desensitization as treatment modalities for Rh immunization. Clin Obstet Gynecol 25:313-319, 1982.
167. Caritis SN, Mueller-Heuback E, Edelstone DI: Effect of betamethasone on analysis of amniotic fluid in the rhesus-sensitized pregnancy. Am J Obstet Gynecol 127:529-532, 1977.
168. Trevett TN Jr, Dorman K, Lamvu G, et al: Antenatal maternal administration of phenobarbital for the prevention of exchange transfusion in neonates with hemolytic disease of the fetus and newborn. Am J Obstet Gynecol 192:478-482, 2005.
169. Neppert J, Pohl E, Mueller-Eckhardt C: Inhibition of immune phagocytosis by human sera with HLA A, B, C and DR but not with DQ or EM type reactivity. Vox Sang 51:122-126, 1986.
170. Neppert J: Rhesus-Du and -D incompatibility in the newborn without haemolytic disease: Inhibition of immune phagocytosis? Vox Sang 53:239, 1987.
171. Dooren MC, Kuijpers RW, Joekes EC, et al: Protection against immune haemolytic disease of newborn infants by maternal monocyte-reactive IgG alloantibodies (anti-HLA-DR). Lancet 339:1067-1070, 1992.
172. Dooren MC, van Kamp IL, Kanhai HH, et al: Evidence for the protective effect of maternal FcR-blocking IgG alloantibodies HLA-DR in Rh D-haemolytic disease of the newborn. Vox Sang 65:55-58, 1993.
173. Eichler H, Zieger W, Neppert J, et al: Mild course of fetal RhD haemolytic disease due to maternal alloimmunisation to paternal HLA class I and II antigens. Vox Sang 68:243-247, 1995.
174. Shepard SL, Noble AL, Filbey D, et al: Inhibition of the monocyte chemiluminescent response to anti-D-sensitized red cells by Fc gamma RI-blocking antibodies which ameliorate the severity of haemolytic disease of the newborn. Vox Sang 70:157-163, 1996.

175. Wiener E, Mawas F, Dellow RA, et al: A major role of class I Fc gamma receptors in immunoglobulin G anti-D-mediated red blood cell destruction by fetal mononuclear phagocytes. Obstet Gynecol 86:157-162, 1995.
176. Whitecar PW, Farb R, Subramanyam L, et al: Paternal leukocyte alloimmunization as a treatment for hemolytic disease of the newborn in a rabbit model. Am J Obstet Gynecol 187:977-980, 2002.
177. Hall AM, Cairns LS, Altmann DM, et al: Immune responses and tolerance to the RhD blood group protein in HLA-transgenic mice. Blood 105:2175-2179, 2005.
178. Bowman JM:. Treatment options for the fetus with alloimmune hemolytic disease. Transfus Med Rev 4:191-207, 1990.
179. Brecher ME: Technical Manual of the American Association of Blood Banks. Bethesda, MD, American Association of Blood Banks, 2002.
180. Bowell PJ, Brown SE, Dike AE, et al: The significance of anti-c alloimmunization in pregnancy. BJOG 93:1044-1048, 1986.
181. Wenk RE, Goldstein P, Felix JK: Alloimmunization by hr'(c), hemolytic disease of newborns, and perinatal management. Obstet Gynecol 67:623-626, 1986.
182. Kozlowski CL, Lee D, Shwe KH, et al: Quantification of anti-c in haemolytic disease of the newborn. Transfus Med 5:37-42, 1995.
183. Hackney DN, Knudtson EJ, Rossi KQ, et al: Management of pregnancies complicated by anti-c isoimmunization. Obstet Gynecol 103:24-30, 2004.
184. Bowman JM, Pollock JM, Manning FA, et al: Severe anti-C hemolytic disease of the newborn. Am J Obstet Gynecol 166:1239-1243, 1992.
185. Joy SD, Rossi KQ, Krugh D, et al: Management of pregnancies complicated by anti-E alloimmunization. Obstet Gynecol 105:24-28, 2005.
186. Trevett TN Jr, Moise KJ Jr: Twin pregnancy complicated by severe hemolytic disease of the fetus and newborn due to anti-g and anti-C. Obstet Gynecol 106:1178-1180, 2005.
187. Daniels G: Blood group antibodies in haemolytic disease of the fetus and newborn. In Hadley A, Soothill P (eds): Alloimmune Disorders in Pregnancy: Anaemia, Thrombocytopenia, and Neutropenia in the Fetus and Newborn, vol. 1. Cambridge, UK: Cambridge University Press, 2002.
188. Caine ME, Mueller-Heubach E: Kell sensitization in pregnancy. Am J Obstet Gynecol 154:85-90, 1986.
189. Bowman JM, Pollock JM, Manning FA, et al: Maternal Kell blood group alloimmunization. Obstet Gynecol 79:239-244, 1992.
190. Berkowitz RL, Beyth Y, Sadovsky E: Death in utero due to Kell sensitization without excessive elevation of the delta OD450 value in amniotic fluid. Obstet Gynecol 60:746-749, 1982.
191. van Dongen H, Klumper FJ, Sikkel E, et al: Non-invasive tests to predict fetal anemia in Kell-alloimmunized pregnancies. Ultrasound Obstet Gynecol 25:341-345, 2005.
192. Rimon E, Peltz R, Gamzu R, et al: Management of Kell isoimmunization: Evaluation of a Doppler-guided approach. Ultrasound Obstet Gynecol 28:814-820, 2006.
193. Bowman JM, Harman FA, Manning CR, et al: Erythroblastosis fetalis produced by anti-k. Vox Sang 56:187-189, 1989.
194. Levine P, Backer M, Wigod M: A human blood group property (Cellano) present in 99.8% of all bloods. Science 109:464-466, 1949.
195. Bryant LB: A case of anti-Cellano (k) with review of the present status of the Kell blood group system. Bulletin of the South Central Association of Blood Banks 8:4-13, 1965.
196. Kulich V: Hemolytic disease of the newborn caused by anti-k antibody. Cesk Pediatr 22:823-826, 1967.
197. Duguid JK, Bromilow IM: Haemolytic disease of the newborn due to anti-k. Vox Sang 58:69, 1990.
198. Stone B, Marsh WL: Hemolytic disease of the newborn caused by anti-M. Br J Haemotol 5:344-347, 1959.
199. Macpherson CR, Zartman ER: Anti-M antibody as a cause of intrauterine death: A follow-up. Am J Clin Pathol 43:544-547, 1965.
200. Matsumoto H, Tamaki Y, Sato S, et al: A case of hemolytic disease of the newborn caused by anti-M: Serological study of maternal blood. Acta Obstet Gynaecol Jpn 33:525-528, 1981.
201. Furukawa K, Nakajima T, Kogure T, et al: Example of a woman with multiple intrauterine deaths due to anti-M who delivered a live child after plasmapheresis. Exp Clin Immunogenet 10:161-167, 1993.
202. Duguid JK, Bromilow IM, Entwistle GD, et al: Haemolytic disease of the newborn due to anti-M. Vox Sang 68:195-196, 1995.
203. Kanra T, Yuce K, Ozcebe IU: Hydrops fetalis and intrauterine deaths due to anti-M. Acta Obstet Gynecol Scand 75:415-417, 1996.
204. De Young-Owens A, Kennedy M, Rose RL, et al: Anti-M isoimmunization: Management and outcome at the Ohio State University from 1969 to 1995. Obstet Gynecol 90:962-966, 1997.
205. Vengelen-Tyler V (ed): Technical Manual of the American Association of Blood Banks. Bethesda, MD, American Association of Blood Banks, 1999.
206. Corfield VA, Moolman JC, Martell R, et al: Polymerase chain reaction-based detection of MN blood group-specific sequences in the human genome. Transfusion 33:119-124, 1993.
207. Mayne KM, Bowell PJ, Green SJ, et al: The significance of anti-S sensitization in pregnancy. Clin Lab Haematol 12:105-107, 1990.
208. Feldman R, Luhby AL, Gromisch DS: Erythroblastosis fetalis due to anti-S antibody. J Pediatr 82:88-91, 1973.
209. Levine P, Ferraro LR, Koch E: Haemolytic disease of the newborn due to anti-S. Blood 7:1030-1037, 1952.
210. Griffith TK: The irregular antibodies: A continuing problem. Am J Obstet Gynecol 137:174-177, 1980.
211. Davie MJ, Smith DS, White UM, et al: An example of anti-s causing mild haemolytic disease of the newborn. J Clin Pathol 25:772-773, 1972.
212. Telischi M, Behzad O, Issitt PD, et al: Hemolytic disease of the newborn due to anti-N. Vox Sang 31:109-116, 1976.
213. Smith G, Knott P, Rissik J, et al: Anti-U and haemolytic disease of the fetus and newborn. BJOG 105:1318-1321, 1998.
214. Burki U, Degan T, Rosenfield R: Stillbirth due to anti-U. Vox Sang 9:209-211, 1964.
215. Austin TK, Finklestein J, Okada DM, et al: Hemolytic disease of newborn infant due to anti-U [Letter]. J Pediatr 89:330-331, 1976.
216. Dhandsa N, Williams M, Joss V, et al: Haemolytic disease of the newborn caused by anti-U. Lancet 2:1232, 1981.
217. Gottschall JL. Hemolytic disease of the newborn with anti-U. Transfusion 21:230-232, 1981.
218. Magaud JP, Jouvenceaux A, Bertrix F, et al: [Perinatal hemolytic disease due to incompatibility in the U system.] Arch Fr Pediatr 38:769-771, 1981.
219. Alfonso JF, de Alvarez RR: Maternal isoimmunization to the red cell antigen U. Am J Obstet Gynecol 81:45-48, 1961.
220. Tuck SM, Studd JW, White JM: Sickle cell disease in pregnancy complicated by anti-U antibody. Case report. BJOG 89:91-92, 1982.
221. Dopp SL, Isham BE: Anti-U and hemolytic disease of the newborn. Transfusion 23:273-274, 1983.
222. Weinstein L, Taylor ES: Hemolytic disease of the neonate secondary to anti-Fya. Am J Obstet Gynecol 121:643-645, 1975.
223. Hessner MJ, Pircon RA, Johnson ST, et al: Prenatal genotyping of the Duffy blood group system by allele-specific polymerase chain reaction. Prenat Diagn 19:41-45, 1999.
224. Hessner MJ, Pircon RA, Johnson ST, et al: Prenatal genotyping of Jk(a) and Jk(b) of the human Kidd blood group system by allele-specific polymerase chain reaction. Prenat Diagn 18:1225-1231, 1998.

Chapter 27

Nonimmune Hydrops

Isabelle Wilkins, MD

Hydrops fetalis is the term used to describe generalized edema in the neonate. This edema is accompanied by collections of fluid in serous spaces. In the past, most cases of hydrops fetalis were caused by severe erythroblastosis due to Rh alloimmunization. Potter[1] was the first to describe nonimmune hydrops fetalis in a group of infants without erythroblastosis whose mothers were Rh-positive.

Since it was first described 60 years ago, nonimmune hydrops (NIH) has become more common than hydrops from alloimmunization. Santolaya and associates[2] reported a series of 76 hydropic fetuses, of which 87% had NIH. Only 4 (4.5%) of 87 cases assessed at a fetal medicine unit reported by Sohan and associates[3] were caused by red cell alloimmunization, and Ismail and coworkers[4] reported 63 prenatally detected cases, of which only 8 (12.7%) had an immune basis. Graves and Baskett[5] examined all babies born at their institution with hydrops and reported that 76% of cases were nonimmune. More recently, Trainor and Tubman reported their experience over three time periods, showing a dramatic increase in the percentage of nonimmune cases of hydrops at delivery, from 0% in 1974 to 80% in 2002.[6]

The incidence of NIH at delivery in published accounts is approximately 1 in 1500 to 1 in 3800.[5,7,8] A large, unselected prenatal ultrasound screening clinic in Finland had a similar rate of 1 in 1700.[9] Trainor and Tubman[6] did not include stillbirths and found a rate of 1.34 per 1000 live births. Reviews from ultrasonography referral centers, however, show an incidence between 1 in 150 and 1 in 766 sonographic examinations.[2,10,11]

NIH is a heterogeneous disorder with a large number of possible causes and associations. Overall, the prognosis is poor; a 52% to 98% perinatal mortality rate is typical.[3,4,9,12] Elucidation of etiology is of primary importance, because treatment and prognosis of this disorder are determined by the underlying fetal condition, but the task may be difficult. Most authors differentiate the rate of prenatal detection of etiology, which is lower than the rate after delivery or at autopsy. Both are important in counseling families and discussing recurrence risks, but only prenatal detection is useful in guiding management and therapy. In most series, cause is found in approximately 51% to 85% of cases before delivery but in up to 95% after delivery, depending in part on parental acceptance of autopsy and karyotyping.[3,4,9,10,12] It is clear that both success in determining etiology and survival statistics differ between early and late gestation, largely because of the different gestational ages at which hydrops of various causes presents. In general, presentation before 24 weeks of gestation occurs in more severe cases, in which the cause is easier to ascertain but perinatal survival is worse.[3,4,9,10-12]

Presenting Signs and Symptoms

Although NIH is a clinical diagnosis concerning the neonate, the condition can be determined antenatally by obstetric sonographic examination, with a success rate of almost 100%. The indication for ultrasonography varies among series. In 1986, Watson and Campbell[13] found that 63% of cases of NIH were discovered on routine ultrasonography, whereas another 30% of patients were referred because of suspected hydramnios. Graves and Baskett[5] found that NIH was less commonly discovered on routine ultrasonography than on ultrasonography ordered for a specific indication. The most common indications in their population were hydramnios, size greater than dates, fetal tachycardia, and maternal pregnancy-induced hypertension. Other frequently cited indications for ultrasound evaluation have included abnormal serum screening, decreased fetal movement, and antenatal hemorrhage.[11,14-15]

Maternal complications of pregnancy are also increased in NIH. Hydramnios, pregnancy-induced hypertension, severe anemia, postpartum hemorrhage, preterm labor, birth trauma, gestational diabetes, a retained placenta, and difficult delivery of the placenta are all frequently mentioned in large series.[5,7,12,15,16]

An uncommon maternal complication of fetal hydrops is called *mirror syndrome*. This condition is rarely a presenting complaint and may develop during conservative management of such pregnancies. Patients generally experience edema and pulmonary edema and may have hypertension and proteinuria. The similarity to severe preeclampsia has led some authors to refer to this condition as pseudotoxemia. The patients may be gravely ill but recover after delivery. The syndrome may also develop after delivery, as it did in two mothers in one series.[12] Although no series exist to direct management, most authors do not advise continuation of the pregnancy.[11,17,18] A case report of fetal hydrops caused by parvovirus infection with concomitant maternal mirror syndrome was self-limited. As the fetal hydrops reversed, so did maternal symptoms, and a term delivery subsequently occurred.[19] Stepan and Faber[20] reported a similar case in which maternal levels of soluble fms-like tyrosine kinase 1 (sFlt1) were extremely elevated initially and dropped after fetal transfusion resulted in resolution of both maternal and fetal symptoms. Espinoza and colleagues[21] investigated levels of soluble vascular endothelial growth factor receptor-1 (sVEGFR-1) in four patients with mirror syndrome. This antiangiogenic factor may be related to the pathogenesis of preeclampsia, and sVEGFR-1 was elevated in these cases.

Ultrasonography

Ultrasound examination is essential to the diagnosis of NIH, and criteria for definition of the disorder in the fetus are based exclusively on ultrasound parameters. The fluid that accumulates may include ascites, pleural effusions, pericardial effusions, and skin edema. Several definitions of fetal NIH have been proposed based on the quantity and distribution of excess fetal water. Variations in these definitions have made direct comparisons among published series inexact. Mahony and coworkers[22] defined hydrops as generalized skin edema with or without an associated serous effusion. Although others have also used this definition,[23] NIH is more commonly defined as edema with one or more effusions, or effusions in at least two spaces; that is, two of the following must be present: ascites, pleural effusion, pericardial effusion, or skin edema.[24,25]

The degree or severity of hydrops is generally subjective. Hutchison and associates[7] described a score based on total number of serous space effusions. Because the only requirement for the definition of NIH was edema, it was possible to have a score of zero (0) with no serous involvement. This score was not predictive of outcome in their series, because the overall perinatal mortality rate was close to 100%. Saltzman and colleagues[26] described a different scoring system, in which each effusion was quantified. With this system, they were able to predict which cases were most likely caused by fetal anemia and which were from other causes. Although they included isoimmunized pregnancies in their series, other forms of anemia followed the same general pattern.

Fluid in one of these spaces may be an early finding in a fetus destined to develop hydrops. At the very least, a careful search for fluid in other serous sites is warranted. Such fetuses should undergo follow-up over time to ensure that hydrops is not developing. In general, these fetuses have a better prognosis than fetuses with hydrops.[27,28]

Fetal Fluid Accumulation

Ascites appears sonographically as an echolucent rim of varying size in the fetal abdomen (Fig. 27-1). A small rim of ascites may be hard to distinguish from a similarly located area of echo dropout common with normal fetuses.[24] One possible distinguishing feature is that a true rim of fluid should be visible all the way around the abdomen in the transverse viewing plane. Longitudinally, the edge of the liver, bladder, or diaphragm may be outlined. When ascites is more marked, the entire liver is outlined and the bowel is compressed (Fig. 27-2). In these more extreme cases, the diagnosis is relatively easy.

Pleural effusions may be unilateral or bilateral. Although the effusions may appear as small rims of fluid outlining the pleural space and diaphragm, more commonly they are large and compress the lung (Fig. 27-3). It is uncommon for a unilateral effusion to shift the mediastinum. In such a case, an extrinsic fluid-filled mass, such as a diaphragmatic hernia or another space-occupying lesion, is likely to be present. Pulmonary hypoplasia is a frequent cause of death in neonates with NIH, and the size of pleural effusions may help to predict this complication.[16]

Pericardial effusions are smaller in total volume and are therefore more difficult to see than ascites or pleural effusions (Fig. 27-4). Some authors[24] have proposed that pericardial effusions indicate cardiac decompensation and that this is the earliest sign of hydrops in fetuses with cardiac lesions. In a group of patients with mixed etiology, Carlson and colleagues[29] found that the biventricular dimension, an indicator of overall cardiac size as measured on M-mode examination, was highly predictive of survival.

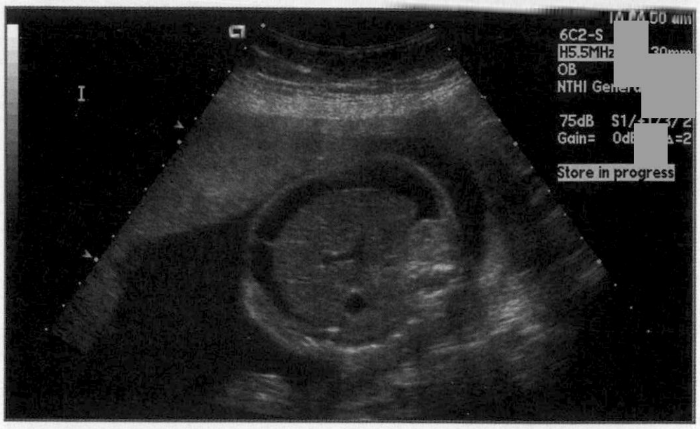

FIGURE 27-1 Transverse image of the fetal abdomen at the level of the stomach. A large rim of ascites is seen within the abdominal wall.

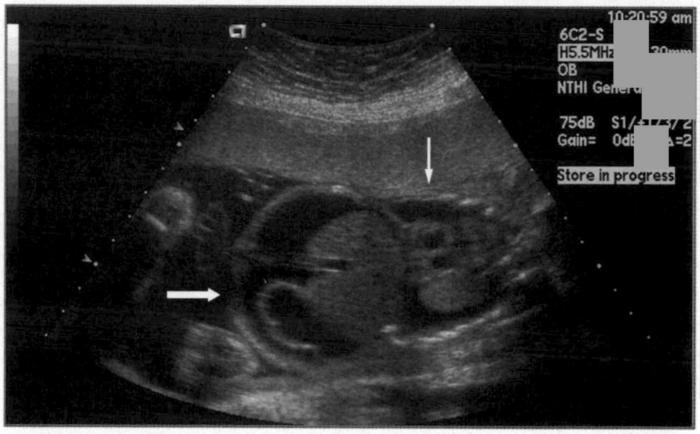

FIGURE 27-2 Longitudinal image of the fetus. Ascitic fluid is seen outlining the liver *(large arrow),* and there is a pleural effusion above the diaphragm *(small arrow).*

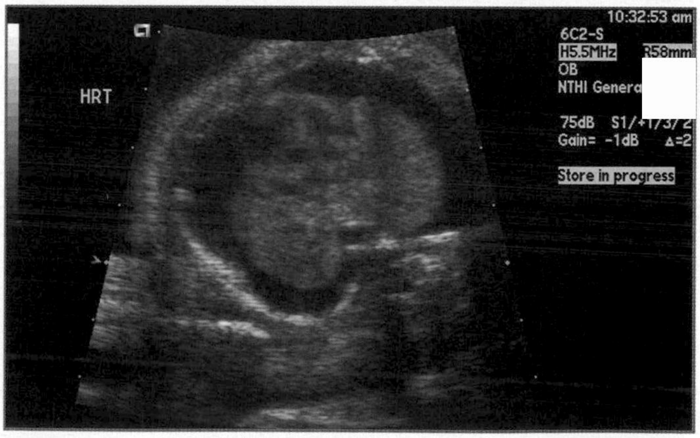

FIGURE 27-3 Transverse image of the fetal chest. Bilateral pleural effusions are seen.

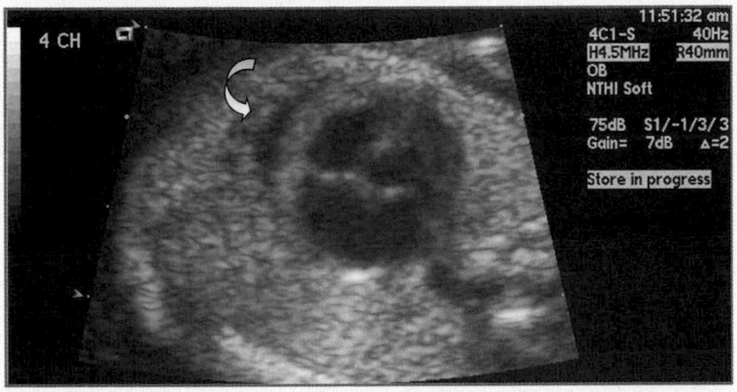

FIGURE 27-4 Transverse image of the fetal chest. Small pericardial effusion *(arrow)*.

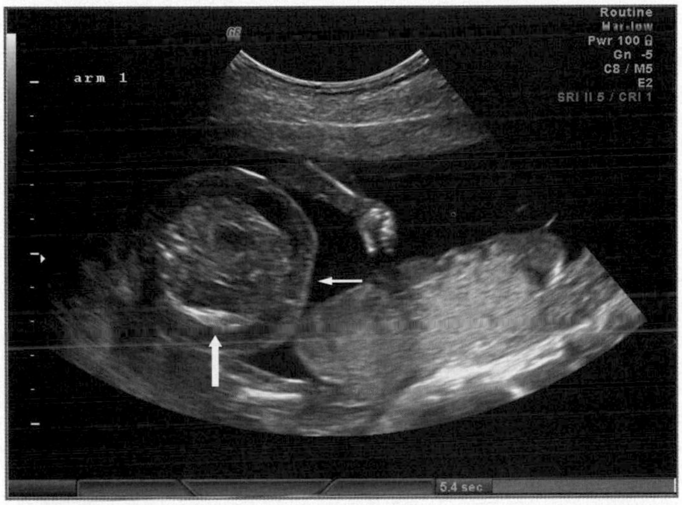

FIGURE 27-5 Transverse image of the fetal chest. Skin edema over fetal chest wall. Rib is marked by *large arrow* and skin edge with *small arrow*.

Skin edema is usually a generalized process, although it is easiest to see with ultrasonography over the chest wall or scalp, where soft tissue is typically thin and any thickness can be appreciated (Fig. 27-5). The usual definition of edema is greater than 5 mm of subcutaneous tissue. This may be misleading if the fetus has redundant skin folds or is macrosomic.

Placental thickening is frequently considered a sign of hydrops as well. Abnormal thickening is usually defined as a thickness of greater than 6 cm,[25,30] although some authors have used a cutoff of 4 cm.[31,32] With hydramnios, the placenta may appear compressed and instead be thin. If therapeutic amniocenteses are performed because of severe hydramnios, the placenta may "thicken" by the end of the procedure, and this occurrence implies that hydrostatic pressure was responsible for the thinned appearance.[33]

According to various authors, hydramnios is present in 40% to 75% of cases of NIH. Although the definition of hydramnios differed among these series, when the condition was present, it was often severe and would therefore have been detected by any quantifying technique. In some cases of fetal hydrops, oligohydramnios is present, and many authors consider this an ominous or late finding. Although oligohydramnios is generally associated with poor pregnancy outcome, its prognosis in NIH depends on the underlying cause rather than simply on this sonographic feature.

Etiology

One of the greatest challenges in the management of a fetus with NIH is ascertaining the cause of the disorder. Causes are numerous, and new associations continually appear in the literature. The causes may be divided into several broad categories that are helpful in organizing an approach to this often-frustrating problem (Table 27-1).

Many of the conditions listed in Table 27-1 are categorized somewhat arbitrarily. For example, many anatomic cardiac lesions have a chromosomal basis. Similarly, viral syndromes that lead to NIH may be associated with fetal anemia, with fetal malformation complexes, or with myocarditis. It is also obvious that some of these syndromes are extremely rare and others are more common. In addition, many of these conditions represent congenital anomalies whereas others are acquired defects. Classifying these conditions differently may be helpful when considering particular problems such as management, recurrence risks, or possible fetal therapy.

Table 27-1 is not a list of etiologic factors but, rather, a list of conditions associated with NIH. The pathophysiology of NIH is well worked out in only a few cases. Furthermore, not all cases have the same pathophysiologic mechanism.

A review by Machin[34] tried to elucidate some of these mechanisms. As he pointed out, hydrops is a common end stage for a variety of diseases reached by several pathways. He proposed five basic disease processes that lead to hydrops: cardiovascular failure, chromosomal abnormalities, thoracic compression, twinning, and fetal anemia. He believed that each of these has a common pathway for the development of hydrops. Furthermore, he suggested that most causes could be classified into one of these large groups.

Cardiovascular Causes

Fetal cardiac abnormalities are among the most common causes of hydrops in most series. Congenital heart disease is a common problem, with an incidence of 8 or 9 per 1000 liveborn infants. Malformations of the cardiovascular system are of varying degrees of complexity and seriousness, but it is not always clear why some of these fetuses experience hydrops and others are born in a well-compensated condition.[35] No forms of congenital heart disease reliably lead to hydrops, although one would expect that the more minor abnormalities are less likely to cause the ultimate decompensation of the fetus. Overall, a structural malformation of the heart with associated fetal hydrops carries an extremely poor prognosis, with a mortality rate approaching 100%.[36,37]

Structural heart disease is diagnosed by means of ultrasonography, with either a targeted ultrasound examination or fetal echocardiography. In general, regardless of the presence of hydrops, cases of cardiac malformation that are diagnosed prenatally have a poor outcome. Crawford and coauthors[37] found only a 17% survival rate in such fetuses. Copel and coworkers[38] suggested that 30% of fetuses with prenatally diagnosed structural congenital heart disease have an abnormal karyotype. For this reason, they recommended that chromosome analysis be obtained whenever this diagnosis is made. Because of the poor prognosis associated with hydrops when an abnormal karyotype is involved, such fetuses usually are not considered candidates for in utero fetal therapy or for active intervention with early delivery and vigorous resuscitation.

Cardiac arrhythmias are also an important cause of hydrops, but the prognosis is entirely different from that for structural heart disease.

TABLE 27-1 CONDITIONS ASSOCIATED WITH NONIMMUNE HYDROPS

Cardiovascular
Malformation
- Left heart hypoplasia
- Atrioventricular canal defect
- Right heart hypoplasia
- Closure of foramen ovale
- Single ventricle
- Transposition of the great vessels
- Ventricular septal defect
- Atrial septal defect
- Tetralogy of Fallot
- Ebstein anomaly
- Premature closure of ductus
- Truncus arteriosus

Tachyarrhythmia
- Atrial flutter
- Paroxysmal atrial tachycardia
- Wolff-Parkinson-White syndrome
- Supraventricular tachycardia

Bradyarrhythmia
Other arrhythmia
High-output failure
- Neuroblastoma
- Sacrococcygeal teratoma
- Large fetal angioma
- Placental chorioangioma
- Umbilical cord hemangioma

Cardiac rhabdomyoma
Other cardiac neoplasia
Cardiomyopathy

Chromosomal
45,X
Trisomy 21
Trisomy 18
Trisomy 13
18q+
13q–
45,X/46,XX
Triploidy
Other

Chondrodysplasias
Thanatophoric dwarfism
Short rib polydactyly
Hypophosphatasia
Osteogenesis imperfecta
Achondrogenesis

Twin Pregnancy
Twin-twin transfusion syndrome
Acardiac twin

Hematologic
α-Thalassemia
Fetomaternal Transfusion
Parvovirus B19 Infection
In Utero Hemorrhage
Glucose-6-Phosphate Dehydrogenase (G6PD) Deficiency
Red Cell Enzyme Deficiencies

Thoracic
Congenital Cystic Adenomatoid Malformation of Lung
Diaphragmatic Hernia
Intrathoracic Mass
Pulmonary Sequestration
Chylothorax
Airway Obstruction
Pulmonary Lymphangiectasia
Pulmonary Neoplasia
Bronchogenic Cyst

Infections
Cytomegalovirus
Toxoplasmosis
Parvovirus B19 (Fifth Disease)
Syphilis
Herpes
Rubella

Malformation Sequences
Noonan Syndrome
Arthrogryposis
Multiple Pterygia
Neu-Laxova Syndrome
Pena-Shokeir Syndrome
Myotonic Dystrophy
Saldino-Noonan Syndrome

Metabolic
Gaucher Disease
GM_1 Gangliosidosis
Sialidosis
Mucopolysaccharidosis Type 4a

Urinary
Urethral Stenosis or Atresia
Posterior Urethral Valves
Congenital Nephrosis (Finnish)
Prune Belly Syndrome

Gastrointestinal
Midgut Volvulus
Malrotation of the Intestines
Duplication of the Intestinal Tract
Meconium Peritonitis
Hepatic Fibrosis
Cholestasis
Biliary Atresia
Hepatic Vascular Malformations

Tachyarrhythmias associated with hydrops usually carry a better prognosis than most other causes of NIH.[25,39] Arrhythmias may be of several types, including tachyarrhythmias, bradyarrhythmias, and dysrhythmias. If an arrhythmia is associated with underlying structural heart disease, the prognosis is as poor as for heart disease without arrhythmia, as described earlier.[40] Bradyarrhythmias with hydrops carry a very poor prognosis, although successful fetal therapy had been described.[41,42]

Premature closure of the foramen ovale is typically idiopathic and can occur at any time during gestation. It can be diagnosed by careful ultrasound examination of the fetal heart, with Doppler studies and color Doppler studies as useful adjuncts to imaging. Usually, this diagnosis is made only after the onset of hydrops, and prognosis is therefore poor.

Premature closure or narrowing of the ductus arteriosus also has been associated with fetal hydrops.[43] In one case, it was associated with other congenital heart disease, a coarctation of the aorta.[44] In other reported cases, the mother was receiving indomethacin for the arrest of preterm labor.[45] Moise and associates[46] described narrowing of the ductus in response to maternal indomethacin ingestion but found it to be measurable and reversible. Vanhaesebrouck and colleagues[47] described NIH with neonatal ileal perforation in fetuses exposed to indomethacin for the arrest of preterm labor.

A variety of other cardiac abnormalities can lead to hydrops. For example, neoplasias such as rhabdomyomas may be present with hydrops. In such cases, one should seek a family history of tuberous sclerosis, because this autosomal dominant disorder may manifest in this fashion.[48,49]

Cardiac failure from myocarditis is responsible for at least some cases of hydrops in fetuses that have congenital infections.[50] Such cases have been documented with fetal parvovirus B19, with cytomegalovirus (CMV), and, much more rarely, with toxoplasmosis. These conditions are discussed later under infectious causes of hydrops.

Various noncardiac lesions can lead to high-output cardiac failure, a presumed mechanism of hydrops. Sacrococcygeal teratomas are large vascular tumors that act as arteriovenous shunts and may be associated with hydrops on this basis.[51,52] The majority of these tumors are well tolerated by the fetus, however, and do not lead to hydrops.[53] Open fetal surgery with resection of the tumor has been attempted in cases associated with fetal hydrops, but only one success has been reported to date.[54]

Placental tumors may also lead to hydrops. These are most commonly chorioangiomas, which are vascular and likely act as arteriovenous shunts.[7,18,55-59]

Other causes of presumed high-output failure associated with fetal hydrops include fetal adrenal neuroblastomas, multiple cases of which have been reported. These rare tumors most likely lead to heart failure based on increased catecholamine release, much as they would in a child with the same lesion. Other angiomas that may lead to hydrops have been described in the cord[60] and in a fetus in the angio-osteohypertrophy syndrome.[61]

Chromosomal Abnormalities

Chromosomal abnormalities are fairly common in cases of fetal hydrops, and they may cause the disorder by any of several mechanisms.[34] Among chromosomally abnormal fetuses with hydrops, cystic hygromas are common.[62] In fact, cystic hygromas are one of the most common causes of hydrops, particularly among fetuses diagnosed before 20 weeks of gestation.[2] The chromosomal abnormality most frequently seen in these fetuses is 45,X, or Turner syndrome. On the other hand, fetuses with this phenotype may also have trisomy 21 or a normal karyotype.[63,64] Among fetuses with a 45,X karyotype, two common structural abnormalities can lead to the development of hydrops. Although one is cystic hygroma, fetuses with this condition also frequently have a tubular coarctation of the aorta. There is some controversy about which of these is the more important mechanism for causing NIH.[34]

Other chromosomal abnormalities have also been described in fetuses with hydrops. The most common are trisomy 21, trisomy 18, trisomy 13, and triploidy. Sex chromosome abnormalities that result in Turner syndrome, such as 45,X/46,XX, have also been reported, as have a large number of more unusual autosomal rearrangements. Structural cardiac lesions are common in aneuploid fetuses and may be associated with hydrops. If no structural cardiac lesion is found, the pathophysiology for the development of hydrops in this situation is unclear. The myeloproliferative disorder common in neonates with Down syndrome has been described in four fetuses with Down syndrome and NIH.[65]

If the karyotype is abnormal, the prognosis is poor, and important information can be given to the parents about recurrence risk and diagnosis in future pregnancies. The overall rate of chromosome abnormality in fetuses with hydrops varies between 7% and 45%, with higher rates among those in whom hydrops is detected before 24 weeks' gestation.[2,4,9,12,42,62,66] Obtaining a fetal karyotype is an essential part of the workup of any fetus with hydrops.

Thoracic Abnormalities

Increases in intrathoracic pressure may lead to the development of hydrops by obstructing venous return and altering cardiovascular hemodynamics. Most of these conditions involve space occupying lesions of the thorax.

Cystic adenomatoid malformation of the lung is divided into several different subtypes, depending on the size and distribution of the cysts. In most cases, if pulmonary hypoplasia is not life-threatening, this lesion is amenable to surgery in the neonate. These fetuses may develop hydrops, however, and this markedly worsens the prognosis.

Most cases of cystic adenomatoid malformation of the lung associated with hydrops involve a single large cyst and a shift of the mediastinum. Continuous drainage of the solitary cyst by means of pleuroamniotic shunt placement or cyst aspiration has been proposed.[67] In cases in which cysts are microscopic or otherwise not amenable to shunt placement and hydrops is present, open fetal surgery has been performed. Although the outcomes have been poor, some of the fetuses have survived; left untreated, they would not have.[67-69] A substantial proportion of prenatally diagnosed cystic adenomatoid malformations resolve spontaneously or regress but do not entirely resolve, including cases with NIH; this has led some to continue expectant management.[70]

Other types of masses or lesions in the chest may be associated with hydrops as well. These include diaphragmatic hernias, hamartomas or other neoplasms of the lung or chest, pulmonary extralobar sequestration syndrome, and various bronchogenic cysts. Diaphragmatic hernia is the most common of these lesions, but it is unusual for affected fetuses to experience hydrops.

Unilateral hydrothorax may present as a space-occupying lesion in the chest and is frequently associated with hydrops. Bilateral hydrothorax may be indistinguishable from other causes of NIH, because one of the features of hydrops is pleural effusion. In such cases, the effusions are the primary event and the hydrops a secondary problem. Many authors have considered unilateral or bilateral fetal hydrothorax to be analogous to neonatal chylothorax.[71,72] Because there are no chylomicrons in the fetus, this is not known with certainty, and in most cases after birth no particular surgery on the presumably abnormal lymphatic system is performed.[73] Overall, these fetuses have a relatively poor prognosis, because pulmonary hypoplasia is frequently present. In the neonate, isolated pleural effusion without hydrops has a much more favorable prognosis, with a 15% mortality rate.[74]

Some authors recommend diagnostic fetal thoracentesis if unilateral or bilateral hydrothorax is suspected. In cases of isolated hydrothorax, lymphocytes predominate in the fluid obtained, although Eddleman and coauthors[75] reported on two cases in which this test was misleading. There are many reports of placement of a pleuroamniotic shunt for continual drainage of this space. The results of such therapy have increased survival to between 40% and 70%.[71,72,74]

The rate of aneuploidy in association with fetal hydrothorax or isolated pleural effusion is high. Rodeck and associates[73] placed shunts before the availability of a fetal karyotype, and one of eight fetuses had Down syndrome. Petrikovsky and colleagues[76] reported three consecutive cases of pleural effusion, all of which involved aneuploid fetuses. However, more recent reports showed a lower rate in apparently isolated cases.[71,72]

Twinning

When one of a set of twins is determined to have fetal hydrops, the differential diagnosis requires special considerations. If it is known that the twins are not monozygotic, the cause is probably unrelated to the twin pregnancy, and the diagnostic approach to the twin with hydrops should be similar to that for any other fetus with the condition. In the case of monozygotic twins, the hydrops is probably related to abnormal vessels in the placenta, resulting in twin-to-twin transfusion syndrome (see Chapter 24).

In the twin-to-twin transfusion syndrome, the fetus with hydrops may be either the donor or the recipient.[15] In the classic situation, the donor twin has growth restriction and oligohydramnios, and the recipient twin has plethora, hydramnios, and perhaps hydrops.[77,78] Presumably, this scenario results from cardiac overload and congestive heart failure; however, it is also possible for the donor twin to have hydrops, in which case the pathophysiology is likely to be related to anemia.[79]

Twin-to-twin transfusion syndrome carries a poor prognosis, particularly if it is found early in gestation or if hydrops is present. Various aggressive therapies have been proposed, including serial amniocenteses, in utero laser ablation of communicating placental vessels, and transabdominal needle septostomy of the dividing membrane. The best treatment is still controversial, because several large series have shown conflicting results, particularly in long-term follow-up of surviving twins.[80-84]

Fetal Anemia

Anemia is a well-known cause of fetal hydrops, and the model used to elucidate the pathophysiology of this condition is alloimmunization. Because immune hydrops has been extensively studied, this anemia is the best-understood mechanism for the development of NIH as well.

One of the most common causes of hydrops in patients from Asia or the eastern Mediterranean region is α-thalassemia.[42,85] This recessive disorder causes formation of abnormal tetramers of the β chain of hemoglobin, which cannot carry oxygen (see Chapter 42). The result is massive tissue hypoxia. Fetuses with this disorder commonly develop hydrops as early as 20 weeks' gestation. Because long-term survival of fetuses with homozygous α-thalassemia is extremely rare, there is no current recommendation for treatment. However, proper diagnosis is important for counseling and prenatal diagnosis in future pregnancies.

Fetomaternal hemorrhage is relatively common and, in rare instances, may be massive enough to cause fetal hydrops.[86,87] In most cases, the cause of the fetomaternal hemorrhage or transfusion is unknown. This diagnosis can be made by use of a Kleihauer-Betke stain to examine peripheral maternal blood for the presence of fetal cells. It is also possible to detect a fetomaternal bleed by an abnormally elevated maternal serum α-fetoprotein level. Although the hemorrhage may be self-limited, if the fetus has developed hydrops, many authors have advocated more aggressive management because of the risk for fetal death. There have now been several case reports of fetuses treated with serial intravascular transfusions with resolution of hydrops and an ultimately good outcome.[87-90]

Fetal hemorrhage with subsequent anemia and hydrops formation has also been reported. This has usually been associated with an intracranial hemorrhage, and, in the absence of a history of trauma, one should suspect a fetal coagulation deficiency such as alloimmune thrombocytopenia.[91,92]

Glucose-6-phosphate dehydrogenase (G6PD) deficiency is a common X-linked condition in African Americans and persons of Mediterranean heritage. This disorder is characterized by hemolytic crises, usually in response to various stimuli including sulfa drugs, aspirin, and fava beans. Female carriers are usually asymptomatic. There are two reports of affected male fetuses' developing anemia and hydrops after maternal ingestion of these substances.[93,94]

A number of inherited erythrocyte enzyme deficiencies can cause fetal anemia and, in rare cases, fetal hydrops.[95,96] Examples include glucose phosphate isomerase deficiency and pyruvate kinase deficiency. These conditions commonly lead to chronic hemolytic anemia, but rarely to severe anemia, in fetal life.

Congenital leukemia can cause anemia and hydrops, and leukemic infiltration of the myocardium has also been demonstrated.[97] Transmission of maternal antibodies to erythroid precursors in a mother who had acquired red blood cell aplasia has been reported. Transfusions to the fetus reversed the hydrops and resulted in a healthy liveborn infant with a normal outcome.[98]

Mari and associates[99] predicted anemia in fetuses with immune hydrops, based on the velocity of blood flow in the middle cerebral artery (MCA). This method was substantiated in subsequent trials and is now widely accepted.[100-102] The same findings appear to be true in fetuses affected by anemia from other causes, including NIH. The most studied model is in parvovirus-induced anemia (see later discussion).[103-106]

Infections

A great deal of literature concerns congenital infection as a cause of NIH. Although many different viruses, bacteria, and parasites cause congenital infection, the effects on the fetus are variable, and no infection predictably results in hydrops fetalis (see Chapter 38). In addition, although researchers have long believed anemia to be the common mechanism for the development of hydrops in these fetuses, myocarditis, hepatitis, or other pathways yet to be elucidated may also be involved.

Syphilis

Congenital syphilis is a well-known cause of fetal hydrops. One can confirm the diagnosis by obtaining a positive serologic test result in the mother. A dark-field examination of amniotic fluid may also be helpful.[107] A fetus with syphilis and hydrops faces a poor prognosis compared to one with a milder case of congenital syphilis. Management remains the same, however: treating the infection in the mother.

Cytomegalovirus

CMV is a common perinatally acquired infection. Although 20% to 30% of maternal primary infections are transmitted to the fetus, fewer result in symptomatic CMV in the fetus or neonate.[108,109] Symptomatic fetuses may show growth restriction, placentomegaly, polyhydramnios or oligohydramnios, hydrops, microcephaly, echogenic bowel, or intracerebral calcifications.[108,110] Ideally, maternal infection is determined by documentation of seroconversion or, alternatively, by rising titers of CMV immunoglobulin (IgG) antibody. Primary infection causes prolonged viral shedding, and a positive maternal urine culture also may be helpful.

Prenatal diagnosis is complicated by the gestational age and the time since maternal infection. In general, multiple parameters are used, including ultrasound findings, amniotic fluid, and fetal blood assays for CMV DNA and CMV-specific IgM in fetal blood after 22 weeks of gestation.[109,110] Blood obtained from the fetus can be tested for CMV-specific IgM if the fetus is past 22 weeks' gestation and is capable of producing IgM. Determination of fetal IgG levels is unhelpful, because these levels may merely reflect transplacental passage of maternal IgG.[109-112] With amniotic fluid culture or polymerase chain reaction (PCR) testing for CMV DNA, gestational age at the time of sampling is important, because many false-negative results are obtained before 20 weeks' gestation. In addition, the time from infection to sampling is important. In the face of a presumptive clinical diagnosis, one should consider repeating amniocentesis, cordocentesis, or both if these have yielded negative results.[112,113]

At present, there is no established in utero antiviral therapy for fetal CMV infection. However a nonrandomized trial of hyperimmune globulin given to women with known transplacental infection showed a decrease in neonatal infection and disease in the treatment group.[114]

Parvovirus

The most frequent manifestation of infection with parvovirus B19 is fifth disease, or erythema infectiosum. This common disorder may be acquired by a pregnant woman from an affected child. It causes a characteristic rash, flu-like symptoms, and arthralgias that may be mild. Fetal infections clearly occur, but the transmission rate is not established.

A recent study from Germany of more than 1000 women with documented seroconversion showed a fetal death rate of 6.3%. All cases of fetal death occurred at less than 20 weeks of gestation, and in that period the fetal death rate was 11%. The risk of NIH was 4%.[115]

Until the recent advent of PCR testing of amniotic fluid and serum, the diagnosis of human parvovirus infection in a fetus with hydrops was difficult.[116,117] Data from older series were based on diagnoses made by isolating virus from fetal blood, detecting parvovirus-specific IgM in fetal serum, or demonstrating virus in fetal tissues.[118,119] Viral particles can be detected by electron microscopy, by PCR, or by finding intranuclear inclusions on cytologic specimens.[50,120-122] Fetal serology may be negative in some cases of fetal infection in which hydrops has developed.[123-125] Easier diagnosis has led to an appreciation of how common this infection is. In a review of published series, Von Kaisenberg and Jonat[126] found that it accounted for 27% of all cases of NIH. Human parvovirus infection may also underlie a substantial portion of NIH cases previously labeled idiopathic.[118,120] The transient nature of this infection and the absence of fetal demise have led many investigators to speculate that the virus may be a causative agent in cases of ascites or hydrops that spontaneously resolve in utero.[125,127]

A characteristic although nonspecific finding in fetuses with this infection and hydrops is elevated maternal serum α-fetoprotein.[128] Data from Carrington and colleagues[123] and from Bernstein and Capeless[129] suggest that a highly elevated maternal serum α-fetoprotein level is a useful marker because it may herald the onset of hydrops in an affected pregnancy. The usual mechanism for the development of hydrops in parvovirus infections is presumably anemia from an aplastic crisis. Parvovirus-infected fetuses undergoing percutaneous umbilical blood sampling or, more recently, MCA velocimetry have been found to be severely anemic.[104,105,123,130] However, the virus has been shown to invade myocardium, and myocarditis may also account for hydropic changes, particularly in less anemic fetuses.[50,131]

Because this virus is not known to be associated with congenital malformations or long-term sequelae, aggressive in utero supportive therapy has been attempted. Transfusions of packed cells to the fetus have resulted in some good outcomes.[115,125,132,133] On reviewing published descriptions of 705 confirmed cases of fetal parvovirus in which 230 fetuses received transfusions, Von Kaisenberg and Jonat[126] concluded that aggressive therapy has a benefit over expectant management. However, more recent long-term follow-up has shown neurodevelopmental abnormalities in survivors unrelated to degree of anemia or hypoxia. The authors speculated that CNS involvement may be a previously unrecognized part of this infection.[134]

Other Infections

Various other infectious agents have been related to hydrops in at least a few cases.[135-141] These include adenovirus, toxoplasmosis, herpes simplex, rubella, Coxsackie virus, influenza, enterovirus, and *Listeria*. In some cases, an infectious process is suspected, but no causative organism can be identified.[142,143]

Metabolic Disease

A variety of genetic metabolic diseases, particularly lysosomal storage diseases, can cause hydrops in the fetus.[144] Gaucher disease, generalized (GM_1) gangliosidosis, Salla disease, sialidosis, mucopolysaccharidosis types 4 and 7, Tay-Sachs disease, and others can all present in this manner.[145-148] Gaucher disease is the most common of these disorders and has been reported the most frequently, but presentation with hydrops is rare.[149] These conditions can recur in subsequent pregnancies because they are typically inherited in an autosomal recessive fashion. Establishing the correct diagnosis is therefore extremely important. This can be accomplished by analysis of oligosaccharides in fetal or neonatal urine or blood, enzyme analysis and carrier testing in the parents, or histologic examination of appropriate fetal tissues.[144,150,151]

Several authors have recently recommended approaches to the diagnostic workup for these disorders based on their experience. Because there are many possible disorders in patients with no family history, they outlined suggested stepwise testing schemes.[152,153]

Other Malformations

A variety of chondrodysplasias may manifest with fetal hydrops. Pretorius and coworkers[154] found all such cases to be associated with fatal dwarfing syndromes. In these cases, the chest is compressed, and the neonates die of respiratory insufficiency. The most common skeletal dysplasias described with fetal hydrops are short-rib polydactyly syndrome, thanatophoric dysplasia, and achondrogenesis. One can diagnose skeletal dysplasia fairly easily with ultrasonography by measuring the extremities relative to head and abdominal size, but classifying the type of chondrodysplasia in a fetus by ultrasonography alone can be difficult. After birth, x-ray studies and examination of other phenotypic features of the neonate can be used to determine the specific type of chondrodysplasia. Because many of the lethal types are inherited in a recessive fashion, the recurrence rate is high. For several of these disorders, the gene responsible has been identified, and the genetic abnormality can be detected on fetal or neonatal tissue specimens.

A number of other genetic syndromes have also been associated with fetal hydrops. These include congenital myotonic dystrophy, arthrogryposis, multiple fetal pterygia, Neu-Laxova syndrome, and Pena-Shokeir syndrome type 1.[62,155,156]

Urinary tract malformations have been described in conjunction with hydrops in numerous reports; however, close examination of these cases reveals that most involved isolated ascites with a urinary tract malformation. This condition, known as urinary ascites, is common, well described, and generally self-limited. It rarely progresses to hydrops.

Various intra-abdominal processes related to the gastrointestinal tract commonly manifest with ascites, but in rare cases they are associated with hydrops. These include meconium peritonitis, small bowel volvulus, and various intestinal atresias.

Other Causes

Diabetes is frequently cited as a cause of NIH, and several large series have included a few cases in which preexisting maternal diabetes was the only etiology.[157] It is not clear whether these fetuses were structurally normal. Other authors found no association between maternal diabetes and NIH.[15]

Several maternal medications have been reported to be associated with NIH in the fetus. Indomethacin may be associated with ductal narrowing, as described earlier. Other reported cases have involved mycophenolate with fetal and neonatal anemia, propylthiouracil (PTU), and enalapril.[158-160]

The list of causes given here is certainly not complete. Numerous case reports have described other syndromes or malformations associated with fetal hydrops. In some of these cases, the association might not be causative or might be unproven, but in others it is more convincing. The literature is constantly being updated, not only with series but with case reports, and this discussion is therefore not exhaustive.

Experimental Management of Idiopathic Cases

Various management strategies have been attempted in cases of NIH of unknown etiology. Shimokawa and associates[161] injected albumin on two occasions into the peritoneal cavity of a fetus with hydrops, and hydrops subsequently resolved. This group later published a series of 21 cases treated with a combination of red blood cell transfusions and serial albumin injections. Improvements occurred only in fetuses without pleural effusions, but within that group, five (72%) of seven fetuses survived.[162]

Lingman and colleagues[163] attempted direct intravascular albumin transfusion on five occasions in a fetus later found to have a lysosomal storage disease. Doppler studies and blood counts before and after the procedures indicated effective plasma expansion and peripheral vasodilatation.

Goldberg and associates[164] placed a peritoneal-amniotic shunt in a second-trimester fetus with NIH of unknown etiology and massive ascites. Although the ascites resolved, other features of hydrops developed, and the fetus ultimately died.

Diagnostic Approach to the Fetus with Hydrops

The workup for a patient with a diagnosis of fetal hydrops should be directed at possible causes. Because the diagnosis is confirmed with ultrasonography, this is frequently the first test performed. During a careful ultrasound examination, the known causes of NIH should be kept in mind. Many of the fetal conditions, congenital anomalies, and malformation sequences that are known to cause hydrops can be found or eliminated on the initial ultrasound examination. Twins, cardiac arrhythmias, and hydrothorax are all examples of obvious ultrasonography-derived diagnoses. The blood-flow velocity of the MCA should be assessed to screen for fetal anemia.

If the examination is unsatisfactory, it should be repeated later to delineate the fetal anatomy as well as possible. Although the underlying diagnosis is far more predictive of outcome than are any specific ultrasonographic parameters, the initial examination can be used to assess the severity of the hydrops and to initiate antenatal testing, if appropriate, depending on gestational age. Assessing the severity of the hydrops is particularly important if the fetus is observed for some length of time or if fetal therapy is attempted. Ultrasound parameters can be longitudinally monitored to predict fetal decompensation or fetal response to in utero therapy.

A history should be taken, with particular attention to ethnic background and any family history of genetic diseases or congenital anomaly, consanguinity, recent maternal infections or exposures, and maternal medications. Once again, careful scrutiny of the listed causes of hydrops gives direction to the types of questions that should be asked of the mother and family.

The initial testing of the mother should include elimination of immune causes of hydrops with blood typing and the indirect Coombs test. A screen for hemoglobinopathies, a Kleihauer-Betke test to look for fetal red blood cells in the maternal circulation, and titers for *t*oxoplasmosis, *o*ther agents, *r*ubella, *c*ytomegalovirus, and *h*erpes simplex (TORCH) are also useful at this time. Some of these tests may not be immediately available, but blood should be drawn and sent to the laboratory.

In addition to careful ultrasonography studies including MCA velocity, fetal echocardiography may be helpful. A fetal karyotype should be obtained in most cases. With the availability of fluorescence in situ hybridization (FISH), rapid karyotyping can be performed on amniotic fluid. If infection is suspected, amniotic fluid can be sent for PCR testing or culture. Fetal blood can also be used for a rapid karyotype, and it can be sent for other tests, such as a complete blood count and platelet count, to rule out fetal anemia or thrombocytopenia. If blood is obtained, serologic studies and cultures can be performed on the specimen.

Fetal serum or amniotic fluid can be frozen or sent for other studies, such as screening for lysosomal storage diseases, if these are suspected. Although the deviation in optical density at 450 nm wavelength (ΔOD450) values are increased in many cases of NIH,[165] this is not clinically useful information, so the study is not usually indicated. Amniotic fluid may be sent for lung-maturity studies if appropriate. A frozen sample of amniotic fluid may be useful for future viral DNA hybridization studies or oligosaccharide analysis if not ordered initially.

Because some test findings are not available promptly, numerous tests may need to be ordered before initial results are available. It is helpful to establish a connection with cooperative laboratory facilities or, if these are not available locally, with reference laboratories to which specimens can be sent.

Management

Management issues are difficult to generalize because they depend on prognosis, gestational age, and presenting signs and symptoms. Before the fetus becomes viable, the prognosis should be explained to the parents, who should be given the option of terminating the pregnancy. If the underlying etiology is amenable to fetal therapy, this should be frankly discussed with the family, but, in general, the parents should be warned that diagnostic error is always possible and that the overall prognosis in NIH is still grim.

Many cases of NIH are detected during the third trimester. If the patient presents in preterm labor or if symptomatic hydramnios exists, difficult decisions need to be made about whether to administer tocolytic medications or to allow labor to continue. It may be warranted to continue tocolysis, as long as the mother is stable, while the fetal workup is being pursued. If a potentially reversible cause of hydrops is found, consultation with neonatology specialists may help guide counseling to the family about the advisability of prolonging the pregnancy and initiating fetal therapy versus proceeding with prompt delivery and postnatal treatment. If a fetal diagnosis with a poor prognosis seems fairly certain, a frank discussion with the family may lead to the discontinuation of tocolytic medication.

If the patient presents with or later shows signs of maternal compromise, such as preeclampsia or antenatal hemorrhage, management should be pursued without regard to fetal outcome, since it is so poor. Management decisions are particularly difficult in idiopathic cases with uncertain prognosis. Even though the overall prognosis is poor in idiopathic cases, every attempt should be made to prolong pregnancies diagnosed during the third trimester to 32 or 34 weeks' gestation, in order to maximize fetal survival, unless there are signs of fetal or maternal decompensation. If significant or symptomatic hydramnios is present, it may be treated with therapeutic amniocenteses, indomethacin, or, more conservatively, bed rest and conventional tocolytic therapy.

Fetal decompensation can be difficult to measure, but the usual biophysical parameters are nonetheless useful. If a fetal reactive heart rate tracing becomes abnormal, this should be interpreted as a sign of acute decompensation. Similarly, oligohydramnios, a decrease in fetal movement, and poor fetal tone are all ominous signs. Unless there is evidence that hydrops is resolving or that treatment has otherwise been effective, there does not seem to be any reason to prolong a pregnancy past 34 weeks' gestation or the attainment of a mature lung profile.

Huhta[166] suggested use of a cardiovascular scoring system to measure the degree of cardiovascular compromise using intracardiac, venous, and umbilical artery Doppler measurements. This method may be used longitudinally to monitor fetuses for decompensation in cases of hydrops.[166,167]

Recurrence Risks

After the delivery of a fetus with NIH, investigation of the cause should continue in the nursery, if necessary. If the fetus is stillborn or dies during the early neonatal period, every attempt should be made to obtain a postmortem examination directed at finding the underlying cause of the problem. Without this information, counseling the patient and her family about future pregnancies is frustrating. Overall, recurrent hydrops fetalis is unusual, and for most families the prognosis is good for a normal pregnancy in the future. However, there are numerous case reports of recurrent pregnancies with hydropic fetuses.[168-173] One must therefore be wary of reassuring families that idiopathic hydrops will not recur, and future pregnancies should be carefully monitored.

Delivery Considerations

Delivery of a fetus with hydrops should be attended by an experienced pediatric team prepared to deal with a sick neonate. Some authors have recommended the liberal use of cesarean section to avoid asphyxia and birth trauma, although no objective data support this approach.[136] Predelivery thoracentesis or paracentesis has also been advocated to enable immediate postnatal resuscitation or, in the case of a large fetal abdominal girth, to facilitate vaginal delivery.[25,79,174,175] A recent series[176] showed increased survival among neonates born later in gestation with normal Apgar scores. Pleural effusion was also associated with a poorer chance for survival. No fetus born in their series before 30 weeks survived.

Immediate problems of the neonate are likely to center on respiratory support and fluid management. Virtually all neonates with hydrops require mechanical ventilation, and edema can make intubation difficult.[177,178]

Postnatal drainage of pleural or peritoneal fluid may be required to maintain oxygenation. Some authors reserve these procedures for extreme cases, whereas others propose a more liberal use of fluid drainage.[177,179,180] Fluid restriction, careful management of electrolytes, judicious use of albumin and diuretics, correction of anemia, and continuous assessment of intravascular volume are all important issues in the first few days of life.

Summary

Although there have been many advances in understanding of the causes of fetal NIH, it remains a difficult clinical problem. Many conditions have been associated with fetal hydrops, but few shed light on the pathophysiology of its development. Once the diagnosis of NIH is established, a careful search for causative fetal pathology should be undertaken. Unfortunately, the results of such a search may not be available at the time when difficult management decisions must be made. Recent advances in fetal therapy have increased the number of fetal conditions for which treatment is possible. However, the overall rates of morbidity in mother and fetus, and of mortality in the fetus, remain high.

References

1. Potter EL: Universal edema of the fetus unassociated with erythroblastosis. Am J Obstet Gynecol 46:130, 1943.
2. Santolaya J, Alley D, Jaffe R, et al: Antenatal classification of hydrops fetalis. Obstet Gynecol 79:256, 1992.
3. Sohan K, Carroll SG, De La Fuente S, et al: Analysis of outcome in hydrops fetalis in relation to gestation age at diagnosis, cause and treatment. Acta Obstet Gynecol Scand 80:726, 2001.
4. Ismail KM, Martin WL, Ghosh S, et al: Etiology and outcome of hydrops fetalis. J Matern Fetal Med 10:175, 2001.
5. Graves GR, Baskett TF: Nonimmune hydrops fetalis: Antenatal diagnosis and management. Am J Obstet Gynecol 148:563, 1984.

6. Trainor B, Tubman R: The emerging pattern of hydrops fetalis: Incidence, aetiology and management. Ulster Med J 75:185-186, 2006.
7. Hutchison AA, Drew JH, Yu VYH, et al: Nonimmunologic hydrops fetalis: A review of 61 cases. Obstet Gynecol 59:347, 1982.
8. Im SS, Rizos N, Joutsi P, et al: Nonimmunologic hydrops fetalis. Am J Obstet Gynecol 148:566, 1984.
9. Heinonen S, Ryynanen M, Kirkinen P: Etiology and outcome of second trimester non-immunologic fetal hydrops. Acta Obstet Gynecol Scand 79:15, 2000.
10. Anandakumar C, Biswas A, Chew SS, et al: Direct fetal therapy for hydrops secondary to congenital atrioventricular heart block. Obstet Gynecol 87:835, 1996.
11. Rose CH, Bofill JA, Le M, Martin RW: Non-immune hydrops fetalis: Prenatal diagnosis and perinatal outcomes. J Miss State Med Assoc 46:99, 2005.
12. McCoy MC, Katz VL, Gould N, et al: Non-immune hydrops after 20 weeks' gestation: Review of 10 years' experience with suggestions for management. Obstet Gynecol 85:578, 1995.
13. Watson J, Campbell S: Antenatal evaluation and management in nonimmune hydrops fetalis. Obstet Gynecol 67:589, 1986.
14. Warsof SL, Nicolaides KH, Rodeck C: Immune and non-immune hydrops. Clin Obstet Gynecol 29:533, 1986.
15. Macafee CAJ, Fortune DW, Beischer NA: Non-immunological hydrops fetalis. J Obstet Gynaecol Br Commonw 77:226, 1970.
16. Castillo RA, Devoe LD, Hadi HA, et al: Nonimmune hydrops fetalis: Clinical experience and factors related to a poor outcome. Am J Obstet Gynecol 155:812, 1986.
17. Van Selm M, Kanhai H, Gravenhorst B: Maternal hydrops syndrome: A review. Obstet Gynecol Surv 46:785, 1991.
18. Dorman SL, Cardwell MS: Ballantyne syndrome caused by a large placental chorioangioma. Am J Obstet Gynecol 173:1632, 1995.
19. Goeden AM, Worthington D: Spontaneous resolution of mirror syndrome. Obstet Gynecol 106:1183, 2005.
20. Stepan H, Faber R: Elevated sFlt1 level and preeclampsia with parvovirus-induced hydrops. N Engl J Med 354:1857-1858, 2006.
21. Espinoza J, Romero R, Nien JK, et al: A role of the anti-angiogenic factor sVEGRF-1 in the "mirror syndrome" (Ballantyne's syndrome). J Matern Fetal Neonatal Med 19:607, 2006.
22. Mahony BS, Filly RA, Callen PW, et al: Severe nonimmune hydrops fetalis: Sonographic evaluation. Radiology 151:757, 1984.
23. Brown BS: The ultrasonographic features of nonimmune hydrops fetalis: A study of 30 successive patients. Can Assoc Radiol J 37:164, 1986.
24. Platt LD, DeVore GR: In utero diagnosis of hydrops fetalis: Ultrasound methods. Clin Perinatol 9:627, 1982.
25. Romero R, Pilu G, Jeanty P, et al: Other anomalies: Nonimmune hydrops fetalis. In Romero R, Pilu G, Jeanty P, et al (eds): Prenatal Diagnosis of Congenital Anomalies. Norwalk, CT, Appleton & Lange, 1988, p 403.
26. Saltzman DH, Frigoletto FD, Harlow BL, et al: Sonographic evaluation of hydrops fetalis. Obstet Gynecol 74:106, 1989.
27. Slesnick TC, Ayres NA, Altman CA, et al: Characteristics and outcomes of fetuses with pericardial effusions. Am J Cardiol 96:599-601, 2005.
28. Favre R, Dreux S, Dommergues M, et al: Nonimmune fetal ascites: A series of 79 cases. Am J Obstet Gynecol 190:407-412, 2004.
29. Carlson DE, Platt LD, Medearis AL, et al: Prognostic indicators of the resolution of nonimmune hydrops fetalis and survival of the fetus. Am J Obstet Gynecol 163:1785, 1990.
30. Chitkara U, Wilkins I, Lynch L, et al: The role of sonography in assessing severity of fetal anemia in Rh- and Kell-isoimmunized pregnancies. Obstet Gynecol 71:393, 1988.
31. Fleischer AC, Killam AP, Boehm FH, et al: Hydrops fetalis: Sonographic evaluation and clinical implications. Radiology 141:163, 1981.
32. Hoddick WK, Mahony BS, Callen PW, et al: Placental thickness. J Ultrasound Med 4:479, 1985.
33. Elliott JP, Urig MA, Clewell WH: Aggressive therapeutic amniocentesis for treatment of twin-twin transfusion synrome. Obstet Gynecol 77:537, 1991.
34. Machin GA: Hydrops revisited: Literature review of 1,414 cases published in the 1980s. Am J Med Genet 34:366, 1989.
35. McFadden DE, Taylor GP: Cardiac abnormalities and nonimmune hydrops fetalis: A coincidental, not causal relationship. Pediatr Pathol 9:11, 1989.
36. Allan LD, Crawford DC, Sheridan R, et al: Aetiology of non-immune hydrops: The value of echocardiography. BJOG 93:223, 1986.
37. Crawford DC, Sunder KC, Allan LD: Prenatal detection of congenital heart disease: Factors affecting obstetric management and survival. Am J Obstet Gynecol 159:352, 1988.
38. Copel JA, Cullen M, Green JJ, et al: The frequency of aneuploidy in prenatally diagnosed congenital heart disease: An indication for fetal karyotyping. Am J Obstet Gynecol 158:409, 1988.
39. Cameron A, Nicholson S, Nimrod C, et al: Evaluation of fetal cardiac dysrhythmias with two-dimensional, M-mode, and pulsed Doppler ultrasonography. Am J Obstet Gynecol 158:286, 1988.
40. Shenker L, Reed KL, Anderson CF, et al: Congenital heart block and cardiac anomalies in the absence of maternal connective tissue disease. Am J Obstet Gynecol 157:248, 1987.
41. Kleinman CS, Nehgme RA: Cardiac arrhythmias in the human fetus. Pediatr Cardiol 25:234-251, 2004.
42. Anandakumar C, Biswas A, Wong YC, et al: Management of non-immune hydrops: 8 Years' experience. Ultrasound Obstet Gynecol 8:196, 1996.
43. Harlass FE, Duff P, Brady K, et al: Hydrops fetalis and premature closure of the ductus arteriosus: A review. Obstet Gynecol Surv 44:541, 1989.
44. Kondo T, Kitazawa R, Noda-Maeda N, Kitazawa S: Fetal hydrops associated with spontaneous premature closure of ductus arteriosus. Pathol Int 56:554-557, 2006.
45. Mogilner BM, Ashkenazy M, Borenstein R, et al: Hydrops fetalis caused by maternal indomethacin treatment. Acta Obstet Gynecol Scand 61:183, 1982.
46. Moise KJ, Huhta JC, Sharif DS, et al: Indomethacin in the treatment of premature labor: Effects on the fetal ductus arteriosus. N Engl J Med 319:327, 1988.
47. Vanhaesebrouck P, Thiery M, Leroy JG, et al: Oligohydramnios, renal insufficiency, and ileal perforation in preterm infants after intrauterine exposure to indomethacin. J Pediatr 113:738, 1988.
48. Ostor A, Fortune DW: Tuberous sclerosis initially seen as hydrops fetalis. Arch Pathol Lab Med 102:34, 1978.
49. King JA, Stamilio DM: Maternal and fetal tuberous sclerosis complicating pregnancy: A case report and overview of the literature. Am J Perinatol 22:103-108, 2005.
50. Naides SJ, Weiner CP: Antenatal diagnosis and palliative treatment of non-immune hydrops fetalis secondary to fetal parvovirus B19 infection. Prenat Diagn 9:105, 1989.
51. Mostoufi-Zadeh M, Weiss LM, Driscoll SH: Nonimmune hydrops fetalis: A challenge in perinatal pathology. Hum Pathol 16:785, 1985.
52. Langer JC, Harrison MR, Schmidt KG, et al: Fetal hydrops and death from sacrococcygeal teratoma: Rationale for fetal surgery. Am J Obstet Gynecol 160:1145, 1989.
53. Gross SJ, Benzie RJ, Sermer M, et al: Prenatal diagnosis and management. Am J Obstet Gynecol 156:393, 1987.
54. Graf JL, Albanese CT, Jennings RW, et al: Successful fetal sacrococcygeal teratoma resection in a hydropic fetus. J Pediatr Surg 35:1489, 2000.
55. Bauer CR, Fojaco RM, Bancalari E, et al: Microangiopathic hemolytic anemia and thrombocythemia in a neonate associated with a large placental chorioangioma. Pediatrics 62:574, 1978.
56. Maidman JE, Yeager C, Anderson V, et al: Prenatal diagnosis and management of nonimmunologic hydrops fetalis. Obstet Gynecol 56:571, 1980.
57. Hirata GI, Masaki D, O'Toole M, et al: Color flow mapping and Doppler velocimetry in the diagnosis and management of a placental chorioangioma associated with nonimmune fetal hydrops. Obstet Gynecol 81:850, 1993.
58. D'Ercole C: Large chorioangioma associated with hydrops fetalis: Prenatal diagnosis and management. Fetal Diagn Ther 11:357, 1996.

59. Russell RT, Carlin A, Ashworth M, Welch CR: Diffuse placental chorioangiomatosis and fetal hydrops. Fetal Diagn Ther 22:183-185, 2007.
60. Seifer DB, Ferguson JE, Behrens CM, et al: Nonimmune hydrops fetalis in association with hemangioma of the umbilical cord. Obstet Gynecol 66:283, 1985.
61. Mor A, Schreyer P, Wainraub Z, et al: Nonimmune hydrops fetalis associated with angio-osteohypertrophy (Klippel-Trenaunay) syndrome. Am J Obstet Gynecol 159:1185, 1988.
62. Holzgreve W, Curry CJ, Golbus MS, et al: Investigation of nonimmune hydrops fetalis. Am J Obstet Gynecol 150:805, 1984.
63. Cullen MT, Gabrielli S, Green JJ, et al: Diagnosis and significance of cystic hygroma in the first trimester. Prenat Diagn 10:643, 1990.
64. Ganapathy R, Guven M, Sethna F, et al: Natural history and outcome of prenatally diagnosed cystic hygroma. Prenat Diagn 24:965-968, 2004.
65. Smrcek JM, Baschat AA, Germer U, et al: Fetal hydrops and hepatosplenomegaly in the second half of pregnancy: A sign of myeloproliferative disorder in fetuses with trisomy 21. Ultrasound Obstet Gynecol 17:403, 2001.
66. Landrum BG, Johnson DE, Ferrara B, et al: Hydrops fetalis and chromosomal trisomies. Am J Obstet Gynecol 154:1114, 1986.
67. Crombleholme TM, Coleman B, Hedrick H, et al: Cystic adenomatoid malformation volume ratio predicts outcome in prenatally diagnosed cystic adenomatoid malformation of the lung. J Pediatr Surg 37:331, 2002.
68. Harrison MR, Adzick NS, Jennings RW, et al: Antenatal intervention for congenital cystic adenomatoid malformation. Lancet 336:965, 1990.
69. Adzick NS, Harrison MR, Crombleholme TM, et al: Fetal lung lesions: Management and outcome. Am J Obstet Gynecol 179:884, 1998.
70. Ierullo AM, Ganapathy R, Crowley S, et al: Neonatal outcome of antenatally diagnosed congenital cystic adenomatoid malformations. Ultrasound Obstet Gynecol 26:150-153, 2005.
71. Smith RP, Illanes S, Denbow ML, Soothill PW: Outcome of fetal pleural effusions treated by thoracoamniotic shunting. Ultrasound Obstet Gynecol 26:63-66, 2005.
72. Picone O, Benachi A, Mandelbrot L, et al: Thoracoamniotic shunting for fetal pleural effusions with hydrops. Am J Obstet Gynecol 191:2047-2050, 2004.
73. Rodeck CH, Fisk NM, Fraser DI, et al: Long-term in utero drainage of fetal hydrothorax. N Engl J Med 319:1135, 1988.
74. Wilson RD, Baxter JK, Johnson MP, et al: Thoracoamniotic shunts: Fetal treatment of pleural effusions and congenital cystic adenomatoid malformations. Fetal Diagn Ther 19:413-420, 2004.
75. Eddleman KA, Levine AB, Chitkara U, et al: Reliability of pleural fluid lymphocyte counts in the antenatal diagnosis of congenital chylothorax. Obstet Gynecol 78:530, 1991.
76. Petrikovsky BM, Shmoys SM, Baker DA, et al: Pleural effusion in aneuploidy. Perinatology 8:214, 1991.
77. Brown DL, Benson CB, Driscoll SG, et al: Twin-twin transfusion syndrome: Sonographic findings. Radiology 170:61, 1989.
78. Blickstein I: The twin-twin transfusion syndrome. Obstet Gynecol 76:714, 1990.
79. Holzgreve W, Holzgreve B, Curry CJR: Nonimmune hydrops fetalis: Diagnosis and management. Semin Perinatol 9:52, 1985.
80. Johnson JR, Rossi KQ, O'Shaughnessy RW: Amnioreduction versus septostomy in twin-twin transfusion syndrome. Am J Obstet Gynecol 185:1044, 2001.
81. Mari G, Roberts A, Detti L, et al: Perinatal morbidity and mortality rates in severe twin-twin transfusion syndrome: Results of the International Amnioreduction Registry. Am J Obstet Gynecol 185:708, 2001.
82. Quintero RA, Bornick PW, Morales WJ, et al: Selective photocoagulation of communicating vessels in the treatment of monochorionic twins with selective growth retardation. Am J Obstet Gynecol 185:689, 2001.
83. Moise KJ: Neurodevelopmental outcome after laser therapy for twin-twin transfusion syndrome. Am J Obstet Gynecol 194:1208, 2006.
84. Lenclen R, Paupe A, Ciaro G, et al: Neonatal outcome in preterm monochorionic twins with twin-to-twin transfusion syndrome after intrauterine treatment with amnioreduction or fetoscopic laser surgery: Comparison with dichorionic twins. Am J Obstet Gynecol 196:450, 2007.
85. Nakayama R, Yamada D, Steinmiller V, et al: Hydrops fetalis secondary to Bart hemoglobinopathy. Obstet Gynecol 67:176, 1986.
86. Owen J, Stedman CM, Tucker TL: Comparison of predelivery versus postdelivery Kleihauer-Betke stains in cases of fetal death. Am J Obstet Gynecol 161:663, 1989.
87. Rubod C, Houfflin V, Belot F, et al: Successful in utero treatment of chronic and massive fetomaternal hemorrhage with fetal hydrops. Fetal Diagn Ther 21:410-413, 2006.
88. Cardwell MS: Successful treatment of hydrops fetalis caused by fetomaternal hemorrhage: A case report. Am J Obstet Gynecol 158:131, 1988.
89. Rouse D, Weiner C: Ongoing fetomaternal hemorrhage treated by serial fetal intravascular transfusions. Obstet Gynecol 76:974, 1990.
90. Thorp JA, Cohen GR, Yeast JD, et al: Nonimmune hydrops caused by massive fetomaternal hemorrhage and treated by intravascular transfusion. Perinatology 9:22, 1992.
91. Bose C: Hydrops fetalis and in utero intracranial hemorrhage. J Pediatr 93:1023, 1978.
92. Daffos F, Forestier F, Muller JY, et al: Prenatal treatment of alloimmune thrombocytopenia. Lancet 2:632, 1984.
93. Perkins RP: Hydrops fetalis and stillbirth in a male glucose-6-phosphate dehydrogenase-deficient fetus possibly due to maternal ingestion of sulfisoxazole. Am J Obstet Gynecol 3:379, 1971.
94. Mentzer WC, Collier E: Hydrops fetalis associated with erythrocyte G-6-PD deficiency and maternal ingestion of fava beans and ascorbic acid. J Pediatr 86:565, 1975.
95. Matthay KK, Mentzer WC: Erythrocyte enzymopathies in the newborn. Clin Haematol 10:31, 1981.
96. Ravindranath Y, Paglia DE, Warrier I, et al: Glucose phosphate isomerase deficiency as a cause of hydrops fetalis. N Engl J Med 316:258, 1987.
97. Gray ES, Balch NJ, Kohler H, et al: Congenital leukaemia: An unusual cause of stillbirth. Arch Dis Child 61:1001, 1986.
98. Oie BK, Hertel J, Seip M, et al: Hydrops foetalis in 3 infants of a mother with acquired chronic pure red cell aplasia: Transitory red cell aplasia in 1 of the infants. Scand J Haematol 33:466, 1984.
99. Mari G, Abuhamad AZ, Uerpairojkit B, et al: Blood flow velocity waveforms of the abdominal arteries in appropriate- and small-for-gestational-age fetuses. Ultrasound Obstet Gynecol 6:15, 1995.
100. Vyas S, Nicolaides KH, Campbell S: Doppler examination of the middle cerebral artery in anemic fetuses. Am J Obstet Gynecol 162:1066, 1990.
101. Mari G, Detti L, Oz U, et al: Long-term outcome in twin-twin transfusion syndrome treated with serial aggressive amnioreduction. Am J Obstet Gynecol 183:211, 2000.
102. Teixeira JM, Duncan K, Letsky E, et al: Middle cerebral artery peak systolic velocity in the prediction of fetal anemia. Ultrasound Obstet Gynecol 15:205, 2000.
103. Delle Chiaie L, Buck G, Grab D, et al: Prediction of fetal anemia with Doppler measurement of the middle cerebral artery peak systolic velocity in pregnancies complicated by maternal blood group alloimmunization or parvovirus B19 infection. Ultrasound Obstet Gynecol 18:232, 2001.
104. Cosmi E, Mari G, Delle Chiaie L, et al: Noninvasive diagnosis by Doppler ultrasonography of fetal anemia resulting from parvovirus infection. Am J Obstet Gynecol 187:1290-1293, 2002.
105. Hernandez-Andrade E, Scheier M, Dezerega V, et al: Fetal middle cerebral artery peak systolic velocity in the investigation of non-immune hydrops. Ultrasound Obstet Gynecol 23:442-445, 2004.
106. Abdel-Fattah SA, Soothill PW, Carroll SG, Kyle PM: Noninvasive diagnosis of anemia in hydrops fetalis with the use of middle cerebral artery Doppler velocity. Am J Obstet Gynecol 185:1411-1415, 2001.
107. Wendel GD: Gestational and congenital syphilis. Clin Perinatol 15:287, 1988.
108. Demmler GJ: Summary of a workshop on surveillance for congenital cytomegalovirus disease. Rev Infect Dis 13:315, 1991.
109. Enders G, Bader U, Lindemann L, et al: Prenatal diagnosis of congenital cytomegalovirus infection in 189 pregnancies with known outcome. Prenat Diagn 21:362-377, 2001.

110. Degani S: Sonographic findings in fetal viral infections: A systematic review. Obstet Gynecol Surv 61:329-336, 2006.
111. Hogge WA, Buffone GJ, Hogge JS: Prenatal diagnosis of cytomegalovirus (CMV) infection: A preliminary report. Prenat Diagn 13:131, 1993.
112. Revello MG, Baldanti F, Furione M, et al: Polymerase chain reaction for prenatal diagnosis of congenital human cytomegalovirus infection. J Med Virol 47:462, 1995.
113. Donner C, Liesnard C, Content J, et al: Prenatal diagnosis of 52 pregnancies at risk for congenital cytomegalovirus infection. Obstet Gynecol 82:481, 1993.
114. Nigro G, Adler SP, LaTorre R et al: Passive immunization during pregnancy for congenital cytomegalovirus infection. N Engl J Med 353:1350-1362, 2005.
115. Enders M, Weidner A, Zoellner I, et al: Fetal morbidity and mortality after acute human parvovirus B19 infection in pregnancy: Prospective evaluation of 1018 cases. Prenat Diagn 24:513-518, 2004.
116. Gentilomi G, Zerbini M, Gallinella G, et al: B19 parvovirus induced fetal hydrops: Rapid and simple diagnosis by detection of B19 antigens in amniotic fluids. Prenat Diagn 18:363, 1998.
117. Dieck D, Lothar Schild R, Hansmann M, et al: Prenatal diagnosis of congenital parvovirus B19 infection: Value of serological and PCR techniques in maternal and fetal serum. Prenat Diagn 19:1119, 1999.
118. Samuels P, Ludmir J: Nonimmune hydrops fetalis: A heterogeneous disorder and therapeutic challenge. Semin Roentgenol 25:353, 1990.
119. Weiner CP, Naides SJ, Pringle K: Fetal survival after human parvovirus B19 infection: Spectrum of intrauterine response in a twin gestation. Am J Perinatol 9:66, 1992.
120. Porter HJ, Khong TY, Evans MF, et al: Parvovirus as a cause of hydrops fetalis: Detection by in situ DNA hybridization. J Clin Pathol 41:381, 1988.
121. Centers for Disease Control and Prevention: Risks associated with human parvovirus B19 infection. MMWR Morb Mortal Wkly Rep 38:81, 1989.
122. Iwa N, Yutani C: Cytodiagnosis of parvovirus B19 infection from ascites fluid of hydrops fetalis. Diagn Cytopathol 13:139, 1995.
123. Carrington D, Whittle MJ, Gibson AAM, et al: Maternal serum alphafetoprotein: A marker of fetal aplastic crisis during intrauterine human parvovirus infection. Lancet 1:433, 1987.
124. Anderson MJ, Khousam MN, Maxwell DJ, et al: Human parvovirus B19 and hydrops fetalis. Lancet 1:535, 1988.
125. Peters MT, Nicolaides KH: Cordocentesis for the diagnosis and treatment of human fetal parvovirus infection. Obstet Gynecol 75:501, 1990.
126. Von Kaisenberg CS, Jonat W: Fetal parvovirus B19 infection. Ultrasound Obstet Gynecol 18:280, 2001.
127. Morey AL, Nicolini U, Welch CR, et al: Parvovirus B19 infection and transient fetal hydrops. Lancet 337:496, 1991.
128. Anand A, Gray ES, Brown T, et al: Human parvovirus infection in pregnancy and hydrops fetalis. N Engl J Med 316:183, 1987.
129. Bernstein IM, Capeless EL: Elevated maternal serum alpha-fetoprotein and hydrops fetalis in association with fetal parvovirus B-19 infection. Obstet Gynecol 74:456, 1989.
130. Rodis JF, Hovick TJ, Quinn DL, et al: Human parvovirus infection in pregnancy. Obstet Gynecol 72:733, 1988.
131. Porter HJ, Quantril AM, Fleming KA: B19 parvovirus infection of myocardial cells. Lancet 1:535, 1988.
132. Soothill P: Intrauterine blood transfusion for non-immune hydrops fetalis due to parvovirus B19 infection. Lancet 336:121, 1990.
133. Sahakian V, Weiner CP, Naides SJ, et al: Intrauterine transfusion treatment of nonimmune hydrops fetalis secondary to human parvovirus B19 infection. Am J Obstet Gynecol 164:1090, 1991.
134. Nagel HT, de Haan TR, Vandenbussche FP, et al: Long-term outcome after fetal transfusion for hydrops associated with parvovirus B19 infection. Obstet Gynecol 109:42-47, 2007.
135. Bain AD, Bowie JH, Flint WF, et al: Congenital toxoplasmosis disease stimulating haemolytic disease of the newborn. J Obstet Gynecol 63:826, 1956.
136. Spahr RC, Botti JJ, MacDonald HM, et al: Nonimmunologic hydrops fetalis: A review of 19 cases. Gynaecol Obstet 18:303, 1980.
137. Robb JA, Benirschke K, Mannino F, et al: Intrauterine latent herpes simplex virus infection: Latent neonatal infection. Hum Pathol 17:1210, 1986.
138. Gembruch U, Niesen M, Hansmann M, et al: Listeriosis: A cause of nonimmune hydrops fetalis. Prenat Diagn 7:277, 1987.
139. Ranucci-Weiss D, Uerpairojkit B, Bowles N, et al: Intrauterine adenoviral infection associated with fetal non-immune hydrops. Prenat Diagn 18:182, 1998.
140. Zornes SL, Anderson PG, Lott RL: Congenital toxoplasmosis in an infant with hydrops fetalis. South Med J 81:391, 1988.
141. Van den Veyver IB, Bowles N, Carpenter RJ, et al: Detection of intrauterine viral infection using the polymerase chain reaction. Mol Genet Metab 63:85, 1998.
142. Zimmer EZ, Gutterman E, Blazer S: Recurrent nonimmune hydrops. J Reprod Med 31:193, 1986.
143. Robertson L, Ott A, Mack L, et al: Sonographically documented disappearance of nonimmune hydrops fetalis associated with maternal hypertension. West J Med 143:382, 1985.
144. Gillan JE, Lowden JA, Gaskin K, et al: Congenital ascites as a presenting sign of lysosomal storage disease. J Pediatr 104:225, 1984.
145. Abu-Dalu KI, Tamary H, Livni N, et al: GM1 gangliosidosis presenting as neonatal ascites. J Pediatr 100:940, 1982.
146. Beck M, Bender SW, Reiter HL, et al: Neuraminidase deficiency presenting as non-immune hydrops fetalis. Eur J Pediatr 143:135, 1984.
147. Bonduelle M, Lissens W, Goossens A, et al: Lysosomal storage diseases presenting as transient or persistent hydrops fetalis. Genet Couns 2:227, 1991.
148. Tasso MJ, Martinez-Gutierrez A, Carrascosa C, et al: GM1-gangliosidosis presenting as nonimmune hydrops fetalis: A case report. J Perinat Med 24:445, 1996.
149. Ginsburg SJ, Groll M: Hydrops fetalis due to infantile Gaucher's disease. J Pediatr 82:1046, 1973.
150. Piraud M, Froissart R, Mandon G, et al: Amniotic fluid for screening of lysosomal storage diseases presenting in utero (mainly as non-immune hydrops fetalis). Clin Chim Acta 248:143, 1996.
151. Groener JEM, de Graaf FL, Poorthuis JHM, et al: Prenatal diagnosis of lysosomal storage diseases using fetal blood. Prenat Diagn 19:930, 1999.
152. Burin MG, Scholz AP, Gus R, et al: Investigation of lysosomal storage disease in nonimmune hydrops fetalis. Prenat Diagn 24:653-657, 2004.
153. Kooper AJ, Janssens PM, de Groot AN, et al: Lysosomal storage diseases in non-immune hydrops fetalis pregnancies. Clin Chim Acta 371:176-182, 2006.
154. Pretorius DH, Rumack CM, Manco-Johnson ML, et al: Specific skeletal dysplasias in utero: Sonographic diagnosis. Radiology 159:237, 1986.
155. Jauniaux E, Van Maldergem L, De Munter C, et al: Nonimmune hydrops fetalis associated with genetic abnormalities. Obstet Gynecol 75:568, 1990.
156. Afifi AM, Bhatia AR, Eyal F: Hydrops fetalis associated with congenital myotonic dystrophy. Am J Obstet Gynecol 166:929, 1992.
157. Poeschmann RP, Verheijen RHM, Van Dongen WJ: Differential diagnosis and causes of nonimmunological hydrops fetalis: A review. Obstet Gynecol Surv 46:223, 1991.
158. Tjeertes IF, Bastiaans DE, van Ganzewinkel CJ, Zegers SH: Neonatal anemia and hydrops fetalis after maternal mycophenolate mofetil use. J Perinatol 27:62-64, 2007.
159. Yanai N, Shveiky D: Fetal hydrops, associated with maternal propylthiouracil exposure, reversed by intrauterine therapy. Ultrasound Obstet Gynecol 23:198-201, 2004.
160. Murki S, Kumar P, Dutta S, Narang A: Fatal neonatal renal failure due to maternal enlapril ingestion. J Matern Fetal Neonatal Med 17:235-237, 2005.
161. Shimokawa H, Hara K, Fukuda A, et al: Idiopathic hydrops fetalis successfully treated in utero. Obstet Gynecol 71:984, 1988.
162. Maeda H, Shimokawa H, Nakano H, et al: Effects of intrauterine treatment on nonimmunologic hydrops fetalis. Fetal Ther 3:198, 1988.
163. Lingman G, Stangenberg M, Legarth J, et al: Albumin transfusion in nonimmune fetal hydrops: Doppler ultrasound evaluation of the acute effects

on blood circulation in the fetal aorta and the umbilical arteries. Fetal Ther 4:120, 1989.
164. Goldberg JD, Mitty H, Dische MR, et al: Prenatal shunting of fetal ascites in nonimmune hydrops fetalis. Am J Perinatol 3:92, 1986.
165. Appelman Z, Blumberg BD, Golabi M, et al: Nonimmune hydrops fetalis may be associated with an elevated delta OD450 in the amniotic fluid. Obstet Gynecol 71:1005, 1988.
166. Huhta JC: Guidelines for the evaluation of heart failure in the fetus with or without hydrops. Pediatr Cardiol 25:274-286, 2004.
167. Hofstaetter C, Hansmann M, Eik-Nes SH, et al: A cardiovascular profile score in the surveillance of fetal hydrops. J Matern Fetal Neonatal Med 19:407-413, 2006.
168. Cumming DC: Recurrent nonimmune hydrops fetalis. Obstet Gynecol 54:124, 1979.
169. Etches PC, Lemons JA: Nonimmune hydrops fetalis: Report of 22 cases including three siblings. Pediatrics 64:326, 1979.
170. Schwartz SH, Viseskul C, Laxova R, et al: Idiopathic hydrops fetalis: Report of 4 patients including 2 affected sibs. Am J Med Genet 8:59, 1981.
171. Battin MR, Yan J, Aftimos S, Roberts A: Congenital chylothorax in siblings. BJOG 107:1516-1518, 2000.
172. Stevenson DA, Pysher TJ, Ward RM, Carey JC: Familial congenital non-immune hydrops, chylothorax, and pulmonary lymphangiectasia. Am J Med Gen A 140:368-372, 2006.
173. Goh SL, Tan JV, Kwek KY, Yeo GS: Recurrent non-immune fetal hydrops: A case report. Ann Acad Med Singapore 35:726-728, 2006.
174. deCrespigny LC, Robinson HP, McBain JC: Fetal abdominal paracentesis in the management of gross fetal ascites. A N Z J Obstet Gynaecol 20:228, 1980.
175. Cardwell MS: Aspiration of fetal pleural effusions or ascites may improve neonatal resuscitation. South Med J 89:177, 1996.
176. Simpson JH, McDevitt H, Young D, Cameron AD: Severity of non-immune hydrops fetalis at birth continues to predict survival despite advances in perinatal care. Fetal Diagn Ther 21:380-382, 2006.
177. Carlton DP, McGillivray BC, Schreiber MD: Nonimmune hydrops fetalis: A multidisciplinary approach. Clin Perinatol 16:839, 1989.
178. Stephenson T, Zuccollo J, Mohajer M: Diagnosis and management of non-immune hydrops in the newborn. Arch Dis Child 70:F151, 1994.
179. Davis CL: Diagnosis and management of nonimmune hydrops. J Reprod Med 27:594, 1982.
180. Ringer SA, Stark AR: Management of neonatal emergencies in the delivery room. Clin Perinatol 16:23, 1989.

Part III

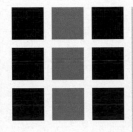

DISORDERS AT THE MATERNAL-FETAL INTERFACE

Chapter 28

Pathogenesis of Spontaneous Preterm Labor

Roberto Romero, MD, and Charles J. Lockwood, MD

Preterm deliveries are those occurring between fetal viability and 37 completed weeks of gestation (menstrual age).[1] Delivery of a previable fetus represents a spontaneous abortion rather than a preterm birth. The precise definition of "viability," however, is a subject of debate because of the increased frequency of survival at very low gestational ages. Some neonates can survive if born around 24 weeks of gestation, but none at 20 weeks; therefore, we propose that preterm birth be defined as one that occurs between 24 and 36 6/7 weeks of gestation. This definition may need to be revised if future technologic advances allow substantial survival at less than 24 weeks of gestation.

A birth weight of 500 g has historically been used to define the lower limit of viability. However, this approach is limited because viable neonates born after 24 weeks may be affected by intrauterine growth restriction (IUGR) and have birth weights of less than 500 g. Conversely, some previable infants may weigh more than 500 g. The threshold of 500 g is valuable if there is uncertainty about gestational age. An accurate definition of preterm birth has implications for the calculation of vital statistics and comparisons of the rates of preterm delivery among different countries and populations, an issue that is often overlooked.

Preterm births can be spontaneous or "indicated." Spontaneous preterm labor can occur with either intact membranes or prelabor (premature) rupture of the fetal membranes (PROM). "Indicated" preterm births are those that result from induced preterm labor or preterm cesarean delivery for maternal or fetal indications, usually because of preeclampsia or IUGR or both. The mechanisms of disease responsible for these two conditions are discussed in other chapters of this text (see Chapter 5).

Of all preterm deliveries, some 25% (reported range, 18.7% to 35.2%) are indicated, and the remainder are spontaneous—45% (23.2% to 64.1%) from preterm labor with intact membranes and 30% (7.1% to 51.2%) from preterm labor after PROM.[2,3] The rate of preterm delivery in the United States has climbed 14% since 1990; this has been attributed to an increased frequency of indicated preterm birth in singleton gestations, an increased number of multiple gestations, and an increased number of older parturients.[4]

Overview of the Mechanisms of Labor

The Common Pathway

The traditional view, which has dominated the study of preterm parturition, is that term and preterm labor are the same processes, albeit occurring at different gestational ages. Indeed, they do share a common pathway, which includes increased uterine contractility, cervical ripening, and membrane rupture.[5] It has been proposed that the fundamental difference between term and preterm labor is that the former results from "physiologic activation" of this common pathway, whereas preterm labor results from a disease process ("pathologic activation") that extemporaneously activates one or more of the components of the common pathway.[6]

The *common pathway of parturition* is defined as the anatomic, biochemical, immunologic, endocrinologic, and clinical events that occur in the mother and fetus in both term and preterm labor.[6] Much clinical emphasis has been placed on the uterine components of the pathway (myometrial contractility, cervical ripening, and membrane rupture) (Fig. 28-1). However, there are systemic changes, such as an increase in the plasma concentration of corticotropin-releasing hormone (CRH) and in the caloric metabolic expenditures, that are also part of the common pathway.[7-10]

Activation of the uterine components of the common pathway of parturition may be synchronous or asynchronous. Synchronous activation results in clinical spontaneous preterm labor. Asynchronous activation results in a different phenotype. For example, predominant activation of the membranes leads to preterm PROM, that of the cervix to cervical insufficiency, and that of myometrium to preterm uterine contractions without cervical change or rupture of membranes (Fig. 28-2).

Spontaneous preterm labor with intact membranes, preterm PROM, and cervical insufficiency can be considered syndromes caused

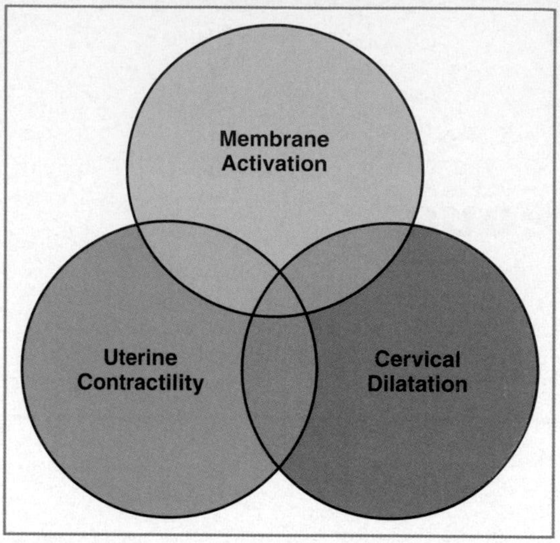

FIGURE 28-1 Uterine components of the common pathway of parturition (preterm and term). (From Romero R, Gomez R, Mazor M, et al: The preterm labor syndrome. In Elder MG, Romero R, Lamont RF (eds). Preterm Labor. New York: Churchill Livingstone, 1997, pp 29-49.)

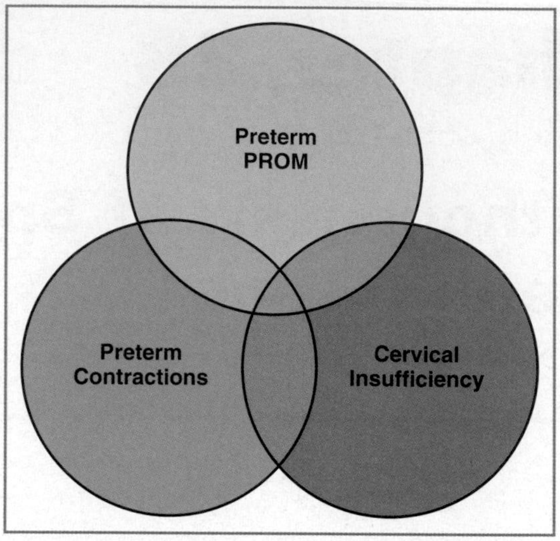

FIGURE 28-2 Clinical manifestations of preterm activation of the common pathway of parturition. Clinical manifestations depend on whether there is synchronous or asynchronous recruitment of the pathway. Cervical insufficiency is the presenting phenotype if activation of the cervix occurs in isolation. Prelabor rupture of membranes (PROM) occurs if decidual/membrane activation is the predominant pathway activated. Isolated activation of the myometrium results in preterm uterine contractions. Synchronous activation of the myometrium and the cervix results in the clinical presentation generally recognized as preterm labor with intact membranes. (From Romero R, Gomez R, Mazor M, et al: The preterm labor syndrome. In Elder MG, Romero R, Lamont RF (eds). Preterm Labor. New York: Churchill Livingstone, 1997, pp 29-49.)

by multiple etiologies with specific pathogenic pathways. This chapter reviews the pathophysiology of the common pathway of parturition and examines the pathologic mechanisms responsible for its activation.

Myometrial Contractility

Although myometrial contractility occurs throughout pregnancy, labor is characterized by a dramatic change in the pattern of uterine contractility, which evolves from "contractures" to "contractions."[6] Nathanielsz and Honnebier[11] and Hsu and colleagues[12] defined *contractures* as epochs of myometrial activity lasting several minutes, associated with a modest increase in intrauterine pressure and fragmented bursts of electrical activity in the electromyogram. In contrast, *contractions* are epochs of myometrial activity of short duration associated with dramatic increases in intrauterine pressure and electromyographic activity. The switch from a predominant contracture pattern to a predominant contraction pattern occurs physiologically during normal labor[13] or can be induced by pathologic events such as food withdrawal, infection, or intra-abdominal surgery.[14-16]

Increased cell-to-cell communication is thought to be responsible for the effectiveness of myometrial contractility during labor. Gap junctions develop in the myometrium just prior to labor and disappear shortly after delivery.[17-21] Gap junction formation and the expression of the gap junction protein, connexin-43, in human myometrium is similar in both term and preterm labor.[22-26] These findings suggest that the appearance of gap junctions and increased expression of connexin-43 may be part of the underlying series of molecular and cellular events responsible for the switch from contractures to contractions before the onset of parturition. Estrogen, progesterone, and prostaglandins have been implicated in the regulation of gap junction formation, and they also influence the expression of connexin-43.[27-29] Lye and others have referred to a set of distinct proteins, called contraction-associated proteins, that are characteristic of this phase of parturition (see Chapter 5).[24,30,31]

Lye and colleagues[32] also proposed that the myometrium undergoes sequential phenotypic remodeling during pregnancy. Their studies were undertaken in rodents but have implications for humans. Three distinct stages of rat gestational myometrial development were recognized:

1. *Proliferative*, in which the number of myocytes increased, as demonstrated by greater proliferation cell nuclear antigen labeling and protein expression in early pregnancy. This phenotype coincided with a higher myometrial expression of antiapoptotic proteins (BCL2 and BCL2L1 [formerly BCL-xL]).
2. *Synthetic*, in which the myometrial cells underwent hypertrophy, as demonstrated by a higher protein/DNA ratio in the second half of pregnancy. This stage coincided with a higher secretion of extracellular matrix (ECM) proteins from the myocytes, in particular collagen I and collagen III, as well as a high concentration of caldesmon (a marker of synthetic phenotype)
3. *Contractile*, which occurred at the end of pregnancy and coincided with low myometrial expression of interstitial matrix proteins and high expression of components of the basement membrane (laminin and collagen IV).

α-Actin was expressed in the myometrium in early pregnancy, whereas γ-actin was highly expressed by myometrium with a contractile phenotype. The switch from a proliferative to a synthetic phenotype appeared to be regulated by caspase 3, and a decrease in progesterone was responsible for the switch from the synthetic to the contractile phenotype.[32] This view is consistent with the proposal of Csapo about the importance of progesterone in the regulation of myometrial contractility at the onset of parturition.[33] Microarray experiments of myometrium in labor indicate an overexpression of genes involved in control of inflammation (Romero et al, unpublished observations). This is consistent with other studies which used subtraction hybridization to identify genes differentially expressed during labor. Interleukin 8 (IL-8) and superoxide dismutase have been found to be differentially regulated.[34]

Cervical Remodeling

The changes in the cervix include: (1) softening, (2) ripening, (3) dilatation, and, after delivery, (4) repair.[35] Sonographic studies have demonstrated that shortening of the cervix occurs before the dramatic increase in uterine contractility that characterizes term and preterm labor. Hence, the regulation of cervical remodeling has become important in the understanding of cervical insufficiency and spontaneous preterm labor.

The molecular and cellular bases for cervical remodeling during pregnancy and parturition are largely dependent on the regulation of extracellular matrix components.[35-41] Softening of the cervix begins in early pregnancy. The tensile strength of the softened cervix appears to be maintained by an increase in collagen synthesis and growth of the cervix. Cervical ripening is characterized by a decreased concentration of collagen and the dispersion of collagen fibrils. The latter has been attributed to glycosaminoglycans, such as decorin and hyaluronan, which promote hydration of cervical tissue and dispersion of the collagen fibers.[36] Dilation of the cervix is an inflammatory phenomenon in which there is an influx of macrophages and neutrophils and matrix degradation.[42-44] Chemokines such as IL-8[45-49] and S100A9[50,51] attract inflammatory cells, which, in turn, release proinflammatory cytokines, including IL-1β[52,53] and tumor necrosis factor-α (TNF-α),[35-54] that can activate the nuclear factor (NF)-κB signaling pathway. NF-κB can block progesterone receptor-mediated actions.[55] Progesterone has been implicated in the regulation of cervical remodeling because (1) administration of antiprogestins to women in the mid-trimester and at term induces cervical ripening;[35,56-60] and (2) the administration of progesterone-receptor antagonists such as mifepristone (RU-486) or onapristone (ZK 98299) to pregnant guinea pigs,[61,62] old-world monkeys,[63] and *Tupaia belangeri* induces cervical ripening.[35] Cervical responsiveness to antiprogestins increases with advancing gestational age,[35] and the effects of antiprogestins in the cervix are not always accompanied by changes in myometrial activity.[35] Indeed, Stys and associates[64] demonstrated a dissociation between the effects of progesterone in the myometrium and those in the cervix. A frequent observation, in animals[62,63] as well as in humans,[65] is that antiprogestins induce cervical ripening but not labor. Indeed, labor may be delayed by days or weeks, or it may not begin at all after cervical ripening has been accomplished in humans.[35] Collectively, these findings suggest that the cervix is a major site of progesterone action. This realization is important, because much of the emphasis in previous years has been on the effect of progesterone on the myometrium. Yet, recent randomized clinical trials suggest that progesterone may be helpful in preventing preterm birth in women with a short cervix.[66-69]

Decidual/Membrane Activation

We use the term *decidual/membrane activation* to refer to a complex set of anatomic and biochemical events that lead to separation of the lower pole of the fetal amniochorionic membranes from the decidua of the lower uterine segment and, eventually, to spontaneous rupture of the membranes and delivery of the placenta.

During pregnancy, the chorioamnionic membranes fuse with the decidua. In preparation for delivery, biochemical events take place to allow separation and postpartum expulsion of the membranes. Fibronectins are a family of important extracellular matrix proteins. The available evidence suggests that degradation of a heavily glycosylated form of cellular fibronectin (i.e., fetal fibronectin) which is present at the chorionic-decidual interface leads to its release into cervical and vaginal secretions immediately before term and preterm parturition.[70-73] Beyond proteolytic degradation of the decidual and amniochorionic extracellular matrix by matrix-degrading enzymes, PROM is also associated with amnion epithelial apoptosis and localized inflammation.[74] Therefore, these processes belong to the common terminal pathway of parturition.

Enzymatic activity of matrix metalloproteinases (MMPs) and other proteases has been implicated in the process of rupture of membranes and parturition with intact membranes (with and without infection).[75-77] Histologic studies of membranes in women with term PROM indicate that membranes that rupture prematurely have a decreased number of collagen fibers, disruption of the normal wavy patterns of these fibers, and deposition of amorphous materials among them.[78] Similar changes have been observed in the membranes apposed to the cervix in women undergoing elective cesarean delivery at term with intact membranes. The implication is that, although spontaneous rupture of membranes normally occurs at the end of the first stage of labor, the process responsible for this phenomenon begins before the onset of labor.

Histologic studies of the site of rupture have demonstrated a zone of altered morphology (ZAM).[79,80] A significant decrease in the amount of collagen type I, III, or V and an increased expression of tenascin have been reported in the ZAM. Tenascin is an extracellular matrix characteristically expressed during tissue remodeling and wound healing. Its identification in the membranes thus signifies the presence of injury and a wound healing–like response. Observations by Bell and colleagues[81,82] suggested that changes in the ZAM are more extensive in the setting of preterm PROM. These morphologic and biochemical observations are consistent with the results of biophysical studies suggesting that rupture of membranes results from the application of acute or chronic stress on localized areas of the membranes that are weaker.

The precise mechanism of decidual/membrane activation remains to be elucidated. As noted, roles for extracellular matrix–degrading enzymes such as the MMPs and apoptosis have been proposed. Several studies have demonstrated increased availability of MMP-1 (interstitial collagenase),[83] MMP-8 (neutrophil collagenase),[84] MMP-9 (gelatinase-B),[85] and neutrophil elastase[86] in the amniotic fluid of women with preterm PROM, compared with women in preterm labor with intact membranes. Plasmin has also been implicated in this process,[73] because this enzyme can degrade type III collagen, fibronectin, and laminin.[87] Other MMPs are likely to be involved, but systematic studies have not been conducted to date.[88-90] A role for tissue inhibitors of MMPs (TIMPs) has also been postulated.[91]

Prostaglandins as Key Activators of the Common Pathway of Parturition

A central question in the understanding of parturition is whether the signals responsible for activation of the common pathway are similar in term and preterm labor. Prostaglandins have been considered the key mediators for the onset of labor,[92-107] because they can induce myometrial contractility,[92,96,105,107] changes in extracellular matrix metabolism associated with cervical ripening,[94,95,99,100,104] and decidual/membrane activation.[5]

Descriptive evidence traditionally invoked to support a role for prostaglandins in the initiation of human labor includes the following: (1) administration of prostaglandins can induce early or late termination of pregnancy (abortion or labor)[103,108-118]; (2) treatment with indomethacin or aspirin can delay spontaneous onset of parturition in animals[119-122]; (3) concentrations of prostaglandins in plasma and amniotic fluid increase during labor[123-130]; (4) intra-amniotic injection of arachidonic acid, the precursor of prostaglandins, induces abortion[101]; (5) amniotic fluid concentrations of prostaglandins increase before the onset of spontaneous labor at term in humans and nonhuman primates[131]; (6) expression of myometrial prostaglandin receptors increases in labor[132,133]; and (7) labor is associated with increased cyclooxygenase-2 (COX-2) expression of messenger RNA (mRNA) and increased activity of this enzyme in amnion (a rate-limiting step in the production of prostaglandins). This increase in amnionic COX-2 activity is accompanied by decreased expression of the prostaglandin-metabolizing enzyme, 15-hydroxy-prostaglandin dehydrogenase (PGDH) in the chorion. This would allow prostaglandins produced in the amnion to traverse the chorion and reach the myometrium, where they can stimulate smooth muscle contractions.[134]

The biochemical mechanisms by which prostaglandins activate the common pathway of parturition are the following: (1) prostaglandins directly promote uterine contractions by increasing sarcoplasmic and transmembrane calcium fluxes and through increased transcription of oxytocin receptors, connexin-43 (gap junctions), and the prostaglandin receptors EP_1 through EP_4 and FP[27,135,136]; (2) prostaglandins induce synthesis of MMPs by fetal membranes and cells within the uterine cervix (as noted, MMPs have been implicated in the mechanisms of membrane rupture and also in cervical ripening)[137,138]; and (3) prostaglandin E_2 (PGE_2) and $PGF_{2\alpha}$ increase the ratio of expression of the progesterone receptor (PR) isoforms, PR-A/PR-B.[139] This may induce a functional progesterone withdrawal. Figure 28-3 describes the molecular mechanisms implicated in the common pathway of parturition.

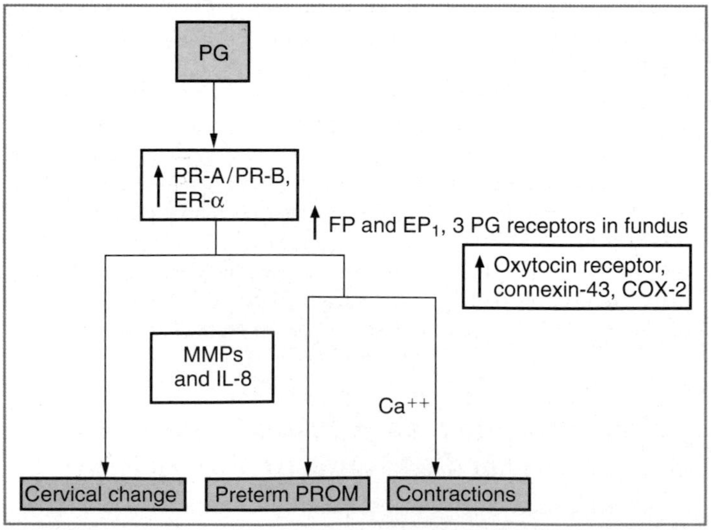

FIGURE 28-3 Molecular mechanisms implicated in the common pathway of parturition. COX-2, cyclooxygenase-2; EP_1, PTGER1, prostaglandin E receptor type 1; ER-α, estrogen receptor-α; FP, PTGFR, prostaglandin F receptor; IL-8, interleukin 8; MMPs, matrix metalloproteinases; PG, prostaglandins; PR, prostaglandin receptor; PROM, premature rupture of membranes.

Spontaneous Preterm Parturition as a "Syndrome"

The current taxonomy of disease in obstetrics is based on the clinical presentation of the mother and not on the mechanisms of disease responsible for the clinical presentation. Neither the term "preterm labor with intact membranes" nor "preterm prelabor rupture of membranes" conveys information about the pathologic process that has led to untimely delivery. This situation is not unique to preterm parturition: it is also the case in preeclampsia, small for gestational age (SGA), fetal death, and other obstetric syndromes.

Generally, the diagnostic labels used in clinical obstetrics simply reflect a collection of symptoms and signs (e.g., abdominal pain due to uterine contractions, leakage of fluid) without information about the mechanisms of disease. The lack of recognition of this is responsible for the failure of any single diagnostic test or treatment to detect, cure, or prevent preterm delivery. To emphasize that preterm labor has multiple causes, we have used the word "syndrome," which is defined as a combination of symptoms or signs that form a distinct clinical picture but can be generated by multiple etiologies. The features of the great obstetric syndromes have been described elsewhere.[140]

We also make a distinction between preterm labor as a multifactorial disorder versus a syndrome. We are unaware of any disease in medicine that is unifactorial. For example, even sickle cell anemia, which is caused by the mutation of a single nucleotide, produces a wide range of clinical manifestations, and environmental factors such as infection or hypoxia can influence the phenotype caused by a single discrete genotype. The term "multifactorial" is often used in genetics to refer to common complex disorders in which the genetic predisposition is attributed to several genes and can be altered by environmental factors. Each of the causes of preterm parturition syndrome fits this definition of multifactorial. For example, in the case of infection, microorganisms can be considered an environmental factor, but the intensity and nature of the host inflammatory response is under genetic control. Thus, gene-environment interactions contribute to the phenotype of infection associated preterm parturition. The same is the case for vascular disease or hemorrhage, stress, and so on. The causes of preterm parturition syndrome are presented in Figure 28-4. The mechanisms of disease for each cause are in the following sections. The molecular signaling pathways implicated in four of these mechanisms are displayed in Figure 28-5.

The Spontaneous Preterm Parturition Syndromes

Infection and Inflammation

Infection is a frequent and important mechanism of disease in preterm delivery. Indeed, it is the only pathologic process for which an unequivocal causal link with preterm parturition has been established. Evidence for causality includes the following: (1) intrauterine infection or systemic administration of microbial products (bacterial endotoxin) to pregnant animals results in spontaneous preterm labor and birth[141-153]; (2) extrauterine maternal infections (malaria,[154,155] pyelonephritis,[156-160] pneumonia,[161-163] and periodontal disease[164-169]) are associated with preterm delivery; (3) subclinical intrauterine infections are consistently associated with preterm labor and preterm birth[170]; (4) pregnant

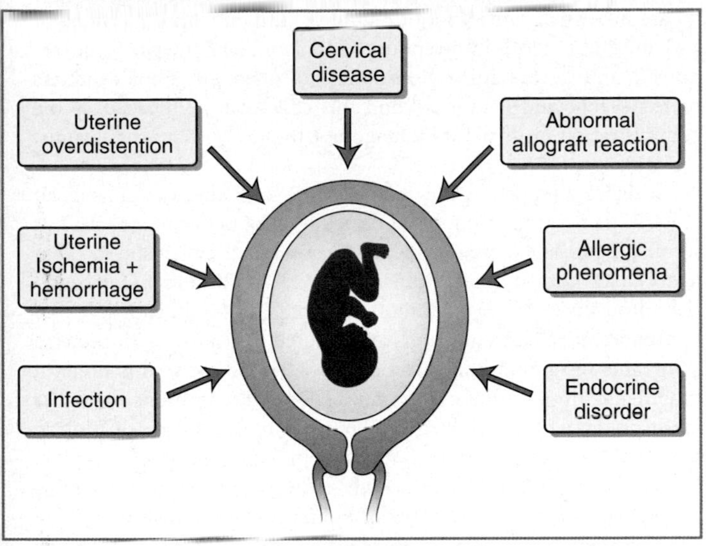

FIGURE 28-4 The preterm parturition syndrome. Multiple pathologic processes can lead to activation of the common pathway of parturition. (Modified from Romero R, Espinoza J, Mazor M, Chaiworapongsa T: The preterm parturition syndrome. In Critchely H, Bennett P, Thornton S (eds): Preterm Birth. London: RCOG Press, 2004, pp 28-60.)

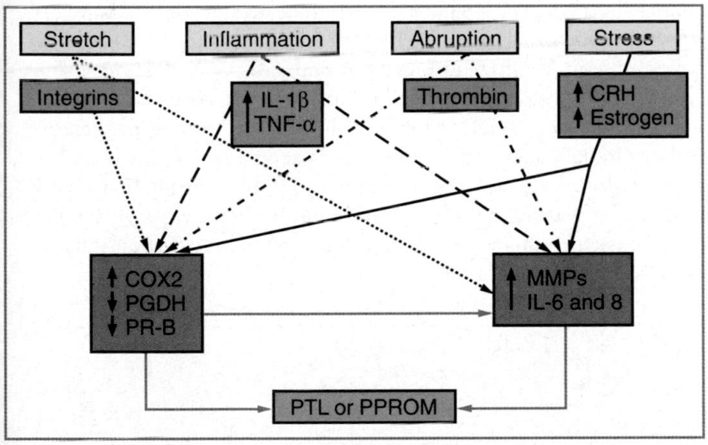

FIGURE 28-5 Principal biochemical mechanisms responsible for the main pathways of preterm parturition. COX2, cyclooxygenase-2; CRH, corticotropin-releasing hormone; IL-1β, interleukin-1β; MMPs, matrix metalloproteinases; PGDH, prostaglandin dehydrogenase; PPROM, preterm premature rupture of membranes; PR-B, progesterone receptor type B; PTL, preterm labor; TNF-α, tumor necrosis factor-α.

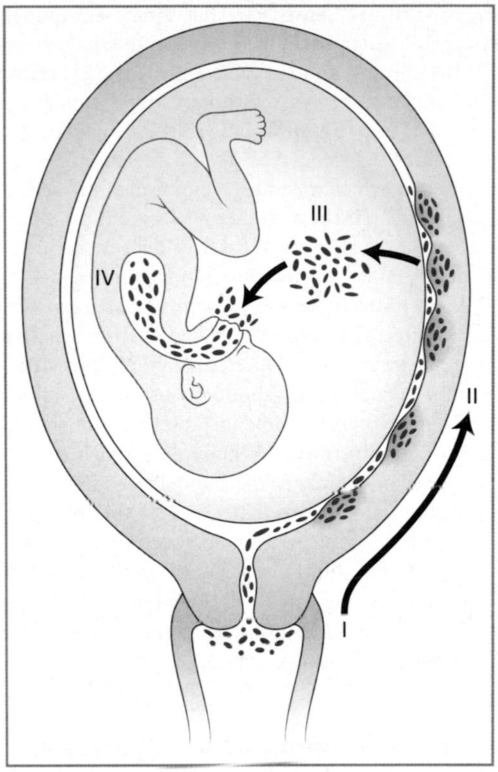

FIGURE 28-6 The pathway of ascending intrauterine infection. Stage I refers to a change in microbial flora in the vagina and/or cervix. In Stage II, microorganisms are located between the amnion and chorion. Stage III represents intra-amniotic infection, and Stage IV is fetal invasion. The most common sites for microbial attack are the skin and the fetal respiratory tract. (Reproduced with permission from Romero R, Mazor M: Infection and preterm labor. Clin Obstet Gynecol 31:553-584, 1988.)

women with intra-amniotic infection[171-173] or inflammation (defined as an elevation of amniotic fluid concentrations of proinflammatory cytokines[174,175] and matrix-degrading enzymes[176] in the mid-trimester) are at risk for subsequent spontaneous preterm birth; (5) antibiotic treatment of ascending intrauterine infections can prevent preterm parturition in experimental models of chorioamnionitis[149,177]; and (6) treatment of asymptomatic bacteriuria prevents preterm birth.[178,179]

Because the amniotic cavity is sterile for bacteria in 99% of cases, detection of microorganisms in the amniotic cavity with either cultivation techniques or molecular microbiologic techniques defines microbial invasion of the amniotic cavity. Microorganisms or their products can elicit an inflammatory response within the amniotic cavity: intra-amniotic inflammation. Inflammation of the chorioamniotic membranes, or histologic chorioamnionitis, can exist without clinical signs of infection (clinical chorioamnionitis). The stages of ascending intrauterine infection are displayed in Figure 28-6.

Microbiologic studies using cultivation techniques suggest that infection may account for 25% to 40% of all preterm births.[180,181] Microbial invasion of the amniotic cavity (MIAC) is present in 12.8%[180] of women with preterm labor with intact membranes, in 32% of those with preterm PROM,[180] and in 51% of patients with acute cervical insufficiency.[182,183] Patients with MIAC are more likely to deliver preterm neonates, have spontaneous rupture of membranes, and develop clinical chorioamnionitis than those with sterile amniotic fluid.[184] The most common organisms found in the amniotic fluid are genital mycoplasmas.[185,186] It is believed that ascending infection is the most common source of microbial invasion of the amniotic cavity, although transplacental infections may also occur. The lower the gestational age at which a patient presents with preterm labor and preterm PROM, the higher the frequency of MIAC.[187,188] Moreover, many of these infections appear to be chronic in nature, because they have been detected in women having mid-trimester amniocentesis for genetic indications.[171-173] Bacterial products such as endotoxin have also been detected in the amniotic cavity of women with preterm labor and preterm PROM.[189,190] Endotoxin has powerful proinflammatory effects in maternal and fetal tissues.[191-193]

Microorganisms are "sensed" by the innate components of the immune system,[194] which include (1) the soluble pattern recognition receptors (PRRs), lectin, and C-reactive protein; (2) transmembrane PRRs, which include scavenger receptors, C-type lectins, and Toll-like receptors (TLRs); and (3) intracellular PRRs, including Nod1 and Nod2, retinoic-induced gene type 1, and melanoma differentiation associated protein 5, which mediate recognition of intracellular pathogens (e.g., viruses).[195] The best-studied PRRs are the TLRs.[194] Ligation of TLR results in activation of NF-κB, which, in turn, leads to the production of cytokines, chemokines, and antimicrobial peptides.[194] Because TLRs are crucial for the recognition of microorganisms, it could be anticipated that defective signaling through this pathway would impair bacteria-induced preterm labor. Consistent with this thesis, a strain of mice bearing a spontaneous mutation for TLR-4 was less likely to deliver preterm after intrauterine inoculation of heat-killed bacteria or administration of lipopolysaccharide than wild-type mice.[151,196] In pregnant women, TLR-2 and TLR-4 are expressed in the amniotic epithelium[197] as well as in decidua.[198] Moreover, spontaneous labor that occurs at term or preterm and is complicated by histologic evidence of chorioamnionitis, regardless of the membrane status (intact or ruptured), is associated with increased mRNA expression of TLR-2 and TLR-4 in the chorioamniotic membranes.[197] These observations suggest that the innate immune system plays a role in parturition.

The Role of Proinflammatory Cytokines

Inflammation and its mediators, chemokines such as IL-8, the proinflammatory cytokines (IL-1β, TNF-α), and other mediators (e.g., platelet activating factor, prostaglandins) are central to preterm parturition induced by infection. IL-1 was the first cytokine implicated in the onset of preterm labor associated with infection.[199] Evidence in support of this concept includes the following: (1) IL-1 is produced by human decidua in response to bacterial products[200]; (2) IL-1α and IL-1β stimulate prostaglandin production by human amnion and decidua[201]; (3) IL-1α and IL-1β concentrations and IL-1–like bioactivity are increased in the amniotic fluid of women with preterm labor and infection[202]; (4) intravenous IL-1β stimulates uterine contractions[203]; and (5) administration of IL-1 to pregnant animals induces preterm labor and delivery,[204] and this effect can be blocked by the administration of its natural antagonist, the IL-1 receptor antagonist (IL-1ra).[205]

Evidence supporting the role of TNF-α in the mechanisms of preterm parturition is similar and includes the following: (1) TNF-α stimulates prostaglandin production by amnion, decidua, and myometrium[148]; (2) human decidua can produce TNF-α in response to bacterial products[206,207]; (3) amniotic fluid TNF-α bioactivity and immunoreactive concentrations are elevated in women with preterm labor and intra-amniotic infection[208]; (4) in women with preterm PROM and intra-amniotic infection, TNF-α concentrations are higher in the presence of labor[208]; (5) TNF-α can stimulate the production of MMPs,[209,210] which have been implicated in membrane rupture[85,211,212]; (6) TNF-α application to the cervix induces changes that resemble cervical ripening[213]; (7) TNF-α can induce preterm parturition when administered systemically to pregnant animals[214,215]; and (8) TNF-α and IL-1β enhance IL-8 expression by decidual cells, and this chemokine is strongly expressed by term decidual cells in the presence of chorioamnionitis.[216] Figure 28-7 displays the mechanisms involved in preterm parturition in the setting of infection.

Other cytokines and chemokines (IL-6,[187,217-221] IL-10,[203,222,223] IL-16,[224] IL-18,[225] colony-stimulating factors,[226-228] macrophage migration inhibitory factor,[229] IL-8,[228,230-234] monocyte chemotactic protein-1,[235] epithelial cell–derived neutrophil-activating peptide-78,[236] and, regulated on activation, normal T-cell expressed and secreted (RANTES)[237]) have also been implicated in infection-induced preterm delivery. The redundancy of the cytokine network implicated in parturition is such that blockade of a single cytokine is insufficient to prevent preterm delivery in the context of infection. For example, preterm labor after exposure to infection can occur in knockout mice for the IL-1 type I receptor, suggesting that IL-1 is sufficient, but not necessary, for the onset of parturition in the context of intra-amniotic infection/inflam-

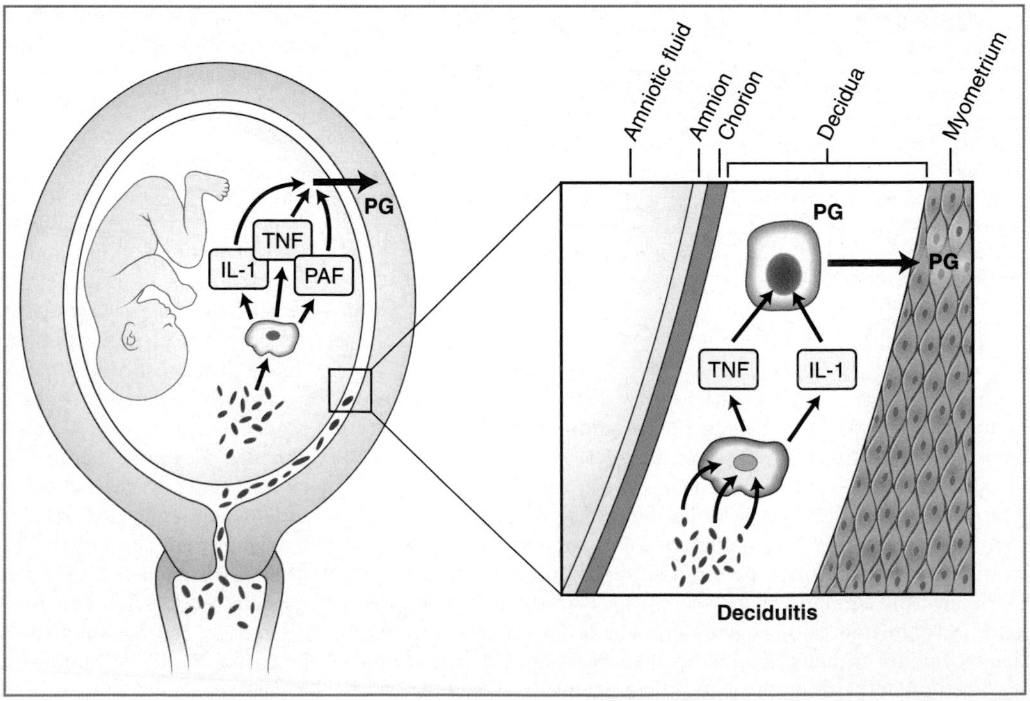

FIGURE 28-7 Cellular and biochemical mechanisms involved in initiation of preterm labor in cases of intrauterine infection. IL-1, interleukin-1; TNF, tumor necrosis factor/cachectin; PG, prostaglandins; PAF, platelet activating factor. (Reproduced with permission from Romero R, Mazor M: Infection and preterm labor. Clin Obstet Gynecol 31:553-584, 1988.)

mation.[238] However, blockade of both signaling pathways (i.e., for IL-1 and TNF-α) in a double-knockout mice model was associated with a decreased rate of preterm birth after the administration of microorganisms.[215]

Anti-inflammatory Cytokines and Preterm Labor

IL-10 is thought to be a key cytokine for the maintenance of pregnancy.[239-241] Its concentrations are increased in intra-amniotic inflammation,[242] suggesting that IL-10 may play a role in dampening the inflammatory response[243-248] and may have therapeutic value.[249-254] In a nonhuman primate model of intrauterine infection, pregnant rhesus monkeys ($n = 13$) were allocated to one of three interventional groups: (1) intra-amniotic IL-1β infusion with maternal dexamethasone intravenously ($n = 4$); (2) intra-amniotic IL-1β + IL-10 ($n = 5$); or (3) intra-amniotic IL-1β administered alone ($n = 5$). Dexamethasone and IL-10 treatment significantly reduced IL-1β–induced uterine contractility ($P < .05$). The amniotic fluid concentrations of TNF-α and leukocyte counts were also decreased by IL-10 treatment ($P < .05$).[203] Furthermore, the administration of IL-10 in animal models of infection has been associated with improved pregnancy outcome.[249,255]

Fetal Involvement in Intrauterine Infection

Carroll and Nicolaides[256] found fetal bacteremia in 33% of fetuses with positive amniotic fluid cultures and in 4% of those with negative amniotic fluid cultures in the context of preterm PROM. Therefore, subclinical fetal infection is far more common than traditionally recognized. Recently, Goldenberg and colleagues[257] reported that 23% of neonates born between 23 and 32 weeks of gestation had positive umbilical blood cultures for genital mycoplasmas.

Inflammation and Fetal Injury: The Fetal Inflammatory Response Syndrome

The fetal inflammatory response syndrome (FIRS) was initially described in pregnancies complicated by preterm labor and preterm PROM.[258,259] It was defined as a fetal plasma concentration of IL-6 greater than 11 pg/mL.[258] Fetuses with an elevated plasma IL-6 concentration had a higher rate of severe neonatal morbidity and a shorter cordocentesis-to-delivery interval than those with an IL-6 concentration lower than 11 pg/mL.[259] These original findings were subsequently confirmed.[259-262] The histopathologic landmarks of FIRS are funisitis and chorionic vasculitis.[263] The disorder can also be diagnosed by measurement of C-reactive protein concentrations in umbilical cord blood.[264] Fetuses with FIRS have more systemic involvement, including hematologic abnormalities (neutrophilia), and a higher median nucleated red blood cell count than those without elevated IL-6.[265] In addition, they have evidence of fetal stress, as determined by the fetal plasma ratio of cortisol to dehydroepiandrosterone sulfate (DHEAS),[266] congenital fetal dermatitis,[267] fetal cardiac dysfunction,[268] involution of the thymus,[269] and abnormalities of the fetal lung[230,232,262,270-274] and brain.[275-304]

Among patients with preterm PROM, elevated fetal plasma IL-6 is associated with the impending onset of preterm labor, regardless of the inflammatory state of the amniotic fluid (Fig. 28-8).[258] This suggests that the human fetus plays a role in initiating the onset of labor. However, maternal-fetal cooperation must occur for parturition to be completed. Fetal inflammation has been linked to the onset of labor in association with ascending intrauterine infection. However, systemic fetal inflammation may occur in the absence of labor if the inflammatory process does not involve the chorioamniotic membranes and decidua. Such instances may take place in the context of hematogenous viral infections or other disease processes (e.g., rhesus alloimmunization).[305]

Gene-Environment Interaction

A gene-environment interaction is said to be present when the risk of a disease (occurrence or severity) among individuals exposed to both the genotype and an environmental factor is either more severe or less severe than that which is predicted from the presence of either the genotype or the environmental exposure alone.[306,307] Evidence in support of a gene-environment interaction in infection-related premature labor was reported by Macones and coworkers[308] in a case-control study in which cases were defined as patients who had a spontaneous preterm delivery (<37 weeks) and controls as women who delivered after 37 weeks. The environmental exposure was clinically diagnosed bacterial vaginosis (symptomatic vaginal discharge, a positive whiff test, and clue cells on a wet preparation). The genotype of interest was TNF-α allele 2, given that carriage of this genotype had been demonstrated by the authors to be associated with spontaneous preterm birth in previous studies.[309] The key observation was that patients with both bacterial vaginosis and the TNF-α allele 2 had an odds ratio of 6.1 (95% confidence interval [CI], 1.9 to 21) for spontaneous preterm delivery and that this odds ratio was higher than for patients with either bacterial vaginosis or carriage of the TNF-α allele alone, suggesting that a gene-environment interaction predisposes to preterm birth.[308,310] Similar interactions may determine the susceptibility to intrauterine infection, microbial invasion of the fetus, and the likelihood of fetal injury.

Uteroplacental Vascular Disease and Decidual Hemorrhage

Vaginal bleeding in the first or second trimester is a risk factor for preterm birth. Bleeding in the first trimester alone is associated with an adjusted risk ratio of 2 (95% CI, 1.6 to 2.5) for preterm delivery.[311] If vaginal bleeding is present in more than one trimester, the odds ratio for preterm PROM is 7.4 (95% CI, 2.2 to 25.6).[312] Therefore, a disorder of uterine hemostasis that manifests clinically as bleeding places the patient at risk for preterm birth. The location of bleeding could be the decidua, specifically the interface between decidual parietalis and chorion or between the basal plate of the placenta and the decidua. The latter, when large enough, is known as abruptio placenta. The typical patient with vaginal bleeding who delivers preterm is a privately insured, white, older, parous, and college-educated patient.[313]

The evidence in support of spiral artery vasculopathy and decidual hemorrhage as a mechanism of disease in spontaneous preterm delivery is the following: (1) abruptio placenta, a lesion of uteroplacental vascular origin is more frequent in women who deliver preterm with intact membranes[314,315] or with PROM than in those who deliver at term[316-318]; (2) the frequency of SGA infants is increased in women who deliver after preterm labor with intact membranes and preterm PROM[319-324] (SGA has generally been attributed to a problem with the uterine vascular supply line, and this could account for both IUGR and abruption-associated preterm parturition); (3) vascular lesions in decidual vessels attached to the placenta have been reported in 34% of women with preterm labor and intact membranes and in 35% of those with PROM, but only in 12% of control patients (term gestations without complications) (such vascular lesions are associated with a mean odds ratio of 3.8 for preterm labor with intact membranes and 4 for PROM)[315]; (4) women with preterm labor and intact membranes and those with preterm PROM have a higher percentage of failure of physiologic transformation in the myometrial segment of the spiral

			n	Procedure-to-delivery interval (median, range, days)
I	AF IL-6 ≤7.9 ng/mL FP IL-6 ≤11 pg/mL	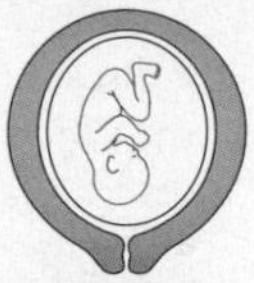	14	5 (0.2–33.6)
II	AF IL-6 >7.9 ng/mL FP IL-6 ≤11 pg/mL	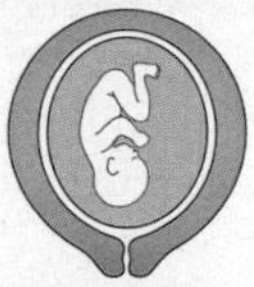	5	7 (1.5–32)
III	AF IL-6 >7.9 ng/mL FP IL-6 >11 pg/mL	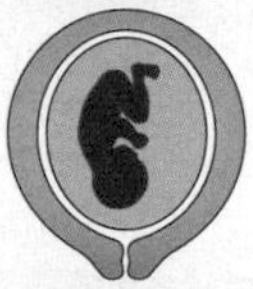	6	1.2 (0.25–2)
IV	AF IL-6 ≤7.9 ng/mL FP IL-6 >11 pg/mL	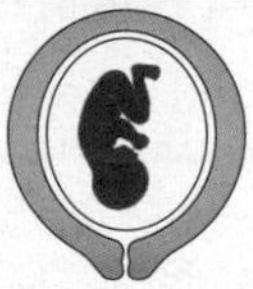	5	0.75 (0.13–1)

FIGURE 28-8 Classification and procedure-to-delivery intervals of patients according to amniotic fluid (AF) and fetal plasma (FP) concentrations of interleukin-6 (IL-6). In the FP, the white color indicates a low concentration of IL-6, and the dark red color represents a high concentration. Likewise, the white color in the AF compartment indicates a low concentration of IL-6, and the gray color indicates a high concentration. (Reproduced with permission from Romero R, Gomez R, Ghezzi F, et al: A fetal systemic inflammatory response is followed by the spontaneous onset of preterm parturition. Am J Obstet Gynecol 179:186-193, 1998.)

arteries than women who deliver at term[325,326]; (5) decidual hemosiderin deposition and retrochorionic hematoma formation is present in 37.5% of patients who deliver preterm after PROM (between 22 and 32 weeks of gestation) than in those who deliver at term (0.8%)[327] (patients with preterm deliveries with intact membranes had decidual hemosiderin in 36% of cases); and (6) patients presenting with preterm labor and intact membranes who go on to have a preterm delivery are more likely to have an abnormal uterine artery velocimetry than patients with an episode of preterm labor who deliver at term.[328-330]

The mechanisms by which uteroplacental ischemia, decidual hemorrhage, or both may activate the common pathway of parturition include the generation of thrombin. Evidence in support of this mechanism has been summarized elsewhere[331] and includes the following: (1) because decidua is a rich source of tissue factor, the primary initiator of coagulation, hemorrhage into the decidua would generate substantial quantities of thrombin, explaining the strong association between abruption and disseminated intravascular coagulation[332]; (2) intrauterine administration of whole blood to pregnant rats stimulates myometrial contractility,[333] but administration of heparinized blood does not (heparin blocks the generation of thrombin)[333]; (3) fresh whole blood stimulates myometrial contractility in vitro, and this effect is partially blunted by incubation with hirudin, a thrombin inhibitor[333]; (4) thrombin stimulates myometrial contractility in a dose-dependent manner[333]; (5) thrombin stimulates the production of MMP-1,[334] urokinase-type plasminogen activator (uPA), and tissue-type plasminogen activator (tPA) by decidualized endometrial stromal cells in culture[335] (MMP-1 can digest collagen directly, whereas uPA and tPA catalyze the transformation of plasminogen into plasmin, which in turn can degrade type III collagen and fibronectin,[336] important components of the extracellular matrix of the chorioamniotic membranes and decidua[337]); (6) thrombin/antithrombin (TAT) complexes, a marker of in vivo generation of thrombin, are increased in the plasma[338] and amniotic fluid[339] of patients with preterm labor and preterm PROM; (7) an elevation of plasma TAT complex concentration in the second trimester is associated with subsequent preterm PROM[340]; and (8) the presence of retroplacental hematoma detected by ultrasound examination in the first trimester is associated with adverse pregnancy outcomes, including preterm delivery and fetal growth restriction.[341]

Additional evidence providing biologic plausibility for a role of thrombin is that the production of MMP-3 mRNA and protein by term decidual cells is normally inhibited by progestins. However, thrombin reverses this inhibition by interacting with the protease-activated receptor type 1 (PAR-1).[342] This is important, because MMP-3 can degrade extracellular matrix located in the decidua and fetal membranes, but it can also activate MMP-1 and MMP-9, which can degrade, respectively, fibrillar collagen and gelatin. Thrombin also binds to PARs and increases expression of MMP-1 mRNA and proteins by decidual cells.[334]

Histologic examination of placentas with abruption frequently show evidence of inflammation.[343,344] Neutrophils in the decidua colocalize with areas of fibrin deposition, suggesting a link between inflam-

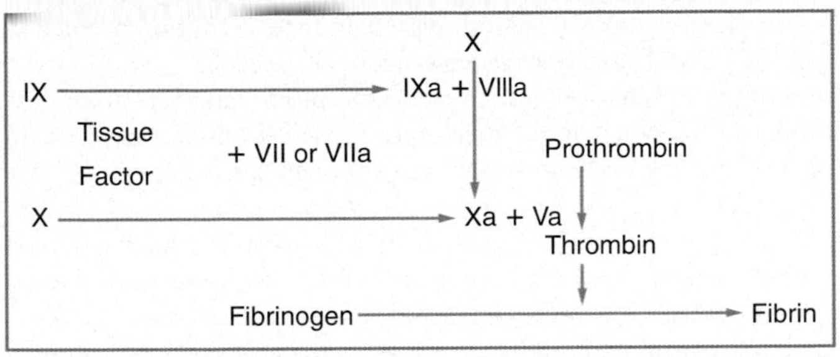

FIGURE 28-9 Tissue factor generates thrombin. The decidua is a rich source of tissue factor, the primary initiator of clotting. Disruption of spiral arteries and/or arterioles permits factor X or IX to be activated by the action of factor VII when complexed with tissue factor. Factor IXa combines with its cofactor VIIa to generate factor Xa indirectly. In either case, Xa binds to its cofactor to convert prothrombin to thrombin, which cleaves fibrinogen to fibrin.

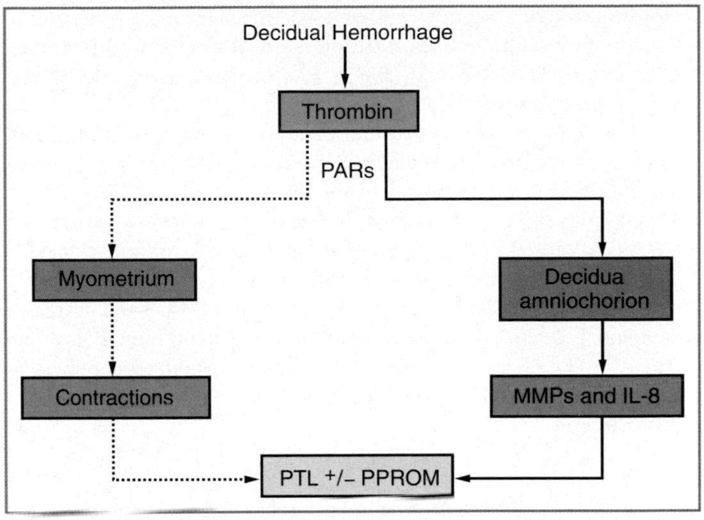

FIGURE 28-10 Mechanisms implicated in abruption-associated preterm labor and delivery. IL-8, interleukin 8; MMPs, matrix metalloproteinases; PARs, protease-activated receptors; PTL, preterm labor; PPROM, preterm premature rupture of membranes.

mation and thrombin generation. Thrombin increases IL-8 mRNA and protein expression by decidual cells. IL-8 is a potent neutrophil chemokine that is capable of attracting neutrophils to the areas of bleeding.[344] Inasmuch as neutrophils are a rich source of MMP-8, MMP-9, elastase,[345] and reactive oxygen radicals,[346-348] these products can contribute to extracellular matrix degradation in the decidual/membrane interface and to membrane rupture.

IL-11 has been demonstrated in the decidua of patients with abruption and preterm PROM. Thrombin induces IL-11 production (mRNA and protein) by decidual cells,[349] and IL-11 can induce PGE_2 production.[349] Therefore, this cytokine provides a link between thrombin generation, inflammation, activation of PARs, and the common pathway of parturition. Figures 28-9 and 28-10 describe the molecular mechanisms implicated in hemorrhage- or vascular-induced preterm labor.

Maternal and Fetal Stress

Maternal stress of exogenous or endogenous origin is modestly associated with an increased risk for preterm delivery.[350-354] The nature and timing of the stressful stimuli can range from a heavy workload to anxiety and depression.[355,356] African-American women with elevated scores for depression have an adjusted odds ratio for preterm delivery of 1.96 (95% CI, 1.04 to 3.72).[357] The absence of similar findings in Hispanic and non-Hispanic white populations suggests an ethnic disparity in the effect of stress in the United States.

The stressful insult could occur in the pre-conceptional period or during pregnancy. Starvation before pregnancy leads to spontaneous preterm delivery in sheep.[358] The precise mechanism whereby stress induces parturition is not known. However, a role for CRH has been proposed. This hormone was originally identified in the hypothalamus but is expressed by the placenta.[359] The maternal plasma CRH concentrations increase during the second half of pregnancy and peak during labor, whereas serum concentrations of the CRH binding protein decline during the third trimester.[360,361]

Smith and colleagues[360,361] demonstrated that the trajectory of CRH serum concentration changes identify women destined for preterm, term, and post-term delivery. The mechanisms regulating the serum concentration and trajectory of CRH have been described as "a placental clock." Because CRH maternal plasma concentrations are elevated in both term and preterm parturition, it would appear that CRH is part of the common pathway of labor.

The mechanisms through which CRH activates the common pathway of parturition include the following: (1) increased production of PGE_2 by amnion, chorion, and placental cells, but not by decidual cells[362-364]; (2) increased production of $PGF_{2\alpha}$ by amnion, decidua, and placental cells, but not by chorion[362-364]; (3) increased expression of MMP-9 by chorion and amnion[365]; (4) stimulation of the release of adrenocorticotropin (ACTH) from the pituitary gland to drive fetal cortisol production[366] (this establishes a feed-forward cycle, because cortisol stimulates production of CRH by the placenta and fetal membranes)[359]; (5) induction of the synthesis of fetal DHEAS by the fetal adrenal zone[367-369] (DHEAS serves as a source for estrogens,[367] which in turn enhance the expression of the oxytocin receptor, COX-2, prostaglandin receptors, and connexin-43)[370-377]; (6) cortisol produced in response to CRH can increase amnion COX-2 expression while inhibiting chorionic PGDH expression[378-381] (resulting in a net bioavailability of prostaglandins); and (7) CRH inhibits progesterone production by the placenta.[382] Figures 28-11 and 28-12 illustrate the molecular mechanisms for stress-associated preterm labor.

As noted, CRH has been implicated in the mechanisms of spontaneous parturition at term. Therefore, this specific pathway may operate in normal term labor as well as in preterm labor. In the former case, placental CRH expression reflects maturation of the fetal hypothalamic-pituitary-adrenal axis; in the latter, it reflects physiologically stressful events occurring at later gestational ages. It may be surmised that some cases of preterm labor occurring close to term resort to the physiologic mechanisms used in term labor after fetal maturation has been accelerated by stressful stimuli.

Uterine Overdistention

Patients with müllerian duct abnormalities,[383] polyhydramnios,[384,385] or multiple gestations[386] are at increased risk for spontaneous preterm labor and delivery. The frequency of preterm delivery in multifetal gestations is 17%, and the mean gestational age at delivery decreases as a function of the number of fetuses: 35.3 weeks for twins, 32.2 weeks for triplets, and 29.9 weeks for quadruplets.[4] Myometrial stretch has been implicated as a key mechanism driving these preterm deliveries.

However, the importance of stretch as a mechanism of activation of the common pathway of parturition is not restricted to the myometrium. Indeed, stretch may play a role in cervical remodeling and membrane rupture.[387]

How does stretch activate the common pathway of parturition? Intra-amniotic pressure remains relatively constant during gestation, despite the continued growth of the fetus, placenta, and uterus.[388,389] This stability of pressure has been attributed to progressive myometrial relaxation caused by the effects of progesterone[390] and nitric oxide.[391] Stretch, however, can induce increased myometrial contractility,[392] prostaglandin release,[393] expression of connexin-43,[26] and increased oxytocin receptors in pregnant and nonpregnant human myometrium.[394] The gene expression of these stretch-induced contraction-associated proteins (CAPs) during pregnancy is inhibited by progesterone.[26]

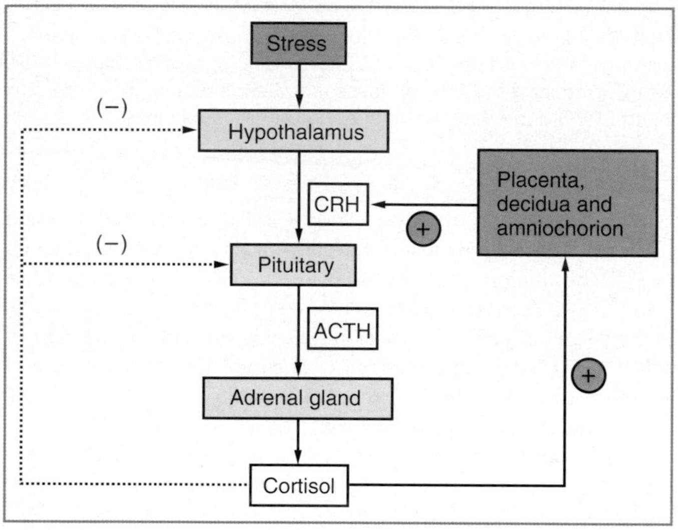

FIGURE 28-11 The fetal hypophysis-pituitary-adrenal-placental axis in pregnancy. ACTH, corticotropin; CRH, corticotropin-releasing hormone.

Mechanical stress in smooth muscle induces activation of integrin receptors[395] and stretch-activated calcium channels,[396,397] phosphorylation of platelet-derived growth factor receptor,[398] and activation of G proteins.[398,399] Mechanical force, once sensed, leads to activation of protein kinase C and mitogen activated protein kinases, increased gene expression of FOS (c-fos) and JUN (c-jun), and enhanced binding activity of transcription factor AP-1, which drives transcription of multiple parturition-associated genes.[24,400-404] Other effects of physical forces relevant to myometrium include increased expression of COX-2, superoxide dismutase, and nitric oxide synthase. The precise nature of the sensing mechanisms of pressure/tension in the myometrium is yet to be determined.

Stretch can also affect the chorioamniotic membranes, which are distended by 40% at 25 to 29 weeks, 60% at 30 to 34 weeks, and 70% at term.[405] Stretching of the membranes in vitro induces histologic changes characterized by elongation of the amnion cells and increased production of collagenase activity and IL-8,[406,407] and stretching of amnion cells in culture results in increased production of PGE_2.[408] Studies using an in vitro cell culture model for fetal membrane distention revealed upregulation of proinflammatory genes, including IL-8 and pre–B-cell colony-enhancing factor (visfatin).[409] Distention of fetal membrane in vitro results in overexpression of four genes, namely IL-8, interleukin enhancer binding factor 2 (ILF2), huntingtin-interacting protein 2, and an interferon-stimulated gene encoding a 54-kDa protein.[410] Collectively, these observations suggest that mechanical forces associated with uterine overdistention may result in activation of mechanisms leading to membrane rupture.

Premature cervical ripening is also a feature of patients with multiple gestations, as well as those with certain müllerian duct anomalies (e.g., incompetent cervix in diethylstilbestrol [DES]-exposed daughters). IL-8,[45,411,412] MMP-1,[104] prostaglandins,[137,413,414] and nitric oxide[415] have been implicated in the control of cervical ripening. Inasmuch as these mediators are produced in response to membrane stretch, they may exert part of their biologic effects in parturition by stimulating extracellular matrix degradation of the cervix.

Figure 28-13 describes the mechanisms by which stretch may activate the common pathway of parturition. It is possible, however, that patients with multiple gestations represent a heterogeneous group.

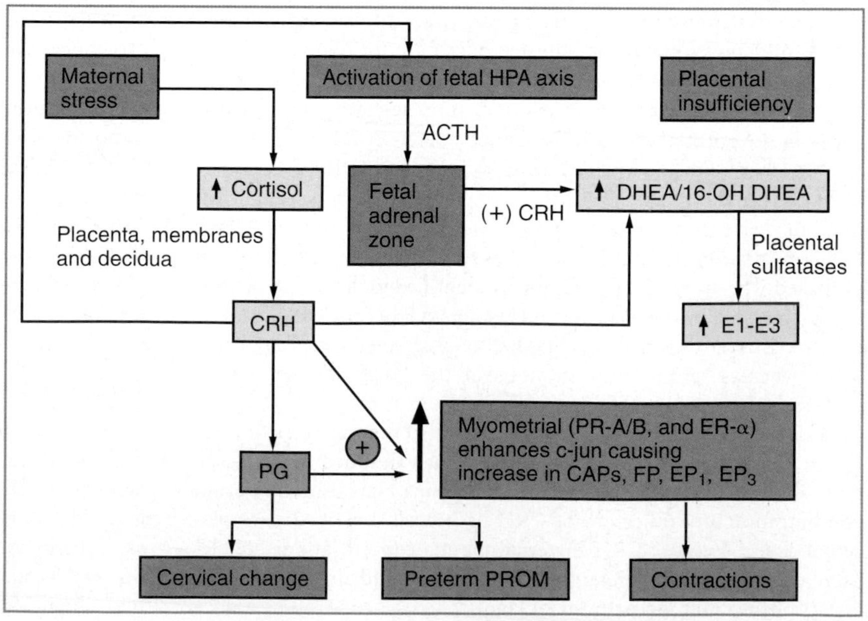

FIGURE 28-12 Proposed pathways by which stress can induce preterm labor. ACTH, corticotropin; CAPs, contraction-associated proteins; CRH, corticotropin-releasing hormone; DHEA, dehydroepiandrosterone; E1-E3, estrone, estradiol, and estriol; EP_1 and EP_3, prostaglandin E receptors types 1 and 3; ER-α, estrogen receptor-α; FP, prostaglandin F receptor; HPA, hypophysis-pituitary-adrenal; PG, prostaglandins; PR, prostaglandin receptor; PROM, premature rupture of membranes.

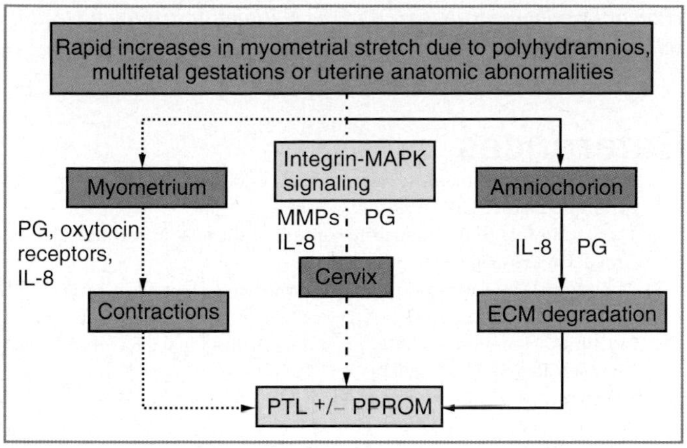

FIGURE 28-13 **Proposed mechanisms by which stretch can induce preterm labor.** ECM, extracellular matrix; IL-8, interleukin 8; MAPK, mitogen-activated protein kinase; MMPs, matrix metalloproteinases; PG, prostaglandins; PTL, preterm labor; PPROM, preterm premature rupture of membranes.

Some such patients have preterm labor associated with infection.[416-418] Others have abnormalities of trophoblast invasion leading to vascular pathology, with or without fetal growth disorders, causing stress or decidual hemorrhage–mediated preterm deliveries. These separate mechanisms of disease may operate alone or in conjunction with uterine overdistention to activate the components of the common pathway.

Allergic Phenomena

Another potential mechanism of disease in preterm labor is an immunologically mediated phenomenon induced by an allergic mechanism. We have previously proposed that an allergic-like immune response (type I hypersensitivity) may be associated with preterm labor.[419] The term "allergy" refers to disorders caused by the response of the immune system to an otherwise innocuous antigen.[420] This "allergen" cross-links immunoglobulin E (IgE) bound to high-affinity receptors on uterine mast cells, causing degranulation of these cells. The products of degranulation initiate inflammation.[421]

Evidence in support of the possibility that an allergic-like phenomenon may operate in preterm labor includes the following: (1) the human fetus is exposed to common allergens such as house-dust mite, which has been detected in amniotic fluid in the mid-trimester of pregnancy and in umbilical cord blood[422]; (2) allergen-specific reactivity has been shown in umbilical cord blood at birth and as early as 23 weeks of gestation[423]; (3) pregnancy is traditionally regarded as a T helper 2 (T_H2) state that favors the production of IgE; (4) the human uterus contains mast cells, the effector cells of allergy[424]; (5) products of mast cell degranulation (i.e., histamine and prostaglandins) may induce myometrial contractility[425,426]; (6) pharmacologic degranulation of mast cells induces myometrial and cervical contractility[427,428]; (7) incubation of myometrial strips from sensitized and nonsensitized animals with an anti-IgE antibody increases myometrial contractility[428]; (8) human myometrial strips obtained from women known to be allergic to ragweed demonstrate increased myometrial contractility when challenged in vitro by the allergen, and, moreover, the sensitivity of the myometrial strips of nonallergic women can be transferred passively by preincubation of the strips with human serum (Robert Garfield, University of Texas, Galveston, personal communication); (9) nonpregnant guinea pigs sensitized with ovalbumin and then challenged with this antigen demonstrate increased uterine tone[428]; (10) traditional descriptions of animals dying of anaphylactic shock have demonstrated enhanced uterine contractility when autopsy was performed immediately after death; (11) severe latex allergy in a pregnant woman after vaginal examination with a latex glove was followed by regular uterine contractions[429]; (12) human decidua contains immune cells capable of identifying local foreign antigens, including macrophages, B cells, T cells,[430,431] and dendritic cells[432]; and (13) we have identified a subgroup of patients with preterm labor who have eosinophils in the amniotic fluid as the predominant white blood cell[419] (under normal circumstances, white blood cells are not present in amniotic fluid; the presence of eosinophils therefore suggests an abnormal immune response, and perhaps they are the markers of an allergic-like response in preterm labor). The antigen eliciting an abnormal immunologic response remains to be identified. Recent evidence suggests that administration of ovalbumin to sensitized pregnant guinea pigs can induce preterm labor and delivery and that this phenomenon can be prevented with treatment with either cromolyn sodium or antihistaminics.[433]

Cervical Disorders

Cervical insufficiency is traditionally considered a cause of mid-trimester abortion. However, accumulating evidence suggests that it can produce a wide spectrum of disease,[434] including the well-recognized recurrent pregnancy loss in the mid-trimester, some forms of preterm labor (presenting with bulging membranes in the absence of significant uterine contractility or rupture of membrane), and probably precipitous labor at term. Cervical disease may be the result of a congenital disorder (i.e., hypoplastic cervix or DES exposure in utero), surgical trauma (i.e., conization resulting in substantial loss of connective tissue) or traumatic damage of the structural integrity of the cervix (i.e., repeated cervical dilation).[435]

Cervical insufficiency in the mid-trimester can be considered an example of asynchronous activation of the mechanisms that induce cervical remodeling. Indeed, it is likely that most cases of "cervical insufficiency" reflect not primary cervical disease leading to premature remodeling but other pathologic processes, such as infection, which has been reported in 50% of patients presenting with acute cervical insufficiency,[183] or recurrent decidual hemorrhage. The reader is referred to a detailed review of this condition and the role of cervical cerclage in the prevention of preterm birth.[436]

Hormonal Disorders: Suspension of Progesterone Action

Progesterone has been considered central to pregnancy maintenance.[437] Progesterone promotes myometrial quiescence, downregulates gap junction formation, inhibits cervical ripening, and decreases the production of chemokines (i.e., IL-8) by the chorioamniotic membranes, which is thought to impede decidual/membrane activation.[65,438-440] Progesterone is considered important for pregnancy maintenance in humans, because inhibition of progesterone action can result in parturition. Administration of progesterone receptor antagonists (i.e., mifepristone or onapristone) to pregnant women, nonhuman primates,[441] and guinea pigs[65] can induce labor or cervical change or both.[437] Therefore, a suspension of progesterone action is believed to be important for the onset of parturition in humans.

In many species, a progesterone withdrawal (a drop in serum progesterone concentration) occurs before spontaneous labor.[442]

However, in humans, nonhuman primates, and guinea pigs, a progesterone withdrawal has not been demonstrated (see Young[443] for a description of the comparative physiology of parturition in mammals).

The mechanism by which, in humans, progesterone action is suspended in the setting of sustained high circulating concentrations of progesterone has eluded discovery. Six potential mechanisms have been posited to explain this paradox: (1) reduced bioavailability of progesterone by binding to a high-affinity protein[444,445]; (2) increased cortisol concentration in late pregnancy, which may compete with progesterone for binding to the glucocorticoid receptor[446]; (3) conversion of progesterone to an inactive form within the target cell before it interacts with its receptor[447,448]; (4) quantitative and qualitative changes in progesterone receptor isoforms (PR-A, PR-B, PR-C)[449-452]; (5) changes in progesterone receptor coregulators[453]; and (6) a functional progesterone withdrawal through NF-κB.[454-456]

Progesterone's actions are mediated by multiprotein complexes, including progesterone receptors, modifying factors (co-regulators and adaptors), and effector proteins (RNA-polymerase, chromatin-remodeling proteins, and RNA-processing factors). In addition, nongenomic mechanisms have recently been proposed.[453]

There is evidence supporting the view that a "functional progesterone withdrawal" occurs locally in intrauterine tissues during human parturition in both term and preterm gestation.[453,457-463] The changes in the ratio of estrogen and progesterone activity could activate the three tissue components of the common pathway of parturition, including myometrium, cervix, and decidual-amniochorionic membranes directly or indirectly through prostaglandin or oxytocin and its receptor systems.[437,450,451,453,457-469] However, the signal eliciting the onset of these hormonal functional changes in human parturition remains to be determined.

The interest in progestins to prevent preterm delivery has been rekindled by several randomized clinical trials, suggesting that progestins may prevent preterm delivery.[470] The initial trials were conducted in women with a previous preterm delivery and used either vaginal progesterone[471] or 17α-hydroxyprogesterone caproate.[67] Subsequently, vaginal progesterone was reported to reduce the rate of preterm birth by 40% in women with a short cervix (≤15 mm).[68] A post hoc analysis of another trial was supportive of this concept.[66,472] The precise mechanisms by which exogenous progestins reduce the rate of preterm birth are unknown. It is possible that exogenous progesterone inhibits cervical remodeling in the mid-trimester of pregnancy through the mechanisms outlined earlier in this chapter.

Summary

It is becoming increasingly evident that preterm labor, preterm PROM, and cervical insufficiency are syndromes caused by multiple pathologic processes leading to increased myometrial contractility, cervical remodeling, and/or membrane activation. The clinical presentation depends on the nature and timing of the insults affecting the various components of the uterine common pathway of parturition. This view has important implications for understanding the biology of preterm parturition, as well as its diagnosis, treatment, and prevention.

Acknowledgment

This work was funded in part by the Intramural Program of the Eunice Kennedy Shriver National Institute of Child Health and Human Development (NICHD) of the National Institutes of Health (NIH).

References

1. Mazaki-Tovi S, Romero R, Kusanovic JP, et al: Recurrent preterm birth. Semin Perinatol 31:142-158, 2007.
2. Parry S, Strauss JF III: Premature rupture of the fetal membranes. N Engl J Med 338:663-670, 1998.
3. Moutquin JM: Classification and heterogeneity of preterm birth. BJOG 110(Suppl 20):30-33, 2003.
4. Martin JA, Hamilton BE, Sutton PD, et al: Births: Final data for 2002. Natl Vital Stat Rep 52:1-113, 2003.
5. Romero R, Mazor M, Munoz H, et al: The preterm labor syndrome. Ann N Y Acad Sci 734:414-429, 1994.
6. Romero R, Gomez R, Mazor M, et al: The preterm labor syndrome. In Elder MG, Romero R, Lamont RF (eds). Preterm Labor. New York: Churchill Livingstone, 1997, pp 29-49.
7. Genazzani AR, Petraglia F, Facchinetti F, et al: Lack of beta-endorphin plasma level rise in oxytocin-induced labor. Gynecol Obstet Invest 19:130-34, 1985.
8. Ohrlander S, Gennser G, Eneroth P: Plasma cortisol levels in human fetus during parturition. Obstet Gynecol 48:381-387, 1976.
9. Petraglia F, Giardino L, Coukos G, et al: Corticotropin-releasing factor and parturition: Plasma and amniotic fluid levels and placental binding sites. Obstet Gynecol 75:784-789, 1990.
10. Randall NJ, Bond K, Macaulay J, et al: Measuring fetal and maternal temperature differentials: A probe for clinical use during labour. J Biomed Eng 13:481-485, 1991.
11. Nathanielsz P, Honnebier M: Myometrial function. In Drife J, Calder A (eds): Prostaglandins and the Uterus. London: Springer-Verlag, 1992, p 161.
12. Hsu HW, Figueroa JP, Honnebier MB, et al: Power spectrum analysis of myometrial electromyogram and intrauterine pressure changes in the pregnant rhesus monkey in late gestation. Am J Obstet Gynecol 161:467-473, 1989.
13. Taylor NF, Martin MC, Nathanielsz PW, et al: The fetus determines circadian oscillation of myometrial electromyographic activity in the pregnant rhesus monkey. Am J Obstet Gynecol 146:557-567, 1983.
14. Binienda Z, Rosen ED, Kelleman A, et al: Maintaining fetal normoglycemia prevents the increase in myometrial activity and uterine 13,14-dihydro-15-keto-prostaglandin F2 alpha production during food withdrawal in late pregnancy in the ewe. Endocrinology 127:3047-3051, 1990.
15. Nathanielsz P, Poore E, Brodie A, et al: Update on molecular events of myometrial activity during pregnancy. In Nathanielsz P, Parer J (eds): Research in Perinatal Medicine. Ithaca, NY: Perinatology, 1987, p 111.
16. Romero R, Avila C, Sepulveda W, et al: The role of systemic and intrauterine infection in preterm labor. In Fuchs A, Fuchs F, Stubblefield P (eds): Preterm Birth: Causes, Prevention, and Management. New York: McGraw-Hill, 1993.
17. Cole WC, Garfield RE, Kirkaldy JS: Gap junctions and direct intercellular communication between rat uterine smooth muscle cells. Am J Physiol 249:C20-C31, 1985.
18. Garfield RE, Sims S, Daniel EE: Gap junctions: Their presence and necessity in myometrium during parturition. Science 198:958-960, 1977.
19. Garfield RE, Sims SM, Kannan MS, et al: Possible role of gap junctions in activation of myometrium during parturition. Am J Physiol 235:C168-C179, 1978.
20. Garfield RE, Hayashi RH: Appearance of gap junctions in the myometrium of women during labor. Am J Obstet Gynecol 140:254-260, 1981.
21. Garfield RE, Puri CP, Csapo AI: Endocrine, structural, and functional changes in the uterus during premature labor. Am J Obstet Gynecol 142:21-27, 1982.

22. Balducci J, Risek B, Gilula NB, et al: Gap junction formation in human myometrium: A key to preterm labor? Am J Obstet Gynecol 168:1609-1615, 1993.
23. Chow L, Lye SJ: Expression of the gap junction protein connexin-43 is increased in the human myometrium toward term and with the onset of labor. Am J Obstet Gynecol 170:788-795, 1994.
24. Lefebvre DL, Piersanti M, Bai XH, et al: Myometrial transcriptional regulation of the gap junction gene, connexin-43. Reprod Fertil Dev 7:603-611, 1995.
25. Orsino A, Taylor CV, Lye SJ: Connexin-26 and connexin-43 are differentially expressed and regulated in the rat myometrium throughout late pregnancy and with the onset of labor. Endocrinology 137:1545-1553, 1996.
26. Ou CW, Orsino A, Lye SJ: Expression of connexin-43 and connexin-26 in the rat myometrium during pregnancy and labor is differentially regulated by mechanical and hormonal signals. Endocrinology 138:5398-5407, 1997.
27. Cook JL, Zaragoza DB, Sung DH, et al: Expression of myometrial activation and stimulation genes in a mouse model of preterm labor: Myometrial activation, stimulation, and preterm labor. Endocrinology 141:1718-1728, 2000.
28. Lye SJ, Nicholson BJ, Mascarenhas M, et al: Increased expression of connexin-43 in the rat myometrium during labor is associated with an increase in the plasma estrogen:progesterone ratio. Endocrinology 132:2380-2386, 1993.
29. Petrocelli T, Lye SJ: Regulation of transcripts encoding the myometrial gap junction protein, connexin-43, by estrogen and progesterone. Endocrinology 133:284-290, 1993.
30. Lye SJ: The initiation and inhibition of labour: Towards a molecular understanding. Semin Reprod Endocrinol 12:284-294, 1994.
31. Lye SJ, Mitchell J, Nashman N, et al: Role of mechanical signals in the onset of term and preterm labor. Front Horm Res 27:165-178, 2001.
32. Lye S, Tsui P, Dorogin A, et al: Myometrial programmning: A new concept underlying the mainteinance of pregnancy and the initiation of labor. In VIIth International Conference on the Extracelullar Matrix of the Female Reproductive Tract and Simpson Symposia, Centre for Reproductive Biology, University of Edinburgh, 2004.
33. Csapo AI: The "see-saw" theory of parturition. Ciba Found Symp (47):159-210, 1977.
34. Chan EC, Fraser S, Yin S, et al: Human myometrial genes are differentially expressed in labor: A suppression subtractive hybridization study. J Clin Endocrinol Metab 87:2435-2441, 2002.
35. Word RA, Li XH, Hnat M, et al: Dynamics of cervical remodeling during pregnancy and parturition: Mechanisms and current concepts. Semin Reprod Med 25:69-79, 2007.
36. Winkler M, Rath W: Changes in the cervical extracellular matrix during pregnancy and parturition. J Perinat Med 27:45-60, 1999.
37. Ludmir J, Sehdev HM: Anatomy and physiology of the uterine cervix. Clin Obstet Gynecol 43:433-439, 2000.
38. Westergren-Thorsson G, Norman M, Bjornsson S, et al: Differential expressions of mRNA for proteoglycans, collagens and transforming growth factor-beta in the human cervix during pregnancy and involution. Biochim Biophys Acta 1406:203-213, 1998.
39. Leppert PC: Anatomy and physiology of cervical ripening. Clin Obstet Gynecol 38:267-279, 1995.
40. Straach KJ, Shelton JM, Richardson JA, et al: Regulation of hyaluronan expression during cervical ripening. Glycobiology 15:55-65, 2005.
41. Obara M, Hirano H, Ogawa M, et al: Changes in molecular weight of hyaluronan and hyaluronidase activity in uterine cervical mucus in cervical ripening. Acta Obstet Gynecol Scand 80:492-496, 2001.
42. Sakamoto Y, Moran P, Bulmer JN, et al: Macrophages and not granulocytes are involved in cervical ripening. J Reprod Immunol 66:161-173, 2005.
43. Hassan SS, Romero R, Haddad R, et al: The transcriptome of the uterine cervix before and after spontaneous term parturition. Am J Obstet Gynecol 195:778-786, 2006.
44. Liggins G: Cervical ripening as an inflammatory reaction. In Ellwood D, Anderson A (eds): The Cervix in Pregnancy and Labour: Clinical and Biochemical Investigations. Edinburgh: Churchill Livingstone, 1981.
45. Sennstrom MK, Brauner A, Lu Y, et al: Interleukin-8 is a mediator of the final cervical ripening in humans. Eur J Obstet Gynecol Reprod Biol 74:89-92, 1997.
46. Sakamoto Y, Moran P, Searle RF, et al: Interleukin-8 is involved in cervical dilatation but not in prelabour cervical ripening. Clin Exp Immunol 138:151-157, 2004.
47. Maradny EE, Kanayama N, Halim A, et al: Effects of neutrophil chemotactic factors on cervical ripening. Clin Exp Obstet Gynecol 22:76-85, 1995.
48. Osmers RG, Blaser J, Kuhn W, et al: Interleukin-8 synthesis and the onset of labor. Obstet Gynecol 86:223-229, 1995.
49. Tornblom SA, Klimaviciute A, Bystrom B, et al: Non-infected preterm parturition is related to increased concentrations of IL-6, IL-8 and MCP-1 in human cervix. Reprod Biol Endocrinol 3:39, 2005.
50. Roth J, Vogl T, Sorg C, et al: Phagocyte-specific S100 proteins: A novel group of proinflammatory molecules. Trends Immunol 24:155-158, 2003.
51. Havelock JC, Keller P, Muleba N, et al: Human myometrial gene expression before and during parturition. Biol Reprod 72:707-719, 2005.
52. Ito A, Hiro D, Ojima Y, et al: Spontaneous production of interleukin-1-like factors from pregnant rabbit uterine cervix. Am J Obstet Gynecol 159:261-265, 1988.
53. Ito A, Leppert PC, Mori Y: Human recombinant interleukin-1 alpha increases elastase-like enzyme in human uterine cervical fibroblasts. Gynecol Obstet Invest 30:239-241, 1990.
54. Kelly RW: Inflammatory mediators and cervical ripening. J Reprod Immunol 57:217-224, 2002.
55. Van der Burg B, Van der Saag PT: Nuclear factor-kappa-B/steroid hormone receptor interactions as a functional basis of anti-inflammatory action of steroids in reproductive organs. Mol Hum Reprod 2:433-438, 1996.
56. Chwalisz K, Shi Shao O, Neff G, et al: The effect of antigestagen ZK 98, 199 on the uterine cervix. Acta Endocrinol 283:113, 1987.
57. Elliott CL, Brennand JE, Calder AA: The effects of mifepristone on cervical ripening and labor induction in primigravidae. Obstet Gynecol 92:804-809, 1998.
58. Giacalone PL, Daures JP, Faure JM, et al: The effects of mifepristone on uterine sensitivity to oxytocin and on fetal heart rate patterns. Eur J Obstet Gynecol Reprod Biol 97:30-34, 2001.
59. Norman J: Antiprogesterones. Br J Hosp Med 45:372-375, 1991.
60. Stenlund PM, Ekman G, Aedo AR, et al: Induction of labor with mifepristone: A randomized, double-blind study versus placebo. Acta Obstet Gynecol Scand 78:793-798, 1999.
61. Chwalisz K, Shao-Qing S, Garfield RE, et al: Cervical ripening in guinea-pigs after a local application of nitric oxide. Hum Reprod 12:2093-2101, 1997.
62. Hegele-Hartung C, Chwalisz K, Beier HM, et al: Ripening of the uterine cervix of the guinea-pig after treatment with the progesterone antagonist onapristone (ZK 98.299): An electron microscopic study. Hum Reprod 4:369-377, 1989.
63. Wolf JP, Sinosich M, Anderson TL, et al: Progesterone antagonist (RU 486) for cervical dilation, labor induction, and delivery in monkeys: Effectiveness in combination with oxytocin. Am J Obstet Gynecol 160:45-47, 1989.
64. Stys SJ, Clewell WH, Meschia G: Changes in cervical compliance at parturition independent of uterine activity. Am J Obstet Gynecol 130:414-418, 1978.
65. Chwalisz K: The use of progesterone antagonists for cervical ripening and as an adjunct to labour and delivery. Hum Reprod (9 Suppl 1):131-161, 1994.
66. DeFranco EA, O'Brien JM, Adair CD, et al: Vaginal progesterone is associated with a decrease in risk for early preterm birth and improved neonatal outcome in women with a short cervix: A secondary analysis from a randomized, double-blind, placebo-controlled trial. Ultrasound Obstet Gynecol 30:697-705, 2007.

67. Meis PJ, Klebanoff M, Thom E, et al: Prevention of recurrent preterm delivery by 17 alpha-hydroxyprogesterone caproate. N Engl J Med 348:2379-2385, 2003.
68. Fonseca EB, Celik E, Parra M, et al: Progesterone and the risk of preterm birth among women with a short cervix. N Engl J Med 357:462-469, 2007.
69. Facchinetti F, Paganelli S, Comitini G, et al: Cervical length changes during preterm cervical ripening: Effects of 17-alpha-hydroxyprogesterone caproate. Am J Obstet Gynecol 196:453-454, 2007.
70. Lockwood CJ, Senyei AE, Dische MR, et al: Fetal fibronectin in cervical and vaginal secretions as a predictor of preterm delivery. N Engl J Med 325:669-674, 1991.
71. Iams JD, Casal D, McGregor JA, et al: Fetal fibronectin improves the accuracy of diagnosis of preterm labor. Am J Obstet Gynecol 173:141-145, 1995.
72. Nageotte MP, Casal D, Senyei AE: Fetal fibronectin in patients at increased risk for premature birth. Am J Obstet Gynecol 170:20-25, 1994.
73. Oshiro B, Edwin S, Silver R: Human fibronectin and human tenascin production in human amnion cells. J Soc Gynecol Invest 3:351A, 1996.
74. Bell SC, Meade EA: Fetal membrane rupture. In Critchley H, Bennett P, Thornton S (eds): Preterm Birth. London: RCOG Press, 2004, pp 195-212.
75. King L, MacDonald P, Casey ML: Regulation of tissue inhibitor of metalloproteinase-1 (TIMP-1) in human amnion. J Soc Gynecol Invest 3:232A, 1996.
76. Romero R, Gomez R, Helming R, et al: Amniotic fluid elastase and secretory leukocyte protease natural inhibitor during labor, rupture of membranes and intrauterine infection. 41st Annual Meeting of the Society for Gynecologic Investigation, Chicago, 1994. Abstract O183, p 183.
77. Vadillo-Ortega F, Hernandez A, Gonzalez-Avila G, et al: Increased matrix metalloproteinase activity and reduced tissue inhibitor of metalloproteinases-1 levels in amniotic fluids from pregnancies complicated by premature rupture of membranes. Am J Obstet Gynecol 174:1371-1376, 1996.
78. Skinner SJ, Liggins GC: Glycosaminoglycans and collagen in human amnion from pregnancies with and without premature rupture of the membranes. J Dev Physiol 3:111-121, 1981.
79. Malak TM, Bell SC: Structural characteristics of term human fetal membranes: A novel zone of extreme morphological alteration within the rupture site. BJOG 101:375-386, 1994.
80. McLaren J, Malak TM, Bell SC: Structural characteristics of term human fetal membranes prior to labour: Identification of an area of altered morphology overlying the cervix. Hum Reprod 14:237-241, 1999.
81. Bell SC, Pringle JH, Taylor DJ, et al: Alternatively spliced tenascin-C mRNA isoforms in human fetal membranes. Mol Hum Reprod 5:1066-1076, 1999.
82. Malak TM, Mulholland G, Bell SC: Morphometric characteristics of the decidua, cytotrophoblast, and connective tissue of the prelabor ruptured fetal membranes. Ann N Y Acad Sci 734:430-432, 1994.
83. Maymon E, Romero R, Pacora P, et al: Evidence for the participation of interstitial collagenase (matrix metalloproteinase 1) in preterm premature rupture of membranes. Am J Obstet Gynecol 183:914-920, 2000.
84. Maymon E, Romero R, Pacora P, et al: Human neutrophil collagenase (matrix metalloproteinase 8) in parturition, premature rupture of the membranes, and intrauterine infection. Am J Obstet Gynecol 183:94-99, 2000.
85. Athayde N, Edwin SS, Romero R, et al: A role for matrix metalloproteinase-9 in spontaneous rupture of the fetal membranes. Am J Obstet Gynecol 79:1248-1253, 1998.
86. Helmig BR, Romero R, Espinoza J, et al: Neutrophil elastase and secretory leukocyte protease inhibitor in prelabor rupture of membranes, parturition and intra-amniotic infection. J Matern Fetal Neonatal Med 12:237-246, 2002.
87. Everts V, van der ZE, Creemers L, Beertsen W: Phagocytosis and intracellular digestion of collagen, its role in turnover and remodelling. Histochem J 28:229-245, 1996.
88. Fortunato SJ, Menon R: Screening of novel matrix metalloproteinases (MMPs) in human fetal membranes. J Assist Reprod Genet 19:483-486, 2002.
89. Reboul P, Pelletier JP, Tardif G, et al: The new collagenase, collagenase-3, is expressed and synthesized by human chondrocytes but not by synoviocytes: A role in osteoarthritis. J Clin Invest 97:2011-2019, 1996.
90. Velasco G, Pendas AM, Fueyo A, et al: Cloning and characterization of human MMP-23, a new matrix metalloproteinase predominantly expressed in reproductive tissues and lacking conserved domains in other family members. J Biol Chem 274:4570-4576, 1999.
91. Maymon E, Romero R, Pacora P, et al: A role for the 72 kDa gelatinase (MMP-2) and its inhibitor (TIMP-2) in human parturition, premature rupture of membranes and intraamniotic infection. J Perinat Med 29:308-316, 2001.
92. Bennett PR, Elder MG, Myatt L: The effects of lipoxygenase metabolites of arachidonic acid on human myometrial contractility. Prostaglandins 33:837-844, 1987.
93. Bleasdale JE, Johnston JM: Prostaglandins and human parturition: regulation of arachidonic acid mobilization. Rev Perinat Med 5:151, 1985.
94. Calder A: Pharmacological management of the unripe cervix in the human. In Naftolin F, Stubblefield P (eds): Dilatation of the Uterine Cervix. New York: Raven Press, 1980, p 317.
95. Calder AA, Greer IA: Pharmacological modulation of cervical compliance in the first and second trimesters of pregnancy. Semin Perinatol 15:162-172, 1991.
96. Carraher R, Hahn DW, Ritchie DM, et al: Involvement of lipoxygenase products in myometrial contractions. Prostaglandins 26:23-32, 1983.
97. Challis JRG: Endocrine control of parturition. Physiol Rev 59:863, 1979.
98. Challis JR, Olson D: Parturition. In Knobil E, Neill J (eds): The Physiology of Reproduction. New York: Raven Press, 1988, p 2177.
99. Ellwood DA, Mitchell MD, Anderson AB, et al: The in vitro production of prostanoids by the human cervix during pregnancy: Preliminary observations. BJOG 87:210-214, 1980.
100. Greer I: Cervical ripening. In Drife J, Calder A (eds): Prostaglandins and the Uterus. London: Springer-Verlag, 1992, p 191.
101. MacDonald PC, Schultz FM, Duenhoelter JH, et al: Initiation of human parturition. I: Mechanism of action of arachidonic acid. Obstet Gynecol 44:629-636, 1980.
102. Mitchell MD: The mechanism(s) of human parturition. J Dev Physiol 6:107-118, 1984.
103. Novy MJ, Liggins GC: Role of prostaglandins, prostacyclin, and thromboxanes in the physiologic control of the uterus and in parturition. Semin Perinatol 4:45-66, 1980.
104. Rajabi M, Solomon S, Poole AR: Hormonal regulation of interstitial collagenase in the uterine cervix of the pregnant guinea pig. Endocrinology 128:863-871, 1991.
105. Ritchie DM, Hahn DW, McGuire JL: Smooth muscle contraction as a model to study the mediator role of endogenous lipoxygenase products of arachidonic acid. Life Sci 34:509-513, 1984.
106. Thorburn GD, Challis JR: Endocrine control of parturition. Physiol Rev 59:863-918, 1979.
107. Wiqvist N, Lindblom B, Wikland M, et al: Prostaglandins and uterine contractility. Acta Obstet Gynecol Scand Suppl 113:23-29, 1983.
108. Ekman G, Forman A, Marsal K, et al: Intravaginal versus intracervical application of prostaglandin E2 in viscous gel for cervical priming and induction of labor at term in patients with an unfavorable cervical state. Am J Obstet Gynecol 147:657-661, 1983.
109. Embrey MP: Induction of abortion by prostaglandins E1 and E2. BMJ 1:258-260, 1970.
110. Gordon-Wright AP, Elder MG: Prostaglandin E2 tablets used intravaginally for the induction of labour. BJOG 86:32-36, 1979.
111. Husslein P: Use of prostaglandins for induction of labor. Semin Perinatol 15:173-181, 1991.
112. Husslein P: Prostaglandins for induction of labour. In Drife J, Calder A (eds): Prostaglandins and the Uterus. London: Springer-Verlag, 1992.
113. Karim SM, Filshie GM: Therapeutic abortion using prostaglandin F2alpha. Lancet 1:157-159, 1970.

114. Macer J, Buchanan D, Yonekura ML: Induction of labor with prostaglandin E2 vaginal suppositories. Obstet Gynecol 63:664-668, 1984.
115. MacKenzie IZ: Prostaglandins and midtrimester abortion. In Drife J, Calder A (eds): Prostaglandins and the Uterus. London: Springer-Verlag, 1992, p 119.
116. World Health Organization Task Force: Repeated vaginal administration of 15-methyl pgf2 alpha for termination of pregnancy in the 13th to 20th week of gestation. Contraception 16:175, 1977.
117. World Health Organization Task Force: Comparison of intra-amniotic prostaglandin f2 alpha and hypertonic saline for second trimester abortion. BMJ 1:1373, 1976.
118. World Health Organization Task Force: Termination of second trimester pregnancy by intramuscular injection of 16-phenoxy-w-17, 18, 19, 20-tetranor PGE methyl sulfanilamide. Int J Gynaecol Obstet 16:175, 1982.
119. Giri SN, Stabenfeldt GH, Moseley TA, et al: Role of eicosanoids in abortion and its prevention by treatment with flunixin meglumine in cows during the first trimester of pregnancy. Zentralbl Veterinarmed A 38:445-459, 1991.
120. Harper MJ, Skarnes RC: Inhibition of abortion and fetal death produced by endotoxin or prostaglandin F2alpha. Prostaglandins 2:295-309, 1972.
121. Keirse MJ: Eicosanoids in human pregnancy and parturition. In Mitchell M (ed): Eicosanoids in Reproduction. Boca Raton, FL: CRC Press, 1990, p 199.
122. Skarnes RC, Harper MJ: Relationship between endotoxin-induced abortion and the synthesis of prostaglandin F. Prostaglandins 1:191-203, 1972.
123. Keirse MJ: Endogenous prostaglandins in human parturition. In Keirse MA, Gravenhorst J (eds): Human Parturition. The Hague, Netherlands: Nijhoff Publishers, 1979, p 101.
124. Romero R, Emamian M, Quintero R, et al: Amniotic fluid prostaglandin levels and intra-amniotic infections. Lancet 1:1380, 1986.
125. Romero R, Emamian M, Wan M, et al: Increased concentrations of arachidonic acid lipoxygenase metabolites in amniotic fluid during parturition. Obstet Gynecol 70:849-851, 1987.
126. Romero R, Emamian M, Wan M, et al: Prostaglandin concentrations in amniotic fluid of women with intra-amniotic infection and preterm labor. Am J Obstet Gynecol 157:1461-1467, 1987.
127. Romero R, Wu YK, Mazor M, et al: Amniotic fluid prostaglandin E2 in preterm labor. Prostaglandins Leukot Essent Fatty Acids 34:141-145, 1988.
128. Romero R, Wu YK, Mazor M, et al: Increased amniotic fluid leukotriene C4 concentration in term human parturition. Am J Obstet Gynecol 159:655-657, 1988.
129. Romero R, Wu YK, Sirtori M, et al: Amniotic fluid concentrations of prostaglandin F2 alpha, 13,14-dihydro-15-keto-prostaglandin F2 alpha (PGFM) and 11-deoxy-13,14-dihydro-15-keto-11, 16-cyclo-prostaglandin E2 (PGEM-LL) in preterm labor. Prostaglandins 37:149-161, 1989.
130. Sellers SM, Mitchell MD, Anderson AB, et al: The relation between the release of prostaglandins at amniotomy and the subsequent onset of labour. BJOG 88:1211-1216, 1981.
131. Romero R, Baumann P, Gonzalez R, et al: Amniotic fluid prostanoid concentrations increase early during the course of spontaneous labor at term. Am J Obstet Gynecol 171:1613-1620, 1994.
132. Brodt-Eppley J, Myatt L: Prostaglandin receptors in lower segment myometrium during gestation and labor. Obstet Gynecol 93:89-93, 1999.
133. Matsumoto T, Sagawa N, Yoshida M, et al: The prostaglandin E2 and F2 alpha receptor genes are expressed in human myometrium and are down-regulated during pregnancy. Biochem Biophys Res Commun 238:838-841, 1997.
134. Mohan AR, Loudon JA, Bennett PR: Molecular and biochemical mechanisms of preterm labour. Semin Fetal Neonatal Med 9:437-444, 2004.
135. Myatt L, Lye SJ: Expression, localization and function of prostaglandin receptors in myometrium. Prostaglandins Leukot Essent Fatty Acids 70:137-148, 2004.
136. Olson DM: The role of prostaglandins in the initiation of parturition. Best Pract Res Clin Obstet Gynaecol 17:717-730, 2003.
137. Denison FC, Calder AA, Kelly RW: The action of prostaglandin E2 on the human cervix: Stimulation of interleukin 8 and inhibition of secretory leukocyte protease inhibitor. Am J Obstet Gynecol 180:614-620, 1999.
138. Yoshida M, Sagawa N, Itoh H, et al: Prostaglandin F(2alpha), cytokines and cyclic mechanical stretch augment matrix metalloproteinase-1 secretion from cultured human uterine cervical fibroblast cells. Mol Hum Reprod 8:681-687, 2002.
139. Madsen G, Zakar T, Ku CY, et al: Prostaglandins differentially modulate progesterone receptor-A and -B expression in human myometrial cells: Evidence for prostaglandin-induced functional progesterone withdrawal. J Clin Endocrinol Metab 89:1010-1013, 2004.
140. Romero R, Espinoza J, Mazor M, et al: The preterm parturition syndrome. In Critchely H, Bennett P, Thornton S (eds): Preterm Birth. London: RCOG Press, 2004, pp 28-60.
141. Elovitz MA, Mrinalini C: Animal models of preterm birth. Trends Endocrinol.Metab 15:479-487, 2004.
142. Fidel PL Jr, Romero R, Wolf N, et al: Systemic and local cytokine profiles in endotoxin-induced preterm parturition in mice. Am J Obstet Gynecol 170:1467-1475, 1994.
143. Gravett MG, Witkin SS, Haluska GJ, et al: An experimental model for intraamniotic infection and preterm labor in rhesus monkeys. Am J Obstet Gynecol 171:1660-1667, 1994.
144. Hirsch E, Saotome I, Hirsh D: A model of intrauterine infection and preterm delivery in mice. Am J Obstet Gynecol 172:1598-1603, 1995.
145. Kullander S: Fever and parturition: An experimental study in rabbits. Acta Obstet Gynecol Scand Suppl 66:77-85, 1977.
146. McDuffie RS Jr, Sherman MP, Gibbs RS: Amniotic fluid tumor necrosis factor-alpha and interleukin 1 in a rabbit model of bacterially induced preterm pregnancy loss. Am J Obstet Gynecol 167:1583-1588, 1992.
147. McKay DG, Wong TC: The effect of bacterial endotoxin on the placenta of the rat. Am J Pathol 42:357-377, 1963.
148. Romero R, Mazor M, Wu YK, et al: Infection in the pathogenesis of preterm labor. Semin Perinatol 12:262-279, 1988.
149. Romero R, Munoz H, Gomez R, et al: Antibiotic therapy reduces the rate of infection-induced preterm delivery and perinatal mortality. Am J Obstet Gynecol 170:390, 1994.
150. Takeda Y, Tsuchiya I: Studies on the pathological changes caused by the injection of the Shwartzman filtrate and the endotoxin into pregnant rabbits. Jap J Exp Med 21:9-16, 1953.
151. Wang H, Hirsch E: Bacterially-induced preterm labor and regulation of prostaglandin-metabolizing enzyme expression in mice: The role of toll-like receptor 4. Biol Reprod 69:1957-1963, 2003.
152. Zahl PA, Bjerknes C: Induction of decidua-placental hemorrhage in mice by the endotoxins of certain gram-negative bacteria. Proc Soc Exp Biol Med 54:329-332, 1943.
153. Gibbs RS, McDuffie RS Jr, Kunze M, et al: Experimental intrauterine infection with *Prevotella bivia* in New Zealand White rabbits. Am J Obstet Gynecol 190:1082-1086, 2004.
154. Gilles HM, Lawson JB, Sibelas M, et al: Malaria, anaemia and pregnancy. Ann Trop Med Parasitol 63:245-263, 1969.
155. Herd N, Jordan T: An investigtion of malaria during pregnancy in Zimbabwe. Afr J Med 27:62, 1981.
156. Hibbard L, Thrupp L, Summeril S, et al: Treatment of pyelonephritis in pregnancy. Am J Obstet Gynecol 98:609-615, 1967.
157. Patrick MJ: Influence of maternal renal infection on the foetus and infant. Arch Dis Child 42:208-213, 1967.
158. Wren BG: Subclinical renal infection and prematurity. Med J Aust 2:596-600, 1969.
159. Cunningham FG, Morris GB, Mickal A: Acute pyelonephritis of pregnancy: A clinical review. Obstet Gynecol 42:112-117, 1973.
160. Kaul AK, Khan S, Martens MG, et al: Experimental gestational pyelonephritis induces preterm births and low birth weights in C3H/HeJ mice. Infect Immun 67:5958-5966, 1999.
161. Benedetti TJ, Valle R, Ledger WJ: Antepartum pneumonia in pregnancy. Am J Obstet Gynecol 144:413-417, 1982.

162. Madinger NE, Greenspoon JS, Ellrodt AG: Pneumonia during pregnancy: Has modern technology improved maternal and fetal outcome? Am J Obstet Gynecol 161:657-662, 1989.
163. Munn MB, Groome LJ, Atterbury JL, et al: Pneumonia as a complication of pregnancy. J Matern Fetal Med 8:151-154, 1999.
164. Goepfert AR, Jeffcoat MK, Andrews WW, et al: Periodontal disease and upper genital tract inflammation in early spontaneous preterm birth. Obstet Gynecol 104:777-783, 2004.
165. Jarjoura K, Devine PC, Perez-Delboy A, et al: Markers of periodontal infection and preterm birth. Am J Obstet Gynecol 192:513-519, 2005.
166. Jeffcoat MK, Geurs NC, Reddy MS, et al: Current evidence regarding periodontal disease as a risk factor in preterm birth. Ann Periodontol 6:183-188, 2001.
167. Offenbacher S, Boggess KA, Murtha AP, et al: Progressive periodontal disease and risk of very preterm delivery. Obstet Gynecol 107:29-36, 2006.
168. Xiong X, Buekens P, Fraser WD, et al: Periodontal disease and adverse pregnancy outcomes: A systematic review. BJOG 113:135-143, 2006.
169. Offenbacher S: Maternal periodontal infections, prematurity, and growth restriction. Clin Obstet Gynecol 47:808-821, 2004.
170. Gomez R, Ghezzi F, Romero R, et al: Premature labor and intra-amniotic infection: Clinical aspects and role of the cytokines in diagnosis and pathophysiology. Clin Perinatol 22:281-342, 1995.
171. Cassell GH, Davis RO, Waites KB, et al: Isolation of *Mycoplasma hominis* and *Ureaplasma urealyticum* from amniotic fluid at 16-20 weeks of gestation: Potential effect on outcome of pregnancy. Sex Transm Dis 10:294-302, 1983.
172. Gray DJ, Robinson HB, Malone J, et al: Adverse outcome in pregnancy following amniotic fluid isolation of *Ureaplasma urealyticum*. Prenat Diagn 12:111-117, 1992.
173. Horowitz S, Mazor M, Romero R, et al: Infection of the amniotic cavity with *Ureaplasma urealyticum* in the midtrimester of pregnancy. J Reprod Med 40:375-379, 1995.
174. Romero R, Munoz H, Gomez R, et al: Two thirds of spontaneous abortion/fetal deaths after genetic amniocentesis are the result of a pre-existing sub-clinical inflammatory process of the amniotic cavity. Am J Obstet Gynecol 172:S261, 1995.
175. Wenstrom KD, Andrews WW, Hauth JC, et al: Elevated second-trimester amniotic fluid interleukin-6 levels predict preterm delivery. Am J Obstet Gynecol 178:546-550, 1998.
176. Yoon BH, Oh SY, Romero R, et al: An elevated amniotic fluid matrix metalloproteinase-8 level at the time of mid-trimester genetic amniocentesis is a risk factor for spontaneous preterm delivery. Am J Obstet Gynecol 185:1162-1167, 2001.
177. Fidel P, Ghezzi F, Romero R, et al: The effect of antibiotic therapy on intrauterine infection-induced preterm parturition in rabbits. J Matern Fetal Neonatal Med 14:57-64, 2003.
178. Romero R, Oyarzun E, Mazor M, et al: Meta-analysis of the relationship between asymptomatic bacteriuria and preterm delivery/low birth weight. Obstet Gynecol 73:576-582, 1989.
179. Smaill F: Antibiotics for asymptomatic bacteriuria in pregnancy. Cochrane Database Syst Rev (2);CD000490, 2001.
180. Goncalves LF, Chaiworapongsa T, Romero R: Intrauterine infection and prematurity. Ment Retard Dev Disabil Res Rev 8:3-13, 2002.
181. Romero R, Salafia CM, Athanassiadis AP, et al: The relationship between acute inflammatory lesions of the preterm placenta and amniotic fluid microbiology. Am J Obstet Gynecol 166:1382-1388, 1992.
182. Mays JK, Figueroa R, Shah J, et al: Amniocentesis for selection before rescue cerclage. Obstet Gynecol 95:652-655, 2000.
183. Romero R, Gonzalez R, Sepulveda W, et al: Infection and labor: VIII. Microbial invasion of the amniotic cavity in patients with suspected cervical incompetence: Prevalence and clinical significance. Am J Obstet Gynecol 167:1086-1091, 1992.
184. Romero R, Espinoza J, Chaiworapongsa T, et al: Infection and prematurity and the role of preventive strategies. Semin Neonatol 7:259-274, 2002.
185. Romero R, Sirtori M, Oyarzun E, et al: Infection and labor: V. Prevalence, microbiology, and clinical significance of intraamniotic infection in women with preterm labor and intact membranes. Am J Obstet Gynecol 161:817-824, 1989.
186. Romero R, Mazor M, Morrotti R, et al: Infection and labor: VII. Microbial invasion of the amniotic cavity in spontaneous rupture of membranes at term. Am J Obstet Gynecol 166:129-133, 1992.
187. Andrews WW, Hauth JC, Goldenberg RL, et al: Amniotic fluid interleukin-6: Correlation with upper genital tract microbial colonization and gestational age in women delivered after spontaneous labor versus indicated delivery. Am J Obstet Gynecol 173:606-612, 1995.
188. Watts DH, Krohn MA, Hillier SL, Eschenbach DA: The association of occult amniotic fluid infection with gestational age and neonatal outcome among women in preterm labor. Obstet Gynecol 79:351-357, 1992.
189. Romero R, Kadar N, Hobbins JC, et al: Infection and labor: The detection of endotoxin in amniotic fluid. Am J Obstet Gynecol 157:815-819, 1987.
190. Romero R, Roslansky P, Oyarzun E, et al: Labor and infection: II. Bacterial endotoxin in amniotic fluid and its relationship to the onset of preterm labor. Am J Obstet Gynecol 158:1044-1049, 1988.
191. Grigsby PL, Hirst JJ, Scheerlinck JP, et al: Fetal responses to maternal and intra-amniotic lipopolysaccharide administration in sheep. Biol Reprod 68:1695-1702, 2003.
192. Jobe AH, Newnham JP, Willet KE, et al: Effects of antenatal endotoxin and glucocorticoids on the lungs of preterm lambs. Am J Obstet Gynecol 182:401-408, 2000.
193. Jobe AH, Newnham JP, Willet KE, et al: Endotoxin-induced lung maturation in preterm lambs is not mediated by cortisol. Am J Respir Crit Care Med 162:1656-1661, 2000.
194. Janeway C, Travers P, Walport M, et al: Innate immunity. In Janeway C, Travers P, Walport M, Schlomchik M (eds): Immunobiology. New York: Garland Science Publishing, 2005, pp 37-102.
195. Hargreaves DC, Medzhitov R: Innate sensors of microbial infection. J Clin Immunol 25:503-510, 2005.
196. Elovitz MA, Wang Z, Chien EK, et al: A new model for inflammation-induced preterm birth: The role of platelet-activating factor and toll-like receptor-4. Am J Pathol 163:2103-2111, 2003.
197. Kim YM, Romero R, Chaiworapongsa T, et al: Toll-like receptor-2 and -4 in the chorioamniotic membranes in spontaneous labor at term and in preterm parturition that are associated with chorioamnionitis. Am J Obstet Gynecol 191:1346-1355, 2004.
198. Krikun G, Lockwood CJ, Abrahams VM, et al: Expression of toll-like receptors in the human decidua. Histol Histopathol 22:847-854, 2007.
199. Romero R, Durum SK, Dinarello CA, et al: Interleukin-1: A signal for the initiation of labor in chorioamnionitis. 33rd Annual Meeting for the Society for Gynecologic Investigation, Toronto, Ontario, 1986.
200. Romero R, Wu YK, Brody DT, et al: Human decidua: A source of interleukin-1. Obstet Gynecol 73:31-34, 1989.
201. Romero R, Durum S, Dinarello CA, et al: Interleukin-1 stimulates prostaglandin biosynthesis by human amnion. Prostaglandins 37:13-22, 1989.
202. Romero R, Brody DT, Oyarzun E, et al: Infection and labor: III. Interleukin-1: A signal for the onset of parturition. Am J Obstet Gynecol 1989;160:1117-1123.
203. Sadowsky DW, Novy MJ, Witkin SS, et al: Dexamethasone or interleukin-10 blocks interleukin-1beta-induced uterine contractions in pregnant rhesus monkeys. Am J Obstet Gynecol 188:252-263, 2003.
204. Romero R, Mazor M, Tartakovsky B: Systemic administration of interleukin-1 induces preterm parturition in mice. Am J Obstet Gynecol 165:969-971, 1991.
205. Romero R, Tartakovsky B: The natural interleukin-1 receptor antagonist prevents interleukin-1-induced preterm delivery in mice. Am J Obstet Gynecol 167:1041-1045, 1992.
206. Casey ML, Cox SM, Beutler B, et al: Cachectin/tumor necrosis factor-alpha formation in human decidua: Potential role of cytokines in infection-induced preterm labor. J Clin Invest 83:430-436, 1989.
207. Romero R, Mazor M, Manogue K, et al: Human decidua: A source of cachectin-tumor necrosis factor. Eur J Obstet Gynecol Reprod Biol 41:123-127, 1991.

208. Romero R, Manogue KR, Mitchell MD, et al: Infection and labor: IV. Cachectin-tumor necrosis factor in the amniotic fluid of women with intraamniotic infection and preterm labor. Am J Obstet Gynecol 161:336-341, 1989.
209. Fortunato SJ, Menon R, Lombardi SJ: Role of tumor necrosis factor-[alpha] in the premature rupture of membranes and preterm labor pathways. Am J Obstet Gynecol 187:1159-1162, 2002.
210. Watari M, Watari H, DiSanto ME, et al: Pro-inflammatory cytokines induce expression of matrix-metabolizing enzymes in human cervical smooth muscle cells. Am J Pathol ;54:1755-1762, 1999.
211. Maymon E, Romero R, Pacora P, et al: Evidence of in vivo differential bioavailability of the active forms of matrix metalloproteinases 9 and 2 in parturition, spontaneous rupture of membranes, and intra-amniotic infection. Am J Obstet Gynecol 183:887-894, 2000.
212. Romero R, Chaiworapongsa T, Espinoza J, et al: Fetal plasma MMP-9 concentrations are elevated in preterm premature rupture of the membranes. Am J Obstet Gynecol 187:1125-1130, 2002.
213. Chwalisz K, Benson M, Scholz P, et al: Cervical ripening with the cytokines interleukin 8, interleukin 1 beta and tumour necrosis factor alpha in guinea-pigs. Hum Reprod 9:2173-2181, 1994.
214. Kajikawa S, Kaga N, Futamura Y, et al: Lipoteichoic acid induces preterm delivery in mice. J Pharmacol Toxicol.Methods 39:147-154, 1998.
215. Hirsch E, Filipovich Y, Mahendroo M: Signaling via the type I IL-1 and TNF receptors is necessary for bacterially induced preterm labor in a murine model. Am J Obstet Gynecol 194:1334-1340, 2006.
216. Lockwood CJ, Arcuri F, Toti P, et al: Tumor necrosis factor-alpha and interleukin-1beta regulate interleukin-8 expression in third trimester decidual cells: Implications for the genesis of chorioamnionitis. Am J Pathol 169:1294-1302, 2006.
217. Cox SM, King MR, Casey ML, et al: Interleukin-1 beta, -1 alpha, and -6 and prostaglandins in vaginal/cervical fluids of pregnant women before and during labor. J Clin Endocrinol Metab 77:805-815, 1993.
218. Gomez R, Romero R, Galasso M, et al: The value of amniotic fluid interleukin-6, white blood cell count, and gram stain in the diagnosis of microbial invasion of the amniotic cavity in patients at term. Am J Reprod Immunol 32:200-210, 1994.
219. Hillier SL, Witkin SS, Krohn MA, et al: NB, Eschenbach DA. The relationship of amniotic fluid cytokines and preterm delivery, amniotic fluid infection, histologic chorioamnionitis, and chorioamnion infection. Obstet Gynecol 81:941-948, 1993.
220. Messer J, Eyer D, Donato L, et al: Evaluation of interleukin-6 and soluble receptors of tumor necrosis factor for early diagnosis of neonatal infection. J Pediatr 129:574-580, 1996.
221. Romero R, Avila C, Santhanam U, et al: Amniotic fluid interleukin 6 in preterm labor: Association with infection. J Clin Invest 85:1392-1400, 1990.
222. Hanna N, Hanna I, Hleb M, et al: Gestational age-dependent expression of IL-10 and its receptor in human placental tissues and isolated cytotrophoblasts. J Immunol 164:5721-5728, 2000.
223. Hanna N, Bonifacio L, Weinberger B, et al: Evidence for interleukin-10-mediated inhibition of cyclo- oxygenase-2 expression and prostaglandin production in preterm human placenta. Am J Reprod Immunol 55:19-27, 2006.
224. Athayde N, Romero R, Maymon E, et al: Interleukin 16 in pregnancy, parturition, rupture of fetal membranes, and microbial invasion of the amniotic cavity. Am J Obstet Gynecol 182:135-141, 2000.
225. Pacora P, Romero R, Maymon E, et al: Participation of the novel cytokine interleukin 18 in the host response to intra-amniotic infection. Am J Obstet Gynecol 183:1138-1143, 2000.
226. Goldenberg RL, Andrews WW, Mercer BM, et al: The preterm prediction study: Granulocyte colony-stimulating factor and spontaneous preterm birth. National Institute of Child Health and Human Development Maternal-Fetal Medicine Units Network. Am J Obstet Gynecol 182:625-630, 2000.
227. Saito S, Kato Y, Ishihara Y, et al: Amniotic fluid granulocyte colony-stimulating factor in preterm and term labor. Clin Chim Acta 208:105-109, 1992.
228. Saito S, Kasahara T, Kato Y, et al: Elevation of amniotic fluid interleukin 6 (IL-6), IL-8 and granulocyte colony stimulating factor (G-CSF) in term and preterm parturition. Cytokine 5:81-88, 1993.
229. Chaiworapongsa T, Romero R, Espinoza J, et al: Macrophage migration inhibitory factor in patients with preterm parturition and microbial invasion of the amniotic cavity. J Matern Fetal Neonatal Med 18:405-416, 2005.
230. Ghezzi F, Gomez R, Romero R, et al: Elevated interleukin-8 concentrations in amniotic fluid of mothers whose neonates subsequently develop bronchopulmonary dysplasia. Eur J Obstet Gynecol Reprod Biol 78:5-10, 1998.
231. Romero R, Ceska M, Avila C, et al: Neutrophil attractant/activating peptide-1/interleukin-8 in term and preterm parturition. Am J Obstet Gynecol 165:813-820, 1991.
232. Yoon BH, Romero R, Jun JK, et al: Amniotic fluid cytokines (interleukin-6, tumor necrosis factor-alpha, interleukin-1 beta, and interleukin-8) and the risk for the development of bronchopulmonary dysplasia. Am J Obstet Gynecol 177:825-830, 1997.
233. Cherouny PH, Pankuch GA, Romero R, et al: Neutrophil attractant/activating peptide-1/interleukin-8: Association with histologic chorioamnionitis, preterm delivery, and bioactive amniotic fluid leukoattractants. Am J Obstet Gynecol 169:1299-1303, 1993.
234. Gonzalez BE, Ferrer I, Valls C, et al: The value of interleukin-8, interleukin 6 and interleukin-1beta in vaginal wash as predictors of preterm delivery. Gynecol Obstet Invest 59:175-178, 2005.
235. Esplin MS, Romero R, Chaiworapongsa T, et al: Monocyte chemotactic protein-1 is increased in the amniotic fluid of women who deliver preterm in the presence or absence of intra-amniotic infection. J Matern Fetal Neonatal Med 17:365-373, 2005.
236. Keelan JA, Yang J, Romero RJ, et al: Epithelial cell-derived neutrophil-activating peptide-78 is present in fetal membranes and amniotic fluid at increased concentrations with intra-amniotic infection and preterm delivery. Biol Reprod 70:253-259, 2004.
237. Athayde N, Romero R, Maymon E, et al: A role for the novel cytokine RANTES in pregnancy and parturition. Am J Obstet Gynecol 181:989-994, 1999.
238. Hirsch E, Muhle RA, Mussalli GM, et al: Bacterially induced preterm labor in the mouse does not require maternal interleukin-1 signaling. Am J Obstet Gynecol 186:523-530, 2002.
239. Krasnow JS, Tollerud DJ, Naus G, et al: Endometrial Th2 cytokine expression throughout the menstrual cycle and early pregnancy. Hum Reprod 11:1747-1754, 1996.
240. Lidstrom C, Matthiesen L, Berg G, et al: Cytokine secretion patterns of NK cells and macrophages in early human pregnancy decidua and blood: Implications for suppressor macrophages in decidua. Am J Reprod Immunol 50:444-452, 2003.
241. Ekerfelt C, Lidstrom C, Matthiesen L, et al: Spontaneous secretion of interleukin-4, interleukin-10 and interferon-gamma by first trimester decidual mononuclear cells. Am J Reprod Immunol 47:159-166, 2002.
242. Greig PC, Herbert WN, Robinette BL, et al: Amniotic fluid interleukin-10 concentrations increase through pregnancy and are elevated in patients with preterm labor associated with intrauterine infection. Am J Obstet Gynecol 173:1223-1227, 1995.
243. Moore KW, de Waal MR, Coffman RL, et al: Interleukin-10 and the interleukin-10 receptor. Annu Rev Immunol 19:683-765, 2001.
244. Murray PJ: Understanding and exploiting the endogenous interleukin-10/STAT3-mediated anti-inflammatory response. Curr Opin Pharmacol 6:379-386, 2006.
245. Trinchieri G: Interleukin-10 production by effector T cells: Th1 cells show self control. J Exp Med 204:239-243, 2007.
246. Berg DJ, Kuhn R, Rajewsky K, et al: Interleukin-10 is a central regulator of the response to LPS in murine models of endotoxic shock and the Shwartzman reaction but not endotoxin tolerance. J Clin Invest 96:2339-2347, 1995.
247. Howard M, Muchamuel T, Andrade S, et al: Interleukin 10 protects mice from lethal endotoxemia. J Exp Med 177:1205-1208, 1993.

248. Lang R, Rutschman RL, Greaves DR, et al: Autocrine deactivation of macrophages in transgenic mice constitutively overexpressing IL-10 under control of the human CD68 promoter. J Immunol 168:3402-3411, 2002.
249. Rodts-Palenik S, Wyatt-Ashmead J, Pang Y, et al: Maternal infection-induced white matter injury is reduced by treatment with interleukin-10. Am J Obstet Gynecol 191:1387-1392, 2004.
250. Chernoff AE, Granowitz EV, Shapiro L, et al: A randomized, controlled trial of IL-10 in humans: Inhibition of inflammatory cytokine production and immune responses. J Immunol 154:5492-5499, 1995.
251. Huhn RD, Radwanski E, Gallo J, et al: Pharmacodynamics of subcutaneous recombinant human interleukin-10 in healthy volunteers. Clin Pharmacol Ther 62:171-180, 1997.
252. Pajkrt D, Camoglio L, Tiel-van Buul MC, et al: Attenuation of proinflammatory response by recombinant human IL-10 in human endotoxemia: Effect of timing of recombinant human IL-10 administration. J Immunol 158:3971-3977, 1997.
253. Chakraborty A, Blum RA, Mis SM, et al: Pharmacokinetic and adrenal interactions of IL-10 and prednisone in healthy volunteers. J Clin Pharmacol 39:624-635, 1999.
254. Wolfberg AJ, Dammann O, Gressens P: Anti-inflammatory and immunomodulatory strategies to protect the perinatal brain. Semin Fetal Neonatal Med 12:296-302, 2007.
255. Terrone DA, Rinehart BK, Granger JP, et al: Interleukin-10 administration and bacterial endotoxin-induced preterm birth in a rat model. Obstet Gynecol 98:476-480, 2001.
256. Carroll SG, Nicolaides KH: Fetal haematological response to intra-uterine infection in preterm prelabour amniorrhexis. Fetal Diagn Ther 10:279-285, 1995.
257. Goldenberg RL, Andrews WW, Goepfert AR, et al: The Alabama Preterm Birth Study: Umbilical cord blood *Ureaplasma urealyticum* and *Mycoplasma hominis* cultures in very preterm newborn infants. Am J Obstet Gynecol 198:43-45, 2008.
258. Gomez R, Romero R, Ghezzi F, et al: The fetal inflammatory response syndrome. Am J Obstet Gynecol 179:194-202, 1998.
259. Romero R, Gomez R, Ghezzi F, et al: A fetal systemic inflammatory response is followed by the spontaneous onset of preterm parturition. Am J Obstet Gynecol 179:186-193, 1998.
260. Chaiworapongsa T, Romero R, Kim JC, et al: Evidence for fetal involvement in the pathologic process of clinical chorioamnionitis. Am J Obstet Gynecol 186:1178-1182, 2002.
261. Witt A, Berger A, Gruber CJ, et al: IL-8 concentrations in maternal serum, amniotic fluid and cord blood in relation to different pathogens within the amniotic cavity. J Perinat Med 33:22-26, 2005.
262. Yoon BH, Romero R, Kim KS, et al: A systemic fetal inflammatory response and the development of bronchopulmonary dysplasia. Am J Obstet Gynecol 181:773-779, 1999.
263. Pacora P, Chaiworapongsa T, Maymon E, et al: Funisitis and chorionic vasculitis: The histological counterpart of the fetal inflammatory response syndrome. J Matern Fetal Med 11:18-25, 2002.
264. Yoon BH, Romero R, Shim JY, et al: C-reactive protein in umbilical cord blood: A simple and widely available clinical method to assess the risk of amniotic fluid infection and funisitis. J Matern Fetal Neonatal Med 14:85-90, 2003.
265. Gomez R, Berry S, Yoon BH, et al: The hematologic profile of the fetus with systemic inflammatory response syndrome. Am J Obstet Gynecol 178:S202, 1998.
266. Yoon BH, Romero R, Jun JK, et al: An increase in fetal plasma cortisol but not dehydroepiandrosterone sulfate is followed by the onset of preterm labor in patients with preterm premature rupture of the membranes. Am J Obstet Gynecol 179:1107-1114, 1998.
267. Kim YM, Romero R, Chaiworapongsa T, et al: Dermatitis as a component of the fetal inflammatory response syndrome is associated with activation of toll-like receptors in epidermal keratinocytes. Histopathology 49:506-514, 2006.
268. Romero R, Espinoza J, Goncalves LF, et al: Fetal cardiac dysfunction in preterm premature rupture of membranes. J Matern Fetal Neonatal Med 16:146-157, 2004.
269. Di Naro E, Cromi A, Ghezzi F, et al: Fetal thymic involution: A sonographic marker of the fetal inflammatory response syndrome. Am J Obstet Gynecol 194:153-159, 2006.
270. Jobe AH: Antenatal associations with lung maturation and infection. J Perinatol 25(Suppl 2):S31-S35, 2005.
271. Speer CP: New insights into the pathogenesis of pulmonary inflammation in preterm infants. Biol Neonate 79:205-209, 2001.
272. Speer CP: Inflammation and bronchopulmonary dysplasia. Semin Neonatol 8:29-38, 2003.
273. Watterberg KL, Demers LM, Scott SM, et al: Chorioamnionitis and early lung inflammation in infants in whom bronchopulmonary dysplasia develops. Pediatrics 97:210-215, 1996.
274. Yoon BH, Romero R, Shim JY, et al: "Atypical" chronic lung disease of the newborn is linked to fetal systemic inflammation. Am J Obstet Gynecol 187:S129, 2002.
275. Alexander JM, Gilstrap LC, Cox SM, et al: Clinical chorioamnionitis and the prognosis for very low birth weight infants. Obstet Gynecol 91:725-729, 1998.
276. Bejar R, Wozniak P, Allard M, et al: Antenatal origin of neurologic damage in newborn infants: I. Preterm infants. Am J Obstet Gynecol 159:357-363, 1988.
277. Dammann O, Leviton A: Infection remote from the brain, neonatal white matter damage, and cerebral palsy in the preterm infant. Semin Pediatr Neurol 5:190-201, 1998.
278. Dammann O, Leviton A: Role of the fetus in perinatal infection and neonatal brain damage. Curr Opin Pediatr 12:99-104, 2000.
279. Dammann O, Kuban KC, Leviton A: Perinatal infection, fetal inflammatory response, white matter damage, and cognitive limitations in children born preterm. Ment Retard Dev Disabil Res Rev 8:46-50, 2002.
280. Dammann O, Leviton A, Gappa M, et al: Lung and brain damage in preterm newborns, and their association with gestational age, prematurity subgroup, infection/inflammation and long term outcome. BJOG 112(Suppl 1):4-9, 2005.
281. Grether JK, Nelson KB: Maternal infection and cerebral palsy in infants of normal birth weight. JAMA 278:207-211, 1997.
282. Nelson KB, Dambrosia JM, Grether JK, et al: Neonatal cytokines and coagulation factors in children with cerebral palsy. Ann Neurol 44:665-675, 1998.
283. Eastman NJ, DeLeon M: The etiology of cerebral palsy. Am J Obstet Gynecol 69:950-961, 1955.
284. Grether JK, Nelson KB, Dambrosia JM, et al: Interferons and cerebral palsy. J Pediatr 134:324-332, 1999.
285. Hagberg B, Hagberg G, Olow I, et al: The changing panorama of cerebral palsy in Sweden: V. The birth year period 1979-82. Acta Paediatr Scand 78:283-290, 1989.
286. Leviton A: Preterm birth and cerebral palsy: Is tumor necrosis factor the missing link? Dev Med Child Neurol 35:553-558, 1993.
287. Leviton A, Paneth N, Reuss ML, et al: Maternal infection, fetal inflammatory response, and brain damage in very low birth weight infants. Developmental Epidemiology Network Investigators. Pediatr Res 46:566-575, 1999.
288. Murphy DJ, Sellers S, MacKenzie IZ, et al: Case-control study of antenatal and intrapartum risk factors for cerebral palsy in very preterm singleton babies. Lancet 346:1449-1454, 1995.
289. Nelson KB, Ellenberg JH: Epidemiology of cerebral palsy. Adv Neurol 19:421-435, 1978.
290. Nelson KB: Can we prevent cerebral palsy? N Engl J Med 349:1765-1769, 2003.
291. O'Shea TM, Klinepeter KL, Dillard RG: Prenatal events and the risk of cerebral palsy in very low birth weight infants. Am J Epidemiol 147:362-369, 1998.
292. Redline RW: Severe fetal placental vascular lesions in term infants with neurologic impairment. Am J Obstet Gynecol 192:452-457, 2005.
293. Verma U, Tejani N, Klein S, et al: Obstetric antecedents of intraventricular hemorrhage and periventricular leukomalacia in the low-birth-weight neonate. Am J Obstet Gynecol 176:275-281, 1997.

294. Wharton KN, Pinar H, Stonestreet BS, et al: Severe umbilical cord inflammation: A predictor of periventricular leukomalacia in very low birth weight infants. Early Hum Dev 77:77-87, 2004.
295. Yoon BH, Romero R, Yang SH, et al: Interleukin-6 concentrations in umbilical cord plasma are elevated in neonates with white matter lesions associated with periventricular leukomalacia. Am J Obstet Gynecol 174:1433-1440, 1996.
296. Yoon BH, Jun JK, Romero R, et al: Amniotic fluid inflammatory cytokines (interleukin-6, interleukin-1beta, and tumor necrosis factor-alpha), neonatal brain white matter lesions, and cerebral palsy. Am J Obstet Gynecol 177:19-26, 1997.
297. Hagberg B, Hagberg G, Beckung E, et al: Changing panorama of cerebral palsy in Sweden: VIII. Prevalence and origin in the birth year period 1991-94. Acta Paediatr 90:271-277, 2001.
298. Hagberg H, Peebles D, Mallard C: Models of white matter injury: Comparison of infectious, hypoxic-ischemic, and excitotoxic insults. Ment Retard Dev Disabil Res Rev 8:30-38, 2002.
299. Hagberg H, Mallard C: Effect of inflammation on central nervous system development and vulnerability. Curr Opin Neurol 18:117-123, 2005.
300. Kaukola T, Satyaraj E, Patel DD, et al: Cerebral palsy is characterized by protein mediators in cord serum. Ann Neurol 55:186-194, 2004.
301. Mallard C, Welin AK, Peebles D, et al: White matter injury following systemic endotoxemia or asphyxia in the fetal sheep. Neurochem Res 28:215-223, 2003.
302. Moon JB, Kim JC, Yoon BH, et al: Amniotic fluid matrix metalloproteinase-8 and the development of cerebral palsy. J Perinat Med 30:301-306, 2002.
303. Yoon BH, Romero R, Kim CJ, et al: High expression of tumor necrosis factor-alpha and interleukin-6 in periventricular leukomalacia. Am J Obstet Gynecol 177:406-411, 1997.
304. Grether JK, Nelson KB, Emery ES III, et al: Prenatal and perinatal factors and cerebral palsy in very low birth weight infants. J Pediatr 128:407-414, 1996.
305. Gotsch F, Romero R, Kusanovic JP, et al: The fetal inflammatory response syndrome. Clin Obstet Gynecol 50:652-683, 2007.
306. Clayton D, McKeigue PM: Epidemiological methods for studying genes and environmental factors in complex diseases. Lancet 358:1356-1360, 2001.
307. Tiret L: Gene-environment interaction: A central concept in multifactorial diseases. Proc Nutr Soc 61:457-463, 2002.
308. Macones GA, Parry S, Elkousy M, et al: A polymorphism in the promoter region of TNF and bacterial vaginosis: Preliminary evidence of gene-environment interaction in the etiology of spontaneous preterm birth. Am J Obstet Gynecol 190:1504-1508, 2004.
309. Roberts AK, Monzon-Bordonaba F, Van Deerlin PG, et al: Association of polymorphism within the promoter of the tumor necrosis factor alpha gene with increased risk of preterm premature rupture of the fetal membranes. Am J Obstet Gynecol 180:1297-1302, 1999.
310. Romero R, Chaiworapongsa T, Kuivaniemi H, et al: Bacterial vaginosis, the inflammatory response and the risk of preterm birth: A role for genetic epidemiology in the prevention of preterm birth. Am J Obstet Gynecol 190:1509-1519, 2004.
311. Williams MA, Mittendorf R, Lieberman E, et al: Adverse infant outcomes associated with first-trimester vaginal bleeding. Obstet Gynecol 78:14-18, 1991.
312. Harger JH, Hsing AW, Tuomala RE, et al: Risk factors for preterm premature rupture of fetal membranes: A multicenter case-control study. Am J Obstet Gynecol 163:130-137, 1990.
313. Strobino B, Pantel-Silverman J: Gestational vaginal bleeding and pregnancy outcome. Am J Epidemiol 129:806-815, 1989.
314. Arias F: Placental insufficiency: An important cause of preterm labor and preterm premature ruptured membranes. 10th Annual Meeting of the Society of Perinatal Obstetricians, Houston, Texas, 1990. Abstract 144.
315. Arias F, Rodriquez L, Rayne SC, et al: Maternal placental vasculopathy and infection: Two distinct subgroups among patients with preterm labor and preterm ruptured membranes. Am J Obstet Gynecol 168:585-591, 1993.
316. Major C, Nageotte M., Lewis D: Preterm premature rupture of membranes and placental abruption: Is there an association between these pregnancy complications? Am J Obstet Gynecol 164:381, 1991.
317. Moretti M, Sibai BM: Maternal and perinatal outcome of expectant management of premature rupture of membranes in the midtrimester. Am J Obstet Gynecol 159:390-396, 1988.
318. Vintzileos AM, Campbell WA, Nochimson DJ, et al: Preterm premature rupture of the membranes: A risk factor for the development of abruptio placentae. Am J Obstet Gynecol 156:1235-1238, 1987.
319. Bukowski R, Gahn D, Denning J, et al: Impairment of growth in fetuses destined to deliver preterm. Am J Obstet Gynecol 185:463-467, 2001.
320. MacGregor SN, Sabbagha RE, Tamura RK, et al: Differing fetal growth patterns in pregnancies complicated by preterm labor. Obstet Gynecol 72:834-837, 1988.
321. Morken NH, Kallen K, Jacobsson B: Fetal growth and onset of delivery: A nationwide population-based study of preterm infants. Am J Obstet Gynecol 195:154-161, 2006.
322. Ott WJ: Intrauterine growth retardation and preterm delivery. Am J Obstet Gynecol 168:1710-1715, 1993.
323. Weiner CP, Sabbagha RE, Vaisrub N, et al: A hypothetical model suggesting suboptimal intrauterine growth in infants delivered preterm. Obstet Gynecol 65:323-326, 1985.
324. Zeitlin J, Ancel PY, Saurel-Cubizolles MJ, et al: The relationship between intrauterine growth restriction and preterm delivery: An empirical approach using data from a European case-control study. BJOG 107:750-758, 2000.
325. Kim YM, Chaiworapongsa T, Gomez R, et al: Failure of physiologic transformation of the spiral arteries in the placental bed in preterm premature rupture of membranes. Am J Obstet Gynecol 187:1137-1142, 2002.
326. Kim YM, Bujold E, Chaiworapongsa T, et al: Failure of physiologic transformation of the spiral arteries in patients with preterm labor and intact membranes. Am J Obstet Gynecol 189:1063-1069, 2003.
327. Salafia CM, Lopez-Zeno JA, Sherer DM, et al: Histologic evidence of old intrauterine bleeding is more frequent in prematurity. Am J Obstet Gynecol 173:1065-1070, 1995.
328. Brar HS, Medearis AL, DeVore GR, et al: Maternal and fetal blood flow velocity waveforms in patients with preterm labor: prediction of successful tocolysis. Am J Obstet Gynecol 159:947-950, 1988.
329. Brar HS, Medearis AL, De Vore GR, et al: Maternal and fetal blood flow velocity waveforms in patients with preterm labor: Relationship to outcome. Am J Obstet Gynecol 161:1519-1522, 1989.
330. Strigini FA, Lencioni G, De Luca G, et al: Uterine artery velocimetry and spontaneous preterm delivery. Obstet Gynecol 85:374-377, 1995.
331. Romero R, Espinoza J, Kusanovic JP, et al: The preterm parturition syndrome. BJOG 113(Suppl 3):17-42, 2006.
332. Lockwood CJ, Krikun G, Papp C, et al: The role of progestationally regulated stromal cell tissue factor and type-1 plasminogen activator inhibitor (PAI-1) in endometrial hemostasis and menstruation. Ann N Y Acad Sci 734:57-79, 1994.
333. Elovitz MA, Saunders T, Ascher-Landsberg J, et al: Effects of thrombin on myometrial contractions in vitro and in vivo. Am J Obstet Gynecol 183:799-804, 2000.
334. Rosen T, Schatz F, Kuczynski E, et al: Thrombin-enhanced matrix metalloproteinase-1 expression: A mechanism linking placental abruption with premature rupture of the membranes. J Matern Fetal Neonatal Med 11:11-17, 2002.
335. Lockwood CJ, Krikun G, Aigner S, et al: Effects of thrombin on steroid-modulated cultured endometrial stromal cell fibrinolytic potential. J Clin Endocrinol.Metab 81:107-112, 1996.
336. Lijnen HR: Matrix metalloproteinases and cellular fibrinolytic activity. Biochemistry (Mosc) 67:92-98, 2002.
337. Aplin JD, Campbell S, Allen TD: The extracellular matrix of human amniotic epithelium: Ultrastructure, composition and deposition. J Cell Sci 79:119-136, 1985.

338. Chaiworapongsa T, Espinoza J, Yoshimatsu J, et al: Activation of coagulation system in preterm labor and preterm premature rupture of membranes. J Matern Fetal Neonatal Med 11:368-373, 2002.
339. Gomez R, Athayde N, Pacora P, et al: Increased thrombin in intrauterine inflammation. Am J Obstet Gynecol 178:S62, 1998.
340. Rosen T, Kuczynski E, O'Neill LM, et al: Plasma levels of thrombin-antithrombin complexes predict preterm premature rupture of the fetal membranes. J Matern Fetal Med 10:297-300, 2001.
341. Nagy S, Bush M, Stone J, et al: Clinical significance of subchorionic and retroplacental hematomas detected in the first trimester of pregnancy. Obstet Gynecol 102:94-100, 2003.
342. Mackenzie AP, Schatz F, Krikun G, et al: Mechanisms of abruption-induced premature rupture of the fetal membranes: Thrombin enhanced decidual matrix metalloproteinase-3 (stromelysin-1) expression. Am J Obstet Gynecol 191:1996-2001, 2004.
343. Darby MJ, Caritis SN, Shen-Schwarz S: Placental abruption in the preterm gestation: An association with chorioamnionitis. Obstet Gynecol 74:88-92, 1989.
344. Lockwood CJ, Toti P, Arcuri F, et al: Mechanisms of abruption-induced premature rupture of the fetal membranes: Thrombin-enhanced interleukin-8 expression in term decidua. Am J Pathol 167:1443-1449, 2005.
345. Lathbury LJ, Salamonsen LA: In-vitro studies of the potential role of neutrophils in the process of menstruation. Mol Hum Reprod 6:899-906, 2000.
346. Karlsson A, Dahlgren C: Assembly and activation of the neutrophil NADPH oxidase in granule membranes. Antioxid Redox Signal 4:49-60, 2002.
347. Britigan BE, Cohen MS, Rosen GM: Detection of the production of oxygen-centered free radicals by human neutrophils using spin trapping techniques: A critical perspective. J Leukoc Biol 41:349-362, 1987.
348. McCord JM, Fridovich I: The biology and pathology of oxygen radicals. Ann Intern Med 89:122-127, 1978.
349. Cakmak H, Schatz F, Huang ST, et al: Progestin suppresses thrombin- and interleukin-1beta-induced interleukin-11 production in term decidual cells: Implications for preterm delivery. J Clin Endocrinol Metab 90:5279-5286, 2005.
350. Lockwood CJ: Stress-associated preterm delivery: The role of corticotropin-releasing hormone. Am J Obstet Gynecol 180:S264-S266, 1999.
351. Wadhwa PD, Culhane JF, Rauh V, et al: Stress, infection and preterm birth: A biobehavioural perspective. Paediatr Perinat Epidemiol 15(Suppl 2):17-29, 2001.
352. Wadhwa PD, Culhane JF, Rauh V, et al: Stress and preterm birth: Neuroendocrine, immune/inflammatory, and vascular mechanisms. Matern Child Health J 5:119-125, 2001.
353. Challis JR, Smith SK: Fetal endocrine signals and preterm labor. Biol Neonate 79:163-167, 2001.
354. Hobel CJ: Stress and preterm birth. Clin Obstet Gynecol 47:856-880, 2004.
355. Mozurkewich EL, Luke B, Avni M, Wolf FM: Working conditions and adverse pregnancy outcome: A meta-analysis. Obstet Gynecol 95:623-635, 2000.
356. Copper RL, Goldenberg RL, Das A, et al: The preterm prediction study: Maternal stress is associated with spontaneous preterm birth at less than thirty-five weeks' gestation. National Institute of Child Health and Human Development Maternal-Fetal Medicine Units Network. Am J Obstet Gynecol 175:1286-1292, 1996.
357. Orr ST, James SA, Blackmore PC: Maternal prenatal depressive symptoms and spontaneous preterm births among African-American women in Baltimore, Maryland. Am J Epidemiol 156:797-802, 2002.
358. Bloomfield FH, Oliver MH, Hawkins P, et al: A periconceptional nutritional origin for noninfectious preterm birth. Science 300:606, 2003.
359. Challis JR, Lye SJ, Gibb W, et al: Understanding preterm labor. Ann N Y Acad Sci 943:225-234, 2001.
360. McLean M, Bisits A, Davies J, et al: A placental clock controlling the length of human pregnancy. Nat Med 1:460-463, 1995.
361. Smith R, Nicholson RC: Corticotrophin releasing hormone and the timing of birth. Front Biosci 12:912-918, 2007.
362. Jones SA, Brooks AN, Challis JR: Steroids modulate corticotropin-releasing hormone production in human fetal membranes and placenta. J Clin Endocrinol Metab 68:825-830.
363. Jones SA, Challis JR: Steroid, corticotrophin-releasing hormone, ACTH and prostaglandin interactions in the amnion and placenta of early pregnancy in man. J Endocrinol 125:153-159, 1990.
364. Jones SA, Challis JR: Effects of corticotropin-releasing hormone and adrenocorticotropin on prostaglandin output by human placenta and fetal membranes. Gynecol Obstet Invest 29:165-168, 1990.
365. Li W, Challis JR: Corticotropin-releasing hormone and urocortin induce secretion of matrix metalloproteinase-9 (MMP-9) without change in tissue inhibitors of MMP-1 by cultured cells from human placenta and fetal membranes. J Clin Endocrinol Metab 90:6569-6574, 2005.
366. Lockwood CJ, Radunovic N, Nastic D, et al: Corticotropin-releasing hormone and related pituitary-adrenal axis hormones in fetal and maternal blood during the second half of pregnancy. J Perinat Med 24:243-251, 1996.
367. Mastorakos G, Ilias I: Maternal and fetal hypothalamic-pituitary-adrenal axes during pregnancy and postpartum. Ann N Y Acad Sci 997:136-149, 2003.
368. Parker CR Jr, Stankovic AM, Goland RS: Corticotropin-releasing hormone stimulates steroidogenesis in cultured human adrenal cells. Mol Cell Endocrinol 155:19-25, 1999.
369. Chakravorty A, Mesiano S, Jaffe RB: Corticotropin-releasing hormone stimulates P450 17alpha-hydroxylase/17,20-lyase in human fetal adrenal cells via protein kinase C. J Clin Endocrinol Metab 84:3732-3438, 1999.
370. Wu WX, Ma XH, Zhang Q, et al: Regulation of prostaglandin endoperoxide H synthase 1 and 2 by estradiol and progesterone in nonpregnant ovine myometrium and endometrium in vivo. Endocrinology 138:4005-4012, 1997.
371. Di WL, Lachelin GC, McGarrigle HH, et al: Oestriol and oestradiol increase cell to cell communication and connexin43 protein expression in human myometrium. Mol Hum Reprod 7:671-679, 2001.
372. Geimonen E, Boylston E, Royek A, et al: Elevated connexin-43 expression in term human myometrium correlates with elevated c-Jun expression and is independent of myometrial estrogen receptors. J Clin Endocrinol Metab 83:1177-1185, 1998.
373. Kimura T, Takemura M, Nomura S, et al: Expression of oxytocin receptor in human pregnant myometrium. Endocrinology 137:780-785, 1996.
374. Richter ON, Kubler K, Schmolling J, et al: Oxytocin receptor gene expression of estrogen-stimulated human myometrium in extracorporeally perfused non-pregnant uteri. Mol Hum Reprod 10:339-346, 2004.
375. Wu WX, Ma XH, Zhang Q, et al: Characterization of topology-, gestation- and labor-related changes of a cassette of myometrial contraction-associated protein mRNA in the pregnant baboon myometrium. J Endocrinol 171:445-453, 2001.
376. Helguera G, Olcese R, Song M, et al: Tissue-specific regulation of Ca(2+) channel protein expression by sex hormones. Biochim Biophys Acta 1569:59-66, 2002.
377. Matsui K, Higashi K, Fukunaga K, et al: Hormone treatments and pregnancy alter myosin light chain kinase and calmodulin levels in rabbit myometrium. J Endocrinol 97:11-19, 1983.
378. Economopoulos P, Sun M, Purgina B, et al: Glucocorticoids stimulate prostaglandin H synthase type-2 (PGHS-2) in the fibroblast cells in human amnion cultures. Mol Cell Endocrinol 117:141-147, 1996.
379. Patel FA, Clifton VL, Chwalisz K, Challis JR: Steroid regulation of prostaglandin dehydrogenase activity and expression in human term placenta and chorio-decidua in relation to labor. J Clin Endocrinol Metab 84:291-299, 1999.
380. Zakar T, Hirst JJ, Mijovic JE, et al: Glucocorticoids stimulate the expression of prostaglandin endoperoxide H synthase-2 in amnion cells. Endocrinology 136:1610-1619, 1995.

381. Sun K, Ma R, Cui X, et al: Glucocorticoids induce cytosolic phospholipase A2 and prostaglandin H synthase type 2 but not microsomal prostaglandin E synthase (PGES) and cytosolic PGES expression in cultured primary human amnion cells. J Clin Endocrinol Metab 88:5564-5571, 2003.
382. Yang R, You X, Tang X, et al: Corticotropin-releasing hormone inhibits progesterone production in cultured human placental trophoblasts. J Mol Endocrinol 37:533-540, 2006.
383. Ludmir J, Samuels P, Brooks S, et al: Pregnancy outcome of patients with uncorrected uterine anomalies managed in a high-risk obstetric setting. Obstet Gynecol 75:906-910, 1990.
384. Hill LM, Breckle R, Thomas ML, et al: Polyhydramnios: Ultrasonically detected prevalence and neonatal outcome. Obstet Gynecol 69:21-25, 1987.
385. Phelan JP, Park YW, Ahn MO, et al: Polyhydramnios and perinatal outcome. J Perinatol 10:347-350, 1990.
386. Besinger R, Carlson N: The physiology of preterm labor. In Keith L, Papiernik E, Keith D, Luke B (eds): Multiple Pregnancy: Epidemiology, Gestation and Perinatal Outcome. London: Parthenon Publishing, 1995, p 415.
387. Levy R, Kanengiser B, Furman B, et al: A randomized trial comparing a 30-mL and an 80-mL Foley catheter balloon for preinduction cervical ripening. Am J Obstet Gynecol 191:1632-1636, 2004.
388. Fisk NM, Ronderos-Dumit D, Tannirandorn Y, et al: Normal amniotic pressure throughout gestation. BJOG 99:18-22, 1992.
389. Sideris IG, Nicolaides KH: Amniotic fluid pressure during pregnancy. Fetal Diagn Ther 5:104-108, 1990.
390. Speroff L, Glass RH, Kase NG: The endocrinology of pregnancy. In Mitchell C (ed): Clinical Gynecologic Endocrinology and Infertility. Baltimore: Williams & Wilkins, 1994, p 251-290.
391. Sladek SM, Westerhausen-Larson A, Roberts JM: Endogenous nitric oxide suppresses rat myometrial connexin 43 gap junction protein expression during pregnancy. Biol Reprod 61:8-13, 1999.
392. Laudanski T, Rocki W: The effects on stretching and prostaglandin F2alpha on the contractile and bioelectric activity of the uterus in rat. Acta Physiol Pol 26:385-393, 1975.
393. Kloeck FK, Jung H: In vitro release of prostaglandins from the human myometrium under the influence of stretching. Am J Obstet Gynecol 115:1066-1069, 1973.
394. Ou CW, Chen ZQ, Qi S, et al: Increased expression of the rat myometrial oxytocin receptor messenger ribonucleic acid during labor requires both mechanical and hormonal signals. Biol Reprod 59:1055-1061, 1998.
395. Tzima E, del Pozo MA, Shattil SJ, et al: Activation of integrins in endothelial cells by fluid shear stress mediates Rho-dependent cytoskeletal alignment. EMBO J 20:4639-4647, 2001.
396. Farrugia G, Holm AN, Rich A, et al: A mechanosensitive calcium channel in human intestinal smooth muscle cells. Gastroenterology 117:900-905, 1999.
397. Holm AN, Rich A, Sarr MG, et al: Whole cell current and membrane potential regulation by a human smooth muscle mechanosensitive calcium channel. Am J Physiol Gastrointest Liver Physiol 279:G1155-G1161, 2000.
398. Hu Y, Bock G, Wick G, Xu Q: Activation of PDGF receptor alpha in vascular smooth muscle cells by mechanical stress. FASEB J 12:1135-1142, 1998.
399. Li C, Xu Q: Mechanical stress-initiated signal transductions in vascular smooth muscle cells. Cell Signal 12:435-445, 2000.
400. Mitchell JA, Lye SJ: Regulation of connexin43 expression by c-fos and c-jun in myometrial cells. Cell Commun Adhes 8:299-302, 2001.
401. Mitchell JA, Lye SJ: Differential expression of activator protein-1 transcription factors in pregnant rat myometrium. Biol Reprod 67:240-246, 2002.
402. Oldenhof AD, Shynlova OP, Liu M, et al: Mitogen-activated protein kinases mediate stretch-induced c-fos mRNA expression in myometrial smooth muscle cells. Am J Physiol Cell Physiol 283:C1530-C1539, 2002.
403. Piersanti M, Lye SJ: Increase in messenger ribonucleic acid encoding the myometrial gap junction protein, connexin-43, requires protein synthesis and is associated with increased expression of the activator protein-1, c-fos. Endocrinology 136:3571-3578, 1995.
404. Shynlova OP, Oldenhof AD, Liu M, et al: Regulation of c-fos expression by static stretch in rat myometrial smooth muscle cells. Am J Obstet Gynecol 186:1358-1365, 2002.
405. Millar LK, Stollberg J, DeBuque L, et al: Fetal membrane distention: Determination of the intrauterine surface area and distention of the fetal membranes preterm and at term. Am J Obstet Gynecol 182:128-134, 2000.
406. Maehara K, Kanayama N, Maradny EE, et al: Mechanical stretching induces interleukin-8 gene expression in fetal membranes: A possible role for the initiation of human parturition. Eur J Obstet Gynecol Reprod Biol 70:191-196, 1996.
407. Maradny EE, Kanayama N, Halim A, et al: Stretching of fetal membranes increases the concentration of interleukin-8 and collagenase activity. Am J Obstet Gynecol 174:843-849, 1996.
408. Kanayama N, Fukamizu H: Mechanical stretching increases prostaglandin E2 in cultured human amnion cells. Gynecol Obstet Invest 28:123-126, 1989.
409. Nemeth E, Tashima LS, Yu Z, et al: Fetal membrane distention: I. Differentially expressed genes regulated by acute distention in amniotic epithelial (WISH) cells. Am J Obstet Gynecol 182:50-59, 2000.
410. Nemeth E, Millar LK, Bryant-Greenwood G: Fetal membrane distention: II. Differentially expressed genes regulated by acute distention in vitro. Am J Obstet Gynecol 182:60-67, 2000.
411. Barclay CG, Brennand JE, Kelly RW, et al: Interleukin-8 production by the human cervix. Am J Obstet Gynecol 169:625-632, 1993.
412. el Maradny E, Kanayama N, Halim A, et al: Interleukin-8 induces cervical ripening in rabbits. Am J Obstet Gynecol 171:77-83, 1994.
413. Calder AA: Prostaglandins and biological control of cervical function. Aust N Z J Obstet Gynaecol 34:347-351, 1994.
414. Stjernholm YM, Sahlin L, Eriksson HA, et al: Cervical ripening after treatment with prostaglandin E2 or antiprogestin (RU486): Possible mechanisms in relation to gonadal steroids. Eur J Obstet Gynecol Reprod Biol 84:83-88, 1999.
415. Ekerhovd E, Weijdegard B, Brannstrom M, et al: Nitric oxide induced cervical ripening in the human: Involvement of cyclic guanosine monophosphate, prostaglandin F(2 alpha), and prostaglandin E(2). Am J Obstet Gynecol 186:745-750, 2002.
416. Mazor M, Hershkovitz R, Ghezzi F, et al: Intraamniotic infection in patients with preterm labor and twin pregnancies. Acta Obstet Gynecol Scand 75:624-627, 1996.
417. Romero R, Shamma F, Avila C, et al: Infection and labor: VI. Prevalence, microbiology, and clinical significance of intraamniotic infection in twin gestations with preterm labor. Am J Obstet Gynecol 163:757-761, 1990.
418. Yoon BH, Park KH, Koo JN, et al: Intra-amniotic infection of twin pregnancies with preterm labor. Am J Obstet Gynecol 176:535. 1997.
419. Romero R, Mazor M, Avila C, et al: Uterine "allergy": A novel mechanism for preterm labor. Am J Obstet Gynecol 164:375. 1991.
420. Holgate ST: The epidemic of allergy and asthma. Nature 402:B2-B4, 1999.
421. Corry DB, Kheradmand F: Induction and regulation of the IgE response. Nature 402:B18-B23, 1999.
422. Holloway JA, Warner JO, Vance GH, et al: Detection of house-dust-mite allergen in amniotic fluid and umbilical-cord blood. Lancet 356:1900-1902, 2000.
423. Jones AC, Miles EA, Warner JO, et al: Fetal peripheral blood mononuclear cell proliferative responses to mitogenic and allergenic stimuli during gestation. Pediatr Allergy Immunol 7:109-116, 1996.
424. Rudolph MI, Reinicke K, Cruz MA, et al: Distribution of mast cells and the effect of their mediators on contractility in human myometrium. BJOG 100:1125-1130, 1993.

425. Padilla L, Reinicke K, Montesino H, et al: Histamine content and mast cells distribution in mouse uterus: The effect of sexual hormones, gestation and labor. Cell Mol Biol 36:93-100, 1990.
426. Rudolph MI, Bardisa L, Cruz MA, et al: Mast cells mediators evoke contractility and potentiate each other in mouse uterine horns. Gen Pharmacol 23:833-836, 1992.
427. Bytautiene E, Vedernikov YP, Saade GR, et al: Endogenous mast cell degranulation modulates cervical contractility in the guinea pig. Am J Obstet Gynecol 186:438-445, 2002.
428. Garfield RE, Bytautiene E, Vedernikov YP, et al: Modulation of rat uterine contractility by mast cells and their mediators. Am J Obstet Gynecol 183:118-125, 2000.
429. Shingai Y, Nakagawa K, Kato T, et al: Severe allergy in a pregnant woman after vaginal examination with a latex glove. Gynecol Obstet Invest 54:183-184, 2002.
430. Bulmer JN, Pace D, Ritson A: Immunoregulatory cells in human decidua: Morphology, immunohistochemistry and function. Reprod Nutr Dev 28:1599-1613, 1988.
431. Lachapelle MH, Miron P, Hemmings R, et al: Endometrial T, B, and NK cells in patients with recurrent spontaneous abortion: Altered profile and pregnancy outcome. J Immunol 156:4027-4034, 1996.
432. Kammerer U, Schoppet M, McLellan AD, et al: Human decidua contains potent immunostimulatory CD83(+) dendritic cells. Am J Pathol 157:159-169, 2000.
433. Bytautiene E, Romero R, Vedernikov YP, et al: Induction of premature labor and delivery by allergic reaction and prevention by histamine H1 receptor antagonist. Am J Obstet Gynecol 191:1356-1361, 2004.
434. Iams JD, Johnson FF, Sonek J, et al: Cervical competence as a continuum: A study of ultrasonographic cervical length and obstetric performance. Am J Obstet Gynecol 172:1097-1103, 1995.
435. Romero R, Mazor M, Gomez R: Cervix, incompetence and premature labor. Fetus 3:1, 1993.
436. Romero R, Espinoza J, Erez O, et al: The role of cervical cerclage in obstetric practice: Can the patient who could benefit from this procedure be identified? Am J Obstet Gynecol 194:1-9, 2006.
437. Mesiano S: Roles of estrogen and progesterone in human parturition. Front Horm Res 27:86-104, 2001.
438. Stjernholm Y, Sahlin L, Akerberg S, et al: Cervical ripening in humans: Potential roles of estrogen, progesterone, and insulin-like growth factor-I. Am J Obstet Gynecol 174:1065-1071, 1996.
439. Gorodeski IG, Geier A, Lunenfeld B, et al: Progesterone (P) receptor dynamics in estrogen primed normal human cervix following P injection. Fertil Steril 47:108-113, 1987.
440. Kelly RW, Leask R, Calder AA: Choriodecidual production of interleukin-8 and mechanism of parturition. Lancet 339:776-777, 1992.
441. Puri CP, Patil RK, Elger WA, et al: Effects of progesterone antagonist ZK 98.299 on early pregnancy and foetal outcome in bonnet monkeys. Contraception 41:197-205, 1990.
442. Bernal AL: Overview of current research in parturition. Exp Physiol 86:213-222, 2001.
443. Young IR: The comparative physiology of parturition in mammals. In Smith R (ed): The enodocrinology of parturition. Basel: Reinhardt Druck, 2001, p 10-30.
444. Schwarz BE, Milewich L, Johnston JM, et al: Initiation of human parturition: V. Progesterone binding substance in fetal membranes. Obstet Gynecol 48:685-689, 1976.
445. Westphal U, Stroupe SD, Cheng SL: Progesterone binding to serum proteins. Ann N Y Acad Sci 286:10-28, 1977.
446. Karalis K, Goodwin G, Majzoub JA: Cortisol blockade of progesterone: A possible molecular mechanism involved in the initiation of human labor. Nat Med 2:556-660, 1996.
447. Milewich L, Gant NF, Schwarz BE, et al: Initiation of human parturition: VIII. Metabolism of progesterone by fetal membranes of early and late human gestation. Obstet Gynecol 50:45-48, 1977.
448. Mitchell BF, Wong S: Changes in 17 beta,20 alpha-hydroxysteroid dehydrogenase activity supporting an increase in the estrogen/progesterone ratio of human fetal membranes at parturition. Am J Obstet Gynecol 168:1377-1385, 1993.
449. How H, Huang ZH, Zuo J, et al: Myometrial estradiol and progesterone receptor changes in preterm and term pregnancies. Obstet Gynecol 86:936-940, 1995.
450. Mesiano S, Chan EC, Fitter JT, et al: Progesterone withdrawal and estrogen activation in human parturition are coordinated by progesterone receptor A expression in the myometrium. J Clin Endocrinol Metab 87:2924-2930, 2002.
451. Pieber D, Allport VC, Hills F, et al: Interactions between progesterone receptor isoforms in myometrial cells in human labour. Mol Hum Reprod 7:875-879, 2001.
452. Condon JC, Hardy DB, Kovaric K, et al: Up-regulation of the progesterone receptor (PR)-C isoform in laboring myometrium by activation of nuclear factor-kappaB may contribute to the onset of labor through inhibition of PR function. Mol Endocrinol 20:764-775, 2006.
453. Zakar T, Hertelendy F: Progesterone withdrawal: key to parturition. Am J Obstet Gynecol 196:289-296, 2007.
454. Allport VC, Pieber D, Slater DM, et al: Human labour is associated with nuclear factor-kappaB activity which mediates cyclo-oxygenase-2 expression and is involved with the "functional progesterone withdrawal." Mol Hum Reprod 7:581-586, 2001.
455. Belt AR, Baldassare JJ, Molnar M, et al: The nuclear transcription factor NF-kappaB mediates interleukin-1beta-induced expression of cyclooxygenase-2 in human myometrial cells. Am J Obstet Gynecol 181:359-366, 1999.
456. Kalkhoven E, Wissink S, Van der Saag PT, et al: Negative interaction between the RelA(p65) subunit of NF-kappaB and the progesterone receptor. J Biol Chem 271:6217-6224, 1996.
457. Merlino AA, Welsh TN, Tan H, et al: Nuclear progesterone receptors in the human pregnancy myometrium: Evidence that parturition involves functional progesterone withdrawal mediated by increased expression of progesterone receptor-A. J Clin Endocrinol Metab 92:1927-1933, 2007.
458. Karteris E, Zervou S, Pang Y, et al: Progesterone signaling in human myometrium through two novel membrane G protein-coupled receptors: Potential role in functional progesterone withdrawal at term. Mol Endocrinol 20:1519-1534, 2006.
459. Oh SY, Kim CJ, Park I, et al: Progesterone receptor isoform (A/B) ratio of human fetal membranes increases during term parturition. Am J Obstet Gynecol 193:1156-1160, 2005.
460. Sheehan PM, Rice GE, Moses EK, et al: 5-Beta-dihydroprogesterone and steroid 5 beta-reductase decrease in association with human parturition at term. Mol Hum Reprod 11:495-501, 2005.
461. Word RA, Landrum CP, Timmons BC, et al: Transgene insertion on mouse chromosome 6 impairs function of the uterine cervix and causes failure of parturition. Biol Reprod 73:1046-1056, 2005.
462. Dong X, Shylnova O, Challis JR, et al: Identification and characterization of the protein-associated splicing factor as a negative co-regulator of the progesterone receptor. J Biol Chem 280:13329-13340, 2005.
463. Brown AG, Leite RS, Strauss JF III: Mechanisms underlying "functional" progesterone withdrawal at parturition. Ann N Y Acad Sci 1034:36-49, 2004.
464. Mesiano S: Myometrial progesterone responsiveness and the control of human parturition. J Soc Gynecol Investig 11:193-202, 2004.
465. Garfield RE, Puri CP, Csapo AI: Endocrine, structural, and functional changes in the uterus during premature labor. Am J Obstet Gynecol 142:21-27, 1982.
466. Condon JC, Jeyasuria P, Faust JM, et al: A decline in the levels of progesterone receptor coactivators in the pregnant uterus at term may antagonize progesterone receptor function and contribute to the initiation of parturition. Proc Natl Acad Sci U S A 100:9518-9523, 2003.
467. Stjernholm-Vladic Y, Wang H, Stygar D, et al: Differential regulation of the progesterone receptor A and B in the human uterine cervix at parturition. Gynecol Endocrinol 18:41-46, 2004.
468. Bethin KE, Nagai Y, Sladek R, et al: Microarray analysis of uterine gene expression in mouse and human pregnancy. Mol Endocrinol 17:1454-1469, 2003.

469. Haluska GJ, Wells TR, Hirst JJ, et al: Progesterone receptor localization and isoforms in myometrium, decidua, and fetal membranes from rhesus macaques: Evidence for functional progesterone withdrawal at parturition. J Soc Gynecol Investig 9:125-136, 2002.
470. Romero R: Prevention of spontaneous preterm birth: The role of sonographic cervical length in identifying patients who may benefit from progesterone treatment. Ultrasound Obstet Gynecol 30:675-686, 2007.
471. da Fonseca EB, Bittar RE, Carvalho MH, et al: Prophylactic administration of progesterone by vaginal suppository to reduce the incidence of spontaneous preterm birth in women at increased risk: A randomized placebo-controlled double-blind study. Am J Obstet Gynecol 188:419-424, 2003.
472. O'Brien JM, Adair CD, Lewis DF, et al: Progesterone vaginal gel for the reduction of recurrent preterm birth: Primary results from a randomized, double-blind, placebo-controlled trial. Ultrasound Obstet Gynecol 30:687-696, 2007.

Chapter 29

Preterm Labor and Birth

Jay D. Iams, MD, Roberto Romero, MD, and Robert K. Creasy, MD

Preterm birth is the principal unsolved problem in perinatal medicine. In 2005, one of every eight births in the United States was preterm—more than 525,000 infants. Advances in care have improved outcomes for preterm infants, but prematurity is still the most common underlying cause of perinatal[1] and infant[2] morbidity and mortality. Surviving infants may experience lifelong consequences, including neurodevelopmental, respiratory, gastrointestinal, and other morbidities. The rate of preterm birth has risen by more than one third since the 1980s, even as the perinatal mortality rate has decreased.

Preterm births are preceded by numerous clinical conditions that fall into two broad categories, according to whether one or more steps of the parturitional process (cervical ripening, membrane and decidual activation, and coordinated uterine contractility) has or has not begun. The first group, often called *spontaneous preterm births,* includes preterm labor with intact membranes, preterm premature rupture of the membranes (pPROM) before labor begins, preterm cervical effacement or insufficiency, and some instances of uterine bleeding of uncertain origin. The second group, called *indicated preterm births,* comprises preterm births that are medically initiated because of maternal or fetal compromise. These categories are sometimes indistinct in clinical practice but are useful to organize intervention strategies. The pathophysiology of preterm parturition is discussed in Chapter 28. This chapter addresses the overall problem of preterm birth, including the epidemiology and burden of disease for all preterm neonates and specific care for the clinical syndrome of preterm labor. Clinical care for pregnancies complicated by cervical insufficiency or pPROM is discussed in Chapters 30 and 31, respectively. Newborn and childhood complications of preterm birth are discussed in Chapter 58.

The Problem of Preterm Birth

Definitions

A birth before 259 days (37 weeks) from the first day of the last normal menstrual period, or 245 days after conception, is commonly defined as *preterm.* The appropriate lower limit of gestational age separating preterm birth from spontaneous abortion is controversial and varies from 20 weeks or earlier in the United States to 23 to 24 weeks in Europe.[3] The 20-week boundary was derived historically from quickening, the first signs of fetal movement, but pathologic and epidemiologic studies suggest that 16 to 17 weeks may be a more appropriate boundary, in that pregnancies ending between 16 and 20 weeks are associated with increased risk of preterm birth in subsequent pregnancies.[4-7]

Infants who weigh less than 2500 g at birth, regardless of gestational age, are designated as *low birth weight* (LBW). Infants who weigh less than 1500 g are called *very low birth weight* (VLBW), and those below 1000 g are *extremely low birth weight* (ELBW).

LBW and preterm infants have in the past been considered together, but advances in pregnancy dating increasingly allow outcomes related to gestational age to be distinguished from outcomes related to birth weight. This is important, because perinatal and infant morbidities vary substantially according to gestational age and maturity as well as birth weight (see also Chapters 34 and 58).[8] The current dual system, wherein obstetric data are recorded by gestational age but neonatal and infant data are analyzed by birth weight, has been identified as an impediment to optimal care by the Institute of Medicine.[9] Data relating outcomes to percentiles of weight for gestational age are needed to identify and understand the causes and consequences of both prematurity and abnormal growth and to allow the fetal and neonatal patient to receive optimal care before and after birth.

The proportion of LBW infants who are preterm versus term varies among developed and underdeveloped nations.[10] In underdeveloped countries, LBW infants are commonly growth restricted due to chronic maternal illness and/or malnutrition regardless of their gestational age (see Chapter 34). In developed nations, the majority of LBW infants are preterm. Indeed, some preterm infants weigh more than 2500 g at birth.[8]

Incidence of Preterm and Low-Birth-Weight Infants

Preterm Birth

Births before 37 weeks in the United States have increased by one third over the last 25 years. The rate was 9.4% in 1981, 10.6% in 1990, 12.7% in 2005, and 12.8% in 2006.[11]

Approximately 75% of preterm births occur between 34 and 36 weeks (Fig. 29-1). Although these late preterm infants experience significant morbidity, the great majority of perinatal mortality and most serious morbidity occurs among the 16% of preterm infants (<3.5% of all births) who are born before 32 weeks' gestation.

Low Birth Weight

Rates of LBW have increased in parallel with the rising preterm birth rate. The overall LBW rate, including singleton and multiple gestations of all races, was 6.7% in 1984, 7.7% in 2001, and 8.2% in 2005. The incidence of VLBW births (<1500 g) increased from 1.16% in 1981, to 1.27% in 1990, and to 1.49% in 2005, related primarily to the increase in multiple gestations.[11]

There is substantial international variation in the LBW rate (Fig. 29-2), owing not only to differences in the actual rates but also to limitations in collecting data and to variations in the definitions and methods used to ascertain birth information.

Ascertainment of Preterm Birth and Low Birth Weight

Reported rates of preterm birth and, to a lesser extent, LBW are influenced by factors that must be understood to use this data appropriately: the variability of definitions, and the prevalence of ultrasound.

Available data are influenced by definitions of preterm and LBW that vary internationally and within the United States, where definitions may differ by state. The lower boundary of gestational age is usually 20 weeks in the United States, but it varies from 20 to 24 weeks in reports from other countries.[12-14] The definition of LBW is universally accepted as a birth weight of less than 2500 g, but the lower boundary of 500 g is variable and in practice may be affected by cultural and religious beliefs and whether the infant shows signs of life.

Determination of gestational age by ultrasound measurement of fetal structures has superior accuracy over other methods when used in the first 12 to 20 weeks of pregnancy (see discussion by G. Alexander in reference 9, pp. 604-643). As the availability and quality of prenatal ultrasound services has increased, the distribution of gestational age has shifted to the left, reducing the number of post-term births and providing a corresponding increase in deliveries before 37 weeks of gestation (Fig. 29-3).

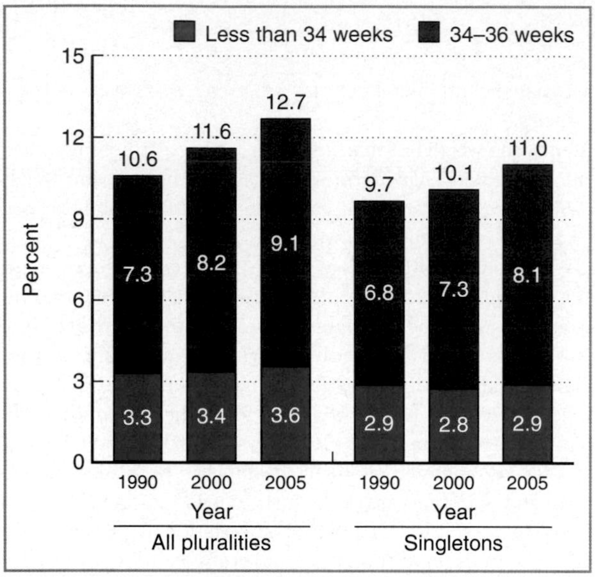

FIGURE 29-1 **Preterm birth rates for all births and for singletons only: United States, 1990, 2000, and 2005.** (From Hamilton BE, Martin JA, Sutton PD, et al: Births: Final data for 2005. Natl Vital Stat Rep 56[6]:4, 2007.)

Rising Incidence of Preterm Birth

Regardless of the definitions chosen and the methods used to determine gestational age, the true incidence of preterm birth has increased in developed countries. There are two major reasons for the increase: the increased number of late preterm births (between 34 and 36 weeks' gestation) and the increased number of multifetal gestations.

In 1990, 7.3% of births occurred between 34 and 36 weeks; that rate has risen steadily, to 9.1% in 2005. In addition to the rise related to improved gestational dating by ultrasound, there has been a true increase in the number of preterm births between 34 and 36 weeks that are intentional or indicated (see earlier discussion). These indicated preterm births are the result of a decision to end the pregnancy for medical or obstetric reasons[15] (Fig. 29-4; see Fig. 29-6).

Increased multifetal gestations are related to fertility therapies.[16-18] Rates of preterm birth for infants born in multifetal pregnancies between 1990 and 2004 are shown in Figure 29-5. The rise in preterm births related to fertility therapies is discussed later in this chapter and in Chapter 25.

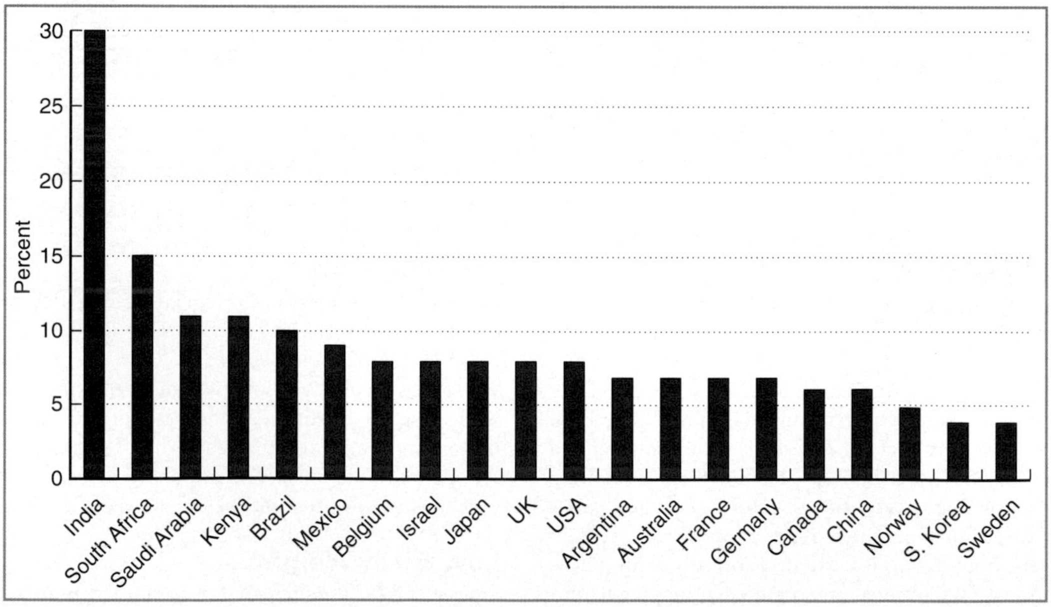

FIGURE 29-2 **Percentage of low-birth-weight infants, by country.** (Data from 2002 [latest available] from World Health Organization, http://www.who.int/whosis/database/core/core_select_process.cfm [accessed November 5, 2007].)

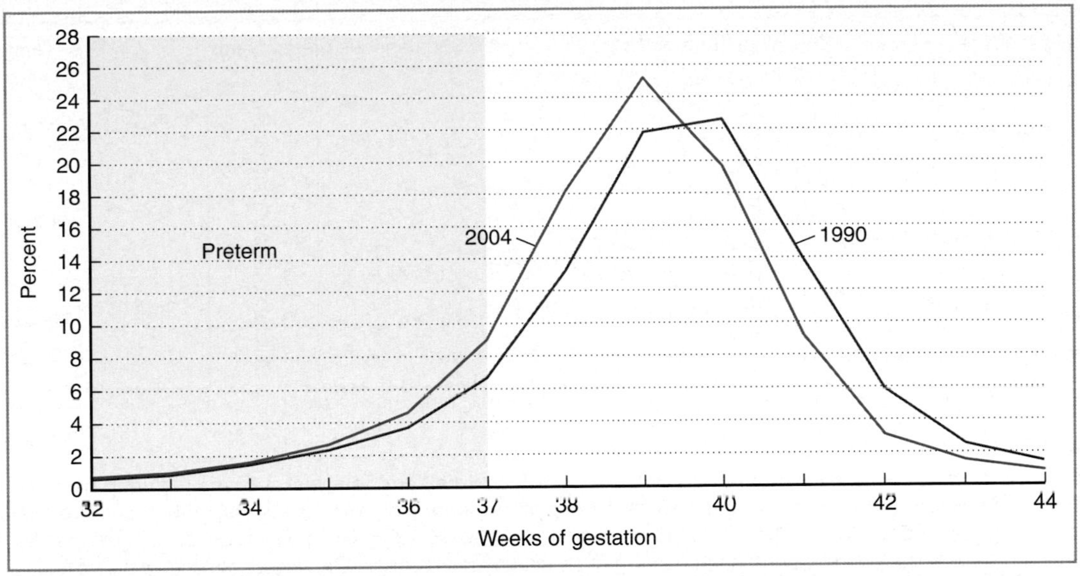

FIGURE 29-3 Distribution of births by gestational age (32-44 weeks): United States, 1990 and 2004. (From Martin JA, Hamilton BE, Sutton PD, et al: Births: Final data for 2004. Natl Vital Stat Rep 55(1):80-81, 2006.)

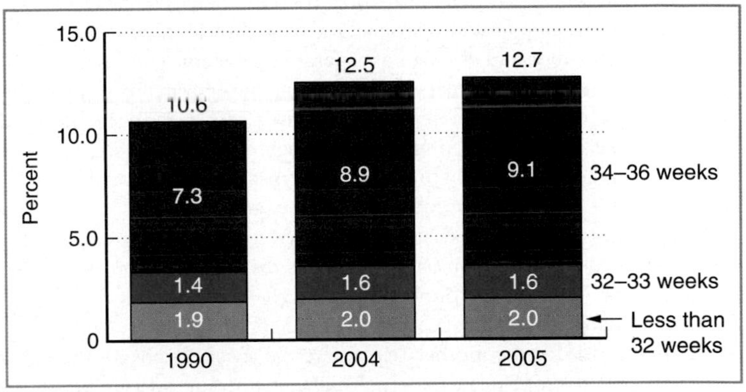

FIGURE 29-4 Percentage of preterm births: United States, 1990, 2004, 2005. The figures for 2005 are based on preliminary data. (From Martin JA, Hamilton BE, Sutton PD, et al: Births: Final data for 2004. Natl Vital Stat Rep 55(1):80-81, 2006.)

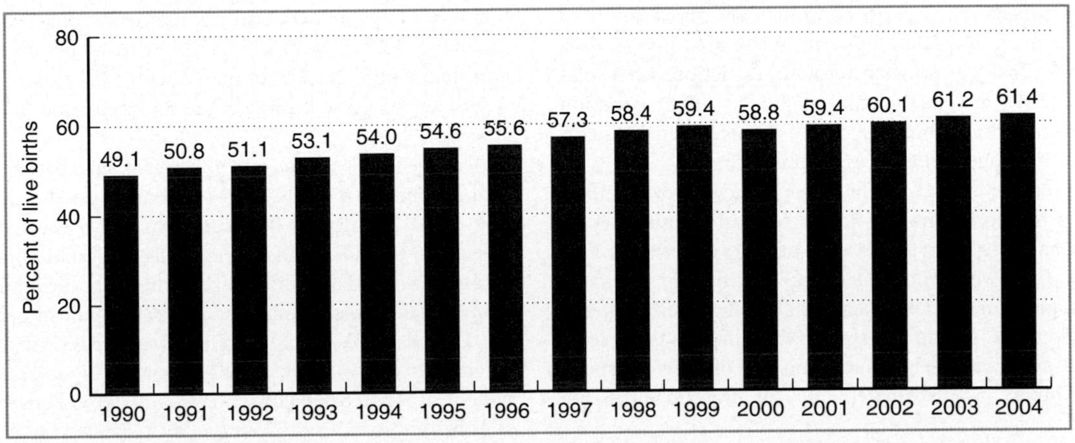

FIGURE 29-5 Rates of preterm birth in multifetal pregnancies, 1990 through 2004. (From March of Dimes Peristats 2007: Rates of preterm birth in multifetal pregnancies 1990-2004. Available at http://www.marchofdimes.com/peristats/.)

The Clinical Presentations of Preterm Birth

Preterm birth has been called "multifactorial" because of the numerous obstetric and medical conditions that accompany it. Traditional obstetric taxonomy has not distinguished the *clinical presentations* of preterm parturition (e.g. preterm labor, pPROM, cervical insufficiency, amnionitis and/or vaginal bleeding) from *causative mechanisms* such as infection, hemorrhage, uterine distention, trauma, or fetal compromise, or from *risk factors* (e.g., multiple gestation, preeclampsia, abruptio

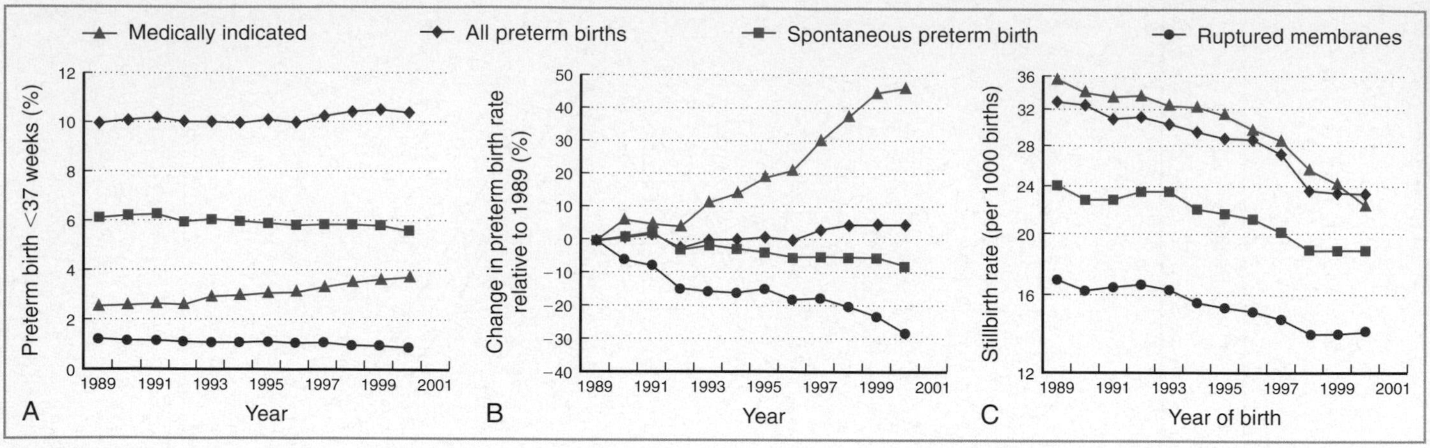

FIGURE 29-6 Temporal changes in singleton preterm births (<37 weeks) overall and in preterm births resulting from ruptured membranes, medically indicated preterm labor, and spontaneous preterm labor in the United States and in stillbirths, all races, 1989-2000. **A,** Rates in each group by year. **B,** The percentage change in rates relative to 1989. **C,** Temporal trends in stillbirth rates. (Adapted from Ananth CVP, Joseph KSM, Oyelese YM, et al: Trends in preterm birth and perinatal mortality among singletons: United States, 1989 through 2000. Obstet Gynecol 105:1084-1091, 2005.)

placentae, placenta previa, fetal growth restriction, maternal diabetes, hypertension, pyelonephritis). Designation of a clinical presentation such as preterm labor and pPROM as separate pathogenic entities has impaired understanding of the pathways leading to preterm birth. It is more useful to understand preterm birth in the two broad categories mentioned—as the result of preterm pathologic initiation of one or more steps in the parturitional process, or as a means to resolve maternal or fetal risk related to continuing the pregnancy.

The concept of spontaneous versus indicated preterm birth offered by Meis and colleagues is consistent with this distinction.[19] *Indicated* preterm deliveries, which account for about 25% of preterm births in the United States, follow medical or obstetric conditions that would create undue risk for the mother (e.g., maternal sepsis, hypoxia), the fetus (e.g., poorly controlled maternal diabetes, intrauterine growth restriction), or both (e.g., maternal hypertension, placenta previa or abruption) if the pregnancy were to continue. The most common diagnoses preceding an indicated preterm birth are preeclampsia (40%), fetal distress (25%), intrauterine growth restriction (10%), placental abruption (7%), and fetal demise (7%).[19,20] Other common causes include pregestational and gestational diabetes, renal disease, Rh sensitization, and congenital malformations.[21,22]

Spontaneous preterm births, on the other hand, follow preterm labor, pPROM, or related diagnoses such as cervical insufficiency or amnionitis when labor begins in the absence of overt maternal or fetal illness that would otherwise require delivery. Risk factors associated with spontaneous preterm birth include genital tract colonization and infection, nonwhite race, multiple gestation, bleeding in the second trimester, low pre-pregnancy weight, and a history of previous spontaneous preterm birth.[23] Approximately 75% of preterm births are spontaneous.[19,24,25]

The distinction between indicated and spontaneous preterm births is not always clear but provides a framework for evaluation of trends and causes of preterm delivery. For example, an increase in indicated preterm births accounts for much of the recent rise in late preterm births and in the overall preterm birth rate in the United States (Fig. 29-6A,B). This increase has been accompanied by a decline in fetal mortality (see Fig. 29-6C), especially after 28 weeks, suggesting that the increased rate of preterm births may reflect improved prenatal care.

Consequences of Preterm Birth

(See Also Chapter 58)

Definitions of Perinatal and Infant Mortality

The *perinatal mortality rate* is the total of fetal deaths after 20 weeks' gestation plus neonatal deaths through the first 28 days of life, per 1000 births (live births + fetal deaths) after 20 weeks' gestation.[1] Preterm birth is the leading cause of perinatal and infant mortality for infants born to women of all races and ethnic backgrounds, and particularly for non-Hispanic black women.[2,26]

The *infant mortality rate* is the number of deaths of live-born infants before 1 year of age per 1000 live births. Figure 29-7 displays the relative contribution of prematurity-related conditions to overall infant mortality in 2004 according to maternal race or ethnicity.[26] Infant mortality increases markedly as gestational age and birth weight decline. In 2001, 41% of all infants born alive before 28 weeks of gestation died within 1 year, compared with 5% of those born at 28 to 31 weeks, 1% of those born at 32 to 35 weeks, and 0.3% of those born at term.[27]

Despite the rise in the rate of preterm birth between 1990 and 2004, fetal and infant mortality rates declined over the same time interval (Fig. 29-8). The decline in perinatal mortality was related primarily to a decrease in fetal deaths after 28 weeks' gestation, corresponding to an increased rate of indicated preterm birth during this time (see Fig. 29-6). Fetal deaths account for more than half of perinatal deaths. In the United States in 2004, there were 25,655 fetal deaths (50.3% between 20 and 27 weeks, and 49.7% after 27 weeks), and 18,602 neonatal deaths (79.8% before 7 days and 20.2% between 7 and 28 days after birth).[1]

Factors Affecting Perinatal, Infant, and Childhood Mortality and Morbidity

(See Also Chapter 58)

DATA COLLECTION

Reports of survival and morbidity vary according to the denominator employed. Obstetric data sets include all living fetuses at entry to

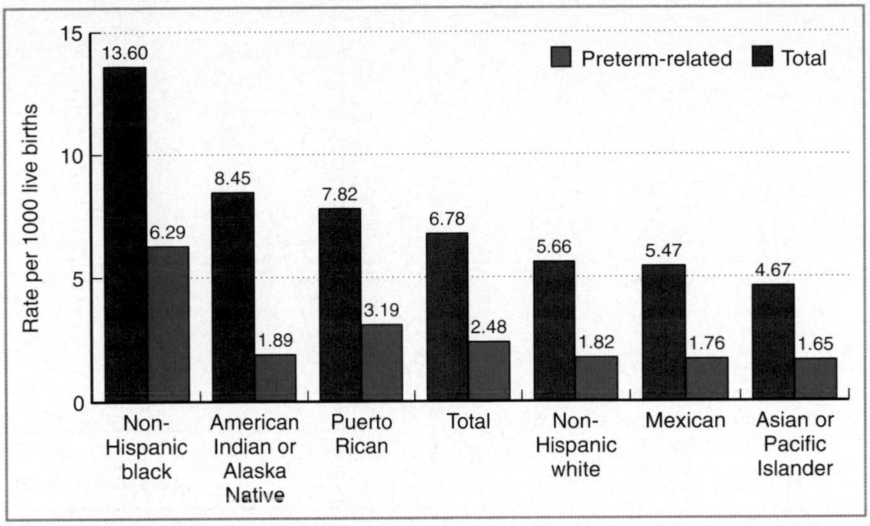

FIGURE 29-7 Total and preterm-related infant mortality rates by race or ethnicity of mother: United States, 2004. Preterm-related deaths are those in which the infant was born preterm (<37 completed weeks of gestation) and the underlying cause of death was assigned to one of the following categories from the *International Classification of Diseases, Tenth Revision:* K550, P000, P010, P011, P015, P020, P021, P070-Po73, P102, P220-229, P250-279, P280, P281, P360-P369, P520-P523, P77. The categories of American Indian or Alaska Native and Asia or Pacific Islander include persons of Hispanic and non-Hispanic origin. (From MacDorman M, Callaghan WM, Mathews TJ, et al: Trends in Preterm-Related Infant Mortality by Race and Ethnicity: United States, 1999-2004. National Center for Health Statistics, 2007. Available at http://www.cdc.gov/nchs/products/pubs/pubd/hestats/infantmort99-04/infantmort99-04.htm [accessed February 28, 2008].)

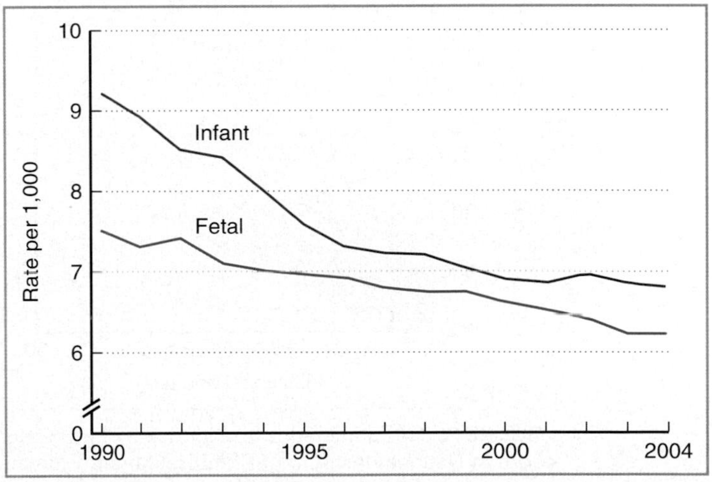

FIGURE 29-8 Fetal and infant mortality rates: United States, 1990-2004. The infant mortality rate is the number of infant deaths per 1000 live births. The fetal mortality rate is the number of fetal deaths occurring after 20 weeks' gestation per 1000 births (live births + fetal deaths). (From MacDorman MF, Munson ML, Kirmeyer S: Fetal and Perinatal Mortality—United States, 2004. Natl Vital Stat Rep 56[3]:1-19, 2007.)

the obstetric suite,[28] whereas neonatal data sets exclude intrapartum and delivery room deaths and thus report rates based on newborns admitted to the nursery.[29,30] Rates of survival and morbidity at the same gestational age and/or birth weight are therefore somewhat higher in neonatal data sets and in data from tertiary care centers.

GESTATIONAL AGE

Before delivery, gestational age is the strongest predictor of survival and morbidity for the infant. The perinatal mortality rate is strongly related to gestational age at birth, especially between 22 and 32 weeks, as was shown in data from one large center in Figure 29-9.[31] Although mortality declines sharply after 32 weeks, infants born between 32 and 36 weeks still have increased rates of adverse outcomes. A French study of outcomes at 5 years of age for infants born between 30 and 34 weeks found a progressive decline in rates of perinatal mortality and neonatal morbidity with advancing gestational age at birth. Rates of cerebral palsy and cognitive impairment at 5 years of age also declined with advancing gestational age at birth.[32]

Neonatal mortality rates at 34, 35, and 36 weeks were 1.1, 1.5, and 0.5 per 1000 live births, respectively, compared with 0.2 per 1000 live births at 39 weeks, in a report from Parkland Hospital.[33] Five percent of infants born at 34 weeks required neonatal intensive care, compared with 2% of those born at 35 weeks, 1.1% at 36 weeks, 0.6% at 37 weeks, and 0.5% at 39 weeks. More than three quarters of late preterm births followed preterm labor or ruptured membranes, with the remainder caused by obstetric complications.

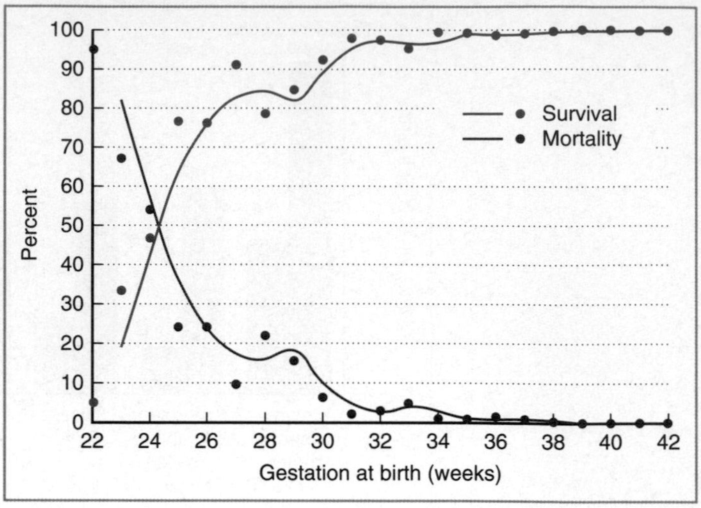

FIGURE 29-9 Survival by gestational age among live-born resuscitated infants. Results of a community-based evaluation of 8523 deliveries, 1997-1998, Shelby County, Tennessee. Curves smoothed by 2-point average. (From Mercer BM: Preterm premature rupture of the membranes. Obstet Gynecol 101:178, 2003, Figure 1.)

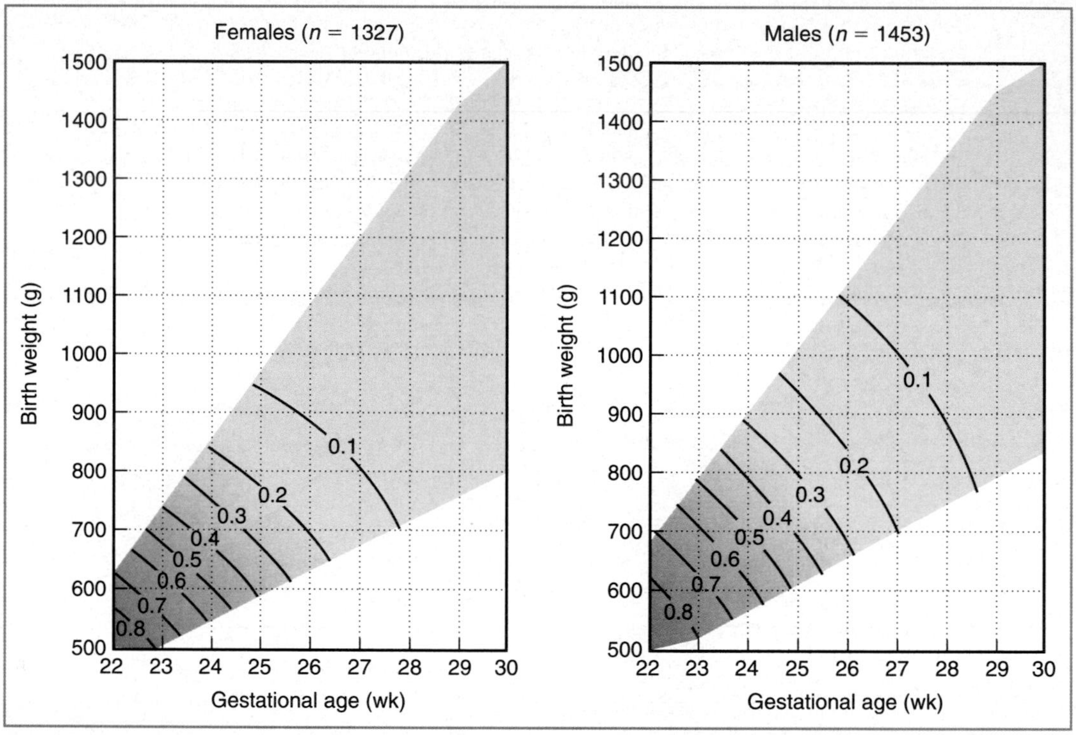

FIGURE 29-10 Estimated mortality risk by birth weight and gestational age based on singleton infants born in National Institute of Child Health and Human Development (NICHD) Neonatal Research Network centers between January 1, 1995, and December 31, 1996. Numeric values represent age- and weight-specific mortality rates and are expressed as decimal fractions (e.g., 0.7 = 70%). (From Lemons JA, Bauer CR, Oh W, et al: Very low birth weight outcomes of the National Institute of Child Health and Human Development Neonatal Research Network, January 1995 through December 1996. NICHD Neonatal Research Network. Pediatrics 107:E1, 2001. Used with permission of the American Academy of Pediatrics.)

BIRTH WEIGHT

After delivery, birth weight and gender can be combined with gestational age to predict mortality, as shown in Figure 29-10 for infants born alive between 22 and 30 weeks' gestation.[29] A recent study combined gestational age, birth weight, gender, treatment with antenatal steroids, and multiple versus singleton gestation to generate improved estimates of neonatal outcomes for infants with birth weights of 400-1000 grams.[34]

Very Low Birth Weight Infants. Regionalized care for high-risk mothers and infants, antenatal fetal treatment with glucocorticoids, neonatal administration of exogenous pulmonary surfactant, and improved ventilator technology have produced survival rates that now exceed 90%, and survival without major morbidity in more than 80% of infants born at 28 weeks' gestation or weighing 1000 g at birth.

Rates of survival with and without morbidity for VLBW infants (500 to 1500 g) born into tertiary neonatal intensive care units in the

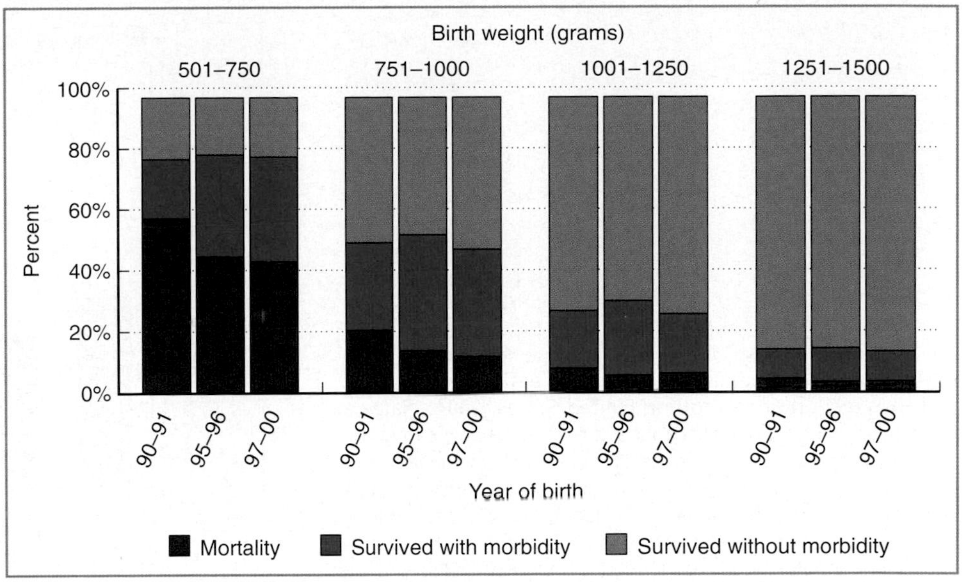

FIGURE 29-11 Changes in mortality, morbidity, and morbidity-free survival over time. Comparison of mortality, morbidity, and morbidity-free survival for very low birthweight infants cared for in twelve National Institute of Child Health and Human Development (NICHD) Neonatal Research Network Centers in 1990-1991, 1995-1996, and 1997-2000 by 250-g birth weight intervals, based on the total number of singleton infants born in the centers. (From Fanaroff AA, Stoll BJ, Wright LL, et al; NICHD Neonatal Research Network: Trends in neonatal morbidity and mortality for very low birthweight infants. Am J Obstet Gynecol 196:147.e1-147.e8, 2007.)

United States did not change appreciably from 1990 to 2000 (Fig. 29-11).[35]

Extremely Low Birth Weight Infants. Increasing attention has been paid to infants born at the periviable thresholds of age (22 to 25 weeks) and weight (400 to 600 g). In a study of singleton births between 1991 and 1996, 56.1% of 406 infants born at 24 weeks and 68% of 454 infants born at 25 weeks survived to hospital discharge.[30] Data from the Vermont Oxford and National Institute of Child Health and Human Development (NICHD) Neonatal Research Networks indicate that rates of survival and morbidity for infants born between 23 and 25 weeks' gestation are unlikely to improve any further. Survival rates for babies born into the tertiary nurseries of the NICHD Neonatal Research Network between 1996 and 2000 improved from 20% to 30% at 23 weeks but only marginally at 24 weeks (from 58% to 60%) and 25 weeks (from 75% to 80%).[36] In the Vermont Oxford data, mortality and morbidity declined steadily between 1991 and 1995 for infants weighing 501 to 1500 g but did not change between 1995 and 1999.[37] The American Academy of Pediatrics[38] and the American College of Obstetricians and Gynecologists (ACOG)[39] issued joint statements on perinatal care at the limits of viability in 2002, with recommendations based on the data reported by Lemons and colleagues in 2001[29] (see also Chapter 58).

Survival among infants born weighing less than 500 g is rare. A Vermont Oxford Network study reported that 48% of 4172 infants with birth weights between 401 and 500 g and a mean gestational age of 23.3 weeks died in the delivery room.[40] Among the 17% who survived to hospital discharge, the mean gestational age was more than 25 weeks, and significant morbidity was universal. Notably, the risk of neonatal mortality does not exceed 50% for babies of any ethnicity or race until the gestational age at birth is less than 24 weeks and birth weight is less than 500 g.[41]

MATERNAL RACE

Perinatal deaths vary significantly by maternal race and ethnicity. The perinatal mortality rate in 2004 for infants born to non-Hispanic black women in the United States was 20.3 (per 1000 live births + fetal deaths), compared with 10 for all other racial and ethnic groups (Fig. 29-12).[1]

The relationship of maternal race to risk of neonatal mortality is complex. African-American infants have a greater overall perinatal mortality rate than do whites or Hispanics. This higher risk is related to increased risk of stillbirth at all gestational ages and increased risk of neonatal mortality for infants born at term and post-term. However, neonatal mortality rates for black preterm and LBW infants are lower than for other ethnic groups.[41]

OTHER FACTORS

Mortality rates for preterm and VLBW infants are lower if the child is female (odds ratio [OR], 0.42; 95% confidence interval [CI], 0.29 to 0.61), is growth restricted (OR, 0.58; CI, 0.38 to 0.88), or was treated with antenatal corticosteroids (OR, 0.52; CI, 0.36 to 0.76), compared with infants at the same gestational age who are male, were normally grown, or did not receive antenatal steroids.[42,43] Intrauterine infection adversely influences survival and morbidity.[43] Mortality rates also vary among neonatal intensive care units, despite similar care practices and patient demographics.[44] Therefore, local statistics are preferred when counseling patients.

Perinatal Morbidity

Preterm infants are at risk for specific diseases related to the immaturity of various organ systems and the cause and circumstances of preterm birth. Common complications in premature infants include respiratory distress syndrome (RDS), intraventricular hemorrhage (IVH), bronchopulmonary dysplasia (BPD), patent ductus arteriosus (PDA), necrotizing enterocolitis (NEC), sepsis, apnea, and retinopathy of prematurity (ROP).

The frequency of major morbidity rises as gestational age decreases, especially before 32 weeks. There is wide geographic variation in the frequency of neonatal morbidities, especially for VLBW infants.[44] Typical rates for the most common morbidities among survivors are shown according to gestational age in Figure 29-13, from a single center,[31] and by birth weight in Table 29-1, from a tertiary care network.[35]

Long-Term Outcomes

Major neonatal morbidities related to preterm birth that carry lifetime consequences include chronic lung disease, grades III and IV IVH,

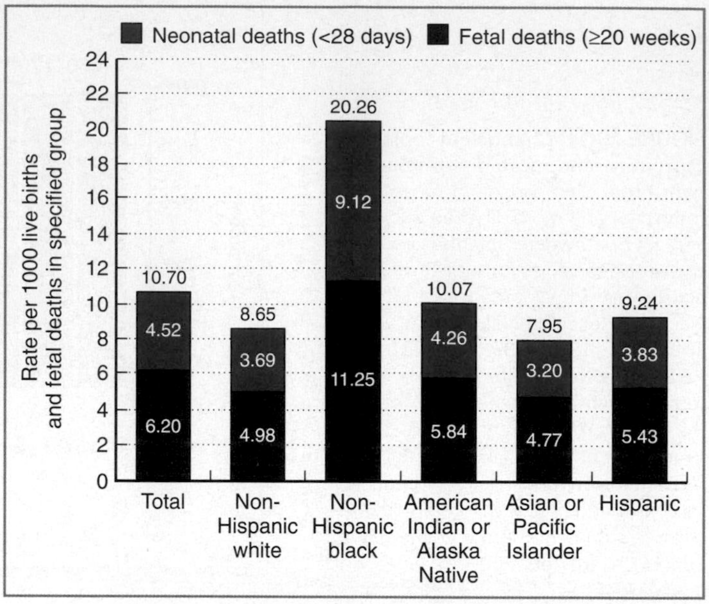

FIGURE 29-12 Perinatal mortality rates, definition II, by race and Hispanic origin of mother: United States, 2004. Rates for non-Hispanic white, non-Hispanic black, and Hispanic categories exclude data from Oklahoma, which did not report Hispanic origin for fetal deaths. Rates for subtotals do not add exactly to totals because of slight differences in the denominators used for rate computations. (From MacDorman MF, Munson ML, Kirmeyer S: Fetal and Perinatal Mortality—United States, 2004. Natl Vital Stat Rep 56[3]:1-19, 2007.)

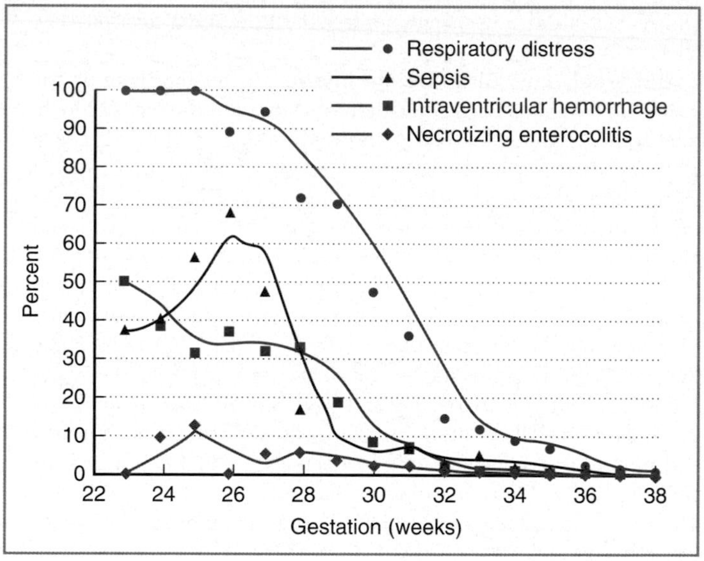

FIGURE 29-13 Acute morbidity by gestational age among surviving infants. Results of a community-based evaluation of 8523 deliveries, 1997-1998, Shelby County, Tennessee. Curves smoothed by 2-point average. (From Mercer BM: Preterm premature rupture of membranes. Obstet Gynecol 101:178, 2003, Figure 2.)

NEC, and vision and hearing impairment. Increased rates of cerebral palsy, neurosensory impairment, reduced cognition and motor performance, academic difficulties, and attention deficit disorders are reported for preterm infants and rise in frequency as the gestational age at birth declines.[28,45-47] Approximately one third of cerebral palsy cases have been attributed to early preterm birth (<32 weeks of gestation).[48] A study of 308 surviving infants born before 25 weeks found that almost all had some disability at age 6 years: 22% had severe neurocognitive disabilities (cerebral palsy, IQ >3 standard deviations below the mean, blind, or deaf), 24% had moderate disability, 34% had mild disability, and 20% had no neurocognitive disability.[47]

Health care workers regularly overestimate the likelihood and severity of neurologic morbidity in infants born preterm.[49] This is important, because these expectations may adversely influence outcomes (Figs. 29-14 and 29-15).[50,51]

Self-esteem among prematurely born infants followed to adolescence does not differ from that among persons born at term. Although 24% of 132 adolescents who weighed less than 1 kg at birth had significant sensory deficits, they did not differ from controls of normal birth weight in their self-perception of global self-worth, scholastic or job competence, or social acceptance.[52]

Epidemiology and Risk Factors for Preterm Birth

Spontaneous preterm birth is similar to other multifactorial disorders, such as cancer or heart disease, wherein multiple endogenous and exogenous risk factors interact to cause disease. In the case of spontaneous preterm birth, such interaction generates the premature and often asynchronous initiation of one or more steps in parturition. Thus, the risk factors for preterm labor are similar to those for pPROM and cervical insufficiency.

TABLE 29-1 PERCENTAGE OF VERY-LOW-BIRTH-WEIGHT INFANTS SURVIVING WITH SELECTED NEONATAL MORBIDITIES*

	501-750 g (*n* = 4,046)	751-1,000 g (*n* = 4,266)	1,001-1,250 g (*n* = 4,557)	1,251-1,500 g (*n* = 5,284)	501-1,500 g (*n* = 18,153)
Survived	55 (38-76)	88 (74-94)	94 (91-97)	96 (93-99)	85 (79-93)
Survived without morbidity	35	57	78	89	70
Survived with Morbidity†					
Overall	65 (48-80)	43 (27-63)	22 (10-33)	11 (5-19)	30 (21-43)
BPD alone	42 (15-61)	25 (5-42)	11 (1-21)	4 (0-9)	17 (4-26)
Severe IVH‡	5 (0-13)	6 (2-17)	5 (<1-8)	4 (0-12)	5 (2-10)
NEC alone	3 (0-16)	3 (1-13)	3 (<1-8)	2 (0-5)	3 (<1-7)
BPD and severe IVH	10 (3-17)	4 (2-11)	2 (0-5)	<1 (0-2)	3 (1-6)
BPD and NEC	4 (0-9)	3 (0-6)	<1 (0-2)	<1 (0-2)	2 (<1-3)
NEC and severe IVH	<1 (0-5)	<1 (0-2)	<1 (0-1)	<1 (0-<1)	<1 (0-1)
BPD and severe IVH and NEC	1 (0-3)	<1 (0-3)	<1 (0-<1)	<1 (0-<1)	<1 (0-<1)

*Data shown as % (range) for infants born in all participating National Institute of Child Health and Human Development (NICHD) Neonatal Research Network centers between January 1, 1998, and December 31, 2002.
†Morbidity is defined as a diagnosis of BPD, IVH grade III or IV, or proven NEC.
‡Severe IVH is defined as grade III (blood in the ventricles with ventriculomegaly) or grade IV (blood/echodensity in the parenchyma).
BPD, bronchopulmonary dysplasia; IVH, intraventricular hemorrhage; NEC, necrotizing enterocolitis.
From Fanaroff AA, Stoll BJ, Wright LL, et al; NICHD Neonatal Research Network. Trends in neonatal morbidity and mortality for very low birthweight infants. Am J Obstet Gynecol 196:147.e1-147.e8, 2007.

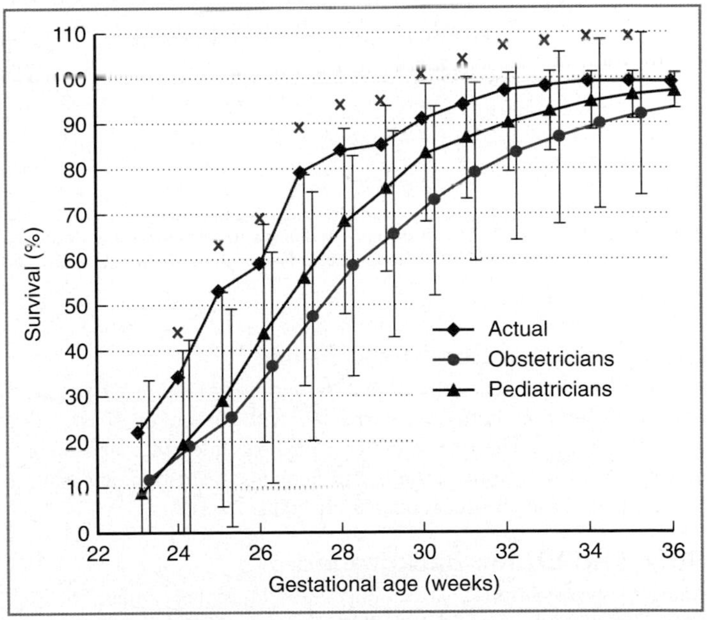

FIGURE 29-14 Estimated versus actual survival rates. Comparison of actual rates of survival of infants born preterm with rates estimated by obstetricians and pediatricians. Error bars represent ±1 standard deviation. ×, $P < .05$. (From Morse SB, Haywood JL, Goldenberg RL, et al: Estimation of neonatal outcome and perinatal therapy use. Pediatrics 105:1046-1050, 2000.)

Maternal Characteristics

Familial Risk

Studies showing familial risk patterns suggest that there is a genetic predisposition for preterm birth. Women whose sisters have had a preterm birth have a 1.8-fold higher risk of preterm delivery,[53] and grandparents of women who deliver preterm are more likely to have been preterm themselves than the grandparents of women who deliver at term.[54] Genetic association studies have discovered polymorphisms in several genes in the mother and the fetus associated with spontaneous preterm birth[55-57] and LBW.[58] Gene-environment interaction was identified in a study wherein neither maternal bacterial vaginosis (BV) nor maternal carriage of an allele of the tumor necrosis factor-α (TNF-α) gene was associated with spontaneous preterm birth if present alone, but the combination significantly increased risk of preterm birth.[59] Another study demonstrated that a polymorphism in the interleukin 6 (IL-6) gene was related to an increased risk of spontaneous preterm birth in African-American women with BV but was not linked to preterm birth risk in African-American women who did not have BV or in Caucasian women regardless of BV status.[55] An interaction between maternal smoking and a genetic polymorphism that increases the likelihood of LBW has also been identified.[58] These studies support a role for gene-environment interactions in the pathogenesis of spontaneous preterm birth. Studies to date have employed the candidate gene approach to study DNA variants of biologically suspected genes, but these are being replaced by whole genome association studies which hold promise for improved understanding of the genetic basis of preterm birth and its sequelae.[60,61]

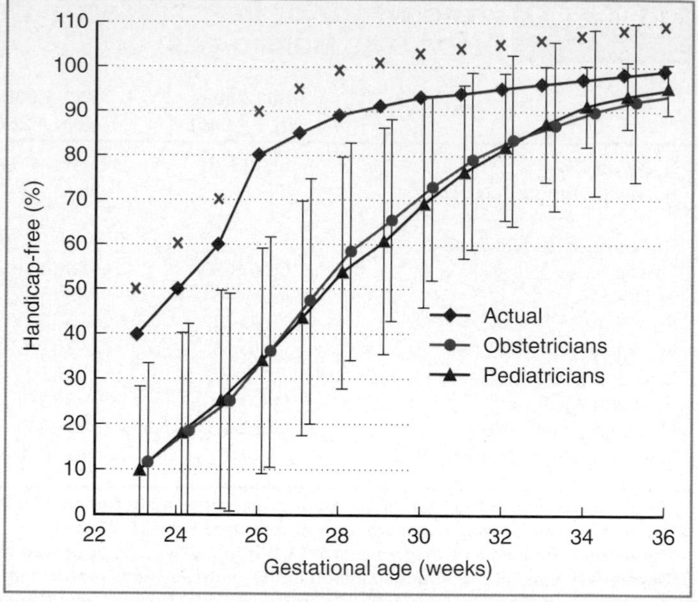

FIGURE 29-15 Estimated versus actual rates of freedom from handicap. Comparison of actual rates of survival free from handicap of infants born preterm with rates estimated by obstetricians and pediatricians. Error bars represent ±1 standard deviation. ×, P < .05. (From Morse SB, Haywood JL, Goldenberg RL, et al: Estimation of neonatal outcome and perinatal therapy use. Pediatrics 105:1046-1050, 2000.)

TABLE 29-2 RISK OF PRETERM BIRTH (%) BY MATERNAL RACE AND EDUCATION

Years of Education	Non-Hispanic Black	Non-Hispanic White	Asian or Pacific Islander	Native American (American Indian and Eskimo)	Hispanic
<8	19.6	11.0	11.5	14.8	10.7
8-12	16.8	9.9	10.5	11.8	10.4
13-15	14.5	8.3	9.1	9.9	9.3
≥16	12.8	7.0	7.5	9.4	8.4

Data from Behrman RE, Stith Butler A (eds); Institute of Medicine Committee on Understanding Preterm Birth and Assuring Healthy Outcomes: Preterm Birth: Causes, Consequences, and Prevention. Washington, DC: National Academies Press, 2007.

Education and Economic Status

Low socioeconomic and educational status, low or high maternal age, and single marital status are correlated with an increased risk of preterm birth.[62,63] The rate of preterm birth declines with advancing education for all ethnic groups but remains higher among non-Hispanic blacks at all educational levels (Table 29-2).

Race and Ethnic Background

Rates of preterm birth are almost twofold higher among black (African-American, and Afro-Caribbean) women (16% to 18%) than in Asian, Hispanic, and white women in the United States and Great Britain. Preterm births before 32 weeks are also significantly increased in black women compared with women from other racial or ethnic groups (Fig. 29-16).[64]

Rates of preterm and LBW infants remain higher for black women, compared with white, Asian, or Hispanic women, after controlling for social disadvantage[65] and education. Remarkably, preterm birth rates are higher for well-educated, non-Hispanic black women than for poorly educated, non-Hispanic white, Asian, or Hispanic women (see Table 29-2).

Rates of preterm birth among Arab-American women are the same or lower than among non-Hispanic white women, despite increased socioeconomic risk.[66] Rates of preterm delivery among black women born outside the United States are generally lower than among African-American women or among Afro-Caribbean women living in the United Kingdom,[67] suggesting a risk induced or enhanced by residence in the United States or Britain. Acute or short-term stress in pregnancy has a weak relationship to the risk of preterm birth, but chronic stress, such as might be experienced by persons of color, has a stronger link to preterm birth (see later discussion).

Maternal Behaviors and Environment

Maternal smoking is related to poor pregnancy outcomes such as growth restriction, placental abruption, infant mortality, and preterm birth, but the relationship to preterm birth is modest.[68-70] A population-based study of more than 300,000 singleton births found a dose-related association between spontaneous preterm birth and smoking more than 10 cigarettes per day (OR, 1.7).[71] Smoking is important because of its high prevalence (20% to 25% of pregnant women smoke) and the potential for successful intervention.[72] The mechanisms by which smoking is related to preterm birth are unclear, but nicotine and carbon monoxide are vasoconstrictors that decrease uteroplacental blood flow. The observed decrease in fetal weight is not surprising.

Substance abuse may be linked to preterm birth risk through concurrent exposure to lifestyle-related risk factors such as limited prenatal care, nutritional deficits, genital tract infections, and cigarette smoking. Marijuana has not been independently related to preterm birth. Initial reports associating cocaine with preterm birth due to abruption may have been influenced by ascertainment bias; the magnitude of the risk of preterm birth among cocaine users is now con-

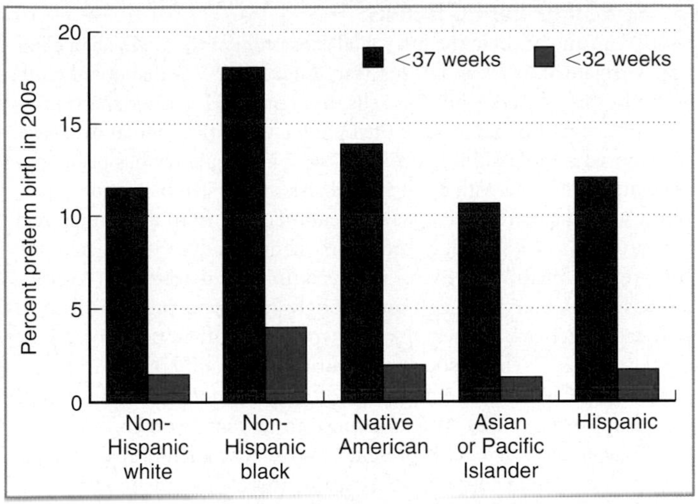

FIGURE 29-16 Rates of preterm birth, by race/ethnicity of mother: United States, 2005. (From Hamilton BE, Martin JA, Ventura SJ: Births: Preliminary data for 2005. Health E-Stats. Natl Vital Stat Rep 55, 2006.)

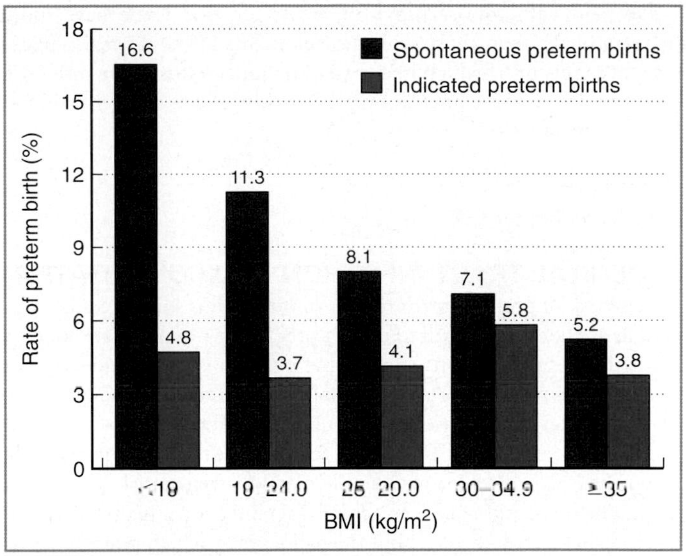

FIGURE 29-17 Comparison of rates of spontaneous and indicated preterm birth by maternal body-mass index (BMI). (Adapted from Hendler I, Goldenberg RL, Mercer BM, et al: The Preterm Prediction Study: Association between maternal body mass index [BMI] and spontaneous preterm birth. Am J Obstet Gynecol 192:882-886, 2005.)

sidered uncertain.[9] Maternal alcohol consumption has a complex association with preterm birth, with some studies showing no relationship or even a modest reduction in the rate of preterm birth among light drinkers[20,73] and others confirming an increased risk related to regular and heavy alcohol intake.[73,74]

Psychological Factors

Stress during pregnancy is a topic of great public interest, but evidence to address this concern is inadequate. Studies relating preterm birth risk to stress in pregnancy suffer from methodologic variation but generally report a modest relationship, with relative risks (RR) of 1.3 to 1.4 for stressful life events such as death of a family member, loss of employment, or divorce.[75,76] Stress is often accompanied by other known risk factors, such as socioeconomic disadvantage, smoking, or African-American ethnicity. Lu and Chen found that adding stress to a statistical model of risk factors for preterm birth in 33,542 women had little effect on the observed relationship between race and preterm birth; they concluded that stressful life events, even events immediately preceding or during pregnancy, do not significantly contribute to racial and ethnic disparities in preterm birth.[77] Evidence that *chronic* stress is related to preterm birth risk is more robust[78] and suggests that stress may increase risk by altering immunologic function.[79-83] Chronic stress related to racism is a potential explanation for the disparity in preterm birth rates between African-American or Afro-Caribbean women and women of other ethnic backgrounds.[83]

Depression before and during pregnancy is being recognized as a risk factor for adverse pregnancy outcomes including preterm birth. Clinical depression occurs in as many as 15% to 35% of women. The reported relationship between depression and risk of preterm birth is modest (less than twofold).[84,85] Risk factors for depression are similar to those related to preterm birth and include non-Hispanic black race, young age, limited education, and exposure to stressful life events.[86] Depressed mood has been reported to correlate with reduced natural killer cell activity and increased plasma concentrations of proinflammatory cytokines,[87] so alterations in immune response may partially mediate the relationship between depression and preterm birth.

Maternal Physical Activity

Work and physical activity have been studied in relation to risk of preterm birth, with conflicting results. Although rates of preterm birth are lower in women who are employed compared with those who are unemployed, the risk among employed women may be increased by work that is physically demanding or stressful. In a European study, the risk of preterm birth was not related to employment per se but was increased among women who worked more than 42 hr/wk (OR, 1.33; CI, 1.1 to 1.6) or who were required to stand for more than 6 hr/day (OR, 1.26; CI, 1.1 to 1.5).[88] Work while standing was associated with preterm birth (OR, 1.56; CI, 1.04 to 2.60) in a study from Guatemala,[89] but this finding was not observed by researchers from North Carolina, where the risk of preterm birth was higher in women who worked nights compared with those who worked days.[90] There are no data to relate specific work tasks to preterm birth risk.

Coitus during pregnancy commonly leads to a transient increase in uterine activity[91] and is an opportunity to acquire genital tract infections, but self-reported sexual activity was not related to the risk of preterm birth in a study of women with a prior preterm birth.[92] The practice of douching before or during pregnancy has been suggested to increase the risk of preterm birth, but the association is confounded by the higher prevalence of BV in African-American women, who are more likely to practice douching.[93,94]

Nutritional Status

The risk of preterm birth has been related to maternal nutritional status during pregnancy, as measured by body mass index (BMI), nutritional intake, and serum markers of nutritional status.[95-97] For example, a low pre-pregnancy BMI is associated with higher risks of spontaneous preterm birth, whereas obesity may be protective (Fig. 29-17).[95] One study found that a low BMI was more strongly related to preterm birth risk among African-American and Hispanic women than among white women.[98]

Women with low serum iron, folate, or zinc levels have more preterm births than those with measurements in the normal range.[97] The mechanisms by which maternal nutritional status might influence preterm birth risk are unclear but may involve effects on uterine blood flow or resistance to infection.[97,99,100]

Infections

(See Also Chapter 28)

GENITAL TRACT INFECTION AND COLONIZATION

The risk of preterm birth related to infection is sometimes considered as a risk that is acquired during pregnancy—an accurate concept for extragenital infections such as pyelonephritis or pneumonia, but one that does not fully apply to genital tract colonization and infection. Pre-pregnancy colonization of the upper and lower genital tract and the maternal immune response to that colonization are increasingly recognized as important aspects of infection-related risk of preterm birth. The correlation between genital tract infection and preterm birth has long been recognized,[101] but the pathways by which infection leads to preterm birth have not, until recently, been understood to involve activation of the innate immune system. Microorganisms are recognized by pattern-recognition receptors such as Toll-like receptors, which, in turn, elicit the release of inflammatory chemokines and cytokines such as IL-8, IL-1β, and TNF-α. During intrauterine infection, microbial products and proinflammatory cytokines stimulate the production of prostaglandins and other inflammatory mediators as well as matrix-degrading enzymes. Prostaglandins stimulate uterine contractility, and degradation of extracellular matrix in the fetal membranes leads to pPROM.[60,102] The contribution of infection to preterm birth has been estimated to be 25% to 40% based on microbiologic studies, but this may be an underestimate, because intrauterine infection is difficult to detect with conventional culture techniques. For example, molecular microbiologic studies based on the polymerase chain reaction (PCR) have revealed evidence of *Ureaplasma urealyticum* in amniotic fluid samples with negative cultures.[103-106]

Intrauterine colonization and infection can occur in the decidua, the chorioamnionic space, or the amniotic cavity. Because microbial colonization is more common in the chorioamnion than within the amniotic cavity, amniotic fluid cultures underestimate the contribution of infection to preterm birth. However, bacteria are known to be present in the chorioamnion in women who deliver healthy infants at term,[107] indicating that bacteria in the chorioamnion do not always generate an inflammatory response that leads to preterm labor and birth. The most common pathway by which microorganisms gain access to the choriodecidua and amniotic cavity is probably ascent from the vagina and the cervix, but the timing of this spread is uncertain. It may occur before or during pregnancy.[108] Regardless of when colonization occurs, intrauterine inflammation is postulated to cause clinical symptoms, such as vaginal discharge, cervical effacement, ruptured membranes, or labor, only when microbial counts increase as the membranes try to adhere to the decidua in the second trimester.[61,102] This phenomenon is consistent with the strong association between increased concentrations of fetal fibronectin, the choriodecidual "glue," in vaginal fluid between 13 and 22 weeks' gestation, with spontaneous preterm birth in the second trimester.[109] The microorganisms most commonly recovered from the amniotic cavity and chorioamnion are genital mycoplasma species, especially *U. urealyticum,* and other organisms of low virulence, consistent with the chronicity of intrauterine infections and the frequent lack of overt clinical signs of infection.[102]

SPECIFIC INFECTIONS

BV, an alteration in the microbial ecosystem of the vagina, is a clinical correlate of lower and upper tract infection. BV is diagnosed clinically by the presence of clue cells, a vaginal pH greater than 4.5, a profuse white discharge, and a fishy odor when the vaginal discharge is exposed to potassium hydroxide.[110] BV in pregnancy has been consistently associated with an increased risk of preterm birth, but apparently only as a marker, because eradication of BV from the genital tract of pregnant women does not consistently reduce the likelihood of preterm birth.[111,112] BV is more commonly detected in African-American women, and is more strongly related to preterm birth in African-American women than in women of other racial or ethnic backgrounds.[113] This association is unrelated to differences in sexual behaviors.[114] Moreover, eradication of BV does not reduce the risk of preterm birth in either African-American or white women.[112,115]

Trichomonas vaginalis is present in 3.1% of women of reproductive age, and it is more common in African-American women (13%) than in other groups.[116] It has been associated with a modest increase in the risk of preterm birth (RR, 1.3) in some studies[117] but not in all.[118]

Sexually transmitted infections, including *Chlamydia trachomatis* (in the presence of a maternal immune response),[119] syphilis, and gonorrhea, confer an increased risk of preterm birth of approximately twofold,[120] but eradication of these organisms does not reduce that risk, again suggesting involvement of host factors.

Clinical markers of genital tract infection that correlate with an increased risk of preterm birth include the detection of BV and an increased level of fetal fibronectin in cervicovaginal fluid after 22 weeks' gestation.[121]

Extragenital infections including pyelonephritis, asymptomatic bacteriuria, pneumonia, and appendicitis are associated with preterm birth.[122,123]

PERIDONTAL DISEASE

Maternal periodontal disease has been linked to an increased risk of preterm birth,[124] but the basis for the association is uncertain.[125] It most likely results from shared variations in the inflammatory response to microorganisms in the oral and genital tracts.[126-129] Goepfert and colleagues demonstrated that, after adjusting for other factors, periodontal disease was not related to increased intrauterine bacterial colonization, histologic chorioamnionitis, or cord blood cytokine levels.[130]

The biologic pathway explaining the relationship between periodontal disease and preterm birth is unknown. Variations in host response to microbial colonization related to genetic polymorphisms or concurrent environmental exposures, or both, have been proposed as contributors to the disparate rates of preterm birth among ethnic groups, particularly in relation to infection-driven preterm birth,[58,131] and may apply to other inflammation at extragenital sites, such as periodontal inflammation.

Reproductive History

Prior Spontaneous Preterm Birth

Although most women who experience a preterm birth will deliver at term in subsequent pregnancies, the recurrence risk for spontaneous preterm birth is twofold or higher. This yields an actual risk that ranges from 15% to 20% to more than 50% to 60% when maternal race, ethnicity, and the number and gestational age of prior preterm deliveries are considered.[4,132-137] The recurrence risk rises in women of all races as the number of prior preterm births increases, with a twofold rise

TABLE 29-3 RISK OF PRETERM BIRTH IN SUBSEQUENT PREGNANCIES

First Birth	Second Birth	Subsequent Preterm Birth (%)
Not preterm		4.4
Preterm		17.2
Not preterm	Not preterm	2.6
Preterm	Not preterm	5.7
Not preterm	Preterm	11.1
Preterm	Preterm	28.4

From Bakketeig LS, Hoffman HJ: Epidemiology of preterm birth: Results from a longitudinal study of births in Norway. In Elder MG, Hendricks CH (eds): Preterm Labor. London, Butterworths, 1981, p. 17.

for each prior preterm birth.[23] The most recent birth is the most predictive, as was demonstrated in a Norwegian study (Table 29-3).

The risk increases further as the gestational age of the index preterm birth declines, especially with gestational age before 32 weeks.[4,9] A prior preterm birth as early as 16 to 18 weeks has been found to confer an increased risk in subsequent pregnancies.[7,9,138]

The risk of recurrence is almost twofold higher for non-Hispanic black women than for any other group. Adams and colleagues related maternal race and gestational age of the initial preterm birth to recurrence risk.[137] If the first preterm birth occurred before 32 weeks, the risk of recurrent preterm birth was 28% for white women but 36% for African-American women.

When multiple risk factors occur in African-American women, recurrence rates approximating 50% have been reported.[139,140] In a placebo-controlled trial of 17α-hydroxyprogesterone caproate (17P) to reduce the risk of preterm birth, 54% of women in the placebo arm delivered before 37 weeks, and 30.7% delivered before 35 weeks. The mean gestational age at delivery in the qualifying pregnancy was 31.3 ± 4.2 weeks; 46% of subjects had more than one prior preterm birth, and 59% were African-American.[139] In another study of 611 women with one (75%) or more (25%) prior preterm births, 40% delivered before 37 weeks, and 25% delivered before 35 weeks of gestation. One quarter of the subjects in this trial were African-American.[140] These rates are consistent with prior studies showing a 1.5- to 2-fold increased risk for each risk factor (African-American race, more than one prior preterm birth, and gestational age <32 weeks)[4,7,9,135] and with prior observational studies.[141]

The mechanisms of recurrence are not clear but have been related to short cervix,[135] infection,[142] and short inter-pregnancy interval. After adjusting for confounding variables, a short interval between pregnancies is associated with a twofold increased risk of preterm birth.[143-145] A short interpregnancy interval is more common among women whose first birth was preterm.

Prior preterm birth of twins confers an increased risk of preterm birth in a subsequent singleton pregnancy that is related to the gestational age at delivery of the index twin pregnancy.[136,146,147] Menard and coworkers[146] studied the outcome of singleton pregnancies after a twin pregnancy and found a 40% risk of preterm birth in a subsequent singleton gestation if the twin birth occurred before 30 weeks' gestation, a modestly increased risk when the twin birth was at 30 to 33 weeks, and no increased risk if the twin birth occurred between 33 and 37 weeks. Facco and colleagues[147] found a fivefold increased risk of preterm birth in women who had previously delivered preterm twins, compared with women whose twin pregnancy was delivered at term.

Prior Indicated Preterm Birth

Women with indicated preterm births also have an increased risk of another indicated preterm birth, because the underlying condition (e.g., maternal diabetes, hypertension) often persists.[4,148] Unexplained fetal growth restriction can also be recurrent.[149,150]

Uterine Anomalies

Women with müllerian duct fusion anomalies have an increased risk of pregnancy loss, with clinical presentations that vary according to uterine anatomy, cervical involvement, and placental implantation site.[151,152] Preterm births are reported in 25% to 50% of pregnancies among women with uterine malformations.[153,154] Among 246 pregnancies in 130 women with uterine anomalies, 20.3% were delivered preterm, 8.5% delivered in the second trimester, and 25% were first trimester losses.[154] The preterm birth rate was particularly increased (approximately 35%) in women with bicornuate, didelphys, or arcuate uteri, compared to those with septate or subseptate uteri (approximately 15%) in this report. Müllerian fusion anomalies may involve the cervix as well as the uterine cavity, so the clinical presentation may include cervical insufficiency, bleeding related to abnormal placental implantation, and preterm labor. Clinical presentations leading to preterm birth in a study of 61 women with uterine anomalies included preterm labor in 39%, pPROM in 13.7%, and abruption in 5.9%.[155] Prenatal exposure to diethylstilbestrol is associated with an increased risk of preterm labor and birth related to the typical T-shaped uterine anomaly.[156]

Pregnancy Termination

A history of elective abortion has been related to an increased risk of preterm birth in subsequent pregnancies.[157-159] In one study, a history of elective abortion was associated with an increased risk for subsequent preterm birth between 22 and 32 weeks of gestation (OR, 1.5; CI, 1.1 to 2.0). Women with more than one elective termination had a higher risk, especially for preterm births before 28 weeks' gestation.[159] Another case-control survey of 2938 preterm and 4781 term births in 10 countries reported that women with a history of induced abortions were significantly more likely to have a subsequent spontaneous preterm delivery. A prior elective abortion did not affect the risk of subsequent indicated preterm birth. The risk of preterm birth increased with the number of abortions, and the strength of the association increased with decreasing gestational age at birth.[158] In another study of 12,432 women, rates of preterm delivery were compared according to the occurrence and number of previous induced abortions; other risk factors were controlled. Previous induced abortion was associated with an increased risk of preterm birth (OR, 1.4; CI, 1.1 to 1.8), and the risk of preterm delivery increased with the number of previous induced abortions (OR, 1.3; CI, 1.0 to 1.7 for one previous abortion, and OR, 1.9; CI, 1.2 to 2.8 for two or more).[160]

The magnitude of the risk of preterm birth related to elective abortion is small but appears to be real. The association could be related to cervical injury but may also be the result of colonization of the upper genital tract. This possibility was suggested by a study that compared subsequent pregnancy outcomes in women who had a prior surgical versus medical abortion and found no difference in the rate of subsequent preterm birth between the two groups.[161] No comparison was made with preterm birth in women without a history of pregnancy termination.

Cervical Surgery

Women treated for cervical intraepithelial neoplasia (CIN) with a loop electrosurgical excision procedure (LEEP), or with cervical conization using either laser or cold knife, have an increased risk of later preterm birth. The largest studies of this relationship have come from Scandinavian registries in which long term follow-up is possible.[162-164] Among 8210 women treated surgically for CIN between 1986 and 2003, the risk of preterm birth before 37 weeks of gestation was increased after cervical conization (RR, 1.99; CI, 1.81 to 2.20), as were the risks for birth between 28 and 31 weeks (RR, 2.86; CI, 2.22 to 3.70) and before 28 weeks (RR, 2.10; CI, 1.47 to 2.99). Risks of LBW and perinatal death were also increased after conization (RR, 2.06; CI, 1.83 to 2.31, and RR, 1.74; CI, 1.30 to 2.32, respectively). A Danish cohort of 11,088 women was monitored from 1991 through 2004; of 14,982 deliveries in the cohort, 542 occurred between 21 and 37 weeks. The rate of preterm birth was 3.5% in women with no previous LEEP and 6.6% in women previously treated with LEEP (OR, 1.8; CI, 1.1 to 2.9). A smaller study from a colposcopy clinic in New Zealand reported an increased risk of pPROM after treatment for CIN, particularly with laser procedures.[165]

Current Pregnancy Characteristics

Bleeding

Vaginal bleeding related to placental abruption or previa often leads to preterm delivery, but first- and second-trimester bleeding of uncertain origin is also significantly associated with subsequent spontaneous preterm birth, especially if the bleeding is recurrent or persistent.[166,167] The mechanism by which bleeding is associated with preterm birth occurring weeks later is uncertain, but it is one of several observations suggesting that injury at the maternal-fetal interface increases the risk of later preterm birth (see Chapter 28). For example, an increase in maternal serum α-fetoprotein not explained by structural fetal anomalies is a marker of fetomaternal bleeding that confers an increased risk of preterm birth[168-170]; this suggests that occult placental hemorrhage may lead to eventual preterm delivery presenting as pPROM, growth restriction, or concealed abruption. First-trimester bleeding in singleton pregnancies after assisted reproductive technology (ART) has been associated with an increased risk of preterm birth. In a review of 1432 singleton pregnancies conceived after ART, women with first-trimester bleeding had increased rates of pPROM (OR, 2.44; CI, 1.38 to 4.31), preterm birth before 37 weeks (OR, 1.64; CI, 1.05 to 2.55), and before 32 weeks preterm birth (OR, 3.05; CI, 1.12 to 8.31).[171]

Similarly, the rate of preterm birth is increased when one fetus in a multifetal gestation is lost, a finding noted among surviving singletons in multifetal gestation conceived by in vitro fertilization (IVF)[172] but not in spontaneously conceived pregnancies.[173] The risk of preterm birth is increased further in higher-order multiple gestations intentionally reduced to twins compared with spontaneous twins.[174] These reports suggest that disturbance of the intrauterine environment in the first or early second trimester is associated with increased subsequent risk of preterm parturition.

Assisted Reproductive Technologies

Preterm birth is more common in pregnancies conceived after ovulation induction and ART, including IVF and gamete and zygote intrafallopian transfer, frozen embryo transfer, and donor embryo transfer.[175] The increased rate of preterm birth after ART is observed in singleton as well as multifetal pregnancies. A review of pregnancy outcome of singletons conceived after in vitro fertilization found increased rates of perinatal mortality (OR, 2.40; CI, 1.59 to 3.63), preterm birth before 37 weeks' gestation (OR, 1.93; CI, 1.36 to 2.74) and before 33 weeks' gestation (OR, 2.99; CI, 1.54 to 5.80), as well as increased rates of VLBW (OR, 3.78; CI, 4.29 to 5.75), small for gestational age (OR, 1.59; CI, 1.20 to 2.11), and congenital malformations (OR, 1.41; CI, 1.06 to 1.88), compared with spontaneously conceived singleton infants.[176] Other meta-analyses have drawn similar conclusions: perinatal mortality, preterm birth, LBW and VLBW, and small for gestational age are all increased approximately twofold for singleton infants born after IVF.[177-179] A review of 27 studies found a threefold increased risk of birth before 32 weeks in singleton pregnancies conceived after IVF (RR, 3.27; CI, 2.03 to 5.28).[180]

Medical stimulation of ovulation (e.g., with clomiphene) is associated with an increased rate of multifetal gestation but was not, until recently, linked to an increased rate of preterm birth in singletons. Ombelet and associates[181] reported a threefold increase in births of infants before 32 weeks and weighing less than 1500 g, and a twofold increase in births before 37 weeks and weighing less than 2500 g, among women who conceived after controlled ovarian stimulation compared with spontaneous conception. The mechanisms for this observation are not known.

Multiple Gestation

(See Also Chapter 25)

Multifetal gestations have a sixfold increased risk of preterm delivery compared with singleton pregnancies. The risk increases with fetal number. Between 15% and 20% of all preterm infants are the product of the 2% to 3% of pregnancies that are multifetal. Almost 60% of twins are born preterm, most often after spontaneous labor or pPROM before 37 weeks' gestation. The remainder deliver preterm because of maternal or fetal conditions such as preeclampsia or growth restriction. Almost all higher-multiple gestations deliver preterm. Rates of preterm and LBW in multifetal pregnancies in 2004 are shown in Table 29-4.

The risk of early birth rises with the number of fetuses, suggesting uterine overdistention and fetal signaling as potential pathways to early initiation of labor. Nevertheless, many women with twins deliver after 37 weeks of gestation, suggesting that uterine stretch or distention is variably accommodated according to maternal characteristics including cervical length, physical activity, uterine tone, and other risk factors.[182-185]

The rate of preterm birth in twins has increased since 1990 (Fig. 29-18).[11] Rates of preterm birth were similar for twin pregnancies resulting from ART ($n = 231$) compared with spontaneously conceived twins ($n = 430$).[186]

Uterine Factors

UTERINE VOLUME

Increased uterine volume caused by excessive amniotic fluid or multiple gestation is a strong risk factor for preterm birth, conferring a relative risk of 6 or greater.[19]

UTERINE CONTRACTIONS

Uterine contraction frequency is related to the risk of preterm birth.[91,187,188] However, uterine contractions do not predict preterm birth well in singletons because of the wide variation in contraction frequency in normal pregnancy and the large overlap in contraction frequency between women who do and do not deliver preterm.[188] Newman and colleagues reported similar results in a study limited to twins.[185]

CERVICAL LENGTH

Digital examination is the traditional method used to detect cervical maturation and changes that predict preterm birth. As labor

TABLE 29-4 PERCENTAGE OF PRETERM AND LOW-BIRTH-WEIGHT BIRTHS BY NUMBER OF FETUSES

Births	Twin	Triplet	Quad	Quint
Gestational Age				
<32 wk	11.8	35.9	64.9	81.4
<37 wk	59.7	93.0	95.9	100
Mean age (±SD)	35.2 ± 3.6	32.1 ± 3.9	29.7 ± 4.5	28.4 ± 2.7
Birth Weight				
<1.5 kg	10.2	33.2	65.1	84.9
<2.5 kg	56.6	94.1	98.4	100
Mean weight (±SD)	2.333 ± 0.634	1.700 ± 0.559	1.276 ± 0.552	1.103 ± 0.383

From Martin JA, Hamilton BE, Sutton PD, et al: Births: Final data for 2004. Natl Vital Stat Rep 55(1):80-81, 2006.

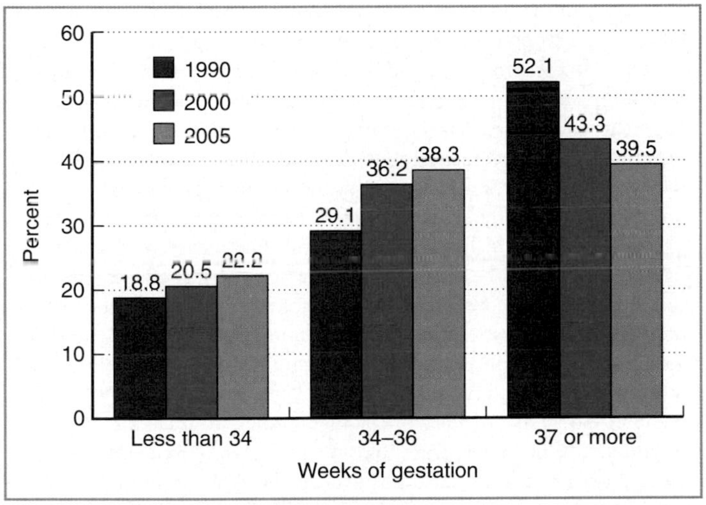

FIGURE 29-18 **Gestational age distribution of twin births: United States, 1990, 2000, and 2005.** (From Hamilton BE, Martin JA, Sutton PD, et al: Births: Final data for 2005. Natl Vital Stat Rep 56[6]:4, 2007.)

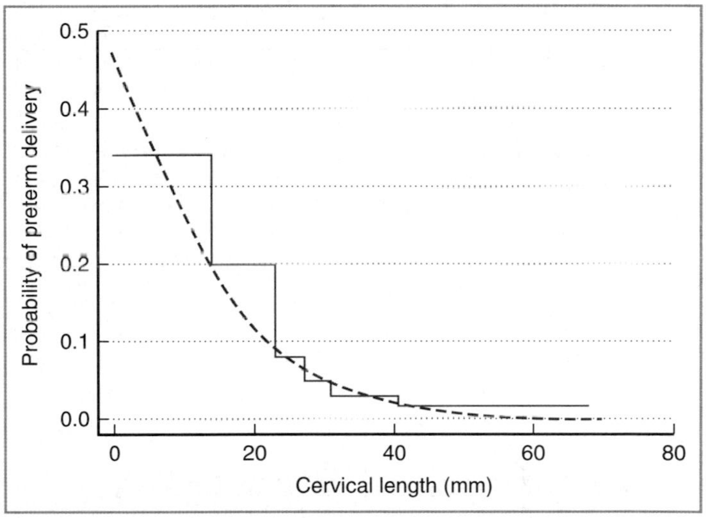

FIGURE 29-19 **Probability of spontaneous preterm delivery based on cervical length.** Estimated probability of spontaneous preterm delivery before 35 weeks of gestation from the logistic-regression analysis *(dashed line)* and observed frequency of spontaneous preterm delivery *(solid line)* according to cervical length measured by transvaginal ultrasonography at 24 weeks. (From Iams JD, Goldenberg RL, Meis PJ, et al: The length of the cervix and the risk of spontaneous premature delivery. N Engl J Med 334:567-573, 1996.)

approaches, the cervix shortens, softens, rotates anteriorly, and dilates. Although emphasis is usually placed on dilation, softening and shortening were the features of the digital examination that most strongly correlated with preterm delivery in a study of 589 nulliparous women.[189] A short cervix detected by ultrasonography is a risk factor for spontaneous preterm delivery[190-193] (Fig. 29-19).[191]

The predictive value of cervical length measurements is influenced by the gestational age at measurement. Cervical effacement in normal parturition begins at about 32 weeks, limiting the utility of cervical length measurements thereafter to excluding preterm labor in women with symptoms. Cervical length measurements before 14 to 15 weeks have no relationship to risk of preterm birth.[194] Cervical length in the second trimester has been most studied. The 50th, 10th, and 3rd percentiles between 16 and 22 weeks are approximately 40, 30, and 25 mm[192,195] when measured endovaginally with a standardized technique[196]; between 22 and 32 weeks, these percentile values are 35, 25, and 15 mm, respectively.[191,193] In an observational study of 2915 women,[191] a cervical length of 25 mm or less (the 10th percentile) at 22 to 24 weeks' gestation was associated with an RR of 6.5 (CI, 4.5 to 9.3) for preterm birth before 35 weeks and an RR of 7.7 (CI, 4.5 to 13.4) for preterm birth before 32 weeks. Serial measurements improve predictive value, but additional observations of funneling and dynamic changes do not.[197,198]

The RR and positive predictive value of cervical length measurements below the 5th percentile are influenced only slightly by a prior history of preterm birth[199,200] but such a history increases the predictive value for longer cervical lengths.[196,201,202] Berghella and associates[203] published regression analyses that demonstrate variation in predictive value of cervical length by gestational age in women with a prior preterm birth. Figure 29-20 displays the likelihood of preterm birth before 32 weeks in a woman with a previous preterm birth.[204]

Cervical insufficiency due to congenital cervical weakness, surgery, or trauma is characterized by ultrasonographic evidence of cervical shortening that is indistinguishable from cervical effacement caused by preterm activation of parturition, so the relative contribution of biophysical versus biochemical causes of short cervix and subsequent preterm birth is not clear (see Chapter 30). Regardless of cause, cervical

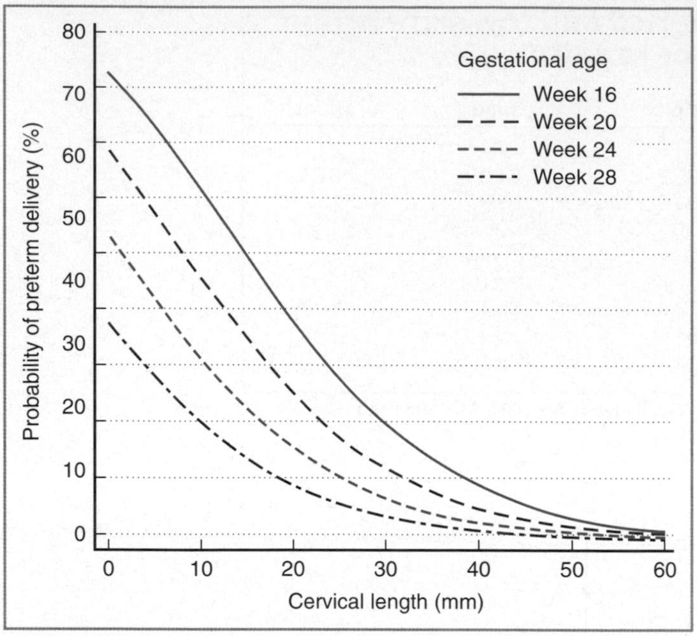

FIGURE 29-20 Predicted probability of delivery before 32 weeks of gestation, by cervical length (mm) and time of measurement (week of pregnancy), in women with a prior preterm birth. (From Berghella V. Gestational age at cervical length measurement and incidence of preterm birth. Obstet Gynecol 110:311-317, 2007.)

effacement or shortening detected by digital or ultrasound examination indicates an increased risk of preterm birth that rises as cervical length decreases.

Interventional Strategies

Efforts to prevent the morbidity and mortality associated with preterm birth may be categorized as *tertiary* (initiated after the process of parturition has begun, with a goal of preventing delivery or improving outcomes for preterm infants), *secondary* (aimed at eliminating or reducing risk in women with known risk factors), or *primary* (directed to all women before or during pregnancy to prevent and reduce risk).

Most obstetric care for preterm birth has been focused on tertiary interventions such as regionalized perinatal care, tocolysis, antenatal corticosteroids, antibiotics, and optimal timing of indicated preterm birth. These measures are intended to reduce the burden of prematurity-related illness and have minimal, if any, effect on the incidence of preterm birth. Chapter 23 describes appropriate use of antenatal glucocorticoids as a tertiary strategy to reduce perinatal morbidity and mortality regardless of the clinical presentation leading to preterm birth. This section describes clinical management of preterm labor. Chapters 30, 31, and 34 address clinical management of the related conditions of cervical insufficiency, pPROM, and fetal growth restriction, respectively.

Treatment of symptomatic preterm labor is directed at arresting labor long enough to transfer the mother to the appropriate hospital for delivery and to allow administration of corticosteroids, two interventions that consistently have been shown to reduce perinatal mortality and morbidity. Other interventions directed at reducing neonatal and infant morbidity and mortality include predelivery antibiotics and neuroprotectants.

Diagnosis of Preterm Labor

Diagnosis and treatment of preterm labor is challenging, because the sequence and timing of events that precede preterm labor are incompletely understood. Because the progression from subclinical preterm parturition to overt preterm labor is often gradual, standard criteria for the diagnosis of preterm labor (uterine contractions accompanied by cervical change) lack precision. The result is overdiagnosis in as many as 40% of women diagnosed with preterm labor and enrollment of women who are not in labor into trials of agents to arrest preterm labor.[205] Moreover, women who were treated to prevent or arrest preterm labor and were thought to have been treated successfully may not have required treatment at all; the true result of treatment is confidently known only for those whose treatment was unsuccessful. Reliable studies of methods to prevent or arrest preterm labor will not be possible until more accurate diagnostic criteria are established.

Preterm labor must be considered whenever abdominal or pelvic symptoms occur after 16 to 20 weeks' gestation. Limitation of this diagnosis to women presenting after 20 weeks is a historical custom at odds with epidemiologic and biologic evidence reviewed previously. Symptoms including pelvic pressure, increased vaginal discharge, backache, and menstrual-like cramps occur commonly during normal pregnancy, and they suggest preterm labor more by their persistence than their severity. Contractions may be painful or painless, depending on the resistance offered by the cervix. Contractions against a closed, uneffaced cervix are likely to be painful, but recurrent pressure or tightening may be the only symptoms when cervical effacement precedes the onset of contractions.[206] The traditional criteria—persistent uterine contractions accompanied by dilation and/or effacement of the cervix—are reasonably accurate if the contraction frequency is six or more per hour and cervical dilation is 3 cm or greater and/or effacement is 80% or greater, or if membranes rupture or bleeding occurs.[207,208] When lower thresholds for contraction frequency and cervical change are used, false-positive diagnosis is common,[205,207] but sensitivity does not necessarily increase.[209] Accurate diagnosis of early preterm labor is difficult, because the symptoms[210] and signs[91] of preterm labor occur commonly in normal women who do not deliver preterm, and because digital examination of the cervix in early labor (<3 cm dilation and <80% effacement) is not highly reproducible.[211-213]

Women with symptoms whose cervical dilation is less than 2 cm and/or whose effacement is less than 80% present a diagnostic challenge. In a clinical trial to identify women with true preterm labor, 179 women with preterm contractions and minimal cervical dilation were randomly assigned to receive either intravenous hydration and observation without intervention or observation after a single dose of 0.25 mg subcutaneous terbutaline.[214] Intravenous hydration did not decrease preterm contractions. Women whose contractions recurred despite transient cessation after terbutaline were more often found to be in preterm labor, leading the authors to conclude that a single dose of subcutaneous terbutaline is an efficient method of identifying true preterm labor.

Diagnostic accuracy can be improved by transvaginal sonographic measurement of cervical length and/or testing for fetal fibronectin in cervicovaginal fluid.[215-220] Both tests improve diagnostic accuracy by reducing false-positive diagnosis. Transabdominal sonography has poor reproducibility for cervical measurement and should not be used clinically without confirmation by a transvaginal ultrasound,[221] but a cervical length of 30 mm or more by endovaginal sonography suggests that preterm labor is unlikely in symptomatic women if the examination is properly performed. Similarly, a negative fibronectin test in women with symptoms before 34 weeks' gestation and cervical dilation of less than 3 cm can also reduce the rate of false-positive diagnosis if the result is returned promptly and the clinician is willing to act on a negative test result by not initiating treatment.[213,216,220]

Clinical markers for high risk of imminent preterm delivery in women with symptoms include ruptured membranes, vaginal bleeding, and cervical dilation beyond 2 cm.[222] Among women with intact membranes, no bleeding, and cervical dilation less than 3 cm, the combination of a positive fibronectin test and a sonographic cervical length of less than 30 mm predicted increased risk of delivery within 48 hours (26%); the risk was less than 7% if only one or neither test is positive.[223] The presence of debris or "sludge" in amniotic fluid near the internal os on transvaginal sonography has also been associated with increased risk of delivery within 48 hours[224] and with intra-amniotic infection[225] in women with symptoms of preterm labor.

Management of Preterm Labor

Treatments to Reduce Morbidity and Mortality

REGIONALIZATION OF CARE

Regionalization of perinatal care reduces morbidity and mortality for preterm infants, especially those born before 32 weeks of gestation[226,227] (see Chapter 58).

ANTENATAL CORTICOSTEROIDS

As discussed in Chapter 23, antenatal treatment with glucocorticoids has been shown to reduce perinatal mortality and morbidity in appropriately conducted trials and in clinical practice. Current guidelines support a single course of antenatal steroids for women at risk of preterm birth. Optimal implementation of antenatal steroid treatment is complicated by difficulty in judging the imminence of preterm birth. Because benefit is maximized by a full course of treatment and is conferred for a period of weeks after treatment, we favor administration of betamethasone or dexamethasone as soon as there is a demonstrated risk of preterm birth in the current pregnancy. We do not administer steroids solely because of a historical risk factor such as prior preterm birth, but we do consider giving steroids at the first evidence of preterm parturition after 24 weeks in the current pregnancy (e.g., bleeding, cervical change demonstrated by digital or ultrasound examination, positive test for fetal fibronectin) in women with multiple gestation or prior preterm birth. We believe that the advantage of assured receipt of steroids outweighs the likelihood that the benefit of treatment will wane before delivery.

ANTIBIOTICS

Women with preterm labor should be treated with antibiotics to prevent neonatal group B streptococcal (GBS) infection (see Chapter 38). Because preterm infants have an increased risk of neonatal GBS infection, compared to infants born at term, intrapartum prophylaxis with penicillin or ampicillin is recommended.[228] There is also evidence that infants born to women with pPROM have reduced perinatal morbidity when antepartum antibiotic prophylaxis has been administered (see Chapter 31).[23,229] Antibiotic therapy for women with preterm labor with intact membranes has not been effective in prolonging pregnancy or reducing morbidity[230-234] and should be limited to prophylaxis of GBS transmission or treatment of a specific pathogen.

NEUROPROTECTANTS

Phenobarbital given to the mother does not reduce neonatal IVH when given alone or in combination with vitamin K.[235-237]

Antenatal maternal treatment with magnesium has been inconsistently associated in observational studies with reduced rates of IVH, cerebral palsy, and perinatal mortality in premature infants.[238-243] A randomized, placebo-controlled trial of antenatal magnesium conducted in 1062 women and infants delivered before 30 weeks' gestation found significantly lower rates of gross motor dysfunction and non-significant trends toward reduced rates of mortality and cerebral palsy in surviving infants in the treated group at 2 years of age.[244] There were no significant adverse effects in infants exposed to antenatal magnesium sulfate. A randomized comparison of magnesium to placebo given before preterm birth as a neuroprotectant to 573 women and their 688 fetuses reported no evidence of harm related to magnesium.[245] Another randomized, double-masked, placebo-controlled trial conducted in 2241 women with imminent preterm birth (91% with pPROM) before 32 weeks' gestation found a 55% reduction (RR, 0.45; CI, 0.23 to 0.87) in cerebral palsy at age 2 years among survivors who received antenatal magnesium just before delivery; 95.6% of the enrolled infants were followed-up.[246] The rate of death before 2 years was similar in magnesium- versus placebo-treated infants (RR, 1.12; CI, 0.85 to 1.47). These data suggest that there may be a role for prenatally administered magnesium sulfate as a neuroprotectant for infants born before 32 weeks' gestation.

Contraindications to Arrest of Labor

Maternal contraindications to tocolysis include hypertension, bleeding, and cardiac disease. Preterm labor accompanied by maternal hypertension may occur in response to fetal stress or distress, uterine ischemia, or occult placental abruption. Vaginal bleeding may occur because of cervical effacement and dilation but is rarely more than spotting. Because thrombin stimulates uterine contractions, both placenta previa and abruption may be accompanied by uterine contractions. Tocolysis is always contraindicated when hemorrhage is significant, but if bleeding is modest and believed to occur in response to contractions, tocolysis may be considered to achieve time for corticosteroids in the setting of extreme prematurity. Such treatment should be undertaken only in hospitals with experience and appropriate laboratory and consultative support, because even low doses of β-mimetic agents and calcium channel blockers may impair the maternal cardiovascular response to hypotension, and prostaglandin inhibitors affect maternal platelet function. Cardiac disease is a contraindication because of the risks of tocolytic drugs in these patients.

Fetal contraindications to tocolysis include gestational age of 36 weeks or more, fetal demise or lethal anomaly, chorioamnionitis, and evidence of acute or chronic fetal compromise.

Tocolytic Therapy

GOALS OF TOCOLYSIS

Tocolytic agents act to inhibit uterine muscle contractions after the parturitional process is well established and therefore have limited opportunity to prevent preterm birth. The goal of tocolysis is to reduce neonatal morbidity and mortality by delaying delivery long enough to allow administration of corticosteroids and maternal in utero transport to an appropriately equipped hospital. Tocolytic drugs are used for this purpose in women with risk of imminent preterm birth due to active preterm labor and, in selected instances, in women with pPROM.

The appropriate benchmark to assess the efficacy of tocolytic agents is improved health outcome for infants born to women with preterm parturition, but most studies have insufficient power to assess the effect of treatment on this end point. One placebo-controlled trial of transdermal nitroglycerin treatment for preterm labor before 28 weeks reported a significant decrease in composite neonatal morbidity in infants born to treated mothers,[247] but such trials are uncommon, so meta-analyses and surrogate end points (e.g., delay in delivery) are more commonly used to assess efficacy and safety. The Cochrane Collaboration (http://www.cochrane.org [accessed February 28, 2008]) regularly conducts meta-analyses of tocolytic drugs; the most recent Cochrane Review concluded that calcium channel blockers such as nifedipine and the oxytocin antagonist atosiban can delay delivery by 2 to 7 days with a favorable ratio of risk to benefit.[248,249] The Cochrane analyses concluded that β-mimetic drugs can delay delivery by 48 hours but have greater side effects than other agents,[250] that magnesium sulfate is ineffective,[251] and that there are insufficient data regarding cyclooxygenase (COX) inhibitors to support conclusions.[252]

These reviews form the basis for clinical algorithms, but they are limited by the design and size of the original research studies. For example, a randomized trial[253] of nifedipine (an agent listed as potentially effective in the Cochrane Review) versus magnesium sulfate (an agent listed as ineffective) illustrates the issues that complicate interpretation of the literature on tocolysis:

1. Randomized trials most often compare two agents to one another, not to placebo, in the belief that placebo treatment is unacceptable.
2. Contraction frequency and cervical change determined by digital examination are the standard entry criteria, but these characteristics have low specificity and sensitivity, and thus lead to the enrollment of women who will deliver at term without treatment in as many as 40% of instances.[205,207,208]
3. The sample size is too small to address health outcomes such as rates of neonatal or infant morbidity, so a surrogate end point, such as prolongation of pregnancy, is used.

These issues so complicate interpretation of this trial[253] that the results have been interpreted to show that nifedipine is superior to magnesium (same efficacy, fewer side effects, and shorter neonatal intensive care unit stay) and that magnesium has efficacy that is "equal" to that of nifedipine. Neither may be true. Rather, the most appropriate interpretation of this and other comparative studies of tocolytics is that, because parturition is a gradual process with an accelerated phase of active labor, it is extremely difficult for researchers to identify the appropriate population and equally difficult to identify the appropriate moment to use tocolysis. Selection of the "best" tocolytic drug is therefore probably less important than selecting the patient for whom labor would otherwise progress to delivery.

CHOOSING A TOCOLYTIC AGENT

The key process in actin-myosin interaction, and therefore in contraction, is myosin light-chain phosphorylation. This reaction is controlled by myosin light-chain kinase (MLCK). The activity of tocolytic agents is related to regulation of the interactions of this enzyme with calcium and with cyclic adenosine monophosphate (cAMP). Calcium is essential for the activation of MLCK and binds to the kinase as calmodulin-calcium complex. Intracellular calcium levels are the product of calcium influx across the cell membrane and release of calcium from intracellular storage sites. Depolarization leads to calcium influx through specific calcium channels that are voltage dependent. This is the site of action of the calcium channel blockers. Calcium can also enter through voltage-independent mechanisms, most notably the calcium-magnesium–adenosine triphosphatase (Ca^{++}, Mg^{++}-ATPase) system. Magnesium ions may interact here to compete with calcium for the voltage-dependent channels. Calcium is stored within cells in the sarcoplasmic reticulum and in mitochondria. Progesterone and cAMP promote calcium storage at these sites, whereas prostaglandin $F_{2\alpha}$ ($PGF_{2\alpha}$) and oxytocin stimulate calcium release. Cyclic AMP directly inhibits MLCK function via phosphorylation. Levels of cAMP are increased by the action of adenylate cyclase, which is stimulated by β-mimetic agents. Thus, β-mimetic tocolytics act through adenylate cyclase to increase cAMP, which inhibits MLCK activity, both by direct phosphorylation and by reducing intracellular free calcium through inhibiting calcium release from storage vesicles. The β-mimetics also interact with surface receptors on the trophoblast to increase cAMP, which in this tissue increases production of progesterone.

Smooth muscle cells contract in a coordinated and effective manner by intercellular communication via gap junctions. Estrogens and progesterone regulate the formation of gap junctions and the concentration of oxytocin receptors.

Tocolytic drugs may be safely used when standard protocols are followed. Selection of the appropriate tocolytic requires consideration of the efficacy, risks, and side effects to identify the optimal agent for each patient. No tocolytic drug is currently approved in the United States for the indication of arresting labor. Drugs marketed for other indications, such as asthma (β-agonists), hypertension (calcium channel blockers), and anti-inflammatory/analgesic agents (nonsteroidal anti-inflammatory drugs [NSAIDs]) are used as tocolytics within rules of the U.S. Food and Drug Administration (FDA) that allow physicians to prescribe medications for "off-label" use.

CALCIUM CHANNEL BLOCKERS

Calcium channel blockers, marketed to treat hypertension, angina, and arrhythmias, are increasingly being used as tocolytic agents. The pharmacologic effect likely occurs by inhibition of the voltage-dependent channels of calcium entry into smooth muscle cells, acting to decrease intracellular calcium and to decrease release of stored calcium from intracellular storage sites. Nifedipine is the calcium blocker most commonly used as a tocolytic agent. Calcium channel blockers are rapidly absorbed after oral administration. Pharmacokinetics in pregnancy are similar to those in the nonpregnant state. Nifedipine appears in plasma within a few minutes after oral administration, reaches peak concentrations at 15 to 90 minutes, and has a half-life of 81 minutes.[254] Placental transfer occurs within 2 to 3 hours after administration of oral nifedipine. The duration of action in the mother of a single dose is up to 6 hours. There are no placebo-controlled trials of calcium channel blockers as tocolytics. The Cochrane Collaboration meta-analyses support the use of calcium channel blockers as short-term tocolytics over other available agents because of their relatively greater contraction suppression and fewer side effects than other agents in 12 reported trials.[248] Rates of birth occurring within 7 days after treatment (RR, 0.76; CI, 0.60 to 0.97) and before 34 weeks' gestation (RR, 0.83; CI, 0.69 to 0.99) were significantly reduced with calcium channel blockers, as were the rates of neonatal morbidities, including respiratory distress (RR, 0.63; CI, 0.46 to 0.88), NEC (RR, 0.21; CI, 0.05 to 0.96), IVH (RR, 0.59; CI, 0.36 to 0.98), and jaundice (RR, 0.73; CI, 0.57 to 0.93), when compared with treatment with other tocolytics. Fewer women treated with calcium channel blockers ceased treatment due to adverse drug reactions (RR, 0.14; CI, 0.05 to 0.36).

Maternal Effects. Hypotension and headache are the most common side effects of nifedipine. Pretreatment with fluids may reduce the incidence of maternal side effects such as headache (20%), flushing (8%), dizziness, and nausea (6%). Most side effects are mild, but myocardial infarction was documented in a healthy young woman 45 minutes after a second dose of nifedipine.[255] Nifedipine is less likely to be discontinued because of maternal side effects than either magnesium sulfate or β-mimetic agents.[248,253,256] Simultaneous or sequential use of calcium channel blockers with β-mimetics is not recommended because of effects on heart rate and blood pressure. Concurrent administration of magnesium with calcium channel blockers may cause skeletal muscle blockade.[257] As with other tocolytics, maternal pulmonary edema has been reported.[258]

Fetal Effects. Early studies in animals reported fetal hypotension, but a study in women treated with calcium channel blockers for preterm labor revealed no changes in the fetal middle cerebral artery, renal artery, ductus arteriosus, umbilical artery, or maternal vessels.[259] There is one report of fetal death in a patient treated with nifedipine for tocolysis.[260] Oei, in summarizing the European experience with nifedipine, advised the following precautions: "calcium channel blockers should not be combined with intravenous β-agonists. Secondly, intravenous nicardipine or high oral doses of nifedipine (≥150 mg/day) should be avoided in cases of cardiovascular compromised pregnant women and/or multiple gestations. In all cases, blood pressure should be monitored and cardiotocography recorded during the administration of immediate release Tablets, and chewing the Tablets should be avoided."[261]

Treatment Protocol. When used as a tocolytic, nifedipine is commonly given orally as a 10- to 20-mg initial dose, repeated every 3 to 6 hours until contractions are rare, then followed by long-acting formulations of 30 or 60 mg every 8 to 12 hours for 48 hours while antenatal steroids are being administered. Serious maternal and fetal side effects are more likely with short-acting preparations when the drug is initiated, and they are more likely in women with hypertension or other cardiovascular disorders. The long-acting preparations have fewer side effects, but headache and hypotension still occur.

Summary of Calcium Channel Blockers. Nifedipine has been used increasingly as a tocolytic because significant maternal and fetal side effects are uncommon and oral administration is convenient. However, efficacy is not established by placebo-controlled trials, and the ideal dosage regimen is not clear. Nifedipine should not be combined with magnesium or β-mimetics, and it should be avoided in the presence of intrauterine infection, maternal hypertension, or cardiac disease.

CYCLOOXYGENASE INHIBITORS

Prostaglandin synthesis is reduced by inhibition of COX by NSAIDs. Prostaglandins mediate the final pathways of uterine muscle contraction, causing an increase in free intracellular calcium levels in myometrial cells and increased activation of MLCK. Gap junction formation is enhanced by prostaglandins. Prostaglandins given to pregnant women can ripen the cervix or induce labor, depending on the dosage and route of administration. COX, also known as prostaglandin synthase, converts arachidonic acid to prostaglandin G_2. Prostaglandin synthesis is increased when the COX-2 form of this enzyme is induced by cytokines, bacterial products such as phospholipases and endotoxins, and corticosteroids.

NSAIDs vary in activity, potency, and side effects. Indomethacin, the NSAID most often used as a tocolytic, crosses the placenta. Unlike aspirin, indomethacin binds reversibly to COX, so that inhibition lasts only until the drug is excreted. Umbilical artery serum concentrations equal maternal levels within 6 hours after oral administration. The half-life in the mother is 4 to 5 hours; it is 15 hours in a full-term infant but is significantly longer in preterm infants.

The Cochrane Review concluded that indomethacin administration was associated with a significant reduction in births before the 37th week, as well as increased gestational age and increased birth weight, but noted that there were insufficient data to determine fetal safety.[252]

Maternal Effects. Prostaglandin inhibition has multiple side effects because of the abundance of prostaglandin-mediated physiologic functions. Serious maternal side effects are uncommon when the agent is used in a brief course of tocolysis. Gastrointestinal side effects such as nausea, heartburn, and vomiting are common but usually mild. Less common but more serious complications include gastrointestinal bleeding, prolonged bleeding time,[262] thrombocytopenia, and asthma in aspirin-sensitive patients. Prolonged treatment with NSAIDs can lead to renal injury, especially if other nephrotoxic drugs are used. Hypertensive women uncommonly experience an acute increase in blood pressure after taking indomethacin. The antipyretic effect of an NSAID may obscure a clinically significant fever. Maternal contraindications to indomethacin tocolysis include renal or hepatic disease, active peptic ulcer disease, poorly controlled hypertension, asthma, and coagulation disorders.

Fetal and Neonatal Effects. Although the maternal side effect profile is mostly benign, serious fetal and neonatal complications of COX inhibitors can occur if the drugs are used outside established protocols. In actual practice, such complications have been rare, but treatment guidelines must be followed carefully. The major fetal side effects are constriction of the ductus arteriosus, oligohydramnios, and neonatal pulmonary hypertension. Ductal constriction may occur because the formation of prostacyclin and PGE_2, which maintain ductal vasodilation, is inhibited by indomethacin.[263] Transient ductal constriction has been reported in as many as 50% of fetuses of women treated with indomethacin before 32 weeks of pregnancy, usually after several days of therapy. This typically resolves within 24 hours after the medication is discontinued without sequelae.[264,265] However, persistent ductal constriction and irreversible right-sided heart failure have been reported.[266]

Primary pulmonary hypertension in the neonate, a potentially fatal illness, has been associated with fetal exposure to NSAIDs[267] including ibuprofen, naproxen, aspirin, and indomethacin. Although maternal indomethacin treatment within 16 hours of birth was blamed for a single case of neonatal pulmonary hypertension,[268] neither a case-control series in which 75 exposed fetuses were matched with 150 controls[269] nor a literature review and meta-analysis that compared outcomes in 1621 infants treated with indomethacin in utero with 4387 unexposed infants found significant differences in neonatal morbidity when maternal indomethacin therapy was used in protocols that limited use to 48 hours or less taken before 32 weeks' gestation.[270,271] This reassuring information does not mitigate the potential fetal risks of NSAID treatment for longer than 48 hours before 32 weeks or for any duration after 32 weeks, nor the risks associated with prolonged or repeated maternal-fetal exposure to NSAIDs at any time during pregnancy.

Oligohydramnios may accompany indomethacin tocolysis, because indomethacin inhibits the normal prostaglandin inhibition of antidiuretic hormone and also exerts direct effects on fetal renal blood flow. These effects are dose related and reversible, but they are not inconsequential: Neonatal renal insufficiency and death after several weeks of antenatal maternal treatment has been reported.[272] Sulindac is an NSAID that has less placental transfer than indomethacin. but amniotic fluid index, hourly fetal urine production, and ductal blood flow were equally reduced in a randomized comparison of sulindac, indomethacin. and nimesulide, another NSAID.[273]

Other complications, including NEC, small-bowel perforation, PDA, jaundice, and IVH, have been observed when indomethacin was used in a clinical setting only after other agents had failed and without limit on the duration or gestational age of treatment.[274] No association with IVH has been reported in studies where standard protocols were used.[269,270,275]

Because of the effect of NSAIDs on fetal urine production and amniotic fluid volume, indomethacin has been used when preterm labor is associated with polyhydramnios.[276] Uterine activity and pain associated with degenerating uterine fibroids in pregnancy also respond well to indomethacin.

Fetal contraindications to the use of indomethacin include growth restriction, renal anomalies, chorioamnionitis, oligohydramnios, ductal dependent cardiac defects, and twin-twin transfusion syndrome.

Treatment Protocol. Indomethacin is well absorbed orally. The usual regimen is a 50-mg oral loading dose followed by 25 to 50 mg by mouth every 6 hours. Therapy is limited to 48 hours and to pregnancies before 32 weeks' gestation because of concern about side effects described earlier.

Amniotic fluid volume and fetal renal anatomy should be assessed before indomethacin is used for tocolysis. Treatment beyond 48 hours may be considered in extraordinary circumstances but requires surveillance of amniotic fluid volume and ductal flow. Repeated courses should be avoided if possible. Treatment should be discontinued if delivery is imminent.

Summary of Indomethacin. Indomethacin is an effective tocolytic agent that is generally well tolerated by the mother. Concern about fetal side effects has appropriately limited the use of indomethacin to brief courses of therapy in patients with preterm labor before 32 weeks' gestation.

OXYTOCIN ANTAGONISTS

Oxytocin stimulates contractions in labor at term by inducing conversion of phosphatidylinositol to inositol triphosphate, which binds to a protein in the sarcoplasmic reticulum, causing release of calcium into the cytoplasm. Oxytocin receptor antagonists compete with oxytocin for binding to receptors in the myometrium and decidua, to prevent or reduce calcium release. The oxytocin receptor antagonist, atosiban, inhibits spontaneous and oxytocin-induced contractions but does not affect prostaglandin-induced contractions. Maternal side effects are uncommon, because oxytocin receptors are located only in the uterus and breast. Oxytocin antagonists cross the placenta but do not affect fetal cardiovascular or acid-base status.

Atosiban was evaluated in a randomized, placebo-controlled trial in which 531 women with preterm labor between 200/7 and 336/7 gestational weeks were treated with either intravenous and subcutaneous atosiban or intravenous and subcutaneous placebo.[277] Women in either study arm with persistent contractions and progressive cervical change 1 hour after entry were treated openly with a tocolytic agent of the clinician's choice. The interval from enrollment to delivery did not differ between the two groups (26 versus 21 days, $P = .6$). However, among 424 women who enrolled after 28 weeks' gestation, those treated with atosiban were more likely to remain undelivered without requiring an alternate tocolytic at 24 hours (73% versus 58%; OR, 1.93; CI, 1.30 to 2.86), at 48 hours (67% versus 56%; OR, 1.62; CI, 1.62 to 2.37), and at 7 days (62% versus 49%; OR, 1.70; CI, 1.17 to 2.46). There were no differences in pregnancy prolongation for subjects enrolled between 20 and 28 weeks. The FDA did not approve atosiban because of an unexpected finding of more perinatal deaths among infants born to women enrolled into the atosiban arm before 26 weeks. It is not clear whether the difference in outcomes was related to the drug or to an inexplicably larger number of women with gestational age less than 26 weeks who were randomized to the atosiban arm. As in other placebo-controlled tocolytic trials, the rate of "successful" treatment in the placebo group was greater than 50%, indicating the difficulty in distinguishing active preterm labor from preterm parturition.

In another trial that compared subcutaneous infusions of atosiban with placebo infusion,[278] there were no differences in the rates of preterm birth before 28, 32, or 37 weeks' gestation, but the interval from the start of maintenance infusion therapy to the first recurrence of preterm labor was longer for the atosiban group. An international study group compared the efficacy and side effect profile of atosiban with those of ritodrine.[279] Efficacy in delaying delivery for 48 hours (about 85% for both drugs) and for 7 days (about 75% for both drugs) was similar, but cardiovascular side effects were much less common for atosiban (4%) than for ritodrine (84%).

The most recent Cochrane Review noted that atosiban treatment was associated with an increased number of infants born weighing less than 1500 g in the treatment group, compared with the group receiving placebo (RR, 1.96; CI, 1.15 to 3.35; 2 trials, 575 infants) but resulted in fewer maternal drug reactions requiring alternative treatment (RR, 0.04; CI, 0.02 to 0.11; 4 trials, 1035 women). Evidence for the efficacy of atosiban to improve infant outcomes was deemed insufficient.[249]

Atosiban is widely used in Europe. In an open, randomized trial of atosiban compared with routinely used tocolytic agents conducted in 585 women, prolongation of pregnancy for 48 hours was equal in both groups, but significantly more women receiving atosiban remained undelivered at 48 hours without requiring an alternative tocolytic (77.6% versus 56.6%; $P < .001$). Maternal side effects were less common in women receiving atosiban.[280]

Summary of Atosiban. Atosiban has minimal side maternal effects and efficacy that is comparable to that of other tocolytics. Although it is commonly used in Europe, it was not approved by the U.S. FDA due to concerns about fetal outcomes in women treated before 26 weeks that may or may not have been related to the drug.

NITRIC OXIDE DONORS

Nitric oxide (NO) acts to maintain normal smooth muscle tone. NO is synthesized during the oxidation of L-arginine to L-citrulline, a reaction catalyzed by nitric oxide synthase (NOS). The interaction between NO and soluble guanylyl cyclase (sGC) links extracellular stimuli of NO formation to synthesis of cyclic guanosine 3′,5′-monophosphate (cGMP) in target cells. The increase in cGMP content in smooth muscle cells activates MLCK, which causes smooth muscle relaxation. NO donors such as nitroglycerin inhibit spontaneous oxytocin- and prostaglandin-induced activity.

Glyceryl trinitrate (GTN) has been studied as an acute uterine relaxant to allow uterine manipulation for external cephalic version or ex utero fetal surgery and also as a tocolytic agent. Studies of GTN as a tocolytic have produced mixed results. Intravenous GTN was less effective in arresting contractions and had more side effects than magnesium sulfate in a study of 31 subjects.[281] In a randomized trial that compared transdermal GTN with ritodrine in 245 women with preterm labor, 74% of participants in both treatment arms delivered after 37 weeks.[282] Treatment was discontinued in 25% of the GTN group due to maternal hypotension. Headache was frequent, occurring in 30% of GTN-treated women. The Cochrane Review summarized four randomized trials that compared NO to placebo, no treatment, or other tocolytics and found that NO treatment of preterm labor was associated with fewer deliveries before 37 weeks, but there were insufficient data to assess newborn outcomes.[283]

A subsequent randomized trial compared β-mimetic tocolysis with GTN plus rescue β-mimetic tocolysis for persistent contractions in 235 women at 24 to 35 weeks' gestation in whom preterm parturition was confirmed by a positive finding of cervicovaginal fetal fibronectin or ruptured membranes. There was no significant difference in the time to delivery using Kaplan-Meier curves ($P = .451$).[284] In another placebo-controlled trial of NO tocolysis before 28 weeks, also published since the Cochrane Review, composite neonatal morbidity was significantly reduced in infants born to mothers treated with NO.[247] This is one of the few studies to report improved neonatal outcome, but these studies are insufficient to recommend NO donors until additional, larger studies are reported.

Headache and hypertension are the most commonly reported maternal side effects. Fetal side effects are uncommonly reported but might be expected because of the drug's effect on maternal blood pressure. Kahler and colleagues investigated maternal and fetal blood flow with Doppler ultrasound in women treated for preterm labor with GTN patches at a dosage of 0.8 mg/hr and found no effect on blood flow in any fetal organ.[285]

Summary of Nitric Oxide. Nitric oxide donors have not been widely used for tocolysis but deserve further investigation. Current data do not support use outside clinical trials.

MAGNESIUM SULFATE

Pharmacology. Magnesium acts by competition with calcium either at the motor end plate (reducing excitation by affecting acetylcholine release and sensitivity at the motor end plate)[286] or at the cell membrane (reducing calcium influx into the cell at depolarization). Myometrial contractility is inhibited when maternal serum levels of magnesium are 5 to 8 mg/dL.[287] Deep tendon reflexes may be lost when concentrations reach 9 to 13 mg/dL, and respiratory depression defects occur at 14 mg/dL. Magnesium is excreted almost entirely by the kidney, with at least 75% of the infused dose of magnesium (for the treatment of preeclampsia) excreted during the infusion and at least 90% excreted within 24 hours.[288] As magnesium is reabsorbed in the loop of Henle by a transport-limited mechanism, the glomerular filtration rate affects excretion significantly. Increases in maternal serum magnesium also result in maternal hypocalcemia (the total calcium level falling by approximately 25%) and an increase in parathyroid hormone but no change in maternal phosphate or calcitonin level. Hypocalcemia is usually asymptomatic. Magnesium ions cross the placenta rapidly, with fetal and newborn levels increasing proportionately with maternal levels.[289] The mean half-life of neonatal hypermagnesemia secondary to maternal therapy may be as long as 40 hours.[288]

Evidence to support magnesium sulfate as an effective tocolytic is weak.[290,291] The Cochrane Library reviewers found no significant advantage regarding the rates of delivery within 48 hours or before 34 or 37 weeks in studies of women treated with magnesium.[251] Two small, randomized trials compared magnesium with nifedipine[253] and celecoxib;[292] both found no difference in the percentage of women who delivered within 48 hours.

Despite the limited evidence of benefit, magnesium has been a common choice because of its familiarity and presumed safety relative to β-mimetics and other tocolytics. This rationale for choosing magnesium sulfate has been challenged by reviews that emphasized the paucity of data to support any benefit[293-296] and by concerns about fetal safety (discussed later). Direct evidence of improved fetal, neonatal, and/or infant outcomes attributable to magnesium tocolysis is absent, and indirect support from comparative trials and secondary analyses is weak.[251,290,293,295,296]

Maternal Effects. Magnesium has a low rate of serious maternal side effects, but flushing, nausea, vomiting, dry mouth, headache, blurred vision, generalized muscle weakness, diplopia, and shortness of breath occur, together with maternal sense of loss of control. Chest pain and pulmonary edema have been reported with a frequency similar to that seen with β-mimetics.[297] If renal function is impaired (and magnesium excretion is thus reduced), hypermagnesemia leading to respiratory impairment is more likely. Theoretically, high serum magnesium concentrations could alter the amount of muscle relaxant needed during general anesthesia. Magnesium should not be used as a tocolytic in women with myasthenia gravis. Hypocalcemia may be asymptomatic, or it may manifest as hand contractures.[298] Prolonged treatment has been associated with maternal osteoporosis.[299] Neuromuscular blockade is possible if magnesium is used concurrently with nifedipine tocolysis.

Neonatal Effects. Magnesium crosses the placenta and achieves serum levels comparable to maternal levels, but serious short-term neonatal complications are uncommon if the duration of maternal therapy does not exceed 48 hours. Neonatal lethargy, hypotonia, and respiratory depression may occur. Prolonged magnesium tocolysis has also been associated with neonatal bone demineralization.[300]

The Magnesium Sulfate Controversy. Large studies (described earlier) that demonstrated the neuroprotectant benefits of magnesium sulfate have overcome and refuted an early report about possible adverse neonatal and infant effects of antenatal magnesium treatment.[241] This report described 9 infant deaths among 85 infants born to 75 mothers: three deaths, occurring at 41, 96, and 141 days of life, were attributed to sudden infant death syndrome; one infant died of congenital anomalies at 24 days of life; two deaths occurred in a twin pair born at 26 weeks with the twin-twin transfusion syndrome (an in utero death in the donor twin and neonatal death at 3 days of age in the recipient twin); another infant, one of twins born at 25 weeks, died at 260 days of age; another born at 33 weeks died at 16 days of age in the emergency department; and another died in the delivery room of a subepicardial bleed. Subsequent randomized trials, however, have enrolled more than 30 times as many subjects without evidence of increased neonatal or infant mortality related to magnesium and have demonstrated a reduction in moderate to severe cerebral palsy in surviving infants.[238,243-246,300,301]

Treatment Protocol. Magnesium sulfate must be given parenterally to achieve serum levels above the normal range. Therapeutic dosage regimens are similar to those used for intravenous seizure prophylaxis of preeclampsia. The customary clinical protocol for magnesium sulfate begins with a loading dose of 4 to 6 g magnesium sulfate in 10% to 20% percent solution (60 mL of 10% magnesium sulfate in 5% dextrose in 0.9% normal saline) given over 30 minutes.[297] This is followed by a maintenance dose of 2 g/hr (40 g of magnesium sulfate added to 1 L 5% dextrose in 0.9% normal saline or Ringer lactate at 50 mL/hr). The intravenous rate is increased by 1 g/hr until the patient has fewer than one contraction per 10 minutes or until a maximum dose of 4 g/hr is reached. Some centers choose 3 g/hr as the upper limit. Intravenous fluids are restricted to 125 mL/hr. Fluid status should be followed closely. Deep tendon reflexes and vital signs, including respiratory rate, should be recorded hourly. Magnesium levels may be obtained to answer safety concerns, but the infusion should be reduced or stopped without waiting for drug level results if respiration or urine output declines. Calcium gluconate should be readily available to reverse the effects of magnesium.

Once contractions have decreased to fewer than 1 every 10 to 15 minutes or have ceased, the infusion may be discontinued without first tapering the infusion rate. Magnesium is sometimes continued until an arbitrary end point is reached (e.g., 12 hours after contractions ceased) or until a steroid course is completed, but this approach is unsupported by data.

If renal function is normal, magnesium is excreted rapidly in the urine. Magnesium should be administered cautiously in women with evidence of renal impairment, such as oliguria or serum creatinine levels higher than 0.9 mg/dL. Magnesium sulfate should not be used in patients with myasthenia gravis, because the magnesium ion competes with calcium.

Summary of Magnesium Sulfate. Magnesium sulfate is a familiar agent, but its tocolytic efficacy is poor. Magnesium may be a useful choice if the diagnosis of preterm labor is early and uncertain and in patients in whom other agents are contraindicated (e.g., those with insulin-dependent diabetes).

β-MIMETIC TOCOLYTICS

β-Sympathomimetic drugs, including terbutaline, ritodrine, and others, have been widely used as tocolytics. These agents act to relax smooth muscle in the bronchial tree, blood vessels, and myometrium through stimulation of the β-receptors. β-Receptors are divided into β_1 and β_2 subtypes. The β_1-receptors are largely responsible for the cardiac effects, while β_2-receptors mediate smooth muscle relaxation, hepatic glycogen production, and islet cell release of insulin. Variable ratios of β_2- to β_1-receptors occur in body tissues. Stimulation of β_1-receptors in the heart, vascular system, and liver accounts for the side effects of these drugs. The most commonly used β-mimetic in the United States is terbutaline (marketed as a drug for asthma), but others, including albuterol, fenoterol, hexoprenaline, metaproterenol, nylidrin, orciprenaline, and salbutamol, are used in other countries. Although ritodrine was approved by the FDA for tocolysis in 1980, it did not achieve wide use because of frequent maternal side effects and is no longer marketed. Terbutaline has a rapid effect when given subcutaneously (3 to 5 minutes). Published protocols often employ subcutaneous administration, with a usual dose of 0.25 mg (250 μg) every 4 hours.[302]

A single subcutaneous dose of terbutaline to arrest contractions during the initial evaluation of preterm contractions may aid in the diagnosis of preterm labor. In one study,[214] women whose contractions persisted or recurred after a single subcutaneous dose were more likely to have true preterm labor; those whose contractions ceased were probably not in labor. In a Cochrane Database analysis of 1332 women enrolled into 11 randomized, placebo-controlled trials of β-mimetic drugs, treated subjects were less likely to deliver within 48 hours (RR, 0.63; CI, 0.53 to 0.75), but not within 7 days.[250] Perinatal and neonatal mortality and perinatal morbidity were not reduced by β-mimetic treatment in this analysis. Side effects requiring change or cessation of treatment were frequent. Other reviews have reported similar conclusions.[303]

Maternal side effects of the β-mimetic drugs are common and diverse due to the abundance of β-receptors in the body. Maternal tachycardia, chest discomfort, palpitation, tremor, headache, nasal congestion, nausea and vomiting, hyperkalemia, and hyperglycemia are significantly more common in women treated with β-mimetics.[250] Most side effects are mild and of limited duration, but serious maternal cardiopulmonary and metabolic complications have been reported.

Cardiopulmonary Complications of β-Mimetics. The β-mimetic agents can produce a mild (5 to 10 mm Hg) fall in diastolic blood pressure, and the extensive peripheral vasodilatation may make it difficult for the patient to mount a normal response to hypovolemia. Exclusion of women with any history of heart disease or significant hemorrhage and limitation of infusion rates to maintain maternal heart rate at less than 130 beats/min are important steps to avoid cardiac complications. Symptomatic arrhythmias and myocardial ischemia have occurred during β-agonist tocolytic therapy; myocardial infarction leading to death has been reported.[304] Tocolysis should be discontinued and oxygen administered whenever a woman reports chest pain during tocolytic therapy. Premature ventricular contractions, premature nodal contractions, and atrial fibrillation noted in association with β-mimetic therapy usually respond to discontinuation of the drug and oxygen administration. Baseline or routine electrocardiograms before or during treatment are not helpful. Nonetheless, an electrocardiogram is indicated if there is no response to oxygen and cessation of β-mimetic therapy. Pulmonary edema has been reported with all tocolytics, including β-mimetic therapy. Restriction of the duration of treatment to less than 24 hours, maintenance of careful attention to fluid status, and detection of complicating conditions such as intrauterine infection may reduce this risk.

Metabolic Complications. β-Mimetic agents induce transient hyperglycemia and hypokalemia during treatment. Measurement of glucose and potassium before therapy is initiated and on occasion during the first 24 hours of treatment may be appropriate to identify significant hyperglycemia (>180 mg/dL) or hypokalemia (<2.5 mEq/L.). These metabolic changes are mild and transient, but prolonged treatment (>24 hours) may rarely induce significant alterations in maternal blood sugar, insulin levels, and energy expenditure.[305] The risk of abnormal glucose metabolism is further increased by simultaneous treatment with corticosteroids. Other agents should probably be chosen for women with pregestational diabetes, and, in most cases, for those with gestational diabetes as well.

Neonatal Effects. Neonatal hypoglycemia, hypocalcemia, and ileus may occur after treatment with β-mimetics and can be clinically significant if the maternal infusion is not discontinued 2 hours or more before delivery.

Given their potential for clinically significant side effects and the availability of alternative choices, the β-sympathomimetic agents should not be used in women with known or suspected heart disease, severe preeclampsia or eclampsia, pregestational or gestational diabetes requiring insulin, or hyperthyroidism. These drugs are contraindicated if suspected preterm labor is complicated by maternal fever, fetal tachycardia, leukocytosis, or other signs of possible chorioamnionitis.

Long-term or maintenance use of β-mimetic drugs has been advocated to suppress contractions and thereby prevent preterm labor, but tachyphylaxis or desensitization of the adrenergic receptor occurs after prolonged exposure to β-agonists, so that increasing dosages are required to sustain a response.

Continuous subcutaneous infusion of terbutaline has been reported to have fewer side effects at lower doses than oral administration.[306] Although these protocols suppressed contractions, they had no effect on rates of preterm birth or perinatal morbidity in randomized, placebo-controlled trials.[307,308] The Cochrane Review did not support terbutaline infusion to prolong pregnancy,[309] nor did the most recent ACOG practice bulletin.[218]

Summary of β-Mimetic Tocolysis. β-Mimetic drugs were once commonly used as tocolytics but are being replaced by agents with better safety and side effect profiles. Terbutaline has relatively few serious side effects when given as a single subcutaneous injection of 0.25 mg to facilitate maternal transfer or to initiate tocolysis while another agent with a slower onset of action is being given, Long-term oral or subcutaneous treatment has not been shown in controlled trials to reduce either prematurity or neonatal morbidity.

CLINICAL USE OF TOCOLYTIC DRUGS

Tocolytic therapy is employed in several clinical circumstances. In caring for a woman with active contractions and advanced cervical effacement with the goal of arresting labor to allow time for maternal transfer, antenatal steroids, and GBS prophylaxis, treatment with subcutaneous terbutaline or oral nifedipine may stop contractions promptly, after which nifedipine may be continued or another agent started. Treatment may be continued at least until contractions occur less frequently than four times per hour without additional cervical change. If labor has been difficult to stop in a patient with complete cervical effacement, acute treatment may be continued for 48 hours while steroid therapy is completed.

If contractions persist despite therapy, the wisdom of tocolytic treatment should be reevaluated. If cervical dilation has progressed beyond 4 cm, treatment should be discontinued in most instances. Persistent contractions despite ongoing tocolysis raise the possibility of placental abruption or intra-amniotic infection. Amniocentesis should be considered.

If fetal well-being can be confirmed (by a normal fetal biophysical profile including normal fluid volume, or by amniocentesis showing a negative amniotic fluid Gram stain, and/or normal amniotic fluid glucose), the accuracy of the original diagnosis should be reconsidered, remembering that significant effacement, softness, and development of the lower uterine segment are the features of the digital examination that most reliably indicate preterm labor. If a fibronectin swab was collected before therapy was begun, it should be sent for analysis. A positive fibronectin test is not confirmatory, but a negative result, if collected before performance of a digital examination, suggests that preterm birth is unlikely (4%) within 2 weeks.[216,223] Alternately, a transvaginal cervical ultrasound examination may be performed. A cervical length of 30 mm or more essentially excludes the diagnosis of preterm labor except in cases of acute abruption.[215]

Initiating treatment with a second agent is often considered when contractions persist. Serum levels are not clinically helpful to adjust the dose of tocolytics. A change to a second agent or combination therapy with multiple agents may slow contractions, but this approach often results in increased side effects as well. Sustained treatment with multiple tocolytics increases the risk of significant side effects and should in general be avoided.

Care after Acute Treatment for Preterm Labor

Continued suppression of contractions after acute tocolysis does not reduce the rate of preterm birth.[310-312] Meta-analyses of the relevant data found no evidence of prolongation of pregnancy or decline in the frequency of preterm birth.[309,313] Outpatient monitoring of uterine contractions and associated care did not improve the rate of delivery before 37 weeks, birth weight, or gestational age at delivery.[314,315]

The duration of hospitalization for preterm labor is influenced by the dilation, effacement and sonographic length of the cervix, ease of tocolysis, gestational age, obstetric history, distance from hospital, and the availability of home and family supportive care. Risk factors that may complicate or increase the risk of recurrent preterm labor, such as a positive genital culture for chlamydia or gonorrhea, urinary tract infection, and anemia, should be addressed before the woman is discharged from hospital care. Social issues such as homelessness, availability of child care, or protection from an abusive partner are important determinants of a patient's ability to comply with medical care and must also be considered before the patient is released from the hospital.

Prevention of Preterm Birth

Great persistence will be required to address the health consequences of preterm birth, because the public significantly underestimates the magnitude of the problem.[316] Primary prevention of the morbidity and mortality of preterm birth is an increasingly compelling strategy as the limitations of tertiary care are recognized. Secondary care for women at risk is a strategy limited to removal rather than avoidance of risk.

Until the multiple pathways that contribute to preterm parturition are better understood, attempts during pregnancy (secondary and tertiary prevention) to prevent preterm birth must accommodate the possibility that prolongation of pregnancy intended to promote maturation might in some cases allow continued exposure to a suboptimal or even hazardous intrauterine environment. Indeed, preterm birth is not a health outcome but instead a surrogate end point for optimal fetal, infant, and lifelong health.[9,317] Indicated preterm birth, by definition, is undertaken to improve maternal and/or fetal and neonatal health, in contrast to presumed fetal benefit for continuing the pregnancy in spontaneous preterm parturition. However, the distinction between indicated and spontaneous preterm birth may be artificial, because factors leading to labor and membrane rupture are understood to include intrauterine inflammation related to microbial infection, uterine vascular compromise, and/or decidual hemorrhage, all of which may contribute to neonatal and infant morbidity as much if not more than fetal immaturity does. Strategies to prevent preterm birth undertaken before conception are not complicated by such concerns.

Prematurity Prevention in Routine Prenatal Care

More than 50% of preterm births occur in pregnancies without obvious risk.[135,318] Prevention of these preterm births might be addressed by incorporating preventive measures into routine prenatal care or by screening apparently low-risk women for specific risk factors, or both. Most North American studies have focused on the content of prenatal care for women with evident risk of preterm birth, but prematurity prevention as part of routine prenatal care has received less attention.[319] European prenatal care, in contrast, emphasizes primary prevention of risk during pregnancy for all pregnant women, including social and financial support for low-risk women.[320] This approach was associated with reduced rates of preterm birth in France in an observational report.[321,322] Efforts to apply the European approach in the United States that emphasized identification and care of women with risk did not reduce the preterm birth rate in randomized trials.[323,324]

Access to Prenatal Care

Early entry into care is associated with low rates of preterm birth, but the relationship is probably based on the high rate of preterm birth among women who receive no prenatal care rather than the content of care received. Early access to prenatal care did not influence the rate of preterm birth among women enrolled in the First- And Second-Trimester Evaluation of Risk (FASTER) study of prenatal diagnostic techniques in the first and second trimesters.[325] Rates of preterm birth remained notably high among African-American women despite early entry into prenatal care in this study.

Nutritional Supplements for All Pregnant Women

Protein and calorie supplementation during pregnancy was not beneficial for preventing preterm birth when evaluated in controlled trials.[326] Calcium supplementation did not reduce the rate of preeclampsia or that of preterm birth in a randomized trial involving 4589 healthy, nulliparous women.[327] In this study, rates of birth before 37 and 34 weeks were not different, nor was the incidence of pPROM. A review of 10 trials including 14,751 women found no effect of calcium supplementation on the risk of preterm birth (RR, 0.81; CI, 0.64 to 1.03), even though preeclampsia was less frequent in calcium-treated subjects (RR, 0.48; CI, 0.33 to 0.69; 12 trials, 15,206 women).[328]

The rates of spontaneous preterm birth before 37, 34, and 28 weeks' gestation were also not improved by supplemental vitamin C and vitamin E given to prevent preeclampsia in a randomized trial conducted in 1877 healthy women.[329] In another trial, supplemental docosahexaenoic acid given to 291 women in the third trimester did not reduce the rate of preterm birth.[330] Prophylaxis of preterm birth with supplemental Ω-3 polyunsaturated fatty acids in women with a history of preterm delivery is discussed later.

Smoking Cessation

Smoking cessation programs are more likely to be well received in pregnancy.[331] A brief (<15 minutes) counseling session with a trained provider offering pregnancy-specific counseling was found to reduce smoking rates in pregnant women.[332] The reduction was modest but clinically significant (RR, 1.7; CI, 1.3 to 2.2). Persistent attention to smoking reduction and cessation in prenatal visits is emphasized in most programs. Smoking cessation in pregnancy may be more successful when specific funding for this service is available.[332] One program reported successful results in 3569 indigent women who received care coordination, nutritional counseling, or psychosocial counseling to address specific risks including smoking and inadequate weight gain.[333] Women who stopped smoking had fewer LBW infants than women who continued to smoke (8.5% versus 13.7%). The rate of LBW was lower in women who achieved adequate weight gain than in those who did not (6.7% versus 17.2%). A Cochrane Review concluded that smoking cessation programs in pregnancy reduce the rate of preterm birth (RR, 0.84; CI, 0.72 to 0.98).[334]

Periodontal Care

The risk of preterm birth rises with increased severity of periodontal disease and when periodontal disease progresses in pregnancy,[124] but the basis for the association is uncertain. It most likely results from shared variations in the inflammatory response to microorganisms in the oral and genital tracts.[128,129] Periodontal care has been advocated as an intervention to reduce preterm birth, but recent randomized trials did not find lower rates of preterm birth in women treated for periodontal disease.[127,335,336]

Screening Low-Risk Women to Reduce Risk

ASYMPTOMATIC BACTERIURIA

Screening and treatment for asymptomatic bacteriuria prevents pyelonephritis[337] and has been reported to reduce the rate of preterm birth, but the optimal screening and treatment protocols to prevent preterm birth have not been studied recently.[123,338]

GENITAL INFECTIONS

Because genital tract colonization and infection have been consistently associated with risk of preterm birth, screening and treatment for organisms including *U. urealyticum*,[339] GBS,[340] and *T. vaginalis*[118,341] have been studied; however, no beneficial effect on the incidence of preterm birth was demonstrated, even when the targeted organism was eradicated. Indeed, screening and treatment of trichomonas may increase the risk of preterm birth.[118,341]

Routine screening of all pregnant women for BV, with treatment intended to reduce preterm birth, has been extensively studied with mixed results.[111,115,342-351] BV carriage has been associated with a positive screening test for fetal fibronectin.[121,352] Although a secondary analysis suggested that antibiotic treatment might reduce the rate of preterm birth in women with BV who also have a positive fibronectin screen,[353] the rate of preterm birth was not reduced by antibiotic treatment of women with a positive fetal fibronectin result who were treated with antibiotics in a randomized trial.[354] Therefore, despite the consistent linkage of maternal BV to risk of preterm birth and the ability of antimicrobial therapy to eradicate BV, screening and treatment for BV does not reliably reduce the occurrence of preterm birth in low-risk women[111,351] and is not recommended in these patients.[217,355]

Screening to Assess Risk of Preterm Birth

SCORING SYSTEMS

Systems to identify women without apparent risk who will deliver preterm begin with individual characteristics such as low pre-pregnancy weight (BMI <19.6 kg/m^2), African-American ethnicity, social risk, depression, and genitourinary colonization as noted earlier, each with a modest relative risk of 1.5- to 2-fold. Risk scoring systems combining these factors have been devised but have a sensitivity of about 25%, even when a history of preterm birth is included.[23] Improved sensitivity has been sought by adding markers of the parturitional process, including biochemical markers in maternal serum (α-fetoprotein, alkaline phosphatase, corticotropin-releasing hormone, relaxin) or in cervical fluid (fetal fibronectin, granulocyte colony-stimulating factor, interleukins) or biophysical markers such as cervical change determined by digital or ultrasound measurement, or combinations of these.[135,352,356-359] Although studies of these markers have helped to define the parturitional process, they are insufficiently sensitive for clinical use.

FETAL FIBRONECTIN

Fetal fibronectin, a glycoprotein thought to act as an adherent at the maternal-fetal interface, is uncommonly present in cervicovaginal secretions in the late second and early third trimesters.[352,360] Asymptomatic women with a positive test for fetal fibronectin have an increased risk of preterm birth before 35 weeks, and particularly within 2 weeks after a positive test.[352,361] This association is believed to be related to disruption of the maternal-fetal decidual interface by inflammation. Although the sensitivity of the fibronectin test for spontaneous birth before 35 weeks approximates 25%, the sensitivity of the test at 22 to 24 weeks for births before 28 weeks was 65% in one study.[135] For this reason, a placebo-controlled trial of metronidazole and erythromycin was conducted in women with a positive test for fetal fibronectin at 21 to 26 weeks' gestation.[354] Preterm birth rates before 37, 35, and 32 weeks were unaffected by antibiotic treatment, with ORs of 1.17 (CI, 0.80 to 1.70), 0.92 (CI, 0.54 to 1.56), and 1.94 (CI, 0.83 to 4.52), respectively. No other interventions for women with a positive fetal fibronectin test have been evaluated in controlled trials. Screening of low-risk women with fetal fibronectin testing is not recommended.[217]

CERVICAL EXAMINATION

Changes in the cervix may precede overt uterine activation and therefore may be used to identify women in whom the parturitional process has begun. Evaluation of the cervix by digital or ultrasound assessment has been shown to identify women with increased risk for preterm birth,[190-193,213] but, because preterm cervical ripening occurs over a period of weeks, the sensitivity to predict imminent preterm birth is modest (25% to 30% for digital examination and 35% to 40% for endovaginal sonography). Interventions undertaken to reduce the risk of preterm birth in response to evidence of cervical effacement have, in the absence of contractions, targeted presumed cervical insufficiency, but cerclage for short cervix in women without a previous early birth is apparently ineffective.[362,363] A placebo-controlled, randomized trial conducted in women with sonographic evidence of short cervix (≤15 mm) found that cerclage had no effect on the rate of preterm birth.[362] However, in another trial that enrolled similar women, treatment with vaginal progesterone significantly reduced the frequency of births before 34 weeks, compared with placebo.[364] These studies have not yet been confirmed by others but represent clear progress. The apparent success of medical over surgical treatment for short cervix suggests that the causes of preterm cervical ripening are more likely biochemical than biophysical.

COMBINED TESTING

The combination of digital examination, fetal fibronectin testing, and cervical sonography in nulliparous and low-risk multiparous women was assessed in a secondary analysis of data from the Preterm Prediction Study.[365] The sensitivity of cervical sonography was 39% for birth before 35 weeks in these low-risk, asymptomatic women. Sensitivities for the more widely available and less costly tests, digital examination and fibronectin, were less than 25%. The combination of serum markers for preterm birth with cervicovaginal fetal fibronectin and ultrasound measurement of cervical length showed improved sensitivity and positive predictive value[356] but, in the absence of an intervention, has no clinical application.

Prevention of Preterm Birth in Women with Clinical Risk Factors

Indicated Preterm Birth

Strategies to prevent indicated preterm births target women with medical disorders and women with risk factors for preeclampsia, such as nulliparity, twin gestation, diabetes, chronic hypertension, and a history of preeclampsia or growth restriction. Numerous trials of various agents (low-dose aspirin,[366,367] antioxidant vitamins C and E,[368] and fish oil[369,370]) have been conducted to test their effects on the rates of preeclampsia, fetal growth restriction, and preterm birth. Cochrane Reviews of these interventions[371] have found only modest benefit for antiplatelet drugs, chiefly low-dose aspirin, namely

- An 8% reduction in the risk of preterm birth from a review of 29 trials that enrolled a total of 31,151 women (RR, 0.92; CI, 0.88 to 0.97)
- A 10% reduction in small-for-gestational-age infants in a review of 36 trials that enrolled 23,638 women (RR, 0.90; CI, 0.83 to 0.98)
- A 14% reduction in fetal or neonatal deaths in a review of 40 trials that enrolled 33,098 women (RR, 0.86; CI, 0.76 to 0.98)

Although a Cochrane Review found a significant reduction in preeclampsia in women treated with supplemental calcium, there was no effect on the rate of preterm birth (RR, 0.81; CI, 0.64 to 1.03; 10 trials, 14,751 women) or on the rate of perinatal death (RR, 0.89; CI, 0.73 to 1.09; 10 trials, 15,141 babies).[328] A similar review of the use of antioxidants to prevent preeclampsia found a slight decrease in preeclampsia but no evidence of a corresponding reduction in the risk of preterm birth.[372]

Spontaneous Preterm Birth

Secondary interventions to reduce spontaneous preterm birth have been studied in women with a history of spontaneous preterm birth alone,[139] in women with a prior preterm birth who also have a current pregnancy risk factor or marker (e.g., BV, short cervix),[373-375] and in women with no prior history who have a major clinical risk factor in the current pregnancy (e.g., multiple gestation,[387] short cervix).[364]

Without a clear understanding of pathophysiology, these trials have been designed to answer clinical questions such as whether a given intervention can reduce the rate of preterm birth in women with historical or current risk factors. Interventions have been selected for study because of their presumed participation in a putative causal pathway. Women enrolled are selected for study because they are easily identified by a history of preterm birth or an inexpensive screening test without necessarily knowing whether they possess the risk factor addressed by the intervention being studied. Therefore, an unknown fraction of subjects in these trials receive an intervention that has no opportunity to exert a beneficial effect, leaving the interpretation of the results open to debate.[377,378] Furthermore, although an effective intervention may interrupt a causal pathway (e.g., an antibiotic may eliminate a genital microorganism), the ultimate clinical outcome may be determined as much by host and environmental factors as by the treatment tested.[131] Finally, the timing of an intervention may determine its clinical efficacy, as may be the case for antibiotic trials.[379]

Analysis from both primary hypothesis-testing and secondary hypothesis-generating studies of variable size and quality have been reported. Interventions tested include reduced maternal activity, nutritional supplements, augmented prenatal care and surveillance, antibiotic prophylaxis, progestational supplements, and cervical cerclage.

MODIFICATION OF MATERNAL ACTIVITY

Restriction of physical activity, including bed rest, limited work, and reduced sexual activity, are frequently recommended to reduce the likelihood of preterm birth in pregnancies at risk of indicated and spontaneous birth, despite the absence of benefit in the literature.[380] Yost and colleagues found no relationship between coitus and risk of recurrent preterm birth,[92] but limitation of sexual and physical activity has not been tested since recent advances in understanding the pathophysiology of preterm parturition. Neither bed rest nor coital abstinence has, for example, been studied in women with short cervix or in the outpatient setting.

NUTRITIONAL SUPPLEMENTS

The preterm birth rate is low in populations with a high dietary intake of Ω-3 polyunsaturated fatty acids (PUFA), which reduce levels of proinflammatory cytokines. Dietary supplementation with PUFAs has been associated with reduced production of inflammatory mediators thought to participate in inflammation-driven parturition. A randomized trial of Ω-3 supplements conducted in women at risk for preterm birth found a 50% decrease in preterm births,[369] and a subsequent randomized trial of supplemental fish oil also reported a significant reduction in recurrent preterm birth (RR, 0.54; CI, 0.30 to 0.98).[370] However, a randomized, placebo-controlled trial of supplemental Ω-3 PUFAs in 852 women with a prior preterm birth found no effect of Ω-3 supplementation on birth or spontaneous birth before 37 or 35 weeks (RR, 0.91; CI, 0.77 to 1.07). The treatment groups did not differ when stratified by fish intake (RR, 0.92; CI, 0.78 to 1.08). In this study, all participants in both arms were treated with 17α-hydroxyprogesterone caproate (17P).[381] In a secondary analysis of data from this study, women enrolled in the trial whose diet included fish once or more per month had a significantly reduced rate of spontaneous preterm birth compared to women who consumed fish less often than once per month (RR, 0.62; CI, 0.45 to 0.86), regardless of their study assignment—a hypothesis that will need to be tested in future studies (Table 29-5).

TABLE 29-5 EFFECTS OF OMEGA-3 POLYUNSATURATED FATTY ACID (PUFA) SUPPLEMENTATION AND CONSUMPTION OF FISH ON PRETERM BIRTH

	PUFA (*n* = 434)	Placebo (*n* = 418)	*P* (PUFA vs Placebo)	Fish ≥1 Meal/Month	Fish <1 Meal/Month	*P* (Fish Intake)
PTB <37 wk	37.8%	41.6%	0.25	35.9%	48.6%	0.0005
sPTB <37 wk	29.0%	31.8%	0.38	37.2%	37.9%	0.002
PTB <35 wk	18.9%	19.9%	0.72	17.2%	24.5%	0.014

PTB, preterm birth; sPTB, spontaneous preterm birth.

From Harper M; for NICHD MFMU Network: Randomized controlled trial of omega-3 fatty acid supplementation for recurrent preterm birth. Society for Maternal-Fetal Medicine: 2008 28th Annual Meeting, abstract 3. Am J Obstet Gynecol 196(6 Suppl S):S2, 2007.

TABLE 29-6 EFFECT OF 17α-HYDROXYPROGESTERONE CAPROATE (17P) ON SPONTANEOUS PRETERM BIRTH (sPTB)

	N*	% sPTB <37 wk	% sPTB <35 wk	% sPTB <32 wk
Placebo	153	54.9	30.7	19.6
17P	306	36.3	20.6	11.4

*Randomization of 17P vs placebo was 2:1.

From Meis PJ, Klebanoff M, Thom E, et al: Prevention of recurrent preterm delivery by 17-alpha-hydroxyprogesterone caproate. N Engl J Med 348:2379-2385, 2003.

ENHANCED CARE FOR WOMEN WITH RISK

Although perhaps helpful in adolescents,[382,383] enhanced prenatal care including social support, home visits, and education has not been an effective strategy to decrease preterm births.[384-388] Reports suggesting that frequent provider-initiated contact and daily uterine contraction assessment for women with a prior preterm birth might reduce recurrence risk were overturned by a large, controlled trial that found no reduction in preterm birth for these measures and, in fact, reported an excess of care without benefit.[315] A Cochrane analysis similarly found no benefit for enhanced prenatal care in women with increased risk.[389]

ANTIBIOTIC TREATMENT

Although screening and treatment of low-risk women for genital tract organisms to reduce preterm birth is not effective, antibiotic treatment for women with a prior preterm birth who also have BV remains controversial. This strategy was suggested by secondary analyses of data in two trials, one that enrolled women at risk for preterm birth,[373] in which benefit was found only in women with BV, and another that enrolled women with BV,[343] in which benefit was limited to women with a prior preterm birth. Other trials of treatment for BV-positive women have produced conflicting results, perhaps because of variations in the timing, dosage, and antibiotic employed.[390-392] Arguments favoring antibiotic screening and treatment of at-risk women were summarized by Lamont,[379] who argued that clindamycin should be used before 20 weeks' gestation to treat women with a prior preterm birth who have BV. Others have emphasized the increased rate of preterm birth in women treated with metronidazole[118,354,392] and the generally negative results of a recent Cochrane Review of 15 trials involving 5888 women.[111] The reviewers concluded that, although antimicrobial treatment can eradicate BV in pregnancy, it does not reduce the risk of preterm birth or pPROM before 37 weeks for all women or for women with a prior preterm birth. However, they did note evidence that treatment before 20 weeks of gestation may reduce the risk of preterm birth.

One potential reason for the failure of antibiotics to reduce preterm birth is that they may not effectively prevent or treat chorioamnionitis. Placental histology studies from two antibiotic trials found no difference in histologic chorioamnionitis between women randomized to receive antibiotics versus placebo.[393,394] Another likely explanation is that host factors including diet, smoking, and genetic variants in inflammatory response influence the risk of infection-related preterm birth, regardless of antibiotic treatment.[131,395]

The data produced by these trials suggest that the contribution to preterm birth of microorganisms colonizing and infecting the genital tract varies significantly among women, probably because of genetic and behavioral influences that must be further elucidated before antimicrobial agents can be used effectively and safely to prevent preterm birth. The appropriate role for antimicrobial therapy to reduce the risk of preterm birth cannot be determined until questions about the roles of concurrent exposures (e.g., smoking), host factors (e.g., genetic polymorphisms), and selection and timing of treatment are answered.[131,377,395]

PROGESTATIONAL AGENTS

Progesterone supplementation for women at risk for preterm birth has been investigated based on several plausible mechanisms of action, including reduced gap junction formation and oxytocin antagonism leading to relaxation of smooth muscle, maintenance of cervical integrity, and anti-inflammatory effects.[396] Small studies performed in women with recurrent miscarriage and preterm birth were reviewed by Keirse, who found no support for the view that 17P protects against miscarriage but suggested that it does reduce the occurrence of preterm birth.[397] This observation prompted two randomized trials of progestational agents in women with risk factors for preterm birth.[139,398] In a trial that enrolled 142 women with a history of preterm birth or other risk factors to receive placebo or 100 mg progesterone suppositories daily beginning at 24 weeks of gestation, the rate of preterm birth before 37 weeks was 28.5% in the placebo arm and 13.5% in the progesterone arm.[398] In the second study, weekly intramuscular injection of 250 mg of 17P was compared with placebo in a randomized trial that enrolled 459 women with a prior spontaneous preterm birth.[139] Women treated with 17P were significantly less likely to deliver before 37, 35, and 32 weeks (Table 29-6).

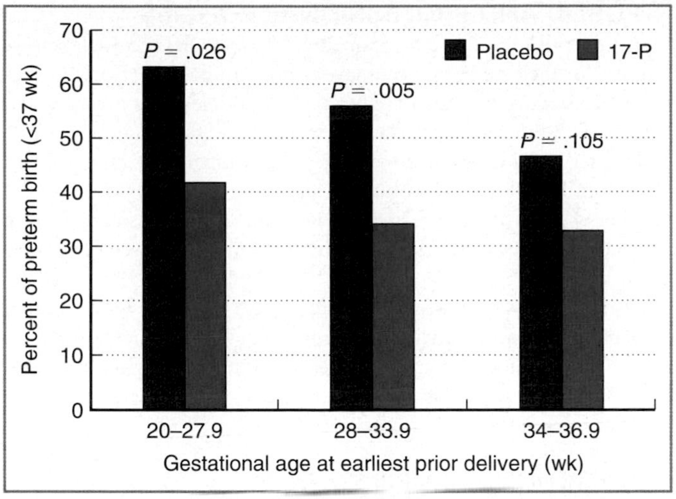

FIGURE 29-21 Effect of 17α-hydroxyprogesterone caproate (17-P) in women with a prior spontaneous preterm birth, by gestational age at the prior delivery. (From Spong CY, Meis PJ, Thom EA, et al: Progesterone for prevention of recurrent preterm birth: Impact of gestational age at previous delivery. Am J Obstet Gynecol 193:1127-1131, 2005.)

Secondary analyses of this study revealed a stronger beneficial effect for women whose qualifying preterm birth was before 34 weeks[399] (Fig. 29-21) and for women with more than one prior preterm birth.[400] The rate of preterm birth before 37 weeks in the placebo group was deemed by some to be higher than expected,[401] but, as noted previously, the recurrence rate was not surprising given the demographics and obstetric history of the women enrolled: 59% of subjects in both groups were African-American, the mean gestational age of the qualifying preterm birth was 31 weeks in both groups, and 32% of women enrolled had more than one prior preterm birth—all factors that increase the risk of recurrence beyond the usual twofold risk associated with a prior preterm birth. The groups differed in the mean number of previous preterm deliveries (1.6 in the placebo group versus 1.4 in the 17P group; $P = .007$), a difference that might have influenced the recurrence rate of 55%.

Meta-analyses of these studies combined with data from earlier trials concluded that the risk of recurrent preterm birth was reduced by 40% to 55% (RR, 0.58; CI, 0.48 to 0.70[402] and RR, 0.45; CI, 0.25 to 0.80[403]). However, these trials were not sufficiently powered to detect effects on neonatal or infant outcomes.[402,404]

Subsequent trials have enrolled women with short cervix (<15 mm) regardless of other historical or current risk,[364] women with twins,[376] and women with prior preterm birth.[140] In a randomized trial that enrolled women with short cervix, those who received vaginal progesterone had a significantly reduced rate of preterm birth before 34 weeks (19%), compared with women who received placebo (41%).[364] However, in another randomized trial conducted in 600 women with twin pregnancies, 17P had no effect on the rate of preterm birth.[376] A third study tested the effect of progesterone vaginal gel on the preterm birth rate in 659 women with a prior preterm birth, specifically taking care not to enroll women who were likely to receive a cerclage.[140] A cervical length measurement was obtained at entry to characterize the a priori risk of women enrolled; the mean cervical length at 18 to 20 weeks was 37 mm, indicating a population with a modest risk of preterm birth (studies indicate that cervical length is superior to obstetric history to predict recurrent PTB). Progesterone did not decrease the frequency of preterm birth at or before 32 weeks, the primary outcome in this study. A secondary analysis of data from this trial suggested that the benefit of progesterone prophylaxis might be limited to women with short cervical length,[405] consistent with another study that enrolled women with short cervix.[364]

The optimal clinical protocols for progesterone have not been developed. Recent small studies have suggested that initiation of prophylaxis after 20 weeks may be beneficial,[406] that discontinuation of prophylaxis may increase the risk of preterm birth,[407] and that treatment after an episode of preterm labor for women with short cervix might be helpful.[408] None of these studies have been large enough to influence current practice, but they do support further investigation to define the appropriate role for this treatment.

The beneficial effect of supplemental progesterone compounds is not universally observed in women with a prior preterm birth, indicating that some pathways to recurrent preterm birth are not affected by this therapy. The absence of effect in twin pregnancy,[376] coupled with reductions in preterm births among women with historical risk[139,398] and short cervix,[364] suggests that the effect may be related to modulation of inflammation or cervical ripening more than an effect on uterine contractility.

The safety of progesterone supplementation is supported by a review of outcomes of pregnancies treated before 1990,[409] by a review of animal studies,[410] and, more recently, by a thorough neurodevelopmental evaluation of children at 4 years of age born in women treated in the NICHD trial.[411] Data in the studies cited here do not show increased rates of fetal growth restriction or stillbirth, but, because prolongation of pregnancy due to progesterone prophylaxis may arise from its anti-inflammatory actions, potential risks related to that action must be a concern.[412]

The potential benefit of wide clinical use of progesterone supplementation awaits further study. Although the rate of preterm birth may not decline appreciably if treatment is limited to those with a prior preterm birth,[413] the savings generated by treating only those women have been estimated at more than $2 billion annually in the United States alone.[414,415]

CERVICAL CERCLAGE

A short cervical length in midpregnancy is associated with an increased risk of early delivery[190-192] and is linked particularly to recurrent preterm birth.[135,196] Cervical length is inversely related to risk of preterm birth, the risk rising as the cervical length decreases. The finding of a short cervix, variably defined as a measurement lower than the 10th or the 3rd percentile (25 or 15 mm, respectively, in the second trimester), may indicate the early onset of parturition in response to biochemical influences of paracrine, endocrine, or inflammatory origin; the biophysical effects of uterine stretch or contractions; or insufficient cervical strength. Because these congenital, biochemical, and biophysical factors may occur in any individual, alone or in combination, to produce a short cervix, the value of any intervention in response to a short cervix has been difficult to determine. Cerclage has been performed in this setting to correct a presumed structural deficiency, but the results have been inconsistent.

The ability of cervical cerclage to prolong pregnancy has been studied in observational and randomized trials,[362,363,374,375,416-429] from which the following conclusions emerge:

- Cervical cerclage in women with a short cervix (<15 mm) who do not have a prior preterm birth does not reduce the rate of spontaneous preterm birth.[362,363]

- Although cerclage may benefit women with short cervix who have a prior preterm birth, the evidence is not conclusive. Selection of the appropriate candidates for cerclage is uncertain.[363,374,375,417-423]
- Prophylactic cerclage for women with a history of preterm birth who are without sonographic demonstration of short cervix in the current pregnancy is not justified by the current literature. There is evidence that these women can be monitored by serial sonographic examination of the cervix, followed by cerclage if the cervix shortens.[416,421,422,430,431]

In a meta-analysis of data from four trials,[363] women with a history of preterm birth who also had a short cervix (defined as <2.5 cm) in the current pregnancy were most likely to benefit from cerclage. In these patients, the risk of birth before 35 weeks was reduced with cerclage treatment (RR, 0.63; CI, 0.48 to 0.85). There was no benefit of cerclage treatment for women with a short cervix who did not have a prior preterm birth (RR, 0.84; CI, 0.60 to 1.17) in this analysis. The risk of preterm birth was actually increased in women with twins and short cervix who were treated with cerclage (RR, 2.15; CI, 1.15 to 4.01).

The efficacy of cerclage thus appears to vary according to the cause of the short cervix. In a study of women with prior preterm birth, the risk of recurrent preterm birth was decreased by cerclage treatment when the level of IL-8 in cervical secretions was low but increased in women treated with cerclage who had an elevated cervical IL-8.[432] These studies suggest that cerclage may reduce the risk of preterm birth in women with a prior preterm birth only when there is ultrasound demonstration of short cervix, and then only when preterm cervical effacement has occurred in the absence of inflammation. No clinical test for cervical inflammation is available. Until such a diagnosis can be made, prophylactic cerclage should be reserved for women who are believed to have anatomic insufficiency, rather than either early delivery history or sonographic findings alone.

Prematurity Prevention Before Pregnancy

Prevention of Risk among Women of Reproductive Age

Pre-conceptional interventions are attractive, because many risk factors are difficult to address successfully in pregnancy.[6]

PUBLIC EDUCATIONAL INTERVENTIONS

The public inaccurately perceives that the problems of preterm infants have been overcome by improved neonatal care.[316] Increased awareness of preterm birth as the leading cause of infant mortality offers an opportunity to raise public awareness of avoidable risk factors.[2] For example, greater public and professional knowledge of evidence suggesting that repeated uterine instrumentation may confer an increased risk of subsequent preterm birth might affect decision making about these procedures.[158,159,162,165] Use of laminaria has been reported to reduce the risk of subsequent preterm birth in women undergoing second-trimester dilation and evacuation.[433]

Similarly, broader public knowledge of the increased risk of preterm birth in singleton gestations conceived with ART might, if coupled with information about the consequences of prematurity, influence fertility care.[434-436] Such educational efforts could be modeled after successful efforts to reduce the prevalence of smoking.

PUBLIC AND PROFESSIONAL POLICIES

In contrast to public education strategies, policies adopted by government or medical bodies can have a more immediate effect. Policies adopted to reduce the risk of higher-order multiple gestation have been successful in Europe, Australia, and the United States. Rates of triplet and higher-order multiple pregnancies wee rising rapidly in the United States until 1998, when voluntary adoption of limitations on the number of embryos transferred was promoted by professional groups. The rate of higher-order multiples then fell by 50% between 1996 and 2003.[437,438]

Social policies to improve pregnancy outcomes have been adopted by many European countries.[320] Minimum paid pregnancy leave of 14 weeks, time off for prenatal visits, exemption from night shifts, and protection from workplace hazards, including complete work leave if necessary, are among the strategies employed.

NUTRITIONAL SUPPLEMENTS

Women considering a pregnancy are routinely advised to initiate supplementation with prenatal vitamins before conception, chiefly to reduce risk of birth defects.[439] A randomized, placebo-controlled trial of vitamin supplementation that enrolled women before conception and continued through the first 2 months of pregnancy found no effect of vitamins on the preterm birth rate.[440]

SMOKING

The attributable risk of cigarette smoking exceeds 25% for preterm birth[441] and approximates 5% for infant mortality.[442] An overall decrease in maternal smoking before conception might be expected to reduce preterm births, but preterm birth rate in the United States rose from 11.6% to 12.5% between 2000 and 2004, a time when smoking among women aged 18 to 44 years declined from 25.5% to 21.7%.[16] Reduced prevalence of smoking would nevertheless have multiple health benefits for pregnant women and infants.

Pre-conceptional Care for Women with Risk

Pre-conceptional interventions to reduce risk of preterm birth typically target women with a previous preterm birth.[443] The upper gestational age boundary for a preterm birth is commonly 37 weeks, and the risk of recurrence declines as the gestational age of the index preterm birth approaches 37 weeks.[4] The lowest gestational age for which an increased risk of preterm birth is observed in subsequent pregnancies is optimal for clinical use and was determined to be 17 to 18 weeks for spontaneous preterm births in studies of data from the Preterm Prediction Study. Previous births before 17 weeks did not confer an increased risk of recurrent preterm delivery.[4,138,443]

As noted earlier. the risk of recurrence is increased for both spontaneous and indicated preterm births.[137,142,148] Risk increases as the gestational age of the previous preterm birth declines and as the number of preterm births increases.[4] Careful review of records from prior pregnancies may be helpful to establish the gestational age of the index birth, estimate the recurrence risk, and identify risks amenable to intervention, including some that may require pre-conceptional intervention (e.g., correction of müllerian anomalies)[444] and others that could determine care choices during pregnancy (e.g., prophylactic progesterone or cerclage). Pre-pregnancy medical risk factors have been identified in as many as 40% of preterm births,[445] suggesting that women with these risks might benefit from pre-conceptional control of diabetes, seizures, asthma, or hypertension.

Internatal care for women with prior preterm birth has been proposed,[446] but evidence that these steps can actually influence the preterm birth rate is lacking. A randomized trial of inter-conceptional home visits and counseling by midwives did not reduce preterm birth and LBW in a study of 1579 women.[447] Based on the hypothesis that pre-conceptional microbial colonization of the endometrium might increase the risk of preterm birth, a randomized, placebo-controlled trial of inter-conceptional antimicrobial treatment was performed in women with a prior early preterm birth.[448] Study participants received metronidazole and azithromycin or placebo at 3-month intervals until their next pregnancy occurred. The rate of recurrent preterm birth was not influenced by antibiotic treatment. The proportion of women enrolled in this study whose qualifying preterm birth was related to infection is not known.[377]

References

1. MacDorman MF, Munson ML, Kirmeyer S: Fetal and Perinatal Mortality—United States, 2004. Natl Vital Stat Rep 56(3):1-19, 2007.
2. Callaghan WD, MacDorman MF, Rasmussen SA, et al: The contribution of preterm birth to infant mortality rates in the United States. Pediatrics 118:1566-1573, 2006.
3. Morrison JJ, Rennie JM: Clinical, scientific and ethical aspects of fetal and neonatal care at extremely preterm periods of gestation. BJOG 104:1341-1350, 1997.
4. Mercer BM, Goldenberg RL, Moawad A, et al: The Preterm Prediction Study: Effect of gestational age and cause of preterm birth on subsequent pregnancy outcome. Am J Obstet Gynecol 181:1216-1221, 1999.
5. Sebire NJ: Choriodecidual inflammatory syndrome (CoDIS) is the leading, and under recognised, cause of early preterm delivery and second trimester miscarriage. Med Hypoth 56:497-500, 2001.
6. Mercer B, Milluzzi B, Collin M: Periviable birth at 20-26 weeks of gestation: Proximate causes, previous obstetric history and recurrence risk. Am J Obstet Gynecol 193:1175-1180, 2005.
7. Edlow AG, Srinivas SK, Elovitz MA: Second-trimester loss and subsequent pregnancy outcomes: What is the real risk? Am J Obstet Gynecol 197:581.e1-581.e6, 2007.
8. Gardosi J: Customized fetal growth standards: Rationale and clinical application. Semin Perinatol 28:33-40, 2004.
9. Behrman RE, Stith Butler A (eds): Institute of Medicine Committee on Understanding Preterm Birth and Assuring Healthy Outcomes. Preterm Birth: Causes, Consequences, and Prevention. Washington, DC: National Academies Press, 2007.
10. Villar J, Belizan JM: The relative contribution of prematurity and fetal growth retardation to low birth weight in developing and developed societies. Am J Obstet Gynecol 143:793-798, 1982.
11. Hamilton BE, Martin JA, Sutton PD, et al: Births: Final data for 2005. Natl Vital Stat Rep 56(6):4, 2007.
12. Craig ED, Mantell CD, Ekeroma AJ, et al: Ethnicity and birth outcome: New Zealand trends 1980-2001. Part 1: Introduction, Methods, Results and Overview. Aust N Z J Obstet Gynaecol 44:530-536, 2004.
13. Lefebvre F, Glorieux J, St Laurent-Gagnon T: Neonatal survival and disability rate at age 18 months for infants born between 23 and 28 weeks of gestation, Am J Obstet Gynecol 174:833-838, 1996.
14. Burke C, Morrison JJ: Perinatal factors and preterm delivery in an Irish obstetric population. J Perinat Med 28:49-53, 2000.
15. Ananth CVP, Joseph KSM, Oyelese YM, et al: Trends in preterm birth and perinatal mortality among singletons: United States, 1989 through 2000. Obstet Gynecol 105:1084-1091, 2005.
16. Martin JA, Hamilton BE, Sutton PD, et al: Births: Final data for 2004. Natl Vital Stat Rep 55(1):80-81, 2006.
17. Wright VC, Schieve LA, Reynolds MA, et al: Assisted reproductive technology surveillance, United States, 2000. MMWR Morb Mortal Wkly Rep 52(SS-9):1-16, 2003.
18. March of Dimes Peristats 2007: Rates of preterm birth in multifetal pregnancies 1990-2004. Available at http://www.marchofdimes.com/peristats/ (accessed April 24, 2008).
19. Meis P, Michielutte R, Peters T, et al: Factors associated with preterm birth in Cardiff, Wales. Am J Obstet Gynecol 173:597-602, 1995.
20. Meis P, Goldenberg R, Mercer B, et al: The Preterm Prediction Study: Risk factors for indicated preterm births. Am J Obstet Gynecol 178:562-567, 1998.
21. Ananth CV, Vintzeleos AM: Maternal-fetal conditions necessitating a medical intervention resulting in preterm birth. Am J Obstet Gynecol 195:1557-1563, 2006.
22. Dolan SM, Gross SJ, Merkatz IR, et al: The contribution of birth defects to preterm birth and low birth weight. Obstet Gynecol 110:318-324, 2007.
23. Mercer BM, Goldenberg RL, Das A, et al: The Preterm Prediction Study: A clinical risk assessment system. Am J Obstet Gynecol 174:1885-1895, 1996.
24. Ananth CV, Vintzileos AM: Epidemiology of preterm birth and its clinical subtypes. J Matern Fetal Neonatal Med 19:773-782, 2006.
25. Morken NH, Källen K, Jacobsson B: Outcomes of preterm children according to type of delivery onset: A nationwide population-based study. Paediatr Perinat Epidemiol 21:458-464, 2007.
26. MacDorman M, Callaghan WM, Mathews TJ, et al: Trends in Preterm-Related Infant Mortality by Race and Ethnicity: United States, 1999-2004. National Center for Health Statistics, 2007. Available at http://www.cdc.gov/nchs/products/pubs/pubd/hestats/infantmort99-04/infantmort99-04.htm (accessed February 28, 2008).
27. Martin JA, Hamilton BE, Sutton PD, et al: Births: Final data for 2002. Natl Vital Stat Rep 52(10):16, 2003.
28. Wood NS, Marlow N, Costeloe K, et al: Neurologic and developmental disability after extremely preterm birth. EPICure Study Group. N Engl J Med 343:378-384, 2000.
29. Lemons JA, Bauer CR, Oh W, et al: Very low birth weight outcomes of the National Institute of Child Health and Human Development Neonatal Research Network, January 1995 through December 1996. Pediatrics 107:e1, 2001.
30. Effer SB, Moutquin J-M, Farine D, et al: Neonatal survival rates in 860 singleton live births at 24 and 25 weeks gestational age: A Canadian multicentre study. BJOG 109:740-745, 2002.
31. Mercer BMM: Preterm premature rupture of the membranes. Obstet Gynecol 101:178-193, 2003.
32. Marret S, Ancel PY, Marpeau L, et al: Neonatal and 5 year outcomes after birth at 30-34 weeks of gestation. Obstet Gynecol 110:72-80, 2007.
33. McIntire DD, Leveno KJ: Neonatal mortality and morbidity rates in late preterm births compared with births at term. Obstet Gynecol 111:35-41, 2008.
34. Available at http://www.nichd.nih.gov/about/org/cdbpm/pp/prog_epbo/epbo_case.cfm, and based on data from Tyson JE, Parikh NA, Langer J, et al: Intensive care for extreme prematurity: Moving beyond gestational age. N Engl J Med 358:1672-1681, 2008.
35. Fanaroff AA, Stoll BJ, Wright LL, et al; NICHD Neonatal Research Network: Trends in neonatal morbidity and mortality for very low birthweight infants. Am J Obstet Gynecol 196:147.e1-147.e8, 2007.
36. Fanaroff AA, Hack M, Walsh MC: The NICHD neonatal research network: Changes in practice and outcomes during the first 15 years. Semin Perinatol 27:281-287, 2003.
37. Horbar JD, Badger GJ, Carpenter JH, et al: Trends in mortality and morbidity for very low birth weight infants, 1991-1999. Pediatrics 110:143-151, 2002.
38. MacDonald H: Perinatal care at the threshold of viability. Pediatrics 110:1024-1027, 2002.
39. Clinical Management Guidelines for Obstetrician-Gynecologists, No. 38: Perinatal Care at the Threshold of Viability. Obstet Gynecol 100:617-624, 2002.
40. Lucey JF, Rowan CA, Shiono P, et al: Fetal infants: The fate of 4172 infants with birth weights of 401 to 500 grams—The Vermont Oxford Network experience (1996-2000). Pediatrics 113:1559-1566, 2004.
41. Alexander GR, Kogan M, Bader D, et al: US birth weight/gestational age-specific neonatal mortality: 1995-1997. Rates for whites, Hispanics, and blacks. Pediatrics 111:e61-e66, 2003.
42. Tyson J, Younes N, Verter J, et al: Viability, morbidity, and resource use among newborns of 501- to 800-g birth weight. JAMA 276:1645-1651, 1996.

43. Barton L, Hodgman J, Pavlova Z: Causes of death in the extremely low birth weight infant. Pediatrics 102:446-451, 1999.
44. Vohr BR, Wright LL, Dusick AM, et al: Center differences and outcomes of extremely low birth weight infants. Pediatrics 113:781-789, 2004.
45. Hack M, Flannery DJ, Schluchter M, et al: Outcomes in young adulthood for very-low-birth-weight infants. N Engl J Med 346:149-157, 2002.
46. Bhutta AT, Cleves MA, Casey PH, et al: Cognitive and behavioral outcomes of school-aged children who were born preterm: A meta-analysis. JAMA 288:728-737, 2002.
47. Marlow N, Wolke D, Bracewell MA, et al; for the EPICure Study Group: Neurologic and developmental disability at six years of age after extremely preterm birth. N Engl J Med 352:9-19, 2005.
48. Winter S, Autry A, Boyle C, et al: Trends in the prevalence of CP in a population based study. Pediatrics 10:1220-1225, 2002.
49. Morse SB, Haywood JL, Goldenberg RL, et al: Estimation of neonatal outcome and perinatal therapy use. Pediatrics 105:1046-1050, 2000.
50. Bottoms SF, Paul RH, Iams JD, et al: Obstetric determinants of neonatal survival of extremely low birth weight infants. Am J Obstet Gynecol 176:960-966, 1997.
51. Shankaran S, Fanaroff A, Wright L, et al: Risk factors for early death among extremely low-birth-weight infants. Am J Obstet Gynecol 186:796-802, 2002.
52. Saigal S, Lambert M, Russ C, Hoult L: Self-esteem of adolescents who were born prematurely. Pediatrics 109:429-433, 2002.
53. Winkvist A, Mogren I, Hogberg U: Familial patterns in birth characteristics: Impact on individual and population risks. Int J Epidemiol 27:248-254, 1998.
54. Porter TF, Fraser AM, Hunter CY, et al: The risk of preterm birth across generations. Obstet Gynecol 90:63-67, 1997.
55. Engel SA, Erichsen HC, Savitz DA, et al: Risk of spontaneous preterm birth is associated with common proinflammatory cytokine polymorphisms. Epidemiology 16:469-477, 2005.
56. Menon R, Velez DR, Simhan H, et al: Multilocus interactions at maternal tumor necrosis factor-alpha, tumor necrosis factor receptors, interleukin-6 and interleukin-6 receptor genes predict spontaneous preterm labor in European-American women. Am J Obstet Gynecol 194:1616-1624, 2006.
57. Crider KS, Whitehead N, Buus RM: Genetic variation associated with preterm birth: A HuGE review. Genet Med 7:593-604, 2005.
58. Wang X, Zuckerman B, Pearson C, et al: Maternal cigarette smoking, metabolic gene polymorphism, and infant birth weight. JAMA 287:195-202, 2002.
59. Macones GA, Parry S, Elkousy M, et al: A polymorphism in the promoter region of TNF and bacterial vaginosis: Preliminary evidence of gene-environment interaction in the etiology of spontaneous preterm birth. Am J Obstet Gynecol 190:1504-1508, 2004.
60. Harvesting the fruits of the human genome. Nat Genet 27:227-228, 2001.
61. Romero R, Espinoza J, Gotsch F, et al: The use of high-dimensional biology (genomics, transcriptomics, proteomics, and metabolomics) to understand the preterm parturition syndrome. BJOG 113:118-135, 2006.
62. Smith LK, Draper ES, Manktelow BN, et al: Socioeconomic inequalities in very preterm birth rates. Arch Dis Child Fetal Neonatal Educ 92:F11-F14, 2007.
63. Thompson JM, Irgens LM, Rasmussen S, Daltveit AK: Secular trends in socio-economic status and the implications for preterm birth. Paediatr Perinat Epidemiol 20:182-187, 2006.
64. Hamilton BE, Martin JA, Ventura SJ: Births: Preliminary data for 2005. Health E-Stats. Natl Vital Stat Rep 55, 2006.
65. Goldenberg RL, Cliver SP, Mulvihill FX, et al: Medical, psychosocial, and behavioral risk factors do not explain the increased risk for low birth weight among black women. Am J Obstet Gynecol 175:1317-1324, 1996.
66. El Reda DK, Grigorescu V, Posner SF, et al: Lower rates of preterm birth in women of Arab ancestry: An epidemiologic paradox—Michigan, 1993-2002. Matern Child Health J 11:622-627, 2007.
67. David RJ, Collins JW Jr: Differing birth weight among infants of U.S-born blacks, African-born blacks, and U.S.-born whites. N Engl J Med 337:1209-1214, 1997.
68. Cnattingius S: The epidemiology of smoking during pregnancy: Smoking prevalence, maternal characteristics, and pregnancy outcomes. Nicotine Tob Res 6(Suppl 2):S125-S140, 2004.
69. Tikkanen M, Nuutila M, Hiilesmaa V, et al: Clinical presentation and risk factors of placental abruption. Acta Obstet Gynecol Scand 85:700-705, 2006.
70. Nabet C, Lelong N, Ancel PY, et al: Smoking during pregnancy according to obstetric complications and parity: Results of the EUROPOP study. Eur J Epidemiol 22:715-721, 2007.
71. Kyrklund-Blomberg NB, Cnattingius S: Preterm birth and maternal smoking: Risks related to gestational age and onset of delivery. Am J Obstet Gynecol 179:1051, 1998.
72. Savitz DA, Dole N, Terry JW, et al: Smoking and pregnancy outcome among African American and white women in central North Carolina. Epidemiology 12:636, 2001.
73. Albertsen K, Andersen A-MN, Olsen J, et al: Alcohol consumption during pregancy and the risk of preterm delivery. Am J Epidemiol 159:155-161, 2004.
74. Sokol RJ, Janisse JJ, Louis JM, et al: Extreme prematurity: An alcohol-related birth effect. Alcohol Clin Exp Res 31:1031-1037, 2007.
75. Savitz DA, Pastore LM: Causes of prematurity. In McCormick MC, Siegel JE (eds): Prenatal Care: Effectiveness and Implementation. Cambridge, UK: Cambridge University Press, 1999.
76. Dole N, Savitz DA, Hertz-Picciotto I, et al: Maternal stress and preterm birth. Am J Epidemiol 157:14-24, 2003.
77. Lu MC, Chen B: Racial and ethnic disparities in preterm birth: The role of stressful life events. Am J Obstet Gynecol 191:691-699, 2004.
78. Rich-Edwards JW, Grizzard TA: Psychosocial stress and neuroendocrine mechanisms in preterm delivery. Am J Obstet Gynecol 192(Suppl):S30-S35, 2005.
79. Kiecolt-Glaser JK, McGuire L, Robles TF, et al: Psychoneuroimmunology: Psychological influences on immune function and health. J Consult Clin Psychology 70:537-547, 2002.
80. Glaser R, Kiecolt-Glaser J: Stress-induced immune dysfunction:implications for health. Nat Rev Immunol 5:243-251, 2005.
81. Ruiz RJR, Fullerton JC, Dudley DJM: The interrelationship of maternal stress, endocrine factors and inflammation on gestational length. Obstet Gynecol Surv 58:415-428, 2003.
82. Annells MF, Hart PH, Mullighan CG, et al: Interleukins-1, -4, -6, -10, tumor necrosis factor, transforming growth factor-β, FAS, and mannose-binding protein C gene polymorphisms in Australian women: Risk of preterm birth. Am J Obstet Gynecol 191:2056, 2004.
83. Hogue CR, Bremner JD: Stress model for research into preterm delivery among black women. Am J Obstet Gynecol 192:s47-s55, 2005.
84. Gavin NI, Gaynes BN, Lohr KN, et al: Perinatal depression: A systematic review of prevalence and incidence. Obstet Gynecol 106:1071-1083, 2005.
85. Dayan J, Creveuil C, Marks MN, et al: Prenatal depression, prenatal anxiety, and spontaneous preterm birth: A prospective cohort study among women with early and regular care. Psychosom Med 68:938-946, 2006.
86. Orr ST, James SA, Prince CB: Maternal prenatal depressive symptoms and spontaneous preterm births among African-American women in Baltimore, Maryland. Am J Epidemiol 156:797-802, 2002.
87. Gennaro S, Fehder W, Nuamah IF, et al: Caregiving to very low birthweight infants: A model of stress and immune response. Brain Behav Immun 11:201-215, 1997.
88. Saurel-Cubizolles MJ, Zeitlin J, Lelong N, et al; for the EUROPOP Group: Employment, working conditions and preterm birth: Results from the EUROPOP case-control survey. J Epidemiol Community Health 58:395-401, 2004.
89. Launer LJ, Villar J, Kestler E, et al: The effect of maternal work on fetal growth and the duration of pregnancy: A prospective study. BJOG 97:62-70, 1990.
90. Pompeii LA, Savitz DA, Evenson KR, et al: Physical exertion at work and the risk of preterm delivery and small for gestational age birth. Obstet Gynecol 106:1279-1288, 2005.

91. Moore TM, Iams JD, Creasy RK, et al: Diurnal and gestational patterns of uterine activity in normal human pregnancy. Obstet Gynecol 83:517-523, 1994.
92. Yost NP, Owen J, Berghella V, et al: Effect of coitus on recurrent preterm birth. Obstet Gynecol 107:793-797, 2006.
93. Fiscella K, Franks P, Kendrick JS, et al: Risk of preterm birth that is associated with vaginal douching. Am J Obstet Gynecol 186:1345-1350, 2002.
94. Misra DP, Trabert B: Vaginal douching and risk of preterm birth among African American women. Am J Obstet Gynecol 196:140, 2007.
95. Hendler I, Goldenberg RL, Mercer BM, et al: The Preterm Prediction Study: Association between maternal body mass index (BMI) and spontaneous preterm birth. Am J Obstet Gynecol 192:882-886, 2005.
96. Scholl TO: Iron status during pregnancy: Setting the stage for mother and infant. Am J Clin Nutr 81:1218S-1222S, 2005.
97. Neggers Y, Goldenberg RL: Some thoughts on body mass index, micronutrient intakes and pregnancy outcome. J Nutr 133:1737S-1740S, 2003.
98. Simhan HN, Bodnar LM: Prepregnancy body mass index, vaginal inflammation, and the racial disparity in preterm birth. Am J Epidemiol 163:459-466, 2006.
99. Goldenberg RL: The plausibility of micronutrient deficiency in relationship to perinatal infection. J Nutr 133:1645S-1648S, 2003.
100. Goldenberg RL, Tamura T: Prepregnancy weight and pregnancy outcome. JAMA 275:1127-1128, 1996.
101. Knox IC Jr, Hoerner JK: The role of infection in premature rupture of the membranes. Am J Obstet Gynecol 59:190-194, 1950.
102. Goldenberg RL, Hauth JC, Andrews WW: Intrauterine infection and preterm delivery. N Engl J Med 342:1500-1507, 2000.
103. Jalava J, Mantymaa ML, Ekblad U, et al: Bacterial 16S rDNA polymerase chain reaction in the detection of intra-amniotic infection. BJOG 103:664-669, 1996.
104. Hitti J, Riley DE, Krohn MA, et al: Broad-spectrum bacterial rDNA polymerase chain reaction assay for detecting amniotic fluid infection among women in premature labor. Clin Infect Dis 24:1228-1232, 1997.
105. Gardella C, Riley DE, Hitti J, et al: Identification and sequencing of bacterial rDNAs in culture-negative amniotic fluid from women in premature labor. Am J Perinatol 21:319-323, 2004.
106. Yoon BH, Romero R, Lim JH, et al: The clinical significance of detecting *Ureaplasma urealyticum* by the polymerase chain reaction in the amniotic fluid of patients with preterm labor. Am J Obstet Gynecol 189:919-924, 2003.
107. Steel JH, Malatos S, Kennea N, et al: Bacteria and inflammatory cells in fetal membranes do not always cause preterm labor. Pediatr Res 57:404-411, 2005.
108. Andrews WW, Goldenberg RL, Hauth JC, et al: Endometrial microbial colonization and plasma cell endometritis after spontaneous or indicated preterm versus term delivery. Am J Obstet Gynecol 193:739-745, 2005.
109. Goldenberg RL, Klebanoff M, Carey JC, et al: Vaginal fetal fibronectin measurements from 8 to 22 weeks' gestation and subsequent spontaneous preterm birth. Am J Obstet Gynecol 183:469-475, 2000.
110. Nugent RP, Krohn MA, Hillier SL: Reliability of diagnosing bacterial vaginosis is improved by a standardized method of gram stain interpretation. J Clin Microbiol 29:297-301, 1991.
111. McDonald HM, Brocklehurst P, Gordon A: Antibiotics for treating bacterial vaginosis in pregnancy. Cochrane Database Syst Rev (1):CD000262, 2007.
112. Okun N, Gronau KA, Hannah ME: Antibiotics for bacterial vaginosis or *Trichomonas vaginalis* in pregnancy: A systematic review. Obstet Gynecol 105:857-868, 2005.
113. Hitti J, Nugent R, Boutain D, et al: Racial disparity in risk of preterm birth associated with lower genital tract infection. Paediatr Perinat Epidemiol 21:330-337.
114. Goldenberg R, Klebanoff M, Nugent R, et al; for the Vaginal Infections in Pregnancy Study Group: Bacterial colonization of the vagina in four ethnic groups. Am J Obstet Gynecol 174:1618-1621.
115. Carey JC, Klebanoff MA, Hauth JC, et al: Metronidazole to prevent preterm delivery in pregnant women with asymptomatic bacterial vaginosis. National Institute of Child Health and Human Development Network of Maternal-Fetal Medicine Units. N Engl J Med 342:534-540, 2000.
116. Sutton M, Sternberg M, Koumans EH, et al: The prevalence of *Trichomonas vaginalis* infection among reproductive-age women in the United States, 2001-2004. Clin Infect Dis 45:1319-1326, 2007.
117. Cotch MF, Pastorek JG 2nd, Nugent RP, et al: *Trichomonas vaginalis* associated with low birth weight and preterm delivery. Sex Transm Dis 24:353-360, 1997.
118. Klebanoff MA, Carey JC, Hauth JC, et al: Failure of metronidazole to prevent preterm delivery among pregnant women with asymptomatic *Trichomonas vaginalis* infection. N Engl J Med 345:487-493, 2001.
119. Sweet RL, Landers DL, Walker C, et al: *Chlamydia trachomatis* infection and pregnancy outcome. Am J Obstet Gynecol 156:824-833, 1987.
120. Donders GG, Desmyter J, De Wet DH, et al: The association of gonorrhea and syphilis with premature birth and low birth weight. Genitourin Med 69:98-101, 1993.
121. Goldenberg RL, Thom E, Moawad AH, et al: The Preterm Prediction Study: Fetal fibronectin, bacterial vaginosis, and peripartum infection. Obstet Gynecol 87:656-660, 1996.
122. Goldenberg RL, Culhane JF, Johnson DC: Maternal infection and adverse fetal and neonatal outcomes. Clin Perinatol 32:523-559, 2005.
123. Romero R, Oyarzun E, Mazor M, et al: Meta-analysis of the relationship between asymptomatic bacteriuria and preterm delivery/low birth weight. Obstet Gynecol 73:576-582, 1989.
124. Offenbacher S, Boggess KA, Murtha AP, et al: Progressive periodontal disease and risk of very preterm delivery. Obstet Gynecol 107:29-36, 2006.
125. Offenbacher S, Jared HL, O'Reilly PG, et al: Potential pathogenic mechanisms of periodontitis associated pregnancy complications. Ann Periodontol 3:233-250, 1998.
126. Klebanoff M, Searle K: The role of inflammation in preterm birth: Focus on periodontitis. BJOG 113(Suppl 3):43-45, 2006.
127. Moore S, Ide M, Coward PY, et al: A prospective study to investigate the relationship between periodontal diseases and adverse pregnancy outcome. Br Dent J 197:251-258, 2004.
128. Pretorius C, Jagatt A, Lamont RF: The relationship between periodontal disease, bacterial vaginosis, and preterm birth. J Perinat Med 35:93-99, 2007.
129. Stamilio DM, Chang JJ, Macones GA: Periodontal disease and preterm birth: Do the data have enough teeth to recommend screening and preventive treatment? Am J Obstet Gynecol 196:93-94, 2007.
130. Goepfert AR, Jeffcoat M, Andrews WW, et al: Periodontal disease and upper genital tract inflammation in early spontaneous preterm birth. Am J Obstet Gynecol 104:777-783, 2004.
131. Romero RM, Chaiworapongsa TM, Kuivaniemi HM, et al: Bacterial vaginosis, the inflammatory response and the risk of preterm birth: A role for genetic epidemiology in the prevention of preterm birth. Am J Obstet Gynecol 190:1509-1519, 2004.
132. Bakketeig LS, Hoffman HJ, Harley EE: The tendency to repeat gestational age and birth weight in successive births. Am J Obstet Gynecol 135:1086-1103, 1979.
133. Bakketeig LS, Hoffman HJ: Epidemiology of preterm birth: Results from a longitudinal study of births in Norway. In Elder MG, Hendricks CH (eds): Preterm Labor. London, Butterworths, 1981.
134. Carr-Hill RA, Hall MH: The repetition of spontaneous preterm labour. BJOG 92:921-928, 1985.
135. Goldenberg RL, Iams JD, Mercer BM, et al: The Preterm Prediction Study: The value of new vs standard risk factors in predicting early and all spontaneous preterm births. NICHD MFMU Network. Am J Public Health 88:233-238, 1998.
136. Bloom SL, Yost NP, McIntire DD, et al: Recurrence of preterm birth in singleton and twin pregnancies. Obstet Gynecol 98:379-385, 2001.
137. Adams MM, Elam-Evans LD, Wilson HG, et al: Rates of and factors associated with recurrence of preterm delivery. JAMA 283:1591-1596, 2000.
138. Iams JD, Goldenberg RL, Mercer BM, et al: The Preterm Prediction Study: Recurrence risk of spontaneous preterm birth. Am J Obstet Gynecol 178:1035, 1998.

139. Meis PJ, Klebanoff M, Thom E, et al: Prevention of recurrent preterm delivery by 17-alpha-hydroxyprogesterone caproate. N Engl J Med 348:2379-2385, 2003.
140. O'Brien JM, Adair CD, Lewis DF, et al: Progesterone vaginal gel for the reduction of recurrent preterm birth: Primary results from a randomized, double-blind, placebo-controlled trial. Ultrasound Obstet Gynecol 30:687-696, 2007.
141. Kaltreider DF, Kohl S: Epidemiology of preterm delivery. Clin Obstet Gynecol 23:17-31, 1980.
142. Goldenberg RL, Andrews WW, Faye-Petersen O, et al: The Alabama Preterm Birth Project: Placental histology in recurrent spontaneous and indicated preterm birth. Am J Obstet Gynecol 195:792-796, 2006.
143. Rawling JS, Rawlings VB, Read JA: Prevalence of low birth weight and preterm delivery in relation to the interval between pregnancies among white and black women. N Engl J Med 332:69-74, 1995.
144. Zhu BP, Rolfs RT, Nangle BE, et al: Effect of the interval between pregnancies on perinatal outcomes. N Engl J Med 340:589-594, 1999.
145. Smith GC, Pell JP, Dobbie R: Interpregnancy interval and risk of preterm birth and neonatal death: Retrospective cohort study. BMJ 327:313, 2003.
146. Menard MK, Newman RB, Keenan A, et al: Prognostic significance of prior preterm twin delivery on subsequent singleton pregnancy. Am J Obstet Gynecol 174:1429-1432, 1996.
147. Facco FL, Nash K, Grobman WA: Are women who have had a preterm twin delivery at greater risk of preterm birth in a subsequent singleton pregnancy? Am J Obstet Gynecol 197:253.e1-253.e3, 2007.
148. Ananth CV, Getahun D, Peltier MR, et al: Recurrence of spontaneous versus medically indicated preterm birth. Am J Obstet Gynecol 195:643-650, 2006.
149. Berghella V: Prevention of recurrent fetal growth restriction. Obstet Gynecol 110:904-912, 2007.
150. Krupa FG, Faltin D, Cecatti JG, et al: Predictors of preterm birth. Int J Gynaecol Obstet 94:5-11, 2006.
151. Rackow BW, Arici A: Reproductive performance of women with mullerian anomalies. Curr Opin Obstet Gynecol 19:229-237, 2007.
152. Lin PJ: Reproductive outcomes in women with uterine anomalies. J Womens Health 13:33-39, 2004.
153. Raga F, Bauset C, Remohi J, et al: Reproductive impact of congenital müllerian anomalies. Hum Reprod 12:2277, 1997.
154. Zlopaša G, Škrablin S, Kalafatić D, et al: Uterine anomalies and pregnancy outcome following resectoscope metroplasty. Int J Gynecol Obstet 98:129-133, 2007.
155. Ahdoot K, Clunie G, Chelmow D, et al: Uterine anomalies and obstetric outcome. Am J Obstet Gynecol 191(abstr. 245):S76, 2004.
156. Kaufman RH, Adam E, Hatch EE, et al: Continued follow-up of pregnancy outcomes in diethylstilbestrol-exposed offspring. Obstet Gynecol 96:483, 2000.
157. Martius JA, Steck T, Oehler MK, et al: Risk factors associated with preterm (<37 + 0 weeks) and early preterm birth (<32 + 0 weeks): Univariate and multivariate analysis of 106,345 singleton births from the 1994 statewide perinatal survey of Bavaria. Eur J Obstet Reprod Biol 80:183-189, 1998.
158. Ancel PY, Lelong N, Papiernik E, et al; for EUROPOP. History of induced abortion as a risk factor for preterm birth in European countries: Results of the EUROPOP survey. Hum Reprod 19:734-740, 2004.
159. Moreau C, Kaminski M, Ancel PY, et al; for the EPIPAGE Group. Previous induced abortions and the risk of very preterm delivery: Results of the EPIPAGE study. BJOG 112:430-437, 2005.
160. Henriet L, Kaminski M: Impact of induced abortions on subsequent pregnancy outcome: The 1995 French national perinatal survey. BJOG 108:1036-1042, 2001.
161. Virk J, Zhang J, Olsen J: Medical abortion and the risk of subsequent adverse pregnancy outcomes. N Engl J Med 357:648-653, 2007.
162. Jakobsson M, Gissler M, Sainio S, et al: Preterm delivery after surgical treatment for cervical intraepithelial neoplasia. Obstet Gynecol 109:309-313, 2007.
163. Nøhr B, Tabor A, Frederiksen K, et al: Loop electrosurgical excision of the cervix and the subsequent risk of preterm delivery. Acta Obstet Gynecol Scand 86:596-603, 2007.
164. Sjøborg KD, Vistad I, Myhr SS, et al: Pregnancy outcome after cervical cone excision: A case-control study. Acta Obstet Gynecol Scand 86:423-428, 2007.
165. Sadler L, Saftlas A, Wang W, et al: Treatment for cervical intraepithelial neoplasia and risk of preterm delivery. JAMA 291:2100-2106, 2004.
166. Ekwo EE, Gosselink CA, Moawad A: Unfavorable outcome in penultimate pregnancy and premature rupture of membranes in successive pregnancy. Obstet Gynecol 80:166-172, 1992.
167. Yang J, Hartmann KE, Savitz DA, et al: Vaginal bleeding during pregnancy and preterm birth. Am J Epidemiol 160:118-125, 2004.
168. Burton BK: Elevated maternal serum alpha-fetoprotein: Interpretation and follow-up. Clin Obst Gynecol 31:293-305, 1988.
169. Krause TG, Christens P, Wohlfahrt J, et al: Second-trimester maternal serum alpha-fetoprotein and risk of adverse pregnancy outcome. Obstet Gynecol 97:277-282, 2001.
170. Chandra S, Scott H, Dodds L, et al: Unexplained elevated maternal serum α-fetoprotein and/or human chorionic gonadotropin and the risk of adverse outcomes. Am J Obstet Gynecol 189:775-781, 2003.
171. De Sutter P, Bontinck J, Schutysers V, et al: First-trimester bleeding and pregnancy outcome in singletons after assisted reproduction. Hum Reprod 21:1907-1911, 2006.
172. Chasen ST, Luo G, Perni SC, et al: Are in vitro fertilization pregnancies with early spontaneous reduction high risk? Am J Obstet Gynecol 195:814-817, 2006.
173. Shebl O, Ebner T, Sommergruber M, et al: Birth weight is lower for survivors of the vanishing twin syndrome: A case-control study. Fertil Steril 2007 Oct 9 [Epub ahead of print].
174. Cheang CU, Huang LS, Lee TH, et al: A comparison of the outcomes between twin and reduced twin pregnancies produced through assisted reproduction. Fertil Steril 88:47-52, 2007.
175. American College of Obstetricians and Gynecologists: Perinatal Risks Associated with Assisted Reproductive Technology. Committee Opinion No. 324. Obstet Gynecol 106:1143-1146, 2005.
176. McDonald SD, Murphy K, Beyene J, et al: Perinatel outcomes of singleton pregnancies achieved by in vitro fertilization: A systematic review and meta-analysis. J Obstet Gynaecol Can 27:449-459, 2005.
177. Schieve LA, Ferre C, Peterson HB, et al: Perinatal outcome among singleton infants conceived through assisted reproductive technology in the United States. Obstet Gynecol 103:1144-1153, 2004.
178. Jackson RA, Gibson KA, Wu YW, et al: Perinatal outcomes in singletons following in vitro fertilization: A meta-analysis. Obstet Gynecol 103:551-563, 2004.
179. McGovern PG, Llorens AJ, Skurnick JH, et al: Increased risk of preterm birth in singleton pregnancies resulting from in vitro fertilization-embryo transfer or gamete intrafallopian transfer: A meta-analysis. Fertil Steril 82:1514-1520, 2004.
180. Helmerhorst FM, Perquin DA, Donker D, et al: Perinatal outcome of singletons and twins after assisted conception: A systematic review of controlled studies. BMJ 328:261, 2004.
181. Ombelet W, Martens G, De Sutter P, et al: Perinatal outcome of 12,021 singleton and 3108 twin births after non–IVF-assisted reproduction: A cohort study. Hum Reprod 21:1025-1032, 2006.
182. Yang JH, Kuhlman K, Daly S, et al: Prediction of preterm birth by second trimester cervical sonography in twin pregnancies. Ultrasound Obstet Gynecol 15:288-291, 2000.
183. Imseis HM, Albert TA, Iams JD: Identifying twin gestations at low risk for preterm birth with a transvaginal ultrasonographic cervical measurement at 24 to 26 weeks' gestation. Am J Obstet Gynecol 177:1149-1155, 1997.
184. Goldenberg RL, Iams JD, Miodovnik M, et al: The Preterm Prediction Study: Risk factors in twin gestations. Am J Obstet Gynecol 175:1047-1053, 1996.
185. Newman RB, Iams JD, Das A, et al: A prospective masked observational study of uterine contraction frequency in twins. Am J Obstet Gynecol 195:1564-1570, 2006.
186. Sciscione A; for the NICHD MFMU Network: Perinatal outcomes in women with twin gestations who conceived spontaneously versus by

assisted reproductive techniques (ART). Society for Maternal-Fetal Medicine: 2008 28th Annual Meeting, abstract 260. Am J Obstet Gynecol 196(6 Suppl S):S84, 2007.
187. Nageotte MP, Dorchester W, Porto M, et al: Quantitation of uterine activity preceding preterm, term, and postterm labor. Am J Obstet Gynecol 158:1254-1259, 1988.
188. Iams JD, Newman RB, Thom EA, et al: Frequency of uterine contractions and the risk of spontaneous preterm delivery. N Engl J Med 346:250-255, 2002.
189. Copper RL, Goldenberg RL, Dubard MB, et al: Cervical examination and tocodynamometry at 28 weeks' gestation: Prediction of spontaneous preterm birth. Am J Obstet Gynecol 172:666-671, 1995.
190. Andersen HF, Nugent CE, Wanty SD, et al: Prediction of risk for preterm delivery by ultrasonographic measurement of cervical length. Am J Obstet Gynecol 163:859-867, 1990.
191. Iams JD, Goldenberg RL, Meis PJ, et al: The length of the cervix and the risk of spontaneous premature delivery. N Engl J Med 334:567-573, 1996.
192. Taipale P, Hiilesmaa V: Sonographic measurement of uterine cervix at 18-22 weeks' gestation and the risk of preterm delivery. Obstet Gynecol 92:902-907, 1998.
193. Heath V, Southall T, Souka A, et al: Cervical length at 23 weeks of gestation: Prediction of spontaneous preterm delivery. Ultrasound Obstet Gynecol 12:312-317, 1998.
194. Berghella V, Talucci M, Desai A: Does transvaginal sonographic measurement of cervical length before 14 weeks predict preterm delivery in high-risk pregnancies? Ultrasound Obstet Gynecol 21:140-144, 2003.
195. Hibbard JU, Tart M, Moawad AH: Cervical length at 16-22 weeks' gestation and risk for preterm delivery. Obstet Gynecol 96:972-978, 2000.
196. Iams JD, Johnson FF, Sonek J, et al: Cervical competence as a continuum: A study of ultrasonographic cervical length and obstetric performance. Am J Obstet Gynecol 172:1097-1103, 1995.
197. Owen J, Yost N, Berghella V, et al: Mid-trimester endovaginal sonography in women at high risk for spontaneous preterm birth. JAMA 286:1340-1348, 2001.
198. Berghella V, Owen J, MacPherson C, et al: Natural history of cervical funneling in women at high risk for spontaneous preterm birth. Obstet Gynecol 109:863-869, 2007.
199. Yost NP, Owen J, Berghella V, et al: Number and gestational age of prior preterm births does not modify the predictive value of a short cervix. Am J Obstet Gynecol 191:241-246, 2004.
200. Durnwald CP, Walker H, Lundy JC, et al: Rates of recurrent preterm birth by obstetrical history and cervical length. Am J Obstet Gynecol 193:1170-1174, 2005.
201. de Carvalho MH, Bittar RE, Brizot Mde L, et al: Prediction of preterm delivery in the second trimester. Obstet Gynecol 105:532-536, 2005.
202. To MS, Skentou CA, Royston P, et al: Prediction of patient-specific risk of early preterm delivery using maternal history and sonographic measurement of cervical length: A population-based prospective study. Ultrasound Obstet Gynecol 27:362-367, 2006.
203. Berghella V, Roman A, Daskalakis C, et al: Gestational age at cervical length measurement and incidence of preterm birth. Obstet Gynecol 110:311-317, 2007.
204. Berghella V: Gestational age at cervical length measurement and incidence of preterm birth. Obstet Gynecol 110:311-317, 2007.
205. King JF, Grant A, Keirse MJNC: Beta-mimetics in preterm labour: An overview of the randomized controlled trials. BJOG 95:211, 1988.
206. Olah KS, Gee GH: The prevention of prematurity: Can we continue to ignore the cervix? BJOG 99:278, 1992.
207. Hueston WJ: Preterm contractions in community settings: II. Predicting preterm birth in women with preterm contractions. Obstet Gynecol 92:43-46, 1998.
208. Macones GA, Segel SY, Stamilio DM, et al: Prediction of delivery among women with early preterm labor by means of clinical characteristics alone. Am J Obstet Gynecol 181:1414-1418, 1999.
209. Peaceman AM, Andrews WW, Thorp JM, et al: Fetal fibronectin as a predictor of preterm birth in patients with symptoms: A multicenter trial. Am J Obstet Gynecol 177:13-18, 1997.
210. Iams JD, Johnson FF, Parker M: A prospective evaluation of the signs and symptoms of preterm labor. Obstet Gynecol 84:227, 1994.
211. Jackson GM, Ludmir J, Bader TJ: The accuracy of digital examination and ultrasound in the evaluation of cervical length. Obstet Gynecol 79:214, 1992.
212. Berghella V, Tolosa JE, Kuhlman K, et al: Cervical ultrasonography compared with manual examination as a predictor of preterm delivery. Am J Obstet Gynecol 177:723-730, 1997.
213. Matijevic R, Grgic O, Vasili O: Is sonographic assessment of cervical length better than digital examination in screening for preterm delivery in a low-risk population? Acta Obstet Gynecol Scand 85:1342-1347, 2006.
214. Guinn DA, Goepfert AR, Owen J, et al: Management options in women with preterm uterine contractions: A randomized clinical trial. Am J Obstet Gynecol 177: 814-818, 1997.
215. Leitich H, Brumbauer M, Kaider A, et al: Cervical length and dilation of the internal os detected by vaginal ultrasonography as markers for preterm delivery: A systematic review. Am J Obstet Gynecol 181:1465-1472, 1999.
216. Leitich H, Egarter C, Kaider A, et al: Cervicovaginal fetal fibronectin as a marker for preterm delivery: A meta-analysis. Am J Obstet Gynecol 180:1169-1176, 1999.
217. American College of Obstetricians and Gynecologists: Assessment of risk factors for preterm birth. ACOG Practice Bulletin No. 31. Obstet Gynecol 98:709-716, 2001.
218. American College of Obstetricians and Gynecologists: Management of preterm labor. ACOG Practice Bulletin No. 43. Obstet Gynecol 101:1039-1047, 2003.
219. Iams JD: Prediction and early detection of preterm labor. Obstet Gynecol 101:402-412, 2003.
220. Incerti M, Ghidini A, Korker V, Pezzullo JC: Performance of cervicovaginal fetal fibronectin in a community hospital setting. Arch Gynecol Obstet 275:347-351, 2007.
221. Mason GC, Maresh MJA: Alterations in bladder volume and the ultrasound appearance of the cervix. BJOG 97:457-458, 1990.
222. Macones GA, Segel SY, Stamilio DM, et al: Predicting delivery within 48 hours in women treated with parenteral tocolysis. Obstet Gynecol 93:432-436, 1999.
223. Gomez R, Romero R, Medina L, et al: Cervicovaginal fibronectin improves the prediction of preterm delivery based on sonographic cervical length in patients with preterm uterine contractions and intact membranes. Am J Obstet Gynecol 192:350-359, 2005.
224. Bujold E, Pasquier JC, Simoneau J, et al: Intra-amniotic sludge, short cervix, and risk of preterm delivery. J Obstet Gynaecol Can 28:198-202, 2006.
225. Espinoza J, Gonçalves LF, Romero R, et al: The prevalence and clinical significance of amniotic fluid "sludge" in patients with preterm labor and intact membranes. Ultrasound Obstet Gynecol 25:346-352, 2005.
226. Yeast J, Poskin M, Stockbauer J, et al: Changing patterns in regionalization of perinatal care and the impact on neonatal mortality. Am J Obstet Gynecol 178:131-135, 1998.
227. Towers CV, Bonebrake R, Padilla G, et al: The effect of transport on the rate of severe intraventricular hemorrhage in very low birth weight infants. Obstet Gynecol 95:291-295, 2000.
228. Schrag S, Gorwitz R, Fultz-Butts K, et al: Prevention of perinatal group B streptococcal disease. Revised guidelines from CDC. MMWR Recomm Rep 16;51(RR-11):1-22, 2002.
229. Kenyon S, Taylor D, Tarnow-Mordi W: Broad-spectrum antibiotics for preterm, prelabour rupture of fetal membranes: The ORACLE I randomised trial. Lancet 357:979-988, 2001.
230. Newton ER, Dinsmoor MJ, Gibbs RS: A randomized, blinded, placebo-controlled trial of antibiotics in idiopathic preterm labor. Obstet Gynecol 74:562-566, 1989.
231. Newton E, Shields L, Ridgway LI, et al: Combination antibiotics and indomethacin in idiopathic preterm labor: A randomized double-blind clinical trial. Am J Obstet.Gynecol 165:1753-1759, 1991.

232. Romero R, Sibai B, Caritis S, et al: Antibiotic treatment of preterm labor with intact membranes: A multicenter, randomized, double-blinded, placebo-controlled trial. Am J Obstet Gynecol 169:764-767, 1993.
233. Norman K, Pattinson R, de Souza J, et al: Ampicillin and metronidazole treatment in preterm labour: A multicentre, randomised controlled trial. BJOG 101:404-408, 1994.
234. Gordon M, Samuels P, Shubert P, et al: A randomized, prospective study of adjunctive ceftizoxime in preterm labor. Am J Obstet.Gynecol 172:1546-1552, 1995.
235. Shankaran S, Papile LA, Wright LL, et al: The effect of antenatal phenobarbital therapy on neonatal intracranial hemorrhage in preterm infants. N Engl J Med 337:466-471, 1997.
236. Thorp JA, Ferrette-Smith D, Gaston LA, et al: Combined antenatal vitamin K and phenobarbital therapy for preventing intracranial hemorrhage in newborns less than 34 weeks' gestation. Obstet Gynecol 86:1-8, 1995.
237. Nelson KB: Can we prevent cerebral palsy? N Engl J Med 349:1765-1769, 2003.
238. Nelson KB, Grether J: Effect of MgSO4 therapy on cerebral palsy rates in infants <1500 grams. J Pediatr 95:263, 1995.
239. Grether JK, Hoogstrate J, Selvin S, Nelson KB: Magnesium sulfate tocolysis and risk of neonatal death. Am J Obstet Gynecol 178:1-6, 1998.
240. Grether JK, Hoogstrate J, Walsh-Greene E, et al: Magnesium sulfate for tocolysis and risk of spastic cerebral palsy in premature children born to women without preeclampsia. Am J Obstet Gynecol 183:717-725, 2000.
241. Mittendorf R, Covert R, Boman J, et al: Is tocolytic magnesium sulphate associated with increased total paediatric mortality? Lancet 350:1517-1518, 1997.
242. Paneth N, Jetton J, Pinto-Martin J, et al: Magnesium sulfate in labor and risk of neonatal brain lesions and cerebral palsy in low birth weight infants. The Neonatal Brain Hemorrhage Study Analysis Group. Pediatrics 99:E1, 1997.
243. Schendel DE, Berg CJ, Yeargin-Allsopp M, et al: Prenatal magnesium sulfate exposure and the risk for cerebral palsy or mental retardation among very low-birth-weight children aged 3 to 5 years. JAMA 276:1805-1810, 1996.
244. Crowther CA, Hiller JE, Doyle LW, et al: Effect of magnesium sulfate given for neuroprotection before preterm birth: A randomized controlled trial. JAMA 290:2669-2676, 2003.
245. Marret S, Marpeau L, Zupan-Simunek V, et al; for the PREMAG trial group: Magnesium sulphate given before very-preterm birth to protect infant brain: The randomised controlled PREMAG trial. BJOG 114:310-318, 2007.
246. Rouse D; for NICHD MFMU Network: A randomized controlled trial of magnesium sulfate for the prevention of cerebral palsy. Society for Maternal-Fetal Medicine: 2008 28th Annual Meeting, abstract 1. Am J Obstet Gynecol 196(6 Suppl S):S2, 2007.
247. Smith GN, Walker MC, Ohlsson A, et al; for the Canadian Preterm Labour Nitroglycerin Trial Group: Randomized double blind placebo controlled trial of transdermal nitroglycerin for preterm labor. Am J Obstet Gynecol 196:37.e1-37.e8, 2007.
248. King JF, Flenady VJ, Papatsonis DNM, et al: Calcium channel blockers for inhibiting preterm labour. Cochrane Database Syst Rev (1):CD002255, 2003.
249. Papatsonis D, Flenady V, Cole S, et al: Oxytocin receptor antagonists for inhibiting preterm labour. Cochrane Database Syst Rev (3):CD004452, 2005.
250. Anotayanonth S, Subhedar NV, Garner P, et al: Betamimetics for inhibiting preterm labour. Cochrane Database Syst Rev (4):CD004352, 2004.
251. Crowther CA, Hiller JE, Doyle LW: Magnesium sulphate for preventing preterm birth in threatened preterm labour. Cochrane Database Syst Rev (4):CD001060, 2002.
252. King J, Flenady V, Cole S, et al: Cyclo-oxygenase (COX) inhibitors for treating preterm labour. Cochrane Database Syst Rev (2):CD001992, 2005.
253. Lyell DJ, Pullen K, Campbell L, et al: Magnesium sulfate compared with nifedipine for acute tocolysis of preterm labor. Obstet Gynecol 110:61-67, 2007.
254. Ferguson JE, Schutz T, Pershe R, et al: Nifedipine pharmacokinetics during preterm labor tocolysis. Am J Obstet Gynecol 161:1485-1490, 1989.
255. Oei SG, Oei SK, Brolmann HA: Myocardial infarction during nifedipine therapy for preterm labor. N Engl J Med 340:154, 1999.
256. Tsatsaris V, Papasonis D, Goffinet F, et al: Tocolysis with nifedipine or beta-adrenergic agonists: A meta-analysis. Obstet Gynecol 97:840, 2001.
257. Ben-Ami M, Giladi Y, Shalev E: The combination of magnesium sulphate and nifedipine: A cause of neuromuscular blockade. Br.J Obstet Gynaecol 101:262-263, 1994.
258. Abbas OM, Nassar AH, Kanj NA, et al: Acute pulmonary edema during tocolytic therapy with nifedipine. Am J Obstet Gynecol 195:e3-e4, 2006.
259. Mari G, Kirshon B, Moise KJ Jr, et al: Doppler assessment of the fetal and uteroplacental circulation during nifedipine therapy for preterm labor. Am J Obstet Gynecol 161:1514-1518, 1989.
260. van Veen AJ, Pelinck MJ, van Pampus MG, et al: Severe hypotension and fetal death due to tocolysis with nifedipine. BJOG 112:509-510, 2005.
261. Oei SG: Calcium channel blockers for tocolysis: A review of their role and safety following reports of serious adverse events. Eur J Obstet Gynecol Reprod Biol 126:137-145, 2006.
262. Lunt CC, Satin AJ, Barth WH Jr, et al: The effect of indomethacin tocolysis on maternal coagulation status. Obstet Gynecol 84:820-822, 1994.
263. Moise KJ Jr: Effect of advancing gestational age on the frequency of fetal ductal constriction in association with maternal indomethacin use. Am J Obstet Gynecol 168:1350-1353, 1993.
264. Moise KJ Jr, Huhta JC, Sharif DS, et al: Indomethacin in the treatment of premature labor: Effects on the fetal ductus arteriosus. N Engl J Med 319:327-331, 1988.
265. Vermillion ST, Scardo JA, Lashus AG, et al: The effect of indomethacin tocolysis on fetal ductus arteriosus constriction with advancing gestational age. Am J Obstet Gynecol 177:256-259, 1997.
266. Mohen D, Newnham JP, D'Orsogna L: Indomethacin for the treatment of polyhydramnios: A case of constriction of the ductus arteriosus. Aust N Z J Obstet Gynaecol 32:243-246, 1992.
267. Alano MA, Ngougmna E, Ostrea EM Jr, et al: Analysis of nonsteroidal antiinflammatory drugs in meconium and its relation to persistent pulmonary hypertension of the newborn. Pediatrics 107:519-523, 2001.
268. Tarcan A, Gürakan B, Yildirim S, et al: Persistent pulmonary hypertension in a premature newborn after 16 hours of antenatal indomethacin exposure. J Perinat Med 32:98-99, 2004.
269. Vermillion ST, Newman RB: Recent indomethacin tocolysis is not associated with neonatal complications in preterm infants. Am J Obstet Gynecol 181:1083-1086, 1999.
270. Loe SM, Sanchez-Ramos L, Kaunitz AM: Assessing the neonatal safety of indomethacin tocolysis: A systematic review with meta-analysis. Obstet Gynecol 106:173-179, 2005.
271. Savage AH, Anderson BL, Simhan HN: The safety of prolonged indomethacin therapy. Am J Perinatol 24:207-213, 2007.
272. van der Heijden BJ, Carlus C, Narcy F, et al: Persistent anuria, neonatal death, and renal microcystic lesions after prenatal exposure to indomethacin. Am J Obstet Gynecol 171:617-623, 1994.
273. Sawdy RJ, Lye S, Fisk NM, et al: A double-blind randomized study of fetal side effects during and after the short-term maternal administration of indomethacin, sulindac, and nimesulide for the treatment of preterm labor. Am J Obstet Gynecol 188:1046-1051, 2003.
274. Norton ME, Merrill J, Cooper BA, et al: Neonatal complications after the administration of indomethacin for preterm labor. N Engl J Med 329:1602-1607, 1993.
275. Suarez RD, Grobman WA, Parilla BV: Indomethacin tocolysis and intraventricular hemorrhage. Obstet Gynecol 97:921-925, 2001.
276. Mamopoulos M, Assimakopoulos E, Reece EA, et al: Maternal indomethacin therapy in the treatment of polyhydramnios. Am J Obstet Gynecol 162:1225-1229, 1990.
277. Romero R, Sibai BM, Sanchez-Ramos L, et al: An oxytocin receptor antagonist (atosiban) in the treatment of preterm labor: A randomized, double-blind, placebo-controlled trial with tocolytic rescue. Am J Obstet Gynecol 182:1173-1183, 2000.

278. Valenzuela GJ, Sanchez-Ramos L, Romero R, et al: Maintenance treatment of preterm labor with the oxytocin antagonist atosiban. The Atosiban PTL-098 Study Group. Am J Obstet Gynecol 182:1184-1190, 2000.
279. Moutquin JM, Sherman D, Cohen H, et al: Double-blind, randomized, controlled trial of atosiban and ritodrine in the treatment of preterm labor: A multicenter effectiveness and safety study. Am J Obstet Gynecol 182:1191-1199, 2000.
280. Husslein P, Cabero Ruara L, Dudenhausen JW, et al: Atosiban versus usual care for the management of preterm labor. J Perinat Med 36:305-313, 2007.
281. El-Sayed YY, Riley ET, Holbrook RH Jr, et al: Randomized comparison of intravenous nitroglycerin and magnesium sulfate for treatment of preterm labor. Obstet Gynecol 93:79, 1999.
282. Lees CC, Lojacono A, Thompson C, et al: Glyceryl trinitrate and ritodrine in tocolysis: An international multicenter randomized study. GTN Preterm Labour Investigation Group. Obstet Gynecol 94:403-408, 1999.
283. Duckitt K, Thornton S: Nitric oxide donors for the treatment of preterm labour. Cochrane Database Syst Rev (3):CD002860, 2002.
284. Bisits A, Madsen G, Knox M, et al: The Randomized Nitric Oxide Tocolysis Trial (RNOTT) for the treatment of preterm labor. Am J Obstet Gynecol 191:683-690, 2004.
285. Kahler C, Schluessner E, Moller A, et al: Nitric oxide donors: Effects on fetoplacental blood flow. Eur J Obstet Gynecol 115:10-14, 2004.
286. Saris NE, Mervaala E, Karppanen H, et al: Magnesium: An update on physiological, clinical and analytical aspects. Clin Chim Acta 294:1, 2000.
287. Taber EB, Tan L, Chao CR, et al: Pharmacokinetics of ionized versus total magnesium in subjects with preterm labor and preeclampsia. Am J Obstet Gynecol 186:1017, 2002.
288. Idama TO, Lindow SW: Magnesium sulfate: A review of clinical pharmacology applied to obstetrics. BJOG 105:260, 1998.
289. Cruikshank DP, Pitkin RM, Reynolds WA, et al: Effects of magnesium sulphate treatment on perinatal calcium metabolism: I. Maternal and fetal responses. Am J Obstet Gynecol 134:243, 1979.
290. Berkman ND, Thorp JM Jr, Lohr KN, et al: Tocolytic treatment for the management of preterm labor: A review of the evidence. Am J Obstet Gynecol 188:1648-1659, 2003.
291. Ramsey PS, Rouse DJ: Magnesium sulfate as a tocolytic agent. Semin Perinatol 25:236-247, 2001.
292. Borna S, Saeidi FM: Celecoxib versus magnesium sulfate to arrest preterm labor: Randomized trial. J Obstet Gynecol Res 33:631-634, 2007.
293. King JF: Tocolysis and preterm labour. Curr Opin Obstet Gynecol 16:459-463, 2004.
294. Grimes DA, Nanda K: Magnesium sulfate tocolysis: Time to quit. Obstet Gynecol 108:986-989, 2006.
295. Simhan HN, Caritis SN: Prevention of preterm delivery. N Engl J Med 357:477-487, 2007.
296. Giles W, Bisits A: Preterm labour: The present and future of tocolysis. Best Pract Res Clin Obstet Gynaecol 21:857-868, 2007.
297. Elliott JP: Magnesium sulfate as a tocolytic agent. Am J Obstet Gynecol 147:277-284, 1983.
298. Koontz SL, Friedman SA, Schwartz ML: Symptomatic hypocalcemia after tocolytic therapy with magnesium sulfate and nifedpine. Am J Obstet Gynecol 190:1773-1776, 2004.
299. Hung JW, Tsai MY, Yang BY, et al: Maternal osteoporosis after prolonged magnesium sulfate tocolysis therapy: A case report. Arch Phys Med Rehabil 86:146-149, 2005.
300. Nassar AH, Sakhel K, Maarouf H, et al: Adverse maternal and neonatal outcome of prolonged course of magnesium sulfate tocolysis. Acta Obstet Gynecol Scand 85:1099-1103, 2006.
301. Rouse DJ, Hirtz DG, Thom E: Association between use of antenatal magnesium sulfate in preterm labor and adverse health outcomes in infants. Am J Obstet Gynecol 188:295, 2003.
302. Stubblefield PG, Heyl PS: Treatment of premature labor with subcutaneous terbutaline. Obstet Gynecol 59:457-462, 1982.
303. Gyetvai K, Hannah ME, Hodnett ED, et al: Tocolytics for preterm labor: A systematic review. Obstet Gynecol 94:869-877, 1999.
304. Benedetti TJ: Maternal complications of parenteral beta-sympathomimetic therapy for premature labor. Am J Obstet Gynecol 145:1-6, 1983.
305. Smigaj D, Roman-Drago NM, Amini SB, et al: The effect of oral terbutaline on maternal glucose metabolism and energy expenditure in pregnancy. Am J Obstet Gynecol 178:1041-1047, 1998.
306. Elliott JP, Istwan NB, Rhea D, et al: The occurrence of adverse events in women receiving continuous subcutaneous terbutaline therapy. Am J Obstet Gynecol 191:1277-1282, 2004.
307. Wenstrom KD, Weiner CP, Merrill D, et al: A placebo-controlled randomized trial of the terbutaline pump for prevention of preterm delivery. Am J Perinatol 14:87-91, 1997.
308. Guinn DA, Goepfert AR, Owen J, et al: Terbutaline pump maintenance therapy for prevention of preterm delivery: A double-blind trial. Am J Obstet Gynecol 179:874-878, 1998.
309. Nanda K, Cook LA, Gallo MF, Grimes DA: Terbutaline pump maintenance therapy after threatened preterm labor for preventing preterm birth. Cochrane Database Syst Rev (4):CD003933, 2002.
310. Iams JD, Johnson FF, O'Shaughnessy RW: Ambulatory uterine activity monitoring in the post-hospital care of patients with preterm labor. Am J Perinatol 7:170-173, 1990.
311. Nagey DA, Bailey-Jones C, Herman AA: Randomized comparison of home uterine activity monitoring and routine care in patients discharged after treatment for preterm labor. Obstet Gynecol 82:319-323, 1993.
312. Brown HL, Britton KA, Brizendine EJ, et al: A randomized comparison of home uterine activity monitoring in the outpatient management of women treated for preterm labor. Am J Obstet Gynecol 180:798-805, 1999.
313. Sanchez-Ramos L, Huddleston JF: The therapeutic value of maintenance tocolysis: An overview of the evidence. Clin Perinatol 30:841-854, 2003.
314. The Collaborative Home Uterine Monitoring Study (CHUMS) Group: A multicenter randomized controlled trial of home uterine monitoring: Active versus sham device. Am J Obstet Gynecol 173:1120-1127, 1995.
315. Dyson DC, Danbe KH, Bamber JA, et al: Monitoring women at risk for preterm birth. N Engl J Med 338:15-19, 1998.
316. Massett HA, Greenup M, Ryan CE, et al: Public perceptions about prematurity: A national survey. Am J Prev Med 24:120-127, 2003.
317. Joseph KS: Theory of obstetrics: An epidemiologic framework for justifying medically indicated early delivery. BMC Pregnancy Childbirth 7:4, 2007.
318. Herron MA, Katz M, Creasy RC: Evaluation of a preterm birth prevention program: Preliminary report. Obstet Gynecol 59:452-456, 1982.
319. White DE, Frazer-Lee NJ, Tough S, et al: The content of prenatal care and its relationship to preterm birth in Alberta, Canada. Health Care Women Int 27:777-792, 2006.
320. Di Renzo GC, Moscioni P, Perazzi A, et al: Social policies in relation to employment and pregnancy in European countries. Prenat Neonat Med 3:147-156, 1998.
321. Papiernik E, Bouyer J, Dreyfus J, et al: Prevention of preterm births: A perinatal study in Haguenau, France. Pediatrics 76:154-158, 1985.
322. Papiernik E: Preventing preterm birth: Is it really impossible? A comment on the IOM report on preterm birth. Matern Child Health J 11:407-410, 2007.
323. Collaborative Group on Preterm Birth Prevention: Multicenter randomized, controlled trial of a preterm birth prevention program. Am J Obstet Gynecol 169:352-366, 1993.
324. Hueston WJ, Knox MA, Eilers G, et al: The effectiveness of preterm-birth prevention educational programs for high-risk women: A meta-analysis. Obstet Gynecol 86:705-712, 1995.
325. Healy AJ, Malone FD, Sullivan LM, et al: Early access to prenatal care: Implications for racial disparity in perinatal mortality. Obstet Gynecol 107:625-631, 2006.
326. Kramer MS, Kakuma R: Energy and protein intake in pregnancy. Cochrane Database Syst Rev (4):CD000032, 2003.
327. Levine RJ, Hauth JC, Curet LB, et al: Trial of calcium to prevent preeclampsia. N Engl J Med 337:69-76, 1997.

328. Hofmeyr GJ, Atallah AN, Duley L: Calcium supplementation during pregnancy for preventing hypertensive disorders and related problems. Cochrane Database Syst Rev (3):CD001059, 2006.
329. Rumbold AR, Crowther CA, Haslam RR, et al: Vitamins C and E and the risks of preeclampsia and perinatal complications. N Engl J Med 354:1796-1806, 2006.
330. Smuts CM, Huang M, Mundy D, et al: A randomized trial of docosahexanoic acid supplementation during the third trimester of pregnancy. Obstet Gynecol 101:469-479, 2003.
331. Fiore MC, Bailey WC, Cohen SJ, et al: Treating tobacco use and dependence. Clinical practice guideline. Rockville, MD: U.S. Department of Health and Human Services, Public Health Service, 2000.
332. Petersen R, Garrett JM, Melvin CL, et al: Medicaid reimbursement for prenatal smoking intervention influences quitting and cessation. Tob Control 15:30-34, 2006.
333. Ricketts SA, Murray EK, Schwalberg R: Reducing low birth weight by resolving risks: results from Colorado's prenatal plus program. Am J Pub Health 95:1952-1957, 2005.
334. Lumley J, Oliver SS, Chamberlain C, et al: Interventions for promoting smoking cessation during pregnancy. Cochrane Database Syst Rev (4): CD001055, 2004.
335. Michalowicz BS, Hodges JS, Di Angelis AJ, et al: Treatment of periodontal disease and the risk of preterm birth. N Engl J Med 355:1885-1894, 2006.
336. Vergnes J-N, Sixou M: Preterm low birthweight and maternal periodontal status: A meta-analysis. Am J Obstet Gynecol 196:135.e1-135.e7, 2007.
337. Smaill F: Antibiotics for asymptomatic bacteriuria in pregnancy. Cochrane Database Syst Rev (2):CD000490, 2001.
338. Elder HA, Santamarina BA, Smith S, et al: The natural history of asymptomatic bacteriuria during pregnancy: The effect of tetracycline on the clinical course and the outcome of pregnancy. Am J Obstet Gynecol 111:441-446, 1971.
339. Eschenbach DA, Nugent RP, Rao VR, et al: A randomized placebo-controlled trial of erythromycin for the treatment of U urealyticum to prevent premature delivery. Am J Obstet Gynecol 164:734, 1991.
340. Klebanoff MA, Regan JA, Rao VR, et al: Outcome of the Vaginal Infections and Prematurity Study: Results of a clinical trial of erythromycin among pregnant women colonized with group B streptococci. Am J Obstet Gynecol 172:1540, 1995.
341. Kigozi GG, Brahmbhatt H, Wabwire-Mangen F, et al: Treatment of trichomonas in pregnancy. Am J Obstet Gynecol 189:1398-1400, 2003.
342. Joesoef MR, Hillier SL, Wiknojosastro G, et al: Intravaginal clindamycin treatment for bacterial vaginosis: Effects on preterm delivery and low birth weight. Am J Obstet Gynecol 173:1527, 1995.
343. McDonald HM, O'Loughlin JA, Vigneswaran R, et al: Impact of metronidazole therapy on preterm birth in women with bacterial vaginosis flora (*Gardnerella vaginalis*): A randomised, placebo controlled trial. BJOG 104:1391-1397, 1997.
344. Rosenstein IJ, Morgan DJ, Lamont RF, et al: Effect of intravaginal clindamycin cream on pregnancy outcome and on abnormal vaginal microbial flora of pregnant women. Infect Dis Obstet Gynecol 8:158-165, 2000.
345. Kurkinen-Raty M, Vuopala S, Koskela M, et al: A randomised controlled trial of vaginal clindamycin for early pregnancy bacterial vaginosis. BJOG 107:1427-1432, 2000.
346. Kekki M, Kurki T, Pelkonen J, et al: Vaginal clindamycin in preventing preterm birth and peri-partal infections in asymptomatic women with bacterial vaginosis. Obstet Gynecol 97:643, 2001.
347. Ugwumadu A, Manyonda I, Reid F, Hay P: Effect of early oral clindamycin on late miscarriage and preterm delivery in asymptomatic women with abnormal vaginal flora and bacterial vaginosis: A randomised controlled trial. Lancet 361:983-988, 2003.
348. Lamont RF, Duncan SLB, Mandal D, et al: Intravaginal clindamycin to reduce preterm birth in women with abnormal genital tract flora. Obstet Gynecol 101:516-522, 2003.
349. Kiss H, Petricevic L, Husslein P: Prospective randomised controlled trial of an infection screening programme to reduce the rate of preterm delivery. BMJ 329:371-375, 2004.
350. Larsson PG, Fahraeus L, Carlsson B, et al: Late miscarriage and preterm birth after treatment with clindamycin: A randomised consent design study according to Zelen. BJOG 113:629-637, 2006.
351. Riggs MA, Klebanoff MA: Treatment of vaginal infections to prevent preterm birth: A meta-analysis. Clinical Obstet Gynecol 47:796-807, 2004.
352. Goldenberg RL, Mercer BM, Meis PJ, et al: The Preterm Prediction Study: Fetal fibronectin testing and spontaneous preterm birth. Obstet Gynecol 87:643-648, 1996.
353. Hendler I, Andrews WW, Carey CJ, et al: The relationship between resolution of asymptomatic bacterial vaginosis and spontaneous preterm birth in fetal fibronectin-positive women. Am J Obstet Gynecol 197:488.e1-488.e5, 2007.
354. Andrews WW, Sibai BM, Thom EA, et al: Randomized clinical trial of metronidazole plus erythromycin to prevent spontaneous preterm delivery in fetal fibronectin-positive women. Obstet Gynecol 101:847-855, 2003.
355. Centers for Disease Control and Prevention: Sexually transmitted diseases treatment guidelines 2006. Available at http://www.cdc.gov/STD/bv/STDFact-BacterialVaginosis.htm#pregnant (accessed April 24, 2008).
356. Goldenberg RL, Iams JD, Mercer BM, et al: The Preterm Prediction Study: Toward a multiple-marker test for spontaneous preterm birth. Am J Obstet Gynecol 185:643-651, 2001.
357. Moawad AH, Goldenberg RL, Mercer B, et al: The Preterm Prediction Study: The value of serum alkaline phosphatase, alpha-fetoprotein, plasma corticotropin-releasing hormone, and other serum markers for the prediction of spontaneous preterm birth. Am J Obstet Gynecol 186:990-996, 2002.
358. Goldenberg RL, Goepfert AR, Ramsey PS: Biochemical markers for the prediction of preterm birth. Am J Obstet Gynecol 192:S36-S46, 2005.
359. Vogel I, Thorsen P, Curry A, et al: Biomarkers for the prediction of preterm delivery. Acta Obstet Gynecol Scand 84:516-625, 2005.
360. Lockwood CJ, Senyei AE, Dische MR, et al: Fetal fibronectin in cervical and vaginal secretions as a predictor of preterm delivery. N Engl J Med 325:669-674, 1991.
361. Goldenberg RL, Mercer BM, Iams JD, et al: The Preterm Prediction Study: Patterns of cervicovaginal fetal fibronectin as predictors of spontaneous preterm delivery. Am J Obstet Gynecol 177:8-12, 1997.
362. To MS, Alfirevic Z, Heath VC, et al: Cervical cerclage for prevention of preterm delivery in women with short cervix: Randomised controlled trial. Lancet 363:1849-1853, 2004.
363. Berghella V, Odibo A, To MS, et al: Cerclage for short cervix on ultrasonography: Meta-analysis of trials using individual patient data. Obstet Gynecol 106:181-189, 2005.
364. Fonseca EB, Celik E, Parra M, et al: Progesterone and the risk of preterm birth among women with a short cervix. N Engl J Med 357:462-469, 2007.
365. Iams JD, Goldenberg RL, Mercer BM, et al: The Preterm Prediction Study: Can low risk women destined for spontaneous preterm birth be identified? Am J Obstet Gynecol 184:652-655, 2001.
366. Sibai BM, Caritis SN, Thom E, et al: Prevention of preeclampsia with low-dose aspirin in healthy, nulliparous pregnant women. N Engl J Med 329:1213-1218, 1993.
367. Caritis S, Sibai B, Hauth J, et al: Low-dose aspirin to prevent preeclampsia in women at high risk. N Engl J Med 338:701-705, 1998.
368. Poston L, Briley AL, Seed PT, et al: Vitamin C and vitamin E in pregnant women at risk for pre-eclampsia (VIP trial): Randomised placebo-controlled trial. Lancet 367:1145-1154, 2006.
369. Olsen SF, Sorenson JD, Secher NJ, et al: Randomized controlled trial of effect of fish-oil supplementation on pregnancy duration. Lancet 339:1003-1007, 1992.
370. Olsen SF, Secher NJ, Tabor A, et al: Randomised clinical trials of fish oil supplementation in high risk pregnancies. Fish Oil Trials In Pregnancy (FOTIP) Team. BJOG 107:382-395, 2000.
371. Duley L, Henderson-Smart DJ, Meher S, King JF: Antiplatelet agents for preventing pre-eclampsia and its complications. Cochrane Database Syst Rev (4):CD004659, 2003.

372. Rumbold A, Duley L, Crowther C, et al: Antioxidants for preventing pre-eclampsia. Cochrane Database Syst Rev (4)CD004227, 2005.
373. Hauth JC, Goldenberg RL, Andrews WW, et al: Reduced incidence of preterm delivery with metronidazole and erythromycin in women with bacterial vaginosis. N Engl J Med 333:1732-1736, 1995.
374. Althuisius SM, Dekker GA, Hummel P, et al: Final results of the Cervical Incompetence Prevention RAndomized Cerclage Trial (CIPRACT): Therapeutic cerclage with bed rest versus bed rest alone. Am J Obstet Gynecol 185:1106-1112, 2001.
375. Rust OA, Atlas RO, Reed J, et al: Revisiting the short cervix detected by transvaginal ultrasound in the second trimester: Why cerclage therapy may not help. Am J Obstet Gynecol 185:1098-1105, 2001.
376. Rouse DJ, Caritis SN, Peaceman AM, et al: A trial of 17 alphahydroxyprogesterone caproate to prevent prematurity in twins. N Engl J Med 357:454-461, 2007.
377. Espinoza J, Erez O, Romero R: Preconceptional antibiotic treatment to prevent preterm birth in women with a previous preterm delivery. Am J Obstet Gynecol 194:630-637, 2006.
378. Romero R, Espinoza J, Erez O, et al: The role of cervical cerclage in obstetric practice: Can the patient who could benefit from this procedure be identified? Am J Obstet Gynecol 194:1-9, 2006.
379. Lamont RF: Can antibiotics prevent preterm birth: The pro and con debate. BJOG 112(Suppl 1):67-73, 2005.
380. Sosa C, Althabe F, Belizán J, et al: Bed rest in singleton pregnancies for preventing preterm birth. Cochrane Database Syst Rev (1):CD003581, 2004.
381. Harper M; for NICHD MFMU Network: Randomized controlled trial of omega-3 fatty acid supplementation for recurrent preterm birth. Society for Maternal-Fetal Medicine: 2008 28th Annual Meeting, abstract 3. Am J Obstet Gynecol 196(6 Suppl S):S2, 2007.
382. Olds DL, Henderson CR Jr, Tatelbaum R, et al: Improving delivery of prenatal care and outcomes of pregnancy: A randomized trial of nurse home visitation. Pediatrics 77:16-28, 1986.
383. Quinlivan JA, Evans SF: Teenage antenatal clinics may reduce the rate of preterm birth: A prospectice study. BJOG 111:571-578, 2004.
384. Bryce RL, Stanley FJ, Garner RB: Randomized controlled trial of antenatal social support to prevent preterm birth. BJOG 98:1001-1008, 1991.
385. Villar J, Farnot U, Barros F, et al: A randomized trial of psychosocial support during high risk pregnancies. N Engl J Med 327:1266-1271, 1992.
386. Collaborative Working Group on Prematurity: Multicenter randomized controlled trial of a preterm birth prevention trial. Am J Obstet Gynecol 169:352-366, 1993.
387. Kitzman H, Olds DL, Henderson CR Jr, et al: Effect of prenatal and home visitation by nurses on pregnancy outcomes, childhood injuries, and repeated childbearing: A randomized study. JAMA 278:644-652, 1997.
388. Klerman LV, Ramey SL, Goldenberg RL, et al: A randomized trial of augmented prenatal care for multiple-risk, Medicaid-eligible African American women. Am J Public Health 91:105-111, 2001.
389. Hodnett ED, Fredericks S: Support during pregnancy for women at increased risk of low birth weight babies. Cochrane Database Syst Rev (3): CD000198, 2003.
390. Gichangi PB, Ndinya-Achola JO, Ombete J, et al: Antimicrobial prophylaxis in pregnancy: A randomized, placebo-controlled trial with cefetamet-pivoxil in pregnant women with a poor obstetric history. Am J Obstet Gynecol 177:680-684, 1997.
391. Vermeulen GM, Bruinse HW: Prophylactic administration of clindamycin 2% vaginal cream to reduce the incidence of spontaneous preterm birth in women with an increased recurrence risk: A randomised placebo-controlled double-blind trial. BJOG 106:652-657, 1999.
392. Shennan A, Crawshaw S, Briley A, et al: A randomised controlled trial of metronidazole for the prevention of preterm birth in women positive for cervicovaginal fetal fibronectin: The PREMET Study. BJOG 113:65-74, 2006.
393. Goldenberg RL, Mwatha A, Read JS, et al: The HPTN 024 study: The efficacy of antibiotics to prevent chorioamnionitis and preterm birth. Am J Obstet Gynecol 194:650-661, 2006.
394. Ugwumadu A, Reid F, Hay P, et al: Oral clindamycin and histologic chorioamnionitis in women with abnormal vaginal flora. Obstet Gynecol 107:863-868, 2006.
395. Esplin MS: Preterm birth: A review of genetic factors and future directions for genetic study. Obstet Gynecol Surv 61:800-806, 2006.
396. Sfakianaki AK, Norwitz ER: Mechanisms of progesterone action in inhibiting prematurity. J Matern Fetal Neonatal Med 19:763-772, 2006.
397. Keirse MJ: Progestogen administration in pregnancy may prevent preterm delivery. BJOG 97:149-154, 1990.
398. da Fonseca EB, Bittar RE, Carvalho MH, Zugaib M: Prophylactic administration of progesterone by vaginal suppository to reduce the incidence of spontaneous preterm birth in women at increased risk: A randomized placebo-controlled double-blind study. Am J Obstet Gynecol 188:419-424, 2003.
399. Spong CY, Meis PJ, Thom EA, et al: Progesterone for prevention of recurrent preterm birth: Impact of gestational age at previous delivery. Am J Obstet Gynecol 193:1127-1131, 2005.
400. Meis PJ, Klebanoff M, Dombrowski MP, et al: Does progesterone treatment influence risk factors for recurrent preterm delivery? Obstet Gynecol 106:557-561, 2005.
401. Thornton JG: Progesterone and preterm labor: Still no definite answers. N Engl J Med 357:499-501, 2007.
402. Dodd JM, Flenady V, Cincotta R, Crowther CA: Prenatal administration of progesterone for preventing preterm birth. Cochrane Database Syst Rev (1):CD004947, 2006.
403. Sanchez-Ramos L, Kaunitz AM, Delke I: Progestational agents to prevent preterm birth: A meta-analysis of randomized controlled trials. Obstet Gynecol 10:273-279, 2005.
404. Mackenzie R, Walker M, Armson A, et al: Progesterone for the prevention of preterm birth among women at increased risk: A systematic review and meta-analysis of randomized controlled trials. Am J Obstet Gynecol 194:1234-1242, 2006.
405. DeFranco EA, O'Brien JM, Adair CD, et al: Vaginal progesterone is associated with a decrease in risk for early preterm birth and improved neonatal outcome in women with a short cervix: A secondary analysis from a randomized, double-blind, placebo-controlled trial. Ultrasound Obstet Gynecol 30:697-705, 2007.
406. How HY, Barton JR, Istwan NB, et al: Prophylaxis with 17 alpha-hydroxyprogesterone caproate for prevention of recurrent preterm delivery: Does gestational age at initiation of treatment matter? Am J Obstet Gynecol 197:260.e1-260.e4, 2007.
407. Rebarber A, Ferrara LA, Hanley ML, et al: Increased recurrence of preterm delivery with early cessation of 17-alpha-hydroxyprogesterone caproate. Am J Obstet Gynecol 196:224.e1-224.e4, 2007.
408. Facchinetti F, Paganelli S, Comitini G, et al: Cervical length changes during preterm cervical ripening: Effects of 17-alpha-hydroxyprogesterone caproate. Am J Obstet Gynecol 196:453.e1-453.e4, 2007.
409. Meis PJ; Society for Maternal-Fetal Medicine: 17-Hydroxyprogesterone for the prevention of preterm delivery. Obstet Gynecol 105:1128-1135, 2005.
410. Christian MS, Brent RL, Calda P: Embryo-fetal toxicity signals for 17alpha-hydroxyprogesterone caproate in high-risk pregnancies: A review of the non-clinical literature for embryo-fetal toxicity with progestins. J Matern Fetal Neonatal Med 20:89-112, 2007.
411. Northen AT, Norman GS, Anderson K, et al: Follow-up of children exposed in utero to 17 alpha-hydroxyprogesterone caproate compared with placebo. Obstet Gynecol 110:865-872, 2007.
412. Elovitz MA, Mrinalini C: The use of progestational agents for preterm birth: Lessons from a mouse model. Am J Obstet Gynecol 195:1004-1010, 2006.
413. Petrini JR, Callaghan WM, Klebanoff M: Estimated effect of 17 alpha hydroxy-progesterone caproate on preterm birth in the United States. Obstet Gynecol 105:267-272, 2005.
414. Bailit JL, Votruba ME: Medical cost savings associated with 17 alpha-hydroxyprogesterone caproate. Am J Obstet Gynecol 196:219.e1-219.e7, 2007.

415. Armstrong J: 17-Progesterone for preterm birth prevention: A potential $2 billion opportunity. Am J Obstet Gynecol 196:194-195, 2007.
416. Guzman ER, Forster JK, Vintzileos AM, et al: Pregnancy outcomes in women treated with elective versus ultrasound-indicated cervical cerclage. Ultrasound Obstet Gynecol 12:323-327, 1998.
417. Berghella V, Daly SF, Tolosa JE, et al: Prediction of preterm delivery with transvaginal ultrasonography of the cervix in patients with high-risk pregnancies: Does cerclage prevent prematurity? Am J Obstet Gynecol 181:809-815, 1999.
418. Althuisius SM, Dekker GA, van Geijn HP, et al: Cervical Incompetence Prevention RAndomized Cerclage Trial (CIPRACT): Study design and preliminary results. Am J Obstet Gynecol 183:823-829, 2000.
419. Hassan SS, Romero R, Maymon E, et al: Does cervical cerclage prevent preterm delivery in patients with a short cervix? Am J Obstet Gynecol 184:1325-1329, 2001.
420. Althuisius S, Dekker G, Hummel P, et al: Cervical Incompetence Prevention RAndomized Cerclage Trial (CIPRACT): Effect of therapeutic cerclage with bed rest vs. bed rest only on cervical length. Ultrasound Obstet Gynecol 20:163-167, 2002.
421. Berghella V, Haas S, Chervoneva I, et al: Patients with prior second-trimester loss: Prophylactic cerclage or serial transvaginal sonograms? Am J Obstet Gynecol 187:747-751, 2002.
422. To MS, Palaniappan V, Skentou C, et al: Elective cerclage vs. ultrasound-indicated cerclage in high-risk pregnancies. Ultrasound Obstet Gynecol 19:475-477, 2002.
423. Berghella V, Odibo AO, Tolosa JE: Cerclage for prevention of preterm birth in women with a short cervix found on transvaginal ultrasound examination: A randomized trial. Am J Obstet Gynecol 191:1311-1317, 2004.
424. Lazar P, Gueguen S, Dreyfus J, et al: Multicentred controlled trial of cervical cerclage in women at moderate risk of preterm delivery. BJOG 91:731-735, 1984.
425. Rush RW, Isaacs S, McPherson K, et al: A randomized controlled trial of cervical cerclage in women at high risk of spontaneous preterm delivery. BJOG 91:724-730, 1984.
426. Final report of the Medical Research Council/Royal College of Obstetricians and Gynaecologists multicentre randomised trial of cervical cerclage. MRC/RCOG Working Party on Cervical Cerclage. BJOG 100:516-523, 1993.
427. Kurup M, Goldkrand JW: Cervical incompetence: Elective, emergent, or urgent cerclage. Am J Obstet Gynecol 181:240-246, 1999.
428. Guzman ER, Ananth CV: Cervical length and spontaneous prematurity: Laying the foundation for future interventional randomized trials for the short cervix. Ultrasound Obstet Gynecol 18:195-199, 2001.
429. Althuisius SM, Dekker GA, Hummel P, van Geijn HP: Cervical Incompetence Prevention RAndomized Cerclage Trial: Emergency cerclage with bed rest versus bed rest alone. Am J Obstet Gynecol 189:907-910, 2003.
430. Groom KM, Bennett PR, Golara M, et al: Elective cervical cerclage versus serial ultrasound surveillance of cervical length in a population at high risk for preterm delivery. Eur J Obstet Gynecol Reprod Biol 112:158-161, 2004.
431. Higgins SP, Kornman LH, Bell RJ, et al: Cervical surveillance as an alternative to elective cervical cerclage for pregnancy management of suspected cervical incompetence. Aust N Z J Obstet Gynaecol 44:228-232, 2004.
432. Sakai M, Shiozaki A, Tabata A, et al: Evaluation of effectiveness of prophylactic cerclage of a short cervix according to interleukin-8 in cervical mucus. Am J Obstet Gynecol 194:14-19, 2006.
433. Kalish RB, Chasen ST, Rosenzweig LB, et al: Impact of midtrimester dilation and evacuation on subsequent pregnancy outcome. Am J Obstet Gynecol 187:882-885, 2002.
434. Allen VM, Wilson RD, Cheung A; Genetics Committee of the Society of Obstetricians and Gynaecologists of Canada (SOGC); Reproductive Endocrinology Infertility Committee of the Society of Obstetricians and Gynaecologists of Canada (SOGC). Pregnancy outcomes after assisted reproductive technology. J Obstet Gynaecol Can 28:220-250, 2006.
435. Reddy UM, Wapner RJ, Rebar RW, et al: Infertility, assisted reproductive technology, and adverse pregnancy outcomes: Executive summary of a National Institute of Child Health and Human Development workshop. Obstet Gynecol 109:967-977, 2007.
436. Johnson B, Chavkin W: Policy efforts to prevent ART-related preterm birth. Matern Child Health J 11:219-225, 2007.
437. Jain T, Missmer SA, Hornstein MD: Trends in embryo-transfer practice and in outcomes of the use of assisted reproductive technology in the United States. N Engl J Med 350:1639-1645, 2004.
438. Min JK, Claman P, Hughes E, et al: Guidelines for the number of embryos to transfer following in vitro fertilization. J Obstet Gynaecol Can 28:799-813, 2006.
439. American College of Obstetricians and Gynecologists. The Importance of Preconception Care in the Continuum of Women's Health Care. ACOG Committee Opinion No. 313. Obstet Gynecol 106:665-666, 2005.
440. Czeizel AE, Dudas I, Metnecki J: Pregnancy outcomes in a randomised controlled trial of periconceptional multivitamin supplementation: Final report. Arch Gynecol Obstet 255:131-139, 1994.
441. Shah NR, Bracken MB: A systematic review and meta-analysis of prospective studies in the association between maternal cigarette smoking and preterm delivery. Am J Obstet Gynecol 182:465-472, 2000.
442. Salihu HM, Pierre-Louis BJ, Alexander GR: Levels of excess infant deaths attributable to maternal smoking during pregnancy in the United States. Matern Child Health J 7:219-227, 2003.
443. Mazaki-Tovi S, Romero R, Kusanovic JP, et al: Recurrent preterm birth. Semin Perinatol 31:142-158, 2007.
444. Patton PE, Novy MJ, Lee DM, Hickok LR: The diagnosis and reproductive outcome after surgical treatment of the complete septate uterus, duplicated cervix and vaginal septum. Am J Obstet Gynecol 190:1669-1675, 2004.
445. Haas JS, Fuentes-Afflick E, Stewart AL, et al: Pre-pregnancy health status and the risk of preterm delivery. Arch Pediatr Adolesc Med 159:58-63, 2005.
446. Lu MC, Kotelchuck M, Culhane JF, et al: Preceonception care between pregnancies: The content of internatal care. Matern Child Health J 10: S107-S122, 2006.
447. Lumley J, Donohue L: Aiming to increase birth weight: A randomised trial of pre-pregnancy information, advice and counselling in inner-urban Melbourne. BMC Public Health 6:299, 2006.
448. Andrews WW Goldenberg RL, Hauth JC, et al: Inter-conceptional antibiotics to prevent spontaneous preterm birth: A randomized trial. Am J Obstet Gynecol 194:617-623, 2006.

Chapter 30

Cervical Insufficiency

Jay D. Iams, MD

Definitions of Cervical Competence and Insufficiency

The definition of cervical competence is functional: The task of the cervix is first to retain the conceptus until maturity and later to dilate sufficiently to allow delivery of the mature infant. The ability to perform these functions repeatedly in successive pregnancies is *cervical competence*. Cervical *insufficiency* describes a presumed physical weakness of cervical tissue that causes or contributes to the loss of an otherwise healthy pregnancy, usually in the second trimester. Anatomic, biochemical, and clinical evidence has consistently supported the belief that some percentage of second-trimester births are primarily or perhaps exclusively caused by congenital or acquired structural weakness of the cervix. However, the incidence, pathophysiology, clinical presentation, and management of the disorder have been difficult to distinguish from those of preterm cervical effacement and dilation caused by factors other than insufficient cervical strength. As described in Chapters 28 and 29, cervical strength or competence appears to be one of many continuous variables that influence the process of preterm parturition, including uterine volume, intrauterine microbial colonization, decidual hemorrhage, and genetic and environmental factors. The term *cervical insufficiency* is applied when participation by other variables is not clinically evident. Although this definition is conceptually straightforward, it is difficult to apply in practice because similar results from the history, symptoms, physical and sonographic examinations, and laboratory evaluation of women with cervical insufficiency are shared by many women with preterm parturition for whom cervical weakness is not the principal cause, and importantly, for whom cerclage is not likely to be beneficial. Indeed, an operational definition of cervical insufficiency is a pregnancy in which a cervical cerclage is likely to improve pregnancy outcome, but there are currently no definitive tests for the diagnosis.

The contribution of cervical insufficiency to spontaneous preterm parturition remains controversial. Studies described in Chapter 29 addressed the benefit of cervical cerclage for women with a prior spontaneous preterm birth and commonly omitted women thought to have "true" cervical insufficiency. Recognizing that the distinction between cervical insufficiency and early spontaneous preterm birth has become increasingly uncertain, this chapter focuses on pregnancy outcomes and treatment of women with structural abnormalities of the cervix.

The Cervix in Pregnancy

Anatomy

The uterine cervix and corpus are derived from fusion of the distal müllerian ducts and subsequent central atrophy.[1] The cervix is primarily fibrous tissue with some (10% to 15%) smooth muscle.[2] The cervicoisthmic zone of histologic transition from fibrous to muscular tissue may be narrow (1 to 2 mm) or relatively wide (5 to 10 mm).[2] The proportion of cervical smooth muscle ranges from 29% in the upper third to 6.4% in the lower third.[3] The muscular uterine isthmus distends and elongates between the 12th and 20th weeks of gestation, consistent with ultrasound studies of the cervix and lower segment during the same period.[4]

Cervical Remodeling during Pregnancy

Biochemical Changes

The cervix changes soon after conception and continues to remodel throughout pregnancy and the puerperium. Cervical remodeling has been described as occurring in four phases: softening, ripening, dilation, and repair (Figure 30-1).[5] Endocervical endothelial cells proliferate during pregnancy and supply cervical mucus and defensins to protect the upper tract from microorganisms. Collagen synthesis increases in early gestation, but collagen concentrations decline as the cervix ripens and the water content of the cervix increases before labor. Abnormalities of cervical remodeling may contribute to the clinical syndrome of cervical insufficiency.

Ultrasonographic Appearance of the Cervix in Normal Pregnancy

Understanding of cervical function in pregnancy has been enhanced by ultrasound images of the cervix over the course of pregnancy. Measurements of the cervix before pregnancy and in the first trimester of pregnancy do not correlate with pregnancy outcomes and are not useful to identify reduced function.[6] Normative values of cervical length have been established in the second and third trimesters of pregnancy, as measured by transvaginal ultrasonography, and are normally distrbuted.[4,7-12] The median and 10th percentiles of length before 20 weeks' gestation are approximately 40 and 30 mm, respectively.[11,12] Between 22 and 32 weeks, the 10th, 50th, and 90th percentiles are 25, 35, and 45 mm, respectively. Parity does not influence cervical length.[10]

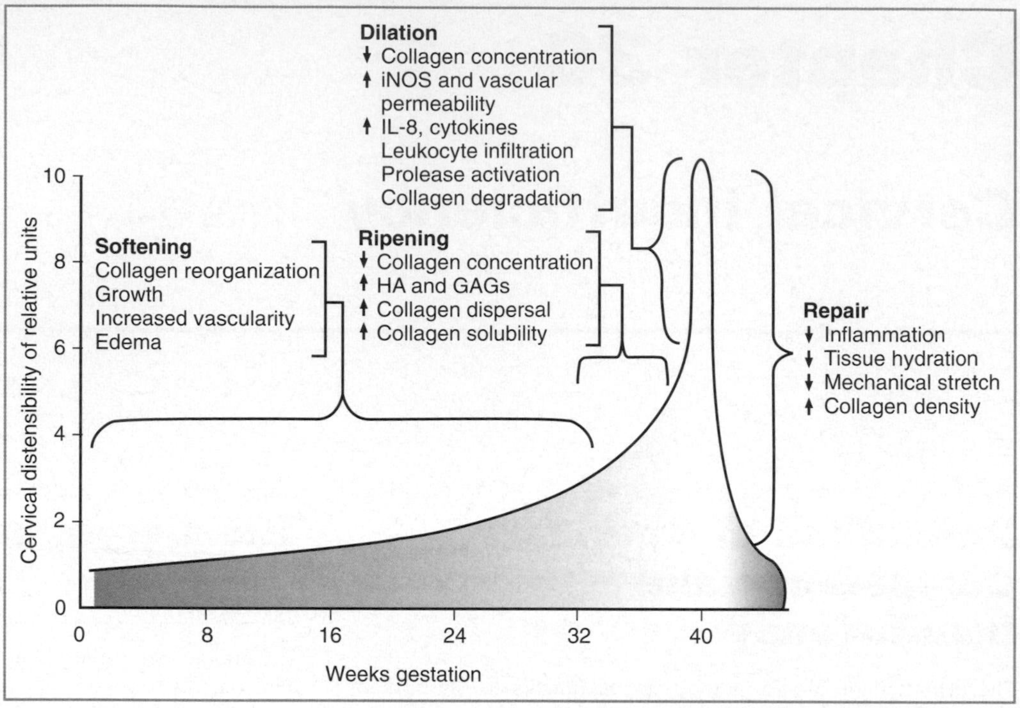

FIGURE 30-1 **Stages of cervical function during pregnancy and the puerperium.** Although the process occurs as a continuum, each stage is characterized by unique biochemical and cellular events. GAGs, glycosaminoglycans; HA, hyaluronan; IL-8, interleukin 8; iNOS, induced nitric oxide synthase. (From Word RA, Li, X-H, Hnat M, et al: Dynamics of cervical remodeling during pregnancy and parturition: Mechanisms and current concepts. Semin Reprod Med 25:69-79, 2007.)

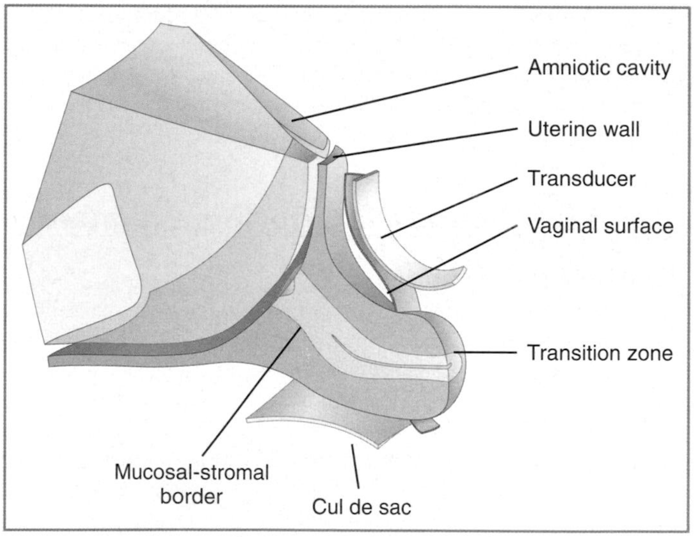

FIGURE 30-2 **Schematic diagram of uterine and cervical structures imaged by endovaginal sonography.** (Courtesy of Dr. Michael House, Tufts–New England Medical Center.)

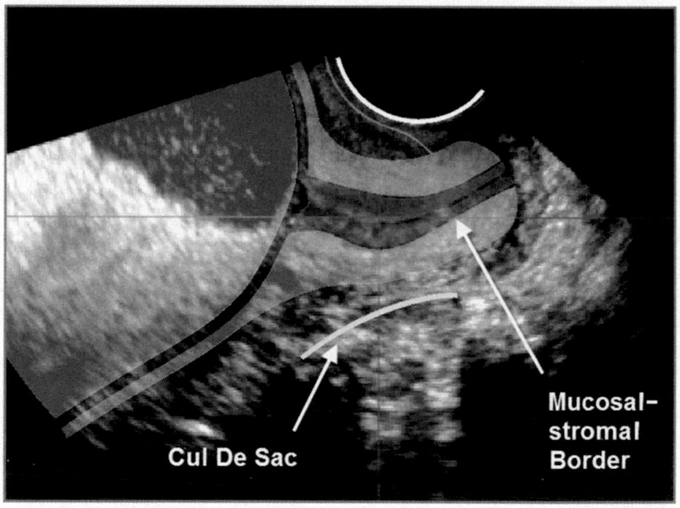

FIGURE 30-3 **Cervix and cervical canal schematic superimposed on endovaginal ultrasound image.** Arrows point to mucosal-stromal border and posterior vaginal cul de sac (pink line). (Courtesy of Dr. Michael House, Tufts–New England Medical Center.)

Measurements are obtained with an endovaginal transducer, as shown in Figures 30-2, 30-3, and 30-4.

Cervical effacement precedes decidual activation at term and for most preterm births by a period of several weeks (4 to 8 weeks or even longer). Effacement begins at the internal cervical os and proceeds caudad according to the T-Y V-U sequence described by Zilianti and colleagues.[9] The process of effacement usually proceeds incrementally, but it can occasionally be seen by real-time ultrasound to be dynamic; that is, the internal os is seen to open and close, giving the appearance of a funnel. Representative endovaginal ultrasound images that display the progressive effacement seen in normal pregnancy are shown in Figures 30-5, 30-6, and 30-7.

The cervix begins to efface normally at about 32 to 34 weeks' gestation, in preparation for birth at term. These same changes often precede spontaneous deliveries in the second and third trimesters regardless of clinical presentation, often without uterine contractions. Therefore, a short or funneled cervix may be observed with ultrasound well in advance of delivery, regardless of gestational age, and regardless of the presumed mechanism—structural weakness, biochemically induced changes in the cervical stroma, or biophysical effects of uterine contractions.

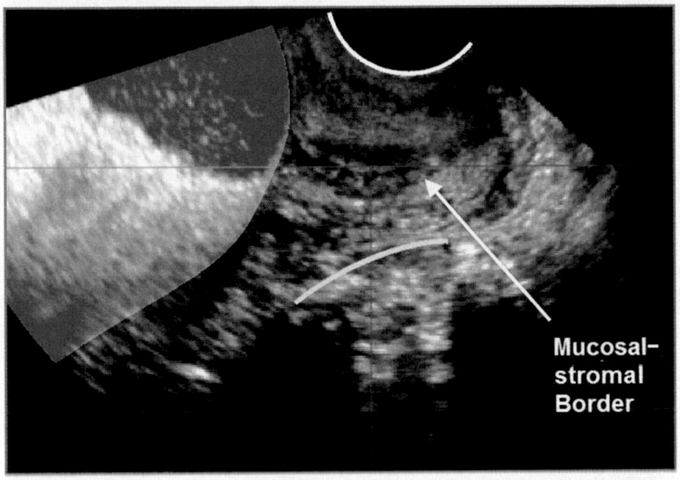

FIGURE 30-4 Endovaginal image of the cervix. Arrow points to mucosal-stromal border. Pink line indicates posterior vaginal cul de sac. (Courtesy of Dr. Michael House, Tufts–New England Medical Center.)

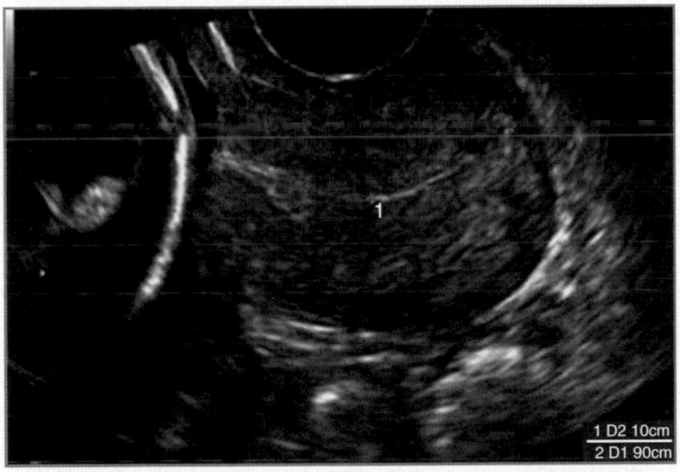

FIGURE 30-5 Endovaginal ultrasound image of a normal cervix at 24 weeks' gestation. The closed portion of the cervical canal is measured from the external os, identified as the most distal point at which anterior and posterior walls of the canal touch, to the internal os, identified as the most proximal point where the walls touch. The cervix in this image is measured in two segments because of the curved canal, a normal finding. The length is 40 mm, the 75th percentile. The internal os is closed, forming a "T" relationship to the canal.

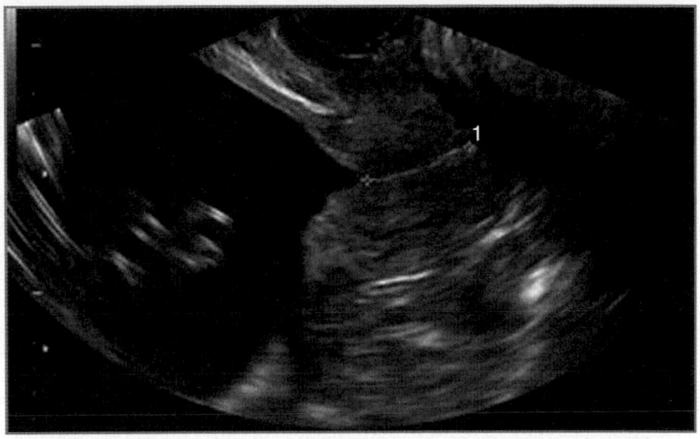

FIGURE 30-6 Endovaginal ultrasound image of a cervix at 25 weeks' gestation, showing Y-shaped funneling at the internal os. The cervical length is 21.3 mm, approximately the 5th percentile.

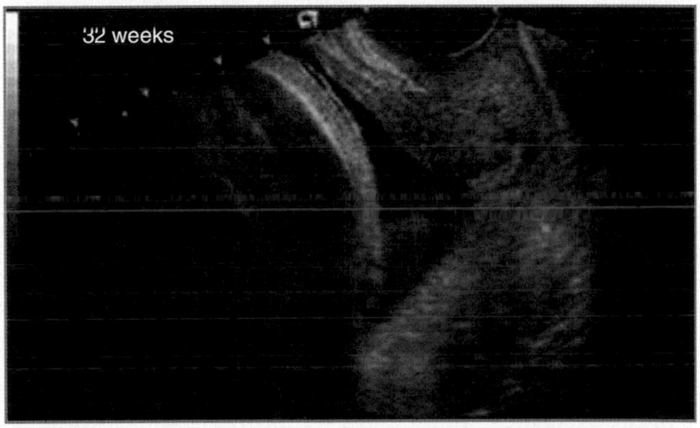

FIGURE 30-7 Endovaginal ultrasound image of the cervix at 32 weeks' gestation, showing substantial effacement where the V shape has almost become a U. The cervix was 1 cm dilated by digital examination. The patient was an outpatient who was not in labor.

Causes of Cervical Dysfunction

Congenital Causes

Collagen

Primary disorders of the cervicoisthmic junction may result from developmental abnormalities in the muscular isthmus and the upper cervix or from derangement of the cervical fibrous tissue resulting in decreased cervical resistance. Concentrations of smooth muscle relative to collagen fibers are higher in women with cervical insufficiency than in women who have no history of preterm birth.[13] Cervical biopsy specimens obtained from normal women after parturition[14] revealed a 12-fold decrease in mechanical strength, a 50% reduction in the concentrations of collagen and sulfated glycosaminoglycans, a 35% reduction in hyaluronic acid, an increase in collagen extractability, and a fivefold increase in collagenolytic activity compared with tissue obtained from normal nonpregnant women. In contrast, cervical biopsy specimens obtained in the second trimester from pregnant women with a history of cervical insufficiency revealed normal collagen concentrations but high collagen extractability and collagenolytic activity—higher than normal postpartum values.[14] Significantly lower concentrations and increased extractability of hydroxyproline were observed in cervical tissue obtained from nonpregnant women with cervical insufficiency in their first pregnancy, compared with cervical tissue from normal parous controls.[15]

Alterations in the regulation of type I collagen expression may influence cervical ripening,[16] and genetic disorders affecting collagen function (e.g., Ehlers-Danlos syndrome) have been associated with increased risk of preterm birth.[17] Familial disorders of collagen are more prevalent than is usually recognized[18] and may explain familial aggregation of cervical insufficiency. In a study of 121 women with, and 165 women without, cervical insufficiency, more than 25% of the former group had a first-degree relative with the same diagnosis, a finding associated with polymorphisms in the genes for collagen type Iα1 and transforming growth factor-β.[19] Familial collagen disorders may therefore contribute to cervical insufficiency.

Biologic Variation in Length

Cervical length, as measured by endovaginal ultrasound in the second trimester of pregnancy, is normally distributed.[10-12] The risk of preterm birth increases as the cervical length in the second trimester decreases (Fig. 30-8).

Individual variation in cervical function is suggested by a rising risk of spontaneous preterm birth before 35 weeks as cervical length declines, especially in the lower quartile of the bell-curve distribution.[10-12] Although this relationship may result from exogenous factors unrelated to inherent cervical strength, short cervical length has been specifically linked to repetitive preterm birth.[20,21] Women with a short cervix during pregnancy are more likely to have a history of preterm birth.[21] Moreover, the gestational age of a prior delivery has been related to cervical length in a subsequent pregnancy: The earlier the gestational age of the previous birth, the shorter the cervix in the current pregnancy.[20] Additional evidence of biologic variation in the cervical competence comes from studies that relate cervical length above the 50th percentile to a decreased risk of spontaneous preterm birth in women with twin and triplet pregnancies.[22-25]

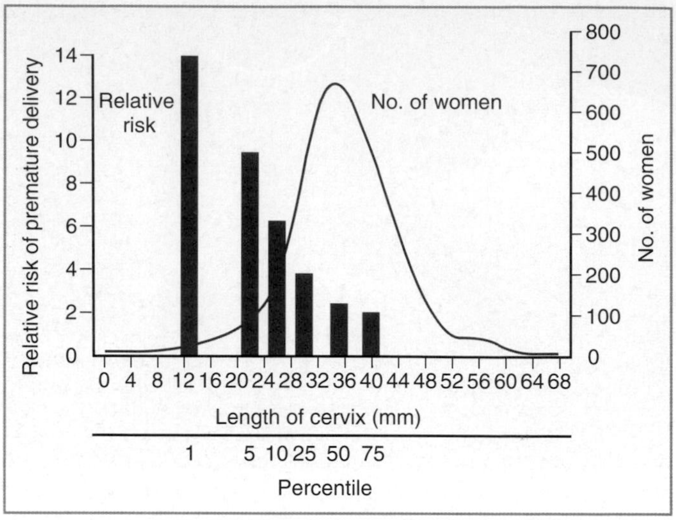

FIGURE 30-8 Distribution of subjects among percentiles for cervical length measured by transvaginal ultrasonography at 24 weeks of gestation *(solid line)* and relative risk of spontaneous preterm delivery before 35 weeks of gestation according to percentiles for cervical length *(bars)*. The risks among women with values equal to or less than the 1st, 5th, 10th, 25th, 50th, and 75th percentiles for cervical length are compared with the risk among women with values greater than the 75th percentile. (From Iams JD, Goldenberg RL, Meis PJ, et al: The length of the cervix and the risk of spontaneous preterm delivery. N Engl J Med 334:567, 1996.)

Uterine Anomalies

Müllerian fusion anomalies may involve the cervix as well as the uterine cavity. Congenital structural uterine abnormalities have been associated with an increased incidence of reproductive loss for multiple reasons, including apparent cervical insufficiency. Case series describing pregnancy outcomes in women with uncorrected uterine anomalies indicate higher rates of preterm birth in women with bicornuate, didelphys, or arcuate uteri, compared to those with septate or subseptate uteri.[26-34] Endovaginal sonography in women with uterine anomalies can reveal cervical duplication or altered uterine anatomy not visible on speculum examination or laparoscopy.

Teratogens: Diethylstilbestrol

Poor pregnancy outcome and structural genital tract abnormalities have been reported in women who were exposed to diethylstilbestrol (DES) in utero,[35] due at least in part to cervical insufficiency attributed to DES exposure.[36] The risk of second-trimester pregnancy loss in DES-exposed women compared with unexposed controls was increased fourfold to fivefold (6.3% to 7.1%, compared to 1.6% in controls).[35] Other possible causes for adverse pregnancy outcomes in DES progeny include upper genital tract abnormalities of uterine cavity shape (e.g., a T-shape) and intrauterine defects such as synechiae and diverticulae.[37]

Acquired Causes

Trauma

OBSTETRIC INJURY

Cervical injury may occur during labor or at the time of delivery. The cervix may be lacerated or stretched beyond tolerance, or it may heal poorly. Women delivered by cesarean section after an arrested second stage of labor can present in the next pregnancy with cervical insufficiency.[38] The mechanism is not clear, but two hypotheses may explain this observation: (1) a prolonged second stage may injure the cervix directly by stretch and trauma, or (2) the low transverse uterine incision may heal poorly in this setting. Cervical injury might also occur during cesarean delivery should the incision extend vertically into the cervix. Poor healing is more common when cofactors such as obesity, smoking, hemorrhage, and infection are present.

DILATION AND CURETTAGE

Mechanical dilation of the cervix before gynecologic procedures or abortion has been blamed for cervical insufficiency,[39] but injury sufficient to alter cervical function is uncommon when performed by an experienced operator with the use of laminaria.[40-42] The risk of preterm birth after pregnancy termination is discussed in Chapter 29.

CERVICAL BIOPSY AND ABLATION OF NEOPLASIA

Diagnosis and treatment of intraepithelial neoplasia requiring cervical biopsy, laser ablation, loop electrosurgical excision procedure (LEEP), or cold knife conization are clearly linked to an increased risk of subsequent preterm birth (see Chapter 29).[43-47] Whether the increase is related to an increased rate of cervical insufficiency, to other effects

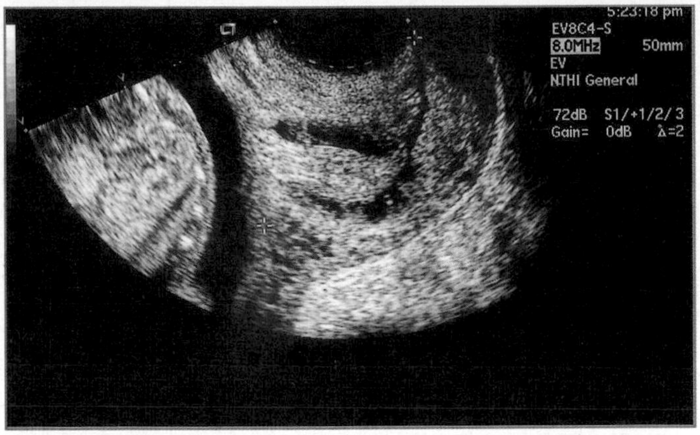

FIGURE 30-9 Cervical polyp. Endovaginal ultrasound image of a cervix with a broad-based cervical polyp.

on cervical function, or to uterine microbial colonization is not known.

Biochemical Influences

Endocrine, paracrine and inflammatory stimuli can effect biochemical changes in cervical structure and function during pregnancy. Softening occurs normally in pregnancy[5] and progresses to ripening, but these events may be prematurely triggered in women with preterm parturition, leading not only to increased risk of preterm labor and ruptured membranes but also to a clinical presentation consistent with cervical insufficiency.[48] The inflammatory cytokine interleukin 8 (IL-8) participates in cervical ripening as a neutrophil chemotactic factor.[49] Increased levels of IL-8 in cervical fluid are associated with increased risk of preterm birth and with failure of cerclage treatment in women with previous preterm birth and short cervix.[50] Weiner and coworkers demonstrated that proteomic markers in amniotic fluid associated with intrauterine inflammation or decidual hemorrhage predicted failure of rescue cerclage.[51]

INTRACERVICAL INFLAMMATION

Anecdotal evidence suggests that an inflamed cervical polyp or necrotic intracervical myoma can cause preterm cervical ripening that may resolve spontaneously or progress to preterm delivery (Fig. 30-9). These instances raise the possibility that other causes of intracervical inflammation, such as microbial infection, may contribute to preterm cervical effacement as well.

Diagnosis of Cervical Insufficiency

History

The diagnosis of cervical insufficiency has traditionally been made by an obstetric history of recurrent painless dilation of the cervix prior to preterm birth in the second trimester. This classic picture was once thought to be the only true presentation, distinct from other causes of early preterm delivery. However, asymptomatic effacement and dilation of the cervix may precede various clinical presentations.[52] Evaluation to identify cervical insufficiency has in the past focused on exclusion of alternative explanations, such as preterm labor, ruptured membranes, discharge, or bleeding, that are now recognized as presenting symptoms and signs of the preterm parturition syndrome (see Chapters 28 and 29), in which a complex interaction of factors can lead to preterm cervical ripening as early as 16 weeks' gestation, often with minimal symptoms. Prior obstetrical taxonomy assigned causation to the clinical presentation (e.g., preterm labor or preterm ruptured membranes *versus* cervical insufficiency) rather than to the underlying pathologic mechanisms that are now understood to be primarily biochemical.[53] For this reason, although a history of painful contractions against an uneffaced cervix argues against cervical insufficiency, presentation with cervical dilation and minimal symptoms is no longer accepted as unique to cervical insufficiency. Cervical insufficiency is characterized clinically more by *recurrent* midpregnancy delivery than by the absence of contractions or infection. A history of short labors, progressively earlier deliveries in successive pregnancies, advanced dilation at the time of first presentation, and prior cervical surgery or injury also suggest cervical insufficiency. Women ultimately diagnosed with cervical insufficiency often describe feelings of pelvic pressure, premenstrual symptoms, and increased vaginal discharge for several days before presentation, sometimes including an office or hospital visit at which the cervix was noted to be closed by digital examination.

Women with atypical obstetric histories that include births at term as well as second-trimester losses may also have cervical insufficiency. In some, the explanation may come from a cervical injury at the time of a prior term birth, or there may be an obvious nonrepetitive cause, but an undiagnosed uterine anomaly should also be considered. The duration of pregnancy in such cases may be determined by the uterine horn in which the pregnancy implants or by the placental implantation site on an incomplete uterine septum.

Physical Examination

Physical examination of the cervix in women who are not pregnant does not identify cervical insufficiency. Speculum examination may reveal cervical lacerations or the effects of previous cervical surgery, but correlation of findings with subsequent pregnancy outcome is poor. Substantial cervical tissue often lies above the lateral vaginal fornices, inaccessible to clinical examination, so that cervical performance in pregnancy is often normal in women with little or no cervix apparent at the vaginal apex.

Serial digital and speculum examinations have been employed to monitor patients with suspected cervical insufficiency, but effacement often precedes palpable or visible dilation of the canal. Initial findings on digital examination are progressive softening and thinning, followed by eventual dilation. Speculum examination first reveals a thin discharge and, with patience and fundal pressure or a Valsalva maneuver, membranes may be visible. Visible or even bulging membranes may be observed in women with no history of problems. Not surprisingly, a closed cervix does not exclude the diagnosis, because cervical effacement and dilation begin at the internal os. Digital examination is less reproducible than ultrasound examination of the cervix.[54-57]

Digital and speculum examination findings can supplement a diagnosis of cervical insufficiency based on maternal history, but they are not themselves definitive, because the same cervical status can result from causes other than structural weakness. Cervical dilation of 1 cm or more appears to be an optimal threshold for placement of cerclage.[58]

Diagnostic Tests

There are no accepted tests or criteria to detect cervical insufficiency outside of pregnancy. Measurement of resistance to the passage of a cervical dilator or Foley balloon and the hysterographic appearance of the cervix have been proposed but have not been helpful clinically.

Ultrasonography

The sonographic appearance of the cervix before conception and in early pregnancy does not offer any consistent evidence of subsequent insufficiency.

Ultrasound examination to detect incompetent cervix in pregnancy was first performed with transabdominal transducers.[59-61] The abdominal technique requires a full maternal bladder to visualize the cervix[62] and thus introduces unpredictable measurement artifact.[63,64] Transvaginal ultrasound examinations produce a more consistent and more accurate image of the cervix while avoiding the confounding effect of a full maternal bladder.[64-66] Figures 30-3 through 30-7, 30-9, and 30-10 depict images generated by placing the endovaginal probe in the anterior vaginal fornix. The details of cervical measurement are important. The standard method employs endovaginal sonography and the "shortest best" technique of caliper placement, in which initial measurements are ignored until the same length is generated repeatedly with the least pressure applied to the cervix to obtain a good image of the endocervical canal.[7,10-12,20,67] Alternative methods produce longer measurements that are not reproducible.[68]

When these studies were first reported, cervical competence was viewed as comprising only two categories: competent or incompetent. The observation of funneling at the internal os in the absence of apparent uterine activity was believed to indicate cervical insufficiency, and ultrasound findings of funneling with a short residual cervix were proposed as diagnostic criteria, especially in women with a history of mid-trimester birth. Subsequent sonographic studies identified progressive cervical effacement that precedes uterine activation by several weeks in both normal and preterm parturition.[7,10-12]

Cervical length is related to the risk of preterm birth.[7,10-12,69,70] The absolute risk of preterm birth varies substantially by population, but an increasing risk of preterm birth as cervical length declines has been consistently reported. Although the risk is strongest for cervical length less than the 10th percentile, there is no threshold value below which a patient always or even usually presents with cervical insufficiency. In a study in which providers were unaware of the cervical ultrasound measurement, more than half of women whose cervical length was less than the 1st percentile (13 mm) at 22 to 24 weeks delivered after 35 weeks (see Fig. 30-8).[10] The association between cervical length and preterm birth is strongest in women with a prior preterm birth and especially strong when the previous preterm birth occurred before 32 weeks.[20,21,71]

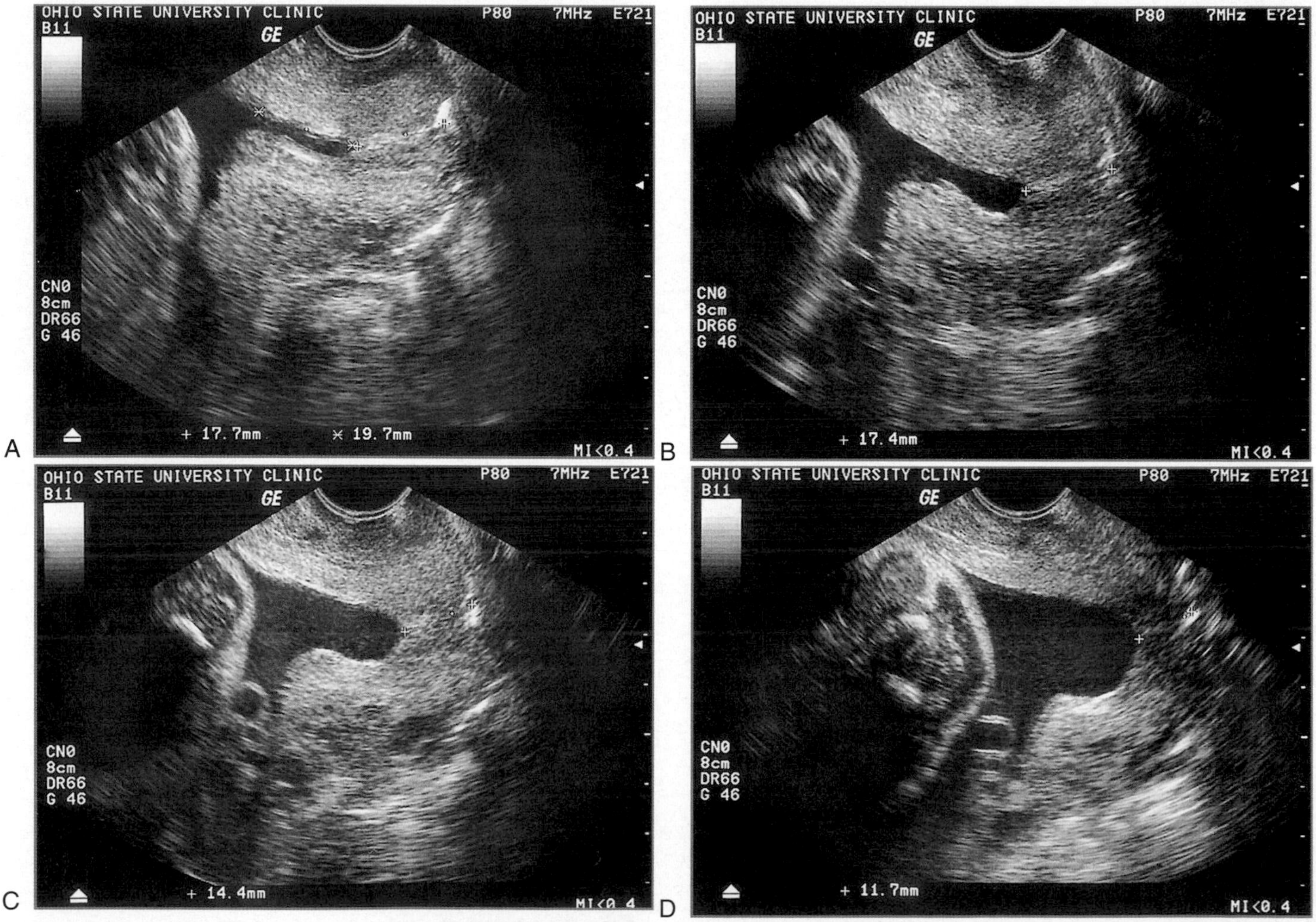

FIGURE 30-10 A sequence of four images obtained over a period of 90 seconds in a patient with a prior preterm birth. **A** through **D**, Progressive cervical change occurs in response to gentle suprapubic pressure. The cervical length measurement is 11.7 mm, the "shortest best" image of the sequence.

Attempts to use a percentile of cervical length, or a combination of length and other sonographic characteristics of the cervix, to distinguish cervical insufficiency from other causes of preterm cervical effacement have not been successful. Although abdominal pressure applied to the fundus or suprapubic area can aid the endovaginal ultrasound examination by revealing the internal os more clearly, funneling, whether spontaneous or in response to increased intra-abdominal pressure, does not define cervical insufficiency or add to the sensitivity or predictive value of cervical length to assess the risk of preterm birth.[72,73] The rate of decrease in cervical length over time[74] and onset of effacement before 20 weeks[71,72,75] are related to an increased risk of early preterm birth but also do not distinguish cervical insufficiency from other causes of preterm delivery.

Clinical Criteria

Attempts to assign a diagnosis of cervical insufficiency based on good response to cerclage therapy in a previous pregnancy have also faltered, first in anecdotes of successful outcomes in women who refused a recommended cerclage, as well as observational studies reporting successful pregnancy outcomes in upwards of 70% of untreated couples with a history of mid-trimester loss,[76,77] and, more recently, in prospective studies of cervical length in women with prior early preterm birth. More than 60% of women with a history of early preterm birth maintain a cervical length greater than 25 mm without treatment and have correspondingly low rates of recurrent preterm birth.[78-81] A recently concluded study performed ultrasound surveillance of cervical length from 16 to 23 weeks in more than 1100 women with a prior preterm birth between 17 and 34 weeks; 70% of these women maintained a cervical length greater than 25 mm and therefore did not qualify for entry into the second phase of the study, a randomized trial of cerclage that will report results in 2009.[82]

The American College of Obstetricians and Gynecologists was unable to identify any level I evidence for its 2003 practice bulletin on cervical insufficiency, in which it endorsed serial transvaginal ultrasound examinations between 16 and 20 weeks for women with historical risk factors for cervical insufficiency.[83] The American College of Radiology 2005 Expert Panel on Women's Imaging report on premature cervical dilation acknowledged the superior images obtained by transvaginal imaging of the cervix, recommended that the cervix be imaged transabdominally during all routine fetal ultrasound examinations in the second trimester, and suggested that women with a short or funneled cervix observed on abdominal ultrasound undergo transvaginal or translabial imaging of cervical length.[84] Diagnostic criteria for cervical insufficiency based on history, physical examination, and imaging studies must therefore be considered as uncertain. Emphasis should be placed on a history of prior cervical trauma, repeated mid-trimester loss, absence of painful contractions, advanced cervical dilation and effacement at presentation, and ultrasound findings of a cervical length of less than the 10th percentile before 24 weeks' gestation.

Treatment of Cervical Insufficiency

When cervical insufficiency was first described,[85,86] surgical correction was proposed by placement of an encircling or cerclage suture or graft, applied before[85,86] or during pregnancy, by either a tranvaginal[87,88] or a transabdominal approach.[89] The cerclage suture has been commonly placed electively between 11 and 15 weeks' gestation, or later in the second trimester in response to physical or ultrasound evidence of cervical dilation. Evidence of benefit for cerclage in initial reports was descriptive.

In addition to cerclage, medical therapies including bed rest, pessaries, antibiotics, anti-inflammatory drugs, and progesterone supplementation have been proposed. As the definition, etiology, and clinical presentation of cervical insufficiency have evolved, the appropriate treatment for women with a history of recurrent midpregnancy deliveries has become increasingly uncertain.

Nonsurgical Treatment

Nonsurgical approaches to the management of cervical insufficiency have been attempted but have not gained widespread acceptance nor proved efficacious in a controlled trial.

Pessaries

Various types of vaginal pessaries have been used in an attempt to change the axis of the cervical canal and prevent alleged gravitational forces from causing cervical dilation and subsequent delivery. A 2000 review of pessaries concluded that there was insufficient evidence to exclude the possibility of benefit.[90] Subsequent observational studies suggested that pessaries may be superior to bed rest and equivalent to surgical cerclage in women with suspected cervical insufficiency.[91-93] There are no randomized trials that compare treatment with pessaries to cerclage.

Medications

Prostaglandin inhibitors have been employed as nonsurgical treatment for cervical insufficiency. A review of indomethacin in controlled trials found that indomethacin might be of benefit in women with short cervix when used before 24 weeks of gestation.[94] Progesterone treatment reduced the risk of preterm birth in asymptomatic women with short cervix (<15 mm),[95] but women with cervical insufficiency were not enrolled in this trial, which is discussed further in Chapter 29.

Surgical Treatment: Cervical Cerclage Procedures

Pre-conceptional Cerclage

Cerclage in the nonpregnant state may be considered if the cervix has a large traumatic defect. Pre-conceptional cerclage placement may complicate management of spontaneous first-trimester abortion or the second-trimester discovery of a serious fetal anomaly. Lash and Lash[86] described a transvaginal procedure to correct a structural defect within the cervix and later[96] reported improved fetal survival after the surgery, compared with prior pregnancies, but fertility was compromised.[97] An alternative procedure was described[98] in which a suture was placed at the level of the internal os after simpler procedures proved unsuccessful. The cervical mucosa was incised and dissected anteriorly and posteriorly to the level of the peritoneal reflection. A nonabsorbable suture was placed circumferentially at the level of the internal os; the uterosacral ligaments and a small amount of cervical tissue, both anteriorly and posteriorly, were included in the suture.

Transabdominal cerclage before conception has been reported in 19 women, all of whom did well.[99]

Cerclage during Pregnancy

The two most commonly performed procedures during pregnancy were reported by Shirodkar[87] and McDonald.[88] If these procedures are

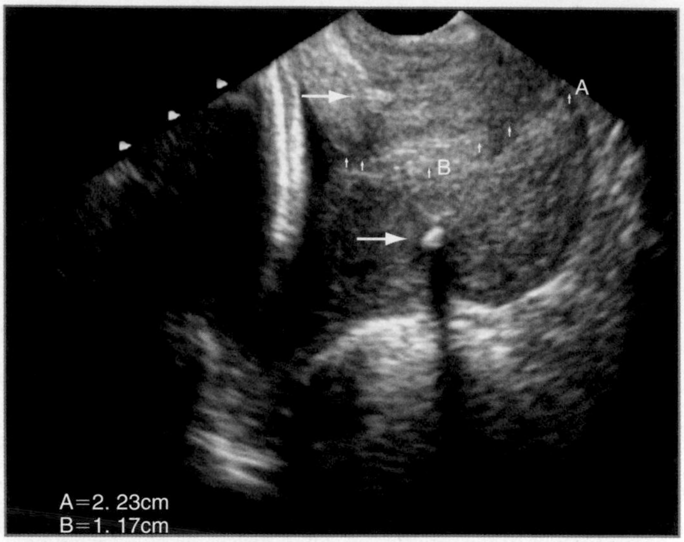

FIGURE 30-11 **Transvaginal cerclage.** Endovaginal ultrasound image of the cervix in a woman with a transvaginal Shirodkar cerclage. *Arrows* point to the 5-mm tape used for the procedure.

unsuccessful or are anatomically difficult, transabdominal cerclage (described later) or a transvaginal procedure using a technique similar to that described by Mann and colleagues[98] are reported to have a high success rate.[100]

Intraoperative ultrasound may aid satisfactory placement of Shirodkar or McDonald cerclage sutures by helping the clinician to judge the site of the suture relative to the internal os and the maternal bladder and rectum (Fig. 30-11). Sonography is performed after the sutures are placed but before the knots are tied.[101] This immediate feedback allows removal and replacement of sutures that are too low or that impinge on adjacent structures.

SHIRODKAR CERCLAGE

Shirodkar[87] used maternal fascia lata as the "suture" material and aneurysm needles to thread the fascia lata strip submucosally, after first incising the vaginal epithelium transversely both anteriorly and posteriorly and reflecting the vesicovaginal and rectovaginal fascia to the level of the internal os. The suture was tied anteriorly, and the anterior and posterior incisions were closed with absorbable material. Since the original report, many modifications have been suggested, including tying the knot posteriorly, leaving the ends of the knot exposed for easier removal, and, most commonly, replacing fascia lata with an inert suture or a 5-mm polyester band mounted on atraumatic needles. Instead of tunneling the suture submucosally, a long, curved Allis clamp may be inserted into the incisions anteriorly and posteriorly, with lateral traction applied on the submucosal tissue to place the cerclage next to the body of the cervix and medial to the uterine vessels. The knot is usually tied anteriorly and tagged to facilitate later removal. The Shirodkar suture may be anchored anteriorly and posteriorly, to avoid slippage or displacement, by including cervical tissue within the cerclage suture or by using a second nonabsorbable suture.

McDONALD CERCLAGE

McDonald[88] described a procedure that requires no submucosal dissection. A purse-string suture is begun anteriorly at the junction of the ectocervix and rugated vagina. Four to six bites of cervix are taken in a circumferential fashion, well into the body of the cervix, avoiding entry into the endocervical canal. Care must be taken to place the suture high on the posterior aspect of the cervix, because this is the most likely site for suture displacement. The suture is tied anteriorly or posteriorly, and the ends are left long enough to facilitate removal at term or at the onset of labor. Variations include use of braided nylon, polyester, or a 5-mm tape. The cervix may be re-entered at the previous point of exit with successive bites to place the suture entirely submucosally, or it may be placed so that it encompasses the cervical serosa.

TRANSABDOMINAL CERVICOISTHMIC CERCLAGE

First described by Benson and Durfee,[89] the transabdominal approach to cerclage placement has become more common as experience has grown.[81,102-107] The original criteria for selection of transabdominal cerclage included a congenitally short or amputated cervix, previously unsuccessful vaginal cerclage with cervical scarring, and cervical distortion or scarring that prevented the transvaginal approach. Transabdominal cerclage has also been recommended after one or more prior vaginal cerclage procedures have failed.[106,108] An explanation for the reported success of the abdominal over the vaginal procedure may come from the novel work of House and Socrate, who created a biomechanical model based on three dimensional ultrasound and magnetic resonance images to study cervical function in pregnancy.[109] Their investigations indicate that the maximum load is born at the internal os,[110] and therefore the cerclage suture is not load-bearing when placed at the midpoint of the cervix, as is often the case with vaginal cerclage.

Suggested timing for abdominal cerclage is between 10 and 14 weeks of gestation, so that uterine manipulation for visualization of both anterior and posterior leaves of the broad ligament can be accomplished easily; however, the procedure has been performed as late as 17 to 18 weeks' gestation.

The operation described by Benson and Durfee[89] may be performed through a Pfannenstiel or vertical incision. The peritoneal reflections are divided transversely, and the bladder is advanced carefully to avoid wide lateral dissection that could injure the massive vascular plexus present during pregnancy. At the level of the uterine isthmus, the space between the ascending and descending branches of the uterine artery is identified and developed by blunt dissection, medial to the uterine arteries and veins and lateral to the connective tissue of the uterine isthmus. Upward traction on the uterine fundus by an assistant exposes the region of the internal os, and the vessels are placed on traction. After the tunnel has been developed in the vascular space bilaterally, the posterior leaf of the broad ligament is punctured bilaterally, and a 5-mm Mersilene tape is passed under direct vision to lie over the posterior peritoneum at the level of the insertions of the uterosacral ligaments. The Mersilene band is tied snugly anteriorly or posteriorly with a square knot, and the cut ends are sutured to the band with fine, nonabsorbable sutures. The peritoneum and abdomen are then closed in routine fashion.

Mahran[102] advocated lateral retraction of the uterine vessels with the operator's fingers while a synthetic 5-mm tape is placed around the cervix from anterior to posterior at the level of the isthmus. The suture is anchored in the cervical tissue both anteriorly and posteriorly (and laterally in the Mackenrodt ligament) and tied posteriorly. This technique minimizes the opportunity for injury to the dilated parametrial venous plexus.

Davis and colleagues[106] reported a retrospective comparison of transvaginal and transabdominal cerclage with the Mahran technique in women with grossly normal cervical anatomy who had a previous transvaginal cerclage with delivery before 33 weeks' gestation. Both

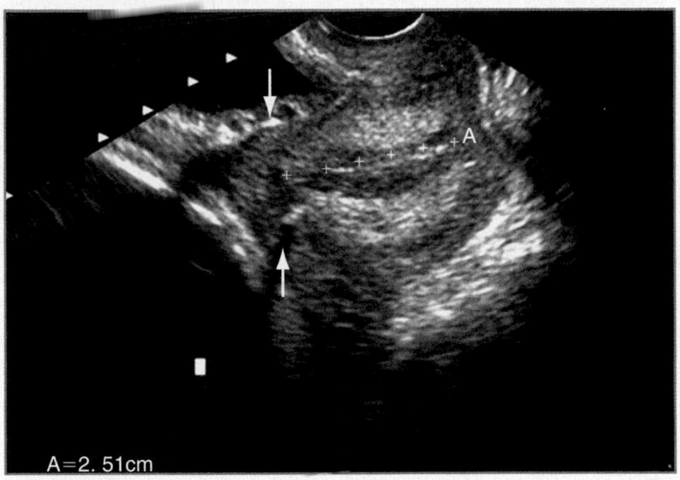

FIGURE 30-12 **Transabdominal cerclage.** Endovaginal ultrasound image of the cervix in a woman with a transabdominal cerclage. *Arrows* point to the 5-mm tape used for the procedure.

delivery before 35 and delivery before 33 weeks' gestation were less common (18% versus 42%; $P = .04$, and 10% versus 38%; $P = .01$, respectively) in the women treated with transabdominal cerclage ($n = 40$) than in those treated with transvaginal cerclage ($n = 24$). The principal difference was a marked reduction in the frequency of preterm ruptured membranes—8% versus 29%, respectively ($P = .03$). Figure 30-12 shows an endovaginal image of the cervix of a woman treated with a transabdominal cerclage. The cerclage is seen near the internal os at a level rarely achieved with a transvaginal procedure.

The transabdominal procedure requires laparotomy for cerclage placement and again for cesarean section. Transabdominal cerclage sutures have been placed laparoscopically[111] and with robotic assistance.[112] The suture may be removed by posterior colpotomy or laparoscopy to allow vaginal delivery, but more often it is left in place, with cesarean section planned before labor. A well-placed cerclage rarely causes symptoms between pregnancies if future childbearing is planned.

Efficacy of Cerclage

The majority of studies describing cerclage treatment are observational, without uniform criteria for diagnosis, choice of treatment, or outcomes. Variation in diagnostic criteria and absence of biomechanical studies have limited the evaluation of efficacy (see previous discussion of biomechanics and abdominal versus vaginal cerclage). Despite the prolonged controversy about the role of cerclage, no randomized trial comparing cerclage with bed rest or no therapy has been reported in women with the classic history. Randomized trials conducted in women with prior preterm birth have excluded those women who were thought to have "true" cervical insufficiency. Randomized trials performed before the advent of transvaginal sonography found little evidence of benefit for cerclage treatment of women with prior preterm birth. Two trials that enrolled women with low to moderate risk of preterm birth found no evidence that McDonald cerclage prolonged gestation or decreased perinatal mortality.[113,114] A multicenter, randomized trial of cervical cerclage in 1292 women with second-trimester loss, preterm delivery, or previous cervical surgery reported fewer deliveries before 33 weeks (13% versus 17%; $P = .03$), fewer infants with birth weights of less than 1500 g (10% versus 13%; $P = .05$), and fewer pregnancy losses including miscarriage, stillbirth, and neonatal death (9% versus 11%; $P = .06$) in women treated with cerclage, but no difference in the percentage of births between 33 and 36 weeks.[115] This trial specifically excluded women thought to have true cervical insufficiency.

Studies of women with clinical risk factors for preterm birth who also had ultrasound documentation of a short cervix were expected to show benefit for cerclage, but descriptive series reported mixed results.[69,72,116-118] The cervical length threshold for cerclage placement ranged from 15 to 30 mm in these studies.

Several randomized trials of cerclage have since been performed in women with risk factors for preterm birth and sonographic evidence of short cervix, again excluding women thought to have cervical insufficiency.[79,119-122] Data from these trials have been combined and analyzed by the original authors into a useful report that suggests that cerclage may reduce the risk of recurrent preterm birth before 35 weeks (relative risk [RR], 0.61; 95% confidence interval [CI], 0.40 to 0.92) in women with a prior preterm birth whose cervical length in the current pregnancy is less than 25 mm, but it appears to provide no benefit for women with a short cervix who have not had a prior preterm birth (RR, 0.84; CI, 0.60 to 1.17).[123,124]

Although these data support consideration of cerclage for women with a prior early preterm birth who have a cervical length of less than 25 mm in the current pregnancy, several recent lines of evidence may modify that conclusion. The first was noted previously: More than two thirds of women with a history of prior preterm birth who are monitored with serial cervical sonography in a subsequent pregnancy do not display a short (<25 mm) cervix and have a low likelihood of recurrent preterm birth without cerclage.[79,80,81,125] Second, among the one third of women with a prior preterm birth who manifest a short cervix in a subsequent pregnancy, an "ultrasound-indicated" cerclage, placed only when the cervix has begun to shorten, is as effective as an early prophylactic cerclage in reducing the risk of recurrent preterm birth.[78-80,126,127] Third, there is evidence that cerclage placement in some women may *increase* the risk of recurrent preterm birth. Sakai and associates[50] studied outcomes in 246 women with a prior preterm birth and a cervical length of 25 mm or less; 165 of these patients were treated with cerclage, and 81 were not, as determined by physician preference. Rates of preterm birth did not differ between these two groups; however, when the data were analyzed according to the level of IL-8 in cervical fluid at enrollment, a different conclusion emerged. Women who had an elevated level of cervical IL-8, indicating cervical inflammation, had *more* preterm births if treated with cerclage, whereas those with a normal level of IL-8 had improved outcomes after cerclage compared with expectant management. Because a clinical test for intracervical inflammation is not available, it is not possible to determine whether a cerclage placed in these circumstances might reduce or increase the risk of preterm birth. Finally, there is evidence from a randomized trial that medical treatment with progesterone for women with a very short cervix (<15 mm) may significantly reduce their risk of preterm birth before 34 weeks, from 44% to 19%.[95] The pathway by which progesterone influences the risk of preterm birth is uncertain, but an anti-inflammatory effect has been proposed. In women with a multiple gestation, cerclage for short cervix has been reported to carry an increased risk for preterm birth (RR, 2.15; CI, 1.15 to 4.01).[123,128]

These reports could be interpreted as suggesting the superiority of one cerclage technique or surgeon over another, or of noncompliance with postoperative care. However, despite strongly voiced anecdotal reports to the contrary, there is no evidence that the Shirodkar technique is more efficacious than the McDonald procedure[129] or that particular operative techniques are essential to good outcome. The more likely explanation for conflicting anecdotal and research results lies in (1) the increasing recognition that preterm cervical shortening is more often a medical than a surgical condition, (2) the inability to identify appropriate candidates for cerclage treatment, and (3) for the few who will benefit, the difficulty in placing a cerclage at the internal cervical os by the vaginal route. Taken together, current research results challenge the wisdom of prophylactic cerclage over selective ultrasound-indicated cerclage, as well as the role of cerclage versus medical treatment for women with a previous preterm birth. The Cochrane Library reviewers found insufficient evidence to support the use of cerclage for women with a prior second-trimester birth or for women with a short cervix.[130] Forthcoming results from a recently concluded trial may aid decisions about selection of candidates for cerclage.

At present, cerclage treatment may be recommended for women with an appropriate obstetric history who also manifest sonographic evidence of cervical change in the current pregnancy. Cerclage is not currently recommended for women with a short cervix who have no history of preterm birth or cervical surgery, nor for women with a prior preterm birth whose cervical length remains greater than the 10th percentile (25 mm). Although prophylactic placement of cerclage at 11 to 14 weeks' gestation may be appropriate in women with convincing histories or prior pregnancies successfully treated with cerclage, the uncertainty of diagnosis and the high likelihood of a good outcome for pregnancy managed with sonographic surveillance and selective cerclage argue against routine placement of prophylactic cerclage in women with a prior preterm birth.

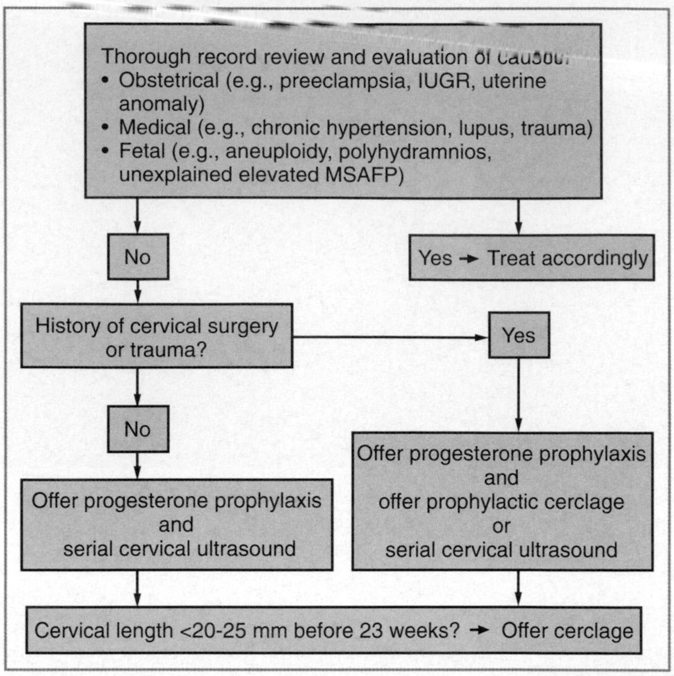

FIGURE 30-13 Care algorithm for women with a history of birth at 16 to 28 weeks. Algorithm of care for women with a prior second-trimester birth used in the Ohio State Prematurity Prevention Program. MSAFP, maternal serum α-fetoprotein.

Clinical Use of Cerclage

Contraindications to cerclage placement at any time during pregnancy include ruptured membranes, evidence of cervical or intrauterine infection, major congenital anomalies of the fetus, vaginal bleeding of undetermined cause, and active labor regardless of etiology.

After contraindications are excluded and the uncertainties regarding cerclage have been discussed with the patient, cerclage placement may be considered in the following situations.

History of Recurrent Mid-trimester Pregnancy Loss

A history of one or more early births between 16 and 30 weeks should generate a thorough review of all previous pregnancies and gynecologic procedures, including pregnancy terminations, cervical LEEP or conization, and cesarean section after a long second stage of labor. A history of cervical surgery followed by a mid-trimester birth requires consideration of cerclage. The index pregnancy should be reviewed to ascertain a history of pelvic pressure, premenstrual symptoms, or increased vaginal discharge in the days preceding the birth. Cervical dilation and effacement at clinical presentation that is out of proportion to clinical symptoms is suggestive, even if it is accompanied by mild uterine activity, ruptured membranes, or vaginal spotting. Presentation with a closed cervix followed by painful labor lasting several hours suggests a diagnosis other than cervical insufficiency. Ultrasound findings of a short or funneled cervix (<25 mm) support but do not establish the diagnosis. Pathology studies of the fetus, placenta, and membranes after a second-trimester birth commonly reveal inflammation, a finding that does not exclude cervical insufficiency but makes it less likely.

Depending on the strength of the history, the options of prophylactic cerclage or serial cervical ultrasound surveillance should be considered, with a preference for the latter as evidence of its safety has accumulated. If prophylactic cerclage is chosen, concerns about exposure of the fetus to medication may be reduced by the use of ultrasound confirmation of fetal viability and conduction anesthesia. For women who choose prenatal diagnosis, serum screening or chorionic villus sampling, or both, may be performed before the cerclage, or an amniocentesis may be elected 2 or more weeks after the cerclage is placed. Prophylactic transabdominal cerclage is reserved for women with poor cervical anatomy who have had an unsuccessful transvaginal cerclage; it may be placed before or after conception.

If sonographic surveillance is chosen, sonography begins at 15 to 16 weeks of gestation, with cerclage placement offered if the cervical length falls to less than 20 to 25 mm before 23 to 24 weeks. The frequency of surveillance is governed by the gestational age at delivery in prior pregnancies and the cervical length, with visits scheduled no less often than every 2 weeks between 15 and 25 weeks' gestation. Women with this history whose cervical length is less than 30 mm before 20 weeks are monitored weekly in our clinic. Our experience is consistent with the literature in that more than 60% of women observed with sonography maintain a cervical length greater than 25 mm and do well without cerclage. Figure 30-13 summarizes the algorithm of care used at Ohio State University Hospital for women with one or more prior second-trimester preterm births.

History of Conization, Loop Electrosurgical Excision Procedure, Diethylstilbestrol Exposure, or Uterine Anomaly without a Prior Preterm Birth

Observation by ultrasound between 15 and 25 weeks is a common choice in this situation. In women with a history of conization, substantial cervical tissue is often visible on ultrasound that is not appreciated by inspection or palpation. The cervical length may be surgically shorter than expected,[44] so observation of progressive effacement or funneling may be better than cervical length as an indicator of risk in these patients. Women with uterine anomalies may have unsuspected cervical duplication or abnormalities that are best found by obtaining coronal and transverse as well as sagittal views of the cervix on endovaginal ultrasound. There is no established protocol for surveillance frequency.

Incidental Ultrasound Observation of Short Cervix

This is an increasingly common scenario for which no evidence-based management exists. Many of these women are identified at the time of a second-trimester ultrasound to assess fetal anatomy. A thorough and confidential reproductive history should be obtained; if risk factors are found, they may be managed accordingly.

Women with incidental short cervix who are nulliparous, or multiparous with a benign obstetric history, are not candidates for cerclage. A randomized trial found no benefit for cerclage,[124] nor did an observational study.[131] Moreover, the risk of preterm birth is increased by cerclage treatment in women with twin pregnancies who are found to have short cervix.[123,128] There is preliminary evidence that treatment with progesterone might reduce the risk of preterm birth in women with an incidental observation of short cervix,[95] but additional studies are required before it can be recommended.

Presentation with Unanticipated Advanced Cervical Dilation on Physical Examination in a Nulliparous or Parous Woman

Symptoms are typically mild or absent, except for pressure and increased discharge. A thorough and confidential history should be obtained, looking specifically for cervical stretch or injury related to delivery or gynecologic disorders, as described earlier. A uterine anomaly should be considered as well.

In contrast to women with ultrasound evidence of short cervix, women who present with advanced dilation detected by digital and speculum examination may benefit from emergent cerclage if no contraindications are present. An observational study of 225 asymptomatic women with cervical dilation of 1 cm or more found improved outcomes for women treated with cerclage compared with bed rest.[58] In a descriptive study of 46 women with bulging membranes, pregnancy outcomes in women treated with cerclage were superior, compared with outcomes in women who refused the procedure.[132] Clinical application of these studies is described later.

Perioperative and Intraoperative Care

Perioperative care for prophylactic cerclage is minimal. In the absence of cervical dilation or effacement, the benefit of adjunctive medications is doubtful. The patient is ordinarily ready to go home after her anesthetic has worn off, with instructions to expect urinary hesitancy, mild abdominal cramping, labial and vaginal discomfort, and light spotting. Women undergoing cerclage after surveillance has revealed short cervix are often treated empirically with antibiotics, nonsteroidal anti-inflammatory drugs, and a period of observation before and after cerclage placement.

If cerclage is performed for a woman with membranes visible at the external os or in the vagina, the prognosis for neonatal survival decreases significantly; however, a cerclage may still be placed if infection and other contraindications can be excluded. A speculum examination should be performed to be certain that the membranes have not ruptured. The patient should be supine or in Trendelenburg position. Uterine activity should be monitored. Infection is a frequent complication; maternal temperature and white blood cell and differential counts should be determined and repeated as necessary to exclude infection.

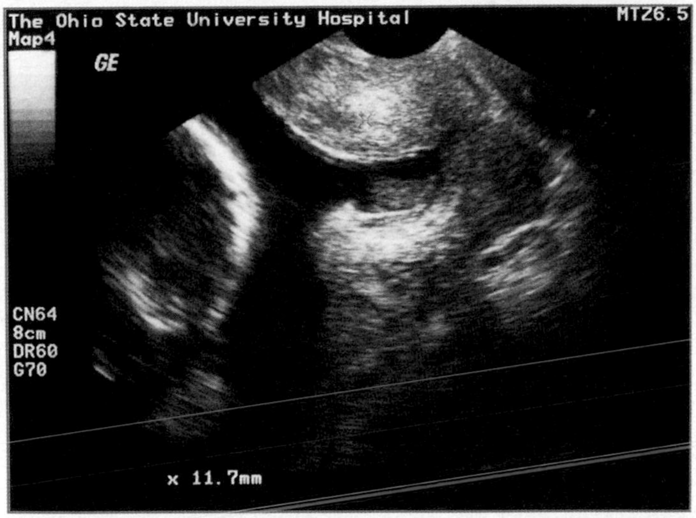

FIGURE 30-14 Amniotic fluid "debris." Endovaginal ultrasound image of cervix with a funnel and debris within the funnel.

Separation of the membranes from the decidua and the presence of "debris" or sludge within the amniotic fluid seen on endovaginal sonography suggest an increased chance of infection and are poor prognostic signs.[51,133-135] Debris or sludge has been determined to be a biofilm, a mechanism employed by low-virulence microorganisms to resist host defenses.[136,137] Amniocentesis to obtain amniotic fluid for aerobic and anaerobic culture, Gram staining, and glucose determination should be considered (Fig. 30-14).

If infection, abruption, and progressive cervical change can be ruled out, prophylactic antibiotics and tocolytics are sometimes employed empirically.[119,121] Reports of candida amnionitis in women treated with antibiotics suggest that a limited duration of prophylaxis may be wise.[138]

The McDonald cerclage is most commonly used if the cervix is well dilated, but the Shirodkar and the Wurm techniques have also been employed. (In the Wurm procedure, nonabsorbable mattress sutures are placed in the cervix from 12 to 6 o'clock and from 3 to 9 o'clock.) Placement of a cervical cerclage of any type under these circumstances is difficult at best. Bulging or prolapsed membranes are easily ruptured intraoperatively. The membranes should be inspected to identify separation or loss of the chorion from the intact amnion. If only the amnion remains, prolongation of pregnancy beyond a few days is unlikely, and consideration should be given to abandoning the procedure. Visible membranes may be replaced into the uterus with gauze on a ring forceps covered by either a condom or a finger cot[139] or with a 16F Foley catheter.[140] The cerclage may then be placed and tied with the catheter in place. The balloon is deflated, and the catheter is withdrawn. Transabdominal amniocentesis may temporarily reduce amniotic fluid volume and assist in spontaneous replacement of the membranes within the uterus.[141] Filling of the maternal bladder with sufficient fluid to compress the lower uterine segment[142] and placement of the cerclage suture with the patient in the knee-chest position[143] have also been reported.

Preoperative dilation of the cervix was the factor most strongly associated with complications and fetal survival in a review of 482 cerclage procedures.[144]

Reported success rates after emergency cerclage—with success defined as reaching "viability"—rose from 10% in 1980[145] to 60% in 1995.[146] Aarts and coworkers summarized data from 13 reports that described 249 patients treated with emergency cerclage procedures performed at a median gestational age of 22.8 weeks. The mean prolongation of pregnancy was 8.1 weeks, and the mean neonatal survival rate was 64% (range, 22% to 100%).[146] Others have found similar results.[147,148]

Often, the only alternative to emergency cerclage in patients with advanced dilation is hospital bed rest. Olatunbosun and associates[149] compared pregnancy outcomes in women treated with emergency cerclage versus bed rest in a nonrandomized study. All patients were enrolled between 20 and 27 weeks of gestation, and all had cervical dilation greater than 4 cm. The perinatal mortality rate did not differ, but the cerclage group spent fewer days in the hospital. There is no consensus about an upper gestational age limit for placement of a cerclage suture, but 24 weeks is commonly used. Prophylaxis against thromboembolism and a dietary and laxative regimen to produce a soft stool may reduce the risks of blood clot and constipation that accompany bed rest, but the emotional and musculoskeletal consequences of bed rest are more difficult to prevent.[150]

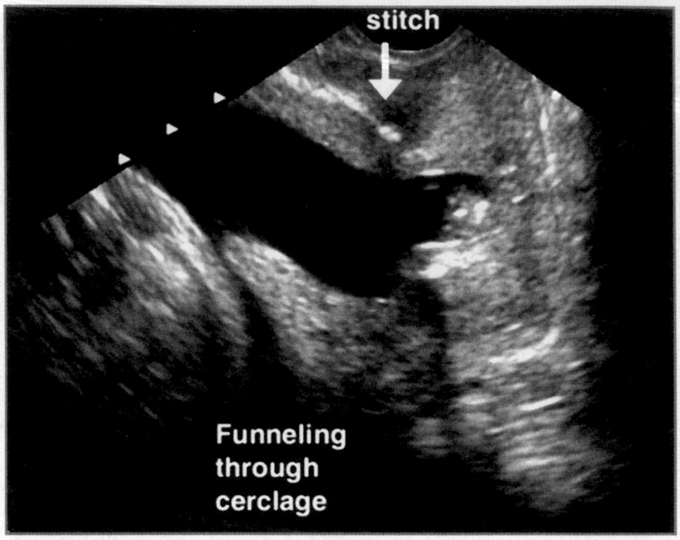

FIGURE 30-15 **Protrusion of the membranes past the plane of the cerclage.** Endovaginal ultrasound image of cervix with membranes funneled past the level of a McDonald cerclage suture. *Arrow* points to the cerclage suture in the anterior cervical lip.

Complications after Cerclage

Morbidity associated with cervical cerclage of all types includes complications related to the procedure itself (anesthetic risks, bleeding, maternal soft tissue injury, spontaneous suture displacement, preterm premature rupture of the membranes [pPROM], and infection) and those related to subsequent delivery (cervical lacerations and fistulas, increased incidence of cesarean section). Ruptured membranes are reported in 1% to 40% of women treated with cerclage. This risk increases with the degree of dilation and effacement and with the gestational age at placement.[144]

Management of pPROM in a patient with a cerclage is controversial. The incidence of infectious complications and poor neonatal outcome was increased in one series when the cerclage was in left in situ after membrane rupture,[151] but two other reports did not find an increased rate of infection or other neonatal or maternal morbidity with delayed removal.[152,153] Deferred removal to prolong pregnancy may be acceptable if pPROM occurs early, but the benefit-to-risk ratio declines as gestational age increases.[154]

Chorioamnionitis resulting from cervical cerclage placement has been reported with varying frequency, from 1%[145] to 6% to 8%.[144] Treadwell and colleagues[144] found that the rate of chorioamnionitis identified on aerobic cultures was significantly associated with cervical dilation (6.2% if the cervix was no more than 2 cm dilated, versus 41.7% if the cervix was >2 cm) and with the timing of the procedure (5.2% if elective versus 14.4% if emergent). The incidence of chorioamnionitis has been reported to be as much as 40% to 50% when anaerobic cultures and research laboratory techniques are used.[155]

Remote sequelae of cervical cerclage procedures include uterine rupture, excessive bleeding with suture removal, cervical dystocia related to scarring at the cerclage site, and cervical lacerations and fistulas. The cervix may not dilate normally in response to labor after a cerclage has been in place, despite its removal at the appropriate time.[145,156] Lindberg[157] reported uterine rupture when labor began before the suture could be removed, a particular concern for women with a prior vertical uterine incision.

Treadwell and coworkers[144] reported an overall incidence of cesarean delivery of 31.8% in 482 patients. Cesarean section for cervical dystocia was more common after Shirodkar than after McDonald cerclage in this series: 11.4% versus 2.6%, respectively ($P < .005$). Cervical lacerations at delivery thought to be related to cerclage have been reported.[144,145] Treadwell and coworkers[144] observed cervical lacerations in 6.2% of patients, more commonly when the cerclage was placed after 18 weeks' gestation. Other maternal morbidity associated with cerclage placement includes vesicovaginal and urethrovaginal fistulas and ulceration of the trigone of the bladder from erosion of the knot of the cerclage.

Postoperative assessment of suture location as well as pregnancy management and outcome can be improved with ultrasonographic assessment of the cervix.[158,159] Both the nylon and Ethibond sutures commonly used in the McDonald procedure (Fig. 30-15) and the 5-mm Mersilene tape used in the Shirodkar procedure (see Fig. 30-11) can be seen easily on transvaginal ultrasonography. The length of the cervix from the plane of the suture to both the internal and external os can be measured. Pregnancy outcomes are better when the membranes do not descend past the plane of the suture and when the cervix is seen to be closed above and below the sutures.[158,159]

Placement of a second cerclage when the first appears to be failing, as indicated by protrusion of the membranes past the plane of the cerclage, can be considered if observed before 20 to 22 weeks' gestation. Patients in whom membrane protrusion is noted with ultrasound after 22 to 24 weeks' gestation are placed on bed rest, usually in the hospital if the membranes are seen to extend below the level of the cerclage on transvaginal sonography (see Fig. 30-15).

Removal can usually be accomplished in the office or clinic without anesthesia if good lighting is provided. Most women expect labor to begin immediately, but that is the exception. An interval of days between removal and the onset of labor does not mean that the diagnosis was incorrect but instead typifies the various etiologies of abnormal cervical competence.

Summary

The clinical syndrome of cervical insufficiency results in early, often recurrent preterm birth in the second trimester. Advanced cervical dilation and effacement with minimal uterine activity is the most typical presentation, but not an exclusive one. The syndrome is the result of the interaction of many factors that affect the strength of the cervix, including biologic variation, obstetric and gynecologic injuries, and inflammation-mediated changes. Diagnosis is difficult and should be based on both the obstetric history and ultrasound evidence of premature effacement. The most effective treatment has not been established. Treatment with cerclage is considered when both historical and ultrasound criteria are met.

References

1. Crosby WM, Hill EC: Embryology of the müllerian duct system. Obstet Gynecol 20:507, 1962.
2. Danforth DN: The fibrous nature of the human cervix and its relation to the isthmic segment in gravid and nongravid uteri. Am J Obstet Gynecol 53:541, 1947.
3. Rorie DK, Newton M: Histological and chemical studies of the smooth muscle in human cervix and uterus. Am J Obstet Gynecol 99:466, 1967.
4. Kushnir O, Vigil DA, Izquierdo L, et al: Vaginal ultrasonographic assessment of cervical length changes during normal pregnancy. Am J Obstet Gynecol 162:991, 1990.
5. Word RA, Li X-H, Hnat M, et al: Dynamics of cervical remodeling during pregnancy and parturition: Mechanisms and current concepts. Semin Reprod Med 25:69-79, 2007.
6. Berghella V, Talucci M, Desai A: Does transvaginal sonographic measurement of cervical length before 14 weeks predict preterm delivery in high-risk pregnancies? Ultrasound Obstet Gynecol 21:140-144, 2003.
7. Andersen HF, Nugent CE, Wanty SD, et al: Prediction of risk for preterm delivery by ultrasonographic measurement of cervical length. Am J Obstet Gynecol 163:859, 1990.
8. Zorzoli A, Soliani A, Perra M, et al: Cervical changes throughout pregnancy as assessed by transvaginal sonography. Obstet Gynecol 84:960, 1994.
9. Zilianti M, Azuaga A, Calderon F, et al: Monitoring the effacement of the uterine cervix by transperineal sonography. J Ultrasound Med 14:719, 1995.
10. Iams JD, Goldenberg RL, Meis PJ, et al: The length of the cervix and the risk of spontaneous preterm delivery. N Engl J Med 334:567, 1996.
11. Taipale P, Hiilesmaa V: Sonographic measurement of uterine cervix at 18-22 weeks' gestation and the risk of preterm delivery. Obstet Gynecol 92:902, 1998.
12. Hibbard JU, Tart M, Moawad AH: Cervical length at 16-22 weeks' gestation and risk for preterm delivery. Obstet Gynecol 96:972, 2000.
13. Buckingham JC, Buethe RA, Danforth DN: Collagen-muscle ratio in clinically normal and clinically incompetent cervices. Am J Obstet Gynecol 91:231, 1965.
14. Rechberger T, Uldbjerg N, Oxlund H: Connective tissue changes in the cervix during normal pregnancy and pregnancy complicated by cervical insufficiency. Obstet Gynecol 71:563, 1988.
15. Petersen LK, Uldbjerg N: Cervical collagen in non-pregnant women with previous cervical insufficiency. Eur J Obstet Gynecol Reprod Biol 67:41, 1996.
16. Iwahashi M, Muragaki Y, Ooshima A, et al: Decreased type I collagen expression in human uterine cervix during pregnancy. J Clin Endocrinol Metab 88:2231-2235, 2003.
17. Leduc L, Wasserstrum N: Successful treatment with the Smith-Hodge pessary of cervical incompetence due to defective connective tissue in Ehlers-Danlos syndrome. Am J Perinatol 9:25-27, 1992.
18. Larsson LG, Mudholkar GS, Baum J, et al: Hypermobility: Prevalence and features in a Swedish population. Br J Rheumatol 32:116-119, 1993.
19. Warren JE, Silver RM, Dalton J, et al: Collagen 1alpha1 and transforming growth factor beta polymorphisms in women with cervical insufficiency. Obstet Gynecol 110:619-624, 2007.
20. Iams JD, Johnson FF, Sonek J, et al: Cervical competence as a continuum: A study of ultrasonographic cervical length and obstetric performance. Am J Obstet Gynecol 172:1097, 1995.
21. Goldenberg RL, Iams JD, Mercer BM, et al: The preterm prediction study: The value of new vs. standard risk factors in predicting early and all spontaneous preterm births. Am J Public Health 88:233, 1998.
22. Imseis HM, Albert TA, Iams JD: Identifying twin gestations at low risk for preterm birth with a transvaginal ultrasonographic cervical measurement at 24 to 26 weeks' gestation. Am J Obstet Gynecol 177:1149, 1997.
23. Ramin KD, Ogburn PL, Mulholland TA, et al: Ultrasonographic assessment of cervical length in triplet pregnancies. Am J Obstet Gynecol 180:1442, 1999.
24. Souka AP, Heath V, Flint S: Cervical length at 23 weeks in twins in predicting spontaneous preterm delivery. Obstet Gynecol 94:540, 1999.
25. To MS, Fonseca EB, Molina FS, et al: Maternal characteristics and cervical length in the prediction of spontaneous early preterm delivery in twins. Am J Obstet Gynecol 194:1360-1365, 2006.
26. Ludmir J, Samuels P, Brooks S, et al: Pregnancy outcome of patients with uncorrected uterine anomalies managed in a high risk setting. Obstet Gynecol 75:906, 1990.
27. Seidman DS, Ben-Rafael Z, Bider D, et al: The role of cervical cerclage in the management of uterine anomalies. Surg Gynecol Obstet 173:384, 1991.
28. Leibovitz Z, Levitan Z, Aharoni A, et al: Cervical cerclage in uterine malformations. Int J Fertil 37:214, 1992.
29. Raga F, Bauset C, Remohi J, et al: Reproductive impact of congenital müllerian anomalies. Hum Reprod 12:2277, 1997.
30. Surico N, Ribaldone R, Arnulfo A, et al: Uterine malformations and pregnancy losses: Is cervical cerclage effective? Clin Exp Obstet Gynecol 27:147, 2000.
31. Woelfer B, Salim R, Banerjee S, et al: Reproductive outcomes in women with congenital uterine anomalies detected by three-dimensional ultrasound screening. Obstet Gynecol 98:1009, 2001.
32. Lin PJ: Reproductive outcomes in women with uterine anomalies. J Womens Health 13:33-39, 2004.
33. Rackow BW, Arici A: Reproductive performance of women with mullerian anomalies. Curr Opin Obstet Gynecol 19:229-237, 2007.
34. Zlopaša G, Škrablin S, Kalafatić D, et al: Uterine anomalies and pregnancy outcome following resectoscope metroplasty. Int J Gynecol Obstet 98:129-133, 2007.
35. Kaufman RH, Adam E, Hatch EE, et al: Continued follow-up of pregnancy outcomes in diethylstilbestrol-exposed offspring. Obstet Gynecol 96:483, 2000.
36. Goldstein DP: Incompetent cervix in offspring exposed to diethylstilbestrol in utero. Obstet Gynecol 52(1 Suppl):73S-75S, 1978.
37. Kaufman RH, Noller K, Adam E, et al: Upper genital tract abnormalities and pregnancy outcome in diethylstilbestrol-exposed progeny. Am J Obstet Gynecol 148:973, 1984.
38. Vyas NA, Vink JS, Ghidini A, et al: Risk factors for cervical insufficiency after term delivery. Am J Obstet Gynecol 195:787-791, 2005.
39. Johnstone FD, Beard RJ, Boyd IE, et al: Cervical diameter after suction termination of pregnancy. BMJ 1(6001):68, 1976.
40. Mandelson MT, Maden CB, Daling JR: Low birth weight in relation to multiple induced abortions. Am J Public Health 82:391, 1992.
41. Zhou W, Sorenson HT, Olsen J: Induced abortion and low birthweight in the following pregnancy. Int J Epidemiol 29:100, 2000.
42. Henriet L, Kaminski M: Impact of induced abortions on subsequent pregnancy outcome: The 1995 French national perinatal survey. BJOG 108:1036, 2001.
43. Kyrgiou M, Koliopoulos G, Martin-Hirsch P, et al: Obstetric outcomes after conservative treatment for intraepithelial or early invasive cervical lesions: Systematic review and meta-analysis. Lancet 367:489-498, 2006.

44. Crane JMG, Delaney T, Hutchens D: Transvaginal ultrsonography in the prediction of preterm birth after treatment for cervical intraepithelial neoplasia. Obstet Gynecol 107:37-44, 2006.
45. Jakobsson M, Gissler M, Sainio S, et al: Preterm delivery after surgical treatment for cervical intraepithelial neoplasia. Obstet Gynecol 109:309-313, 2007.
46. Nøhr B, Tabor A, Frederiksen K, et al: Loop electrosurgical excision of the cervix and the subsequent risk of preterm delivery. Acta Obstet Gynecol Scand 86:596-603, 2007.
47. Sjøborg KD, Vistad I, Myhr SS, et al: Pregnancy outcome after cervical cone excision: A case-control study. Acta Obstet Gynecol Scand 86:423-428, 2007.
48. Romero R, Espinoza J, Erez O, et al: The role of cervical cerclage in obstetric practice: Can the patient who could benefit from this procedure be identified? Am J Obstet Gynecol 194:1-9, 2006.
49. Kelly RW: Inflammatory mediators and cervical ripening. J Reprod Immunol 57:217-224, 2002.
50. Sakai M, Shiozaki A, Tabata M, et al: Evaluation of effectiveness of prophylactic cerclage of a short cervix according to interleukin-8 in cervical mucus. Am J Obstet Gynecol 194:14-19, 2006.
51. Weiner CP, Lee KY, Buhimschi CS, et al: Proteomic biomarkers that predict the clinical success of rescue cerclage. Am J Obstet Gynecol 192:710-718, 2005.
52. Crombleholme WR, Minkoff HL, Delke I, et al: Cervical cerclage: An aggressive approach to threatened or recurrent pregnancy wastage. Am J Obstet Gynecol 146:168, 1983.
53. Romero R, Espinoza J, Kusanovic JP, et al: The preterm parturition syndrome. BJOG 113:17-42, 2006.
54. Gomez R, Galasso M, Romero R, et al: Ultrasonographic examination of the uterine cervix is better than cervical digital examination as a predictor of the likelihood of premature delivery in patients with preterm labor and intact membranes. Am J Obstet Gynecol 171:956-964, 1994.
55. Goldberg J, Newman RB, Rust PF: Interobserver reliability of digital and endovaginal ultrasonographic cervical length measurements. Am J Obstet Gynecol 177:853-858, 1997.
56. Zlatnik FJ, Yankowitz J, Whitham J, et al: Vaginal ultrasound as an adjunct to cervical digital examination in women at risk of early delivery. Gynecol Obstet Invest 51:12-16, 2001.
57. Matijevic R, Grgic O, Vasilj O: Is sonographic assessment of cervical length better than digital examination in screening for preterm delivery in a low-risk population? Acta Obstet Gynecol Scand 85:1342-1347, 2006.
58. Pereira L, Cotter A, Gomez R, et al: Expectant management compared with physical examination indicated cerclage in selected women with a dilated cervix at 14(0/7)-25(6/7) weeks: Results from the EM-PEC international cohort study. Am J Obstet Gynecol 197:483.e1-483.e8, 2007.
59. Sarti DA, Sample WF, Hobel CJ, et al: Ultrasonic visualization of a dilated cervix during pregnancy. Radiology 130:417, 1979.
60. Ayers JWT, DeGrood RM, Compton AA, et al: Sonographic evaluation of cervical length in pregnancy: Diagnosis and management of preterm cervical effacement in patients at risk for premature delivery. Obstet Gynecol 71:939, 1988.
61. Podobnik M, Bulic M, Smiljanic N, et al: Ultrasonography in the detection of cervical incompetency. J Clin Ultrasound 13:383, 1988.
62. Confino E, Mayden KL, Giglia RV, et al: Pitfalls in sonographic imaging of the incompetent uterine cervix. Acta Obstet Gynecol Scand 65:593-597, 1986.
63. Mason GC, Maresh MJA: Alterations in bladder volume and the ultrasound appearance of the cervix. BJOG 97:457, 1990.
64. Andersen HF: Transvaginal and transabdominal ultrasonography of the uterine cervix during pregnancy. J Clin Ultrasound 19:77, 1991.
65. Ludmir J: Sonographic detection of cervical insufficiency. Clin Obstet Gynecol 31:101, 1988.
66. Guzman ER, Rosenberg JC, Houlihan C, et al: A new method using vaginal ultrasound and transfundal pressure to evaluate the asymptomatic incompetent cervix. Obstet Gynecol 83:248, 1994.
67. Yost NP, Bloom SL, Twickler DM, et al: Pitfalls in ultrasonic cervical length measurement for predicting preterm birth. Obstet Gynecol 93:510, 1999.
68. Gramellini D, Fieni S, Molina E, et al: Transvaginal sonographic cervical length changes during normal pregnancy. J Ultrasound Med 21:227, 2002.
69. Heath VCF, Souka AP, Erasmus I, et al: Cervical length at 23 weeks' gestation: The value of Shirodkar suture for the short cervix. Ultrasound Obstet Gynecol 12:318, 1998.
70. Owen J, Yost N, Berghella V, et al: Can shortened midtrimester cervical length predict very early spontaneous preterm birth? Am J Obstet Gynecol. 191:298-303, 2004.
71. Andrews WW, Copper R, Hauth JC, et al: Second-trimester cervical ultrasound: Associations with increased risk for recurrent early spontaneous delivery. Obstet Gynecol 95:222-226, 2000.
72. Owen J, Yost N, Berghella V, et al: Mid-trimester endovaginal sonography in women at high risk for spontaneous preterm birth. JAMA 286:1340-1348, 2001.
73. Berghella V, Owen J, MacPherson C, et al: Natural history of cervical funneling in women at high risk for spontaneous preterm birth. Obstet Gynecol 109:863-869, 2007.
74. Guzman ER, Mellon C, Vintzeleos AM, et al: Longitudinal assessment of endocervical canal length between 15 and 24 weeks' gestation in women at risk for pregnancy loss or preterm birth. Obstet Gynecol 92:31, 1998.
75. MacDonald R, Smith P, Vyas S: Cervical insufficiency: The use of transvaginal sonography to provide an objective diagnosis. Ultrasound Obstet Gynecol 18:211, 2001.
76. Tho PT, Byrd JR, McDonough PG: Etiologies and subsequent reproductive performance in 100 couples with recurrent abortion. Fertil Steril 32:389, 1979.
77. Harger JH: Cervical cerclage: Patient selection, morbidity and success rates. Clin Perinatol 10:321, 1983.
78. Guzman EJ, Forster JK, Vintzeleos AM, et al: Pregnancy outcomes in women treated with elective versus ultrasound-indicated cerclage. Ultrasound Obstet Gynecol 12:323, 1998.
79. Althuisius SM, Dekker GA, van Geijn HP, et al: Cervical Incompetence Prevention Randomized Cerclage Trial (CIPRACT): Study design and preliminary results. Am J Obstet Gynecol 183:823-829, 2000.
80. To MS, Palaniappan V, Skentou C, et al: Elective cerclage vs. ultrasound-indicated cerclage in high risk pregnancies. Ultrasound Obstet Gynecol 19:475, 2002.
81. Groom KM, Bennett PR, Golara M: Elective cervical cerclage versus serial ultrasound surveillance of cervical length in a population at high risk for preterm delivery. Eur J Obstet Gynecol Reprod Biol 112:158-161, 2004.
82. Vaginal Ultrasound Cerclage Trial, NCT 00059683. Available at http://www.clinicaltrials.gov (accessed March 6, 2008).
83. American College of Obstetricians and Gynecologists: Cervical insufficiency. ACOG Practice Bulletin No. 48. Obstet Gynecol 102:1092-1099, 2003.
84. Fleischer AC, Andreotti RF, Bohm-Velez M, et al: Expert Panel on Women's Imaging: Premature cervical dilation. Reston, VA: American College of Radiology, 2005. Available at www.acr.org (accessed April 18, 2008).
85. Palmer R, LaComme JL: La beáance de l'orifice interne, cause d'avortment a repetition une observation de dechirure cervico-isthmique repare chirurgicalement, avec gestation a term consecutive. Gynecol Obstet (Paris) 47:905, 1948.
86. Lash AF, Lash SR: Habitual abortion: The competent internal os of the cervix. Am J Obstet Gynecol 59:68, 1950.
87. Shirodkar VN: A new method of operative treatment for habitual abortions in the second trimester of pregnancy. Antiseptic 52:299, 1955.
88. McDonald IA: Suture of the cervix for inevitable miscarriage. J Obstet Gynaecol Br Commonw 64:346, 1957.
89. Benson RC, Durfee RB: Transabdominal cervicouterine cerclage during pregnancy for the treatment of cervical incompetency. Obstet Gynecol 25:145, 1965.
90. Newcomer J: Pessaries for the treatment of incompetent cervix and premature delivery. Obstet Gynecol Surv 55:443, 2000.
91. Arabin B, Halbesma JR, Vork F, et al: Is treatment with vaginal pessaries an option in patients with a sonographically detected short cervix? J Perinat Med 31:122-133, 2003.

92. Antczak-Judycka A, Sawicki W, Spiewankiewicz B, et al: Comparison of cerclage and cerclage pessary in the treatment of pregnant women with incompetent cervix and threatened preterm delivery. Ginekol Pol 74:1029-1036, 2003.
93. Acharya G, Eschler B, Grønberg M, et al: Noninvasive cerclage for the management of cervical incompetence: A prospective study. Arch Gynecol Obstet 273:283-287, 2006.
94. Berghella V, Rust OA, Althuisius SM: Short cervix on ultrasound: Does indomethacin prevent preterm birth? Am J Obstet Gynecol 195:809-813, 2006.
95. Fonseca EB, Celik E, Parra M, et al: Progesterone and the risk of preterm birth among women with a short cervix. N Engl J Med 357:462-469, 2007.
96. Lash AF: Fertility and reproduction following repair of the incompetent internal os of the cervix. Fertil Steril 11:531, 1960.
97. Lees DH, Sutherst JR: The sequelae of cervical trauma. Am J Obstet Gynecol 120:1050, 1974.
98. Mann EC, McLaren WD, Hoyt OB: The physiology and clinical significance of the uterine isthmus. Am J Obstet Gynecol 81:209, 1961.
99. Groom KM, Jones BA, Edmonds DK, et al: Preconception transabdominal cervicoisthmic cerclage. Am J Obstet Gynecol 191:230-234, 2004.
100. Katz M, Abrahams C: Transvaginal placement of cervicoisthmic cerclage: Report on pregnancy outcome. Am J Obstet Gynecol 192:1989-1992, 2005.
101. Ludmir J, Jackson M, Samuels P: Transvaginal cerclage under ultrasound guidance in cases of severe cervical hypoplasia. Obstet Gynecol 78:1067, 1991.
102. Mahran M: Transabdominal cervical cerclage during pregnancy. Obstet Gynecol 52:502, 1978.
103. Wallenburg HCS, Lotgering FK: Transabdominal cerclage for closure of the incompetent cervix. Eur J Obstet Reprod Biol 25:121, 1987.
104. Novy MJ: Transabdominal cervicoisthmic cerclage: A reappraisal 25 years after its introduction. Am J Obstet Gynecol 164:1635, 1991.
105. Cammarano CL, Herron MA, Parer JT: Validity of indications for transabdominal cervicoisthmic cerclage for cervical insufficiency. Am J Obstet Gynecol 172:1871, 1995.
106. Davis G, Berghella V, Talucci M, et al: Patients with a prior failed transvaginal cerclage: A comparison of obstetrics outcomes with either transabdominal or transvaginal cerclage. Am J Obstet Gynecol 183:836, 2000.
107. Lotgering FK, Gaugler-Senden IP, Lotgering SF, et al: Outcome after transabdominal cervicoisthmic cerclage. Obstet Gynecol 107:779-784, 2006.
108. Debbs RH, DeLa Vega GA, Pearson S, et al: Transabdominal cerclage after comprehensive evaluation of women with previous unsuccessful transvaginal cerclage. Am J Obstet Gynecol 197:317.e1-317.e4, 2007.
109. House M, Socrate S: The cervix as a biomechanical structure. Ultrasound Obstet Gynecol 28:745-749, 2006.
110. House M, Paskaleva AP, Myers K, et al: The biomechanics of cerclage placement: The effect of cerclage position and stress relaxation on cervical stress. Society for Maternal-Fetal Medicine: 2006 26th Annual Meeting, abstract 51. Am J Obstet Gynecol 193(6 Suppl S):S21, 2005.
111. Mingione MJ, Scibetta JJ, Sanko SR, et al: Clinical outcomes following interval laparoscopic transabdominal cervico-isthmic cerclage placement: Case series. Hum Reprod 18:1716-1719, 2003.
112. Barmat L, Glaser G, Davis G, et al: Da Vinci-assisted abdominal cerclage. Fertil Steril 88:1437.e1-1437.e3, 2007.
113. Lazar P, Guegen S, Dreyfus J, et al: Multicentred controlled trial of cervical cerclage in women at moderate risk of preterm delivery. BJOG 91:731, 1984.
114. Rush RW, Issacs S, McPherson K, et al: A randomized controlled trial of cervical cerclage in women at high risk of spontaneous delivery. BJOG 91:724, 1984.
115. MacNaughton MC, Chalmers IG, Dubowitz V, et al: Final report of the Medical Research Council/Royal College of Obstetrics and Gynaecology multicentre randomised trial of cervical cerclage. BJOG 100:516, 1993.
116. Berghella V, Daly SF, Tolosa JE, et al: Prediction of preterm delivery with transvaginal ultrasonography of the cervix in patients with high-risk pregnancies: Does cerclage prevent prematurity? Am J Obstet Gynecol 181:809, 1999.
117. Hibbard JU, Snow J, Moawad AH: Short cervical length by ultrasound and cerclage. J Perinatol 3:161, 2000.
118. Hassan SS, Romero R, Maymon E, et al: Does cervical cerclage prevent preterm delivery in patients with a short cervix? Am J Obstet Gynecol 184:1325, 2001.
119. Althuisius SM, Dekker GA, Hummel P, et al: Final results of the Cervical Incompetence Prevention Randomized Cerclage Trial (CIPRACT): Therapeutic cerclage with bed rest versus bed rest alone. Am J Obstet Gynecol 185:1106-1112, 2001.
120. Rust OA, Atlas RO, Jones KJ, et al: A randomized trial of cerclage versus no cerclage among patients with ultrasonographically detected second-trimester preterm dilatation of the internal os. Am J Obstet Gynecol 183:830, 2000.
121. Rust OA, Atlas RO, Reed J, et al: Revisiting the short cervix detected by transvaginal ultrasound in the second trimester: Why cerclage therapy may not help. Am J Obstet Gynecol 185:1098-1105, 2001.
122. Berghella V, Odibo AO, Tolosa JE: Cerclage for prevention of preterm birth in women with a short cervix found on transvaginal ultrasound examination: A randomized trial. Am J Obstet Gynecol 191:1311-1317, 2004.
123. Berghella V, Odibo A, To MS, et al: Cerclage for short cervix on ultrasonography: Meta-analysis of trials using individual patient data. Obstet Gynecol 106:181-189, 2005.
124. To MS, Alfirevic Z, Heath VC, et al: Cervical cerclage for prevention of preterm delivery in women with short cervix: Randomised controlled trial. Lancet 363:1849-1853, 2004.
125. Higgins SP, Kornman LH, Bell RJ, et al: Cervical surveillance as an alternative to elective cervical cerclage for pregnancy management of suspected cervical incompetence. Aust N Z J Obstet Gynaecol 44:228-232, 2004.
126. Cook CM, Ellwood DA: The cervix as a predictor of preterm delivery in "at-risk" women. Ultrasound Obstet Gynecol 15:109, 2000.
127. Kelly S, Pollock M, Maas B, et al: Early transvaginal ultrasonography versus early cerclage in women with an unclear history of incompetent cervix. Am J Obstet Gynecol 184:1097, 2001.
128. Roman AS, Rebarber A, Pereira L, et al: The efficacy of sonographically indicated cerclage in multiple gestations. J Ultrasound Med 24:763-768, 2005.
129. Odibo AO, Berghella V, To MS, et al: Shirodkar versus McDonald cerclage for the prevention of preterm birth in women with short cervical length. Am J Perinatol 24:55-60, 2007.
130. Drakeley AJ, Roberts D, Alfirevic Z: Cervical stitch (cerclage) for preventing pregnancy loss in women. Cochrane Database Syst Rev (1):CD003253, 2003.
131. Incerti M, Ghidini A, Locatelli A, et al: Cervical length < or = 25 mm in low-risk women: A case control study of cerclage with rest vs rest alone. Am J Obstet Gynecol 197:315.e1-315.e4, 2007.
132. Daskalakis G, Papantoniou N, Mesogitis S, et al: Management of cervical insufficiency and bulging fetal membranes. Obstet Gynecol 107:221-226, 2006.
133. Hassan S, Romero R, Hendler I, et al: A sonographic short cervix as the only clinical manifestation of intra-amniotic infection. J Perinat Med 34:13-19, 2006.
134. Bujold E, Pasquier JC, Simoneau J, et al: Intra-amniotic sludge, short cervix, and risk of preterm delivery. J Obstet Gynaecol Can 28:198-202, 2006.
135. Kusanovic JP, Espinoza J, Romero R, et al: Clinical significance of the presence of amniotic fluid "sludge" in asymptomatic patients at high risk for spontaneous preterm delivery. Ultrasound Obstet Gynecol 30:706-714, 2007.
136. Romero R, Kusanovic JP, Espinoza J, et al: What is amniotic fluid "sludge"? Ultrasound Obstet Gynecol 30:793-798, 2007.
137. Romero R, Schaudinn C, Kusanovic JP, et al: Detection of a microbial biofilm in intraamniotic infection. Am J Obstet Gynecol 198:135.e1-135.e5, 2008.
138. Qureshi F, Jacques SM, Bendon RW, et al: Candida funisitis: A clinicopathologic study of 32 cases. Pediatr Dev Pathol 1:118, 1998.

139. Novy MJ: Combating recurrent abortion and premature delivery with cervical cerclage. [Special issue.] Contemp Obstet Gynecol 25:113, 1985.
140. Holman MR: An aid for cervical cerclage. Obstet Gynecol 42:478, 1973.
141. Locatelli A, Vergani P, Bellini P, et al: Amnioreduction in emergency cerclage with prolapsed membranes: Comparison of two methods for reducing the membranes. Am J Perinatol 16:73, 1999.
142. Sheerer LJ, Lam L, Katz M: A New Technique for Cervical Cerclage in the Presence of Prolapsed Fetal Membranes. Orlando, FL: Society for Perinatal Obstetricians, 1987.
143. Ogawa M, Sanada H, Tsuda A, et al: Modified cervical cerclage in pregnant women with advanced bulging membranes: Knee-chest positioning. Acta Obstet Gynecol Scand 78:779, 1999.
144. Treadwell MC, Bronsteen RA, Bottoms SF: Prognostic factors and complication rates for cervical cerclage: A review of 482 cases. Am J Obstet Gynecol 165:555, 1991.
145. Harger JH: Comparison of success and morbidity in cervical cerclage procedures. Obstet Gynecol 56:543, 1980.
146. Aarts JM, Brons JTJ, Bruinse HW: Emergency cerclage: A review. Obstet Gynecol Surv 50:459, 1995.
147. Benifla JL, Goffinet F, Darai E, et al: Emergency cervical cerclage after 20 weeks' gestation: A retrospective study of 6 years' practice in 34 cases. Fetal Diagn Ther 12:274-278, 1997.
148. Chasen ST, Silverman NS: Mid-trimester emergent cerclage: A ten year single institution review. J Perinatol 18:338, 1998.
149. Olatunbosun OA, al-Nuaim L, Turnell RW: Emergency cerclage compared with bedrest for advanced cervical dilatation during pregnancy. Int Surg 80:170, 1995.
150. Maloni JA, Chance B, Zhang C, et al: Physical and psychosocial side effects of antepartum hospital bed rest. Nurs Res 42:197-203, 1993.
151. Ludmir J, Bader T, Chen L, et al: Poor perinatal outcome associated with retained cerclage in patients with premature rupture of membranes. Obstet Gynecol 84:823, 1994.
152. McElrath TF, Norwitz ER, Lieberman ES, et al: Perinatal outcome after preterm premature rupture of membranes with in situ cervical cerclage. Am J Obstet Gynecol 187:1147-1152, 2002.
153. Jenkins TM, Berghella V, Shlossman PA, et al: Timing of cerclage removal after preterm premature rupture of the membranes: Maternal and neonatal outcomes. Am J Obstet Gynecol 183:847, 2000.
154. O'Connor S, Kuller JA, McMahon MJ: Management of cervical cerclage after preterm premature rupture of membranes. Obstet Gynecol Surv 54:391, 1999.
155. Romero R, Gonzalez R, Sepulveda W, et al: Infection and labor: VIII. Microbial invasion of the amniotic cavity in patients with suspected cervical insufficiency. Am J Obstet Gynecol 167:1086, 1992.
156. Kuhn RJP, Pepperell RJ: Cervical ligation: A review of 242 pregnancies. Aust N Z J Obstet Gynaecol 17:79, 1977.
157. Lindberg BS: Maternal sepsis, uterine rupture, and coagulopathy complicating cervical cerclage. Acta Obstet Gynecol Scand 58:317, 1979.
158. Andersen HF, Karimi A, Sakala EP, et al: Prediction of cervical cerclage outcome by endovaginal sonography. Am J Obstet Gynecol 171:1102, 1994.
159. Guzman ER, Houlihan C, Vintzileos A, et al: The significance of transvaginal ultrasonographic evaluation of the cervix in women treated with emergency cerclage. Am J Obstet Gynecol 175:471, 1996.

Chapter 31

Premature Rupture of the Membranes

Brian M. Mercer, MD

Rupture of the fetal membranes is an integral part of the normal parturition process at term and is inevitable in the process of preterm birth. Spontaneous rupture of the membranes (SROM) at term and preterm can occur any time before or after the onset of contractions. SROM before the onset of contractions is referred to as premature rupture of the membranes (PROM). Membrane rupture at term usually occurs as a result of a physiologic process of progressive membrane weakening. Preterm PROM generally results from pathologic weakening of the fetal membranes, which has several causes. Although delivery after PROM may be required by the presence of advanced labor, intrauterine infection, vaginal bleeding due to placental abruption, or non-reassuring fetal status, the physician often needs to make the decision whether to actively pursue delivery or conservatively manage the pregnancy. Management of PROM hinges on knowledge of gestational age, the neonatal risks related to immediate delivery, and an understanding of the anticipated clinical course and relative risks of intrauterine infection, abruptio placentae, and fetal distress or death from umbilical cord accident or intrauterine infection with conservative management.

Physiology and Pathophysiology of Membrane Rupture

The fetal membranes consist of the amnion, which lines the amniotic cavity, and the thicker chorion, which adheres to the maternal decidua. Initially, the amnion and chorion are separate layers. The amnionic sac is visible on first trimester ultrasound scans until it fuses with the chorion by the end of the 14th week of gestation. Subsequently, the amnion and chorion are connected by a collagen-rich connective tissue layer, with the amnion represented by a single cuboidal epithelial amnion layer and subjacent compact and spongy connective tissue layers, and a thicker chorion consisting of reticular and trophoblastic layers. Together, the amnion and chorion form a stronger unit than either layer individually. Physiologic membrane remodeling occurs with advancing gestational age, reflecting changes in collagen content and type, changes in intercellular matrix, and progressive cellular apoptosis. These changes lead to structural weakening of the membranes, which is more evident in the region of the internal cervical os.[1-8]

Membrane weakening can be stimulated by exposure to local matrix metalloproteinases (e.g., MMP-1, MMP-2, MMP-9), decreased levels of membrane tissue inhibitors of matrix metalloproteinases (e.g., TIMP-1, TIMP-3), and increased poly[ADP-ribose]polymerase (PARP) cleavage.[6,9] Term or preterm uterine contractions can also lead to membrane rupture resulting from increased bursting pressure due to increased intra-amniotic pressure and from "strain hardening" with repeated uterine contractions. If the fetal membranes do not rupture before labor, the work to cause membrane rupture at the internal cervical os decreases with advancing cervical dilatation because of the lack of anchoring to the supportive decidua and enhanced ability to stretch with contractions.[1]

Preterm membrane rupture can arise through a number of pathways that ultimately result in accelerated membrane weakening. Bacterial collagenases and proteases can directly cause fetal membrane tissue weakening.[10] An increase in local host cytokines or an imbalance in the interaction between MMPs and TIMPs in response to microbial colonization can have similar effects.[11] There is specific evidence linking urogenital tract infection and colonization with preterm PROM. Amniotic fluid cultures after PROM are frequently positive (25% to 35%),[12-19] and histologic evaluation in the setting of preterm birth frequently has demonstrated acute inflammation and bacterial contamination along the choriodecidual interface.[20] Although these findings may reflect ascending infection after PROM, it is likely that ascending colonization and infection are directly involved in the pathogenesis of preterm PROM in many cases. Genital tract pathogens that have been associated with PROM include *Neisseria gonorrhoeae, Chlamydia trachomatis, Trichomonas vaginalis,* and group B β-hemolytic streptococcus.[20-26] Although group B streptococcus (GBS) bacteriuria has been associated with preterm PROM and low-birth-weight infants[27] and an association between cervical colonization and preterm PROM is possible,[28] it does not appear that vaginal GBS carriage is associated with preterm PROM.[29,30] Although there is a well-established association between bacterial vaginosis and preterm birth, including that related to preterm PROM,[31,32] it remains unclear whether bacterial vaginosis merely identifies women with a predisposition to abnormal genital tract colonization and inflammation, facilitates ascent of other bacteria to the upper genital tract, or is directly pathogenic and causative of membrane rupture. Physical effects related to preterm contractions and prolapsing membranes with premature cervical dilatation can predispose the fetal membranes to rupture, as can the increased intrauterine pressure seen with polyhydramnios.[4,33] It is likely that certain connective tissue disorders (e.g., Ehlers-Danlos syndrome) can result in intrinsic weakening of the membranes. Clinical associations with preterm PROM include low socioeconomic status, lean maternal body mass (<19.8 kg/m^2), nutritional deficiencies (e.g., copper, ascorbic acid), and prior cervical conization. During pregnancy, maternal cigarette smoking, cervical cerclage, second- and third-trimester bleeding, pulmonary disease, prior episodes of preterm labor or contractions, and uterine overdistention with polyhydramnios or multiple gestations have been linked to preterm PROM.[4,33-45]

Although one or more risk factors may lead to membrane rupture, the ultimate clinical cause of PROM is often not evident at delivery. In some cases, factors leading to membrane rupture are subacute or chronic in nature. Women with a prior preterm birth have increased risk for preterm birth due to PROM in subsequent pregnancies, especially if the prior preterm delivery resulted from PROM.[46] Asymptomatic women with a short cervical length (<25 mm) remote from delivery are also at increased risk for subsequent preterm birth due to preterm labor or PROM. Some women may have polymorphisms for inflammatory proteins that alter their inflammatory response and increase the risk for preterm birth.[47,48]

Prediction and Prevention

Because PROM at term usually is part of the normal parturition process, the focus of efforts has been on the prediction and prevention of preterm birth caused by PROM. Prevention of preterm PROM would be particularly appealing because labor and intrauterine infection or other complications necessitating delivery often ensue soon after membrane rupture occurs. The optimal way to prevent complications from preterm PROM is to prevent its occurrence. Potentially modifiable risk factors for preterm PROM include cigarette smoking, poor nutrition, urinary tract and sexually transmitted infections, acute pulmonary diseases, and severe polyhydramnios.

Other than treatment of infections, it is unknown whether correction of these factors can avert this complication. Although most other risk factors are fixed in that they cannot be removed or remedied in a particular woman, knowledge of risk can help to counsel women about suspicious symptoms and the importance of timely evaluation if preterm PROM occurs. Broad-based preventive strategies such as progesterone supplementation can be considered for those at risk due to less specific risk factors such as a history of spontaneous preterm birth[49,50] (see Chapter 29). Although one study suggested that vitamin C supplementation had value in preventing preterm PROM (7.6% versus 24.5%; $P = .02$), studies in which vitamin C was given alone or with other supplements to women without prior preterm birth as a risk factor indicate a trend toward *increased* preterm birth with such treatments (relative risk [RR] = 1.38; 95% confidence interval [CI], 1.04 to 1.82).[51,52] Vitamin C supplementation to prevent preterm birth due to PROM thus cannot be recommended until there is solid evidence of benefit.

Perhaps the strongest risk factor for preterm PROM is a history of prematurity or PROM.[53] Those with an early preterm birth have the highest risk for a recurrence. A history of preterm birth after PROM confers a 3.3-fold increased risk for recurrent preterm birth due to the same cause (13.5% versus 4.1%; $P < .01$) and a 13.5-fold higher risk of subsequent delivery before 28 weeks (1.8% versus 0.13%; $P < .01$). Because prior obstetric outcome has such a strong influence on subsequent pregnancy outcomes, it is useful to evaluate nulliparas separately from those with prior deliveries. When assessed at 22 to 24 weeks' gestation, medical complications (e.g., pulmonary disease in pregnancy), work during pregnancy, low maternal body mass index (<19.8 kg/m^2), and bacterial vaginosis are associated with preterm birth due to PROM.[46] Identification of a cervical length shorter than 25 mm on transvaginal ultrasound also confers an increased risk of subsequent PROM in nulliparas and multiparas. In this study, nulliparas with a short cervix and a positive cervicovaginal fibronectin screening result at 22 to 24 weeks had a one-in-six chance (16.7%) of delivering a preterm infant because of PROM, and the combination of a prior preterm birth due to PROM, a short cervical length, and a positive fetal fibronectin screening result increased the risk of delivery at less than 35 weeks because of preterm PROM by 10.9-fold (25% versus 2.3%).[46]

Unfortunately, despite knowledge of a broad range of potential risk factors for preterm birth, we are able to predict only a small fraction of women destined to deliver preterm, and most preterm births due to preterm labor or PROM occur in women considered to be at low risk for these events. Ancillary tests such as fetal fibronectin screening or transvaginal cervical sonography should be incorporated into routine practice only after effective interventions to prevent PROM have been identified for those with an abnormal test result. Because most cases of preterm PROM cannot be predicted or prevented, clinical efforts continue to be focused on evaluation and treatment of women who present with symptoms of preterm PROM.

Clinical Course

PROM affects approximately 8% of pregnancies at term, and 95% of these women will deliver within 28 hours of membrane rupture.[54] Preterm PROM is also associated with brief latency from membrane rupture to delivery; delivery within 1 week is the most common outcome after preterm PROM at any gestational age. On average, latency increases with decreasing gestational age at membrane rupture. When PROM occurs before 34 weeks' gestation, 93% of women will deliver within 1 week, and 50% to 60% of those who are managed conservatively will deliver within 1 week.[55,56] With PROM near the limit of viability, 60% to 70% deliver within 1 week, but 1 in 5 will have a latency of 4 or more weeks if they are managed conservatively.[35] Although the likelihood of spontaneous resealing of the membranes after preterm PROM is low (3% to 13%), the prognosis for those with PROM occurring after amniocentesis is much better, with 86% to 94% resealing spontaneously.[44,57,58] In a study of women with PROM after second-trimester amniocentesis, leakage stopped in most cases with conservative management, although a normal fluid volume sometimes took time to re accumulate (in a range of 8 to 51 days).[58]

Complications after Premature Rupture of the Membranes

Maternal Complications

Chorioamnionitis complicates 9% of pregnancies with term PROM, a risk that increases to 24% with membrane rupture lasting longer than 24 hours.[59] The risk of intrauterine infection increases with the duration of membrane rupture and with declining gestational age.[54,55,60-62] Conservative management of PROM provides the opportunity for subclinical deciduitis to progress to overt infection and for ascending infection to occur.[20,54,55,62] Chorioamnionitis can complicate 13% to 60% of cases when PROM occurs remote from term. Endometritis occurs in 2% to 13% of cases.[63,64] Placental abruption is diagnosed in 4% to 12% of pregnancies complicated by PROM and can occur before or after the onset of membrane rupture.[34,65,66] Maternal sepsis (0.8%) leading to death (0.14%) is a uncommon complication of preterm PROM occurring near the limit of viability.[67]

Fetal Complications

The risks to the fetus are primarily those related to intrauterine infection, umbilical cord compression, and placental abruption. Fetal heart rate patterns consistent with umbilical cord compression due to oligohydramnios are commonly seen after PROM.[68] Umbilical cord prolapse can occur after membrane rupture, particularly with fetal malpresentation, which is more common with preterm gestations. Fetal death occurs in 1% to 2% of cases of conservatively managed PROM.[56] The reported incidence of fetal death after PROM at 16 to 28 weeks ranges from 3.8% to 22%.[36,69,70] This particularly high risk of fetal loss may reflect increased susceptibility to umbilical cord compression and hypoxia or intrauterine infection, but it may also reflect less aggressive obstetric interventions for fetal compromise before the limit of viability.

Neonatal Complications

Gestational age at delivery is the primary determinant of the frequency and severity of neonatal complications after PROM. Respiratory distress syndrome, necrotizing enterocolitis, intraventricular hemorrhage, and sepsis are the most common serious acute morbidities, and they are common with early preterm birth. Neonatal sepsis is twofold more common after preterm PROM than after preterm birth due to preterm labor. Neonatal infection can manifest as congenital pneumonia, sepsis, meningitis, and late-onset bacterial or fungal infection. Early preterm birth can lead to long-term complications, including chronic lung disease, visual or hearing difficulties, mental retardation, developmental and motor delay, and cerebral palsy. In general, these long-term morbidities are uncommon with delivery after about 32 weeks' gestation.[71,72] Cerebral palsy and periventricular leukomalacia have been associated with amnionitis,[73] and increased amniotic fluid cytokines and fetal systemic inflammation have been associated with preterm PROM, periventricular leukomalacia, and cerebral palsy.[74-76] This highlights the need for potential neonatal benefit from delayed delivery if conservative management is to be attempted because this delay offers the opportunity for intrauterine infection to develop. Alternatively, early gestational age at birth has been associated with neonatal white matter damage ($P < .001$) after controlling for other factors.[77] Despite the described associations between PROM, intrauterine infection or inflammation, and adverse neurologic outcomes, it has not been shown that immediate delivery after PROM can prevent these morbidities.

In the past, mid-trimester PROM, which encompasses membrane rupture occurring at about 16 to 26 weeks' gestation, was considered as a separate entity from preterm PROM because neonatal death usually could be anticipated with immediate delivery. With current survival rates of about 25% to 85% after delivery at 23 to 26 weeks' gestation, mid-trimester PROM is no longer a relevant clinical entity.[71,72,78-80] Previable PROM occurring before the limit of viability (i.e., before 23 weeks' gestation) is a special circumstance that places the fetus in particular jeopardy. Immediate delivery will result in neonatal death. Conservative management may result in fetal or neonatal loss before viability, and if viability is reached, delivery is likely at an early gestational age, when the risks of long-term sequelae are highest. The neonatal survival rate after PROM occurring before 24 weeks has previously been reported to be approximately 30%, compared with 57% for rupture at 24 to 26 weeks' gestation.[67] In a review of 201 cases from 11 studies, the perinatal survival rate with conservative management of PROM before 23 weeks' gestation was 21%, but there was similar survival after PROM at less than 20 weeks.[81] These reported outcomes of previable PROM may be optimistic because most studies have been retrospective and have included only patients amenable to conservative management.

Fetal lung growth and development can be especially adversely affected when PROM occurs in the early phases of development.[82-87] With PROM occurring during the late pseudoglandular or canalicular stage of pulmonary development, tracheobronchial collapse or loss of intrinsic factors within the tracheobronchial fluid, or both, may lead to failure of the terminal bronchioles and alveoli to develop, with resultant failure of lung growth.[88-91] Pulmonary hypoplasia develops over weeks after membrane rupture occurs. It is most accurately diagnosed pathologically based on radial alveolar counts and lung weights.[92,93] In surviving infants, pulmonary hypoplasia is suggested by a small chest circumference with severe respiratory distress or persistent pulmonary hypertension and radiographic findings such as small, well-aerated lungs with a bell-shaped chest and elevation of the diaphragm.[83,88]

Overall, pulmonary hypoplasia becomes evident in 0% to 26.5% of infants (mean = 5.9%) delivering after PROM at 16 to 26 weeks' gestation. Early PROM before 20 weeks' gestation carries the highest potential for lethal pulmonary hypoplasia (≈50% with PROM before 19 weeks' gestation).[83,86-88,94-96] With PROM at 15 to 16 weeks, an amniotic fluid index of 2 cm or less, and a latency of 28 days, the risk of pulmonary hypoplasia is estimated to be 74% to 82%.[97] Lethal pulmonary hypoplasia is uncommon with PROM after 24 to 26 weeks' gestation (0% to 1.4%) because there has been adequate alveolar development to support extrauterine life by this time.[83,84,98] However, nonlethal pulmonary hypoplasia increases the likelihood of pulmonary barotrauma, including pneumothorax, pneumomediastinum, and the need for high ventilatory pressures because of poor pulmonary compliance.[83,98,99] With prolonged oligohydramnios, restriction deformities can occur in up to 27% of fetuses.[67,83,98-101]

Diagnosis

In more than 90% of cases, the diagnosis of PROM can be confirmed by clinical assessment, including the combination of history, clinical examination, and laboratory evaluation. Because optimal clinical care requires an accurate diagnosis, attention should be paid to confirming the diagnosis when a suspicious history or ultrasound finding of oligohydramnios is identified. Other potentially confounding findings such as urine leakage, increased vaginal discharge with cervical dilatation or membrane prolapse, cervical infection, passage of the mucous plug, and the presence of semen or vaginal douching should be considered.

A sterile speculum examination should be performed to provide confirmatory evidence of membrane rupture and to inspect for cervicitis and for umbilical cord or fetal prolapse, to assess cervical dilatation and effacement, and to obtain cultures, including endocervical *Neisseria gonorrhoeae* and *Chlamydia trachomatis*, and anovaginal *Streptococcus agalactiae* (i.e., GBS), as appropriate. Initially, digital cervical examination should be avoided unless imminent delivery is anticipated because the needed information usually can be obtained with visualization of the cervix. Digital examination can shorten latency between membrane rupture and delivery, and some studies have shown it to introduce vaginal organisms into the cervical canal and to increase the risk of infection.[102-107]

The diagnosis of membrane rupture is confirmed by visualization of fluid passing from the cervical canal. If the diagnosis is not confirmed on initial inspection, the pH of the vaginal side walls or pooled vaginal fluid can be evaluated using Nitrazine paper, which turns blue at a pH above 6.0 to 6.5. Amniotic fluid usually has a pH of 7.1 to 7.3, whereas normal vaginal secretions have a pH of about 4.5 to 6.0. Blood or semen contamination, alkaline antiseptics, and bacterial vaginosis can cause false-positive Nitrazine test results. If further clarification is needed, microscopic inspection can be performed for the presence of arborized crystals (i.e., ferning) (Fig. 31-1) in an air-dried sample collected from the vaginal side walls or pooled vaginal fluid. Ferning results from the interaction of amniotic fluid proteins and salts. Cervical mucus should be avoided during sampling because it can also yield a ferning pattern on microscopy. The fern test is unaffected by meconium and vaginal pH, but it can be falsely positive if there is heavy blood contamination.[108,109] Prolonged leakage with minimal residual fluid can lead to false-negative clinical, Nitrazine, and ferning test results. Re-examination after prolonged recumbency or alternate measures can be considered if initial testing is negative. Assessment of cervicovaginal secretions for fetal fibronectin, prolactin, human chorionic gonadotropin (hCG), and other markers may assist in the diagnosis of PROM. However, these tests usually are not more helpful than the initial measures listed previously, because a positive test result may reflect decidual disruption rather than membrane rupture in some cases and a negative test result cannot exclude the diagnosis unequivocally.

If the diagnosis remains unclear after initial evaluation, documentation of oligohydramnios by ultrasound, in the absence of fetal urinary tract malformations or significant growth restriction, is suggestive of membrane rupture. Ultrasonographically guided amniocentesis with infusion of indigo carmine dye (1 mL of dye in 9 mL of sterile normal saline), followed by observation for passage of blue fluid from the vagina onto a perineal pad, can confirm or disprove the diagnosis of membrane rupture. Amniocentesis in the setting of oligohydramnios can be difficult, and particular attention should be paid to avoidance of the umbilical cord vessels, which can have the appearance of a thin, linear fluid space under this circumstance.

Some women with a history suspicious for membrane rupture but a negative speculum examination result and a normal amniotic fluid volume on ultrasound subsequently return with gross membrane rupture. This pattern may reflect initial transudation of a small amount of fluid across a weakened membrane or minimal leakage around a firmly applied presenting fetal part. Women with a suspicious history and initially negative testing should be encouraged to return for reevaluation if symptoms are persistent or recurrent.

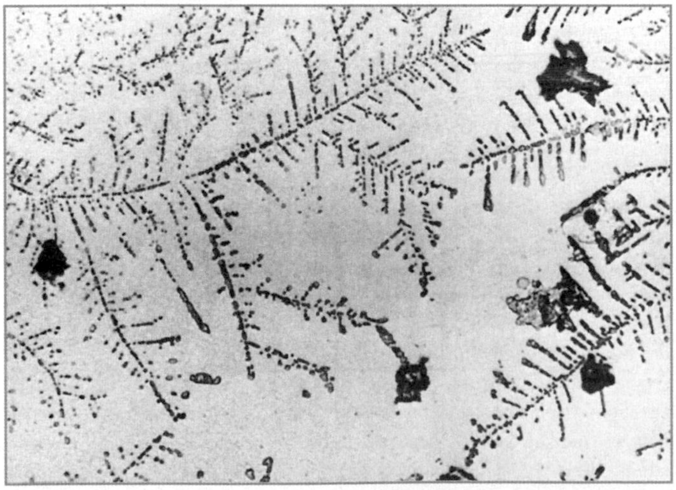

FIGURE 31-1 Ferning. A typical ferning appearance is seen after a swab from the posterior vaginal fornix was smeared on glass slide and the specimen allowed to air dry. The sample was obtained from a patient with premature rupture of the membranes. (Image courtesy of Thomas Garite, University of California at Irvine, Orange, California.)

Management of Premature Rupture of the Membranes

Management of PROM is based primarily on the estimated risks for fetal and neonatal complications with immediate delivery weighed against the potential risks and benefits of conservative management to extend the pregnancy after membrane rupture (Fig. 31-2). The risks of maternal morbidity should also be considered, especially under the circumstance of previable PROM.

Initial Evaluation

After the diagnosis of membrane rupture is confirmed, the duration of membrane rupture should be estimated to assist the pediatric caregivers with subsequent management decisions. Gestational age is established based on the combination of menstrual dates, clinical history, and ultrasound findings, as appropriate. Fetal presentation is assessed, and the patient is evaluated for labor, clinical findings of intrauterine infection, and significant vaginal bleeding. Fetal well-being is assessed by continuous heart rate monitoring if the limit of viability has been reached. After preterm PROM, it is important to evaluate fetal growth and residual amniotic fluid volume by ultrasound, and the potential of fetal abnormalities that can lead to polyhydramnios should be considered. Although narrowing of the biparietal diameter (i.e., dolichocephaly) due to oligohydramnios or breech presentation can result in underestimation of gestational age and fetal weight, ultrasound usually is as reliable after PROM as it is with intact membranes.[110] Tables using fetal head circumference rather than biparietal diameter can be consulted as needed. GBS carrier status should be ascertained if available from culture results within 6 weeks or there has been a positive urine culture in the current pregnancy, and the need for intrapartum prophylaxis should be determined. In the absence of available culture results, a risk factor–based approach should be used for prevention of vertical transmission.[111]

If conservative management is planned, the patient should be cared for in a facility with the ability to provide emergent delivery for placental abruption, fetal malpresentation, or fetal distress. The facility should also have neonatal intensive care facilities and offer acute neonatal resuscitation, because conservative management usually is undertaken only if there is a significant risk of neonatal morbidity and mortality with immediate delivery. Prenatal maternal transfer should be undertaken early in the course of management if these resources are not available. Because of the potential for acute complications, outpatient management usually is not recommended when PROM occurs after the limit of viability.

Term Premature Rupture of the Membranes

There is no substantial fetal benefit to expectant management of pregnancy after membrane rupture at 37 weeks' gestation or later. Expectant management of PROM at term was practiced in the 1980s and early 1990s based on studies suggesting that immediate induction after term PROM might increase the risks of infection and cesarean delivery.[112-115]

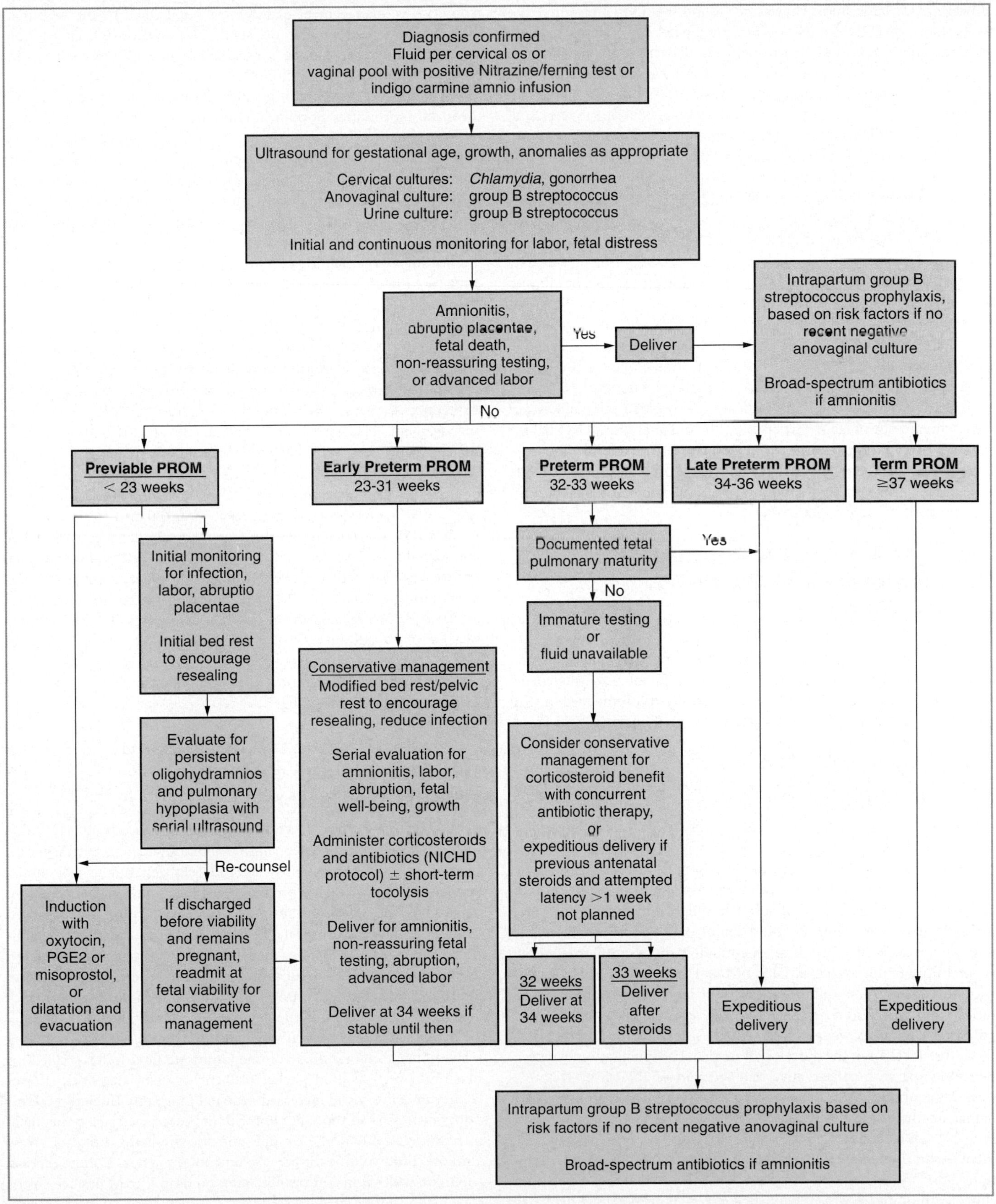

FIGURE 31-2 Algorithm for management of premature rupture of the membranes (PROM). The algorithm includes several alternatives for the approach to term and preterm PROM. NICHD, National Institute of Child Health and Human Development; PGE2, prostaglandin E_2. (Adapted from Mercer BM: Preterm premature rupture of the membranes. Obstet Gynecol 101:178-193, 2003.)

However, four large studies have since found that induction with oxytocin after term PROM does not increase the risks of maternal or neonatal infections, nor does it make cesarean delivery more likely.[54,116-118] In the largest study, oxytocin induction after term PROM reduced the duration of membrane rupture (17.2 versus 33.3 hours; $P < .001$) and the frequencies of chorioamnionitis (4.0% versus 8.6%; $P < .001$) and postpartum febrile morbidity (1.9% versus 3.6%; $P = .008$), without increasing the risk of cesarean delivery (13.7% versus 14.1%) or neonatal infections (2.0% versus 2.8%).[54] Neonatal antibiotic therapy was less common with immediate induction (7.5% versus 13.7%; $P < .001$), likely because of a lower concern regarding the potential for neonatal infection with less frequent prolonged rupture of the membranes and less chorioamnionitis. Meta-analysis of studies comparing prostaglandin induction and conservative management in this setting has found shorter latency, decreased rates of chorioamnionitis, and less frequent neonatal intensive care unit (NICU) admissions with no increase in cesarean delivery rates with prostaglandin administration.[119] Because oxytocin can more easily be discontinued, this choice is somewhat more appealing, given similar efficacy for labor induction.

In summary, available data indicate that women with PROM at term who are not in labor on arrival at the hospital should have labor induced, usually with an oxytocin infusion, to reduce the risk of maternal and neonatal complications. Caregivers should allow an adequate time for the latent phase of labor and minimize digital vaginal examinations until the active phase of labor.

Preterm Premature Rupture of the Membranes at 32 to 36 Weeks' Gestation

Although infants born at 34 to 36 weeks' gestation (i.e., late preterm birth) have a higher risk of complications than term infants, severe acute morbidities and mortality are uncommon, and antenatal corticosteroids for fetal maturation are not typically recommended in this gestational age range.[71,120] Conservative management of PROM at 34 to 36 weeks prolongs pregnancy by only days, significantly increases the risk of chorioamnionitis (16% versus 2%; $P = .001$), and reduces umbilical cord pH (7.35 versus 7.25; $P = .009$), and it has not been shown to improve neonatal outcomes.[121,122] For these reasons, women presenting with late preterm PROM at 34 to 36 weeks should be actively delivered.

With delivery at 32 to 33 weeks' gestation, gestational age–dependent neonatal morbidities, including respiratory distress syndrome, can occur, but the likelihood of survival is high, and chronic morbidities are uncommon. Amniotic fluid can be collected from the vaginal pool at initial sterile speculum examination or by amniocentesis if vaginal fluid is not available. Each of the TDx/TdXFLx FLM II assay (Abbott Laboratories, Abbott Park, IL), the lecithin-to-sphingomyelin ratio (L/S ratio), and the phosphatidylglycerol (PG) test can predict pulmonary maturity when performed on vaginal pool specimens.[123-128] Modest reductions in the duration of neonatal hospital stay and hyperbilirubinemia with conservative management of PROM at 32 to 33 weeks' gestation have been reported.[122] Alternatively, conservative management prolonged pregnancy only briefly (36 versus 14 hours; $P < .001$) in a randomized, controlled trial of conservative management versus immediate induction after PROM at 32 to 36 weeks' gestation. This limited benefit was offset by a 2.5-fold increased risk of chorioamnionitis (27.7% versus 10.9%; $P = .06$), increased neonatal sepsis workups (59.6% versus 28.3%; $P = .003$) and increased neonatal antibiotic treatment for suspected infection (78.7% versus 34.8%; $P < .001$).[129] The potential for occult umbilical cord compression during conservative management of PROM is highlighted by the high incidence of recurrent variable decelerations found during intermittent monitoring (19.4%) among conservatively managed women. In this study, documented fetal pulmonary maturity was a requirement for enrollment, and neither group suffered any significant noninfectious neonatal morbidities. Specific attention to those enrolled at 32 to 33 weeks' gestation revealed similar trends regarding brief latency, increased amnionitis, suspected neonatal sepsis, and antibiotic treatment with conservative management.[130] Based on these findings, the woman with PROM and documented fetal pulmonary maturity at 32 to 33 weeks' gestation is at low risk for complications after immediate delivery and increased risk with conservative management. Amniotic fluid studies documenting pulmonary maturity in this gestational age range are useful to identify women who should be offered expeditious delivery.

If fetal pulmonary testing reveals an immature result or if amniotic fluid cannot be obtained for assessment, conservative management with antenatal corticosteroid administration for fetal maturation is an appropriate choice. Concurrent antibiotic treatment should be given to reduce the risk of intrauterine infection during conservative management (discussed later). There are no data regarding optimal management after antenatal corticosteroid treatment is completed. However, because conservative management increases the risks of chorioamnionitis and prolonged hospitalization and because it is unlikely that conservative management for less than 1 week will result in further significant spontaneous fetal maturation, delivery should be considered if elective delivery is planned within 7 days after antenatal corticosteroid benefit has been achieved. If antenatal corticosteroids are not to be given to accelerate fetal pulmonary maturity after PROM at 32 to 33 weeks, consideration should be given to the potential benefits of expeditious delivery unless conservative management to extend latency for 1 or more weeks will be attempted. These decisions should take into consideration local population-based risks of infection and neonatal morbidities.

Preterm Premature Rupture of the Membranes at 23 to 31 Weeks' Gestation

Because delivery before 32 weeks' gestation is associated with a high risk for perinatal death, severe neonatal morbidities, and long-term sequelae, women with PROM between 23 and 31 weeks' gestation usually should be managed expectantly to prolong pregnancy unless there is evidence of intrauterine infection, suspected placental abruption, advanced labor, or a non-reassuring fetal heart rate pattern. Under certain additional circumstances, delivery may be appropriate despite an early gestational age at membrane rupture (e.g., fetal transverse lie and back up with coexisting advanced cervical dilatation, human immunodeficiency virus infection, primary herpes simplex virus infection).

In women with conservatively managed PROM remote from term, a low initial amniotic fluid volume (amniotic fluid index <5.0 cm or maximum vertical fluid pocket <2.0 cm) is associated with shorter latency to delivery and increased neonatal morbidity (including respiratory distress syndrome) but not with increased maternal or neonatal infection after PROM.[131] Despite this, the predictive value of a low amniotic fluid volume for adverse outcomes is poor. A short cervical length on endovaginal ultrasound after preterm PROM has been associated with shorter latency to delivery.[132-134] The latest study of cervical length in women with preterm PROM found that 83% of women delivered within 7 days if the initial cervical length was 1 to 10 mm, compared with 18% for a cervical length more than 30 mm, but only

41 women were evaluated.[132] However, currently available studies of initial amniotic fluid volume and cervical length assessment in women with preterm PROM have insufficient power and consistency to guide management.

Conservative management includes initial prolonged continuous fetal heart rate and maternal contraction monitoring to assess fetal well-being and identify occult contractions and evidence of umbilical cord compression. If initial testing results are reassuring, the patient can be transferred to an inpatient unit or transferred to a facility capable of emergent delivery and acute neonatal resuscitation for modified bed rest. Because of the high risk of heart rate abnormalities due to umbilical cord compression (32% to 76%), fetal assessment should be performed at least daily for those with initially reassuring test results.[68,135] Continuous monitoring may be appropriate for women with intermittent fetal heart rate decelerations but otherwise reassuring findings. Although the nonstress test and biophysical profile have the ability to confirm fetal well-being in the setting of preterm PROM, fetal heart rate monitoring can identify variable and late decelerations in addition to uterine activity. Biophysical profile testing may also be confounded by the presence of oligohydramnios but can be helpful if the nonstress test is equivocal, particularly remote from term when the fetal heart rate pattern is less likely to be reactive. A nonreactive result for a nonstress test and a biophysical profile score of 6 or less within 24 hours of delivery have been associated with perinatal infection.[136,137] A nonreactive nonstress test subsequent to an initially reactive result should be considered suspicious.

Conservative management requires surveillance for the development of labor, abruptio placentae, and intrauterine infection. Chorioamnionitis confers increased risks of perinatal mortality and intraventricular hemorrhage, and it is diagnosed clinically by the presence of maternal fever above 38.0 °C (100.4 °F) with uterine tenderness or with maternal or fetal tachycardia in the absence of another evident source of infection.[63] After the diagnosis of chorioamnionitis is made, delivery should be pursued and broad-spectrum antibiotics should be initiated because treatment before delivery has been shown to decrease the incidence of neonatal sepsis.[138-140] Although evaluation of the maternal white blood cell count can be helpful if clinical findings are equivocal, the counts can be artificially elevated within 5 to 7 days of antenatal corticosteroid administration. If the diagnosis of chorioamnionitis is suspected but additional confirmation is needed, amniocentesis may yield helpful results.[15,141,142] A glucose concentration below 16 to 20 mg/dL (sensitivity and specificity of 80% to 90% for a positive culture) and a Gram stain positive for bacteria (sensitivity of 36% to 80% and specificity of 80% to 97% for a positive culture) support the presence of intrauterine infection. The presence of leukocytes alone in amniotic fluid after PROM is not well correlated with intrauterine infection. Although a positive amniotic fluid culture supports clinical suspicion of chorioamnionitis (sensitivity of 65% to 85% and specificity of 85%), these results are not likely to be available before the diagnosis is clarified.[17] One study suggested that determination of glucose levels from vaginally collected amniotic fluid may be a simple and noninvasive method for identification of intra-amniotic infection.[143] In this promising study, a vaginal pool glucose value below 5 mg/dL had a 74.2% accuracy rate for identifying women with a positive amniotic fluid culture. Although research has found elevated amniotic fluid interleukin levels to be associated with early delivery and perinatal infectious morbidity,[141] such testing is not available in most clinical laboratories.

Antenatal Corticosteroids

Respiratory distress syndrome is the most common acute morbidity after conservatively managed preterm PROM.[144] Antenatal corticosteroid administration after preterm PROM has been extensively studied, generating several meta-analyses.[145-147] Although early reviews produced conflicting conclusions about the utility of antenatal corticosteroid treatment after PROM, a later meta-analysis concluded that antenatal glucocorticoids significantly reduce the risks of respiratory distress syndrome (20% versus 35.4%), intraventricular hemorrhage (7.5% versus 15.9%), and necrotizing enterocolitis (0.8% versus 4.6%), without increasing the risks of maternal (9.2% versus 5.1%) or neonatal (7.0% versus 6.6%) infections in women with preterm PROM.[147] Multivariate analysis of prospective observational trials suggested a benefit of antenatal corticosteroid use regardless of membrane rupture.[148] Three studies in which prophylactic antibiotics were given concurrent to antenatal corticosteroids found treatment to reduce respiratory distress syndrome (18.4% versus 43.6%; $P = .03$) perinatal mortality (1.3% versus 8.3%; $P = .05$), and composite morbidities (29.3% versus 48.6%; $P < .05$), with no increase in perinatal infections.[149-151]

The National Institutes of Health Consensus Development Panel recommended a single course of antenatal corticosteroids for women with PROM before 30 to 32 weeks' gestation in the absence of intra-amniotic infection.[152] Data regarding repeated weekly courses of antenatal corticosteroids after preterm PROM are conflicting. In a retrospective study that controlled for gestational age and other factors, two or more courses of antenatal corticosteroids were associated with increased early neonatal sepsis (15.3% versus 2% for a single course or 1.5% for no courses; $P < .001$).[153] In another retrospective analysis of repeated antenatal corticosteroids, there was no reduction in respiratory distress syndrome, but intraventricular hemorrhage and amnionitis were less common, and there was a trend toward less sepsis.[154] Respiratory distress syndrome was less common in another retrospective review of repeated courses of antenatal corticosteroids (34.9% versus 45.2%) without an increase in neonatal sepsis (9.9% versus 6.2%).[155]

Based on current evidence that antenatal corticosteroids are effective for induction of fetal pulmonary maturity without increasing the risk of infection and that most women will remain pregnant for the 24 to 48 hours needed to achieve corticosteroid benefit after PROM, a single course of antenatal corticosteroids should be considered when PROM occurs before 32 weeks' gestation and for women with documented pulmonary immaturity at 32 to 33 weeks' gestation. Betamethasone (two doses of 12 mg IM, given 24 hours apart) or dexamethasone (four doses of 6 mg IM, given 12 hours apart) is considered appropriate. Repeated weekly antenatal corticosteroids are not recommended after preterm PROM. The benefits and risks of a single rescue course remote from initial corticosteroid administration remain to be determined.

Adjunctive Antibiotics

Antibiotic therapy is given during conservative management of preterm PROM to treat or prevent ascending decidual infection to prolong pregnancy and to reduce gestational age–dependent morbidity while limiting the risk of neonatal infection. More than two dozen randomized clinical trials have been summarized in several meta-analyses.[56,156,157] In the latest one, antibiotic treatment after preterm PROM significantly reduced chorioamnionitis (relative risk [RR] = 0.57); delivery within 48 hours (RR = 0.71) and within 7 days (RR = 0.80); and reduced infant morbidities, including neonatal infection (RR = 0.68); and major cerebral abnormalities on ultrasound before discharge (RR = 0.82) compared with placebo therapy.[157] The need for surfactant administration (RR = 0.83) and oxygen therapy (RR = 0.88) was also reduced. Antibiotics did not influence the risk of necrotizing enterocolitis (RR = 1.14; CI, 0.66 to 1.97). Oral amoxicillin-clavulanic acid treatment was associated with increased necrotizing enterocolitis (RR = 4.60; 95% CI, 1.98 to 10.72) in this analysis, but oral erythromycin therapy was not (RR = 1.00; CI, 0.56 to 1.80).[157] The study that dominated this meta-analysis included women with PROM up to 36 weeks' gestation and included a population at low risk for necrotizing enterocolitis overall (i.e., 0.5% among controls), and it was the only one of 10 studies that found a significant increase in necrotizing enterocolitis with antibiotic therapy.[158] The meta-analysis found treatment with "all penicillins" (excluding amoxicillin-clavulanic acid) versus placebo to be associated with fewer births within 48 hours and 7 days of PROM, less overall maternal infection and chorioamnionitis, less neonatal infection, fewer positive neonatal blood cultures, and fewer major intracranial cerebral ultrasound abnormalities. Because of the increased risk of neonatal necrotizing enterocolitis with amoxicillin-clavulanate, the study authors recommended erythromycin as a better choice, even though benefits were limited to reduction in delivery at 48 hours, fewer positive neonatal blood cultures, and a reduced need for oxygen therapy.

In a clinical trial with adequate power to evaluate antibiotic therapy during conservative management of women with preterm PROM before 32 weeks' gestation, the National Institutes of Child Health and Human Development Maternal Fetal Medicine Units (NICHD-MFMU) Research Network assigned women with PROM to initial aggressive intravenous therapy for 48 hours (2 g of ampicillin IV every 6 hours and 250 mg of erythromycin IV every 6 hours) followed by oral therapy for 5 days (250 mg of amoxicillin PO every 8 hours and 333 mg of enteric-coated erythromycin base PO every 8 hours) to provide limited-duration, broad-spectrum antimicrobial coverage before delivery.[144,159] GBS screening was performed. GBS carriers were treated with ampicillin for 1 week and again in labor, and they were analyzed separately. Antibiotic treatment increased the likelihood of continued pregnancy after 7 days of treatment by twofold. Benefit persisted for 3 weeks after randomization despite discontinuation of antibiotics at 7 days. Babies born to women treated with ampicillin plus erythromycin had a reduced incidence of one or more major infant morbidities (53% versus 44% rate of composite morbidity, including death, respiratory distress syndrome, early sepsis, severe intraventricular hemorrhage, and severe necrotizing enterocolitis; $P < .05$). Antibiotic therapy also significantly reduced individual gestational age–dependent morbidities, including respiratory distress syndrome (40.5% versus 48.7%), patent ductus arteriosus (11.7% versus 20.2%), chronic lung disease (bronchopulmonary dysplasia: 20.5% versus 13.0%), and stage 3 or 4 necrotizing enterocolitis (2.3% versus 5.8%), with P values of 0.05 or less for each. Chorioamnionitis was reduced with the study's antibiotics (23% versus 32.5%; $P = .01$), and neonatal sepsis (8.4% versus 15.6%; $P = .009$) and pneumonia (2.9% versus 7.0%; $P = .04$) were reduced for those who were not GBS carriers. The antibiotic study group had less neonatal GBS sepsis (0% versus 1.5%; $P = .03$). Two other studies have attempted to determine whether antibiotic therapy of shorter duration could provide similar benefit, but the studies lacked size and power to demonstrate equivalent effectiveness.[160,161]

In summary, broad-spectrum antibiotic (ampicillin-amoxicillin plus erythromycin) therapy for women with preterm PROM before 32 weeks' gestation prolongs pregnancy sufficiently to reduce neonatal gestational age–dependent morbidities and reduce the frequencies of maternal and neonatal infections.[144] An alternative conclusion from the latest meta-analysis is that penicillins other than amoxicillin-clavulanic acid are an acceptable treatment for preterm PROM and that the benefits of erythromycin are limited to brief pregnancy prolongation, less need for oxygen therapy, and fewer positive neonatal blood cultures.[157] This is not inconsistent with the NICHD-MFMU approach. Up to a 7-day course of parenteral and oral therapy using ampicillin-amoxicillin and erythromycin is recommended for women undergoing conservative management of preterm PROM remote from term. Shortages in intravenous and oral antibiotics have led to the need for alternative antibiotic choices. Oral ampicillin, erythromycin, and azithromycin are likely appropriate alternatives if needed.

Adjunctive antibiotic administration to prolong latency must be distinguished from intrapartum prophylaxis to prevent vertical transmission of GBS from mother to baby.[111] Known GBS carriers and those who deliver before carrier status can be determined should receive intrapartum prophylaxis to prevent vertical transmission, regardless of prior antibiotic treatments. Women with a diagnosis of chorioamnionitis should receive broad-spectrum intrapartum antibiotic therapy.

Tocolysis

Evidence from prospective studies of tocolysis after PROM is similar to that from studies of tocolysis for preterm labor with intact membranes.[162-167] After preterm PROM, prophylactic tocolysis with β-agonists before the onset of contractions can prolong pregnancy briefly. Therapeutic tocolysis administered only after contractions occur has not been shown to be effective in prolonging latency. In a retrospective comparison of aggressive tocolysis with limited treatment for contractions only during the first 48 hours, aggressive therapy was not associated with longer latency (3.8 versus 4.5 days; $P = .16$).[167] A report from the Collaborative Study on Antenatal Steroids suggested tocolytic use after PROM was associated with subsequent neonatal respiratory distress syndrome, but the biologic mechanism for this association is unclear.[168]

Overall, the available prospective studies have not found tocolytic treatment after PROM to increase or prevent neonatal morbidities after PROM. Tocolytic therapy has not been studied when antenatal corticosteroids and antibiotics were administered concurrently, and it remains plausible that prophylactic tocolysis could delay delivery long enough to allow antibiotic suppression of subclinical decidual infection and for corticosteroid effects on the fetus. Pending further study in this area, tocolytic therapy should not be considered an expected practice after preterm PROM, but it may be appropriate in pregnancies at high risk for neonatal complications with early preterm birth.

Cervical Cerclage

Preterm PROM complicates about one fourth of pregnancies with a cervical cerclage and one half of pregnancies requiring an emergent cerclage.[43,169,170] Because no prospective studies have been performed regarding management of preterm PROM with a cerclage in situ, recommendations reflect the data available from retrospective cohorts. The risk of adverse perinatal outcomes does not appear to be different when PROM occurs with a cerclage or without one, provided the cerclage is removed on admission after PROM.[171-172]

Several small studies comparing pregnancies of preterm PROM in which the cerclage was retained or removed have yielded consistent patterns.[173-175] No study has found cerclage retention after PROM to reduce the frequency or severity of infant morbidities after preterm PROM, and each has demonstrated statistically insignificant trends toward increased maternal infectious morbidity with only brief pregnancy prolongation. One study found increased infant mortality and mortality due to sepsis with cerclage retention after PROM.[173] One study that compared different practices at two institutions found longer latencies with cerclage retention, but this finding could reflect population or practice differences at these institutions rather than the effect of cerclage retention.[174]

Because cerclage retention after PROM has not been shown to improve perinatal outcomes and there are potential risks related to leaving the cerclage in situ, removal is recommended when PROM occurs, particularly if the indication for initial cerclage placement was not strong. While deferred removal might enhance pregnancy prolongation for corticosteroid administration, the risks and benefits of this approach have not been determined.

Maternal Herpes Simplex Virus Infection

Neonatal herpes simplex infection most commonly results from direct maternal-fetal transmission at delivery, but hematogenous transmission can occur to the fetus in utero in some cases. Neonatal infection rates after primary and secondary maternal infections occur in 34% to 80% and 1% to 5% of cases, respectively,[176,177] and infection can result in mortality rates of 50% to 60% and serious sequelae in up to 50% of survivors.[178,179]

Based on two case series including a total of 35 women with an active maternal genital herpesvirus infection, it has been generally accepted that increasing latency after membrane rupture of more than 4 to 6 hours increases risk of neonatal infection and that cesarean delivery should be performed expeditiously to prevent fetal infection in this setting.[180-182] However, a case series of women with conservatively managed PROM before 32 weeks' gestation coincident to active recurrent herpes simplex virus lesions suggests that conservative management may be considered.[183] Antenatal corticosteroids and antibiotics were not administered, and antiviral therapy was inconsistent in this series. Cesarean delivery was performed for women with active lesions at the time of delivery. After latencies ranging from 1 to 35 days, none of the 26 infants developed neonatal herpes infection (CI, 0% to 10.4%).

Based on these data, conservative management of PROM complicated by recurrent maternal herpes simplex virus infection may be appropriate if membrane rupture occurs remote from term and the potential for mortality or serious sequelae with delivery is considered to be high. Antiviral therapy (e.g., acyclovir) during conservative management can reduce viral shedding and the frequency of recurrence.

Previable Premature Rupture of the Membranes before 23 Weeks' Gestation

Although the cause is often not apparent, clinical antecedents can be helpful in determining the likely outcomes in some cases of previable PROM. Membrane rupture after amniocentesis is associated with cessation of leakage and subsequent successful pregnancy outcomes in most cases. Alternatively, previable PROM in a pregnancy complicated by persistent second-trimester bleeding, oligohydramnios, or an elevated level of maternal serum α-fetoprotein more likely reflects an abnormality of placentation, which carries a poor prognosis.

The patient with previable PROM and no other indication for immediate delivery should be counseled regarding the risks and benefits of expectant management, including a realistic appraisal of potential fetal and neonatal outcomes according to the available information for gestational age–appropriate outcomes.[71,72,184] In addition to the maternal risks of conservative management previously delineated, muscle wasting, bone demineralization, and deep venous thrombosis can also occur with prolonged bed rest, and there are significant financial and social implications of prolonged hospitalization. Prediction of specific neonatal outcomes after previable PROM is extremely difficult because it is not possible to predict extended latency, the ultimate gestational age at delivery, or the degree of neonatal pulmonary hypoplasia at the time of initial presentation with PROM.

For women who decide that the risks of conservative management exceed the potential benefits, delivery can usually be accomplished with vaginal prostaglandin E_2, oral or vaginal prostaglandin E_1 (i.e., misoprostol), with a high-dose oxytocin infusion, or by dilatation and evacuation. The optimal approach depends on the patient's characteristics (e.g., gestational age, evident amnionitis, prior cesarean delivery) and preference, the available facilities, and the physician's experience with these techniques.

Data to guide the management for women who choose conservative management of previable PROM are lacking. There is no consensus about the advantages of inpatient versus outpatient management. Initial inpatient evaluation may include strict bed and pelvic rest to enhance the opportunity for resealing and for early identification of infection and placental abruption. Women who are discharged should be advised to abstain from intercourse and limit physical activity. They should return immediately in case of fever, abdominal pains, suspicious vaginal discharge, or any vaginal bleeding. Hospitalization for the duration of amniotic fluid leakage may be appropriate in some circumstances. Discharged patients are typically readmitted to hospital after the limit of viability has been reached to allow early intervention for infection, placental abruption, labor, and non-reassuring fetal heart rate patterns. Administration of antenatal corticosteroids for fetal maturation at this time is appropriate.

After an initial ultrasound assessment, repeated evaluation can be performed every 1 to 2 weeks to determine whether there is re-accumulation of amniotic fluid and to evaluate lung growth. Persistent, severe oligohydramnios after PROM before 20 weeks is the strongest predictor of subsequent lethal pulmonary hypoplasia. Serial fetal biometric evaluation (e.g., lung length, chest circumference), ratios to adjust for overall fetal size (thoracic to abdominal circumference, thoracic circumference to femur length) and Doppler studies of fetal pulmonary artery and ductus arteriosus waveform modulation with fetal breathing movements can demonstrate whether fetal pulmonary growth has occurred over time. These results have a high predictive value for neonatal mortality due to pulmonary hypoplasia.[88,96,185-190] If pulmonary hypoplasia becomes evident before the limit of viability or there is persistent, severe oligohydramnios, the patient may choose to reconsider her decision regarding ongoing expectant management.

Treatments to seal the membrane defect or restore normal amniotic fluid volume include transabdominal amnioinfusion and membrane sealing with fibrin, platelet, cryoprecipitate, or gel-foam plugs. These methods are described in a review.[191] The maternal risks and fetal benefits of these interventions have not been adequately evaluated, and there are inadequate data to recommend that any of these approaches be incorporated into routine clinical practice.

Summary

When term or preterm PROM occurs, there is the potential for significant perinatal morbidity and mortality, which can be reduced by considered and timely obstetric interventions. Expeditious delivery of the patient with term and late preterm PROM can reduce the risk of perinatal infections without increasing the likelihood of operative delivery. Conservative management of PROM remote from term can reduce infectious and gestational age–dependent morbidities. Regardless of management approach, infants delivered after early preterm or previable PROM are at high risk for perinatal complications, many of which cannot be avoided with current technologies and management algorithms. Attention to early diagnosis and management of complications that occur after PROM can lead to good perinatal outcomes in many cases.

References

1. Kitzmiller J: Preterm premature rupture of the membranes. In Fuchs F, Stubblefield PG (eds): Preterm Birth Causes, Prevention and Management. New York, Macmillan, 1984, p 298.
2. Lei H, Kalluri R, Furth EE, et al: Amnion type IV collagen composition and metabolism: Implications for membrane breakdown. Biol. Reprod 60:176-182, 1999.
3. Lei H, Furth EE, Kalluri R, et al: A program of cell death and extracellular matrix degradation is activated in the amnion before the onset of labor. J Clin Invest 98:1971-1978, 1997.
4. Skinner SJM, Campos GA, Liggins GC: Collagen content of human amniotic membranes: Effect of gestation length and premature rupture. Obstet Gynecol 57:487-489, 1981.
5. Malak TM, Bell SC: Structural characteristic of term human fetal membranes: A novel zone of extreme morphological alteration within the rupture site. BJOG 101:375-386, 1994.
6. El Khwad M, Stetzer B, Moore RM, et al: Term human fetal membranes have a weak zone overlying the lower uterine pole and cervix before the onset of labor. Biol Reprod 72:720-726, 2005.
7. McLaren J, Taylor DJ, Bell SC: Increased incidence of apoptosis in nonlabor affected cytotrophoblast cells in term fetal membranes overlying the cervix. Hum Reprod 14:2:895-900, 1999.
8. McParland PC, Taylor DJ, Bell SC: Mapping of zones of altered morphology and choriodeciduaic connective tissue cellular phenotype in human fetal membranes (amnion and deciduas) overlying the lower uterine pole and cervix before labor at term. Am J Obstet Gynecol 189:1481-1488, 2003.
9. McLaren J, Taylor DJ, Bell SC: Increased concentration of pro-matrix metalloproteinase 9 in term fetal membranes overlying the cervix before labor: Implications for membrane remodeling and rupture. Am J Obstet Gynecol 182:409-416, 2000.
10. Parry S, Strauss JF: Premature rupture of the fetal membranes. N Engl J Med 338:663-670, 1998.
11. Athayde N, Edwin SS, Romero R, et al: A role for matrix metalloproteinase-9 in spontaneous rupture of the fetal membranes. Am J Obstet Gynecol 179:1248-1253, 1998.
12. Garite TJ, Freeman RK, Linzey EM, Braly P: The use of amniocentesis in patients with premature rupture of membranes. Obstet Gynecol 54:226-230, 1979.
13. Cotton DB, Gonik B, Bottoms SF: Conservative vs. aggressive management of preterm rupture of membranes. A randomized trial of amniocentesis. Am J Perinatol 1:322-324, 1984.
14. Romero R, Quintero R, Oyarzun E, et al: Intraamniotic infection and the onset of labor in preterm premature rupture of the membranes. Am J Obstet Gynecol 159:661-666, 1988.
15. Broekhuizen FF, Gilman M, Hamilton PR: Amniocentesis for Gram stain and culture in preterm premature rupture of the membranes. Obstet Gynecol 66:316-321, 1985.
16. Dudley J, Malcolm G, Ellwood D: Amniocentesis in the management of preterm premature rupture of the membranes. Aust N Z J Obstet Gynaecol 31:331-336, 1991.
17. Gauthier DW, Meyer WJ: Comparison of gram stain, leukocyte esterase activity, and amniotic fluid glucose concentration in predicting amniotic fluid culture results in preterm premature rupture of membranes. Am J Obstet Gynecol 167:1092-1095, 1992.
18. Mercer BM, Moretti ML, Prevost RR, Sibai BM: Erythromycin therapy in preterm premature rupture of the membranes: A prospective, randomized trial of 220 patients. Am J Obstet Gynecol 166:794-802, 1992.
19. Carroll SG, Papaioannou S, Davies ET, Nicolaides KH: Maternal assessment in the prediction of intrauterine infection in preterm prelabor amniorrhexis. Fetal Diagn Ther 10:290-296, 1995.
20. Romero R, Mazor M, Wu YK, et al: Infection in the pathogenesis of preterm labor. Semin Perinatol 12:262-279, 1988.
21. Heddleston L, McDuffie RS Jr, Gibbs RS: A rabbit model for ascending infection in pregnancy: Intervention with indomethacin and delayed ampicillin-sulbactam therapy. Am J Obstet Gynecol 169:708-712, 1993.
22. McDonald HM, O'Loughlin JA, Jolley PT, et al: Changes in vaginal flora during pregnancy and association with preterm birth. J Infect Dis 170:724-728, 1994.
23. Regan JA, Chao S, James LS: Premature rupture of membranes, preterm delivery, and group B streptococcal colonization of mothers. Am J Obstet Gynecol 141:184-186, 1981.
24. Alger LS, Lovchik JC, Hebel JR, et al: The association of *Chlamydia trachomatis, Neisseria gonorrhoeae,* and group B streptococci with preterm rupture of the membranes and pregnancy outcome. Am J Obstet Gynecol 159:397-404, 1988.
25. Ekwo EE, Gosselink CA, Woolson R, Moawad A: Risks for premature rupture of amniotic membranes. Int J Epidemiol 22:495-503, 1993.
26. McGregor JA, French JI, Parker R, et al: Prevention of premature birth by screening and treatment for common genital tract infections: Results of a prospective controlled evaluation. Am J Obstet Gynecol 173:157-167, 1995.
27. Regan JA, Klebanoff MA, Nugent RP, et al: Colonization with group B streptococci in pregnancy and adverse outcome. VIP Study Group. Am J Obstet Gynecol 174:1354-1360, 1996.
28. Matorras R, Garcia Perea A, Omeñaca F, et al: Group B streptococcus and premature rupture of membranes and preterm delivery. Gynecol Obstet Invest 27:14-18, 1989.
29. Romero R, Mazor M, Oyarzun E, et al: Is there an association between colonization with group B Streptococcus and prematurity? J Reprod Med 34:797-801, 1989.
30. Kubota T: Relationship between maternal group B streptococcal colonization and pregnancy outcome. Obstet Gynecol 92:926-930, 1998.
31. Romero R, Chaiworapongsa T, Kuivaniemi H, Tromp G: Bacterial vaginosis, the inflammatory response and the risk of preterm birth: A role for genetic epidemiology in the prevention of preterm birth. Am J Obstet Gynecol 190:1509-1519, 2004.
32. Hillier SL, Nugent RP, Eschenbach DA, et al: Association between bacterial vaginosis and preterm delivery of a low-birth-weight infant. The Vaginal Infections and Prematurity Study Group. N Engl J Med 333:1737-1742, 1995.
33. Lavery JP, Miller CE, Knight RD: The effect of labor on the rheologic response of chorioamniotic membranes. Obstet Gynecol 60:87-92, 1982.
34. Meis PJ, Ernest JM, Moore ML: Causes of low birth-weight births in public and private patients. Am J Obstet Gynecol 156:1165-1168, 1987.
35. Tucker JM, Goldenberg RL, Davis RO, et al: Etiologies of preterm birth in an indigent population: Is prevention a logical expectation? Obstet Gynecol 77:343-347, 1991.
36. Taylor J, Garite T: Premature rupture of the membranes before fetal viability. Obstet Gynecol 64:615-620, 1984.
37. Minkoff H, Grunebaum AN, Schwarz RH, et al: Risk factors for prematurity and premature rupture of membranes: A prospective study of the vaginal flora in pregnancy. Am J Obstet Gynecol 150:965-972, 1984.
38. Naeye R: Factors that predispose to premature rupture of the fetal membranes. Obstet Gynecol 60:93-98, 1982.
39. Maradny EE, Kanayama N, Halim A, et al: Stretching of fetal membranes increases the concentration of interleukin-8 and collagenase activity. Am J Obstet Gynecol 174:843-849, 1996.
40. Ekwo EE, Gosselink CA, Moawad A: Unfavorable outcome in penultimate pregnancy and premature rupture of membranes in successive pregnancy. Obstet Gynecol 80:166-172, 1982.
41. Harger JH, Hsing AW, Tuomala RE, et al: Risk factors for preterm premature rupture of fetal membranes: A multicenter case-control study. Am J Obstet Gynecol 163:130-137, 1990.

42. Naeye RL, Peters EC: Causes and consequences of premature rupture of the fetal membranes. Lancet 1:192-194, 1980.
43. Charles D, Edwards WB: Infectious complications of cervical cerclage. Am J Obstet Gynecol 141:1065-1070, 1981.
44. Gold RB, Goyer GL, Schwartz, et al: Conservative management of second trimester post-amniocentesis fluid leakage. Obstet Gynecol 74:745-747, 1989.
45. Hadley CB, Main DM, Gabbe SG: Risk factors for preterm premature rupture of the fetal membranes. Am J Perinatol 7:374-379, 1990.
46. Mercer BM, Goldenberg RL, Meis PJ, et al, and the National Institutes of Child Health and Human Development Maternal Fetal Medicine Units (NICHD-MFMU) Network: The preterm prediction study: Prediction of preterm premature rupture of the membranes using clinical findings and ancillary testing. Am J Obstet Gynecol 183:738-745, 2000.
47. Roberts AK, Monzon-Bordonaba F, Van Deerlin PG, et al: Association of polymorphism within the promoter of the tumor necrosis factor alpha gene with increased risk of preterm premature rupture of the fetal membranes. Am J Obstet Gynecol 180:1297-1302, 1999.
48. Millar LK, Boesche MH, Yamamoto SY, et al: A relaxin mediated pathway to preterm premature rupture of the fetal membranes that is independent of infection. Am J Obstet Gynecol 179:126-134, 1998.
49. Meis PJ, Klebanoff M, Thom E, et al, for the National Institute of Child Health and Human Development Maternal-Fetal Medicine Units Network: Prevention of recurrent preterm delivery by 17 alpha-hydroxyprogesterone caproate. N Engl J Med 348:2379-2385, 2003.
50. da Fonseca EB, Bittar RE, Carvalho MH, Zugaib M: Prophylactic administration of progesterone by vaginal suppository to reduce the incidence of spontaneous preterm birth in women at increased risk: A randomized placebo-controlled double-blind study. Am J Obstet Gynecol 188:419-424, 2003.
51. Casanueva E, Ripoll C, Tolentino M, et al: Vitamin C supplementation to prevent premature rupture of the chorioamniotic membranes: A randomized trial. Am J Clin Nutr 81:859-863, 2005.
52. Rumbold A, Crowther CA: Vitamin C supplementation in pregnancy. Cochrane Database Syst Rev (1):CD004072, 2005.
53. Mercer BM, Goldenberg RL, Moawad AH, et al: for the National Institutes of Child Health and Human Development Maternal Fetal Medicine Units (NICHD-MFMU) Network: The preterm prediction study: Effect of gestational age and cause of preterm birth on subsequent obstetric outcome. Am J Obstet Gynecol 181:1216-1221, 1999.
54. Hannah ME, Ohlsson A, Farine D, et al: Induction of labor compared with expectant management for prelabor rupture of membranes at term. N Engl J Med 334:1005-1010, 1996.
55. Wagner MV, Chin VP, Peters CJ, et al: A comparison of early and delayed induction of labor with spontaneous rupture of membranes at term. Obstet Gynecol 74:93-97, 1989.
56. Mercer B, Arheart K: Antimicrobial therapy in expectant management of preterm premature rupture of the membranes. Lancet 346:1271-1279, 1995.
57. Johnson JWC, Egerman RS, Moorhead J: Cases with ruptured membranes that "reseal." Am J Obstet Gynecol 163:1024-1032, 1990.
58. Borgida AF, Mills AA, Feldman DM, et al: Outcome of pregnancies complicated by ruptured membranes after genetic amniocentesis. Am J Obstet Gynecol 183:937-939, 2000.
59. Gunn GC, Mishell DR, Morton DG: Premature rupture of the fetal membranes: A review. Am J Obstet Gynecol 106:469-482, 1970.
60. Hillier SL, Martius J, Krohn M, et al: A case-control study of chorioamnionic infection and histologic chorioamnionitis in prematurity. N Engl J Med 319:972-978, 1988.
61. Morales WJ: The effect of chorioamnionitis on the developmental outcome of preterm infants at one year. Obstet Gynecol 70:183-186, 1987.
62. Guise JM, Duff P, Christian JS: Management of term patients with premature rupture of membranes and an unfavorable cervix. Am J Perinatol 9:56-60, 1992.
63. Garite TJ, Freeman RK: Chorioamnionitis in the preterm gestation. Obstet Gynecol 59:539-545, 1982.
64. Simpson GF, Harbert GM Jr: Use of β-methasone in management of preterm gestation with premature rupture of membranes. Obstet Gynecol 66:168-175, 1985.
65. Gonen R, Hannah ME, Milligan JE: Does prolonged preterm premature rupture of the membranes predispose to abruptio placentae? Obstet Gynecol 74:347-350, 1989.
66. Vintzileos AM, Campbell WA, Nochimson DJ, Weinbaum PJ: Preterm premature rupture of the membranes: A risk factor for the development of abruptio placentae. Am J Obstet Gynecol 156:1235-1238, 1987.
67. Schucker JL, Mercer BM: Midtrimester premature rupture of the membranes. Semin Perinatol 20:389-400, 1996.
68. Moberg LJ, Garite TJ, Freeman RK: Fetal heart rate patterns and fetal distress in patients with preterm premature rupture of membranes. Obstet Gynecol 64:60-64, 1984.
69. Bengtson JM, VanMarter LJ, Barss VA, et al: Pregnancy outcome after premature rupture of the membranes at or before 26 weeks' gestation. Obstet Gynecol 73:921-926, 1989.
70. Beydoun SN, Yasin SY: Premature rupture of the membranes before 28 weeks: Conservative management. Am J Obstet Gynecol 155:471-479, 1986.
71. Mercer BM: Preterm premature rupture of the membranes. Obstet Gynecol 101:178-193, 2003.
72. Lemons JA, Bauer CR, Oh W, et al: Very low birth weight outcomes of the National Institute of Child Health and Human Development Neonatal Research Network, January 1995 through December 1996. NICHD Neonatal Research Network. Pediatrics 107:E1-E8, 2001.
73. Wu YW, Colford JM Jr: Chorioamnionitis as a risk factor for cerebral palsy: A meta-analysis. JAMA 284:1417-1424, 2000.
74. Yoon BH, Jun JK, Romero R, et al: Amniotic fluid inflammatory cytokines (interleukin-6, interleukin 1b, and tumor necrosis factor-α), neonatal brain white matter lesions, and cerebral palsy. Am J Obstet Gynecol 177:19-26, 1997.
75. Yoon BH, Romero R, Kim CJ, et al: High expression of tumor necrosis factor-alpha and interleukin-6 in periventricular leukomalacia. Am J Obstet Gynecol 177:406-411, 1997.
76. Yoon BH, Romero R, Yang SH, et al: Interleukin-6 concentrations in umbilical cord plasma are elevated in neonates with white matter lesions associated with periventricular leukomalacia. Am J Obstet Gynecol 174:1433-1440, 1996.
77. Locatelli A, Ghidini A, Paterlini G, et al: Gestational age at preterm premature rupture of membranes: A risk factor for neonatal white matter damage. Am J Obstet Gynecol 193:947-951, 2005.
78. Louis JM, Ehrenberg HM, Collin MF, Mercer BM: Perinatal intervention and neonatal outcomes near the limit of viability. Am J Obstet Gynecol 191:1398-1402, 2004.
79. Kilpatrick SJ, Schlueter MA, Piecuch R, et al: Outcome of infants born at 24-26 weeks' gestation. I. Survival and cost. Obstet Gynecol 90:803-808, 1997.
80. Bottoms SF, Paul RH, Iams JD, et al: Obstetric determinants of neonatal survival: Influence of willingness to perform cesarean delivery on survival of extremely low-birth-weight infants. Am J Obstet Gynecol 176:960-966, 1997.
81. Dewan H, Morris JM: A systematic review of pregnancy outcome following preterm premature rupture of membranes at a previable gestational age. Aust N Z J Obstet Gynaecol 41:389-394, 2001.
82. Vergani P, Ghidini A, Locatelli A, et al: Risk factors for pulmonary hypoplasia in second-trimester premature rupture of membranes. Am J Obstet Gynecol 170:1359-1364, 1994.
83. Rotschild A, Ling EW, Puterman ML, Farquharson D: Neonatal outcome after prolonged preterm rupture of the membranes. Am J Obstet Gynecol 162:46-52, 1990.
84. van Eyck J, van der Mooren K, Wladimiroff JW: Ductus arteriosus flow velocity modulation by fetal breathing movements as a measure of fetal lung development. Am J Obstet Gynecol 163:558-566, 1990.
85. Hibbard JU, Hibbard MC, Ismail M, Arendt E: Pregnancy outcome after expectant management of premature rupture of the membranes in the second trimester. J Reprod Med 38:945-951, 1993.

86. Moretti M, Sibai B: Maternal and perinatal outcome of expectant management of premature rupture of the membranes in midtrimester. Am J Obstet Gynecol 159:390-396, 1988.
87. Rib DM, Sherer DM, Woods JR: Maternal and neonatal outcome associated with prolonged premature rupture of membranes below 26 weeks' gestation. Am J Perinatol 10:369-373, 1993.
88. Lauria MR, Gonik B, Romero R: Pulmonary hypoplasia: Pathogenesis, diagnosis, and antenatal prediction. Obstet Gynecol 86:466-475, 1995.
89. Nakayama DK, Glick PL, Harrison ML, et al: Experimental pulmonary hypoplasia due to Oligohydramnios and its reversal by relieving thoracic compression. J Pediatr Surg 18:347-353, 1983.
90. Adzick NS, Harrison MR, Glick PL, et al: Experimental pulmonary hypoplasia and oligohydramnios: Relative contributions of lung fluid and fetal breathing movements. J Pediatr Surg 19:658-663, 1984.
91. Harding R, Hooper SB, Dickson KA: A mechanism leading to reduced lung expansion and lung hypoplasia in fetal sheep during Oligohydramnios. Am J Obstet Gynecol 163:1904-1913, 1990.
92. Askenazi SS, Perlman M: Pulmonary hypoplasia: Lung weight and radial alveolar count as criteria of diagnosis. Arch Dis Child 54:614-618, 1979.
93. Wigglesworth JS, Desai R: Use of DNA estimation for growth assessment in normal and hypoplastic fetal lungs. Arch Dis Child 56:601-605, 1981.
94. Carroll SG, Blott M, Nicolaides KH: Preterm prelabor amniorrhexis: Outcome of live births. Obstet Gynecol 86:18-25, 1995.
95. Moessinger AC, Collins MH, Blanc WA, et al: Oligohydramnios-induced lung hypoplasia: The influence of timing and duration in gestation. Pediatr Res 20:951-954, 1986.
96. Rizzo G, Capponi A, Angelini E, et al: Blood flow velocity waveforms from fetal peripheral pulmonary arteries in pregnancies with preterm premature rupture of the membranes: Relationship with pulmonary hypoplasia. Ultrasound Obstet Gynecol 15:98-103, 2000.
97. Winn HN, Chen M, Amon E, et al: Neonatal pulmonary hypoplasia and perinatal mortality in patients with midtrimester rupture of amniotic membranes: A critical analysis. Am J Obstet Gynecol 182:1638-1644, 2000.
98. Nimrod C, Varela-Gittings F, Machin G, et al: The effect of very prolonged membrane rupture on fetal development. Am J Obstet Gynecol 148:540-543, 1984.
99. Dowd J, Permezel M: Pregnancy outcome following preterm premature rupture of the membranes at less than 26 weeks' gestation. Aust N Z J Obstet Gynaecol 32:120-124, 1992.
100. Hadi HA, Hodson CA, Strickland D: Premature rupture of the membranes between 20 and 25 weeks' gestation: Role of amniotic fluid volume in perinatal outcome. Am J Obstet Gynecol 170:1139-1144, 1994.
101. Blott M, Greenough A: Neonatal outcome after prolonged rupture of the membranes starting in the second trimester. Arch Dis Child 63:1146-1151, 1988.
102. Alexander JM, Mercer BM, Miodovnik M, et al. The impact of digital cervical examination on expectantly managed preterm rupture of membranes. Am J Obstet Gynecol 183:1003-1007, 2000.
103. Lewis DF, Major CA, Towers CV, et al: Effects of digital vaginal examinations on latency period in preterm premature rupture of membranes. Obstet Gynecol 80:630-634, 1992.
104. Munson LA, Graham A, Koos BJ, Valenzuela GJ: Is there a need for digital examination in patients with spontaneous rupture of the membranes? Am J Obstet Gynecol 153:562-563, 1985.
105. Brown CL, Ludwiczak MH, Blanco JD, Hirsch CE: Cervical dilation: Accuracy of visual and digital examinations. Obstet Gynecol 81:215-216, 1993.
106. Imseis HM, Trout WC, Gabbe SG: The microbiologic effect of digital cervical examination. Am J Obstet Gynecol 180:578-580, 1999.
107. Schutte MF, Treffers PE, Kloosterman GJ, Soepatmi S: Management of premature rupture of membranes: The risk of vaginal examination to the infant. Am J Obstet Gynecol 146:395-400, 1983.
108. Reece EA, Chervenak FA, Moya FR, Hobbins JC: Amniotic fluid arborization: Effect of blood, meconium, and pH alterations. Obstet Gynecol 64:248-250, 1984.
109. Rosemond RL, Lombardi SJ, Boehm FH: Ferning of amniotic fluid contaminated with blood. Obstet Gynecol 75:338-340, 1990.
110. Bottoms SF, Welch RA, Zador IE, Sokol RJ: Clinical interpretation of ultrasound measurements in preterm pregnancies with premature rupture of the membranes. Obstet Gynecol 69:358-362, 1987.
111. American College of Obstetricians and Gynecologists (ACOG): Prevention of early-onset group B streptococcal disease in newborns. Committee opinion no. 279, December 2002. Obstet Gynecol 100:1405-1412, 2002.
112. Duff P, Huff RW, Gibbs RS: Management of premature rupture of membranes and unfavorable cervix in term pregnancy. Obstet Gynecol 63:697-702, 1984.
113. Fayez JA, Hasan AA, Jonas HS, Miller GL: Management of premature rupture of the membranes. Obstet Gynecol 52:17-21, 1978.
114. Morales WJ, Lazar AJ: Expectant management of rupture of membranes at term. South Med J 79:955-958, 1986.
115. Van der Walt D, Venter PF: Management of term pregnancy with premature rupture of the membranes and unfavourable cervix. S Afr Med J 75:54-56, 1989.
116. Grant JM, Serle E, Mahmood T, et al: Management of prelabour rupture of the membranes in term primigravidae: Report of a randomized prospective trial. BJOG 99:557-562, 1992.
117. Ladfors L, Mattsson LA, Eriksson M, Fall O: A randomised trial of two expectant managements of prelabour rupture of the membranes at 34 to 42 weeks. BJOG 103:755-762, 1996.
118. Shalev E, Peleg D, Eliyahu S, Nahum Z: Comparison of 12- and 72-hour expectant management of premature rupture of membranes in term pregnancies. Obstet Gynecol 85:1-3, 1995.
119. Tan BP, Hannah ME: Prostaglandins for prelabour rupture of membranes at or near term. Cochrane Database Syst Rev (2):CD000178, 2000.
120. Escobar GJ, Clark RH, Greene JD: Short-term outcomes of infants born at 35 and 36 weeks' gestation: We need to ask more questions. Semin Perinatol 30:28-33, 2006.
121. Naef RW 3rd, Allbert JR, Ross EL, et al: Premature rupture of membranes at 34 to 37 weeks' gestation: Aggressive vs. conservative management. Am J Obstet Gynecol 178:126-130, 1998.
122. Neerhof MG, Cravello C, Haney EI, Silver RK: Timing of labor induction after premature rupture of membranes between 32 and 36 weeks' gestation. Am J Obstet Gynecol 180:349-352, 1999.
123. Edwards RK, Duff P, Ross KC: Amniotic fluid indices of fetal pulmonary maturity with preterm premature rupture of membranes. Obstet Gynecol 96:102-105, 2000.
124. Lewis DF, Towers CV, Major CA, et al: Use of Amniostat-FLM in detecting the presence of phosphatidyl glycerol in vaginal pool samples in preterm premature rupture of membranes. Am J Obstet Gynecol 169:573-576, 1993.
125. Estol PC, Poseiro JJ, Schwarcz R: Phosphatidylglycerol determination in the amniotic fluid from a PAD placed over the vulva a method for diagnosis of fetal lung maturity in cases of premature ruptured membranes. J Perinat Med 20:65-71, 1992.
126. Shaver DC, Spinnato JA, Whybrew D, et al: Comparison of phospholipids in vaginal and amniocentesis specimens of patients with premature rupture of membranes. Am J Obstet Gynecol 156:454-457, 1987.
127. Phillippe M, Acker D, Torday J, et al: The effects of vaginal contamination on two pulmonary phospholipid assays. J Reprod Med 27:283-286, 1982.
128. Golde SH: Use of obstetric perineal pads in collection of amniotic fluid in patients with rupture of the membranes. Am J Obstet Gynecol 146:710-712, 1983.
129. Mercer BM, Crocker L, Boe N, Sibai B: Induction vs. expectant management in PROM with mature amniotic fluid at 32-36 weeks: A randomized trial. Am J Obstet Gynecol 82:775-782, 1993.
130. Mercer BM, in response to Repke JT, Berck DJ: Preterm premature rupture of membranes: A continuing dilemma. Am J Obstet Gynecol 170:1835-1836, 1994.
131. Mercer BM, Rabello YA, Thurnau GR, et al: The NICHD-MFMU antibiotic treatment of preterm PROM study: Impact of initial amniotic fluid volume on pregnancy outcome. Am J Obstet Gynecol 194:438-445, 2006.

132. Tsoi E, Fuchs I, Henrich W, et al: Sonographic measurement of cervical length in preterm prelabor amniorrhexis. Ultrasound Obstet Gynecol 24:550-553, 2004.
133. Rizzo G, Capponi A, Angelini E, et al: The value of transvaginal ultrasonographic examination of the uterine cervix in predicting preterm delivery in patients with preterm premature rupture of membranes. Ultrasound Obstet Gynecol 11:23-29, 1998.
134. Carlan SJ, Richmond LB, O'Brien WF: Randomized trial of endovaginal ultrasound in preterm premature rupture of membranes. Obstet Gynecol 89:458-461, 1997.
135. Smith CV, Greenspoon J, Phelan JP, Platt LD: Clinical utility of the nonstress test in the conservative management of women with preterm spontaneous premature rupture of the membranes. J Reprod Med 32:1-4, 1987.
136. Vintzileos AM, Campbell WA, Nochimson DJ, Weinbaum PJ: The use of the nonstress test in patients with premature rupture of the membranes. Am J Obstet Gynecol 155:149-153, 1986.
137. Hanley ML, Vintzileos AM: Biophysical testing in premature rupture of the membranes. Semin Perinatol 20:418-425, 1996.
138. Sperling RS, Ramamurthy RS, Gibbs RS: A comparison of intrapartum vs. immediate postpartum treatment of intraamniotic infection. Obstet Gynecol 70:861-865, 1987.
139. Gibbs RS, Dinsmoor MJ, Newton ER, Ramamurthy RS: A randomized trial of intrapartum vs. immediate postpartum treatment of women with intra-amniotic infection. Obstet Gynecol 72:823-828, 1988.
140. Gilstrap LC 3rd, Leveno KJ, Cox SM, et al: Intrapartum treatment of acute chorioamnionitis: Impact on neonatal sepsis. Am J Obstet Gynecol 159:579-583, 1988.
141. Romero R, Yoon BH, Mazor M, et al: A comparative study of the diagnostic performance of amniotic fluid glucose, white blood cell count, interleukin-6, and Gram stain in the detection of microbial invasion in patients with preterm premature rupture of membranes. Am J Obstet Gynecol 169:839-851, 1993.
142. Belady PH, Farhouh LJ, Gibbs RS: Intra-amniotic infection and premature rupture of the membranes. Clin Perinatol 24:43-57, 1997.
143. Buhimschi CS, Sfakianaki AK, Hamar BG, et al: A low vaginal "pool" amniotic fluid glucose measurement is a predictive but not a sensitive marker for infection in women with preterm premature rupture of membranes. Am J Obstet Gynecol 194:309-316, 2006.
144. Mercer B, Miodovnik M, Thurnau G, et al: for the NICHD-MFMU Network: Antibiotic therapy for reduction of infant morbidity after preterm premature rupture of the membranes: A randomized controlled trial. JAMA 278:989-995, 1997.
145. Ohlsson A: Treatments of preterm premature rupture of the membranes: A meta-analysis. Am J Obstet Gynecol 160:890-906, 1989.
146. Crowley PA: Antenatal corticosteroid therapy: A meta-analysis of the randomized trials, 1972 to 1994. Am J Obstet Gynecol 173:322-335, 1995.
147. Harding JE, Pang J, Knight DB, Liggins GC: Do antenatal corticosteroids help in the setting of preterm rupture of membranes? Am J Obstet Gynecol 184:131-139, 2001.
148. Wright LL, Verter J, Younes N, et al: Antenatal corticosteroid administration and neonatal outcome in very low birth weight infants: The NICHD Neonatal Research Network. Am J Obstet Gynecol 173:269-274, 1995.
149. Lewis DF, Brody K, Edwards MS, et al: Preterm premature ruptured membranes: A randomized trial of steroids after treatment with antibiotics. Obstet Gynecol 88:801-805, 1996.
150. Pattinson RC, Makin JD, Funk M, et al: The use of dexamethasone in women with preterm premature rupture of membranes—a multicentre, double-blind, placebo-controlled, randomised trial. Dexiprom Study Group. S Afr Med J 89:865-870, 1999.
151. Lovett SM, Weiss JD, Diogo MJ, et al: A prospective, double blind randomized, controlled clinical trial of ampicillin-sulbactam for preterm premature rupture of membranes in women receiving antenatal corticosteroid therapy. Am J Obstet Gynecol 176:1030-1038, 1997.
152. National Institutes of Health Consensus Development Panel: Antenatal corticosteroids revisited: Repeat courses. National Institutes of Health Consensus Development Conference Statement, August 17-18, 2000. Obstet Gynecol 98:144-150, 2001.
153. Vermillion ST, Soper DE, Chasedunn-Roark J: Neonatal sepsis after betamethasone administration to patients with preterm premature rupture of membranes. Am J Obstet Gynecol 181:320-327, 1999.
154. Ghidini A, Salafia CM, Minior VK: Repeated courses of steroids in preterm membrane rupture do not increase the risk of histologic chorioamnionitis. Am J Perinatol 14:309-313, 1997.
155. Abbasi S, Hirsch D, Davis J, et al: Effect of single vs. multiple courses of antenatal corticosteroids on maternal and neonatal outcome. Am J Obstet Gynecol 182:1243-1249, 2000.
156. Egarter C, Leitich H, Karas H, et al: Antibiotic treatment in premature rupture of membranes and neonatal morbidity: A meta-analysis. Am J Obstet Gynecol 174:589-597, 1996.
157. Kenyon S, Boulvain M, Neilson J: Antibiotics for preterm rupture of membranes. Cochrane Database Syst Rev (2):CD001058, 2003.
158. Kenyon SL, Taylor DJ, Tarnow-Mordi W, for the Oracle Collaborative Group: Broad spectrum antibiotics for preterm, prelabor rupture of fetal membranes: The ORACLE I Randomized trial. Lancet 357:979-988, 2001.
159. Mercer BM, Goldenberg RL, Das AF, et al: for the National Institute of Child Health and Human Development Maternal-Fetal Medicine Units Network: What we have learned regarding antibiotic therapy for the reduction of infant morbidity. Semin Perinatol 27.217-230, 2003.
160. Lewis DF, Adair CD, Robichaux AG, et al: Antibiotic therapy in preterm premature rupture of membranes: Are seven days necessary? A preliminary, randomized clinical trial. Am J Obstet Gynecol 188:1413-1416; discussion 1416-1417, 2003.
161. Segel SY, Miles AM, Clothier B, et al: Duration of antibiotic therapy after preterm premature rupture of fetal membranes. Am J Obstet Gynecol 189:799-802, 2003.
162. Christensen KK, Ingemarsson I, Leideman T, et al: Effect of Ritodrine on labor after premature rupture of the membranes. Obstet Gynecol 55:187-190, 1980.
163. Levy DL, Warsof SL: Oral Ritodrine and preterm premature rupture of membranes. Obstet Gynecol 66:621-623, 1985.
164. Weiner CP, Renk K, Klugman M: The therapeutic efficacy and cost-effectiveness of aggressive tocolysis for premature labor associated with premature rupture of the membranes. Am J Obstet Gynecol 159:216-222, 1988.
165. Garite TJ, Keegan KA, Freeman RK, Nageotte MP: A randomized trial of Ritodrine tocolysis vs. expectant management in patients with premature rupture of membranes at 25 to 30 weeks of gestation. Am J Obstet Gynecol 157:388-393, 1987.
166. How HY, Cook CR, Cook VD, et al: Preterm premature rupture of membranes: Aggressive tocolysis vs. expectant management. J Matern Fetal Med 7:8-12, 1998.
167. Combs CA, McCune M, Clark R, Fishman A: Aggressive tocolysis does not prolong pregnancy or reduce neonatal morbidity after preterm premature rupture of the membranes. Am J Obstet Gynecol 190:1723-1731, 2004.
168. Curet LB, Rao AV, Zachman RD, et al: Association between ruptured membranes, tocolytic therapy, and respiratory distress syndrome. Am J Obstet Gynecol 148:263-268, 1984.
169. Treadwell MC, Bronsteen RA, Bottoms SF: Prognostic factors and complication rates for cervical cerclage: A review of 482 cases. Am J Obstet Gynecol 165:555-558, 1991.
170. Harger JH: Comparison of success and morbidity in cervical cerclage procedures. Obstet Gynecol 56:543-548, 1990.
171. Blickstein I, Katz Z, Lancet M, Molgilner BM: The outcome of pregnancies complicated by preterm rupture of the membranes with and without cerclage. Int J Gynaecol Obstet 28:237-242, 1989.
172. Yeast JD, Garite TR: The role of cervical cerclage in the management of preterm premature rupture of the membranes. Am J Obstet Gynecol 158:106-110, 1988.
173. Ludmir J, Bader T, Chen L, et al: Poor perinatal outcome associated with retained cerclage in patients with premature rupture of membranes. Obstet Gynecol 84:823-826, 1994.

174. Jenkins TM, Berghella V, Shlossman PA, et al: Timing of cerclage removal after preterm premature rupture of membranes: Maternal and neonatal outcomes. Am J Obstet Gynecol 183:847-852, 2000.
175. McElrath TF, Norwitz ER, Lieberman ES, Heffner LJ: Perinatal outcome after preterm premature rupture of membranes with in situ cervical cerclage. Am J Obstet Gynecol 187:1147-1152, 2002.
176. Brown ZA, Vontver LA, Benedetti J, et al: Effects on infants of a first episode of genital herpes during pregnancy. N Engl J Med 317:1246-1251, 1987.
177. Chuang T: Neonatal herpes: Incidence, prevention and consequences. Am J Prev Med 4:47-53, 1988.
178. Visintine AM, Nahmias AJ, Josey WE: Genital herpes. Perinatal Care 2:32-41, 1978.
179. Stagno S, Whitley RJ: Herpesvirus infections of pregnancy. Part II. Herpes simplex virus and varicella zoster infections. N Engl J Med 313:1327-1330, 1985.
180. Amstey MS: Management of pregnancy complicated by genital herpes virus infection. Obstet Gynecol 37:515-520, 1971.
181. Nahmias AJ, Josey WE, Naib ZM, et al: Perinatal risk associated with maternal genital herpes simplex virus infection. Am J Obstet Gynecol 110:825-837, 1971.
182. Gibbs RS, Amstey MS, Lezotte DC: Role of cesarean delivery in preventing neonatal herpes virus infection. JAMA 270:94-95, 1993.
183. Major CA, Kitzmiller JL: Perinatal survival with expectant management of midtrimester rupture of membranes. Am J Obstet Gynecol 163:838-844, 1990.
184. American College of Obstetricians and Gynecologists (ACOG): Perinatal care at the threshold of viability. ACOG practice bulletin, no. 38, September 2002. Int J Gynaecol Obstet 79:181-188, 2002.
185. Laudy JA, Tibboel D, Robben SG, et al: Prenatal prediction of pulmonary hypoplasia: Clinical, biometric, and Doppler velocity correlates. Pediatrics 109:250-258, 2002.
186. Yoshimura S, Masuzaki H, Gotoh H, et al: Ultrasonographic prediction of lethal pulmonary hypoplasia: Comparison of eight different ultrasonographic parameters. Am J Obstet Gynecol 175:477-483, 1996.
187. D'Alton M, Mercer B, Riddick E, Dudley D: Serial thoracic vs. abdominal circumference ratios for the prediction of pulmonary hypoplasia in premature rupture of the membranes remote from term. Am J Obstet Gynecol 166:658-663, 1992.
188. Vintzileos AM, Campbell WA, Rodis JF, et al: Comparison of six different ultrasonographic methods for predicting lethal fetal pulmonary hypoplasia. Am J Obstet Gynecol 161:606-612, 1989.
189. van Eyck J, van der Mooren K, Wladimiroff JW: Ductus arteriosus flow velocity modulation by fetal breathing movements as a measure of fetal lung development. Am J Obstet Gynecol 163:558-566, 1990.
190. Blott M, Greenough A, Nicolaides KH, Campbell S: The ultrasonographic assessment of the fetal thorax and fetal breathing movements in the prediction of pulmonary hypoplasia. Early Hum Dev 21:143-151, 1990.
191. Devlieger R, Millar LK, Bryant-Greenwood G, et al: Fetal membrane healing after spontaneous and iatrogenic membrane rupture: A review of current evidence. Am J Obstet Gynecol 195:1512-1520, 2006.

Chapter 32

Post-term Pregnancy

Jamie L. Resnik, MD, and Robert Resnik, MD

In 1902, Ballantyne[1] described the problem of the post-term pregnancy for the first time in modern obstetric terms. Although the language used to describe the entity in early 20th-century Scotland was different from that of today, Ballantyne's words clearly reflected the thinking of his time: "The postmature infant . . . has stayed too long in intrauterine surroundings; he has remained so long in utero that his difficulty is to be born with safety to himself and his mother. The problem of the . . . postmature infant is intranatal."

During the ensuing years, the issue of post-term pregnancy, its risks, and its management generated great interest and controversy. An abundance of older as well as more recent data have firmly established that the fetal risk associated with a prolonged pregnancy is real, albeit small. Consequently, the pregnancy that continues beyond 42 weeks requires careful surveillance.

Definition and Incidence

By definition, a term gestation is one that is completed in 37 to 42 weeks. Pregnancy is considered prolonged, or post-term, when it exceeds 294 days from the last menstrual period (LMP), or 42 weeks. The frequency of this occurrence has been reported to range from 4% to 14%, with only 2% to 7% of pregnancies completing 43 weeks. The chances that parturition will occur precisely at 280 days after the first day of the LMP (40 weeks) is only 5%.

One of the major problems in delineating the extent of risk beyond term is the limited reliability of the LMP as a basis for accurately predicting gestational age. Traditionally, and until the 1990s, most epidemiologic studies pertaining to fetal and neonatal risks of delayed parturition were based on the LMP. Since that time, the use of ultrasound, particularly in the first trimester, has led to much greater precision in pregnancy dating, and data confirm that the LMP is a much less reliable predictor of true gestational age. For example, as early as 1988, Boyd and colleagues[2] showed that the incidence of post-term gestation fell from 7.5% when based on menstrual dating to 2.6% when early ultrasound examination was used. In a subsequent study by Gardosi and colleagues,[3] the post-term delivery rate among women dated by LMP was 9.5% but decreased to 1.5% if ultrasound dating was used. In their study, 71.5% of "post-term" inductions as dated by LMP were not post-term according to ultrasound studies. This finding is consistent with the observations of Taipale and Hiilesmaa,[4] who performed ultrasound examinations at 8 to 16 weeks' gestation in 17,221 women. When ultrasound biometric criteria rather than the LMP were used to determine gestational age, the number of post-term pregnancies fell from 10.3% to 2.7%. Although a second-trimester screening examination performed between 17 and 22 weeks' gestation was reported in one recent study to be more accurate in predicting the delivery date than a first-trimester screen,[5] most reports have tended to agree with the findings of Bennett and associates.[6] These authors randomly assigned women to either a first-trimester (n = 104) or a second-trimester (n = 92) ultrasound examination; 5 of the women in the first group underwent labor induction for a post-term gestation, compared with 12 of those in the second group. In any case, it is clear that use of the LMP alone tends to substantially overestimate the number of post-term gestations and that the widespread use of first-trimester ultrasound examinations, now used for noninvasive genetic screening, will have a great impact on the diagnosis and subsequent management of this entity.

Pathogenesis

Knowledge of the mechanism of parturition is increasing rapidly, and the current understanding of the pertinent molecular, biochemical, and physiologic findings are reviewed in Chapter 5. It is clear that the normal timing of parturition requires the integration and synchrony of numerous factors, including the fetal hypothalamic-pituitary-adrenal axis, the placenta and its membranes, and the myometrium and cervix. Although it is not known specifically why some pregnancies are abnormally prolonged, clues exist from interesting observations of aberrant timing of labor in humans and other species. For example, it has long been known that fetal pituitary defects in Holstein cattle may lead to failure of normal delivery timing.[7] In humans, congenital primary fetal adrenal hypoplasia and placental sulfatase deficiency leading to low estrogen production may result in delayed onset of labor and failure of normal cervical ripening.[8,9]

Whether the primary defect in delayed parturition involves aberrations in fetal endocrine signaling or abnormalities in the setting of the "placental clock" (as was suggested by McLean and colleagues[10]), or whether the myometrial contractile and cervical softening mechanisms are at fault, it is clear from the abundant data currently available that the timing of parturition is determined by complex interactions at the maternal-fetal interface.

Risk Factors

Primiparity has long been known to be more frequently associated with post-term gestation than multiparity. However, there also appears to be an increased frequency of recurrence among women who have had a previous post-term pregnancy. One large cohort study from Denmark has demonstrated that women who delivered post-term in their first pregnancy had an almost threefold increase in the incidence of subsequent post-term pregnancy, compared with those whose first delivery was at term.[11] These findings were recently confirmed by Kistka and coworkers[12] in a study of 368,633 births in Missouri, in which mothers with an initial post-term birth were at increased risk for a subsequent post-term pregnancy (relative risk [RR], 1.88; 95% confidence interval [CI], 1.79 to 1.97). These findings also suggest the possibility of a genetic predisposition, inasmuch as the risk of recurrent post-term pregnancy in the Danish study was not observed if the first and second children had different fathers.

Perinatal Risks

Morbidity and Mortality

Almost all reports up to the present time, even those with inherent limitations imposed by inaccuracies in gestational age determination, suggest an increase in perinatal morbidity and mortality when pregnancy goes beyond 42 weeks' gestation. One of the earliest and most frequently cited studies was provided by the National Birthday Trust of Britain in 1958, which undertook a detailed examination of more than 17,000 births in the United Kingdom from March 3 to March 9 of that year.[13] Their data demonstrated that the perinatal mortality rate began to increase after 42 weeks' gestation, doubling by about 43 weeks, and was four to six times higher at 44 weeks than at term. A more recent study showed that the risks begin to accelerate between 41 and 42 weeks and rise more sharply after that point (Fig. 32-1).[14] Numerous other reports have confirmed this increase in risk.[15-17] Alexander and associates[18] retrospectively evaluated outcomes of more than 27,000 pregnancies with 41 or 42 weeks' gestation, compared with approximately 29,000 completed at 40 weeks' gestation. Length of labor, incidence of prolonged second-stage labor, forceps use, and cesarean delivery were all increased with the longer gestation period. It is not clear, however, whether the observed increase in complications was due to prolonged gestation, routine use of induction at 42 weeks, or both.

In a more recent Norwegian study, in which 17,493 pregnancies with confirmed dates by second-trimester ultrasound were analyzed, 1336 were found to be post-term. The post-term group had twice the perinatal mortality rate (CI, 0.9 to 4.6); the RR of having an Apgar score lower than 7 at 5 minutes was 2.0 (CI, 1.2 to 3.3), and the RR of requiring neonatal intensive care was 1.6 (CI, 1.3 to 2.0).[19] Another prospective cohort study of 27,514 pregnancies from the same country demonstrated that maternal and fetal risks were lowest at 39 weeks' gestation, with increasing rates of maternal and neonatal complications, as well as operative deliveries, as pregnancy proceeded past term.[20] Similar findings were reported in a Danish population.[21]

Abnormal Fetal Growth

Since the report of Clifford[22] and his description of the postmature-dysmature neonate with wasting of subcutaneous tissue, meconium staining, and peeling of skin, many have focused their attention on the problems of the undernourished post-term fetus. In fact, only 10% to 20% of true post-term fetuses exhibit any of the findings described by Clifford. *Macrosomia* is actually a far more common complication, because, under most circumstances, the fetus continues to grow in utero. Twice as many post-term fetuses weigh more than 4000 g, compared with term infants,[17,23] and birth injuries can occur as a result of difficult forceps deliveries and shoulder dystocia. Morbidity also includes cephalohematomas, fractures, and brachial plexus palsy.[24] Study of fetal growth characteristics in 7000 post-term infants confirmed a gradual shift toward higher birth weights and greater head circumference between 273 and 300 days of gestational age.[25] These findings were further reinforced by a study of 519 pregnancies extending beyond 41 weeks, in which 23% of the newborns weighed more than 4000 g and 4% weighed more than 4500 g.[26]

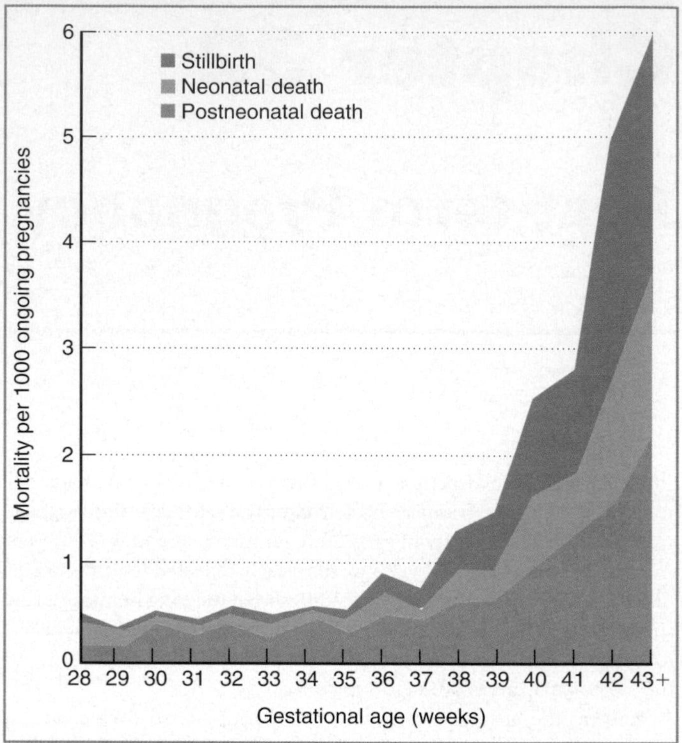

FIGURE 32-1 Perinatal mortality as a function of gestational age. The rates of stillbirth, neonatal, and postneonatal death increase with advancing gestational age beyond 41 weeks. The perinatal mortality is expressed per 1000 ongoing pregnancies. (From Hilder L, Costeloe K, Thilaganathan B: Prolonged pregnancy: Evaluating gestation-specific risks of fetal and infant mortality. BJOG 1998;105:169-173.)

Although the majority of post-term infants are appropriately grown or macrosomic, the risk of a small-for-gestational-age (SGA) infant is also increased in post-term pregnancy. In a population-based study of 510,029 singleton pregnancies from the Swedish Birth Registry, the rate of SGA infants increased from 2.2% in term infants to 3.8% in post-term infants.[27]

Meconium Staining and Pulmonary Aspiration

Almost all studies of post-term gestation report a markedly higher incidence of meconium-stained amniotic fluid, compared with term pregnancies, and the greater risk of meconium aspiration syndrome in these infants is well recognized.[17] Among those infants defined by ultrasound-estimated fetal growth curves to be appropriately sized for gestational age (AGA), those delivered post-term had a threefold higher incidence of meconium aspiration and twice the risk of an Apgar score of less than 4 at 5 minutes, compared with term AGA infants.[27] The presence of oligohydramnios further complicates the risks of meconium staining because of the lack of fluid to dilute the meconium, which results in thicker, more tenacious material in the oropharynx and lower in the respiratory tract.

Fetal Evaluation and Management

When one considers the rapidly accelerating risk of fetal morbidity and mortality between 42 and 43 weeks' gestation and again between 43 and 44 weeks' gestation (see Fig. 32-1), it becomes apparent that no historically derived or laboratory-measured fetal age provides the precision required in the management of the post-term pregnancy. Traditional landmarks, such as LMP, uterine size, and first auscultation of fetal heart tones, can miscalculate gestational age by 2 weeks or more. Even sensitive sonographic determinations, such as crown-to-rump length in the first trimester, demonstrate a range of several days. In fact, in any given gestation, the actual fetal age is known only if the time of ovulation and conception have been studied, as in ovulation induction and in vitro fertilization. Therefore, a gravida thought to be at 41 to 42 weeks or further in gestation, in current practice, either is induced and delivered or undergoes meticulous antenatal monitoring.

Antenatal Fetal Monitoring

Despite the lack of randomized clinical trials, it is generally accepted that careful antepartum and intrapartum fetal monitoring can virtually eliminate fetal post-term mortality and reduce fetal morbidity.[28-32] However, a careful evidence-based literature analysis concluded that data were insufficient to determine whether routine antenatal surveillance *before* 41 weeks' gestation improves outcome or which type of monitoring and frequency are most appropriate.[33] Consequently, most obstetricians initiate antenatal testing at 41 weeks' gestation and repeat the testing twice weekly. This testing consists of either a biophysical profile (BPP) or a nonstress test and assessment of amniotic fluid volume.

In a study of 307 women whose pregnancies had proceeded beyond 294 days, a normal twice-weekly BPP that included normal amniotic fluid volume resulted in no perinatal mortalities, and morbidity was equivalent to that observed in a comparison group undergoing elective labor induction with a favorable cervix.[32] Based on a cumulative experience with 19,221 high-risk pregnancies, the same investigative group recommended delivery if amniotic fluid volume decreases.[34]

The technique used to assess *amniotic fluid volume* and its role in evaluation of the prolonged gestation remains controversial because of conflicting studies regarding which of the two tests of volume (amniotic fluid index [AFI] or single vertical pocket) is the better predictor of outcome and the possibility that the AFI may lead to too many unnecessary interventions. Oligohydramnios is thought to be a marker for fetal complications, including umbilical cord compresssion, hypoxemia, and meconium aspiration, as well as fetal heart rate abnormalities and risk of neonatal admission to an intensive care unit.[35-37] Bochner and coworkers[36] observed an almost 24-fold increase in cesarean delivery for the indication of fetal distress when the maximum vertical amniotic fluid pocket depth was less than 3 cm. The incidence of meconium-stained amniotic fluid in the post-term gestation was 37% among those women with adequate amniotic fluid volume but increased to 71% if the amniotic fluid volume was decreased.[31]

However, a cohort study done in Sweden showed no correlation between an AFI of less than 5 cm and adverse outcome.[38] Similarly, Divon and associates,[39] in a longitudinal assessment of AFI in 139 women with post-term pregnancy, found an increased frequency of abnormal fetal heart rate tracings and meconium staining but no other significant adverse fetal outcome. Alfirevic and colleagues[40] compared both methods with respect to pregnancy intervention in post-term pregnancies and found more frequent abnormal AFIs than abnormal vertical pocket depths, leading to more inductions and fetal monitoring but no difference in perinatal outcome. Morris and colleagues[41] conducted a prospective, double-blinded, cohort study to determine whether an AFI of less than 5 cm or a single vertical pocket of less than 2 cm was superior in predicting adverse perinatal events. They found the AFI to be significantly more associated with birth asphyxia and meconium aspiration, but with poor sensitivity. More recently, Zhang and associates,[42] using data from the Routine Antenatal Diagnostic Imaging with Ultrasound (RADIUS) study, compared a large population of women screened by ultrasound to control subjects and observed that women with isolated oligohydramnios had no greater adverse perinatal events or impaired growth. Another study comparing the two techniques showed that the single vertical pocket method used for antepartum surveillance led to less frequent diagnosis and intervention for oligohydramnios, but without any difference in adverse perinatal outcomes.[43]

Given these disparate findings, it is not difficult to understand why there is no consensus as to the reliability or superiority of either technique for identification of the fetus at risk in prolonged pregnancy. Therefore, it is reasonable to conclude that an AFI of less than 5 cm, particularly if it has been falling sharply over a short time interval, or the absence of a single identifiable vertical pocket of greater than 2 cm, indicates that delivery is warranted. Conversely, it is also reasonable to consider that the finding of a normal amniotic fluid volume implies little fetal risk.

There does not appear to be any value in monitoring Doppler flow velocity in fetal vessels, inasmuch as there is no correlation between the findings and outcome.[44] Zimmerman and associates[45] demonstrated that the sensitivity of umbilical artery velocimetry for predicting poor outcome was 7%.

Fetal Monitoring versus Induction of Labor

Even though antenatal monitoring can virtually eliminate perinatal mortality in the post-term gestation, some morbidity—including meconium staining, increased cesarean delivery for a diagnosis of fetal distress, and macrosomia with its associated complications—still exists. Although the frequency of morbid events is very low, the continuing concern has been addressed by an alternative approach—that of cervical ripening followed by induction at 41 or 42 weeks' gestation.

Comparison of these two management approaches in several randomized controlled trials has yielded generally similar results. Hannah and coauthors[46] studied 3407 women with uncomplicated pregnancies at 41 or more weeks' duration, who were randomly assigned to either elective induction after cervical ripening with prostaglandin E_2 (PGE_2) gel or serial antenatal monitoring (fetal kicks, nonstress test, amniotic fluid). In the monitored group, labor was induced only if there was evidence of compromised fetal status. The authors observed a lower rate of cesarean delivery for a diagnosis of fetal distress in the induction group but no significant difference between the two groups in fetal mortality or morbidity. The same investigators subsequently reported that routine induction was more cost-effective than serial antenatal monitoring.[47] The Maternal-Fetal Medicine Network prospectively evaluated 440 patients, comparing induction with serial monitoring.[48] They observed no fetal deaths in either group, and rates of neonatal morbidity and cesarean delivery were similar. A more recent study from Norway, in which 254 women at 41 weeks' gestation were randomly assigned to an induction or expectant management group, found no differences in neonatal outcomes or mode of delivery.[49]

These combined trials have led to the conclusion that neither approach has a substantive advantage over the other. A small advantage to the induction approach was suggested by the recent Cochrane Review of 19 studies, which determined that a policy of labor induction at 41 weeks resulted in fewer fetal deaths, although the differences and absolute risk were extremely small (1 in 2986 versus 9 in 2953; odds ratio, 0.3; CI, 0.9 to 0.99). There was no significant difference in the cesarean section rate.[50]

Nevertheless, in terms of physician preferences in the United States, induction at 41 weeks has become the mode of practice and the debate moot. A recent survey of 1000 randomly selected members of the American College of Obstetricians and Gynecologists revealed that 73% routinely induce low-risk women at 41 weeks. For women who decline induction, approximately 65% of physicians initiate antenatal testing twice weekly at 41 weeks.[51] It is clear that medical induction rates have increased sharply in the United States. Between 1980 and 1996, the rate of induction doubled (from 12.9% to 25.8%), the most common indication being that of the post-term pregnancy.[52]

Management Summary

It seems appropriate to recommend the following steps to evaluate and manage the post-term gestation:

1. Although there is insufficient evidence because of the low-risk nature of either approach, current obstetric practice dictates that labor induction be offered between 41 and 42 weeks' gestation in the presence of a favorable cervix.
2. If the cervix is unfavorable, alternate approaches include either cervical ripening followed by induction of labor or twice-weekly fetal monitoring. Delivery should be accomplished promptly if there is evidence of fetal compromise.
3. It is prudent to use the BPP, or some modification of the BPP, to determine antenatal fetal condition.

Methods of Labor Induction

The issue of labor induction and cervical ripening agents is addressed in detail in Chapter 36 and is summarized briefly here.

Because normal labor depends on efficient myometrial contractions acting on a compliant cervix to efface and dilate it, methods of labor induction must take into account both components of the uterus. If the cervix is already soft, effaced, and partially dilated, intravenous infusion of oxytocin may be sufficient to stimulate contractions. Conventional practice requires amniotomy to be performed as a first step, because this procedure maximizes the effectiveness of oxytocin. If the cervix is unripe, oxytocin will not cause it to ripen, and amniotomy is inappropriate. Although labor contractions can be stimulated by oxytocin, such a result is futile, because many hours of such contractions are required to produce any sort of change in the cervix, and the ensuing prolonged labor can lead to an increase in obstetric morbidity, including a significant risk of postpartum hemorrhage and an increased risk of cesarean delivery.

The Bishop score,[53] or some suitable modification of it, can be used as a guide to select the most appropriate induction technique. This is especially true in primigravid women. If the Bishop score is lower than 5, amniotomy and oxytocin infusion are associated with an unacceptably high incidence of unsuccessful inductions as well as fetal and maternal complications.[54] In these circumstances, cervical ripening should be undertaken before uterine contractions are provoked. Given the rapidly increasing use of transvaginal ultrasound (TVUS) to assess cervical length and dilatation and its usefulness in the diagnosis of preterm labor, it is not unreasonable to apply this technology to cervical assessment in post-term pregnancy. One study of 240 women, comparing TVUS with digital cervical examination using receiver operating characteristic (ROC) curves, demonstrated that a cervical length of 28 mm was a better predictor of induction success (vaginal delivery within 24 hours) than the Bishop score.[55] However, conflicting findings were reported by Chandra and associates.[56]

The most frequently used current cervical ripening techniques include chemical agents such as PGE_2 (dinoprostone, trade names Prepidil and Cervidil Rx), administered vaginally or intracervically, and misoprostol (Cytotec Rx), administered vaginally or orally. Both appear to be effective in improving the Bishop score and to result in shorter labor times and possibly fewer failed inductions. Misoprostol, in doses of 25 μg given vaginally every 4 hours, appears to be slightly more effective that dinoprostone but is associated with a higher frequency of uterine tachysystole. A recent review of randomized trials performed between 1987 and 2005 compared the two agents and confirmed that misoprostol was superior to dinoprostone at any dose and route of administration in terms of achieving vaginal delivery within 24 hours. There was no difference in the rate of cesarean delivery.[57] This study confirmed an earlier Cochrane database review which concluded that the use of vaginal misoprostol is more effective than conventional methods of cervical ripening and labor induction. Compared with placebo, oxytocin, or intracervical or vaginal PGE_2, misoprostol resulted in increased cervical ripening, decreased use of oxytocin, and increased rates of vaginal delivery. However, misoprostol also caused an increased rate of uterine hyperstimulation.[58]

Vaginal inserts such as balloon catheters also have their advocates for cervical ripening. A systematic review concluded that these mechanical dilators do not compare favorably with chemical inducing agents in terms of delivery success rates but are associated with less uterine hypercontactility.[59]

Developmental Effects of Post-term Gestation

Studies on the development of children from prolonged pregnancies are difficult to evaluate because investigators have not separated neonates asphyxiated in utero and growth-restricted (dysmature) post-term neonates from otherwise normally born neonates. A study of neonatal behavior among 106 dysmature infants revealed an increased number of illnesses and sleep disorders as well as diminished social competence during the first year of life (Vineland Social Maturity Scale). Also, and not unexpectedly, the incidence of fetal distress was high, and those babies who were asphyxiated in utero had a higher incidence of abnormal neurologic signs in the neonatal period.[60] All infants had signs of desquamation of skin and wasting of subcutaneous tissue, however, and the group of children studied was not compared with any post-term children who did not have these physical findings at birth.

Field and coworkers[61] studied a group of 40 dysmature offspring, all of whom had parchment-like skin and long, thin bodies. At birth, their Brazelton interaction and motor scores were lower than in term controls, and at 4 months they scored lower on the Denver Developmental Scale. By 8 months, the Bayley motor scores of the post-term subjects were equivalent to those of control infants, but their mental scores were slightly lower. This study differed in at least one significant way from that of Lovell[60]: The Apgar scores at 5 minutes in the two groups were identical, thus partially correcting for in utero asphyxia.

In a large retrospective review, Zwerdling[23] observed that post-term infants weighing less than 2500 g had a neonatal mortality rate seven times that of post-term infants as a whole. This finding confirmed the additional risk of the dysmature growth pattern in some post-term infants. The increased mortality rate was observed up to 2 years of age, but at 5 years the data on growth and intelligence in Zwerdling's study population revealed no differences between prolonged-gestation and normal-gestation children. These findings were confirmed in a prospective study in which 129 children born of prolonged pregnancy were compared with 184 term controls.[62] At 1 year and again at 2 years of age, there were no differences between the two groups with respect to intelligence scores, physical milestones, or intercurrent illnesses.

One recent cohort study from Denmark linked hospital records of 277,435 pregnancies delivering at term or beyond to cases of childhood epilepsy. The researchers found a slight increase in the incidence of epilepsy as a function of gestational age at or after 43 weeks, but only among those infants delivered by cesarean section or other operative delivery.[63] The risk was not observed after 1 year of life. Whether this finding reflects a problem unique to advanced gestational age or complications that required expedient delivery is unclear.

References

1. Ballantyne JW: The problem of the postmature infant. J Obstet Gynaecol Br Emp 2:36, 1902.
2. Boyd ME, Usher RH, McLean FH, et al: Obstetric consequences of postmaturity. Am J Obstet Gynecol 158:334, 1988.
3. Gardosi J, Vanner T, Francis A: Gestational age and induction of labour for prolonged pregnancy. BJOG 104:792, 1997.
4. Taipale P, Hiilesmaa V: Predicting delivery date by ultrasound and last menstrual period on early gestation. Obstet Gynecol 97:189, 2001.
5. Olesen AW, Thomsen SG: Prediction of delivery date by sonography in the first and second trimesters. Ultrasound Obstet Gynecol 28:292-297, 2006.
6. Bennett KA, Crane JM, O'Shea P, et al: First trimester ultrasound screening is effective in reducing post-term labor induction rates: A randomized controlled trial. Am J Obstet Gynecol 190:1077-1081, 2004.
7. Holm LW: Prolonged pregnancy. Adv Vet Sci 11:159, 1967.
8. France JT, Liggins GC: Placenta sulfatase deficiency. J Clin Endocrinol 29:138, 1969.
9. Fliegner JRH, Schindler I, Brown JB: Low urinary oestriol excretion during pregnancy associated with placental sulphatase deficiency or congenital adrenal hypoplasia. J Obstet Gynaecol Br Commonw 79:810, 1972.
10. McLean M, Bisits S, Davies J, et al: A placental clock controlling the length of human pregnancy. Nat Med 1:460-463, 1995.
11. Olesen AW, Basso O, Olsen J: Risk of recurrence of prolonged pregnancy. BMJ 326:476, 2003.
12. Kistka ZA, Palomar L, Boslaugh SE, et al: Risk for postterm delivery after previous postterm delivery. Am J Obstet Gynecol 196:241.e1-6, 2007.
13. Butler NR, Alberman ED: The Second Report of the 1958 British Perinatal Mortality Survey. Edinburgh, E & S Livingstone, 1969, p 327.
14. Hilder L, Costeloe K, Thilaganathan B: Prolonged pregnancy: Evaluating gestation-specific risks of fetal and infant mortality. BJOG 105:169-173, 1998.
15. Nakano R: Post-term pregnancy: A five year review from Osaka National Hospital. Acta Obstet Gynecol Scand 51:217, 1972.
16. Sachs BP, Friedman EA: Results of an epidemiological study of post-date pregnancy. J Reprod Med 31:162, 1986.
17. Eden R, Seifert L, Winegar A, et al: Perinatal characteristics of uncomplicated post-date pregnancies. Obstet Gynecol 69:296, 1987.
18. Alexander JM, McIntire DD, Leveno UJ: Forty weeks and beyond: Pregnancy outcomes by week of gestation. Obstet Gynecol 96:291, 2000.
19. Nakling J, Backe B: Pregnancy risk increases from 41 weeks of gestation. Acta Obstet Gynecol 85:663-668, 2006.
20. Heimstad R, Romundstad PR, Eik-Nes SH, et al: Outcomes of pregnancies beyond 37 weeks of gestation. Obstet Gynecol 108:500-508, 2006.
21. Olesen AW, Westergaard JG, Olsen J: Perinatal and maternal complications related to post-term delivery: A national regiser-based study, 1978-1993. Am J Obstet Gynecol 189:222-227, 2003.
22. Clifford SH: Postmaturity—with placental dysfunction. J Pediatr 44:1, 1954.
23. Zwerdling MA: Factors pertaining to prolonged pregnancy and its outcome. Pediatrics 40:202, 1967.
24. Usher RH, Boyd ME, McLean FH, et al: Assessment of fetal risk in post-date pregnancies. Am J Obstet Gynecol 158:259, 1988.
25. McLean FH, Boyd ME, Usher RH: Post-term infants: Too big or too small? Am J Obstet Gynecol 164:619, 1991.
26. Pollack RN, Hauer-Pollack G, Divon MY: Macrosomia in post-dates pregnancy: The accuracy of routine ultrasonographic screening. Am J Obstet Gynecol 167:7, 1992.
27. Clausson B, Cnattingius S, Axelsson O: Outcomes of post-term births: The role of fetal growth restriction and malformations. Obstet Gynecol 94:758, 1999.
28. Hauth JC, Goodman MT, Gilstrap LC III, et al: Post-term pregnancy. J Obstet Gynecol 56:467, 1980.
29. Freeman RK, Garite TJ, Modanlou H, et al: Postdate pregnancy: Utilization of contraction stress testing for primary fetal surveillance. Am J Obstet Gynecol 140:128, 1981.
30. Eden R, Gergely RZ, Schifrin BS, et al: Comparison of antepartum testing schemes for the management of the postdate pregnancy. Am J Obstet Gynecol 144:683, 1982.
31. Phelan JP, Platt LP, Yeh S-Y, et al: The role of ultrasound assessment of amniotic fluid volume in the management of the post-date pregnancy. Am J Obstet Gynecol 151:304, 1984.
32. Johnson JM, Harman CR, Lange IR, et al: Biophysical profile scoring in the management of the post-term pregnancy. Am J Obstet Gynecol 154:269, 1986.
33. American College of Obstetricians and Gynecologists: ACOG Practice Patterns: Management of Post-term Gestation. Practice Bulletin No. 55. Washington, DC, ACOG, 2004.
34. Manning FA, Morrison I, Harman CR, et al: Fetal assessment based on fetal biophysical profile scoring: Experience in 19,221 referred high risk pregnancies. II: An analysis of false negative deaths. Am J Obstet Gynecol 157:880, 1987.
35. Leveno KJ, Quirk JG, Cunningham FG, et al: Prolonged pregnancy: I. Observations concerning the causes of fetal distress. Am J Obstet Gynecol 150:465, 1984.
36. Bochner CJ, Medearis Al, Davis J, et al: Antepartum predictors of fetal distress in post-term pregnancy. Am J Obstet Gynecol 157:353, 1987.
37. Tongsong T, Srisomboon J: Amniotic fluid volume as a predictor of fetal distress in post-term pregnancy. Int J Gynaecol Obstet 40:213, 1993.
38. Montan S, Malcus P: Amniotic fluid index in prolonged pregnancy. J Matern Fetal Invest 5:4, 1995.
39. Divon M, Marks AD, Henderson CE: Longitudinal measurement of amniotic fluid index in post-term pregnancies and its association with fetal outcome. Am J Obstet Gynecol 172:142, 1995.
40. Alfirevic Z, Luckas M, Walkinshaw SA, et al: A randomized comparison between amniotic fluid index and maximum pool depth in the monitoring of post-term pregnancy. BJOG 104:207, 1997.

41. Morris JM, Thompson K, Smithey J, et al: The usefulness of ultrasound assessment of amniotic fluid in predicting adverse outcome in prolonged pregnancy: A prospective blinded observational study. BJOG 110:989-994, 2003.
42. Zhang J, Troendle J, Meikle S, et al: Isolated oligohydramnios is not associated with adverse pregnancy outcome. BJOG 111:220-225, 2004.
43. Chauhan SP, Doherty DD, Magann EF, et al: Amniotic fluid index vs single deepest pocket technique during modified biophysical profile: A randomized clinical trial. Am J Obstet Gynecol 191:661-667, 2004.
44. Guidetti DA, Divon MY, Cavalieri RL, et al: Fetal umbilical artery flow velocimetry in post-date pregnancies. Am J Obstet Gynecol 157:1521, 1987.
45. Zimmerman P, Alback T, Koskinen J, et al: Doppler flow velocimetry of the umbilical artery, uteroplacental arteries and fetal middle cerebral artery in prolonged pregnancy. Ultrasound Obstet Gynecol 5:189, 1995.
46. Hannah ME, Hannah WJ, Hellmann J, et al: Induction of labor as compared with serial antenatal monitoring in post-term pregnancy. N Engl J Med 326:1587, 1992.
47. Goeree R, Hannah ME, Hweson S: Cost-effectiveness of induction of labor versus serial antenatal monitoring in the Canadian Multicentre Post-term Pregnancy Trial. Canadian Med Assoc 152:1445, 1995.
48. National Institute of Child Health and Development (NICHD) Network of Maternal-Fetal Medicine Unit: A clinical trial of induction of labor versus expectant management in post-term pregnancy. Am J Obstet Gynecol 170:716, 1994.
49. Heimstad R, Skogvoll E, Mattsson L-A, et al: Induction of labor or serial antenatal fetal monitoring in the post-term pregnancy: A randomized controlled trial. Obstet Gynecol 109:609-617, 2007.
50. Gulmezoglu AM, Crowther CA, Middleton P: Induction of labour for improving birth outcomes for women at or beyond term. Cochrane Database Syst Rev (4):CD004945, 2006.
51. Cleary-Goldman J, Bettes B, Robinson JN, et al: Post-term pregnancy: Practice patterns of contemporary obstetricians and gynecologists. Am J Perinatol 23:15-20, 2006.
52. Yawn BP, Wollan P, McKeon K, et al: Temporal changes in rates and reasons for medical induction of term labor, 1980-1996. Am J Obstet Gynecol 184:611, 2001.
53. Bishop EH: Pelvic scoring for elective induction. Obstet Gynecol 24:266, 1964.
54. Calder AA, Greer CA: Cervical physiology and induction of labor. In Bonnar J (ed): Recent Advances in Obstetrics and Gynecology 17. Edinburgh, Churchill Livingstone, 1992.
55. Pandis GU, Papageorghiou AJ, Ramanathan JG, et al: Preinduction sonographic measurement of cervical length in the prediction of successful induction of labor. Ultrasound Obstet Gynecol 18:623, 2001.
56. Chandra S, Crane JMG, Hutchens D, et al: Transvaginal ultrasound and digital examination in predicting successful labor induction. Obstet Gynecol 98:2, 2001.
57. Crane JM, Butler B, Young DC, et al: Misoprostol compared with prostaglandin E2 for labour induction in women at term with intact membranes and unfavourable cervix: A systematic review. BJOG 113:1366-1376, 2006.
58. Hofmeyr GJ, Gulmezoglu AM: Vaginal misoprostol for cervical ripening and induction of labour. Cochrane Database Syst Rev (1):CD000941, 2003.
59. Boulvain M, Kelly A, Lohse C, et al: Mechanical methods for induction of labour. Cochrane Database Syst Rev (4):CD000941, 2002.
60. Lovell KE: The effect of postmaturity on the developing child. Med J Austr 1:13, 1973.
61. Field TM, Dabiri C, Hallock N, et al: Developmental effects of prolonged pregnancy in the postmaturity syndrome. J Pediatr 90:836, 1977.
62. Shime J, Librach CL, Gare DJ, et al: The influence of prolonged pregnancy on infant development at one and two years of age: A prospective controlled study. Am J Obstet Gynecol 154:341, 1986.
63. Ehrenstein V, Pedersen L, Holsteen V, et al: Postterm delivery and risk for epilepsy in childhood. Pediatrics 119:554-561, 2007.

Chapter 33

Embryonic and Fetal Demise

Michael J. Paidas, MD, and Nazli Hossain, MBBS

Miscarriage is the most common complication of pregnancy.[1] It is estimated that up to one half of women will have at least one miscarriage.[2-4] Several factors contribute to inconsistencies in the definition, evaluation, and management of this pregnancy complication. One rational approach to the topic is to consider pregnancy loss according to gestational age intervals and to consider whether pregnancy loss is an isolated or recurrent phenomenon. Although approximately 15% of clinically recognized pregnancies end in miscarriage, if pregnancy loss from the period of conception is considered, more than 50% of pregnancies are lost.[1,5,6] One percent of couples may have two or more consecutive losses before the third trimester.[7]

Embryonic Losses

Peri-implantation Loss

The earliest pregnancy losses occur in the peri-implantation period. Implantation begins approximately 7 days after ovulation, which is between days 19 and 24 of the preceding menstrual cycle.[8] Implantation has been divided into three stages.[9] The initial stage is blastocyst apposition to the endometrial epithelium. Progesterone-dependent organelles, called pinopodes, appear on the surface of the endometrial epithelium on day 19 to 21 of the menstrual cycle, and they interdigitate with the blastocyst's outer syncytiotrophoblast to mediate initial linkage.[10] The second step in the implantation process is blastocyst adhesion, which is mediated by mucin 1. A subset of women with recurrent miscarriage has reduced levels of mucin-related secretory products.[11]

The third stage of implantation is trophoblast invasion into the uterine endometrium and vasculature and formation of the maternal fetal interface, which is mediated by several decidual-derived paracrine growth and angiogenic factors and by leukocyte-derived cytokines.[12] Theoretically, genetic abnormalities in blastocyst or endometrial cell adhesion or in paracrine signaling may lead to peri-implantational loss. Postimplantation events are characterized by increased expression of decidualized endometrial T_H2 cytokines (i.e., interleukin 4 [IL-4], IL-5, and IL-10) and reduced levels of T_H1 cytokines (i.e., IL-2, interferon γ [IFN-γ], as well as tumor necrosis factor α [TNF-α]).[13] Several immune factors have been implicated in pregnancy loss. Pregnancy should not be characterized as a state of immune suppression, but rather as a state of carefully orchestrated inflammation.[14] Indeed, overexpression of the anti-inflammatory T_H2 phenotype has been found in women with recurrent pregnancy loss.[15] Immune cells such as macrophages and uterine natural killer (uNK) cells may play a crucial role in normal implantation by producing angiogenic and growth factors or cytokines required for blastocyst growth and differentiation and by clearing apoptotic endometrial cells to allow for expansion of the growing embryo and extraembryonic structures.

Trophoblast expresses the nonimmunogenic human leukocyte antigen G (HLA-G), which has been postulated to offer protection against lysis by uNK cells.[16] However, HLA-G protein is not unique to pregnancy; it has been identified in unfertilized oocytes.[17] Although several investigators have reported that the presence of soluble HLA-G molecules in human embryo culture supernatants after in vitro fertilization or intracytoplasmic sperm injection correlates with successful pregnancy outcome,[18,19] others have disputed this finding.[20,21] HLA-G may play a role in early pregnancy, but HLA-G–negative embryos can implant.[22] It is unlikely that HLA-G polymorphisms represent a bona fide cause of early pregnancy loss.

Genetic Abnormalities Causing Embryonic Loss

Aneuploidy is the most common cause of embryonic loss before 10 weeks' gestation. At least one half of all miscarriages are caused by cytogenetic abnormalities. Collectively, the most common error is trisomy, followed by polyploidy and monosomy X.[2,3,23] In a study of chromosomal abnormalities involving first-trimester loss in 96 women, Stern and colleagues[24] found that 83% of karyotypes were abnormal. Pauli and coworkers[25] found the relative distribution of chromosomal abnormalities causing pregnancy loss to be 23% each for monosomy X (45X) and trisomy 21, 21% for trisomy 18, and 8% for trisomy 13.

Aneuploidies are usually the result of errors occurring in the first meiotic oocyte division. The cause of recurrent aneuploid loss in the setting of advanced maternal age is not completely understood. One theory is that continuous exposure to physiological oxidative stress in cycling women leads to progressively poorer oocyte quality. Animal models have demonstrated that excess oxidative stress leads to premature ovarian failure.[26] Another theory holds that there is a progressive maternal age–dependent depletion of oocytes available at the stage of maturation needed to complete normal meiosis.[27] Consistent with this theory, women with at least one trisomic fetus enter menopause at an earlier age compared with women without a similar history.[28] Maternal age–associated shortening of oocyte telomeres has also been suggested as a cause of accelerated embryo fragmentation and apoptosis.[29] Moreover, shortened telomeres can lead to abnormal chiasma formation and nondisjunction, providing a potential explanation of the maternal age–associated embryonic aneuploidy.[30]

Because advanced maternal age is associated with an increased risk of aneuploid offspring, one stochastic approach argues that to increase the chance of euploid live births, superovulation with in vitro fertilization and preimplantation diagnosis should be performed for the common trisomies found in abortus materials. This would theoretically increase the number of available euploid embryos. However, it has been argued that the bulk of these excess oocytes would have been selected out by natural processes. Moreover, several studies have suggested that this approach does not increase live birth rates.[31-33]

Low maternal folate levels have been found in women with miscarriage due to aneuploidy (odds ratio [OR] = 1.95; 95% confidence interval [CI], 1.09 to 3.48) but not when the fetal karyotype is normal (OR = 1.11; 95% CI, 0.55 to 2.24).[34] Folate deficiency may also have a role in meiotic nondisjunction. A meta-analysis suggested that fasting hyperhomocysteinemia is modestly associated with recurrent pregnancy loss (<16 weeks).[35] Folate supplementation can eliminate this potential mechanism. Because of the potential collateral benefits of folate in reducing the occurrence of fetal neural tube defects and its lack of toxicity, we recommend treating patients with unexplained early losses with folate (4 mg/day) beginning in the preconception period.

In addition to the advanced maternal age–associated risk of aneuploid pregnancy loss, other genetic, age-independent factors can predispose to recurrent miscarriage. Approximately 10% of patients with recurrent miscarriage may harbor such a factor.[36] Specific conditions include chromosomal fragility,[37,38] mosaicism, and deletions and large pericentric and paracentric chromosomal inversions.[39,40] A balanced reciprocal translocation or robertsonian translocation in one partner occurs in 4% of couples with recurrent miscarriage.[41] Carriers of the former are phenotypically normal, but 50% to 70% of their gametes and embryos are unbalanced because of abnormal segregation at meiosis.[42] Ironically, couples with a structural chromosomal abnormality who conceive spontaneously have a higher rate of live births (50% to 65%) than those conceiving after in vitro fertilization with preimplantation genetic screening, which is associated with a 29% live birth rate per oocyte retrieval and 38% per embryo transfer.[43]

Embryonic deaths may also be associated with single-gene mutation. Results of these mutations include glycogen storage diseases and hemoglobinopathies.[44] There are also X-linked disorders, which result in death of male fetuses only. These disorders include incontinentia pigmenti and Rett syndrome. The risk of recurrence of Rett syndrome is higher for male fetuses.

Endocrine Disorders Causing Embryonic Loss

Progesterone is required for successful implantation and maintenance of pregnancy. It plays a critical role in endometrial hemostasis and architectural integrity.[45] Progesterone's endometrial effects are mediated by its specific receptor isoforms, A and B, which are structurally identical, except for an additional 165 amino acids in the B isoform. Each isoform is functionally distinct, mediating its physiologic effects without much overlap. Progesterone plays a critical role in regulating migration and proliferation of immune and inflammatory cell populations located in the endometrium.[46] Progesterone may act as an immune suppressant, blocking T_H1 activity and inducing release of T_H2 cytokines (i.e., IL-4 and IL-10).[47] Defective corpus luteum function, or a luteal phase defect, has been implicated in early pregnancy loss for several decades.[48]

Removal of the corpus luteum before 8 weeks' gestation has led to spontaneous abortion.[49] This observation provides the rationale for exogenous progesterone therapy if the corpus luteum is removed early in pregnancy. Conversely, progesterone receptor antagonists given within the first 7 weeks of pregnancy induce abortion.[50] A luteal phase defect is defined as a lag of more than 2 days from the histologic development of the endometrium compared with the day of the menstrual cycle.[51,52] Because out-of-phase endometria can be found in up to 30% of the isolated menstrual cycles of fertile women, the diagnosis of luteal phase defect should be made only if it can be demonstrated in two consecutive cycles.[53]

Many causes have been suggested for the luteal phase defect. They include diminished production of progesterone by the corpus luteum, lower follicle-stimulating hormone (FSH) levels in the follicular phase, abnormal patterns of luteinizing hormone (LH) secretion, decreased ovulatory levels of FSH and LH, and decreased endometrial response to secreted progesterone.[53] Other potential mechanisms include decreased gonadotropin-releasing hormone secretion, inadequate ovarian steroidogenesis, and endometrial receptor defects.[53] Clinical trials have provided mixed results concerning the significance of luteal phase defects and the efficacy of treatment. Daly and colleagues[54] evaluated 33 infertile women with documented luteal phase defects, and 14 women who had biopsy-proven correction of the luteal phase defect did not have miscarriages. However, among the 16 women without correction, there were only four pregnancies that ended in abortion.[54] Balasch and colleagues[55] reported the results of 1492 biopsies in 1055 women. Fifteen of 20 pregnancies in women with an in-phase biopsy result went to term, but so did four of six pregnancies in women with an out-of-phase biopsy result. Moreover, term pregnancy rates were similar in women treated and those untreated for luteal phase defects.[55]

Serum progesterone levels are less invasive and less costly than endometrial biopsy, which is considered to be the gold standard for the diagnosis of luteal phase defect. Progesterone levels of 10 to 12 ng/mL determined 1 week before menses have been used as a marker for luteal phase defects. Unfortunately, progesterone levels do not correlate with endometrial histology.[56] The diagnostic criteria and proposed treatment for this putative disorder require validation.[57]

Thyroid dysfunction resulting in overt hypothyroidism or hyperthyroidism has been implicated in pregnancy loss. However, subclinical hypothyroidism probably is not a cause of early pregnancy loss.[58] Some investigators have shown that antithyroid antibodies and milder forms of thyroid disease have been associated with miscarriage.[59,60] One prospective study investigating the presence of antithyroid antibodies in patients with recurrent abortion found that 19% of affected women demonstrated anti-thyroglobulin or thyroid microsomal antibodies.[61] Pratt and colleagues[62] first reported that euthyroid women with first-trimester pregnancy losses had an increased incidence of antithyroid antibodies. However, they subsequently reported that an increase in nonspecific, multiorgan antibodies was responsible for the apparent increase in antithyroid antibodies.[63] Moreover, clinical outcomes were not significantly different among patients with or without these antibodies. Routine screening of patients with early pregnancy loss for antithyroid antibodies is not recommended, nor are therapies available.

Polycystic ovarian syndrome (PCOS) has been implicated in early pregnancy loss for several decades. Patients with recurrent pregnancy loss have a higher prevalence of polycystic ovaries (40%) compared with 23% of unselected women.[64] One randomized, placebo-controlled trial failed to demonstrate that suppression of LH secretion increased live birth rates.[65] Patients with PCOS and insulin resistance have elevated levels of plasminogen activator inhibitor 1 (PAI-1), reflecting impaired fibrinolysis.[66,67] Elevated levels of PAI-1 may impede trophoblast invasion mediated by urokinase-type plasminogen activator. Homozygosity for the 4G/4G PAI-1 polymorphism, a mutation associated with mild hypofibrinolysis, has been found in higher frequency in patients with PCOS and pregnancy loss than in women with normal-appearing ovaries.[68]

Analysis of follicular fluid from patients with PCOS demonstrates elevated levels of glucose, insulin-like growth factor 1 (IGF-1), and androgens, which can be embryotoxic. Metformin, an insulin-sensitizing agent, has been offered as a targeted therapy to reverse the pathologic endocrine changes associated with PCOS. Although a small, retrospective study demonstrated that treatment of patients with PCOS with metformin reduced the risk for miscarriage,[69] a large, prospective study failed to confirm these results.[70]

Prolactin is a key hormone involved in ovulatory and endometrial development. Elevated prolactin levels have been implicated in pregnancy loss, and treatment with bromocriptine, which suppresses pituitary prolactin secretion, has been associated with improved pregnancy rates.[71]

Mixed Embryonic and Fetal Losses

Immunologic Causes

Analysis of the transcriptome of chromosomally normal chorionic villi from patients with recurrent pregnancy loss has demonstrated aberrant expression of several groups of immunologically relevant genes.[72] Embryonic and unexplained fetal deaths have been associated with complement activation. The median plasma concentration of C5a was higher in patients with fetal death than in normal pregnant women (median of 16 ng/mL [range, 4.5 to 402.5] versus median of 11.6 ng/mL [range, 1.2 to 87.1]; $P < .001$].[73]

Unexplained fetal death in the absence of evidence of infection also has been linked to memory T cells. Blackwell and associates[74] conducted a study to determine whether unexplained fetal death was associated with a change in the proportion of naive-like and memory-like T cells in the maternal blood, as determined by the CD45 isoforms on the surface of $CD4^+$ lymphocytes. Patients with intrauterine fetal death had a higher percentage of $CD45RO^+CD4^+$ T lymphocytes than normal pregnant women (median of 57.7% [range, 35.4 to 78.6] for fetal death versus median of 49.9% [range, 19.1 to 86.8] for normal pregnancy; $P = .004$).[74]

Natural killer (NK) cells are involved in direct killing of virus-infected cells, cytokine production, and immune surveillance.[75] Excessive NK cell activity has been implicated in pregnancy loss, presumably by damaging the implanting blastocyst or interfering with normal placentation.[76] The process is likely mediated by the interaction between surface NK receptors and major histocompatibility class I molecules, including human leukocyte antigens C, E, and G expressed on the surface of the invading trophoblast.[77-79] The existence of discrete populations of peripheral blood and uNK cells has contributed to confusion regarding the role of NK cells and pregnancy loss. Approximately 90% of peripheral NK cells express low levels of CD56 but do express CD16. These CD56(dim) cells are more cytotoxic and express members of the killer immunoglobulin-like receptor (KIR) family. In contrast, D56(bright) cells have low cytotoxicity and do not express KIRs. In the uterus, 90% of the NK cells are CD56(bright)$CD16^-$. There is evidence that uNK cells may modulate the cellular growth, differentiation, and regeneration of the uterine mucosa[80] and promote placental invasion.[81] CD56(bright) cells express the high-affinity IL-2 receptor, higher levels of IFN-γ and TNF-α, granulocyte-macrophage colony-stimulating factor (GM-CSF), IL-10, and IL-13.[82]

Microarray data comparing peripheral NK and uNK cells have demonstrated that several genes are preferentially overexpressed in the uNK cells, suggesting the unique role of these cells.[83] Other gene array data reveal that several cytokines are very abundant in the endometrium: monocyte chemotactic protein 3, eotaxin, fractalkine, macrophage inflammatory protein 1β, 6Ckine, IL-8, hemophiltrate CC chemokine 1 and 4, and macrophage-derived chemokine.[84] In early pregnancy, uNK cells represent 70% of the total leukocyte population. They are rarely seen by 20 weeks' gestation, and they are absent in term decidua.[85]

Peripheral blood NK cell number and activity have been investigated in patients with pregnancy loss. Shakhar and associates[86] found that women with primary recurrent pregnancy loss had the highest levels of NK cell number and activity, whereas secondary aborters had intermediate levels, and control patients had the lowest levels, suggesting that NK cells are involved in pregnancy loss.[86] When patients with recurrent early pregnancy loss were examined prospectively during a subsequent pregnancy, pregnancies ending in loss (with normal fetal karyotype) were characterized by elevated NK cell percentage and activity.[87] Some investigators[88,89] suggested that elevated peripheral NK cells are predictors of pregnancy loss, with levels of more than 18% associated with impending pregnancy loss.[89] This led to the empiric offering of immunophenotype profiling in such patients. However, decidual uNK cell numbers are not increased in spontaneous compared with induced abortion specimens.[90]

Because of the clear differences between uNK and peripheral blood NK cells, the scientific basis for evaluating peripheral blood NK cells in patients with pregnancy loss is highly suspect. Moreover, there is growing evidence that increased decidual uNK cell activity is required for normal placentation,[91] and that reduced decidual uNK cell activity may be associated with preeclampsia and intrauterine growth restriction.[92] There is little evidence to support the assessment of peripheral NK cell activity in recurrent miscarriage patients.

Several studies of women with reproductive failure have been directed at suppressing NK cells with the use of steroids, intravenous immune globulin (IVIG), and TNF-α–blocking drugs. Morikawa and colleagues[93] evaluated the outcome of IVIG treatment in 18 pregnancies from 15 women with four or more consecutive, unexplained miscarriages. They found that 14 treated pregnancies resulted in live births and that 4 resulted in abortions with chromosomal abnormalities. Treatment also reduced preinfusion peripheral blood NK cell activity and NK cell number. However, meta-analysis of 19 such trials did not reveal any significant differences in live birth rates between treated and control groups.[94] The role of NK cells in pregnancy loss remains controversial, and treatments aimed at altering the NK cell status of women are highly investigational. Moreover, there is growing evidence against treatment to suppress decidual uNK cell activity with IVIG.

Absence of blocking antibodies has been offered as an explanation of maternally immunologically mediated pregnancy loss. These blocking antibodies were considered to be maternal antipaternal lymphocytotoxic antibodies. It was posited that excessive HLA sharing by prospective parents would lead to the absence of these antibodies. The proposed consequence was that placental antigens would be exposed to a more cytotoxic maternal immune response. Proposed treatments included infusion of male-partner or third-party leukocytes or extracts of placental trophoblast into the prospective mother to induce antibody production. However, meta-analyses fail to support such approaches.[95] In a double-blind, placebo-controlled, multicenter, randomized clinical trial in which 91 patients with recurrent miscarriage were assigned to immunization with paternal mononuclear cells and 92 were assigned to sterile saline injections, higher numbers of viable pregnancies occurred in the placebo group (41 [48%] of 85 versus 31 [36%] of 86; OR = 0.60; 95% CI, 0.33 to 1.12). This therapy does not have merit.[96]

Uterine Abnormalities

Müllerian fusion defects have been associated with fetal and neonatal losses because of preterm delivery, low birth weight, malpresentation, and abruption.[97,98] There is contradictory evidence linking such defects with embryonic loss. Salim and associates[99] evaluated 509 women with or without a history of three or more consecutive, unexplained pregnancy losses before 14 weeks' gestation using three-dimensional ultrasound. They found major congenital anomalies in 23.8% of women with losses and 5.3% in controls.[99] However, in both groups, the most common anomalies were arcuate and subseptate uteri, which accounted for more than 90% of cases. The former anomaly does not appear to be associated with a higher rate of recurrent abortion and may represent a normal variant.[100] The prevalence of major anomalies was 6.9% among women with recurrent miscarriage, compared with 1.7% in controls.[100] Table 33-1 shows the relative distribution of the major anomalies and their associated miscarriage rates.[101] Various theories have been promulgated to account for the association of uterine anomalies with recurrent miscarriage, including decreased vascularity in the septum, increased inflammation, and a reduction in sensitivity to steroid hormones.[101] However, there is not substantial evidence to favor one putative cause over another. Moreover, there are no controlled, randomized clinical trials of pregnancy outcome after resection of the uterine septum, although reductions in recurrent loss have been reported in several large series.[102,103] Traditional open metroplasty is rarely recommended for bicornuate or didelphys uteri because of the attendant risks of infertility and uterine rupture during pregnancy and because of the more favorable associated pregnancy outcomes.

Although myomas are quite common, they usually do not adversely impact pregnancy.[104] However, submucous myomas that distort the uterine cavity have been posited as causes of recurrent miscarriage and reduced in vitro fertilization success rates.[105] It is plausible that they cause pregnancy loss by a variety of mechanisms, including distorting the overlying endometrium, resulting in a poorly decidualized implantation site; compromising local endometrial blood supply; infarction resulting from rapid growth that outstrips the myomatous blood supply, leading to necrosis and so-called red degeneration that causes production of proinflammatory cytokines; and induction of fetal deformations when they encroach on the space occupied by the developing fetus, typically in the second or third trimester.[106] Hysteroscopic resection may improve fertility, live birth rates, and bleeding patterns.[107] A prospective study is being conducted to correlate the presence of sonographically identified myomas with pregnancy outcomes. Preliminary data on 1313 women have demonstrated that women with myomas had an increased rate of prior miscarriage (OR = 2.17).[108] Endometrial polyps have been posited as causes of recurrent miscarriage, and descriptive series suggest improvements in pregnancy outcomes after hysteroscopic resection.[109]

Based on expert opinion, it seems reasonable to offer patients with recurrent miscarriage screening for uterine defects by sonohysterography. Subsequent magnetic resonance imaging (MRI) or concomitant use of three-dimensional ultrasound can enable differentiation of bicornuate from septate uteri. Operative hysteroscopy can then be employed for the treatment of submucous fibroids, polyps, and septa. However, these recommendations are not based on well-conducted, randomized clinical trials.

Approximately 15% to 30% of women with uterine synechiae (i.e., Asherman syndrome) have recurrent abortions.[110] Lysis under direct hysteroscopic visualization should be offered to these patients. Postoperative management should include estrogen administration and insertion of an intrauterine device or inflated Foley bulb catheter.[110]

Fetal Loss

Fetal death has been defined by the World Health Organization (WHO) as death before complete expulsion or extraction from the mother of the product of conception, irrespective of duration of pregnancy.[1] It has been classified into three groups: early, occurring before 20 completed weeks' gestation; intermediate, occurring between 20 and 27 weeks; and late fetal death, occurring after more than 28 weeks' gestation.[111]

Epidemiology of Second- and Third-Trimester Loss

The rate of stillbirth in United States is higher than the neonatal mortality rate. In 2003, the U.S. rate was 6.23 stillbirths per 1000 live births and fetal deaths after 20 weeks' gestation.[112] The rate of fetal loss at less than 27 weeks' gestation is 3.2 per 1000. It is estimated that approximately one half of the fetal deaths occur at less than 28 weeks' gestation and that only 20% of fetal deaths occur near term. The death rate is two to three times higher for black fetuses compared with white fetuses.[113] An intermediate rate is observed for interracial couples, with a relative risk (RR) of 1.17 (95% CI, 1.10 to 1.26) found when the mother is white and the father is black.[114]

As expected, the fetal death rate is much higher for high-risk pregnancies than for low-risk pregnancies. Smulian and associates[115] compared the fetal death rates for low-risk and high-risk groups. The fetal death rate for low-risk pregnancies was 1.6 per 1000 births. The fetal death rates per 1000 births for high-risk conditions (i.e., abruption, small for gestational age, gestational hypertensive disorders, chronic hypertension, and diabetes) were 61.4, 9.6, 3.5, 7.6, and 3.9, respectively.[115]

The rate of stillbirth is higher in resource-poor countries. A WHO study that included six developing countries found a stillbirth rate of

TABLE 33-1 MÜLLERIAN DUCT ANOMALIES AND THEIR ASSOCIATION WITH MISCARRIAGE

Müllerian Anomaly	Prevalence among Patients with Müllerian Anomalies	Risk of Spontaneous Loss at Less Than 20 Weeks
Septum	55%	65%
Unicornuate uterus	20%	51%
Uterus didelphys	5-7%	43%
Bicornuate uterus	10%	32%

12.5 per 1000 births at the gestational age of more than 28 weeks.[116] Spontaneous preterm delivery and hypertensive disorders were the most common obstetric events leading to perinatal deaths (28.7% and 23.6%, respectively). Pregnancy loss also is associated with increased maternal morbidity, especially in low-income countries.[117] Related problems include maternal infection, increased blood loss, and maternal death.

Advanced maternal age is an important factor contributing to fetal death. Medical disorders such as hypertension, diabetes mellitus, abruptio placentae, and multiple gestations are more commonly associated with advanced maternal age. Even after adjusting for these conditions, advanced maternal age continues to act as an independent risk factor for fetal demise. The risk of stillbirth is increased between 37 and 41 weeks' gestation. Reddy and colleagues[118] studied a cohort of 5,458,735 singleton pregnancies without congenital anomalies and found that the relative risk of stillbirth was higher among women 40 years old or older compared with women between 35 and 39 years old (RR = 1.88 versus 1.32).[118] A retrospective, cohort analysis[119] of singleton births delivered between 1995 and 2000 used the U.S. linked birth and infant death data for women with ages ranging from 15 to 45 years. The relative risks for fetal death at 24 weeks or more and at 32 weeks or more among women between the ages of 35 and 39 years were 1.21 and 1.31, respectively, whereas the relative risks were 1.62 and 1.67, respectively, among women between the ages of 40 and 44 years.[119] These findings have been confirmed in a number of other studies.[120,121]

Hemoglobin concentration has been associated with a risk for stillbirth. In a Swedish population–based, matched case-control study, higher concentrations of hemoglobin in the first trimester were associated with an increased risk for stillbirth. Women with hemoglobin concentrations of 146 g/L or higher were at increased risk for stillbirth (OR = 1.8; 95% CI, 1.0 to 3.3).[122]

Genetic Abnormalities Causing Second- and Third-Trimester Fetal Loss

Chromosomal abnormalities of the fetus are responsible for 6% to 12% of fetal death after 20 weeks' gestation.[24,44,123] The proportion of chromosomal abnormalities is higher in fetuses with structural abnormalities. The most common type of abnormality is aneuploidy, and the most common aneuploidies are trisomies 21, 18, and 13. A genetic abnormality confined to the placenta in the presence of a normal fetal karyotype is associated with fetal death and severe growth retardation. This phenomenon is known as confined placental mosaicism (CPM). Increased maternal age is one of the etiologic factors for CPM; others include mitotic nondisjunction.[44]

Infection Causing Second- and Third-Trimester Fetal Loss

Maternal infection may cause fetal death by several mechanisms. Systemic maternal infection may result in fetal death. It may take the form of maternal high-grade fever, respiratory distress, or other systemic reaction to the illness. In these cases, the fetus is not directly affected but presumably dies because of cardiovascular sequelae of the mother's systemic infection. Examples include fetal death associated with maternal influenza,[77,124] chickenpox infections, and polio.[125] The placenta may be directly infected with the organism, resulting in placental insufficiency and causing fetal death, as occurs with malaria during pregnancy. The biologic basis for susceptibility to malaria in pregnancy was recently advanced by the discovery that erythrocytes infected with *Plasmodium falciparum* accumulate in the placenta through adhesion to molecules such as chondroitin sulfate A.[126]

The fetus may be directly infected through the membranes or placenta with the infectious organism, resulting in damaged fetal organs such as the lung, liver, brain, and heart. An example is infection with parvovirus. Maternal infections associated with fetal death include those caused by spirochetes, protozoa, viruses, and bacteria. Maternal–fetal infections are responsible for 10% to 25% of all fetal deaths. The earlier the gestational age at fetal death, the more likely infection is the etiologic agent. Copper and colleagues[127] found that 19% of fetal deaths were associated with infection at a gestational age less than 28 weeks, whereas only 2% were associated with infection in fetal death at term.

Maternal syphilis is an important cause of intrauterine fetal death, especially in countries with a high prevalence of syphilis. The prevalence of seropositivity in pregnancy is 0.2% to 4.5% in northern Europe and the United States. The rate of maternal syphilis has declined in the United States. From 1992 through 1998, 942 deaths, including 760 stillbirths, were reported among 14,627 cases of congenital syphilis, yielding a case-fatality ratio (i.e., stillborns and deaths/all cases) of 6.4%.[128] The seropositivity for African countries is between 3% and 18%.[129] Most deaths are observed in the second trimester. The organism can cross the placenta as early as 9 to 10 weeks' gestation.[130] Placental infection results in decreasing blood flow in the placenta, causing ischemic changes. Another spirochete responsible for fetal death is the tick-borne spirochete *Borrelia burgdorferi*, which is responsible for Lyme disease. The organism does cross the placenta, and there have been a few case reports of fetal death due to maternal infection.[131]

Other bacterial infections implicated in fetal death include those caused by *Ureaplasma urealyticum*, *Mycoplasma hominis*, group B streptococci, *Klebsiella*, *Escherichia coli*, and *Listeria monocytogenes*. These organisms may reach the fetus by ascending infections spreading from the lower genital tract and then into the decidua and chorion and occasionally into the amniotic fluid. Bacteria may also reach the fetus by hematogenous spread. Most fetal deaths due to bacterial infection occur between 24 and 27 weeks' gestation.[132] Listeriosis in pregnancy, caused by a gram-positive rod, commonly occurs in the third trimester. In humans, this pathogen has the ability to cross the intestinal, placental, and blood-brain barriers, leading to maternal gastroenteritis, fetal infections, and meningoencephalitis, respectively.[133] Pregnant women may present with flulike illness, including fever, chills, and back pain. The diagnosis is usually based on a blood culture if other common causes of fever such as urinary tract infection and pharyngitis have been ruled out. *Listeria* infection during pregnancy may lead to fetal death, preterm labor, or in utero fetal infection. Affected newborns have multiple abscesses in skin and visceral organs, and they die soon after birth.

It is difficult to estimate the true burden of fetal demise caused by viral infections, mainly because of the difficulty in culturing the agent responsible for fetal death. The most common viral infection associated with nonimmune hydrops causing fetal death is parvovirus B19, which is responsible for 1% of fetal deaths in the United States.[127] Maternal infection before 20 weeks' gestation may cause hydrops by infecting fetal erythropoietic tissue or by directly affecting the fetal myocardium.[134] Infection with parvovirus elicits an immune response in the mother, resulting in subsequent protection against maternal and fetal infections. Close-contact exposure of nonimmune women results in maternal infection in about 25% of cases. Of these, about 30% will pass the infection to the fetus. Fetal hydrops or other sequelae occur in only 10% of those affected, and stillbirth occurs in about 1% of cases.[135]

Viruses responsible for fetal death include enterovirus, echovirus, and coxsackievirus, all of which cross the placenta. This group of enteroviruses is associated with spontaneous abortions and stillbirths.[136,137] In a study from Sweden, of 21 women who had stillbirths, 52% were positive for coxsackievirus B, whereas only 22% of controls were positive.[136]

Cytomegalovirus (CMV), a herpes virus, infects 8000 infants each year in the United States.[138] About 10% of affected infants with congenital CMV infection have signs and symptoms at birth, whereas 90% remain asymptomatic but develop sequelae such as sensorineural hearing loss later in life. Maternal CMV infection can be primary or secondary. Lack of maternal immunity in cases of primary CMV infection results in more severe consequences. Symptomatic congenital CMV infection results from the mother becoming infected with CMV during or just before pregnancy. The risk for fetus is greater if the maternal infection occurs earlier in gestation.[139] The rate of congenital CMV infection diagnosis depends on maternal serology (i.e., anti-CMV IgM and low avidity anti-CMV IgG). Viral culture of amniotic fluid or polymerase chain reaction analysis after 20 weeks' gestation, ultrasound diagnosis of fetal abnormalities, and placental enlargement can identify disease and predict long-term sequelae.

Mother-child transmission of congenital CMV infection may be impeded by maternal administration of hyperimmune globulin (HIG) in women with primary CMV infection. Nigro and colleagues[139] have shown that monthly administration of HIG (100 U/kg) until delivery in women with primary infection starting at a gestational age less than 21 weeks significantly reduced the rate of congenital CMV infection compared with women who did not receive HIG (16% versus 56%; $P < .001$). The administration of HIG significantly ($P < .001$) increased CMV-specific IgG concentrations and avidity, decreased NK cells and HLA-DR$^+$ cells, and had no adverse effects.[139]

Placental Abruption Causing Second- and Third-Trimester Fetal Loss

Abruptio placentae is defined as decidual hemorrhage causing premature separation of normally implanted placenta. It complicates 1% of pregnancies. The incidence of abruption is highest between 24 and 28 weeks' gestation and decreases as the gestation advances. Risk factors include maternal substance abuse, hypertension, multiple pregnancy, hydramnios, infections, thrombophilia, and a history of abruption in a prior pregnancy. Inherited thrombophilia associated with placental abruption includes factor V Leiden (FVL) mutation, prothrombin gene mutation, and protein S deficiency.[140]

Placental abruption may be associated with fetal death in cases of severe abruption (>50% separation of the placenta). The diagnosis of abruption is more often made on clinical grounds. Severe cases may be associated with disseminated intravascular coagulopathy (DIC). Only 10% of affected patients show significant coagulopathy. In the event of massive separation, coagulopathy is seen in 20% to 30% of cases. The risk of developing DIC in abruptio placentae depends on the degree of abruption, the time interval between placental abruption and delivery, and the prognosis of the fetus. In less severe abruption, it is assumed that silent placental infarcts cause consumption of coagulation factors such as factor VIII and the release of degradation products. Alternatively, in massive abruption, decidual tissue factor–activated coagulation factors enter into systemic circulation through the uterine veins and cause DIC. Abruptio placentae with fetal compromise has been associated with cardiovascular events in later life in a population-based study.[141] The risk of recurrent stillbirth due to abruption is 9% to 15%.

Fetomaternal Hemorrhage Causing Second- and Third-Trimester Fetal Loss

Abruption can also cause fetomaternal hemorrhage (FMH). Other causes include external cephalic version and maternal trauma, which can lead to fetal death. FMH is responsible for 5% of stillbirths. A small amount of fetomaternal transfusion is of no major consequence, but large bleeds (>30 mL) are associated with clinical consequences that include unexpected anemia at birth.[142]

The American College of Obstetricians and Gynecologists (ACOG) guidelines on stillbirths and neonatal deaths recommend immediate assessment for FMH. The clinical picture consists of decreased fetal movements, a sinusoidal pattern on cardiotocography, and ultrasound evidence of hydrops fetalis. The diagnostic tools include Kleihauer-Betke test, flow cytometry, and Doppler ultrasound of the middle cerebral artery to diagnose fetal anemia.[143,144] The fetus can respond well to an acute blood loss of 40% of blood volume, but larger hemorrhages result in fetal death. Smaller bleeds over a prolonged time allow for cardiovascular adaptation. There is a role for intrauterine blood transfusion in these cases.[145] Anemia at birth is treated with postnatal transfusion. In a series of 48 fetuses described by Rubod and associates,[146] long-term follow-up of these newborns failed to reveal neurologic sequelae (0%; 95% CI, 0.0% to 11.6%).

Medical Conditions Causing Second- and Third-Trimester Fetal Loss

Overall, 10% of fetal deaths are attributed to maternal medical disorders such as preeclampsia, diabetes mellitus, thyroid disorders, systemic lupus erythematosus, intrahepatic cholestasis of pregnancy, and chronic renal diseases. The major contributors are preeclampsia (4% to 9%)[147,148] and diabetes mellitus (2% to 5%). The risk of fetal demise due to hypertensive disorders is greater among African-American women than among white women.[149] Fetal death rates are also higher for women with severe preeclampsia, those with HELLP syndrome (*h*emolysis, *e*levated *l*iver enzymes, and *l*ow *p*latelets), and women with chronic hypertension with superimposed preeclampsia.[150-152] The fetal mortality rate is also high for women with severe preeclampsia before 24 weeks' gestation.[153] The main reasons for fetal mortality in hypertensive disorders include prematurity, intrauterine growth restriction, and abruptio placentae. There has been a decline in fetal deaths from hypertensive disorders because of better medical and obstetric care. This is not true for the developing world, where maternal and fetal mortality rates are higher and hypertension is the second leading cause of maternal mortality.[154] Most fetal deaths linked to maternal hypertensive disorders occur before admission to the hospital.[155] In women having stillbirths due to hypertensive disorders, the risk of recurrence in the next pregnancy is about 14%. The risk of recurrent stillbirth due to hypertension is inversely proportional to the gestational age at the initial fetal death.

Type 1 and type 2 diabetes mellitus are associated with an increased risk of fetal demise. Overall fetal death rates for nondiabetic and diabetic patients were 4.0 and 5.9 per 1000 births, respectively, with an adjusted relative risk of 2.0 (95% CI, 1.8 to 2.2) in a report from the National Center for Health Statistics.[156] This study did not differentiate between gestational and pregestational diabetes. The reasons for fetal death in mothers with diabetes are postulated to be hyperglycemia, ketoacidosis, congenital anomalies, infections, and maternal obesity.[157] Fetal acidosis is the most likely reason for fetal death in the third trimester.[158] A comprehensive, multidisciplinary approach is the key to management of diabetic pregnancies. There is a role for antenatal fetal surveillance of diabetic women. Doppler velocimetry of the maternal and fetal vasculature has been more useful in the surveillance of the fetuses of diabetic mothers than the biophysical profile.[159] The risk of cesarean delivery is also increased among diabetic mothers. Subclinical diabetes and thyroid disorders do not pose an increased risk for recurrent fetal loss.

There has been an increase in the prevalence of obesity in the United States; one in three women is obese.[160] Because obesity has been associated with an increased incidence of stillbirth, this epidemic may be driving higher loss rates even while other sources are being reduced. A meta-analysis of the literature found that the risk of stillbirth was almost twice as high among obese pregnant women as among lean pregnant women.[161] It is not clear whether the relationship between obesity and stillbirth is direct or indirect. Obesity does lead to diabetes mellitus, hypertension, or undiagnosed impaired glucose tolerance, all of which may contribute to stillbirth. Other plausible mechanisms include hyperlipidemia, which leads to reduced prostacyclin secretion and enhanced peroxidase production, which results in platelet aggregation and vasoconstriction.[162]

Multifetal Pregnancy Causing Fetal Loss

The risk of fetal death is increased in the multiple gestations; perinatal mortality is 8-fold to 10-fold higher.[163] The increased perinatal mortality rate is attributed to prematurity, preeclampsia, and abruption and to problems unique to multiple pregnancies, such as cord entanglement in monoamniotic twins and twin-twin transfusion syndrome (TTTS) in monochorionic and diamniotic twins. TTTS is seen in 10% to 15% of monochorionic twins because of a chronic imbalance between interfetal blood flow across vascular anastomoses. TTTS occurs between 15 and 26 weeks' gestation, and it can be diagnosed with ultrasound. The ultrasound features include hydramnios in the recipient twin (deepest vertical pocket of ≥8 cm before 20 weeks and ≥10 cm between 20 and 26 weeks) and oligohydramnios in the donor twin (deepest vertical pocket ≤2 cm). A combination of different markers can help to identify an at-risk monochorionic pregnancy with TTTS. They include increased nuchal translucency (>95th percentile) on ultrasound in at least one fetus at 11 to 14 weeks' gestation, absence of arterio-arterial anastomosis on color Doppler, and velamentous cord insertion. The latter condition has been found in 60% of affected monochorionic twins.[164] The second twin is also at increased risk because of anoxia and premature placental separation during the second stage of labor.

Antiphospholipid Antibody Syndrome Causing Fetal Loss

Antiphospholipid syndrome is defined clinically by the presence of arterial or venous thrombosis, fetal death in the second or third trimester, or thrombocytopenia, coupled with serologic findings such as anticardiolipin antibodies or lupus anticoagulant. The anticardiolipin antibodies are immunoglobulins directed against proteins bound to negatively charged (anionic) phospholipids. Such antibodies are thought to promote uteroplacental thrombosis and fetal death through multiple pathogenic mechanisms, such as interference with the prostacyclin-thromboxane balance and by affecting the adhesion molecules between trophoblast. Antiphospholipid antibodies can interfere with activation of protein C by disruption of the thrombomodulin-thrombin complex and by inhibition of the assembly of the protein C complex. They also can inhibit the activity of protein C directly or through its cofactor protein S and through antibodies directed against the substrates of activated protein C, including factors Va and VIIIa, thereby protecting them from inactivation.[165]

Whether antiphospholipid antibodies can also cause embryonic loss is controversial. The plausible mechanism for early pregnancy losses includes inhibition of endovascular trophoblast invasion, induction of trophoblast apoptosis, and inhibition of trophoblast hormone production. These theories are strengthened by the fact that heparin attenuates trophoblast apoptosis and facilitates trophoblast invasion. Antiphospholipid antibodies are associated with obstetric complications, including fetal loss, abruption, severe preeclampsia, and intrauterine growth restriction.

Inherited Thrombophilia Causing Fetal Loss

Inherited thrombophilia is associated with an increased risk for fetal loss and other placenta-mediated pregnancy complications (Tables 33-2 and 33-3) (see Chapter 40). Most studies showing an association between fetal loss and thrombophilia have done so for losses at more than 10 weeks' gestation and for losses at more than 20 weeks in particular.[166,167] In a meta-analysis, Rey and colleagues[168] found FVL mutation, prothrombin gene mutation, and protein S deficiency to be significantly associated with nonrecurrent late fetal loss. The association is most robust for the FVL mutation, which arises from a point mutation in the factor V gene, causing the substitution of glutamine for arginine at position 506, the site of cleavage for activated protein C, resulting in activated protein C resistance. The European Prospective Cohort on Thrombophilia (EPCOT) study, a multicenter evaluation of patients with inherited thrombophilia, revealed a twofold increased risk for stillbirth for women with combined thrombophilic defects and antithrombin deficiency.[169] Independent of the FVL mutation, activated protein C resistance is associated with second-trimester fetal loss.[170] Combined thrombophilic defects exert a greater influence on fetal loss than only thrombophilia. Women with any of the following factors should be screened for thrombophilia:

TABLE 33-2 DETECTION OF MATERNAL INHERITED THROMBOPHILIA

Thrombophilia	Detection Methods	Reference
Factor V Leiden	Polymerase chain reaction	204
Prothrombin G20201A	Polymerase chain reaction	205
Hyperhomocysteinemia	Fasting assay, enzyme-linked immunosorbent assay	206
Antithrombin deficiency	Functional assay with a cutoff of <60%	205
Protein S deficiency	Measure total free antigen with a cutoff of <45% in pregnant patients	207, 208
Protein C deficiency	Functional assay with a cutoff of <50%	209
Protein Z antigen	Enzyme-linked immunosorbent assay	208

TABLE 33-3 ASSOCIATIONS OF THROMBOPHILIA TYPES WITH NONRECURRENT FETAL LOSS

Thrombophilia	Intrauterine Fetal Death OR (95% CI)
Factor V Leiden mutation	3.26 (1.82-5.83)
Prothrombin 20210A mutation	2.30 (1.09-4.87)
Protein S deficiency	7.39 (1.28-42.83)
Antithrombin deficiency	1.54 (0.97-2.45)
Protein C deficiency	1.41 (0.96-2.07)
Activated protein C resistance	2.07 (0.40-10.67)

Data from Rey E, Kahn SR, David M, et al: Thrombophilic disorders and fetal loss: A meta-analysis. Lancet 361:901-908, 2003.

- Unexplained fetal loss in a current pregnancy
- History of unexplained fetal loss in second or third trimester
- History of recurrent severe preeclampsia or HELLP at less than 36 weeks' gestation
- History of unexplained abruption
- Personal history of thrombosis
- Family history of thrombosis

The risk for stillbirth in the presence of thrombophilia is 3.6 times higher than without the disorder.[171] When attributing fetal death to thrombophilia, it is important to consider objective evidence of placental insufficiency, such as placental infarction, or abnormal Doppler velocimetry. Table 33-3 shows the association of different thrombophilias with fetal death. Fetal genetic risk factors for thrombosis (e.g., FVL mutation, prothrombin gene mutation) have also been found to be associated with fetal death. An increased risk for fetal death in the second trimester in fetal carriers of the FVL mutation has been found in several studies.[172,173]

Thrombophilia may confer an increased likelihood of other pregnancy complications, but the association is weak. There is a lack of evidence for an association between thrombophilia and placenta-mediated thrombophilic complications.[174] Rodger and associates[174] have argued that analysis of case-control, and meta-analyses do not have sufficient power to detect an association between thrombophilia and adverse pregnancy outcomes.[174]

Recurrent Second- and Third-Trimester Fetal Loss

Many of the causes previously discussed are more common causes of isolated stillbirth. However, women who had a stillbirth in a previous pregnancy have a 6-fold to 10-fold increased risk for stillbirth in a subsequent pregnancy. In a population-based study to identify the risk of recurrence of fetal death in a low-risk group of women with a history of fetal death in a prior pregnancy at a gestational age of 20 to 44 weeks, the adjusted risk of stillbirth was almost six times higher among women with a prior stillbirth (hazard ratio [HR] = 5.8; 95% CI, 3.7 to 9.0).[175] These investigators found that recurrence risk increased with earlier gestational ages (20 to 28 weeks) in the prior loss. In an analysis across racial groups in the United States, the same group of investigators found that white women had a lower absolute risk for stillbirth recurrence than black women (19.1 versus 35.9 of 1000; $P < .05$).[176]

The risk of recurrence is different for different etiologic factors. For example, fetal loss due to cord accidents is less likely to recur compared with loss due to placental insufficiency or thrombophilic disorders. Coppens and colleagues[177] did not find any significant difference in subsequent pregnancy outcomes for women with or without FVL and prothrombin gene mutations and first pregnancy loss. The live birth rate for the second pregnancy after early loss (<12 weeks' gestation) was 77% (95% CI, 62 to 87) for carriers and 76% (95% CI, 57 to 89) for noncarriers (RR = 1.0; 95% CI, 0.8 to 1.3). In contrast, they found that after a late first loss (>12 weeks), the live birth rates were 68% (95% CI, 46 to 85) and 80% (95% CI, 49 to 94) for carriers and noncarriers, respectively (RR = 0.9; 95% CI, 0.5 to 1.3).[177]

Diagnostic Considerations for Second- and Third-Trimester Fetal Loss

Chromosomal abnormalities are responsible for 50% of first-trimester losses, 15% of second-trimester losses, and 5% of third-trimester losses.[110] Fetal karyotyping should be performed if either parent is a carrier for a balanced translocation or there is a history of recurrent pregnancy loss or stillbirths in first-degree relatives. ACOG recommends cytogenetic studies for the fetus in the event of dysmorphic features, growth abnormalities, congenital anomalies, and hydrops and when a parent carries a balanced chromosomal rearrangement or has a mosaic karyotype.

The importance of a fetal autopsy in reaching a conclusive diagnosis cannot be underestimated. A fetal autopsy can determine the structural and morphologic abnormalities, and it may help to exclude infection, anemia, and metabolic disorders as causes of fetal death. An autopsy includes invasive and noninvasive components. The noninvasive components include review of premortem medical records, external examination of the fetus and gross and histological examination of the placenta and membranes, cytogenetic and metabolic investigations of cord blood, and radiographs. The invasive diagnosis includes examination and dissection of internal organs. Postmortem fetal MRI can assist in diagnosing the underlying cause without the need for fetal dissection.[178]

Histologic examination of the placenta, although often neglected, is an important tool in reaching a diagnosis of the cause of fetal death. Placental pathology can be helpful in differentiating acute from chronic perinatal stress, in diagnosing specific causes in abnormal pregnancies, and in assessing newborn risks. Maternal infections responsible for fetal death can be evaluated by examination of the placenta. Similarly, thromboembolic events, such as caused by a thrombophilia, can be determined by the placental examination. Placental thrombosis and infarction have been identified in the placenta of thrombophilic women with fetal losses.[173,179] Assessment of maternal TORCH (*t*oxoplasmosis, *o*ther agents, *r*ubella, *c*ytomegalovirus, and *h*erpes simplex) serologies has been traditionally advised, but its utility in the developed world is uncertain. It may be of more significance in areas where these maternal infections are endemic. ACOG guidelines on stillbirth and neonatal deaths recommend screening for parvovirus B-19 IgM and IgG antibodies and syphilis.

Women of reproductive age may use alcohol or other substances such as heroin, cocaine, and amphetamine. The National Institute on Drug Abuse (NIDA), in one of the few large surveys of maternal substance abuse, found that 5.5% of mothers reported taking an illicit substance during gestation.[180] Many of these agents are known to cross human placenta and produce a number of undesirable effects. Drug transfer across the placenta occurs by means of passive diffusion, active transport, and pinocytosis. Movement of a drug across the placenta depends on the size of molecule, solubility, and protein binding. Obstetric complications include placental insufficiency, miscarriage,

TABLE 33-4 RECOMMENDED EVALUATION OF PATIENTS WITH SECOND- OR THIRD-TRIMESTER ISOLATED OR RECURRENT FETAL LOSS

Fetal workup
Fetal autopsy
Placental pathology
Radiograph of fetal skeleton
Maternal workup
Complete blood count
Kleihauer-Betke test
Parvovirus B19 IgG and IgM
Maternal serology for syphilis
Lupus anticoagulant
Anticardiolipin antibodies
Free thyroxine and thyroid-stimulating hormone
Inherited thrombophilia workup (see Table 33-2)

Modified from Silver RM, Varner MW, Reddy U, et al: Work-up of stillbirth: A review of the evidence. Am J Obstet Gynecol 196:433-444, 2007.

intrauterine death, and increased incidence of infectious and sexually transmitted diseases in the drug-abusing mother.[181] The increased risk of obstetric complications may be attributed to a lack of prenatal care for this group of women. Only 25% of women with drug abuse seek antenatal care before labor; for those who do, it occurs mostly in the third trimester.[182] Apart from increased susceptibility to sexually transmitted diseases, pregnant drug abusers also suffer from an increased number of medical problems such as anemia, bacteremia, hypertension, nutritional deficiencies, and tuberculosis. The association of maternal alcohol abuse with fetal alcohol syndrome (e.g., dysmorphic features, impaired intellectual development) is well known. Maternal drug use during pregnancy can be monitored with urine, sweat, oral fluid, or hair testing. Toxicologic screening for substance abuse is done in most medical institutions. Urinary analysis is commonly employed, but measurement of stable metabolites can also be carried out using meconium, hair, and umbilical cord samples. Table 33-4 details the suggested evaluation of second- and third-trimester fetal loss.

Management of Fetal and Embryonic Loss

Delivery of the fetus in a woman with embryonic and fetal demise calls for emotional and medical support by a caring physician. The patient can be counseled by the obstetrician, neonatologist, nurse practitioner, or genetic counselor. It is necessary to talk to parents about their wishes, their fears concerning future pregnancies, and their views about postmortem evaluations. The importance of an autopsy should be emphasized to identify the cause of stillbirth and help determine management of future pregnancies. Mothers should be followed in the postpartum period for depression. For losses after 27 weeks, in the absence of any identifiable cause for stillbirth, parents should be reassured that the risk of recurrence is no greater than 3%.[183] The risk of recurrence is greater for women with losses at less than 27 weeks' gestation.

Most women find it disturbing to carry a nonviable fetus, but others may like to have some time to share the grief with family before proceeding to termination. In both cases, the woman's wishes need to be addressed. There is no urgency to evacuate the uterus if surveillance is offered for infection and coagulopathy. A low serum level of fibrinogen (<100 mg/dL) and a low platelet count are considered evidence of coagulopathy. Earlier studies quoted rates of coagulation abnormalities as high as 25% to 30%, whereas later reports state a much lower rate of coagulopathy associated with fetal demise.[184,185] This change is attributed to early diagnosis by ultrasound. Tables 33-4 and 33-5 detail the suggested evaluation of recurrent fetal and embryonic losses, respectively.

TABLE 33-5 EVALUATION FOR RECURRENT FIRST-TRIMESTER LOSS

Karyotype of miscarried tissue (in all cases of fetal loss)
Parental karyotype
Luteal-phase assessment
Glucose tolerance testing
Thyroid function testing
Uterine cavity assessment by sonohysterography (preferred), hysterosalpingogram, or hysteroscopy
Antiphospholipid antibody screen
Inherited thrombophilias, if losses between 10 and 13 weeks

Management of Embryonic and First-Trimester Fetal Loss

Medical and surgical management can be used for first-trimester loss. Surgical management includes vacuum aspiration, dilatation, and aspiration or curettage. Medical management includes the use of prostaglandins, mifepristone, and methotrexate. These drugs can be used alone or in combination. A Cochrane review on medical management of first-trimester loss found oral misoprostol less effective than vaginal misoprostol (RR = 3.00; 95% CI, 1.44 to 6.24).[186] The oral route was also associated with adverse events such as nausea, vomiting, diarrhea, and shivering. Mifepristone alone is less effective than when combined with prostaglandins (RR = 3.76; 95% CI, 2.30 to 6.15).[186] Misoprostol used in combination with mifepristone reduces the induction-delivery interval compared with that for either agent alone.[187,188] This also is important for women with late fetal demise (>24 weeks' gestation). The optimal doses of misoprostol and mifepristone are not known. A reduced dose (a dose of 200 mg given once) of mifepristone, followed by gemeprost to soften and dilate the cervix and stimulate the uterus to contract, has been found to be cost-effective and efficacious.

Management of Second- and Third-Trimester Fetal Loss

The choice between medical and surgical methods depends on the gestational age of the fetus. Treatment before 14 weeks' gestation has traditionally been surgical, but medical treatments may be equally effective. Surgical treatment in the early part of the second trimester is safe in experienced hands, but the procedure becomes more difficult in the late second and early third trimesters. As the gestation advances, induction of labor becomes a more favorable choice. A Cochrane review found vaginal misoprostol more effective than placebo in the termination of nonviable pregnancies before 24 weeks' gestation.[189] Misoprostol is an effective myometrial stimulant and acts by means of EP-2 and EP-3 prostanoid receptors.[190] It acts through vaginal and oral routes. Vaginally absorbed serum levels are more prolonged and are associated with fewer side effects. Oral misoprostol (400 μg) was found to be less effective than vaginal misoprostol, but this difference was not seen with an 800-μg dose.[189] Sublingual misoprostol has been found equivalent to the vaginal route in inducing complete miscarriage (RR = 1.00; 95% CI, 0.85 to 1.18). Other doses used include 400, 600, and 800 μg. The dose also depends on gestational age. Wet preparations were as effective as the dry preparations.[189]

Other drugs used for medical termination of pregnancy include prostaglandin $F_{2\alpha}$, prostaglandin E_2, ergometrine, and oxytocin. Side effects of misoprostol include nausea, vomiting, diarrhea, shivering, and elevated temperature. These effects are usually dose related and transitory. The toxic dose for humans is not known, and there is no known antidote for the drug. Misoprostol has been associated with maternal death in a case report.[191] It is generally recommended that all prostaglandins for medical induction of labor be avoided in cases of prior cesarean delivery if the uterine size is greater than 24 to 26 weeks' gestation.

Management of Subsequent Pregnancy in Patients with a History of Embryonic or Fetal Loss

Increased antenatal surveillance during future pregnancies is strongly recommended for women with a history of embryonic or fetal loss. Counseling for control or cessation of contributing factors such as weight, smoking, alcohol, and medical conditions (e.g., diabetes mellitus, thyroid disorders, chronic hypertension) plays an important role for this group of women. The risk of recurrent late fetal loss is reduced by 14% with the use of aspirin alone (RR = 0.86; 95% CI, 0.76 to 0.98).[192] In women with antiphospholipid antibodies, thromboprophylaxis with aspirin and heparin increases the live birth rate. In a randomized, double-blind, placebo-controlled study involving 82 patients with recurrent pregnancy loss and without such antibodies by Tulppala and colleagues,[193] use of low dose aspirin alone was not found to have any effect on the live birth rate (RR = 1.00; 95% CI, 0.78 to 1.29).

Similarly, women with known inherited thrombophilia and recurrent fetal loss may benefit from heparin prophylaxis. In an open-label, quasi-random study of 160 patients with prior losses after 10 weeks associated with known thrombophilic defects, Gris and associates[194] compared low-molecular-weight heparin (LMWH) with aspirin. They found an increased live birth rate with the use of LMWH (RR = 10.00; 95% CI, 1.56 to 64.20). Paidas and coworkers[195] found an 80% reduction in fetal loss with the use of heparin in women with FVL or prothrombin gene mutations and prior fetal loss.[195] Brenner and colleagues[196] showed an increased live birth rate (76% versus 28%) with 80 mg of LMWH compared with 40 mg in a cohort of women with known thrombophilia and fetal loss.[196] Although there is a lack of randomized studies, observational studies and historical cohort analyses have shown an increased live birth rate with the use of heparin in women with inherited thrombophilias and adverse pregnancy outcomes.[196,197]

Several trials are being conducted to evaluate the role of heparin in improving maternal and fetal outcomes. These include the Thrombophilia in Pregnancy Prophylaxis Study (TIPPS, ISRCTN87441504), Fragmin in Pregnant Women with a History of Uteroplacental Insufficiency and Thrombophilia (FRUIT, ISRCTN87325378) study, Anticoagulants for Living Fetuses (ALIFE, ISRCTN58496168) study, and Scottish Pregnancy Intervention (SPIN, ISRCTN06774126) study. A consensus panel statement was published to aid clinicians in managing anticoagulant therapy during pregnancy.[198] With respect to preventing adverse pregnancy outcome, the statement authors recognized the limited data that are available. For recurrent and unexplained fetal losses, many authorities offer prophylactic heparin anticoagulation in a subsequent pregnancy if patients are found to have an inherited thrombophilia. In a large, retrospective cohort study, 84 consecutive, multiparous patients with a history of severe preeclampsia and fetal growth restriction were assigned to receive no treatment, low-dose aspirin alone, or low-dose aspirin plus LMWH. The combination of prophylactic heparin and low-dose aspirin protected against an adverse outcome in the index pregnancy.[199] Randomized clinical trials are required to determine the optimal strategy for preventing recurrent adverse outcomes.

Several forms of immunotherapy have been used in the treatment of women with recurrent embryonic or fetal losses because immune aberration was considered to be an etiologic agent. These methods include paternal cell immunization, third-party donor cell immunization, trophoblast membrane infusion, and IVIG. A Cochrane review of the use of immunotherapy for recurrent pregnancy loss did not find any improvement in the live birth rate with the use of immunotherapy compared with placebo.[200]

Progesterone has been used widely for a long time to prevent recurrent losses. A large number of randomized trials have been conducted to evaluate the efficacy of progesterone in the previously described circumstances. A Cochrane review on the use of progesterone for recurrent miscarriage found a statistically significant improvement in the live birth rate among women with a history of recurrent pregnancy loss (OR = 0.39; 95% CI, 0.17 to 0.91).[201] Table 33-6 summarizes the other pharmacologic options available to women with prior fetal loss.

Other measures to improve fetal survival in subsequent pregnancies include increased fetal surveillance by means of nonstress testing, serial ultrasound, Doppler velocimetry for growth-restricted fetuses, and amniotic fluid indices. The decision about when to start antenatal testing depends on maternal age, the maternal and fetal risk factors in ongoing pregnancy, and gestational age at which prior fetal death occurred. Antepartum testing in women with advanced maternal age and prior stillbirth has decreased the number of stillbirths in subsequent pregnancies.[202] In a study of 300 women with a history of stillbirth in previous pregnancies, Weeks and coworkers[203] started antepartum surveillance at 32 weeks' gestation for adverse pregnancy

TABLE 33-6 EFFICACY OF PHARMACOLOGIC THERAPIES FOR RECURRENT PREGNANCY LOSS AND FETAL DEMISE

Pharmacotherapy	Statistical Significance (95% CI)	Reference
Progesterone	OR = 0.39 (0.17-0.91)	201
Aspirin	RR = 1.00 (0.78-1.29)	210
Intravenous immune globulin	OR = 0.98 (0.45-2.13)	94
Paternal leukocyte immunization	OR = 1.05 (0.75-1.47)	94

outcomes and abnormal antepartum test results. They had only one stillbirth in the cohort group. The study authors concluded that antepartum surveillance of healthy pregnant women with a history of stillbirth should begin by 32 weeks' gestation.[203] Surveillance may be started earlier for women with fetal growth restriction or those who have chronic medical diseases such as hypertension. It should include a twice-weekly nonstress test, amniotic fluid index, and biophysical profile. Similarly, ultrasound scans to evaluate growth should be carried out at intervals of 2 weeks. Fetal kick counts should start at 28 weeks' gestation in this group of women. ACOG guidelines also recommend that antepartum surveillance should start at 32 weeks' gestation. There may be a role for elective induction at the completion of 39 weeks' gestation or at 37 to 38 weeks after fetal lung maturity is documented by amniocentesis.

Conclusion

Embryonic and fetal demise are catastrophic events in a couple's lives. Although there may be no optimal workup for determining the cause of fetal demise, investigations such as fetal autopsy, karyotyping the parents and fetus, placental evaluation, and maternal serology for syphilis and antibody screening may provide answers in most cases. Screening for antiphospholipid antibodies is recommended for embryonic and fetal losses. For fetal losses, screening for inherited thrombophilia and antiphospholipid antibodies is recommended in the event that results of the first-tier tests are inconclusive.

References

1. Rai R, Regan L: Recurrent miscarriage. Lancet 368:601-611, 2006.
2. Stirrat GM: Recurrent miscarriage. Lancet 336:673-675, 1990.
3. Stephenson MD, Awartani KA, Robinson WP: Cytogenetic analysis of miscarriages from couples with recurrent miscarriage: A case-control study. Hum Reprod 17:446-451, 2002.
4. Greenwold N, Jauniaux E: Collection of villous tissue under ultrasound guidance to improve the cytogenetic study of early pregnancy failure. Hum Reprod 17:452-456, 2002.
5. Wilcox AJ, Weinberg CR, O'Connor JF, et al: Incidence of early loss of pregnancy. N Engl J Med 319:189-194, 1988.
6. Chard T: Frequency of implantation and early pregnancy loss in natural cycles. Baillieres Clin Obstet Gynaecol 5:179-189, 1991.
7. Regan L: Recurrent miscarriage. BMJ 302:543-544, 1991.
8. Klentzeris LD: The role of endometrium in implantation. Hum Reprod 12(Suppl):170-175, 1997.
9. Enders AC: Trophoblast-uterine interactions in the first days of implantation: Models for the study of implantation events in the human. Semin Reprod Med 18:255-263, 2000.
10. Vitiello D, Patrizio P: Implantation and early embryonic development: Implications for pregnancy. Semin Perinatol 31:204-207, 2007.
11. Serle E, Aplin JD, Li TC, et al: Endometrial differentiation in the peri-implantation phase of women with recurrent miscarriage: A morphological and immunohistochemical study. Fertil Steril 62:989-996, 1994.
12. Norwitz ER, Schust DJ, Fisher SJ: Implantation and the survival of early pregnancy. N Engl J Med 345:1400-1408, 2001.
13. Choudhury SR, Knapp LA: Human reproductive failure. I. Immunological factors. Hum Reprod Update 7:113-134, 2001.
14. Barnea ER: Applying embryo-derived immune tolerance to the treatment of immune disorders. Ann N Y Acad Sci 1110:602-618, 2007.
15. Bates MD, Quenby S, Takakuwa K, et al: Aberrant cytokine production by peripheral blood mononuclear cells in recurrent pregnancy loss? Hum Reprod 17:2439-2444, 2002.
16. Fuzzi B, Rizzo R, Criscuoli L, et al: HLA-G expression in early embryos is a fundamental prerequisite for the obtainment of pregnancy. Eur J Immunol 32:311-315, 2002.
17. Jurisicova A, Casper RF, MacLusky NJ, Librach CL: Embryonic human leukocyte antigen-G expression: Possible implications for human preimplantation development. Fertil Steril 65:997-1002, 1996.
18. Sher G, Keskintepe L, Ginsburg M: sHLA-G expression: Is it really worth measuring? Reprod Biomed Online 14:9-10, 2007.
19. Sher G, Keskintepe L, Batzofin J, et al: Influence of early ICSI-derived embryo sHLA-G expression on pregnancy and implantation rates: A prospective study. Hum Reprod 20:1359-1363, 2005.
20. Sageshima N, Shobu T, Awai K, et al: Soluble HLA-G is absent from human embryo cultures: A reassessment of sHLA-G detection methods. J Reprod Immunol 75:11-22, 2005.
21. Van Lierop MJ, Wijnands F, Loke YW, et al: Detection of HLA-G by a specific sandwich ELISA using monoclonal antibodies G233 and 56B. Mol Hum Reprod 8:776-784, 2002.
22. Bainbridge D, Ellis S, Le Bouteiller P, Sargent I: HLA-G remains a mystery. Trends Immunol 22:548-552, 2001.
23. Kalousek DK: Two different pregnancy outcomes of trisomic zygote rescue through postzygotic mitotic error. Birth Defects Orig Artic Ser 30:295-299, 1996.
24. Strom CM, Ginsberg N, Applebaum M, et al: Analyses of 95 first-trimester spontaneous abortions by chorionic villus sampling and karyotype. J Assist Reprod Genet 9:458-461, 1992.
25. Pauli RM, Reiser CA, Lebovitz RM, Kirkpatrick SJ: Wisconsin Stillbirth Service Program. I. Establishment and assessment of a community-based program for etiologic investigation of intrauterine deaths. Am J Med Genet 50:116-134, 1994.
26. Hu X, Roberts JR, Apopa PL, et al: Accelerated ovarian failure induced by 4-vinyl cyclohexene diepoxide in Nrf2 null mice. Mol Cell Biol 26:940-954, 2006.
27. Warburton D: The effect of maternal age on the frequency of trisomy: Change in meiosis or in utero selection? Prog Clin Biol Res 311:165-181, 1989.
28. Freeman SB, Yang Q, Allran K, et al: Women with a reduced ovarian complement may have an increased risk for a child with Down syndrome. Am J Hum Genet 66:1680-1683, 2000.
29. Keefe DL, Franco S, Liu L, et al: Telomere length predicts embryo fragmentation after in vitro fertilization in women—toward a telomere theory of reproductive aging in women. Am J Obstet Gynecol 192:1256-1260, 2005.
30. Liu L, Blasco M, Keefe DL: Requirement of functional telomeres for metaphase chromosome alignments and integrity of meiotic spindles. EMBO Rep 3:230-234, 2002.
31. Platteau P, Staessen C, Michiels A, et al: Preimplantation genetic diagnosis for aneuploidy screening in women older than 37 years. Fertil Steril 84:319-324, 2005.
32. Rubio C, Rodrigo L, Perez-Cano I, et al: FISH screening of aneuploidies in preimplantation embryos to improve IVF outcome. Reprod Biomed Online 11:497-506, 2005.
33. Rubio C, Pehlivan T, Rodrigo L, et al: Embryo aneuploidy screening for unexplained recurrent miscarriage: A minireview. Am J Reprod Immunol 53:159-165, 2005.
34. George L, Mills JL, Johansson AL, et al: Plasma folate levels and risk of spontaneous abortion. JAMA 288:1867-1873, 2002.
35. Nelen WL, Blom HJ, Steegers EA, et al: Hyperhomocysteinemia and recurrent early pregnancy loss: A meta-analysis. Fertil Steril 74:1196-1199, 2000.
36. Sachs ES, Jahoda MG, Van Hemel JO, et al: Chromosome studies of 500 couples with two or more abortions. Obstet Gynecol 65:375-378, 1985.
37. Toncheva D: Fragile sites and spontaneous abortions. Genet Couns 2:205-210, 1991.
38. Giardino D, Bettio D, Simoni G: 12q13 Fragility in a family with recurrent spontaneous abortions: Expression of the fragile site under different culture conditions. Ann Genet 33:88-91, 1990.

39. Wolf GC, Mao J, Izquierdo L, Joffe G: Paternal pericentric inversion of chromosome 4 as a cause of recurrent pregnancy loss. J Med Genet 31:153-155, 1994.
40. Turczynowicz S, Sharma P, Smith A, Davidson AA: Paracentric inversion of chromosome 14 plus rare 9p variant in a couple with habitual spontaneous abortion. Ann Genet 35:58-60, 1992.
41. Clifford K, Rai R, Watson H, Regan L: An informative protocol for the investigation of recurrent miscarriage: Preliminary experience of 500 consecutive cases. Hum Reprod 9:1328-1332, 1994.
42. Munne S, Escudero T, Sandalinas M, et al: Gamete segregation in female carriers of Robertsonian translocations. Cytogenet Cell Genet 90:303-308, 2000.
43. Braude P, Pickering S, Flinter F, Ogilvie CM: Preimplantation genetic diagnosis. Nat Rev Genet 3:941-953, 2002.
44. Wapner RJ, Lewis D: Genetics and metabolic causes of stillbirth. Semin Perinatol 26:70-74, 2002.
45. Schatz F, Krikun G, Caze R, et al: Progestin-regulated expression of tissue factor in decidual cells: Implications in endometrial hemostasis, menstruation and angiogenesis. Steroids 68:849-860, 2003.
46. Choi BC, Polgar K, Xiao L, Hill JA: Progesterone inhibits in-vitro embryotoxic Th1 cytokine production to trophoblast in women with recurrent pregnancy loss. Hum Reprod 15(Suppl 1):46-59, 2000.
47. Nardo LG, Sallam HN: Progesterone supplementation to prevent recurrent miscarriage and to reduce implantation failure in assisted reproduction cycles. Reprod Biomed Online 13:47-57, 2006.
48. Jones GS: Some newer aspects of the management of infertility. JAMA 141:1123-1129, 1949.
49. Csapo AI, Pulkkinen M: Indispensability of the human corpus luteum in the maintenance of early pregnancy. Luteectomy evidence. Obstet Gynecol Surv 33:69-81, 1978.
50. Peyron R, Aubeny E, Targosz V, et al: Early termination of pregnancy with mifepristone (RU 486) and the orally active prostaglandin misoprostol. N Engl J Med 328:1509-1513, 1993.
51. Noyes RW, Haman JO. Accuracy of endometrial dating; correlation of endometrial dating with basal body temperature and menses. Fertil Steril 4:504-517, 1953.
52. Roberts CP, Murphy AA: Endocrinopathies associated with recurrent pregnancy loss. Semin Reprod Med 18:357-362, 2000.
53. Peters AJ, Lloyd RP, Coulam CB: Prevalence of out-of-phase endometrial biopsy specimens. Am J Obstet Gynecol 166(Pt 1):1738-1745; discussion 1745-1746, 1992.
54. Daly DC, Walters CA, Soto-Albors CE, Riddick DH: Endometrial biopsy during treatment of luteal phase defects is predictive of therapeutic outcome. Fertil Steril 40:305-310, 1983.
55. Balasch J, Ballesca JL, Fabregues F, et al: Transvaginal intratubal insemination, ectopic pregnancy and treatment by single-dose parenteral methotrexate. Hum Reprod 7:1457-1460, 1992.
56. Tyack AJ, Lambadarios C, Parsons RJ, et al: Plasma progesterone and oestradiol-17beta changes during abortion induced by prostaglandin F2alpha. J Obstet Gynaecol Br Commonw 81:52-56, 1874.
57. American College of Obstetricians and Gynecologists. Management of recurrent pregnancy loss. ACOG practice bulletin no. 24, February 2001. Int J Gynaecol Obstet 78:179-190, 2002.
58. Montoro M, Collea JV, Frasier SD, Mestman JH: Successful outcome of pregnancy in women with hypothyroidism. Ann Intern Med 94:31-34, 1981.
59. Stagnaro-Green A, Roman SH, Cobin RH, et al: Detection of at-risk pregnancy by means of highly sensitive assays for thyroid autoantibodies. JAMA 264:1422-1425, 1990.
60. Glinoer D, Soto MF, Bourdoux P, et al: Pregnancy in patients with mild thyroid abnormalities: Maternal and neonatal repercussions. J Clin Endocrinol Metab 73:421-427, 1991.
61. Rushworth FH, Backos M, Rai R, et al: Prospective pregnancy outcome in untreated recurrent miscarriers with thyroid autoantibodies. Hum Reprod 15:1637-1639, 2000.
62. Pratt DE, Kaberlein G, Dudkiewicz A, et al: The association of antithyroid antibodies in euthyroid nonpregnant women with recurrent first trimester abortions in the next pregnancy. Fertil Steril 60:1001-1005, 1993.
63. Pratt D, Novotny M, Kaberlein G, et al: Antithyroid antibodies and the association with non-organ-specific antibodies in recurrent pregnancy loss. Am J Obstet Gynecol 168(Pt 1):837-841, 1993.
64. Rai R, Backos M, Rushworth F, Regan L: Polycystic ovaries and recurrent miscarriage—a reappraisal. Hum Reprod 15:612-615, 2000.
65. Clifford K, Rai R, Watson H, et al: Does suppressing luteinising hormone secretion reduce the miscarriage rate? Results of a randomised controlled trial. BMJ 312:1508-1511, 1996.
66. Craig LB, Ke RW, Kutteh WH: Increased prevalence of insulin resistance in women with a history of recurrent pregnancy loss. Fertil Steril 78:487-490, 2002.
67. Glueck CJ, Awadalla SG, Phillips H, et al: Polycystic ovary syndrome, infertility, familial thrombophilia, familial hypofibrinolysis, recurrent loss of in vitro fertilized embryos, and miscarriage. Fertil Steril 74:394-397, 2000.
68. Regan L, Carrington B, Rasul S, et al: Polycystic ovaries, insulin resistance, hypofibrinolysis, and recurrent miscarriage [abstract 20]. Reprod Sci 12:91A-92A, 2005.
69. Glueck CJ, Wang P, Goldenberg N, Sieve-Smith L: Pregnancy outcomes among women with polycystic ovary syndrome treated with metformin. Hum Reprod 17:2858-2864, 2002.
70. Legro RS, Barnhart HX, Schlaff WD, et al, for the Cooperative Multicenter Reproductive Medicine Network: Clomiphene, metformin, or both for infertility in the polycystic ovary syndrome. N Engl J Med 356:551-566, 2007.
71. Hirahara F, Andoh N, Sawai K, et al: Hyperprolactinemic recurrent miscarriage and results of randomized bromocriptine treatment trials. Fertil Steril 70:246-252, 1998.
72. Baek KH, Choi BC, Lee JH, et al: Comparison of gene expression at the feto-maternal interface between normal and recurrent pregnancy loss patients. Reprod Fertil Dev 14:235-240, 2002.
73. Richani K, Romero R, Soto E, et al: Unexplained intrauterine fetal death is accompanied by activation of complement. J Perinat Med 33:296-305, 2005.
74. Blackwell S, Romero R, Chaiworapongsa T, et al: Unexplained fetal death is associated with changes in the adaptive limb of the maternal immune response consistent with prior antigenic exposure. J Matern Fetal Neonatal Med 14:241-246, 2003.
75. Devi Wold AS, Arici A: Natural killer cells and reproductive failure. Curr Opin Obstet Gynecol 17:237-241, 2005.
76. Loke YW, King A: Human Implantation: Cell Biology and Immnunology. Cambridge, UK, Cambridge University Press, 1995.
77. King A, Allan DS, Bowen M, et al: HLA-E is expressed on trophoblast and interacts with CD94/NKG2 receptors on decidual NK cells. Eur J Immunol 30:1623-1631, 2000.
78. King A, Burrows TD, Hiby SE, et al: Surface expression of HLA-C antigen by human extravillous trophoblast. Placenta 21:376-387, 2000.
79. Verma S, King A, Loke YW: Expression of killer cell inhibitory receptors on human uterine natural killer cells. Eur J Immunol 27:979-983, 1997.
80. King A, Burrows T, Verma S, et al: Human uterine lymphocytes. Hum Reprod Update 4:480-485, 1998.
81. Moffett A, Regan L, Braude P: Natural killer cells, miscarriage, and infertility. BMJ 329:1283-1285, 2004.
82. Cooper MA, Fehniger TA, Turner SC, et al: Human natural killer cells: A unique innate immunoregulatory role for the CD56(bright) subset. Blood 97:3146-3151, 2001.
83. Koopman LA, Kopcow HD, Rybalov B, et al: Human decidual natural killer cells are a unique NK cell subset with immunomodulatory potential. J Exp Med 198:1201-1212, 2003.
84. Jones RL, Hannan NJ, Kaitu'u TJ, et al: Identification of chemokines important for leukocyte recruitment to the human endometrium at the times of embryo implantation and menstruation.J Clin Endocrinol Metab 89:6155-6167, 2004.

85. Trundley A, Moffett A: Human uterine leukocytes and pregnancy. Tissue Antigens 63:1-12, 2004.
86. Shakhar K, Ben-Eliyahu S, Loewenthal R, et al: Differences in number and activity of peripheral natural killer cells in primary versus secondary recurrent miscarriage. Fertil Steril 80:368-375, 2003.
87. Yamada H, Morikawa M, Kato EH, et al: Pre-conceptional natural killer cell activity and percentage as predictors of biochemical pregnancy and spontaneous abortion with normal chromosome karyotype. Am J Reprod Immunol 50:351-354, 2003.
88. Aoki K, Kajiura S, Matsumoto Y, et al: Preconceptional natural-killer-cell activity as a predictor of miscarriage. Lancet 345:1340-1342, 1995.
89. Beer AE, Kwak JY, Ruiz JE: Immunophenotypic profiles of peripheral blood lymphocytes in women with recurrent pregnancy losses and in infertile women with multiple failed in vitro fertilization cycles. Am J Reprod Immunol 35:376-382, 1996.
90. Shimada S, Nishida R, Takeda M, et al: Natural killer, natural killer T, helper and cytotoxic T cells in the decidua from sporadic miscarriage. Am J Reprod Immunol 56:193-200, 2006.
91. Hanna J, Goldman-Wohl D, Hamani Y, et al: Decidual NK cells regulate key developmental processes at the human fetal-maternal interface. Nat Med 12:1065-1074, 2006.
92. Hiby SE, Walker JJ, O'shaughnessy KM, et al: Combinations of maternal KIR and fetal HLA-C genes influence the risk of preeclampsia and reproductive success. J Exp Med 200:957-965, 2004.
93. Morikawa M, Yamada H, Kato EH, et al: Massive intravenous immunoglobulin treatment in women with four or more recurrent spontaneous abortions of unexplained etiology: Down regulation of NK cell activity and subsets. Am J Reprod Immunol 46:399-404, 2001.
94. Scott JR: Immunotherapy for recurrent miscarriage Cochrane Database Syst Rev (1):CD000112, 2003.
95. Porter TF, LaCoursiere Y, Scott JR: Immunotherapy for recurrent miscarriage. Cochrane Database Syst Rev (2):CD000112, 2006.
96. Ober C, Karrison T, Odem RR, et al: Mononuclear-cell immunisation in prevention of recurrent miscarriages: A randomised trial. Lancet 354:365-369, 1999.
97. Ben Rafael Z, Seidman DS, Recabi K, et al: Uterine anomalies. A retrospective, matched, control study. J Reprod Med 36:723-727, 1991.
98. Stein AL, March CM: Pregnancy outcome in women with mullerian duct anomalies. J Reprod Med 35:411-414, 1990.
99. Salim R, Regan L, Woelfer B, et al: A comparative study of the morphology of congenital uterine anomalies in women with and without a history of recurrent first trimester miscarriage. Hum Reprod 18:162-166, 2003.
100. Raga F, Bauset C, Remohi J, et al: Reproductive impact of congenital mullerian anomalies. Hum Reprod 12:2277-2281, 1997.
101. Devi Wold AS, Pham N, Arici A: Anatomic factors in recurrent pregnancy loss. Semin Reprod Med 24:25-32, 2006.
102. Daly DC, Maier D, Soto-Albors C: Hysteroscopic metroplasty: Six years' experience. Obstet Gynecol 73:201-205, 1989.
103. De Cherney AH, Russell JB, Graebe RA, Polan ML: Resectoscopic management of mullerian fusion defect. Fertil Steril 45:726-728, 1986.
104. Vergani P, Ghidini A, Strobelt N, et al: Do uterine leiomyomas influence pregnancy outcome? Am J Perinatol 11:356-358, 1994.
105. Bajeckal N, Li TC: Fibroids, infertility and pregnancy wastage. Hum Reprod 6:614-620, 2000.
106. Simpson JL: Submucous myomas. Clin Obstet Gynecol 50:10-30, 2007.
107. Fernandez H, Sefrioui O, Virelizier C, et al: Hysteroscopic resection of submucosal myomas in patients with infertility. Hum Reprod 6:1489-1492, 2001.
108. Hartmann KE, Herring AH, Savitz DA: Predictors of the presence of uterine fibroids in the first trimester of pregnancy: A prospective cohort study [abstract 789]. J Soc Gynecol Investig 11:340A, 2004.
109. Sanders B: Uterine factors and infertility. J Reprod Med 51:169-176, 2006.
110. Simpson JL: Causes of fetal wastage. Clin Obstet Gynecol 50:10-30, 2007.
111. Petitti DB: The epidemiology of fetal death. Clin Obstet Gynecol 30:253-258, 1987.
112. MacDorman MF, Hoyert DL, Martin JA, et al: Fetal and perinatal mortality, United States, 2003. Natl Vital Stat Rep 55:1-17, 2007.
113. Ferguson R, Myers SA: Population study of the risk of fetal death and its relationship to birthweight, gestational age, and race. Am J Perinatol 11:267-272, 1994.
114. Getahun D, Ananth CV, Selvam N, Demissie K: Adverse perinatal outcomes among interracial couples in the United States. Obstet Gynecol 106:81-88, 2005.
115. Smulian JC, Ananth CV, Vintzileos AM, et al: Fetal deaths in the United States: Influence of high-risk conditions and implications for management. Obstet Gynecol 100:1183-1189, 2002.
116. Ngoc NT, Merialdi M, Abdel-Aleem H, et al: Causes of stillbirths and early neonatal deaths: Data from 7993 pregnancies in six developing countries. Bull World Health Organ 84:699-705, 2006.
117. Goyaux N, Alihonou E, Diadhiou F, et al: Complications of induced abortion and miscarriage in three African countries: A hospital-based study among WHO collaborating centers. Acta Obstet Gynecol Scand 80:568-573, 2001.
118. Reddy UM, Ko CW, Willinger M: Maternal age and the risk of stillbirth throughout pregnancy in the United States. Am J Obstet Gynecol 195:764-770, 2006.
119. Canterino JC, Ananth CV, Smulian J, et al: Maternal age and risk of fetal death in singleton gestations: USA, 1995-2000. J Matern Fetal Neonatal Med 15:193-197, 2004.
120. Hoffman MC, Jeffers S, Carter J, et al: Pregnancy at or beyond age 40 years is associated with an increased risk of fetal death and other adverse outcomes. Am J Obstet Gynecol 196:e11-e13, 2007.
121. Cnattingius S, Forman MR, Berendes HW, Isotalo L: Delayed childbearing and risk of adverse perinatal outcome. A population-based study. JAMA 268:886-890, 1992.
122. Stephansson O, Dickman PW, Johansson A, Cnattingius S: Maternal hemoglobin concentration during pregnancy and risk of stillbirth. JAMA 284:2611-2617, 2000.
123. Froen JF, Arnestad M, Frey K, et al: Risk factors for sudden intrauterine unexplained death: Epidemiologic characteristics of singleton cases in Oslo, Norway, 1986-1995. Am J Obstet Gynecol 184:694-702, 2001.
124. Hardy JB: Fetal consequences of maternal viral infections in pregnancy. Arch Otolaryngol 98:218-227, 1973.
125. Horn P: Pregnancy complicated by anterior poliomyelitis; experience in Los Angeles County Hospital with report of 180 consecutive cases. Ann West Med Surg 5:93-108, 1951.
126. Rogerson SJ, Hviid L, Duffy PE, et al: Malaria in pregnancy: Pathogenesis and immunity. Lancet Infect Dis 7:105-117, 2007.
127. Copper RL, Goldenberg RL, DuBard MB, Davis RO: Risk factors for fetal death in white, black, and Hispanic women. Collaborative Group on Preterm Birth Prevention. Obstet Gynecol 84:490-495, 1994.
128. Gust DA, Levine WC, St Louis ME, et al: Mortality associated with congenital syphilis in the United States, 1992-1998. Pediatrics 109:E79, 2002.
129. Wilkinson D, Sach M, Connolly C: Epidemiology of syphilis in pregnancy in rural South Africa: Opportunities for control. Trop Med Int Health 2:57-62, 1997.
130. Nathan L, Bohman VR, Sanchez PJ, et al: In utero infection with *Treponema pallidum* in early pregnancy. Prenat Diagn 17:119-123, 1997.
131. Elliott DJ, Eppes SC, Klein JD: Teratogen update: Lyme disease. Teratology 64:276-281, 2001.
132. Fretts RC: Etiology and prevention of stillbirth. Am J Obstet Gynecol 193:1923-1935, 2005.
133. Lecuit M: Understanding how *Listeria monocytogenes* targets and crosses host barriers. Clin Microbiol Infect 11:430-436, 2005.
134. Enders M, Weidner A, Zoellner I, et al: Fetal morbidity and mortality after acute human parvovirus B19 infection in pregnancy: Prospective evaluation of 1018 cases. Prenat Diagn 24:513-518, 2004.
135. Brown KE: What threat is human parvovirus B19 to the fetus? A review. BJOG 96:764-767, 1989.

136. Frisk G, Diderholm H: Increased frequency of coxsackie B virus IgM in women with spontaneous abortion. J Infect 24:141-145, 1992.
137. Brady WK, Purdon A Jr: Intrauterine fetal demise associated with enterovirus infection. South Med J 79:770-772, 1986.
138. Fowler KB, Stagno S, Pass RF, et al: The outcome of congenital cytomegalovirus infection in relation to maternal antibody status. N Engl J Med 326:663-667, 1992.
139. Nigro G, Adler SP, La Torre R, Best AM: Passive immunization during pregnancy for congenital cytomegalovirus infection. N Engl J Med 353:1350-1362, 2005.
140. Facchinetti F, Marozio L, Grandone E, et al: Thrombophilic mutations are a main risk factor for placental abruption. Haematologica 88:785-788, 2003.
141. Ray JG, Vermeulen MJ, Schull MJ, Redelmeier DA: Cardiovascular Health After Maternal Placental Syndromes (CHAMPS): Population-based retrospective cohort study. Lancet 366:1797-1803, 2005.
142. Giacoia GP: Severe fetomaternal hemorrhage: A review. Obstet Gynecol Surv 52:372-380, 1997.
143. Savithrisowmya S, Singh M, Kriplani A, et al: Assessment of fetomaternal hemorrhage by flow cytometry and Kleihauer-Betke test in Rh-negative pregnancies. Gynecol Obstet Invest 65:84-88, 2007.
144. Cosmi E, Saccardi C, Mari G: Non-invasive diagnosis of fetomaternal hemorrhage by Doppler assessment of the middle cerebral artery peak systolic velocity: A longitudinal prospective study [abstract P51.01]. Ultrasound Obstet Gynecol 30:648, 2007.
145. Weisberg L, Kingdom J, Keating S, et al: Treatment options in fetomaternal hemorrhage: Four case studies. J Obstet Gynaecol Can 26:893-898, 2004.
146. Rubod C, Deruelle P, Le Goueff F, et al: Long-term prognosis for infants after massive fetomaternal hemorrhage. Obstet Gynecol 110(Pt 1):256-260, 2007.
147. Ananth CV, Savitz DA, Bowes WA Jr: Hypertensive disorders of pregnancy and stillbirth in North Carolina, 1988 to 1991. Acta Obstet Gynecol Scand 74:788-793, 1995.
148. Morrison I, Olsen J: Weight-specific stillbirths and associated causes of death: An analysis of 765 stillbirths. Am J Obstet Gynecol 152:975-980, 1985.
149. Getahun D, Ananth CV, Kinzler WL: Risk factors for antepartum and intrapartum stillbirth: A population-based study. Am J Obstet Gynecol 196:499-507, 2007.
150. Yadav S, Saxena U, Yadav R, Gupta S: Hypertensive disorders of pregnancy and maternal and foetal outcome: A case controlled study. J Indian Med Assoc 95:548-551, 1997.
151. Martin JN Jr, Rinehart BK, May WL, et al: The spectrum of severe preeclampsia: Comparative analysis by HELLP (hemolysis, elevated liver enzyme levels, and low platelet count) syndrome classification. Am J Obstet Gynecol 180(Pt 1):1373-1384, 1999.
152. Sibai BM, Abdella TN, Anderson GD: Pregnancy outcome in 211 patients with mild chronic hypertension. Obstet Gynecol 1983;61:571-576, 1983.
153. Gaugler-Senden IP, Huijssoon AG, Visser W, et al: Maternal and perinatal outcome of preeclampsia with an onset before 24 weeks' gestation. Audit in a tertiary referral center. Eur J Obstet Gynecol Reprod Biol 128:216-221, 2006.
154. Ronsmans C: Maternal mortality: Who, when, where, and why. Lancet 368:1189-1200, 2006.
155. Andrews WW, Cox SM, Sherman ML, Leveno KJ: Maternal and perinatal effects of hypertension at term. J Reprod Med 37:73-76, 1992.
156. Mondestin MA, Ananth CV, Smulian JC, Vintzileos AM: Birth weight and fetal death in the United States: The effect of maternal diabetes during pregnancy. Am J Obstet Gynecol 187:922-926, 2002.
157. Cundy T, Gamble G, Townend K, et al: Perinatal mortality in type 2 diabetes mellitus. Diabet Med 17:33-39, 2000.
158. Bradley RJ, Brudenell JM, Nicolaides KH: Fetal acidosis and hyperlacticaemia diagnosed by cordocentesis in pregnancies complicated by maternal diabetes mellitus. Diabet Med 8:464-468, 1991.
159. Yoon BH, Romero R, Roh CR, et al: Relationship between the fetal biophysical profile score, umbilical artery Doppler velocimetry, and fetal blood acid-base status determined by cordocentesis. Am J Obstet Gynecol 169:1586-1589, 1993.
160. Flegal KM, Carroll MD, Ogden CL, Johnson CL: Prevalence and trends in obesity among US adults, 1999-2000. JAMA 288:1723-1727, 2002.
161. Chu SY, Kim SY, Lau J, et al: Maternal obesity and risk of stillbirth: A metaanalysis. Am J Obstet Gynecol 197:223-228, 2007.
162. Stone JL, Lockwood CJ, Berkowitz GS, et al: Risk factors for severe preeclampsia. Obstet Gynecol 83:357-361, 1994.
163. Luke B, Brown MB: The changing risk of infant mortality by gestation, plurality, and race: 1989-1991 versus 1999-2001. Pediatrics 118:2488-2497, 2006.
164. Fries MH, Goldstein RB, Kilpatrick SJ, et al: The role of velamentous cord insertion in the etiology of twin-twin transfusion syndrome. Obstet Gynecol 81:569-574, 1993.
165. de Groot PG, Horbach DA, Derksen RH: Protein C and other cofactors involved in the binding of antiphospholipid antibodies: Relation to the pathogenesis of thrombosis. Lupus 5:488-493, 1996.
166. Roque H, Paidas MJ, Funai EF, et al: Maternal thrombophilias are not associated with early pregnancy loss. Thromb Haemost 91:290-295, 2004.
167. Lockwood CJ: Inherited thrombophilias in pregnant patients: Detection and treatment paradigm. Obstet Gynecol 99:333-341, 2002.
168. Rey E, Kahn SR, David M, Shrier I: Thrombophilic disorders and fetal loss: A meta-analysis. Lancet 361:901-908, 2003.
169. Preston FE, Rosendaal FR, Walker ID, et al: Increased fetal loss in women with heritable thrombophilia. Lancet 348:913-916, 1996.
170. Lindqvist PG, Svensson P, Dahlback B: Activated protein C resistance—in the absence of factor V Leiden—and pregnancy. J Thromb Haemost 4:361-366, 2006.
171. Lockwood CJ: Heritable coagulopathies in pregnancy. Obstet Gynecol Surv 54:754-765, 1999.
172. Dekker JW, Lind J, Bloemenkamp KW, et al: Inherited risk of thrombosis of the fetus and intrauterine fetal death. Eur J Obstet Gynecol Reprod Biol 117:45-48, 2004.
173. Rai RS, Regan L, Chitolie A, et al: Placental thrombosis and second trimester miscarriage in association with activated protein C resistance. BJOG 103:842-844, 1996.
174. Rodger MA, Paidas M: Do thrombophilias cause placenta-mediated pregnancy complications? Semin Thromb Hemost 33:597-603, 2007.
175. Sharma PP, Salihu HM, Kirby RS: Stillbirth recurrence in a population of relatively low-risk mothers. Paediatr Perinat Epidemiol 21(Suppl 1):24-30, 2007.
176. Sharma PP, Salihu HM, Oyelese Y, et al: Is race a determinant of stillbirth recurrence? Obstet Gynecol 107(Pt 1):391-397, 2006.
177. Coppens M, Folkeringa N, Teune MJ, et al: Outcome of the subsequent pregnancy after a first loss in women with the factor V Leiden or prothrombin 20210A mutations. J Thromb Haemost 5:1444-1448, 2007.
178. Brookes JS, Hagmann C: MRI in fetal necropsy. J Magn Reson Imaging 24:1221-1228, 2006.
179. Dizon-Townson DS, Meline L, Nelson LM, et al: Fetal carriers of the factor V Leiden mutation are prone to miscarriage and placental infarction. Am J Obstet Gynecol 177:402-405, 1997.
180. Huestis MA, Choo RE: Drug abuse's smallest victims: In utero drug exposure. Forensic Sci Int 128:20-30, 2002.
181. Ornoy A: The effects of alcohol and illicit drugs on the human embryo and fetus. Isr J Psychiatry Relat Sci 39:120-132, 2002.
182. Perlmutter JF: Heroin addiction and pregnancy. Obstet Gynecol Surv 29:439-446, 1974.
183. Heinonen S, Kirkinen P: Pregnancy outcome after previous stillbirth resulting from causes other than maternal conditions and fetal abnormalities. Birth 27:33-37, 2000.
184. Maslow AD, Breen TW, Sarna MC, et al: Prevalence of coagulation abnormalities associated with intrauterine fetal death. Can J Anaesth 43:1237-1243, 1996.

185. Duchinski T, Pisarek-Miedzinska D, Szczepanski M: Hemostatic variables in patients with intrauterine fetal death. Int J Gynaecol Obstet 42:3-7, 1993.
186. Kulier R, Gulmezoglu AM, Hofmeyr GJ, et al: Medical methods for first trimester abortion. Cochrane Database Syst Rev (2):CD002855, 2004.
187. Wagaarachchi PT, Ashok PW, Narvekar NN, et al: Medical management of late intrauterine death using a combination of mifepristone and misoprostol. BJOG 109:443-447, 2002.
188. Fairley TE, Mackenzie M, Owen P, Mackenzie F: Management of late intrauterine death using a combination of mifepristone and misoprostol—experience of two regimens. Eur J Obstet Gynecol Reprod Biol 118:28-31, 2005.
189. Neilson JP, Hickey M, Vazquez J: Medical treatment for early fetal death (less than 24 weeks). Cochrane Database Syst Rev (3):CD002253, 2006.
190. Senior J, Marshall K, Sangha R, Clayton JK: In vitro characterization of prostanoid receptors on human myometrium at term pregnancy. Br J Pharmacol 108:501-506, 1993.
191. Henriques A, Lourenco AV, Ribeirinho A, et al: Maternal death related to misoprostol overdose. Obstet Gynecol 109(Pt2):489-490, 2007.
192. Duley L, Henderson-Smart DJ, Meher S, King JF: Antiplatelet agents for preventing pre-eclampsia and its complications. Cochrane Database Syst Rev (2):CD004659, 2007.
193. Tulppala M, Marttunen M, Söderstrom-Anttila V, et al: Low-dose aspirin in prevention of miscarriage in women with unexplained or autoimmune related recurrent miscarriage: Effect on prostacyclin and thromboxane A_2 production. Hum Reprod 12:1567-1572, 1997.
194. Gris JC, Mercier E, Quere I, et al: Low-molecular-weight heparin versus low-dose aspirin in women with one fetal loss and a constitutional thrombophilic disorder. Blood 103:3695-3699, 2004.
195. Paidas M, Ku DH, Triche E, et al: Does heparin therapy improve pregnancy outcome in patients with thrombophilias? J Thromb Haemost 2:1194-1195, 2004.
196. Brenner B, Hoffman R, Carp H, et al, for the LIVE-ENOX Investigators: Efficacy and safety of two doses of enoxaparin in women with thrombophilia and recurrent pregnancy loss: The LIVE-ENOX study. J Thromb Haemost 3:227-229, 2005.
197. Paidas MJ, Ku DH, Langhoff-Roos J, et al: Inherited thrombophilias and adverse pregnancy outcome: Screening and management. Semin Perinatol 29:150-163, 2005.
198. Duhl AJ, Paidas MJ, Ural SH, et al, for the Pregnancy and Thrombosis Working Group. Antithrombotic therapy and pregnancy: Consensus report and recommendations for prevention and treatment of venous thromboembolism and adverse pregnancy outcomes. Am J Obstet Gynecol 197:457.e1-e21, 2007.
199. Urban G, Vergani P, Tironi R, et al: Antithrombotic prophylaxis in multiparous women with preeclampsia or intrauterine growth retardation in antecedent pregnancy. Int J Fertil Womens Med 52:59-67, 2007.
200. Porter TF, LaCoursiere Y, Scott JR: Immunotherapy for recurrent miscarriage. Cochrane Database Syst Rev (2):CD000112, 2006.
201. Oates-Whitehead RM, Haas DM, Carrier JA: Progestogen for preventing miscarriage. Cochrane Database Syst Rev (4):CD003511, 2003.
202. Fretts RC, Elkin EB, Myers ER, Heffner LJ: Should older women have antepartum testing to prevent unexplained stillbirth? Obstet Gynecol 104:56-64, 2004.
203. Weeks JW, Asrat T, Morgan MA, et al: Antepartum surveillance for a history of stillbirth: When to begin? Am J Obstet Gynecol 172(Pt 1):486-492, 1995.
204. Price DT, Ridker PM: Factor V Leiden mutation and the risks for thromboembolic disease: A clinical perspective. Ann Intern Med 127:895-903, 1997.
205. Samama M, Gerotziafas G, Conard J, et al: Clinical aspects and laboratory problems in hereditary thrombophilia. Haemost 29:76-99, 1999.
206. Langman LJ, Ray JG, Evrovski J, et al: Hyperhomocyst(e)inemia and the increased risk of venous thromboembolism: More evidence from a case-control study. Arch Intern Med 160:961-964, 2000.
207. Goodwin AJ, Rosendaal FR, Kottke-Marchant K, et al: A review of the technical, diagnostic, and epidemiologic considerations for protein S assays. Arch Pathol Lab Med 126:1349-1366, 2002.
208. Paidas MJ, Ku DH, Lee MJ, et al: Protein Z, protein S levels are lower in patients with thrombophilia and subsequent pregnancy complications. J Thromb Haemost 3:497-501, 2005.
209. Vossen CY, Preston FE, Conard J, et al: Hereditary thrombophilia and fetal loss: A prospective follow-up study. J Thromb Haemost 2:592-596, 2004.
210. Di Nisio M, Peters L, Middeldorp S: Anticoagulants for the treatment of recurrent pregnancy loss in women without antiphospholipid syndrome. Cochrane Database Syst Rev 2:CD004734, 2005.

Chapter 34

Intrauterine Growth Restriction

Robert Resnik, MD, and Robert K. Creasy, MD

Human pregnancy, similar to pregnancy in other polytocous animal species, can be affected by conditions that restrict the normal growth of the fetus. The growth-restricted fetus is at higher risk for perinatal morbidity and mortality, the risk rising with the severity of the restriction. This chapter reviews the various causes of fetal growth restriction and considers the methods of antepartum recognition and diagnosis along with clinical management. The term intrauterine growth restriction (IUGR), which we first introduced in the third edition of this text, is preferred over intrauterine growth retardation, which frequently connotes mental retardation to the patient.

Definitions

At the beginning of the 20th century all small newborns were thought to be premature, but by the middle of the century the concept of the undernourished neonate arose, and newborns weighing less than 2500 g were then classified by the World Health Organization as low-birth-weight infants. In the 1960s, Lubchenco, Battaglia and colleagues, in a series of classic papers, published detailed graphs of birth weight as a function of gestational age and associated adverse outcomes.[1,2] It was then suggested to classify low-birth-weight neonates into three groups[2,3]:

1. *Preterm neonates*—newborns delivered before 37 completed weeks of gestation who are of appropriate size for gestational age (AGA)
2. *Preterm and growth-restricted neonates*—newborns delivered before 37 completed weeks of gestation who are small for gestational age (SGA)
3. *Term growth-restricted neonates*—newborns delivered after 37 completed weeks of gestation who are SGA. (Not all SGA term neonates are growth restricted; some cases result from the normal distribution of neonatal weight among a normal base population.)

The classification of newborns by birth weight percentile is of prognostic significance in that those of lower percentiles are at increased risk for immediate perinatal morbidity and mortality, as well as subsequent adult disease.

There is continuing debate as to whether the 10th, 5th, or 3rd birth weight percentile should be used as a cutoff for designation of SGA. The lower the percentile, the higher the risk of poor outcome, but also the greater the chance that a neonate with IUGR and poor outcome will not be detected. The *population*-based growth curves that traditionally have been used in the United States define SGA as a birth weight below the 10th percentile for gestational age. However, it has been shown[4] that mortality for infants with birth weights between the 10th and 15th percentile are still increased, with an odds ratio approaching 2. Conversely, many newborns whose weights are below the 10th percentile are perfectly normal and simply constitutionally small. An alternative approach, which has sound physiologic and epidemiologic rationale, is that of using *customized* rather than population-based fetal growth curves.[5] This concept uses optimal birth weight as the end point of a growth curve; it is based on the ability of a fetus to achieve its growth potential, determined prospectively and independently of maternal pathology. This approach uses the known variables affecting fetal weight, such as maternal height, weight, ethnicity, and parity at the beginning of pregnancy, to calculate fetal weight trajectories and optimal fetal weight at delivery. A recent large Spanish study[6] showed that customized birth weight percentiles more accurately reflect the potential for adverse outcome. Indeed, newborns considered to be of low birth weight by the general standards, but not by the customized percentiles, did very well. These findings were confirmed by studies from New Zealand and France.[7-9] Customized growth charts can be downloaded at Gestation Network (http://www.gestation.net [accessed February 5, 2008]).

The reliance on only gestational age and birth weight also neglects the issue of body size and length and the clinical observations that there are two main clinical types of IUGR newborns: (1) the infant who is of normal length for gestational age but whose birth weight is below normal (asymmetrically small), and (2) the neonate whose length and weight are both below normal (symmetrically small). Many SGA newborns are merely constitutionally smaller than others and are not at increased risk for either early or remote morbidity and mortality.

One method to evaluate this issue is the ponderal index,[10,11] which is calculated from the birth weight (in grams) and the crown-heel length (in centimeters):

$$\text{Ponderal index} = (\text{birth weight})/(\text{crown-heel length})^3 \times 100$$

Neonates with a ponderal index of less than the 10th percentile for gestational age are defined as growth restricted. In term infants, this index is not significantly affected by differences in race or sex. The disadvantage of this index is the potential error introduced by cubing the crown-heel length. It is not clear whether asymmetric IUGR and symmetric IUGR are two distinct entities or are merely reflections of the severity of the growth restriction process (excluding chromosomal aberrations and infectious disease).

There is currently no acceptable means, except perhaps by the ponderal index, to classify a newborn whose weight is more than 2500 g as having IUGR. The newborn who weighs 2800 g at birth may be growth restricted if the mother has had three previous infants weighing more than 3700 g, but the classification systems would place such an infant in the normal growth category.[12]

Rate of Fetal Growth

Different standards for fetal growth throughout gestation have been reported. These standards set the normal range, on the basis of statistical considerations, between 2 standard deviations of the mean (2.5th to 97.5th percentile) or between the 10th and 90th percentiles for fixed gestational ages. The standards most widely used in the United States in the 1960s and 1970s were those developed in Denver, Colorado.[1,2] The Denver standards, however, do not reflect the increase in median birth weight that has occurred over the last 4 decades or the birth weight standards for babies born at sea level. More contemporary standards are available from large geographic regions, such as the state of California, based on data from more than 2 million singleton births between 1970 and 1976.[13] Brenner and colleagues[14] used data on black and white infants from Cleveland and aborted fetuses from North Carolina. Ott[15] studied newborns from St. Louis. Arbuckle and associates[16] based their study on more than 1 million singleton births and more than 10,000 twin gestations in Canada between 1986 and 1988, and Alexander and colleagues[17] used information from 3.8 million births in the United States in 1991. A comparison of their 1991 U.S. national data with that of previous reports (Fig. 34-1) reveals that most of the latter underestimated fetal growth beginning at about 32 weeks. For example, the use of the Colorado[1] or California[13] databases would have resulted in only 2.8% and 7.1% of births, respectively, being classified as below the 10th percentile compared with the 1991 data. The gender-specific 10th percentile values from 20 to 44 weeks are listed in Table 34-1.

Data obtained from study of induced abortions and spontaneous deliveries indicate that the rate of fetal growth increases from 5 g/day at 14 to 15 weeks of gestation to 10 g/day at 20 weeks, and to 30 to 35 g/day at 32 to 34 weeks. The total substrate needs of the fetus are thus relatively small in the first half of pregnancy, after which the rate of weight gain rises precipitously. The mean weight gain peaks at approximately 230 to 285 g/wk at 32 to 34 weeks of gestation, after which it decreases, possibly even reaching zero weight gain, or even weight loss, at 41 to 42 weeks of gestation (Fig. 34-2).[13,17] If growth rate is expressed as the percentage of increase in weight over the previous week, however, the percentage of increase reaches a maximum in the first trimester and decreases steadily thereafter.

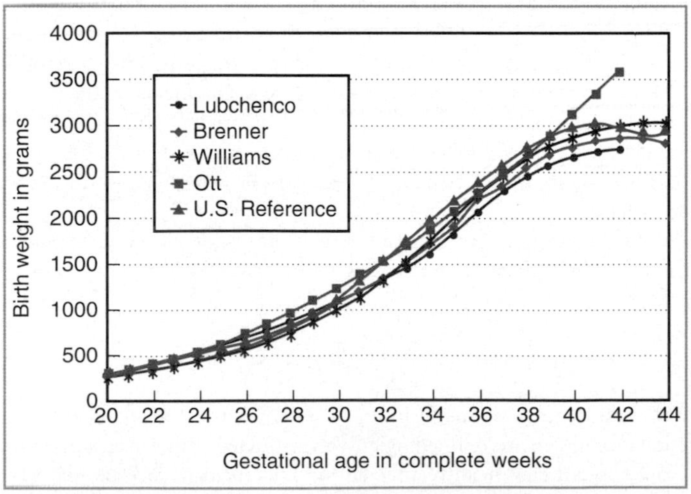

FIGURE 34-1 Fetal weight as a function of gestational age by selected references. (From Alexander GR, Himes JH, Kaufman RB, et al: A United States national reference for fetal growth. Obstet Gynecol 87:167, 1996. Reprinted with permission from the American College of Obstetricians and Gynecologists.)

Incidence of Intrauterine Growth Restriction

The incidence of IUGR varies according to the population under examination, the geographic location, the standard growth curves used as reference, and the percentile chosen to indicate abnormal growth (i.e., the 3rd, 5th, 10th, or 15th).

Approximately one fourth to one third of all infants weighing less than 2500 g at birth have sustained IUGR, and approximately 4% to 8% of all infants born in developed countries and 6% to 30% of those born in developing countries have been classified as growth restricted.[18]

TABLE 34-1 10TH PERCENTILE OF BIRTH WEIGHT (g) FOR GESTATIONAL AGE BY GENDER: UNITED STATES, 1991, SINGLE LIVE BIRTHS TO RESIDENT MOTHERS

Gestational Age (Wk)	Male	Female
20	270	256
21	328	310
22	388	368
23	446	426
24	504	480
25	570	535
26	644	592
27	728	662
28	828	760
29	956	889
30	1117	1047
31	1308	1234
32	1521	1447
33	1751	1675
34	1985	1901
35	2205	2109
36	2407	2300
37	2596	2484
38	2769	2657
39	2908	2796
40	2986	2872
41	3007	2891
42	2998	2884
43	2977	2868
44	2963	2853

From Alexander GR, Himes JH, Kaufman RB, et al: A United States national reference for fetal growth. Obstet Gynecol 87:167, 1996.

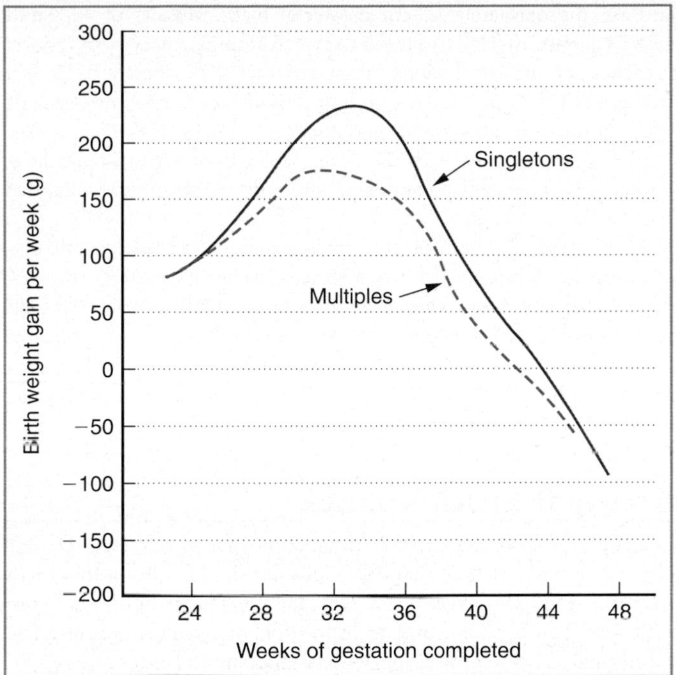

FIGURE 34-2 Median growth rate curves for single and multiple births in California, 1970-1976. (From Williams RL, Creasy RK, Cunningham GC, et al: Fetal growth and perinatal viability in California. Obstet Gynecol 59:624, 1982. Reprinted with permission from the American College of Obstetricians and Gynecologists.)

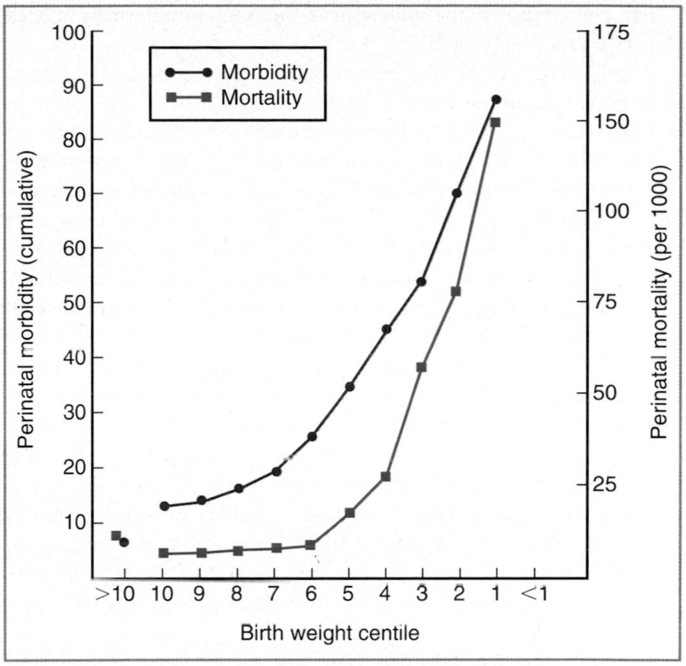

FIGURE 34-3 Morbidity and mortality in 1560 small-for-gestational-age fetuses. (From Manning FA: Intrauterine growth retardation. In Manning FA: Fetal Medicine: Principles and Practice. Norwalk, CT, Appleton & Lange, 1995, p. 312.)

Perinatal Mortality and Morbidity

IUGR is associated with an increase in fetal and neonatal mortality and morbidity rates. Perinatal mortality rates for fetuses and neonates weighing less than the 10th percentile, but between 1500 and 2500 g, were 5 to 30 times greater than those of newborns between the 10th and 90th percentiles; for those weighing less than 1500 g, the rates were 70 to 100 times greater.[13] In addition, for birth weights below the 10th percentile, the fetal and neonatal mortality rates rise as gestation advances if birth weights do not increase.

As depicted in Figure 34-3, Manning showed that perinatal morbidity and mortality increase if birth weights are below the 10th percentile, and markedly so if below the 6th percentile.[19]

In general, fetal mortality rates for IUGR fetuses are 50% higher than neonatal mortality rates, and male fetuses with IUGR have a higher mortality rate than female fetuses. The 10% to 30% increase in incidence of minor and major congenital anomalies associated with IUGR accounts for 30% to 60% of the IUGR perinatal deaths (50% of stillbirths and 20% of neonatal deaths).[20] Infants with symmetric IUGR are more likely to die in association with anomalous development or infection. If, however, in the absence of congenital abnormalities, chromosomal defects, and infection, neonates with symmetric IUGR are probably not at increased risk of neonatal morbidity.[21] The incidence of mortality in the preterm newborn is higher if IUGR is also present.[22] The incidence of intrapartum fetal distress with IUGR approximates 25% to 50%.[23,24]

In addition, IUGR may contribute to perinatal morbidity and mortality by leading to both induced and spontaneous preterm births and the neonatal problems associated with preterm delivery.[25] Specific morbidities are discussed later in this chapter and in Chapter 58.

Long-term sequelae of IUGR, such as various adult diseases including chronic hypertension, heart and lung disease, and type 2 diabetes, are discussed in greater detail in Chapter 59. Lower intelligence quotients, increased mental retardation, and cerebral palsy have also been reported.[26-28]

Etiology of Intrauterine Growth Restriction

IUGR encompasses many different maternal and fetal entities. Some can be detected before birth, whereas others can be found only at autopsy. It is important to discern the cause of IUGR, because in many cases subsequent pregnancies may also be affected.

Genetic Factors

There has been much interest in determining the relative contributions of factors that produce birth weight variation, namely the maternal and fetal genetic factors and the environment of the fetus. Approximately 40% of total birth weight variation is due to the genetic contributions from mother and fetus (approximately half from each), and the other 60% is due to contributions from the fetal environment.[29]

Although both parents' genes affect childhood growth and final adult size, the maternal genes have the main influence on birth weight. The classic horse-pony cross-breeding experiments by Walton and Hammond demonstrated the important role of the mother.[30] Foals of the maternal horse and paternal pony are significantly larger than foals of the maternal pony and paternal horse, and foals of each cross are comparable in size to foals of the pure maternal breed. These results clearly demonstrated the widely held thesis of a maternally related constraint on fetal growth.

Similar conclusions of maternal constraint to growth are reached from family studies in humans. Low and high birth weights recur in families with seemingly otherwise normal pregnancies. Sisters of women with IUGR babies tend to have IUGR babies, a trend that is not seen in their brothers' babies.[31] There is also a greater similarity in birth weight between maternal half siblings and full siblings than between paternal half siblings and full siblings. Mothers of IUGR infants were frequently growth restricted at birth themselves.[32,33] Although the maternal phenotypic expression—particularly maternal height—may affect fetal growth, the evidence for such an influence is not convincing. Social deprivation has also been associated with IUGR, a finding not explained by known physiologic or pathologic factors.[34]

The one definite paternal influence on fetal growth and size at birth is the contribution of a Y chromosome rather than an X chromosome. The male fetus grows more quickly than the female fetus and weighs approximately 150 to 200 g more than the female at birth.[35] There is also a suggestion that paternal size at birth can influence fetal growth, with birth weights potentially increased by 100 to 175 g.[36] Also, the greater the antigenic dissimilarity between the parents, the larger the fetus.

Whether it is genetically determined or not, women who were SGA at birth have double the risk of reduced intrauterine growth in their fetuses.[37] In similar fashion, fetuses destined to deliver preterm have a higher incidence of reduced fetal growth.[25,38] The role of the genetic constitution of mother or fetus in these observations is not clear.

Specific maternal genotypic disorders can cause IUGR, one example being phenylketonuria.[39] Infants born to homozygously affected mothers almost always have IUGR, but whether the reason is an abnormal amount of metabolite crossing from mother to fetus or an inherent problem in the fetus is unknown.

There is a significant association between IUGR and congenital malformations (see later discussion) Such abnormalities can be caused by established chromosomal disorders or by dysmorphic syndromes, such as various forms of dwarfism. Some of these malformations are the expression of a specific gene abnormality with a known inheritance pattern, whereas others are only presumed to be the result of a gene mutation or an adverse environmental influence.

Although in some reports only 2% to 5% of IUGR infants have a chromosomal abnormality, the incidence rises to 20% if IUGR and mental retardation are both present.[40] Birth weights in infants with trisomy 13, 18, and 21 are lower than normal,[41,42] with the decrease in birth weight being less pronounced in trisomy 21. The frequency distribution of birth weights in infants with trisomy 21 is shifted to the left of the normal curve after 34 weeks of gestation, resulting in gestational ages 1 to 1.5 weeks less than normal, and birth weights and lengths are less than in control infants from 34 weeks until term. This effect is more marked after 37 weeks of gestation, but birth weights are still only approximately 1 standard deviation from mean weight. Birth weights in translocation trisomy 21 are comparable to those in primary trisomy 21. Birth weights of newborns who are mosaic for normal and 21-trisomic cells are lower than normal but higher than those of 21-trisomic infants.[29] Newborns with other autosomal abnormalities, such as deletions (chromosomes 4, 5, 13, and 18) and ring chromosome structure alterations, also have had impaired fetal growth.

Although abnormalities of the female (X) and male (Y) sex chromosomes are frequently lethal (80% to 95% result in first-trimester spontaneous abortions), they could be a cause of IUGR in a newborn.[18,28] Infants with XO sex chromosomes have a lower mean birth weight than control infants (approximately 85% of normal for gestational age) and are approximately 1.5 cm shorter at birth. Mosaics of 45,X and 46,XX cells are affected to a lesser degree. Although a paucity of reports prevents definite conclusions, it appears that the repressive effect on fetal growth is increased with the addition of X chromosomes, each of which results in a 200- to 300-g reduction in birth weight.[43]

IUGR is associated with numerous other dysmorphic syndromes, particularly those causing abnormal brain development (see Chapters 1 and 17).

The overall contribution that chromosomal and other genetic disorders make to human IUGR is estimated to be 5% to 20%. Approximately 25% of fetuses with early-onset fetal growth restriction could have chromosomal abnormalities, and karyotyping via cordocentesis can be considered (see Chapter 17). A genetic basis should be considered strongly if IUGR is encountered in association with neurologic impairment or early polyhydramnios.

Congenital Anomalies

In a study of more than 13,000 anomalous infants, 22% had IUGR.[44] Newborns with cardiac malformations are frequently of low birth weight and length for gestation, with the possible exception of those with tetralogy of Fallot and transposition of the great vessels. The subnormal size of many infants with cardiac anomalies (as low as 50% to 80% of normal weight with septal defects) is associated with a subnormal number of parenchymal cells in organs such as the spleen, liver, kidneys, adrenals, and pancreas.[45] The anencephalic fetus is also usually growth restricted.

Approximately 25% of newborns with a single umbilical artery weigh less than 2500 g at birth, and some of these are born preterm.[46] Abnormal umbilical cord insertions into the placenta are also occasionally associated with poor fetal growth.[47] The presence of cord encirclements around the fetal body is also associated with IUGR.[48]

Structural malformations, single umbilical artery, and monozygotic twins are relatively rare and probably account for no more than 1% to 2% of all human instances of IUGR.

Infection

Infectious disease is known to cause IUGR, but the number of organisms having this effect is poorly defined, and the extent of the growth restriction can be variable There is sufficient evidence for a causal relationship between infectious disease and IUGR for two viruses—rubella and cytomegalovirus,[49] and there is evidence for a possible relationship with varicella,[50] severe herpes zoster, and human immunodeficiency virus (HIV) infection, although the latter may be complicated by other problems associated with HIV (see Chapter 38).

With rubella infection, the incidence of IUGR may be as high as 60%, with infected cells remaining viable for many months.[51] There is capillary endothelial damage, hypoplasia, and necrotizing angiopathy in many fetal organs.[52] With cytomegalovirus infection, there is cytolysis, localized necrosis within various fetal organs, and a decrease in cell number.[53]

Although there are no bacterial infections known to cause IUGR, histologic chorioamnionitis is strongly associated with symmetric IUGR between 28 and 36 weeks, and with asymmetric IUGR after 36 weeks of gestation.[54]

Protozoan infections resulting from *Toxoplasma gondii, Plasmodium* sp., or *Trypanosoma cruzi* (Chagas disease) reportedly can cause IUGR.[49]

Although the incidence of maternal infections with various organisms may be as high as 15%, the incidence of congenital infections is estimated to be no more than 5%. It is believed that infectious disease can account for no more than 5% to 10% of human IUGR.

Multiple Gestation

It has long been recognized that multiple pregnancies are associated with a high progressive decrease in fetal and placental weight as the number of offspring increases in humans and in various animal species (see Chapter 25).[55,56] In both singleton and twin gestations, there is a relationship between total fetal mass and maternal mass. The increase in fetal weight in singleton gestations is linear from approximately 22 to 24 weeks until approximately 32 to 36 weeks of gestation.[13,17] During the last weeks of pregnancy, the increase in fetal weight declines, actually becoming negative after 42 weeks in some pregnancies.

If nutrition is adequate in the neonatal period, the slope of the increase in neonatal weight parallels the increase in fetal weight seen before 34 to 38 weeks. The decline in fetal weight increase occurs when the total fetal mass approximates 3000 to 3500 g for either singleton or twin gestations. When growth rate is expressed incrementally, the weekly gain in singletons peaks at approximately 230 to 285 g/wk between 32 and 34 weeks of gestation (see Fig 34-2). In individual twin fetuses, the incremental weekly gain peaks at 160 to 170 g/wk between 28 and 32 weeks of gestation.[13] However, recent studies in triplets have indicated that the growth of individual triplets may continue in a linear fashion well beyond a total combined weight of 3500 g.[57] Others have reported that before 35 weeks of gestation, triplets grow at about the 30th percentile for singletons, and by 38 weeks the average weight of each triplet is at the 10th percentile.[58] Significant birth weight discordance also occurs if there is unequal sharing of the placental mass.[59] If multifetal reduction is performed, there is an increase in IUGR in the surviving fetuses.[60]

The decrease in weight of twin fetuses, frequently with mild IUGR, is usually due to decreased cell size; the exception is severe IUGR associated with monozygosity and vascular anastomoses, wherein cell number also may be decreased.[61] These changes in twins are similar to those seen in IUGR secondary to poor uterine perfusion or maternal malnutrition. Twins with mild IUGR have an acceleration of growth after birth, so that their weight equals the median weight of singletons by 1 year of age. This observation supports the thesis that the etiology of poor fetal growth in twin gestations is an inability of the environment to meet fetal needs, rather than an inherent diminished growth capacity of the twin fetus. The example of twin fetuses supports the thesis derived from normal singleton pregnancies that the human fetus is seldom able to express its full potential for growth.

Many components of the environment can limit fetal growth (see later discussions). Twin-to-twin transfusion secondary to vascular anastomoses in monochorionic-monozygotic twins frequently results in IUGR of one twin, usually the donor (see Chapter 25). Maternal complications associated with IUGR occur more frequently with twins, and the incidence of congenital anomalies is almost twice that of singletons, primarily among monozygotic twin gestations. The incidence of IUGR in twins is 15% to 25%[16,62]; because the incidence of spontaneous multiple gestations approximates 1%, these pregnancies probably account for less than 3% of all cases of human IUGR. The actual incidence could be closer to 5% because of the increase in multiple gestations secondary to assisted reproductive techniques.

Inadequate Maternal Nutrition

Numerous animal studies have demonstrated that undernutrition of the mother caused by protein or caloric restriction can affect fetal growth adversely. However, information from experiments using small animals, in which the fetomaternal mass is much greater than in human pregnancy and the fetal and neonatal growth rate reaches its maximum after birth, must be extrapolated with caution. Nevertheless, such animal studies have engendered important concepts.

Winick[63] reported that there are three phases of fetal growth: cellular hyperplasia, followed by both hyperplasia and hypertrophy, and then predominantly hypertrophy. If there is a decrease in available substrate, the timing of the decrease is reflected in the type of IUGR observed. If the insult occurs early in pregnancy, the fetus is likely to be born with a decrease in cell number and cell size (such as might be observed with severe chronic maternal undernutrition or an inability to increase uteroplacental blood flow during gestation) and to have symmetric IUGR. If the insult occurs late in gestation, such as with twin gestation, the fetus is likely to have a normal cell number but a restriction of cell size (which can be returned to normal with adequate postnatal nutrition) and to have asymmetric IUGR.

The importance of maternal nutrition in fetal growth and birth weight was demonstrated by studies in Russia and Holland, where women suffered inadequate nutrition during World War II. The population in Leningrad underwent a prolonged period of poor nutrition, during which both preconception nutritional status and gestational nutrition were poor and birth weights were reduced by 400 to 600 g.[64] In Holland, a 6 month famine created conditions that permitted evaluation of the effect of malnutrition during each of the trimesters of pregnancy in a group of women previously well nourished.[65] Birth weights declined by approximately 10%, and placental weights by 15%, only when undernutrition occurred in the third trimester with daily caloric intake of less than 1500 kcal. The difference in severity of the IUGR in these two populations suggests the importance of prepregnancy nutritional status, an idea that has been substantiated.[18,66] In addition, animal studies indicate that fetal growth, metabolic and endocrine function, as well as placental status and function in late pregnancy, are significantly altered by the periconception maternal nutritional status, an effect independent of fetal size.[67] More recent studies have shown that inadequate weight gain in pregnancy (defined as <0.27 kg/wk, or <10 kg at 40 weeks, or based on suggested weight gain for body mass indices; see Chapter 10) is associated with an increased risk of IUGR. Weight gain in the second trimester appears to be particularly important.[67] Adequate maternal weight gain by 24 to 28 weeks in multiple pregnancies correlates positively with good fetal growth.[68]

It is still unclear whether it is generalized calorie intake reduction or specific substrate limitation (e.g., protein or key mineral restriction), or both, that is important in producing IUGR (see Chapter 10). Glucose uptake by the fetus is critical, because there is the suggestion that little glucogenesis occurs in the normal fetus. In the IUGR fetus, the maternal-fetal glucose concentration difference is increased as a function of the severity of the IUGR,[69] facilitating glucose transfer across the small placenta. Decreases in zinc content of peripheral blood leukocytes also correlate positively with IUGR,[70] and serum zinc concentrations of less than 60 μg/dL in the third trimester are associated with a fivefold increase in the incidence of low birth weight.[71] Similarly, an association between low serum folate levels and IUGR has been reported.[72] Although there have been numerous studies on supplementation, there is no convincing evidence that high protein intake or caloric supplementation has a beneficial effect on fetal weight. In addition, if a fetus is receiving decreased oxygen delivery as a result of decreased uteroplacental perfusion and has adapted by slowing metabolism and growth, it may not be advisable to increase substrate delivery. This important issue remains unresolved.

Another maternal nutrient that is important to fetal growth is oxygen. It is probably a primary determinant of fetal growth. IUGR infants have a decrease in the partial pressure of oxygen and decreased oxygen saturation values in the umbilical vein and artery.[73] The median birth weight of infants of women living more than 10,000 feet above sea level is approximately 250 g less than that of infants of women living at sea level.[74] Pregnancies complicated by maternal cyanotic heart disease usually result in IUGR, but it is unclear whether abnormal maternal hemodynamics or the reduction in oxygen saturation (by approximately 40% in the umbilical vein) accounts for the poor fetal growth.[75] The association between hemoglobinopathies and IUGR could be due to decreased blood viscosity or decreased fetal oxygenation. Patients with chronic pulmonary disease (e.g., poorly controlled asthma, cystic fibrosis, bronchiectasis) and those with severe kyphoscoliosis may be at increased risk of IUGR.

Environmental Toxins

Maternal cigarette smoking decreases birth weight by approximately 135 to 300 g; the fetus is symmetrically smaller.[76,77] If smoking is stopped before the third trimester, its adverse effect on birth weight is reduced.[77] More disturbing is the reported dose-response relationship between maternal smoking and a smaller infant head size, specifically a circumference of less than 32 cm, as well as a head circumference more than 2 standard deviations below that expected for gestational age.[78] The reason why not all women who smoke have IUGR infants could be a function of maternal genetic susceptibility.[79]

Reduction in birth weight also occurs with maternal alcohol ingestion of as little as one to two drinks per day.[80] Cocaine use in pregnancy similarly decreases birth weight, but there is also a reduction of head circumference that is more pronounced than the reduction in birth weight.[81] Use of other drugs, such as the anticonvulsants phenytoin and trimethadione, warfarin, and heroin, has been implicated in IUGR (see Chapter 20).

Placental Factors

Although placental size does not necessarily equate with function, our inability to clinically properly evaluate human placental function has resulted in studies of the interrelationships of size, morphometry, and clinical outcome. In general, birth weight increases with increasing placental weight in both animals and humans. IUGR without other anomalies is usually associated with a small placenta. Chromosomally normal IUGR newborns have a 24% smaller placenta for gestational age.[82] A small placenta is not always associated with an IUGR newborn, but a large infant from an otherwise normal pregnancy does not have a small placenta. Placental weight increases throughout normal gestation; with IUGR, the placental weight plateaus after 36 weeks or earlier, and the placenta (after being trimmed of the membranes and cord) weighs less than 350 g.[83] As normal gestation advances, there is a greater increase in fetal weight than in placental weight, so there is an increase in the fetal-placental weight ratio in large-for-gestational-age (LGA), AGA, and SGA infants in the last half of gestation. In all three categories, when the fetal-placental weight ratio is greater than 10, there is an increased incidence of depressed newborns; this suggests that it is not only the IUGR fetus that can outgrow the capacity of the placenta to bring about adequate transfer of necessary nutrients.[83]

Adequate trophoblastic invasion of the uterine decidual bed, and the resultant alteration in uterine blood flow, is a vital necessity, not only for the initial establishment and adherence of the pregnancy, but for also the adequate supply of nutrients to the fetus. The trophoblasts invade the decidua and myometrium to anchor the placenta, and a subpopulation of cytotrophoblasts invades the uterine blood vessels at the implantation site, resulting in extensive remodeling of the vessels.[84-87] There is a replacement of endothelium and uterine smooth muscle cells, which leads to a reduction in uterine arterial resistance and an increase in uteroplacental perfusion. Apoptosis plays an integral role in these vascular changes. It has also been suggested that the cytotrophoblast initiates lymphangiogenesis in the pregnant uterus; this is normally lacking in the nonpregnant state.

A number of reports have revealed that, in many cases of IUGR, particularly in early IUGR, the depth of invasion by the cytotrophoblasts is shallow and the endovascular invasion rudimentary; they have thus confirmed the early classic work of Brosens and colleagues,[88] who described reduced trophoblastic invasion and decreased pregnancy-associated alterations in the placental bed of IUGR pregnancies. The detailed morphologic studies of Aherne and Dunnill[89] also demonstrated that the mean surface area and, more importantly, the capillary surface area were reduced in the placentas of IUGR newborns. Apoptosis at the implantation site is increased with IUGR, and this has been suggested to be the mechanism limiting endovascular invasion.[86,90,91] The placental vascular endothelial growth factor (VEGF) and placenta growth factor (PIGF) were reduced, and antagonists were increased, in studies of early IUGR confirmed by Doppler imaging.[92] In summary, early abnormal implantation plays a key role in IUGR, but the exact controlling mechanisms behind the impaired placentation remain to be delineated.

The terminal villi are maldeveloped in IUGR pregnancies when absent end-diastolic flow is demonstrated, indicating that these morphologic changes are associated with increased vascular impedance.[93] When end-diastolic flow, is absent, there are more occlusive lesions of the intraplacental vasculature than when end-diastolic flow is present.[94]

Information from cordocentesis studies has revealed fetal hypoxemia, hypercapnia, acidosis, and hypoglycemia in severe IUGR.[95,96] There is also a decrease in α-aminonitrogen, particularly branched-chain amino acids, in the plasma of the IUGR fetus.[97]

Abnormal insertions of the cord, placental hemangiomas, abruptio placentae, and placenta previa are also associated with IUGR.[98-100]

Maternal Vascular Disease

Substantial evidence from experimental animal studies suggests that alterations in uteroplacental perfusion affect the growth and status of the placenta as well as the fetus. Ligation of the uterine artery of one horn of the pregnant rat results in IUGR of those fetuses nearest the constriction, and fetal and placental weights in guinea pigs, mice, and rabbits are lowest in the middle of each uterine horn, where arterial perfusion is lowest. Repetitive embolization of the uterine vascular bed during the last quarter of gestation in sheep gives rise to localized hyalinization and fibrinoid changes in the placenta[101] and results in a 40% reduction in placental weight and alterations in organ growth patterns similar to those observed in IUGR fetuses from pregnancies complicated by maternal hypertensive disease. In addition, umbilical blood flow is reduced and fetal oxidative metabolism is decreased.[101,102]

It has been strongly suggested in various studies that uteroplacental blood flow is decreased in pregnancies complicated by maternal hypertensive disease. Defective trophoblastic invasion of the uterine vascular bed results in relatively intact musculoelastic vessels that resist the normal decrease in uterine vascular resistance.[103] Clearance of radioactive tracers from the intervillous space is reduced in preeclamptic patients.[104,105] Because maternal body mass and plasma volume are correlated, reduced plasma volume or prevention of plasma volume expansion could lead to decreased cardiac output and uterine perfusion and a resultant decrease in fetal growth.[106,107] Alternatively, it may be that abnormal placentation comes first.

The importance of normal trophoblastic invasion leading to normal maternal cardiovascular changes has been indicated by central maternal cardiovascular studies. IUGR below the 3rd percentile at 25 to 37 weeks of gestation is associated with reduced maternal systolic function, increased vascular resistance, and probable lack of volume expansion in otherwise normotensive patients.[108]

Uteroplacental flow-velocity waveform studies, using Doppler methods in pregnancies complicated by hypertension, have shown a higher incidence of IUGR in pregnancies in which abnormal waveforms were recorded. These abnormal waveforms are thought to reflect abnormally increased resistance to blood flow.[109,110] High-resistance hypertension is associated with a marked decrease in fetal weight compared with low-resistance hypertension.[111] Increasing uteroplacental resistance, recorded with this methodology, has been positively correlated with fetal hypoxemia as determined by cordocentesis in IUGR fetuses.[95]

As discussed in Chapter 40, there is conflicting evidence as to whether the congenital thrombophilias contribute to the clinical development of IUGR, with most recent studies suggesting the lack of an association.[112-115]

There are only fragmentary suggestions relating abnormal anatomic uterine vascular anatomy and IUGR. IUGR may occur at a higher frequency if the pregnancy is in a unicornuate uterus; vascular abnormalities are likely but unproven in such cases.[116] Patients with two (rather than the usual one) ascending uterine arteries on each side of the uterus also have a higher rate of IUGR.[117] However, pregnancy after bilateral ligation of the internal iliac and ovarian arteries, or after embolization of leiomyomata, is not associated with IUGR.[118,119]

Because exercise can affect uterine perfusion, this subject has been studied extensively. A moderate regimen of weight-bearing exercise in early pregnancy probably enhances fetal growth.[120] However, high levels of exercise (>50% of prepregnancy levels) in middle and late pregnancy result mainly in a symmetric reduction in fetal growth and neonatal fat mass.[121] In assessing levels of aerobic activity, neonates born to women in the highest quartile weighed 600 g less than those in the lowest quartile, an effect mainly seen in taller women.[122]

Clinical maternal vascular disease and the presumed decrease in uteroplacental perfusion can account for at least 25% to 30% of IUGR infants. Undiagnosed decreased perfusion could also be the cause of IUGR in an otherwise normal pregnancy, such as with recurrent idiopathic fetal growth restriction. A history of a previous low-birth-weight infant is significantly associated with the subsequent birth of an infant with decreased weight, decreased ponderal index, and decreased head circumference.[123] This finding of symmetric growth restriction is in contrast to the asymmetric IUGR usually seen with maternal vascular disease.

Vascular disease becomes more prevalent with advancing age. In one recent large study, after controlling for confounding variables, the incidence of SGA births was increased more in nulliparous patients than in multiparous patients older than 30 years of age.[124]

Maternal and Fetal Hormones

In general, there is limited transfer of the various circulating maternal hormones into the fetal compartments (see Chapters 46 through 48).

Although the effects of hypothyroidism or hyperthyroidism on fetal size are not striking, studies in subhuman primates indicate that, when the mother and fetus are athyroid, there is retarded osseous development and reduced protein synthesis in the fetal brain.[125]

Maternal diabetes without vascular disease is frequently associated with excessive fetal size (see Chapter 46). Although insulin does not cross the placenta, fetal hyperinsulinemia as well as hyperplasia of the pancreatic islet cells is seen frequently with maternal diabetes. These changes are thought to occur as a result of maternal hyperglycemia, which leads to fetal hyperglycemia and an increased response of the fetal pancreas. Fetal hypoinsulinemia produced experimentally in the rhesus monkey results in IUGR; rarely, infants have been born with severe IUGR and requiring insulin treatment at birth, suggesting hypoinsulinemia in utero.[126,127] If nutrient transfer becomes limited owing to placental disease secondary to maternal vascular disease, the fetus of the diabetic mother can sustain IUGR.

Even though human growth hormone is present early in gestation, there is minimal evidence that it regulates fetal weight, although a deficiency could retard skeletal growth.[128] Convincing evidence is also lacking that adrenal hormones have a role in producing IUGR in humans.

Several small polypeptides with in vitro growth-promoting activity have been purified (e.g., insulin-like growth factor 1 [IGF-1], IGF-2), but the exact role of these peptides and their binding proteins as fetal growth factors and their potential relationship to IUGR are currently not well understood.

Leptin (from Greek *leptos*, "thin") is a polypeptide hormone discovered in 1994. It has been shown to moderate feeding behavior and adipose stores. It is produced predominantly by adipocytes but can also be produced by the placenta, because neonatal levels fall dramatically after birth.[128] Reported concentrations in IUGR have varied, and the exact role that this hormone plays in fetal growth remains to be clarified.

Diagnosis of Intrauterine Growth Restriction

Determination of Cause

An attempt should be made to determine the cause of fetal aberrant growth before delivery in order to provide appropriate counseling; perform ultrasonographic evaluation for fetal growth velocity, delineate anatomy and function; and obtain neonatal consultation.

The various disorders associated with suboptimal fetal growth were addressed earlier in this chapter and are summarized in Table 34-2. Often, the cause is readily apparent. Among patients with significant chronic hypertensive disease, those who take prescribed medications known to be associated with prenatal growth deficiency, and those whose fetuses have congenital or chromosomal abnormalities, the diagnosis is easily established and management plans can be made. At times, however, the causal factors can be more elusive. For example, growth restriction associated with preeclampsia may antedate the appearance of hypertension or proteinuria by several weeks. In many instances, a careful history, maternal examination, and ultrasound evaluation reveal the etiology.

History and Physical Examination

Clinical diagnosis of IUGR by physical examination alone is inaccurate; often, the diagnosis is not made until after delivery. Most clinical

TABLE 34-2 DISORDERS AND OTHER FACTORS ASSOCIATED WITH INTRAUTERINE GROWTH RESTRICTION*

Maternal Factors
Hypertensive disease, chronic or preeclampsia
Renal disease
Severe nutritional deficiencies (e.g., inflammatory bowel disease, markedly inadequate pregnancy weight gain in the underweight woman, malnutrition)
Pregnancy at high altitude
Specific prescribed medications (e.g., antiepileptics)
Smoking, alcohol use, illicit drug use
Fetal Factors
Multiple gestations
Placental abnormalities
Infections
Aneuploidy or structural abnormalities

***Growth is also strongly influenced by maternal prepregnancy weight and by ethnicity, which must be considered when evaluating overall growth (by use of customized versus population-based growth curves).**

studies demonstrate that, with the use of physical examination alone, the diagnosis of IUGR is missed or incorrectly made almost half the time. Techniques such as measurement of the symphysis-fundal height are helpful in screening for abnormal fetal growth and documenting continued growth if they are performed repeatedly by the same observer, but they are not sensitive enough for accurate detection of most infants with IUGR.[129,130]

Despite the inaccuracy of such indicators, fetal assessment and specific aspects of the patient's risk factors increase the clinician's index of suspicion about suboptimal fetal growth, without which more definitive laboratory investigation might not be considered. As discussed earlier, maternal disease entities such as hypertension, in particular severe preeclampsia and chronic hypertension with superimposed preeclampsia, carry a high incidence of IUGR. The diagnosis of a multiple gestation suggests the likelihood of diminished fetal growth relative to gestational age, as well as preterm birth. Additional maternal risk factors include documented rubella or cytomegalovirus infection, heavy smoking, heroin or cocaine addiction, alcoholism, and poor nutritional status both before conception and during pregnancy combined with inadequate weight gain during pregnancy.

Ultrasonography

Currently, ultrasonographic evaluation of the fetus is the preferred and accepted modality for the diagnosis of inadequate fetal growth. It offers the advantages of reasonably precise estimations of fetal weight, determination of interval fetal growth velocity, and measurement of several fetal dimensions to describe the pattern of growth abnormality. Use of these ultrasound measurements requires accurate knowledge of gestational age. Accordingly, if a patient is known to be at risk for a fetal growth abnormality, the crown-to-rump length should be determined during the first trimester.

Measurements of biparietal diameter, head circumference, abdominal circumferences, and femur length allow the clinician to use accepted formulas to estimate fetal weight and to determine whether a fetal growth aberration represents an asymmetric, symmetric, or mixed pattern[131] (Fig. 34-4). As discussed previously, intrinsic fetal insults occurring early in pregnancy (e.g., infection, exposure to certain drugs or other chemical agents, chromosomal abnormalities, other congenital malformations) are likely to affect fetal growth at a time of development when cell division is the predominant mechanism of growth. Consequently, musculoskeletal dimensions and organ size may be adversely affected, and a symmetric pattern of aberrant growth is observed. Given this set of circumstances, one might expect to find that the femur length and head circumference are small for a given gestational age, as are the abdominal circumference and overall fetal weight, all of which are characterized as *symmetric* IUGR. Symmetric IUGR accounts for approximately 20% to 30% of all growth-restricted fetuses.

At the other end of the spectrum, an extrinsic insult occurring later in pregnancy, usually characterized by inadequate fetal nutrition due to placental insufficiency, is more likely to result in *asymmetric* growth restriction. In this type, femur length and head circumference are spared, but abdominal circumference is decreased because of subnormal hepatic growth, and there is a paucity of subcutaneous fat. The most common disorders that limit the availability of fetal substrates for metabolism are the hypertensive complications of pregnancy, which are associated with decreased uteroplacental perfusion, and placental infarcts, which limit the trophoblastic surface area available for substrate transfer. In fact, a falloff in the interval growth of the *abdominal circumference* is one of the earliest findings in extrinsic or asymmetric IUGR[132,133]; conversely, the finding of an abdominal circumference in the normal range for gestational age markedly decreases the likelihood of IUGR. Frequently, these patterns of growth abnormality merge, particularly after long-standing fetal nutritional deprivation.

Distinguishing between symmetric and asymmetric IUGR is also of considerable clinical significance and may provide useful information for both diagnostic and counseling purposes. For example, a diagnosis of symmetric IUGR in early pregnancy suggests a poor prognosis when the diagnostic possibilities are considered (e.g., fetal infection, aneuploidy); conversely, asymmetric IUGR observed in the third trimester, particularly if it is associated with maternal hypertension or placental dysfunction, usually imparts a more favorable prognosis with careful fetal evaluation, appropriate delivery timing, and skillful neonatal management.

Considerable attention has been directed at early ultrasound findings that may provide for the early prediction of IUGR. In a study of 976 women whose pregnancies were the product of assisted reproductive technologies, the risk of delivering an SGA fetus decreased as a function of increasing crown-rump length in the first trimester.[134] This confirmed previous findings suggesting that suboptimal growth in the first trimester is associated with IUGR.[135]

Efforts have also been made to correlate Doppler findings in the uterine artery with subsequent pregnancy complications, including IUGR. Utilizing transvaginal color Doppler at 23 weeks' gestation, Papageorghiou and colleagues observed that increases in the uterine artery pulsatility index and "notching" were associated with subsequent development of IUGR, although the predictive value was low.[136] In a more recent study of uterine artery pulsatility index at 11 to 14 weeks' gestation, a value greater than the 95th percentile predicted SGA with accuracy in 23% of the cases, and with increased sensitivity if the maternal serum concentration of plasma-associated pregnancy protein A (PAPP-A) was low. However, this parameter did not reach statistical significance.[137] The eventual practical role that uterine artery Doppler ultrasound may play in the prediction of IUGR, if any, awaits more extensive evaluation.

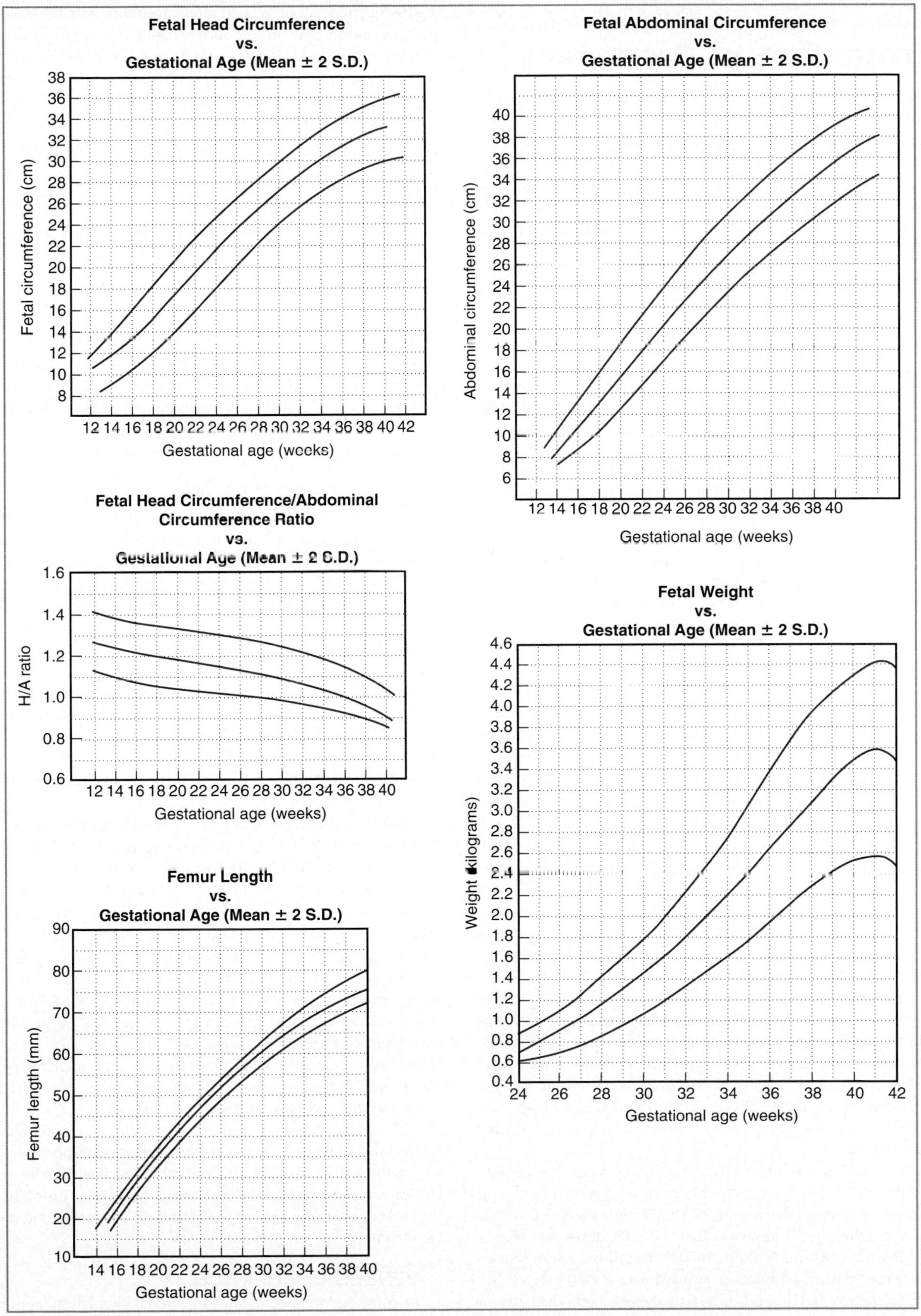

FIGURE 34-4 Composite of fetal body measurements used for serial evaluations of fetal growth.

Management of Pregnancy

The cornerstones of management for the pregnancy complicated by IUGR are surveillance of fetal growth velocity and function (well-being) and determination of appropriate delivery timing. Delivery at or near term is usually indicated if fetal growth has continued to be adequate and antenatal testing results have been normal. Management is far more challenging remote from term and requires use of the biophysical profile (BPP), measurement of amniotic fluid volume (AFV), and Doppler assessment of the fetal circulation, combined with good clinical judgment. The comments in the following sections pertain primarily to the use of antenatal testing in the *preterm* fetus with IUGR.

Antenatal Fetal Testing

The various diagnostic modalities used for fetal assessment are discussed in detail in Chapter 21, but specific points are reemphasized here.

Biophysical Profile and Amniotic Fluid Volume

The BPP is appealing, inasmuch as it provides a multidimensional survey of fetal physiologic parameters. In particular, AFV assessment is an important aspect of the BPP, because oligohydramnios is a frequent finding in the IUGR pregnancy caused by placental insufficiency. This is presumably a result of diminished fetal blood volume, renal blood flow, and urinary output. Human fetal urinary production rates can be measured with considerable accuracy,[138] and three separate studies have shown decreased rates in the presence of fetal growth restriction.[139-141]

The significance of AFV with respect to fetal outcome has been well documented. Manning and coworkers reported the diagnostic value of AFV measurement in discriminating normal from aberrant fetal growth. Among 91 patients with normal AFV, 86 delivered infants whose birth weights were appropriate for gestational age. In contrast, 26 of 29 patients with decreased AFV delivered growth-restricted infants.[142] Severe oligohydramnios is associated with a high risk of fetal compromise.[143,144]

It is likely that the chronic hypoxic state frequently observed in the fetus with IUGR is responsible for diverting blood flow from the kidney to other organs that are more critical during fetal life (see Chapters 12 and 14). Nicolaides and associates[141] observed reduced fetal urinary flow rates in IUGR, and the degree of reduction was well correlated with the degree of fetal hypoxemia as reflected by fetal blood Po_2 measured after cordocentesis.

The most appropriate technique for assessment of AFV, as well as the arguments for and against each technique, are addressed in Chapters 21 and 32. It is reasonable to conclude at this time that a single vertical pocket smaller than 2 cm, or an amniotic fluid index of less than 5 cm, or both, suggests that there is a clinically significant decrease in AFV; conversely, a normal AFV is very reassuring with respect to fetal well-being and also suggests the possibility of a normal but constitutionally small fetus.

There is a paucity of evidence from randomized trials to validate the use of the BPP.[145] However, its usefulness was suggested by several large observational reports. In a study of 19,221 high-risk pregnancies, Manning and colleagues[146] observed that the fetal death rate after a normal BPP score (≥8) was 0.726 in 1000 births; only 14 such fetuses died. Of the total patient population, approximately 4380 pregnancies were complicated by IUGR, and only 4 of those infants died after a normal test, yielding a false-negative test rate of less than 1 in 1000. In a subsequent analysis of perinatal morbidity and mortality among patients monitored with the BPP, a highly significant inverse correlation was observed for IUGR and last test score. If the last test score was 8 or higher, only 3.4% of 6500 high-risk patients had infants with IUGR. Conversely, if the last test score was 4 or 2, the incidence of IUGR increased to 29% and 41%, respectively.[147]

Doppler Ultrasound Assessment of the Fetal Vasculature

ARTERIAL CIRCULATION

There has been great interest in the role of Doppler assessment of the fetal arterial and venous circulation in predicting and evaluating fetal growth restriction as well as other fetal complications (see Chapter 21). It is now clear that umbilical arterial velocimetry is of considerable value in predicting perinatal outcome in the fetus with IUGR, and it is the only modality validated by randomized trials. A substantial pathologic correlation helps to explain the increased vascular resistance in IUGR. Specifically, fetuses demonstrating an absence of end-diastolic flow exhibited maldevelopment of the placental terminal villous tree. The correlations among placental pathology, abnormal umbilical artery velocimetry, and IUGR were reviewed by Kingdom and coworkers.[148]

Several randomized trials have been reported which, taken together, demonstrated a decrease in perinatal deaths when umbilical arterial Doppler assessment was used in conjunction with other types of antenatal testing.[149-151] A meta-analysis of 12 randomized, controlled trials showed that clinical action guided by umbilical Doppler velocimetry reduced the odds of perinatal death by 38% and decreased the risk of inappropriate intervention in pregnancies thought to be at risk of IUGR.[152] Although the authors hypothesized that this beneficial effect depended on the incidence of absent end-diastolic velocity rather than simply decreased flow, the number of studies with sufficient data was inadequate to draw this conclusion. A recent retrospective cohort study of 151 IUGR fetuses comparing abnormal umbilical artery Doppler, a "nonreactive" nonstress test, and a BPP value of 6 or less confirmed that abnormal Doppler flow was the best predictor of adverse outcome.[153]

Therefore, umbilical artery velocimetry plays a significant role in the management of IUGR. A normal velocimetry result in the suspect small fetus is usually indicative of a constitutionally small but otherwise normal baby,[154] although a normal finding is also observed in the chromosomally or structurally abnormal fetus.[155] Diminished end-diastolic flow is rarely associated with significant neonatal morbidity, but the absence or reversal of end-diastolic flow predicts significantly increased perinatal morbidity and mortality and long-term poor neurologic outcome, compared with continuing diastolic flow.[156,157] Furthermore, markedly diminished end-diastolic flow can be observed at very premature gestational ages, well before the BPP demonstrates abnormalities. Consequently, abnormal umbilical velocimetry findings should be interpreted in conjunction with other tests of fetal well-being and in the context of the gestational age.

There also has been interest in the evaluation of middle cerebral artery flow, inasmuch as the normal adaptive response to hypoxia within the fetus is to increase cerebral blood flow ("brain-sparing"). However, the results from several studies have been contradictory, and the focus of attention has been on umbilical artery flow and the venous circulation.

VENOUS CIRCULATION

In contrast to abnormalities in arterial circulation, abnormalities observed in the venous circulation presumably reflect central cardiac failure, and multiple current studies suggest that specific aberrations of flow through the ductus venous and umbilical vein are indicative of imminent fetal demise, as well as substantial morbidity among survivors. The temporal sequence of Doppler-measured flow abnormalities in the arterial and venous circulations of the IUGR fetus has been delineated.[158,159] The fetus with severe IUGR first demonstrates changes in the umbilical and middle cerebral arteries. This is followed by alterations in the venous circulation, including the ductus venosus (abnormalities in the atrial portion of the flow) and the umbilical vein (pulsatile flow). These changes and their pathophysiology have been summarized in detail by Baschat and Harman.[160] What has become clear is that abnormal venous Doppler waveforms in the preterm IUGR fetus are indicative of poor acid-base status and outcome.[161,162] Therefore, the challenge for the clinician is to try to optimize delivery timing in the very preterm fetus, before significant abnormalities in the venous circulation occur.

Antepartum Therapy

Maternal hyperoxia has been shown to increase umbilical P_{O_2} and pH in the hypoxemic, acidotic, growth-restricted fetus.[163] Among surviving fetuses, there was also an improvement in mean velocity of blood flow through the thoracic aorta. In support of these findings, Battaglia and coworkers treated 17 of 36 women whose pregnancies were complicated by IUGR with maternal hyperoxia and confirmed improvement in both blood gases and Doppler flow. They also observed a significant improvement in perinatal mortality in the oxygen-treated patients.[164] However, the evidence is inconclusive regarding whether chronic maternal oxygen therapy is of value, and any differences reported in outcome could be due to more advanced gestational age in oxygen-treated groups.[165]

Nutritional supplements, including antioxidants such as vitamins C and E, have not been shown to be effective in reducing the risk of IUGR.[166] There has also been considerable interest in the role of fish oil supplements, but a Cochrane Database Review of six trials revealed no significant difference in the proportion of SGA infants in treated versus untreated groups.[167]

The role of low-dose aspirin remains controversial, and most studies have examined subsets of women treated for the prevention of preeclampsia. A meticulous analysis of the current data revealed a 10% reduction in SGA infants, but this strong trend did not achieve statistical significance.[168] This subject was recently reviewed by Berghella.[169]

Timing of Delivery

The prohibitive perinatal morbidity and mortality rates among IUGR infants were discussed previously. Controversy continues with regard to the timing of delivery for such infants to ensure that neurologic damage or fetal intrauterine death does not occur because of chronic oxygen deprivation. This problem is underscored by the fact that, if deaths among congenitally infected and anomalous infants are excluded, the perinatal risk is still higher for growth-restricted infants than for AGA newborns. Although opinions vary as to the role of preterm versus term delivery of the IUGR fetus, it is usually prudent to deliver the growth-restricted infant close to term, as long as growth continues and antenatal tests are reassuring. Tests of fetal lung maturation may be of value if the course of action is not entirely clear. In the case of the preterm fetus, delivery is indicated in the presence of worsening maternal hypertensive disease, failure of continuing growth, or reversal of umbilical artery flow as assessed by Doppler ultrasound. The preterm fetus (<34 weeks' gestation) should receive the benefit of corticosteroids for lung maturation.

The Growth Restriction Intervention Trial (GRIT) study underscored the difficulty in selecting the most appropriate delivery time to prevent morbidity.[170] In a randomized trial of 548 preterm IUGR pregnancies (24 to 36 weeks' gestation) in which fetal compromise was identified but uncertainty regarding delivery persisted, approximately half of the pregnancies were delivered and the other half continued until the clinical course was clear. There was no difference in mortality between the two groups. However, among infants with less than 31 weeks' gestation, severe disabilities were observed in 13% of the immediate deliveries, compared with 5% of those that were delayed.

The overall findings and guidelines for evaluation and management of the fetus with IUGR are summarized in Table 34-3.

TABLE 34-3 EVALUATION AND MANAGEMENT OF THE FETUS WITH INTRAUTERINE GROWTH RESTRICTION

	Constitutionally Small Fetus	Fetus with Structural or Chromosome Abnormality or Fetal Infection	Substrate Deprivation or Uteroplacental Insufficiency
Growth rate and pattern	Usually below but parallel to normal; symmetric	Markedly below normal; symmetric	Variable; usually asymmetric
Anatomy	Normal	Usually abnormal	Normal
Amniotic fluid volume	Normal	Normal or hydramnios; decreased in the presence of renal agenesis or urethral obstruction	Low
Additional evaluation	None	Karyotype; specific testing for viral DNA in amniotic fluid as indicated	Fetal lung maturity testing as indicated
Additional laboratory evaluation of fetal well-being	Normal BPP/UAV	BPP variable; normal UAV	BPP score decreases; UAV evidence of vascular resistance
Continued surveillance and timing of delivery	None; anticipate term delivery	Dependent on etiology	BPP and UAV; delivery timing requires balance of gestational age and BPP/UAV findings; fetal lung maturity testing often helpful

BPP, biophysical profile; IUGR, intrauterine growth restriction; UAV, umbilical artery velocimetry.
From Resnik R: Intrauterine growth restriction. Obstet Gynecol 99:490, 2002.

Intrapartum Management

It has long been recognized that lower Apgar scores and meconium aspiration, as well as other manifestations of poor oxygenation during labor, occur with greater frequency among IUGR infants. The problem of intrapartum asphyxia has been further elucidated by studies demonstrating the acid-base status of growth-restricted infants at the time of delivery. If moderate-to-severe metabolic acidosis is defined as an umbilical artery buffer base value of less than 37 mEq/L (normal, >40 mEq/L), almost 50% of IUGR neonates show signs of acidosis at the time of delivery.[171] These findings document the problems of oxygenation during labor in such fetuses and emphasize that meticulous fetal surveillance is required during this critical period.

Consequently, the clinician should proceed to cesarean delivery if there is evidence of deteriorating fetal status or an unripe cervix or if there is any indication of additional fetal compromise during labor.

Neonatal Complications and Long-term Sequelae

The growth-restricted fetus can experience numerous complications in the neonatal period related to the etiology of the growth insult as well as antepartum and intrapartum factors. These include neonatal asphyxia, meconium aspiration, hypoglycemia and other metabolic abnormalities, and polycythemia (see Chapter 58). After correction for gestational age, a large population-based outcomes analysis showed that the premature IUGR infant is at increased risk of mortality, necrotizing enterocolitis, and need for respiratory support at 28 days of age.[172] This observation takes on more significance inasmuch as prematurity and IUGR frequently coexist.

Beyond the neonatal period, data by Low and colleagues[173] showed that fetal growth restriction has a deleterious effect on cognitive function, independent of other variables. With the use of numerous standardized tests to evaluate learning ability, and excluding those children with genetic or major organ system malformations, they found that almost 50% (37/77) of SGA children had learning deficits at ages 9 to 11 years. Blair and Stanley[174] also reported a strong association between IUGR and spastic cerebral palsy in newborns born after 33 weeks of gestation. This association was highest in IUGR infants who were short, thin, and of small head size. Newborns who were at or above the 10th percentile for weight but had abnormal ponderal indices were also at risk for spastic cerebral palsy.[175] In a recent Danish autopsy study, investigators observed a significantly lower cell number in the cortex of IUGR fetuses and infants compared with normal controls, a finding that may, in part, explain the clinical observations.[176] Other investigators have reported more favorable neurologic outcomes in IUGR infants.[177,178]

There is currently substantial research effort to explore the role of IUGR and adult disease: the so-called "fetal origins of disease" hypothesis. This subject is addressed in Chapter 11. The epidemiologic studies of Barker's group have indicated that IUGR is a significant risk factor for the subsequent development of chronic hypertension, ischemic heart disease, type 2 diabetes, and obstructive lung disease.[179] Maternal and fetal malnutrition seem to have both short- and long-term effects. The concept of programming during intrauterine life, however, needs to include a host of other factors, such as the genotype of both mother and fetus, maternal size and obstetric history, and postnatal and lifestyle factors.

References

1. Lubchenco LO, Hansman C, Boyd E: Intrauterine growth as estimated from liveborn birth-weight data at 24 to 42 weeks of gestation. Pediatrics 32:793, 1963.
2. Battaglia FC, Lubchenco LO: A practical classification of newborn infants by weight and gestational age. J Pediatr 71:159, 1967.
3. Yerushalmy J: Relation of birth weight, gestational age, and the rate of intrauterine growth to perinatal mortality. Clin Obstet Gynecol 13:107, 1970.
4. Seeds JW, Peng T: Impaired fetal growth and risk of fetal death: Is the tenth percentile the appropriate standard? Am J Obstet Gynecol 178:658, 1998.
5. Gardosi J: Customized fetal growth standards: Rationale and clinical application. Semin Perinatol 28:33, 2004.
6. Figueras F, Figueras J, Meler E, et al: Customized birthweight standards accurately predict perinatal morbidity. Arch Dis Child Fetal Neonatal Educ 92: F277-F280, 2007.
7. Groom KM, Poppe KK, North RA, et al: Small-for-gestational age infants classified by customized or population birthweight centiles: Impact of gestational age at delivery. Am J Obstet Gynecol 197:239.e1-239.e5, 2007.
8. McCowan LM, Harding JE, Stewart AW: Customized birthweight centiles predict SGA pregnancies with perinatal morbidity. BJOG 112:1026-1033, 2005.
9. Ego A, Subtil D, Grange G, et al: Customized versus population-based birth weight standards for identifying growth restricted infants: A French multicenter study. Am J Obstet Gynecol 194:1042-1049, 2006.
10. Miller HC, Hassanein K: Diagnosis of impaired fetal growth in newborn infants. Pediatrics 48:511, 1971.
11. Daikoku NH, Johnson JWC, Graf C, et al: Patterns of intrauterine growth retardation. Obstet Gynecol 54:211, 1979.
12. Brar HS, Rutherford SP: Classification of intrauterine growth retardation. Semin Perinatol 12:2, 1988.
13. Williams RL, Creasy RK, Cunningham GC, et al: Fetal growth and perinatal viability in California. Obstet Gynecol 59:624, 1982.
14. Brenner WE, Edelman DA, Hendricks CH: A standard of fetal growth for the United States of America. Am J Obstet Gynecol 126:555, 1976.
15. Ott W: Intrauterine growth retardation and preterm delivery. Am J Obstet Gynecol 168:710, 1993.
16. Arbuckle TE, Wilkins R, Sherman GJ: Birth weight percentiles by gestational age in Canada. Obstet Gynecol 81:39, 1993.
17. Alexander GR, Himes JH, Kaufman RB, et al: A United States national reference for fetal growth. Obstet Gynecol 87:163, 1996.
18. Kramer MS: Determinants of low birth weight: Methodological assessment and meta-analysis. Bull WHO 65:663, 1987.
19. Manning FA: Intrauterine growth retardation. In Manning FA: Fetal Medicine: Principles and Practice. Norwalk, CT, Appleton & Lange, 1995, p 307.
20. Ounsted M, Moar V, Scott WA: Perinatal morbidity and mortality in small-for-dates babies: The relative importance of some maternal factors. Early Hum Dev 5:367, 1981.
21. Dashe JS, McIntire DD, Lucas MJ, et al: Effects of symmetric and asymmetric fetal growth on pregnancy outcomes. Obstet Gynecol 96:321, 2000.
22. Piper JM, Xenakais E-J, McFarland M, et al: Do growth-retarded premature infants have different rates of perinatal morbidity and mortality than appropriately grown premature infants? Obstet Gynecol 87:169, 1996.
23. Spinello A, Capuzzo E, Egbe TO, et al: Pregnancies complicated by intrauterine growth retardation. J Reprod Med 40:209, 1995.
24. Minior VK, Divon MY: Fetal growth restriction at term: Myth or realty. Obstet Gynecol 92:57, 1998.
25. Morken N-H, Kallen K, Jacobsson B: Fetal growth and onset of delivery: A nationwide population-based study of preterm infants. Am J Obstet Gynecol 195:154, 2006.
26. Blair E, Stanley F: Intrauterine growth and spastic cerebral palsy: I. Association with birth weight for gestational age. Am J Obstet Gynecol 162:229, 1990.

27. Goldenberg RL, DuBard MB, Cliver SP, et al: Pregnancy outcomes and intelligence at age 5 years. Am J Obstet Gynecol 175:1511, 1996.
28. Wienerroither H, Steiner H, Tomaselli J, et al: Intrauterine blood flow and long term intellectual, neurologic and social development. Obstet Gynecol 97:449, 2001.
29. Polani PE: Chromosomal and other genetic influences on birth weight variation. In Elliot K, Knight J (eds): Size at Birth. Amsterdam, Associated Scientific Publishers, 1974.
30. Walton A, Hammond J: The maternal effects on growth and conformation in the Shire horse-Shetland pony crosses. Proc R Soc Biol 125:311, 1938.
31. Johnstone F, Inglis L: Familial trends in low birth weight. BMJ 3:659, 1974.
32. Ounsted M, Ounsted C: Maternal regulations of intrauterine growth. Nature 187:777, 1966.
33. Simpson JW, Lawless RW, Mitchell AC: Responsibility of the obstetrician to the fetus: 2. Influence of prepregnancy weight and pregnancy weight gain on birth weight. Obstet Gynecol 45:481, 1975.
34. Wilcox MA, Smith SJ, Johnson IR, et al: The effect of social deprivation on birthweight, excluding physiologic and pathologic effects. BJOG 102:918, 1995.
35. Thomson AM, Billewicz WZ, Hytten FE: The assessment of fetal growth. J Obstet Gynaecol Br Commonw 75:906, 1968.
36. Klebanoff MA, Mednick BR, Schulsinger C, et al: Father's effect on infant birth weight. Am J Obstet Gynecol 178:1022, 1998.
37. Klebanoff MA, Schulsinger C, Mednick BR, et al: Preterm and small-for-gestational-age birth across generations. Am J Obstet Gynecol 176:521, 1997.
38. Bukowski R, Gahn D, Denning J, et al: Impairment of growth in fetuses destined to deliver preterm. Am J Obstet Gynecol 185:463, 2001.
39. Saugstad LF: Birth weights in children with phenylketonuria and in their siblings. Lancet 1:809, 1972.
40. Snijders RJM, Sherrod C, Gosden CM, et al: Fetal growth retardation: Associated malformations and chromosomal abnormalities. Am J Obstet Gynecol 168:547, 1993.
41. Chen ATL, Chan Y-K, Falek A: The effects of chromosome abnormalities on birth weight in man: II. Autosomal defects. Hum Hered 22:209, 1972.
42. Peuschel SM, Rothman KJ, Ogilvy JD: Birth weight of children with Down's syndrome. Am J Ment Defic 80:442, 1976.
43. Barlow P: The influence of inactive chromosomes on human development: Anomalous sex chromosome complements and the phenotype. Hum Genet 17:105, 1973.
44. Khoury MJ, Erickson D, Cordero JE, et al: Congenital malformation and intrauterine growth retardation: A population study. Pediatrics 82:83, 1988.
45. Naeye RL: Unsuspected organ abnormalities associated with congenital heart disease. Am J Pathol 47:905, 1965.
46. Froehlich LA, Fujikura R: Significance of a single umbilical artery. Am J Obstet Gynecol 94:174, 1966.
47. Feldman DM, Borgida AF, Trymbulak WP, et al: Clinical implications of velamentous cord insertion in triplet gestations. Am J Obstet Gynecol 186:809, 2002.
48. Sornes T: Umbilical cord encirclements and fetal growth restriction. Obstet Gynecol 86:725, 1995.
49. Klein JO, Remington JS: Current concepts of infections of the fetus and newborn infant. In Remington JS, Klein JO (eds): Infectious Diseases of the Fetus and Newborn Infant, 4th ed. Philadelphia, WB Saunders, 1995.
50. Alkalay AL, Pomerance JJ, Rimoin DL: Fetal varicella syndrome. J Pediatr 111:320, 1987.
51. Peckham CS: Clinical laboratory study of children exposed in utero to maternal rubella. Arch Dis Child 47:571, 1972.
52. Preblud SR, Alford CA Jr: Rubella. In Remington JS, Klein JO (eds): Infectious Diseases of the Fetus and Newborn Infant, 3rd ed. Philadelphia, WB Saunders, 1990.
53. Naeye RL: Cytomegalovirus disease: The fetal disorder. Am J Clin Pathol 47:738, 1967.
54. Williams MC, O'Brien WF, Nelson RN, et al: Histologic chorioamnionitis is associated with fetal growth restriction in term and preterm infants. Am J Obstet Gynecol 183:1094, 2000.
55. Barcroft J, Kennedy JA: The distribution of blood between the fetus and placenta in sheep. J Physiol 95:173, 1939.
56. McKeown T, Record RG: Observations on foetal growth in multiple pregnancy in man. J Endocrinol 8:386, 1952.
57. Jones JS, Newman RB, Miller MC: Cross-sectional analysis of triplet birth weight. Am J Obstet Gynecol 164:135, 1991.
58. Elster AD, Bleyl JL, Craven TE: Birth weight standards for triplets under modern obstetric care in the United States, 1984-1989. Obstet Gynecol 77:387, 1991.
59. Fick AL, Feldstein VA, Norton ME, et al: Unequal placental sharing aand birth weight discordance in monochorionic diamniotic twins. Am J Obstet Gynecol 195:178, 2006.
60. Silver RK, Helford BT, Russell TL, et al: Multifetal reduction increases the risk of preterm delivery and fetal growth restriction: A case control study. Fertil Steril 67:30, 1997.
61. Naeye RL, Benirschke K, Hagstrom JWC, et al: Intrauterine growth of twins as estimated from liveborn birth weight data. Pediatrics 37:409, 1966.
62. Secher NJ, Kaern J, Hansen PK: Intrauterine growth in twin pregnancies: Prediction of fetal growth retardation. Obstet Gynecol 66:63, 1985.
63. Winick M: Cellular changes during placental and fetal growth. Am J Obstet Gynecol 109:166, 1971.
64. Antonov AN: Children born during siege of Leningrad in 1942. J Pediatr 30:250, 1947.
65. Stein Z, Susser M: The Dutch famine, 1944-1945, and the reproductive process: I. Effects on six indices at birth. Pediatr Res 9:70, 1975.
66. Abrams B, Newman V: Small-for-gestational-age birth: Maternal predictors and comparison with risk factors of spontaneous preterm delivery in the same cohort. Am J Obstet Gynecol 164:785, 1991.
67. Oliver MH, Hawkes P, Harding JE: Periconceptual undernutrition alters growth trajectory and metabolic and endocrine responses to fasting in late-gestation fetal sheep. Pediatr. Res 57:591, 2005.
68. Luke B, Nugent C, van de Ven C, et al: The association between maternal factors and perinatal outcome in triplet pregnancies. Am J Obstet Gynecol 187:752, 2002.
69. Marconi AM, Paolin C, Buscaglia M, et al: The impact of gestational age and fetal growth on the maternal-fetal glucose concentration differences. Obstet Gynecol 87:937, 1996.
70. Wells JL, James DK, Luxton R, et al: Maternal leukocyte zinc deficiency at start of third trimester as a predictor of fetal growth retardation. BMJ 294:1054, 1987.
71. Neggers YH, Cutter GR, Alvarez JO, et al: The relationship between maternal serum zinc levels during pregnancy and birthweight. Early Hum Dev 25:75, 1991.
72. Goldenberg RL, Tamura T, Cliver SP, et al: Serum folate and fetal growth retardation: A matter of compliance? Obstet Gynecol 79:71, 1992.
73. Lackman F, Capewell V, Gagnon R, et al: Fetal umbilical cord oxygen values and birth to placental weight ratio in relation to size at birth. Am J Obstet Gynecol 185:674, 2001.
74. Lichty JA, Ting RY, Bruns PD, et al: Studies of babies born at high altitude. Am J Dis Child 93:666, 1957.
75. Novy MJ, Peterson EN, Metcalfe J: Respiratory characteristics of maternal and fetal blood in cyanotic congenital heart disease. Am J Obstet Gynecol 100:821, 1968.
76. Wen SW, Goldenberg RL, Cutter GR, et al: Smoking, maternal age, fetal growth and gestational age at delivery. Am J Obstet Gynecol 162:53, 1990.
77. Cliver SP, Goldenberg RL, Cutter GR, et al: The effect of cigarette smoking on neonatal anthropometric measurements. Obstet Gynecol 85:625, 1995.
78. Kallen K: Maternal smoking during pregnancy and infant head circumference at birth. Early Hum Dev 58:197, 2000.

79. Wang X, Zuckerman B, Pearson C, et al: Maternal cigarette smoking, metabolic gene polymorphism and infant birth weight. JAMA 287:195, 2002.
80. Mills JL, Graubard BI, Harley EE, et al: Maternal alcohol consumption and birthweight: How much drinking during pregnancy is safe? JAMA 252:1875, 1984.
81. Little BB, Snell LM: Brain growth among fetuses exposed to cocaine in utero: Asymmetrical growth retardation. Obstet Gynecol 77:361, 1991.
82. Heinonen S, Taipale P, Saarikoski S: Weights of placenta from small-for-gestational-age infants revisited. Placenta 86:428, 2001.
83. Molteni RA, Stys SJ, Battaglia FC: Relationship of fetal and placental weight in human beings: Fetal/placental weight ratios at various gestational ages and birth weight distributions. J Reprod Med 21:327, 1978.
84. Fisher SJ: The placental problem: Linking abnormal cytotrophoblast differentiation to the maternal symptoms of preeclampsia. Reprod Biol Endocrinol 2:53, 2004.
85. Kaufman P, Black S, Huppertz B: Endovascular trophoblast invasion: Implications for the pathogenesis of intrauterine growth retardation and peeeclampsia. Biol Reprod 69:1, 2003.
86. Red-Horse K, Rivera J, Schanz A, et al: Cytotrophoblast induction of arterial apoptosis and lymphangiogenesis in an in vivo model of human placentation. J Clin Invest 116:2643, 2006.
87. Huppertz B, Kadyrov M, Kingdom JCP: Apoptosis and its role in the trophoblast. Am J Obstet Gynecol 195:29, 2006.
88. Brosens I, Dixon HG, Robertson WB: Fetal growth retardation and the arteries of the placental bed. BJOG 84:656, 1977.
89. Aherne W, Dunnill MS: Quantitative aspects of placental structure. J Pathol Bacteriol 91:123, 1966.
90. Ishihara N, Matsuo H, Murakoshi H, et al: Increased apoptosis in syncytiotrophoblast in human term placentas complicated by either preeclampsia or intrauterine growth retardation. Am J Obstet Gynecol 186:158, 2002.
91. Levy R, Smith SD, Yusuf K, et al: Trophoblast apoptosis from pregnancies complicated by fetal growth restriction is associated with enhanced p53 expression. Am J Obstet Gynecol 186:1056, 2002.
92. Crispi F, Dominguez C, Llurba E, et al: Placental growth factors and uterine artery Doppler findings for characterization of different subsets in preeclampsia and in intrauterine growth restriction. Am J Obstet Gynecol 195:201, 2006.
93. Krebs C, Marca LM, Leiser RL, et al: Intrauterine growth restriction with absent end-diastolic flow velocity in the umbilical artery is associated with maldevelopment of the placental terminal villous tree. Am J Obstet Gynecol 175:1534, 1996.
94. Salafia CM, Pezzullo JC, Minior VK, et al: Placental pathology of absent and reversed end-diastolic flow in growth restricted fetuses. Obstet Gynecol 90:830, 1997.
95. Soothill PW, Nicolaides KH, Bilardo K, et al: Uteroplacental blood velocity index and umbilical venous PO_2, PCO_2, pH, lactate and erythroblast count in growth retarded fetuses. Fetal Ther 1:174, 1986.
96. Soothill PW, Nicolaides KH, Campbell S: Prenatal asphyxia, hyperlactiacidemia, hypoglycemia and erythroblastosis in growth retarded fetuses. BMJ 294:1046, 1987.
97. Cetin I, Corbetta C, Sereni LP, et al: Umbilical amino acid concentrations in normal and growth-retarded fetuses sampled in utero by cordocentesis. Am J Obstet Gynecol 162:253, 1990.
98. Shanklin DR: The influence of placental lesions and the newborn infant. Pediatr Clin North Am 17:25, 1970.
99. Ananth CV, Wilcox AJ: Placental abruption and perinatal mortality in the United States. Am J Epidemiol 153:332, 2001.
100. Ananth CV, Demissie K, Smulian JC, et al: Relationship among placenta previa, fetal growth restriction and preterm delivery: A population based study. Obstet Gynecol 98:299, 2001.
101. Creasy RK, Barrett CT, de Swiet M, et al: Experimental intrauterine growth retardation in the sheep. Am J Obstet Gynecol 112:566, 1972.
102. Clapp JF III, Szeto HH, Larrow R, et al: Fetal metabolic response to experimental placental vascular damage. Am J Obstet Gynecol 140:446, 1981.
103. Kong TY, DeWolf F, Robertson WB, et al: Inadequate maternal vascular response to placentation in pregnancies complicated by preeclampsia and small-for-gestational age infants. BJOG 93:1049, 1986.
104. Dixon HG, Browne JCM, Davey DA: Choriodecidual and myometrial blood flow. Lancet 2:369, 1963.
105. Kaar K, Joupilla P, Kuikka J, et al: Intervillous blood flow in normal and complicated late pregnancy measured by means of an intravenous Xe133 method. Acta Obstet Gynecol Scand 59:7, 1980.
106. Rosso P, Donoso E, Braun S, et al: Hemodynamic changes in underweight pregnant women. Obstet Gynecol 79:908, 1992.
107. Duvekot JJ, Cheriex EC, Pieters FAA, et al: Maternal volume homeostasis in early pregnancy in relation to fetal growth restriction. Obstet Gynecol 85:361, 1995.
108. Bamfo JE, Kametas NA, Turan O, et al: Maternal cardiac function in fetal growth. BJOG 113:784, 2006.
109. Fleischer A, Schulman H, Farmakides G, et al: Uterine artery Doppler velocimetry in pregnant women with hypertension. Am J Obstet Gynecol 154:806, 1986.
110. Campbell S, Bewley S, Cohen-Overbeek T: Investigation of the uteroplacental circulation by Doppler ultrasound. Semin Perinatol 11:362, 1987.
111. Easterling TR, Benedetti TJ, Carlson KC, et al: The effect of maternal hemodynamics on fetal growth in hypertensive pregnancies. Am J Obstet Gynecol 165:902, 1991.
112. Infante-Rivard C, Rivard GE, Yotov WV, et al: Absence of association of thrombophilia polymorphisms with intrauterine growth restriction. N Engl J Med 347:19-25, 2002.
113. Dizon-Townson D, Miller C, Sibai B, et al: The relationship of the factor V Leiden mutation and pregnancy outcomes for the mother and fetus. Obstet Gynecol 106:517-524, 2005.
114. Franchi F, Cetin I, Todros T, et al: Intrauterine growth restriction and genetic predisposition to thrombophilia. Haematologica 89:444-449, 2004.
115. Salomon O, Seligsohn U, Steinberg DM, et al: The common prothrombotic factors in nulliparous do not compromise blood flow in the feto-maternal circulation and are not associated with preeclampsia or intrauterine growth restriction. Am J Obstet Gynecol 191:2002-2009, 2004.
116. Andrews MC, Jones HW Jr: Impaired reproductive performance of the unicornuate uterus: Intrauterine growth retardation, infertility, and recurrent abortion in five cases. Am J Obstet Gynecol 144:173, 1982.
117. Burchell RC, Creed F, Rasoulpour M, et al: Vascular anatomy of the human uterus and pregnancy wastage. BJOG 85:698, 1978.
118. Shinagawa S, Nomura Y, Kudoh S: Full-term deliveries after ligation of bilateral internal iliac arteries and infundibulopelvic ligaments. Acta Obstet Gynecol Scand 60:439, 1981.
119. Pron G, Mocarski E, Bennett J, et al: Pregnancy after uterine artery embolization for leiomyomata: The Ontario Multicenter Trial. Obstet Gynecol 105:67, 2005.
120. Clapp JF, Kim H, Burciu B, et al: Beginning regular exercise in early pregnancy: Effect upon fetoplacental growth. Am J Obstet Gynecol 183:1484, 2000.
121. Clapp JF, Kim H, Burciu B, et al: Continuing regular exercise during pregnancy: Effect of exercise volume on fetoplacental growth. Am J Obstet Gynecol 186:142, 2002.
122. Perkins CCD, Pivarnik JM, Paneth N, et al: Physical activity and fetal growth during pregnancy. Obstet Gynecol 109:81, 2007.
123. Goldenberg RL, Hoffman HJ, Cliver SP, et al: The influence of previous low birth weight or birth weight, gestational age, and anthropometric measurement in the current pregnancy. Obstet Gynecol 79:276, 1992.
124. Cnattingius S, Forman MR, Poerendes HW, et al: Effect of age, parity and smoking on pregnancy outcome: A population based study. Am J Obstet Gynecol 168:16, 1993.
125. Thorburn GD: The role of the thyroid gland and kidneys in fetal growth. In Elliot K, Knight J (eds): Size at Birth. Amsterdam, Associated Scientific Publishers, 1974.

126. Liggins GC: The influence of the fetal hypothalamus and pituitary on growth. In Elliot K, Knight J (eds): Size at Birth. Amsterdam, Associated Scientific Publishers, 1974.
127. Sherwood WG, Chance GW, Hill DE: A new syndrome of pancreatic agenesis. Pediatr Res 8:360, 1974.
128. Henson MC, Castracane VD: Leptin in pregnancy. Biol Reprod 74:218, 2006.
129. Neilson JP: Symphysis-fundal height measurement in pregnancy. Cochrane Database Syst Rev (2):CD000944, 2000.
130. Mongelli M, Gardosi J: Symphysis-fundus height and pregnancy characteristics in ultrasound-dated pregnancies. Obstet Gynecol 94:591-594, 1999.
131. Hadlock FP, Harrist RB, Carpenter RD, et al: Sonographic estimation of fetal weight. Radiology 150:535, 1984.
132. Snijders RJ, Nicolaides KH: Fetal biometry at 14-40 weeks gestation. Ultrasound Obstet Gynecol 4:34, 1994.
133. Chang TC, Robson SC, Boys RJ, et al: Prediction of the small-for-gestational age infant: Which ultrasonic measurement is best? Obstet Gynecol 80:1030, 1992.
134. Bukowski R, Smith GC, Malone FD, et al: Fetal growth in early pregnancy and risk of delivering low birth weight infant: Prospective cohort study. BMJ 334:836, 2007.
135. Smith GC, Smith MF, McNay MB, et al: First trimester growth and the risk of low birth weight. N Engl J Med 339:1817, 1998.
136. Papageorghiou AT, Yu CK, Bindra R, et al: The Fetal Medicine Foundation Second Trimester Screening Group: Multicenter screening for pre-eclampsia and fetal growth restriction by transvaginal uterine artery Doppler at 23 weeks of gestation. Ultrasound Obstet Gynecol 18:441, 2001.
137. Pilalis A, Souka AP, Antsaklis P, et al: Screening for preeclampsia and fetal growth restriction by uterine artery Doppler and PAPP-A at 11-14 weeks gestation. Ultrasound Obstet Gynecol 29:135, 2007.
138. Rabinowitz R, Peters MT, Sanjay V, et al: Measurement of fetal urine production in normal pregnancy by real time ultrasonography. Am J Obstet Gynecol 161:1264, 1989.
139. Wladimiroff JW, Campbell S: Fetal urine production rates in normal and complicated pregnancies. Lancet 2:151, 1974.
140. Kurjak A, Kirkinen P, Latin V, et al: Ultrasonic assessment of fetal kidney function in normal and complicated pregnancies. Am J Obstet Gynecol 141:266, 1981.
141. Nicolaides KH, Peters MT, Vyas S: Relation of rate of urine production to oxygen tension in small-for-gestational age fetuses. Am J Obstet Gynecol 162:387, 1990.
142. Manning FA, Hill LM, Platt LD: Qualitative amniotic fluid volume determination by ultrasound: Antepartum detection of intrauterine growth retardation. Am J Obstet Gynecol 139:254, 1981.
143. Chamberlain PF, Manning FA, Morrison I, et al: Ultrasound evaluation of amniotic fluid: I. The relationship of marginal and decreased amniotic fluid volume to perinatal outcome. Am J Obstet Gynecol 150:245, 1984.
144. Bastide A, Manning FA, Harman C, et al: Ultrasound evaluation of amniotic fluid: Outcome of pregnancies with severe oligohydramnios. Am J Obstet Gynecol 154:895, 1986.
145. Alfirevic Z, Neilson JP: Biophysical profile for fetal assessment in high risk pregnancies. Cochrane Database Syst Rev (2):CD000038, 2000.
146. Manning FA, Morrison I, Harman CR, et al: Fetal assessment based on fetal biophysical profile scoring: Experience in 19,221 high-risk pregnancies. Am J Obstet Gynecol 157:880, 1987.
147. Manning FA, Harman CR, Morrison I, et al: Fetal assessment based on fetal biophysical profile scoring. Am J Obstet Gynecol 162:703, 1990.
148. Kingdom JCP, Burrell SJ, Kaufmann P: Pathology and clinical implications of abnormal umbilical artery Doppler waveforms. Ultrasound Obstet Gynecol 9:271, 1997.
149. Almstrom H, Axelsson O, Cnattingius S, et al: Comparison of umbilical artery velocimetry and cardiotacography for surveillance of small-for-gestational-age fetuses: A multicenter randomized controlled trial. Lancet 340:936, 1992.
150. Omtzigt AM, Reuwer PJ, Bruinse HW: A randomized controlled trial on the clinical value of umbilical Doppler velocimetry in antenatal care. Am J Obstet Gynecol 170:625, 1994.
151. Pattison RC, Norman K, Odendal HJ: The role of Doppler velocimetry in the management of high-risk pregnancies. BJOG 101:114, 1994.
152. Alfirevic Z, Neilson JP: Doppler ultrasonography in high-risk pregnancies: Systematic review with meta-analysis. Am J Obstet Gynecol 172:1379, 1995.
153. Gonzalez JM, Stamillo DM, Ural S, et al: Relationship between abnormal fetal testing and adverse perinatal outcomes in intrauterine growth restriction. Am J Obstet Gynecol 196:e48, 2007.
154. Ott WJ: Intrauterine growth restriction and Doppler ultrasonography. J Ultrasound Med 19:661, 2000.
155. Wladimiroff JW, vd Wijngaard JA, Degani S, et al: Cerebral and umbilical arterial waveforms in normal and growth-retarded pregnancies. Obstet Gynecol 69:705, 1987.
156. Karsdorp VH, van Vugt JM, van Geijn HP, et al: Clinical significance of absent or reversed end-diastolic velocity waveforms in the umbilical artery. Lancet 334:1664, 1994.
157. Valcamonico A, Danti L, Frusca T, et al: Absent end-diastolic velocity in umbilical artery: Risk of neonatal morbidity and brain damage. Am J Obstet Gynecol 170:796, 1994.
158. Ferrazzi E, Bozzo M, Rigano S, et al: Temporal sequence of abnormal Doppler changes in the peripheral and central circulatory systems of the severely growth-restricted fetus. Ultrasound Obstet Gynecol 19:140, 2002.
159. Baschat AA, Gembruch U, Harman CR: The sequence of changes in Doppler and biophysical parameters as severe fetal growth restriction worsens. Ultrasound Obstet Gynecol 18:571, 2001.
160. Baschat AA, Harman CR: Antenatal assessment of the growth restricted fetus. Curr Opin Obstet Gynecol 13:161, 2001.
161. Schwarze A, Gembruch U, Krapp M, et al: Qualitative venous Doppler flow waveform analysis in preterm intrauterine growth-restricted fetuses with ARED flow in the umbilical artery-correlation with short term outcome. Ultrasound Obstet Gynecol 25:573, 2005.
162. Turan S, Turan OM, Berg C, et al: Computerized fetal heart rate analysis, Doppler ultrasound and biophysical profile score in the prediction of acid-base status of growth-restricted fetuses. Ultrasound Obstet Gynecol 30:750, 2007.
163. Nicolaides KH, Bradley RJ, Soothill PW, et al: Maternal oxygen therapy for intrauterine growth retardation. Lancet 1:942, 1987.
164. Battaglia C, Artini PG, d'Ambrogio G, et al: Maternal hyperoxygenation in the treatment of intrauterine growth retardation. Am J Obstet Gynecol 167:430, 1992.
165. Gulmezoglu AM, Hofmeyer GJ: Maternal oxygen administration for suspected and impaired fetal growth. Cochran Database Syst Rev (2): CD000137, 2000.
166. Rumbold AR, Crowther CA, Haslam RR, et al: ACTS Study Group. Vitamins C and E and the risks of reeclampsia and perinatal complications. N Engl J Med 354:1796, 2006.
167. Makrides M, Duley L, Olsen SAF: Marine oil, and other prostaglandin precursor, supplementation for pregnancy uncomplicated by preeclampsia or intrauterine growth restriction. Cochrane Database Syst Rev (3): CD003402, 2006.
168. Duley L, Henderson-Smart DJ, Meher S, et al: Antiplatelet agents for preventing pre-eclampsia and its complications. Cochrane Database Syst Rev (2):CD004659, 2007.
169. Berghella V: Prevention of recurrent fetal growth restriction. Obstet Gynecol 110:904, 2007.
170. Thornton JG, Hornbuckle J, Vail A, et al: Infant wellbeing at 2 years of age in the Growth Restriction Intervention Trial (GRIT): Multicentered randomised controlled trial. Lancet 364:513, 2004.
171. Low JA, Boston RW, Pancham SR: Fetal asphyxia during the intrapartum period in growth-retarded infants. Am J Obstet Gynecol 113:351, 1972.
172. Garite TJ, Clark R, Thorp JA: Intrauterine growth restriction increases morbidity and mortality among premature neonates. Am J Obstet Gynecol 191:481, 2004.

173. Low JA, Handley-Derry MH, Burke SO, et al: Association of intrauterine fetal growth retardation and learning deficits at age 9 to 11 years. Am J Obstet Gynecol 167:1499, 1992.
174. Blair E, Stanley F: Intrauterine growth and spastic cerebral palsy: I. Association with birth weight and gestational age. Am J Obstet Gynecol 162:229, 1990.
175. Blair E, Stanley F: Intrauterine growth and spastic cerebral palsy: II. The association with morphology at birth. Early Hum Dev 28:91, 1992.
176. Samuelsen GB, Pakkenberg B, Bogdanovic N, et al: Severe cell reduction in the future brain cortex in human growth-restricted fetuses and infants. Am J Obstet Gynecol 197;56.e1-56.e7, 2007.
177. Paz I, Laor A, Gale R, et al: Term infants with fetal growth restriction are not all at increased risk for low intelligence scores at 17 years. J Pediatr 138:87, 2001.
178. McCowan LME, Pryor J, Harding JE: Perinatal predictors of neurodevelopmental outcome in small-for-gestational-age children at 18 months of age. Am J Obstet Gynecol 186:1069, 2002.
179. Barker DJP, Robinson RJ (eds): Fetal and Infant Origins of Adult Disease. London, British Medical Journal, 1992.

Chapter 35

Pregnancy-Related Hypertension

James M. Roberts, MD, and Edmund F. Funai, MD

Classification of Hypertensive Disorders

Interpreting epidemiologic studies of the hypertensive disorders of pregnancy is difficult because the terminology is inconsistent.[1] Several systems of nomenclature are in use around the world. The system prepared by the National Institutes of Health (NIH) Working Group on Hypertension in Pregnancy,[2] although imperfect, has the advantage of clarity and is available in published form for investigators throughout the world. The NIH system has four main classes: chronic hypertension, preeclampsia and eclampsia, preeclampsia superimposed on chronic hypertension, and gestational hypertension.

Chronic Hypertension

Chronic hypertension is defined as hypertension that is observable before pregnancy or that is diagnosed before the 20th week of gestation. Hypertension is defined as a persistent blood pressure greater than 140/90 mm Hg. Hypertension for which a diagnosis is confirmed for the first time during pregnancy and that persists beyond the 84th day after delivery is also classified as chronic hypertension.

Preeclampsia and Eclampsia

The diagnosis of preeclampsia is determined by increased blood pressure accompanied by proteinuria. The diagnosis requires a systolic pressure of 140 mm Hg or higher or a diastolic pressure of 90 mm Hg or higher. Diastolic blood pressure is defined as the Korotkoff phase V value (i.e., disappearance of sounds). Gestational blood pressure elevation should be determined by at least two measurements, with the repeat blood pressure performed in a manner that reduces the likelihood of artifact and patient anxiety.[3] Absent from the diagnostic criteria is the former inclusion of an increment of 30 mm Hg in systolic or 15 mm Hg in diastolic blood pressure, even when absolute values are below 140/90 mm Hg. This definition was excluded because available evidence shows that women in this group are not likely to suffer increased adverse outcomes.[4,5] Nonetheless, women who have an increase of 30 mm Hg in systolic or 15 mm Hg in diastolic blood pressure warrant close observation, especially if proteinuria and hyperuricemia (i.e., uric acid ≥ 5.5 mg/dL)[6] are also present.[3]

Proteinuria is defined as the urinary excretion of at least 300 mg of protein in a 24-hour specimen. This usually correlates with 30 mg/dL of protein (i.e., 1+ dipstick reading) or more in a random urine determination. Because of the discrepancy between random protein determinations and 24-hour urine protein values in women with preeclampsia (which can be higher or lower),[7-9] the diagnosis should be based on a 24-hour urine specimen or on a timed collection corrected for creatinine excretion if a 24-hour collection is not feasible.[3]

Preeclampsia occurs as a spectrum but is arbitrarily divided into mild and severe forms. This terminology is useful for descriptive purposes but does not indicate specific diseases, nor should it indicate arbitrary cutoff points for therapy. The diagnosis of severe preeclampsia is confirmed when any of the following criteria are met[10]:

- Blood pressure of 160 mm Hg systolic or higher or 110 mm Hg diastolic or higher on two occasions at least 6 hours apart while the patient is on bed rest
- Proteinuria of 5 g or higher in a 24-hour urine specimen or 3+ or greater on two random urine samples collected at least 4 hours apart
- Oliguria of less than 500 mL in 24 hours
- Cerebral or visual disturbances
- Pulmonary edema or cyanosis
- Epigastric or right upper quadrant pain
- Impaired liver function
- Thrombocytopenia
- Fetal growth restriction

Eclampsia is the occurrence of seizures that cannot be attributed to other causes in a woman with preeclampsia.

Edema occurs in too many normal pregnant women to be discriminant and has been abandoned as a marker in preeclampsia by the National High Blood Pressure Education Program and by other classification schemes.[11,12] Edema of the hands and face occurs in 10% to 15% of women whose blood pressure remains normal throughout pregnancy.[13] Edema can be massive in women with severe preeclampsia, rendering the patient virtually unrecognizable (Fig. 35-1).

Preeclampsia Superimposed on Chronic Hypertension

There is ample evidence that preeclampsia can occur in women who are already hypertensive and that the prognosis for mother and fetus is much worse with both conditions than with either alone. Distinguishing superimposed preeclampsia from worsening chronic hypertension tests the skills of the clinician. For clinical management, the principles of high sensitivity and unavoidable overdiagnosis are appro-

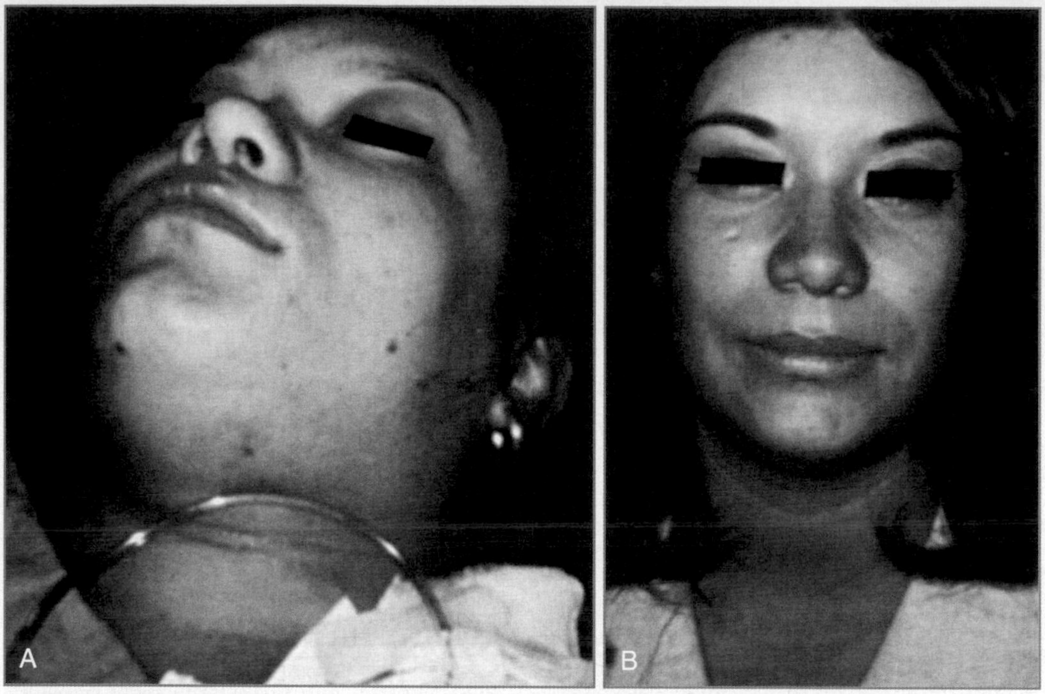

FIGURE 35-1 **Facial edema in severe preeclampsia.** Markedly edematous facies of this severely preeclamptic woman **(A)** is especially evident when compared with her appearance 6 weeks after delivery **(B)**.

priate, especially with advancing gestational age. The suspicion of superimposed preeclampsia mandates close observation, with delivery indicated by the overall assessment of maternal and fetal well-being rather than by any fixed end point. The diagnosis of superimposed preeclampsia is highly likely with the following findings:

1. In women with documented hypertension and no proteinuria before 20 weeks' gestation
   - New-onset proteinuria, defined as the urinary excretion of 0.3 g of protein or more in a 24-hour specimen
2. In women with hypertension and proteinuria before 20 weeks' gestation
   - A sudden increase in proteinuria
   - A sudden increase in blood pressure in a woman whose blood pressure has previously been well controlled
   - Objective evidence of involvement of multiple organ systems, such as thrombocytopenia (platelet count < 100,000/mm^3), an increase in liver transaminases to abnormal levels,[3] or sudden worsening of renal function

Gestational Hypertension

A woman who has no proteinuria and a blood pressure elevation detected for the first time during pregnancy is classified as having gestational hypertension. This is a provisional diagnosis that includes women with preeclampsia who have not yet manifested proteinuria and women who do not have preeclampsia. The hypertension may be accompanied by other concerning signs or symptoms that can influence management. A final determination that the woman does not have preeclampsia can be made only after delivery. If preeclampsia has not developed and blood pressure has returned to normal by 12 weeks after delivery, the diagnosis of transient hypertension of pregnancy can be assigned. If blood pressure elevation persists, the diagnosis is chronic hypertension. The diagnosis of gestational hypertension is used during pregnancy only until a more specific diagnosis can be assigned after delivery.[3]

Problems with Classification

The degree of blood pressure elevation that constitutes gestational hypertension is controversial. Because average blood pressure in women younger than 30 years is 120/60 mm Hg, the standard definition of hypertension (i.e., blood pressure >140/90 mm Hg) is judged by some to be too high,[14] resulting in the suggestion that women with blood pressure increases greater than 30 mm Hg systolic or 15 mm Hg diastolic should be observed closely even if absolute blood pressure has not exceeded 140/90 mm Hg.[3]

Blood pressures measured in early pregnancy to diagnose chronic hypertension are problematic. Blood pressure usually decreases early in pregnancy, reaching its nadir at about the time women often present for obstetric care (Fig. 35-2). The decrease averages 7 mm Hg for diastolic and systolic readings. In some women, blood pressure may decline by more than 7 mm Hg; in others, the early decline and subsequent return of blood pressure to pre-pregnant levels in late gestation may satisfy criteria for a diagnosis of preeclampsia. Women with hypertension before pregnancy have a greater decrease in blood pressure in early pregnancy than do normotensive women,[15] and they are more likely to be misdiagnosed as preeclamptic according to blood pressure criteria.

The diagnosis of chronic hypertension based on the failure of blood pressure to return to normal by 84 days after delivery can be in error. In a long-range, prospective study by Chesley,[16] many women who remained hypertensive 6 weeks after delivery were normotensive at long-term follow-up. Neither proteinuria nor hypertension is specific

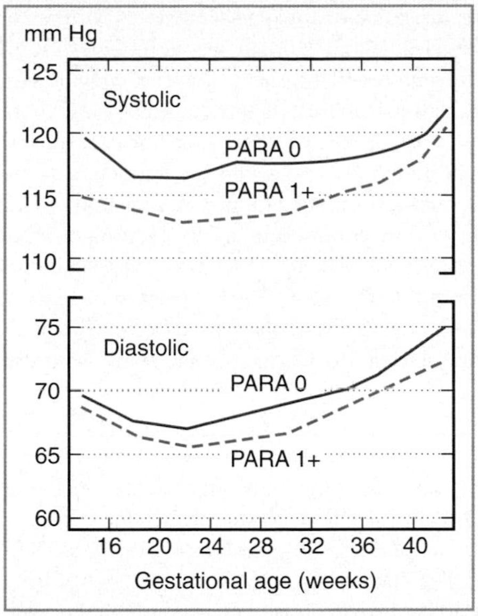

FIGURE 35-2 Blood pressure correlated with gestational age. The mean blood pressure was plotted against gestational age for 6000 white women between the ages of 25 and 34 years who delivered singleton term infants. (From Christianson R, Page EW: Studies on blood pressure during pregnancy: Influence of parity and age. Am J Obstet Gynecol 125:509, 1976. Courtesy of the American College of Obstetricians and Gynecologists.)

TABLE 35-1 RENAL BIOPSY FINDINGS IN PATIENTS WITH A CLINICAL DIAGNOSIS OF PREECLAMPSIA

Biopsy Findings	Primigravidas (*n* = 62)	Multigravidas (*n* = 152)
Glomeruloendotheliosis with or without nephrosclerosis	70%	14%
Normal histology	5%	53%
Chronic renal disease, chronic glomerulonephritis, or chronic pyelonephritis	25%	21%
Arteriolar nephrosclerosis	0%	12%

Modified from McCartney CP: Pathological anatomy of acute hypertension of pregnancy. Circulation 30(Suppl II):37, 1964; by permission of the American Heart Association, Inc.

to preeclampsia, and their presence in pregnancy can have other explanations.

Renal biopsy specimens from women with preeclampsia demonstrate these diagnostic difficulties (Table 35-1).[17] Of 62 women with a diagnosis of preeclampsia in their first pregnancies, 70% had a glomerular lesion believed to be characteristic of the disorder, but 24% had evidence of chronic renal disease that was not previously suspected. Renal biopsy specimens of multiparous women with a clinical diagnosis of superimposed preeclampsia also demonstrate the uncertainty of diagnosis. Of 152 subjects, only 3% had the characteristic glomerular lesion, but 43% had evidence of preexisting renal or vascular disease.

Preeclampsia has a clinical spectrum ranging from mild to severe forms. The illness in affected women does not begin with eclampsia or the severe manifestations of preeclampsia. Rather, the disease progresses at various rates. In most cases, progression is slow, and the disorder may remain mild. In others, the disease can progress rapidly, changing from mild to severe over days to weeks or, in fulminant cases, progressing in days or hours.

In a series of eclamptic women analyzed by Chesley,[18] 25% had evidence of only mild preeclampsia in the days preceding convulsions. For purposes of clinical management, overdiagnosis must be accepted because prevention of the serious complications of preeclampsia and eclampsia requires increased sensitivity and early treatment, primarily through the timing of delivery. For this reason, studies of preeclampsia are necessarily confounded by inclusion of women diagnosed as preeclamptic who have another cardiovascular or renal disorder.

HELLP Syndrome

The pathophysiologic changes of preeclampsia can occur in the absence of hypertension and proteinuria. This is not surprising, because the traditional diagnostic criteria have more historical than pathophysiologic relevance.[18] This situation presents a challenge to clinicians and demands that they remain alert to the possibility of preeclampsia in pregnant women with signs and symptoms that may be explained by reduced organ perfusion. One clear setting in which this occurs is the HELLP syndrome (*h*emolysis, *e*levated *l*iver enzymes, and *l*ow *p*latelets), a combination of findings that defines a reasonably consistent syndrome.[19]

For management purposes, it is appropriate to consider HELLP as a variant of preeclampsia, but they may be different entities. Women with HELLP are more often older, white, and multiparous than preeclamptic women. Not all women with HELLP have hypertension.[20] From a pathophysiologic perspective, changes in the renin-angiotensin system characteristic of preeclampsia are not present in HELLP.[21] Nonetheless, progression of the disease and its termination with delivery argue for an observation and management strategy similar to that for preeclampsia.

Preeclampsia and Eclampsia

Epidemiology of Preeclampsia and Eclampsia

Despite the difficulties in clinical diagnosis, there exists a disorder unique to pregnancy characterized by poor perfusion of many vital organs (including the fetoplacental unit) that is completely reversible with the termination of pregnancy. Pathologic, pathophysiologic, and prognostic findings indicate that preeclampsia is not merely an unmasking of preexisting, underlying hypertension. Although the unique nature of preeclampsia has been well documented for many years, controversies in therapy persist because of management strategies based on principles used to treat hypertension in nonpregnant individuals. The successful management of preeclampsia requires an understanding of the pathophysiologic changes in this condition and recognition that the signs of preeclampsia (i.e., increased blood pressure and proteinuria) are only signs and do not cause the other features of preeclampsia.

Women at Risk

Preeclampsia occurs in about 4% of pregnancies that continue past the first trimester. Nulliparity is the most common feature of women who develop preeclampsia. At least two thirds of cases occur in the first pregnancy that progresses beyond the first trimester. Other risk factors for preeclampsia are similar in nulliparous and parous women.[22]

Although preeclampsia was thought to be more common among women of lower socioeconomic status, this impression may be a consequence of the associations of preeclampsia with age, race, and parity. Studies of pregnant women in Scotland[23] from Aberdeen,[24] Finland,[25] and Israel[26] found that preeclampsia was not related to socioeconomic status. Eclampsia, in contrast, is clearly more common in women of lower socioeconomic status,[23,25,26] related to the lack of availability of quality obstetric care for indigent women. Remarkably, preeclampsia and eclampsia were once thought to occur more frequently in women of higher socioeconomic status.[18]

There is a relationship between the extremes of childbearing age and the incidence of eclampsia and preeclampsia. Because most first pregnancies occur in young women, most cases of preeclampsia and eclampsia occur in this age group, but the association with young maternal age is lost when parity is considered. In the studies cited,[23,25,26] a higher incidence of preeclampsia was found in older women independent of parity.

The relationship of preeclampsia and eclampsia to race is complicated by the higher prevalence of chronic hypertension in African Americans and the difficulty in differentiating preeclampsia from unrecognized preexisting chronic hypertension. Some studies indicate a relationship.[26,27] In a small case-control study of carefully defined preeclampsia, black race was a significant risk factor only in nulliparous women (odds ratio [OR] = 12.3; 95% confidence interval [CI], 1.6 to 100.8).[28] Other studies support a more modest increased risk in African-American women.[29,30] Studies that include the more severe forms of preeclampsia more often suggest an increased incidence among African-American women.[28]

In contrast, the incidence of rigorously defined preeclampsia did not differ by race after other risk factors were controlled in two large, prospective trials of medical prophylaxis that enrolled 2947[31] and 4314[32] nulliparous women. Maternal nonwhite race appears to be related more to the severity than the incidence of disease.

A diverse array of medical disorders that often coexist with pregnancy, including diabetes, chronic hypertension, chronic renal disorders, and rheumatologic conditions, have been associated with preeclampsia. The existence and severity of diabetes have been associated with an increased risk for preeclampsia, and diabetic microvascular disease further increases this risk. This relationship has been found in Sweden[33] and in the United States.[34] Both studies[33,34] demonstrated that the risk of preeclampsia was approximately 20% and 21% in 491 and 462 pregnancies, respectively. This estimate is far more modest than the 50% incidence reported in historical cohorts.[18] The preeclampsia risk increased according to the severity of disease, with an 11% to 12% risk among women with class B diabetes and 21% to 23% with class C and D diabetes. Microvascular disease increased this risk to 36% to 54% in diabetics with class F or R disease.[33,34]

Chronic renal insufficiency and hypertension are well-recognized risk factors. Of women with hypertension antedating pregnancy, 25% develop preeclampsia.[35,36] Renal insufficiency with[33,37] and without diabetes[38-40] also is an important risk factor.[38,40]

Connective tissue disorders such as systemic lupus erythematosus[41,42] and antiphospholipid antibody syndrome[43-45] have been reported as risk factors for preeclampsia. With lupus, the risk is particularly elevated with hypertension or nephropathy.[46,47] However, data concerning an association between isolated antiphospholipid antibodies and preeclampsia have been conflicting, with some studies demonstrating no relationship[48,49] and others confirming the association.[44,50]

Obesity is a risk factor for preeclampsia.[28,51] In the National Institute of Child Health and Human Development (NICHD) study of aspirin to prevent preeclampsia in low-risk pregnancies,[31] the incidence of preeclampsia increased with maternal body mass index. Even in women of normal weight, there is a linear relationship between pre-pregnancy body mass index and the frequency of preeclampsia.[52] The mechanism may be related to increased insulin resistance, because preeclampsia is more common in another setting of increased insulin resistance: gestational diabetes.[53] With a threefold increased risk for obese women and with 35% to 50% of women of reproductive age in the United States being obese, obesity has become a major attributable risk factor for preeclampsia, which is associated with more than one third of cases of preeclampsia.

Certain conditions of pregnancy increase the risk of preeclampsia. The incidence is increased among parous and nulliparous women with multiple gestations, although to a larger degree in the latter.[36,54] In a study of 34,374 pregnancies with singleton, twin, triplet, or quadruplet pregnancies, the incidence of preeclampsia increased with each additional fetus. The incidences were 6.7%, 12.7%, 20.0%, and 19.6%, respectively.[55] The disease process may be initiated earlier and may be more severe in these cases.[54]

Preeclampsia affects 70% of women with large, rapidly growing hydatidiform moles and occurs earlier than usual during gestation.[56] In cases of preeclampsia occurring before 24 weeks' gestation, hydatidiform mole should be suspected and sought.

An interesting variant of preeclampsia is the *mirror syndrome*, in which the mother's peripheral edema mirrors the fetal hydrops. It occurs with fetal hydrops, although not with erythroblastosis uncomplicated by hydrops. The incidence approaches 50% of pregnancies complicated by hydrops. The mirror syndrome is not confined to hydrops resulting from isoimmunization. In one series, mirror syndrome occurred in 9 of 11 pregnancies with hydropic infants of nonimmune origin.[57] This condition can manifest early in pregnancy with severe signs and symptoms of preeclampsia, and it has resolved with treatment of the underlying process.[58-60] Proteinuria is massive, and blood pressure elevation and edema are marked. Eclampsia occurs rarely (see Chapter 26).

Short-Term Prognosis for Preeclampsia

PERINATAL MORTALITY

The perinatal mortality rate is increased in infants of preeclamptic women.[61-63] In a study that examined 10,614,679 singleton pregnancies in the United States from 1995 to 1997 after 24 weeks' gestation, the relative risk for fetal death was 1.4 for infants born to women with any of the gestational hypertensive disorders and 2.7 for those born to women with chronic hypertensive disorders compared with low-risk controls. Causes of perinatal death are placental insufficiency and abruptio placentae,[64] which cause intrauterine death before or during labor, and prematurity. Predictably, the mortality rate is higher for infants of women with more severe forms of the disorder. At any level of disease severity, the perinatal mortality rate is greatest for women with preeclampsia superimposed on preexisting vascular disease.

The stillbirth rate attributable to preeclampsia has declined dramatically in the past 35 years. However, infants born of preeclamptic pregnancies continue to have an approximately twofold increased risk for neonatal death.[65] Although neonatal survival rates have improved dramatically, delivery before 34 weeks' gestation continues to be associated with an increased risk of long-range neurologic disability (see Chapter 58).

Growth restriction is more common in infants born to preeclamptic women (see Chapter 34) and more pronounced with increasing severity and earlier diagnosis.[66] As with perinatal mortality, intrauterine growth restriction (IUGR) is more common in infants of chronically hypertensive women with superimposed preeclampsia.[67]

The dramatic decrease in perinatal mortality rate among infants of preeclamptic women is the result in part of improved medical and obstetric management, including improved assessment of fetal well-being in the antepartum and intrapartum periods. The primary effect on the perinatal mortality rate, however, has come from improvements in neonatal care.

MATERNAL MORTALITY

Maternal death associated with preeclampsia predominantly results from complications of abruptio placentae, hepatic rupture, and eclampsia. Historically, the mortality rate of eclamptic women was most effectively reduced by avoiding iatrogenic complications related to overmedication and overzealous attempts at vaginal delivery. In series from the late 19th century, when immediate delivery was the practice, the mortality rate of eclamptic women was 20% to 30%. Expectant management with profound maternal sedation with narcotics and hypnotics in the early 20th century was associated with a 10% to 15% mortality rate. The change to magnesium as the exclusive agent in the 1920s and 1930s resulted in a maternal mortality rate of 5%. Although magnesium was undoubtedly helpful, the primary factor responsible for improved mortality was decreased maternal sedation.[18] The currently used combination of magnesium sulfate ($MgSO_4$) and antihypertensive drugs as sole pharmacologic agents, followed by timely delivery, has produced a maternal mortality rate of almost zero[68,69] because of an appreciation of the profound pathophysiologic abnormalities of preeclampsia, careful cardiopulmonary monitoring, and limitation of unproven interventions.

RECURRENCE IN SUBSEQUENT PREGNANCIES

Data from classic series indicate that the likelihood of recurrent preeclampsia is influenced by the certainty of the clinical diagnosis in the first pregnancy. Of 225 women with hypertension during pregnancy chosen for study without regard to parity, 70% had a recurrence of preeclampsia in their next pregnancy.[70] In a study of primiparas with severe preeclampsia, the recurrence rate was 45% .[71] Because the diagnosis in these studies was based solely on clinical findings, these groups probably included patients with unrecognized preexisting blood pressure elevation or underlying renal or cardiovascular disease.

Recurrence rates were reported in 2006 for 896 parous women in Iceland according to standardized diagnostic criteria in both pregnancies (i.e., National High Blood Pressure Criteria[3]). The rates of recurrence differed substantially by the diagnosis in the first pregnancy, as seen in Table 35-2.[72]

To determine the subsequent pregnancy outcomes of women who clearly had preeclampsia, Chesley and colleagues[74] followed 270 women with eclampsia for more than 40 years; only two were lost to follow-up. Among 187 women who had eclampsia in the first pregnancy, 33% had a hypertensive disorder in any subsequent pregnancy. In most, the condition was not severe, but 5% had recurrent eclampsia. Twenty women with eclampsia as multiparas had recurrent hypertension in 50% of subsequent pregnancies.

Women with a clinical diagnosis of preeclampsia have increased risk for hypertensive disorders in subsequent pregnancies. The chances of recurrence decrease as the likelihood of true preeclampsia increases. If the condition does recur, it will usually not be worse, and if preeclampsia truly arose de novo, it probably will be less severe in subsequent pregnancies. Some women, however, are normotensive between pregnancies but have recurrent preeclampsia. The risk of such recurrence is increased when preeclampsia occurs in the late second or early third trimester.[73] The recurrence of severe preeclampsia or eclampsia in one pregnancy predicts its likely recurrence in subsequent pregnancies.

Preeclampsia and Cardiovascular Disease in Later Life

Evidence that preeclampsia is associated with long-term maternal health consequences is based on the work of Chesley and coworkers,[74] who followed a cohort of white women with eclampsia in their first pregnancy and reported no increased risk of subsequent chronic hypertension. However, mortality was twofold to fivefold higher over the next 35 years among women with eclampsia in any pregnancy after the first (Fig. 35-3). The findings of Chesley and colleagues[74] led to speculation that multiparous women with preeclampsia or eclampsia were more likely to have had unrecognized underlying chronic hypertension and that this, not preeclampsia, caused the subsequent increase in mortality. Sibai and associates[71] also found that women with recurrent preeclampsia were more likely to develop chronic hypertension. These studies are the basis for a statement by The National High Blood Pressure Education Program's Working Group on High Blood Pressure during Pregnancy that recurrent hypertension in pregnancy, preeclampsia in a multipara, and early-onset disease in any pregnancy may all herald increased future health risks.[2]

Women with idiopathic preeclampsia (i.e., preeclampsia occurring in nulliparous women without underlying renal or cardiovascular disease, including chronic hypertension) were not thought to have increased risk of later vascular disease until a report from Norway[75] found modest (1.65-fold) increased cardiovascular mortality for nulliparous women with preeclampsia at term and an eightfold increased risk when preeclampsia was severe enough to lead to preterm delivery.

TABLE 35-2 TYPE OF RECURRENT HYPERTENSION DURING THE SECOND PREGNANCY BY TYPE OF HYPERTENSION IN THE FIRST PREGNANCY

	Second Pregnancy*					
First Pregnancy	Normal	Gestational Hypertension	Preeclampsia	Chronic Hypertension	Superimposed Preeclampsia	All Recurrences
Gestational hypertension (*n* = 511)	153 (29.9%)	239 (46.8%)	25 (4.9%)	82 (16%)	12 (2.3%)	358 (70.1%)
Preeclampsia/eclampsia (*n* = 151)	63 (41.7%)	52 (34.4%)	17 (11.3%)	16 (10.6%)	3 (2%)	88 (58.3%)
Chronic hypertension (*n* = 200)	24 (12%)	69 (34.5%)	6 (3%)	91 (45.5%)	10 (5%)	176 (88%)
Superimposed preeclampsia (*n* = 34)	2 (5.9%)	10 (29.4%)	4 (11.8%)	14 (41.2%)	4 (11.8%)	32 (94%)
Total (*N* = 896)	242 (27%)	370 (41.3%)	52 (5.8%)	203 (22.7%)	29 (3.2%)	654 (73%)

*No women had eclampsia in the second pregnancy.

From Hjartardottir S, Leifsson BG, Geirsson RT, Steinthorsdottir V: Recurrence of hypertensive disorder in second pregnancy. Am J Obstet Gynecol 194:916-920, 2006.

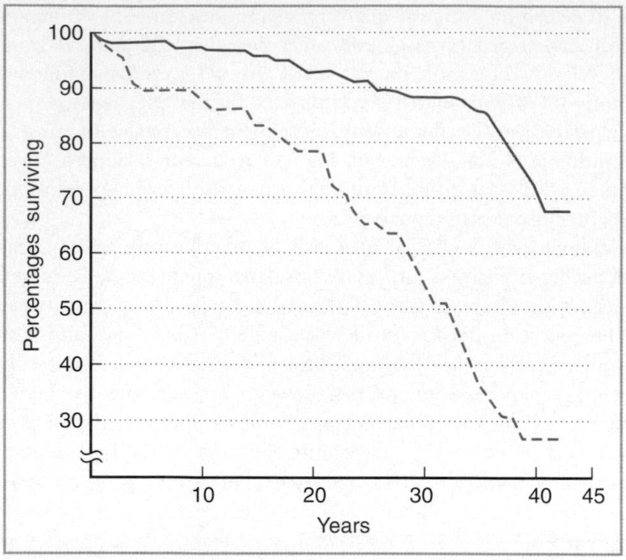

FIGURE 35-3 Eclampsia survivorship. Survival times are plotted for women with eclampsia in the first pregnancy *(solid line)* and those with eclampsia in a later pregnancy *(dashed line)*. Survival of women with first-pregnancy eclampsia was not different from survival of a control group. (From Chesley LC, Annitto JE, Cosgrove RA: The remote prognosis of eclamptic women: Sixth periodic report. Am J Obstet Gynecol 124:446, 1976, Courtesy of the American College of Obstetricians and Gynecologists.)

Scottish investigators reported a fourfold increased risk of subsequent hypertension in nulliparous women with preeclampsia[2,76,77] (OR = 3.98; CI, 2.82 to 5.61). Funai and colleagues[78] described excess long-term mortality in women with prior preeclampsia that was largely attributed to a threefold increase in deaths due to cardiovascular disease. Other reports support a link between preeclampsia and maternal ischemic heart disease,[79,80] which is sometimes evident 20 years after the preeclamptic pregnancy and coincident with the onset of menopause.[78,80] A family history of cardiovascular disease increases the association between preeclampsia and cardiovascular outcomes.[81] Obesity is a known risk factor for preeclampsia and cardiovascular disease. Although controlling for obesity attenuates the increased risk of death for postmenopausal women, this risk is not fully explained by obesity alone.[82]

The relationships among obesity, insulin resistance, and preeclampsia are part of an interesting relationship of preeclampsia to the metabolic or insulin resistance syndrome.[83] This syndrome predisposes to cardiovascular disease in later life and consists of obesity, hypertension, dyslipidemia (i.e., increased low-density lipoprotein [LDL] cholesterol, decreased high-density lipoprotein [HDL] cholesterol, and increased triglycerides), and increased uric acid, all of which are found in women with preeclampsia.[83] Other conditions predisposing to later-life cardiovascular disease—including elevated levels of homocysteine,[84] evidence of androgen excess (including polycystic ovarian syndrome),[85] elevated testosterone levels,[86] male fat distribution (i.e., increased waist-to-hip ratio),[87] and lipoprotein lipase mutations[88]—are also linked to an increased risk for preeclampsia.

Women who appear normal years after a preeclamptic pregnancy may nevertheless demonstrate subtle metabolic and cardiovascular abnormalities. Compared with women with uncomplicated pregnancies, formerly preeclamptic women have evidence of endothelial dysfunction,[89,90] higher blood pressures,[89] increased insulin resistance,[91] dyslipidemia,[92] altered angiogenic factors,[93] and increased antibodies to the angiotensin-2 receptor.[94] These data may explain the common risk factors for preeclampsia and cardiovascular disease, but alternative explanations, such as that preeclampsia causes vascular injury that increases cardiovascular risk or that normal pregnancies have a protective effect, cannot be excluded.

TABLE 35-3 SIGNS AND SYMPTOMS OF PREECLAMPSIA OR ECLAMPSIA

Cerebral	Blurred vision
Headache	Amaurosis
Dizziness	Gastrointestinal
Tinnitus	Nausea
Drowsiness	Vomiting
Change in respiratory rate	Epigastric pain
Tachycardia	Hematemesis
Fever	Renal
Visual	Oliguria
Diplopia	Anuria
Scotomata	Hematuria
	Hemoglobinuria

Clinical Presentation

Preeclampsia can manifest with a wide spectrum of disease, ranging from life-threatening neurologic, renal, hepatic, and coagulation abnormalities to mild findings of preeclampsia with minimal end-organ involvement. The fetus may be severely compromised by the maternal condition and by extreme preterm delivery or only minimally affected. These variations have puzzled clinicians and researchers for many years. An understanding of the pathophysiology of the disorder provides insight into the diverse clinical presentations.

Symptoms

Most women with early preeclampsia are asymptomatic. The absence of symptoms is the rationale for frequent obstetric visits in late pregnancy. In most cases, signs such as increased blood pressure and proteinuria antedate overt symptoms.

The various symptoms associated with preeclampsia, especially preeclampsia of increasing severity, are listed in Table 35-3. Because preeclampsia is a disease of generalized poor perfusion, the diversity of symptoms related to many organ systems is not surprising. Symptoms suggesting hepatic, neurologic, and visual involvement are particularly worrisome. They include epigastric pain, "stomach upset," and pain penetrating to the back. Headache and mental confusion indicate poor cerebral perfusion and may be precursors of convulsions. Visual symptoms ranging from scotomata to blindness indicate retinal arterial spasm and edema. Symptoms suggesting congestive heart failure or abruptio placentae also represent significant complications of preeclampsia. Other symptoms, such as tightness of hands and feet and paresthesias resulting from medial or ulnar nerve compression, may alarm the patient but have little prognostic significance.

Signs

Signs of preeclampsia usually antedate symptoms. The most common sequence is increased blood pressure followed by proteinuria.[18]

BLOOD PRESSURE CHANGE

An increase in blood pressure is required for the diagnosis of preeclampsia. Blood pressure variation in normal pregnancy can lead to misdiagnosis. In clinical practice, the serious effects of preeclampsia on the mother and fetus warrant such overdiagnosis. The primary pathophysiologic alteration, poor tissue perfusion resulting from vasospasm, is revealed more by blood pressure changes than by absolute blood pressure levels. Although a diagnosis of preeclampsia is not made without absolute blood pressure increases to 140 mm Hg systolic or 90 mm Hg diastolic, women who reach this level from a low early pregnancy value typically manifest more vasospasm than those for whom 140/90 mm Hg represents a smaller increase.

Although maternal and fetal risks rise with increasing blood pressure,[95] serious complications can occur in women who experience only modest blood pressure elevation. In two series, 20% of women with eclampsia never had a systolic blood pressure above 140 mm Hg.[18,96] In a large, prospective study from the United Kingdom, there were 383 confirmed cases of eclampsia, of which 77% were hospitalized before seizures occurred. Of these, 38% of the cases were not preceded by documented proteinuria or hypertension.[97] Others have noticed similar findings.[98,99]

PROTEINURIA

Among the diagnostic signs of preeclampsia, proteinuria in the presence of hypertension is the most reliable indicator of fetal jeopardy. In two studies of preeclampsia, the perinatal mortality rate tripled for women with proteinuria,[100] and the amount of proteinuria correlated with increased perinatal mortality rate and the number of growth-restricted infants.[101] A later study demonstrated that the risk for delivering a small for gestational age fetus was higher in women with hypertension and proteinuria (52%) compared with women with new-onset gestational hypertension (15%) or chronic hypertension (12%). The perinatal mortality rate was fourfold higher with proteinuria and hypertension than in pregnancies complicated by hypertension alone.[102]

RETINAL CHANGES

Retinal vascular changes on funduscopic examination occur in retinal arterioles in at least 50% of women with preeclampsia, and they are important because they correlate best with renal biopsy-proven changes of preeclampsia.[103] Localized retinal vascular narrowing is visualized as segmental spasm, and the generalized narrowing is indicated by a decrease in the ratio of arteriolar-venous diameter from the usual 3:5 to 1:2 or even 1:3. It can occur in all vessels or, in early stages, in single vessels.[104] Preeclampsia does not cause chronic arteriolar changes; the presence of arteriolar sclerosis detected by increased light reflex, copper wiring, or arteriovenous nicking indicates preexisting vascular disease.

HYPERREFLEXIA

Although hyperreflexia is given much clinical attention and deep tendon reflexes are increased in many women before seizures, convulsions can occur in the absence of hyperreflexia,[68] and many pregnant women are consistently hyperreflexic without being preeclamptic. Changes, or lack thereof, in deep tendon reflexes are not part of the diagnosis of preeclampsia.

OTHER SIGNS

Other signs that occur less commonly in preeclampsia are indicators of involvement of specific organs in the preeclamptic process. Women with marked edema may have ascites and hydrothorax, and those with congestive heart failure display increased neck vein distention, gallop rhythm, and pulmonary rales. Hepatic capsular distention, manifested by hepatic enlargement and tenderness, is a particular concern, as is disseminated intravascular coagulation (DIC) sufficient to cause petechiae or generalized bruising and bleeding.

Laboratory Findings

Major changes revealed by laboratory studies occur in severe preeclampsia and eclampsia. In the patient with mild preeclampsia, changes in most of these indicators may be minimal or absent.

RENAL FUNCTION STUDIES

Serum Uric Acid Concentration and Urate Clearance. Uric acid is the most sensitive laboratory indicator of preeclampsia available to clinicians. A decrease in uric acid clearance precedes a measurable decrease in the glomerular filtration rate (GFR). Hypertension with hyperuricemia but without proteinuria was associated with growth restriction as commonly as hypertension and proteinuria without elevated uric acid in one series.[105] Although increased serum uric acid concentration is often attributed to altered renal function, an alternative view favors increased production caused by oxidative stress.[106] An elevated uric acid level may itself have pathogenic effects.[107] Table 35-4 shows normal uric acid levels during gestation and levels associated with preeclampsia.

Serum Creatinine Concentration and Creatinine Clearance. Creatinine clearance is decreased in most patients with severe preeclampsia, but it can be normal in women with mild disease. Serial serum creatinine determinations may indicate decreased clearance, but single values are not helpful unless markedly elevated because of the wide range of normal values. The serum creatinine concentration varies as a geometric function of creatinine clearance so that small changes in glomerular filtration are best determined by measurements of creatinine clearance.

TABLE 35-4 PLASMA URATE CONCENTRATIONS IN NORMOTENSIVE AND HYPERTENSIVE PREGNANT WOMEN

	Normotensive Patients			Hypertensive Patients		
Weeks of Gestation	mmol/L	SD*	mg/dL	mmol/L	SD*	mg/dL
24-28	0.18	(20%)	3.02	0.24	(20%)	4.03
29-32	0.18	(35%)	3.02	0.28	(25%)	4.7
33-36	0.20	(30%)	3.36	0.30	(20%)	5.04
37-40	0.26	(20%)	4.4	0.31	(23%)	5.28
41-42	0.25	(24%)	4.2	0.32	(12%)	5.38

*Each number in parentheses is the standard deviation given as a percentage of the mean values shown. Values for hypertensive and normotensive women are statistically different at all gestational ages ($P < .05$).

Modified from Shuster E, Weppelman B: Plasma urate measurements and fetal outcome in preeclampsia. Gynecol Obstet Invest 12:162, 1981.

LIVER FUNCTION TESTS

Although most tests of liver function are not highly predictive of severity of preeclampsia,[18] the association between microangiopathic anemia and elevations in aspartate aminotransferase (AST) and alanine aminotransferase (ALT) carries an especially disturbing prognosis for the mother and infant.[19,108] These findings usually correlate with the severity of disease and, when associated with hepatic enlargement, may be a sign of impending hepatic rupture.

COAGULATION FACTORS

Although overt DIC is rare, subtle evidence of activation of the coagulation cascade occurs in many women with preeclampsia. The average platelet count in the patient with mild preeclampsia is similar to the platelet count in normal pregnant women.[109] However, careful platelet counts performed sequentially may reveal decreased platelets in many patients.[110] Highly sensitive indicators of activation of the clotting system, reduced serum concentrations of antithrombin III,[111] a decrease in the ratio of factor VIII bioactivity to factor VIII antigen,[112] and subtle indicators of platelet dysfunction, including alteration of turnover,[6] activation,[113] size,[114] and content,[115] exist in even mild preeclampsia and may antedate clinically evident disease.

METABOLIC CHANGES

Preeclampsia is characterized by an increase in the insulin resistance of normal pregnancy. Signs of the insulin resistance syndrome are exaggerated.[110] Levels of circulating lipids already elevated in normal pregnancy[116] are accentuated in women with preeclampsia.[117] Triglycerides and fatty acid levels are elevated, changes that antedate clinically evident disease by weeks to months.[118,119] Levels of the cardioprotective HDL cholesterol are reduced in preeclamptic women,[120] whereas levels of a variant of LDL cholesterol (i.e., small, dense cholesterol that is strongly associated with cardiovascular disease) are increased.[121,122] These changes resolve after delivery.

Pathologic Changes in Preeclampsia

The pathologic changes found in organs of women dying of eclampsia and in biopsy specimens from women with preeclampsia provide strong evidence that preeclampsia is not merely an unmasking of essential hypertension or a variant of malignant hypertension. These findings also indicate that the elevation of blood pressure probably does not have primary pathogenetic importance.

Brain

Cerebral edema, once thought to be a common finding in women dying of eclampsia, was uncommon among postmortem examinations performed within 2 to 3 hours of death.[123] However, studies using computed tomography again raised the possibility that cerebral edema is an important pathophysiologic event in some women with preeclampsia.[124] Noninvasive studies of cerebral blood flow and resistance suggest that vascular barotrauma and loss of cerebral vascular autoregulation contribute to the pathogenesis of cerebral vascular pathology in cases of preeclampsia or eclampsia.[125]

Liver

Gross lesions of the liver are visible in about 60% of women dying of eclampsia, and one third of the remaining livers are microscopically abnormal. Many early investigators thought that the hepatic changes were pathognomonic for eclampsia,[126] but similar changes have been described in women dying of abruptio placentae.[127]

Two temporally and etiologically distinct hepatic lesions have been described.[123] Initially, hemorrhage into the hepatic cellular columns results from vasodilatation of arterioles, producing dislocation and deformation of the hepatocytes in their stromal sleeves (Fig. 35-4). Later, intense vasospasm causes hepatic infarction, ranging from small to large areas beginning near the sinusoids and extending into the area near the portal vessels (Fig. 35-5). Hemorrhagic changes are present in 66% and necrotic changes in 40% of eclamptic women and in about one half as many preeclamptic women. Hyalinization and thrombosis of hepatic vessels have been cited as evidence of DIC, but they may be the result of hemorrhage.

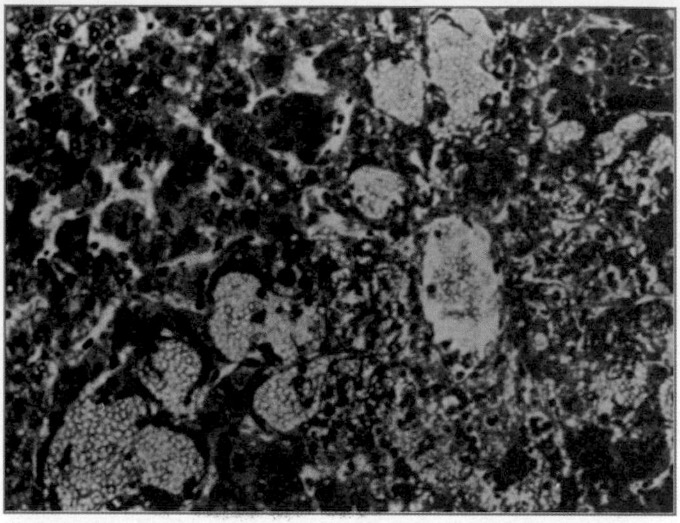

FIGURE 35-4 Hemorrhagic hepatic lesions in eclampsia. Hemorrhage into the periportal area occurred with crescentic compression of liver cells. (From Sheehan HL, Lynch JB: Pathology of Toxemia in Pregnancy. London, Churchill Livingstone, 1973.)

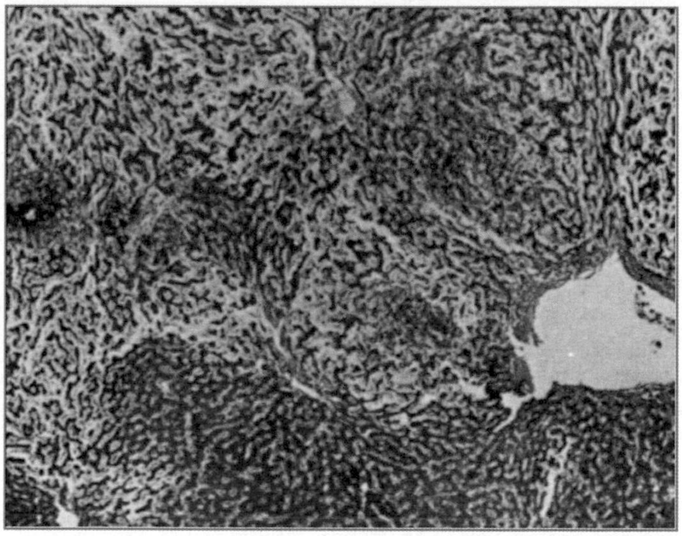

FIGURE 35-5 Hepatic infarction in eclampsia. Hepatic infarction caused by intense vasospasm manifests as small to large areas beginning near the sinusoids and extending into the area near the portal vessels. (From Sheehan HL, Lynch JB: Pathology of Toxemia in Pregnancy. London, Churchill Livingstone, 1973.)

Kidney

The pathologic renal changes of preeclampsia and eclampsia are clearly different from those seen in other hypertensive or renal disorders.

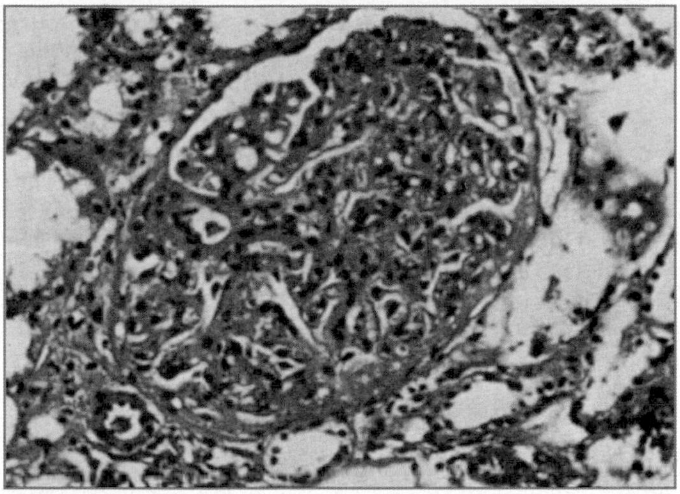

FIGURE 35-6 **Glomerular changes in preeclampsia are identified by light microscopy.** The enlarged glomerulus completely fills Bowman's capsule. Diffuse edema of the glomerular wall is indicated by the vacuolated appearance. The visible capillary loops are extremely narrow, and there are virtually no red blood cells in the capillary tuft.

Glomerular, tubular, and arteriolar changes have been described. The glomerular lesion is considered by some to be pathognomonic of preeclampsia and eclampsia, but identical changes have been seen in placental abruption without evident preeclampsia.[128] This change is not seen in any other form of hypertension.

GLOMERULAR CHANGES

Changes seen by light microscopy in glomeruli that are characteristic of preeclampsia include[103] decreased glomerular size, with protrusion of the glomerular tuft into the proximal tubule. The diameter of the glomerular capillary lumen is decreased and contains few blood cells. The endothelial-mesangial cells have increased cytoplasmic volume and can contain lipoid droplets (Fig. 35-6).

Electron microscopic examination of glomeruli provides more evidence that the primary pathologic change occurs in endothelial cells, which are greatly increased in size and can occlude the capillary lumen; their cytoplasm contains electron-dense material.[129] The basement membrane bordering the epithelial cell may be slightly thickened, and it also contains electron-dense material. The epithelial cell podocytes are not altered (Fig. 35-7). These changes are collectively called *glomerular capillary endotheliosis.*

Characteristic glomerular changes occur in 70% of primiparas but in only 14% of multiparas with a diagnosis of preeclampsia.[17] The more likely the diagnosis of preeclampsia, the more common the glomerular lesion. As the clinical condition worsens, the magnitude of the glomerular lesion increases. The glomerular lesions are reversible after delivery and are not present in subsequent biopsy specimens obtained 5 to 10 weeks later.[103]

The glomerular changes correlate more consistently with proteinuria than with hypertension, suggesting that proteins identified immunohistochemically may be trapped in the glomerulus. These staining patterns are not found in other renal disorders with proteinuria. The glomerular changes of preeclampsia can be mimicked in animal studies by reducing the renal concentration of vascular endothelial growth factor (VEGF), which usually exists in high concentration in this tissue by increasing the synthesis of the VEGF antagonist soluble Fms-like tyrosine kinase 1 (sFlt1).[130]

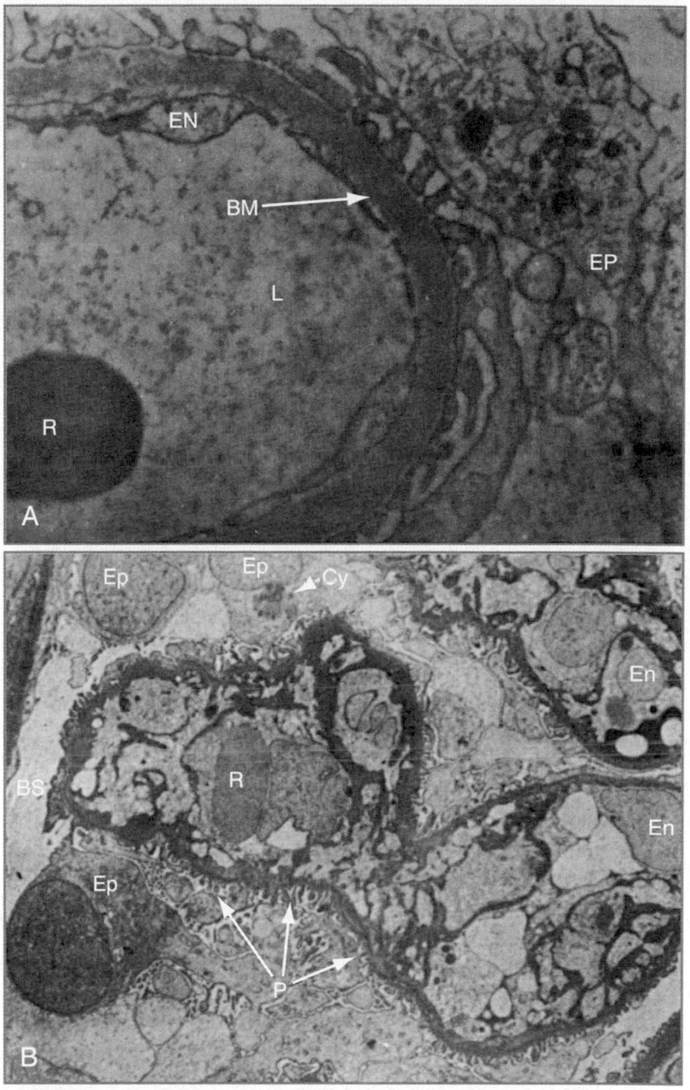

FIGURE 35-7 **Electron photomicrographs of renal glomeruli.** **A,** Normal anatomy. **B,** Biopsy specimen from a preeclamptic woman. Endothelial cells (En) are markedly enlarged, obstruct the capillary lumen, and contain electron-dense inclusions. The basement membrane (BM) is slightly thickened with inclusions, but the epithelial foot processes (EP) are normal. BM, basement membrane; BS, Bowman's space; Cy, cytoplasmic inclusions; EN, capillary endothelial cells that line the glomeruli; Ep, renal epithelial cells; L, capillary lumen containing red blood cells; P, podocytes; R, red blood cell. (From McCartney CP: Pathological anatomy of acute hypertension of pregnancy. Circulation 30[Suppl II]:37, 1964. By permission of the American Heart Association, Inc.)

NONGLOMERULAR CHANGES

Pathologic changes in renal tubules include dilatation of proximal tubules with thinning of the epithelium,[123] tubular necrosis,[103] enlargement of the juxtaglomerular apparatus,[131] and hyaline deposition in renal tubules.[123] Fat deposition in women with prolonged heavy proteinuria has been reported.[123] Necrosis of the loop of Henle, a change that correlates with the degree of hyperuricemia, has also been described.[131]

Thickening of renal arterioles may be seen in preeclampsia, especially in women with preexisting hypertension. Unlike the glomerular

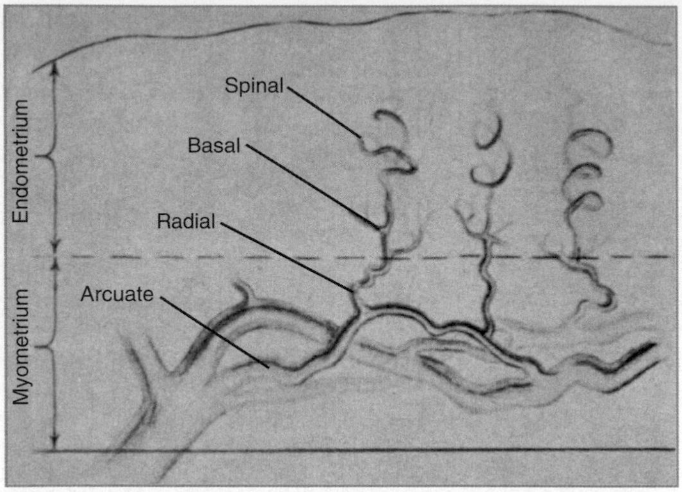

FIGURE 35-8 Schematic representation of uterine arteries. The characteristic changes occur in the decidual vessels supplying the placental site in a normal pregnancy. (From Okkels H, Engle ET: Studies of the finer structure of the uterine vessels of the *Macacus* monkey. Acta Pathol Microbiol Scand 15:150, 1938.)

lesion, it does not regress after delivery,[103] suggesting that the arteriolar change results from coincident disease, not preeclampsia.

Vascular Changes in the Placental Site

The characteristic changes in the decidual vessels supplying the placental site in normal pregnancy are depicted in Figure 35-8. In normal pregnancy, the spiral arteries (Fig. 35-9) increase greatly in diameter.[132] Morphologically, the endothelium is replaced by trophoblast, and the internal elastic lamina and smooth muscle of the media are replaced by trophoblast and an amorphous matrix-containing fibrin (see Fig. 35-9).[133] These changes occur originally in the decidual portion of the spiral arteries but extend into the myometrium as pregnancy advances and can even involve the distal portion of the uterine radial artery. The basal arteries are not affected. These morphologic changes are considered to be a vascular reaction to the trophoblast, occurring directly or humorally, that results in increased perfusion of the placental site.

In placental-site vessels of women with preeclampsia, the normal physiologic changes do not occur, or they are limited to the decidual portion of the vessels. Myometrial segments of spiral arteries retain the nonpregnant component of intima and smooth muscle, and the diameter of these arteries is about 40% that of vessels in normal pregnancy.[134] Spiral arterioles in decidua and myometrium and basal and radial arterioles may become necrotic, with components of the normal vessel wall replaced by amorphous material and foam cells, a change called *acute atherosis* (Fig. 35-10).[135] This lesion is best seen in the basal arteries because they do not undergo the normal changes of pregnancy. It is also present in decidual and myometrial spiral arteries and can progress to vessel obliteration. The obliterated vessels correspond to areas of placental infarction.

Failed vascular remodeling and atherotic changes may be seen with fetal growth restriction in women without clinical evidence of preeclampsia. Atherotic changes occur in decidual vessels of some diabetic women,[136] and failed vascular remodeling is present in about one third of women who experience preterm labor.[137] It appears that abnormal invasion may be necessary but is not sufficient to cause preeclampsia.

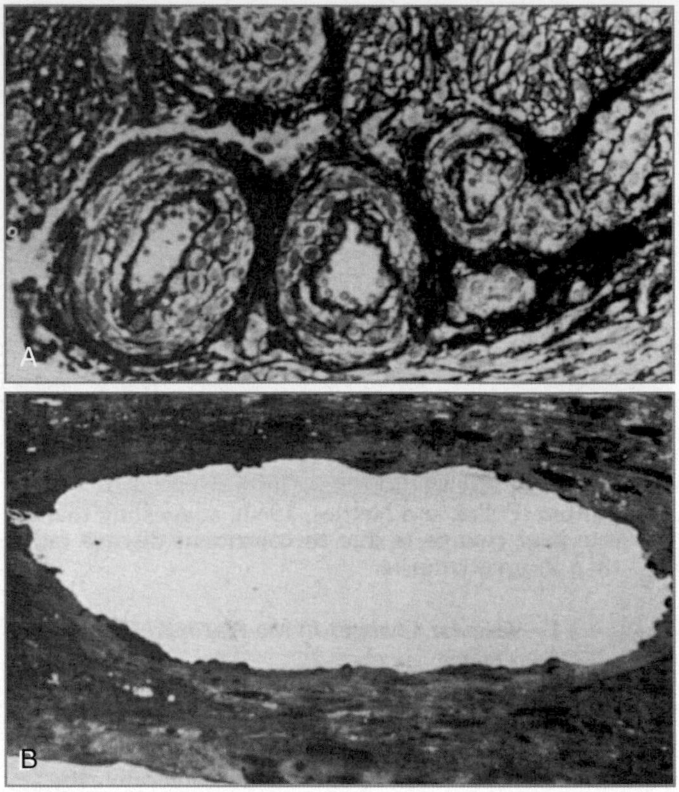

FIGURE 35-9 Spiral arterial changes in normal pregnancy. **A,** In the section of spiral arterioles at the junction of the endometrium and myometrium in a nonpregnant woman, notice the inner elastic lamina and smooth muscle. **B,** In a section of a spiral arteriole at the same scale and from the same location during pregnancy, notice the markedly increased diameter and absence of inner elastic lamina and smooth muscle. (From Sheppard BL, Bonnar J: Uteroplacental arteries and hypertensive pregnancy. In Bonnar J, MacGillivray I, Symonds G [eds]: Pregnancy Hypertension. Baltimore, University Park Press, 1980, p 205.)

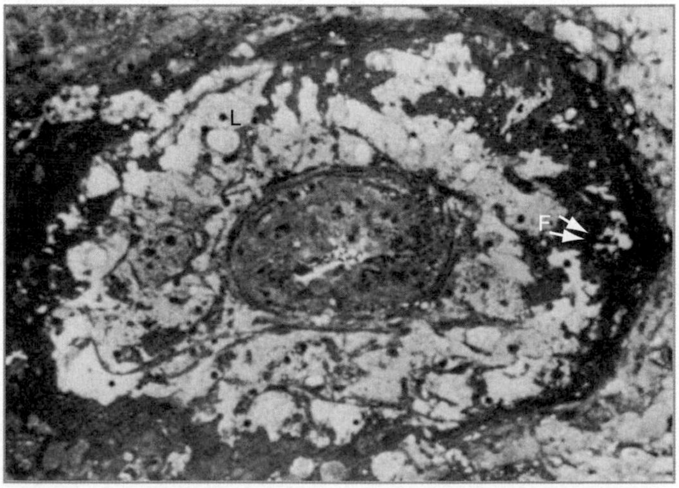

FIGURE 35-10 Atherosis. Numerous lipid-laden cells (L) and fibrin deposition (F) are present in the media of this occluded decidual vessel. (From Sheppard BL, Bonnar J: Uteroplacental arteries and hypertensive pregnancy. In Bonnar J, MacGillivray I, Symonds G [eds]: Pregnancy Hypertension. Baltimore, University Park Press, 1980, p 205.)

Changes characteristic of preeclampsia have been observed in the decidual vessels of one in seven primiparous women and in a lower percentage of multiparous women at the time of first-trimester abortion.[138,139] These findings suggest that disordered placentation precedes the clinical presentation of preeclampsia. The cause of the decidual vascular lesions is unknown. The appearance of the atherotic vessels resembles vessels in transplanted kidneys that have undergone rejection, suggesting an immunologic cause, which is consistent with findings of a study that demonstrated components of complement (e.g., C3) in decidual vessels with the lesion.[140]

The vascular remodeling of spiral arteries supplying the intervillous space is intimately related to normal trophoblast invasion.[141] The expression of adhesion molecules and their receptors that characterizes implantation is abnormal in preeclampsia.[142] The trophoblast that lines the decidual vessels of normal pregnant women begins to express molecules usually present only on endothelium,[143] a phenomenon that does not occur in preeclampsia.[144] Potential mechanisms responsible for the normal and abnormal changes include decidually produced cytokines[145-147] and local oxygen tension.[148,149] There may be interactions of specific molecules on trophoblast and maternal decidual cells that drive invasion. Invasive cytotrophoblasts express a human leukocyte antigen (HLA) molecule (HLA-C) that is minimally heterogeneous. Interaction of this molecule with a receptor on maternal decidual cells, killer immunoglobulin receptors (KIRs), causes various degrees of activation of the trophoblast cell, depending on the combination of KIR and HLA-C subtypes. Mothers with the minimally activating KIR subtype who have a fetus with a specific HLA-C subtype (HLA-C2) have an increased frequency of preeclampsia. This is not an immune interaction because the relationship persists regardless of maternal HLA-C subtype. Researchers propose that this combination does not favor trophoblast invasion and vascular remodeling. Population studies indicate that populations in which HLA-C2 is common have a reduced frequency of the specific inhibitory KIR subtype and vice versa.[150]

Placental Pathologic Changes

Ultrastructural examination of placentas from women with preeclampsia reveals an abnormal syncytiotrophoblast containing areas of cell death and degeneration. Viable-appearing syncytiotrophoblast is also abnormal, with decreased density of microvilli, dilated endoplasmic reticulum, and decreased pinocytotic and secretory activity. The cells of the villous cytotrophoblast cells are increased in number and have higher mitotic activity. The basement membrane of the trophoblast is irregularly thickened, with fine fibrillary inclusions.[151]

The changes may be caused by local hypoxia. Similar syncytiotrophoblastic changes are present in placental segments maintained under hypoxic conditions in vitro.[152] The cytotrophoblastic alterations are also consistent with hypoxia. The cytotrophoblasts comprise the stem cells of the trophoblast and responds to damage by proliferation. The trophoblast of the preeclamptic placenta is characterized by increased apoptosis and necrosis,[153,154] possibly caused by hypoxia or hypoxia reperfusion injury,[155] and this may be the origin of the increased circulating syncytiotrophoblast microparticles in preeclampsia.[156]

Summary of Pathologic Changes in Preeclampsia

Structural changes associated with preeclampsia and eclampsia lead to two important conclusions. First, preeclampsia is not an alternate form of malignant hypertension. The renal changes in preeclamptic and eclamptic women and the structural changes in other organs of women dying of eclampsia differ from the alterations caused by malignant hypertension. Second, the pathologic findings indicate that the primary pathology is poor tissue perfusion, not blood pressure elevation. The histologic data support the clinical impression that the poor perfusion results from profound vasospasm, which increases total peripheral resistance and blood pressure.

Pathophysiologic Changes in Preeclampsia

Preeclampsia can cause changes in virtually all organ systems. Several organ systems are consistently and characteristically involved, and these are discussed in the following sections.

Cardiovascular Changes

Blood pressure is the product of cardiac output and systemic vascular resistance. Cardiac output is increased by up to 50% in normal pregnancy, but blood pressure does not usually increase, indicating that systemic vascular resistance decreases. Blood pressure is lower in the first half of pregnancy than in the postpartum period, when cardiac output returns to nonpregnant levels (see Fig. 35-2). Some women destined to develop preeclampsia have a higher cardiac output before clinically evident disease. However, cardiac output is reduced to prepregnancy levels with the onset of clinical preeclampsia.[157,158] Although some studies suggest increased cardiac output,[159] most have found normal or slightly reduced cardiac output in women with untreated preeclampsia.[160] Increased systemic vascular resistance is the mechanism for the increase in blood pressure in clinical preeclampsia.

There is substantial evidence that arteriolar narrowing occurs in preeclampsia. Changes in the caliber of retinal arterioles correlate with the clinical severity of the disorder and with renal biopsy-confirmed diagnosis of preeclampsia.[103] Similar findings occur in vessels of the nail bed and conjunctiva. Measurements of forearm blood flow indicate higher resistance in preeclamptic than in normal pregnant women.[161,162] It is unlikely that this effect is determined by the autonomic nervous system. Although normal pregnant women are exquisitely sensitive to the interruption of autonomic neurotransmission by ganglionic blockade and high spinal anesthesia, preeclamptic women are less sensitive.[163] This finding suggests that the arteriolar constriction of preeclampsia is not maintained by the autonomic nervous system and that humoral factors are implicated. The increased sympathetic activity in preeclampsia, however, raises questions about these older findings.[164] Assays of concentrations of recognized endogenous vasoconstrictors are limited to determinations of catecholamines and angiotensin II. Results suggest minimal or no change in catecholamines, whereas circulating angiotensin II concentrations are lower in preeclamptic women.[165]

Levels of endothelin-1, a vasoconstrictor produced by endothelial cells, are increased in the blood of preeclamptic women[166] at concentrations much lower than those necessary to stimulate vascular smooth muscle contraction in vitro. It is not clear whether these circulating concentrations reflect endothelial production sufficient to stimulate local vasoconstriction or low concentrations of endothelin potentiate contractile responses to other agonists.

As indicated by the older term *toxemia*, early investigators suspected that preeclampsia was caused by circulating humors. Early reports suggesting etiologic agents such as pressor substances in blood, decidual extracts, placental extracts, and amniotic fluid of preeclamptic patients have not been replicated. The explanation for the pressor effects was, in some studies, normal endogenous pressors; in others, the explanation was faulty methodology and failure to recognize the immunologic difference between the source of the extract and the

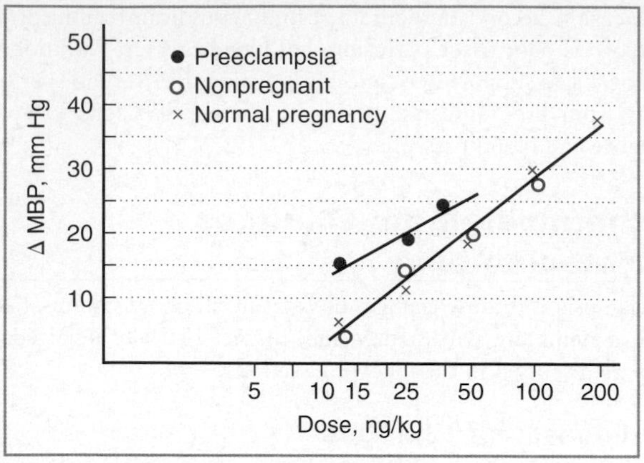

FIGURE 35-11 Mean dose-response graphs for norepinephrine. Women with preeclampsia have an increased sensitivity to all endogenous pressors. MBP, mean blood pressure. (From Talledo OE, Chesley LC, Zuspan FP: Renin-angiotensin system in normal and toxemic pregnancies. III. Differential sensitivity to angiotensin II and norepinephrine in toxemia of pregnancy. Am J Obstet Gynecol 100:218, 1968. Courtesy of the American College of Obstetricians and Gynecologists.)

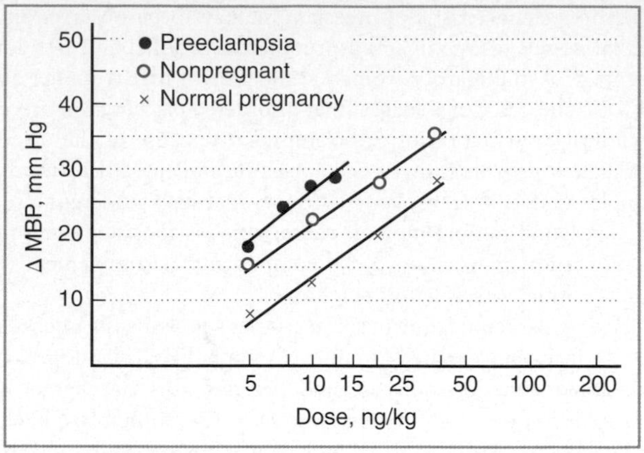

FIGURE 35-12 Mean dose-response graphs for angiotensin. Preeclamptic women are much more sensitive to angiotensin II than normal pregnant and nonpregnant women. MBP, mean blood pressure. (From Talledo OE, Chesley LC, Zuspan FP: Renin-angiotensin system in normal and toxemic pregnancies. III. Differential sensitivity to angiotensin II and norepinephrine in toxemia of pregnancy. Am J Obstet Gynecol 100:218, 1968. Courtesy of the American College of Obstetricians and Gynecologists.)

animals tested. In other experiments, no defect is obvious. The hypothesis that arteriolar constriction of preeclampsia is caused by new circulating pressors has largely been abandoned.[18]

A more compelling explanation for vasospasm in preeclampsia is increased response to normal concentrations of endogenous pressors. Women with preeclampsia have higher sensitivity to all the endogenous pressors that have been tested. They are exquisitely sensitive to vasopressin.[167,168] Vasopressin can elicit marked blood pressure elevation, seizures, and oliguria in some patients.[168] Sensitivity to epinephrine[169] and norepinephrine[170] is also increased (Fig. 35-11). The most striking difference is seen in the sensitivity of the preeclamptic woman to angiotensin II. Normal pregnant women are less sensitive to angiotensin II than nonpregnant women, requiring approximately 2.5 times as much angiotensin to raise the blood pressure by a similar increment.[171] In contrast, preeclamptic women are much more sensitive to angiotensin II than are normal pregnant and nonpregnant women (Fig. 35-12).[170]

In a classic study, angiotensin II sensitivity was significantly increased many weeks before the development of elevated blood pressure (Fig. 35-13).[172] Although resistance to angiotensin II does not decrease to nonpregnant levels until 32 weeks' gestation, significant differences in sensitivity between women who later become hypertensive and those who remain normotensive have been observed as early as 14 weeks. However, a large British study did not confirm this classic finding,[173] perhaps reflecting the heterogeneity of preeclampsia.[174]

The decreased sensitivity of normal pregnant women to angiotensin II and the lower systemic vascular resistance in normal pregnancy suggest that arteriolar narrowing in preeclamptic women may result from decreased levels of circulating or local vasodilator substances, rather than from increased levels of circulating pressors. This attractive hypothesis, however, is not consistent with the unchanged sensitivities to norepinephrine, epinephrine, and vasopressin in normal pregnancy.[168-170]

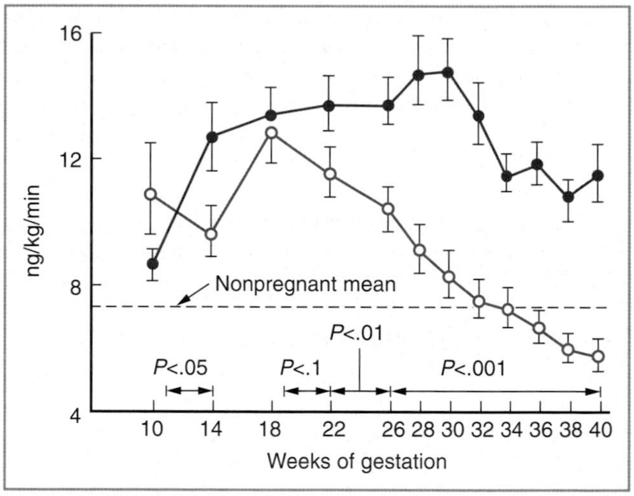

FIGURE 35-13 Angiotensin sensitivity throughout pregnancy. The dose of angiotensin II necessary to increase diastolic blood pressure 20 mm Hg in women who developed elevated blood pressure in late pregnancy *(blue line, open circles)* was compared with the dose for those who remained normotensive *(red line, solid circles)*. The graph demonstrates that a significantly lower dose was required in the former group as early as 10 to 14 weeks' gestation. (From Gant NF, Daley GL, Chand S, et al: A study of angiotensin II pressor response throughout primigravid pregnancy. J Clin Invest 49:82, 1973. With permission of the American Society for Clinical Investigation.)

Coagulation Changes

The syndrome of DIC occurs in preeclampsia and has been suggested as a primary pathogenetic factor[175] (see Chapter 40). Activation of the coagulation system manifests as the intravascular disappearance of procoagulants, intravascular appearance of degradation products of fibrin, and end-organ damage from the formation of microthrombi.[176] In the most advanced form of DIC, procoagulants—especially fibrinogen and platelets—decrease to a degree sufficient to produce spontaneous hemorrhage. In milder forms, only highly sensitive indicators of clotting system activation are present. Decreasing platelet concentrations is such a sign but may be evident only by serial observations.[96] Sensitive indicators of intravascular coagulation, such as an elevated level of fibrin degradation products; increased platelet turnover,[6] volume,[114] and activation[177]; reduced platelet content[178]; increased platelet content in plasma[179]; reduced levels of antithrombin III[111]; and a reduced ratio of factor VIII activity to factor VIII antigen,[180] are common when concentrations of procoagulants remain normal. Subtle signs of platelet dysfunction,[6,114,177-179] reduced antithrombin III,[111] and reduction in the ratio of factor VIII bioactivity to factor VIII antigen[112] are present in women with mild preeclampsia and may precede its clinical signs.

Abnormalities of blood coagulation sufficient to make a diagnosis of DIC are present in approximately 10% of women with severe preeclampsia or eclampsia.[181] Results of highly sensitive assays of coagulation activation suggest, however, that abnormalities of the coagulation system are present in many patients with mild to moderate preeclampsia. Coagulation changes are thought to be secondary rather than primary pathogenetic factors[182] because levels of procoagulants are usually normal, and another early sign of preeclampsia—increased serum uric acid—may precede changes in coagulation.[110]

The cause of the change in coagulation factors is uncertain. Vascular damage resulting from vasospasm may initiate DIC[182] and probably contributes to activation of the clotting system in severe preeclampsia. Signs of endothelial dysfunction also antedate clinical disease,[183] and activation of platelets and other components of the coagulation cascade is a well recognized consequence of endothelial dysfunction.[184] Vascular changes in the implantation site that appear to antedate blood pressure elevation may be pathogenetically important.

Whether coagulation changes measured in preeclamptic patients represent true DIC or a localized consumption of procoagulants in the intervillous space is not clear. Microthrombi and the presence of fibrin antigen have been inconsistently observed in liver, placenta, and kidney.[185-187] Early coagulation changes such as factor VIII activity-antigen ratios and platelet count correlate better with the fetal outcome as measured by mortality and growth restriction rates than with the clinical severity of preeclampsia. Identical coagulation changes occur in normotensive women with growth-restricted fetuses,[188] suggesting that localized coagulation in the intervillous space is important. Similarly, an increased concentration of fibrin antigen has been reported in the placentas of preeclamptic patients.[185]

Endothelial Cell Dysfunction

There is increasing support for endothelial dysfunction as a pathophysiologic component of preeclampsia.[183,189,190] Alterations of glomerular endothelial cells are a consistent feature of preeclampsia. Levels of cellular fibronectin,[191,192] growth factors,[193] vascular cell adhesion molecule 1 (VCAM-1),[194] factor VIII antigen, and peptides released from injured endothelial cells are increased in preeclamptic women before the appearance of clinical disease.[112] Examination showed that the endothelial function of vessels of preeclamptic women was impaired in vitro.[195,196]

The endothelium is a complex tissue with many important functions. Prevention of coagulation and modulation of vascular tone have special relevance to preeclampsia. Intact vascular endothelium is resistant to thrombus formation.[197] With vascular injury, endothelial cells can initiate coagulation by the intrinsic pathway (i.e., contact activation)[198] or by the extrinsic pathway (i.e., tissue factor).[199] Platelet adhesion can also occur after injury with exposure of subendothelial components, such as collagen[200] and microfibrils.

Endothelium profoundly influences the response of vascular smooth muscle to vasoactive agents. The response to some agents[201] can change from dilation to constriction with the removal of endothelium. Prostacyclin, a highly potent vasodilator, is produced by endothelium. Vessels from preeclamptic women and the umbilical vessels of their neonates generate less prostacyclin than similar vessels from normal pregnant women.[202-204] If potent inhibitors preventing the synthesis of all prostaglandins (including prostacyclin) are administered to pregnant women, the usual resistance to the vasoconstrictor effect of angiotensin II is abolished.[205] Conversely, if aspirin is used as an inhibitor of prostaglandin synthesis in a manner determined to specifically reduce contractile prostanoids (e.g., thromboxane A_2) much more than prostacyclin, the increased angiotensin II sensitivity of preeclamptic women is reduced.[206]

Nitric oxide (NO) is another bioactive material produced by normal endothelium.[207] Its release is stimulated by several hormones and neurotransmitters and by hydrodynamic shear stress. NO is quite labile and acts synergistically with prostacyclin as a local vasodilator and inhibitor of platelet aggregation. Current thinking favors NO as an endogenous vasodilator of pregnancy. Administration of inhibitors of NO synthesis reduces blood flow much more strikingly in pregnant than in nonpregnant women.[208] Production of NO is reduced with endothelial cell injury. Information about NO production in preeclampsia is conflicting,[209-214] in part because of the use of blood concentrations of NO metabolites to determine production in the setting of the reduced renal function of preeclampsia.[215] Two studies have documented reduced urinary NO excretion in preeclampsia,[212,216] and another found increased excretion.[217] Perhaps the most compelling data are from estimates of the tissue concentrations of nitrotyrosine (i.e., product of the interaction of NO and superoxide). Nitrotyrosine residues are increased in the placenta[218] and vessels[219] of women with preeclampsia. It is posited that the placenta directly or indirectly produces factors that alter endothelial function. Candidate molecules include the following:

- Cytokines[220] (with increasing evidence that endothelial dysfunction is part of a generalized increased inflammatory response[221])
- Placental fragments (i.e., syncytiotrophoblast microvillous membranes)[222]
- Free radicals
- Reactive oxygen species[223]

The latter hypothesis—that oxidative stress causes endothelial dysfunction—is especially interesting in view of the similarities of the lipid changes of preeclampsia to those of atherosclerosis,[118] an endothelial disorder in which oxidative stress is thought to play a key role.[224]

The information available indicates that endothelial cell dysfunction can alter vascular responses and intravascular coagulation in a manner consistent with the pathophysiologic abnormalities of preeclampsia. Evidence is accumulating that endothelial injury may play a central role in the pathogenesis of preeclampsia.

Renal Function Changes

Renal function changes characteristic of women with preeclampsia or eclampsia include decreased glomerular filtration and proteinuria. Changes in components of the renin-angiotensin system probably differ from those of normal pregnancy. Sodium excretion is decreased, resulting in fluid retention and edema.

GLOMERULAR FUNCTIONAL CHANGES

Glomerular Filtration Rate. Decreased glomerular filtration frequently complicates preeclampsia, and it is explained only partially by decreased renal plasma flow (RPF). The filtration fraction (GFR/RPF) may be decreased[18] because of intrarenal redistribution of blood flow.[225] A more obvious explanation is glomeruloendotheliosis, in which the occlusion of glomerular capillaries by swollen endothelial cells probably renders many glomeruli nonfunctional.

Protein Leakage. The pathogenesis of proteinuria in preeclampsia is primarily explained by glomerular changes. The normal absence of protein in urine results from a relative impermeability of glomeruli to large protein molecules and from the tubular resorption of smaller proteins that cross the glomeruli. As glomerular damage occurs, permeability to proteins increases. As damage increases, so does the size of the protein molecule that can cross the glomerular membrane. Increased permeability results in decreased selectivity. With minimal glomerular damage or tubular dysfunction, only small protein molecules are excreted, but with greater damage, large and small proteins are present in urine.

In women with preeclampsia, selectivity is low, indicating increased permeability and glomerular damage.[226] The well-known clinical observation that the magnitude of proteinuria in preeclamptic women varies greatly over time was quantitated by Chesley,[227] who noticed hourly variation in the urinary creatinine-to-protein ratio in women with preeclampsia that was not present in the urine of individuals with other proteinuric conditions.

Because structural glomerular changes are constant, proteinuria in preeclamptic women must in part depend on a varying functional cause (e.g., a variation in the intensity of the renal vascular spasm). That vascular spasm can cause proteinuria has been demonstrated by measuring urinary excretion of protein in individuals subjected to the cold pressor test. Immersing a patient's hand in ice water for 60 seconds increases blood pressure by more than 16 mm Hg (systolic and diastolic), and an increase in protein excretion almost invariably occurs.[228]

RENAL TUBULAR FUNCTIONAL CHANGES

Uric Acid Clearance. Three separate processes are involved in the renal excretion of urate. Urate is completely filtered at the glomerulus. It is not bound to plasma proteins under physiologic conditions,[229] and glomerular urate concentration is equal to renal arterial plasma concentration. Urate is secreted and reabsorbed by renal tubules. Most urate (98%) is reabsorbed, and about 80% of excreted urate is accounted for by urate secretion. Both processes occur predominantly in the proximal tubule. Reabsorption occurs to a greater extent than secretion, and urate clearance is about 10% of creatinine clearance.[230]

Abnormalities of uric acid clearance have long been recognized as a consistent phenomenon in preeclampsia[231] and have been regarded as a function of decreased glomerular filtration.[232] Several studies have demonstrated the discrepancy between uric acid clearance and both inulin clearance and creatinine clearance.[233,234] Serial studies also reveal that decreased uric acid clearance precedes decreases in the GFR.[235]

Urate clearance is decreased by hypovolemia, presumably as a result of nonspecific stimulation of proximal tubular reabsorption.[236] Plasma volume depletion is coincident with urate clearance changes,[237] suggesting that volume change may account for the abnormality in urate clearance. However, the correlation between the degree of volume depletion and the decrease in urate clearance is poor.[237]

Angiotensin II infusion decreases urate clearance even in the presence of normal blood volume.[238] The increase in angiotensin II sensitivity seen in preeclampsia may account for the change in renal function. Local effects of angiotensin II may also be important because this substance can be produced locally,[239] unassociated with increased circulating angiotensin II.

In summary, uric acid clearance changes earlier in preeclamptic pregnancy than does the GFR, suggesting a tubular rather than a glomerular functional explanation. Although the exact mechanism for the urate clearance change is not established, the common feature in the suggested mechanisms is decreased renal perfusion; however, increased production by poorly perfused tissue cannot be excluded.[106,240]

Urinary Concentrating Capacity. Although the issue is not fully settled, the tubular concentrating capacity is probably unchanged in normal pregnancies.[241] Assali and associates[242] suggested that urinary concentrating ability is decreased in hypertensive women. The limitations of these studies include the failure to account for parallel changes in the concentrating capacity and GFR[243] and the use of specific gravity—an unreliable estimate of osmolality—as the measure of concentration.[18]

Normal pregnant women were found to have decreased capacity to concentrate urine (measured as osmolar concentration and corrected for the GFR) in response to vasopressin administration, a decrease similar to that seen in pregnant women who were or later became hypertensive.[244] Conflicting study results suggesting that tubular concentrating capacity is unchanged in normal pregnancy are confounded by a failure to correct for the increased GFR of normal pregnancy, which concomitantly increases concentrating capacity.[243]

Excretion of Phenolsulfonphthalein. Because phenolsulfonphthalein is secreted by proximal tubular cells, its excretion can be used as an indicator of proximal tubular function.[235] However, phenolsulfonphthalein excretion is altered independently of tubular secretory capacity with increased[245] or decreased[246] renal plasma flow or reduced GFR[247] and with increased urinary dead space (a problem pertinent in pregnancy). When these factors are controlled, reduced phenolsulfonphthalein excretion precedes changes in the GFR and clinically evident disease in women with preeclampsia.[235]

Renin-Angiotensin-Aldosterone System. The renin-angiotensin-aldosterone system (RAAS) is important in pressure and volume regulation in normal pregnancy (Fig. 35-14).[248] Dramatic changes occur in the RAAS during pregnancy.[249] The following components are increased:

- Angiotensinogen (i.e., renin substrate)
- Plasma renin activity[250]

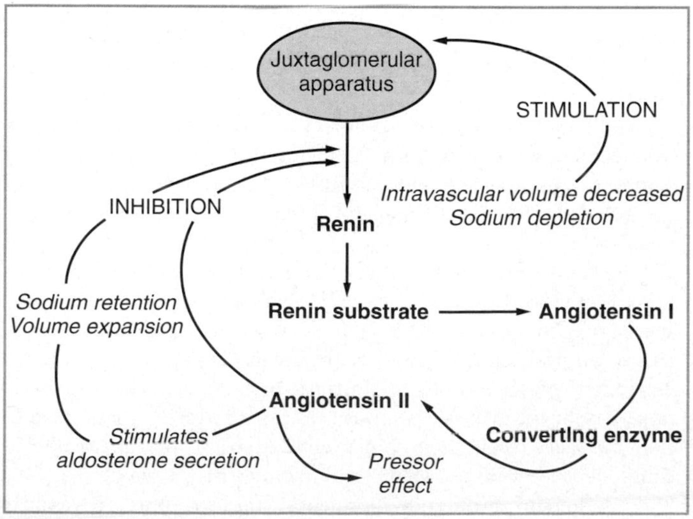

FIGURE 35-14 Schematic representation of the renin-angiotensin system. The system regulates pressure and volume in normal pregnancies, and abnormalities contribute to preeclampsia.

- Plasma renin concentration
- Angiotensin II concentration[250,251]
- Aldosterone[252]

Abnormalities of the RAAS have been proposed as causal factors in preeclampsia[253] because angiotensin II is a potent vasoconstrictor, it influences aldosterone secretion and consequent sodium retention, and at high concentrations, it can cause proteinuria. Myometrium and chorion can synthesize renin, which is stimulated in experimental animals by uterine ischemia.[254]

Most investigators agree that the angiotensinogen level remains elevated in preeclampsia.[250,255] The plasma renin activity and plasma renin concentration are reduced in preeclampsia compared with normal pregnancy.[256] In a prospective study of women with chronic hypertension, plasma renin activity was lower when superimposed preeclampsia developed (i.e., diagnostic blood pressure increase and proteinuria) than in chronic hypertensive women without superimposed preeclampsia and in normal pregnant women. Concentrations were similar in early pregnancy in all groups and decreased only slightly before the increase in blood pressure.[257]

The reduced renin activity in preeclampsia suggests suppression of renin release. This is puzzling in view of the reduced plasma volume that is characteristic of preeclampsia. There is no apparent nonphysiologic suppression of renin activity, because usual physiologic perturbations result in appropriately increased and decreased concentrations of plasma renin activity (i.e., renin is increased with upright posture and head-up tilt[258] and falls with volume expansion[259]). Despite the reduced content of the vascular compartment in preeclampsia, the intense vasoconstriction characteristic of preeclampsia results in a physiologic perception of overfill, suppressing renin release. The reduced renin activity in preeclampsia results in reduced angiotensin II[165] and aldosterone concentrations[260] compared with concentrations in normal pregnancy.

Attempts to test the role of the renin-angiotensin system (RAS) by using angiotensin II antagonists or by converting enzyme inhibitors have not clarified this point. Administration of the angiotensin antagonist (1-Sar-8-Ile-angiotensin II) to pregnant hypertensive women increases blood pressure,[261] and because this antagonist is a partial agonist, the increase in blood pressure may reflect the increased angiotensin sensitivity of hypertensive pregnant women. The administration of the angiotensin antagonist saralasin[262] or the angiotensin-converting enzyme inhibitor SQ 20,881[263] in the postpartum period did not have significant effects on blood pressure in a mixed group of women with hypertension.

Interest in the role of the RAS in preeclampsia has increased as the effects of angiotensin on responses other than blood pressure have been recognized.[264] The activation of NADPH oxidase in several tissues by angiotensin II can generate oxidative stress.[264-266] Hypoxia-inducing factors (HIFs) induce molecules responsible for many of the responses to hypoxia. These factors are upregulated in the placenta of a woman with preeclampsia[267] and can be activated by angiotensin II.[268] Antibodies to angiotensin II that activate angiotensin receptors and likely increase the sensitivity of these receptors to angiotensin II are present in women with preeclampsia.[269]

Studies indicate that no simple relationship exists between components of the RAS and preeclampsia. The significance, however, of reduced plasma renin activity, plasma renin concentration, and angiotensin II concentration on blood pressure and sodium excretion in this group of women—who show apparent volume constriction and who are exquisitely sensitive to angiotensin II—deserves elucidation.

Atrial Natriuretic Factor. Atrial natriuretic factor (ANF), a peptide produced in response to atrial stretch with hypervolemia, regulates intravascular volume by several mechanisms. ANF increases sodium excretion and the egress of fluid from the intravascular compartment. Although the reduced plasma volume of preeclampsia predicts reduced ANF concentration, the concentration is increased,[270] and the increase precedes clinical disease.[271] The stimulus for this increase is unclear, but the paradoxical finding of increased circulating ANF levels and reduced renin concentration with reduced plasma volume in preeclamptic women suggests that the reduced plasma volume is increased relative to the constricted vascular compartment.

Changes in Sodium Excretion. Sodium retention has long been considered an integral part of the pathophysiology of preeclampsia. Women with eclampsia and severe preeclampsia have very little chloride and sodium in the urine.[272] After delivery, however, chloride excretion increases dramatically. Infusion of hypertonic saline into preeclamptic women results in excretion of the infused sodium at about one half of the rate seen in normal pregnant women.[167] Similar results occur in women with glomeruloendotheliosis identified on renal biopsy.[273] Most studies of exchangeable sodium have indicated an increase in total body sodium in preeclamptic patients.[274,275]

The cause of sodium retention in preeclamptic women is difficult to determine because of the enormous number of factors that influence sodium excretion in normal pregnancy and because of the many demonstrated anomalies of renal function in preeclampsia that can cause sodium retention (Table 35-5). Any or all of the demonstrated changes in plasma volume, angiotensin sensitivity, and renal function may act on several of the factors listed in Table 35-5 to cause sodium retention.

Several investigators have considered the increased sodium retention to be a primary factor inciting the pathogenetic changes in pre-

TABLE 35-5 FACTORS AFFECTING SODIUM BALANCE IN NORMAL PREGNANCY

Factors Affecting Glomerular Filtration
Blood pressure in critical areas of the kidney
Relative tonus of afferent and efferent glomerular arterioles
Plasma oncotic pressure
Intrarenal redistribution of blood flow
Central nervous system effects
Factors Affecting Tubular Reabsorption
Aldosterone
Progesterone (an aldosterone antagonist)
Renal vascular resistance
Perfusion pressure in peritubular capillaries
Oncotic pressure in peritubular capillaries
Non-reabsorbable anions in the filtrate
Velocity of flow in tubules
Reabsorptive capacity of tubules
Estrogens (stimulate sodium reabsorption, possibly indirectly, by effects on vascular permeability)
Plasma sodium concentration
Hematocrit (viscosity effects)
Changes of plasma volume
Angiotensin
Sympathetic nervous system
Possibly a natriuretic hormone ("third factor")

Modified from Chesley LC: Hypertensive Disorders in Pregnancy. New York, Appleton-Century-Crofts, 1978.

eclampsia. Although this possibility cannot be definitely excluded, it is not likely for several reasons:

1. Angiotensin sensitivity precedes obvious fluid retention by months.
2. Thiocyanate space, an indicator of sodium space, does not reliably predict preeclampsia.[276]
3. Restriction of dietary sodium or increasing sodium excretion with diuretics does not affect the occurrence of preeclampsia.[277-279]

SUMMARY OF RENAL FUNCTION CHANGES

Renal function changes in preeclampsia are consistent and characteristic. Changes in tubular function precede the more widely appreciated changes in glomerular function. These functional changes return to normal within weeks to months after the conclusion of pregnancy. Prospective, sequential studies of renal function indicate that some of these changes antedate the clinical diagnosis of preeclampsia, but they do not necessarily antedate other indicators of preeclampsia such as changes in coagulation and plasma volume. They are therefore unlikely to be causal abnormalities. Although the cause of renal functional changes is not clear, they may be explained by systemic or regional abnormalities of renal perfusion.

Immunologic Changes and Activation of Inflammatory Responses

Epidemiologic and laboratory observations suggest that fetal-maternal immunologic interactions may be etiologically important in the pathogenesis of preeclampsia. The increased incidence of preeclampsia in first pregnancies and the protective effect even of miscarriage suggest that maternal exposure to fetal antigens may be protective, an effect that appears to be lost if the father is not the same man who fathered the prior pregnancy.[280,281] The increased risk of preeclampsia with a new father is affected by the interpregnancy interval, which tends to be longer in pregnancies with new fathers. This finding is compatible with an immunoprotective effect of antigen exposure, which is also lost when antigen exposure is minimal for a prolonged period.[282] Exposure to paternal components of fetal antigen through sexual activity with the potential father before the first pregnancy is also associated with reduced risk of preeclampsia.[283,284] The pathologic changes in decidual vessels at the placental site in preeclampsia are similar to the vascular changes of acute immunologic rejection.[140]

Several immunologic mechanisms have been suggested.[285,286] Preeclampsia may be an immune complex disease. There is an efflux of fetal antigen into the maternal circulation during pregnancy. If the maternal antibody response is adequate, the complexes are cleared by the reticuloendothelial system, and no damage occurs. If the antibody response or clearance mechanisms are inadequate,[287] the pathologic immune complexes formed can cause vasculitis, glomerular damage, and activation of the coagulation system. An inadequate maternal antibody response also can be suggested by HLA typing that demonstrates an increased concordance of the major histocompatibility antigens in maternal-paternal pairs that result in preeclamptic pregnancies.[286] However, preeclampsia is less common in consanguineous marriages, a finding incompatible with this concept.[288] Alternatively, the maternal antibody system may be overwhelmed by an excess of fetal antigen, a theory supported by the increased incidence of preeclampsia when trophoblastic tissue is increased (e.g., twins, hydatidiform mole, hydropic placenta). Few data support this concept.

Actual measurements of immune complexes in women with preeclampsia are inconsistent because of broadly different methodologies and definitions of preeclampsia. Increased immune complexes are a feature of normal pregnancy, with further increases in women with mild preeclampsia and significant elevations observed in women with severe preeclampsia.[289]

Another hypothesis about the immunologic cause of preeclampsia is that vascular changes in the spiral arterioles of the placental implantation site are the result of an allograft rejection between mother and fetus. However, who is rejecting whom?[286] Should the spiral arteries lined with trophoblast be thought of as fetal vessels, with the fetus rejecting the mother, or as maternal vessels, with the mother rejecting the fetus?

If preeclampsia represents a rejection of the fetus by the mother, the protective effect of previous exposure to antigen indicates that the preeclamptic mother has a deficit of blocking antibodies or of suppressor cell function. The recognition of a unique HLA antigen, HLA-G, on the trophoblast[290] suggests other possible causes of rejection of the fetus. HLA-G is a class I antigen present almost exclusively on the cytotrophoblast with minimal heterogeneity. Unlike classic HLA antigens, which exhibit numerous epitopes, fetal HLA-G in the trophoblast is likely to be identical in most fetuses, and the fetus would exhibit the same antigen as that expressed by the mother during her fetal life. Because an immune cell (i.e., natural killer lymphocyte) found in maternal decidua in high numbers is postulated to destroy cells not bearing HLA antigens, a reduced level of HLA-G may render the fetus a target for these cells. Unusual epitopes of HLA-G also can activate maternal immune defenses. Although there are suggestions that polymorphisms of HLA-G may be more common in preeclampsia,[291] the data are minimal, and findings are not universally accepted.[292]

If preeclampsia represents a rejection of the mother by the fetus, the preeclamptic mother would have to be deficient in the capacity to destroy fetal immune cells. These alternative hypotheses—one requiring active intervention and the other passive intervention by the maternal immune system—should give disparate results in in vitro testing of maternal immune function. The experimental evidence available is not consistent enough to confirm or to contradict either hypothesis.

The innate immune response system may also play a role.[293] Normal pregnancy is associated with an activation of inflammatory response that is similar to that seen in sepsis. This inflammatory response is further increased in preeclampsia.[294] Materials released from the placenta, perhaps microvillus particles associated with aponecrosis, interact with maternal immune cells to produce inflammatory activation.[295] Increased release of these materials in preeclampsia is posited to augment the immune response with secondary pathogenetic effects of this inflammatory activation.

An immunologic cause of preeclampsia is consistent with much that is known about the disorder. Increased delineation of the changes in the immunologic activity in preeclampsia may provide insight into the cause of preeclampsia and normal fetal-maternal compatibility during pregnancy.

Oxidative Stress

Oxidative stress occurs when there is an excess of active oxygen products beyond the capacity of buffering mechanisms, antioxidants, and antioxidant enzymes. This phenomenon can occur with excess production of reactive oxygen products or with deficiency of antioxidant mechanisms.[296] Reactive oxygen products can damage proteins, lipids, and DNA, and the endothelium is particularly vulnerable. Levels of lipid markers of oxidative stress are increased in women with preeclampsia.[297,298] Lipid oxidation products, protein products of oxidation, protein carbonyls,[299] and nitrotyrosine are present in the circulation, blood vessels,[219] and placenta[218] of preeclamptic women and their fetuses. Reduced levels of antioxidants[300,301] and increased levels of antibodies to oxidized LDL cholesterol[302] are found in excess in women with preeclampsia. These changes are not likely the result of preeclampsia, because reduced antioxidants and increased lipid peroxidation products are present in women destined to develop preeclampsia.[303,304]

The excess oxidative species relevant to preeclampsia have several origins. Transition metals such as iron catalyze the formation of reactive oxygen species, and free iron and redox active copper[305] are increased in the blood of women with preeclampsia.[306] Reduced tissue perfusion sufficient to result in hypoxia and followed by restored perfusion and reoxygenation leads to the formation of reactive oxygen species.[307] This mechanism is compatible with pregnancy and preeclampsia. Uterine and placental blood flow is not privileged, and flow is reduced when blood is shunted to other organs during exercise, eating, and other normal activities. In late pregnancy, uterine and placental blood flow is reduced profoundly by postural effects on uterine perfusion. All of these changes are reversible and are followed by restored perfusion. In normal pregnancy, reduced placental perfusion as described is not sufficient to generate free radicals. In preeclampsia, however, free radicals are generated in the intervillous space.[218,308] Reduced placental perfusion may result in maternal systemic disease as the products of oxidative stress are transferred to the maternal circulation.[309]

Genetics of Preeclampsia

The tendency of preeclampsia and eclampsia to occur in daughters and sisters of women with preeclampsia is frequently overlooked. In Aberdeen, Scotland, the incidence of proteinuric preeclampsia was increased fourfold among sisters of women who had preeclampsia in their first pregnancy compared with sisters of women who did not.[310] The incidence of preeclampsia was 15% among mothers but only 4% among mothers-in-law of preeclamptic women.[311] Chesley and Cooper[312] evaluated preeclampsia in the first pregnancy of sisters, daughters, granddaughters, and daughters-in-law of women who had been eclamptic. The incidence of preeclampsia was 37% among sisters, 26% among daughters, and 16% among granddaughters. The incidence was 6% among daughters-in-law. The fetal genome is also related to the occurrence of preeclampsia. Men who have fathered preeclamptic pregnancies are more likely to father preeclamptic pregnancies with new partners than are men who have never been fathers in preeclamptic pregnancies.[317] Men born to preeclamptic pregnancies are more likely to be fathers of preeclamptic pregnancies than are men who are born of non-preeclamptic pregnancies.[314]

What is inherited in preeclampsia? Possibilities include immunologic differences, features that compromise implantation, and an increased response to the systemic insult caused by reduced placental perfusion. Examinations of candidate genes support all possibilities. In some populations, certain HLA types are more common in the mother and the fetus from preeclamptic pregnancies.[315,316] A variant of the angiotensinogen gene—reported to be more common in some studies[317-319]—is speculated to influence blood pressure and spiral artery remodeling.[320] Gene variants potentially leading to aberrations of endothelial function are more common in preeclamptic women.[321-323] Mutations leading to increased risk factors for later-life cardiovascular disease, including function-perturbing mutations of lipoprotein lipase genes[88] and methylene tetrahydrofolate reductase (MTHFR, an enzyme abnormality associated with increased circulating homocysteine),[322] are associated with preeclampsia. As is common in studies of genetic polymorphisms, the results vary according to the population studied.[324] Although these and other studies[325] support the genetic heterogeneity of preeclampsia,[174] the literature may be underpowered and subject to publication bias.[326]

In the Genetics of Preeclampsia study of 1000 paternal, maternal, and fetal triads, none of the usual candidates was related to preeclampsia.[326] The results of linkage analyses to perform hypothesis-free testing of genetic associations have varied. Associations of preeclampsia have been found with loci on chromosomes 2p,[327,328] 2q,[327,328] 4q,[325,329] 9,[329] and 10[330] in different populations. A novel study from the Netherlands[330] combined physical localization of a candidate gene with a search for functionally relevant genes in this chromosomal region. This methodology identified *STOX1*, a paternally imprinted gene involved in trophoblast differentiation. As a paternally imprinted gene, *STOX1* is active only when coming from the mother. A mutated version of this gene was consistently present in affected sisters in preeclamptic pedigrees. Although *STOX1* was localized to chromosome 10 in the Netherlands study, a paralogue of this gene, *STOX2*, is located on chromosome 4q, close to the suggestive region identified in genome-wide searches in Finland and Australia. The use of high-throughput genetic and gene expression and proteomic studies is just beginning to be applied to the study of preeclampsia.[326]

Management of Preeclampsia

Philosophy of Management

The optimal philosophy of management is a product of the current knowledge about the pathophysiologic changes of and prognosis for preeclampsia. Three principles can be applied.

First, delivery is always appropriate therapy for the mother but may not be so for the fetus. Because we do not understand its cause, attempts to prevent preeclampsia by conventional medical approaches have been understandably unsuccessful. The primary goal of therapy is to prevent maternal morbidity and mortality. Preeclampsia is progressive at variable rates, and careful antepartum observation can identify the woman at risk. Preeclampsia is completely reversible and begins to abate with delivery. If only maternal well-being were considered, delivery of all preeclamptic women, regardless of severity of process or stage of gestation, would be appropriate. Expectant management is appropriate in some circumstances to attain an optimal outcome for the fetus. The goal of any therapy for preeclampsia other than delivery must be improved rates of perinatal and long-term mortality and morbidity for the fetus, infant, and child.

Second, the signs and symptoms of preeclampsia are not pathogenetically important. The pathologic and pathophysiologic changes of preeclampsia indicate that poor perfusion, caused at least in part by vasospasm, is the major factor leading to the derangement of maternal physiologic function and ultimately leading to perinatal mortality and morbidity. This same abnormality causes increased total peripheral resistance, with subsequent elevation of blood pressure and decreased renal perfusion leading to sodium retention and edema. The proteinuria of preeclampsia is at least partially explained by vasospasm and by reversible glomerular damage. Attempts to treat preeclampsia by natriuresis or by lowering blood pressure do not alleviate the important pathophysiologic changes. Natriuresis may be counterproductive and may adversely affect fetal outcome because the plasma volume is already reduced in preeclamptic women.

Third, the pathogenic changes of preeclampsia are present long before clinical criteria for diagnosis are evident. Changes in vascular reactivity, plasma volume, and renal function antedate—in some cases by months—the increases in blood pressure, protein excretion, and sodium retention. Irreversible changes affecting fetal well-being therefore may be present before the clinical diagnosis is made. This likely explains the failure of dietary, pharmacologic, and postural therapy instituted after the recognition of clinical disease to reduce perinatal morbidity and mortality. The only rationale for therapy other than immediate delivery is to palliate the maternal condition to allow fetal maturation, and even this rationale is controversial.

Delivery

Delivery is the definitive treatment for preeclampsia.

DELIVERY REMOTE FROM TERM

Delivery in the setting of severe preeclampsia usually is chosen for the maternal and fetal indications described previously. Fetal indications for intervention include the following:

- Non-reassuring fetal test results
- Estimated fetal weight less than the 5th percentile for gestational age
- Oligohydramnios (i.e., amniotic fluid index below 5.0 cm or maximal vertical pocket of fluid less than 2.0 cm)
- Persistent absent or reversed diastolic flow on umbilical artery Doppler velocimetry in a growth-restricted fetus

Delivery should be considered for all women with severe preeclampsia who have reached a favorable gestational age, which usually is defined as more than 32 to 34 weeks' gestation.

DELIVERY AT OR NEAR TERM

The treatment of choice for preeclampsia at term is delivery. Expectant management may be considered when preeclampsia is diagnosed at less than 32 to 34 weeks' gestation, even if disease is severe. However, as gestational age approaches 34 weeks, short- and long-term neonatal outcomes are excellent, and the potential benefits of expectant management become less compelling. At 34 to 37 weeks, decisions regarding delivery are not guided by good evidence, and clinical judgment must consider the neonatal prognosis, severity of maternal disease, and the wishes of the patient.

ROUTE OF DELIVERY

Delivery is usually accomplished by the vaginal route, with cesarean delivery reserved for obstetric indications. The decision to expedite delivery in the setting of severe preeclampsia does not mandate immediate cesarean birth.[331] Cervical ripening agents may be used if the cervix is not favorable before induction[332] and if the fetus can be satisfactorily monitored; however, a prolonged induction is best avoided, especially in the presence of IUGR or oligohydramnios. The rate of vaginal delivery after labor induction decreases to about 33% at less than 28 to 34 weeks' gestation because of the high frequency of non-reassuring fetal heart rate tracings and failure of induction.[333] Some physicians recommend scheduled cesarean delivery for women with severe preeclampsia with a pregnancy of less than 30 weeks' gestation and with an unfavorable Bishop score.[334]

After the decision for delivery is made, induction should be carried out aggressively and expeditiously. Cesarean delivery should be reserved for obstetric indications. Because the probability of fetal compromise in preeclampsia is high, it is mandatory in all vaginal deliveries that the fetus be monitored adequately. When feasible, internal monitoring is preferable to allow determination of variability; however, external monitoring, if technically good, is adequate until internal monitoring is possible. Magnesium sulfate may reduce fetal heart rate variability,[335] but if normal variability was never evident, fetal scalp blood sampling may be necessary to ensure that decreased variability is not related to fetal compromise. For the woman with marked hepatic capsular distention, cesarean delivery is indicated if vaginal delivery is not imminent. Even several extra hours can threaten the life of the mother, and liver rupture is difficult to predict and to treat. In some cases of severe preeclampsia, especially those with HELLP syndrome, rapidly worsening thrombocytopenia or other signs of maternal instability may preclude a trial of labor.

Regional anesthesia offers its usual advantages for vaginal and cesarean delivery but does carry the possibility of extensive sympatholysis with consequent decreased cardiac output, hypotension, and impairment of already compromised uteroplacental perfusion. This problem can be avoided by meticulous attention to anesthetic technique and volume expansion. Regional anesthesia is not a rational means of lowering blood pressure because it does so at the expense of cardiac output. Similarly, although analgesia with narcotics is not contraindicated and may be used when necessary, attempting to manage or prevent eclampsia with profound maternal sedation has been ineffective and even dangerous.

Antepartum Management

When preeclampsia is suspected, a careful evaluation of mother and fetus is essential. Maternal blood pressure, laboratory values, and fetal well-being should be assessed. If the diagnosis of preeclampsia is confirmed, maternal seizure prophylaxis should be considered, blood pressure should be controlled to a level that minimizes risk of maternal stroke, and plans for delivery should be made according to the gestational age.

ASSESSMENT AND MONITORING OF THE MOTHER AND FETUS

Maternal Monitoring. There are two goals for antepartum monitoring of the mother:

- Recognizing the condition early, because infants of mothers with even mild preeclampsia are at increased risk for adverse outcomes.
- Gauging the rate of progression of the condition to prevent severe morbidity by delivery and to determine whether fetal well-being can be monitored safely by the usual intermittent observations

Ideally, identification of early changes allows intervention before the advent of clinical symptoms. Although many hemodynamic, volume, and metabolic changes antedate the diagnostic clinical signs in women destined to develop preeclampsia, none is sensitive enough to be clinically useful.[7,33,112,167,235,336-338] The increased blood pressure response to angiotensin II[172,339,340] in women destined to have elevated blood pressure in late pregnancy was once the gold standard against which other predictors were judged, but a large study failed to confirm the predictive value of the test,[112,173] and it is neither simple nor safe enough for extensive clinical use. Abnormal uterine artery Doppler velocimetry in the second trimester has a positive predictive value for preeclampsia of about 20%. Although useful for research identification of subjects, the low sensitivity and positive predictive value limit its use in clinical care.[341] The role of Doppler velocimetry in patient management remains uncertain. Other suggested markers include angiogenic and antiangiogenic factors, but clinical use awaits additional evaluation.[342]

Clinical management is dictated by the overt clinical signs of preeclampsia. Proteinuria—the most valid clinical indicator of preeclampsia—is often a late change, sometimes even preceded by seizures, and it is therefore not useful for early recognition of disease. Although rapid weight gain and edema of the hands and face suggest fluid and sodium retention characteristic of preeclampsia, they are not universally present in or uniquely characteristic of preeclampsia. These signs are at most a reason for close observation of blood pressure and urinary protein levels. Early recognition of preeclampsia is necessarily based primarily on diagnostic blood pressure increases in the late second and early third trimesters compared with pressures in early pregnancy. Blood pressure changes without proteinuria undoubtedly occur in some normal women and in some with underlying renal or vascular disease. Because the goal of early diagnosis is to identify patients requiring more careful observation, overdiagnosis is preferable to underdiagnosis.

After blood pressure changes diagnostic of preeclampsia occur, evidence of multiorgan involvement should be sought through laboratory assessment. A 24-hour or timed urine specimen should be collected,[343] regardless of findings on urine dipstick evaluation.[9] Because of the hectic protein excretion characteristic of the disorder,[344] 24-hour urine collections may reveal excretion of more than 300 mg of protein, even with only trace proteinuria identified on the dipstick evaluation.[9] Platelet count and liver enzyme tests should also be obtained.[2] To rule out fulminant progression, repeated examination of pressure and urinary protein is suggested within 24 hours. The frequency of subsequent observations is determined by these initial observations and the ensuing clinical progression. If the condition appears stable, once- or twice-weekly observations may be appropriate. Any evidence of progression merits more frequent observations, perhaps in the hospital. The appearance of proteinuria is an especially important sign of progression and requires frequent observation.

If deterioration in laboratory findings, symptoms, or clinical signs occurs, the decision to continue the pregnancy is determined day by day. Subjective evidence of central nervous system involvement (i.e., headache, disorientation, and visual symptoms) and hepatic distention (i.e., abdominal pain and right upper quadrant or epigastric tenderness) indicates worsening preeclampsia. Important clinical signs are blood pressure, urinary output, and fluid retention as evidenced by daily weight increase.

Laboratory studies are performed at intervals of no less often than every 48 hours. Tests should include a platelet count and fibrin split products, urinary protein excretion and serum creatinine levels, and serum levels of transaminases.

Fetal Observation. Assessment of fetal well-being is required to determine whether continuing the pregnancy is safe (see Chapter 21). With the diagnosis of gestational hypertension, fetal assessment for size by sonography and for function by nonstress testing is indicated. After the diagnosis of preeclampsia is made, it is mandatory to monitor the fetal condition. Ultrasound evaluation of fetal weight and amniotic fluid volume and a nonstress test of the fetal heart rate should be performed. Alternatively, a complete biophysical profile may be performed. Doppler velocimetry is not recommended unless fetal growth restriction is identified.

As long as the maternal condition is mild and stable, weekly monitoring of the fetus appears to be adequate. Unfortunately, no test of fetal well-being is satisfactory when the mother's condition is unstable, and testing should be repeated whenever the maternal status changes. Management of fetal growth restriction, a common complication of preeclampsia, is discussed in Chapter 34. Amniotic fluid testing for fetal lung maturity (see Chapter 23) may aid the decision to deliver the fetus with growth restriction. Fetal jeopardy, rather than lung maturity, is the fetal criterion to determine delivery when preeclampsia occurs remote from term.

Expectant Management of Severe Preeclampsia Remote from Term

Prolonged expectant antepartum management of women with severe preeclampsia is not practiced in most centers. With improvements in neonatal care, many clinicians regard delivery of women with severe preeclampsia beyond 32 to 34 weeks' gestation to be in the best interests of the mother and fetus. When gestational age is critical (<32 weeks), the physician may consider control of maternal blood pressure along with meticulous observation of maternal and fetal conditions. This approach requires personnel and facilities for very close assessment of both patients.

The initial evaluation and management of a woman suspected to have severe preeclampsia between 24 and 32 to 34 weeks' gestation includes the following components:

- The pregnant woman is admitted to the hospital.
- A course of antenatal corticosteroids is administered (see Chapter 23). Barring rapid deterioration of the maternal or fetal status, reasonable efforts should be made to delay delivery for 48 hours to complete a full course of antenatal corticosteroids. Neonates from preeclamptic pregnancies may have a reduced incidence of respiratory distress syndrome, but this does not justify withholding antenatal corticosteroid therapy.[345,346]
- Seizure prophylaxis is undertaken with magnesium sulfate.
- Blood pressure is monitored at least every 1 to 2 hours.
- Fluid intake and urine output are strictly monitored.
- A 24-hour urine collection is used to determine protein excretion and creatinine clearance.
- Laboratory studies include a complete blood cell count with a platelet count and smear and determinations of electrolytes, creatinine, ALT, AST, lactic acid dehydrogenase (LDH), uric acid, and albumin. A coagulopathy profile (i.e., prothrombin time [PT], partial thromboplastin time [PTT], and fibrinogen) should be obtained if the ALT and AST values are more than twice normal or if the platelet count is less than 100,000 cells/μL.
- Assessment of fetal well-being includes a nonstress test, amniotic fluid volume determination, and estimation of fetal size. If growth restriction is recognized, umbilical artery Doppler velocimetry is suggested.

After the complete assessment of the fetus and mother, the safety and potential utility of expectant management should be reassessed daily. Several factors mandate delivery regardless of gestational age. Under these circumstances, the initial dose of antenatal steroids should be administered, but pregnancy should not be unnecessarily prolonged to give the second dose.

CONTRAINDICATIONS TO EXPECTANT MANAGEMENT

Immediate delivery should be considered if any of the following conditions are present:

- Maternal hemodynamic instability (e.g., shock)
- Non-reassuring fetal test results (e.g., persistently abnormal fetal heart rate testing, estimated fetal weight less than the 5th percentile for gestational age, oligohydramnios with amniotic

fluid index <5.0 cm or maximal vertical pocket <2.0 cm, persistent absent or reversed diastolic flow on umbilical artery Doppler velocimetry in a growth-restricted fetus)
- Persistent, severe hypertension unresponsive to medical therapy
- Persistent headache, visual aberrations, or epigastric or right upper quadrant pain
- Eclampsia
- Pulmonary edema
- Renal failure with a marked rise in serum creatinine (i.e., serum creatinine concentration increased by 1 mg/dL over baseline) or urine output less than 0.5 mL/kg/hr for 2 hours that is unresponsive to hydration with two intravenous boluses of 500 mL of fluid
- Laboratory abnormalities (e.g., rapid increase in aminotransferases that exceeds twice the upper limit of normal, progressive decrease in the platelet count to less than 100,000 cells/μL, coagulopathy in the absence of an alternative explanation) that worsen over a period of 6 to 12 hours
- Abruptio placentae
- Gestational age more than 34 weeks
- HELLP syndrome (Some studies have reported that serious maternal complications in the setting of expectant management of HELLP syndrome are uncommon with careful maternal monitoring.[347,348] However, the aim of expectant management is to improve neonatal morbidity and mortality, and it has not been shown that overall perinatal outcome is improved with expectant management compared with pregnancies delivered after a course of corticosteroids. Expectant management remains an investigational approach.[349,350])
- Patient who does not want to undergo risks of expectant management

If the fetus and mother have none of these signs or symptoms and the informed woman agrees, expectant management may be considered.

CANDIDATES FOR EXPECTANT MANAGEMENT

In women with severe preeclampsia remote from term, the decision to continue pregnancy beyond that required for corticosteroids depends on the results of frequent maternal and fetal assessment and continual review of the ongoing risks of conservative management versus the benefit of further fetal maturation. These women should be cared for in a hospital setting and cared for by or in consultation with a maternal-fetal medicine specialist. In this environment, expectant management of severe preeclampsia remote from term may be considered in four circumstances.

The first is transient abnormal laboratory test results. Asymptomatic women before 34 weeks' gestation with severe preeclampsia on the basis of laboratory abnormalities that improve or resolve within 24 to 48 hours after hospitalization may be managed expectantly.[351,352] If initial laboratory abnormalities include elevated liver function test results (e.g., ALT, AST) less than twice the upper limit of normal, a platelet count of less than 100,000 cells/μL but greater than 75,000 cells/μL, and coagulopathy in the absence of an alternative explanation, it is reasonable to delay delivery, administer antenatal corticosteroids, and repeat laboratory tests every 6 to 12 hours. If the laboratory values show a trend toward improvement, or if they resolve, expectant management may be continued until a more favorable gestational age. Delivery is warranted if liver function test values or platelet counts deteriorate or coagulopathy occurs.

The second reason to consider expectant management of severe preeclampsia remote from term is severe preeclampsia based solely on proteinuria. In the absence of other features of severe preeclampsia, proteinuria greater than 5 g in 24 hours is not an indication for delivery. Several clinical studies have shown that neither the rate of increase nor the amount of proteinuria affects maternal or perinatal outcome in the setting of preeclampsia.[353,354] For this reason, after the threshold of 300 mg in 24 hours for the diagnosis of preeclampsia has been exceeded, 24-hour urinary protein estimations do not bear repeating.

The third reason is severe preeclampsia based solely on fetal growth restriction. Women with severe preeclampsia based only on the presence of IUGR in the setting of preeclampsia may be managed expectantly if they meet the following criteria[355]:

- Mild IUGR, defined as an estimated fetal weight between the 5th and 10th percentile for gestational age (see Chapter 34)
- Gestational age less than 32 weeks
- Reassuring fetal test results, defined as a reassuring nonstress test result, adequate amniotic fluid volume (AFI > 5.0 cm or maximal vertical pocket >2.0 cm), and no persistent absent or reversed diastolic flow on umbilical artery Doppler velocimetry (see Chapter 21)

These women should be admitted to the hospital for close maternal surveillance and daily fetal testing.[356] The admission-to-delivery interval in such pregnancies averages only 3 days, and more than 85% of these women require delivery within 1 week of presentation.[350,355]

The fourth reason to consider expectant management is severe preeclampsia based solely on blood pressure criteria. Two studies have established a precedent for expectant management of patients with severe preeclampsia by blood pressure criteria alone in pregnancies less than 32 weeks with reassuring fetal testing.[351,352]

COMPONENTS OF EXPECTANT MANAGEMENT

Expectant management of severe preeclampsia is not associated with any direct maternal benefits. The mother is assuming a small but significant risk to her own health to delay delivery until a more favorable gestational age is reached for her child.

If the contraindications to expectant management described previously are absent, the following protocol may minimize the risk of maternal and fetal complications:

- Close supervision of the mother and fetus is crucial because it is impossible to predict the clinical course the disease will take after admission.[349]
- The mother is hospitalized until delivery.
- The patient is kept on bed rest with bathroom privileges.
- Blood pressure is monitored every 2 to 4 hours while the patient is awake.
- Maternal symptoms are assessed every 2 to 4 hours while she is awake.
- Fluid intake and urine output are strictly recorded.
- Complete blood cell count, electrolyte determinations, and liver and renal function tests are performed at least twice weekly, if not daily.
- The mother is given antenatal corticosteroids, if not previously given.
- Regular assessment of fetal well-being (at least daily nonstress tests with a biophysical profile if nonreactive)[3]
- Delivery occurs after 32 to 34 weeks' gestation, depending on the clinical scenario.

If abnormal laboratory test results are obtained on admission, tests should be repeated every 6 to 12 hours. Delivery should be considered if there is no trend toward improvement within 12 hours of admission or if the condition worsens after an initial improvement.

There is no standardized protocol for fetal assessment in this setting. We perform fetal kick counts and nonstress tests at least daily, ultrasound assessment of amniotic fluid volume once or twice per week, ultrasound estimation of fetal growth every 10 to 14 days, and weekly Doppler velocimetry of the umbilical artery if the fetus is growth restricted.

Several management strategies with no proven benefit in the setting of severe preeclampsia are often recommended, but they are best avoided. They include the routine use of continuous fetal heart rate monitoring, routine initiation of antihypertensive therapy (antihypertensive therapy should be avoided, with the exception of women with chronic hypertension and those being managed according to standard protocols for severe preeclampsia by blood pressure criteria only remote from term),[352] prolonged (>48 hours) antepartum administration of magnesium sulfate for seizure prophylaxis, serial 24-hour urine collections for protein quantitation, and routine assessment of fetal lung maturity. However, the latter may be useful between 30 and 34 weeks when there is contradictory or equivocal evidence of maternal or fetal deterioration.

Postpartum administration of intravenous dexamethasone does not reduce the severity or duration of disease. The serendipitous observation that women who had received antepartum steroids appeared to evidence improvement in the HELLP syndrome[357] stimulated several retrospective and observational studies.[358-363] These studies and a small, randomized, controlled trial[364] suggest improvement in laboratory findings and prolongation of pregnancy. The determination of appropriate dosing and whether the benefit of therapy exceeds risks await larger, randomized, controlled trials. Its benefit for patients with HELLP syndrome remains controversial.[365]

OUTCOMES OF EXPECTANT MANAGEMENT

Several studies have shown that with close monitoring, pregnancies complicated by severe preeclampsia could be managed expectantly and extended by 5 to 19 days, on average, with good maternal and neonatal outcomes. However, pregnancies with a growth-restricted fetus typically deliver in 3 to 5 days.[351,352,366,367]

Intrapartum Management

The intrapartum management of women with preeclampsia tests the obstetric and medical skills of the health care team. The patient with severe preeclampsia or eclampsia is acutely ill, with functional derangements of many organ systems.[368] Improved appreciation of the gravity of this situation and enhanced methods of maternal monitoring have reduced mortality rates. One study from the United Kingdom demonstrated a significant reduction in maternal death due to eclampsia from 15.1% in the 1940s to less than 3.9% after 1950.[368] Failure to recognize and appropriately manage this grave condition probably accounts for most deaths. Even mildly preeclamptic women can experience an acceleration of disease during labor.

Baseline information should be obtained to determine renal function, coagulation status, and liver function. Determination of the serum protein concentration informs the choice of appropriate fluid administration. Some investigators advocate the use of intensive cardiovascular monitoring, with Swan-Ganz catheters or with central venous pressure catheters in all women with severe preeclampsia or eclampsia (see Chapter 57). Such a practice is probably indicated in oliguric patients whose urinary output does not improve with a modest fluid challenge. The major problems to be managed are those of high blood pressure, intravascular volume, and convulsions. Less commonly, patients with DIC and myocardial dysfunction require treatment.

SEIZURE PROPHYLAXIS AND TREATMENT

Most seizures occur during the intrapartum and postpartum periods, when the preeclamptic process is most likely to accelerate. In the Magpie study, 10,000 preeclamptic women were randomized to receive magnesium sulfate or placebo. Magnesium sulfate clearly reduced the risk of eclampsia in this trial,[369] and it was shown in separate trials to be superior for this purpose to other prophylactic medications, including phenytoin[370,371] and diazepam.[372,373]

Despite the demonstrated efficacy of magnesium sulfate, it is difficult to select preeclamptic women for whom the risks of seizure exceed the risk of prophylaxis. In the Magpie study, treatment was effective and safe even in developing countries, but most of these women had significant disease. Twenty-five percent were defined as having severe preeclampsia, and 75% required antihypertensive therapy. Although the use of magnesium prophylaxis in so-called mild preeclampsia is controversial, the incidence of eclampsia increased by 50% in a large obstetric service when magnesium prophylaxis was limited to women with severe disease.[374] A review of eclamptic patients from another large U.S. center indicates the difficulty in selecting preeclamptic women with disease severe enough to warrant therapy. None of the clinical signs and symptoms considered to be prognostic of seizures was absolutely reliable. Seventeen percent of women who had seizures did not have headache, 80% did not have epigastric pain, and 20% had normal deep tendon reflexes (Table 35-6). The lack of absolute correlation with proteinuria is consistent with the observations by Chesley and Chesley[276] more than 50 years ago that 24% of patients do not have proteinuria before seizures.

Most U.S. investigators recommend prophylactic anticonvulsant therapy for all women with a blood pressure elevation diagnostic of preeclampsia, regardless of whether other signs and symptoms, including proteinuria, are present. This approach includes women for whom the risks of treatment may exceed the risks from seizures. The first requirement for anticonvulsant prophylaxis is that the agent and dosage schedule must be extremely safe for the mother. Safety for the fetus and neonate is the next criterion.

Magnesium Sulfate. Magnesium sulfate offers considerable advantages for prophylaxis in women with preeclampsia. Its pharmacokinetic processes during pregnancy are well established, as are its efficacy and safety for the mother and fetus.

TABLE 35-6 FREQUENCY OF SYMPTOMS PRECEDING ECLAMPSIA

Symptom	Frequency (%)
Headache	83
Hyperreflexia	80
Proteinuria	80
Edema	60
Clonus	46
Visual signs	45
Epigastric pain	20

Adapted from Sibai BM, Lipshitz J, Anderson GD, Dilts PV Jr: Reassessment of intravenous $MgSO_4$ therapy in preeclampsia-eclampsia. Obstet Gynecol 57:199-202, 1981; with permission from the American College of Obstetricians and Gynecologists.

TABLE 35-7 EFFECTS ASSOCIATED WITH VARIOUS SERUM MAGNESIUM LEVELS

Effect	Serum Level (mEq/L)
Anticonvulsant prophylaxis	4-6
Electrocardiographic changes	5-10
Loss of deep tendon reflexes	10
Respiratory paralysis	15
Cardiac arrest	>25

TABLE 35-8 SAFETY AND EFFICACY OF INTRAVENOUS MAGNESIUM SULFATE THERAPY

Factor	Number (%)
Number of women treated	1870
Number of women with seizures	11 (0.6)
Number with seizure morbidity	1 (0.05)
Number with morbidity from treatment	0 (0)

Adapted from Sibai BM, Lipshitz J, Anderson GD, Dilts PV Jr: Reassessment of intravenous $MgSO_4$ therapy in preeclampsia-eclampsia. Obstet Gynecol 57:199-202, 1981; with permission from the American College of Obstetricians and Gynecologists.

The volume of distribution of magnesium is greater than that of sucrose, indicating that the distribution of this ion goes beyond extracellular fluid and enters bones and cells.[375] Magnesium circulates largely unbound to protein and is almost exclusively excreted in urine. It is reabsorbed in the proximal tubule by a process limited by transport maximum (T_{max}), and its excretion increases as the filtered load increases above the T_{max}.[376] In women with normal renal function, the half-time for excretion is about 4 hours.[375] Because excretion depends on delivery of a filtered load of magnesium that exceeds the T_{max}, the half-time of excretion is prolonged in women with a decreased GFR.

The clinically relevant effects of elevated serum magnesium concentrations are related primarily to the membrane effects. Magnesium slows or blocks neuromuscular and cardiac conducting system transmission, decreases smooth muscle contractility, and depresses central nervous system irritability. These actions produce the desired anticonvulsant effect and cause decreased uterine and myocardial contractility, depressed respirations, and interference with cardiac conduction. These effects occur at different serum magnesium concentrations (Table 35-7). Doses of magnesium sulfate sufficient for anticonvulsant therapy cause little change in blood pressure.

Depression of deep tendon reflexes occurs at serum concentrations lower than those associated with adverse cardiac and respiratory effects. The presence of deep tendon reflexes indicates that the serum magnesium concentration is not dangerously high. If deep tendon reflexes are lost, the serum magnesium concentration may be greater than 10 mEq/L, but brisk deep tendon reflexes do not signify inadequate magnesium dosage. Any attempt to titrate magnesium therapy until deep tendon reflexes are eliminated is irrational and dangerous.

In the United States, magnesium sulfate is routinely given intravenously, rather than by more painful intramuscular injections. A typical loading dose is 4 to 6 g given intravenously over about 15 to 30 minutes, followed by 1 to 2 g/hr as a continuous infusion. Magnesium is administered by continuous infusion because intermittent bolus infusions result in only transient elevations of magnesium level. To ensure consistent infusion and to avoid inadvertent administration of large doses of magnesium, mechanically controlled infusion is mandatory. In all patients, deep tendon reflexes should be checked regularly (at least every 2 hours) to make sure they remain present, and the respiratory rate must be monitored.

The rate of infusion is modified for patients with compromised renal function. If the maternal creatinine level is greater than 1.0 mg/dL, serum magnesium levels should be obtained and the infusion rate limited to no more than 1 g/hr if there is further evidence of renal impairment. If overdosage occurs, especially with apnea, calcium gluconate (10 mL of a 10% solution injected intravenously over 3 minutes) is an effective antidote. The "therapeutic concentrations" of magnesium have been empirically determined and are the levels attained with dosages found to be usually effective and safe (Table 35-8). No study has compared magnesium concentrations in patients successfully or unsuccessfully treated with $MgSO_4 \cdot 7\ H_2O$. We do not recommend titrating levels to any specific therapeutic range, and there is no evidence that levels greater than 6 mEq/L increase efficacy. Magnesium is not a perfect anticonvulsant, and some women have convulsions even with high serum concentrations.[377]

Based on extensive experience, intravenous administration of magnesium at doses up to 2 g/hr appears to be safe if renal function is normal. In the Magpie study, doses of 1 g/hr given intravenously were effective without serious complications in 5000 treated women; some were treated in underdeveloped nations.

Magnesium sulfate therapy at effective anticonvulsant doses is safe for the fetus and neonate. Neonatal serum magnesium concentrations are almost identical to those of the mother.[378] Although amniotic fluid magnesium concentrations increase with prolonged infusion because of fetal renal excretion, fetal serum magnesium levels do not increase, and there is no evidence of cumulative effects on the neonate of prolonged magnesium administration for seizure prophylaxis.

In a study of 118 infants of mothers treated with magnesium sulfate, the average serum magnesium concentration was 3.7 mEq/L. There was no correlation of magnesium levels with Apgar scores.[379] Administration of magnesium to the mother may have additional beneficial effects for the fetus, which are being tested in controlled trials (see Chapter 29).

Phenytoin. Phenytoin is an effective anticonvulsant with pharmacologic effects that would not be predicted to produce adverse effects on the fetus or neonate. In several small studies, there were no obvious adverse fetal or maternal effects.[380,381] Although phenytoin is not as effective as magnesium for prophylaxis or treatment of eclampsia,[372,382] it can be used safely when magnesium is inappropriate, such as in women with myasthenia gravis or markedly compromised renal function. Phenytoin nonetheless does have potential severe adverse effects that may be magnified by unfamiliarity of obstetric personnel with its use.

Anticonvulsant Therapy. Magnesium is more effective than phenytoin or benzodiazepam to treat eclamptic seizures.[372] An initial infusion of 4 g can be administered safely intravenously over as little as 5 minutes, and intravenous $MgSO_4$ can be administered at 1 to 2 g/hr to maintain therapeutic serum magnesium levels. If a patient already receiving magnesium has an eclamptic seizure, it is safer to terminate seizures with another agent, such as 5 to 10 mg of diazepam (Valium), 4 mg of lorazepam (over 2 to 5 minutes),[383] or a short-acting barbiturate, such as pentobarbital (125 mg given intravenously). If these measures fail, general anesthesia may be necessary to terminate the seizures.

TABLE 35-9 DRUGS FOR TREATMENT OF HYPERTENSIVE EMERGENCIES

	Time Course of Action						
Drug	Onset	Maximum	Duration	Intramuscular Dosage	Intravenous Dosage	Interval between Doses	Mechanism
Hydralazine	10-20 min	20-40 min	3-8 hr	10-50 mg	5-25 mg	3-6 hr	Direct dilatation of arterioles
Sodium nitroprusside	0.52-2 min	1-2 min	3-5 min	—	IV solution: 0.01 g/L; IV infusion rate: 3-4 μg/kg/min		Direct dilatation of arterioles and veins
Labetalol	1-2 min	10 min	6-16 hr	—	20-50 mg	3-6 hr	α- and β-Adrenergic blocker
Nifedipine	5-10 min	10-20 min	4-8 hr	—	10 mg orally	4-8 hr	Calcium channel blocker

Most seizures terminate spontaneously within 1 to 2 minutes. The most important measures for any seizure before pharmacologic therapy is initiated are prevention of injury and protection of the airway to prevent aspiration.

ANTIHYPERTENSIVE THERAPY

Antihypertensive agents are not administered routinely to women with preeclampsia. There is no evidence that administration of these agents has beneficial fetal effects. The suggestion that lowering blood pressure reduces the risk of seizures has not been tested. The goal of antihypertensive treatment is prevention of intracranial bleeding and stroke.

Therapy is reserved for women in whom blood pressure is elevated to more than 160 mm Hg systolic or more than 105 to 110 mm Hg diastolic, which are the levels associated with intracranial bleeding or stroke.[384,385] The goal of blood pressure control is not to attain normal blood pressure but merely to reduce blood pressure to a level that can provide a margin of maternal safety (i.e., 135 to 145 mm Hg systolic and 95 to 100 mm Hg diastolic) without compromising adequate uterine perfusion. These patients have elevated blood pressure with reduced plasma volume. Overly aggressive treatment lowers maternal cardiac output and uterine perfusion and may result in iatrogenic fetal distress.

Several agents available for reducing blood pressure rapidly are described in Table 35-9. Not listed in this table are potent diuretic agents that lower blood pressure rapidly by depleting plasma volume, because the use of these agents in the plasma volume–depleted patient may reduce maternal cardiac output and uterine perfusion.

Hydralazine. The agent most widely used to reduce blood pressure in women with severe preeclampsia is hydralazine. As a direct vasodilator, it offers two major advantages. First, vasodilation with hydralazine results in a reflex increase in cardiac output and increased uterine blood flow as blood pressure decreases. Second, the increase in cardiac output blunts the hypotensive effect and makes it difficult to overdose the patient. The important side effects of hydralazine are headache and epigastric pain, which may be confused with worsening preeclampsia.

The pharmacokinetic profile of hydralazine is outlined in Table 35-9. The onset of action occurs in 10 to 20 minutes, and peak action occurs 20 minutes after administration, even when the agent is given intravenously. The duration of action is 3 to 8 hours. The use of continuous intravenous infusions of hydralazine is not sensible because minute-to-minute control cannot be attained. An alternative approach is to administer the drug as a bolus infusion, repeated at 20-minute intervals until the desired control is attained and then repeated as necessary. A test dose of 1 mg is given over 1 minute, and blood pressure is determined to avoid idiosyncratic hypotensive effects; 4 mg is then infused over 2 to 4 minutes. After 20 minutes, the blood pressure is determined, and the following criteria for action are taken into account:

- If there was no effect from the first dose of hydralazine, the dose is repeated.
- If a suboptimal effect was obtained, a second, smaller dose is given.
- If diastolic blood pressure is between 90 and 100 mm Hg, therapy is not repeated until diastolic blood pressure increases to 105 mm Hg.

Other Drugs. In rare instances, hydralazine may not effectively lower blood pressure to the desired level. If blood pressure control is not adequate after the administration of 20 mg of hydralazine, other hypotensive agents must be used.

The calcium entry blocker nifedipine has been taken orally in doses of 10 mg, which may be repeated after 30 minutes if needed to lower blood pressure rapidly. For maintenance dosing, 10 to 20 mg can then be given every 3 to 6 hours as needed. It is quite effective and well tolerated; headache is the most common side effect.[386]

Labetalol, a mixed α-adrenergic and β-adrenergic antagonist, also is useful for reducing blood pressure acutely. It is given intravenously as a bolus infusion, beginning with 10 mg and followed by repeated doses that may be increased up to twofold (e.g., 20 mg, 40 mg, 80 mg), with doubling every 10 minutes as needed (up to 300 mg) for blood pressure control.[387] The major reservation about the use of labetalol is that, unlike the vasodilators hydralazine and nifedipine, it does not reduce afterload. There are theoretical disadvantages with using labetalol for managing cardiac failure associated with the hypertension of preeclampsia.

Methyldopa (formerly designated α-methyldopa) is a safe and well-tested drug. However, its delayed onset of action (4 to 6 hours), even when administered intravenously, limits its usefulness for hypertensive emergencies. On the basis of side effects and experience, nifedipine or labetalol are preferred when hydralazine is ineffective.

MANAGEMENT OF OLIGURIA

In preeclamptic women, oliguria can have a prerenal or renal origin (see Chapters 44 and 57). Even though plasma volume is decreased in preeclamptic patients, the use of fluids is controversial. Excessive fluid infusion can lead to congestive heart failure and perhaps cerebral edema[388]; nevertheless, oliguria can be corrected in many patients by fluid infusion.

To avoid complications, the physician should not prescribe hypotonic fluids. They worsen the dilutional decreases in serum osmolality that may occur with any of the following: oliguria from renal causes, elevated antidiuretic hormone (ADH) level in response to stress, and oxytocin treatment.

Fluids must be administered with the understanding that oliguria may have a renal origin and that the patient is at risk for fluid overloading. Because acute renal failure resulting in permanent renal damage is rare in pregnancy (whereas pulmonary edema is a common event on some obstetric services), oliguria should be defined conservatively as less than 20 to 30 mL/hr for 2 hours.

If there are no clinical signs or history suggesting congestive heart failure, 1000 mL of isotonic crystalloid can safely be infused in 1 hour. If urine output increases, fluid infusion is maintained at 100 mL of isotonic crystalloid per hour. If the oliguria does not resolve, further fluid infusion should be guided by central venous or, preferably, pulmonary wedge pressures (see Chapter 57).

Relatively small amounts of intrapartum and postpartum blood loss can result in profound hypovolemia and shock in patients who already have compromised blood volumes. A large peripheral line should be in place at all times in case rapid replacement of blood volume becomes necessary.

MANAGEMENT OF LESS COMMON PROBLEMS

Disseminated Intravascular Coagulation. Evidence of DIC is an important indicator of severity and progression of preeclampsia. DIC is measurable by the usual clinical tests in 20% of severely preeclamptic and eclamptic women and is sufficient to cause coagulation problems in less than 10%.

Definitive therapy for DIC is removal of the inciting factor. In preeclampsia, whether the cause of the coagulation disorder is endothelial cell damage, release of thromboplastic materials, vasospasm with attendant microangiopathic changes, or local consumption of procoagulants in the choriodecidual space, the inciting factor is pregnancy related, and definitive therapy is termination of the pregnancy. The long-range follow-up of women with preeclampsia indicates that all organ system functions return to normal. It is unlikely that occlusion of the microvasculature by thrombi in mild forms of DIC causes permanent damage.

Evidence of early DIC is not by itself an absolute indication for immediate delivery. With rapidly deteriorating renal or hepatic function or DIC complicated by spontaneous hemorrhage, however, delivery should be expeditious.

The experience with heparin anticoagulation, which has been used to maintain pregnancies in women with symptomatic DIC or as a prophylactic measure to prevent DIC, indicates that these approaches are not effective.[389] The use of heparin during labor in women in whom DIC necessitates delivery has not been studied extensively. The experiences already cited, however, indicate that the approach may be dangerous.

If procoagulants decrease to a level associated with spontaneous hemorrhage, appropriate procoagulant therapy should be given before delivery. This should be done whether the anticipated mode of delivery is vaginal or cesarean (see Chapter 40).

Pulmonary Edema. Pulmonary edema occurs in a small number of women with preeclampsia. In the past, this complication was associated with high rates of maternal mortality. The pathogenesis of pulmonary edema often is iatrogenic fluid overload, but it can be cardiogenic or involve transudation of fluid into alveoli. The noncardiogenic variety results from decreased colloid oncotic pressure or a pulmonary vascular leakage, and it can occur in the antepartum, intrapartum, or postpartum period. Delayed onset of pulmonary edema requires special awareness because the edema usually occurs during postpartum diuresis, when most concerns about the complications of preeclampsia are diminishing.

Management of pulmonary edema requires intensive monitoring, with the capability to assess pulmonary and cardiac function accurately and to perform mechanical ventilation as needed (see Chapter 57). With accurate assessment of cardiopulmonary function and aggressive treatment, the mortality resulting from pulmonary edema in preeclampsia has been greatly reduced.[390]

Postpartum Management in Preeclampsia

Delivery does not immediately reverse the pathophysiologic changes of preeclampsia, and it is necessary to continue palliative therapy for various periods. Some of the constraints on therapy, however, are eliminated by delivery of the fetus. Approximately one third of convulsions occur in the postpartum period, most within 24 hours and virtually all within 48 hours, although there are rare exceptions. Most physicians advocate continuing anticonvulsant therapy for 24 hours after delivery. For simplicity, magnesium sulfate therapy is usually continued, but because there is no need to consider fetal effects, any safe anticonvulsant regimen is reasonable at this time.

Anticonvulsant efficacy rather than sedation is the goal, and barbiturate anticonvulsants in usual therapeutic doses require days to achieve effective levels. Similarly, phenytoin must be administered intravenously in large doses to achieve therapeutic levels within hours, with the attendant dangers of cardiac arrhythmia. Serum magnesium concentrations decrease with increased urinary output, and with puerperal diuresis, it is extremely unlikely that the serum magnesium concentration is therapeutic at usual doses. Despite this drawback, convulsions rarely occur in the postpartum period, suggesting that rapid diuresis indicates resolution of the preeclamptic process and that therapy may no longer be required.

On the basis of these considerations, it appears reasonable to discontinue magnesium sulfate therapy when diuresis occurs before 24 hours after delivery. Some investigators recommend continuing magnesium sulfate administration for longer than 24 hours in selected patients, but it is difficult to determine the basis on which this selection can be made. In one randomized trial limited to women with mild preeclampsia, there was no difference in seizure risk when magnesium was discontinued after only 12 hours.[391] Unfortunately, this study was limited by a relatively small sample, and it is likely that any future studies will be similarly underpowered because of the rarity of the outcome.

Hypertension may take considerably longer than 24 to 48 hours to resolve. Women who are hypertensive 6 weeks after delivery may be normotensive at long-term follow-up.[74] The indications for therapy are similar to those for the antepartum period. The patient with blood pressure greater than 160 mm Hg systolic or 105 mm Hg diastolic after delivery should be treated; the fetus no longer influences therapeutic choices. If rapid blood pressure control is necessary, sodium nitroprusside is more effective and better tolerated than hydralazine. Diuretics and conventional oral antihypertensive agents can be started to achieve smooth control. The woman who remains hypertensive (>100 mm Hg diastolic pressure) should be sent home with continued antihypertensive therapy.

Patients with lesser elevations require no therapy. The choice of drugs is based on the usual step method of antihypertensive therapy. The patient sent home with a therapeutic regimen must be warned about symptoms of hypotension, and she must be seen at weekly intervals, because the need for therapy diminishes rapidly in some cases.

Therapies No Longer Recommended

Strict sodium restriction and diuretic therapy have no role in the prevention or treatment of preeclampsia. In women with marked sodium retention as manifested by significant edema, modest sodium restriction may not alter the course of the disease but can reduce discomfort. Diuretics should not be given because plasma volume is already decreased, and further volume depletion can affect the fetus adversely. Attempts to modify the progression of the disease by volume expansion have not been conclusively shown to be helpful and require more thorough evaluation before being used in routine management of preeclampsia.[392]

Sodium nitroprusside is a potent, short-acting, direct vasodilator that allows excellent moment-to-moment blood pressure control. However, because elevated fetal concentrations of serum cyanide, sometimes to toxic levels, have been reported in animal studies,[393] this agent is rarely used in humans.

Diazoxide is a thiazide analogue that has no diuretic effect, but it is an extremely potent antihypertensive agent, acting as a direct vasodilator. It is rarely used because of effects on maternal and fetal carbohydrate metabolism and its profound and slowly reversible effect on blood pressure.

There is little evidence that therapeutic efforts alter the underlying pathophysiology of preeclampsia. Therapeutic intervention for clinically evident preeclampsia is palliative. At best, it may slow the progression of the condition, but it is more likely to allow continuation of the pregnancy. Bed rest is a usual and reasonable recommendation for the woman with mild preeclampsia, although its efficacy is not clearly established.[394] Prophylactic hospitalization with increased bed rest may reduce the incidence of preeclampsia for women at high risk identified by increased angiotensin sensitivity.[395] It is unclear, however, which of the several behavioral modifications involved in hospital residence is important. Anecdotal reports of clinical improvement with bed rest must be tempered by the recognition of the unpredictable course of preeclampsia.

Follow-up Assessment for Preeclampsia

Because the early recognition and treatment of significant blood pressure elevation reduce morbidity, all women with a clinical diagnosis of preeclampsia deserve long-range follow-up. Decisions for evaluation and treatment should be deferred until 12 weeks after delivery because some women who are hypertensive at 6 weeks are normotensive years later. The woman who is normotensive 12 weeks after delivery should be advised of her increased risk for hypertension in later life[77] and should be counseled to have her blood pressure checked at least yearly. Because of the association between preeclampsia and later cardiovascular disease,[78] formal assessment of cardiovascular risk factors in such patients is prudent.

Prevention of Preeclampsia

Since the preeclamptic syndrome was first recognized, prevention has been attempted. Sodium restriction and nutrient supplements have been unsuccessful.[18] Randomized, controlled trials based on several hypotheses for preventing preeclampsia have been performed. The sequence of studies for each intervention has been similar, with initial small, single-center studies suggesting benefit and subsequent larger, well-powered studies finding no significant benefit.[36,396-398]

Aspirin trials to prevent preeclampsia are a prototype. More than 35,000 women have been included in randomized, controlled trials of various sizes and quality to determine the benefit of aspirin.[399] Small, single-center studies suggested benefit,[400-402] but larger, multicenter trials showed no effect.[36,403] One potential explanation is publication bias in favor of positive results. Results also might have varied because of the heterogeneity of preeclampsia, with benefit of therapy evident in only a subset.

A meta-analysis of trials that enrolled a large number of pregnant women found benefit for antiplatelet treatment (i.e., aspirin) to reduce the frequency of the diagnosis of preeclampsia, preterm delivery, and growth-restricted infants.[399,404] There was a modest reduction of the incidence of preeclampsia (17%), with 72 women needing treatment to prevent one case of preeclampsia. There was a 14% reduction in the rate of fetal and neonatal deaths, with a number needed to treat of 243 to prevent one death. The investigators concluded that antiplatelet agents such as aspirin have moderate benefits when used for prevention of preeclampsia and its consequences.

Using another analytical strategy, meta-analysis of individual patient data, the Perinatal Antiplatelet Review of International Studies (PARIS) Collaborative Group attempted to differentiate the success of aspirin in subsets according to maternal diagnosis, dosage of aspirin, and time when therapy was initiated. Although the group did confirm a reduction in preterm birth and the incidence of preeclampsia by 10% with aspirin, they did not identify any particular subgroups for whom aspirin was more effective. There was no difference in perinatal death for women treated with prophylactic aspirin.[405]

The estimated number of women to treat to prevent one case of preterm birth in this study was 500 for low-risk pregnancies (incidence of 2%) and 50 for high-risk pregnancies when the estimated incidence of preeclampsia was 20%. Decisions about the choice of aspirin with this degree of efficacy must consider the short-term adverse effects on the mother and infant, which have not been evident in the large number of women treated, and the long-term outcome, which is largely unknown.[406]

Calcium supplementation to prevent preeclampsia was initiated with similar enthusiasm. Calcium was tested in a large, randomized, controlled trial in the United States[396] based on initial studies and meta-analyses.[407] The conclusion of this study was unequivocal, finding no evidence that 2 g of supplemental calcium administered to pregnant women from early gestation onward reduced the incidence of preeclampsia, altered blood pressure, or affected fetal weight. A review of published studies concluded that any benefit of calcium was related to low calcium intake before pregnancy in some women.[408] Based on this rationale, the World Health Organization conducted a trial of calcium supplementation in populations with low calcium intake. Treatment did not reduce the diagnosis of preeclampsia but did reduce adverse outcomes.[409] Calcium administration has therefore been proposed as useful in low calcium consuming populations.[410]

Oxidative stress has been suggested as important in preeclampsia. The results of antioxidant therapy are similar to those with calcium and aspirin; an initial small trial of antioxidant vitamins C and E suggested benefit,[411] but a subsequent, larger trial did not.[397] There was concern about the safety of this therapy for the fetus because an excess of low-birth-weight infants (but not IUGR or premature infants) occurred in the antioxidant-treated group. The largest trial of low-risk women is ongoing, with results expected in 2008. This study initiated antioxidant treatment far earlier in pregnancy than the other studies (start date at 9 to 16 weeks), with 40% of women enrolled before 12 weeks, whereas the other studies began at an average of 18 weeks. This may be relevant because oxidative stress is known to accompany the establishment of the intervillous circulation at 8 to 10 weeks' gestation.[412] The primary outcome in this study is a composite outcome of maternal and fetal morbidity. Final decisions about efficacy and safety await the conclusion of this trial.[408]

The results of these studies of prophylaxis raise several important points:

- Randomized clinical trials of appropriate population and size to achieve sufficient power must guide clinical management. Nonetheless, the success in small trials and the failure in large, multicenter trials may be related to the heterogeneity of patients with preeclampsia.[174] Prophylaxis may be effective in a specific subset of women (e.g., calcium supplementation in women with low average calcium intake).
- Because the diagnosis of preeclampsia is based on signs that usually have minimal causal significance, prophylactic therapy should be aimed at the pathophysiology and judged by effects on perinatal outcome.
- The aspirin and calcium data suggest that initiation of therapy before disease is clinically evident may be successful if specific interventions can be applied to appropriately selected subjects.

Chronic Hypertension

Differentiation of chronic hypertension from preeclampsia is complex but essential. Even more important is the difficult discrimination between exacerbation of preexisting hypertension and the onset of superimposed preeclampsia. The rate of progression and the effect on the mother and fetus of these conditions are different in the two diseases. Management of hypertension in early pregnancy requires early recognition of blood pressure elevation, baseline testing to aid in the later diagnosis of superimposed preeclampsia, and meticulous maternal and fetal observation. If a decision is made to use antihypertensive therapy, antihypertensive drugs must be chosen on the basis of considerations specific to pregnancy.

Epidemiology

The prevalence of chronic hypertension increases with advancing age. In whites, the risk increases from 0.6% (18 to 29 years old) to 4.6% (30 to 39 years old). In African-American women, the risks increased to 2% and 22.3%, respectively.[413] Preeclampsia occurs in 25% of hypertensive women, compared with 4% in previously normotensive women.

Pathogenesis

Effects of Chronic Hypertension on the Mother

Blood pressure elevation during pregnancy without the superimposition of preeclampsia has the same impact as blood pressure increases in any other 10-month period. Systolic and diastolic blood pressures that exceed 160 and 105 mm Hg, respectively, increase the risk of morbidity even over this short period.

Maternal morbidity and mortality rates are greater among women with superimposed preeclampsia than among those with preeclampsia arising de novo. Blood pressure elevation with superimposed preeclampsia is also greater, increasing the possibility of intracranial bleeding. Two thirds of cases of eclampsia occur in first pregnancies, but two thirds of maternal deaths due to eclampsia occur in pregnancies other than the first pregnancy, in which underlying hypertension is a more common predisposing factor.[414]

One review of 28 women with preeclampsia and stroke examined blood pressures before the event. The range of systolic values ranged from 159 to 198 mm Hg, and the range for diastolic values was much greater, from 81 to 133 mm Hg (mean, 98 mm Hg). Only five women had diastolic values greater than 105 mm Hg.[385] Morbidity is difficult to predict by blood pressure, although it seems to be significantly increased when systolic pressures exceed 160 mm Hg and may be increased when diastolic pressures exceed 100 mm Hg.[385] The National High Blood Pressure Education Program Working Group on High Blood Pressure in Pregnancy has recommended initiating therapy when systolic pressures exceed 150 to 160 mm Hg and diastolic pressures exceed 100 to 110 mm Hg.

Effects of Chronic Hypertension on the Fetus

The perinatal mortality rate for infants born to hypertensive mothers increases as maternal blood pressure rises.[101] Without antihypertensive therapy, a woman with a systolic pressure of 200 mm Hg or a diastolic pressure of 120 mm Hg had only a 50% chance of bearing a living infant. The perinatal mortality rate is strikingly higher in hypertensive women with proteinuria, indicating the impact of superimposed preeclampsia on the fetus.

The perinatal mortality rate for infants of women with superimposed preeclampsia is greater than for infants of women in whom the condition arises de novo.[415] There are two explanations for this difference.

First, the decidual vessels of women with even mild preexisting hypertension demonstrate vascular changes similar to the changes in renal arterioles seen in women with long-standing hypertension.[416] Decreased uteroplacental perfusion resulting from this change may be additive and perhaps synergistic with the decidual vascular changes of preeclampsia. The decidual vascular changes likely explain the higher incidence of abruptio placentae among women with superimposed preeclampsia.

Second, preeclampsia appears earlier in pregnancies of hypertensive women than in those of normotensive women. Fetal growth restriction is common in infants of hypertensive women, and it increases in frequency and severity with increasing maternal blood pressure.[101]

Some investigators suggest that hypertension without preeclampsia has no adverse effect on the fetus,[286,417] but this observation ignores the effects of growth restriction. In a study of almost 300 pregnancies of women with chronic hypertension, perinatal death occurred only in growth-restricted infants.[418]

Diagnosis

Chronic hypertension is defined as hypertension that is observable before pregnancy or that is diagnosed before the 20th week of gestation. Hypertension is defined as a blood pressure greater than 140/90 mm Hg. If the diagnosis of hypertension is confirmed for the first time during pregnancy and it persists beyond the 84th day after delivery, it is classified as chronic hypertension.

Pharmacologic Management of Hypertension

Antihypertensive Therapy in the Reduction of Maternal and Fetal Morbidity and Mortality

Antihypertensive therapy reduces maternal mortality as effectively during pregnancy as at any other time. Lowering of markedly elevated blood pressure (>100 mm Hg diastolic pressure) can reduce the risk of morbid events even over 10 months, whereas the impact of such reduction on the minimal morbidity associated with less elevated pressures is unlikely. Antihypertensive therapy for women with mild to moderate hypertension can reduce the risk for severe hypertension in later pregnancy.[419]

It has been postulated that antihypertensive therapy for the mother and fetus might reduce the incidence of superimposed preeclampsia, but there has been no evidence of that effect in large trials of antihypertensive therapy administered during pregnancy. A Cochrane review indicates no effect of antihypertensive therapy on the perinatal mortality rate, but antihypertensive therapy was begun in the first trimester in only 2 of 46 studies included in the review.[419] Because pathologic and pathophysiologic changes are present as early as 14 weeks' gestation, it is possible that therapy was begun too late to have any effect on preeclampsia or fetal outcomes. There is no evidence that antihypertensive therapy increased perinatal mortality rates in any of these studies.[420,421] If therapy is indicated for maternal considerations (diastolic pressure >100 mm Hg), it is safe for the fetus if the choice of drug is appropriate.[422]

There is some suggestion that antihypertensive therapy may be associated with an increased risk of small infants. This increase is small and driven largely by therapy with β-blockers, specifically atenolol.[423]

Overview of Therapy for Hypertension in Pregnancy

Antihypertensive therapy can be used safely in pregnancy when indicated by the maternal condition. Therapy reduces the maternal risks of markedly elevated pressures, and in women with mild to moderate hypertension, it prevents severe hypertension later in pregnancy. The decision to use antihypertensive therapy is based on maternal considerations.

Antihypertensive medication is reserved for women with diastolic pressures above 90 mm Hg. Women using hypertensive therapy when they become pregnant, regardless of pretreatment blood pressure, are best served by continuation of therapy. There is no evidence that antihypertensive therapy presents a substantial risk to the fetus, and discontinuation of therapy may adversely affect long-range compliance with drug therapy, increasing the risk to the mother.

Perhaps in no other area of medicine is therapy with the potential for benefit or danger to two individuals so poorly evaluated. There is virtually no information from large, randomized, controlled trials about the fetal and maternal benefits and risks of antihypertensive therapy for mild to moderate chronic hypertension in pregnancy.

Choice of Antihypertensive Agents

EFFECT ON THE FETUS

Fetal considerations, particularly teratogenic concerns, influence the choice of antihypertensive agents (see Chapter 20). Few of the available antihypertensive agents have been associated with morphologic teratogenic effects; exceptions are the angiotensin-converting enzyme (ACE) inhibitors (discussed later). Because development does not end with gross organ development, long-term follow-up of infants and children treated in utero is needed. Such information is available only for methyldopa. Children of mothers treated with this agent during pregnancy showed no signs of neurologic or somatic abnormalities when examined at age 7 years.[424]

Maternal drug therapy can have pharmacologic effects on the fetus. For example, maternal treatment with propranolol reduced fetal and maternal cardiac output in animal studies.[425] Because of the potential pharmacokinetic differences between mother and fetus, appropriate dosage for the mother may be excessive for the fetus.[426] Drug effects of minimal importance to the mother and fetus may be of great importance to the infant.

EFFECT ON UTERINE BLOOD FLOW

Maternal medication may affect fetal well-being by altering uterine blood flow. Antihypertensive drugs act by reducing cardiac output or systemic vascular resistance, which may affect blood flow to the uterus. Optimal drug choice in pregnancy avoids agents that reduce uterine and therefore uteroplacental blood flow. Agents that reduce cardiac output are best avoided because they almost inevitably reduce uterine blood flow. Antihypertensive drugs that act on total peripheral resistance may increase, decrease, or have no effect on uterine perfusion, depending on the pattern of blood flow redistribution.

Reliable information on the effects of antihypertensive drugs on human uterine blood flow is scant. Data on the potential effects of these drugs are based on studies in pregnant animals in which it was assumed that humans and sheep respond identically or in which blood flow to the kidney—an exquisitely autoregulated organ that usually receives 10% of cardiac output—was compared with blood flow to the uterus, an organ whose perfusion increases 500-fold over several months. With these limitations, Table 35-10 outlines the available information about antihypertensive agents used in pregnancy.

USE OF DRUGS

Two common classes of antihypertensive medications—diuretics and β-adrenergic blockers—warrant comment.

Diuretics. The indiscriminate use of diuretic agents during pregnancy has appropriately been condemned and is no longer common. In an epidemiologic assessment of 8000 pregnancies, a small but significant increase in perinatal mortality rate was demonstrated in women receiving continued or intermittent diuretic therapy, especially when the drug was begun late in pregnancy.[427] Lack of expansion of intravascular volume during pregnancy also has adverse prognostic significance.[337,428] In women taking diuretics from early pregnancy onward, plasma volume does not expand as much as in normal pregnancy.[429,430] Because of this, some physicians have recommended that diuretics be avoided entirely during pregnancy.[286,431] However, diuretics are used frequently in nonpregnant patients for antihypertensive therapy, and their efficacy, safety, and infrequency of side effects are extensively documented.[432] The combination of diuretics with other antihypertensive drugs allows the use of lower doses of the other agents by preventing sodium retention.

Despite these theoretical concerns, when continuous diuretic therapy is begun before 24 to 30 weeks' gestation, there is no evidence of an increased perinatal mortality rate or decreased neonatal weights.[277,279] However, diuretic therapy should never be instituted if there is any evidence of reduced uteroplacental perfusion, such as fetal growth restriction or preeclampsia. Diuretic therapy increases the serum concentration of uric acid and thereby renders uric acid determinations invalid for evaluating superimposed preeclampsia.

β-Adrenergic Antagonists. β-Adrenergic antagonists are the initial antihypertensive agents for nonpregnant patients in many settings. These agents lower blood pressure by reducing cardiac output and perhaps by interfering with renin release.

Infants born to women treated with β-blockers in pregnancy are more often growth restricted compared with infants born to women treated with placebo or other antihypertensive drugs.[433,434] Most growth-restricted infants were born to women who received atenolol.[423] β-Adrenergic antagonists vary according to their β_1-adrenergic subtype-specific (e.g., metoprolol, atenolol) and lipid solubility. For

TABLE 35-10 ANTIHYPERTENSIVE AGENTS USED IN PREGNANCY

Agent	Mechanism	Cardiac Output	Renal Blood Flow	Side Effects: Maternal	Side Effects: Neonatal
Thiazide	Initial: decreased plasma volume and cardiac output	Decreased	Decreased	Electrolyte depletion, serum uric acid increase, thrombocytopenia, hemorrhagic pancreatitis	Thrombocytopenia
	Later: decreased total peripheral resistance	Unchanged	Unchanged or increased		
Methyldopa	False neurotransmission, central nervous system effect	Unchanged	Unchanged	Lethargy, fever, hepatitis, hemolytic anemia, positive Coombs test result	
Hydralazine	Direct peripheral vasodilation	Increased	Unchanged or increased	Flushing, headache, tachycardia, palpitations, lupus syndrome	
Prazosin	Direct vasodilator and cardiac effects	Increased or unchanged	Unchanged	Hypotension with first dose; little information on use in pregnancy	
Clonidine	Central nervous system effects	Unchanged or increased	Unchanged	Rebound hypertension; little information on use in pregnancy	
Propranolol	β-Adrenergic blockade	Decreased	Decreased	Increased uterine tone with possible decrease in placental perfusion	Depressed respiration
Labetalol	α- and β-Adrenergic blockade	Unchanged	Unchanged	Tremulousness, flushing, headache	See propranolol
Reserpine	Depletion of norepinephrine from sympathetic nerve endings	Unchanged	Unchanged	Nasal stuffiness, depression, increased sensitivity to seizures	Nasal congestion, increased respiratory tract secretions, cyanosis, anorexia
Enalapril	Angiotensin-converting enzyme inhibitor	Unchanged	Unchanged	Hyperkalemia, dry cough	Neonatal anuria
Nifedipine	Calcium channel blocker	Unchanged	Unchanged	Orthostatic hypotension, headache, tachycardia	None demonstrated in humans

example, atenolol more readily crosses the placenta compared with metoprolol. Some of the β-adrenergic antagonists, such as oxprenolol, also have β-agonist effects. The decision, both theoretical and empiric, about the safety and efficacy of these drugs requires evaluation of the pharmacologic characteristics of each drug rather than consideration of them as a class.

Labetalol. Unlike atenolol, labetalol possesses both α-adrenergic and β-adrenergic antagonist activity. It is commonly used during pregnancy for acute treatment of preeclampsia and as therapy for chronic hypertension. Although some reports have suggested potential growth restriction,[433] other studies have not.[435,436] Experience has not identified it as a teratogen (see Pharmacologic Recommendations, later).

Hydralazine. Although hydralazine seems to be an ideal antihypertensive drug for pregnant women, side effects, including headache and palpitations caused by reflex increase in cardiac output, usually prevent its use in effective dosages for chronic hypertension. Tachyphylaxis has been described with hydralazine, making its use limited to short-term blood pressure control.

Methyldopa. Methyldopa, the drug used in the largest study and the only drug whose safety for infants has been demonstrated in long-range follow-up assessments, is the benchmark of antihypertensive therapy in pregnancy. It frequently causes drowsiness, however, especially when used in the large doses necessary when diuretics are not used concomitantly, and occasionally to a degree that is incapacitating, particularly for ambulatory patients.[437] In the original examination of infants whose mothers received methyldopa, there was a small but statistically significant decrease in head circumference, although this effect was not found in follow-up studies.[424]

Other Drugs. Several other antihypertensive drugs are available that may offer theoretical advantages for use in pregnancy. More data are required about the efficacy and the immediate and long-range safety of these drugs in pregnancy.

One agent that is widely used in nonpregnant patients is enalapril, an ACE inhibitor. Unexplained fetal death in pregnant ewes and rabbit does treated with another ACE inhibitor, captopril, have been borne out by clinical experience. Although there are no reports of fetal death, renal agenesis and neonatal renal dysfunction have been reported.[438] This class of drugs is now considered pregnancy category X. There is less experience with angiotensin II receptor blockers (ARBs) such as losartan and telmisartan, although case reports suggest problems similar to those with ACE inhibitors.[439-441] ACE inhibitors and ARBs should be discontinued before pregnancy or as soon as pregnancy is detected.[442]

Pharmacologic Recommendations

ACE inhibitors and ARBs should be discontinued during pregnancy. No other drugs are absolutely contraindicated.

The drug regimens suggested in the following paragraphs are preferred because of the available information regarding efficacy, side effects, and long-term follow-up. If a woman has established excellent blood pressure control, however, especially after unsuccessful trials of other agents, she should continue the successful regimen on becoming pregnant. Women receiving atenolol should switch to another β-adrenergic antagonist of equivalent efficacy, such as metoprolol.

The use of diuretic therapy is associated with few acute adverse effects and potentiates other drug effects. Although the use of diuretics from early pregnancy onward appears safe,[277-279] theoretical concerns raised by the effects of these agents on plasma volume militate against their use as initial therapy. Diuretics are also contraindicated for women with evidence of decreased uterine perfusion manifested as IUGR or preeclampsia. If the pregnancy is less than 30 weeks' gestation, these drugs appear safe despite theoretical concerns. The initial dose should be 25 mg of hydrochlorothiazide equivalent, increasing at 2- to 4-day intervals to 50 mg/day. Sodium restriction should be avoided, and dietary potassium should be supplemented when diuretics are used.

Because of its established efficacy and fetal safety, methyldopa has for many years been chosen to initiate antihypertensive therapy in pregnancy. The initial dosage is 250 mg taken at night and then 250 mg twice daily, increasing to a maximum of 1 g twice daily. If the maximal dose is not tolerated or does not control blood pressure, another agent should be added (not substituted). The addition of a diuretic usually dramatically increases the efficacy of methyldopa.

Labetalol or nifedipine is commonly added to methyldopa therapy when a second agent is required, and they are increasingly used as first-line therapy. If three drugs appear to be necessary to control blood pressure, consultation with a cardiologist or nephrologist is prudent. Used as a primary or secondary agent, labetalol is begun at 100 mg taken twice each day; it is given up to 2.4 g per day in divided doses, but the typical maximal dosage is 400 to 600 mg twice each day. Nifedipine may be given 10 to 30 mg three times each day or as 30 to 60 mg once each day in sustained-release form.

Obstetric Management of Hypertension

Obstetric management of the woman with chronic hypertension comprises the following measures:

- Recognizing superimposed preeclampsia early in the pregnancy
- Monitoring fetal well-being
- Excluding pheochromocytoma

Early in pregnancy, studies of renal function (i.e., creatinine clearance and 24-hour protein excretion), a serum urate determination, and a platelet count should be performed. These baseline studies may aid in differentiating exaggeration of the usual blood pressure changes of pregnancy from superimposed preeclampsia later in pregnancy. Because preeclampsia occurs at earlier gestational ages in hypertensive women, these patients should be seen more frequently, such as every other week at 24 to 26 weeks' gestation and weekly after 30 weeks.

Ultrasonographic evaluation of the fetus between 18 and 24 weeks' gestation allows accurate dating and provides a baseline for determining incremental growth when there is suspicion of growth restriction. Because precise knowledge of the gestational age may become critical if early delivery is needed, a first-trimester ultrasound scan to establish accurately the due date is prudent.

Most hypertensive pregnant women have essential hypertension. Thorough evaluation for most secondary forms of hypertension is best reserved for the postpartum period because of the obfuscation of many of these forms by physiologic changes of pregnancy and because of the risks of diagnostic procedures to the mother and fetus.

Pheochromocytoma is a potentially lethal complication, especially during the intrapartum period. This condition can be simply, accurately, and inexpensively diagnosed in many individuals with fixed hypertension by determination of the serum or urinary catecholamine concentration. Hypertensive women in whom this analyte has not been measured in the past should undergo this determination in early pregnancy.

Coarctation of the aorta is a rare cause of hypertension in women of reproductive age. It can be detected readily by determination of a lag between radial and femoral pulses, which should be measured as part of the physical examination of hypertensive patients.

Extensive antenatal fetal surveillance should be employed for pregnancies with preeclampsia or growth-restricted infants.[3] Because of the controversy surrounding uncomplicated hypertension and perinatal mortality and because the origin of the increased mortality is placental insufficiency, many clinicians employ some form of antenatal surveillance for uncomplicated cases in the third trimester.

References

1. Rippman E: Pra-eklampsie oder Schwangerschaftsspatgestose? Gynaecologia 167:178, 1969.
2. Gifford R, August P, Cunningham G, et al: The National High Blood Pressure Education Program Working Group on High Blood Pressure in Pregnancy. Bethesda, National Institutes of Health and National Heart, Lung, and Blood Institute, 2000.
3. Report of the National High Blood Pressure Education Program Working Group on High Blood Pressure in Pregnancy. Am J Obstet Gynecol 183: S1-S22, 2000.
4. North RA, Taylor RS, Schellenberg JC: Evaluation of a definition of pre-eclampsia. BJOG 106:767-773, 1999.
5. Zhang J, Klebanoff MA, Roberts JM: Prediction of adverse outcomes by common definitions of hypertension in pregnancy. Obstet Gynecol 97:261-267, 2001.
6. Inglis TC, Stuart J, George AJ, Davies AJ: Haemostatic and rheological changes in normal pregnancy and pre-eclampsia. Br J Haematol 50:461-465, 1982.
7. Abuelo JG: Validity of dipstick analysis as a method of screening for proteinuria in pregnancy. Am J Obstet Gynecol 169:1654, 1993.
8. Kuo VS, Koumantakis G, Gallery ED: Proteinuria and its assessment in normal and hypertensive pregnancy. Am J Obstet Gynecol 167:723-728, 1992.
9. Meyer NL, Mercer BM, Friedman SA, Sibai BM: Urinary dipstick protein: A poor predictor of absent or severe proteinuria. Am J Obstet Gynecol 170(Pt 1):137-141, 1994.
10. American College of Obstetricians and Gynecologists (ACOG): Diagnosis and management of preeclampsia and eclampsia. ACOG practice bulletin no. 33, January 2002. Obstet Gynecol 99:159-167, 2002.
11. Brown MA, Lindheimer MD, de Swiet M, et al: The classification and diagnosis of the hypertensive disorders of pregnancy: Statement from the International Society for the Study of Hypertension in Pregnancy (ISSHP). Hypertens Pregnancy 20:IX-XIV, 2001.
12. Helewa ME, Burrows RF, Smith J, et al: Report of the Canadian Hypertension Society Consensus Conference. 1. Definitions, evaluation and classification of hypertensive disorders in pregnancy. CMAJ 157:715-725, 1997.
13. Thomson AM, Hytten FE, Billewicz WZ: The epidemiology of oedema during pregnancy. J Obstet Gynaecol Br Commonw 74:1-10, 1967.
14. Vartran C: Hypertension in pregnancy: A new look. Proc R Soc Med 59:841, 1966.
15. Chesley L, Annitto J: Pregnancy in the patient with hypertensive disease. Am J Obstet Gynecol 53:372, 1947.

16. Chesley L: Toxemia of pregnancy in relation to chronic hypertension. West J Surg Obstet Gynecol 64:284, 1956.
17. McCartney CP: Pathological anatomy of acute hypertension of pregnancy. Circulation 30(Suppl 2):37-42, 1964.
18. Chesley L: Hypertensive Disorders in Pregnancy. New York, Appleton-Century-Crofts, 1978.
19. Weinstein L: Syndrome of hemolysis, elevated liver enzymes, and low platelet count: A severe consequence of hypertension in pregnancy. Am J Obstet Gynecol 142:159-167, 1982.
20. Egerman RS, Sibai BM: HELLP syndrome. Clin Obstet Gynecol 42:381-389, 1999.
21. Bussen SS, Sutterlin MW, Steck T: Plasma renin activity and aldosterone serum concentration are decreased in severe preeclampsia but not in the HELLP syndrome. Acta Obstet Gynecol Scand 77:609-613, 1998.
22. Funai EF, Paltiel OB, Malaspina D, et al: Risk factors for pre-eclampsia in nulliparous and parous women: The Jerusalem perinatal study. Paediatr Perinat Epidemiol 19:59-68, 2005.
23. Nelson T: A clinical study of preeclampsia. Parts I and II. J Obstet Gynaecol Br Emp 62:48, 1955.
24. Lawlor DA, Morton SM, Nitsch D, Leon DA: Association between childhood and adulthood socioeconomic position and pregnancy induced hypertension: Results from the Aberdeen children of the 1950s cohort study. J Epidemiol Community Health 59:49-55, 2005.
25. Vara P, Timonen S, Lokki O: Toxaemia of late pregnancy. A statistical study. Acta Obstet Gynecol Scand 44(Suppl):3-45, 1965.
26. Davies AM, Czaczkes JW, Sadovsky E, et al: Toxemia of pregnancy in Jerusalem. I. Epidemiological studies of a total community. Isr J Med Sci 6:253-266, 1970.
27. Vollman RF: Rates of toxemia by age and parity. In Die Spät Gestose (E- and H-Gestose). Basel, Schwabe, 1970, p 338.
28. Eskenazi B, Fenster L, Sidney S: A multivariate analysis of risk factors for preeclampsia. JAMA 266:237-241, 1991.
29. Mittendorf R, Lain KY, Williams MA, Walker CK: Preeclampsia. A nested, case-control study of risk factors and their interactions. J Reprod Med 41:491-496, 1996.
30. Knuist M, Bonsel GJ, Zondervan HA, Treffers PE: Risk factors for preeclampsia in nulliparous women in distinct ethnic groups: A prospective cohort study. Obstet Gynecol 92:174-178, 1998.
31. Sibai BM, Gordon T, Thom E, et al: Risk factors for preeclampsia in healthy nulliparous women: A prospective multicenter study. The National Institute of Child Health and Human Development Network of Maternal-Fetal Medicine Units. Am J Obstet Gynecol 172(Pt 1):642-648, 1995.
32. Sibai BM, Ewell M, Levine RJ, et al: Risk factors associated with preeclampsia in healthy nulliparous women. The Calcium for Preeclampsia Prevention (CPEP) Study Group. Am J Obstet Gynecol 177:1003-1010, 1997.
33. Hanson U, Persson B: Outcome of pregnancies complicated by type 1 insulin-dependent diabetes in Sweden: Acute pregnancy complications, neonatal mortality and morbidity. Am J Perinatol 10:330-3333, 1993.
34. Sibai BM, Caritis S, Hauth J, et al: Risks of preeclampsia and adverse neonatal outcomes among women with pregestational diabetes mellitus. National Institute of Child Health and Human Development Network of Maternal-Fetal Medicine Units. Am J Obstet Gynecol 182:364-369, 2000.
35. Sibai BM, Lindheimer M, Hauth J, et al: Risk factors for preeclampsia, abruptio placentae, and adverse neonatal outcomes among women with chronic hypertension. National Institute of Child Health and Human Development Network of Maternal-Fetal Medicine Units. N Engl J Med 339:667-671, 1998.
36. Caritis S, Sibai B, Hauth J, et al: Low-dose aspirin to prevent preeclampsia in women at high risk. National Institute of Child Health and Human Development Network of Maternal-Fetal Medicine Units. N Engl J Med 338:701-705, 1998.
37. Purdy LP, Hantsch CE, Molitch ME, et al: Effect of pregnancy on renal function in patients with moderate-to-severe diabetic renal insufficiency. Diabetes Care 19:1067-1074, 1996.
38. Hou SH, Grossman SD, Madias NE: Pregnancy in women with renal disease and moderate renal insufficiency. Am J Med 78:185-194, 1985.
39. Jones DC, Hayslett JP: Outcome of pregnancy in women with moderate or severe renal insufficiency. N Engl J Med 335:226-232, 1996.
40. Cunningham FG, Cox SM, Harstad TW, et al: Chronic renal disease and pregnancy outcome. Am J Obstet Gynecol 163:453-459, 1990.
41. Egerman RS, Ramsey RD, Kao LW, et al: Hypertensive disease in pregnancies complicated by systemic lupus erythematosus. Am J Obstet Gynecol 193:1676-1679, 2005.
42. Chakravarty EF, Colon I, Langen ES, et al: Factors that predict prematurity and preeclampsia in pregnancies that are complicated by systemic lupus erythematosus. Am J Obstet Gynecol 192:1897-1904, 2005.
43. Branch DW, Silver RM, Blackwell JL, et al: Outcome of treated pregnancies in women with antiphospholipid syndrome: An update of the Utah experience. Obstet Gynecol 80:614-620, 1992.
44. Yasuda M, Takakuwa K, Tokunaga A, Tanaka K: Prospective studies of the association between anticardiolipin antibody and outcome of pregnancy. Obstet Gynecol 86(Pt 1):555-559, 1995.
45. Lima F, Khamashta MA, Buchanan NM, et al: A study of sixty pregnancies in patients with the antiphospholipid syndrome. Clin Exp Rheumatol 14:131-136, 1996.
46. Packham DK, Lam SS, Nicholls K, et al: Lupus nephritis and pregnancy. Q J Med 83:315-324, 1992.
47. Julkunen H, Kaaja R, Palosuo T, et al: Pregnancy in lupus nephropathy. Acta Obstet Gynecol Scand 72:258-263, 1993.
48. Lockwood CJ, Romero R, Feinberg RF, et al: The prevalence and biologic significance of lupus anticoagulant and anticardiolipin antibodies in a general obstetric population. Am J Obstet Gynecol 161:369-373, 1989.
49. Harris EN, Spinnato JA: Should anticardiolipin tests be performed in otherwise healthy pregnant women? Am J Obstet Gynecol 165(Pt 1):1272-1277, 1991.
50. Branch DW, Porter TF, Rittenhouse L, et al: Antiphospholipid antibodies in women at risk for preeclampsia. Am J Obstet Gynecol 184:825-832; discussion 832-834, 2001.
51. Stone JL, Lockwood CJ, Berkowitz GS, et al: Risk factors for severe preeclampsia. Obstet Gynecol 83:357-361, 1994.
52. Bodnar LM, Ness RB, Markovic N, Roberts JM: The risk of preeclampsia rises with increasing prepregnancy body mass index. Ann Epidemiol 15:475-482, 2005.
53. Roach VJ, Hin LY, Tam WH, et al: The incidence of pregnancy-induced hypertension among patients with carbohydrate intolerance. Hypertens Pregnancy 19:183-189, 2000.
54. Sibai BM, Hauth J, Caritis S, et al: Hypertensive disorders in twin versus singleton gestations. National Institute of Child Health and Human Development Network of Maternal-Fetal Medicine Units. Am J Obstet Gynecol 182:938-942, 2000.
55. Day MC, Barton JR, O'Brien JM, et al: The effect of fetal number on the development of hypertensive conditions of pregnancy. Obstet Gynecol 106(Pt 1):927-931, 2005.
56. Page E: The relation between hydatid moles, relative ischemia of the gravid uterus, and placental origin of eclampsia. Am J Obstet Gynecol 37:291, 1939.
57. Scott JS: Pregnancy toxaemia associated with hydrops foetalis, hydatidiform mole and hydramnios. J Obstet Gynaecol Br Emp 65:689-701, 1958.
58. Midgley DY, Harding K: The mirror syndrome. Eur J Obstet Gynecol Reprod Biol 88:201-202, 2000.
59. Duthie SJ, Walkinshaw SA: Parvovirus associated fetal hydrops: Reversal of pregnancy induced proteinuric hypertension by in utero fetal transfusion. BJOG 102:1011-1013, 1995.
60. Rana S, Venkatesha S, DePaepe M, et al: Cytomegalovirus-induced mirror syndrome associated with elevated levels of circulating antiangiogenic factors. Obstet Gynecol 109(Pt 2):549-552, 2007.
61. Plouin PF, Chatellier G, Breart G, et al: Frequency and perinatal consequences of hypertensive disease of pregnancy. Adv Nephrol Necker Hosp 15:57-69, 1986.
62. Smulian JC, Ananth CV, Vintzileos AM, et al: Fetal deaths in the United States. Influence of high-risk conditions and implications for management. Obstet Gynecol 100:1183-1189, 2002.

63. Conde-Agudelo A, Belizan JM, Diaz-Rossello JL: Epidemiology of fetal death in Latin America. Acta Obstet Gynecol Scand 79:371-378, 2000.
64. Naeye RL, Friedman EA: Causes of perinatal death associated with gestational hypertension and proteinuria. Am J Obstet Gynecol 133:8-10, 1979.
65. Basso O, Rasmussen S, Weinberg CR, et al: Trends in fetal and infant survival following preeclampsia. JAMA 296:1357-1362, 2006.
66. Odegard RA, Vatten LJ, Nilsen ST, et al: Preeclampsia and fetal growth. Obstet Gynecol 96:950-955, 2000.
67. Lopez-Llera M, Hernandez Horta JL: Perinatal mortality in eclampsia. J Reprod Med 8:281-287, 1972.
68. Sibai BM, McCubbin JH, Anderson GD, et al: Eclampsia. I. Observations from 67 recent cases. Obstet Gynecol 58:609-613, 1981.
69. Pritchard JA, Pritchard SA: Standardized treatment of 154 consecutive cases of eclampsia. Am J Obstet Gynecol 123:543-552, 1975.
70. Berman S: Observations in the toxemic clinic, Boston Lying-In Hospital, 1923-1930. Obstet Gynecol 203:361, 1930.
71. Sibai BM, el-Nazer A, Gonzalez-Ruiz A: Severe preeclampsia-eclampsia in young primigravid women: Subsequent pregnancy outcome and remote prognosis. Am J Obstet Gynecol 155:1011-1016, 1986.
72. Hjartardottir S, Leifsson BG, Geirsson RT, Steinthorsdottir V: Recurrence of hypertensive disorder in second pregnancy. Am J Obstet Gynecol 194:916-920, 2006.
73. Sibai BM, Mercer B, Sarinoglu C: Severe preeclampsia in the second trimester: Recurrence risk and long-term prognosis. Am J Obstet Gynecol 165(Pt 1):1408-1412, 1991.
74. Chesley SC, Annitto JE, Cosgrove RA: The remote prognosis of eclamptic women. Sixth periodic report. Am J Obstet Gynecol 124:446-459, 1976.
75. Irgens HU, Reisaeter L, Irgens LM, Lie RT: Long term mortality of mothers and fathers after pre-eclampsia: Population based cohort study. BMJ 323:1213-1217, 2001.
76. Chesley LC, Annitto JE, Cosgrove RA: The remote prognosis of eclamptic women. Sixth periodic report. Am J Obstet Gynecol 124:448, 1976.
77. Wilson BJ, Watson MS, Prescott GJ, et al: Hypertensive diseases of pregnancy and risk of hypertension and stroke in later life: Results from cohort study. BMJ 326:845, 2003.
78. Funai EF, Friedlander Y, Paltiel O, et al: Long-term mortality after preeclampsia. Epidemiology 16:206-215, 2005.
79. Smith GC, Pell JP, Walsh D: Pregnancy complications and maternal risk of ischaemic heart disease: A retrospective cohort study of 129,290 births. Lancet 357:2002-2006, 2001.
80. Arnadottir GA, Geirsson RT, Arngrimsson R, et al: Cardiovascular death in women who had hypertension in pregnancy: A case-control study. BJOG 112:286-292, 2005.
81. Ness RB, Markovic N, Bass D, et al: Family history of hypertension, heart disease, and stroke among women who develop hypertension in pregnancy. Obstet Gynecol 102:1366-7131, 2003.
82. Samuels-Kalow ME, Funai EF, Buhimschi C, et al: Prepregnancy body mass index, hypertensive disorders of pregnancy, and long-term maternal mortality. Am J Obstet Gynecol 197:490 e1-e6, 2007.
83. Barden AE, Beilin LJ, Ritchie J, et al: Does a predisposition to the metabolic syndrome sensitize women to develop pre-eclampsia? J Hypertens 17:1307-1315, 1999.
84. Powers RW, Evans RW, Majors AK, et al: Plasma homocysteine concentration is increased in preeclampsia and is associated with evidence of endothelial activation. Am J Obstet Gynecol 179(Pt 1):1605-1611, 1998.
85. Fridstrom M, Nisell H, Sjoblom P, Hillensjo T: Are women with polycystic ovary syndrome at an increased risk of pregnancy-induced hypertension and/or preeclampsia? Hypertens Pregnancy 18:73-80, 1999.
86. Acromite MT, Mantzoros CS, Leach RE, et al: Androgens in preeclampsia. Am J Obstet Gynecol 180(Pt 1):60-63, 1999.
87. Sattar N, Clark P, Holmes A, et al: Antenatal waist circumference and hypertension risk. Obstet Gynecol 97:268-271, 2001.
88. Hubel CA, Roberts JM, Ferrell RE: Association of pre-eclampsia with common coding sequence variations in the lipoprotein lipase gene. Clin Genet 56:289-296, 1999.
89. Agatisa PK, Ness RB, Roberts JM, et al: Impairment of endothelial function in women with a history of preeclampsia: An indicator of cardiovascular risk. Am J Physiol Heart Circ Physiol 286:H1389-H1393, 2004.
90. Chambers JC, Ueland PM, Obeid OA, et al: Improved vascular endothelial function after oral B vitamins: An effect mediated through reduced concentrations of free plasma homocysteine. Circulation 102:2479-2483, 2000.
91. Laivuori H, Tikkanen MJ, Ylikorkala O: Hyperinsulinemia 17 years after preeclamptic first pregnancy. J Clin Endocrinol Metab 81:2908-2911, 1996.
92. Hubel CA, Snaedal S, Ness RB, et al: Dyslipoproteinaemia in postmenopausal women with a history of eclampsia. BJOG 107:776-784, 2000.
93. Wolf M, Hubel CA, Lam C, et al: Preeclampsia and future cardiovascular disease: Potential role of altered angiogenesis and insulin resistance. J Clin Endocrinol Metab 89:6239-6243, 2004.
94. Hubel CA, Wallukat G, Wolf M, et al: Agonistic angiotensin II type 1 receptor autoantibodies in postpartum women with a history of preeclampsia. Hypertension 49:612-617, 2007.
95. Buchbinder A, Sibai BM, Caritis S, et al: Adverse perinatal outcomes are significantly higher in severe gestational hypertension than in mild preeclampsia. Am J Obstet Gynecol 186:66-71, 2002.
96. Dieckman W: The Toxemias of Pregnancy, 2nd ed. St Louis, CV Mosby, 1952.
97. Douglas KA, Redman CW: Eclampsia in the United Kingdom. BMJ 309:1395-400, 1994.
98. Sibai BM: Eclampsia. VI. Maternal-perinatal outcome in 254 consecutive cases. Am J Obstet Gynecol 163:1049-1054; discussion 1054-1055, 1990.
99. Conde-Agudelo A, Kafury-Goeta AC: Epidemiology of eclampsia in Colombia. Int J Gynaecol Obstet 61:1-8, 1998.
100. Macgillivray I: Some observations on the incidence of pre-eclampsia. J Obstet Gynaecol Br Emp 65:536-539, 1958.
101. Tervila L, Goecke C, Timonen S: Estimation of gestosis of pregnancy (EPH-gestosis). Acta Obstet Gynecol Scand 52:235-443, 1973.
102. Ferrazzani S, Caruso A, De Carolis S, et al: Proteinuria and outcome of 444 pregnancies complicated by hypertension. Am J Obstet Gynecol 162:366-371, 1990.
103. Pollak VE, Nettles JB: The kidney in toxemia of pregnancy: A clinical and pathologic study based on renal biopsies. Medicine (Baltimore) 39:469-526, 1960.
104. Jaffe G, Schatz H: Ocular manifestations of preeclampsia. Am J Ophthalmol 103(Pt 1):309-315, 1987.
105. Roberts JM, Bodnar LM, Lain KY, et al: Uric acid is as important as proteinuria in identifying fetal risk in women with gestational hypertension [see comment]. Hypertension 46:1263-1269, 2005.
106. Many A, Hubel CA, Roberts JM: Hyperuricemia and xanthine oxidase in preeclampsia, revisited. Am J Obstet Gynecol 174(Pt 1):288-291, 1996.
107. Johnson RJ, Kang DH, Feig D, et al: Is there a pathogenetic role for uric acid in hypertension and cardiovascular and renal disease? Hypertension 41:1183-1190, 2003.
108. Martin JN Jr, Blake PG, Perry KG Jr, et al: The natural history of HELLP syndrome: Patterns of disease progression and regression. Am J Obstet Gynecol 164(Pt 1):1500-1509; discussion 1509-1513, 1991.
109. Burrows RF, Kelton JG: Thrombocytopenia at delivery: A prospective survey of 6715 deliveries. Am J Obstet Gynecol 162:731-734, 1990.
110. Redman CW, Bonnar J, Beilin L: Early platelet consumption in pre-eclampsia. BMJ 1:467-469, 1978.
111. Weiner CP, Brandt J: Plasma antithrombin III activity: An aid in the diagnosis of preeclampsia-eclampsia. Am J Obstet Gynecol 142:275-281, 1982.
112. Redman CW, Denson KW, Beilin LJ, et al: Factor-VIII consumption in pre-eclampsia. Lancet 2:1249-1252, 1977.
113. Lok CA, Nieuwland R, Sturk A, et al: Microparticle-associated P-selectin reflects platelet activation in preeclampsia. Platelets 18:68-72, 2007.
114. Hutt R, Ogunniyi SO, Sullivan MH, Elder MG: Increased platelet volume and aggregation precede the onset of preeclampsia. Obstet Gynecol 83:146-149, 1994.

115. Hayashi M, Inoue T, Hoshimoto K, et al: Characterization of five marker levels of the hemostatic system and endothelial status in normotensive pregnancy and pre-eclampsia. Eur J Haematol 69:297-302, 2002.
116. Knopp R: Lipid Metabolism in Pregnancy. New York, Springer-Verlag, 1991.
117. Hubel C, Roberts J: Lipid metabolism and oxidative stress. In Lindheimer M, Roberts J, Cunningham F (eds): Chesley's Hypertensive Disorders in Pregnancy. Stamford, CT, Appleton & Lange, 1999, p 453.
118. Hubel CA, McLaughlin MK, Evans RW, et al: Fasting serum triglycerides, free fatty acids, and malondialdehyde are increased in preeclampsia, are positively correlated, and decrease within 48 hours post partum. Am J Obstet Gynecol 174:975-982, 1996.
119. Lorentzen B, Endresen M, Clausen T, et al: Fasting serum free fatty acids and triglycerides are increased before 20 weeks of gestation in women who later develop preeclampsia. Hypertens Pregnancy 13:103, 1994.
120. Rosing U, Samsioe G, Olund A, et al: Serum levels of apolipoprotein A-I, A-II and HDL-cholesterol in second half of normal pregnancy and in pregnancy complicated by pre-eclampsia. Horm Metab Res 21:376-382, 1989.
121. Hubel CA, Shakir Y, Gallaher MJ, et al: Low-density lipoprotein particle size decreases during normal pregnancy in association with triglyceride increases. J Soc Gynecol Investig 5:244-250, 1998.
122. Sattar N, Bendomir A, Berry C, et al: Lipoprotein subfraction concentrations in preeclampsia: Pathogenic parallels to atherosclerosis. Obstet Gynecol 89:403-408, 1997.
123. Sheehan H, Lynch J: Pathology of Toxemia in Pregnancy. London, Churchill Livingstone, 1973.
124. Naheedy MH, Biller J, Schiffer M, et al: Toxemia of pregnancy: Cerebral CT findings. J Comput Assist Tomogr 9:497-501, 1985.
125. Belfort MA, Varner MW, Dizon-Townson DS, et al: Cerebral perfusion pressure, and not cerebral blood flow, may be the critical determinant of intracranial injury in preeclampsia: A new hypothesis. Am J Obstet Gynecol 187:626-634, 2002.
126. Schmorl G: Zur pathologischen Anatomie Untersuchung uber Puerperal-Eklampsie. Verhandl Dtsch Gesellsch Gyneakol 1901:203, 1901.
127. Sheehan H: Pathologic lesions in the hypertensive toxaemias of pregnancy. In Hammond J, Browne F, Wolstenholm G (eds): Toxaemias of Pregnancy, Human and Veterinary. Philadelphia, Blakiston, 1950, p 16.
128. Thomson D, Paterson WG, Smart GE, et al: The renal lesions of toxaemia and abruptio placentae studied by light and electron microscopy. J Obstet Gynaecol Br Commonw 79:311-320, 1972.
129. Spargo B, McCartney CP, Winemiller R: Glomerular capillary endotheliosis in toxemia of pregnancy. Arch Pathol 68:593-599, 1959.
130. Maynard SE, Min JY, Merchan J, et al: Excess placental soluble fms-like tyrosine kinase 1 (sFlt1) may contribute to endothelial dysfunction, hypertension, and proteinuria in preeclampsia [see comment]. J Clin Invest 111:649-658, 2003.
131. Altchek A, Albright NL, Sommers SC: The renal pathology of toxemia of pregnancy. Obstet Gynecol 31:595-607, 1968.
132. Ramsey E, Harris H: Comparison of uteroplacental vasculature and circulation in the rhesus monkey and man. Carnegie Contrib Embryol 38:59-70, 1966.
133. Brosens IA, Robertson WB, Dixon HG: The role of the spiral arteries in the pathogenesis of preeclampsia. Obstet Gynecol Annu 1:177-191, 1972.
134. Khong TY, De Wolf F, Robertson WB, Brosens I: Inadequate maternal vascular response to placentation in pregnancies complicated by pre-eclampsia and by small-for-gestational age infants. BJOG 93:1049-1059, 1986.
135. Zeek PM, Assali NS: Vascular changes in the decidua associated with eclamptogenic toxemia of pregnancy. Am J Clin Pathol 20:1099-1109, 1950.
136. Kitzmiller JL, Watt N, Driscoll SG: Decidual arteriopathy in hypertension and diabetes in pregnancy: Immunofluorescent studies. Am J Obstet Gynecol 141:773-779, 1981.
137. Arias F, Rodriquez L, Rayne SC, Kraus FT: Maternal placental vasculopathy and infection: Two distinct subgroups among patients with preterm labor and preterm ruptured membranes. Am J Obstet Gynecol 168:585-591, 1993.
138. Lichtig C, Deutsch M, Brandes J: Immunofluorescent studies of the endometrial arteries in the first trimester of pregnancy. Am J Clin Pathol 83:633-636, 1985.
139. Nadji P, Sommers SC: Lesions of toxemia in first trimester pregnancies. Am J Clin Pathol 59:344-349, 1973.
140. Kitzmiller JL, Benirschke K: Immunofluorescent study of placental bed vessels in pre-eclampsia of pregnancy. Am J Obstet Gynecol 115:248-251, 1973.
141. Cross JC, Werb Z, Fisher SJ: Implantation and the placenta: Key pieces of the development puzzle. Science 266:1508-1518, 1994.
142. Zhou Y, Damsky CH, Chiu K, et al: Cytotrophoblast expression of integrin extracellular matrix receptors is altered in preeclampsia. In Soars MJ, Handwerger S, Talamantes F (eds): Trophoblast Cells: Pathways for Maternal-Embryonic Communication. New York, Springer-Verlag, 1993, p 109.
143. Zhou Y, Fisher SJ, Janatpour M, et al: Human cytotrophoblasts adopt a vascular phenotype as they differentiate. A strategy for successful endovascular invasion? J Clin Invest 99:2139-2151.
144. Zhou Y, Damsky CH, Fisher SJ: Preeclampsia is associated with failure of human cytotrophoblasts to mimic a vascular adhesion phenotype. One cause of defective endovascular invasion in this syndrome? J Clin Invest 99:2152-2164, 1997.
145. Caniggia I, Grisaru-Gravnosky S, Kuliszewsky M, et al: Inhibition of TGF-beta 3 restores the invasive capability of extravillous trophoblasts in preeclamptic pregnancies. J Clin Invest 103:1641-1650, 1999.
146. Librach CL, Feigenbaum SL, Bass KE, et al: Interleukin-1 beta regulates human cytotrophoblast metalloproteinase activity and invasion in vitro. J Biol Chem 269:17125-17131, 1994.
147. Bass KE, Morrish D, Roth I, et al: Human cytotrophoblast invasion is up-regulated by epidermal growth factor: Evidence that paracrine factors modify this process. Dev Biol 164:550-561, 1994.
148. Caniggia I, Winter J, Lye SJ, Post M: Oxygen and placental development during the first trimester: Implications for the pathophysiology of preeclampsia. Placenta 21(Suppl A):S25-S30, 2000.
149. Genbacev O, Joslin R, Damsky CH, et al: Hypoxia alters early gestation human cytotrophoblast differentiation/invasion in vitro and models the placental defects that occur in preeclampsia. J Clin Invest 97:540-550, 1996.
150. Hiby SE, Walker JJ, O'Shaughnessy KM, et al: Combinations of maternal KIR and fetal HLA-C genes influence the risk of preeclampsia and reproductive success. J Exp Med 200:957-965, 2004.
151. Jones CJ, Fox H: An ultrastructural and ultrahistochemical study of the human placenta in maternal pre-eclampsia. Placenta 1:61-76, 1980.
152. Fox H, Kharkongor NF: The effect of hypoxia on human trophoblast in organ culture. J Pathol 101:v, 1970.
153. Allaire AD, Ballenger KA, Wells SR, et al: Placental apoptosis in preeclampsia. Obstet Gynecol 96:271-276, 2000.
154. Huppertz B, Kingdom J, Caniggia I, et al: Hypoxia favours necrotic versus apoptotic shedding of placental syncytiotrophoblast into the maternal circulation. Placenta 24:181-190, 2003.
155. Hung TH, Skepper JN, Charnock-Jones DS, Burton GJ: Hypoxia-reoxygenation: A potent inducer of apoptotic changes in the human placenta and possible etiological factor in preeclampsia. Circ Res 90:1274-1281, 2002.
156. Goswami D, Tannetta DS, Magee LA, et al: Excess syncytiotrophoblast microparticle shedding is a feature of early-onset pre-eclampsia, but not normotensive intrauterine growth restriction. Placenta 27:56-61, 2006.
157. Bosio PM, McKenna PJ, Conroy R, O'Herlihy C: Maternal central hemodynamics in hypertensive disorders of pregnancy. Obstet Gynecol 94:978-984, 1999.
158. Easterling TR, Benedetti TJ, Schmucker BC, Millard SP: Maternal hemodynamics in normal and preeclamptic pregnancies: A longitudinal study. Obstet Gynecol 76:1061-1069, 1990.
159. Mabie WC, Ratts TE, Sibai BM: The central hemodynamics of severe preeclampsia. Am J Obstet Gynecol 161(Pt 1):1443-1448, 1989.

160. Wallenburg H: Hemodynamics in hypertensive pregnancy. In Rubin P (ed): Hypertension in Pregnancy. Handbook of Hypertension, vol 10. Amsterdam, Elsevier, 1988, p 66.
161. Duncan SL, Ginsburg J: Arteriolar distensibility in hypertensive pregnancy. Am J Obstet Gynecol 100:222-229, 1968.
162. Spetz S: Peripheral circulation in pregnancy complicated by toxaemia. Acta Obstet Gynecol Scand 44:243-257, 1965.
163. Assali NS, Prystowsky H: Studies on autonomic blockade. I. Comparison between the effects of tetraethylammonium chloride (TEAC) and high selective spinal anesthesia on blood pressure of normal and toxemic pregnancy. J Clin Invest 29:1354-1366, 1950.
164. Schobel HP, Grassi G: Hypertensive disorders of pregnancy: A dysregulation of the sympathetic nervous system? J Hypertens 16:569-570, 1998.
165. Hanssens M, Keirse MJ, Spitz B, van Assche FA: Angiotensin II levels in hypertensive and normotensive pregnancies. BJOG 98:155-161, 1991.
166. Taylor RN, Varma M, Teng NN, Roberts JM: Women with preeclampsia have higher plasma endothelin levels than women with normal pregnancies. J Clin Endocrinol Metab 71:1675-1677.
167. Chesley LC, Valenti C: The evaluation of tests to differentiate preeclampsia from hypertensive disease. Am J Obstet Gynecol 75:1165-1173, 1958.
168. Dieckman W, Michel H: Vascular-renal effects of posterior pituitary extracts in pregnant women. Am J Obstet Gynecol 33:131, 1937.
169. Zuspan FP, Nelson GH, Ahlquist RP: Epinephrine infusions in normal and toxemic pregnancy. I. Nonesterified fatty acids and cardiovascular alterations. Am J Obstet Gynecol 90:88-98, 1964.
170. Talledo O, Chesley L, Zuspan F: Renin-angiotensin system in normal and toxemic pregnancies: III. Differential sensitivity to angiotensin II and norepinephrine in toxemia of pregnancy. Am J Obstet Gynecol 100:218, 1968.
171. Schwarz R, Retzke U: Cardiovascular response to infusions of angiotensin II in pregnant women. Obstet Gynecol 38:714-718, 1971.
172. Gant NF, Daley GL, Chand S, et al: A study of angiotensin II pressor response throughout primigravid pregnancy. J Clin Invest 52:2682-2689, 1973.
173. Kyle PM, Buckley D, Kissane J, et al: The angiotensin sensitivity test and low-dose aspirin are ineffective methods to predict and prevent hypertensive disorders in nulliparous pregnancy. Am J Obstet Gynecol 173(Pt 1):865-872, 1995.
174. Ness RB, Roberts JM: Heterogeneous causes constituting the single syndrome of preeclampsia: A hypothesis and its implications. Am J Obstet Gynecol 175:1365-1370, 1996.
175. McKay DG: Hematologic evidence of disseminated intravascular coagulation in eclampsia. Obstet Gynecol Surv 27:399-417, 1972.
176. Bell WR: Disseminated intravascular coagulation. Johns Hopkins Med J 146:289-299, 1980.
177. Janes SL, Kyle PM, Redman C, Goodall AH: Flow cytometric detection of activated platelets in pregnant women prior to the development of preeclampsia. Thromb Haemost 74:1059-1063, 1995.
178. Douglas JT, Shah M, Lowe GD, et al: Plasma fibrinopeptide A and betathromboglobulin in pre-eclampsia and pregnancy hypertension. Thromb Haemost 47:54-55, 1982.
179. Socol ML, Weiner CP, Louis G, et al: Platelet activation in preeclampsia. Am J Obstet Gynecol 151:494-497, 1985.
180. Denson KW: The ratio of factor VIII-related antigen and factor VIII biological activity as an index of hypercoagulability and intravascular clotting. Thromb Res 10:107-119, 1977.
181. Roberts JM, May WJ: Consumptive coagulopathy in severe preeclampsia. Obstet Gynecol 48:163-166, 1976.
182. Pritchard JA, Cunningham FG, Mason RA: Coagulation changes in eclampsia: Their frequency and pathogenesis. Am J Obstet Gynecol 124:855-864, 1976.
183. Roberts JM: Endothelial dysfunction in preeclampsia. Semin Reprod Endocrinol 16:5-15, 1998.
184. Nachman RL: The 1994 Runme Shaw Memorial Lecture: Thrombosis and atherogenesis—molecular connections. Ann Acad Med Singapore 24:281-289, 1995.
185. Matter L, Faulk W: Fibrinogen degradation products and factor VIII consumption in normal pregnancy and preeclampsia: Role of the placenta. In Bonnar M, MacGillivray I, Symonds M (eds): Pregnancy Hypertension. Baltimore, University Park Press, 1980, p 327.
186. Arias F, Mancilla-Jimenez R: Hepatic fibrinogen deposits in pre-eclampsia. Immunofluorescent evidence. N Engl J Med 295:578-582, 1976.
187. Vassali P, Morris R, McCluskey R: The pathogenic role of fibrin deposition in the glomerular lesions of toxemia of pregnancy. J Exp Med 118:467, 1963.
188. Whigham KA, Howie PW, Shah MM, Prentice CR: Factor VIII related antigen/coagulant activity ratio as a predictor of fetal growth retardation: A comparison with hormone and uric acid measurements. BJOG 87:797-803, 1980.
189. Roberts JM, Redman CW: Pre-eclampsia: More than pregnancy-induced hypertension. Lancet 341:1447-1451, 1993.
190. Roberts JM, Taylor RN, Musci TJ, et al: Preeclampsia: An endothelial cell disorder. Am J Obstet Gynecol 161:1200-1204, 1989.
191. Taylor RN, Crombleholme WR, Friedman SA, et al: High plasma cellular fibronectin levels correlate with biochemical and clinical features of preeclampsia but cannot be attributed to hypertension alone. Am J Obstet Gynecol 165(Pt 1):895-901, 1991.
192. Lockwood CJ, Peters JH: Increased plasma levels of ED1+ cellular fibronectin precede the clinical signs of preeclampsia. Am J Obstet Gynecol 162:358-362, 1990.
193. Taylor RN, Heilbron DC, Roberts JM: Growth factor activity in the blood of women in whom preeclampsia develops is elevated from early pregnancy. Am J Obstet Gynecol 163(Pt 1):1839-1844, 1990.
194. Krauss T, Kuhn W, Lakoma C, Augustin HG: Circulating endothelial cell adhesion molecules as diagnostic markers for the early identification of pregnant women at risk for development of preeclampsia. Am J Obstet Gynecol 177:443-449, 1997.
195. Cockell AP, Poston L: Flow-mediated vasodilatation is enhanced in normal pregnancy but reduced in preeclampsia. Hypertension 30(Pt 1):247-251, 1997.
196. Knock GA, Poston L: Bradykinin-mediated relaxation of isolated maternal resistance arteries in normal pregnancy and preeclampsia. Am J Obstet Gynecol 175:1668-1674, 1996.
197. Rodgers GM, Greenberg CS, Shuman MA: Characterization of the effects of cultured vascular cells on the activation of blood coagulation. Blood 61:1155-1162, 1983.
198. Wiggins RC, Loskutoff DJ, Cochrane CG, et al: Activation of rabbit Hageman factor by homogenates of cultured rabbit endothelial cells. J Clin Invest 65:197-206, 1980.
199. Maynard JR, Dreyer BE, Stemerman MB, Pitlick FA: Tissue-factor coagulant activity of cultured human endothelial and smooth muscle cells and fibroblasts. Blood 50:387-396, 1977.
200. Baumgartner H, Hardenschild C: Adhesion of platelets to subendothelium. Ann N Y Acad Sci 201:22, 1977.
201. Furchgott RF: Role of endothelium in responses of vascular smooth muscle. Circ Res 53:557-573, 1983.
202. Dadak C, Kefalides A, Sinzinger H, Weber G: Reduced umbilical artery prostacyclin formation in complicated pregnancies. Am J Obstet Gynecol 144:792-795, 1982.
203. Remuzzi G, Marchesi D, Zoja C, et al: Reduced umbilical and placental vascular prostacyclin in severe pre-eclampsia. Prostaglandins 20:105-110, 1980.
204. Bussolino F, Benedetto C, Massobrio M, Camussi G: Maternal vascular prostacyclin activity in pre-eclampsia. Lancet 2:702, 1980.
205. Everett RB, Worley RJ, MacDonald PC, Gant NF: Effect of prostaglandin synthetase inhibitors on pressor response to angiotensin II in human pregnancy. J Clin Endocrinol Metab 46:1007-1010, 1978.
206. Sanchez-Ramos L, O'Sullivan MJ, Garrido-Calderon J: Effect of low-dose aspirin on angiotensin II pressor response in human pregnancy. Am J Obstet Gynecol 156:193-194, 1987.
207. Moncada S, Palmer RM, Higgs EA: Nitric oxide: Physiology, pathophysiology, and pharmacology. Pharmacol Rev 43:109-142, 1991.

208. Williams DJ, Vallance PJ, Neild GH, et al: Nitric oxide-mediated vasodilation in human pregnancy. Am J Physiol 272(Pt 2):H748-H752, 1997.
209. Pathak N, Sawhney H, Vasishta K, Majumdar S: Estimation of oxidative products of nitric oxide (nitrates, nitrites) in preeclampsia. Aust N Z J Obstet Gynaecol 39:484-487, 1999.
210. Smarason AK, Allman KG, Young D, Redman CW: Elevated levels of serum nitrate, a stable end product of nitric oxide, in women with preeclampsia. BJOG 104:538-543, 1997.
211. Silver RK, Kupferminc MJ, Russell TL, et al: Evaluation of nitric oxide as a mediator of severe preeclampsia. Am J Obstet Gynecol 175(Pt 1):1013-1017, 1996.
212. Davidge ST, Stranko CP, Roberts JM: Urine but not plasma nitric oxide metabolites are decreased in women with preeclampsia. Am J Obstet Gynecol 174:1008-1013, 1996.
213. Curtis N, Gude N, King R, et al: Nitric oxide metabolites in normal human pregnancy and preeclampsia. Hypertens Pregnancy 14:339, 1995.
214. Seligman SP, Buyon JP, Clancy RM, et al: The role of nitric oxide in the pathogenesis of preeclampsia. Am J Obstet Gynecol 171:944-948, 1994.
215. Roberts JM: Plasma nitrites as an indicator of nitric oxide production: Unchanged production or reduced renal clearance in preeclampsia? Am J Obstet Gynecol 176:954-955, 1997.
216. Begum S, Yamasaki M, Mochizuki M: Urinary levels of nitric oxide metabolites in normal pregnancy and preeclampsia. J Obstet Gynaecol Res 22:551-559, 1996.
217. Ranta V, Viinikka L, Halmesmaki E, Ylikorkala O: Nitric oxide production with preeclampsia. Obstet Gynecol 93:442-445, 1999.
218. Myatt L, Rosenfield RB, Eis AL, et al: Nitrotyrosine residues in placenta. Evidence of peroxynitrite formation and action. Hypertension 28:488-493, 1996.
219. Roggensack AM, Zhang Y, Davidge ST: Evidence for peroxynitrite formation in the vasculature of women with preeclampsia. Hypertension 33:83-89, 1999.
220. Greer IA, Lyall F, Perera T, et al: Increased concentrations of cytokines interleukin-6 and interleukin-1 receptor antagonist in plasma of women with preeclampsia: A mechanism for endothelial dysfunction? Obstet Gynecol 84:937-940, 1994.
221. Redman CW, Sargent IL: Latest advances in understanding preeclampsia. Science 308:1592-1594, 2005.
222. Smarason AK, Sargent IL, Starkey PM, Redman CW: The effect of placental syncytiotrophoblast microvillous membranes from normal and preeclamptic women on the growth of endothelial cells in vitro. BJOG 100:943-949, 1993.
223. Hubel CA, Roberts JM, Taylor RN, et al: Lipid peroxidation in pregnancy: New perspectives on preeclampsia. Am J Obstet Gynecol 161:1025-1034, 1989.
224. Witztum JL: The oxidation hypothesis of atherosclerosis. Lancet 344:793-795, 1994.
225. Hollenberg NK, Epstein M, Rosen SM, et al: Acute oliguric renal failure in man: Evidence for preferential renal cortical ischemia. Medicine (Baltimore) 47:455-474, 1968.
226. Katz M, Berlyne GM: Differential renal protein clearance in toxaemia of pregnancy. Nephron 13:212-220, 1974.
227. Chesley L: Renal function tests in the differentiation of Bright's disease from so-called specific toxemia of pregnancy. Surg Gynecol Obstet 67:481, 1938.
228. Chesley LC, Markowitz I, Wetchler BB: Proteinuria following momentary vascular constriction. J Clin Invest 18:51-58, 1939.
229. Farrell P: Protein binding of urate ions in vitro and in vivo. In Edwards D (ed): Drugs and the Kidney. Progress in Biochemistry and Pharmacology, vol 9. Basel, S Karger, 1974.
230. Emmerson B: Effect of drugs on the renal handling of urate. In Edwards D (ed): Drugs and the Kidney. Progress in Biochemistry and Pharmacology, vol 9. Basel, S Karger, 1974.
231. Stander H, Cadden J: Blood chemistry in preeclampsia and eclampsia. Am J Obstet Gynecol 28:856, 1934.
232. Schaffer N, Dill L, Cadden J: Uric acid clearance in normal pregnancy and preeclampsia. J Clin Invest 22:201, 1943.
233. Hayashi T: Uric acid and endogenous creatinine clearance studies in normal pregnancy and toxemias of pregnancy. Am J Obstet Gynecol 71:859-870, 1956.
234. Seitchik J: Observations on the renal tubular reabsorption of uric acid. I. Normal pregnancy and abnormal pregnancy with and without preeclampsia. Am J Obstet Gynecol 65:981-985, 1953.
235. Gallery ED, Gyory AZ: Glomerular and proximal renal tubular function in pregnancy-associated hypertension: A prospective study. Eur J Obstet Gynecol Reprod Biol 9:3-12, 1979.
236. Suki W, Hull A, Rector FJ, et al: Mechanism of the effect of thiazide diuretics on calcium and uric acid. J Clin Invest 46:1121, 1967.
237. Gallery E, Saunders D, Boyce E, et al: Relation between plasma volume and uric acid in the development of hypertension in pregnancy. In Bonnar M, MacGillivray I, Symonds M (eds): Pregnancy Hypertension. Baltimore, University Park Press, 1980, p 175.
238. Ferris TF, Gorden P: Effect of angiotensin and norepinephrine upon urate clearance in man. Am J Med 44:359-365, 1968.
239. Sokabe H: Phylogeny of the renal effects of angiotensin. Kidney Int 6:263-271, 1974.
240. Parks DA, Granger DN: Xanthine oxidase: Biochemistry, distribution and physiology. Acta Physiol Scand Suppl 548:87-99, 1986.
241. Kaitz AL: Urinary concentrating ability in pregnant women with asymptomatic bacteriuria. J Clin Invest 40:1331-1338, 1961.
242. Assali NS, Kaplan SA, Fomon SJ, Douglass RA Jr: Renal function studies in toxemia of pregnancy; excretion of solutes and renal hemodynamics during osmotic diuresis in hydropenia. J Clin Invest 32:44-51, 1953.
243. Steele TW, Gyory AZ, Edwards KD: Renal function in analgesic nephropathy. BMJ 2:213-216, 1969.
244. Gallery EDM, Gyory AZ. Urinary concentration, white blood cell excretion, acid excretion, and acid-base status in normal pregnancy: Alterations in pregnancy-associated hypertension. Am J Obstet Gynecol 135:27-36, 1979.
245. Ochwadt BK, Pitts RF: Disparity between phenol red and Diodrast clearances in the dog. Am J Physiol 187:318-322, 1956.
246. Heidland A, Reidl E: Klinisch-experimentelle Untersuchung uber den renalen Phenolsulfonphthalein-Transport. Arch Klin Med 214:163, 1968.
247. Healy JK, Edwards KD, Whyte HM: Simple tests of renal function using creatinine, phenolsulphonphthalein, and pitressin. J Clin Pathol 17:557-563, 1964.
248. Ehrlich EN, Lindheimer MD: Sodium metabolism, aldosterone and the hypertensive disorders of pregnancy. J Reprod Med 8:106-110, 1972.
249. Brown MA, Wang J, Whitworth JA: The renin-angiotensin-aldosterone system in pre-eclampsia. Clin Exp Hypertens 19:713-726, 1997.
250. Weir RJ, Paintin DB, Brown JJ, et al: A serial study in pregnancy of the plasma concentrations of renin, corticosteroids, electrolytes and proteins and of haematocrit and plasma volume. J Obstet Gynaecol Br Commonw 78:590-602, 1971.
251. Gordon RD, Symonds EM, Wilmshurst EG, Pawsey CG: Plasma renin activity, plasma angiotensin and plasma and urinary electrolytes in normal and toxaemic pregnancy, including a prospective study. Clin Sci 45:115-127, 1973.
252. Bay WH, Ferris TF: Factors controlling plasma renin and aldosterone during pregnancy. Hypertension 1:410-415, 1979.
253. Langford HG, Pickering GW: The action of synthetic angiotensin on renal function in the unanesthetized rabbit. J Physiol 177:161-173, 1965.
254. Ferris TF, Stein JH, Kauffman J: Uterine blood flow and uterine renin secretion. J Clin Invest 51:2827-2833, 1972.
255. Tapia HR, Johnson CE, Strong CG: Renin-angiotensin system in normal and in hypertensive disease of pregnancy. Lancet 2:847-850, 1972.
256. Nicholson E, Gallery E, Brown M, et al: Renin activation in normal and hypertensive human pregnancy. Clin Exp Hypertens B 6:435, 1988.
257. August P, Lenz T, Ales KL, et al: Longitudinal study of the renin-angiotensin-aldosterone system in hypertensive pregnant women: Deviations related to the development of superimposed preeclampsia. Am J Obstet Gynecol 163(Pt 1):1612-1621, 1990.
258. Brown M, Zammit V, Adsett D: Stimulation of active renin release in normal and hypertensive pregnancy. Clin Sci 79:505, 1990.

259. Brown MA, Gallery ED, Ross MR, Esber RP: Sodium excretion in normal and hypertensive pregnancy: A prospective study. Am J Obstet Gynecol 159:297-307, 1988.
260. Brown MA, Zammit VC, Mitar DA, Whitworth JA: Renin-aldosterone relationships in pregnancy-induced hypertension. Am J Hypertens 5(Pt 1):366-371, 1992.
261. Saruta T, Nakamura R, Nagahama S, et al: Effects of angiotensin II analog on blood pressure, renin and aldosterone in women on oral contraceptives and toxemia. Gynecol Obstet Invest 12:11-20, 1981.
262. Pipkin F, Oats J, Symonds E: The effect of a specific AII antagonist (saralasin) on blood pressure in the immediate puerperium. In Bonnar M, MacGillivray I, Symonds M (eds): Pregnancy Hypertension. Baltimore, University Park Press, 1980, p 75.
263. Sullivan JM, Palmer ET, Schoeneberger AA, et al: SQ 20,881: Effect on eclamptic–pre-eclamptic women with postpartum hypertension. Am J Obstet Gynecol 131:707-715, 1978.
264. Wolf G: Free radical production and angiotensin. Curr Hypertens Rep 2:167-173, 2000.
265. Griendling KK, Ushio-Fukai M: Reactive oxygen species as mediators of angiotensin II signaling. Regul Pept 91:21-27, 2000.
266. Jaimes EA, Galceran JM, Raij L: Angiotensin II induces superoxide anion production by mesangial cells. Kidney Int 54:775-784, 1998.
267. Rajakumar A, Whitelock KA, Weissfeld LA, et al: Selective overexpression of the hypoxia-inducible transcription factor, HIF-2alpha, in placentas from women with preeclampsia. Biol Reprod 64:499-506, 2001.
268. Richard DE, Berra E, Pouyssegur J: Nonhypoxic pathway mediates the induction of hypoxia-inducible factor 1alpha in vascular smooth muscle cells. J Biol Chem 275:26765-26771, 2000.
269. Wallukat G, Homuth V, Fischer T, et al: Patients with preeclampsia develop agonistic autoantibodies against the angiotensin AT1 receptor. J Clin Invest 103:945-952, 1999.
270. Irons DW, Baylis PH, Butler TJ, Davison JM: Atrial natriuretic peptide in preeclampsia: Metabolic clearance, sodium excretion and renal hemodynamics. Am J Physiol 273(Pt 2):F483-F487, 1997.
271. Malee MP, Malee KM, Azuma SD, et al: Increases in plasma atrial natriuretic peptide concentration antedate clinical evidence of preeclampsia. J Clin Endocrinol Metab 74:1095-1100, 1992.
272. Zangmeister W: Untersuchungen uber die Blutbeschaffenheit und die Harnsekretion bei Eklampsie. Z Geburtschilfe Gynaekol 50:385, 1903.
273. Sarles HE, Hil SS, LeBlanc AL, et al: Sodium excretion patterns during and following intravenous sodium chloride loads in normal and hypertensive pregnancies. Am J Obstet Gynecol 102:1-7, 1968.
274. Chesley L: Sodium retention and preeclampsia. Am J Obstet Gynecol 95:127, 1966.
275. Dieckman W, Pottinger R: Total exchangeable sodium and space in normal and preeclamptic patients determined with sodium22. Am J Obstet Gynecol 74:816, 1957.
276. Chesley L, Chesley E: An analysis of some factors associated with the development of preeclampsia. Am J Obstet Gynecol 45:748, 1943.
277. Kraus GW, Marchese JR, Yen SS: Prophylactic use of hydrochlorothiazide in pregnancy. JAMA 198:1150-1154, 1966.
278. Weseley AC, Douglas GW: Continuous use of chlorothiazide for prevention of toxemia of pregnancy. Obstet Gynecol 19:355-358, 1962.
279. Flowers CE Jr, Grizzle JE, Easterling WE, Bonner OB: Chlorothiazide as a prophylaxis against toxemia of pregnancy. A double-blind study. Am J Obstet Gynecol 84:919-929, 1962.
280. Trupin LS, Simon LP, Eskenazi B: Change in paternity: A risk factor for preeclampsia in multiparas. Epidemiology 7:240-244, 1996.
281. Need JA: Pre-eclampsia in pregnancies by different fathers: Immunological studies. BMJ 1:548-549, 1975.
282. Basso O, Christensen K, Olsen J: Higher risk of pre-eclampsia after change of partner. An effect of longer interpregnancy intervals? Epidemiology 12:624-629, 2001.
283. Robillard PY, Hulsey TC: Association of pregnancy-induced-hypertension, pre-eclampsia, and eclampsia with duration of sexual cohabitation before conception. Lancet 347:619, 1996.
284. Marti J, Herrman U: Immunogestosis: A new concept of "essential" EPH gestosis, with special consideration of the primigravid patient. Am J Obstet Gynecol 128:489, 1977.
285. Dekker GA, Sibai BM: The immunology of preeclampsia. Semin Perinatol 23:24-33, 1999.
286. Redman CW: Treatment of hypertension in pregnancy. Kidney Int 18:267-278, 1980.
287. Feinberg BB, Jack RM, Mok SC, Anderson DJ: Low erythrocyte complement receptor type 1 (CR1, CD35) expression in preeclamptic gestations. Am J Reprod Immunol 54:352-357, 2005.
288. Stevenson AC, Davison BC, Say B, et al: Contribution of fetal/maternal incompatibility to aetiology of pre-eclamptic toxaemia. Lancet 2:1286-1289, 1971.
289. Feinberg BB: Preeclampsia: The death of Goliath. Am J Reprod Immunol 55:84-98, 2006.
290. Kovats S, Main EK, Librach C, et al: A class I antigen, HLA-G, expressed in human trophoblasts. Science 248:220-223, 1990.
291. O'Brien M, McCarthy T, Jenkins D, et al: Altered HLA-G transcription in pre-eclampsia is associated with allele specific inheritance: Possible role of the HLA-G gene in susceptibility to the disease. Cell Mol Life Sci 58:1943-1949, 2001.
292. Aldrich C, Verp MS, Walker MA, Ober C: A null mutation in HLA-G is not associated with preeclampsia or intrauterine growth retardation. J Reprod Immunol 47:41-48, 2000.
293. Sacks G, Sargent I, Redman C: An innate view of human pregnancy. Immunol Today 20:114-118, 1999.
294. Sacks GP, Studena K, Sargent K, Redman CW: Normal pregnancy and preeclampsia both produce inflammatory changes in peripheral blood leukocytes akin to those of sepsis. Am J Obstet Gynecol 179:80-86, 1998.
295. Redman CW, Sacks GP, Sargent IL: Preeclampsia: An excessive maternal inflammatory response to pregnancy. Am J Obstet Gynecol 180(Pt 1):499-506, 1999.
296. Hubel CA: Oxidative stress in the pathogenesis of preeclampsia. Proc Soc Exp Biol Med 222:222-235, 1999.
297. Maseki M, Nishigaki I, Hagihara M, et al: Lipid peroxide levels and lipids content of serum lipoprotein fractions of pregnant subjects with or without pre-eclampsia. Clin Chim Acta 115:155-161, 1981.
298. Sekiba K, Yoshioka T: Changes of lipid peroxidation and superoxide dismutase activity in the human placenta. Am J Obstet Gynecol 135:368-371, 1979.
299. Zusterzeel PL, Rutten H, Roelofs HM, et al: Protein carbonyls in decidua and placenta of pre-eclamptic women as markers for oxidative stress. Placenta 22:213-219, 2001.
300. Hubel CA, Kagan VE, Kisin ER, et al: Increased ascorbate radical formation and ascorbate depletion in plasma from women with preeclampsia: Implications for oxidative stress. Free Radic Biol Med 23:597-609, 1997.
301. Mikhail MS, Anyaegbunam A, Garfinkel D, et al: Preeclampsia and antioxidant nutrients: Decreased plasma levels of reduced ascorbic acid, alpha-tocopherol, and beta-carotene in women with preeclampsia. Am J Obstet Gynecol 171:150-157, 1994.
302. Branch DW, Mitchell MD, Miller E, et al: Pre-eclampsia and serum antibodies to oxidised low-density lipoprotein. Lancet 343:645-646, 1994.
303. Chappell LC, Seed PT, Kelly FJ, et al: Vitamin C and E supplementation in women at risk of preeclampsia is associated with changes in indices of oxidative stress and placental function. Am J Obstet Gynecol 187:777-784, 2002.
304. Chappell LC, Seed PT, Briley A, et al: A longitudinal study of biochemical variables in women at risk of preeclampsia. Am J Obstet Gynecol 187:127-136, 2002.
305. Kagan VE, Tyurin VA, Borisenko GG, et al: Mishandling of copper by albumin: Role in redox-cycling and oxidative stress in preeclampsia plasma. Hypertens Pregnancy 20:221-241, 2001.
306. Entman SS, Moore RM, Richardson LD, Killam AP: Elevated serum iron in toxemia of pregnancy. Am J Obstet Gynecol 143:398-404, 1982.
307. Many A, Roberts JM: Increased xanthine oxidase during labour—implications for oxidative stress. Placenta 18:725-726, 1997.

308. Many A, Hubel CA, Fisher SJ, et al: Invasive cytotrophoblasts manifest evidence of oxidative stress in preeclampsia. Am J Pathol 156:321-331, 2000.
309. Roberts JM, Hubel CA: Is oxidative stress the link in the two-stage model of pre-eclampsia? Lancet 354:788-789, 1999.
310. Adams E, MacGillivray I: Long-term effect of pre-eclampsia on blood pressure. Lancet 2:1373-1375, 1961.
311. Sutherland A, Cooper DW, Howie PW, et al: The incidence of severe pre-eclampsia amongst mothers and mothers-in-law of pre-eclamptics and controls. BJOG 88:785-791, 1981.
312. Chesley LC, Cooper DW: Genetics of hypertension in pregnancy: Possible single gene control of pre-eclampsia and eclampsia in the descendants of eclamptic women. BJOG 93:898-908, 1986.
313. Lie RT, Rasmussen S, Brunborg H, et al: Fetal and maternal contributions to risk of pre-eclampsia: Population based study. BMJ 316:1343-1347, 1998.
314. Esplin MS, Fausett MB, Fraser A, et al: Paternal and maternal components of the predisposition to preeclampsia. N Engl J Med 344:867-872, 2001.
315. Johnson N, Moodley J, Hammond M: HLA status of the fetus born to African women with eclampsia. Clin Exp Hypertens Pregnancy B 9:311, 1990.
316. Kilpatrick DC, Gibson F, Livingston J, Liston WA: Pre-eclampsia is associated with HLA-DR4 sharing between mother and fetus. Tissue Antigens 35:178-181, 1990.
317. Ward K, Hata A, Jeunemaitre X, et al: A molecular variant of angiotensinogen associated with preeclampsia. Nat Genet 4:59-61, 1993.
318. Arngrimsson R, Purandare S, Connor M, et al: Angiotensinogen: A candidate gene involved in preeclampsia? Nat Genet 4:114-115, 1993.
319. Wilton A, Kaye J, Guo G, et al: Is angiotensinogen a good candidate gene for preeclampsia? Hypertens Pregnancy 14:251, 1995.
320. Morgan T, Craven C, Nelson L, et al: Angiotensinogen T235 expression is elevated in decidual spiral arteries. J Clin Invest 100:1406-1415, 1997.
321. Sohda S, Arinami T, Hamada H, et al: Methylenetetrahydrofolate reductase polymorphism and pre-eclampsia. J Med Genet 34:525-526, 1997.
322. Grandone E, Margaglione M, Colaizzo D, et al: Factor V Leiden, C > T MTHFR polymorphism and genetic susceptibility to preeclampsia. Thromb Haemost 77:1052-1054, 1997.
323. Arngrimsson R, Hayward C, Nadaud S, et al: Evidence for a familial pregnancy-induced hypertension locus in the eNOS-gene region. Am J Hum Genet 61:354-362, 1997.
324. Roberts JM, Cooper DW: Pathogenesis and genetics of pre-eclampsia. Lancet 357:53-56, 2001.
325. Harrison GA, Humphrey KE, Jones N, et al: A genomewide linkage study of preeclampsia/eclampsia reveals evidence for a candidate region on 4q. Am J Hum Genet 60:1158-1167, 1997.
326. Chappell S, Morgan L: Searching for genetic clues to the causes of pre-eclampsia. Clin Sci 110:443-458, 2006.
327. Arngrimsson R, Siguroardottir S, Frigge ML, et al: A genome-wide scan reveals a maternal susceptibility locus for pre-eclampsia on chromosome 2p13. Hum Mol Genet 8:1799-1805, 1999.
328. Moses EK, Lade JA, Guo G, et al: A genome scan in families from Australia and New Zealand confirms the presence of a maternal susceptibility locus for pre-eclampsia, on chromosome 2. Am J Hum Genet 67:1581-1585, 2000.
329. Laivuori H, Lahermo P, Ollikainen V, et al: Susceptibility loci for pre-eclampsia on chromosomes 2p25 and 9p13 in Finnish families. Am J Hum Genet 72:168-177, 2003.
330. Lachmeijer AM, Arngrimsson R, Bastiaans EJ, et al: A genome-wide scan for preeclampsia in the Netherlands. Eu J Hum Genet 9:758-764, 2001.
331. Coppage KH, Polzin WJ: Severe preeclampsia and delivery outcomes: Is immediate cesarean delivery beneficial? Am J Obstet Gynecol 186:921-923, 2002.
332. Nassar AH, Adra AM, Chakhtoura N, et al: Severe preeclampsia remote from term: Labor induction or elective cesarean delivery? Am J Obstet Gynecol 179:1210-1213, 1998.
333. Alexander JM, Bloom SL, McIntire DD, Leveno KJ: Severe preeclampsia and the very low birth weight infant: Is induction of labor harmful? Obstet Gynecol 93:485-488, 1999.
334. Sibai BM: Diagnosis and management of gestational hypertension and preeclampsia. Obstet Gynecol 102:181-192, 2003.
335. Stallworth JC, Yeh SY, Petrie RH: The effect of magnesium sulfate on fetal heart rate variability and uterine activity. Am J Obstet Gynecol 140:702-706, 1981.
336. Browne F: The early signs of preeclampsia toxaemia, with special reference to the order of their appearance, and their interrelation. J Obstet Gynaecol Br Emp 40:1160, 1933.
337. Arias F: Expansion of intravascular volume and fetal outcome in patients with chronic hypertension and pregnancy. Am J Obstet Gynecol 123:610-616, 1975.
338. Gallery ED, Hunyor SN, Ross M, Gyory AZ: Predicting the development of pregnancy-associated hypertension. The place of standardised blood-pressure measurement. Lancet 1:1273-1275, 1977.
339. Nakamura T, Ito M, Matsui K, et al: Significance of angiotensin sensitivity test for prediction of pregnancy-induced hypertension. Obstet Gynecol 67:388-394, 1986.
340. Oney T, Kaulhausen H: The value of the angiotensin sensitivity test in the early diagnosis of hypertensive disorders in pregnancy. Am J Obstet Gynecol 142:17-20, 1982.
341. Chien PF, Arnott N, Gordon A, et al: How useful is uterine artery Doppler flow velocimetry in the prediction of pre-eclampsia, intrauterine growth retardation and perinatal death? An overview. BJOG 107:196-208, 2000.
342. Myatt L, Miodovnik M: Prediction of preeclampsia. Semin Perinatol 23:45-57, 1999.
343. Adelberg AM, Miller J, Doerzbacher M, Lambers DS: Correlation of quantitative protein measurements in 8-, 12-, and 24-hour urine samples for the diagnosis of preeclampsia. Am J Obstet Gynecol 185:804-807, 2001.
344. Chesley L: The variability of proteinuria in the hypertensive complications of pregnancy. J Clin Invest 18:617, 1939.
345. Perlman JM, Risser RC, Gee JB: Pregnancy-induced hypertension and reduced intraventricular hemorrhage in preterm infants. Pediatr Neurol 17:29-33, 1997.
346. American College of Obstetricians and Gynecologists (ACOG): Antenatal corticosteroid therapy for fetal maturation. ACOG committee opinion. Int J Gynaecol Obstet 78:95-97, 2002.
347. Visser W, Wallenburg HC: Temporising management of severe pre-eclampsia with and without the HELLP syndrome. BJOG 102:111-117, 1995.
348. van Pampus MG, Wolf H, Westenberg SM, et al: Maternal and perinatal outcome after expectant management of the HELLP syndrome compared with pre-eclampsia without HELLP syndrome. Eur J Obstet Gynecol Reprod Biol 76:31-36, 1998.
349. Sibai BM: Diagnosis, controversies, and management of the syndrome of hemolysis, elevated liver enzymes, and low platelet count. Obstet Gynecol 103(Pt 1):981-991, 2004.
350. Sibai BM, Barton JR: Expectant management of severe preeclampsia remote from term: Patient selection, treatment, and delivery indications. Am J Obstet Gynecol 196:514 e1-e9, 2007.
351. Odendaal HJ, Pattinson RC, Bam R, et al: Aggressive or expectant management for patients with severe preeclampsia between 28-34 weeks' gestation: A randomized controlled trial. Obstet Gynecol 76:1070-1075, 1990.
352. Sibai BM, Mercer BM, Schiff E, Friedman SA: Aggressive versus expectant management of severe preeclampsia at 28 to 32 weeks' gestation: A randomized controlled trial. Am J Obstet Gynecol 171:818-822, 1994.
353. Schiff E, Friedman SA, Kao L, Sibai BM: The importance of urinary protein excretion during conservative management of severe preeclampsia. Am J Obstet Gynecol 175:1313-1316, 1996.
354. Hall DR, Odendaal HJ, Steyn DW, Grove D: Urinary protein excretion and expectant management of early onset, severe pre-eclampsia. Int J Gynaecol Obstet 77:1-6, 2002.

355. Chammas MF, Nguyen TM, Li MA, et al: Expectant management of severe preterm preeclampsia: Is intrauterine growth restriction an indication for immediate delivery? Am J Obstet Gynecol 183:853-858, 2000.
356. Chari RS, Friedman SA, O'Brien JM, Sibai BM: Daily antenatal testing in women with severe preeclampsia. Am J Obstet Gynecol 173:1207-1210, 1995.
357. Magann EF, Martin RW, Isaacs JD, et al: Corticosteroids for the enhancement of fetal lung maturity: Impact on the gravida with preeclampsia and the HELLP syndrome. Aust N Z J Obstet Gynaecol 33:127-131, 1993.
358. Magann EF, Martin JN Jr. Complicated postpartum preeclampsia-eclampsia. Obstet Gynecol Clin North Am 22:337-356, 1995.
359. Martin JN Jr, Perry KG Jr, Blake PG, et al: Better maternal outcomes are achieved with dexamethasone therapy for postpartum HELLP (hemolysis, elevated liver enzymes, and thrombocytopenia) syndrome. Am J Obstet Gynecol 177:1011-1017, 1997.
360. O'Brien JM, Milligan DA, Barton JR: Impact of high-dose corticosteroid therapy for patients with HELLP (hemolysis, elevated liver enzymes, and low platelet count) syndrome. Am J Obstet Gynecol 183:921-924, 2000.
361. O'Brien JM, Shumate SA, Satchwell SL, et al: Maternal benefit of corticosteroid therapy in patients with HELLP (hemolysis, elevated liver enzymes, and low platelet count) syndrome: Impact on the rate of regional anesthesia. Am J Obstet Gynecol 186:475-479, 2002.
362. Tompkins MJ, Thiagarajah S: HELLP (hemolysis, elevated liver enzymes, and low platelet count) syndrome: The benefit of corticosteroids. Am J Obstet Gynecol 181:304-309, 1999.
363. Yalcin OT, Sener T, Hassa H, et al: Effects of postpartum corticosteroids in patients with HELLP syndrome. Int J Gynaecol Obstet 61:141-148, 1998.
364. Magann EF, Bass D, Chauhan SP, et al: Antepartum corticosteroids: Disease stabilization in patients with the syndrome of hemolysis, elevated liver enzymes, and low platelets (HELLP). Am J Obstet Gynecol 171:1148-1153, 1994.
365. Barrilleaux PS, Martin JN Jr, Klauser CK, et al: Postpartum intravenous dexamethasone for severely preeclamptic patients without hemolysis, elevated liver enzymes, low platelets (HELLP) syndrome: A randomized trial. Obstet Gynecol 105:843-848, 2005.
366. Hall DR, Odendaal HJ, Kirsten GF, Smith J, Grove D: Expectant management of early onset, severe pre-eclampsia: Perinatal outcome. BJOG 107:1258-1264, 2000.
367. Haddad B, Deis S, Goffinet F, et al: Maternal and perinatal outcomes during expectant management of 239 severe preeclamptic women between 24 and 33 weeks' gestation. Am J Obstet Gynecol 190:1590-1595; discussion 1595-1597, 2004.
368. Leitch CR, Cameron AD, Walker JJ: The changing pattern of eclampsia over a 60-year period. BJOG 104:917-922, 1997.
369. Altman D, Carroli G, Duley L, et al: Do women with pre-eclampsia, and their babies, benefit from magnesium sulphate? The Magpie trial: A randomised placebo-controlled trial. Lancet 359:1877-1890, 2002.
370. Lucas MJ, Leveno KJ, Cunningham FG: A comparison of magnesium sulfate with phenytoin for the prevention of eclampsia. N Engl J Med 333:201-205, 1995.
371. Duley L, Henderson-Smart D: Magnesium sulphate versus phenytoin for eclampsia. Cochrane Database Syst Rev (4):CD000128, 2003.
372. Which anticonvulsant for women with eclampsia? Evidence from the Collaborative Eclampsia Trial. Lancet 345:1455-1463, 1995.
373. Duley L, Henderson-Smart D: Magnesium sulphate versus diazepam for eclampsia. Cochrane Database Syst Rev (4):CD000127, 2003.
374. Alexander JM, McIntire DD, Leveno KJ, Cunningham FG: Selective magnesium sulfate prophylaxis for the prevention of eclampsia in women with gestational hypertension. Obstet Gynecol 108:826-832, 2006.
375. Chesley LC: Parenteral magnesium sulfate and the distribution, plasma levels, and excretion of magnesium. Am J Obstet Gynecol 133:1-7, 1979.
376. Massey S: Pharmacology of magnesium. Annu Rev Pharmacol Toxicol 17:67, 1977.
377. Chesley LC, Tepper I: Plasma levels of magnesium attained in magnesium sulfate therapy for preeclampsia and eclampsia. Surg Clin North Am 37:353-367, 1957.
378. Pritchard JA: The use of the magnesium ion in the management of eclamptogenic toxemias. Surg Gynecol Obstet 100:131-140, 1955.
379. Pritchard JA, Stone SR: Clinical and laboratory observations on eclampsia. Am J Obstet Gynecol 99:754-765, 1967.
380. Appleton MP, Kuehl TJ, Raebel MA, et al: Magnesium sulfate versus phenytoin for seizure prophylaxis in pregnancy-induced hypertension. Am J Obstet Gynecol 165(Pt 1):907-913, 1991.
381. Crowther C: Magnesium sulphate versus diazepam in the management of eclampsia: A randomized controlled trial. BJOG 97:110-117, 1990.
382. Lucas MJ, Leveno KJ, Cunningham FG: Magnesium sulfate versus phenytoin for the prevention of eclampsia-reply. N Engl J Med 333:1639, 1995.
383. Prasad K, Al-Roomi K, Krishnan PR, Sequeira R: Anticonvulsant therapy for status epilepticus. Cochrane Database Syst Rev (4):CD003723, 2005.
384. Lindenstrom E, Boysen G, Nyboe J: Influence of systolic and diastolic blood pressure on stroke risk. A prospective observational study. Am J Epidemiol 142:1279-1290, 1995.
385. Martin JN Jr, Thigpen BD, Moore RC, et al: Stroke and severe preeclampsia and eclampsia: A paradigm shift focusing on systolic blood pressure [see comment]. Obstet Gynecol 105:246-254, 2005.
386. Greer I, Walker J, Bjornsson S, et al: Second line therapy with nifedipine in severe pregnancy induced hypertension. Clin Exp Hypertens B 8:277, 1989.
387. Mabie WC, Gonzalez AR, Sibai BM, Amon E: A comparative trial of labetalol and hydralazine in the acute management of severe hypertension complicating pregnancy. Obstet Gynecol 70(Pt 1):328-333, 1987.
388. Benedetti TJ, Quilligan EJ: Cerebral edema in severe pregnancy-induced hypertension. Am J Obstet Gynecol 137:860-862, 1980.
389. Howie PW, Prentice CR, Forbes CD: Failure of heparin therapy to affect the clinical course of severe pre-eclampsia. BJOG 82:711-717, 1975.
390. Cotton DB, Benedetti TJ: Use of the Swan-Ganz catheter in obstetrics and gynecology. Obstet Gynecol 56:641-645, 1980.
391. Ehrenberg HM, Mercer BM: Abbreviated postpartum magnesium sulfate therapy for women with mild preeclampsia: A randomized controlled trial. Obstet Gynecol 108:833-838, 2006.
392. Goodlin RC, Cotton DB, Haesslein HC: Severe edema-proteinuria-hypertension gestosis. Am J Obstet Gynecol 132:595-598, 1978.
393. Naulty J, Cefalo RC, Lewis PE: Fetal toxicity of nitroprusside in the pregnant ewe. Am J Obstet Gynecol 139:708-711, 1981.
394. Mathews DD: A randomized controlled trial of bed rest and sedation or normal activity and non-sedation in the management of non-albuminuric hypertension in late pregnancy. BJOG 84:108-114, 1977.
395. Hauth JC, Cunningham FG, Whalley PJ: Management of pregnancy-induced hypertension in the nullipara. Obstet Gynecol 48:253-259, 1976.
396. Levine RJ, Hauth JC, Curet LB, et al: Trial of calcium to prevent pre-eclampsia. N Engl J Med 337:69-76, 1997.
397. Poston L, Briley AL, Seed PT, et al, for the Vitamins in Pre-eclampsia Trial: Vitamin C and vitamin E in pregnant women at risk for pre-eclampsia (VIP trial): Randomised placebo-controlled trial [see comment]. Lancet 367:1145-1154, 2006.
398. Rumbold AR, Crowther CA, Haslam RR, et al: Vitamins C and E and the risks of preeclampsia and perinatal complications [see comment]. N Engl J Med 354:1796-1806, 2006.
399. Duley L, Henderson-Smart DJ, Knight M, King JF: Antiplatelet agents for preventing pre-eclampsia and its complications. Cochrane Database Syst Rev (1):CD004659, 2004.
400. Beaufils M, Uzan S, Donsimoni R, Colau JC: Prevention of pre-eclampsia by early antiplatelet therapy. Lancet 1:840-842, 1985.
401. Hauth JC, Goldenberg RL, Parker CR Jr, et al: Low-dose aspirin therapy to prevent preeclampsia. Am J Obstet Gynecol 168:1083-1091; discussion 1091-1093, 1993.
402. Schiff E, Peleg E, Goldenberg M, et al: The use of aspirin to prevent pregnancy-induced hypertension and lower the ratio of thromboxane A_2 to prostacyclin in relatively high risk pregnancies. N Engl J Med 321:351-356, 1989.

403. Collaborative Low-dose Aspirin Study in Pregnancy (CLASP) Collaborative Group: A randomised trial of low-dose aspirin for the prevention and treatment of pre-eclampsia among 9364 pregnant women. CLASP (Collaborative Low-dose Aspirin Study in Pregnancy) Collaborative Group. Lancet 343:619-629, 1994.
404. Duley L, Henderson-Smart DJ, Meher S, King JF: Antiplatelet agents for preventing pre-eclampsia and its complications. Cochrane Database Syst Rev (2):CD004659, 2007.
405. Askie LM, Duley L, Henderson-Smart DJ, et al: Antiplatelet agents for prevention of pre-eclampsia: A meta-analysis of individual patient data. Lancet 369:1791-1798, 2007.
406. Roberts JM, Catov JM: Aspirin for pre-eclampsia: Compelling data on benefit and risk. Lancet 369:1765-1766, 2007.
407. Bucher HC, Guyatt GH, Cook RJ, et al: Effect of calcium supplementation on pregnancy-induced hypertension and preeclampsia: A meta-analysis of randomized controlled trials. JAMA 275:1113-1117, 1996.
408. Villar J, Belizan JM: Same nutrient, different hypotheses: Disparities in trials of calcium supplementation during pregnancy. Am J Clin Nutr 71:1375S-1379S, 2000.
409. Villar J, Abdel-Aleem H, Merialdi M, et al: World Health Organization randomized trial of calcium supplementation among low calcium intake pregnant women. Am J Obstet Gynecol 194:639-649, 2006.
410. Hofmeyr GJ, Atallah AN, Duley L: Calcium supplementation during pregnancy for preventing hypertensive disorders and related problems. Cochrane Database Syst Rev (1):CD001059, 2002.
411. Chappell LC, Seed PT, Briley AL, et al: Effect of antioxidants on the occurrence of pre-eclampsia in women at increased risk: A randomised trial. Lancet 354:810-816, 1999.
412. Burton GJ, Jauniaux E: Placental oxidative stress: From miscarriage to preeclampsia. J Soc Gynecol Investig 11:342-352, 2004.
413. Sibai BM: Chronic hypertension in pregnancy. Obstet Gynecol 100:369-377, 2002.
414. Neutra R, Neff R: Fetal death in eclampsia. II. The effect of non-therapeutic factors. BJOG 82:390-396, 1975.
415. Lin CC, Lindheimer MD, River P, Moawad AH: Fetal outcome in hypertensive disorders of pregnancy. Am J Obstet Gynecol 142:255-260, 1982.
416. Robertson WB, Brosens I, Dixon HG: The pathological response of the vessels of the placental bed to hypertensive pregnancy. J Pathol Bacteriol 93:581-592, 1967.
417. Sibai BM, Abdella TN, Anderson GD: Pregnancy outcome in 211 patients with mild chronic hypertension. Obstet Gynecol 61:571-576, 1983.
418. Rey E, Couturier A: The prognosis of pregnancy in women with chronic hypertension. Am J Obstet Gynecol 171:410-416, 1994.
419. Abalos E, Duley L, Steyn DW, Henderson-Smart DJ: Antihypertensive drug therapy for mild to moderate hypertension during pregnancy [update of Cochrane Database Syst Rev (2):CD002252, 2001]. Cochrane Database Syst Rev (1):CD002252, 2007.
420. Naden RP, Redman CW: Antihypertensive drugs in pregnancy. Clin Perinatol 12:521-538, 1985.
421. Roberts JM, Perloff DL: Hypertension and the obstetrician-gynecologist. Am J Obstet Gynecol 127:316-325, 1977.
422. Kincaid-Smith P, Bullen M, Mills J: Prolonged use of methyldopa in severe hypertension in pregnancy. BMJ 1:274-276, 1966.
423. Duley L, Meher S, Abalos E: Management of pre-eclampsia. BMJ 332:463-468, 2006.
424. Ounsted M, Cockburn J, Moar VA, Redman CW: Maternal hypertension with superimposed pre-eclampsia: Effects on child development at $7^1/_2$ years. BJOG 90:644-649, 1983.
425. Oakes G, Walker A, Ehrenkranz R, et al: Effect of propranolol infusion on the umbilical and uterine circulations of pregnant sheep. Am J Obstet Gynecol 126:1038, 1976.
426. Rane A, Tomson G: Prenatal and neonatal drug metabolism in man. Eur J Clin Pharmacol 18:9-15, 1980.
427. Christianson R, Page E: Diuretic drugs and pregnancy. Obstet Gynecol 48:647, 1976.
428. Soffronoff EC, Kaufmann BM, Connaughton JF: Intravascular volume determinations and fetal outcome in hypertensive diseases of pregnancy. Am J Obstet Gynecol 127:4-9, 1977.
429. Sibai BM, Grossman RA, Grossman HG: Effects of diuretics on plasma volume in pregnancies with long-term hypertension. Am J Obstet Gynecol 150:831-835, 1984.
430. Sibai B, Abdella T, Anderson G, et al: Plasma volume Findings in pregnant women with mild hypertension: Therapeutic considerations. Am J Obstet Gynecol 15:539, 1983.
431. Feitelson PJ, Lindheimer MD: Management of hypertensive gravidas. J Reprod Med 8:111-116, 1972.
432. Jandhyala B, Clarke D, Buckley J: Effects of prolonged administration of certain antihypertensive agents. J Pharm Sci 63:1497, 1974.
433. Sibai BM, Gonzalez AR, Mabie WC, Moretti M: A comparison of labetalol plus hospitalization versus hospitalization alone in the management of preeclampsia remote from term. Obstet Gynecol 70(Pt 1):323-327, 1987.
434. Easterling TR, Brateng D, Schmucker B, et al: Prevention of preeclampsia: A randomized trial of atenolol in hyperdynamic patients before onset of hypertension. Obstet Gynecol 93(Pt 1):725-733, 1999.
435. Plouin PF, Breart G, Maillard F, et al: Comparison of antihypertensive efficacy and perinatal safety of labetalol and methyldopa in the treatment of hypertension in pregnancy: A randomized controlled trial. BJOG 95:868-876, 1988.
436. Pickles CJ, Symonds EM, Broughton Pipkin F: The fetal outcome in a randomized double-blind controlled trial of labetalol versus placebo in pregnancy-induced hypertension. BJOG 96:38-43, 1989.
437. Redman CW, Beilin LJ, Bonnar J: Treatment of hypertension in pregnancy with methyldopa: Blood pressure control and side effects. BJOG 84:419-426, 1977.
438. Rosa FW, Bosco LA, Graham CF, et al: Neonatal anuria with maternal angiotensin-converting enzyme inhibition. Obstet Gynecol 74(Pt 1):371-374, 1989.
439. Pietrement C, Malot L, Santerne B, et al: Neonatal acute renal failure secondary to maternal exposure to telmisartan, angiotensin II receptor antagonist. J Perinatol 23:254-255, 2003.
440. Serreau R, Luton D, Macher MA, et al: Developmental toxicity of the angiotensin II type 1 receptor antagonists during human pregnancy: A report of 10 cases. BJOG 112:710-712, 2005.
441. Saji H, Yamanaka M, Hagiwara A, Ijiri R: Losartan and fetal toxic effects. Lancet 357:363, 2001.
442. Burrows RF, Burrows EA: Assessing the teratogenic potential of angiotensin-converting enzyme inhibitors in pregnancy. Aust N Z J Obstet Gynaecol 38:306-311, 1998.

Part IV

MATERNAL COMPLICATIONS

Chapter 36

Clinical Aspects of Normal and Abnormal Labor

John M. Thorp, Jr., MD

Normal Labor and Its Limits

The proper management of labor and delivery depends on a thorough understanding of the biology of normal labor. Given the inherent limitations in our knowledge of human labor, the astute clinician must take care to not draw firm conclusions and be willing to change his or her practice. Moreover, effective recognition and management of labor abnormalities requires knowledge of the limits of labor and of the physiologic response of both the mother and the fetus to the stresses of labor and delivery.

Uterine contractions occur throughout normal pregnancy. These contractions are irregular in timing and intensity, discoordinate in distribution, and, for the most part, entirely painless. Such uterine activity continues in normal pregnancy until late in the third trimester, when the contractions become more frequent, of greater and more consistent intensity, and more coordinated. Also, during the latter part of the third trimester, effacement (shortening) and dilation of the cervix begin. At the end of this largely painless phase, clinical labor begins, defined as the onset of painful uterine contractions associated with effacement and dilation of the cervix.

The precise onset of this combination of events frequently cannot be ascertained, and for practical purposes clinicians must rely on the patient's best estimate of when her labor contractions began or when they became regular in consistency and intensity. The specific onset of cervical effacement and dilation can rarely be documented in cases of spontaneous onset of labor; not uncommonly, both effacement and dilation occur late in the third trimester, before the onset of regular or noticeable uterine contractions. Therefore, the precise onset of labor is difficult to determine, and much of what is written about false labor, prodromal labor, and the latent phase of labor is influenced by this uncertainty.

Hendricks and colleagues,[1] who reported the findings of serial cervical examinations of 303 patients in the third trimester, studied these prelabor changes of the cervix. Cervical dilation began earlier and was of greater magnitude in multiparas than in primiparas. Cervical effacement, on the other hand, began earlier and was of greater magnitude in primiparas. These authors introduced the concept of the "cervical coefficient," which is the product of cervical dilation (in centimeters) and the percentage of effacement. They found that, at any point in prelabor, the cervical coefficient is relatively the same for all patients regardless of parity. The mean cervical dilation during the last 3 days before the onset of labor is 1.8 cm for nulliparas and 2.2 cm for multiparas. Their study stressed the importance of the prelabor preparation of the cervix and its influence on the duration of labor. It also pointed out the difficulty of using a specific time for onset of labor if it is defined as the beginning of cervical dilation.

Categorization of Labor Events

By convention, labor is divided into three stages:

1. *First stage:* from onset of labor to full dilation of the cervix
2. *Second stage:* from full dilation of the cervix to delivery of the infant
3. *Third stage:* from delivery of the infant to delivery of the placenta

Pritchard and MacDonald[2] described a fourth stage of labor, comprising the hour immediately following delivery of the placenta.

One of the most thorough evaluations of the first stage of labor was that by Friedman,[3] conveniently summarized in a monograph. His graphostatistical analysis of labor in term patients[3,4] depicted the relationship between the duration of labor and dilatation as a sigmoid curve, reflecting its exponential nature. He divided the first stage of labor into two major phases:

1. *Latent phase:* from the onset of regular uterine contractions to the beginning of the active phase
2. *Active phase:* from the time at which the rate of cervical dilation begins to change rapidly (usually at about 3 to 4 cm of dilation) to full dilation

Data from several thousand patients, in whom cervical dilation and the station of the presenting fetal part were documented throughout labor, were used to establish normal limits of labor for nulliparous and multiparous patients. A group of nulliparas and a group of multiparas were selected in whom there were no apparent complications of labor and who delivered normal infants. From these cases, the norms for "ideal" labor were determined (Table 36-1). Descent of the fetal head in relationship to the ischial spines was found to begin well before the

TABLE 36-1 CHARACTERISTICS OF LABOR IN NULLIPARAS AND MULTIPARAS*

	Nulliparas		Multiparas	
Characteristic	All Patients	Ideal Labor	All Patients	Ideal Labor
Duration of first stage (hr)				
Latent phase	6.4 ± 5.1	6.10 ± 4.0	4.80 ± 4.9	4.50 ± 4.2
Active phase	4.6 ± 3.6	3.40 ± 1.5	2.40 ± 2.2	2.10 ± 2.0
Total	11.0 ± 8.7	9.50 ± 5.5	7.20 ± 7.1	6.60 ± 6.2
Maximum rate of descent (cm/hr)	3.3 ± 2.3	3.60 ± 1.9	6.60 ± 4.0	7.00 ± 3.2
Duration of second stage (hr)	1.1 ± 0.8	0.76 ± 0.5	0.39 ± 0.3	0.32 ± 0.3

***Mean ± SD.**
Data from Friedman EA: Labor: Clinical Evaluation and Management, 2nd ed. New York, Appleton-Century-Crofts, 1978.

second stage. The rate of descent increased late in the first stage and continued linearly into the second stage of labor until the perineal floor was reached. Data for the maximum rate of descent and the length of the second stage of labor in all patients are also given in Table 36-1.

Friedman[3,4] formulated a series of definitions that have been incorporated into routine obstetric care. For example, he defined no cervical dilation for 2 hours as an arrest of the active phase of labor and a rate of dilation in the active phase of 1.2 cm/hr as a protracted active phase. His work has helped generations of obstetricians conceptualize progress in labor and has provided a standardized model for intervention.

Are Friedman's labor curve and definitions applicable to populations a half century later? Numerous studies done in the last decade indicate that the pattern of labor progression is different from what was observed in the 1950s[5-9] and that the clinical cutoff points for intervention and the duration of those interventions derived from Friedman's work are no longer clinically useful.[10,11] Zhang, Troendle, and Yancey,[12] in a landmark paper using a statistical approach based on likelihood, demonstrated how different contemporary labor progression is from that described in earlier years. Differences include the following: (1) a gradual rather than an abrupt transition from latent to active-phase labor; (2) a length of active labor of 5.5 hours, rather than the 2.5 hours described by Friedman; (3) no deceleration phase; (4) the common occurrence of at least 2 hours elapsing in the active phase without cervical dilation; and (5) the 5th percentile for rate of dilation being less than 1 cm/hr.

The findings of Zhang's group[12] appear in Table 36-2 and Figure 36-1. The figure allows comparison of Friedman's labor curves to those generated from contemporary practice. Rouse and colleagues[11] incorporated this finding of slower rates of progression in modern labor into a demonstration that showed that extending the minimum period of oxytocin augmentation for active-phase labor arrest, from 2 to at least 4 hours, was both effective and safe. The curves from both eras are plots of dilation against time and mimic an exponential mathematical equation. Like a compound interest curve, they begin slowly and rise more quickly as time elapses. The exponential nature of this biologic function can exasperate the patience of the laboring woman, her family, and caregivers. It lends biologic support to the age-old adage, "Patience is the virtue of the obstetrician."

TABLE 36-2 EXPECTED TIME INTERVAL AND RATE OF CHANGE AT EACH STAGE OF CERVICAL DILATION*

Cervical Dilation (cm)			
From	To	Time Interval (hr)	Rate of Cervical Dilation (cm/hr)
2	3	3.2 (0.6, 15.0)	0.3 (0.1, 1.8)
3	4	2.7 (0.6, 10.1)	0.4 (0.1, 1.8)
4	5	1.7 (0.4, 6.6)	0.6 (0.2, 2.8)
5	6	0.8 (0.2, 3.1)	1.2 (0.3, 5.0)
6	7	0.6 (0.2, 2.2)	1.7 (0.5, 6.3)
7	8	0.5 (0.1, 1.5)	2.2 (0.7, 7.1)
8	9	0.4 (0.1, 1.3)	2.4 (0.8, 7.7)
9	10	0.4 (0.1, 1.4)	2.4 (0.7, 8.3)

***Median (5th, 95th percentiles).**
Data from Zhang J, Troendle J, Yancey MK: Reassessing the labor curve in nulliparous women. Am J Obstet Gynecol 187:824, 2002. Printed with permission from CV Mosby.

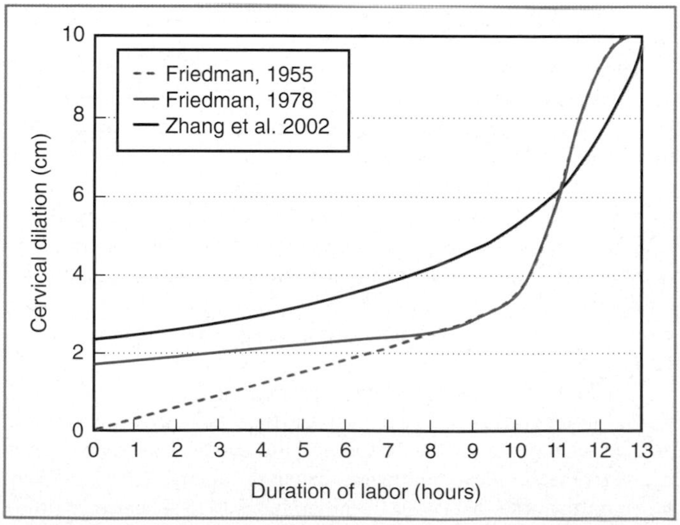

FIGURE 36-1 Comparison between Friedman's labor curves and the modern-day pattern of cervical dilation. (Data from Zhang J, Troendle J, Yancey MK: Reassessing the labor curve in nulliparous women. Am J Obstet Gynecol 187:824, 2002. Printed with permission from CV Mosby.)

Role of the Maternal Pelvis

The intelligent management of labor depends on an understanding of its mechanism as well as the norms and limits of its progress. One of the most important and helpful studies for understanding the mechanism of labor was that of Caldwell and associates.[13] This report was the culmination of a study of more than 1000 radiographic examinations of the pelvis and fetal head performed before, during, or after labor, in relation to the known details of delivery and the facts ascertained by vaginal examination. Many of the findings of this and later studies by the same authors[14] were incorporated in a monograph by Steer.[15] Although a complete review of these important works is beyond the scope of this text, a study of their contributions will substantially increase the reader's understanding of the influence of the pelvic architecture on normal and abnormal labor. Several of the important findings of these studies are worth reemphasizing here.

With a gynecoid or android type of pelvis, the fetal head engages in the transverse position 60% to 70% of the time. The anthropoid pelvis predisposes to engagement in the occiput anterior or posterior position. After the fetal head enters the pelvis in the transverse position, it is carried downward and backward until it impinges on the sacrum low in the midpelvis. It is at this point that internal rotation begins.

Internal rotation usually occurs in the midpelvis. Anterior rotation of the fetal head is practically complete when the head makes contact with the lower aspects of the pubic rami.

The common occurrence of engagement and descent predominantly in the posterior pelvis is usually associated with a normal progress of labor and spontaneous delivery; when engagement and descent occur predominantly in the forepelvis, however, there is a higher incidence of abnormal progress of labor and a higher rate of operative delivery. If the fetal head is descending in the posterior pelvis, the cervix usually is felt posteriorly in the vagina. If the cervix is palpated in a forward position, closer to the symphysis than to the sacrum, engagement and descent in the forepelvis must be suspected.

The increasing use of the vacuum extractor and the cesarean operation for delivery after second-stage arrest of labor has contributed to the lessening of emphasis on knowledge about pelvic types and their influence on descent and rotation of the fetal head. The relationship between pelvic architecture and the position of the fetal head, however, often allows useful prediction or explanation of abnormal labor, especially in the descent phase.

A careful clinical examination frequently discloses the essential dimensions and shape of the pelvis. In general, the characteristics of the anterior segment of the inlet correspond to those of the anterior portion of the lower pelvis:

- A subpubic arch with a well-rounded apex and ample space between the ischial tuberosities is associated with a gynecoid anterior segment at the inlet.
- A subpubic arch with a narrow angle and straight rami, convergent sidewalls, and prominent spines is associated with a narrowed, android anterior segment at the inlet.
- A narrow subpubic arch with straight sidewalls is characteristic of an anthropoid anterior segment at the inlet.
- A wide subpubic arch with straight or divergent sidewalls and a wide interspinous diameter is associated with a flat anterior segment at the inlet.

The posterior segment can best be characterized by palpation of the sacrospinous ligament and the sacrosciatic notch. A narrow notch, associated with a short sacrosciatic ligament (less than 2 fingerbreadths), suggests an android posterior segment. A sacrosciatic ligament length of 2 to 3 fingerbreadths suggests a gynecoid posterior segment. If the ligament is directed backward and the spines are close together, the posterior segment of the inlet is probably anthropoid. If the ligament is directed laterally and the spines are far apart, the posterior segment of the inlet is likely to be flat.

The pelvic configuration can be assessed at the time of a pelvic examination when the patient is admitted to the labor unit, or it can be determined as part of the initial examination when the patient registers for prenatal care. The advantages of performing the assessment when the patient is hospitalized in labor are the increased relevance of the information at that time and the probability that the individual performing the examination will incorporate the results into a comprehensive assessment of the labor.

Documentation of Labor Progression

One of the most important aspects of the management of labor is accurate and thorough documentation of the progress of labor or the lack of it. Most authorities agree that a graphic display of intrapartum data that allows prompt visualization of the status and progress of cervical dilation and, in some cases, descent of the presenting part is an essential adjunct to intrapartum patient monitoring. This can be accomplished with a simple record of cervical dilation plotted against time on ruled graph paper or by a more comprehensive recording of all intrapartum data related in graphic form to the progress of cervical dilation.

If the data about effacement and dilation of the cervix and station and position of the presenting part are recorded only in narrative form, early and significant abnormalities of labor may not be recognized as soon as they would if a more visual display of labor progress were available. This is especially important if more than one attendant monitors the patient, as frequently occurs in a labor that is longer than normal or a labor that overlaps a change of shift in the hospital. Tabular and graphic displays of intrapartum data are entirely in keeping with the concept that labor and delivery are worthy of intensive surveillance, and they afford a convenient method of reviewing labor events in situations of an untoward fetal or maternal outcome.

The crucial factor in the evidence-based management of labor is the timing of interventions such as amniotomy, stimulation of contractions with oxytocin, operative delivery, or, in much of the world, transfer from home to a unit for those interventions. A World Health Organization trial performed in multiple labor units across the world, in which a graphical "partogram" was relied on to time interventions, demonstrated reductions in prolonged labors, in the frequency of emergency abdominal delivery, and in the use of oxytocin augmentation.[16] Therefore, visual representation of dilation versus time can help clinicians improve the care of patients in labor.

The compulsiveness, form, and orderliness of documentation of labor events need not interfere with compassionate, family-centered care of a woman in labor. In fact, the challenge of modern obstetrics is to manage a pregnancy with the least interference and yet maintain the capability of recognizing and correcting incipient complications at the earliest possible moment.

Management of Labor Abnormalities

Abnormalities of the First Stage

In attempting to extend Friedman's work[3,4] into contemporary practice, with its longer duration of normal labors, the modern obstetrician

TABLE 36-3 FACTORS ASSOCIATED WITH FAILURE TO PROGRESS IN THE FIRST STAGE OF LABOR

Factor	Odds Ratio	95% Confidence Interval
Premature rupture of membranes	3.8	3.2-4.5
Nulliparity	3.8	3.3-4.3
Labor induction	3.3	2.9-3.7
Maternal age >35 yr	3.0	2.6-3.6
Fetal weight >4 kg	2.2	1.8-2.7
Hypertensive disorder	2.1	1.8-2.6
Hydramnios	1.9	1.5-2.3
Fertility treatment	1.8	1.4-2.4

Modified from Sheiner E, Levy A, Feinstein O, et al: Risk factors and outcomes of failure to progress during the first stage of labor: A population-based study. Acta Obstet Gynecol Scand 81:224, 2002, table IV. Printed with permission from Blackwell Munksgaard.

is faced with confusing definitions, the applicability of which in the individual case cannot be certain. Other than the recommendations of Rouse and colleagues[11] to prolong augmentation in the face of second-stage arrest, we know of no new clinical guidelines for obstetricians to use. Moreover, Friedman's management suggestions were made without experimental verification of the hypotheses underlying his thinking. Until such desperately needed investigations are completed, however, Friedman's framework[3]—in which he described labor abnormalities, identified associated problems, detailed the prognosis for the mother and fetus, and recommended a course of management—remains clinically useful.

Friedman[3] reported that abnormalities of the first stage of labor occurred in 8% of parturients, with a much higher incidence among primiparas than among nulliparas. Philpott and Castle[17] found that 11% of primiparas experienced abnormal labor progress in the first stage and required oxytocin augmentation. In a population-based study of 92,918 women, Sheiner and associates[18] found that failure to progress complicated 1.3% of all labors and resulted in abdominal deliveries. Independent risk factors are listed in Table 36-3.

Prolonged Latent Phase

On the basis of the 95th percentile limit of the distribution of latent-phase duration in the primiparous population, 20 hours is considered the definition of an abnormal latent phase. For multiparas, 14 hours is the corresponding definition of prolonged latent phase. Sometimes it is difficult to ascertain the difference between a prolonged latent phase and so-called "false" labor. Friedman[3] found that prolongation of the latent phase was associated with excessive sedation, prematurely administered epidural anesthesia, unfavorable cervical status, or myometrial dysfunction.

Although early studies suggested that prolongation of the latent phase was not associated with increased perinatal mortality and was not the harbinger of other abnormalities of labor,[19] subsequent studies showed otherwise. In a study of 10,979 patients in San Francisco, Chelmow and colleagues[20] found that prolonged latent phase of labor, defined as longer than 12 hours for nulliparous patients and longer than 6 hours for multiparous patients, was associated with an increased risk for subsequent labor abnormalities, cesarean delivery, low Apgar scores, and need for neonatal resuscitation. These risks for adverse outcomes remained significantly elevated even when the data were controlled for other labor abnormalities, prolonged rupture of membranes, meconium-stained amniotic fluid, parity, and epidural use. In addition to the increased risk of cesarean delivery, these authors found that a prolonged latent phase of labor in patients who delivered vaginally was associated with an approximately twofold increased incidence of third-degree and fourth-degree lacerations, febrile morbidity, and intrapartum blood loss.

One of the major problems with evaluation and management of the latent phase of labor is knowing at what hour labor began. For this reason, some authorities have used the time of admission to the hospital as a convenient starting point for judging when to intervene in the progress of labor.[17,21,22] Friedman,[3] however, regarded the onset of regular contractions as the beginning of labor and recommended intervention when the duration of the latent phase of labor reached 20 hours in the primipara. He found that either adequate sedation ("therapeutic narcosis") or oxytocin augmentation resulted in the resumption of normal cervical dilation. Because most patients are exhausted after 20 hours of labor, Friedman preferred therapeutic narcosis over oxytocin augmentation. For narcosis, he recommended morphine sulfate, 15 to 20 mg, with 10 to 15 mg more if the first dose has not made the patient somnolent and thereby inhibited uterine contractions. The obvious advantage of this therapy is that the patient awakens rested and refreshed and prepared for the active phase of labor.

Critics of this approach, especially O'Driscoll and Meagher,[22] argued that waiting out 20 hours of latent phase before considering the labor to be abnormal only promotes exhaustion and discourages the patient. They advocated a protocol for active management of labor, which has been practiced and evaluated at the National Maternity Hospital in Dublin. This involves several important features:

1. Patients are admitted to the labor unit only when they are experiencing painful uterine contractions as well as complete effacement of the cervix, ruptured membranes, or passage of blood-stained mucus.
2. Amniotomy is performed soon after admission for patients who have intact membranes.
3. Oxytocin augmentation of labor is performed if the progress of labor is less than 1 cm/hr over a 2-hour period. Oxytocin infusion is begun at 4 mU/min and is increased by 6 mU/min every 15 minutes until there are seven contractions per 15 minutes. The oxytocin infusion rate does not exceed 40 mU/min.
4. Continuous electronic fetal heart rate monitoring is used only if there is meconium-stained amniotic fluid and after fetal scalp pH has been performed to rule out fetal acidosis.
5. A nurse-midwife is in constant attendance with the patient throughout labor.
6. The patient is assured that if her labor exceeds 12 hours, cesarean delivery will probably be performed.
7. The progress of labor is documented on a simple graphic form, and the senior obstetrician in charge of the unit reviews all cases daily. A partogram, as described earlier, is used to time interventions.
8. This approach to the management of labor is confined to nulliparas.

The active management protocol, with minor modifications, has been evaluated in several obstetric services in the United States as well as in other countries. These studies have consistently demonstrated a small but significant shortening of labor associated with active management. Although most of these studies have also demonstrated a decrease in the incidence of cesarean delivery for dystocia,[23-26] the largest prospective and best-designed controlled trial showed no difference in the incidence of cesarean delivery for dystocia[27] but did show shortened labor and a decreased incidence of maternal infection with the active management protocol.

Holmes and associates[28] clearly demonstrated that women who present to the hospital with less than 3 cm dilation are more likely to undergo cesarean section or operative vaginal delivery than women presenting with more advanced dilation. Interestingly, they found that women presenting with less than 3 cm dilation had spent less time at home (2.0 versus 4.5 hours) since the onset of painful uterine contractions. Their results imply that women who present with reduced cervical dilation could have intrinsically different labors than those who present with more advanced dilation. Murphy and coworkers[29] and Falzone and colleagues[30] made similar observations, noting that nulliparous women presenting in labor with unengaged and particularly floating (above −3/3 station) fetal heads had higher risks for obstetric intervention.

Protraction Disorders

Protraction disorders are those in which progress of cervical dilation and descent of the fetal head occur at a slower than normal rate in the active phase of labor. The rate of cervical dilation for nulliparas should be at least 1.2 cm/hr; for multiparas, it should be 1.5 cm/hr or faster. These criteria for minimum rates of cervical change represent the 95th percentiles for each parity category. For descent of the fetal head, the rate for nulliparas should be 1.0 cm/hr or faster; for multiparas, it should be 2.0 cm/hr.

Friedman[3] found protraction disorders in primiparas to be associated frequently with cephalopelvic disproportion (CPD), use of conduction anesthesia, and fetal malposition. Whether these factors are related in a cause-and-effect manner is not known. Moreover, he found oxytocin augmentation and therapeutic narcosis to be of little value in these cases. Friedman also noted unusually high neonatal mortality and morbidity rates when this labor abnormality was terminated by mid-forceps delivery; however, the diagnosis of a primary dysfunctional labor (i.e., persisting at a cervical dilation rate of less than 1.2 cm/hr) is usually made in retrospect, after oxytocin augmentation has been used and found not to increase the dilation rate.

The experiences of Beazley and Kurjak[21] and those of O'Driscoll and Meagher[22] suggested that an early, more active use of oxytocin, as described in the active management of labor, effectively corrects most protraction disorders, although these authors did not specifically separate protraction disorders from arrest disorders. Those who advocate the active management of labor explain that the use of x-ray pelvimetry is unnecessary in the nulliparous patient, because rupture of the uterus does not occur with the recommended oxytocin augmentation. Therefore, in nulliparous patients with suboptimal progress of labor of any cause, it is safe to use a trial of oxytocin to determine whether labor will progress to completion.

Ganström and associates[31] demonstrated significant differences in collagen content and collagen remodeling in the cervix and lower uterine segment in patients with protracted labors compared with those having normal labors. This finding may explain why some patients with protracted labor do not respond to oxytocin augmentation.

Arrest Disorders

Friedman[3] defined an arrest disorder as the cessation of either cervical dilation or descent of the fetal head in the active phase of labor for longer than 2 hours. In their pure form, arrest disorders differ from protraction abnormalities in that, before the arrest of progress, the rate of cervical dilation or descent of the fetal head is normal. Arrest of progress can also complicate a protraction disorder. In either situation, Friedman[3] found that 45% of the cases of arrest disorder were associated with CPD. Philpott and Castle[32] also found that patients whose labor progress crossed the "action line" (i.e., those with protraction or arrest disorders) had smaller pelvic measurements and more often required cesarean delivery for CPD.

Because of the frequent association between arrest disorders and CPD, Friedman[3] recommended radiographic cephalopelvimetry followed by cesarean delivery for those with CPD and oxytocin augmentation for the remainder. He found that 80% of women with arrest disorders who did not have CPD delivered after oxytocin augmentation. Philpott and Castle[32] and O'Driscoll and Meagher[22] found that radiographic studies are not required, especially in primiparas, and that a trial of oxytocin augmentation is indicated in all protraction and arrest disorders. With careful monitoring of mother and fetus and discontinuation of augmentation if there is no progress after 4 to 6 hours, patients are not in danger. This is the approach of most, if not all, obstetric services in the United States; radiographic cephalopelvimetry is seldom used in the management of abnormal labor in vertex presentations.[33-35]

A notable exception is the use of the fetal-pelvic index by Thurnau and Morgan.[36] This technique combines ultrasound measurement of the fetal head circumference (HC) and abdominal circumference (AC) and radiographic measurement of the maternal pelvic inlet circumference (IC) and midpelvic circumference (MC). The fetal-pelvic index is the sum of the two greatest positive circumference differences (i.e., HC − IC, HC − MC, AC − IC, or AC − MC). A positive fetal-pelvic index value indicates the presence of fetal-pelvic disproportion, and a negative fetal-pelvic index value indicates the absence of fetal-pelvic disproportion. This index had a 94% positive predictive value for cesarean delivery of patients with abnormal labor patterns. These authors also found the fetal-pelvic index to be useful in predicting the success of induction of labor[37] and the success of women attempting vaginal birth after previous cesarean delivery.[38] Ferguson and colleagues[39] were not able to confirm the efficacy of the fetal-pelvic index, and the method is not widely used.

Using labor progression guidelines based on the slower labor curves characteristic of modern parturients, Rouse and colleagues[10] demonstrated the effectiveness of a new protocol to treat arrest disorders. Their protocol had three principal elements:

- An intent to achieve a sustained uterine contraction pattern of greater than 200 Montevideo units as measured by an intrauterine pressure catheter
- A minimum of 4 hours of oxytocin-augmented labor arrest with a contraction pattern of greater than 200 Montevideo units before proceeding to abdominal delivery for active-phase arrest (more liberal than the original Friedman[3] cutoff of 2 hours)
- For patients who cannot achieve a sustained uterine contraction pattern of greater than 200 Montevideo units, administration of a minimum of 6 hours of oxytocin augmentation before proceeding to cesarean delivery for active-phase labor arrest

The researchers demonstrated not only the effectiveness (92% vaginal delivery rate) but also the safety of this approach, with no serious adverse maternal or perinatal effects. The only cost of liberalization of the minimums was an increased risk of maternal infection, with the risk proportional to the time elapsed.

The recommendations of Rouse and colleagues[10] raise the issue of whether intrauterine pressure catheters are useful tools for clinicians managing labor abnormalities. Lucidi and colleagues[40] reviewed the literature in 2001 and noted that there were no clinical trials testing the utility of this device. Noteworthy is the absence of this technique from the routines of the active management protocols described heretofore. It would seem that partograms have a much stronger evidence basis than measurement of uterine contractibility to guide the timing of obstetric interventions.

Several authors have evaluated the effect of ambulation on the progress of labor. Flynn and coworkers[41] found that patients who ambulated had more rapid labor with fewer instances of fetal distress than a similar number of patients who labored in bed. Williams and associates,[42] studying 48 patients who ambulated, could find no differences in duration of labor or frequency of fetal distress compared with control patients. Read and colleagues[43] studied 14 patients whose labors were regarded as requiring augmentation because of lack of progress attributed to inadequate contractions. In the eight patients who were randomized to an ambulation study protocol, progress of labor was as rapid as in six control patients whose labors were augmented with oxytocin.

These studies suggest that ambulation is not detrimental to the progress of labor or the well-being of the fetus. It has not been established, however, whether ambulation is clearly beneficial or whether it is a substitute for pharmacological augmentation of labor in cases of abnormal progress.

Abnormalities of the Second Stage

Abnormalities of Rotation and Descent

Textbooks of obstetrics traditionally have discussed the first and second stages of labor as if they were separate clinical and biological entities, which, in fact, they are not. Descent and rotation of the fetal head frequently occur before complete dilation of the cervix, a phenomenon that is clear to most clinicians and that was confirmed by the studies of Friedman.[3] In addition to showing slower rates of cervical dilation than did Friedman, the contemporary data of Zhang, Troendle, and Yancey[12] showed a slower rate of fetal head descent. As demonstrated in Table 36-4 and Figure 36-2, it can take up to 3 hours to descend from +1/3 to +3/3 station and an additional 30 minutes for delivery. Again, there is a clear need for practice guidelines to incorporate these new data.

Arrest of descent and rotation, whether it occurs before or after complete dilation of the cervix, is a matter of concern and requires evaluation. Arbitrary limits on the duration of the second stage of labor probably resulted from the misinterpretation of the data presented by Hellman and Prystowsky.[44] In that study, patients whose second stage of labor was longer than 2 hours were at increased risk for perinatal and maternal morbidity. This observation was interpreted by many clinicians to mean that delivery of the fetus should be accomplished, by whatever means, before 2 hours of the second stage had elapsed. This interpretation occasionally resulted in traumatic midforceps operations or unnecessary cesarean deliveries, not to mention overzealous use of the vacuum extractor. The reader should note that their recommendation of a 2-hour second stage limit antedates electronic fetal monitoring.

Cohen[45] demonstrated that, if patients with fetal distress or traumatic delivery are excluded, the duration of the second stage bears no relationship to perinatal outcome. If there are no serious fetal heart rate abnormalities, if the mother is well hydrated and reasonably comfortable, and if there is some progress in descent or rotation of the fetal head (regardless of how slow), there is no need for operative delivery. Similarly, Menticoglou and associates[46] confirmed that the duration of the second stage of labor is in itself not related to untoward outcomes. Hansen and coauthors,[47] in a trial of active versus passive pushing in the second stage, found that second-stage lengths of up to 4 to 9 hours had no harmful effects. Moreover, delayed pushing was better tolerated by patients and was associated with fewer fetal heart rate decelerations.

After the cervix is dilated more than 7 cm, descent or rotation of the fetal head can be expected. If this does not occur, uterine contrac-

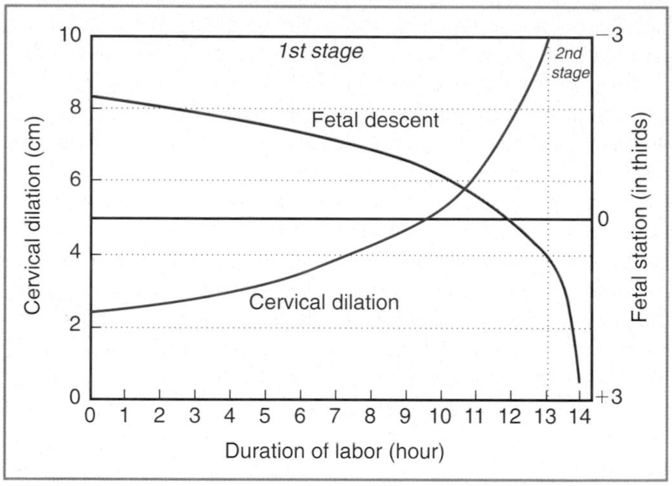

FIGURE 36-2 Patterns of cervical dilation *(left scale)* and fetal descent *(right scale)* in nulliparas. (From Zhang J, Troendle J, Yancey MK: Reassessing the labor curve in nulliparous women. Am J Obstet Gynecol 187:824, 2002. Printed with permission from CV Mosby.)

TABLE 36-4 EXPECTED TIME INTERVAL AND RATE OF DESCENT AT EACH STAGE OF STATION*

Station (in Thirds)		First and Second Stages		Second Stage Only	
From†	To	Time Interval (hr)	Rate (cm/hr)†	Time Interval (hr)	Rate (cm/hr)
−2	−1	7.9 (0.9, 65)	0.2 (0.03, 1.8)	—	—
−1	0	1.8 (0.1, 23)	0.9 (0.07, 12)	—	—
0	+1	1.4 (0.1, 13)	1.2 (0.12, 12)	—	—
+1	+2	0.4 (0.04, 3.8)	4.4 (0.44, 42)	0.27 (0.02, 2.93)	6.2 (0.57, 3.9)
+2	+3	0.1 (0.02, 0.9)	12.8 (1.9, 83)	0.11 (0.02, 0.63)	15.2 (2.6, 83)

*Median (5th, 95th percentiles).
†Measurement has been converted from thirds to fifths.
Data from Zhang J, Troendle J, Yancey MK: Reassessing the labor curve in nulliparous women. Am J Obstet Gynecol 187:824, 2002. Printed with permission from CV Mosby.

tions, if they are not adequate, should be augmented with oxytocin. Manual examination to determine the position of the fetal head and the dimensions and shape of the pelvis often helps at this point. Posterior presentation, brow presentation, marked degrees of asynclitism, and very large infants are associated with longer labors, even with adequate contractions.

The Mueller-Hillis maneuver[48] also may help. The obstetrician applies pressure to the uterine fundus with one hand and detects descent of the fetal head with the examining finger in the vagina. If the fetal head descends 1 cm or more with fundal pressure, the prognosis for vaginal delivery is good; if no descent occurs, the prognosis for delivery is poor. This maneuver is not predictive of outcome if it is performed early in labor,[49] but it is helpful late in the first stage or in the second stage of labor.[48]

Shoulder Dystocia

Shoulder dystocia occurs in 0.24% to 2.00% of vaginal deliveries.[50-53] This wide range of prevalence estimates highlights the lack of a standard definition. The cause is impingement of the biacromial diameter of the fetus against the symphysis pubis anteriorly and the sacral promontory posteriorly. Why the shoulders do not descend in the oblique diameters of the pelvis is unclear, although sometimes the fetus is simply too large. Although the risk of shoulder dystocia rises with increasing birth weight, 40% to 50% of cases occur in infants whose birth weight is less than 4000 g.

Risk factors for shoulder dystocia[50,54-56] include fetal macrosomia, diabetes, a history of shoulder dystocia in a previous birth, and prolonged second stage of labor. Other factors that have been inconsistently reported as increasing the risk[52,53,57] include a history of macrosomia or post-term pregnancy, multiparity, obesity, and operative vaginal delivery from the midpelvis. In 50% of cases of shoulder dystocia, no risk factors are identified.

Maternal morbidity from shoulder dystocia includes postpartum hemorrhage and rectal injuries. The morbidity for the infant is attributable to asphyxia from delay in delivery or to trauma from the maneuvers used to deliver the fetus. Infant morbidity related to trauma includes brachial plexus and phrenic nerve injuries and fractures of the humerus and clavicle.[58] The most serious traumatic morbidity is brachial plexus injury (Erb palsy), which occurs in 10% to 20% of infants born after shoulder dystocia.[52,58] If they are recognized early, 80% to 90% of brachial plexus injuries recover completely with proper physical therapy and, in some situations, neurosurgical management.[59] For this reason, permanent neurological injury is rare, occurring in 1 or 2 of every 10,000 births. This low prevalence greatly limits the ability to conduct prospective prevention studies.

Most brachial plexus injuries resulting from shoulder dystocia involve the arm and shoulder that are in the anterior pelvis at the time of delivery. The brachial plexus is believed to be injured when excessive downward traction and lateral extension of the fetal head and neck occur during the attempt to deliver the anterior shoulder[53]; however, there are exceptions to this cause of brachial plexus injury.[60] Some infants with brachial plexus injuries were born by vaginal delivery in which there was no evidence of shoulder dystocia.[61] Also, brachial plexus palsy can involve the arm that was in the posterior pelvis at the time of delivery.[62] Furthermore, Erb palsy has occurred in infants born by cesarean delivery.[63,64] Finally, several reports have described brachial plexus injuries in newborns in whom other physical findings and electromyographic tests confirmed that the lesions occurred before the onset of labor.[65,66] It is postulated that these injuries resulted from chronic nerve compression due to malposition in utero.[67,68] The presence of a permanent injury does not imply that the delivering clinician applied excessive force despite the *res ipsa loquitur* argument seen in so many torts arising from these births.

PREVENTION OF SHOULDER DYSTOCIA

Prevention of shoulder dystocia by prophylactic induction of labor is not effective.[69] Primary cesarean delivery can prevent shoulder dystocia in a small proportion of patients when several predisposing factors are present, such as multiparity, gestational diabetes, and an estimated fetal weight in excess of 4500 g. Rouse and Owen,[70] using decision analytic techniques, concluded that prophylactic cesarean delivery for sonographically detected fetal macrosomia to prevent shoulder dystocia is a Faustian bargain. Use of either 4000 or 4500 g as the cutoff point for abdominal delivery would require more than 1000 cesarean sections to prevent one permanent injury to the brachial plexus. Also, if arrest of descent of the fetal head occurs during labor along with other risk factors for shoulder dystocia, operative vaginal delivery should be avoided.

MANAGEMENT OF SHOULDER DYSTOCIA

Conventional wisdom dictates that the most effective treatment includes prompt recognition that delivery of the shoulders will be difficult and avoidance of excessive downward traction on the fetal head when attempting to deliver the anterior shoulder. Retraction of the fetal head immediately on its delivery (turtle sign) is an early warning that delivery of the shoulders may be difficult. Studies using simulated models of the fetus and pelvis demonstrated that obstetricians frequently underestimate the amount of traction they apply to the fetal head.[71,72]

Several maneuvers have been useful in resolving shoulder dystocia. Hyperflexion of the mother's thighs, known as the McRoberts maneuver, flattens the lumbosacral curve, thereby removing the sacral promontory as an obstruction to the inlet.[73,74] The knee-chest position tends to accomplish the same end. Suprapubic pressure can be applied in conjunction with the McRoberts maneuver.

Rubin[75] described rotating the fetal shoulders into the oblique position by inserting the fingers of one hand vaginally behind the most accessible shoulder (usually the posterior) and pushing the shoulder toward the fetal chest. This is a substantial improvement on the commonly described Woods maneuver, which involves pushing the shoulder toward the fetal back.[76]

If these maneuvers are not successful, the posterior arm of the fetus can be delivered if the obstetrician inserts one hand posteriorly, grasps the elbow, and draws the arm across the chest of the fetus.[77] This maneuver may result in fracture of the humerus or the clavicle, which is a consistently remedial injury and preferable to a brachial plexus injury of the opposite arm. Finally, replacement of the fetal head in the uterus followed by cesarean delivery—the Zavanelli maneuver—could be necessary in rare instances.[78]

Although the soft tissue of the perineum does not contribute to shoulder dystocia, many protocols recommend a wide episiotomy to facilitate performing one or more of the described maneuvers.

The successful management of shoulder dystocia is a matter of considerable obstetric judgment and skill. There is an inverse relationship between the incidence of brachial plexus injuries from shoulder dystocia and the experience of the obstetrician.[79] Shoulder dystocia culminating in an injury that is permanent (1 in 10,000 births) is so rare[80] that all of the recommendations on prevention are based on accumulated wisdom and opinion rather than evidence-based medicine. Athukorala and coauthors demonstrated the paucity of evidence for interventions in their systematic review[81] and pointed to the flimsy foundation underlying any obstetrician who would criticize another's management of shoulder dystocia or say that any particular approach in his or her own hands would have prevented an injury.

Abnormalities of the Third Stage

Placental Separation and Control of Uterine Bleeding

The third stage of labor is defined as the time from delivery of the infant to delivery of the placenta. For all practical purposes, one should include the hour after the delivery of the placenta in the third stage of labor, because it is during this time that the patient is at greatest risk for postpartum hemorrhage.

After the infant is born, the uterus contracts, and placental separation occurs by cleavage along the plane of the decidua basalis. Placental separation usually is complete by the time two contractions have occurred, although several additional contractions may be necessary to accomplish expulsion of the placenta from the uterus. Large venous sinuses are exposed after separation of the placenta, and control of bleeding from these sinuses depends primarily on contraction of uterine muscle and only secondarily on coagulation and thrombus formation in the placental site. The average blood loss during a normal vaginal delivery is about 600 mL.[82] In the young, healthy parturient, acute blood loss is well tolerated because of the increased blood volume of pregnancy and the decrease in vascular volume that occurs with the reduction of the uteroplacental circulation at the time of birth.

Management of the placenta in the third stage is a matter of debate among qualified obstetricians. Elective manual removal of the placenta, if performed promptly, has been associated with no increase in puerperal morbidity. Advantages include immediate identification of retained placental fragments and intrauterine extensions of cervical lacerations and shortened time of placental removal.[83,84] Manual removal, however, is not a painless procedure in the unanesthetized patient, and it is unnecessarily invasive in most cases. Gentle massage of the uterine fundus encourages uterine contractions and helps one to detect changes in the shape of the uterus that signal placental separation. Vigorous fundal massage accomplishes nothing, is painful, and could, if combined with excessive traction on the umbilical cord of a placenta implanted in the fundus of the uterus, promote uterine inversion.

The prophylactic administration of a uterotonic medication to reduce blood loss, either immediately after delivery of the infant or after delivery of the placenta, is a generally accepted practice, and prospective trials show that it decreases blood loss and reduces the need for therapeutic oxytocics.[85] These trials also found no difference in effectiveness of ergot preparations compared with oxytocin, although there were nonsignificant trends toward an increased need for manual removal of the placenta and for blood transfusions and an increase in blood pressure associated with the use of ergot alkaloids. Intravenous oxytocin is the drug of choice on most obstetric services. Prophylactic administration of the thermostabile prostaglandin E_1 analog, misoprostol, has been used to reduce bleeding in the third stage of labor.[86-89]

Retained Placenta

If the placenta has not been delivered with gentle umbilical cord traction and uterine massage after 30 minutes, it should be removed manually under general anesthesia or after a tocolytic drug has been given intravenously in combination with sufficient parenteral analgesia. Nitroglycerin is particularly useful in this situation as a tocolytic.[90] It may be given by translingual spray (400-μg premetered spray, 1 to 2 sprays repeated every 3 to 5 minutes for a maximum of three doses in 15 minutes) or by intravenous injection (50 to 150 μg, repeated in 30 to 60 seconds if blood pressure is stable).

In rare instances, placental retention is caused by placenta accreta, the result of defective decidua basalis. It is characterized by the attachment and growth of chorionic villi directly into the myometrium. If the placenta cannot be removed manually and placenta accreta is suspected, hysterectomy is usually required to avoid catastrophic hemorrhage. The etiology of placenta accreta is not known, but there is a strong association with implantation of the placenta in the lower uterine segment, placenta previa, and prior cesarean delivery.

A report of 22 cases of placenta accreta by Read and coworkers[91] suggested that, in cases of focal or partial placenta accreta without excessive blood loss, conservative management may be successful. The conservative approach includes curettage of the retained placenta or suturing of the bleeding site (in cases of cesarean delivery); it should be considered only if preservation of fertility is of utmost importance and with the awareness that hysterectomy will be necessary if the conservative approach does not promptly control the blood loss. Descargues and associates[92] described the role of prophylactic, selective embolization of the uterine arteries in cases of abnormal placentation diagnosed before delivery.

The episiotomy and vaginal or cervical lacerations are also sources of blood loss in the third stage of labor. Careful inspection of the vagina and cervix immediately after delivery allows one to identify lacerations of these structures so that they can be repaired promptly. Prompt repair also facilitates the management of an unexpected hemorrhage in the immediate recovery period by allowing the obstetrician to promptly attend to uterine atony.

Postpartum Hemorrhage

In the event of an immediate postpartum hemorrhage, the patient's vital signs should be monitored frequently, adequate intravenous lines should be established promptly, adequate fluid replacement should be started with infusion of lactated Ringer solution, and preparations should be made for blood transfusion. Thereafter, a prompt review should be made seeking possible sources of hemorrhage, including uterine atony; cervical, vaginal, or uterine lacerations; coagulopathies (spontaneous or iatrogenic); adherent placenta (accreta); and uterine inversion. Real-time ultrasound scanning is helpful in identifying retained portions of placenta or residual blood clots within the uterus.

Because the usual source of hemorrhage is uterine atony, intravenous oxytocin should be given in amounts adequate to compensate for the decreased sensitivity of the postpartum uterus to this drug.[93] Usually, 20 to 30 units of oxytocin in 1000 mL of fluid, given at an infusion rate not to exceed 100 mU/min, suffices. Because this amount of oxytocin far exceeds the threshold for its maximum antidiuretic effect,[94] it must be recognized that fluid overloading is a potential danger in these patients. Bolus injections of oxytocin could cause hypotension and should be avoided, especially in patients who are at risk for volume depletion from hemorrhage.[95] Methylergonovine or ergonovine maleate, given in doses of 0.2 mg intramuscularly, is often effective in maintaining uterine tonus, but such drugs should not be given intravenously because of the danger of hypertension, central nervous system vasospasm, and hemorrhage.[96]

Increasingly, the 15-methyl analog of prostaglandin $F_{2\alpha}$ (carboprost tromethamine) is being used to treat uterine atony if oxytocin infusion is not successful.[97] The recommended dose is 250 μg intramuscularly, which can be repeated within a few minutes if the first injection does not suffice. Prostaglandin, particularly prostaglandin $F_{2\alpha}$, should be used with great caution, if at all, in patients with cardiovascular disease or asthma.

Based on its demonstrated effectiveness as a prophylactic measure against hemorrhage when given in the third stage of labor equivalent to oxytocin and Methergine, misoprostol has been used to manage severe postpartum hemorrhage. Abdel-Aleem and colleagues[98] gave 1000 μg of misoprostol rectally, and Adekanmi and associates[99] administered 800 μg of misoprostol into the uterus transvaginally to control hemorrhage. Both authors reported successes after failure of conventional pharmacotherapy.

In some cases, uterine atony and uterine hemorrhage persist despite all measures taken to enhance uterine contractions and after other possible sources of vaginal or cervical hemorrhage have been excluded. In these situations, exploratory laparotomy is often necessary (see Chapter 57).

During preparation for laparotomy, one can take several measures that may adequately control the hemorrhage and avoid an operative procedure:

- Use of a large Foley catheter balloon as a tamponade to halt bleeding from a low placental implantation site[100]
- Packing of the uterine cavity with sterile gauze (although no well-designed study has been undertaken to prove that packing is effective, retrospective evidence indicates that this measure can control hemorrhage resulting from atony in some cases[101])
- For some patients, selective embolization of pelvic vessels to control hemorrhage adequately, in hospitals where the necessary facilities and personnel are available[102]

If all of these procedures have been tried in vain, laparotomy is performed with one or more of the following goals: (1) to identify any sources of occult intra-abdominal bleeding, such as unexpected uterine laceration; (2) to control the bleeding by appropriate arterial ligations; (3) in the most extreme and refractory cases, to perform hysterectomy.

When laparotomy is performed for postpartum hemorrhage, the patient should be placed in semilithotomy position. Sterile drapes should be applied in such a way that one observer can, with a sterile speculum, examine the vagina and cervix to determine when the bleeding has ceased. If major uterine lacerations are not found, the uterine arteries should be ligated by the method described by O'Leary and O'Leary[103] (see Chapter 57). If this measure does not control uterine bleeding, the hypogastric arteries should be ligated. In 1997, B-Lynch and colleagues[104] described a "brace" suturing technique that results in closure of the uterine blood supply. Other authors have confirmed the effectiveness of this uterine-conserving technique in small case series.[105,106] The Hayman technique is a simpler way to "brace" suture the uterus.[106]

Burchell[107] described the pelvic vascular supply and demonstrated that the transient decreases in blood pressure and blood flow through regional vessels that occur at the time of internal iliac artery ligation are responsible for the control of hemorrhage. Because of the ample collateral circulation, there appear to be no long-term consequences of hypogastric artery ligation, and women have delivered normal infants in subsequent pregnancies after undergoing this procedure. Occasionally, a patient complains of mild bladder dysfunction and buttock pain in the immediate postoperative period, but these symptoms are transient.

In cases of extensive postpartum hemorrhage, the use of a central venous pressure line or a Swan-Ganz catheter facilitates more accurate monitoring of the cardiovascular status of the patient and avoids serious errors of hydration and pulmonary edema[108,109] (see Chapter 57).

Inversion of the Uterus

Inversion of the uterus, a rare but dramatic complication of the third stage of labor and the immediate puerperium, must be recognized and corrected promptly to avoid serious long-term morbidity.[110] Uterine inversion is probably related to fundal implantation of the placenta, which results in thinning of the uterine wall in the area of implantation. Fundal implantation occurs in only 10% of all pregnancies but has been found in virtually all reported cases of acute puerperal uterine inversion in which the site of placental implantation was recorded.[110,111] The thin fundal area of the myometrium invaginates as the placenta separates, whereupon the inversion proceeds, with the uterus virtually delivering itself inside out. With this scenario in mind, one can easily imagine that vigorous fundal pressure or excessive cord traction could contribute to the tendency to inversion in a uterus predisposed by fundal implantation of the placenta.

Complete uterine inversion occurs when the inverted fundus extends beyond the cervix, usually looking like a beefy-red mass at the vaginal introitus. Incomplete inversions occur when the inverted fundus has not extended beyond the external cervical os. These cases are not as obvious and may be detected only by bimanual or visual examination of the cervix. In cases of postpartum hemorrhage in which the uterine fundus cannot be palpated abdominally, incomplete uterine inversion should be suspected.

Tocolytic drugs, including magnesium sulfate,[112] β-mimetic compounds,[113] and nitroglycerin[114] have been used to assist in reinversion of the uterus. Because of the extensive blood loss and shock that often are associated with uterine inversion, an anesthesiologist should be summoned as soon as the diagnosis is recognized so that general anesthesia can be available if reinversion using tocolysis fails.

The technique of reinversion is the same whether it is accomplished with intravenous tocolysis or general anesthesia. The uterus is reinverted with gentle but firm and persistent pressure applied on the fundus to elevate it into the vagina.[115] In most cases, this technique, which presumably results in reinversion by indirect traction on the round ligaments when the uterus is elevated into the abdomen, is successful. Authorities disagree about whether the placenta, which is often attached to the inverted fundus, should be removed before attempts to reinvert the fundus are made. The practical matter is that the Johnson technique for reinversion[115] is easier if the placenta is not in place.

If the diagnosis is made and reinversion is accomplished promptly, there are no long-term sequelae. If the complication is unrecognized and reinversion is delayed, tissue edema magnifies the constriction of the cervix around the inverted fundus, making reinversion difficult. Tissue necrosis and damage to the bladder or urethra could ensue.

If the Johnson method of reinversion is not successful, laparotomy should be performed. The first step is to grasp the round ligaments about 1 inch into the inverted uterus and exert traction while an assistant elevates the uterus with a hand in the vagina. This procedure, described by Huntington,[116] may fail because the inverted fundus is too tightly trapped below the cervical ring, in which case the Haultain[117] procedure may be performed. In the Haultain procedure, a longitudinal incision is made posteriorly through the inverted fundus, allowing ample room to reinvert the fundus. The incision is then closed, leaving the equivalent of a classic cesarean incision on the posterior surface of the uterus. If uterine inversion is recognized and treated promptly, an operative procedure is rarely necessary to accomplish reinversion.

The third stage of labor and the immediate puerperal recovery period are a crucial time for the parturient. Occasionally, uterine hemorrhage goes undetected or is recognized but treated inadequately. Acute tubular necrosis, pituitary necrosis, and adult respiratory distress syndrome—all recognized complications of puerperal shock and hypoxia—can be avoided by careful observation of all patients during this time and by deliberate and aggressive management of hemorrhage if it occurs.

Induction of Labor

Induction of labor is elective (i.e., performed for the convenience of the patient or professional staff) or is indicated for medical, obstetric, or fetal complications of pregnancy.

Between 1989 and 1998 in the United States, there was an increase in the incidence of induction of labor, from 9% to 19% of all births (Fig. 36-3).[118,119] In 1998, the incidence of induction of labor varied widely from region to region, from 10.9% in Hawaii to 41.6% in Wisconsin. Also, the increase in the incidence of indicated induction was significantly smaller than the overall increase (70% to 100% increase), suggesting that the rate of elective induction increased more rapidly than did the rate of indicated induction.

Nicholson and colleagues[120] and Caughey and colleagues[121] questioned the conventional wisdom that induction is a risk factor for abdominal delivery. They pointed out that comparisons between women induced at a given gestational age and those in spontaneous labor at that age overestimate the risk of cesarean section, because the real comparison group for induced women should be the entire cohort awaiting spontaneous labor. Analysis of cohorts with their novel approach indicated that induction reduces the risk of abdominal delivery compared to expectant management, which is the real choice a woman and her obstetrician face. Verification of this inversion of conventional wisdom in prospective trials would radically change the practice of contemporary obstetrics.

Elective Induction

Elective induction of labor is often justified on one or more of the following grounds:

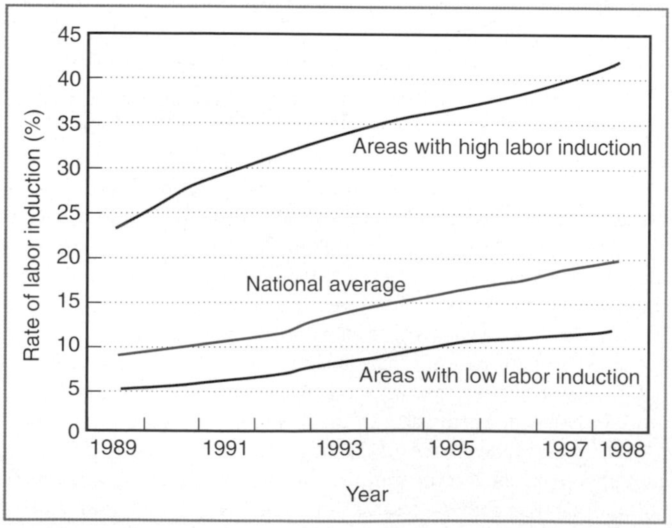

FIGURE 36-3 **Rate of labor induction in the United States, 1989-1998.** (From Zhang J, Yancey MK, Henderson CE: U.S. national trends in labor induction, 1989-1998. J Reprod Med 47:121, 2002. Printed with permission from the Journal of Reproductive Medicine.)

- To assure the patient that the physician with whom she has good rapport will be present during delivery
- To ensure that labor will occur when maximum physician, nursing, and support personnel coverage is available in case of labor complications
- To enable the patient to plan for care of her home and other children and allow her partner to make suitable arrangements to be with her during labor and delivery

The studies by Keettel at the University of Iowa between 1957 and 1966 established the safety of elective induction of labor in patients who were at term and whose cervix was partially effaced and dilated at least 2 cm.[122] Subsequent studies confirmed this salutary experience.[123,124] Follow-up studies of children for as long as 8 years found no evidence of neurodevelopmental abnormalities related to elective induction of labor.[125,126]

There are two major risks of elective induction of labor: an increased risk for cesarean delivery and an increased risk for neonatal respiratory morbidity. Elective induction of labor at term is associated with a twofold increased incidence of cesarean delivery compared with spontaneous labor.[127,128] This increase is confined almost entirely to nulliparous women and, more specifically, to those in whom the induction of labor is attempted when the cervix is not well effaced and somewhat dilated.[129,130] This risk can be minimized by restricting elective induction of labor to patients with a favorable or ripe cervix.

An objective classification for selection of patients who are "favorable" for induction of labor[131] is shown in Table 36-5. Bishop found that a pelvic score of 9 or greater, in the term multipara, was associated with no failed inductions of labor in his series and that the average duration of labor was 4 hours. Although the criteria for successful induction of labor as described by Bishop applied only to multiparous women, subsequent studies showed the usefulness of Bishop's scoring system in nulliparous patients.[132] There is a 50% risk of failed induction of labor in nulliparous women at term for whom the Bishop pelvic score is 5 or less. Lange and colleagues,[133] in a study of induction of labor in 808 patients, found that dilatation was the most important of the five components in the Bishop score and recommended that it be scored at twice the value given by Bishop. Most experienced obstetricians would agree with this. Transvaginal ultrasound examination of the cervix does not improve on the Bishop score in predicting the success of induction of labor.[134,135] The presence of fetal fibronectin (fFN) in cervical and vaginal secretions is an additional means for predicting the success of induction of labor.[136,137] The role that vaginal

TABLE 36-5 PELVIC SCORING TABLE FOR SELECTION OF PATIENTS FOR ELECTIVE INDUCTION*

	Points Assigned			
Factor	**0**	**1**	**2**	**3**
Dilation (cm)	0	1-2	3-4	5-6
Effacement (%)	0-30	40-50	60-70	80
Station	−3	−2	−1 or 0	+1 or +2
Consistency	Firm	Medium	Soft	—
Position	Posterior	Middle	Anterior	—

***The total pelvic score is obtained by adding the points scored for each factor.**
Adapted from Bishop EH: Pelvic scoring for elective induction. Obstet Gynecol 24:266, 1964.

fFN can play in selecting patients for elective induction of labor has yet to be determined.[138]

Amniotomy is often successful in inducing labor in patients who have a favorable cervix, although the mechanism of action is not entirely clear. Mitchell and associates[139] showed that artificial rupture of the membranes is followed by a substantial increase in plasma prostaglandins. In one of the largest studies of elective induction of labor, Keettel[122] found that, if the patient was at term with a vertex presentation, the fetal vertex was engaged in the pelvis, and the cervix was at least 2 cm dilated and partially effaced, only 3.4% of patients required oxytocin infusion after amniotomy to induce labor successfully. If the use of oxytocin is necessary, it should be given by intravenous infusion, preferably by constant infusion pump, with monitoring of the fetal heart rate, uterine contractions, and maternal vital signs. Whether induction is elective or indicated, adequate stimulation of uterine contractions is important in reducing the incidence of failed induction of labor. Rouse and associates[11] and Lin and Rouse[140] showed the effectiveness of requiring a minimum of 12 hours of oxytocin stimulation after membrane rupture before failed labor induction is diagnosed.

The second major risk of elective induction of labor is neonatal respiratory morbidity.[141,142] This is caused, in part, by surfactant deficiency resulting from unexpected delivery of a premature infant. Consequently, scrupulous attention to confirmation of gestational age is necessary. The following criteria should be fulfilled before a patient is considered a candidate for induction:

1. A well-established ovulation date, which can be determined by one of the following:
   a. A regular menstrual history prior to the last menstrual period; the last menstrual period should not be considered normal if it occurred after cessation of oral contraceptive use
   b. Basal body temperature chart demonstrating a biphasic rise
   c. Clomiphene induction of ovulation followed by early confirmation of ovulation in pregnancy
   d. Artificial insemination or in vitro fertilization and embryo transfer
2. Examination of the patient by the 14th week of pregnancy in which the uterine size was consistent with estimated gestational dates
3. Sonographic estimation of fetal weight performed before 20 weeks' gestation
4. Bishop pelvic score of 6 or greater

Using these criteria, the patient should be considered for elective induction of labor at 40 weeks (280 ± 3 days) after the last menstrual period, if the menstrual interval is 28 days, or at 266 days ± 3 days after the suspected ovulation date.

For some infants who develop respiratory morbidity after elective induction of labor, the cause is that birth takes place before the occurrence of the normal events associated with parturition that prepare the fetus for the transition to extrauterine life.[143] One of the critical transition phenomena is a decrease in fetal lung fluid associated with the spontaneous onset of labor.[144,145] If this does not occur, the most common manifestation in the newborn is "wet lung syndrome," which clears spontaneously in a few hours. In some infants, the respiratory morbidity is more serious, involving persistence of the fetal circulation and requiring mechanical ventilation.[146]

Waiting until the pregnancy is at 40 weeks' gestation and the cervix is well effaced and partially dilated before induction of labor can minimize the risks of cesarean delivery and neonatal respiratory morbidity. If an obstetrics service concludes that elective induction of labor is permissible, the professional staff, including physicians and nurses from labor and delivery and the nursery, should collectively agree on criteria for patient selection and draw up a protocol for the labor induction procedure. After such guidelines of care are established, elective induction of labor should undergo periodic review to determine the degree of compliance with the guidelines and to identify any related maternal or perinatal morbidity.

Indicated Induction

Induction of labor is indicated if prolongation of pregnancy is dangerous for either the mother or the fetus and there are no contraindications to amniotomy or the augmentation of uterine contractions. Maternal indications include the following:

- Severe pregnancy-induced hypertension
- Fetal death
- Chorioamnionitis

Fetal indications for pregnancy termination include any condition in which a variety of fetal tests demonstrate significant fetal jeopardy in any of the following settings:

- Diabetes mellitus
- Post-term pregnancy, especially in association with oligohydramnios
- Hypertensive complications of pregnancy
- Intrauterine growth restriction
- Isoimmunization
- Chorioamnionitis
- Premature rupture of the membranes with established fetal maturity

Induction of labor is contraindicated any time that spontaneous labor and delivery would be more dangerous for the mother or fetus than abdominal delivery. Such conditions include

- Acute severe fetal distress
- Shoulder presentation
- Floating fetal presenting part
- Uncontrolled hemorrhage
- Placenta previa
- Previous uterine incision that would preclude a trial of labor

The following are relative contraindications to induction of labor:

- Grand multiparity (five or more previous pregnancies beyond 20 weeks' gestation)
- Multiple pregnancy
- Suspected CPD
- Breech presentation
- Inability to adequately monitor the fetal heart rate throughout labor

The relative contraindications are all controversial, and there are mitigating circumstances under which induction of labor might be attempted in any of them.

If the cervical status is favorable and the vertex is well engaged (Bishop pelvic score ≥6), the preferred method of labor induction is amniotomy, followed, if necessary, by a closely monitored oxytocin infusion. If the cervical status is not favorable, as is common when delivery is indicated for maternal or fetal complications, several methods may improve cervical effacement and dilatation.

Danforth[147] was among the first to study the effect of pregnancy on the cervix and to describe the histology of cervical softening and effacement. The cervix is composed largely of connective tissue, including types I, III, and IV collagen, and only 10% to 15% smooth muscle.[148] Before the onset of labor, the collagen content of the cervix decreases by 30% to 50% as the content of water and noncollagen and nonelastin proteins increases. The process of cervical ripening involves the production of cytokines (tumor necrosis factor α, interleukin 1β [IL-1β], IL-6, IL-8) and the extravasation of neutrophils into the cervical stroma. Degranulation of the neutrophils releases proteases that are involved in the modification of cervical collagen.[149] The proteolytic enzymes are responsible for degrading cross-linked, newly synthesized collagen and thereby contribute to the rearrangement of collagen cells that is a hallmark of cervical softening. Apoptosis of smooth muscle cells in the cervix may also contribute to cervical ripening.[150] That this process is a genetically determined, timed event may explain the length of gestation. Although the specific endocrine and biomolecular mechanisms of cervical ripening (including the role of prostaglandins) are not fully understood, the result of this phenomenon is softening, thinning, and early dilation of the cervix.

Multiple drugs and devices have been used to enhance cervical ripening: oxytocin, estrogen, corticosteroids, hyaluronidase, breast stimulation, sexual intercourse, relaxin, castor oil, prostaglandin E_1 (PGE_1) and E_2 (PGE_2), mifepristone, hydrophilic cervical inserts, balloon catheters, and extra-amniotic saline infusion. Systematic reviews of the studies of most of these methods are included in the Cochrane Database. Table 36-6 lists methods that have been found to be ineffective or unsafe or for other reasons not commonly used. Table 36-7 summarizes the findings of the systematic reviews in the Cochrane Database regarding methods of cervical ripening that are presently in common use and for which there is some evidence of both efficacy and safety. The end points of the studies on cervical ripening included changes in effacement and dilatation of the cervix, time of delivery after the medication or device was applied, and incidence of cesarean delivery. Vaginal applications of PGE_2, which are available in the United States as dinoprostone (Prepidil and Cervidil), have been shown to be effective in promoting cervical ripening.[151]

Misoprostol (PGE_1), originally approved for use in preventing gastric ulcers induced by nonsteroidal anti-inflammatory drugs, has proved to be an effective cervical ripening agent when applied intravaginally in doses of 25 or 50 µg. A meta-analysis by Hofmeyr and Gulmezoglu[152] found that misoprostol was more effective in cervical

TABLE 36-6 CERVICAL RIPENING—METHODS EITHER INEFFECTIVE OR NOT IN COMMON USE

Method of Cervical Ripening	Online Source	No. of Trials in Review	Major Findings
Oxytocin	Kelly & Tan, (3):CD003246, 2001	58	Less effective than intracervical or intravaginal PGE_2
Estrogen	Thomas, Kelly, & Kavanagh, (4): CD003393, 2001	6	Insufficient data to determine efficacy
Corticosteroids	Kavanagh, Kelly, & Thomas, (2): CD003100, 2001 (updated 2006)	2	Insufficient data to determine efficacy; not recommended for clinical practice
Hyaluronidase	Kavanagh, Kelly, & Thomas, (2): CD003097, 2001 (updated 2005)	8	Insufficient data to determine efficacy
Breast stimulation	Kavanagh, Kelly, & Thomas, (4): CD003392, 2001 (updated 2005)	6	Effective in increasing incidence of women in labor within 72 hours, but safety issues not fully evaluated
Sexual intercourse	Kavanagh, Kelly, & Thomas, (2): CD003093, 2001	6	Insufficient data to determine efficacy
Castor oil	Kelly, Kavanagh, & Thomas, (2): CD003099, 2001	1	No reduction in cesarean delivery rate; high incidence of side effects
Relaxin	Kelly, Kavanagh, & Thomas, (2): CD003103, 2001	4	Improves cervical softening and effacement but does not increase success of induction of labor; not clinically useful
Extra-amniotic prostaglandin	Hutton & Mozurkewich, (2): CD003092, 2001	10	Compared with intravaginal or intracervical PGE_2 or Foley catheter, no difference in outcomes
Intravenous prostaglandin	Luckas & Bricker, (4):CD002864, 2000	13	No more effective than IV oxytocin, with more side effects and uterine hyperstimulation
Stripping (sweeping) membranes	Boulvain, Stan, & Irion, (4): CD000451, 1997 (updated 2004)	22	Does not produce clinically important benefits; safe but associated with patient discomfort
Mifepristone	Neilson, (4):CD002865, 2000	7	Insufficient data to determine efficacy
Oral PGE_1	Alfirevic & Weeks, (4):CD001338, 2000 (updated 2005)	41	No evidence for greater efficacy than intravaginal PGE_1; doses $\geq$100 µg increase the incidence of side effects and uterine hyperstimulation
Oral PGE_2	French, (2):CD003098, 2001	19	No more effective than IV oxytocin, with more side effects

From Cochrane Database of Systemic Reviews. Available at http://www.cochrane.org/reviews/index.htm.

TABLE 36-7 CERVICAL RIPENING—METHODS COMMONLY USED

Method of Cervical Ripening	Online Source	No. Trials in Review	Major Findings
Mechanical methods (laminaria Foley catheter)	Boulvain et al, (4):CD001233, 2001	45	Compared with intravaginal and intracervical PGE_2, no reduction in cesarean delivery rate and lower incidence of uterine hyperstimulation
Intravaginal and intracervical PGE_2	Boulvain, Kelly, Irion, (1): CD006971, 2008	52	Compared with placebo, increased incidence of vaginal delivery within 24 hr but no decrease in cesarean delivery
Intravaginal PGE_1	Hofmeyr & Gülmezoglu, (1): CD000941, 1998 (updated 2002)	70	Compared with vaginal or cervical PGE_2, increased incidence of vaginal delivery within 24 hr, with no difference in cesarean delivery rate and a higher incidence of uterine hyperstimulation

From Cochrane Database of Systemic Reviews. Available at http://www.cochrane.org/reviews/index.htm.

ripening and induction of labor than intravaginal or intracervical PGE_2. Although intravaginal misoprostol in doses of 25 μg compared with 50 μg results in greater need for oxytocin augmentation, there is less uterine hyperstimulation; therefore, the most commonly recommended regimen is 25 μg repeated every 4 hours. In April 2002, the manufacturer of misoprostol (Cytotec) revised the drug labeling information to acknowledge use of the medication for cervical ripening and induction of labor, although the U.S. Food and Drug Administration has not formally approved the drug for this use.

A systematic review of the studies of various cervical inserts, including laminaria tents and balloon catheters, found that these devices (compared with intravaginal PGE_2) achieved a lower rate of delivery within 24 hours, resulted in no difference in cesarean delivery rate, and were less likely to cause uterine hyperstimulation.[153] Small studies found that the use of the Foley catheter compared favorably with intravaginal PGE_1 (misoprostol) for cervical ripening,[154] but larger prospective trials are needed to confirm this impression.

Although randomized trials have shown that prostaglandins in general, and misoprostol specifically, result in cervical ripening as manifest in a significant increase in the Bishop pelvic score, they have not demonstrated a significant decrease in the incidence of failed induction of labor or a decrease in the risk of cesarean delivery after induction of labor in nulliparous patients. This suggests that failed induction of labor could be the result of several incomplete mechanisms of parturition, of which cervical ripening is but one manifestation.

Abnormal Presentations

Breech Presentation

Breech presentation occurs in approximately 3% to 4% of all deliveries. Its incidence decreases with advancing gestation. Weisman,[155] using periodic radiographic examination throughout pregnancy, found that 24% of fetuses were in breech presentation at 18-22 weeks of gestation, 8% at 28 to 30 weeks, 7% at 34 weeks, and 2.8% at 38 to 40 weeks. It is generally agreed that higher rates of neonatal morbidity and mortality are associated with breech presentation than with cephalic presentation at all gestational ages and birth weights.[156] There is less agreement about what can be done to eliminate the risk for the infant in breech presentation at the time of delivery.

Part of the problem could be inherent in the etiology of breech presentation itself. Term breech presentation is associated with fundal-cornual implantation of the placenta, which occurs in only 7% of all pregnancies.[157] This association suggests that breech presentation often is related to a space problem in the uterus: Given the fundal-placental implantation, an otherwise normal fetus finds it more comfortable to assume a breech position. Other studies have suggested that breech presentation could result from abnormal motor ability or diminished muscle tone in the fetus.

Braun and colleagues,[158] reporting from a dysmorphology clinic, showed that the expected incidence of breech presentation (corrected for gestational age) was higher in fetuses with a variety of congenital disorders. Specifically, infants with neuromuscular disorders had an inordinately high rate of breech presentation at delivery.[159,160] Furthermore, McBride and associates[161] found that 100 children delivered in a breech presentation at term and studied at 5 years of age scored less well on motor skills than children delivered in cephalic presentations, regardless of the method by which the breech delivery was accomplished. These results suggested that, at least in some cases, the fetus remains in a breech position because it is less capable of movement within the uterus. If these concepts are accurate, the outcome for the fetus in a breech presentation could depend to a great extent on the reason for the breech position rather than the eventual mode of delivery.

Risks to the fetus inherent in breech presentation during labor and delivery include the following:

- Prolapse of the umbilical cord (especially in the footling breech)
- Trapping of the after-coming head by the incompletely dilated cervix (particularly in preterm infants weighing less than 1500 g and in CPD)
- Trauma resulting from extension of the head or nuchal position of the arms

Wright[162] was the first to suggest that a policy of cesarean delivery for all breech presentations would result in the lowest possible perinatal morbidity and mortality rates. Nevertheless, most patients with a term breech presentation were delivered vaginally until the mid-1970s, when the cesarean delivery rate began to increase as a result of the concern for fetal well-being. At one university center, the rate of cesarean delivery for term breech presentation abruptly increased, from 13% in the years 1970 to 1975 to 54% in 1976 to 1977.[163] In that study, a detailed analysis of the eight perinatal deaths that occurred among patients with a term breech presentation who delivered vaginally after having documented criteria for safe vaginal delivery found that six of the deaths would have been prevented by planned cesarean delivery. After 1975, the rate of cesarean delivery for breech presentation increased among most obstetric services in the United States. Data combined largely from retrospective cohort studies comparing vaginal with cesarean birth for patients with term breech presentations showed a small but statistically significant increase in risk of perinatal mortality and morbidity in patients who had vaginal deliveries.[164-166]

In 2000, Hannah and colleagues[167] published the results of a large multicenter, randomized, controlled trial comparing planned vaginal delivery with planned cesarean delivery in patients with a breech presentation at term. This study of 2088 subjects was terminated when an independent data monitoring committee found statistically significant evidence that perinatal morbidity and mortality were greater with planned vaginal delivery, without any significant differences in maternal mortality or serious morbidity. There were several limitations to this study: (1) fewer than 10% of women underwent x-ray pelvimetry (thought by many authorities to be essential in screening patients for safe vaginal delivery); (2) the frequency and use of oxytocin for induction or augmentation of labor were not controlled for in the regression analyses; and (3) most importantly, 22% of patients who delivered vaginally were not attended by an obstetrician, whereas this was true for only one of the patients delivered by cesarean section.[168-170] These and other limitations notwithstanding, the results of this study confirmed the mounting evidence from most of the retrospective studies that even with careful screening of patients with a breech presentation for a trial of labor, the risk of perinatal death and serious morbidity is slightly but significantly greater for planned vaginal delivery than for planned cesarean delivery.

In light of these findings, the ACOG[171] recommended that, if external version is not successful in a woman with a breech presentation at term, the patient should be advised to undergo a planned cesarean delivery. This recommendation does not apply to patients with breech presentation of a second twin.

Long-term developmental outcome (5 years) of surviving infants delivered vaginally in a breech presentation does not differ significantly from that of infants delivered by cesarean section because of breech presentation.[161,172,173]

Breech Vaginal Delivery

Some authorities still take the position that, in the presence of a qualified obstetrician, a patient who fulfills criteria for safe vaginal delivery of a breech presentation can be offered this option.[168,174,175] Because of the declining frequency of breech delivery, however, fewer obstetricians are acquiring the requisite skills to safely allow a trial of labor and vaginal delivery for patients with breech presentations. Criteria for allowing a trial of labor in a breech presentation are as follows:

- Frank or complete breech presentation
- Estimated fetal weight of 2000 to 3800 g
- Normal gynecoid pelvis with adequate measurements
- Flexed fetal head

Safe vaginal delivery of a breech presentation depends, to a great extent, on the experience, judgment, and skill of the obstetrician. If an obstetrician is unsure about his or her skills for vaginal delivery with a breech presentation, cesarean delivery is preferred.

Most authorities agree that radiographic pelvimetry has a place in selecting patients for a trial of labor when there is a breech presentation. Potter and coworkers[176] studied 13 term infants without congenital defects who died from intracranial injury as a result of vaginal breech delivery. In 7 of the 13 mothers, pelvic radiographs (five of which were obtained in the puerperium) revealed diminished pelvic capacity. In the remaining six patients, radiographs were not obtained.

Beischer[177] reviewed the outcome of term breech radiographs. Thirteen patients were delivered by cesarean section; all infants survived. Among the 51 infants delivered vaginally, there were 4 deaths, 3 of which were the result of tentorial tears. That study, together with the report of Todd and Steer[178] of 1006 term breech deliveries, suggested that vaginal delivery is not safe with radiographic pelvic measurements of less than the following:

- Anteroposterior diameter of the inlet, 11 cm
- Widest transverse of the inlet, 12 cm
- Interspinous diameter, 9 cm

Any other encroachment on the space below the inlet also contraindicates vaginal delivery. Pelvimetry performed with computed tomography exposes the fetus to substantially less radiation and is performed with greater facility in most hospitals than conventional x-ray pelvimetry.[179,180] Also, pelvimetry by magnetic resonance imaging has been used for breech presentation, but the cost and the greater time required for this procedure make it less practical than pelvimetry via computed tomography.[181]

Not uncommonly, patients are found to be in labor with an unexpected breech presentation. This will continue to occur despite the increasing practice of planned cesarean delivery for all patients with a term breech presentation. In a study by Zatuchni and Andros,[182] clinical screening of patients with breech presentations at term identified mothers who safely accomplished a vaginal delivery. Screening criteria did not include radiographic pelvimetry. On admission to the hospital in labor, patients were evaluated according to a "diagnostic index" (Table 36-8). In a prospective study of 139 patients with term breech presentations, which excluded patients with a prolapsed umbilical cord, severe congenital anomaly, or uterine bleeding, the authors found that perinatal mortality and morbidity occurred only in patients with an index of 3 or lower and that cesarean delivery of all patients with such an index would have resulted in an abdominal delivery rate of 21.5%.

The method of pain control for a vaginal breech delivery is another controversial issue. Conduction anesthesia has been used with good results,[183] and a case can be made that it prevents the mother from pushing uncontrollably in the second stage and allows for an easier and more comfortable application of the Piper forceps to the after-coming head. In a study of 643 singleton term breech presentations, however, epidural analgesia was associated with longer duration of labor, increased need for augmentation of labor with oxytocin, and a significantly higher rate of cesarean delivery in the second stage of labor.[184] An anesthesiologist can be of great assistance if there is difficulty in the delivery of nuchal arms or the after-coming head.

Fetal monitoring is essential during labor with a breech presentation. Because the fetal abdomen and the insertion of the umbilical cord are in the lower uterine segment during the late first stage and the second stage of labor, significant variable decelerations are more likely to be encountered than with cephalic presentation. For this reason, membranes should be left intact as long as possible, to provide some hydraulic protection against umbilical cord compression. Vaginal breech deliveries are more often associated with significant fetal acidosis than cephalic presentations.[185] Therefore, one must exercise careful

TABLE 36-8 PROGNOSTIC INDEX FOR VAGINAL BREECH DELIVERY*

	Points Assigned		
Factor	**0**	**1**	**2**
Parity	0	>1	—
Gestational age (wk)	39	38	37
Estimated fetal weight	>8 lb (3630 g)	7 lb 1 oz to 7 lb 15 oz (3176–3629 g)	<7 lb (3175 g)
Previous breech deliveries (birth weight >2500 g)	0	1	2
Dilation (cm)	2	3	4
Station	–3 or higher	–2	–1 or lower

*The index is obtained by adding the points scored for each factor.
Adapted from Zatuchni GI, Andros GJ: Prognostic index for vaginal delivery in breech presentation at term: Prospective study. Am J Obstet Gynecol 98:854, 1967.

judgment as to when to intervene for "fetal distress." Fetal blood samples can be obtained from the buttock if there is a suspected or ominous fetal heart rate pattern; if the pH obtained between contractions is lower than 7.20 early in the second stage, abdominal delivery should be considered.

The use of oxytocin for induction of labor or augmentation of abnormal labor in a breech presentation is controversial. In the randomized, controlled trial by Hannah and associates,[167] a disproportionate number (64%) of the perinatal deaths in the intended vaginal delivery arm occurred in labors that were induced or augmented with oxytocin. If oxytocin is used, it must be administered with extraordinary caution.

Skillful, atraumatic delivery, regardless of the route of birth, is essential in keeping infant morbidity to a minimum. Milner[186] showed that application of forceps to the after-coming head was associated with a reduced rate of neonatal mortality from breech delivery. The well-illustrated publication by Piper and Bachman,[187] describing the use of the forceps designed by Piper and presenting in detail the method of breech delivery, should be standard reading for all physicians planning to assist in the vaginal delivery of a breech presentation. Even when the delivery is cesarean, forceps should be available (use of Piper forceps is not necessary), and they should be applied through the uterine incision to the after-coming head if there is any difficulty with its extraction. Calvert[188] found that infants in breech presentation born by cesarean section had a higher incidence of birth asphyxia than a comparable group of infants in cephalic presentation born by cesarean. A uterine incision does not ensure an atraumatic delivery of an infant, especially one in a breech presentation.

External Version

External version substantially reduces the incidence of term breech presentation.[189,190] If the procedure is performed at 36 weeks' gestation, the success rate is approximately 65%. Complications that require immediate delivery, including placental separation and umbilical cord compression, occur in 1% to 2% of patients. The procedure is performed late in gestation and with cesarean delivery capability available, so that prompt delivery can be accomplished if persistent umbilical cord compression or premature separation of the placenta occurs. Tocolytic medications have been used in most series to prevent uterine contractions during the procedure, and the evidence shows that their use improves the success rate of external version.[191] Some have found that the use of epidural analgesia, either with the initial attempt or after a first attempt has failed, improves the success rate of external version, but the extant studies are not large enough to determine the safety of this practice or its cost-effectiveness.[192-194]

Overall, for patients who undergo external version of a breech presentation at 36 weeks' gestation, the risk of cesarean delivery is reduced by 50%. In addition to a reduced morbidity risk for mother and infant, cost savings are substantial.[195] Chan and coauthors[196] compared delivery outcomes in pregnancies that had undergone successful external cephalic version for breech presentation with singleton vertex presentations without external version. After successful external version, patients had significantly higher rates of instrumental delivery and emergency cesarean delivery. The higher risk of operative delivery was the result of an increase in several major indications: fetal heart rate abnormalities, failure of labor to progress, and failed induction of labor. It is apparent that external cephalic version, even when successful, does not eliminate all of the risks inherent in breech presentation.

Contraindications to external version include the following:

- Uterine anomalies
- Third-trimester bleeding
- Multiple gestation
- Oligohydramnios
- Evidence of uteroplacental insufficiency
- A nuchal cord as identified by ultrasonography
- Previous cesarean delivery or other significant uterine surgery
- Obvious CPD

Primiparity, maternal obesity, advanced gestation, anterior implantation of the placenta, and excessive fetal weight have been associated with decreased success of external version but are not in themselves contraindications.

The procedure should be performed in a hospital in which cesarean delivery can be accomplished if unrelenting fetal distress occurs. A real-time ultrasonographic scan is performed to confirm the breech presentation; to detect multiple gestation, oligohydramnios, or fetal abnormalities; and to measure fetal dimensions.

Following a reactive nonstress test, a tocolytic drug is administered (terbutaline sulfate, 0.25 mg subcutaneously). (Some obstetricians prefer to first attempt version without tocolysis, proceeding with external version under tocolysis if this is unsuccessful.) After the uterus relaxes, the version is attempted. One person can elevate and laterally displace the breech while a second person manipulates the fetal head in the opposite direction. Mineral oil on the abdomen facilitates movement of the hands during the procedure. A forward roll is attempted; if this is unsuccessful, a backward roll is tried. The fetal heart rate should be monitored intermittently with Doppler or real-time scanning. Fetal bradycardia occurs in about 20% of cases but almost always subsides after the manipulation ceases. External fetal heart rate monitoring is continued for 1 hour, after which the patient is discharged. Patients who are Rh-negative and who have a negative antibody titer should be given 1 unit (300 μg) of Rh immune globulin because of the risk of fetal-maternal transfusion associated with version (6% to 28%).[197,198]

Transverse Lie (Shoulder Presentation)

Transverse lie occurs in approximately 1 of every 300 deliveries.[199] Cruikshank and White,[200] reporting on 118 shoulder presentations, found that prematurity (38%) and high parity (87% of patients had already borne three or more infants) were the two most frequently associated conditions. Premature rupture of membranes (30%) and placenta previa (10%) are also more common in transverse lie than in longitudinal presentation. The high perinatal mortality rates (3.9% to 24%) associated with transverse lie[199] are almost surely a result of the high prevalence of low-birth-weight infants in shoulder presentations, although prolapse of the umbilical cord occasionally results in perinatal death of a term infant in transverse lie. These accidents typically happen unexpectedly, when spontaneous rupture of the membranes occurs outside the hospital setting. In such cases, the patient is usually admitted to the hospital with a severely asphyxiated or dead fetus.

The diagnosis can usually be made by palpation of the abdomen. Not infrequently, the patient notes that the fetus is in an unusual position and draws this fact to the physician's attention. The fetal position can be confirmed by real-time ultrasonography.

Management of the patient with a confirmed diagnosis of transverse lie depends on the length of gestation, the size of the fetus, the position of the placenta, and whether the membranes have ruptured. If the patient is in labor with a transverse lie and the expected fetal weight and gestational age are below those compatible with a reasonable (10%) chance of survival, no intervention is necessary beyond attempts to stop labor in the interest of increasing fetal weight and maturity before delivery. A fetus of this size (usually <600 g) eventually is delivered vaginally in shoulder presentation *(conduplicato corpore)* without undue trauma to the mother. If the gestational age or expected fetal weight is such that the chance for neonatal survival, in the absence of severe asphyxia or trauma, is greater than 10%, cesarean delivery is usually necessary, especially if the membranes are ruptured or placenta previa is present.

The role of external version in the management of transverse lie is highly controversial. Before 36 to 37 weeks' gestation in patients who are not in labor, external version should not be attempted because of the danger of cord entanglement or placental trauma and the difficulty of maintaining the normal axial lie after version. Moreover, there is the possibility that spontaneous version to a longitudinal lie will occur with additional growth and maturity of the fetus or with the onset of contractions. However, if a transverse lie is identified at or beyond 36 to 37 weeks' gestation in a patient with intact membranes, and CPD and placenta previa are not present, external version often results in a longitudinal lie and a normal vaginal delivery.

Edwards and Nicholson[201] demonstrated the benefits of a policy of admitting to the hospital all patients beyond 37 weeks' gestation in whom "unstable lie" is diagnosed. Their protocol in such patients was to search for etiologic factors and then, provided CPD and placenta previa were excluded, to perform external version followed by induction of labor after 38 weeks' gestation. In 102 cases so managed, 86 patients delivered vaginally, with only 1 case of cord prolapse and no perinatal deaths. In contrast, in 50 cases of unstable lie at or beyond 37 weeks' gestation in which the onset of spontaneous labor was awaited, there were 10 cases of prolapsed cord and 4 perinatal deaths. This experience suggests that, when a transverse or oblique lie is identified at or beyond 37 weeks' gestation, thorough etiologic evaluation and admission to the hospital should be considered.

If fetal mobility is restricted by well-advanced labor or the absence of amniotic fluid, or if placenta previa or CPD is detected, abdominal delivery in transverse lie is mandatory. Most authorities advise a low vertical or classic uterine incision in such cases, although Cruikshank and White[200] found an extraordinarily high maternal morbidity rate (severe intraperitoneal infection, 21%; maternal death, 8.3%) associated with classic incisions for delivery in shoulder presentations. The low transverse incision often suffices in cases of a back-up transverse lie, and the high transverse incision described by Durfee[202] can be used in cases of a back-down shoulder presentation.

Finally, a technique of intra-abdominal version to allow the use of a low transverse incision has been described.[203] Use of a transverse rather than a vertical incision decreases the overall maternal morbidity of cesarean delivery by reducing acute puerperal complications associated with vertical incisions and by allowing the option of managing subsequent pregnancies with a trial of labor and vaginal delivery. However, uterine incision should always be chosen with the primary purpose of abdominal delivery in mind (i.e., to avoid fetal trauma and asphyxia).

Deflection Abnormalities

Brow and face presentations are manifestations of different degrees of deflection of a cephalic presentation and therefore can be considered together. Seeds and Cefalo[199] reviewed the literature regarding brow and face presentations. Each occurs with a frequency of about 1 in 500 deliveries, although the incidence probably would be higher if all fetal presentations were assessed carefully early in labor. About 50% of such diagnoses are not made until the second stage of labor; many of the deflection problems detected early in labor correct themselves spontaneously as labor progresses.

With the exception of anencephaly, which almost always results in a face presentation, fetal anomalies do not seem to account for deflection problems in labor. Commonly reported etiologic factors in brow and face presentations include

- CPD
- Increased parity
- Prematurity
- Premature rupture of membranes

Apart from prematurity and anencephaly, the major problem associated with deflection presentations is dysfunctional labor in brow presentations. Friedman[3] found that face presentation, contrary to generally held clinical impressions, did not appear to affect the course of labor significantly in either nulliparas or multiparas.

Brow presentation, in contrast, was associated with abnormalities of descent and longer second stage of labor compared with vertex presentation in matched controls. This is not surprising, because in brow presentation the largest dimension of the head, the mento-occipital diameter, must negotiate the inlet of the pelvis. Consequently, successful descent, rotation, and delivery of a brow presentation in the term infant depend on conversion to either a face or a vertex presentation. Moreover, it is often the delay in labor associated with this conversion that results in a more careful assessment of fetal position and the recognition of a brow presentation. Perinatal mortality rates for brow and face presentations are higher than for vertex presentations, but the differences can be accounted for by fetal anomalies (anencephaly), prematurity, and asphyxia and trauma associated with manipulation during vaginal delivery.

Management begins with recognition of the abnormality. Awareness and diagnosis of deflection problems are enhanced by an emphasis on careful vaginal examination and a description of the position and characteristics of the presenting fetal part as an essential element in labor monitoring. If, on vaginal examination, the lambdoid sutures and posterior fontanelle cannot easily be identified as occupying a central position in the pelvis, an abnormal presentation or deflection of a cephalic presentation must be suspected. Palpation of the anterior fontanelle or one of the orbits clearly identifies a deflection problem. Furthermore, in cases of abnormal descent or prolonged second stage of labor, deflection of the fetal head should be considered one of the possible causes, and the patient should be reevaluated with this in mind.

If deflection of the fetal head is identified in association with abnormal progression of labor, CPD must be suspected. Friedman[3] found that 10.9% of patients with brow presentation had clinical and radiographic evidence of CPD, compared with 2.7% of controls with vertex presentations. If progress of labor is arrested and CPD is suspected, cesarean delivery is indicated. If labor progresses and there is evidence of resolution of a brow presentation to either a face or vertex presentation, labor should be managed with the expectation of vaginal delivery. If labor is arrested and there are poor uterine contractions in the absence of CPD, the use of a carefully monitored course of oxytocin augmentation may be warranted. Seeds and Cefalo[199] suggested that radiographic pelvimetry be considered in these situations to exclude CPD.

Most brow presentations convert spontaneously to either a face or a vertex presentation, and 70% to 90% of face presentations result in spontaneous delivery. If the brow presentation fails to convert or the face presentation rotates to a persistent mentum posterior, cesarean delivery is required. If uncorrectable fetal distress occurs, labor should be terminated by abdominal delivery. It is generally agreed that rotating the fetal head or converting its deflection position either manually or with forceps is excessively dangerous to fetus and mother.

Compound Presentation

A compound presentation exists if an extremity is adjacent to the presenting part. This complication of labor occurs in approximately 1 of every 1000 deliveries and is associated with high rates of prematurity (31% to 61%) and fetal mortality (16% to 22%).[200,204,205] Cord prolapse, which occurs in 11% to 20% of cases, is the most common intrapartum complication.[199] The vertex-arm combination is the most frequent compound presentation and has the best prognosis.

Management includes early diagnosis and fetal monitoring, with retraction of the presenting extremity and normal vaginal delivery occurring in most cases. If fetal distress or cord prolapse occurs or labor progress ceases, abdominal delivery should be accomplished promptly. Stimulation or manipulation of the presenting extremity to encourage retraction within the uterus is controversial.

Cruikshank and White[200] reported that, of 32 compound presentations, the presenting extremity could be manually replaced in 16 cases, resulting in uneventful vaginal delivery in 15 of the patients. On the other hand, Seeds and Cefalo,[199] in their review of the literature regarding compound presentation, advised against manipulation of the prolapsed part. Indeed, spontaneous retraction of the extremity occurs so frequently that attempts to replace it may not be necessary and, in certain cases, may encourage prolapse of the umbilical cord.

Operative Delivery

Cesarean Delivery

The evolution of cesarean delivery as a safe procedure with extraordinarily low maternal and fetal mortality rates is one of the most important developments in modern perinatal medicine. Maternal mortality rates from cesarean operations in the 19th century were 85% or greater, with the operation being performed only in the most extraordinary circumstances to save the life of the mother.[206] By the early decades of the 20th century, several important innovations in surgical care had occurred, including aseptic technique, reliable anesthesia, and the control of hemorrhage by proper suturing of tissue planes as well as ligation of severed blood vessels. Specifically for the cesarean operation, introduction of the low-segment incision, which allows exclusion of the uterine wound from the peritoneal cavity, dramatically decreased the risk of postoperative peritonitis as a complication of puerperal endometritis.[207]

The later additions of blood transfusion and antibiotic therapy further reduced the morbidity and mortality of cesarean delivery, to the extent that, in 1950, D'Esopo published a remarkable study reporting 1000 consecutive cesarean deliveries without a single maternal death.[208] The decrease in maternal morbidity of cesarean delivery made the operation a reasonable alternative for delivery of the fetus at increased risk for asphyxia or trauma from labor and vaginal delivery. This decrease, together with more sophisticated methods of detecting chronic and acute fetal distress (e.g., ultrasonography, continuous fetal heart monitoring, fetal scalp blood sampling) changed the indications for and frequency of cesarean section for delivery.

Before 1960, cesarean deliveries comprised fewer than 5% of births and were performed primarily for maternal indications such as placenta previa, radiographically documented CPD, failure of induction of labor in severe preeclampsia, and repeat cesarean delivery.[209] After 1960, with the emergence of fetal diagnostic and monitoring techniques, cesarean delivery rates gradually increased worldwide and were more commonly performed for fetal indications.[210,211] The rate and duration of the increase varied; in the United States, the rate of cesarean delivery reached a peak of 23.5% in 1988.[212] Four indications were found to account for 90% of the increase in the United States: dystocia, repeat cesarean delivery, breech presentation, and "fetal distress."[213] Although new indications for cesarean delivery, such as fetal spinal or abdominal wall abnormalities and prevention of vertical transmission of certain infectious diseases, played a small role in this increase, a more important effect was a lowered threshold for the standard indications.[214] Fear of litigation also played a role in the rise in cesarean delivery rates, not only in the United States but also in the United Kingdom.[215] Although it has been suggested that the rate of cesarean delivery is linked to physician reimbursement, the increase in cesarean delivery rates in countries that have global obstetric fees (e.g., Australia) suggests that financial incentive alone cannot account for the rise in cesarean delivery rates.[216]

In some countries, such as Brazil and Chile, the increase in the cesarean delivery rate has been well beyond that which could be accounted for by obstetric or medical indications.[217,218] In these countries, the increase has occurred largely as a result of an increase in prelabor elective cesarean delivery, presumably for the convenience of patients or doctors. This phenomenon has occurred primarily, though not exclusively, among women in upper income levels. There is debate as to whether this has resulted from a patient population that is well educated in the risks and benefits of vaginal versus cesarean delivery and exercising their right of patient autonomy or a patient population that has been overly influenced and biased by health care providers to choose cesarean delivery.[219]

In the 1990s, interest emerged in the role of cesarean delivery to prevent pelvic floor dysfunction that has been attributed to vaginal birth. The risk of urinary incontinence at 6 months after delivery is twofold greater for women who have a spontaneous vaginal delivery than for those who have a cesarean delivery.[220] In a large, multicenter, prospective, randomized, controlled trial of planned prelabor cesarean delivery compared with planned vaginal delivery in women with a term breech presentation, urinary incontinence was less common at 3 months after cesarean delivery (relative risk, 0.62; 95% confidence interval [CI], 0.41 to 0.93).[221] The long-term effects of vaginal delivery on urinary continence are less clear-cut. Buchsbaum and colleagues[222] found no significant difference in the incidence of urinary incontinence in nulliparous versus parous postmenopausal women. In a large, population-based study in Australia, MacLennan and associates[223] found that the incidence of long-term pelvic floor dysfunction, including urinary incontinence, was greater in women who had operative vaginal deliveries than in those who had cesarean deliveries. However, there was no difference in incidence of pelvic floor dysfunction with cesarean versus spontaneous vaginal delivery.

Sultan and colleagues[224] found that forceps delivery and episiotomy were risk factors for anal sphincter lacerations, whereas vacuum-assisted delivery and cesarean delivery were protective.[224] Other studies found that cesarean delivery was associated with a reduced incidence of fecal incontinence if it was performed before onset of the second stage of labor.[225] Associations between the method of delivery and long-term anal sphincter function are less clear. Nygarrd and associates,[226] in a 30-year follow-up study of anal incompetence, found that the aging process was as important as obstetric events.

Notwithstanding the mounting evidence of an untoward effect of vaginal delivery (especially forceps delivery) on postpartum pelvic floor dysfunction, prospective randomized trials with adequate follow-up are necessary to adequately evaluate the effect of various methods of delivery on long-term pelvic floor function. There is currently insufficient evidence to recommend elective cesarean delivery to prevent long-term urinary or anal incontinence.

Finally, a number of the common risk factors for cesarean delivery—fetal macrosomia, advanced maternal age, increased maternal body mass index, gestational diabetes, multiple pregnancy, and dystocia in nulliparous women—are increasing in frequency, especially in developed countries.

Cesarean delivery rates vary widely worldwide, from as low as 5% in Bolivia to as high as 40% in Chile.[216] In the United States, the rate of cesarean deliveries declined 8% between 1991 and 1996 but has steadily increased thereafter, primarily because of a decline in vaginal births after previous cesarean deliveries,[227] reaching 29.1% of all births in 2004 (National Center for Health Statistics preliminary birth data for 2004, available at http://www.cdc.gov/nchs/births.htm [accessed February 8, 2008]).

It seems unlikely that the cesarean delivery rate in the United States or in most developed countries will ever be as low as 15%, which is the goal of the World Health Organization.[228] The cesarean delivery rate will not reach this level and is likely to increase gradually for the following reasons:

- There is a heightened sensitivity to, and lowered threshold for, using cesarean delivery for the traditional indications.
- There is an increased proportion of pregnant women whose pregnancies are complicated by the conditions for which cesarean delivery is necessary.
- There are evolving new indications for cesarean delivery, albeit indications that are variously supported by reliable evidence.
- Emphasis on patient autonomy in making decisions about method of delivery will result in women's vulnerability to bias and non–evidence-based information about the relative risks and benefits of cesarean delivery.
- The benefits of a trial of labor for women with a previous cesarean delivery are equivocal.
- Fear of litigation will persist in the absence of tort reform.

Visco and colleagues from the University of North Carolina conducted a systematic evidence review on the topic of cesarean delivery on maternal request.[229] After a review of 1406 articles, they concluded that the evidence about this approach to childbirth is "significantly limited" and that the literature confounded by having studied *actual* route of delivery rather than *planned* route. They could make no conclusions on the effectiveness and safety of cesarean delivery on maternal request and called for the establishment of a CRT code that could document this indication. A 2006 NIH consensus conference came to similar conclusions (the final statement and video from that event are available at http://consensus.nih.gov [accessed February 8, 2008]).

Another factor that tends to increase the rate of cesarean delivery is the waning enthusiasm for a trial of labor in women who have had a previous cesarean delivery. This has occurred as a result of an increase in the number, if not the incidence, of untoward fetal and maternal consequences of uterine rupture. In the 1980s, the incidence of vaginal birth after a previous cesarean (VBAC) increased in response to initiatives to control the rising cesarean delivery rate. Consequently, more physicians experienced one or more cases of uterine rupture, even though the incidence of symptomatic scar separation remained constant at about 0.5%. Relatively large population-based, retrospective studies have found the overall risk of serious maternal complications (e.g., uterine rupture, hysterectomy) to be twofold to threefold higher for a trial of labor after a previous cesarean compared with a repeat elective cesarean delivery.[230,231] In a large, population-based study from Scotland comparing perinatal outcomes (not related to congenital abnormalities) for women who had a trial of labor after a previous cesarean delivery, compared with those who had an elective repeat cesarean delivery, the risk of delivery-related perinatal death in the former group (12.9/10,000) was 11 times greater than with repeat cesarean.[232]

Complications of Cesarean Delivery

MATERNAL COMPLICATIONS

Although cesarean delivery is a reasonably safe surgical procedure, it is generally regarded as being associated with higher risks of morbidity and mortality than vaginal delivery. Data from the Professional Activities Survey of the Commission of Professional and Hospital Activities for the year 1978, which included about 1 million births and 100,000 cesarean deliveries, showed the rates of maternal death per 100,000 births to be 9.8 for vaginal deliveries, 40.0 for all cesarean deliveries, and 18.4 for "repeat" cesarean deliveries.[213] Others have documented lower risks for cesarean delivery. Sachs and colleagues,[233] reviewing cesarean delivery–related mortality in Massachusetts in the period 1954 to 1985, found that the rate of death directly related to cesarean birth was 5.8 per 100,000 procedures. Frigoletto and coworkers[234] reported on 10,231 consecutive cesarean deliveries at Boston Hospital for Women between 1968 and 1978 without a single maternal death. Varying definitions of maternal mortality and failure to control for the confounding influences of parity, maternal age, and medical and obstetric complications account for some of the differences in maternal mortality rates associated with cesarean delivery. In a study of 250,000 deliveries, Lilford and associates[235] found a sevenfold relative risk of death associated with cesarean compared with vaginal delivery when preexisting medical conditions were excluded. The same authors found that the relative risk of dying from a nonelective cesarean birth compared with an elective cesarean birth when preexisting medical conditions were excluded was 1.5. A population-based study in Washington State (1987-1997) that controlled for parity, maternal age, severe preeclampsia, and deaths unrelated to pregnancy found no significant increase in maternal mortality related to cesarean delivery.[236]

It is apparent that the risks of morbidity and mortality of cesarean delivery are influenced by the associated medical complications in the patient requiring abdominal delivery and the skill of the medical team performing the procedure. Serious intraoperative complications occur in approximately 2% of cesarean deliveries and include anesthesia accidents (e.g., problems with intubation, drug reactions, aspiration pneumonitis), hemorrhage, bowel or bladder injury, amniotic fluid embolism, and air embolism.[237]

Frequently, cesarean delivery must be performed under emergency conditions soon after the patient is admitted to the hospital. Patient anxiety, obesity, an incompletely emptied stomach, acute hemorrhage from a placental accident, low blood volume and constricted vascular space in association with pregnancy-induced hypertension, and hypotension secondary to vena caval and aortic compression by the pregnant uterus are just a few of the problems frequently encountered in patients requiring emergency cesarean delivery. These problems challenge even the most skilled anesthesiologist. On some occasions, an emergency cesarean delivery must be performed with such haste that sterile and surgical techniques are compromised. Urinary tract injuries, which occur in 1 or 2 per 1000 deliveries, are 10 times more common in cesarean deliveries than in operative vaginal deliveries.[238] Most of the injuries that occur with cesarean delivery are simple bladder lacerations that are promptly identified and repaired without sequelae. Bowel injuries are often associated with intra-abdominal adhesions from previous cesarean deliveries or other abdominal surgeries. Some intraoperative complications, such as amniotic fluid embolus syndrome and air embolus, are extremely rare and usually not preventable.

The following are postpartum maternal complications associated with cesarean delivery:

- Atelectasis
- Endomyometritis
- Urinary tract infection
- Abdominal wound hematoma formation, dehiscence, infection, or necrotizing fasciitis
- Thromboembolic disease
- Bowel dysfunction—adynamic ileus, pseudo-obstruction of the cecum (Ogilvie syndrome), and sigmoid volvulus

Duff[239] found that, with the use of prophylactic antibiotics, the rate of febrile puerperal complications for cesarean delivery was 5% to 10% in a university obstetric service (see Chapter 38). Watson and colleagues[240] found that febrile morbidity occurred in only 2.3% of high-risk private patients who underwent cesarean delivery. The rate of febrile morbidity in patients undergoing cesarean delivery without labor was only 0.5%. These studies emphasized the fact that low socioeconomic status and labor are important risk factors for postpartum febrile morbidity after cesarean delivery.

Postcesarean endomyometritis is a polymicrobial infection characterized by abdominal pain, malaise, anorexia, fever, uterine tenderness, and malodorous lochia. Prompt diagnosis and proper selection of antibiotic therapy for patients who become symptomatic with endomyometritis is important. In a systematic review of 47 trials comparing various antibiotic regimens for treatment of puerperal endometritis, French and Smaill[241] found that the combination of clindamycin and gentamicin administered intravenously was more effective than other regimens. Regimens with activity against penicillin-resistant anaerobic bacteria were superior to those without this coverage. Furthermore, they found that oral follow-up treatment was not necessary once the clinical signs indicated improvement.

Postcesarean bacteriuria occurs in approximately 11% of patients and is related largely to routine urethral catheterization.[242] Studies have shown that the risk of urinary tract infection after cesarean delivery can be reduced substantially by eliminating catheterization or by using intermittent rather than indwelling catheterization.[243,244]

Wound hematomas are usually caused by faulty hemostasis and respond to drainage of the hematoma. The use of prophylactic antibiotics has substantially decreased the incidence of postcesarean abdominal wound infections, which now occur in 3% or less of cesarean deliveries.[245,246] Cesarean deliveries performed in the second stage of labor carry greater risk for wound infection, and obesity and the use of suprafascial drains are also risk factors. Obese women are at increased risk for development of necrotizing fasciitis, one of the most serious and potentially fatal consequences of wound infection.[247] Between 25% and 30% of wound infections are caused by *Staphylococcus aureus*; these infections do not usually originate from wound contamination from the endometrium. For this reason, attention to sterile technique and proper wound care are essential for patients undergoing cesarean delivery.

Puerperal deep venous thrombosis occurs in 1% to 2% of patients delivered by cesarean section.[248] Although pulmonary embolism is rare, it is one of the major causes of maternal mortality. Obesity, prolonged operative procedures, endometritis, and any inherited thrombophilia are risk factors. Treatment is intravenous heparinization followed by treatment with oral anticoagulants, the duration of which depends on the severity of the disease and whether the patient is found to have an inherited thrombophilia. Postoperative pelvic thrombophlebitis is a diagnosis made by exclusion when puerperal fever does not respond to antibiotic therapy but resolves with heparin treatment. Ovarian vein thrombosis can be recognized in patients with postoperative abdominal pain and a palpable tender mass extending from the lower quadrant into the flank, usually on the right side. Prophylactic heparinization is commonly used in the United Kingdom and Europe for both elective and emergency cesarean deliveries, but in the United States it is used only in patients at high risk for thromboembolism.[249,250] There is no consensus as to whether an evaluation for inherited thrombophilia should be recommended for all patients with postcesarean deep venous thrombosis or pulmonary embolism. Clearly, such testing is in order if there is a family history of thromboembolism.

Postoperative adynamic ileus is not uncommon after cesarean section, especially if the bowel has been manipulated during the surgery. Kammen and colleagues,[251] in a study of 21 patients who had abdominal radiographs because of obstructive symptoms after cesarean delivery, found radiographic signs of distal colonic obstruction in 15. All 21 patients had rapid clinical and radiographic improvement on conservative management, confirming the eventual diagnosis of transient postoperative ileus. A more serious problem is postcesarean pseudocolonic obstruction with marked dilation of the cecum (Ogilvie syndrome). Although the etiology and pathogenesis of this syndrome is not clear, early recognition and surgical decompression are necessary to avoid rupture of the cecum.[252]

Prophylactic antibiotics, regional anesthesia, early ambulation, and intermittent rather than indwelling urethral catheterization all have contributed to reducing the incidence of postcesarean febrile complications.

The incidence of long-term complications of cesarean delivery is more difficult to document. These complications include the following:

- Cesarean delivery in a subsequent pregnancy
- Uterine rupture in a subsequent pregnancy
- Placenta previa or placenta accreta in a subsequent pregnancy
- Ectopic pregnancy
- Infertility
- Bowel obstruction resulting from intra-abdominal adhesions
- Decision to limit family size
- Fewer subsequent pregnancies

In the United States, the incidence of repeat cesarean delivery is greater than 75%. Among women who have a trial of labor after a previous cesarean delivery in which a low-transverse uterine incision was used, the risk of uterine rupture is 0.5% to 1.0%.[253] This risk has remained remarkably constant for decades. The risk is substantially increased after the classic (i.e., fundal) cesarean incision. Ananth and associates,[254] in a systematic review of 36 studies published from 1950 through 1996, found that women who had a cesarean delivery were at twofold to threefold greater risk for placenta previa in the subsequent pregnancy compared with women who had a vaginal delivery, and the risk increased with the number of prior cesarean deliveries (see Chapter 37). A more recent, population-based, retrospective study of births in the state of Washington found a somewhat lower but statistically significant risk of placenta previa (odds ratio [OR], 1.4; CI, 1.1 to 1.6) for the next pregnancy after a first-birth cesarean.[255] Some authors also have found an association between previous cesarean delivery and placenta accreta in subsequent pregnancies, but this association is more difficult to document because of the rarity of placenta accreta[256] (see Chapter 37). Although there is controversy as to whether there is an increased risk of ectopic pregnancy after cesarean delivery, there are a number of reports of ectopic pregnancies occurring in the uterine incision.[257-259] Somewhat less controversial is the increased risk of infertility for patients delivered by cesarean.[260] Postcesarean infertility is not explained by increased maternal age or by voluntary infertility, but it may be related to fallopian tube damage from postpartum infection.

NEONATAL COMPLICATIONS

It appears that the safest, most atraumatic method of delivery for an infant is by cesarean section, and the increase in cesarean delivery rates after 1960 undoubtedly was fueled, in part, by concerns about the dangers to the fetus of labor and vaginal delivery in certain situations. Nevertheless, abdominal delivery is also associated with uncommon but significant dangers to the infant, including the following:

- Fetal asphyxia resulting from uteroplacental hypoperfusion induced by conduction anesthesia or maternal position
- Neonatal respiratory morbidity
- Scalpel lacerations

Maternal hypotension and its deleterious effect on uteroplacental perfusion are well-known dangers of the supine position. Conduction anesthesia, by blocking vasoconstriction in the lower extremities through the sympathetic nervous system, can further reduce cardiac output and further compromise uterine blood flow. Corke and associates[261] demonstrated that even brief (2-minute) episodes of hypotension result in umbilical blood gas values consistent with metabolic acidosis.

Cesarean delivery has long been recognized to be associated with an increase in neonatal respiratory morbidity at all gestational ages.[262-264] The frequency of this complication, its specific etiology and pathophysiology, and the mortality rate associated with it are all matters of dispute. The incidence of severe respiratory morbidity in infants born by elective cesarean delivery near term is inversely related to gestational age. Wax and colleagues[146] found that infants born by elective cesarean delivery at 37 and 38 weeks' gestation had greatly increased risks, of severe respiratory morbidity requiring mechanical ventilation (38-fold and 13-fold, respectively), compared with those born at 39 or 40 weeks' gestation. This syndrome could be related to a number of problems, without a clear-cut and similar pathophysiology in each case, but the common denominator is cesarean delivery, especially when it is performed in the absence of labor. Morrison and coauthors,[265] in a study of 33,289 deliveries at or after 37 weeks of gestation, found that the incidence of neonatal respiratory morbidity was significantly higher for the group delivered by cesarean section before labor (35.5/1000) compared with cesarean section during labor (12.2/1000) (OR, 2.9; CI, 1.9 to 4.4).

Some cases of respiratory morbidity after cesarean delivery are due to true iatrogenic prematurity, in which inaccurate gestational dates result unexpectedly in a premature infant. Even careful attention to the duration of pregnancy and the use of amniotic fluid tests of fetal lung maturity have not completely eliminated this problem. Schreiner and colleagues[266] and Heritage and Cunningham[267] suggested that neonatal respiratory disease after elective repeat cesarean delivery—usually manifested as mild transient tachypnea of the newborn (wet lung syndrome)—is, in its most severe form, persistence of the fetal circulation. These observations, together with the studies of Boon and associates[268] demonstrating the reduced air volume in the lungs of infants delivered by cesarean section compared with those delivered vaginally, suggest that the neonatal respiratory disease after cesarean delivery is caused by incomplete adaptation of the fetal lung to extrauterine respiration. The specific sequence and timing for this adaptation to extrauterine cardiorespiratory status are unknown; nor is it known whether the physiologic and mechanical events of labor and delivery are necessary to complete pulmonary adaptation. The higher incidence of neonatal respiratory morbidity associated with repeat cesarean delivery in patients not in labor compared with those who are in labor suggests that labor is the signal that crucial physiologic changes have occurred to prepare a fetus for extrauterine life.

Accidental lacerations of the fetus occur in 1% to 2% of cesarean deliveries.[269,270] The frequency of these accidents appears to be related to the experience of the surgeon, the most common situation being a well-thinned-out lower uterine segment in a patient who has ruptured membranes; in such cases, the uterus at the incision site may be only 2 or 3 mm thick. Usually, these inadvertent scalpel lacerations of the fetus are of only cosmetic importance, but we know of one infant who died as a result of a thrombosis of the sagittal sinus secondary to a scalpel incision incurred during cesarean delivery.

Cesarean delivery also imparts added risks for infants of future pregnancies, including fetal death resulting from antepartum rupture of uterine incisions and neonatal respiratory disease associated with subsequent elective cesarean delivery.[229]

Indications for Cesarean Delivery

Reducing the frequency of maternal and neonatal complications of cesarean delivery begins with a proper respect for the dangers of the procedure and careful selection of patients to be delivered in this manner. In general, cesarean delivery is indicated any time delivery must be accomplished and induction of labor, a trial of labor, additional labor, or vaginal delivery of the fetus is deemed to be of greater risk to the mother or the fetus than abdominal delivery. This straightforward generalization, although constituting a more rational approach than a simple list of absolute indications for the operation, does not do justice to the complexities of the decision in each case.

As the fetal indications for cesarean delivery have multiplied, so have the dilemmas of balancing the benefits and risks of operation for the mother and the fetus. For example, in placenta previa, vaginal delivery subjects both mother and fetus to unacceptable risks of exsanguination, and cesarean delivery is clearly in the best interests of both patients. In the case of a difficult mid-forceps delivery for fetal distress or failure of progress in the second stage of labor, the fetus will most certainly benefit from an expeditious abdominal delivery, but the mother's risks from cesarean versus vaginal delivery are a matter of serious debate. At the other end of the spectrum is the case of a footling breech presentation or genital herpes simplex infection, in which the operation is performed entirely for the benefit of the fetus, with no advantages to the mother apart from the reassurance that it may help her infant. Countless other situations could be used as examples of the difficult decision that faces both physician and patient when evaluating the proper method of delivery. One of the most recent examples, ironically, is the interest in nulliparous patients being considered as candidates for elective cesarean delivery in the absence of the usual indications for abdominal delivery. Studies that have linked postpartum urinary and anal incontinence to vaginal delivery have encouraged some women, especially nulliparas, and their obstetricians to consider elective cesarean delivery at term to reduce the risk of pelvic floor dysfunction. Harer[271] summarized the arguments in support of such a practice. As noted earlier in this chapter, however, there is insufficient evidence from adequate prospective trials to determine the long-term consequences of alternative methods of delivery on pelvic floor function or to support a recommendation for elective cesarean section to reduce the risks of urinary and anal sphincter incontinence.

The Consensus Development Statement on Cesarean Childbirth[213] did much to clarify the indications for cesarean delivery and to draw attention to specific situations in which the need for cesarean delivery can be reduced by thorough evaluation of the patient and the facility.

The problem of dystocia, which includes both proven CPD and the less well-defined problem of "failure of labor to progress," was found to account for 30% of the increase in cesarean delivery rates in the United States. Studies by Silbar[272] and by Seitchik and colleagues[273] found that the increase in cesarean birth rate for dystocia resulted, in part, from an increased incidence of large infants and a consequent absolute increase in fetal-pelvic disproportion. Continuous electronic fetal heart rate monitoring contributed to the increase in cesarean delivery for "dystocia." Haverkamp and associates,[274] in a prospective, controlled study, found that cesarean delivery was more often performed for dystocia when continuous labor and fetal monitoring data were available, compared with documentation of uterine contractions and fetal heart rate data via palpation and auscultation by a nurse at the bedside. In the absence of data about absolute intrauterine pressure values and subtle fetal heart rate decelerations, it is tempting to speculate that there is longer and more vigorous oxytocin augmentation of desultory labors before cesarean section is considered in the group monitored by a bedside nurse. Or perhaps the nurse at the bedside allays anxiety and thereby contributes to a normal labor pattern and less fetal distress.

The diagnosis of fetal distress, which accounted for 10% to 15% of the increase in cesarean delivery rate in the studies described, is often made in the context of a labor that is not progressing normally. Zalar and Quilligan[275] found that the use of fetal scalp blood sampling substantially reduced the number of cesarean deliveries performed for presumed fetal distress. Moreover, as experience is gained with reading fetal monitoring tracings, one is less likely to perform operative deliveries for abnormal but not necessarily ominous fetal heart rate changes. Consequently, judicious interpretation of continuous fetal heart rate monitoring data and persistent attention to factors that will improve the fetal environment often allow the additional time needed for successful labor and vaginal delivery. Garite and colleagues[276] found that continuous fetal pulse oximetry in labor resulted in a 50% reduction in the number of cesarean deliveries for nonreassuring fetal status, compared with continuous electronic fetal heart rate monitoring in control subjects, but the overall rate of cesarean section was not reduced, because the number of abdominal deliveries for dystocia increased.

Bloom and coworkers[277] randomly assigned 5341 nulliparous women in labor to either "open" or "masked" fetal pulse oximetry. Clinicians had access to oximetry data in the "open" arm and did not in the "masked" arm. There were no differences in the overall rate of cesarean delivery, nor in the rates of abdominal delivery for dystocia or fetal distress; a planned subanalysis of cases with nonreassuring fetal heart rate tracings also demonstrated no differences. This trial called into question the value of fetal pulse oximetry in helping patients forego abdominal delivery or improving the health of newborns.

The waning enthusiasm for midpelvic forceps deliveries has contributed to the increased number of cesarean deliveries in the "dystocia" category.

Vaginal Birth after Cesarean Section

Before 1980, abdominal delivery after a previous cesarean section accounted for 25% to 30% of the increase in cesarean delivery rate.[213] However, previous cesarean delivery performed through a low transverse uterine incision for a nonrecurring indication (presumed CPD not included) need not be an indication for a subsequent cesarean delivery. In hospitals with appropriate facilities (i.e., services and staff available for prompt emergency cesarean birth), a patient who has undergone previous cesarean delivery can be allowed a trial of labor.

In a meta-analysis of 31 studies that included 11,417 patients with a trial of labor after a previous low-transverse cesarean delivery, Rosen and associates[278] found that maternal febrile morbidity was significantly lower after a trial of labor than after an elective repeat cesarean. Although the combined rate of rupture or dehiscence of the uterine wound was the same in the two groups, the odds ratio for perinatal death in all patients with a trial of labor, compared with those who had undergone elective cesarean delivery, was 2.1 (CI, 1.3 to 3.4). The intended route of delivery, the presence of an unknown type of scar, and the use of oxytocin made no difference in the rate of uterine wound dehiscence.

In a study of 6138 patients with one previous low-transverse cesarean birth, McMahon and colleagues[230] found that major maternal complications (defined as need for hysterectomy, uterine rupture, or serious operative injury) occurred more often in women with a trial of labor than in those who delivered by repeat elective cesarean (OR, 1.8; CI, 1.1 to 3.0). All of the major complications occurred in women with unsuccessful vaginal birth.

Consequently, the overall risk associated with a trial of labor after a previous cesarean delivery will be decreased by selecting women who have a high probability (>80%) of successful vaginal delivery. Women likely to have a successful VBAC are those who are younger than 35 years of age, whose fetus weighs less than 4000 g, and whose previous cesarean delivery was performed for a reason other than failure of descent in the second stage of labor.

Small series have addressed the question of the safety of VBAC in patients with breech presentation,[279] twin gestation,[280] or post-term pregnancy.[281] Although each of these reports noted no greater incidence of complications in those circumstances than for VBAC in singleton pregnancies with a vertex, term presentation, the small number of patients in each series demands continued caution in recommending VBAC for such patients.

Intrapartum rupture of a low-transverse uterine scar, which occurs in 0.5% to 1% of women who undertake a trial of labor after a cesarean delivery, is a serious emergency and can result in perinatal death.[282] Furthermore, serious puerperal morbidity is more common in women who undergo cesarean delivery after a trial of labor than in those who undergo a repeat elective abdominal delivery.[230] After being fully informed about the risks and benefits of a trial of labor and VBAC, women are not universally enthusiastic. More than 25% choose to undergo another elective cesarean delivery if given the chance.[283]

Landon and associates[284] reported on a cohort study of more than 30,000 women in which women with one prior cesarean delivery underwent either elective repeat cesarean delivery or a trial of labor. The prevalence of symptomatic uterine rupture was 0.7%. No infant in the repeat cesarean group but 12 of the infants in the trial of labor group suffered encephalopathy, and 7 of those 12 cases were associated with uterine rupture (for a rate of 0.46 per 1000 trials of labor). The rates of endometritis and of transfusion were higher in the trial of labor group, but there were no differences in the rates of hysterectomy or maternal death. This contemporary cohort is useful in counseling patients and demonstrates the low absolute risks associated with either approach.

Reducing Morbidity of Cesarean Delivery

When cesarean delivery must be performed, the following measures ensure the lowest morbidity and mortality risks for mother and infant:

- Anesthesia administered by a skilled anesthesiologist
- Attention to maternal position and blood volume in the peripartum period
- Prophylactic antibiotics
- Use of a transverse uterine incision whenever possible
- Awaiting the onset of labor whenever possible in cases of repeat cesarean delivery
- Presence of a person skilled in newborn resuscitation

Equally good neonatal and maternal outcomes from cesarean delivery can be obtained with spinal, epidural, or general anesthesia or with local infiltration, provided that it is administered by a skilled person who is fully aware of the unique physiologic problems of the pregnant patient and her fetus.[285-287] There are, however, maternal and fetal risks associated with each method of anesthesia.

SPINAL ANESTHESIA

Spinal anesthesia is associated with the highest incidence of hypotension and should always be accompanied by uterine displacement, maternal prehydration, and (more controversially) prophylactic ephedrine administration. Lindblad and associates[288] used Doppler ultrasound to estimate fetal aortic and umbilical blood flow in women during cesarean delivery with intrathecal anesthesia. They found that, if maternal blood pressure was maintained within the normal range with preload infusion of lactated Ringer solution and ephedrine, fetal blood flow was unaffected for 30 minutes after induction. After this time, the pulsatility index in the fetal vessels decreased. Most important for the obstetrician is the awareness that, with spinal anesthesia, the time from onset of anesthesia to delivery of the infant is directly related to the degree of fetal metabolic acidosis resulting from uteroplacental hypoperfusion.[289] Simply because the patient is alert is no reason to procrastinate in delivering the infant. There is perhaps as much, if not more, need for prompt delivery of the infant after spinal anesthesia as there is with general anesthesia.

EPIDURAL ANESTHESIA

Epidural anesthesia is associated with maternal hypotension less often than is spinal anesthesia. Jouppila and colleagues,[290] however, found that epidural anesthesia was associated with a decreased clearance of xenon 133 (presumed to reflect decreased uteroplacental perfusion), especially when hypotension occurs. One major disadvantage of epidural block for cesarean delivery is the time required for the onset of operative anesthesia, which could preclude its use in many emergency situations. Quinn and Kilpatrick's study[291] of fetal outcomes in 212 consecutive cesarean deliveries demonstrated that regional anesthesia is satisfactory for urgent cesarean deliveries provided that delivery is not required within 20 minutes. Inhalation anesthesia was needed if the time interval from decision to delivery was less than 20 minutes.

GENERAL ANESTHESIA

General anesthesia, which has the advantage of rapid onset, is also associated with decreased uteroplacental perfusion during induction of the anesthesia.[292] Pulmonary aspiration of gastric contents (Mendelson syndrome) is always a major threat with general anesthesia, and this risk is accentuated by the delayed gastric emptying in patients in labor; Cohen[293] reviewed this subject. There is evidence that the particulate antacids, which are commonly used preoperatively to neutralize gastric acidity, may themselves cause pulmonary damage if aspirated, and their use has not eliminated Mendelson syndrome. A nonparticulate antacid such as sodium citrate, given 10 to 45 minutes before anesthesia, alone or in combination with a histamine$_2$ (H_2) receptor blocker such as ranitidine, should significantly decrease the risk of aspiration without contributing added hazard.[294] Perhaps the most important safeguard against the aspiration syndrome is skillful intubation while cricoid pressure is applied.

In patients given general anesthesia, as well as those given conduction anesthesia, prompt delivery of the infant is important, the crucial time being that from incision of the uterus to delivery.[295] Delivery of the infant within 90 seconds of making the uterine incision reduces the risk of fetal hypoxemia from altered uteroplacental and umbilical blood flow.

If regional anesthesia is used, adequate volume replacement is important in preventing hypotension. Prehydration with 1000 mL of saline or injection of lactated Ringer solution frequently compensates for vasodilation after onset of anesthesia. The supine position is a well known but frequently neglected danger in all pregnant women in the third trimester.[296] Often, during preparation for surgery and administration of the anesthetic agent, the patient is placed flat on her back. Appropriate wedges, left lateral tilt of the table, and even operating with the patient in the lateral position have been shown to prevent supine hypotension and reduce fetal asphyxia.

Bloom and colleagues,[297] using the previously described registry,[284] demonstrated that more than 93% of abdominal deliveries could be accomplished with a regional technique, with a low failure rate (3.0%). Risk factors for needing general anesthesia included maternal size, increasing preoperative risk scores, and short interval from decision to incision. One maternal death was caused by an anesthetic complication (fluid intubation). This large series attests to the preferability and safety of regional anesthesia in contemporary obstetrics.

In addition to the use of regional anesthesia and early ambulation, the widespread use of prophylactic antibiotics for patients undergoing a cesarean delivery has reduced the risk of puerperal morbidity (see Chapter 38). The use of prophylactic antibiotics for cesarean delivery was the subject of two extensive systematic reviews. Smaill and Hofmeyr[298] reviewed 81 trials and found a significant reduction of puerperal endometritis and wound infection among women treated with prophylactic antibiotics for cesarean delivery, compared with women who did not receive such treatment. Hopkins and Smaill[299] reviewed 47 trials comparing various antibiotic regimens used as prophylaxis for cesarean delivery. Ampicillin and first-generation cephalosporins were equally effective in reducing puerperal endometritis. Multiple-dose regimens were of no greater efficacy than single-dose treatments, and there was no significant difference in outcome with systemic versus lavage administration. Also, there was no advantage for the use of antibiotics with a broader range of activity. Although there is no conclusive evidence regarding optimal timing of administration, most obstetricians administer the medication after the umbilical cord is clamped, in the interest of avoiding unnecessary exposure of the infant to an antibiotic. Finally, antibiotic prophylaxis reduces morbidity in elective cesarean delivery as well as in cesarean delivery performed during labor.

In the past, the extraperitoneal approach to cesarean delivery was used if chorioamnionitis was suspected.[300,301] It appears that this operative technique is no longer widely taught or used, and the risks and benefits of this approach, compared with the standard intraperitoneal approach, have not been delineated.

The advantages of the transverse compared with the vertical uterine incision for cesarean delivery were first recognized by Kerr,[302] who showed that low vertical incisions almost always extended into the thicker muscle layers of the fundus and were more frequently complicated by improper healing and subsequent rupture. Also, if the entire uterine incision could be covered by bladder peritoneum, the risk of postoperative ileus, peritonitis, and subsequent adhesions and bowel obstruction was reduced.

The advantages of awaiting onset of labor before performing a subsequent cesarean delivery are the elimination of iatrogenic prematurity and reduction of the risk of neonatal respiratory illness. Awaiting the onset of labor also results in thinning of the lower uterine segment, which decreases blood loss and facilitates development of the bladder flap during the procedure.

Finally, the presence of a professional skilled in neonatal resuscitation is essential, especially when cesarean delivery is performed for fetal distress. It is not only courteous but also often vitally important to inform the pediatrician or nursery personnel as early as possible of an impending cesarean delivery. Special equipment, drugs, and blood products may need to be assembled for a sick neonate. It is a disservice to the mother to perform a major operation in the interest of fetal well-being and not follow up with the most expert care of the newborn.

Cesarean hysterectomy is occasionally lifesaving, especially in cases of uncontrolled hemorrhage from the site of a placenta previa, placenta accreta, or ruptured uterus. Cesarean hysterectomy could also be the treatment of choice in the woman with chorioamnionitis who desires sterilization and in whom cesarean delivery is indicated. For other indications, such as cervical intraepithelial neoplasia and a request for sterilization with a subsequent cesarean delivery, the operation is associated with sufficient morbidity to make its usefulness in these situations doubtful.

In a review of cesarean hysterectomy including 3913 operations, Park and Duff[303] found the following complication rates: maternal mortality, 0.71%; bladder injury, 3%; vesicovaginal fistula, 0.4%; ureteral injury, 0.25%; and intraperitoneal bleeding requiring reoperation, 0.97%. Supracervical cesarean hysterectomy is justified in cases of life-threatening hemorrhage if the patient's vital signs are unstable. Complete removal of the cervix is one of the most difficult and time-consuming aspects of the cesarean hysterectomy procedure, especially if there has been substantial effacement and dilation of the cervix.

Obstetric Forceps Delivery

Obstetric forceps were first used by members of the Chamberlen family in the 17th century but were not widely accepted until 100 years later.[304] William Smellie was the first to systematically teach the principles of forceps deliveries. It is clear that he also was fully aware of the potential dangers of the instruments; in the introduction to Volume II of *Treatise on the Theory and Practice of Midwifery*,[305] he wrote, "If these expedients (forceps) are used prematurely when the nature of the case does not absolutely require such assistance, the mischief that may ensue will often over balance the service for which they were intended and this consideration is one of my principal motives for publishing this second volume."

In 1988, the American College of Obstetricians and Gynecologists (ACOG)[306] issued a Committee Opinion establishing new definitions for obstetric forceps. These definitions, which were incorporated in the 1991 ACOG Technical Bulletin entitled Operative Vaginal Delivery,[307] were divided into three categories:

1. Outlet forceps
   a. Scalp is visible at the introitus without separating labia
   b. Fetal skull has reached pelvic floor
   c. Sagittal suture is in anteroposterior diameter or right or left occiput anterior or posterior position
   d. Fetal head is at or on perineum
   e. Rotation does not exceed 45 degrees
2. Low forceps
   a. Leading point of fetal skull is at station at +2 cm or lower and not on the pelvic floor
   b. Rotation is less than or equal to 45 degrees (left or right occiput anterior to occiput anterior or left or right occiput posterior to occiput posterior)
   c. Rotation is greater than 45 degrees
3. Mid-forceps
   a. Station is above +2 cm but head is engaged

This classification reflects what has been widely recognized among practicing obstetricians, that there are two types of forceps deliveries: low forceps deliveries, which are usually simple and uncomplicated for both mother and infant, and mid-forceps deliveries, which sometimes are difficult and can cause substantial trauma to either patient.

Hagadorn-Freathy and colleagues[308] prospectively evaluated forceps deliveries, comparing outcomes as designated by the ACOG criteria published in 1965.[309] When the older classification was used, there was no difference in outcome between outlet forceps and mid-forceps deliveries. When the deliveries were reclassified according to the more recent criteria, however, mid-forceps deliveries were associated with lower cord pH values and a higher incidence of fetal injury, compared with outlet or low forceps deliveries. In a review of operative vaginal deliveries, Bowes and Katz[310] found that serious short-term maternal and perinatal morbidity are increased in forceps delivery if the vertex is above +2 cm station in the pelvis, compared with +2 station or lower.

A retrospective, population-based study of 583,340 live-born singleton infants in California found that, among patients in labor for whom spontaneous vaginal delivery did not occur, there was no statistically significant difference in the incidence of neonatal intracranial hemorrhage between delivery by vacuum extraction, delivery by forceps, and cesarean delivery.[311] Another important finding of this study was that the incidence of serious neonatal morbidity was significantly greater when cesarean delivery was performed after a failed attempt at vaginal delivery with either forceps or vacuum extractor, compared with cesarean delivery after a trial of operative vaginal delivery. There were multiple limitations to this study, including lack of information about the level of experience of those who performed the operative deliveries. Such limitations notwithstanding, the study suggested that, if spontaneous delivery cannot be accomplished safely for the mother or infant and the circumstances are not favorable for a relatively easy operative vaginal delivery, the patient should be delivered by cesarean. This contention is supported by evidence that many modern residency training programs in obstetrics and gynecology are not providing sufficient skill in the safe use of forceps.[312]

Few studies with long-term follow-up of infants delivered with forceps have been published. Friedman and colleagues[313] published results from a collaborative perinatal project in which children delivered by mid-forceps demonstrated lower intelligence quotient (IQ) scores and a higher prevalence of suspected speech, language, and hearing abnormalities than did children born spontaneously. McBride and coworkers[161] studied 700 5-year-old children, all of whom were born at term, including 175 born by mid-forceps delivery. Using a variety of neurologic, hearing, visual acuity, and development tests, these authors found no differences related to method of delivery among the children who had been born in cephalic presentation. Dierker and associates[314] compared 110 children 2 years of age or older who had been delivered by mid-forceps with a similar number of children of the same age delivered by cesarean section. They found five cases of abnormal development among the children delivered by mid-forceps and seven cases among those delivered by cesarean section.

Seidman and coauthors[315] related obstetric interventions to medical examinations and intelligence tests performed on more than 32,000 17-year-old men and women inducted into the Israeli Defense Forces. The mean intelligence scores for those delivered by forceps or vacuum extractor were not statistically different from those delivered spontaneously or by cesarean section.

In a retrospective study of 3417 children, Wesley and coworkers[316] found no association of forceps delivery (versus spontaneous delivery) with decreased IQ score at 5 years of age. The studies that demonstrated no untoward long-term effect of operative vaginal delivery are those in which the infants were born after 1970. A more conservative attitude about forceps, which has characterized the period since the late 1970s, may have been responsible for the salutary outcomes noted in recent studies of both short-term and long-term effects of operative vaginal delivery.

Mid-forceps deliveries, as defined by the 1991 ACOG criteria, should be undertaken with caution and with a willingness to abandon the procedure in favor of cesarean delivery if there is difficulty with proper application of the instrument or if the head does not easily descend or rotate. The use and teaching of midforceps delivery under the appropriate circumstances and by an adequately trained individual is in accord with current recommendations of the ACOG.[317]

Patel and Murphy[318] reviewed the role of forceps in modern practice. Their 2004 review concluded that (1) most women prefer spontaneous delivery; (2) obstetricians increasingly choose cesarean section if problems arise during the second stage of labor; (3) injury to the pelvic floor and trauma to the baby are more common with forceps, whereas hemorrhage and maternal-infant separation occur more often after abdominal delivery; and (4) forceps delivery results in less morbidity in subsequent pregnancies. The authors bemoaned the decline in forceps skills among junior clinicians and advocated further research regarding the long-term sequelae of forceps operations.

Vacuum Extraction

Malmström introduced the vacuum extractor into modern obstetrics in 1954.[319] Since that time, it has largely replaced the use of obstetric forceps in Scandinavia and continental Europe, and it is used with increasing frequency in the United States.[320] Bowes and Katz[310] reviewed the use of the vacuum extractor for obstetric delivery. The indications for its use are virtually the same as those for the use of forceps:

- Arrest of labor in the second stage
- Maternal indication for shortening of the second stage of labor (e.g., cardiovascular or cerebrovascular disease, maternal exhaustion)
- Fetal distress
- Elective low pelvic delivery

Contraindications for use of the vacuum extractor include the following:

- CPD
- Face or brow presentation
- Breech presentation
- Unengaged fetal head
- Premature infant
- Incompletely dilated cervix

Maternal complications of vacuum extractor delivery, including cervical and vaginal trauma, are generally less frequent and less severe than those of forceps delivery, and this is one of the major advantages of the instrument. Minor fetal complications include cephalhematomas and retinal hemorrhages, which are usually benign and self-limited. More serious complications, such as subgaleal hemorrhage (4%) and intracranial hemorrhage (2.5%), are usually associated with prolonged labor and fetal asphyxia but are probably less common than in forceps deliveries performed under the same circumstances.

Johanson and Menon[321] performed a systematic review of nine randomized, controlled trials comparing the vacuum extractor with forceps for assisted vaginal delivery. They concluded that failure to deliver the infant occurred more often with the vacuum extractor than with the forceps. The vacuum extractor was associated with significantly less maternal pelvic trauma but with a greater risk for neonatal cephalhematomas and retinal hemorrhages. A 5-year follow-up study of 278 infants who were involved in a randomized, controlled trial of vacuum extraction versus forceps delivery found no statistical difference in long-term untoward effects between the two methods.[322] Almost all studies have found a substantial increase in risk of maternal and fetal morbidity when failure to deliver with the vacuum extractor is followed by an attempt to deliver with forceps. For example, Towner and colleagues[311] found that use of both vacuum extraction and forceps resulted in a rate of intracranial hemorrhage that was 7.4 times greater than with spontaneous delivery, and 3.4 times greater than with use of the vacuum extractor as the sole instrument. Also, Gardella and associates[323] compared 3741 combined vacuum and forceps deliveries with the same number of vacuum-only and forceps-only deliveries. There was a significant increase in both neonatal and maternal injury with sequential use of the instruments. A recommendation to avoid the combination of vacuum extractor followed by forceps is in accord with the current guidelines on operative vaginal delivery published by ACOG.[317]

Two major advantages of the vacuum extractor are the ease with which it can be applied and the need for less anesthesia than is required for forceps delivery. Moreover, it is far easier to teach and to learn the appropriate skill required to use the vacuum extractor safely than to acquire a similar level of skill with forceps delivery. Many of the studies that established the effectiveness and safety of the vacuum extractor compared with obstetric forceps were conducted with the Malmström metal cup or the Bird modification of the Malmström device. Currently, a variety of both rigid and soft polyethylene or silicone vacuum cups are the preferred instruments for vacuum extraction and the ones most commonly used in residency training programs in the United States.[320] Randomized trials of soft versus rigid vacuum extractor cups show that soft cups have lower success rates than rigid cups but are less likely to cause maternal and fetal trauma.[324]

The collective evidence of the comparative efficacy and safety of vacuum extraction versus forceps has led some authorities to recommend the vacuum extractor as the instrument of first choice for operative vaginal delivery.[325]

Analgesia and Anesthesia for Low-Risk Labor and Vaginal Delivery

History

An interesting monograph by Caton[326] and a shorter account by Caton and colleagues[327] chronicled the history of pain relief for childbirth during the past two centuries. It is safe to say that the plight of women in labor has improved dramatically since the 16th century, when Eufame MacLayne, a woman of some station, was tried by due process, convicted of an act contrary to divine law, chained to a stake atop Castle Hill, and burned. Her only crime was having received "a certain medicine for the relief of pain in childbirth."[328] Until the 18th century, labor was conducted without the use of effective analgesia or anesthesia. The birth process was simply acknowledged to be a painful, traumatic, and often frightening experience that was to be endured with the aid of only crude and unproven potions. James Simpson, who held the Chair of Midwifery at the University of Edinburgh, was the first to administer chloroform to a woman in labor and became a champion of obstetric anesthesia.[329] His work, and especially his care of Queen Victoria, who enjoyed the birth of one of her many children with the assistance of chloroform, changed both public and professional attitudes about the benefits of providing pain relief for women during labor. Modern obstetric units, many with the service of full-time obstetric anesthesiologists, provide a wide range of options for pain management, including psychophysiologic methods, parenteral analgesia, and regional analgesia.

One of the most important assets of a modern facility offering a full range of perinatal services is the presence of a qualified obstetric anesthesiologist. The physiologic changes that characterize pregnancy result in metabolic, respiratory, and cardiovascular phenomena not encountered in the nonpregnant state. These changes, together with the presence of the fetus in utero, are a challenge for the anesthesiologist. Furthermore, high-risk obstetric patients frequently have fetal or maternal problems that further complicate the already difficult task of administering anesthesia to two patients simultaneously (see Chapter 56).

The choice of drug and anesthetic technique for labor and delivery depends on the skill and experience of the person who performs the procedure, the progress of labor, other complications of pregnancy or labor, and the desires of the patient. With proper antenatal psychological preparation, many patients require minimal, if any, analgesia or anesthesia throughout labor, and healthy infants are born in most of these cases. Nothing should be done to discourage such a practice. Furthermore, everything should be done to facilitate birthing in quiet, pleasant, and friendly surroundings in which a friend or family members accompany the parturient. There is considerable evidence that a supportive birth attendant (doula) reduces the need for analgesia and anesthesia and, in some populations, reduces the incidence of dystocia.[189,330]

Analgesia

Sedatives and narcotic analgesics are frequently administered alone or in combination in the first stage of labor. There is increasing evidence that opioids given systemically do not relieve the pain of labor.[331,332] These drugs do reduce anxiety and result in sedation. All drugs of this type rapidly appear in the fetal circulation when administered to the mother. Predictably, there will be some sedation of the infant, depending on the specific drug given, the amount, the time, and the route of administration.

The drug most commonly used for pain is meperidine in doses of 50 to 100 mg intramuscularly or 25 to 50 mg intravenously. To enhance its effect, provide additional sedation, and prevent nausea, physicians may prescribe a phenothiazine such as promethazine, 25 mg, as well. The half-life of meperidine is increased and is more variable in pregnant women than in nonpregnant subjects. Furthermore, fetal hypoxia reduces the clearance of meperidine from fetal blood.[333] If the neonate appears depressed as the result of the administration of meperidine to the mother, injection of the narcotic antagonist naloxone may be indicated (0.1 mg/kg intravenously or intramuscularly). Other analgesics, such as butorphanol, nalbuphine, and fentanyl, all of which cause less respiratory depression, are used frequently for intrapartum pain control.[334-336]

Systematic reviews of parenteral opioids for relief of labor pain published by Elbourne and Wiseman[337] and Bricker and Lavender[338] included 48 trials comparing a variety of parenteral opioids with placebo, with each other, and with regional analgesia. These reviews concluded that epidural analgesia provides more effective pain relief than does parenteral analgesia. However, there is no clear evidence any one medication or one method of administration used for parenteral analgesia is superior to another. Long-term effects of parenteral opioids used during labor have not been studied extensively, although there is some concern about genetic imprinting at birth for later self-destructive behavior and drug addiction.[339]

Paracervical Block

Paracervical block was a popular form of anesthesia for the first stage of labor until it was implicated in several fetal deaths and was shown to be associated with fetal bradycardia in 25% to 35% of cases.[340-342] In some cases, death was related to direct injection of large doses of local anesthetic agents into the fetus, whereas the fetal bradycardia was probably a response to rapid uptake of the drug from the highly vascular paracervical space.

Although not advocated with enthusiasm by most authorities, this form of anesthesia is still used, especially in hospitals in which epidural anesthesia is not available. If paracervical block is used wisely in low-risk patients, it is safe and effective for the first stage of labor.[343] The anesthetic should be administered with great care to avoid direct fetal injection, and using the smallest amount of drug possible. Chloroprocaine (1% to 2%), rather than lidocaine or mepivacaine, should be used if repeated doses will be required.[344] Anyone using paracervical block anesthesia should read the excellent account of this method by Chestnut.[345]

Pudendal Block

Pudendal block is a common form of anesthesia used for vaginal delivery. When successful, it provides adequate pain relief for episiotomy, spontaneous delivery, forceps or vacuum extraction delivery from a low pelvic station, and repair of perineal, vaginal, or cervical lacerations. Because the local anesthetic agent is injected well away from the parauterine vasculature, uteroplacental blood flow and fetal heart rate are not affected to the same degree as in paracervical block. Occasionally, vaginal hematomas can be caused by pudendal nerve block, but the most dreaded complication is a retropsoas or pelvic abscess.[346,347] It is surprising that this complication does not occur more frequently, inasmuch as the injection is made through a nonsterile field. The infrequency of infections in the Alcock canal is probably a consequence of the prolonged compression of the paravaginal tissues by the fetal head, which prevents hematoma formation.

The success of pudendal nerve block depends on a clear understanding of the anatomy of the pudendal nerve and surrounding structures. The anatomic study by Klink[348] clarified the course of the pudendal nerve, described the variations of the nerve and its branches, and discussed the anatomy in relation to the performance of successful regional anesthesia. This article, with its helpful illustrations, is an excellent resource.

Low Spinal Anesthesia

Low spinal anesthesia, often called saddle block, is an effective means of anesthesia. It is relatively simple to perform and provides prompt, reliable pain relief that is adequate for spontaneous delivery or instrument delivery from the low pelvic or midpelvic station. It usually consists of 4 mg of tetracaine administered in a hyperbaric solution at the L4-L5 interspace with the patient sitting.

Although this technique is intended to anesthetize only the "saddle region," the level of anesthesia sometimes is as high as the T10 dermatome. Because of the ease of administration and the reliability of this form of anesthesia, it has been a favorite of obstetricians practicing in hospitals in which anesthesiologists are available only for cesarean delivery or other emergencies. As a result of the profound sympathetic block that occurs with spinal anesthesia, however, saddle block can be associated with profound hypotension and a decrease in uteroplacental perfusion. Furthermore, it can interfere with the voluntary abdominal pushing effort far more than epidural anesthesia, frequently resulting in delivery of the infant by forceps. The popularity of this form of obstetric anesthesia is waning because it is being replaced by epidural anesthesia and because many patients insist on unmedicated, natural delivery.

Epidural Analgesia and Anesthesia

Epidural anesthesia is being used with increasing frequency, especially in hospitals where anesthesiologists are available to patients in labor 24 hours a day. In experienced hands, epidural anesthesia has an excellent safety record.[349] Although it is the most difficult form of anesthesia to administer, it has the advantage of providing excellent pain relief for the first and second stages of labor and for delivery without altering the consciousness of the mother. Bupivacaine and chloroprocaine are the drugs most commonly used, the former providing more prolonged anesthesia but with a greater delay in onset. The use of combinations of local anesthetics and narcotics also provides excellent analgesia with less motor blockade.[350]

Continuous lumbar epidural anesthesia has been associated with late decelerations in fetal heart rate suggestive of decreased uteroplacental perfusion in as many as 20% of cases. This is more common with bupivacaine than with chloroprocaine or lidocaine.[351] Also, the use of oxytocin to augment labor in cases in which continuous epidural anesthesia is used has been reported to increase the frequency of late decelerations noted on fetal monitoring.[352] When uterine hypertonus or maternal hypotension is associated with the augmentation of contractions in patients with epidural anesthesia, fetal heart rate patterns indicating uteroplacental insufficiency occur in as many as 70% of cases.[353] Prehydration of the mother and avoidance of the supine position[354] can reduce the incidence of uteroplacental insufficiency with epidural anesthesia. The use of drug mixtures of local anesthetics and analgesics results in less motor block; this allows women who have epidural anesthesia to be more mobile during labor, and they are less likely to be confined to the supine position.

Thorp and Breedlove[355] reviewed the benefits and risks of epidural analgesia for labor and delivery. Both retrospective and prospective controlled trials have demonstrated that epidural analgesia results in longer labors and a higher incidence of operative vaginal delivery and cesarean delivery than intravenous analgesia. Some studies have suggested that the untoward effect of epidural analgesia on labor occurs primarily in patients in whom the epidural is placed when the cervix is dilated less than 5 cm[356]; however, controlled trials by Chestnut and coauthors[357,358] established that the time of onset of epidural analgesia did not affect length of labor or method of delivery. In a retrospective, case-controlled study, Thompson and colleagues[359] showed that those patients who had abnormal labor progress after epidural analgesia often had abnormal labor curves before placement of the epidural block.

Zhang and associates[360] used a unique approach to determine whether epidural analgesia prolongs labor and increases the risk of cesarean delivery. A natural experiment occurred wherein the incidence of labor epidural anesthesia was suddenly increased from 1% to 84% in a brief period of time while other conditions remained unchanged. There was no resultant change in overall rate of abdominal delivery, rate of abdominal delivery for dystocia, rate of instrumental delivery, or length of the first stage of labor. The second stage of labor was prolonged by a mean of 25 minutes. Moreover, on-demand epidural analgesia did not increase the risk of fetal head malposition.[361] The work of these authors confirmed the important studies of others[362-364] in finding that labor epidural analgesia does not increase the risk of cesarean delivery or the use of oxytocin or operative vaginal delivery. The only consistent effect of epidural analgesia is prolongation of the second stage of labor. Therefore, fear of increasing the risk of dystocia should not be used to limit patients' access to this effective analgesic technique.

The relationship between epidural analgesia for labor and delivery and chronic back pain after delivery is controversial. Retrospective studies found an association between epidural analgesia for labor and chronic back pain.[365] However, a more recent prospective study, in which women were monitored for 1 year after delivery, found no statistically significant difference in the incidence of persistent back pain among those who did or did not receive epidural analgesia during labor.[366]

Another problem encountered with epidural analgesia or anesthesia for labor is an increased incidence of intrapartum fever.[367] Fever occurs in approximately 30% of laboring patients after 4 to 5 hours of continuous epidural anesthesia. The specific cause of the febrile response is not known, although it could be related to the autonomic block that occurs with epidural anesthesia. Nevertheless, a clinical dilemma occurs in differentiating a "benign" febrile response to the epidural from intra-amniotic infection. As a consequence, most patients who develop a fever in labor are treated with antibiotics, and their infants are evaluated and treated for suspected sepsis.[368] At present, there is no clear-cut way to avoid this problem.

An additional benefit of epidural anesthesia for patients undergoing cesarean delivery is that opioids can be injected into the epidural space to provide prolonged postoperative analgesia.[369] The rare occurrence of serious respiratory depression (1 in 1200 cases) appears to be the only major complication. Transient nausea, urinary retention, and pruritus have also been reported in patients treated with epidural opioids.

Lieberman and O'Donoghue,[370] in a comprehensive systematic review of the unintended effects of epidural analgesia during labor, drew attention to the many unanswered questions that remain despite the large number of studies that have been performed. Because many such studies lacked proper randomization to eliminate selection bias, there is a need for trials comparing epidural analgesia with other forms of analgesia wherein randomization occurs during pregnancy rather than after labor begins. Nevertheless, Lieberman and O'Donoghue contended that current evidence supports the recommendation that women (especially nulliparous women) considering epidural analgesia for labor should be told the following:

- They are less likely to have a spontaneous vaginal delivery.
- The duration of their labor is likely to be longer.
- They will have an increased risk of instrument-assisted delivery, which is associated with an increased risk for serious perineal laceration.
- They are at greater risk of developing a fever during labor, which could lead to an evaluation and treatment of their infant for suspected sepsis.

There is evidence that the use of epidural anesthesia for pain control in labor is related to the size of the delivery service in hospitals in the United States.[371] In 1997, the use of epidural analgesia in labor was 50% among obstetric services with more than 1500 births per year, compared with 21% among obstetric units with fewer than 500 births per year. Clearly, this must reflect the more frequent availability of 24-hour coverage by anesthesiologists on the obstetric units of the larger hospitals. Proposed solutions to increase the availability of epidural anesthesia for women in labor include allowing certified registered nurse anesthetists (CRNAs) or adequately trained obstetricians to perform epidural anesthesia. Either of these innovations has economic and medicolegal ramifications that must be considered.

Labor Monitoring

The term "fetal monitoring" has become almost synonymous with continuous electronic fetal monitoring (see Chapter 22). The more comprehensive term, labor monitoring, means the conduct and management of the labor event from its onset to its completion. The primary goal of labor monitoring is to achieve delivery of a healthy infant from a healthy mother with as little trauma as possible. A secondary goal is to accomplish this delivery in a manner that is not degrading to the mother and that enhances and strengthens family relationships in a way that is consistent with the cultural and personal expectations of the patient. In a narrower context, this latter goal has been defined as "reducing bonding failure."[372] Certainly, a healthy and supportive family unit augments the growth and development of the newborn. To accomplish these goals requires attention to all the details of the labor and delivery process as they relate to a specific patient's medical, obstetric, and psychosocial situation.

One of the paradoxes of modern obstetric care is that the technologic advances that have contributed substantially to the identification and correction of the pathophysiologic abnormalities of labor may depersonalize the labor event and even introduce phenomena that alter maternal and fetal physiology and create substantial maternal and family anxiety. The outcry against such depersonalization has come from many quarters and has resulted in reexamination of the management of labor and delivery. Indeed, it has been found that many of the traditional hospital obstetric practices, such as the perineal shave, enemas, and isolation of the patient from her family and friends, are not beneficial. More liberal use of ambulation and positions of comfort in labor and delivery have been found to be physiologically beneficial. Furthermore, the presence of family members or supportive friends may decrease anxiety, shorten the duration of labor, and reduce the need for medications.

Perhaps the most important figure in this entire scenario is the bedside nurse in the labor and delivery unit. The nurse's role is to bridge the gap between the most sophisticated obstetric technology and the expectations and needs of the patient and her family. The nurse must thoroughly understand the physiology and pathophysiology of labor; must be able to collect, record, and interpret the data throughout the labor; and must anticipate both maternal and fetal problems. Furthermore, the nurse must provide timely communications to the physicians responsible for the patient's care and frequently must intelligibly and compassionately help to interpret the course of labor to the patient and her family. This implies a one-to-one nurse-patient ratio for patients in active labor. All of these goals should be accomplished in a facility in which there can be an immediate response to a fetal or maternal emergency in the form of prompt delivery or resuscitation if necessary.

References

1. Hendricks CH, Brenner WE, Kraus G: The normal cervical dilatation pattern in late pregnancy and labor. Am J Obstet Gynecol 106:1065, 1970.
2. Pritchard JA, MacDonald PC (eds): Williams' Obstetrics, 16th ed. New York, Appleton-Century-Crofts, 1980, p 426.

3. Friedman EA: Labor: Clinical Evaluation and Management, 2nd ed. New York, Appleton-Century-Crofts, 1978.
4. Friedman EA: Primigravid labor: A graphicostatistical analysis. Obstet Gynecol 6:567, 1955.
5. Kilpatrick SJ, Laros RK Jr: Characteristics of normal labor. Obstet Gynecol 74:85, 1989.
6. Albers LL, Schiff M, Gorwoda JG: The length of active labor in normal pregnancies. Obstet Gynecol 87:355, 1996.
7. Rinehart BK, Terrone DA, Hudson C, et al: Lack of utility of standard labor curves in the prediction of progression during labor induction. Am J Obstet Gynecol 182:1520, 2000.
8. Impey L, Hobson J, O'Herligy C: Graphic analysis of actively managed labor: Prospective computation of labor progression in 500 consecutive nulliparous women in spontaneous labor at term. Am J Obstet Gynecol 183:438, 2000.
9. Kelly G, Peaceman AM, Colangelo L, et al: Normal nulliparous labor: Are Friedman's definitions still relevant? [Abstract.] Am J Obstet Gynecol 182: S129, 2000.
10. Rouse DJ, Owen J, Hauth JC: Active-phase labor arrest: Oxytocin augmentation for at least 4 hours. Obstet Gynecol 93:323, 1999.
11. Rouse DJ, Owen J, Hauth JC: Criteria for failed labor induction: Prospective evaluation of a standardized protocol. Obstet Gynecol 96:671, 2000.
12. Zhang J, Troendle J, Yancey MK: Reassessing the labor curve in nulliparous women. Am J Obstet Gynecol 187:824, 2002.
13. Caldwell WE, Moloy HC, D'Esopo DA: Further studies on the mechanism of labor. Am J Obstet Gynecol 30:763, 1935.
14. Caldwell WE, Moloy HC, D'Esopo DA: The more recent conceptions of the pelvic architecture. Am J Obstet Gynecol 40:558, 1940.
15. Steer CM (ed): Moloy's Evaluation of the Pelvis in Obstetrics. Philadelphia, WB Saunders, 1959.
16. World Health Organisation Maternal and Safe Motherhood Programme. World Health Organisation partograph in management of labour. Lancet 343:1399, 1994.
17. Philpott RH, Castle WM: Cervicographs in the management of labour in primigravidae: I. The alert line for detecting abnormal labor. J Obstet Gynaecol Br Commonw 79:592, 1972.
18. Sheiner E, Levy A, Feinstein U, et al: Risk factors and outcome of failure to progress during the first stage of labor: A population-based study. Acta Obstet Gynecol Scand 81:222, 2002.
19. Friedman EA: Labor: Clinical Evaluation and Management, 1st ed. New York, Appleton-Century-Crofts, 1967.
20. Chelmow D, Kilpatrick SJ, Laros RK Jr: Maternal and neonatal outcomes after prolonged latent phase. Obstet Gynecol 81:486, 1993.
21. Beazley JM, Kurjak A: The influence of a partograph on the active management of labour. Lancet 2:348, 1972.
22. O'Driscoll K, Meagher D: Active Management of Labour. Philadelphia, WB Saunders, 1980.
23. Akoury HA, Brodie G, Caddick R, et al: Active management of labor and operative delivery in nulliparous women. Am J Obstet Gynecol 158:255, 1988.
24. Turner MJ, Brassil M, Gordon H: Active management of labor associated with a decrease in the cesarean section rate in nulliparas. Obstet Gynecol 71:150, 1988.
25. Boylan P, Frankowski R, Rountree R, et al: The effect of active management of labor on the incidence of caesarean section for dystocia in nulliparae. Am J Perinatol 8:373, 1991.
26. Lopez-Zeno JA, Peaceman AM, Adashek JA, et al: A controlled trial of a program for the active management of labor. N Engl J Med 326:450, 1992.
27. Frigoletto FD, Leiberman E, Lang JM, et al: A clinical trial of active management of labor. N Engl J Med 333:485, 1995.
28. Holmes P, Oppenheimer L, Wen S: The relationship between cervical dilatation at initial presentation in labour and subsequent intervention. BJOG 108:1120, 2001.
29. Murphy K, Shah L, Cohen W: Labor and delivery in nulliparous women who present with an unengaged fetal head. J Perinatol 18:122, 1998.
30. Falzone S, Chauhan S, Mobley J, et al: Unengaged vertex in nulliparous women in active labor. J Reprod Med 43:676, 1998.
31. Ganström L, Ekman G, Malmström A: Insufficient remodeling of the uterine connective tissue in women with protracted labour. BJOG 98:1212, 1991.
32. Philpott RH, Castle WM: Cervicographs in the management of labour in primigravidae: II. The action line and treatment of abnormal labor. J Obstet Gynaecol Br Commonw 79:599, 1972.
33. O'Brien WF, Cefalo RC: Evaluation of x-ray pelvimetry and abnormal labor. Clin Obstet Gynecol 25:157, 1982.
34. Parsons MT, Spellacy WN: Prospective randomized study of x-ray pelvimetry in the primigravida. Obstet Gynecol 66:76, 1985.
35. Floberg J, Belfrage P, Ohlsen H: Influence of pelvic outlet capacity on labor: A prospective pelvimetry study of 1429 unselected primiparas. Acta Obstet Gynaecol Scand 66:121, 1987.
36. Thurnau GR, Morgan MA: Efficacy of the fetal-pelvic index as a predictor of fetal-pelvic disproportion in women with abnormal labor patterns that require labor augmentation. Am J Obstet Gynecol 159:1168, 1988.
37. Morgan MA, Thurnau GR: Efficacy of the fetal-pelvic index in patients requiring labor inductions. Am J Obstet Gynecol 159:621, 1988.
38. Thurnau GR, Scates DH, Morgan MA: The fetal-pelvic index: A method of identifying fetal-pelvic disproportion in women attempting vaginal birth after previous cesarean delivery. Am J Obstet Gynecol 165:353, 1991.
39. Ferguson JE, Newberry YG, DeAngelis GA, et al: The fetal-pelvic index has minimal utility in predicting fetal-pelvic disproportion. Am J Obstet Gynecol 179:1186, 1998.
40. Lucidi RS, Chez RA, Creasy RK: The clinical use of intrauterine pressure catheters. J Matern Fetal Med 10:420, 2001.
41. Flynn AM, Kelly J, Hollins G, et al: Ambulation in labor. BMJ 2:591, 1978.
42. Williams RM, Thom MH, Studd JW: A study of the benefits and acceptability of ambulation in spontaneous labour. BJOG 87:122, 1980.
43. Read JA, Miller FC, Paul RH: Randomized trial of ambulation versus oxytocin for labor enhancement: A preliminary report. Am J Obstet Gynecol 139:669, 1981.
44. Hellman LM, Prystowsky H: Duration of the second stage of labor. Am J Obstet Gynecol 63:1223, 1952.
45. Cohen WR: Influence of the duration of second stage of labor on perinatal outcome and puerperal morbidity. Obstet Gynecol 49:266, 1977.
46. Menticoglou SM, Manning F, Harman C, et al: Perinatal outcome in relation to second-stage duration. Am J Obstet Gynecol 173:906, 1995.
47. Hansen S, Clark S, Foster J: Active pushing versus passive fetal descent in the second stage of labor: A randomized controlled trial. Obstet Gynecol 99:29, 2002.
48. March MR, Adair CD, Veille J-C, et al: The modified Mueller-Hillis maneuver in predicting abnormalities in second stage of labor. Int J Gynaecol Obstet 55:105, 1996.
49. Thorp JM, Pahel-Short L, Bowes WA Jr: The Mueller-Hillis maneuver: Can it be used to predict dystocia? Obstet Gynecol 82:519, 1993.
50. Acker DB, Sachs BP, Friedman EA: Risk factors for shoulder dystocia in the average infant. Obstet Gynecol 67:614, 1986.
51. Gross SJ, Shime J, Farine D: Shoulder dystocia: Predictors and outcome: A five-year review. Am J Obstet Gynecol 156:1408, 1987.
52. Nocon JJ, McKenzie DK, Thomas LJ, et al: Shoulder dystocia: An analysis of risks and obstetric maneuvers. Am J Obstet Gynecol 168:1732, 1993.
53. Basket TF, Allen AC: Perinatal implications of shoulder dystocia. Obstet Gynecol 86:14, 1995.
54. Benedetti TJ, Gabbe SG: Shoulder dystocia: A complication of fetal macrosomia and prolonged second stage of labor with midpelvic delivery. Obstet Gynecol 52:526, 1978.
55. Smith RB, Lane C, Pearson JF: Shoulder dystocia: What happens at the next delivery? BJOG 101:713, 1994.
56. Lewis DF, Raymond RC, Perkins MB, et al: Recurrence rate of shoulder dystocia. Am J Obstet Gynecol 172:1369, 1995.

57. McFarland M, Hod M, Piper JM, et al: Are labor abnormalities more common in shoulder dystocia? Am J Obstet Gynecol 173:1211, 1995.
58. Al-Najashi S, Al-Suleiman SA, El-Yahai A, et al: Shoulder dystocia: A clinical study of 56 cases. Aust N Z J Obstet Gynaecol 29:129, 1989.
59. Sloof ACJ: Obstetric brachial plexus lesions and their neurosurgical treatment. Microsurgery 16:30, 1995.
60. DeMott RK: Brachial plexus deficits with and without shoulder dystocia. Am J Obstet Gynecol 195:630, author reply 631, 2006.
61. Jennet RJ, Tarby TJ, Kreinick CJ: Brachial plexus palsy: An old problem revisited. Am J Obstet Gynecol 166:1673, 1992.
62. Hankins GDV, Clark SL: Brachial plexus palsy involving the posterior shoulder at spontaneous vaginal delivery. Am J Perinatol 14:44, 1995.
63. McFarland LV, Raskin M, Daling J, et al: Erb/Duchenne's palsy: A consequence of fetal macrosomia and method of delivery. Obstet Gynecol 68:784, 1986.
64. Morrison JC, Sanders JR, Magann EF, et al: The diagnosis and management of dystocia of the shoulder. Surg Gynecol Obstet 175:515, 1992.
65. Dunn DW, Engle WA: Brachial plexus palsy: Intrauterine onset. Pediatr Neurol 1:365, 1985.
66. Koenigsberger MR: Brachial plexus palsy at birth: Intrauterine or due to birth trauma? Ann Neurol 8:228, 1980.
67. Sandmire H, DeMott R. Erb's palsy causation: A historical perspective. Birth 29:52, 2002.
68. Gherman R, Ouzounian J, Goodwin T: Brachial plexus palsy: An in utero injury? Am J Obstet Gynecol 180:1303, 1999.
69. Gonen O, Rosen DJD, Dolfin Z, et al: Induction of labor versus expectant management in macrosomia: A randomized study. Obstet Gynecol 89:913, 1997.
70. Rouse DJ, Owen J: Prophylactic cesarean delivery for fetal macrosomia diagnosed by means of ultrasonography: A Faustian bargain? Am J Obstet Gynecol 181:332, 1999.
71. Allen R, Sorab J, Gonik B: Risk factors for shoulder dystocia: An engineering study of clinician-applied forces. Obstet Gynecol 77:352, 1991.
72. Allen RH, Bankoski BR, Butzin CA, et al: Comparing clinician applied leads for routine, difficult, and shoulder dystocia deliveries. Am J Obstet Gynecol 171:1621, 1994.
73. Gonik B, Stringer CA, Held B: An alternate maneuver for management of shoulder dystocia. Am J Obstet Gynecol 145:882, 1983.
74. Gonik B, Allen R, Sorab J: Objective evaluation of the shoulder dystocia phenomenon: Effect of maternal pelvic orientation of force reduction. Obstet Gynecol 74:44, 1989.
75. Rubin A: Management of shoulder dystocia. JAMA 188:835, 1964.
76. Woods CE: A principle of physics as applicable to shoulder dystocia. Am J Obstet Gynecol 45:796, 1943.
77. Barnum CG: Dystocia due to the shoulders. Am J Obstet Gynecol 50:439, 1949.
78. O'Leary JA: Cephalic replacement for shoulder dystocia: Present status and future role of the Zavanelli maneuver. Obstet Gynecol 82:847, 1993.
79. Acker DB, Gregory KD, Sachs BP, et al: Risk factors for Erb-Duchenne palsy. Obstet Gynecol 71:389, 1988.
80. Chauhan SP, Rose CH, Gherman RB, et al: Brachial plexus injury: A 23-year experience from a tertiary center. Am J Obstet Gynecol 192:1795, discussion 1800, 2005.
81. Athukorala C, Middleton P, Crowther CA: Intrapartum interventions for preventing shoulder dystocia. Cochrane Database Syst Rev (4):CD005543, 2006.
82. Pritchard JA: Changes in the blood volume during pregnancy and delivery. Anesthesiology 26:393, 1965.
83. Thomas WO: Manual removal of the placenta. Am J Obstet Gynecol 86:600, 1963.
84. Blanchette H: Elective manual exploration of the uterus after delivery: A study and review. J Reprod Med 19:13, 1977.
85. Elbourne DR, Prendiville WJ, Carroli G, et al: Prophylactic use of oxytocin in the third stage of labour. Cochrane Database Syst Rev (4):CD001808, 2001.
86. Walley R, Wilson J, Crane J, et al: A double-blind placebo controlled randomised trial of misoprostol and oxytocin in the management of the third stage of labour. BJOG 107:1111, 2000.
87. Ng PS, Chan A, Sin WK, et al: A multicentre randomized controlled trial of oral misoprostol and i.m. syntometrine in the management of the third stage of labour. Hum Reprod 16:31, 2001.
88. Gulmezoglu A, Villar J, Ngoc N, et al: WHO multicentre randomised trial of misoprostol in the management of the third stage of labour. Lancet 358:689, 2001.
89. Lokugamage A, Sullivan K, Niculescu I, et al: A randomized study comparing rectally administered misoprostol versus Syntometrine combined with an oxytocin infusion for the cessation of primary postpartum hemorrhage. Acta Obstet Gynecol Scand 80:835, 2001.
90. DeSimone CA, Norris MC, Leighton BL: Intravenous nitroglycerin aids manual extraction of retained placenta. Anesthesiology 73:787, 1990.
91. Read JA, Cotton DB, Miller FC: Placenta accreta: Changing clinical aspects and outcome. Obstet Gynecol 56:31, 1980.
92. Descargues G, Douvrin F, Degre S, et al: Abnormal placentation and selective embolization of the uterine arteries. Eur J Obstet Gynecol 99:47, 2001.
93. Hendricks CH: Uterine contractility at delivery and in the puerperium. Am J Obstet Gynecol 83:890, 1962.
94. Munsick RA: Renal hemodynamic effects of oxytocin in antepartal and postpartal women. Am J Obstet Gynecol 108:729, 1970.
95. Hendricks CH, Brenner WE: Cardiovascular effects of oxytocic drugs used postpartum. Am J Obstet Gynecol 108:751, 1970.
96. Browning DJ: Serious side effects of ergometrine and its use in routine obstetric practice. Med J Aust 1:957, 1974.
97. Buttino L Jr, Garite TJ: The use of 15 methyl F2 alpha prostaglandin (Prostin 15M) for the control of postpartum hemorrhage. Am J Perinatol 3:241, 1986.
98. Abdel-Aleem H, Nashar I, Abdel-Aleem A: Management of severe postpartum hemorrhage with misoprostol. Int J Gynecol Obstet 72:75, 2001.
99. Adekanmi O, Purmessur S, Edwards G, et al: Intrauterine misoprostol for the treatment of severe recurrent atonic secondary postpartum haemorrhage. BJOG 108:541, 2001.
100. Bowen LW, Beeson JH: Use of a large Foley catheter balloon to control postpartum hemorrhage resulting from a low placental implantation: A report of two cases. J Reprod Med 30:623, 1985.
101. Hester JD: Postpartum hemorrhage and re-evaluation of uterine packing. Obstet Gynecol 45:501, 1975.
102. Vedantham S, Goodwin SC, McLucas B, et al: Uterine artery embolization: An underused method of controlling hemorrhage. Am J Obstet Gynecol 176:938, 1997.
103. O'Leary JL, O'Leary JA: Uterine artery ligation for control of postcesarean section hemorrhage. Obstet Gynecol 43:849, 1974.
104. B-Lynch C, Coker A, Lawal A, et al: The B-Lynch surgical technique for the control of massive postpartum haemorrhage: An alternative to hysterectomy? Five cases reported. BJOG 104:372, 1997.
105. Ferguson JE, Bourgeois FJ, Underwood P: B-Lynch suture for postpartum hemorrhage. Obstet Gynecol 95:1020, 2000.
106. Hayman RG, Arulkumaran S, Steer PJ: Uterine compression sutures: Surgical management of postpartum hemorrhage. Obstet Gynecol 99:502, 2002.
107. Burchell RC: Physiology of internal iliac artery ligation. J Obstet Gynaecol Br Commonw 75:642, 1968.
108. Swan HJC: Balloon flotation catheters: Their use in hemodynamic monitoring in clinical practice. JAMA 233:865, 1975.
109. Berkowitz RL, Rafferty TD: Pulmonary artery flow-directed catheter use in the obstetric patient. Obstet Gynecol 55:507, 1980.
110. Watson P, Besch N, Bowes WA Jr: Management of acute and subacute puerperal inversion of the uterus. Obstet Gynecol 55:12, 1980.
111. McCullagh WM III: Inversion of the uterus: A report of three cases and an analysis of 223 recently recorded cases. J Obstet Gynaecol Br Emp 32:280, 1925.
112. Grossman RA: Magnesium sulfate for uterine inversion. J Reprod Med 26:261, 1981.

113. Catanzarite VA, Moffitt KD, Baker ML, et al: New approaches to the management of acute uterine inversion. Obstet Gynecol 68:78, 1986.
114. Altabef KM, Spencer JT, Zinberg S: Intravenous nitroglycerin for uterine relaxation of an inverted uterus. Am J Obstet Gynecol 166:1237, 1992.
115. Johnson AB: A new concept in the replacement of the inverted uterus and a report of nine cases. Am J Obstet Gynecol 57:557, 1949.
116. Huntington JL: Acute inversion of the uterus. Boston Med Surg J 15:376, 1921.
117. Haultain FWN: The treatment of chronic uterine inversion by abdominal hysterotomy with a successful case. BMJ 2:974, 1901.
118. Zhang J, Yancey MK, Henderson CE: U.S. national trends in labor induction, 1989-1998. J Reprod Med 47:120, 2002.
119. MacDorman MF, Mathews TJ, Martin JA, et al: Trends and characteristics of induced labour in the United States, 1989-1998. Paediatr Perinat Epidemiol 16:263, 2002.
120. Nicholson JM, Kellar LC, Cronholm PF, Macones GA. Active management of risk in pregnancy at term in an urban population: An association between a higher induction of labor rate and a lower caesarean delivery rate. Am J Obstet Gynecol 191:1516-1528, 2004.
121. Caughey AB, Nicholson JM, Cheng YW, et al: Induction of labor and cesarean delivery by gestational age. Am J Obstet Gynecol 195:700-705, 2006.
122. Keettel WC: Inducing labor by rupturing membranes. Postgrad Med 44:199, 1968.
123. Cole RA, Howie PW, MacNaughton MC: Elective induction of labour: A randomized prospective trial. Lancet 1:767, 1975.
124. Tylleskär J, Finnstrom O, Leijon I, et al: Spontaneous labor and elective induction: A prospective randomized study. I: Effects on mother and fetus. Acta Obstet Gynecol Scand 58:513, 1979.
125. Black BP, McBride WG: Children born after elective induction of labour. Med J Aust 2:362, 1979.
126. Friedman EA, Sachtleben MR, Wallace BA: Infant outcome following labor induction. Am J Obstet Gynecol 133:718, 1979.
127. Maslow AS, Sweeny A: Elective induction of labor as a risk factor for cesarean delivery among low-risk women at term. Obstet Gynecol 95:917, 2000.
128. Seyb ST, Berka RJ, Socol ML, et al: Risk of cesarean delivery with elective induction of labor at term in nulliparous women. Obstet Gynecol 94:600, 1999.
129. Dublin S, Lydon-Rochelle M, Kaplan RC, et al: Maternal and neonatal outcomes after induction of labor without an identified indication. Am J Obstet Gynecol 183:986, 2000.
130. Heinberg EM, Wood RA, Chambers RB: Elective induction of labor in multiparous women. Does it increase the risk of cesarean section? J Reprod Med 47:399, 2002.
131. Bishop EH: Pelvic scoring for elective induction. Obstet Gynecol 24:266, 1964.
132. Macer JA, Macer CL, Chan LS: Elective induction versus spontaneous labor: A retrospective study of complications and outcome. Am J Obstet Gynecol 166:1690, 1992.
133. Lange AP, Secher NJ, Westergaard JG, et al: Prelabor evaluation of inducibility. Obstet Gynecol 60:137, 1982.
134. Ware V, Raynor BD: Transvaginal ultrasonographic cervical measurement as a predictor of successful labor induction. Am J Obstet Gynecol 182:1030, 2000.
135. Watson WJ, Stevens D, Welter S, et al: Factors predicting successful labor induction. Obstet Gynecol 88:990, 1996.
136. Garite T, Casal D, Garcia-Alonso A, et al: Fetal fibronectin: A new tool for the prediction of successful induction of labor. Am J Obstet Gynecol 175:1516, 1996.
137. Bailit JL, Downs SM, Thorp JM: Reducing the cesarean delivery risk in elective inductions of labor: A decision analysis. Paediatr Perinatal Epidemiol 16:90, 2002.
138. Sciscione A, Hoffman MK, DeLuca S, et al. Fetal fibronectin as a predictor of vaginal birth in nulliparas undergoing preinduction cervical ripening. Obstet Gynecol 106:980, 2005.
139. Mitchell MD, Flint APF, Bibby J, et al: Rapid increases in plasma prostaglandin concentrations after the vaginal examination and amniotomy. BMJ 2:1183, 1977.
140. Lin MG, Rouse DJ. What is a failed labor induction? Clin Obstet Gynecol 49:585, 2006.
141. Maisels MJ, Rees R, Marks K, et al: Elective delivery of the term fetus: An obstetrical hazard. JAMA 238:2036, 1977.
142. Madar J, Richmond S, Hey E: Surfactant-deficient respiratory distress after elective delivery at "term." Acta Paediatr 88:1244, 1999.
143. Gluckman PD, Sizonenko SV, Bassett NS: The transition from fetus to neonate: An endocrine perspective. Acta Paediat Suppl 88:7, 1999.
144. Bland RD: Lung liquid clearance before and after birth. Sem Perinatol 12:124, 1988.
145. McCray PB Jr, Bettencourt JD: Prostaglandins stimulate fluid secretion in human lung fluid. J Develop Physiol 19:29, 1993.
146. Wax JR, Herson V, Carignan E, et al: Contribution of elective delivery to severe respiratory distress at term. Am J Perinatol 19:81, 2002.
147. Danforth DN: The fibrous nature of the cervix and its relation to the isthmic segment in gravid and nongravid uteri. Am J Obstet Gynecol 53:541, 1947.
148. Leppert PC: Anatomy and physiology of cervical ripening. Clin Obstet Gynecol 38:267, 1995.
149. Winkler M, Rath W: Changes in the cervical extracellular matrix during pregnancy and parturition. J Perinat Med 27:45, 1999.
150. Allaire AD, D'Andrea N, Truong P, et al: Cervical stroma apoptosis in pregnancy. Obstet Gynecol 97:399, 2001.
151. Kelly AJ, Kavanagh J, Thomas J: Vaginal prostaglandin (PGE2 and PGF2a) for induction of labour at term. Cochrane Database Syst Rev (2): CD003101, 2001.
152. Hofmeyr GJ, Gülmezoglu AM: Vaginal misoprostol for cervical ripening and induction of labor. Cochrane Database Syst Rev (1):CD000941, 1998 (updated 2002).
153. Boulvain M, Kelly A, Lohse C, et al: Mechanical methods for induction of labour. Cochrane Database Syst Rev (4):CD001233, 2001.
154. Sciscione AC, Nguyen L, Manley J, et al: A randomized comparison of transcervical Foley catheter to intravaginal misoprostol for preinduction cervical ripening. Obstet Gynecol 97:603, 2001.
155. Weisman AI: An antepartum study of fetal polarity and rotation. Am J Obstet Gynecol 48:550, 1944.
156. Brenner WE, Bruce RD, Hendricks CH: The characteristics and perils of breech presentation. Am J Obstet Gynecol 118:700, 1974.
157. Stevenson CS: The principal cause of breech presentation in single term pregnancies. Am J Obstet Gynecol 60:41, 1950.
158. Braun FHT, Jones KL, Smith DW: Breech presentation as an indicator of fetal abnormality. J Pediatr 86:419, 1975.
159. Axelrod FB, Leistner HL, Porges RF: Breech presentation among infants with familial dysautonomia. J Pediatr 84:107, 1974.
160. Ralis ZA: Traumatizing effect of breech delivery on infants with spina bifida. J Pediatr 87:613, 1975.
161. McBride WG, Black BP, Brown CJ, et al: Method of delivery and developmental outcome at five years of age. Med J Aust 1:301, 1979.
162. Wright RC: Reduction of perinatal mortality and morbidity in breech delivery through routine use of cesarean delivery. Obstet Gynecol 14:758, 1959.
163. Bowes WA Jr, Taylor ES, O'Brien M, et al: Breech delivery: Evaluation of the method of delivery on perinatal results and maternal morbidity. Am J Obstet Gynecol 135:965, 1979.
164. Bingham P, Lilford RJ: Management of the selected term breech presentation: Assessment of the risks of selected vaginal delivery versus cesarean section for all cases. Obstet Gynecol 69:965, 1987.
165. Cheng M, Hannah M: Breech delivery at term: A critical review of the literature. Obstet Gynecol 82:605, 1993.
166. Hannah M, Hannah W: Cesarean section or vaginal birth for breech presentation at term. BMJ 312:1451, 1996.
167. Hannah ME, Hannah WJ, Hewson SA, et al: Planned caesarean section versus planned vaginal birth for breech presentation at term: a randomized multicentre trial. Lancet 356:1375, 2000.

168. Hauth JC, Cunningham FG: Vaginal breech delivery is still justified. Obstet Gynecol 99:1115, 2002.
169. Somerset D: Term breech trial does not provide unequivocal evidence. BMJ 324:50, 2002.
170. Keirse MJNC: Evidence-based childbirth only for breech babies? Birth 29:55, 2002.
171. American College of Obstetricians and Gynecologists: Mode of Term Singleton Breech Delivery. ACOG Committee Opinion 265. Washington, DC, ACOG, 2001.
172. Danielian PJ, Wang J, Hall MH: Long-term outcome by method of delivery of fetuses in breech presentation at term: Population based follow up. BMJ 312:1451, 1996.
173. Munstedt K, von Georgi R, Reucher S, et al: Term breech and long-term morbidity: Cesarean section versus vaginal delivery. Eur J Obstet Gynecol Reprod Biol 96:163, 2001.
174. Irion O, Almagbaly PH, Morabia A: Planned vaginal delivery versus elective caesarean section: A study of 705 singleton term breech presentations. BJOG 105:710, 1998.
175. Kayem G, Goffinet F, Clèment D, et al: Breech presentation at term: Morbidity and mortality according to the type of delivery at Port Royal Maternity Hospital from 1993 through 1999. Eur J Obstet Gynecol Reprod Biol 102:137, 2002.
176. Potter MG, Heaton CH, Douglas GW: Intrinsic fetal risk in breech delivery. Obstet Gynecol 15:158, 1960.
177. Beischer NA: Pelvic contraction in breech presentation. J Obstet Gynaecol Br Commonw 73:421, 1966.
178. Todd WD, Steer CM: Term breech: Review of 1006 term breech deliveries. Obstet Gynecol 22:583, 1963.
179. Kopelman JN, Duff P, Karl RT, et al: Computed tomographic pelvimetry in the evaluation of breech presentation. Obstet Gynecol 68:455, 1986.
180. Christian SS, Brady K, Read JA, et al: Vaginal breech delivery: A five-year prospective evaluation of a protocol using computed tomographic pelvimetry. Am J Obstet Gynecol 163:848, 1990.
181. Van Loon AJ, Mantinoh A, Thiun CJ, et al: Pelvimetry by magnetic resonance imaging in breech presentation. Am J Obstet Gynecol 163:1256, 1990.
182. Zatuchni GI, Andros GJ: Prognostic index for vaginal delivery in breech presentation at term: Prospective study. Am J Obstet Gynecol 98:854, 1967.
183. Crawford JS: Appraisal of lumbar epidural blockade in patients with singleton fetus presenting by breech. J Obstet Gynaecol Br Commonw 81:867, 1974.
184. Chadha YC, Mahmood TA, Dick MJ, et al: Breech delivery and epidural analgesia. BJOG 99:96, 1992.
185. Hill JG, Eliot BW, Campbell AJ, et al: Intensive care of the fetus in breech labor. BJOG 83:271, 1976.
186. Milner RDG: Neonatal mortality of breech deliveries with and without forceps to the after-coming head. BJOG 82:783, 1975.
187. Piper EB, Bachman C: The prevention of fetal injuries in breech delivery. JAMA 92:217, 1929.
188. Calvert JP: Intrinsic hazard of breech presentation. BMJ 281:1319, 1980.
189. Zhang J, Bernask JW, Leybovich E, et al: Continuous labor support from labor attendant for primiparous women: A meta-analysis. Obstet Gynecol 88:739, 1996.
190. Hofmeyr GJ, Kulier R: External cephalic version for breech presentation at term. Cochrane Database Syst Rev (2):CD000083, 1996.
191. Hofmeyr GJ, Gyte G: Interventions to help external cephalic version for breech presentation. Cochrane Database Syst Rev (3):CD000184, 1996 (updated 2003).
192. Schorr SJ, Speights SE, Ross EL, et al: A randomized trial of epidural anesthesia to improve external cephalic version success. Am J Obstet Gynecol 177:1133, 1997.
193. Neiger R, Hennessy MD, Patel M: Reattempting failed external cephalic version under epidural anesthesia. Am J Obstet Gynecol 179:1136, 1998.
194. Rozenberg P, Goffinet F, de Spirlet M, et al: External cephalic version with epidural anaesthesia after failure of a first trial with beta-mimetics. BJOG 107:406, 2000.
195. Mauldin JG, Mauldin PD, Feng T, et al: Determining the clinical efficacy and cost savings of successful external cephalic version. Am J Obstet Gynecol 175:1639, 1996.
196. Chan LY-S, Leung TY, Fok WY, et al: High incidence of obstetric interventions after successful external cephalic version. BJOG 109:627, 2002.
197. Marcus RG, Crewe-Brown H, Krawitz S, et al: Fetomaternal hemorrhage following successful and unsuccessful attempts at external version. BJOG 82:578, 1975.
198. Gjode P, Rasmussen TB, Jorgenson J: Feto-maternal bleeding during attempts at external version. BJOG 87:571, 1980.
199. Seeds JW, Cefalo RC: Malpresentations. Clin Obstet Gynecol 25:145, 1982.
200. Cruikshank DP, White CA: Obstetric malpresentations: Twenty years' experience. Am J Obstet Gynecol 116:1097, 1973.
201. Edwards RL, Nicholson HO: The management of the unstable lie in late pregnancy. J Obstet Gynaecol Br Commonw 76:713, 1969.
202. Durfee RB: Low classical cesarean section. Postgrad Med 51:219, 1972.
203. Pelosi MA, Apuzzio J, Fricchione D, et al: The intra-abdominal version technique for delivery of transverse lie by low segment cesarean section. Am J Obstet Gynecol 136:1009, 1979.
204. Breen JL, Wiesmeier E: Compound presentations: A survey of 131 patients. Obstet Gynecol 32:419, 1968.
205. Weissberg SM, O'Leary JA: Compound presentation of the fetus. Obstet Gynecol 41:60, 1973.
206. Eastman NJ: The role of frontier America in the development of cesarean section. Am J Obstet Gynecol 24:919, 1932.
207. Frank F: Suprasymphyseal delivery and its relation to other operations in the presence of contracted pelvis. Arch Gynaecol 81:46, 1907.
208. D'Esopo DA: A review of cesarean section at Sloan Hospital for Women 1942-1947. Am J Obstet Gynecol 59:77, 1950.
209. Smith EF, MacDonald FA: Cesarean section: An evaluation of current practice in the New York Lying-In Hospital. Obstet Gynecol 6:593, 1953.
210. Notzon FC, Placek PJ, Taffels M: Comparison of national cesarean-section rates. N Engl J Med 316:386, 1987.
211. Notzon FC: International differences in the use of obstetric interventions. JAMA 263:3286, 1990.
212. Curtin SC, Kozak LJ, Gregor KD: U.S. cesarean and VBAC rates stalled in the mid-1990s. Birth 27:54-57, 2000.
213. Rosen MG (Chairman): Report of the Consensus Task Force on Cesarean Childbirth. NIH Publication No. 82-2067. Bethesda, MD, National Institutes of Health, 1981.
214. Leitch CR, Walker JJ: The rise in cesarean section rate: The same indications but a lower threshold. BJOG 105:621, 1998.
215. Notzon FC, Cnattingius S, Bergsjø P, et al: Cesarean section delivery in the 1980s: International comparison by indication. Am J Obstet Gynecol 170:495, 1994.
216. Walker R, Turnbull D, Wilkinson C: Strategies to address global cesarean section rates: A review of the evidence. Birth 29:28, 2002.
217. Belizan JM, Althabe F, Barros FC, et al: Rates and implications of cesarean sections in Latin America ecological study. BMJ 319:1397, 1999.
218. Potter JE, Berquó E, Perpétuo IHO, et al: Unwanted caesarean sections among public and private patients in Brazil: Prospective study. BMJ 323:1155, 2001.
219. Béhague DP, Victoria CG, Barros FC: Consumer demand for caesarean sections in Brazil: Population based birth cohort study linking ethnographic and epidemiological methods. BMJ 324:942, 2002.
220. Farrell SA, Allen VM, Baskett TF: Parturition and urinary incontinence in primiparas. Obstet Gynecol 97:350, 2001.
221. Hannah ME, Hannah WJ, Hodnett ED, et al: Outcomes at 3 months after planned cesarean vs planned vaginal delivery for breech presentation at term. The International Randomized Term Breech Trial. JAMA 287:1822, 2002.

222. Buchsbaum GM, Chin M, Glantz C, et al: Prevalence of urinary incontinence and associated risk factors in a cohort of nuns. Obstet Gynecol 100:226, 2002.
223. MacLennan AH, Taylor AW, Wilson DH, et al: The prevalence of pelvic floor disorders and their relationship to gender, age, parity and mode of delivery. BJOG 107:1460, 2000.
224. Sultan AH, Kamm MA, Hudson CN, et al: Anal-sphincter disruption during vaginal delivery. N Engl J Med 329:1905, 1993.
225. Fynes M, Donnelly VS, O'Connell PR, et al: Cesarean delivery and anal sphincter injury. Obstet Gynecol 92:496, 1998.
226. Nygaard IE, Rao SS, Dawson JD: Anal incontinence after anal sphincter disruption: A 30-year retrospective cohort study. Obstet Gynecol 89:896, 1997.
227. Ventura SJ, Martin JA, Curtin SC, et al: Births: Final data for 1999. Natl Vital Stat Rep 49:1, 2001.
228. World Health Organization: Appropriate technology for birth. Lancet 2:436, 1985.
229. Visco AG, Viswanathan M, Lohr KN, et al. Cesarean delivery on maternal request: A systematic evidence review of maternal and neonatal outcomes. Obstet Gynecol 108:1517, 2006.
230. McMahon MJ, Luther ER, Bowes WA Jr, et al: Comparison of a trial of labor with an elective second cesarean section. N Engl J Med 335:689, 1996.
231. Lydon-Rochelle M, Holt VL, Easterling TR, et al: Risk of uterine rupture during labor among women with a prior cesarean delivery. N Engl J Med 345:3, 2001.
232. Smith GC, Cameron AD, Dobbie R: Risk of perinatal death associated with labor after previous cesarean delivery in uncomplicated term pregnancies. JAMA 287:2684, 2002.
233. Sachs BP, Yeh J, Acker D, et al: Cesarean section-related maternal mortality in Massachusetts, 1954-1985. Obstet Gynecol 71:385, 1988.
234. Frigoletto FD Jr, Ryan KJ, Phillippe M: Maternal mortality rate associated with cesarean section: An appraisal. Am J Obstet Gynecol 136:969, 1980.
235. Lilford RJ, Van Coeverden De Groot HA, Moore PJ, et al: The relative risks of caesarean section (intrapartum and elective) and vaginal delivery: A detailed analysis to exclude the effects of medical disorders and other acute pre-existing physiological disturbance. BJOG 97:883, 1990.
236. Lydon-Rochelle M, Holt V, Easterling TR, et al: Cesarean delivery and postpartum mortality among primiparas in Washington State, 1987-1996. Obstet Gynecol 97:169, 2001.
237. Neilsen TF, Hökegård K-H: Cesarean section and intraoperative surgical complications. Acta Obstet Gynecol Scand 63:103, 1984.
238. Rajasekar D, Hall M: Urinary tract injuries during obstetric intervention. BJOG 104:731, 1997.
239. Duff P: Prophylactic antibiotics for cesarean delivery: A simple cost-effective strategy for prevention of postoperative morbidity. Am J Obstet Gynecol 157:794, 1987.
240. Watson WJ, George RJ, Welter S, et al: High-risk obstetric patients: Maternal morbidity after cesareans. J Reprod Med 42:267, 1997.
241. French LM, Smaill FM: Antibiotic regimens for endometritis after delivery. Cochrane Database Syst Rev (2):CD001067, 2000 (updated 2004).
242. Buchholz NP, Daly-Grandeau E, Huber-Buchholz M-M: Urological complications associated with caesarean section. Eur J Obstet Gynecol 56:161, 1994.
243. Tangtrakul S, Taechaiya S, Suthutvoravat S: Post-caesarean section urinary tract infection: A comparison between intermittent and indwelling catheterization. J Med Assoc Thailand 77:244, 1994.
244. Barnes JS: Is it better to avoid urethral catheterization at hysterectomy and caesarean section? Aust N Z J Obstet Gynaecol 38:315, 1998.
245. Emmons SL, Krohn M, Jackson M, et al: Development of wound infections among women undergoing cesarean section. Obstet Gynecol 72:559, 1988.
246. Roberts S, Maccato M, Faro S, et al: The microbiology of post-cesarean wound morbidity. Obstet Gynecol 81:383, 1993.
247. Gallup DG, Freedman MA, Meguiar RV, et al: Necrotizing fasciitis in gynecologic and obstetric patients: A surgical emergency. Am J Obstet Gynecol 187:305, 2002.
248. Bergqvist A, Bergqvist D, Hallbooki T: Acute deep vein thrombosis (DVT) after cesarean section. Acta Obstet Gynecol Scand 58:473, 1979.
249. Stirrup CA, Lucas DN, Cox MC, et al: Maternal anti-factor Xa activity following subcutaneous unfractionated heparin after caesarean section. Anaesthesia 56:855, 2001.
250. Tulley L, Gates S, Brocklehurst P: Surgical techniques used during cesarean section operations: Results of a national survey of practice in the UK. Eur J Obstet Gynecol Reprod Biol 102:120, 2002.
251. Kammen BF, Sevine MS, Rubesin SE, et al: Adynamic ileus after cesarean section mimicking intestinal obstruction: Fndings on abdominal radiographs. Br J Radiol 73:951, 2001.
252. Ravo B, Pollane M, Ger R: Pseudo-obstruction of the colon following cesarean section: A review. Dis Colon Rectum 26:440, 1983.
253. Flamm BL, Goings JR, Liu Y, et al: Elective repeat cesarean delivery versus trial of labor: A prospective multicenter study. Obstet Gynecol 83:927, 1994.
254. Ananth CV, Smulian JC, Vintzileous AM: The association of placenta previa with history of cesarean delivery and abortion. Am J Obstet Gynecol 177:1071, 1997.
255. Lydon-Rochelle M, Holt VL, Easterling TR, et al: First-birth cesarean and placental abruption or previa at second birth. Obstet Gynecol 97:765, 2001.
256. Clark SL, Koonings PP, Phelan JP: Placenta previa/accreta and prior cesarean section. Obstet Gynecol 66:89, 1985.
257. Kendrick JS, Tierney EF, Lawson HW, et al: Previous cesarean delivery and the risk of ectopic pregnancy. Obstet Gynecol 87:297, 1996.
258. Hemminki E, Meriläinen J: Long-term effects of cesarean sections: Ectopic pregnancies and placental problems. Am J Obstet Gynecol 174:1569, 1996.
259. Haimov-Kochman R, Sciaky-Tamir Y, Yancii N, et al: Conservative management of two ectopic pregnancies implanted in previous uterine scars. Ultrasound Obstet Gynecol 19:616, 2002.
260. Hemminki E: Impact of caesarean section on future fertility: A review of cohort studies. Paediatr Perinat Epidemiol 10:366, 1996.
261. Corke BC, Datta S, Ostheimer GW, et al: Spinal anesthesia for cesarean section: The influence of hypotension on neonatal outcome. Anaesthesia 37:658, 1982.
262. Clifford SH: A consideration of the obstetrical management of premature labor. N Engl J Med 210:570, 1934.
263. Usher R, McLean F, Maughan GB: Respiratory distress syndrome in infants delivered by cesarean section. Am J Obstet Gynecol 88:806, 1964.
264. Van den Berg A, Van Elberg RM, van Geijn HP, et al: Neonatal respiratory morbidity following elective caesarean section in term infants: A 5-year retrospective study and review of the literature. Eur J Obstet Gynecol Reprod Biol 98:9, 2001.
265. Morrison JJ, Rennie JM, Milton PJ: Neonatal respiratory morbidity and mode of delivery at term: Influence of timing of elective caesarean section. BJOG 102:101, 1995.
266. Schreiner RL, Stevens DC, Smith WL, et al: Etiology of the respiratory distress following elective cesarean section. [Abstract 107.] Pediatr Res 13:505, 1979.
267. Heritage CK, Cunningham MD: Association of elective repeat cesarean delivery and persistent pulmonary hypertension of the newborn. Am J Obstet Gynecol 152:627, 1985.
268. Boon AW, Milner AD, Hopkin IE: Lung volumes and lung mechanics in babies born vaginally and by elective and emergency lower segmental cesarean section. J Pediatr 98:812, 1981.
269. Gerber AH: Accidental incision of the fetus during cesarean delivery. Int J Gynaecol Obstet 12:46, 1974.
270. Smith JF, Hernandez C, Wax JR: Fetal laceration injury at cesarean delivery. Obstet Gynecol 90:344, 1997.
271. Harer WB Jr: A guest editorial: Quo vadis cesarean delivery? Obstet Gynecol Surv 57:61, 2002.
272. Silbar EL: Factors related to the increasing cesarean section rates for cephalopelvic disproportion. Am J Obstet Gynecol 154:1095, 1986.
273. Seitchik J, Holden AEC, Castillo M: Amniotomy and oxytocin treatment of functional dystocia and route of delivery. Am J Obstet Gynecol 155:585, 1986.

274. Haverkamp AD, Orleans M, Langendoerfer S, et al: A controlled trial of the differential effects of intrapartum fetal monitoring. Am J Obstet Gynecol 134:399, 1979.
275. Zalar RW, Quilligan EJ: The influence of scalp sampling on the cesarean section rate for fetal distress. Am J Obstet Gynecol 135:239, 1979.
276. Garite TJ, Dildy GA, McNamara H, et al: A multicenter controlled trial of fetal pulse oximetry in the intrapartum management of nonreassuring fetal heart rate patterns. Am J Obstet Gynecol 183:1049, 2000.
277. Bloom SL, Spong CY, Thom E, et al: for the NIHHD Maternal-Fetal Medicine Units Network: Fetal pulse oximetry and caesarean delivery. N Engl J Med 355:2195, 2006.
278. Rosen MG, Dickinson JC, Westhoff CL: Vaginal birth after cesarean: A meta-analysis of morbidity and mortality. Obstet Gynecol 77:465, 1991.
279. Sarno AP, Phelan JP, Ahn MO, et al: Vaginal birth after cesarean delivery: Trial of labor in women with breech presentation. J Reprod Med 34:831, 1989.
280. Strong TH, Whelan JP, Ahn MO, et al: Vaginal birth after cesarean delivery in twin gestation. Am J Obstet Gynecol 161:29, 1989.
281. Yeh S, Huang X, Whelan JP: Postterm pregnancy after previous cesarean section. J Reprod Med 29:41, 1984.
282. Scott JR: Mandatory trial of labor after cesarean delivery: An alternative viewpoint. Obstet Gynecol 77:881, 1991.
283. Joseph GF Jr, Steman CM, Robichaux AG: Vaginal birth after cesarean section: The impact of patient resistance to a trial of labor. Am J Obstet Gynecol 164:1441, 1991.
284. Landon MB, Hauth JC, Leveno KJ, et al; for the NICHHD Maternal-Fetal Medicine Units Network: Maternal and perinatal outcomes associated with a trial of labor after prior caesarean delivery. N Engl J Med 351:2581, 2004.
285. Datta S, Alper MH: Anesthesia for cesarean section. Anesthesiology 53:142, 1980.
286. Reisner LS: Anesthesia for cesarean section. Clin Obstet Gynecol 23:517, 1980.
287. Abboud TK, Nagappala S, Murakawa K, et al: Comparison of the effects of general and regional anesthesia for cesarean section on neonatal neurologic and adaptive capacity scores. Anesth Analg 64:996, 1985.
288. Lindblad A, Bernow J, Marsal K: Fetal blood flow during intrathecal anaesthesia for elective caesarean section. Br J Anesth 61:376, 1988.
289. Crawford JS: Maternal and cord blood at delivery: II. Parameters of respiratory exchange: Elective cesarean section. Am J Obstet Gynecol 93:37, 1965.
290. Jouppila R, Jouppila P, Kuikka J, et al: Placental blood flow during cesarean section under lumbar extradural anesthesia. Br J Anaesth 50:275, 1978.
291. Quinn AJ, Kilpatrick A: Emergency caesarean section during labour: Response time and type of anaesthesia. Eur J Obstet Gynecol Reprod Biol 54:25, 1994.
292. Jouppila P, Kuikka J, Jouppila R, et al: Effect of induction of general anesthesia for cesarean section on intervillous blood flow. Acta Obstet Gynecol Scand 58:249, 1979.
293. Cohen S: The aspiration syndrome. Clin Obstet Gynaecol 9:235, 1982.
294. Stuart HC, An AF, Rubidium SJ, et al: Acid aspiration prophylaxis for emergency caesarean section. Anaesthesia 51:415, 1996.
295. Crawford JS, Burton M, Davies P: Anaesthesia for section: Further refinements of a technique. Br J Anaesth 45:726, 1973.
296. Marx GF, Bassell GM: Hazards of the supine position in pregnancy. Clin Obstet Gynaecol 9:255, 1982.
297. Bloom SL, Spong CY, Weiner SJ, et al; for the NICHHD Maternal-Fetal Medicine Units Network: Complications of anesthesia for caesarean delivery. Obstet Gynecol 106:281, 2005.
298. Smaill F, Hofmeyr GJ: Antibiotic prophylaxis for cesarean section. Cochrane Database Syst Rev (2):CD000933, 1999 (updated 2002).
299. Hopkins L, Smaill F: Antibiotic prophylaxis regimens and drugs for cesarean section. Cochrane Database Syst Rev (2):CD001136, 1999.
300. Hanson H: Revival of the extraperitoneal cesarean section. Am J Obstet Gynecol 130:102, 1978.
301. Perkins RP: Role of extraperitoneal cesarean section. Clin Obstet Gynecol 25:583, 1980.
302. Kerr JMM: The technic of cesarean section with special reference to the lower uterine segment incision. Am J Obstet Gynecol 12:729, 1926.
303. Park RC, Duff WP: Role of cesarean hysterectomy in modern obstetric practice. Clin Obstet Gynecol 23:601, 1980.
304. Graham H: Eternal Eve: The History of Gynaecology and Obstetrics. Garden City, NY, Doubleday, 1951, pp 171-213.
305. Johnstone RW: William Smellie: The Master of British Midwifery. London, E & S Livingstone, 1952.
306. American College of Obstetricians and Gynecologists: Obstetrics Forceps. ACOG Committee Opinion 59. Washington, DC, ACOG, 1988.
307. American College of Obstetricians and Gynecologists: Operative Vaginal Delivery. ACOG Technical Bulletin 152. Washington, DC, ACOG, 1991.
308. Hagadorn-Freathy AS, Yeomans ER, Hankins GDV: Validation of the 1988 ACOG forceps classification system. Obstet Gynecol 77:356, 1991.
309. American College of Obstetricians and Gynecologists: Manual of Standards in Obstetric-Gynecologic Practice, 2nd ed. Washington, DC, ACOG, 1965.
310. Bowes WA Jr, Katz VL: Operative vaginal delivery: Forceps and vacuum extractor. Curr Prob Obstet Gynecol Fertil 17:83, 1994.
311. Towner D, Castro MA, Eby-Wilkens E, et al: Effect of mode of delivery in nulliparous women on neonatal intracranial injury. N Engl J Med 341:1709, 1999.
312. Robson S, Pridmore B: Have Kielland forceps reached their "use by" date? Aust N Z J Obstet Gynaecol 39:301, 1999.
313. Friedman EA, Sachtleben-Murray MR, Dahrouge D: Long-term effects of labor and delivery on offspring: A match-pair analysis. Am J Obstet Gynecol 150:941, 1984.
314. Dierker LJ Jr, Rosen MG, Thompson K, et al: Midforceps deliveries: Long-term outcome of infants. Am J Obstet Gynecol 154:764, 1986.
315. Seidman DS, Laor A, Gale R, et al: Long-term effects of vacuum and forceps deliveries. Lancet 337:1583, 1991.
316. Wesley BD, van den Berg BJ, Reece EA: The effect of forceps delivery on cognitive development. Am J Obstet Gynecol 169:1091, 1993.
317. American College of Obstetricians and Gynecologists: Operative Vaginal Delivery. ACOG Practice Bulletin 17. Washington, DC, ACOG, 2000.
318. Patel RR, Murphy DJ: Forceps delivery in modern obstetric practice. BMJ 328:1302, 2004.
319. Malmström T: Vacuum extractor: An obstetrical instrument. Acta Obstet Gynecol Scand 33:S1, 1954.
320. Bofill JA, Rust OA, Perry KG Jr, et al: Forceps and vacuum delivery: A survey of North American residency programs. Obstet Gynecol 88:622, 1996.
321. Johanson RB, Menon V: Vacuum extraction versus forceps for assisted vaginal delivery. Cochrane Database Syst Rev (3):CD000224, 1997 (updated 1998).
322. Johanson RB, Heycock E, Carter J, et al: Maternal and child health after assisted vaginal delivery: Five-year follow-up of a randomized controlled study comparing forceps and ventouse. BJOG 106:544, 1999.
323. Gardella C, Taylor M, Benedetti T, et al: The effect of sequential use of vacuum and forceps for assisted vaginal delivery on neonatal and maternal outcomes. Am J Obstet Gynecol 185:896, 2001.
324. Johanson R, Menon V: Soft versus rigid vacuum extractor cups for assisted vaginal delivery. Cochrane Database Syst Rev (2):CD000446, 1998 (updated 2000).
325. Chalmers JA, Chalmers I: The obstetric vacuum extractor is the instrument of first choice for operative vaginal delivery. BJOG 96:505, 1989.
326. Caton D: What a Blessing She Had Chloroform: The Medical and Social Response to the Pain of Childbirth from 1800 to the Present. New Haven, Yale University Press, 1999.
327. Caton D, Frölich MA, Euliano TY: Anesthesia for childbirth: Controversy and change. Am J Obstet Gynecol 186:S25, 2002.
328. Atkinson DT: Magic, Myth and Medicine. Cleveland, World Publishing, 1956, p 271.
329. Speert H: Obstetric and Gynecologic Milestones, Illustrated. New York, Parthenon, 1996, p 498.
330. Kennell J, Klaus M, McGrath S, et al: Continuous emotional support during labor in a US hospital. JAMA 265:2197, 1991.

331. Olofsson CH, Ekblom A, Ekman-Ordeberg G, et al: Analgesic efficacy of intravenous morphine in labour pain: A reappraisal. Int J Obstet Anesth 5:176, 1996.
332. Olofsson CH, Ekblom A, Ekman-Ordeberg G, et al: Lack of analgesic effect of systemically administered morphine or pethidine on labour pain. BJOG 103:968, 1996.
333. Barrier G, Sureau C: Effects of anaesthetic and analgesic drugs on labour, fetus, and neonate. Clin Obstet Gynaecol 9:351, 1982.
334. Podlas J, Breland BD: Patient-controlled analgesia with nalbuphine during labor. Obstet Gynecol 70:202, 1987.
335. Atkinson BD, Truitt LJ, Rayburn WF, et al: Double-blind comparison of intravenous butorphanol (Stadol) and fentanyl (Sublimaze) for analgesia during labor. Am J Obstet Gynecol 171:993, 1994.
336. Rayburn WF, Smith CV, Parriott JE, et al: Randomized comparison of meperidine and fentanyl during labor. Obstet Gynecol 74:604, 1989.
337. Elbourne D, Wiseman RA: Types of intra-muscular opioids for maternal pain relief in labour. Cochrane Database Syst Rev (2):CD001237, 2000 (updated 2006).
338. Bricker L, Lavender T: Parenteral opioids for labor pain relief: A systematic review. Am J Obstet Gynecol 186:S94, 2002.
339. Nyberg K, Buka SL, Lipsitt LD: Perinatal medication as a potential risk factor for adult drug abuse in a North American cohort. Epidemiology 11:715, 2000.
340. Rosefsky JB, Petersiel ME: Perinatal deaths associated with mepivacaine paracervical-block anesthesia in labor. N Engl J Med 278:530, 1968.
341. Goddard WB: Fetal monitoring in a private hospital: Observations of fetal bradycardia following paracervical block anesthesia. Am J Obstet Gynecol 109:1145, 1971.
342. Freeman RK, Gutierrez NA, Ray ML, et al: Fetal cardiac response to paracervical block anesthesia: I. Obstet Gynecol 113:583, 1972.
343. Rosen M: Paracervical block for labor analgesia: A brief historic review. Am J Obstet Gynecol 186:D127, 2002.
344. Freeman DW, Arnold NI: Paracervical block with low doses of chloroprocaine: Fetal and maternal effects. JAMA 231:56, 1975.
345. Chestnut DH: Alternative regional anesthetic techniques: Paracervical block, lumbar sympathetic block, pudendal block, and perineal infiltration. In Chestnut DH (ed): Obstetric Anesthesia: Principles and Practice. St. Louis, Mosby, 1994, pp 420-425.
346. Wenger DR, Gitchell RG: Severe infections following pudendal block anesthesia: Need for orthopedic awareness. J Bone Joint Surg Am 55:202, 1973.
347. Svancarik W, Cairina O, Schaefer G Jr, et al: Retropsoas and subgluteal abscesses following paracervical and pudendal anesthesia. JAMA 237:892, 1977.
348. Klink EW: Perineal nerve block: An anatomic and clinical study in the female. Obstet Gynecol 1:137, 1953.
349. Leighton BL, Halpern SH: The effects of epidural analgesia on labor, maternal, and neonatal outcomes: A systematic review. Am J Obstet Gynecol 186:S69, 2002.
350. Lysak SZ, Eisenach JC, Dobson CE II: Patient-controlled epidural analgesia during labor: A comparison of three solutions with a continuous infusion control. Anesthesiology 72:44, 1990.
351. Abboud TK, Khoo SS, Miller F, et al: Maternal, fetal, and neonatal responses after epidural anesthesia with bupivacaine, 2-chloroprocaine, or lidocaine. Anesth Analg 61:638, 1982.
352. McDonald JS, Bjorkman LL, Reed EC: Epidural analgesia for obstetrics: A maternal, fetal, and neonatal study. Am J Obstet Gynecol 120:1055, 1974.
353. Schifrin BS: Fetal heart rate patterns following epidural anaesthesia and oxytocin infusion during labour. J Obstet Gynaecol Br Commonw 79:332, 1972.
354. Collins KM, Bevan DR, Beard RW: Fluid loading to reduce abnormalities of fetal heart rate and maternal hypotension during epidural analgesia in labour. BMJ 2:1460, 1978.
355. Thorp JA, Breedlove G: Epidural analgesia in labor: An evaluation of risks and benefits. Birth 23:63, 1996.
356. Thorp JA, Eckert LO, Ang MS, et al: Epidural analgesia and cesarean section for dystocia: Risk factors in nulliparas. Am J Perinatol 8:402, 1991.
357. Chestnut DH, McGrath JM, Vincent RD Jr, et al: Does early administration of epidural analgesia affect obstetric outcome in nulliparous women who are in spontaneous labor? Anesthesiology 80:1201, 1994.
358. Chestnut DH, Vincent RD Jr, McGrath JM, et al: Does early administration of epidural analgesia affect obstetric outcome in nulliparous women who are receiving intravenous oxytocin? Anesthesiology 80:1193, 1994.
359. Thompson TT, Thorp JM Jr, Mayer D, et al: Does epidural anesthesia cause dystocia? J Clin Anesth 70:58, 1998.
360. Zhang J, Yancey M, Klebanoff M, et al. Does epidural analgesia prolong labor and increase risk of cesarean delivery? A natural experiment. Am J Obstet Gynecol 185:128, 2001.
361. Yancey M, Zhang J, Schweitzer D, et al: Epidural analgesia and fetal head malposition at vaginal delivery. Obstet Gynecol 97:608, 2001.
362. Bofill JA, Vincent RD, Ross EL, et al: Nulliparous active labor, epidural analgesia, and cesarean delivery for dystocia. Am J Obstet Gynecol 177:1465, 1997.
363. Sharma SK, Sidawi JE, Ramin SM, et al: Cesarean delivery: A randomized trial of epidural versus patient-controlled meperidine analgesia during labor. Anesthesiology 87:487, 1997.
364. Ramin SM, Gambling DR, Lucas MJ, et al: Randomized trial of epidural versus intravenous analgesia during labor. Obstet Gynecol 86:783, 1995.
365. MacArthur C, Lewis M, Knox EG, et al: Epidural anaesthesia and long term backache after childbirth. BMJ 301:9, 1990.
366. Macarthur AJ, Macarthur C, Weeks SK: Is epidural anesthesia in labor associated with chronic low back pain? A prospective cohort study. Anesth Analg 85:1066, 1997.
367. Fusi L, Steer PJ, Maresh MJA, et al: Maternal pyrexia associated with the use of epidural analgesia in labour. Lancet 1:1250, 1989.
368. Lieberman E, Lang JM, Frigoletto F Jr, et al: Epidural analgesia, intrapartum fever, and neonatal sepsis evaluation. Pediatrics 99:415, 1997.
369. Cousins ML, Mather LE: Intrathecal and epidural administration of opioids. Anesthesiology 61:276, 1984.
370. Lieberman E, O'Donoghue C: Unintended effects of epidural analgesia during labor: A systematic review. Am J Obstet Gynecol 186:S31, 2002.
371. Marmor TR, Krol DM: Labor pain management in the United States: Understanding patterns and the issues of choice. Am J Obstet Gynecol 186:S173, 2002.
372. Ounsted C, Roberts JS, Gordon M, et al: Fourth goal of perinatal medicine. BMJ 284:879, 1982.
373. Boulvain M, Kelly A, Irion O: Intracervical prostaglandins for induction of labour. Cochrane Database Syst Rev (1):CD006971, 2008.

Chapter 37

Placenta Previa, Placenta Accreta, Abruptio Placentae, and Vasa Previa

Andrew D. Hull, MD, and Robert Resnik, MD

Bleeding in the later stages of pregnancy has been described as "third-trimester bleeding" or "antepartum hemorrhage." Late pregnancy bleeding is a significant cause of maternal and fetal morbidity, fetal mortality, and preterm delivery. Traditional accounts of such bleeding have addressed placenta previa, abruptio placentae, and vasa previa, although in fact the only thing that these clinical problems have in common is that they all are concerned, to a greater or lesser extent, with hemorrhage. The etiology, management, and complications of each are quite distinct. In the past, uncertainty in precise diagnosis of the cause of late pregnancy bleeding has led to these conditions being considered together, but the universal availability of ultrasound technology has eliminated much of the diagnostic dilemma.

Bleeding during the second half of pregnancy complicates about 6% of all pregnancies. Placenta previa is ultimately documented in 7% of cases, and evidence of significant placental abruption is found in 13%. In the remaining 80% of cases, the bleeding can be ascribed to either early labor or local lesions of the lower genital tract or no source can be identified.[1] Faced with a woman with late pregnancy bleeding, the clinician must rapidly reach a firm diagnosis and management plan to ensure the optimum outcome for mother and baby. Ultrasonography, electronic fetal monitoring, and, frequently, evaluation of the function of the maternal coagulation system make up the foundation on which both diagnosis and management are developed. Clinical assessment must occur simultaneously with imaging and fetal assessment.

In asymptomatic patients who are without antenatal bleeding but have been identified by prenatal ultrasound as having risk factors (placenta previa, placenta accreta, or vasa previa), timing of delivery is the most important clinical decision that has to be made.

Placenta Previa

Definition and Epidemiology

Advances in the precision of sonographic diagnosis, particularly transvaginal ultrasound (TVUS) technology, as well as an increased understanding of the changing relationship between the placenta and the internal cervical os as pregnancy advances, have rendered traditional definitions and classifications of placenta previa obsolete. *Placenta previa* exists when the placenta covers the cervix either completely or partially or extends close enough to the cervix to cause bleeding when the cervix dilates or the lower uterine segment effaces. The term "low-lying placenta" should be reserved for cases in which the placenta is seen on transabdominal ultrasound to extend into the lower uterine segment but its precise limits have not been defined, and for cases identified before the third trimester. TVUS allows location of the placenta in relation to the internal cervical os with great precision. When such studies are performed, the placenta may be classified as a *complete previa* if it completely covers the internal os. The term *marginal placenta previa* should be used if the placental edge lies 2.5 cm or closer to the internal os. It has been shown that when the placenta is more than 2 to 3 cm from the cervix, there is no increased risk of bleeding.[2] A definitive diagnosis of placenta previa should be avoided in asymptomatic patients before the third trimester, because many cases of placenta previa identified early in pregnancy will resolve as pregnancy advances.

Placenta previa affects about 1 (0.5%) of every 200 pregnancies at term.[3] There is some evidence that the incidence of placenta previa is increasing.[4] This increase may be related to the increasing rate of cesarean section observed in all developed countries. A single prior cesarean section or a prior pregnancy complicated by placenta previa increases the incidence of placenta previa in a subsequent pregnancy to as high as 5%,[1,5,6] rising even further with a history of more prior cesarean deliveries.[7] Advanced maternal age increases the incidence of placenta previa to 2% after 35 years of age and 5% after age 40.[7] Multiparity, prior suction curettage, and smoking are all associated with higher risks of placenta previa.[8-10] The relative risks for these associated factors are summarized in Table 37-1.

Pathogenesis

The underlying cause of placenta previa is unknown. There is a clear association between placental implantation in the lower uterine segment and prior endometrial damage and uterine scarring from curettage, surgical insult, prior placenta previa, and multiple prior pregnancies.

At least 90% of placentas identified as being "low lying" in early pregnancy will ultimately resolve by the third trimester.[11] The term "placental migration" is widely used to describe this phenomenon. The placenta clearly does not move; rather, it is likely that the placenta grows toward the better blood supply at the fundus, a process known as trophotropism, leaving the distal portions of the placenta, closer to the relatively poor blood supply of the lower segment, to regress and atrophy. As the uterus grows and expands to accommodate the developing fetus, there is differential growth of the lower segment, and this may further increase the distance between the lower edge of the placenta and the cervix.

Bleeding from placenta previa may occur before labor as a result of development of the lower uterine segment and effacement of the cervix with advancing gestation. Prelabor uterine contractions may also produce bleeding, as may intercourse or injudicious vaginal examination. Once labor begins, significant bleeding will occur as the cervix dilates and the placenta is forced to separate from the underlying decidua.

Diagnosis

The classic history for placenta previa is that of painless third-trimester bleeding. Several small "herald bleeds" may occur in advance of major hemorrhage, but in up to 10% of cases there is no bleeding until the onset of labor. Some women experience pain secondary to uterine contractions. Bleeding may be provoked by labor, examination, or intercourse but it usually has no identifiable precipitating cause. The patient is more likely to have a fetus with an abnormal lie, inasmuch as the placenta previa may prevent the fetus from establishing normal polarity. All women presenting with painless vaginal bleeding after 20 weeks' gestation should be assumed to have a placenta previa until proven otherwise. Transabdominal ultrasound should be quickly utilized to screen for placenta previa. Unless the placenta is clearly fundal and the lower segment is clear, TVUS should then be performed. Transabdominal ultrasound has been shown to be inferior to TVUS for definitive placental localization.[12,13] Concerns regarding the potential for TVUS to provoke bleeding are unfounded, and several studies have confirmed the safety of a careful TVUS approach (Fig. 37-1).[7,13,14] The placement of the transvaginal probe should be observed continuously on the ultrasound monitor during insertion, to avoid placing the probe into a potentially dilated cervix. If a transvaginal probe is unavailable, translabial imaging using a regular abdominal probe can produce excellent results, with better visualization of the relationship between the cervix and placenta than is obtained from transabdominal scanning.[15] A digital or speculum examination to inspect the cervix for local causes of bleeding should not be performed until placenta previa has been excluded by ultrasonography.

In the unusual setting of significant late pregnancy bleeding where ultrasound is not available and the diagnosis is not clear, there is still a place for the "double-setup" examination. The patient is taken to the operating room, where preparations are made for a cesarean delivery. A vaginal examination is then performed, beginning in the vaginal fornices and avoiding placing the fingers directly in the cervix. If a placenta previa is detected, cesarean section is then performed. If no placenta previa is found, a search for other causes of third-trimester bleeding ensues.

TABLE 37-1 RISK FACTORS AND RELATIVE RISKS OF PLACENTA PREVIA

Risk Factor	Increased Risk	Reference
Previous placenta previa	83×	Monica and Lilja, 1995
Previous cesarean section	1.5-153×	Herschkowitz et al, 1995; Hemminki and Merilainen, 1996
Previous suction curettage for abortion	1.33×	Taylor et al, 1994
Age > 35 yr	4.73×	Iyasu et al, 1993
Age > 40 yr	93×	Ananth et al, 1996
Multiparity	1.1-1.73×	Williams and Mittendorf, 1993
Nonwhite race (all)	0.33×	Iyasu et al, 1993
Asian race	1.93×	Iyasu et al, 1993
Cigarette smoking	1.4-33×	Handler et al, 1994; Ananth, Savits, and Luther, 1996; Chelmow et al, 1996

Implications of Early Pregnancy Diagnosis

The routine use of ultrasonography in the first and second trimesters of pregnancy has led to the frequent observation of a low-lying placenta or a previa.

Transabdominal ultrasound tends to over-diagnose low-lying placenta, especially when the bladder is empty.[16] Even with TVUS, the findings may not correlate with the placental position at term. Several reports confirm that up to 10 times as many women are found to have

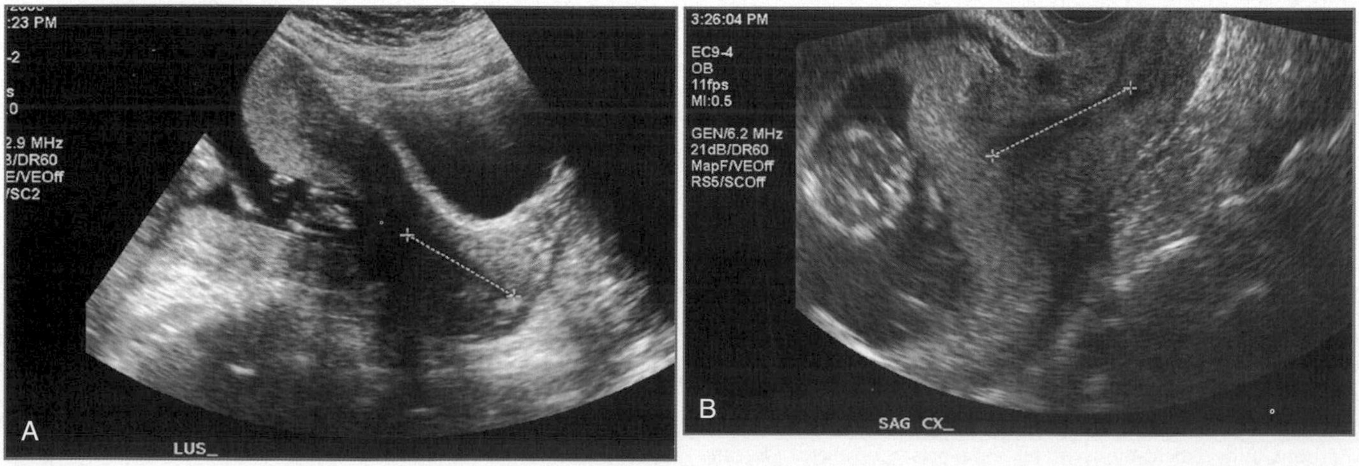

FIGURE 37-1 Ultrasound study performed at 18 weeks' gestation for fetal anatomy survey. **A,** Transabdominal ultrasound shows an apparent "low-lying placenta." **B,** Transvaginal ultrasound shows that the placenta completely covers the cervix.

a placenta previa in the second or first trimester than at delivery.[14,17-21] The earlier in pregnancy a diagnosis of placenta previa is made, the less likely it is that the finding will persist at delivery.[22] The likelihood of persistence to term of a placenta previa found in the second trimester is also related to the degree to which the placenta overlies the cervix[14,17-21] and the thickness of the placental edge.[23] It is recommended that a follow-up ultrasound study be performed between 28 and 32 weeks' gestation to further evaluate the placental position. If there appears to be a significant change in the position of the placental edge over time, a final study should be done at 36 weeks, before making a final decision as to the appropriate route of delivery.

Management

Any woman with vaginal bleeding after 20 weeks' gestation should be assessed on a labor and delivery unit. The primary focus should be on hemodynamic assessment of the mother and assessment of fetal well-being. Vital signs are obtained, and electronic fetal monitoring initiated. One or two large-gauge intravenous lines should be placed, and maternal blood should be sent for determination of the hematocrit and type and screen. For substantial bleeding episodes, 2 to 4 units of blood should be cross-matched. Obstetric units might consider the use of an "Obstetric Hemorrhage Protocol" to facilitate access to the resources of the hospital blood bank for this and any other obstetric hemorrhage (Table 37-2). Rh immune globulin is administered, when appropriate, to Rh-negative, nonimmunized women.

Once the patient is stabilized and fetal condition has been assessed, the definitive cause of the bleeding can be addressed. If the diagnosis is clearly placenta previa and the patient is at or beyond 36 weeks' gestation, delivery is appropriate. If bleeding is excessive or continues, or if there are concerns about the condition of the fetus, the patient should be delivered regardless of gestational age. In all other cases, management may be conservative and has been shown to be safe,[24,25] with prolongation of pregnancy by an average of 4 weeks after the initial bleeding episode. The closer it is to a gestational age of 36 weeks, the less likely it is that a significant prolongation of pregnancy will be gained.[26] Betamethasone to enhance fetal lung maturation should be administered to patients who are at less than 34 weeks' gestation if expectant management is planned.

There is controversy regarding the role of tocolytics in the setting of hemorrhage from placenta previa. Both β-mimetics and magnesium sulfate[27-29] have been used in this setting and appear to be associated with significant prolongation of pregnancy without adverse effects.

After the initial presentation with bleeding, patients should remain in hospital until they are free of bleeding for at least 48 hours. Some may then be considered for home management. Several studies have addressed the issue of safety of outpatient management in a controlled setting at home.[25,30-33] With the exception of one report of an increase in perinatal mortality and morbidity and earlier gestational age,[34] it appears to be a safe approach. Patients selected for home management should be asymptomatic with regard to bleeding and abdominal pain, be able to remain at home with limited activity, and have adequate support as well as adequate access to transport to a nearby hospital if bleeding recurs. A second significant bleeding episode usually results in readmission until delivery.

Several strategies have been proposed to reduce the risk of hemorrhage in women with a known placenta previa. Bed rest, reduced activity, and avoidance of intercourse are commonly mandated and seem logical, although there is no conclusive evidence to support these measures. Cervical cerclage was evaluated in two small prospective studies[35,36] without clear benefit and is not recommended.

All women whose placenta lies within 2 cm of the cervix, as documented by a late third-trimester TVUS scan, should be delivered by cesarean section.[37-39] An asymptomatic woman whose placenta lies more than 2 cm from the cervical os can be allowed to labor safely.[16] It should be noted that the presence of a low-lying placenta, even if it does not cause intrapartum bleeding, increases the risk of postpartum hemorrhage because of lower uterine segment atony.

Cesarean section for placenta previa should be performed by the most experienced team available because of the substantial risk of intraoperative hemorrhage.[40] In most instances, a lower uterine segment incision is appropriate. If the placenta is anterior, it is necessary to clamp the umbilical cord immediately to prevent excessive blood loss caused by disruption of the placenta during entry. A vertical incision is also reasonable in such cases and may be preferable if the fetus is premature or if a transverse lie exists.[41] Postpartum hemorrhage may occur from the placental implantation site secondary to atony and may require the use of additional pharmacologic agents to control blood loss, such as methylergonovine maleate (Methergine), 15-methyl prostaglandin $F_{2\alpha}$ (Hemabate), and high-dose oxytocin, used either singly or in combination. The B-Lynch suture[42] or local suturing of the placental bed may be needed to control bleeding. In rare cases of refractory hemorrhage, hysterectomy may be required.

Among women known to have a placenta previa who do not require very early delivery, elective delivery should be performed before significant bleeding has occurred. It is reasonable to plan on delivery at or just after 36 weeks' gestation, because there is little fetal advantage after that time, when weighed against the risk of a sudden and possibly excessive bleeding episode. The alternative is to perform an amniocentesis to confirm lung maturity before delivery, but the risk of hemorrhage with delayed delivery usually outweighs the risk of fetal lung immaturity at that gestational age.

The selection of anesthesia to be used for cesarean section in cases of placenta previa should be decided by the obstetrician and anesthesiologist involved with the delivery, in concert with the patient. In the United Kingdom, regional anesthesia was preferred by most obstetric

TABLE 37-2 OBSTETRIC HEMORRHAGE PROTOCOL

Blood is immediately drawn and set up for
- Type and cross-matching
- Hematocrit
- Coagulation studies (PT/PTT/fibrinogen)
- Wall clot (blood is drawn into a plain tube and set aside—should clot within 6 min)

An ABG determination may be requested to assess acute blood loss (typically, every increment in base deficit of −1 to −2 requires 1 unit of PRBCs to correct it)

Four units of type-specific or O-negative blood are made immediately available.

The laboratory immediately starts to cross-match 4 units of blood and stays 4 units ahead of blood use.

Two units of FFP are thawed and made available.

One 10-pack of platelets is made available.

The blood bank is alerted to provide further units of blood, FFP, and platelets as needed.

Further samples for ABGs and other laboratory studies are drawn as required.

ABGs, arterial blood gases; FFP, fresh-frozen plasma; PRBCs, packed red blood cells; PT, prothrombin time; PTT, partial thromboplastin time.

anesthesiologists in a survey[43] and was used in 60% of cases in a retrospective series.[44] Regional anesthesia is associated with lower operative blood loss and less need for transfusion than general anesthesia,[3,45] probably because many inhaled anesthetics cause uterine relaxation.

Complications

Placenta Accreta

One of the most serious complications of placenta previa is the development of *placenta accreta*. This condition involves trophoblastic invasion beyond the normal boundary established by the Nitabuch fibrinoid layer. If invasion extends into the myometrium, the term *placenta increta* is used; placental invasion beyond the uterine serosa (at times involving the bladder or other pelvic organs and vessels) is termed *placenta percreta*. Histologic examples of normal placental implantation and placenta accreta are shown in Figure 37-2.

Placenta accreta is associated positively with advanced maternal age, smoking, and parity, but the strongest recognized association is with placenta previa and prior uterine surgery.[46,47] In patients with placenta previa, the risk of accreta is 10% to 25% with one prior cesarean section and exceeds 50% with two or more prior cesareans.[48-50] Prevalence appears to be similar in women with these risk factors undergoing second-trimester pregnancy termination.[51]

The diagnosis of placental invasion of the myometrium usually can be made by ultrasound,[52-54] with a reported sensitivity and specificity for the diagnosis of approximately 0.8 and 0.95, respectively.[53,55,56] Magnetic resonance imaging (MRI) has also been used to confirm the diagnosis or better delineate the presence or extent of accreta.[53] MRI is also useful in the presence of a posterior placenta and in the assessment of deep myometrial, parametrial, and bladder involvement.[55,57]

The ultrasound appearance of a normal placental attachment site is shown in Figure 37-3A. Normal attachment is characterized by a homogeneous appearance of the placenta and a hypoechoic boundary

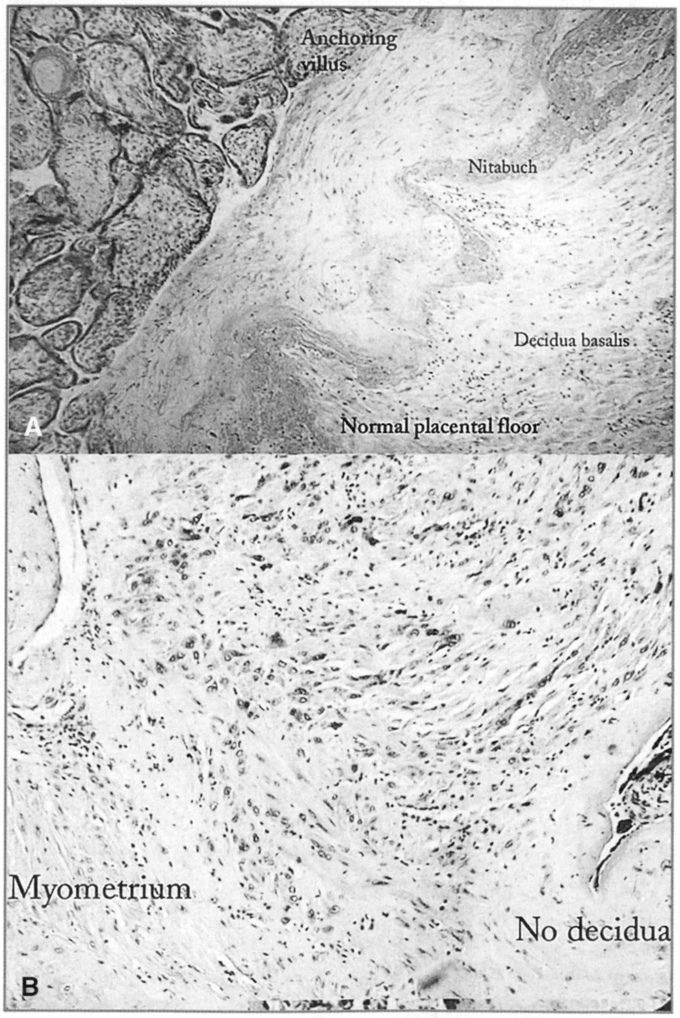

FIGURE 37-2 Histologic appearance of normal placental implantation and placenta accreta. **A,** Histologic section of a normal placental attachment site. Trophoblastic tissue with anchoring villi encroach but do not go through the Nitabuch membrane. **B,** Representative histologic section of placenta accreta, demonstrating invasion of trophoblasts into the myometrial tissue.

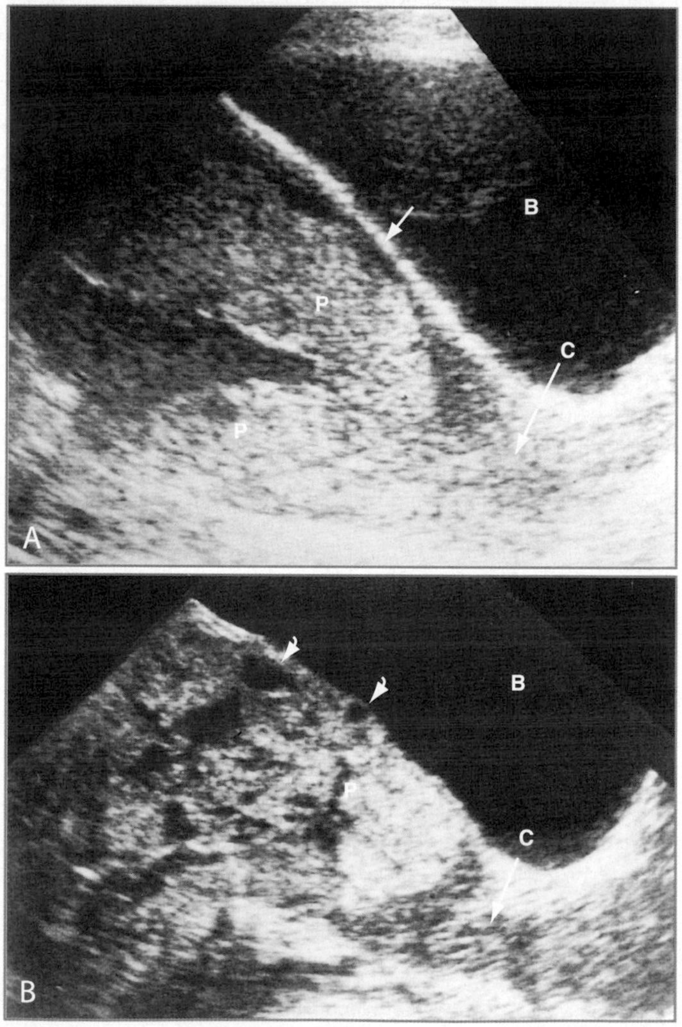

FIGURE 37-3 Ultrasound appearance of a normal placental attachment site and placenta accreta. **A,** Normal placental attachment in an anterior placenta previa. A hypoechoic area separates the bladder wall and the placental tissue, representing myometrium and myometrial vasculature. **B,** Characteristic ultrasound appearance of placenta accreta. Note the lack of a hypoechoic area, as well as obliteration of the well-delineated bladder wall. In addition, there are intraplacental sonolucent spaces *(arrows)* adjacent to the involved uterine wall. B, bladder; C, cervix; P, placenta.

between the placenta and the bladder that represents the myometrium and the normal retroplacental myometrial vasculature. The bladder wall is intact throughout. In contrast, placental accreta is associated with loss of the normal hypoechoic boundary, and there are usually intraplacental sonolucent spaces adjacent to the involved uterine wall (see Fig. 37-3B). Color-flow and power Doppler sonography have also been reported to facilitate the diagnosis.[58-60] Chou and associates[60] evaluated 80 women with placenta previa to determine the accuracy of color-flow Doppler ultrasonography in distinguishing between uncomplicated placenta previa and placenta accreta. Using their criteria, the antepartum diagnosis of accreta was made in 16 of the 80 women studied and was confirmed histopathologically in 14. The sensitivity and specificity for diagnosis were 0.82 and 0.97, respectively. Although it is clear that larger numbers of patients must be studied by these various modalities to more accurately determine the sensitivities and specificities of diagnosis, various types of ultrasonography and MRI appear to hold promise in making or excluding the diagnosis in most cases.

It is important, if at all possible, to make the diagnosis before delivery, because intraoperative hemorrhage can be massive, and placenta accreta has been reported to be the most common indication for emergency peripartum hysterectomy.[61,62] In an effort to diminish blood loss, it is recommended that delivery be accomplished through a fundal incision followed by clamping of the cord. The placenta is allowed to remain in situ while the surgeons proceed to a total abdominal hysterectomy. This may require very complex surgical technique and planning, and a pelvic surgeon capable of wide resection of the lower uterine segment and parametrial areas should be available, as well as ample transfusion capability.

Although published reports are not extensive, it has been suggested that balloon occlusion of the aorta or internal iliac vessels may help to prevent excessive blood loss during resection of the lower uterine segment. This involves preoperative placement of balloon-tipped catheters retrograde through the femoral arteries immediately before surgery. The catheters are guided under fluoroscopic direction into the internal iliac arteries and inflated during the dissection. However, the value and safety of this approach have been challenged with the recent reports of no proven benefit and embolic complications.[63,64] Nevertheless, the placement of catheters does provide the opportunity to manage potential postoperative bleeding with angiographic embolization rather than reexploration.

Conservative management may be an option if there is suspicion of a small focal accreta, if there is a fundal location after a myomectomy or classic cesarean section, or with a posteriorly implanted placenta. A few reports have suggested leaving the uterus and placenta in situ and using methotrexate postoperatively.[65-67] However, the numbers of reported cases are very few, and hemorrhagic and infectious complications have usually resulted. Consequently, a definitive surgical approach to this serious obstetric complication is strongly recommended.

Neonatal Complications

It has been suggested that repetitive bleeding from placenta previa is associated with fetal growth impairment,[68] although this has been disputed.[26] Pregnancies complicated by placenta previa have also been reported to be associated with higher rates of fetal anomalies,[69] neurodevelopmental delay,[70] and sudden infant death syndrome (SIDS).[71] The reasons for these findings are unknown.

As might be expected, placenta previa and previa accreta are a cause of preterm birth due to the need for iatrogenic preterm delivery. Accreta has also been reported to have a negative influence on fetal growth (odds ratio, 5.05 compared with controls).[72]

Vasa Previa

Definition and Epidemiology

Vasa previa is a rare but potentially catastrophic complication in which fetal vessels run through the fetal membranes and are at risk of rupture with consequent fetal exsanguination. It is estimated that vasa previa affects between 1 in 1275 and 1 in 8333 pregnancies.[73,74]

Pathogenesis

Vasa previa may occur because the insertion of the umbilical cord into the placenta is velamentous, with the umbilical vessels coursing through the fetal membranes before inserting into the placental disk and the unsupported vessels then overlying the cervix. It may also result from the presence of a bilobed or succenturiate placenta with the vessels connecting the placenta similarly overlying the cervix.[16] If the condition goes unrecognized, it is associated with a fetal mortality rate of almost 60%. In addition to a succenturiate placenta[75] and velamentous insertion, other risk factors include a low-lying placenta observed in the second trimester,[76] multiple gestation, and in vitro fertilization.[77]

Diagnosis

The key to reducing fetal loss from vasa previa is prenatal diagnosis.[16] Many cases of vasa previa are identified only at the time of vessel rupture in labor. Vaginal bleeding is followed by fetal distress and death if emergent delivery cannot be effected in time. Because the entire fetal cardiac output passes through the cord, it can take less than 10 minutes for total exsanguination to occur. Electronic fetal monitoring may show an initial tachycardia, rapidly followed by decelerations, bradycardia, and a preterminal sinusoidal rhythm.[78] If a cesarean delivery can be accomplished immediately and with sufficient rapidity, good newborn outcome can be obtained by aggressive postnatal transfusion therapy.[79]

It has been suggested that the blood from the vagina may be tested to confirm its fetal origin, using the Apt or Kleihauer-Betke tests or electrophoresis.[80] In actual practice, such tests are either unavailable or cannot be done quickly enough to be of any value. Occasionally, fetal vessels have reportedly been felt through the membranes during vaginal examination or visualized on amnioscopy; such observations are really only of historical interest in modern practice.

It is now well established that vasa previa may be diagnosed prenatally using ultrasound.[81,82] Routine obstetric ultrasound should include an assessment of the placental site and number of placental lobes and an evaluation of the placental cord insertion site. In all cases in which a multilobed or succenturiate placenta or a low-lying placenta or velamentous cord insertion is identified using transabdominal ultrasound, a detailed examination of the lower uterine segment and cervix should be performed using TVUS. Gray-scale ultrasound can identify placental cord insertion in most cases, but color or power Doppler makes the process easier and should be used (Figs. 37-4 and 37-5).[81-84] There have been several studies evaluating this approach for prenatal detection of vasa previa,[81,82,84,85] all of which showed high specificity and sensitivity of detection with little impact on the length of scan time. More importantly, in cases in which vasa previa was detected prenatally, there were no fetal deaths from the condition. A recent retrospective, multicenter study showed newborn survival rates of 97% in prenatally detected cases of vasa previa and a fetal loss rate of 56% in cases not identified before the commencement of labor.[86] Newer imaging modalities such

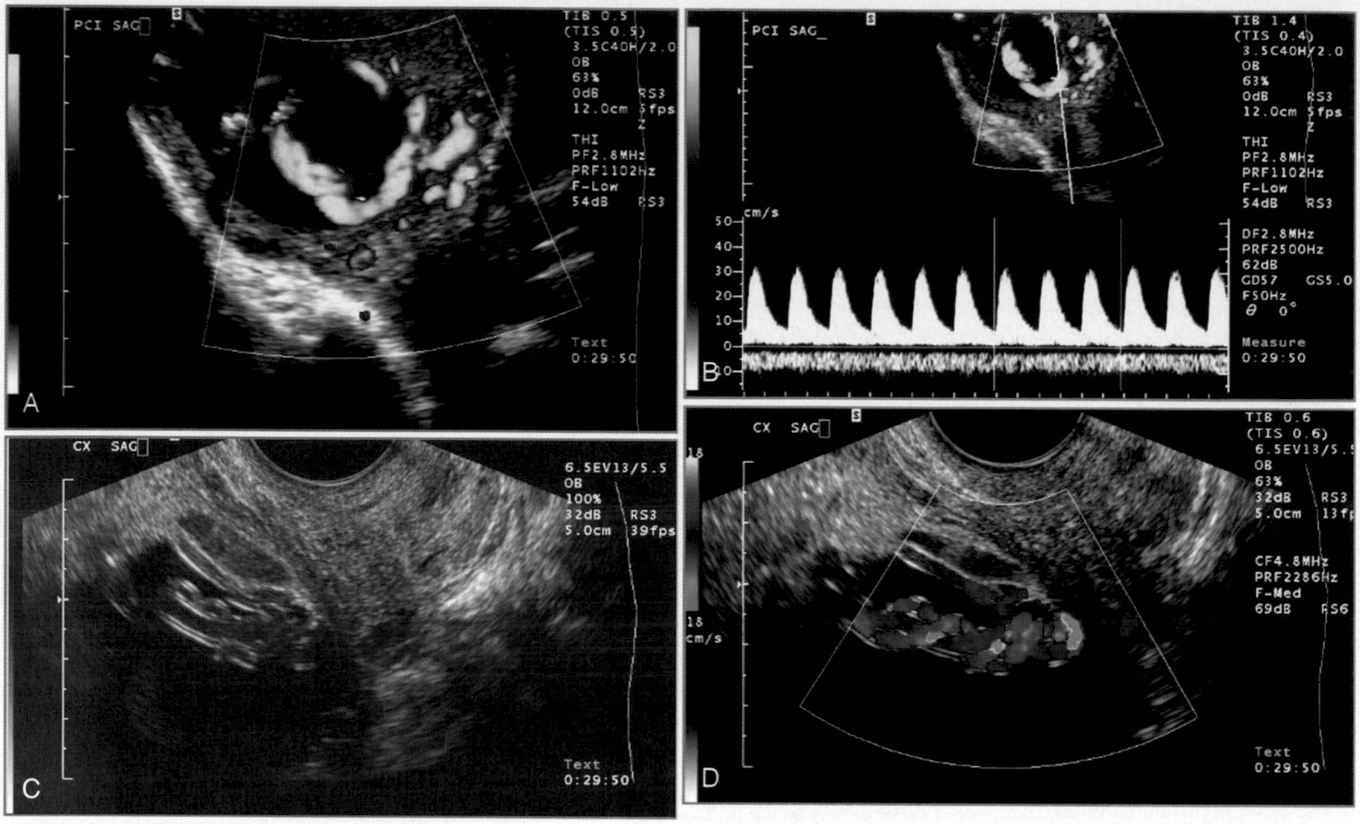

FIGURE 37-4 Vasa previa identified at 18 weeks' gestation on routine ultrasound studies. **A,** Transabdominal power Doppler identifies the umbilical cord possibly overlying the cervix. **B,** A fetal arterial waveform using power and pulse-wave Doppler. **C,** Vasa previa in gray scale on transvaginal ultrasound. **D,** Confirmation of the vasa previa using color Doppler transvaginally.

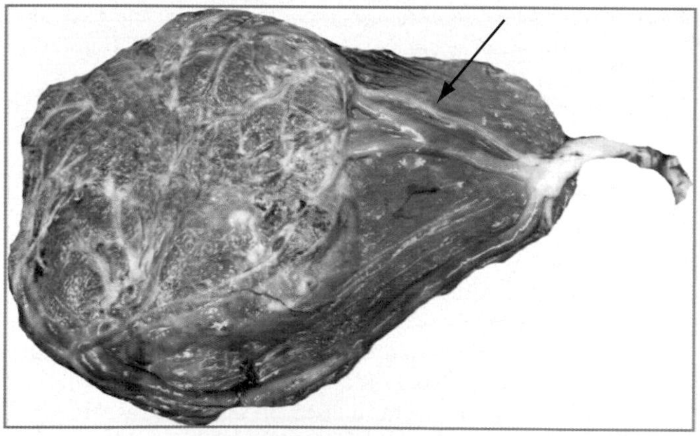

FIGURE 37-5 Vasa previa. The placenta from the case identified in Figure 37-4. The patient was delivered by elective cesarean section at 34 weeks. *Arrow* shows velamentous cord insertion.

as MRI[87] and three-dimensional ultrasound have been described in the evaluation of vasa previa.[87-89] MRI is of little practical use in routine cases. Although transvaginal three-dimensional power Doppler provides an excellent means of visualizing the entire lower uterine segment for the evaluation of vasa previa, similar information may be obtained by careful use of a two-dimensional vaginal probe. Such imaging combined with maternal positional change, the use of the Trendelenburg position, and gentle manual elevation of the fetal presenting part aid in visualizing the fetal vessels. The latter technique is particularly useful because the vessels may be compressed by the presenting part and thus difficult to visualize.

Management

There is no uniformity of opinion as to the optimal management strategy for pregnancies with a prenatally diagnosed vasa previa, particularly in regard to the timing of elective delivery. It has been suggested that patients be hospitalized at 30 to 32 weeks and delivered at 35 to 36 weeks' gestation without confirmation of lung maturity by amniocentesis.[16] This approach is based on the 10% risk of membrane rupture before labor and the high associated fetal mortality rate. Our approach has been to assess cervical length weekly from at least 30 weeks using TVUS. If the cervix is 2.5 cm in length or greater, out-of-hospital management continues. The patient is administered betamethasone just before 34 weeks' gestation and is delivered by cesarean section between 34 and 35 weeks, without additional testing for fetal lung maturity.

Prevention of Adverse Outcomes

A significant reduction in fetal mortality should be possible with a diligent search as previously described. Public and professional awareness has been heightened by such organizations as The International Vasa Previa Foundation (http://www.vasaprevia.com [accessed February 8, 2008]). However, a high index of suspicion by the attending physician and a meticulous approach to diagnosis provide the best opportunity for a favorable outcome.

Abruptio Placentae

Definition and Epidemiology

Abruptio placentae is the premature separation of a normally sited placenta before birth, after 20 weeks' gestation. It is a particularly hazardous condition associated with significant maternal and fetal morbidity and mortality. About 1% of all pregnancies are complicated by clinically recognized abruption.[90-93] The degree of abruption ranges across a broad clinical spectrum, from minor degrees of placental separation, with little effect on maternal or fetal outcome, to major abruption associated with fetal death and maternal morbidity. Abruption sufficient to cause fetal death occurs in about 1 of every 420 deliveries.[94] If placentas are routinely examined after delivery, evidence of abruption may be found in almost 4% of cases, most of which were unrecognized and of no apparent clinical consequence. There has been an increase of almost 25% in the rate of clinically detected abruption in the United States in recent decades, with a disproportionate increase seen among African-American women.[95]

The incidence of abruption peaks between 24 and 26 weeks' gestation.[96] Approximately 10% of all preterm births occur because of abruption,[90] and the infant outcomes are associated with increased rates of perinatal asphyxia,[97] intraventricular hemorrhage, periventricular leukomalacia,[98] and cerebral palsy[99] when compared with gestational age–matched controls. Perinatal mortality in pregnancies complicated by abruption may be declining overall,[93,100] but the rate continues to be higher than in gestational age–matched controls without abruption.[96] Placental separation is strongly associated with preterm premature rupture of the membranes (pPROM), in both a causal and a consequential manner.[101] Most pregnancies complicated by abruption result in the delivery of an infant weighing less than the 10th percentile for gestational age,[102-104] suggesting a common pathway linking abruption to placental dysfunction and intrauterine growth retardation (IUGR).

Pathogenesis

Abruption results from bleeding between the decidua and placenta (Fig. 37-6). The hemorrhage dissects the decidua apart, with loss of the corresponding placental area for gaseous exchange and provision of fetal nutrition. The process may be self-limited or ongoing with further dissection of the decidua. Dissection can lead to external bleeding if it reaches the placental edge and tracks down between the fetal membranes; circumferential dissection leading to near-total separation of the placenta can occur, particularly with concealed abruption. The underlying event in many cases of abruption is thought to be vasospasm of abnormal maternal arterioles. Some cases may result from venous hemorrhage into areas of the decidua that have become necrotic secondary to thrombosis. Long-standing predisposition to abruption may be inferred from the finding that women destined to suffer abruption have low levels of pregnancy-associated plasma protein A (PAPP-A).[105] Evidence of preexisting placental pathology in women with abruption includes poor trophoblastic invasion,[106] inadequate remodeling of the uterine circulation as reflected by abnormal uterine artery Doppler flow,[107] and the well-established associations among preeclampsia, IUGR, and abruption—all of which may be regarded as primary placental disorders. Abruption may also occur secondary to acute shearing forces affecting the placenta-decidua interface, such as those that occur with trauma—particularly rapid deceleration injuries (motor vehicle accidents) and the sudden decompression of an overdistended uterus that occurs with membrane rupture in polyhydramnios or delivery of a multiple gestation.

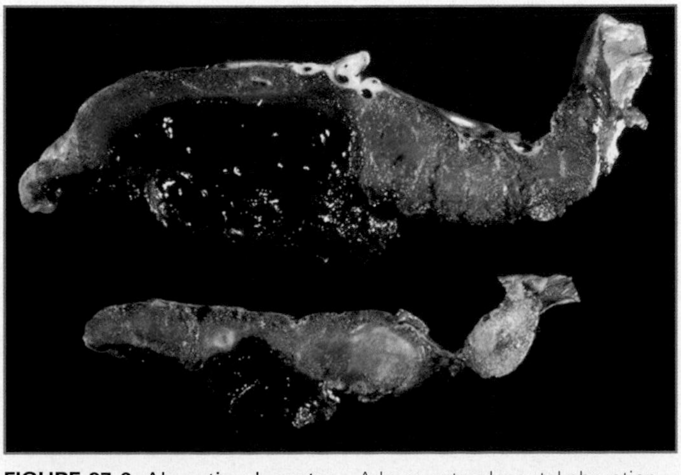

FIGURE 37-6 Abruptio placentae. A large retroplacental abruption at 30 weeks' gestation is shown.

As the abruption process continues, loss of placental function results in fetal hypoxia and may end in fetal death. The acute hemorrhage activates the coagulation cascade, and, with ongoing bleeding, disseminated intravascular coagulation (DIC) may result. Continued bleeding, with maternal hypovolemia and poor tissue perfusion, aggravates the DIC and results in a downward spiral into hemorrhagic shock. Bleeding into the myometrial tissue can lead to a Couvelaire uterus which becomes atonic and increases the risk of uterine hemorrhage after delivery.

Risk Factors and Associations for Abruption

The most important risk factor for abruption is a history of abruption in a prior pregnancy.[108] One meta-analysis showed an increase of up to 20-fold in the risk of abruption if a prior pregnancy had been similarly affected.[109] With two prior pregnancies complicated by abruption, the risk of recurrence is 25%.[94]

Maternal hypertension is also a significant risk factor for abruption. Chronic hypertension is associated with a fivefold increase in risk, which rises to eightfold with superimposed preeclampsia.[96] Preeclampsia alone is also strongly linked to abruption and to the severity of abruption.[110] It seems plausible that preeclampsia and abruption share many underlying pathologic mechanisms.

Perhaps the most readily preventable risk factor for abruption is cigarette smoking. Cigarette smokers are up to 2.5 times more likely to have an abruption than nonsmokers,[111-115] and they have twice the perinatal mortality of nonsmokers.[116] There is a dose-response relationship between the number of cigarettes smoked and the risk of abruption.[115,117,118] Even women who stop smoking before pregnancy are at increased risk. Substance abuse is closely linked to abruption—any agent that causes vasospasm or transient severe hypertension may be causative.[119,120] In the United States, as many as 10% of pregnant women who are cocaine and crack cocaine users will experience placental abruption.[121] Multiparity is also positively correlated with a small increase in the risk of abruption.[1,102] The apparent association between maternal age and abruption is not significant when parity is taken into account.

There has been substantial recent interest in the possible association between thrombophilic disorders and abruption. Some retrospective studies of abruption have found increased rates of thrombophilia.[122,123]

However, both retrospective[124] and prospective case-control studies[125] of women with the factor V Leiden mutation showed no increase in abruption risk. It is established that hyperhomocysteinemia is associated with abruption,[123] although, in the absence of hyperhomocysteinemia, the specific *MTHFR* gene mutations themselves do not appear to be associated with an increased risk.[126,127]

Motor vehicle accidents are the most common traumatic event associated with abruption, and clinical evidence of abruption may not be apparent for 24 hours or longer after the trauma. Women with vaginal bleeding or contractions after a motor vehicle accident should be observed for at least 24 hours; those who are asymptomatic can safely be discharged after 6 hours of monitoring.[128,129]

Membrane rupture may precede or follow chronic retroplacental bleeding or an acute abruption, and women with ruptured membranes should be monitored carefully for this possibility.[109,130] Those with early pregnancy bleeding who have a subchorionic hematoma visible on ultrasound are also at increased risk for both pPROM and abruption.[131]

Screening tests performed for other indications may identify groups of women who are at increased risk for abruption but may have no other high-risk factors. These tests include maternal first- and second-trimester serum screening for aneuploidy. Women with PAPP-A levels below the 5th percentile at the time of first-trimester serum screening for trisomy 21 have an increased risk of abruption,[105] but low levels of human chorionic gonadotropin (hCG) in the first trimester are not similarly associated.[132] In one study of routine uterine artery Doppler velocimetry performed at 11 to 14 weeks' gestation as a screen for IUGR and preeclampsia, a pulsatility index higher than the 95th percentile or a PAPP-A value lower than the 10th percentile predicted 43% of pregnancies with a subsequent abruption.[133] In an earlier study of uterine artery Doppler ultrasound, persistent notching of the waveform after 24 weeks was associated with increased risk for abruption as well as IUGR and preeclampsia.[107]

Women with otherwise unexplained elevated serum levels (>2 multiples of the median [MOM]) of α-fetoprotein (AFP) on second-trimester serum screening for trisomy 21 have long been thought to be at increased risk for a wide range of adverse pregnancy outcomes, including abruption.[134,135] However, a recent case-matched, prospective study found elevated AFP levels to be associated with an increased risk of abruption but no increase in the frequency of IUGR, preterm delivery, low birth weight, or fetal death.[136] A recent attempt to establish a critical cutoff value for elevated AFP and increased risk of abruption stressed the low specificity and high false-positive rate of the test.[136]

Elevated hCG values at the time of second-trimester serum screening have similarly been associated with adverse pregnancy outcome, including abruption.[137] Previously, a value greater than 2.0 MOM was thought to be significant in this context, but one recent case-controlled study showed that the threshold should be set at 3.0 MOM. Even at that level, a positive test had poor predictive value and was not associated with increased risk of abruption.[138] Abnormal inhibin values do not appear to be predictive of abruption.

Diagnosis

The diagnosis of placental abruption is made based on clinical findings. The classic presentation is that of vaginal bleeding, usually accompanied by abdominal (uterine) pain. Examination often reveals uterine tenderness, and contractions may be present. About 10% of abruptions are concealed, with no vaginal bleeding. If bleeding is present, the amount is often a poor guide to the degree of separation, because there is usually a mixed picture of apparent and concealed hemorrhage. Fetal compromise is a common finding, and if more than 50% of the placenta is involved, fetal death is likely. Massive concealed abruption often manifests with severe pain, a hard uterus, and a dead fetus; such a picture may occur in association with severe preeclampsia or the recent use of a vasoactive drug such as cocaine.[139] If abruption occurs in a posteriorly located placenta, severe back pain may be the only symptom; it may be worsened by abdominal palpation that pushes the fetus against the placenta. Abruption may precipitate preterm labor, and it should always be considered in the differential diagnosis for a patient in apparent idiopathic preterm labor.

Although ultrasonography is an integral part of the diagnostic approach to late pregnancy bleeding, its utility is primarily for the exclusion of placenta previa as the cause of hemorrhage. At least 50% of abruptions produce no findings on ultrasound.[140-142] What is visualized by ultrasound depends on the site, scale, and timing of bleeding. In early acute abruptions, blood and clot retained within the uterus appear as hyperechoic or isoechoic collections relative to placental echogenicity.[143] In cases that remain undelivered, the hematomas resolve over several weeks, becoming hypoechoic and then sonolucent, usually by 2 weeks after the event.[143] Intrauterine clot may "jiggle" when bounced by the transducer—the "jello" sign. An acute abruption with obvious vaginal bleeding, in which little or no blood is retained within the uterus, may have no specific sonographic findings. Therefore, the absence of ultrasound findings never excludes an abruption.

Cardiotocography is an integral part of the evaluation for late pregnancy bleeding. Abruption is commonly accompanied by uterine contractions that may not be appreciated clinically, particularly after trauma.[144] Fetal heart rate tracings may exhibit a variety of abnormal patterns, including variable and late decelerations, poor variability, prolonged bradycardia, or a sinusoidal pattern; these are not specific to abruption and reflect underlying evolving fetal asphyxia.

Kleihauer-Betke testing is of no diagnostic value in abruption: It may be negative with proven abruption[128,129,145] or positive when no abruption has occurred. Its only value in this setting is to guide Rh immune globulin dosing in Rh-negative women who are thought to have sustained an abruption.

Chronic abruption-oligohydramnios sequence (CAOS) is a term that was coined to describe women who present with bleeding attributed to abruption and go on to develop oligohydramnios without evidence of ruptured membranes.[146] Twenty-four patients were described, all of whom delivered preterm (average gestational age, 28 weeks). For the most part, the earlier the onset of bleeding, the earlier the delivery. More than half of the women went on to develop pPROM before delivery and after the development of oligohydramnios.

Management

The key to optimizing maternal and fetal outcome in abruptio placentae is the individualization of care. Precise management depends on the extent of maternal and/or fetal compromise and the gestational age. Decision making should be rapid but methodical; delay in diagnosis and inappropriate triage leads to significantly increased perinatal mortality.[147] Twenty percent of all fetal deaths from abruption occur after presentation to the hospital, and 30% of those deaths occur within 2 hours after admission.

Initial assessment should focus on maternal hemodynamic status (remembering that blood pressure may be elevated in the setting of preeclampsia) and fetal well-being. Maternal vital signs should be measured frequently, because they may change suddenly as the abruption evolves. Electronic fetal monitoring should begin immediately and be continuous throughout further assessment and management. A large-gauge intravenous line should be placed (two lines if the patient is hemodynamically unstable). Initial laboratory studies should include a baseline complete blood count and platelet count, type and screen and cross-match where appropriate, blood urea nitrogen and electrolytes, coagulation studies, and a wall clot. These studies serve as useful baseline references. An indwelling bladder catheter should be placed to allow urinary output to be closely monitored. In unstable or critically ill patients, management may be aided by placement of a central venous pressure line (preferably with a Cordis introducer) or an arterial line. The involvement of the obstetric anesthetic team should be sought early.

After these steps are taken, attention should be directed at excluding a placenta previa (by ultrasound examination) and deciding on the timing and route of delivery. Maternal or fetal compromise mandates immediate delivery, usually by cesarean section unless the patient is in an advanced stage of labor. If the event occurs after 34 weeks' gestation, delivery should not be delayed, because the risks of conservative management outweigh any considerations of prematurity of the fetus. Between 20 and 34 weeks, if mother and fetus are stable, an attempt at conservative management may be considered.[148,149] Betamethasone should be administered to enhance fetal lung maturity in all such cases. The patient should be monitored closely, because she continues to be at risk of an evolving process. The use of tocolytics is controversial; in most cases, they should not be used. Although studies addressing this issue have found no increase in adverse fetal or maternal events,[27,141,148-150] no prospective trial has been performed.

If the patient has sustained a mild separation at a premature gestational age and is asymptomatic without evidence of bleeding, discharge home may be considered as an alternative to prolonged hospitalization. Either way, a clear management plan for delivery should be developed based on subsequent events or the reaching of an arbitrary gestational age (usually 37 weeks). The evaluation of patients undergoing expectant management should include regular assessment of fetal growth and tests of well-being, because these fetuses are at increased risk for IUGR.

If an abruption occurs after 34 weeks' gestation and maternal and fetal condition permit, vaginal delivery is preferred. Amniotomy should be performed, and, if needed, an oxytocin infusion should be started. Labor usually progresses rapidly, even without augmentation. However, if progress is slow or maternal or fetal status deteriorates, cesarean section should be performed. If abruption has resulted in fetal death, vaginal delivery is preferred unless there are other obstetric contraindications or the mother is hemodynamically unstable.

Coagulopathy develops in about 10% of abruptions. It usually is related to the severity of the event and is particularly likely to occur if there is fetal demise or massive hemorrhage. An aggressive approach should be used to maintain maternal blood volume and oxygen-carrying capacity, including the use of component therapy (fresh-frozen plasma and platelets). The coagulation tests most frequently used, and the component replacement therapy for women with DIC, are summarized in Tables 37-3 and 37-4.

TABLE 37-3 COAGULATION TESTS USED IN THE DIAGNOSIS OF ABRUPTIO PLACENTAE

Test	What It Measures	Normal Value	Value in Abruption
Bleeding time	Vascular integrity and platelet function	1-5 min	Usually normal; test is of little clinical use in diagnosing abruption
Whole blood clotting time	Platelet function Fibrinolytic activity	Clot formation: 4-8 min Clot retraction: <1 hr Clot lysis: none in 24 hr	Clot formation abnormality indicates severe deficiency Abnormal retraction with thrombocytopenia
Fibrinogen	Fibrinogen level	400-650 mg/100 mL	Usually decreased
Platelet count	Number of platelets	>140,000/mm^3	Usually decreased
Fibrin degradation products	Fibrin and fibrinogen degradation products	<10 μg/mL	Almost always elevated; most sensitive test
Euglobulin clot lysis time	Fibrinolytic activity	None in 2 hr	Difficult to interpret with low fibrinogen levels
Prothrombin time	Factors II, V, VII, X	10-12 sec	Normal to prolonged
Partial thromboplastin time	Factors II, V, XIII, IX, X, XI	24-38 sec	Normal to prolonged
Thrombin time	Factors I, II Circulating split products Heparin effect	16-20 sec	Parallels fall in fibrinogen; good marker of abruption severity
Red blood cell morphology	Microangiopathic hemolysis	Absence of distortion or fragmentation	Presence of distortion or fragmentation is uncommon but indicates risk of renal cortical necrosis

TABLE 37-4 BLOOD REPLACEMENT PRODUCTS

Component	Volume per Unit (mL)*	Factors Present	Effect of 1 Unit
Fresh whole blood	500	RBCs; all procoagulants	↑ Hematocrit 3%
Packed RBCs	200	RBCs only	↑ Hematocrit 3%
Fresh-frozen plasma	200-400	All procoagulants; no platelets	↑ Fibrinogen 25 mg/dL
Cryoprecipitate	20-50	Fibrinogen; factors VIII, XIII	↑ Fibrinogen 15-25%
Platelet concentrate	35-60	Platelets; small amounts of fibrinogen; factors V, VIII	↑ Platelet count approximately 8000/mm^3

RBCs, red blood cells.
***Volume depends on individual blood bank.**

Prevention

A prior abruption increases the risk of abruption in a subsequent pregnancy up to 20-fold.[151] Modification of risk factors includes treatment of chronic hypertension, smoking cessation, and avoidance of substance abuse. Women with hyperhomocysteinemia should be treated with folate.

References

1. Ananth CV, Wilcox AJ, Savitz DA, et al: Effect of maternal age and parity on the risk of uteroplacental bleeding disorders in pregnancy. Obstet Gynecol 88:511-516, 1996.
2. Iyasu S, Saftlas AK, Rowley DL, et al: The epidemiology of placenta previa in the United States, 1979 through 1987. Am J Obstet Gynecol 168:1424-1429, 1993.
3. Frederiksen MC, Glassenberg R, Stika CS: Placenta previa: A 22-year analysis. Am J Obstet Gynecol 180:1432-1437, 1999.
4. Hemminki E, Merilainen J: Long-term effects of cesarean sections: Ectopic pregnancies and placental problems. Am J Obstet Gynecol 174:1569-1574, 1996.
5. Hershkowitz R, Fraser D, Mazor M, Leiberman JR: One or multiple previous cesarean sections are associated with similar increased frequency of placenta previa. Eur J Obstet Gynecol Reprod Biol 62:185-188, 1995.
6. Monica G, Lilja C: Placenta previa, maternal smoking and recurrence risk. Acta Obstet Gynecol Scand 74:341-345, 1995.
7. Timor-Tritsch IE, Yunis RA: Confirming the safety of transvaginal sonography in patients suspected of placenta previa. Obstet Gynecol 81:742-744, 1993.
8. Williams MA, Mittendorf R: Increasing maternal age as a determinant of placenta previa: More important than increasing parity? J Reprod Med 38:425-428, 1993.
9. Taylor VM, Kramer MD, Vaughan TL, Peacock S: Placenta previa and prior cesarean delivery: How strong is the association? Obstet Gynecol 84:55-57, 1994.
10. Handler AS, Mason ED, Rosenberg DL, Davis FG: The relationship between exposure during pregnancy to cigarette smoking and cocaine use and placenta previa. Am J Obstet Gynecol 170:884-889, 1994.
11. Wexler P, Gottesfeld KR: Early diagnosis of placenta previa. Obstet Gynecol 54:231-234, 1979.
12. Smith RS, Lauria MR, Comstock CH, et al: Transvaginal ultrasonography for all placentas that appear to be low-lying or over the internal cervical os. Ultrasound Obstet Gynecol 9:22-24, 1997.
13. Leerentveld RA, Gilberts EC, Arnold MJ, Wladimiroff JW: Accuracy and safety of transvaginal sonographic placental localization. Obstet Gynecol 76:759-762, 1990.
14. Rosati P, Guariglia L: Clinical significance of placenta previa detected at early routine transvaginal scan. J Ultrasound Med 19:581-585, 2000.
15. Hertzberg BS, Bowie JD, Carroll BA, et al: Diagnosis of placenta previa during the third trimester: Role of transperineal sonography. AJR Am J Roentgenol 159:83-87, 1992.
16. Oyelese Y, Smulian JC: Placenta previa, placenta accreta, and vasa previa. Obstet Gynecol 107:927-941, 2006.
17. Becker RH, Vonk R, Mende BC, et al: The relevance of placental location at 20-23 gestational weeks for prediction of placenta previa at delivery: Evaluation of 8650 cases. Ultrasound Obstet Gynecol 17:496-501, 2001.
18. Taipale P, Hiilesmaa V, Ylostalo P: Transvaginal ultrasonography at 18-23 weeks in predicting placenta previa at delivery. Ultrasound Obstet Gynecol 12:422-425, 1998.
19. Hill LM, Dinofrio DM, Chenevey P: Transvaginal sonographic evaluation of first-trimester placenta previa. Ultrasound Obstet Gynecol 5:301-303, 1995.
20. Mustafa SA, Brizot ML, Carvalho MH, et al: Transvaginal ultrasonography in predicting placenta previa at delivery: A longitudinal study. Ultrasound Obstet Gynecol 20:356-359, 2002.
21. Lauria MR, Smith RS, Treadwell MC, et al: The use of second-trimester transvaginal sonography to predict placenta previa. Ultrasound Obstet Gynecol 8:337-340, 1996.
22. Dashe JS, McIntire DD, Ramus RM, et al: Persistence of placenta previa according to gestational age at ultrasound detection. Obstet Gynecol 99:692-697, 2002.
23. Ghourab S: Third-trimester transvaginal ultrasonography in placenta previa: Does the shape of the lower placental edge predict clinical outcome? Ultrasound Obstet Gynecol 18:103-108, 2001.
24. Cotton DB, Read JA, Paul RH, Quilligan EJ: The conservative aggressive management of placenta previa. Am J Obstet Gynecol 137:687-695, 1980.
25. Love CD, Wallace EM: Pregnancies complicated by placenta praevia: What is appropriate management? BJOG 103:864-867, 1996.
26. Brenner WE, Edelman DA, Hendricks CH: Characteristics of patients with placenta previa and results of "expectant management." Am J Obstet Gynecol 132:180-191, 1978.
27. Towers CV, Pircon RA, Heppard M: Is tocolysis safe in the management of third-trimester bleeding? Am J Obstet Gynecol 180:1572-1578, 1999.
28. Besinger RE, Moniak CW, Paskiewicz LS, et al: The effect of tocolytic use in the management of symptomatic placenta previa. Am J Obstet Gynecol 172:1770-1775; discussion 1775-1778, 1995.
29. Sharma A, Suri V, Gupta I: Tocolytic therapy in conservative management of symptomatic placenta previa. Int J Gynaecol Obstet 84:109-113, 2004.
30. Droste S, Keil K: Expectant management of placenta previa: Cost-benefit analysis of outpatient treatment. Am J Obstet Gynecol 170:1254-1257, 1994.
31. Mouer JR: Placenta previa: Antepartum conservative management, inpatient versus outpatient. Am J Obstet Gynecol 170:1683-1685; discussion 1685-1686, 1994.
32. Rosen DM, Peek MJ: Do women with placenta praevia without antepartum haemorrhage require hospitalization? Aust N Z J Obstet Gynaecol 34:130-134, 1994.
33. Wing DA, Paul RH, Millar LK: Management of the symptomatic placenta previa: A randomized, controlled trial of inpatient versus outpatient expectant management. Am J Obstet Gynecol 175:806-811, 1996.
34. D'Angelo LJ, Irwin LF: Conservative management of placenta previa: A cost-benefit analysis. Am J Obstet Gynecol 149:320-326, 1984.
35. Arias F: Cervical cerclage for the temporary treatment of patients with placenta previa. Obstet Gynecol 71:545-548, 1988.
36. Cobo E, Conde-Agudelo A, Delgado J, et al: Cervical cerclage: An alternative for the management of placenta previa? Am J Obstet Gynecol 179:122-125, 1998.
37. Oppenheimer LW, Farine D, Ritchie JW, et al: What is a low-lying placenta? Am J Obstet Gynecol 165:1036-1038, 1991.
38. Bhide A, Prefumo F, Moore J, et al: Placental edge to internal os distance in the late third trimester and mode of delivery in placenta praevia. BJOG 110:860-864, 2003.
39. Dawson WB, Dumas MD, Romano WM, et al: Translabial ultrasonography and placenta previa: Does measurement of the os-placenta distance predict outcome? J Ultrasound Med 15:441-446, 1996.
40. Royal College of Obstetricians and Gynaecologists. Placenta Praevia and Placenta Praevia Accreta Diagnosis and Management. Clinical Green Top Guidelines No. 27. London, RCOG, 2005.
41. Boehm FH, Fleischer AC, Barrett JM: Sonographic placental localization in the determination of the site of uterine incision for placenta previa. J Ultrasound Med 1:311-314, 1982.
42. Lynch BC, Coker A, Lawal AH, et al: The B-Lynch surgical technique for the control of massive postpartum haemorrhage: An alternative to hysterectomy? Five cases reported. BJOG 104:372-375, 1997.
43. Bonner SM, Haynes SR, Ryall D: The anaesthetic management of caesarean section for placenta praevia: A questionnaire survey. Anaesthesia 50:992-994, 1995.
44. Parekh N, Husaini SW, Russell IF: Caesarean section for placenta praevia: A retrospective study of anaesthetic management. Br J Anaesth 84:725-730, 2000.

45. Hong JY, Jee YS, Yoon HJ, Kim SM: Comparison of general and epidural anesthesia in elective cesarean section for placenta previa totalis: Maternal hemodynamics, blood loss and neonatal outcome. Int J Obstet Anesth 12:12-16, 2003.
46. Usta IM, Hobeika EM, Musa AA, et al: Placenta previa-accreta: Risk factors and complications. Am J Obstet Gynecol 193:1045-1049, 2005.
47. Silver RM, Landon MB, Rouse DJ, et al: Maternal morbidity associated with multiple repeat cesarean deliveries. Obstet Gynecol 107:1226-1232, 2006.
48. Clark SL, Koonings PP, Phelan JP: Placenta previa/accreta and prior cesarean section. Obstet Gynecol 66:89, 1985.
49. Chattopadhyay SK, Kharif H, Sherbeeni MM: Placenta previa and accreta after previous cesarean section. Eur J Obstet Gynaecol Reprod Biol 52:151, 1993.
50. Lira Plascencia J, Ibarguengoitia Ochoa F, Arqueta Z, et al: Placenta praevia/accreta and previous cesarean section: Experience of five years at the Mexico National Institute of Perinatology. Gynecol Obstet Mex 63:337, 1995.
51. Rashbaum WK, Gates EJ, Jones J, et al: Placenta accreta encountered during dilation and evacuation in the second trimester. Obstet Gynecol 85:701, 1995.
52. Comstock CH: Antenatal diagnosis of placenta accreta: A review. Ultrasound Obstet Gynecol 26:89-96, 2005.
53. Warshak CR, Eskander R, Hull AD, et al: Accuracy of ultrasonography and magnetic resonance imaging in the diagnosis of placenta accreta. Obstet Gynecol 108:573-581, 2006.
54. Grosvenor A, Silver R, Porter TF, et al: Optimal management of placenta accreta. Am J Obstet Gynecol 195(6 Suppl 1):S82, 2006.
55. Levine D, Hulka CA, Ludmir J, et al: Placenta accreta: Evaluation with color Doppler US, power Doppler US, and MI imaging. Radiology 205:773, 1997.
56. Finberg HJ, Williams JW: Placenta accreta: Prospective sonographic diagnosis in patients with placenta previa and previous cesarean section. J Ultrasound Med 11:333-343, 1992.
57. Maldjian C, Adam R, Pelosi M, et al: MRI appearance of placenta percreta and placenta accreta. Magn Reson Imaging 17:965-971, 1999.
58. Lerner JP, Deane S, Timor-Tritsch IE: Characterization of placenta accreta using transvaginal sonography and color Doppler imaging. Ultrasound Obstet Gynecol 5:198, 1995.
59. Twickler DM, Lucas MJ, Balis AB, et al: Color flow mapping for myometrial invasion in women with a prior cesarean delivery. J Matern Fetal Med 9:330, 2000.
60. Chou MM, Tseng JJ, Ho ES, et al: Three dimensional color power Doppler imaging in the assessment of uteroplacental neovascularization in placenta previa increta/percreta. Am J Obstet Gynecol 185:1257, 2001.
61. Zelop CM, Harlow BL, Frigoletto FD, et al: Emergency peripartum hysterectomy. Am J Obstet Gynecol 168:1443-1448, 1993.
62. Kwee A, Bots ML, Visser GH, et al: Emergency peripartum hysterectomy: A prospective study in the Netherlands. Eur J Obstet Gynecol Reprod Biol 124:187-192, 2006.
63. Bodner LJ, Nosher JL, Gribbin C, et al: Balloon-assisted occlusion of the internal iliac arteries in patients with placenta accrete/percreta. Cardiovasc Intervent Radiol 29:354-361, 2006.
64. Shrivastava V, Nageotte M, Major C, et al. Case-control comparison of cesarean hysterectomy with and without prophylactic placement of intrafascular balloon catheters for placenta accreta. Am J Obstet Gynecol 197:40231-40235, 2007.
65. Jaffe R, DuBeshter B, Sherer DM, et al: Failure of methotrexate treatment for term placenta percreta. Am J Obstet Gynecol 171:558, 1994.
66. Matthews NM, McCowan LM, Patten P: Placenta previa accreta with delayed hysterectomy. Aust N Z J Obstet Gynaecol 36:476, 1996.
67. Mussalli GM, Shah J, Berch DJ, et al: Placenta accreta and methotrexate therapy: Three case reports. J Perinatal 20:331, 2000.
68. Varma TR: Fetal growth and placental function in patients with placenta praevia. J Obstet Gynaecol Br Commonw 80:311-315, 1973.
69. Crane JM, van den Hof MC, Dodds L, et al: Neonatal outcomes with placenta previa. Obstet Gynecol 93:541-544, 1999.
70. Spinillo A, Fazzi E, Stronati M, et al: Early morbidity and neurodevelopmental outcome in low-birthweight infants born after third trimester bleeding. Am J Perinatol 11:85-90, 1994.
71. Li DK, Wi S: Maternal placental abnormality and the risk of sudden infant death syndrome. Am J Epidemiol 149:608-611, 1999.
72. Gielchinsky Y, Mankuta D, Rojansky N, et al: Perinatal outcome of pregnancies complicated by placenta accrtea. Obstet Gynecol 104:527-530, 2004.
73. Fung TY, Lau TK: Poor perinatal outcome associated with vasa previa: Is it preventable? A report of three cases and review of the literature. Ultrasound Obstet Gynecol 12:430-433, 1998.
74. Oyelese KO, Turner M, Lees C, Campbell S: Vasa previa: An avoidable obstetric tragedy. Obstet Gynecol Surv 54:138-145, 1999.
75. Lijoi AF, Brady J: Vasa previa diagnosis and management. J Am Board Fam Pract 16:543-548, 2003.
76. Francois K, Mayer S, Harris C, Perlow JH: Association of vasa previa at delivery with a history of second-trimester placenta previa. J Reprod Med 48:771-774, 2003.
77. Schachter M, Tovbin Y, Arieli S, et al: In vitro fertilization is a risk factor for vasa previa. Fertil Steril 78:642-643, 2002.
78. Antoine C, Young BK, Silverman F, et al: Sinusoidal fetal heart rate pattern with vasa previa in twin pregnancy. J Reprod Med 27:295-300, 1982.
79. Schellpfeffer MA: Improved neonatal outcome of vasa previa with aggressive intrapartum management: A report of two cases. J Reprod Med 40:327-332, 1995.
80. Vandrie DM, Kammeraad LA: Vasa previa: Case report, review and presentation of a new diagnostic method. J Reprod Med 26:577-580, 1981.
81. Catanzarite V, Maida C, Thomas W, et al: Prenatal sonographic diagnosis of vasa previa: Ultrasound findings and obstetric outcome in ten cases. Ultrasound Obstet Gynecol 18:109-115, 2001.
82. Lee W, Lee VL, Kirk JS, et al: Vasa previa: Prenatal diagnosis, natural evolution, and clinical outcome. Obstet Gynecol 95:572-576, 2000.
83. Daly-Jones E, Hollingsworth J, Sepulveda W: Vasa praevia: Second trimester diagnosis using colour flow imaging. BJOG 103:284-286, 1996.
84. Sepulveda W, Rojas I, Robert JA, et al: Prenatal detection of velamentous insertion of the umbilical cord: A prospective color Doppler ultrasound study. Ultrasound Obstet Gynecol 21:564-569.
85. Nomiyama M, Toyota Y, Kawano H: Antenatal diagnosis of velamentous umbilical cord insertion and vasa previa with color Doppler imaging. Ultrasound Obstet Gynecol 12:426-429, 1998.
86. Oyelese Y, Catanzarite V, Prefumo F, et al: Vasa previa: The impact of prenatal diagnosis on outcomes. Obstet Gynecol 103:937-942, 2004.
87. Nimmo MJ, Kinsella D, Andrews HS: MRI in pregnancy: The diagnosis of vasa previa by magnetic resonance imaging. Bristol Med Chir J 103:12, 1988.
88. Canterino JC, Mondestin-Sorrentino M, Muench MV, et al: Vasa previa: Prenatal diagnosis and evaluation with 3-dimensional sonography and power angiography. J Ultrasound Med 24:721-724, quiz 725; 2005.
89. Oyelese Y, Chavez MR, Yeo L, et al: Three-dimensional sonographic diagnosis of vasa previa. Ultrasound Obstet Gynecol 24:211-215, 2004.
90. Ananth CV, Berkowitz GS, Savitz DA, Lapinski RH: Placental abruption and adverse perinatal outcomes. JAMA 282:1646-1651, 1999.
91. Ananth CV, Wilcox AJ: Placental abruption and perinatal mortality in the United States. Am J Epidemiol 153:332-337, 2001.
92. Salihu HM, Bekan B, Aliyu MH, et al: Perinatal mortality associated with abruptio placenta in singletons and multiples. Am J Obstet Gynecol 193:198-203, 2005.
93. Rasmussen S, Irgens LM, Bergsjo P, Dalaker K: The occurrence of placental abruption in Norway 1967-1991. Acta Obstet Gynecol Scand 75:222-228, 1996.
94. Pritchard JA, Mason R, Corley M, Pritchard S: Genesis of severe placental abruption. Am J Obstet Gynecol 108:22-27, 1970.
95. Ananth CV, Oyelese Y, Yeo L, et al: Placental abruption in the United States, 1979 through 2001: Temporal trends and potential determinants. Am J Obstet Gynecol 192:191-198, 2005.

96. Oyelese Y, Ananth CV: Placental abruption. Obstet Gynecol 108:1005-1016, 2006.
97. Perlman JM, Risser R: Can asphyxiated infants at risk for neonatal seizures be rapidly identified by current high-risk markers? Pediatrics 97:456-462, 1996.
98. Gibbs JM, Weindling AM: Neonatal intracranial lesions following placental abruption. Eur J Pediatr 153:195-197, 1994.
99. Spinillo A, Fazzi E, Stronati M, et al: Severity of abruptio placentae and neurodevelopmental outcome in low birth weight infants. Early Hum Dev 35:45-54, 1993.
100. Naeye RL, Harkness WL, Utts J: Abruptio placentae and perinatal death: A prospective study. Am J Obstet Gynecol 128:740-746, 1977.
101. Rosen T, Schatz F, Kuczynski E, et al: Thrombin-enhanced matrix metalloproteinase-1 expression: A mechanism linking placental abruption with premature rupture of the membranes. J Matern Fetal Neonatal Med 11:11-17, 2002.
102. Hibbard BM, Jeffcoate TN: Abruptio placentae. Obstet Gynecol 27:155-167, 1966.
103. Sheiner E, Shoham-Vardi I, Hallak M, et al: Placental abruption in term pregnancies: Clinical significance and obstetric risk factors. J Matern Fetal Neonatal Med 13:45-49, 2003.
104. Ananth CV, Smulian JC, Srinivas N, et al: Risk of infant mortality among twins in relation to placental abruption: Contributions of preterm birth and restricted fetal growth. Twin Res Hum Genet 8:524-531, 2005.
105. Dugoff L, Hobbins JC, Malone FD, et al: First-trimester maternal serum PAPP-A and free-beta subunit human chorionic gonadotropin concentrations and nuchal translucency are associated with obstetric complications: A population-based screening study (the FASTER Trial). Am J Obstet Gynecol 191:1446-1451, 2004.
106. Dommisse J, Tiltman AJ: Placental bed biopsies in placental abruption. BJOG 99:651-654, 1992.
107. Harrington K, Cooper D, Lees C, et al: Doppler ultrasound of the uterine arteries: The importance of bilateral notching in the prediction of pre-eclampsia, placental abruption or delivery of a small-for-gestational-age baby. Ultrasound Obstet Gynecol 7:182-188, 1996.
108. Toivonen S, Heinonen S, Anttila M, et al: Obstetric prognosis after placental abruption. Fetal Diagn Ther 19:336-341, 2004.
109. Ananth CV, Savitz DA, Williams MA. Placental abruption and its association with hypertension and prolonged rupture of membranes: A methodologic review and meta-analysis. Obstet Gynecol 88:309-318, 1996.
110. Golditch IM, Boyce NE Jr: Management of abruptio placentae. JAMA 212:288-293, 1970.
111. Cnattingius S: Maternal age modifies the effect of maternal smoking on intrauterine growth retardation but not on late fetal death and placental abruption. Am J Epidemiol 145:319-323.
112. Kramer MS, Usher RH, Pollack R, et al: Etiologic determinants of abruptio placentae. Obstet Gynecol 89:221-226, 1997.
113. Castles A, Adams EK, Melvin CL, et al: Effects of smoking during pregnancy: Five meta-analyses. Am J Prev Med 16:208-215, 1999.
114. Ananth CV, Savitz DA, Luther ER: Maternal cigarette smoking as a risk factor for placental abruption, placenta previa, and uterine bleeding in pregnancy. Am J Epidemiol 144:881-889, 1996.
115. Ananth CV, Smulian JC, Vintzileos AM: Incidence of placental abruption in relation to cigarette smoking and hypertensive disorders during pregnancy: A meta-analysis of observational studies. Obstet Gynecol 93:622-628, 1999.
116. Raymond EG, Mills JL: Placental abruption: Maternal risk factors and associated fetal conditions. Acta Obstet Gynecol Scand 72:633-639, 1993.
117. Kyrklund-Blomberg NB, Gennser G, Cnattingius S: Placental abruption and perinatal death. Paediatr Perinat Epidemiol 15:290-297, 2001.
118. Misra DP, Ananth CV: Risk factor profiles of placental abruption in first and second pregnancies: Heterogeneous etiologies. J Clin Epidemiol 52:453-461, 1999.
119. Kennare R, Heard A, Chan A: Substance use during pregnancy: Risk factors and obstetric and perinatal outcomes in South Australia. Aust N Z J Obstet Gynaecol 45:220-225, 2005.
120. Addis A, Moretti ME, Ahmed Syed F, et al: Fetal effects of cocaine: An updated meta-analysis. Reprod Toxicol 15:341-369, 2001.
121. Hoskins IA, Friedman DM, Frieden FJ, et al: Relationship between antepartum cocaine abuse, abnormal umbilical artery Doppler velocimetry, and placental abruption. Obstet Gynecol 78:279-282, 1991.
122. Kupferminc MJ, Eldor A, Steinman N, et al: Increased frequency of genetic thrombophilia in women with complications of pregnancy. N Engl J Med 340:9-13, 1999.
123. Goddijn-Wessel TA, Wouters MG, van de Molen EF, et al: Hyperhomocysteinemia: A risk factor for placental abruption or infarction. Eur J Obstet Gynecol Reprod Biol 66:23-29, 1996.
124. Prochazka M, Happach C, Marsal K, et al: Factor V Leiden in pregnancies complicated by placental abruption. BJOG 110:462-466, 2003.
125. Dizon-Townson D, Miller C, Sibai B, et al: The relationship of the factor V Leiden mutation and pregnancy outcomes for mother and fetus. Obstet Gynecol 106:517-524, 2005.
126. Jaaskelainen E, Keski-Nisula L, Toivonen S, et al: MTHFR C677T polymorphism is not associated with placental abruption or preeclampsia in Finnish women. Hypertens Pregnancy 25:73-80, 2006.
127. Jarvenpaa J, Pakkila M, Savolainen ER, et al: Evaluation of factor V Leiden, prothrombin and methylenetetrahydrofolate reductase gene mutations in patients with severe pregnancy complications in northern Finland. Gynecol Obstet Invest 62:28-32, 2006.
128. Dahmus MA, Sibai BM: Blunt abdominal trauma: Are there any predictive factors for abruptio placentae or maternal-fetal distress? Am J Obstet Gynecol 169:1054-1059, 1993.
129. Towery R, English TP, Wisner D: Evaluation of pregnant women after blunt injury. J Trauma 35:731-735; discussion 735-736, 1993.
130. Major CA, de Veciana M, Lewis DF, Morgan MA: Preterm premature rupture of membranes and abruptio placentae: Is there an association between these pregnancy complications? Am J Obstet Gynecol 172:672-676, 1995.
131. Ball RH, Ade CM, Schoenborn JA, Crane JP: The clinical significance of ultransonographically detected subchorionic hemorrhages. Am J Obstet Gynecol 174:996-1002, 1996.
132. Yaron Y, Ochshorn Y, Heifetz S, et al: First trimester maternal serum free human chorionic gonadotropin as a predictor of adverse pregnancy outcome. Fetal Diagn Ther 17:352-356, 2002.
133. Pilalis A, Souka AP, Antsaklis P, et al: Screening for pre-eclampsia and fetal growth restriction by uterine artery Doppler and PAPP-A at 11-14 weeks' gestation. Ultrasound Obstet Gynecol 29:135-140, 2007.
134. Katz VL, Chescheir NC, Cefalo RC: Unexplained elevations of maternal serum alpha-fetoprotein. Obstet Gynecol Surv 45:719-726, 1990.
135. Jauniaux E, Gulbis B, Tunkel S, et al: Maternal serum testing for alpha-fetoprotein and human chorionic gonadotropin in high-risk pregnancies. Prenat Diagn 16:1129-1135, 1996.
136. Tikkanen M, Hamalainen E, Nuutila M, et al: Elevated maternal second-trimester serum alpha-fetoprotein as a risk factor for placental abruption. Prenat Diagn 27:240-243, 2007.
137. Van Rijn M, van der Schouw YT, Hagenaars AM, et al: Adverse obstetric outcome in low- and high- risk pregnancies: Predictive value of maternal serum screening. Obstet Gynecol 94:929-934, 1999.
138. Towner D, Gandhi S, El Kady D: Obstetric outcomes in women with elevated maternal serum human chorionic gonadotropin. Am J Obstet Gynecol 194:1676-1681; discussion 1681-1682, 2006.
139. Nyberg DA, Mack LA, Benedetti TJ, et al: Placental abruption and placental hemorrhage: Correlation of sonographic findings with fetal outcome. Radiology 164:357-361, 1987.
140. Glantz C, Purnell L: Clinical utility of sonography in the diagnosis and treatment of placental abruption. J Ultrasound Med 21:837-840, 2002.
141. Sholl JS: Abruptio placentae: Clinical management in nonacute cases. Am J Obstet Gynecol 156:40-51, 1987.
142. Jaffe MH, Schoen WC, Silver TM, et al: Sonography of abruptio placentae. AJR Am J Roentgenol 137:1049-1054, 1981.
143. Nyberg DA, Cyr DR, Mack LA, et al: Sonographic spectrum of placental abruption. AJR Am J Roentgenol 148:161-164, 1987.

144. Warner MW, Salfinger SG, Rao S, et al: Management of trauma during pregnancy. Aust N Z J Surg 74:125-128, 2004.
145. Emery CL, Morway LF, Chung-Park M, et al: The Kleihauer-Betke test: Clinical utility, indication, and correlation in patients with placental abruption and cocaine use. Arch Pathol Lab Med 119:1032-1037, 1995.
146. Elliott JP, Gilpin B, Strong TH Jr, Finberg HJ: Chronic abruption-oligohydramnios sequence. J Reprod Med 43:418-422, 1998.
147. Knab DR. Abruptio placentae: An assessment of the time and method of delivery. Obstet Gynecol 52:625-629, 1978.
148. Bond AL, Edersheim TG, Curry L, et al: Expectant management of abruptio placentae before 35 weeks gestation. Am J Perinatol 6:121-123, 1989.
149. Combs CA, Nyberg DA, Mack LA, et al: Expectant management after sonographic diagnosis of placental abruption. Am J Perinatol 9:170-174, 1992.
150. Saller DN Jr, Nagey DA, Pupkin MJ, Crenshaw MC Jr: Tocolysis in the management of third trimester bleeding. J Perinatol 10:125-128, 1990.
151. Rasmussen S, Irgens LM, Dalaker K: Outcome of pregnancies subsequent to placental abruption: A risk assessment. Acta Obstet Gynecol Scand 79:496-501, 2000.

Chapter 38

Maternal and Fetal Infections

Patrick Duff, MD, Richard L. Sweet, MD, and Rodney K. Edwards, MD, MS

Infectious disease is the single most common problem encountered by the obstetrician. Some conditions, such as urinary tract infections, endometritis, and mastitis, pose a risk primarily to the mother. Other disorders, such as group B streptococcal (GBS) infection, herpes simplex infection, rubella, cytomegalovirus infection, and toxoplasmosis are of principal concern because of the risk of fetal or neonatal complications. Still others, such as human immunodeficiency virus (HIV) infection and syphilis, may cause serious morbidity for both mother and baby.

This chapter reviews the twenty-nine most common infections that occur during pregnancy. Each section considers the epidemiology, pathogenesis, diagnosis, and treatment of an individual infectious disease with which the obstetrician should be familiar.

Candidiasis (Monilial Vaginitis)

Vulvovaginal candidiasis (VVC) is primarily caused by *Candida albicans*. Other species, such as *Candida glabrata*, *Candida parapsilosis*, *Candida tropicalis*, and *Candida lusitaniae*, are responsible for fewer than 10% of cases. *C. albicans* is a saprophytic yeast that exists as part of the endogenous flora of the vagina. The organism is present in the vagina of approximately 25% to 30% of sexually active women.[1] It may become an opportunistic pathogen, especially if host defense mechanisms are compromised. However, the biologic mechanisms that allow this commensal microorganism to become a pathogen are not completely understood.[2] Systemic candidiasis is a rare event in gravid patients, occurring only in the presence of disease entities causing significant debilitation (e.g., sepsis, malignancy). VVC is a much more common infection and is the second most common cause of vaginitis after bacterial vaginosis.

Epidemiology

Seventy-five percent of women will have at least one episode of VVC during their life, and 40% to 45% will have two or more episodes.[1] *C. albicans* is the predominant yeast isolated (>90% of cases) from patients with VVC, with other species (i.e., *C. glabrata*, *C. parapsilosis*, and *C. tropicalis*) being less commonly recovered. In the past, it was believed that non-*albicans* species were becoming increasingly common, especially in cases of recurrent VVC. However, in a recent study, Sobel and colleagues[3] reported that *C. albicans* was recovered from 401 (94%) of 425 women with recurrent VVC.

Predisposing factors associated with vaginal colonization with *C. albicans* include diabetes mellitus, pregnancy, obesity, recent use of antibiotics, steroids, and immunosuppression. Pregnancy is associated with not only increased colonization but also increased susceptibility to infection and lower cure rates. Previously, oral contraceptives were thought to increase colonization of yeast in the vagina. However, with the advent of low-dose oral contraceptives, no increase in *Candida* isolation among oral contraceptive users has been noted.[4]

Other risk factors for *C. albicans* have been described. In a population of women attending a sexually transmitted disease (STD) clinic, Eckert and associates[5] reported that the principal risk factors were condom use, luteal phase of the menstrual cycle, sexual frequency greater than four times per month, recent antibiotic use, young age, past gonococcal infection, and absence of current bacterial vaginosis. Recently, Beigi and coworkers[6] noted additional risk factors, including marijuana use, use of depo-medroxyprogesterone acetate, sexual activity within the past 5 days, concurrent *Lactobacillus* colonization, and concurrent GBS colonization.

Symptomatic VVC affects 15% of pregnant women. The hormonal environment of pregnancy, in which high levels of estrogen produce an increased concentration of vaginal glycogen, accounts for the increased frequency of symptomatic infection in gravid patients. In addition, suppression of cell-mediated immunity in pregnancy may decrease the ability to limit fungal proliferation.

Pathogenesis

As mentioned previously, the pathogenesis by which *C. albicans* evolves from a commensal microorganism colonizing the vagina to the pathogenic microbe involved in vulvovaginal vaginitis, invasive *Candida* infections, and disseminated candida sepsis is poorly understood. Kalo-Klein and Witkin[7] suggested that hormonal status may modulate the immune system, and, as a result, influence the pathogenicity of *Candida* species. They noted that the host responses to *C. albicans* were decreased in the luteal phase. Recently, Giraldo and colleagues[8] reported that a variant (gene polymorphism) in the gene coding for the mannose-binding lectin (MBL), a critical component of the mucosal innate immune system, was more frequently found in women with recurrent VVC than in those with acute VVC or controls.

The pathogenesis of invasive candidiasis is similar to that associated with bacterial microorganisms. Initially, there must be colonization resulting from adhesion of *C. albicans* to the skin or vaginal mucosa; this is followed by penetration of epithelial barriers, resulting in locally invasive or widely disseminated disease.[9]

Congenital candidiasis characteristically manifests at birth or within the first 24 hours after birth. It usually results from an intrauterine infection or heavy maternal vaginal colonization at the time of labor and delivery. The potential mechanisms for intrauterine *Candida* infection are quite similar to those of bacterial intra-amniotic infection, including hematogenous spread from mother to fetus, invasion of intact membranes, and ascending infection following rupture of the membranes.[9,10] In contrast to bacterial neonatal sepsis, the presence of an intrauterine foreign body, most commonly a cerclage suture, is a recognized risk factor for congenital candidiasis. VVC has not been associated with preterm birth, preterm labor, low birth weight, or premature rupture of the membranes (PROM).[10,11]

Recurrent VVC is defined as four or more episodes of symptomatic VVC in 1 year. Recurrent VVC occurs in a small percentage of women (<5%). The pathogenesis of recurrent VVC is poorly understood, and the majority of those affected do not have any apparent predisposing or underlying conditions. *C. glabrata* and other non-*albicans Candida* species are recovered from in 10% to 20% of women with recurrent VVC.[12,13]

Diagnosis

The clinical manifestations in pregnancy are similar to those in the nonpregnant state; they include pruritus and burning, dysuria, dyspareunia, fissures, excoriations with secondary infection, and pruritus ani. The vaginal discharge is usually thick, white, and curdlike.

The diagnosis of VVC can be made in a woman who had signs and symptoms of vaginitis when either (1) a 10% potassium hydroxide (KOH) wet preparation or Gram staining of a vaginal discharge sample reveals yeasts or pseudohyphae, or (2) a culture discloses yeast.[12] The vaginal pH in women with VVC is normal (<4.5). Women with a positive KOH wet mount should be treated for VVC. Women who have negative KOH smear despite clinical signs and symptoms suggestive of VVC should have vaginal cultures for yeast. In patients with recurrent VVC, the laboratory should be requested to identify the species of *Candida* recovered.

The clinical manifestations of congenital candidiasis range from superficial skin infection and oral infection to severe systemic disease with hemorrhage and necrosis of the heart, lungs, kidneys, and other organs. The most common route of infection is by direct contact during delivery through an infected vagina. Oropharyngeal candidiasis of the neonate (thrush) is the most frequent manifestation of congenital infection.

Treatment

The regimens recommended by the Centers for Disease Control and Prevention (CDC) for the treatment of VVC are listed in Table 38-1.[12] Short-course topical formulations (i.e., single-dose and 1- to 3-day regimens) effectively treat uncomplicated VVC, providing relief of symptoms and negative cultures in 80% to 90% of patients who complete therapy. Intravaginal preparations of butoconazole, clotrimazole, miconazole, and tioconazole are available over the counter (OTC). According to the CDC, women who previously were diagnosed with VVC are not necessarily more likely to accurately diagnose themselves. Therefore, women whose symptoms persist after use of an OTC preparation or who have a recurrence of symptoms within 2 months should be assessed with office-based testing.[12]

VVC is not usually acquired through sexual intercourse, so treatment of sex partners is not recommended. Treatment of partners should be considered for women who have recurrent VVC and for male sex partners with balanitis.[12]

The CDC recommends that topical azole therapies be the first line of treatment in pregnancy for VVC. These topical medications should be applied for 7 days. For complicated cases of VVC, a longer duration of initial therapy (e.g., 7 to 14 days of topical therapy or a 100-mg, 150-mg, or 200-mg oral dose of fluconazole every third day for a total

TABLE 38-1 RECOMMENDED REGIMENS FOR TREATMENT OF VULVOVAGINAL CANDIDIASIS IN PREGNANT AND NONPREGNANT WOMEN

Antifungal Agent	Formulation	Regimen
Intravaginal Agents		
Butoconazole	2% cream*	5 g intravaginally for 3 days
	2% cream (Butoconazole 1—sustained release)	5 g single intravaginal application
Clotrimazole	1% cream*	5 g intravaginally for 7-14 days
	100 mg vaginal tablet	One tablet qd for 7 days
	100 mg vaginal tablet	Two tablets at one time daily for 3 days
Miconazole	2% cream*	5 g intravaginally for 7 days
	100 mg vaginal suppository*	One suppository qd for 7 days
	200 mg vaginal suppository*	One suppository qd for 3 days
	1200 mg vaginal suppository*	One suppository qd for 1 day
Nystatin	100,000-unit vaginal tablet	One tablet qd for 14 days
Tioconazole	6.5% ointment*	5 g intravaginally in a single application
Terconazole	0.4% cream	5 g intravaginally for 7 days
	0.8% cream	5 g intravaginally for 3 days
	80 mg vaginal suppository	One suppository qd for 3 days
Oral Agent		
Fluconazole	150 mg oral tablet	One tablet in single dose

*Over-the-counter preparation.

From Centers for Disease Control and Prevention: Sexually Transmitted Diseases Treatment Guidelines, 2006. MMWR Recommendations and Reports 55(RR-11):1-94, 2006.

of 3 doses) should be considered. Fluconazole is a U.S. Food and Drug Administration (FDA) class C drug. It should be reserved for highly select patients, such as those who are allergic to topical antifungal medications or who have recurrent persistent infection.[12]

Trichomoniasis

Clinical Presentation

Trichomonas vaginalis is a common cause of vaginitis, with infection often characterized by intense pruritus, strong odor, and dysuria. Physical examination typically shows a malodorous, yellow-green, frothy discharge. However, variations of the gross appearance occur in approximately 50% of cases, with many women showing minimal or no symptoms. The diagnosis may be confirmed by microscopic examination of a smear of the discharge diluted with saline. The examination reveals many leukocytes and bacteria; trichomonads are recognized by their size (slightly larger than leukocytes) and active flagella. The sensitivity of wet mount is only 60% to 70%.[14] Cultures for *Trichomonas* are more sensitive than wet mount, and commercial systems are available to facilitate culture of this parasite. There currently are two point-of-care diagnostic tests available, the OSOM Trichomonas Rapid Test (Genzyme Diagnostics, Cambridge, MS) and the Affirm VP III (Becton Dickenson, San Jose, CA). These tests have better sensitivity than wet mount, but false-positive results may be a problem, especially in low-prevalence populations.

The prevalence of *T. vaginalis* vaginitis in pregnancy ranges from less than 10% to 50%, depending on the patient population. Consequently, it has been difficult to establish whether the incidence of this vaginal infection truly is increased in pregnant women.

Adverse Effects in Pregnancy

An increased rate of PROM at term has been linked to positive genital tract cultures for *T. vaginalis* (27.5% with infection versus 12.8% without; $P < .03$).[15] In the large National Institutes of Health infection and prematurity study, *T. vaginalis* infection at midpregnancy was associated significantly with low birth weight (odds ratio [OR], 1.3; 95% confidence interval [CI], 1.1 to 1.5), preterm delivery (OR, 1.3; CI, 1.1 to 1.4), and PROM (OR, 1.4, CI, 1.1 to 1.6), even after adjustment for confounding factors and other microbes.[16] In addition, trichomoniasis has been associated with increased rates of HIV transmission.[17,18]

Treatment

The recommended treatment for trichomoniasis is oral metronidazole, 2 g in a single dose. An alternative regimen is metronidazole, 500 mg orally twice a day for 7 days.[12] No consistent association has been demonstrated between use of metronidazole in pregnancy and teratogenesis or mutagenesis in infants.[19] Tinidazole, another nitroimidazole drug, recently was approved by the FDA for treatment of trichomoniasis (2 g orally in a single dose). However, metronidazole should be favored for the treatment of pregnant women because of its superior safety profile. Topical agents often are unsuccessful in relieving symptoms or in eradicating this protozoon.

Among women with asymptomatic trichomoniasis in pregnancy, treatment in the second trimester (two 2.0 g doses 48 hours apart at 16 to 23 weeks, repeated at 24 to 29 weeks) did not result in better pregnancy outcomes than did placebo. Indeed, those given metronidazole had a significantly higher frequency of preterm delivery.[20] Accordingly, although symptomatic pregnant women with trichomoniasis should be treated to relieve symptoms, routine screening and treatment are not recommended.

Bacterial Vaginosis

Epidemiology and Pathogenesis

This infection was formerly called nonspecific vaginitis, *Gardnerella vaginalis* vaginitis, or *Haemophilus vaginalis* vaginitis; *bacterial vaginosis* (BV) is the preferable term. The condition is marked by a major shift in vaginal flora from the normal predominance of lactobacilli to a predominance of anaerobes, which are increased 100-fold compared with normal secretions. *G. vaginalis* is present in 95% of cases but also is present in 30% to 40% of normal women. *Mycoplasma hominis* in vaginal secretions is increased significantly in cases of BV.

BV is the most common type of infectious vaginitis. Between 10% and 30% of pregnant women fulfill the criteria, but half of them are asymptomatic.

Diagnosis

Clinically, the primary symptoms are discharge and odor. Itching usually is not prominent. Diagnosis of BV is based on the presence of three of the following four clinical features: (1) an amine-like or fishy odor that may be accentuated after addition of KOH or after coitus (owing to the alkaline pH of semen); (2) a thin, homogeneous, gray or white discharge; (3) an elevated pH (≥4.5); and (4) on wet mount, true "clue" cells (squamous epithelial cells so heavily stippled with bacteria that their borders are obscured). Typically in cases of BV, clue cells account for more than 20% of epithelial cells, and there are few leukocytes. An experienced observer will note an increase in numbers and kinds of bacteria and a reduction in numbers of lactobacilli. A Gram stain of vaginal secretions also demonstrates the shift in bacteria and clue cells.

Adverse Effects in Pregnancy

Evidence consistently has associated BV with increased likelihoods of preterm delivery,[21-24] clinical chorioamnionitis,[25] histologic chorioamnionitis,[26] and endometritis.[27] The risk for preterm delivery among women with BV has varied (OR, 1.4 to 8) but has been significant in all populations studied.

Treatment

In nonpregnant women, the most consistent cure rates (90%) have been achieved with metronidazole (e.g., 500 mg twice a day for 7 days). Lower cure rates (60% to 80%) are observed with a single 2.0-g dose of metronidazole. Oral clindamycin (300 mg twice a day for 7 days) is effective in treating nonpregnant patients and appears to be safe in pregnancy. Vaginal clindamycin cream (2%) and metronidazole gel (0.75%) also are effective in nonpregnant women. However, the preferred regimens in pregnancy are shown in Table 38-2. There is no longer an exclusion for use of metronidazole in any trimester of pregnancy. A recent meta-analysis showed no evidence of teratogenesis.[12,28-30]

In view of the consistent association of BV with adverse pregnancy outcomes, clinical treatment trials have been undertaken. Three trials, all conducted in patients who were considered to be at high risk (on the basis of either a previous preterm birth or other high-risk demographic features), revealed improvement in outcome with prenatal treatment of BV (Table 38-3). In a group of women who experienced a spontaneous preterm birth due to preterm labor or PROM during a previous pregnancy, treatment of BV with oral metronidazole led to a significant reduction in preterm birth, low birth weight, and PROM ($P < .05$ for each).[31] In a prospective, two-phase trial involving 1260 women, treatment of BV significantly decreased preterm birth ($P < .05$).[32] Finally, among women at risk because of a previous preterm birth or low maternal weight, treatment with a combination of metronidazole and erythromycin significantly improved pregnancy outcome compared to placebo in patients who had BV ($P < .006$); in those patients without BV, pregnancy outcome was not improved.[33]

In a treatment trial of women at low risk of preterm delivery, oral metronidazole (twice daily for 2 days at 24 weeks, with repeat treatment, if needed, at 29 weeks) led to no reduction in preterm birth overall but produced a significant reduction in the subgroup of women with a previous preterm birth.[34] In the Maternal-Fetal Medicine Units Network treatment trial of women with asymptomatic BV, the treatment regimen also was short (two 2.0-g doses at 16 to 24 weeks and again at 24 to 30 weeks, with the repeat treatment at least 14 days after the initial doses). Use of metronidazole in this regimen led to no significant improvement overall or in any subgroup (e.g., women with a previous preterm birth).[35] These studies are summarized in Figure 38-1. In view of these disparate results, the American College of Obstetricians and Gynecologists (ACOG)[36] concluded in 2001, "Currently, there are insufficient data to suggest [that] screening and treating women at either low or high risk will reduce the overall rate of preterm birth."

However, Goldenberg and colleagues[37] reached a different conclusion, taking into consideration the metronidazole regimen used. We agree with their recommendation of treatment with oral metronidazole for at least 7 days in women at high risk (e.g., those with previous preterm birth). Screening and treatment of these high-risk women should occur at the first prenatal visit. Recommendations for management of BV in pregnancy are presented in Table 38-4.

TABLE 38-2 CDC-RECOMMENDED REGIMENS FOR TREATING BACTERIAL VAGINOSIS

Metronidazole 500 mg PO bid for 7 days
OR
Metronidazole 250 mg PO tid for 7 days
OR
Clindamycin 300 mg PO bid for 7 days

Gonorrhea

Gonorrhea, which is caused by the gram-negative diplococcus, *Neisseria gonorrhoeae*, is probably the oldest known STD. Almost 340,000 new infections with *N. gonorrhoeae* were reported in the United States in 2005,[38] making gonorrhea the second most commonly reported communicable disease in the nation.

Epidemiology

The CDC received 339,593 reports of gonorrhea in 2005. However, even this volume of reports underestimates the incidence, and public health experts estimate that 600,000 new cases of *N. gonorrhoeae* infection occur each year in the United States. From 1975 through 1997, there was a dramatic decrease of 74% in reported cases of gonorrhea. In 1998, an 8.9% increase occurred, followed by plateauing of the number of reported cases.[38,39]

In 2003, for the first time, the reported gonorrhea rate was higher among women (118.8 per 100,000 population than among men (113 per 100,000).[40] Disappointingly, in 2005, both the number of reported cases and the prevalence rate of gonorrhea increased for the first time

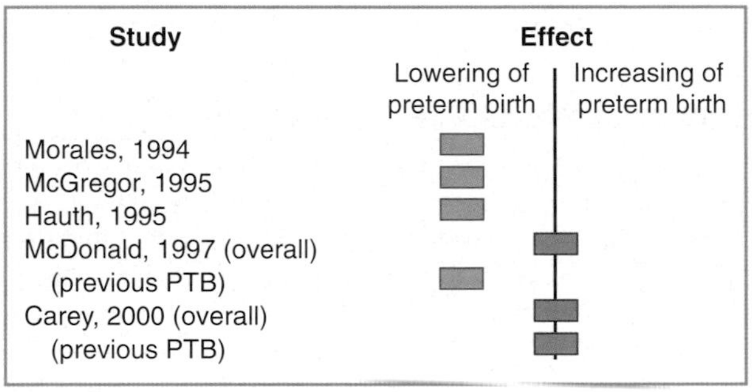

FIGURE 38-1 Bacterial vaginosis treatment trials. Summary of treatment trials of bacterial vaginosis in pregnancy to prevent preterm birth.

TABLE 38-3 STUDIES OF BACTERIAL VAGINOSIS IN PREGNANCY IN PATIENTS AT HIGH RISK FOR PRETERM DELIVERY

Study	Design	Study Population	Preterm Birth: Antibiotic Treatment (%)	Preterm Birth: No Treatment or Placebo (%)	Significance (*P*)
Morales et al, 1994	Randomized, placebo-controlled	80 women with previous spontaneous preterm birth in Florida	18	39	<.05
Hauth et al, 1995	Randomized, placebo-controlled	258 women with previous preterm birth or low maternal weight in Alabama	31	49	.006
McGregor et al, 1995	Nonrandomized, two-phase trial	1260 women in Colorado with a 15% preterm birth rate	9.8	18.8	.02

Modified from Gibbs RS, Eschenbach DA: Use of antibiotics to prevent preterm birth. Am J Obstet Gynecol 177:375, 1997.

in almost a decade. In a recent cross-sectional cohort study, The National Longitudinal Study of Adolescent Health reported that the overall prevalence of gonorrhea in the United States was 0.43% (CI, 0.29% to 0.63%).[41] The prevalence of gonorrhea in pregnancy ranges from 0% to 10%, with marked variations according to risk status and geographic locale.[42]

TABLE 38-4 RECOMMENDATIONS FOR MANAGEMENT OF BACTERIAL VAGINOSIS IN PREGNANCY

Symptomatic pregnant women with BV can be treated safely in any trimester with oral metronidazole or clindamycin.
Routine screening and treatment of BV in asymptomatic women at low risk for preterm birth *cannot* be endorsed (USPTF: D recommendation).
Screening for BV may be considered in asymptomatic women at high risk for preterm birth, such as those with previous preterm birth. Women who test positive should be treated.
The value of rescreening and retreating is unclear.

BV, bacterial vaginosis; USPTF, U.S. Preventive Services Task Force.

A number of risk factors for gonorrhea among sexually active women have been elucidated. Young age is the greatest risk factor, with sexually active women younger than 25 years of age being at highest risk for gonorrhea infection. Other risk factors for gonorrhea include previous gonococcal infection, presence of other STDs, multiple sex partners, new sex partners, inconsistent condom use, drug use, and commercial sex work. Nonwhite race, low socioeconomic status, inner-city dwelling, and unmarried status are additional risk factors for infection with *N. gonorrhoeae* (Figs. 38-2 and 38-3).[12]

Pathogenesis

Transmission of *N. gonorrhoeae* occurs almost solely by sexual contact, and the risk of transmission from an infected male to a female partner is 50% to 90% with a single exposure.[43] The incubation period is 3 to 5 days.

Infection with *N. gonorrhoeae* in pregnancy is a major concern. Although gonococcal ophthalmia neonatorum has been recognized since the late 19th century as a significant consequence of maternal infection with *N. gonorrhoeae*, it is only in the last 40 years that an association has been recognized between maternal infection with *N. gonorrhoeae* and disseminated gonococcal infection (DGI), amniotic

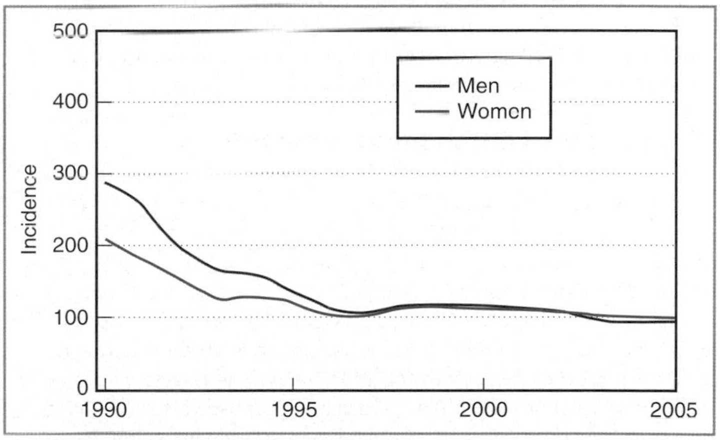

FIGURE 38-2 **Incidence of gonorrhea per 100,000 population, by sex—United States, 1990-2005.** The overall incidence of gonorrhea in the United States has declined since 1975 but increased in 2005 for the first time since 1999. In 2005, incidence was slightly higher among women than among men.

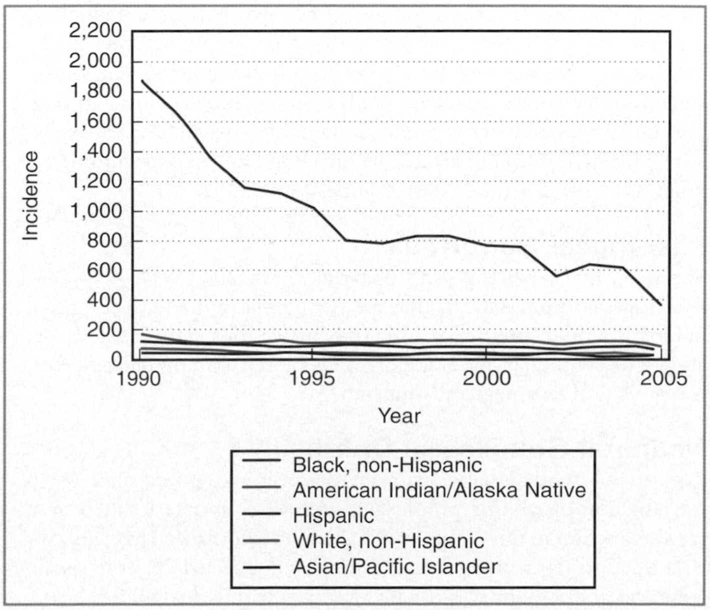

FIGURE 38-3 **Gonorrhea incidence per 100,000 population, by race/ethnicity—United States, 1990-2005.** Gonorrhea incidence among blacks decreased considerably during the 1990s, but blacks continue to have the highest rate among all races/ethnicities. In 2005, gonorrhea incidence among non-Hispanic blacks was approximately 18 times greater than among non-Hispanic whites.

infection syndrome, and perinatal complications including PROM, chorioamnionitis, preterm delivery, intrauterine growth restriction, neonatal sepsis, and postpartum endometritis.[4]

Adherence of *N. gonorrhoeae* to the mucosal epithelium of the genital tract is the initial step in the pathogenesis of gonococcal infection. Attachment of *N. gonorrhoeae* is mediated by pili and other surface proteins (e.g., porin protein, opacity-associated proteins, reduction-modifiable protein). Lipopolysaccharides, immunoglobulin A, and iron-repressible proteins are additional gonococcal virulence factors. Once *N. gonorrhoeae* attaches to mucosal cells, it enters the cell via endocytosis. Subsequently, the organism releases endotoxin, resulting in widespread cell damage.[44]

Clinical Manifestations

Anogenital Gonorrhea

The clinical manifestations of gonococcal infection are dependent on the site of inoculation and whether the infection remains localized or spreads systematically. The overwhelming majority of women with *N. gonorrhoeae* infection are asymptomatic. This observation is particularly true in pregnancy. The endocervix is the primary site of infection. When symptoms develop, they usually include vaginal discharge and dysuria. On examination, a mucopurulent discharge is usually apparent in the endocervical canal. Inflammation of the Skene or Bartholin glands may occur. In patients who engage in rectal intercourse, a mucopurulent proctitis may also be apparent.

Disseminated Gonococcal Infection

DGI is an important presentation of gonorrhea in pregnancy. Pregnant women, especially during the second and third trimester, appear to be at increased risk for disseminated infection, which has two stages. The early, bacteremic stage is characterized by chills, fever, and typical skin lesions. The lesions appear initially as small vesicles, which become pustules and develop a hemorrhagic base. The center becomes necrotic. Such lesions can occur anywhere on the body but are most frequently present on the volar aspects of the arms, hands, and fingers. They fade without residual scarring. Blood cultures are positive for *N. gonorrhoeae* in 50% of patients in whom culture is done during the bacteremic stage. DGI is occasionally complicated by perihepatitis and rarely by endocarditis or meningitis. Joint symptoms are frequently present during this stage, as well as in the second, septic arthritis phase. This stage is characterized by a purulent synovial effusion. The knees, ankles, and wrists are most commonly involved. Blood cultures during this stage are usually sterile. Gonococci may be isolated from the septic joints during the second stage. The infection may become chronic or progress to septic arthritis and joint destruction.[12]

Pharyngeal Gonorrhea

The majority of patients with pharyngeal infections with *N. gonorrhoeae* are asymptomatic. If they are symptomatic, the most common finding is a mild sore throat and erythema; lesions and exudates may also be present. Pharyngeal gonorrhea is more common during pregnancy than in nonpregnant women.[45]

Neonatal Gonococcal Ophthalmia

Gonococcal ophthalmia neonatorum has been recognized since 1881. Introduction of routine prophylaxis with silver nitrate resulted in a rapid reduction in this complication. Most newborns who have gonorrhea acquire it during passage through an infected cervical canal. Gonococcal ophthalmia is usually observed within 4 days after birth, but incubation periods of up to 21 days have been reported. A frank purulent conjunctivitis occurs and usually affects both eyes. Untreated gonococcal ophthalmia can rapidly progress to corneal ulceration, resulting in corneal scarring and blindness.

Gonococcal Infection in Pregnancy and in the Neonate

The effects of gonorrheal infection on both mother and fetus were not fully appreciated until 4 decades ago.[4,46,47] Studies at that time identified an association between untreated maternal endocervical gonorrhea and perinatal complications, including PROM, preterm delivery, chorioamnionitis, neonatal sepsis, and maternal postpartum sepsis.

The amniotic infection syndrome is an additional manifestation of gonococcal infection in pregnancy. This condition is characterized by placental, fetal membrane, and umbilical cord inflammation that occurs after PROM and is associated with infected oral and gastric aspirate, leukocytosis, neonatal infection, and maternal fever. Preterm delivery is common, and perinatal morbidity may be significant.[46]

Diagnosis

The diagnosis of infection with *N. gonorrhoeae* requires sampling of potentially infected sites. Available methods include culture, nucleic acid hybridization tests, and nucleic acid amplification tests (NAATs).[48] Unlike for *Chlamydia trachomatis* infection, the CDC has not provided guidance with respect to general or targeted screening for gonorrhea infection.[49] Even in the absence of formal guidelines, gonorrhea screening has been implemented in conjunction with routine chlamydial screening. Implementation of these joint screening protocols has been shown to be cost-effective.

Screening for gonorrhea during pregnancy is clearly cost-effective if the prevalence exceeds 1%. Therefore, the CDC recommends that all pregnant women at risk for gonorrhea, as well as those living in an area where the prevalence of *N. gonorrhoeae* is high, be tested for *N. gonorrhoeae* at their first prenatal visit.[12] Targeted patients include

1. Partners of men with gonorrhea or urethritis
2. Patients known to have other STDs, including HIV infection
3. Patients with multiple sex partners
4. Young, unmarried inner-city women
5. Intravenous drug users
6. Women with symptoms or signs of lower genital tract infection.

The CDC and the ACOG recommend that at-risk women be rescreened for *N. gonorrhoeae* during the third trimester.[12,50] A recent study demonstrated the value of a repeat screen in the third trimester for *N. gonorrhoeae* among at-risk women who had an initial negative early pregnancy screen.[42] In this study, 38 (5.1%) of 751 at-risk women had gonorrhea (based on a positive DNA direct assay) at their first prenatal visit. An additional 19 women (2.5%) were newly positive at their third-trimester screen. In other words, approximately one third of at-risk women tested positive for *N. gonorrhoeae* only on the repeat third-trimester screen.

Several reliable nonculture assays for detection of *N. gonorrhoeae* have become available and are increasingly being used.[48] They include nonamplified DNA probe tests (discussed later) and NAATs such as polymerase chain reaction (PCR), ligase chain reaction (LCR), transcription-mediated amplification (TMA), and strand displacement assay (SDA). These newer technologies compare favorably to culture with selective media. For nonamplified DNA probes, the sensitivity ranges from 89% to 97%, and the specificity is 99%. For NAATs, the sensitivity and specificity are both excellent (>99%). Whereas the introduction of dual, single-swab NAATs for detection of *C. trachomatis* and *N. gonorrhoeae* has simplified testing and facilitated expansion of STD screening to nontraditional settings, there is a downside to single-swab NAATs.[51] First, the prevalence of *N. gonorrhoeae* is substantially lower than that of *C. trachomatis*, especially in most community-based settings.[52] As a result, when providers intend to screen primarily for *C. trachomatis*, they are also screening for *N. gonorrhoeae*. The potential for false-positive *N. gonorrhoeae* test results increases because the positive predictive value of a test decreases as the prevalence of disease decreases. Second, as NAATs replace culture assays, fewer isolates are available for antibiotic susceptibility testing. As a result, monitoring of trends in antimicrobial susceptibility of *N. gonorrhoeae*, a major public health issue, may be compromised.

Treatment

The treatment of gonococcal infection in pregnant women is similar to that in nonpregnant women, with the exception that tetracycline should not be used for concomitant chlamydial infection. Both asymptomatic and symptomatic infections should be treated.

The treatment of gonococcal infection in the United States has been influenced by two factors. First, there has been increasing prevalence and spread of infections caused by antibiotic-resistant *N. gonorrhoeae*, such as penicillinase-producing *N. gonorrhoeae*, tetracycline-resistant *N. gonorrhoeae*, and chromosomally mediated *N. gonorrhoeae*, which is resistant to multiple antibiotics. Moreover, in recent years, quinolone resistant *N. gonorrhoeae* (QRNG) has emerged as a major public health problem.[12,53] QRNG continues to spread and increase in prevalence, making treatment of gonorrhea with quinolones such as ciprofloxacin inadvisable in many geographic areas and populations. According to the CDC,[12] resistance to ciprofloxacin usually indicates resistance to other quinolones. QRNG is common in parts of Europe, the Middle East, Asia, and the Pacific and is becoming increasingly common in the United States. For example, in California the rate of QRNG increased from less than 1% in 1999 to more than 20% in the second half of 2003.[54] Similarly high rates of QRNG have been reported in Hawaii.[55] As a result, in 2005, the CDC advised that quinolones should not be used in California or Hawaii.[56] In 2004, 6.8% of isolates collected by CDC's Gonococcal Isolate Surveillance Project (GISP)[57] were resistant to ciprofloxacin. QRNG was more common among men who have sex with men (MSM) than among heterosexual men (23.9% versus 2.9%).[39,58] Subsequently, the prevalence of QRNG increased in other areas of the United States, leading to changes in recommended treatment regimens by other states and local areas. In a 2007 update to its Sexually Transmitted Diseases Treatment Guidelines, the CDC announced that quinolones are no longer recommended for the treatment of gonorrheal infections.[407]

The second factor that influences treatment recommendations is the high frequency (20% to 50%) of coexisting chlamydial infection in women infected with *N. gonorrhoeae*. This finding has led to the recommendation that women treated for gonococcal infection should also be treated routinely for chlamydia.[12] Current CDC recommendations for the treatment of *N. gonorrhoeae* in pregnancy are listed in Tables 38-5 and 38-6.

Ceftriaxone in a single intramuscular injection of 125 mg provides sustained, high bactericidal levels in blood and is safe and effective for treatment of uncomplicated gonorrhea, curing 98.9% of urethral, cervical, and anorectal infections.[12,59] The antimicrobial spectrum of cefixime is similar to that of ceftriaxone, but the 400-mg dose does not achieve as high or as sustained serum levels as the 125-mg ceftriaxone dose. Cefixime, in a 400 mg oral dose, cures 97.4% of uncomplicated urethral, cervical, and anogenital gonorrhea.[59] Ciprofloxacin is safe, is inexpensive, and can be administered orally, but it is no longer universally effective against *N. gonorrhoeae* in the United States. The same holds true for ofloxacin and levofloxacin. In addition, quinolones should not be used during pregnancy.

TABLE 38-5 RECOMMENDATIONS FOR THE TREATMENT OF UNCOMPLICATED GONORRHEA OF THE CERVIX, URETHRA, AND RECTUM

Recommended Regimens (in addition to treatment for chlamydial infection if not ruled out)
Ceftriaxone* 125 mg IM in a single dose
Cefixime* 400 mg PO in a single dose
Alternative Regimens
Spectinomycin* 2 g IM in a single dose
Single-dose cephalosporin* regimens

*Recommended for use in pregnancy.
From Centers for Disease Control and Prevention: Update to CDC's Sexually Transmitted Diseases Treatment Guidelines, 2006: Fluoroquinolones No Longer Recommended for Treatment of Gonococcal Infections. MMWR Morb Mortal Wkly Rep 56(14):332-336, 2007.

TABLE 38-6 RECOMMENDATIONS FOR THE TREATMENT OF COMPLICATED GONORRHEA (DISSEMINATED GONOCOCCAL INFECTION, MENINGITIS, ENDOCARDITIS)

Recommended Regimen
Ceftriaxone* 1 g IM or IV q24h
Alternative Regimens
Cefotaxime* 1 g IV q8h
Ceftizoxime* 1 g IV q8h
Spectinomycin* 2 g IM q12h

*Recommended for use in pregnancy.
From Centers for Disease Control and Prevention: Update to CDC's Sexually Transmitted Diseases Treatment Guidelines, 2006: Fluoroquinolones No Longer Recommended for Treatment of Gonococcal Infections. MMWR Morb Mortal Wkly Rep 56(14):332-336, 2007.

Several alternative antimicrobial agents are suggested by the CDC for treatment of uncomplicated gonococcal infections of the cervix, urethra, and anorectum. Spectinomycin is effective (cure rate >98%), but it is expensive and is available only as an injection. In addition, it is not readily available any longer. During pregnancy, it is useful for patients who are allergic to cephalosporins. Alternative single-dose cephalosporins include ceftizoxime 500 mg IM, cefoxitin 2 g IM with probenecid 1 g orally, and cefotaxime 500 mg IM. Alternative single-dose oral quinolones (not recommended for pregnancy) include gatifloxacin 400 mg, norfloxacin 800 mg, and lomefloxacin 400 mg. The CDC suggests that cefpodoxime and cefuroxime axetil as additional oral alternatives for treatment of uncomplicated urogenital gonorrhea.[12]

As noted by the CDC, effective management of STDs such as gonorrhea requires treatment of the woman's current sex partner or partners to prevent reinfection. Patients should be instructed to refer their sex partners for evaluation and treatment. Alternatively, patient-delivered treatment for sex partners is also effective.[12,60]

Pregnant women should not be treated with quinolones or tetracyclines. Pregnant women infected with *N. gonorrhoeae* should be treated with one of the recommended or alternative cephalosporins. Those who cannot tolerate cephalosporins should be treated with spectinomycin 2 g IM as a single dose, if it is available. Either amoxicillin or azithromycin is recommended as treatment for presumed concomitant chlamydial infection during pregnancy.[12]

Patients with DGI should be hospitalized for initial therapy (see Table 38-6). In addition, patients with DGI should be evaluated clinically for evidence of endocarditis or meningitis. All of the recommended and alternative regimens for DGI should be continued for 24 to 48 hours after improvement begins. At that time, therapy may be switched to cefixime, 400 mg orally twice daily. With gonococcal meningitis and endocarditis, the recommended regimen is ceftriaxone 1 to 2 g IV every 12 hours. Meningitis requires 10 to 14 days of therapy, and treatment for endocarditis should be continued for a minimum of 4 weeks.[12]

With use of recommended treatment, follow-up testing to document eradication of gonorrhea is no longer recommended. Instead, rescreening in 2 to 3 months to identify reinfection is suggested. If other antimicrobial agents are used for the treatment of *N. gonorrhoeae*, follow-up assessment is suggested. Follow-up cultures should be obtained from the infected site 3 to 7 days after completion of treatment. Specimens should be obtained from the anal canal as well as the endocervix; failure to obtain a specimen from the anal canal results in missing 50% of resistant *N. gonorrhoeae* strains. With NAATs, repeat testing should be performed 3 weeks after treatment. Patients who have symptoms that persist after treatment should be evaluated by culture, and isolated organisms should be tested for antimicrobial susceptibility.[12]

Prevention

Primary prevention of gonorrhea requires adopting safe sex practices, including condom use; limiting the number of sexual partners; and ensuring that sexual partners are evaluated and treated. The increasing frequency of asymptomatic gonorrhea infection in women makes screening for *N. gonorrhoeae* during the antepartum period an important aspect of preventing the perinatal morbidity associated with this organism. At-risk patients should be rescreened in the third trimester. Instillation of a prophylactic agent into the eyes of all newborn infants is recommended to prevent gonococcal ophthalmia neonatorum. The recommended agents are erythromycin (0.5%) ophthalmic ointment, tetracycline (1%) ophthalmic ointment, and silver nitrate (1%) aqueous solution.

Chlamydial Infection

C. trachomatis infection is the most common bacterial STD in the United States, with an estimated 3 million new infections annually. The estimated cost of untreated chlamydial infection and their sequelae is more than $2 billion annually.[12,61]

In women, untreated chlamydial infection results in substantial adverse reproductive effects, including pelvic inflammatory disease and its sequelae of tubal factor infertility, ectopic pregnancy, and chronic pelvic pain. Chlamydial infection during pregnancy is associated with several adverse maternal outcomes, including preterm delivery, premature rupture of the membranes, low birth weight, and neonatal death.[4,62] Untreated *C. trachomatis* infection also may result in neonatal conjunctivitis or pneumonia or both.[4,63]

C. trachomatis may be differentiated on a serologic basis into 15 recognized serotypes. Three of these serotypes (L1, L2, L3) cause lymphogranuloma venereum. The other serotypes cause endemic blinding trachoma (A, B, Ba, and C) or inclusion conjunctivitis, newborn pneumonia, urethritis, cervicitis, endometritis, pelvic inflammatory disease, and the acute urethral syndrome (strains D through K).[4]

Epidemiology

As noted by Peipert,[64] the prevalence of *C. trachomatis* infection depends on the characteristics of the population studied. Prevalence rates in the United States vary significantly, ranging from 4% to 12% among family planning clinic attendees, from 2% to 7% among college students, and from 6% to 20% among STD clinic attendees.[4] Recently, in the National Longitudinal Study of Adolescent Health,[65] the overall prevalence of chlamydial infection was found to be 4.19%, with women (4.74%; CI, 3.93% to 5.71%) more likely to be infected than men (3.67%; CI, 2.93% to 4.58%). In 2005, more than 975,000 cases of chlamydial genital infection were reported to the CDC, almost 50,000 more than in 2004. The CDC estimates that the true frequency of chlamydial infection each year is 3 million cases, the majority of which are not reported to public health officials.[61]

The prevalence of *C. trachomatis* infection among pregnant women is about 2% to 3% but may be higher in certain high-risk populations.[4] Among pregnant women, risk factors for chlamydial infection include the following:

1. Unmarried status
2. Age younger than 25 years
3. Multiple sex partners
4. New sex partner in past 3 months
5. Black race
6. Presence of another STD
7. Partners with nongonococcal urethritis
8. Presence of mucopurulent endocervicitis
9. Sterile pyuria (acute urethral syndrome)
10. Resident of socially disadvantaged community
11. Late or no prenatal care

Detection rates as high as 25% to 30% have been reported in screening and prospective studies of such populations. In the Preterm Prediction Study of the National Institute of Child Health and Human Development Maternal-Fetal Medicine Units Network, the overall prevalence of *C. trachomatis* among pregnant women was 11%.[6] In an interesting follow-up study, Sheffield and colleagues[66] demonstrated that chlamydial infection resolved spontaneously in almost half of infected pregnant women, especially in older women and with increasing time since diagnosis.

Infants born to women with a chlamydial infection of the cervix are at a 60% to 70% risk of acquiring the infection during passage through the birth canal. Approximately 25% to 50% of exposed infants acquire conjunctivitis in the first 2 weeks of life, and 10% to 20% develop pneumonia within 3 or 4 months.[4]

Pathogenesis

Chlamydiae are obligate intracellular bacteria separated into their own order, Chlamydiales, on the basis of a unique growth cycle that distinguishes them from all other microorganisms. This cycle involves infection of the susceptible host cell by a chlamydia-specific phagocytic process, so that these organisms are preferentially ingested. After attachment and ingestion, the chlamydiae remain in a phagosome throughout the growth cycle, but surface antigens of chlamydiae appear to inhibit phagolysosomal fusion. These two virulence factors—enhanced ingestion and inhibition of phagolysosomal fusion—attest to an exquisitely adapted parasitism.

Once in the cell, the chlamydial *elementary body*, which is the infectious particle, changes to a metabolically active replicating form called the *reticulate body*, which synthesizes its own macromolecules and divides by binary fission. Chlamydiae are energy parasites; because they do not synthesize their own adenosine triphosphate, energy-rich compounds must be supplied to them by the host cell. By the end of the growth cycle (approximately 48 hours), most reticulate bodies have reorganized into elementary bodies, which are released through mechanical disruption of the host cell to initiate new infection cycles.

Chlamydia are unique bacteria that do not stain with Gram stain. In many respects, they are similar to other bacteria: They contain DNA and RNA, are susceptible to certain antibiotics, have a rigid cell wall similar in structure and content to those of gram-negative bacteria, and multiply by binary fission. However, they differ from other bacteria and resemble viruses in being obligate intracellular parasites. They may be regarded as bacteria that have adapted to an intracellular environment. They need viable cells for multiplication and survival.[4]

Adverse Pregnancy Outcome

Controversy exists as to whether maternal cervical *C. trachomatis* infection is associated with adverse pregnancy outcome. Although some studies have demonstrated an association of maternal chlamydial infection with preterm birth, low birth weight, PROM, and perinatal death,[67-69] others have failed to confirm such an association.[4,70] Harrison[71] and Sweet[72] and their colleagues demonstrated that a subgroup of infected women in whom immunoglobulin M (IgM) antibody was present were at significantly increased risk for PROM, preterm birth, and delivery of a low-birth-weight infant. These authors postulated that IgM seropositivity reflected recent acquisition and acute chlamydial infection, which may play a more important role than chronic infection.[62]

In additional attempts to address the role of *C. trachomatis* in adverse pregnancy outcome, researchers have undertaken treatment studies of chlamydial infection in pregnant women. In a historical control study, Ryan and colleagues[73] reported that untreated chlamydia-infected pregnant women in a high-prevalence population (21% positive) had a significantly increased incidence of PROM and of low-birth-weight infants and decreased perinatal survival compared with treated women or women not infected with chlamydia. Similarly, Cohen and coworkers[74] reported that treatment of chlamydial infection resulted in decreased rates of preterm delivery, PROM, preterm labor, and fetal growth restriction. There were experimental design flaws or limitations in both studies. However, because it is unethical to conduct a prospective, randomized, placebo-controlled trial in which some patients are not treated, these studies are the best available to date.

The role of cervical chlamydial infection in producing postpartum endometritis is also controversial. Early studies in the ophthalmology literature demonstrated an association between inclusion conjunctivitis in newborns and an increased risk for postpartum infection in their mothers. In a prospective study, Wager and associates[75] demonstrated that pregnant women with chlamydial cervical infection at their initial prenatal visit were at increased risk for endometritis after vaginal delivery. However, multiple other studies have failed to confirm such an association.[71,72,76-78]

Diagnosis

Until recently, the optimum diagnostic test for chlamydial infection was tissue culture. However, culture requires cold storage, a susceptible tissue culture cell line, a 1-week waiting time for results, and substantial technical expertise. In addition, culture is expensive and, with the advent of NAATs, has been shown to be relatively insensitive (65% to 85%).

Before the introduction of NAATs, antigen-detection methods were widely used. To a large extent, these antigen detection tests have now been replaced by DNA/RNA based methods, both nonamplified and amplified types. Nonamplified tests such as the Gen-Probe PACE-2 assay (Gen-Probe, San Diego, CA) use DNA/RNA hybridization technology. In a large multicenter study, Black and coauthors[79] reported that the sensitivity of PACE-2 ranged from 60.8% to 71.6%, and the specificity ranged from 99.5% to 99.6%. An important advantage of DNA probe–based testing is that it can be used in conjunction with a probe for the detection of *N. gonorrhoeae* in a single swab. Additional advantages include ease of transport, ability to batch specimens, and decreased cost. As a result, by the late 1990s, the DNA probe became the most widely used diagnostic test for *C. trachomatis* infection in the United States.

More recently, DNA/RNA amplification technology has been introduced into clinical practice. NAATs have excellent sensitivity and specificity for chlamydial testing. Currently, clinically available NAATs include tests based on PCR (Roche Molecular Systems, Branchburg, NJ), TMA (AMP.CT Gen-Probe), and SDA (Bectun Dickenson, Sparks, MD). LCR-based tests (Abbott Laboratories, Chicago) are no longer available. NAATs have performed better than culture, antigen detection, or DNA probe techniques for detection of *C. trachomatis.*[12,80,81] A major advantage of NAATs is their ability to identify patients with a low inoculum of *C. trachomatis*. Moreover, NAATs have demonstrated excellent sensitivity and specificity for detecting chlamydia in urine specimens, allowing noninvasive screening for *C. trachomatis*. However, use of a vaginal swab has been shown to have equivalent or better sensitivity and specificity and is better accepted by patients, especially when patient-obtained specimens are used.[82-84]

According to the CDC, all pregnant women should be routinely tested for *C. trachomatis* at their first prenatal visit.[12] Women younger than 25 years of age and those at increased risk for chlamydial infection also should be retested during the third trimester to prevent maternal postnatal complications and chlamydial infection in the infant. In addition, the CDC suggests that first-trimester screening might prevent the adverse effects of chlamydial infection during pregnancy (e.g., preterm birth, PROM, low birth weight).

Treatment

Screening of sexually active women for chlamydial infection is a national priority in the United States.[85,86] Identification and treatment of women infected with *C. trachomatis* prevent horizontal transmission to sex partners and vertical transmission of *C. trachomatis* to infants during birth.[12] In addition, treatment of chlamydial infection early in pregnancy seems to reduce the rate of adverse pregnancy outcomes (e.g., preterm birth, intrauterine growth restriction, low birth weight, PROM).[4,64]

TABLE 38-7 TREATMENT RECOMMENDATIONS FOR CHLAMYDIAL INFECTION IN PREGNANT WOMEN

Recommended Regimens
Azithromycin 1 g PO in a single dose
Amoxicillin 500 mg PO tid for 7 days
Alternative Regimens
Erythromycin base 500 mg PO qid for 7 days
Erythromycin base 250 mg PO qid for 14 days
Erythromycin ethylsuccinate 800 mg PO qid for 7 days
Erythromycin ethylsuccinate 400 mg PO qid for 14 days

From Centers for Disease Control and Prevention. Sexually Transmitted Diseases Treatment Guidelines, 2006. MMWR Recommendations and Reports 55(RR-11):1-94, 2006.

The CDC recommendations for treatment of chlamydial infection in pregnant women are listed in Table 38-7. Doxycycline, ofloxacin, and levofloxacin are recommended for nonpregnant women but are contraindicated in pregnancy. In 2006, azithromycin, as a single 1-g dose, was added to the list of recommended regimens for treatment of chlamydial infection during pregnancy. Single-dose therapy with azithromycin definitely improves patient compliance.[12]

Amoxicillin, 500 mg orally three times daily for 7 days, was initially demonstrated to be effective for treatment of chlamydial infection during pregnancy by Crombleholme and colleagues.[87] Multiple studies have since confirmed the efficacy and safety of amoxicillin, including a Cochrane Collaboration review of 11 randomized trials for the treatment of chlamydia during pregnancy.[88]

Although erythromycin regimens were once the mainstay for treatment of chlamydial infection during pregnancy, the frequent gastrointestinal side effects associated with erythromycin, which lead to noncompliance, have relegated them to alternative status.[12] In a recent observational cohort, Rahangdale and coworkers[89] reported that the treatment efficacy for erythromycin was 64%, compared to 97% for azithromycin and 95% for amoxicillin. Erythromycin estolate is contraindicated in pregnancy due to drug-related hepatotoxicity. The lower dose, 14-day regimens for erythromycin can be used if gastrointestinal tolerance is an issue, especially for women who are allergic to amoxicillin and azithromycin.

Unlike in nonpregnant women and men, repeat testing (preferably by NAATs) 3 weeks after completion of therapy is recommended for all pregnant women to ensure cure, in light of the sequelae that can occur in the mother and newborn infant if chlamydial infection persists. Sex partners should be referred for evaluation, testing, and treatment. The CDC suggests that, if concerns exist that sex partners will not seek evaluation and treatment, consideration should be given for delivery of antibiotic therapy (either a prescription or medication) by female patients to their sex partners. This approach decreases the rate of persistent or recurrent chlamydia compared with standard partner referral.[12,90,91]

Prevention

Primary prevention of chlamydial infection requires decreasing the risk of exposure to men infected with *C. trachomatis*. Although abstinence would accomplish this, it is often not a practical approach. Mutual monogamous relationships and safe sexual behaviors (e.g., condom use) are effective. A chlamydia vaccine may be developed in the future.

Secondary prevention requires population-based screening for chlamydia and treatment of infected women and their sex partners. As discussed previously, routine screening of all pregnant women at the first prenatal visit and screening of all nonpregnant women 25 years of age and younger is recommended. In addition, women older than 25 years of age who are at increased risk for chlamydial infection (e.g., multiple sex partners, new sex partner recently, previous chlamydial infection, other STDs) should be screened. This approach has been shown to both reduce the prevalence of chlamydial infection and decrease the risk of complications such as pelvic inflammatory disease and perinatal transmission.[86]

Human Papillomavirus Infection

Human papilloma virus (HPV) is a double-stranded DNA virus that is a member of the papovavirus family. More than 100 HPV types have been identified; of these, 35 primarily infect the genital tract. HPV is the most common sexually transmitted infection in the United States, with approximately 6.2 million new HPV infections occurring each year.[92]

HPV infection may result in either clinically apparent, grossly visible disease (e.g., genital warts) or subclinical disease. The majority of HPV infections are asymptomatic, unrecognized, or subclinical. The common genital HPV types can be divided into two major categories based on their oncogenic potential. HPV types in the low oncogenic risk group include types 6, 11, 42, 43, and 44. These types are associated with genital warts, condylomata, and some cases of low-grade squamous intraepithelial lesions. The high oncogenic risk group includes types 16, 18, 20, 31, 45, 54, 55, 56, 64, and 68. These high-risk types are frequently detected in women with high-grade squamous intraepithelial neoplasia and invasive cancers. The majority of the clinically apparent lesions are the classic genital warts (condyloma acuminatum). An estimated 1% of sexually active adults are diagnosed annually with genital warts.

Epidemiology

Sexual transmission is the primary route for transmission of HPV, and both urogenital and anorectal infections are seen.[4] The highest-risk groups for HPV infection are sexually active adolescents and young adults, with 75% of new HPV infections occurring among those 15 to 24 years old. HPV is highly contagious, and transmission rates are high, with approximately 65% of sexual contacts becoming infected. Although it is rare, perinatal transmission, especially of HPV types 6 and 11, can occur.[4]

Risk factors for HPV infection include early onset of sexual activity, multiple sexual partners, increased frequency of intercourse, exposure to sex partner with genital warts, failure to use condoms, and cigarette smoking.[4] In addition, Winer and colleagues[93] observed that smoking, oral contraceptive use, and report of a new male partner—in particular, one the patient knew for less than 8 months before sex occurred or one who reports having other partners—were predictive of new HPV infection. Furthermore, pregnancy is associated with an increased presence of HPV infection and genital warts, and immunosuppressive states (e.g., HIV infection with low $CD4^+$ T-cell count) result in increased viral titers of HPV and more rapid progression of HPV disease–associated cervical intraepithelial neoplasia (CIN).[4]

Respiratory papillomatosis (laryngeal papilloma) is a rare disease in the neonate that is caused by HPV-6 and HPV-11. Laryngeal papillomas can be particularly troublesome, because they may produce respiratory distress secondary to obstruction and because recurrence after treatment is common. Transplacental and intrapartum transmission of HPV can occur, as well as infection via contact during the neonatal period.[4]

Because genital papillomavirus infection is so common and respiratory papillomatosis is rare, the risk of intrapartum transmission is low, perhaps on the order of 1 case of juvenile respiratory papillomatosis per 1000 children born to infected mothers. Watts and associates[94] reported that, among 151 pregnant women evaluated for HPV by clinical, colposcopic, and PCR tests at less than 20, 34, and 36 weeks of gestation, 112 (74%) had evidence of HPV. HPV was identified in only 3 (4%) of 80 infants born to women with HPV detected at 34 to 36 weeks' gestation, but it also was found in 5 (8%) of 63 infants born to women in whom HPV DNA was not detected. Tenti and coworkers[95] also demonstrated that pregnant women with latent HPV infection have a low potential for transmitting the virus to the oropharyngeal mucosa of their newborns. Although these authors reported that HPV DNA was detected in 11 neonates born vaginally to HPV-positive women (vertical transmission rate, 30%; CI, 15.9% to 47%), all infants tested negative by 5 weeks after birth and remained so throughout the 18-month follow-up period. These findings suggest that the infants who were HPV-positive at birth were contaminated and not infected.

Other recent studies have supported the finding that the risk of perinatal transmission of HPV is low.[96,97] Of these, the most informative was the study by Smith and colleagues.[96] They detected HPV type specific concordance in only 1 mother/infant pair among the 6 (3.7%) infants born to 164 mothers with cervical HPV infection. In addition, a third of the HPV-positive newborns were born to mothers who tested negative for HPV DNA during pregnancy.

Pathogenesis

Genital HPV infections are transmitted primarily by sexual activity. Clinical lesions and subclinical infections occur in the urogenital and anorectal areas. As noted previously, the infectivity rate is high, with transmission occurring to sexual partners in approximately 65% of cases. The average incubation period is 2 to 3 months.

The HPV viral genome consists of three major regions; two protein-encoding regions (early and late gene regions) and a noncoding upstream regulatory region (URR). The URR controls transcription of both the early and the late region, resulting in regulation of viral proteins and production of infectious particles. The early region contains open reading frames (ORFs), which are transcriptional units that encode for a series of proteins designated E_1, E_2, E_4, E_5, E_6, and E_7. Early region gene expression controls replication, transcription, and cellular transformation of viral DNA. Most importantly, it also plays a role in unregulated cellular proliferation. Whereas E_6 and E_7 encode proteins involved in viral replication, they are the oncogenic genes and also code proteins critical for host cell immortalization and transformation. The late gene region contains two ORFs (L_1 and L_2), which encode structural proteins responsible for production of the viral capsid. The L_1 protein is the key component of the recently introduced HPV vaccine and is highly immunogenic.[98]

Acute HPV infection occurs when microtrauma secondary to sexual intercourse allows virus to enter the skin or mucosa of the genital tract. The postpubertal adolescent cervix is characterized by a large transformation zone which is more susceptible to minor trauma during sexual intercourse and whose immature columnar epithelial cells are particularly susceptible to HPV. This may explain why young, sexually active adolescents are at the greatest risk for acquiring HPV

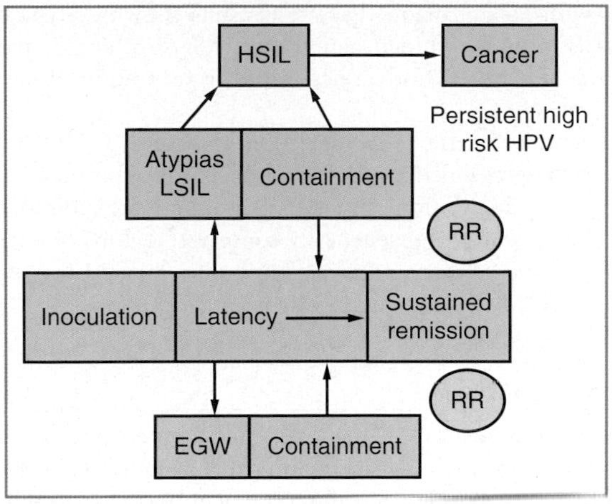

FIGURE 38-4 Natural history of human papillomavirus infection. EGW, external genital warts; HPV, human papillomavirus infection; HSIL, high-grade squamous intraepithelial lesion; LSIL, low-grade intraepithelial lesion; RR, recurrences.

infection. HPV enters cells in the basal layer of the epithelium and matures as it passes through the parabasal, spinous, and granular layers of the epithelium.[93,99]

Following acute HPV infection, several clinical scenarios can occur (Fig. 38-4). Latent viral infection occurs when the HPV genome is stabilized as a nonintegrated episome and remains in host cells without causing clinical or morphologic changes in the squamous epithelium of the genital tract. Latency can lead to sustained remission, which is the case in the vast majority of HPV infections. Alternatively, active infection may occur, depending on the type of HPV present. Low-risk HPV types, especially 6 and 11, cause proliferation of squamous epithelial cells with resultant formation of genital warts. High-risk oncogenic HPV types may become integrated into the host genome, resulting in CIN. CIN may progress to precancerous lesions (CIN 2 and 3) and, ultimately, to invasive cervical cancer. Alternatively, CIN may resolve spontaneously, especially CIN 1 and, to a lesser extent, CIN 2.

Diagnosis

Genital Warts

The diagnosis of genital warts is usually made by visual inspection. Biopsy is required only in certain circumstances: (1) the diagnosis is uncertain; (2) the lesions do not respond to standard therapy; (3) the disease worsens during therapy; (4) the patient is immunocompromised; or (5) the warts are pigmented, indurated, fixed, bleeding, or ulcerated. Use of HPV nucleic acid tests is not recommended in the routine diagnosis and management of visible genital warts.[12]

Asymptomatic Human Papillomavirus Infection

Because HPV cannot be cultured, detection of asymptomatic infection requires identification of viral nucleic acid (DNA or RNA) or capsid protein.[12,100] Only the Digene Hybrid Capture 2 (HC 2) High-Risk HPV DNA Test (Qiagen Digene, Gaithersburg, MD) is approved by the U.S. FDA for clinical use. This test uses liquid nucleic acid hybridization to detect 13 high-risk HPV types (16, 18, 31, 33, 35, 39, 45, 51, 52, 56, 58, 59, and 68). Type-specific results are not reported; rather, the specimen is identified as positive or negative for high-risk HPV. In particular, the HC2 High-Risk HPV test is approved for triage of women with Papanicolaou (Pap) test results showing atypical squamous cells of undetermined significance (ASC-US) and, in combination with the Pap test, for cervical cancer screening in women older than 30 years of age.

Less sensitive methods for detection of suspected HPV infection include cytologic evidence of HPV (koilocytosis), colposcopy, biopsy, and acetic acid application. Although they are not available for clinical use, PCR assays targeting genetically conserved regions of the L_1 gene and HPV serologic assays to detect antibodies to the L_1 viral protein have been used in research and epidemiologic studies.

Treatment

Options for treatment of genital warts during pregnancy are limited. The safety of podophyllin resin, podofilox, or imiquimod in pregnancy has not been established. Trichloracetic acid (TCA) or bichloracetic acid (BCA), 80% to 90% solution, may be used on a weekly basis. Alternatively, the lesions may be excised by scissors, scalpel, curettage, or electrosurgery. Cryosurgery can be used to treat vaginal lesions.[12] Treatment should be limited to patients who have multiple, confluent lesions.

As noted by the CDC, it is unclear whether cesarean delivery prevents juvenile-onset recurrent respiratory papillomatosis.[12,101] Therefore, cesarean delivery should not be performed solely to prevent transmission of HPV infection to the newborn. Cesarean delivery should be considered if obstruction of the pelvic outlet is likely or if vaginal delivery would result in excessive bleeding because of multiple confluent lesions.

Prevention

Transmission of HPV occurs through contact with infected genital skin, mucous membranes, or body fluids from a sexual partner with clinical or subclinical HPV infection. As with other STDs, preventing the spread of HPV to a susceptible population is more cost-effective than secondary prevention. Prevention of HPV transmission incorporates the following approaches: (1) abstinence (most effective, but may not be practical); (2) long-term mutual monogamy with a single partner; (3) limiting the number of sexual partners; (4) limiting sexual contacts to men who have been abstinent for a longer period of time; (5) having a circumcised partner; (6) using latex condoms; and (7) receiving the HPV vaccine.

The most exciting new development for prevention of HPV infection is the introduction into clinical practice of prophylactic HPV vaccines. The first such vaccine to become available was the quadrivalent HPV vaccine, Gardisil (Merck & Co., Whitehouse Station, NJ), which protects against HPV types 6, 11, 16, and 18.[100,102]

Neither routine surveillance for HPV infection nor partner notification is deemed useful for HPV prevention. The rationale for this conclusion is that HPV is so prevalent that most partners are already infected. In addition, no prevention or treatment strategies are recommended for partners. Similarly, no treatment strategies or prevention strategies are recommended for prevention of perinatal transmission of HPV. Therefore, cesarean delivery for prevention of HPV infection in newborns is not indicated.

Urinary Tract Infection

Urinary tract infections (UTIs) are a major public health problem in the United States, affecting approximately 11 million women annually, with an associated direct cost of $1.6 billion.[103] In women, UTIs are divided into five major categories[104,105] (Table 38-8).

TABLE 38-8 CLASSIFICATION OF URINARY TRACT INFECTIONS

Asymptomatic bacteriuria (ASB)
Acute uncomplicated cystitis
Recurrent cystitis
Acute uncomplicated pyelonephritis
Complicated urinary tract infection
Multiple frequent recurrences
High probability of drug-resistant uropathogen
Increased risk for sepsis syndrome

Women are 14 times more likely to develop UTIs than men. Presumably, this female predominance is the result of several factors, including (1) a shorter urethra in women; (2) continuous contamination of the external one third of the urethra by pathogenic bacteria from the vagina and rectum; (3) failure of females to empty their bladders as completely as males; and (4) movement of bacteria into the female bladder during sexual intercourse.[4]

UTI is the most common medical complication of pregnancy. UTIs occur in up to 20% of pregnancies and account for 10% of antepartum hospitalizations.[4,106] Among pregnant women, almost all UTIs fall into three categories: (1) ASB; (2) acute cystitis; and (3) acute pyelonephritis. Of critical importance is the recognition that the normal physiologic changes associated with pregnancy (e.g., progesterone effect on ureteral smooth muscle peristalsis, obstruction of the ureters by the enlarging uterus) predispose pregnant women with ASB to the development of acute pyelonephritis. Moreover, UTIs in pregnancy place the fetus and mother at risk for substantial morbidity and even mortality.[4,104]

Asymptomatic Bacteriuria

Epidemiology

Obstetricians have long recognized the serious nature of symptomatic UTIs in pregnancy. However, it was not until the early 1960s that Kass demonstrated that significant bacteriuria can occur in the absence of symptoms or signs of UTI.[107] He established quantitative bacteriology as the indispensable laboratory aid for the diagnosis, follow-up, and confirmation of cure of UTI. From these studies evolved the commonly accepted definition of ASB: the presence of 10^5 or more colonies of a bacterial organism per milliliter of urine on two consecutive clean, midstream-voided specimens in the absence of signs or symptoms of UTI. Persistent ASB was identified in 6% of pregnant patients. Acute pyelonephritis developed in 40% of the patients with ASB who received placebo, but pyelonephritis rarely occurred when bacteriuria was eliminated. Kass also noted that rates of neonatal death and prematurity were two to three times greater in bacteriuric women receiving placebo than in nonbacteriuric women or bacteriuric women whose infection was eliminated by antibiotics. He concluded that detection of material bacteriuria would identify patients at risk for pyelonephritis and premature delivery and maintained that pyelonephritis in pregnancy could be prevented by detection and treatment of bacteriuria in early pregnancy. Moreover, Kass estimated that 10% of premature births could be prevented by such a program.[107]

Most cases of ASB in pregnancy are detected at the initial prenatal visit, and relatively few pregnant women acquire bacteriuria after the initial visit. Thus, the bacteriuria antedates the pregnancy. The prevalence of ASB in pregnant women ranges from 2% to 11%, with the majority of investigations reporting 4% to 7%. An increased prevalence of bacteriuria in females has been associated with lower socioeconomic status, diminished availability of medical care, and increased parity. Recently, Thurman and coworkers determined that sickle cell trait carriers are not more susceptible than other pregnant women to ASB.[108]

Untreated ASB during pregnancy often leads to acute pyelonephritis. Women with ASB in early pregnancy are at a 20- to 30-fold increased risk of developing acute pyelonephritis during pregnancy, compared to pregnant women without bacteriuria.[109] Studies performed in the 1960s, using sulfonamides or nitrofurantoin, demonstrated that antimicrobial treatment of ASB during pregnancy significantly reduced the risk of developing pyelonephritis, from about 20% to 35% to between 1% and 4%. Before the advent of universal screening for ASB in early pregnancy, the reported rate of acute pyelonephritis in pregnancy was 3% to 4%; afterward, it was 1% to 2%.[110,111] Similarly, studies in Europe assessing the implementation of screening and treatment programs for ASB in pregnant women demonstrated a significant reduction in the rate of acute pyelonephritis in pregnancy.[112,113] For this reason, it is important that the presence of bacteriuria be identified. Other claims, such as that ASB predisposes the patient to anemia, preeclampsia, and chronic renal disease, are controversial and unproven.

Kass[107] initially reported an association between ASB and prematurity and observed that eradication of bacteriuria with antimicrobial therapy significantly reduced the rate of preterm delivery. He proposed that early detection and treatment of bacteriuria would prevent 10% to 20% of preterm births. Subsequently, numerous studies demonstrated conflicting results regarding bacteriuria and prematurity. Kincaid-Smith and Bullen[114] suggested the hypothesis that underlying renal disease is the major cause of the excessive risk of prematurity or low birth weight among bacteriuric pregnant women. The many different definitions for prematurity used in the literature contributed to this confusion.

More recent studies, including meta-analyses, demonstrated an association between ASB and low birth weight and preterm delivery.[115-118] Bacteriuria is only one of many factors that may influence the onset of premature labor. Because both the incidence of bacteriuria in pregnancy and the incidence of prematurity vary inversely with socioeconomic status, any relationship between bacteriuria and gestational length and birth weight may be complex and difficult to establish. In an attempt to resolve this controversy, Romero and colleagues[115] used the technique of meta-analysis to assess the relationship between ASB and preterm delivery and/or low birth weight. Meta-analysis confirmed a statistically significant increased risk for low-birth-weight infants among bacteriuric women. Their study also demonstrated a significant association between bacteriuria and preterm delivery and showed a statistically significant reduction in the incidence of low birth weight among bacteriuric women treated in eight placebo-controlled treatment trials.

Meis and colleagues[117] demonstrated in a multivariate analysis that bacteriuria significantly increased the occurrence of preterm birth (relative risk, 2.03; CI, 1.50 to 2.75). Schieve and colleagues,[116] in an analysis of 150,000 births in the University of Illinois Perinatal Network database, reported that women with antepartum UTI were at increased risk for delivering preterm and low-birth-weight infants. With multivariate analysis, the odds ratios were 1.4 (CI, 1.2 to 1.6) and 1.3 (CI, 1.1 to 1.4) for low-birth-weight and preterm birth, respectively. Moreover, Smaill[118] reported a meta-analysis of treatment versus placebo trials for ASB in pregnancy that demonstrated a one-third reduction in the rate of low-birth-weight infants (from 15% to 10%) in women whose bacteriuria was treated. Therefore, it appears that maternal ASB is a risk factor for preterm delivery and low birth weight and that this risk can be reduced by screening and treatment of ASB in pregnant women.[119] With recognition that ASB increases the risk for developing acute pyelonephritis and preterm delivery and low birth weight, the ACOG and the U.S. Preventive Services Task Force recommend screening to detect ASB in pregnancy.[120,121]

Symptomatic UTI is more often found in pregnant women than in nonpregnant women. This observation suggests that some factors present during gestation allow bacteria to replicate in the urine and ascend to the upper urinary tract. Several findings support this view.[4] The normal female urinary tract undergoes dramatic physiologic and anatomic changes during pregnancy. Briefly, a decrease in ureteral muscle tone and activity results in a lower rate of passage of urine throughout the urinary collecting system. The upper ureters and renal pelves become dilated, resulting in a physiologic hydronephrosis of pregnancy. These changes are caused by the effects of progesterone on muscle tone and peristalsis and, more important, by mechanical obstruction of the enlarging uterus. Changes in the bladder also occur in pregnancy, including decreased tone, increased capacity, and incomplete emptying, all of which predispose to vesicoureteric reflux. Hypotonia of the vesicle musculature, vesicoureteric reflux, and dilation of the ureters and renal pelves result in static columns of urine in the ureters, facilitating the ascending migration of bacteria to the upper urinary tract after bladder infection is established. The hypokinetic collecting system reduces urine flow, and urinary stasis occurs, predisposing to infection.

Alterations in the physical and chemical properties of urine during pregnancy exacerbate bacteriuria, further predisposing to ascending infection. Because of the increased excretion of bicarbonate, urinary pH rises, encouraging bacterial growth. Glycosuria, which is common in pregnancy, favors an increase in the rate of bacterial multiplication. The increased urinary excretion of estrogens may also be a factor in the pathogenesis of symptomatic UTI during pregnancy. In animal experiments, estrogen enhances the growth of strains of *Escherichia coli* that cause pyelonephritis and predispose to renal leukocyte migration, phagocytosis, and complement activity. The cumulative effect of these physiologic factors is an increased risk that infection in the bladder may ascend to the kidneys.

Pathogenic characteristics of microorganisms such as *E. coli* are major determinants of UTI. These include pili (adherence), K antigen (antiphagocytic activity), hemolysin (cytotoxicity), and antimicrobial resistance. Host susceptibility factors include anatomic or functional abnormalities of the urinary tract and uroepithelial and vaginal epithelial cells with increased attachment of uropathogenic *E. coli*. Women who do not secrete the ABO blood group antigens are particularly likely to harbor pathogenic *E. coli* in the urogenital epithelium.

Pathogenesis

In general, the urinary tract is sterile, with the exception of the distal urethra, which is often colonized with bacteria from the skin and vaginal and anal flora. Ascension of bacteria from the urethra into the bladder results in ASB. Bacteria associated with ASB derive from the normal flora of the gastrointestinal tract, vagina, and periurethral area. In addition, instrumentation of the urinary tract (e.g., bladder catheterization) may introduce bacteria into the bladder of patients without prior colonization. In women with ASB, bacteria persist in the urinary tract but do not elicit sufficient enough host response to result in either symptoms or eradication of the bacteria from the urinary tract. Factors such as host susceptibility, bacterial virulence, incomplete bladder emptying, obstruction, or presence of a foreign body (e.g., catheter) predispose to persistence of bacteria.[109]

As noted in many studies, *E. coli* is overwhelmingly the most frequent microorganism recovered in patients with ASB, including pregnant women.[4] Other gram-negative enterobacteria (e.g., *Klebsiella, Proteus*) and gram-positive bacteria such as *Staphylococcus saprophyticus*, GBS, and the enterococcus cause the remaining cases of ASB in young, sexually active women.

A series of studies compared genetic markers or phenotypic expression of potential bacterial virulence factors among *E. coli* strains isolated from various types of UTIs.[109,122,123] One of those publications[123] focused on *E. coli* isolates from pregnant women. Among patients with ASB, *E. coli* strains demonstrated a lower frequency of genetic markers or phenotypic expression of virulence factors than did those recovered from patients with acute cystitis or acute pyelonephritis.

Several studies have shown that the incidence of ASB in nonpregnant women is comparable to the incidence in pregnant women in the same locale.[107-109] It appears that most women in whom bacteriuria is first discovered during pregnancy have acquired ASB earlier in life. Although pregnancy per se does not cause any major increase in incidence of bacteriuria, it does predispose to the development of acute pyelonephritis in bacteriuric patients.

Diagnosis

Although the diagnosis of ASB was originally based on obtaining two consecutive midstream urine cultures containing at least 100,000 colony-forming units per milliliter (CFU/mL) of a uropathogen, a single positive urine specimen is used for clinical diagosis.[4,124] Urine cultures are relatively expensive and require 24 to 48 hours for results. Therefore, inexpensive, rapid, office-based screening tests have undergone clinical testing. These include microscopic urinalysis, nitrite and leukocyte esterase dipstick, Gram stain, Uricult dip slide, Cult-Dip Plus, and Uristat test. However, although it is more costly than rapid tests, urine culture remains the screening test of choice for detecting ASB in pregnancy.[4,124-126]

Recent investigations have reconfirmed the lack of sensitivity and specificity of alternate methodologies for the diagnosis of ASB, particularly in pregnant women.[127,128] As noted by McNair and colleagues,[127] the potential serious sequelae of undiagnosed and untreated ASB mandate that urine culture be used to detect ASB in pregnant women. Both the U.S. Preventive Services Task Force and the Infectious Disease Society of America (IDSA) concur with this recommendation.[109,121] Although there is consensus that all pregnant women should be screened for ASB by urine culture at least once in early pregnancy, no recommendation has been made for or against repeated screening of culture-negative women in later pregnancy. Our approach is not to rescreen culture-negative, asymptomatic women later in pregnancy unless there is a history of recurrent UTIs.

Treatment

Detection and treatment of ASB give the obstetrician an opportunity to prevent significant medical complications of pregnancy. Screening at the original antenatal visit, appropriate treatment, and eradication of bacteriuria significantly reduce the frequency of antenatal acute pyelonephritis. Clinical trials demonstrate that treatment of ASB reduces the risk of acute pyelonephritis in pregnancy by 80% to 90%, to about 1% to 4%.[129-131] In addition, screening and treatment of ASB significantly reduce the risks for preterm delivery and delivery of a low-birth-weight infant.[115-118]

Treatment should be designed to maintain sterile urine throughout pregnancy, using the shortest possible course of antimicrobial agents in order to minimize the cost and the toxic effects of these drugs in mother and fetus. Because most antibacterial agents are excreted by glomerular filtration, therapeutic concentrations are readily achieved in the urine. In fact, the concentration of these drugs in urine greatly exceeds that required for the treatment of most UTIs. Even drugs that do not reach therapeutic concentrations in serum, such as nitrofurantoin, reach significant concentrations in urine.[132]

No single agent is clearly better than another. At present, it is generally accepted that short courses of treatment are preferable, because (1) the duration of initial therapy does not affect the recurrence rate, (2) a short course minimizes the adverse drug effects in mother and fetus, (3) emergence of resistant bacteria is discouraged, (4) patient compliance is enhanced, and (5) costs are kept to a minimum.

Although a 3-day course of antibiotic therapy is recommended for the treatment of uncomplicated UTI in nonpregnant women, until recently a 7-day course was preferred for pregnant women.[105] However, a Cochrane Collaboration systematic review concluded that there was insufficient evidence to recommend a duration of antimicrobial therapy for pregnant women among the single-dose, 3-day, 4-day, and 7-day treatment regimens.[133] Most experts prefer the 7-day approach. Treatment of ASB is empiric, and in vitro susceptibility testing is not recommended for the initial positive culture.[4]

A wide variety of antimicrobial agents have been used successfully for management of ASB in pregnancy (Table 38-9). These include β-lactam antibiotics such as ampicillin and cephalosporins which do not pose any significant risk to the fetus. Other commonly used antibiotics include short-acting sulfonamides, nitrofurantoin, and trimethoprim-sulfamethoxazole.

TABLE 38-9 ANTIMICROBIAL TREATMENT OF ASYMPTOMATIC BACTERIURIA AND ACUTE CYSTITIS DURING PREGNANCY

Antimicrobial Agent	Regimen
Single-Dose Treatments**	
Ampicillin*	2 g
Amoxicillin*	3 g
Nitrofurantoin monohydrate macrocrystals (Macrobid)	200 mg
Trimethoprim-sulfamethoxazole DS	320/1600 mg
3-Day or 7-Day Treatments	
Ampicillin*	250 mg qid
Amoxicillin*	500 mg tid
Cephalexin*	250-500 mg qid
Nitrofurantoin monohydrate macrocrystals	100 mg bid
Sulfisoxazole	Initial 2 g dose, then 1 g qid
Trimethoprim-sulfamethoxazole DS	160/800 mg bid
Suppressive Therapy	
Nitrofurantoin monohydrate macrocrystals	100 mg qhs (duration of pregnancy)
Trimethoprim-sulfamethoxazole DS	160/800 qhs (duration of pregnancy)

*Only in geographic areas with low levels of resistance to *Escherichia coli*.

**Should not be used in pregnancy because of unacceptably high rate of failure.

DS, double strength.

The quinolones are not approved for use during pregnancy because of concerns regarding their teratogenic effect on fetal cartilage. However, use of fluoroquinolones for resistant microorganisms is appropriate. In such instances, ciprofloxacin 250 mg twice daily or levofloxacin 250 mg daily may be used. Use of ampicillin or amoxicillin has been questioned for treatment of UTIs, because the predominant etiologic organism is *E. coli*, and resistance rates of *E. coli* to ampicillin in the United States are 30% or greater.[105] Of additional concern is the decreased susceptibility of *E. coli* to trimethoprim-sulfamethoxazole, which ranges from 5% to 15% depending on the geographic area.[105,134-136]

When short courses of therapy are prescribed for ASB during pregnancy, continuous surveillance for recurrent bacteriuria by repeat urine cultures is essential. It is appropriate to treat recurrent ASB with antimicrobial agents on the basis of the microorganism's sensitivities for the remainder of the pregnancy and for at least 2 weeks after delivery. Alternatively, a short course of therapy with urine culture screening at each prenatal visit may be instituted. Persistent ASB should necessitate continuous antimicrobial therapy for the duration of pregnancy. A single daily dose of nitrofurantoin, 100 mg, preferably after the evening meal, is recommended. Alternatively, short-acting sulfonamide preparations such as trimethoprim-sulfamethoxazole may be prescribed.

Prevention

Because ASB antedates pregnancy and typically is not acquired during pregnancy, there is no prevention strategy available. Recurrent ASB has been noted in up to 30% of pregnant women.[137] Close monitoring with frequent urine cultures after diagnosis and treatment of ASB in early pregnancy can prevent recurrent or persistent ASB. Most importantly, diagnosis, treatment, and eradication of ASB in pregnant women substantially reduce the occurrence of acute pyelonephritis and reduce the incidence of preterm births.

Cystitis in Pregnancy

Acute cystitis is a distinct syndrome characterized by urinary urgency, frequency, dysuria, and suprapubic discomfort in the absence of systemic symptoms such as high fever and costovertebral angle tenderness. Gross hematuria may be present; the urine culture is invariably positive for bacterial growth. The gold standard for diagnosing acute cystitis, in the past, has been a quantitative culture containing at least 100,000 CFU/mL. Stamm and coworkers[138] demonstrated that a urine culture positive for bacterial growth with more than 100 CFU/mL, in combination with symptoms of dysuria and frequency, is sufficient to confirm the diagnosis of cystitis, particularly if the urine sample was obtained by catheterization.

Epidemiology

The incidence of acute cystitis among pregnant women ranges from 0.3% to 1.3%.[123] Harris and Gilstrap[139] reported a recurrence rate of 1.3% for cystitis during pregnancy. Although increased diagnosis and treatment of ASB reduced the incidence of pyelonephritis at their institution, the incidence of acute cystitis remained constant. On initial screening urine cultures, 64% of the patients who ultimately developed cystitis had negative cultures; in contrast, only a minority of those patients with ASB and acute pyelonephritis had negative cultures. The authors noted that the recurrence pattern in patients with acute cystitis was also different from that in patients with either bacteriuria or acute pyelonephritis. Disease recurred in 75% of patients with acute pyelonephritis who were not given suppressive antimicrobial therapy, compared with only 17% of patients with acute cystitis.

Acute cystitis tends to occur during the second trimester.[139] This also differs from the pattern seen with ASB (in which almost all cases are diagnosed in the first trimester) or with acute pyelonephritis (diagnosed in the first and third trimesters). In addition, acute cystitis does not increase the risk for preterm birth, low birth weight, or acute pyelonephritis.[4,104,124] In fact, the only morbidity associated with acute cystitis in pregnancy is the discomfort that occurs with symptomatic UTI.

Pathogenesis

As reported by Scholes and associates,[140] the major risk factors for acute cystitis in young women are a history of prior acute cystitis and frequent or recent sexual activity. By 24 years of age, approximately 1 in 3 women have experienced at least one episode of acute cystitis, and 30% to 40% have one or more recurrences.[141] Nonsecretors of ABO blood group antigens are at increased risk for recurrent cystitis.[142]

As in ASB, the microorganisms associated with acute cystitis originate from the flora of the gastrointestinal tract, vagina, and periurethral area and ascend via the urethra to colonize and infect the bladder. The most common bacteria isolated from the urine of women with acute cystitis is *E. coli* (80% to 85%), followed by *S. saprophyticus*, other gram-negative enterobacteria (e.g., *Klebsiella pneumoniae*, *Proteus mirabilis*), GBS, and the enterococcus.[4]

Diagnosis

In nonpregnant women, the diagnosis of acute uncomplicated cystitis relies on symptoms of dysuria, urgency, and frequency plus evidence of pyuria (microscopic or dipstick). In pregnancy, culture confirmation is recommended.[4] Once cystitis is suspected, either a catheterized specimen or a clean-catch midstream specimen for urinalysis and culture should be obtained before treatment with antibiotics. However, because of the symptomatology of acute cystitis and the danger of upward extension of the infection to the kidney, it is not advisable to await the results of culture. The constellation of symptoms and demonstration of white blood cells and bacteria on urinalysis should be sufficient grounds for beginning therapy.

Urine dipstick testing has replaced microscopy because it is cheaper, faster, and more convenient. The presence of either nitrite or leukocyte esterase is considered a positive result, with a sensitivity of 75% and a specificity of 82%.[144] Whereas a positive result is highly predictive of UTI, a negative dipstick test does not rule out an infection in acutely symptomatic women.[143] A clean midstream urine or catheter specimen with greater than 10^2 bacteria per milliliter obtained from an acutely dysuric woman is diagnostic of acute cystitis.[138]

Treatment

Pregnant women with acute cystitis should receive immediate therapy with an antibiotic agent. The organisms most commonly isolated in acute cystitis are *E. coli*, other gram-negative facultative organisms, *S. saprophyticus*, and GBS. The duration of therapy in cystitis should be 3 to 7 days. Single-dose therapy is not recommended in pregnancy. The antimicrobial agents used to treat cystitis in pregnancy are similar to those for ASB and are summarized in Table 38-9. Relief of symptoms occurs in more than 90% of women within 72 hours after treatment initiation.[144]

In pregnant women with acute cystitis, a "test of cure" urine examination should be performed 1 to 2 weeks after completion of therapy. If it is positive, a different regimen than that used initially should be started. Continuous prophylaxis (at bedtime) is recommended for women who have three or more symptomatic UTIs in a 12-month period. Either nitrofurantoin or trimethoprim-sulfamethoxazole is recommended. Postcoital prophylaxis is an alternative option.[4]

Prevention

Because the risk for acute cystitis is not associated with the presence of ASB, screening for and treatment of ASB early in pregnancy does not reduce the incidence of acute cystitis in pregnancy. Moreover, one of the major risk factors for acute cystitis, use of a diaphragm and spermicide for contraception, is not an issue during pregnancy. However, recurrent acute cystitis can be prevented with daily antibiotic prophylaxis. Nitrofurantoin and trimethoprim-sulfamethoxazole are acceptable alternatives.

Acute Pyelonephritis

Acute pyelonephritis is one of the most common medical complications of pregnancy.[4,144] Despite recommendations for routine screening of pregnant women and treatment of ASB, the incidence of acute pyelonephritis in pregnancy ranges from 1% to 2.5%. In a recent large prospective cohort at Parkland Hospital, the incidence of antepartum acute pyelonephritis was 14 per 1000 deliveries.[144] Recurrence during the same pregnancy is frequent, occurring in 10% to 18% of cases. In addition, acute pyelonephritis in pregnancy can cause significant maternal morbidity and, in rare instances, maternal and fetal mortality.[4,106,144]

Epidemiology

As noted, the incidence of acute pyelonephritis in pregnancy ranges from 1% to 2.5%. The incidence varies depending on several factors, including population characteristics, prevalence of ASB, whether routine screening with culture and treatment of ASB occurs, and whether patients receive prenatal care, especially early first-trimester assessment.

The major risk factors for acute pyelonephritis are previous episodes of acute pyelonephritis and the presence of ASB.[4] In the absence of routine screening and treatment of ASB, up to 40% of pregnant women with ASB will develop acute pyelonephritis. Therefore, screening and treatment of ASB dramatically reduce the incidence of pyelonephritis. With universal screening, the reported incidence is 1% to 2%,[110,111,145] Among pregnant women not receiving suppressive antimicrobial therapy to prevent acute pyelonephritis for the duration of pregnancy, recurrence has been noted in up to 60%; with suppressive therapy, the recurrence rate is less than 10%.[4,145] Other predisposing factors for acute pyelonephritis during pregnancy include obstructive and neurologic diseases affecting the urinary tract and the presence of ureteral or renal calculi.

Recently, Hill and coworkers[144] examined the incidence of risk factors among women with acute antepartum pyelonephritis. Overall, 13% had at least one maternal risk factor for antepartum pyelonephritis. As demonstrated in the older literature, the most common risk factor was a previous history of pyelonephritis and ASB. Other factors include young maternal age and nulliparity.

Pathogenesis

Although ASB is no more frequent in pregnant than in nonpregnant women, acute pyelonephritis is a much more frequent sequela during pregnancy. Several factors during pregnancy facilitate bacterial replication in urine and ascent to the upper urinary tract. In the bladder, there is decreased tone, increased capacity, and incomplete emptying; as a consequence, there is a predisposition for vesicoureteric reflux to occur. Moreover, the physiologic hydronephrosis of pregnancy, caused by the effects of progesterone on muscle tone and peristalsis in the ureters and the mechanical obstruction of the enlarging uterus, facilitates ascent of bacteria into the upper urinary tract.[4]

Alterations in the physical and chemical properties of urine during pregnancy also facilitate ascending infection. Bacterial growth is enhanced by the elevated urinary pH during pregnancy. Glycosuria is more frequent and also enhances bacterial growth. The increased urinary excretion of estrogen also may play a role in the pathogenesis of acute antepartum pyelonephritis. Estrogen has been shown to accelerate the growth of strains of *E. coli* that cause pyelonephritis.[4,146,147]

Pathogenic mechanisms also exist in the microorganisms associated with acute pyelonephritis. The requisite first step for establishing colonization or infection in the urinary tract is bacterial adherence to urogenital epithelium. *E. coli* attaches to uroepithelium via two adhesions: P fimbriae (pap encoded adhesions) and type 1 pili. The prevalence of *E. coli* strains expressing P fimbriae from patients with acute pyelonephritis (75% to 100%) is significantly greater than among fecal strains from persons without UTI. On the other hand, type 1 pili are almost universally expressed among uropathogenic and fecal commensal *E. coli* strains.[148]

The most common bacteria associated with acute pyelonephritis are *E. coli*, *Klebsiella* species, and *Enterobacter* species. Dunlow and Duff[149] reported that, in a group of women with antepartum pyelonephritis, *E. coli* (80%) was the dominant pathogen, with *K. pneumoniae* (7.4%), *Staphylococcus aureus* (6.7%), and *P. mirabilis* (2%) isolated much less frequently. More recently, Hill and colleagues[144] observed that the predominant microorganisms recovered from patients with acute antepartum pyelonephritis were *E. coli* (70%), *Klebsiella-Enterobacter* (3%), *Proteus* (2%), and gram-positive bacteria, including GBS (10%).

Diagnosis

Acute pyelonephritis is characterized by fever, chills, flank pain, dysuria, urgency, and frequency. Nausea and vomiting may also be present. On physical examination, fever and costovertebral angle tenderness are often present. Laboratory abnormalities include pyuria and bacteriuria. White blood cell casts are highly predictive of acute pyelonephritis. The diagnosis is ultimately confirmed by a positive urine culture.[4]

As noted by Sheffield and Cunningham,[104] the clinical findings of acute pyelonephritis in pregnancy are similar to those described in nonpregnant women. Onset of symptoms is usually abrupt. Fever is universal, and the diagnosis is suspect if it is absent. In 50% of cases occurring during pregnancy, pyelonephritis is unilateral and on the right side. Unilateral left side and bilateral infections are each present in 25% of cases. Most likely, right urethral obstruction secondary to uterine dextrorotation explains the right-sided predominance seen in pregnancy.

Although 10% to 20% of pregnant women with acute pyelonephritis are bacteremic, the usefulness of obtaining routine blood cultures in suspected cases of acute uncomplicated pyelonephritis has been questioned.[150,151] The rationale for this new approach includes the facts that blood cultures are expensive, the bacterium isolated is invariably the organism recovered from the urine culture, and change of antibiotics usually is based on lack of clinical response rather than culture results.

Pyelonephritis is not only a serious risk for preterm labor and delivery but also a serious threat to maternal well-being. Up to 20% of pregnant women with acute pyelonephritis develop evidence of multiorgan system involvement secondary to endotoxemia and the sepsis syndrome.[4,152,153] The primary pathogenic mechanism results from endothelial activation followed by capillary fluid leakage and extravasation, with resultant decreased perfusion of vital organs. This vascular derangement worsens the hypovolemia that is often present as a result of fever and vomiting, leading to hypotension.

Multiple sepsis-related complications have been reported in pregnant women with acute pyelonephritis. Anemia, caused by hemolysis initiated by endotoxemia, occurs in 23% to 66% of these patients. Rarely, evidence of disseminated intravascular coagulation (DIC) may be present. With severe sepsis, DIC is common and is associated with potentially serious complications (e.g., purpura fulminans).[4,152,153]

Before the recognition that aggressive fluid resuscitation is a critical component of the management of acute pyelonephritis in pregnancy, approximately 20% of pregnant women with acute pyelonephritis had transient renal dysfunction, as documented by decreased creatinine clearance.[154] More recently, with aggressive fluid resuscitation, the rate of renal dysfunction is 7%.[144] Although renal dysfunction may be transient, it is important to recognize its presence so that nephrotoxic antimicrobial agents (e.g., aminoglycosides) can be withheld, used with caution, or not used at all. In addition, antibiotics that are excreted by the kidney should be administered in reduced dosages.

Cunningham and coworkers[153] initially reported that acute pyelonephritis of pregnancy may be complicated by adult respiratory distress syndrome (ARDS). Acute respiratory insufficiency, the most common serious complication of severe sepsis, develops in 2% to 8% of pregnant women with acute pyelonephritis.[4,155] Hill and associates[144] reported that 7% of pregnant women with acute pyelonephritis developed respiratory insufficiency. The pathophysiology involves cytokine inflammatory injury to vascular endothelium, which leads to increased alveolar membrane permeability. ARDS should be suspected in patients who present with dyspnea, tachypnea, hypoxemia, or a chest radiograph suggestive of pulmonary edema or ARDS.

Towers and colleagues[155] identified several risk factors for ARDS in patients with antepartum pyelonephritis: elevated maternal heart rate (>110 beats/min); use of a tocolytic agent; use of ampicillin as the sole antibiotic; temperature 103° F or higher within the first 24 hours; and fluid overload. More recently, in a study of 440 cases of acute antepartum pyelonephritis, Hill and coworkers[144] reported that women with respiratory insufficiency received more intravenous fluids during the first 48 hours and had higher maximum temperatures, higher heart rates, lower hematocrits, and higher rates of septicemia. Moreover, tachypnea was present only in patients with respiratory insufficiency. Fortunately, most cases with pulmonary capillary injury respond to oxygen supplementation and diuresis. However, intubation and mechanical ventilation are required in severe cases. The cytokine inflammatory response may also lead to uterine contractions.[124]

Treatment

The management of acute uncomplicated pyelonephritis in pregnant women has changed dramatically since the 1990s. Traditionally, patients with acute uncomplicated pyelonephritis were hospitalized and treated with parenteral antimicrobial therapy, but more recent studies have demonstrated that, for women with mild to moderate disease, oral therapy on an outpatient basis is appropriate. In addition, the duration of therapy has been reduced from 6 weeks to 2 weeks.[156-158]

Hooton[156] outlined factors that should be considered when selecting agents for empiric treatment of uncomplicated acute pyelonephritis:

1. Antimicrobial spectrum of the agent
2. Pharmacokinetics allowing for infrequent dosing intervals
3. Prevalence of resistance among uropathogens in the geographic area
4. Duration of adequate urinary and renal tissue levels
5. Effect of antimicrobial agent on the fecal and vaginal flora
6. Adverse side effects
7. Cost
8. Public health concerns regarding development of resistance

Limited information has been published to assist in determining optimal antimicrobial regimens and duration of therapy for treatment of acute uncomplicated pyelonephritis in pregnant women. Moreover, the management of acute pyelonephritis has become more complex with the trend for increasing resistance of uropathogens, especially resistance to β-lactam antibiotics (e.g., ampicillin) and trimethoprim-sulfamethoxazole.[136,156]

For purposes of treatment, patients with acute uncomplicated pyelonephritis may be stratified into two groups: those with severe disease, who require hospitalization and parenteral antibiotics, and those with mild to moderate disease, who can be treated on an outpatient basis with oral agents. As described in the IDSA guidelines, mild disease is characterized by low-grade fever, normal or slightly elevated white blood cell count, and absence of nausea and vomiting.[136] Patients requiring hospitalization are those with high fevers, high white blood cell counts, vomiting, dehydration, evidence of sepsis, or no response during an initial period of observation.

The management of acute pyelonephritis in pregnant women follows many of the same principles used for nonpregnant women, with several important differences. In general, fluoroquinolones should be avoided in pregnancy, unless no alternative antimicrobial agent is available. Second, although earlier studies suggested that outpatient oral therapy is an acceptable alternative for mild to moderate pyelonephritis,[151,159,160] most experts currently recommend that pregnant women with acute pyelonephritis be initially assessed during a 12- to 24-hour hospital stay before a decision is made about outpatient management. Finally, because of the potential for renal dysfunction and respiratory insufficiency in pregnant women with acute pyelonephritis, careful monitoring of renal function, urinary output, and respiratory status, including pulse oximetry, is necessary.

Management of acute pyelonephritis in pregnancy is outlined in Table 38-10. Because of the frequency of dehydration, respiratory

TABLE 38-10 MANAGEMENT OF ACUTE PYELONEPHRITIS IN PREGNANT WOMEN

In-hospital observation with assessment for 12-24 hr
- Urinalysis and urine culture
- Complete blood count, serum creatinine, electrolytes
- Frequent monitoring of vital signs (especially for onset of tachypnea)
- Monitoring of urine output (consider Foley catheter)
- Intravenous crystalloid fluid resuscitation to maintain urine output at ≥30-50 mL/hr
- Chest radiograph and arterial blood gas analysis in patients with dyspnea or tachypnea
- Intravenous antimicrobial therapy

Patients who respond to initial parenteral antimicrobial and fluid resuscitation may be discharged after 12-24 hr of observation with oral antimicrobial agent to complete 14 days of therapy

Patients with high fever, signs of respiratory insufficiency, poor urine output, evidence of sepsis, or inability to tolerate oral medication require hospitalization insufficiency, and renal dysfunction associated with acute pyelonephritis in pregnancy, aggressive fluid resuscitation with crystalloid solutions such as lactated Ringer solution or normal saline is critical. Fluid resuscitation must be balanced with the risk of pulmonary edema, so close monitoring of respiratory status with pulse oximetry is imperative. Blood cultures should be obtained from patients who have evidence of sepsis or septic shock or who fail to respond to initial therapy.

Vital signs, including respiratory rate, and urine output should be closely monitored. Tachypnea, hypotension, and oliguria are signs of impending sepsis or septic shock. In gestations beyond 24 weeks, uterine activity and fetal heart rate should be monitored closely. If uterine contractions persist despite rehydration, tocolytic therapy should be considered, with due consideration to the synergistic cardiovascular effects of tocolytics and sepsis. Use of a cooling blanket or acetaminophen or both reduces cardiovascular stress. This is important in early pregnancy, secondary to possible teratogenic effects of hyperthermia.[104] Similarly, if preterm labor is a concern, untreated hyperthermia increases the metabolic needs of the fetus.

A number of antimicrobial regimens may be used to treat acute pyelonephritis in pregnancy (Table 38-11). Given the high incidence of resistance by *E. coli* to ampicillin and first-generation cephalosporins (cephalexin, cefazolin), these agents are not recommended.[4] Ceftriaxone, 1 to 2 g IV as a single daily dose, is effective and, given its extended spectrum, provides excellent coverage against the major uropathogens (except *Enterococcus*). After discharge, ceftriaxone can be continued as a single daily dose of 1 to 2 g as home parenteral therapy. Alternatively, an oral cephalosporin or trimethoprim-sulfamethoxazole can be given, depending on the results of susceptibility studies. Some authors favor an initial combination of ampicillin plus gentamicin.[104] Patients should respond within 48 hours. For patients who do not respond, investigation for urinary obstruction or complications of renal infection (e.g., perinephric abscess) should be undertaken. Once hospitalized patients are afebrile and asymptomatic for 24 to 48 hours, they may be discharged to complete a 14-day course of therapy.

TABLE 38-11 ANTIMICROBIAL TREATMENT OF ACUTE PYELONEPHRITIS IN PREGNANT WOMEN

Agent	Dosage
Outpatient Regimens (14 days)	
Amoxicillin	500 mg tid
Amoxicillin-clavulanate	875/125 mg bid
Trimethoprim-sulfamethoxazole DS	160/800 mg bid
Parenteral Regimens	
Ceftriaxone	1-2 g q24h
Cefepime	2 g q8h
Cefotetan	2 g q12h
Cefotaxime	1-2 g q8h
Trimethoprim-sulfamethoxazole	2 mg/kg q6h
Ampicillin	2 g q6h
PLUS Gentamicin	3-5 mg/kg/day (qd or in 3 divided doses)
Cefazolin	1-2 g q8h
PLUS Gentamicin	3-5 mg/kg/day in 3 divided doses or 7 mg/kg of ideal body weight q24h
OR Aztreonam	1-2 g q8 to 12h (in lieu of gentamicin)
Ampicillin-sulbactam	1.5 g q6h
Piperacillin-tazobactam	3.75 g q6-8h

DS, double strength.

Administration of aminoglycosides requires particular caution. Although they are rare with the dosage and duration of aminoglycosides used in the treatment of acute uncomplicated pyelonephritis, both maternal and fetal nephrotoxicity and ototoxicity have been reported, especially with prolonged use. The more frequent occurrence of renal dysfunction in pregnant women with acute pyelonephritis should raise additional concerns regarding the use of aminoglycosides[4] Therefore, unless the causative microorganism is resistant to other antimicrobials or the patient is allergic to other agents, aminoglycoside use is best avoided. A possible exception is the pregnant woman with severe septic shock, for whom an aminoglycoside should be used to provide coverage against more resistant gram-negative enterobacteria such as *Pseudomonas aeruginosa*, *Enterobacter* species., or *Citrobacter* species. In pregnant women receiving an aminoglycoside, serum levels should be monitored to ensure adequate serum concentrations and prevent toxicity. Either multidose gentamicin (3-5 mg/kg/24 hours in 3 divided doses) or single-dose gentamicin daily regimen is appropriate.

Prevention

Both secondary and tertiary prevention strategies are critical to prevent acute pyelonephritis during pregnancy. As previously noted, the major factors associated with development of acute pyelonephritis in pregnancy are the presence of ASB which antedates the pregnancy and the physiologic changes of pregnancy that predispose to ascent of bacteria to the upper urinary tract.

There are no known methods of primary prevention for acute pyelonephritis. However, screening for, and eradication of, bacteriuria early in pregnancy substantially reduces the incidence of acute pyelonephritis. Daily nighttime suppressive therapy after treatment of acute pyelonephritis significantly reduces the risk for recurrent acute pyelonephritis during pregnancy or immediately after delivery.

After completion of therapy for acute pyelonephritis during pregnancy, 30% to 40% of women have recurrent bacteriuria. If this is left untreated, approximately 25% develop recurrent pyelonephritis. Harris and Gilstrap[139] reported that, among patients not receiving suppressive antimicrobial regimens for the duration of pregnancy, 60% had a recurrent episode of acute pyelonephritis. In the group maintained on suppressive therapy, the recurrence rate was only 2.7%. Other studies have reported a similar high rate of recurrence in pregnant women after an episode of acute pyelonephritis if they did not receive suppressive therapy.[161]

The recommended drug for suppression after treatment of acute pyelonephritis in pregnancy is nitrofurantoin, 100 mg at bedtime for the duration of the pregnancy. Alternatively, trimethoprim-sulfamethoxazole 160/800 mg daily at bedtime may be given, recognizing that the sulfa moiety in the sulfamethoxazole confers a small risk of kernicterus in the newborn if given in the third trimester. An acceptable alternative to daily suppressive therapy is to obtain urine cultures every 2 weeks for the duration of pregnancy in order to detect and promptly treat recurrent bacteriuria.[162] Although recurrent or persistent bacteriuria was found to be more common with this latter approach, the rates of acute pyelonephritis were similar in the urine culture group and the suppressive therapy group. Daily suppressive therapy is more cost-effective than frequent reculturing.

Chorioamnionitis

Bacterial infection of the amniotic cavity is a major cause of perinatal mortality and maternal morbidity. Indeed, in the last few years, significant associations between clinical intra-amniotic infection and long-term neurologic development in the newborn, including cerebral palsy, have been reported (see Chapter 58).

A number of terms for this infection have been used, including "clinical chorioamnionitis," "amnionitis," "intrapartum infection," "amniotic fluid infection," and "intra-amniotic infection." The term *clinical chorioamnionitis* is invoked to distinguish the clinical syndrome of fever and uterine tenderness from ASB colonization, subclinical infection of the amniotic cavity, or histologic inflammation of the placenta and fetal membranes in the absence of maternal symptoms.

Clinical chorioamnionitis occurs in 0.5% to 10% of pregnancies.[163] Histologic chorioamnionitis occurs more frequently than does clinically evident infection, being present in up to 20% of term deliveries and more than half of preterm deliveries.

Pathogenesis

With the onset of labor or with rupture of the membranes, bacteria from the lower genital tract are able to ascend into the amniotic cavity. This is the most common pathway for development of clinical chorioamnionitis. Occasional cases occurring in the absence of membrane rupture or labor support a less frequent hematogenous or transplacental route of infection. For example, fulminating clinical chorioamnionitis with intact membranes may be caused by *Listeria monocytogenes*. Less commonly, the infection may develop as a consequence of obstetric procedures, such as cervical cerclage, amniocentesis, or percutaneous umbilical blood sampling. The absolute risk of chorioamnionitis is low with all of these procedures, occurring in 2% to 8% of patients after cerclage, in fewer than 1% after amniocentesis, and in up to 5% after intrauterine transfusion. Bacteria also may reach the amniotic cavity from extragenital sources such as the urinary tract or periodontal tissue.

Epidemiology

Clinical chorioamnionitis is a leading risk factor for neonatal sepsis. Yancey and coworkers[164] found this infection to have by far the highest odds ratio (OR, 25) for suspected or proven neonatal sepsis, compared with other obstetric risk factors such as preterm delivery, rupture of membranes more than 12 hours, postpartum endometritis, or maternal carriage of GBS.

Risk factors for clinical chorioamnionitis are largely obstetric conditions in patients experiencing protracted labor. They include

- Low parity
- Prolonged labor
- Prolonged rupture of membranes
- Multiple vaginal examinations in labor
- Internal fetal monitoring
- Maternal BV[165-169]
- Microbiology

As with other pelvic infections, clinical chorioamnionitis is usually polymicrobial in origin. The most common organisms found in the amniotic fluid of women with chorioamnionitis are *Bacteroides* species (25%), *G. vaginalis* (24%), GBS (12%), other aerobic streptococci (13%), *E. coli* (10%), and other aerobic gram-negative rods (10%).[170]

A role for genital mycoplasmas has been suggested by case reports of their isolation from amniotic fluid of clinically infected patients and by a controlled study reporting that 35% of fluid specimens from patients with chorioamnionitis yielded *M. hominis*, whereas only 8% of matched control fluids had this organism ($P < .001$).[171]

Present evidence suggests a small role, if any, for *C. trachomatis* in amniotic fluid infections. This organism rarely is isolated in cases of clinical chorioamnionitis, and no significant antibody changes to *C. trachomatis* have been noted in sera of women with this infection. Pregnant women with cervical *C. trachomatis* infections do not have higher rates of intrapartum fever.[72,172]

Diagnosis

The clinical diagnosis of chorioamnionitis requires a high index of suspicion. Usual laboratory indicators of infection, such as positive stains for organisms or leukocytes and positive cultures, are found much more frequently than is clinically evident infection. Diagnosis typically is based on the signs of maternal fever, maternal or fetal tachycardia, uterine tenderness, foul odor of the amniotic fluid, and leukocytosis. Bacteremia occurs in approximately 10% of the cases. Because peripheral blood leukocytosis occurs commonly in normal labor, a high white blood cell count (>15,000/mL) supports, but is not diagnostic of, infection.

Direct examination of the amniotic fluid, via amniocentesis or aspiration through an intrauterine pressure catheter, may provide important diagnostic information. Positive amniotic fluid Gram stains for bacteria or leukocytes occur significantly more often in women with clinical chorioamnionitis than in matched controls.[170] In patients with suspected amnionitis, low amniotic fluid glucose levels are a good predictor of a positive amniotic fluid culture but a poorer predictor of clinical chorioamnionitis. If the amniotic fluid glucose concentration is greater than 20 mg/dL, the likelihood of a positive culture is less than 2%. If the glucose level is less than 5 mg/dL, the likelihood of a positive culture rises to approximately 90%.[173,174] Although the test is not readily available to the clinician, an elevated concentration of interleukin 6 (IL-6) in the amniotic fluid is the most sensitive and specific marker for predicting a positive amniotic fluid culture.[174]

Management

If acute chorioamnionitis is strongly suspected, most experts agree that prompt institution of intravenous antibiotics and delivery of the fetus are required. However, specific points of management details remain unresolved.

Regarding the timing of delivery, excellent maternal-neonatal outcome has been reported without the use of arbitrary time limits. Gibbs and colleagues[170] reported on a policy in which cesarean delivery was performed only for standard obstetric indications and not for the presence of clinical chorioamnionitis alone. The mean time from diagnosis to delivery was between 3 and 5 hours, and more than 90% of patients were delivered within 12 hours after diagnosis. Those who were delivered vaginally had lower rates of morbidity. No critical interval from diagnosis of chorioamnionitis to delivery could be identified.

Three studies demonstrated a significant advantage for intrapartum rather than immediate postpartum antibiotic treatment (Table 38-12). In a nonrandomized trial, Sperling and coworkers[175] reported a lower incidence of neonatal sepsis when antibiotic treatment was

TABLE 38-12 RATES OF NEONATAL SEPSIS AFTER INTRAPARTUM VERSUS NEONATAL ANTIBIOTIC TREATMENT IN CASES OF INTRA-AMNIOTIC INFECTION

		Rate of Neonatal Sepsis (%)		
Study	*N*	Intrapartum Treatment	Neonatal Treatment	*P*
Sperling et al, 1987	257	2.8	19.6	.001
Gibbs et al, 1988	45	0	21	.03
Gilstrap et al, 1988	273	1.5	5.7	.06

begun at the time of diagnosis, compared with treatment begun immediately after delivery. Gilstrap and colleagues[176] found an almost fourfold reduction in neonatal sepsis with use of intrapartum treatment (5.7% versus 1.5%, $P = .06$). In a randomized trial, Gibbs and colleagues[177] used ampicillin (2 g intravenously every 6 hours) plus gentamicin (1.5 mg/kg every 8 hours), initiating treatment either intrapartum or immediately postpartum. In addition, clindamycin was used after umbilical cord clamping if cesarean delivery was performed, because of the high failure rate of ampicillin and gentamicin alone in women delivered abdominally. Maternal outcome was improved, and confirmed neonatal sepsis was decreased by intrapartum treatment. Other regimens employing an extended-spectrum penicillin (e.g., ampicillin plus a β-lactamase inhibitor) or other agents with similar activity may be equally effective, but no comparative trials have been performed.

The duration of postpartum antibiotic therapy needed for patients with clinical chorioamnionitis was addressed in a randomized clinical trial by Edwards and Duff.[178] They showed that one additional dose of a broad-spectrum combination of antibiotics (ampicillin plus gentamicin) was sufficient postpartum therapy for women with clinical chorioamnionitis. As mentioned previously, it is imperative that a drug with excellent anaerobic coverage (e.g., clindamycin, metronidazole) be given intraoperatively to women undergoing cesarean delivery.

Short-Term Outcome

Since 1979, reports from systematically collected data on the outcome of mothers and neonates in pregnancies complicated by intra-amniotic infection have shown a vastly improved perinatal outcome compared with older studies. Maternal outcome is excellent, with no deaths, few cases of septic shock, and rare pelvic abscesses. The cesarean delivery rate is increased twofold to threefold in all studies, usually because of dystocia. Perinatal mortality is increased in cases of clinical chorioamnionitis, but little of the excess mortality can be attributed to infection per se. Among term infants born after clinical chorioamnionitis, perinatal mortality is less than 1%.

Yoder and colleagues[179] published a case-control study of 67 patients with microbiologically confirmed clinical chorioamnionitis at term. There was only one perinatal death, which was unrelated to infection. Cerebrospinal fluid cultures were negative in all 49 infants sampled, and there was no clinical evidence of meningitis. Chest radiographs were interpreted as "possible" pneumonia in 20% and as "unequivocal" pneumonia in only 4%. Neonatal bacteremia was documented in 8%. There was no significant difference in the frequency of low Apgar scores between the chorioamnionitis and control groups.

TABLE 38-13 META-ANALYSIS OF CHORIOAMNIONITIS AS A RISK FACTOR FOR CEREBRAL PALSY AND CYSTIC PERIVENTRICULAR LEUKOMALACIA

Diagnosis	*N*	RR (95% CI)
Preterm Infants		
Cerebral Palsy		
Clinical chorioamnionitis	11	1.9 (1.4-2.5)
Histologic chorioamnionitis	5	1.6 (0.9-2.7)
Cystic PVL		
Clinical chorioamnionitis	6	3.0 (2.2-4.0)
Histologic chorioamnionitis	7	2.1 (1.5-2.9)
Term Infants		
Cerebral Palsy		
Clinical chorioamnionitis	2	4.7 (1.3-16.2)
Histologic chorioamnionitis	1	8.9 (1.9-40)

CI, confidence interval; PVL, periventricular leukomalacia; RR, relative risk.

Data from Grether JK, Nelson KB: Maternal infection and cerebral palsy in infants of normal birth weight. JAMA 278:207, 1997; Wu YW, Colford JM Jr: Chorioamnionitis as a risk factor for cerebral palsy: A meta-analysis. JAMA 284:1417, 2000.

Preterm neonates born to mothers with clinical chorioamnionitis experience a higher frequency of complications than do those born to mothers without this disorder. Garite and Freeman[180] noted that the perinatal death rate was significantly higher in 47 preterm neonates with chorioamnionitis than in 204 uninfected neonates with similar birth weights (13% versus 3%, $P < .05$). The group with chorioamnionitis also included a significantly higher number with respiratory distress syndrome (34% versus 16%, $P < .01$) and infection (17% versus 7%, $P < .05$).

Patients with clinical chorioamnionitis are more likely to require cesarean delivery, often for uterine dysfunction, inadequate uterine response to oxytocin, or abnormal labor progress even when uterine activity is adequate. And, when the combination of prematurity and chorioamnionitis occurs, the risk of serious sequelae in the neonate is increased.

Long-Term Outcome

There is increasing evidence that intrauterine infection is associated with increased risks of respiratory distress syndrome, periventricular leukomalacia, and cerebral palsy. The unifying hypothesis for these varying morbidities is that intra-amniotic infection leads to fetal infection and to an overexuberant fetal production of cytokines, which leads in turn to pulmonary and brain cell damage. The "fetal inflammatory response syndrome" has been likened to the systemic inflammatory response syndrome in adults. Several studies have linked maternal infection with cerebral palsy and with cystic necrosis of the white matter in preterm and term infants. Intrauterine exposure to maternal infection is associated with an increased risk of cerebral palsy (OR, 9.3) in infants of normal birth weight.[181] The results of a recent meta-analysis are summarized in Table 38-13.

Amniotic fluid concentrations of the inflammatory cytokines, IL-1β, IL-6, and tumor necrosis factor are higher in preterm infants with periventricular leukomalacia than in those without such lesions.[182] In addition, the presence of cerebral palsy at 3 years of age is more common in infants delivered preterm with funisitis or elevated amniotic fluid concentrations of IL-6 or IL-8.[183] Among preterm infants, respiratory distress syndrome has been significantly associated with high levels of tumor necrosis factor in amniotic fluid, with positive cultures of amniotic fluid, and with severe histologic chorioamnionitis, even after adjustment for birth weight, infant gender, race, and mode of delivery. These observations collectively have aroused renewed interest in the importance of the long-term effects of intrauterine infection, as well as strategies to avoid their serious complications.[184] These issues also are addressed in Chapter 58.

Prevention

Numerous approaches have been tested as preventive techniques. Chlorhexidine vaginal washes during labor[185,186] and selected infection-control measures[168] have been ineffective. Antepartum treatment of BV has not been shown to decrease the rate of chorioamnionitis.[187] Use of broad-spectrum antibiotics in patients with preterm labor but intact membranes appears to be ineffective overall in decreasing chorioamnionitis.[188]

Intrapartum prophylaxis to prevent neonatal GBS sepsis decreases the frequency of chorioamnionitis. Use of a screening-based strategy (which results in more women receiving antibiotics) compared with a risk-based strategy produces lower rates of chorioamnionitis.[189] In addition, active management of labor,[190] induction of labor (compared with expectant management) after PROM at term,[191] and use of antibiotics in selected patients with PROM[192-195] have each been shown to decrease the rate of chorioamnionitis.

Episiotomy Infection

Although episiotomy and vaginal laceration repair are commonly performed after a vaginal delivery, infection is an infrequent complication. Shy and Eschenbach[196] classified episiotomy infections according to the extent of the structures involved (Fig. 38-5). The same classification may be used for infections of perineal lacerations.

Simple Episiotomy Infection

A localized infection may involve only the skin and subcutaneous tissue (including the Camper fascia of the perineum) adjacent to the episiotomy. Signs are local edema and erythema with exudate; more extensive findings should raise the suspicion of a deeper infection. Treatment consists of opening, exploring, and débriding the perineal wound. Drainage alone usually is adequate, but appropriate antibiotics should be given if there is marked superficial cellulitis or isolation of group A streptococci. The episiotomy incision should not be immediately resutured. Most episiotomy wounds heal by granulation. Wounds involving the external anal sphincter or rectal mucosa may be repaired after the field is free of infection.

Recently, there has been considerable interest in early repair of episiotomy dehiscence. Such dehiscence usually is associated with infection. Early repair requires prompt and meticulous débridement at the time of diagnosis, followed by antibiotics and frequent cleansing. When the tissue appears healthy (usually after about 1 week or longer),

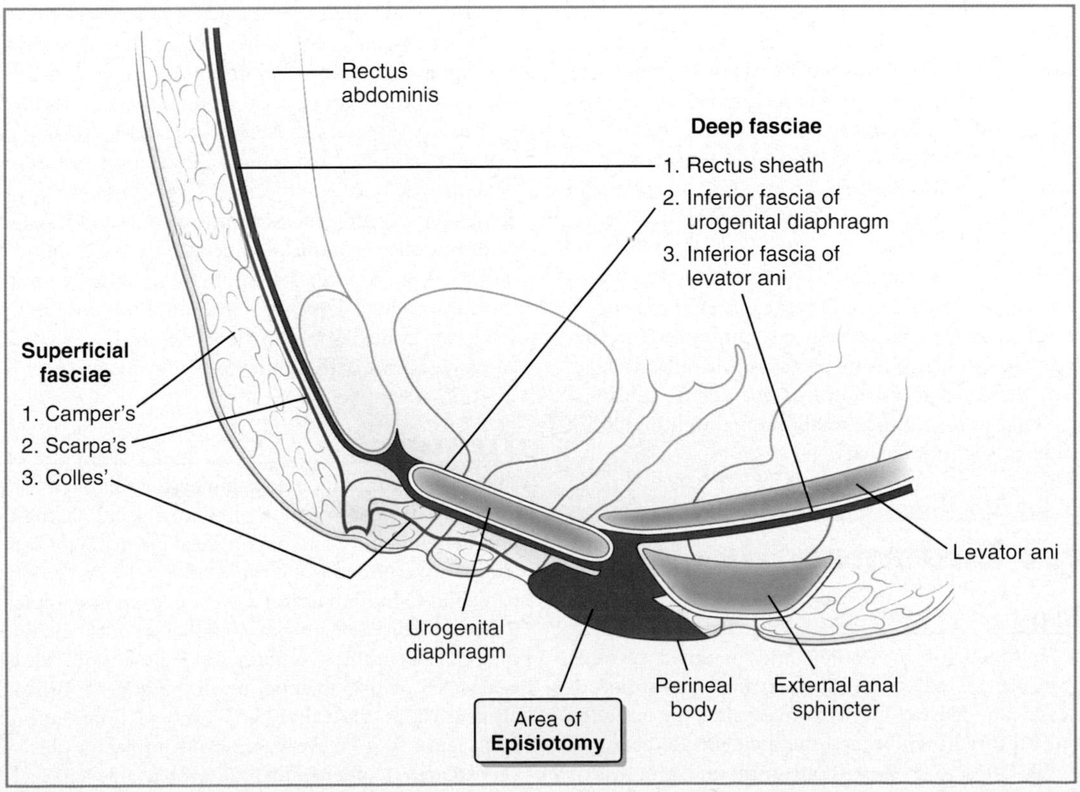

FIGURE 38-5 Structures potentially involved in episiotomy. Paramedian sagittal section of the fascial layers of the perineum. (From Shy KK, Eschenbach DA: Fatal perineal cellulitis from an episiotomy site. Obstet Gynecol 54:292, 1979. Reprinted with permission of the American College of Obstetricians and Gynecologists.)

a definitive repair can be undertaken. For fourth-degree lacerations, a bowel preparation should be given before the repair. Such repair is an attractive option compared with the delay of 2 to 3 months recommended in older literature.[197-200]

Necrotizing Fasciitis

With necrotizing fasciitis, both layers of the superficial perineal fascia (i.e., the Camper and Colles fascias) become necrotic, and infection spreads along the fascial planes to the abdominal wall, thigh, and/or buttock. Typically, the deep perineal fascia (i.e., inferior fascia of the urogenital diaphragm) is not involved. Skin findings are variable but initially include edema and erythema without clear borders. Later, there is progressive, brawny edema of the skin. The skin becomes blue or brown, and bullae or frank gangrene may occur. As the infection progresses, there may be either loss of sensation or hyperesthesia.

Associated findings include marked hemoconcentration, although often after fluid replacement the patient is anemic. Hypocalcemia also may develop, because of the saponification of fatty acids. Traditionally, this infection has been associated with group A streptococci, but anaerobic bacteria also play an important role.

For therapy to be effective, appropriate antibiotics must be combined with adequate débridement. Indications for surgical exploration include extension beyond the labia, unilateral or markedly asymmetric edema, signs of systemic toxicity or deterioration, and failure of the infection to resolve within 24 to 48 hours. At surgery, necrotizing fasciitis may be recognized by separation of the skin from the deep fascia, absence of bleeding along incision lines, and a serosanguineous discharge. Dissection must be wide enough to remove all necrotic tissue.

Myonecrosis

Myonecrosis is an infection that involves the muscle beneath the deep fascia. It often is the result of a myotoxin elaborated by *C. perfringens*, but it occasionally can result from an extension of necrotizing fasciitis. Onset may be early and typically is accompanied by severe pain. Treatment of this condition also consists of extensive débridement and high-dose antibiotics, including penicillin, if clostridia infection is suspected.

Clinicians should recognize that not all puerperal vulvar edema signifies serious perineal infection. In fact, most cases of vulvar edema result from less serious causes, such as hematoma, prolonged bearing-down in labor, generalized edema from preeclampsia, allergic reactions, or trauma. In these instances, however, the edema usually is bilateral, does not extend to the buttock or abdominal wall, and is not accompanied by signs of systemic toxicity.

Puerperal Endometritis

Epidemiology

The frequency of endometritis in women after planned cesarean delivery ranges from 5% to 15%, depending on maternal socioeconomic status. If cesarean delivery is performed after an extended period of labor and ruptured membranes, the incidence of endometritis is approximately 30% to 35% without antibiotic prophylaxis and approximately 15% with prophylaxis. In highly indigent patient populations, the frequency of postcesarean endometritis may be even higher.[201]

Pathogenesis

Endometritis is a polymicrobial infection caused by microorganisms that are part of the normal vaginal flora. These aerobic and anaerobic bacteria gain access to the upper genital tract, peritoneal cavity, and bloodstream as a result of vaginal examinations during labor and manipulations during surgery. The most common pathogens are GBS, anaerobic gram-positive cocci (streptococci and peptostreptococci species), anaerobic gram-negative bacilli (predominantly *E. coli*, *K. pneumoniae*, and *Proteus* species), and anaerobic gram-negative bacilli (principally *Bacteroides* and *Prevotella* species). *C. trachomatis* is not a common cause of early-onset puerperal endometritis but has been implicated in late-onset infection. The genital mycoplasmas, *M. hominis* and *Ureaplasma urealyticum*, may be pathogenic in some patients, but they usually are present in association with other, more highly virulent bacteria.[201,202]

The principal risk factors for endometritis are cesarean delivery, young age, low socioeconomic status, extended duration of labor, extended duration of ruptured membranes, and multiple vaginal examinations. Preexisting infection of the lower genital tract due to gonorrhea, GBS, or BV also predisposes to ascending infection after delivery.[203]

Diagnosis

Patients with endometritis typically have a fever of 38° C or higher within 36 hours after delivery. Associated findings include malaise, tachycardia, lower abdominal pain and tenderness, uterine tenderness, and malodorous lochia. A small number of patients have a tender, indurated, inflammatory mass in the broad ligament, posterior cul-de-sac, or retrovesical space.

The initial differential diagnosis of puerperal fever should include endometritis, atelectasis, pneumonia, viral syndrome, pyelonephritis, and appendicitis. Distinction among these disorders usually can be made on the basis of physical examination and selected laboratory tests such as a peripheral white blood cell count, urinalysis and culture, and, in some patients, chest radiography. Blood cultures are indicated for patients who have a poor initial response to therapy or for those who are immunocompromised or are at increased risk for bacterial endocarditis. Cultures of the lower genital tract and endometrium are rarely indicated. Such cultures are difficult to obtain without contamination from lower genital tract flora. In addition, by the time these culture results are available, most patients already have responded to treatment and have been discharged from the hospital.

Treatment

The most commonly used regimen for treatment of puerperal endometritis is the combination of clindamycin (900 mg IV every 8 hours) plus gentamicin (7.5 mg/kg of ideal body weight every 24 hours). An alternative regimen is metronidazole (500 mg IV every 12 hours) plus penicillin (5 million units IV every 6 hours) or ampicillin (2 g IV every 6 hours) plus gentamicin (7 mg/kg of ideal body weight every 24 hours). Both of these combination regimens provide excellent coverage against all of the potential pelvic pathogens. Broad-spectrum single agents such as cefotetan (2 g IV every 12 hours), ticarcillin plus clavulanic acid (3.1 g IV every 6 hours), ampicillin plus sulbactam (3 g IV every 6 hours), piperacillin plus tazobactam (3.375 g IV every 6 hours), imipenem-cilastatin (500 mg IV every 6 hours), or ertapenem (1 g IV every 24 hours) may be used for treatment of endometritis. However, in most hospital formularies, these broad-spectrum single agents are more expensive than the generic combination regimens listed earlier.[204]

Once intravenous antibiotics are begun, approximately 90% to 95% of patients experience defervescence within 48 to 72 hours. Once the patient has been afebrile and asymptomatic for approximately 24 hours, parenteral antibiotics should be discontinued, and the patient should be discharged. As a general rule, an extended course of oral antibiotics is not necessary after discharge.[205] There are at least two exceptions to this general rule. First, patients who have had a vaginal delivery and who defervescence within 24 hours are candidates for early discharge. In these individuals, a short course of an oral antibiotic such as amoxicillin-clavulanate (875 mg orally every 12 hours) may be substituted for continued parenteral therapy. Second, patients who have had a staphylococcal bacteremia may require a more extended period of administration of parenteral and oral antibiotics.[204]

Patients who fail to respond to the antibiotic therapy outlined here usually have one of two problems. The first is a resistant organism. In patients who are treated with clindamycin plus gentamicin, the principal resistant organism is enterococcus. This organism can be adequately covered by adding ampicillin or penicillin to the treatment regimen. For those who are taking a broad-spectrum single agent, potential weaknesses in coverage include some aerobic and some anaerobic gram-negative bacilli. These patients should be changed to the triple-drug regimen (clindamycin or metronidazole, plus penicillin or ampicillin, plus gentamicin).

The second major cause of treatment failure is an abdominal wound infection. Some patients have an actual incisional abscess. In these cases, the wound should be opened to effect drainage, and an antibiotic that has excellent antistaphylococcal coverage should be added to the treatment regimen. Most experts prefer an agent such as nafcillin (2 g IV every 6 hours). Some women do not have frank pus in the incision but rather an extensive cellulitis in the soft tissue around the incision. In these patients, the wound does not have to be opened. However, an antistaphylococcal antibiotic should be added to the treatment regimen.[204]

Other possible causes of a poor response to treatment include pelvic abscess, septic pelvic vein thrombophlebitis, and drug reaction. The management of pelvic abscess and septic pelvic vein thrombophlebitis is discussed in the following sections. Drug reaction should be suspected if the patient has a peripheral blood eosinophilia and if the temperature elevation corresponds with the time of drug administration. In these individuals, discontinuation of the antibiotic usually results in prompt resolution of fever.

Prevention

Ideally, the best approach to endometritis is prevention of infection. In this regard, prophylactic antibiotics clearly are of proven value in reducing the frequency of postcesarean endometritis, particularly in women having surgery after an extended period of labor and ruptured membranes. The most appropriate agent for prophylaxis is a limited-spectrum (first-generation) cephalosporin such as cefazolin. Cefazolin should be administered in an intravenous dose of 1 g immediately after the neonate's umbilical cord is clamped. Although extended-spectrum penicillins and cephalosporins are effective for prophylaxis, they offer no advantage over cefazolin and are several times more expensive. In addition, widespread use of these drugs for prophylaxis ultimately may limit their usefulness for treatment of an established infection. Patients who have an immediate hypersensitivity reaction to β-lactam antibiotics should receive a single dose of clindamycin (900 mg IV) plus gentamicin (1.5 mg/kg IV) immediately after the umbilical cord is clamped. Although these antibiotics are used for treatment of overt infections, their administration still is warranted in penicillin-allergic patients who are at high risk for postoperative infection.[204,205]

Another important method for preventing endometritis is to remove the placenta by gentle traction on the umbilical cord rather than manually. Several investigators[206,207] have confirmed that, when other factors are controlled, manual removal of the placenta significantly increases the frequency of postcesarean endometritis.

Wound Infection

Epidemiology and Pathogenesis

Wound infection after cesarean delivery usually occurs in association with endometritis rather than as an isolated condition. Approximately 3% to 5% of women with postcesarean endometritis have a concurrent wound infection. The principal risk factors for this complication are low socioeconomic status, extended duration of labor, extended duration of ruptured membranes, preexisting infection such as chorioamnionitis, obesity, insulin dependent diabetes, an immunodeficiency disorder, corticosteroid or immunosuppressive therapy, and poor surgical technique. The major organisms that cause postcesarean wound infection are *S. aureus*, aerobic streptococci, and aerobic and anaerobic gram-negative bacilli.[208]

Diagnosis

The diagnosis of wound infection should be of paramount consideration in a woman who has had a poor initial clinical response to antibiotic therapy for endometritis. Clinical examination usually shows erythema, induration, and tenderness at the margins of the abdominal incision and pus exudes from within the incision. Some patients have an extensive cellulitis without actual purulent drainage.

Clinical examination usually is sufficient to establish the correct diagnosis. Culture of the wound exudate should be performed routinely because of the possibility of a methicillin-resistant *Staphylococcus aureus* (MRSA) infection.[209]

Treatment

If frank pus or significant serosanguineous effusion is present in the incision, the wound must be opened and drained completely. Antibiotic therapy should be modified to provide coverage against staphylococci. Nafcillin, 2 g IV every 6 hours, is an appropriate drug for this purpose. In patients who are allergic to β-lactam antibiotics, vancomycin, 1 g IV every 12 hours, is an acceptable alternative.[204]

Once the wound is opened, it should be repacked two to three times daily with gauze dampened with saline. A clean dressing should be applied, and the wound should initially be allowed to heal by secondary intention. After all signs of infection have resolved and healthy granulation tissue is apparent, a secondary closure may be considered. Antibiotics should be continued until the base of the wound is clean and all signs of cellulitis have resolved. Patients usually can be treated on an outpatient basis once the acute signs of infection have subsided.

Necrotizing fasciitis is an uncommon but extremely serious complication of abdominal wound infection. It has also been reported in association with infection of the episiotomy site (see earlier discussion). This condition is particularly likely to occur in patients who have insulin-dependent diabetes, cancer, or an immunodeficiency disorder.

Multiple bacterial pathogens, particularly anaerobes, have been isolated from patients with necrotizing fasciitis.

This condition should be suspected if the margins of the wound become discolored, cyanotic, and devoid of sensation. When the wound is opened, the subcutaneous tissue is easily dissected free of the underlying fascia, but muscle tissue is not affected. If the diagnosis is uncertain, a tissue biopsy specimen should be performed and examined immediately by frozen section.

Necrotizing fasciitis is a life-threatening condition that requires aggressive medical and surgical management. Broad-spectrum antibiotics with activity against all potential pathogens should be administered. The patient's intravascular volume should be maintained with infusions of crystalloid, and electrolyte abnormalities should be promptly corrected. Of greatest importance, the wound must be completely débrided and all necrotic tissue removed. In many instances, the required dissection is extensive and is best managed in consultation with an experienced general or plastic surgeon.

Pelvic Abscess

Epidemiology and Pathogenesis

With the advent of modern antibiotics, pelvic abscesses after cesarean or vaginal delivery have become extremely rare. As with wound infections, pelvic abscesses, when they do occur, usually develop in women who initially had postcesarean endometritis. The frequency of pelvic abscess as a complication of endometritis is less than 1%.[201]

Pelvic abscesses typically are located in the anterior or posterior cul-de-sac or within the leaves of the broad ligament. The bacteria usually isolated from abscess cavities are anaerobic gram-positive organisms such as *Peptococci* and *Peptostreptococci* species, anaerobic gram-negative bacilli (particularly *Bacteroides* and *Prevotella* species), and aerobic gram-negative bacilli such as *E. coli*, *Klebsiella*, and *Proteus* species.[202,203]

Diagnosis

Patients who have a pelvic abscess typically experience persistent fever despite appropriate antibiotic therapy for endometritis. In addition, they usually have malaise, tachycardia, tachypnea, lower abdominal pain and tenderness, and a palpable pelvic mass. The peripheral white blood cell count usually is elevated (>20,000/mm^3), and there is a shift toward immature cell forms. The diagnosis of pelvic abscess may be confirmed by ultrasound, computed tomographic (CT) scanning, or magnetic resonance imaging (MRI).[210] The latter two tests are slightly more sensitive, but more expensive, than ultrasound.

Treatment

Patients who develop an abscess after delivery usually require surgical drainage in addition to broad-spectrum antibiotic therapy. If the abscess is located in the posterior cul-de-sac, colpotomy drainage may be feasible. For abscesses located anterior or lateral to the uterus, drainage may be accomplished by CT- or ultrasound-guided placement of a catheter drain. If access to the abscess cavity is limited by the interposition of bowel, or if the abscess is extensive, open laparotomy is indicated.[207]

Patients also must receive antibiotics that have excellent activity against multiple aerobic and anaerobic pathogens. One regimen that has been tested extensively in obstetric patients with serious infections is the combination of penicillin (5 million units IV every 6 hours) or ampicillin (2 g IV every 6 hours), plus gentamicin (7 mg/kg of ideal body weight every 24 hours), plus clindamycin (900 mg IV every 8 hours) or metronidazole (500 mg IV every 12 hours). If the patient is allergic to β-lactam antibiotics, vancomycin (1 g IV every 12 hours) can be substituted for penicillin or ampicillin. Aztreonam (1 g IV every 8 hours) can be used in lieu of gentamicin if the patient is at risk for nephrotoxicity. Alternatively, broad-spectrum agents, such as one of the carbapenems—imipenem-cilastatin (500 mg IV every 6 hours), meropenem (1 g IV every 8 hours), or ertapenem (1 g IV every 24 hours)—provide excellent coverage against the usual pathogens responsible for an abscess. Intravenous antibiotics should be continued until the patient has been afebrile and asymptomatic for a minimum of 24 to 48 hours. Thereafter, the patient should be treated with a combination of oral antibiotics that cover the major pathogens.[204] One appropriate regimen is ofloxacin (400 mg every 24 hours) or levofloxacin (750 mg every 24 hours) plus metronidazole (500 mg twice daily) to complete a total treatment course of 10 to 14 days.[12]

Septic Shock

Epidemiology and Pathogenesis

The term "severe sepsis" refers to infection-induced organ dysfunction or hypoperfusion abnormalities. *Septic shock* implies hypotension that is not reversed with fluid resuscitation and which is associated with multiorgan dysfunction.[208] In obstetric patients, the most common predisposing conditions for septic shock are septic abortion, acute pyelonephritis, chorioamnionitis, and puerperal endometritis. Fewer than 2% of patients with any of these conditions develop septic shock. The most common pathogenic organisms are *E. coli*, *K. pneumoniae*, and *Proteus* species. Highly virulent, drug-resistant organisms such as *Pseudomonas*, *Enterobacter*, and *Serratia* species are uncommon except in immunosuppressed patients.[209]

Aerobic gram-negative bacilli such as *E. coli* have a complex lipopolysaccharide in their cell wall, termed endotoxin. When released into the systemic circulation, endotoxin causes a variety of immunologic, hematologic, neurohormonal, and hemodynamic derangements that ultimately result in multiple-organ dysfunction.[211-213]

In the early stages of septic shock, patients usually are restless, disoriented, tachycardic, and hypotensive. Although hypothermia may be present initially, most patients subsequently have a high fever. The skin may be warm and flushed owing to a preliminary phase of vasodilation. Later, extensive vasoconstriction occurs, and the skin becomes cool and clammy. Cardiac arrhythmias may develop, and signs of myocardial ischemia may occur. Jaundice, typically due to hemolysis, may be evident. Urinary output decreases, and spontaneous bleeding from the genitourinary tract or venipuncture sites may occur as a result of a coagulopathy. ARDS is a common complication of sepsis and is usually manifested by dyspnea, stridor, cough, tachypnea, bilateral rales, and wheezing. In addition to these systemic signs and symptoms, affected patients also may have specific findings related to their primary site of infection, such as uterine tenderness in women with endometritis or chorioamnionitis or flank tenderness in patients with pyelonephritis.[212,213]

Diagnosis

The differential diagnosis of septic shock in obstetric patients includes hypovolemic and cardiogenic shock, diabetic ketoacidosis, anaphylactic reaction, anesthetic reaction, and pulmonary embolism. Distinction among these disorders usually can be made on the basis of a detailed history and physical examination and selected laboratory studies. The white blood cell count initially may be decreased in septic shock but subsequently becomes elevated. The hematocrit may be decreased if blood loss has occurred. The platelet count and serum fibrinogen concentration are typically decreased. Serum concentration of fibrin degradation products is usually elevated. The prothrombin time and activated partial thromboplastin time (aPTT) are frequently prolonged. Serum concentrations of transaminase enzymes and bilirubin often are increased. The blood urea nitrogen and serum creatinine concentrations are also increased.

Septic patients should have a chest radiograph to determine whether pneumonia or ARDS is present. In addition, a CT scan, MRI, or ultrasound study may be of value in localizing an abscess. Patients also require continuous electrocardiographic monitoring to detect arrhythmias or signs of myocardial ischemia. Blood samples for culture should be obtained, one drawn percutaneously and one drawn through each vascular device that has been in place longer than 48 hours.[211]

Treatment

The first priority in treatment is fluid resuscitation with isotonic crystalloids such as Ringer lactate solution or normal saline or colloids. There is no firm evidence that one type of solution is better than another, although crystalloids are used more commonly. Intravenous fluid administration should be titrated in accordance with the patient's pulse, blood pressure, and urine output. If the initial fluid infusion is not successful in restoring hemodynamic stability, a right-sided heart catheter should be inserted to monitor pulmonary artery wedge pressure. Treatment goals of fluid resuscitation include a central venous pressure of 8 to 12 mm Hg, a mean arterial pressure of 65 mm Hg or higher, urine output of 0.5 mL/kg or greater, and a mixed venous oxygen saturation of 70% or greater.[211]

The "7-3 rule" is helpful in guiding fluid resuscitation. Ringer lactate or normal saline should be infused at a rate of 10 mL/min for 15 minutes. If the pulmonary capillary wedge pressure (PCWP) does not increase by more than 3 mm Hg, the bolus should be repeated. If the PCWP increases by 7 mm Hg or more, the fluid bolus should be withheld. The optimal PCWP in septic patients is 12 to 16 mm Hg.[213] Transfusion of red blood cells is indicated to maintain a hemoglobin concentration of 7.0 to 9.0 g/L.

If fluid resuscitation alone does not restore adequate tissue perfusion, dopamine should be administered (starting dose, 1 to 3 μg/kg/min) to stimulate myocardial contractility and improve the perfusion of central organs. In some patients with persistent low cardiac output and low blood pressure in the face of adequate fluid resuscitation, dobutamine should be added to the vasopressor therapy to improve cardiac output. In addition, such patients should be treated with intravenous corticosteroids (hydrocortisone, 200 to 300 mg/day for 7 days in 3 or 4 divided doses or by continuous infusion).[211,214]

Patients in septic shock also should be treated with broad-spectrum antibiotics. The triple combination of penicillin or ampicillin, plus clindamycin or metronidazole, plus gentamicin (in the doses specified earlier for treatment of pelvic abscess) is an excellent initial regimen. Alternatively, a broad-spectrum antibiotic such as imipenem-cilastatin (500 mg IV every 6 hours), meropenem (1 g IV every 8 hours), ertapenem (1 g IV every 24 hours), piperacillin-tazobactam (3.375 g IV every 6 hours), ampicillin-sulbactam (3 g IV every 6 hours), or ticarcillin-clavulanic acid (3.1 g IV every 6 hours) can be administered. The duration of antibiotic therapy should be 5 to 10 days, depending on the rapidity of the patient's response.[204]

Patients also may require surgery to evacuate retained, infected products of conception, to drain a pelvic abscess, or to remove an infected intravascular catheter. Indicated surgery never should be delayed because the patient is unstable, because operative intervention may be precisely the step necessary to reverse septic shock.

The patient's core temperature should be maintained as close to normal as possible by use of antipyretics and a cooling blanket. Coagulation abnormalities should be corrected. Insulin should be administered as needed to maintain euglycemia. Granulocyte colony-stimulating factor may be indicated for severely neutropenic patients. Severely ill patients should receive prophylaxis for deep venous thrombosis with either unfractionated or fractionated heparin. They also should receive stress ulcer prophylaxis with histamine$_2$ (H_2) blockers.[211,214]

In addition, treatment with activated protein C (24 μg/kg/min for 96 hours) may be of value in decreasing mortality and minimizing organ dysfunction in severely ill patients.[214] Activated protein C ultimately reduces inflammation by inhibiting platelet aggregation, neutrophil recruitment, and degranulation of mast cells.

Patients should be given oxygen supplementation and observed closely for evidence of ARDS, which is one of the major causes of mortality in patients with severe sepsis.[215] Oxygenation should be monitored by means of a pulse oximeter or radial artery catheter. If evidence of respiratory failure develops, the patient should be intubated promptly and supported with mechanical ventilation and positive end-expiratory pressure.[211,215]

The prognosis in patients with septic shock clearly depends on the severity of the patient's underlying illness. In otherwise healthy patients, mortality should not exceed 15%. The prognosis for complete recovery is excellent, provided that the patient receives timely therapy.[215,216]

Septic Pelvic Vein Thrombophlebitis

Epidemiology and Pathogenesis

Like pelvic abscess, septic pelvic vein thrombophlebitis is extremely rare in modern obstetrics, occurring in approximately 1 of every 2000 pregnancies overall and in fewer than 1% of patients who have puerperal endometritis.[217] Septic pelvic vein thrombophlebitis occurs in two distinct forms. The most commonly described disorder is acute thrombosis of one (usually the right) or both ovarian veins (ovarian vein syndrome).[218] Affected patients typically develop a moderate temperature elevation in association with lower abdominal pain during the first 48 to 96 hours after delivery. The pain usually localizes to the side of the affected vein but may radiate into the groin, upper abdomen, or flank. In addition, nausea, vomiting, and abdominal bloating may be present.

On physical examination, the patient usually is found to have tachycardia. Tachypnea, dyspnea, and even stridor may be evident if septic pulmonary embolization has occurred. The abdomen is tender, and bowel sounds often are decreased or absent. Most patients have voluntary and involuntary guarding, and 50% to 70% have a tender, rope-like mass that originates near one cornua and extends laterally and cephalad toward the upper abdomen. The principal conditions that should be considered in the differential diagnosis of ovarian vein syndrome are acute pyelonephritis, nephrolithiasis, appendicitis, broad-ligament hematoma, adnexal torsion, and pelvic abscess.

The second presentation of septic pelvic vein thrombophlebitis has been termed "enigmatic fever."[219] These patients usually have been treated initially for presumed puerperal endometritis. Subsequently, they experience some subjective improvement, with the exception of persistent fever. They do not appear to be seriously ill, and positive findings are limited to persistent fever and tachycardia. Disorders that must be considered in the differential diagnosis of enigmatic fever are drug reaction, viral syndrome, recrudescence of connective tissue disease, and pelvic abscess.

Diagnosis

CT and MRI are the diagnostic tests of greatest value in confirming the diagnosis of pelvic vein thrombophlebitis.[220] These tests are most sensitive in detecting large thrombi in the major pelvic vessels. They are not as useful in identifying thrombi in smaller vessels. In some cases, the diagnosis is one of exclusion and is confirmed by observing the patient's response to an empiric trial of heparin.[217]

Treatment

The traditional treatment for patients with presumed septic pelvic vein thrombophlebitis is therapeutic anticoagulation with intravenous heparin. The dose of heparin should be adjusted to maintain the aPTT at approximately two times normal. Alternatively, medication may be adjusted to achieve a serum heparin concentration of 0.2 to 0.7 IU/mL. Intravenous heparin should be continued for 7 to 10 days, depending on the response to treatment. Long-term anticoagulation with oral agents probably is unnecessary unless the patient has massive clotting throughout the pelvic venous plexus or has sustained a pulmonary embolism. Patients should be given broad-spectrum antibiotics, such as those used for treating pelvic abscess, throughout the period of heparin administration.[217,221]

Once medical therapy is initiated, there is usually objective evidence of a response within 48 to 72 hours. If no improvement is noted, surgical intervention may be considered. The surgical approach should be tailored to the specific intraoperative findings. In most instances, treatment requires only ligation of the affected vessels. Extension of the thrombosis along the vena cava to the point of origin of the renal veins may require embolectomy. Excision of the infected vessel and removal of the ipsilateral adnexa and uterus are indicated only in the presence of a well-defined abscess. Consultation should be obtained from an experienced vascular surgeon if surgical intervention becomes necessary.[221]

Mastitis

Epidemiology and Pathogenesis

Mastitis occurs in 5% to 10% of lactating women.[223] The principal causative organisms are *S. aureus* and *Viridans streptococci*. These organisms are part of the mother's skin flora and are introduced into the milk ducts when the infant suckles.[222,223]

Diagnosis

Affected women initially experience malaise, followed by a relatively high fever (39° C or higher) and chills. Thereafter, an erythematous, tender area appears in the affected breast. In addition, patients also may experience pain and tenderness in the ipsilateral axilla, and the milk from the infected breast may be discolored. In a small percentage of patients, an actual abscess forms within the affected breast.[224]

The diagnosis of mastitis is usually established on the basis of the patient's symptoms and clinical examination findings. Culture of milk from the infected breast is not helpful. However, if an abscess is suspected on physical examination, the contents should be drained and cultured, particularly in light of the recent increase in methicillin-resistant staphylococcal infections.

Treatment

Mastitis usually can be treated successfully with oral antibiotics that have excellent coverage against staphylococci and streptococci. Initially, sodium dicloxacillin, 500 mg orally four times daily, is preferable. In a woman with a history of a mild allergic reaction to penicillin, cephalexin, 500 mg orally four times daily, may be substituted for sodium dicloxacillin. With a history of a serious immediate hypersensitivity reaction to penicillin, clindamycin, 300 mg orally every 6 hours, is an appropriate alternative. The duration of antibiotic therapy depends on the patient's response to treatment but usually should extend for approximately 7 to 10 days.[204]

There are no reports to suggest that nursing from the infected breast is contraindicated. Therefore, the patient should be encouraged to continue nursing once the tenderness in the affected breast has decreased.

Hospitalization and treatment with intravenous antibiotics should be considered for immunosuppressed patients and for those who are at particular risk for having complications should staphylococcal bacteremia develop (e.g., patients with prosthetic heart valves). In addition, women with a breast abscess should be hospitalized for intravenous antibiotic therapy and surgical drainage. Appropriate intravenous drugs include nafcillin (2 g every 6 hours), cefazolin (1 g every 8 hours), or vancomycin (1 g every 12 hours). Other agents with excellent antistaphylococcal coverage include linezolid (600 mg every 12 hours) and quinupristin/dalfopristin (7.5 mg/kg every 8 hours). These latter two drugs are extremely expensive and should not routinely be used as first-line agents.[204]

Prevention

In an effort to prevent mastitis, lactating women should be advised to take measures to prevent drying and cracking of the nipples. Specifically, they should avoid the use of alcohol-based products for cleaning the nipples and should apply a moisturizing agent such as lanolin to the nipple and areola after nursing.

Cytomegalovirus Infection

Epidemiology and Pathogenesis of Maternal and Fetal Infection

Cytomegalovirus (CMV) is a DNA virus that is a member of the herpesvirus family. Like other members of this family, CMV may remain latent in host cells after the initial infection. Recurrent infection is usually caused by reactivation of an endogenous latent virus rather than reinfection with a new viral strain.[225,226]

CMV is not highly contagious; close personal contact is required for infection to occur. Horizontal transmission may result from transplantation of an infected organ or transfusion of infected blood, sexual contact, or contact with contaminated saliva or urine. Vertical transmission may occur as a result of transplacental infection, exposure to contaminated genital tract secretions during delivery, or breastfeeding. The incubation period of CMV ranges from 28 to 60 days.[227]

Among young children, the most important risk factor for infection is close contact with playmates (e.g., from handling toys that are contaminated by infected saliva).[228,229] Most children who acquire CMV infection are asymptomatic. When clinical manifestations are present, they include malaise, low-grade fever, lymphadenopathy, and hepatosplenomegaly. Most immunocompetent adults with CMV also are asymptomatic or have only mild symptoms suggestive of a flulike illness. However, in an immunosuppressed patient, CMV infection can be quite serious.

The diagnosis of CMV infection is confirmed by viral culture. The highest concentrations of virus are in urine, seminal fluid, saliva, and breast milk, with most cultures becoming positive within 72 to 96 hours. PCR methodology permits identification of viral antigen within 24 hours.[225,227]

Serologic methods also are of value in establishing the diagnosis of CMV infection. Positive IgM titers usually decline rapidly over a period of 30 to 60 days, but they can remain elevated for many months. There is no single IgG titer that clearly differentiates acute from recurrent infection. However, a fourfold or greater change in the IgG titer over 2 weeks usually is consistent with recent acute infection. Another useful test for differentiating acute from recurrent infection is assessment of the avidity of IgG antibody. Low- to moderate-avidity IgG antibody, combined with the presence of IgM antibody, is consistent with acute infection. If high-avidity IgG antibody is present, the patient typically has recurrent infection.[230,231]

Approximately 50% to 80% of adult women in the United States have serologic evidence of past CMV infection. However, the presence of antibodies is not perfectly protective against either reinfection or vertical transmission of infection from mother to fetus. Therefore, pregnant women with either recurrent or primary infection pose a risk to their fetus.[229,232]

Antepartum (congenital) infection results from hematogenous dissemination of virus across the placenta and poses the greatest risk to the fetus. Dissemination is much more likely in the presence of a primary maternal infection. Among women who acquire primary CMV infection during pregnancy, approximately half will infect their fetus. The overall risk of congenital infection is greatest when maternal infection occurs in the third trimester, but the probability of severe fetal injury is highest when it occurs in the first trimester.

Approximately 5% to 15% of infants who develop congenital CMV infection as a result of primary maternal infection are symptomatic at birth. The most common clinical manifestations of severe neonatal infection are hepatosplenomegaly, intracranial calcifications, jaundice, growth restriction, microcephaly, chorioretinitis, hearing loss, thrombocytopenia, hyperbilirubinemia, and hepatitis. Approximately 30% of severely infected infants die, and 80% of survivors have major morbidity. Among the 85% to 90% of infants with congenital CMV infection who are asymptomatic at birth, 10% to 15% subsequently develop hearing loss, chorioretinitis, or dental defects within the first 2 years of life.[229,232]

Pregnant women who experience recurrent or reactivated CMV infection are much less likely to transmit infection to their fetus. If recurrent infection develops in pregnancy, approximately 5% to 10% of infants become infected; however, none of these neonates will be symptomatic at birth. The most common sequelae are hearing loss, visual deficits, and mild developmental delays.[232-235]

Perinatal infection can occur during delivery as a result of exposure to infected genital tract secretions. Infection also can occur as a result of breastfeeding. However, when the virus is acquired in one of these ways, infants rarely have major abnormalities.

Diagnosis of Congenital Infection

The most sensitive and specific test for diagnosing congenital CMV infection is the identification of CMV in amniotic fluid by either culture or PCR.[234,235] This test is of greater accuracy than cordocentesis for two major reasons. First, it can be performed at gestational ages when sampling of cord blood is technically not possible (<20 weeks). Second, fetal anti-CMV–specific IgM antibody is usually not apparent until 23 weeks' gestation or later, which may be many weeks after infection occurred.

Identification of the virus in amniotic fluid by culture or PCR does not necessarily delineate the severity of fetal injury. Fortunately, sonography is invaluable in providing information about the condition of the fetus. The principal sonographic findings suggestive of serious fetal injury are microcephaly, ventriculomegaly, intercerebral calcification, fetal hydrops, growth restriction, and oligohydramnios. Less common findings include fetal heart block, echogenic bowel, meconium peritonitis, renal dysplasia, ascites, and pleural effusions.

Treatment

Until recently, no consistently effective therapy for congenital CMV infection was available. However, in 2005, Nigro and colleagues[236] published a prospective cohort study from eight medical centers describing the use of hyperimmune globulin as treatment and prophylaxis for congenital CMV infection. Of 157 women with confirmed primary CMV infection, 148 were asymptomatic and were identified by routine serologic screening; 8 women had symptomatic viral infection, and 1 was identified because her fetus had abnormal ultrasound findings. Forty-five women had had a primary infection longer than 6 weeks before enrollment, underwent amniocentesis, and had CMV detected in amniotic fluid by PCR or culture. Thirty-one of these women received intravenous treatment with CMV-specific hyperimmune globulin (200 U/kg of maternal body weight). Nine of the 31 received one or two additional infusions into either the amniotic fluid or the umbilical cord because their fetuses had persistent abnormalities on ultrasound. Fourteen women declined treatment; 7 of these women had infants who were acutely symptomatic at the time of delivery. In contrast, only 1 of the 31 treated women had an infant with clinical disease at birth (adjusted OR, 0.02, $P < .001$).

In this same investigation,[236] 84 additional women did not have an amniocentesis because their infection occurred within 6 weeks before enrollment, their gestational age was less than 20 weeks, or they declined amniocentesis. Thirty-seven of these women received hyperimmune globulin, 100 U/kg every month until delivery, and 47 declined treatment. Six of the treated women delivered infected infants, as did 19 of the untreated women (adjusted OR, 0.32, $P = .04$). No adverse effects of hyperimmune globulin were noted in either group receiving immunotherapy.

This report by Nigro and colleagues had several shortcomings.[237] The design of the study was neither randomized nor controlled. There are at least some biologic reasons to question whether the remarkable success reported by the authors will be maintained in larger, randomized studies. The authors also did not address the financial and logistic issues associated with screening large obstetric populations for CMV infection, triaging the inevitable patients with false-positive results, offering amniocentesis and targeted sonography to women who seroconvert, and then treating at-risk patients with hyperimmune globulin. Nevertheless, the authors' observations are extremely interesting and offer the best available therapy for this dangerous perinatal infection.

Prevention

Ideally, preventive measures should be employed to ensure that women do not contract CMV infection during pregnancy. One simple measure is using CMV-negative blood products when transfusing pregnant women or fetuses. In addition, women should be encouraged to use careful hand washing techniques after handling infant diapers and toys. They also should adopt safe sexual practices if they are not already engaged in a mutually faithful, monogamous sexual relationship.[225,228,237]

Group B Streptococcal Infection

The hemolytic streptococci cause a variety of infections and are significant causes of perinatal morbidity and mortality. In 1933, Lancefield used serologic techniques to subdivide β-hemolytic streptococci into specific groups, designated A, B, C, D, and E. Only groups A, B, and D commonly are involved in human disease.

Group A β-hemolytic streptococcus (*Streptococcus pyogenes*) long has been recognized as a major pathogen in perinatal sepsis.[238] Several case series have documented fulminant puerperal infection, with multisystem dysfunction, resulting from group A streptococci.[239]

The Lancefield group B streptococci, GBS (*Streptococcus agalactiae*) can be classified into five major serotypes on the basis of antigenic structure. They originally were thought to be commensal organisms. By the 1960s GBS had been linked to neonatal infections, and by the 1970s they had emerged as the leading cause of neonatal sepsis. Today, GBS still are among the leading organisms in perinatal sepsis and have become the focus of national prevention strategies. In 1995, in surveillance areas set up by the CDC, the rate of perinatal sepsis was 1.3 per 1000 liveborn infants, accounting for an estimated 7000 to 8000 cases per year in the United States.[240] Outcome has improved dramatically in recent years, but morbidity still is substantial, particularly in preterm infants. One data set showed an overall case fatality rate of 4%, 2% in term infants but 16% in preterm infants.

GBS have been reported to cause 1% to 5% of UTIs in pregnancy. In addition, a characteristic early onset of puerperal endometritis has been associated with these organisms.

Epidemiology

Asymptomatic rectovaginal colonization with GBS occurs in approximately 20% of pregnant women. The choice of culture medium is a crucial determinant of the prevalence of GBS. The highest yield occurs when a selective medium, such as LIM or Trans-Vag broth, is used as an enriching step before plating on sheep's blood agar.

The single greatest risk factor for colonization with GBS in a newborn is being born to a colonized mother. Without intervention, more than half of infants born to colonized mothers will become colonized.[241] Also, 16% to 45% of nursery personnel are carriers of GBS infection, and nosocomial acquisition in newborns is common. There clearly is an association between heavy growth of GBS in the maternal genital tract and the development of GBS sepsis in neonates. Yet, a surprisingly high percentage of neonates with GBS sepsis (perhaps 25%) are born to women with light colonization. Therefore, focusing solely on heavily colonized women in preventive approaches is inadequate.

The documented colonization rate for GBS has been far higher than the attack rate in terms of neonatal infection. Overall, sepsis develops in only 1% of infants of colonized mothers. The following are risk factors for GBS neonatal sepsis[242]:

- Prematurity (or low birth weight as its surrogate)
- Maternal intrapartum fever (presumably as a result of chorioamnionitis)
- Membrane rupture for longer than 18 hours
- A previous infant infected with GBS disease
- GBS bacteriuria in this pregnancy

Because of the preponderance of term infants overall, 70% to 80% of cases of neonatal GBS infection in the United States occur in infants born after 36 weeks' gestation.[243,244] Today, approximately half of cases are early in onset (first week of life). Previously, before implementation of intrapartum antibiotic prophylaxis (IAP), at least three quarters of cases were of the early-onset variety.[243,244] The most common diagnosis with early-onset disease is bacteremia (89%); meningitis but not bacteremia is diagnosed in 10%, and both bacteremia and meningitis in 1%.[243]

Clinical Manifestations in the Neonate

Two clinically distinct neonatal GBS infections have been identified: early- and late-onset disease.[245]

Early-Onset Infection

Early-onset infection appears within the first week of life, usually within 48 hours. It is characterized by rapid clinical deterioration and a high mortality rate. The association between gestational age and early-onset GBS infection is shown in Table 38-14. In its most fulminant form, early-onset GBS infection manifests as septic shock accompanied by respiratory distress and leads to death within several hours despite appropriate antibiotic therapy. In less severe disease, the clinical findings are similar to those seen in respiratory distress syndrome. Although pulmonary disease predominates in early-onset disease, meningitis may be present in 10% to 30% of cases. The case fatality rate for early-onset disease is now approximately 4.5%.[243] Current nationwide prevention strategies have decreased the number of cases of early-onset GBS sepsis by an estimated 3900 per year and the number of deaths by 200 per year.[246]

TABLE 38-14 EARLY-ONSET GROUP B STREPTOCOCCAL DISEASE, BY GESTATIONAL AGE, 1993-1998

Gestational Age (Wk)	% of Cases	Case Fatality Rate (%)
≤33	9	30
34-36	8	10
≥37	83	2

Data from Schrag SJ, Zywicki S, Farley MM, et al: Group B streptococcal disease: The era of intrapartum antibiotic prophylaxis. N Engl J Med 342:15, 2000.

Late-Onset Infection

Late-onset infection with GBS occurs more insidiously, usually after the first week of life. In the majority of infants, meningitis is the predominant clinical manifestation. Although the mortality rate in late-onset GBS infection is lower (2%) than with early-onset disease, up to 50% of babies with meningitis subsequently demonstrate neurologic sequelae. Late-onset disease may result in localized infections involving the middle ear, sinuses, conjunctiva, breasts, lungs, bones, joints, or skin. Meningitis appears to be related to the serotype of GBS. More than 80% of early-onset GBS infections in which meningitis is present are caused by Lancefield type III organisms; in late-onset disease, 95% of meningitis is attributable to this subtype.

Although early-onset disease is acquired mainly via transmission from the mother's genital tract either before or during parturition, such a route of transmission is not implicated in late-onset disease. Nosocomial transmission of GBS can occur in the nursery from colonized nursing staff or from other infants. Current prevention strategies have not decreased the number of cases of late-onset GBS disease in newborns.[243,246]

Clinical Manifestations in the Mother

GBS is a major cause of puerperal infection. Features of GBS puerperal infection include the development of a high fever within 12 hours after delivery, tachycardia, abdominal distention, and endometritis. Some patients have no localizing signs early in the course of the infection.

Diagnosis

The diagnosis of maternal asymptomatic genitourinary or gastrointestinal colonization with GBS can be confirmed by culture. Several rapid diagnostic tests are available for detection of GBS from maternal sources, but most methods are insufficiently sensitive. Some newer PCR-based tests seem to be an exception to that statement.[247,248]

Most colonized neonates are asymptomatic, and the clinical manifestations of neonatal infection are not sufficient for diagnosis in the absence of a positive culture. The diagnosis should be suspected if the clinical manifestations occur in the setting of a risk factor for infection.

Treatment

Penicillin G remains the drug of choice for symptomatic GBS infection in both mother and neonate if the infecting organism has been identified. In most instances, however, treatment must be initiated before the availability of culture results. In these instances, a broad-spectrum approach for empirically treating the mother with chorioamnionitis or puerperal sepsis and the neonate with sepsis is required. Ampicillin frequently is used in such situations and provides adequate treatment for GBS infection. Alternative drugs for patients with a contraindication to penicillin are a cephalosporin in those not at risk for immediate penicillin hypersensitivity or vancomycin in patients who are at risk (e.g., those with immediate urticaria or bronchospasm as manifestations of penicillin allergy). Because of rising resistance, clindamycin and erythromycin no longer can be relied upon to treat GBS infection unless susceptibility to these antibiotics has been demonstrated for a given isolate.

Prevention

Because of the severity of early-onset GBS neonatal infection, major efforts have been directed toward use of IAP in gravid women whose genital tracts are colonized with GBS. Strategies can be classified as antepartum, intrapartum, neonatal, and immunologic.

Antepartum Strategies

Antepartum strategies to reduce maternal carrier rates generally have been unsuccessful owing to recolonization and are therefore not recommended.

Intrapartum Strategies

Intrapartum strategies have been the most attractive to date from both clinical and cost-effectiveness perspectives.

To standardize a national approach, in 1996, the CDC published recommendations that were also endorsed by the ACOG. These recommendations have been disseminated widely and have resulted in dramatic decreases in early-onset neonatal GBS sepsis.[244,246] In 2002, these guidelines were revised, based on several studies, including a large case-control series.[246,247] The main changes in the 2002 guidelines are recommendation of the screen-based approach only, a change in the recommended alternative antibiotics for penicillin-allergic patients, and provision of more specific recommendations for selected clinical scenarios. These guidelines are summarized here (Fig. 38-6).

1. All pregnant women should be screened at 35 to 37 weeks' gestation for vaginorectal GBS colonization. IAP should be given at the time of labor or rupture of membranes to those identified as GBS carriers. GBS colonization in a previous pregnancy does not obviate need for screening in subsequent pregnancies; colonization in a previous pregnancy is not an indication for IAP in subsequent deliveries.
2. GBS bacteriuria: Give IAP to women with GBS in urine in any concentration.
   a. Prenatal screening at 35 to 37 weeks is not necessary in these patients.
   b. Treat bacteriuria by usual standards of care.
3. Women with previous birth of infant with GBS disease should receive IAP; prenatal screening is not necessary for these women.
4. If the result of the GBS culture is not known at the time of labor, give IAP under any of the following circumstances:
   a. Less than 37 weeks' gestation
   b. Rupture of membranes at least 18 hours earlier
   c. Temperature at or greater than 100.4° F (38.0° C)
5. In cases of onset of labor or rupture of membranes earlier than 37 weeks with "significant risk for imminent preterm delivery," treat as follows:
   a. If the patient had a negative screening culture for GBS within the past 4 weeks, IAP is not indicated.
   b. If colonization status is unknown at admission, perform screening culture and initiate IAP; if the culture is negative, stop IAP.
6. Specimens

   Collection

   a. Collect specimen from distal vagina and the anorectum.
   b. Specimen may be collected by patient or provider.
   c. Do not use a speculum.
   d. Transport medium is acceptable.
   e. Label the specimen "GBS culture."

   Laboratory processing

   f. Inoculate into selective broth medium (e.g., LIM, Trans-Vag)
   g. Methods have been provided for susceptibility testing to clindamycin and erythromycin for GBS isolates from penicillin-allergic women.

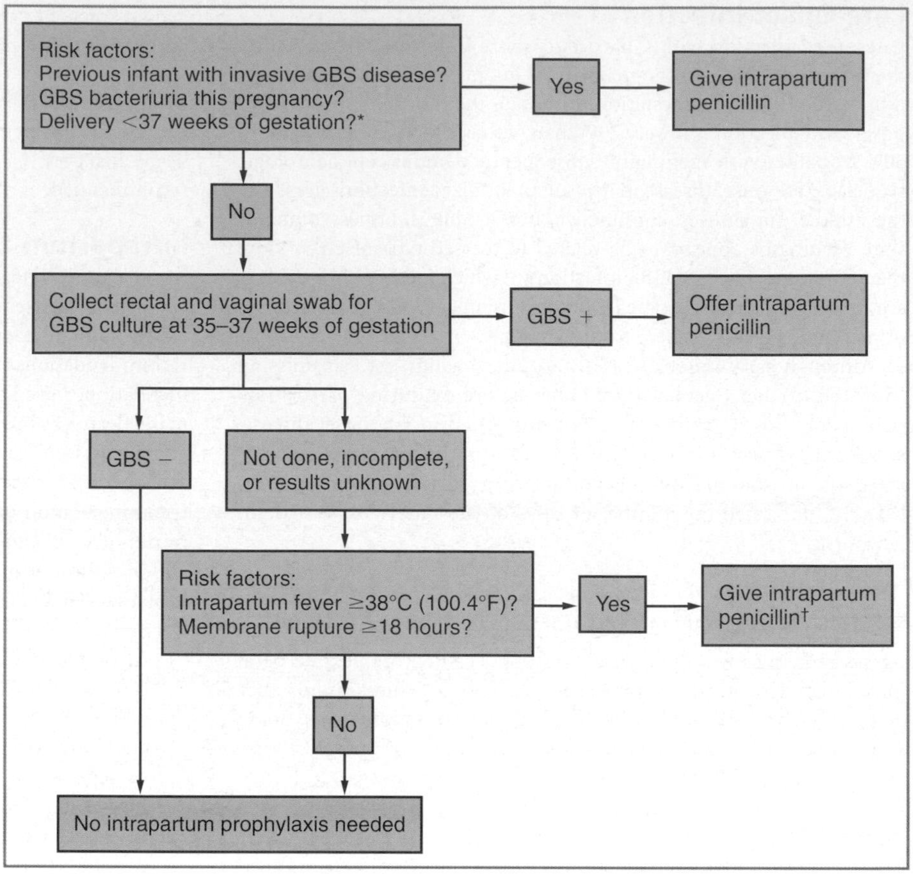

FIGURE 38-6 Algorithm for prevention of early-onset group B streptococcal (GBS) disease in neonates, with prenatal screening at 35 to 37 weeks. *If membranes rupture before 37 weeks' gestation and the mother has not begun labor, collect GBS culture and administer antibiotics until cultures are completed and the results are negative. †Broader-spectrum antibiotics may be considered at the physician's discretion, based on clinical indications (e.g., ampicillin plus gentamicin to treat clinical chorioamnionitis). (Adapted from Centers for Disease Control and Prevention: Prevention of perinatal group B streptococcal disease: A public health perspective. MMWR Morb Mortal Wkly Rep 45[RR-7]:1, 1996.)

   h. Laboratories "should report results to site of delivery and provider."
7. Inform patients of results and recommend IAP.
   a. In the absence of GBS bacteriuria, do not treat GBS genital colonization before the intrapartum period.
8. For cesarean delivery before rupture of membranes and before labor, IAP is not indicated.
9. Penicillin G is the drug of choice.
   a. The recommended dose for penicillin G is 5 million units initially, then 2.5 million units every 4 hours intravenously until delivery.
   b. Ampicillin remains an alternative.
   c. When ampicillin is used, the dose is 2 g intravenously initially, followed by 1 g every 4 hours until delivery.
   d. For penicillin allergy, clindamycin is no longer a drug of choice, unless susceptibility has been documented. Erythromycin no longer should even be considered as an alternate drug because of the high rate of resistance.
10. For patients with penicillin allergy, treat as follows:
   a. If not at high risk for anaphylaxis, the drug of choice is cefazolin, 2 g intravenously, then 1 g every 8 hours until delivery.
   b. If at high risk for anaphylaxis and GBS is susceptible: The drug of choice is clindamycin, 900 mg intravenously every 8 hours.
   c. If at high risk for anaphylaxis and GBS is resistant to clindamycin or of unknown susceptibility: The drug of choice is vancomycin, 1 g every 12 hours.
11. Routine use of prophylaxis for newborns whose mothers received IAP is not recommended. Antibiotics should be given to infants only if sepsis is suspected clinically.
12. Other items:
   a. Consider establishing surveillance.
   b. Improve laboratory protocols for isolation and reporting.
   c. Ensure communication.
   d. Educate staff.

The guidelines suggest penicillin G as the drug of choice for IAP and list ampicillin as an "acceptable alternative." Concern about ampicillin's broader spectrum of activity is the reason for this recommendation. However, when evaluated in a randomized clinical trial, IAP with either ampicillin or penicillin significantly increased the likelihood of recovery of ampicillin-resistant gram-negative organisms from the lower genital tract, and there was no difference between the two drugs for this effect.[249] Because of these data, we believe that the choice of whether to use penicillin or ampicillin for IAP should be based on cost and availability.

Another caveat involves the technique for collection of the screening culture. The guidelines call for sampling the vagina and rectum. However, two thirds of women report at least mild pain associated with collection of the rectal sample.[250] Furthermore, Jamie and colleagues[251] evaluated whether there was any advantage to sampling the vagina and rectum, compared with sampling the vagina and perianal skin. They found no difference in culture positivity in a cohort of 200 women. Therefore, it seems reasonable to obtain samples for screening cultures for GBS colonization from the distal vagina and perianal skin.

Neonatal Strategies

Measures to prevent GBS infection in the newborn have focused on the reports of decreases in neonatal early-onset disease when penicillin is given at birth. Although initial reports were encouraging, most trials in low-birth-weight infants have not found this approach to be effective. These results are not surprising in view of Boyer and Gotoff's observation[252] that up to 40% of neonates in whom GBS sepsis develops are already bacteremic at birth, suggesting that a single dose of penicillin after delivery may be "too little and too late."

Immunologic Strategies

The immunologic approach is appealing, but a vaccine has not yet been developed. Such a vaccine would need to be polyvalent to cover all serotypes involved in early-onset sepsis. One limitation of this approach is that it would not be optimally protective for infants born before 32 weeks of gestation because of modest placental transfer of maternal antibody before that time. Thus, the most vulnerable infants would be left with minimal protection. Nevertheless, it is estimated that a vaccine approach would prevent up to 90% of cases of neonatal GBS infection.[253]

Summary

No current approach is foolproof. However, the application of IAP has resulted in a significant reduction in the rate of early-onset neonatal GBS infection. In 2004, the rate was 0.34 per 1000 live births, less than a third of the rate only 10 years before.

Herpes Simplex Infection

Herpes simplex virus (HSV) may infect the mother, the newborn, or, on rare occasions, the fetus. In the adult, typical lesions are vesicular or ulcerative, involving only the skin and mucous membranes. More widespread infection involving the central nervous system (CNS) is an extremely unusual adult complication and most often develops in people with underlying debilitating disease. On the other hand, because of an incompletely developed immune system, the newborn is subject to systemic, and frequently lethal, disease.

Epidemiology

In adults, the virus commonly causes infection of the oral cavity, skin, and lower genital tract. In the past, HSV type 1 (HSV-1) was said to be responsible for infection of the mouth and of the skin above the waist, and HSV-2 was implicated in infection of the genitalia and of the skin below the waist. However, both viruses can cause either genital or oropharyngeal lesions, which are indistinguishable clinically. Furthermore, in some populations, HSV-1 has been reported to account for 30% to 40% of new cases of genital herpes,[254] but genital HSV-1 recurs much less commonly than genital HSV-2.[254,255]

Genital herpes is spread by sexual contact. The prevalence of serum antibodies to HSV-2 is increasing in the United States. Between 1988 and 1994, 21.9% of the population age 12 years or older was found to be seropositive, representing a 30% increase since the period 1976 to 1980 and corresponding to 45 million cases of infection.[256] The disease does not appear to be more severe or more protracted in pregnancy.

Clinically, there are three syndromes of genital herpes:

1. *First-episode primary genital herpes* is the clinical presentation in a patient without antibodies to either HSV-1 or HSV-2. Its clinical manifestations include severe local symptoms, with lesions lasting 3 to 6 weeks, regional adenopathy, constitutional symptoms, and, in a small percentage of cases, viral meningitis. However, it should be noted that as many as two thirds of women with HSV-2 antibodies have acquired the infection asymptomatically.[257] This observation represents a major change from previous concepts.
2. *First-episode nonprimary genital herpes* is the initial clinical episode with either HSV-1 or HSV-2 in a patient who has antibodies to the other viral serotype. Because the antibody response is directed against epitopes within areas of homology in the glycoprotein G expressed by each viral type, there is some cross-reactivity. Therefore, the presentation is more similar to recurrent episodes.
3. *Recurrent genital herpes infections* are much milder and shorter, with lesions lasting 3 to 10 days. The course of the infection is shorter, owing to the preexisting presence of antibody to the viral serotype causing the recurrent infection.

When primary genital herpes occurs in pregnancy, there is a high risk of fetal and neonatal involvement, but this risk mainly exists with infection late in pregnancy. Brown and coworkers[258] found that serious morbidity occurred in 6 of 15 infants born to women with primary infection in pregnancy and in 4 of 5 born to mothers with primary infection in the third trimester. However, the same group showed that, overall, maternal seroconversion to HSV-2 during pregnancy does not result in greater risks of low birth weight, preterm delivery, fetal growth restriction, stillbirth, or neonatal death.[259] When recurrent episodes occur during pregnancy, there appears to be no increase in abortion or low-birth-weight infants.[257]

Transplacental infection of the fetus resulting in congenital infection is a rare complication of maternal infection, presumably arising from primary infections with viremia. Only a few such documented cases have been reported.[260]

A major perinatal problem is neonatal herpes infection. Exact estimates of its frequency are subject to error, because up to 50% of infants with culture-proven fatal disease do not show typical lesions on the skin or mucous membranes. In addition, recent treatment recommendations probably have decreased the incidence of neonatal disease. The disease manifests at the end of the first week of life. The presentation may include skin lesions, cough, cyanosis, tachypnea, dyspnea, jaundice, seizures, and DIC.

Neonatal herpes is acquired perinatally from an infected lower maternal genital tract, most commonly during a vaginal delivery. In a study by Brown and colleagues,[259] only those women with very recent infection (i.e., presence of virus in the genital tract but without development of type-specific antibody) had infected infants. In that situation, the risk was high (four of nine cases). The risk is considerably lower among women with recurrent, clinically evident infection—in the range of 1% to 2%. In one study, the incidence of infection in infants born vaginally to women with asymptomatic recurrent infection was 0 in 34 cases.[261] However, asymptomatically infected patients can give birth to seriously infected neonates. In a referral nursery, 70% of mothers of infected infants had asymptomatic infections. Among infants with disseminated herpes, the risk of death or serious sequelae exceeds 40%, even with antiviral therapy.[262]

Diagnosis

The clinical diagnosis of genital herpes is based on the typical painful crops of vesicles and ulcers in various stages of progression. With primary infection, tender inguinal adenopathy, fever, and other, more marked constitutional symptoms may occur. Primary genital herpes lesions resolve without scarring after 3 to 6 weeks. The frequency of clinically detectable recurrences varies widely among individuals, but about 50% of patients have recurrent disease within 6 months. Recurrences are milder, with fewer lesions, fewer constitutional symptoms, and a shorter course (usually 3 to 10 days).

Because many patients present with genital herpes infection after the vesicles have evolved into ulcers, clinical diagnosis based on the classic presentation of grouped, painful vesicles has a low sensitivity and specificity. Furthermore, making the diagnosis of genital herpes has social and future implications. Therefore, first-episode infections should be confirmed by laboratory tests.

The "gold standard" diagnostic test to detect the presence of herpes virus infection has been the viral culture. The virus grows rapidly, and most positive cultures are identifiable at 48 to 72 hours. Culture of vesicular fluid has the highest yield, and the sensitivity of culture decreases with increasing duration of active lesions. The diagnosis of herpes infection can be made using the Tzanck smear or Papanicolaou smear. However, neither of these tests can differentiate among HSV-1, HSV-2, and varicella-zoster virus infection, and neither of them has a high sensitivity or specificity.

PCR to detect HSV DNA probably is the most useful diagnostic test available. Results are available in a matter of hours, and PCR exceeds culture in identifying positive cases. With the use of PCR, the frequency of asymptomatic viral shedding of HSV particles has been shown to be eight times higher than previously reported using culture.[263-265]

Previously, HSV antibody tests could not discriminate infection with HSV-1 from that with HSV-2. Newer IgG assays that are specific to the respective glycoprotein G of each type now allow clinicians to distinguish between these infections.[266] However, the role of serologic testing in making the diagnosis of genital herpes is controversial. Furthermore, cost-effectiveness analyses regarding whether pregnant women should be screened for serologic evidence of prior HSV-2 infection have had mixed results.[267,268]

Treatment

During clinically evident episodes, treatment consists of supportive measures such as oral analgesics, hygiene, and topical anesthetics. Secondary infections such as candidiasis also should be treated. Many women find that frequent bathing, followed by thorough drying of the affected area with a hair dryer, provides temporary relief.

Acyclovir, an antiviral agent with excellent activity against herpes infection, is a specific inhibitor of viral thymidine kinase. It is available in topical, oral, and intravenous preparations. In nonpregnant individuals, all of these forms have been of value in decreasing the duration of symptoms and of viral shedding in primary genital infection, but oral therapy seems to be superior to topical therapy and equivalent to intravenous therapy for treatment of non–life-threatening infections. The oral form is effective in shortening recurrences significantly (400 mg orally three times daily for 5 days) and in suppressing frequent recurrences (400 mg orally twice daily). Such suppressive therapy with acyclovir has been demonstrated to be safe and effective for 6 years or more.[269]

For treatment of genital herpes, valacyclovir (Valtrex) and famciclovir (Famvir) have the advantage of better absorption and a longer half-life than acyclovir. Both are indicated for the treatment of recurrent genital herpes, and valacyclovir is indicated for the treatment of first-episode infections. Both drugs are more expensive than acyclovir.

Management of Herpes Infection in Pregnancy

Because of the severity of neonatal herpes infection and the lack of satisfactory therapy, the only current way of preventing neonatal infection is to avoid contact between the fetus and the infected maternal lower genital tract by means of cesarean delivery. Accordingly, cesarean delivery is recommended when typical herpes lesions are present at labor, regardless of the time since membrane rupture.[12,270,271]

In 1986, Arvin and colleagues[272] reported HSV cultures in a series of 515 pregnant women with recurrent herpes infection. Seventeen women had positive antepartum cultures, but none was positive at delivery. Of 354 asymptomatic mothers, 5 (1.4%) had positive results at delivery, but none had positive antepartum cultures. The likelihood of asymptomatic shedding at delivery was 1.3%. Brown and colleagues[259] published a cohort study that included more than 40,000 women. Testing for HSV included both culture and PCR. From the 202 women from whom HSV was isolated at the time of labor, 10 infants developed HSV infection. Those born by cesarean delivery were less likely to develop HSV infection than those born vaginally (1.2% versus 7.7%; $P = .047$).

For gravidas with recurrent genital herpes, treatment with acyclovir (400 mg three times daily) starting at 36 weeks' gestation decreases the proportion of patients with clinical lesions at the time of labor and lessens the need for cesarean delivery.[273] Such an approach has been shown to be cost-effective.[274]

There are no data supporting a risk to the fetus from maternal administration of acyclovir, valacyclovir, or famciclovir. However, we believe that acyclovir should be the drug of choice for suppression of recurrent genital herpes during the third trimester, because this drug has been the most extensively studied.

Current recommendations for prenatal and intrapartum care include the following:

1. Obstetricians should ask all pregnant women about a history of genital herpes.
2. If the diagnosis of genital herpes has not been previously confirmed by culture or PCR, specimens should be obtained during an active episode of apparent HSV infection.
3. Serial cultures beginning at 34 to 36 weeks are *not* recommended for *asymptomatic* women with a history of herpes infection.
4. The patient with a history of genital herpes should be instructed to come to the hospital early in labor or immediately if PROM has occurred. The patient also should be informed of the low risk of asymptomatic infection at delivery (1%) and the low risk of neonatal infection after delivery through an asymptomatically infected genital tract.
5. When the patient arrives in labor or with membrane rupture, a careful pelvic examination should be performed. If no lesions are present, the delivery can be managed normally. If lesions are observed, cesarean delivery is recommended to prevent neonatal herpes.

Women with nongenital herpes do not require any special precautions during labor and delivery, apart from barrier isolation of the infected skin, gown and glove precautions, and proper disposal of linen and dressings. Precautions should be taken to avoid contact of the newborn with the infected maternal skin. After the lesions have become encrusted, the mother may handle and feed her infant.

Human Immunodeficiency Virus Infection

Epidemiology

HIV infection is caused by an RNA retrovirus. Two major strains of the virus have been identified, HIV-1 and HIV-2; each major strain has several substrains. HIV-1 infection is more widely prevalent throughout the world. HIV-2 infection is uncommon in the United States except among patients who have traveled to areas of the world where this infection is endemic (e.g., sub-Saharan Africa) or who have shared needles with, or had sex with, someone from that area of the world.[275]

In the United States, HIV infection is more common in African-American and Hispanic women than in Caucasians. The most common mechanism of transmission of infection is heterosexual contact. Intravenous drug use also is an extremely important mechanism of transmission. Transmission through organ donation, artificial insemination, or blood transfusion is exceedingly rare. Important risk factors for sexual transmission of HIV infection include multiple sexual partners; receptive anal intercourse; unprotected intercourse; concurrent STDs, especially those that cause genital ulcers; sexual contact with an uncircumcised male; severe illness in the infected partner; sex during menstruation; and bleeding during intercourse (e.g., from sexual assault).[276]

Pathogenesis

HIV infection typically evolves through four major stages. The first stage of infection is the *acute retroviral illness*.[277] Within several weeks after exposure, the patient typically develops a severe flulike illness characterized by malaise, poor appetite, weight loss, low-grade fever, and generalized lymphadenopathy. Over a period of several weeks, this phase of the illness gradually resolves, and the patient enters the *latent phase of infection*. In this phase of the infection, the viral load in the plasma tends to be relatively low, and the virus is primarily concentrated in lymphatic tissue, where it replicates at a slow rate. With appropriate anti-retroviral therapy and supportive care, the latent phase of illness may extend beyond 10 years in many patients. Over time, however, the viral load progressively increases, and patients enter a *symptomatic phase* of the infection. Eventually, all infected patients develop *acquired immunodeficiency syndrome (AIDS)*, albeit at a much slower rate than in the early years of the HIV epidemic.

Diagnosis

Opportunistic diseases are the hallmark of HIV infection. The most common serious opportunistic disease in women is *Pneumocystis jiroveci* pneumonia; second most common is *Mycobacterium avium-intracellulare* infection. Other important opportunistic diseases include tuberculosis, toxoplasmosis, CMV infection, candidiasis, and non-Hodgkin lymphoma.[278]

The initial screening test for HIV infection should be the enzyme immunoassay (EIA) for HIV-1 and HIV-2. If this test is positive, a confirmatory test such as the Western blot or immunofluorescent assay (IFA) should be performed. If both tests are positive, the probability of a false-positive sequence is extremely low.

The CDC now recommends universal screening for HIV infection in pregnant women. The "opt out" strategy is the one most likely to ensure compliance with screening. With this strategy, HIV testing is considered part of the routine prenatal laboratory panel. Patients must specifically decline the screening test; otherwise, it is routinely performed.

Treatment

In the absence of any intervention, the risk of perinatal transmission of HIV infection is approximately 25%.[279] With the interventions outlined in this section, perinatal transmission should be reduced to less than 2%.[280] Most cases of transmission occur at the time of delivery. Antenatal transmission is possible, typically as a result of invasive antepartum procedures such as amniocentesis or chorionic villus sampling. Postnatal transmission also can occur from breastfeeding. The principal risk factors for perinatal transmission of HIV infection are

- History of previously affected infant
- Severe maternal disease
- Preterm delivery
- Intrapartum blood exposure as a result of events such as vaginal lacerations, episiotomy, or instrumental delivery
- Time since rupture of membranes greater than 4 hours
- Invasive antepartum procedures
- Chorioamnionitis
- Concurrent STDs
- Vaginal delivery in the presence of an elevated viral load

At the time of her first prenatal appointment, the HIV-infected patient should have a $CD4^+$ count and viral load measurement to assess her degree of immunosuppression. She should be screened for all other STDs, such as gonorrhea, chlamydia, syphilis, hepatitis B, and hepatitis C. She also should be tested for tuberculosis. If her $CD4^+$ count is greater than 200 cells/mm^3, the purified protein derivative (PPD) should be a reliable screening test. If the $CD4^+$ count is less than 200/mm^3, a negative test may be the result of anergy, and such patients should have a chest radiograph to be certain that tuberculosis is not present. Patients should be tested for toxoplasmosis and CMV infection as well, because both can cause serious perinatal infection, which can be successfully treated with either antibiotics or immunotherapy.

In an effort to prevent opportunistic infections, the HIV-positive pregnant woman should be vaccinated for pneumococcal infection, influenza, hepatitis A and B, and meningococcal infection. She also should receive prophylactic antibiotics to protect against other pathogens.[278] If her $CD4^+$ count is less than 200/mm^3 and she previously has had an infection with *P. jiroveci*, she should receive trimethoprim-sulfamethoxazole-DS, 1 tablet daily. This medication also provides protection against toxoplasmosis infection. If her tuberculin skin test is positive and her chest radiograph shows no evidence of active disease, she should receive prophylaxis with isoniazid (INH), 300 mg orally each day, plus pyridoxine, 50 mg daily. The latter drug is administered to prevent peripheral neurotoxicity from isoniazid. If the patient's $CD4^+$ count falls to a range of 50 to 75 cells/mm^3, she should receive prophylaxis against *M. avium-intracellulare* with azithromycin, 1200 mg orally each week. If a patient has recurrent candidiasis, she can be treated with fluconazole, 150 mg orally, each day. If her $CD4^+$ count falls to less than 50/mm^3, she also should receive prophylaxis with fluconazole to prevent cryptococcal infection. A patient with recurrent herpes simplex infection should receive prophylaxis with acyclovir, 400 mg PO twice daily.

The single most important intervention is treatment with highly active antiretroviral therapy (HAART).[281,282] The ACTG-076 trial[279] was the first to demonstrate that treatment of pregnant women with prophylactic zidovudine is highly effective in reducing the rate of perinatal transmission of HIV infection. In that trial, the observed frequency of transmission was reduced from 26% in the placebo group to 8% in those patients who received zidovudine. Subsequent uncontrolled studies showed that treatment of the mother with combination chemotherapy reduces the rate of perinatal transmission to less than 2%.[280]

The antiretroviral agents currently available are summarized in Table 38-15. The combination of zidovudine (300 mg) and lamivudine

TABLE 38-15 DRUGS FOR TREATMENT OF HUMAN IMMUNODEFICIENCY VIRUS INFECTION

Agent	Usual Adult Dose	Major Adverse Effects
Nucleotide Analogue		
Tenofovir (Viread)	300 mg qd	GI irritation, elevation in transaminase concentrations, decrease in serum carnitine, nephrotoxicity
Nucleoside Analogues		
Abacavir (Ziagen)	300 mg bid	Hypersensitivity reaction
Didanosine (DDI, Videx) or Videx EC	200 mg bid 400 mg qd	Pancreatitis and peripheral neuropathy
Emtricitabine (Emtriva)	200 mg qd	Headache, diarrhea, nausea, rash, hyperpigmentation, hepatitis
Lamivudine (3TC, Epivir)	150 mg bid or 300 mg qd	Marrow suppression
Stavudine (d4T, Zerit)	40 mg bid	Peripheral sensory neuropathy
Zalcitabine (ddC, Hivid)	0.75 mg q8h	Peripheral neuropathy, pancreatitis
Zidovudine (AZT, Retrovir)	300 mg bid	Marrow suppression
Combination Nucleoside Analogues		
Combivir (zidovudine + lamivudine)	1 tablet bid	Marrow suppression
Trizivir (zidovudine + lamivudine + abacavir)	1 tablet bid	Marrow suppression
Non-nucleoside Reverse Transcriptase Inhibitors		
Delavirdine (Rescriptor)	400 mg tid	Rash, hepatitis
Efavirenz (Sustiva)	600 mg qd	Rash, CNS changes. **Drug is teratogenic and should not be used in pregnancy.**
Nevirapine (Viramune)	200 mg bid	Rash, hepatitis
Unique Triple Combination		
Atripla (efavirenz + emtricitabine + tenofovir)	Single daily dose: 600/200/300 mg	Lactic acidosis, severe hepatomegaly, steatosis
Protease Inhibitors		
Amprenavir (Agenerase)	1200 mg bid	Rash and GI irritation
Atazanavir (Reyataz)	400 mg qd	Hyperbilirubinemia, prolonged Q-T interval, hyperlipidemia
Darunavir (Prezista)—must be given with ritonavir)	600/100 mg bid	Diarrhea, nausea, headache, increased transaminase activity, increased serum lipids
Indinavir (Crixivan)	800 mg tid	Nephrolithiasis, GI upset
Lopinavir/ritonavir (Kaletra)	3 gelatin capsules (133.3/33.3 mg) bid	Diarrhea, nausea, fatigue, headache, asthenia
Nelfinavir (Viracept)	1250 mg bid	Diarrhea, fatigue, poor concentration
Ritonavir (Norvir)	100-400 mg bid	GI irritation, seizures, hepatitis, diabetes, marrow suppression
Tipranavir (Aptivus)—must be given with ritonavir	500/200 mg bid	Hepatitis, diarrhea, nausea, vomiting, abdominal pain
Saquinavir:		GI irritation, peripheral neuropathy, headache, rash
Hard gel cap (Invirase)	400 or 1000 mg bid	
Soft gel cap (Fortovase)	1200 mg tid	
Fusion Inhibitor		
Enfuvirtide (Fuzeon)	90 mg bid	GI irritation, rash, hypotension, injection site reaction

CNS, central nervous system; GI, gastrointestinal tract.

(150 mg) (Combivir, twice daily) plus ritonavir (400 mg) and lopinavir (100 mg) (Kaletra, twice daily) is recommended. The patient's response to treatment should be evaluated by obtaining serial measurements of viral load. If a clear response to treatment has not occurred within 12 to 16 weeks, the patient should have viral genotyping to determine whether she has a resistant organism. If resistance is identified, the entire antiviral regimen should be changed in accordance with the susceptibility pattern identified.

If the therapy reduces the patient's viral load to less than 1000 copies/mL, vaginal delivery is acceptable, provided that there are no other indications for cesarean delivery. During labor, every precaution should be taken to minimize contact between the infant's skin and mucous membranes and contaminated maternal blood and genital tract secretions. Specifically, amniotomy, scalp monitoring, scalp pH assessment, episiotomy, and instrumental delivery should be avoided if at all possible. Although all of these agents have potentially serious side effects in the mother, only efavirenz is clearly teratogenic in the fetus.

If the patient does not have an optimal response to therapy and her viral load remains greater than 1000 copies/mL, she should be delivered by cesarean at approximately 38 weeks' gestation, before the onset of labor and rupture of membranes. Amniocentesis should not be routinely performed before this procedure, because it poses a small risk of transmitting HIV infection to the infant.

Regardless of the method of delivery, the patient should receive intravenous zidovudine during delivery (2 mg/kg for 1 hour, then 1 mg/kg/hr until delivery). For patients scheduled for cesarean delivery, the infusion should begin approximately 4 hours before surgery. Infants delivered to infected mothers typically are treated with antiretroviral agents for at least 6 weeks after delivery.[283-287]

If the HIV status of the patient is unknown and she is admitted in labor, a rapid serologic screening should be performed. Current assays should yield reliable results within 1 hour. Management of seropositive patients and their infants should proceed as outlined earlier until definitive testing is completed.[288,289]

Listeriosis

Epidemiology and Pathogenesis

Listeriosis is an infection caused by *L. monocytogenes*, a motile, non–spore-forming, gram-positive bacillus. Although seven species of *Listeria* are recognized, *L. monocytogenes* is the principal human pathogen. Patients who are immunocompromised and pregnant women and their newborns are particularly susceptible to infection with *L. monocytogenes*. Of concern to the obstetrician is the association between maternal listerial infection and stillbirth, preterm labor, and fetal infection. High perinatal morbidity and mortality rates have been reported for listerial infection in pregnancy.[290-294]

As with GBS infection, neonatal listeriosis has been divided into two serologically and clinically distinct types. *Early-onset* disease, associated with serotypes Ia and IVb, takes the form of a diffuse sepsis with involvement of multiple organs, including the lungs, liver, and CNS. Early-onset listeriosis is associated with a high rate of stillbirth and a high neonatal mortality rate. It appears to occur more frequently in low-birth-weight infants. *Late-onset* listeriosis manifests as meningitis, usually in term infants born to mothers with uneventful perinatal courses. Neurologic sequelae, such as hydrocephalus and mental retardation, are common with late-onset disease. In addition, a mortality rate approaching 40% has been reported.[290-294]

It is possible that an ascending route of infection from cervical colonization with *L. monocytogenes* plays a role in the pathogenesis of neonatal infection. However, the more important and more common route of infection is hematogenous dissemination of the organism through the placenta, which leads to placental abscesses and ultimately to fetal septicemia.

Human listeriosis manifests in both epidemic and sporadic forms. The *epidemic* form is associated with contamination of food and food products. Foods that particularly pose a risk include fresh, unpasteurized cheeses (e.g., Mexican "queso fresco") and processed meats such as hot dogs.[295] Cherubin and colleagues[293] reviewed more than 120 cases of listeriosis. They identified pregnancy and neonatal status as two of the major risk factors for this disease. Indeed, the deaths associated with listeriosis occurred predominantly among premature and stillborn infants delivered to infected pregnant women. Moreover, the earlier the stage of gestation when infection manifested, the higher the risk of fetal death. Listerial infection tends to adversely affect immunocompromised adults and fetuses or neonates with immature immune systems.

The *sporadic* form of listeriosis occurs more commonly than the epidemic form. The incidence of listeriosis appears to be decreasing. The crude incidence in 2003 was 3.1 cases per 1 million population. The decrease in the last decade is thought to be the result of a lower prevalence of *L. monocytogenes* contamination of ready-to-eat foods.[296]

Diagnosis

Many pregnant women with listeriosis are asymptomatic. When symptomatic, they present with a flulike syndrome characterized by fever, chills, malaise, myalgias, back pain, and upper respiratory complaints. Such symptoms occur in two thirds of cases.[297] The viral-like prodrome characterizes the bacteremic stage of listeriosis. Gellin and Broome[291] suggested that this is probably the time when the placenta and fetus are seeded with *L. monocytogenes*. Maternal infection tends to be mild and is not associated with significant morbidity. However, diffuse sepsis may occur on occasion. No specific clinical manifestations have been demonstrated that help to distinguish listeriosis from other infections that may occur during pregnancy. Therefore, pregnant women presenting with these symptoms in the late second or early third trimester should be evaluated for possible listeriosis.

Early-onset neonatal listeriosis occurs in infants who are infected in utero, often before the start of labor, and manifests during the first few hours to days of life. Late-onset neonatal listeriosis occurs in term infants who appear healthy at birth and manifest infection several days to weeks after delivery.[291] Meningitis is more common than sepsis with late-onset disease. Either intrapartum transmission or nosocomial transmission after delivery can result in late-onset infection.[291]

Because of the high mortality rate associated with both early- and late-onset neonatal listerial infection, it is crucial that the obstetrician maintain a high index of suspicion that any febrile illness in pregnancy may be due to *L. monocytogenes*. In patients with these symptoms, cervical and blood cultures should be obtained for *L. monocytogenes* as soon as possible. Because colonies of *L. monocytogenes* may be mistaken on the Gram stain for diphtheroids and therefore ignored, it is important to inform the microbiologist that listerial infection is a concern. In febrile pregnant women, a Gram stain revealing gram-positive pleomorphic rods with rounded ends is highly suggestive of, and should be presumed to be, *L. monocytogenes*.

Treatment

Penicillin G and ampicillin are effective in vivo against *L. monocytogenes*. Current opinion holds that optimal therapy includes a combination of ampicillin plus an aminoglycoside. Maternal treatment consists of ampicillin (1 to 2 g intravenously every 4 to 6 hours) and gentamicin (2 mg/kg intravenously every 8 hours). For the newborn, the ampicillin dosage is 200 mg/kg/day in 4 to 6 divided doses. The duration of treatment is usually 1 week. A single case report has suggested that, following documentation by amniocentesis of intrauterine listerial infection, antibiotic treatment without immediate delivery may be successful and may result in a normal healthy fetus.[298,299] An earlier study[300] also suggested that rapid diagnosis and aggressive antibiotic management in the antenatal patient with listeriosis may reduce the complications of this illness. In addition, these authors reviewed reported cases of listerial septicemia and antepartum antibiotic use: There was one maternal death, and 16 of 20 infants survived. These data compared favorably to the perinatal mortality rate of 33% to 73% observed in cases of untreated maternal disease.

Mumps

Epidemiology and Pathogenesis

The diagnosis of mumps is usually made on the basis of clinical examination. Mumps is an acute, generalized nonexanthmatous infection with a predilection for the parotid and salivary glands. The infection also can affect the brain, pancreas, and gonads. Mumps is caused by an RNA virus that is a member of the paramyxovirus family. It is transmitted by saliva and respiratory droplet contamination and has been recovered from salivary and respiratory secretions from 7 days before the onset of parotitis until 9 days afterward. The usual incubation period is 14 to 18 days.

Diagnosis

The prodrome of mumps consists of fever, malaise, myalgias, and anorexia. Parotitis follows within 24 hours and is characterized by swollen and tender parotid glands. In most cases, parotitis is bilateral. The submaxillary glands are involved less often and almost never without parotid gland involvement. The sublingual glands rarely are affected. Although mumps usually is a self-limited and complication-free disease, it can cause aseptic meningitis, pancreatitis, mastitis, thyroiditis, myocarditis, nephritis, and arthritis.

Adverse Effects in Pregnancy

Mumps in pregnant women is generally benign and no more severe than in nonpregnant patients. Aseptic meningitis in pregnant patients is neither more common nor more severe. Mortality in association with mumps is extremely rare in both pregnant and nonpregnant patients.

Mumps during the first trimester is associated with a twofold increase in the incidence of spontaneous abortion. There is no association between maternal mumps infection and preterm delivery, fetal growth restriction, or perinatal mortality.[301]

Whether mumps infection may result in congenital disease remains controversial.[302] Despite animal studies in which mumps virus induced congenital malformations, definitive evidence of a teratogenic potential for mumps virus in humans has not been reported. Siegal[303] noted that the rate of congenital malformations in infants born to women who had mumps during pregnancy (2 of 117) was no different than the rate in infants born to uninfected mothers (2 of 123). The predominant concern has been the postulated association between maternal mumps infection and the development of subsequent congenital cardiac abnormalities, specifically endocardial fibroelastosis.[304] The issue remains unresolved.

Treatment

The treatment of mumps both in pregnant and nonpregnant patients is symptomatic. Analgesics, bed rest, and application of cold or heat to the parotid glands are useful. Maternal mumps is not an indication for termination of pregnancy. The live-attenuated mumps vaccine is effective in preventing primary mumps. Ninety-five percent of vaccinated susceptible subjects develop antibodies without clinically adverse reactions. The duration of protection afforded by immunization is not known.

Although mumps vaccine virus has been recovered from fetal and placental tissue when vaccination occurred during pregnancy, there is no evidence that the vaccine virus is teratogenic in humans. Nevertheless, given the innocuous nature of mumps in pregnancy, immunization with the mumps live-virus vaccine in pregnancy is contraindicated on the theoretical grounds that the developing fetus might be harmed. However, mumps vaccination should not be considered an indication for pregnancy termination. Women vaccinated with mumps vaccine should not become pregnant for at least 1 month.

Parvovirus Infection

Epidemiology and Pathogenesis

Parvovirus infection is a rare, but potentially extremely serious, perinatal complication. The infection is caused by a DNA organism, the B19 parvovirus. The virus is transmitted primarily by respiratory droplets and infected blood products. Immunity to parvovirus increases progressively throughout childhood and young adult life. Approximately 50% to 60% of women of reproductive age have evidence of prior infection, and immunity is long-lasting.[305,306]

The incubation period for parvovirus is 10 to 20 days. The most common clinical manifestation of infection is erythema infectiosum (fifth disease). Erythema infectiosum is usually manifested by a low-grade fever, malaise, myalgias, arthralgias, and a "slapped cheek" facial rash. An erythematous, lacelike rash also may extend onto the torso and upper extremities. In children, parvovirus infection also can cause transient aplastic crisis. This same disorder may occur in adults who have an underlying hemaglobinopathy.[306]

When maternal parvovirus infection occurs during pregnancy, the virus can cross the placenta and infect red cell progenitors in the fetal bone marrow. The virus attaches to the i antigen on red cell stem cells and suppresses erythropoiesis, thereby resulting in severe anemia and high-output congestive heart failure. This same antigen also is present on fetal myocardial cells, and, in some fetuses, the viral infection causes a cardiomyopathy that further contributes to heart failure.[306]

The most obvious manifestation of congenital infection is hydrops fetalis. The risk of hydrops is directly related to the gestational age at which maternal infection occurs. If infection develops during the first 12 weeks of gestation, the risk of hydrops varies from less than 5% to approximately 10%. If infection occurs during weeks 13 through 20, the risk of infection decreases to 5% or less. If infection occurs beyond the 20th week of gestation, the risk of fetal hydrops is 1% or less.[307-309]

Diagnosis

The best way to confirm the diagnosis of maternal parvovirus infection is through serologic testing. Table 38-16 illustrates the possible combinations of serologic test results that may occur in women who are being evaluated for possible parvovirus infection.

Once maternal infection is confirmed, the fetus should be evaluated for evidence of anemia. The best test for assessment of anemia is ultrasound assessment of middle cerebral artery (MCA) via Doppler velocimetry. Serial examinations should be performed for at least 8 weeks

TABLE 38-16 POSSIBLE RESULTS OF SEROLOGIC TESTS FOR PARVOVIRUS AFTER DOCUMENTED EXPOSURE

IgM	IgG	Interpretation
Negative	Negative	Susceptible
Negative	Positive	Prior immunity—protected against second infections
Positive	Negative	Acute infection—within previous 7 days
Positive	Positive	Subacute infection >7 days and <120 days

Ig, immunoglobulin.

after documentation of maternal seroconversion, because the incubation period for fetal infection may be longer than that observed in children and adults.

The most obvious ultrasound manifestation of fetal anemia is hydrops. However, by the time sonographic evidence of hydrops is present, the fetal hematocrit is likely to be less than 20%. Therefore, a more precise way to detect evolving fetal anemia is to assess Doppler velocimetry in the fetal MCA.[310] Increases in peak systolic velocity in this vessel correlate well with fetal hematocrit. If velocimetry indicates fetal anemia, a cordocentesis should be performed to determine the fetal hematocrit. If anemia is confirmed, an intrauterine blood transfusion should be performed.

Treatment

Two retrospective studies have demonstrated that intrauterine transfusion is lifesaving in the setting of congenital parvovirus infection. The first investigation was published by Fairley and collegues.[311] They reviewed 66 cases of fetal hydrops caused by parvovirus infection. Twenty-six fetuses were dead at the time of diagnosis, and two were electively aborted. Twelve of the 38 live fetuses had an intrauterine transfusion, three of whom died. Among the 26 fetuses who did not receive an intrauterine transfusion, 13 died. The odds ratio for fetal death in infants who received a transfusion was 0.14 (CI, 0.02 to 0.96). A second important study was published by Rodisand associates.[312] They surveyed specialists in maternal-fetal medicine and reported the outcomes of 460 cases of parvovirus infection. Twenty-seven of 164 fetuses who received an intrauterine transfusion died. Of the 296 fetuses who did not receive an intrauterine transfusion, 138 died. The observed difference in outcome was highly significant ($P < .001$). Although cases of spontaneous resolution of fetal hydrops have been reported, the studies presented here clearly support a firm recommendation for intrauterine transfusion (Level II—2 evidence, "A" recommendation).

Infants who survive intrauterine infection with parvovirus usually have an excellent long-term prognosis.[313] However, isolated case reports have been published documenting neurologic morbidity and prolonged, transfusion-dependent anemia.[314,315] More recently, Nagel and colleagues[316] reported an 8-year follow-up of 16 hydropic fetuses who received intrauterine transfusions for congenital parvovirus infection and survived. Eleven (68%) of the children were normal, and 5 (32%) had delayed psychomotor development. In light of these reports, a third-trimester ultrasound to reassess fetal growth and evaluate the anatomy of the CNS, together with long-term surveillance for neurologic problems, seems to be a prudent course of management.

Rubella

Epidemiology

Rubella (also called "German measles" or "3-day measles") is caused by an RNA virus. Rubella infection develops primarily in young children and adolescents and is most common in the springtime. Major epidemics of rubella occurred in the United States in 1935 and 1964; minor sporadic epidemics occurred approximately every 7 years until the late 1960s. With licensure of an effective vaccine in 1969, the frequency of rubella declined markedly. In 1999, the incidence of rubella was 0.1 per 100,000.[317] Persistence of this infection appears to be caused by failure to vaccinate susceptible individuals rather than by a lack of immunogenicity of the vaccine.[318]

The rubella virus is spread by respiratory droplets. From the upper respiratory tract, the virus travels quickly to the cervical lymph nodes and then is disseminated hematogenously throughout the body. The incubation period is approximately 2 to 3 weeks. The virus is present in blood and nasopharyngeal secretions for several days before appearance of the characteristic rash and continues to be shed from the nasopharynx for several days after appearance of the rash. Therefore, the patient may be contagious for a period of 7 to 10 days.[318]

Antibody against rubella does not normally appear in the serum until after the rash has developed. Acquired immunity to rubella usually lasts for life. Second infections have occurred after both natural infections and vaccination, but recurrent infections usually are not associated with serious illness, viremia, or congenital infection.

Clinical Presentation

Most infections with rubella are subclinical. Of those individuals who do show symptoms, most have mild constitutional symptoms such as malaise, headache, myalgias, and arthralgias. The principal clinical manifestation of rubella is a widely disseminated, nonpruritic, erythematous, maculopapular rash. Postauricular adenopathy and mild conjunctivitis also are common. These clinical manifestations usually are short-lived and typically resolve within 3 to 5 days.

Diagnosis

The differential diagnosis of rubella includes rubeola, roseola, other viral exanthems, and drug reaction. Rubella usually can be distinguished from these other conditions on the basis of the characteristic rash and serologic testing. Serum IgM antibody concentration reaches a peak 7 to 10 days after the onset of illness and then declines over a period of 4 weeks. The serum concentration of IgG rises more slowly, but antibody levels persist throughout the lifetime of the individual.[318]

Congenital Rubella Infection

Because of the success of rubella vaccination campaigns, the incidence of congenital rubella syndrome (CRS) in the United States has declined dramatically. Fewer than 50 cases of congenital rubella occur each year. However, approximately 10% to 20% of women in the United States remain susceptible to rubella, and their fetuses are at risk for serious injury should infection occur during pregnancy.[319]

Rubella virus crosses the placenta by hematogenous dissemination, and the frequency of congenital infection is critically dependent on the time of exposure to the virus. The fetus is not at risk from infection before the time of conception. However, approximately 50% to 80% of infants exposed to the virus within 12 weeks after conception will manifest signs of congenital infection. The rate of congenital infection declines sharply with advancing gestational age, so that very few fetuses are affected if infection occurs beyond 18 weeks of gestation.[320,321]

The four most common anomalies associated with CRS are deafness (affecting 60% to 75% of fetuses), eye defects such as cataracts or retinopathy (10% to 30%), CNS defects (10% to 25%), and cardiac malformations (10% to 20%). The most common cardiac abnormality is patent ductus arteriosus, although supravalvular pulmonic stenosis is perhaps the most pathognomonic. Other possible abnormalities include microcephaly, mental retardation, pneumonia, fetal growth restriction, hepatosplenomegaly, hemolytic anemia, and thrombocytopenia.[320-323]

A variety of tests have been proposed for the diagnosis of CRS. Fetal blood, obtained by cordocentesis, can be used to determine the total and viral-specific IgM concentration. However, cordocentesis technically is difficult before 20 weeks' gestation, and fetal immunoglobulins usually cannot be detected before 22 to 24 weeks. Chorionic villi, fetal blood, and amniotic fluid samples all can be tested via PCR for rubella antigen. Because of its lower complication rate, amniocentesis is the procedure of choice. Although these tests can demonstrate that rubella virus is present in the fetal compartment, they do not indicate the degree of fetal injury. Furthermore, the possibility of false-positive test results cannot be excluded. Accordingly, detailed ultrasound examination is the best test to determine whether serious fetal injury has occurred as a result of maternal rubella infection. Possible anomalies detected by ultrasound include growth restriction, microcephaly, CNS abnormalities, and cardiac malformations.

The prognosis for infants with CRS is guarded. Approximately 50% of affected individuals have to attend schools for the hearing-impaired. An additional 25% require at least some special schooling because of hearing impairment, and only 25% are able to attend mainstream schools.[322]

Prevention of Rubella Infection

Ideally, women of reproductive age should have a preconception appointment when they are contemplating pregnancy. At that time, they should be evaluated for immunity to rubella. If serologic testing demonstrates that they are susceptible, they should be vaccinated with rubella vaccine before conception occurs. If preconception counseling is not possible, patients should have a test for rubella at the time of their first prenatal appointment. Women who are susceptible to rubella should be counseled to avoid exposure to other individuals who may have viral exanthems.

If a susceptible woman subsequently is exposed to rubella, serologic tests should be obtained to determine whether acute infection has occurred. If acute infection is documented by identification of IgM antibody, the patient should be counseled about the risk of CRS. The diagnostic tests for detection of congenital infection should be reviewed, and the patient should be offered the option of pregnancy termination, depending on the assessed risk of serious fetal injury.

Pregnant women who are susceptible to rubella should be vaccinated immediately after delivery. The rubella vaccine is available in monovalent, bivalent (measles-rubella), and trivalent (measles-mumps-rubella) forms. Approximately 95% of patients who receive rubella vaccine seroconvert, and antibody levels persist for at least 18 years in more than 90% of vaccinees.

Adverse effects of vaccination are minimal, even in adults. Fewer than 25% of patients experience mild constitutional symptoms such as low-grade fever and malaise. Fewer than 10% of vaccinees have arthralgias, and fewer than 1% develop frank arthritis. Other complaints, such as pain and paresthesias, have been rare. Women who have received the vaccine cannot transmit infection to susceptible contacts, such as young children in the home, and vaccinated women may breastfeed their infants. In addition, the vaccine can be administered in conjunction with immunoglobulin preparations such as Rh immune globulin.[319,323] Women who receive rubella vaccine should practice secure contraception for at least 1 month after vaccination.[324]

To decrease the occurrence of rubella, recommended public health policies include vaccinating all children aged 12 to 15 months or older and all adolescents and adults not known to be immune, unless they are pregnant or have other contraindications to vaccination. Also, all prenatal patients should be screened as early as possible in pregnancy.[318] Contraindications to vaccination include febrile illness, immunosuppression, and pregnancy. Precautions also are necessary in the rare individual with neomycin allergy.

Rubeola

Epidemiology

The measles (rubeola) virus is a single-stranded RNA paramyxovirus that closely is related to the canine distemper virus. The wild virus is pathogenic only for primates, and humans are the only natural host.

The virus is spread by respiratory droplets and is highly contagious. Between 75% and 90% of susceptible contacts become infected after exposure. Before a measles vaccine was available, essentially all children experienced natural measles infection. Since licensure of the first measles vaccine in 1963, the incidence of infection has decreased by almost 99%. As expected, children younger than 10 years of age have shown the greatest decline in incidence. During the mid-1980s, almost 60% of reported cases affected children older than 10 years of age, compared with only 10% of cases occurring during the period from 1960 to 1964.[325]

In recent years, two major types of measles outbreaks have occurred in the United States. One type has developed among unvaccinated preschoolers, including children younger than 15 months of age. Another type has occurred among previously vaccinated school-age children and college students. Approximately one third of the cases in the latter type of outbreak have been in individuals who were previously vaccinated. Presumably, these cases result from either *primary failure* to respond to the first vaccine or *secondary failure*, a situation in which an adequate serologic response develops initially but immunity wanes over time.[325,326]

The clinical manifestations of measles usually appear within 10 to 14 days after exposure. The most common signs and symptoms are fever, malaise, coryza, sneezing, conjunctivitis, cough, photophobia, and Koplik spots (blue-gray specks on a red base that develop on the buccal mucosa opposite the second molars). Patients typically develop a generalized nonpruritic maculopapular rash that begins on the face and neck and then spreads to the trunk and extremities. It usually lasts for approximately 5 days and subsequently recedes in the same sequence in which it appeared. The duration of illness is approximately 7 to 10 days (hence, the name, the "10-day measles"). Patients are contagious from 1 to 4 days before the onset of coryza until several days after appearance of the rash. Immunity to measles should be lifelong after wild virus infection and is mediated by both humoral and cell-mediated mechanisms.

Although measles is typically a minor illness, some patients develop serious sequelae. Otitis media occurs in 7% to 9% of infected patients; bronchiolitis and pneumonia affect 1% to 6%. A severe form of hepatitis also may occur. In a report by Atmar and associates,[327] 7 (54%) of 13 pregnant women with measles developed hepatitis.

Encephalitis occurs in approximately 1 in every 1000 cases of measles. It results from both viral infection of the CNS and a hypersensitivity reaction to the systemic viral infection. Measles encephalitis may lead to permanent neurologic impairment, including mental retardation; the mortality rate from this complication is approximately 15% to 33%. Another unusual, but extremely serious, complication of measles is subacute sclerosing panencephalitis. This complication occurs in 0.5 to 2 cases per 1000. It usually develops about 7 years after the acute measles infection and is more common in children who had measles before the age of 2 years. The disorder is characterized by progressive neurologic debilitation and has an almost uniformly fatal outcome.[325,327]

A final complication is *atypical measles*. This disorder is a severe form of measles reinfection that affects young adults previously vaccinated with the formalin-inactivated killed measles vaccine that was distributed in the United States from 1963 to 1967. Affected patients have extremely high antibody titers to measles, and they experience high fever, pneumonitis, pleural effusion, and a coarse maculopapular, hemorrhagic, or urticarial rash. Although the disease usually is self-limited, atypical measles can lead to hepatic, cardiac, and renal failure. Interestingly, affected patients are not contagious to others.[325,328]

Five clinical criteria should be present to establish the diagnosis of measles: fever of 38.3° C or higher, characteristic rash lasting longer than 3 days, cough, coryza, and conjunctivitis. Although the virus can be cultured, the mainstay of diagnostic tests is detection of antibody to measles. The hemagglutination inhibition assay and the enzyme-linked immunosorbent assay (ELISA) are the most useful serologic tests for determination of a patient's susceptibility to measles and for confirmation of infection. The serologic confirmation of acute measles virus infection is based on detection of IgM-specific antibody or a fourfold change in the IgG titer in acute and convalescent sera. The acute titer for IgG antibody should be obtained within 3 days after the onset of the rash, and the convalescent titer should be obtained 10 to 20 days later.

Obstetric Considerations

Several reports have documented an increase in maternal mortality associated with measles infection during pregnancy; most deaths have been caused by pulmonary complications. In one of the earliest investigations, Christensen and colleagues[329] described an epidemic of measles in Greenland in 1951. Four (4.8%) of 83 pregnant women who developed measles died. An unspecified number of these women also had active tuberculosis. In the report by Atmar and associates,[327] one (8%) of 13 pregnant women with measles died because of severe respiratory infection. Eberhart-Phillips and coworkers[330] evaluated 58 pregnant women with measles. Thirty-five (60%) required hospitalization, 15 (26%) developed pneumonia, and 2 (3%) died.

Reports also have described a slight increase in the frequency of preterm delivery and spontaneous abortion among women who developed measles during pregnancy. In the study by Eberhart-Phillips and colleagues,[330] 13 (26%) of 50 women with continuing pregnancies delivered preterm. Fortunately, the frequency of congenital anomalies is not increased significantly in women who contract measles during pregnancy.

Although congenital anomalies are rare, infants of mothers who are acutely infected at the time of delivery are at risk for *neonatal measles*. This infection typically develops within the first 10 days of life and results from transplacental transmission of the virus. The mortality rate in preterm and term infants with neonatal measles has been reported to be as high as 60% and 20%, respectively.[331]

Preventive Measures

Ideally, all women of reproductive age should have evidence of immunity to measles before attempting pregnancy. Originally, public health officials thought that a single injection of live measles vaccine when a child was approximately 15 months of age provided lifelong immunity. As noted previously, however, several recent outbreaks of measles have occurred due to secondary vaccine failures. Accordingly, the Advisory Committee on Immunization Practices (ACIP) recommends that all individuals who have not been infected with the live virus receive a second dose of the vaccine at 4 to 6 years of age. If this second dose is not administered in childhood, it should be administered before a woman plans her first pregnancy. There are only three contraindications to use of the live measles vaccine: pregnancy, severe febrile illness, and history of anaphylactic reaction to egg protein or neomycin.[332]

If a susceptible pregnant woman is exposed to measles, she should immediately receive passive immunoprophylaxis with immune globulin, 0.25 mL/kg intramuscularly, up to a maximum dose of 15 mL. If she develops measles despite immunoprophylaxis, she should be observed for evidence of serious complications such as otitis media, hepatitis, encephalitis, and pneumonia. Secondary bacterial infections should be treated promptly with antibiotics. Administration of aerosolized ribavirin may be of benefit to patients with severe viral pneumonitis.[333]

The affected patient should be counseled that the risk of injury to her fetus is very low. The most effective method of evaluating the fetus for in utero infection is detailed ultrasound examination. Findings suggestive of in utero infection include microcephaly, growth restriction, and oligohydramnios. If the mother developed measles within 7 to 10 days of delivery, the neonate should receive intramuscular immunoglobulin in a dose of 0.25 mL/kg. These infants subsequently should receive the live measles vaccine when they are 15 months of age.[333]

Syphilis

Syphilis is a chronic systemic infection resulting from the spirochete *Treponema pallidum*. It has been recognized for several centuries that primary, secondary, and early latent syphilis in pregnant women cause infection of the fetus, with resultant stillbirths, congenital abnormalities, and active disease at birth. Because of this significant morbidity, great emphasis has been placed on routine screening of all pregnant women for syphilis. Acquisition is usually through sexual contact.

Epidemiology

Since the startling prediction in 1937 by United States Surgeon General Thomas Parran that 10% of Americans would be infected with syphilis during their lives, the rates of primary and secondary syphilis have dramatically decreased, finally reaching a nadir in 2000 (Fig. 38-7).[334] This striking decline was associated with the institution of public health control measures and the availability of penicillin. The generally downward trend in the syphilis rate was temporarily interrupted in the late 1970s and early 1980s when the rates of primary and secondary syphilis began increasing, in large part due to increases among men having sex with men. After the advent of the HIV/AIDS epidemic and public health efforts promoting safer sex, the rates of syphilis resumed their downward trend.

However, in the late 1980s another transient epidemic of primary and secondary syphilis occurred in the United States.[4] Coincident with this rise was a dramatic increase in reported cases of congenital syphilis.[335] After a low of 108 cases of congenital syphilis in 1978, there were 350 cases reported in 1986, and 3850 cases in 1992, with an incidence rate of 100 per 100,000 live births (Fig. 38-8). Almost 90% of congenital syphilis cases occurred among blacks or Hispanics, and 50% of the cases occurred among mothers receiving no prenatal care. Reasons for this dramatic upsurge include exchange of drugs (e.g., "crack" cocaine) for sex; decreased funding for syphilis control; treatment of penicillinase-producing *N. gonorrhoeae* with spectinomycin, which

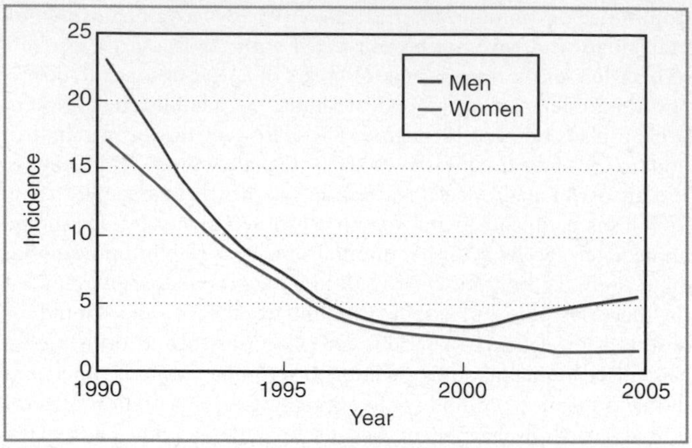

FIGURE 38-7 Incidence of primary and secondary syphilis per 100,000 population, by sex—United States, 1990-2005. During 2004-2005, the incidence of primary and secondary syphilis in the United States increased slightly, from 2.7 to 3.0 cases per 100,000 (from 0.8 to 0.9 per 100,000 in women, and from 4.7 to 5.1 per 100,000 in men).

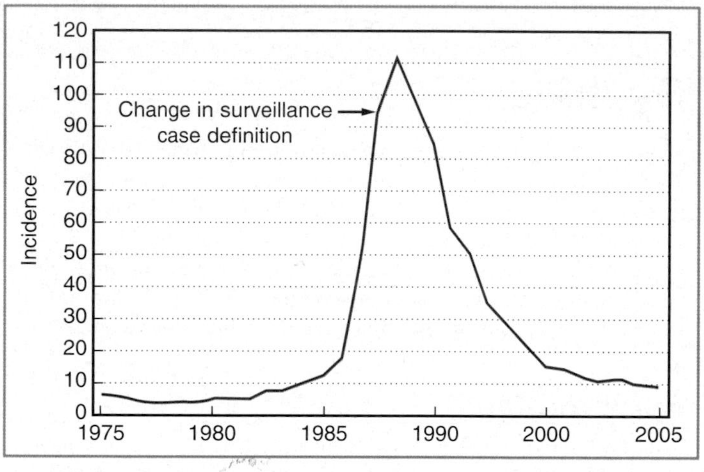

FIGURE 38-8 Incidence of congenital syphilis (per 100,000 live births) among infants aged 0 to 12 months—United States, 1975-2005. The incidence of congenital syphilis has declined since 1991. In 2005, the rate was 8.0 cases per 100,000 live births.

does not treat incubating syphilis; and the use of revised reporting guidelines for congenital syphilis, which were introduced in 1989.

Following this latest epidemic, the rates of primary and secondary syphilis fell from their peak in 1990 (18.4 cases per 100,000 population and more than 112,000 reported cases of primary and secondary syphilis) to a nadir in 2000 (2.1 cases per 100,000 population and fewer than 6000 reported cases of primary and secondary syphilis). This was the lowest rate since syphilis reporting began in 1941. Concomitant with the plummeting rates of primary and secondary syphilis, the rates of congenital syphilis also dramatically fell, declining from 3850 cases in 1992 to 451 cases in 2002.[336]

As a result of this dramatic decline in syphilis rates, the CDC launched the National Syphilis Elimination Plan in 1999. However, this plan for elimination of syphilis in the United States has proved overly optimistic.[337-339]

Pathogenesis

T. pallidum is efficiently transmitted during sexual contact, and syphilis is acquired in 50% to 60% of partners after a single sexual exposure to an infected individual with early syphilis. Spirochetes may gain access through any break in the skin or via microscopic tears in genital tract mucosal surfaces, which occur almost universally during sexual intercourse. The mean incubation time is 21 days, with a range of 10 to 90 days.[4]

The primary stage of syphilis is characterized by the chancre, which appears at the site of entry for *T. pallidum*. The chancre is a painless, nontender, ulcerated lesion with a raised border and an indurated base. The most common site for the chancre is the genital area. In men, the lesion is easily apparent, and syphilis is often diagnosed in its primary stage. In women, the lesion most commonly is on the cervix or in the vagina and is not recognized. Therefore, the chancre often escapes detection in women, and it is unusual to diagnose the primary stage of syphilis in females. Usually only a single chancre is present, but multiple chancres occur in up to 30% of cases. Painless inguinal lymphadenopathy is frequently present. The primary chancre, even without treatment, heals spontaneously in 3 to 6 weeks.

After resolution of the primary stage, the patient enters the secondary or spirochetemia (bacteremia) stage of syphilis. Syphilis always disseminates during the secondary stage. Any organ can potentially be infected, especially the CNS. Although the secondary stage of syphilis is characterized by involvement of all major organ systems by *T. palladium*, it manifests most commonly with skin and mucous membrane lesions. These clinical manifestations of secondary syphilis include a generalized maculopapular rash that begins on the trunk and proximal extremities and spreads to the entire body, especially involving the palms and soles; mucous patches; condyloma latum; and generalized lymphadenopathy. These mucocutaneous lesions are highly contagious.

Even without treatment, the manifestations of secondary syphilis spontaneously clear within 2 to 6 weeks, and the latent stage of syphilis is entered, in which there is no apparent clinical disease. In the era before the availability of penicillin, about 25% of such patients had a recrudescence of secondary syphilis. Because these relapses usually occurred within 1 year, the term "early latent period" was applied to this time period. In the late latent stage (>1 year), patients are not contagious by sexual transmission, but the spirochete may still be transplacentally transmitted to a fetus.[340,341]

Without treatment, one third of patients progress and develop tertiary syphilis, characterized by involvement of the cardiovascular, central nervous, or musculoskeletal, and/or various organ systems with gummas (late benign tertiary syphilis).[340] One half of patients with tertiary syphilis develop late benign syphilis (gummas), one fourth develop cardiovascular disease, and one fourth have neurologic disease. The cardiovascular manifestations of tertiary syphilis include aortic aneurysm and aortic insufficiency. In the CNS, tertiary disease produces general paresis, tabes dorsalis, optic atrophy, and meningovascular syphilis. The Argyll-Robertson pupil (i.e., pupil does not react to light but accommodates) is virtually pathognomonic of tertiary syphilis. The pathogenesis of tertiary syphilis is based on the tropism of *T. pallidum* for arterioles, which results in obliterative endarteritis with subsequent tissue destruction.

Congenital Syphilis

The clinical spectrum in congenital syphilis includes stillbirth, neonatal death, nonimmune hydrops, clinically apparent syphilis during the early months of life (early congenital syphilis), and the classic stigmata of late congenital syphilis (see Table 38-17).[4] The most severe adverse pregnancy outcomes occur with primary or secondary syphilis. Pregnant women diagnosed with syphilis are usually in the latent stage and have had the disease for longer than 1 year. Consequently, about two thirds of infants with early congenital syphilis are asymptomatic at birth and do not develop evidence of active disease for 3 to 8 weeks. Chancres do not occur unless the disease is acquired at the time of passage through the birth canal. The characteristic manifestations of early congenital syphilis (onset at <2 years of age) include a maculopapular rash that may progress to desquamation or formation of vesicles and bullae, snuffles (a flulike syndrome associated with a nasal discharge), mucous patches in the oral pharyngeal cavity, hepatosplenomegaly, jaundice, lymphadenopathy, pseudoparalysis of Parrot due to osteochondritis, chorioretinitis, and iritis.[341]

Untreated or incompletely treated early congenital syphilis will progress to the classic manifestations of late congenital syphilis. These include Hutchinson teeth, mulberry molars, interstitial keratitis, eighth-nerve deafness, saddle nose, rhagades, saber shins, and neurologic manifestations (mental retardation, hydrocephalus, general paresis, optic nerve atrophy, and Clutton joints). These stigmata associated with late congenital syphilis are the result of scarring induced by early lesions or reactions to persistent inflammation.[341]

T. pallidum can cross the placenta and infect the fetus as early as the 6th gestational week.[342] Clinical manifestations are not apparent until after 16 weeks of gestation, when fetal immunocompetence develops. Therefore, the risk to the fetus is present throughout pregnancy, and the degree of risk is related to the quantity of spirochetes in the maternal bloodstream. Transmission may also occur intrapartum via contact with active genital lesions in the mother. Women with primary or secondary syphilis are more likely to transmit infection to their offspring than are women with latent disease. Maternal primary syphilis and secondary syphilis are associated with a 50% probability of congenital syphilis and a 50% rate of perinatal death; early latent syphilis, with a 40% risk of congenital syphilis and a 20% mortality rate; and late latent syphilis, with a 10% risk of congenital syphilis.[343,344] Similar high rates of morbidity and mortality among the infants of mothers with untreated syphilis of less than 4 years' duration were reported in 1959 by Inraham,[345] who noted a perinatal death rate of 43% (29% stillborn, and 14% neonatal); among liveborn infants, 41% had congenital syphilis.

Experience during the syphilis epidemic in the late 1980s and early 1990s confirmed that untreated syphilis is associated with significant and frequent adverse effects on pregnancy. Ricci and associates[346] reported that, among 56 cases of congenital syphilis, 19 (35%) were stillbirths, and the perinatal mortality rate was 464 per 1000 live births. Preterm labor and delivery were significantly more common, infants with congenital syphilis had significantly lower birth weights, and 21% had intrauterine growth restriction. McFarlin and coworkers[335] reviewed 253 cases of maternal syphilis. They reported a preterm delivery rate of 28%; 10 (13.9%) of 72 cases of congenital syphilis were stillbirths. In addition, the manifestations of congenital syphilis are usually less severe in association with long-standing maternal disease than with early syphilis of less than 1 year's duration. Coles and colleagues,[347] in a review of 322 cases of congenital syphilis in upstate New York from 1989 to 1992, reported that 31 (10%) stillbirths and 59 (19%) newborns with clinical evidence of congenital syphilis were documented. Factors believed to contribute to the development of congenital syphilis included infection late in pregnancy, treatment less than 30 days before delivery, misdiagnosis or inappropriate treatment of the mother, and no serologic testing during pregnancy.

Diagnosis

The most definitive methods for diagnosing early syphilis are dark-field microscope examination or direct fluorescent antibody tests of lesion exudates or tissue.[12] A presumptive diagnosis can be made using serologic testing. The serologic tests are classified into two types: nonspecific tests for reagin-type antibodies and specific antitreponemal antibody tests.

Nonspecific antibody tests include the Venereal Disease Research Laboratory (VDRL) test and the rapid plasma reagin (RPR) test. These are used for screening. All pregnant women should be screened at the initial prenatal visit. High-risk patients should be rescreened at 28 weeks of gestation. In areas with high rates of congenital syphilis, rescreening at admission in labor is also recommended. In populations in which prenatal care is less than optimal, RPR-card test screening is recommended at the time pregnancy is diagnosed, with treatment of patients who have a reactive test. The CDC recommends that any woman who delivers a stillborn infant after 20 weeks of gestation should be screened for syphilis. In addition, the CDC advises that no infant should leave the hospital without the maternal serostatus for syphilis having been assessed at some time in pregnancy.[12]

Treponema-specific tests are employed for confirming the diagnosis of syphilis in patients who have reactive VDRL or RPR results. These tests include the fluorescent treponemal antibody absorption (FTA-ABS) test and the *T. pallidum* particle agglutination (TP-PA) test.

Usually the nonspecific test result becomes nonreactive after treatment. In some patients, a low titer may persist for a long time, in some cases for life. Once reactive, specific treponemal tests usually remain positive for life. In pregnancy, it is best to consider all seropositive women as infected unless an adequate treatment history is documented and sequential serologic antibody titers have declined.

It is critical to recognize that when the syphilitic chancre first appears, both the nonspecific test results and the treponemal-specific test results may be nonreactive. Therefore, lesions suspicious for syphilis should be sampled for detection of spirochetes and submitted to the laboratory for dark-field examination and fluorescent-antibody staining.

Although the CNS is involved in almost half of the patients with early syphilis, fewer than 10% of patients with untreated syphilis progress to symptomatic late neurosyphilis. If patients are treated appropriately for early syphilis, neurosyphilis should be extremely rare. The CDC has stated that, unless clinical signs or symptoms of neurologic involvement are present, lumbar puncture is not recommended for routine evaluation in primary or secondary syphilis. In patients with latent syphilis, prompt CSF examination should be performed if any of the following conditions is present[12]:

1. Clinical evidence of neurologic involvement (e.g., cognitive dysfunction, motor or sensory deficits, ophthalmic or auditory symptoms, cranial nerve palsies, symptoms or signs of meningitis)
2. Evidence of active tertiary syphilis (e.g., aortitis, gummas, iritis)
3. Treatment failure
4. HIV infection with latent syphilis or syphilis of unknown duration

Recently, it has been suggested that only HIV-infected patients with neurologic manifestations or a serum RPR result of 1/32 or greater require a lumbar puncture.[348] Marra and colleagues[349] studied 326 patients with syphilis in an attempt to define clinical and laboratory features that identify patients with neurosyphilis. Sixty-five patients (20.1%) had neurosyphilis. In multivariate analysis, an RPR titer of 1/32 or greater increased the odds of neurosyphilis almost 11-fold in HIV-uninfected individuals and almost sixfold among HIV-infected patients. In HIV-infected subjects, a $CD4^+$ of 350 cells/mL or less conferred a 3.10-fold increased odds of neurosyphilis.

No single test is adequate to diagnose neurosyphilis in all patients. Therefore, the diagnosis is based on various combinations of tests, including reactive serologic tests, abnormal CSF cell count, elevated protein, and/or a reactive CSF VDRL, with or without clinical manifestations. CSF studies demonstrating pleocytosis, elevated protein levels, and a reactive CSF VDRL are diagnostic of neurosyphilis. On occasion, however, results may be nonreactive when neurosyphilis is present. Recently, it has been suggested that increased levels of tau protein may be useful in discriminating neurosyphilis from syphilis without nervous system involvement.[350]

The diagnosis of reinfection or persistence of active syphilis can be made in patients previously known to have syphilis by following the titer of the quantitative VDRL. With successful therapy, the VDRL titer should decrease and become negative or very low within 6 to 12 months in early syphilis and within 12 to 24 months in late syphilis (>1 year's duration). A rising titer indicates the need for further diagnostic measures, such as a lumbar puncture, and appropriate treatment.

The diagnosis of congenital syphilis is easily confirmed in the clinically apparent case in which a jaundiced, hydropic baby with florid disease and a large, edematous placenta are delivered and laboratory studies confirm the presence of the disease. However, most infected newborns are asymptomatic at birth. Although the cord blood may give a positive nonspecific test result for syphilis, the diagnosis of congenital syphilis is complicated by the transplacental transfer of maternal nontreponemal and treponemal IgG antibodies to the fetus.[12]

As a result, the interpretation of reactive serologic tests for syphilis in infants is difficult. Therefore, treatment decisions must be frequently made on the basis of (1) identification of syphilis in the mother; (2) adequacy (or lack thereof) of maternal treatment; (3) presence of clinical, laboratory or radiologic evidence of syphilis in the infant; and (4) comparison of maternal (at delivery) and infant nontreponemal serologic titers using the same test and same laboratory.[12] Any infant with a positive VDRL result but no clinical evidence of syphilis should have serial monthly quantitative VDRL tests for at least 9 months. A rising titer indicates active disease and the need for therapy. Infected infants may be asymptomatic and the serum VDRL may be normal if maternal infection occurred late in pregnancy.

In 1998, the CDC implemented a new case definition for congenital syphilis surveillance (Table 38-17). A diagnosis of congenital syphilis can be confirmed by identifying spirochetes in suspicious lesions, body fluids, or tissues with dark-field microscopy, silver staining, immunofluorescence, or PCR for *T. pallidum* DNA.[351] Several new laboratory tests have been introduced to facilitate the diagnosis of congenital syphilis. These include PCR and the rabbit infectivity test (RIT).

TABLE 38-17 CONGENITAL SYPHILIS CASE DEFINITION

Confirmed Case

Infant in whom *Treponema palladium* is identified by dark-field microscopy, fluorescent antibody, or other specific stains in specimens from lesions, placenta, umbilical cord, or autopsy material

Presumptive Case

1. Any infant whose mother had untreated* or inadequately treated syphilis at delivery, regardless of signs or symptoms†

OR

2. Any infant or child who has a reactive treponemal test for syphilis and any one of the following:
   a. Evidence of congenital syphilis on physical examination
   b. Evidence of congenital syphilis on long-bone radiography
   c. **Reactive CSF VDRL test**
   d. Elevated CSF white blood cell count (>5/mm^3) or protein concentration (>5 mg/dL)
   e. Reactive test for FTA-ABS-19S-IgM antibody

CSF, cerebrospinal fluid; FTA-ABS, fluorescent treponemal antibody absorption; IgM, immunoglobulin M; VDRL, Venereal Disease Research Laboratory.

*On penicillin therapy or penicillin given <30 days before delivery.

†Clinical signs in an infant include hepatosplenomegaly, characteristic skin rash, condyloma lata, snuffles, jaundice, pseudoparalysis, anemia, thrombocytopenia, and edema. Stigmata in children older than 2 years of age include interstitial keratitis, nerve deafness, anterior bowing of shins, frontal bossing, mulberry molars, Hutchinson teeth, saddle nose, rhagades, and Clutton joints.

From Centers for Disease Control and Prevention: Congenital Syphilis Case Definition. Atlanta, GA: U.S. Department of Health and Human Services, CDC, 1998.

Treatment

All pregnant women who have a history of sexual contact with a person with documented syphilis, dark-field microscope confirmation of the presence of spirochetes, or serologic evidence of syphilis via a specific treponemal test should be treated. In addition, patients in whom the diagnosis cannot be ruled out with certainty or those who have been previously treated but now show evidence of reinfection, such as dark-field microscope confirmation or a fourfold rise in titer on a quantitative nontreponemal test, should receive appropriate treatment.

Treatment schedules for syphilis recommended by CDC in 2006 are shown in Table 38-18. Penicillin administered parenterally is the preferred treatment for all stages of syphilis.[12]

The preparation of penicillin used and the length of treatment are determined by the stage and clinical manifestations of the disease. Although several alternatives to penicillin might be effective in nonpregnant penicillin-allergic patients, parenteral penicillin G is the only therapy with documented efficacy for syphilis during pregnancy. In pregnancy, parenteral penicillin G is effective for treating maternal infection, preventing transmission to the fetus, and treating established fetal infection. Therefore, the CDC recommends that pregnant patients with syphilis in any stage who are allergic to penicillin should be desensitized and treated with penicillin.[12]

Desensitization is a relatively safe and straightforward procedure that can be accomplished orally or intravenously. Oral desensitization is generally believed to be safer and easier to perform. Patients should be desensitized in a hospital setting, because serious IgE-mediated allergic reactions can occur. Desensitization can be accomplished in approximately 4 hours (Table 38-19), after which the first dose of penicillin is administered. After desensitization, patients must be maintained on penicillin continuously for the duration of their therapeutic course.

Although erythromycin was at one time considered an alternative to penicillin for the treatment of syphilis during pregnancy, its efficacy for treatment of syphilis in the fetus and for prevention of transmis-

TABLE 38-18 CDC-RECOMMENDED TREATMENT OF SYPHILIS DURING PREGNANCY, 2006

Diagnosis	Treatment
1. Primary, secondary, and early latent syphilis (<1 yr)	Benzathine penicillin G, 2.4 million units IM in a single dose
2. Late latent syphilis (>1 yr), latent syphilis of unknown duration, and tertiary syphilis	Benzathine penicillin G, 7.2 million units total, administered as 3 doses of 2.4 million units IM each at 1-wk intervals
3. Neurosyphilis	Aqueous crystalline penicillin G, 18-24 million units per day administered as 3-4 million units IV every 4 hr or by continuous infusion for 10-14 days OR Procaine penicillin, 2.4 million units IM daily, plus probenecid 500 mg PO qid, both for 10-14 days
4. Penicillin-allergic	Pregnant women with a history of penicillin allergy should have allergy confirmed and then be desensitized

Modified from Centers for Disease Control and Prevention. Sexually Transmitted Diseases Treatment Guidelines, 2006. MMWR Recommendations and Reports 55(RR-11):22-35, 2006.

TABLE 38-19 ORAL DESENSITIZATION PROTOCOL FOR PATIENTS WITH A POSITIVE SKIN TEST FOR PENICILLIN ALLERGY*

Penicillin V Suspension Dose†	Amount (Units/mL)‡	mL	Units	Cumulative Dose (Units)
1	1,000	0.1	100	100
2	1,000	0.2	200	300
3	1,000	0.4	400	700
4	1,000	0.8	800	1,500
5	1,000	1.6	1,600	3,100
6	1,000	3.2	3,200	6,300
7	1,000	6.4	6,400	12,700
8	10,000	1.2	12,000	24,700
9	10,000	2.4	24,000	48,700
10	10,000	4.8	48,000	96,700
11	80,000	1.0	80,000	176,700
12	80,000	2.0	160,000	336,700
13	80,000	4.0	320,000	656,700
14	80,000	8.0	640,000	1,296,700

***Observation period: 30 minutes before parenteral administration of penicillin.**
†Interval between doses, 15 minutes; elapsed time, 3 hours and 45 minutes; cumulative dose, 1.3 million units.
‡The specific amount of drug is diluted in approximately 30 mL of water and then administered orally.
From Wendel GO Jr, Stark BJ, Jamison RB, et al: Penicillin allergy and desensitization in serious infections during pregnancy. N Engl J Med 312:1229-1232, 1985. Reprinted with permission from the New England Journal of Medicine.

sion is inadequate. Although doxycycline and tetracycline are alternatives for nonpregnant patients, they usually are not used in pregnancy.

Concern has been raised as to whether the recommended regimens of penicillin are optimal in pregnancy. Several reports demonstrated worrisome instances of treatment failures despite adherence to recommended guidelines.[335,352] A high maternal VDRL titer at the time of diagnosis, unknown duration of infection, treatment within 4 weeks of delivery, and ultrasound signs of fetal syphilis (e.g., hepatomegaly, fetal hydrops, placentomegaly) are associated with failure to prevent congenital syphilis.

Because of these reports demonstrating a high failure rate for treatment of syphilis in pregnancy, some experts recommend additional therapy.[12] A second dose of benzathine penicillin G (2.4 million units intramuscularly) may be given 1 week after the initial dose for pregnant women with primary, secondary, or early latent syphilis. During the second half of pregnancy, management of syphilis may be facilitated by sonographic assessment for evidence of congenital syphilis. Sonographic signs of fetal or placental syphilis (e.g., hepatomegaly, ascites, hydrops, a thickened placenta) indicate a greater risk for fetal treatment failure.[353]

Syphilis can involve the CNS during any stage of disease. Therefore, any patient with syphilis who demonstrates clinical evidence of neurologic involvement should have a lumbar puncture to assess the CSF for evidence of neurosyphilis. Patients with neurosyphilis should be treated with high doses of aqueous penicillin G, as noted in Table 38-17.

Obstetric caregivers should be aware that women treated for syphilis during the second half of pregnancy are at risk for preterm labor or fetal distress if the Jarisch-Herxheimer reaction occurs. The Jarisch-Herxheimer reaction occurs commonly during the treatment of early syphilis; among 33 pregnant women, the reaction complicated therapy in 100% and 60% of patients treated for primary or secondary syphilis, respectively.[354] The Jarisch-Herxheimer reaction characteristically includes fever, chills, myalgia, headache, hypotension, and transient worsening of cutaneous lesions. It commences within several hours after treatment and resolves by 24 to 36 hours. Among pregnant women, the most frequent findings are fever (73%), uterine contractions (67%), and decreased fetal movement (67%). Transient late decelerations were observed in 30% of monitored fetuses.

Because of these findings, sonographic assessment of the fetus before initiating therapy for early syphilis in the last half of pregnancy has been recommended.[355] If the results are normal, ambulatory treatment may be initiated. If abnormal findings suggesting fetal infection are identified, hospitalization for treatment and fetal monitoring is recommended. Sanchez and Wendel[352] demonstrated that, in the presence of severe fetal compromise before treatment, early delivery with treatment of the mother and neonate after delivery may yield an improved outcome.

For primary and secondary syphilis, patients should be re-examined clinically and serologically at 6 months and 12 months after treatment. A two-dilution (fourfold) decline in the nontreponemal titer at 1 year after treatment is used to define response.[356] Patients with signs or symptoms that persist or recur and those with a sustained fourfold increase in the nontreponemal test titer have probably failed treatment or become reinfected. They should be re-treated, be assessed for HIV infection, and undergo analysis of the CSF. For re-treatment, weekly injections of benzathine penicillin G 2.4 million units IM for 3 weeks is suggested.[12]

With latent syphilis, quantitative nontreponemal titers should be repeated at 6, 12, and 24 months. Patients with a normal CSF examination should be re-treated for latent syphilis if (1) titers increase fourfold, (2) an initially high titer (≥1:32) fails to decline at least fourfold (i.e., two dilutions) within 12 to 24 months after therapy, or (3) signs or symptoms of syphilis develop. There is limited information available concerning either clinical response or follow-up in patients treated for tertiary syphilis.[12]

In pregnant women treated for syphilis, the CDC recommends repeating serologic titers at 28 to 32 weeks' gestation, and again at delivery, and following the recommendations described earlier for the stage of disease. Alternatively, serologic titers can be checked monthly in women who are at high risk for reinfection or who live in a geographic area where the prevalence of syphilis is high.[12]

Congenital syphilis is unusual if the mother received adequate treatment with penicillin during pregnancy. Infants should be treated for presumed congenital syphilis if they were born to mothers in the following categories:

1. Mothers who have untreated syphilis at delivery
2. Mothers who have serologic evidence of relapse or reinfection after treatment (i.e., a rise in titer by at least fourfold)
3. Mothers who were treated for syphilis during pregnancy with nonpenicillin regimens
4. Mothers who were treated for syphilis less than 1 month before delivery
5. Mothers who do not have a well-documented history of treatment of syphilis
6. Mothers who do not demonstrate an adequate response (fourfold decrease) of nontreponemal antibody titers despite appropriate penicillin treatment
7. Mothers who were treated for syphilis appropriately before pregnancy but had insufficient serologic follow-up to ensure response to treatment.

Any child with symptomatic congenital syphilis should undergo a lumbar puncture, complete blood count, and long-bone radiography before treatment. If these results are normal, a single intramuscular dose of benzathine penicillin G (50,000 units/kg) should be given. With abnormal results or if compliance is not ensured, the infant should be given a 10-day course of either aqueous crystalline penicillin G (50,000 units/kg IV every 12 hours for the first 7 days of life, and then every 8 hours for the next 3 days) or procaine penicillin (50,000 units/kg/day IM).[12]

Prevention

Serologic screening of all pregnant women during the early stages of pregnancy is recommended. In geographic areas with a high prevalence of syphilis and in patients at high risk, serologic testing should be repeated at 28 to 32 weeks' gestation and at delivery.[12]

Toxoplasmosis

Epidemiology and Pathogenesis

Toxoplasma gondii is a protozoan that has three distinct life forms: trophozoite, cyst, and oocyst. The life cycle of this organism is dependent on wild and domestic cats, which are the only known host for the oocyst. The oocyst is formed in the intestine of the cat and subsequently is excreted in feces. Mammals, such as cows, ingest the oocyst, which is disrupted in the animal's intestine, releasing the invasive trophozoite. The trophozoite then is disseminated throughout the body, ultimately forming cysts in brain and muscle.[357]

Human infection occurs when infected meat is ingested or oocysts are ingested via contamination by cat feces. Infection rates are highest in areas of poor sanitation and crowded living conditions. Stray cats and domestic cats that eat raw meat are most likely to carry the parasite. The cyst is completely destroyed by heating.

Approximately half of all adults in the United States have antibody to this organism. Immunity is usually long-lasting except in immunosuppressed patients. The prevalence of antibody is highest in lower socioeconomic classes. The frequency of seroconversion during pregnancy is approximately 5%, and about 3 in 1000 infants show evidence of congenital infection. Clinically significant infection occurs in only 1 in 8000 pregnancies. Clinical manifestations of infection are the result of direct organ damage and the subsequent immunologic response to parasitemia and cell death. Immunity to this infection is mediated primarily through T lymphocytes.[357]

Diagnosis

Most infections in humans are asymptomatic. Even in the absence of symptoms, however, patients may have evidence of multiorgan involvement, and clinically apparent disease can develop after a long period of asymptomatic infection. Symptomatic toxoplasmosis usually manifests as an illness similar to mononucleosis.

In contrast to infection in the immunocompetent host, toxoplasmosis can be a devastating infection in the immunosuppressed patient. In these individuals, dysfunction of the CNS is the most common manifestation of infection. Findings typically include encephalitis, meningoencephalitis, and intracerebral abscess. Pneumonitis, myocarditis, and generalized lymphadenopathy also occur commonly.

Routine screening for toxoplasmosis in pregnancy is not indicated. However, immunosuppressed patients, women who have contact with outdoor cats, and patients with suspicious symptoms should be tested. The diagnosis of toxoplasmosis in the mother is best confirmed by serology. Serologic tests suggestive of an acute infection include identification of IgM-specific antibody, demonstration of an extremely high IgG antibody titer, and documentation of IgG seroconversion from negative to positive. Clinicians should be aware that serologic assays for toxoplasmosis are not well standardized. Therefore, if initial laboratory tests suggest an acute maternal infection, additional evaluation, as detailed in the following paragraphs, is indicated before concluding that the fetus is at risk for serious injury.[357,358]

Approximately 40% of neonates born to mothers with acute toxoplasmosis have evidence of infection. Congenital infection is most likely to occur when maternal infection develops during the third trimester. The risk of injury to the fetus is greatest, however, when maternal infection occurs in the first trimester.

The usual clinical manifestations of congenital toxoplasmosis include a disseminated purpuric rash, enlargement of the spleen and liver, ascites, chorioretinitis, uveitis, periventricular calcifications, ventriculomegaly, seizures, and mental retardation. Chronic or latent infection in the mother is unlikely to be associated with serious fetal injury.

The most valuable test for confirmation of congenital toxoplasmosis is detection of toxoplasmic DNA in amniotic fluid using the PCR methodology. In an important initial investigation, Hohlfeld and associates[359] identified 34 infants with confirmed congenital toxoplasmosis. Amniotic fluid specimens from all affected pregnancies were positive by PCR, and test results were available within 1 day after specimen collection. In a subsequent investigation, Romand and colleagues[360] reported that the PCR test for toxoplasmic DNA had an overall sensitivity of 64% (CI, 53% to 75%). No false-positive results were noted, and the positive predictive value was 100%. Once amniocentesis has confirmed toxoplasmic infection, targeted ultrasound examination is indicated to look for specific findings suggestive of severe fetal injury.

Treatment

In the immunocompetent adult, toxoplasmosis usually is an asymptomatic or self-limited illness that does not require treatment. Immunocompromised patients should be treated with a combination of oral sulfadiazine (4-g loading dose followed by 1 g four times daily) plus pyrimethamine (50 to 100 mg initially, then 25 mg daily). Extended courses of treatment may be necessary to cure the infection.

When acute toxoplasmosis occurs during pregnancy, treatment is indicated, because maternal therapy reduces the risk of congenital infection and decreases the late sequelae of infection. Pyrimethamine is not recommended for use during the first trimester of pregnancy because of possible teratogenicity. Sulfonamides may be used alone, but single-agent therapy appears to be less effective than combination therapy. Spiramycin has been used extensively in European countries with excellent success. It is available in the United States through special permission from the CDC.[358]

Aggressive early treatment of infants with congenital toxoplasmosis is indicated and consists of combination therapy with pyrimethamine, sulfadiazine, and leucovorin for 1 year. Early treatment reduces, but does not eliminate, the late sequelae of toxoplasmosis such as chorioretinitis. Early treatment of the neonate appears to be comparable in effectiveness to in utero therapy.[361]

In pregnant women, prevention of toxoplasmosis is of paramount importance. Pregnant women should be advised to avoid contact with cat litter if at all possible. If they must change the litter, they should wear gloves and wash their hands afterward. They should always wash their hands after preparing meat for cooking, and they should never eat raw or rare beef, fowl, or pork. Meat should be cooked thoroughly until the juices are clear. Fruits and vegetables also should be washed carefully to remove possible contamination by oocysts.

Varicella-Zoster Virus Infection

Epidemiology and Pathogenesis

The varicella-zoster virus (VZV) is a DNA organism that is a member of the herpesvirus family. The organism causes varicella (chickenpox) and herpes zoster infection (shingles). Varicella is of great importance in pregnancy because it poses risks to the mother, fetus, and neonate.[362] Herpes zoster infection can be a painful and somewhat debilitating condition, especially in an immunosuppressed patient. However, because it occurs in a patient who already has antibody against VZV, herpes zoster poses essentially no risk to the fetus or neonate and is not discussed further in this chapter.

Varicella occurs in approximately 1 to 5 cases per 10,000 pregnancies. The infection is transmitted by respiratory droplets and by direct contact with vesicular lesions. The incubation period of the organism is 10 to 14 days. Varicella is among the most highly contagious of any viral infection.[363]

Diagnosis

The typical clinical manifestation of varicella is a disseminated, pruritic, vesicular rash. The lesions typically occur in crops and evolve in sequential fashion from vesicle to pustule, eventually crusting over to form a dry scab. Varicella is almost always a mild, self-limited infection in children. However, approximately 20% of infected adults develop pneumonia, and approximately 1% develop encephalitis. Both of these complications can cause serious morbidity and even mortality. The diagnosis can be confirmed by identification of anti-VZV IgM antibody.[363]

Treatment

All pregnant women should be questioned about prior varicella at the time of their first prenatal appointment. If they have a well-defined history of infection, they should be reassured that second infections are extremely unlikely and that, should a second infection occur, the risk to the fetus is negligible. Women who are not certain of prior exposure should have an anti-VZV IgG assay. Approximately 75% of individuals who are uncertain about their prior history actually have definitive serologic evidence of immunity. Women who do not have antibody against varicella should be cautioned about the need to avoid exposure to people who have vesicular viral eruptions.[364,365]

If a susceptible pregnant patient is exposed to someone with varicella, she should be treated within 72 to 96 hours with one of two agents to prevent active infection. The most extensively tested regimen is intramuscular varicella zoster immune globulin (VZIG), 1 vial per 10 kg of weight up to a maximum of 5 vials.[366] However, the U.S. company that manufactured this agent has discontinued its production, and securing the product through international manufacturers is problematic. An alternative method of prophylaxis is to administer oral acyclovir (800 mg, five times daily for 7 days) or oral valacyclovir (1000 mg, three times daily for 7 days).[367]

Pregnant women who develop varicella despite immunoprophylaxis should be treated with oral acyclovir or valacyclovir in the same dose as outlined for prophylaxis. Patients who have evidence of pneumonia, encephalitis, or disseminated infection and those who are immunosuppressed should be hospitalized and treated with intravenous acyclovir (10 mg/kg infused over 1 hour every 8 hours for 10 days).[363,366,368]

Acute varicella infection during pregnancy has been associated with spontaneous abortion, intrauterine fetal death, and congenital anomalies. However, these complications are rare. Investigations, have shown that the frequency of fetal anomalies was less than 1% when maternal infection occurred in weeks 1 through 12 of pregnancy and 2% or less when infection occurred in weeks 13 through 20.[369,370]

The most valuable test to identify fetal injury due to congenital varicella is targeted ultrasound examination. Possible findings include intrauterine growth restriction, microcephaly, ventriculomegaly, echogenic foci in the fetal liver, and limb anomalies.[363]

Neonatal varicella, as opposed to congenital varicella infection, occurs when the mother develops acute varicella during the period from 5 days before to 2 days after delivery. If infection occurs at this time, there is no opportunity for protective antibody to cross the placenta. The manifestations of neonatal varicella include disseminated mucocutaneous lesions, visceral infection, pneumonia, and encephalitis. In the absence of timely antiviral chemotherapy, up to 30% of infected infants die of complications of neonatal varicella. Infants born during this window of time must avoid contact with vesicular lesions on the mother's skin. These infants, and any infants with suspected exposure in the nursery or postpartum ward also should receive immunoprophylaxis with VZIG or treatment with antiviral agents such as acyclovir or valacyclovir.[363]

Prevention

In an effort to prevent the serious conditions noted here, all women of reproductive age should be vaccinated for varicella if they have not already acquired natural immunity. The varicella vaccine (Varivax) is a live virus vaccine that is highly immunogenic. Individuals aged 1 to 12 years should receive one dose of the vaccine subcutaneously. Individuals older than 12 years of age require two subcutaneous doses, administered 4 to 6 weeks apart. Contraindications to the vaccine include pregnancy, an immunodeficiency disorder, high-dose corticosteroid therapy, untreated tuberculosis, severe systemic illness, and an allergy to neomycin, which is one component of the vaccine.[365,371,372] The CDC guidelines[366] indicate that the vaccine may be considered in breastfeeding mothers, although there is little information about whether the vaccine virus is excreted in breast milk. Vaccine recipients pose minimal risk of transmitting infection to susceptible contacts if no rash develops after the vaccination. If a rash does develop, there is a very small risk of transmission to susceptible contacts.[365]

Viral Influenza

Epidemiology

Influenza is caused by an RNA virus of the myxovirus family. Three antigenically different influenza viruses have been identified.[373] Type A influenza is responsible for most epidemics and is associated with severe clinical presentation. Type B influenza is less frequently associated with epidemics and tends to cause milder clinical disease. Type C is the least frequent type and, as a result, is not accounted for in the annual influenza vaccine.

Influenza is of major clinical importance, both in the United States and worldwide. In the United States, the disease causes 30,000 to 40,000 excess deaths and approximately 200,000 hospitalizations annually.[374,375] Pregnant women suffer disproportionate morbidity and mortality during influenza pandemics.[376]

Influenza virus is characterized by low-level alterations of the surface proteins of influenza A (hemagglutinin A and neuraminidase). This antigenic drift allows the virus to change enough to evade the host's immune system response and cause the yearly epidemics. At approximately 20- to 40-year intervals, a more profound change of the surface proteins occurs, possibly as a result of genetic recombination, and leads to a substantially different surface protein configuration. It is this antigenic shift that imparts the novel properties for a virulent strain of influenza virus associated with pandemics. The aggressive nature of pandemic influenza also results, in part, from the lack of relevant immunity in the population to this novel surface protein configuration.[376]

Three influenza pandemics occurred in the last century: 1918, 1957, and 1968. Of these, two were major in nature. The pandemic of 1918 was responsible for between 30 and 50 million deaths worldwide and 500,000 deaths in the United States. The Asian influenza pandemic of 1957-1958 also caused substantial morbidity and mortality.[377]

The influenza A strains responsible for all three of these great pandemics originated in Southeast Asia. Great concern has arisen that another pandemic of influenza will soon occur because of the emergence of a new influenza A strain (avian H5N1) in that region.[378] According to the World Health Organization, this virus has caused almost 100 deaths and has a case mortality rate of 55%.[379] Although cases in humans have been reported, to date efficient human-to-human transmission has not occurred. Given the natural history of genetic shifting and evolution of the influenza virus, the ease of rapid worldwide travel, and the crowded living conditions in many areas of the world, it may only be a matter of time before a pandemic on the scale of the 1918 influenza pandemic (or greater) occurs.[376]

Annually, in the United States, influenza is responsible for 82 million infections and health care costs estimated at billions of dollars.[380] Epidemics in the United States occur during the winter months (November through March). The rates of infection are highest in children, who are a major reservoir for spread of infection to adults, including pregnant women. The rates of serious illness and death are highest among persons 65 years of age and older, children younger than 2 years of age, and people of any age who have medical conditions that place them at increased risk for complications of influenza.[381]

Pathogenesis

The influenza virus is transmitted primarily by respiratory droplets and, to a limited extent, by direct contact. The incubation period is relatively short, 1 to 5 days. Influenza occurs most commonly in the late fall and winter, and epidemics recur with regularity because the virus mutates in important ways from year to year. Immunity to the strains that caused infection in one year does not necessarily provide protection against strains that circulate in subsequent years.

Influenza can range in severity from a mild respiratory infection to a life-threatening pneumonia. The illness typically begins abruptly with prodromal symptoms of malaise, myalgia, and headache in association with fever. Subsequently, the patient develops a dry, nonproductive cough, coryza, mild dyspnea, and sore throat. On physical examination, the temperature is elevated and the pharynx is inflamed; auscultation of the chest discloses rales and rhonchi. In some patients, a secondary bacterial pneumonia develops, and their cough then becomes productive of purulent sputum.[382]

Influenza virus infects the ciliated columnar epithelial cells of the respiratory tract, with resultant cellular necrosis and sloughing. Consequently, either the upper or the lower respiratory tract may be a site of infection.

In pregnancy, the major concern is the increased risk for development of life-threatening pneumonia.[373,376] Influenza virus has not been associated with an increased risk of spontaneous abortion, stillbirth, or congenital anomalies. However, an infant delivered to an acutely infected patient may develop neonatal influenza as a result of close personal contact with the mother after delivery. In addition, mothers with severe respiratory infections may have an increased risk of preterm labor. In previous reports of influenza pandemics, pregnant women experienced increased morbidity and mortality compared with non-pregnant patients.[383-385]

Neuzil and coauthors[386] assessed the impact of influenza on pregnant women during nonpandemic "flu" seasons. They reported that the relative risk for hospitalization with cardiorespiratory complications in pregnant women, compared with nonpregnant women, was 1.4 at 14 to 20 weeks' gestation, rising to 4.7 in weeks 37 through 42. Moreover, women in the third trimester had a hospitalization rate similar to that of nonpregnant women with high-risk medical conditions.

Diagnosis

The presence of the clinical manifestations described earlier is highly suggestive of influenza. The diagnosis can be confirmed by culture of the virus from respiratory secretions and by documentation of characteristic rises in serum antibody to influenza A and B. Chest radiography also may be of great value in assessing the severity of the pulmonary infection.

Treatment

The management of influenza in pregnant women is similar to that in nonpregnant persons, consisting of symptomatic relief, with bed rest, analgesia, liberal fluid intake, and fever control with acetaminophen (650 mg PO every 4 to 6 hours, maximum 4 g/24 hours). Patients should be reevaluated immediately if signs of worsening pneumonia or preterm labor develop. In addition, if they have disabling symptoms, they should be offered treatment with either zanamivir (10 mg twice daily for 5 days) or oseltamivir (75 to 150 mg PO twice daily for 5 days).[387] Although amantidine is effective in nonpregnant patients, it has been associated with teratogenic effects in animals and is not recommended for use in pregnancy.[373] If pneumonia occurs in a pregnant woman with influenza, prompt hospitalization with broad-spectrum antibiotic coverage for bacteria that cause superinfection (e.g., *S. aureus, Streptococcus pneumoniae, Haemophilus influenzae*) is required. Respiratory support is indicated in the presence of inadequate oxygenation, retention of carbon dioxide, or excessively labored breathing.

Prevention

The key to the prevention of influenza is vaccination. Immunization is 70% to 90% effective in either preventing influenza or diminishing the severity of illness. The ACIP[381,388] recommends annual vaccination for

1. Children aged 6 to 59 months
2. Women who will be pregnant during flu season
3. Persons aged 50 years or older
4. Children and adolescents (aged 6 months to 18 years) who are receiving long-term aspirin therapy
5. Adults and children with chronic disorders of pulmonary or cardiovascular systems
6. Adults and children who have required medical follow-up or hospitalization in the past year for chronic metabolic diseases (e.g., diabetes mellitus), renal dysfunction, hemoglobinopathies, or immunodeficiency
7. Persons having any condition that compromises respiratory function or increases risk of aspiration
8. Residents of nursing homes and other chronic care facilities
9. Persons living with or caring for individuals at high risk for influenza-related complications
10. Health care workers

The vaccine contains killed, inactivated virus and is safe for use in pregnancy. Since 2004, the CDC has recommended universal vaccination for all pregnant women regardless of gestational age.[381] Roberts and colleagues[388] recently demonstrated that universal vaccination with inactivated trivalent influenza vaccine is cost-saving in pregnant women. The recently available live, attenuated intranasal influenza vaccine is contraindicated during pregnancy.[381,389]

Viral Hepatitis

Hepatitis A

Hepatitis A is the second most common form of viral hepatitis in the United States. The infection is caused by an RNA virus that is transmitted by fecal-oral contact. The incubation period ranges from 15 to 50 days. Infections in children are usually asymptomatic; infections in adults are usually symptomatic. The disease is most prevalent in areas of poor sanitation and close living.[390]

The typical clinical manifestations of hepatitis include low-grade fever, malaise, poor appetite, right upper quadrant pain and tenderness, jaundice, and acholic stools. The diagnosis is best confirmed by detection of IgM antibody specific for the hepatitis A virus.

Hepatitis A does not cause a chronic carrier state. Perinatal transmission virtually never occurs, and, therefore, the infection does not pose a major risk to either the mother or the baby. The exception is the development of fulminant hepatitis and liver failure in the mother, but such a situation is extremely rare.[390]

Hepatitis A can be prevented by administration of an inactivated vaccine. Two formulations of the vaccine are available: Vaqta and Havrix. Both vaccines require an initial intramuscular injection, followed by a second dose 6 to 12 months later. The vaccine should be offered to the following individuals in the following categories[391]:

- International travelers
- Children in endemic areas
- Intravenous drug users
- Individuals who have occupational exposure (e.g., workers in a primate laboratory)
- Residents and staff of chronic care institutions
- Individuals with liver disease
- Homosexual men
- Individuals with clotting factor disorders

Standard immune globulin provides reasonably effective passive immunization for hepatitis A if it is given within 2 weeks after exposure. The standard intramuscular dose of immune globulin is 0.02 mg/kg.[392]

Hepatitis E

Hepatitis E is caused by an RNA virus. The epidemiology of hepatitis E is similar to that of hepatitis A. The incubation period averages 45 days. The disease is rare in the United States but is endemic in developing countries of the world. In these countries, maternal infection with hepatitis E often has an alarmingly high mortality rate, in the range of 10% to 20%. This is probably less the result of virulence of the microorganism and more related to poor nutrition, poor general health, and lack of access to modern medical care.[390]

The clinical presentation of acute hepatitis E is similar to that of hepatitis A. The diagnosis can be established with the use of electron microscopy to identify viral particles in the stool of infected patients. The most useful diagnostic test, however, is serology.

Hepatitis E does not cause a chronic carrier state. Perinatal transmission can occur but is extremely rare.[393]

Hepatitis B

Hepatitis B is caused by a DNA virus that is transmitted parenterally and via sexual contact. The infection also can be transmitted perinatally from an infected mother to her infant.

Acute hepatitis B occurs in 1 or 2 of every 1000 pregnancies in the United States. The chronic carrier state is more frequent, occurring in 6 to 10 of 1000 pregnancies. Worldwide, more than 400 million individuals are chronically infected with hepatitis B virus. In the United States alone, approximately 1.25 million people are chronically infected.[390]

Approximately 90% of patients who acquire hepatitis B mount an effective immunologic response to the virus and completely clear their infection. Fewer than 1% of infected patients develop fulminate hepatitis and die. Approximately 10% of patients develop a chronic carrier state. Some individuals with chronic hepatitis B infection ultimately develop severe chronic liver disease such as chronic active hepatitis, chronic persistent hepatitis, cirrhosis, or hepatocellular carcinoma. This sequela is particularly likely in patients who are coinfected with hepatitis D or hepatitis C or both.[390]

The diagnosis of hepatitis B is best confirmed by serologic tests. Patients with acute hepatitis B are positive for the hepatitis B surface antigen and positive for IgM antibody to the core antigen. Patients with chronic hepatitis B are positive for the surface antigen and positive for IgG antibody to the core antigen. Acutely or chronically infected patients may or may not be positive for the hepatitis B e antigen. If this latter antigen is present, it denotes active viral replication and a high level of infectivity.[394]

In the absence of intervention, approximately 20% of mothers who are seropositive for hepatitis B surface antigen will transmit infection to their neonates. Approximately 90% of mothers who are positive for both the surface antigen and the e antigen transmit infection. Fortunately, excellent immunoprophylaxis for prevention of perinatal transmission of hepatitis B infection is now available. Infants delivered to seropositive mothers should receive hepatitis B immune globulin within 12 hours after birth. Before their discharge from the hospital, these infants also should begin the hepatitis B vaccination series. The CDC now recommends universal vaccination of all infants for hepatitis B. In addition, the vaccine should be offered to all women of reproductive age.[394,395]

Hepatitis D (Delta Virus Infection)

Hepatitis D is an RNA virus that is dependant on coinfection with hepatitis B for replication. Therefore, the epidemiology of hepatitis D is essentially identical to that of hepatitis B. Patients with hepatitis D may have two types of infection. Some have acute hepatitis D and hepatitis B (coinfection). These individuals typically clear their infection and have a good long-term prognosis. Others have chronic hepatitis D infection superimposed on chronic hepatitis B infection (superinfection). These women are particularly likely to develop chronic liver disease.[390]

The diagnosis of hepatitis D can be established by identifying the delta antigen in liver tissue or serum. However, the most useful diagnostic tests are detection of IgM and/or IgG antibody in serum.[390]

As noted, hepatitis D can cause a chronic carrier state in conjunction with hepatitis B infection. Perinatal transmission of hepatitis D occurs but is uncommon. Moreover, the immunoprophylaxis outlined for hepatitis B is highly effective in preventing transmission of hepatitis D.[390,394]

Hepatitis C

Hepatitis C is caused by an RNA virus. The virus may be transmitted parenterally, via sexual contact, and perinatally. In many patient populations, hepatitis C is as common or more common than hepatitis B. Chronic hepatitis C infection now is the number one indication for liver transplantation in the United States.[390,396-398]

Hepatitis C is usually asymptomatic, at least in its initial stages. The diagnosis is best confirmed by serologic testing. The initial screening test should be an EIA. The confirmatory test is a recombinant immunoblot assay (RIBA). Seroconversion may not occur for up to 16 weeks after infection. In addition, although these immunologic tests have been available for many years, they still do not consistently and precisely distinguish between IgM and IgG antibody.[390]

In patients who have a low serum concentration of hepatitis C RNA and who do not have coexisting HIV infection, the risk of perinatal transmission of hepatitis C is less than 5%. If the patient's serum concentration of hepatitis C RNA is high or she is coinfected with HIV, or both, the perinatal transmission rate may approach 25%.[399,400] Several small, nonrandomized, uncontrolled cohort studies (level II evidence) support a role for elective cesarean delivery before the onset of labor and rupture of membranes in selected women who have detectable hepatitis C virus RNA. For women who have undetectable serum concentrations of RNA, vaginal delivery appears to be a reasonable plan of management.[401,402]

Hepatitis G

Hepatitis G is caused by an RNA virus that is related to the hepatitis C virus. Hepatitis G is more prevalent, but less virulent, than hepatitis C. Many patients who have hepatitis G are coinfected with hepatitis A, B, C, and/or HIV. Coinfection with hepatitis G does not adversely effect the prognosis of these other infections.[403-406]

Most patients with hepatitis G are asymptomatic. The diagnosis is best established by detection of the virus on PCR and identification of antibody on ELISA testing.

Hepatitis G can cause a chronic carrier state, and perinatal transmission has been documented. However, the clinical effects of infection in both mother and baby appear to be minimal. Accordingly, patients should not routinely be screened for this infection, and no special treatment is indicated even if infection is confirmed.[390]

Table 38-20 summarizes the key features of each form of hepatitis.

TABLE 38-20 HEPATITIS IN PREGNANCY: SUMMARY OF KEY FEATURES

Infection	Mechanism of Transmission	Best Diagnostic Test	Carrier State	Perinatal Transmission	Vaccine	Remarks
Hepatitis A	Fecal-oral	Antibody detection	No	No	Yes	Passive immunization with immune globulin
Hepatitis E	Fecal-oral	Antibody detection	No	Rare	No	High maternal mortality in developing countries
Hepatitis B	Parenteral, sexual contact	Antigen detection	Yes	Yes	Yes	Passive immunization with hepatitis B immune globulin
Hepatitis D	Parenteral, sexual contact	Antibody detection	Yes	Yes	Prevented by hepatitis B vaccine	Virus cannot replicate in absence of hepatitis B infection
Hepatitis C	Parenteral, sexual contact	Antibody detection	Yes	Yes	No	Cesarean delivery for women with detectable serum hepatitis C virus RNA
Hepatitis G	Parenteral, sexual contact	Antibody detection	Yes	Yes	No	No clinical significance of infection

References

1. Sobel JD, Faro S, Force RW, et al: Vulvovaginal candidiasis: Epidemiology, diagnostic, and therapeutic considerations. Am J Obstet Gynecol 178:203-211, 1998.
2. Witkin SS, Giraldo PC, Linhares J: New insights into the immune pathogenesis of recurrent vulvovaginal candidiasis. Int J Gynecol Obstet 12:114-118, 2000.
3. Sobel JD, Wiesenfeld HC, Martens M, et al: Maintenance fluconazole therapy for recurrent vulvovaginal candidiasis. N Engl J Med 351:876-883, 2004.
4. Sweet RL, Gibbs RS: Infectious Diseases of the Female Genital Tract. Philadelphia, Lippincott Williams & Wilkins, 2002.
5. Eckert LO, Hawes SE, Stevens CE, et al: Vulvovaginal candidiasis: Clinical manifestations, risk factors, management algorithm. Obstet Gynecol 92:757-765, 1998.
6. Beigi RH, Meyn LA, Moore DM, et al: Vaginal yeast colonization in nonpregnant women: A longitudinal study. Obstet Gynecol 104:926-930, 2004.
7. Kalo-Klein A, Witkin SS: Candida albicans: Cellular immune system interactions during different stages of the menstrual cycle. Am J Obstet Gynecol 161:1132-1136, 1989.
8. Giraldo PC, Babula O, Goncalves KS, et al: Mamooc binding lectin gene polymorphism, vulvovaginal candidiasis, and bacterial vaginosis. Obstet Gynecol 109:1123-1128, 2007.
9. Bendel CM: Candidiasis. In Remington JS, Klein JO, Wilson CB, et al (eds): Infectious Diseases of the Fetus and Newborn Infant. Philadelphia, Elsevier Saunders, 2006, p 1107.
10. Rogue H, Abdelhak Y, Young BK: Intro-amniotic candidiasis: Case report and meta-analysis of 54 cases. J Perinat Med 27:253-262, 1999.
11. Darmstadt GI, Dinulos JG, Miller Z: Congenital cutaneous candidiasis: Clinical presentation, pathogenesis, and management guidelines. Pediatrics 105:438-444, 2000.
12. Centers for Disease Control and Prevention: Sexually transmitted diseases treatment guidelines, 2006. MMWR Morb Mortal Wkly Rep 55(RR-11):54-56, 2006.
13. Rex JH, Walsh TJ, Sobel JD, et al: Practice guidelines for the treatment of candidiasis. Clin Infect Dis 30:662-678, 2000.
14. Wise W, Patel SR, Patel SC, et al: A meta-analysis of the Papanicolaou smear and wet mount for the diagnosis of vaginal trichomoniasis. Am J Med 108:301, 2000.
15. Minkoff H, Grunebaum AN, Schwarz RH, et al: Risk factors for prematurity and premature rupture of membranes: A prospective study of the vaginal flora in pregnancy. Am J Obstet Gynecol 150:965, 1984.
16. Cotch MF, Pastorek JG II, Nugent RP, et al: *Trichomonas vaginalis* associated with low birth weight and preterm delivery: The Vaginal Infections and Prematurity Study Group. Sex Transm Dis 24:353, 1997.
17. Laga M, Manoka A, Kivuvu M, et al: Non-ulcerative sexually transmitted diseases as risk factors for HIV-1 transmission in women: Results from a cohort study. AIDS 7:95, 1993.
18. McClelland RS, Langare L, Hassan WM, et al: Infection with *Trichomonas vaginalis* increases the risk of HIV-1 acquisition. J Infect Dis 195:698, 2007.
19. Burtin P, Taddio A, Ariburnu O, et al: Safety of metronidazole in pregnancy: A meta-analysis. Am J Obstet Gynecol 172:525, 1995.
20. Klebanoff MA, Carey JC, Hauth JC, et al: Failure of metronidazole to prevent preterm delivery among pregnant women with asymptomatic *Trichomonas vaginalis* infection. N Engl J Med 345:487, 2001.
21. Gravett MG, Hummel D, Eschenbach DA, et al: Preterm labor associated with subclinical amniotic fluid infection and with bacterial vaginosis. Obstet Gynecol 67:229, 1986.
22. Gravett MG, Preston-Nelson HP, DeRouen T, et al: Independent associations of bacterial vaginosis and *Chlamydia trachomatis* infection with adverse pregnancy outcome. JAMA 256:1899, 1986.
23. Martius J, Krohn MA, Hillier SL, et al: Relationships of vaginal *Lactobacillus* species, cervical *Chlamydia trachomatis*, and bacterial vaginosis to preterm birth. Obstet Gynecol 71:89, 1988.
24. Hillier SL, Nugent RP, Eschenbach DA, et al: Association between bacterial vaginosis and preterm delivery of a low-birth-weight infant. N Engl J Med 333:2737, 1995.
25. Silver HM, Sperling RS, St Clair PJ, et al: Evidence relating bacterial vaginosis to intraamniotic infection. Am J Obstet Gynecol 161:808, 1989.
26. Hillier SL, Martius J, Kohn M, et al: A case-control study of chorioamnionitic infection and histology of chorioamnionitis in prematurity. N Engl J Med 319:972, 1988.
27. Newton ER, Prihoda TJ, Gibbs RS: A clinical and microbiologic analysis of risk factors for puerperal endometritis. Obstet Gynecol 75:402, 1990.
28. Caro-Paton T, Carvajal A, Martin de Diego I, et al: Is metronidazole teratogenic? A meta-analysis. Br J Clin Pharmacol 44:179, 1997.
29. Piper JM, Mitchel EF, Ray WA: Prenatal use of metronidazole and birth defects: No association. Obstet Gynecol 82:348, 1993.
30. Burtin P, Taddio A, Ariburnu O, et al: Safety of metronidazole in pregnancy: A meta-analysis. Am J Obstet Gynecol 172:525, 1995.
31. Morales WJ, Schorr S, Albritton J: Effect of metronidazole in patients with preterm birth in preceding pregnancy and bacterial vaginosis: A placebo-controlled, double-blind study. Am J Obstet Gynecol 171:345, 1994.
32. McGregor JA, French JI, Parker R, et al: Prevention of premature birth by screening and treatment for common genital tract infections: Results of a prospective controlled evaluation. Am J Obstet Gynecol 173:157, 1995.

33. Hauth JC, Goldenberg RL, Andrews WW, et al: Reduced incidence of preterm delivery with metronidazole and erythromycin in women with bacterial vaginosis. N Engl J Med 333:1732, 1995.
34. McDonald HM, O'Loughlin JA, Vigneswaran R, et al: Impact of metronidazole therapy on preterm birth in women with bacterial vaginosis flora (*Gardnerella vaginalis*): A randomised, placebo controlled trial. BJOG 104:1391, 1997.
35. Carey JC, Klebanoff MA, Hauth JC, et al: Metronidazole to prevent preterm delivery in pregnant women with asymptomatic bacterial vaginosis. N Engl J Med 342:534, 2000.
36. American College of Obstetricians and Gynecologists: Assessment of Risk Factors for Preterm Birth. ACOG Practice Bulletin No. 31. Washington, DC, ACOG, 2001.
37. Goldenberg RL, Hauth JC, Andrews WW: Intrauterine infection and preterm delivery. N Engl J Med 342:1500, 2000.
38. Centers for Disease Control and Prevention. Sexually Transmitted Disease Surveillance, 2004. Atlanta, GA: U.S. Department of Health and Human Services, CDC, National Center for HIV, STD, and TB Prevention, 2005.
39. Centers for Disease Control and Prevention: Summary of Notifiable Diseases, United States, 2002. MMWR Morb Mortal Wkly Rep 51:1-84, 2004.
40. Centers for Disease Control and Prevention: Summary of Notifiable Diseases—United States, 2003. MMWR Morb Mortal Wkly Rep 52:1-85, 2005.
41. Miller WC, Ford CA, Morris M, et al: Prevalence of chlamydial and gonococcal infection among young adults in the United States. JAMA 291:2229-2236, 2004.
42. Miller JM, Maupin RT, Mestad RE, Nsuami M: Initial and repeated screening for gonorrhea during pregnancy. Sex Transm Dis 30:728-730, 2003.
43. Hooper RB: Cohort study of venereal disease: The risk of gonorrhea transmission from infected women to men. Am J Epidemiol 108:136, 1989.
44. Sweet RL: Sexually transmitted diseases. In Bieber EJ, Sanfilippo JS, Horowitz IR (eds): Clinical Gynecology. Philadelphia, Churchill Livingstone, 2006, pp 259-284.
45. Corman LC, Levison MF, Knight R, et al: The high frequency of pharyngeal gonococcal infection in a prenatal clinic population. JAMA 230:568, 1974.
46. Handsfield HH, Hodson A, Holmes KK: Neonatal gonococcal infection: I. Orogastric contamination with *Neisseria gonorrhoeae.* JAMA 225:697-701, 1973.
47. Amstey MS, Steadman KT: Symptomatic gonorrhea and pregnancy. J Am Vener Dis Assoc 3:14-16, 1976.
48. Daris JD, Riley PK, Petess CW, et al: A comparison of ligase chain reacton to polymerase chain reaction in the detection of *Chlamydia trachomatis* endocervical infections. Infect Dis Obstet Gynecol 6:57-60, 1998.
49. Bernstein KT, Mehta SD, Rompalo AM, et al: Cost-effectiveness of screening strategies for gonorrhea among females in private sector care. Obstet Gynecol 107:813-821, 2006.
50. American College of Obstetricians and Gynecologists: Gonorrhea and Chlamydial Infections. Technical Bulletin No. 190. Washington, DC, ACOG, 1994.
51. Katz AR, Effler PV, Ohye RG, et al: False-positive gonorrhea test results with a nucleic acid amplification test: The impact of low prevalence on positive predictive value. Clin Infect Dis 38:814-819, 2004.
52. Dicker LW, Mosure DJ, Berman SM, et al: Gonorrhea prevalence and co-infection with chlamydia in women in the United States, 2000. Sex Transm Dis 30:472-476, 2003.
53. Tapsall JW: What management is there for gonorrhea in the post quinolone era? Sex Transm Dis 33:8-10, 2006.
54. Bauer HM, Mark KE, Samuel M, et al: Prevalence of and associated risk factors for fluoroquinolone-resistant *Neisseria gonorrhoeae* in California, 2000-2003. Clin Infect Dis 41:795-803, 2005.
55. Newna LM, Wang SA, Ohye RG, et al: The epidemiology of fluoroquinolone-resistant *Neisseria gonorrhoeae* in Hawaii, 2001. Clin Infect Dis 38:649-654, 2004.
56. Centers for Disease Control and Prevention: Increases in fluoroquinolone-resistant *Neisseria gonorrhoeae*—Hawaii and California, 2001. MMWR Morb Mortal Wkly Rep 51:1041-1044, 2005.
57. Centers for Disease Control and Prevention: Sexually transmitted diseases surveillance 2004 supplement: Gonococcal Isolate Surveillance Project (GISP) annual report, 2004. Atlanta, GA, U.S. Department of Health and Human Services, CDC, National Center for HIV, STD, and TB Prevention, 2005.
58. Centers for Disease Control and Prevention: Increases in fluoroquinolone-resistant *Neisseria gonorrhoeae* among men who have sex with men—United States, 2003, and Revised recommendations for gonorrhea treatment, 2004. MMWR Morb Mortal Wkly Rep 53:335-338, 2004.
59. Moran JS, Levine WC: Drugs of choice for the treatment of uncomplicated gonococcal infections. Clin Infect Dis 20(Suppl 1):547-565, 1995.
60. Golden MR, Whittington WLH, Handsfield HH, et al: Effect of expedited treatment of sex partners on recurrent or persistent gonorrhea or chlamydial infection. N Engl J Med 352:676-685, 2005.
61. Centers for Disease Control and Prevention: Summary of notifiable diseases—United States, 2005. MMWR Morb Mortal Wkly Rep 54(53):1-92, 2007.
62. Andrews WW, Goldenberg RI, Mercer B, et al: The Preterm Prediction Study: Association of second trimester genitourinary chlamydial infection with subsequent spontaneous preterm birth. Am J Obstet Gynecol 183:662-668, 2000.
63. Jain S: Perinatally acquired *Chlamydia trachomatis* associated morbidity in young infants. J Matern Fetal Med 8:130-133, 1999.
64. Peipert JF: Genital chlamydial infections. N Engl J Med 349:2424-2430, 2003.
65. Miller WC, Ford CA, Morris MS, et al: Prevalence of chlamydial and gonococcal infections among young adults in the United States. JAMA 291:2229-2236, 2004.
66. Sheffield JS, Andrews WW, Klebanoff MA, et al: Spontaneous resolution of asymptomatic *Chlamydia trachomatis* in pregnancy. Obstet Gynecol 105:557-562, 2005.
67. Gravett MG, Nelson HP, DeRouen T, et al: Independent associations of bacterial vaginosis and *Chlamydia trachomatis* infection with adverse pregnancy outcome. JAMA 256:1899-1903, 1986.
68. Alger LS, Lovchik JC, Hebel JR, et al: The association of *Chlamydia trachomatis, Neisseria gonorrhoeae*, and group B streptococci with preterm rupture of the membranes and pregnancy outcome. Am J Obstet Gynecol 159:397-404, 1988.
69. Claman P, Toye B, Peeling RW, et al: Serologic evidence of *Chlamydia trachomatis* infection and risk of preterm birth. Can Med Assoc J 153:259-262, 1995.
70. Iams JD, Romero R: Preterm birth. In Gabbe SG, Niebyl JR, Simpson JL (eds): Obstetrics. Normal and Problem Pregnancies (5th ed.). Philadelphia, Churchill Livingstone, 2007, pp 668-712.
71. Harrison HR, Alexander ER, Weinstein L, et al: Cervical *Chlamydia trachomatis* and mycoplasmal infections in pregnancy: epidemiology and outcomes. JAMA 250:1721-1727, 1983.
72. Sweet RL, Landers D, Walker C, et al: *Chlamydia trachomatis* infection and pregnancy outcome. Am J Obstet Gynecol 156:824-833, 1987.
73. Ryan GM, Abdella TN, McNeeley SG, et al: *Chlamydia trachomatis* infection in pregnancy and effect of treatment on outcome. Am J Obstet Gynecol 162:34-39, 1990.
74. Cohen I, Veille C, Calkins BM: Improved pregnancy outcome following successful treatment of chlamydial infection. JAMA 263:3160-3163, 1990.
75. Wager GP, Martin DH, Koutsky L, et al: Puerperal infectious morbidity: Relationship to route of delivery and to antepartum *Chlamydia trachomatis* infection. Am J Obstet Gynecol 138:1028-1033, 1980.
76. Blanco JD, Diaz KC, Lipscomb KA, et al: *Chlamydia trachomatis* isolation in patients with endometritis after cesearean section. Am J Obstet Gynecol 152:278-279, 1985.
77. Berman SM, Harrison HR, Boyce WT, et al: Low birth weight, prematurity and postpartum endometritis: Association with pronatal cervical *Myco-*

plasma hominis and *Chlamydia trachomatis* infections. JAMA 257:1189-1194, 1987.
78. McGregor JA, French JL, Richter R, et al: Antenatal microbiologic and maternal risk factors associated with prematurity. Am J Gynecol 163:1580-1591, 1990.
79. Black CM, Marrazo J, Johnson RE, et al: Head-to-head multicenter comparison of DNA probe and nucleic acid amplification tests for *Chlamydia trachomatis* infection in women performed with an improved reference standard. J Clin Microbiol 40:3757-3763, 2002.
80. Sweet RL, Wiesenfeld HC, Uhrin M, et al: Comparison of EIA, culture and polymerase chain reaction for *Chlamydia trachomatis* in a sexually transmitted diseases clinic. J Infect Dis 170:500-501, 1994.
81. Centers for Disease Control and Prevention: Screening tests to detect *Chlamydia trachomatis* and *Neisseria gonorrhoeae* infections, 2002. MMWR Morb Mortal Wkly Rep 51(RR-15), 2002.
82. Wiesenfeld HC, Heine RP, Rideout A, et al: The vaginal introitus: A novel site for *Chlamydia trachomatis* testing in women. Am J Obstet Gynecol 174:1542-1546, 1996.
83. Schachter J, Chernesky MA, Willis DE, et al: Vaginal swabs are the specimens of choice when screening for *Chlamydia trachomatis* and *Neisseria gonorrhoeae*: Result from a multicenter evaluation of the APTMA assays for both infections. Sex Transm Dis 32:725-728, 2005.
84. Hsieh Y-H, Howell MR, Gaydos JC, et al: Preference among female Army recruits for use of self-administered vaginal swabs or urine to screen for *Chlamydia trachomatis* genital infections. Sex Transm Dis 30:769-773, 2003.
85. U.S. Preventive Services Task Force: Screening for chlamydial infections: Recommendations and rationale. Am J Prev Med 20:90-94, 2001.
86. Scholes D, Stergachis A, Heidrich FE, et al: Prevention of pelvic inflammatory disease by screening for cervical chlamydial infection. N Engl J Med 334:1362-1366, 1996.
87. Crombleholme WR, Schachter J, Grossman M, et al: Amoxicillin therapy for *Chlamydia trachomatis* in pregnancy. Obstet Gynecol 75:752-756, 1990.
88. Brocklehurst P, Rooney G: Interventions for testing genital *Chlamydia trachomatis* infection in pregnancy. Cochrane Database Syst Rev (2): CD000054, 2000.
89. Rahangdale L, Guerry S, Baver HM, et al: An observational cohort study of *Chlamydia trachomatis* treatment in pregnancy. Sex Transm Dis 33:106-110, 2006.
90. Schillinger JA, Kissenger P, Calvert H, et al: Patient-delivered partner treatment with azithromycin to prevent repeated *Chlamydia trachomatis* infections among women: A randomized, controlled trial. Sex Transm Dis 30:49-56, 2003.
91. Golden MR, Whittington WLH, Handsfield HH, et al: Effect of expedited treatment of sex partners on recurrent or persistent gonorrhea or chlamydial infection. N Engl J Med 352:676-685, 2005.
92. Cates W Jr: Estimates of the incidence and prevalence of sexually transmitted diseases in the United States. American Social Health Panel. Sex Transm Dis 26:S2-S7, 1999.
93. Winer RL, Lee S-K, Hughes JP, et al: Genital human papillomavirus infection: Incidence and risk factors in a cohort of female university students. Am J Epidemiol 157:218-226, 2003.
94. Watts DH, Koutsky LA, Holmes KK, et al: Low risk of perinatal transmission of human papillomavirus: Results of a prospective cohort study. Am J Obstet Gynecol 178:365-373, 1998.
95. Tenti P, Zappatore R, Migliora P, et al: Perinatal transmission of human papillomavirus from gravidas with latent infections. Obstet Gynecol 93:475-479, 1999.
96. Smith EM, Ritchie JM, Yankowitz J, et al: Human papillomavirus prevalence and types in newborns and parents: Concordance and modes of transmission. Sex Transm Dis 31:57-62, 2004.
97. Shah K, Kashima H, Polk BF, et al: Rarity of cesarean delivery in cases of juvenile-onset respiratory papillomatosis. Obstet Gynecol 68:795-799, 1986.
98. Briston RE, Montz FJ: Human papillomavirus: Molecular based screening applications in cervical neoplasia. A primer for primary care physicians. Prim Care Update Ob/Gyns 5:238-246, 1995.
99. Ruger KM, Kahn JA: Human papillomavirus and adolescent girls. Curr Womens Health Rep 2:468-475, 2002.
100. Centers for Disease Control and Prevention: Quadrivalent human papillomavirus vaccine: Recommendations of the Advisory Committee on Immunization Practices (ACIP). MMWR Morb Mortal Wkly Rep 56(RR-02):1-24, 2007.
101. Puranen M, Yliskoski M, Saarikoski S, et al: Vertical transmission of human papillomavirus from infected mothers to their newborn babies and persistence of virus into childhood. Am J Obstet Gynecol 174:694-699, 1996.
102. Garland, SM, Hernandez-Avila M, Wheeler CM, et al: Quadrivalent vaccine against human papillomavirus to prevent anogenital diseases. N Engl J Med 356:1928-1943, 2007.
103. Foxman B, Barlow R, D'Arcy H, et al: Urinary tract infection: Self-reported incidence and associated costs. Ann Epidemiol 10:509-515, 2000.
104. Sheffield JS, Cunningham FG: Urinary tract infection in women. Obstet Gynecol 106:1085-1092, 2005.
105. Stamm WE, Hooton TM: Management of urinary tract infections in adults. N Engl J Med 329:1328-1334, 1993.
106. Bacak SJ, Callaghan WM, Dietz PM, et al: Pregnancy-associated hospitalizations in the United States, 1999-2000. Am J Obstet Gynecol 192:592-597, 2005.
107. Kass EH: The role of asymptomatic bacteriuria in the pathogenesis of pyelonephritis. In Quinn EL, Kass EH (eds): Biology of Pyelonephritis. Boston, Little, Brown, 1960, pp 399-412.
108. Thurman AR, Steed LL, Hulsey T, et al: Bacteriuria in pregnant women with sickle cell trait. Am J Obstet Gynecol 194:1366-1370, 2006.
109. Nicolle LE: Asymptomatic bacteriuria: When to screen and when to treat. Infect Dis Clin North Am 17:367-394, 2003.
110. Harris RE: The significance of eradication of bacteriuria during pregnancy. Obstet Gynecol 53:71-73, 1979.
111. Andrews WW, Cox SM, Gilstrap LC: Urinary tract infections in pregnancy. Int Urogynecol J 1:155-163, 1990.
112. Gratacos E, Torres P-J, Vila J, et al: Screening and treatment of asymptomatic bacteriuria in pregnancy prevent pyelonephritis. J Infect Dis 169:1390-1392, 1994.
113. Uncu Y, Uncu G, Esmer A, Bilgel N: Should asymptomatic bacteriuria be screened in pregnancy? Clin Exp Obstet Gynecol 29:281-285, 2002.
114. Kinçaid-Smith P, Bullen M: Bacteriuria in pregnancy. Lancet 1:395-399, 1965.
115. Romero R, Oyarzun E, Mazor M, et al: Meta-analysis of the relationship between asymptomatic bacteriuria and preterm delivery/low birthweight. Obstet Gynecol 73:576-582, 1989.
116. Schieve LA, Handler A, Hershow R, et al: Urinary tract infection during pregnancy: Its associations with maternal morbidity and perinatal outcome. Am J Public Health 84:405-410, 1994.
117. Meis PJ, Michielutte R, Peters TJ, et al: Factors associated with preterm birth in Cardiff, Wales. Am J Obstet Gynecol 173:597-602, 1995.
118. Smaill F: Antibiotic versus no treatment for asymptomatic bacteriuria. In Pre-Cochrane Reviews: The Cochrane Pregnancy and Childbirth Database. Issue 2. Oxford, BMJ Publishing Group, 1995.
119. Mittendorf R, Williams MA, Kass EH: Prevention of preterm delivery and low birth weight associated with asymptomatic bacteriuria. Clin Infect Dis 14:927, 1992.
120. American Academy of Pediatrics and American College of Obstetricians and Gynecologists: Guidelines for Perinatal Care, 5th ed. Elk Grove Village, IL, AAP, and Washington, DC, ACOG, 2002, p 90.
121. Preventive Services Task Force (US): Guide to Clinical Preventative Services, 2nd ed. Washington, DC, U.S. Department of Health and Human Services, 1996.
122. Svanborg C, Godaly G: Bacterial virulence in urinary tract infection. Infect Dis Clin North Am 11:513-529, 1997.

123. Stenquist K, Sandberg T, Lidin-Janson G, et al: Virulence factors of *Escherichia coli* in urinary isolates from pregnant women. J Infect Dis 156:870-877, 1987.
124. Millar LK, Cox SM: Urinary tract infections complicating pregnancy. Infect Dis Clin North Am 11:13-26, 1997.
125. Rouse DJ, Andrews WW, Goldenberg RL, et al: Screening and treatment of asymptomatic bacteriuria of pregnancy to prevent pyelonephritis: A cost-effectiveness and cost-benefit analysis. Obstet Gynecol 86:119-123, 1995.
126. Hooton TM, Stamm WE: Diagnosis and treatment of uncomplicated urinary tract infection. Infect Dis Clin North Am 11:551-581, 1997.
127. McNair RD, MacDonald R, Dooley SL, et al: Evaluation of the centrifuged and Gram-stained smear, urinalysis, and reagent strip testing to detect asymptomatic bacteriuria in obstetric patients. Am J Obstet Gynecol 182:1076-1079, 2000.
128. Bachman JW, Heise RH, Naessons JM, et al: A study of various tests to detect asymptomatic urinary tract infections in an obstetric population. JAMA 270:1971-1974, 1993.
129. LeBlanc AL, McGanity WJ: The impact of bacteriuria in pregnancy: A survey of 1300 pregnant patients. Biol Med (Paris) 22:336-347, 1964.
130. Brumfitt W: The effects of bacteriuria in pregnancy on maternal and fetal health. Kidney Int 8(Suppl):113-119, 1975.
131. Little PJ: The incidence of urinary infection in 5000 pregnant women. Lancet 4:925-928, 1966.
132. Whalley PJ, Cunningham FG: Short-term versus continuous antimicrobial therapy for asymptomatic bacteriuria in pregnancy. Obstet Gynecol 49:262-265, 1977.
133. Villar J, Lydon-Rochelle MT, Gulmezoglu AM, et al: Duration of treatment for asymptomatic bacteriuria during pregnancy. Cochrane Database Syst Rev (2):CD000491, 2000.
134. Jamie, WE, Edwards RK, Duff P: Antimicrobial susceptibility of gram-negative uropathogens isolated from obstetric patients. Infect Dis Obstet Gynecol 10:123-126, 2002.
135. Gupta K, Scholes D, Stamm WE: Increasing prevalence of antimicrobial resistance among uropathogens causing acute uncomplicated cystitis. JAMA 281:736-738, 1999.
136. Warren JW, Abrutyn E, Hebel JR, et al: Guidelines for antimicrobial treatment of uncomplicated acute bacterial cystitis and pyelonephritis in women. Clin Infect Dis 29:745-758, 1999.
137. Whalley P: Bacteriuria of pregnancy. Am J Obstet Gynecol 97:723-738, 1967.
138. Stamm WE, Counts GW, Running KR, et al: Diagnosis of coliform infection in acutely dysuric women. N Engl J Med 307:463-468, 1982.
139. Harris RE, Gilstrap LC: Prevention of recurrent pyelonephritis during pregnancy. Obstet Gynecol 44:637-641, 1974.
140. Scholes D, Hooton TM, Roberts PL, et al: Risk factors for recurrent urinary tract infection in young women. J Infect Dis 182:1177-1182, 2000.
141. Hooton TM, Besser R, Foxman B, et al: Acute uncomplicated cystitis in an era of increasing antibiotic resistance: A proposed approach to empirical therapy. Clin Infect Dis 39:75-80, 2004.
142. Sheinfeld J, Schaeffer AJ, Cordon-Cardo C, et al: Association of the Lewis blood-group phenotype with recurrent urinary tract infections in women. N Engl J Med 320:773-777, 1989.
143. Hurlbut TA 3rd, Littenberg B: The diagnostic accuracy of rapid dipstick tests to predict urinary tract infection. Am J Clin Pathol 96:582-588, 1991.
144. Hill JB, Sheffield JS, McIntire DD, et al: Acute pyelonephritis in pregnancy. Obstet Gynecol 105:18-23, 2005.
145. Cunningham FG, Morris, GB, Mickal A: Acute pyelonephritis of pregnancy: A clinical review. Obstet Gynecol 42:112-117, 1973.
146. Andriole V, Cohn GL: The effect of diethylstilbestrol on the susceptibility of rats to hematogenous pyelonephritis. J Clin Infest 43:1136-1145, 1964.
147. Harle EMG, Bullen JJ, Thompson DA: Influence of estrogen on experimental pyelonephritis caused by *Escherichia coli*. Lancet 2:283-286, 1975.
148. Johnson JR: Virulence factors in *Escherichia coli* urinary tract infection. Clin Microbiol Rev 4:80-128, 1999.
149. Dunlow S, Duff P: Prevalence of antibiotic-resistant uropathogens in obstetric patients with acute pyelonephritis. Obstet Gynecol 76:241-244, 1990.
150. MacMilllan MC, Grimes DA: The limited usefulness of urine and blood cultures in treating pyelonephritis in pregnancy. Obstet Gynecol 78:745-748, 1991.
151. Wing DA, Hendershott CM, Debuque L, et al: Outpatient treatment of acute pyelonephritis in pregnancy after 24 weeks. Obstet Gynecol 94:683-688, 1999.
152. Cox SM, Shelburne P, Mason R, et al: Mechanisms of hemolysis and anemia associated with acute antepartum pyelonephritis. Am J Obstet Gynecol 164:587-590, 1991.
153. Cunningham FG, Lucas MJ, Hankins GDV: Pulmonary injury complicating antepartum pyelonephritis. Am J Obstet Gynecol 156:797-807, 1987.
154. Gilstrap LC, Cunningham FG, Whalley PJ: Acute pyelonephritis in pregnancy: An anterospective study. Obstet Gynecol 57:409-413, 1981.
155. Towers CV, Kaminskas CM, Garite TJ, et al: Pulmonary injury associated with antepartum pyelonephritis: Can patients at risk be identified? Am J Obstet Gynecol 164:974-980, 1991.
156. Hooton TM: The current management strategies for community-acquired urinary tract infection. Infect Dis Clin North Am 17:303-332, 2003.
157. Bergeron MG: Treatment of pyelonephritis in adults. Med Clin North Am 79:619-649, 1997.
158. Safrin S, Siegal D, Black D: Pyelonephritis in adult women: Inpatient versus outpatient therapy. Am J Med 85:793-798, 1988.
159. Angel JL, O'Brien WF, Finan MA, et al: Acute pyelonephritis in pregnancy: A prospective study of oral versus intravenous antibiotic therapy. Obstet Gynecol 76:28-32, 1990.
160. Millar LK, Wing DA, Paul RH, et al: Outpatient treatment of pyelonephritis in pregnancy: A randomized controlled trial. Obstet Gynecol 86:560-564, 1995.
161. VanDorsten JP, Lenke RR, Schifrin BS: Pyelonephritis in pregnancy: The role of in-hospital management and nitrofurantoin suppression. J Reprod Med 32:897-900, 1987.
162. Lenke RR, VanDorsten JP, Schifrin BS: Pyelonephritis in pregnancy: A prospective randomized trial to prevent recurrent disease evaluating suppressive therapy with nitrofurantoin and close surveillance. Am J Obstet Gynecol 146:953-957, 1983.
163. Gibbs RS, Duff P: Progress in pathogenesis and management of clinical intra-amniotic infection. Am J Obstet Gynecol 164:1317, 1991.
164. Yancey MK, Duff P, Kubilis P, et al: Risk factors for neonatal sepsis. Am J Obstet Gynecol 87:188, 1996.
165. Newton ER, Prihoda TJ, Gibbs RS: Logistic regression analysis of risk factors for intra-amniotic infection. Obstet Gynecol 73:571, 1989.
166. Newton ER, Piper J, Peairs W: Bacterial vaginosis and intraamniotic infection. Am J Obstet Gynecol 175:672, 1997.
167. Soper DE, Mayhall CG, Dalton HP: Risk factors for intraamniotic infections: A prospective epidemiologic study. Am J Obstet Gynecol 161:562, 1989.
168. Soper DE, Mayhall CG, Froggatt JW: Characterization and control of intra-amniotic infection in an urban teaching hospital. Am J Obstet Gynecol 175:304, 1996.
169. Gibbs RS: Chorioamnionitis and bacterial vaginosis. Am J Obstet Gynecol 169:460, 1993.
170. Gibbs RS, Blanco JD, St. Clair PJ, et al: Quantitative bacteriology of amniotic fluid from patients with clinical intra-amniotic infection at term. J Infect Dis 145:1, 1982.
171. Blanco JD, Gibbs RS, Malherbe H, et al: A controlled study of genital mycoplasmas in amniotic fluid from patients with intra-amniotic infection. J Infect Dis 147:650, 1983.
172. Schachter J (ed): Chlamydial Infections. Amsterdam, Elsevier, 1982.
173. Kiltz RJ, Burke MS, Porreco RP: Amniotic fluid glucose concentration as a marker for intra-amniotic infection. Am J Obstet Gynecol 78:619, 1991.

174. Romero R, Yoon BH, Mazor M, et al: The diagnostic and prognostic value of amniotic fluid white blood cell count, glucose, interleukin-6, and Gram stain in patients with preterm labor and intact membranes. Am J Obstet Gynecol 169:805, 1993.
175. Sperling RS, Ramamurthy S, Gibbs RS: A comparison of intrapartum versus immediate postpartum treatment of intra-amniotic infection. Obstet Gynecol 70:861, 1987.
176. Gilstrap LC, Leveno KJ, Cox SM: Intrapartum treatment of acute chorioamnionitis: Impact on neonatal sepsis. Am J Obstet Gynecol 159:579, 1988.
177. Gibbs RS, Dinsmoor MJ, Newton ER, et al: A randomized trial of intrapartum vs. immediately postpartum treatment of intra-amniotic infection. Obstet Gynecol 72:823, 1988.
178. Edwards RK, Duff P: Single additional dose postpartum therapy for women with chorioamnionitis. Obstet Gynecol 102:957, 2003.
179. Yoder RP, Gibbs RS, Blanco JD, et al: A prospective controlled study of maternal and perinatal outcome after intra-amniotic infection at term. Am J Obstet Gynecol 145:695, 1983.
180. Garite TJ, Freeman RK: Chorioamnionitis in the preterm gestation. Obstet Gynecol 59:539-545, 1982.
181. Grether JK, Nelson KB: Maternal infection and cerebral palsy in infants of normal birth weight. JAMA 278:207, 1997.
182. Yoon BH, Romero R, Yang SH, et al: Interleukin-6 concentrations in umbilical cord plasma are elevated in neonates with periventricular white matter lesions associated with periventricular leukomalacia. Am J Obstet Gynecol 174:1433, 1996.
183. Yoon BH, Romero R, Park JS, et al: Fetal exposure to an intra-amniotic inflammation and the development of cerebral palsy at the age of three years. Am J Obstet Gynecol 182:675, 2000.
184. Hitti J, Krohn MA, Patton D, et al: Amniotic fluid tumor necrosis factor-α and the risk of respiratory distress syndrome among preterm infants. Am J Obstet Gynecol 177:50, 1997.
185. Rouse DJ, Hauth JC, Andrews WW, et al: Chlorhexidine vaginal irrigation for the prevention of prepartal infection: A placebo-controlled randomized clinical trial. Am J Obstet Gynecol 176:617, 1997.
186. Sweeten KM, Eriksen NJ, Blanco JD: Chlorhexidine versus sterile water vaginal wash during labor to prevent peripartum infection. Am J Obstet Gynecol 176:426, 1997.
187. Carey JC, Klebanoff MA, Hauth JC, et al: Metronidazole to prevent preterm delivery in pregnant women with asymptomatic bacterial vaginosis. N Engl J Med 342:534, 2000.
188. Egarter C, Leitich H, Husslein P, et al: Adjunctive antibiotic treatment in preterm labor and neonatal morbidity: A meta-analysis. Obstet Gynecol 88:303, 1996.
189. Locksmith GJ, Clark P, Duff P: Maternal and neonatal infection rates with three different protocols for prevention of group B streptococcal disease. Am J Obstet Gynecol 180:416, 1999.
190. Lopez-Zeno JA, Peaceman AM, Adashek JA, et al: A controlled trial of a program for the active management of labor. N Engl J Med 326:450, 1992.
191. Mozurkewich EL, Wolf FM: Premature rupture of membranes at term: A meta-analysis of three management schemes. Am J Obstet Gynecol 89:1035, 1997.
192. Mercer BM, Arheart KL: Antimicrobial therapy in expectant management of preterm premature rupture of the membranes. Lancet 346:1271, 1995.
193. Egarter C, Leitich H, Kara H, et al: Antibiotic treatment in preterm premature rupture of membranes and neonatal morbidity: A meta-analysis. Am J Obstet Gynecol 174:589, 1996.
194. Mercer BM, Miodovnik M, Thurnau G, et al: Antibiotic therapy for reduction of infant morbidity after preterm premature rupture of the membranes. JAMA 278:989, 1997.
195. Kenyon SL, Taylor DJ, Tarnow-Mordi W, et al: Broad-spectrum antibiotics for spontaneous preterm labour: The ORACLE II randomised trial. Lancet 357:989, 2001.
196. Shy KK, Eschenbach DA: Fatal perineal cellulitis from an episiotomy site. Obstet Gynecol 54:292, 1979.
197. Hauth JC, Gilstrap LC III, Ward SC, et al: Early repair of an external sphincter ani muscle and rectal mucosal dehiscence. Obstet Gynecol 67:806, 1986.
198. Hankins GDV, Hauth JC, Gilstrap LC III, et al: Early repair of episiotomy dehiscence. Obstet Gynecol 75:48, 1990.
199. Ramin SM, Ramus RM, Little BB, et al: Early repair of episiotomy dehiscence associated with infection. Am J Obstet Gynecol 167:1104, 1992.
200. Ramin SM, Gilstrap LC III: Episiotomy and early repair of dehiscence. Clin Obstet Gynecol 37:816, 1994.
201. Duff P. Pathophysiology and management of postcesarean endometritis. Obstet Gynecol 67:269-276, 1986.
202. Watts DH, Eschenbach DA, Kenny GE: Early postpartum endometritis: The role of bacteria, genital mycoplasmas, and *Chlamydia trachomatis*. Obstet Gynecol 73:52-60, 1989.
203. Newton ER, Prihoda TJ, Gobbs RS. A clinical and microbiologic analysis of risk factors for puerperal endometritis. Obstet Gynecol 75:402-406, 1990.
204. Duff P: Antibiotic selection in obstetrics: Making cost-effective choices. Clin Obstet Gynecol 45:59-72, 2002.
205. Soper DE, Kemmer CT, Conover WB: Abbreviated antibiotic therapy for the treatment of postpartum endometritis. Obstet Gynecol 69:127-130, 1987.
206. Atkinson MW, Owen J, Wren A, Hauth JC: The effect of manual removal of the placenta on post-cesarean endometritis. Obstet Gynecol 87:99-102, 1996.
207. Lasley DS, Eblen A, Yancey MK, Duff P: The effect of placental removal on the incidence of post-cesarean infection. Am J Obstet 176:1250-1254.
208. Gibbs RS, Blanco JD, St. Clair PJ: A case-control study of wound abscess after cesarean delivery. Obstet Gynecol 62:498-501, 1983.
209. Chen KT, Huard RC, Della-Latta P, Saiman L: Prevalence of methicillin-sensitive and methicillin resistant *Staphylococcus aureus* in pregnant women. Obstet Gynecol 108:482-487, 2006.
210. Knochel JG, Koehler PR, Lee TG, Welch DM: Diagnosis of abdominal abscess with computed tomography, ultrasound, and 111In leukocyte scans. Radiology 137:425-432, 1980.
211. Dellinger RP, Carlet JM, Masur H, et al: Surviving Sepsis Campaign guidelines for management of severe sepsis and septic shock. Crit Care Med 32:858-873, 2004.
212. Mabie WC, Barton JR, Sibai B: Septic shock in pregnancy. Obstet Gynecol 90:553-561, 1997.
213. American College of Obstetricians and Gynecologists: Septic Shock. ACOG Technical Bulletin No. 204. Washington, DC, ACOG, 1995.
214. Russell JA: Management of sepsis. N Engl J Med 355:1699-1713, 2006.
215. Wheeler AP, Bernard GR: Treating patients with severe sepsis. N Engl J Med 340:207-214, 1999.
216. Hotchkiss RS, Karl IE: The pathophysiology and treatment of sepsis. N Engl J Med 348:138-150, 2003.
217. Duff P, Gibbs RS: Pelvic vein thrombophlebitis: Diagnostic dilemma and therapeutic challenge. Obstet Gynecol Surv 38:365-373, 1983.
218. Munsick RA, Gillanders LA: A review of the syndrome of puerperal ovarian vein thrombophlebitis. Obstet Gynecol Surv 36:57-66, 1981.
219. Dunn LJ, Van Voorhis LW: Enigmatic fever and pelvic thrombophlebitis. N Engl J Med 276:265-268, 1967.
220. Brown CLL, Lowe TE, Cunningham FG, et al: Puerperal pelvic vein thrombophlebitis: Impact on diagnosis and treatment using x-ray computed tomography and magnetic resonance imaging. Obstet Gynecol 68:789-794, 1986.
221. Duff P: Septic pelvic vein thrombophlebitis. In Pastorek JG (ed): Obstetric and Gynecologic Infectious Disease. New York, Raven Press, 1994, pp 165-170.
222. Ripley D: Mastitis. Prim Care Update Ob/Gyns 6:88-92, 1999.
223. Hager WD: Puerperal mastitis. Contemporary Ob-Gyn (September):27-31, 1989.
224. Milligan DA, Duff P: Puerperal mastitis. In Pastorek JG (ed): Obstetric and Gynecologic Infectious Disease. New York, Raven, 1994, pp 445-454.
225. Duff P: Cytomegalovirus infection in pregnancy. Infect Dis Obstet Gynecol 2:146-152, 1994.

226. Brown HL, Abernathy MP: Cytomegalovirus infection. Semin Perinatol 22:260-266, 1998.
227. Betts RF: Cytomegalovirus infection epidemiology and biology in adults. Semin Perinatol 7:22-30, 1983.
228. Adler SP: Cytomegalovirus and child day care. N Engl J Med 321:1290-1296, 1989.
229. Stagno S, Pass RF, Dworsky ME, et al: Congenital cytomegalovirus infection. N Engl J Med 306:945-949, 1982.
230. Baker DA: New screening tests: HSV, CMV, HBV, HCV, parvovirus, and HIV. OBG Management, October 2005.
231. Guerra B, Simonazzi G, Banfi A, et al: Impact of diagnostic and confirmatory tests and prenatal counseling on the rate of pregnancy termination among women with positive cytomegalovirus immunoglobulin M antibody titers. Am J Obstet Gynecol 196:221.e1-221.e6, 2007.
232. Fowler KB, Stagno S, Pass RF, et al: The outcome of congenital cytomegalovirus infection in relation to maternal antibody status. N Engl J Med 326:663-667, 1992.
233. Fowler KB, Stagno S, Pass RF: Maternal immunity and prevention of congenital cytomegalovirus infection. JAMA 289:1008-1111, 2003.
234. Donner C, Liesnard C, Content J: Prenatal diagnosis of 52 pregnancies at risk for congenital cytomegalovirus infection. Obstet Gynecol 82:481-486, 1993.
235. Azam AZ, Vial Y, Fawer CL, et al: Prenatal diagnosis of congenital cytomegalovirus infection. Obstet Gynecol 97:443-448, 2001.
236. Nigro G, Adler SP, LaTorre R, et al: Passive immunization during pregnancy for congenital cytomegalovirus infection. N Engl J Med 353:1350-1362, 2005.
237. Duff P: Immunotherapy for congenital cytomegalovirus infection. N Engl J Med 353:1402-1404, 2005.
238. Gardner SW, Yow MD, Leeds LJ, et al: Failure of penicillin to eradicate group B streptococcal colonization in the pregnant woman. Am J Obstet Gynecol 135:1062, 1979.
239. Silver RM, Heddleston LN, McGregor JA, et al: Life-threatening puerperal infection due to group A streptococci. Obstet Gynecol 79:894, 1992.
240. American College of Obstetricians and Gynecologists: Prevention of Early-Onset Group B Streptococcal Disease in Newborns. ACOG Technical Bulletin No. 173. Washington, DC, ACOG, 1996.
241. Silver HM, Gibbs RS, Gray BM, et al: Risk factors for perinatal group B streptococcal disease after amniotic fluid colonization. Am J Obstet Gynecol 163:19, 1990.
242. Centers for Disease Control and Prevention: Prevention of perinatal group B streptococcal disease: A public health perspective. MMWR Morb Mortal Wkly Rep 45(RR-7):1, 1996.
243. Centers for Disease Control and Prevention: Decreasing the incidence of perinatal group B streptococcal disease—United States, 1993-1995. MMWR Morb Mortal Wkly Rep 46:473, 1997.
244. Centers for Disease Control and Prevention: Early-onset and late-onset neonatal group B streptococcal disease—United States, 1996-2004. MMWR Morb Mortal Wkly Rep 54:1205, 2005.
245. Baker CJ: Summary of the workshop on perinatal infections due to group B streptococcus. J Infect Dis 136:137, 1977.
246. Schrag SJ, Gorwitz R, Fultz-Butts K, et al: Prevetion of perinatal group B streptococcal disease: Revised guidelines from CDC. MMWR Recomm Rep 51:1, 2002.
247. Bergeron MG, Ke D, Menard C, et al: Rapid detection of group B streptococci in pregnant women at delivery. N Engl J Med 343:175, 2000.
248. Davies HD, Miller MA, Faro S, et al: Multicenter study of a rapid molecular-based assay for the diagnosis of group B streptococcus colonization in pregnant women. Clin Infect Dis 39:1129, 2004.
249. Edwards RK, Clark P, Sistrom CL, et al: Intrapartum antibiotic prophylaxis: 1. Relative effects of recommended antibiotics on gram-negative pathogens. Obstet Gynecol 100:534, 2002.
250. Orafu C, Gill P, Nelson K, et al: Perianal versus anorectal specimens: Is there a difference in group B streptococcal detection? Obstet Gynecol 99:1036, 2002.
251. Jamie WE, Edwards RK, Duff P: Vaginal-perianal compared with vaginal-rectal cultures for identification of group B streptococci. Obstet Gynecol 104:1058, 2004.
252. Boyer KM, Gotoff SP: Prevention of early-onset neonatal group B streptococcal disease with selective intrapartum chemoprophylaxis. N Engl J Med 314:1665, 1986.
253. Coleman RT, Sherer DM, Maniscalco WM: Prevention of neonatal group B streptococcal infections: Advances in maternal vaccine development. Obstet Gynecol 80:301, 1992.
254. Brown ZA, Selke S, Zeh J, et al: The acquisition of herpes simplex virus during pregnancy. N Engl J Med 337:509, 1997.
255. Lafferty WE, Coombs RW, Benedetti J, et al: Recurrences after oral and genital herpes simplex virus infection: Influence of site of infection and viral type. N Engl J Med 316:1444, 1987.
256. Fleming DT, McQuillan GM, Johnson RE, et al: Herpes simplex virus type 2 in the United States, 1976-1994. N Engl J Med 337:1105, 1997.
257. Kulhanjian JA, Soroush V, Au DS, et al: Identification of women at unsuspected risk of primary infection with herpes simplex virus type 2 during pregnancy. N Engl J Med 326:916, 1992.
258. Brown ZA, Vantuer LA, Benedetti J, et al: Effects on infants of a first episode of genital herpes in pregnancy. N Engl J Med 317:1246, 1987.
259. Brown, ZA, Wald A, Ashley-Morrow R, et al: Effect of serological status and cesarean delivery on transmission rates of herpes simplex virus from mother to infant. JAMA 289:203, 2003.
260. Hutto C, Arvin A, Jacobs R, et al: Intrauterine herpes simplex virus infections. Pediatrics 110:97, 1987.
261. Prober CG, Sullender WM, Yasukawa LL, et al: Low risk of herpes simplex virus infections in neonates exposed to the virus at the time of vaginal delivery to mothers with recurrent genital herpes simplex virus infections. N Engl J Med 316:240, 1987.
262. Whitley R, Arvin A, Prober C, et al: Predictors of morbidity and mortality in neonates with herpes simplex virus infections. N Engl J Med 324:450, 1991.
263. Nahass GT, Goldstein BA, Zhu WY, et al: Comparison of Tzanck smear, viral culture, and DNA diagnostic methods in detection of herpes simplex and varicella-zoster infection. JAMA 268:2541, 1992.
264. Cone RW, Hobson AC, Brown Z, et al: Frequent detection of genital herpes simplex virus DNA by polymerase chain reaction among pregnant women. JAMA 272:792, 1994.
265. Rogers BB, Josephson SL, Mak SK, et al: Polymerase chain reaction amplification of herpes simplex virus DNA from clinical samples. Obstet Gynecol 79:464, 1992.
266. Ashley-Morrow R, Nollkamper J, Robinson N, et al: Performance of Focus ELISA tests for herpes simplex virus type 1 (HSV-1) and HSV-2 antibodies among women in ten diverse geographic locations. Clin Microbiol Infect 10:530, 2004.
267. Baker D, Brown Z, Hollier LM, et al: Cost-effectiveness of herpes simplex virus type 2 serologic testing and antiviral therapy in pregnancy. Am J Obstet Gynecol 191:2074, 2004.
268. Thung SF, Grobman WA: The cost-effectiveness of routine antenatal screening for maternal herpes simplex virus-1 and -2 antibodies. Am J Obstet Gynecol 192:483, 2005.
269. Fife KH, Crumpacker SC, Mertz GJ, et al: Recurrence and resistance patterns of herpes simplex virus following cessation of > or = 6 years of chronic suppression with acyclovir. J Infect Dis 169:1338, 1994.
270. American College of Obstetricians and Gynecologists: Perinatal Herpes Simplex Infections. ACOG Technical Bulleletin No. 22. Washington, DC, 1988.
271. Gibbs RS, Amstey MS, Sweet RS, et al: Management of genital herpes infection in pregnancy. Obstet Gynecol 71:779, 1988.
272. Arvin AM, Hensleigh PA, Prober CG, et al: Failure of antepartum maternal cultures to predict the infant's risk of exposure to herpes simplex virus at delivery. N Engl J Med 315:796, 1986.
273. Brocklehurst P, Kinghorn G, Carney O, et al: A randomized placebo controlled trial of suppressive acyclovir in late pregnancy in women with recurrent genital herpes infection. BJOG 105:275, 1998.

274. Randolph AG, Hartshorn RM, Washington AE, et al: Acyclovir prophylaxis in late pregnancy to prevent neonatal herpes: A cost-effectiveness analysis. Obstet Gynecol 88:603, 1996.
275. O'Brien TR, George JR, Holmberg SD: Human immunodeficiency virus type 2 infection in the United States. JAMA 267:2775, 1992.
276. Minkoff HL: Human immunodeficiency virus infection in pregnancy. Semin Perinatol 22:293-308, 1998.
277. Hammer SM: Management of newly diagnosed HIV infection. N Engl J Med 353:1702-1710, 2005.
278. Kovacs JA, Masur H: Prophylaxis against opportunistic infections in patients with human immunodeficiency virus infection. N Engl J Med 342:1416-1429, 2000.
279. Connor EM, Sperling RS, Gelber R, et al: Reduction of maternal-infant transmission of human immunodeficiency virus type 1 with zidovudine treatment. N Engl J Med 331:1173-1180, 1994.
280. Minkoff H: Human immunodeficiency virus infection in pregnancy. Obstet Gynecol 101:797-810, 2003.
281. Minkoff H, Augenbraun M: Antiretroviral therapy for pregnant women. Am J Obstet Gynecol 176:478-489, 1997.
282. Public Health Service Task Force Perinatal HIV Guidelines Working Group: Summary of the updated recommendations from the Public Health Service Task Force to reduce perinatal human immunodeficiency virus-1 transmission in the United States. Obstet Gynecol 99:1117-1126, 2002.
283. American College of Obstetricians and Gynecologists: Human Immunodeficiency Virus Infections in Pregnancy. ACOG Educational Bulletin No. 232. Washington, DC, ACOG, 1997.
284. American College of Obstetricians and Gynecologists: Scheduled Cesarean Delivery and the Prevention of Vertical Transmission of HIV Infection. Committee Opinion No. 234. Washington, DC: ACOG, 2000.
285. The International Perinatal HIV Group: The mode of delivery and the risk of vertical transmission of human immunodeficiency virus type 1. N Engl J Med 340:977-987, 1999.
286. Mandlebrot L, LeChanadec J, Benebi A, et al: Perinatal HIV-1 transmission: Interaction between zidovudine prophylaxis and mode of delivery in the French perinatal cohort. JAMA 280:55-60, 1998.
287. The European Mode of Delivery Collaboration: Elective cesarean section versus vaginal delivery in prevention of vertical HIV-1 transmission: A randomized clinical trial. Lancet 353:1035-1039, 1999.
288. Minkoff H, O'Sullivan MJ: The case for rapid HIV testing during labor. JAMA 279:1743-1744, 1998.
289. Watts DH: Management of human immunodeficiency virus infection in pregnancy. N Engl J Med 346:1879-1891, 2002.
290. Ahlfors C, Goertzman BW, Holsted CC, et al: Neonatal listeriosis. Am J Dis Child 131:405, 1977.
291. Gellin BG, Broome CV: Listeriosis. JAMA 261:1313, 1989.
292. McLauchlin J: Human listeriosis in Britain, 1967-1985: A summary of 722 cases. I: Listeriosis during pregnancy and in the newborn. Epidemiol Infect 104:181, 1990.
293. Cherubin CE, Appleman MD, Heseltine PN, et al: Epidemiologic spectrum and current treatment of listeriosis. Rev Infect Dis 13:1180, 1991.
294. Bortolussi R, Schlech WF: Listeriosis. In Remington JS, Klein JO (eds): Infectious Diseases of the Fetus and Newborn Infant. Philadelphia, WB Saunders, 2001, p 1157.
295. MacDonald PDM, Whitwan RE, Boggs JD, et al: Outbreak of listeriosis among Mexican immigrants as a result of consumption of illicitly produced Mexican-style cheese. Clin Infect Dis 40:677, 2005.
296. Voetsch AC, Angulo FJ, Jones TF, et al: Reduction in the incidence of invasive listeriosis in foodborne diseases active surveillance network sites, 1996-2003. Clin Infect Dis 44:513, 2007.
297. Boucher M, Yonekura ML: Perinatal listeriosis (early onset): Correlation of antenatal manifestations and neonatal outcome. Obstet Gynecol 68:593, 1986.
298. Kalstone C: Successful antepartum treatment of listeriosis. Am J Obstet Gynecol 164:571, 1991.
299. Lorber B: Listeriosis. Clin Infect Dis 24:1, 1997.
300. Katz VL, Weinstein L: Antepartum treatment of *Listeria monocytogenes* septicemia. South Med J 75:1353, 1982.
301. Monif GRG: Maternal mumps infection during gestation: Observations in the progeny. Am J Obstet Gynecol 119:549, 1974.
302. Gershon A: Chickenpox, measles and mumps. In Remington JS, Klein JO (eds): Infectious Diseases of the Fetus and Newborn Infant. Philadelphia, WB Saunders, 1990.
303. Siegal M: Congenital malformations following chickenpox, measles, mumps, and hepatitis: Results of a chart study. JAMA 226:1521, 1973.
304. St. Geme JW Jr, Noren GR, Adams P: Proposed embryopathic relationship between mumps virus and primary endocardial fibroelastosis. N Engl J Med 275:339, 1966.
305. Kumar ML. Human parvovirus B19 and its associated diseases. Clin Perinatol 18:209-224, 1991.
306. Markenson GR, Yancey MK: Parvovirus B19 infections in pregnancy. Semin Perinatol 22:309-317, 1998.
307. Centers for Disease Control and Prevention: Risks associated with human parvovirus B19 infection. MMWR Morb Mortal Wkly Rep 38:81-97, 1989.
308. Harger JH, Adler SP, Koch WC, et al: Prospective evaluation of 618 pregnant women exposed to parvovirus B19: Risks and symptoms. Obstet Gynecol 91:413-420, 1998.
309. Public Health Laboratory Service Working Party on Fifth Disease: Prospective study of human parvovirus (B19) infection in pregnancy. BMJ 300:1166-1171, 1990.
310. Oepkes D, Seaward G, Vandenbussche FPHA, et al: Doppler ultrasonography versus amniocentesis to predict fetal anemia. N Engl J Med 355:155-164, 2006.
311. Fairley CK, Smoleniec JS, Caul OE, et al: Observational study of effect of intrauterine transfusions on outcome of fetal hydrops after parvovirus B19 infection. Lancet 346:1335-1337, 1995.
312. Rodis JF, Borgida AF, Wilson M, et al: Management of parvovirus infection in pregnancy and outcomes of hydrops: A survey of members of the Society of Perinatal Obstetricians. Am J Obstet Gynecol 179:985-988, 1998.
313. Rodis JF, Rodner C, Hansen AA, et al: Long-term outcome of children following human parvovirus B19 infection. Obstet Gynecol 91:125-128, 1998.
314. Brown KE, Green SW, deMayolo JA: Congenital anemia after transplacental B19 parvovirus infection. Lancet 343:895-896, 1994.
315. Conry JA, Torok T, Andrews I: Perinatal encephalopathy secondary to in utero human parvovirus B19 (HPV) infection [Abstract]. Neurology 43: A346, 1993.
316. Nagel HTC, de Haan TR, Vandenbussche FPHA, et al: Long-term outcome after fetal transfusion for hydrops associated with parvovirus B19 infection. Obstet Gynecol 109:42-47, 2007.
317. Reef SE, Frey TK, Theall K, et al: The changing epidemiology of rubella in the 1990s: On the verge of elimination and new challenges for control and prevention. JAMA 287:464, 2002.
318. American College of Obstetricians and Gynecologists: Rubella and pregnancy. ACOG Technical Bulletin No. 171. Washington, DC, ACOG, 1992.
319. Centers for Disease Control and Prevention: Rubella prevention: Recommendations of the Immunization Practices Advisory Committee (ACIP). MMWR Morb Mortal Wkly Rep 39:1, 1990.
320. Miller E, Cradock-Watson JE, Pollock TM: Consequences of confirmed maternal rubella at successive stages of pregnancy. Lancet 2:781, 1982.
321. Munro ND, Sheppard S, Smithells RW, et al: Temporal relations between maternal rubella and congenital defects. Lancet 2:201, 1987.
322. McIntosh EDG, Menser MA: A fifty-year follow-up of congenital rubella. Lancet 340:414, 1992.
323. Centers for Disease Control and Prevention: Rubella and congenital rubella syndrome—United States, January 1, 1991-May 7, 1994. MMWR Morb Mortal Wkly Rep 43:391, 1994.
324. Centers for Disease Control and Prevention: Revised ACIP recommendation for avoiding pregnancy after receiving a rubella-containing vaccine. MMWR Morb Mortal Wkly Rep 50:1117, 2001.

325. National Vaccine Advisory Committee: The measles epidemic: The problems, barriers, and recommendations. JAMA 266:1547, 1991.
326. Hersh BS, Markowitz LE, Maes EF, et al: The geographic distribution of measles in the United States, 1980 through 1989. JAMA 267:1936, 1992.
327. Atmar RL, Englund JA, Hammill H: Complications of measles during pregnancy. Clin Infect Dis 14:217, 1992.
328. Atkinson WL, Hadler SC, Redd SB, et al: Measles surveillance—United States, 1991. MMWR Morb Mortal Wkly Rep 41:1, 1992.
329. Christensen PE, Schmidt H, Bang HO, et al: An epidemic of measles in southern Greenland, 1951. Acta Med Scand 144:450, 1953.
330. Eberhart-Phillips JE, Frederick PD, Baron RC, et al: Measles in pregnancy: A descriptive study of 58 cases. Obstet Gynecol 82:797, 1993.
331. Centers for Disease Control and Prevention: Measles prevention: Supplementary statement. MMWR Morb Mortal Wkly Rep 38:11, 1989.
332. Stein SJ, Greenspoon JS: Rubeola during pregnancy. Obstet Gynecol 78:925, 1991.
333. Centers for Disease Control and Prevention: Measles prevention: Recommendations of the Immunization Practices Advisory Committee (ACIP). MMWR Morb Mortal Wkly Rep 38:1, 1989.
334. Parran T: Shadow on the Land. New York, Reynal & Hitchcock, 1937.
335. McFarlin BL, Bottoms SF, Dock BS, et al: Epidemic syphilis: Maternal factors associated with congenital infection. Am J Ostet Gynecol 170:535-540, 1994.
336. Centers for Disease Control and Prevention: Congenital syphilis—United States, 2002. MMWR Morb Mortal Wkly Rep 53:716-719, 2004.
337. Centers for Disease Control and Prevention: Primary and secondary syphilis—United States, 2003-2004. MMWR Morb Mortal Wkly Rep 55:269-273, 2006.
338. Centers for Disease Control and Prevention: Congenital syphilis. United States, 2000. MMWR 50:573-577, 2001.
339. Centers for Disease Control and Prevention: The National Plan to Eliminate Syphilis from the United States. Atlanta, GA: U.S. Department of Health and Human Services, CDC, 2006.
340. Youmans JB: Syphilis and other venereal diseases. Med Clin North Am 48:571-582, 1964.
341. Ingall D, Sanchez PJ, Bakes CJ: Syphilis. In Remington JS, Klein JO, Wilson CB, et al (eds): Infectious Diseases of the Fetus and Newborn Infant. Philadelphia, Elsevier Saunders, 2006, pp 545-580.
342. Harter CA, Benirschke K: Fetal syphilis in the first trimester. Am J Obstet Gynecol 124:705-711, 1976.
343. Fiumara NJ, Fleming WL, Downing JG, et al: The incidence of prenatal syphilis at the Boston City Hospital. N Engl J Med 247:48-52, 1952.
344. Fiumara NJ, Lessell S: Manifestations of late congenital syphilis: An analysis of 271 patients. Arch Dermatol 102:78-83, 1970.
345. Inraham NR: The value of penicillin alone in the prevention and treatment of congenital syphilis. Acta Derm Venereal Suppl (Stockh) 31:60-87, 1959.
346. Ricci, JM, Fojaco RM, O'Sullivan MJ: Congenital syphillis: The University of Miami/Jackson Memorial Medical Center experience, 1986-1988. Obstet Gynecol 74:687-693, 1989.
347. Coles FB, Hipp SS, Silberstein GS, et al: Congenital syphilis surveillance in upstate New York, 1989-1992: Implications for prevention and clinical management. J Infect Dis 171:732-735, 1995.
348. Libois A, DeWit S, Poll B, et al: HIV and syphilis: When to perform a lumbar puncture. Sex Transm Diseases 34:141-144, 2007.
349. Marra CM, Maxwell CL, Smith SL, et al: Cerebrospinal fluid abnormalities in patients with syphilis: Association with clinical and laboratory features. J Infect Dis 189:369-376, 2004.
350. Paraskevas GP, Kapaki E, Kararizou E, et al: Cerebrospinal fluid tau protein is increased in neurosyphilis: A discrimination from syphilis without nervous system involvement? Sex Transm Dis 34:220-223, 2007.
351. Genest DR, Choi-Hong SR, Tate JE, et al: Diagnosis of congenital syphilis from placental examination: Comparison of histopathology, Steiner stain, and polymerase chain reaction for *Treponema pallidum* DNA. Hum Pathol 27:366-372, 1996.
352. Sanchez PJ, Wendel GD: Syphilis in pregnancy. Clin Perinatal 24:71-90, 1997.
353. Hollier LM, Harstad TW, Sanchez PJ, et al: Fetal syphilis: Clinical and laboratory characteristics. Obstet Gynecol 97:947-953, 2001.
354. Klein VR, Cox SM, Mitchell MD, et al: The Jarisch-Herxheimer reaction complicating syphilotherapy in pregnancy. Obstet Gynecol 75:375-380, 1990.
355. Hollier LM, Cox SM: Syphilis. Semin Perinatol 22:323-331, 1998.
356. Rolfs RT, Joesoef MR, Hendershot EF, et al: A randomized trial of enhanced therapy for early syphilis in patients with and without human immunodeficiency virus infection: The Syphilis and HIV Study Group. N Engl J Med 337:307-314, 1997.
357. Egerman RS, Beazley D: Toxoplasmosis. Semin Perinatol 22:332-338, 1998.
358. Daffos F, Forestier F, Capella-Pavlousky M, et al: Prenatal management of 746 pregnancies at risk for congenital toxoplasmosis. N Engl J Med 318:271-275, 1988.
359. Hohlfield P, Daffos F, Costa JM, et al: Prenatal diagnosis of congenital toxoplasmosis with a polymerase-chain-reaction test on amniotic fluid. N Engl J Med 331:695-699, 1994.
360. Romand S, Wallon M, Franck J, et al: Prenatal diagnosis using polymerase chain reaction on amniotic fluid for congenital toxoplasmosis. Obstet Gynecol 97:296-300, 2001.
361. Guerina NG, Hsu HW, Meissner H, et al: Neonatal serologic screening and early treatment for congenital *Toxoplasma gondii* infection. N Engl J Med 330:1858-1863, 1994.
362. Duff P: Varicella: Five priorities for clinicians. Infect Dis Obstet Gynecol 1:163-165, 1994.
363. Chapman S, Duff P: Varicella in pregnancy. Semin Perinatol 17:403-409, 1993.
364. McGregor JA, Mark S, Crawford GP, Levin MJ: Varicella zoster antibody testing in the care of pregnant women exposed to varicella. Am J Obstet Gynecol 157:281-284, 1987.
365. Smith WJ, Jackson LA, Watts DH, Koepsell TD: Prevention of chickenpox in reproductive-age women: Cost-effectiveness of routine prenatal screening with postpartum vaccination of susceptibles. Obstet Gynecol 92:535-545, 1998.
366. Centers for Disease Control and Prevention: Prevention of varicella. MMWR Morb Mortal Wkly Rep 45(Suppl):1-37, 1996.
367. Asano Y, Yoshikawa T, Suga S, et al: Postexposure prophylaxis of varicella in family contact by oral acyclovir. Pediatrics 92:219-222, 1993.
368. Wallace MR, Bowler WA, Murray NB, et al: Treatment of adult varicella with oral acyclovir: A randomized placebo-controlled trial. Am Intern Med 117:358-363, 1992.
369. Enders G, Miller E, Cradock-Watson J, et al: Consequences of varicella and herpes-zoster in pregnancy: Prospective study of 1739 cases. Lancet 343:1547-1551, 1994.
370. Pastuszak AL, Levy M, Schick B, et al: Outcome after maternal varicella infection in the first 20 weeks of pregnancy. N Engl J Med 330:901-905, 1994.
371. Duff P: Varicella vaccine. Infect Dis Obstet Gynecol 4:63-65, 1996.
372. Vazquez M, LaRussa PS, Gershon AA, et al: The effectiveness of the varicella vaccine in clinical practice. N Engl J Med 344:955-960, 2001.
373. Sweet RL, Gibbs RS: Prenatal infections. In Sweet RL, Gibbs RS (eds): Infectious Diseases of the Female Genital Tract. Philadelphia, Lippincott Williams & Wilkins, 2006, pp 449-500.
374. Patriarca PA, Strikas RA: Influenza vaccine for healthy adults? N Engl J Med 333:933-934, 1995.
375. Poland GA: If you could halve the mortality rate, would you do it? Clinical Infect Dis 35:378-380, 2002.
376. Beigi RH: Pandemic influenza and pregnancy: A call for preparedness planning. Obstet Gynecol 109:1193-1196, 2007.
377. Garcia-Sastre A, Whitley RJ: Lessons learned from reconstructing the 1918 influenza pandemic. J Infect Dis 194:S127-S132, 2006.
378. Morgan A: Avian influenza: An agricultural perspective. J Infect Dis 194: S139-S146, 2006.

379. Poland GA: Vaccines against avian influenza—A race against time. N Engl J Med 354:1411-1413, 2006.
380. Simonsen L, Fukuda K, Schonberger LB, et al: The impact of influenza epidemics on hospitalizations. J Infect Dis 181:831-837, 2000.
381. Centers for Disease Control and Prevention: Influenza vaccine recommendations. MMWR Morb Mortal Wkly Rep 55:1-42, 2006.
382. Rhoton-Vlasak A: Viral influenza in women. Prim Care Update OB/Gyns 6:107, 1999.
383. Harris JW: Influenza occurring in pregnant women: A statistical study of thirteen hundred and fifty cases. JAMA 72:978-980, 1919.
384. Freeman DW, Barno A: Deaths from Asian influenza associated with pregnancy. Am J Obstet Gynecol 78:1172-1175, 1959.
385. Finland M: Influenza complicating pregnancy. In Charles D, Finland M (eds): Obstetrics and Perinatal Infections. Philadelphia, Lee & Febiger, 1973, pp 355-398.
386. Neuzil KM, Reed GW, Mitchel EF, et al: Impact of influenza on actue cardiopulmonary hospitalizations in pregnant women. Am J Epidemiol 148:1094-1102, 1998.
387. Anonymous. Two neuroaminidase inhibitors for treatment of influenza. Med Lett Drugs Ther 41:91, 1999.
388. Roberts S, Hollier LM, Sheffield J, et al: Cost-effectiveness of universal influenza vaccination in a pregnant population. Obstet Gynecol 107:1323-1329, 2006.
389. Munoz EM, Griesinger AJ, Wehmannen OA, et al: Safety of influenza vaccination during pregnancy. Am J Obstet Gynecol 192:1098-1106, 2005.
390. Duff P: Hepatitis in pregnancy. Semin Perinatol 22:277-283, 1998.
391. Duff B, Duff P: Hepatitis A vaccine: Ready for prime time. Obstet Gynecol 91:468-471, 1998.
392. Centers for Disease Control and Prevention: Prevention of Hepatitis A through active or passive transmission. MMWR Morb Mortal Wkly Rep 45:1-29, 1996.
393. Khuroo MS, Kamili S, Jameel S: Vertical transmission of hepatitis E virus. Lancet 345:1025-1026, 1995.
394. Centers for Disease Control and Prevention: Hepatitis B virus: A comprehensive strategy for eliminating transmission in the United States through universal childhood vaccination. MMWR Morb Mortal Wkly Rep 40:1-25, 1991.
395. Poland GA, Jacobson RM: Prevention of hepatitis B with the hepatitis B vaccine. N Engl J Med 351:2832-2838, 2004.
396. Leikin EL, Reirus JF, Schnell E, et al: Epidemiologic predictors of hepatitis C virus infection in pregnant women. Obstet Gynecol 84:529-534, 1994.
397. Bohman VR, Stettler W, Little BB, et al: Seroprevalence and risk factors for hepatitis C virus antibody in pregnant women. Obstet Gynecol 80:609-613, 1992.
398. Lauer GM, Walter BD: Hepatitis C virus infection. N Engl J Med 345:41-52, 2001.
399. Ohto H, Terazawa S, Sasaki N, et al: Transmission of hepatitis C virus from mothers to infants. N Engl J Med 330:744-750, 1994.
400. Steininger C, Kundi M, Jatzko G, et al: Increased risk of mother-to-infant transmission of hepatitis C virus by intrapartum infantile exposure to blood. J Infect Dis 187:345-351, 2003.
401. Gibb DM, Goodall RL, Dunn DT, et al: Mother-to-child transmission of hepatitis C virus: Evidence for preventable peripartum transmission. Lancet 356:904-907, 2000.
402. Zanetti AR, Paccagnini S, Principi N, et al: Mother-to-infant transmission of hepatitis C virus. Lancet 345:289-291, 1995.
403. Jarvis LM, Davidson F, Hanley JP, et al: Infection with hepatitis G virus among recipients of plasma products. Lancet 348:1352-1355, 1996.
404. Kew MC, Kassionides C: HGV: Hepatitis G virus or harmless G virus. Lancet 348(Suppl):10, 1996.
405. Alter MJ, Gallagher M, Morris TT, et al: Acute non-A-E hepatitis in the United States and the role of hepatitis G infection. N Engl J Med 336:741-746, 1997.
406. Miyakawa Y, Mayuma M: Hepatitis G virus: A true hepatitis virus or an accidental tourist? N Engl J Med 336:795-796, 1997.
407. Centers for Disease Control and Prevention: Update to CDC's Sexually Transmitted Diseases Treatment Guidelines, 2006: Fluoroquinolones No Longer Recommended for Treatment of Gonococcal Infections. MMWR Morb Mortal Wkly Rep 56(14):332-336, 2007.

Chapter 39

Cardiac Diseases

Daniel G. Blanchard, MD, and Ralph Shabetai, MD

Diagnosis of Heart Disease in Pregnancy

Pregnant women with heart disease are at higher risk for cardiovascular complications during pregnancy and also have a higher incidence of neonatal complications.[1] However, the significant hemodynamic changes that accompany pregnancy make the diagnosis of certain forms of cardiovascular disease difficult. During normal pregnancies, women frequently experience dyspnea, orthopnea, easy fatigability, dizzy spells, and, occasionally, even syncope. On physical examination, dependent edema, rales in the lower lung fields, visible neck veins, and cardiomegaly are commonly found. Systolic murmurs occur in more than 95% of pregnant women, and internal mammary flow murmurs and venous hums are common. A third heart sound (S_3 gallop) is often present.[2] Nevertheless, certain findings indicate heart disease in pregnancy and should suggest the presence of a significant cardiovascular abnormality. These symptoms include severe dyspnea, syncope with exertion, hemoptysis, paroxysmal nocturnal dyspnea, and chest pain related to exertion. Physical signs of organic heart disease include a fourth heart sound (S_4 gallop), cyanosis, clubbing, diastolic murmurs, sustained cardiac arrhythmias, and loud, harsh systolic murmurs.[3]

If there is a strong suspicion of heart disease during pregnancy, confirmatory diagnostic tests should be initiated. The changes of normal pregnancy must be recognized so that the findings are not misinterpreted. For example, nonspecific ST segment and T-wave abnormalities and shifts in the electrical axis can occur.[4] Pregnancy also produces changes in the echocardiogram, including alterations in cardiac dimensions and performance. The internal dimensions of all the cardiac chambers are increased, and slight regurgitation through the four valves is frequently observed. The ejection fraction (EF) and stroke volume are concomitantly larger, and the cardiac output is increased.[5] A small pericardial effusion can be a normal finding in pregnant women.[6] Both radiographic and radionuclide diagnostic procedures should be avoided during pregnancy unless the procedure is deemed essential for the health and safety of the mother.

Pre-Conception Counseling

If a woman plans to become pregnant but knows that she has heart disease, she and her physicians must be fully aware of several fundamental principles. The cardiovascular system undergoes specific adaptations to meet the increased demands of the mother and fetus during pregnancy. The most important of these are increases in blood volume, cardiac output, and heart rate. These adaptations exacerbate the symptoms and clinical signs of heart disease and may necessitate significant escalation in treatment.

Cardiac risk varies among the specific forms of heart disease and also with severity. During prepregnancy counseling, the physician should describe the nature of the heart disease in terms comprehensible to the prospective parents. The risk to the woman, which can vary from negligible to prohibitive, should be spelled out as clearly as possible.[7] On this basis, the patient may be advised either that the contemplated pregnancy is safe, will be uncomfortable and will necessitate treatment, carries a significantly increased risk, or would be extremely dangerous and should not be undertaken.

In the case of certain cardiac conditions, the patient should be strongly advised to undergo the necessary treatment before pregnancy and to allow several months to elapse before becoming pregnant. Examples in this category include the following:

- Large intracardiac shunt (atrial or ventricular septal defect) with mild to moderate pulmonary hypertension
- Patent ductus arteriosus (PDA) with mild to moderate pulmonary hypertension
- Severe coarctation of the aorta
- Severe mitral stenosis or regurgitation
- Severe aortic stenosis or regurgitation
- Tetralogy of Fallot
- Various congenital malformations and acquired heart diseases

Again, it is imperative that the palliative procedure be carried out before pregnancy is undertaken and that a year or so elapse before pregnancy occurs. Flexibility in clinical judgment is necessary, however. A woman with moderately severe valvular disease may require a prosthetic valve in the future. In such a case, the patient should be advised to have her family before valve replacement—with its associated anticoagulant risk—is required[8] (see Pregnancy in Patients with Artificial Heart Valves, later). The valvular heart lesions associated with high and low maternal and fetal risk during pregnancy are listed in Tables 39-1 and 39-2.

As previously noted, some cardiac disorders are so serious in nature that the physiologic changes of a superimposed pregnancy pose prohibitive risks to the mother; they carry such a high maternal mortality risk that pregnancy is contraindicated. In such circumstances, patients must be strongly cautioned against becoming pregnant. If such a patient is seen for the first time when she is already pregnant, termination of the pregnancy is recommended. The most serious of the cardiac

TABLE 39-1 VALVULAR HEART LESIONS ASSOCIATED WITH HIGH MATERNAL AND/OR FETAL RISK DURING PREGNANCY

Severe AS with or without symptoms
AR with NYHA functional class III-IV symptoms
MS with NYHA functional class II-IV symptoms
MR with NYHA functional class III-IV symptoms
Aortic and/or mitral valve disease resulting in severe pulmonary hypertension (pulmonary pressure greater than 75% of systemic pressures)
Aortic and/or mitral valve disease with significant LV dysfunction (EF < 40%)
Mechanical prosthetic valve requiring anticoagulation
Marfan syndrome with or without AR

AR, aortic regurgitation; AS, aortic stenosis; EF, ejection fraction; LV, left ventricular; MR, mitral regurgitation; MS, mitral stenosis; NYHA, New York Heart Association.
Reproduced with permission from Bonow RO, Carabello B, DeLeon AC, et al: ACC/AHA 2006 guidelines for the management of patients with valvular heart disease. Circulation 114:84, 2006.

TABLE 39-2 VALVULAR HEART LESIONS ASSOCIATED WITH LOW MATERNAL AND FETAL RISK DURING PREGNANCY

Asymptomatic AS with low mean gradient (<25 mm Hg and aortic valve area >1.5 cm²) in the presence of normal LV systolic function (EF > 50%)
NYHA functional class I or II AR with normal LV systolic function
NYHA functional class I or II MR with normal LV systolic function
MVP with no MR or mild to moderate MR with normal LV systolic function
Mild MS (mitral valve area >1.5 cm², gradient <5 mm Hg) without severe pulmonary hypertension
Mild to moderate pulmonary valve stenosis

AR, aortic regurgitation; AS, aortic stenosis; EF, ejection fraction; LV, left ventricular; MR, mitral regurgitation; MS, mitral stenosis; MVP, mitral valve prolapse; NYHA, New York Heart Association.
Reproduced with permission from Bonow RO, Carabello B, DeLeon AC, et al: ACC/AHA 2006 guidelines for the management of patients with valvular heart disease. Circulation 114:84, 2006.

disorders are those involving pulmonary hypertension, particularly those associated with a right-to-left shunt in cardiac blood flow (Eisenmenger syndrome). Low cardiac output states and entities in which there is an increased risk of aortic dissection (Marfan syndrome) also represent an extraordinarily high risk of maternal mortality. These high-risk maternal cardiovascular disorders are listed in Table 39-3.

In some women with specific dangerous cardiovascular diseases, pregnancy is contraindicated because of the substantial risk of maternal death.[9] Examples include the following:

- Dilated cardiomyopathy or left ventricular dysfunction (EF < 40%) of any cause
- Severe pulmonary hypertension of any cause
- Marfan syndrome, especially with aortic root dilation (diameter > 4 cm)

TABLE 39-3 HIGH-RISK MATERNAL CARDIOVASCULAR DISORDERS

Disorder	Estimated Maternal Mortality Rate (%)
Aortic valve stenosis	10-20
Coarctation of the aorta	5
Marfan syndrome	10-20
Peripartum cardiomyopathy	15-60
Severe pulmonary hypertension	50
Tetralogy of Fallot	10

If a patient with one of these disorders presents when she is already pregnant, she should be strongly urged to consider early termination. A carefully planned suction curettage before 13 weeks' gestation would place such a patient at minimal risk. Termination of pregnancy beyond 13 weeks increases the risk to the mother, because many of the cardiovascular alterations that occur in pregnancy have taken place.

Infective endocarditis often causes rapid and serious deterioration of the cardiac status, posing a major threat to the life and health of the mother and, therefore, of the fetus as well. Scrupulous attention to prophylaxis against endocarditis is critical during pregnancy. Pregnant women must pay meticulous attention to their dental health; if they have cardiac lesions susceptible to infective endocarditis, neglect of antibacterial prophylaxis could have dire consequences. In general, women with valvular heart disease should have antibiotic prophylaxis at the time of delivery.[10,11]

The prospective parents will want to know not only about the risk to the health and life of the future mother but also about the fetal risks. One of the most important questions is whether the mother's heart disease is hereditary and, if so, what is the risk that the infant will be born with the same defect. A detailed family cardiac history must be obtained before pregnancy, especially if the prospective mother has heart disease.

Some of the cardiomyopathies, especially hypertrophic forms, may be inherited in a mendelian manner.[12] Familial dilated cardiomyopathy has also been described. Approximately 20% of idiopathic dilated cardiomyopathy is inherited.[13] There is a strong familial tendency in certain congenital malformations, such as PDA and arterial septal defect (ASD). Additionally, mothers with congenital heart disease may have children with unrelated congenital malformations: this risk appears to be approximately 5%.[3,14] Also, pregnant women with advanced heart disease, especially those with low cardiac output or severe hypoxia, experience a greatly increased incidence of spontaneous abortion, stillbirths, and small or deformed children.[9] For most pregnant women with heart disease, vaginal delivery (with a low threshold for forceps or vacuum assistance) is recommended. Elective cesarean section is recommended in cases of Marfan syndrome or aortic aneurysm of any cause.[3]

Today's prospective mother wants to know about the risks to her fetus of drugs, other therapies, and diagnostic tests that are used to treat heart disease. Echocardiography poses no threat to the fetus, but radiation incurred with radionuclide angiography, cardiac catheterization with contrast angiography, or computed tomography pose a potential hazard to the fetus. If these studies are required, they should be performed before pregnancy occurs; they should be repeated thereafter only if mandated for the safety of the mother, and pelvic shielding should be used.

Maternal infection with the virus that causes German measles (rubella) is associated with a high risk of congenital malformation of the fetal heart as well as PDA. If the patient has not had German measles as a child and has never been inoculated against it and her antibody titer confirms the absence of immunity, she should be vaccinated some months before becoming pregnant.

Every pregnant woman who is known or thought to have heart disease should, at a minimum, be evaluated once by a cardiologist who understands the cardiovascular adaptations to pregnancy. The cardiologist will prescribe necessary diagnostic studies and treatments and, of equal importance, will not allow unnecessary ones. The effects of heart disease can often be ameliorated by correcting coexisting medical problems, such as anemia, chronic infection, anxiety, thyroid dysfunction, hypertension, and arrhythmia.

Cardiovascular Adaptations to Pregnancy

Increased Blood Volume

The cardiovascular alterations observed in pregnancy are discussed in detail in Chapter 7 but are reviewed here briefly. It is worthwhile to reconsider and emphasize some of the most important cardiovascular changes that occur during pregnancy, because they may significantly alter the course of cardiac disease or may themselves be influenced by a specific disorder.

Blood volume and cardiac output increase during pregnancy.[15] The uterus hypertrophies, endometrial vascularization is greatly increased, and the placenta becomes a highly vascular structure that functions to some extent as an arteriovenous shunt. In addition, generalized arteriolar dilation develops, mediated most probably by estrogen. These mechanisms combine to lower systemic vascular resistance and increase the pulse pressure. The total blood volume rises steadily during the first trimester and is increased by almost 50% by the 30th week, remaining more or less constant thereafter.[16] Several mechanisms are responsible for increasing blood volume in pregnancy, including steroid hormones of pregnancy, elevated plasma renin activity, and elevated plasma aldosterone levels. Human placental lactogen, atrial natriuretic factor, and other peptides may also play significant roles in governing changes of blood volume in pregnancy. Hypervolemia also occurs with trophoblastic disease, indicating that a fetus is not essential for its development. Heart rate increases by 10 to 20 beats/min. In a normal pregnancy, blood pressure does not increase, because the increased intravascular volume is balanced by decreased peripheral vascular resistance mediated by the placenta. Plasma volume tends to increase more than the red blood cell mass, accounting for a "physiologic anemia" that is common in pregnancy. Treatment with iron corrects the anemia which, if left untreated, may become significant (hematocrit as low as 33% and hemoglobin 11 g/dL).

Cardiac Output

Cardiac output rises during the first few weeks of pregnancy and is 30% to 45% above the nonpregnant level by the 20th week, remaining there until term.[15] The increase in cardiac output in the first trimester begins rapidly and peaks between the 20th and 26th week. Early in pregnancy, the dominant factor is elevated stroke volume; later, increased heart rate predominates.[17] In late pregnancy, the enlarged uterus partially impedes venous return by compressing the inferior vena cava, accounting for lower cardiac output. This is one reason why some obstetricians prefer to manage labor with the patient in the left decubitus position.

Cardiac Performance

Echocardiographic studies have shown increases in the left ventricular fiber shortening velocity and in EF. These changes do not necessarily indicate increased myocardial contractility but may simply be the result of decreased peripheral vascular resistance and increased preload. In any case, stroke volume is increased, and cardiac output is further augmented by the 10% to 15% increase in heart rate that characterizes normal pregnancy.[18]

Demands on the cardiovascular system increase significantly during labor and delivery. Pain increases sympathetic tone, and uterine contractions induce wide swings in the systemic venous return. With placental separation, autotransfusion of at least 500 mL takes place, placing an acute load on the diseased heart, unless offset by blood loss. These large shifts in blood volume can precipitate, on the one hand, shock, and on the other, pulmonary edema in women with severe heart disease.

If a chest radiograph is obtained in a pregnant woman, the cardiac silhouette often appears slightly enlarged owing to the combined effects of volume overload and elevation of the diaphragm. Routine echocardiographic studies have demonstrated that a small, silent pericardial effusion is quite common.[6]

Electrocardiographic Changes

The mean QRS axis may shift to the left[19] as a result of the elevated diaphragm. In later pregnancy, the axis may shift to the right when the fetus descends into the pelvis. Minor ST segment and T-wave changes may be observed, usually in lead III but sometimes aVF as well. Less often, T inversions may appear transiently in the left precordial leads. Occasionally, small Q waves may accompany T-wave inversion in leads III and aVF. These changes are seldom of sufficient magnitude to raise the question of ischemic heart disease, which in any case is relatively uncommon in pregnancy, especially if the mother is young and free from symptoms. Extrasystoles and supraventricular tachycardia are more common during pregnancy. Symptoms of palpitations are common during pregnancy but only rarely signify the presence of organic heart disease.

General Guidelines for Management

During treatment of all pregnant patients with heart disease, priority must be given to maternal health, but all possible therapeutic measures should also be taken to protect the developing fetus. The aspects of management are outlined in Table 39-4.

Because pregnancy increases the demands on the heart, physical exertion frequently must be restricted, especially if it causes symptoms. Some women with certain forms of cardiac disease, such as significant mitral stenosis and cardiomyopathy, tolerate pregnancy poorly and cannot endure physical exertion. They may require strict bed rest for the duration of the pregnancy, particularly during the last trimester. Women with heart disease have a limited ability to increase cardiac output to meet increased metabolic demands and should minimize the demands placed on the heart from physical activity.

TABLE 39-4 CARDIAC DISEASE IN PREGNANCY: ASPECTS OF MANAGEMENT

Activity restriction
Diet modification
Team approach for medical care
Infection control
Immunizations
Prophylaxis against bacterial endocarditis
Prophylaxis against rheumatic fever
Interruption of pregnancy
Counseling
Contraception or sterilization
Cardiovascular surgery
Cardiovascular drugs

Cardiovascular Drugs

Some of the drugs commonly used in the management of cardiovascular disease have potentially harmful effects on the developing embryo and fetus. For example, there is no question that oral anticoagulants are potential teratogens when administered in the first trimester (see Chapter 20 and later discussion in this chapter). The "warfarin embryopathy syndrome," consisting of nasal hypoplasia, optic atrophy, digital abnormalities, and mental impairment, occurs in a minority of cases. The actual risk of warfarin embryopathy is difficult to estimate and has ranged from 4% to 67% in various reports.[20,21] A risk of 4% to 10% seems more reasonable.[22] There is some evidence that embryopathy is less likely if the warfarin dose is 5 mg/day or less.[23] The fetal risks continue beyond the first trimester, because warfarin increases the possibility of both fetal and intrauterine bleeding.

Anticoagulation presents a significant practical problem in the management of atrial fibrillation, systemic or pulmonary embolism, thrombophlebitis, and pulmonary hypertension in pregnancy. The most vexing problem arises in the setting of prosthetic heart valves[10,11] (discussed later). In the case of mechanical valve prostheses, warfarin appears to be superior to heparin in preventing valvular thrombosis. Although heparin is safer for the fetus, there is probably an increased risk for the mother.[20,24] This is a complex medical issue, and no randomized trial to determine the optimal anticoagulant therapy for women with a prosthetic valve has been conducted. Therefore, recommendations are based on smaller studies and on clinical judgment.[10,11] No single regimen is likely to be applicable to all such cases, because the issue is complicated by the type and generation of the prosthetic valve, the cardiac rhythm, and the size and contractility of the cardiac chambers.

β-Adrenergic blocking agents, used for the treatment of hypertension and tachyarrhythmia, have been associated with neonatal respiratory depression, sustained bradycardia, and hypoglycemia when administered late in pregnancy or just before delivery. However, if they are used judiciously in selected cases (e.g., in women with cardiomyopathy and heart failure), β-blockers are usually well tolerated.

The thiazide diuretics are another class of drugs that can produce harmful effects on the fetus—especially if they are used in the third trimester or for extended periods—and may impair normal expansion of plasma volume. Rarely, severe neonatal electrolyte imbalance, jaundice, thrombocytopenia, liver damage, and even death have been reported.

There have been numerous reports of fetal and neonatal renal complications after the use of angiotensin-converting enzyme (ACE) inhibitors during pregnancy.[25,26] These complications suggest a profound and deleterious effect on fetal renal function, leading to decreased renal function and oligohydramnios, as well as neonatal renal failure. ACE inhibitors are absolutely contraindicated during pregnancy. Another class of antihypertensive drugs, the angiotensin receptor blockers, also may affect fetal renal function and are likewise absolutely contraindicated in pregnancy.

The indications and possible adverse effects of commonly prescribed cardioactive drugs during pregnancy are summarized in Table 39-5.

Team Approach to Medical Care

Medical care for pregnant women with heart disease is best provided through the cooperative efforts of a cardiologist who is familiar with the hemodynamic changes of pregnancy and an obstetrician. Frequent visits to both specialists, along with open consultations, can provide the patient with consistent advice and reassurance and can circumvent the worry and anxiety created by confusing and conflicting information. In addition, the anesthesiologist needs to be consulted during the antepartum period to outline the anticipated approach to intrapartum management, a time of maximum risk for most of these women. The role of the anesthesiologist and the approach to women with pregnancies complicated by cardiac disease are summarized in Chapter 56.

Congenital Heart Disease

A number of simple congenital malformations are compatible with a normal or nearly normal pregnancy. Congenital malformations previously associated with high maternal morbidity and mortality and fetal wastage now frequently end with a satisfactory outcome because of palliative or corrective surgery. Despite recent advances, however, women with congenital heart disease who become pregnant still have a significant risk of miscarriage, cardiac complications, and premature delivery.[27]

The care of adults with congenital heart malformation is an important and growing branch of cardiology[7,28,29] that requires the cooperative efforts of medical and pediatric cardiologists, cardiac surgeons, and, in the case of pregnancy, obstetricians and anesthesiologists.[30,31]

Left-to-Right Shunt

Atrial Septal Defect

ASD may be undiscovered before pregnancy, because symptoms are often absent and the physical findings are not blatant. Other causes of left-to-right shunt, such as PDA and ventricular septal defect (VSD), are more likely to be discovered and treated in infancy or childhood. Physicians should be alert to the higher possibility of uncorrected defects in women who have immigrated from an undeveloped country.

Closure of uncomplicated large ostium secundum ASD is straightforward and safe and usually is curative. Therefore, the procedure should be done before pregnancy. Many ASDs can now be closed percutaneously, using a "clamshell" or "umbrella" device inserted via a transvenous catheter.[32] If the patient is unwilling to undergo ASD closure, she can be advised that the lesion is unlikely to complicate pregnancy and labor, provided that pulmonary hypertension is not present.[3]

TABLE 39-5 INDICATIONS FOR AND POSSIBLE ADVERSE EFFECTS OF COMMONLY PRESCRIBED CARDIOACTIVE DRUGS ON MOTHER AND FETUS

Drug	Use in Pregnancy	Potential Side Effects	Breastfeeding	Risk Category*
Adenosine	Maternal and fetal arrhythmias	No side effects reported; data on use during first trimester are limited	Data NA	C
Amiodarone	Maternal arrhythmias	IUGR, prematurity, congenital goiter, hypothyroidism and hyperthyroidism, transient bradycardia, prolonged QT in the newborn	Not recommended	C
ACEIs and angiotensin receptor blockers	Hypertension	Oligohydramnios, IUGR, prematurity, neonatal hypotension, renal failure, anemia, death, skull ossification defect, limb contractures, patent ductus arteriosus	Compatible	X
β-Blockers	Hypertension, maternal arrhythmias, myocardial ischemia, mitral stenosis, hypertrophic cardiomyopathy, hyperthyroidism, Marfan syndrome	Fetal bradycardia, low placental weight, possible IUGR, hypoglycemia; no information on carvedilol	Compatible; monitoring of infant's heart rate recommended	Acebutolol: B Labetalol: C Metoprolol: C Propranolol: C Atenolol: D
Digoxin	Maternal and fetal arrhythmias, heart failure	No evidence for unfavorable side effects on the fetus	Compatible	C
Diltiazem	Myocardial ischemia, tocolysis	Limited data; increased incidence of major birth defects	Compatible	C
Disopyramide	Maternal arrhythmias	Limited data; may induce uterine contraction and premature delivery	Compatible	C
Diuretics	Hypertension, congestive heart failure	Hypovolemia leads to reduced uteroplacental perfusion, fetal hypoglycemia, thrombocytopenia, hyponatremia, hypokalemia; thiazide diuretics can inhibit labor and suppress lactation	Compatible	C
Flecainide	Maternal and fetal arrhythmias	Limited data; 2 cases of fetal death after successful treatment of fetal SVT reported, but relation to flecainide uncertain	Compatible	C
Heparin	Anticoagulation	None reported	Compatible	C
Hydralazine	Hypertension	None reported	Compatible	C
Lidocaine	Local anesthesia, maternal arrhythmias	No evidence for unfavorable fetal effects; high serum levels may cause CNS depression at birth	Compatible	C
Nifedipine	Hypertension, tocolysis	Fetal distress related to maternal hypotension reported	Compatible	C
Nitrates	Myocardial infarction and ischemia, hypertension, pulmonary edema, tocolysis	Limited data; use is generally safe; few cases of fetal heart rate deceleration and bradycardia have been reported	Data NA	C
Procainamide	Maternal and fetal arrhythmias	Limited data; no fetal side effects reported	Compatible	C
Propafenone	Fetal arrhythmias	Limited data; fetal death reported after direct intrauterine administration in fetuses with fetal hydrops	Data NA	C
Quinidine	Maternal and fetal arrhythmias	Minimal oxytocic effect, high doses may cause premature labor or abortion; transient neonatal thrombocytopenia and damage to eighth nerve reported	Compatible	C
Sodium nitroprusside	Hypertension, aortic dissection	Limited data; potential thiocyanate fetal toxicity, fetal mortality reported in animals	Data NA	C
Sotalol	Maternal arrhythmias, hypertension, fetal tachycardia	Limited data; 2 cases of fetal death and 2 cases of significant neurologic morbidity in newborns reported, as well as bradycardia in newborns	Compatible; monitoring of infant's heart rate recommended	B
Verapamil	Maternal and fetal arrhythmias, hypertension, tocolysis	Limited data; other than 1 case of fetal death of uncertain cause, no adverse fetal or newborn effects reported	Compatible	C
Warfarin	Anticoagulation	Crosses placental barrier; fetal hemorrhage in utero, embryopathy, CNS abnormalities	Compatible	X

ACE, angiotensin-converting enzyme inhibitor; CNS, central nervous system; IUGR, intrauterine growth retardation; NA, not available; SVT, supraventricular tachycardia.

***U.S. Food and Drug Administration classification of drug risk. B: Either animal reproduction studies have not demonstrated a fetal risk but there are no controlled studies in pregnant women, or animal reproduction studies have shown an adverse effect that was not confirmed in controlled studies in women. C: Either studies in animals have revealed adverse effects on the fetus and there are no controlled studies in women, or studies in women and animals are not available. Drug should be given only if the potential benefits justify the potential risks to the fetus. D: There is positive evidence of human fetal risk, but the benefits from use in pregnant women may be acceptable despite the risk. X: Studies in animals or human beings have demonstrated fetal abnormalities. The risk of the use of the drug in pregnant women clearly outweighs any possible benefit. The drug is contraindicated in women who are or may become pregnant.**

Source: Drug Information for the Health Care Professional (USDPI Vol 1). Micromedex, 23rd ed, January 1, 2003. (Adapted and modified from Elkayam U. Pregnancy and cardiovascular disease. In Zipes DP, Libby P, Bonow RO, Braunwald E (eds): Braunwald's Heart Disease: A Textbook of Cardiovascular Medicine, 7th ed. Philadelphia: Elsevier, 2005, p 1965.)

Metcalfe and colleagues[33] reported one maternal death among 219 pregnancies in 113 women with ASD. Peripheral vasodilation, if anything, reduces the left-to-right shunt.[17] Because ASD in young women is not associated with heart failure, diuretics and extreme limitation of intravenous infusion are not warranted. A small percentage of patients with ASD have atrial flutter or fibrillation, which usually is paroxysmal. This arrhythmia can be managed along conventional lines, often with digoxin if necessary. The prospective mother should be informed that closure of the defect does not prevent atrial fibrillation once the arrhythmia has occurred.

ASD can be difficult to diagnose during pregnancy. The murmur associated with ASD may be inconspicuous, being a pulmonary ejection systolic murmur and therefore not unlike the physiologic murmur of pregnancy. However, the second heart sound is widely split and may be fixed throughout the respiratory cycle, a distinctly abnormal finding. The electrocardiogram (ECG) shows incomplete right bundle branch block and, in the case of the much more common ostium secundum defect, right axis deviation. In the less common ostium primum defect, marked left axis deviation accompanies incomplete right bundle branch block. The chest radiograph shows right atrial and right ventricular enlargement, prominent pulmonary arteries, and plethoric lung fields. Echocardiography establishes or confirms the diagnosis (Fig. 39-1), obviating the need for cardiac catheterization in many cases.

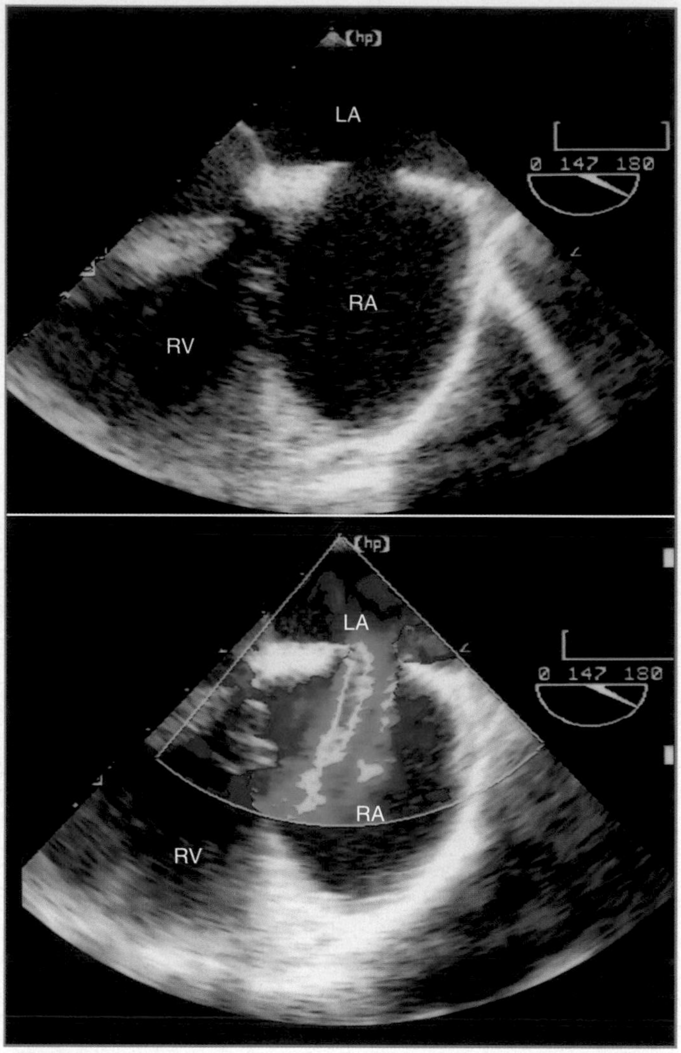

FIGURE 39-1 Transesophageal echocardiographic image of atrial septal defect (ostium secundum). In the upper panel, a large defect in the interatrial septum is present. In the lower panel, the blue/yellow color represents blood flow from the left atrium (LA) into the right atrium (RA). RV, right ventricle.

Complicated Atrial Septal Defect

If atrial arrhythmias recur frequently—and especially if the heart rate is difficult to control—catheter ablation is successful in restoring normal sinus rhythm without the need for antiarrhythmic drugs. In most cases, this procedure should not be done until after delivery because of the extensive radiation exposure that is needed. In rare instances, pregnancy and labor may be associated with a paradoxical systemic embolus resulting from a thrombus migrating from the inferior vena cava across the ASD into the left atrium.

In the uncommon event that the patient is more than 35 years old and has an uncorrected large ASD, the likelihood of chronic atrial fibrillation, right ventricular dysfunction, and pulmonary hypertension rises significantly. Pregnancy is not advised if any of these sequelae is present. If the patient insists on going through with the pregnancy, prolonged bed rest will be required, and vigorous treatment of heart failure may be needed. The maternal risk is increased, and there is significant risk of fetal loss. Although warfarin is generally recommended for chronic atrial fibrillation, its use is best avoided (especially in the first trimester); aspirin would be a reasonable compromise. Severe pulmonary hypertension is an uncommon feature of an ostium secundum ASD but is a contraindication to pregnancy. The ostium primum ASD, which is associated with Down syndrome and poses a risk of endocarditis, is more often associated with severe pulmonary hypertension. Infective endocarditis rarely, if ever, complicates a simple ostium secundum ASD; therefore, prophylaxis during labor is not warranted.

Ventricular Septal Defect

The clinical spectrum and risk of VSD may range from so mild that it has little or no effect on pregnancy to so high that maternal or fetal death can occur. Small defects in the muscular ventricular septum frequently close spontaneously during childhood. However, these defects occasionally persist, allowing a small left-to-right shunt, manifested by a loud pansystolic murmur along the left sternal border accompanied by a coarse thrill. The chest radiograph is often normal, as is the ECG. The echocardiogram is usually diagnostic (Fig. 39-2). These findings constitute the maladie de Roger. Prophylaxis against infective endocarditis is indicated, but otherwise this lesion has no effect on pregnancy or labor.

When the defect is in the membranous septum, spontaneous closure is rare. In the absence of significant pulmonary vascular disease, the same pansystolic murmur and thrill are found. If the shunt is large, however, the lung fields are plethoric on chest radiography, and the heart and pulmonary arteries are enlarged. The classic ECG shows a pattern of biventricular hypertrophy. In such cases, flow through the pulmonary vascular bed is usually at least twice the systemic cardiac output. Patients with a relatively large, uncomplicated left-to-right shunt through a VSD tolerate pregnancy well and, in this respect, are comparable to patients with ASD. However, prophylaxis against endocarditis is essential in cases of VSD.

Here it is appropriate to detour from clinical description to pathophysiology. Pulmonary vascular resistance is calculated as the pressure drop across the pulmonary vascular bed divided by the flow through it:

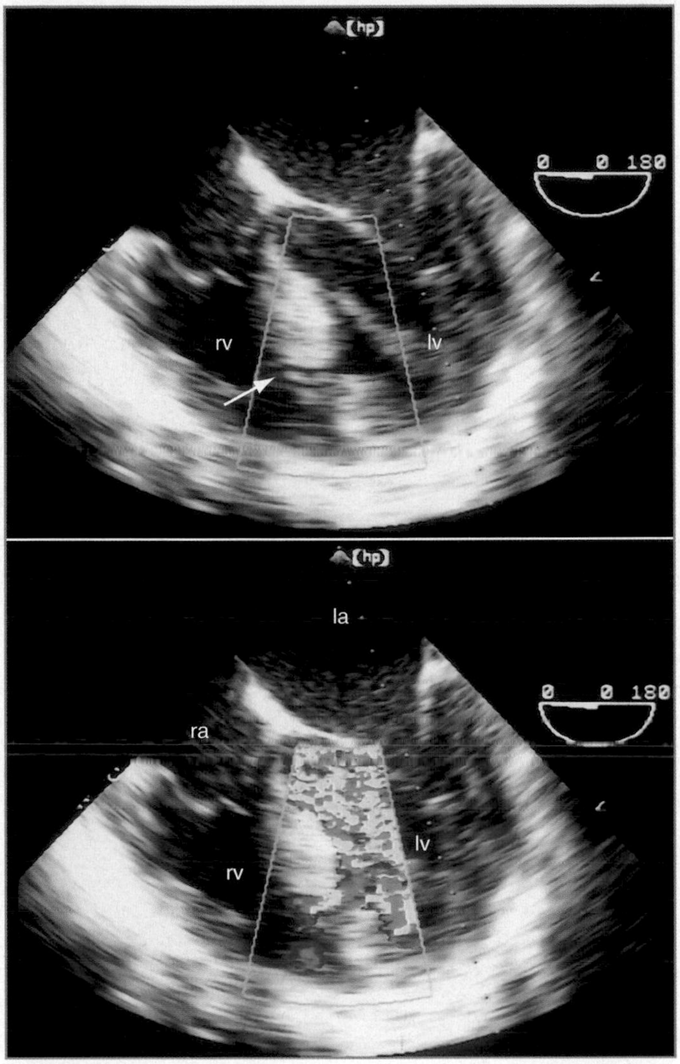

FIGURE 39-2 Transesophageal echocardiographic image of a small muscular ventricular septal defect. In the upper panel, a small communication is seen *(arrow)* between the right ventricle (rv) and left ventricle (lv). In the lower panel, color imaging confirms blood flow between the two chambers. la, left atrium; ra, right atrium.

$$R = (MPAP - MPCWP)/Q_{pulm}$$

where R is pulmonary vascular resistance in Wood units; MPAP and MPCWP (in mm Hg) are the mean pulmonary arterial and capillary wedge pressures, respectively; and Q_{pulm} is total flow through the right heart and pulmonary circulation (i.e., cardiac output plus left-to-right shunt) in liters per minute.

Resistance can be described in Wood units or in dyne·s/cm^5. The Wood unit has the merit of simplicity and is derived from clinical units of pressure and flow. The more fundamental but less friendly dyne·s/cm^5 can be obtained by multiplying Wood units by 80. Normal pulmonary vascular resistance is 0.5 to 1.5 units. When a clinician is faced with a pregnant woman with pulmonary hypertension, the key to her risk during pregnancy lies in the pulmonary vascular resistance. High flow, by itself, can be the mechanism for pulmonary hypertension without dangerous elevation in the resistance. This mechanism can be appreciated by rewriting the resistance equation to read

$$P = Q \cdot R$$

where P is the pressure drop and Q is the flow across the pulmonary vascular bed.

A patient at one extreme may have a large shunt with pulmonary flow of 20 L/min and an R of 3 units, yielding an MPAP of 55 mm Hg (assuming a normal MPCWP of 5 mm Hg). At the other extreme, a patient with pulmonary vascular disease may have a pulmonary blood flow of 7 L/min and an R of 7 units, yielding an MPAP of 44 mm Hg. The higher the pulmonary vascular resistance (R), the greater the maternal risk. The risk is prohibitive when R reaches the systemic level (approximately 15 Wood units). In borderline cases (e.g., patients with R between 5 and 8 units), a pulmonary arteriolar vasodilating agent is sometimes administered to determine whether the increased resistance is partially reversible or completely irreversible. An increase in pulmonary vascular resistance of 3 to 4 units is considered mild, 5 to 7 units is moderate, and more than 8 units is severe.

VSD may be associated with considerable increase in pulmonary vascular resistance, reflecting occlusive disease of the small pulmonary arteries and arterioles. This development, if it is to occur, usually does so in childhood; unless corrected, it leads to the Eisenmenger syndrome (discussed later). However, a small number of adults may survive with VSD and pulmonary vascular resistance that is significantly elevated but falls short of the Eisenmenger syndrome. Such patients are at high risk for death during pregnancy or labor, and there is a high risk of fetal impairment or loss. The patient should be told that early therapeutic abortion would be the safest option, and that later pregnancy would be hazardous and would require intensive care, with physical exercise strictly curtailed and prolonged bed rest enforced. The combination of decreased physical activity, pulmonary hypertension, and pulmonary vascular disease would constitute a sound rationale for instituting anticoagulation, which is another reason why pregnancy is better avoided or terminated.

Some authorities strongly advise that delivery be effected prematurely by means of cesarean section and urge sterilization at the same operation. The dangers must be thoroughly understood by women in this category who insist on continuing pregnancy.

Patent Ductus Arteriosus

The loud, continuous or machinery murmur of typical PDA with a large left-to-right shunt and no pulmonary vascular disease is so striking that the lesion is almost invariably detected and corrected in infancy or childhood. Occasionally, however, women of childbearing age or pregnant women from underdeveloped countries may present with a PDA. If the left-to-right shunt is large, the circulation is hyperdynamic, with a wide arterial pulse pressure, low arterial diastolic pressure, and hyperactive precordium. The heart may be somewhat enlarged to clinical and radiologic examination, and the ECG may show left ventricular hypertrophy. The echocardiogram is useful for demonstrating a shunt between the two great vessels (Fig. 39-3). The signs of hyperdynamic circulation resulting from the PDA are exaggerated by pregnancy.

Because the murmur of PDA is systolic-diastolic, it is commonly referred to as a “continuous” murmur, although it usually peaks late in systole. Because of its characteristics, the murmur is also referred to as a “machinery” murmur. It is maximal in the left infraclavicular region. It must be distinguished from a venous hum, which is loudest in the neck rather than the infraclavicular area. Venous hum is common in pregnant women, and it changes dramatically with changes in the position of the head.

Division or occlusion of the PDA should be accomplished before pregnancy is undertaken. Currently, most PDAs can be closed by the insertion of an occluder device delivered via a percutaneous intravas-

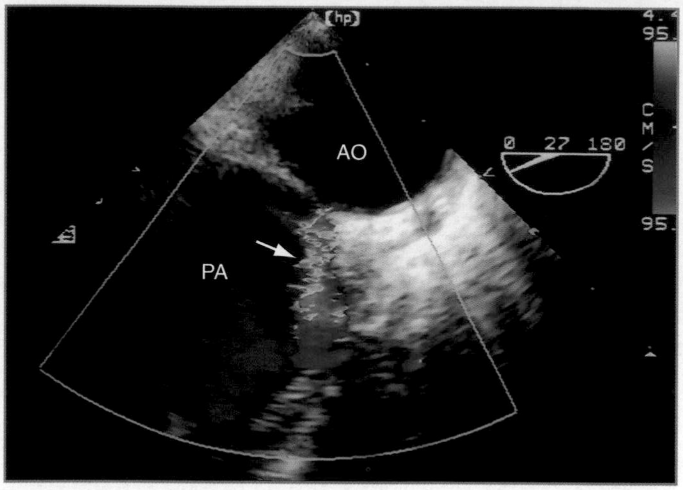

FIGURE 39-3 **Transesophageal echocardiographic image of a patent ductus arteriosus.** A communication is present between the proximal portion of the descending aorta (AO) and the pulmonary artery (PA). Color imaging (*arrow*) confirms blood flow from the aorta into the PA.

cular catheter.[34] If a patient does become pregnant before PDA occlusion, an uncomplicated left-to-right shunt can be managed safely. Endocarditis is a risk in patients with PDA, and antibiotic prophylaxis is required. Embolic complications of infective endocarditis and endarteritis secondary to PDA may take the form of infected pulmonary emboli. The patient becomes febrile with respiratory symptoms, and the chest radiograph shows multiple opacities and infiltrates.

The leading cause of Eisenmenger syndrome is a large VSD, followed in prevalence by a large PDA. As with VSD, individuals with PDA may sustain severe increases in pulmonary vascular resistance with the corresponding pulmonary hypertension and right ventricular hypertrophy, yet fall short of Eisenmenger physiology. The maternal risk during pregnancy is high in this situation, similar to that encountered in VSD with equivalent pathology. Treatment is the same as in VSD with Eisenmenger syndrome. When the pulmonary pressure rises, the aortopulmonary shunt decreases, and the murmur becomes progressively quieter and shorter, until it finally disappears.

In general, the woman with uncomplicated PDA tolerates pregnancy well. If pulmonary hypertension supervenes, the risk to the mother becomes significant. Therefore, if pulmonary hypertension is suspected and documented, termination of pregnancy is strongly recommended.

Eisenmenger Syndrome

Eisenmenger syndrome is characterized by a congenital communication between the systemic and pulmonary circulations and increased pulmonary vascular resistance, either to systemic level (so that there is no shunt across the defect) or exceeding systemic (allowing right-to-left shunting). As mentioned, the most common underlying defect is a large VSD, followed in prevalence by a large PDA. Eisenmenger pathophysiology is less common in ASD. Occasionally, this type of pathophysiology develops in other, less common defects. By the time the syndrome is fully developed, it is often difficult clinically to diagnose the underlying defect. For this discussion, the VSD serves as a good model (Fig. 39-4).

Eisenmenger pathophysiology develops only if the defect is large and is not restrictive, resulting in equal systolic pressure in the two

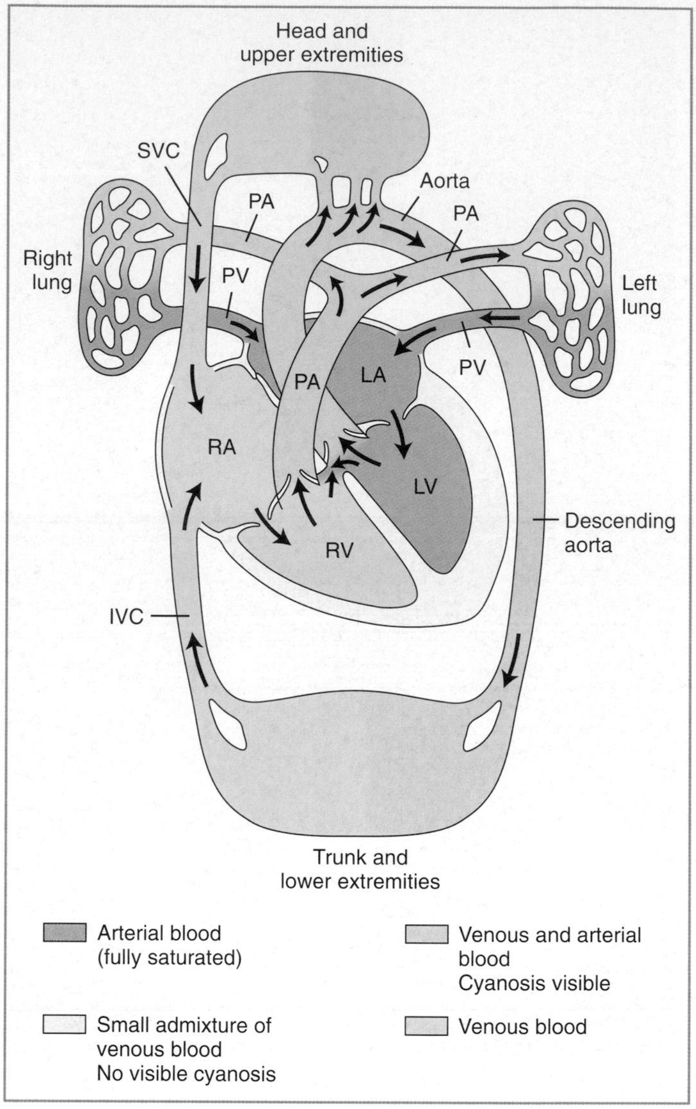

FIGURE 39-4 **Eisenmenger complex.** Here the cause of right-to-left shunt across the ventricular septal defect is increased pulmonary vascular resistance arising in the small pulmonary arteries and arterioles. IVC, inferior vena cava; LA, left atrium; LV, left ventricle; PA, pulmonary artery; PV, pulmonary vein; RA, right atrium; RV, right ventricle; SVC, superior vena cava. (Reprinted by permission of the publisher. From Taussig HB: Congenital Malformations of the Heart. Cambridge, Mass, Harvard University Press, 1960. Copyright © 1960 by the Commonwealth Fund by the President and Fellows of Harvard College.)

ventricles. It is more common in girls and develops at a young age. Therefore, when increased pulmonary vascular resistance is detected in a child with a large VSD, operative closure must be done as soon as possible to prevent the development of Eisenmenger pathophysiology. Once this has appeared, pulmonary hypertension is irreversible, and the VSD is consequently inoperable (unless lung transplantation is performed as well).

The major clues that pulmonary vascular resistance is increasing are (1) diminution of evidence of a left-to-right shunt and (2) the appearance of progressively severe pulmonary hypertension. The pansystolic murmur of VSD or the continuous murmur of PDA is replaced by a short ejection systolic murmur. The lungs are no longer plethoric but show large central pulmonary arteries and small peripheral arteries characteristic of severe pulmonary hypertension. Because the shunt has disappeared, the radiographic cardiothoracic ratio returns to normal but the main pulmonary segment is prominent. There is usually a striking right ventricular heave, a loud and palpable pulmonary valve closure sound, and an ejection sound in early systole. When concentric ventricular hypertrophy gives way to dilatation and right-sided heart failure, evidence of tricuspid regurgitation appears. Until then, the mean venous pressure is normal but the amplitude of the a wave may be increased, reflecting decreased right ventricular diastolic compliance.

If pulmonary vascular resistance is significantly higher than systemic levels, right-to-left shunting of blood occurs and causes cyanosis and clubbing of the fingers and toes. This shunting of deoxygenated blood into the systemic circulation leads to hypoxemia and triggers a reactive erythrocytosis as the system attempts to increase peripheral oxygen delivery. This increases blood viscosity and can cause sludging and decreased flow of blood, especially in small vessels. A high hematocrit value, however, is not an automatic indication for serial phlebotomy, because this approach can lead to iron deficiency and microcytosis. Tissue hypoxia may then actually worsen, a particularly undesirable result in pregnancy. Phlebotomy is reserved for patients without evidence of iron deficiency on laboratory testing who have symptoms of hyperviscosity, including headache, dizziness, visual disturbance, myalgia, and bleeding diathesis. Quantitative volume replacement is necessary during phlebotomy.

Attempted surgical correction of a congenital cardiac shunt after Eisenmenger syndrome is present usually results in the death of the patient.[35] Many patients ultimately die of right-sided heart failure, pulmonary hypertension, or pulmonary hemorrhage.[36]

The woman with Eisenmenger syndrome must be informed that pregnancy carries a mortality risk of about 50%.[37] Even if the mother survives, the outcome for the fetus is likely to be poor, because the fetal mortality rate exceeds 50% in cyanotic women with Eisenmenger syndrome.[36] Sudden death may occur at any time, but labor, delivery, and particularly the early puerperium seem to be the most dangerous periods.[38] Any significant fall in venous return, regardless of cause, impairs the ability of the right heart to pump blood through the high, fixed pulmonary vascular resistance. Hypotension and shock can occur quickly and are often unresponsive to medical therapy.

The major physiologic difficulty in pulmonary hypertension is maintenance of adequate pulmonary blood flow. Any event or condition that decreases venous return, such as vasodilation on the systemic side of the circulation from epidural anesthesia or pooling of blood in the lower extremities from vena caval compression, decreases preload to the right ventricle and pulmonary blood flow. Therefore, management during pregnancy centers on the maintenance of pulmonary blood flow. If the patient insists on continuing her pregnancy, limitation of physical activity is essential, as is the use of pressure-graded elastic support hose, low-flow home oxygen therapy, and monthly monitoring of blood and platelet counts. Because of the precarious physiologic balance, a planned delivery should be performed with intensive care monitoring, including a Swan-Ganz catheter and provisions for skilled obstetric anesthesia care. Anesthetic considerations for this entity are discussed in Chapter 56.

On a more optimistic note, a report published in 1995 described 13 pregnancies in 12 women with Eisenmenger syndrome who elected not to accept advice to terminate pregnancy.[39] Mean systolic pulmonary arterial pressure was 113 mm Hg. Three spontaneous abortions, one premature labor, and two maternal deaths occurred. The seven patients who reached the end of the second trimester were hospitalized until term, treated with oxygen and heparin, and delivered by cesarean section. One patient died a month after delivery. Most of the infants were small, and one died. Despite this better-than-average outcome, pregnancy should not be encouraged in women with Eisenmenger syndrome or in those with a systemic level of pulmonary hypertension of any cause.

Primary Pulmonary Hypertension

Severe idiopathic ("primary") pulmonary hypertension, like the Eisenmenger syndrome, carries a high risk in pregnancy, and the same principles apply to its management. Pregnancy is not advised in women with this condition, because the mortality rate approaches 50%.[40]

Severe pulmonary hypertension can result from taking appetite-suppressing drugs. The fenfluramine-phentermine regimen ("fen-phen") was a notorious culprit[41] and was withdrawn from the market. Treatment strategies include vasodilators, sometimes by chronic intravenous infusion, and nitric oxide inhalation. In some 25% of cases, pulmonary arterial pressure is lowered by prostacyclin infusion.[42] This response predicts a favorable response to chronic oral nifedipine administration and a good prognosis. Balloon atrial septostomy,[43,44] through the foramen ovale or via transseptal puncture, can be used, in extreme cases of pulmonary hypertension, to relieve right heart pressure, usually as a bridge to transplantation.

Congenital Obstructive Lesions

Some congenital cardiac malformations are characterized by obstruction to left or right ventricular outflow. The more common examples include pulmonary stenosis, aortic stenosis, and coarctation of the aorta. The hypoplastic left heart syndrome seldom allows survival to childbearing age, and those who do survive usually have undergone a major palliative procedure, such as construction of a ventriculoaortic conduit with a prosthetic valve, that would constitute a strong contraindication to pregnancy.

Mitral Stenosis

Congenital mitral stenosis is a rare malformation. When it is associated with an ASD, it constitutes the Lutembacher syndrome. Survival to childbearing age is usual. Both lesions tend to promote atrial fibrillation. Ideally, the mitral valve and the atrial defect should be repaired before pregnancy.

Aortic Stenosis

(see also the later section on aortic stenosis under Aortic Valve Disease)

Bicuspid aortic valve is one of the more common congenital malformations that may lead to aortic stenosis, regurgitation, or both (Fig. 39-5). Often, aortic stenosis is not present during early life but progresses over time because of valve calcification and gradual restriction in leaflet motion. The bicuspid valve may occur as an isolated defect or in combination with other congenital anomalies, most commonly aortic coarctation. Congenital aortic stenosis, on the other hand, can be severe at birth and may cause severe left ventricular hypertrophy

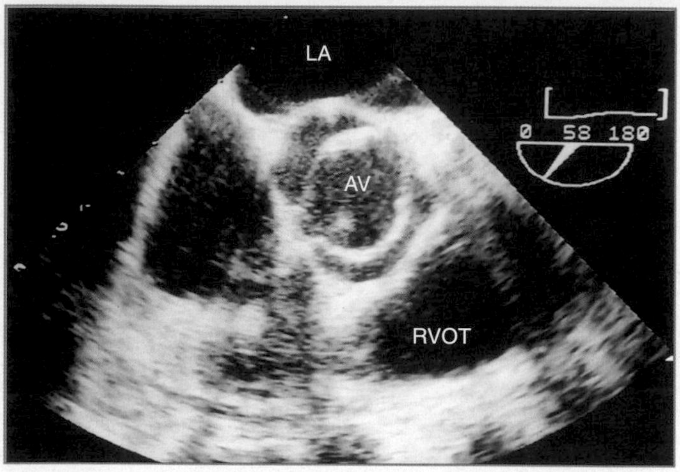

FIGURE 39-5 **Transesophageal echocardiographic image of a bicuspid aortic valve.** During systole, only two aortic valve (AV) leaflets are seen. LA, left atrium; RVOT, right ventricular outflow tract.

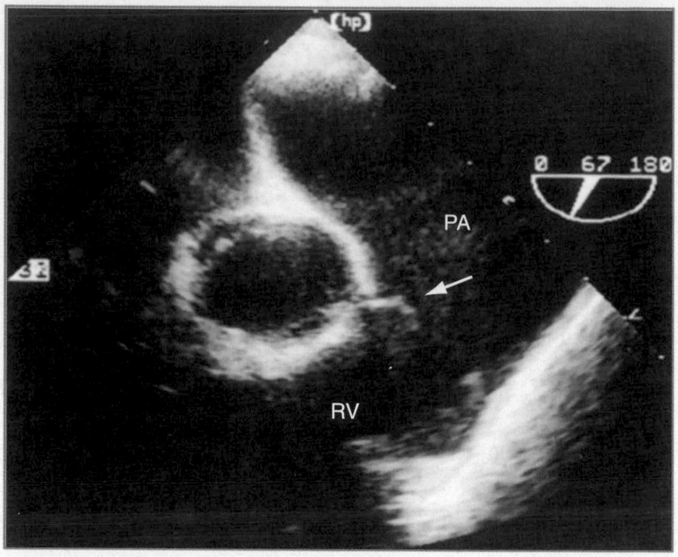

FIGURE 39-6 **Transesophageal echocardiographic image of pulmonic stenosis.** The pulmonic valve leaflets exhibit characteristic doming *(arrow)*. PA, pulmonary artery; RV, right ventricle.

that limits the ability of the heart to respond to demands for increased cardiac output.

In the syndrome of severe congenital aortic stenosis, the pulses are of slow upstroke and diminished amplitude. Unlike adults with acquired aortic stenosis, children and young adults with congenital aortic stenosis have an abnormally loud aortic valve closure sound. Left ventricular ejection is prolonged, so that the aortic valve closure sound may occur after the pulmonary valve closure sound. Therefore, splitting of the second heart sound is paradoxical and is heard in expiration instead of inspiration. Often a loud ejection sound is heard in early systole. The duration of the ejection murmur and the time to its peak intensity increase with worsening severity of aortic stenosis.

The ECG shows severe left ventricular hypertrophy. The chest radiograph is characterized by poststenotic dilatation of the aorta. Although some patients complain of dyspnea, chest pain, and syncope, others remain asymptomatic. The lesion can be recognized and its severity assessed by Doppler echocardiography.

Critical calcific aortic stenosis is usually treated by aortic valve replacement in older patients, but aortic valve repair is often possible in younger women of childbearing age with congenital aortic stenosis. If aortic stenosis is severe—and especially if it is symptomatic—the woman should be advised against becoming pregnant. She should be advised that, if the aortic valve must be replaced, pregnancy and labor would be difficult and dangerous because of the need for anticoagulant treatment after a mechanical prosthesis is implanted. Maternal mortality rates as high as 17% have been reported,[45] although more recent data have suggested a somewhat lower risk. However, these studies also emphasize the adverse effects of severe maternal aortic stenosis on fetal outcomes, including increased rates of preterm delivery and intrauterine growth restriction.[46] If aortic stenosis is moderate in severity, the patient should be advised to complete her pregnancies before the aortic valve is replaced. Labor can be managed in such cases without a high maternal or fetal risk, but assisted shortening of the second stage of labor is recommended.[47]

Strict limits on physical exertion and prolonged periods of bed rest may be required. Left ventricular failure may appear and may necessitate the use of diuretic agents and digitalis. Rarely, even in the presence of severe aortic stenosis, heart failure may be due to another cause (e.g., peripartum cardiomyopathy).[48] Prophylaxis against bacterial endocarditis at delivery is recommended.

Vasodilators, helpful in patients with heart failure of other etiology, are dangerous in patients with aortic stenosis, because the impeded left ventricle may not be able to fill the dilated peripheral vascular bed. It should be remembered that the lowered systemic vascular resistance of pregnancy adversely affects aortic stenosis. The obstructed left ventricle is limited in its ability to fill the dilated peripheral bed, a situation that can lead to syncope or more serious manifestations of limited, relatively fixed cardiac output.

Pulmonic Stenosis

The murmur of pulmonic stenosis is loud and is often accompanied by a thrill. The lesion is usually detected in early childhood and is likely to have been corrected before the childbearing age. Expectant mothers who have not had adequate health supervision in childhood may have unrecognized pulmonary stenosis.

The diagnosis is suggested by a long, harsh systolic murmur over the upper left sternal border that is usually preceded by an ejection sound. The venous pressure is normal, but there are striking a waves in the jugular venous pulse. The pulmonary valve closure sound is usually too soft to hear when pulmonary stenosis is severe. Severe pulmonary stenosis causes massive concentric right ventricular hypertrophy; this is manifested by a left parasternal heave and by tall R waves and deeply inverted T waves in the right precordial leads of the ECG. Tall, pointed P waves are also present, denoting right atrial enlargement.

Right ventricular enlargement and poststenotic dilatation of the main and left pulmonary arteries are seen on the chest radiograph, which also may show slightly diminished peripheral pulmonary vasculature. Echocardiography demonstrates limited opening of the pulmonic valve leaflets (Fig. 39-6), right ventricular hypertrophy, and abnormally high velocity of blood flow in the pulmonary artery. Doppler echocardiography also allows calculation of the right ventricular pressure and the systolic pressure gradient across the valve. These pressures can also be measured directly in the hemodynamics laboratory (Fig. 39-7).

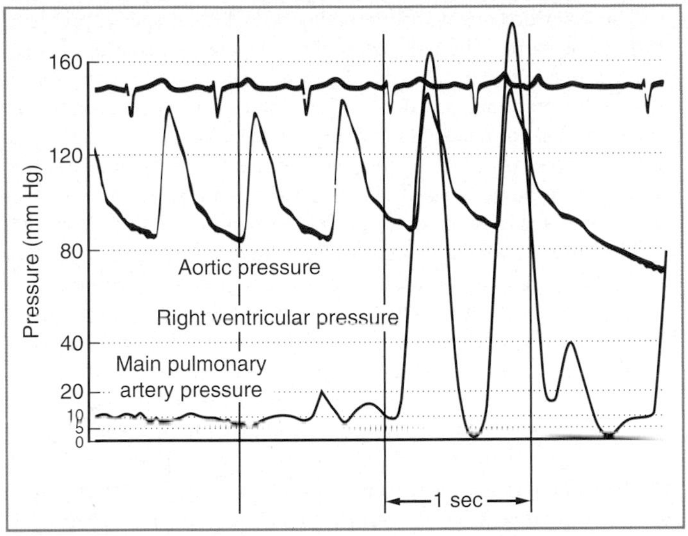

FIGURE 39-7 Pressure tracings in severe pulmonary stenosis. Pulmonary pressure is extremely low and appears damped. Right ventricular pressure is suprasystemic. (From Shabetai R, Adolph RJ: Principles of cardiac catheterization. In Fowler NO [ed]: Cardiac Diagnosis and Treatment. Hagerstown, MD: Harper & Row, 1980, p 106.)

Pulmonic stenosis is generally well tolerated so that neither pregnancy nor labor poses a significant threat.[49] Prophylaxis against infective endocarditis is necessary. More severe pulmonary stenosis requires treatment. Unlike aortic stenosis, however, critical pulmonary stenosis does not require valve replacement or open repair. Most cases are treated successfully with transvenous balloon valvuloplasty.[50] Ideally, this should be carried out before pregnancy is undertaken; if a woman does become pregnant and develops intractable right-sided heart failure, the procedure can still be safely performed (but at some risk to the fetus). Extreme pulmonary stenosis (right ventricular systolic pressure > systemic systolic pressure) is a contraindication to pregnancy until the lesion is adequately treated.

Right-to-Left Shunt without Pulmonary Hypertension (Tetralogy of Fallot)

The congenital cyanotic heart diseases discussed so far have been associated with a communication between the pulmonary and systemic circulations and pulmonary vascular resistance sufficiently high to cause a right-to-left shunt. However, cyanosis occurs in other congenital malformations, in which there is a defect between the right and left sides of the heart but also right ventricular outflow obstruction (Figs. 39-8 and 39-9). Examples include the tetralogy of Fallot and tricuspid atresia.

Tetralogy of Fallot is used to illustrate this class of congenital malformation of the heart, because it is by far the most common form of cyanotic congenital heart disease encountered in pregnancy. Moreover, the offspring of a mother with tetralogy of Fallot has a 2% to 13% chance of inheriting the condition.[51] The syndrome includes (1) a large defect high in the ventricular septum; (2) pulmonary stenosis, which may be at the valve itself but more commonly is in the infundibulum of the right ventricle; (3) dextroposition of the aorta so that the aortic orifice sits astride the VSD and overrides, at least in part, the right ventricle; and (4) right ventricular hypertrophy (Fig. 39-10).

A wide spectrum of clinical presentations may be present, depending on the relative size of the VSD and the degree of right ventricular

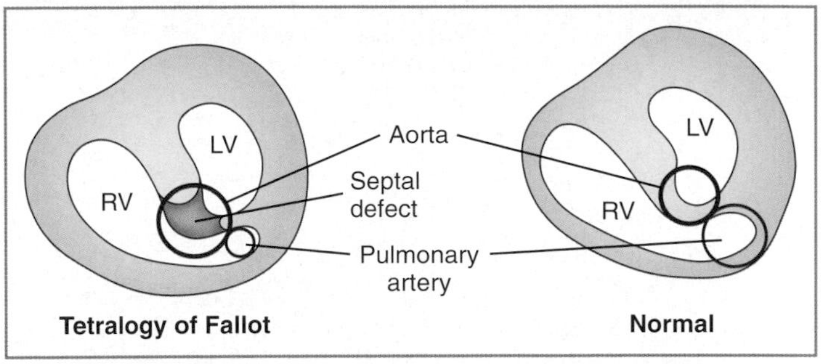

FIGURE 39-8 Tetralogy of Fallot. The anatomic pathology *(left)* compared with normal *(right)*. Note the ventricular septal defect, the aorta (which overrides the defect), the pulmonary stenosis, and the right ventricular hypertrophy. LV, left ventricle; RV, right ventricle. (Reprinted by permission of the publisher. From Taussig HB: Congenital Malformations of the Heart. Cambridge, Mass, Harvard University Press, 1960. Copyright © 1960 by the Commonwealth Fund of the President and Fellows of Harvard College.)

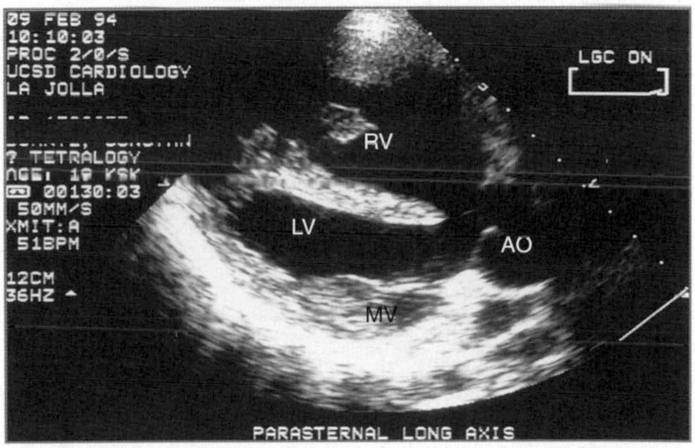

FIGURE 39-9 Transthoracic echocardiographic image of tetralogy of Fallot. A large ventricular septal defect is present, and the aorta (AO) overrides the interventricular septum. LV, left ventricle; MV, mitral valve; RV, right ventricle.

outflow obstruction that diverts blood flow through the VSD. In the typical case, right and left ventricular systolic pressures are equal but the pulmonary artery pressure is exceedingly low. A loud, long systolic murmur is audible along the left sternal border. The murmur is caused by an abnormal flow pattern through the obstructed right ventricular outflow tract. The pulmonary valve closure sound is usually inaudible. Patients are usually cyanotic and often have significant clubbing of the fingers and toes. The hematocrit value is greatly elevated because of the severe erythrocytosis. Phlebotomy is not indicated to treat the hematocrit level per se but is indicated if symptoms of hyperviscosity occur. Ignoring this important therapeutic principle leads to a microcytic anemia that further complicates pregnancy. The ECG shows severe right ventricular hypertrophy. The chest radiograph is characterized by a normal-sized heart and a concavity in the region where the pulmonary artery should be (Fig. 39-11). As in all malformations of this general type, the lung fields are oligemic, showing small vessels throughout.

Most adults born with the tetralogy of Fallot and lesions with similar pathophysiology have undergone surgical treatment before reaching young adulthood. Children raised in undeveloped countries are an important exception. Many patients have had surgery to close

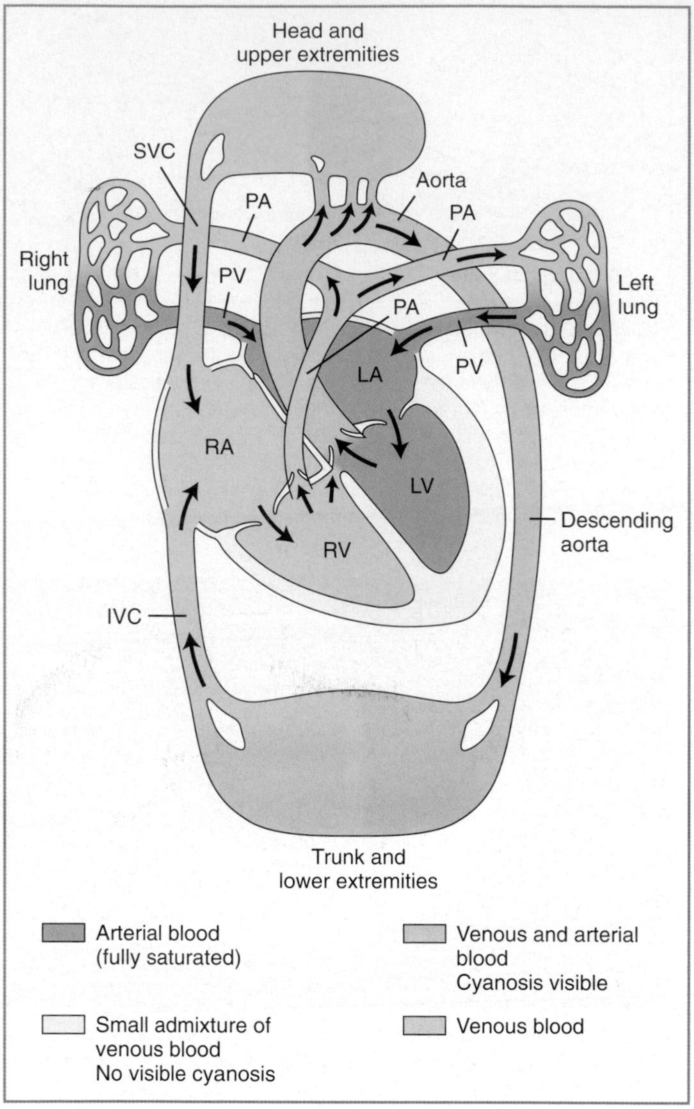

FIGURE 39-10 Tetralogy of Fallot. Blood shunts from left to right through the ventricular septal defect because its flow to the lungs is impeded by pulmonary stenosis; this results in cyanosis. IVC, inferior vena cava; LA, left atrium; LV, left ventricle; PA, pulmonary artery; PV, pulmonary vein; RA, right atrium; RV, right ventricle; SVC, superior vena cava. (Reprinted by permission of the publisher. From Taussig HB: Congenital Malformations of the Heart. Cambridge, Mass, Harvard University Press, 1960. Copyright © 1960 by the Commonwealth Fund by the President and Fellows of Harvard College.)

the VSD and relieve the pulmonary stenosis, constituting virtual "total repair" and rendering them potentially safe candidates for pregnancy and delivery. However, the operation is not curative. Significant arrhythmia and conduction defects that may eventually lead to the need for electronic cardiac pacing or an implantable defibrillator may occur years after an apparently successful operation. Other sequelae and residua include only partial relief of the right ventricular outflow obstruction and pulmonic regurgitation. This latter problem is usually well tolerated early but may lead to right-sided heart failure, necessitating reoperation. In addition, women with repaired tetralogy of Fallot and significant pulmonic regurgitation have a higher risk of decompensation during pregnancy.[52]

The cyanotic patient with tetralogy of Fallot has special problems during pregnancy. The reduced systemic vascular resistance of pregnancy causes more blood to shunt from right to left, leaving less to flow to the pulmonary circulation. This intensifies hypoxemia and can lead to syncope or death. Maintenance of venous return is crucial. The most dangerous times for these women are late pregnancy and the early puerperium, because venous return is impeded by the large gravid uterus near term and by peripheral venous pooling after delivery. Pressure-graded elastic support hose are recommended. Blood loss during labor may compromise venous return, and blood volume must be promptly and adequately restored. Anesthetic considerations during delivery are discussed in detail in Chapter 56. Antibiotic prophylaxis should be used in these susceptible patients at delivery.

Because of the combined high maternal risk and high incidence of fetal loss, pregnancy is discouraged in women with uncorrected tetralogy of Fallot. The prognosis is particularly bleak in those women with a history of repeated syncopal episodes, a hematocrit level greater than 60%, or a right ventricular systolic pressure greater than 120 mm Hg. If a young woman with untreated tetralogy of Fallot requests prepregnancy counseling, she should be advised to undergo surgical correction before pregnancy. Pregnancy does not represent a significantly increased risk for patients in whom the VSD has been patched and the pulmonary stenosis corrected.

Coarctation of the Aorta

Coarctation of the aorta is a congenital defect in the area of the aorta where the ligamentum arteriosum and the left subclavian artery insert (the distal portion of the aortic arch). The malformation may be simple or complex, and it is either isolated or associated with PDA and other malformations, notably aortic stenosis and aortic regurgitation secondary to a bicuspid aortic valve. It may also occur in women with Turner syndrome. The lesion should be detected and treated surgically or by balloon dilation in infancy or childhood, but it may be present in women who are, or want to become, pregnant.

Typical features include the following:

- Upper extremity hypertension but lower extremity hypotension
- Visible and palpable collateral arteries in the scapular area
- A late systolic murmur, usually loudest over the interscapular region
- Femoral pulses that lag behind the carotid pulses and are of diminished amplitude
- Notching of the inferior rib borders seen on the chest radiograph and resulting from erosion by arterial collaterals that bridge the coarctation

Electrocardiographic evidence of severe left ventricular hypertrophy strongly suggests associated aortic stenosis. Surgical grafting or percutaneous intravascular balloon dilation reduces the upper extremity hypertension, but blood pressure does not always return to normal, and hypertension may recur in later life.

Whenever possible, the operation should be performed before pregnancy; otherwise, the maternal mortality rate is approximately 3%. Coarctation is associated with congenital berry aneurysm of the circle of Willis and hemorrhagic stroke. The risk of stroke may increase during labor because of transient elevations in blood pressure. Patients are at risk for aortic dissection and infective endocarditis involving an abnormal aortic valve; these risks increase during pregnancy.[53] Hypertension often worsens as well.[54] Coarctation is also associated with an increased frequency of preeclampsia.[31] The operation does not

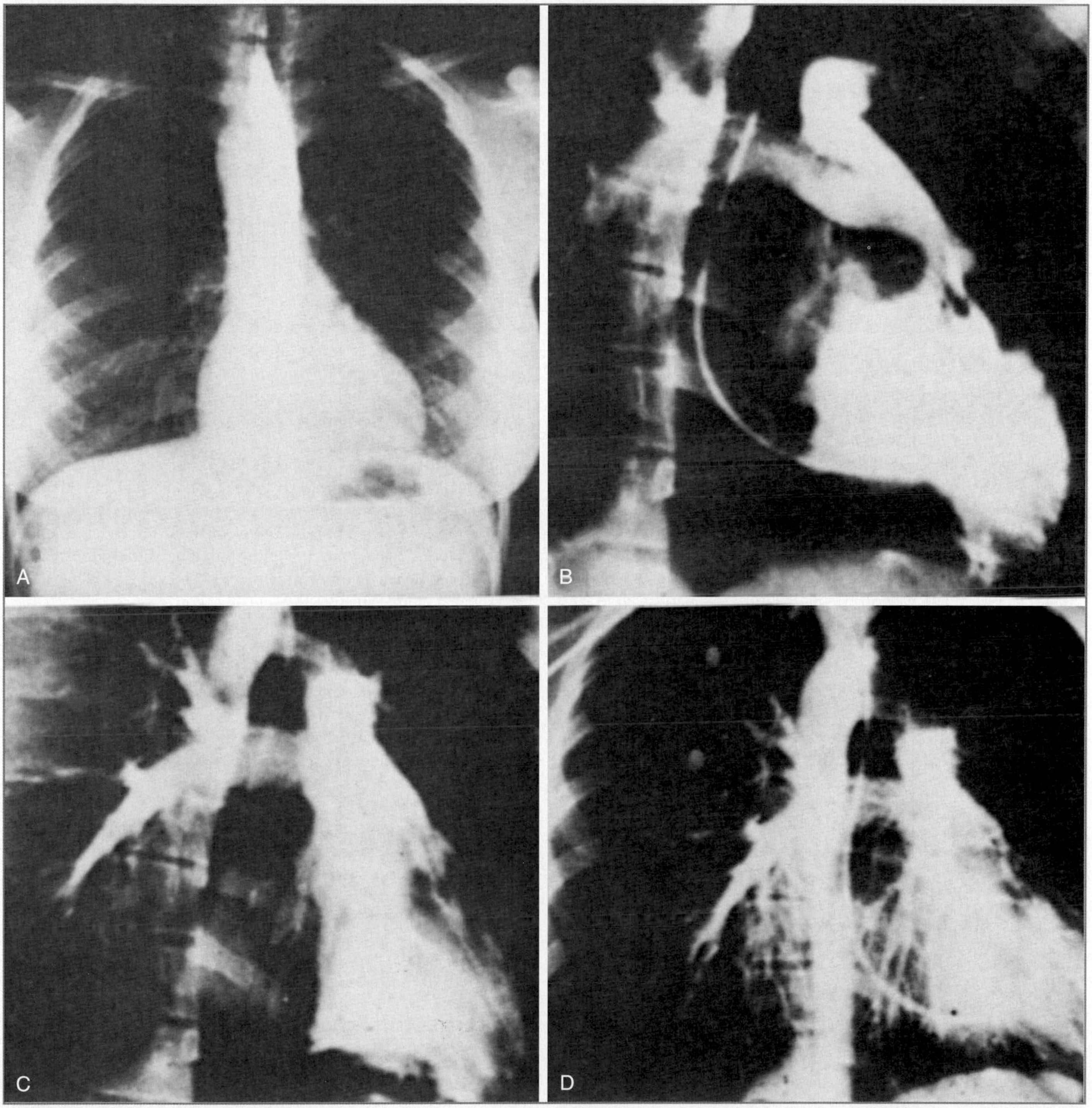

FIGURE 39-11 Tetralogy of Fallot. **A,** Chest radiograph. Note concavity in the area of the pulmonary artery, oligemic lungs, and right aortic arch. **B,** Right ventriculogram. Note the narrow right ventricular outflow tract. **C,** Further clarification of the pulmonary arteries. The left ventricle is slightly opacified via the ventricular septal defect. **D,** The associated right-sided aortic arch is now visible. (From Shabetai R, Adolph RJ: Principles of cardiac catheterization. In Fowler NO [ed]: Cardiac Diagnosis and Treatment. Hagerstown, MD: Harper & Row, 1980, p 106.)

require cardiopulmonary bypass and can be carried out with safety for the mother and with less fetal risk than accompanies open heart surgery with cardiopulmonary bypass. Although transvascular balloon dilation of aortic coarctation is a viable option for children and infants with coarctation, its use in adults is controversial.[55] The procedure is well accepted for treatment of postsurgical renarrowing of the coarctation, but de novo balloon angioplasty carries a risk of aortic dissection and rupture. A number of centers are now performing balloon dilation with stent implantation for adults with unoperated aortic coarctation, but large, multicenter studies are currently not available.[56]

If delivery must be undertaken in cases of unoperated coarctation, blood pressure can be titrated with β-adrenergic–blocking agents delivered by intravenous drip.

Other Congenital Cardiac Malformations

Ebstein Anomaly

Ebstein anomaly is a malformation of the tricuspid valve in which the septal leaflet is displaced apically and the anterior leaflet is abnormally large in size. The deformed tricuspid valve apparatus may be significantly incompetent or stenotic, depending on the location of the anomalously placed cusps of the valve. In some cases, the malformation causes impediment to right ventricular outflow.

The clinical features are easily recognized by a cardiologist, and the echocardiogram is characteristic and reliable (Fig. 39-12). This syndrome is frequently associated with anomalous atrioventricular conduction pathways and with the Wolff-Parkinson-White syndrome. Patients may also have an ASD with right-to-left shunting and cyanosis. Supraventricular arrhythmias are also common.

The most favored treatment is reconstruction of the tricuspid valve, for which satisfactory techniques have now been developed. The operation should be performed before pregnancy is undertaken. Interruption of anomalous conduction pathways also can be performed during surgery.

The Mayo Clinic group[57] reported on 111 pregnancies in 44 women with Ebstein anomaly resulting in 95 live births, although most of the infants had low birth weight. Vaginal delivery was performed in 89% and cesarean section in 9%; 23 deliveries were premature. Nineteen pregnancies ended with spontaneous abortion, and seven ended with therapeutic abortion. Congenital heart disease occurred in 6% of the children of mothers with Ebstein anomaly.

Congenital Atrioventricular Block

Congenital atrioventricular block differs somewhat from heart block in adults. The pacemaker is usually junctional, and therefore the QRS complex is normal or only slightly widened and the ventricular rate is more rapid than in acquired complete atrioventricular block. Although these patients appear to do well during childhood and young adulthood, the lesion is associated with an unexpectedly high mortality rate. Therefore, treatment with a pacemaker is indicated in many of the cases.[58] The pacemaker used should be dual-chamber and rate-responsive, so that normal cardiovascular dynamics at rest and exercise will be preserved. Patients who are untreated or who have received a pacemaker are at slight to no increased risk during pregnancy.

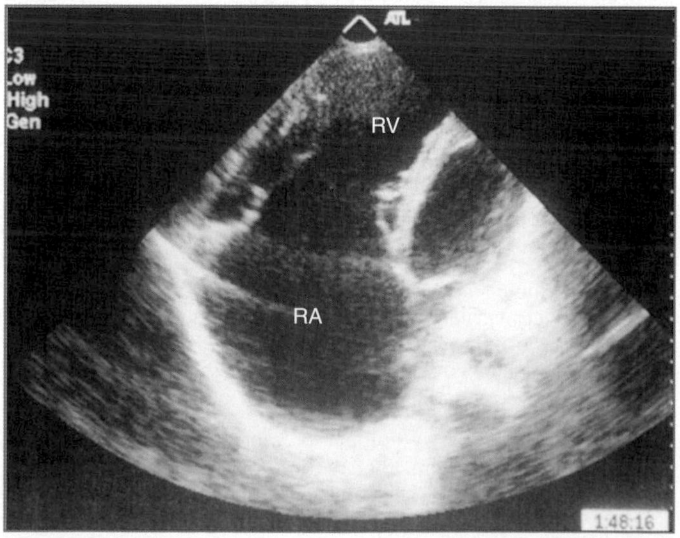

FIGURE 39-12 Ebstein anomaly. The right atrium (RA) and right ventricle (RV) are markedly dilated, and the tricuspid valve is displaced toward the cardiac apex.

Additional Malformations

A number of other malformations may be present in women of childbearing age, including

- Other left-to-right or right-to-left shunts
- Transposition of the great vessels
- Truncus arteriosus
- Single-ventricle double-outlet right ventricle
- Various obstructive lesions

The malformations may be multiple and complex. Survival to adulthood depends on at least partial correction, which may have been furnished by surgical operation or may be part of the malformation. For example, in D-type transposition of the great vessels, the aorta arises from the right ventricle and the pulmonary artery from the left. Survival requires a shunt at some level (ASD, VSD, or PDA) so that oxygenated blood can enter the systemic circulation.

Some of these women with untreated and delicately balanced lesions bear children, but usually this is not wise to attempt. Transposition of the great vessels is now treated by anastomosis of the aorta to the morphologic left ventricle and of the pulmonary artery to the morphologic right ventricle. Lesions such as single ventricle may be palliated by the Fontan procedure, in which venous return is connected directly to the pulmonary circulation, bypassing the right side of the heart. Neither procedure constitutes a cure, but successful pregnancy can occur.

In summary, patients should be evaluated and tracked by a cardiologist who is experienced in congenital heart disease and by a maternal-fetal medicine specialist with knowledge and experience in managing pregnancy in women with congenital cardiac lesions.[7,31]

Rheumatic Heart Disease

Rheumatic Fever

Rheumatic fever is now distinctly uncommon in the United States, Canada, Western Europe, and Great Britain, but it is still prevalent in less economically developed countries. Young female immigrants to the Western world constitute a large proportion of the patients with a history of rheumatic fever. These women are at risk of developing rheumatic valvular heart disease 10 to 20 years after the initial episode of rheumatic fever.

Chronic Rheumatic Heart Disease

In the United States, acute rheumatic fever with carditis has been uncommon for many years, and chronic rheumatic heart disease, which manifests years to decades after the episode of acute rheumatic fever, is becoming uncommon among the native childbearing population. Control of rheumatic fever has largely shifted the burden of

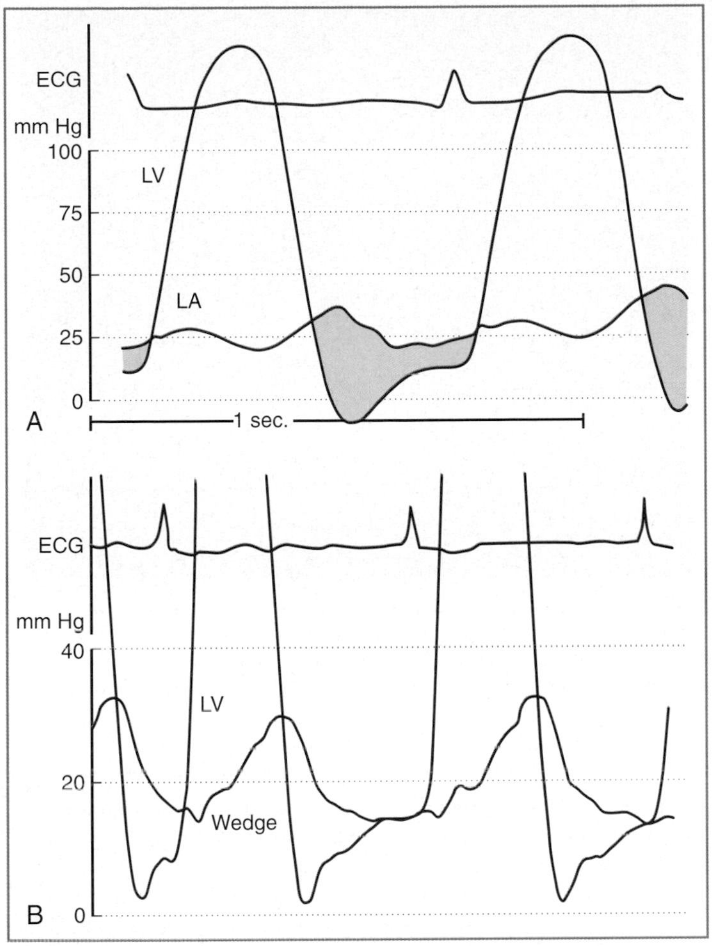

FIGURE 39-13 Hemodynamics of mitral valve disease. **A,** Mitral stenosis. The diastolic pressure gradient *(shaded area)* between the left atrium (LA) and left ventricle (LV) persists to end-diastole. **B,** Mitral regurgitation. Note the large systolic pressure wave of the pulmonary wedge pressure tracing. The diastolic pressure gradient is limited to early diastole. ECG, electrocardiogram.

rheumatic heart disease from teenagers to women in the third and fourth decades of life.

The characteristic lesion of rheumatic heart disease is mitral stenosis, and the next most common manifestation is the combination of mitral stenosis with aortic regurgitation. The mitral valve may become both stenotic and incompetent, and the valve may calcify. Pure mitral regurgitation is almost always nonrheumatic, except in young people with acute carditis. Similarly, aortic valve disease without mitral involvement is seldom rheumatic. Tricuspid regurgitation is a late secondary manifestation that occurs secondary to pulmonary hypertension and right ventricular enlargement.

Mitral Stenosis

The principal features are enlargement of the left atrium and right ventricle, a diastolic murmur at the cardiac apex, and pulmonary hypertension. Inflow to the left ventricle is impeded by the narrowed valve and can be accomplished only by an increased level of pressure in the left atrium (Figs. 39-13 and 39-14). The faster the heart rate, the less time in diastole, and the less time for ventricular filling. Left atrial pressure therefore is further elevated by tachycardia. Atrial fibrillation

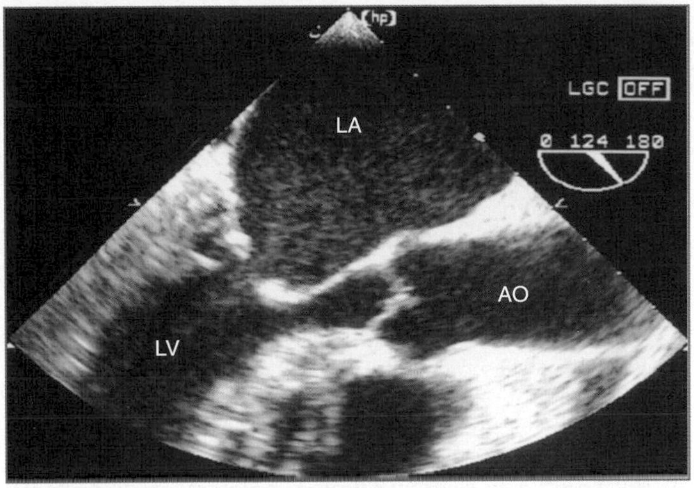

FIGURE 39-14 Transesophageal echocardiographic image of mitral stenosis. During diastole, opening of the mitral valve is restricted by scarring and fusion of the leaflet tips. Characteristic doming of the leaflet is also present. AO, aorta; LA, left atrium; LV, left ventricle.

eventually supervenes, causing a fall in cardiac output and escalation of left atrial hypertension, especially if the ventricular rate is not controlled. Atrial fibrillation substantially increases the probability of thrombus in the left atrial appendage and the threat of a subsequent embolic stroke.

Effect of Pregnancy

Pregnancy drastically stresses the circulation in women with severe mitral stenosis. The increased blood volume, heart rate, and cardiac output raise left atrial pressure to a level that causes severe pulmonary congestion, leading to progressive exertional dyspnea, orthopnea, paroxysmal nocturnal dyspnea, and pulmonary edema. Women who have not been receiving antenatal care often present initially with severe pulmonary edema during pregnancy. In long-standing cases, severe right-sided heart failure develops. Infective endocarditis, pulmonary embolism, and massive hemoptysis may also occur. The maternal risk for death is highest in the third trimester and in the puerperium.[10,11]

Significant Mitral Stenosis without Heart Failure

Patients who have mitral stenosis without heart failure should be advised to undergo percutaneous balloon mitral valvuloplasty and to postpone pregnancy until after full recovery from the procedure. If they do not follow this advice and do become pregnant, one reasonable course in the first trimester may be pregnancy termination, followed by mitral valve operation and subsequent pregnancy planning. If this is not acceptable, the patient can be advised to remain under frequent close supervision by the cardiologist and obstetrician and to accept long periods of rest, prohibition of strenuous activity, salt restriction, and diuretic treatment. If this type of regimen is followed closely and is expertly supervised, maternal mortality is low.[10,11] Atrial fibrillation signals the need for digitalis, a β-adrenergic blocking agent, or a calcium channel blocking agent to maintain a normal heart rate. More than one of these drugs may be needed to achieve the desired result without side effects. For patients with atrial fibrillation and significant mitral stenosis, anticoagulant treatment is recommended.

Depending on her course, the woman may have to spend many weeks in bed and should be admitted to the hospital well in advance of labor. The supine posture should be avoided as much as possible, and delivery in the left lateral decubitus position is desirable. The lithotomy position, with the patient on her back and her feet elevated in stirrups, is an invitation to pulmonary edema. The crisis of pulmonary edema may appear despite good management. Sedation (to drop the heart rate and promote cardiac filling and output) and diuretic treatment must then be followed by prompt delivery if the fetus is viable.

Percutaneous balloon valvuloplasty is a nonsurgical means to dilate mitral stenosis and is the current treatment of choice for most patients with symptomatic mitral stenosis.[59,60] The procedure can be done during pregnancy if heart failure is severe, and it appears to be safer for the fetus than open mitral commissurotomy.[61] Lead shielding should be used, because fluoroscopy is required to guide the balloon into the mitral orifice. Balloon valvuloplasty should be used with caution during pregnancy, and it should be reserved for women who are unresponsive to aggressive medical therapy.[10,11] If possible, the procedure should be put off at least until after the first trimester. Patients with confirmed mitral stenosis and right-sided heart failure with severe pulmonary congestion should avoid pregnancy until after the valvular disease is corrected, because the risk of maternal mortality is high.

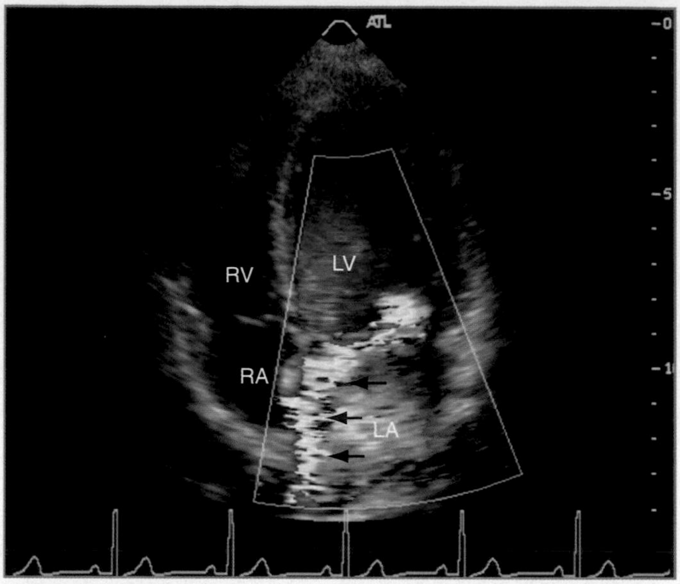

FIGURE 39-15 Transthoracic echocardiographic image of severe mitral regurgitation. During systole, the mitral valve does not coapt properly, and an eccentric jet of mitral regurgitation is present *(arrows).* LA, left atrium; LV, left ventricle; RA, right atrium; RV, right ventricle.

Mitral Valve Prolapse

In the past, a degree of prolapse of the mitral valve was considered so prevalent in the general population,[62] particularly among young women, that authorities differed as to whether mitral valve prolapse (MVP) should be considered a normal variant or abnormal. More exacting echocardiographic criteria have yielded more realistic and much lower estimates of the prevalence of MVP (perhaps 1% of the female population).[63]

True MVP occurs because portions of the mitral valve apparatus are redundant and, therefore, the leaflets balloon into the left atrium during systole. The leaflets may remain coapted during systole, or they may separate, causing a variable degree of mitral regurgitation. More severe prolapse may be caused by myxomatous degeneration of the mitral leaflets. These abnormalities of connective tissue may be isolated to the mitral valve, or they may be a part of Marfan syndrome (see later discussion). MVP (and sometimes tricuspid valve prolapse) may be associated with congenital malformations, notably ASD.

Mitral regurgitation may be absent, intermittent, or permanent and may be of any degree of severity. Severe mitral regurgitation greatly enlarges the left atrium (Fig. 39-15) and ventricle and eventually leads to left ventricular failure and pulmonary hypertension, the latter less severe than with mitral stenosis.

Past reports have associated MVP with a number of disorders, including stroke, dysautonomia, panic attacks, anxiety, and transient ischemic attacks,[64,65] but more recent studies[66,67] have discounted almost all of these associations. The syndrome of myxomatous mitral valve degeneration with prolapse and mitral regurgitation is quite uncommon, and many women who were diagnosed with MVP more than 10 years ago do not have any actual pathology. For this reason, it may be prudent to order an echocardiogram for any woman who was diagnosed with MVP a number of years ago if she has no symptoms or signs of mitral regurgitation. This may prevent needless and repeated exposure to antibiotics (e.g., before dental procedures).

Some women with MVP complain of chest pain, which can be suggestive of angina pectoris. Although the coronary arteriogram is normal, T-wave inversions, especially in leads II, III, and aVF, are found in a small proportion, and the treadmill exercise test may induce ST-segment depression, indistinguishable from ischemia.[68]

In most cases, the diagnosis of MVP is made by the physician providing pre-conception counseling and antenatal care. The examination reveals a systolic click occurring between the first and second heart sounds. The click may or may not be followed by a midsystolic or late systolic murmur. The click and murmur vary with the patient's posture and hydration status. In most patients, no other abnormality is found on clinical examination. Unless significant mitral regurgitation is present, the patient should be told that pregnancy, labor, and delivery will be safe and unaffected by the prolapse.

Patients with MVP and significant mitral regurgitation are far fewer in number than those with simple prolapse. The murmur is louder, longer, and may become pansystolic. Clinical and laboratory evidence of enlargement of the left atrium and ventricle increases with increasing severity and duration of regurgitation. Even modest impairment of left ventricular function, especially if it is progressive, indicates that pregnancy may well precipitate heart failure and cannot be lightly undertaken. More obvious left ventricular dysfunction (e.g., EF < 40%) indicates that the woman should be strongly advised to avoid pregnancy. She should then be referred for complete cardiologic evaluation[2] and surgery to address the mitral regurgitation. In most cases of MVP, the valve can be repaired rather than replaced. It is important to appreciate that left ventricular function deteriorates after mitral valve replacement but may improve after mitral valve repair.[69] Thereafter, if the result is good and ventricular function is significantly improved, pregnancy may be undertaken successfully.

Chest pain and arrhythmias are best managed with β-adrenergic blockers such as atenolol or metoprolol. If symptoms are unusually pronounced, thyroid function tests should be checked as well. Because the gravid uterus and vasodilation may add to postural hypotension, the patient should be informed that she may experience lightheadedness, dizziness, or fainting with prolonged standing during pregnancy.

Mitral Regurgitation Not Caused by Prolapse

In younger women, mitral regurgitation may be a result of rheumatic or congenital disease. In older women, mitral regurgitation is more often a manifestation of hypertension, ischemia, idiopathic myocardial disease, or infective endocarditis.

Most of the information regarding mitral regurgitation in prolapse also applies here. In older women, the valve is more likely to be calcified; fewer of the valves are amenable to repair and must be replaced. The problems posed by prosthetic valves in pregnant women are discussed later in this chapter; the hemodynamics are illustrated in Figure 39-13, and echocardiography is illustrated in Figure 39-15.

In patients with far-advanced left ventricular dysfunction or failure who have severe mitral regurgitation, it can be difficult to determine which is the cause and which the result. In either case, the patient with a greatly enlarged and hypokinetic ventricle must be advised against becoming pregnant. Most of the pregnancy would be spent in bed, the course would be punctuated by episodes of uncompensated congestive heart failure (any of which could prove fatal or require therapeutic abortion), and the risk to the fetus would exceed 50%.

Pregnancy in patients with mild or moderate mitral regurgitation can be managed safely with a conservative regimen of reduced physical activity, salt restriction, and low doses of a diuretic agent. Low-dose digoxin may be helpful if atrial fibrillation supervenes. As mentioned previously, severe mitral regurgitation indicates a need for repair or replacement of the valve when symptoms and/or early evidence of declining ventricular function appear.[2,70] Clearly, surgical treatment is best undertaken before pregnancy. If the woman is already pregnant, the physician should make every effort to help her to carry the pregnancy to term using strict medical measures. This course is particularly important if clinical, radiologic, and echocardiographic criteria suggest that the valve is irreparable and would require replacement.

Aortic Valve Disease

Aortic Stenosis

(see also the earlier section on aortic stenosis under Congenital Obstructive Lesions)

The etiologic mechanism of aortic stenosis commonly is degeneration, often of a congenitally bicuspid valve. The problem may be encountered in women a decade or more older than those with rheumatic or congenital aortic valve disease. The combination of aortic and mitral stenosis is usually caused by rheumatic heart disease. Critical aortic stenosis leads to severe left ventricular hypertrophy and, eventually, to left ventricular failure. Before overt heart failure develops, syncope or even sudden death may occur.

The characteristic findings include an ejection systolic murmur that is harsher and longer and peaks later than the normal ejection murmur of pregnancy. It is usually loudest at the second right intercostal space. If aortic stenosis is severe, the pulse upstroke is slow, and left ventricular hypertrophy is evident on the ECG. The echocardiogram is a more sensitive and more specific marker of left ventricular hypertrophy. Doppler echocardiographic measurement of blood flow velocity through the aortic valve permits reliable estimation of the systolic pressure drop across the valve, as well as calculation of the valve area. The hemodynamics are illustrated in Figure 39-16. The left ventricle in women remodels differently than in men. The concentric hypertrophy is more pronounced, the cavity is smaller, and systolic function is supranormal.

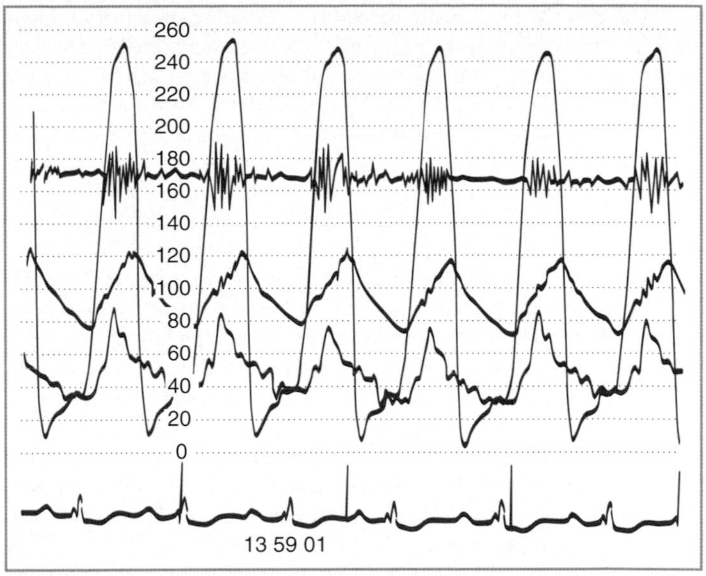

FIGURE 39-16 Hemodynamic data in aortic stenosis. Left ventricular pressure is 250/40 mm Hg (normal, 120/10 mm Hg). Aortic systolic pressure is 130 mm Hg lower than the left ventricular pressure and shows a slow upstroke and vibrations representing the systolic thrill. The record above the aortic pressure tracing is a phonocardiogram showing the systolic murmur. Also shown is the pulmonary wedge pressure (lowest pressure tracing), which is elevated to equal the left ventricular diastolic pressure. The bottom tracing is the electrocardiogram. (From Shabetai R, Adolph RJ: Principles of cardiac catheterization. In Fowler NO [ed]: Cardiac Diagnosis and Treatment. Hagerstown, MD: Harper & Row, 1980, p 106.)

The left ventricle does not dilate until the ventricle fails, and so a dilated ventricle in aortic stenosis is an ominous sign that calls for rapid intervention. In general, aortic valve replacement is preferred to percutaneous balloon aortic valvuloplasty, but open heart surgery presents a high risk to the fetus. For this reason, some have advised balloon aortic valvuloplasty for treatment of aortic stenosis during pregnancy,[71] but valve replacement will almost certainly have to be done soon after delivery.

Hemodynamic monitoring is recommended during labor in patients with moderate to severe aortic stenosis. Vaginal delivery is preferred, with assisted second stage of labor. If cesarean section is performed, some have suggested that general anesthesia is preferred.[72] See Chapter 56 for more details regarding anesthesia management.

Pregnancy in women with a mechanical aortic valve replacement must be undertaken with great caution and meticulous management, because continuous anticoagulation is necessary (see Pregnancy in Patients with Artificial Heart Valves, later).

Aortic Regurgitation

The etiologic mechanism of aortic regurgitation is commonly rheumatic heart disease, in which case mitral stenosis often coexists. Other diseases, such as Marfan syndrome, bicuspid aortic valve, infective endocarditis, and systemic lupus erythematosus, also may cause severe aortic regurgitation. This valvular lesion imposes a volume rather than a pressure overload on the heart and, as such, is usually well tolerated in pregnancy and labor.[15]

The diagnosis is usually based on the finding of a typical, high-pitched, blowing diastolic murmur and can be quantified by Doppler echocardiography. Both pregnancy and aortic regurgitation contribute to hypervolemia and peripheral vasodilatation. A prolonged course without decompensation is characteristic of chronic aortic regurgitation; once heart failure appears, however, the course may progress rapidly downhill.

Traditionally, aortic valve replacement is not recommended until symptoms of heart failure (most notably exertional dyspnea) occur or left ventricular dysfunction/enlargement is seen on echocardiography. Repair of aortic regurgitation is much less successful than repair of mitral regurgitation. For a woman who is contemplating pregnancy, the need for aortic valve replacement constitutes the grounds on which the medical advisor should caution against pregnancy and make the patient fully understand the consequences of choosing otherwise. If left ventricular dysfunction and heart failure are absent, carefully supervised pregnancy is in order, and the woman should be encouraged to complete her family before cardiac dysfunction and the need for valve replacement arise.

In many cases, the cause of aortic regurgitation is unclear. Special care must be taken to rule out aortic aneurysm or dissection, especially if aortic regurgitation is associated with Marfan syndrome or coarctation of the aorta, because these conditions can result in aortic rupture and constitute strong reasons to advise against pregnancy.

Drug-Induced Valvular Heart Disease

A recently recognized cause of deformity and regurgitation of the cardiac valves is ingestion of the drug combination, fenfluramine-phentermine. The revelation of this side effect led to withdrawal of this drug combination from the market in the late 1990s. The mechanism of the effect of these drugs is unclear, and there is evidence that valvular lesions may sometimes gradually improve after discontinuation of the drugs.[73] In some cases, however, valve surgery has been necessary.[74]

Cardiomyopathy

Cardiomyopathy is a disorder of myocardial structure or function. A number of forms exist, and several types that are seen in pregnant women are discussed here.

Dilated Cardiomyopathy

In dilated cardiomyopathy, the cardiac chambers are severely dilated and the left ventricle is diffusely hypokinetic. Left ventricular wall tension is increased, and systolic pump function progressively declines. Consequently, cardiac output falls and filling pressures increase; both of these changes cause progressive dyspnea, edema, and fatigue. Serious ventricular arrhythmia develops in most cases.

Despite advances in treatment, the 5-year survival rate in patients with dilated cardiomyopathy and symptomatic heart failure approaches 50%. In some cases, however, improvement or even return to normal has been noted. Both ACE inhibitors and β-adrenergic blocking agents (most notably carvedilol) have been shown to slow the deterioration of left ventricular function in patients with congestive heart failure and occasionally to actually improve the left ventricular EF.[75] In addition, some of the patients who recover may have had unrecognized myocarditis that did not progress to cardiomyopathy. Dilated cardiomyopathy may be the outcome of an autoimmune response to a myocardial injury, most commonly viral myocarditis. The exact role of alcohol is unclear, but it is at least a major aggravating factor in some cases.

Patients may have symptoms and signs of heart failure for which no cause can be found on clinical and laboratory examination. Weight is increased, the jugular venous pressure is elevated, and the heart is enlarged. An S_3 gallop is often present, frequently accompanied by the murmurs of mitral and tricuspid regurgitation, which develop as a consequence of cardiac dilatation. The ECG is usually abnormal, often showing left ventricular hypertrophy or left bundle branch block. Echocardiography shows enlargement and hypocontractility of the ventricles. The patients are subject to mural thrombus in the cardiac chambers with a consequent risk of stroke or pulmonary embolism. Established dilated cardiomyopathy, even when heart failure is compensated, is a contraindication to pregnancy.

It was formerly thought that dilated cardiomyopathy was sporadic and not familial, but inherited cases have now been observed. It is estimated that 20% of cases are genetic in origin.[13] Therefore, if an extensive family history of heart failure is present, the prospective mother and father should be informed of the potential risk of genetic transmission.

In a young woman with severe dilated cardiomyopathy, manifested by greatly impaired ventricular function and drastically reduced exercise capacity, cardiac transplantation should be considered. Successful pregnancy has been reported in women who have undergone heart or heart-lung tranplantation.[76-78]

Peripartum Cardiomyopathy

Peripartum cardiomyopathy is a form of dilated cardiomyopathy that occurs in the last month of pregnancy or during the first 5 months after delivery, in the absence of previous heart disease.[79] The incidence in the United States is 1 case per 3000 to 4000 live births. Additional diagnostic criteria include a left ventricular EF of less than 45% and, most importantly, the absence of other identifiable causes of heart failure.[80] Whether the peripartum or postpartum state somehow constitutes the original myocardial insult or is an aggravating factor in individuals susceptible to cardiomyopathy for other reasons is not known.[81] It has been suggested that some cases are caused by active myocarditis,[82] but other investigators have reported that the incidence of myocarditis is the same in idiopathic and peripartum cardiomyopathy.[83] It is also possible that the stress of pregnancy may "unmask" an underlying cardiomyopathic process that might otherwise have manifested later in life.[84] This devastating disease can affect previously healthy young women and can cause unexpected sudden death.[85]

The clinical course of peripartum cardiomyopathy is frustratingly variable and difficult to predict.[86] About 20% of patients have a dramatic and fulminant downhill course and can be saved only with cardiac transplantation. Others, perhaps 30% to 50%, have partial recovery with persistence of some degree of cardiac dysfunction. The rest show remarkable recovery.[81] Apparently, the initial degree of left ventricular dysfunction does not predict the long-term outcome.[87] A recent study showed that cardiac function improved gradually over a 5-year period.[88]

Women who recover from peripartum cardiomyopathy must be informed that cardiomyopathy may recur with a subsequent pregnancy. For some time, this risk has been believed to be 50%.[87] However, one report of four women who had peripartum cardiomyopathy with a previous pregnancy but whose hearts remained normal clinically and by echocardiography in a subsequent pregnancy indicated that the risk may be less.[89] The largest study to date of patients with a history of peripartum cardiomyopathy who subsequently became pregnant[90] showed that heart failure recurred in 20% of those patients whose EF had normalized after the previous pregnancy. None of these patients died during the study period. However, heart failure recurred in 40% of the patients who had persistent left ventricular dysfunction after their previous pregnancy, and the maternal mortality in this group was 19%. A study from Haiti of 15 women with peripartum cardiomyopathy showed a recurrence rate of almost 50% during a subsequent pregnancy.[91] Therefore, the risk of recurrent heart failure is high in women with peripartum cardiomyopathy, especially in those who do not have complete recovery of left ventricular function.

Treatment is similar to that for other patients with heart failure. Because ACE inhibitors are contraindicated during pregnancy hydralazine is the vasodilator of choice. If cardiac dysfunction is severe, anticoagulation is usually recommended, given the prothrombotic tendency of pregnancy. Low-molecular-weight heparin (LMWH) is probably preferred to unfractionated heparin (warfarin is not recommended).[86]

Idiopathic Hypertrophic Cardiomyopathy

Hypertrophic cardiomyopathy, which is usually inherited as an autosomal dominant trait with variable penetrance but sometimes is caused by a spontaneous mutation, is being recognized with increasing frequency. The phenotypes vary greatly. Left ventricular outflow tract obstruction may or may not be present, and the hypertrophy may be either symmetrical or asymmetrical. The chief symptoms are angina, dyspnea, arrhythmia, and syncope. Sudden death is a feature mostly confined to patients in whom the diagnosis is established in childhood or youth, patients with a history of syncope or ventricular arrhythmia, and patients with a family history of hypertrophic cardiomyopathy and sudden death. Recent research has shown that certain specific genetic defects place patients at great risk for sudden death.

When the disease is first detected in older adults, the course is more benign and sudden death is rare. Left ventricular hypertrophy is often apparent on clinical examination and ECG and is invariably present on the echocardiogram. The echocardiographic findings are often diagnostic and include marked thickening of the ventricular septum, usually with less thickness of the other walls of the left ventricle (asymmetrical hypertrophy), and abnormal systolic anterior movement of the mitral valve (Fig. 39-17). The internal dimensions of the left ventricle are normal to small, and its contractility is increased.

An important feature in many cases is obstruction of the space between the ventricular septum and the anterior leaflet of the mitral valve. This space constitutes the left ventricular outflow tract. Outflow obstruction by the anterior mitral valve leaflet is worsened by increased inotropy, decreased heart size, and diminished peripheral vascular resistance. The normal fall in peripheral vascular resistance that accompanies pregnancy tends to increase outflow tract obstruction, although this effect may be compensated for by the physiologic increase in blood volume. In addition, vena caval obstruction in late pregnancy and blood loss at delivery, both of which may result in hypotension, can have a similar deleterious effect. Outflow tract obstruction may also be worsened by the increases in circulating catecholamine levels frequently encountered during labor and delivery. The Valsalva maneuver during the second stage of labor may greatly diminish heart size and increase outflow tract obstruction. Despite all these problems, however, most pregnant women with hypertrophic cardiomyopathy do tolerate labor and delivery.[92]

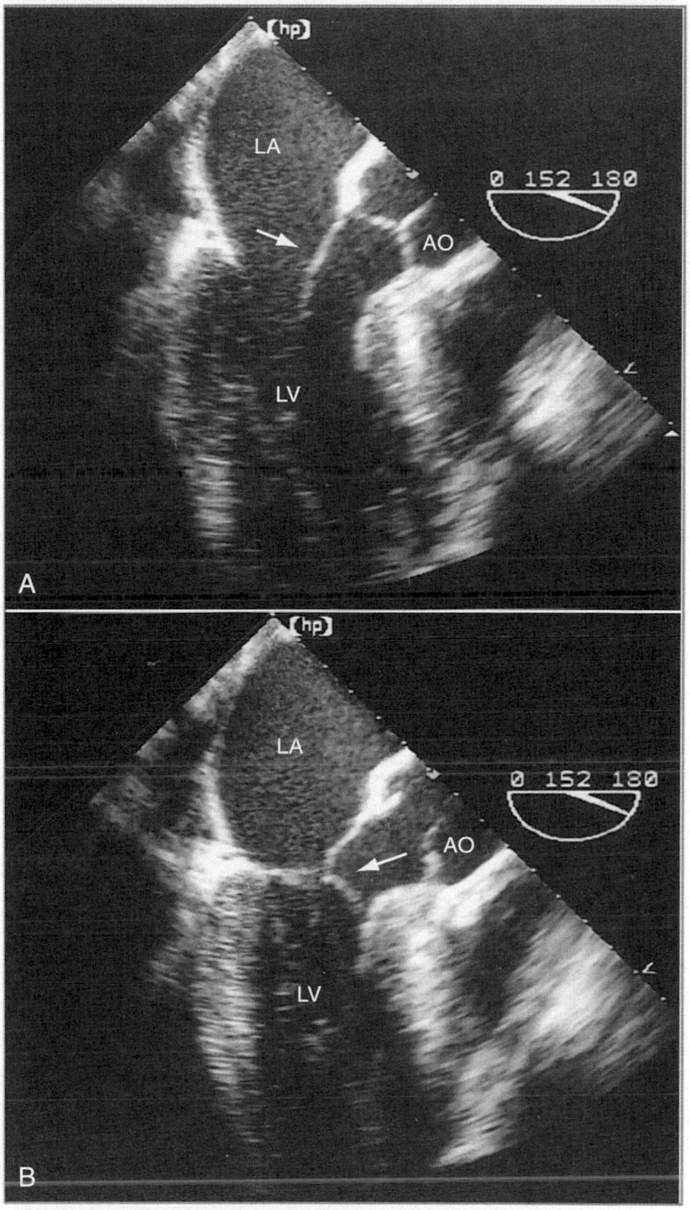

FIGURE 39-17 Transesophageal echocardiographic images of hypertrophic cardiomyopathy. **A,** During diastole the anterior leaflet of the mitral valve *(arrow)* is in a normal position. **B,** During systole the leaflet *(arrow)* is pulled by Venturi forces into the left ventricular outflow tract, causing obstruction to outflow. AO, aorta; LA, left atrium; LV, left ventricle.

There is a complex interplay between the hemodynamics of the cardiomyopathy and those of pregnancy, neither of which is constant. Exacerbation of symptoms[93] and even sudden death[94] have been reported during pregnancy in women with obstructive cardiomyopathy. Treatment is aimed at avoiding hypovolemia, maintaining venous return, and diminishing the force of myocardial contraction by avoiding anxiety, excitement, and strenuous activity.

Because left ventricular diastolic compliance can be greatly reduced in this disease, excessive or too rapid volume repletion can induce pulmonary edema. β-Adrenergic blockade is considered first-line pharmacologic therapy for symptomatic hypertrophic cardiomyopathy and can be continued or instituted during pregnancy. The dose should be the minimal effective dose needed to avoid excessive slowing of the fetal heart.

Esmolol can be given intravenously if the patient first presents with severe symptoms. Volume replacement and vasopressor therapy may be needed, along with β-adrenergic blockers. Calcium channel blockers, such as verapamil, have been shown to be effective in reducing symptoms, but they must be used cautiously because they can cause pulmonary edema in severe cases. Nifedipine, because of its vasodilator properties, is best avoided.

Vaginal delivery is almost always appropriate in the absence of an obstetric indication for abdominal delivery. Impaired venous return is highly undesirable in hypertrophic cardiomyopathy and can be ameliorated by managing the second stage of labor with the patient in the left lateral decubitus position.

Acquired Immunodeficiency Syndrome

Myocarditis or cardiomyopathy is frequently discovered on postmortem examination of patients with acquired immunodeficiency syndrome (AIDS).[95,96] Symptomatic myocardial disease, although considerably less common, also occurs. If patients with full-blown AIDS are screened for cardiac involvement (e.g., by echocardiography), cardiac or pericardial involvement is found in almost 75% of the cases.[97] In some cases, these abnormalities are transient.[98] Myocarditis is usually caused by opportunistic infection, but in some cases hybridization studies have proved direct AIDS infection. Clinical findings range from occult ventricular dysfunction to severe uncompensated heart failure. Rarely, even Kaposi sarcoma has been detected in the heart or pericardium. Pericardial effusion, often occult, is one of the more common cardiac manifestations and suggests a worse prognosis.[99] Malignant lymphoma involving the myocardium and endocardium has been reported as well. In the current era of highly-active antiretroviral therapy (HAART), myocardial involvement has become considerably less common in patients with human immunodeficiency virus (HIV) infection. However, some classes of antiretroviral drugs appear to cause dyslipidemia, and this can lead to an increased risk of coronary artery disease (CAD) and subsequent myocardial infarction.[100]

Cardiac failure ranks low on the list of problems faced by the physician managing pregnancy complicated by AIDS. Nevertheless, physicians need to be on guard lest severe dilated cardiomyopathy, myocarditis, or cardiac tamponade develop, and the pregnant woman must be treated appropriately to prevent transmission of HIV to her offspring (see Chapter 38.)

Coronary Artery Disease

Because premenopausal women enjoy substantial protection against coronary atherosclerosis,[15] ischemic heart disease is rarely relevant to obstetric practice. However, CAD may be found in women of childbearing age when other risk factors, such as insulin-dependent diabetes, smoking, or severe dyslipidemia, overwhelm the natural protection they should normally enjoy. Lupus erythematosus, especially when treated with steroidal agents, may precipitate premature CAD. Coronary atherosclerosis appears in a significant proportion of patients who have received a cardiac transplant[101] and may be observed in familial lipid disorders. In the latter instance, the exact nature of the lipid disorder must be defined by detailed analysis of the patient's lipid chemistry and lipoproteins to enable the physician to provide an accurate forecast of the risk that the infant would inherit the lipid disorder and premature CAD. In women with CAD or severe dyslipidemia, oral contraceptives may be detrimental.[102] In addition, spasm of anatomically normal coronary arteries leading to myocardial infarction has been reported.[103] Finally, as mentioned earlier, women with HIV infection may develop dyslipidemia on HAART, which can increase the risk of CAD.[100]

Spontaneous coronary artery dissection is quite rare and occurs chiefly in young women during or soon after pregnancy.[104,105] Treatment has included placement of a stent, emergency coronary bypass operation, and thrombolysis.[106-109] Although coronary artery dissection is very uncommon, it is extremely important to consider this diagnosis whenever a woman presents with severe chest pain in the peripartum period. If the coronary artery dissection remains undetected, massive myocardial infarction and even death can occur. If the diagnosis is made expediently, however, outcome appears to be quite good, and long-term survival is expected.[110]

Management of Stable Angina Pectoris

Women with CAD who experience angina pectoris only at high levels of exertion should be treated with β-adrenergic blocking drugs, aspirin, and lipid-lowering agents. In this setting, the likelihood of significant complications during pregnancy, labor, or delivery is low. If there is any question regarding the severity of myocardial ischemia, however, stress testing should be performed before pregnancy is attempted. Similarly, a woman who previously sustained a myocardial infarction but recovered without heart failure, significant left ventricular dysfunction, or unstable angina pectoris can also be advised that her pregnancy and labor should be relatively uncomplicated.

The major indications that pregnancy and labor would pose a significant risk to a woman with ischemic heart disease are the presence of overt heart failure, significant enlargement or dysfunction of the left ventricle, and ischemia at rest or provoked by mild exertion.

Severe Myocardial Ischemic Syndromes: Unstable Angina

The diagnosis of severe ischemia may be confirmed if angina occurs at rest or with mild exertion. This unstable angina frequently, but not necessarily, follows a period of classic stable angina pectoris. Unstable angina is a clear warning of the imminence of a major ischemic event, such as acute myocardial infarction or a fatal ventricular arrhythmia. Starting a pregnancy under these circumstances is not advisable, and aggressive treatment (including coronary angiography followed by percutaneous coronary intervention or coronary artery bypass surgery) is recommended. If the outcome is satisfactory, pregnancy can then be considered.

In some women with CAD, the clinical picture is less dramatic but a treadmill exercise test demonstrates that profound and dangerous ischemia can be precipitated by minimal exertion. If the treadmill test provokes an abnormal response at a low level of exercise, and particularly if this response is accompanied by either angina pectoris or a fall in blood pressure, the woman is at high risk for a serious and possibly fatal myocardial ischemic event and must not undertake pregnancy unless the myocardium can be revascularized.

Pregnant women who develop unstable ischemia require aggressive treatment in an intensive care unit. If the ischemia proves intractable, percutaneous coronary intervention (e.g., stenting) or bypass graft surgery will be necessary.[111] If possible, the coronary bypass operation should be performed without cardiopulmonary bypass to help decrease the risk to the fetus.[112]

Myocardial Infarction

Acute myocardial infarction complicates about 1 in 10,000 pregnancies.[113] The highest incidence appears to occur in the third trimester and in older (>33 years) multigravidas. The maternal mortality rate is high (about 20%), and death usually occurs at the time of infarction or during labor and delivery.[114] Coronary angiography in this population demonstrated atherosclerosis in about 40% of cases, coronary thrombosis without atherosclerosis in 20%, and coronary dissection in 16%, but 30% had normal coronary arteries.[114] Treatment of acute myocardial infarction during pregnancy should include use of heparin and β-blockers (unless acute heart failure is present). The use of thrombolytics in pregnancy is controversial, because there is increased risk of maternal hemorrhage. Therefore, percutaneous coronary intervention (with stenting) is probably the procedure of choice. Obviously, this exposes the fetus to radiation, and so extensive lead shielding should be used.

A remote myocardial infarction, followed by recovery without angina, major left ventricular dysfunction, or heart failure, should have little influence on pregnancy or labor. Patients should wait a year after an infarction before undertaking pregnancy. In many cases, coronary arteriography should be done first so that, if critical coronary stenoses are found, myocardial revascularization can be performed. Severe left ventricular damage and heart failure are contraindications to pregnancy.

For remote myocardial infarction without evidence of ischemia, heart failure, or severe left ventricular dysfunction, simple electrocardiographic monitoring suffices during labor. If a large myocardial infarction has occurred during pregnancy, then arterial blood pressure, central venous pressure, pulmonary arterial and pulmonary wedge pressure, and cardiac output should be monitored invasively. Monitoring should be continued until after the completion of labor, because maternal preload abruptly increases with the birth, after which substantial loss of blood can accompany delivery of the placenta.

Heart Failure

Chronic heart failure is a syndrome that develops when the heart cannot meet the metabolic requirements of the normally active individual. It may be defined as ventricular dysfunction causing dyspnea, fatigue, and sometimes arrhythmia. The lesion may be an intrinsic myocardial abnormality. Examples include myocarditis, the various cardiomyopathies, ischemic heart disease, other specific myocardial disorders (e.g., amyloidosis), and metabolic abnormalities (e.g., myxedema). The myocardial response to chronic pressure overload is concentric hypertrophy with increased thickness of the ventricular walls; the response to chronic volume overload is dilation (eccentric hypertrophy). Contractile power is eventually diminished with either type of overload, resulting in decreased pump function of the heart. Causes include valvular disease, systemic and pulmonary hypertension, and congenital malformations. The clinical manifestations result in part from the abnormal loading conditions and in part from the damaged myocardium.

Manifestations

The principal manifestations of heart failure are caused by increased left and right ventricular diastolic pressure, which engenders pulmonary and systemic congestion, and reduced cardiac output (during exercise or, in severe cases, at rest as well). The combined effects of inadequate cardiac output and congestion are dyspnea, fatigue, and edema. In the later stages of heart failure, these changes lead to progressive dysfunction of vital organs, principally the liver and kidneys. The prognosis of severe uncorrectable heart failure is quite poor, and pregnancy is absolutely contraindicated.

The critical clinical features that enable physicians to diagnose and monitor the course of heart failure are body weight, jugular venous pressure, the S_3, cardiac size, radiologic evidence of pulmonary congestion, pulmonary rales, and peripheral edema. Echocardiography is an extremely useful tool for evaluating left ventricular function and prognosis in heart failure[115] and should be performed without delay if heart failure is suspected. Circulating B-type natriuretic peptide (BNP) is increased in congestive heart failure. Serum BNP levels provide an effective, inexpensive, and quickly available test for heart failure. The degree of BNP increase correlates with the severity of heart failure.[116]

The presence of heart failure greatly limits physical activity and warrants several or all of the following treatments:

- Continuous, usually escalating courses of diuretic drugs
- β-Adrenergic receptor blockers
- ACE inhibitors (or, if these are not well tolerated, angiotensin receptor blockers)—note that these agents are contraindicated during pregnancy and should be replaced by hydralazine
- Salt restriction
- Digoxin

If heart failure is first discovered during pregnancy, episodes of cardiac decompensation that do not respond to adjustment of orally administered medicine necessitate admission to an intensive care unit. There, the effects of treatment on cardiac output, pulmonary arterial pressure, systemic venous pressure, and pulmonary wedge pressure, along with the maternal and fetal ECGs, can be monitored. If the hemodynamic parameters and clinical condition indicate continuing deterioration despite maximal medical therapy, emergency abdominal delivery may be necessary.

Asymptomatic Left Ventricular Dysfunction

There is a remarkable lack of correlation between symptoms of heart failure and objective evidence of left ventricular dysfunction.[117] For example, patients with chronic heart disease after myocardial infarction may have a considerably enlarged and extremely hypokinetic ventricle and yet be relatively free from symptoms. For this reason, any woman who has sustained myocardial damage should have left ventricular function assessed by echocardiography before deciding on pregnancy.

Cardiac Transplantation

Some women with advanced heart failure become successful recipients of a cardiac transplant. Successful pregnancy and delivery in patients with cardiac transplantation have been reported.[78] Medical treatment after transplantation is complex because of the immunosuppressive drug regimen, the frequent endomyocardial biopsies, and the uncertain long-term prognosis. Women should delay pregnancy for at least 1 year after cardiac transplantation, by which time the risk of acute rejection and the intensity of immunosuppression and biopsy surveys are considerably less.

Disturbances of Cardiac Rhythm

Isolated supraventricular and ventricular extrasystoles are very common, and no treatment is necessary. Pre-conception counseling is simplified by a clear appreciation of several general principles.

Arrhythmia that occurs in the absence of organic heart disease is almost always benign and is therefore not an indication for pharmacologic treatment unless the woman finds the symptoms intolerable. Reassuring her of the benign nature of this symptom is often all that is required. Sustained symptomatic arrhythmia, however, requires treatment, which can be pharmacologic or procedural (e.g., transcatheter ablation of an anomalous conduction pathway, insertion of an implantable cardiac defibrillator).

Pregnancy and labor should be safe except in the group with sustained ventricular arrhythmia, with its attendant risk of cardiac arrest and need for vigorous treatment. Pharmacologic treatment for serious arrhythmia is likely to include newly introduced agents, such as amiodarone or sotalol, for which there is at best limited knowledge of potentially unfavorable effects on the fetus. Ideally, pregnancy should be postponed until the arrhythmia has been eliminated or at least controlled, preferably by nonpharmacologic means. If antiarrhythmic drugs must be used, whenever possible they should be those that have been used for several decades, allowing prediction of the fetal risk.

High-grade atrioventricular conduction disturbance, especially if it is symptomatic, is treated by artificial pacing, which should not influence pregnancy, labor, or the fetus. Electrical cardioversion or defibrillation of the mother's heart does not disturb or damage the fetal heart.[118]

It is clearly desirable to evaluate disturbances of cardiac rhythm and conduction before pregnancy, proceeding to full electrophysiologic testing if indicated. This plan avoids exposing a fetus to potentially toxic antiarrhythmic agents and the radiation associated with electrophysiologic investigation.

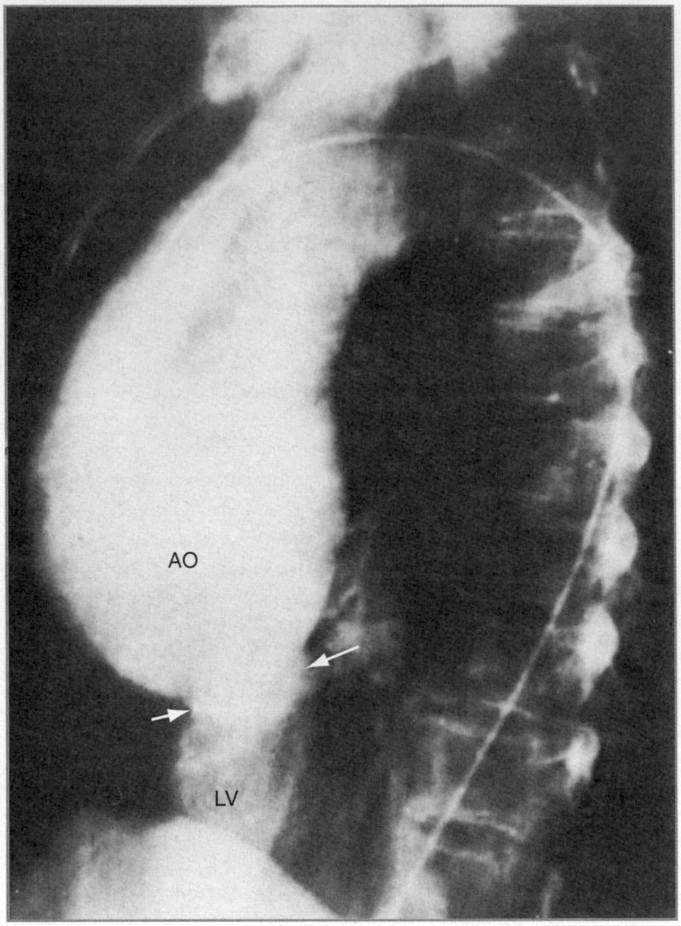

FIGURE 39-18 Aortic aneurysm. Aortogram showing an aneurysm of the ascending aorta (AO) with regurgitation of contrast through an incompetent aortic valve *(arrows)* into the left ventricle (LV). (From Shabetai R, Adolph RJ: Principles of cardiac catheterization. In Fowler NO [ed]: Cardiac Diagnosis and Treatment. Hagerstown, MD: Harper & Row, 1980, p 106.)

Marfan Syndrome

Marfan syndrome is variably expressed and inherited as an autosomal dominant trait. If it is left untreated, life expectancy is reduced by half in those who exhibit the classic syndrome. The basic defect is one of connective tissue, particularly fibrillin, and connective tissue weakness in the aorta causes the dangerous complications, most notably aortic dissection.[119]

Symptoms and signs may include dyspnea and chest pain, an aortic diastolic murmur, and a midsystolic click. The best diagnostic test, and apparently the most critical one for determining the outcome of pregnancy, is the echocardiogram. More than 90% of patients have evidence of MVP, and 60% have echocardiographic evidence of aortic root dilatation.[120]

Pregnancy is particularly dangerous for patients with this syndrome, because there appears to be a high risk of aortic rupture and dissection, especially if dilatation of the aortic root is present.[47] Women with an aortic diameter exceeding 40 mm are at greatest risk of death during pregnancy.[121] The physician should also make sure the woman understands the 50% risk of genetic transmission of Marfan syndrome to her children.

Deficiency of elastic tissue is the cause of myxomatous degeneration of the aortic and mitral valves and cystic medial necrosis of the aorta (Figs. 39-18 and 39-19). This abnormality translates to large aneurysms of the aortic root, multiple aneurysms elsewhere along the course of the aorta and great vessels, and severe aortic and mitral regurgitation with resulting heart failure. Surgery is indicated for rapidly expanding aneurysm or if dissection is evident. Pregnancy is poorly tolerated under these conditions, and labor may precipitate rupture of an aneurysm or aortic dissection.

If a woman with Marfan syndrome chooses to become pregnant, therapy is directed at markedly limiting physical activity, preventing hypertensive complications, and decreasing the pulsatile forces on the aortic wall with the use of a β-blocker. Long-acting β-blockers are indicated before, during, and after pregnancy in women with Marfan syndrome.[122] Once the aortic root diameter reaches 50 to 55 mm, most authorities recommend prophylactic aortic valve and root replacement because of the high risk of aortic dissection. Abdominal delivery is recommended to avoid the hemodynamic stress of labor.

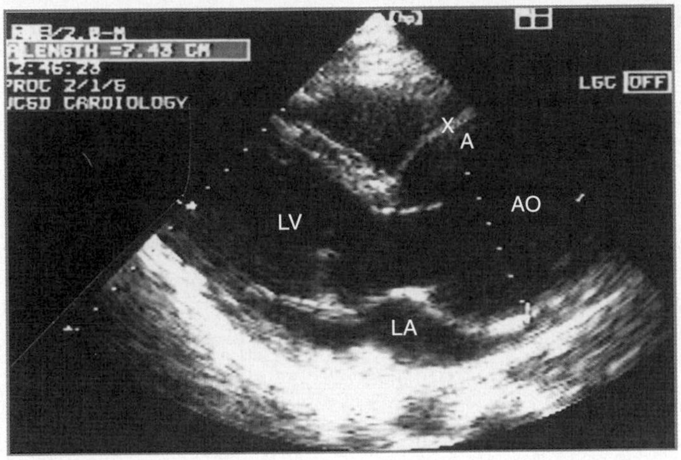

FIGURE 39-19 **Marfan syndrome.** The echocardiogram shows a markedly dilated aortic root, measuring 7.4 cm in diameter (normal, ≤3.5 cm). A, annulus diameter (7.43 cm); AO, aorta; LA, left atrium; LV, left ventricle.

Pregnancy in Patients with Artificial Heart Valves

Pregnancy in women with artificial heart valves is one of the most complex and challenging areas where cardiology and obstetrics intersect, and it could be the topic of an entire chapter itself. The discussion here covers three basic groups of patients:

1. Women contemplating pregnancy who are likely to need a valve replacement in the medium- to long-term future, such as women with moderate aortic or pulmonic stenosis, severe but asymptomatic mitral or aortic regurgitation with normal myocardial function, or mild to moderate mitral stenosis
2. Women who wish to become pregnant but have severe valve disease that must be addressed expediently, including those with severe aortic or mitral stenosis, severe mitral regurgitation with cardiac dysfunction, or severe aortic regurgitation with cardiac dysfunction
3. Women with mechanical valve replacements who become pregnant.

The only group for whom no management controversy exists is the first.[123] Without question, women who are likely to need valve surgery in several years should be strongly encouraged to complete their childbearing as quickly as possible—so that they will not become members of the second or third group.

Women in the second group require valve replacement before pregnancy. In most adult patients younger than 70 years of age (but not in women who wish to become pregnant), mechanical prosthetic valves would be favored over biologic prostheses, because biologic valves have a shorter life span and deteriorate much more quickly than mechanical valves. This difference appears even more pronounced in younger patients; it was once thought that pregnancy itself hastened biologic valve deterioration, but this does not appear to be true.[124] In any case, younger patients with biologic valves will almost certainly require repeat surgery. With mechanical valves, however, the patient faces the requirement for lifelong anticoagulation and the resultant small increase in risk of bleeding.

It is important to note that the anticoagulant of choice with a mechanical valve is warfarin, not heparin. Although heparin is clearly safer for the fetus,[125] it is not equivalent to warfarin in preventing thromboembolic complications (especially during the prothrombotic state of pregnancy). This has been shown in several studies and appears to be most striking in the case of single tilting-disk mechanical prostheses.[8,24] Therefore, many experts agree that women who require valve surgery before pregnancy should receive a bioprosthetic valve—even though repeat surgery will be necessary in the future—because these valves have a much lower thromboembolic risk and do not usually require systemic anticoagulation. Women with normally functioning biologic valve replacements tolerate pregnancy well.

Management of the last group (i.e., women with mechanical cardiac valves who become pregnant) is the most difficult. A woman with a mechanical prosthetic heart valve should be counseled strongly that pregnancy is risky, primarily because of the risk of embolic phenomena. If the patient decides to proceed with pregnancy, warfarin is superior to heparin for preventing thromboemboli with mechanical valves. However, warfarin is teratogenic and carries a 4% to 10% risk of warfarin embryopathy.[126,127] This risk appears to be dose dependent as well.[23] For these reasons, the U.S. manufacturer of Coumadin (warfarin) states that the drug is absolutely contraindicated during pregnancy. Although warfarin is used during pregnancy in Europe (after the first 12 weeks) and is recommended until the 35th week of pregnancy, American physicians face a particularly difficult dilemma because of the manufacturer's contraindication (even though this contradicts guidelines from acknowledged expert panels).[2,10,11] In addition, many pregnant women would prefer to put themselves rather than the fetus at risk. Therefore, subcutaneous or intravenous heparin is used during pregnancy in many American women with mechanical heart valves, even though thromboembolic risk is higher.[127,128] During treatment with heparin or LMWH, the activated partial thromboplastin time (or anti-Xa heparin levels) must be monitored frequently. In addition, the dose must be adjusted as the patient gains weight during pregnancy. There is some evidence that LMWH is superior to unfractionated heparin in nonpregnant patients with mechanical prostheses,[129] and this approach has been used successfully in a number of pregnant patients.[130,131] However, in a recent small study of enoxaparin in pregnant women with prosthetic heart valves, two of eight patients developed prosthetic valve thrombosis leading to maternal and fetal death.[132] It is unclear but possible that these women did not receive adequate dosing of enoxaparin. Randomized trials have not been performed, and more information is needed before LMWH can be recommended over unfractionated heparin in this setting.[133]

Tables 39-6 and 39-7 show two currently proposed protocols for anticoagulation in the pregnant woman with a mechanical heart valve. Most authorities recommend using heparin through the first trimester, although continuous use of warfarin until week 35 is an option in high-risk patients (those with first-generation tilting-disk prostheses in the mitral position).[10,11] The joint American College of Cardiology (ACC)/American Heart Association (AHA) Guidelines for the Management of Patients with Valvular Heart Disease[2] stress the importance of discussing the risks and benefits of various anticoagulation approaches with the patient, because she must be a full partner in her medical care. She must be informed that if she chooses to change from warfarin to heparin during the first trimester (or for the entire pregnancy), she has a higher risk of both thrombosis and bleeding, and any risk to her jeopardizes the baby as well. Table 39-6, from Elkayam and

TABLE 39-6 RECOMMENDED APPROACH FOR ANTICOAGULATION PROPHYLAXIS IN WOMEN WITH PROSTHETIC HEART VALVES (PHV) DURING PREGNANCY

Higher Risk*	Lower Risk†
Warfarin (INR 2.5-3.5) for 35 wk *followed by* UFH (mid-interval aPTT >2.5) or LMWH (pre-dose anti-Xa ≈ 0.7) + ASA 80-100 mg qd **OR** UFH (aPTT 2.5-3.5) or LMWH (pre-dose anti-Xa ≈ 0.7) for 12 wk *followed by* Warfarin (INR 2.5-3.5) to 35th wk *then* UFH (mid-interval aPTT >2.5) or LMWH (pre-dose anti-Xa ≈ 0.7) + ASA 80-100 mg qd	SC UFH (mid-interval aPTT, 2.0-3.0) or LMWH (pre-dose anti-Xa ≈ 0.6) for 12 wk *followed by* Warfarin (INR 2.5-3.0) for 35 wk *then* SC UFH (mid-interval aPTT 2.0-3.0) or LMWH (pre-dose anti-Xa ≈ 0.6) **OR** SC UFH (mid-interval aPTT 2.0-3.0) or LMWH (pre-dose anti-Xa ≈ 0.6) throughout pregnancy

aPTT, activated partial thromboplastin time; ASA, acetylsalicylic acid; INR, international normalized ratio; LMWH, low-molecular-weight heparin; SC, subcutaneous; UFH, unfractionated heparin.
***First-generation PHV (e.g., Starr-Edwards, Bjork-Shiley) in the mitral position, atrial fibrillation, history of thromboembolism on anticoagulation.**
†Second-generation PHV (e.g., St. Jude Medical, Medtronic-Hall) and any mechanical PHV in the aortic position.
Reproduced with permission from Elkayam U, Bitar F: Valvular heart disease and pregnancy. Part II: Prosthetic valves. J Am Coll Cardiol 46:403, 2005.

TABLE 39-7 RECOMMENDATIONS OF THE SEVENTH ACCP CONSENSUS CONFERENCE ON ANTITHROMBOTIC THERAPY FOR PROPHYLAXIS IN PATIENTS WITH MECHANICAL HEART VALVES

1. Aggressive adjusted-dose UFH, q12h SC throughout pregnancy; mid-interval aPTT time maintained at >2× control levels, or anti-Xa heparin level maintained at 0.35 to 0.70 IU/mL

OR

2. LMWH throughout pregnancy, in doses adjusted according to weight or as necessary to maintain a 4-h postinjection anti-Xa heparin level of about 1.0 IU/mL

OR

3. UFH or LMWH, as above, until the 13th week; then change to warfarin until the middle of the third trimester, then restart UFH or LMWH therapy until delivery

ACCP, American College of Chest Physicians; aPTT, activated partial thromboplastin time; LMWH, low-molecular-weight heparin; SC, subcutaneous; UFH, unfractionated heparin.
Data from Bates SM, Greer IA, Hirsh J, Ginsberg JC: Use of antithrombotic agents during pregnancy: The seventh ACCP conference on antithrombotic and thrombolytic therapy. Chest 126:627S, 2004.

Bitar,[11] stratifies treatment options by risk of thrombosis and recommends consideration of continuing warfarin throughout the pregnancy (until week 35) for patients with first-generation valves in the mitral position, atrial fibrillation, or a history of previous embolic events. The treatment options in Table 39-7, from the American College of Chest Physicians[134] are simpler, but they do not differentiate on the basis of the type of mechanical valve or its position (aortic versus mitral). Consultation and close follow-up during pregnancy with an experienced cardiologist is strongly recommended, as well as meticulous attention to blood coagulation testing. Because preterm labor occurs frequently in this group,[24] warfarin should be replaced by therapeutic doses of subcutaneous heparin beginning at the 35th week of gestation. If labor occurs while a patient is taking warfarin, cesarean section is recommended to avoid fetal cerebral hemorrhage during vaginal delivery.[2]

All patients with prosthetic heart valves require antibiotic prophylaxis for dental and surgical procedures and at delivery. Prevention of prosthetic valve endocarditis is essential, because the mortality rate can reach 40%. The patient who experiences endocarditis with a prosthetic valve must receive aggressive antibiotic therapy and often will require valve replacement. Obviously, the risk to the fetus is exorbitant.

Cardiac Surgery during Pregnancy

Whenever possible, any woman who requires cardiac surgery should undergo the procedure before becoming pregnant. Nevertheless, as explained previously, in rare instances a patient may require surgery during pregnancy. Valvular surgery has been performed successfully during pregnancy for many years, and patients have also undergone coronary artery bypass surgery and emergency aortic dissection repair. Cardiac surgery during pregnancy does not appear to increase the maternal mortality risk.[135,136] There is, however, a 10% to 15% risk of fetal mortality because of the nonpulsatile blood flow and hypotension associated with conventional cardiopulmonary bypass. Therefore, whenever possible, cardiac surgery should be performed without cardiopulmonary bypass. In addition, hypothermia should be avoided, because this appears to be especially dangerous to the fetus. In one study, fetal mortality was decreased by half when normothermic perfusion was used instead of hypothermic perfusion.[136] Hypothermia stimulates uterine contractions and impairs oxygen delivery to the fetus, mandating careful monitoring of the uterus and the fetal heart. The deleterious effect of hypothermia on umbilical blood flow has been documented by transvaginal ultrasonography.[137]

Experimental studies suggest that fetal survival can be improved by the use of pulsatile perfusion, but results are not yet clear. If bypass is required for cardiac surgery at an immature gestational age, high-flow high-pressure normothermic perfusion should be instituted.[138] If possible, surgery should be postponed until the third trimester, when the fetal risk is considerably reduced. Fetal bradycardia is often seen during surgery and may require rapid treatment, usually with intravenous nitroprusside. In addition, preterm labor occurs more frequently in women undergoing cardiac surgery.

During surgery and in the immediate postoperative period, these patients should be monitored very closely. In general, use of intra-arterial and Swan-Ganz catheters and electrocardiographic monitoring of the woman and the fetus is recommended. Transesophageal echocardiography is also helpful in some cases and provides direct assessment of valvular and ventricular function. Maintenance of acceptable arterial oxygen levels and normal blood pressure, plus avoidance of hypothermia, are of utmost importance to the fetus.

The Use of Prophylactic Antibiotics to Prevent Infective Endocarditis in Pregnant Women with Heart Disease

The most recent recommendations from the American Heart Association (AHA) regarding the use of prophylactic antibiotics represent a major departure from previous guidelines and are summarized here because of the importance of this information to those caring for women with heart disease. The most prominent aspect of the new guidelines is that antibiotics to prevent infective endocarditis (IE) are now recommended *only* for those patients deemed to be at the highest risk. These high risk cardiac conditions include:

1. Prosthetic heart valve or prosthetic material used for cardiac valve repair
2. Previous IE
3. Congenital heart disease (CHD)
   Unrepaired CHD, including palliative shunts and conduits
   Completely repaired congenital heart defect with prosthetic material or device, whether replaced by surgery or by catheter intervention, during the first 6 months after the procedure (during the process of endothelialization)
   Repaired CHD with residual defects at the site or adjacent to the site of a prosthetic patch or prosthetic device (which inhibit endothelialization)
4. Cardiac transplantation recipients who develop cardiac valvulopathy

The reader is referred to the AHA publication for additional details and the consensus panel's rationale.[139]

References

1. Siu SC, Colman JM, Sorensen S, et al: Adverse neonatal and cardiac outcomes are more common in pregnant women with cardiac disease. Circulation 105:2179, 2002.
2. Bonow RO, Carabello B, DeLeon AC, et al: ACC/AHA 2006 guidelines for the Management of Patients with Valvular Heart Disease. Circulation 114:84, 2006.
3. Thorne SA: Pregnancy in heart disease. Heart 90:450, 2004.
4. Schwartz DB, Schamroth L: The effect of pregnancy on the frontal plane QRS axis. J Electrocardiol 12:279, 1979.
5. Rubler S, Damani PM, Pinto ER: Cardiac size and performance during pregnancy estimated with echocardiography. Am J Cardiol 40:534, 1977.
6. Haiat R, Halphen C: Silent pericardial effusion in late pregnancy: A new entity. Cardiovasc Intervent Radiol 7:267, 1984.
7. Stout K: Pregnancy in women with congenital heart disease: The importance of evaluation and counselling. Heart 91:713, 2005.
8. Born D, Martinez EE, Almeid PAM, et al: Pregnancy in patients with prosthetic heart valves: The effects of anticoagulation on mother, fetus and neonate. Am Heart J 124:413, 1992.
9. Siu SC, Sermer M, Colman JM, et al: Prospective multicenter study of pregnancy outcomes in women with heart disease. Circulation 96:2789, 2001.
10. Elkayam U, Bitar F: Valvular heart disease and pregnancy. Part I: Native valves. J Am Coll Cardiol 46:223, 2005.
11. Elkayam U, Bitar F: Valvular heart disease and pregnancy. Part II: Prosthetic valves. J Am Coll Cardiol 46:403, 2005.
12. Bjarnason I, Jonsson S, Hardarson T: Mode of inheritance of hypertrophic cardiomyopathy in Iceland. Br Heart J 47:122, 1982.
13. McMinn TR, Ross J Jr: Hereditary dilated cardiomyopathy. Clin Cardiol 18:7, 1995.
14. Corone P, Bonaiti C, Feingold J, et al: Familial congenital heart disease: How are the various types related? Am J Cardiol 51:942, 1983.
15. Sullivan JM, Ramanathan KB: Management of medical problems in pregnancy: Severe cardiac disease. N Engl J Med 313:304, 1985.
16. Elkayam U, Gleicher N: Hemodynamics and cardiac function during normal pregnancy and the puerperium. In Elkayam U, Gleicher N (eds): Cardiac Problems in Pregnancy. New York, Liss, 1990.
17. Metcalfe J, Ueland K: Maternal cardiovascular adjustments to pregnancy. Progr Cardiovasc Dis 16:363, 1974.
18. Katz R, Karliner JS, Resnik R: Effects of a natural volume overload state (pregnancy) on left ventricular performance in normal human subjects. Circulation 58:434, 1978.
19. Carruth JE, Mivis SB, Brogan DR, et al: The electrocardiogram in normal pregnancy. Am Heart J 102:1075, 1981.
20. Sbarouni E, Oakley CM: Outcome of pregnancy in women with valve prostheses. Br Heart J 71:196, 1994.
21. Wong V, Cheng CH, Chan KC: Fetal and neonatal outcome of exposure to anticoagulants during pregnancy. Am J Med Genet 45:17, 1993.
22. Hirsh J, Fuster V: Guide to anticoagulant therapy. Part 2: Oral anticoagulants. Circulation 89:1469, 1994.
23. Vitale N, De Feo M, De Santo LS, et al: Dose-dependent fetal complications of warfarin in pregnant women with mechanical heart valves. J Am Coll Cardiol 33:1637, 1999.
24. Salazar E, Izaguirre R, Verdejo J, et al: Failure of adjusted doses of subcutaneous heparin to prevent thromboembolic phenomena in pregnant patients with mechanical cardiac valve prostheses. J Am Coll Cardiol 27:1698, 1996.
25. Rosa FW, Bosco LA, Graham CF, et al: Neonatal anuria with maternal angiotensin-converting enzyme inhibition. Obstet Gynecol 74:371, 1989.
26. Scott AA, Purohit DM: Neonatal renal failure: A complication of maternal antihypertensive therapy. Am J Obstet Gynecol 160:1223, 1989.
27. Drenthen W, Pieper PG, Roos-Hesselink JW, et al: Outcome in pregnancy in women with congenital heart disease: A literature review. J Am Coll Cardiol 49:2303, 2007.
28. Skorton DJ, Cheitlin MD, Freed MD, et al: Guidelines for training in adult cardiovascular medicine: Core Cardiology Training Symposium (COCATS). J Am Coll Cardiol 25:31, 1995.
29. Warnes C: Establishing an adult congenital heart disease clinic. Am J Card Imaging 9:11, 1995.
30. Perloff JK: Special facilities for the comprehensive care of adults with congenital heart disease. In Perloff JK, Child JS (eds): Congenital Heart Disease in Adults. Philadelphia, Saunders, 1991, p 7.
31. Uebing A, Steer PJ, Yentis SM, Gatzoulis MA: Pregnancy and congenital heart disease. BMJ 332:401, 2006.
32. Aeschbacher BC, Chatterjee T, Meier B: Transesophageal echocardiography to evaluate success of transcatheter closure of large secundum atrial

septal defects in adults using the buttoned device. Mayo Clin Proc 75:913, 2000.

33. Metcalfe J, McAnulty JH, Ueland K: Cardiac Disease and Pregnancy: Physiology and Management. Boston, Little, Brown, 1986, p 223.
34. Rashkind WJ, Mullins CE, Hellenbrand WE, et al: Nonsurgical closure of patent ductus arteriosus: Clinical application of the Rashkind PDA Occluder System. Circulation 75:583, 1987.
35. Wood P: The Eisenmenger syndrome or pulmonary hypertension with reversed central shunt. BMJ 701:755, 1958.
36. Yentis SM, Steer PJ, Plaat F. Eisenmenger's syndrome in pregnancy: Maternal and fetal mortality in the 1990s. BJOG 105:921, 1998.
37. Gleicher N, Midwall J, Hochberger D, et al: Eisenmenger's syndrome and pregnancy. Obstet Gynecol Surv 34:721, 1979.
38. Spinnato JA, Kraynack BJ, Cooper MW: Eisenmenger's syndrome in pregnancy: Epidural anesthesia for elective cesarean section. N Engl J Med 304:1215, 1981.
39. Avila WS, Grinberg M, Snitcowsky R, et al: Maternal and fetal outcome in pregnant women with Eisenmenger's syndrome. Eur Heart J 16:460, 1995.
40. McCaffrey RM, Dunn LJ: Primary pulmonary hypertension in pregnancy. Obstet Gynecol Surv 19:567, 1964.
41. Abenhaim L, Moride Y, Brenot F, et al: Appetite suppressant drugs and the risk of primary pulmonary hypertension. N Engl J Med 335:609, 1996.
42. Barst RJ, Rubin LJ, Long WA, et al: A comparison of continuous intravenous epoprostenol (prostacyclin) with conventional therapy for primary pulmonary hypertension: The Primary Pulmonary Hypertension Study Group [see comments]. N Engl J Med 334:296, 1996.
43. Rothman A, Beltran D, Kriett JM, et al: Graded balloon dilation atrial septostomy as a bridge to lung transplantation in pulmonary hypertension. Am Heart J 125:1763, 1993.
44. Thanopoulos BD, Georgakopoulos D, Tsaousis GS, et al: Percutaneous balloon dilatation of the atrial septum: Immediate and midterm results. Heart 76:502, 1996.
45. Arias F, Pineda J: Aortic stenosis in pregnancy. J Reprod Med 20:229, 1978.
46. Hameed A, Karaalp IS, Tummala PP, et al: The effect of valvular heart disease on maternal and fetal outcome. J Am Coll Cardiol 37:893, 2001.
47. Elkayam U, Ostrzega E, Shotan A, et al: Cardiovascular problems in pregnant women with the Marfan syndrome. Ann Intern Med 123:117, 1995.
48. Purcell IF, Williams DO: Peripartum cardiomyopathy complicating severe aortic stenosis. Int J Cardiol 52:163, 1995.
49. Hameed A, Yuodim K, Mahboob A, et al: Effect of the severity of pulmonary stenosis on pregnancy outcome: A case-control study. Am J Obstet Gynecol 191:93, 2004.
50. Stanger P, Cassidy SC, Girod DA, et al: Balloon pulmonary valvuloplasty: Results of the valvuloplasty and angioplasty register. Am J Cardiol 65:775, 1990.
51. Morris CD, Menashe VD: Recurrence of congenital heart disease in offspring of parents with surgical correction. Clin Res 33:68A, 1985.
52. Meijer JM, Pieper PG, Drenthen W, et al: Pregnancy, fertility, and recurrence risk in corrected tetralogy of Fallot. Heart 91:801, 2005.
53. Barash PG, Hobbins JC, Hook R, et al: Management of coarctation of the aorta during pregnancy. J Thorac Cardiovasc Surg 69:781, 1975.
54. Beauchesne LM, Connolly HM, Ammash NM, et al: Coarctation of the aorta: Outcome of pregnancy. J Am Coll Cardiol 38:1728, 2001.
55. Ovaert C, McCrindle BW, Nykanen D, et al: Balloon angioplasty of native coarctation: Clinical outcomes and predictors for success. J Am Coll Cardiol 35:988, 2000.
56. Inglessis I, Landzberg MJ: Interventional catheterization in adult congenital heart disease. Circulation 115:1622, 2007.
57. Connolly HM, Warnes CR: Ebstein's anomaly: Outcome of pregnancy. J Am Coll Cardiol 23:1194, 1994.
58. Reid JM, Coleman EN, Doig W: Complete congenital heart block: Report of 35 cases. Br Heart J 48:236, 1982.
59. Kalra GS, Arora R, Khan JA, et al: Percutaneous mitral commissurotomy for severe mitral stenosis during pregnancy. Cathet Cardiovasc Diagn 33:28, 1994.
60. Lefevre T, Bonan R, Serra A, et al: Percutaneous mitral valvuloplasty in surgical high risk patients. J Am Coll Cardiol 17:348, 1991.
61. de Souza JAM, Martinez EE, Ambrose JA, et al: Percutaneous balloon mitral valvuloplasty in comparison with open mitral valve commissurotomy for mitral stenosis during pregnancy. J Am Coll Cardiol 37:900, 2001.
62. Devereux RB, Perloff JK, Reichek N, et al: Mitral valve prolapse. Circulation 54:3, 1976.
63. Levine RA, Handschumacher MD, Sanfilippo AJ, et al: Three-dimensional echocardiographic reconstruction of the mitral valve, with implications for the diagnosis of mitral valve prolapse. Circulation 80:589, 1989.
64. Hartman N, Kramer R, Brown T, et al: Panic disorder in patients with mitral valve prolapse. Am J Psychiatry 139:669, 1982.
65. Perloff JK, Child JS, Edwards JE: New guidelines for the clinical diagnosis of mitral valve prolapse. Am J Cardiol 57:1124, 1986.
66. Freed LA, Levy D, Levine RA, et al: Prevalence and clinical outcome of mitral-valve prolapse. N Engl J Med 341:1, 1999.
67. Gilon D, Buananno FS, Leavitt M, et al: Lack of evidence of an association between mitral-valve prolapse and stroke in young patients. N Engl J Med 341:8, 1999.
68. Butman S, Chandraratna PA, Milne N, et al: Stress myocardial imaging in patients with mitral valve prolapse: Evidence of a perfusion abnormality. Cathet Cardiovasc Diagn 8:243, 1982.
69. Bach DS, Bolling SF: Early improvement in congestive heart failure after correction of secondary mitral regurgitation in end-stage cardiomyopathy. Am Heart J 129:1165, 1995.
70. Otto CM: Evaluation and management of chronic mitral regurgitation. N Engl J Med 345:740, 2001.
71. Banning AP, Pearson JF, Hall RJ: Role of balloon dilatation of the aortic valve in pregnant patients with severe aortic stenosis. Br Heart J 70:544, 1993.
72. Silversides CK, Colman JM, Sermer M, et al: Early and intermediate-term outcomes of pregnancy with congenital aortic stenosis. Am J Cardiol 91:1386, 2003.
73. Mast ST, Jollis JG, Ryan T, et al: The progression of fenfluramine-associated valvular heart disease assessed by echocardiography. Ann Intern Med 134:261, 2001.
74. Connolly HM, Crary JL, McGoon MD, et al: Valvular heart disease associated with fenfluramine-phentermine. N Engl J Med 337:581, 1997.
75. Hunt SA, Abraham WT, Chin MH, et al: ACC/AHA guideline update for the diagnosis and management of chronic heart failure in the adult. J Am Coll Cardiol 46:1116-43, 2005.
76. Baron O, Hubaut J, Galetta D, et al: Pregnancy and heart-lung transplantation. Heart Lung Transplant 21:914, 2002.
77. Troche V, Ville Y, Fernandez H: Pregnancy after heart or heart-lung transplantation: A series of 10 pregnancies. BJOG 105:454, 1998.
78. Morini A, Spina V, Aleandri V, et al: Pregnancy after heart transplant: Update and case report. Hum Reprod 13:749, 1998.
79. Pearson GD, Veille JC, Rahimtoola S, et al: Peripartum cardiomyopathy: NHLBI/NIH workshop recommendations and review. JAMA 283:1183, 2000.
80. Hibbard JU, Lindheimer M, Lang RM: A modified definition for peripartum cardiomyopathy and prognosis based on echocardiography. Obstet Gynecol 94:311, 1999.
81. Sliwa K, Fett J, Elkayam U. Peripartum cardiomyopathy. Lancet 368:687, 2006.
82. Van Hoeven KH, Kitsis RN, Katz SD, et al: Peripartum versus idiopathic dilated cardiomyopathy in young women: A comparison of clinical, pathologic and prognostic features. Int J Cardiol 40:57, 1993.
83. Rezeq MN, Rickenbacher PR, Fowler MB, et al: Incidence of myocarditis in peripartum cardiomyopathy. Am J Cardiol 74:474, 1994.
84. Lampert MB, Weinert L, Hibbard J, et al: Contractile reserve in patients with peripartum cardiomyopathy and recovered left ventricular function. Am J Obstet Gynecol 176:189, 1997.

85. McIndor AK, Hammond EJ, Babington PCB: Peripartum cardiomyopathy presenting as a cardiac arrest at induction of anaesthesia for emergency caesarean section. Br J Anaesth 75:97, 1995.
86. Reimold SC, Rutherford JD: Peripartum cardiomyopathy. N Engl J Med 344:1629, 2001.
87. Cole P, Cook F, Plappert T: Longitudinal changes in left ventricular architecture and function in peripartum cardiomyopathy. Am J Cardiol 60:811, 1987.
88. Fett JD, Christie LG, Carraway RD, et al: Five-year prospective study of the incidence and prognosis of peripartum cardiomyopathy at a single institution. Mayo Clin Proc 80:1602, 2005.
89. St John Sutton M, Cole P, Plappert M: Effects of subsequent pregnancy on left ventricular function in peripartum cardiomyopathy. Am Heart J 121:1776, 1991.
90. Elkayam U, Tummala PP, Rao K, et al: Maternal and fetal outcomes of subsequent pregnancies in women with peripartum cardiomyopathy. N Engl J Med 344:1567, 2001.
91. Fett JD, Christie LG, Murphy JG: Outcome of subsequent pregnancy after peripartum cardiomyopathy: A case series from Haiti. Ann Int Med 145:30, 2006.
92. Oakley GDG, McGarry K, Limb DG, et al: Management of pregnancy in patients with hypertrophic cardiomyopathy. BMJ 1:1749, 1979.
93. Tessler MJ, Hudson R, Naugler-Colville MA, et al: Pulmonary oedema in two parturients with hypertrophic obstructive cardiomyopathy (HOCM). Can J Anaesth 37:469, 1990.
94. Pelliccia F, Cianfroca C, Gaudio C, et al: Sudden death during pregnancy in hypertrophic cardiomyopathy. Eur Heart J 13:421, 1992.
95. Bestetti RB: Cardiac involvement in the acquired immune deficiency syndrome. Int J Cardiol 22:143, 1989.
96. Lewis W: AIDS: Cardiac findings from 115 autopsies. Progr Cardiovasc Dis 32:207, 1989.
97. Raffanti SP, Chiaramida AJ, Sen P, et al: Assessment of cardiac function in patients with the acquired immunodeficiency syndrome. Chest 93:592, 1988.
98. Blanchard DG, Hagenhoff C, Chow L, et al: Reversibility of cardiac abnormalities in human immunodeficiency virus (HIV)-infected individuals: A serial echocardiographic study. J Am Coll Cardiol 17:270, 1991.
99. Heidenreich PA, Eisenberg MJ, Kee LL, et al: Pericardial effusion and AIDS: Incidence and survival. Circulation 92:3229, 1995.
100. The DAD Study Group: Class of antiretroviral drugs and the risk of myocardial infarction. N Engl J Med 356:1723, 2007.
101. Johnson DE, Alderman EL, Schroeder JS, et al: Transplant coronary artery disease: Histopathologic correlation with angiographic morphology. J Am Coll Cardiol 17:449, 1991.
102. Ratnoff OD, Kaufman R: Arterial thrombosis in oral contraceptive users. Arch Intern Med 142:447, 1982.
103. Maekawa K, Ohnish H, Hirase T, et al: Acute myocardial infarction during pregnancy caused by coronary artery spasm. J Intern Med 235:489, 1994.
104. Klutstein MW, Tzivoni D, Bitran D, et al: Treatment of spontaneous coronary artery dissection: Report of three cases. Cathet Cardiovasc Diag 40:372, 1997.
105. Vilke GM, Mahoney G, Chan TC: Postpartum coronary artery dissection. Ann Emerg Med 32:260, 1998.
106. Kearney P, Singh H, Hutter J, et al: Spontaneous coronary artery dissection: A report of three cases and review of the literature. Postgrad Med J 69:940, 1993.
107. Efstratiou A, Singh B: Combined spontaneous postpartum coronary artery dissection and pulmonary embolism with survival. Cathet Cardiovasc Diagn 31:29, 1994.
108. Porras MC, Gill JZ: Intracoronary stenting for postpartum coronary artery dissection. Ann Intern Med 128:873, 1998.
109. Thistlethwaite PA, Tarazi RY, Giordano FJ, et al: Surgical management of spontaneous left main coronary artery dissection. Ann Thorac Surg 66:258, 1998.
110. Koul AK, Hollander G, Moskovits N, et al: Coronary artery dissection during pregnancy and the postpartum period: Two case reports and a review of the literature. Cathet Cardiovasc Intervent 52:88, 2001.
111. Garry D, Leikin E, Fleisher AG, et al: Acute myocardial infarction in pregnancy with subsequent medical and surgical management. Obstet Gynecol 87:802, 1996.
112. Silberman S, Fink D, Berko RS, et al: Coronary artery bypass surgery during pregnancy. Eur J Cardiothorac Surg 10:925, 1996.
113. Mabie WC, Freire MV: Sudden chest pain and cardiac emergencies in the obstetric patient. Obstet Gynecol Clin North Am 22:19, 1995.
114. Roth A, Elkayam U: Acute myocardial infarction associated with pregnancy. Ann Intern Med 125:751, 1996.
115. Xie G-Y, Berk MR, Smith MD, et al: Prognostic value of Doppler transmitral flow patterns in patients with congestive heart disease. J Am Coll Cardiol 24:132, 1994.
116. Maisel AS, Krishnaswany P, Nowalk RM, et al: Rapid measurement of B-type natriuretic peptide in the emergency diagnosis of heart failure. N Engl J Med 347:161, 2002.
117. Engler R, Ray R, Higgins CB, et al: Clinical assessment and follow up of functional capacity in patients with chronic congestive cardiomyopathy. Am J Cardiol 49:1832, 1982.
118. Schroeder JS, Harrison DC: Repeated cardioversion during pregnancy: Treatment of refractory paroxysmal atrial tachycardia during 3 successive pregnancies. Am J Cardiol 27:445, 1971.
119. Pyeritz RE, McKusick VA: The Marfan syndrome: Diagnosis and management. N Engl J Med 300:772, 1979.
120. Brown OR, DeMots H, Kloster FE, et al: Aortic root dilatation and mitral valve prolapse in Marfan's syndrome: An echocardiographic study. Circulation 52:651, 1975.
121. Pyeritz RE: Maternal and fetal complications of pregnancy in Marfan syndrome. Am J Med 71:784, 1981.
122. Shores J, Berger KR, Murphy EA, et al: Progression of aortic dilatation and the benefit of long-term beta-adrenergic blockade in Marfan's syndrome. N Engl J Med 330:1335, 1994.
123. Oakley CM: Anticoagulants in pregnancy. Br Heart J 74:107, 1995.
124. Salazar E, Espinola N, Roman L, et al: Effect of pregnancy on the duration of bovine pericardial bioprostheses. Am Heart J 137:714, 1999.
125. Ginsberg JS, Hirsh J, Turner DC: Risks to the fetus of anticoagulant therapy during pregnancy. Thromb Haemost 61:197, 1989.
126. Ayhan A, Yapar EG, Yuce K, et al: Pregnancy and its complications after cardiac valve replacement. Int J Gynaecol Obstet 35:117, 1991.
127. Chan WS, Anand S, Ginsberg JS: Anticoagulation of pregnant women with mechanical heart valves. Arch Intern Med 160:191, 2000.
128. Evans W, Laifer SA, McNanley TJ, et al: Management of thromboembolic disease associated with pregnancy. J Matern Fetal Med 6:21, 1997.
129. Montalescot G, Polle V, Collet JP, et al: Low molecular weight heparin after mechanical heart valve replacement. Circulation 101:1083, 2000.
130. Arnaout MS, Kazma H, Khalil A, et al: Is there a safe anticoagulation protocol for pregnant women with prosthetic valves? Clin Exp Obstet Gynecol 25:101, 1998.
131. Elkayam U: Pregnancy through a prosthetic heart valve. J Am Coll Cardiol 33:1642, 1999.
132. Ginsberg JS, Chan WS, Bates SM, Kaatz S: Anticoagulation of pregnant women with mechanical heart valves. Arch Intern Med 163:694, 2003.
133. Shapira Y, Sagie A, Battler A: Low-molecular-weight heparin for the treatment of patients with mechanical heart valves. Clin Cardiol 25:323, 2002.
134. Bates SM, Greer IA, Hirsh J, Ginsberg JC: Use of antithrombotic agents during pregnancy: The seventh ACCP conference on antithrombotic and thrombolytic therapy. Chest 126:627S, 2004.
135. Strickland RA, Oliver WC Jr, Chantigian RC, et al: Anesthesia, cardiopulmonary bypass, and the pregnant patient. Mayo Clin Proc 66:411, 1991.
136. Pomini F, Mercogliano D, Cavalletti C, et al: Cardiopulmonary bypass in pregnancy. Ann Thorac Surg 61:259, 1996.

137. Goldstein I, Jacobi P, Gutterman E, et al: Umbilical artery flow velocity during maternal cardiopulmonary bypass. Ann Thorac Surg 60:1116, 1995.
138. Parry AJ, Westaby S: Cardiopulmonary bypass during pregnancy. Ann Thorac Surg 61:1865, 1996.
139. Wilson W, Taubert KA, Gewitz M, et al: Prevention of infective endocarditis: Guidelines from the American Heart Association: A guideline from the American Heart Association Rheumatic Fever, Endocarditis, and Kawasaki Disease Committee, Council on Cardiovascular Disease in the Young, and the Council on Clinical Cardiology, Council on Cardiovascular Surgery and Anesthesia, and the Quality of Care and Outcomes Research Interdisciplinary Working Group. Circulation 116:1736-1754, 2007.

Chapter 40

Coagulation Disorders in Pregnancy

Charles J. Lockwood, MD, and Robert M. Silver, MD

Disorders of the hemostatic system can lead to both hemorrhage and thrombosis. The former can result from inherited and acquired defects in hemostasis and platelets, and the latter is greatly increased in the presence of inherited and acquired defects in the endogenous anticoagulant system.[1,2] In addition to their association with thrombosis, the leading cause of maternal death in the United States, inherited and acquired thrombophilias as well as certain bleeding dyscrasias, have also been associated with adverse pregnancy outcomes. This chapter reviews the hemostatic system and its modulators and then discusses the various common inherited and acquired disorders of platelet function, coagulation, and anticoagulation and their impact on both mother and fetus.

The Hemostatic System

The hemostatic system is designed to ensure that hemorrhage is avoided in the setting of vascular injury while the fluidity of blood is maintained in the intact circulation. After vascular injury, activation of the clotting cascade and simultaneous platelet adherence, activation, and aggregation are required to form the optimal fibrin-platelet plug and thus avoid bleeding. The system is held in check by a potent series of anticoagulant proteins as well as a highly regulated fibrinolytic system. Pregnancy presents an additional challenge to this system, because the risk of hemorrhage during placentation and in the third stage of labor is high, and the risk of thrombosis in the highly vulnerable uteroplacental and intervillous circulations is also great. Through a series of local and systemic adaptations, the vast majority of pregnant women are able to balance these paradoxical requirements and achieve uncomplicated pregnancies.

Platelet Plug Formation

After vascular injury, platelets rolling and flowing in the bloodstream are arrested at sites of endothelial disruption by the interaction of collagen with von Willebrand factor (vWF). Attachment to collagen exposes sites on the vWF molecule that permit it to bind to the platelet glycoprotein Ib/IX/V complex (GpIb-IX-V) receptor.[3] Abnormal platelet adhesion and bleeding can result from mutations in GpIb-X-V (e.g., Bernard-Soulier disease) or from defects in the vWF gene (von Willebrand disease [vWD]). Platelets can also adhere to subendothelial collagen via their GpIa-IIa ($\alpha_2\beta_1$ integrin) and GpVI receptors. Deficiencies in either receptor cause mild bleeding diatheses.

Adherent platelets are activated by collagen after binding to the GpVI receptor.[4] This triggers receptor phosphorylation, leading to activation of phospholipase C, which causes the generation of inositol triphosphate and 1,2,-diacylglycerol. The former triggers a calcium flux, and the latter activates protein kinase C, which, in turn, triggers platelet secretory activity and activates various signaling pathways. Such signaling promotes activation of the GpIIb-IIIa ($\alpha_{IIB}\beta_3$ integrin) receptor, a crucial step in subsequent platelet aggregation (see later discussion). Thus, collagen serves to promote both platelet adhesion and platelet activation. However, maximal platelet activation requires binding of thrombin to platelet type 1 and 4 protease-activated receptors (PAR-1, PAR-4).[5] Platelet activation is also mediated by receptor binding to thromboxane A_2 (TXA_2) and adenosine diphosphate (ADP), which are released by adjacent activated platelets. Collagen and these circulating agonists induce calcium-mediated formation of platelet pseudopodia, promoting further adhesion.

Platelet secretory activity includes the release of α-granules containing vWF, vitronectin, fibronectin, thrombospondin, partially activated factor V, fibrinogen, β-thromboglobulin, and platelet-derived growth factor. These factors either enhance adhesion or promote clotting. Secretory activity also includes the release of dense granules containing ADP and serotonin, which enhance, respectively, platelet activation and vasoconstriction in damaged vessels. Calcium flux promotes the synthesis of TXA_2 by the sequential action of phospholipase A_2, cyclooxygenase-1 (COX-1) and TXA_2 synthase and its passive diffusion across platelet membranes to promote both vasoconstriction and, as noted, activation of adjacent platelets.[4] Inherited disorders of α-granule homeostatic and release proteins result in gray platelet syndrome, whereas deficiencies in dense granule–related genes are associated with Wiskott-Aldrich, Chediak-Higashi, Hermansky-Pudlak, and thrombocytopenia–absent radius syndrome. Inhibition of COX-1–mediated TXA_2 synthesis by nonsteroidal anti-inflammatory drugs (NSAIDs) also can also impair platelet function.

Platelet aggregation follows activation-induced conformational changes in the platelet membrane GpIIb-IIIa receptor, so-called inside-out signaling. The receptor forms a high-affinity bond to divalent fibrinogen molecules. The same fibrinogen molecule is also able to bind to adjacent platelet GpIIb-IIIa receptors.[6] Because these receptors are abundant (40,000 to 80,000 copies), large platelet rosettes quickly form, reducing blood flow and sealing vascular leaks.[4] Mutations in the GpIIb-IIIa gene cause the bleeding dyscrasia known as Glanzmann thrombasthenia. Figure 40-1 presents a schematic review of platelet function.

Platelet activation and aggregation are prevented in intact endothelium via the latter's elaboration of prostacyclin, nitric oxide, and ADPase as well as by active blood flow. Cyclic adenosine monophosphate (cAMP) inhibits platelet activation, and this is the basis for the

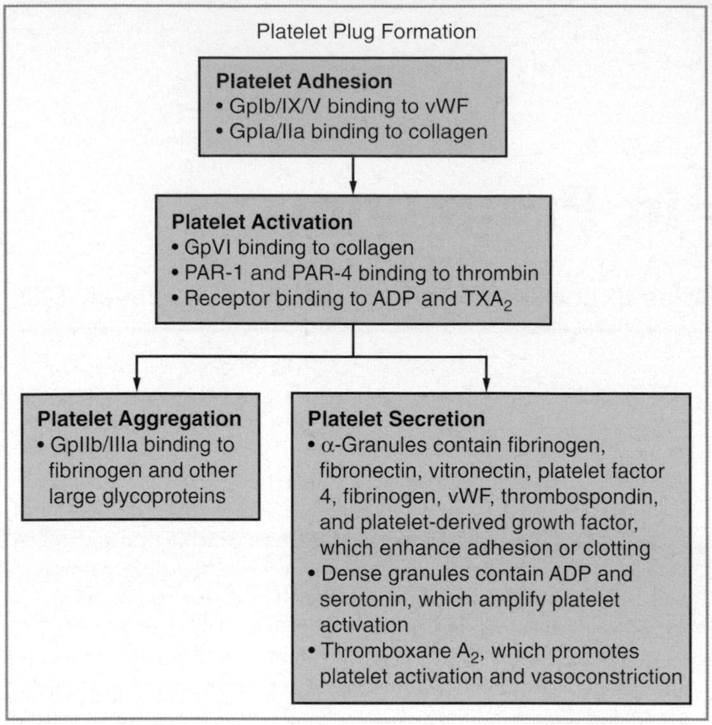

FIGURE 40-1 Schematic review of platelet function. ADP, adenosine diphosphate; Gp, glycoprotein; PAR, protease-activated receptor; TXA_2, thromboxane A_2; vWF, von Willebrand factor.

therapeutic effects of dipyridamole. Normal pregnancy is associated with a modest decline in platelet number[7] and with evidence of progressive platelet activation.[8]

Fibrin Plug Formation

Effective hemostasis requires the synergistic interaction of the clotting cascade with platelet activation and aggregation. This synergism is in part mechanical, because fibrin and platelets together form an effective hemostatic plug after significant vascular disruption. However, biochemical synergism also occurs, because activated platelets contribute clotting factors and form an ideal surface for clot propagation. Conversely, optimal platelet activation and subsequent aggregation require exogenous thrombin generation (see Fig. 40-1). Therefore, the avoidance of hemorrhage ultimately depends on the interplay between platelets and the coagulation cascade.

Understanding of the coagulation component of hemostasis has evolved rapidly in the past two decades. Clotting is no longer thought of as a seemingly infinite cascade of enzymatic reactions occurring in the blood but rather as a highly localized cell surface phenomenon.[9] Clotting is initiated when subendothelial (extravascular) cells expressing tissue factor (TF), a cell membrane–bound glycoprotein, come into contact with circulating factor VII. Intrauterine survival is not possible in the absence TF.[10] TF is primarily expressed on the cell membranes of perivascular smooth muscle cells, fibroblasts, and tissue parenchymal cells, but not on healthy endothelial cells. However, TF also circulates in the blood in very low concentrations, as part of cell-derived microparticles or in a truncated soluble form.[8,11]

After vascular disruption and in the presence of ionized calcium, perivascular cell TF comes into contact with plasma factor VII on negatively charged (anionic) cell membrane phospholipids. Factor VII is unique in that it has low intrinsic clotting activity. In addition, it may autoactivate after binding to TF or be activated by thrombin or factors IXa or Xa.[12] Activation of factor VII to VIIa increases its catalytic activity more than 100-fold, and its promiscuous activation potential ensures that factor VIIa will be readily available to initiate clotting.

The complex of TF and factor VII(a) can activate both factor X and factor IX. Factor Xa remains active as long as it is bound to TF-VIIa in the cell membrane–bound prothrombinase complex. However, when factor Xa diffuses away from the site of vascular injury, it is rapidly inhibited by tissue factor pathway inhibitor (TFPI) or antithrombin (AT). This serves to prevent inappropriate propagation of the clot throughout the vascular tree.[9] Factor Xa ultimately binds to its cofactor, Va, which is generated from its inactive form by the action of factor Xa itself or by thrombin. Partially activated factor Va can also be delivered to the site of clot initiation after its release from platelet α-granules (Fig. 40-2A).[8] The Xa/Va complex catalyzes the conversion of prothrombin (factor II) to thrombin (factor IIa). Thrombin, in turn, converts fibrinogen to fibrin, and, as noted, activates platelets (see Fig. 40-2A).

Following this initial TF-mediated reaction, the clotting cascade is amplified by clotting reactions that occur on adjacent activated platelets.[9] Locally generated factor IXa diffuses to adjacent activated platelet membranes, or to perturbed endothelial cell membranes, where it binds to factor VIIIa. This cofactor is not only directly activated by thrombin but is released from its vWF carrier molecule through the action of thrombin.[9] The factor IXa/VIIIa complex can then generate factor Xa at these sites to further drive thrombin generation (see Fig. 40-2B). The significant hemorrhagic sequelae of hemophilia underscore the vital role played by platelet surface factor IXa-VIIIa–mediated factor Xa generation in ensuring hemostasis.[9]

The clotting cascade can also be amplified via the activation of factor XI to XIa by thrombin on activated platelet surfaces; factor XIa also activates factor IX (see Fig. 40-2C). The lack of significant hemorrhagic sequelae in patients with factor XI deficiency emphasizes that this mechanism is of lesser importance in the maintenance of hemostasis. Factor XIa has been describing as serving a "booster function" in coagulation.[9]

A third, theoretical coagulation amplification pathway may be mediated by circulating TF-bearing microparticles that bind to activated platelets at sites of vascular injury through the interaction between P-selectin glycoprotein ligand-1 on the microparticles and P-selectin on activated platelets (see Fig. 40-2C).[13] Taken together factor IXa, factor XIa, and TF-platelet surface events lead to additional factor Xa generation and thence to enhanced production of thrombin and fibrin. They also reflect the synergism that exists between platelet activation and the coagulation cascade.

The stable hemostatic plug is finally formed only when fibrin monomers self-polymerize and are cross-linked by thrombin-activated factor XIIIa (see Fig. 40-2D). This last reaction highlights the dominant role that thrombin plays in the coagulation cascade: Thrombin activates platelets, generates fibrin, and activates the crucial clotting cofactors V and VIII, as well as the key clotting factors VII, XI, and XIII. This accounts for the primacy of antithrombin factors in preventing inappropriate intravascular clotting (i.e., thrombosis).

Prevention of Thrombosis: The Anticoagulant System

As noted, the hemostatic system not only must prevent hemorrhage after vascular injury but also must maintain the fluidity of the circula-

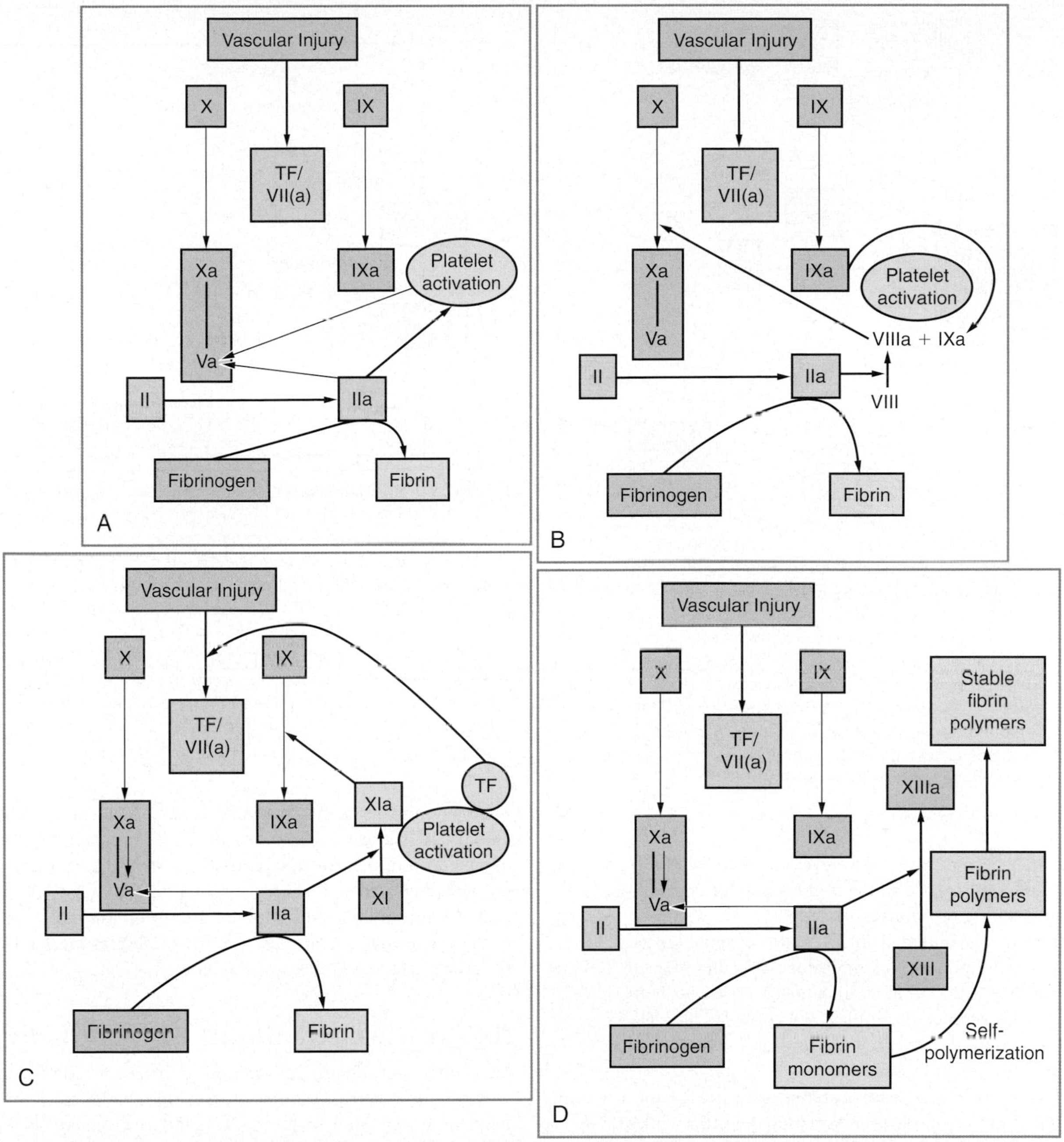

FIGURE 40-2 Fibrin plug formation. **A,** After vascular disruption, plasma factor VII binds to tissue factor (TF) to form the TF/VII(a) complex, which activates both factor X and factor IX. Factor Xa binds to factor Va, which has been activated by thrombin (factor IIa) or released from platelet α-granules. The Xa/Va complex catalyzes the conversion of prothrombin (factor II) to thrombin, which, in turn, converts fibrinogen to fibrin and activates platelets. **B,** The clotting cascade is amplified by clotting reactions that occur on adjacent activated platelets. Locally generated factor IXa binds to factor VIIIa, which is activated by thrombin. The factor IXa/VIIIa complex then generates factor Xa. **C,** Coagulation is further boosted by the thrombin-mediated activation of factor XI to factor XIa, which also activates factor IX. Circulating TF-bearing microparticles may also bind to activated platelets at sites of vascular injury. **D,** The stable hemostatic plug is finally formed when fibrin monomers self-polymerize and are cross-linked by thrombin-activated factor XIIIa.

tion in an intact vasculature. Indeed, thrombotic disease is a consequence of inappropriate and/or excess thrombin generation. As was the case with avoiding hemorrhage, avoidance of thrombosis is again dependent on the synergistic interaction of platelets and the coagulant system. As noted earlier, clotting is initiated locally at sites of vascular injury and amplified by the arrival, adherence, and activation of platelets. This local coagulation reaction is relatively protected from the dampening effects of circulating endogenous anticoagulants, both because of its intensity and because it is shielded by the initial layer of adherent and activated platelets. However, maximal platelet activation occurs only after stimulation by both subendothelial collagen and thrombin, so, as additional platelets aggregate on top of the initial layer

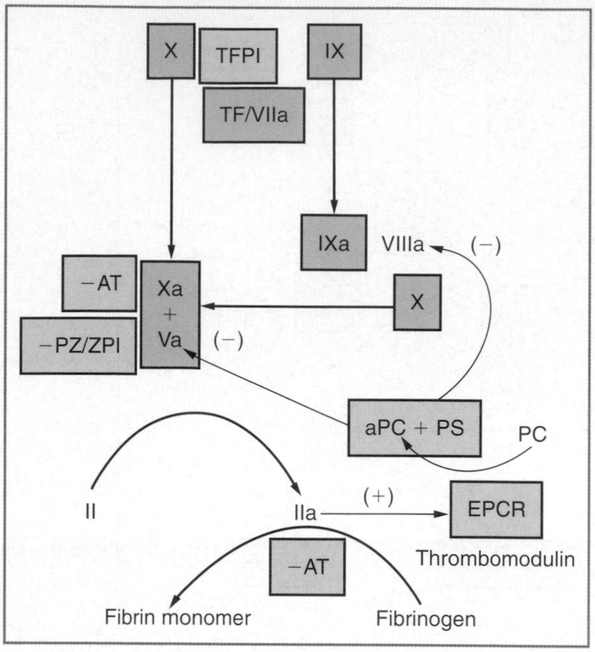

FIGURE 40-3 **The anticoagulant system.** Tissue factor pathway inhibitor (TFPI) binds with tissue factor (TF), factor VIIa, and factor Xa to form the prothrombinase complex. Thrombin, after binding to thrombomodulin, can activate protein C (PC) when bound to the endothelial protein C receptor (EPCR). Activated protein C (aPC) then binds to its cofactor, protein S (PS), to inactivate factors VIIIa and Va. Factor Xa is inhibited by the protein Z-dependent protease inhibitor (ZPI) when complexed to its cofactor, protein Z (PZ). Antithrombin (AT) potently inhibits both factor Xa and thrombin.

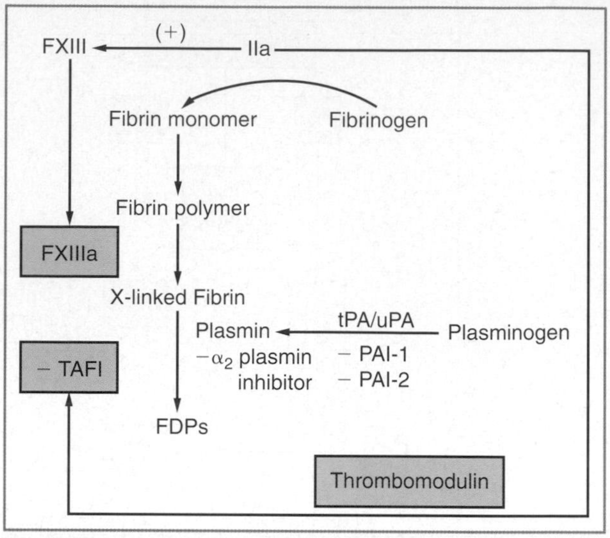

FIGURE 40-4 **Fibrinolysis.** The cross-linked fibrin polymer (X-linked Fibrin), which was stabilized by thrombin (factor IIa)-activated factor XIIIa, is degraded to fibrin degradation products (FDPs) by the action of plasmin, which is generated by the proteolysis of plasminogen via tissue-type plasminogen activator (tPA) and urokinase-type plasminogen activator (uPA). To prevent excessive fibrinolysis, plasmin is inhibited by α_2-plasmin inhibitor, and tPA and uPA are inhibited by plasminogen activator inhibitor type 1 (PAI-1) and type 2 (PAI-2). In addition, thrombin-activated fibrinolytic inhibitor (TAFI), which is activated by the thrombin-thrombomodulin complex, cleaves terminal lysine residues from fibrin to render it resistant to plasmin.

of platelets, they become progressively less activated, and their clotting reaction becomes more susceptible to the action of circulating inhibitors, thus attenuating the clotting cascade.[9]

Prevention of disseminated intravascular coagulation (DIC) ultimately requires the presence of inhibitor molecules (Fig. 40-3). The first inhibitory molecule is TFPI which forms a complex with TF, VIIa, and Xa (the prothrombinase complex).[14] As noted earlier, TFPI is most effective distal to the initial site of clotting, and it can be bypassed by the generation of factors IXa and XIa.

Paralleling its pivotal role in initiating the hemostatic reaction, thrombin also plays a central role in initiating the anticoagulant system. Thrombin binds to thrombomodulin, and the resultant conformational change permits thrombin to activate protein C (PC) when bound to damaged endothelium or the endothelial protein C receptor (EPCR). Activated protein C (aPC) then binds to its cofactor, protein S (PS), to inactivate factors VIIIa and Va. However, this process is far less efficient at blocking thrombin generation on activated platelets, possibly because platelet-derived, partially activated factor Va is resistant to aPC/PS inactivation.[15] Therefore, additional anticoagulant reactions are required. Factor Xa can be efficiently inhibited by the protein Z–dependent protease inhibitor (ZPI) when complexed to its cofactor, protein Z (PZ).[16] ZPI also inhibits factor XIa in a process that does not require PZ. Deficiencies of PZ can promote both intracerebral bleeding and systemic thrombosis, the latter predominating in the setting of coexistent inherited thrombophilias.

The most potent inhibitor of both factor Xa and thrombin is antithrombin (AT, previously known as antithrombin III or ATIII) (see Fig. 40-3). Antithrombin bound to vitronectin can bind thrombin or factor Xa. The resultant conformational change facilitates AT binding to endothelial surface heparanoids or exogenous heparin, which augments thrombin inactivation more than 1000-fold.[17] Although thrombin generated at the initial site of vascular injury is relatively "protected" from AT, thrombin produced more distally on the surface of activated platelets is readily susceptible.[9] Similar inhibitory mechanisms utilize heparin cofactor II and α_2-macroglobulin.

Restoration of Blood Flow: Fibrinolysis

Fibrinolysis permits the restoration of circulatory fluidity and serves as another barrier to thrombosis (Fig. 40-4). The cross-linked fibrin polymer is degraded to fibrin degradation products (FDPs) by the action of plasmin embedded in the fibrin clot.[18] Plasmin is, in turn, generated by the proteolysis of plasminogen via tissue-type plasminogen activator (tPA), which is also embedded in fibrin. Endothelial cells also synthesize a second plasminogen activator, urokinase-type plasminogen activator (uPA), whose primary function is cell migration and extracellular matrix remodeling.

Fibrinolysis is, in turn, modulated by a series of inhibitors. Plasmin is inhibited by α_2-plasmin inhibitor, which, like plasmin and plasminogen, is bound to the fibrin clot, where it is positioned to prevent premature fibrinolysis. Platelets and endothelial cells release type-1 plasminogen activator inhibitor (PAI-1) in response to thrombin binding to PARs. The PAI-1 molecule inhibits both tPA and uPA. In pregnancy, the decidua is also a very rich source of PAI-1,[19] and the placenta can synthesize another antifibrinolytic molecule, PAI-2. Fibrinolysis can also be inhibited by thrombin-activated fibrinolytic inhibitor (TAFI). This carboxypeptidase cleaves terminal lysine residues from fibrin to render it resistant to plasmin. TAFI is activated by the thrombin-thrombomodulin complex.[20] In the initial stages of clotting, platelets and endothelial cells release PAI-1, but, after a delay, endothelial cells release tPA and uPA to promote fibrinolysis. This biologic process permits sequential clotting followed by fibrinolysis to restore vascular patency.

The fibrinolytic system can also interact with the coagulation cascade. FDPs inhibit the action of thrombin, and this is a major source of hemorrhage in DIC. Moreover, PAI-1 bound to vitronectin and heparin also inhibits thrombin and factor Xa activity.[21]

The Effect of Pregnancy on Hemostasis

As noted, pregnancy and delivery present unique and paradoxical challenges to a woman's hemostatic system. They also present one of the greatest risks for venous thromboembolism (VTE) that most young women will face. Profound alterations in both local uterine and systemic clotting, anticoagulant, and fibrinolytic systems are required to meet this enormously complex challenge. The uterine decidua is ideally positioned to regulate hemostasis during placentation and the third stage of labor. Progesterone augments expression of TF[22] and PAI-1[19] on perivascular decidualized endometrial stromal cells. The crucial importance of the decidua in the maintenance of puerperal hemostasis is highlighted by the massive hemorrhage that accompanies obstetric conditions associated with impaired decidualization (e.g., ectopic and cesarean scar pregnancy, placenta previa, and accreta). That decidual TF plays the primary role in mediating puerperal hemostasis is demonstrated by the observation that transgenic TF knockout mice rescued by the expression of low levels of human TF have a 14% incidence of fatal postpartum hemorrhage despite far less invasive placentation.[23]

The extraordinarily high level of TF expression in human decidua can also serve a pathologic function if local hemostasis proves inadequate to contain spiral artery damage and hemorrhage into the decidua occurs (i.e., abruption). This bleeding results in intense generation of thrombin and occasionally in frank hypofibrinogenemia and DIC. However, thrombin can also bind to decidual PAR-1 receptors to promote production of matrix metalloproteinases and cytokines, contributing to the tissue breakdown and inflammation associated with abruptio placenta and preterm premature rupture of the membranes.[24-27]

Pregnancy also induces systemic changes in the hemostatic system. It is associated with a doubling in concentration of fibrinogen and increases of 20% to 1000% in factors VII, VIII, IX, and X as well as vWF.[28] Levels of prothrombin and factor V remain relatively unchanged, and levels of factor XI decline modestly. The net effect is an increase in thrombin-generating potential. Pregnancy is also associated with 60% to 70% declines in free PS levels, which nadir at delivery due to hormonally induced increases in levels of its carrier protein, the complement 4B–binding protein.[29] As a consequence, pregnancy is associated with an increased resistance to aPC. These effects are exacerbated by cesarean delivery and infection, which drive further reduction in the concentration of free PS. Levels of PAI-1 increase threefold to fourfold during pregnancy, and plasma PAI-2 values, which are negligible before pregnancy, reach high concentrations at term.[30] Thus, pregnancy is associated with increased clotting potential, decreased anticoagulant activity, and decreased fibrinolysis.[30]

Pregnancy is also associated with venous stasis in the lower extremities resulting from compression of the inferior vena cava and pelvic veins by the enlarging uterus as well as a hormone-mediated increase in deep vein capacitance secondary to increased circulating levels of estrogen and local production of prostacyclin and nitric oxide. Pregnancy is also frequently associated with obesity, insulin resistance, and hyperlipidemia, all of which further increase levels of PAI-1.[31]

Disorders Promoting Thrombosis in Pregnancy

Acquired Thrombophilias: Antiphospholipid Antibodies

The combination of VTE, obstetric complications, and antiphospholipid antibodies (APA) defines the antiphospholipid antibody syndrome (APS).[32] These antibodies are directed against proteins bound to negatively charged surfaces, usually anionic phospholipids. Therefore, APAs can be detected (1) by screening for antibodies that directly bind protein epitopes such as β_2-glycoprotein-1, prothrombin, annexin V, aPC, PS, protein Z, ZPI, tPA, factor VII(a), and XII, the complement cascade constituents C4 and CH50, and oxidized low-density lipoproteins, or (2) by indirectly assessing antibodies that react to proteins present in an anionic phospholipid matrix (e.g., cardiolipin, phosphatidylserine), or (3) by assessing the downstream effects of these antibodies on prothrombin activation in a phospholipid milieu (i.e., lupus anticoagulants).[33]

The diagnosis of APS has been a controversial topic. A recent consensus conference proposed the criteria outlined in Table 40-1.[34] In brief, APS requires the presence of at least one clinical criterion (confirmed thrombosis or pregnancy morbidity) and one laboratory criterion (lupus anticoagulant [LA], anticardiolipin (ACA), or anti-β_2-glycoprotein-1 antibody). However, the presence of thrombosis must take into account confounding variables that lessen the certainty of the diagnosis (see Table 40-1). Uteroplacental insufficiency may be recognized by the sequelae of nonreassuring fetal surveillance tests suggestive of fetal hypoxemia, abnormal Doppler flow velocimetry waveform analysis suggestive of fetal hypoxemia, oligohydramnios (amniotic fluid index ≤5 cm), or birth weight less than the 10th percentile. Classification of APS should not be made if less than 12 wk or more than 5 years separates the positive APA test and the clinical manifestation.

Venous thrombotic events associated with APA include deep venous thrombosis (DVT) with or without acute pulmonary emboli; cerebral vascular accidents and transient ischemic attacks are the most common arterial events. At least half of patients with APA have systemic lupus erythematosus (SLE). A meta-analysis of 18 studies examining the thrombotic risk among SLE patients with LA, found odds ratios (OR) of 6.32 (95% confidence interval [CI], 3.71 to 10.78) for a VTE episode and 11.6 (CI, 3.65 to 36.91) for recurrent VTE.[35] By contrast, ACAs were associated with lower ORs of 2.50 (CI, 1.51 to 4.14) for an acute VTE and 3.91 (CI, 1.14 to 13.38) for recurrent VTE. A meta-analysis of studies involving more than 7000 patients in the general population identified a range of ORs for arterial and venous thromboses in patients with LA: 8.6 to 10.8 and 4.1 to 16.2, respectively.[33] The comparable numbers for ACA were 1 to 18 and 1 to 2.5. Therefore, there appears to be a consistently greater risk of VTE associated with LA compared with isolated ACA. Recurrence risks of up to 30% have been reported in affected patients, so long-term prophylaxis is required.[36] The risk of VTE in pregnancy and the puerperium accruing to affected patients is poorly studied but may be as high as 5% despite treatment.[37]

As noted, APA are associated with obstetric complications including fetal loss, abruption, severe preeclampsia, and intrauterine growth

TABLE 40-1 REVISED CLASSIFICATION CRITERIA FOR DIAGNOSIS OF THE ANTIPHOSPHOLIPID ANTIBODY SYNDROME (APS)*

Clinical Criteria

1. Vascular thrombosis†: One or more clinical episodes of arterial, venous, or small-vessel thrombosis, in any tissue or organ confirmed by objective, validated criteria (i.e., unequivocal findings of appropriate imaging studies or histopathology).
2. Pregnancy morbidity:
   a. One or more unexplained deaths of a morphologically normal fetus at or beyond 10 weeks of gestation, with normal fetal morphology documented by ultrasound or by direct examination of the fetus, or
   b. One or more premature births of a morphologically normal neonate before the 34th week of gestation because of (i) eclampsia or severe preeclampsia or (ii) recognized uteroplacental insufficiency, or
   c. Three or more unexplained consecutive euploid spontaneous abortions before 10 weeks of gestation, with maternal anatomic or hormonal abnormalities and paternal and parental chromosomal causes excluded.

Laboratory Criteria‡

1. Lupus anticoagulant (LA) present in plasma, on two or more occasions at least 12 wk apart, detected according to the guidelines of the ISTH Scientific Subcommittee on Lupus Anticoagulants/Phospholipid-Dependent Antibodies.
2. Anticardiolipin antibody (aCL) of IgG and/or IgM isotype in serum or plasma, present in medium or high titer (i.e., >40 GPL or MPL, or >99th percentile), on two or more occasions, at least 12 wk apart, measured by a standardized ELISA.
3. Anti-β_2-glycoprotein-1 antibody of IgG and/or IgM isotype in serum or plasma (in titer >99th percentile), present on two or more occasions, at least 12 wk apart, measured by a standardized ELISA, according to recommended procedures.

***APS is present if at least one clinical criterion and one laboratory criterion are met.**

†Coexisting inherited or acquired factors for thrombosis are not reasons for excluding patients from APS trials. However, two subgroups of APS patients should be recognized, according to (1) the presence or (2) the absence of additional risk factors for thrombosis. Indicative (but not exhaustive) of such factors are age (>55 yr in men, >65 yr in women); presence of any of the established risk factors for cardiovascular disease (hypertension, diabetes mellitus, elevated LDL or low HDL cholesterol, cigarette smoking, family history of premature cardiovascular disease, BMI ≥30 kg/m^2, microalbuminuria, estimated GFR <60 mL/min), inherited thrombophilias, oral contraceptive use, nephrotic syndrome, malignancy, immobilization, and surgery. Patients who fulfill criteria should be stratified according to contributing causes of thrombosis.

‡Investigators are strongly advised to classify APS patients in studies into one of the following categories: I, more than one laboratory criteria present (any combination); IIa, LA present alone; IIb, aCL antibody present alone; IIc, Anti-β_2 glycoprotein-1 antibody present alone.

APA, antiphospholipid antibody; BMI, body mass index; ELISA, enzyme-linked immunosorbent assay; GFR, glomerular filtration rate; GPL, IgG phospholipid units; HDL, high-density lipoprotein; IgG, immunoglobulin G; IgM, immunoglobulin M; ISTH, International Society on Thrombosis and Hemostasis; LDL, low-density lipoprotein; MPL, IgM phospholipid units.

Modified from Miyakis S, Lockshin MD, Atsumi D, et al: International consensus statement on an update of the classification criteria for definite antiphospholipid syndrome (APS). J Thromb Haemost 4:295-306, 2006.

restriction (IUGR). LA are associated with fetal loss after the first trimester, with ORs ranging from 3.0 to 4.8, and ACA display a wider range of ORs, 0.86 to 20.0.[33] It is controversial whether APA are associated with recurrent (more than three) early (<10 weeks) spontaneous abortions in the absence of stillbirth. At least 50% of pregnancy losses in patients with APA occur after the 10th week of gestation.[38] Moreover, compared with patients who have unexplained first-trimester spontaneous abortions without APA, those with antibodies more often have demonstrable embryonic cardiac activity (86% versus 43%; $P < .01$).[39]

The association between APA and infertility also is uncertain. Increased levels of APA have been reported in women with infertility.[40,41] However, a meta-analysis of seven studies of affected patients undergoing in vitro fertilization found no significant association between APA and either clinical pregnancy (OR, 0.99; CI, 0.64 to 1.53) or live birth rate (OR, 1.07; CI, 0.66 to 1.75).[42] Finally, there is also no evidence that treating patients who have APA with anticoagulant medications improves outcomes of in vitro fertilization.[43]

Women with APS who have pregnancies reaching viability are at increased risk for obstetric outcomes associated with abnormal placentation such as preeclampsia and IUGR. Up to 50% of pregnancies in women with APS develop preeclampsia, and one third have IUGR.[37] Abnormal fetal heart rate tracings prompting cesarean delivery are also common. Conversely, most cases of preeclampsia and IUGR occur in women without APA. Although increased positive tests for APA have been reported in women with preeclampsia, especially in severe disease with onset before 34 weeks' gestation[44] and IUGR, most large retrospective and prospective studies have not found an association between these conditions and APA.[45] This is not surprising, given the common occurrence of preeclampsia and IUGR and the relative infrequency of APS.

A myriad of mechanisms have been proposed for APA-mediated arterial and venous thrombosis. Direct inhibition of the anticoagulant effects of anionic phospholipid-binding proteins such as β_2-glycoprotein-1 and annexin V has been shown.[46,47] In addition, APA appear to inhibit thrombomodulin, aPC, and AT activity; to induce TF, PAI-1, and vWF expression in endothelial cells; and to augment platelet activation. Recently, APA induction of complement activation has been suggested to play a role in fetal loss, with heparin preventing such aberrant activation.[48]

Contemporary management of affected patients during pregnancy requires treatment with either unfractionated heparin or low-molecular-weight heparin (LMWH) plus low-dose aspirin (LDA) at 50 to 80 mg/day. Rai and colleagues conducted a randomized, controlled trial among 90 APA-positive women with a history of recurrent fetal loss who received either LDA alone or LDA plus 5000 U of unfractionated heparin SQ every 12 hours until either recurrent loss or 34 weeks of gestation.[39] The live birth rate was significantly higher with combined heparin and LDA than with LDA alone: 71% (32/45) versus 42% (19/45) (OR, 3.37; CI, 1.40 to 8.10). Interestingly, 90% of the losses occurred in the first trimester, and there was no difference in outcome between the two groups for women whose pregnancies advanced beyond 13 weeks' gestation. Similar results were found in a nonrandomized trial by Kutteh.[49] On the other hand, Farquharson and coworkers found no advantage to adding LMWH to LDA.[50] However, this latter study has been criticized because of the very low levels of APA present in affected patients as well as imperfect randomization. Meta-analysis found that unfractionated heparin plus LDA (two trials; $N = 140$) significantly reduced pregnancy loss compared with LDA alone (relative risk [RR], 0.46; CI, 0.29 to 0.71) and that there was no advantage of high-dose over low-dose unfractionated heparin (one trial; $N = 50$).[51] Another meta-analysis found that enoxaparin treatment resulted in an increased live birth rate, compared with LDA (RR, 10.0; CI, 1.56 to 64.20).[52] Three studies of LDA alone versus placebo included in the meta-analysis showed no significant reduction in pregnancy loss (RR, 1.05; CI, 0.66 to 1.68).[51]

Adverse pregnancy outcomes can still occur despite treatment. Backos and associates conducted a prospective observational study of 150 women treated with LDA and either unfractionated heparin (5000 U given SQ every 12 hours) or enoxaparin (20 mg daily) from the time of positive embryonic cardiac activity to either pregnancy loss or 34 weeks of gestation.[53] The live birth rate was 71%. However, 27% of the patients miscarried (mostly in the first trimester), and gestational hypertension occurred in 17%, abruption in 7%, and IUGR in 15%.

Intravenous immune globulin (IVIG) has been reported to improve outcome in women with APS for whom treatment with heparin and LDA has failed.[54] The efficacy of the combination of LDA and LMWH in affected patients was compared with that of IVIG for the prevention of recurrent fetal loss in a study including 40 women,[55] who were randomized to receive either LMWH (5700 IU/day SQ) and LDA or IVIG (400 mg/kg IV for 2 days, followed by 400 mg/kg every month). Although the clinical characteristics of the two groups were similar at the time of randomization, women receiving LMWH and LDA had a higher live birth rate (84%) than those receiving IVIG alone (57%). Moreover, IVIG plus heparin and LDA was also not superior to heparin and LDA alone in another small, randomized trial.[56] Therefore, IVIG is not recommended as first-line therapy for APS.

Given these small study sizes and heterogeneous therapies employed, recommendations for treatment are difficult to make. It is unlikely that a patient with no history of VTE who has repetitive early losses and borderline positive APA levels reflects the same degree of risk or need for intense therapy as a patient with high levels of APA, prior VTE, and recurrent growth-retarded stillbirths. It is unclear whether the former patient requires any therapy, but the latter patient needs therapeutic unfractionated heparin or LMWH with LDA.[57] Tincani and associates reported on a survey of members of the International Advisory Board of the 10th International Congress on Antiphospholipid Antibodies. The consensus of the group was that treatment for APA-positive pregnant patients should be LMWH and LDA.[57] The dosage and frequency of LMWH depends on the situation, including the patient's body weight and past history. Patients with previous thromboses should receive two injections per day. The use of IVIG should be restricted to patients with pregnancy losses despite conventional treatment (see later discussion for details of heparin dosing).

Inherited Thrombophilias

Inherited thrombophilias have been linked to VTE. However, the occurrence of VTE in patients with an inherited thrombophilia is highly dependent on the presence of other predisposing factors, especially a personal or family history of VTE. Even more controversial is the association between inherited thrombophilias and adverse pregnancy outcomes.

Factor V Leiden Mutation

Present in about 5% of the European population and 3% of African-Americans, factor V Leiden (FVL) is the most common of the serious heritable thrombophilias.[58] The mutation is virtually absent in African blacks, Chinese, Japanese, and other Asians. The mutation causes a substitution of glutamine for arginine at position 506, the site of proteolysis and inactivation by aPC/PS, and FVL is the leading cause of aPC resistance. The heterozygous state is symptomatic, with a fivefold increased risk of VTE, but homozygous patients have a 25-fold increased risk (Table 40-2). FVL is associated with about 40% of VTE events in pregnant patients.[59] However, given the low prevalence of VTE in pregnancy (1/1400) and the high incidence of the mutation in the European-derived population, the risk of VTE among FVL heterozygotes without a personal history of VTE or an affected first-degree relative is less than 0.3%.[59] Nevertheless, the risk is at least 10% among pregnant women who have either a personal history of VTE or an affected first-degree relative.[60] Pregnant homozygous patients without a personal history of VTE or an affected first-degree relative have a 1.5% risk for VTE in pregnancy; if there is a personal or family history

TABLE 40-2 INHERITED THROMBOPHILIAS AND THEIR ASSOCIATION WITH VENOUS THROMBOEMBOLISM (VTE) IN PREGNANCY

		Probability of VTE (%) without or with a Personal History of VTE or a First-Degree Relative with VTE		
Thrombophilia	**Relative Risk of VTE (95% CI)**	Without	With	**Ref. No.**
FVL (homozygous)	25.4 (8.8-66)	1.5	17	46
FVL (heterozygous)	5.3 (3.7-7.6)	0.20-0.26	10	45, 46
PGM (homozygous)	NA	2.8	>17	46
PGM (heterozygous)	6.1 (3.4-11.2)	0.37	>10	45, 46
FVL/PGM (compound heterozygous)	84 (19-369)	4.7	NA	46
Antithrombin deficiency (<60% activity)	119	3.0-7.2	>40%	46, 47
Protein S deficiency (<55% activity)	NA	<1	6.6	46, 47
Protein C deficiency (<50% activity)	13.0 (1.4-123)	0.8-1.7	2-8	46, 47

CI, confidence interval; FVL, factor V Leiden mutation; NA, not available; PGM, prothrombin gene mutation.

of VTE, the risk is 17% (see Table 40-2). Screening can be done by assessing aPC resistance using a second-generation coagulation assay followed by genotyping for the FVL mutation if aPC resistance is found in a pregnant or nonpregnant woman. Alternatively, patients can simply be genotyped for FVL.

The College of American Pathologists Consensus Conference on Thrombophilia compared 16 case-control studies reporting a link between FVL and unexplained recurrent fetal loss and 6 studies failing to establish such an association and concluded that the latter studies were smaller and tended to include patients with early first-trimester losses.[61,62] In a meta-analysis of 31 studies, FVL was associated with early (<13 weeks) pregnancy loss, with an OR of 2.01 (CI, 1.13 to 3.58), but it was more strongly associated with late (>19 weeks), nonrecurrent fetal loss, with an OR of 3.26 (CI, 1.82 to 5.83).[63] A case-control study noted an even stronger link between FVL and recurrent fetal losses after 22 weeks' gestation (OR, 7.83; CI, 2.83 to 21.67).[64] Dudding and Attia conducted a meta-analysis and found no significant association between FVL and first-trimester loss but an OR of 2.4 (CI, 1.1 to 5.2) for isolated (nonrecurrent) third-trimester fetal loss, which increased to 10.7 (CI, 4.0 to 28.5) for two or more second- or third-trimester fetal losses.[65] Similarly, Lissalde-Lavigne and associates reported the results of a case-control study nested in the 32,700 Nimes Obstetricians and Haematologists (NOHA) First study cohort.[66] Multivariate analysis revealed an association between FVL and pregnancy loss after 10 weeks (OR, 3.46; CI, 2.53 to 4.72) but not for losses occurring between 3 and 9 weeks. These studies strongly suggest that FVL is associated with fetal (>9 weeks) and not embryonic (<9 weeks) losses.

The association between FVL and late, compared with early, pregnancy losses was also demonstrated by a large European retrospective cohort study involving 571 women with thrombophilia having 1524 pregnancies, compared with 395 controls having 1019 pregnancies.[67] There was a statistically significant association between any inherited thrombophilia and stillbirth (OR, 3.6; CI, 1.4 to 9.4) but not spontaneous abortion (OR, 1.27; CI, 0.94 to 1.71). The same trend was noted for FVL, with an OR for stillbirth of 2.0 (CI, 0.5 to 7.7) compared with 0.9 for spontaneous abortion (CI, 0.5 to 1.5). These same investigators then monitored a subset of 39 thrombophilic and 51 control patients who had no previous history of fetal loss and did not receive anticoagulation during the prospective follow-up aspect of the study.[68] They reported a modestly increased overall risk of fetal loss in a subsequent pregnancy among women with thrombophilia (7/39 versus 7/51; RR, 1.4; CI, 0.4 to 4.7) and also among those with FVL (RR, 1.4; CI, 0.3 to 5.5). However, this study lacked power to exclude the usually reported twofold to threefold higher rates of loss associated with FVL, because there were only 21 patients. Nevertheless, given the trends, the authors concluded that "Women with thrombophilia appear to have an increased risk of fetal loss, although the likelihood of a positive outcome is high in both women with thrombophilia and in controls."[68]

In a retrospective cohort study, Roque and colleagues evaluated 491 patients with a history of various adverse pregnancy outcomes for a variety of thrombophilias and reported that the presence of FVL was paradoxically protective against losses before 10 weeks of gestation (OR, 0.23; CI, 0.07 to 0.77) but was significantly associated with losses after 14 weeks (OR, 3.71; CI, 1.68 to 8.23).[69] Moreover, women who experienced only euploid losses were not more likely to have an identified thrombophilia than women who experienced only aneuploid early losses (OR, 1.03; CI, 0.38 to 2.75). Consistent with this protective effect of FVL on early pregnancy is the observation that implantation rates after in vitro fertilization were substantially higher among FVL carriers than among noncarriers (90% versus 49%; $P = .02$).[70]

Early pregnancy is associated with a low-oxygen environment, with intervillous oxygen pressures of 17.9 ± 6.9 mm Hg at 8 to 10 weeks, rising to 60.7 ± 8.5 mm Hg at 12 to 13 weeks.[71] Trophoblast plugging of the spiral arteries has been demonstrated in placental histologic studies before 10 weeks of gestation, and low Doppler flow is noted in the uteroplacental circulation before 10 weeks.[72] Indeed, the undetectable levels of superoxide dismutase in trophoblast before 10 weeks of gestation are consistent with a hypoxic state.[73] Therefore, if FVL or other thrombophilias are associated with early pregnancy loss, it is most likely through mechanisms other than placental thrombosis. Also, because a majority of early pregnancy losses are associated with aneuploidy, thrombophilias are likely to play a far lesser role in such cases. In contrast, uteroplacental thrombosis after 9 weeks would be expected to reduce oxygen and nutrient delivery to a progressively larger embryo, accounting for the apparent link between FVL and the other maternal thrombophilias and later adverse pregnancy outcomes.

The correlation between FVL and other later adverse pregnancy events is more controversial. Kupferminc and associates studied 110 women and reported a link between FVL and severe preeclampsia (OR, 5.3; CI, 1.8 to 15.6).[74] However, multiple case-control studies have failed to demonstrate a link between FVL and moderate or severe preeclampsia.[75-77] Dudding and Attia's meta-analysis estimated a 2.9-fold (CI, 2.0 to 4.3) increased risk of severe preeclampsia among FVL carriers.[65] Similarly, Lin and August conducted a meta-analysis of 31 studies involving 7522 patients and reported pooled ORs of 1.81 (CI, 1.14 to 2.87) for FVL and all preeclampsia and 2.24 (CI, 1.28 to 3.94) for FVL and severe preeclampsia.[78] However, Kosmas and coauthors evaluated 19 studies involving 2742 hypertensive women and 2403 controls and reported that, whereas the studies published before 2000 found a modest association between FVL and preeclampsia (OR, 3.16; CI, 2.04 to 4.92), those published after 2000 did not (OR, 0.97; CI, 0.61 to 1.54).[79] This suggests a reporting bias. Therefore, there is not sufficient evidence to conclude that FVL is associated with an increased occurrence of preeclampsia, although there is inadequate power to rule out an association between this thrombophilia and severe, early-onset preeclampsia.

Kupferminc and colleagues also reported a modest association between FVL and abruption (OR, 4.9; CI, 1.4 to 17.4).[74] A second case-control study found that 17 of 27 patients with abruption had aPC resistance, compared with 5 of 29 control subjects (OR, 8.16; CI, 3.6 to 12.75), and 8 cases were found to have the FVL mutation, compared with one control.[80] Prochazka and associates conducted a retrospective case-control study among 180 women with placental abruption and 196 controls and found a significantly increased incidence of FVL carriage among cases compared with controls (14.1% versus 5.1%; OR, 3.0; CI, 1.4 to 6.7).[81] Alfirevic and coworkers conducted a meta-analysis that revealed a strong association between placental abruption and both homozygosity and heterozygosity for the FVL mutation (OR, 16.9; CI, 2.0 to 141.9, and OR, 6.7; CI, 2.0 to 21.6, respectively).[82] Therefore, there appears to be evidence of an association between FVL carriage and placental abruption, although large case-control and retrospective cohort studies are needed to confirm this link.

There is less consistent evidence for an association between FVL and IUGR. Martinelli and coauthors reported a strong association between FVL and IUGR (OR, 6.9; CI, 1.4 to 33.5).[83] However, multiple, large case-control and cohort studies have reported no statistically significant association between FVL and IUGR of less than the 10th or less than the 5th percentile.[74,77,84] Howley and colleagues conducted a systematic review of studies describing the association between FVL and IUGR; among 10 case-control studies meeting selection criteria, there was a significant association between FVL and IUGR (OR, 2.7;

CI, 1.3 to 5.5).[85] However, no association was found among five cohort studies, of which three were prospective and two retrospective (RR, 0.99; CI, 0.5 to 1.9). The authors suggested that the putative association between IUGR and FVL was most likely driven by small, poor-quality studies that demonstrated extreme associations.

In summary, there appears to be a modest association between FVL and fetal loss after 10 weeks, and particularly with isolated losses after 22 weeks. There is a possible association between FVL and abruption. However, no clear association exists between FVL and either preeclampsia or IUGR, although studies have been underpowered to definitely exclude a link with severe early-onset preeclampsia or severe IUGR. It also is noteworthy that two prospective cohort studies found no association between FVL and any adverse obstetric outcome, including pregnancy loss, preeclampsia, and IUGR,[86,87] but these studies were underpowered to draw firm conclusions. It is important to note that, although thrombophilia may be sufficient to cause pregnancy loss and perhaps abruption, most affected individuals without such prior obstetric complications are at low risk for subsequent adverse pregnancy outcomes.

Other Factor V Mutations

Other mutations in the factor V gene have been variably linked to maternal VTE and adverse pregnancy outcomes. The factor V HR2 haplotype causes decreased factor V cofactor activity in the aPC-mediated degradation of factor VIIIa; however, a meta-analysis demonstrated no statistically significant association between the HR2 haplotype and risk of VTE (OR, 1.15; CI, 0.98 to 1.36).[88] There are conflicting reports about the linkage of the factor V HR2 haplotype and recurrent pregnancy loss. Zammiti and associates reported no association with losses before 8 weeks, but homozygosity for the factor V HR2 haplotype was associated with significant and independent risks of pregnancy loss during weeks 8 and 9, which increased during weeks 10 to 12 and culminated after 12 weeks.[89] In contrast, Dilley and colleagues found no association between carriage of the factor V HR2 haplotype and pregnancy loss.[90] The sample sizes of these studies were too small to draw firm conclusions from, nor can conclusions be reached about the link between factor V HR2 haplotype and other adverse pregnancy outcomes.

Two other mutations in the factor V gene that occur at the second aPC cleavage site, factor V R306G Hong Kong and factor V R306T Cambridge, have also been described but do not appear to be strongly associated with VTE.[91] There are inadequate data to assess any linkage between these mutations and adverse pregnancy outcomes.[89]

Prothrombin Gene Mutation

The prothrombin G20210A polymorphism is a point mutation causing a guanine→adenine switch at nucleotide position 20210 in the 3′-untranslated region of the gene.[58] This nucleotide switch results in increased translation, possibly due to enhanced stability of messenger RNA (mRNA). As a consequence, there are increased circulating levels of prothrombin. Although the mutation is present in only 2% to 3% of the European population, it is associated with 17% of VTEs in pregnancy.[59] However, as was the case with FVL, the risk of VTE in pregnant patients who are heterozygous for the prothrombin G20210A gene mutation (PGM) but who are without a personal or strong family history of VTE is less than 0.5%.[59] Pregnant PGM-heterozygous patients with such a history have at least a 10% risk of VTE.[60] PGM-homozygous patients without a personal or strong family history have a 2.8% risk for VTE in pregnancy, whereas such a history probably confers a risk of at least 20% (see Table 40-2). Because the combination of FVL and PGM has synergistic hypercoagulable effects, compound heterozygotes are at greater thrombotic risk than either FVL or PGM homozygotes. Pregnant patients who are compound heterozygotes without a personal or strong family history have a 4.7% risk of VTE.[59,60]

The PGM has been associated with an increased risk of pregnancy loss in multiple case-control studies. One such study reported the presence of the PGM in 7 of 80 patients with recurrent miscarriage, compared with 2 of 100 control patients (9% versus 2%; $P = .04$; OR, 4.7; CI, 0.9 to 23).[92] Finan and associates also found an association between PGM and recurrent abortion, with an OR of 5.05 (CI, 1.14 to 23.2).[93] However, other studies have failed to identify a link.[94,95] A 2004 meta-analysis of seven studies evaluating the correlation between PGM and recurrent pregnancy loss, defined as two or more losses in the first or second trimester, found a combined OR of 2.0 (CI, 1.0 to 4.0).[96] Analogous to FVL, the association between PGM and pregnancy loss increases with increasing gestational age. In the meta-analysis by Rey and colleagues, an association was reported between PGM and recurrent loss before 13 weeks' gestation (OR, 2.3; CI, 1.2 to 4.79), but, as with FVL, a stronger association was observed between PGM and recurrent fetal loss before 25 weeks (OR, 2.56; CI, 1.04 to 6.29).[63] Therefore, PGM appears to fit the pattern displayed by FVL carriers of progressively greater risk of fetal loss with advancing gestation; however, these risks remain quite modest.

There are more limited data on the association between PGM and abruption. The case-control study of Kupferminc and associates found an association between the PGM and abruptio placenta (OR, 8.9; CI, 1.8 to 43.6),[74] whereas Prochazka and colleagues found no such link.[81] Meta-analyses suggested a strong link between PGM heterozygosity and placental abruption (OR, 28.9; CI, 3.5 to 236.7).[82] It can be concluded that there is probably a link between the PGM and abruptio placentae.

The link between the PGM and other adverse pregnancy events is far less certain. Kupferminc and colleagues found an association between the PGM and IUGR of less than the 5th percentile (OR, 4.6; CI, 1 to 20) but no link between the PGM and severe preeclampsia.[74] Martinelli and coworkers noted a strong association between PGM and IUGR in their case-control study (OR, 5.9; CI, 1.2 to 29.4).[83] In contrast, the large case-control study of Infante-Rivard and colleagues reported no link in heterozygotes between PGM and IUGR, with an OR of 0.92 (CI, 0.36 to 2.35).[84] Similar results have been observed by other workers.[74,80] A number of other case-control studies and meta-analyses have failed to establish a link between PGM and either preeclampsia or severe preeclampsia.[77,78,97,98]

Therefore, although most individual studies are limited by small sample size, case-control design, and the potential for selection biases (as was the case with FVL), there may be a weak association between the PGM and fetal loss as well as abruptio placenta. However, there does not appear to be a significant link between PGM and IUGR or preeclampsia.

Hyperhomocysteinemia

Hyperhomocysteinemia can result from a number of mutations in the methionine metabolic pathway. Homozygosity for mutations in the methylene tetrahydrofolate reductase (MTHFR) gene is by far the most common cause. Homozygosity for the MTHFR C677T polymorphism is present in 10% to 16% of all Europeans, and that for the A1298C mutation occurs in 4% to 6%.[99] Importantly, about 40% of whites are heterozygous for this polymorphism, and most heterozygotes have normal levels of homocysteine. Moreover, because homocysteine levels decrease in pregnancy and U.S. diets are replete with folic acid supplementation, hyperhomocysteinemia is extremely rare even among homozygotes. In addition, although hyperhomocysteinemia is a risk factor for VTE (OR, 2.5; CI, 1.8 to 3.5),[100] MTHFR mutations per se do not appear to convey an increased risk for VTE in either nonpregnant[101] or pregnant women.[102]

As with thrombotic risk, meta-analyses suggest that elevated fasting homocysteine levels are more strongly associated with recurrent pregnancy loss (<16 weeks) than are MTHFR mutations, with an OR of 2.7 (CI, 1.4 to 5.2) versus 1.4 (CI, 1.0 to 2.0), respectively.[103] The Hordaland Homocysteine Study assessed the relationship between plasma homocysteine values in 5883 women and their prior 14,492 pregnancy outcomes.[104] When the authors compared the upper with the lower quartile of plasma homocysteine levels, elevated levels trended toward an association with preeclampsia (OR, 1.32; CI, 0.98 to 1.77), very low birth weight (OR, 2.01; CI, 1.23 to 3.27), and stillbirth (OR, 2.03; CI, 0.98 to 4.21), although none of these associations reached statistical significance.[105] In contrast, a clear association was demonstrated between placental abruption and homocysteine levels greater than 15 μmol/L (OR, 3.13; CI, 1.63 to 6.03), and a weaker but significant association was observed between homozygosity for the C677T MTHFR mutation and abruption (OR, 1.6; CI, 1.4 to 4.8). Indeed, a meta-analysis of these two risk factors found that hyperhomocysteinemia had a larger pooled OR for abruption (5.3; CI, 1.8 to 15.9) than did homozygosity for the MTHFR mutation (2.3; CI, 1.1 to 4.9).[106]

These studies strongly suggest that hyperhomocysteinemia, but not simply the presence of the MTHFR mutations, is linked to VTE and adverse pregnancy outcomes. Moreover, whereas homozygosity for MTHFR mutations is very common (10% to 20% in European populations), hyperhomocysteinemia is quite rare. Therefore, screening for this disorder should be limited, requiring a fasting homocysteine level greater than 12 μmol/L to be considered positive in pregnant patients.[146]

Antithrombin Deficiency

Deficiency of AT is both the rarest and the most thrombogenic of the heritable thrombophilias. More than 250 mutations have been identified in the AT gene, producing a highly variable phenotype. In general, disorders can be classified into three types: type 1, those associated with reductions in both antigen and activity; type 2, those associated with normal levels of antigen but decreased activity; and type 3, the very rare homozygous deficiency associated with little or no activity.[58,108] Complicating matters further, patients can develop acquired AT deficiency due to liver impairment, increased consumption of AT associated with sepsis or DIC, or increased renal excretion in severe nephrotic syndrome. However, both inherited and acquired AT deficiencies are associated with VTE.

Because screening for AT deficiency is done by assessing activity, its prevalence varies with the activity cutoff level employed, ranging from 0.02% to 1.1%. The recommended cutoff for "abnormality" is 50% activity, which is associated with a prevalence of 0.04% (1/2500 people).[108] Although it increases the risk of VTE up to 25-fold in the nonpregnant state,[108] because of its rarity AT deficiency is associated with only 1% to 8% of VTE episodes.[58] Pregnancy may increase its thrombogenic potential substantially (see Table 40-2). Moreover, use of a less stringent threshold yields a higher prevalence of AT deficiency in patients with VTE. For example, in one study, 19.3% of pregnant women with VTE had less than 80% AT activity,[59] but many of these cases may have been acquired due to clot-associated AT consumption. Conversely, the overall risk of VTE in pregnancy associated with AT deficiency has been variably reported as 3% to 48%.[30,60,109,110] The risk of VTE in pregnancy among AT-deficient patients most likely varies also with a personal or family history (from 3% to 7% without such a history to as much as 40% with such a history).[60]

In the largest retrospective cohort study, AT deficiency was associated with a significantly increased risk of stillbirth after 28 weeks' gestation (OR, 5.2; CI, 1.5 to 18.1) but had a more modest association with miscarriage before 28 weeks (OR, 1.7; CI, 1.0 to 2.8).[67] Given its rarity, there is a paucity of evidence concerning the link between AT deficiency and other adverse pregnancy outcomes. Roque and associates found it to be associated with increased risks of IUGR (OR, 12.93; CI, 2.72 to 61.45), abruption (OR, 60.01; CI, 12.02 to 300.46), and preterm delivery (OR, 4.72; CI, 1.22 to 18.26).[69]

Protein C Deficiency

Deficiency of PC results from more than 160 distinct mutations, producing a highly variable phenotype. As was the case with AT deficiency, PC deficiency can be associated with either reductions in both antigen and activity (type 1) or normal levels of antigen but decreased activity (type 2).[58] The very rare homozygous PC deficiency results in neonatal purpura fulminans and a requirement for lifelong anticoagulation.[111] Activity levels can be ascertained by either a functional (clotting) or chromogenic assay.

Estimates of prevalence and thrombotic risk reflect the cutoff values employed. Most laboratories use activity cutoff values of 50% to 60%, which are associated with prevalence estimates of 0.2% to 0.3% and RRs for VTE of 6.5 to 12.5.[58,68,108] The risk of VTE in pregnancy among PC-deficient patients has been reported to range from 2% to 8%.[30,112,113] Because of its rarity, there are few reports linking PC deficiency to adverse pregnancy outcomes, and those that exist involve too few patients to draw any firm conclusions. In their case-control study, Roque and colleagues reported a strong link between PC deficiency and abruption (OR, 13.9; CI, 2.21 to 86.9) and between PC deficiency and preeclampsia (OR, 6.85; CI, 1.09 to 43.2).[69] A meta-analysis also reported a strong association of this deficiency and preeclampsia/eclampsia (OR, 21.5; CI, 1.1 to 414.4) but not stillbirth.[82] It is biologically plausible that PC deficiency should pose risks of fetal loss and abruption analogous to those associated with FVL. However, given the very small sample sizes, no firm conclusions can be drawn regarding the link between PC deficiency and either preeclampsia or IUGR.

Protein S Deficiency

More than 130 mutations have been linked to deficiency of PS.[58] The great majority of affected patients can be characterized as having low levels of both total and free PS antigen (type 1) or as having only a low free PS level due to enhanced binding to the complement 4B–binding protein (type 2a). The latter condition is frequently caused by a serine 460 to proline mutation (protein S Heerlen), which has been associated with either FVL or PC mutation in about half of affected patients.[114] As with PC deficiency, homozygous PS deficiency results in neonatal purpura fulminans.[111]

Screening for PS deficiency can be done with an activity assay, but this approach is associated with substantial interassay and intra-assay variability, in part because of frequently changing physiologic levels of complement 4B–binding protein.[115] Detection of free PS antigen levels lower than 55% in a nonpregnant woman is consistent with the diagnosis.[115] However, Paidas and colleagues found far lower levels in normal pregnancy, with suggested cutoff levels for free PS of 29% for the first and second trimesters and 23% for the third trimester.[29] With such criteria, the prevalence of true PS deficiency is low (0.03% to 0.13%) in the nonpregnant state and rises up to 3% in the pregnant state, but its degree of thrombogenicity is modest (OR, 2.4; CI, 0.8 to 7.9).[29,58,115] Among those patients with PS deficiency and a strong family history of VTE, the risk of VTE in pregnancy is 6.6% (see Table 40-2).[112]

The meta-analysis by Rey and colleagues reported an association between PS deficiency and recurrent late (>22 weeks or <25 weeks) fetal loss (OR, 14.7; CI, 1.0 to 2181) as well as nonrecurrent fetal losses at greater than 22 weeks (OR, 7.4; CI, 1.3 to 43).[63] A second meta-analysis suggested an even stronger link between PS deficiency and stillbirth (OR, 16.2; CI, 5.0 to 52.3), IUGR (OR, 10.2; CI, 1.1 to 91.0), and preeclampsia/eclampsia (OR, 12.7; CI, 4 to 39.7), but not abruption.[82] Again, the small sample sizes limit the ability to draw firm conclusions.

Protein Z-Dependent Protease Inhibitor and Protein Z Deficiency

Two nonsense mutations in the coding region of the ZPI gene have been identified to occur more often in patients with VTE (4.4%) than in controls (0.8%) (OR, 5.7; CI, 1.25 to 26.0).[116] Deficiency of PZ (activity <5th percentile) has been associated with strokes but not with VTE.[117] PZ deficiency was linked to late fetal loss (10 to 16 weeks' gestation) in one study (OR, 6.7; CI, 3.1 to 14.8)[118] but not in another.[119] Paidas and associates prospectively compared PZ levels in 103 patients with subsequent normal pregnancy outcome and 106 women with various adverse pregnancy outcomes including fetal loss, IUGR, preeclampsia, and abruption; they noted lower first-trimester PZ levels among the patients with subsequent adverse outcomes (1.81 ± 0.7 versus 2.21 ± 0.8 μg/mL; $P < .001$).[29] There were also lower PZ levels in affected patients in the second trimester (1.5 ± 0.4 versus 2.0 ± 0.5 μg/mL; $P < .0001$) and in the third trimester (1.6 ± 0.5 versus 1.9 ± 0.5 μg/mL; $P < .0002$). However, it is unclear whether low PZ levels were causative or whether PZ was reduced as a result of other thrombophilias or the ongoing uteroplacental pathologic processes. Although PZ deficiency may have its own pathogenic potential, its presence with other thrombophilic mutations in patients with prior fetal loss may also confer resistance to heparin therapy.[119]

Mutations in Fibrinolytic Pathway Genes

Two polymorphisms, 675 4G/5G and A844G, in the promoter region of the PAI-1 gene have been described.[120] Homozygosity for the 4G/4G allele in the PAI-1 gene results in the presence of four instead of five consecutive guanine nucleotides in the promoter region, producing a site that is too small to permit repressor binding. Conversely, the A844G polymorphism affects a consensus sequence binding site for the regulatory protein Ets, enhancing PAI-1 gene transcription. The prevalence of the 4G/4G genotype in the general population is high, ranging from 23.5% to 32.3%.[121,122] Moreover, most studies have not found any independent relationship between the 4G/4G polymorphism and the development of VTE in unselected patients.[123-125] However, the 4G/4G genotype has been linked to a further increased risk for VTE when it is present in patients with PS deficiency or FVL, suggesting that it plays an additive but not independent role in the genesis of VTE.[126,127] No relationship has been demonstrated between the A844G polymorphism and VTE.[123]

There are limited data on the association between the 4G/4G allele and adverse pregnancy outcomes. No statistically significant association was found between isolated homozygosity for the 4G/4G mutation and recurrent spontaneous abortion in several small studies.[128,129] However, endothelial expression of PAI-1 is induced by angiotensin II, and generation of the latter molecule is increased by a deletion (D)/insertion (I) polymorphism in the angiotensin I–converting enzyme (ACE) gene. Buchholz and associates observed a significant increase in the combination of the PAI-1 4G/4G and ACE D/D genotypes among patients with recurrent spontaneous abortion compared with controls (13.6% versus 4.7%; OR, 3.2; $P = .01$).[121]

Moreover, a possible association exists between the 4G/4G allele and later adverse pregnancy outcomes. Yamada and coworkers described a modest association between 4G/4G homozygosity and the occurrence of severe preeclampsia (OR, 1.62; CI, 1.02 to 2.57).[130] Glueck and colleagues conducted a case-control study and observed that compared to patients with either the 5G/5G or the 4G/5G allele, those who were homozygous for the 4G/4G allele had greater rates of prematurity (14% versus 3%; $P = .001$), second- and third-trimester deaths (9% versus 2%; $P = .004$), and IUGR (4% versus 0.4%; $P = .012$).[131] However, caution must be exercised in the interpretation of these data, because the occurrence of adverse outcomes was lower in the control group than would be expected in the general population, and 30% of patients who were homozygous for the 4G/4G mutation had coexisting thrombophilias.[131] As was the case for the association between 4G/4G homozygosity and VTE, this mutation may be more likely to be linked with adverse pregnancy outcomes when it occurs simultaneously with other thrombophilic disorders or with triggers of increased PAI-1 expression such as the ACE D/D genotype and disorders linked to insulin resistance (e.g., obesity, type 2 diabetes, hyperlipidemia, polycystic ovary syndrome).

Polymorphisms have been described in the TAFI and tPA genes, but no clear link has been established for either with increased VTE risk or adverse pregnancy outcomes.

Other Thrombophilic Mutations

The -455GtoA polymorphism in the fibrinogen β gene leads to increased plasma fibrinogen levels but an unclear thrombotic risk.[132] Both the apolipoprotein B R3500Q and E2/E3/E4 polymorphisms and the platelet receptor gene polymorphisms GpIIIa L33P and GpIa 807CtoT also offer an uncertain VTE risk, although they may contribute to coronary and cerebral artery thrombosis, particularly in the presence of other risk factors such as smoking, hypertension, obesity, and diabetes. The common hereditary hemochromatosis gene (HFE gene C282Y mutation) does not appear to be a risk factor for VTE, even when it is present in patients with FVL.[133] An analysis of links between fetal loss and β-fibrinogen -455GtoA, between apolipoprotein B R3500Q and E2/E3/E4, and between GpIIIa L33P and HFE C282Y found no significant associations.[134]

Polymorphisms have also been described in the thrombomodulin, TFPI, and endothelial PC receptor genes, but they are of no or unknown thrombogenic potential.[58] The Val34Leu polymorphism in the factor XIII gene is associated with increased activation by thrombin and a potentially thrombotic phenotype[135] but confers uncertain risks for VTE and adverse pregnancy outcome.

Summary

A great number of potentially thrombophilic polymorphisms are being uncovered, at an ever-increasing pace. Although most of these mutations do not appear to be highly thrombogenic when present in isolation, they may exert an additive or even a synergistic effect on the thrombogenicity of other disorders. This might account for the finding of a very modest association between a given thrombophilic state (e.g., FVL, PS deficiency) and the isolated occurrence of VTE or adverse pregnancy outcomes in low-risk populations together with a far higher concordance rate within certain families.

Screening for Thrombophilias

Screening and Prevention of Venous Thromboembolism

The presence of a known thrombophilia increases the recurrence risk of VTE among pregnant women. Brill-Edwards and associates prospectively evaluated 125 pregnant women with a prior VTE, 95 of whom were tested for acquired and inherited thrombophilias (including APAs, FVL, and PGM) and for PC, PS and AT deficiencies.[136] Antenatal heparin was withheld in all patients, but postpartum anticoagulation was provided. The overall antepartum recurrence rate for VTE was 2.4% (CI, 0.2% to 6.9%), but no recurrences were observed in the 44 women who had no evidence of thrombophilia and whose previous episode of thrombosis was associated with temporary risk factors that included pregnancy itself. Among the 51 women who had a thrombophilia or whose previous VTE was considered idiopathic, the antepartum recurrence rate was 5.9% (CI, 1.2% to 16.2%), and among the 25 thrombophilic patients the recurrence risk was 16% (4 patients) (OR, 6.5; CI, 0.8 to 56.3). Therefore, there appears to be evidence-based justification to test pregnant patients with a prior history of VTE associated with temporary and reversible risk factors (e.g., fractures, prolonged immobilization, cancer), because the presence of a thrombophilic state would be an indication for antepartum as well as postpartum thromboprophylaxis. Conversely, women with a prior VTE associated with a nonrecurring risk factor who are without thrombophilia or other current major risk or susceptibility factors (e.g., need for prolonged bed rest, obesity, current superficial thrombophlebitis) may not need antepartum prophylactic heparin therapy during pregnancy.[136] However, because thrombotic events during pregnancy in such women have been reported on rare occasions,[110] the risks and benefits of antepartum thromboprophylaxis should be discussed with the patient. Also, such patients should receive postpartum prophylaxis, because most pregnancy-associated fatal pulmonary embolisms occur in the postpartum period. In this setting, knowledge of the thrombophilic state affects management.

The 7th American College of Chest Physicians Guidelines for the Antenatal and Peripartum Management of Thrombophilia suggest that the occurrence of VTE in nonpregnant patients who are receiving estrogen-containing contraceptives is comparable with such events occurring in pregnancy. In either case they would recommend antepartum and postpartum prophylaxis in a subsequent pregnancy, regardless of thrombophilia status in women who had a VTE during a prior pregnancy or while taking estrogen-containing contraceptives.[137] Similarly, consideration should also be given to screening of pregnant women who have a strong family history (i.e., affected first-degree relative) of VTE. Given the greater than 10% risk of VTE in pregnancy among patients with such a history and a thrombophilia (see Table 40-2), thromboprophylaxis, although of unproven efficacy, is a reasonable option. Cost-effective screens should be initially limited to the most common and most thrombogenic disorders, including FVL and PGM. Negative results should lead to evaluation of fasting homocysteine levels and PC, PS, and AT deficiencies.

The dosing regimen to be employed varies with the severity of the thrombophilia, the patient's family history, and the nature of the prior VTE episodes. In general, for patients with a personal or strong family history of VTE and a lesser thrombogenic thrombophilia (e.g., FVL, PGM, hyperhomocysteinemia refractory to folate therapy, PC or PS deficiency), antepartum prophylaxis with either mini-dose unfractionated heparin or low-dose LMWH is effective in preventing DVT in pregnant patients at risk. The standard regimen of unfractionated heparin used in pregnancy consists of 5000 units administered SQ every 12 hours, increased by 2500 units in the second and third trimesters. However, Barbour and associates observed that this standard unfractionated heparin regimen was inadequate to achieve the desired anti-factor Xa therapeutic range in 5 of 9 second-trimester pregnancies and in 6 of 13 third-trimester pregnancies.[138] Therefore, assessment of anti-factor Xa levels may be important.

Alternatively, prophylaxis can employ LMWH. Regimens can include dalteparin 5000 U SQ, given every 12 hours or once a day, or enoxaparin 30 mg SQ, every 12 hours or 40 mg SQ once a day. Whereas monitoring of anti-factor Xa levels is not necessary in nonpregnant patients, given the absence of data in pregnancy, the greater variability in heparin binding, and the increased volume of distribution and/or metabolism and excretion in pregnancy, we recommend serial measurements of anti-factor Xa levels, with a goal of 0.1 to 0.2 U/mL at 4 hours after each injection.

For patients with highly thrombogenic thrombophilias (e.g., homozygotes or compound heterozygotes for FVL and PGM, patients with AT deficiency or APS with prior VTE) who have a personal or strong family history of VTE, and for patients with recurrent VTE, therapeutic (high-dose) unfractionated heparin or LMWH should be used. The goal of unfractionated heparin therapy is to obtain and maintain an activated partial thromboplastin time (aPTT) of 1.5 to 2.5 times control values or a plasma heparin concentration of 0.2 to 0.4 U/mL, or an anti-factor Xa concentration of 0.4 to 0.7 U/mL. The aPTT should not be used to guide unfractionated heparin therapy in patients with prolonged aPTT due to LAs. Therapeutic LMWH therapy consists of enoxaparin 1 mg/kg SQ twice daily or a comparable dose of dalteparin (e.g., 10,000 U SQ every 12 hours). Barbour and colleagues evaluated whether the standard therapeutic doses of dalteparin maintained peak therapeutic levels of anticoagulation during pregnancy and reported that 85% (11/13) of patients required an upward dosage adjustment.[139] Therefore, we recommend titrating either agent to maintain factor Xa levels at 0.6 to 1.0 U/mL 4 hours after injection. For patients with highly thrombogenic thrombophilias in the absence of a personal or strong family history of VTE, we recommend using an intermediate or "high prophylactic" dose of LMWH, titrating the dose to maintain factor Xa levels at 0.4 to 0.6 U/mL.

Regardless of whether the patient is receiving prophylactic, therapeutic, or high prophylactic doses of LMWH, we recommend switching to the comparable dose of unfractionated heparin at 36 weeks, to permit application of neuraxial anesthesia if desired or indicated during labor or delivery. Both heparin and LMWH are associated with an increased risk for osteopenia. Although of unproven benefit, it seems prudent to advise axial skeleton weight-bearing exercise and calcium supplementation. These medications also increase the risk for heparin-induced thrombocytopenia, which paradoxically is associated with thrombosis. With therapeutic doses of LMWH and with any dose of unfractionated heparin, platelet counts should be obtained after 3 to 4 days of therapy and intermittently for the first 3 weeks of treatment.[140]

Postpartum thromboprophylaxis is also required. Warfarin is considered safe to take while breast feeding. Warfarin is started within 24 hours of commencing heparin therapy. Doses are determined by monitoring the international normalized ratio (INR). To avoid paradoxical thrombosis and skin necrosis from warfarin's early, predominantly anti-PC effect, it is critical to maintain these women on therapeutic doses of unfractionated heparin or LMWH for a minimum of 5 days and until the INR is in the therapeutic range (2.0 to 3.0) for 2 consecutive days.

Screening and Prevention of Adverse Pregnancy Outcomes

As can be discerned from the preceding review, there appears to be a modest and consistent association between the major inherited thrombophilias (including FVL, PGM, elevated fasting homocysteine levels and PC, PS, and AT deficiency) and fetal loss after 10 weeks, and particularly isolated losses after 22 weeks. There is also a possible association between these thrombophilic states and abruption. However, no clear association exists between FVL or the other major thrombophilias and either preeclampsia or IUGR, although studies have been underpowered to definitely exclude a link with severe early-onset preeclampsia and/or severe (<5th percentile) IUGR.

There are few studies examining the effectiveness of anticoagulation therapy in patients harboring inherited thrombophilias who have experienced recurrent fetal loss or other adverse pregnancy outcomes. Kupferminc and associates treated pregnant thrombophilic women who had a prior history of severe preeclampsia, abruption, IUGR, or stillbirth with enoxaparin 40 mg/day and LDA, plus folate supplementation for those patients found to be homozygous for the MTHFR mutation.[141] They reported that, compared to their prior pregnancies, patients receiving LMWH plus LDA had an increased mean gestational age at delivery (32.1 [±5.0] versus 37.6 [±2.3] weeks) and also increased birth weight of their infants (1175 [±590] versus 2719 [±526] g) ($P < .0001$ for both comparisons).

In a prospective cohort study, Folkeringa and colleagues assessed the effects of anticoagulant drugs on fetal loss in women with AT, PC, or PS deficiency.[142] Of 37 women with a deficiency, 26 (70%) received thromboprophylaxis during pregnancy, with no fetal losses, compared to 45% fetal loss in deficient women not receiving thromboprophylaxis ($P = .001$). The adjusted RR of fetal loss with versus without thromboprophylaxis was 0.07 (CI, 0.001 to 0.7).

Gris and colleagues conducted a randomized trial of anticoagulation in 160 women who had had one unexplained fetal loss after 10 weeks of gestation and who were heterozygous for FVL, PGM, or PS deficiency.[119] All patients were given 5 mg folic acid daily before conception; once pregnant, they were randomized to receive either LDA (100 mg daily) or enoxaparin (40 mg daily) beginning in the 8th week. Uncomplicated live births were noted in 28.8% of the LDA group and in 86.2% of the enoxaparin group ($P < .0001$; OR, 15.5; CI, 7 to 34). Enoxaparin proved superior to LDA among FVL patients. PZ deficiency and/or positive anti-PZ antibodies was associated with poorer outcomes. Although these results are impressive, this study has been criticized because of its lack of blinding and the high loss rate in the LDA-only group.

In summary, observational, prospective cohort, and randomized, controlled trials all suggest that LMWH with or without LDA reduces the recurrence risk of fetal loss in thrombophilic patients. Based on these findings, the following recommendations can be made:

1. Women with hyperhomocysteinemia should receive folic acid supplementation regardless of their antecedent VTE or obstetric history, given its low toxicity. For those with a history of VTE or recurrent fetal loss in whom folate does not correct the metabolic disorder, prophylactic unfractionated heparin or LMWH should be considered.
2. As noted earlier, patients in the highly thrombogenic thrombophilia group (AT deficiency, homozygous or compound heterozygous FVL or PGM), regardless of their obstetric history, should be offered "high prophylactic" doses of LMWH, with the dose titrated to maintain factor Xa levels at 0.4 to 0.6 U/mL (if there is no personal or strong family history of VTE) or to maintain therapeutic doses of LMWH (if there is such a history).
3. Pregnant women with less thrombogenic thrombophilias (e.g., heterozygous FVL or PGM, PC or PD deficiency, hyperhomocysteinemia unresponsive to folate therapy) who have no personal or strong family history of VTE but unexplained fetal loss after 9 weeks can be offered antepartum prophylaxis after full informed consent is obtained regarding the unproven efficacy of this treatment. They should receive postpartum thromboprophylaxis if they require a cesarean delivery, because most fatal acute pulmonary emboli occur during this period.
4. It is unclear whether patients with recurrent abruption in the absence of other known risk factors (e.g., smoking, renal disease, hypertension, uterine anomalies) should be offered antepartum prophylaxis.
5. At this time, there appears to be no justification for offering antepartum thromboprophylaxis to asymptomatic, otherwise low-risk women with lesser thrombophilias who have recurrent preeclampsia or IUGR. However, given the possible association between inherited thrombophilias and later adverse pregnancy outcomes, it is reasonable to consider close maternal/fetal surveillance appropriate in this population. Fetal growth may be monitored with serial ultrasound examinations (every 4 to 6 weeks) beginning at 20 weeks' gestation. Doppler flow studies of the umbilical artery may be used as a fetal assessment tool in the setting of IUGR. Nonstress testing and biophysical profiles may be appropriate at 36 weeks or earlier, as clinically indicated. Early delivery may be indicated for deteriorating maternal or fetal condition. Surveillance can be decreased if there is no evidence of placental insufficiency.

Acquired Platelet Disorders

Idiopathic Thrombocytopenic Purpura

Also known as primary immune or autoimmune thrombocytopenic purpura, idiopathic thrombocytopenic purpura (ITP) is a syndrome of immunologically mediated thrombocytopenia that is characterized by increased platelet destruction. Immunoglobulin G (IgG) antibody binds to platelets, rendering them more susceptible to sequestration and premature destruction in the reticuloendothelial system, especially the spleen. The rate of destruction exceeds the compensatory ability of the bone marrow to produce new platelets, leading to thrombocytopenia.

In adults, ITP is usually chronic. It may coexist with pregnancy, because the disease usually manifests in the second to third decade of life and has a female preponderance of 2 : 1.[143] In fact, ITP is the most common autoimmune bleeding disorder encountered during pregnancy. The overall course of ITP is not consistently influenced by pregnancy (although, rarely, women experience repeated flares with each pregnancy); however, pregnancy may be adversely affected by ITP, and the primary risk is hemorrhage in the peripartum period. Because the placenta selectively transports maternal IgG antiplatelet antibodies into the fetal circulation, fetal thrombocytopenia also may occur.

DIAGNOSIS

Most women with ITP have a history of petechiae, ecchymoses, easy bruising, menorrhagia, or other bleeding manifestations. The diagnosis is primarily one of exclusion and is based on the history, physical examination, complete blood count (CBC), and examination of the peripheral blood smear.[144] The CBC is normal except for thrombocytopenia (platelet count <100,000/μL), and the smear may show an increased proportion of slightly enlarged platelets. The history and physical examination usually exclude other causes of thrombocytopenia. Rarely, a bone marrow biopsy is required to clarify the diagnosis. Typical bone marrow findings include increased numbers of immature megakaryocytes. Although the issue is controversial, many authorities do not routinely perform this procedure in typical cases of ITP, especially in women younger than 40 years of age.[143]

It can be difficult to distinguish ITP from other causes of maternal thrombocytopenia. The condition most commonly confused with ITP is incidental thrombocytopenia of pregnancy, also known as "essential" or "gestational" thrombocytopenia. Incidental thrombocytopenia of pregnancy is mild (platelets >70,000 cells/μL), asymptomatic, and often first noted by the clinician after a CBC obtained as part of a routine automated prenatal screening test.[145,146] In contrast to ITP, incidental thrombocytopenia of pregnancy is common. It occurs in up to 5% of pregnant women and accounts for more than 70% of maternal thrombocytopenia.[146,147] Individuals with incidental thrombocytopenia have no prior history of thrombocytopenia and are not at risk for bleeding complications or fetal thrombocytopenia. No special care is required for these women. Other causes of maternal thrombocytopenia that should be considered are preeclampsia, pseudothrombocytopenia due to laboratory artifact, SLE, APS, human immunodeficiency virus (HIV) or hepatitis C virus infection, drug-induced thrombocytopenia, thrombotic thrombocytopenia, immunodeficiency states, hereditary thrombocytopenias, and DIC.

Numerous direct and indirect assays of antiplatelet antibodies have been developed to confirm the diagnosis of ITP. Most patients with ITP have platelet-associated immunoglobulin, and many also have circulating unbound antiplatelet antibodies. Levels of direct (platelet-associated) IgG have a strong inverse correlation with the maternal platelet count and intravascular platelet life span.[148] Nonetheless, a negative result does not exclude a diagnosis of ITP.[149] Concentrations of indirect (circulating) antiplatelet antibodies less reliably predict maternal platelet counts. Although assays for direct and indirect antiplatelet antibodies are widely available, they are not recommended for the routine evaluation of maternal thrombocytopenia or ITP.[144] Assays for antiplatelet antibodies are hampered by a variety of problems, including the use of several different assays, a large degree of interlaboratory variation, and a high background rate of platelet-associated IgG. Furthermore, women with ITP cannot be distinguished from those with incidental thrombocytopenia of pregnancy on the basis of antiplatelet antibody testing.[150]

MATERNAL CONSIDERATIONS

The goal of maternal therapy during pregnancy is to minimize the risk of hemorrhage and to restore a normal platelet count. Asymptomatic pregnant women with ITP and platelet counts greater than 50,000/μL do not require treatment. In nonpregnant patients, most authorities recommend treatment if the platelet count is lower than 10,000/μL or in the presence of bleeding, but it is controversial whether a particular platelet count (e.g., <50,000/μL or <30,000/μL) is sufficient indication for therapy during pregnancy in asymptomatic women. A reasonable approach is to aim for a platelet count greater than 30,000/μL throughout pregnancy and greater than 50,000/μL near term.

The American Society of Hematology ITP Practice Guideline Panel[151] recommends treating pregnant women with platelet counts between 10,000 and 30,000/μL during the second or third trimester. More aggressive treatment is often pursued close to the estimated due date, in anticipation of potential bleeding, surgery, or need for regional anesthesia. Some anesthesiologists may require a platelet count greater than 80,000/μL before deeming the woman's condition safe for placement of an epidural catheter.[152]

Glucocorticoid Drugs. Glucocorticoid drugs have been the cornerstone of ITP therapy in pregnancy. Prednisone, 1 to 1.5 mg/kg/day, or the therapeutic equivalent, is the initial treatment of choice. Improvement usually occurs within 3 to 7 days and reaches a maximum within 2 to 3 weeks. Some increase in the platelet count occurs in 50% to more than 70% of patients, depending on the duration and intensity of therapy.[144] Complete remission has been reported in 5% to 30% of cases.[144] If platelet counts become normal, the steroid dose can be tapered by 10% to 20% per week until the lowest dosage required to maintain the platelet count higher than 50,000/μL is reached.

It is uncertain how steroids improve platelet counts and decrease bleeding in patients with ITP. Proposed mechanisms of action[153] include increased platelet production, decreased production of antiplatelet antibodies and platelet-associated IgG, decreased clearance of antibody-coated platelets by the reticuloendothelial system, and decreased capillary fragility. Adverse effects of steroid use in pregnancy are well known and include glucose intolerance, osteoporosis, hypertension, psychosis, and moon facies. Accordingly, the dose and duration of therapy should be minimized.

Intravenous Immune Globulin. IVIG is used in cases of ITP refractory to corticosteroids as well as in urgent circumstances, such as preoperatively, in the peripartum period, or when the platelet count is less than 10,000/μL (or <30,000/μL in a bleeding patient). IVIG is a pooled concentrate of immunoglobulins collected from many donors. High doses of IVIG (1000 mg/kg/day for 2 to 5 days) usually induce a peak platelet count within 7 to 9 days. More than 80% of patients treated with this regimen will have a peak platelet count greater than 50,000/μL, and in 30% of patients the duration of the response lasts for more than 30 days.[154,155] Although the mechanism of action is unclear, it seems to involve depression of antiplatelet antibody production, interference with antibody attachment to platelets, inhibition of macrophage receptor-mediated immune complex clearance, and blockage of Fc receptors in the reticuloendothelial system.[155-157] In responders, only 2 or 3 days of IVIG therapy may be needed, and higher doses of 800 or 1000 mg/kg may suffice as a single or double infusion.[158]

Although IVIG had previously been associated with occasional hepatitis C transmission, the current purification process eliminates the risk of blood-borne infections. HIV transmission has never been associated with IVIG use. Untoward effects of IVIG include headache, chills, nausea, liver dysfunction, alopecia, transient neutropenia, flushing, autoimmune hemolytic anemia, and anaphylactic reactions in patients with IgA deficiencies.[159] There are no known adverse fetal effects. IVIG is extremely expensive, and for that reason its use is best reserved for urgent cases and for ITP refractory to corticosteroids. Examples include a platelet count less than 5000/μL despite treatment with steroids for several days, active bleeding, and extensive and progressive purpura.[143]

Platelet Transfusions. Platelet transfusions should be considered only as a temporary measure to control life-threatening hemorrhage or to prepare a patient for cesarean delivery or other surgery. Survival of transfused platelets is decreased in patients with ITP, because antiplatelet antibodies also bind to platelets. Therefore, the usual elevation in platelets of approximately 10,000/μL per unit of platelet concentrate is not achieved in patients with ITP. A transfusion of 8 to 10 packs is sufficient in most cases.

Splenectomy. Complete remission is obtained in 80% of patients with ITP who undergo splenectomy. This operation, which removes the major sites of platelet destruction and antiplatelet antibody production, is usually avoided during pregnancy because of risks to the fetus and technical difficulties with the procedure. Nonetheless, splenectomy can be safely accomplished during pregnancy if necessary, ideally in the second trimester. It also has been combined with cesarean delivery at term without reported morbidity. Splenectomy (during pregnancy) is appropriate for women with platelet counts lower than 10,000/μL who are bleeding and have not responded to IVIG and steroids.[144]

Rhesus Immune Globulin. Anti-Rh(D) immune globulin has been successfully used to treat ITP in RhD-positive individuals. Indeed, immune globulin against Rh(D) (75 μg per kilogram of maternal weight) works as well as corticosteroids at initial presentation.[160] It is more costly than steroids but has fewer side effects. Anti-Rh(D) is not typically used during pregnancy because of a theoretic risk of fetal erythrocyte destruction, although it would most likely bind maternal red blood cells before reaching the fetal circulation. Cases of successful and safe use of anti Rh(D) during pregnancy (in RhD-positive women) have been reported.[161]

Other drugs used to treat ITP, such as vinca alkaloids, colchicine, cyclophosphamide, and danazol, are best avoided in pregnancy because of the potential for adverse effects on the fetus. Azathioprine may be considered in refractory cases.

FETAL CONSIDERATIONS

Because the placenta is permeable to circulating maternal antiplatelet IgG, fetal thrombocytopenia may occur with maternal ITP. Occasionally, this results in minor clinical bleeding, such as purpura, ecchymoses, hematuria, or melena. In rare cases, fetal thrombocytopenia can lead to intracranial hemorrhage (ICH), resulting in severe neurologic impairment or death. Indeed, concern for ICH and its avoidance has become the central issue in the obstetric management of ITP.

Clinicians have tried a variety of strategies intended to minimize fetal bleeding problems in women with ITP. It is now clear that maternal medical therapies such as IVIG[162] and steroids[162-164] do not reliably prevent fetal thrombocytopenia. On the basis of reports of ICH associated with vaginal birth,[165] some clinicians recommended cesarean delivery for women with ITP.[166] Others have proposed that cesarean delivery be reserved for fetuses with platelet counts lower than 50,000/μL.[167] This tactic was prompted by observations that hemorrhagic complications are extremely rare in infants with platelet counts greater than 50,000/μL, and the risk of fetal bleeding is inversely proportional to the platelet count.[163,168] With this plan, however, a method is needed to determine which fetuses are thrombocytopenic—ideally, one that is noninvasive, reproducible, and sensitive in identifying at-risk fetuses. No such test is available.

Maternal characteristics and serologic findings, including thrombocytopenia, previous splenectomy, and platelet-associated antibodies, do not correlate strongly with neonatal thrombocytopenia.[146,169] Fetal thrombocytopenia is uncommon in the absence of circulating antiplatelet antibodies,[170] but exceptional cases have been reported.[171] In addition, positive results have a low positive predictive value,[170] and assays for indirect antiplatelet antibodies can be difficult to perform.

Good correlation has been reported between neonatal platelet counts and the platelet count of infants born previously to a woman with ITP.[164] However, older siblings are not always available for comparison, and concordance among sibling platelet counts is imperfect.[164] Furthermore, discordant platelet counts have been detected in twin gestations complicated by ITP.[169,172] Therefore, no historical factor or maternal blood test can accurately predict the fetal platelet count in all cases.

Some investigators have advocated the use of fetal scalp sampling during labor to directly measure the fetal platelet count.[167,173] Vaginal delivery is permitted if the platelet count is greater than 50,000/μL; otherwise, the birth is by cesarean delivery. This method is attractive because it involves negligible risk to mother and fetus and uses an assay (platelet count) that is widely available and inexpensive. Indeed, fetal scalp sampling has allowed 80% of fetuses with platelet counts greater than 50,000/μL to safely deliver vaginally.[169] The major drawback is the occasional occurrence of falsely low platelet counts, resulting in unnecessary cesarean deliveries.[174-176] Further, fetal scalp sampling cannot always easily be accomplished if there is limited cervical dilation or a high presenting part.

These problems can be circumvented with the use of cordocentesis to determine the fetal platelet count. This method results in accurate platelet counts and can be performed before labor.[162,177,178] The procedure is usually deferred until fetal maturity is present. As with scalp sampling, the delivery route is based on the fetal platelet count. However, cordocentesis cannot always be accomplished in the late third trimester,[177,178] the skills required are not available in all centers, and the procedure is expensive. Cordocentesis also may result in serious complications.[176] Hemorrhage at the puncture site, cord hematoma, and cord spasm with fetal bradycardia contribute to an overall associated mortality rate of 2.7%.[179] Procedure-related complications have been reported in about 4% to 5% of cordocenteses in patients with presumed ITP.[180] In several instances, fetuses with normal platelet counts were delivered by cesarean section or incurred serious morbidity. Bleeding is more likely in the presence of severe thrombocytopenia.[181,182] The true incidence of complications may be even higher: procedure-related complications often go unreported, and reporting centers tend to have the most expertise with the procedure and are likely to have lower complication rates than other facilities.[179]

Problems with fetal scalp sampling and cordocentesis have prompted reevaluation of the efficacy of these procedures in the management of pregnancies complicated by ITP.[163,183,184] In addition, several reports have suggested that hemorrhagic complications in thrombocytopenic neonates are unrelated to the route of delivery.[163,168,176,185] In a review of 474 neonates born to mothers with ITP, 29% of thrombocytopenic infants delivered vaginally suffered clinically apparent bleeding, compared with 30% of those delivered by cesarean section.[163] A careful analysis of the literature also suggests that no case of ICH has been directly attributable to intrapartum events.[176,184]

Another important consideration is the relative infrequency of ICH in infants born to mothers with ITP. For example, in a comprehensive population-based study of almost 16,000 pregnancies complicated by ITP, there were no cases of ICH.[147] The only three infants with ICH had alloimmune, not autoimmune, thrombocytopenia. These observations were confirmed in retrospective analyses of ITP in pregnancy. The proportion of infants with platelet counts lower than 50,000/μL is about 15%, and this may be an overestimate of the risk because of publication bias. Serious bleeding complications occurred in 22 of 688 neonates,[180] and only 6 (0.87%) had ICH. None of the cases of ICH were clearly demonstrated to be caused by intrapartum events. In one review of 288 ITP pregnancies wherein fetal platelet counts were determined at the time of delivery, there were no cases of ICH or perinatal death.[168]

In summary, obstetric management of ITP remains controversial, but most investigators now believe that fetal scalp sampling, cordocentesis, and cesarean delivery contribute to cost and morbidity without preventing neonatal bleeding complications. Therefore, it is recommended that ITP be managed without determination of the fetal platelet count and that cesarean delivery be reserved for the usual obstetric indications.[163,168,176,184] In contrast, others have found that the potential 1% risk of ICH warrants cesarean delivery in selected cases.[144,186] Those clinicians who favor interventional management use fetal scalp sampling to determine the fetal platelet count in pregnancies most at risk for thrombocytopenia (e.g., when there is a sibling with severe thrombocytopenia). The use of cordocentesis in the obstetric management of ITP is difficult to justify.

Delivery should be accomplished in a setting in which platelets, fresh-frozen plasma, and IVIG are available. A neonatologist or pediatrician familiar with the disorder should be present to promptly treat any hemorrhagic complications in the neonate. The platelet count of the affected newborn usually falls after delivery, and the lowest platelet count is not reached for several days.[187] Most infants are asymptomatic, and the thrombocytopenia is self-limited. Nonetheless, daily platelet counts should be obtained for several days. Although breastfeeding early in the puerperium may theoretically cause neonatal thrombocytopenia, many women with ITP have done so without clinical sequelae.

Neonatal Alloimmune Thrombocytopenia

In contrast to the minimal fetal risks in maternal ITP, fetal/neonatal alloimmune thrombocytopenia (NAIT) is a serious and potentially life-threatening condition that affects 0.2 to 1.0 of every 1000 live births in white people.[188-190] Rates vary by ethnicity, and African Americans appear to be affected less frequently.[191] The disorder occurs as the result of maternal alloimmunization against fetal platelet antigens that are lacking on the mother's own platelets; it is analogous to the hemolytic anemia caused by maternal alloimmunization against fetal erythrocyte antigens.

Several polymorphic, diallelic platelet antigen systems are responsible for NAIT. Many of these antigen systems were simultaneously identified in different parts of the world and given several names. To minimize confusion, uniform nomenclature has been adopted to describe these antigen systems as human platelet antigens (e.g., HPA-1), with alleles designated as "a" or "b."[192] The most frequent cause of NAIT in whites is sensitization against HPA-1a, also known as PLAT or Zwa. The antigens HPA-1a (PLAl) and HPA-lb (PLA2) are the product of polymorphic alleles that differ by a single base-pair change in the gene encoding the platelet glycoprotein GpIIIa (integrin β_3).[193] In turn, this causes a substitution of proline for leucine in the protein, resulting in antigenically distinct conformations. Of all white people, 97% are HPA-1a positive; 69% are homozygous HPA-1a, and 28% are heterozygous.[194] Several other antigens, including HPA-lb, HPA-5b (Br), HPA-3b (Bak), and HPA-4b (Yuk), also may cause NAIT (Table 40-3). In Asians, sensitization against HPA-4 is the most common cause of NAIT.

Although approximately 1 in 42 pregnancies is incompatible for HPA-1a, NAIT develops in only 1 of every 20 to 40 of these cases. In some instances,[195] the disorder remains subclinical because the antiplatelet antibodies are not potent enough to induce thrombocytopenia in the infant.[196] In addition to antigen exposure, there appears to be a need for an immunologic susceptibility to HPA-la sensitization. The human leukocyte antigen (HLA) class II determinant, Dw52a, appears to be a requirement for the development of antibodies against HPA-1a.[197] Associations between sensitization to other platelet antigens and HLA phenotypes are less well characterized, although DR6 has been linked to anti-HPA-5.[198] In contrast to rhesus isoimmunization, NAIT can occur during a first pregnancy without prior exposure to the offending antigen. The diagnosis is usually made after birth in an infant with unexplained severe thrombocytopenia, often associated with ecchymoses or petechiae.[188,199] The most serious bleeding complication is ICH, which occurs in 10% to 20% of infants with NAIT.[199,200] Fetal ICH due to NAIT can occur in utero,[201] and 25% to 50% of cases of ICH are detected by sonography before delivery.[201] Characteristic sonographic findings include evidence of intracranial hematoma or hemorrhage and porencephalic cysts. Obstructive hydrocephalus also may be present. As with red cell alloimmunization, the condition tends to worsen throughout pregnancy, as well as in subsequent pregnancies.[200,202,203] NAIT should be suspected in cases of otherwise unexplained fetal or neonatal thrombocytopenia, in utero or ex utero ICH, or porencephaly. Serologic evaluation should be performed in an experienced laboratory with special interest and expertise in NAIT.

In most cases, the diagnosis of NAIT can be determined by testing the parents; testing of fetal or neonatal blood is confirmatory and occasionally helpful. Appropriate assays include serologic confirmation of maternal antiplatelet antibodies that are specific for paternal or fetal/neonatal platelets. In addition, individuals should undergo platelet typing with zygosity testing. This can be determined serologically or with DNA-based tests, because the genes and polymorphisms for HPAs recognized to cause NAIT are well characterized. This is particularly useful for obstetric management, because fetal HPA typing can be accomplished with amniocytes.[204] Chorionic villus sampling should be avoided, because it may exacerbate the alloimmune reaction.

TABLE 40-3 PLATELET-SPECIFIC ALLOANTIGENS THAT ARE ASSOCIATED WITH ALLOIMMUNE THROMBOCYTOPENIA

HPA System Name	Antigen	Familiar Name
Polymorphisms of GpIIIa		
HPA-1	HPA-1a	$P1^{A1}$, Zw^a
	HPA-1b	$P1^{A1}$, Zw^b
HPA-4	HPA-4a	Pen^a, Yuk^b
	HPA-4b	Pen^b, Yuk^a
HPA-6	HPA-6bw	Ca, Tu
HPA-7	HPA-7bw	Mo
HPA-8	HPA-8w	Sr-a
HPA-10	HPA-10bw	La(a)
HPA-11	HPA-11bw	Gro(a)
HPA-14	HPA-14bw	Oe(a)
HPA-16	HPA-16bw	Duv(a)
Polymorphisms of GpIIb		
HPA-3	HPA-3a	Bak^a, Lek
	HPA-3b	Bak^b
HPA-9	HPA-9bw	Max^a
Polymorphisms of GpIa		
HPA-5	HPA-5a	Br^b, Zavb
	HPA-5b	Br^a, Zava
HPA-13	HPA-13bw	Sit(a)
Polymorphisms of GpIb		
HPA-2	HPA-2b	Ko^a, Sib-a
HPA-12	HPA-12bw	Ly(a)
Other probable platelet alloantigen specificities		
HPA-15	HPA-15a	Gov a
	HPA-15b	Gov b

Gp, glycoprotein; HPA, human platelet antigen.
Modified from Mark E. Brecher (ed): Platelet and granulocyte antigens and antibodies. In Technical Manual, 15th ed. Bethesda, MD: American Association of Blood Banks. Reprinted with permission from Berkowitz RL, Bussel JB, McFarland JG: Alloimmune thrombocytopenia: State of the art 2006. Am J Obstet Gynecol 195:907-13.a, 2006.

Occasionally, results are ambiguous, and in some cases, an antigen incompatibility cannot be identified. The management of such difficult cases is best individualized and underscores the need for consultation with physicians and laboratories familiar with the disorder.

The natural history of NAIT is difficult to ascertain, because it is usually unrecognized during first affected pregnancies, and subsequent pregnancies are influenced by therapeutic interventions. Nonetheless, several observations can be made from a large cohort of 107 fetuses with NAIT (97 with HPA-la incompatibility) who were followed with serial cordocenteses to determine the fetal platelet count:[205]

1. The recurrence risk of NAIT is extremely high and is 100% if the fetus has the HPA-la antigen in sensitized HPA-la-negative mothers.
2. Fetal thrombocytopenia caused by HPA-la sensitization is often severe and can occur early in gestation. Of the patients studied, 50% had initial platelet counts of less than 20,000/μL. This included 21 (46%) of 46 fetuses tested before 24 weeks' gestation.
3. A history of a sibling with antepartum ICH is a risk factor for the development of severe thrombocytopenia. However, neither a sibling platelet count nor a sibling with ICH recognized after delivery reliably predicts the initial fetal platelet count.
4. Thrombocytopenia uniformly worsens in untreated fetuses. Seven fetuses in this cohort had initial platelet counts higher than 80,000/μL and were not treated. All demonstrated rapid and substantial decreases in their platelet counts.

NAIT associated with antigens other than HPA-la is less well studied. In the large series reported by Bussel and colleagues, thrombocytopenia associated with anti-HPA-la was more severe than NAIT caused by other antigen incompatibilities.[205] Therefore, data regarding HPA-la incompatibility cannot be generalized to other causes of NAIT.

The explicit goal of the obstetric management of pregnancies at risk for NAIT is to prevent ICH and its associated complications. As with ITP, antepartum management is controversial and few randomized data are available to guide therapy. In contrast to ITP, however, the dramatically higher frequency of ICH associated with NAIT justifies more aggressive interventions. Also, therapy must be initiated antenatally because of the risk of in utero ICH. If the diagnosis is uncertain, the risk of NAIT should be confirmed by documentation of platelet incompatibility or maternal antiplatelet antibodies specific for paternal or fetal platelets. It is unnecessary to repeat testing in a family with a case of previously confirmed NAIT. Antibody titers are poorly predictive of risk to the current pregnancy and need not be obtained once the diagnosis is secure. If the father is heterozygous for the offending antigen, fetal genotyping should be accomplished with amniocytes. This strategy can prevent additional expensive and risky interventions in approximately 50% of cases.

If the fetus is considered to be at risk, most investigators recommend cordocentesis to determine the fetal platelet count. This strategy avoids treatment of fetuses with normal platelet counts and provides feedback about treatment response in cases of thrombocytopenia. The drawback is the modest but clinically important risk of fetal hemorrhage after cordocentesis in the setting of severe NAIT.[182,191] Because of this risk, a case could be made to initiate therapy without knowledge of the fetal platelet count. It is controversial whether the benefits of fetal blood sampling outweigh the risks in most cases. Many clinicians now transfuse between 5 and 15 mL of packed, washed, and irradiated maternal platelets (obtained by plateletpheresis) at the time of cordocentesis.[182] Although the efficacy of this approach is unproved, it may decrease the risk of bleeding complications at the time of the procedure. It is important to distinguish this use of platelets from platelet transfusions intended as primary therapy (see later discussion).

The optimal timing of the initial cordocentesis is controversial. ICH can occur early in gestation,[206] prompting some authorities to recommend fetal blood sampling as soon as the procedure is technically feasible (18 to 20 weeks). Such cases are rare, however, and the consequences of bleeding complications from cordocentesis are potentially more grave at previable gestational ages. Fetal blood sampling can probably be safely delayed until 24 to 26 weeks in most cases. Further studies should resolve some of these issues. Meanwhile, it seems prudent to individualize the management of each case, depending on the pertinent antigen and the severity of NAIT during previously affected pregnancies.

Proposed therapies to increase the fetal platelet count and prevent ICH include maternal treatment with steroids and IVIG,[189,207-210] fetal treatment with IVIG,[211-213] and fetal platelet transfusions.[203] However, no therapy is effective in all cases.

The administration of IVIG directly to the fetus has not consistently raised fetal platelet counts[216]; however, because only a small number of patients have been treated, lack of efficacy has not been proved. Platelet transfusions are effective,[217] but the short half-life of transfused platelets necessitates weekly procedures. The potential risks involved with multiple transfusions and the potential for increased sensitization[191,217,218] limit the attractiveness of this treatment. Platelet transfusions are perhaps best reserved for severe cases refractory to other therapies.

Administration of IVIG to the mother appears to be the most consistently effective antenatal therapy for NAIT. Bussel and colleagues demonstrated that weekly infusions of 1 g/kg maternal weight of IVIG often stabilize or increase the fetal platelet count.[189,207,209] In a study of 55 women with NAIT and thrombocytopenic fetuses, between 62% and 85% of fetuses responded to IVIG therapy, depending on how "response" was defined.[207] No fetus suffered ICH. In fact, ICH is extremely rare in pregnancies treated with IVIG, occurring in only 1 of more than 100 cases managed by Bussel and his collaborators.[202] The mechanism of action is uncertain but may be related to placental Fc receptor blockade preventing active transport of antiplatelet antibodies across the placenta.[219]

Bussel and coworkers[207] also showed that low-dose dexamethasone therapy does not improve fetal platelet counts beyond the effect achieved with IVIG. Fetal platelet counts increased to a similar degree in NAIT patients randomized to treatment with either IVIG alone or IVIG plus 1.5 mg/day of dexamethasone.[207] In contrast, 5 of 10 patients with no response to IVIG had increased fetal platelet counts after the addition of 60 mg/day of prednisone.[207] They also noted that fewer than half of fetuses with platelet counts lower than 20,000/μL responded to the initial dose of IVIG.

This led to a subsequent parallel set of randomized trials, in which patients were stratified by level of risk for severe thrombocytopenia and ICH. The first trial, conducted in 40 women with either a prior infant with ex utero ICH or a current fetus with a platelet count of less than 20,000/μL, randomized treatment IVIG 1 g/kg/wk plus prednisone 1 mg/kg/day versus IVIG 1 mg/kg/wk alone, after a cordocentesis at 20 weeks.[220] IVIG and steroids increased the mean platelet count over 3 to 8 weeks by 67,100/μL, compared with 17,300/μL for IVIG alone ($P < .001$). Moreover, the difference in treatment was more profound in the subgroup of cases with initial fetal platelet counts lower than 10,000/μL. In these cases, IVIG and prednisone increased the platelet count in 82% of cases, compared with 18% for IVIG alone.[200]

Thirty-nine women at lower risk for fetal ICH (i.e., no prior infant with ICH and current fetal platelet count >20,000/μL) were randomized to treatment with IVIG (1 g/kg/wk) or lower-dose prednisone (0.5 mg/kg/day). There was no significant difference in fetal response to these two regimens.[200] The same group also treated 15 women who had prior infants with in utero ICH with IVIG, 1 or 2 g/kg/wk, beginning at 12 weeks' gestation. Therapy was intensified (increased IVIG and/or adding steroids) if there was severe thrombocytopenia at 20 weeks. All fetuses responded adequately to intensified therapy, except one that had in utero ICH at 19 weeks' gestation.[189]

Berkowitz, Bussel, and colleagues reported further results of a recent randomized clinical trial comparing outcome in "standard risk (no prior infant with ICH)" pregnancies for NAIT treated with IVIG 2 g/kg/wk versus IVIG 1 g/kg/wk plus 0.5 mg/kg/day of prednisone.[200] Outcomes were similar and excellent in both groups, with no cases of ICH. Empiric therapy was started at 20 weeks' gestation, and cordocentesis was done once at 32 weeks. Salvage therapy (either adding steroids or increasing the dose of IVIG) was done if the platelet count was lower than 50,000/μL.[200]

Most authorities recommend cesarean delivery for fetuses with platelet counts of less than 50,000/μL.[191] As discussed in the section on ITP, vaginal delivery has never been shown to cause ICH, and cesarean delivery has never prevented it. Furthermore, the use of 50,000/μL as a cutoff is entirely arbitrary. Nonetheless, the substantial rate of ICH probably justifies cesarean delivery in pregnancies with severe NAIT.

In summary, according to the available current data, it seems appropriate to stratify treatment based on the level of risk for NAIT. In families with prior in utero ICH, empiric treatment early in pregnancy is advised. In women who previously delivered infants with ex utero ICH, or who currently have a fetus with a platelet count lower than 20,000/μL, appropriate treatment is IVIG and glucocorticoids. However, lower doses of IVIG (or glucocorticoids) may be used in lower-risk cases. It is controversial whether the information obtained from assessment of fetal platelet count by cordocentesis justifies the risk of that procedure.[191,220,221] There appears to be value in adjusting the initial treatment based on fetal platelet count—increasing the dose of IVIG or adding glucocorticoids, or both—in cases of treatment failure.[191,207,220] Therefore, we consider assessment of the fetal platelet count between 24 and 32 weeks' gestation in fetuses at risk based on genotyping or paternal testing. The procedure can usually be safely delayed until the fetus reaches viability. Cordocentesis may be especially helpful in cases that are not caused by HPA-1a, because the recurrence risk is less and the clinical course less predictable. The fetal platelet count may be again determined at term to guide the route of delivery, as outlined, if vaginal birth is desired. Alternatively, a platelet count of greater than 100,000/μL at 32 weeks can be used as a threshold to allow vaginal delivery at term.[200] This strategy usually limits the number of cordocenteses to no more than two or three per pregnancy. Empiric treatment without cordocentesis also is a reasonable option, and care should be individualized after appropriate counseling regarding pros and cons of cordocentesis.

There are no data to support population-wide screening for potential HPA incompatibility.[191] Studies are ongoing to address the efficacy and cost-effectiveness of such programs. Another clinical dilemma is the patient whose sister has had a pregnancy with NAIT. It may be worthwhile to assess platelet antigen incompatibility, HLA phenotype, and (in cases at risk based on these tests) fetal platelet count in such patients. However, we have not found such testing to be useful. Instead, we reassure such women that their prospective risk of NAIT is low and that we are unsure about the clinical relevance of such testing.

Thrombotic Thrombocytopenic Purpura and Hemolytic Uremic Syndrome

Thrombotic thrombocytopenic purpura (TTP) and hemolytic uremic syndrome (HUS) are thrombotic microangiopathies that are characterized by thrombocytopenia, hemolytic anemia, and multisystem organ failure. They are rare entities, but they may occur during pregnancy, are life-threatening, and can be difficult to distinguish from the HELLP syndrome (*h*emolysis, *e*levated *l*iver enzymes, and *l*ow *p*latelets). The incidence is estimated to be 1:25,000 births.[222] Early diagnosis and treatment are critical, because mortality may be reduced by 90%.[223]

TTP is characterized by central nervous system (CNS) abnormalities, severe thrombocytopenia, and intravascular hemolytic anemia. The most common CNS abnormalities are headache, altered consciousness, seizures, and sensory-motor deficits. Renal dysfunction and fever also may occur. Individuals with HUS have renal involvement as the major finding, as well as thrombocytopenia and hemolytic anemia. The conditions are difficult to distinguish from each other, because up to 50% of patients with HUS have CNS abnormalities, and renal dysfunction may occur in up to 80% of those with TTP. For this reason, the two disorders are often considered as a single entity.[224,225]

The pathophysiology of both conditions is abnormal and profound intravascular platelet aggregation leading to multiorgan ischemia. In HUS, this occurs predominantly in the kidney. The inciting event in TTP is uncertain. One possibility is an abnormal immune response, because the condition is associated with several autoimmune disorders. It is more common in women, consistent with many other autoimmune conditions. Other possibilities are medications such as chemotherapy agents, viral infection, and perhaps pregnancy itself, although many individuals have no risk factors. Larger than average vWF multimers appear to contribute to the pathophysiology, promoting abnormal platelet aggregation.[226] A plasma enzyme termed ADAMTS13 cleaves these vWF multimers, thereby preventing the formation of platelet clumps. ADAMTS13 activity may be absent in patients with TTP, making it a risk factor for the condition.[227] Deficiency in ADAMTS13 may be congenital,[228] or it may be acquired through the development of autoantibodies.[229] HUS is most often seen in children after a diarrheal illness caused by *Escherichia coli.* Hemolysin from Shiga toxin–negative *E. coli* O26 attaches to receptors in renal epithelium, leading to endothelial injury, platelet activation/aggregation, and ischemia.[230] In adults, HUS is often precipitated by pregnancy, chemotherapy, or bone marrow transplantation. The recurrence risk is higher in adults and in patients who do not have infectious diarrhea as an inciting event.

The diagnosis of these conditions is clinical, because there is no laboratory "gold standard." CBC and peripheral blood smear confirms thrombocytopenia and microangiopathic hemolytic anemia (schistocytes, helmet cells, and burr cells). Lactate dehydrogenase and bilirubin are elevated, indicating hemolysis. Serum creatinine and blood urea nitrogen may be elevated, especially in HUS. Clotting studies are typically normal early in the disease process. However, secondary DIC may occur after tissue necrosis. Large multimers of vWF may be present in cases of TTP, and renal biopsy may show microvascular occlusions and intraglomerular platelet aggregates in HUS. ADAMTS13 activity may be decreased in both TTP and HUS.[227] However, in many centers, results may not be available in a timely fashion.[231] Both disorders are hard to distinguish from preeclampsia.[231,232] Potential clinical signs and laboratory tests to differentiate these conditions are shown in Table 40-4.[233] The distinction between preeclampsia and TTP or HUS is

TABLE 40-4 CLINICAL CHARACTERISTICS AND LABORATORY FINDINGS IN TTP, HUS, AND SEVERE PREECLAMPSIA/HELLP SYNDROME

	TTP	HUS	Preeclampsia/HELLP
Neurologic symptoms	+++	+/–	+/–
Fever	++	+/–	–
Hypertension	+/–	+/–	+/–
Renal dysfunction	+/–	+++	+/–
Skin lesions (purpura)	+	–	–
Platelets	↓↓↓	↓↓	↓
PT/PTT	↔	↔	↓ or ↔
Fibrinogen	↔	↔	↓ or ↔
BUN/Cr	↑	↑↑↑	↑
AST/ALT	↔	↔	↑
LDH	↑↑↑	↑↑↑	↑
Multimeric forms of vWF	+	+	–
ADAMTS13 activity	↓↓↓	↓↓↓ ???	–

+ = mild symptoms present; ++ = moderate symptoms present; +++ = severe symptoms present; +/– = mild or no symptoms present; – = no symptoms present; ↓ = mildly decreased; ↓↓ = moderately decreased; ↓↓↓ = severely decreased; ↑ = mild elevation; ↑↑↑ = severe elevation; ↔ = no change.

ADAMTS13, von Willebrand factor–cleaving protease; ALT, alanine aminotransferase; AST, aspartate aminotransferase; BUN, blood urea nitrogen; Cr, creatinine; HELLP, hemolysis, elevated liver enzymes, and low platelets; HUS, hemolytic uremic syndrome; LDH, lactate dehydrogenase; PT, prothrombin time; PTT, partial thromboplastin time; TTP, thrombotic thrombocytopenic purpura; vWF, von Willebrand factor.

Modified from Esplin MS, Branch DW: Diagnosis and management of thrombotic microangiopathies during pregnancy. Clin Obstet Gynecol 42:360, 1999.

critical, because the former will improve with delivery, but TTP and HUS require additional therapy.

Plasmapheresis has been reported to substantially increase the survival rate with TTP to about 80%.[234,235] Efficacy is less certain for HUS, but good outcomes have been reported.[233,235] The mechanism of action is unclear but may involve removal of platelet-aggregating agents, such as large vWF multimers, or autoantibodies against ADAMTS13. Additional treatment includes infusion of platelet-poor or cryoprecipitate-poor fresh-frozen plasma (30 mL/kg/day), which may replace ADAMTS13, thus reducing vWF multimer size and reducing platelet aggregation. Platelet transfusions should be avoided, because it may precipitate the disease.[223] However, red blood cell transfusion is often necessary. Glucocorticoids or other immunosuppressive therapy may be useful (potentially to reduce antibodies to ADAMTS13) and is recommended for patients who do not respond immediately to plasma exchange.[227] Efficacy is uncertain. Treatment should continue for several days after recovery. Refractory cases may benefit from cytotoxic immunosuppressive agents. These therapies are generally accepted for TTP. Therapy is similar for HUS, although efficacy is less certain. Individuals with HUS often require dialysis as well.

About 10% to 25% of TTP cases occur during pregnancy or the postpartum period. Indeed, pregnancy is considered to be a risk factor for TTP and HUS, perhaps because of physiologic reduction in ADAMTS13 levels, general hypercoagulability, and synergistic features with preeclampsia.[236,237] HUS is more likely to occur in the peripartum or postpartum period. If TTP or HUS manifests during pregnancy, there is a risk of up to 33% for fetal mortality.[238,239] Fetal death is caused by previable delivery, severe maternal illness, and placental insufficiency. If TTP or HUS occurs early in gestation, aggressive treatment with plasma infusions, plasmapheresis, and steroids should be initiated. Delivery of the fetus should be considered in refractory cases, because improvement has been reported in sporadic cases.[233] At later gestational ages, delivery becomes a more attractive option. It is important to consider TTP and HUS in cases of apparent preeclampsia or HELLP syndrome that do not improve without 48 to 72 hours after delivery.

It also is important to counsel women about the recurrence risk for these conditions. In a small series of women with TTP or HUS in pregnancy, half had a least one recurrence.[222] Long-term morbidity and mortality were substantial. However, good outcomes have been reported in subsequent pregnancies in women with prior TTP or HUS associated with pregnancy.[240,241] Serial and prophylactic plasma exchange may be useful in women with prior TTP or HUS and persistent severely reduced ADAMTS13 activity.[241]

Drug-Induced Thrombocytopenia and Functional Platelet Defects

Some drugs, such as heparin and quinidine, can cause thrombocytopenia. Functional platelet defects occur when there are normal numbers of platelets that do not function properly. Drugs are a common cause of this condition. Examples include aspirin, NSAIDs, antimicrobial agents such as carbenicillin, and glyceryl guaiacolate, which is present in some cold remedies.

Congential Platelet Disorders

Von Willebrand Disease

vWD occurs in 1.3% of individuals, making it the most common inherited bleeding disorder.[242,243] The condition is caused by abnormal platelet adhesion resulting from deficiencies or abnormalities in vWF. There are three types. Type I, the most common variety, accounts for 80% of cases; it is usually inherited in an autosomal dominant fashion and is characterized by deficiencies in structurally normal factor VIII and vWF. In type I vWD, platelets fail to aggregate in the presence of ristocetin. Type II vWD is less common and may be transmitted in an autosomal recessive fashion. There are several subtypes of type II vWD, which is notable for vWF that does not function normally. Type IIA involves a deficiency of normal high-molecular-weight multimers of vWF, with consequent decreased affinity for platelets. Type IIB is characterized by vWF with an increased affinity for platelets due to an increased affinity for GpIb. The clinical disorder is similar to that caused by pseudo-vWD, which results from defective GpIb and also leads to hyperactive platelet binding to vWF. Type IIM is notable for morphologically and qualitatively abnormal vWF with reduced interaction with GpIb. Type IIN is caused by vWF with impaired binding to factor VIII. Type III also is an autosomal recessive trait and is the least common of the three types. Individuals with type III vWD have severe deficiencies of vWF/factor VIII. vWD and its subtypes may be diagnosed with a variety of laboratory studies, as summarized in Table 40-5.[244,245]

A primary treatment for many women with vWD is desmopressin (DDAVP), which increases plasma factor VIII and vWF levels (Table 40-6).[246,247] Response to DDAVP is highly variable among women with vWD, although most of those with type I disease have a favorable

TABLE 40-5 CONGENITAL BLEEDING AND PLATELET DISORDERS

Disorders	Definition	Diagnostic Assays
Hemophilia A		
Severe	Factor VIII <2%	Prolonged aPTT, low factor VIII
Mild	Factor VIII 2-25%	Prolonged aPTT, low factor VIII
Carrier	Factor VIII ≈50%	aPTT usually normal, low factor VIII
Hemophilia B		
Severe	Factor IX <2%	Prolonged aPTT, low factor IX
Mild	Factor IX 2-25%	Prolonged aPTT, low factor IX
Carrier	Factor IX ≈50%	aPTT usually normal, low factor IX
Factor VII deficiency	Low factor VII	Prolonged INR, low factor VII
Factor X deficiency	Low factor X	Prolonged aPTT, prolonged INR, low factor X
Factor XI deficiency	Low factor XI	Prolonged aPTT, low factor XII
Factor XII deficiency	Low factor XII	Prolonged aPTT, low factor XII
Factor XIII deficiency	Low factor XIII	Normal aPTT and INR, low factor XIII
Hypofibrinogenemia	Low fibrinogen	Low fibrinogen
vWD Types I and III	Deficient (type I) or absent (type III) vWF	Absent vWF:RCoF and RIPA; platelets aggregate with bovine plasma
Type IIA	Qualitatively abnormal vWF: lack of HMW multimers	Multimeric analysis
Type IIB	Qualitatively abnormal vWF; spontaneously binds platelets; lack of HMW multimers	Platelets aggregate to 0.5 mg/mL of ristocetin; multimeric analysis ↓ platelets
Pseudo-vWD	Platelets spontaneously bind GpIb-IX-V complex	Absent vWF:RCoF activity; differentiated from vWD by no clumping to bovine plasma
Bernard-Soulier syndrome	Platelet GpIb is defective	Absent vWF:RCoF activity; differentiated from vWD by no clumping to bovine plasma
Secretion defects	Arachidonic acid and prostaglandin pathway abnormalities	Aspirin/NSAIDs are common causes; abnormal response to collagen, arachidonic acid; normal primary wave only
Storage pool deficiencies	Abnormal function or component deficiency of platelet granules (α, δ, or both)	Primary wave only; decreased collagen assay; variable arachidonic acid assay; mepacrine labeling
Glanzmann thrombasthenia	GpIIb-IIIa is absent, present in minimal amounts, or qualitatively abnormal	Platelets not activated by ADP, collagen, or arachidonic acid

ADP, adenosine diphosphate; aPTT, activated partial thromboplastin time; Gp glycoprotein; HMW, high molecular weight; INR, international normalized ratio; NSAIDs, nonsteroidal anti-inflammatory drugs; RCoF, ristocetin cofactor; RIPA, ristocetin-induced platelet agglutination; vWD, von Willebrand disease; vWF, von Willebrand factor.

response. Some women with type IIA vWD also respond well to DDAVP. However, the drug should be avoided in women with type IIB disease, because it may cause thrombocytopenia.[248] Patients with type III disease rarely respond. Ideally, an individual's response to DDAVP should be tested under nonurgent circumstances. A typical dose is 0.3 μg/kg to a maximum of 20 μg SQ or diluted in 50 to 100 mL of normal saline and given intravenously over 30 minutes. If the patient is not pregnant, the drug may be administered on day 1 of menses. A subjective decrease in flow is considered a positive response. If the patient is pregnant or not bleeding, the response is gauged by assessing a change in platelet count and vWF:ristocetin cofactor (RCoF) peak activity at 90 minutes after the administration of DDAVP. Adverse effects of DDAVP include headache, flushing, changes in blood pressure, fluid retention, and hyponatremia. The drug is pregnancy category B.

Replacement of clotting factors is the other standard treatment for VWD. In cases with factor VIII:c or vWF levels less than 50 IU/dL, prophylactic treatment should be given to cover invasive procedures and delivery.[247] Patients with low vWF levels and either known positive responses to DDAVP or type I disease should be given prophylactic treatment with a single dose of DDAVP, either 60 minutes before anticipated delivery or at the time of cord clamping.[247] Additional doses are of uncertain benefit and may be harmful. Special attention must be given to the possibility of fluid retention and hyponatremia when using DDAVP near the time of childbirth.[243] Women who do not respond to DDAVP may be treated with factor VIII/vWF plasma concentrate in the form of plasma, cryoprecipitate, Humate-P, and Koate. These products are typically labeled with vWF:Ac concentrations indicating functional activity: 1 IU/kg of vWF:Ac increases the plasma level by 2.0 U/dL. Ideally, vWF:Ac levels should be 50% of normal (50 IU/dL) in prophylactic settings; 100% of normal is the goal in cases of bleeding or surgery. This level should be maintained for at least 3 days after vaginal delivery or 5 days after cesarean delivery.[247] Tranexamic acid also may be useful in controlling or preventing postpartum hemorrhage.[247]

Pregnancy is not contraindicated in women with vWD, but they should be informed of the potential for bleeding.[243,244] A recent large epidemiologic study estimated the OR of postpartum hemorrhage for women with vWD to be 1.5 (CI, 1.1 to 2.0).[249] The OR for needing a blood transfusion was 4.7 (CI, 3.2 to 7.0), and 5 of 4067 women died (a rate 10-fold higher than in the general population).[249] The antepartum period is an ideal time to characterize the type of vWD and the response to DDAVP. If possible, a multidisciplinary team including a hematologist, obstetrician, and anesthesiologist should coordinate care and a management plan.[247] Prenatal diagnosis is possible in many cases, and genetic counseling should be offered to affected families (Table 40-7). This is especially pertinent for patients who are at risk of having a fetus with severe type III disease. At times, genetic testing of amnio-

TABLE 40-6 TREATMENT OF CONGENITAL BLEEDING AND PLATELET DISORDERS

Disorder	Threshold for Treatment	Treatment
Hemophilia A	Bleeding; before delivery/procedures if factor VIII level <50 IU/dL	Factor VIII concentrate, cryoprecipitate, DDAVP
Hemophilia B	Bleeding; before delivery/procedures if factor IX level <50 IU/dL	Factor IX concentrate, cryoprecipitate
Factor VII deficiency	Bleeding; before delivery/procedures if factor VII level <50 IU/dL	rFVIIa, factor VII concentrate
Factor X deficiency	Bleeding; possibly before delivery/procedures	Factor IX concentrate, FFP
Factor XI deficiency	Bleeding; before delivery/procedures if factor XI level <15 IU/dL	Factor XI concentrate, FFP (do not exceed peak factor XI levels of 70 IU/dL)
Factor XII deficiency	?	?
Factor XIII deficiency	Bleeding; pregnancy	Factor XIII concentrate, FFP, cryoprecipitate (keep XIIIa antigen or activity >10% of normal)
Hypofibrinogenemia	Bleeding; fibrinogen <150 mg/dL; pregnancy	FFP, cryoprecipitate (keep fibrinogen >100 mg/dL)
vWD		
Type I	Bleeding	DDAVP (if favorable response), tranexamic acid, FFP, cryoprecipitate, Humate-P, Koate (goals are >50 IU/dL of vWF:Ac)
Type IIA	Bleeding; operative delivery; procedures	DDAVP (if favorable response), transexamic acid, FFP, cryoprecipitate, Humate-P, Koate (goal is >50 IU/dL of vWF:Ac)
Type IIB	Bleeding; operative delivery; procedures	FFP, cryoprecipitate, Humate-P, Koate (goal is >50 IU/dL of vWF:Ac); DDAVP is contraindicated
Type IIN	Bleeding; operative delivery; procedures	FFP, cryoprecipitate, Humate-P, Koate (goal is >50 IU/dL of vWF:Ac)
Type IIM	Bleeding; operative delivery; procedures	FFP, cryoprecipitate, Humate-P, Koate (goal is >50 IU/dL of vWF:Ac)
Type III	Bleeding; all deliveries; procedures	FFP, cryoprecipitate, Humate-P, Koate (goal is >50 IU/dL of vWF:Ac); DDAVP is not effective
Bernard-Soulier syndrome	Bleeding (prophylaxis for delivery is controversial)	Platelet transfusion (possibly DDAVP, transexaminic acid, immune suppression, rFVIIa)
Storage pool deficiencies	Bleeding (prophylaxis for delivery is controversial)	Platelet transfusion; ? DDAVP
Glanzmann thrombasthenia	Bleeding; delivery; procedures	Platelet transfusion, rFVIIa

DDAVP, desmopressin; FFP, fresh-frozen plasma; rFVIIa, recombinant activated factor VII; vWD, von Willebrand disease; vWF, von Willebrand factor.

cytes or chorionic villi is possible in cases of known mutations or restriction fragment length polymorphisms.[250,251] Also, cordocentesis to perform functional assays on fetal blood may be diagnostic, although results can be unreliable due to variable penetrance, and the risk of bleeding at cordocentesis is increased in affected cases.[252,253] It may be helpful to assess levels of vWF antigen (vWF:Ag), vWF:Ac, and factor VIII:c on a serial basis (e.g., on the initial visit, at 28 and 34 weeks' gestation, and before invasive procedures and delivery).[247] VIII/vWF concentrates, DDAVP, skilled anesthesia personnel, and hematology consultation should be available at delivery.

Neuraxial anesthesia is considered to be contraindicated in most women with vWD, but safe use of regional anesthesia has been reported in a few women with mild type I disease.[254,255] Regional anesthesia is thought to be safe if factor VIII and vWF:RCoF levels are greater than 50 IU/dL, although this is unproven.[243,247] Cesarean delivery has been advised by some authorities in an attempt to avoid fetal bleeding.[256] However, the procedure is of unproven efficacy and bleeding has been reported in affected infants born by cesarean.[256] Given the unproven efficacy and the risk of maternal hemorrhage, elective cesarean delivery is not routinely advised in cases of vWD.[244,247] However, traumatic delivery, such as vacuum or rotational forceps, should be avoided. Neonates born to mothers with vWD should be tested to determine their vWF status. There is an increased risk of hemorrhage after delivery, even several weeks later. Frequent patient contact, monitoring of vFW levels, and prolonged prophylaxis may reduce this risk, but this also is unproven.[243]

Bernard-Soulier Syndome

Bernard-Soulier syndrome is usually transmitted in an autosomal recessive fashion; therefore, a family history is rare, although a variant appears to be autosomal dominant. Affected individuals have mucocutaneous bleeding due to a defect or deficiency in the platelet glycoproteins (GpIb-IX-V) that form a transmembrane complex that binds vWF.[257] The result is platelets that cannot bind to subendothelial surface. Laboratory diagnosis includes a decreased number of relatively large platelets, absent ristocetin response, a failure of platelets to aggregate in response to bovine plasma, and decreased platelet GpIb-IX-V complex density as measured by flow cytometry.[258] Successful treatment requires platelet transfusion.

Prenatal diagnosis is possible in many cases and should be offered to families with a prior affected child. Because of previous platelet transfusions, affected mothers often are at risk for NAIT. Cesarean delivery is controversial and should be reserved for obstetric indications.[244,259] Regional anesthesia is considered to be contraindicated. Prophylactic platelet transfusion before delivery in this setting is also controversial because of the risk of alloimmune thrombocytopenia. This risk must be weighed against frequent hemorrhagic complications related to delivery, especially postpartum complications.[259] The use of

TABLE 40-7 PRENATAL DIAGNOSIS OF CONGENITAL BLEEDING AND PLATELET DISORDERS*

Disorder	Tissue Required	Tests	Comment
Hemophilia A	Amniocytes, fetal blood	Fetal gender; factor VIII mutation analysis, linkage analysis (if family mutation is known); cord blood factor VIII levels	Because of the risk of bleeding, cordocentesis is reserved for cases in which genetic testing is nondiagnostic.
Hemophilia B	Amniocytes, fetal blood	Fetal gender; factor IX mutation analysis, linkage analysis (if family mutation is known); cord blood factor IX levels	Because of the risk of bleeding, cordocentesis is reserved for cases in which genetic testing is nondiagnostic.
Factor VII deficiency	Amniocytes, fetal blood	Factor VII mutation analysis, linkage analysis (if family mutation is known); cord blood factor VII levels	Because of the risk of bleeding, cordocentesis is reserved for cases in which genetic testing is nondiagnostic.
Factor X deficiency	Amniocytes, fetal blood	Factor X mutation analysis, linkage analysis (if family mutation is known); cord blood factor X levels	Because of the risk of bleeding, cordocentesis is reserved for cases in which genetic testing is nondiagnostic.
vWD (types I and III)	Amniocytes or fetal blood	Mutation analysis, linkage analysis if family mutation known; vWF:RCoF	Because of the risk of bleeding, cordocentesis is reserved for cases in which genetic testing is nondiagnostic.
vWD (type II)	Amniocytes or fetal blood	Mutation analysis, linkage analysis if family mutation known; vWF:RCoF	Because of the risk of bleeding, cordocentesis is reserved for cases in which genetic testing is nondiagnostic.
Bernard-Soulier syndrome	Amniocytes or fetal blood	Mutation analysis, linkage analysis if family mutation known; vWF: RCoF; bovine plasma	Because of the risk of bleeding, cordocentesis is reserved for cases in which genetic testing is nondiagnostic. Cordocentesis is extremely hazardous if fetus is positive for the mutation.
Glanzmann thrombasthenia	Amniocytes or fetal blood	Mutation analysis, linkage analysis if family mutation known; functional assays; anti-GpIIb-IIIa antibody binding	Because of the risk of bleeding, cordocentesis is reserved for cases in which genetic testing is nondiagnostic. Cordocentesis is extremely hazardous if fetus is positive for the mutation.
Gray platelet syndrome	Fetal blood	Microscopic analysis	Normal fetal platelets have α-granules.
Wiscott-Aldrich syndrome	Amniocytes or fetal blood	Mutation analysis, linkage analysis if family mutation known; platelet size/volume	Because of the risk of bleeding, cordocentesis is reserved for cases in which genetic testing is nondiagnostic.
Chediak-Higashi syndrome	Fetal blood	Peroxidase stain of neutrophils	Proven successful in feline model.
Hermansky-Pudlak syndrome	Amniocytes	Mutation analysis, linkage analysis if family mutation known	—

***Genes and some mutations have been identified for deficiencies of factors X, XI, XII, XIII, and fibrinogen. Therefore, prenatal diagnosis using amniocytes may be possible. Cordocentesis also may be informative through the direct measurement of factor levels.**
Gp, glycoprotein; RCoF, ristocetin cofactor; vWD, von Willebrand disease; vWF, von Willebrand factor.

HLA and platelet antigen–matched platelets may reduce this risk. Several other strategies may reduce the risk of bleeding, or may be used to treat bleeding after delivery, in women with Bernard-Soulier syndrome. These include DDAVP, antifibrinolytic therapy with tranexamic acid, immune suppression to prolong platelet survival, and recombinant activated factor VII (rFVIIa).[259-262] The optimal dose of rFVIIa is uncertain, but a dose of 90 to 120 μg/kg body weight, repeated every 2 hours (if there is a good response), has been recommended.[259]

Disorders of Platelet Secretion

Disorders of platelet secretion include several rare conditions characterized by platelet storage pool deficiencies. These disorders involve deficient or abnormal platelet granules or their contents.

GRAY PLATELET SYNDROME

Gray platelet syndrome is caused by a deficiency of α-granules in platelets and megakaryocytes. Platelet α-granules contain vWF, platelet factor 4, and platelet-derived growth factor. Characteristic gray-appearing platelets are noted on peripheral smear or marrow aspirate after staining with Romanowsky solution. Treatment includes platelet transfusion. Good pregnancy outcome was reported in a patient with gray platelet syndrome after platelet transfusion.[263]

DELTA STORAGE POOL DISEASE

Delta (δ) storage pool disease involves a deficiency in dense granules (δ granules) in platelets containing ADP. Diagnosis is made by electron microscopy or by an adenosine triphosphate (ATP)-to-ADP ratio greater than 3 : 1 in inactive platelets. Other syndromes associated with δ storage pool disease include the Chediak-Higashi, Wiskott-Aldrich, thrombocytopenia with absent radii (TAR), and Hemansky-Pudlak syndromes. Most patients with δ-storage pool diseases respond to platelet transfusion, although some may respond to DDAVP. Rarely, individuals have congenital or acquired abnormalities of d and a granules, termed αδ storage pool disease. A case of an uncomplicated pregnancy without treatment was reported in a patient with Chediak-Higashi syndrome.[264] Wiscott-Aldrich syndrome is an X-linked immunodeficiency syndrome that is associated with early mortality. Prenatal diagnosis is possible and should be offered to affected families.[265]

Thrombocytopenia associated with TAR typically resolves at 1 year of life. Prenatal diagnosis of the syndrome has been reported.[266] Several pregnancies have been reported in women with Hermansky-Pudlak syndrome.[267,268] This autosomal recessive condition is characterized by oculocutaneous albinism, platelet storage pool deficiency, and the accumulation of ceroid (a yellow, granular substance) in reticuloendothelial cells. It is common in some areas of Puerto Rico.[267,268]

GLANZMANN THROMBASTHENIA

Glanzmann thrombasthenia is an abnormality in the quantity or quality (or both) of the platelet membrane glycoprotein, GpIIb-IIIa.[269] The disease is transmitted in an autosomal dominant fashion and has been reported to occur most often in Iraqi-Jewish and Arab populations in Israel, in Southern India, and among European Gypsies.[270,271] Patients with type 1 Glanzmann thrombasthenia lack detectable GpIIb-IIIa, whereas those with type 2 disease have only 10% to 20% of normal platelet surface GpIIb-IIIa.

These patients are at lifelong risk for bleeding, often requiring frequent platelet transfusions. Accordingly, many develop alloimmune antibodies against platelet antigens, causing their pregnancies to be at risk for NAIT (see earlier discussion).[272] Women with a history of multiple platelet transfusions should undergo evaluation for parental platelet antigen incompatibility and the presence of specific anti-platelet antibodies for fetal antigens. Cordocentesis has been particularly risky in affected pregnancies and is best avoided if possible. This makes prenatal diagnosis more difficult. In cases of known mutations, fetal genotype may be obtained from amniocytes or chorionic villi (avoid chorionic villus sampling if the patient has antibodies).

The primary intrapartum treatment for Glanzmann thrombasthenia is platelet transfusion.[273,274] If possible, type-specific platelets should be used to avoid platelet alloimmunization. If pooled platelets must be used in sensitized women, immunosuppressive therapy may prolong the lifespan and effectiveness of the platelets. Cesarean delivery should be reserved for the usual obstetric indications, including alloimmune thrombocytopenia. Postpartum hemorrhage is common. Hormonal treatment and prolonged use of uterotonic agents may reduce the risk of this complication, although this approach is of unproven efficacy. The use of rFVIIa appears to be safe and relatively effective in patients with Glanzmann thrombasthenia,[274-276] and it may prove to be an important tool for the treatment of this disease during pregnancy.

Bleeding Disorders

Acquired Bleeding Disorders

Factor VIII Inhibitors

The development of antibodies against factor VIII is a rare but serious acquired bleeding disorder. The inciting event is unknown, but the condition often manifests in the postpartum period.[277] Clinical features are similar to those seen in hemophilia. Diagnosis is made by prolonged clotting times that do not normalize in response to mixing studies with normal plasma. Demonstration of a specific factor VIII inhibitor and documentation of low levels of factor VIII in the plasma confirm the diagnosis. Hemorrhage may be severe and may respond to activated prothrombin complex concentrate or rFVIIa.[276,277] Mild cases often respond to DDAVP and factor VIII concentrates.[277] Plasmapheresis may be helpful in refractory cases. The disease typically regresses spontaneously over time. Although IgG antibodies to factor VIII may develop, infants are rarely affected. The condition usually remits spontaneously, with or without the use of immunosuppressive therapy.[277]

Congenital Bleeding Disorders

Hemophilia A (Factor VIII Deficiency) and Hemophilia B (Factor IX Deficiency)

Hemophilia A and B are caused by congenital deficiencies of factor VIII and IX, respectively. They are inherited in an X-linked recessive fashion. Therefore, affected females are uncommon. Heterozygous carriers are usually asymptomatic. Rarely, a heterozygous female has clinical symptoms of bleeding, perhaps because of skewed X inactivation of the X chromosome containing the normal gene. Symptoms tend to be mild, and serious hemorrhage during labor and delivery is rare. Treatment may be accomplished with factor VIII concentrate or cryoprecipitate for hemophilia A and factor IX concentrate or fresh-frozen plasma for hemophilia B.[247]

Pregnancy issues often focus on the fetus/neonate, because 50% of male offspring born to female carriers will be affected. Carrier detection of hemophilia A may be accomplished using assays for factor VIII and is reliable during pregnancy. Prenatal diagnosis is feasible through factor VIII and IX gene mutation analysis or linkage analysis (or both).[251] Rarely, cordocentesis may be used to detect an affected fetus by testing levels of factors VIII and IX (which are normally lower in a fetus than in an adult). However, this approach is reserved for cases in which genetic testing is not diagnostic, because the procedure is risky.[247]

Levels of factor VIII or IX, or both, should be assessed at the initial pregnancy visit, at 28 and 34 weeks of gestation, and again at delivery.[247] Recombinant factor VIII and IX should be used as the treatment of choice in pregnant carriers of hemophilia A and B, respectively. Treatment should be initiated in the setting of bleeding or factor VIII or IX levels lower than 50 IU/dL.[247] DDAVP may be helpful in women with hemophilia A, but not in those with hemophilia B. Regional anesthesia should be safe in women with normal coagulation studies and factor levels greater than 50 IU/dL. Vaginal delivery has not been shown to increase bleeding in affected male infants. However, fetal scalp electrodes, operative vaginal delivery, and circumcision should be avoided in male infants born to carriers of hemophilia A. Postnatal diagnosis may be established in newborns through assays of maternal and cord blood. Carriers of hemophilia B are detected by factor IX assay. Levels of factor IX in carriers are usually decreased, although they may be normal. Delivery issues with hemophilia B are similar to those for hemophilia A.

Other Factor Deficiencies

Deficiencies of factors VII, X, XI, and XIII are uncommon hereditary bleeding disorders. Factor VII, X, and XIII deficiencies are probably autosomal recessive traits, whereas factor XI deficiency appears to be an incompletely autosomal-recessive trait. Replacement with rFVIIa is the treatment of choice for women with factor VII deficiency.[278] Factor X–deficient women may be treated with fresh-frozen plasma or factor IX concentrates to treat active bleeding.[279,280] Prophylactic transfusion may be useful before vaginal or cesarean delivery.[279,281] Individuals who are homozygous for factor XI deficiency have levels less than 20% of normal, whereas heterozygotes have levels that are 30% to 65% of normal.[282] Bleeding does not always correlate with factor XI concentrations, and heterozygotes may have minor bleeding problems. Most women do not experience hemorrhage during delivery,[283,284] and it may be possible to stratify patients with the condition into bleeding and nonbleeding phenotypes.[284] Prophylactic treatment is not required for all deliveries, and treatment may be reserved for excessive bleeding.[283,284] This may be accomplished with fresh-frozen plasma given as a 10 mL/kg load followed by 5 mL/kg per day, or through direct replacement with factor XI concentrate.

Factor XIII deficiency is rare but can lead to severe bleeding such as ICH after minor trauma and abnormal wound healing. Life-threatening umbilical cord stump hemorrhage has occurred in affected newborns. An increased risk of recurrent pregnancy loss also has been reported in women with factor XIII deficiency.[285] This is thought to be the result of decidual bleeding, and successful pregnancy rarely occurs without treatment. Diagnosis is made by assessment of factor XIII (A and S subunits) or by dissolution of clot in 5-molar urea. Treatment includes transfusion with factor XIII concentrate, fresh-frozen plasma, cryoprecipitate, and/or whole blood. Small amounts of plasma may provide adequate factor XIII for hemostasis. Although of uncertain efficacy, maintenance of XIIIA-antigen (Ag) or XIII-activity (act) at 10% is advised.[285] This may require the administration of 1 vial of XIIIA concentrate (250 IU) every 7 days in early pregnancy, followed by 2 vials every 7 days after 23 weeks gestation.[285,286] Extra replacement (e.g., 4 vials) may be helpful at the time of delivery.[285]

Hypofibrinogenemia/Afibrinogenemia

Congenital hypofibrinogenemia is a rare, autosomal-dominant condition characterized by bleeding as well as obstetric problems such as abruption, postpartum hemorrhage, and recurrent pregnancy loss.[287,288] The condition is defined as the presence of structurally normal fibrinogen in concentrations of less than 150 mg/dL.[287] Miscarriage at midgestation appears to be caused by perigestational hemorrhage.[288] This is supported by data from transgenic mice lacking fibrinogen, who suffer uniform pregnancy loss at day 10.[289] Pregnancy loss in these mice is corrected by the addition of fibrinogen. Dysfibrinogenemia has been weakly associated with hypercoagulability, rather than hypocoagulability. Successful pregnancies in women with hypofibrinogenemia have been reported with the use of fresh-frozen plasma or cryoprecipitate to maintain fibrinogen levels greater than 100 to 150 mg/dL.[287,288] Each unit of cryoprecipitate contains about 300 mg of fibrinogen, which raises the plasma concentration by approximately 6 mg/dL.

Factor XII deficiency

Factor XII is involved in both coagulation and fibrinolysis, and deficient individuals have been reported to be at increased risk for both bleeding and thrombosis. However, it is not clear that this condition increases the risk for either bleeding or thrombosis.[290] The condition is of interest because it is associated with recurrent pregnancy loss.[291,292]

Plasminogen Activator Inhibitor 1 Deficiency

Individuals with elevated levels of PAI-1 are at increased risk for thrombosis and possibly for pregnancy loss. In contrast, deficiency of PAI-1 has been reported to be associated with an increased risk of bleeding.[293] The condition often manifests as menorrhagia and may be responsive to aminocaproic acid.[293] Indeed, low PAI-1 activity has been reported in 23% of patients referred for evaluation of bleeding diathesis, compared with 10% of controls (OR, 2.75; CI, 1.39 to 5.42).[294] It may prove to be an important cause of abnormal bleeding. There are few data regarding pregnancy in women with PAI-1 deficiency.

References

1. Martinelli I, Mannucci PM, De Stefano V, et al: Different risks of thrombosis in four coagulation defects associated with inherited thrombophilia: A study of 150 families. Blood 92:2353-2358, 1998.
2. Nurden AT, Nurden P: Inherited disorders of platelets: an update. Curr Opin Hematol 13:157-162, 2006.
3. Ruggeri ZM, Dent JA, Saldivar E: Contribution of distinct adhesive interactions to platelet aggregation in flowing blood. Blood 94:172-178, 1999.
4. Abrams CS: Intracellular signaling in platelets. Curr Opin Hematol 12:401-405, 2005.
5. Bevers EM, Comfurius P, Hemker HC, et al: On the procoagulant activity of platelets stimulated by collagen and thrombin. Thromb Res 33:553-554, 1984.
6. Pytela R, et al: Platelet membrane glycoprotein IIb/IIIa: Member of a family of Arg-Gly-Asp—Specific adhesion receptors. Science 231:1559-1562, 1986.
7. Sill PR, Lind T, Walker W: Platelet values during normal pregnancy. Br J Obstet Gynaecol 92:480-483, 1985.
8. Wallenburg HC, van Kessel PH: Platelet lifespan in normal pregnancy as determined by a nonradioisotopic technique. Br J Obstet Gynaecol 85:33-36, 1978.
9. Monroe DM, Hoffman M: What does it take to make the perfect clot? Arterioscler Thromb Vasc Biol 26:41-48, 2006.
10. Mackman N: Role of tissue factor in hemostasis, thrombosis, and vascular development. Arterioscler Thromb Vasc Biol 24:1015-1022, 2004.
11. Giesen PL, Nemerson Y: Tissue factor on the loose. Semin Thromb Hemost 26:379-384, 2000.
12. Neuenschwander PF, Fiore MM, Morrissey JH: Factor VII autoactivation proceeds via interaction of distinct protease-cofactor and zymogen-cofactor complexes: Implications of a two-dimensional enzyme kinetic mechanism. J Biol Chem 268:21489-21492, 1993.
13. Falati S, Liu Q, Gross P, et al: Accumulation of tissue factor into developing thrombi in vivo is dependent upon microparticle P-selectin glycoprotein ligand 1 and platelet P-selectin. J Exp Med 197:1585-1598, 2003.
14. Broze GJ Jr: The rediscovery and isolation of TFPI. J Thromb Haemost 1:1671-1675, 2003.
15. Oliver JA, Monroe DM, Churen FC, et al: Activated protein C cleaves factor Va more efficiently on endothelium than on platelet surfaces. Blood 100:539-546, 2002.
16. Broze GJ Jr: Protein Z-dependent regulation of coagulation. Thromb Haemost 86:8-13, 2001.
17. Preissner KT, Zwicker L, Muller-Berghaus G: Formation, characterization and detection of a ternary complex between S protein, thrombin and antithrombin III in serum. Biochem J 243:105-111, 1987.
18. Ranby M, Brandstrom A: Biological control of tissue plasminogen activator-mediated fibrinolysis. Enzyme 40:130-143, 1988.
19. Schatz F, Lockwood CJ: Progestin regulation of plasminogen activator inhibitor type 1 in primary cultures of endometrial stromal and decidual cells. J Clin Endocrinol Metab 77:621-625, 1993.
20. Bouma BN, Meijers JC: New insights into factors affecting clot stability: A role for thrombin activatable fibrinolysis inhibitor (TAFI; plasma procarboxypeptidase B, plasma procarboxypeptidase U, procarboxypeptidase R). Semin Hematol 41(1 Suppl 1):13-19, 2004.
21. Urano T, Ihara H, Takada Y, et al: The inhibition of human factor Xa by plasminogen activator inhibitor type 1 in the presence of calcium ion, and its enhancement by heparin and vitronectin. Biochim Biophys Acta 1298:199-208, 1996.
22. Lockwood CJ, Krikun G, Rahman M, et al: The role of decidualization in regulating endometrial hemostasis during the menstrual cycle, gestation, and in pathological states. Semin Thromb Hemost 33:111-117, 2007.
23. Erlich J, Parry GC, Fearns C, et al: Tissue factor is required for uterine hemostasis and maintenance of the placental labyrinth during gestation. Proc Natl Acad Sci USA 96:8138-8143, 1999.
24. Mackenzie AP, Schatz F, Krikun G, et al: Mechanisms of abruption-induced premature rupture of the fetal membranes: Thrombin enhanced

decidual matrix metalloproteinase-3 (stromelysin-1) expression. Am J Obstet Gynecol 191:1996-2001, 2004.
25. Lockwood CJ, Toti P, Arcuri F, et al: Mechanisms of abruption-induced premature rupture of the fetal membranes: Thrombin-enhanced interleukin-8 expression in term decidua. Am J Pathol 167:1443-1449, 2005.
26. Cakmak H, Schatz F, Huang ST, et al: Progestin suppresses thrombin- and interleukin-1beta-induced interleukin-11 production in term decidual cells: Implications for preterm delivery. J Clin Endocrinol Metab 90:5279-5286, 2005.
27. Matta P, Lockwood CJ, Schatz F, et al: Thrombin regulates monocyte chemoattractant protein-1 expression in human first trimester and term decidual cells. Am J Obstet Gynecol 196:268e1-268e8, 2007.
28. Bremme KA: Haemostatic changes in pregnancy. Best Pract Res Clin Haematol 16:153-168, 2003.
29. Paidas MJ, Ku DH, Lee MJ, et al: Protein Z, protein S levels are lower in patients with thrombophilia and subsequent pregnancy complications. J Thromb Haemost 3:497-501, 2005.
30. Hellgren M: Hemostasis during normal pregnancy and puerperium. Semin Thromb Hemost 29:125-130, 2003.
31. Juhan Vague I, Alessi MC, Vague P: Increased plasma plasminogen activator inhibitor 1 levels: A possible link between insulin resistance and atherothrombosis. Diabetologia 34:457-462, 1991.
32. Wilson WA, Gharari AE, Koike T, et al: International consensus statement on preliminary classification criteria for definite antiphospholipid syndrome: Report of an international workshop. Arthritis Rheum 42:1309-1311, 1999.
33. Galli M, Luciani D, Bertolini G, et al: Anti-beta 2-glycoprotein I, antiprothrombin antibodies, and the risk of thrombosis in the antiphospholipid syndrome. Blood 102:2717-2723, 2003.
34. Miyakis S, Lockshin MD, Atsumi D, et al: International consensus statement on an update of the classification criteria for definite antiphospholipid syndrome (APS). J Thromb Haemost 4:295-306, 2006.
35. Wahl DG, Guillemin F, de Maistre E, et al: Risk for venous thrombosis related to antiphospholipid antibodies in systemic lupus erythematosus: A meta-analysis. Lupus 6:467-473, 1997.
36. Crowther MA, Ginsberg JS, Julian J, et al: A comparison of two intensities of warfarin for the prevention of recurrent thrombosis in patients with the antiphospholipid antibody syndrome. N Engl J Med 349:1133-1138, 2003.
37. Branch DW, Silver RM, Blackwell JL, et al: Outcome of treated pregnancies in women with antiphospholipid syndrome: An update of the Utah experience. Obstet Gynecol 80:614-620, 1992.
38. Branch DW, Silver RM: Criteria for antiphospholipid syndrome: Early pregnancy loss, fetal loss, or recurrent pregnancy loss? Lupus 5:409-413, 1996.
39. Rai RS, Clifford K, Cohen H, et al: High prospective fetal loss rate in untreated pregnancies of women with recurrent miscarriage and antiphospholipid antibodies. Hum Reprod 10:3301-3304, 1995.
40. Birkenfeld A, Mukaida T, Minichiello L, et al: Incidence of autoimmune antibodies in failed embryo transfer cycles. Am J Reprod Immunol 31:65-68, 1994.
41. Birdsall MA, Lockwood GM, Ledger WL, et al: Antiphospholipid antibodies in women having in-vitro fertilization. Hum Reprod 11:1185-1189, 1996.
42. Hornstein MD, Davis OK, Massey JB, et al: Antiphospholipid antibodies and in vitro fertilization success: A meta-analysis. Fertil Steril 73:330-333, 2000.
43. Stern C, Chamley L, Norris H, et al: A randomized, double-blind, placebo-controlled trial of heparin and aspirin for women with in vitro fertilization implantation failure and antiphospholipid or antinuclear antibodies. Fertil Steril 80:376-383, 2003.
44. Branch DW, Andres R, Digrek B, et al: The association of antiphospholipid antibodies with severe preeclampsia. Obstet Gynecol 73:541-545, 1989.
45. Lee RM, Brown MA, Branch DW, et al: Anticardiolipin and anti-beta2-glycoprotein-I antibodies in preeclampsia. Obstet Gynecol 102:294-300, 2003.
46. Field SL, Brighton TA, McNeil HP, et al: Recent insights into antiphospholipid antibody-mediated thrombosis. Baillieres Best Pract Res Clin Haematol 12:407-422, 1999.
47. Rand JH, Wu XX, Andree HA, et al: Pregnancy loss in the antiphospholipid-antibody syndrome: A possible thrombogenic mechanism. N Engl J Med 337:154-160, 1997.
48. Girardi G, Redecha P, Salmon JE: Heparin prevents antiphospholipid antibody-induced fetal loss by inhibiting complement activation. Nat Med 10:1222-1226, 2004.
49. Kutteh WH: Antiphospholipid antibody-associated recurrent pregnancy loss: Treatment with heparin and low-dose aspirin is superior to low-dose aspirin alone. Am J Obstet Gynecol 174:1584-1589, 1996.
50. Farquharson RG, Quenby S, Greaves M: Antiphospholipid syndrome in pregnancy: A randomized, controlled trial of treatment. Obstet Gynecol 100:408-413, 2002.
51. Empson M, Lassere M, Craig J, et al: Prevention of recurrent miscarriage for women with antiphospholipid antibody or lupus anticoagulant. Cochrane Database Syst Rev (2):CD002859, 2005.
52. Di Nisio M, Peters L, Middeldorp S: Anticoagulants for the treatment of recurrent pregnancy loss in women without antiphospholipid syndrome. Cochrane Database Syst Rev (2):CD004734, 2005.
53. Backos M, Rai R, Baxter N, et al: Pregnancy complications in women with recurrent miscarriage associated with antiphospholipid antibodies treated with low dose aspirin and heparin. Br J Obstet Gynaecol 106:102-107, 1999.
54. Clark AL, Branch DW, Silver RM, et al: Pregnancy complicated by the antiphospholipid syndrome: Outcomes with intravenous immunoglobulin therapy. Obstet Gynecol 93:437-441, 1999.
55. Triolo G, Ferrante A, Ciccia F, et al: Randomized study of subcutaneous low molecular weight heparin plus aspirin versus intravenous immunoglobulin in the treatment of recurrent fetal loss associated with antiphospholipid antibodies. Arthritis Rheum 48:728-731, 2003.
56. Branch DW, Peaceman AM, Druzin M, et al: A multicenter, placebo-controlled pilot study of intravenous immune globulin treatment of antiphospholipid syndrome during pregnancy. The Pregnancy Loss Study Group. Am J Obstet Gynecol 182(1 Pt 1):122-127, 2000.
57. Tincani A, Branch W, Levy RA, et al: Treatment of pregnant patients with antiphospholipid syndrome. Lupus 12:524-529, 2003.
58. Franco RF, Reitsma PH: Genetic risk factors of venous thrombosis. Hum Genet 109:369-384, 2001.
59. Gerhardt A, Scharf RE, Beckmann MW, et al: Prothrombin and factor V mutations in women with a history of thrombosis during pregnancy and the puerperium. N Engl J Med 342:374-380, 2000.
60. Zotz RB, Gerhardt A, Scharf RE: Inherited thrombophilia and gestational venous thromboembolism. Best Pract Res Clin Haematol 16:243-259, 2003.
61. Press RD, Bauer KA, Kujorich JL, et al: Clinical utility of factor V Leiden (R506Q) testing for the diagnosis and management of thromboembolic disorders. Arch Pathol Lab Med 126:1304-1318, 2002.
62. Brenner BR, Nowak-Gottl U, Kosch A, et al: Diagnostic studies for thrombophilia in women on hormonal therapy and during pregnancy, and in children. Arch Pathol Lab Med 126:1296-1303, 2002.
63. Rey E, Kahn SR, David M, et al: Thrombophilic disorders and fetal loss: A meta-analysis. Lancet 361:901-908, 2003.
64. Gris JC, Quere I, Monpeyroux F, et al: Case-control study of the frequency of thrombophilic disorders in couples with late foetal loss and no thrombotic antecedent: The Nimes Obstetricians and Haematologists Study 5 (NOHA5). Thromb Haemost 81:891-899, 1999.
65. Dudding TE, Attia J: The association between adverse pregnancy outcomes and maternal factor V Leiden genotype: A meta-analysis. Thromb Haemost 91:700-711, 2004.
66. Lissalde-Lavigne G, Fabbro-Peray P, Quere I, et al: Factor V Leiden and prothrombin G20210A polymorphisms as risk factors for miscarriage during a first intended pregnancy: The matched case-control "NOHA First" study. J Thromb Haemost 3:2178-2184, 2005.
67. Preston FE, Rosendaal FR, Walker ID, et al: Increased fetal loss in women with heritable thrombophilia. Lancet 48:913-916, 1996.

68. Vossen CY, Preston FE, Conard J, et al: Hereditary thrombophilia and fetal loss: A prospective follow-up study. J Thromb Haemost 2:592-596, 2004.
69. Roque H, Paidas MJ, Funai EF, et al: Maternal thrombophilias are not associated with early pregnancy loss. Thromb Haemost 91:290-295, 2004.
70. Gopel W, Ludwig M, Junge AK, et al: Selection pressure for the factor-V-Leiden mutation and embryo implantation. Lancet 358:1238-1239, 2001.
71. Rodesch F, Simon P, Donner C, et al: Oxygen measurements in endometrial and trophoblastic tissues during early pregnancy. Obstet Gynecol 80:283-285, 1992.
72. Jaffe R: Investigation of abnormal first-trimester gestations by color Doppler imaging. J Clin Ultrasound 21:521-526, 1993.
73. Watson AL, Skepper JN, Jauniaux E, et al: Susceptibility of human placental syncytiotrophoblastic mitochondria to oxygen-mediated damage in relation to gestational age. J Clin Endocrinol Metab 83:1697-1705, 1998.
74. Kupferminc MJ, Eldor A, Steinman N, et al: Increased frequency of genetic thrombophilia in women with complications of pregnancy. N Engl J Med 340:9-13, 1999.
75. Currie L, Peek M, McNiven M, et al: Is there an increased maternal-infant prevalence of factor V Leiden in association with severe pre-eclampsia? BJOG 109:191-196, 2002.
76. van Pampus MG, Wolf H, Koopman MM, et al: Prothrombin 20210 G: A mutation and factor V Leiden mutation in women with a history of severe preeclampsia and (H)ELLP syndrome. Hypertens Pregnancy 20:291-298, 2001.
77. D'Elia AV, Driul L, Giacomello R, et al: Frequency of factor V, prothrombin and methylenetetrahydrofolate reductase gene variants in preeclampsia. Gynecol Obstet Invest 53:84-87, 2002.
78. Lin J, August P: Genetic thrombophilias and preeclampsia: A meta-analysis. Obstet Gynecol 105:182-192, 2005.
79. Kosmas IP, Tatsioni A, Ioannidis JP: Association of Leiden mutation in factor V gene with hypertension in pregnancy and pre-eclampsia: A meta-analysis. J Hypertens 21:1221-1228, 2003.
80. Wiener-Megnagi Z, Ben-Shlomo I, Goldberg Y, Shalev E: Resistance to activated protein C and the Leiden mutation: High prevalence in patients with abruptio placentae. Am J Obstet Gynecol 179:1565-1567,1998.
81. Procházka M, Lubuský M, Slavík L, et al: Frequency of selected thrombophilias in women with placental abruption. Aust N Z J Obstet Gynaecol 47(4):297-301, 2007.
82. Alfirevic Z, Roberts D, Martlew V: How strong is the association between maternal thrombophilia and adverse pregnancy outcome? A systematic review. Eur J Obstet Gynecol Reprod Biol 101:6-14, 2002.
83. Martinelli P, Grandone E, Colaizzo D, et al: Familial thrombophilia and the occurrence of fetal growth restriction. Haematologica 86:428-431, 2001.
84. Infante-Rivard C, Rivard GE, Yotov WV, et al: Absence of association of thrombophilia polymorphisms with intrauterine growth restriction. N Engl J Med 347:19-25, 2002.
85. Howley HE, Walker M, Rodger MA: A systematic review of the association between factor V Leiden or prothrombin gene variant and intrauterine growth restriction. Am J Obstet Gynecol 192:694-708, 2005.
86. Lindqvist PG, Svensson PJ, Marsaal K, et al: Activated protein C resistance (FV:Q506) and pregnancy. Thromb Haemost 81:532-537, 1999.
87. Dizon-Townson D, Miller C, Sibai B, et al: The relationship of the factor V Leiden mutation and pregnancy outcomes for mother and fetus. Obstet Gynecol 106:517-524, 2005.
88. Castaman G, Faioni EM, Tosetto A, et al: The factor V HR2 haplotype and the risk of venous thrombosis: A meta-analysis. Haematologia 88:1182-1189, 2003.
89. Zammiti W, Mtiraoui N, Mercier E, et al: Association of factor V gene polymorphisms (Leiden; Cambridge; Hong Kong and HR2 haplotype) with recurrent idiopathic pregnancy loss in Tunisia: A case-control study. Thromb Haemost 95:612-617, 2006.
90. Dilley A, Benito C, Hooper WC, et al: Mutations in the factor V, prothrombin and MTHFR genes are not risk factors for recurrent fetal loss. J Matern Fetal Neonatal Med 11:176-182, 2002.
91. Franco RF, Maffei FH, Lourenco D, et al: Factor V Arg306→Thr (factor V Cambridge) and factor V Arg306→Gly mutations in venous thrombotic disease. Br J Haematol 103:888-890, 1998.
92. Foka ZJ, Lambropoulos AF, Saravelos H, et al: Factor V Leiden and prothrombin G20210A mutations, but not methylenetetrahydrofolate reductase C677T, are associated with recurrent miscarriages. Hum Reprod 15:458-462, 2000.
93. Finan RR, Tamim H, Ameen G, et al: Prevalence of factor V G1691A (factor V-Leiden) and prothrombin G20210A gene mutations in a recurrent miscarriage population. Am J Hematol 71:300-305, 2002.
94. Carp H, Salomon O, Seidman D, et al: Prevalence of genetic markers for thrombophilia in recurrent pregnancy loss. Hum Reprod 17:1633-1637, 2002.
95. Jivraj S, Rai R, Underwood J, et al: Genetic thrombophilic mutations among couples with recurrent miscarriage. Hum Reprod 21:1161-1165, 2006.
96. Kovalevsky G, Gracia CR, Berlin JA, et al: Evaluation of the association between hereditary thrombophilias and recurrent pregnancy loss: A meta-analysis. Arch Intern Med 164:558-563, 2004.
97. Morrison ER, Miedzybrodzka ZH, Campbell DM, et al: Prothrombotic genotypes are not associated with pre-eclampsia and gestational hypertension: Results from a large population-based study and systematic review. Thromb Haemost 87:779-785, 2002.
98. Livingston JC, Barton JR, Park V, et al: Maternal and fetal inherited thrombophilias are not related to the development of severe preeclampsia. Am J Obstet Gynecol 185:153-157, 2001.
99. Peng F, Labelle LA, Rainey BJ, et al: Single nucleotide polymorphisms in the methylenetetrahydrofolate reductase gene are common in US Caucasian and Hispanic American populations. Int J Mol Med 8:509-511, 2001.
100. den Heijer M, Rosendaal FR, Blom HJ, et al: Hyperhomocysteinemia and venous thrombosis: A meta-analysis. Thromb Haemost 80:874-877, 1998.
101. Domagala TB, Adamek L, Nizankowska E, et al: Mutations C677T and A1298C of the 5,10-methylenetetrahydrofolate reductase gene and fasting plasma homocysteine levels are not associated with the increased risk of venous thromboembolic disease. Blood Coagul Fibrinolysis 13:423-431, 2002.
102. McColl MD, Ellison J, Reid F, et al: Prothrombin 20210 G→A, MTHFR C677T mutations in women with venous thromboembolism associated with pregnancy. BJOG 107:565-569, 2000.
103. Nelen WL, Blom HJ, Steegers EA, et al: Hyperhomocysteinemia and recurrent early pregnancy loss: A meta-analysis. Fertil Steril 74:1196-1199, 2000.
104. Vollset SE, Refsum H, Irgens LM, et al: Plasma total homocysteine, pregnancy complications, and adverse pregnancy outcomes: The Hordaland Homocysteine study. Am J Clin Nutr 71:962-968, 2000.
105. Nurk E, Tell GS, Refsum H, et al: Associations between maternal methylenetetrahydrofolate reductase polymorphisms and adverse outcomes of pregnancy: The Hordaland Homocysteine Study. Am J Med 117:26-31, 2004.
106. Ray JG, Laskin CA: Folic acid and homocyst(e)ine metabolic defects and the risk of placental abruption, pre-eclampsia and spontaneous pregnancy loss: A systematic review. Placenta 20:519-529, 1999.
107. Castanon MM, Lauricella AM, Kordich L, et al: Plasma homocysteine cutoff values for venous thrombosis. Clin Chem Lab Med 45:232-236, 2007.
108. Carraro P: Guidelines for the laboratory investigation of inherited thrombophilias: Recommendations for the first level clinical laboratories. Clin Chem Lab Med 41:382-391, 2003.
109. Conard J, Horellon MH, Van Dreden P, et al: Thrombosis and pregnancy in congenital deficiencies in AT III, protein C or protein S: Study of 78 women. Thromb Haemost 63:319-320, 1990.
110. De Stefano V, Martinelli I, Rossi E, et al: The risk of recurrent venous thromboembolism in pregnancy and puerperium without antithrombotic prophylaxis. Br J Haematol 135:386-391, 2006.

111. Marlar RA, Neumann A: Neonatal purpura fulminans due to homozygous protein C or protein S deficiencies. Semin Thromb Hemost 16:299-309, 1990.
112. Friederich PW, Sanson BJ, Simioni P, et al: Frequency of pregnancy-related venous thromboembolism in anticoagulant factor-deficient women: Implications for prophylaxis. Ann Intern Med 125:955-960, 1996.
113. Hellgren M, Tengborn L, Abildgaard U: Pregnancy in women with congenital antithrombin III deficiency: Experience of treatment with heparin and antithrombin. Gynecol Obstet Invest 14:127-141, 1982.
114. Borgel D, Duchemin J, Alhenc-Gelas M, et al: Molecular basis for protein S hereditary deficiency: Genetic defects observed in 118 patients with type I and type IIa deficiencies. The French Network on Molecular Abnormalities Responsible for Protein C and Protein S Deficiencies. J Lab Clin Med 128:218-227, 1996.
115. Goodwin AJ, Rosendaal FR, Kottke-Marchant K, et al: A review of the technical, diagnostic, and epidemiologic considerations for protein S assays. Arch Pathol Lab Med 126:1349-1366, 2002.
116. Water N, Tan T, Ashton F, et al: Mutations within the protein Z-dependent protease inhibitor gene are associated with venous thromboembolic disease: A new form of thrombophilia. Br J Haematol 127:190-194, 2004.
117. Vasse M, Guegan-Massardier E, Borg JY, et al: Frequency of protein Z deficiency in patients with ischaemic stroke. Lancet 357:933-934, 2001.
118. Gris JC, Quere I, Dechaud H, et al: High frequency of protein Z deficiency in patients with unexplained early fetal loss. Blood 99:2606-2608, 2002.
119. Gris JC, Mercier E, Quere I, et al: Low-molecular-weight heparin versus low-dose aspirin in women with one fetal loss and a constitutional thrombophilic disorder. Blood 103:3695-3699, 2004.
120. Morange PE, Henry M, Tregouet D, et al: The A844G polymorphism in the PAI-1 gene is associated with a higher risk of venous thrombosis in factor V Leiden carriers. Arterioscler Thromb Vasc Biol 20:1387-1391, 2000.
121. Buchholz T, Lohse P, Rogenhofer N, et al: Polymorphisms in the ACE and PAI-1 genes are associated with recurrent spontaneous miscarriages. Hum Reprod 18:2473-2477, 2003.
122. Varela ML, Adamczuk YP, Forastiero RR, et al: Major and potential prothrombotic genotypes in a cohort of patients with venous thromboembolism. Thromb Res 104:317-324, 2001.
123. Gubric N, Stegnar M, Peternel P, et al: A novel G/A and the 4G/5G polymorphism within the promoter of the plasminogen activator inhibitor-1 gene in patients with deep vein thrombosis. Thromb Res 84:431-443, 1996.
124. Ridker PM, Hennekens CH, Lindpaintner K, et al: Arterial and venous thrombosis is not associated with the 4G/5G polymorphism in the promoter of the plasminogen activator inhibitor gene in a large cohort of US men. Circulation 95:59-62, 1997.
125. Stegnar M, Uhrin P, Peternel P, et al: The 4G/5G sequence polymorphism in the promoter of plasminogen activator inhibitor-1 (PAI-1) gene: Relationship to plasma PAI-1 level in venous thromboembolism. Thromb Haemost 79:975-979, 1998.
126. Zöller B, Garcia de Frutos P, Dahlbäck B: A common 4G allele in the promoter of the plasminogen activator inhibitor-1 (PAI-1) gene as a risk factor for pulmonary embolism and arterial thrombosis in hereditary protein S deficiency. Thromb Haemost 79:802-807, 1998.
127. Junker R, Nabavi DG, Wolff E, et al: Plasminogen activator inhibitor-1 4G/4G genotype is associated with cerebral sinus thrombosis in factor V Leiden carriers. Thromb Haemost 80:706-707, 1998.
128. Wolf CE, Haubelt H, Pauer HU, et al: Recurrent pregnancy loss and its relation to FV Leiden, FII G20210A and polymorphisms of plasminogen activator and plasminogen activator inhibitor. Pathophysiol Haemost Thromb 33:134-137, 2003.
129. Dossenbach-Glaninger A, van Trotsenburg M, Dossenbach M, et al: Plasminogen activator inhibitor 1 4G/5G polymorphism and coagulation factor XIII Val34Leu polymorphism: impaired fibrinolysis and early pregnancy loss. Clin Chem 49:1081-1086, 2003.
130. Yamada N, Arinami T, Yamakawa-Kobayashi K, et al: The 4G/5G polymorphism of the plasminogen activator inhibitor-1 gene is associated with severe preeclampsia. J Hum Genet 45:138-141, 2000.
131. Glueck CJ, Phillips H, Cameron D, et al: The 4G/4G polymorphism of the hypofibrinolytic plasminogen activator inhibitor type 1 gene: An independent risk factor for serious pregnancy complications. Metabolism 49:845-852, 2000.
132. van der Bom JG, de Maat MP, Bots ML, et al: Elevated plasma fibrinogen: Cause or consequence of cardiovascular disease? Arterioscler Thromb Vasc Biol 18:621-625, 1998.
133. Brown K, Luddington R, Taylor SA, et al: Risk of venous thromboembolism associated with the common hereditary haemochromatosis Hfe gene (C282Y) mutation. Br J Haematol 105:95-97, 1999.
134. Hefler L, Jirecek S, Heim K, et al: Genetic polymorphisms associated with thrombophilia and vascular disease in women with unexplained late intrauterine fetal death: A multicenter study. J Soc Gynecol Investig 11:42-44, 2004.
135. Kobbervig C, Williams E: FXIII polymorphisms, fibrin clot structure and thrombotic risk. Biophys Chem 112:223-228, 2004.
136. Brill-Edwards P, Ginsberg JS, Gent M, et al: Recurrence of clot in this pregnancy study group: Safety of withholding heparin in pregnant women with a history of venous thromboembolism. N Engl J Med 343:1439-1444, 2000.
137. Blickstein D: The 7th American College of Chest Physicians Guidelines for the Antenatal and Peripartum Management of Thrombophilia: A Tutorial. Obstet Gynecol Clin North Am 33:499-505, 2006.
138. Barbour LA, Smith JM, Marlar RA: Heparin levels to guide thromboembolism prophylaxis during pregnancy. Am J Obstet Gynecol 173:1869-1873, 1995.
139. Barbour LA, Oja JL, Schultz LK: A prospective trial that demonstrates that dalteparin requirements increase in pregnancy to maintain therapeutic levels of anticoagulation. Am J Obstet Gynecol 191:1024-1029, 2004.
140. Warkentin TE, Greinacher A: Heparin-induced thrombocytopenia: Recognition, treatment, and prevention. The seventh ACCP conference on Antithrombotic and Thrombolytic Therapy. Chest 126(3 Suppl):311S-317S, 2004.
141. Kupferminc MJ, Fait G, Many A, et al: Low-molecular-weight heparin for the prevention of obstetric complications in women with thrombophilias. Hypertens Pregnancy 20:35-44, 2001.
142. Folkeringa N, Brouwer JL, Korteweg FJ, et al: Reduction of high fetal loss rate by anticoagulant treatment during pregnancy in antithrombin, protein C or protein S deficient women. Br J Haematol 136:656-661, 2007.
143. Cines DB, Blanchette VS: Immune thrombocytopenic purpura. N Engl J Med 346:995-1008, 2002.
144. George JN, Woolf SH, Raskob GE, et al: Idiopathic thrombocytopenic purpura: A practice guideline developed by explicit methods for the American Society of Hematology. Blood 88:3, 1996.
145. Burrows RF, Kelton JG: Incidentally detected thrombocytopenia in healthy mothers and their infants. N Engl J Med 319:142, 1988.
146. Burrows RF, Kelton JG: Thrombocytopenia at delivery: A prospective survey of 6715 deliveries. Am J Obstet Gynecol 162:731.a, 1990.
147. Burrows BF, Kelton JG: Fetal thrombocytopenia and its relation to maternal thrombocytopenia. N Engl J Med 329:1463.a, 1993.
148. George JN, El-Harake MA, Raskob GE: Chronic idiopathic thromboeytopenic purpura. N Engl J Med 331:1207, 1994.
149. Raife TJ, Olsen JD, Lentz SR: Platelet antibody testing in idiopathic thrombocytopenic purpura. Blood 89:1112-1114, 1996.
150. Lescale KB, Eddleman KA, Cines DB, et al: Antiplatelet antibody testing in thrombocytopenic pregnant women. Am J Obstet Gynecol 114:1014, 1996.
151. American Society of Hematology ITP Practice Guideline Panel: Diagnosis and treatment of idiopathic thrombocytopenic purpura: Recommendations of the American Society of Hematology. Ann Intern Med 126:319, 1997.

152. Webert KE, Mittai R, Sigouin C, et al: A retrospective 11-year analysis of obstetric patients with idiopathic thrombocytopenic purpura. Blood 102:4306-4311, 2003.
153. Martin JN, Morrison JC, Files JC: Autoimmune thrombocytopenic purpura: Current concepts and recommended practices. Am J Obstet Gynecol 150:86, 1984.
154. Imbach P, Jungi TW: Possible mechanisms of intravenous immunoglobulin: Treatment in childhood idiopathic thrombocytopenic purpura. Blood 46:117, 1983.
155. Bussel JB, Pham LC: Intravenous treatment with gamma globulin in adults with immune thrombocytopenia purpura: Review of the literature. Vox Sang 52:206, 1987.
156. Barton JC, Saleh MN: Case report: Immune thrombocytopenia: Effects of maternal gammaglobulin infusion in maternal and fetal serum, platelet, and monocyte IgG. Am J Med Sci 293:112, 1987.
157. Fehr J, Hofmann V, Kappeler U: Transient reversal of thrombocytopenia in idiopathic thrombocytopenic purpura by high-dose intravenous gamma globulin. N Engl J Med 306:1254, 1982.
158. Newland AC: The use and mechanisms of action of intravenous immune globulin: An update. Br J Haematol 72:301, 1989.
159. Ben-Chetrit E, Putterman C: Transient neutropenia induced by intravenous immune globulin. N Engl J Med 326:270, 1992.
160. Newman GC, Novoa MV, Fodero EM, et al: A dose of 75 μg/kg/d of i.v. anti-D increases the platelet count more rapidly and for a longer period of time than 50 μg/kg/d in adults with immune thrombocytopenic purpura. Br J Haematol 112:1076-1078, 2001.
161. Michel M, Novoa MV, Bussel JB: Intravenous anti-D as a treatment for immune thrombocytopenic purpura (ITP) during pregnancy. Br J Haematol 123:142-146, 2003.
162. Kaplan C, Daffos F, Forestier F, et al: Fetal platelet counts in thrombocytopenic pregnancy. Lancet 336:979, 1990.
163. Cook RL, Miller RC, Katz VL, Cefalo RC: Immune thrombocytopenic purpura in pregnancy: A reappraisal of management. Obstet Gynecol 78:578, 1991.
164. Christiaens CCML, Nieuwenhuis HK, Von Dens Borne AEGKr, et al: Idiopathic thrombocytopenic purpura in pregnancy: A randomized trial on the effect of antenatal low dose corticosteroids on neonatal platelet count. Br J Obstet Gynaecol 97:893, 1990.
165. Jones RW, Asher MI, Rutherford CJ, Munro HM: Autoimmune (idiopathic) thrombocytopenic purpura in pregnancy and the newborn. Br J Obstet Gynaecol 84:679, 1977.
166. Carloss H, McMillan R, Crosby WH: Management of pregnancy in women with immune thrombocytopenic purpura. JAMA 224:2756, 1980.
167. Ayromlooi J: A new approach to the management of immunologic thrombocytopenic purpura in pregnancy. Am J Obstet Gynecol 130:235, 1978.
168. Burrows RF, Kelton JC: Pregnancy in patients with idiopathic thrombocytopenic purpura: Assessing the risks for the infant at delivery. Obstet Gymecol Surv 48:781.b, 1993.
169. Scott JR, Rote NS, Cruikshank DP: Antiplatelet antibodies and platelet counts in pregnancies complicated by autoimmune thrombocytopenic purpura. Am J Obstet Gynecol 145:932, 1983.
170. Samuels P, Russel JB, Braitman LE, et al: Estimation of the risk of thrombocytopenia in the offspring of pregnant women with presumed immune thrombocytopenia purpura. N Engl J Med 323:229, 1990.
171. Rauch AE, Mycek JA, Mills CR, et al: Risk of hrombocytopenia in offspring of mothers with presumed immune thrombocytopenic purpura. N Engl J Med 326:1841, 1990.
172. Moise KJ, Cotton DB: Discordant fetal platelet counts in a twin gestation complicated by idiopathic thrombocytopenic purpura. Am J Obstet Gynecol 156:1141, 1987.
173. Scott JR, Cruikshank DP, Kochenour NK, et al: Fetal platelet counts in the obstetric management of immunologic thrombocytopenic purpura. Am J Obstet Gynecol 136:495, 1980.
174. Wahbeh CJ, Eden RD, Killam AP, Gall SA: Pregnancy and immune thrombocytopenic purpura. Am J Obstet Gynecol 149:238, 1984.
175. Christiaens GCML, Helmerhorst FM: Validity of intrapartum diagnosis of fetal thrombocytopenia. Am J Obstet Gynecol 157:864, 1987.
176. Payne SD, Resnik R, Moore TR, et al: Maternal characteristics and risk of severe neonatal thrombocytopenia and intra-cranial hemorrhage in pregnancies complicated by autoirnmune thrombocytopenia. Am J Obstet Gynecol 177:149, 1997.
177. Moise KJ Jr, Carpenter RJ Jr, Cotton DB, et al: Percutaneous umbilical cord blood sampling in the evaluation of fetal platelet counts in pregnant patients with autoimmune thrombocytopenic purpura. Obstet Gynecol 72:346, 1988.
178. Scioscia AL, Grannum PAT, Copel JA, Hobbins JC: The use of percutaneous umbilical blood sampling in immune thrombocytopenic purpura. Am J Obstet Gynecol 159:1066, 1988.
179. Ghidini A, Sepulveda W, Lockwood CJ, Romero R: Complications of fetal blood sampling. Am J Obstet Gvnecol 168:1339, 1993.
180. Silver RM: Management of idiopathic thrombocytopenic purpura in pregnancy. Clin Obstet Gynecol 41:436, 1998.
181. Segal NI, Manning FA, Harman CR, Menticoglou S: Bleeding after intravascular transfusion: Experimental and clinical observations. Am J Obstet Gynecol 165:1.414, 1991.
182. Paidas MJ, Berkowitz RL, Lynch L, et al: Alloimmune thrombocytopenia: Fetal and neonatal losses related to cordocentesis. Am J Obstet Gynecol 172:475, 1995.
183. Burrows RF, Kelton JG: Low fetal risks in pregnancies associated with idiopathic thrombocytopenic purpura. Am J Obstet Gynecol 163:1147.b, 1990.
184. Silver RM, Branch DW, Scott JR: Maternal thrombocytopenia in pregnancy: Time for a reassessment. Am J Obstet Gynecol 173:479, 1995.
185. Laros RK, Kagan R: Route of delivery for patients with immune thrombocytopenia. Am J Obstet Gynecol 148:901, 1984.
186. Skupski DW, Bussel JB: Further insights into autoimmune thrombocytopenia and pregnancy. Am J Obstet Gynecol 174:1944, 1996.
187. Kelton JG, Inwood MJ, Barr RM, et al: The prenatal prediction of thrombocytopenia in infants of mothers with clinically diagnosed immune thrombocytopenia. Am J Obstet Gynecol 144:449, 1992.
188. Blanchette VS, Chen L, Defreidberg A, et al: Alloimmunization to the PLAT platelet antigen: Results of a prospective study. Br J Haematol 14:209, 1990.
189. Bussel JB, Berkowitz RL, McFarland JG, et al: Antenatal treatment of neonatal alloimmune thrombocytopenia. N Engl J Med 319:1374, 1988.
190. Williamson LM, Hacket G, Rennie J, et al: The natural history of fetomaternal alloimmunization to the platelet specific antigen HPA-1a (PlA1, Zwa) as determined by antenatal screening. Blood 92:2280-2287, 1998.
191. Berkowitz RL, Bussel JB, McFarland JG: Alloimmune thrombocytopenia: State of the art 2006. Am J Obstet Gynecol 195:907-13.a, 2006.
192. Von dens Borne AEG, Decary F: Nomenclature of platelet-specific antigens. Transfusion 30:477, 1990.
193. Newman PJ, Derbes RS, Aster RH: The human platelet alloantigens, PLA' and PLA2, are associated with a leucine33/proline33 amino acid polymorphism in membrane glycoprotein IIIA and are distinguishable by DNA typing. J Clin Invest 83:1778, 1989.
194. Shulman NR, Jordan JV: Platelet immunology. In Colman RW Hirsh J, Marder VJ, Salzman EW (eds): Hemostasis and Thrombosis: Basic Principles and Clinical Practice. Philadelphia: JB Lippincott, 1982, pp 274-342.
195. Shulman NR, Marder VJ, Heller MC, Collier EM: Platelet and leukocyte isoantigens and their antibodies: Serologic, physiologic and clinical studies. Prog Hematol 4:222, 1964.
196. Tanning E, Sldbsted L: The frequency of platelet alloantibodies in pregnant women and the occurrence and management of neonatal alloimmune thrombocytopenic purpura. Obstet Gynecol Surv 45:521, 1990.
197. Valentin N, Vergracht A, Bignon JD, et al: HLA-DRw52a is involved in alloimmunization against PLA1 antigen. Hum Immunol 27:73, 1990.
198. Mueller-Eckhardt C, Mueller-Eckhardt G, Willen-Ohff H, et al: A new immune response marker for immunization against the platelet alloantigen Br. Vox Sang 57:90.a, 1989.
199. Mueller-Eckhardt C, Kiefel V, Grubert A, et al: 347 cases of suspected neonatal alloimmune thrombocytopenia. Lancet i:363.b, 1989.

200. Berkowitz R, Bussel JB, Hung C, Wissert M: A randomized prospective treatment trial for patients with "standard risk" alloimmune thrombocytopenia (AIT). Am J Obstet Gynecol 195:S23, 2006.
201. Herman JH, Jumbelic MI, Ancona RJ, Kiclder TS: In utero cerebral hemorrhage in alloimmune thrombocytopenia. Am J Pediatr Hematol Oncol 8:312, 1986.
202. Bussel JB, Skupski DW, MacFarland JG: Fetal alloimmune thrombocytopenic: Consensus and controversy. J Matern Fetal Med 5:281.b, 1996.
203. Kaplan C, Forestier F, Cox WL, et al: Management of alloimmune thrombocytopenia: Antenatal diagnosis and in utero transfusion of maternal platelets. Blood 72:340, 1988.
204. McFarland JG, Aster RH, Bussel JB, et al: Prenatal diagnosis of neonatal alloimmune thrombocytopenia using allele-specific oligonucleotide probes. Blood 78:2276, 1991.
205. Bussel JB, Zabusky MR, Berkowitz RL, McFarland JG: Fetal alloimmune thrombocytopenia. N Engl J Med 337:22-26, 1997.
206. Giovangrandi Y, Daffos E, Kaplan C, et al: Very early intracranial hemorrhage in alloimmune thrombocytopenia. Lancet 11:310, 1990.
207. Bussel JB, Berkowitz RL, Lynch L, et al: Antenatal management of alloimmune thrombocytopenia with intravenous-γ-globulin: A randomized trial of the addition of low dose steroid to intravenous-γ-globulin. Am J Obstet Gynecol 174:1414.a, 1996.
208. Mir N, Samson D, House MJ, et al: Failure of antenatal high-dose immunoglobulin to improve fetal platelet count in neonatal alloimmune thrombocytopenia. Vox Sang 55:188, 1988.
209. Lynch L, Bussel JB, McFarland JC, et al: Antenatal treatment of alloimmune thrombocytopenia. Obstet Gynecol 80:67, 1992.
210. Marzusch K, Shcnaidt M, Dietl J, et al: High-dose immunoglobulin in the antenatal treatment of neonatal alloimmune thrombocytopenia: Case report and review. Br J Obstet Gynaecol 99:260, 1992.
211. Nicolini U, Tannirandorn Y, Gonzalez P, et al: Continuing controversy in alloimmune thrombocytopenia: Fetal hyperimmunoglobulinemia fails to prevent thrombocytopenia. Am J Obstet Gynecol 163:1144, 1990.
212. Bowman J, Harman C, Menrigolou S, Pollack J: Intravenous fetal transfusion of immunoglobulin for alloimmune thrombocytopenia. Lancet 340:1034, 1992.
213. Zimmerman R, Huch A: In utero fetal therapy with immunoglobulin for alloimmune thrombocytopenia. Lancet 340:606, 1992.
214. Nicoliru U, Bedeck CH, Kochenour NK, et al: In-utero platelet transfusion for alloimmune thrombocytopenia [Letter]. Lancet 2:506, 1988.
215. Murphy MF, Pullon HW II, Metcalfe P, et al: Management of fetal alloimmune thrombocytopenia by weekly in utero platelet transfusions. Vox Sang 58:45, 1990.
216. Silver RM, Porter TF, Branch DW, et al: Neonatal alloimmune thrombocytopenia: Antenatal management. Am J Obstet Gynecol 182:1233, 2000.
217. Overton TG, Duncan KR, Jolley M, et al: Serial platelet transfusion for fetal alloimmune thrombocytopenia: Platelet dynamics and perinatal outcome. Am J Obstet Gynecol 186:826-831, 2002.
218. Birchall JE, Murphy MF, Kaplan C, Kroll H: European collaborative study of the antenatal management of feto-maternal alloimune thrombocytopenia. Br J Haematol 122:175-288, 2003.
219. Morgan CL, Cannell GR, Addison RS, Minchinton RM: The effect of intravenous immunoglobulin on placental transfer of a platelet-specific antibody: Anti-PL. Transfus Med 1:209, 1991.
220. Berkowitz RL, Kolb A, McFarland JG, et al: Parallel randomized trials of risk-based therapy for fetal alloimmune thrombocytopenia. Obstet Gynecol 107:91-6.b/?, 2006.
221. Thung SF, Grobman WA: The cost effectiveness of empiric intravenous immunoglobulin for the antepartum treatment of fetal and neonatal alloimune thrombocytopenia. Am J Obstet Gynecol 193:1094-1099, 2005.
222. Dashe JS, Ramin SM, Cunningham FG: The long term consequences of thrombotic microangiopathy (thrombotic thrombocytopenic purpura and hemolytic uremic syndrome) in pregnancy. Obstet Gynecol 91:662, 1998.
223. Bell WR, Braine HG, Ness PM, et al: Improved survival in thrombocytopenic purpura-hemolytic uremic syndrome. N Engl J Med 325:398, 1991.
224. Remuzzi G: HUS and TTP: Variable expression of a single entity [Clinical conference]. Kidney Int 32:292, 1987.
225. Vesey SK, George JN, Lammle B, et al: ADAMTS13 activity in thrombotic thombocytoepnic purpura-hemolytic uremic syndrome: Relation to presenting features and clinical outcomes in a prospective cohort of 142 patients. Blood 101:60, 2003.
226. Furlan M, Robles R, Galbusera M, et al: Von Willebrand factor-cleaving protease in thrombotic thrombocytopenic purpura and the hemolytic uremic syndrome. N Engl J Med 339:1578-1584, 1998.
227. George JN: ADAMTS13, thrombotic thrombocytopenic purpura, and hemolytic syndrome. Curent Hematol Rep 4:167, 2005.
228. Levy GG, Nichols WC, Lian EC, et al: Mutations in a member of the ADAMTS gene family cause thrombotic thrombocytopenicpurpura. Nature 413:488, 2001.
229. Starke R, Machin S, Scully M, et al: The clinical utility of ADAMTS13 activity, antigen and autoantibody assays in thrombotic thrombocytopenic purpura. Br J Haematol 136:649, 2006.
230. Gordjani N, Sutor AH, Zimmerhackl LB, Brandis M: Hemolytic uremic syndromes in childhood. Semin Thromb Hemost 23:281, 1997.
231. Rehberg JF, Briery C, Hudson WT, et al: Thrombotic thrombocytopenic purpura masquerading as hemolysis, elevated liver enzymes, low platelets (HELLP) syndrome in late pregnancy. Obstet Gyncol 108:817, 2006.
232. Brostrom S, Bergman OJ: Thrombotic thrombocytopenic purpura: A difficult differential diagnosis in pregnancy. Acta Obstet Gynecol Scand 79:84, 2000.
233. Esplin MS, Branch DW: Diagnosis and management of thrombotic microangiopathies during pregnancy. Clin Obstet Gynecol 42:360, 1999.
234. Rock GA, Shumak KH, Buskard NA, et al: Comparison of plasma exchange with plasma infusion in the treatment of thrombotic thrombocytopenic purpura. Canadian Apheresis Study Group [see comments]. N Engl J Med 325:393, 1991.
235. Rock G, Shumak KH, Kelton J, et al: Thrombotic thrombocytopenic purpura: Outcome in 24 patients with renal impairment treated with plasma exchange. Transfusion (Paris) 32:710, 1992.
236. George JN: The association of pregnancy with thrombotic thrombocytopenic purpura-hemolytic syndrome. Curr Opin Hematol 10:339, 2003.
237. Sanchez-Luceros, A, Farias CE, Amaral MM, et al: von Willebrand factor-cleaving protease (ADAMTS13) activity in normal non-pregnant women, pregnant and post-delivery women. Thromb Haemost 92:1320, 2004.
238. Egerman RS, Witlin AG, Friedman SA, et al: Thrombotic thrombocytopenic purpura and hemolytic uremic syndrome in pregnancy: Review of 11 cases. Am J Obstet Gynecol 175:950, 1996.
239. Castella M, Pujol M, Julia A, et al: Thombotic thrombocytopenic purpura and pregnancy: A review of 10 cases. Vox Sanguinis 87:287, 2004.
240. Vesely SK, Li X, McMinn JR, et al: Pregnancy outcomes after recovery from thrombotic thrombocytopenic purpura-hemolytic uremic syndrome. Transfusion 44:1149, 2004.
241. Scully M, Starke R, Lee R, et al: Successful management of pregnancy in women with a history of thrombotic thrombocytopaenic purpura. Blood Coagul Fibrinolysis 17:459, 2006.
242. Bloom AL: von Willebrand factor: Clinical features of inherited and acquired disorders. Mayo Clin Proc 66:743, 1991.
243. James AH: Von Willebrand disease. Obstet Gynecol Surv 61:136, 2006.
244. Fausett B, Silver RM: Congenital disorders of platelet function. Clin Obstet Gynecol 42:390, 1999.
245. Roque H, Funai E, Lockwood CJ: Von Willebrand disease and pregnancy. J Matern Fetal Med 9:257, 2000.
246. Phillips MD, Santhouse A: von Willebrand disease: Recent advances in pathophysiology and treatment. Am J Med Sci 316:77, 1998.
247. Lee CA, Chi C, Pavord SR, et al: The obstetric and gynaecological management of women with inherited bleeding disorders: Review with guidelines produced by a taskforce of UK Haemophilia Centre Doctor's Organization. Haemophilia 12:301, 2006.

248. Holmberg L, Nillson IM, Borge L, et al: Plaetlet aggregation induced by 1-desamino-8-D-arginine vasoporessin (DDAVP) in type IIB von Willebrand disease. N Engl J Med 309:816, 1983.
249. James AH, Jamison MG: Bleeding events and other complications during pregnancy and childbirth in women with von Willebrand disease. J Thromb Haemost 5:1165-1169, 2007.
250. Peake IR, Bowen D, Bignell P, et al: Family studies and prenatal diagnosis in severe von Willebrand disease by polymerase chain reaction amplification of a variable number tandem repeat region of the von Willebrand factor gene. Blood 76:555, 1990.
251. Peyvandi F, Jayandharan G, Chandy M, et al: Genetic diagnosis of haemophilia and other inherited bleeding disordes. Haemophilia 12:82, 2006.
252. Rothschild C, Forestier F, Daffos F, et al: Prenatal diagnosis in type IIA von Willebrand disease. Nouv Rev Fr Hematol 32:125, 1990.
253. Shetty S, Ghosh K: Robustness of factor assays following cordocentesis in the prenatal diagnosis of hemophilia and other bleeding disorders. Haemophilia 13:172, 2007.
254. Sage DJ: Epidurals, spinals, and bleeding disorders in pregnancy: A review. Anesth Intensive Care 18:319, 1990.
255. Marrache D, Mercier FJ, Boyer-Newman C, et al: Epidural analgesia for parturients with type 1 von Willebrand disease. Int J Obstet Anesth 16:231-235, 2007.
256. Chediak JR, Alban GM, Maxey B: von Willebrand's disease and pregnancy: Management during delivery and outcome of offspring. Am J Obstet Gynecol 155:618, 1986.
257. Berndt MC, Gregory C, Chong BH, et al: Additional glycoprotein defects in Bernard-Soulier's syndrome: Confirmation of genetic basis by parental analysis. Blood 62:800, 1983.
258. Lopez JA, Andrews RK, Afshar-Kharghan V, Berndt MC: Bernard-Soulier syndrome. Blood 91:4397, 1998.
259. Prabu P, Parapia LA: Bernard-Soulier syndrome in pregnancy. Clin Lab Haematol 28:198, 2006.
260. Peaceman AM, Katz AR, Laville M: Bernar-Soulier syndrome complicating pregnancy: A case report. Obstet Gynecol 73:457, 1989.
261. Saade G, Homsi R, Seoud M: Bernard-Soulier syndrome in pregnancy: A report of four pregnancies in one patient, and review of the literature. Eur J Obstet Gynecol Reprod Biol 40:149, 1991.
262. Kaleelrahman M, Minford A, Parapia LA: Use of recombinant factor VIIa in inherited platelet disorders. Br J Haematol 125:95, 2004.
263. Edozien LC, Jip J, Mayers FN: Platelet storage pool deficiency in pregnancy. Br J Clin Pract 49:220, 1995.
264. Price FV, Legro RS, Watt-Morse M, Kaplan SS: Chediak-Higashi syndrome in pregnancy. Obstet Gynecol 79:804-806, 1992.
265. Siminovitch KA: Prenatal diagnosis and genetic analysis of Wiskott-Aldrich syndrome. Prenat Diagn 23:1014, 2003.
266. Shelton SD, Paulyson K, Kay HH: Prenatal diagnosis of thrombocytopenia absent radius (TAR) syndrome and vaginal delivery. Prenat Diagn 19:54, 1999.
267. Reiss RE, Copel JA, Roberts NS, Hobbins JC: Hermansky-Pudlak syndrome in pregnancy: Two case studies. Am J Obstet Gynecol 153:564, 1985.
268. Wax JR, Rosengren S, Spector E, et al: DNA diagnosis and management of Hermansky-Pudlak syndrome in pregnancy. Am J Perinat 18:159, 2001.
269. Seligsohn U, Mibashan RS, Rodeck CH, et al: Prenatal diagnosis of Glanzmann's thrombasthenia [Letter]. Lancet 2:1419, 1985.
270. Reichert N, Seligsohn U, Ramot B: Clinical and genetic aspects of Glanzmann's thrombasthenia in Israel: A report of 22 cases. Thromb Diath Hemorrh 3:806, 1975.
271. Walters JP, Hall JS: Glanzmann's thrombasthenia and pregnancy. West Indian Med J 39:256, 1990.
272. Leticee N, Kaplan C, Lemery D: Pregnancy in mother with Glanzmann's thrombasthenia and isoantibody against GPIIb-IIIa: Is there a foetal risk? Eur J Obstet Gynecol Reprod Biol 121:139, 2005.
273. Sherer DM, Lerner R: Glanzmann's thrombasthenia in pregnancy: A case and review of the literature. Am J Perinatol 16:297, 1999.
274. Kale A, Bayhan G, Yalinkaya A, et al: The use of recombinant factor VIIa in a primagravida with Glanzmann's thrombasthenia during delivery. J Perinat Med 32:456, 2004.
275. Poon MC, d'Orion R, Hann I, et al: Use of recombinant factor VIIa (NovoSeven) in patients with Glanzmann thrombasthenia. Semin Hematol 38:21, 2001.
276. Franchini M, Lippi G, Franchi M: The use of recombinant activated factor VII in obstetric and gynaecological hemorrhage. BJOG 114:8, 2006.
277. Franchini M: Postpartum acquired factor VII inhibitors. Am J Hematol 81:768, 2006.
278. Kulkarni AA, Lee CA, Kadir RA: Pregnancy in women with congenital factor VII deficiency. Haemophilia 12:413, 2006.
279. Romagnolo C, Burati S, Ciaffoni S, et al: Severe factor X deficiency in pregnancy: Case report and review of the literature. Haemophilia 10:665, 2004.
280. Uprichard J, Perry DJ: Factor X deficiency. Blod Rev 16:97-110, 2002.
281. Bofill JA, Young RA, Perry KG: Successful pregnancy in a woman with severe factor X deficiency. Obstet Gynecol 88:723, 1996.
282. Leiba H, Ramot B, Many A: Heredity and coagulation studies in ten families with factor XI deficiency. Br J Haematol 11:654, 1965.
283. Salomon O, Steinberg DM, Tamarin I, et al: Plasma replacement therapy during labor is not mandatory for women with severe factor XI deficiency. Blood Coagul Fibrinolysis 16:37, 2005.
284. Myers B, Pavrod S, Kean L, et al: Pregnancy outcome in factor XI deficiency: Incidence of miscarriage, antenatal and postnatal hemorrhage in 33 women with factor XI deficiency. BJOG 114:643, 2007.
285. Asahina T, Kobayashi T, Takeuchi K, et al: Congenital blood coagulation factor XIII deficiency and successful deliveries: A review of the literature. Obstet Gynecol Surv 62:255, 2007.
286. Kobayashi T, Terao T, Kojima T, et al: Congenital factor XIII deficiency with treatment of factor XIII concentrate and normal vaginal delivery. Gynecol Obstet Invest 29:235, 1990.
287. Frenkel E, Duskin C, Herman A, et al: Congenital hypofibrinogenemia in pregnancy: Report of two cases and review of the literature. Obstet Gynecol Surv 59:775, 2004.
288. Funai EF, Klein SA, Lockwood CJ: Successful pregnancy outcome in a patient with both congenital hypofibrinogenemia and protein S deficiency. Obstet Gynecol 20:858, 1997.
289. Iwaki T, Sandoval-Cooper MJ, Pavia M, et al: Fibrinogen stabilizes placental-maternal attatchment during embryonic development in the mouse. Am J Pathol 160:1021, 2002.
290. Girolami A, Randi ML, Gavasso S, et al: The occasional venous thromboses seen in patients with severe (homozygous) FXII deficiency are probably due to associated risk factors: A study of prevalence in 21 patients and review of the literature. J Thromb Thrombolysis 17:139, 2004.
291. Girolami A, Zocca N, Girolami B, et al: Pregnancies and oral contraceptive therapy in severe (homozygous) FXII deficiency: A study in 12 patients and review of the literature. J Thromb Thrombolysis 18:209, 2004.
292. Sotiriadis A, Makrigiannakis A, Stefos T, et al: Fibrinolytic defects and recurrent miscarriage. Obstet Gynecol 109:1146, 2007.
293. Repine T, Osswald M: Menorrhagia due to a qualitative deficiency of plasminogen activator inhibitor-1: Case report and literature review. Clin Appl Thrombosis/Hemostasis 10:293-296, 2004.
294. Agren A, Wiman B, Stiller V, et al: Evaluation of low PAI-1 activity as a risk factor for hemorrhagic diathesis. J Thromb Haemost 4:201-208, 2006.

Chapter 41

Thromboembolic Disease in Pregnancy

Charles J. Lockwood, MD

Venous thromboembolism (VTE) is the leading cause of maternal mortality in the United States, accounting for almost 20% of pregnancy-related deaths in the past decade.[1] A retrospective cohort study of 268,525 patients over a 19-year period reported a prevalence of VTE of 1 per 1627 births; of these cases, 77% were deep venous thromboses (DVTs), and 23% were acute pulmonary emboli (PE).[2] No antecedent history of VTE was present in 86% of these patients. Moreover, among nonpregnant adults who have a fatal PE, 65% (95% confidence intervals [CI], 40.8% to 84.6%) die within 1 hour after onset.[3] These findings underscore the need for a high index of suspicion, a sensitive and rapid diagnostic algorithm, and expeditious initiation of treatment in pregnant women with suspected VTE.

Among pregnant women, 98.4% of DVTs are localized to the lower extremities, with the left leg affected in 82% of cases.[2] The occurrence of DVT is more common in the antepartum than in the postpartum period (74% versus 26%; $P < .001$), with a mean gestational age at diagnosis of 16.8 ± 2.4 weeks. Nearly 50% of antepartum DVTs are detected by 15 weeks, 38% between 16 and 30 weeks, and only 12% after 30 weeks. In contrast, most PEs are diagnosed in the postpartum period (60.5%) and are strongly associated with cesarean delivery (relative risk [RR], 30.3; $P < .001$).[2]

Risk Factors

Pregnancy Is a Prothrombotic State

Normally, VTE is a disease of aging, occurring in fewer than 1 of every 10,000 healthy women before 40 years of age.[4] However, the risk of VTE is increased sixfold in pregnancy. Pregnancy induces this prothrombotic state in a number of ways. Compared to nonpregnant women of reproductive age, pregnancy is associated with increases of 20% to 1000% in plasma concentrations of fibrinogen; factors VII, VIII, IX, X, and XII; and von Willebrand factor.[5] In addition, activity of the anticoagulant factor, protein S, declines, on average, to 39% of normal in the second trimester and 31% of normal in the third trimester.[6] As a consequence, pregnancy is associated with an increase in resistance to activated protein C. The net effect of these changes is an increase in thrombin generation, as measured by increased levels of fibrinopeptide A and the thrombin-antithrombin complex.[7] Protein S levels drop even further after cesarean delivery or infection, helping to account for the high prevalence of PE after cesarean deliveries. Levels of plasminogen activator inhibitor 1 (PAI-1), which inhibits clot lysis, increase threefold to fourfold during pregnancy, whereas plasma PAI-2 values, which are negligible before pregnancy, reach high concentrations at term.[5] Thus, pregnancy is associated with increased thrombin-generating potential, decreased endogenous anticoagulant effects, and impaired fibrinolysis.

The occurrence of VTE in pregnancy is also promoted by venous stasis in the lower extremities resulting from compression of the inferior vena cava and pelvic veins by the enlarging uterus, compression of the left common iliac vein by the right iliac artery,[8] and increases in deep vein capacitance caused by increased circulating levels of progesterone and local endothelial production of prostacyclin and nitric oxide.[9,10]

Risk Factors Not Specific to Pregnancy

Additional risk factors for VTE that may be more common in pregnancy include trauma, infection, obesity, severe proteinuria, and prolonged bed rest. Maternal age greater than 35 years doubles the risk of VTE in pregnancy.[11] One study found that, among patients undergoing cesarean delivery who developed a PE, 36% were older than 35 years of age, and 55% were obese (body mass index >29).[12]

Antiphospholipid antibody (APA) syndrome is associated with a 1% to 5% risk of VTE in pregnancy and the puerperium despite thromboprophylaxis.[13,14] In a case-control study of 30 pregnant women with VTE versus matched controls who were subsequently analyzed for APA, the prevalence of these antibodies was substantially increased in cases compared with controls (27% versus 3%; $P = .026$).[15]

The presence of an inherited thrombophilic disorder also increases the risk of VTE during pregnancy, particularly in the setting of a personal or strong family history. For example, the factor V Leiden (FVL) mutation is present in 40% of pregnant patients with VTE.[16,17] However, because the prevalence of VTE in pregnancy is low (1/1600) and the incidence of heterozygosity for FVL in European populations is high (5%), the actual risk of VTE among gravidas who are without a personal history of VTE or an affected first-degree relative is less than 0.2% to 0.3%.[16,17] With such a history, the risk of VTE in the antepartum or postpartum period is greater than 10%. Similar observations have been made for the other common inherited thrombophilias (see Chapter 40 and Table 41-1).

The presence of a thrombophilia can also affect the recurrence risk for VTE among pregnant women. Brill-Edwards and colleagues prospectively followed 125 pregnant women with a prior VTE, 95 of whom were tested for thrombophilias, including FVL; the prothrombin G20210A gene mutation (PGM); protein C, protein S, and antithrombin deficiencies; and the APAs, anticardiolipin antibodies, and lupus anticoagulant.[23] The authors withheld antepartum thrombopro-

TABLE 41-1 INHERITED THROMBOPHILIAS AND THEIR ASSOCIATION WITH VENOUS THROMBOEMBOLISM IN PREGNANCY

Thrombophilia	% VTE in Pregnancy	% Thrombophilia in European Populations	Relative Risk or Odds Ratio (95% CI)	Probability of VTE in Patients without Personal or Family History of VTE (%)	Probability of VTE with a Personal or Strong Family History of VTE (%)	References
FVL (homozygous)	<1	0.06+	25.4 [8.8-66]	1.5	17	16-19
FVL (heterozygous)	40-44	5	6.9 [3.3-15.2]	0.26	10	16,17
PGM (homozygous)	<1	0.02+	NA	2.8	>17	18
PGM (heterozygous)	17	3	9.5 [2.1-66.7]	0.37	>10	16,17
FVL/PGM (compound heterozygous)	<1	0.15	84 [19-369]	4.7	NA	16,17
Antithrombin deficiency	1-8	0.04	119	3.0-7.2	>40	16-21
Protein S deficiency	12.4	0.03-0.13	2.4 [0.8-7.9]	<1	6.6	16-18, 21
Protein C deficiency	<10	0.2-0.3	6.5-12.5	0.8-1.7	NA	16,18, 22

+, calculated based on a Hardy-Weinberg equilibrium; CI, confidence interval; FVL, factor V Leiden; NA, not applicable; PGM, prothrombin G20210A gene mutation; VTE, venous thromboembolism.

phylaxis but employed it in the postpartum period. They noted an overall antepartum recurrence rate of 2.4% (CI, 0.2% to 6.9%) but no recurrences in the 44 women without a detectable thrombophilia whose previous VTE was associated with a temporary risk factor (among which the authors included pregnancy itself). In contrast, the recurrence risk for VTE among the 25 thrombophilic patients was 16% (4 patients) (odds ratio [OR], 6.5; CI, 0.8 to 56.3). Therefore, it would appear prudent to test pregnant patients who have a history of a VTE associated with a transient risk factor (e.g., fracture) for thrombophilias. Similarly, consideration should be given to screening pregnant women who have a strong family history (i.e., affected first-degree relative) of VTE, particularly if they are likely to be exposed to other risk factors such as prolonged mobilization or cesarean delivery.

Diagnosis and Evaluation of Venous Thromboembolism in Pregnancy

The clinical signs and symptoms of VTE are neither sensitive nor specific. Indeed, three quarters of patients in whom the diagnosis of either DVT or PE is suspected are unaffected.[24] Conversely, many of those ultimately diagnosed with VTE do not have classic features. To make an early diagnosis, clinicians must exercise a high index of suspicion and approach the diagnosis in a systematic fashion.

Deep Venous Thrombosis

Clinical Presentation

Only a third of patients with unilateral lower extremity edema, erythema, warmth, pain, tenderness, and a positive Homan sign—the traditional hallmarks of DVT—prove to have the diagnosis when objective diagnostic tests are performed.[25] Differential diagnoses include a ruptured or strained muscle or tendon, cellulitis, knee joint injury, Baker cyst, cutaneous vasculitis, superficial thrombophlebitis, and lymphedema. The positive predictive value of these signs and symptoms increases substantially in patients at increased risk. However, there is no risk assessment model that has been validated in pregnancy.

TABLE 41-2 DVT CLINICAL CHARACTERISTIC SCORE

Item No.	Description	Score
1	Immobilization due to cast or paresis	+1
2	Bed rest for >3 days or major surgery within 12 wk requiring general or regional anesthesia	+1
3	Localized tenderness along deep venous system	+1
4	Entire leg swollen	+1
5	Asymmetric calf swelling >3 cm measured 10 cm below tibial tuberosity	+1
6	Pitting edema only in symptomatic leg	+1
7	Collateral nonvaricose superficial veins	+1
8	Active cancer	+1
9	Prior documented DVT	+1
10	Alternative diagnosis at least as likely as DVT	−2

*Patients with a score <2 are considered unlikely, and those with a score ≥2 are considered likely, to have deep venous thrombosis (DVT). Adapted from Wells PS, Anderson DR, Rodger M, et al: Evaluation of D-dimer in the diagnosis of suspected deep-vein thrombosis. N Engl J Med 349:1227-1235, 2003.

Wells and associates introduced and validated a simple model in nonpregnant patients (Table 41-2).[26] In the Wells model, 46% of nonpregnant patients were categorized as likely to have a DVT (score = 2), and, of these patients, 28% (CI, 24% to 32%) were found to have either proximal DVT or PE. In contrast, of the 54% who were categorized as unlikely to have a DVT, only 6% (CI, 4% to 8%) proved to have a proximal DVT or PE. Therefore, the first step in diagnosing DVT is risk ascertainment.

Venous Ultrasonography

Venous ultrasonography (VUS) with or without color Doppler imaging has become the primary diagnostic modality for evaluating pregnant patients who are at risk for DVT. The test is performed by placing the ultrasound transducer over the common femoral vein, beginning at the inguinal ligament, and then moving down the leg to sequentially image the greater saphenous vein, the superficial femoral vein, and then the popliteal vein to its trifurcation with the deep veins of the calf. Calf veins are then insonated. Pressure is applied with the probe to determine whether the vein under examination is compressible. The most accurate ultrasonic criterion for diagnosing DVT is noncompressibility of the venous lumen in a transverse plane under gentle probe pressure using duplex and color flow Doppler.[25] The sensitivity and specificity of VUS are reported to be 90% to 100% for proximal vein thromboses.[27] Meta-analysis suggests that VUS is also effective at screening for calf vein DVT, with a sensitivity of 92.5% (CI, 81.8% to 97.9%) and a specificity of 98.7% (CI, 95.5% to 99.9%), yielding an overall accuracy of 97.2% (CI, 93.9% to 99.0%).[28] Even though there is a paucity of data on the performance of VUS in pregnancy, it has become the gold standard for DVT detection in the nonpregnant state.[29]

Magnetic Resonance Venography

It appears that magnetic resonance (MR) imaging may be superior to VUS, and perhaps the equivalent of contrast venography, for diagnosing DVT. The sensitivity of MR imaging for the diagnosis of proximal leg vein DVT has been reported to be 100% (CI, 87% to 100%); the specificity, 100% (CI, 92% to 100%); and the overall accuracy, 96% (CI, 89% to 99%).[30] Moreover, MR venography is significantly more sensitive and more accurate than sonography for the detection of pelvic and calf DVT. The published literature suggests that the range of sensitivity for MR imaging in the diagnosis of DVT is 80% to 100%, and its specificity is 90% to 100%, with median published rates of 100% for both.[31]

Contrast Venography

Before improvements in sonographic imaging technology and the introduction of MR venography, contrast venography was the gold standard for the diagnosis of DVT. The procedure involved injecting a contrast agent into a superficial vein on the dorsum of the foot and allowing it to circulate into the deep venous system while radiographic images were obtained of the lower leg, thigh, and pelvis. The diagnosis required intraluminal filling defects observed on two or more views or an abrupt cutoff of contrast material. It was the most sensitive test for calf vein DVTs. Although accurate, it was expensive, invasive, and painful and risked radiation exposure. In addition, the contrast medium could potentially induce renal compromise and chemical phlebitis.

D-dimer Assays

Laboratory evaluation of D-dimer concentrations has been advocated as an exclusionary test for DVT in low-risk nonpregnant women. A D-dimer study is very likely to be positive in a patient with DVT, but it is also commonly positive in patients with uncomplicated pregnancies. Conversely, if a D-dimer assay is negative in a pregnant patient with suspected DVT, the diagnosis is even less likely than with a comparable negative finding in the nonpregnant state. Recently developed D-dimer assays include two rapid enzyme-linked immunosorbent assays (ELISAs) (Instant-IA D-Dimer, Stago, Asnières, France, and VIDAS DD, bioMérieux, Marcy-l'Etoile, France) and a rapid whole blood assay (SimpliRED D-Dimer, Agen Biomedical, Brisbane, Australia). In nonpregnant patients, the sensitivity of the rapid ELISAs is greater than 95% and that of the SimpliRED D-dimer assay is reportedly 85%.[32] In nonpregnant patients, there appears to be utility in combining a sensitive D-dimer assay with a noninvasive imaging test. Wells and associates reported that, when the whole blood assay for D-dimer (SimpliRED) was used in combination with impedance plethysmography (IPG), two clinically useful patterns emerged in 70% of at-risk patients.[33] The first pattern was a normal IPG and a negative D-dimer assay, which had a negative predictive value for DVT of 97% overall and 99% for proximal vein DVT. The second pattern was the combination of a positive D-dimer and an abnormal IPG, which had a positive predictive value of 93% for any DVT and 90% for proximal DVT. However, if the D-dimer and IPG results were discordant, it was not possible to reliably exclude or diagnose DVT, and such discordant results occurred in 28% of patients. Extrapolation of these findings to pregnancy is difficult, not only because of the high "false-positive" rate of D-dimer testing (>50%)[34] but because IPG is rarely performed anymore.

A number of investigators have argued that, given the high rate of false-positive results on D-dimer testing in pregnancy, it can be used as a screening test in low-risk patients, because a negative D-dimer result in a pregnant woman would have an exceedingly high negative predictive value. Morse measured D-dimer values in 48 women, aged 17 to 36 years, at 16, 26, and 34 weeks of gestation and compared these values to those of 34 healthy, nonpregnant controls.[34] Morse found a progressive increase in D-dimer concentrations across gestation (191 ± 25 ng/mL at 16 weeks, 393 ± 72 ng/mL at 26 weeks, and 544 ± 96 ng/mL at 34 weeks), all of which were significantly higher than the values in nonpregnant women (140 ± 58 ng/mL). Because the cutoff value for normal D-dimer levels at the author's hospital was 280 ng/mL, most pregnant patients would be considered positive. The author recommended new threshold ranges for 16 to 26 weeks (<465 ng/mL) and for 27 to 34 weeks (<640 ng/mL) of gestation.

There is preliminary evidence that the combination of VUS and D-dimer values measured by the SimpliRED D-dimer test may be useful in diagnosing DVT in pregnancy.[35] Based on the initial VUS and D-dimer results, women were categorized into one of four groups and managed accordingly. Group 1 (VUS normal, D-dimer normal) comprised 31 patients who had routine follow-up until 6 weeks postpartum; none of these patients developed objectively diagnosed VTE (CI, 0% to 9.2%). In group 2 (VUS normal, D-dimer abnormal), 4 (22%) of 18 women were diagnosed with DVT on serial VUS at 3 and 7 days, and, of the 14 (78%) with negative serial VUS, none developed VTE during follow-up (CI, 0% to 19.3%). In patients for whom VUS was equivocal (group 3), venography was performed. If the VUS result was positive (group 4), DVT was diagnosed. The authors concluded that the finding of a normal VUS together with a normal D-dimer result or an abnormal D-dimer result coupled with reassuring serial VUS findings allows the safe exclusion of DVT in pregnant patients, but that larger confirmatory studies were needed.

Testing Algorithms for Deep Venous Thrombosis in Pregnancy

The cornerstone of the evaluation of pregnant patients for possible DVT is a VUS. However, D-dimer assessment can be employed either as an initial screen in low-risk patients or as an adjunct to VUS. Figure 41-1 outlines a diagnostic paradigm which assumes the availability of a sensitive D-dimer assay and clinical risk assessment. In this paradigm, low-risk patients are given a D-dimer test. If the result is negative, they are discharged for routine follow-up. If the D-dimer test is positive, they undergo a VUS. Patients with moderate or high risk on clinical assessment proceed directly to VUS. If the VUS result is positive, DVT is diagnosed and the patient is treated. If it is negative and the patient remains symptomatic, serial VUS testing can be performed in 3 days, 7 days, or both. If the repeat VUS findings are positive, the patient is treated. If both VUS studies are negative, the patient has routine follow-up. In particularly high-risk settings (e.g., known

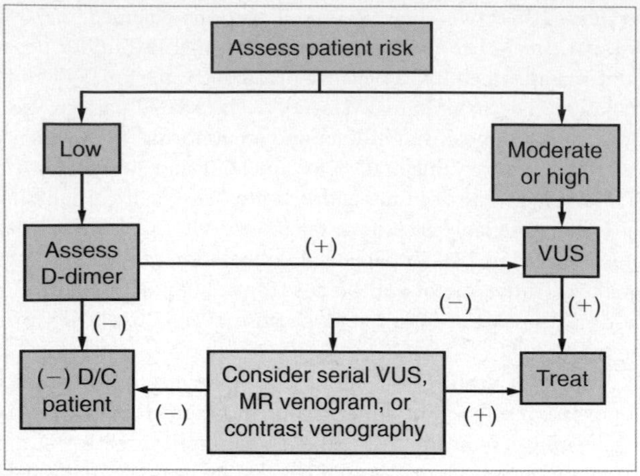

FIGURE 41-1 **Testing algorithm for deep venous thrombosis in pregnancy, assuming availability of D-dimer test and clinical assessment.** D/C, discharge patient; MR, magnetic resonance; VUS, venous ultrasonography.

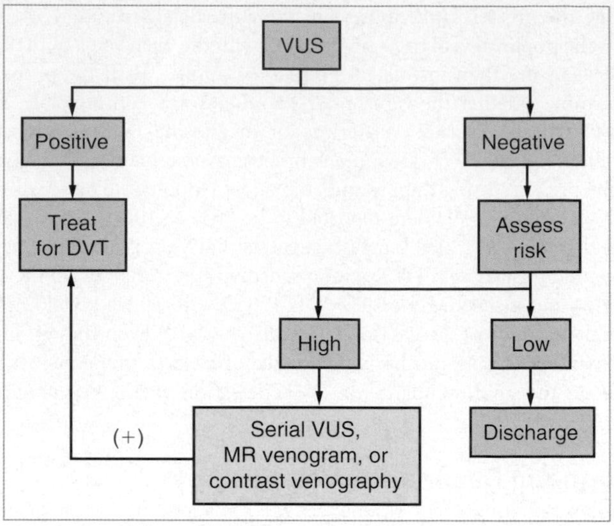

FIGURE 41-2 **Testing algorithm for deep venous thrombosis (DVT) in pregnancy with venous ultrasonography (VUS) as the initial test.** MR, magnetic resonance.

thrombophilia, suspected iliac vein thrombus), more definitive diagnostic tests can be performed, such as an MR or contrast venogram if the D-dimer is positive and the initial VUS is negative. The problem with this approach is that, as noted previously, the majority of pregnant women after 16 weeks' gestation will have a positive D-dimer assay if a nonpregnant threshold is used. Moreover, there has been no validation of higher D-dimer thresholds in pregnancy, and there are no validated risk scoring systems. Importantly, the Wells criteria may not be appropriate in pregnancy, which is intrinsically a high-risk state.

Figure 41-2 assumes the use of a VUS as the initial test, with patients subsequently triaged based on the VUS result or clinical risk assessment determining the need for additional evaluations. A positive VUS result prompts treatment. Follow-up of a negative VUS result depends on the patient's risk category. If it is low, the patient is discharged to routine follow-up. If it is moderate or high, she undergoes serial VUS or, if the index of suspicion is high enough, MR or contrast venography.

The diagnostic scheme in Figure 41-3 utilizes VUS and D-dimer testing without formal clinical risk assessment to triage patients. The combination of a negative D-dimer result and a negative VUS study is associated with a very low risk of DVT, and such patients are discharged to routine follow-up. A positive VUS, which is virtually always associated with a positive D-dimer test, prompts treatment. However, a negative VUS result combined with a positive D-dimer test is followed with either serial VUS or MR or contrast venography, depending on the clinician's index of suspicion. It should be noted that D-dimer testing is likely to be completely irrelevant in puerperal and postoperative patients, because these patients have very high false-positive rates.[36,37] The diagnostic approach outlined in Figure 41-2 should be employed in those settings.

The diagnosis of recurrent DVT in pregnancy presents a diagnostic challenge, because VUS findings remain abnormal after an initial thrombus for up to 1 year in as many as 50% of patients.[32] In this setting, an increase of more than 4 mm in the compressed diameter of a previously involved vein has been reported to provide strong evidence of recurrent thrombosis, but this observation requires confirmation.[38] In such cases, strong consideration should be given to D-dimer assessment and adjunct imaging with MR or contrast venography. A

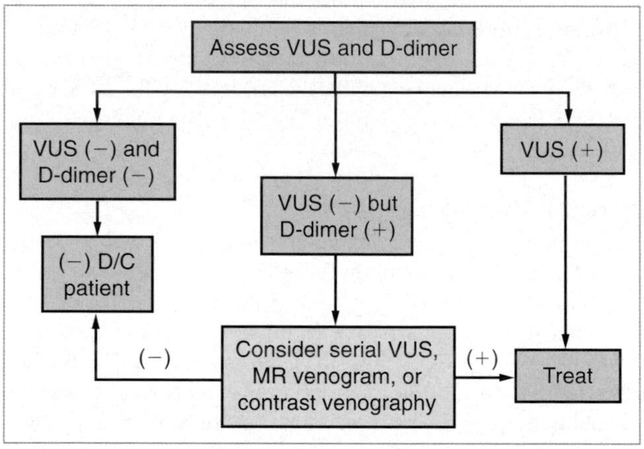

FIGURE 41-3 **Testing algorithm for deep venous thrombosis in pregnancy, using venous ultrasonography (VUS) and D-dimer testing without formal clinical risk assessment.** D/C, discharge; MR, magnetic resonance.

negative D-dimer finding would be very reassuring, whereas observation of an intraluminal filling defect on MR or contrast venography would be diagnostic of recurrent DVT.[32]

Acute Pulmonary Embolus

Clinical Findings

In nonpregnant women, the classic presentation of PE includes tachypnea (>20 breaths/min) and tachycardia (>100 beats/min), either of which is present in 90% of cases.[39] Additional common symptoms include dyspnea and pleuritic chest pain. In contrast, lightheadedness and syncope are rare and are indicative of massive emboli.[40] In the nonpregnant state, the nonspecific nature of these signs and symptoms is a result of the common comorbidities found in older patients, including viral and bacterial pneumonia, postoperative atelectasis, pneumothorax, exacerbation of chronic obstructive lung disease, congestive heart failure, lung cancer, musculoskeletal chest wall pain, esophageal

TABLE 41-3 PULMONARY EMBOLISM RISK SCORE*

Scoring Factor	Points
Clinical signs and symptoms of DVT	+3.0
Alternative diagnosis deemed less likely than PE	+3.0
Heart rate >100 beats/min	+1.5
Immobilization or surgery in previous 4 wk	+1.5
Prior VTE	+1.5
Hemoptysis	+1.0
Active cancer	+1.0

*Clinical probability of PE is low with a cumulative score <2.0, intermediate with a score of 2.0-6.0, and high with a score >6.0.
DVT, deep venous thrombosis; PE, pulmonary embolism; VTE, venous thromboembolism.
Adapted from Fedullo PF, Tapson VF: Clinical practice: The evaluation of suspected pulmonary embolism. N Engl J Med 349:1247-1256, 2003.

spasm, pericarditis, pleuritis, and anxiety. Although these comorbidities are far less common in otherwise young and healthy pregnant women, pregnancy itself can be associated with dyspnea, tachycardia, lightheadedness, orthostatic presyncope, and various chest wall complaints. Therefore, a high index of suspicion is required.

The initial step in the evaluation of any patient is risk assessment. Table 41-3 outlines one scoring system used in nonpregnant patients, in which patients in the low-probability group had a prevalence of PE of 10% or less, those in the intermediate group had a prevalence of about 30%, and those in the high-probability group had a prevalence of PE of 70% or more.[40] This system has not been validated in pregnant patients. Furthermore, given the thrombogenic nature of pregnancy and the puerperal state, particularly after cesarean delivery, it may be prudent to consider all pregnant patients as being at high risk.

Nonspecific Diagnostic Tests

CHEST RADIOGRAPHY

Chest radiographs can play an important role in the evaluation of pregnant patients with suspected PE. Given concerns about excess breast irradiation during computed tomographic pulmonary angiography (CTPA), and because ventilation-perfusion (V/Q) studies have exceptionally high negative predictive values in otherwise healthy pregnant women, some investigators have advocated obtaining an initial chest radiograph to triage patients to either CTPA or V/Q scan.[41] If the radiograph is normal, a V/Q scan is obtained; if it is abnormal (e.g., infiltrates, which could compromise the V/Q study by causing matched ventilation-perfusion abnormalities), a CTPA is ordered. Abnormal findings on radiography may also be consistent with a PE. Such findings, which include pleural effusion, pulmonary infiltrates, atelectasis, and elevated hemidiaphragm, underscore the need for CTPA, because it can diagnose a broad range of lung pathology. However, chest radiography is rarely directly diagnostic of a PE, because the classic radiographic findings of pulmonary infarction, such as Hampton's hump or decreased vascularity (Westermark sign), are rarely seen.[31]

ELECTROCARDIOGRAPHY

In nonpregnant patients, electrocardiographic (ECG) changes are present in 87% of patients with documented PE who are otherwise without underlying cardiopulmonary disease.[42] However, truly characteristic ECG changes usually reflect the hemodynamic sequelae of acute cor pulmonale characteristic of a massive PE (i.e., $S_1Q_3T_3$ pattern, right bundle branch block, P-wave pulmonale, or right axis deviation) and therefore are rare.[42] Moreover, such changes are not universal, even among critically ill patients. Constantini and associates reported changes characteristic of right ventricular strain including an S_1Q_3 pattern in 67% of such patients, with a "septal embolic pattern" in 53%, and either anterior lead T-wave inversion or new right bundle branch block in only 16%.[43] However, there are no data on ECG changes in pregnant women with PE. Moreover, pregnancy-induced physiologic changes mimic left heart strain (e.g., T inversions in the left precordial leads) and, therefore, may mask PE-induced right heart strain changes. Conversely, some physiologic changes may simulate PE changes (e.g., physiologic Q waves in leads 3 and aVF), leading to false-positive results. For these reasons, the screening value of ECG in the setting of maternal acute PE is probably low. However, assessment of the maternal ECG may have utility in making decisions about how aggressively to pursue secondary diagnostic studies (see Testing Algorithms for Pulmonary Embolism, later).

ARTERIAL BLOOD GASES

In young, nonpregnant patients, assessments of arterial blood gases and oxygen saturation are of limited value in the setting of acute PE, because PO_2 values higher than 80 mm Hg are found in 29% of such patients who are younger than 40 years of age.[44] Given that PO_2 levels are even higher in pregnant women, the test is likely to produce even more false-negative results in pregnancy. However, as was the case with maternal ECG, assessment of maternal oxygen saturation may have utility in making decisions about how aggressively to pursue secondary diagnostic studies (see Testing Algorithms for Pulmonary Embolism, later).

ECHOCARDIOGRAPHY

More than 80% of nonpregnant patients with acute PE have echocardiographic or Doppler abnormalities, including dilated and hypokinetic right ventricle and tricuspid regurgitation.[45,46] Because young, pregnant women are unlikely to have cardiorespiratory comorbidities that can mimic these findings (e.g., chronic obstructive pulmonary disease), maternal echocardiography may be useful in pregnant women with suspected PE. Optimal screening requires transesophageal echocardiography with or without contrast enhancement.[47] Indeed, there is a report in which intraoperative transesophageal echocardiography was used to diagnose a right atrial thrombus during a cesarean delivery.[48]

Specific Diagnostic Tests

VENTILATION-PERFUSION SCANNING

In nonpregnant adults, V/Q scanning has largely been replaced by CTPA. In younger, otherwise healthy, pregnant women, V/Q scans have superior PE diagnostic characteristics compared with their use in older, nongravid patients, who frequently have cardiorespiratory comorbidities.[41] Because of this improved accuracy in pregnancy, and given concerns about the extent of maternal breast irradiation with CTPA, V/Q scans may still have a limited role in ruling out PE in select pregnant and puerperal patients.[41] The perfusion component of a V/Q scan requires injecting human albumin macroaggregates labeled with radioactive isotopes (e.g., technetium 99m) into the bloodstream, where they are deposited in the pulmonary capillary bed and imaged by a photoscanner. The ventilation component requires inhalation of radiolabeled (e.g., xenon 133) aerosols whose distribution in the alveolar space is assessed by a gamma camera. Comparison of the perfusion and ventilation scans produces characteristic patterns that can be used to assign diagnostic probabilities.

The chief limitation of V/Q scanning in nonpregnant patients is that only 30% to 40% of older patients with preexisting lung disease who have large matched V/Q defects are subsequently shown to have a PE, leading to false-positive results.[25] Fortunately, pregnant patients are generally free of chronic lung disease. Moreover, as noted earlier, the proportion of nondiagnostic V/Q scans can be further reduced by obtaining an initial chest radiograph and triaging pregnant patients with an abnormal result to CTPA.[41] Furthermore, although fetal radiation exposure is higher with V/Q scanning than with CTPA (0.11 to 0.22 mGy versus 0.003 to 0.08 mGy),[49] all of these exposures are exceedingly low, and the risk of subsequent leukemogenesis is estimated at 1 case per 16,000 fetuses exposed to 1 mGy of radiation. Moreover, half-dose perfusion scans can be employed in young, healthy, pregnant women. Such half-doses result in breast irradiation levels of 0.25 mGy, which is 140-fold lower than the exposure from CTPA (i.e., 35 mGy per breast).[41]

The diagnostic efficacy of V/Q scanning for PE was assessed by the multicenter Prospective Investigation of Pulmonary Embolism Diagnosis (PIOPED) in 931 nonpregnant adults.[50] In this study, patients with high-probability scans were found by definitive testing (e.g., pulmonary contrast angiography) to have PE in 87% of cases, but only 41% of patients with PE had high-probability scans (sensitivity, 41%; specificity, 97%). In contrast, 33% of patients with intermediate-probability scans had a PE, and PE was present in only 14% of patients with low-probability scans and 4% of those with negative scans. Investigators also found that PE can be present in a substantial percentage of high-risk patients with nondiagnostic V/Q scans. One study found that, among high-risk women, the prevalence of PE in those with low and intermediate probability on V/Q scanning was 40% and 66%, respectively.[31] Conversely, 44% of low-risk patients with a high-probability V/Q scan did not have a PE. These findings underscore the value of first determining the patient's clinical risk category if V/Q scanning is to be used as a first-line screening method. This is problematic in pregnancy, because there are no validated risk scoring systems.

The efficacy of V/Q scanning in pregnancy was assessed by Chan and coworkers.[51] They evaluated 120 consecutive pregnant women having 121 V/Q scans for suspected PE. All V/Q results were reinterpreted by two independent experts. Eight of the patients (6.6%) were already receiving treatment for VTE before their V/Q scan. Of the remaining 113 scans, 83 (73.5%) were interpreted as normal, 28 (24.8%) as nondiagnostic, and 2 (1.8%) as high-probability. None of the 104 women who did not receive treatment because of a reassuring scan (i.e., 80 with normal and 24 with nondiagnostic results) had a subsequent VTE over a follow-up period of more than 20 months. This study suggested that the negative predictive value of V/Q scanning is higher in pregnancy than among older, nonpregnant patients.

COMPUTED TOMOGRAPHIC PULMONARY ANGIOGRAPHY

CTPA has become the gold standard for the diagnosis of PE in nonpregnant patients.[41] Cross and colleagues compared CTPA to V/Q scans for the initial investigation of patients with suspected PE and observed that definitive diagnoses of various etiologies were more frequent with CTPA (90% versus 54%; $P < .001$).[52] However, although CTPA more often demonstrated nonembolic lesions responsible for the patients' symptoms, there was no difference in the detection rate of PE between the two groups. Meta-analysis of 23 studies demonstrated very low 3-month rates of subsequent VTE (1.4%; CI, 1.1% to 1.8%) and fatal PE (0.51%; CI, 0.33% to 0.76%) after a negative CTPA study.[53] These results compare very favorably with both a negative contrast pulmonary angiogram and a negative (normal or near-normal) V/Q scan.

It had been argued that CTPA is less accurate with small, isolated subsegmental, peripheral vessels and horizontally oriented vessels in the right middle lobe. However, newer technology using spiral computed tomographic scanners with multiple detector rows and 1-mm slices appears to improve the accuracy of CTPA for diagnosing subsegmental infarcts and may reduce false-negative results to 5%.[54] In addition, traditional contrast pulmonary angiograms have relatively poor interobserver agreement (45% to 66%) for diagnosis of subsegmental PE.[55,56] Therefore, CTPA appears to be of comparable or superior efficacy to contrast angiography.

MAGNETIC RESONANCE ARTERIOGRAPHY

Meaney and colleagues compared standard conventional intravenous contrast pulmonary angiography with magnetic resonance angiography (MRA) during the pulmonary arterial phase of the cardiac cycle after an intravenous bolus of gadolinium and observed that MRA had an overall sensitivity of 100%, a specificity of 95% (CI, 87% to 100%), and positive and negative predictive values of 87% (CI, 74% to 100%) and 100%, respectively.[57] Oudkerk and associates conducted a prospective study of MRA in which conventional contrast pulmonary angiography results were available for 118 patients at risk for PE.[58] The prevalence of PE was 30%, and MRA identified 27 of 35 patients with angiographically confirmed PE (sensitivity, 77%; CI, 61% to 90%). The sensitivity of MRA for isolated subsegmental, segmental, and central or lobar PE was 40%, 84%, and 100%, respectively. In fact, MRA identified PE in two patients with normal angiograms. Given its lack of radiation exposure, and if its efficacy is confirmed by larger studies, MRA may become the primary diagnostic test, where it is available, for ruling out PE in pregnancy.

CONVENTIONAL CONTRAST PULMONARY ARTERIOGRAPHY

Pulmonary arteriography was long considered the gold standard for the diagnosis of PE, with sensitivities and specificities of 100% by definition. However, as noted earlier, interobserver agreement decreases with smaller peripheral lesions. To perform the study, a catheter is usually placed in the right femoral, basilic, or right internal jugular vein. A PE is diagnosed by the finding of an intraluminal filling defect on two views of a pulmonary artery. The procedure has a 0.5% mortality rate and a complication rate of 3%, including sequelae of contrast injections and catheter placement such as respiratory failure (0.4%), renal failure (0.3%), cardiac perforation (1%), and groin hematoma requiring transfusion (0.2%). In light of these risks, pulmonary arteriography has fallen out of favor given the relative safety and efficacy of the other available tests.[40,59,60] Moreover, contrast pulmonary arteriography is relatively contraindicated in the presence of a significant hemorrhagic risk (e.g., disseminated intravascular coagulation, thrombocytopenia) and in patients with renal insufficiency. Left bundle branch blocks require the use of a temporary pacemaker during the procedure to avoid induction of complete heart block.[31]

Pulmonary arteriography from the brachial vein route generates 0.5 mGy (0.05 rad) of fetal exposure, whereas the femoral vein approach generates 2.2 to 3.3 mGy (0.22 to 0.33 rad) of fetal exposure, making the former the preferable route in pregnancy.[61] Concerns also exist regarding the development of fetal goiter after maternal exposure to iodinated contrast material. Therefore, the fetal heart rate should be assessed biweekly to rule out hypothyroidism, and, if delivery occurs proximate to the test, neonatal thyroid function should be checked during the first week after the procedure.[62] Given the high sensitivity and specificity of CTPA and MRA, as well as the relatively high maternal morbidity and concerns with both fetal irradiation and iodinated contrast exposure attendant on contrast pulmonary arteriography, the latter has fallen into disuse as a tool for diagnosing PE in pregnancy.

EVALUATION OF LOWER EXTREMITIES FOR VENOUS THROMBOSIS

Approximately 75% of patients with PE have imaging evidence of DVT, and two thirds of those lesions are present in the proximal vein. However, only a quarter of patients with symptomatic PE have symptomatic DVT.[63] Therefore, in stable patients before definitive diagnostic imaging, and in high-risk pregnant patients in whom CTPA, V/Q scanning, or MRA is not diagnostic, detection of leg vein DVT by VUS can establish the need for anticoagulation.[64]

D-DIMER ASSAYS AS A SCREEN FOR PULMONARY EMBOLISM

A negative D-dimer concentration (<500 ng/mL) has been advocated as a "rule-out" test in patients with low probability of PE because of its high (95%) negative predictive value.[31] Kearon and colleagues observed that, among patients at low clinical risk for PE, none of those with a negative D-dimer result and no additional diagnostic testing had a subsequent VTE, compared with 1 patient with VTE among 182 with negative D-dimer result who had additional testing.[65] They concluded that, for patients with a low probability of PE whose D-dimer result is negative, additional diagnostic testing can be withheld without increasing the frequency of VTE.

Meta-analysis of studies examining the accuracy of D-dimer determinations in the diagnosis of PE demonstrate a mean sensitivity of 95% (CI, 88.0% to 100%), a specificity of 45% (CI, 38% to 53%), and positive and negative likelihood ratios of 1.74 (CI, 1.55 to 1.91) and 0.11 (CI, 0.03 to 0.39), respectively.[66] The quantitative rapid ELISA had a sensitivity of 98% (CI, 88.0% to 100%), a specificity of 40% (CI, 29% to 50%), and positive and negative likelihood ratios of 1.62 (CI, 1.38 to 1.91) and 0.05 (CI, 0.00 to 4.15), respectively. The whole blood D-dimer assay kit yielded a sensitivity of 82% (CI, 74 to 91), a specificity of 63% (CI, 54% to 71%), and positive and negative likelihood ratios of 2.21 (CI, 1.81 to 2.70) and 0.28 (CI, 0.18 to 0.43), respectively. The authors concluded that a negative result on quantitative rapid ELISA was as diagnostically useful as a normal V/Q scan for excluding PE. As was discussed for the use of D-dimer assays in the diagnosis of DVT, the specificity and positive predictive value for D-dimer assays in the workup of patients at risk for PE are likely to be far lower in pregnant, puerperal, and postoperative patients, whereas the sensitivity and negative predictive value should be higher in these settings.

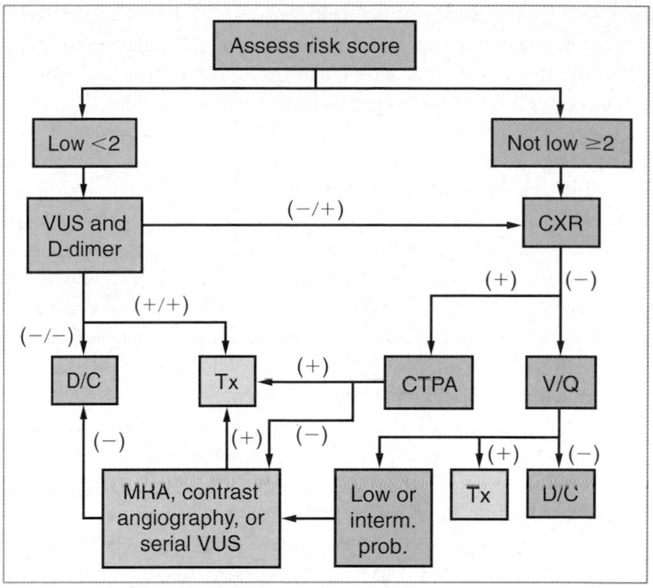

FIGURE 41-4 Testing algorithm for pulmonary emboli with initial triage based on clinical probability. CTPA, computed tomographic pulmonary angiography; CXR, chest radiography; D/C, discharge; interm. prob., intermediate probability; MRA, magnetic resonance angiography; Tx, treatment; V/Q, ventilation-perfusion studies; VUS, venous ultrasonography.

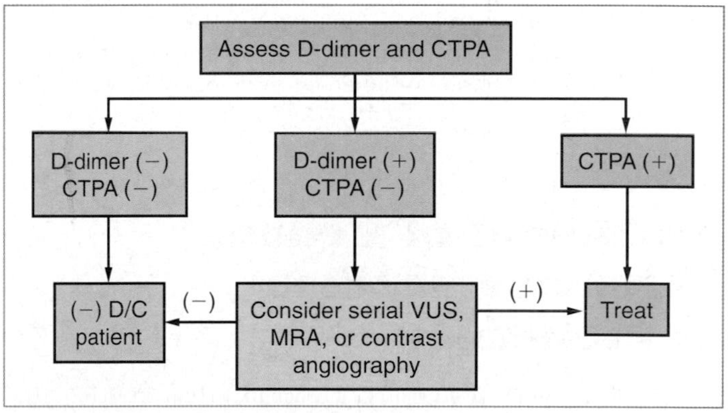

FIGURE 41-5 Testing algorithm for pulmonary emboli with triage based on results from D-dimer testing and computed tomographic pulmonary angiography (CTPA). D/C, discharge; MRA, magnetic resonance angiography; VUS, venous ultrasonography.

Testing Algorithms for Pulmonary Embolism

There is considerable controversy regarding the optimal paradigm for diagnosing PE in pregnancy. Clinical risk assessment tools have not been validated for pregnant patients. D-dimer testing is likely to be associated with a very high false-positive rate. Moreover, as noted earlier, concern has been expressed regarding the relatively high radiation exposure to maternal breasts after CTPA. Conversely, V/Q scans deliver higher radiation doses to the fetus, have limited application in the setting of cardiorespiratory comorbidities, and are frequently no longer available in contemporary radiology practices. MRA may prove to be the ideal alternative, but there are currently too few studies to recommend its widespread use, even where the technology is available.

Two general strategies emerge. The first (Fig. 41-4) seeks to minimize radiation exposure to both the fetus and maternal breasts by performing an initial triage based on clinical probability. Patients who are deemed to be at low risk then undergo both VUS and D-dimer testing; those at high risk and those with a positive D-dimer test receive chest radiography followed by either CTPA or V/Q scanning. This approach would be favored in nonacute settings with equivocal signs and symptoms. The second approach (Fig. 41-5) seeks to maximize the speed and sensitivity of the diagnosis and should be used for patients who are more symptomatic or where there is a high index of suspicion. In this paradigm, triage is done with D-dimer testing and CTPA.

In Figure 41-4, patients should be minimally symptomatic and preferably should have reassuring oxygen saturation values (>80%). The workup commences with a risk assessment (see Table 41-3). Patients who are considered to be at low clinical risk (i.e., risk score <2) should have a VUS and D-dimer test. Obviously, if the VUS result is positive, treatment should be initiated. If both the D-dimer and the VUS studies are negative, the patient can be discharged to routine follow-up. If the VUS is negative but the D-dimer test is positive, the patient is regarded as if she had a clinical risk assessment that was not low (i.e., ≥2). In these latter patients, the workup commences with a chest radiograph. If the results are positive, the patient proceeds to a CTPA. If this is positive for PE, treatment is immediately commenced. If the CTPA is negative, consideration can be given to a serial VUS if not already done. If other ancillary tests are not reassuring (e.g., low oxygen saturation, abnormal ECG), then consideration should be given to an MRA or contrast angiogram. Alternatively, if the chest radiograph is negative, a V/Q scan is performed. If this is negative or normal, the patient can be discharged to routine follow-up. If the V/Q scan indicates a high probability of PE, treatment should begin. If the V/Q scan returns an intermediate or low probability of PE, then consideration can be given to a serial VUS if not already done, or, if other ancillary tests are not reassuring, an MRA or contrast angiogram can be done.

The paradigm in Figure 41-5 should be used for women with more pronounced symptoms or unfavorable signs (e.g., oxygen saturation values <80%, abnormal ECG). The workup begins with D-dimer determination and CTPA. In patients with a high pretest probability of PE or who are very symptomatic, anticoagulation should be commenced as soon as the blood sample is sent to the laboratory for D-dimer determination. If both the D-dimer and CTPA studies are negative, the patient is at very low risk and can be discharged to routine follow-up, though the cause of her symptoms must be identified (e.g., pneumonia, pulmonary edema, cardiomyopathy, esophagitis). If the CTPA is positive, then anticoagulant treatment is begun or continued. If the CTPA is negative and the D-dimer value is positive or the index of suspicion remains high because of low oxygen saturation or an abnormal ECG, consideration should be given to a serial VUS, MRA, or contrast angiography.

Treatment of Venous Thromboembolism in Pregnancy

Patients with new-onset VTE during pregnancy should receive therapeutic anticoagulation for at least 4 months during the pregnancy, followed by prophylactic therapy continuing for at least 6 weeks after delivery. During pregnancy, either unfractionated heparin or low-molecular-weight heparin (LMWH) is the anticoagulant of choice, given its efficacy and safety profile. Neither formulation crosses the placenta, and neither poses teratogenic risks. After delivery, oral anticoagulation with warfarin may be started and is considered safe in breastfeeding mothers. The primary risks of long-term heparin therapy in pregnancy are hemorrhage and osteoporosis.

Heparin Therapy

Therapeutic Unfractionated Heparin

The initial intravenous unfractionated heparin dosage for pregnant patients with acute VTE should be determined with the use of a weight-based nomogram, and subsequent dosage modifications should be predicated on the activated partial thromboplastin time (aPTT) (Table 41-4). This regimen has been shown in nonpregnant patients to reduce recurrence rates.[67]

TABLE 41-4 ADMINISTRATION OF INTRAVENOUS HEPARIN USING A WEIGHT-BASED NOMOGRAM*

aPTT Value	Adjustment
<35 sec (<1.2 × control)	Repeat 80 U/kg bolus, then increase infusion rate by 4 U/kg/hr
35-45 sec (1.2-1.5 × control)	Repeat 40 U/kg bolus, then increase infusion rate by 2 U/kg/hr
46-70 sec (1.6-2.3 × control)	No change in dosing
71-90 sec (2.4-3.0 × control)	Decrease infusion rate by 2 U/kg/hr
>90 sec (>3.0 × control)	Stop infusion for 1 hr, then restart original dose decreased by 3 U/kg/hr

*Give bolus of 80 U/kg of body weight, followed by a maintenance dose of 18 U/kg/hr. Assess aPTT values every 4-6 hr and make adjustments made based on the aPTT values obtained.
aPTT, activated partial thromboplastin time.
Adapted from Raschke RA, Reilly BM, Guidry JR, et al: The weight-based heparin dosing nomogram compared with a "standard care" nomogram: A randomized controlled trial. Ann Intern Med 119:874-881, 1993.

The overall goal is to obtain and maintain an aPTT of 1.5 to 2.5 × control values. The aPTT should not be used to guide unfractionated heparin therapy in patients with prolonged aPTT values due to the presence of lupus anticoagulants. In these patients, plasma heparin activity can be measured by either a protamine sulfate or an anti-factor Xa chromogenic assay. Target plasma heparin concentrations of 0.2 to 0.4 U/mL are equivalent to anti-factor Xa concentrations of 0.4 to 0.7 U/mL. The usual duration of intravenous heparin therapy is 5 days, although patients with large iliofemoral thromboses or massive PEs should receive heparin for 7 to 10 days or until clinical improvement is noted.[31] After hospital discharge, therapeutic doses of unfractionated heparin are administered subcutaneously every 8 to 12 hours to maintain the aPTT at 1.5 to 2 × control values 6 hours after the injection. This therapy should be continued for 20 weeks and then followed by prophylactic dosing until delivery.

The standard prophylactic regimen of unfractionated heparin used in pregnancy consists of 5000 units administered subcutaneously every 12 hours, increased by 2500 U in the second and third trimesters. However, Barbour and associates observed that this standard heparin regimen was inadequate to achieve the desired anti-factor Xa therapeutic range in 5 of 9 second-trimester pregnancies and in 6 of 13 third-trimester pregnancies.[68] Therefore, careful assessment of anti-factor Xa levels 4 to 6 hours after injection is required to properly adjust the dosage.

If vaginal or cesarean delivery occurs more than 4 hours after a prophylactic dose of unfractionated heparin, the patient is not at significant risk for hemorrhagic complications. Patients receiving unfractionated heparin who experience bleeding or require rapid reversal of the anticoagulant to effect delivery can be administered protamine sulfate by slow intravenous infusion of less than 20 mg/min, with no more than 50 mg given over 10 minutes. The amount of protamine needed to neutralize heparin is derived by determining the amount of residual heparin in the circulation, assuming a half-life for intravenously administered heparin of 45 minutes. Full neutralization of heparin activity would require 1 mg protamine sulfate per 100 units of residual circulating heparin. If the heparin was administered subcutaneously, repeated small infusions of protamine are required.

Finally, antithrombin concentrates may be used in antithrombin-deficient patients in the peripartum period.

One of the most serious potential complications of heparin therapy is heparin-induced thrombocytopenia (HIT). This condition arises in 3% of nonpregnant patients given initial heparin therapy. Type 1 HIT (HIT-1) occurs within days after initial heparin exposure, results from benign platelet clumping in vitro, is self-limited, is not associated with a significant risk of hemorrhage or thrombosis, and does not require cessation of therapy. In contrast, type 2 HIT is a rare, immunoglobulin-mediated syndrome paradoxically associated with venous and arterial thrombosis that occurs 5 to 14 days after initiation of therapy. Monitoring for HIT should include every-other-day platelet counts for 2 weeks.[69] Because it can be difficult to distinguish the two entities, a 50% decline in platelet count from its pretreatment high should prompt cessation of therapy. The diagnosis of HIT-2 is confirmed by serotonin release assays, heparin-induced platelet aggregation assays, flow cytometry, or solid phase immunoassays.[70] If it is confirmed, all forms of heparin, including intravenous flushes, must be avoided.

Low-Molecular-Weight Heparin

In nonpregnant patients, the mainstay of acute treatment of VTE is now LMWH. Meta-analyses of 22 studies including 8867 nonpregnant patients suggest that LMWH has fewer thrombotic complications than unfractionated heparin (3.6% versus 5.4%; OR, 0.68; CI, 0.55 to 0.84; 18 trials), produces a greater reduction in thrombus size (53% versus 45%, OR, 0.69, CI, 0.59 to 0.81; 12 trials), and results in fewer major hemorrhages (1.2% versus 2.0%; OR, 0.57; CI, 0.39 to 0.83; 19 trials) and fewer deaths (4.5% versus 6.0%; OR, 0.76; CI, 0.62 to 0.92; 18 trials).[71] However, comparable data have not been assembled for pregnant patients. Nevertheless, LMWH is now commonly employed to treat acute VTE in pregnancy and also as prophylaxis.

The initial therapeutic dose of LMWH varies with the specific agent. Two agents have been approved by the U.S. Food and Drug Administration (FDA) for the treatment of acute VTE: enoxaparin and tinzaparin. Enoxaparin is given at a dose of 1 mg/kg administered subcutaneously twice daily (i.e., every 12 hours). For tinzaparin, the dose is 175 IU/kg administered subcutaneously once daily. A third LMWH, dalteparin, has also been used off-label at doses of 100 U/kg every 12 hours. Barbour and colleagues evaluated whether the standard therapeutic doses of dalteparin maintained peak therapeutic levels of anticoagulation during pregnancy; in 85% of patients, dosage adjustments were required to maintain peak anti-Xa activity between 0.5 and 1.0 IU/mL.[72] Given these data and the fact that pregnancy presents a period of rapidly changing volumes of distribution and fluctuating concentrations of heparin-binding proteins, it appears prudent to monitor anti-Xa activity during therapeutic treatment with LMWH in pregnant patients and to adjust the doses to maintain a therapeutic level (i.e., anti-factor Xa levels of 0.6 to 1.2 U/mL) 4 hours after an injection.

As with unfractionated heparin, treatment should continue for 20 weeks, and then prophylactic dosages should be given (e.g., enoxaparin, 40 mg SQ every 12 hr; dalteparin, 5000 U SQ once daily). There is controversy as to whether prophylactic LMWH warrants surveillance with anti-factor Xa levels. If surveillance is undertaken, the goal should be an anti-factor Xa level between 0.1 to 0.2 U/mL 4 hours after an injection.

Patients with antithrombin deficiency, and patients who are homozygotes or compound heterozygotes for the FVL or PGM mutation and have a prior VTE or affected first-degree relative, require therapeutic anticoagulation throughout pregnancy. In our practice, pregnant patients with these highly thrombogenic thrombophilias who are without a personal or strong family history of VTE should receive subtherapeutic doses of LMWH, with the goal of maintaining anti-factor Xa levels of 0.3 to 0.7 U/mL 4 hours after injection.

Regional anesthesia is contraindicated within 24 hours after therapeutic LMWH administration because of the risk of epidural hematoma; therefore, we recommend switching to unfractionated heparin at 36 weeks, or earlier if preterm delivery is expected. However, vaginal or cesarean delivery occurring more than 12 hours after a prophylactic dose or 24 hours after a therapeutic dose of LMWH should not be associated with treatment-induced hemorrhage. If shorter intervals are encountered, protamine may partially reverse the anticoagulant effects of LMWH. The dosage is 1 mg of protamine for every 100 anti-Xa units of LMWH, but anti-factor Xa activity can be only partially (80%) reversed.[73]

The risk of HIT-2 appears to be far lower in patients receiving LMWH compared to unfractionated heparin, and it is lower still for obstetric patients receiving prophylactic LMWH therapy.[74,75] However, platelet counts should still be obtained every 2 or 3 days from day 4 to day 14.[69]

Postpartum Anticoagulation

Unfractionated heparin or LMWH can be restarted 4 to 6 hours after vaginal delivery or 6 to 12 hours after cesarean delivery. Postpartum patients should be started immediately on warfarin. The initial doses of warfarin should be 5 mg daily for 2 days. Subsequent doses are determined by monitoring the international normalized ratio (INR). To avoid paradoxical thrombosis and skin necrosis from warfarin's initial anti-protein C effect, it is critical to maintain these women on therapeutic doses of unfractionated heparin for a minimum of 5 days and until the INR has been at therapeutic levels (2.0 to 3.0) for 2 consecutive days. After an uncomplicated initial VTE during pregnancy, without other high-risk conditions such as APA syndrome or antithrombin deficiency, therapy should be continued in the postpartum period for 3 to 6 months. Because warfarin does not significantly accumulate in breast milk and does not induce an anticoagulant effect in the infant, it is not contraindicated in breastfeeding mothers.

Management of warfarin overdoses or hemorrhagic complications is guided by the severity of the problem. For example, if patients are found to have elevated INRs (>3.0) without bleeding, vitamin K can be given orally. However, if mild bleeding is present, vitamin K can be administered subcutaneously.[76] Normalization of the INR can occur within 6 hours after a 5-mg oral or subcutaneous dose of vitamin K. Larger doses have a more rapid onset but render patients resistant to re-anticoagulation with warfarin. In the setting of significant hemorrhage, fresh-frozen plasma will replenish clotting factors and can be used with subcutaneous vitamin K to reverse the effects of warfarin.

Complex Presentations

Type 2 Heparin-Induced Thrombocytopenia

In patients with a history or new presentation of HIT-2, heparin and LMWH are contraindicated. Fondaparinux presents an excellent alternative. It is a synthetic heparin pentasaccharide that complexes with the antithrombin binding site for heparin to permit the selective inactivation of factor Xa but not thrombin. Excretion is renal, and the drug has a 15-hour half-life after a once-daily subcutaneous injection. Buller and associates conducted a randomized, double-blind trial of fondaparinux, administered subcutaneously once a day at a dose of 5.0 mg for patients weighing less than 50 kg, 7.5 mg for those weighing 50 to 100 kg, and 10.0 mg for those weighing more than 100 kg, versus enoxaparin among 2205 patients with acute symptomatic DVT.[77] No differences in recurrent VTE were observed between the two groups. Fondaparinux is considered a pregnancy class B agent by the FDA. It has been used in a small number of pregnant patients without adverse sequelae, although it has been found to be present in umbilical-cord plasma at concentrations approximately 10% of those in the maternal plasma.[78] These levels are well below those required for effective anticoagulation. However, fondaparinux use in pregnant women is best limited to those patients with no obvious therapeutic alternatives, such as patients with HIT-2 or severe allergic reaction to heparin.

Thromboprophylaxis in Pregnant Patients with Mechanical Heart Valves

There remains considerable controversy concerning optimal management of VTE in pregnant women with mechanical heart valves. These patients are given warfarin when in the nonpregnant state. However, warfarin is loosely bound to albumin, readily crosses the placenta, and is associated with an increased rate of birth defects (OR, 3.86; CI, 1.86 to 8.00) with exposure between 8 and 12 weeks' gestation.[79] The classic fetal warfarin syndrome includes nasal hypoplasia, stippled epiphysis, and characteristic central nervous system defects including agenesis of the corpus callosum, Dandy-Walker malformation, midline cerebellar atrophy, and ventral midline dysplasia with optic atrophy. Maternal warfarin therapy after 12 weeks' gestation has been associated with fetal and placental hemorrhage which can occur throughout pregnancy.

For these reasons, the agent is usually avoided during pregnancy. However, it may be appropriate to use warfarin in pregnant patients who have a mechanical heart valve. Meta-analysis suggests that, when warfarin is used throughout pregnancy the cumulative risk of embryopathy in 6.4% (CI, 4.6% to 8.9%), but the risk of valvular thrombosis is quite low (3.9%; CI, 2.9% to 5.9%).[80] In contrast, a regimen consisting of unfractionated heparin from 6 to 12 weeks, followed by warfarin until 36 weeks and then by unfractionated heparin until delivery, appears to reduce fetal risks but is associated with a substantially increased risk of valve thrombosis (9.2%; CI, 5.9% to 13.9%).

Warfarin is best employed in pregnant patients with mechanical heart valves when the dosage can be kept lower than 5 mg/day, because cohort studies suggest that this dose is associated with a lower rate of fetal complications.[81] If warfarin is used in this setting, the target INR should be 2.5 to 3.5. Low-dose aspirin should be used as an adjunct to warfarin, based on a study of antithrombotic therapy in high-risk patients with mechanical valves.[82] Warfarin therapy should be stopped by 36 weeks, and unfractionated heparin should then be administered subcutaneously every 8 to 12 hours, with doses adjusted to keep the aPTT value at 2 × control or the anti-Xa heparin level at 0.35 to 0.70 U/mL.

No large clinical studies exist to guide use of LMWH in pregnant patients with mechanical heart valves. However, the manufacturer of enoxaparin (Lovenox, Aventis, Bridgewater, NJ) specifically recommends against its use in this setting, based on a small number of reports to the FDA of valvular thrombosis in pregnant women so treated. The Anticoagulation in Prosthetic Valves and Pregnancy Consensus Report Panel and Scientific Roundtable analyzed these reported cases of valvular thrombosis in pregnant patients receiving LMWH for mechanical heart valve prostheses in 2002 and concluded that virtually all such cases were associated with underdosing or inadequate monitoring.[83] Further, the panel recommended enoxaparin therapy in such patients in lieu of warfarin, beginning at a dose of 1 mg/kg SQ every 12 hours. They also recommended weekly monitoring of peak antifactor Xa levels 4 hours after injection, as well as monitoring trough levels immediately before the next dose. Dose adjustments should be made to insure that trough levels remain between 0.5 and 1.2 U/mL.[83] In addition, the use of low-dose aspirin was recommended for such patients.[83] These patients should be extensively counseled about the risks and benefits of these different regimens to both their own health and that of their fetus.

Thrombolytic Therapy

Although the mortality rate for expeditiously diagnosed and treated uncomplicated PE is less than 2% to 7%,[84] rates higher than 50% have been reported for patients who were hemodynamically unstable at the time of presentation.[85] This has led to more aggressive use of thrombolytic therapy in patients with massive PE. However, meta-analysis of 9 randomized, controlled trials comparing thrombolytic agents versus intravenous heparin in patients with PE found thrombolytic therapy offered no statistically significantly different effect on mortality (RR, 0.63; CI, 0.32 to 1.23) or on recurrence of PE (RR, 0.59; CI, 0.30 to 1.18) compared with heparin, but such therapy was associated with a significantly increased risk of major hemorrhage (RR, 1.76; CI, 1.04 to 2.98).[86]

Pregnancy poses special concerns for thrombolytic therapy given the risk of abruption and puerperal hemorrhage. Turrentine and colleagues reviewed the outcomes of 172 pregnancies treated with thrombolytic therapy and reported a maternal mortality rate of 1.2%, a fetal loss rate of 6%, and maternal hemorrhagic complications in 8%.[87] Although the data are limited, the risk of hemorrhage in the postpartum period appears to be limited to those treated within 8 hours of delivery.[88] Therefore, given the lack of clear benefit and potentially unique risks in decompensated pregnant patients refractory to heparin therapy, surgical thrombolectomy may be the preferred option.

Prevention

Nonpharmacologic Prevention

A Cochrane review of randomized, controlled trials indicated that use of graduated compression stockings in hospitalized patients with prolonged medical immobilization, or application of such stockings from before surgery until discharge or restoration of full mobility, reduced the occurrence of DVT from 27% to 13% (OR, 0.34; CI, 0.25 to 0.46).[89] A cohort study suggested that use of graduated elastic compression stockings also reduced the prevalence of VTE in puerperal patients, from 4.3% to 0.9%.[90] In addition, graduated elastic compression stockings have been shown to increase femoral vein flow velocity in late pregnancy.[91]

Meta-analysis in nonpregnant patients with high or moderate risk suggests that intermittent pneumatic compression devices decrease the relative risk of DVT by 62% compared with placebo, by 47% compared with graduated compression stockings, and by 48% compared with low-dose unfractionated heparin.[92] Because graduated elastic compression stockings and pneumatic compression stockings have no hemorrhagic risk and have been shown to be an effective means of DVT prophylaxis in surgical patients and possibly in pregnant patients, they should be strongly considered for prophylaxis in high-risk pregnant patients (e.g., obesity, thrombophilia, strong family history) who are admitted for labor and/or delivery or who require prolonged bed rest, and also in all pregnant patients undergoing an elective or repeat cesarean delivery without prior labor. Caution must be exercised in their immediate preoperative use after labor, because DVT may have already formed and could be theoretically dislodged by either device.

Finally, in pregnancy, left-lateral decubitus positioning during the third trimester may also reduce the risk of VTE.

Pharmacologic Prevention

As noted, among pregnant patients who have had a previous VTE, recurrence risks are highly dependent on the presence of a thrombophilia and the nature of the risk factors associated with the prior thrombus.[26] Whereas VTE recurrences were not observed in women without detectable thrombophilias whose previous VTE was associated with a temporary risk factor, 16% of thrombophilic patients who did not receive thromboprophylaxis during pregnancy had a recurrent VTE.[26] However, even the former group of patients require postpartum thromboprophylaxis. In addition, it has been argued that thrombophilic patients who are without a personal history of VTE but who have an affected first-degree relative should also receive thromboprophylaxis during pregnancy and the postpartum period. Those with highly thrombogenic thrombophilias (e.g., antithrombin deficiency, homozygosity or compound heterozygosity for the FVL or PGM mutation) should receive both therapeutic or subtherapeutic doses of LMWH throughout pregnancy and postpartum anticoagulation. However, such therapy does not appear to be justified during the antepartum period in patients with less thrombogenic thrombophilias (e.g., heterozygosity for FVL or PGM, protein C deficiency, protein S deficiency) who are without a personal or strong family history of VTE. However, these patients should receive postpartum anticoagulation if they require a cesarean delivery, to reduce the risk of a fatal PE.

A very limited number of studies have assessed the value of perioperative thromboprophylaxis in cesarean delivery.[93,94] However, perioperative thromboprophylaxis with low-dose unfractionated heparin may be appropriate for patients undergoing cesarean delivery who have a history of VTE and known highly thrombogenic thrombophilia, as well as those with mechanical heart valve prostheses.

Inferior Vena Cava Filters

Inferior vena cava filters are designed for use in patients in whom anticoagulation is absolutely contraindicated, such as those with a hemorrhagic stroke, recent or current hemorrhage, or recent surgery. This intervention appears to be appropriate in patients who have recurrent PE despite adequate anticoagulation and in those in whom a PE would probably be lethal (e.g., patients with pulmonary hypertension). Pregnant patients with a history of HIT-2 were traditional candidates for inferior vena caval filters, but the use of fondaparinux during pregnancy and the direct thrombin inhibitors (e.g., Lepirudin) in the postpartum period has rendered this indication less absolute.[95] Although the use of filters is generally discouraged in younger patients, retrievable filters have been employed successfully in pregnant women and may prove ideal in this setting.[96]

Summary

Acute PE remains a leading cause of maternal morbidity and mortality. Periods of maximal risk include the immediate puerperal perioperative period. Additional risk factors include prior VTE, positive family history, obesity, thrombophilias, infection, trauma, and immobilization. The prompt diagnosis of VTE requires assessment of clinical risk followed by initiation of the proper diagnostic algorithm. Treatment requires prompt initiation of unfractionated heparin or LMWH. Prevention includes identification of high-risk patients and both nonpharmacologic and pharmacologic interventions.

References

1. Chang J, Elam-Evans LD, Berg CJ, et al: Pregnancy-related mortality surveillance—United States, 1991-1999. MMWR Surveill Summ 52:1-8, 2003.
2. Gherman RB, Goodwin TM, Leung B, et al: Incidence, clinical characteristics, and timing of objectively diagnosed venous thromboembolism during pregnancy. Obstet Gynecol 94:730-734, 1999.
3. Stein PD, Henry JW: Prevalence of acute pulmonary embolism among patients in a general hospital and at autopsy. Chest 108:978-981, 1995.
4. Cushman M: Epidemiology and risk factors for venous thrombosis. Semin Hematol 44:62-69, 2007.
5. Bremme KA: Haemostatic changes in pregnancy. Best Pract Res Clin Haematol 16:153-168, 2003.
6. Paidas MJ, Ku DH, Lee MJ, et al: Protein Z, protein S levels are lower in patients with thrombophilia and subsequent pregnancy complications. J Thromb Haemost 3:497-501, 2005.
7. de Boer K, ten Cate JW, Sturk A, et al: Enhanced thrombin generation in normal and hypertensive pregnancies. Am J Obstet Gynecol 160:95-100, 1989.
8. Cockett FB, Thomas ML, Negus D: Iliac vein compression: Its relation to iliofemoral thrombosis and the post-thrombotic syndrome. BMJ 2:14-19, 1967.
9. Edouard DA, Pannier BM, London GM, et al: Venous and arterial behavior during normal pregnancy. Am J Physiol 274:H1605-H1612, 1998.
10. Carbillon L, Uzan M, Uzan S: Pregnancy, vascular tone, and maternal hemodynamics: A crucial adaptation. Obstet Gynecol Surv 55:574-581, 2000.
11. Macklon NS, Greer IA: Venous thromboembolic disease in obstetrics and gynaecology: The Scottish experience. Scott Med J 41:83-86, 1996.
12. Chisaka H, Utsunomiya H, Okamura K, Yaegashi N: Pulmonary thromboembolism following gynecologic surgery and cesarean section. Int J Gynaecol Obstet 84:47-53, 2004.
13. Clark CA, Spitzer KA, Crowther MA, et al: Incidence of postpartum thrombosis and preterm delivery in women with antiphospholipid antibodies and recurrent pregnancy loss. J Rheumatol 34:996-996, 2007.
14. Branch DW, Silver RM, Blackwell JL, et al: Outcome of treated pregnancies in women with antiphospholipid syndrome: An update of the Utah experience. Obstet Gynecol 80:614-620, 1992.
15. Ogunyemi D, Cuellar F, Ku W, Arkel Y: Association between inherited thrombophilias, antiphospholipid antibodies, and lipoprotein A levels and venous thromboembolism in pregnancy. Am J Perinatol 20:17-24, 2003.
16. Gerhardt A, Scharf RE, Beckmann MW, et al: Prothrombin and factor V mutations in women with a history of thrombosis during pregnancy and the puerperium. N Engl J Med 342:374-380, 2000.
17. Zotz RB, Gerhardt A, Scharf RE: Inherited thrombophilia and gestational venous thromboembolism. Best Pract Res Clin Haematol 16:243-259, 2003.
18. Friederich PW, Sanson BJ, Simioni P, et al: Frequency of pregnancy-related venous thromboembolism in anticoagulant factor-deficient women: implications for prophylaxis. Ann Intern Med 125:955-960, 1996.
19. Franco RF, Reitsma PH: Genetic risk factors of venous thrombosis. Hum Genet 109:369-384, 2001.
20. Carraro P, European Communities Confederation of Clinical Chemistry and Laboratory Medicine, Working Group on Guidelines for Investigation of Disease: Guidelines for the laboratory investigation of inherited thrombophilias: Recommendations for the first level clinical laboratories. Clin Chem Lab Med 41:382-391, 2003.
21. Goodwin AJ, Rosendaal FR, Kottke-Marchant K, Bovill EG: A review of the technical, diagnostic, and epidemiologic considerations for protein S assays. Arch Pathol Lab Med 126:1349-1366, 2002.

22. Conard J, Horellou MH, Van Dreden P, et al: Thrombosis and pregnancy in congenital deficiencies in AT III, protein C or protein S: Study of 78 women. Thromb Haemost 63:319-320, 1990.
23. Brill-Edwards P, Ginsberg JS, Gent M, et al; Recurrence of Clot in This Pregnancy Study Group: Safety of withholding heparin in pregnant women with a history of venous thromboembolism. N Engl J Med 343:1439-1444.
24. Ginsberg JS: Management of venous thromboembolism. N Engl J Med 335:1816-1828, 1996.
25. Hirsh J, Hoak J: Management of deep vein thrombosis and pulmonary embolism: A statement for healthcare professionals from the Council on Thrombosis (in consultation with the Council on Cardiovascular Radiology), American Heart Association. Circulation 93:2212-2245, 1996.
26. Wells PS, Anderson DR, Rodger M, et al: Evaluation of D-dimer in the diagnosis of suspected deep-vein thrombosis. N Engl J Med 349:1227-1235, 2003.
27. Kassai B, Boissel JP, Cucherat M, et al: A systematic review of the accuracy of ultrasound in the diagnosis of deep venous thrombosis in asymptomatic patients. Thromb Haemost 91:655-666, 2004.
28. Gottlieb RH, Widjaja J, Tian L, et al: Calf sonography for detecting deep venous thrombosis in symptomatic patients: Experience and review of the literature. J Clin Ultrasound 27:415-420, 1999.
29. Andrews EJ Jr, Fleischer AC: Sonography for deep venous thrombosis: Current and future applications. Ultrasound Q 21:213-225, 2005.
30. Evans AJ, Sostman HD, Witty LA, et al: Detection of deep venous thrombosis: Prospective comparison of MR imaging and sonography. J Magn Reson Imaging 6:44-51, 1996.
31. Tapson VF, Carroll BA, Davidson BL, et al: The diagnostic approach to acute venous thromboembolism: Clinical practice guideline. American Thoracic Society. Am J Respir Crit Care Med 160:1043-1066, 1999.
32. Hirsh J, Lee AY: How we diagnose and treat deep vein thrombosis. Blood 99:3102-3110, 2002.
33. Wells PS, Brill-Edwards P, Stevens P, et al: D-dimer testing for deep venous thrombosis: A metaanalysis. Circulation 91:2184-2187, 1995.
34. Morse M: Establishing a normal range for D-dimer levels through pregnancy to aid in the diagnosis of pulmonary embolism and deep vein thrombosis. J Thromb Haemost 2:1202-1204, 2004.
35. Chan WS, Chunilal SD, Lee AY, et al: Diagnosis of deep vein thrombosis during pregnancy: A pilot study evaluating the role of d-dimer and compression leg ultrasound during pregnancy. Blood 100:275A, 2002.
36. Epiney M, Boehlen F, Boulvain M, et al: D-dimer levels during delivery and the postpartum. J Thromb Haemost 3:268-271, 2005.
37. Koh SC, Pua HL, Tay DH, Ratnam SS: The effects of gynaecological surgery on coagulation activation, fibrinolysis and fibrinolytic inhibitor in patients with and without ketorolac infusion. Thromb Res 79:501-514, 1995.
38. Prandoni P, Cogo A, Bernardi E, et al: A simple ultrasound approach for detection of recurrent proximal-vein thrombosis. Circulation 88:1730-1735, 1993.
39. Stein PD, Terrin ML, Hales CA, et al: Clinical, laboratory, roentgenographic, and electrocardiographic findings in patients with acute pulmonary embolism and no pre-existing cardiac or pulmonary disease. Chest 100:598-603, 1991.
40. Fedullo PF, Tapson VF: Clinical practice: The evaluation of suspected pulmonary embolism. N Engl J Med 349:1247-1256, 2003.
41. Scarsbrook AF, Gleeson FV: Investigating suspected pulmonary embolism in pregnancy. BMJ 334:418-419, 2007.
42. The Urokinase Pulmonary Embolism Trial: A national cooperative study. Circulation 47(Suppl 2):1-108, 1973.
43. Costantini M, Bossone E, Renna R, et al: Electrocardiographic features in critical pulmonary embolism: Results from baseline and continuous electrocardiographic monitoring. Ital Heart J 5:214-216.
44. Green RM, Meyer TJ, Dunn M, Glassroth J: Pulmonary embolism in younger adults. Chest 101:1507-1511, 1992.
45. Come PC: Echocardiographic evaluation of pulmonary embolism and its response to therapeutic interventions. Chest 101:151S-162S, 1992.
46. Kasper W, Meinertz T, Kersting F, et al: Echocardiography in assessing acute pulmonary hypertension due to pulmonary embolism. Am J Cardiol 45:567-572, 1980.
47. Pruszczyk P, Torbicki A, Pacho R, et al: Noninvasive diagnosis of suspected severe pulmonary embolism: Transesophageal echocardiography versus spiral CT. Chest 112:722-728, 1997.
48. Adachi T, Umezaki I, Okano H, et al: Placenta previa totalis complicated with pulmonary embolism during cesarean section: A case report. Semin Thromb Hemost 31:321-326, 2005.
49. Winer-Muram HT, Boone JM, Brown HL, et al: Pulmonary embolism in pregnant patients: Fetal radiation dose with helical CT. Radiology 224:487-492, 2002.
50. The PIOPED Investigators: Value of the ventilation/perfusion scan in acute pulmonary embolism: Results of the Prospective Investigation Of Pulmonary Embolism Diagnosis (PIOPED). JAMA 263:2753-2759, 1990.
51. Chan WS, Ray JG, Murray S, et al: Suspected pulmonary embolism in pregnancy: Clinical presentation, results of lung scanning, and subsequent maternal and pediatric outcomes. Arch Intern Med 162:1170-1175, 2002.
52. Cross JJ, Kemp PM, Walsh CG, et al: A randomized trial of spiral CT and ventilation perfusion scintigraphy for the diagnosis of pulmonary embolism. Clin Radiol 53:177-182, 1998.
53. Moores LK, Jackson WL Jr, Shorr AF, Jackson JL: Meta-analysis: Outcomes in patients with suspected pulmonary embolism managed with computed tomographic pulmonary angiography. Ann Intern Med 141:866-874, 2004.
54. Remy-Jardin M, Remy J, Baghaie F, et al: Clinical value of thin collimation in the diagnostic workup of pulmonary embolism. AJR Am J Roentgenol 175:407-411, 2000.
55. Diffin D, Leyendecker JR, Johnson SP, et al: Effect of anatomic distribution of pulmonary emboli on interobserver agreement in the interpretation of pulmonary angiography. AJR Am J Roentgenol 171:1085-1089, 1998.
56. Stein PD, Henry JW, Gottschalk A: Reassessment of pulmonary angiography for the diagnosis of pulmonary embolism: Relation of interpreter agreement to the order of the involved pulmonary arterial branch. Radiology 210:689-691, 1999.
57. Meaney JF, Weg JG, Chenevert TL, et al: Diagnosis of pulmonary embolism with magnetic resonance angiography. N Engl J Med 336:1422-1427, 1997.
58. Oudkerk M, van Beek EJ, Wielopolski P, et al: Comparison of contrast-enhanced magnetic resonance angiography and conventional pulmonary angiography for the diagnosis of pulmonary embolism: A prospective study. Lancet 359:1643-1647, 2002.
59. Mills SR, Jackson DC, Older RA, et al: The incidence, etiologies, and avoidance of complications of pulmonary angiography in a large series. Radiology 136:295-299, 1980.
60. Dalen JE, Brooks HL, Johnson LW, et al: Pulmonary angiography in acute pulmonary embolism: Indications, techniques, and results in 367 patients. Am Heart J 81:175-185, 1971.
61. Brent RL: The effect of embryonic and fetal exposure to x-ray, microwaves, and ultrasound: Counseling the pregnant and nonpregnant patient about these risks. Semin Oncol 16:347-368, 1989.
62. Webb JA, Thomsen HS, Morcos SK; Members of Contrast Media Safety Committee of European Society of Urogenital Radiology (ESUR): The use of iodinated and gadolinium contrast media during pregnancy and lactation. Eur Radiol 15:1234-1240, 2005.
63. Kearon C: Diagnosis of pulmonary embolism. CMAJ 168:183-194, 2003.
64. Stein PD, Hull RD, Saltzman HA, Pineo G: Strategy for diagnosis of patients with suspected pulmonary embolism. Chest 103:1553-1559, 1993.
65. Kearon C, Ginsberg JS, Douketis J, et al; Canadian Pulmonary Embolism Diagnosis Study (CANPEDS) Group: An evaluation of D-dimer in the diagnosis of pulmonary embolism: A randomized trial. Ann Intern Med 144:812-821, 2006.
66. Stein PD, Hull RD, Patel KC, et al: D-dimer for the exclusion of acute venous thrombosis and pulmonary embolism: A systematic review. Ann Intern Med 140:589-602, 2004.

67. Raschke RA, Reilly BM, Guidry JR, et al: The weight-based heparin dosing nomogram compared with a "standard care" nomogram: A randomized controlled trial. Ann Intern Med 119:874-881, 1993.
68. Barbour LA, Smith JM, Marlar RA: Heparin levels to guide thromboembolism prophylaxis during pregnancy. Am J Obstet Gynecol 173:1869-1873, 1995.
69. Warkentin TE, Greinacher A: Heparin-Induced thrombocytopenia: Recognition, treatment, and prevention. The Seventh ACCP Conference on Antithrombotic and Thrombolytic Therapy. Chest 126:311S-337S, 2004.
70. Walenga JM, Jeske WP, Fasanella AR, et al: Laboratory diagnosis of heparin-induced thrombocytopenia. Clin Appl Thromb Hemost 5(Suppl 1):S21-S27, 1999.
71. Dongen C, Belt A, Prins M, Lensing A: Fixed dose subcutaneous low molecular weight heparins versus adjusted dose unfractionated heparin for venous thromboembolism. Cochrane Database Syst Rev (4):CD001100, 2004.
72. Barbour LA, Oja JL, Schultz LK: A prospective trial that demonstrates that dalteparin requirements increase in pregnancy to maintain therapeutic levels of anticoagulation. Am J Obstet Gynecol 191:1024-1029, 2004.
73. Holst J, Lindblad B, Bergqvist D, et al: Protamine neutralization of intravenous and subcutaneous low-molecular-weight heparin (tinzaparin, Logiparin): An experimental investigation in healthy volunteers. Blood Coagul Fibrinolysis 5:795-803, 1994.
74. Fausett MB, Vogtlander M, Lee RM, et al: Heparin-induced thrombocytopenia is rare in pregnancy. Am J Obstet Gynecol 185:148-152, 2001.
75. Lepercq J, Conard J, Borel-Derlon A, et al: Venous thromboembolism during pregnancy: A retrospective study of enoxaparin safety in 624 pregnancies. BJOG 108:1134-1140, 2001.
76. Ansell J, Hirsh J, Poller L, et al: The pharmacology and management of the vitamin K antagonists. The Seventh ACCP Conference on Antithrombotic and Thrombolytic Therapy. Chest 126:204S-233S, 2004.
77. Buller HR, Davidson BL, Decousus H, et al; Matisse Investigators. Fondaparinux or enoxaparin for the initial treatment of symptomatic deep venous thrombosis: A randomized trial. Ann Intern Med 140:867 873, 2004.
78. Dempfle CE: Minor transplacental passage of fondaparinux in vivo. N Engl J Med 350:1914-1915, 2004.
79. Schaefer C, Hannemann D, Meister R, et al: Vitamin K antagonists and pregnancy outcome: A multi-centre prospective study. Thromb Haemost 95:949-957, 2006.
80. Chan WS, Anand S, Ginsberg JS: Anticoagulation of pregnant women with mechanical heart valves: A systematic review of the literature. Arch Intern Med 160:191-196, 2000.
81. Vitale N, De Feo M, De Santo LS, et al: Dose-dependent fetal complications of warfarin in pregnant women with mechanical heart valves. J Am Coll Cardiol 33:1637-1641, 1999.
82. Ginsberg JS, Chan WS, Bates SM, Kaatz S: Anticoagulation of pregnant women with mechanical heart valves. Arch Intern Med 163:694-698, 2003.
83. The Anticoagulation in Prosthetic Valves and Pregnancy Consensus Report Panel and Scientific Roundtable: Anticoagulation and enoxaparin use in patients with prosthetic heart valves and/or pregnancy. Fetal-Maternal Medicine Consensus Reports 3:1, 2002.
84. Dolovich LR, Ginsberg JS, Douketis JD, et al: A meta-analysis comparing low-molecular-weight heparins with unfractionated heparin in the treatment of venous thromboembolism: Examining some unanswered questions regarding location of treatment, product type, and dosing frequency. Arch Intern Med 160:181-188, 2000.
85. Goldhaber SZ, Visani L, De Rosa M: Acute pulmonary embolism: Clinical outcomes in the International Cooperative Pulmonary Embolism Registry (ICOPER). Lancet 353:1386-1389, 1999.
86. Thabut G, Thabut D, Myers RP, et al: Thrombolytic therapy of pulmonary embolism: A meta-analysis. J Am Coll Cardiol 40:1660-1667, 2002.
87. Turrentine MA, Braems G, Ramirez MM: Use of thrombolytics for the treatment of thromboembolic disease during pregnancy. Obstet Gynecol Surv 50:534-541, 1995.
88. Fagher B, Ahlgren M, Astedt B: Acute massive pulmonary embolism treated with streptokinase during labor and the early puerperium. Acta Obstet Gynecol Scand 69:659-661, 1990.
89. Amarigiri SV, Lees TA: Elastic compression stockings for prevention of deep vein thrombosis. Cochrane Database Syst Rev (3):CD001484, 2000.
90. Zaccoletti R, Zardini E: Efficacy of elastic compression stockings and administration of calcium heparin in the prevention of puerperal thromboembolic complications. Minerva Ginecol 44:263-266, 1992.
91. Norgren L, Austrell C, Nilsson L: The effect of graduated elastic compression stockings on femoral blood flow velocity during late pregnancy. Vasa 24:282-285, 1995.
92. Vanek VW: Meta-analysis of effectiveness of intermittent pneumatic compression devices with a comparison of thigh-high to knee-high sleeves. Am Surg 64:1050 1058, 1998.
93. Burrows RF, Gan ET, Gallus AS, et al: A randomised double-blind placebo controlled trial of low molecular weight heparin as prophylaxis in preventing venous thrombolic events after caesarean section: A pilot study. BJOG 108:835-839, 2001.
94. Gates S, Brocklehurst P, Ayers S, Bowler U; Thromboprophylaxis in Pregnancy Advisory Group: Thromboprophylaxis and pregnancy: Two randomized controlled pilot trials that used low-molecular-weight heparin. Am J Obstet Gynecol 191:1296-1303, 2004.
95. Hirsh J, O'Donnell M, Weitz JI: New anticoagulants. Blood 105:453-463, 2005.
96. Ferraro F, D'Ignazio N, Matarazzo A, et al: Thromboembolism in pregnancy: A new temporary caval filter. Minerva Anestesiol 67:381-385, 2001.

Chapter 42

Anemia and Pregnancy

Sarah J. Kilpatrick, MD, PhD

Anemia is defined as a hemoglobin (Hb) value less than the lower limit of normal that is not explained by the state of hydration. This definition has physiologic validity, in that it is the amount of Hb per unit volume of blood that determines the oxygen-carrying capacity of blood. The normal Hb level for the adult female is 14.0 ± 2.0 g/dL.[1] Based on this normal value, 20% to 60% of prenatal patients will be found to be anemic at some time during their pregnancy. In one study, 32% of women presenting at less than 7 weeks' gestation had an Hb value lower than 12 g/dL, suggesting that the prevalence of anemia is high.[2] Because of the normal hemodilution that occurs during pregnancy, the Centers for Disease Control and Prevention defines anemia in pregnancy as an Hb concentration lower than 11 g/dL in the first and third trimesters, or lower than 10.5 g/dL in the second trimester.[3] Some women with mild anemia will be missed using this definition.

Clinical Presentation

Symptoms caused by anemia are those resulting from tissue hypoxia, the cardiovascular system's attempts to compensate for the anemia, or an underlying disease. Tissue hypoxia produces fatigue, lightheadedness, weakness, and exertional dyspnea. Cardiovascular compensation leads to a hyperdynamic circulation, with attendant symptoms of palpitations and tachycardia. Clinical conditions commonly associated with anemia in pregnancy include multiple pregnancy, trophoblastic disease, chronic renal disease, chronic liver disease, and chronic infection. In obstetric patients, however, anemia is most commonly discovered not because of symptoms but because a complete blood count (CBC) is obtained as part of routine laboratory evaluation, either at the initial prenatal visit or at repeat screening at 24 to 28 weeks' gestation.

Evaluation of Anemia

Anemia is not a diagnosis; rather, like fever or edema, it is a sign. The key issue in the evaluation of anemia is to define the underlying mechanism or pathologic process. Although a mild anemia caused by iron deficiency during pregnancy is of little consequence to either the mother or the fetus, a similarly mild anemia caused by carcinoma of the colon has grave implications. One must also keep in mind the genetic implications of many anemias, such as the hemoglobinopathies and hereditary spherocytosis.

Table 42-1 presents a classification of anemia based on the pathophysiologic mechanism involved. Although a mechanistic classification of anemia provides an exhaustive catalog of diagnoses, it does not lend itself to a systematic investigation of an individual patient. Rather, when the patient is anemic one wants to know (1) the morphology of the anemia and (2) the reticulocyte count. Determining the answers to these questions allows one to make a first approximation of a specific diagnosis and to answer the following questions:

1. What is the mechanism of the anemia?
2. Is there an underlying disease?
3. What is appropriate treatment?

The CBC and the reticulocyte count provide the answers to the first two questions. These data allow a morphologic classification of the anemia and indicate whether the marrow is hyperproliferative or hypoproliferative. The patient's Hb value is determined by converting the pigment to cyanmethemoglobin and quantitating the amount spectrophotometrically. The remainder of the values are obtained by flow cytometry with an electronic cell counter.

Based on the size of the red blood cells (RBCs), anemia can be classified as microcytic, normocytic, or macrocytic. The appearance of the RBCs may also provide a clue to the mechanism of the anemia. For example, hypochromic microcytic cells associated with a low reticulocyte count suggests iron deficiency, thalassemia trait, sideroblastic anemia, or lead poisoning. Oval macrocytes combined with a low reticulocyte count and hypersegmented polymorphonuclear leukocytes suggest megaloblastic anemia (vitamin B_{12} or folate deficiency). Oval microcytes and an elevated reticulocyte count are characteristic of hereditary spherocytosis. Various poikilocytes, such as sickle cells, acanthocytes, target cells, and schistocytes, suggest sickle cell disease, acanthocytosis, Hb C disease, and mechanical RBC destruction, respectively. Although the CBC is an excellent first step in the approximate diagnosis of anemia, additional studies are usually necessary to confirm the diagnosis. Table 42-2 lists laboratory studies frequently used in the evaluation of an anemic patient.

Serum Hb and serum haptoglobin levels are useful in defining intravascular hemolysis. If serum haptoglobin is absent or low in conjunction with an elevated serum Hb, the presence of intravascular hemolysis is established. Further studies are necessary to rule in or rule out specific causes of intravascular hemolysis, such as severe autoimmune hemolytic anemia (direct Coombs test), paroxysmal nocturnal hemoglobinuria (PNH) (osmotic fragility), and hemoglobinopathies including sickle cell disease and thalassemia major (Hb electrophoresis).

Total bilirubin is elevated modestly in hemolytic anemia (rarely in excess of 4 mg/dL). The increase results predominantly from an

TABLE 42-1 ANEMIA CLASSIFIED BY PATHOPHYSIOLOGIC MECHANISM

I. Dilutional (expansion of the plasma volume)
  A. Pregnancy
  B. Hyperglobulinemia
  C. Massive splenomegaly
II. Decreased RBC production
  A. Bone marrow failure
    1. Decreased building blocks or stimulation
      a. Iron, protein
      b. Chronic infection, chronic renal disease
    2. Decreased erythron
      a. Hypoplasia (hereditary, drugs, radiation, toxins)
      b. Marrow replacement (tumor, fibrosis, infection)
  B. Ineffective production
    1. Megaloblastic (vitamin B_{12} and folate deficiency, myelodysplasia, erythroleukemia)
    2. Normoblastic (refractory anemia, thalassemia)
III. Increased RBC loss
  A. Acute hemorrhage
  B. Hemolysis
    1. Intrinsic RBC disorders
      a. Hereditary
        (1) Hemoglobinopathies
        (2) RBC enzyme deficiency
        (3) Membrane defects
        (4) Porphyrias
      b. Acquired
        (1) Paroxysmal nocturnal hemoglobinuria
        (2) Lead poisoning
    2. Extrinsic RBC disorders
      a. Immune
      b. Mechanical
      c. Infection
      d. Chemical agents
      e. Burns
      f. Hypersplenism
      g. Liver disease

RBC, red blood cell.

TABLE 42-2 LABORATORY STUDIES USEFUL IN EVALUATION OF ANEMIA

Laboratory Study	Reference Range
Red blood cell (RBC) count	4.0-5.2 × 10^{12}/L
Mean corpuscular volume (MCV)	80-100 μm^3
Mean corpuscular hemoglobin concentration (MCHC)	31-36 g/dL
Reticulocyte count	48-152 × 10^9/L (0.5-1.5%)
Serum (free) hemoglobin	1.0-5 mg/dL
Serum haptoglobin	30-200 mg/dL
Total bilirubin	0.1-1.2 mg/dL
Direct Coombs test	Negative
Hb electrophoresis	>98% A
	<3.5% A_2
	<2% F
Serum ferritin	>20 µg/L
Plasma iron	33-102 µg/dL
Plasma total iron-binding capacity	194-372 µg/dL
Transferrin saturation	16-60%
Folate level	
Serum	>20 µg/L
Red blood cells	165 ng/mL
Serum vitamin B_{12}	190-950 ng/L
Anti-intrinsic factor antibody (AIF)	Negative

increase in the indirect fraction. However, significant hemolysis can occur without an elevation in the bilirubin. Therefore, the bilirubin level is helpful only when it is elevated.

The direct Coombs test uses anti-human immunoglobulin to detect immunoglobulins attached to the surface of RBCs. A positive test indicates an immune cause for a hemolytic anemia. In such cases, it is important to search for underlying causes for autoimmunity, such as connective tissue disease, lymphoma, carcinoma, and sarcoidosis. The diagnosis and management of glucose-6-phosphate dehydrogenase (G6PD) deficiency and of the various hemoglobinopathies are discussed later in this chapter.

The free erythrocyte protoporphyrin (FEP),[4] plasma iron, plasma total iron-binding capacity (TIBC),[5] and serum ferritin level[6,7] are useful in establishing a diagnosis of iron deficiency. Protoporphyrin is generated in the penultimate step of heme synthesis, with iron subsequently incorporated into protoporphyrin to create heme. Iron deficiency causes elevated FEP. Serum ferritin correlates closely with body iron stores, and many investigators support the use of serum ferritin as the best single test in patients with anemia to make a diagnosis of iron deficiency anemia.[6,8] A ferritin level of 12 µg/L or lower is consistent with iron deficiency anemia. Plasma iron and serum ferritin levels are both increased after ingestion of iron.[9,10] Therefore, iron therapy must be discontinued for 24 to 48 hours before these studies are carried out. In iron deficiency, the FEP increases approximately fivefold. Iron is transported in the plasma bound to transferrin. In the iron-deficient state, the plasma iron decreases, the TIBC increases, and the percent of iron saturation decreases. In contrast, with chronic infection, both the plasma iron and the TIBC are decreased, but the percent saturation remains normal.

Serum folate, RBC folate, and serum vitamin B_{12} levels are useful in defining the cause of macrocytic anemia. Because the RBC folate more accurately reflects the body's folate stores, many laboratories no longer offer the serum folate determination. The presence of serum intrinsic factor antibodies is specific for pernicious anemia. However, they are undetectable in approximately 40% of cases, so the absence of these antibodies does not rule out a diagnosis of pernicious anemia.

Although a bone marrow aspiration or biopsy can add much useful information, it is rarely done today in pregnant anemic women. In addition to providing a ratio of myeloid to erythroid production (normal, approximately 3:1), it provides a measure of iron stores, allows a differential count of myeloid and erythroid precursors, provides evidence of infiltration with neoplasm, and allows histologic and bacteriologic confirmation of infection.

Normal Hematologic Events Associated with Pregnancy

Blood Volume Changes

During pregnancy, there is normally a 36% increase in the blood volume, the maximum being reached at 34 weeks' gestation.[11] The plasma volume increases by 47%, but the RBC mass increases only by 17%; the latter reaches its maximum at term. As shown in Figure 42-1,

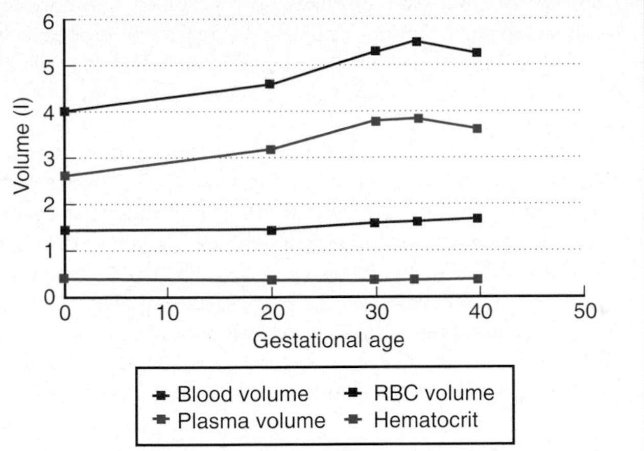

FIGURE 42-1 Hematologic changes during pregnancy. RBC, red blood cell. (Redrawn from Peck TM, Arias F: Hematologic changes associated with pregnancy. Clin Obstet 22:785, 1979.)

this disparity produces a relative hemodilution throughout pregnancy, which reaches its maximum between 28 and 34 weeks. Although this dilutional effect lowers the Hb, hematocrit (Hct), and RBC count, it causes no change in the mean corpuscular volume or in the mean corpuscular Hb concentration. Therefore, serial evaluation of these two indices is useful in differentiating dilutional anemia from progressive iron deficiency anemia during pregnancy: In the former, the indices do not change; in the latter, they decrease progressively.

Iron Kinetics

The classic study by Scott and Pritchard shows that iron stores in healthy women are marginal at best.[12] These authors evaluated iron stores in the bone marrow of healthy, white college students who had never been pregnant and had never donated blood. Approximately two thirds had minimal iron stores. In another study, Pritchard and colleagues demonstrated that almost 50% of healthy primigravidas had minimal iron stores in the marrow during the first trimester.[13]

The major reason for poor iron stores is thought to be menstrual loss. Data from Monsen and associates indicated that the usual menstrual loss is 25 to 30 mL of whole blood.[14] This is equivalent to 12 to 15 mg of elemental iron, because each milliliter of blood contains 0.5 mg of iron. To meet the iron loss for menses alone, a woman must absorb 1.5 to 2.0 mg of elemental iron from her diet each day. Because only 10% of dietary iron is usually absorbed, and the average diet contains only 6 mg/1000 kilocalories, a woman's iron balance is precarious at best.

Pregnancy presents substantial demands on iron balance, exceeding that saved by 9 months of amenorrhea.[13] Table 42-3 lists the iron requirements for pregnancy. If available iron stores are insufficient to meet the demands of pregnancy, iron-deficient erythropoiesis results. In a prospective study of 35 nonanemic women, ferritin levels were measured before and during pregnancy to determine the relationship of iron stores to developing anemia.[15] Approximately 60% of the women with a ferritin concentration less than 20 μg/L before pregnancy were anemic by 20 weeks' gestation, compared with 25% of women with normal prepregnancy ferritin levels. Fenton and colleagues used serum ferritin levels to evaluate iron stores in pregnant women and found significantly higher ferritin levels in women who were receiving iron supplementation than in those who were not.[16] The usual sequence of events in regard to iron deficiency is an absence of iron in the marrow followed by the development of abnormal plasma iron studies (transferrin, ferritin, or FEP). The RBCs first become microcytic, then hypochromic. Finally, anemia develops.

TABLE 42-3 IRON REQUIREMENTS FOR PREGNANCY

Required for	Average (mg)	Range (mg)
External iron loss	170	150-200
Expansion of red blood cell mass	450	200-600
Fetal iron	270	200-370
Iron in placenta and cord	90	30-170
Blood loss at delivery	150	90-310
Total requirement	980	580-1340
Requirement less red blood cell expansion	840	440-1050

Most women enter pregnancy with marginal iron stores. Pregnancy places a large demand on iron balance that cannot be met with the usual diet. In the absence of supplementation, iron deficiency develops. Supplementation with 60 mg of elemental iron per day during the second and third trimesters meets the daily requirement. The Institute of Medicine recommends that supplementation be offered only to women whose serum ferritin level is less than 20 μg/L.[17] Although this is a valid recommendation scientifically, the high cost of the screening limits its applicability.

The fetal compartment preferentially obtains iron, folate, and vitamin B_{12} from—and at the expense of—the mother.[18-20] Maternal iron is transferred to the fetus via serum transferrin. Transferrin binds to receptors in placental syncytiotrophoblast, where the iron is released and subsequently binds to ferritin in placenta cells. It is then transferred to apotransferrin, which enters into the fetal circulation as holotransferrin. If maternal iron status is low, placental transferrin receptors increase to facilitate more uptake of iron by the placenta.[21]

Folate

Folic acid, a water-soluble vitamin, is widely available in the diet. Dietary folates are, in fact, a family of compounds that appear as polyglutamates. In humans, the only source of folate is the diet, and absorption occurs primarily in the proximal jejunum. Before folate can be absorbed, it must be reduced to the monoglutamate form.[22] Pancreatic conjugases within the intestine are responsible for this process. The activity of conjugase is decreased by use of anticonvulsants, oral contraceptives, alcohol, or sulfa drugs.[23] Therefore, in addition to an absolute diminution in dietary intake, the combination of increased need (e.g., multiple pregnancy, hemolytic anemia) and decreased absorption can lead to folate deficiency.[20,24,25]

The folate requirement of 50 μg/day for a nonpregnant woman increases to 300 to 500 μg/day during pregnancy.[13,26] Because adequate folate intake before and during the first weeks of pregnancy reduces the occurrence of neural tube defects, all women considering pregnancy should consume 400 μg of folate per day.[27] One study estimated that a folate supplementation of 400 μg/day would reduce the risk of neural tube defects by 36%, and that 5 mg/day would reduce the risk by 85%.[28] If a previous pregnancy was complicated by a neural tube defect, the mother's intake of folate should be 4 mg/day in the next pregnancy, starting at least 4 weeks before conception and continuing through the first 3 months of pregnancy.[27,29] When folate depletion occurs, the usual sequence of events is a decreased serum folate, hypersegmentation of polymorphonuclear leukocytes, a decrease in RBC folate, the appearance of ovalocytes in the blood, development of an abnormal marrow, and, finally, anemia.[22]

Vitamin B_{12}

Vitamin B_{12}, also abundantly available in the diet, is bound to animal protein. Absorption requires hydrochloric acid and pepsin to free the cobalamin molecule from protein. Intrinsic factor is also essential for absorption. After absorption, transport occurs via binding to transcobalamin II. Most of the vitamin B_{12} is stored in the liver, and individuals typically have a 2- to 3-year store available.[5]

Morphologic Classification of Anemia

Microcytic Anemia

The microcytic anemias are characterized by abnormal Hb synthesis with normal RBC production. A logical progression of diagnostic steps requires, first, that iron deficiency anemia be ruled out. If iron deficiency anemia is diagnosed rather than ruled out, it is important to consider gastrointestinal bleeding as the cause, although it is rare in pregnant women. This can be accomplished by testing the stool for the presence of occult blood with guaiac or other equally sensitive reagent. If a microcytic anemia is not the result of iron deficiency, one must seek another cause, such as hemoglobinopathy, chronic infection, or one of the sideroblastic anemias. For this purpose, the following tests should be considered:

- Hb electrophoresis
- Plasma iron and TIBC
- FEP
- DNA probing for α-genes
- Bone marrow examination

As noted, iron deficiency anemia is associated with decreased serum iron, increased TIBC (>400 μg/dL), reduced serum ferritin concentration (<30 μg/L), and elevated FEP. Anemia of chronic disorders is associated with decreased serum iron and elevated FEP but paradoxically normal or increased ferritin and decreased TIBC. If the serum iron and TIBC are normal or increased and FEP is normal, the patient usually has thalassemia or a sideroblastic anemia. Hb electrophoresis and DNA probes are used to define the thalassemias, and ring sideroblasts are present in the bone marrow of individuals with hereditary or acquired sideroblastic anemia.

Normocytic Anemia

Because of the diverse nature of normocytic anemia, it is the most difficult type to evaluate. The reticulocyte count varies according to whether RBC production is increased, normal, or decreased. If erythropoiesis is increased, one must differentiate between hemorrhage and an increased rate of destruction. The blood smear may reveal a type of RBC shape that can be virtually diagnostic. Fragmented cells are seen in microangiopathic hemolysis—as in the HELLP syndrome (*h*emolysis, *e*levated *l*iver enzymes, *l*ow *p*latelets) and thrombotic thrombocytopenic purpura—and in association with prosthetic heart valves. Other types of poikilocytes identified include sickle cells, target cells, stomatocytes, ovalocytes, spherocytes, elliptocytes, and acanthocytes.

The Coombs test differentiates immune from nonimmune causes of hemolysis. Immune hemolysis is related to alloantibodies, drug-induced antibodies, and autoantibodies. Nonimmune causes of hemolysis include various hemoglobinopathies, hereditary disorders of the RBC membrane (spherocytosis and elliptocytosis), hereditary deficiency of an RBC enzyme, and the porphyrias. Acquired nonimmune hemolysis is caused by either PNH or lead poisoning.

Bone marrow examination is essential for the evaluation of patients who have hypoproliferative anemias with normal iron studies. If erythropoiesis is megaloblastic, folate or vitamin B_{12} deficiency is a likely cause. If it is sideroblastic, both acquired and hereditary forms of sideroblastic anemia must be considered.

Finally, if erythropoiesis is normoblastic, etiologic mechanisms fall into two major categories. The first category has myeloid-to-erythroid production ratios greater than 4:1 and includes aplasia, bone marrow infiltration, effects of chronic diseases, and endocrine disorders such as hypothyroidism and hypopituitarism. In the second category, there is ineffective erythropoiesis, usually associated with a myeloid to erythroid production ratio lower than 2:1.

Macrocytic Anemia

Macrocytic anemia is associated with either (1) an increased rate of RBC production and release of less than fully mature RBCs or (2) disorders of impaired DNA synthesis. Early use of a bone marrow examination is helpful in pointing the investigation in the correct direction. If maturation is megaloblastic, abnormal serum vitamin B_{12} and RBC folate levels allow a diagnosis of vitamin B_{12} or folate deficiency. If a diagnosis of folate deficiency is confirmed, the various causes of decreased deconjugation of the polyglutamate and malabsorption must be considered. If anti-intrinsic factor antibodies are present, a diagnosis of pernicious anemia is ensured. If anti-intrinsic factor antibodies are absent, a Schilling test is required to differentiate between pernicious anemia and a small-bowel malabsorption syndrome. The Schilling test is performed by oral loading with cobalt 58—labeled cobalamin. Urinary excretion of cobalamin measured over 24 hours is then assessed. If abnormal excretion is noted (<10%), the test is repeated with ^{58}Co-labeled cobalamin bound to intrinsic factor. If pernicious anemia is present, excretion will normalize; if malabsorption is the cause, excretion will remain reduced.

Anemia and Perinatal Morbidity and Mortality

Fetal Effects of Maternal Anemia

Although it has been traditionally taught that significant maternal anemia is associated with suboptimal fetal outcome, data supporting this concept are scarce. Most recent studies, including a meta-analysis, reported a significant relationship between anemia early in pregnancy and preterm delivery but no significant association with small-for-gestational-age (SGA) neonates.[30-33] Earlier studies reporting on maternal anemia and poor fetal outcome produced conflicting data.[34-37] Studies in sheep showed that fetal oxygen consumption is maintained until the maternal Hct was reduced by more than 50%.[38] Therefore, maternal anemia needs to be severe to affect the fetus.

Elevated Hb early in pregnancy has also been associated with poor perinatal outcome, including stillbirth and SGA neonates.[39,40] In a case-control study, women with stillbirths had a significantly higher incidence of Hb higher than 14.5 g/dL than did control women without stillbirths.[40] Although the mechanism for this association is unknown, the authors hypothesized that high Hb may be a marker of inadequate plasma-volume expansion and hence reduced blood flow to the intervillous space. An alternate hypothesis was offered by Sagen and associates, who believed that these data were evidence of chronic hypoxia.[39]

In Africa, Asia, and Latin America, the relative risk of maternal mortality with severe anemia (Hb < 4.7 g/dL) was significantly elevated at 3.5.[41] In a case series of 130 women with a Hb less than 5 g/dL in the third trimester in India, more than half had a preterm delivery, and more than 25% had postpartum hemorrhage, sepsis, or a stillbirth. Further, eight women died.[42] However, these studies and others are fraught with confounders, including hemorrhage at delivery and lack of access to care, so it is difficult to know whether the key factor associated with these deaths was the baseline anemia. Therefore, although profound maternal anemia can have adverse effects on the fetus, the margin of safety appears to be large. It may be that the prevalence of severe anemia is too low in industrialized countries to see consistent associations with poor fetal or maternal outcomes.

Although there is no association between maternal third-trimester Hb and cord-blood Hb, maternal Hb and/or ferritin were significantly associated with cord-blood ferritin.[21,43] In several studies, the umbilical cord-blood ferritin levels of infants whose mothers were iron deficient were reduced, compared with those of infants whose mothers were not iron deficient.[16,44] Yet, infants whose ferritin levels were low were not anemic and had normal iron kinetics, and their serum ferritin values were not in the iron-deficient range. In a study of newborns of women with severe folate deficiency, Pritchard and colleagues found normal neonatal levels of folate.[13] Even more interesting, Colomer found that 1-year-old infants had a 5.7-fold increased risk of anemia if their mothers were anemic at delivery, compared with nonanemic mothers, even after the data were controlled for feeding practices and socioeconomic status.[45] In another interesting trial, iron supplementation in women who were not anemic in the first trimester was associated with a significant reduction in the incidence of birth weight less than 2500 g and in incidence of SGA neonates.[46] This trial randomized nonanemic women to receive 30 mg ferrous sulfate or placebo by 20 weeks' gestation. Almost 17% of the placebo-treated women but only 4% of the iron-treated women had low-birth-weight neonates, and 18% and 7%, respectively, had babies that were SGA. These provocative results, indicating that improved iron reserves enhance fetal growth independent of anemia status, may be generalizable only to populations with a high incidence of smoking, because 36% to 40% of the women in each group smoked. However, another randomized trial of routine versus indicated (Hb < 10 g/dL) treatment with iron revealed no difference in perinatal outcome or long-term outcome, including subsequent pregnancies.[47]

Genetic Implications

Many of the hemolytic anemias are inherited as either autosomal-dominant or recessive traits. Therefore, once the correct diagnosis has been made, the genetic implications should be thoroughly discussed with the patient and her partner. If appropriate, the discussion should include antenatal diagnosis.

Specific Anemias

Space does not allow a detailed discussion of the diagnosis and treatment of literally hundreds of different anemias. Instead, a scheme of diagnostic studies that are useful in evaluating any anemia and a discussion of specific anemias that are commonly seen during pregnancy are presented.

Iron Deficiency Anemia

Iron deficiency is the cause of 75% of all anemias in pregnancy, and its prevalence may be as high as 47%.[18 50] Clinical symptoms include easy fatigue, lethargy, and headache. Pica, which may involve the ingestion of clay, dirt, ice, or starch, is a classic manifestation of iron deficiency and was significantly associated in one study with lower maternal Hb but not with adverse pregnancy outcomes.[51] Clinical findings include pallor, glossitis, and cheilitis. Koilonychia has been associated with iron deficiency anemia but is a rare finding. The laboratory characteristics of iron deficiency anemia are a microcytic, hypochromic anemia with evidence of depleted iron stores, low plasma iron, high TIBC, low serum ferritin, and/or elevated FEP. If a bone marrow examination is performed, stainable iron is found to be markedly depleted or absent. Although iron supplementation has not been shown to alter perinatal outcome, the Centers for Disease Control and Prevention strongly recommends screening and treatment of iron deficiency anemia in pregnancy.[6,52,53] The rationale is that treatment maintains maternal iron stores and may be beneficial for neonatal iron stores.[6]

The specific treatment is oral iron, most commonly ferrous sulfate, 325 mg one to three times daily. Other iron preparations are more expensive and do not offer any advantage over ferrous sulfate if equal amounts of elemental iron are given. Reticulocytosis should be observed after 7 to 10 days of therapy, and the Hb can rise by as much as 1 g/wk in severely anemic individuals. Absorption from the gastrointestinal tract can be enhanced by the administration of 500 mg of ascorbic acid with each dose of iron. Gastrointestinal side effects associated with iron therapy include nausea, vomiting, abdominal cramps, diarrhea, and constipation. These symptoms correspond to the dose of elemental iron ingested; if symptoms are troublesome, the dose of iron should be reduced. Ferrous sulfate syrup (300 mg/5 mL) is an effective way of tailoring the dose to the patient's tolerance. Once the anemia has resolved, the patient should continue to receive iron therapy for an additional 6 months to replace iron stores.

Parenteral administration of iron is rarely indicated and should be reserved for patients with a malabsorption syndrome and those who refuse to take oral iron and are significantly anemic (Hb < 8.5 g/dL).[54] There are currently three parenteral forms of iron approved for use in the United States: iron dextran, sodium ferric gluconate, and iron sucrose.[55] These are usually given intramuscularly or intravascularly, and, because severe anaphylaxis can occur in 1% of patients, a test dose should be administered first. In the absence of any reaction, daily injections of 2 mL (100 mg) can be administered until the full dose is reached. Iron dextran contains 50 mg of iron per milliliter and comes in 2-mL ampules. The required dose of iron dextran needed to correct anemia and replenish stores can be calculated as follows[56]:

1. Milligrams of Fe needed = Hb deficit (in g/dL) × lean body wt (lb) + 1000, where the Hb deficit is calculated for women as 12 minus the patient's Hb value

2. Milliliters of iron dextran needed = mg of Fe needed ÷ 50 mg/mL

Iron sucrose and sodium ferric gluconate preparations appear to have fewer adverse events, including anaphylaxis, in part because of lower molecular weights.[55-57] In a recent study, oral iron was compared with intravenous iron sucrose in a randomized trial of pregnant women with Hb values of 8 to 10 g/dL.[58] The increase in Hb (2 g/dL) was the same in both groups at day 30. In another, partially randomized study comparing oral iron with intramuscular iron dextran in anemic women, there was no significant difference in term Hb levels but a significant increase in ferritin in the group treated with intramuscular iron, compared with orally treated women.[59] In contrast, another randomized trial comparing oral to intravenous iron sucrose found that the latter was associated with a significantly larger increase in Hb at 2 and 4 weeks and at delivery.[60] However, at delivery, there was less than 1 mg/dL difference between the mean Hb values in the two groups. The authors reported no serious side effects in either group.

Subcutaneous erythropoietin with or without oral iron therapy or intravenous iron sucrose has been used successfully to treat severe iron deficiency anemia in pregnancy, with no significant risks to the mother.[61-63] In one study in women for whom oral iron therapy had failed and who had an Hb value lower than 8.5 g/dL, the addition of erythropoietin to oral iron was associated with normalization of Hb in 2 weeks in 73% of the women.[62] Darbepoetin alfa, which has a longer half-life than erythropoietin, has also been used to successfully treat anemia after renal transplantation in a pregnant patient.[64]

Megaloblastic Anemia

Megaloblastic anemia is the second most common nutritional anemia seen during pregnancy. Most commonly, folate deficiency is the cause, but a deficiency in vitamin B_{12} must also be considered. The etiology of these anemias are poor nutrition and or decreased absorption. With the increase in pregnancies occurring after bariatric surgery, it is possible that bariatric surgery may become a common cause of folate or B_{12} deficiency in pregnancy in the United States.[65]

Patients with folate deficiency present with the typical symptoms of anemia plus roughness of the skin and glossitis. The CBC reveals a macrocytic or normocytic, normochromic anemia with hypersegmentation of the polymorphonuclear leukocytes. The reticulocyte count is normal or low, and the white blood cell and platelet counts are frequently decreased. Bone marrow examination is not usually necessary for diagnosis, but if it is done, megaloblastic erythropoiesis is noted. The RBC folate level is decreased to less than 165 ng/mL (serum folate to less than 2 μg/L), and the vitamin B_{12} level is normal. Treatment consists of oral folic acid administered in a dose of 1 mg/day. Parenteral folic acid may be indicated for individuals with malabsorption. A reticulocyte response should be seen in 48 to 72 hours, and the platelet count should normalize within a few days. The neutrophils normalize after 1 to 2 weeks.

In addition to anemia, women with vitamin B_{12} deficiency may also manifest neurologic defects relating to damage to the posterior columns of the spinal cord. It is critical that individuals with vitamin B_{12} deficiency not be treated with folic acid alone. Such treatment may well improve the anemia but has absolutely no salutary effect on the neuropathy and, in fact, may make it worse. As with folate deficiency, vitamin B_{12} deficiency is associated with dietary deficiency, an increased requirement, or both. Except in strict vegetarians who avoid all animal products, dietary deficiency is rare.

The most common causes of vitamin B_{12} deficiency are autoimmune inhibition of intrinsic factor production (pernicious anemia), inadequate production of intrinsic factor after gastrectomy, and the presence of a malabsorption syndrome. The morphologic features of B_{12} deficiency are similar to those of folate deficiency. In this instance, the serum vitamin B_{12} level is low and the folate level is normal. Because ineffective erythropoiesis is a prominent feature, evidence of low-grade hemolysis may be present (increased bilirubin and decreased haptoglobin). The measurement of anti-intrinsic factor antibodies is useful. Treatment consists of an intramuscular dose of 1000 μg (1 mg) of vitamin B_{12} every day for 1 week, then 1 mg every week for 4 weeks, and then 1 mg every month for the remainder of the patient's life in cases of pernicious anemia. A prompt reticulocyte response is anticipated after 3 to 5 days of therapy.

Hereditary Spherocytosis and Elliptocytosis

Spherocytosis is the most common form of inherited hemolytic anemia. The inheritance is autosomal-dominant with variable penetrance. Hereditary spherocytosis (HS) is characterized by a structural defect in the erythrocyte membrane caused by several different molecular defects in the membrane proteins, including spectrin deficiency and ankyrin deficinecy.[66] The classic characteristic is an increased RBC osmotic fragility. The prevalence of the disorder is 2-3/10,000, which implies around 1000 pregnancies annually in women with spherocytosis. A hemolytic crisis can be precipitated by many conditions, such as infection, trauma, and pregnancy itself.[67] A relationship between increased hemolysis and increased maternal blood volume and splenic blood flow has been proposed. An alternative suggestion is an increased osmotic fragility during the third trimester of pregnancy.[68]

The diagnosis is suspected on the basis of family history and findings in the CBC and reticulocyte count that suggest a hyperproliferative anemia. Confirmation is obtained with the osmotic fragility test. Prenatal care of women with hereditary spherocytosis who have not had a splenectomy requires vigilance for hemolytic crisis and folate supplementation to ensure adequate marrow function.[69] A hemolytic crisis can be treated conservatively with replacement transfusions or with splenectomy. Because splenectomy is mechanically difficult to accomplish during the third trimester of pregnancy, it is sometimes preceded by delivery. In the absence of severe, untreated anemia, spherocytosis does not contribute to perinatal morbidity or mortality.

Hereditary elliptocytosis, also inherited as an autosomal-dominant trait, is a milder hemolytic state also caused by a structural defect in the RBC wall. The signs and symptoms are similar to those of spherocytosis but are not as severe. Most cases detected during pregnancy have been successfully treated with supportive therapy alone.[70]

Autoimmune Hemolytic Anemia

There are two major types of antibodies responsible for autoimmune hemolytic anemia: warm-reactive and cold-reactive. Most warm-reactive antibodies are of the immunoglobulin G (IgG) class and are directed against some component of the Rh system on the surface of the RBC. In contrast, most cold-reactive antibodies are IgM; they are usually anti-I or anti-i. Autoimmune hemolytic anemia with warm-reactive antibodies is frequently seen in association with various hematologic malignancies (chronic lymphocytic leukemia, lymphoma), lupus erythematosus, viral infections, and drug ingestion. Penicillin and α-methyldopa have been reported to cause autoimmune hemolytic anemia. Cold-reacting antibodies can be seen in association with mycoplasmal infections, infectious mononucleosis, and lymphoreticular neoplasms.

In a large number of cases, no specific inciting event can be identified.[71] The diagnosis is suspected when a hyperproliferative, macrocytic anemia is identified. The stained smear of peripheral blood often reveals microcytes, polychromatophilia, poikilocytosis, and the presence of normoblasts. Leukocytosis is frequently seen and is a result of marrow hyperactivity. The critical study to confirm the diagnosis is a positive direct Coombs test. There are several case reports in the literature describing pregnancy-induced hemolytic anemia in which no etiology could be discerned, the disease was diagnosed during pregnancy, and spontaneous remission occurred after delivery.[72,73] The most recent report described a woman who had hemolytic anemia diagnosed in three separate pregnancies that was not responsive to either steroids or intravenous IgG therapy but resolved after delivery in all pregnancies.[72]

Treatment of autoimmune hemolytic anemia is directed toward both the hemolytic process and the underlying disease. Blood transfusion, corticosteroid therapy, immunosuppression, and splenectomy are the most frequently used measures. In cases with warm-reactive antibodies, corticosteroid should be tried initially, because approximately 80% of patients respond dramatically. Splenectomy is an effective form of treatment in approximately 60% of patients with warm-reactive antibodies. If the disease is refractory to both corticosteroid therapy and splenectomy, a trial of immunosuppression is warranted. The treatment of cold-reactive antibodies depends on the severity of the hemolytic process. In patients with mild anemia, avoidance of cold temperatures is all that is required. Corticosteroid therapy and splenectomy are usually not effective if the majority of the RBC breakdown is intravascular. In patients with severe anemia, a trial of immunosuppression or plasmapheresis should be considered.

Gluose-6-Phosphate Dehydrogenase Deficiency

More than 20 different hereditary RBC enzyme defects have been described, most with an associated hemolytic anemia. Of these, only G6PD deficiency occurs with more than occasional frequency. The genetic locus controlling G6PD synthesis is on the X chromosome, and males with an abnormal gene may suffer hemolysis, especially if they are exposed to oxidant drugs that stress the pentose phosphate pathway of the erythrocyte. Female heterozygotes are generally clinically unaffected by similar exposure. The G6PD activity of the RBCs in heterozygous females is usually intermediate between the activity in hemizygous males and that in normal subjects. However, some female carriers have normal G6PD activity, whereas others have activity that falls within the range seen in affected males. It has been proposed that this is consistent with the Lyon hypothesis, that one of the two X chromosomes of every female cell is randomly inactivated in early embryonic life and continues to be inactive throughout all cell divisions.[74] Therefore, a few heterozygous women may be severely deficient in G6PD activity, but most have sufficient activity to withstand added stress on this critical metabolic pathway in erythrocytes.

The ethnic groups in which variants of the deficiency occur with greatest frequency are blacks, Mediterranean populations, Sephardic and Asiatic Jews, and selected Asian populations. Of African-American males in the United States, 12% are reported to be deficient in G6PD activity. Most affected individuals are hematologically normal unless they have been exposed to certain drugs or chemicals or have experienced metabolic disturbances or infections that precipitate an acute hemolytic episode. Most affected African Americans carry a variant with these properties. Their hemolytic episodes are relatively mild. Greeks, Sardinians, and Sephardic Jews are more likely to carry G6PD Mediterranean, in which hemolysis is characteristically more severe and favism (hemolysis induced by ingestion of fava beans) occurs. The G6PD-deficient African-American population has not been reported to experience favism.

It is relatively unusual for a pregnant woman to experience severe sequelae of G6PD deficiency. However, Silverstein and associates reported Hct levels lower than 30% in 62% of 180 G6PD-deficient women.[75] Prudence would argue against exposure of a known carrier to precipitants of hemolysis. Sulfonamides, sulfones, some antimalarials, nitrofurans, naphthalene, probenecid, para-aminosalicylic acid–isoniazid, and nalidixic acid are among the medications and commonly occurring environmental chemicals known to precipitate RBC destruction in at-risk individuals.

One report suggested an increased incidence of low-birth-weight infants born to G6PD-deficient mothers, but no correction for the effects of anemia or urinary tract infection was employed.[76] Affected male infants born of carrier females have a higher incidence of neonatal hyperbilirubinemia, sometimes severe, than normal infants, and careful observation of those at risk is strongly advised.[77] The incidence of severe jaundice in G6PD-deficient newborn males is approximately 5%, rising to 50% if there is a history of an icteric sibling.

If a hemolytic episode occurs during pregnancy because of G6PD deficiency in a female heterozygote or the very rare homozygote, management should include prompt discontinuation of any medication or other agent that may be responsible, treatment of any intercurrent illness, and, if clinically indicated, transfusion support. In patients with the variant common among African Americans, even in the male hemizygote, the G6PD activity of young RBCs is much higher than in RBCs that have circulated for weeks and months. Old cells may be totally devoid of activity. Hence, the hemolytic episode, recognized early, is generally relatively mild and can be limited to the oldest population of circulating RBCs if the inciting agent is eliminated. A comprehensive review of G6PD deficiency was published by Beutler.[74]

Aplastic and Hypoplastic Anemia

Aplastic anemia is characterized by pancytopenia in the presence of a hypocellular bone marrow. If it is left untreated, patients usually die from infection or bleeding. Three mechanisms have been postulated to explain the development of aplastic anemia: (1) insufficient stem cells resulting from an intrinsic defect or a reduction in number after exposure to a noxious agent, (2) the presence of a suppressor substance that inhibits the maturation of the myeloid precursors, and (3) development of an autoimmune reaction that causes death of the stem cells.

Agents such as benzene, ionizing radiation, nitrogen mustard, antimetabolites, antimitotic agents, certain antibiotics, and toxic chemicals predictably lead to marrow aplasia. In another category are agents such as chloramphenicol, anticonvulsants, analgesics, and gold salts, which induce aplasia only occasionally. Finally, hundreds of agents of various types have been implicated in several cases as causes of aplastic anemia. In about 50% of the cases, however, careful search does not reveal any causative agent.

Holly described eight patients with hypoplastic anemia detected during pregnancy that remitted spontaneously after delivery.[78] The bone marrow was described as hypocellular with an increase in megakaryocytes. There are now many case reports and series of pregnancy-associated aplastic anemia, although they present a spectrum of clinical and bone marrow findings that makes it difficult to substantiate the existence of an aplastic anemia specifically related to pregnancy.[79-84] Many papers used the criteria delineated by Snyder and coworkers[84] as evidence that the disease was pregnancy related: identification of the disease after the onset of pregnancy; no other etiology of aplastic anemia; decrease in all blood cell counts and in Hb; and hypoplastic bone marrow. However, recovery from the aplastic anemia was not universally documented after delivery, which raises the question of whether it is truly pregnancy related.[80,82]

Patients with aplastic anemia seek medical attention because of symptoms related to profound anemia, bleeding, or infection. The CBC reveals pancytopenia with a hypoproliferative reticulocyte count. Examination of the bone marrow reveals hypoplasia with normoblastic erythropoiesis. Severe aplastic anemia is fatal for more than 50% of affected patients.[85]

Bone marrow transplantation is now the treatment of choice, and long-term survival of 50% to 70% of patients can be expected. Alternatives include antithymocyte globulin, immunosuppressive therapy, and other supportive therapy described later in this section.[86] Survivors have had successful pregnancies after bone marrow transplantation.[87-90] The largest series examined pregnancy outcomes in 146 pregnancies occurring after treatment for aplastic anemia in 41 women.[89] The outcomes in cases treated with total-body irradiation and bone marrow transplantation were compared with those in cases treated with high-dose chemotherapy and bone marrow transplantation. The data demonstrated no increase in the incidence of congenital anomalies in infants. However, total-body irradiation was associated with an increased risk of spontaneous abortion. Twenty-five percent of the pregnancies ended with a preterm delivery or delivery of a low-birth-weight infant. A more recent paper described pregnancy outcomes of 36 women with aplastic anemia who had been treated with immunosuppression before their pregnancy.[91] Only 11 of these women had complete remission before they became pregnant, and 19% of the total group had a relapse of their aplastic anemia during pregnancy that required transfusion. Two women died, one of whom also had PNH, and two women had eclampsia. The majority of the pregnancies resulted in live births, with a 14% prematurity rate. Several patients were treated with cyclosporine or corticosteroids during their pregnancy.

During pregnancy, supportive therapy remains the major objective, because bone marrow transplantation is still relatively contraindicated in pregnancy. In recent years, with modern supportive therapy, the maternal mortality rate has been 15% or less, and more than 90% of patients survive in remission.[80,82] Treatment consists of maintenance of Hb levels through periodic transfusion, prevention and treatment of infection, stimulation of hematopoiesis with androgens, splenectomy, intravenous immune globulin (IVIG), and intravenous steroids.[92] Two case reports described successful pregnancies with a combination of RBC and platelet transfusions, cyclosporine, human granulocyte colony-stimulating factor, high-dose intravenous prednisone, and intravenous immunoglobulin.[79,83] In a series of 14 women diagnosed during pregnancy, all of whom were treated with transfusions only, there were no deaths, and 10 of the women had normal pregnancy outcomes.[82] The four abnormal outcomes were spontaneous abortion, preterm delivery, preeclampsia, and intrauterine growth restriction (IUGR). Androgen therapy can be effective at stimulating erythropoiesis; however, androgens are contraindicated during pregnancy unless the fetus is demonstrated to be male. Androgenic agents commonly used include the anabolic steroids, oxymetholone, nandrolone decanoate, or testosterone enanthate. Adrenocorticosteroids have also been widely used with some benefit. However, the remission rate with steroids is only 12%.

Because of anecdotal reports of complete remission after pregnancy termination, it is tempting to consider therapeutic abortion. However, thorough examination of the available literature indicates that abortion or premature termination of pregnancy is not associated with a more favorable outcome. The only reason to terminate pregnancy prematurely is inability to treat the patient satisfactorily during pregnancy with transfusion alone and a consequent need to proceed to marrow transplantation.

Paroxysmal Nocturnal Hemoglobinuria

PNH was named for its characteristic nighttime hemolysis with dark early-morning urine. Hemolysis in PNH occurs as a result of a somatic mutation in the phosphatidylinositol glycan class A *(PIGA)* gene on the X chromosome. This enzyme mediates formation of phosphatidylinositol anchors for various transmembrane proteins, including inhibitors of the complement proteins.[93] These latter proteins normally are present in the RBC and protect against complement activation. Their reduction renders RBCs susceptible to intravascular hemolysis by complement. PNH usually begins insidiously, and there is no familial tendency. Considerable variability exists in severity of the disease, and the classic presentation of hemoglobinuria is seen in only 25% of patients. Exacerbations of the hemolytic process are precipitated by infection, menstruation, transfusion, surgery, and ingestion of iron.

The most serious complications are marrow aplasia, thrombosis, and infection. Thrombosis accounts for 50% of deaths in nonpregnant patients and often involves intra-abdominal vessels, including Budd-Chiari syndrome resulting from hepatic vein thrombosis.[94,95] Although anemia is the most prominent hematologic feature of PNH, leukopenia and thrombocytopenia also occur frequently. The diagnosis is based on tests including the sucrose hemolysis and acidified serum lysis tests, which demonstrate the sensitivity of the patient's RBCs to complement.

There are two excellent reviews of PNH in pregnancy.[93,96] A review of 20 case reports and series encompassing 33 pregnancies in 24 women revealed several interesting features. One third of these cases were diagnosed for the first time during pregnancy, and 12% of the pregnancies were complicated by thromboembolism with three fourths of the patients having Budd-Chiari syndrome or hepatic vein thrombus.[96] Half of these women died. In addition, there were two maternal deaths from infection, which means that the maternal mortality rate in this summary of 24 women with PNH was 17%. In addition, 73% had anemia or hemolysis during pregnancy, and 27% developed thrombocytopenia. In another review, the most common complication was venous thrombosis.[93] Although at least two pregnant or puerperal women developed a thromboembolism despite receiving thromboprophylaxis, experts continue to recommend thromboprophylaxis.[93,96] This may be particularly challenging if the patient develops thrombocytopenia. There is one case report of a successful labor epidural placement in a woman with PNH and a platelet count of 64,000/mL.[97]

The optimal treatment of PNH is replacement of the abnormal stem cells with cells capable of producing the normal cellular components. This has been accomplished by bone marrow transplantation. The major therapeutic modalities during pregnancy are iron therapy, transfusions, corticosteroids, and androgen treatment (if the fetus is male).[93,98,99] Iron can be administered orally to replace the considerable amount lost in the urine. However, in patients with significant iron deficiency, such treatment may lead to a burst of erythropoiesis, with delivery of a cohort of cells susceptible to the lytic action of complement. If a hemolytic episode follows iron therapy, it should be treated with either suppression of erythropoiesis by transfusion or suppression of hemolysis with corticosteroids. When acute hemolytic episodes occur, treatment is aimed at diminishing hemolysis and preventing complications.

Hemoglobinopathies

The hemoglobinopathies can be broadly divided into two general types. In the thalassemia syndromes, normal Hb is synthesized at an abnormally slow rate. In contrast, the structural hemoglobinopathies occur because of a specific change in the amino acid content of Hb. These structural changes may have either no effect or profound effects on the function of Hb, including instability of the molecule, reduced solubility, methemoglobinemia, and increased or decreased oxygen affinity.

Thalassemia Syndromes

The thalassemia syndromes are named and classified by the type of chain that is inadequately produced. The two most common types are α-thalassemia and β-thalassemia, both of which affect the synthesis of Hb A. Reduced synthesis of γ or δ chains and combinations in which two or more globin chains are affected are relatively rare. In each instance, the thalassemia is a quantitative disorder of globin synthesis.

α-Thalassemia

In patients with α-thalassemia, one or more structural genes are physically absent from the genome. The various α-thalassemia genotypes are summarized in Figure 42-2. In blacks, the most common two-gene deletion state consists of one gene missing on each chromosome. In Asians, most often both genes are missing from the same chromosome. In the homozygous stage, all four genes are deleted and no chains are produced. In such cases, the fetus is unable to synthesize normal Hb F or any adult hemoglobins. This deficiency results in high-output cardiac failure, hydrops fetalis, and stillbirth.[100]

The most severe form of α-thalassemia compatible with extrauterine life is Hb H disease, which results from deletion of three α genes. In these patients, abnormally high quantities of both Hb H (β_4) and Hb Barts (γ_4) accumulate. Because Hb H precipitates within the RBC, the cell is removed by the reticuloendothelial system, leading to a moderately severe hemolytic anemia. In α-thalassemia minor (also called α-thalassemia-1), two genes are deleted, resulting in a mild hypochromic, microcytic anemia that must be differentiated from iron deficiency. A single gene deletion (α-thalassemia 2) is clinically undetectable and is called the "silent carrier" state.

The diagnosis of α-thalassemia is presumptive by exclusion of iron deficiency and β-thalassemia. Although α-thalassemia-1 minor does not present a hazard to the adult, there are serious genetic implications when a mating of two individuals with the trait occurs. Under these circumstances, one must make a specific diagnosis by using restriction endonuclease techniques or a DNA probe before undertaking antenatal diagnosis.[101]

β-Thalassemia

β-Thalassemia is autosomal-recessive and is more common in people of Mediterranean, Middle Eastern, and Asian descent. The underproduction of β-globulin chains is caused by point mutations with single nucleotide substitution or oligonucleotide addition or deletion.[102] The

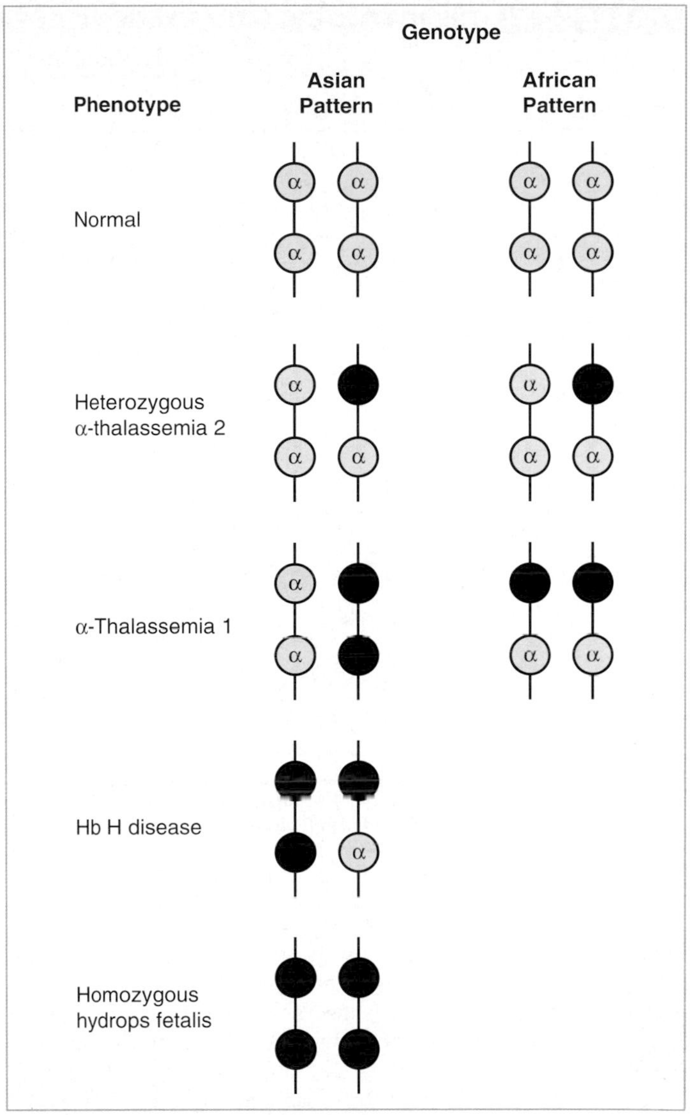

FIGURE 42-2 Genotypes of the various α-thalassemia syndromes. Hb H, hemoglobin H.

β-globin gene is on chromosome 11. In homozygous β-thalassemia, α-chain production is unimpeded, and these highly unstable chains accumulate and eventually precipitate; markedly ineffective erythropoiesis and severe hemolysis result in a condition known as β-thalassemia major or Cooley anemia. There is variation in severity depending on whether homozygous for reduced (β^+) or absent (β^0) β-globin synthesis (see Table 42-4). The fetus is protected from severe disease by α-chain production. However, this protection disappears rapidly after birth, with the affected infant becoming anemic by 3 to 6 months of age. The infant has splenomegaly and requires blood transfusions every 3 to 4 weeks. Death typically occurs by the third decade of life and is usually secondary to myocardial hemochromatosis. Female infants surviving until puberty are usually amenorrheic and have severely impaired fertility.[103,104]

β-Thalassemia minor (also called β-thalassemia trait) results in a variable degree of illness, depending on the rate of β-chain production. The characteristic findings include a relatively high RBC membrane rigidity, moderate to marked microcytosis, and a peripheral smear resembling that observed in iron deficiency. Hb electrophoresis char-

TABLE 42-4 HEMATOLOGIC AND CLINICAL ASPECTS OF THE THALASSEMIA SYNDROMES

	Hemoglobin (Hb) Pattern*				
Condition	**Hb Level**	**Hb A_2**	**HB F**	**Other Hb**	**Clinical Severity**
Homozygotes					
α-Thalassemia	↓↓↓↓	0	0	80% Hb Barts, remainder Hb H and H Portland, some Hb A	Hydrops fetalis
β^+-Thalassemia	↓↓↓	Variable	↑↑	Some Hb A	Moderately severe Cooley anemia
β^0-Thalassemia	↓↓↓↓	Variable	↑↑↑	No Hb A	Severe Cooley anemia
$\delta\beta^0$-Thalassemia	↓↓	0	100%	No Hb A	Thalassemia intermedia
Heterozygotes					
α-Thalassemia silent carrier	N	N	N	1-2% Hb Barts in cord blood at birth	N
α-Thalassemia trait	↓	N	N	5% Hb Barts in cord blood at birth	Very mild
Hb H disease	↓↓	N	N	4-30% Hb H in adults; 25% Hb Barts in cord blood	Thalassemia intermedia
β^+-Thalassemia	↓ to ↓↓	↑	↑	None	Mild
β^0-Thalassemia	↓ to ↓↓	↓	↑↑↑	None	Mild

***Number of arrows indicates relative intensity of increase or decrease.**
↑, increased; ↓, decreased; β^+, reduced β-globin synthesis; β^0, absent β-globin synthesis; $\delta\beta^0$, both δ- and β-globin synthesis reduced or absent; N, normal.

acteristically shows an elevation of Hb A_2. β-Thalassemia trait does not impair fertility, and the incidence of prematurity, low-birth-weight infants, and infants of abnormal size for gestational age is identical to that in normal women.[105,106] Nineteen women with β-thalassemia major or intermedia (e.g., the compound heterozygous state) were followed through 22 pregnancies; 21 viable infants were delivered.[107] These patients all had intensive treatment, including transfusions and iron-chelating agents, if necessary, before pregnancy or if their Hb concentration was greater than 7 g/dL. In addition, all women had a prepregnancy cardiac echocardiogram showing a left ventricular ejection fraction greater than 55%. These results suggest that women with well-managed, stable β-thalassemia can do very well during pregnancy.[107] The clinical characteristics and hematologic findings of the various thalassemias are summarized in Table 42-4.

Because of increased Asian immigration, the number of β-thalassemia cases in the United States has risen, so maternal screening of appropriate women is important.[108] In California, cases of β-thalassemia major, Hb E/β-thalassemia, and other combined structural Hb abnormalities are more common than phenylketonuria or galactosemia.[108] A suggestion for easy antenatal maternal screening for α- and β-thalassemia is shown in Figure 42-3.[105,109] Prenatal diagnosis, including preimplantation genetic diagnosis, is now available for β-thalassemia by polymerase chain reaction techniques of mutation detection on fetal blood or fetal DNA obtained from amniocentesis or chorionic villus sampling.[102,110-113]

Structural Hemoglobinopathies

To date, several hundred variants of α, β, γ, and δ chains have been identified. Most differ from normal chains by only one amino acid.

TABLE 42-5 FREQUENCY OF THE MOST COMMON HEMOGLOBINOPATHIES IN ADULT AFRICAN AMERICANS

Hemoglobinopathy	Abbreviated Name	Frequency
Sickle cell trait	Hb SA	1:122
Sickle cell anemia	Hb SS	1:708
Sickle cell–hemoglobin C disease	Hb SC	1:757
Hemoglobin C disease	Hb CC	1:4790
Hemoglobin C trait	Hb CA	1:41
Hemoglobin S–β-thalassemia	Hb S-β-thal	1:1672
Hemoglobin S-high F	Hb S-HPFH	1:3412

The nomenclature and frequency of the most common hemoglobinopathies among African Americans are depicted in Table 42-5.[114] Confirmation of a diagnosis of a specific hemoglobinopathy requires identification of the abnormal Hb by means of Hb electrophoresis.

Sickle Cell Trait

Traditionally, women with sickle cell trait have been thought to do well during pregnancy and labor. However, new studies have reported conflicting results about increased morbidities in women with sickle trait.[115-117] A case-control study from Mississippi, in which women with or without the trait were matched for race, reported a significant decrease in gestational age at birth (33 versus 35 weeks), lower mean birth weight, and an increased rate of fetal death (9.7% versus 3.5%) in the women with sickle cell trait.[116] Of interest, 42% of the fetal

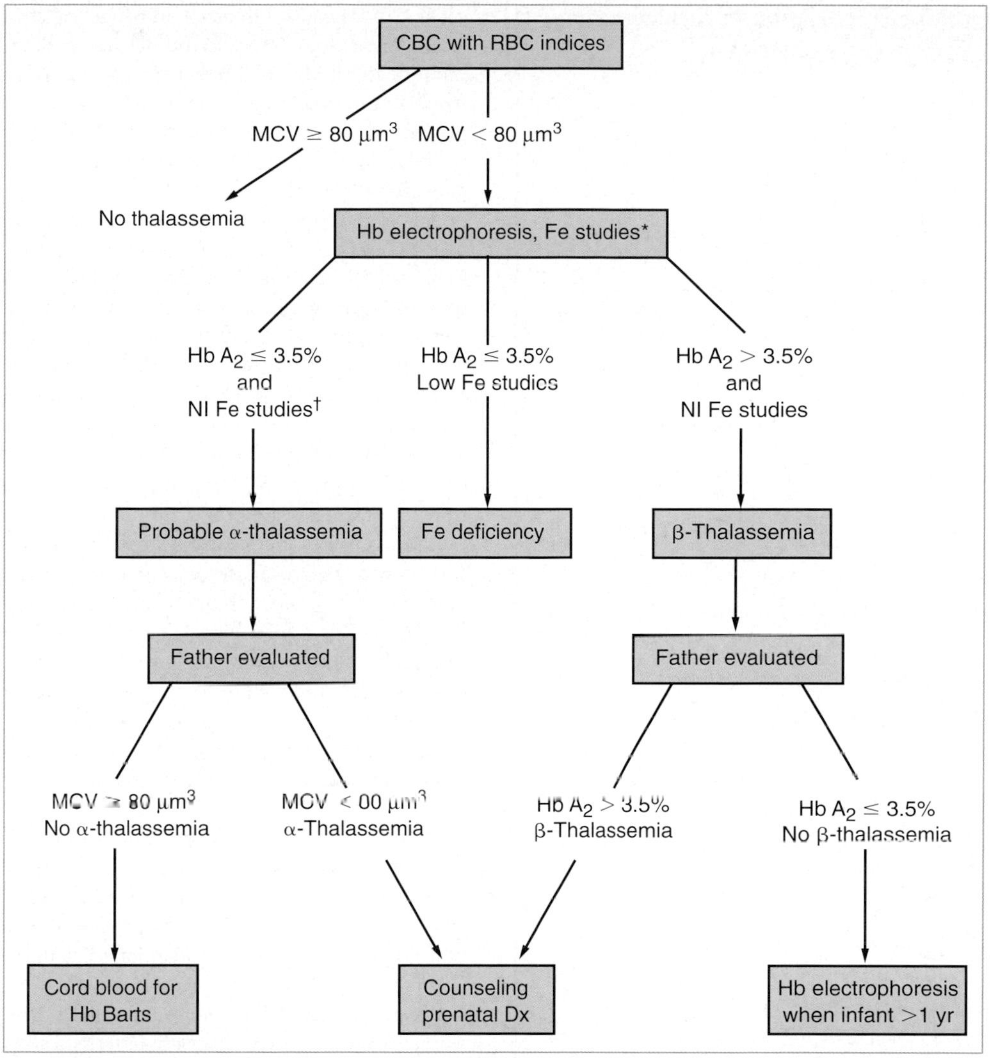

FIGURE 42-3 Maternal screening for α- and β-thalassemia. *May be serum Fe, total Fe binding capacity. †Percent transferrin saturation >15 or ferritin >12 µg/L. CBC, complete blood count; Dx, diagnosis; Fe, iron; Hb, hemoglobin; Nl, normal; MCV, mean corpuscular volume; RBC, red blood cell.

deaths in the sickle cell trait group were early deaths (16 to 20 weeks). In contrast, in a large cohort study of all African-American deliveries at one institution that compared those with and without maternal sickle cell trait, the trait was found to have a significant protective effect for preterm delivery at less than 32 weeks (0.9% versus 4.5%).[115] This protective effect was even more apparent in women with multiple gestations, with 0% versus 22% delivering before 32 weeks.

Because there is an increased rate of urinary tract infection among women with sickle cell trait, pregnant patients should be repeatedly screened for asymptomatic bacteriuria.[118-120] Recently, in a large case-control study of women with or without sickle cell trait who were matched for race, age, gestational age, and entry into prenatal care, there was no significant difference in the incidence of positive urine cultures (22% versus 19%).[117] However, pyelonephritis was significantly more common in the women with sickle cell trait (2.4% versus 0.7%). Another study suggested that the risk of preeclampsia was increased to 25% in those with the trait, compared with 10% in a sickle-negative control group.[121] These patients may become iron deficient, and iron supplementation during pregnancy is indicated.

Sickle Cell Anemia

Patients with sickle cell anemia (SCA) suffer from lifelong complications, in part as a result of the markedly shortened life span of their RBCs. Virtually all signs and symptoms of SCA are secondary to hemolysis, vaso-occlusive disease, or an increased susceptibility to infection (Table 42-6). Clinical manifestations may affect growth and development, with growth restriction and skeletal changes secondary to expansion of the marrow cavity. Painful crises may occur in the long bones, abdomen, chest, or back. The cardiovascular manifestations are those of a hyperdynamic circulation, and pulmonary signs may be secondary to either infection or vaso-occlusion. In addition to painful vaso-occlusive episodes, patients may exhibit hepatomegaly, signs and symptoms of hepatitis, cholecystitis, and painful splenic infarcts. Genitourinary signs include an impairment in concentrating ability (hyposthenuria), hematuria, and pyelonephritis.

Whether pregnancy in women with SCA is associated with more maternal complications is controversial. One comparison of pregnancy outcomes between women with and without SCA revealed no significant differences. Rates of maternal morbidity from SCA were the same during pregnancy as in the nonpregnant state.[122] However,

TABLE 42-6 CLINICAL MANIFESTATIONS OF SICKLE CELL ANEMIA

- I. Growth and development
  - A. Retarded growth
  - B. Skeletal changes
  - C. Decreased life span
- II. Sickle cell crisis
  - A. Painful vaso-occlusive episodes: bones, abdomen, chest, and back
- III. Cardiovascular manifestations of hyperdynamic circulation
  - A. Cardiomegaly
  - B. Systolic murmurs
  - C. Failure
- IV. Pulmonary signs
  - A. Infection: pneumococcus, mycoplasma, hemophilus, salmonella
  - B. Vascular occlusion
- V. Abdominal involvement
  - A. Painful vaso-occlusive episodes
  - B. Hepatomegaly
  - C. Hepatitis
  - D. Cholecystitis
  - E. Splenic infarction
- VI. Bone and joint changes
  - A. Bone marrow infarction
  - B. Osteomyelitis: salmonella
  - C. Arthritis
- VII. Genitourinary signs
  - A. Hyposthenuria
  - B. Hematuria
  - C. Pyelonephritis
- VIII. Neurologic manifestations
  - A. Vascular occlusion
  - B. Convulsions
  - C. Hemorrhage
  - D. Visual disturbances
- IX. Ocular manifestations
  - A. Conjunctival vessel changes
  - B. Vitreous hemorrhage

another study showed a significant increase in antepartum admissions, preterm labor or preterm premature rupture of membranes, and postpartum infection in women with versus those without SCA.[123] In two studies, there was no difference in the incidence of preeclampsia in women with and without SCA.[123,124] Series examining maternal deaths have been too small to determine whether there is an increased risk with SCA; however, pulmonary embolus or acute chest syndrome or both was the cause in 5 of 7 deaths.[125]

It is not known whether the frequency of painful crises in women with SCA changes with pregnancy. In one large study, the average number of crises per patient per pregnancy was 1 to 2, and other studies have suggested that 20% to 50% of affected pregnant women had crises.[122,124,126,127] Treatment is largely symptomatic, with the major objectives being to end a painful crisis and to combat infection. Hydration, oxygen therapy, and pain management are the cornerstones of managing a pain crisis. Acute chest syndrome is one of the most severe complications of SCA and can be very difficult to treat. It has been reported to occur in up to 20% of pregnancies.[122,124,128] Urinary tract and pulmonary infections should be diagnosed promptly and treated vigorously with appropriate antibiotics. Transfusion therapy has been used widely for years in the treatment of symptomatic patients. Partial exchange transfusions or prophylactic transfusions have been advocated.[129,130] The goal of partial exchange transfusions is to keep the Hb A level higher than 50% and the Hct greater than 25%.[131] A prospective, randomized study of 72 patients with SCA showed no significant difference in perinatal outcome between women who were treated with prophylactic transfusions and those who received transfusions only if their Hb level fell to less than 6 g/dL or the Hct to less than 18%.[127] However, this study did report a significant decrease in crises during pregnancy, from 50% to 14%, in the group receiving prophylactic transfusions. Sixty-six patients with sickle cell–Hb C disease and 23 with sickle cell–β-thalassemia received transfusions for hematologic reasons only and experienced similar perinatal outcomes.[127] However, the benefits attained must be balanced against a 25% incidence of alloimmunization and 20% occurrence of delayed transfusion reaction.

Several studies documented no relationship between maternal anemia and risk for IUGR or perinatal death in women with SCA.[124,132] The use of prophylactic transfusions should be individualized. An excellent review of SCA in nonpregnant individuals suggested that transfusion is indicated for symptomatic acute anemia, severe symptomatic chronic anemia, acute chest syndrome with hypoxia, and surgery with general anesthesia and may be useful for severe protracted pain episodes.[133] Most observers believe that the prepregnancy course of a woman is a good index of how she will fare during pregnancy. Although fetal outcomes are generally good in pregnancies complicated by SCA, there continues to be an increased risk of prematurity and IUGR.[122,123,134,135] The most recent series showed an incidence of IUGR and preterm delivery of 45% each, and both were significantly more common in women with SCA than in the control group without SCA.[123]

Serial ultrasound studies should be done throughout pregnancy to confirm normal fetal growth. There are no prospective studies on the use of antepartum fetal testing in women with SCA, so this should be instituted at the discretion of the physician. In addition, preimplantation genetic diagnosis with polymerase chain reaction assays is available for SCA.[110]

In general, prenatal vitamins without iron should be given to women who are receiving multiple transfusions. But all women with SCA should have an additional folic acid supplement of 1.0 mg/day prescribed. The pneumococcal vaccine should be given if the patient has not had the vaccine within the past year. During labor and delivery, the patient must remain well oxygenated and hydrated. If an exchange transfusion protocol has been used and the Hb A level is greater than 40%, painful crises are distinctly unusual.[136] Finally, a recent retrospective study of 40 women with SCA reported that the initial prenatal white blood cell count was significantly higher in those women who subsequently developed SCA-related complications (11.2×10^9/L) during their pregnancy than in those who did not develop complications (8×10^9/L).[137]

Hemoglobin Sickle C Disease

Women who are doubly heterozygous for both the Hb S and the Hb C genes are said to have Hb SC disease. Hb electrophoresis reveals approximately 60% Hb C and 40% Hb S. Patients with Hb SC disease typically have a normal habitus, a healthy childhood, and a normal life span. If a systematic screening program has not been used, the condition may first be detected in many women during the latter part of pregnancy, when a complication occurs. At the beginning of pregnancy, most women are mildly anemic and splenomegaly is present. Examination of a peripheral blood smear shows numerous target cells. Hb electrophoresis ensures the correct diagnosis.[138,139]

During pregnancy, 40% to 60% of patients with Hb SC disease present as if they had SCA. In contrast to patients with SCA, those with

Hb SC disease frequently experience rapid and severe anemic crises resulting from splenic sequestration. These patients also have a greater tendency to experience bone marrow necrosis with the release of fat-forming marrow emboli. The clinical manifestations of Hb SC disease are otherwise similar to those of SCA but milder, and the general management of symptomatic patients is identical. Considerations for the management of labor are the same as with SCA. In a recent report, women with Hb SC disease had a significantly increased risk of antepartum admission, IUGR, and postpartum infection compared to women without sickle disease, but these risks were only half as great as those of the women with SCA.[123] Similarly, Serjeant and associates reported that the rates of miscarriage, live-born delivery, and newborn weight less than 2500 g in women with Hb SC disease were similar to those in women with normal Hb and significantly better than those in women with SCA.[140] Rates of pain crises, acute chest syndrome, and urinary tract infections were similar in women with Hb SC disease and those with SCA.[140]

Hemoglobin S-β-Thalassemia

Patients with Hb S-β-thalassemia are heterozygous for the sickle cell and the β-thalassemia genes, and in general about 10% of sickle cell disease is caused by Hb S-β-thalassemia.[111] In addition to decreased β-chain production, there is a variably increased production of Hb F and Hb A_2. Because of this variable production rate, Hb electrophoresis reveals a spectrum of Hb concentrations. Hb S may account for 70% to 95% of the Hb present, with Hb F rarely exceeding 20%.[141] Because of the thalassemia influence, the Hb S concentration exceeds the Hb A concentration. This is in sharp contrast to patients with sickle cell trait, in whom Hb A levels exceed the concentration of Hb S.

The diagnosis is made in an anemic patient by demonstrating increased Hb A_2 and Hb F levels in association with a level of Hb S exceeding that of Hb A. The peripheral smear reveals hypochromia and microcytosis with anisocytosis, poikilocytosis, basophilic stippling, and target cells. The clinical manifestations of this disorder parallel those of SCA but are generally milder. Painful crises may occur; however, these patients have a normal body habitus and frequently enjoy an uncompromised life span. The role of exchange transfusion should be similar to that in patients with SCA; that is, exchange transfusion should be reserved for the woman who experiences painful crises or whose anemia leads to an Hct lower than 25%.

Hemoglobin C Trait and Disease

Hb C trait is an asymptomatic trait without reproductive consequences. Target cells are found in the peripheral smear, but anemia is not present. Hb C disease, the homozygous state, is a mild disorder that usually is discovered during a medical evaluation. Mild hemolytic anemia with an Hct in the range of 25% to 35% is characteristic. The RBCs show microspherocytes and characteristic targeting. No increased morbidity or mortality is associated with pregnancy, and no specific therapy is indicated.

Hemoglobin E Disease

The recent immigration of Southeast Asians to the United States has resulted in an increase in the number of individuals with Hb E trait and disease. The clinical and laboratory manifestations of the various Hb E syndromes are outlined in Table 42-7.[142,143] Most individuals have a mild microcytic anemia that is of no clinical significance, and no treatment is necessary. However, patients who are homozygous for Hb E have a greater degree of microcytosis and are frequently anemic. Target cells are prominent. As with Hb C trait and disease, no specific therapy is required, and reproductive outcome is normal.

Anemias Associated with Systemic Disease

The normal bone marrow has the capacity to increase its RBC production sixfold to eightfold in response to anemia. This compensatory mechanism, which is responsible also for the increase in RBC mass in normal pregnancy, is triggered by tissue hypoxia and mediated by erythropoietin. The response may be absent or blunted in some circumstances, most commonly in chronic disorders. Chronic infections, rheumatoid arthritis, and other inflammatory states are characterized by a mild normocytic, normochromic anemia (or sometimes a hypochromic, microcytic anemia) with low serum iron concentration, low transferrin level, inappropriately low reticulocyte count, and generous but poorly utilized stores of reticuloendothelial iron. Although the bone marrow is normally cellular, it does not respond appropriately to the mildly accelerated RBC destruction typical of chronic inflammation. Studies thus far have not determined whether the defect in erythropoiesis can be attributed to inadequate erythropoietin secretion. In the absence of pregnancy, the Hb concentration in these chronic states is frequently 9 to 10 g/dL, and the Hct concentration is approximately 30%. The hydremia of pregnancy may lower these values somewhat.

A similar but frequently more complicated anemia accompanies renal failure. Here, more often perhaps than in chronic inflammatory states, blood loss and hemolysis are contributory factors, and the serum iron and transferrin changes noted earlier are less regular. In

TABLE 42-7 VARIOUS GENOTYPES OF HEMOGLOBIN E AND THEIR PHENOTYPIC EXPRESSION*

			Hb Electrophoresis (%)				
Genotype	**Degree of Anemia**	**MCV†**	**A + A_2**	**E**	**F**	**S**	**Phenotype Expression**
A/E	0	↓	68	30	<2	0	None
E/E	0 to +	↓↓	<4	94	<2	0	None
E/α-thal	+ to ++	↓	50	15	35	0	None
S/E	++	↓	0	40	0	60	None
E/β^+-thal	++	↓↓	10	60	30	0	Splenomegaly
E/β^0-thal	+++	↓↓	0	60	40	0	Splenomegaly

*Number of + symbols indicates relative severity of anemia.
†Number of arrows indicates relative amount of decrease.
Hb, hemoglobin; MCV, mean corpuscular volume.

many of these situations, diminished erythropoietin is important in the pathogenesis.

Renal failure and chronic inflammation are rare in pregnancy, so management of the associated anemias is seldom a clinical problem in obstetric patients. Occasionally, however, it is the anemia that calls attention to the underlying disease. These anemias do not respond to hematinic agents or steroid hormones (unless the adrenal steroids play some role in controlling the underlying disease, as in rheumatoid arthritis or lupus). Erythropoietin is useful in treating chronic renal disease and can often obviate the need for repeated RBC transfusion.[144]

References

1. Laros RK Jr (ed): Blood Disorders in Pregnancy. Philadelphia: Lea & Febiger, 1986.
2. Wiebe ER, Trouton KJ, Eftekhari A: Anemia in early pregnancy among Canadian women presenting for abortion. Int J Gynaecol Obstet 94:60-61, 2006.
3. Centers for Disease Control and Prevention: Current trends: CDC criteria for anemia in children and childbearing-aged women. MMWR Morb Mortal Wkly Rep 38:400-404, 1989.
4. Schifman RB, Thomasson JE, Evers JM: Red blood cell zinc protoporphyrin testing in iron-deficiency anemia in pregnancy. Am J Obstet Gynecol 157:304, 1987.
5. Ho CH, Yuan CC, Yeh SH: Serum ferritin, folate and cobalamin levels and their correlation with anemia in normal full-term pregnant women. Eur J Obstet Gynecol Reprod Biol 26:7, 1987.
6. Haram K, Nilsen ST, Ulvik RJ: Iron supplementation in pregnancy: Evidence and controversies. Acta Obstet Gynaecol Scand 80:683, 2001.
7. Puolakka A, Janne O, Pararinen A, et al: Serum ferritin in the diagnosis of anemia during pregnancy. Acta Obstet Gynaecol Scand 95(Suppl):57, 1980.
8. Alper BS, Kimber R, Reddy AK: Using ferritin levels to determine iron-deficiency anemia in pregnancy. J Fam Practice 49:829, 2000.
9. Seligman PA, Caskey JH, Frazier JI, et al: Measurements of iron absorption from prenatal multivitamin-mineral supplements. Obstet Gynecol 61:356, 1983.
10. Taylor DJ, Mallen C, McDougall N, et al: Effect of iron supplement on serum ferritin levels during and after pregnancy. BJOG 89:1011, 1982.
11. Peck TM, Arias F: Hematologic changes associated with pregnancy. Clin Obstet 22:785, 1979.
12. Scott DE, Pritchard JA: Iron deficiency in healthy young college women. JAMA 199:147, 1967.
13. Pritchard JA, Whalley PJ, Scott DE: The influence of maternal folate and iron deficiency on intrauterine life. Am J Obstet Gynecol 104:388, 1969.
14. Monsen ER, Kuhn JH, Finch CA: Iron status of menstruating females. Am J Clin Nutr 20:842, 1967.
15. Casanueva E, Pfeffer F, Drijanski A, et al: Iron and folate status before pregnancy and anemia during pregnancy. Ann Nutr Metab 47:60-63, 2003.
16. Fenton V, Cavill J, Fisher J: Iron stores in pregnancy. Br J Haematol 37:145, 1977.
17. Institute of Medicine: Iron Deficiency Anemia: Recommended Guidelines for Prevention, Detection and Management among U.S. Children and Women of Childbearing Age. Washington, DC: National Academy Press, 1993.
18. Galbraith GMP, Galbraith RM, Temple A, et al: Demonstration of transferrin receptors on human placental trophoblast. Blood 55:240, 1980.
19. Okuyama T, Tawada T, Furuya H, et al: The role of transferrin and ferritin in the fetal-maternal-placental unit. Am J Obstet Gynecol 152:344, 1985.
20. Johan E, Magnus EM: Plasma and red blood cell folate during normal pregnancy. Acta Obstet Gynaecol Scand 60:247, 1981.
21. Allen LH: Anemia and iron deficiency: Effects on pregnancy outcome. Am J Clin Nutr 71(5 Suppl):1280S-1284S, 2000.
22. Herbert V, Colman N, Spivack M: Folic acid deficiency in the United States: Folate assays in a prenatal clinic. Am J Obstet Gynecol 123:175, 1975.
23. Shojania AM, Hornady GJ: Oral contraceptives and folate absorption. J Lab Clin Med 82:869, 1973.
24. Iyengar L: Folic acid absorption in pregnancy. BJOG 82:20, 1975.
25. Pritchard JA, Whalley PJ, Scott DE: Infants of mothers with megaloblastic anemia due to folate deficiency. JAMA 211:1982, 1970.
26. Kitay DZ: Folic acid deficiency in pregnancy. Am J Obstet Gynecol 104:1067, 1969.
27. Centers for Disease Control and Prevention: Recommendations for the use of folic acid to reduce the number of cases of spina bifida and other neural tube defects. MMWR Morb Morta Wkly Rep 41:001, 1992.
28. Wald NJ, Law MR, Morris JK, et al: Quantifying the effect of folic acid. Lancet 358:2069, 2001.
29. American College of Obstetricians and Gynecologists: Folic Acid for the Prevention of Recurrent Neural Tube Defects. ACOG Committee Opinion No. 252. Washington, DC: ACOG, 2003.
30. Bondevik GT, Lie RT, Ulstein M, et al: Maternal hematological status and risk of low birth weight and preterm delivery in Nepal. Acta Obstet Gynecol Scand 80:402, 2001.
31. Levy A, Fraser D, Katz M, et al: Maternal anemia during pregnancy is an independent risk factor for low birthweight and preterm delivery. Eur J Obstet Gynecol Reprod Biol 122:182-186, 2005.
32. Scanlon KS, Yip R, Schieve LA, Cogswell ME: High and low hemoglobin levels during pregnancy: Differential risks for preterm birth and small for gestational age. Obstet Gynecol 96:741, 2000.
33. Xiong X, Buekens P, Alexander S, et al: Anemia during pregnancy and birth outcome: A meta-analysis. Am J Perinatol 17:137, 2000.
34. Goldenberg RL, Tamura T, DuBard M, et al: Plasma ferritin and pregnancy outcome. Am J Obstet Gynecol 175:1356, 1996.
35. Klebanoff MA, Shiono PH, Shelby JV, et al: Anemia and spontaneous preterm birth. Am J Obstet Gynecol 59:164, 1991.
36. Lu ZM, Goldenberg RL, Cliver SP, et al: The relationship between maternal hematocrit and pregnancy outcome. Obstet Gynecol 77:190, 1991.
37. Scholl TO, Hediger ML, Fischer RL, et al: Anemia vs. iron deficiency: Increased risk of preterm delivery in a prospective study. Am J Clin Nutr 55:985, 1992.
38. Paulone ME, Edelstone DI, Shedd A: Effects of maternal anemia on utero-placental and fetal oxidative metabolism in sheep. Am J Obstet Gynecol 156:230, 1987.
39. Sagen N, Nilsen ST, Kim HC, et al: Maternal hemoglobin concentration is closely related to birth weight in normal pregnancies. Acta Obstet Gynecol 63:245, 1984.
40. Stephansson O, Dickman PW, Johansson A, et al: Maternal hemoglobin concentration during pregnancy and risk of stillbirth. JAMA 284:2611, 2000.
41. Brabin BJ, Hakimi M, Pelletier D: An analysis of anemia and pregnancy-related maternal mortality. J Nutrition 131:604S, 2001.
42. Patra S, Pasrija S, Trivedi SS, Puri M: Maternal and perinatal outcome in patients with severe anemia in pregnancy. Int J Gynaecol Obstet 91:164-165, 2005.
43. Milman N, Agger AO, Nielsen OJ: Iron status markers and serum erythropoietin in 120 mothers and newborn infants. Acta Obstet Gynaecol Scand 73:200-204, 1994.
44. Singla PN, Tyagi M, Shankar R, et al: Fetal iron status in maternal anemia. Acta Paediatr 85:1327, 1996.
45. Colomer J, Colomer C, Gutierrez D, et al: Anaemia during pregnancy as a risk factor for infant iron deficiency: Report from the Valencia Infant Anaemia Cohort (VIAC) study. Paediatr Perinat Epidemiol 4:196-204, 1990.
46. Cogswell M, Parvanta I, Ickes L, et al: Iron supplementation during pregnancy, anemia, and birth weight: A randomized controlled trial. Am J Clin Nutr 78:773-781, 2003.

47. Hemminki E, Merilainen J: Long term follow-up of mothers and their infants in a randomized trial on iron prophylaxis during pregnancy. Am J Obstet Gynecol 173:205, 1995.
48. Jaime-Perez JC, Gomez-Almaguer D: Iron stores in low-income pregnant Mexican women at term. Arch Med Res 33:81, 2002.
49. Sifakis S, Pharmakides G: Anemia in pregnancy. Ann N Y Acad Sci 900:125-36, 2000.
50. Swensen AR, Harnack LJ, Ross JA: Nutritional assessment of pregnant women enrolled in the Special Supplemental Program for Women, Infants, and Children (WIC). J Am Diet Assoc 101:903, 2001.
51. Rainville AJ: Pica practices of pregnant women are associated with lower maternal hemoglobin level at delivery. J Am Diet Assoc 101:318, 2001.
52. Centers for Disease Control and Prevention: Recommendations to prevent and control iron deficiency anemia in the United States. MMWR Morb Mortal Wkly Rep 47:1, 1998.
53. Sloan NL, Jordan E, Winkoff B: Effects of iron supplementation on maternal hematologic status in pregnancy. Am J Public Health 92:288, 2002.
54. Hamstra RD, Block MH, Schocket AL: Intravenous iron dextran. JAMA 233:1726, 1980.
55. Fishbane S: Safety in iron management. Am J Kidney Dis 41(5 Suppl):18-26, 2003.
56. Fairbanks VF: Manual of Clinical Hematology. Philadelphia: Lippincott Williams & Wilkins, 2002, Chapter 2 (Iron-Deficiency Anemia), pp 17-39.
57. Bashiri A, Burstein E, Sheiner E, Mazor M: Anemia during pregnancy and treatment with intravenous iron: Review of the literature. Eur J Obstet Gynecol Reprod Biol 110:2-7, 2003.
58. Bayoumeu F, Subiran-Buisset C, Baka NE, et al: Iron therapy in iron deficiency anemia in pregnancy: Intravenous route versus oral route. Am J Obstet Gynecol 186:518, 2002.
59. Sharma JB, Jain S, Mallika V, et al: A prospective, partially randomized study of pregnancy outcomes and hematologic responses to oral and intramuscular iron treatment in moderately anemic pregnant women. Am J Clin Nutr 79:116-122, 2004.
60. Al RA, Unlubilgin E, Kandemir O, et al: Intravenous versus oral iron treatment of anemia in pregnancy. Obstet Gynecol 106:1335-1340, 2005.
61. Breymann C, Visca E, Huch R, et al: Efficacy and safety of intravenously administered iron sucrose with and without adjuvant recombinant human erythropoietin for the treatment of resistant iron-deficiency anemia during pregnancy. Am J Obstet Gynecol 184:662, 2001.
62. Sifakis S, Angelakis E, Vardaki E, et al: Erythropoietin in the treatment of iron deficiency anemia during pregnancy. Gynecol Obstet Invest 51:150, 2001.
63. Vora M, Gruslin A: Erythropoietin in obstetrics. Obstet Gynecol Surv 53:500, 1998.
64. Goshorn J, Youell TD. Darbepoetin alfa treatment for post-renal transplantation anemia during pregnancy. Am J Kidney Dis 46:E81-E86, 2005.
65. Kominiarek M, Kilpatrick SJ: Bariatric surgery and the OB GYN patient. Contemporary Obstet Gynecol:76-88, 2005.
66. Gallagher PG, Forget BG: Hematologically important mutations: spectrin and ankyrin variants in hereditary spherocytosis. Blood Cells Mol Dis 24:539-543, 1998.
67. Moore A, Sherman MM, Strongin MJ: Hereditary spherocytosis with hemolytic crisis during pregnancy. Obstet Gynecol 47:19S, 1976.
68. Magid MS, Perkins M, Gottfried EL: Increased erythrocyte osmotic fragility in pregnancy. Am J Obstet Gynecol 144:910, 1982.
69. Maberry MC, Mason RA, Cunningham FG, et al: Pregnancy complicated by hereditary spherocytosis. Obstet Gynecol 79:735, 1992.
70. Breckenridge RL, Riggs JA: Hereditary elliptocytosis with hemolytic anemia complicating pregnancy. Am J Obstet Gynecol 101:861, 1968.
71. Sacks DA, Platt L, Johnson CS: Autoimmune hemolytic anemia during pregnancy. Am J Obstet Gynecol 140:942, 1981.
72. Kumar R, Advani AR, Sharan J, et al: Pregnancy induced hemolytic anemia: An unexplained entity. Ann Hematol 80:623-626, 2001.
73. Starkson NF, Bell WR, Kickler TS: Unexplained hemolytic anemia associated with pregnancy. Am J Obstet Gynecol 146:617-622, 1983.
74. Beutler E: Glucose-6-phosphate dehydrogenase deficiency. N Engl J Med 324:169, 1991.
75. Silverstein E, Roadman C, Byers RH, et al: Hematologic problems in pregnancy: III. Glucose-6-phosphate dehydrogenase deficiency. J Reprod Med 12:153, 1974.
76. Perkins RP: The significance of glucose-6-phosphate dehydrogenase deficiency in pregnancy. Am J Obstet Gynecol 125:215, 1976.
77. Weng YH, Chou YH, Lien RI: Hyperbilirubinemia in healthy neonates with glucose-6-phosphate dehydrogenase deficiency. Early Hum Dev 71:129-136, 2003.
78. Holly RG: Hypoplastic anemia in pregnancy. Obstet Gynecol 1:533, 1953.
79. Ascarelli MH, Emerson ES, Bigelow CL, et al: Aplastic anemia and immune-mediated thrombocytopenia: Concurrent complications encountered in the third trimester of pregnancy. Obstet Gynecol 91:803, 1998.
80. Deka D, Malhotra N, Sinha A, et al: Pregnancy associated aplastic anemia: Maternal and fetal outcome. J Obstet Gynaecol Res 29:67-72, 2003.
81. Fleming AF: Hypoplastic anaemia in pregnancy. Clin Haematol 2:477, 1973.
82. Kwon JY, Lee Y, Shin JC, et al: Supportive management of pregnancy-associated aplastic anemia. Int J Gynaecol Obstet 95:115-120, 2006.
83. Ohba T, Yoshimura T, Araki M, et al: Aplastic anemia in pregnancy: Treatment with cyclosporine and granulocyte-colony stimulating factor. Acta Obstet Gynecol 78:458, 1999.
84. Snyder TE, Lee LP, Lynch S: Pregnancy-associated hypoplastic anemia: A review. Obstet Gynecol Surv 46:264, 1991.
85. Lynch RE, Williams DM, Reading JC, et al: The prognosis in aplastic anemia. Blood 45:517, 1975.
86. Kojima S, Nakao S, Tomonaga M, et al: Consensus conference on the treatment of aplastic anemia. Int J Hematol 72:118, 2000.
87. Deeg HJ, Kennedy MS, Sanders JR, et al: Successful pregnancy after marrow transplantation for severe aplastic anemia and immunosuppression with cyclosporine. JAMA 250:647, 1983.
88. Doney K, Storb R, Buckner CD, et al: Marrow transplantation for treatment of pregnancy-associated aplastic anemia. Exp Hematol 13:1080, 1985.
89. Sanders JE, Hawley J, Levy W, et al: Pregnancies following high-dose cyclophosphamide with or without high-dose busulfan or total-body irradiation and bone marrow transplantation. Blood 87:3045, 1996.
90. Schmidt H, Ehninger G, Dopfer R, et al: Pregnancy after bone marrow transplantation for severe aplastic anemia. Bone Marrow Transplant 2:329, 1987.
91. Tichelli A, Socie G, Marsh J, et al; European Group for Blood and Marrow Transplantation Severe Aplastic Anaemia Working Party: Outcome of pregnancy and disease course among women with aplastic anemia treated with immunosuppression. Ann Intern Med 137:164-172, 2002.
92. McGuire WA, Yang HH, Bruno E, et al: Treatment of antibody-mediated pure red-cell aplasia with high-dose intravenous gamma globulin. N Engl J Med 317:1004, 1987.
93. Fieni S, Bonfanti L, Gramellini D, et al: Clinical management of paroxysmal nocturnal hemoglobinuria in pregnancy: A case report and updated review. Obstet Gynecol Surv 61:593-601, 2006.
94. Bjorge L, Ernst P, Haram KO: Paroxysmal nocturnal hemoglobinuria in pregnancy. Acta Obstet Gynaecol Scand 82:1067-1071, 2003.
95. Thome SD, Petz LD: Manual of Clinical Hematology. Philadelphia: Lippincott Williams & Wilkins, 2002, Chapter 4 (Hemolytic Anemia: Hereditary and Acquired), pp 90-117.
96. Ray JG, Burows RF, Ginsberg JS, Burrows EA: Paroxysmal nocturnal hemoglobinuria and the risk of venous thrombosis: Review and recommendations for management of the pregnant and nonpregnant patient. Haemostasis 30:103-117, 2000.
97. Stocche RM, Garcia LV, Klamt JG: Labor analgesia in a patient with paroxysmal nocturnal hemoglobinuria with thromboxytopenia. Reg Anesth Pain Med 26:79-82, 2001.
98. Hurd WW, Miodovnik M, Stys SJ: Pregnancy associated with paroxysmal nocturnal hemoglobinuria. Obstet Gynecol 60:742, 1982.

99. Solal-Celigny P, Tertian G, Fernandez H, et al: Pregnancy and paroxysmal nocturnal hemoglobinuria. Arch Intern Med 148:593, 1988.
100. Higgs DR, Vickers MA, Wilkie AOM, et al: A review of the molecular genetics of the human α-globin gene cluster. Blood 73:1081, 1989.
101. Old JM: Prenatal diagnosis of hemoglobinopathies. In Milunsky A (ed): Genetic Disorders and the Fetus: Diagnosis, Prevention and Treatment, 4th ed. Baltimore: Johns Hopkins University Press, 1998, p 581.
102. Cao A, Saba L, Galanello R, et al: Molecular diagnosis and carrier screening for β thalassemia. JAMA 178:1273, 1997.
103. Fosburg MT, Nathan DG: Treatment of Cooley's anemia. Blood 76:435, 1990.
104. Kazazian HH, Boehm CD: Molecular basis and prenatal diagnosis of β-thalassemia. Blood 72:1107, 1988.
105. Alger LS, Golbus MS, Laros RK Jr: Thalassemia and pregnancy. Am J Obstet Gynecol 134:662, 1979.
106. Fleming AF, Lynch W: Beta-thalassemia minor during pregnancy with particular reference to iron status. J Obstet Gynaecol Br Comm 76:451, 1967.
107. Aessopos A, Karabatsos F, Farmakis D, et al: Pregnancy in patients with well-treated β-thalassemia: Outcome for mothers and newborn infants. Am J Obstet Gynecol 180:360, 1999.
108. Lorey F, Cunningham G: Impact of Asian immigration on thalassemia in California. Ann N Y Acad Sci 859:442, 1998.
109. Kilpatrick SJ, Laros RK: Thalassemia in pregnancy. Clin Obstet Gynecol 38:485, 1995.
110. De Rycke M, Van de Velde H, Sermon K, et al: Preimplantation genetic diagnosis for sickle-cell anemia and for beta-thalassemia. Prenat Diagn 21:214, 2001.
111. Rappaport VJ, Velazquez M, Williams K: Hemoglobinopathies in pregnancy. Obstet Gynecol Clin North Am 31:287-317, 2004.
112. Traeger-Synodinos J, Vrettou C, Palmer G, et al: An evaluation of PGD in clinical genetic services through 3 years application for prevention of β-thalassaemia major and sickle cell thalassaemia. Mol Hum Reprod 9:301-307, 2003.
113. Vrettou C, Traeger-Synodinos J, Tzetis M, et al: Real-time PCR for single-cell genotyping in sickle cell and thalassemia syndromes as a rapid, accurate, reliable, and widely applicable protocol for preimplantation genetic diagnosis. Hum Mutat 23:513-521, 2004.
114. Motulsky AG: Frequency of sickling disorders in U.S. blacks. N Engl J Med 288:31, 1973.
115. Bryant A, Cheng Y, Lyell D, et al: Presence of the sickle cell trait and preterm delivery in African-American women. Obstet Gynecol 109:870-874, 2007.
116. Taylor MY, Wyatt-Ashmead J, Gray J, et al: Pregnancy loss after first-trimester viability in women with sickle cell trait: Time for a reappraisal? Am J Obstet Gynecol 194:1604-1608, 2006.
117. Thurman AR, Steed LL, Hulsey T, Soper DE: Bacteriuria in pregnant women with sickle cell trait. Am J Obstet Gynecol 194:1366-1370, 2006.
118. Blattner P, Dar H, Nitowski HM: Pregnancy outcome in women with sickle cell trait. JAMA 238:1392, 1977.
119. Whalley PJ, Pritchard JA, Richards JR: Sickle cell trait and pregnancy. JAMA 186:1132, 1963.
120. Whalley PJ, Martin FG, Pritchard JA: Sickle cell trait and urinary tract infections during pregnancy. JAMA 189:903, 1964.
121. Larrabee KD, Monga M: Women with sickle cell trait are at increased risk for preeclampsia. Am J Obstet Gynecol 177:425, 1997.
122. Smith JA, Espeland M, Bellevue R, et al: Pregnancy in sickle cell disease: Experience of the Cooperative Study of Sickle Cell Disease. Obstet Gynecol 87:199, 1996.
123. Sun PM, Wilburn W, Raynor D, et al: Sickle cell disease in pregnancy: Twenty years of experience at Grady Memorial Hospital, Atlanta, Georgia. Am J Obstet Gynecol 184:1127, 2001.
124. Serjeant G, Loy LL, Crowther M, et al: Outcome of pregnancy in homozygous sickle cell disease. Obstet Gynecol 103:1278-1285, 2004.
125. Hassell K: Pregnancy and sickle cell disease. Hematol Oncol Clin North Am 19:903-916, 2005.
126. Howard RJ, Tuck SM, Pearson TC: Pregnancy in sickle cell disease in the UK: Results of a multicentre survey of the effect of prophylactic blood transfusion on maternal and fetal outcome. BJOG 102:947-951, 1995.
127. Koshy M, Burd L, Wallace D, et al: Prophylactic red-cell transfusion in pregnant patients with sickle cell disease. N Engl J Med 319:1447, 1988.
128. Koshy M, Burd L: Management of pregnancy in sickle cell syndromes. Hematol Oncol North Am 5:585-596, 1991.
129. Cunningham FG, Pritchard JA, Mason RA, et al: Prophylactic transfusion of normal red blood cells during pregnancy complicated by sickle cell hemoglobinopathies. Am J Obstet Gynecol 135:994, 1979.
130. Francis RB, Johnson CS: Vascular occlusion in sickle cell disease: Current concepts and unanswered questions. Blood 77:1405, 1991.
131. Rust OA, Perry KG: Pregnancy complicated by sickle hemoglobinopathy. Clin Obstet Gynecol 38:472, 1995.
132. Powars D, Sandhu M, Niland-Weiss J, et al: Pregnancy in sickle cell disease. Obstet Gynecol 67:217-228, 1986.
133. Steinberg MH: Management of sickle cell disease. N Engl J Med 340:1021, 1999.
134. Cunningham FG, Pritchard JA, Mason RA: Pregnancy and sickle cell hemoglobinopathies. Obstet Gynecol 62:419, 1983.
135. Morrison JC, Wiser WL: The use of prophylactic partial exchange transfusion in pregnancies associated with sickle cell hemoglobinopathies. Obstet Gynecol 48:510, 1976.
136. Morrison JC, Whybrew WD, Bucovary ET: Use of partial exchange transfusion preoperatively in patients with sickle cell hemoglobinopathies. Am J Obstet Gynecol 132:59, 1978.
137. Litos M, Sarris I, Bewley S, et al: White blood cell count as a predictor of the severity of sickle cell disease during pregnancy. Eur J Obstet Gynecol Reprod Biol 133:169-172, 2007.
138. Laros RK Jr: Sickle cell hemoglobin C disease in pregnancy. Pa Med 70:73, 1967.
139. Maberry MC, Mason RA, Cunningham FG, et al: Pregnancy complicated by hemoglobin CC and C-β-thalassemia disease. Obstet Gynecol 76:324, 1990.
140. Serjeant G, Hambleton I, Thame M: Fecundity and pregnancy outcome in a cohort with sickle cell-haemoglobin C disease followed from birth. Int J Gynaecol Obstet 112:1308-1314, 2005.
141. Laros RK Jr, Kalstone C: Sickle cell beta-thalassemia and pregnancy. Obstet Gynecol 37:67, 1971.
142. Ferguson JE, O'Reilly RA: Hemoglobin E and pregnancy. Obstet Gynecol 66:136, 1985.
143. Wong SC, Ali MAM: Hemoglobin E disease. Am J Hematol 13:15, 1982.
144. Erslev AJ: Erythropoietin. N Engl J Med 324:1339, 1991.

Chapter 43

Malignancy and Pregnancy

David Cohn, MD, Bhuvaneswari Ramaswamy, MD, and Kristie Blum, MD

Cancer occurring during pregnancy is not rare. Approximately 1 of 1000 pregnant women is diagnosed with a new malignancy each year in the United States.[1] Cancer is one of the leading causes of nonaccidental deaths in the United States in women between the ages of 15 and 34, and it is the leading cause of death in the women between the ages of 35 and 54 years.[2] The most common malignancies in women 15 to 34 years old are malignant melanoma, breast cancer, leukemia, cervical cancer, central nervous system tumors, and non-Hodgkin lymphoma. Lung, colorectal, and ovarian cancer also are common in 35- to 54-year-old women.[1] Melanoma is estimated to occur in 1 of 1000, cervical cancer in 1 of 2000, Hodgkin lymphoma in 1 of 3000, breast cancer in 1 of 3000, ovarian cancer in 1 of 18,000, and leukemia in 1 of 75,000 pregnancies. The current social trend of delaying pregnancy into the later reproductive years will result in more cancers being diagnosed during gestation.

The management of cancer in pregnancy is challenging, posing ethical and medical dilemmas. Limited prospective data are available, which hinders the decision-making process. The goal of cancer therapy in pregnant women is to provide the best cancer care for the patient while minimizing the potential harm to the fetus.

Cancers in pregnancy are often categorized by the time of diagnosis: those discovered during the antenatal period, at the time of delivery, or up to 1 year after birth. More than 50% of cancers complicating pregnancy are found within 1 year after delivery, and more than 25% are found in the antenatal period. Few are found at delivery.[3]

When a malignant neoplasm is diagnosed in pregnancy, the health of the mother and fetus must be considered. When cancer is diagnosed early in a desired pregnancy, the clinical situation is complex. If delaying treatment will not affect the maternal prognosis, treatment may be deferred until the fetus has achieved maturity. If the prognosis is expected to worsen with delayed treatment, the risks and benefits of more immediate treatment must be weighed against the risks to the pregnancy and the fetus. Given the complex management involved in the care of a pregnant patient with cancer, a multidisciplinary team is essential to ensure that the mother, family, and all members of the health care team are well informed about the risks, benefits, and alternatives of the treatment choices and modalities. In addition to the medical aspects of the care, management must be individualized to balance the ethical, moral, spiritual, and cultural issues that complicate such a diagnosis.

Factors such as the hormonal milieu, increased vascularity, altered lymphatic drainage, and immune adaptations in pregnancy have historically been thought to increase the risk of malignancy and to increase the likelihood of a more aggressive course with poorer outcomes than would be expected in a nonpregnant woman. However, there is no evidence to suggest that pregnancy directly or indirectly affects the incidence or outcome of cancer. This chapter addresses the issues related to the diagnosis and care for a pregnant patient with cancer.

Ovarian and Cervical Malignancies

Ovarian Cancer

Epidemiology, Diagnosis, and Tumor Types

One of 18,000 pregnancies is complicated by an ovarian malignancy.[4-6] Approximately 1 of 1000 pregnant women undergo exploratory surgery to evaluate an adnexal mass, and 1% to 3% of these masses are malignant.[7,8] This incidence is lower than among nonpregnant women, probably because pregnancy occurs in younger women, in whom most ovarian masses are corpus luteum cysts or other benign simple cysts and most ovarian neoplasms are teratomas or cystadenomas.[9-11] Most ovarian malignancies found in pregnancy are germ cell tumors, but the incidence of epithelial ovarian malignancies identified during pregnancy may increase as women defer childbearing into later in their reproductive years.

Rarely, a woman presents with an advanced ovarian malignancy requiring extensive cytoreduction. If the malignancy is diagnosed when the fetal prognosis allows delivery or the patient does not wish to continue the pregnancy, immediate surgical exploration for cytoreduction and subsequent adjuvant treatment should be undertaken. If the pregnancy is desired and the fetus cannot be delivered, management is complex. In selected patients, antepartum bilateral oophorectomy and cytoreduction can be performed, with the pregnancy continuing and adjuvant treatment delayed until delivery. Management must be individualized for each patient based on her desire for future fertility, gestational age, and extent of disease. In selected patients, antepartum neoadjuvant (before surgery) chemotherapy administered until fetal maturity, followed by cytoreductive surgery at abdominal delivery, may be considered.

Germ cell cancers are the most common ovarian malignancy diagnosed in pregnancy; up to 30% of malignancies in pregnancy are dysgerminomas. They most often manifest with torsion. The serum level of maternal lactate dehydrogenase (LDH), the tumor marker for dysgerminomas, is not altered by pregnancy, and it can serve as a marker for the disease during pregnancy.[12]

TABLE 43-1 COMPONENTS OF COMPREHENSIVE SURGICAL STAGING OF GYNECOLOGIC CANCERS

Sampling of pelvic cytology or ascites
Ipsilateral salpingo-oophorectomy
Hysterectomy and contralateral salpingo-oophorectomy (eliminated in selected patients)
Peritoneal biopsies (e.g., anterior and posterior cul-de-sac, pelvic side walls, abdominal gutters, diaphragms)
Biopsies of adhesions or other abnormalities
Omentectomy
Bilateral pelvic lymphadenectomy
Bilateral aortic lymphadenectomy

Standard management of a suspected ovarian dysgerminoma during pregnancy is surgery. Unilateral oophorectomy for diagnosis with comprehensive surgical staging (Table 43-1) and preservation of the contralateral ovary and uterus is recommended. Because 15% of dysgerminomas are bilateral, inspection of the contralateral ovary with biopsy or removal of abnormalities should be performed for therapeutic and prognostic reasons. Wedge resection or biopsy of a normal-appearing contralateral ovary is unnecessary because of the risk of increased adhesion formation and possible infertility. Patients with advanced dysgerminoma require chemotherapy with bleomycin, etoposide, and cisplatin (BEP regimen).

The prognosis for women with early-stage dysgerminoma is excellent. With advanced disease, approximately 10% of tumors will recur, but most are cured with chemotherapy or radiation therapy. The cure rate for women with early-stage disease is excellent.

Endodermal sinus tumors (i.e., yolk sac tumors) of the ovary are rare, aggressive tumors that confer a poor prognosis. These tumors are marked by increased serum levels of maternal α-fetoprotein (AFP), which may be elevated in normal and abnormal pregnancies. Nevertheless, an extremely elevated AFP level in an apparently normal pregnancy may be associated with an endodermal sinus tumor. Because of their aggressive nature, surgery is indicated for the diagnosis of an endodermal sinus tumor, and adjuvant chemotherapy is administered to all women with this diagnosis.

Sex cord–stromal tumors (mainly granulosa cell tumors and Sertoli-Leydig cell tumors) are rare ovarian cancers in reproductive-age women and therefore rare in pregnancy. Independent of pregnancy, these tumors manifest with evidence of hormone excess (i.e., virilization or hyperestrogenism). During pregnancy, they more commonly manifest with hemorrhagic rupture leading to hemoperitoneum. Management includes unilateral oophorectomy and surgical staging. Adjuvant therapy is reserved for patients with advanced or recurrent disease.

For patients with ovarian cancer diagnosed during pregnancy, oncologic outcomes appear to be similar to those for patients who are not pregnant. However, the therapeutic plan must be modified by pregnancy in some circumstances.

Management of Adnexal Masses Occurring during Pregnancy

In the United States, 10% of women undergo surgery for an ovarian mass during their lifetime, and up to 20% of these masses are identified as malignant.[13] The common use of obstetric ultrasound has led to increased discovery of adnexal masses complicating gestation. Masses once found at the time of abdominal delivery, during the postpartum period, or later are now incidentally detected during a first or second trimester ultrasound examination. Approximately 0.2% to 2% of pregnancies are complicated by an adnexal mass, and 1% to 3% of these are malignant.[4,9,14-18] These estimates are uncertain because many masses incidentally discovered may regress, are not reported, or may not require or receive any intervention. Although many ovarian masses diagnosed during pregnancy are benign cysts that undergo spontaneous regression by the second trimester, some of these masses persist through the second trimester and beyond, potentially causing pregnancy-related complications and requiring surgical evaluation and intervention.

Approximately 75% of adnexal masses complicating pregnancy are simple cysts measuring less than 5 cm in diameter, and the remaining one fourth are simple or complex masses that exceed 5 cm in diameter. During pregnancy, 70% of ovarian masses spontaneously resolve by the early second trimester, becoming undetectable by 14 to 15 weeks' gestational age.[9,16] Functional cysts are the most common, and dermoid cysts (i.e., benign cystic teratomas) are the most common neoplasm encountered in pregnancy. Other common benign masses include paraovarian cysts, endometriomas, leiomyomas, and benign neoplasms such as cystadenomas.[8-11]

Adnexal masses larger than 8 cm in diameter are more often complicated by pain, torsion, rupture, or internal hemorrhage than smaller lesions. Preterm labor, preterm premature rupture of membranes, obstruction of labor, and fetal death have rarely been observed.[19-21] Ovarian torsion occurs most commonly in the late first or early second trimester, when the uterus is growing out of the true pelvis and in the puerperium and when the uterus undergoes rapid involution. If clinical signs or symptoms consistent with torsion, rupture, or hemorrhage occur, emergent surgery is indicated independent of gestational age. In the case of an ovarian tumor larger than 8 cm in diameter in a woman who does not undergo surgery, the clinician and patient must be aware of the increased risk of complications and their symptoms.

In the non-emergent setting, the radiographic and ultrasonographic characteristics of the mass commonly have been used to guide management. In masses that appear simple and cystic in nature and are less than 6 cm in diameter, the risk of malignancy is low (<1%); these can be observed without surgery.[9-11,19] Surgical exploration should be performed for masses that persist into the second trimester, are rapidly enlarging, exceed 8 cm in diameter, or appear malignant.[13] Because levels of cancer antigen 125 (CA 125) levels usually are elevated during the beginning of pregnancy and persist throughout pregnancy, serum testing is unreliable for evaluating the risk of an epithelial malignancy. If the source of the mass is not clear, magnetic resonance imaging can be employed to differentiate ovarian from extraovarian masses.

Surgical exploration for an ovarian mass is optimally undertaken at 16 to 20 weeks' gestation, when physiologic cysts have regressed and, if an oophorectomy is required, when the placenta has become hormonally functional and independent of the corpus luteum. If the mass is discovered in the late third trimester, evaluation, management, and surgical exploration may be deferred until or after delivery in some circumstances. If delivery is abdominal, diagnosis and potential staging can be undertaken at the time of cesarean section; if delivery is vaginal, surgery may be postponed, depending on the nature and appearance of the mass.

Cervical Cancer

According to the National Cancer Institute, an estimated 11,070 new cases of cervical cancer are expected to be diagnosed in the United

States in 2008, with an estimated 3870 deaths from the disease.[22] Invasive cervical cancer in pregnancy is uncommon, comprising only approximately 1% of total cervical cancers diagnosed, but pre-invasive cervical neoplasia is common in reproductive-age women, occurring in 5 to 50 cases per 1000 pregnancies.[23-25] The incidence of cervical cancer has declined because of implementation of the Papanicolaou (Pap) smear to screen for cervical dysplasia and cancer. The practicing obstetrician-gynecologist is more likely to encounter an abnormal Pap smear than invasive cervical cancer during pregnancy. Although Pap smears and routine screening are readily available in most developed countries, most women diagnosed with cervical cancer have not had appropriate screening. Pregnancy and prenatal care affords an opportunity to screen and treat many patients who would otherwise not access the health care system.

Cervical Intraepithelial Neoplasia

As many as 5% of pregnancies may be complicated by an abnormal Pap smear result.[25] Cervical cytology and physical examination are the principal forms of cervical cancer screening during pregnancy. Although endocervical curettage should be avoided during pregnancy to prevent direct or indirect injury to the pregnancy, an endocervical brush should be employed to increase the adequacy of the smear. This can increase the incidence of spotting after collection, but it appears to have no effect on the risk for serious adverse outcomes related to the pregnancy.[26] During pregnancy, the goal of evaluation of an abnormal Pap smear result and cervical dysplasia is determination of the extent of neoplasia; the aim is to rule out invasive cancer and allow therapy for pre-invasive disease to be deferred until after delivery.

The Bethesda system is the standard classification system for cervical neoplasia. It is used to guide the management of patients with abnormal cervical cytology. Atypical squamous cells of uncertain significance (ASC-US) should be managed as in the nonpregnant state. Options include repeat cytologic examination at a close interval follow-up visit, immediate colposcopy, or triage with high-risk human papillomavirus (HPV) testing. Patients with an ASC-US Pap results without evidence of HPV infection can be evaluated after delivery. ASC smears in which a high-grade lesion cannot be excluded (ASC-H) usually are managed with colposcopy, although some clinicians use HPV status to triage these smears. Women who are found to have low- or high-grade squamous intraepithelial lesions (LSILs or HSILs) should undergo colposcopy to evaluate the extent and severity of neoplasia.[27]

Pap smears revealing atypical glandular cells (AGCs), although rare in pregnancy, also warrant colposcopic examination. Pregnancy complicates the cytologic interpretation of AGC, because sloughed decidual cells, endocervical gland hyperplasia, and cells demonstrating an Arias-Stella reaction, all of which are benign, can occur in normal pregnancy. Compared with nonpregnant patients, for whom AGC is associated with malignancy in as many as 25% of cases, AGC found in pregnancy is less likely to indicate malignancy. However, the inability to perform an endocervical curettage and endometrial sampling limits the evaluation of AGC during pregnancy.

Colposcopic evaluation in pregnancy is facilitated by the eversion of the transformation zone. The procedure should be performed whenever indicated by the cytology results, regardless of pregnancy. The purpose of colposcopy in pregnancy is to exclude the presence of malignancy. Biopsies should be performed for any suspicious lesions seen at the time of colposcopic evaluation. Biopsies should be done only for the most suspicious areas, and taking many samples at one examination should be avoided.[28] Colposcopic diagnostic accuracy, with or without biopsy, is 95% to 99%, and complications are rare.[29] The most common complication associated with colposcopically directed biopsy is hemorrhage resulting from the increased vascularity of the cervix during pregnancy. Bleeding can be stopped by direct pressure to the site, with application of Monsel's (ferric subsulfate) solution, silver nitrate, vaginal packing, and rarely, suture ligation of vessels. Colposcopy and biopsy do not jeopardize the pregnancy as long as endocervical curettage is avoided. Observation without therapy is appropriate for pregnant women with cervical dysplasia if invasive cervical cancer has been excluded by colposcopy (with or without biopsies).[29-34] This approach is supported by the American College of Obstetricians and Gynecologists (ACOG).[35] Inadequate colposcopic evaluation is indication for further evaluation with a cone biopsy in the nonpregnant patient, but pregnant women with an unsatisfactory initial colposcopic result may undergo repeat colposcopy in 6 to 12 weeks. Because the transformation zone undergoes further eversion as pregnancy progresses, a later examination may be satisfactory.[36] Treatment for cervical dysplasia such as laser therapy, cryotherapy, loop electrosurgical excision procedure (LEEP), and cone biopsy may therefore be deferred until the postpartum period. In women with biopsy-proven dysplasia identified during pregnancy who have no evidence of invasion by colposcopy, management may consist of serial colposcopy examinations with intermittent cervical cytology and expectant management of the pregnancy. Because regression of cervical dysplasia after pregnancy has been reported, withholding definitive treatment of this disease (in the absence of invasive cervical cancer) is appropriate. At 6 months after delivery, almost 70% of cervical intraepithelial neoplasia (CIN) II and III lesions resolved,[33] which is higher than the rate for the nonpregnant population.[33,37] For this reason, delay of definitive therapy until after delivery is appropriate in a patient without evidence of invasive cervical cancer; however, the maximum interval from delivery until postpartum evaluation and management of cervical dysplasia has not been determined. Cervical cytology, colposcopy, directed biopsies, and endocervical curettage usually are performed around the 6-week postpartum evaluation.

In the pregnant state, LEEP and cone biopsies should be reserved for the exclusion of invasive disease. Risks of these procedures in pregnancy include cramping, bleeding, infection, premature preterm rupture of membranes, spontaneous abortion, preterm labor, and pregnancy loss. Complication rates are similar for LEEP and cone biopsy.[38] If a LEEP or cone biopsy is indicated to rule out malignancy, the safest time to perform them seems to be in the middle of the second trimester, between 14 and 20 weeks, or after fetal maturity is documented. In an effort to minimize preterm delivery after cone biopsy, some physicians have advocated concurrent MacDonald cerclage at the time of cone biopsy. Although there were no complications in the largest study of this strategy, only 17 patients were evaluated.[39]

For patients with cervical dysplasia diagnosed during pregnancy without any clinical evidence of invasive cervical cancer, the route of delivery is not affected by the dysplasia. However, some physicians have documented an increased rate of spontaneous remission of cervical cancer after vaginal delivery compared with cesarean delivery[40]; others have not found this to be the case.[41]

Cervical Carcinoma

The occurrence of cervical carcinoma in pregnancy is rare, comprising only 1% of all cervical cancers diagnosed annually. However, because cervical cytology and examination are typically performed at the first prenatal visit, cervical cancer is one of the most common cancers diagnosed during pregnancy. Manifestation of cervical cancer during pregnancy is similar to that outside pregnancy, and most women present without symptoms. When detected in pregnancy, cervical cancer is usually stage I disease due to increased surveillance. The most common symptom of cervical cancer in pregnancy is bleeding, especially after coitus. It is imperative for clinicians caring for pregnant women to recognize that vaginal bleeding is not necessarily related to the pregnancy and can be caused by other illnesses.

Pregnancy was once believed to alter the course of cervical cancer compared with nonpregnant cohorts, but there is no difference in survival or disease characteristics when matched cohorts are studied.[37,42,43] However, when compared with nonpregnant counterparts, pregnant women with cervical cancer are much more likely to have stage I disease, and most have stage IB disease.[42,44-47] Because of the physiologic and anatomic changes of pregnancy, induration or nodularity at the inferior cardinal ligament is less prominent, leading to underestimation of the stage and degree of tumor involvement. Nonetheless, pregnancy does not affect the survival rate for cervical cancer. The overall survival rate is 80% compared with 82% in nonpregnant patients.[48]

According to the International Federation of Gynecology and Obstetrics (FIGO), clinical staging of cervical cancer can include intravenous pyelography, chest radiography, cystoscopy, and sigmoidoscopy. Although not included in the FIGO staging system, intravenous contrast–enhanced computed tomography (CT) has often been used for staging and treatment planning. The use and timing of these staging studies during pregnancy must be considered carefully because of the ionizing radiation used with CT and fluoroscopy (for barium enema and cystoscopy; see Table 43-2). Chest radiography is acceptable during pregnancy with appropriate abdominal and pelvic shielding. In some case reports, magnetic resonance imaging (MRI), which has been shown to be safe during pregnancy, has been used to define the extent of extracervical tumor spread.[49,50]

After a stage has been established, management must be individualized. A multidisciplinary team, which may include a perinatologist, neonatologist, radiation oncologist, and gynecologic oncologist, must be recruited to counsel the patient regarding treatment options related to the stage, fetal status, and gestational age and to determine her desire to continue her pregnancy. In certain circumstances, treatment of the cancer is recommended despite the potential lethality of the therapy on the pregnancy. In others, treatment can be delayed until after delivery or until a gestational age when delivery will not produce significant morbidity.

In pregnant women with a cervical biopsy suggesting microinvasive cervical cancer, a cervical cone biopsy must be performed to definitively establish the diagnosis. Women with stage IA1 cervical cancer (<3 mm of invasion, <7 mm of tumor breadth) can be followed with periodic colposcopy and cytology, and the infant can be delivered when obstetrically indicated. Definitive management is deferred to the intrapartum (with cesarean hysterectomy) or postpartum period. Surgical treatment for stage IA1 cervical cancer may include cervical conization (with negative margins) or extrafascial hysterectomy, depending on the desire for future fertility. Cone biopsy during pregnancy carries additional risks over that performed outside of pregnancy. The timing of cone biopsy during pregnancy is controversial, with some physicians reporting fetal loss rates approximating 25% when conization is performed during the first trimester,[51] whereas others have described the relative safety of early conization.[52] Most agree, however, that the rates of fetal loss are less than 10% in the second trimester and nonexistent in the third trimester. Blood loss associated with cone biopsy increases with increasing gestational age. For that reason, care must be taken in determining when a cone biopsy should be performed during pregnancy. Limited data exist regarding the role of the LEEP during pregnancy.[38,53] The initial investigation of this technique was associated with maternal and fetal morbidity, blood transfusion, inadequate specimens, and residual disease in the conization specimen.[38] Further investigation of the relative safety and efficacy of LEEP compared with knife conization in pregnancy is required. When "microinvasive" cervical cancer is suggested by a cervical biopsy or invasive disease is suspected at colposcopy but not confirmed on biopsy, cervical conization is necessary, regardless of the duration of pregnancy. The procedure is optimally performed in the operating room, with a knife, after the period of organogenesis has passed and after appropriate counseling about the risks of fetal loss and transfusion. After conization with negative margins in a woman with confirmed pre-invasive disease or microinvasive carcinoma, follow-up colposcopy and possibly cytology can be used to monitor disease progression during pregnancy, with no alteration in the intrapartum management. In women who have completed childbearing, cesarean hysterectomy or postpartum hysterectomy can be considered. Although controversial, patients with cervical adenocarcinoma in situ or stage IA1 cervical adenocarcinoma with negative cone biopsy margins probably can be managed conservatively during their pregnancy, because most studies demonstrate a low risk of parametrial and lymphatic metastasis with early invasive cervical adenocarcinoma.[54-56] However, there is a paucity of data regarding this disease during pregnancy.[57] Women with positive margins for dysplasia after conization during pregnancy must be counseled regarding the risk of current invasive disease, with management based on the risk and benefits of observation, repeat conization, or definitive therapy for possible invasive cervical cancer during pregnancy.

In women with stage IA2 or IB cervical cancer, identical oncologic outcomes have been reported with radiation therapy or radical hysterectomy and lymphadenectomy in addition to adjuvant radiation therapy (possibly with concurrent radiosensitizing chemotherapy). The advantage of primary surgical management includes the ability to preserve ovarian function and to avoid the potential negative impact on sexual function imparted by radiation therapy. The diagnosis of a stage IA2 or IB cervical cancer during pregnancy does not change the potential therapies recommended. The initiation of treatment is the critical issue in the management of early cervical cancer during pregnancy, specifically related to the potential risk of delay of definitive therapy on cancer outcomes to minimize fetal morbidity and mortality. Case reports and small case series suggest that a moderate delay in definitive therapy is associated with oncologic outcomes similar to those treated promptly. Sood and colleagues[58] described 11 women whose definitive treatment for stage IA and IB cervical cancers was delayed by an average of 16 weeks (range, 3 to 32 weeks). All 11 women remained without evidence of disease and without apparent negative outcomes related to the delay in definitive therapy during pregnancy. These and other reports of small series with a variety of treatment strategies suggest that a moderate delay of definitive therapy does not incur excessive risk. For this reason, women who are diagnosed with early cervical cancer at or beyond 20 weeks of their pregnancy are commonly offered the option of delaying therapy until delivery later in pregnancy or after birth. Women diagnosed with an early cervical cancer before 20 weeks should be informed of the risk of adverse oncologic outcomes related to delay of definitive therapy for their cervical cancer. However, the degree of risk is uncertain given the small number of patients for whom this management strategy has been reported. Thorough documentation of the risks of a decision to delay definitive treatment is imperative.

Immediate treatment options include radiation therapy or radical hysterectomy and lymphadenectomy for stage IA2 or IB disease. Irradiation usually leads to spontaneous abortion at a dose of 4000 cGy; evacuation of the uterus before therapy or in the absence of miscarriage from radiation therapy can be considered. For women who choose to delay therapy for fetal development, coordination of care with the perinatologist, neonatologist, and gynecologic oncologist is critical to determine the appropriate gestational age for delivery that balances the maternal oncologic risks with the fetal risks of prematurity. Delivery, depending on the clinical extent of the cancer, followed by pelvic irradiation in 2 to 3 weeks is one option. Alternatively, cesarean delivery followed immediately by radical hysterectomy and lymphadenectomy is often recommended for reproductive-age women with early cervical cancer to preserve ovarian and vaginal function compared with radiation therapy. At surgery, it may be appropriate to move the ovaries out of the potential radiation field (i.e., oophoropexy) in women who may need postoperative adjuvant teletherapy.

For women with advanced cervical cancer who present in the second half of pregnancy, delay of therapy for fetal maturity carries a small but unquantifiable risk of adverse cancer outcome. Cesarean delivery (to avoid delivery through a cervical tumor[59]) followed by radiation therapy with concurrent chemotherapy usually is recommended. In the first trimester and early second trimester, delay of therapy may increase the risk of a poor oncologic outcome, and it is therefore recommended to begin treatment at the time of diagnosis with ultimate sacrifice of the pregnancy as an unavoidable outcome. Evacuation of the uterus can be performed before irradiation or after radiation therapy if spontaneous miscarriage does not ensue. The anatomic distortion that occurs in pregnancy must be considered when planning radiotherapy to ensure the appropriate treatment fields. Patients who refuse immediate therapy for advanced cervical cancer during the first half of a pregnancy must be counseled regarding the potential impact on tumor growth and spread and the worsened prognosis. In selected patients, neoadjuvant chemotherapy (to decrease the risk of cancer progression during pregnancy) can be considered with definitive chemoradiotherapy initiated after delivery. However, there are limited data to support this management strategy.[60-62]

For women who delay definitive therapy for their cervical cancer until the postpartum period, the mode of delivery remains controversial. For early-stage disease, there is no consensus on whether vaginal delivery affects survival and prognosis. However, delivery through a bulky and friable cervical cancer leads to the potential risk of hemorrhage. Cervical cancer may recur at the episiotomy site, typically within 6 months of delivery.[63,64] For these reasons, vaginal delivery should be reserved for appropriately counseled and carefully selected women with intraepithelial lesions and early-stage cancers. Women with cervical cancer who have delivered vaginally with episiotomy who later develop a lesion in the episiotomy should undergo biopsy to rule out recurrence at this site. For women with early cervical cancer whose primary therapy will be surgical, abdominal delivery with concurrent hysterectomy (i.e., extrafascial hysterectomy or radical hysterectomy and lymphadenectomy, depending on the tumor stage) is recommended.

In selected women with early cervical cancer, radical excision of the cervix (i.e., radical trachelectomy) and lymphadenectomy can be considered for definitive treatment of stage I cervical cancer with the potential to maintain future fertility. This procedure is usually performed independent of pregnancy, but it has been reported during pregnancy.[65] After radical trachelectomy, oncologic outcomes appear favorable in women with small squamous lesions without lymphovascular invasion. Although most women who attempt pregnancy after radical trachelectomy are able to conceive, pregnancy rates are decreased because of cervical dysfunction. The risk of preterm delivery is increased after radical trachelectomy, although most women deliver at term. Overall, approximately 2% develop recurrence, and 56% deliver a viable pregnancy (28% are term, and 28% are preterm).[66-71]

Treatment of Cancer during Pregnancy

Radiation Therapy

Radiation during pregnancy may be used for diagnosis or therapy. Diagnostic radiation for cancer during pregnancy, in the form of x-rays, is used in chest radiography, CT for evaluation or staging of a cancer, and fluoroscopic techniques such as intravenous pyelography (IVP), retrograde pyelography, and barium enema. Radiographic imaging is often necessary for cancer during pregnancy. The known risks of diagnostic radiation have to be balanced with the expected benefits of such imaging. Units of radiation are expressed as rad, gray (Gy), milligray (mGy), or centigray (cGy). These interchangeable terms are units of absorbed dose and reflect the amount of energy deposited into a mass of tissue. One gray equals 100 rad. As it relates to pregnancy, the absorbed dose is the dose received by the entire fetus. Diagnostic radiation doses are less than 1 mGy (<0.1 cGy), and therapeutic radiation for cervical cancer delivers more than 4000 cGy to the fetus.

Because there is no dose of diagnostic radiation that is completely safe for the fetus, radiography should be avoided if possible during fetal development and minimized at all times during pregnancy. However, fetal tolerance to the level of radiation encountered in diagnostic procedures is greater than generally understood. Rarely does diagnostic radiography exceed the threshold of fetal tolerance during a pregnancy (Table 43-2). At the time of conception, exposure of 10 cGy usually results in embryologic death. If the embryo survives, radiation-induced noncancer health effects are unlikely. At all stages of gestation, radiation-induced noncancer health effects are not detectable for fetal doses below 5 cGy. From 16 weeks' gestation to birth, radiation-induced

TABLE 43-2 APPROXIMATE FETAL DOSES FROM COMMON DIAGNOSTIC RADIOGRAPHIC PROCEDURES

Examination	Mean Dose (cGy)
Conventional x-ray examinations	
Abdomen (KUB)	0.24
Chest	0.001
Intravenous urogram (IVP)	0.73
Lumbar spine	0.34
Pelvis	0.17
Hip	0.13
Skull	<0.001
Thoracic spine	<0.001
Dental films	<0.001
Fluoroscopic examinations	
Barium meal (upper gastrointestinal)	3.9
Voiding cystourethrogram	4.6
Cardiac catheterization	0.1
Computed tomography	
Abdomen with contrast	2
Abdomen without contrast	1
Pelvis with contrast	2
Pelvis without contrast	1
Chest	<0.01
Head	<0.01

noncancer health effects are unlikely below 50 cGy. The risk of childhood cancer from prenatal radiation exposure is related to the amount of prenatal radiation exposure above the usual background. At a dose up to 5 cGy, the incidence of childhood cancer is 0.3% to 1%; at a dose of 5 to 50 cGy, the incidence is 1% to 6%; and at a dose higher than 50 cGy, the incidence is more than 6%.[72] At a dose of 5 to 50 cGy between 8 and 15 weeks after conception, growth retardation and mental retardation can occur, with severe mental retardation occurring in up to 20% of cases. At this dose, there are no noncancer health effects expected with exposure at 16 weeks to term. At doses higher than 50 cGy, these noncancer health effects are expected to be more severe and more common than with lower doses, and the health effects can occur even with exposure from 16 to 25 weeks. After 25 weeks, prenatal radiation exposure with doses higher than 50 cGy leads to fetal death in a dose-dependent manner.[73,74] Given the rarity of diagnostic radiation dosages beyond the thresholds of fetal exposure, therapeutic abortion is rarely recommended for this reason alone. When many radiographic studies are required, the fetal radiation dose should be monitored. Increased use of MRI and ultrasonography, imaging modalities that do not employ ionizing radiation, may avoid concerns related to the fetal risks of imaging studies.

Therapeutic radiation for cervical cancer during pregnancy is lethal to a fetus. Radiation exposure while the fetus is in the uterus leads to fetal death, usually followed by spontaneous abortion. Pelvic radiotherapy for cervical cancer leads to sterility as a result of the direct cytotoxic effect on the endometrium and ovarian injury by standard pelvic doses for treating this cancer (usually more than 4500 cGy). The threshold values for permanent and temporary sterility have not been clearly defined, but the risk of sterility is related to ovarian reserve (i.e., age at exposure) and dose. In women 40 years of age or older, 600 cGy can induce menopause. Adolescent girls treated with 2000 cGy fractionated over 5 to 6 weeks have a 95% likelihood of permanent sterility. With conventional therapeutic doses of radiation for cervical cancer, any field that includes the ovaries will cause sterility. Although the uterine effects cannot be avoided, transposing the ovaries out of the pelvic radiation field can preserve function in many women undergoing pelvic radiotherapy for cervical cancer.

Chemotherapy

The teratogenic effect of chemotherapy is inarguable. The effects of chemotherapeutic medications vary according to their mechanism of action and the gestational age of the fetus during their administration. Although there are few data regarding the use of cytotoxic chemotherapy during pregnancy for the treatment of gynecologic cancers, there is considerable literature about the use of these agents for treatment of pregnant women with lymphomas and leukemias. These data indicate that fetal exposure to chemotherapeutic agents within 2 weeks after conception leads to spontaneous abortion or no effect, with subsequent normal development. Chemotherapeutic agents kill rapidly dividing cells nonselectively in carcinomas and the embryo or fetus.[11,75] The most susceptible period is the first trimester, when organogenesis occurs.[76] During organogenesis, exposure to most cytotoxic chemotherapeutics carries a high incidence of congenital malformations.[77] Numerous uncontrolled, observational reports describe good fetal and maternal outcomes with administration of chemotherapy during the second and third trimesters[78-82] but increased intrauterine growth restriction, low birth weight, spontaneous abortion, and preterm labor are also reported.[77,80,83]

Chemotherapy around the time of delivery may cause concerns because of the risks of maternal myelosuppression with resultant neutropenia and thrombocytopenia. Furthermore, there may not be sufficient time for excretion of chemotherapy agents and their active metabolites from the fetus in time for delivery. The infant, after separation from the excretional function of the placenta and without mature hepatorenal excretion mechanisms, may experience adverse effects after birth. Other factors, such as maternal nutritional status, can alter protein-binding and serum free-drug concentration, and the expanded plasma volume experienced during pregnancy also affects the pharmacokinetics of a chemotherapeutic agent. To minimize the maternal and fetal risks associated with chemotherapy in proximity to delivery, a careful delivery plan with input from the obstetrician, perinatologist, neonatologist, and oncologists involved must be made.

If chemotherapy for a gynecologic cancer is required during pregnancy, ovarian function is usually preserved, and future fertility should not be jeopardized. Long-term follow-up of children who were exposed to anti-neoplastic agents in utero found that exposed offspring usually have normal birth weights, educational performance, and reproductive capacity.[84-87]

Surgical Principles

Pregnant women are not immune to processes that require surgical intervention. Because of their relative youth and general good health, pregnant women tolerate surgical procedures well, and obstetric outcomes are usually good after uncomplicated surgical procedures. Among 5405 women undergoing non-obstetric surgical procedures, most were performed in the second trimester.[88] The rates of stillbirth and congenital anomalies were not different from those for pregnancies not associated with surgery, but low birth weight and preterm delivery were more common. An increased risk of preterm delivery has been reported after surgery in the first trimester, and it was increased with longer procedure times.[89] If surgery is required during pregnancy, it should be performed when possible during the second trimester and under controlled circumstances. Urgent procedures performed in pregnancy should be carried out in an efficient, effective manner. In particular, abdominal surgery during pregnancy carries increased fetal risk compared with extra-abdominal surgery.

Laparoscopic surgery is feasible and relatively safe during pregnancy.[90-94] Laparoscopic procedures are associated with less pain in the postoperative period, reduced use of analgesics and tocolytics, and overall shorter length of bed rest and hospitalization compared with laparotomy. The most common indications for laparoscopic surgery during pregnancy are cholecystectomy, evaluation of an adnexal mass, and appendectomy.[95] Surgical risks inherent to minimally invasive surgery do not appear to be increased in pregnancy, and laparoscopic techniques in pregnant patients should not differ greatly from that of open procedures. As with open procedures, fetal heart tones should be obtained before and after the procedure. Continuous intraoperative fetal heart rate monitoring, if technically feasible, may be helpful to ensure satisfactory uterine blood flow in procedures when maternal blood loss is anticipated. A sustained fall in fetal heart rate may indicate decreased uterine perfusion that can be restored by repositioning the patient to relieve aortocaval compression or by expanding the intravascular volume. Nasogastric or orogastric decompression can be used to minimize insertion of ports into the stomach, and the patient should be placed in a leftward tilt to minimize aortocaval compression. The pneumoperitoneum should be established through an open technique to minimize the risk of uterine perforation or laceration. Although rare, insertion of the Veress needle to establish the pneumoperitoneum into the uterus has led to fetal loss through the development of a pneumoamnion.[96] Ancillary ports should be placed carefully. Because of an intra-abdominal space that is progressively compromised, laparoscopy usually should be avoided after the late second trimester; however, this situation should be evaluated on a case-by-case basis. One possible risk of laparoscopy is that the developing fetus may be exposed to acidosis caused by maternal absorption of the carbon dioxide gas with subsequent hypercarbia and serum conversion to carbonic acid. Studies of fetal sheep in response to insufflation have demonstrated that these animals have adequate compensatory response and placental reserve to tolerate insufflation, although one pregnant ewe died during establishment of the pneumoperitoneum.[97,98] There have been no human reports of fetal loss attributable to acidosis caused by pneumoperitoneum, and this risk may be theoretical. With any surgical approach during pregnancy (open or minimally invasive), the gravid uterus should be manipulated as little as possible to minimize the risk of spontaneous preterm labor, ruptured membranes, or other complications. Prophylactic tocolytics at the time of surgery in the second trimester do not decrease the risk of preterm labor or preterm delivery in these patients, but it may be beneficial in the third trimester.[89]

Gestational Trophoblastic Neoplasia

Gestational trophoblastic neoplasia (GTN) is a spectrum of pregnancy-related conditions that have the potential for local invasion, distant metastasis, and death from disease. These conditions arise from abnormal fertilization and manifest as a missed abortion, as a miscarriage, or are concurrent with or follow a normal gestation. During the past 50 years, significant strides have been made in the diagnosis and treatment of GTN, and it is the most successfully treated gynecologic cancer and one of the most curable solid tumors in women. The full discussion of the diagnosis and treatment of GTN is beyond the scope of this text but can be found in texts of gynecologic oncology.

GTN is described here as it relates to ongoing pregnancies. As a pregnancy-related cancer, GTN can be diagnosed and followed with serum levels of β-human chorionic gonadotropin (β-hCG). Using transvaginal ultrasonography, an intrauterine pregnancy can be diagnosed when the β-hCG level is 1500 to 2000 IU/mL (for singleton gestations). The threshold for transabdominal ultrasonography is higher—approximately 6500 IU/mL. When an abnormal pregnancy is diagnosed, GTN must be considered. The histologic spectrum of GTN includes partial and complete molar pregnancies, gestational choriocarcinoma, and placental-site trophoblastic tumors. Molar pregnancy occurs in 1 of every 1000 pregnancies in the United States, and it is more common in women at the extremes of age for reproduction. Women most often present with amenorrhea, followed by vaginal bleeding in the first trimester. With the increasing use of transvaginal ultrasound in early pregnancy, it is rare for molar pregnancies to manifest later in the course of the disease, when hyperthyroidism, severe hyperemesis, and hypertension may occur. Often, patients complain of passage of vesicles from the uterus. These vesicles are usually seen on transvaginal ultrasound, and in the absence of a gestational sac or fetal parts, a diagnosis of partial molar pregnancy is usually made. Clinically, the uterus is larger than expected because of the molar pregnancy or the resultant ovarian thecal lutein cysts. Included in the differential diagnosis of a positive serum β-hCG level in the absence of an intrauterine or extrauterine pregnancy must be that of phantom β-hCG syndrome,[99] in which circulating serum factors such as heterophilic antibodies or nonactive forms of β-hCG interact with the β-hCG antibody to create false-positive β-hCG results. These findings may lead to inappropriate initiation of therapy for GTN. This false β-hCG reading can be excluded by running a simultaneous urine sample for β-hCG, because these serum factors are not excreted in the urine. Alternatively, the serum can be serially diluted, with the expectation of a linear decrease in β-hCG levels in the case of a true-positive result. Because not all β-hCG testing platforms are susceptible to this false-positive result, the use of an alternative platform may exclude phantom β-hCG syndrome.[99,100]

Molar pregnancy may coexist with a normal gestation in 1 of 20,000 to 100,000 pregnancies.[101] Coordinated care among the obstetrician, perinatologist, neonatologist, and gynecologic oncologist must ensue. These pregnancies are associated with a higher incidence of complications such as fetal death, vaginal bleeding, pre-eclampsia, and persistent GTN after evacuation. Historically, early pregnancy termination has been recommended to avoid subsequent complications. However, in the largest reported series,[101] 60% of women who chose to continue a normal pregnancy coexistent with a complete molar pregnancy experienced spontaneous abortion or fetal demise before 24 weeks, and 40% delivered a live infant at 24 weeks or later (most after 32 weeks). The rate of persistent GTN requiring chemotherapy was not different in women undergoing early pregnancy termination compared with those who did not terminate and no different from that experienced by patients with a singleton complete molar event in this series.[101]

Pregnancy and Solid Tumors

Breast Cancer in Pregnancy

Gestational or pregnancy-associated breast cancer is defined as breast cancer that is diagnosed during pregnancy, in the first postpartum year, or any time during lactation. Physiologic changes in the breast make the diagnosis of breast cancer during pregnancy a challenge. Nevertheless, any discrete lump felt in the breast should be investigated further by a specialist breast team.

Epidemiology

Breast cancer is one of the most common malignancies encountered in pregnant women. The reported incidence ranges from 1.3[102] to 3.3[2] cases per 10,000 live births. Although only 0.2% to 3.8% of breast cancers diagnosed in women younger than age 50 are pregnancy associated, almost 10% to 20% of breast cancers diagnosed in women in their 30s are discovered during pregnancy.[103,104] This pattern of prevalence is likely to change in the future with an increase in gestational breast cancers as more women delay childbearing.

Clinical Presentation and Diagnosis

The most common clinical presentation of breast cancer in pregnant and nonpregnant women is a painless lump in the breast. Occasionally, refusal by an infant to nurse from a lactating breast may signify an occult carcinoma, and it has been described as the milk rejection sign.[105] The physiologic changes in the breast during pregnancy and lactation result in engorgement and increased nodularity, which makes it a challenge for the patient and clinician to identify these tumors by palpation. Such challenges result in diagnostic delays of 2 months or longer, which in part is responsible for the advanced stage at diagnosis in pregnant or lactating women. In a mathematical model assessing tumor progression over time, a 1-month delay in the treatment of primary tumor increased the risk of axillary metastases by 0.9% to 1.8%.[106] Clinicians therefore should perform a thorough

TABLE 43-3 DIFFERENTIAL DIAGNOSIS OF A BREAST MASS IN A PREGNANT OR LACTATING WOMAN

Breast cancer
Lactating adenoma
Fibrocystic disease
Milk retention cyst
Abscess
Lipoma
Hamartoma
Leukemia or lymphoma
Phyllodes tumors
Sarcoma

breast examination at the initial prenatal visit and without hesitation thereafter.

The differential diagnosis of a breast mass in a pregnant or lactating woman is provided in Table 43-3. Although 80% of breast biopsies obtained from pregnant women are benign, it is important to biopsy any lump that is present for 2 to 4 weeks.[107]

IMAGING

Mammography has a high false-negative rate during pregnancy, with sensitivity rates ranging from 63% to 78% in some studies.[108,109] Mammography during pregnancy is safe because the average glandular dose to the breast for a two-view mammogram (200 to 400 mrad) results in a negligible radiation dose of only 0.4 mrad to the fetus.[110,111] Radiation exposure is expressed as gray (Gy) units (1 Gy = 1000 mGy = 100 rad; 1 rad = 10 mGy). Fetal exposures less than 5 rad (50 mGy) are not thought to cause malformation (see Chapter 20),[62] and mammography still has a place in the evaluation of a breast mass in pregnancy.

Ultrasound is usually the preferred imaging modality to evaluate a breast mass in a pregnant woman. It is inexpensive, safe for the fetus, and can distinguish between solid and cystic lesions in 97% of patients.[112-114] If lymph nodes are palpable, axillary sonography with ultrasound-guided fine-needle aspiration biopsy should be done as part of staging evaluation.

The American Cancer Society recommends screening MRI for women who have an approximately 20% to 25% or greater lifetime risk of breast cancer,[115] but there are no published data regarding the use of MRI to diagnose breast cancer during pregnancy. Although gadolinium-enhanced MRI is more sensitive than mammography for detecting invasive breast cancer, its use in pregnant women is limited by its passage across the placenta and reported association with fetal abnormalities in rats. MRI therefore is not recommended for the diagnosis of breast cancer during pregnancy. For postpartum women at the time of diagnosis, gadolinium-enhanced breast MRI may be considered if necessary.[110,116] MRI may be used for staging evaluation in a pregnant woman as long as contrast is avoided (staging evaluation is discussed later).

BIOPSY

Core-needle biopsy is the preferred method of tissue confirmation in pregnant women with suspected breast cancer.[107] This can be performed under local anesthesia and has no risks unique to pregnancy. Although fine-needle aspiration can be used, the proliferative changes induced by pregnancy may result in an indeterminate score requiring additional evaluation for diagnosis.[117,118] The accuracy of interpretation of fine-needle aspiration biopsy depends on an experienced pathologist who is aware that the woman is pregnant.

One of the known, albeit rare, complications of such biopsies during lactation is the development of milk fistula.[119] Suspending breastfeeding before the biopsy decreases the incidence of milk fistula.

STAGING

Evaluation. The tumor, node, and metastasis (TNM) staging system of the American Joint Committee on Cancer is appropriate for pregnant and nonpregnant women with breast cancer. Women with gestational breast cancer often present with later-stage disease than women who are not pregnant, which is attributable to the delay in diagnosis. A thorough history and physical examination of the breast and axilla are required to determine whether the woman needs a comprehensive staging workup.

Axillary Staging. Clinically palpable lymph nodes should be evaluated by ultrasound-guided fine-needle aspiration biopsy for pathologic confirmation. Sentinel lymph node biopsy has emerged as the standard technique in staging clinically node-negative women with early-stage breast cancer. Sentinel lymph node biopsy has not been fully evaluated in gestational breast cancer. Isosulphan blue dye should not be administered to pregnant women. Some small studies have reported that the use of double-filtered technetium sulfur colloid to map sentinel lymph nodes in pregnancy is safe, but no supporting larger studies have been reported.[110,120,121] Sentinel lymph node biopsy is not recommended in women with gestational breast cancer outside of a clinical trial.[122]

Distant Metastases. The three most common sites of distant metastases in breast cancer are the lung, liver, and bone. As with nonpregnant women, women with gestational breast cancer who are asymptomatic and are clinically node negative do not require further formal staging because the yield in such patients is low. Complete radiologic staging evaluation should be considered in women with symptoms, women with clinically palpable nodes, and women with T3 or T4 lesions. Chest radiographs can be performed safely in pregnancy with abdominal shielding. Chest CT scans should be avoided. If further evaluation of the chest is required, MRI (without gadolinium) of the thorax is preferred. Abdominal ultrasound is the safest method to look for liver metastases in pregnancy, although MRI without contrast can be done if necessary.[110] CT of the abdomen and pelvis is not preferred in pregnant women because fetal radiation exposure approximates 250 mrad. For bony metastasis, low-dose bone scans or MRI without contrast of the thoracic and lumbar spine is recommended.[123] Baker and colleagues[124] reported a "low-dose" bone scan with a fetal exposure of only 0.08 rad, compared with the standard 0.19 rad of conventional bone scan. Maternal hydration and frequent voiding is required to reduce the fetal exposure to radiation resulting from accumulation of radionuclides in the maternal bladder. Plain skeletal radiographs including the spine and pelvis are acceptable and safe options for evaluation of bone with less than 1 rad (0.01 Gy) of exposure to the fetus. The other alternative to identify metastatic bony lesions is noncontrast MRI of thoracic and lumbar spine. MRI is also the most sensitive and safe way to scan the brain for metastatic lesions.

Among the blood tests routinely obtained, alkaline phosphatase is not helpful. The level normally doubles or even quadruples during pregnancy, and it therefore cannot be used as an indicator for metastases.[125]

Pathology of Gestational Breast Cancer

Most breast cancers in pregnancy are poorly differentiated, infiltrating, ductal carcinomas.[126] Women with breast cancer in pregnancy have larger tumors and more frequent nodal involvement, metastasis, and vascular invasion.[104,127,128] Women with gestational breast cancers have a higher incidence of inflammatory breast cancer and are 2.5 times more likely to have distant metastatic disease.[129] Breast cancers that have estrogen or progesterone receptors are less common (25%) during pregnancy compared with the rate of 55% to 60% in nonpregnant premenopausal women.[103,112,126,127] The high levels of circulating estrogen and progesterone in pregnancy may bind all the hormone receptor sites or downregulate them, resulting in negative receptor status in hormone binding assay. One series suggested that the proportion of hormone receptor positive tumors in pregnant women is closer to the nonpregnant state when immunohistochemical methods are used.[130] Amplification of the *HER2* gene or increased expression of its ERBB2 protein (i.e., the oncoprotein fragment p105 is used in assays) is observed in approximately one fourth of breast cancers. Few studies have reported the incidence of this gene amplification in pregnant women with breast cancer, but most have quoted a higher incidence. For example, one series found that 7 (58%) of 12 gestational breast cancers were HER2 positive compared with 16% of age-matched nonpregnant controls.[130] However, the percentage of HER2-positive tumors was similar to that for nonpregnant breast cancer patients in a prospective series of pregnant breast cancer patients.[126]

Treatment

The treatment of breast cancer during pregnancy should closely follow the guidelines recommended for women who are not pregnant. Treatment should be administered with a curative intent with minimal delay. Therapeutic decisions should be individualized, taking into consideration the gestational age, stage of the disease, and the preferences of the patient and her family. Abortion is usually not recommended but may be considered for an individual patient during treatment planning. Care by her obstetrician, perinatologist, and oncology team should be coordinated as described previously for women with leukemia, lymphoma, or solid tumors.

LOCOREGIONAL TREATMENT

Surgery is the definitive treatment for pregnancy-associated breast cancer. Mastectomy with axillary dissection is traditionally considered the best choice for stage I, II, and some stage III breast cancers when the patient chooses to continue the pregnancy.[131,132] Mastectomy eliminates the need for breast radiation therapy in stage I and II disease and therefore minimizes the risk associated with fetal radiation exposure. If breast reconstruction is desired, it should be delayed until after delivery because prolonged surgery may increase fetal complications.

Breast-conservation surgery is a treatment option for women diagnosed in the late second trimester or early third trimester. Lumpectomy with axillary dissection is feasible in pregnancy. In such cases, radiation therapy to the entire ipsilateral breast is delayed until after delivery.[133] In women who present with locally advanced-stage disease, neoadjuvant chemotherapy can be considered before definitive surgery. The feasibility of breast-conservation surgery depends on the clinical response (Fig. 43-1).

Axillary dissection is an essential component of treatment and staging because nodal metastases are commonly found in pregnancy-associated breast cancer. Choice of systemic therapy also depends on comprehensive staging of the nodal involvement. Although sentinel lymph node biopsy is the preferred method of axillary staging in women with clinically node-negative breast cancer, the safety and reliability of this procedure in pregnant women have not been established. Sentinel lymph node biopsy is not recommended for pregnant women with early-stage breast cancer.[122]

Adjuvant radiation therapy improves local control of breast cancer and survival. The risks of teratogenicity and induction of childhood malignancies and hematologic disorders complicate but do not

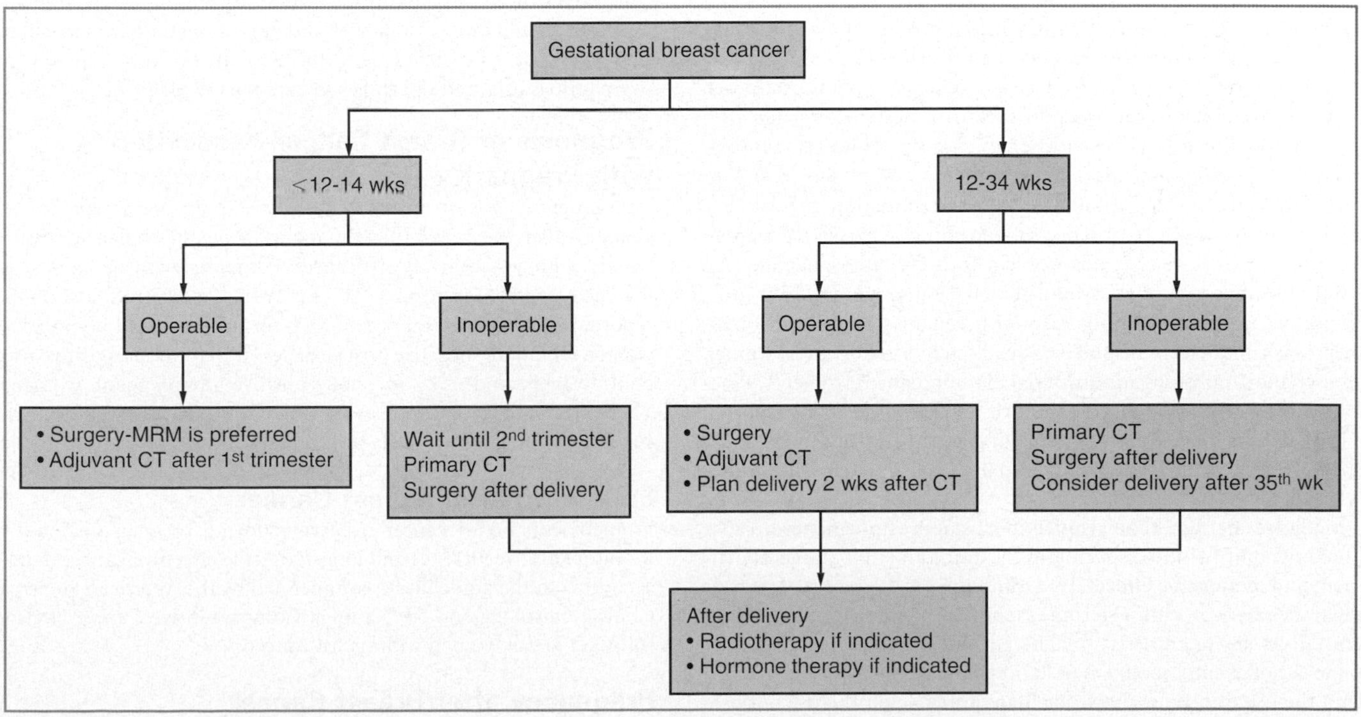

FIGURE 43-1 Algorithms for treatment of breast cancer in pregnancy. Neoadjuvant chemotherapy can be considered before definitive surgery for women who present with locally advanced stage disease. Breast conservation surgery depends on the clinical response to therapy. CT, chemotherapy; MRM, modified radical mastectomy.

preclude the use of radiation therapy in the management of breast cancer in pregnancy.[134] In selected and appropriately counseled women, radiotherapy of breast cancer is possible with fetal doses that fall below the customary threshold for malformations of 5 rad. The excess childhood cancer risk has been estimated as 6.57 cases per 10,000 children per rad per year.[135] For a typical treatment regimen approximating 50 Gy (5000 rad), radiation of the maternal breast or chest wall has been estimated to expose the fetus to as little as 0.1% to 0.3% of the total dose, or 0.05 to 0.15 Gy of the total dose,[121] or as much as 3.9 to 15 rad in the first trimester and 20 rad in late third trimester.[136] Some experts do not recommend radiation therapy during pregnancy,[137,138] but each patient should be counseled based on her own circumstances.

SYSTEMIC THERAPY

Adjuvant chemotherapy is recommended for all premenopausal patients with node-positive breast cancer or with tumors greater than 1 to 2 cm in diameter that are poorly differentiated. Most of the pregnancy-associated breast cancers fit in this category. All chemotherapeutic agents used in breast cancer have been categorized by the U.S. Food and Drug Administration as category D or X, indicating that teratogenic effects have occurred in humans (see Chapter 20). Information regarding the effects of chemotherapy administered during pregnancy is largely compiled from case reports and small case series. Dosing of chemotherapy during pregnancy is complicated by increased plasma volume, increased hepatorenal clearance, decreased serum albumin, and decreased gastric emptying, which increases absorption.[139]

Chemotherapy exposure during the first trimester, the period of organogenesis, carries the greatest risk for spontaneous abortion, fetal death due to chromosomal, and congenital abnormalities. Chemotherapy is usually deferred during this period as long as the health of the mother is not compromised because of the treatment delay.[140-142]

The incidence of congenital malformation is low if chemotherapy is administered to women in second or third trimester.[123,127,128,131,139,143] One review reported a 1.3% risk of fetal malformation for 150 women given chemotherapy in the second or third trimester, compared with a risk of 16% in first-trimester chemotherapy.[144] However, approximately 50% of infants exposed to chemotherapy in the second or third trimester manifest intrauterine growth retardation, prematurity, and low birth weight.[145,146] The most commonly used regimen in gestational breast cancer is doxorubicin with cyclophosphamide (AC regimen) with or without 5-fluorouracil (FAC regimen). The only prospective study of chemotherapy in pregnant women with breast cancer was conducted with the FAC regimen in a cohort of 24 women and used the same doses administered to nonpregnant women.[132] Chemotherapy was not given in the first trimester, and the study reported no birth defects in the infants. The median gestational age in this study was 38 weeks. It is unclear whether in utero exposure to anthracyclines is cardiotoxic to the fetus.

Methotrexate should be avoided in all stages of pregnancy because of the possibility of third spacing in the amniotic fluid and its abortifacient and teratogenic effects.[142,144] Although several case reports have shown the safety of administering taxanes during pregnancy, the long-term effects are unknown.[147,148] The current international guidelines for the use of chemotherapy in gestational breast cancer do not recommend the use of taxanes.[149] No data are available on the use of dose-dense therapy in pregnancy, and it is not recommended. Chemotherapy should be avoided for 3 to 4 weeks before delivery to avoid infectious complications due to transient myelosuppression.

Addition of trastuzumab to adjuvant chemotherapy has made a significant impact on disease-free and overall survival in women with HER2-overexpressing breast cancers. Only four case reports of the use of trastuzumab in pregnancy have been published.[150-154] Reversible oligohydramnios and reversible maternal heart failure were described. No fetal abnormalities have so far been reported.

For women who have hormone receptor–positive breast cancer during pregnancy, therapy with tamoxifen or other selective estrogen receptor modulators is deferred until after delivery. These agents have been associated with vaginal bleeding, spontaneous abortion, birth defects, and fetal death.[155-157] Long-term effects of tamoxifen on female offspring are unknown.

Use of antiemetics such as promethazine, ondansetron, or dexamethasone is considered safe during pregnancy. Granulocyte colony-stimulating growth factor and erythropoietin have been safely used in pregnant patients, and their use should follow the general guidelines.

Monitoring of Pregnancy and Timing of Delivery

Pregnant women with breast cancer should be monitored closely by their obstetrician and oncologist. Gestational age should be accurately determined to plan the timing of chemotherapy and delivery. If possible, delivery should be planned 3 to 4 weeks after chemotherapy, allowing time for the recovery of cell counts. The timing of delivery is related to the maternal condition, need for further therapy, and expected neonatal and infant outcomes. As a general rule, women receiving chemotherapy should be cautioned against breastfeeding while receiving chemotherapy.

Termination of Pregnancy

Early termination of pregnancy does not improve the outcome of breast cancer in pregnancy.[158] Some series suggest inferior outcomes in pregnant women with breast cancer who undergo elective termination compared with those who continue with the pregnancy.[159] Termination decisions should be individualized and depend on the patient's willingness to accept a possible risk to the fetus from cancer therapy, her overall prognosis, and the ability to care for the offspring.

Prognosis of Breast Cancer Associated with Pregnancy

The prognosis of breast cancer occurring during pregnancy has changed over the years. Current reports suggest similar survival of women with gestational breast cancers compared with age- and stage-matched control groups.[128,158,160] In 1994, Petrek and associates[161] reported a 5-year survival rate of 82% for pregnant and nonpregnant women with node-negative breast cancer, 47% for node-positive pregnant women, and 59% for node-positive nonpregnant women.[161] There are, however, other case-control studies that showed decreased survival for pregnant women with breast cancer.[129,162]

Follow-up after Breast Cancer

Women with breast cancer occurring during pregnancy should be monitored for recurrence and long-term side effects of cancer therapy according to the guidelines recommended by the American Society of Clinical Oncology and the National Comprehensive Cancer Network (NCCN) for all women with breast cancer.

Pregnancy after Breast Cancer

The impact of future pregnancy in young women with breast cancer is uncertain. Three large, registry-based studies have concluded that women who become pregnant after successful treatment of breast cancer do not have worse prognosis with regard to their cancer.[143,163-165] Reports that the outcome of early breast cancer is improved in women with a subsequent pregnancy suggest a possible antitumor effect of pregnancy.[166-168] Most recurrences of breast cancer occur within the first 2 years after initial treatment, and oncologists therefore recommend a delay of 2 to 3 years before contemplating pregnancy.[169]

Malignant Melanoma in Pregnancy

Malignant melanoma occurs in 2.8 of 1000 deliveries[170] and accounts for 8% of all gestational malignant tumors. Concerns regarding the possible relationship between melanoma and pregnancy arose from early reports of poor outcome of melanoma in pregnant women.[171] Melanoma occurring during pregnancy may be more advanced and is more likely located in sites associated with poorer prognosis.[172-174] Head, neck, and truncal lesions occurred in 43% of pregnant patients, compared with 38% of nonpregnant controls, but other reports found no increase in poor prognostic locations in pregnancy.[175] Pregnancy has been associated with increased tumor thickness in some reports.[175-177] There may be a hormonal induction of proliferation of the cancerous melanoma cells in pregnancy, but no specific pregnancy-related hormone has been identified. The effect of pregnancy on tumor site and thickness remains unclear.

Historically, melanoma in pregnancy has been associated with a poorer prognosis, with several controlled studies reporting a decrease in survival rates compared with those for nonpregnant women.[173,174,178,179] However, when matched for site and stage, no significant difference in survival is observed. Trapeznikov and coworkers[179] reported the only study showing a difference in survival rate despite matching by age, tumor site, and stage. At 10 years of follow-up, there was a statistically different survival rate of 26% for the pregnant group and 43% for the nonpregnant group in this study.[179]

Other studies have not observed any significant differences in survival rates in pregnant women, but some report a shorter disease-free survival for pregnant women,[175-177,180,181] perhaps because of the shorter follow-up period in these studies. Three large, case-control studies of the prognosis of melanoma diagnosed during pregnancy did not show any difference in survival.[182-184] O'Meara and colleagues[184] used the records from the California Cancer Registry between 1991 and 1999 and reported no difference in survival between 303 patients with pregnancy-associated melanoma and 1799 age-matched nonpregnant controls.

Surgery is the only effective cure for melanoma. Recommendations should be based on the same prognostic factors established for a nonpregnant patient. In a pregnant woman diagnosed with early-stage melanoma, there is no reason to delay surgery. Chemotherapy does not offer sufficient benefit to the mother to warrant risk to the fetus. In pregnant women presenting with metastatic disease, the decision regarding termination of pregnancy and initiating systemic therapy should be individualized according to the prognosis and the patient's wishes. Although melanoma is not the most common malignancy manifesting in pregnancy, it is the most common cancer to metastasize to the placenta.

Colon Cancer in Pregnancy

Colorectal cancer in pregnancy presents a diagnostic, therapeutic, and ethical challenge. Colorectal cancer in pregnancy is a rare event, with a reported incidence of 0.008% (1 in 13,000) pregnancies.[185] Approximately 300 cases have been reported in the literature. The mean age of diagnosis of colorectal cancer in pregnancy is 31 years (range, 16 to 48 years).[186] The management of colorectal cancer in pregnancy raises several ethical and medicolegal issues because the treatment goals for the mother often conflict with the interests of the fetus. The diagnosis is particularly difficult because the common signs and symptoms of colon cancer are often attributed to the pregnancy. This results in advanced stages of the disease at diagnosis, with a correspondingly poor prognosis. Enhanced awareness among the medical community is needed to diagnose colon cancer earlier in pregnancy and thereby improve outcomes. A team approach involving experts in obstetrics, neonatology, gastrointestinal surgery, and medical oncology is required for optimal management.

Clinical Presentation

Common presenting signs and symptoms of colon cancer include abdominal pain, anemia, nausea, vomiting, constipation, abdominal mass, weight loss, and rectal bleeding. Many of these symptoms occur normally in pregnancy, and others, such as weight loss and an abdominal mass, can be masked by pregnancy.[187] This diagnostic challenge often leads to delayed diagnosis and evaluation and to a poor prognosis for colorectal cancer in pregnancy. A review of 41 cases of colorectal cancer in pregnancy demonstrated that all the patients presented with Duke class B or greater disease.[186]

Predisposing Factors

Colorectal cancer is rare in young patients, and colorectal cancer in pregnancy designates a special group of young women who must have predisposing factors leading to this condition. Predisposing factors for colon cancer include hereditary nonpolyposis colorectal cancer (HNPCC) (i.e., Lynch syndrome), familial adenomatous polyposis, Gardner's syndrome, Peutz-Jeghers syndrome, and long-standing inflammatory bowel disease. However, in their review of 19 pregnant patients with colorectal cancer, Girard and coworkers[185] attributed these predisposing factors to only four patients.

Factors such as steroid hormones, TP53 protein abnormality, and cyclooxygenase-2 (COX-2) enzyme levels have been implicated in colorectal cancer in pregnancy. Between 20% and 54% of colon cancers have estrogen receptors, and some studies have also demonstrated progesterone receptors.[188] The role these hormones play in the progression of colon cancers has been related to the interaction between their receptors and other growth-signaling pathways.[189] However, data to support an etiologic role of hormone receptors in colon cancer and circulating hormones are conflicting.

Diagnosis

Colonoscopy is the procedure of choice to obtain a biopsy and confirm a diagnosis in a nonpregnant patient with suspected colorectal cancer. However, pregnancy is a relative contraindication to colonoscopy. Possible adverse effects of colonoscopy in pregnant women include placental abruption from mechanical pressure to the uterus, fetal exposure to potential teratogenic medications, and fetal injury resulting from maternal hypoxia or hypotension.[190] The patient and her family should be fully informed about all potential risks to the mother and fetus, and informed consent should be obtained. The risks may be minimized with gentle abdominal compression during colonic intubation, use of meperidine instead of benzodiazepines, administering oxygen to the mother, and antenatal fetal monitoring.[191]

Pregnant patients with persistent gastrointestinal symptoms should be evaluated by a specialist gastroenterologist with sigmoidoscopy as an alternate to colonoscopy. Most cases of colorectal carcinomas in pregnancy are rectal carcinomas; 86% of colorectal carcinomas diagnosed in pregnancy were below the peritoneal reflection in one review.[173] The serum level of carcinoembryonic antigen (CEA) is a reliable laboratory test used for the diagnosis, prognosis, and monitoring of the colorectal cancer in pregnancy.[192] Unfortunately, it is not a useful tool for screening because of its low sensitivity and specificity. Abdominal CT used for staging of colon cancer is contraindicated in pregnancy. Alternatives include ultrasound and MRI without contrast to assess the extent of the cancer in the abdomen and pelvis in a pregnant woman. Ultrasound has a sensitivity of 75% for detecting hepatic metastatic lesions.

Treatment

Management of colorectal cancer in pregnancy is influenced by the gestational age, tumor stage, and need for elective or emergent surgery. There are no universally accepted guidelines for treatment. Goals of care are prompt initiation of treatment of the cancer and delivery of the infant as soon as neonatal outcomes are optimized. When colorectal cancer is diagnosed in the first 20 weeks of pregnancy, the recommended treatment is surgical removal of the tumor. Colon cancer is rarely detected before 20 weeks' gestation, which explains the paucity of data on fetal outcome after colonic or rectal resections. Anecdotal reports have described birth of normal infants after such resections. Because of the controversial data regarding the risks of such resections to the pregnancy, termination of pregnancy and resection of the tumor constitute the recommended treatment.[193] Delaying surgery until after delivery may result in significant tumor progression and is not recommended.

When the diagnosis is made after 20 weeks of pregnancy, surgery may be delayed until the fetal prognosis has improved. However, delay can result in progression of the cancer, increasing the mother's risks. The patient should be fully informed about these risks before making a decision to postpone surgery.

Colorectal cancer in pregnancy may be complicated by ovarian metastases, which are reported in 25% in pregnant patients but only 3% to 8% in nonpregnant patients.[194,195] Prophylactic bilateral salpingo-oophorectomy simultaneous with resection is recommended by some, but it is associated with an increased risk for spontaneous abortion. Bilateral wedge biopsies of the ovaries may be performed during surgery for pathologic examination and subsequent removal if the ovaries are involved.[196]

Adjuvant chemotherapy is recommended for stage II or III colorectal cancer. Chemotherapy cannot be administered in the first trimester but can be considered in the second or third trimesters. The most commonly used agent is 5-fluorouracil, but its use in pregnancy has been associated with fetal abnormalities.[197] Irinotecan, oxaliplatin, bevacizumab, and cetuximab are all newer agents used in the management of colorectal cancer, but experience with these agents in pregnancy is not well documented. Adjuvant radiation therapy is indicated in the management of Dukes B and C rectal cancers, but it is contraindicated in pregnancy. Radiation therapy should be employed postoperatively after delivery or elective abortion.

Prognosis

Colorectal cancer in pregnancy is associated with a poor prognosis. There are no reports of 5-year survivors of colorectal cancer diagnosed in pregnancy. Despite the poor prognosis, the stage-for-stage survival of women with colorectal cancer in pregnancy is similar to that of the general population.[186] Delay in diagnosis and advanced-stage disease at presentation most likely explain the overall poor prognosis in pregnancy. Gestational colon cancer also appears to worsen the pregnancy outcomes. Woods and associates[198] reported that 78% of pregnancies in women with colon cancer resulted in live births; deaths were attributed to prematurity and intrauterine demise.

Hematologic Malignancies during Pregnancy

Diagnosis and management of acute and chronic leukemias, non-Hodgkin lymphoma (NHL), and Hodgkin lymphoma (HL) arising within the setting of pregnancy are difficult. Approximately 1 of 1000 to 6000 pregnancies[199] and 1 of 75,000[200] pregnancies are complicated by lymphoma or leukemia, respectively. Because hematologic malignancy during pregnancy is rare and clinical trials in pregnancy are complicated by ethical dilemmas, there are few data to guide decisions about imaging, therapy, maternal toxicities, and gestational and postnatal complications.

Therapeutic options include observation, radiotherapy, chemotherapy, and termination of pregnancy. Several retrospective studies suggest that chemotherapy can often be safely administered during the second and third trimesters of pregnancy, and it should be considered in women with potentially curable and life-threatening leukemias and lymphomas.[199,200] In women with aggressive and curable hematologic malignancies, delay in therapy can prevent remission, contribute to future disease relapse, and hasten maternal death.[200] Chemotherapy during the second and third trimesters should therefore be considered for pregnant women with acute leukemia, HL, and Burkitt and diffuse, large B-cell NHL. When chemotherapy poses a high risk to the fetus (e.g., in the first trimester in women with few clinical manifestations) or when the hematologic malignancy is incurable (e.g., indolent NHL, chronic leukemias), fetal toxicity can be limited by deferring treatment until later stages of the pregnancy or by using palliative chemotherapy or steroids during pregnancy. Regardless of the therapeutic approach, the management of a pregnant patient with a hematologic malignancy requires careful coordination and collaboration among medical oncologists, perinatologists, and neonatologists.

Hodgkin Lymphoma in Pregnancy

Epidemiology, Diagnosis, and Staging

HL is the fourth most common malignancy complicating pregnancy.[201] The relative frequency of HL in pregnancy is a function of the high incidence of HL in persons 15 to 34 years old. HL typically manifests as enlarging lymphadenopathy, favoring the lymph nodes of the neck, mediastinum, and axilla. A contiguous pattern of spread of HL between lymphatic channels of the upper neck, chest, and mediastinum has been described,[202] with lymph node involvement tracking from the neck to the mediastinum and axilla before involvement of intra-abdominal nodes or the spleen. Patients with mediastinal adenopathy often notice increasing shortness of breath or cough, symptoms common in normal pregnancies, which may delay diagnosis in pregnant women. Isolated subdiaphragmatic lymphadenopathy rarely occurs.

Diagnosis of HL requires excisional or core-needle biopsy, because the malignant Reed-Sternberg cells are often missed on fine-needle aspiration. Staging for HL follows the Ann Arbor staging system (Table 43-4) and usually requires CT of the chest, abdomen, and pelvis; bone marrow biopsy; and ^{18}F-fluorodeoxyglucose positron emission tomography (FDG-PET). Bone marrow biopsy can be performed safely during pregnancy, but the fetal risks associated with ionizing radiation preclude the use of abdominal pelvic CT and PET in pregnant women. Typical staging of pregnant patients consists of a CT chest with appropriate abdominal shielding and the use of abdominal

TABLE 43-4 ANN ARBOR STAGING SYSTEM FOR HODGKIN LYMPHOMA AND NON-HODGKIN LYMPHOMA

Stage*	Description
I	Involvement of a single lymph node region or lymphoid structure or involvement of a single extralymphatic site (I_E)
II	Involvement of two or more lymph node regions on the same side of the diaphragm, which may be accompanied by localized, contiguous involvement of an extralymphatic site or organ (II_E)
III	Involvement of lymph node regions on both sides of the diaphragm, which may also be accompanied by involvement of the spleen (III_S) or by localized contiguous involvement of an extralymphatic site or organ (III_E)
IV	Diffuse or disseminated involvement of one or more extralymphatic organs or tissues, with or without lymph node involvement

***The absence or presence of fever (>38 °C), unexplained weight loss (>10% of body weight), or night sweats should be indicated by the suffix letters A or B, respectively (e.g., IIA, IIIB).**

MRI to detect intra-abdominal adenopathy. Because multiagent chemotherapy is used to treat early-stage and advanced-stage HL, accurate staging is less critical for the pregnant patient because the chemotherapy treats disease above and below the diaphragm. Few patients receive radiotherapy alone.

PET has been incorporated into response definitions for HL and aggressive NHL.[203] The use of PET improves the sensitivity of traditional staging methods, and its results have prognostic significance during therapy.[204-206] However, because it is contraindicated during pregnancy, PET scan can be delayed until the completion of therapy and after delivery. Although a pretherapy PET scan can facilitate the interpretation of post-therapy PET scans, a PET scan is not required at diagnosis for the management of patients with classic HL because it is routinely avid for FDG.[203] At the conclusion of therapy, a PET scan is essential for persons with HL to confirm a complete remission of a disease for which residual mediastinal masses may represent fibrosis or persistent disease. PET negativity correlates with disease-free survival.[204-206] Although a PET scan cannot be used to stage a pregnant patient, it is performed for all patients after delivery on completion of therapy.

Therapy

Therapeutic options for pregnant patients with HL depend on clinical features, maternal wishes, fetal risks, the gestational age at diagnosis, and potential complications. Pregnancy was associated with poor patient outcomes in HL, late presentation, minimal response to therapy, and short progression-free and overall survival times.[207-209] However, these reports were likely confounded by delayed diagnosis and inferior therapy, because later series incorporating multiagent chemotherapy regimens into the treatment of pregnant patients demonstrated response and survival outcomes comparable to those for nonpregnant patients.[208,210-213]

CHEMOTHERAPY

During the first trimester, in women with painless adenopathy and without respiratory compromise or B symptoms (e.g., fevers, night sweats, weight loss >10% [see Table 43-4]), therapy may be deferred until after the first trimester to minimize the risk of fetal teratogenicity from chemotherapy. In women with symptoms, palliative measures such as corticosteroids or single-agent chemotherapy (i.e., vinblastine) may be necessary to control symptoms until the second trimester. Chemotherapy in the first trimester has been associated with fetal malformations, an increased risk of spontaneous abortion, and stillbirth.[214-218] In particular, antimetabolites (e.g., fluorouracil, gemcitabine, fludarabine, cytarabine) or alkylating agents (e.g., busulfan, chlorambucil, cyclophosphamide, ifosfamide) should be avoided in the first trimester because of their teratogenic effects.[199,218-220] Fortunately, the front-line chemotherapy regimen commonly used to treat HL is doxorubicin (Adriamycin), bleomycin, vinblastine, and dacarbazine (ABVD), consisting of antitumor antibiotics and antimicrotubule agents. In some series, ABVD has been administered during the first trimester without fetal complications.[84,221] However, because data to support the safe use of ABVD in the first trimester are limited and the potential for teratogenesis is significant, ABVD should be offered only during the first trimester after appropriate counseling when the health of the mother is at risk due to rapidly progressive disease. Palliative treatment of symptoms with steroids, single-agent treatment with vinblastine, or delayed therapy until the second trimester are preferable options.

Therapy for HL during the second and third trimester consists primarily of chemotherapy. ABVD appears safe in the second and third trimesters of pregnancy,[84,221] and because HL is potentially curable, the regimen should be offered to all patients unless delivery is expected within 2 to 3 weeks. Prolonged treatment delays may ultimately affect the prognosis of the mother and increase the risk for future relapse. Unlike the first trimester, in which the potential fetal effects of chemotherapy include malformations and demise, multiagent chemotherapy in the second and third trimesters primarily results in lower birth weights, with rare reports of cardiac toxicity related to anthracycline (Adriamycin) therapy and neonatal myelosuppression complicated by respiratory distress or enterocolitis.[218,222] One trial correlated cardiac toxicity with higher doses of the anthracycline, with a dose per cycle of Adriamycin exceeding 70 mg/m^2 associated with a 30-fold increase in fetal events.[218] Fortunately, with the ABVD regimen, the Adriamycin dose per cycle is only 50 mg/m.^{2} In at least one series with long-term follow-up of 3 to 19 years, children born to women who received chemotherapy in their first, second, and third trimesters did not experience neurologic, psychologic, or immunologic effects, and they did not develop secondary malignancies.[221] These reports offer some reassurance that standard doses of ABVD are likely safe in the second and third trimesters of pregnancy.

RADIOTHERAPY

Before the advent of the ABVD chemotherapy, radiotherapy with abdominal shielding was occasionally employed for the treatment of pregnant women with early-stage HL confined to the neck, mediastinum, or axilla. However, radiotherapy as a single modality has fallen out of favor in treating nonpregnant and pregnant patients because chemotherapy alone or combined-modality regimens (e.g., ABVD and involved field radiotherapy) have become the standard of care for early-stage and advanced-stage HL. Combined-modality regimens are more effective than radiation alone in early-stage HL, require limited doses and fields of radiation, and may have fewer late toxicities than previously employed extended fields of radiation.[223] Because most pregnant women cannot be adequately evaluated for intra-abdominal involvement because PET scans and abdominal CT are contraindicated, radiotherapy alone may undertreat patients with undetected stage III or IV disease. Extended fields and higher doses of radiation have been associated with second malignancies, including breast and lung cancers, and with late cardiovascular disease in HL survivors.[224-226] Radiotherapy fields encompassing the mediastinum or axilla ultimately include breast tissue and potentially increase the risk for late secondary breast cancers, particularly in women younger than 30 years old.[224] Radiotherapy alone therefore is only considered for selected patients (pregnant and nonpregnant) with stage I or II HL confined to the neck without B symptoms. In this setting, fetal exposure usually is less than 0.1 Gy (10 rad) with abdominal shielding.[227,228] Mediastinal radiation or mantle field irradiation (neck and mediastinum) typically leads to fetal radiation doses of 0.03 to 0.25 Gy, exceeding the recommended fetal radiation exposure of 0.1 Gy. When this dose is required for therapy, chemotherapy should be employed during pregnancy and, if necessary, radiotherapy delayed until after delivery.[227,228] Despite the fetal and maternal risks associated with radiotherapy, some patients will ultimately require radiotherapy for early-stage disease as part of combined-modality therapy regimens or to treat sites of initially bulky disease, where radiotherapy can minimize the risk of relapse.[229] In these patients, ABVD chemotherapy is offered during the second and third trimesters of pregnancy, with radiotherapy withheld until the postpartum period.

Non-Hodgkin Lymphoma in Pregnancy

Epidemiology, Diagnosis, and Staging

The incidence of NHL during pregnancy is low, although the incidence of NHL in the general population has been steadily rising since the 1980s, increasing the likelihood of diagnosis during pregnancy.[230] Studies of NHL during pregnancy are complicated by the number of subtypes of NHL—at least 30 using the World Health Organization classification system of lymphoid malignancies[231]—including B-cell, T-cell, NK-cell, and plasma cell neoplasms. As a result, the presenting features of the disease depend on the histologic subtype. Aggressive B-cell NHL subtypes (i.e., diffuse, large B-cell; primary mediastinal B-cell; and Burkitt lymphomas)[207,232,233] more commonly occur during pregnancy because these diseases more frequently affect younger patients than indolent or T-cell subtypes. However, indolent NHL, including follicular and marginal zone lymphomas, T-cell lymphoma, and multiple myeloma, have been reported during pregnancy.[234-245]

Diffuse, large B-cell lymphoma is perhaps the most common NHL during pregnancy, followed by Burkitt lymphoma. Diffuse, large B-cell lymphoma comprises 30% to 40% of all NHLs and can occur at any age. Common clinical presentations include lymphadenopathy, a mediastinal mass, involvement of a single extranodal site (e.g., bones, lung, liver), and B symptoms.[199,231] Primary mediastinal large-cell lymphoma is a clinical variant of diffuse, large B-cell lymphoma that has a female predominance, a large anterior mediastinal mass associated with dense fibrosis, and often involvement of other extranodal sites.[231,246] A patient's presenting features often are related to compressive symptoms from the mediastinal mass, including dyspnea on exertion or superior vena cava syndrome.

Burkitt lymphoma is uncommon in adults, representing only 1% to 2% of all NHL subtypes, but it accounts for 30% to 50% of all childhood lymphomas.[218] The median age of adult patients at presentation is 30 years, and as a result, Burkitt lymphoma is the second most common NHL manifesting during pregnancy.[247] Burkitt NHL frequently manifests in extranodal sites, often with intra-abdominal masses arising from the mesenteric lymph nodes, bowel, kidney, liver, spleen, or ovaries. A high incidence of breast, cervical, uterine, and ovarian involvement by Burkitt NHL is reported in pregnant patients.[233,244,248-252] Involvement of these organs is observed in nonpregnant patients with Burkitt lymphoma; however, the increased blood flow to the breast, ovary, cervix, and uterus during pregnancy may also contribute to this presentation.

Similar to HL, the diagnosis of NHL during pregnancy requires core-needle or excisional biopsy because fine-needle aspiration is often insufficient to confirm the subtype of NHL.[253] Routine staging of NHL, as in HL, follows the Ann Arbor staging system (see Table 43-4) and requires CT scans of the chest, abdomen, and pelvis; bone marrow biopsy; and occasionally a PET scan. Bone marrow biopsy, CT of the chest (with abdominal shielding), and MRI of the abdomen are typically employed for the pregnant patient with NHL to minimize fetal radiation exposure. PET, which is routinely performed for patients with aggressive NHL to determine therapeutic response and prognosis,[203-206] can be deferred until the end of therapy and after delivery.

Therapy

Historically, coincident pregnancy at the time of a diagnosis of NHL was associated with poor patient outcomes.[207,208,254-256] This may be attributed to the higher frequency of aggressive NHL subtypes in pregnant patients and to a reluctance to treat pregnant patients with the multiagent chemotherapy regimens necessary for long-term cure. The rarity of NHL and the variety of subtypes of NHL have made accurate assessment of outcomes during pregnancy difficult because of the unique prognosis, clinical outcome, and therapeutic approach for each NHL subtype. In retrospective series, pregnancy did not adversely influence patient outcomes when multiagent chemotherapy was administered during the second and third trimesters.[217,232,257]

TREATMENT OF DIFFUSE, LARGE B-CELL NON-HODGKIN LYMPHOMA

Chemotherapy is the mainstay of therapy for most aggressive NHL subtypes. In nonpregnant patients with diffuse, large B-cell lymphoma, an approach of three to six cycles of rituximab, cyclophosphamide, Adriamycin, vincristine, and prednisone (RCHOP regimen) with additional involved radiotherapy for early-stage or bulky NHL is potentially curative. RCHOP has been safely administered during the second and third trimesters of pregnancy, with limited toxicity to the mother or fetus, with the exception of decreased birth weight and fetal B-cell depletion.[258,259] Rituximab, an anti-CD20 monoclonal antibody, specifically targets malignant and normal B cells bearing CD20. This agent can deplete normal B cells in treated patients for 3 to 6 months; however, this has not been associated with an increased incidence of infections.[260] This same B-cell depletion is observed in infants whose mothers receive rituximab while pregnant, and the effect may persist for up to 4 months after birth with no consequent increase in infections.[259]

Because of the potential teratogenic effects of chemotherapy in the first trimester, combination chemotherapy with RCHOP is usually reserved until later trimesters for pregnant women with diffuse, large B-cell and primary mediastinal large-cell NHL. However, both are potentially curable malignancies, and therapy in the second and third trimesters should be considered after appropriate counseling. Deferring all therapy until after delivery can potentially compromise outcome because these aggressive lymphomas progress quickly, and the likelihood of cure decreases with advanced stages. For women with symptoms during the first trimester, palliative steroids may be administered until later stages of pregnancy, when chemotherapy administration is less risky. Radiotherapy is frequently administered after chemotherapy for women with early-stage or bulky disease, and it can be delayed until after delivery.

TREATMENT OF BURKITT NON-HODGKIN LYMPHOMA

Treatment of Burkitt NHL during pregnancy is quite challenging. This malignancy is curable in up to 84% of young patients, but Burkitt lymphoma has a doubling time of 25 hours and can rapidly progress to involve the bone marrow or central nervous system, making observation until after delivery almost impossible. Alkylating agents, antimetabolites, antimicrotubule agents, and antitumor antibiotics are all incorporated into typical Burkitt lymphoma regimens, which include methotrexate, Adriamycin, cyclophosphamide, vincristine, ifosfamide, cytarabine, etoposide, and intrathecal chemotherapy.[247] Treatment with less aggressive regimens, including RCHOP, may adversely affect patient outcome. Therapy after relapse is frequently ineffective. Patients who relapse or progress during initial treatment require stem cell transplantation. Optimal and immediate treatment at diagnosis with multiagent chemotherapy is critical and potentially curative.

Although some series have reported safely administering these multiagent regimens containing cyclophosphamide, doxorubicin, etoposide, vincristine, methotrexate, ifosfamide, and cytarabine (i.e., CODOX-M/IVAC regimen) during pregnancy,[257] such series are limited. Other physicians have recommended palliating the patient with RCHOP until delivery, at which time aggressive, multiagent regimens can be administered.[258] These approaches may result in increased risk to the fetus or a increased risk of relapse for the mother. All options, including termination of the pregnancy, must be weighed. Potential toxicities and disease outcomes must be discussed with the mother and the obstetric, oncology, and pediatric physicians. Treatment options during pregnancy for women with Burkitt NHL must be determined on an individual basis, but if the pregnancy is allowed to continue, strong consideration should be given to administration of multiagent chemotherapy with a clear understanding of the potential fetal risks associated with this approach, because this malignancy is potentially curable and can progress within days. However, because of the limited data regarding toxicities associated with these multiagent regimens, including profound and prolonged myelosuppression, termination of pregnancy is often recommended.

Leukemia in Pregnancy

Epidemiology and Diagnosis

Acute leukemia complicates about 1 in 75,000 pregnancies.[200,261] Several subtypes of acute leukemia are recognized. They are separated on the basis of their cell of origin (i.e., myeloid and lymphoid) and cytogenetic abnormalities.[231] The most commonly encountered acute leukemias during pregnancy include acute myeloid leukemia (AML), acute promyelocytic leukemia (APL), and acute lymphoid leukemia (ALL). Presenting features include elevated white blood cell counts, neutropenia, anemia, thrombocytopenia, disseminated intravascular coagulation with associated bleeding or thrombosis (in APL) and occasionally lymphadenopathy (in ALL). The diagnosis of acute leukemia during pregnancy requires peripheral blood examination and bone marrow biopsy with flow cytometry and cytogenetic analysis.

Therapy

In a retrospective review of 37 women presenting with acute leukemia during pregnancy, the median age at diagnosis was 30 years (range, 19 to 45 years), and the gestational age at diagnosis was 23 weeks (range, 5 to 37 weeks).[261] Twenty-four percent of patients presented during the first trimester, 27% in the second, and 49% during the third. Four (11%) of these cases were APL, 6 (16%) were ALL, and 27 (73%) were AML. In all cases, chemotherapy was initiated immediately, with therapeutic abortion recommended to the women presenting in the first trimester. Multiagent chemotherapy consisted of anthracycline (i.e., idarubicin or Adriamycin) and cytarabine for AML; anthracycline, cytarabine, and all-*trans*-retinoic acid for APL; and anthracyclines, vincristine, cyclophosphamide, prednisone, and asparaginase for ALL. Ninety-two percent achieved a complete remission, and the 3-year disease-free survival reached 65%, which was similar to the rate for the nonpregnant population. Overall, 11 infants who were exposed to chemotherapy during the second or third trimesters were delivered, and all developed normally, with no growth or developmental abnormalities or infectious complications.

A second large case series described the outcomes of 51 pregnant women diagnosed with acute leukemia between 1968 and 1986.[262] In this series, AML accounted for 51% of cases, ALL for 33%, and APL for 8.5%, with 26% of patients presenting during the first trimester, 32% during the second, and 42% in the third. For the 43 women diagnosed in the second and third trimesters, 1 spontaneous abortion, 1 elective abortion, 2 stillbirths, 1 low-birth-weight infant, 18 premature births, and 20 term deliveries were reported. Only one congenital malformation (i.e., adherence of the iris to the cornea) occurred, and 3 of 39 infants had transient cytopenias. For 15 women treated during the first trimester, three infants had low birth weights, seven infants were premature, one was stillborn, two were delivered at term, and three abortions occurred. One infant had esophageal atresia and anomalous inferior vena cava and eventually developed a neuroblastoma and thyroid carcinoma at age 14.

Fetal risk was highest with chemotherapy exposure in the first trimester; however, combination chemotherapy must be considered for acute leukemia patients who are pregnant because of the likelihood of rapid disease progression and maternal complications without therapy. Potential risks from acute leukemia and its treatment during pregnancy include preterm delivery, low birth weight, disseminated intravascular coagulation, and maternal or fetal bleeding and infection because of thrombocytopenia and neutropenia.

References

1. Wingo PA, Tong T, Bolden S: Cancer statistics, 1995. Cancer J Clin 45:8-30, 1995; erratum 127-128.
2. Antonelli NM, Dotters DJ, Katz VL, Kuller JA: Cancer in pregnancy: A review of the literature. Part I. Obstet Gynecol Surv 51:125-134, 1996.
3. Smith LH, Danielsen B, Allen ME, Cress R: Cancer associated with obstetric delivery: Results of linkage with the California cancer registry. Am J Obstet Gynecol 189:1128-1135, 2003.
4. Creasman WT, Rutledge F, Smith JP: Carcinoma of the ovary associated with pregnancy. Obstet Gynecol 38:111-116, 1971.
5. Zhao XY, Huang HF, Lian LJ, Lang JH: Ovarian cancer in pregnancy: A clinicopathologic analysis of 22 cases and review of the literature. Int J Gynecol Cancer 16:8-15, 2006.
6. Sayedur Rahman M, Al-Sibai MH, Rahman J, et al: Ovarian carcinoma associated with pregnancy. A review of 9 cases. Acta Obstet Gynecol Scand 81:260-264, 2002.
7. Jacob JH, Stringer CA: Diagnosis and management of cancer during pregnancy. Semin Perinatol 14:79-87, 1990.
8. Whitecar MP, Turner S, Higby MK: Adnexal masses in pregnancy: A review of 130 cases undergoing surgical management. Am J Obstet Gynecol 181:19-24, 1999.

9. Leiserowitz GS, Xing G, Cress R, et al: Adnexal masses in pregnancy: How often are they malignant? Gynecol Oncol 101:315-321, 2006.
10. Thornton JG, Wells M: Ovarian cysts in pregnancy: Does ultrasound make traditional management inappropriate? Obstet Gynecol 69:717-721, 1987.
11. Hogston P, Lilford RJ: Ultrasound study of ovarian cysts in pregnancy: Prevalence and significance. BJOG 93:625-628, 1986.
12. Schmeler KM, Mayo-Smith WW, Peipert JF, et al: Adnexal masses in pregnancy: Surgery compared with observation. Obstet Gynecol 105(Pt 1):1098-1103, 2005.
13. American College of Obstetricians and Gynecologists (ACOG): Management of adnexal masses. Practice bulletin. Obstet Gynecol 110:201-214, 2007.
14. Roberts JA: Management of gynecologic tumors during pregnancy. Clin Perinatol 10:369-382, 1983.
15. Ueda M, Ueki M: Ovarian tumors associated with pregnancy. Int J Gynaecol Obstet 55:59-65, 1996.
16. Bernhard LM, Klebba PK, Gray DL, Mutch DG: Predictors of persistence of adnexal masses in pregnancy. Obstet Gynecol 93:585-589, 1999.
17. Hermans RH, Fischer DC, van der Putten HW, et al: Adnexal masses in pregnancy. Onkologie 26:167-172, 2003.
18. Agarwal N, Parul, Kriplani A, et al: Management and outcome of pregnancies complicated with adnexal masses. Arch Gynecol Obstet 267:148-152, 2003.
19. Bromley B, Benacerraf B: Adnexal masses during pregnancy: Accuracy of sonographic diagnosis and outcome. J Ultrasound Med 16:447-454, 1997.
20. Struyk AP, Treffers PE: Ovarian tumors in pregnancy. Acta Obstet Gynecol Scand 63:421-424, 1984.
21. Hess LW, Peaceman A, O'Brien WF, et al: Adnexal mass occurring with intrauterine pregnancy: Report of fifty-four patients requiring laparotomy for definitive management. Am J Obstet Gynecol 158:1029-1034, 1988.
22. Jemal A, Siegel R, Ward E, et al: Cancer statistics, 2008. CA Cancer J Clin 58:71-96, 2008.
23. Jolles CJ: Gynecologic cancer associated with pregnancy. Semin Oncol 16:417-424, 1989.
24. Hacker NF, Berek JS, Lagasse LD, et al: Carcinoma of the cervix associated with pregnancy. Obstet Gynecol 59:735-746, 1982.
25. Campion MJ, Sedlacek TV: Colposcopy in pregnancy. Obstet Gynecol Clin North Am 20:153-163, 1993.
26. Paraiso MF, Brady K, Helmchen R, Roat TW: Evaluation of the endocervical Cytobrush and Cervex-Brush in pregnant women. Obstet Gynecol 84:539-543, 1994.
27. Massad SL, Wright TC, Cox TJ, et al: Managing abnormal cytology results in pregnancy. J Low Genit Tract Dis 9:146-148, 2005.
28. Wright TC Jr, Cox JT, Massad LS, et al: 2001 Consensus guidelines for the management of women with cervical cytological abnormalities. JAMA 287:2120-2129, 2002.
29. Economos K, Perez Veridiano N, Delke I, et al: Abnormal cervical cytology in pregnancy: A 17-year experience. Obstet Gynecol 81:915-918, 1993.
30. Benedet JL, Boyes DA, Nichols TM, Millner A: Colposcopic evaluation of pregnant patients with abnormal cervical smears. BJOG 84:517-521, 1977.
31. DePetrillo AD, Townsend DE, Morrow CP, et al: Colposcopic evaluation of the abnormal Papanicolaou test in pregnancy. Am J Obstet Gynecol 121:441-445, 1975.
32. Woodrow N, Permezel M, Butterfield L, et al: Abnormal cervical cytology in pregnancy: Experience of 811 cases. Aust N Z J Obstet Gynaecol 38:161-165, 1998.
33. Yost NP, Santoso JT, McIntire DD, Iliya FA: Postpartum regression rates of antepartum cervical intraepithelial neoplasia II and III lesions. Obstet Gynecol 93:359-362, 1999.
34. Palle C, Bangsboll S, Andreasson B: Cervical intraepithelial neoplasia in pregnancy. Acta Obstet Gynecol Scand 79:306-310, 2000.
35. American College of Obstetricians and Gynecologists (ACOG): Clinical management guidelines for obstetrician-gynecologists: Cervical cytology screening. Practice bulletin no. 45, August 2003 (replaces committee opinion 152, March 1995). Obstet Gynecol 102:417-427, 2003.
36. American College of Obstetricians and Gynecologists (ACOG): Management of abnormal cervical cytology and histology. Practice bulletin no. 66, September 2005. Obstet Gynecol 106:645-664, 2005.
37. Kiguchi K, Bibbo M, Hasegawa T, et al: Dysplasia during pregnancy: A cytologic follow-up study. J Reprod Med 26:66-72, 1981.
38. Robinson WR, Webb S, Tirpack J, et al: Management of cervical intraepithelial neoplasia during pregnancy with LOOP excision. Gynecol Oncol 64:153-155, 1997.
39. Goldberg GL, Altaras MM, Block B: Cone cerclage in pregnancy. Obstet Gynecol 77:315-317, 1991.
40. Ahdoot D, Van Nostrand KM, Nguyen NJ, et al: The effect of route of delivery on regression of abnormal cervical cytologic findings in the postpartum period. Am J Obstet Gynecol 178:1116-1120, 1998.
41. Kaneshiro BE, Acoba JD, Holzman J, et al: Effect of delivery route on natural history of cervical dysplasia. Am J Obstet Gynecol 192:1452-1454, 2005.
42. Hopkins MP, Morley GW: The prognosis and management of cervical cancer associated with pregnancy. Obstet Gynecol 80:9-13, 1992.
43. Zemlickis D, Lishner M, Degendorfer P, et al: Maternal and fetal outcome after invasive cervical cancer in pregnancy. J Clin Oncol 9:1956-1961, 1991.
44. Monk BJ, Montz FJ: Invasive cervical cancer complicating intrauterine pregnancy: Treatment with radical hysterectomy. Obstet Gynecol 80:199-203, 1992.
45. Duggan B, Muderspach LI, Roman LD, et al: Cervical cancer in pregnancy: Reporting on planned delay in therapy. Obstet Gynecol 82(Pt 1):598-602, 1993.
46. Greer BE, Easterling TR, McLennan DA, et al: Fetal and maternal considerations in the management of stage I-B cervical cancer during pregnancy. Gynecol Oncol 34:61-65, 1989.
47. Senekjian EK, Hubby M, Bell DA, et al: Clear cell adenocarcinoma (CCA) of the vagina and cervix in association with pregnancy. Gynecol Oncol 24:207-219, 1986.
48. van der Vange N, Weverling GJ, Ketting BW, et al: The prognosis of cervical cancer associated with pregnancy: A matched cohort study. Obstet Gynecol 85:1022-1026, 1995.
49. Hannigan EV: Cervical cancer in pregnancy. Clin Obstet Gynecol 33:837-845, 1990.
50. Hricak H, Gatsonis C, Chi DS, et al: Role of imaging in pretreatment evaluation of early invasive cervical cancer: Results of the intergroup study American College of Radiology Imaging Network 6651–Gynecol Oncol Group 183. J Clin Oncol 23:9329-9337, 2005.
51. Averette HE, Nasser N, Yankow SL, Little WA: Cervical conization in pregnancy. Analysis of 180 operations. Am J Obstet Gynecol 106:543-549, 1970.
52. Hannigan EV, Whitehouse HH 3rd, Atkinson WD, Becker SN: Cone biopsy during pregnancy. Obstet Gynecol 60:450-455, 1982.
53. Mitsuhashi A, Sekiya S: Loop electrosurgical excision procedure (LEEP) during first trimester of pregnancy. Int J Gynaecol Obstet 71:237-239, 2000.
54. Kasamatsu T, Okada S, Tsuda H, et al: Early invasive adenocarcinoma of the uterine cervix: Criteria for nonradical surgical treatment. Gynecol Oncol 85:327-332, 2002.
55. Poynor EA, Marshall D, Sonoda Y, et al: Clinicopathologic features of early adenocarcinoma of the cervix initially managed with cervical conization. Gynecol Oncol 103:960-965, 2006.
56. Bull-Phelps SL, Garner EI, Walsh CS, et al: Fertility-sparing surgery in 101 women with adenocarcinoma in situ of the cervix. Gynecol Oncol 107:316-319, 2007.
57. Lacour RA, Garner EI, Molpus KL, et al: Management of cervical adenocarcinoma in situ during pregnancy. Am J Obstet Gynecol 192:1449-1451, 2005.
58. Sood AK, Sorosky JI, Krogman S, et al: Surgical management of cervical cancer complicating pregnancy: A case-control study. Gynecol Oncol 63:294-298, 1996.

59. Baloglu A, Uysal D, Aslan N, Yigit S: Advanced stage of cervical carcinoma undiagnosed during antenatal period in term pregnancy and concomitant metastasis on episiotomy scar during delivery: A case report and review of the literature. Int J Gynecol Cancer 17:1155-1159, 2007.
60. Tewari K, Cappuccini F, Gambino A, et al: Neoadjuvant chemotherapy in the treatment of locally advanced cervical carcinoma in pregnancy: A report of two cases and review of issues specific to the management of cervical carcinoma in pregnancy including planned delay of therapy. Cancer 82:1529-1534, 1998.
61. Caluwaerts S, Van Calsteren K, Mertens L, et al: Neoadjuvant chemotherapy followed by radical hysterectomy for invasive cervical cancer diagnosed during pregnancy: Report of a case and review of the literature. Int J Gynecol Cancer 16:905-908, 2006.
62. Bader AA, Petru E, Winter R: Long-term follow-up after neoadjuvant chemotherapy for high-risk cervical cancer during pregnancy. Gynecol Oncol 105:269-272, 2007.
63. Cliby WA, Dodson MK, Podratz KC: Cervical cancer complicated by pregnancy: Episiotomy site recurrences following vaginal delivery. Obstet Gynecol 84:179-182, 1994
64. Goldman NA, Goldberg GL: Late recurrence of squamous cell cervical cancer in an episiotomy site after vaginal delivery. Obstet Gynecol 101(Pt 2):1127-1129, 2003.
65. Ungar L, Smith JR, Palfalvi L, Del Priore G: Abdominal radical trachelectomy during pregnancy to preserve pregnancy and fertility. Obstet Gynecol 108(Pt 2):811-814, 2006.
66. Burnett AF, Roman LD, O'Meara AT, Morrow CP: Radical vaginal trachelectomy and pelvic lymphadenectomy for preservation of fertility in early cervical carcinoma. Gynecol Oncol 88:419-423, 2003.
67. Roman LD: Pregnancy after radical vaginal trachelectomy: Maybe not such a risky undertaking after all. Gynecol Oncol 98:1-2, 2005.
68. Abu-Rustum NR, Sonoda Y, Black D, et al: Fertility-sparing radical abdominal trachelectomy for cervical carcinoma: Technique and review of the literature. Gynecol Oncol 103:807-813, 2006.
69. Plante M, Renaud MC, Hoskins IA, Roy M: Vaginal radical trachelectomy: A valuable fertility-preserving option in the management of early-stage cervical cancer. A series of 50 pregnancies and review of the literature. Gynecol Oncol 98:3-10, 2005.
70. Schlaerth JB, Spirtos NM, Schlaerth AC: Radical trachelectomy and pelvic lymphadenectomy with uterine preservation in the treatment of cervical cancer. Am J Obstet Gynecol 188:29-34, 2003.
71. Bernardini M, Barrett J, Seaward G, Covens A: Pregnancy outcomes in patients after radical trachelectomy. Am J Obstet Gynecol 189:1378-1382, 2003.
72. Giles D, Hewitt D, Stewart A, Webb J: Malignant disease in childhood and diagnostic irradiation in utero. Lancet 271:447, 1956.
73. Lowe SA: Diagnostic radiography in pregnancy: Risks and reality. Aust N Z J Obstet Gynaecol 44:191-196, 2004.
74. Streffer C, Shore R, Konermann G, et al: Biological effects after prenatal irradiation (embryo and fetus). A report of the International Commission on Radiological Protection. Ann ICRP 33:5-206, 2003.
75. Williams SF, Schilsky RL: Antineoplastic drugs administered during pregnancy. Semin Oncol 27:618-622, 2000.
76. Beeley L: Adverse effects of drugs in the first trimester of pregnancy. Clin Obstet Gynaecol 8:261-274, 1981.
77. Doll DC, Ringenberg QS, Yarbro JW: Management of cancer during pregnancy. Arch Intern Med 148:2058-2064, 1988.
78. Henderson CE, Elia G, Garfinkel D, et al: Platinum chemotherapy during pregnancy for serous cystadenocarcinoma of the ovary. Gynecol Oncol 49:92-94, 1993.
79. King LA, Nevin PC, Williams PP, Carson LF: Treatment of advanced epithelial ovarian carcinoma in pregnancy with cisplatin-based chemotherapy. Gynecol Oncol 41:78-80, 1991.
80. Malfetano JH, Goldkrand JW: Cis-platinum combination chemotherapy during pregnancy for advanced epithelial ovarian carcinoma. Obstet Gynecol 75(Pt 2):545-547, 1990.
81. Sood AK, Shahin MS, Sorosky JI: Paclitaxel and platinum chemotherapy for ovarian carcinoma during pregnancy. Gynecol Oncol 83:599-600, 2001.
82. Mendez LE, Mueller A, Salom E, Gonzalez-Quintero VH: Paclitaxel and carboplatin chemotherapy administered during pregnancy for advanced epithelial ovarian cancer. Obstet Gynecol 102(Pt 2):1200-1202, 2003.
83. Sutcliffe SB: Treatment of neoplastic disease during pregnancy: Maternal and fetal effects. Clin Invest Med 8:333-338, 1985.
84. Aviles A, Neri N: Hematological malignancies and pregnancy: A final report of 84 children who received chemotherapy in utero. Clin Lymphoma 2:173-177, 2001.
85. Partridge AH, Garber JE: Long-term outcomes of children exposed to antineoplastic agents in utero. Semin Oncol 27:712-726, 2000.
86. Zemlickis D, Lishner M, Degendorfer P, et al: Fetal outcome after in utero exposure to cancer chemotherapy. Arch Intern Med 152:573-576, 1992.
87. Garber JE: Long-term follow-up of children exposed in utero to antineoplastic agents. Semin Oncol 16:437-444, 1989.
88. Mazze RI, Kallen B: Reproductive outcome after anesthesia and operation during pregnancy: A registry study of 5405 cases. Am J Obstet Gynecol 161:1178-1185, 1989.
89. Kort B, Katz VL, Watson WJ: The effect of nonobstetric operation during pregnancy. Surg Gynecol Obstet 177:371-376, 1993.
90. Soriano D, Yefet Y, Seidman DS, et al: Laparoscopy versus laparotomy in the management of adnexal masses during pregnancy. Fertil Steril 71:955-960, 1999.
91. Akira S, Yamanaka A, Ishihara T, et al: Gasless laparoscopic ovarian cystectomy during pregnancy: Comparison with laparotomy. Am J Obstet Gynecol 180(Pt 1):554-557, 1999.
92. Al-Fozan H, Tulandi T: Safety and risks of laparoscopy in pregnancy. Curr Opin Obstet Gynecol 14:375-379, 2002.
93. Mathevet P, Nessah K, Dargent D, Mellier G: Laparoscopic management of adnexal masses in pregnancy: A case series. Eur J Obstet Gynecol Reprod Biol 108:217-222, 2003.
94. Stepp KJ, Tulikangas PK, Goldberg JM, et al: Laparoscopy for adnexal masses in the second trimester of pregnancy. J Am Assoc Gynecol Laparosc 10:55-59, 2003.
95. Lachman E, Schienfeld A, Voss E, et al: Pregnancy and laparoscopic surgery. J Am Assoc Gynecol Laparosc 6:347-351, 1999.
96. Friedman JD, Ramsey PS, Ramin KD, Berry C: Pneumoamnion and pregnancy loss after second-trimester laparoscopic surgery. Obstet Gynecol 99:512-513, 2002.
97. Hunter JG, Swanstrom L, Thornburg K: Carbon dioxide pneumoperitoneum induces fetal acidosis in a pregnant ewe model. Surgical endoscopy 9:272-277, 1995; discussion 277-279.
98. Barnard JM, Chaffin D, Droste S, Tierney A, Phernetton T: Fetal response to carbon dioxide pneumoperitoneum in the pregnant ewe. Obstet Gynecol 85(Pt 1):669-674, 1995.
99. American College of Obstetricians and Gynecologists (ACOG): Avoiding inappropriate clinical decisions based on false-positive human chorionic gonadotropin test results. Committee opinion no. 278, November 2002. Obstet Gynecol 100(Pt 1):1057-1059, 2002.
100. Cole LA: Phantom hCG and phantom choriocarcinoma. Gynecol Oncol 71:325-329, 1998.
101. Sebire NJ, Foskett M, Paradinas FJ, et al: Outcome of twin pregnancies with complete hydatidiform mole and healthy co-twin. Lancet 359:2165-2166, 2002.
102. Smith LH, Danielsen B, Allen ME, Cress R: Cancer associated with obstetric delivery: Results of linkage with the California cancer registry. Am J Obstet Gynecol 189:1128-1135, 2003.
103. Wallack MK, Wolf JA Jr, Bedwinek J, et al: Gestational carcinoma of the female breast. Curr Probl Cancer 7:1-58, 1983.
104. Anderson BO, Petrek JA, Byrd DR, et al: Pregnancy influences breast cancer stage at diagnosis in women 30 years of age and younger. Ann Surg Oncol 3:204-211, 1996.
105. Saber A, Dardik H, Ibrahim IM, Wolodiger F: The milk rejection sign: A natural tumor marker. Am Surgeon 62:998-999, 1996.

106. Nettleton J, Long J, Kuban D, et al: Breast cancer during pregnancy: Quantifying the risk of treatment delay. Obstet Gynecol 87:414-418, 1996.
107. Collins JC, Liao S, Wile AG: Surgical management of breast masses in pregnant women. J Reprod Med 40:785-788, 1995.
108. Liberman L, Giess CS, Dershaw DD, et al: Imaging of pregnancy-associated breast cancer. Radiology 191:245-248, 1994.
109. Ahn BY, Kim HH, Moon WK, et al: Pregnancy- and lactation-associated breast cancer: Mammographic and sonographic findings. J Ultrasound Med 22:491-499, 2003.
110. Nicklas AH, Baker ME: Imaging strategies in the pregnant cancer patient. Semin Oncol 27:623-632, 2000.
111. Kopans D: Mammography and radiation risk. In Janower ML, Linton OW (eds): Radiation Risk: A Primer. Reston, Va, American College of Radiology 1996, p 21.
112. Ishida T, Yokoe T, Kasumi F, et al: Clinicopathologic characteristics and prognosis of breast cancer patients associated with pregnancy and lactation: Analysis of case-control study in Japan. Jpn J Cancer Res 83:1143-1149, 1992.
113. Samuels TH, Liu FF, Yaffe M, Haider M: Gestational breast cancer. Can Assoc Radiol J 49:172-180, 1998.
114. Kopans DB, Feig SA, Sickles EA: Malignant breast masses detected only by ultrasound: A retrospective review [comment]. Cancer 77:208-209, 1996.
115. Saslow D, Boetes C, Burke W, et al: American Cancer Society guidelines for breast screening with MRI as an adjunct to mammography. CA Cancer J Clin 57:75-89, 2007.
116. Garel C, Brisse H, Sebag G, et al: Magnetic resonance imaging of the fetus. Pediatr Radiol 28:201-211, 1998.
117. Bottles K, Taylor RN: Diagnosis of breast masses in pregnant and lactating women by aspiration cytology. Obstet Gynecol 66(Suppl):76S-78S, 1985.
118. Gupta RK: Fine needle aspiration cytodiagnosis of primary and metastatic squamous cell carcinoma of the breast. Acta Cytol 41:692-696, 1997.
119. Schackmuth EM, Harlow CL, Norton LW: Milk fistula: A complication after core breast biopsy. AJR Am J Roentgenol 161:961-962, 1993.
120. Morita ET, Chang J, Leong SP: Principles and controversies in lymphoscintigraphy with emphasis on breast cancer. Surg Clin North Am 80:1721-1739, 2000.
121. Mondi MM, Cuenca RE, Ollila DW, et al: Sentinel lymph node biopsy during pregnancy: Initial clinical experience. Ann Surg Oncol 14:218-221, 2007.
122. Lyman GH, Giuliano AE, Somerfield MR, et al: American Society of Clinical Oncology guideline recommendations for sentinel lymph node biopsy in early-stage breast cancer [see comment]. J Clin Oncol 23:7703-7720, 2005.
123. Gwyn K, Theriault R: Breast cancer during pregnancy. Oncology (Williston Park) 15:39-46, 2001; discussion 46, 49-51.
124. Baker J, Ali A, Groch MW, et al: Bone scanning in pregnant patients with breast carcinoma. Clin Nucl Med 12:519-524, 1987.
125. Knox TA: Evaluation of abnormal liver function in pregnancy. Semin Perinatol 22:98-103, 1998.
126. Middleton LP, Amin M, Gwyn K, et al: Breast carcinoma in pregnant women: Assessment of clinicopathologic and immunohistochemical features. Cancer 98:1055-1060, 2003.
127. Reed W, Hannisdal E, Skovlund E, et al: Pregnancy and breast cancer: A population-based study. Virchows Arch 443:44-50, 2003.
128. Ibrahim EM, Ezzat AA, Baloush A, et al: Pregnancy-associated breast cancer: A case-control study in a young population with a high-fertility rate. Med Oncol 17:293-300, 2000.
129. Bonnier P, Romain S, Dilhuydy JM, et al: Influence of pregnancy on the outcome of breast cancer: A case-control study. Societe Francaise de Senologie et de Pathologie Mammaire Study Group. Int J Cancer 72:720-727, 1997.
130. Elledge RM, Ciocca DR, Langone G, McGuire WL: Estrogen receptor, progesterone receptor, and HER-2/neu protein in breast cancers from pregnant patients [see comment]. Cancer 71:2499-2506, 1993.
131. Woo JC, Yu T, Hurd TC: Breast cancer in pregnancy: A literature review. Arch Surg 138:91-98, 2003; discussion 99.
132. Berry DL, Theriault RL, Holmes FA, et al: Management of breast cancer during pregnancy using a standardized protocol. J Clin Oncol 17:855-861, 1999.
133. Kuerer HM, Gwyn K, Ames FC, Theriault RL: Conservative surgery and chemotherapy for breast carcinoma during pregnancy [see comment]. Surgery 131:108-110, 2002.
134. Kal HB, Struikmans H: Radiotherapy during pregnancy: Fact and fiction. Lancet Oncol 6:328-333, 2005.
135. Greskovich JF Jr, Macklis RM: Radiation therapy in pregnancy: Risk calculation and risk minimization. Semin Oncol 27:633-645, 2000.
136. Antypas C, Sandilos P, Kouvaris J, et al: Fetal dose evaluation during breast cancer radiotherapy. Int J Radiat Oncol Biol Phys 40:995-999, 1998.
137. Mayr NA, Wen BC, Saw CB: Radiation therapy during pregnancy. Obstet Gynecol Clin North Am 25:301-321, 1998.
138. Fenig E, Mishaeli M, Kalish Y, Lishner M: Pregnancy and radiation. Cancer Treat Rev 27:1-7, 2001.
139. Cardonick E, Iacobucci A: Use of chemotherapy during human pregnancy [see comment]. Lancet Oncol 5:283-291, 2004.
140. Germann N, Goffinet F, Goldwasser F: Anthracyclines during pregnancy: Embryo-fetal outcome in 160 patients. Ann Oncol 15:146-150, 2004.
141. Murray CL, Reichert JA, Anderson J, Twiggs LB: Multimodal cancer therapy for breast cancer in the first trimester of pregnancy: A case report. JAMA 252:2607-2608, 1984.
142. Ebert U, Loffler H, Kirch W: Cytotoxic therapy and pregnancy. Pharmacol Ther 74:207-220, 1997.
143. Sutton R, Buzdar AU, Hortobagyi GN: Pregnancy and offspring after adjuvant chemotherapy in breast cancer patients. Cancer 65:847-850, 1990.
144. Doll DC, Ringenberg QS, Yarbro JW: Antineoplastic agents and pregnancy. Semin Oncol 16:337-346, 1989.
145. Zemlickis D, Lishner M, Degendorfer P, et al: Maternal and fetal outcome after breast cancer in pregnancy. Am J Obstet Gynecol 166:781-787, 1992.
146. Giacalone PL, Laffargue F, Benos P: Chemotherapy for breast carcinoma during pregnancy: A French national survey. Cancer 86:2266-2272, 1999.
147. Gonzalez-Angulo AM, Walters RS, Carpenter RJ Jr, et al: Paclitaxel chemotherapy in a pregnant patient with bilateral breast cancer. Clin Breast Cancer 5:317-319, 2004.
148. Gadducci A, Cosio S, Fanucchi A, et al: Chemotherapy with epirubicin and paclitaxel for breast cancer during pregnancy: Case report and review of the literature. Anticancer Res 23:5225-5229, 2003.
149. Loibl S, von Minckwitz G, Gwyn K, et al: Breast carcinoma during pregnancy. International recommendations from an expert meeting [see comment]. Cancer 106:237-246, 2006.
150. Bader AA, Schlembach D, Tamussino KF, et al: Anhydramnios associated with administration of trastuzumab and paclitaxel for metastatic breast cancer during pregnancy. Lancet Oncol 8:79-81, 2007.
151. Fanale MA, Uyei AR, Theriault RL, et al: Treatment of metastatic breast cancer with trastuzumab and vinorelbine during pregnancy. Clin Breast Cancer 6:354-356, 2005.
152. Kelly HL, Collichio FA, Dees EC: Concomitant pregnancy and breast cancer: Options for systemic therapy. Breast Dis 23:95-101, 2005.
153. Waterston AM, Graham J: Effect of adjuvant trastuzumab on pregnancy. J Clin Oncol 24:321-322, 2006.
154. Watson WJ: Herceptin (trastuzumab) therapy during pregnancy: Association with reversible anhydramnios. Obstet Gynecol 105:642-643, 2005.
155. Cullins SL, Pridjian G, Sutherland CM: Goldenhar's syndrome associated with tamoxifen given to the mother during gestation. JAMA 271:1905-1906, 1994.
156. Isaacs RJ, Hunter W, Clark K: Tamoxifen as systemic treatment of advanced breast cancer during pregnancy—case report and literature review. Cynecol Oncol 80:405-408, 2001.
157. Tewari K, Bonebrake RG, Asrat T, Shanberg AM: Ambiguous genitalia in infant exposed to tamoxifen in utero. Lancet 350:183, 1997.
158. Nugent P, O'Connell TX: Breast cancer and pregnancy. Arch Surg 120:1221-1224, 1985.

159. Clark RM, Chua T: Breast cancer and pregnancy: The ultimate challenge. Clin Oncol (R Coll Radiol) 1:11-18, 1989.
160. Reed W, Sandstad B, Holm R, Nesland JM: The prognostic impact of hormone receptors and c-erbB-2 in pregnancy-associated breast cancer and their correlation with BRCA1 and cell cycle modulators. Int J Surg Pathol 11:65-74, 2003.
161. Petrek JA, Dukoff R, Rogatko A: Prognosis of pregnancy-associated breast cancer [see comment]. Cancer 67:869-872, 1991.
162. Tretli S, Kvalheim G, Thoresen S, Host H: Survival of breast cancer patients diagnosed during pregnancy or lactation. Br J Cancer 58:382-384, 1988.
163. Danforth DN Jr. How subsequent pregnancy affects outcome in women with a prior breast cancer. Oncology (Williston Park) 5:23-30, 1991; discussion 30-31, 35.
164. Kroman N, Mouridsen HT: Prognostic influence of pregnancy before, around, and after diagnosis of breast cancer. Breast 12:516-521, 2003.
165. von Schoultz E, Johansson H, Wilking N, Rutqvist LE: Influence of prior and subsequent pregnancy on breast cancer prognosis. J Clin Oncol 13:430-434, 1995.
166. Sankila R, Heinavaara S, Hakulinen T: Survival of breast cancer patients after subsequent term pregnancy: "Healthy mother effect." Am J Obstet Gynecol 170:818-823, 1994.
167. Ariel IM, Kempner R: The prognosis of patients who become pregnant after mastectomy for breast cancer. Int Surg 74:185-187, 1989.
168. Gelber S, Coates AS, Goldhirsch A, et al: Effect of pregnancy on overall survival after the diagnosis of early-stage breast cancer [see comment]. J Clin Oncol 19:1671-1675, 2001.
169. Helewa M, Levesque P, Provencher D, et al: Breast cancer, pregnancy, and breastfeeding. J Obstet Gynaecol Can 24:164-184, 2002.
170. Smith RS, Randall P: Melanoma during pregnancy. Obstet Gynecol 34:825-829, 1969.
171. Pack GT, Scharnagel IM: The prognosis of malignant melanoma in pregnant women. Cancer 4:324-334, 1951.
172. George PA, Fortner JG, Pack GT: Melanoma with pregnancy. A report of 115 cases. Cancer 13:854-859, 1960.
173. Houghton AN, Flannery J, Viola MV: Malignant melanoma of the skin occurring during pregnancy. Cancer 48:407-410, 1981.
174. Shiu MH, Schottenfeld D, Maclean B, Fortner JG: Adverse effect of pregnancy on melanoma: A reappraisal. Cancer 37:181-187, 1976.
175. MacKie RM, Bufalino R, Morabito A, et al, for The World Health Organisation Melanoma Programme: Lack of effect of pregnancy on outcome of melanoma [see comment]. Lancet 337:653-655, 1991.
176. McManamny DS, Moss AL, Pocock PV, Briggs JC: Melanoma and pregnancy: A long-term follow-up. BJOG 96:1419-1423, 1989.
177. Reintgen DS, McCarty KS Jr, Vollmer R, et al: Malignant melanoma and pregnancy. Cancer 55:1340-1344, 1985.
178. Kjems E, Krag C: Melanoma and pregnancy. A review. Acta Oncol 32:371-378, 1993.
179. Trapeznikov NN, Khasanov ShR, Iavorskí VV: Melanoma of the skin and pregnancy [in Russian]. Vopr Onkol 33:40-46, 1987.
180. Slingluff CL Jr, Reintgen DS, Vollmer RT, Seigler HF: Malignant melanoma arising during pregnancy. A study of 100 patients. Ann Surg 211:552-557, 1990; discussion 558-559.
181. Wong DJ, Strassner HT: Melanoma in pregnancy. Clinical Obstet Gynecol 33:782-791, 1990.
182. Daryanani D, Plukker JT, De Hullu JA, et al: Pregnancy and early-stage melanoma [see comment]. Cancer 97:2248-2253, 2003.
183. Lens MB, Rosdahl I, Ahlbom A, et al: Effect of pregnancy on survival in women with cutaneous malignant melanoma. J Clin Oncol 22:4369-4375, 2004.
184. O'Meara AT, Cress R, Xing G, et al: Malignant melanoma in pregnancy. A population-based evaluation. Cancer 103:1217-1226, 2005.
185. Girard RM lJ, Baillot R: Carcinoma of the colon associated with pregnancy: Report of a case. Dis Colon Rectum 24:473-475, 1981.
186. Bernstein MA, Madoff RD, Caushaj PF: Colon and rectal cancer in pregnancy. Dis Colon Rectum 36:172-178, 1993.
187. Heise RH, Van Winter JT, Wilson TO, Ogburn PL Jr: Colonic cancer during pregnancy: Case report and review of the literature. Mayo Clin Proc 67:1180-1184, 1992.
188. Slattery ML, Samowitz WS, Holden JA: Estrogen and progesterone receptors in colon tumors. Am J Clin Pathol 113:364-368, 2000.
189. Korenaga D, Orita H, Maekawa S, et al: Relationship between hormone receptor levels and cell-kinetics in human colorectal cancer. Hepatogastroenterology 44:78-83, 1997.
190. Cappell MS: Colon cancer during pregnancy. Gastroenterol Clin North Am 32:341-383, 2003.
191. Cappell MS, Colon VJ, Sidhom OA: A study of eight medical centers of the safety and clinical efficacy of esophagogastroduodenoscopy in 83 pregnant females with follow-up of fetal outcome with comparison control groups. Am J Gastroenterol 91:348-354, 1996.
192. Lamerz R, Ruider H: Significance of CEA determinations in patients with cancer of the colon-rectum and the mammary gland in comparison to physiological states in connection with pregnancy. Bull Cancer 63:575-586, 1976.
193. Walsh C, Fazio VW: Cancer of the colon, rectum, and anus during pregnancy. The surgeon's perspective. Gastroenterol Clin North Am 27:257-267, 1998.
194. Mason MH 3rd, Kovalcik PJ: Ovarian metastases from colon carcinoma. J Surg Oncol 17:33-38, 1981.
195. Pitluk H, Poticha SM: Carcinoma of the colon and rectum in patients less than 40 years of age. Surg Gynecol Obstet 157:335-337, 1983.
196. Nesbitt JC, Moise KJ, Sawyers JL: Colorectal carcinoma in pregnancy. Arch Surg 120:636-640, 1985.
197. Stephens JD, Golbus MS, Miller TR, et al: Multiple congenital anomalies in a fetus exposed to 5-fluorouracil during the first trimester. Am J Obstet Gynecol 137:747-749, 1980.
198. Woods JB, Martin JN Jr, Ingram FH, et al: Pregnancy complicated by carcinoma of the colon above the rectum. Am J Perinatol 9:102 110, 1992.
199. Traulle C, Coiffier B: Lymphoma and pregnancy. In Canellos G, Lister T, Young B (eds): The Lymphomas, 2nd ed. Philadelphia, Saunders Elsevier; 2006, pp 536-541.
200. Lichtman M, Liesveld J: Acute myelogenous leukemia. In Beutler E, Lichtman M, Coller B, et al (eds): Williams Hematology, 6th ed. New York, McGraw-Hill, 2001, p 1065.
201. Weisz B, Schiff E, Lishner M: Cancer in pregnancy: Maternal and fetal implications. Hum Reprod Update 7:384-393, 2001.
202. Rosenberg S, Kaplan H: Evidence of an orderly progresssion in the spread of Hodgkin's disease. Cancer Res 26:1225-1231, 1966.
203. Juweid M, Stroobants S, Hoekstra O, et al: Use of positron emission tomography for response assessment of lymphoma: Consensus of the imaging subcommitted of international harmonization project in lymphoma. J Clin Oncol 25:571-578, 2007.
204. Haioun C, Itti E, Rahmouni A, et al: [18F]fluoro-2-deoxy-D-glucose positron emission tomography (FDG-PET) in aggressive lymphoma: An early prognostic tool for predicting patient outcome. Blood 106:1376-1381, 2005.
205. Hutchings M, Loft A, Hansen M, et al: FDG-PET after two cycles of chemotherapy predicts treatment failure and progression-free survival in Hodgkin lymphoma. Blood 107:52-59, 2006.
206. Jerusalem G, Beguin Y, Fassotte MF, et al: Whole-body positron emission tomography using ^{18}F-fluorodeoxyglucose for posttreatment evaluation in Hodgkin's disease and non-Hodgkin's lymphoma has higher diagnostic and prognostic value than classical computed tomography scan imaging. Blood 94:429-433, 1999.
207. Pohlman B, Macklis R: Lymphoma and pregnancy. Semin Oncol 27:657-666, 2000.
208. Gelb A, van de Rijn M, Warnke R, Kamel O: Pregnancy-associated lymphomas. A clinicopathologic study. Cancer 78:304-310, 1996.
209. Southman C, Diamond H, Craver L: Pregnancy during Hodgkin's disease. Cancer 9:1141-1146, 1956.
210. Barry R, Diamond H, Craver L: Influence of pregnancy on the course of Hodgkin's disease. Am J Obstet Gynecol 84:445-454, 1962.

211. Gobbi P, Attardo-Parrinello A, Danesino M, et al: Hodgkin's disease and pregnancy. Hematologica 69:336-341, 1984.
212. Nisce L, Tome M, He S, et al: Management of co-exisitng Hodgkin's disease and pregnancy. Am J Clin Oncol 9:146-151, 1986.
213. Lishner M, Zemlickis D, Degendrofer P, et al: Maternal and fetal outcome following Hodgkin's disease in pregnancy. Br J Cancer 65:114-117, 1992.
214. Ebert U, Loffler H, Kirch W: Cytotoxic therapy and pregnancy. Pharmacol Ther 74:207-220, 1997.
215. Wiebe V, Sipila P: Pharmacology of anti-neoplastic agents in pregnancy. Crit Rev Oncol Hematol 16:75-112, 1994.
216. Zemlickis D, Lishner M, Degendrofer P, et al: Fetal outcome after in utero exposure to cancer chemotherapy. Arch Intern Med 152:573-576, 1992.
217. Dilek I, Topcu N, Demir C, et al: Hematological malignancy and pregnancy: A single-institution experience of 21 cases. Clin Lab Hematol 28:170-176, 2006.
218. Germann N, Goffinet F, Goldwasser F: Anthracyclines during pregnancy: Embryo-fetal outcome in 160 patients Ann Oncol 15:146-150, 2004.
219. Doll D, Ringenberg Q, Yarbro J: Anti-neoplastic agents and pregnancy. Semin Oncol 16:337-346, 1989.
220. Glantz J: Reproductive toxicity of alkylating agents. Obstet Gynecol Surv 49:709-715, 1994.
221. Aviles A, Diaz-Maqueo JC, Talavera A, et al: Growth and development of children of mothers treated with chemotherapy during pregnancy: Current status of 43 children. Am J Hematol 36:243-248, 1991.
222. Garcia EL, Valcarcel M, Santiago-Borrero P: Chemotherapy during pregnancy and its effects on the fetus—neonatal myelosuppression: Two case reports. J Perinatol 19:230-233, 1999.
223. Koontz BF, Kirkpatrick JP, Clough RW, et al: Combined-modality therapy versus radiotherapy alone for treatment of early-stage Hodgkin's disease: Cure balanced against complications. J Clin Oncol 24:605-611, 2006.
224. Ng AK, Bernardo MV, Weller E, et al: Second malignancy after Hodgkin disease treated with radiation therapy with or without chemotherapy: Long-term risks and risk factors. Blood 100:1989-1996, 2002.
225. Ng AK, Bernardo MP, Weller E, et al: Long-term survival and competing causes of death in patients with early-stage Hodgkin's disease treated at age 50 or younger. J Clin Oncol 20:2101-2108, 2002.
226. Dores GM, Metayer C, Curtis RE, et al: Second malignant neoplasms among long-term survivors of Hodgkin's disease: A population-based evaluation over 25 years. J Clin Oncol 20:3484-3494, 2002.
227. Mazonakis M, Varveris H, Fasoulaki M, Damilakis J: Radiotherapy of Hodgkin's disease in early pregnancy: Embryo dose measurements. Radiother Oncol 66:333-339, 2003.
228. Kal HB, Struikmans H: Radiotherapy during pregnancy: Fact and fiction. Lancet Oncol 6:328-333, 2005.
229. Meyer RM, Gospodarowicz MK, Connors JM, et al: Randomized comparison of ABVD chemotherapy with a strategy that includes radiation therapy in patients with limited-stage Hodgkin's lymphoma: National Cancer Institute of Canada Clinical Trials Group and the Eastern Cooperative Oncology Group. J Clin Oncol 23:4634-4642, 2005.
230. Reis L, Eisner M, Kosary C, et al (eds): SEER Cancer Statistics Review, 1975-2001. Bethesda, Md, National Cancer Institute, 2004.
231. Jaffe E, Harris N, Stein H, Vardiman J (eds): World Health Organization Classification of Tumors. Lyon, IARC Press; 2001.
232. Lishner N, Zemlickis D, Sutcliff S, et al: Non-Hodgkin's lymphoma and pregnancy. Leuk Lymphoma 14:411-413, 1994.
233. Kirkpatrick AW, Bailey DJ, Weizel HA: Bilateral primary breast lymphoma in pregnancy: A case report and literature review. Can J Surg 39:333-335, 1996.
234. Kimby E, Sverrisdottir A, Elinder G: Safety of rituximab therapy during the first trimester of pregnancy: A case history. Eur J Haematol 72:292-295, 2004.
235. Amitay-Layish I, David M, Kafri B, et al: Early-stage mycosis fungoides, parapsoriasis en plaque, and pregnancy. Int J Dermatol 46:160-165, 2007.
236. Malik S, Oliver R, Odejinmi F: A rare association with hypercalcemia Pregnancy and multiple myeloma. J Obstet Gynaecol 26:693-695, 2006.
237. Iyengar P, Reid-Nicholson M, Moreira AL: Pregnancy-associated anaplastic large-cell lymphoma of the breast: A rare mimic of ductal carcinoma. Diagn Cytopathol 34:298-302, 2006.
238. Niitsu N, Kohri M, Togano T, et al: Development of hepatosplenic gamma-delta T-cell lymphoma with pancytopenia during early pregnancy: A case report and review of the literature. Eur J Haematol 73:367-371, 2004.
239. Forthman CL, Ponce BA, Mankin HJ: Multiple myeloma with a pathologic fracture during pregnancy. A case report. J Bone Joint Surg Am 86:1284-1288, 2004.
240. Ravikanti L, Singh V: Subcutaneous panniculitic T-cell lymphoma presenting as pyrexia of unknown origin in pregnancy: A case report and literature review. Aust N Z J Obstet Gynaecol 43:166-168, 2003.
241. Maglione A, Di Giorgio G, Petruzzelli F, Longo MP: Multiple myeloma diagnosed during early pregnancy: A case report. Eur J Obstet Gynecol Reprod Biol 111:214-215, 2003.
242. Echols KT, Gilles JM, Diro M: Mycosis fungoides in pregnancy: Remission after treatment with alpha-interferon in a case refractory to conventional therapy: A case report. J Matern Fetal Med 10:68-70, 2001.
243. Castelo-Branco C, Torne A, Cararach V, Iglesias X: Mycosis fungoides and pregnancy. Oncol Rep 8:197-199, 2001.
244. Wang PH, Chao KC, Lin G, et al: Primary malignant lymphoma of the cervix in pregnancy. A case report. J Reprod Med 44:630-632, 1999.
245. Yamamoto O, Tajiri M, Asahi M: Lymphomatoid papulosis associated with pregnancy. Clin Exp Dermatol 22:141-143, 1997.
246. van Besien K, Kelta M, Bahaguna P: Primary mediastinal B-cell lymphoma: A review of pathology and management. J Clin Oncol 19:1855-1864, 2001.
247. Blum KA, Lozanski G, Byrd JC: Adult Burkitt leukemia and lymphoma. Blood 104:3009-3020, 2004.
248. Illes A, Banyai A, Jenei K, et al: Bilateral primary malignant lymphoma of the breast during pregnancy. Haematologia (Budap) 27:99-105, 1996.
249. Selvais PL, Mazy G, Gosseye S, et al: Breast infiltration by acute lymphoblastic leukemia during pregnancy. Am J Obstet Gynecol 169:1619-1620, 1993.
250. Barnes MN, Barrett JC, Kimberlin DF, Kilgore LC: Burkitt lymphoma in pregnancy. Obstet Gynecol 92(Pt 2):675-678, 1998.
251. Antic N, Colovic M, Cemerikic V, et al: Disseminated Burkitt's-like lymphoma during pregnancy. Med Oncol 17:233-236, 2000.
252. Magloire LK, Pettker CM, Buhimschi CS, Funai EF: Burkitt's lymphoma of the ovary in pregnancy. Obstet Gynecol 108(Pt 2):743-745, 2006.
253. Hehn ST, Grogan TM, Miller TP: Utility of fine-needle aspiration as a diagnostic technique in lymphoma. J Clin Oncol 22:3046-3052, 2004.
254. Aviles A, Diaz-Maqueo J, Torras V, et al: Non-Hodgkin's lymphomas and pregnancy: Presentation of 16 cases. Gynecol Oncol 37:335-337, 1990.
255. Ward E, Weiss R: Lymphoma and pregnancy. Semin Oncol 16:397-409, 1989.
256. Dhedin N, Coiffier B: Lymphoma and pregnancy. In Canellos G, Lister T, Young B (eds): The Lymphomas. New York, Elsevier, 1993, pp 549-556.
257. Lam MS: Treatment of Burkitt's lymphoma during pregnancy. Ann Pharmacother 40:2048-2052, 2006.
258. Friedrichs B, Tiemann M, Salwender H, et al: The effects of rituximab treatment during pregnancy on a neonate. Hematologica 91:1426-1427, 2006.
259. Herold M, Schnohr S, Bittrich H: Efficacy and safety of combined rituximab chemotherapy during pregnancy. J Clin Oncol 19:3439, 2001.
260. Maloney DG, Grillo-Lopez AJ, White CA, et al: IDEC-C2B8 (Rituximab) anti-CD20 monoclonal antibody therapy in patients with relapsed low-grade non-Hodgkin's lymphoma. Blood 90:2188-2195, 1997.
261. Chelghoum Y, Vey N, Raffoux E, et al: Acute leukemia during pregnancy. Cancer 104:110-117, 2005.
262. Reynoso E, Shepherd F, Messner H, et al: Acute leukemia during pregnancy: The Toronto Leukemia Study Group experience with long-term follow-up of children exposed in utero to chemotherapeutic agents. J Clin Oncol 5:1098-1106, 1987.

Chapter 44

Renal Disorders

David J. Williams, PhD, and John M. Davison, MD

Among the many physiologic changes that occur in normal pregnancy, few are as profound as those affecting the urinary system.[1] These healthy alterations and various diagnostic pitfalls for the unwary clinician are discussed in Chapter 7. Improvements in our knowledge about gestational physiology in antenatal care generally, technology for fetal surveillance, and neonatology services have meant better care and outcomes for women with renal problems and their newborns.[2,3] With this is mind, this chapter focuses on urinary tract infection (UTI), acute and chronic renal disease in pregnancy, and the management of pregnant women on dialysis or with renal allografts.

Urinary Tract Infection

The incidence of asymptomatic bacteriuria (i.e., significant growth of a uropathogen in the absence of symptoms) is 2% to 10%, which is the same during pregnancy as it is in sexually active nonpregnant women.[4] However, the structural and immunologic changes to the urothelium of the renal tracts during pregnancy[5] make it more likely that a lower UTI will ascend to cause acute pyelonephritis.[4,5] During pregnancy, 12.5% to 30% of women with untreated asymptomatic bacteriuria develop acute pyelonephritis,[4,6-8] a serious infection with significant morbidity for the mother and fetus.

Diagnosis of Urinary Tract Infections

During pregnancy, symptoms suggesting a UTI are dysuria and offensive-smelling urine. Others usually associated with a UTI are urinary frequency, nocturia, urge incontinence, and strangury (i.e., the urge to pass urine having just done so), but these symptoms are also found in healthy pregnant women.

Microscopy and culture of a freshly voided midstream urine sample allow quantification of pyuria (i.e., leukocytes in the urine) and growth of a urinary pathogen. A bacterial UTI is the most common cause of pyuria and is considered significant if microscopy of a sample of unspun midstream urine reveals more than 10 leukocytes per microliter. Urine culture is conventionally recognized as significant if there is growth of more than 10^5 colony-forming units per milliliter (CFU/mL) of a single recognized uropathogen, in association with pyuria.[9] Low counts of bacteriuria[10] (2^4 to 10^4 CFU/mL) may still be significant if symptomatic women have a high fluid intake or are infected with a slow-growing organism. If left untreated, most symptomatic women with low-count bacteriuria will have 10^5 CFU/mL 2 days later.[9] During pregnancy, the most common uropathogens are bowel commensals, *Escherichia coli* (70% to 80%), *Klebsiella*, *Proteus*, *Enterobacter*, and *Staphylococcus saprophyticus*.

If urine from a symptomatic pregnant woman is cloudy and positive on dipstick testing for nitrite (produced by most uropathogens) and leukocyte esterase (produced by white blood cells), a UTI is likely and empiric treatment can be started.[9] These urine sticks are not sensitive enough to be used for screening for asymptomatic bacteriuria in early pregnancy,[10] and microscopy and culture of a clean catch midstream urine sample is necessary. Hematuria and proteinuria are unreliable indicators of a UTI, but they are important signs of renal disease (discussed later).

Asymptomatic Bacteriuria

Maternal and Fetal Risks

During pregnancy, untreated asymptomatic bacteriuria will develop into acute pyelonephritis in up to 30% of women, but if treated, less than 1% of pregnant women develop pyelonephritis.[4,6,7] A systematic review of 14 studies confirmed that antibiotic treatment of asymptomatic bacteriuria significantly reduced the incidence of pyelonephritis compared with placebo or no treatment (odds ratio [OR], 0.25; 95% confidence interval [CI], 0.14 to 0.48).[11] After successful treatment of asymptomatic bacteriuria, monthly screening of midstream urine is necessary, because about 30% of women will have a relapse of bacteriuria, making them vulnerable to acute pyelonephritis again.[4]

Asymptomatic bacteriuria has been associated with an increased risk of preterm delivery and low birth weight.[12] Treatment of asymptomatic bacteriuria has been shown to reduce the incidence of low-birth-weight infants (OR, 0.66; 95% CI, 0.49 to 0.89)[11] but have no effect on preterm delivery.[6] It has been suggested that the underlying renal pathology, which is commonly associated with bacteriuria, is responsible for poor pregnancy outcomes.[6] Additional good-quality studies are needed to settle this issue.

Management of Asymptomatic Bacteriuria

Contrary to much published advice, not all pregnant women need to be screened for asymptomatic bacteriuria. There are two main reasons. First, the prevalence of asymptomatic bacteriuria varies between populations, and where it is low (<2.5%), it is hard to justify the cost-effectiveness of screening. In populations in which the prevalence of asymptomatic bacteriuria is more than 5%, the case for screening is much stronger.[7] Second, approximately 1% to 2% of the 90% to 98% of asymptomatic women who test negative for bacteriuria in the first trimester will develop a symptomatic UTI.[8,13] This means that one third of all women who develop a UTI in late pregnancy would have been missed on first-trimester screening.[8,13] Women at increased risk for pyelonephritis or renal impairment should be screened for asymptomatic bacteriuria every 4 to 6 weeks throughout pregnancy.

Treatment of Urinary Tract Infections

There is no consensus about the optimal treatment of asymptomatic bacteriuria[14] or the empiric treatment of symptomatic UTIs in pregnancy.[15] Most urinary infections during pregnancy (approximately 75%) are caused by *E. coli*, which is usually sensitive to nitrofurantoin (89%), trimethoprim with or without sulfamethoxazole (87%), ampicillin (72%), or cephalosporins.[16,17] Until well-structured trials are done, the most cost-effective treatment for asymptomatic bacteriuria or a first episode of cystitis is nitrofurantoin monohydrate macrocrystals (100 mg twice daily for 3 days) or trimethoprim (200 mg twice daily for 3 days).[17] Nitrofurantoin should be avoided after the onset of labor in patients with glucose-6-phosphate dehydrogenase deficiency, although no well-documented cases of hemolysis in neonates have been recorded,[18] and trimethoprim should be avoided in the first trimester because it is a folic acid antagonist associated with an increased risk of neural tube defect.[19]

Screening for recurrent infections should begin 1 week after completion of initial treatment and then be done every 4 to 6 weeks for the remainder of pregnancy. Recurrent infections or a first infection in a pregnant woman at high risk for pyelonephritis should be treated with a 7- to 10-day course of an antibiotic that reflects antibacterial sensitivities.[17] Women who have had two episodes of asymptomatic bacteriuria or cystitis should be considered for low-dose antibiotic prophylaxis—guided by the sensitivities of the most recent infective organism—for the remainder of pregnancy and until 4 to 6 weeks after birth.[20] Suitable regimens for long-term antibiotic prophylaxis include nitrofurantoin (50 to 100 mg each night), amoxicillin (250 mg each night), cephalexin (125 to 250 mg each night), or trimethoprim (100 to 150 mg each night).[20] These women should also be investigated for structural abnormalities of the renal tracts or renal calculus using ultrasonography.

Acute Pyelonephritis

The same uropathogens that cause asymptomatic bacteriuria and cystitis are responsible for acute pyelonephritis.[21] The prevalence of asymptomatic bacteriuria in a pregnant population dictates the incidence of acute pyelonephritis. Screening and treating a high-risk population for asymptomatic bacteriuria reduces the incidence of acute pyelonephritis to less than 1%.[8,11] Unless acute pyelonephritis is treated promptly, there is considerable maternal and fetal morbidity.[21]

Maternal Symptoms and Signs

Most women with acute pyelonephritis present in the second or third trimester.[21] More than 80% of women present with backache, fever, rigors and costovertebral angle tenderness, and about one half have lower urinary tract symptoms, nausea, and vomiting.[21] Bacteremia occurs in 15% to 20% of pregnant women with acute pyelonephritis,[21] and a small proportion of these women will develop septic shock and increased capillary leak, leading to pulmonary edema.[22] It is important, however, to differentiate the hypotension due to reduced intravascular volume (i.e., fever, nausea, and vomiting) from that caused by septic shock. Women with pyelonephritis at risk for serious complications are those who present with the highest fever (>39.4 °C) and tachycardia (>110 beats/min) at 20 weeks' gestation or later and who have received tocolytic agents and injudicious fluid replacement.[23]

Fetal Risks

Acute pyelonephritis can trigger uterine contractions and preterm labor.[24] Antibiotic treatment of pyelonephritis reduces uterine activity, but patients with recurrent infection or marked uterine activity are at increased risk for preterm labor.[24] Because uterine activity often occurs in the absence of cervical change and because tocolysis with β-mimetics aggravates the cardiovascular response to endotoxemia,[23] tocolytic therapy should be used with care and only in those with cervical changes.[25]

Management of Acute Pyelonephritis

Women suspected of acute pyelonephritis from their history, symptoms, and signs should be admitted to the hospital. Laboratory tests should include a full blood cell count, serum creatinine concentration, levels of electrolytes, and urine culture. If there are systemic symptoms or septic shock, a blood culture may be useful. Pregnant women with pyelonephritis and septic shock need intensive care. For these women, assessment of the state of hydration is critical and often requires invasive hemodynamic monitoring with a central venous pressure line. This can optimize fluid balance, aiming for a urine output greater than 30mL/hr to minimize renal impairment and reduce the risk of pulmonary edema. Intravenous antibiotics should be started empirically (discussed later) until the sensitivities of blood and urine cultures are known. These women often have transient renal impairment, thrombocytopenia, and hemolysis, suggesting that the alveolar capillary endothelium is damaged by endotoxin.[22] A blood film and lactate dehydrogenase concentration can be used to diagnose hemolysis.

Trials investigating the outpatient management of pyelonephritis in pregnancy have identified a group of women who can be managed at home.[25] These women should be less than 24 weeks' gestation, be relatively healthy, and understand the importance of compliance. They should have an initial period of observation in the hospital to demonstrate an ability to take oral fluids and receive intramuscular cefuroxime or ceftriaxone. After satisfactory laboratory tests, they can go home and are seen again within 24 hours for a second intramuscular dose of cephalosporin. They then start a 10-day course of oral cephalexin (500 mg four times daily) or appropriate antibiotic with regular outpatient follow-up.[24] Following this regimen, 90% of women will improve as outpatients, and 10% will require hospital admission because of sepsis or recurrent pyelonephritis. Women with acute pyelonephritis who are beyond 24 weeks' gestation should be admitted for at least 24 hours to observe the maternal condition as described earlier and to monitor uterine activity and the fetal heart rate.[25]

Gram-negative bacteria causing pyelonephritis in pregnancy are often resistant to ampicillin,[26] and intravenous cefuroxime (750 mg to 1.5 gm, depending on severity of condition, every 8 hours) is an effective first choice until culture sensitivities are known.[15] Women allergic to β-lactam antibiotics can be given intravenous gentamicin (1.5 mg/kg every 8 hours) for the initial treatment of acute pyelonephritis. A single-dose regimen (7 mg/kg every 24 hours) should be avoided during pregnancy to reduce the very small risk of cranial nerve VIII damage to the fetus.[17] Serum concentrations of gentamicin should be measured and dose adjustments made according to identified levels. Intravenous antibiotics should be continued until the patient has been afebrile for 24 hours. Oral antibiotics should then be given for 7 to 10 days, according to bacterial sensitivities, or if not available, as if for symptomatic lower UTI.[17]

Failure of these measures to improve the maternal clinical condition within 48 to 72 hours suggests an underlying structural abnormality. Ultrasonography is an easy but inconclusive way of excluding stones. If clinical suspicion is high, a plain abdominal radiograph can identify 90% of renal stones, and a one-shot intravenous urogram (IVU) at 20 to 30 minutes can identify the remainder.[25] The risk to the fetus from radiation of one or two radiographs is minimal, especially when compared with the clinical benefit of identifying an obstructed, nonfunctioning kidney. Urinary tract obstruction can also be detected using magnetic resonance urography, especially during the second and third trimesters.[27]

After one episode of pyelonephritis, pregnant women should have monthly urine cultures to screen for a recurrence.[25] The risk of recurrent pyelonephritis can be reduced with antimicrobial prophylaxis chosen according to the sensitivities of initial bacterial infection[20,28] or with nitrofurantoin (100 mg every night) continued until 4 to 6 weeks after delivery.[25]

Acute Renal Failure in Pregnancy

Acute renal failure has become a rare but serious complication of pregnancy. In early pregnancy, acute renal failure is associated with septic abortion (a complication largely confined to the developing world) and dehydration related to hyperemesis gravidarum. Around the time of delivery, acute renal failure is most commonly caused by gestational syndromes such as preeclampsia and abruptio placentae (Table 44-1). However, pregnancy is a prothrombotic state that is associated with heightened inflammation[29] and major changes to the vascular endothelium,[30] particularly the glomerular capillary endothelium.[31] These physiologic changes predispose pregnant women to acute glomerular capillary thrombosis. Whereas nonpregnant patients who suffer an acute prerenal insult (e.g., hemorrhage, dehydration, septic shock) may develop transient acute tubular necrosis if inadequately treated, the same prerenal insult in pregnancy is more likely to develop into renal cortical necrosis with permanent renal impairment. This is even more likely to occur if a prerenal insult coexists with a pregnancy-related condition that induces a consumptive coagulopathy or endothelial damage (e.g., preeclampsia).

Management is aimed at identification and correction of the precipitating insult and optimal fluid resuscitation, which is best guided by monitoring the central venous pressure and pulmonary artery wedge pressure. If oliguria persists despite euvolemia with deteriorating renal function or fluid overload, fluid restriction followed by renal replacement therapy is indicated.

TABLE 44-1 CAUSES OF ACUTE RENAL FAILURE IN PREGNANCY

Most common causes	Severe preeclampsia
	Placental abruption
Causes in early pregnancy	Septic abortion
	Hyperemesis gravidarum
	Ovarian hyperstimulation syndrome
Rare causes	Amniotic fluid embolus
	Hemolytic uremic syndrome/ thrombotic thrombocytopenic purpura
	Acute fatty liver of pregnancy
	Acute obstruction of renal tracts

Preeclampsia

Preeclampsia and the Kidney

Preeclampsia rarely causes acute renal failure severe enough to require dialysis.[32] In a cohort of South African women with severe preeclampsia and renal impairment, 7 (10%) of 72 required temporary dialysis, and none developed chronic renal failure.[32] All women with severe preeclampsia who needed dialysis had hemorrhage, which often was caused by abruptio placentae.[32] Preeclampsia causing mild transient renal impairment (serum creatinine up to 125 μmol/L or 1.41 mg/dL) is common, but with appropriate management, there should be complete recovery of renal function.

Women with preexisting renal disease are more vulnerable to preeclampsia, especially when it is associated with chronic hypertension[33] (see Chapter 35). A meta-analysis of trials investigating the effectiveness of low-dose aspirin (50 to 150 mg/day) in pregnant women with moderate to severe renal disease revealed a significant reduction in the risk of preeclampsia and perinatal death.[34]

Conversely, 2% to 5% of women with preeclampsia are later found to have underlying renal disease,[35] but if preeclampsia is severe, up to 20% of women will have chronic kidney disease (CKD).[36] Women who have had preeclampsia should therefore be checked for persistent postpartum hypertension and proteinuria. Gestational hypertension usually resolves within 3 months of delivery, but severe proteinuria due to preeclampsia can take up to 12 months to disappear. Women who have had preeclampsia are more likely to have persistent microalbuminuria compatible with microvascular disease and are at increased risk for cardiovascular disease in later life.[37,38]

Women who develop high levels of proteinuria (>10 g/24 hr) tend to have earlier-onset preeclampsia and deliver at an earlier gestational age compared with preeclamptic women who have less marked proteinuria (<5 g/24 hr).[39] After correction for prematurity, however, massive proteinuria (>10 g/24 hr) has no significant effect on neonatal outcome.[39] Increasing proteinuria is not therefore an indication for delivery. We suggest that pregnant women who develop a proteinuria level of more than 1 to 3 g in 24 hours accompanied by other maternal risk factors for thrombosis should be considered for thromboprophylaxis with enoxaparin (40 mg SC each day) or Fragmin (5000 units SC each day).

The diagnosis of preeclampsia is difficult if there is chronic hypertension and preexisting proteinuria, especially because these two parameters become increasingly marked in late pregnancy. Hyperuricemia and intrauterine growth restriction are common features of preeclampsia and chronic renal impairment, but the presence of increased levels of hepatic transaminases and thrombocytopenia support a diagnosis of preeclampsia.[40]

Preeclampsia: Management of Renal Impairment and Fluid Balance

The cure for severe preeclampsia is delivery of the infant and placenta. Delivery may halt the general progression of preeclampsia, but postpartum maternal renal function usually deteriorates before improving.[32] It is advisable to recommend delivery for women who have preeclampsia and an increase in the serum creatinine concentration from about 70 μmol/L (0.79 mg/dL) to more than 120 μmol/L (1.36 mg/dL) to prevent ongoing renal impairment.

Fluid balance is critical to the management of acute renal failure during pregnancy. Too little intravascular fluid leads to prerenal failure, which is especially damaging to chronically impaired kidneys, whereas too much fluid risks pulmonary edema, adult respiratory distress syndrome, and maternal death.[41] Transient oliguria (<100 mL over 4 hours) is a common observation in the first 24 hours after a healthy pregnancy. If a preeclamptic woman is not obviously hypovolemic and has a serum urea level of 5 mmol/L or less and serum creatinine level of 90 µmol/L or less, repeated fluid challenges to increase urine output are unnecessary and increase the maternal risk of pulmonary edema. Women with severe preeclampsia and renal impairment (i.e., serum creatinine level of more than 120 µmol/L or 1.36 mg/dL) should have their fluid balance guided by a central venous pressure catheter or, when available, a pulmonary artery flotation catheter on a high-dependency unit familiar with this equipment.[42] The rate of fluid replacement should take account of central venous filling pressure, pulmonary wedge pressure, hourly urine output, and insensible loses. After the patient is euvolemic, the rate of intravenous fluid replacement should equal the previous hours' urine output plus insensible losses; this is usually 30 mL/hr if the patient is afebrile. The amount of intravenous fluid replacement can be reduced after the mother can take oral fluid and her renal impairment starts to improve. Intravenous fluid regimens that stick to a fixed hourly replacement can lead to fluid overload in oliguric women and to reduced intravascular volume in those having a diuresis. Fluid replacement should include blood to replace blood loses and then isotonic sodium chloride or compound sodium lactate (i.e., Hartmann's solution). Dextrose solutions are hypotonic and lead to maternal hyponatremia (5% dextrose contains only 30 mmol/L of NaCl, compared with 150 mmol/L of NaCl in a 0.9% sodium chloride solution).

Low-dose "renal" dopamine infusion (3 µg/kg/min) was previously used to increase renal blood flow in people with acute renal failure, but it is no longer thought to be beneficial. It is recommended that once hypovolemia has been corrected, as judged by the central venous pressure or pulmonary wedge pressure, preeclamptic women with oliguria (<200 mL/12 hr) and a serum urea level higher than 14 mmol/L (39 mg/dL) and serum creatinine level higher than 500 mmol/L (5.65 mg/dL) may benefit from a furosemide infusion (5 mg/hr) in an effort to prevent fluid overload and hemodialysis.[43]

After acute tubular necrosis is established with oliguria and a rising serum creatinine level despite adequate intravascular volume and blood pressure, fluid intake should be restricted to avoid fluid overload. In these circumstances, dialysis is indicated. There are no good studies that have followed up women with acute renal failure related to preeclampsia, but those with the most severe renal impairment will undoubtedly be left with a degree of permanent renal impairment that may not manifest until later life.[32]

Hypertension due to preeclampsia is caused by vasoconstriction around a reduced plasma volume.[40] For this reason and despite the lack of evidence from randomized trials, women with severe preeclampsia often receive plasma volume expansion before therapeutic vasodilation. Unless there are signs of pulmonary edema (i.e., basal crackles and $PO_2 < 95\%$ on air), 500 mL of colloid or crystalloid given over 30 to 60 minutes or 250 mL per hour until the pulmonary wedge pressure is 10 to 12 mm Hg can improve maternal and fetal well-being in cases of severe preeclampsia.[45,46] A vasodilator given alone can cause profound hypotension that may threaten maternal renal, cerebral, and uteroplacental blood flow.

Hemolytic Uremic Syndrome and Thrombotic Thrombocytopenic Purpura

Hemolytic uremic syndrome (HUS) and thrombotic thrombocytopenic purpura (TTP) are similar syndromes (designated HUS/TTP). They are characterized by microangiopathic hemolytic anemia and thrombocytopenia. The congenital and acquired forms of HUS/TTP are more common in late pregnancy.[46] Women with HUS/TTP develop platelet thrombi attached to von Willebrand factor multimers in end-organ microvessels. This typically results in a multiorgan disorder with abdominal ischemia and renal or neurologic impairment.[47] A plasma metalloprotease (ADAMTS13), which normally cleaves von Willebrand factor multimers to prevent microthrombi, is deficient in some women with congenital HUS/TTP,[48] and antibodies that neutralize ADAMTS13 have been found in women with acquired HUS/TTP.[49]

HUS/TTP is more common in women (approximately 70% of cases) and more common in association with pregnancy (approximately 13% of cases).[46] During pregnancy, the levels of ADAMTS13 fall progressively.[50] This may explain why women with a congenital deficiency of ADAMTS13 or with other risk factors for thrombosis (e.g., obesity, thrombophilia) are predisposed to peripartum HUS/TTP.

Hemolytic Uremic Syndrome, Thrombotic Thrombocytopenic Purpura, and Preeclampsia

Preeclampsia shares many similarities with HUS/TTP. Both syndromes occur most frequently in the third trimester or immediately after delivery. It is, however, important to differentiate them, because management is different. Women with HUS/TTP often present with gastrointestinal or neurologic abnormalities,[46] and they are more likely to have severe renal impairment, hemolysis, and thrombocytopenia compared with women who have preeclampsia. Because disseminated intravascular coagulation (DIC) is rare in HUS/TTP, the prothrombin time and kaolin clotting time are usually normal.[47] Women with preeclampsia are also more likely to have elevated levels of hepatic transaminases, heavy proteinuria, and abnormal clotting compared with women with HUS/TTP.[40] However, in many women, the distinction between preeclampsia and HUS/TTP can be determined only by the course of the illness after delivery,[51] but acute renal failure due to preeclampsia usually becomes transiently worse before improving.[32]

Management of Hemolytic Uremic Syndrome and Thrombotic Thrombocytopenic Purpura

Maternal survival from HUS/TTP greatly improved since treatment with plasmapheresis (i.e., infusion of fresh plasma and removal of old plasma).[52] Until recently, it was unclear why plasmapheresis worked, but the discovery of antibodies to ADAMTS13 (removed with old plasma) and a congenital deficiency of ADAMTS13 (replenished with infusion of fresh plasma) gives reason to this process. However, severe deficiency of ADAMTS13, which is not a routine laboratory measurement, is not present in all cases of HUS/TTP, and plasmapheresis is effective in pregnant women who have milder deficiencies of ADAMTS13.[53]

Steroids are often added to the plasma exchange regimen and are a rationale choice for acquired HUS/TTP with an autoimmune pathology, but there are no randomized, controlled trials of their use. Antiplatelet regimens with aspirin and dipyridamole may also be beneficial in conjunction with plasma exchange.[54] Conversely, administration of platelets to thrombocytopenic patients with HUS/TTP can result in a precipitous decline in clinical status.

Acute Renal Cortical Necrosis

In the developed world, acute renal cortical necrosis (ARCN) has become a rare complication of pregnancy. The reduced incidence of septic abortion and improved management of peripartum obstetric emergencies have prevented prerenal impairment developing into acute tubular necrosis and then renal cortical necrosis. In the developing world, however, obstetric emergencies are still responsible for most cases of ARCN.[55] Acute renal failure after septic abortion or peripartum obstetric emergencies developed into ARCN in 20% of women after a prolonged period of acute tubular necrosis.[56]

ARCN is most commonly caused by abruption of the placenta with hemorrhage, amniotic fluid embolus, and sepsis associated with DIC.[57] After hemorrhage or sepsis with hypotension, prerenal failure without adequate resuscitation leads to acute tubular necrosis. If anuria persists for longer than a week, ARCN should be suspected. A definitive diagnosis can be made with renal biopsy, but it is often missed because of the patchy nature of cortical necrosis. Selective renal angiography can confirm the diagnosis, but it introduces another nephrotoxic agent and is usually unnecessary. Because of the serious nature of the precipitating illness and the limited availability of renal replacement therapy in the developing world, the maternal mortality rate is still high.[56]

For women who survive the acute illness, renal function usually returns slowly over the next 6 to 24 months. Long-term renal function depends on the extent of cortical necrosis, which is often incomplete. Hyperfiltration through remnant glomeruli usually leads to a subsequent progressive decline in renal function.

Acute Fatty Liver of Pregnancy

Acute fatty liver of pregnancy (AFLP) causes reversible peripartum liver and renal impairment in 1 of 5000 to 10,000 pregnancies.[58] The diagnosis is based on clinical and laboratory findings of impaired liver, renal function, and clotting function, rather than on histologic or radiologic evidence of a fatty liver.[58] Women with AFLP usually present with nausea, vomiting, and abdominal cramps. Impaired renal function and reduced plasma antithrombin levels are early findings of AFLP that may precede liver dysfunction.[58] In established cases of AFLP, depressed function of the liver with prolonged prothrombin time, hypoglycemia, and DIC are more markedly abnormal than levels of liver transaminases, which may only be moderately elevated.[58] In a series of 28 women with AFLP, other ubiquitous laboratory findings at the time of delivery were elevated levels of serum total bilirubin (mean, 7.5 mg/dL), serum creatinine (mean, 205 mmol/L or 2.3 mg/dL), and uric acid (mean, 11 mg/dL).[58]

A recessively inherited fetal inborn error of mitochondrial fatty acid oxidation may explain up to 20% of AFLP cases.[59] Mitochondrial fatty acid oxidation is important for normal renal and liver function and may therefore explain the dual vulnerability of these organs in women with AFLP.

In women with AFLP, maternal renal impairment is aggravated by hypotension from hemorrhage, which is most likely to follow an emergency operative delivery.[58,60] The combination of renal dysfunction, hemorrhage, and DIC resulting from liver failure during pregnancy or after delivery requires intensive care with a multidisciplinary team of hepatologists, nephrologists, intensive care specialists, and obstetricians. Management is supportive and aimed at maintaining adequate fluid balance for renal perfusion, replacing blood, correcting the coagulopathy with fresh frozen plasma and possibly with antithrombin concentrate and fresh platelets. Hypoglycemia should be corrected with 10% dextrose solutions. Temporary dialysis may be necessary, but with good supportive care, recovery of normal renal and liver function is usual.[58] Perinatal survival in association with AFLP is improving, but it depends on the early recognition of the maternal condition, close fetal surveillance, timely delivery, and excellent neonatal care.

Nephrotoxic Drugs during Pregnancy

Nonsteroidal anti-inflammatory drugs (NSAIDs), including the more selective cyclooxygenase-2 (COX-2) inhibitors, when given to the mother in the peripartum period, reduce renal blood flow and have been associated with acute renal impairment in the mother and fetus.[61] Women with reduced intravascular volume, especially with preexisting renal impairment, are particularly vulnerable and should be prescribed NSAIDs with caution. Aminoglycosides are also nephrotoxic and should be prescribed with care and attention to drug plasma levels in women with mild renal impairment.

Acute Renal Obstruction in Pregnancy

The renal tracts may be obstructed during pregnancy by renal calculi (discussed later), congenital renal tract abnormalities, or a gestational overdistention syndrome. Women born with congenital obstructive uropathies at the pelviureteral junction (PUJ) or vesicoureteric junction (VUJ) are at increased risk of urine outflow obstruction in the second half of pregnancy, even if they have had surgical correction in childhood.[62] Congenital abnormalities of the lower urinary tracts, including the bladder and urethra, are varied and usually require extensive surgical correction in childhood. During pregnancy, these women are at increased risk for recurrent urine infections and, less commonly, for outflow obstruction requiring temporary nephrostomy or a ureteric stent.[63]

Women with a single kidney and urologic abnormalities are particularly vulnerable to develop post-renal failure in relation to gestational obstruction of their solitary kidney. An incomplete obstruction can cause renal impairment with an apparently good urine output. High backpressures compress and damage the renal medulla, leading to a loss of renal concentrating ability and production of dilute urine that is passed through an incomplete obstruction. It is also important for the obstetrician to remember that a congenitally single kidney is often associated with other abnormalities of the genital tracts, such as a unicornuate uterus.[64]

During pregnancy, the renal tracts can rarely and spontaneously become grossly overdistended. If untreated, overdistention occasionally can lead to rupture of the kidney or renal tracts.[65] Women with overdistention of the renal tracts initially present with severe loin pain, most commonly on the right side and radiating to the lower abdomen. The pain is positional and inconstant; it is characteristically relieved by lying on the opposite side and tucking the knees up to the chest. A palpable tender flank mass may suggest renal tract rupture.[65] Rupture of the kidney almost always occurs in a previously diseased kidney, usually in association with a benign hamartoma or renal abscess.[65] Urinalysis can reveal gross or microscopic hematuria. A renal ultrasound can detect a hydronephrotic kidney with a grossly dilated pelvicaliceal system. Occasionally, a urinoma is evident around the kidney, indicating rupture of the renal pelvis that can sometimes seal spontaneously.

The pain from the overdistention syndrome varies from mild to very severe. Women with mild symptoms can usually be managed with advice on positional relief and regular analgesia. Women with severe unremitting pain, hematuria, and grossly distended renal tracts on ultrasound in the absence of structural or infected masses usually have immediate pain relief after decompression of the system with a ureteric stent or nephrostomy. Rupture of the kidney necessitates immediate surgery and almost invariably an emergency nephrectomy.[65]

Chronic Kidney Disease

Normal Pregnancy and Renal Assessment

The glomerular filtration rate (GFR), measured as 24-hour creatinine clearance, increases by more than 50% shortly after conception. Serum creatinine (and urea nitrogen levels, which average 70 µmol/L (0.8 mg/dL) and 5 mmol/L (13 mg/dL), respectively, in nonpregnant women, decrease to mean values of 50 µmol/L (0.6 mg/dL) and 3 mmol/L (9 mg/dL) in pregnant women. Near term, a 15% to 20% decrement in GFR occurs, which affects serum creatinine levels minimally.

Serum creatinine values of 80 µmol/L (0.9 mg/dL) and urea nitrogen of 6 mmol/L (14 mg/dL), which are acceptable in nonpregnant subjects, are suspect in pregnant women. However, the physician should use caution in assessing renal function by serum creatinine levels alone, because the creatinine is filtered and secreted by the kidney, and the ratio of creatinine to inulin clearance normally falls to between 1.1 and 1.2. As renal disease progresses, a greater portion of urinary creatinine is formed as a result of secretion (clearance ratios rise to between 1.4 and 1.6 when the serum creatinine level is 1.4). The GFR may be overestimated by 50%.

Formulas (e.g., the Cockroft-Gault formula) that use serum creatinine in relation to age, height, and weight to calculate GFR should not be used in pregnancy because weight or body size does not reflect kidney size. The use of estimated GFR (eGFR) from the Modification of Diet in Renal Disease (MDRD) formula, whereby the serum creatinine value is adjusted for age, gender, and race, cannot be recommended for use in pregnancy because it significantly underestimates the GFR.[66] Ideally, evaluation of renal function in pregnancy should be based on the clearance of creatinine rather than its serum concentration. Creatinine levels may increase by up to 12 µmol/L (0.15 mg/dL) shortly after ingestion of cooked meat (because cooking converts preformed creatine into creatinine), and the timing of the blood sample during a clearance period must take into account meals and their content.

Renal Dysfunction and Preconception Counseling

CKD is often clinically and biochemically silent until renal impairment is advanced. Symptoms are unusual until GFR declines to less than 25% of normal, and more than 50% of renal function can be lost before the serum creatinine level rises above 120 µmol/L (1.36 mg/dL). However, women who become pregnant with a serum creatinine level above 125 µmol/L (1.4 mg/dL) are at increased risk for an accelerated decline in renal function and poor pregnancy outcome.[67-70]

CKD is universally classified into five stages according to the level of renal function (i.e., GFR) (Table 44-2). CKD stages 3 through 5 (GFR < 60 mL/min) affect approximately 1 in 250 women of childbearing age (20 to 39 years),[71] but due to reduced fertility and an increased rate of early miscarriage, pregnancy in these women is less common. Studies of CKD in pregnancy have mostly classified women on the basis of serum creatinine values, but we estimate that approximately 1 of 750 pregnancies are complicated by CKD stages 3, 4, or 5.[72,73] Some women are discovered to have CKD for the first time during pregnancy. Approximately 20% of women who develop early preeclampsia (≤30 weeks' gestation), especially those with heavy proteinuria, have previously unrecognized CKD.[74]

TABLE 44-2 STAGES OF CHRONIC KIDNEY DISEASE

Stage	Description	GFR*
1	Kidney damage with normal or increased GFR	≥90
2	Kidney damage with mildly decreased GFR	60-89
3	Moderately decreased GFR	30-59
4	Severely decreased GFR	15-29
5	Kidney failure	<15 or dialysis

*Glomerular filtration rate (GFR) reported as mL/min/1.73 m^2.
From the National Kidney Foundation: K/DOQI clinical practice guidelines for chronic kidney disease: Evaluation, classification and stratification. Am J Kidney Dis 39(Suppl 1):S1-S266, 2002.

Women with CKD are less able to make the renal adaptations characteristic of and essential to healthy pregnancy. Their inability to boost renal hormones often leads to normochromic normocytic anemia, reduced plasma volume expansion, and vitamin D deficiency.[75,76] The gestational rise in GFR is impaired in women with moderate renal impairment and usually absent in those with a serum creatinine level higher than 200 µmol/L (2.26 mg/dL).[68,77,78] If preeclampsia develops there is often a mild deterioration in renal function, but the addition of a prerenal insult, such as significant peripartum hemorrhage, can seriously threaten maternal renal function.

Renal Dysfunction and the Impact of Pregnancy

Mild Renal Impairment: Chronic Kidney Disease Stages 1 and 2

Most women with CKD who become pregnant have mild renal dysfunction, and pregnancy usually succeeds without affecting renal prognosis. However, complications such as preeclampsia, intrauterine fetal growth restriction, and preterm birth are more common (Table 44-3).[69,68]

A case-controlled study of 360 women with primary glomerulonephritis and only mild pre-pregnancy renal dysfunction (serum creatinine level less than 110 µmol/L), minimal proteinuria (<1 g/24 hr), and absent or well-controlled hypertension, showed that pregnancy had little or no adverse effect on long-term (up to 25 years) maternal renal function.[79] The situation is quite different for women who have moderate to severe renal impairment (CKD stages 3, 4, or 5).

Moderate to Severe Renal Impairment: Chronic Kidney Disease Stages 3 through 5

Small, mainly uncontrolled, retrospective studies have shown that women with the worst pre-pregnancy renal function are at greatest risk for an accelerated decline in renal function caused by pregnancy (see Table 44-3). Proteinuria and hypertension add to this risk.[68,70,77,80,81] One retrospective series of women with CKD (87 pregnancies) found that those with initially moderate renal impairment (serum creatinine level of 124 to 168 mmol/L or 1.4 to 1.9 mg/dL) had a 40% risk of a pregnancy-related decline in renal function, which persisted after delivery in about one half of those affected, whereas 13 (65%) of 20 women with severe renal impairment (i.e., serum creatinine level higher than 177 mmol/L or 2.0 mg/dL) had a decline in renal function

TABLE 44-3 PRE-PREGNANCY RENAL FUNCTION IN CHRONIC RENAL DISEASE WITH ESTIMATES FOR PREGNANCY OUTCOME (>24 WEEKS) AND IMPACT ON MATERNAL RENAL FUNCTION

Serum Creatinine Level µmol/L (mg/dL)	IUGR (%)	Preterm Delivery (%)	Preeclampsia (%)	Perinatal Deaths (%)	Loss of Renal Function* Pregnancy (%)	Persists after Delivery (%)	ESRF in 1 Year (%)
<125 (<1.4)	25	30	22	1	2	—	—
125-180 (1.4-2.0)	40	60	40	5	40	20	2
>180 (>2.0)	65	>95	60	10	70	50	35

*Estimates are based on literature from 1985 to 2007, with all pregnancies attaining at least 24 weeks' gestation.
ESRF, end-stage renal function; IUGR, intrauterine growth restriction.
Data from references 67-70, 72, 77, 78, 83, 165-169.

during the third trimester that persisted in almost all and deteriorated to end-stage renal failure in 7 (35%) of 20.[67,82]

The first *prospective* study to assess the rate of decline of maternal renal function before and after pregnancy in 49 women with pre-pregnancy CKD stages 3 to 5 confirmed these earlier observations.[70] Specifically, women with a pre-pregnancy eGFR less than 40 mL/min/1.73 m^2 and proteinuria level of more than 1 g in 24 hours, but not either factor alone, showed an accelerated decline in renal function after their pregnancy compared with before pregnancy. Chronic hypertension, which predisposes women to preeclampsia, may explain why those with milder renal dysfunction also have a gestational decline in renal function. This risk is reduced when hypertension is controlled.

Impact of Chronic Kidney Disease on Perinatal Outcome

Maternal hypertension, proteinuria, and recurrent urinary infection often coexist in women with CKD, and it is difficult to apportion the contribution that each factor makes to a poor pregnancy outcome. It appears, however, that each factor is individually and cumulatively detrimental to fetal outcome.[67,70,76,77] Although women with severe renal impairment have the greatest difficulty conceiving, the highest rate of miscarriage, and poorest fetal outcome, there is a spectrum of poor outcomes, including preeclampsia, fetal growth restriction, preterm delivery, and perinatal death, correlating with the level of renal dysfunction.[68,69,70,78,83]

Preconception Counseling

Initiating and sustaining pregnancy are related to the degree of functional impairment. Fertility is diminished as renal function falls. When the preconception serum creatinine level exceeds 280 µmol/L (3 mg/L), corresponding to a GFR of less than 25 mL/min, normal pregnancy is unusual; however, successes have been documented in women with moderate to severe disease, including some treated with dialysis because of accelerated maternal renal deterioration.[84]

Ideally, pregnancy is probably best restricted to women with preconception serum creatinine levels below 180 µmol/L (2 mg/dL) and a diastolic blood pressure of 90 mm Hg or less. If the patient has hypertension requiring more than one drug for control, prognosis becomes substantially poorer. Some clinicians extend this limit to 250 µmol/L (2.8 mg/dL), whereas others believe it should be no higher than 140 µmol/L (1.5 mg/dL). Whatever level is used, we reiterate that degrees of impairment not causing symptoms or disrupting homeostasis in nonpregnant individuals can still jeopardize pregnancy. Clinical complications such as hypertension, proteinuria, and infection increase the risk of complications at all levels of renal impairment.

A question should be asked: Is pregnancy advisable? If a woman with chronic renal disease wishes to have a family, the sooner she starts, the better. In some of these patients, renal function continues to decline with time. Women are not always counseled before conception. A patient with suspected or known renal disease may present already pregnant, and the question then becomes whether to continue the pregnancy.

Ideally, all women with CKD should be made aware of the risks pregnancy may have on their own long-term renal function and pregnancy outcome before they conceive. Folic acid (400 mg daily) should be given as usual around conception until at least 12 weeks' gestation. Low-dose aspirin (50 to 150 mg/day) should be started in early pregnancy to reduce risk of preeclampsia and improve perinatal outcome.[34] Regular drugs should be reviewed so that fetotoxic drugs (e.g., angiotensin-converting enzyme [ACE] inhibitors, angiotensin II receptor blockers) can be stopped as soon as pregnancy is confirmed.[85]

There are reports of women with severe chronic renal failure having successful pregnancies managed without dialysis.[86] In one woman, the serum creatinine level was 700 µmol/L (8 mg/dL) at the time of spontaneous delivery.[87] Dialysis has also been instituted prophylactically during pregnancy to increase the chances of a successful outcome.[88] Nevertheless, we believe that these women should not take additional health risks. The aim should be to preserve what little renal function remains and to achieve renal rehabilitation by dialysis and transplantation, after which the question of pregnancy can be considered if appropriate.

The literature that forms the basis of our views is primarily *retrospective*. Most patients described had only mild dysfunction, and women with greater dysfunctional disease were limited in number. Confirmation of any preconception guidelines requires definitive observational trials that must be prospective.

Antenatal Strategy and Decision Making

Patients should be seen at least at 2-week intervals or less until 32 weeks' gestation, after which assessment should be weekly. Routine serial antenatal observations should be supplemented with the following:

1. Assessment of renal function using serum creatinine levels and protein excretion using the protein to creatinine ratio on a spot urine sample on approximately a monthly basis

2. Careful monitoring of blood pressure for early detection of hypertension and treatment to keep blood pressure at 140/90 mm Hg or less
3. Early detection of superimposed preeclampsia, with checks of blood urea nitrogen, full blood cell count, liver function tests, blood pressure, and proteinuria
4. Biophysical assessment of fetal size, development, and well-being
5. Early detection of asymptomatic bacteriuria or confirmation of UTI every month

Renal Function

If renal function deteriorates, reversible causes should be sought, such as a UTI, subtle dehydration, or electrolyte imbalance, which is occasionally precipitated by inadvertent diuretic therapy. Near term, a 15% to 20% decrement in function, which affects serum creatinine levels minimally, is permissible. Failure to detect a reversible cause of a significant decrement is reason to end the pregnancy by elective delivery. When proteinuria occurs and persists but blood pressure is normal and renal function is preserved, the pregnancy can be allowed to continue.

Blood Pressure

Most of the specific risks of hypertension appear to be mediated through superimposed preeclampsia. There is still controversy about the incidence of preeclampsia in women with preexisting renal disease. The diagnosis cannot be made with certainty on clinical grounds alone because hypertension and proteinuria may be manifestations of the underlying renal disease. Treatment of hypertension in pregnancy is considered in Chapter 35.

High blood pressure in the presence of an underlying kidney disorder is treated more aggressively than are other hypertensive complications of pregnancy. This is done because such actions preserve function longer. Although diastolic levels of 100 mm Hg or less may be permissible in many pregnant women with underlying essential hypertension, a diastolic goal of 90 mm Hg or less should be set for patients with renal disease.

Fetal Surveillance and Timing of Delivery

Serial assessment of fetal well-being is essential because renal disease can be associated with intrauterine growth restriction, and when complications do arise, the judicious moment for intervention is influenced by fetal status. Current technology should minimize the risk of intrauterine fetal death and neonatal morbidity and mortality. Regardless of gestational age, most infants weighing 1500 g or more are better off in a special care nursery than in a hostile intrauterine environment. Deliberate preterm delivery may be necessary if renal function deteriorates substantially or for the usual maternal and fetal causes, such as uncontrollable hypertension, and signs adduced by monitoring of fetal jeopardy.

Renal Biopsy

Percutaneous renal biopsy is usually avoided in pregnancy because the plethoric kidney appears to be more prone to bleeding, especially in hypertensive pregnant women.[89] Renal biopsy, although not usually required for the diagnosis and management of preeclampsia, may be indicated if there is reason to suspect a renal lesion that could be successfully treated, especially in early pregnancy and up to 32 weeks' gestation, whilst permitting the pregnancy to continue.

Postpartum Care

It can take up to 3 months (occasionally longer) for the physiologic changes of pregnancy to disappear. During that time, close monitoring of fluid balance, renal function, and blood pressure and a further review of drug therapy are necessary. Breastfeeding should be encouraged in women with CKD, but is sometimes not possible for those with severe CKD. Information is still lacking on whether some immunosuppressive drugs appear in breast milk, but prednisolone, azathioprine, and ACE inhibitors are barely detectable in breast milk. Women who have heavy proteinuria associated with preeclampsia should be followed until the proteinuria disappears or a diagnosis of renal disease is made.

Problems Associated with Specific Kidney Diseases

In 1991, Imbasciati and Ponticelli[90] reviewed outcomes for more than 1000 patients with a variety of specific disorders, which were usually documented by kidney biopsy. In this review and in other editorials,[3] therapeutic abortions were excluded from calculation of pregnancy success rates and the discussion of the underlying factors.

Acute and Chronic Glomerulonephritis

The acute form of glomerulonephritis is a rare complication of pregnancy, and it can be mistaken for preeclampsia. For patients with chronic glomerulonephritis, one view warns of aggravation because of the hypercoagulable state accompanying pregnancy, with patients more prone to superimposed preeclampsia or hypertensive crises earlier in pregnancy. The consensus, however, is that if renal function is stable and hypertension is absent, most pregnancies are successful.[76] In a review of 906 pregnancies in 557 women, these generalizations were endorsed[90] and several specific issues were highlighted:

- Complications developed more frequently in women who already had some dysfunction or hypertension in early pregnancy.
- De novo hypertension or worsening of preexisting hypertension occurred in 25% of pregnancies but usually reverted after delivery, suggesting superimposed preeclampsia, a diagnosis that is not easy to confirm in this group of patients.
- In 10% of pregnancies, hypertension persisted after delivery, especially in patients with focal and segmental glomerulosclerosis, membranoproliferative glomerulonephritis, and IgA nephropathy.
- Higher rates of fetal loss observed in these women can be accounted for by the greater prevalence of severe hypertension and renal insufficiency.

Other, smaller series have endorsed these points. For example, pregnancy is well tolerated without effect on the course of the disease if blood pressure is normal and the GFR is higher than 70 mL/minute before conception.[76,91] With hypertension, the rate of live births is reduced if hypertension exists before pregnancy or is not well controlled during gestation.

Hereditary nephritis, an uncommon disorder, may first manifest or become exacerbated during pregnancy, but most gestations succeed. One variant of hereditary nephritis involves disordered platelet morphology and function. In these cases, pregnancy has been successful but was sometimes complicated by bleeding problems, especially at delivery.

Chronic Pyelonephritis

Chronic pyelonephritis (i.e., tubulointerstitial disease) in pregnancy may be infectious or noninfectious. The prognosis in pregnancy is similar to that for patients with glomerular disease; the outcome is best for patients with adequate renal function and normal blood pressure. Compared with nonpregnant women, pregnant women have a higher frequency of symptomatic infections, but these patients may have a more benign antenatal course than do women with glomerular disease.

Reflux Nephropathy

The term *reflux nephropathy* is used to describe renal morphologic and functional changes that relate to past (and usually present) vesicoureteric reflux, which often is complicated by recurrent infection. Opinions were once controversial, but with preserved renal function and no hypertension, fetal and maternal outcomes appear to be excellent.[77] For these patients, vigilance is still necessary to detect and treat UTIs (28% to 65%), with many physicians advocating prophylactic antibiotics. Unfortunately, reflux nephropathy is often associated with hypertension and moderate or severe renal dysfunction by the time these patients reach childbearing age, and such a scenario adversely affects pregnancy outcome. Specific obstetric concerns about affected patients include severe intrauterine growth restriction and the risk of sudden, rapid worsening of hypertension and renal function with accelerated progression to renal failure.[92]

Urolithiasis

The prevalence of urolithiasis in pregnancy is 0.03% to 0.35%.[93] Renal and ureteric calculi cause nonuterine abdominal pain severe enough to necessitate hospital admission during pregnancy. Most calculi are calcium oxalate (the more benign type), but occasionally, the more malicious struvite stones (e.g., staghorn) are seen. Uric acid and cystine are much less common.

Management should be conservative initially, with adequate hydration, appropriate antibiotic therapy, and pain relief with systemic analgesics. Most women pass their stones spontaneously. The use of continuous segmental (T11 to L2) epidural block has been advocated, as in nonpregnant patients with ureteric colic, and it may favorably influence spontaneous passage of the stones. With good pain relief, patients micturate without difficulty, move without assistance, and are less at risk for thromboembolic problems than if they are drowsy, nauseated, and bedridden with pain.

When there are complications that may require surgical intervention, pregnancy should not be a deterrent to limited IVU, even though the clinician may be reluctant to consider radiologic investigation. Specific clinical criteria should be met before a limited IVU is undertaken: microscopic hematuria, recurrent urinary tract symptoms, and sterile urine culture when pyelonephritis is suspected. The presence of two of these criteria indicates a diagnosis of calculi in 60% of women.[94]

Magnetic resonance urography can be used to avoid radiation exposure.[95] Another approach involves the cystoscopic placement of an intraureteral tube, or stent, between the bladder and kidney under local anesthesia.[96] The stent retains its position because it has a pigtail or J-like curve at each end (double-J), and it can be changed every 8 weeks to prevent encrustation. Early empiric use for presumed stone obstruction in pregnant women with flank pain is recommended by some, especially when hydration, analgesia, and antibiotics do not resolve pain or fever, and when the pregnancy is over, the usual x-ray evaluation is obtained and standard management resumed.[97]

Sonographically guided percutaneous nephrostomy is another effective and safe method of treating gravidas with ureteric colic or symptomatic obstructive hydronephrosis. The procedure is rapid, requires minimal anesthesia, and is preferable to retrograde stenting or more invasive surgery.

In patients with cystinuria, assiduous maintenance of high fluid intake is the mainstay of management. Although D-penicillamine appears relatively safe, it should be used only for severe cases, such as when urinary cystine excretion is known to be very high.[98]

Autosomal Dominant Polycystic Kidney Disease

Autosomal dominant polycystic kidney disease (ADPKD) is the most common genetic renal disorder, but it may remain undetected during pregnancy. Careful questioning for a history of familial problems and the use of ultrasonography may lead to earlier detection. Patients do well when functional impairment is minimal and hypertension is absent, as is often the case in childbearing years.[99] They do, however, have an increased incidence of hypertension late in pregnancy and a higher rate of perinatal mortality compared with that in pregnancies of sisters unaffected by this autosomal dominant disease.

Women with advanced renal failure are best advised against pregnancy, although use of prophylactic dialysis has been advocated, despite lack of controlled studies, for this type of patient.[100] If one or the other prospective parent has evidence of polycystic renal disease, the couple may seek genetic counseling. There is a 50% chance of transmitting the disease to the offspring, which is caused by two identified genes: *PKD1* (85%) and *PKD2* (15%). DNA probe techniques can make the diagnosis of ADPKD, but a significant number of ADPKD mutations are caused by multiple amino acid substitutions, which need to be interpreted with caution.[101]

Diabetic Nephropathy

Because many patients have had diabetes since childhood, they probably already have microscopic changes in the kidneys.[102] During pregnancy, diabetic women have an increased prevalence of covert bacteriuria (and may be more susceptible to symptomatic UTI), peripheral edema, and preeclampsia.[84]

Most women with diabetic nephropathy who become pregnant still have good renal function and demonstrate normal GFR increments (with perhaps significant proteinuria), and pregnancy does not accelerate renal deterioration.[103] There is, however, a report of diabetic women with moderate renal dysfunction (serum creatinine level above 125 μmol/L or ≤1.4 mg/dL) whose renal function permanently deteriorated in pregnancy compared with the changes before and afterward.[104] Such changes occurred despite good metabolic control and might have been related to hypertension, which often accelerates in the third trimester regardless of intensified treatment.[105] However, there were no controls for this study. The condition of diabetic patients with creatinine levels above 1.4 mg/dL who do not become pregnant often progresses rapidly to further renal failure.

Hypertension should be treated more intensively in diabetics. As with other renal disorders during pregnancy, we believe that more aggressive antihypertensive therapy is a reasonable objective. These patients often are treated with "renoprotecting" ACE inhibitors or angiotensin receptor blockers prescribed before conception, but these drugs should be stopped as soon as possible after conception to avoid teratogenic effects that become evident after 6 weeks' gestation.[85]

Systemic Lupus Erythematosus

Systemic lupus erythematosus (SLE) is a relatively common disease and has a predilection for women of childbearing age. Its coincidence with pregnancy poses complex clinical problems because of the profound disturbance of the immunologic system, multiorgan involvement, and complicated immunology of pregnancy itself.[84] The outcome of pregnancy for women with SLE is variable and to some extent unpredictable, so careful monitoring, especially for those women with lupus nephritis, is required (see Chapter 51).

Decisions regarding the status of the disease and the importance of having a child to the patient and her partner should be made on an individual basis. Most pregnancies succeed, especially when the maternal disease has been in complete clinical remission for 6 months before conception, even if there were marked pathologic changes in the original renal biopsy and heavy proteinuria in the early stages of the disease.[106] Continued signs of disease activity or increasing renal dysfunction reduces the likelihood of an uncomplicated pregnancy and the clinical course thereafter.

The effects of gestation on SLE activity and on the course of lupus nephritis have long been debated. Taking into account extrarenal manifestations and renal changes, at least 50% of women show some change in clinical status, often called a *lupus flare*.[107] Some increments in proteinuria or blood pressure may result from preeclampsia. Women with lupus nephritis and renal insufficiency (serum creatinine level higher than 125 μmol/L or 1.4 mg/dL) that antedates pregnancy have worse outcomes.

Lupus nephritis may sometimes become manifest during pregnancy, and when accompanied by hypertension and renal dysfunction, it may be mistaken for preeclampsia. Some patients experience relapse, occasionally severely in the puerperium; therefore, some clinicians prescribe or increase immunosuppression at this time.[108] It is our practice to increase immunosuppression only if there are signs of increased disease activity.

SLE serum contains an array of autoantibodies (i.e., lupus serum factor) against nucleic acids, nucleoproteins, cell-surface antigens, and phospholipids. Antiphospholipid antibodies exert a complicated effect on the coagulation system.[109] This led to the definition of a lupus anticoagulant, which is found in 5% to 10% of patients with SLE (see Chapter 40). Because treatment with low-molecular-weight heparin and aspirin may lead to successful pregnancies, it is important to screen for lupus anticoagulant in women with SLE and especially in those with a history of recurrent intrauterine death or thrombotic episodes to identify this particular cohort.

Periarteritis Nodosa

In contrast to lupus nephritis, the outcome of pregnancy in women with renal involvement as a result of periarteritis nodosa is very poor, largely because of the associated hypertension, which frequently is malignant. Many cases in the literature have involved maternal demise. However, this dismal prognosis is based primarily on selected anecdotal studies, and a few successful pregnancies have been reported. Still, until more data are available (perhaps through a registry), consideration of early therapeutic termination must be made in the best interests of maternal health.

Systemic Sclerosis

Scleroderma is a term that includes a heterogeneous group of limited and systemic conditions causing hardening of the skin. Systemic sclerosis implies involvement of skin and other sites, particularly certain internal organs. Renal involvement is thought to occur in about 60% of these patients, usually within 3 to 4 years of diagnosis. Manifestation may take one of three forms: sudden onset of malignant hypertension, rapidly progressive renal failure, or slowly increasing azotemia.[110]

The combination of systemic sclerosis and pregnancy is unusual because the disease occurs most often in the fourth and fifth decades, and affected patients are usually infertile. When it has its onset in pregnancy, there is a greater tendency for deterioration. Patients with scleroderma and no evidence of renal involvement before conception have developed severe kidney disease during gestation. There are also instances in which pregnancy has been uneventful and successful, but marked reactivation occurred unexpectedly in the puerperium. Most maternal deaths involve rapidly progressive scleroderma with severe pulmonary complications, infections, hypertension, and renal failure.

The extent of systemic involvement is probably more important than the duration of the disease, and limited, mild disease carries a better prognosis. Sclerosis usually spares the abdominal wall skin, but there is one report of hydronephrosis, presumed to have been caused by thickened skin and decreased abdominal wall compliance, in a twin pregnancy complicated by polyhydramnios.[111]

Wegener Granulomatosis

Information on the outcome of pregnancy in women with Wegener granulomatosis is scarce. Proteinuria (with or without hypertension) is common, and reports have described complicated and uneventful pregnancies.[112] Experience with cyclophosphamide (Cytoxan) in pregnancy is limited, and the risks to the embryo and fetus must be weighed in relation to the course of the disease if such therapy were to be withheld from the mother.

Previous Urinary Tract Surgery

Permanent urinary diversion is still used in the management of patients with congenital lower urinary tract defects, but its use for neurogenic bladder has declined since the introduction of self-catheterization. The most common complication of pregnancy is urinary infection. Premature labor occurs in 20%, and the use of prophylactic antibiotics throughout pregnancy may reduce its incidence. Decline in renal function may occur, invariably related to infection or intermittent obstruction, or both. With an ileal conduit, elevation and compression by the expanding uterus can cause outflow obstruction, whereas with a ureterosigmoid anastomosis, actual ureteral obstruction may occur. The changes usually reverse after delivery.

The mode of delivery is dictated by obstetric factors. Abnormal presentation accounts for a cesarean section rate of 25%. Vaginal delivery is safe, but because the continence of a ureterosigmoid anastomosis depends on an intact anal sphincter, this area must be protected with a mediolateral episiotomy.

During the past decade, urinary tract reconstruction by means of augmentation cystoplasty, with or without artificial genitourinary sphincter, has become more common. Deterioration of renal function and urinary tract obstruction or infection can occur at any time in pregnancy. Delivery by cesarean section is recommended for these gravidas because of the potential for disruption of the continence mechanism.

Solitary Kidney

Some patients have a congenital absence of one kidney or marked unilateral renal hypoplasia. Most, however, have had a previous nephrectomy because of pyelonephritis (with abscess or hydronephrosis), unilateral tuberculosis, congenital abnormalities, or a tumor. It is important to know the indication for and the time elapsed since the nephrectomy. In patients with an infectious or a structural renal problem, sequential pre-pregnancy investigation is needed to detect any persistent infection.

It makes no difference whether the right or left kidney remains, as long as it is located in the normal anatomic position. If function is normal and stable, women with this problem seem to tolerate pregnancy well despite the superimposition of GFR increments on already hyperfiltering nephrons. Single kidneys are most often associated with the rare instances of acute renal failure as a result of obstruction during pregnancy.

Ectopic kidneys (usually pelvic) are more vulnerable to infection and are associated with decreased fetal salvage, probably because of associated malformations of the urogenital tract. If infection occurs in a solitary kidney during pregnancy and does not quickly respond to antibiotics, termination may have to be considered for preservation of renal function.

Nephrotic Syndrome

The most common cause of nephrotic syndrome in late pregnancy is preeclampsia. Other causes include proliferative or membranoproliferative glomerulonephritis, lipid nephrosis, lupus nephritis, hereditary nephritis, diabetic nephropathy, renal vein thrombosis, and amyloidosis. Some of these conditions do not respond to steroids and may even be aggravated by them; this emphasizes the importance of a tissue diagnosis before steroid therapy is begun.[113]

If renal function is adequate and hypertension is absent, there should be few complications during pregnancy and good fetal outcome. However, physiologic changes occurring during gestation may mimic aggravation or exacerbation of disease. Increments in renal hemodynamics and increases in renal vein pressure may enhance protein excretion during pregnancy. Serum albumin levels usually decrease by 0.5 to 1.0 g/dL during normal pregnancy, and further decreases due to nephrotic syndrome may enhance the tendency toward fluid retention. Care must be taken with the use of diuretics to treat edema because reduced intravascular volume may reduce uteroplacental perfusion or aggravate the increased tendency to thrombotic episodes.

Human Immunodeficiency Virus—Associated Nephropathy

During the past 25 years, there have been increasing numbers of reports about a nephrotic syndrome and severe renal impairment in patients infected with the human immunodeficiency virus (HIV).[114] The condition is characterized by severe proteinuria, by bright echogenic kidneys, and often by rapid progression to end-stage renal disease. The distinctive features seen on histologic evaluation of renal biopsy are a collapsing glomerulosclerosis, visceral epithelial cell hypertrophy, and cystic tubular degenerative changes.[114] The incidence of this HIV-associated nephropathy appears to be increasing, particularly in the African-American population and in cases of intravenous drug abuse. Although few cases of this nephropathy have been reported in pregnant women, with the rising incidence of acquired immunodeficiency syndrome (AIDS), especially among black African women, this form of renal disease should be considered in HIV-infected patients presenting with severe proteinuria.

Factors Affecting Prognosis

Effects of Specific Disorders on Fetal Outcome

The problems associated with the specific disorders discussed in this section are summarized in Table 44-4. In general, we suggest that preserved renal function and the absence of hypertension before conception predict successful fetal outcome and few maternal complications, regardless of the nature of the disorder. These conclusions often are based on poorly controlled, retrospective data, underscoring the need for registries and for prospectively acquired data; there is only one such study.[70]

Effect of Pregnancy on Renal Disease/Remote Prognosis

Pregnancy does not adversely affect the natural history of the renal lesion if kidney dysfunction is minimal and hypertension is absent at conception, with the exception of certain collagen disorders. An important factor in remote prognosis is the sclerotic effect that hyperfiltration might already have had in the residual (intact) glomeruli of kidneys of patients with renal insufficiency. Further progressive loss of renal function can ensue in pregnancy, but this is not the case in animals when pregnancy is superimposed on experimental glomerulonephritis.[115]

The superimposition of pregnancy hyperfiltration on the compensatory changes already present in a single kidney may lessen the lifespan of the kidney. The crux of this hypothesis is the implication that increases in glomerular pressure or glomerular plasma flow cause sclerosis within the glomerulus and that in pregnancy further physiologic hyperfiltration augments the damage. In health, it seems unlikely that there are long-term renal sequelae.[115] More human and animal research is needed because patients with renal disease can have unpredicted, accelerated, and irreversible renal decline in pregnancy or immediately afterward, and the mechanisms are unknown.

Hemodialysis Patients and Pregnancy

It has been several decades since the first description of conception and successful delivery in a patient on chronic hemodialysis, and additional case reports and registry data have been published since then.[116-119] Any optimism must be tempered by the thought that clinicians are reluctant to publish failures or disasters, and consequently, the true incidence of unsuccessful pregnancies in women on dialysis cannot be determined. The high surgical abortion rate in these patients, although decreased from 40% in 1989 to 18% today, still indicates that those who become pregnant do so accidentally, probably because they are unaware that pregnancy is a possibility.

TABLE 44-4 CHRONIC RENAL DISEASE AND PREGNANCY

Renal Disease	Effects
Chronic glomerulonephritis and focal glomerular sclerosis (FGS)	Incidence of high blood pressure late in gestation is increased, but there usually is no adverse effect if renal function is preserved and hypertension is absent before gestation. Some disagree, believing coagulation changes in pregnancy exacerbate disease, especially immunoglobulin A (IgA) nephropathy, membranoproliferative glomerulonephritis, and FGS.
IgA nephropathy	Some cite risks of sudden escalating or uncontrolled hypertension and renal deterioration. Most find good outcomes when renal function is preserved.
Chronic pyelonephritis (infectious tubulointerstitial disease)	Bacteriuria occurs in pregnancy and may lead to exacerbation.
Reflux nephropathy	In the past, some emphasized risks of sudden escalating hypertension and worsening of renal function. Consensus now is that results are satisfactory when preconception function is only mildly affected and hypertension is absent. Vigilant screening for urinary tract infections is necessary.
Urolithiasis	Ureteral dilatation and stasis do not seem to affect natural history, but infections can become more frequent. Stents have been successfully placed, and sonographically controlled ureterostomy has been performed during gestation.
Polycystic kidney disease	Functional impairment and hypertension are usually minimal in childbearing years.
Diabetic nephropathy	There are no adverse effects of the renal lesion. Frequencies of infections, edema, and preeclampsia increase.
Systemic lupus erythematosus	Prognosis is most favorable if disease is in remission 6 or more months before conception. Some authorities increase steroid dosage in the immediate postpartum period.
Periarteritis nodosa	Fetal prognosis is poor. Disease is associated with maternal death. Therapeutic abortion should be considered.
Scleroderma	For onset during pregnancy, there can be rapid overall deterioration. Reactivation of quiescent scleroderma can occur during pregnancy and after delivery.
Previous urologic surgery	Depending on the original reason for surgery, there may be other malformations of the urogenital tract. Urinary tract infection is common during pregnancy, and renal function may undergo reversible decrease. No significant obstructive problem, but cesarean section may be necessary in case of abnormal presentation or to avoid disruption of the continence mechanism if artificial sphincters or neourethras are present.
After nephrectomy, solitary and pelvic kidney	Pregnancy is well tolerated. Condition may be associated with other malformations of the urogenital tract. Dystocia rarely occurs with a pelvic kidney.

Counseling and Early Pregnancy Assessment

Despite irregular or absent menstruation and impaired infertility, women on dialysis should use contraception if they wish to avoid pregnancy.[120] The introduction of recombinant human erythropoietin (rHuEPO) for the treatment of women with renal failure appears to be associated in some cases with return of normal menses (and ovulation), probably because of improved overall health.[121]

There are substantial arguments against pregnancy, not least of which are the risks to the patient (e.g., severe hypertension, cardiac failure, maternal death) and the fact that even when therapeutic termination of pregnancy is excluded, there is at the very best only a 40% to 50% likelihood of a successful outcome.[122] If only data since the late 1990s are considered, fetal survival seems to be improving, although maternal risk remains formidable (Table 44-5).[116]

Early diagnosis of pregnancy is difficult. A missed period is usually ignored. The mistake the clinician may make is failure to consider the possibility of pregnancy, and many of these patients have not been given contraception counseling. Resistance to rHuEPO or progression of anemia (i.e., hematocrit decrease by 8% of prepregnancy levels) can be a useful clue to early diagnosis of pregnancy. Urine pregnancy tests are unreliable, and definitive diagnosis and estimation of gestational age are best accomplished by sonar technology.

TABLE 44-5 ESTIMATES FOR PREGNANCY COMPLICATIONS AND OUTCOMES IN DIALYSIS PATIENTS

Complication or Outcome	Incidence or Timing*
Polyhydramnios	40%
Intrauterine growth restriction	90%
Preterm delivery	85%
Average gestational age at delivery	33 wk
Hypertension/preeclampsia	70%
(Severe)	15%
Surviving infant	
Conceived on dialysis	50%
Conceived before dialysis	75%

***Estimates are based on literature from 1992 to 2007, with all pregnancies attaining at least 24 weeks' gestation.**
Data from references 2, 88, 121, 123-127, 163, 164.

Antenatal Strategy and Decision Making

For a successful outcome, scrupulous attention must be paid to blood pressure control, fluid balance, increased hours of dialysis, and provision of good nutrition. Excellent publications should be consulted for more details.[116,123-127]

Dialysis Policy

Some patients show apparent increments in GFR even though the level of renal function is too poor to sustain life without hemodialysis, whereas other women remain completely anuric.[128] Women with some residual renal function and satisfactory daily urine volumes, in whom dialysis control is easier, are more likely to become pregnant and to sustain pregnancy.

Management of dialysis during pregnancy should mimic the physiologic changes of healthy pregnancy as closely as possible. This aim can be capsulated in seven points:

1. Maintain serum urea at less than 20 mmol/L (60 mg/dL), although some would argue lower (e.g., 15 mmol/L [<45 mg/dL]). This is likely to necessitate almost daily dialysis from the end of the first trimester
2. Avoid hypotension during dialysis, which could be damaging to the fetus. In late pregnancy, the gravid uterus and the supine posture may aggravate this by decreasing venous return.
3. Ensure good control of blood pressure, but consider excess fluid as a cause of hypertension.
4. Ensure minimal fluctuations in fluid balance, and limit volume changes.
5. Scrutinize carefully for preterm labor, because dialysis or uterine contractions with or without significant changes in fetal hemodynamics are associated.[127]
6. Watch calcium levels closely, and avoid hypercalcemia.
7. Limit interdialysis weight gain to about 1 kg until late pregnancy. After midpregnancy, the physician should take the classic 0.5 kg/wk weight gain into account when considering dry weight. This means at least a 50% increase in hours and frequency of dialysis. Frequent dialysis renders dietary management and control of weight gain much easier.

In one report from Saudi Arabia of 27 pregnancies in 22 women, only 10 went beyond 28 weeks' gestation, and 8 of these were successful.[124] Comparing the pregnancies that ended before 28 weeks with those that went beyond, the researchers found no significant differences in blood pressure, hemoglobin, creatinine levels, type of dialysate, obstetric history, or duration on hemodialysis, but the dialysis hours were significantly longer for the successful group.

Intensified Anemia Management

Patients with severe renal insufficiency are usually anemic. This anemia is aggravated further in pregnancy, and increased erythropoietin therapy and even blood transfusion may be needed, especially before delivery. Caution is necessary because erythropoietin therapy or transfusion may exacerbate hypertension and impair the ability to control circulatory overload, even with extra dialysis. Fluctuations in blood volume can be minimized if packed red cells are transfused during dialysis.

It appears that genetically engineered erythropoietin (rHuEPO) is well tolerated in pregnancy.[121,130] The theoretical risks of hypertension alluded to previously and thrombotic complications have not been cited. Invariably, rHuEPO requirements to maintain a target hematocrit of 30% increase until delivery[131] may attain 300 IU/kg/wk.[126] No adverse effects have been identified in neonates in whom normal hematologic indices and erythropoietin concentrations for gestational age suggest that rHuEPO does not have significant transplacental effects.

Unnecessary blood sampling should be avoided when there is anemia or a lack of venipuncture sites. The protocol for various tests usually performed in a particular unit should be followed strictly, with no more blood removed per venipuncture than is absolutely necessary.

Hypertension

Because patients with hypertension may have abnormal lipid profiles and possibly accelerated atherogenesis, it is difficult to predict the cardiovascular capacity to tolerate pregnancy. Diabetic women receiving dialysis who have become pregnant are those in whom cardiovascular problems are most evident. In these and other women with renal disease, a normotensive state at conception is reassuring. Unfortunately, blood pressure tends to be labile, and hypertension is a common problem, although it may be possible to help control it by dialysis.

Ensuring Good Maternal Nutrition

Despite more frequent dialysis, relatively free dietary intake should be discouraged. A daily oral intake of 70 g of protein, 1500 mg of calcium, 50 mM of potassium, and 80 mM of sodium is advised, with supplements of dialyzable vitamins, particularly folic acid. Vitamin D supplementation can be difficult to judge in patients who have had parathyroidectomy. In addition, the placenta produces hydroxyvitamin D, which is one reason why oral supplementation may have to be curtailed. All of this poses risks for fetal nutrition in addition to the fact that the exact impact of the uremic environment is difficult to assess. The use of parenteral nutrition supplementation in pregnancy in these gravidas has been advocated.[132]

Fetal Surveillance and Timing of Delivery

What has been said with regard to chronic renal disease applies here as well. Cesarean section should be necessary only for purely obstetric reasons. It could be argued that elective cesarean section in all cases may minimize potential problems during labor. Preterm labor is generally the rule and may commence during hemodialysis.[133] The role of cesarean section in this situation needs to be carefully considered.

Peritoneal Dialysis Patients and Pregnancy

Since 1976, continuous ambulatory peritoneal dialysis (CAPD) and continuous cycling peritoneal dialysis have been used more frequently in the management of patients with all forms of renal insufficiency. Several features of peritoneal dialysis make it an attractive approach for the management of renal failure in pregnancy:

- Maintenance of a more stable environment for the fetus in terms of fluid and electrolyte concentrations
- Avoidance of episodes of abrupt hypotension, a frequent occurrence during hemodialysis, which can cause fetal distress
- Continuous allowance for extracellular fluid volume control so that blood pressure control is augmented
- Better blood sugar control in patients with diabetes mellitus with the use of intraperitoneal insulin

Nevertheless, there appears to be no differences in outcome because of mode of renal replacement therapy (i.e., hemodialysis versus peritoneal dialysis), and there may even be greater infertility in patients receiving CAPD.[88,116] Peritoneal dialysis may not be able to keep up with the physiologic changes of pregnancy to the same extent as daily hemodialysis.

Peritonitis, which can be a severe complication of CAPD, accounts for most therapy failures in nonpregnant populations. Peritonitis superimposed on a pregnancy can present a confusing diagnostic picture and a whole series of treatment problems.

Renal Transplant Patients and Pregnancy

After transplantation, renal and endocrine functions return rapidly, and normal sexual activity can ensue.[134] About 1 in 50 women of childbearing age with a functioning renal transplant becomes pregnant. Of the conceptions, 40% do not go beyond the initial trimester because of spontaneous or therapeutic abortion. More than 90% of pregnancies that continue past the first trimester end successfully (Table 44-6).[75]

Allografting has been performed when the surgeons were unaware that the recipient was in early pregnancy.[135] Obstetric success in such cases does not negate the importance of contraception counseling for all patients with renal failure and the exclusion of pregnancy before transplantation.

Counseling and Early Pregnancy Assessment

A woman should be counseled from the time the various treatments for renal failure and the potential for optimal rehabilitation are discussed. Information regarding potential reproductive capacity must be included. Even after transplantation, stress will still be a major factor in everyday life, which will always have a baseline of uncertainty. Couples who want a child should be encouraged to discuss all the implications, including the harsh realities of maternal prospects of survival.[136]

Preconception Guidelines

Individual centers have their own guidelines.[137,138] For most, a wait of 12 to 18 months after transplantation is advised. This has turned out to be good advice, because by then, the patient will have recovered from the major surgery and any sequelae, graft function will have stabilized, and immunosuppression is likely to be at maintenance levels. If function is well maintained at 24 months, there also is a high probability of allograft survival at 5 years.

A suitable set of guidelines is given here, but the criteria are only relative:

1. Good general health for 12 to 18 months after transplantation, with comorbid factors under control
2. Stature compatible with good obstetric outcome
3. No or minimal proteinuria.
4. Absence of or well-controlled hypertension
5. No evidence of graft rejection
6. Absence of pelvicalyceal distention on a recent IVU or renal ultrasound
7. Stable renal function with a serum creatinine level of 180 μmol/L (2 mg/dL) or less and preferably less than 125 μmol/L (1.4 mg/dL)[139,140]
8. Drug therapy reduced to maintenance levels for prednisone (≤15 mg/day), azathioprine (≤2 mg/kg/day), cyclosporine (≤5 mg/kg/day), and tacrolimus (≤0.1 to 0.2 mg/kg/day)

Experience with newer immunosuppressive drugs (e.g., mycophenolate mofetil, sirolimus) is minimal, and current advice is to avoid their use in pregnancy unless stopping them would seriously endanger maternal health. Further information is keenly awaited about outcomes with the use of newer agents.

Pregnancy in the female transplant population and its ethical dilemmas have been comprehensively discussed in several publications, particularly those from a Consensus Conference on Reproductive Issues and Transplantation.[138,141,142] These issues do apply to all women with potentially serious medical conditions and their partners who want to become parents.

Ectopic Pregnancy

Ectopic pregnancy occurs in at least 0.5% of all conceptions. The diagnosis can be difficult because irregular bleeding and amenorrhea accompany deteriorating renal function or even an intrauterine pregnancy. Patients who have had previous urologic surgery, peritoneal dialysis, and pelvic inflammatory disease are at higher risk for ectopic pregnancy because of pelvic adhesions. Intrauterine contraceptive devices have a higher failure rate in immunosuppressed women. The main clinical problem is that symptoms of genuine pelvic pathology are erroneously attributed to the transplant.

Antenatal Strategy and Decision Making

Patients must be monitored as high-risk cases by an obstetrician and an experienced transplantation nephrologist. Management requires attention to serial assessment of renal function, diagnosis and treat-

TABLE 44-6 PRE-PREGNANCY RENAL FUNCTION IN RENAL TRANSPLANT RECIPIENTS WITH ESTIMATES FOR PREGNANCY OUTCOME (>24 WEEKS) AND IMPACT ON MATERNAL RENAL FUNCTION

Serum Creatinine Level μmol/L (mg/dL)	IUGR (%)	Preterm Delivery (%)	Preeclampsia (%)	Perinatal Deaths (%)	Loss of Renal Function*		
					Pregnancy (%)	Persists after Delivery (%)	ESRF in 1 year (%)
<125 (<1.4)	30	35	24	3	15	4	—
125-160 (1.4-1.85)	50	70	45	7	20	7	10
>160 (>1.85)	60	90	60	12	45	35	70

*Estimates are based on literature from 1991 to 2007, with all pregnancies attaining at least 24 weeks' gestation.
ESRF, end-stage renal function; IUGR, intrauterine growth restriction.
Data from references 139, 140, 145, 148, 158, 166, 170-177.

ment of rejection, blood pressure control, early diagnosis or prevention of anemia, treatment of any infection, and meticulous assessment of fetal well-being.

Antenatal visits should be at least at every 2 weeks up to 32 weeks and weekly thereafter. The following tests should be undertaken monthly:

- Complete blood cell count, including platelets
- Blood urea nitrogen
- Creatinine level
- Electrolyte levels
- Urate levels
- Twenty-four-hour creatinine clearance and protein excretion
- Midstream urine specimens for microscopy and culture

Liver function tests, plasma protein, and calcium and phosphate levels should be checked at 6-week intervals. Tests for cytomegalovirus and herpesvirus should be performed during each trimester if the initial findings are negative (see Chapter 38). Although immunosuppressive therapy is usually maintained at pre-pregnancy levels, adjustments may be needed if there are decreases in the maternal white blood cell and platelet counts. Hematinic agents should be prescribed if the various hematologic indices show deficiency.

Allograft Function

Serial data on renal function are needed to supplement routine antenatal observations (discussed earlier). The anatomic changes and the increased and then sustained GFR characteristic of early pregnancy are evident, even though the allograft is ectopic, denervated, potentially damaged by previous ischemia, and immunologically different from both recipient and fetus. The better the pre-pregnancy GFR, the greater the increment in pregnancy, and graft gender has no significant effect on the hyperfiltration response.[143] Transient reductions in GFR can occur during the third trimester and usually do not represent a deteriorating situation with permanent impairment. In 15% of patients, significant renal functional impairment develops during pregnancy and may persist after delivery. Because a gradual decline in function is common in nonpregnant patients, it is difficult to delineate a specific effect of pregnancy.

Subclinical chronic rejection with declining renal function may occur after an episode of acute rejection or if immunosuppression becomes suboptimal. Whether cyclosporine is more nephrotoxic in pregnancy compared with the blunting of augmentation in GFR in the nonpregnant patient is unknown. We recommend keeping cyclosporine and tacrolimus levels at the lower end of the therapeutic range during pregnancy, which usually necessitates a small rise in drug dose. Increases in proteinuria, often to abnormal levels, occur near term in 40% of patients; this regresses after delivery and, in the absence of hypertension, is not significant.

Allograft Rejection

Serious rejection episodes occur in 6% of pregnant allograft recipients. Although this incidence of rejection is no greater than that expected for nonpregnant transplant patients, it is unusual because it has been assumed that the privileged immunologic state of pregnancy could be beneficial. Rejection can occur in the puerperium and may be caused by return to a normal immune state (despite immunosuppression) or possibly by a rebound effect from the altered immunoresponsiveness of pregnancy.

Chronic rejection may be a problem in all recipients, having a progressive subclinical course. Whether a pregnancy influences the course of subclinical chronic rejection is unknown. No factors consistently predict which patients will experience allograft rejection during pregnancy. Some have hypothesized a nonimmune contribution to chronic graft failure because of the damaging effect of hyperfiltration through remnant nephrons, which is perhaps even exacerbated during pregnancy. From the clinical viewpoint, several points are important. Because rejection is difficult to diagnose, when any of the clinical hallmarks are present (e.g., fever, oliguria, deteriorating renal function, renal enlargement, tenderness), the diagnosis should be considered. Although ultrasonography may prove helpful in the nonpregnant setting, in the pregnant state, without renal biopsy, rejection cannot be distinguished from acute pyelonephritis, recurrent glomerulopathy, possibly severe preeclampsia, and even cyclosporine nephrotoxicity. Renal biopsy is indicated before aggressive anti-rejection therapy is instigated.

Immunosuppression

Immunosuppressive therapy is usually maintained at pre-pregnancy levels, but adjustments may be needed if the maternal leukocyte or platelet count decreases.[144,145] When white blood cell counts are maintained within physiologic limits for pregnancy, the neonate usually is born with a normal blood count. Azathioprine liver toxicity has been seen occasionally during pregnancy, and it responds to dose reduction. The National Transplantation Pregnancy Registry (NTPR), maintained by Vincent T. Armenti at Thomas Jefferson University in Philadelphia, is accruing data.[146,147]

Numerous adverse effects are attributed to cyclosporine in nonpregnant transplant recipients, including renal toxicity, hepatic dysfunction, chronic hypertension, tremor, convulsions, diabetogenic effects, hemolytic uremic syndrome, and neoplasia. In pregnancy, some of the maternal adaptations that normally occur may theoretically be blunted or abolished by cyclosporine, especially plasma volume expansion and renal hemodynamic augmentation. Data suggest that patients treated with cyclosporine have more hypertension (≈70%) and smaller infants (20% to 50%), but it is still too early for definitive conclusions.[140,148]

Newer agents such as mycophenolate mofetil (MMF/CellCept) and lymphocyte immune globulin (Atgam) are being prescribed more frequently for transplant recipients,[149] but there is little information about these agents in pregnancy. Orthodione (OKT3) is an IgG that crosses the placenta, but data are limited.[150] Some of the agents were originally considered to have a rescue role only for kidney and kidney-pancreas transplantations, but they are being used as primary immunosuppressants.[149]

Hypertension and Preeclampsia

At least 50% of patients have significant hypertension requiring medication before pregnancy (see Chapter 35). All medications should be reviewed. The appearance of hypertension or worsening of chronic hypertension in the third trimester, its relationship to deteriorating renal function, and the possibility of chronic underlying pathology and preeclampsia are diagnostic problems. Escalating hypertension, particularly before 28 weeks' gestation, is associated with adverse perinatal outcome,[151] which may be linked to covert cardiovascular changes that accompany or are aggravated by chronic hypertension. Preeclampsia is diagnosed clinically in about 30% of pregnancies with transplants.

Infections

Patients should be carefully monitored for all types of infection throughout pregnancy. Prophylactic antibiotics must be given before any surgical procedure, however trivial. The various viral infections that may be involved in these patients are discussed in Chapter 38.

Diabetes Mellitus

Pregnancies are increasingly reported in women whose renal failure was caused by juvenile onset type 1 diabetes mellitus. Pregnancy complications occur with at least twice the frequency seen in the nondiabetic patient, and this may result from the presence of generalized cardiovascular pathology, which is part of the metabolic risk factor syndrome.[152] Successful pregnancies are increasingly reported after confirmed pancreas-kidney allografting.

Fetal Surveillance and Timing of Delivery

The points given for chronic renal disease are equally applicable to transplantation patients. Preterm delivery is common (45% to 60%) because of intervention for obstetric reasons and the common occurrence of preterm labor or preterm rupture of membranes. Preterm labor frequently is associated with poor renal function.[144] However, gestational age is the crucial confounding variable associated with renal dysfunction and hypertension, and it needs adjusting when assessing influence on birth weight.

Vaginal delivery should be the aim, and there usually is no mechanical injury to the transplant. Unless there are specific obstetric problems, spontaneous onset of labor can be awaited.[153]

Management during Labor

Careful monitoring of maternal fluid balance, cardiovascular status, and temperature is essential, and aseptic technique is important for every procedure. Surgical induction of labor (i.e., amniotomy) and episiotomy warrant antibiotic coverage. Pain relief is conducted as for healthy women. Augmentation of steroids is necessary to cover delivery.

Role of Cesarean Section

The kidney does not usually obstruct the birth canal. Cesarean section is necessary for the usual obstetric reasons. Several factors are important when choosing the delivery route. Transplant recipients may have pelvic osteodystrophy related to previous renal failure (and dialysis) or prolonged steroid therapy, particularly before puberty. Antenatal diagnosis of these problems is important and permits the planning of elective cesarean delivery.

If there is a question of disproportion or kidney compression, simultaneous IVU and x-ray pelvimetry can be performed (with limitation of the IVU to one to three films) at 36 weeks' gestation. When a cesarean section is performed, a lower segment approach is usually feasible, although previous urologic surgery or peritonitis may make this difficult.

Pediatric Management

Immediate Problems

More than 50% of liveborn infants have no neonatal problems. Preterm delivery is common (45% to 60%), small-for-gestational-age (SGA) infants are delivered in 30% to 50% of cases, and the two factors occasionally coexist. Although management is the same as in neonates of other mothers, some specific problems exist. Adrenocortical insufficiency due to the maternal steroid therapy potentially increases the risk of overwhelming neonatal infection. There are anecdotal data associating tacrolimus with oligoanuria and hypokalemia in the neonate.[133]

Breastfeeding

There are substantial benefits to breastfeeding. It could be argued that because the infant has been exposed to immunosuppressive agents and their metabolites in pregnancy, breastfeeding should not be allowed. Little is known, however, about the quantities of these agents and their metabolites in breast milk and whether the levels are biologically trivial or substantial. Cyclosporine levels in breast milk are usually greater than those in a simultaneously taken blood sample. Until the many uncertainties are resolved, breastfeeding should not be encouraged or perhaps limited to 1 month in the first instance and the neonate monitored for healthy growth and well-being after that time. Azathioprine does not appear in breast milk,[154] but cyclosporine and tacrolimus do.[155]

Long-Term Assessment

Azathioprine can cause abnormalities in the chromosomes of leukocytes, which may take almost 2 years to disappear spontaneously. The sequelae could be eventual development of malignant tumors in affected offspring, autoimmune complications, or abnormalities in the reproductive performance in the next generation.[145] There are some worrisome animal data. For instance, fertility problems affect the female offspring of mice that have received low doses of 6-mercaptopurine, the major metabolite of azathioprine (equivalent to 3 mg/kg). These offspring subsequently proved to be sterile; if they conceived, they had smaller litters and more dead fetuses than did unexposed dams, with the inference that exposure in utero may not affect otherwise normal females until they attempt childbearing.[156] The long-term sequelae of in utero exposure to the newer immunosuppressants are unknown. However, to date, information about general progress in early childhood has been good.[157]

Maternal Follow-up after Pregnancy

The ultimate measure of transplant success is the long-term survival of the patient and the graft. Because it is only 30 years since this procedure became widely employed in the management of end-stage renal failure, few long-term data from sufficiently large series exist from which to draw conclusions. The long-term results for renal transplantation come from a period when many aspects of management would be unacceptable by current standards. Average survival figures for large numbers of patients worldwide indicate that about 90% of recipients of kidneys from related living donors are alive 5 years after transplantation. With cadaver kidneys, the figure is approximately 60%. If renal function was normal 2 years after transplantation, the survival rate increased to about 80%. This is why women are counseled to wait 1 to 2 years before considering a pregnancy, although the emerging view is that 1 year is sufficient.[138,141]

A major concern is that the mother may not survive or remain well enough to rear the child she bears. Pregnancy occasionally and sometimes unpredictably causes irreversible declines in renal function. However, the consensus is that pregnancy has no effect on graft function or survival provided graft function before pregnancy is satisfactory (ideally, a serum creatinine level less than 125 μmol/L or 1.4 mg/dL).[140,158] Repeated pregnancies do not adversely affect graft function or fetal development, provided that renal function is well preserved at the time of conception.[159,160] If the pre-pregnancy serum creatinine level is higher than 150 μmol/L (1.8 mg/dL) and there is drug-treated hypertension during pregnancy, there is poorer graft survival after pregnancy.[140]

Many women choose parenthood in an effort to reestablish a normal life and possibly in defiance of the sometimes negative attitudes of the medical establishment. More long-term studies are needed to assess this area, especially with the advent of newer immunosuppressive drugs, so that counseling can be based on recorded experience rather than clinical anecdote.

Contraception

It is unwise to offer the option of sterilization at the time of transplantation; this decision should not take place at that time. Oral contraceptives may cause or aggravate hypertension or thromboembolism and can produce subtle changes in the immune system, but this does not necessarily contraindicate their use.

An intrauterine contraceptive device (IUD) may aggravate menstrual problems, which may obscure signs and symptoms of abnormalities of early pregnancy, such as threatened abortion and ectopic pregnancy. The increased risk of pelvic infection associated with the IUD in an immunosuppressed patient makes this method worrisome. Because insertion or replacement of an IUD can be associated with bacteremia of vaginal origin, antibiotic coverage is essential at this time. The efficacy of the IUD may be reduced by immunosuppressive and anti-inflammatory agents, possibly because of modification of the leukocyte response. Careful counseling and follow-up are essential.

Gynecologic Problems

There is a danger that symptoms resulting from genuine pelvic pathology may be erroneously attributed to the transplant because of its location near the pelvis. Patients may be at slightly higher risk for ectopic pregnancy because of pelvic adhesions resulting from previous urologic surgery, pelvic inflammatory disease, or the overzealous use of IUDs. Diagnosis can be overlooked because irregular bleeding and amenorrhea may be associated with deteriorating renal function and intrauterine pregnancy.

Transplant recipients receiving immunosuppressive therapy have a malignancy rate estimated to be 100 times greater than normal, and the female genital tract is no exception.[161] This association is probably related to factors such as loss of immune surveillance, chronic immunosuppression allowing tumor proliferation, and prolonged antigenic stimulation of the reticuloendothelial system. Regular gynecologic assessment is essential. Management should be on conventional lines, with the outcome unlikely to be influenced by stopping or reducing immunosuppression.

Summary

Changes in the urinary tract during normal pregnancy are so marked that norms in the nonpregnant state cannot be used for obstetric management. Awareness of all gestational alterations is essential if kidney problems in pregnancy are to be suspected or detected and then handled correctly.

Lower urinary infections are no more common in pregnancy compared with sexually active nonpregnant women, but lower UTIs are more likely to ascend to cause pyelonephritis. Asymptomatic bacteriuria should be screened for every 4 to 6 weeks in women who have renal disease and treated. If there is more than one UTI, low-dose antibiotic prophylaxis should be given for the remainder of the pregnancy and until 6 weeks after delivery.

Most women with mild and moderate renal disease tolerate pregnancy well and have a successful obstetric outcome without adverse effect on the natural history of the underlying renal lesion. Crucial determinants are renal functional status at conception, the presence or absence of hypertension, and the type of renal disease. There have been disagreements regarding pregnancy outcome in the presence of focal glomerular sclerosis, IgA nephropathy, mesangioproliferative glomerulonephritis, and reflux disease, although the evidence seems to favor the importance of renal function before pregnancy. Patients with certain collagen disorders (especially periarteritis nodosa and scleroderma) do poorly. In general, prognosis is good if renal dysfunction is minimal and hypertension is absent.

Pregnancy in women receiving dialysis treatment can be excessively complicated. Increased frequency and duration of dialysis are needed to increase the likelihood of a successful pregnancy outcome. There is high fetal wastage at all stages of pregnancy, but especially in the first trimester. In the absence of severe maternal problems, the hazards of pregnancy in renal transplant recipients are minimal, and successful obstetric outcome is the rule.

The key to management of acute renal failure in pregnancy is to identify the cause of renal impairment and treat it. This often necessitates premature delivery in favor of maternal health.

References

1. Jeyabalan A, Conrad KP: Renal function during normal pregnancy and preeclampsia. Front Biosci 12:2425, 2007.
2. Hou S: Historical perspective of pregnancy in chronic renal disease. Adv Chronic Kidney Dis 14:116, 2007.
3. Lindheimer MD, Davison JM: Pregnancy and CKD: Any progress? Am J Kidney 49:729, 2007.
4. Little PJ: The incidence of urinary infection in 5000 pregnant women. Lancet 2:925-928, 1966.
5. Nowicki B: Urinary tract infection in pregnant women: Old dogmas and current concepts regarding pathogenesis. Curt Infect Dis Rep 4:529-535, 2000.
6. Kincaid Smith P, Bullen M: Bacteriuria in pregnancy. Lancet 191:359-399, 1965.
7. Campbell-Brown M, McFadyen IR, Seal DV, Stephenson ML: Is screening for bacteriuria in pregnancy worthwhile? BMJ 294:1579-1582, 1987.
8. Cunningham FG, Lucas MJ: Urinary tract infections complicating pregnancy. Baillieres Clin Obstet Gynaecol 8:353-373, 1994.
9. Tomson C: Urinary tract infection. In Warrell DA, Cox TM, Firth J, Benz EJ (eds): Oxford Textbook of Medicine, 4th ed. Oxford, UK, Oxford University Press, 2003, pp 420-433.
10. Tincello DG, Richmond DH: Evaluation of reagent strips in detecting asymptomatic bacteriuria in early pregnancy: Prospective case series. BMJ 316:435-437, 1998.
11. Smaill F, Vazquez JC: Antibiotics for asymptomatic bacteriuria in pregnancy. Cochrane Database Syst Rev (2):CD000490, 2007.
12. Romero R, Oyarzun E, Mazor M, et al: Meta-analysis of the relationship between asymptomatic bacteriuria and preterm delivery/low birth weight. Obstet Gynecol 73:576-582, 1989.
13. Whalley P: Bacteriuria of pregnancy. Am J Obstet Gynecol 97:723-738, 1967.
14. Villar J, Lydon-Rochelle MT, Gulmezoglu AM, Roganti A: Duration of treatment for asymptomatic bacteriuria during pregnancy. Cochrane Database Syst Rev (2):CD000491, 2000.
15. Vazquez JC, Villar J: Treatments for symptomatic urinary tract infections during pregnancy. Cochrane Database Syst Rev (3):CD002256, 2003.
16. Jamie WE, Edwards RK, Duff P: Antimicrobial susceptibility of gram-negative uropathogens isolated from obstetric patients. Infect Dis Obstet Gynecol 10:123-126, 2002.
17. Duff P: Antibiotic selection in obstetrics: Making cost-effective choices. Clin Obstet Gynecol 45:59-72, 2002.
18. Gait JE: Hemolytic reactions to nitrofurantoin in patients with glucose-6-phosphate dehydrogenase deficiency: Theory and practice. DICP 24:1210-1213, 1990.

19. Hernandez-Diaz S, Werler MM, Walker AM, Mitchell AA: Neural tube defects in relation to use of folic acid antagonists during pregnancy. Am J Epidemiol 153:961-968, 2001.
20. Dwyer PL, O'Reilly M: Recurrent urinary tract infection in the female. Curr Opin Obstet Gynecol 14:537-543, 2002.
21. Gilstrap LC, Cunningham FG, Whalley PJ: Acute pyelonephritis in pregnancy: An anterospective study. Obstet Gynecol 57:409-413, 1981.
22. Cunningham FG, Lucas, Hankins GD: Pulmonary injury complicating antepartum pyelonephritis. Am J Obstet Gynecol 156:797-807, 1987.
23. Towers CV, Kaminskas CM, Garite TJ, et al: Pulmonary injury associated with antepartum pyelonephritis: Can patients at risk be identified? Am J Obstet Gynecol 164:974-978, 1991.
24. Millar LK, DeBuque L, Wing DA: Uterine contraction frequency during treatment of pyelonephritis in pregnancy and subsequent risk of preterm birth. J Perinat Med 31:41-46, 2003.
25. Wing DA: Pyelonephritis in pregnancy. Treatment options for optimal outcomes. Drugs 61:2087-2096, 2001.
26. Dunlow SG, Duff P: Prevalence of antibiotic-resistant uropathogens in obstetric patients with acute pyelonephritis. Obstet Gynecol 76:241-245, 1990.
27. Spencer JA, Chahal R, Kelly A, et al: Evaluation of painful hydronephrosis in pregnancy: Magnetic resonance urographic patterns in physiological dilatation versus calculous obstruction. J Urol 171:256-260, 2004.
28. Sandberg T, Brorson JE: Efficacy of long-term antimicrobial prophylaxis after acute pyelonephritis in pregnancy. Scand J Infect Dis 23:221-223, 1991.
29. Redman CW, Sacks GP, Sargent IL: Preeclampsia: An excessive maternal inflammatory response to pregnancy. Am J Obstet Gynecol 180:499-506, 1999.
30. Poston L, Williams DJ: Vascular function in normal pregnancy and preeclampsia. In Hunt BJ, Poston L, M Schachter, Halliday A (eds): An Introduction to Vascular Biology. Cambridge, UK, Cambridge University Press, 2002, pp 198-425.
31. Spargo B, McCartney CP, Winemiller R: Glomerular capillary endotheliosis in toxaemia of pregnancy. Arch Pathol 593-599, 1959.
32. Drakely AJ, Le Roux PA, Anthony J, Penny J: Acute renal failure complicating severe pre-eclampsia requiring admission to an obstetric intensive care unit. Am J Obstet Gynecol 186:253-256, 2002.
33. Fink JC, Schwartz SM, Benedetti TJ, Stehman-Breen CO: Increased risk of adverse maternal and infant outcomes among women with renal disease. Paediatr Perinat Epidemiol 12:277-287, 1998.
34. Coomarasamy A, Honest H, Papaioannou S, et al: Aspirin for prevention of preeclampsia in women with historical risk factors: A systematic review. Obstet Gynecol 101:1319-1332, 2003.
35. Reiter L, Brown MA, Whitworth JA: Hypertension in pregnancy: The incidence of underlying renal disease and essential hypertension. Am J Kidney Dis 24:883-887, 1994.
36. Murakami S, Saitoh M, Kubo T, et al: Renal disease in women with severe preeclampsia or gestational proteinuria. Obstet Gynecol 96:945-949, 2000.
37. Bar J, Kaplan B, Wittenberg C, et al: Microalbuminuria after pregnancy complicated by pre-eclampsia. Nephrol Dial Transplant 14:1129-1132, 1999.
38. Bellamy L, Casas JP, Hingorani AD, Williams DJ: Pre-eclampsia and the risk of cardiovascular disease and cancer in later life: A systematic review and meta-analysis. BMJ 335:974, 2007.
39. Newman MG, Robichaux AG, Stedham CM, et al: Perinatal outcomes in preeclampsia that is complicated by massive proteinuria. Am J Obstet Gynecol 188:264-268, 2003.
40. Williams DJ, de Swiet M: Pathophysiology of pre-eclampsia. Intensive Care Med 23:620-629, 1997.
41. Confidential Enquiry into Maternal and Child Health (CEMACH): Why Mothers Die 2000-2002. Available at http://www.cemach.org.uk (accessed January 15, 2008).
42. Gilbert WM, Towner DR, Field NT, Anthony J: The safety and utility of pulmonary artery catheterization in severe preeclampsia and eclampsia. Am J Obstet Gynecol 182:1397-1403, 2000.
43. Keiseb J, Moodley J, Connolly CA: Comparison of the efficacy of continuous furosemide and low-dose dopamine infusion in preeclampsia/eclampsia related oliguria in the immediate postpartum period. Hypertens Pregnancy 21:225-234, 2002.
44. Boito SME, Struijk PC, Pop GAM, et al: The impact of maternal plasma volume expansion and antihypertensive treatment with intravenous dihydralazine on fetal and maternal haemodynamics during pre-eclampsia: A clinical, echo-Doppler and viscometric study. Ultrasound Obstet Gynecol 23:327-332, 2004.
45. Visser W, Wallenberg HCS: Maternal and perinatal outcome of temporizing management in 254 consecutive patients with severe pre-eclampsia remote from term. Eur J Obstet Gynecol Reprod Biol 63:147-154, 1995.
46. George JN: The association of pregnancy with thrombotic thrombocytopenic purpura-hemolytic uremic syndrome. Curr Opin Hematol 10:339-344, 2003.
47. Yarranton H, Machin SJ: An update on the pathogenesis and management of acquired thrombotic thrombocytopenic purpura. Curr Opin Neurol 16:367-373, 2003.
48. Bianchi V, Robles R, Alberio L, et al: Von Willebrand factor-cleaving protease (ADAMTS13) in thrombocytopenic disorders: A severely deficient activity is specific for thrombotic thrombocytopenic purpura. Blood 100:710-713, 2002.
49. Tsai HM, Lian EC: Antibodies to von Willebrand factor-cleaving protease in acute thrombotic thropurpura. N Engl J Med 339:1585-1594, 1998.
50. Mannucci PM, Canciani MT, Forza I, et al: Changes in health and disease of the metalloprotease that cleaves von Willebrand factor. Blood 98:2730-2735, 2001.
51. McMinn JR, George JN: Evaluation of women with clinically suspected thrombotic thrombocytopenic purpura-hemolytic uremic syndrome during pregnancy. J Clin Apheresis 16:202-209, 2001.
52. Rock GA, Shumak KH, Buskard NA, et al: Comparison of plasma exchange with plasma infusion in the treatment of thrombotic thrombocytopenic purpura. Canadian Apheresis Study Group. N Engl J Med 325:393-397, 1991.
53. Vesely SK, George JN, Lammle B, et al: ADAMTS13 activity in thrombotic thrombocytopenic purpura-hemolytic uremic syndrome: Relation to presenting features and clinical outcomes in a prospective cohort of 142 patients. Blood 102:60-68, 2003.
54. Bobbio-Pallavicini E, Gugliotta R, Centurioni R, et al: Antiplatelet agents in thrombotic thrombocytopenic purpura (TTP): Results of a randomised multicenter trial by the Italian Cooperative group for TTP. Haematologica 82:429-435, 1997.
55. Chugh KS, Jha V, Sakhuja V, Joshi K: Acute renal cortical necrosis—a study of 113 patients. Ren Fail 16:37-47, 1994.
56. Prakash J, Triathi K, Pandey LK, et al: Renal cortical necrosis in pregnancy-related acute renal failure. J Indian Med Assoc 94:227-229, 1996.
57. Pertuiset N, Grunfeld JP: Acute renal failure in pregnancy. Baillieres Clin Obstet Gynaecol 8:333-351, 1994.
58. Castro MA, Fassett MJ, Reynolds TB, et al: Reversible peripartum liver failure: A new perspective on the diagnosis, treatment, and cause of acute fatty liver of pregnancy, based on 29 consecutive cases. Am J Obstet Gynecol 181:389-395, 1999.
59. Yang Z, Yamada J, Zhao Y, et al: Prospective screening for pediatric mitochondrial trifunctional protein defects in pregnancies complicated by liver disease. JAMA 288:2163-2166, 2002.
60. Pereira SP, O'Donohue J, Wendon J, Williams R: Maternal and perinatal outcome in severe pregnancy-related liver disease. Hepatology 26:1258-1262, 1997.
61. Steiger RM, Boyd EL, Powers DR, et al: Acute maternal renal insufficiency in premature labor treated with indomethacin. Am J Perinatol 10:381-383, 1993.
62. Mor Y, Leibovitch I, Fridmans A, et al: Late post-reimplantation ureteral obstruction during pregnancy: A transient phenomenon. J Urol 170:845-848, 2003.
63. Greenwell TJ, Venn SN, Creighton S, et al: Pregnancy after lower urinary tract reconstruction for congenital abnormalities. BJU Int 92:773-777, 2003.

64. Bingham C, Ellard S, Cole TR, et al: Solitary functioning kidney and diverse genital tract malformations associated with hepatocyte nuclear factor-1beta mutations. Kidney Int 61:1243-1251, 2002.
65. Meyers SJ, Lee RV, Munschauer RW: Dilatation and nontraumatic rupture of the urinary tract during pregnancy: A review. Obstet Gynecol 66:809-815, 1985.
66. Smith MC, Moran P, Ward MK, Davison JM: Assessment of glomerular filtration rate during pregnancy using the MDRD formula. BJOG 115:109-112, 2008.
67. Jones DC, Hayslett JP: Outcome of pregnancy in women with moderate or severe renal insufficiency. N Engl J Med 335:226, 1996.
68. Jungers P, Chauveau D, Choukronn G, et al: Pregnancy in women with impaired renal function. Clin Nephrol 47:281, 1997.
69. Fischer MJ, Lehnerz SD, Hebert JR, Parikh CR: Kidney disease is an independent risk factor for adverse fetal and maternal outcomes in pregnancy. Am J Kidney Dis 43:415-423, 2004.
70. Imbasciati E, Gregorini G, Cabiddu G, et al, on behalf of the Collaborative Group Rene e Gravidanza of the Societa Italiana di Nefrolgia. Pregnancy in CKD stages 3-5: Maternal and fetal outcomes. Am J Kidney 49:753, 2007.
71. Centers for Disease Control and Prevention (CDC): Prevalence of chronic kidney disease and associated risk factors—United States, 1999-2004. MMWR Morb Mortal Wkly Rep 56:161-165, 2007.
72. Trevisan G, Ramos JG, Martins-Costa S, et al: Pregnancy in patients with chronic renal insufficiency at Hospital de Clinicas of Porto Alegre, Brazil. Ren Fail 26:29-34, 2004.
73. Fischer MJ: Chronic kidney disease and pregnancy: Maternal and fetal outcomes. Adv Chronic Kidney Dis 14:132-145, 2007.
74. Murakami S, Saitoh M, Kubo T, et al: Renal disease in women with severe preeclampsia or gestational proteinuria. Obstet Gynecol 96:945-949, 2000.
75. Davison JM, Baylis C: Pregnancy in patients with underlying renal disease. In Davison AM, Cameron JC, Grunfeld JP, Ponticelli C, et al (eds): Oxford Textbook of Clinical Nephrology. Oxford, UK, Oxford University Press, 2005, p 2243.
76. Williams D: Renal disorders. In James DK, Steer PJ, Weiner CP, Gonik B (eds): High Risk Pregnancy: Management Options, 3rd ed. Philadelphia, Elsevier, 2006, pp 1098-1124.
77. Jungers P, Houillier P, Chauveau D, et al: Pregnancy in women with reflux nephropathy. Kidney Int 50:593, 1996.
78. Cunningham FG, Cox SM, Harstad TW, et al: Chronic renal disease and pregnancy outcome. Am J Obstet Gynecol 163:453, 1990.
79. Jungers P, Houillier P, Forget D, et al: Influence of pregnancy on the course of primary chronic glomerulonephritis. Lancet 346:1122-1124, 1995.
80. Holley JL, Bernardini J, Quadri KHM, et al: Pregnancy outcomes in a prospective matched control study of pregnancy and renal disease. Clin Nephrol 45:77-82, 1996.
81. Hemmelder MH, de Zeeuw D, Fidler V, de Jong PE: Proteinuria: A risk factor for pregnancy-related renal function decline in primary glomerular disease? Am J Kidney Dis 26:187-192, 1995.
82. Epstein FH: Pregnancy and renal disease. N Engl J Med 335:277, 1996.
83. Rashid M, Rashid HM: Chronic renal insufficiency in pregnancy. Saudi Med J 24:709, 2003.
84. Jungers P, Chauveau D: Pregnancy in renal disease. Kidney Int 52:871, 1997.
85. Cooper WO, Hernandez-Diaz S, Arbogast PG, et al: Major congenital malformations after first-trimester exposure to ACE inhibitors. N Engl J Med 354:2443-2451, 2006.
86. Grunebaum AN, Minkoff H: Twin gestation and perinatal follow-up in a woman with severe chronic renal failure managed without dialysis: A case report. J Reprod Med 32:463, 1987.
87. Vogt K, Kensch G, Baumann U, et al: Successful pregnancy in advanced renal failure without dialysis. Paediatr Nephrol 3:189, 1989.
88. Okundaye IB, Abrinko P, Hou SH: Registry of pregnancy in dialysis patients. Am J Kidney Dis 31:766, 1998.
89. Lupton MGF, Williams DJ: The ethics of research on pregnant women: Is maternal consent sufficient? BJOG 111:1307-1312, 2004.
90. Imbasciati E, Ponticelli C: Pregnancy and renal disease: Predictors for fetal and maternal outcome. Am J Nephrol 11:353, 1991.
91. Abe S: Pregnancy in glomerulonephritic patients with decreased renal function. Hypertens Pregnancy 15:305, 1996.
92. Mansfield JT, Snow BW, Cartright PC, Wadsworth K: Complications of pregnancy in women after childhood reimplantation for vesicoureteral reflux: An update with 25 years follow-up. J Urol 154:787, 1995.
93. Butler EL, Cox SM, Eberts EG, et al: Symptomatic nephrolithiasis complicating pregnancy. Obstet Gynecol 96:753, 2000.
94. Miller DR, Kakkis J: Prognosis, management and outcome of obstructive renal disease in pregnancy. J Reprod Med 27:199, 1982.
95. Spencer JA, Chahal R, Kelly A, et al: Evaluation of painful hydronephrosis in pregnancy: Magnetic resonance urographic patterns in physiological dilatation versus calculus obstruction. J Urol 171:256-260, 2004.
96. Loughlin KR, Bailey RB: Internal ureteral stents for conservative management of ureteral calculi during pregnancy. N Engl J Med 315:1647, 1986.
97. Butler EL, Cox SM, Eberts EG, Cunningham FG: Symptomatic nephrolithiasis complicating pregnancy. Obstet Gynecol 96:753-756, 2000.
98. Gregory MC, Mansell MA: Pregnancy and cystinuria. Lancet 2:1158, 1983.
99. Chapman AB, Johnson AM, Gabow PA: Pregnancy outcome and its relationship to progression of renal failure in autosomal dominant polycystic renal disease. J Am Soc Nephrol 5:1178, 1994.
100. Alcalay M, Blau A, Barkai G, et al: Successful pregnancy in a patient with polycystic disease and advanced renal failure: The use of prophylactic dialysis. Am J Kidney 19:382, 1992.
101. Garcia-Gonzalez MA, Jones JG, Allen SK, et al: Evaluating the clinical utility of a molecular genetic test for polycystic kidney disease. Mol Genet Metab 92.160-167:2007.
102. Hayslett JP, Reece EA: Managing diabetic patients with nephropathy and other vascular complications. Baillieres Clin Obstet Gynaecol 8:405, 1994.
103. Combs GA, Kitzmiller JL: Diabetic nephropathy and pregnancy. Clin Obstet Gynecol 34:505, 1991.
104. Purdy LP, Hantsch CE, Molitch ME, et al: Effect of pregnancy on renal function in patients with moderate-to-severe diabetic renal insufficiency. Diabetes Care 19:1067, 1996.
105. Gordon M, Landon MB, Samuels P, et al: Perinatal outcome and long term follow up associated with modern management of diabetic nephropathy. Obstet Gynecol 87:401, 1996.
106. Rahman FZ, Rahman J, Al-Suleiman SA, Rahman MS: Pregnancy outcome in lupus nephropathy. Arch Gynecol Obstet 271:222-226, 2005.
107. Petri M: Systemic lupus erythematosus and pregnancy. Rheum Dis Clin North Am 20:87-118, 1994.
108. Huong DL, Wechsler B, Vauthier-Brouzes D, et al: Pregnancy in past or present lupus nephritis: A study of 32 pregnancies from a single centre. Ann Rheum Dis 60:599-604, 2001.
109. Cowchock FS, Reece EA, Bulasan D, et al: Repeated fetal losses associated with antiphospholipid antibodies: A collaborative randomised trial comparing prednisone with low dose heparin treatment. Am J Obstet Gynecol 166:1318, 1992.
110. Magmon R, Fejgin M: Scleroderma in pregnancy. Obstet Gynecol Surv 44:530, 1989.
111. Moore M, Saffran JE, Barol HSB, et al: Systemic sclerosis and pregnancy complicated by obstructive uropathy. Am J Obstet Gynecol 153:893, 1985.
112. Murty GE, Davison JM, Cameron DS: Wegener's granulomatosis complicating pregnancy: First report of a case with a tracheostomy. J Obstet Gynaecol 10:399, 1991.
113. Uribe LG, Thakur VD, Krane NK: Steroid-responsive nephrotic syndrome with renal insufficiency in the first trimester of pregnancy. Am J Obstet Gynecol 164:568, 1991.
114. Han Tm, Naicker S, Ramdial PK, Assounqa AG: A cross-sectional study of HIV-seropositive patients with varying degrees of proteinuria in South Africa. Kidney Int 69:2243-2250, 2006.
115. Baylis C: Glomerular filtration and volume regulation in gravid animal models. Baillieres Clin Obstet Gynaecol 1:789, 1994.

116. Okundaye I, Abrinko P, Hou S: Registry of pregnancy in dialysis patients. Am J Kidney Dis 31:766-773, 1998.
117. Chao A, Huang J-Y, Lien R, et al: Pregnancy in women who undergo long-term hemodialysis. Am J Obstet Gynecol 187:152-156, 2002.
118. Hou S: Pregnancy in dialysis patients: Where do we go from here? Semin Dial 16:376, 2003.
119. Hou S: Historical perspective of pregnancy in chronic kidney disease. Adv Chronic Kidney Dis 14:116-118, 2007.
120. Schmidt RJ, Holley JL: Fertility and contraception in end-stage renal disease. Adv Ren Replace Ther 5:38-44, 1998.
121. Braga J, Marques R, Blanco A, et al: Maternal and perinatal implications of the use of recombinant erythropoietin. Acta Obstet Gynecol Scand 75:449, 1996.
122. Hou S, Firanek C: Management of the pregnant dialysis patient. Adv Ren Replace Ther 5:24, 1998.
123. Redrow M, Cherem L, Elliott J, et al: Dialysis in the management of pregnant patients with renal insufficiency. Medicine (Baltimore) 67:199, 1988.
124. Souqiyyeh MZ, Huraib SO, Mohd Saleh A, et al: Pregnancy in chronic hemodialysis patients in the Kingdom of Saudi Arabia. Am J Kidney 19:235, 1992.
125. Bagon JA, Vernaeve H, De Muylder X, et al: Pregnancy and dialysis. Am J Kidney 31:756, 1998.
126. Haase M, Morgera S, Bamberg C, et al: A systematic approach to managing dialysis patients—the importance of an intensified haemodiafiltration protocol. Nephrol Dial Transplant 20:2537-2542, 2005.
127. Moranne O, Samouelian V, Lapeyre F, et al: A systematic approach to managing pregnant dialysis patients—the importance of an intensified haemodiafiltration protocol [author reply]. Nephrol Dial Transplant 21:1443, 2006.
128. Amoah E, Arab H: Pregnancy in a hemodialysis patient with no residual renal function. Am J Kidney 17:585, 1991.
129. Oosterhof H, Navis CJ, Go JG, et al: Pregnancy in patients on haemodialysis: Fetal monitoring by Doppler velocimetry of the umbilical artery. BJOG 100:1140, 1993.
130. McGregor E, Stewart G, Junor BJR: Successful use of recombinant human erythropoietin in pregnancy. Nephrol Dial Transplant 6:292, 1991.
131. Maruyama H, Arakawa M: Diagnostic clue to pregnancy in hemodialysis patients: Progressive anemia resistant to erythropoietin. J Am Soc Nephrol 8:A1130, 1997.
132. Brookhyser J, Wiggins K: Medical nutrition in pregnancy and kidney disease. Adv Ren Replace Ther 5:53, 1998.
133. Blowey DL, Warady BA: Neonatal outcome in pregnancies associated with renal replacement therapy. Adv Ren Replace Ther 5:45, 1998.
134. Anantharam P, Schmidt RJ: Sexual function in chronic kidney disease. Adv Chronic Kidney 14:119, 2007.
135. Lockwood GM, Ledger WL, Barlow DH: Successful pregnancy outcome in a renal transplant patient following in vitro fertilization. Hum Reprod 10:1528, 1995.
136. Stotland NL, Stotland NE: The mother and the burning building syndrome. Obstet Gynecol Surv 53:1, 1997.
137. Lindheimer MD, Katz AI: Pregnancy in the renal transplant patient. Am J Kidney 19:173, 1994.
138. McKay DB, Josephson MA: Pregnancy in recipients of solid organs—effects on mother and child. N Engl J Med 354:1281, 2006.
139. Crowe AV, Rustom R, Gradden C, et al: Pregnancy does not adversely affect renal transplant function. Q J Med 92:631,1999.
140. Sibanda N, Briggs JD, Davison JM, et al: Pregnancy after organ transplantation: A report from the UK Transplant Pregnancy Registry. Transplantation 83:1301, 2007.
141. McKay DB, Josephson MA, Armenti VT, et al: Reproduction and transplantation: Report on the AST Consensus Conference on Reproductive Issues and Transplantation. Am J Transplant 5:1592-1599, 2005.
142. Ross LF: Ethical considerations related to pregnancy in transplant recipients. N Engl J Med 354:1313, 2006.
143. Smith MC, Ward MK, Davison JM: Sex and the pregnant kidney: Does renal allograft gender influence gestational renal adaptation in renal transplant recipients? Transplant Proc 36:2639-2642, 2004.
144. Armenti VT, Moritz MJ, Davison JM: Drug safety issues in pregnancy following transplantation and immunosuppression: Effects and outcomes. Drug Saf 19:219, 1998.
145. Armenti VT, Moritz MJ, Davison JM: Immunosuppression in pregnancy: Choices for infant and maternal health. Drugs 62:2361, 2002.
146. Armenti VT, Radomski JS, Moritz MJ, et al: Report from National Transplantation Pregnancy Registry (NTPR): Outcome of pregnancy after transplantation. Clin Transpl 10:131, 2003.
147. Armenti VT, Moritz MJ, Davison JM: Pregnancy following transplantation. In James DK, Steel J, Weiner CP, Gonik B (eds): High Risk Pregnancy: Management Options, 3rd ed. Philadelphia, Elsevier Science, 2006, p 1174.
148. Fischer T, Neumayer HH, Fischer R, et al: Effect of pregnancy on long-term kidney function in renal transplant recipients treated with cyclosporine and with azathioprine. Am J Transplant 5:2732, 2005.
149. Andrews PA: Renal transplantation. BMJ 324:530, 2002.
150. Ghandour FZ, Knauss TC, Hricik DE: Immunosuppressive drugs in pregnancy. Adv Ren Replace Ther 5:31,1998.
151. Sturgiss SN, Davison JM: Perinatal outcome in renal allograft recipients: Prognostic significance of hypertension and renal function before and during pregnancy. Obstet Gynecol 78:573, 1991.
152. Dimeny E, Fellström B: Metabolic abnormalities in renal transplant recipients: Risk factors and prediction of graft dysfunction? Nephrol Dial Transplant 12:21, 1997.
153. Hussey MJ, Pombar X: Obstetric care for renal allograft recipients or for women treated with hemodialysis or peritoneal dialysis during pregnancy. Adv Ren Replace Ther 5:3, 1998.
154. Gardner SJ, Gearry RB, Roberts RL, et al: Exposure to thiopurine drugs through breast milk is low based on metabolic concentrations in mother-infant pairs. Brit J Clin Pharmacol 62:453, 2006.
155. French AE, Soldin SJ, Soldin OP, et al: Milk transfer and neonatal safety of tacrolimus. Ann Pharmacother 37:815, 2003.
156. Reimers TJ, Sluss PM: 6-Mercaptopurine treatment of pregnant mice: Effects on second and third generations. Science 202:65, 1978.
157. Willis FR, Findlay CA, Gorrie MJ, et al: Children of renal transplant recipient mothers. Paediatr Child Health 36:230-235, 2000.
158. Bar J, Ben Harousch A, Mor E, et al: Pregnancy after renal transplantation—effect on 15 year graft survival. Hypertens Pregnancy 23(Suppl 1):126, 2004.
159. Ehrich JHH, Loirat C, Davison JM, et al: Repeated successful pregnancies after kidney transplantation in 102 women. Nephrol Dial Transplant 11:1312, 1996.
160. Owda AK, Abdalla AH, Al-Sulaiman, MH, et al: No evidence of functional deterioration of renal graft after repeated pregnancies a report on 3 women with 17 pregnancies. Nephrol Dial Transplant 13:1281, 1998.
161. Newstead CG: Assessment of risk of cancer after renal transplantation. Lancet 351:610, 1998.
162. National Kidney Foundation. K/DOQI clinical practice guidelines for chronic kidney disease: Evaluation, classification and stratification. Am J Kidney Dis 39(Suppl 1):S1-S266, 2002.
163. Chan WS, Okun N, Kjellstrand CM: Pregnancy in chronic dialysis: A review and analysis of the literature. Int J Artif Organs 21:259-268, 1998.
164. Reddy SS, Holley JL: Management of the pregnant chronic dialysis patient. Adv Chronic Kidney Dis 14:146-155, 1007.
165. Hou S, Grossman SD, Madias NE, et al: Pregnancy in women with renal disease and moderate renal insufficiency. Am J Med 78:185-194, 1985.
166. Haugen G, Fauchald P, Sodal G, et al: Pregnancy outcome in renal allograft recipients: Influence of ciclosporin A. Eur J Obstet Gynecol Reprod Biol 21;39:25-29, 1991.
167. Abe S: The influence of pregnancy on the long-term renal prognosis of IgA nephropathy. Clin Nephrol 41:61-64, 1994.
168. Bar J, Ben-Rafael Z, Padoa A, et al: Prediction of pregnancy outcome in subgroups of women with renal disease. Clin Nephrol 53:437-444; 2000.

169. Modena A, Hoffman M, Tolosa JE: Chronic renal disease in pregnancy: A modern approach to predicting outcome. Am J Obstet Gynecol 193:S86, 2006.
170. Fischer T, Neumayer HH, Fischer R, et al: Effect of pregnancy on long-term kidney function in renal transplant recipients treated with cyclosporine and with azathioprine. Am J Transplant 5:2732-2739, 2005.
171. Davison JM: Towards long-term graft survival in renal transplantation: Pregnancy. Nephrol Dial Transplant 10(Suppl 1):85-89, 1995.
172. Sturgiss SN, Davison JM: Effect of pregnancy on the long-term function of renal allografts: An update. Am J Kidney Dis 26:54-56, 1995.
173. Nojima M, Ihara H, Ichikawa Y, et al: Influence of pregnancy on graft function after renal transplantation. Transplant Proc 28:1582-1585, 1996.
174. Toma H, Tanabe K, Tokumoto T, et al: Pregnancy in women receiving renal dialysis or transplantation in Japan: A nationwide survey. Nephrol Dial Transplant 14:1511-1516, 1999.
175. Miranda CT, Melarango C, Camara NO, et al: Adverse effects of pregnancy on renal allograft function. Transplant Proc 34:506-507, 2002.
176. Thompson BC, Kingdon EJ, Tuck SM, et al: Pregnancy in renal transplant recipients: The Royal Free Hospital experience. QJM 96:837-844, 2003.
177. Rahamimov R, Ben-Haroush A, Wittenberg C, et al: Pregnancy in renal transplant recipients: Long-term effect on patient and graft survival. A single-center experience. Transplantation 81:660-664, 2006.

Chapter 45

Respiratory Diseases in Pregnancy

Janice E. Whitty, MD, and Mitchell P. Dombrowski, MD

Proper functioning of the cardiorespiratory system is imperative to achieve adequate oxygenation of maternal and fetal tissues. The maternal cardiorespiratory system undergoes significant changes during gestation to optimize oxygen delivery to the fetus and maternal tissues. Pulmonary disease is one of the most frequent maternal complications during pregnancy, and it may result in significant morbidity or mortality for the mother and her fetus. Depending on the specific diagnosis, other maternal complications of pregnancy may have an adverse or positive impact on the pulmonary function of the gravida.

In this chapter, we briefly review the physiologic adaptations of the respiratory system that occur during gestation. Specific respiratory diseases that occur in pregnancy and the effects of the disease on pregnancy and pregnancy on the disease are discussed. The obstetrician should realize that most diagnostic tests useful in evaluating pulmonary function during gestation are not harmful to the fetus and, if indicated, should be performed. Most medications used to treat respiratory disease in pregnancy are also well tolerated by the fetus. With few exceptions, the diagnostic and treatment algorithms for respiratory disease closely resemble those used for a nonpregnant woman.

Physiologic Changes of the Respiratory System

Because there is no increase in respiratory rate, the increase in maternal minute ventilation results from an increase in tidal volume.[1] The almost 50% increase in tidal volume occurs at the expense of an 18% decrease in the functional residual capacity. The resulting hyperventilation of pregnancy results in a compensated respiratory alkalosis (i.e., arterial partial pressure of carbon dioxide [$PaCO_2$] ≤ 30 mm Hg) and a modest increase in arterial oxygenation tension (i.e., 101 to 104 mm Hg).[2] The $PaCO_2$ decreases early in pregnancy in parallel with the change in ventilation; however, a further progressive decrease in $PaCO_2$ may occur.[3] The decrease in $PaCO_2$ is even greater at altitudes where the mother exhibits compensatory hyperventilation in an attempt to maintain the arterial partial pressure of oxygen as high as possible. The decrease in $PaCO_2$ is matched by an equivalent increase in renal excretion of and decrease in plasma bicarbonate concentration; therefore, arterial pH is not altered from the normal nonpregnant level of about 7.4.

It has been suggested that the hyperventilation of pregnancy results primarily from progesterone acting as a respiratory stimulant.[4] Because hyperventilation has been observed during the luteal phase of the menstrual cycle and progesterone can produce similar changes in nonpregnant women, it is likely that this phenomenon results from progestational influences.[5,6] The $PaCO_2$ is linearly and inversely related to the log of the progesterone concentration.[7] Wilbrand and colleagues[8] reported that progesterone lowers the carbon dioxide threshold of the respiratory center. During pregnancy, the sensitivity of the respiratory center increases[9] so that an increase in $PaCO_2$ of 1 mm Hg increases ventilation by 6 L/min in pregnancy, compared with 1.5 L/min in the nonpregnant state.[1,10,11] It is possible that progesterone acts as a primary stimulant to the respiratory center independently of any change in carbon dioxide sensitivity or threshold.[4] In addition to stimulating ventilation, progesterone may also increase levels of carbonic anhydrase B in the red blood cell.[12] Schenker and associates[13] reported that carbonic anhydrase levels increase in pregnant patients and in women taking oral contraceptives. An increase in the carbonic anhydrase level facilitates carbon dioxide transfer and tends to decrease $PaCO_2$ independently of any change in ventilation. This respiratory stimulant effect of progesterone has been used in the treatment of respiratory failure and emphysema.[6,14,15]

During gestation, ventilation is increased by the rise in tidal volume from approximately 500 to 700 mL in each breath.[1,16-18] Because there is no change in respiratory rate, minute ventilation rises from about 7.5 to 10.5 L/min.[11,17,19] Minute ventilation increases in the first trimester and remains at that level throughout pregnancy. The physiologic dead space is increased by about 60 mL in pregnancy. This may result from dilation of the small airways.[11] Residual volume is reduced by about 20%,[16] from 1200 to 1000 mL.[20-22] The vital capacity, which is the maximum volume of gas that can be expired after a maximum inspiration, does not change in pregnancy.[16,21-25]

Anatomic Changes of the Respiratory System

Observed changes in the configuration of the chest during pregnancy are in keeping with the findings of no change in vital capacity and a reduction in residual volume. The effect of pregnancy on pulmonary mechanics has been compared with the effect of a pneumoperitoneum. In both situations, the residual lung volume is decreased, but ventilation remains unimpaired. Radiologic studies performed early in pregnancy have shown that the subcostal angle increases from 68 to 103 degrees before there is any mechanical pressure from the enlarging uterus.[26] The level of the diaphragm rises by about 4 cm, and the transverse diameter of the chest increases by 2 cm.[27-29] These changes account for the decrease in residual volume because the lungs are relatively compressed during forced expiration; however, the excursion of the diaphragm in respiration increases by about 1.5 cm in pregnancy compared with the nonpregnant state.[29,30]

Oxygen Delivery and Consumption

Oxygen Delivery

All tissues require oxygen for the combustion of organic compounds to fuel cellular metabolism. The cardiopulmonary system delivers a continuous supply of oxygen and other essential substrates to tissues. Oxygen delivery depends on oxygenation of blood in the lungs, oxygen-carrying capacity of the blood, and cardiac output.[31] Under normal conditions, oxygen delivery exceeds oxygen consumption by about 75%.[32] The amount of oxygen delivered is determined by the cardiac output (CO, L/min) times the arterial oxygen content (CaO_2, mL/O_2/min):

$$\text{Oxygen delivery} = CO \times CaO_2 \times 10 \text{ (700 to 1400 mL/min)}$$

The arterial oxygen content is determined by the amount of oxygen that is bound to hemoglobin (i.e., arterial blood saturation with oxygen [SaO_2]) and by the amount of oxygen that is dissolved in plasma (i.e., arterial partial pressure of oxygen [$PaO_2 \times 0.0031$]):

$$CaO_2 = (\text{hemoglobin} \times 1.34 \times SaO_2) + (PaO_2 \times 0.0031)$$
$$\text{(16 to 22 mL } O_2\text{/dL)}$$

As can be seen in this formula, the amount of oxygen dissolved in plasma is negligible, and the arterial oxygen content therefore depends largely on hemoglobin concentration and arterial oxygen saturation. Oxygen delivery can be impaired by conditions that affect arterial oxygen content or cardiac output (flow), or both. Anemia leads to low arterial oxygen content because of a lack of hemoglobin binding sites for oxygen. Carbon monoxide poisoning likewise decreases oxyhemoglobin because of blockage of binding sites for oxygen. The patient with hypoxemic respiratory failure does not have sufficient oxygen available to saturate the hemoglobin molecule. Desaturated hemoglobin is altered structurally such that it has a diminished affinity for oxygen.[33]

The amount of oxygen available to tissues also is affected by the affinity of the hemoglobin molecule for oxygen. The oxyhemoglobin dissociation curve (Fig. 45-1) and the conditions that influence the binding of oxygen negatively or positively must be considered when attempts are made to maximize oxygen delivery.[34] An increase in the plasma pH level or a decrease in temperature or the concentration of 2,3-diphosphoglycerate can increase hemoglobin affinity for oxygen, shifting the curve to the left and resulting in diminished tissue oxygenation. If the plasma pH level, temperature, or 2,3-diphosphoglycerate level increases, hemoglobin affinity for oxygen decreases, and more oxygen is available to tissues (see Fig. 45-1).[34]

In certain clinical conditions, such as septic shock and adult respiratory distress syndrome, there is maldistribution of flow relative to oxygen demand, leading to diminished delivery and consumption of oxygen. The release of vasoactive substances is hypothesized to result in the loss of normal mechanisms of vascular autoregulation, producing regional and microcirculatory imbalances in blood flow.[35] This mismatching of blood flow with metabolic demand causes excessive blood flow to some areas and relative hypoperfusion of other areas, limiting optimal systemic use of oxygen.[35] The patient with diminished cardiac output resulting from hypovolemia or pump failure is unable to distribute oxygenated blood to tissues. Therapy directed at increasing the volume with normal saline or with blood if the hemoglobin

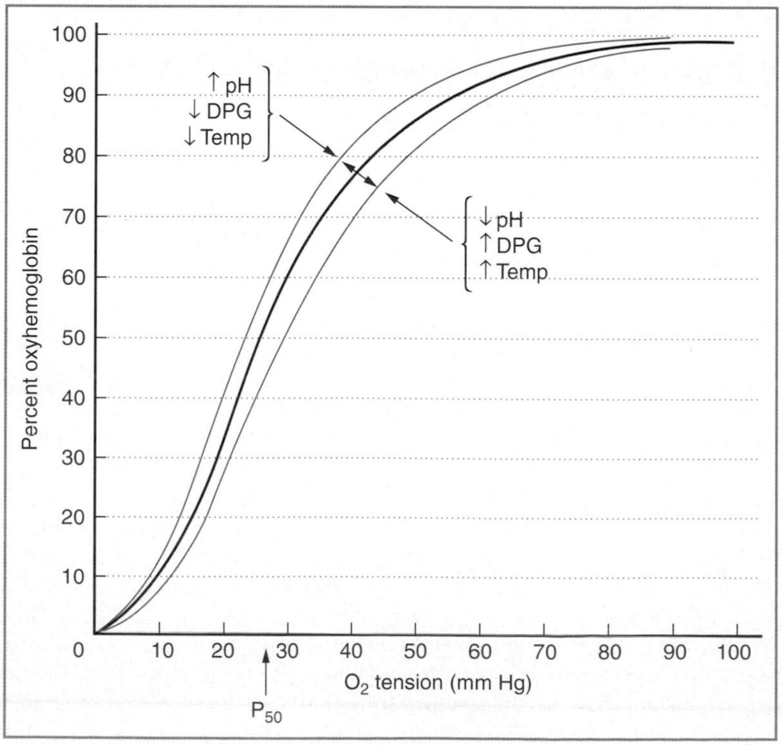

FIGURE 45-1 The oxygen-binding curve for human hemoglobin A under physiologic conditions *(red curve)*. The affinity is shifted by changes in pH, diphosphoglycerate (DPG) concentration, and temperature. P_{50} is the oxygen tension at one-half saturation.

level is less than 10 g/dL increases delivery of oxygen in the hypovolemic patient. The patient with cardiac failure may benefit from inotropic support and afterload reduction in addition to supplementation of intravascular volume.

Relationship of Oxygen Delivery to Consumption

Oxygen consumption is the product of the arteriovenous oxygen content difference ($C_{(a-v)}O_2$) and cardiac output (CO). Under normal conditions, oxygen consumption is a direct function of the metabolic rate[36]:

$$\text{Oxygen consumption} = C_{(a-v)}O_2 \times CO \times 10$$
$$(180 \text{ to } 280 \text{ mL/min})$$

The oxygen extraction ratio is the fraction of delivered oxygen that actually is consumed:

$$\text{Oxygen extraction ratio} = O_2 \text{ consumption}/O_2 \text{ delivery } (0.25)$$

The normal oxygen extraction ratio is about 25%. A rise in the oxygen extraction ratio is a compensatory mechanism used when oxygen delivery is inadequate for the level of metabolic activity. A subnormal value suggests flow maldistribution, peripheral diffusion defects, or functional shunting.[36] As the supply of oxygen is reduced, the fraction extracted from blood increases and oxygen consumption is maintained. If a severe reduction in oxygen delivery occurs, the limits of oxygen extraction are reached, tissues are unable to sustain aerobic energy production, and consumption decreases. The level of oxygen delivery at which oxygen consumption begins to decrease is called *critical oxygen delivery* (Fig. 45-2).[37] At the critical oxygen delivery level, tissues begin to use anaerobic glycolysis, with resultant lactate production and metabolic acidosis.[37] If oxygen deprivation continues, irreversible tissue damage and death ensue.

Mixed Venous Oxygenation

The mixed venous oxygen tension and mixed venous oxygen saturation ($S\bar{v}O_2$) are parameters of tissue oxygenation.[37] The normal mixed venous oxygen tension is 40 mm Hg with a saturation of 73%. Saturations less than 60% are abnormally low. These parameters can be measured directly by obtaining a blood sample from the distal port of the pulmonary artery catheter. The $S\bar{v}O_2$ also can be measured continuously with special pulmonary artery catheters equipped with fiberoptics. Mixed venous oxygenation is a reliable parameter in the patient with hypoxemia or low cardiac output, but findings must be interpreted with caution. When the $S\bar{v}O_2$ is low, oxygen delivery can be assumed to be low. However, normal or high $S\bar{v}O_2$ values do not guarantee that tissues are well oxygenated. In conditions such as septic shock and adult respiratory distress syndrome, the maldistribution of systemic flow may lead to an abnormally high $S\bar{v}O_2$ value in the face of severe tissue hypoxia.[35] The oxygen dissociation curve must be considered when interpreting the $S\bar{v}O_2$ as an indicator of tissue oxygenation.[33] Conditions that result in a left shift of the curve cause the venous oxygen saturation to be normal or high, even when the mixed venous oxygen content is low. $S\bar{v}O_2$ is useful for monitoring trends in a particular patient, because a significant decrease occurs when oxygen delivery has decreased because of hypoxemia or a decrease in cardiac output.

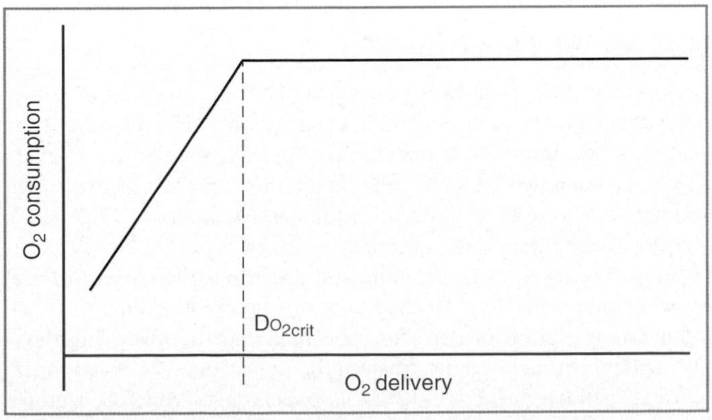

FIGURE 45-2 Relationship of oxygen consumption (Vo_2) and oxygen delivery (Do_2). At the point of critical oxygen delivery, tissues begin to use anaerobic glycolysis, with resultant lactate production and metabolic acidosis. If the oxygen deprivation continues, irreversible tissue damage and death ensue.

Oxygen Delivery and Consumption in Pregnancy

The physiologic anemia of pregnancy results in a reduction in the hemoglobin concentration and arterial oxygen content. Oxygen delivery is maintained at or above normal despite this because of the 50% increase in cardiac output. The pregnant woman therefore depends on cardiac output for maintenance of oxygen delivery more than the nonpregnant patient.[38] Oxygen consumption increases steadily throughout pregnancy and is greatest at term, reaching an average of 331 mL/min at rest and 1167 mL/min with exercise.[11] During labor, oxygen consumption increases by 40% to 60%, and cardiac output increases by about 22%.[39,40] Because oxygen delivery normally far exceeds consumption, the normal pregnant patient usually is able to maintain adequate delivery of oxygen to herself and her fetus, even during labor. When a pregnant patient has low oxygen delivery, she very quickly can reach the critical oxygen delivery level during labor, compromising herself and her fetus. The obstetrician therefore must make every effort to optimize oxygen delivery before allowing labor to begin in the compromised patient.

Pneumonia in Pregnancy

Pneumonia is fortunately a rare complication of pregnancy, occurring in 1 of 118 to 2288 deliveries.[41,42] However, pneumonia contributes to considerable maternal mortality and is reportedly the most common non-obstetric infection to cause maternal mortality in the peripartum period.[43] Maternal mortality was as high as 24% before the introduction of antibiotic therapy.[44] Research reports have documented a dramatic decrease in maternal mortality from 0% to 4% with modern management and antibiotic therapy.[42,45,46] Preterm delivery is a significant complication of pneumonia complicating pregnancy. Even with antibiotic therapy and modern management, preterm delivery continues to occur for 4% to 43% of gravidas who have pneumonia.[42,45,46]

The increasing incidence of pneumonia in pregnancy may reflect the declining general health status of certain segments of the childbearing population (e.g., morbid obesity).[46] The epidemic of human immunodeficiency virus (HIV) infection has increased the number of potential mothers who are at risk for opportunistic lung infections.

HIV infection is also associated with increased risks of invasive pneumococcal disease (odds ratio [OR] = 41.8) and Legionnaire disease (OR = 41.8).[47] HIV infection further predisposes the pregnant woman to the infectious complications of acquired immunodeficiency syndrome (AIDS).[47,48] Reported incidence rates range from 97 to 290 cases per 1000 HIV-infected persons per year. HIV-infected persons are 7.8 times more likely to develop pneumonia than non-HIV-infected individuals with similar risk factors. Women with medical conditions that increase the risk for pulmonary infection, such as cystic fibrosis (CF), are living to childbearing age more frequently than in the past. This disorder contributes to the increased incidence of pneumonia in pregnancy.

Pneumonia can complicate pregnancy at any time during gestation and may be associated with preterm birth, poor fetal growth, and perinatal loss. In an early report, 17 of 23 patients developed pneumonia between 25 and 36 weeks' gestation.[49] In that series, seven gravidas delivered during the course of their acute illness, and there were two maternal deaths. Another report described 39 cases of pneumonia in pregnancy.[45] Sixteen gravidas presented before 24 weeks' gestation, 15 between 25 and 36 weeks' gestation, and 8 after 36 weeks' gestation. Twenty-seven patients in this series were followed to completion of pregnancy; only two required delivery during the acute phase of pneumonia. Of these 27 patients, 3 suffered a fetal loss, and 24 delivered live fetuses, although there was one neonatal death resulting from prematurity.

Madinger and associates[42] reported 25 cases of pneumonia occurring among 32,179 deliveries and observed that fetal and obstetric complications were much more common than in earlier studies. Preterm labor complicated 11 of 21 gestations. Eleven patients had pneumonia at the time of delivery. Preterm delivery was more likely for women who had bacteremia, needed mechanical ventilation, and had a serious underlying maternal disease. In addition to the complication of preterm labor, there were three perinatal deaths in this series. Berkowitz and LaSala[46] reported 25 patients with pneumonia complicating pregnancy; 14 women had term deliveries, 1 delivered preterm, 3 had a voluntary termination of pregnancy, 3 had term deliveries of growth-restricted infants, and 4 were lost to follow-up. Birth weight was significantly lower in the study group in this series (2770 ± 224 g versus 3173 ± 99 g in the control group; $P < .01$). In this series, pneumonia complicated 1 of 367 deliveries. The investigators attributed the increase in the incidence of pneumonia in this population to a decline in general health status, including anemia, a significant incidence of cocaine use (52% versus 10% of the general population), and HIV positivity (24% versus 2% of the general population) in the study group.

Bacteriology

Most series describing pneumonia complicating pregnancy have used incomplete methodologies to diagnose the etiologic pathogens for pneumonia, relying primarily on cultures of blood and sputum. In most cases, no pathogen was identified; however, pneumococcus and *Haemophilus influenzae* remain the most common identifiable causes of pneumonia in pregnancy.[42,45,46] Because comprehensive serologic testing has rarely been done, the true incidence of viral, *Legionella*, and *Mycoplasma* pneumonia in pregnancy is difficult to estimate. The data presented by Benedetti, Madinger, Berkowitz, and their respective colleagues all support pneumococcus as the predominant pathogen causing pneumonia in pregnancy and *H. influenzae* as the second most common organism.[42,45,46] In the series of Berkowitz and LaSala,[46] one patient was infected with *Legionella* species.

Pneumonia in pregnancy has several causes, including mumps, infectious mononucleosis, swine influenza, influenza A, varicella, coccidioidomycosis, and other fungi.[50] Varicella pneumonia can complicate primary varicella infections in 5.2% to 9%[51] of infections in pregnancy, compared with 0.3% to 1.8% in the nonpregnant population.[52] Influenza A has a higher mortality rate among pregnant women than among nonpregnant patients.[53] The increase in virulence of viral infections reported in pregnancy may result from the alterations in maternal immune status that characterize pregnancy, including reduced lymphocyte proliferative response, reduced cell-mediated cytotoxicity by lymphocytes, and a decrease in the number of helper T lymphocytes.[53,54] Viral pneumonias can also be complicated by superimposed bacterial infection, particularly pneumococcus.

Aspiration Pneumonia

Mendelson syndrome describes chemical pneumonitis resulting from the aspiration of gastric contents in pregnancy. Chemical pneumonitis can be superinfected with pathogens present in the oropharynx and gastric juices, primarily anaerobes and gram-negative bacteria.[45] Mendelson's original report of aspiration[55] consisted of 44,016 nonfasted obstetric patients between 1932 and 1945, and more than one half had received "operative intervention" with ether by mask without endotracheal intubation. He described aspiration in 66 cases (rate of 1 case per 667 patients). Although several of the patients were critically ill from their aspirations, most recovered within 24 to 36 hours, and only two died from this complication (rate of 1 death per 22,008 patients). A review described 37,282 vaginal deliveries; 85% were performed with general anesthesia by mask and without intubation, and 65% to 75% had ingested liquids or solid food within 4 hours of onset of labor.[56] The investigators found five mild cases of aspiration (1 per 7456 patients) with no sequelae.[56] Another report described one occurrence of "mild aspiration" without adverse outcome among 1870 women undergoing nonintubated peripartum surgery with intravenous ketamine, benzodiazepines, barbiturates, fentanyl, or some combination of these drugs.[57] Soreide and colleagues[58] observed four episodes of aspiration each during 36,800 deliveries and 3600 cesarean sections with no mortality. Based on these data, most hospitals permit free intake of clear liquids during labor. The risk of aspiration, pneumonia, and death from general anesthesia appears to be very low. This may reflect the use of modern techniques and therapy to reduce gastric pH.

Bacterial Pneumonia

Streptococcus pneumoniae (pneumococcus) is the most common bacterial pathogen that causes pneumonia in pregnancy; *H. influenzae* is the next most common. These pneumonias typically manifest as an acute illness accompanied by fever, chills, and a purulent, productive cough and are seen as a lobar pattern on the chest radiograph (Fig. 45-3). Streptococcal pneumonia produces a "rusty" sputum, with gram-positive diplococci on Gram stain, and it demonstrates asymmetrical consolidation with air bronchograms on the chest radiograph.[54] *H. influenzae* is a gram-negative coccobacillus that produces consolidation with air bronchograms, often in the upper lobes.[54] Less common bacterial pathogens include *Klebsiella pneumoniae*, which is a gram-negative rod that causes extensive tissue destruction with air bronchograms, pleural effusion, and cavitation seen on the chest radiograph. Patients with *Staphylococcus aureus* pneumonia present with pleuritis, chest pain, purulent sputum, and consolidation without air bronchograms identified on the chest radiograph.[54]

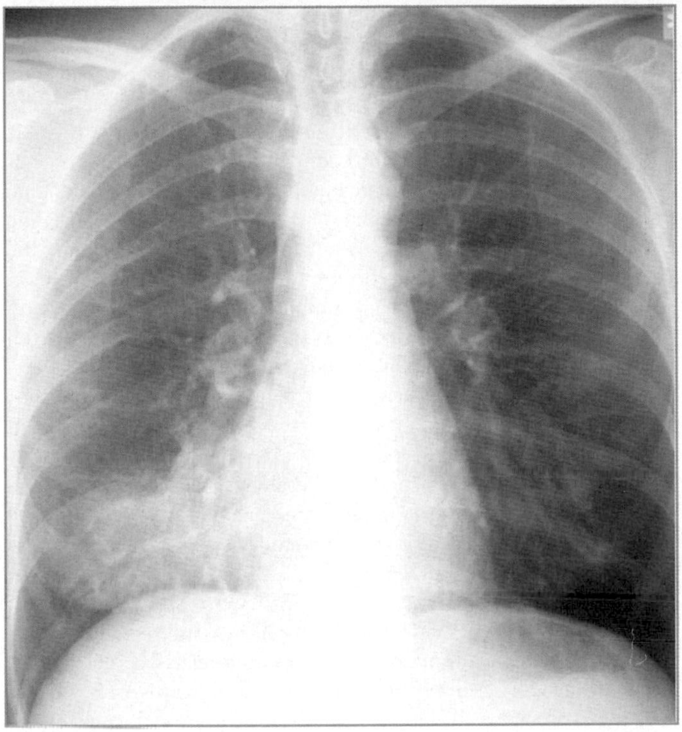

FIGURE 45-3 Right lower lobe pneumonia. Lobar consolidation in the right lower lobe is consistent with pneumococcal pneumonia.

Patients infected with atypical pneumonia pathogens, such as *Mycoplasma pneumoniae*, *Legionella pneumophila*, and *Chlamydia pneumoniae* (TWAR agent), present with gradual onset of symptoms. They have a lower fever, appear less ill, have mucoid sputum, and have a patchy or interstitial infiltrate seen on the chest radiograph. The severity of the findings on the chest radiograph usually is out of proportion to the mild clinical symptoms. *M. pneumoniae* is the most common organism responsible for atypical pneumonia and is best detected by the presence of cold agglutinins in about 70% of cases.

The normal physiologic changes in the respiratory system associated with pregnancy result in a loss of ventilatory reserve. Coupled with the immunosuppression that accompanies pregnancy, this puts the mother and fetus at great risk from respiratory infection. Any gravida suspected of having pneumonia should be managed aggressively. The pregnant patient should be admitted to the hospital and a thorough investigation undertaken to determine the cause. One study examined 133 women admitted with pneumonia during pregnancy using protocols based on the British Thoracic Society and American Thoracic Society admission guidelines for management of nonpregnant individuals. The investigators reported that if the American Thoracic Society guidelines were used, 25% of the pregnant women with pneumonia could have avoided admission. Using the American criteria, none of the gravidas who would have been managed as an outpatient had any complications. If the British Thoracic Society guidelines had been used; 66% of the pregnant women in this group would have been assigned to outpatient therapy. However, 14% would have required readmission for complications. Most of the 133 women who were hospitalized with pneumonia in this study did not receive a chest radiograph for confirmation of the diagnosis. This limits the value of the study for guiding admission criteria for pneumonia in pregnancy. Until additional information is available, admission for all pregnant women with pneumonia is still recommended.

The workup should include a physical examination, arterial blood gas determinations, a chest radiograph, sputum Gram stain and culture, and blood cultures. Several studies have called into question the use of cultures to identify the microbes of community-acquired pneumonia. Success rates for identification of the bacterial cause with cultures range from 2.1% to approximately 50%. Review of available clinical data reflects an overall reliance on clinical judgment and the patient's response to treatment to guide therapy. Other tests are available to identify the cause of pneumonia that do not require culture and are more sensitive and specific. An assay approved by the U.S. Food and Drug Administration (FDA) for pneumococcal urinary antigen has been assessed in several studies. The sensitivity for identifying pneumococcal disease in adults is reportedly 60% to 90%, with a specificity close to 100%. In one study, the pneumococcal antigen was detected in 26% of patients in whom no pathogens had been identified. This finding suggests that cases that are undiagnosed by standard test can be identified with the assay. In this study, 10% of samples from patients with pneumonia caused by other agents were positive on the pneumococcal assay, indicating a potential problem with specificity. If the response to therapy directed at pneumococcus is inadequate, coverage for other potential pathogens should be added.

The test for *Legionella* urinary antigen has a sensitivity of 70% and specificity of 90% for serogroup 1. This is especially useful in the United States and Europe, because about 85% of *Legionella* isolates are serogroup 1. *Legionella* is a common cause of severe community-acquired pneumonia. The urinary antigen for serogroup 1 should be considered for any patient requiring admission into an intensive care unit for pneumonia.

Percutaneous-transthoracic needle aspiration has been advocated as a valuable and safe method to increase the chance of establishing the causative agent for pneumonia. This test should be reserved for use in compromised individuals, suspected tuberculosis in the absence of a productive cough, selected cases of chronic pneumonia, pneumonia associated with neoplasm or a foreign body, suspected *Pneumocystis jiroveci* pneumonia, and suspected conditions that necessitate lung biopsy. Cold agglutinins and *Legionella* titers may also be useful. Empiric antibiotic coverage should be started, usually with a third-generation cephalosporin such as ceftriaxone or cefotaxime. *Legionella* pneumonia has a high mortality rate and sometimes manifests with consolidation, mimicking pneumococcal pneumonia. It is recommended that a macrolide, such as azithromycin, be added to the empiric therapy. Dual coverage has been demonstrated to improve response to therapy even for abbreviated macrolide regimens. This may reflect the added anti-inflammatory effect of the macrolides. Azithromycin administration is an independent predictor of a positive outcome and reduced length of hospital stay for patients with mild to moderate community-acquired pneumonia. The use of macrolides to treat community-acquired pneumonia should be limited when possible, because their use has also been associated with increased penicillin resistance by *S. pneumoniae*.

When admission for pneumonia is required, there is evidence that inpatient and 30-day mortality rates have been reduced when antibiotics are administered in less than 8 hours. Current U.S. federal standards require that the first dose of antibiotics be administered within 4 hours of arrival to the hospital. After the results of the sputum culture, blood cultures, Gram stain, and serum studies are obtained and a pathogen has been identified, antibiotic therapy can be directed toward the identified cause. The third-generation cephalosporins are effective agents for most pathogens causing a community-acquired pneumonia. They are also effective against penicillin-resistant *S. pneumoniae*. The quinolones as a class should be avoided in pregnancy because they may damage developing fetal cartilage. However, with the emergence of highly resistant bacterial pneumonia, their use may be lifesaving and therefore justified in specific circumstances. The respiratory quinolones are effective against highly penicillin-resistant *S. pneumoniae* strains, and their use does not increase resistance. The respiratory quinolones include levofloxacin, gatifloxacin, and moxifloxacin. These are ideal agents for community-acquired pneumonia because they are highly active against penicillin-resistant strains of *S. pneumoniae.* They are also active against *Legionella* and the other atypical pulmonary pathogens. Another advantage is a favorable pharmacokinetic profile, such that blood or lung levels are the same whether the drug is administered orally or intravenously. Arguments against more extensive respiratory quinolone use are based on concerns about the potential for developing resistance, the variable incidence of *Legionella*, and cost. An additional caveat is that the respiratory quinolones are only partially effective against *Mycobacterium tuberculosis.* Evaluation for this infection should be done when considering the use of quinolones for pneumonia.

In addition to antibiotic therapy, oxygen supplementation should be given. Frequent arterial blood gas measurements should be obtained to maintain partial pressure of oxygen at 70 mm Hg, a level necessary to ensure adequate fetal oxygenation. Arterial saturation also can be monitored with pulse oximetry. When the gravida is afebrile for 48 hours and has signs of clinical improvement, an oral cephalosporin can be started and intravenous therapy discontinued. A total of 10 to 14 days of treatment should be completed.

Pneumonia in pregnancy can be complicated by respiratory failure requiring mechanical ventilation. If this occurs, team management should include the obstetrician, maternal-fetal medicine specialist, and intensivist. In addition to meticulous management of the gravida's respiratory status, the patient should be maintained in the left lateral recumbent position to improve uteroplacental perfusion. The viable fetus should be monitored with continuous fetal monitoring. If positive end-expiratory pressure greater than 10 cm H_2O is required to maintain oxygenation, central monitoring with a pulmonary artery catheter should be instituted to adequately monitor volume status and maintain maternal and uteroplacental perfusion. There is no evidence documenting that elective delivery results in overall improvement in respiratory function,[59] and elective delivery should be reserved for the usual obstetric indications. However, if there is evidence of fetal compromise or profound maternal compromise and impending demise, delivery should be accomplished.

Pneumococcal polysaccharide vaccination prevents pneumococcal pneumonia in otherwise healthy populations with an efficacy of 65% to 84%. The vaccine is safe in pregnancy and should be administered to high-risk gravidas. Those at high risk include individuals with sickle cell disease with autosplenectomy, patients who have a surgical splenectomy, and individuals who are immunosuppressed. An additional advantage to maternal immunization with the pneumococcal vaccine is that several studies have demonstrated there is significant transplacental transmission of vaccine-specific antibodies in infants at birth and at 2 months. Colostrum and breast milk antibodies are also significantly increased in women who have received the pneumococcal vaccine.

Viral Pneumonias

Influenza

An estimated 4 million cases of pneumonia and influenza occur annually in the United States, and it is the sixth leading cause of death.[60] In contrast to the general population, pregnant women seem to be at higher risk for influenza pneumonia.[61,62] Epidemiologic data from the 1918 to 1919 influenza A pandemic revealed a maternal mortality rate that approached 50% for pregnant women with influenza pneumonia.[63,64] Three types of influenza virus can cause human disease—A, B, and C—but most epidemic infections are caused by influenza A.[50] Influenza A typically has an acute onset after a 1- to 4-day incubation period and first manifests as high fever, coryza, headache, malaise, and cough. In uncomplicated cases, results of the chest examination and chest radiograph are normal.[50] If symptoms persist longer than 5 days, especially in a pregnant woman, complications should be suspected. Pneumonia may complicate influenza as the result of secondary bacterial infection or viral infection of the lung parenchyma.[50] In the epidemic of 1957, autopsies demonstrated that pregnant women died most commonly of fulminant viral pneumonia, whereas nonpregnant patients died most often of secondary bacterial infection.[65]

A large, nested, case-control study evaluated the rate of influenza-related complications over 17 influenza seasons among women enrolled in the Tennessee Medicaid system. This study demonstrated a high risk for hospitalization for influenza-related reasons in low-risk pregnant women during the last trimester of pregnancy. The study authors estimated that 25 of 10,000 women in the third trimester during the influenza season are hospitalized with influenza-related complications. A later, matched-cohort study using the administrative database of pregnant women enrolled in the Tennessee Medicaid system examined pregnant women between the ages of 25 and 44 years with respiratory hospitalization during the 1985 to 1993 influenza seasons. In this population of pregnant women, those with asthma accounted for one half of all respiratory-related hospitalizations during the influenza season. Among pregnant women with diagnosis of asthma, 6% required respiratory hospitalization during the influenza season (OR = 10.63; 95% confidence interval [CI], 8.61 to 13.83) compared with women without a medical comorbidity. This study detected no significant increases in adverse perinatal outcome associated with respiratory hospitalization during flu season.

Primary influenza pneumonia is characterized by rapid progression from a unilateral infiltrate to diffuse bilateral disease. The gravida may develop fulminant respiratory failure requiring mechanical ventilation and positive end-expiratory pressure. Aggressive therapy is indicated when pneumonia complicates influenza in pregnancy. Antibiotics should be started and directed at the likely pathogens that can cause secondary infection, including *S. aureus*, pneumococcus, *H. influenzae*, and certain enteric gram-negative bacteria. Antiviral agents, such as oseltamivir and zanamivir, should also be considered.[66] It has been recommended that the influenza vaccine be given routinely to gravidas in the second and third trimester of pregnancy to prevent the occurrence of influenza and the development of pneumonia. Women at high risk for pulmonary complications, such as those with asthma, chronic obstructive pulmonary disease, cystic fibrosis, and splenectomy, should be vaccinated regardless of the trimester to prevent the occurrence of influenza and the development of secondary pneumonia. In addition to maternal protection, prospective studies have demonstrated higher cord blood antibody levels to influenza in infants born to mothers immunized during pregnancy. There is a delay in the onset and decrease in severity of influenza in infants born with higher antibody levels.

Varicella

Varicella-zoster virus is a DNA virus that usually causes a benign, self-limited illness in children, but it may infect up to 2% of all adults.[67] Varicella infection occurs in 0.7 of every 1000 pregnancies.[68] Pregnancy may increase the likelihood of varicella pneumonia, complicating the primary infection.[52] Treatment with acyclovir is safe in pregnancy. In one report,[52] there was one intrauterine fetal death. Another report[51] documented a 5.2% incidence of varicella pneumonia among gravidas with varicella-zoster infection. The investigators also reported that gravidas who smoke or manifest more than 100 skin lesions are more likely to develop pneumonia.[51] Varicella pneumonia occurs most often in the third trimester, and the infection is likely to be severe.[52,68,69] The maternal mortality rate for varicella pneumonia may be as high as 35% to 40%, compared with 11% to 17% for nonpregnant individuals.[52,69] Although one review reported a decreased mortality rate, with only three deaths among 28 women with varicella pneumonia,[68] another study documented a maternal mortality rate of 35%.[52] However, a later report documented 100% survival among 18 gravidas with varicella pneumonia who were treated with acyclovir.[51] In this report, there was one intrauterine fetal death at 25 weeks' gestation in a woman with varicella. In one report of 312 pregnancies, there was no increase in the number of birth defects and no consistent pattern of congenital abnormalities. In another report, 17 other infants were delivered beyond 36 weeks, and there was no evidence of neonatal varicella.[51]

Varicella pneumonia usually manifests 2 to 5 days after the onset of fever, rash, and malaise and is heralded by the onset of pulmonary symptoms, including cough, dyspnea, pruritic chest pain, and hemoptysis.[52] The severity of the illness may vary from asymptomatic radiographic abnormalities to fulminant pneumonitis and respiratory failure (Fig. 45-4).[52,70]

All gravidas with varicella pneumonia should be aggressively treated with antiviral therapy and admitted to the intensive care unit for close observation or intubation if indicated. Acyclovir, a DNA polymerase inhibitor, should be started. The early use of acyclovir was associated with an improved hospital course after the 5th day and a lower mean temperature, lower respiratory rate, and improved oxygenation.[57] Treatment with acyclovir is safe in pregnancy. Among 312 pregnancies, there was no increase in the number of birth defects and no consistent

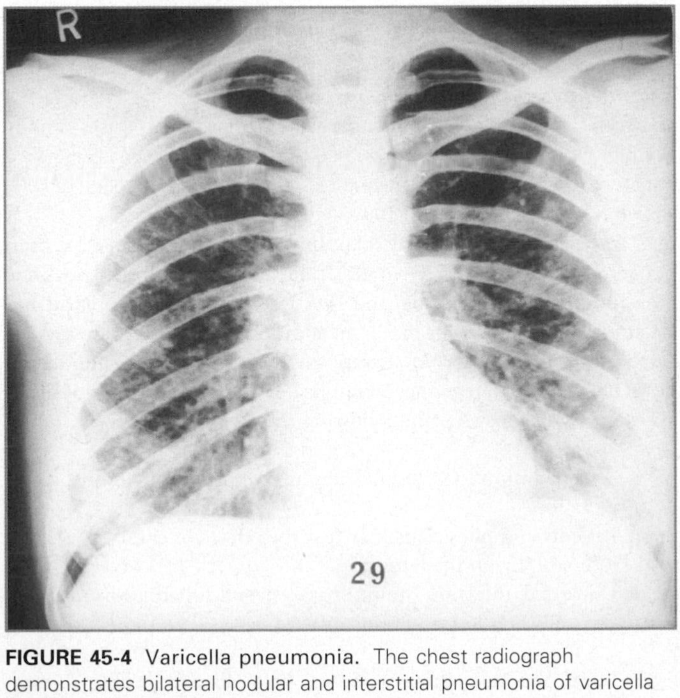

FIGURE 45-4 Varicella pneumonia. The chest radiograph demonstrates bilateral nodular and interstitial pneumonia of varicella pneumonia.

pattern of congenital abnormalities.[71] A dose of 7.5 mg/kg given intravenously every 8 hours has been recommended.[72]

Varicella vaccine is an attenuated live virus vaccine that was added to the universal childhood immunization schedule in the United States in 1995. The program of universal childhood vaccination against varicella in the United States has resulted in a sharp decline in the rate of death from varicella. However, varicella vaccine is not recommended for use in pregnancy. The overall decline in incidence of adult varicella infection because of childhood vaccination will likely result in a decreased incidence of varicella infection and varicella pneumonia during pregnancy.

A study[73] assessed the risk of congenital varicella syndrome and other birth defects in offspring of women who inadvertently received varicella vaccine during pregnancy or within 3 months of conception. Fifty-eight women received their first dose of varicella vaccine during the first or second trimester. No cases (0%) of congenital varicella syndrome were identified among 56 live births (CI, 0 to 15.6). Among the prospective reports of live births, five congenital anomalies were identified in the susceptible cohort or the sample population as a whole. The investigator suggested that although the numbers in the study were small, the results should provide some reassurance to health care providers and women with inadvertent exposure before or during pregnancy.

Pneumocystis jiroveci

Infection with the HIV virus significantly increases the risk for pulmonary infection. *S. pneumoniae* and *H. influenzae* are the most commonly isolated organisms.[73] One report[74] also identified *Pseudomonas aeruginosa* as a significant cause of bacterial pneumonia in HIV-infected individuals. *Pneumocystis* pneumonia, an AIDS-defining illness, occurs more frequently when the helper T-cell count ($CD4^+$) is less than 200 cells/mm^3. *Pneumocystis jiroveci* pneumonia (PJP), formerly designated *Pneumocystis carinii* pneumonia (PCP), is the most common of the serious opportunistic infections in pregnant women infected with HIV.[75,76] *P. jiroveci* is the number one cause of pregnancy-associated AIDS deaths in the United States.[77] Initial reports of PJP in pregnancy described a 100% maternal mortality rate.[47,75,78-80] However, in a 2001 review of 22 cases of PJP in pregnancy, the mortality rate was 50% (11 of 22 patients).[81] However, the mortality rate is still higher than that reported for HIV-infected nonpregnant individuals.[81] In that series, respiratory failure developed in 13 patients, and 59% required mechanical ventilation. The survival rate of gravidas requiring mechanical ventilation was 31%. In this series, maternal and fetal outcomes were better in cases of PJP that occurred during the third trimester of pregnancy.

A high index of suspicion is necessary when gravidas at risk for HIV infection present with symptoms such as weight loss, fatigue, fever, tachypnea, dyspnea, and nonproductive cough.[75] The onset of disease can be insidious, including normal radiographic findings, and it can then proceed to rapid deterioration.[75] When the chest radiograph is positive, it typically exhibits bilateral alveolar disease in the perihilar regions and lower lung fields (Fig. 45-5), which can progress to include the entire parenchyma.[75] Diagnosis can be accomplished by means of sputum silver stains, bronchial aspiration, or bronchoscope-directed biopsy.[82] Lung biopsy is recommended for definitive diagnosis.[78]

Therapy for PJP in pregnancy includes trimethoprim-sulfamethoxazole (TMP-SMX), which is a category C drug. Gravidas with a history of PJP, a $CD4^+$ lymphocyte count of less than 200/mm^3, or oral pharyngeal candidiasis should receive prophylaxis.[83] TMP-SMX is the drug of choice and may provide cross protection against toxoplasmosis and other bacterial infections.[84] The usual dose is one double-strength

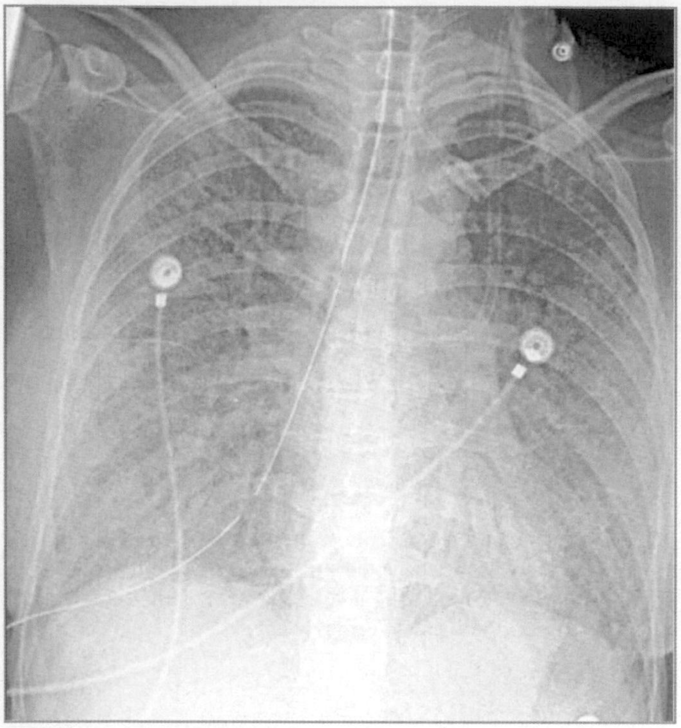

FIGURE 45-5 *Pneumocystis jiroveci* pneumonia (PJP). Bilateral alveolar disease is consistent with PJP pneumonia.

tablet (150 mg/m² of TMP and 750 mg/m² of SMX given three times each week). Adverse reactions such as drug allergy, nausea, fever, neutropenia, anemia, thrombocytopenia, and elevated transaminase levels have been reported in 20% to 30% of nonpregnant individuals receiving TMP-SMX therapy.[84] Complete blood cell count with a differential cell count and liver function tests should be obtained every 6 to 8 weeks to monitor for toxicity. Other regimens used for prophylaxis for individuals with intolerance to TMP-SMX include aerosolized pentamidine (300 mg every month by Respirgard II nebulizer) or dapsone (100 mg once daily). Hussain and colleagues[85] found that the survival rate for patients treated with SMX alone was 71% (5 of 7 patients) and that the rate with SMX and steroids was 60% (3 of 5 patients); the overall survival rate for both groups was 66.6% (8 of 12 patients). The investigators concluded that PJP has a more aggressive course during pregnancy, with increased morbidity and mortality.[85] However, treatment with SMX compared with other therapies may result in improved outcome. They also caution that withholding appropriate PJP prophylaxis may adversely affect maternal and fetal outcomes.[85]

PJP is a devastating opportunistic infection in pregnant women who are infected with HIV. The maternal mortality rate is extremely high, and prophylaxis with TMP-SMX is indicated during the antepartum period for individuals with a CD4⁺ cell count less than 200/mm³ or a history of oropharyngeal candidiasis and for individuals with a prior history of PJP infection. Initiation of therapy during the antepartum period can also prevent the rare occurrence of perinatally transmitted PJP.[84] When a gravida is demonstrating symptoms consistent with a possible infection, a diligent search should be conducted to quickly identify PJP as the cause of pneumonia. When PJP is untreated, the maternal mortality rate can approach 100%. In summary, PJP pneumonia remains a dreaded complication of HIV infection and an AIDS-defining illness. There is a very high maternal and fetal mortality rate when PJP complicates pregnancy. Primary prophylaxis against *Pneumocystis* pneumonia with TMP-SMX in HIV-infected adults, including pregnant women and patients receiving highly active antiretroviral therapy, should begin when the CD4⁺ cell count is less than 200 cells/mm³ or there is a history of oropharyngeal candidiasis. Prophylaxis should be discontinued when the CD4⁺ cell count increases to more than 200 cells/mm³ for a period of 3 months.

Tuberculosis in Pregnancy

Tuberculosis kills more than 1 million women per year worldwide, and it is estimated that 646 million women and girls are already infected with tuberculosis. In women between 15 and 44 years old in developing countries, tuberculosis is the third most common cause of morbidity and mortality combined, and tuberculosis kills more women than any other infectious disease, including malaria and AIDS.

Case-notification rates from countries with a high prevalence of tuberculosis suggest that tuberculosis may be less common among females.[86] Epidemiologic information shows differences between men and women in prevalence of infection, rate of progression from infection to disease, incidence of clinical disease, and mortality resulting from tuberculosis. Seventy percent more smear-positive male than female tuberculosis patients are diagnosed every year and reported to the World Health Organization.[86] Differences between males and females have also been shown in the development and outcome of active disease, with female cases having a higher progression from infection to disease and a higher case-fatality rate.[87] The conclusion of a research workshop on gender and tuberculosis was that a combination of biologic and social factors is responsible for these differences.[86]

The incidence of tuberculosis in the United States began to decline in the early part of the 20th century and fell steadily until 1953, when the introduction of isoniazid led to a dramatic decrease in the number of cases, from 84,000 cases in 1953 to 22,255 cases in 1984.[88] However, since 1984, there have been significant changes in tuberculosis morbidity trends. From 1985 through 1991, reported cases of tuberculosis increased by 18%, representing approximately 39,000 more cases than expected had the previous downward trend continued. This increase results from many factors, including the HIV epidemic, deterioration in the health care infrastructure, and more cases among immigrants.[88,89] Between 1985 and 1992, the number of tuberculosis cases among women of childbearing age increased by 40%.[90] One report described tuberculosis-complicated pregnancies in 94.8 cases per 100,000 deliveries between 1991 and 1992.[91]

The emergence of drug-resistant tuberculosis has become a serious concern. In New York City in 1991, 33% of tuberculosis cases were resistant to at least one drug, and 19% were resistant to isoniazid and rifampin. Multidrug resistance is an additional problem. Many centers advocate directly observed therapy in the treatment of multidrug-resistant disease. Pregnancy complicates treatment of multidrug-resistant tuberculosis for the following reasons:

- Several antimycobacterial drugs are contraindicated during gestation.
- Patients and physicians may fear the effects of chest radiography on the fetus.
- Untreated, infectious, multidrug-resistant tuberculosis may be vertically and laterally transmitted.[92]

In one report,[92] three patients had disease resulting from multidrug-resistant *M. tuberculosis*, and one had disease resulting from multidrug-resistant *Mycobacterium bovis*. Only one patient began retreatment during pregnancy because her organism was susceptible to three antituberculosis drugs that were considered nontoxic to the fetus. Despite concern about teratogenicity of the second-line antituberculosis medications, careful timing of treatment initiation resulted in clinical cure for the mothers, regardless of some complications because of chronic tuberculosis or therapy. In this series, all infants were born healthy and remained free of tuberculosis.[92]

Diagnosis

Most gravidas with tuberculosis in pregnancy are asymptomatic. All gravidas at high risk for tuberculosis (Table 45-1) should be screened with subcutaneous administration of intermediate-strength purified protein derivative (PPD). If anergy is suspected, control antigens such as candidal, mumps, or tetanus toxoids should be used.[93] The sensitivity of the PPD is 90% to 99% for exposure to tuberculosis. The tine test should not be used for screening because of its low sensitivity.

The onset of the recent tuberculosis epidemic stimulated the need for rapid diagnostic tests using molecular biology methods to detect *M. tuberculosis* in clinical specimens. Two direct amplification tests have been approved by the FDA, the *Mycobacterium tuberculosis* Direct (MTD) Test (Gen-Probe, San Diego, CA) and the Amplicor *Mycobacterium tuberculosis* (MTB) Test (Roche Diagnostic Systems, Branchburg, NJ). Both tests amplify and detect *M. tuberculosis* 16S ribosomal DNA.[94] When testing acid-fast stained smear–positive respiratory specimens, each test has a sensitivity of greater than 95% and a specificity of essentially 100% for detecting the *M. tuberculosis* complex.[95,96] When testing acid-fast stained smear–negative respiratory specimens, the specificity remains greater than 95%, but the sensitivity ranges from 40% to 77%.[95,96] These tests are FDA approved only for testing acid-fast stained smear–positive respiratory specimens obtained from untreated patients or those who have received no more than 7 days of antituberculosis therapy. The PPD remains the most commonly used screening test for tuberculosis.

Immigrants from areas where tuberculosis is endemic may have received the bacillus Calmette-Guérin (BCG) vaccine, and they are likely to have a positive response to the PPD. However, this reactivity should wane over time. The PPD should be used to screen these patients for tuberculosis unless their skin tests are known to be positive.[93] If BCG vaccine was given 10 years earlier and the PPD is positive with a skin test reaction of 10 mm or more, the individual should be considered infected with tuberculosis and managed accordingly.[93]

TABLE 45-1 HIGH-RISK FACTORS FOR TUBERCULOSIS

Human immunodeficiency virus infection
Close contact with persons known or suspected to have tuberculosis
Medical risk factors known to increase risk for disease if infected
Birth in a country with high tuberculosis prevalence
Medically underserved status
Low income
Alcohol addiction
Intravenous drug use
Residency in a long-term care facility (e.g., correctional institutions, mental institutions, nursing homes and facilities)
Health professionals working in high-risk health care facilities

Women with a positive PPD skin test result must be evaluated for active tuberculosis with a thorough physical examination for extrapulmonary disease and a chest radiograph after they are beyond the first trimester.[54] Symptoms of active tuberculosis include cough (74%), weight loss (41%), fever (30%), malaise and fatigue (30%), and hemoptysis (19%).[97] Individuals with active pulmonary tuberculosis may have radiographic findings, including adenopathy, multinodular infiltrates, cavitation, loss of volume in the upper lobes, and upper medial retraction of hilar markings (Fig. 45-6). The finding of acid-fast bacilli in early morning sputum specimens confirms the diagnosis of pulmonary tuberculosis. At least three first-morning sputum samples should be examined for the presence of acid-fast bacilli. If sputum cannot be produced, sputum induction, gastric washings, or diagnostic bronchoscopy may be indicated.

Extrapulmonary tuberculosis occurs in up to 16% of cases in the United States; however, the pattern may occur in 60% to 70% of all patients with AIDS.[98] Extrapulmonary sites include lymph nodes, bone, kidneys, intestine, meninges, breasts, and endometrium. Extrapulmonary tuberculosis appears to be rare in pregnancy.[99] Extrapulmonary tuberculosis that is confined to the lymph nodes has no effect on obstetric outcomes, but tuberculosis at other extrapulmonary sites does adversely affect the outcome of pregnancy.[100] Jana and colleagues[100] documented that tuberculosis lymphadenitis did not affect the course of pregnancy, labor, or perinatal outcome. However, compared with control women, the 21 women with tubercular involvement of other extrapulmonary sites had higher rates of antenatal hospitalization (24% versus 2%; $P < .0001$), infants with low Apgar scores (≤6) soon after birth (19% versus 3%; $P = .01$), and low-birth-weight (<2500 g) infants (33% versus 11%; $P = .01$). Rarely, mycobacteria

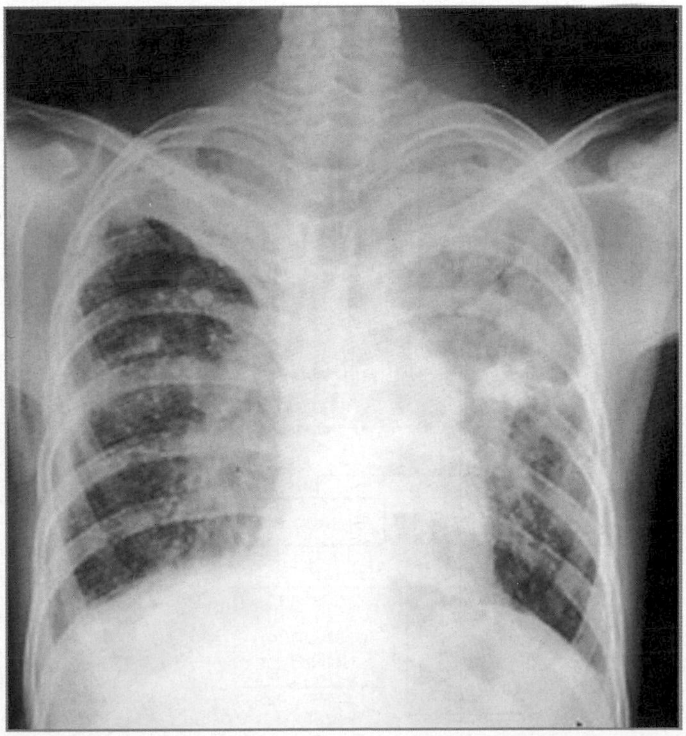

FIGURE 45-6 Chest radiograph of pulmonary tuberculosis. Radiographic findings may include adenopathy, multinodular infiltrates, cavitation, loss of volume in the upper lobes, and upper medial retraction of hilar markings.

invade the uteroplacental circulation, and congenital tuberculosis results.[49,90,101] The diagnosis of congenital tuberculosis is based on one of the following factors[90]:

- Demonstration of primary hepatic complex or cavitating hepatic granuloma by percutaneous liver biopsy at birth
- Infection of the maternal genital tract or placenta
- Lesions seen in the first week of life
- Exclusion of the possibility of postnatal transmission by a thorough investigation of all contacts, including attendants

Prevention

Most gravidas with a positive PPD result in pregnancy are asymptomatic and have no evidence of active disease; they are classified as infected without active disease. The risk of progression to active disease is highest in the first 2 years of conversion. It is important to prevent the onset of active disease while minimizing maternal and fetal risk. An algorithm for management of the positive PPD is presented in Figure 45-7.[102,103] In women with a known recent conversion (2 years) to a positive PPD result and no evidence of active disease, the recommended prophylaxis is isoniazid (300 mg/day), starting after the first trimester and continuing for 6 to 9 months.[54] Under base-case assumptions in a Markov decision-analysis model, the fewest cases of tuberculosis within the cohort occurred with antepartum treatment (1400 per 100,000), compared with no treatment (3300 per 100,000) or postpartum treatment (1800 per 100,000).[104] Antepartum treatment resulted in a marginal increase in life expectancy because of the prevented isoniazid-related hepatitis and deaths, compared with no treatment or postpartum treatment. Antepartum treatment was the least expensive.[104] Isoniazid should be accompanied by pyridoxine (vitamin B_6) supplementation (50 mg/day) to prevent the peripheral neuropathy that is associated with isoniazid treatment. Women with an unknown or prolonged duration of PPD positivity (>2 years) should receive isoniazid (300 mg/day) for 6 to 9 months after delivery. Isoniazid prophylaxis is not recommended for women older than 35 years who have an unknown or prolonged PPD positivity in the absence of active disease. The use of isoniazid is discouraged in this group because of an increased risk for hepatotoxicity. Isoniazid is associated with hepatitis in pregnant and nonpregnant adults. However, monthly monitoring of liver function tests may prevent this adverse outcome. Among individuals receiving isoniazid, 10% to 20% will develop mildly elevated values detected on liver function tests. These changes resolve after the drug is discontinued.[105]

Treatment

The gravida with active tuberculosis should be treated initially with isoniazid (300 mg/day) combined with rifampin (600 mg/day) (Table 45-2).[106] Resistant disease results from initial infection with resistant strains (33%) or can develop during therapy.[107] The development of resistance is more likely in individuals who are noncompliant with therapy. If resistance to isoniazid is identified or anticipated, 2.5 g of ethambutol per day should be added, and the treatment period should

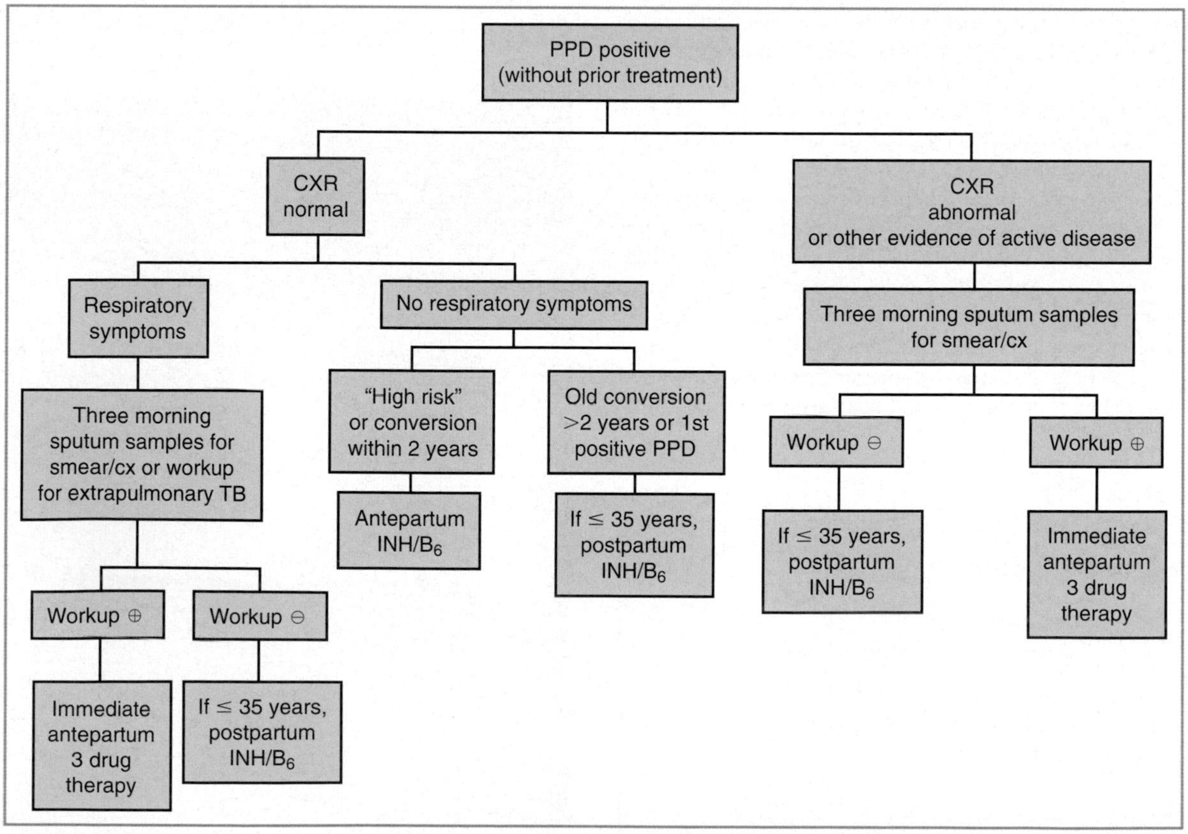

FIGURE 45-7 **Algorithm for the management of a patient with a positive purified protein derivative (PPD) result.** In women with known conversion within the past 2 years to a positive PPD result and no evidence of active disease, the recommended prophylaxis is 300 mg of isoniazid per day, starting after the first trimester and continuing for 6 to 9 months. B_6, pyridoxine; cx, culture; CXR, chest radiograph; INH, isoniazid, TB, tuberculosis.

TABLE 45-2 ANTITUBERCULOSIS DRUGS

Drug	Dosage Route	Daily Dose	Weekly Dose	Major Adverse Reactions
First-Line Drugs (for Initial Treatment)				
Isoniazid	PO, IM	10 mg/kg, up to 300 mg	15 mg/kg, up to 900 mg	Hepatic enzyme elevation, peripheral neuropathy hepatitis, hypersensitivity
Rifampin	PO	10 mg/kg, up to 600 mg	10 mg/kg, up to 600 mg	Orange discoloration of secretions and urine; nausea, vomiting, hepatitis, febrile reaction, purpura (rare)
Pyrazinamide	PO	15-30 mg/kg, up to 2 g	50-70 mg/kg, twice	Hepatotoxicity, hyperuricemia, arthralgias, rash, gastrointestinal upset
Ethambutol	PO	15 mg/kg, up to 2.5 g	50 mg/kg	Optic neuritis (decreased red-green color discrimination, decreased visual acuity), rash
Streptomycin	IM	15 mg/kg, up to 1 g	25-30 mg/kg, up to 1 g	Ototoxicity, nephrotoxicity
Second-Line Drugs (Daily Therapy)				
Capreomycin	IM	15-30 mg/kg, up to 1 g		Auditory, vestibular, and renal toxicity
Kanamycin	IM	15-30 mg/kg, up to 1 g		Auditory and renal toxicity, rare vestibular toxicity
Ethionamide	PO	15-20 mg/kg, up to 1 g		Gastrointestinal disturbance, hepatotoxicity, hypersensitivity
p-Amino-salicylic acid	PO	150 mg/kg, up to 1 g		Gastrointestinal disturbance, hypersensitivity, hepatotoxicity, sodium load
Cycloserine	PO	15-20 mg/kg, up to 1 g		Psychosis, convulsions, rash

IM, intramuscularly; PO, orally.

be extended to 18 months.[108] Ethambutol is teratogenic in animals; however, this effect has not been seen in humans.

The most common side effect of ethambutol therapy is optic neuritis. Streptomycin should be avoided during pregnancy because it is associated with cranial nerve VIII damage in neonates.[109] Antituberculous agents not recommended for use in pregnancy include ethionamide, streptomycin, capreomycin, kanamycin, cycloserine, and pyrazinamide.[54] However, case reports documenting the use of these antituberculous agents in pregnancy revealed no adverse fetal or neonatal effects. There were no congenital abnormalities, and pregnancy outcomes for the individuals treated were good. Untreated tuberculosis has been associated with higher morbidity and mortality rates among pregnant women. The management of the gravida with multidrug-resistant tuberculosis should be individualized. The patient should be counseled about the small risk of teratogenicity and understand that the risk of postpartum transmission of tuberculosis to the infant may be higher among those born to patients with drug-resistant tuberculosis. In patients with active disease at the time of delivery, separation of the mother and newborn should be accomplished to prevent infection of the newborn.

Women who are being treated with antituberculous drugs may breastfeed. Only 0.75% to 2.3% of isoniazid and 0.05% of rifampin are excreted into breast milk. Ethambutol excretion into breast milk is also minimal. However, if the infant is concurrently taking oral antituberculous therapy, excessive drug levels may be reached in the neonate, and breastfeeding should be avoided. Breastfed infants of women taking isoniazid should receive a multivitamin supplement that includes pyridoxine.[54] Neonates of women taking antituberculous therapy should have a PPD skin test at birth and again when 3 months old. Infants born to women with active tuberculosis at the time of delivery should receive isoniazid prophylaxis (10 mg/kg/day) until maternal disease has been inactive for 3 months as evidenced by negative maternal sputum cultures.[54] Infants of women with multidrug-resistant tuberculosis should probably be placed with an alternative caregiver until there is no evidence of active disease in the mother. The newborn should also receive BCG vaccine and isoniazid prophylaxis.[92] Active tuberculosis in the neonate should be treated appropriately with isoniazid and rifampin immediately on diagnosis or with multiagent therapy if drug-resistant organisms are identified. Infants and children who are at high risk for intimate and prolonged exposure to untreated or ineffectively treated persons should receive the BCG vaccine.[110]

In summary, high-risk gravidas should be screened for tuberculosis and treated appropriately with isoniazid prophylaxis for infection without overt disease and with dual antituberculous therapy for active disease. The newborn also should be screened for evidence of tuberculosis. Proper screening and therapy will lead to a good outcome for the mother and infant in most cases.

Asthma in Pregnancy

Asthma may be the most common potentially serious medical condition to complicate pregnancy.[111] Asthma is characterized by chronic airway inflammation with increased airway responsiveness to a variety of stimuli and airway obstruction that is partially or completely reversible.[111] Approximately 4% to 8% of pregnancies are complicated by asthma.[112,113] The prevalence and morbidity rates for asthma are increasing, although the mortality rate has decreased in recent years.

Insight into the pathogenesis of asthma has changed with the recognition that airway inflammation occurs in almost all cases. The medical management for asthma emphasizes treatment of airway inflammation to decrease airway responsiveness and prevent asthma symptoms.

Diagnosis

The enlarging uterus elevates the diaphragm about 4 cm, reducing the functional residual capacity. However, there are no significant alterations in forced vital capacity, peak expiratory flow rate (PEFR), or forced expiratory volume in 1 second (FEV_1) in normal pregnancies. Shortness of breath at rest or with mild exertion is common and is often referred to as physiologic dyspnea of pregnancy. Asthma is characterized by paroxysmal or persistent symptoms, including breathlessness, chest tightness, cough, and sputum production. The diagnosis of asthma is based on a history of symptoms and results of spirometry. Patients with asthma have improved FEV_1 after administration of a short-acting, inhaled β_2-agonist and increased sensitivity to inhaled methacholine, although this test is not usually performed during pregnancy.

In 2004, the National Asthma Education and Prevention Program (NAEPP) Working Group on Asthma and Pregnancy[114] defined mild intermittent, mild persistent, moderate persistent, and severe persistent asthma according to daytime and nighttime symptoms (e.g., wheezing, cough, dyspnea) and objective tests of pulmonary function. The most commonly used pulmonary function parameters are the PEFR and FEV_1. The NAEPP guidelines suggest classifying asthma *severity* in patients not on symptom-controlling drugs and asthma *control* in patients on symptom-controlling medications (Table 45-3).[115] Pregnant patients with mild asthma according to symptoms and pulmonary function who nonetheless required regular medications to control their asthma are similar to those with moderate asthma with respect to asthma exacerbations; those requiring regular systemic corticosteroids to control asthma symptoms were similar to severe asthmatics with respect to exacerbations.[116]

Effects of Pregnancy on Asthma

Asthma has been associated with considerable maternal morbidity. In a large, prospective study of pregnant women, those with mild asthma had an exacerbation rate of 12.6% and hospitalization rate of 2.3%; those with moderate asthma had an exacerbation rate of 25.7% and hospitalization rate of 6.8%; and severe asthmatics had an exacerbation rate of 51.9% and hospitalization rate of 26.9%.[116] The effects of pregnancy on asthma vary. In a large, prospective study, 23% improved and 30% became worse during pregnancy.[116] One of the most important conclusions of this study is that pregnant women with mild or even well-controlled asthma should be monitored by PEFR and FEV_1 testing during pregnancy.

Effects of Asthma on Pregnancy

Existing studies on the effects of asthma on pregnancy have had inconsistent results in regard to maternal and perinatal outcomes. For example, asthma has been associated with increased perinatal mortality,[117] hyperemesis gravidarum,[118] hemorrhage,[112,118,119] hypertension or preeclampsia,[118-125] preterm birth,[118,122,123,126-128] hypoxia at birth,[118] low birth weight,[118,129] increased cesarean section,[119,121,122,126,129] small-for-gestational-age status or intrauterine growth restriction,[122,123,130] gestational diabetes,[119,126] and anomalies.[122]

In contrast, asthma has *not* been associated with prematurity,[112,117,129-132] malformations,[112,118,121,123,131] birth injury,[118] increased perinatal mortality,[118] reduced gestational age,[120,121,133-135] reduced mean birth weight,[120,121,129,134-136] perinatal death,[119,121,131,135,137] low Apgar score,[121] neonatal respiratory difficulty,[121] antepartum or postpartum hemorrhage,[123,129,133] perinatal complications,[124,129] gestational hypertension or preeclampsia,[126,130,131,138] intrauterine growth restriction,[126,131] increased cesarean section,[112,132,137] low birth weight,[121,132,133,136,137] gestational diabetes,[112,124] or respiratory distress syndrome.[112]

Many of these studies have methodologic inadequacies, including low power, variable inclusion criteria, little or no information regarding asthma management or control, and time frames that do not reflect current management. Some positive findings may result from nonexistent or inadequate control for confounders such as oral corticosteroid treatment, ethnicity, smoking status, obesity, socioeconomic status, and hypertension. Another potential explanation for inconsistencies is that most of these studies did not classify asthma severity. Classification of asthma severity has important clinical implications in regard to asthma morbidity and tailoring optimal treatment regimens.[139,140] Asthma medications and poor asthma control leading to hypoxia may explain some of these observations.[141] Some data support a relationship between poor asthma control, as indicated by hospitalization for exacerbations or decreased FEV_1 values, and low birth weight and low ponderal index.[137,141,142] Studies have shown that women with more severe asthma may have the greatest risk for complications during pregnancy,[122,126,127,143] whereas better-controlled asthma is associated with decreased risks.[131,144,145] Poor control of asthma during pregnancy may be caused by the physician's reluctance to prescribe medications during pregnancy. Women with asthma significantly reduce their medications, especially inhaled and rescue corticosteroids, during the first trimester.[146]

There is considerable consistency among prospective studies of the effects of asthma during pregnancy. Eight prospective studies reporting maternal and neonatal outcomes with at least 100 subjects

TABLE 45-3 CLASSIFICATION OF ASTHMA SEVERITY AND CONTROL IN PREGNANT PATIENTS

	Well Controlled*	Not Well Controlled*		Very Poorly Controlled*
Signs and Symptoms	Intermittent†	Mild Persistent†	Moderate Persistent†	Severe Persistent†
Symptom frequency/short-acting β-agonist use	≤2 days per week	>2 days per week, but not daily	Daily symptoms	Throughout the day
Nighttime awakening	≤2 times per month	>2 times per month	>1 time per week	≥4 times per week
Interference with normal activity	None	Minor limitation	Some limitation	Extremely limited
FEV_1 or peak flow (percent predicted/personal best)	>80%	>80%	60-80%	<60%

*Asthma control: assess in patients on long-term-control medications to determine whether step-up, step-down, or no change in therapy is indicated.
†Asthma severity: assess severity for patients who are not on long-term-control medications, see Table 45-7 to determine starting controller therapy based on severity.
FEV_1, forced expiratory volume in 1 second.

in locations at or near sea level have been published in the English literature.[121,124,131-133,137,144,145,147] These studies show that a gravida with mild or moderate asthma can have excellent maternal and perinatal outcomes (Table 45-4). These findings do not contradict the possibility that suboptimal control of asthma during pregnancy is associated with increased risk to the mother or infant.[145] Lower FEV_1 values during pregnancy are significantly associated with increased risks for low birth weight and prematurity.[148] The two largest studies indicate that classification of asthma severity with therapy tailored according to asthma severity can result in excellent perinatal and maternal outcomes.[144,145] This generally confirms the findings of two earlier and smaller prospective cohort studies[131,133] in which asthma was managed by asthma specialists.

There are important caveats when interpreting this literature. Prospective studies have tended to find fewer significant adverse associations, possibly because of better asthma surveillance and treatment. The excellent maternal and perinatal outcomes were achieved at centers that tended to actively manage asthma during pregnancy. Women who enroll in research studies tend to be more compliant and better motivated than the general public. The lack of finding more adverse outcomes among women with severe asthma may also be a function of the relatively small numbers of this cohort and the resulting lack of power to find adverse outcomes that were statistically significant. Nonetheless, these prospective studies are reassuring in their consensus of good pregnancy outcomes among women with asthma. However, they do not suggest that asthma should be considered to be a benign condition, because active asthma management was a part of these studies and might have positively influenced outcomes.

Management Approaches

The ultimate goal of asthma therapy during pregnancy is to maintain adequate oxygenation of the fetus by prevention of hypoxic episodes in the mother. Other goals include achievement of minimal or no maternal symptoms day or night, minimal or no exacerbations, no limitations of activities, maintenance of normal or near-normal pulmonary function, minimal use of short-acting β_2-agonists, and minimal or no adverse effects from medications. Consultation or comanagement with an asthma specialist is appropriate for evaluation of the role of allergy and irritants, complete pulmonary function studies, or evaluation of the medication plan if there are complications in achieving the goals of therapy or the patient has severe asthma. A team approach is helpful if more than one clinician is managing the asthma and the pregnancy. The effective management of asthma during pregnancy relies on four integral components: objective assessment, trigger avoidance, patient education, and pharmacologic therapy.

Objective Measures for Assessment and Monitoring

Subjective measures of lung function by the patient or physician provide an insensitive and inaccurate assessment of airway hyperresponsiveness, airway inflammation, and asthma severity. The FEV_1 value after a maximal inspiration is the single best measure of pulmonary function. When adjusted for confounders, a mean FEV_1 less than 80% of the predicted value has been significantly associated with increased preterm delivery at less than 32 weeks and less than 37 weeks and with a birth weight less than 2500 g.[148] However, measurement of

TABLE 45-4 PROSPECTIVE COHORT STUDIES REPORTING OBSTETRIC AND NEONATAL OUTCOMES

Outcomes	Dombrowski et al, 2004[145] (N = 1739)	Bracken et al, 2003[144] (N = 872)	Stenius-Aarniala et al, 1996[133] (N = 504)	Schatz et al, 1995[131] (N = 486)	Mihrshani et al, 2003[124] (N = 340)	Jana et al, 1995[137] (N = 182)	Stenius-Aarniala and Teramo, 1988[121] (N = 181)	Minerbi-Codish et al, 1998[132] (N = 101)
Preterm, < 32 weeks	No	NR	NR	NR	NR	NR	NR	NR
Preterm, < 37 weeks	No (yes if severe)	No (yes if oral steroids)	No	No	No	No	NR	No
Preeclampsia	No	No (yes if daily symptoms)	No	No	No	NR	Yes	No
Cesarean delivery	Yes (if moderate or severe)	NR	Yes (if elective)	NR	No	No	Yes	No
Gestational diabetes	No (yes if severe)	NR	No	No	NR	NR	No	No
Small for gestational age	No	No (yes if daily symptoms)	NR	No	NR	NR	NR	No
Malformation	No	NR	No	No	NR	No	NR	No
Antenatal hemorrhage	NR	NR	No	NR	NR	No	No	NR
Postnatal hemorrhage	No	NR	NR	NR	NR	NR	NR	NR
RDS/HMD	No	NR	NR	No	NR	NR	No	NR
NEC	No	NR	NR	No	NR	NR	NR	NR
Perinatal death	No	NR	No	No	NR	No	No	NR
NICU admission	No	NR	No	NR	No	NR	No	NR

HMD, hyaline membrane disease; NEC, necrotizing enterocolitis; NICU, neonatal intensive care unit; No, no significant association; NR, not reported; RDS, respiratory distress syndrome; Yes, significantly increased.

FEV_1 requires a spirometer. The PEFR correlates well with the FEV_1, and it can be measured reliably with inexpensive, disposable, portable peak flow meters.

PEFR monitoring by the patient provides valuable insight to the course of asthma throughout the day, assesses circadian variation in pulmonary function, and helps detect early signs of deterioration so that timely therapy can be instituted. Patients with persistent asthma should be evaluated at least monthly, and those with moderate to severe asthma should have daily PEFR monitoring.[114] The typical PEFR in pregnancy should be 380 to 550 L/min. She should establish her "personal best" PEFR and then calculate her individualized PEFR zones. The green zone is more than 80% of the personal best PEFR, yellow zone is between 50% and 80% of the personal best value, and red zone is less than 50% of the personal best PEFR.

Avoiding or Controlling Asthma Triggers

Limiting adverse environmental exposures during pregnancy is important for controlling asthma. Irritants and allergens that provoke acute symptoms also increase airway inflammation and hyperresponsiveness. Avoiding or controlling such triggers can reduce asthma symptoms, airway hyperresponsiveness, and the need for medical therapy. Association of asthma with allergies is common; 75% to 85% of patients with asthma have positive skin test results for common allergens, including animal dander, house dust mites, cockroach antigens, pollens, and molds. Other common nonimmunologic triggers include tobacco smoke, strong odors, air pollutants, food additives such as sulfites, and certain drugs, including aspirin and β-blockers. Another trigger can be strenuous physical activity. For some patients, exercise-induced asthma can be avoided with inhalation of albuterol 5 to 60 minutes before exercise.

Specific measures for avoiding asthma triggers include removing carpeting, using an allergen-impermeable mattress and pillow covers, weekly washing of bedding in hot water, avoiding tobacco smoke, inhibiting mite and mold growth by reducing humidity, and leaving the house when it is vacuumed. Animal dander control includes weekly bathing of the pet, keeping furry pets out of the bedroom, or removing the pet from the home. Cockroaches can be controlled by poison or bait traps and eliminating exposed food or garbage.

Patient Education

Patients should be made aware that controlling asthma during pregnancy is especially important for the well-being of the fetus. The pregnant woman should understand that she can reduce symptoms by limiting asthma triggers. She should have a basic understanding of the medical management during pregnancy, including self-monitoring of PEFRs and the correct use of inhalers. The patient should be instructed on proper PEFR technique. She should make the measurement while standing, take a maximum inspiration, and observe the reading on the peak flow meter.

Pharmacologic Therapy

The goals of asthma therapy include relieving bronchospasm, protecting the airways from irritant stimuli, mitigating pulmonary and inflammatory responses to an allergen exposure, and resolving the inflammatory process in the airways, leading to improved pulmonary function with reduced airway hyperresponsiveness. The step-care approach uses the least amount of drug intervention necessary to control a patient's severity of asthma.

It is safer for pregnant women with asthma to be treated with asthma medications than it is for them to have asthma symptoms and exacerbations.[114] Current pharmacologic therapy emphasizes treatment of airway inflammation to decrease airway hyperresponsiveness and prevent asthma symptoms. Typical dosages of commonly used asthma medications are listed in Table 45-5. Low, medium, and high doses of inhaled corticosteroids are provided in Table 45-6.

TABLE 45-5 TYPICAL DOSAGES OF ASTHMA MEDICATIONS

Drug	Dosage
Albuterol MDI	2-6 puffs as needed
Salmeterol DPI	1 puff bid
Fluticasone and salmeterol (Advair) DPI	1 inhalation bid, dose depends on severity of asthma
Montelukast	10-mg tablet at night
Zafirlukast	20 mg twice daily
Prednisone	20-60 mg/day for active symptoms
Theophylline	Start at 200 mg PO bid, target serum levels of 5-12 μg/mL (decrease dosage by one half if treated with erythromycin or cimetidine)
Ipratropium MDI	2-3 puffs q6h
Ipratropium nebulizer	1 mL (0.25 mg) q6h
Cromolyn MDI	2 puffs qid

DPI, dry powder inhaler; MDI, metered-dose inhaler; PO, orally.

Although it is assumed that asthma medications are equally effective during pregnancy, differences in maternal physiology and pharmacokinetics may affect the absorption, distribution, metabolism, and clearance of medications during pregnancy. Endocrinologic and immunologic changes during pregnancy include elevations in free plasma cortisol, possible tissue refractoriness to cortisol,[149] and changes in cellular immunity.[150]

STEP THERAPY

The step-care approach to therapy increases the number and frequency of medications with increasing asthma severity (Table 45-7). Based on the severity of asthma, medications are considered to be *preferred* or *alternative*. Patients not optimally responding to treatment should be stepped up to more intensive medical therapy. After control is achieved and sustained for several months, a step-down approach can be considered, but it should be undertaken cautiously and gradually to avoid compromising the stability of the asthma control. For some patients, it may be prudent to postpone until after birth attempts to reduce therapy that is effectively controlling the patient's asthma.[114] For a patient who had a favorable response to an alternative drug before becoming pregnant, it is preferable to maintain the therapy that successfully controlled the asthma before pregnancy. However, when initiating new treatment for asthma during pregnancy, preferred medications should be considered rather than alternative treatment options.[114]

A burst of oral corticosteroids is indicated for exacerbations not responding to initial β_2-agonist therapy, regardless of asthma severity. Patients who require increasing inhaled albuterol therapy to control their symptoms may benefit from oral corticosteroids. In such cases, a short course of oral prednisone (40 to 60 mg/day) for 1 week followed by 7 to 14 days of tapering may be effective.

INHALED CORTICOSTEROIDS

Inhaled corticosteroids are the preferred treatment for the management of all levels of persistent asthma during pregnancy.[114] Because almost all patients have airway inflammation, inhaled corticosteroids

TABLE 45-6 COMPARATIVE DAILY DOSES FOR INHALED CORTICOSTEROIDS

Drug	Dose Conversion*	Low Dose	Medium Dose	High Dose
Beclomethasone HFA	40 μg/puff	2-6 puffs	>6-12 puffs	>12 puffs
	80 μg/puff	1-3 puffs	>3-6 puffs	>6 puffs
Budesonide	200 μg/inhalation	1-3 puffs	>3-6 puffs	>6 puffs
Flunisolide	250 μg/puff	2-4 puffs	4-8 puffs	>8 puffs
Fluticasone HFA	44 μg/puff	—	2-6 puffs	—
	110 μg/puff	2 puffs	2-4 puffs	>4 puffs
	220 μg/puff	1-2 puffs	—	>2 puffs
Fluticasone DPI	50 μg/inhalation	2-6 puffs	—	—
	100 μg/inhalation	1-3 puffs	3-5 puffs	>5 puffs
	250 μg/inhalation	1 puff	2 puffs	>2 puffs
Mometasone	200 μg/inhalation	1 puff	2 puffs	>2 puffs
Triamcinolone	75 μg/puff	4-10 puffs	10-20 puffs	>20 puffs

*The dose of total daily puffs is usually divided as a twice/day regimen.
DPI, dry powder inhaler; HFA, hydrofluoroalkane.
From National Asthma Education and Prevention Program Full Report of the Expert Panel: Guidelines for the Diagnosis and Management of Asthma, 2007. Available at http://www.nhlbi.nih.gov/guidelines/asthma/asthsumm.pdf (accessed January 2008).

TABLE 45-7 STEP-CARE THERAPY FOR ASTHMA DURING PREGNANCY

Type of Asthma	Preferred Management	Alternative Management
Mild intermittent	No daily medications, albuterol as needed	—
Mild persistent	Low dose inhaled corticosteroid	Cromolyn, leukotriene receptor antagonist, or theophylline (serum level of 5-12 μg/mL)
Moderate persistent	Low-dose inhaled corticosteroid and salmeterol, medium-dose inhaled corticosteroid, or (if needed) medium-dose inhaled corticosteroid and salmeterol	Low-dose or (if needed) medium-dose inhaled corticosteroid and a leukotriene receptor antagonist or theophylline (serum level of 5-12 μg/mL)
Severe persistent	High-dose inhaled corticosteroid and salmeterol and (if needed) oral corticosteroid	High-dose inhaled corticosteroid and theophylline (serum level of 5-12 μg/mL) and (if needed) oral corticosteroid

have been advocated as first-line therapy for those with mild asthma.[151] The use of inhaled corticosteroids among nonpregnant asthmatics has been associated with a marked reduction in fatal and near-fatal episodes of asthma.[152] Inhaled corticosteroids produce clinically important improvements in bronchial hyperresponsiveness that appear dose related[153] and include prevention of increased bronchial hyperresponsiveness after seasonal exposure to allergen.[154,155] Continued administration is effective in reducing the immediate pulmonary response to an allergen challenge. In a prospective, observational study of 504 pregnant women with asthma, 177 patients were not initially treated with inhaled budesonide or inhaled beclomethasone.[133] This cohort had a 17% rate of acute exacerbation rate compared with only a 4% rate among those treated with inhaled corticosteroids from the start of pregnancy.

The NAEPP Working Group reviewed 10 studies that included 6113 patients who took inhaled corticosteroids during pregnancy for asthma.[114] There is no evidence linking inhaled corticosteroid use with increases in congenital malformations or adverse perinatal outcomes. Included among these studies was the Swedish Medical Birth Registry that had 2014 infants whose mothers had used inhaled budesonide in early pregnancy.[156] Because there are more data on using budesonide during pregnancy than on using other inhaled corticosteroids, the NAEPP considered budesonide to be a preferred medication. However, if a woman's asthma is well controlled by a different inhaled corticosteroid before pregnancy, it seems reasonable to continue that medication during pregnancy. All inhaled corticosteroids are labeled by the FDA as pregnancy class C, except budesonide, which is class B.

INHALED β_2-AGONISTS

Inhaled β_2-agonists are recommended for all degrees of asthma during pregnancy.[114,157] Albuterol has the advantage of a rapid onset of effect in the relief of acute bronchospasm by means of smooth muscle relaxation, and it is an excellent bronchoprotective agent for pretreatment before exercise. Salmeterol and formoterol are long-acting preparations.

The β_2-agonists are associated with tremor, tachycardia, and palpitations. They do not block the development of airway hyperresponsiveness.[158] Comparison of an inhaled glucocorticoid, budesonide, with the inhaled terbutaline raised the question about whether routine use of terbutaline may result in increased airway hyperresponsiveness.[151] Increased frequency of bronchodilator use may indicate the need for additional anti-inflammatory therapy; chronic use of short-acting β_2-agonists has been associated with an increased risk of death.[157,159] The β_2-agonists appear to be safe based on a NAEPP review of six published studies of a total of 1599 women with asthma who took β_2-agonists during pregnancy.[114] In a large, prospective study, no significant relationship was found between the use of inhaled β_2-agonists (n = 1828) and adverse pregnancy outcomes.[160]

CROMOLYN

Cromolyn sodium is virtually devoid of significant side effects. It blocks the early and late phases of pulmonary response to an allergen challenge, and it prevents the development of airway hyperresponsiveness.[158] Cromolyn does not have any intrinsic bronchodilator or antihistaminic activity. Compared with inhaled corticosteroids, the time to maximal clinical benefit is longer for cromolyn. Cromolyn appears to be less effective than inhaled corticosteroids in reducing objective and subjective manifestations of asthma. Cromolyn appears to be safe during pregnancy[160] and is an alternative treatment for mild persistent asthma.[114]

THEOPHYLLINE

Theophylline is an alternative treatment for mild persistent asthma and an adjunctive treatment for the management of moderate and severe persistent asthma during pregnancy.[114] Subjective symptoms of adverse theophylline effects, including insomnia, heartburn, palpitations, and nausea, may be difficult to differentiate from typical pregnancy symptoms. High doses have caused jitteriness, tachycardia, and vomiting in mothers and neonates.[161,162] Dosing guidelines have recommended that serum theophylline concentrations be maintained at 5 to 12 μg/mL during pregnancy.[114] Theophylline can have significant interactions with other drugs, which can cause decreased clearance with resultant toxicity. For instance, cimetidine can cause a 70% increase in serum levels, and erythromycin use can increase theophylline serum levels by 35%.[163]

The main advantage of theophylline is the long duration of action, 10 to 12 hours with the use of sustained-release preparations, which is especially useful in the management of nocturnal asthma.[164] Theophylline is indicated only for chronic therapy and is not effective for the treatment of acute exacerbations during pregnancy.[165] Theophylline has anti-inflammatory actions[166] that may be mediated by inhibition of leukotriene production and its capacity to stimulate prostaglandin E_2 production.[167] Theophylline may potentiate the efficacy of inhaled corticosteroids.[168]

The NAEPP reviewed eight human studies that had a total of 660 women with asthma who took theophylline during pregnancy.[114] These studies and clinical experience confirm the safety of theophylline at a serum concentration of 5 to 12 μg/mL during pregnancy. In a randomized, controlled trial, there were no differences in asthma exacerbations or perinatal outcomes in a cohort receiving theophylline compared with the cohort receiving inhaled beclomethasone.[169] However, the theophylline cohort had significantly more reported side effects, discontinuation of the study medication, and an increased proportion of those with an FEV_1 less than 80% of the predicted value.

LEUKOTRIENE MEDIATORS

Leukotrienes are arachidonic acid metabolites that have been implicated in transducing bronchospasm, mucous secretion, and increased vascular permeability.[170] Bronchoconstriction associated with aspirin ingestion can be blocked by leukotriene receptor antagonists.[171] Treatment with the leukotriene receptor antagonist montelukast (Singulair) has significantly improved pulmonary function as measured by FEV_1.[170] The leukotriene receptor antagonists zafirlukast (Accolate) and montelukast are pregnancy category B drugs. There are minimal data regarding the efficacy or safety of these agents during human pregnancy. Leukotriene receptor antagonists provide an alternative treatment for mild persistent asthma and an adjunctive treatment for the management of moderate and severe persistent asthma during pregnancy.[114]

ORAL CORTICOSTEROIDS

The NAEPP Working Group reviewed eight human studies, including one report of two meta-analyses.[114] Most subjects in these studies did not take oral corticosteroids for asthma, and the length, timing, and dose of exposure to the drug were not well described. The panel concluded that findings from the evidence are conflicting. Oral corticosteroid use during the first trimester of pregnancy is associated with a threefold increased risk for isolated cleft lip with or without cleft palate. Because the background incidence is about 0.1%, the excess risk attributable to oral steroids is 0.2% to 0.3%.[172] Oral corticosteroid use during pregnancy by patients who have asthma has been associated with an increased incidence of preeclampsia, preterm delivery, and low birth weight.[126,131,144,160,172] A prospective study found that use of systemic corticosteroids resulted in a deficit of about 200 g in birth weight compared with controls and those exclusively treated with β_2-agonists.[173] However, it is difficult to separate the effects of the oral corticosteroids on these outcomes from the effects of severe or uncontrolled asthma.

Because of the uncertainties in these data and the definite risks of severe, uncontrolled asthma to the mother and fetus, the NAEPP Working Group recommends the use of oral corticosteroids when indicated for the long-term management of severe asthma or exacerbations during pregnancy.[114] For the treatment of acute exacerbations, methylprednisolone or other corticosteroids may be given at a dose of 120 to 180 mg per day in three or four divided doses; after the PEFR reaches 70% of the personal best value, the daily dosage of parenteral or oral corticosteroid, such as prednisone, can be dropped to 60 to 80 mg per day.[114]

Management of Allergic Rhinitis Exacerbating Asthma

Rhinitis, sinusitis, and gastroesophageal reflux may exacerbate asthma symptoms, and their management should be considered an integral aspect of asthma care. Intranasal corticosteroids are the most effective medications for control of allergic rhinitis. Loratadine (Claritin) or cetirizine (Zyrtec) are recommended second-generation antihistamines. Because oral decongestant ingestion during the first trimester has been associated with gastroschisis, inhaled decongestants or inhaled corticosteroids should be considered before use of oral decongestants.[114] Immunotherapy is considered safe during pregnancy, but because of the risk of anaphylaxis, initiation of immunotherapy is not recommended during pregnancy.

Antenatal Management

Patients with moderate or severe asthma should be considered to be at risk for pregnancy complications. Adverse outcomes can be increased by underestimation of asthma severity and undertreatment of asthma. The first prenatal visit should include a detailed medical history with attention to medical conditions that can complicate the management of asthma, including active pulmonary disease. The patient should be questioned about her smoking history and the presence and severity of symptoms, episodes of nocturnal asthma, the number of days of work missed, and emergency care visits due to asthma. Asthma severity should be determined (see Table 45-3). The type and amount of asthma medications, including the number of puffs of β_2-agonists used each day, should be determined.

Gravidas with moderate or severe asthma should have scheduling of prenatal visits based on clinical judgment. In addition to routine care, monthly or more frequent evaluations of asthma history (i.e., emergency visits, hospital admissions, symptom frequency, severity, nocturnal symptoms, and medication dosages and compliance) and pulmonary function (i.e., FEV_1 or PEFR) are recommended. Patients should be instructed on proper dosing and administration of their asthma medications.

Daily peak flow monitoring should be considered for patients with moderate to severe asthma and especially for patients who have difficulty perceiving signs of worsening asthma.[114] It may be helpful to maintain an asthma diary containing a daily record of symptoms, peak flow measurements, activity limitations, medical contacts initiated, and regular and as-needed medications taken. Identifying and avoiding asthma triggers can lead to improved maternal well-being and less need for medications. Specific recommendations can be made for appropriate environmental controls based on the patient's history of exposure and, when available, skin test reactivity to asthma triggers.

Women who have moderate or severe asthma during pregnancy may benefit from additional fetal surveillance in the form of ultrasound examinations and antenatal fetal testing. Because asthma has been associated with intrauterine growth restriction and preterm birth, it is useful to establish pregnancy dating accurately by first-trimester ultrasound when possible. In the opinion of the NAEPP Working Group,[114] the evaluation of fetal activity and growth by serial ultrasound examinations may be considered for women who have suboptimally controlled asthma, for those with moderate to severe asthma (starting at 32 weeks), and after recovery from a severe asthma exacerbation. The intensity of antenatal surveillance of fetal well-being should be considered on the basis of the severity of the asthma and any other high-risk features of the pregnancy. All patients should be instructed to be attentive to fetal activity.

TABLE 45-8 HOME MANAGEMENT OF ACUTE ASTHMA EXACERBATIONS

Initial Approach
Use albuterol MDI at a dose of 2-4 puffs (or single nebulizer treatment), and measure PEFR.
Poor Response
If PEFR < 50% of predicted, severe wheezing and shortness of breath occur, or fetal movement is decreased, repeat albuterol at a dose of 2-4 puffs by MDI and obtain emergency care.
Incomplete Response
If PEFR is 50-80% of predicted or if wheezing and shortness of breath persist, repeat albuterol treatment at a dose of 2-4 puffs by MDI at 20-minute intervals up to two more times.
If repeat PEFR is 50-80% of predicted or if fetal movement is decreased, contact caregiver or go for emergency care.
Good Response
If PEFR > 80% of predicted, there is no wheezing or shortness of breath, and the fetus is moving normally, patient may continue inhaled albuterol at a dose of 2-4 puffs by MDI every 3-4 hours as needed.

MDI, metered-dose inhaler; PEFR, peak expiratory flow rate.
Modified from National Asthma Education and Prevention Program (NAEPP) expert panel report (NAEPP 04): Managing asthma during pregnancy: Recommendations for pharmacologic treatment 2004 update. NHLBI, NIH publication no. 05-3279. Available at http://www.nhlbi.nih.gov/health/prof/lung/asthma/astpreg/astpreg_qr.pdf (accessed January 2008).

Home Management of Asthma Exacerbations

An asthma exacerbation that causes minimal problems for the mother may have severe sequelae for the fetus. An abnormal fetal heart rate tracing may be the initial manifestation of an asthmatic exacerbation. A maternal Po_2 value of less than 60 mm Hg or hemoglobin saturation of less than 90% may be associated with profound fetal hypoxia. Asthma exacerbations in pregnancy should be aggressively managed. Patients should be given an individualized guide for decision making and rescue management, and they should be educated to recognize signs and symptoms of early asthma exacerbations, such as coughing, chest tightness, dyspnea, or wheezing, or by a 20% decrease in the PEFR. Early recognition enables prompt institution of home rescue treatment to avoid maternal and fetal hypoxia.

Patients should use inhaled albuterol (two to four puffs) every 20 minutes for up to 1 hour (Table 45-8). The response is considered to be good if symptoms are resolved or become subjectively mild, normal activities can be resumed, and the PEFR is more than 70% of the personal best value. The patient should seek further medical attention if the response is incomplete or if fetal activity is decreased.

Hospital and Clinic Management

The principal goal of hospital and clinic management should be the prevention of hypoxia. Measurement of oxygenation by pulse oximetry is essential, and arterial blood gas determinations should be obtained if oxygen saturation remains less than 95%. Chest radiographs usually are not needed. Continuous electronic fetal monitoring should be initiated if gestation has advanced to point of potential fetal viability. Albuterol (2.5 to 5 mg every 20 minutes for three doses and then 2.5 to 10 mg every 1 to 4 hours as needed or 10 to 15 mg/hr administered continuously) should be delivered by nebulizer driven with oxygen.[114] Occasionally, nebulized treatment is not effective because the patient is moving air poorly; in such cases, terbutaline (0.25 mg) can be administered subcutaneously every 15 minutes for three doses. The patient should be assessed for general level of activity, color, pulse rate, use of accessory muscles, and airflow obstruction determined by auscultation and FEV_1 or PEFR before and after each bronchodilator treatment. Guidelines for the management of asthma exacerbations are given in Table 45-9.

Labor and Delivery Management

Asthma medications should not be discontinued during labor and delivery. Although asthma is usually quiescent during labor, consideration should be given to assessing PEFRs on admission and at 12-hour intervals. The patient should be kept hydrated and should receive adequate analgesia to decrease the risk of bronchospasm. If systemic corticosteroids have been used in the previous 4 weeks, intravenous corticosteroids (e.g., 100 mg of hydrocortisone every 8 hours) should be administered during labor and for the 24-hour period after delivery to prevent an adrenal crisis.[114] An elective delivery should be postponed if the patient is having an exacerbation.

It is rarely necessary to perform a cesarean section for an acute asthma exacerbation. Maternal compromise and fetal compromise usually respond to aggressive medical management. Occasionally, delivery may improve the respiratory status of a patient with unstable asthma who has a mature fetus. Prostaglandin E_2 or E_1 can be used for cervical ripening, the management of spontaneous or induced abortions, or postpartum hemorrhage, although the patient's respiratory status should be monitored.[174] Carboprost (15-methyl $PGF_{2\alpha}$) and ergonovine and methylergonovine (Methergine) can cause bronchospasm.[175] Magnesium sulfate is a bronchodilator, but indomethacin can induce bronchospasm in the aspirin-sensitive patient. There are no reports of the use of calcium channel blockers for tocolysis among

TABLE 45-9 EMERGENCY DEPARTMENT AND HOSPITAL-BASED MANAGEMENT OF ASTHMA EXACERBATION

Initial Assessment and Treatment

Obtain a history, perform an examination (e.g., auscultation, use of accessory muscles, heart rate, respiratory rate), assess PEFR or FEV_1 and oxygen saturation, and obtain other tests as indicated.

Initiate fetal assessment; consider fetal monitoring or BPP, or both, if the fetus is potentially viable.

For severe exacerbations (i.e., FEV_1 or PEFR < 50% with severe symptoms at rest), administer high-dose albuterol by nebulizer every 20 minutes or continuously for 1 hour and provide inhaled ipratropium bromide and a systemic corticosteroid.

Give albuterol by MDI or nebulizer, providing up to three doses in the first hour.

Administer an oral corticosteroid if there was no immediate response or the patient recently was treated with a systemic corticosteroid.

Administer oxygen to maintain a saturation level greater than 95%.

Repeat assessment of symptoms, the physical examination, and assessment of PEFR and oxygen saturation.

Continue albuterol every 60 minutes for 1 to 3 hours, provided there is improvement.

Repeat Assessment

Evaluate the symptoms, perform a physical examination, assess PEFR and oxygen saturation, and obtain other tests as needed.

Continue fetal assessment.

Good Response

Values for FEV_1 or PEFR are 70% of normal or greater.

Response is sustained for 60 minutes after the last treatment.

Patient is not in distress.

Results of the physical examination are normal.

Fetal status is reassuring.

Patient is discharged to her home.

Incomplete Response

Values for FEV_1 or PEFR are between 50% and 70% of normal.

Symptoms are mild or moderate.

Continue fetal assessment until the patient is stabilized.

Monitor the FEV_1 or PEFR, oxygen saturation, and pulse.

Continue inhaled albuterol and oxygen.

Administer inhaled ipratropium bromide.

Administer a systemic (oral or intravenous) corticosteroid.

The decision for hospitalization is individualized.

Poor Response

Values for FEV_1 or PEFR are less than 50%.

Values for P_{CO_2} are greater than 42 mm Hg.

Results of the physical examination include severe symptoms, drowsiness, and confusion.

Continue fetal assessment.

Admit the patient to the intensive care unit.

Impending or Actual Respiratory Arrest

Admit the patient to the intensive care unit.

Perform intubation and mechanical ventilation with 100% oxygen.

Administer nebulized albuterol plus inhaled ipratropium bromide.

Administer an intravenous corticosteroid.

Intensive Care Unit

Administer inhaled albuterol hourly or continuously plus inhaled ipratropium bromide.

Administer an intravenous corticosteroid.

Administer oxygen.

Intubation and mechanical ventilation may be necessary.

Continue fetal assessment until the patient is stabilized.

Discharge to Home

Continue treatment with albuterol.

Administer an oral systemic corticosteroid if indicated.

Initiate or continue inhaled corticosteroid until review at medical follow-up.

Provide patient education.

Review the patient's medicine use.

Review or initiate an action plan.

Recommend close medical follow-up.

BPP, biophysical profile; FEV_1, forced expiratory volume in 1 second; MDI, metered-dose inhaler; P_{CO_2}, carbon dioxide partial pressure; PEFR, peak expiratory flow rate.

Modified from National Asthma Education and Prevention Program (NAEPP) expert panel report (NAEPP 04): Managing asthma during pregnancy: Recommendations for pharmacologic treatment—2004 update. NHLBI, NIH publication no. 05-3279. Available at http://www.nhlbi.nih.gov/health/prof/lung/asthma/astpreg/astpreg_qr.pdf (accessed January 2008).

patients with asthma, although an association with bronchospasm has not been observed with wide clinical use.

Lumbar anesthesia has the benefit of reducing oxygen consumption and minute ventilation during labor.[176] Fentanyl may be a better analgesic than meperidine, which causes histamine release, but meperidine is rarely associated with the onset of bronchospasm during labor. A 2% incidence of bronchospasm has been reported with regional anesthesia.[177] Ketamine is useful for induction of general anesthesia because it can prevent bronchospasm.[178] Communication between the obstetric, anesthetic, and pediatric caregivers is important for optimal care.

Breastfeeding

Only small amounts of asthma medications enter breast milk. Prednisone, theophylline, antihistamines, beclomethasone, β_2-agonists, and cromolyn are not considered to be contraindications for breastfeeding.[114,179] However, among sensitive individuals, theophylline may cause toxic effects in the neonate, including vomiting, feeding difficulties, jitteriness, and cardiac arrhythmias.

Overview of Asthma during Pregnancy

Asthma is an increasingly common problem during pregnancy. Mild and moderate asthma can be associated with excellent maternal and perinatal pregnancy outcomes, especially if patients are managed according to contemporary NAEPP recommendations. Severe and poorly controlled asthma may be associated with increased prematurity, the need for cesarean delivery, preeclampsia, and growth restriction. Severe asthma exacerbations can result in maternal morbidity and mortality and can have commensurate adverse pregnancy outcomes. The management of asthma during pregnancy should be based on objective assessment, trigger avoidance, patient education, and step therapy. Asthma medications should be continued during pregnancy and while breastfeeding.

Restrictive Lung Disease in Pregnancy

Clinical Manifestations

Restrictive ventilatory defects occur when lung expansion is limited because of alterations in the lung parenchyma or because of abnormalities in the pleura, chest wall, or the neuromuscular apparatus.[180] These conditions are characterized by a reduction in lung volumes and an increase in the ratio of FEV_1 to forced vital capacity.[181] The interstitial lung diseases include idiopathic pulmonary fibrosis, sarcoidosis, hypersensitivity pneumonitis, pneumomycosis, drug-induced lung disease, and connective tissue disease. Additional conditions that cause a restrictive ventilatory defect include pleural and chest wall diseases and extrathoracic conditions such as obesity, peritonitis, and ascites.[181]

Restrictive lung disease in pregnancy has not been well studied. Consequently, little is known about the effects of restrictive lung disease on the outcome of pregnancy or the effects of pregnancy on the disease process. One study presented data on nine pregnant women with interstitial and restrictive lung disease who were prospectively managed.[182] Diagnoses included idiopathic pulmonary fibrosis, hypersensitivity pneumonitis, sarcoidosis, kyphoscoliosis, and multiple pulmonary emboli. Three of the gravidas had severe disease characterized by a vital capacity of no more than 1.5 L (50% of predicted) or a diffusing capacity of no more than 50% of predicted. Five of the patients had exercise-induced oxygen desaturation, and four patients required supplemental oxygen. In this group, one patient had an adverse outcome and was delivered at 31 weeks. She subsequently required mechanical ventilation for 72 hours. All other patients were delivered at or beyond 36 weeks with no adverse intrapartum or postpartum complications. All infants were at or above the 30th percentile for growth.[182] The investigators concluded that restrictive lung disease was well tolerated in pregnancy. However, exercise intolerance is common, and these patients may require early oxygen supplementations.[182]

Sarcoidosis

Sarcoidosis is a systemic granulomatosis disease of undetermined origin that often affects young adults. Pregnancy outcome for most patients with sarcoidosis is good.[183,184] In one study, 35 pregnancies in 18 patients with sarcoidosis were evaluated retrospectively.[183] There was no effect of the disease process during pregnancy in nine patients, improvement was demonstrated in six patients, and there was a worsening of the disease in three patients. During the postpartum period, no relapse occurred in 15 patients; however, progression of the disease continued in 3 women. Another retrospective study assessed 15 pregnancies complicated by maternal sarcoidosis over a 10-year period.[184] Eleven of these patients remained stable, two experienced disease progression, and two died because of complications of severe sarcoidosis. In this group, factors indicating a poor prognosis included parenchymal lesions identified on the chest radiograph, advanced radiographic staging, advanced maternal age, low inflammatory activity, requirement for drugs other than steroids, and the presence of extrapulmonary sarcoidosis.[184] Both patients who succumbed during gestation had severe disease at the onset of pregnancy. The overall cesarean section rate was 40%, and 4 (27%) of 15 infants weighed less than 2500 g. None of the patients developed preeclampsia. One explanation for the commonly observed improvement in sarcoidosis may be the increased concentration of circulating corticosteroids during pregnancy. However, because sarcoidosis improves spontaneously in many nonpregnant patients, the improvement may be coincident with pregnancy.

Maycock and associates[185] reported 16 pregnancies in 10 patients with sarcoidosis. Eight of these patients showed improvement in at least some of the manifestations of sarcoidosis during the antepartum period. In two patients, no effect was seen. A recurrence of the abnormal findings was observed in the postpartum period within several months after delivery in approximately one half of the patients. Some had new manifestations of sarcoidosis not previously observed. Another study examined 17 pregnancies in 10 patients and concluded that pregnancy had no consistent effect on the course of the disease.[186] Scadding[187] separated patients into three categories based on characteristic patterns of their chest radiographs. When the lesions on the chest radiograph had resolved before pregnancy, radiographs remained normal throughout gestation. In women with radiographic changes before pregnancy, resolution continued throughout the prenatal period. Patients with inactive fibrotic residual disease had stable chest radiographs, and those with active disease tended to have partial or complete resolution of those changes during pregnancy. However, most patients in the latter group experienced exacerbation of the disease within 3 to 6 months after delivery.

Patients with pulmonary hypertension complicating restrictive lung disease may have a mortality rate as high as 50% during gestation. These patients need close monitoring during the labor, delivery, and postpartum periods. Invasive monitoring with a pulmonary artery catheter may be indicated to optimize cardiorespiratory function. Gravidas with restrictive lung disease, including pulmonary sarcoidosis, may benefit from early institution of steroid therapy for evidence of worsening pulmonary status. Individuals with evidence of severe disease need close monitoring and may require supplemental oxygen therapy during gestation.

During labor, consideration should be given to the early use of epidural anesthesia if it is not contraindicated. The early institution of pain management in this population can minimize pain, decrease the sympathetic response, and decrease oxygen consumption during labor and delivery. The use of general anesthesia should be avoided, if possible, because these patients may develop pulmonary complications after general anesthesia, including pneumonia and difficulty weaning from the ventilator. Close fetal surveillance throughout gestation is indicated because impaired oxygenation may lead to impaired fetal growth and the development of fetal heart rate abnormalities during labor and delivery.

An additional consideration is the need to counsel all women with restrictive lung disease about the potential for continued impairment of their respiratory status during pregnancy, particularly if their respiratory status is deteriorating when they conceive. The individual with clinical signs consistent with pulmonary hypertension or severe restrictive disease should be cautioned about the possibility of maternal mortality resulting from worsening pulmonary function during gestation.

In summary, although the literature on restrictive lung disease in pregnancy is limited, it supports the conclusion that most patients with restrictive lung disease complicating pregnancy, including those with pulmonary sarcoidosis, can have a favorable pregnancy outcome. However, the clinician should keep in mind that patients with restrictive lung disease can have worsening of their clinical condition and may succumb during gestation.

Cystic Fibrosis in Pregnancy

CF involves the exocrine glands and epithelial tissues of the pancreas, sweat glands, and mucous glands in the respiratory, digestive, and reproductive tracts. Chronic obstructive pulmonary disease, pancreatic exocrine insufficiency, and elevated levels of sweat electrolytes are present in most patients with CF.[188] The disease is genetically transmitted with an autosomal recessive pattern of inheritance. The CF gene was identified and cloned in 1989. The gene is localized to chromosome 7, and the molecular defect accounting for most cases has been identified.[189,190,191] In the United States, approximately 4% of the white population are heterozygous carriers of the CF gene. The disease occurs in 1 of 3200 white live births.[192]

Morbidity and mortality in patients with CF usually result from progressive chronic bronchial pulmonary disease. Pregnancy and the attendant physiologic changes can stress the pulmonary, cardiovascular, and nutritional status of women with CF. The purpose of this section is to familiarize the obstetrician and gynecologist with the physiologic effects of this complex disease, the impact of the disease on pregnancy, and the effect of pregnancy on the disease.

Survival for patients with CF has increased dramatically since 1940. According to the Cystic Fibrosis Foundation's Patient Registry (www.cff.org), survival in 2006 had increased to 37 years. More than 40% of all people with CF in the United States are 18 years or older.[188] This increase in survival of patients with CF likely reflects earlier diagnosis and intervention and the advances in antibiotic therapy and nutritional support. Because of the improvements in care, more women with CF are entering reproductive age. Unlike men with CF who are infertile for the most part, women with CF are often fertile.

The first case of CF complicating pregnancy was reported in 1960, and a total of 13 pregnancies in 10 patients with CF were reported in 1966.[193,194] Cohen and colleagues[195] conducted a survey of 119 CF centers in the United States and Canada and identified a total of 129 pregnancies in 100 women by 1976. Hilman and colleagues[188] surveyed 127 CF centers in the United States between 1976 and 1982. A total of 191 pregnancies were reported during this period in women with CF who were between 16 and 36 years old, with a mean age of 22.6 years.[188] The annual number of CF pregnancies reported to the Cystic Fibrosis Patient Registry doubled between 1986 and 1990, with 52 pregnancies reported in 1986, compared with 111 pregnancies reported in 1990. In 2006 209 women with CF were pregnant. Because the number of women with CF achieving pregnancy is steadily increasing, it is imperative that the obstetrician be familiar with the disease.

Effect of Pregnancy on Cystic Fibrosis

The physiologic changes associated with pregnancy are well tolerated by healthy gravidas, but those with CF may adapt poorly. During pregnancy, there is an increase in resting minute ventilation, which at term may approach 150% of control values.[196] Enlargement of the abdominal contents and upward displacement of the diaphragm leads to a decrease in functional residual volume and a decrease in residual volume.[196] Pregnancy is also accompanied by subtle alterations in gas exchange with widening of the alveolar-arterial oxygen gradient that is most pronounced in the supine position.[196] Alterations in pulmonary function are of little consequence in the normal pregnant woman, but in the gravida with CF, these changes may contribute to respiratory decompensation that can lead to an increase in morbidity and mortality for the mother and the fetus. Women with CF and advanced lung disease also may have pulmonary hypertension.

Nutritional requirements are increased during pregnancy, with approximately 300 kcal/day in additional fuel needed to meet the requirements of mother and fetus.[197] Most patients with CF have pancreatic exocrine insufficiency. Digestive enzymes and bicarbonate ions are diminished, resulting in maldigestion, malabsorption, and malnutrition.[197] Gastrointestinal manifestations of CF include steatorrhea, abdominal pain, distal intestinal obstruction syndrome, and rectal prolapse. Gastroesophageal reflux, peptic ulcer disease, acute pancreatitis, and intussusception occur to different degrees in patients with CF. Partial or complete obstruction of the gastrointestinal tract in older children and adults, also known as distal obstruction syndrome, can be precipitated by dehydration, a change in eating habits, a change in enzyme brand or dose, or immobility. It is treated with a combination of laxatives and enemas. Patients with CF are encouraged to eat a diet that provides 120% to 150% of the recommended energy intake of normal age- and sex-matched controls. This is only a guideline, because in practice, the energy requirement for a patient with CF is that of their ideal body weight when malabsorption has been minimized. Research done by the United Kingdom Dieticians Cystic Fibrosis Interest Group found that women with CF who received preconception counseling had a significantly greater mean maternal weight gain and significantly heavier infants than women who had not received preconception advice.[198]

Grand and colleagues[194] reported 13 pregnancies in 10 women with CF. Of these, five women had a progressive decline in their pulmonary function, two of whom died of cor pulmonale in the immediate postpartum period. Pregnancy was well tolerated in 5 of 10 women, 2 of whom went on to have subsequent pregnancies that were similarly well tolerated.[194] In this study, the pregravid pulmonary status of the patient was the most important predictor of outcome. However, there was no quantification of pulmonary function. A case report by Novy and colleagues[199] described pulmonary function and gas exchange in a pregnant woman with CF. The patient had severe disease as evidenced by a vital capacity of only 0.72 L and a PaO_2 of 50 mm Hg at presentation. The patient suffered a progressive increase in residual volume and decline in vital capacity that was accompanied by worsening hypoxemia and hypercapnia, resulting in respiratory distress and right-sided heart failure in the early postpartum period.[199] Based on the experience with this patient and a review of the literature, the investigators recommended therapeutic abortion for any patient demonstrating progressive pulmonary deterioration and hypoxemia despite maximal medical management.[199]

In 1980, Cohen and associates[195] described 100 patients and a total of 129 pregnancies. Ninety-seven pregnancies (75%) were completed, and 89% of these women delivered viable infants. Twenty-seven percent of these fetuses were delivered preterm. There were 11 perinatal deaths and no congenital anomalies. In this study, 65% of patients required antibiotic therapy before delivery. In 1983, Palmer and colleagues[200] retrospectively reviewed the pre-pregnancy status of eight women with CF who subsequently completed 11 pregnancies. They found that five women tolerated pregnancy without difficulty but that three had irreversible deterioration in their clinical status. The investigators identified four maternal factors that predicted outcome: clinical status (i.e., Shwachman score), nutritional status (i.e., percent of predicted weight for height), the extent of chest radiologic abnormalities (i.e., Brasfield chest radiographic score), and the magnitude of pulmonary function impairment. Women with good clinical study results, good nutritional status (i.e., within 15% of their predicted ideal body weight for height), nearly normal chest radiographs, and only mild obstructive lung disease tolerated pregnancy well without deterioration.[200]

Several reports suggest that patients with mild CF, good nutritional status, and less impairment of lung function tolerate pregnancy well. However, those with poor clinical status, malnutrition, hepatic dysfunction, or advanced lung disease are at increased risk from pregnancy.[201-203] Kent and Farquharson[203] reviewed the literature and reported 217 pregnancies. In this series, the frequency of preterm delivery was 24.3%, and the perinatal death rate was 7.9%. Poor outcomes were associated with a maternal weight gain of less than 4.5 kg and a forced vital capacity of less than 50% of the predicted value. Edenborough and colleagues[204] also described pregnancies in women with CF. There were 18 live births (81.8%), one third of which were preterm deliveries, and 18.2% of patients had abortions. There were four maternal deaths within 3.2 years after delivery. In this series, lung function was available before delivery, immediately after delivery, and after pregnancy. The investigators demonstrated a decline of 13% in FEV_1 and 11% in forced vital capacity during pregnancy. Most patients returned to baseline pulmonary function after pregnancy. Although most of the women in this series tolerated pregnancy well, those with moderate to severe lung disease (i.e., FEV_1 < 60% of the predicted value) more often had preterm infants and had increased loss of lung function compared with those with milder disease.[204]

In two other series, pre-pregnancy FEV_1 was found to be the most useful predictor of outcomes in pregnant women with CF.[204,205] There was also a positive correlation of pre-pregnancy FEV_1 with maternal survival. For the 72 pregnancies identified, the outcomes were known for 69; there were 48 live births (70%), of which 22 were premature (46%); 14 therapeutic abortions (20%); and 7 miscarriages (10%). There were no stillbirths, neonatal deaths, or early maternal deaths. Three major fetal anomalies were seen, but no infant had CF. Another report similarly documented the outcome of 72 pregnancies with CF.[206]

Pulmonary involvement in CF includes chronic infection of the airways and bronchiectasis. There is selective infection with certain microorganisms, such as *S. aureus*, *H. influenzae*, *P. aeruginosa*, and *Burkholderia cepacia*. In one report, three of four deaths during pregnancy occurred in gravidas colonized with *B. cepacia*.[207] Gilljam and associates[208] reported outcomes for a cohort of pregnancies for women with CF from 1963 to 1998. For 92 pregnancies in 54 women, there were 11 miscarriages and 7 therapeutic abortions. Forty-nine women gave birth to 74 children. The mean follow-up time was 11 ± 8 years. One patient was lost to follow-up shortly after delivery, and one was lost after 12 years. The overall mortality rate was 19% (9 of 48 patients). Absence of *B. cepacia* ($P < .001$), pancreatic sufficiency ($P = .01$), and pre-pregnancy FEV_1 more than 50% of the predicted value ($P = .03$) were associated with better survival rates. When adjusted for the same parameters, pregnancy did not affect survival compared with the entire adult female CF population. The decline in FEV_1 was comparable with that in the total CF population. Three women had diabetes mellitus, and seven developed gestational diabetes. There were six preterm infants and one neonatal death. CF was diagnosed in two children. Gilljam and coworkers[208] concluded that the maternal and fetal outcomes were good for most women with CF. Risk factors for mortality are similar to those for the nonpregnant CF population. Pregnancies should be planned so that there is an opportunity for counseling and optimization of the medical condition. Good communication between the CF team and the obstetrician is important.[208]

A recent review of 10 pregnancies in 10 cystic fibrosis lung transplant recipients document 9 live births and 1 therapeutic abortion. Five were preterm births but all were well at follow-up. Three transplant recipients developed rejection during the pregnancy. One woman had evidence of rejection prior to conception. All 4 women died within 38 months of delivery. Pregnancy CF in lung transplant patients is feasible but carries a high risk of maternal mortality.[209]

Counseling Pregnant Women with Cystic Fibrosis

Women with CF should be advised about the potential adverse affects of pregnancy on maternal health status. Factors that may predict poor outcome include pre-pregnancy evidence of poor nutritional status, significant pulmonary disease with hypoxemia, and pulmonary hypertension. Liver disease and diabetes mellitus are also poor prognostic factors. Gravidas with poor nutritional status, pulmonary hypertension (e.g., cor pulmonale), and deteriorating pulmonary function early in gestation should consider therapeutic abortion, because the risk of maternal mortality may be unacceptably high.

The woman with CF who is considering pregnancy should consider the need for strong psychosocial and physical support after delivery. The rigors of child rearing may add to the risk of maternal deterioration during this period. Her family should be willing to provide physical and emotional support and should be aware of the potential for deterioration in the mother's health and the potential for maternal mortality. The need for care of a potentially preterm, growth-restricted neonate, with all of its attendant morbidities and potential mortality, should be discussed. Long term, the woman and her family should consider the fact that her life expectancy may be shortened by CF, and plans should be made for rearing of the child in the event of maternal death.

Management of the Pregnancy Complicated by Cystic Fibrosis

Care of the gravida with CF should be a coordinated team effort. Physicians familiar with the complications and management of CF should be included, as well as a maternal-fetal medicine specialist and neonatal team.

The gravida should be assessed for potential risk factors, such as severe lung disease, pulmonary hypertension, poor nutritional status, pancreatic failure, and liver disease, preferably before attempting gestation but certainly during the early months of pregnancy. Gravidas should be advised to be 90% of ideal body weight before conception if possible. A weight gain of 11 to 12 kg is recommended.[188] Frequent monitoring of weight; levels of blood glucose, hemoglobin, total protein, serum albumin, and fat-soluble vitamins A and E; and the prothrombin time is suggested.[188] At each visit, the history of caloric intake and symptoms of maldigestion and malabsorption should be taken, and pancreatic enzymes should be adjusted if needed. Patients who are unable to achieve adequate weight gain through oral nutritional supplements may be given nocturnal enteral nasogastric tube feeding. In this situation, the risk of aspiration should be considered, especially in patients with a history of gastroesophageal reflux, which is common in CF.[188] If malnutrition is severe, parenteral hyperalimentation may be necessary for successful completion of the pregnancy.[210]

Baseline pulmonary function should be assessed, preferably before conception. Assessment should include forced vital capacity, FEV_1, lung volumes, pulse oximetry, and arterial blood gas measurements, if indicated. These values should be serially monitored during gestation, and deterioration in pulmonary function should be addressed immediately. An echocardiogram can assess the patient for underlying pulmonary hypertension and cor pulmonale. If pulmonary hypertension or cor pulmonale is diagnosed, the gravida should be advised about the high risk of maternal mortality.

Early recognition and prompt treatment of pulmonary infections is important in the management of the pregnant woman with CF. Treatment includes intravenous antibiotics in the appropriate dose, keeping in mind the increased clearance of these drugs because of pregnancy and CF. Plasma levels of aminoglycosides should be monitored and adjusted as indicated by the results. Chest physical therapy and bronchial drainage are also important components of the management of pulmonary infections in CF. Because *P. aeruginosa* is the most frequently isolated bacterium associated with chronic endobronchitis and bronchiectasis, antibiotic regimens should include coverage for this organism.

If the patient with CF has pancreatic insufficiency and diabetes mellitus, careful monitoring of blood glucose levels and insulin therapy are indicated. Pancreatic enzymes may need to be replaced to optimize the patient's nutritional status. Because of malabsorption of fats and frequent use of antibiotics, the CF patient is prone to vitamin K deficiency. The prothrombin time should be checked regularly, and parenteral vitamin K should be administered if the prothrombin time is elevated.

The fetus of a woman with CF is at risk for uteroplacental insufficiency and intrauterine growth restriction. The maternal nutritional status and weight gain during pregnancy affect fetal growth. Nonstress testing should be started at 32 weeks' gestation or sooner if there is evidence of fetal compromise. If there is evidence of severe fetal compromise, delivery should be accomplished. Likewise, evidence of profound maternal deterioration, such as a marked and sustained decline in pulmonary function, development of right-sided heart failure, refractory hypoxemia, and progressive hypercapnia and respiratory acidosis, may be maternal indications for early delivery. If the fetus is potentially viable, the administration of betamethasone may be beneficial. Vaginal delivery should be attempted when possible.

Labor, delivery, and the postpartum period can be particularly dangerous for the patient with CF. The augmentation in cardiac output stresses the cardiovascular system and can lead to cardiopulmonary failure in the patient with pulmonary hypertension and cor pulmonale. These patients are also more likely to develop right-sided heart failure. Heart failure should be treated with aggressive diuresis and supplemental oxygen. Management may be optimized by insertion of a pulmonary artery catheter to monitor right- and left-sided filling pressures. Pain control can reduce the sympathetic response to labor and tachycardia. This benefits the patient who is demonstrating pulmonary or cardiac compromise. In the patient with a normal partial thromboplastin time, insertion of an epidural catheter for continuous epidural analgesia may be beneficial. This is also useful in the event a cesarean delivery is indicated because general anesthesia and its possible effects on pulmonary function can be avoided. If general anesthesia is needed, preoperative anticholinergic agents should be avoided because they tend to promote drying and inspissation of airway secretions. Close fetal surveillance is essential because the fetus might have been suffering from uteroplacental insufficiency during gestation and is more prone to develop evidence of compromise during labor. Delivery by cesarean section should be reserved for the usual obstetric indications.

In summary, more women with CF are living to childbearing age and are capable of conceiving. Clinical experience has demonstrated that pregnancy in women with mild CF is well tolerated. Women with severe disease have an associated increase in maternal and fetal morbidity and mortality. The potential risk to any one individual with CF desiring pregnancy should be assessed and discussed in detail with the patient and her family.

References

1. Prowse CM, Gaensler EAL: Respiratory and acid base changes during pregnancy. Anesthesiology 26:31, 1965.
2. Templeton A, Kelman GR: Maternal blood-gases, (PAO_2–PaO_2), physiological shunt and VD/VT in normal pregnancy. Br J Anaesth 48:1001, 1976.
3. Boutourline-Young H, Boutourline-Young E: Alveolar carbon dioxide levels in pregnant, parturient and lactating subjects. J Obstet Gynaecol Br Emp 63:509, 1956.
4. Skatrud JB, Dempsey JA, Kaiser DG: Ventilatory response to medroxyprogesterone acetate in normal subjects: Time course and mechanism. J Appl Physiol 44:939, 1978.
5. Goodland RL, Pommerenke WT: Cyclic fluctuations of the alveolar carbon dioxide tension during the normal menstrual cycle. Fertil Steril 3:394, 1952.
6. Lyons HA, Huang CT: Therapeutic use of progesterone in alveolar hypoventilation associated with obesity. Am J Med 44:881, 1968.
7. Machida GL: Influence of progesterone on arterial blood and CSF acid-base balance in women. J Appl Physiol 51:1433, 1981.
8. Wilbrand U, Porath CH, Matthaes P, et al: Der einfluss der Ovarialsteroide auf die Funktion des Atemzentrums. Arch Gynakol 191:507, 1959.
9. Lyons HA, Antonio R: The sensitivity of the respiratory center in pregnancy and the administration of progesterone. Trans Assoc Am Physicians 72:173, 1959.
10. Eng M, Butler J, Bonich JJ: Respiratory function in pregnant obese women. Am J Obstet Gynecol 123:241, 1975.
11. Pernoll ML, Metcalfe J, Kovach PA, et al: Ventilation during rest and exercise in pregnancy and postpartum. Respir Physiol 25:295, 1975.

12. Paciorek J, Spencer N: An association between plasma progesterone and erythrocyte carbonic anhydrase I concentration in women. Clin Sci 58:161, 1980.
13. Schenker JG, Ben-Yoseph Y, Shapira E: Erythrocyte carbonic anhydrase B levels during pregnancy and use of oral contraceptives. Obstet Gynecol 39:237, 1972.
14. Cullen JH, Brum VC, Reid TWH: The respiratory effects of progesterone in severe pulmonary emphysema. Am J Med 27:551, 1959.
15. Sutton FD, Zwillich CW, Creagh CE, et al: Progesterone for outpatient treatment of Pickwickian syndrome. Ann Intern Med 83:476, 1975.
16. Cugell DW, Frank NR, Gaensler EA, Badger TL: Pulmonary function in pregnancy: Serial observations in normal women. Am Rev Tuberc 67:568, 1953.
17. Lehmann V, Fabel H: Lungenfunktionsuntersuchungen an Schwangeren. I. Lungenvolumina. Z Geburtshilfe Perinatol 177:387, 1973.
18. Puranik BM, Kaore SB, Kurhade GA, et al: A longitudinal study of pulmonary function tests during pregnancy. Indian J Physiol Pharmacol 38:129, 1994.
19. Knuttgen HG, Emerson K: Physiological response to pregnancy at rest and during exercise. J Appl Physiol 36:549, 1974.
20. Gazioglu K, Kaltreider NL, Rosen M, et al: Pulmonary function during pregnancy in normal women and in patients with cardiopulmonary disease. Thorax 25:445, 1970.
21. Lehmann V, Fabel H: Lungenfunktionsuntersuchungen an Schwangeren. II. Ventilation, Atemmechanik und Diffusionkapazitt. Z Geburtshilfe Perinatol 177:397, 1973.
22. Milne JA: The respiratory response to pregnancy. Postgrad Med J 55:318, 1979.
23. Heidenreich J, Kafarnik D, Westenburger U, et al: Statische und Dynamische Ventilationgrossen in der Schwangerschaft und im Wochenbett. Arch Gynakol 210:208, 1971.
24. Sims CD, Chamberlain GVP, de Swiet M: Lung function tests in bronchial asthma during and after pregnancy. BJOG 88:434, 1976.
25. Alaily AB, Carrol KB: Pulmonary ventilation in pregnancy. BJOG 85:518, 1978.
26. Thomson KJ, Cohen ME: Studies on the circulation in normal pregnancy. II. Vital capacity observations in normal pregnant women. Surg Gynecol Obstet 66:591, 1938.
27. Klaften E, Palugyay J: Verleichende Untersuchungen über Lage und Ausdehnung von Herz und Lunge in der Schwangerschaft und im Wochenbett. Arch Gynakol 131:347, 1927.
28. Klaften E, Palugyay J: Zur Physiologie der Atmung in der Schwangerschaft. Arch Gynakol 129:414, 1926.
29. Mobius WV: Abrung und Schwangerschaft. Munch Med Wochenschr 103:1389, 1961.
30. McGinty AP: The comparative effect of pregnancy and phrenic nerve interruption on the diaphragm and their relation to pulmonary tuberculosis. Am J Obstet Gynecol 35:237, 1938.
31. Barcroft J: On anoxemia. Lancet 11:485, 1920.
32. Cain SM: Peripheral uptake and delivery in health and disease. Clin Chest Med 4:139, 1983.
33. Bryan-Brown CW, Baek SM, Makabali G, et al: Consumable oxygen: Oxygen availability in relation to oxyhemoglobin dissociation. Crit Care Med 1:17, 1973.
34. Perutz MF: Hemoglobin structure and respiratory transport. Sci Am 239:92, 1978.
35. Rackow EC, Astiz M: Pathophysiology and treatment of septic shock. JAMA 266:548, 1991.
36. Shoemaker WC, Ayres S, Grenvik A, et al: Textbook of Critical Care, 2nd ed. Philadelphia, WB Saunders, 1989.
37. Shibutani K, Komatsu T, Kubal K, et al: Critical level of oxygen delivery in anesthetized man. Crit Care Med 11:640, 1983.
38. Barron W, Lindheimer M: Medical Disorders During Pregnancy. St. Louis, CV Mosby, 1991, p 234.
39. Gemzell CA, Robbe H, Strom G, et al: Observations on circulatory changes and muscular work in normal labor. Acta Obstet Gynaecol Scand 36:75, 1957.
40. Ueland K, Hansen JM: Maternal cardiovascular hemodynamics. II. Posture and uterine contractions. Am J Obstet Gynecol 103:1, 1969.
41. Oxhorn H: The changing aspects of pneumonia complicating pregnancy. Am J Obstet Gynecol 70:1057, 1955.
42. Madinger NE, Greenspoon JS, Gray-Ellrodt A: Pneumonia during pregnancy: Has modern technology improved maternal and fetal outcome? Am J Obstet Gynecol 161:657, 1989.
43. Kaunitz AM, Hughes JM, Grimes DA, et al: Causes of maternal mortality in the United States. Obstet Gynecol 65:605, 1985.
44. Finland M, Dublin TD: Pneumococcic pneumonias complicating pregnancy and the puerperium. JAMA 112:1027, 1939.
45. Benedetti TJ, Valle R, Ledger W: Antepartum pneumonia in pregnancy. Am J Obstet Gynecol 144:413, 1982.
46. Berkowitz K, LaSala A: Risk factors associated with the increasing prevalence of pneumonia during pregnancy. Am J Obstet Gynecol 163:981, 1990.
47. Koonin LM, Ellerbrock TV, Atrash HK, et al: Pregnancy-associated deaths due to AIDS in the United States. JAMA 261:1306, 1989.
48. Dinsmoor MJ: HIV infection and pregnancy. Med Clin North Am 73:701, 1989.
49. Hopwood HG: Pneumonia in pregnancy. Obstet Gynecol 25:875, 1965.
50. Rodrigues J, Niederman MS: Pneumonia complicating pregnancy. Clin Chest Med 13:679, 1992.
51. Harger JH, Ernest JM, Thurnau GR, et al: Risk factors and outcome of varicella-zoster virus pneumonia in pregnant women. J Infect Dis 185:422, 2002.
52. Haake DA, Zakowski PC, Haake DL, et al: Early treatment with acyclovir for varicella pneumonia in otherwise healthy adults: Retrospective controlled study and review. Rev Infect Dis 12:788, 1990.
53. McKinney WP, Volkert P, Kaufman J: Fatal swine influenza pneumonia during late pregnancy. Arch Intern Med 150:213, 1990.
54. American College of Obstetricians and Gynecologists (ACOG): Pulmonary disease in pregnancy. ACOG technical bulletin no. 224. Washington, DC, American College of Obstetricians and Gynecologists, 1996.
55. Mendelson CL: The aspiration of stomach contents into the lungs during obstetric anesthesia. Am J Obstet Gynecol 52:191, 1946.
56. Krantz ML, Edwards WL: The incidence of nonfatal aspiration in obstetric patients. Anesthesiology 30:84, 1973.
57. Ezri T, Szmuk P, Stein A, et al: Peripartum general anesthesia without tracheal intubation: Incidence of aspiration pneumonia. Anaesthesia 55:421, 2000.
58. Soreide E, Bjornestad E, Steen PA: An audit of perioperative aspiration pneumonitis in gynaecological and obstetric patients. Acta Anaesth Scand 40:14, 1996.
59. Tomlinson MW, Caruthers TJ, Whitty JE, et al: Does delivery improve maternal condition in the respiratory-compromised gravida? Obstet Gynecol 91:108, 1998.
60. National Center for Health Statistics: National hospital discharge survey: Annual summary 1990. Vital Health Stat 13:1, 1992.
61. Kort BA, Cefalo RC, Baker VV: Fatal influenza A pneumonia in pregnancy. Am J Perinatol 3:179, 1986.
62. Mullooly JP, Barker WH, Nolan TF Jr: Risk of acute respiratory disease among pregnant women during influenza A epidemics. Public Health Rep 101:205, 1986.
63. Harris JW: Influenza occurring in pregnant women. JAMA 72:978, 1919.
64. Freeman DW, Barno A: Deaths from Asian influenza associated with pregnancy. Am J Obstet Gynecol 78:1172, 1959.
65. Hollingsworth HM, Pratter MR, Irwin RS: Acute respiratory failure in pregnancy. J Intensive Care Med 4:11, 1989.
66. Prevention and Control of Influenza: Recommendations of the Advisory Committee on Immunization Practices (ACIP). MMWR 56:1-54, 2007.
67. Cox SM, Cunningham FG, Luby J: Management of varicella pneumonia complicating pregnancy. Am J Perinatol 7:300, 1990.
68. Esmonde TG, Herdman G, Anderson G: Chickenpox pneumonia: An association with pregnancy. Thorax 44:812, 1989.
69. Smego RA, Asperilla MO: Use of acyclovir for varicella pneumonia during pregnancy. Obstet Gynecol 78:1112, 1991.

70. Harris RE, Rhades ER: Varicella pneumonia complicating pregnancy: Report of a case and review of literature. Obstet Gynecol 25:734, 1965.
71. Andrews EB, Yankaskas BC, Cordero JF, et al: Acyclovir in pregnancy registry: Six years' experience. Obstet Gynecol 79:7, 1992.
72. Brown ZA, Baker DA: Acyclovir therapy during pregnancy. Obstet Gynecol 73:526, 1989.
73. Pickard RE: Varicella pneumonia in pregnancy. Am J Obstet Gynecol 101:504, 1968.
74. Afessa B, Green B: Bacterial pneumonia in hospitalized patients with HIV infection. The pulmonary complications, ICU support, and prognostic factors of hospitalized patients with HIV (PIP) study. Chest 117:1017, 2000.
75. Minkoff H, deRegt R, Landesman S, Schwarz R: *Pneumocystis carinii* associated with acquired immunodeficiency syndrome in pregnancy: A report of three maternal deaths. Obstet Gynecol 67:284, 1986.
76. Armstrong D: Aerosol pentamidine. Ann Intern Med 109:852, 1988.
77. Stratton P, Mofenson LM, Willoughby AD: Human immunodeficiency virus infection in pregnant women under care at AIDS clinical trials in the United States. Obstet Gynecol 79:364, 1992.
78. Jensen LP, O'Sullivan MJ, Gomez-del-Rio M, et al: Acquired immunodeficiency (AIDS) in pregnancy. Am J Obstet Gynecol 148:1145, 1984.
79. Antoine C, Morris M, Douglas G: Maternal and fetal mortality in acquired immunodeficiency syndrome. N Y State J Med 86:443, 1986.
80. Kell PD, Barton SE, Smith DE, et al: A maternal death caused by AIDS. Case report. BJOG 98:725, 1991.
81. Ahmad H, Mehta NJ, Manikal VM, et al: *Pneumocystis carinii* pneumonia in pregnancy. Chest 120:666, 2001.
82. Clinton M, Niederman M, Matthay R: Maternal pulmonary disorders complicating pregnancy. In Reece EA, Hobbins JC, Mahoney MJ, et al (eds): Medicine of the Fetus and Mother. Philadelphia, Lippincott, 1992, p 317.
83. Hicks ML, Nolan GH, Maxwell SL, et al: Acquired immuno-deficiency syndrome and *Pneumocystis carinii* infection in a pregnant woman. Obstet Gynecol 76:480, 1990.
84. Bardeguez AD: Management of HIV infection for the childbearing age woman. Clin Obstet Gynecol 39:344, 1996.
85. Hussain A, Mehta NJ, Manikal VM, et al: *Pneumocystis carinii* pneumonia in pregnancy. Chest 120:666, 2001.
86. Diwan VK, Thorson A: Sex, gender and tuberculosis. Lancet 353:1000, 1999.
87. Holmes CB, Hausler H, Numm P: A review of sex differences in the epidemiology of tuberculosis. Int J Tuberc Lung Dis 2:96, 1998.
88. Initial therapy for tuberculosis in the era of multidrug resistance—recommendations of the advisory council for the elimination of tuberculosis. MMWR Morb Mortal Wkly Rep 42:536, 1993.
89. Frieden TR, Sterling T, Pablos-Mendez A, et al: The emergence of drug-resistant tuberculosis in New York City. N Engl J Med 328:521, 1993.
90. Cantwell MF, Shehab AM, Costello AM: Brief report: Congenital tuberculosis. N Engl J Med 330:1051, 1994.
91. Margono F, Mroveh J, Garely A, et al: Resurgence of active tuberculosis among pregnant women. Obstet Gynecol 83:911, 1994.
92. Nitta AT, Milligan D: Management of four pregnant women with multidrug-resistant tuberculosis. Clin Infect Dis 28:1298, 1999.
93. Centers for Disease Control: The use of preventive therapy for tuberculosis infection in the United States. MMWR Morb Mortal Wkly Rep 39:9, 1990.
94. Griffith DE: Mycobacteria as pathogens of respiratory infection. Infect Dis Clin North Am 12:593, 1998.
95. American Thoracic Society Workshop: Rapid diagnostic tests for tuberculosis—what is the appropriate use? Am J Respir Crit Care Med 155:1804, 1997.
96. Barnes PF: Rapid diagnostic tests for tuberculosis, progress but no gold standard. Am J Respir Crit Care Med 155:1497, 1997.
97. Good JT, Iseman MD, Davidson PT, et al: Tuberculosis in association with pregnancy. Am J Obstet Gynecol 140:492, 1981.
98. American Thoracic Society: Mycobacteriosis and the acquired immunodeficiency syndrome. Am Rev Respir Dis 136:492, 1987.
99. Hamadeh MA, Glassroth J: Tuberculosis and pregnancy. Chest 101:1114, 1992.
100. Jana N, Vasishta K, Saha SC, et al: Obstetrical outcomes among women with extrapulmonary tuberculosis. N Engl J Med 341:645, 1999.
101. Vallejo JC, Starke JR: Tuberculosis and pregnancy. Clin Chest Med 13:693, 1992.
102. Sackoff JE, Pfeiffer MR, Driver CR, et al: Tuberculosis prevention for non-US-born pregnant women. Am J Obstet Gynecol 194:451, 2006.
103. Riley L: Pneumonia and tuberculosis in pregnancy. Infect Dis Clin North Am 11:119, 1997.
104. Boggess KA, Myers ER, Hamilton CD: Antepartum or postpartum isoniazid treatment of latent tuberculosis infection. Obstet Gynecol 96:757, 2000.
105. Robinson CA, Rose NC: Tuberculosis: Current implications and management in obstetrics. Obstet Gynecol Surv 51:115, 1999.
106. Myers JP: New recommendations for the treatment of tuberculosis. Curr Opin Infect Dis 18:133, 2005.
107. Van Rie A, Warren R, Richardson M, et al: Classification of drug-resistant tuberculosis in an epidemic era. Lancet 356:22, 2000.
108. Fox CW, George RB: Current concepts in the management and prevention of tuberculosis in adults. J La State Med Soc 144:363, 1992.
109. Robinson GC, Cambion K: Hearing loss in infants of tuberculosis mothers treated with streptomycin during pregnancy. N Engl J Med 271:949, 1964.
110. Rendig EK Jr: The place of BCG vaccine in the management of infants born to tuberculosis mothers. N Engl J Med 281:520, 1969.
111. Schatz M, Zeiger RS, Hoffman CP: Intrauterine growth is related to gestational pulmonary function in pregnant asthmatic women. Kaiser-Permanente Asthma and Pregnancy Study Group. Chest 98:389, 1990.
112. Alexander S, Dodds L, Armson BA: Perinatal outcomes in women with asthma during pregnancy. Obstet Gynecol 92:435, 1998.
113. Kwon HL, Belanger K, Bracken M. Asthma prevalence among pregnant and childbearing-aged women in the United States: Estimates from national health surveys. Ann Epidemiol 13:317, 2003.
114. National Asthma Education and Prevention Program: Expert Panel Report: Managing asthma during pregnancy: Recommendations for pharmacologic treatment—2004 update. NHLBI, NIH publication no. 05-3279. Available at http://www.nhlbi.nih.gov/health/prof/lung/asthma/astpreg/astpreg_qr.pdf (accessed January 2008).
115. National Asthma Education and Prevention Program: Full Report of the Expert Panel: Guidelines for the Diagnosis and Management of Asthma, 2007. Available at http://www.nhlbi.nih.gov/health/prof/lung/asthma/astpreg/astpreg_full.pdf (accessed January 2008).
116. Schatz M., Dombrowski MP, Wise R, et al, for the NICHD Maternal-Fetal Medicine Units Network, and NHLBI. Asthma morbidity during pregnancy can be predicted by severity classification. J Allergy Clin Immunol 112:28, 2003.
117. Gordon M, Niswander KR, Brerendes H, Kantor AG: Fetal morbidity following potentially anoxigenic obstetric conditions. VII. Bronchial asthma. Am J Obstet Gynecol 106:421, 1970.
118. Bahna SL, Bjerkedal T: The course and outcome of pregnancy in women with bronchial asthma. Acta Allergol 27:397, 1972.
119. Wen SW, Demissie K, Liu S: Adverse outcomes in pregnancies of asthmatic women: Results from a Canadian population. Ann Epidemiol 11:7, 2001.
120. Dombrowski MP, Bottoms SF, Boike GM, Wald J: Incidence of preeclampsia among asthmatic patients lower with theophylline. Am J Obstet Gynecol 155:265, 1986.
121. Stenius-Aarniala BS, Teramo PK: Asthma and pregnancy: A prospective study of 198 pregnancies. Thorax 43:12, 1988.
122. Demisse K, Breckenridge MB, Rhoads GG: Infant and maternal outcomes in the pregnancies of asthmatic women. Am J Respir Crit Care Med 158:1091, 1998.
123. Liu S, Wen SW, Demissie K, et al: Maternal asthma and pregnancy outcomes: A retrospective cohort study. Am J Obstet Gynecol 184:90, 2001.
124. Mihrshani S, Belousov E, Marks GB, Peat J: Pregnancy and birth outcomes in families with asthma. J Asthma 40:181, 2003.

125. Rudra CB, Williams MA, Frederick IO, Luthy DA: Maternal asthma and risk of preeclampsia, a case-control study. J Reprod Med 51:94, 2006.
126. Perlow JH, Montgomery D, Morgan MA, et al: Severity of asthma and perinatal outcome. Am J Obstet Gynecol 167:963, 1992.
127. Kallen B, Rydhstroem H, Aberg A: Asthma during pregnancy–a population based study. Eur J Epidemiol 16:167, 2000.
128. Sorensen TK, Dempsey JC, Xiao R, et al: Maternal asthma and risk of preterm delivery. Ann Epidemiol 13:267, 2003.
129. Lao TT, Huengsburg M: Labour and delivery in mothers with asthma. Eur J Obstet Gynecol Reprod Biol 35:183, 1990.
130. Mabie WC, Barton JR, Wasserstrum N, Sibai BM: Clinical observations an asthma in pregnancy. J Matern Fetal Med 1:45, 1992.
131. Schatz M, Zeiger RS, Hoffman CP, et al: Perinatal outcomes in the pregnancies of asthmatic women: A prospective controlled analysis. Am J Respir Crit Care Med 151:1170, 1995.
132. Minerbi-Codish I, Fraser D, Avnun L, et al: Influence of asthma in pregnancy on labor and the newborn. Respiration 65:130, 1998.
133. Stenius-Aarniala BSM, Hedman J, Teramo KA: Acute asthma during pregnancy. Thorax 51:411, 1996.
134. Olesen C, Thrane N, Nielsen GL, et al: A population-based prescription study of asthma drugs during pregnancy: Changing the intensity of asthma therapy and perinatal outcomes. Respiration 68:256, 2001.
135. Norjavaara E, de Verdier MG: Normal pregnancy outcomes in a population-based study including 2968 pregnant women exposed to budesonide. J Allergy Clin Immunol 111:736, 2003.
136. Doucette JT, Bracken MB: Possible role of asthma in the risk of preterm labor and delivery. Epidemiology 4:143, 1993.
137. Jana N, Vasishta K, Saha SC, Khunnu B: Effect of bronchial asthma on the course of pregnancy, labour and perinatal outcome. J Obstet Gynaecol 21:227, 1995.
138. Lehrer S, Stone J, Lapinski R, et al: Association between pregnancy-induced hypertension and asthma during pregnancy. Am J Obstet Gynecol 168:1463, 1993.
139. National Asthma Education Program Report of the Working Group on Asthma and Pregnancy: Management of asthma during pregnancy. NIH publication no. 93-3279A. Bethesda, National Institutes of Health, September 1993.
140. National Asthma Education and Prevention Program Expert Panel Report 2: Guidelines for the Diagnosis and Management of Asthma. NHLBI, NIH Publication no. 97-4051. Bethesda, National Institutes of Health and National Heart, Lung, and Blood Institute, April 1997.
141. Schatz M, Dombrowski M: Asthma and allergy during pregnancy: Outcomes of pregnancy in asthmatic women. Immunol Asthma Clin North Am 20:1, 2000.
142. Fitzsimons R, Greenberger PA, Patterson R: Outcome of pregnancy in women requiring corticosteroids for severe asthma. J Allergy Clin Immunol 78:349, 1986.
143. Greenberger PA, Patterson R: The outcome of pregnancy complicated by severe asthma. Allergy Proc 9:539, 1988.
144. Bracken MB, Triche EW, Belanger K, et al: Asthma symptoms, severity, and drug therapy: A prospective study of effects on 2205 pregnancies. Obstet Gynecol 1024:739, 2003.
145. Dombrowski MP, Schatz M, Wise R, et al, for the National Institute of Child Health and Human Development (NICHD) Maternal-Fetal Medicine Units Network and the National Heart, Lung, and Blood Institute (NHLBI): Asthma during pregnancy. Obstet Gynecol 103:5, 2004.
146. Enriquez R, Pingsheng W, Griffen MR, et al: Cessation of asthma medication in early pregnancy. Am J Obstet Gynecol 195:149, 2006.
147. Triche EW, Saftlas AF, Belanger D, et al: Association of asthma diagnosis, severity, symptoms, and treatment with risk of preeclampsia. Obstet Gynecol 104:585, 2004.
148. Schatz MS, Dombrowski MP, Wise R, et al, for the National Institute of Child Health and Human Development (NICHD) Maternal-Fetal Medicine Units Network and the National Heart, Lung, and Blood Institute (NHLBI): Spirometry is related to perinatal outcomes in pregnant women with asthma. Am J Obstet Gynecol 194:120, 2006.
149. Nolten W, Rueckert P: Elevated free cortisol index in pregnancy: Possible regulatory mechanisms. Am J Obstet Gynecol 139:492, 1981.
150. Bailey K, Herrod H, Younger R, Shaver D: Functional aspects of T-lymphocyte subsets in pregnancy. Obstet Gynecol 66:211, 1985.
151. Haahtela T, Jarvinen M, Kava T, et al: Comparison of β_2-agonist, terbutaline, with an inhaled corticosteroid, budesonide, in newly detected asthma. N Engl J Med 325:338, 1991.
152. Ernst P, Spitzer WO, Suissa S, et al: Risk of fatal and near-fatal asthma in relation to inhaled corticosteroid use. JAMA 268:3462, 1992.
153. Kraan J, Koeter GH, van der Mark TW, et al: Dosage and time effects of inhaled budesonide on bronchial hyperactivity. Am Rev Respir Dis 137:44, 1988.
154. Lowhagen O, Rak S: Modification of bronchial hyperreactivity after treatment with sodium cromoglycate during pollen season. J Allergy Clin Immunol 75:460, 1985.
155. Woolcock AJ, Jenkins C: Corticosteroids in the modulation of bronchial hyperresponsiveness. Immunol Allergy Clin North Am 10:543, 1990.
156. Kallen B, Rydhstroem H, Aberg A: Congenital malformations after use of inhaled budesonide in early pregnancy. Obstet Gynecol 93:392, 1999.
157. Sears MR, Taylor DR, Print CG, et al: Regular inhaled β-agonist treatment in bronchial asthma. Lancet 336:1391, 1990.
158. Cockcroft DW, Murdock KY: Comparative effects of inhaled salbutamol, sodium cromoglycate, and beclomethasone dipropionate on allergen-induced early asthmatic responses, last asthmatic responses, and increased bronchial responsiveness to histamine. J Allergy Clin Immunol 79:734, 1987.
159. Spitzer WO, Suissa S, Ernst P, et al: The use of beta-agonists and the risk of death and near death from asthma. N Engl J Med 326:501, 1992.
160. Schatz M, Dombrowski MP, Wise R, et al, for the NICHD Maternal-Fetal Medicine Units Network and the NHLBI: The relationship of asthma medication use to perinatal outcomes. J Allergy Clin Immunol 113:104, 2004.
161. Arwood LL, Dasta JF, Friedman C: Placental transfer of theophylline: Two case reports. Pediatrics 63:844, 1979.
162. Yeh TF, Pildes RS: Transplacental aminophylline toxicity in a neonate [letter]. Lancet 1:910, 1977.
163. Hendeles L, Jenkins J, Temple R: Revised FDA labeling guideline for theophylline oral dosage forms. Pharmacotherapy 15:409, 1995.
164. Joad JP, Ahrens RC, Lindgren SD, Weinberger MM: Relative efficacy of maintenance therapy with theophylline, inhaled albuterol, and the combination for chronic asthma. J Allergy Clin Immunol 79:78, 1987.
165. Wendel PJ, Ramin SM, Barnett-Hamm C, et al: Asthma treatment in pregnancy: A randomized controlled study. Am J Obstet Gynecol 175:150, 1996.
166. Pauwels R, Van Renterghem D, Van der Straeten M, et al: The effect of theophylline and enprofylline on allergen-induced bronchoconstriction. J Allergy Clin Immunol 76:583, 1985.
167. Juergens UR, Degenhardt V, Stober M, Vetter H: New insights in the bronchodilatory and anti-inflammatory mechanisms of action of theophylline. Arzneimittelforschung 49:694, 1999.
168. Evans DJ, Taylor DA, Zetterstrom O, et al: A comparison of low-dose inhaled budesonide plus theophylline and high-dose inhaled budesonide for moderate asthma. N Engl J Med 337:1412, 1997.
169. Dombrowski MP, Schatz M, Wise R, et al, for the National Institute of Child Health and Human Development (NICHD) Maternal-Fetal Medicine Units Network and the National Heart, Lung, and Blood Institute (NHLBI): Randomized trial of inhaled beclomethasone dipropionate versus theophylline for moderate asthma during pregnancy. Am J Obstet Gynecol 190:737, 2004.
170. Knorr B, Matz J, Bernstein JA, et al: Montelukast for chronic asthma in 6 to 14 year old children. JAMA 279:1181, 1998.
171. Wenzel SE: New approaches to anti-inflammatory therapy for asthma. Am J Med 104:287, 1998.
172. Park-Wyllie L, Mazzotta P, Pastuszak A, et al: Birth defects after maternal exposure to corticosteroids: Prospective cohort study and meta-analysis of epidemiological studies. Teratology 62:385, 2000.

173. Bakhireva LN, Jones KL, Schatz M, et al: Asthma medication use in pregnancy and fetal growth. J Allergy Clin Immunol 116:503, 2005.
174. Towers CV, Briggs GG, Rojas JA: The use of prostaglandin E_2 in pregnant patients with asthma. Am J Obstet Gynecol 190:1777, 2004.
175. Crawford JS: Bronchospasm following ergonovine. Anesthesiology 35:397, 1980.
176. Hägerdal M, Morgan CW, Sumner AE, Gutsche BB: Minute ventilation and oxygen consumption during labor with epidural analgesia. Anesthesiology 59:425, 1983.
177. Fung DL: Emergency anesthesia for asthma patients. Clin Rev Allergy 3:127, 1985.
178. Hirshman CA, Downes H, Farbood A, Bergman NA: Ketamine block of bronchospasm in experimental canine asthma. Br J Anaesth 51:713, 1979.
179. American Academy of Pediatrics Committee on Drugs: Transfer of drugs and other chemicals into human milk. Pediatrics 84:924, 1989.
180. West JB: Pulmonary Pathophysiology. Baltimore, Williams & Wilkins, 1978, p 92.
181. King TE Jr: Restrictive lung disease in pregnancy. Clin Chest Med 13:607, 1992.
182. Boggess KA, Easterling TR, Raghu G: Management and outcome of pregnant women with interstitial and restrictive lung disease. Am J Obstet Gynecol 173:1007, 1995.
183. Agha FP, Vade A, Amendola MA, et al: Effects of pregnancy on sarcoidosis. Surg Gynecol Obstet 155:817, 1982.
184. Haynes de Regt R: Sarcoidosis and pregnancy. Obstet Gynecol 70:369, 1987.
185. Maycock RL, Sullivan RD, Greening RR, et al: Sarcoidosis and pregnancy. JAMA 164:158, 1957.
186. Reisfield DR: Boeck's sarcoid and pregnancy. Am J Obstet Gynecol 75:795, 1958.
187. Scadding JG: Sarcoidosis. London, Eyre & Spottiswoode, 1967.
188. Hilman BC, Aitken ML, Constantinescu M: Pregnancy in patients with cystic fibrosis. Clin Obstet Gynecol 39:70, 1996.
189. Kerem B, Rommens JM, Buchanan JA, et al: Identification of the cystic fibrosis gene: Genetic analysis. Science 245:1073, 1989.
190. Riordan JR, Rommens JM, Kerem B, et al: Identification of the cystic fibrosis gene: Cloning and characterization of complementary DNA. Science 245:1066, 1989.
191. Rommens JM, Iannuzzi MC, Kerem B, et al: Identification of the cystic fibrosis gene: Chromosome walking and jumping. Science 245:1059, 1989.
192. Kotloff RM, FitzSimmons SC, Fiel SB: Fertility and pregnancy in patients with cystic fibrosis. Clin Chest Med 13:623, 1992.
193. Siegel B, Siegel S: Pregnancy and delivery in a patient with CF of the pancreas: Report of a case. Obstet Gynecol 16:439, 1960.
194. Grand RJ, Talamo RC, di Sant'Agnese PA, et al: Pregnancy in cystic fibrosis of the pancreas. JAMA 195:993, 1966.
195. Cohen LF, di Sant'Agnese PA, Friedlander J: Cystic fibrosis and pregnancy: A national survey. Lancet 2:842, 1980.
196. Weinberger SE, Weiss ST, Cohen WR, et al: Pregnancy and the lung. Am Rev Respir Dis 121:559, 1980.
197. Rush D, Johnstone FD, King JC: Nutrition and pregnancy. In Burrows GN, Ferris TF (eds): Medical Complications During Pregnancy, 3rd ed. Philadelphia, WB Saunders, 1988.
198. Dowsett J: An overview of nutritional issues for the adult with cystic fibrosis. Nutrition 16:566, 2000.
199. Novy MJ, Tyler JM, Shwachman H, et al: Cystic fibrosis and pregnancy. Report of a case with a study of pulmonary function and arterial blood gases. Obstet Gynecol 30:530, 1967.
200. Palmer J, Dillon-Baker C, Tecklin JS, et al: Pregnancy in patients with cystic fibrosis. Ann Intern Med 99:596, 1983.
201. Corkey CW, Newth CJ, Corey M, Levison H: Pregnancy in cystic fibrosis: A better prognosis in patients with pancreatic function? Am J Obstet Gynecol 140:737, 1981.
202. Canny GJ, Corey M, Livingstone RA, et al: Pregnancy and cystic fibrosis. Obstet Gynecol 77:850, 1991.
203. Kent NE, Farquharson DF: Cystic fibrosis in pregnancy. Can Med Assoc J 149:809, 1993.
204. Edenborough FP, Stableforth DE, Webb AK, et al: Outcome of pregnancy in women with cystic fibrosis. Thorax 50:170, 1995.
205. Olson GL: Cystic fibrosis in pregnancy. Semin Perinatol 21:307, 1997.
206. Edenborough FP, Mackenzie WE, Stableforth DE: The outcome of 72 pregnancies in 55 women with cystic fibrosis in the United Kingdom 1977-1996. BJOG 107:254, 2000.
207. Tanser SJ, Hodson ME, Geddes DM: Case reports of death during pregnancy in patients with cystic fibrosis—three out of four patients were colonized with *Burkholderia cepacia*. Respir Med 94:1004, 2000.
208. Gilljam M, Antoniou M, Shin J, et al: Pregnancy in cystic fibrosis. Chest 118:85, 2000.
209. Gyi KM, Hodson ME, Yacoub MY: Pregnancy in cystic fibrosis lung transplant recipients: Case series and review. J Cystic Fibrosis 5:171-175, 2006.
210. Cole BN, Seltzer MH, Kassabian J, et al: Parenteral nutrition in a pregnant cystic fibrosis patient. JPEN J Parenter Enteral Nutr 11:205, 1987.

Chapter 46

Diabetes in Pregnancy

Thomas R. Moore, MD, and Patrick Catalano, MD

Global and National Prevalence of Diabetes

Worldwide Perspective on Diabetes

An epidemic of diabetes and obesity is sweeping the globe, largely because of marked shifts in dietary practices and physical activity. In 2000, 171 million persons on the planet were known to have diabetes, and by 2030, this figure is expected to increase to 366 million. More than 80% of people with diabetes worldwide live in low- and middle-income countries. During the next 2 decades, the world population is expected to increase by 37%, but the prevalence of diabetes will increase by 114%. In India, sub-Saharan Africa, and Latin America, diabetes prevalence is projected to increase by 150% to 160%.[1]

In the United States and other developed economies, the rise in diabetes prevalence is projected to be higher than 50%. As shown in Figure 46-1, in 2005, 20.8 million people (7% of the population) have been diagnosed with some form of diabetes. Another 6.2 million with diabetes are undiagnosed. Of women 20 years or older, 8.8% have overt diabetes, but there is a strong predilection for this disease among ethnic groups. Higher-than-expected rates of pregestational diabetes in women of childbearing age have been reported for 13.3% of non-Hispanic blacks, 9.5% of Hispanic and Latino Americans, and 12.8% of Native Americans.[2]

Epidemiology of Diabetes in U.S. Women

Studies suggest that the prevalence of diabetes among women of childbearing age is increasing in the United States.[3,4] Continued immigration among populations with high rates of type 2 diabetes and the impact of changes in diet (i.e., increased calories and fat content) and lifestyle (i.e., sedentary) have brought marked increases in the percentage of patients with preexisting diabetes who will become pregnant in the future. A virtual epidemic of childhood obesity is occurring in the United States, bringing with it a sharp rise in childhood and adolescent diabetes. This trend will have a profound impact on obstetrics and pediatrics in the next 2 decades and beyond.[5] Increased outreach efforts to provide care to the populations experiencing rising rates of pregestational diabetes will be necessary if a significant increase in maternal and newborn morbidity is to be avoided. When offspring of diabetic mothers are compared with weight-matched controls, the risk of serious birth injury is doubled, the likelihood of cesarean section is tripled, and the incidence of newborn intensive care unit admission is quadrupled.[6]

Before the 20th century, pregnancy in the diabetic woman portended death of mother or child, or both. In the 21st century, centers providing meticulous metabolic and obstetric surveillance report perinatal loss rates approaching but still higher than those seen in the nondiabetic population.[7,8] Nevertheless, major problems with fetal and maternal management persist. Stillbirth rates have fallen dramatically but remain threefold or fourfold greater than rates for the normoglycemic population. Congenital fetal anomalies, many of them life threatening and debilitating, remain three to four times more common in diabetic pregnancies than in nondiabetic pregnancies.[9] Macrosomia and birth injury occur 10 times more frequently in diabetic fetuses. Studies indicate that the magnitude of such risks is proportional to the degree of maternal hyperglycemia.[10,11] To a great extent, the excessive fetal and neonatal morbidity of diabetes in pregnancy is preventable or at least reducible by meticulous prenatal and intrapartum care. This chapter reviews the pathophysiology of this complex group of disorders and identifies the obstetric interventions that can improve outcome.

Classification and Pathobiology of Diabetes Mellitus

Diagnostic and classification criteria for diabetes were issued by the American Diabetes Association (ADA) in 1997.[12] These criteria were further modified in 2003 regarding the diagnosis of impaired fasting glucose.[13] This nomenclature is useful because it categorizes patients according to the underlying pathophysiology, although we recognize that the criteria are not as mutually exclusive as once thought. The classification includes four clinical types:

1. Type 1 diabetes, formerly referred to as insulin-dependent or juvenile-onset diabetes.
2. Type 2 diabetes, formerly referred to as non–insulin-dependent or adult-onset diabetes
3. Other specific types of diabetes related to a variety of genetic-, drug-, or chemical-induced diabetes
4. Gestational diabetes mellitus

An alternative classification that is commonly used in obstetrics was proposed by Priscilla White when she was at the Joslin Clinic in Boston in 1932.[14] This classification (Table 46-1) was based on the duration of the disease and secondary vascular damage to retinal, renal, and cardiovascular structures. Because the White classification is primarily descriptive and because it does not reflect the increase in type 2 diabetes in the population and the discovery of better-defined genetic causes, the ADA classification is preferred. The pathophysiology of the various types of diabetes is discussed subsequently.

Type 1 Diabetes

Type 1 diabetes accounts for approximately 5% to 10% of patients diagnosed with diabetes in the general population. However, type 1 diabetes may represent a slightly greater fraction of women in the reproductive age group because of the relatively earlier age of onset of type 1 diabetes compared with type 2 diabetes. Type 1 diabetes results from a cellular-mediated autoimmune destruction of the beta cells of the pancreas. Markers of the immune response include islet cell autoantibodies, autoantibodies to insulin, autoantibodies to glutamic acid decarboxylase (GAD2, formerly designated GAD65), and autoantibodies to the tyrosine phosphatase IA-2 and IA-2β. One and usually more of these autoantibodies are present in 85% to 90% of individuals with elevated fasting glucose and type 1 diabetes.[15]

Autoimmune destruction of beta cells has many genetic predispositions and is related to environmental factors. Although viruses were initially implicated, the environmental conditions leading to auto destruction of the beta cells remain largely undefined. Most evidence indicates a genetic predisposition related to an individual's human leukocyte antigen (HLA) associations with linkage to *DQA* and *DQB* genes. Type 1 diabetes is concordant in 33% to 50% of monozygotic twins, suggesting that environmental triggers are required to initiate the disease process in genetically predisposed individuals.

Type 1 diabetes usually is characterized by an abrupt clinical onset after a period of immune destruction of the beta cells that might have been in progress for some time. The beta cell destruction continues after the clinical onset of diabetes, usually leading to an absolute insulinopenia with resultant life-long requirements for insulin replacement. Although type 1 diabetes was previously referred to as juvenile-onset diabetes, it can occur at virtually any age. The disease is particularly common in whites, especially those of Northern European ancestry, and Sardinians.

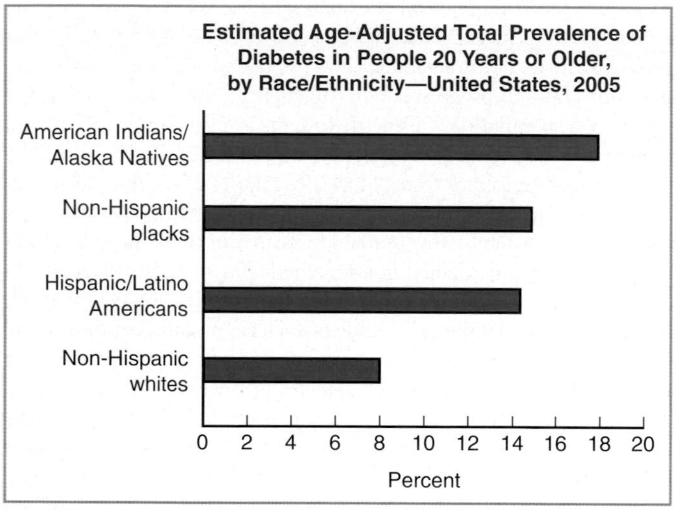

FIGURE 46-1 Estimated prevalence of diabetes in the United States 2005. For American Indians/Alaska Natives, the estimate of total prevalence was calculated using the estimate of diagnosed diabetes from the 2003 outpatient database of the Indian Health Service and the estimate of undiagnosed diabetes from the 1999-2002 National Health and Nutrition Examination Survey (NHANES). For the other groups, the 1999-2002 NHANES estimates of total prevalence (diagnosed and undiagnosed) were projected to the year 2005. (Printed with permission from http://diabetes.niddk.nih.gov/dm/pubs/statistics/index.htm#age.)

Type 2 Diabetes

Type 2 diabetes involves a loss of balance between insulin sensitivity and insulin (i.e., beta cell) response. The relationship between these two factors can be expressed as the disposition index (i.e., the normal inverse relationship between the two factors can be expressed as a constant).[16] A decline in the disposition index is associated with the development of type 2 diabetes. Both insulin resistance and beta cell dysfunction exist in individuals who develop type 2 diabetes. There is little agreement about whether the beta cell function is an independent event or is coincident with decreased insulin sensitivity and whether the abnormalities are causally linked.

The decreased insulin sensitivity and inadequate insulin response leads to an increase in circulating glucose concentrations, and the decreased insulin sensitivity in individuals with type 2 diabetes results in the inability of insulin to suppress lipolysis in adipose tissue. Many predisposing factors are related to decreased insulin sensitivity (i.e., increased insulin resistance). They include obesity, a sedentary lifestyle, family history and genetics, puberty, advancing age, and of particular concern to the obstetrician, the intrauterine environment. Although it

TABLE 46-1 THE WHITE CLASSIFICATION OF DIABETES IN PREGNANCY

White Class	Age at Onset (Years)		Duration (Years)	Complications
A	Any		Any	Diagnosed before pregnancy; no vascular disease
B	≥20	or	<10	No vascular disease
C	10-19	or	10-19	No vascular disease
D	<10	or	≥20	Background retinopathy only or hypertension
E				Calcification of pelvic arteries (no longer used)
F				Nephropathy (>500 mg of proteinuria per day)
H				Arteriosclerotic heart disease
R				Proliferative retinopathy or vitreous hemorrhage
T				After renal transplantation

Adapted from Hare JW, White P: Gestational diabetes and the White classification. Diabetes Care 3:394, 1980. Copyright © 1980 by the American Diabetes Association.

TABLE 46-2 CRITERIA FOR THE DIAGNOSIS OF DIABETES

Symptoms of diabetes and a casual plasma glucose level ≧200 mg/dL (11.1 mmol/L). Casual is defined as any time of day without regard to time since the last meal. The classic symptoms of diabetes include polyuria, polydipsia, and unexplained weight loss.
or
Fasting plasma glucose level ≧126 mg/dL (7.0 mmol/L). Fasting is defined as no caloric intake for at least 8 hours.
or
Two-hour plasma glucose ≧200 mg/dL (11.1 mmol/L) during an oral glucose tolerance test. The test should be performed as described by the World Health Organization, using a glucose load containing the equivalent of 75-g anhydrous glucose dissolved in water.

Adapted from American Diabetes Association: Clinical practice recommendations: Standards of medical care for diabetes—2007. Diabetes Care 30:S4-S41, 2007.

was formerly believed that type 2 diabetes was primarily a disorder of older individuals (accounting for its being called adult-onset diabetes), there has been a significant increase in the prevalence of type 2 diabetes since 1990. At the turn of the 21st century, an estimated 13.8 million people had a diagnosis of diabetes, 5 million people had undiagnosed diabetes, and 41 million people had prediabetes.[17]

Although it is not in the scope of this chapter to review the spectrum of possible causes of type 2 diabetes, the increase in obesity in the general population is a contributing factor; it is estimated that approximately two thirds of the population in the United States are overweight or obese.[18] Obesity, particularly central obesity, which is estimated by waist circumference, is a well-described risk factor. This increase in visceral obesity affects hepatic metabolic function and is a rich source of cytokines and inflammatory factors, which are recognized as contributing to increasing insulin resistance.

Criteria for the diagnosis of diabetes in nonpregnant adults are shown in Table 46-2. Although the 75-g, 2-hour oral glucose tolerance test (OGTT) is the most sensitive and specific diagnostic test for type 2 diabetes, because of the ease of administration and reproducibility, the fasting glucose test is often used as a first-line diagnostic test,[19] particularly in the nongravid population. Because the onset of type 2 diabetes is usually insidious, hyperglycemia not sufficient to make the diagnostic criteria for type 2 diabetes is often categorized as impaired fasting glucose (IFG) (100 mg/dL to 125 mg/dL) or, if the 75-g OGTT is employed, as impaired glucose tolerance (IGT) (2-hour glucose level of 140 mg/dL to 199 mg/dL). The IFG and IGT have been officially designated *prediabetes*, and prediabetic individuals are at high risk for the development of type 2 diabetes.[19]

Gestational Diabetes Mellitus

Gestational diabetes mellitus (GDM) as defined by the Fourth International Workshop-Conference on Gestational Diabetes as "carbohydrate intolerance of various degrees of severity, with onset or first recognition during pregnancy."[20] This definition does not preclude the possibility that glucose intolerance might have predated the pregnancy or that medications might be needed for optimal glucose control. The underlying pathophysiology of GDM in most instances is similar to that observed for type 2 diabetes: an inability to maintain an adequate insulin response because of the significant decreases in insulin sensitivity with advancing gestation. About 2% to 13% of women diagnosed as having GDM have detectable antibodies directed against specific beta cell antigens.[21,22] Some of these deficiencies are population dependent. Other patients diagnosed with GDM have genetic variants that have been identified as causes of diabetes in the general population, including autosomal dominant (discussed later) and maternal or mitochondrial inheritance patterns.[23,24]

It is estimated that as many as 3% to 9% of the population of pregnant women will be diagnosed with GDM.[15] This translates into approximately 135,000 cases of GDM per year in the United States alone. This is not surprising, because in many respects, GDM is the harbinger of type 2 diabetes for many women, based on the underlying pathophysiology of GDM and the increase in obesity in women of reproductive age. Similarly, there is an increase in the incidence of GDM in women immigrating to the United States, presumably because of changes in diet and lifestyle. Clinical recognition of GDM is important because therapy can reduce pregnancy complications and potentially reduce long-term sequelae in the offspring.

Genetic and Other Causes of Diabetes

The ADA's fourth classification of diabetes includes specific types of diabetes attributed to "other causes." These causes include genetic defects in insulin action, diseases of the exocrine pancreas (e.g., cystic fibrosis), and drug- or chemical-induced diabetes, such as in the treatment of human immunodeficiency virus (HIV) infection or after organ transplantation.[19] One of the well characterized genetic defects is often included under the heading of maturity-onset diabetes of the young (MODY) (i.e., the glucokinase [GK] mutation). In 1998, Hattersley and colleagues[25] described the various phenotypic permutations associated with the mutations of the glucokinase gene. Glucokinase phosphorylates glucose to glucose-6 phosphate in the pancreas and liver. A heterozygous glucokinase mutation results in hyperglycemia, usually with a mildly elevated fasting glucose and abnormal OGTT result. This occurs because of a defect in the sensing of glucose by the beta cell, resulting in decreased insulin release, and to a lesser degree because of reduced hepatic glycogen synthesis. In pregnancy, it is estimated that 3% of women with GDM and an elevated fasting glucose level greater than 110 mg/dL have this mutation. If the heterozygous mutation is present in the fetus, then the altered glucose sensing by the fetal pancreas will result in a decrease in insulin secretion. In the fetus, insulin is a primary stimulus for growth, and any defect in fetal insulin secretion results in decreased fetal growth and possible growth restriction. Depending on whether the mother or fetus, or both, have a defect in the glucokinase gene, the phenotype of the infant can vary from intrauterine growth restriction (IUGR) through normal fetal growth and to macrosomia.

Maternal-Fetal Metabolism in Normal and Diabetic Pregnancy

There are significant changes in maternal metabolism in normal pregnancy. These include changes in maternal nutrient metabolism (i.e., carbohydrate, lipid, and protein metabolism) and changes in factors such as energy expenditure. The overall goal of these maternal metabolic adaptations is to prepare the pregnant woman to meet the increased energy needs of the mother and growth of the fetus in the latter third of pregnancy, when approximately 70% of fetal growth takes place.[26] The alterations in maternal metabolism are relatively uniform during pregnancy unless there are major perturbations such as starvation conditions. The metabolic changes during pregnancy therefore take place on the background of a woman's pregestational metabolic status. For example, if a woman is healthy and lean before conception, there is an increased need to store adipose tissue in early pregnancy to meet the increased energy demands of late gestation and to develop insulin resistance in late gestation to provide nutrients for the growing fetus. If a woman is obese before conception, there is little need to gain additional adipose tissue, but there is the requirement to provide nutrients for the fetus in late gestation.

Normal Glucose-Tolerant Pregnancy

Glucose homeostasis is primarily a balance between insulin resistance and insulin secretion. The alterations in insulin resistance affect endogenous glucose production (primarily hepatic glucose metabolism) and peripheral glucose metabolism, which takes place in skeletal muscle. In the lean pregnant woman with normal glucose tolerance, there is a significant 30% increase in basal hepatic glucose production by the third trimester of pregnancy (Fig. 46-2). This is associated with a significant increase in basal or fasting insulin concentrations.[27] The decrease in fasting glucose concentrations most likely is the result of increasing plasma volumes in early gestation and increased fetoplacental use in late pregnancy. In the postprandial state, the increasing insulin concentrations enhance glucose uptake into skeletal muscle and adipose tissue, and they almost completely suppress hepatic glucose production. Although this is the case in lean women, obese women with normal glucose tolerance have a decreased ability for insulin to completely suppress hepatic glucose production in late pregnancy.[28] These data support the concept of decreased insulin sensitivity in late gestation that is more severe in obese women compared with non-obese counterparts.

Peripheral insulin resistance is defined as the decreased ability of insulin to affect glucose uptake primarily in skeletal muscle and to a lesser degree in adipose tissue. Various methods are used to assess insulin sensitivity in vivo, including mathematical models of fasting glucose and insulin modeling (e.g., homeostasis model assessment [HOMA],[29] OGTT[30]), the intravenous glucose tolerance test (i.e., Bergman minimal model),[31] and what many consider to be the gold standard: the hyperinsulinemic-euglycemic clamp.[32] Most of these measures have identified a significant 50% to 60% decrease in insulin sensitivity in late gestation.[33] The changes in insulin sensitivity during gestation are a reflection of a woman's pregravid insulin sensitivity status. Lean women usually have greater pregravid insulin sensitivity compared with overweight or obese women. These differences manifest before pregnancy, and when evaluated against the metabolic background of pregnancy, the relationships are similar in late pregnancy, albeit reduced by approximately 50% to 60% (Fig. 46-3). The decreases in insulin sensitivity in late pregnancy are accompanied by an increase in insulin response. The increased insulin response to a glucose load increases approximately threefold compared with pregravid measures (Fig. 46-4).

Diabetic Pregnancy

Alterations in glucose metabolism in women with diabetes have been most extensively examined in women with GDM, although the alterations in glucose metabolism in women with type 2 diabetes are most likely very similar but with increased insulin resistance and further decompensation of beta cell function. In lean and obese women with GDM with mildly elevated fasting glucose levels, there is a similar increase in basal endogenous glucose production, as was observed in subjects with normal glucose tolerance, although fasting insulin concentrations, particularly in late gestation, are greater than observed in normal glucose-tolerant women.[28,34] However, during insulin infusion during euglycemic clamps, the ability of insulin to suppress endogenous glucose production is decreased (approximately 80% versus 95%) in GDM compared with a matched control group. There is also a sig-

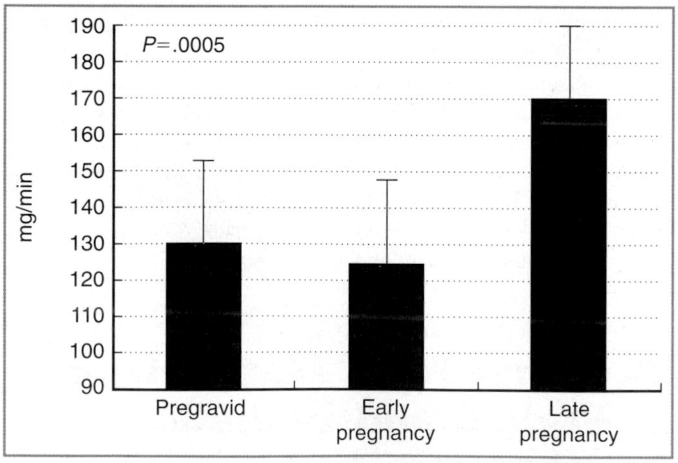

FIGURE 46-2 Alterations in glucose production. Longitudinal changes in total basal endogenous (primarily hepatic) glucose production (mean ± SD) from pregravid through early gestation (12 to 14 weeks) and late gestation (34 to 36 weeks). (Adapted from Catalano PM, Tyzbir ED, Wolfe RR, et al: Longitudinal changes in basal hepatic glucose production and suppression during insulin infusion in normal pregnant women. Am J Obstet Gynecol 167:913-919, 1992.)

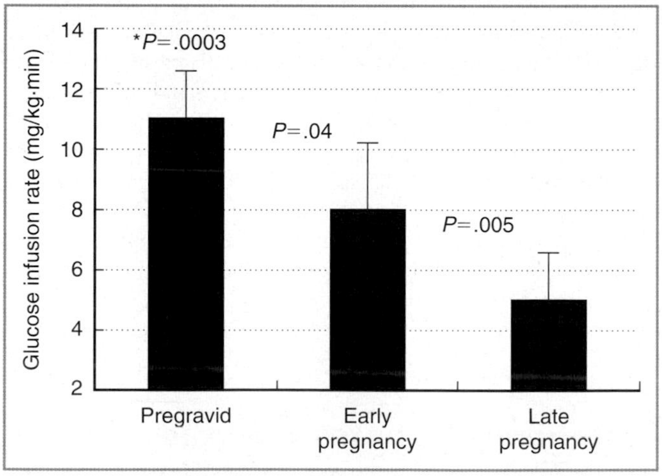

FIGURE 46-3 Alterations in insulin resistance. Longitudinal changes in glucose infusion rate (i.e., insulin sensitivity) in lean women from pregravid through early (12 to 14 weeks) and late (34 to 36 weeks) pregnancy during hyperinsulinemic-euglycemic clamp (mean ± SD). The *asterisk* indicates change over time from pregravid status through late pregnancy (ANOVA). (Adapted from Catalano PM, Tyzbir ED, Roman NM, et al: Longitudinal changes in insulin release and insulin resistance in non-obese pregnant women. Am J Obstet Gynecol 165:1667-1672, 1991.)

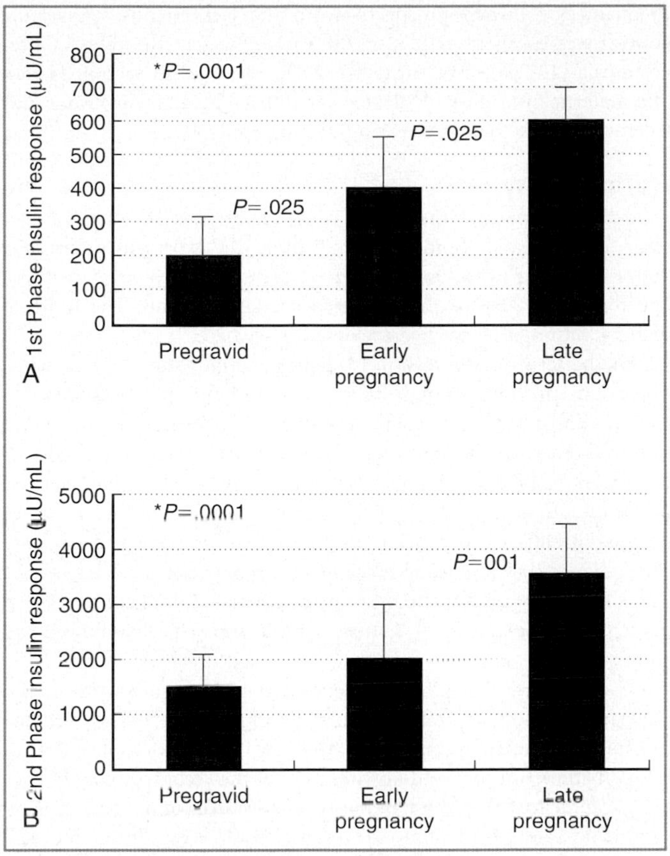

FIGURE 46-4 **Increased insulin response.** Changes in first **(A)** and second **(B)** phase pregravid through early (12 to 14 weeks) and late (34 to 36 weeks) pregnancy insulin response during an intravenous glucose tolerance test (mean ± SD). The *asterisk* indicates change over time from pregravid status through late pregnancy (ANOVA). (Adapted from Catalano PM, Tyzbir ED, Roman NM, et al: Longitudinal changes in insulin release and insulin resistance in non-obese pregnant women. Am J Obstet Gynecol 165:1667-1672, 1991.)

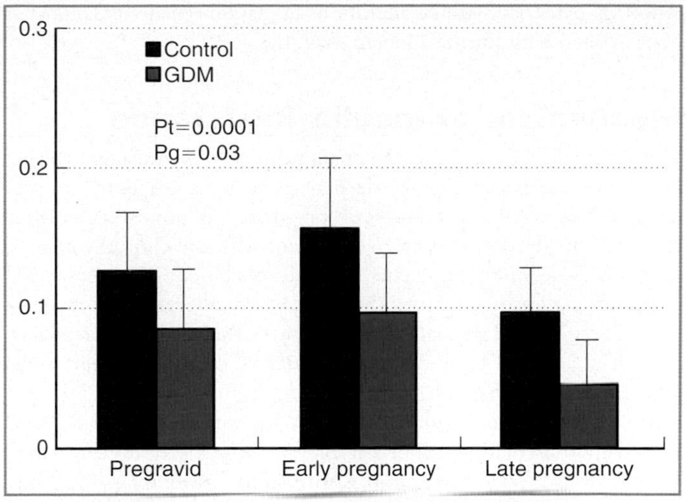

FIGURE 46-5 **Alterations in insulin sensitivity.** Longitudinal changes in insulin sensitivity during clamp 40 mU·m^{-2}·min^{-1} insulin infusion in obese women (mean ± SD). GDM, gestational diabetes mellitus; Pg, difference between groups; Pt, individual longitudinal changes with time. (Adapted from Catalano PM, Huston L, Amini SB, Kalhan SC: Longitudinal changes in glucose metabolism during pregnancy in obese women with normal glucose tolerance and gestational diabetes. Am J Obstet Gynecol 180:903-916, 1999.)

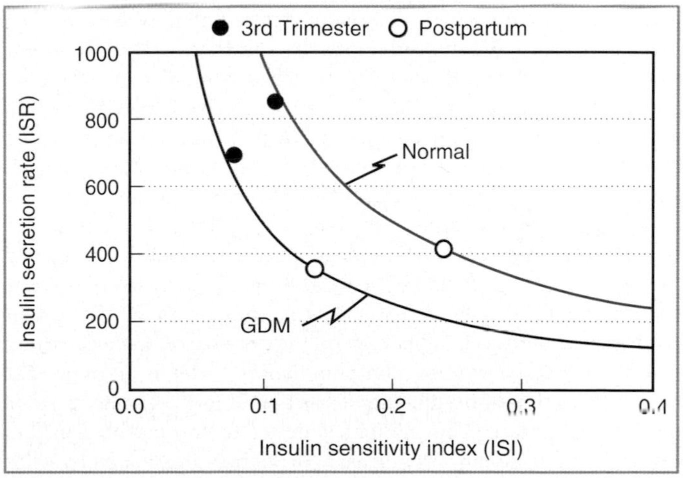

FIGURE 46-6 **Insulin sensitivity and secretion relationships in normal women and women with gestational diabetes mellitus.** Prehepatic insulin secretion was assessed during steady-state hyperglycemia using plasma insulin and C-peptide concentrations and C-peptide kinetics in individual patients. (Printed with permission from Buchanan TA: Pancreatic β-cell defects in gestational diabetes: Implications for the pathogenesis and prevention of type 2 diabetes. J Clin Endocrinol Metab 86:989-993, 2001.)

nificant decrease in insulin sensitivity in women who go on to develop GDM, when estimated before conception or after delivery,[35] compared with a matched control group. During pregnancy, the percent decrease in insulin sensitivity is approximately the same as the percent change in a matched control group (i.e., approximately 50% to 60%). The decreased insulin sensitivity observed during pregnancy in the woman who develops GDM is a function of her pregravid metabolic status, and clinically, the increased glucose concentrations represent the inability of pancreatic beta cells to normalize glucose levels (Fig. 46-5).

The relationship between insulin sensitivity and insulin response has been characterized by Bergman and colleagues[16] as a hyperbolic curve or, when multiplied, as the *disposition index.* A curve that is "shifted to the left" can be plotted for individuals who go on to develop GDM (Fig. 46-6). Whether the insulin resistance precedes the beta cell defect or they occur concomitantly is not known with certainty. However, Buchanan[36] proposed that insulin resistance caused the beta cell dysfunction in susceptible individuals. The increased risk of type 2 diabetes in women who formerly had GDM may be a function of decreasing insulin sensitivity (i.e., worsening insulin resistance) exacerbated by increasing age, adiposity, and the inability of the beta cells to fully compensate.

The data on the changes on glucose metabolism in women with type 1 diabetes are not as well examined. Schmitz and coworkers[37] evaluated the longitudinal changes in insulin sensitivity in women with type 1 diabetes in early and late pregnancy and after delivery. There was a 50% decrease in insulin sensitivity in late gestation. There was no significant difference in insulin sensitivity in these women in early pregnancy or within 1 week of delivery compared with nonpregnant women with type 1 diabetes. Based on the available data, women with type 1 diabetes have similar alterations in insulin sensitivity compared with women with normal glucose tolerance.

Mechanism of Insulin Resistance

The mechanisms related to the changes in insulin resistance during pregnancy are better characterized because of research in the past decade. The insulin resistance of pregnancy is almost completely reversed shortly after delivery,[38] consistent with the clinically marked decrease in insulin requirements. The placenta has long been suspected of producing hormonal factors related to these alterations in metabolism. The placental mediators of insulin resistance in late pregnancy have been ascribed to alterations in maternal cortisol concentrations and placenta-derived hormones such as human placental lactogen (HPL), progesterone, and estrogen.[39-41] Kirwan and associates[42] reported that circulating tumor necrosis factor-α (TNF-α) concentrations had an inverse correlation with insulin sensitivity as estimated from clamp studies. Among leptin, HPL, cortisol, human chorionic gonadotropin, estradiol, progesterone, and prolactin, TNF-α was the only significant predictor of the changes in insulin sensitivity from the pregravid period through late gestation. TNF-α and other cytokines are produced by the placenta, and 95% of these molecules are transported to maternal rather than fetal circulations.[42] Other factors, such as circulating free fatty acids, may contribute to the insulin resistance of pregnancy.[43]

Studies in human skeletal muscle and adipose tissue have demonstrated defects in the post-receptor insulin-signaling cascade during pregnancy. Friedman and colleagues showed that women in late pregnancy have reduced insulin receptor substrate-1 (IRS-1) concentrations compared with those of matched nonpregnant women.[44] Downregulation of the IRS-1 protein closely parallels insulin's decreased ability to induce additional steps in the insulin signaling cascade that result in the transporter (GLUT-4) arriving at the cell surface to allow glucose to enter the cell. Downregulation of IRS-1 closely parallels the decreased ability of insulin to stimulate 2-deoxyglucose uptake in vitro in pregnant skeletal muscle. During late pregnancy in women with GDM, in addition to decreased IRS-1 concentrations, the insulin receptor-β (i.e., component of the insulin receptor within the cell rather than on the cell surface) has a decreased ability to undergo tyrosine phosphorylation.[44] This is an important step in the action of insulin after it has bound to the insulin receptor on the cell surface. This additional defect in the insulin-signaling cascade is not found in pregnant or nonpregnant women with normal glucose tolerance and results in a 25% lower glucose transport activity. TNF-α also acts by means of a serine/threonine kinase, thereby inhibiting IRS-1 and tyrosine phosphorylation of the insulin receptor.[45] These post-receptor defects may contribute in part to the pathogenesis of GDM and an increased risk for type 2 diabetes in later life.

Complications of Diabetes during Pregnancy

Maternal Morbidity

Women with pregestational diabetes are at risk for a number of obstetric and medical complications. The relative risk of these problems is proportional to the duration and severity of disease. Evers and coworkers reported the maternal morbidity of a cohort of 323 type 1 diabetic pregnancies followed prospectively in the Netherlands.[46] Glycemic control was excellent (Hb A_{1c} ≤7.0% in 75%), but the rates of preeclampsia (12.7%), preterm delivery (32%), cesarean section (44%), and maternal mortality (60 deaths per 100,000 pregnancies) were considerably higher than in the nondiabetic population.

Retinopathy

Diabetic retinopathy is the leading cause of blindness between the ages of 24 and 64 years.[47] Some form of retinopathy is present in virtually 100% of women who have had type 1 diabetes for 25 years or more; approximately 20% of these women are legally blind. The topic of diabetic retinopathy has been reviewed elsewhere.[48]

The pattern of progression of diabetic retinopathy is predictable, proceeding from mild nonproliferative abnormalities, which are associated with increased vascular permeability, to moderate and severe nonproliferative diabetic retinopathy, which is characterized by vascular closure, to proliferative diabetic retinopathy, which is characterized by the growth of new blood vessels on the retina and posterior surface of the vitreous. It has been proposed that pregnancy accelerates these changes, although the mechanism is controversial.[49] Trials have not shown any acceleration in microvascular complications when pregnant and nonpregnant diabetic subjects were closely followed and compared.[50]

Vision loss resulting from diabetic retinopathy results from several mechanisms. First, central vision may be impaired by macular edema or capillary nonperfusion. Second, the new blood vessels of proliferative diabetic retinopathy and contraction of the accompanying fibrous tissue can distort the retina and lead to tractional retinal detachment, producing severe and often irreversible vision loss. Third, the new blood vessels may bleed, adding the further complication of preretinal or vitreous hemorrhage.

FACTORS AFFECTING PROGRESSION OF RETINOPATHY DURING PREGNANCY

Although past studies suggested that rapid induction of glycemic control in early pregnancy stimulated retinal vascular proliferation,[51] later investigations indicate that the severity and duration of diabetes before pregnancy have a greater effect. Temple and colleagues[52] studied 179 women with pregestational type 1 diabetes, performing dilated fundal examination at the first prenatal visit, 24 weeks, and 34 weeks. Progression to proliferative diabetic retinopathy occurred in only 2.2%, and moderate progression occurred in 2.8%. However, progression was significantly greater in women who had had diabetes for more than 10 years (10% versus 0%; $P = .007$) and in women with moderate to severe background retinopathy before pregnancy (30% versus 3.7%; $P = .01$). In the European Diabetes (EURODIAB) Prospective Complications Study, 793 potentially childbearing women at baseline completed the follow-up, and 21% gave birth. Duration of diabetes and high HbA_{1c} levels at recruitment were significant risk factors for retinopathy progression, whereas giving birth was not.[50]

OPHTHALMOLOGIC MANAGEMENT DURING PREGNANCY

Screening for retinopathy by a qualified ophthalmologist is recommended before pregnancy and again during the first trimester for patients with pregestational diabetes because of the demonstrated effectiveness of laser photocoagulation therapy in arresting progression. Patients with minimal disease should be re-examined once or twice during the pregnancy and at 3 and 6 months after delivery. Those with significant retinal pathology may require monthly follow-up.[53]

Nephropathy

Diabetes is the most common cause of end-stage renal disease in the United States and Europe. In the United States, diabetic nephropathy accounts for about 45% of new cases of this condition. In 2003, the cost for treatment of diabetic patients with end-stage renal disease was in excess of $55,000 annually per person and more than $5 billion in aggregate.[54] About 20% to 40% of patients with type 1 or type 2 diabetes develop evidence of nephropathy over time, but the rate and extent of progression are highly individual.[53]

The pathophysiology of diabetic renal disease is incompletely understood, but several factors play a role, including genetic susceptibility, control of hyperglycemia, and the duration and severity of coexisting hypertension. Additional insults, such as repeated urinary tract infections, excessive glycogen deposition, and papillary necrosis, all hasten deterioration of renal function. The kidney is normal at the onset of diabetes, but within a few years, glomerular basement membrane thickening can be identified. By 5 years, there is expansion of the glomerular mesangium, resulting in diffuse diabetic glomerulosclerosis. All patients with marked mesangial expansion exhibit proteinuria exceeding 400 mg in 24 hours. The peak incidence of nephropathy occurs after about 16 years of diabetes.

CATEGORIES OF DIABETIC NEPHROPATHY

Categories of diabetic nephropathy are distinguished by the level of urinary protein excretion. Table 46-3 shows normal values and the current clinical criteria for microalbuminuria and nephropathy. Screening for microalbuminuria can be performed by three methods: measurement of the albumin to creatinine ratio in a random spot collection; 24-hour collection with creatinine, allowing the simultaneous measurement of creatinine clearance; and timed (e.g., 4-hour or overnight) collection. The first method is preferred because it is the easiest to carry out in an ambulatory setting, and it provides adequately accurate information. The other methods are rarely used.[55]

EFFECT OF PREGNANCY ON PROGRESSION OF NEPHROPATHY

Although some clinicians discourage pregnancy in women with diabetic renal disease because of concerns of permanent renal deterioration as a result of the pregnancy, recent data consistently indicate that pregnancy does not measurably alter the time course of diabetic renal disease.

Progression of diabetic nephropathy is closely related to the degree of glycemic control. To the extent that most women have better glycemic control during pregnancy, delay or slowing of renal function deterioration can be expected. A study of renal function for 4 years before and 4 years after pregnancy in 11 patients with diabetic nephropathy[56] showed that the gradual rise in serum creatinine over that period was unaffected by the intervening pregnancy. Imbasciati and coworkers[57] performed a longitudinal study of 58 women with chronic renal disease, following each through pregnancy. The mean serum creatinine level was 6 mg/dL at the start of the study and 6 mg/dL after delivery. Although they found that women with glomerular filtration rates less than 40 mL/min and with proteinuria greater than 1 g/day had increased risk of delivering a child with a birth weight less than 2500 g (odds ratio [OR] = 5.1; 95% confidence interval [CI], 1.03 to 25.6), the association was not related to renal disease, hypertension, and maternal age. When the cohort was taken as a whole, even those with lower glomerular filtration rates and higher levels of proteinuria had similarly modest changes in renal function when after- and before-pregnancy indices were compared.[57]

Rossing and colleagues[58] evaluated the effect of pregnancy on deterioration of renal function in 93 women older than 20 years. They compared groups of never-pregnant and ever-pregnant women who received similar medical therapy and who had similar degrees of renal function at the start of the study. The results are shown in Figure 46-7. Based on this excellent prospective study, it is evident that pregnancy neither alters the time course of renal disease nor increases the likelihood of transition to end-stage renal disease.

COURSE OF DIABETIC NEPHROPATHY DURING PREGNANCY

In general, patients with underlying renal disease before pregnancy can be expected to experience various degrees of deterioration during pregnancy. The physiologic changes associated with normal pregnancy increase renal blood flow and glomerular filtration by 30% to 50%. Most women with preexisting diabetic nephropathy experience this improvement in renal function, especially during the second trimester.[59] During the third trimester, however, when mean arterial pressure and peripheral vascular resistance typically increase, women with diabetic microvascular disease may experience marked diminution of renal function, an exacerbation in hypertension, and in many cases, preeclampsia. The third-trimester increase in maternal blood pressure and serum creatinine concentration are among the most common

TABLE 46-3 CATEGORIES OF DIABETIC RENAL DISEASE

Category*	Albumin-to-Creatinine Ratio (μg/mg)†
Normal	<30
Microalbuminuria	30-299
Nephropathy	≥300

*Categories of diabetic nephropathy are distinguished by the level of urinary protein excretion. Two of three collections in a 3- to 6-month period should be abnormal for a diagnosis of microalbuminuria or nephropathy.
†The ratio of albumin to creatinine was determined by random spot collection.
Adapted from American Diabetes Association. Standards of medical care in diabetes. Diabetes Care 28(Suppl 1):S4-S36, 2005.

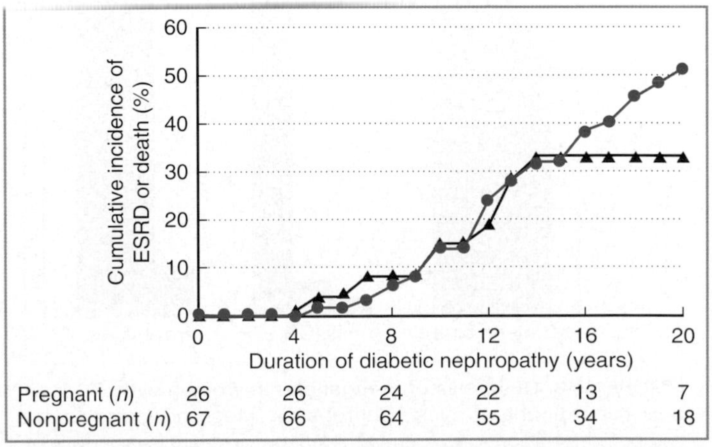

FIGURE 46-7 End-stage renal disease. Cumulative incidence of end-stage renal disease (ESRD) in ever-pregnant *(triangles)* and never-pregnant *(circles)* groups. (From Rossing K, Jacobsen P, Hommel E, et al: Pregnancy and progression of diabetic nephropathy. Diabetologia 45:36, 2002.)

precipitating events leading to indicated preterm delivery in diabetic women. Although delivering the fetus to interrupt the precipitous rise in blood pressure may result in premature birth, this is usually preferable to the risk of maternal renal failure or stroke (discussed later).

Reece and colleagues[60] reviewed the outcomes of 315 pregnant women with preexisting diabetic nephropathy. Of these, 17% ultimately developed end-stage renal disease, and 5% died as a result of renal insufficiency. During pregnancy, proteinuria and mean arterial pressure significantly increased from the first to the third trimester ($P < .05$). Another study by Purdy and coworkers[61] demonstrated a rise in the mean serum creatinine level from 1.8 mg/dL before pregnancy to 2.5 mg/dL in the third trimester. Renal function was stable in 27%, transiently worsened during pregnancy in 27%, and demonstrated a permanent decline in 45%. Proteinuria increased during pregnancy in 79%, and exacerbation of hypertension or preeclampsia occurred in 73%.

Ekbom and colleagues[62] compared the outcomes of pregnancies in women with microalbuminuria or overt nephropathy and those without. Their results (Fig. 46-8) indicate that the likelihood of preterm delivery is considerably increased for women with microalbuminuria, mainly because of preeclampsia.

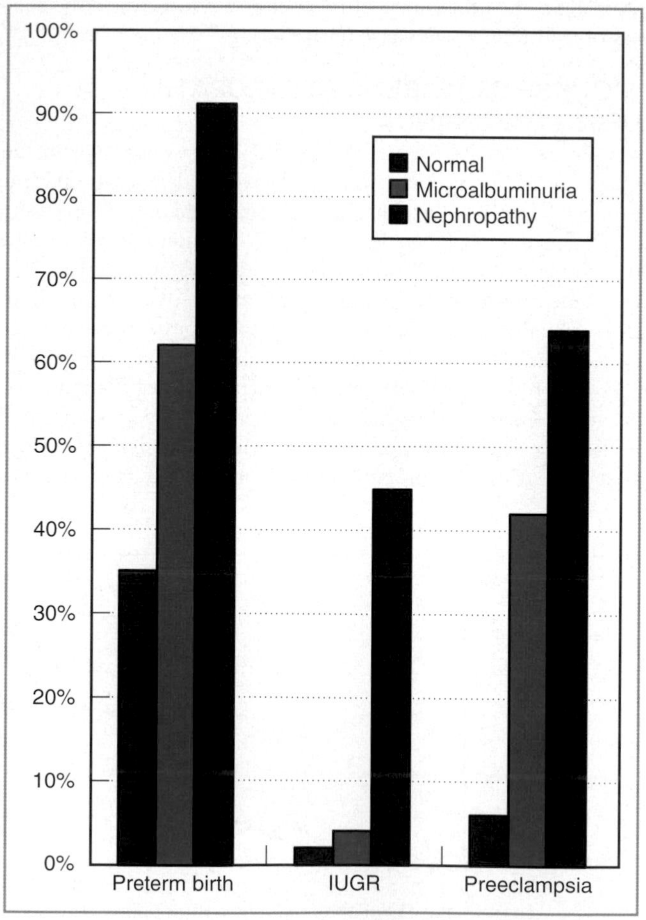

FIGURE 46-8 **Outcomes of pregnancies in women with microalbuminuria or overt nephropathy.** Pregnancy outcomes are compared for diabetic women with underlying renal disease. IUGR, intrauterine growth restriction. (Adapted from Ekbom P, Damm P, Feldt-Rasmussen U, et al: Pregnancy outcome in type 1 diabetic women with microalbuminuria. Diabetes Care 24:1739, 2001. Copyright © American Diabetes Association. Reprinted with permission from the American Diabetes Association.)

RENAL DIALYSIS IN DIABETIC PREGNANT WOMEN

Although women receiving dialysis for end-stage renal disease are often amenorrheic or at least anovulatory, pregnancies have become increasingly common[63] during therapy (3% to 7%).[64] Unfortunately, the prognosis for pregnancy in diabetic women with end-stage renal disease continues to be exceedingly poor, with fetal loss rates remaining in the range of 30% to 50% over the past decade. Neonatal death rates are between 5% and 15%, and less than one half of pregnancies among women with end-stage renal disease result in viable children. About 60% of births are premature, often because of uncontrollable hypertension, renal failure, or fetal growth failure.[65] Of the 20% to 25% of pregnancies ending in live births, 40% of babies are severely growth restricted.

A major practical problem with achieving a successful pregnancy outcome while on hemodialysis is proper maintenance of maternal vascular volume. Dialysis teams are accustomed to removing significant vascular volume at each session. However, during a normal pregnancy, there is a progressive expansion in vascular volume of at least 20% to 30% above nonpregnant values from 8 to 30 weeks' gestation. This volume augmentation is required to maintain uteroplacental perfusion and fetal growth. Pregnancies in which vascular volume does not increase appropriately have a high incidence of fetal growth restriction and stillbirths. Difficulties with vascular underfill (e.g., hypertension, poor fetal growth, asphyxia) and overfill (e.g., hypertension) are common in pregnant patients on hemodialysis and often are difficult to rectify.

The poor prognosis associated with hemodialysis combined with other considerations has prompted increased interest in continuous ambulatory peritoneal dialysis. Several successful pregnancy series have been reported.[65-67] Although fluid and chemical balance is constant and heparinization is not necessary, intrauterine deaths, abruption, prematurity, hypertension, and fetal distress still occur. The best strategy for most diabetic women on dialysis desiring pregnancy is to undergo kidney transplantation.

RENAL TRANSPLANTATION

Successful pregnancy after renal transplantation is now a reality. Davison's[67] review of 1569 pregnancies in women with renal allografts found that of the 60% of pregnancies that continued beyond the first trimester, 92% resulted in a viable infant. Preeclampsia occurred in 30%, preterm delivery in about 50%, and IUGR in 20%. Patients with the worst renal function had the poorest pregnancy outcomes. Similar results were reported by Yassaee and Moshiri.[68] The most common maternal complications in 95 pregnancies were anemia in 65%, and preeclampsia in 47%. Three patients lost their graft, and six had impaired kidney allograft function 2 years after pregnancy.[68]

In a historical cohort study, 86 women who had at least one post-transplantation pregnancy were compared with 125 who had no pregnancy after renal transplantation. Patients were matched for age, cause of end-stage renal disease, treatment protocol, and first serum creatinine level. The 5-year patient and graft survival rates were not significantly different between the study groups. Among the women with at least one pregnancy, only 10% had serum creatinine levels above 1.5 mg/dL at the end of 46 months of follow-up, compared with 28% of the never-pregnant group.[69] Based on these findings, it appears that perinatal outcomes are better in patients who have undergone renal transplantation than in those with end-stage renal disease who are on dialysis.

Cardiovascular Complications

Cardiovascular complications experienced by pregnant women with diabetes include chronic hypertension, pregnancy-induced hypertension, and rarely, atherosclerotic heart disease. In composite studies of all types of diabetic pregnancies, the incidence of hypertensive disorders during pregnancy varies from 15% to 30%,[70,71] with the rate of hypertension increased fourfold over that for the nondiabetic population.[72]

CHRONIC HYPERTENSION

Chronic hypertension (i.e., blood pressure at or above 140/90 mm Hg before 20 weeks' gestation)[73] complicates 10% to 20% of pregnancies in diabetic women and up to 40% of those in diabetic women with preexisting renal or retinal vascular disease.[74] The perinatal problems encountered with chronic hypertension include IUGR, maternal stroke, preeclampsia, and abruptio placentae. In pregestational diabetes, the prevalence of chronic hypertension increases with duration of diabetes and is closely associated with nephropathy.[72,75]

The Diabetes in Early Pregnancy (DIEP) study reported that women with type 1 diabetes have higher mean blood pressures throughout pregnancy than do normal controls.[76] In a significant proportion of patients, this difference is probably evidence of underlying renal compromise. Preexisting chronic hypertension should be suspected when the diabetic patient's systolic blood pressure exceeds 130/80 mm Hg before the third trimester. The diagnosis is strengthened by finding a failure of mean blood pressure to decline normally in the late second trimester, elevation in the blood urea nitrogen level above 10 mg/dL, serum creatinine concentration above 1 mg/dL, creatinine clearance less than 100 mL/min, or a combination of these factors.

PREECLAMPSIA

Preeclampsia is more common among women with diabetes, occurring four times as frequently in women with pregestational diabetes as in those without diabetes.[72] The risk of developing preeclampsia is proportional to the duration of diabetes before pregnancy and the existence of nephropathy and hypertension; more than one third of pregnant women who have had diabetes for more than 20 years develop this condition. As is shown in Figure 46-9, patients with White class B diabetes have a risk profile similar to that of nondiabetic patients, but women with evidence of renal or retinal vasculopathy (classes D, F, or R) have a 50% excess risk of hypertensive complications over the rate observed for those with no hypertension. Women with diabetic nephropathy have similar rates of preeclampsia.

Renal function assessments should be performed in each trimester in women with overt diabetic vascular disease and in those who have had diabetes for more than 10 years. Significant proteinuria, plasma uric acid levels above 6 mg/dL, or evidence of HELLP syndrome (*h*emolysis, *e*levated *l*iver enzymes, and *l*ow *p*latelets) should prompt a workup for preeclampsia.

HEART DISEASE

Although coronary heart disease is rarely encountered in pregnant women with diabetes, a study by Airaksinen and colleagues[77] suggests that such women may have preclinical cardiomyopathy and autonomic neuropathy. The diabetic women studied had less than the expected increase in left ventricular size and stroke volume in pregnancy, lower heart rate increases, and smaller increments in cardiac output.

Although uncommon, atherosclerotic heart disease (White class H) may afflict diabetic patients in the later reproductive years. Patients with this complication have a mean age of 34 years and exhibit other evidence of diabetic vascular involvement (White class D or R).[78] For diabetic women with cardiac involvement, pregnancy outcome is

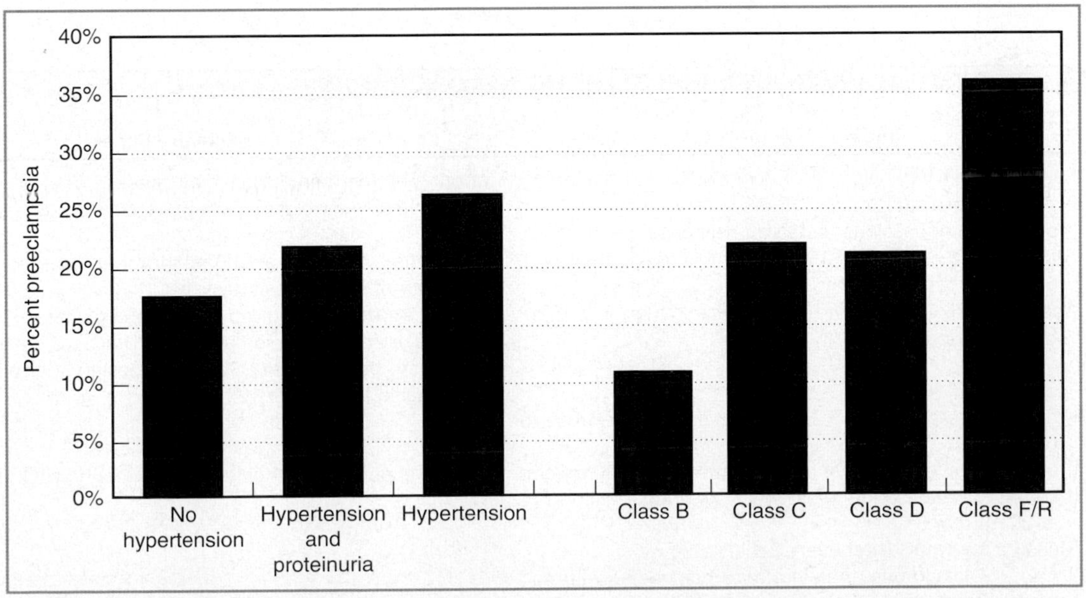

FIGURE 46-9 Likelihood of preeclampsia in diabetic pregnancy by White's class and preexisting hypertension. The risk of developing preeclampsia is proportional to the duration of diabetes before pregnancy and the existence of nephropathy and hypertension. (From Sibai BM, Caritis S, Hauth J, et al: Risks of preeclampsia and adverse neonatal outcomes among women with pregestational diabetes mellitus. National Institute of Child Health and Development Network of Maternal-Fetal Medicine Units. Am J Obstet Gynecol 182:364, 2000.)

dismal, with a maternal mortality rate of 50% or higher and perinatal loss rates approaching 30%.[79] Recognition of cardiac compromise in pregnant women with diabetes may be difficult because of the decrease in exercise tolerance that occurs during normal pregnancy. Compromised cardiac function may also be difficult to detect in patients restricted to bed rest for hypertension or poor fetal growth. It is prudent to obtain a detailed cardiovascular history in all diabetic patients and to consider electrocardiography and maternal echocardiography in patients who have type 1 diabetes and are older than 30 years or in patients who have had diabetes for 10 years or more. With intensive monitoring, successful pregnancy is possible, albeit hazardous for women with significant cardiac disease.[80]

Diabetic Ketoacidosis

Diabetic ketoacidosis (DKA) during pregnancy is a medical emergency for the mother and fetus. Pregnant women with type 1 diabetes are at increased risk for DKA, although the incidence and morbidity of this complication have decreased from 20% or more in the older literature to approximately 2% in later reports.[81] The rate of intrauterine fetal death, formerly as high as 35% with DKA during pregnancy, has dropped to 10% or less.

Precipitating factors for ketoacidosis include pulmonary, urinary, or soft tissue infections; poor compliance; and unrecognized new onset of diabetes. Because severe DKA threatens the life of the mother and fetus, prompt treatment is essential. Fetal well-being in particular is in jeopardy until maternal metabolic homeostasis is reestablished. High levels of plasma glucose and ketones are readily transported to the fetus, which may be unable to secrete sufficient quantities of insulin to prevent DKA in utero.

DKA evolves from inadequate insulin action and functional hypoglycemia at the target tissue level. This leads to increased hepatic glucose release but decreased or absent tissue disposal of glucose. Glucose-lacking tissues release ketone bodies, and vascular hyperglycemia promotes osmotic diuresis. Over time, the diuresis causes profound vascular volume depletion and loss of electrolytes. The release of stress hormones (i.e., catecholamines, glucagon, growth hormone, and cortisol) further impairs insulin action and contributes to insulin resistance. Left unchecked, this cycle of dehydration, tissue hypoglycemia, and electrolyte depletion can lead to multisystem collapse, coma, and death.

Early in the illness, hyperglycemia and ketosis are moderate. If hyperglycemia is not corrected, diuresis, dehydration, and hyperosmolality follow. Pregnant women in the early stages of ketoacidosis respond quickly to appropriate treatment of the initiating cause (e.g., broad-spectrum antibiotics), additional doses of regular insulin, and volume replacement.

Patients with advanced DKA usually present with typical findings, including hyperventilation, normal or obtunded mental state (depending on severity of the acidosis), dehydration, hypotension, and a fruity odor to the breath. Abdominal pain and vomiting may be prominent symptoms. The diagnosis of DKA is confirmed by the presence of hyperglycemia (glucose >200 mg/100 mL) with positive test results for serum ketones at a level of 1:4 or greater.

As many as one third of patients in the early or very late stages of DKA may have initial blood glucose levels less than 200 mg/dL.[82] A pregnant diabetic patient with a history of poor food intake or vomiting for more than 12 to 16 hours should have a thorough workup for DKA, including a complete blood cell count and electrolyte determinations. A serum bicarbonate level below 18 mg/dL should prompt performance of an arterial blood gas analysis. In all cases of DKA, the diagnosis is confirmed by arterial blood gases demonstrating a metabolic acidemia (i.e., base excess of −4 or lower).[83]

Table 46-4 contains a protocol for treatment of DKA. The important steps in management should include the following:

- Search for and treat the precipitating cause. Typical initiators include pyelonephritis and pulmonary or gastrointestinal viral infections.
- Perform vigorous and sustained volume resuscitation. The patient will continue to generate vascular volume deficits

TABLE 46-4 TREATMENT PROTOCOL FOR DIABETIC KETOACIDOSIS*

Measures	Initial Phase (6-24 hr)	Recovery Phase
General	Search for initiating cause of ketoacidosis. Insert bladder catheter. If patient is unconscious, establish nasogastric tube.	Continue treatment of initiating cause. Remove bladder catheter when vascular volume is replaced.
Fluids	Administer 0.9% NaCl at 1000 mL/hr × 2 hr and then 500 mL/hr until 5-8 L infused.	Continue 0.9% NaCl at 100 mL/hr for at least 48 hours to avoid return of ketoacidosis.
Insulin	Administer 20 U of insulin by IV bolus and then 5-10 U/hr by IV infusion.	When acidosis is resolved and plasma glucose <160 mg/dL, reduce insulin infusion to 0.7-2.0 U/hr. Return to patient's prior SC insulin dosing after plasma glucose is stable for at least 12 hr.
Glucose	When plasma glucose is <250 mg/dL, add 5% dextrose to 0.9% NaCl.	
Potassium	If serum K^+ level is normal or low, infuse KCl at 20 mEq/hr. If serum K^+ level is high, wait until K^+ is normal, then KCl at 20 mEq/hr. Measure serum K^+ level every 2-4 hr.	Use oral potassium supplementation for 1 week.
Bicarbonate	If pH is <7.1, add one ampule of bicarbonate (50 mEq) to IV; repeat until pH >7.1.	

***These are general guidelines. Because there may be wide variation in individual patient needs, there is no substitute for careful monitoring of each patient, particularly in the initial phase of therapy.**

IM, intramuscular; IV, intravenous; KCl, potassium chloride; NaCl, sodium chloride; SC, subcutaneous.

Adapted from American College of Obstetricians and Gynecologists (ACOG): Clinical management guidelines for obstetrician-gynecologists. ACOG practice bulletin no. 60, March 2005. Pregestational diabetes mellitus. Obstet Gynecol 105:675-685, 2005.

until her glucose levels and acidosis are largely resolved. A physiologic fluid such as 0.9% NaCl with 20 mEq/L of potassium should be used and continued until the acidosis is substantially corrected (base excess of −2 or less). This usually requires an infusion at 1 to 2 L/hr for the first 1 to 2 hours, followed by reduced rates (150 to 200 mL/hr) until the base deficit approaches a normal level.

- Place a bladder catheter to monitor urine output.
- Use insulin to correct hyperglycemia. Although intermittent injections can be used, a continuous infusion of regular or short-acting insulin (i.e., lispro or aspart) allows frequent adjustments. When giving insulin as a continuous infusion, 1 to 2 units/hr gradually corrects the patient's glucose abnormality over 4 to 8 hours. Attempts to normalize plasma glucose levels rapidly (i.e., in less than 2 to 3 hours) may result in hypoglycemia and further physiologic counterregulatory responses.
- Monitor serum bicarbonate levels and arterial blood gas base deficits every 1 to 3 hours to guide management. Even when the plasma glucose level is normalized, acidemia may persist, as evidenced by continuing abnormalities in the patient's electrolyte concentrations. Unless volume therapy is continued until the patient's electrolyte stores and plasma concentrations have substantially returned to normal, DKA may reappear, and the cycle of metabolic derangement will be renewed.

When DKA occurs after 24 weeks' gestation, fetal status should be continuously monitored by fetal heart rate monitoring or a biophysical profile, or both. However, even when fetal status is questionable during the phase of therapeutic volume and plasma glucose correction, emergency cesarean section should be avoided. Usually, correction of the maternal metabolic disorder is effective in normalizing fetal status. Nevertheless, if a reasonable effort has been expended in correcting the maternal metabolic disorder and the fetal status remains a concern, delivery should not be delayed.

Fetal Morbidity and Mortality

Perinatal mortality in diabetic pregnancy has decreased 30-fold since the discovery of insulin in 1922 and the institution of intensive obstetric and infant care in the 1970s. Improved techniques of maintaining maternal euglycemia have led to later timing of delivery and reduced iatrogenic respiratory distress syndrome. Nevertheless, the perinatal mortality rates reported for diabetic women remain approximately twice those observed in the nondiabetic population (Table 46-5). Congenital malformations, respiratory distress syndrome, and extreme prematurity account for most perinatal deaths in diabetic pregnancies.

TABLE 46-5 PERINATAL MORTALITY RATES IN DIABETIC PREGNANCY*

Group	Gestational	Overt	Normal†
Fetal mortality rate (%)*	4.7	10.4	5.7
Neonatal mortality rate (%)*	3.3	12.2	4.7
Perinatal mortality rate (%)*	8.0	22.6	10.4

*Mortality rates = deaths per 1000 live births.
†Normal was determined from California data from 1986; figures were corrected for birth weight, sex, and race.

Miscarriage

Studies of miscarriage rates from a decade ago indicated an increased incidence of spontaneous abortion among women with pregestational diabetes, especially those with poor glucose control during the periconceptional period. Given the well-documented association between congenital anomalies and hyperglycemia, such a finding is not surprising. Sutherland and Pritchard[84] reported the outcomes of 164 diabetic pregnancies managed with relaxed glycemic control and found a spontaneous abortion rate of almost double the expected rate. Miodovnik and coworkers[85] studied spontaneous abortion in diabetic pregnancy prospectively and found an increasing rate among patients with more advanced classes of diabetes (rates for classes C, D, and F were 25%, 44%, and 22%, respectively). Later studies of populations with better glycemic control report miscarriage rates similar to those in the nondiabetic population,[86,87] indicating that diabetic women with excellent glycemic control have a risk of miscarriage equivalent to those without diabetes.

These studies can be used to encourage patients who have not yet conceived to achieve excellent glycemic control. Patients presenting in early pregnancy with normal glycohemoglobin values can be reassured that the overall elevation in risk of miscarriage is modest. However, for patients with glycohemoglobin values 2 to 3 standard deviations above the norm, intense early pregnancy surveillance is indicated.

Congenital Anomalies

Among women with overt diabetes before conception, the risk of a structural anomaly in the fetus is increased fourfold to eightfold,[88] compared with the 1% to 2% risk for the general population. In a cohort study of 2359 pregnancies in women with pregestational diabetes, the major congenital anomaly rate was 4.6% overall, with 4.8% for type 1 diabetes and 4.3% for type 2 diabetes, more than double the expected rate. Neural tube defects were increased 4.2-fold and congenital heart disease by 3.4-fold. Of all anomalies confirmed in the neonate, only 65% were diagnosed antenatally.[9] The typical congenital anomalies observed in diabetic pregnancies and their frequency of occurrence are listed in Table 46-6.

There is no increase in birth defects among offspring of diabetic fathers and nondiabetic women and women who develop gestational diabetes after the first trimester, indicating that glycemic control during embryogenesis is the main factor in the genesis of diabetes-associated birth defects. A classic report by Miller and coauthors[89] compared the frequency of congenital anomalies in patients with normal or high first-trimester maternal glycohemoglobin levels and found only a 3.4% rate of anomalies with an Hb A_{1c} value less than 8.5%, whereas the rate

TABLE 46-6 CONGENITAL MALFORMATIONS IN INFANTS OF INSULIN-DEPENDENT DIABETIC MOTHERS

Anomaly	Approximate Relative Risk	Percent Risk (%)
All cardiac defects	18	8.5
All central nervous system anomalies	16	5.3
Anencephaly	13	
Spina bifida	20	
All congenital anomalies	8	18.4

Adapted from Becerra JE, Khoury MJ, Cordero JF, et al: Diabetes mellitus during pregnancy and the risks for specific birth defects: A population based case-control study. Pediatrics 85:1, 1990.

of malformations in patients with poorer glycemic control in the periconceptional period (Hb A_{1c} above 8.5) was 22.4%. Lucas and coworkers[90] reported an overall malformation rate of 13.3% in 105 diabetic patients. However, the risk of delivering a malformed infant was zero with an Hb A_1 value less than 7%, 14% with Hb A_1 between 7.2% and 9.1%, 23% with Hb A_1 between 9.2% and 11.1%, and 25% with Hb A_1 greater than 11.2%.

PATHOGENESIS

The mechanism by which hyperglycemia disturbs embryonic development is multifactorial. The potential teratologic role of disturbances in the metabolism of inositol, prostaglandins, and reactive oxygen species has been established.[91] Embryonic hyperglycemia may promote excessive formation of oxygen radicals in susceptible fetal tissues, which are inhibitors of prostacyclin.[92] The resulting overabundance of thromboxanes and other prostaglandins may then disrupt the vascularization of developing tissues. In support of this theory, addition of prostaglandin inhibitors to mouse embryos in culture medium prevented glucose-induced embryopathy.[93] The pathogenic role of free radical species in teratogenesis with diabetes has been underscored by demonstrating the effect of dietary antioxidants experimentally. High doses of vitamins C and E decreased fetal dysmorphogenesis to nondiabetic levels in rat pregnancy and rat embryo culture.[94,95]

PREVENTION

Because the critical time for teratogenesis is during the period 3 to 6 weeks after conception, nutritional and metabolic intervention must be instituted preconceptionally to be effective. Several clinical trials of preconceptional metabolic care have demonstrated that malformation rates equivalent to those in the general population can be achieved with meticulous glycemic control.[96] Although studies of dietary folate and vitamin C supplementation have demonstrated success in reducing the incidence of congenital anomalies in experimental diabetes in rats,[97] the efficacy of a high-antioxidant diet in preventing diabetes-induced structural anomalies in humans has not been adequately explored. Preconceptional management of pregestational diabetics is discussed in the following sections.

Intrauterine Growth Restriction

Although the weights of infants of diabetic mothers (IDMs) usually are skewed into the upper range, IUGR occurs with significant frequency in diabetic pregnancies, especially in women with underlying vascular disease. Additional factors that increase the risk for IUGR in a diabetic pregnancy include the higher incidence of structural anomalies and maternal hypertension.

Asymmetrical IUGR is encountered most frequently in diabetic patients with vasculopathy (i.e., retinal, renal, or chronic hypertension).[88] This association suggests that uteroplacental vasculopathy may promote restricted fetal growth in these patients.[98] Patients with poor glycemic control and frequent episodes of ketosis and hypoglycemia are also prone to preeclampsia and poor fetal growth. Whether fetal growth restriction results from poor maternal-placental blood flow or intrinsically poor placental function is unresolved.[99]

Fetal Obesity

Macrosomia has been defined using various criteria, which include birth weight greater than the 90th percentile, birth weight greater than 4000 g, and estimates of neonatal adiposity based on body composition measures. As early as 1923, research by Moulton[100] described variability in weight among various mammalian species that was attributed to the amount of adipose tissue or fat mass rather than lean body mass. Using autopsy data and chemical analysis of 169 stillbirths, Sparks[101] described a relatively comparable rate of accretion of lean body mass in fetuses that were small for gestational age (SGA), average for gestational age (AGA), and large for gestational age (LGA), but he found considerable variation in the accretion of fetal fat in utero. The human fetus at term has the greatest percent of body fat (approximately 10% to 12%) compared with other mammals.[102]

GROWTH DYNAMICS

The increased growth of the mother is composed primarily of total body water and adipose tissue in early gestation.[26] Relative to the fetoplacental unit, the human placenta attains most of its growth by the middle of the second trimester. In contrast, approximately 70% of fetal growth occurs over the last third of gestation (1000 g at 28 weeks to 3500 g at term). Yang and associates[6] reported that IDMs with diabetes still have an increased relative risk (RR) of being LGA (RR = 3.59; 95% confidence interval [CI], 1.55 to 5.84) compared with the infants of women with normal glucose tolerance.[100] Ogata and colleagues,[103] using serial ultrasound measures of the fetus of women with diabetes, described an increase in the rate of abdominal circumference growth after 24 weeks' gestation. The increase in growth appears to affect primarily insulin-sensitive tissues such as the subcutaneous fat included in measures of abdominal circumference.[104] Ninety-five percent of the variance in fetal abdominal circumference can be accounted for by subcutaneous fat rather than intra-abdominal measures such as liver size. This is consistent with the inability of the fetal liver to store much glycogen in early third trimester. Reece and coworkers[105] showed that fetuses of diabetic mothers have normal growth of lean body mass such as head and skeletal growth, even when there is marked hyperglycemia. In longitudinal ultrasound studies, Bernstein and associates[106] reported that fetal fat and lean body mass demonstrate unique growth profiles. These unique ultrasound profiles potentially provide a more sensitive marker of abnormal fetal growth, particularly in infants of women with diabetes based on the increased fat mass rather than lean mass of these neonates.[106] At delivery, body composition studies by Catalano and colleagues[107] have shown that birth weight alone, even when AGA, may not be a sensitive enough measure of fetal growth in the infant of the diabetic mother. They reported that although there were no significant differences in birth weight or lean body mass, the infants of women with GDM had increased fat mass and percent body fat compared with a normoglycemic control group (Table 46-7).

PATHOPHYSIOLOGY OF FETAL OVERGROWTH

Maternal Glucose Concentrations. Because glucose is the most easily measured nutrient and marker of diabetes, most studies evaluating the effect of diabetes on fetal growth have used measures of glucose as a reference. Findings from the DIEP indicate that birth weight correlated best with second- and third-trimester postprandial glucose measures. When 2-hour postmeal glucose measures averaged 120 mg/dL or less, approximately 20% of infants were macrosomic. In contrast, when 2-hour postprandial glucose measures averaged up to 160 mg/dL, the rate of macrosomia reached 35%.[108] Similarly, Combs and coworkers[109] reported that macrosomia was significantly associated with postprandial glucose levels between 29 and 32 weeks' gestation.[109] In contrast, Persson and associates[110] showed that fasting glucose concentrations account for 12% of the variance in birth weight and correlated best with estimates of neonatal fat. Uvena and colleagues[111] found the strongest correlation was between fasting glucose and neonatal adiposity, rather than postprandial measures.

Fetal Insulin Concentrations. Based on the early work of Pedersen,[112] fetal insulin has long been considered a principal driving

TABLE 46-7 NEONATAL ANTHROPOMETRICS OF NEWBORNS OF WOMEN WITH GESTATIONAL DIABETES MELLITUS AND NORMAL GLUCOSE TOLERANCE

Feature Measured*	GDM (n = 195)	NGT (n = 220)	*P* Value
Weight (g)	3398 ± 550	3337 ± 549	.26
Fat free mass (g)	2962 ± 405	2975 ± 408	.74
Fat mass (g)	436 ± 206	362 ± 198	.0002
Body fat (%)	2.4 ± 4.6	10.4 ± 4.6	.0001
Skinfold			
Triceps	4.7 ± 1.1	4.2 ± 1.0	.0001
Subscapular	5.4 ± 1.4	4.6 ± 1.2	.0001
Flank	4.2 ± 1.2	3.8 ± 1.0	.0001
Thigh	6.0 ± 1.4	5.4 ± 1.5	.0001
Abdominal wall	3.5 ± 0.9	3.0 ± 0.8	.0001

*Data are presented as the mean ± SD.
GDM, gestational diabetes mellitus; NGT, normal glucose tolerance.
Adapted from Catalano PM, Thomas A, Huston-Presley L, Amini SB: Increased fetal adiposity: A very sensitive marker of abnormal in utero development. Am J Obstet Gynecol 189:1698-1704, 2003.

factor of in utero fetal growth. Experimental data gathered from non-human primates by Susa and coworkers[113] showed that in the rhesus monkey when implanted with an Alzet pump, which delivered continuous, increasing insulin concentrations to the fetus independent of the mother's metabolic condition, there was evidence of fetal overgrowth.[111] In contrast, when genetic mutations such as glucokinase deficiencies existed only in the fetus, the inability of the beta cell to respond to increasing glucose concentrations results in fetal growth restriction.[25] Many studies have confirmed the correspondence of increased cord insulin concentrations with fetal macrosomia. Schwartz and associates[114] found that umbilical cord insulin concentrations at delivery correlated with the degree of macrosomia. Cordocentesis studies in late third trimester showed that the ratio of fetal plasma insulin to glucose and the degree of macrosomia were strongly correlated.[115] Krew and colleagues[116] reported that amniotic fluid C-peptide measures at term had a strong correlation with fetal adiposity but not lean body mass.

The relationship between elevated insulin concentrations and fetal macrosomia exists in late pregnancy, and there is evidence of altered metabolic function in early gestation. Carpenter and colleagues[117] reported that elevated amniotic fluid insulin concentrations obtained from normoglycemic patients at 14 to 20 weeks' gestation and adjusted for maternal age and weight correlated with the likelihood of subsequently diagnosed GDM (OR = 1.9; CI, 1.3 to 2.4). Each increase in amniotic fluid insulin multiple of the median (MOM) was associated with a threefold increase in fetal macrosomia.[117] These data support the concept that the underlying pathophysiology of GDM and fetal macrosomia may exist earlier in gestation than is routinely screened for and that it is consistent with subclinical pregravid maternal metabolic disturbances.

Growth Factors. There has been considerable interest in the role of insulin-like growth factors (IGFs) and fetal growth. Members of the IGF family have been implicated in abnormalities of increased and decreased fetal growth in humans. IGF-1 and the ratio of IGF-2 to the IGF-2 soluble receptor have been positively correlated with the Ponderal index.[118] However, there is also direct evidence using rodent knockout models. Baker and coworkers[119] reported that null mutations for the *IGF1* or *IGF2* gene decreases neonatal weight by 40% in mice. The effect of both genes is additive.[119] Liu and associates[120] previously reported that IGF-1, IGF-2, and IGF-binding protein-3 (IGFBP-3) were significantly elevated in women with type 1 and 2 diabetes compared with a control group. These data are consistent with the findings of other investigators, including data for women with type 1 and 2 diabetes.[121,122] Roth and colleagues[123] reported that cord levels of IGF-1 were significantly greater in macrosomic IDMs than in nonmacrosomic infants of glucose-tolerant or diabetic mothers. Radaelli and coworkers[124] showed that there was a strong negative correlation between maternal circulating IGFBP-1 and lean body mass in the infants. The study authors speculated that IGFBP-1 might influence fetal growth by affecting IGF mediated placental nutrient transport, particularly of glucose or amino acids rather than lipids. Decreased IGFBP-1 levels are in keeping with a potential negative transcriptional regulation of the *IGFBP1* gene by insulin.[124]

Maternal Obesity. Obesity is an epidemic in developed countries and the developing world.[125] In the United States, the prevalence of obesity, defined as a body mass index (BMI = weight/height^2) greater than 30 rose to 30.5% in 2000, compared with 22.9% from 1994 through 1998. The proportion of the population meeting the definition of overweight (BMI > 25) increased from 55.9% to 64.5% during the same period.[18] The risk of obesity is disproportionate among the races, increasing most among African Americans and Hispanics, the same populations at risk for type 2 diabetes. Several studies suggest that maternal obesity before conception has an independent effect on fetal macrosomia. Vohr and associates[126] analyzed various risk factors for neonatal macrosomia in women with overt and GDM compared with obese and normal weight controls.[126] Multiple regression analyses revealed the pre-pregnancy weight and weight gain were significant predictors for infants of GDM and control mothers. In an effort to better understand the potential independent effect of maternal obesity on growth of infants of GDM and normoglycemic women, Catalano and colleagues[127] performed a stepwise logistic regression analysis on data for 220 infants of mothers with normal glucose tolerance and 195 infants of GDM (Table 46-8). Gestational age at term had the strongest correlation with birth weight and lean body mass. In contrast, maternal pregravid BMI had the strongest correlation (approximately 7%) with fat mass and percent body fat. Although almost 50% of the subjects had GDM, only 2% fraction of the variance was correlated to fat mass.[127] These data support an independent effect of maternal pregravid obesity on fetal growth, particularly fat mass, independent of GDM.

Other Fuels. Many factors are related to fetal overgrowth of the infant of a woman with diabetes. The significant decreases in insulin sensitivity in late gestation affect glucose and lipid and amino acid metabolism. Although we clinically concentrate on glucose, other nutrients most probably contribute to fetal overgrowth. This concept is consistent with the hypothesis of fuel-mediated teratogenesis first proposed by Freinkel in 1980.[128] Circulating amino acid concentrations reflect the balance between protein breakdown and synthesis. Duggleby and Jackson[129] estimated that there is a 15% increase in protein synthesis during the second trimester and a further 25% increase in the third trimester compared with levels in nonpregnant women. These differences appear to have a strong relationship to fetal growth, particularly lean body mass. Butte and coworkers[130] and Metzger and associates[131] independently reported higher amino acid concentrations in women with GDM compared with a normoglycemic control group. Zimmer and colleagues[132] reported no significant difference in amino acid turnover in women with GDM and a control group. However, the

TABLE 46-8 STEPWISE REGRESSION ANALYSIS OF FACTORS RELATING TO FETAL GROWTH AND BODY COMPOSITION IN INFANTS OF WOMEN WITH GESTATIONAL DIABETES MELLITUS (n = 195) AND NORMAL GLUCOSE TOLERANCE (n = 220)

Factor	r^2	Δr^2	P value
Birth Weight			
Estimated gestational age	0.114	—	
Pregravid weight	0.162	0.048	
Weight gain	0.210	0.048	
Smoking (–)	0.227	0.017	
Parity	0.239	0.012	.0001
Lean Body Mass			
Estimated gestational age	0.122	—	
Smoking (–)	0.153	0.031	
Pregravid weight	0.179	0.026	
Weight gain	0.212	0.033	
Parity	0.225	0.013	
Maternal height	0.241	0.016	
Paternal weight	0.250	0.009	.0001
Fat Mass*			
Pregravid BMI	0.066	—	
Estimated gestational age	0.136	0.070	
Weight gain	0.171	0.035	
Group (GDM)	0.187	0.016	.0001
Percent Body Fat*			
Pregravid BMI	0.072	—	
Estimated gestational age	0.116	0.044	
Weight gain	0.147	0.031	
Group (GDM)	0.166	0.019	.0001

***Pregravid maternal obesity has the strongest correlation with neonatal measures of fat mass/% body fat in contrast to lean body mass.**
BMI, body mass index; GDM, gestational diabetes mellitus.
Adapted from Catalano PM, Ehrenberg HM: The short and long term implications of maternal obesity on the mother and her offspring. BJOG 113:1126-1133, 2006.

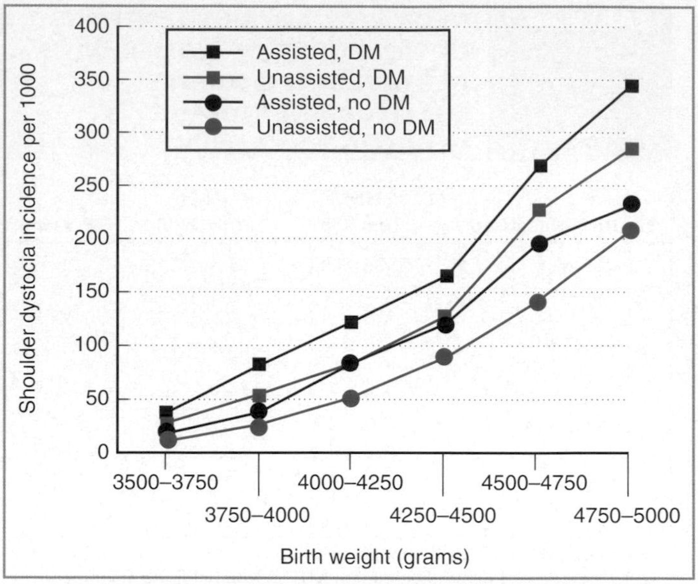

FIGURE 46-10 **Risk of shoulder dystocia by diabetes status and instrumental delivery.** Shoulder dystocia occurred more often in diabetic deliveries requiring operative vaginal assistance and in fetuses above the 90th percentile of birth weight for age. DM, diabetes mellitus. (From Nesbitt TS, Gilbert WM, Herrchen B: Shoulder dystocia and associated risk factors with macrosomic infants born in California. Am J Obstet Gynecol 179:476, 1998.)

investigators found that hyperinsulinemia was required to maintain normal amino acid turnover in the GDM women.[132] Kalhan and coworkers[133] reported that leucine turnover and oxidation were greater in the obese woman with GDM compared with less obese control subjects. The increased insulin concentrations required to maintain appropriate amino acid levels in the woman with diabetes may be another manifestation of the increased insulin resistance in pregnant women with GDM.

Knopp and associates[134] found that there is a twofold to fourfold increase in triglyceride concentrations and a 25% to 50% increase in cholesterol during gestation. This group also reported a further increase in triglyceride and high-density lipoprotein cholesterol concentrations in type 2 and GDM patients.[135] Similarly, Xiang and colleagues[43] described increased basal free fatty acid concentrations in Hispanic women with GDM in the third trimester compared with a matched control group.[136] Knopp and coworkers[137] also reported that mid-trimester triglyceride concentrations were a better predictor of macrosomia than glucose values during the glucose tolerance test. Similarly, Kitajima and colleagues[138] examined lipid profiles in women with an abnormal glucose challenge test in pregnancy and reported that the triglycerides had a significant correlation with birth weight, even after adjusting for significant covariables. Although lipid transport from the mother to fetus is not well understood, maternal lipid metabolism may play a significant role in fetal growth, particularly in accrual of adipose tissue.

Birth Injury

Birth injury is more common among the offspring of diabetic mothers, and macrosomic fetuses are at the highest risk.[139] The most common birth injuries associated with diabetes are brachial plexus palsy, facial nerve injury, humerus or clavicle fracture, and cephalhematoma. Athukorala and associates[140] studied women with gestational diabetes and found a positive relationship between the severity of maternal fasting hyperglycemia and the incidence of shoulder dystocia, with a doubling of risk with each 1-mmol increase in the fasting plasma glucose value on the OGTT. Shoulder dystocia occurred more often in diabetic deliveries requiring operative vaginal assistance (RR = 9.58; CI, 3.70 to 24.81: $P < .001$) and in fetuses above the 90th percentile of birth weight for age (RR = 4.57; CI, 1.74 to 12.01; $P < .005$) (Fig. 46-10).

Most of the birth injuries occurring in infants of diabetic pregnancy are associated with difficult vaginal delivery and shoulder dystocia. Although shoulder dystocia occurs in 0.3% to 0.5% of vaginal deliveries among normal pregnant women, the incidence is twofold to fourfold higher for women with diabetes because the excessive fetal fat deposition associated with hyperglycemia in poorly controlled diabetic pregnancy causes the fetal shoulder and abdominal widths to become massive.[140] Although one half of shoulder dystocias occur in infants of normal birth weight (2500 to 4000 g), the incidence of shoulder dystocia rises 10-fold to 5% to 7% among infants weighing 4000 g or more. However, if maternal diabetes is present, the risk at each birth-weight class is increased fivefold.[141] These risks are further magnified if a forceps or vacuum delivery is performed.[142]

The level of glycemic control is strongly correlated with the risk of shoulder dystocia and birth injury, presumably because increasing levels of hyperglycemia are associated with greater fetal fat deposition. Athukorola and colleagues[140] reported a positive correlation between the severity of maternal fasting hyperglycemia and the risk of shoulder dystocia, with each 1-mmol increase in the fasting value in the OGTT associated with an increasing relative risk of 2.09 (CI, 1.03 to 4.25).

Although it would be desirable to predict shoulder dystocia on the basis of warning signs during labor such as labor protraction, a suspected macrosomic infant, or the need for midpelvic forceps delivery, less than 30% of these events can be predicted from clinical factors.[143]

Neonatal Morbidity and Mortality

Polycythemia and Hyperviscosity

Polycythemia (i.e., central venous hemoglobin concentration >20 g/dL or hematocrit >65%) occurs in 5% to 10% of IDMs and is apparently related to glycemic control. Hyperglycemia is a powerful stimulus for fetal erythropoietin production, which is probably mediated by decreased fetal oxygen tension.[144] Untreated, neonatal polycythemia may promote vascular sludging, ischemia, and infarction of vital tissues, including the kidneys and central nervous system.

Neonatal Hypoglycemia

Approximately 15% to 25% of neonates delivered from women with diabetes during gestation develop hypoglycemia during the immediate newborn period.[145] Neonatal hypoglycemia is less common when tight glycemic control is maintained during pregnancy[146] and in labor.

A detailed study by Taylor and associates[147] found no correlation between the likelihood of neonatal hypoglycemia and Hb A_{1c}, whereas mean maternal glucose levels during labor were strongly predictive. Because unrecognized postnatal hypoglycemia may lead to neonatal seizures, coma, and brain damage, it is imperative that the neonatal team caring for the neonate follow a protocol of frequent postnatal glucose monitoring until metabolic stability is ensured.

Neonatal Hypocalcemia and Hyperbilirubinemia

Low levels of serum calcium (<7 mg/100 mL) have been reported in up to 50% of IDMs during the first 3 days of life, although later series record an incidence of 5% or less with better-managed pregnancies.[148] Neonatal hyperbilirubinemia occurs in approximately 25% of IDMs, a rate approximately double that for normal infants, with prematurity and polycythemia being the primary contributing factors. Close monitoring of the newborn of diabetic pregnancy is necessary to avoid the further morbidity of kernicterus, seizures, and neurologic damage.

Hypertrophic and Congestive Cardiomyopathy

In some macrosomic, plethoric infants of mothers with poorly controlled diabetes, a thickened myocardium and significant asymmetrical septal hypertrophy has been described.[149] The prevalence of clinical and subclinical asymmetrical septal hypertrophy in IDMs has been estimated to be as high as 30% at birth, with resolution by 1 year of age.[150] Kjos and colleagues[151] found that cardiac dysfunction associated with this entity often leads to respiratory distress, which may be mistaken for hyaline membrane disease.

IDMs who manifest cardiac dysfunction in the neonatal period may have congestive or hypertrophic cardiomyopathy. This condition is often asymptomatic and unrecognized. Echocardiograms show a hypercontractile, thickened myocardium, often with septal hypertrophy disproportionate to the ventricular free walls.[152] The ventricular chambers are often smaller than normal, and there may be anterior systolic motion of the mitral valve, producing left ventricular outflow tract obstruction.

Neonatal septal hypertrophy may be a response to chronic hyperglycemia. The maternal level of IGF-1, which is elevated in suboptimally controlled diabetic pregnancy, is significantly elevated in neonates with asymmetrical septal hypertrophy. Because IGF-1 does not cross the placenta, it may exert its action through binding to the IGF-1 receptor on the placenta.[153] Halse and coworkers[154] found that the level of B-type natriuretic protein (BNP), a marker for congestive cardiac failure, is elevated in neonates whose mothers had poor glycemic control during the third trimester.

Septal hypertrophy can be identified with sonography in the prenatal period. Cooper and coworkers[155] performed serial fetal echocardiography on 61 pregnant, diabetic women, demonstrating excessive ventricular septal thickness in the fetuses that were diagnosed postnatally with asymmetrical septal hypertrophy. When the newborns with asymmetrical septal hypertrophy were compared with normal infants, birth weights (4009 versus 3457 g; $P < .01$) and maternal glycosylated hemoglobin levels (6.7% versus 5.7%) were higher in infants with cardiomyopathy.

Respiratory Distress Syndrome

Until recently, respiratory distress syndrome was the most common and most serious disease in IDMs. In the 1970s, improved prenatal maternal management for diabetes and new techniques in obstetrics for timing and mode of delivery resulted in a dramatic decline in its incidence, from 31% to 3%.[156] However, even when matched by gestational week of pregnancy, IDMs are more than 20 times as likely as infants from normal pregnancies to develop respiratory distress syndrome.[157]

The increased susceptibility to respiratory distress may result from altered production of alveolar surfactant or abnormal pulmonary function. Kulovich and Gluck[158] reported delayed timing of phospholipid production in diabetic pregnancy, as indicated by a delay in the appearance of phosphatidylglycerol in the amniotic fluid. In their study, maturational delay occurred only in gestational diabetes (White class A patients); fetuses of women with other forms of diabetes showed normal or accelerated maturation of pulmonary phospholipid profiles.

Although some investigators have failed to demonstrate a delay in lung maturation in diabetic pregnancy,[159,160] most reports in the literature indicate a significant biochemical and physiologic delay in IDMs. Tyden and colleagues[161] and Landon and coworkers[162] reported that fetal lung maturity occurred later in pregnancies with poor glycemic control (mean plasma glucose level >110 mg/dL), regardless of class of diabetes, when the infants were stratified by maternal plasma glucose levels. These findings were confirmed by Moore,[163] who demonstrated no differences in the rate of rise of the amniotic fluid lecithin-to-sphingomyelin ratio among types of diabetes or degree of glucose control but found that amniotic fluid phosphatidylglycerol was delayed approximately 1.5 weeks in women with pregestational or GDM diabetes compared with controls (Fig. 46-11). The delay in phosphatidylglycerol was associated with an earlier and higher peak in the level of phosphatidyl inositol, suggesting that elevated maternal plasma levels of myoinositol in diabetic women may inhibit or delay the production of phosphatidylglycerol in the fetus.

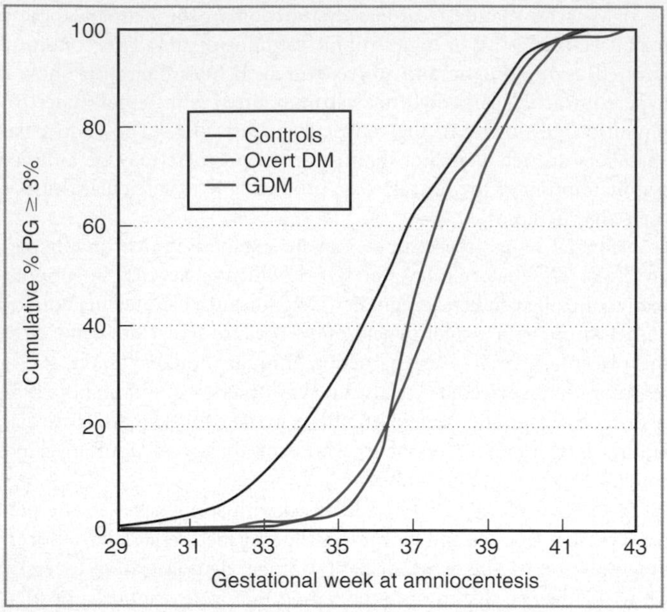

FIGURE 46-11 Delay in fetal pulmonary phosphatidyl glycerol. The delay in fetal pulmonary phosphatidyl glycerol was associated with a sustained peak in phosphatidyl inositol in diabetic pregnancy, suggesting that elevated maternal plasma levels of myoinositol in a diabetic woman may inhibit or delay the production of phosphatidyl glycerol in the fetus. DM, diabetes mellitus; GDM, gestational diabetes mellitus; PG, phosphatidyl glycerol. (From Moore TR: A comparison of amniotic fluid fetal pulmonary phospholipids in normal and diabetic pregnancy. Am J Obstet Gynecol 186:641, 2002.)

It is possible that poor neonatal respiratory performance in the IDM may have a histologic basis in addition to a biochemical cause. Kjos and coauthors[151] identified respiratory distress in 3.4% of infants delivered of diabetic women, but surfactant-deficient airway disease accounted for less than one third of cases, with transient tachypnea, hypertrophic cardiomyopathy, and pneumonia responsible for most.

The near-term infant of a mother with poorly controlled diabetes is more likely to have neonatal respiratory dysfunction than is the infant of a nondiabetic mother. The observations of Moore[163] indicate that the average nondiabetic fetus achieves pulmonary maturity at 34 to 35 weeks' gestation, with more than 99% of normal newborns having a mature phospholipid profile by 37 weeks. In diabetic pregnancy, however, it cannot be assumed that lung maturity exists until approximately 10 days after the nondiabetic time (38.5 gestational weeks). Any delivery contemplated before 38.5 weeks' gestation for other than the most urgent fetal and maternal indications should be preceded by documentation of pulmonary maturity by amniocentesis. The neonatal complications of the offspring of diabetic pregnancy is discussed further in Chapter 58.

Long-Term Risks for the Fetus of the Obese Mother

Although much has been written about the increased risk of the metabolic syndrome (i.e., obesity, hypertension, insulin resistance, and dyslipidemia) in infants born SGA, evidence points toward an increase in adolescent and adult obesity in infants born LGA or macrosomic. There has been abundant evidence linking higher birth weights to increased obesity of adolescents and adults for at least 25 years.[164] Large cohort studies such as the Nurses Health Study[165] and the Health Professional Follow-up Study[166] report a J-shaped curve (i.e., a slightly greater BMI among subjects born small but a much greater prevalence of overweight and obesity in those born large).[167] The increased prevalence of adolescent obesity is related to an increased risk of the metabolic syndrome. The increased incidence of obesity accounts for much of the 33% increase in type 2 diabetes, particularly among the young. Between 50% and 90% of adolescents with type 2 diabetes have a BMI greater than 27,[168] and 25% of obese children between 4 and 10 years old have impaired glucose tolerance.[169] The epidemic of obesity and subsequent risk for diabetes and components of the metabolic syndrome may begin in utero with fetal overgrowth and adiposity, rather than undergrowth.

A retrospective cohort study by Whitaker[170] enrolling more than 8400 children in the United States in the early 1990s reported that children who were born to obese mothers (based on BMI in the first trimester) were twice as likely to be obese when they were 2 years old. If a woman had a BMI of 30 or more in the first trimester, the prevalences of childhood obesity (BMI > 95th percentile based on criteria of the Centers for Disease Control and Prevention [CDC]) at ages 2, 3, and 4 years were 15.1%, 20.6%, and 24.1%, respectively. This was between 2.4 and 2.7 times the prevalence of obesity observed in children of mothers whose BMI values were in the normal range (18.5 to 24.9). This effect was only slightly modified by birth weight.

There is an independent effect of maternal pregravid weight and diabetes on birth weight and on the adolescent risk of obesity. Langer and colleagues[171] reported that in obese women with GDM whose glucose was well controlled on diet alone, the odds of fetal macrosomia (birth weight >4000 g) were significantly increased (OR = 2.12) compared with women with well-controlled (diet only) GDM and normal BMIs. Similar results were reported for women with GDM who were poorly controlled with diet or with insulin. In well-controlled, insulin-requiring women with GDM, there was no significant increased risk of macrosomia with increasing pregravid BMI. Dabelea and associates[172] reported that the mean adolescent BMI was 2.6 kg/m^2 greater in sibling offspring of diabetic pregnancies compared with the index siblings born when the mothers previously had normal glucose tolerance. Both maternal pregravid obesity and the presence of maternal diabetes may independently affect the risk of adolescent obesity in the offspring.

This risk of developing the metabolic syndrome in adolescents was addressed by Boney and colleagues[173] in longitudinal cohort study of AGA and LGA infants of women with normal glucose tolerance and GDM. The metabolic syndrome was defined as the presence of two or more of the following components: obesity, hypertension, glucose intolerance, and dyslipidemia. Maternal obesity was defined as a pregravid BMI higher than 27.3. Children who were LGA at birth had an increased hazard ratio (HR) for metabolic syndrome (HR = 2.19; CI, 1.25 to 3.82; $P = .01$) by age 11 years, as did children of obese women (HR = 1.81; CI, 1.03 to 3.19; $P = .04$). The presence of maternal GDM was not independently significant, but the risk for developing metabolic syndrome was significantly different between LGA and AGA offspring of GDM by age 11 years (RR = 3.6).

Childhood Neurologic Abnormalities

Several reports have suggested childhood neurodevelopmental abnormalities in offspring of diabetic mothers. Rizzo and colleagues[174] compared the offspring of 201 mothers with diabetes with 83 children of normal mothers and correlated subsequent childhood obesity in the offspring of diabetic mothers with internalizing behavior problems, somatic complaints, anxiety or depression, and social problems. Ornoy and associates[175] assessed IQ scores on the Wechsler Intelligence Scale for Children–Revised (WISC-R) and Bender tests of the children born to diabetic mothers. No differences were found between the study groups in various sensorimotor functions compared with controls, but the children of diabetic mothers performed less well than controls in fine and gross motor functions, and they scored lower on the Pollack taper test, which is designed to detect inattention and hyperactivity. These investigators also found a negative correlation between the severity of maternal hyperglycemia, as assessed by glycosylated hemoglobin levels in the third trimester, and performance on neurodevelopmental and behavioral tests.

Preconceptional Management of Women with Pregestational Diabetes

Although widely underused,[176] preconceptional care programs have consistently been associated with decreased morbidity and mortality.[177] Patients enrolled in preconceptional diabetes-management programs obtain earlier prenatal care and have lower Hb A_{1c} values in the first trimester.[178] A comparison of outcomes among women participating in a intensive preconceptional program with outcomes among women receiving standard care demonstrated lower perinatal mortality (0% versus 7%) and reduced congenital anomalies (2% versus 14%). When the preconceptional program was discontinued because of a lack of funds, the congenital anomaly rate increased by more than 50%.[7]

Risk Assessment

Several factors should be considered in preconceptional diabetes risk assessment (Table 46-9):

- Glycemic control should be assessed directly from glucose logs and by glycosylated hemoglobin levels.
- For patients who have had diabetes for 10 years or longer, an electrocardiogram, an echocardiogram, and microalbuminuria and serum creatinine studies should be performed.
- Because retinopathy can progress during pregnancy, the patient should establish a relationship with a qualified ophthalmologic provider. A baseline retinal evaluation should be completed within the year before conception, with laser photocoagulation performed if needed. Previous laser treatment is not a contraindication to pregnancy and may avoid significant hemorrhage during pregnancy.
- Thyroid function (i.e., thyroid-stimulating hormone and free thyroxine) should be evaluated and corrected as necessary in all patients with pregestational diabetes because of the frequent coincidence of autoimmune thyroid disease and diabetes.
- A daily prenatal vitamin that provides 1 mg of folic acid should be prescribed for a minimum of 3 months before conception, because folate supplementation significantly reduces the risk of congenital neural tube defects.
- The patient's occupational, financial, and personal situation should be reviewed, because job and family pressures can become barriers to achieving and maintaining excellent glycemic control. In patients with pre-pregnancy hypertension or proteinuria, particular emphasis should be given to defining support systems that permit extended bed rest in the third trimester, if it becomes necessary.
- The patient's preconception medications should be reviewed and altered to avoid teratogenicity and potential embryonic toxicity. Statins are pregnancy category X drugs and should be discontinued before conception. Angiotensin-converting enzyme (ACE) inhibitors and angiotensin receptor blockers (ARBs) should be discontinued before conception because of first trimester teratogenicity and fetal renal toxicity in the second half of pregnancy. Among oral antidiabetic agents used by reproductive-aged women, metformin and acarbose are classified as pregnancy category B drugs, although systematic data on safety are lacking. All other agents are category C drugs, and unless the potential risks and benefits of oral antidiabetic agents in the preconception period have been

TABLE 46-9 PRECONCEPTIONAL EVALUATION OF THE DIABETIC PATIENT

Procedure	Tests	Recommendations
Medical history, family history, review of symptoms	Selected patients: fasting and postprandial C-peptide determinations to clarify type of diabetes	Avoid pregnancy until Hb A_{1c} value is in the normal, nonpregnant range
Physical examination findings		
Hypertension	ECG, cardiac, renal evaluation	Antihypertensive medications
Retinopathy	Retinal evaluation	Ophthalmology consultation
Goiter	T_4, thyroid-stimulating hormones, antibodies	
Neuropathy		Vascular, podiatric evaluations
Obesity		Exercise, weight loss
Proteinuria	24-hr urine for protein, creatinine	Nephrology consultation if renal function abnormal
Diabetes assessment		
Glycemic control	Hb A_{1c} Home glucose monitoring Stable glycemic profile	
Nutrition		Dietitian consultation
Occupational and family life assessment		Help prepare patient for lifestyle commitments necessary for tight glycemic control

ECG, electrocardiogram; Hb, hemoglobin; T_4, thyroxine.

carefully weighed, they usually should be discontinued in pregnancy.

Metabolic Management

The goal of preconceptional metabolic management is to achieve an Hb A_{1c} level within the normal range before conception using a safe and reliable medication regimen that permits a smooth transition through the first trimester. The patient should be skilled in managing her glucose levels in a narrow range well before pregnancy begins, so that the inevitable insulin adjustments necessitated by the appetite, metabolic, and activity changes of early pregnancy can be accomplished smoothly.

A regimen of regular monitoring of preprandial and postprandial capillary glucose levels should be instituted. Although there are no data indicating that postprandial glucose monitoring is required before pregnancy to achieve adequate control, monitoring these levels increases the preconceptional woman's awareness of the interaction of dietary content and quality with postprandial glycemic excursions.[179] The insulin regimen should result in a smooth glucose profile throughout the day, with no hypoglycemic reactions between meals or at night.

Oral Hypoglycemic Agents

A longitudinal trial in the United Kingdom of intensified metabolic therapy in nonpregnant women with type 2 diabetes[180] demonstrated that oral agents were more effective than insulin in lowering Hb A_{1c} levels. This effect was attributed to improved compliance and fewer hypoglycemic reactions. For this and other reasons, most women with type 2 diabetes use one or more oral agents for glycemic control—typically metformin and a sulfonylurea or thiazolidinediones. Details of the mechanism of action and pharmacology of these oral hypoglycemic agents are discussed later. Despite the absence of evidence of teratogenicity for most of these compounds, none is recommended for use in pregnancy. Standard practice is to transition these patients to insulin management preconceptionally.

A possible exception is the use of metformin in infertile patients with polycystic ovary syndrome who are otherwise oligo-ovulatory. These patients have higher conception and lower miscarriage rates with metformin treatment.[181] Although two small series documenting the apparent safety of continuing metformin during pregnancy have been published,[182,183] discontinuing metformin after pregnancy is established is recommended.

Metformin readily crosses the placenta, exposing the fetus to concentrations approaching those in the maternal circulation. The sequelae of such exposure (i.e., effects on neonatal obesity and insulin resistance) remain unknown. A study of perfused human placental lobules from gestational diabetic and normoglycemic women demonstrated that metformin was readily transferred from the maternal to the fetal circulation.[184]

A more direct assessment of maternal and fetal pharmacodynamics was performed by Charles and coworkers[185] by obtaining maternal blood in the third trimester from metformin takers with gestational or type 2 diabetes. Cord blood also was obtained. Mean metformin concentrations in cord and maternal plasma were 0.81 and 1.2 mg/L, respectively. The maternal plasma half-life is 5.1 hours. Because these pharmacokinetics are similar to those in nonpregnant patients, no dosage adjustment is warranted.[185]

With regard to teratogenicity associated with metformin use in pregnancy, Gilbert and associates performed a meta-analysis of eight available studies. The malformation rate in the disease-matched control group was approximately 7.2%, statistically significantly higher than the rate found in the metformin group (1.7%). After adjustment for confounders, first-trimester metformin treatment was associated with a statistically significant 57% reduction in birth defects.[186]

In a study of women with type 2 diabetes mellitus, 93 of whom took metformin (61 in the first trimester and 32 throughout the pregnancy) and 121 of whom did not take metformin, there was no difference between the metformin and control groups in the rate of preeclampsia (13% versus 14%; $P = .84$), perinatal loss (3% versus 2%; $P = .65$), or neonatal morbidity, including rate of prematurity (23% versus 22%; $P = .7$), admission to the neonatal unit (40% versus 48%; $P = .27$), respiratory distress (9% versus 18%; $P = .07$), and neonatal hypoglycemia (20% versus 31%; $P = .08$).[187]

The concentrations of metformin in breast milk are generally low, and the mean infant exposure to metformin has been reported in the range of 0.28% to 1.08% of the weight-normalized maternal dose. No adverse effects on blood glucose of nursing infants have been reported.[188]

Antihypertensive Medications

Hypertension is a common comorbidity of diabetes and is found in 20% to 30% of women who have had diabetes for longer than 10 years. Although treatment of modest degrees of hypertension (<160 mm Hg systolic) during pregnancy has not been shown to be beneficial in improving perinatal outcome,[74] treatment in nonpregnant diabetic women is recommended when blood pressure is consistently higher than 130/80 mm Hg.[19] The U.K. Prospective Diabetes Study and the Hypertension Optimal Treatment trial demonstrated improved outcomes, especially in preventing stroke, in patients assigned to lower blood pressure targets. Patients frequently enter the preconceptional period taking one or more antihypertensive medications.[189] In preconceptional and pregnant patients with diabetes and chronic hypertension, blood pressure target goals of 110/65 to 129/79 mm Hg are recommended in the interest of long-term maternal health and minimizing impaired fetal growth.[19]

None of the commonly used antihypertensive medications (e.g., calcium channel blockers, β-blockers, methyldopa) is teratogenic. ACE inhibitors deserve special mention because in nonpregnant subjects with diabetic nephropathy, they have been shown to ameliorate proteinuria and delay progression to end-stage renal disease. These medications are therefore considered first-line agents for diabetic women with significant proteinuria.[180] Many women with type 1 diabetes present for consultation preconceptionally or even in early pregnancy while taking these medications. It is not clear whether these medications have teratogenic effects when used in the first trimester, but use in the second trimester and beyond can cause a marked reduction in fetal renal blood flow, resulting in oligohydramnios and even frank fetal renal failure.[190] These medications should not be used during pregnancy, especially after the first trimester. Similar concerns exist for other agents in this family (i.e., ARBs and angiotensin receptor antagonists).[191]

Diagnosing Diabetes

Overt Diabetes

Patients with type 1 diabetes are typically diagnosed during an episode of hyperglycemia, ketosis, and dehydration. Type 1 diabetes is rarely diagnosed during pregnancy. The diagnosis of type 2 diabetes cannot be accomplished during pregnancy because of the overlap with early-onset gestational diabetes. Although the finding of an elevated Hb A_{1c} level in early pregnancy may be suggestive, definitive diagnosis of type 2 diabetes must be made after pregnancy. The diagnostic criteria recommended by the ADA for diabetes are listed in Table 46-2.

Hyperglycemia not sufficient to meet the diagnostic criteria for diabetes is categorized as IFG or IGT, depending on whether it is identified through a fasting plasma glucose level or a 75-g, 2-hour OGTT[19]:

IFG: fasting plasma glucose level of 100 to 125 mg/dL (5.5 to 6.9 mmol/L)
IGT: 2-hour plasma glucose level of 140 to 199 mg/dL (7.8 to 11 mmol/L)

Patients with IFG or IGT before pregnancy should be considered at extremely high risk for developing GDM. GDM patients whose postpartum testing results in the diagnosis of IFG or IGT are at significant risk for the disease evolving into frank diabetes within 5 to 10 years.

Patients with IFG or IGT should be counseled regarding weight loss and provided instruction for increasing physical activity. Monitoring for the development of diabetes in those with prediabetes should be performed every 1 to 2 years. Screening for and appropriate treatment for other cardiovascular risk factors (e.g., tobacco use, hypertension, dyslipidemia) is important. There is insufficient evidence to support the use of drug therapy in women with IFG or IGT.

Gestational Diabetes

Risk Factor Screening

Risk factor assessment for GDM should be performed at the first prenatal visit. High-risk clinical characteristics include the following:

- Age older than 35 to 40 years
- Obesity (BMI > 30)
- History of GDM
- Delivery of a previous LGA infant
- Polycystic ovary syndrome
- A strong family history of diabetes

Patients with these risk factors should receive plasma glucose screening without delay. High-risk women not found to have GDM at the initial screening should be tested again between 24 and 28 weeks' gestation.

Previously, screening of all pregnant women for GDM was recommended, but the ADA[192] modified this recommendation such that screening can be omitted for low-risk women meeting all of the criteria listed in Table 46-10. This policy is based on the findings of Naylor and colleagues,[193] who reported that women with one or no risk factors had a 0.9% risk of GDM, whereas 4% to 7% of those with two to five risk factors were diagnosed with GDM, resulting in a sensitivity of approximately 80% with a false-positive rate of 13%.

One- or Two-Step Screening

The diagnosis of GDM is based on a positive OGTT result. Guidelines issued by the Fourth International Workshop-Conference on Gestational Diabetes Mellitus[194] and reaffirmed by the Fifth International Conference[195] and the American College of Obstetricians and Gynecologists (ACOG)[196] recommend the use of the Carpenter and Coustan diagnostic criteria for the 3-hour, 100-g glucose OGTT (Table 46-11). However, these expert bodies also acknowledge the alternative use of a single-step, 2-hour, 75-g glucose OGTT.

TABLE 46-10 LOW-RISK CRITERIA FOR GESTATIONAL DIABETES SCREENING

Age ≤25 years*
Weight normal before pregnancy
Member of an ethnic group with a low prevalence of diabetes (e.g., northern European whites)
No known diabetes in first-degree relatives
No history of abnormal glucose tolerance
No history of poor obstetric outcome

***All criteria must be met to omit screening for gestational diabetes mellitus.**

American Diabetes Association: Gestational diabetes mellitus: A position statement. Diabetes Care 27(Suppl 1):S88, 2004.

TABLE 46-11 THREE-HOUR 100-GRAM ORAL GLUCOSE TOLERANCE TEST FOR GESTATIONAL DIABETES

Test Prerequisites

1-hr, 50-g glucose challenge result ≥135 mg/dL
Overnight fast of 8-14 hr
Carbohydrate loading for 3 days, including ≥150 g of carbohydrate
Seated, not smoking during the test
Two or more values must be met or exceeded for a diagnosis of GDM

Assessment for Gestational Diabetes Mellitus	Plasma Glucose Level after a 100-g Glucose Load mg/dL (mmol/L)
Fasting	95 (5.3)
1 hr	180 (10.0)
2 hr	155 (8.6)
3 hr	140 (7.8)

ONE-STEP OPTION

The one-step, 75-g glucose, 2-hour OGTT, which is commonly used outside the United States, is no longer recommended because of its inferior detection rate of GDM. Mello and colleagues[197] compared the diagnostic efficiency of the 75-g, 2-hour OGTT with the 3-hour, 100 g-OGTT and found that the 2-hour test was less than one half as sensitive in diagnosing GDM (5% versus 12%).

The current one-step option involves direct administration of the 3-hour, 100-g glucose OGTT. Two or more values must be met or exceeded for the diagnosis of GDM. The critical cutoff values for the 3-hour OGTT are listed in Table 46-11. Direct, one-step administration of the 3-hour, 100-g OGTT test should be considered in women with prior GDM, especially those with additional risk factors such as obesity.

TWO-STEP OPTION

In the two-step approach, a screening glucose challenge test (GCT) is administered using 50 g of glucose in the fasting or nonfasting state.

TABLE 46-12 SENSITIVITY AND COST ASSOCIATED WITH UNIVERSAL AND SELECTIVE SCREENING WITH VARIOUS GLUCOSE CHALLENGE THRESHOLDS

	Threshold Value for 1-hr, 50-g Glucose Challenge	
Factor	**130 mg/dL**	**140 mg/dL**
Sensitivity (%)	100	79
Percent of population (%) requiring OGTT	22	13
	Threshold Value (mg/dL)	**Sensitivity (%)**
Universal	140	90
	130	100
Risk factors + age ≥25 yr	140	85
	130	95

OGTT, oral glucose tolerance test.
Adapted from Coustan DR, Nelson C, Carpenter MW, et al: Maternal age and screening for gestational diabetes: A population based study. Obstet Gynecol 73:557, 1989.

For those whose plasma glucose value obtained after 1 hour exceeds a critical threshold value, a 100-g, 3-hour OGTT is administered, using the diagnostic criteria listed in Table 46-11.

THRESHOLD VALUE FOR THE GLUCOSE CHALLENGE TEST

The sensitivity of the GDM testing regimen depends on the threshold value used for the 50-g GCT. Recommendations from the ADA[19] and ACOG[196] explain that using a threshold value of 140 mg/dL results in approximately 80% detection of GDM, whereas using a threshold of 130 mg/dL results in 90% detection. A potential disadvantage of using the lower value of 130 mg/dL is an approximate doubling in the number of OGTTs performed. The Canadian study,[193] based on receiver-operator curve analysis, calculated that diagnostic efficiency was optimized when a GCT threshold of 130 mg/dL was used for intermediate-risk women (i.e., two to four risk factors) and 128 mg/dL for higher-risk women. These issues are summarized in Table 46-12.

A threshold plasma glucose value of 130 mg/dL is recommended for use in practices with a significant proportion of higher-risk gravidas (e.g., multiracial, obese). This approach provides excellent test sensitivity for GDM (>90%) with acceptable cost. Definitive randomized trials regarding cost-effectiveness with respect to perinatal outcomes and neonatal costs have not yet been performed.[198]

MAXIMUM VALUE FOR THE GLUCOSE CHALLENGE TEST

The risk of GDM is approximately proportional to the result of the 1-hour GCT. Dooley and coworkers[199] found that among nonwhite women, the risk of GDM with a 1-hour glucose value of 200 mg/dL or more is greater than 90%. Bobrowski and colleagues[200] reported that all patients with a screening result above 216 mg/dL had a positive 3-hour OGTT result. Most experts omit the 3-hour OGTT for patients with GCT results of 200 mg/dL or greater and manage the patient as a gestational diabetic.

SINGLE ABNORMAL VALUE ON THE 3-HOUR ORAL GLUCOSE TOLERANCE TEST

A fasting plasma glucose level exceeding 126 mg/dL should be considered highly suspicious for diabetes in pregnant and nonpregnant patients. Individuals with fasting plasma glucose levels above 126 mg/dL should have another fasting test; if the result of the second test is high, GDM is confirmed.

Patients with a single abnormal OGTT value are at increased risk for infants with macrosomia and neonatal morbidity. Berkus and colleagues[201] followed 764 patients with GDM, stratified by the number of abnormal values on their OGTTs. Patients with one or more abnormal OGTT values had double the incidence of macrosomic infants (23% to 27% versus 13%; $P < .01$). When Langer and coworkers[202] compared perinatal outcomes in patients with a single abnormal OGTT value with normal women and with aggressively managed GDM patients, they found the incidence of macrosomia to be more than threefold higher in the single abnormal value group than in the normal (34% versus 9%) and GDM (34% versus 12%) groups. Neonatal morbidity was fivefold higher in the single abnormal OGTT value group (15%) compared with the control and GDM groups (3%).

McLaughlin and colleagues[203] reviewed the perinatal outcomes of 14,036 women who had normal 1-hour or 3-hour glucose levels using standard criteria (i.e., 1-hour GCT cutoff of 140 mg/dL and 3-hour OGTT [see Table 46-11]). Of these, 3% had a single elevated value on the 3-hour test. Comparing the single elevated value group to those with all normal values, higher rates of cesarean delivery, preeclampsia, chorioamnionitis, birth weights higher than 4000 g and 4500 g, and neonatal intensive care unit admission were recorded (adjusted OR = 1.6, 1.5, 1.5, 1.7, 2.2, and 1.5, respectively; $P < .03$).[203]

These results underscore the problems associated with the methods used to identify patients with GDM. The relationships among carbohydrate metabolism, macrosomia, and neonatal morbidity create a continuum that defies a single, clear-cut criterion for diagnosis in all populations. The recommended schemes identify at most 90% of pregnancies susceptible to hyperglycemia and fetal macrosomia. The astute clinician should approach women with several GDM risk factors and a single abnormal OGTT value with caution. When in doubt, a trial of capillary glucose testing may help to clarify the patient's metabolic status.

Other Tests for Gestational Diabetes

Several investigators have searched for a single, nonglucose blood test that can accurately predict the results of the OGTT. Because of the proportional relationship of glycated proteins and long-term plasma glucose concentrations, fructosamine and Hb A_{1c} screening have been evaluated. Roberts and colleagues[204] suggested that fructosamine screening for GDM could produce a sensitivity of 85% with a specificity of 95%. A positive relationship between fructosamine levels and macrosomia was demonstrated.[205,206] However, subsequent studies have reported significantly lower sensitivities.[207,208]

Inferior sensitivity and predictive values have been reported for glycohemoglobin measurements (i.e., Hb A_1 and Hb A_{1c}) by Shah and colleagues,[209] Baxi and associates,[210] and Artal and coworkers[211] (22%, 63%, and 74%, respectively). A study by Agarwal and associates[212] assessed the use of lower cutoffs for fructosamine and Hb A_{1c} to exclude subjects from further GDM screening and higher cutoffs for one-step diagnosis. The lower cutoffs achieved sensitivities of 90% and negative predictive values of more than 85%. However, the upper cutoff values did not achieve acceptable positive predictive values to be useful for diagnosing GDM. Thus the role of these tests would be to identify patients rather than to screen for GDM, but using them would impose

TABLE 46-13 PREVALENCE OF GESTATIONAL DIABETES IN VARIOUS NATIONAL AND ETHNIC GROUPS

Study	Population	Prevalence (%)
Harris et al, 1997	Native American (Cree)	8.3
Henry et al, 1993	Australian	7.8
	Vietnamese	4.3
Nahum et al, 1993	African American	7.5
	White	4.7
	Asian	4.2
Lopez-de la Pena et al, 1997	Mexican	6.9
Yalcin et al, 1996	Turkish	6.6
Rith-Najarian et al, 1996	Native American (Chippewa)	5.8
Fraser et al, 1994	Israeli	5.7
	Bedouin	2.4
Rizvi et al, 1992	Pakistani	3.5
Miselli et al, 1994	Italian	2.3
Serirat et al, 1992	Thai	2.2
Jang et al, 1995	Korean	2.2
Mazze et al, 1992	White, Minnesota	1.5

an additional step and cost on the diagnostic regimen. Although screening with glycosylated proteins could theoretically reduce the number of two-step diagnostic procedures, their lack of sensitivity in diagnosis and the additional time and cost have left these studies of limited use in screening for GDM.

Timing of Gestational Diabetes Screening

FIRST-TRIMESTER SCREENING

The timing of glucose tolerance testing during pregnancy is critical, because delayed diagnosis increases the duration of deranged maternal metabolism and accelerated fetal growth. However, because the prevalence of GDM increases with advancing gestation due to rising insulin resistance mediated by placental hormones, testing too early can overlook some patients who will develop disease later.

A surprising percentage of patients (6% to 20%) with GDM can be diagnosed in the first trimester. Most have significant risk factors for glucose intolerance. Moses and associates[213] assessed the prevalence of GDM in patients with various risk factors. GDM was identified in 6.7% overall, in 8.5% of women 30 years old or older, in 12.3% of women with a BMI of 30 or more, and in 11.6% of women with a family history of diabetes. A combination of risk factors predicted GDM in 61% of cases compared with 4.8% of those without risk factors. The additional effect of ethnicity on the prevalence of GDM is summarized in Table 46-13.

Risk factor assessment for GDM (i.e., maternal age, ethnicity, obstetric and family history, body habitus, prior GDM, prior IGT, prior macrosomic infant, or unexplained stillbirth) should be performed at the first prenatal visit of all pregnant women. Patients with any of these risk factors (Table 46-14) should undergo screening as soon as feasible, and if results are negative, tests should be repeated at 24 to 28 weeks' gestation.

THIRD-TRIMESTER SCREENING

Because the insulin resistance that causes hyperglycemia increases as the third trimester progresses, early testing may miss some patients who later become glucose-intolerant. Performing the test too late in

TABLE 46-14 RISK FACTORS FOR GESTATIONAL DIABETES

Patients with any of these factors should be screened for GDM at the first prenatal visit:

- Maternal age >25 yr
- Previous macrosomic infant
- Previous unexplained fetal demise
- Previous pregnancy with GDM
- Strong immediate family history of NIDDM or GDM
- Obesity (>90 kg)
- Fasting glucose >140 mg/dL (7.8 mM) or random glucose >200 mg/dL (11.1 mM)

GDM, gestational diabetes mellitus; NIDDM, non–insulin-dependent diabetes mellitus.

the third trimester limits the time in which metabolic intervention can take place. For this reason, it is recommended that glucose tolerance testing be performed in all patients at 24 to 28 weeks' gestation.[214]

Whether administered at 12 or 26 weeks, the GCT can be performed without regard to recent food intake (i.e., nonfasting state). Coustan and coworkers[215] have shown that tests performed in fasting subjects are more likely to yield falsely elevated results than are tests conducted between meals. This finding was confirmed by Sermer and colleagues.[216]

Metabolic Management of Women with Pregestational Diabetes

The primary goals of metabolic management (i.e., glycemic monitoring, dietary regulation, and insulin therapy) in diabetic pregnancy are to prevent or minimize the postnatal sequelae of diabetes—macrosomia, shoulder dystocia, birth injury, and postnatal metabolic instability—in the newborn. A secondary goal is to reduce the risk of pediatric and adult metabolic syndrome in the offspring. If this goal is to be achieved, glycemic control must be instituted early and aggressively.

Principles of Medical Nutritional Therapy

There is a surprising lack of well-controlled research on the optimal diet for lean or obese women with diabetes. Most recommendations regarding dietary therapy are based on common sense and experience. Because women with all types of diabetes experience inadequate insulin action after feeding, the goal of medical nutritional therapy is to avoid single, large meals containing foods with a high percentage of simple carbohydrates that release glucose rapidly from the maternal gut. Three major meals and three snacks are preferred, because this multiple-feeding regimen limits the amount of calories presented to the bloodstream during any given interval. The use of nonglycemic foods that release calories from the gut slowly also improves metabolic control. Examples include foods with complex carbohydrates and fiber, such as whole-grain breads and legumes. Carbohydrates should account for no more than 50% of the diet, with protein and fats equally accounting for the remainder.[19]

Medical nutritional therapy should be supervised by a trained professional—ideally, a registered dietitian. In many programs, dietary counseling is capably provided by a certified diabetes educator. In any case, formal dietary assessment and counseling should be provided at several points during the pregnancy to design a dietary prescription that can provide adequate quantity and distribution of calories and nutrients to meet the needs of the pregnancy and support achieving the plasma glucose targets that have been established. For obese women (BMI > 30 kg/m^2), a 30% to 33% calorie restriction (to 25 kcal/kg of actual weight per day or less) has been shown to reduce hyperglycemia and plasma triglycerides with no increase in ketonuria.

Moderate restriction of dietary carbohydrates to 35% to 40% of calories has been shown to decrease maternal glucose levels and improve maternal and fetal outcomes.[217] In a nonrandomized study, subjects with low-carbohydrate intake (<42%) frequently required the addition of insulin for glucose control (RR = 0.14; $P < .05$), had a significantly lower rate of macrosomia (RR = 0.22; $P < .04$), and had a lower rate of cesarean deliveries for cephalopelvic disproportion and macrosomia (RR = 0.15; $P < .04$).

Low-Glycemic Foods

Manipulation of the type of carbohydrate in the diet can provide additional benefits in glycemic control. Crapo and coauthors[218] compared the blood glucose excursions induced by the ingestion of 50 g of carbohydrate from dextrose, rice, potatoes, corn, and bread. They observed that the highest glucose response occurred with dextrose and potatoes, with much lower peaks occurring after intake of corn and rice. This led to the concept of classifying foods by their glycemic index related to their tendency to induce hyperglycemia. In general, low-glycemic foods, such as complex (rather than simple) carbohydrates and those with higher soluble fiber content, are associated with a more gradual release of glucose into the bloodstream.

Formal dietary consultation at periodic intervals during the pregnancy improves metabolic control. Timing and content of meals should be reviewed at each visit together with the patient's individual food preferences. In all pregnant women, the continuing fetal consumption of glucose from the maternal bloodstream results in a steady downward drift in maternal glucose levels unless feeding occurs. In patients taking insulin or oral hypoglycemics, prolonged periods (>4 hours) without food intake increase the risk of hypoglycemic episodes. In these patients, a rather rigid schedule of three meals plus snacks at mid-morning, mid-afternoon, and bedtime is often necessary to achieve smooth control. Because insulin resistance changes dynamically during pregnancy, the dietary prescription must be continually adjusted according to the patient's weight gain, insulin requirement, and pattern of exercise.

Avoiding Nocturnal Hypoglycemia

Unopposed intermediate-acting insulin action during the hours of sleep frequently results in severe nocturnal hypoglycemia at 3 to 4 AM in individuals with type 1 diabetes. Reducing the insulin dose to avoid this complication typically leads to unacceptably high glucose levels on rising at 6 to 7 AM, whereas adding a bedtime snack helps to moderate the effect of bedtime insulin and to sustain glucose levels during the night. The snack should contain a minimum of 25 g of complex carbohydrate and enough protein or fat to help prolong release from the gut during the hours of sleep.

Avoiding Ketosis

The issue of maternal ketosis and its potential effect on childhood mental performance is a source of continuing controversy. Churchill and associates[219] reported that ketonuria during pregnancy is associated with impairment of neuropsychological development of offspring. This report has resulted in admonitions to avoid caloric reduction in any pregnant woman. The methodology in Churchill and associates' study has been criticized, however, because the ketonuria data were obtained from many different hospitals by having a nurse obtain a single urine sample for ketone testing on the day of delivery.

Coetzee and colleagues[220] found morning ketonuria in 19% of women with insulin-independent diabetes on a 1000-calorie diet, 14% of those on a 1400- to 1800-calorie diet, and 7% of normal pregnant women on a free diet. There were no untoward neonatal events in infants of any of the ketonuric mothers. Rizzo and coworkers[174] studied 223 pregnant women with diabetes and their offspring and 35 with normal glucose tolerance and found no relationship between maternal hypoglycemia and intellectual function of the offspring.

There may be a difference between starvation ketosis and the ketosis that develops with poorly controlled diabetes. Ketonuria develops in 10% to 20% of normal pregnancies after an overnight fast and may protect the fetus from starvation in the nondiabetic mother. In the final analysis, significant maternal ketonemia resulting in maternal acidemia is probably unfavorable for the mother and fetus. The small degrees of ketosis occurring in many pregnant women, including those with diabetes, are unlikely to lead to measurable deficits in the newborn.

Principles of Glucose Monitoring

Glycohemoglobin

Measurements of glycosylated hemoglobin have proved to be a useful index of glycemic control over the long term (4 to 6 weeks), providing a numeric index of the patient's overall compliance.[221] Although assessing Hb A_{1c} levels every 4 to 6 weeks during pregnancy rarely alters management significantly, it can provide the patient with a score by which she can rate the success of her hourly efforts to keep her blood glucose levels within a narrow range. Glycohemoglobin levels are too crude to guide the adjustments to insulin.

Self-Monitoring of Blood Glucose

The availability of capillary glucose chemical test strips has revolutionized the management of diabetes, and they should be considered the standard of care for pregnancy monitoring. The discipline of measuring and recording blood glucose levels before and after meals has a positive effect on improving glycemic control.[222]

TIMING OF CAPILLARY GLUCOSE MONITORING

The frequency and timing of self-monitoring of blood glucose should be individualized (Table 46-15). However, because postprandial values have the strongest correlation with fetal growth, checking after meals is essential. The DIEP study reported that when postprandial glucose values averaged 120 mg/dL, approximately 20% of infants were macrosomic, whereas a modest 30% rise in postprandial glucose levels to a mean level of 160 mg/dL resulted in a 35% rate of macrosomia.[223] Similar results emphasizing postprandial blood glucose monitoring were reported by de Veciana and associates,[224] who randomized diabetic women to use of preprandial or postprandial blood glucose levels for dietary and insulin management. The women managed using postprandial levels had markedly better results than did those managed using preprandial levels. In the postprandial group, with the mean (± standard deviation) change in the glycosylated hemoglobin value greater (−3 ± 2.2% versus 0.6 ± 1.6%; $P < .001$), the birth weights were lower (3469 ± 668 g versus 3848 ± 434 g; $P = .01$), and the rates of

TABLE 46-15 TIMING OF HOME CAPILLARY GLUCOSE MONITORING

Capillary Glucose Assessment	Advantage	Disadvantage
Preprandial	Permits prospective adjustment of food intake, supplementation of preprandial insulin	Preprandial or fasting glucose levels correlate poorly with fetal morbidity. Significant postprandial hyperglycemia may go undetected.
Postprandial	Permits supplementation of insulin to reduce postprandial glucose overshoots; improved postprandial control correlates with improved fetal or neonatal outcome	Results are obtained after food intake.
Bedtime	Permits adjustment of calories at bedtime snack, adjustment of bedtime insulin	
3-4 AM	Enables detection of nocturnal hypoglycemia	Interrupts sleep, may increase stress

neonatal hypoglycemia (3% versus 21%; $P = .05$) and macrosomia (12% versus 42%; $P = .01$) were lower.

With these facts in mind, a typical glucose monitoring schedule involves capillary glucose checks on rising in the morning, 1 or 2 hours after breakfast, before and after lunch, before dinner, and at bedtime. For patients taking intermediate- or long-acting medication at bedtime, a capillary glucose level between 3 and 4 AM (the lowest glucose level of the day) two to three times per week is helpful in interpreting the glucose values in the morning.

The clinician should be aware of the specific type of capillary glucose reflectance meter being used by the patient, because plasma glucose values are 10% to 15% less than those measured in whole blood from the same sample. Most of the newer reflectance meters are calibrated for plasma glucose readings. The target glucose values used in management depend on the type of meter used.

TARGET CAPILLARY GLUCOSE LEVELS

Controversy exists about whether the target glucose levels to be maintained during diabetic pregnancy should be designed to limit macrosomia or to closely mimic nondiabetic pregnancy profiles. The Fifth International Workshop-Conference on Gestational Diabetes[195] recommends the following:

Fasting plasma glucose level of 90 to 99 mg/dL (5.0 to 5.5 mmol/L)

and

1-hour postprandial plasma glucose level less than 140 mg/dL (<7.8 mmol/L)

or

2-hour postprandial plasma glucose level less than 120 to 127 mg/dL (<6.7 to 7.1 mmol/L)

Only recently have data been reported that describe normal glucose variations during pregnancy in nondiabetic gravidas. The profiles described by Cousins and colleagues[225] (Fig. 46-12) are derived from highly controlled studies in which volunteer subjects were fed test meals with specific caloric content on a rigid schedule. Parretti and coworkers[226] profiled normal pregnant women twice monthly preprandially and postprandially during the third trimester. Testing was done with capillary glucose meters, and the women followed an ad libitum diet. The results of the 95th percentile of the plasma glucose excursions are shown in Figure 46-13. Fasting and premeal plasma glucose levels are usually below 80 mg/dL and often below 70 mg/dL. Peak postprandial plasma glucose values rarely exceed 110 mg/dL.

Yogev and colleagues[227] obtained continuous glucose information from nondiabetic pregnant women using a sensor that monitored

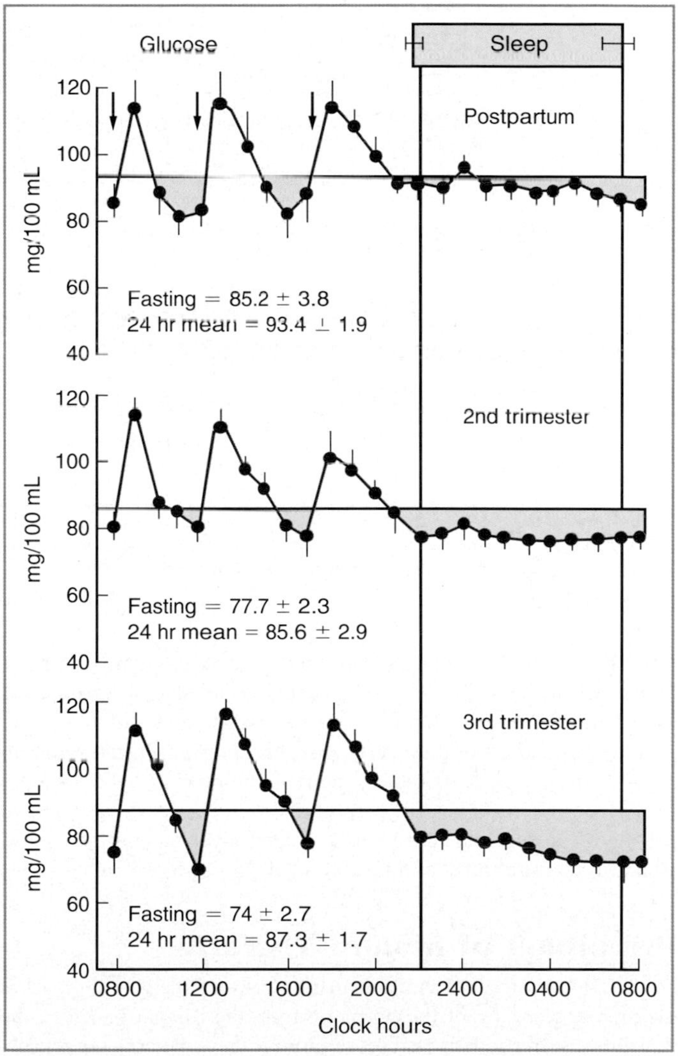

FIGURE 46-12 **Glucose variations during pregnancy.** Profile of blood glucose over 24 hours in the second and third trimesters of pregnancy, with postpartum observations used as a control. *Error bars* represent standard error. *Arrows* indicate time of test meal administration. (From Cousins L, Rigg L, Hollingsworth D, et al: The 24-hour excursion and diurnal rhythm of glucose, insulin and C peptide in normal pregnancy. Am J Obstet Gynecol 136:483, 1980.)

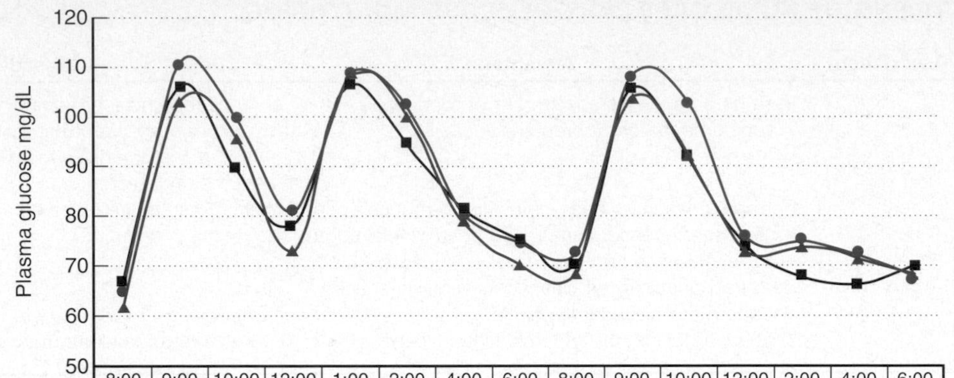

	8:00 AM	9:00 AM	10:00 AM	12:00 AM	1:00 PM	2:00 PM	4:00 PM	6:00 PM	8:00 PM	9:00 PM	10:00 PM	12:00 AM	2:00 AM	4:00 AM	6:00 AM
28 Weeks	67	106	89	78	106	95	81	75	70	106	91	74	68	66	70
32 Weeks	62	103	95	73	109	100	79	70	69	104	92	73	74	72	68
36 Weeks	65	111	99	81	108	102	80	75	73	108	103	76	75	73	68

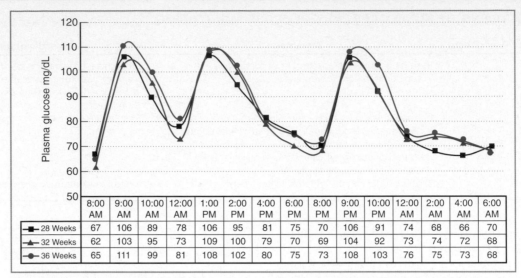

FIGURE 46-13 Diurnal plasma glucose profile in normoglycemic third-trimester gravidas. The numbers represent the 95th percentile values. (Adapted from Parretti E, Mecacci F, Papini M, et al: Third-trimester maternal glucose levels from diurnal profiles in nondiabetic pregnancies: Correlation with sonographic parameters of fetal growth. Diabetes Care 24:1317, 2001. Copyright © American Diabetes Association. Reprinted with permission from the American Diabetes Association.)

TABLE 46-16 AMBULATORY GLUCOSE VALUES IN PREGNANT WOMEN WITH NORMAL GLUCOSE TOLERANCE

Study	Subjects (*N*)	Fasting (mg/dL)	Postprandial Level at 60 min (mg/dL)	Postprandial Peak (mg/dL)
Parretti et al, 2001	51	69 (57-81)	108 (96-120)	
Yogev et al, 2004	57	75 (51-99)	105 (79-131)	110 (68-142)*

***The time of the peak postprandial glucose concentration was 70 minutes (range, 44 to 96).**
Adapted from Metzger BE, Buchanan TA, Coustan DR, et al: Summary and recommendations of the Fifth International Workshop-Conference on Gestational Diabetes Mellitus. Diabetes Care 30:S251-S260, 2007.

interstitial fluid glucose levels, and they found results similar to those of Parretti and coworkers.[226] The range of normal glucose levels occurring in nondiabetic pregnancy is summarized in Table 46-16.

In consideration of these facts, the target plasma glucose values to be used during pregnancy management of women with diabetes should range from 65 to 95 mg/dL preprandially and never exceed 130 to 140 mg/dL postprandially at 1 hour.[226] Superb glycemic control requires attention to preprandial and postprandial glucose levels.

Principles of Insulin Therapy

Despite the fact that no available insulin delivery method approaches the precise secretion of the hormone from the human pancreas, the judicious use of modern insulins can mimic these patterns remarkably well. The goal of exogenous insulin therapy during pregnancy must be to achieve diurnal glucose excursions similar to those of nondiabetic pregnant women. Given that in normal pregnant women, postprandial blood glucose excursions are maintained within a relatively narrow range (70 to 120 mg/dL), the task of reproducing this profile is daunting and requires meticulous daily attention by both patient and physician.

As pregnancy progresses, the increasing fetal demand for glucose results in lower fasting and between-meal blood glucose levels, increasing the risk of symptomatic hypoglycemia. Upward adjustment of short-acting insulins to control postprandial glucose surges within the target range only exacerbates the tendency to interprandial hypoglycemia. Any insulin regimen for pregnant women requires combinations and timing of insulin injections different from those that would be effective in the nonpregnant state. The regimens must be modified continually as the patient progresses from the first to the third trimester and as insulin resistance rises. The regimen should always be matched to the patient's unique physiology, work, rest, and food intake schedule.

Types of Insulin

The types of insulin frequently used in diabetes control are listed in Table 46-17. Several newer insulins are available for use, but most have not been extensively evaluated in pregnancy. They include the short-acting insulins lispro (Humalog) and aspart (Novolog) and the newer, very-long-acting, molecularly modified insulins detemir (Levemir) and glargine (Lantus). The activity profiles of the intermediate- and long-acting insulins are shown in Figure 46-14.[228]

Typical Insulin Regimens

Flexibility is important in dosing and adjusting insulin during pregnancy. Although most patients find it necessary to organize their mealtimes and physical activity around their insulin regimen, changing the timing of insulin injections and types of insulin is frequently necessary

TABLE 46-17 INSULIN PREPARATIONS AND PHARMACOKINETICS

Insulin Preparation	Time to Peak Action (hr)*	Total Duration of Action (hr)*	Comment
Insulin lispro (Humalog)	1	2	Onset within 10 min of injection; no need to delay meal onset after injection
Insulin aspart (Novolog)	1	2	Onset within 10 min of injection; no need to delay meal onset after injection
Regular insulin	2	4	Good coverage of individual meals if injected 20 min before eating; increased risk of postprandial hypoglycemia with unopposed action 2-3 hr after eating.
NPH insulin	4	8	Provides intermediate-acting control; give on rising and at bedtime; risk of 3 AM hypoglycemia
Insulin glargine (Lantus)	5	<24	Prolonged flat action profile; limited pregnancy experience; increased risk of nocturnal hypoglycemia or undertreatment during the day

***Times are approximate in typical pregnant women with diabetes.**

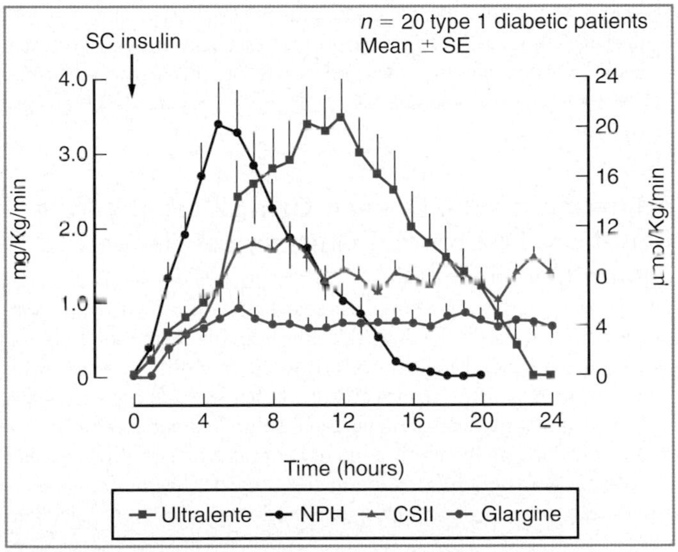

FIGURE 46-14 Activity profiles of intermediate- and long-acting insulins. The kinetics of NPH, Ultralente, glargine (Lantus), and continuous subcutaneous insulin infusion with lispro insulin are graphed. The curves show the glucose infusion rate necessary to maintain plasma glucose at 130 mg/dl. CSII, continuous subcutaneous insulin infusion; SC, subcutaneous; SE, standard error. (From Lepore M, Pampanelli S, Fanelli C, et al: Pharmacokinetics and pharmacodynamics of subcutaneous injection of long-acting human insulin analog glargine, NPH insulin, and Ultralente human insulin and continuous subcutaneous infusion of insulin lispro. Diabetes 49:2142, 2000. Copyright © American Diabetes Association. Reprinted with permission from the American Diabetes Association.)

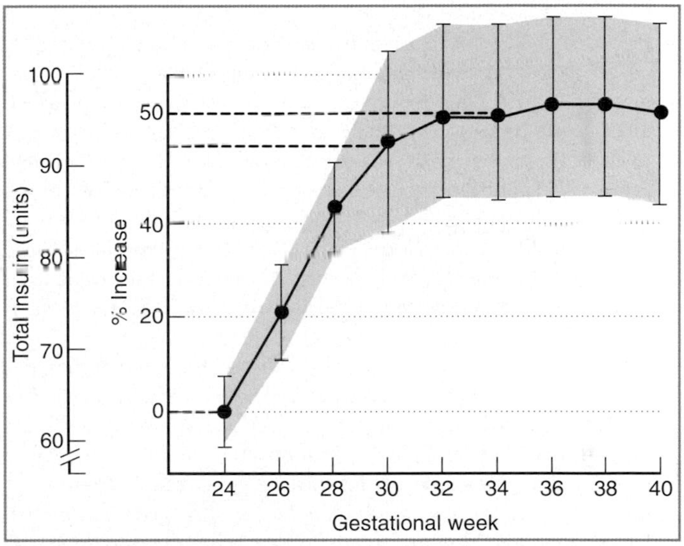

FIGURE 46-15 Progressive insulin requirements. The insulin requirements of women with gestational diabetes change throughout pregnancy. (From Langer O: Maternal glycemic criteria for insulin therapy in gestational diabetes mellitus. Diabetes Care 21(Suppl 2): B91, 1998.)

to match lifestyle and occupational needs and to optimize glycemic control. The following guidelines and examples can help in managing and adjusting insulin during pregnancy:

1. In the first trimester, reduce the insulin dose by 10% to 25% to avoid hypoglycemia. Reduced physical activity and caloric intake associated with the appetite changes and fatigue of early pregnancy lead to increased insulin effectiveness and interprandial hypoglycemia. It is typical to reduce insulin progressively from the 6th to the 14th week and then to begin restoring it as the insulin resistance mediated by rising placental hormones returns in the second trimester. Jovanovic and colleagues[108] reported from the DIEP study that a significant 18% increase in mean weekly dosage was observed between weeks 3 and 7 ($P < .0001$), followed by a significant 9% decline from week 7 through week 15 ($P < .0001$). In women with pregestational diabetes, continual downward adjustment in insulin is typically required from the first prenatal visit until approximately 14 to 16 weeks, after which requirements begin to rise steadily.
2. A typical total insulin dose is 0.7 units/kg in the first trimester, but this must be increased progressively with pregnancy duration from the second trimester onward. In women with type 1 diabetes, insulin increases are usually 20% to 30% over nonpregnant baseline by the end of pregnancy (Figure 46-15).[229] In insulin-resistant type 2 patients, 30% to 150% increases are not unusual. Insulin requirements normally plateau after 35 weeks' gestation and often drop significantly after 38 weeks.

3. The kinetics of NPH insulin are such that care must be taken to time peak action at 5 to 7 AM and avoid peaking at 4 AM, when maternal glucose levels are lowest. For many women, whose bedtime may be at 8 or 9 PM, NPH peaks early and exposes the mother and fetus to nocturnal hypoglycemia. It is often better to administer NPH at a set time between 10 and 11 PM, not the less accurate timing of "bedtime," to optimize needed insulin action during the hours of 5 to 7 AM.
4. A combination of short- and intermediate-acting insulins is employed to maintain glucose levels in an acceptable range. A typical regimen involves intermediate-acting insulin (NPH) before breakfast and at bedtime, with injections of regular or short-acting insulin before breakfast and before dinner. Two thirds of insulin is given in the morning and one third in the afternoon and at bedtime. For example, the regimen may be 20 units of NPH and 10 units of regular insulin in the morning, 8 units of regular insulin with dinner, and 8 units of NPH at 10 PM. The AM dose of NPH covers the periods before and after lunch. Avoid NPH injections at dinnertime because the peak occurs at 2 to 3 AM, creating symptomatic hypoglycemia.
5. Preprandial doses of regular insulin sufficient to keep 1-hour postprandial plasma glucose levels below 130 mg/dL may result in hypoglycemia 2 to 4 hours later (e.g., regular insulin before breakfast often causes hypoglycemia at 10 AM). When regular insulin is used to cover the major meals, snacks are essential in the late morning, the late afternoon, and before bedtime to avoid interprandial hypoglycemia. This interprandial hypoglycemia effect is intensified if the regular insulin injection is not given at least 20 to 30 minutes before the meal. This precaution is particularly relevant for hospitalized patients (because meals do not always arrive on schedule) and when taking meals in restaurants.
6. The short-acting insulins lispro or aspart are preferred during diabetic pregnancy. Lispro is manufactured by inverting a short amino acid sequence within the insulin molecule, resulting in a significantly faster onset of action. Lispro injections immediately before meals reduce the risk of hangover hypoglycemia because of the short duration of action. Using an in vitro perfusion model, Holcberg and colleagues[230] reported that lispro does not cross the human placenta. Compared with regular human insulin, the peak serum lispro concentration is three times higher, time to peak is 4.2 times faster, the absorption rate constant is double, and the duration of action is one half as long.[228] These kinetics allow the patient to inject insulin just before eating, rather than having to delay 20 to 30 minutes to allow regular insulin to begin its effect. Compared with regular insulin, lispro reduced postprandial hyperglycemia and decreased the rate of mild hypoglycemic episodes; it was also associated with lower predelivery Hb A_{1c} values and received higher patient satisfaction scores.[231] Similar findings have been reported when insulin aspart was compared with regular insulin.[232] In summary, lispro or aspart can be substituted 1 : 1 for regular insulin, and each is highly effective when given before meals in reducing postprandial glycemia while avoiding insulin hangover, which increases patient compliance. Short-acting insulins are effective when used in the insulin pump (discussed later).[233] With regard to safety and effectiveness, small studies have indicated equivalent perinatal outcomes.[234,235] Mathieson and coworkers[236] reported similar perinatal outcomes but improved maternal glycemic control in pregnant women randomized to aspart or regular insulin, demonstrating significantly lower mean postprandial plasma glucose levels with aspart (P = .003). A more detailed study of glucose dynamics after administration of aspart or regular insulin to women with gestational diabetes by Pettitt and associates[237] found that glucose areas under the curve were significantly lower with insulin aspart (180-min area, 7.1 $mg \cdot h \cdot dL^{-1}$; P = .018) but not with regular insulin (30.2 $mg \cdot h \cdot dL^{-1}$; P = .997) or with no insulin (29.4 $mg \cdot h \cdot dL^{-1}$), indicating the potential for improved glycemic control with short-acting insulins compared with regular insulin.
7. The use of insulin glargine during pregnancy is problematic because of its 20- to 26-hour duration. In three large comparative trials of nonpregnant subjects, glargine decreased glycosylated hemoglobin or fasting blood glucose levels, or both, to an extent similar to that seen with NPH insulin. A lower incidence of hypoglycemia, especially at night, was reported in most trials with insulin glargine compared with NPH insulin.[238] Experience is limited in pregnancy, but the few studies existing demonstrate satisfactory results.[239,240] Although the relatively flat activity profile of glargine is attractive, the dose must be regulated to keep basal insulin action during the night from causing hypoglycemia. During the day, when insulin resistance and insulin requirements are higher, the nocturnal basal rate is usually inadequate, and NPH must be added. As shown in Figure 46-14, the nocturnal low glucose level (typically at 4 AM) decreases as the third trimester progresses. Great care must be exercised in using glargine to avoid severe nocturnal hypoglycemia. Glargine appears to be safe for use during embryogenesis if glucose control is adequate.[241]

Adjusting Insulin Dosage Using Carbohydrate Counting, Preprandial Glucose Levels, and Insulin Corrections

Intermediate- and long-acting insulins should be adjusted no more frequently than weekly or biweekly to maintain preprandial plasma glucose levels in the target range (70 to 105 mg/dL). However, with short-acting insulins, glycemic control is better when the patient is able to vary, within a reasonable range, the insulin dose she uses to cover a meal, depending on its calorie content (or grams of carbohydrate) and the plasma glucose level existing at the time she begins eating. This often means varying short-acting insulin dosage with every injection.

CARBOHYDRATE COUNTING

Patients with pregestational diabetes are usually taught to count the grams of carbohydrate in their meals and adjust the short-acting insulin dosage accordingly. A typical meal containing 60 grams of carbohydrate may require 4 to 6 units of lispro (ratio of 1 unit of insulin to grams of carbohydrate of 1 : 15) in the nonpregnant individual. In the first trimester, a typical ratio is approximately 1 : 12. However, by the second trimester, more insulin is required (1 : 10 to 1 : 6), and in the third trimester, especially in patients with some degree of insulin resistance, ratios fall to 1 : 6 or even 1 : 2. The clinician should anticipate these increases in insulin as pregnancy progresses, because the patient often interprets these changes as errors or failure.

Carbohydrate counting has limits in accuracy (e.g., miscalculation of carbohydrate content, individual differences in glucose uptake dynamics), which may result in erratic control. During pregnancy, women who relatively strictly regiment their food quantity, content, and timing, so that carbohydrate calculations are within a reasonably narrow range, have better control.

PREPRANDIAL GLUCOSE LEVELS

Given the same calorie content of a meal, achieving target postprandial plasma glucose levels requires more insulin if the preprandial glucose level is higher. Allowing patients to add 2 units of lispro when the preprandial glucose level exceeds 120 mg/dL and to reduce lispro dosage by 2 units when the preprandial glucose level is below 80 mg/dL provides smoother control and avoids undesired postprandial glycemic excursions when the preprandial glucose is outside the target range.

INSULIN CORRECTIONS

Women with pregestational diabetes are frequently taught how to perform preprandial and postprandial insulin corrections. A typical regimen is to add 1 to 2 units of lispro for every 50 mg/dL that the glucose level is out of target range. A preprandial glucose level of 130 mg/dL would require 1 unit of lispro over the prescribed dose for that meal. As pregnancy progresses, corrections increase from 1 per 50 mg/dL to 1 per 20 mg/dL. However, the patient must be instructed not to take more than 4 to 6 correction units in a single bolus during pregnancy and instead retest glucose in 1 to 2 hours and apply an additional correction at that time.

Use of the Insulin Pump

Most of the principles described to enhance and smooth glycemic control by manipulating timing, quantity, and type of insulin can be used with greater facility with continuous, subcutaneous insulin infusion delivered by a programmable pump. These devices, which infuse insulin by means of a convenient catheter placed into the subcutaneous tissue near the abdomen, can be programmed to provide varying basal and bolus levels of insulin, which change smoothly even while the patient sleeps or exercises.

The effectiveness of continuous, subcutaneous insulin infusion in pregnancy is well established.[242-244] Hieronimus and colleagues[245] compared outcomes of 33 pregnant women managed with insulin pumps with 23 receiving multiple injections and reported similar Hb A_{1c} levels and rates of macrosomia and cesarean deliveries. Lapolla and coworkers[246] reported a small cohort of 25 women treated with insulin pumps in pregnancy compared with conventional insulin treatment ($n = 68$) and found no differences in glycemic control or perinatal outcome.

Use of continuous, subcutaneous, programmable insulin infusion has several advantages over conventional intermittent insulin administration, including the convenience of changing basal rates automatically when the patient is asleep or otherwise occupied and providing adjustable boluses discreetly from a pump worn under the clothing without the need for needles, syringes, and medication vials. Because pump malfunctions, precipitation of insulin inside the pump mechanism, abscess formation, and poor uptake from the infusion site can occur unexpectedly, successful insulin pump use requires a meticulous patient, a knowledgeable diabetologist or perinatologist, and prompt availability of emergency counseling and assistance on a 24-hour basis.[247]

A properly designed insulin pump infusion scheme allows convenient tailoring of the insulin administration profile to the patient's individual metabolic and lifestyle rhythms. A sample regimen is shown in Table 46-18. The lowest infusion rate of the day is between 11 PM and 4 AM, when it is set at about 70% of the mean rate needed during the day. The basal rate must be increased to 1.3 to 1.5 times the mean daily rate between 5 AM and 10 AM to provide extra insulin coverage for the high insulin-resistance period as the day begins (i.e., dawn effect). For the remainder of the day (10 AM to 11 PM), a steady mean infusion rate is usually sufficient. Insulin boluses, programmed to limit the postprandial excursion to 130 mg/dL or less at 1 hour, are given as often as needed. The enhanced ability for the patient to administer extra insulin doses without syringes and insulin vials is of great value in improving the smoothness of glycemic control.

Starting Insulin with Gestational Diabetes

Clinicians and patients are reluctant to start insulin in patients with gestational diabetes, but this intervention may be essential if macrosomia is to be reduced or avoided. Because the period of maximum fetal growth velocity (200 g/wk) and fat accretion occurs at approximately 33.5 weeks' gestation, delaying definitive therapy with repeated attempts to correct a suboptimal glucose profile with dietary adjustments may, by 33 to 34 weeks, have missed the time when glycemic intervention is most effective in modulating fetal growth. It is reasonable to allow a 1- to 2-week trial of dietary management before resorting to other measures, but waiting longer does not significantly increase the likelihood of good control. McFarland and colleagues[248] have shown that approximately 50% of patients achieve good glycemic control during the first 2 weeks of dietary therapy, but by the 4th week, only an additional 10% attain acceptable blood glucose levels.

The value of insulin administration in gestational diabetes was assessed by Crowther and associates,[249] who randomized 1000 women with gestational diabetes to insulin treatment or no medical therapy in the Australian Carbohydrate Intolerance Study in Pregnant Women (ACHOIS trial). Controls with normal OGTT results were included in the trial. In the insulin group, glucose levels were maintained at less than 99 mg/dL before meals and less than 126 mg/dL 2 hours postprandially. The rate of serious perinatal complications was significantly lower among the infants of 490 women in the intervention group than among the infants of 510 women in the routine-care group (1% versus 4%; RR adjusted for maternal age, race or ethnic group, and parity = 0.33; CI, 0.14 to 0.75; $P = .01$). The intervention group had a significantly higher rate of labor induction than the routine-care group (39% versus 29%), but the rates of cesarean delivery were similar. Cord plasma glucose levels were higher in women receiving routine care compared with controls, but it was normalized by treatment for mild GDM ($P = .01$). At 3 months after delivery, the

TABLE 46-18 TYPICAL SECOND-TRIMESTER CONTINUOUS ADMINISTRATION PROFILE USING A SUBCUTANEOUS INSULIN INFUSION PUMP

Time	Basal Rate	Bolus (U)	Comment
12 midnight	0.6 U/hr		Lower basal rate for sleep
5 AM	1.5 U/hr		Higher basal rate opposes the "dawn effect" of rising serum glucose from 4 to 6 AM
7 AM		8	Prebreakfast bolus
9 AM	1.0 U/hr		Lower basal rate to match increased physical activity, decreased insulin needs
12 noon		4	Prelunch bolus
6 PM		4	Predinner bolus
10 PM	0.6 U/hr		Lower basal rate for sleep

intervention group had lower rates of depression and higher quality-of-life scores.

With regard to newborn outcomes in the ACHOIS trial, umbilical cord serum insulin and insulin to glucose ratio were similar between the three groups, but leptin concentration, an indicator of fat mass, was lower in treated women with GDM compared with routine care ($P = .02$), suggesting that treatment of GDM using diet, blood glucose monitoring, and insulin, if necessary, influences the fetal adipoinsular axis, which may reduce the risk of childhood and adult obesity late in life.[250]

Jovanovic-Peterson and colleagues[251] reported a protocol in which GDM patients were treated with insulin if any fasting glucose level exceeded 90 mg/dL or postprandial glucose level exceeded 120 mg/dL. Over a period of 6 years, this protocol resulted in a decrease in the rate of macrosomic infants from 18% to 7% and a drop in the cesarean rate from 30% to 20%. Buchanan and associates[252] used ultrasound screening of fetal abdominal circumference in 303 diet-controlled GDM patients at 28 weeks to identify early macrosomia that might benefit from insulin treatment. When pregnancies with a fetal abdominal circumference above the 75th percentile were randomized to continued diet or twice-daily insulin therapy, birth weights and percentage of macrosomic infants were reduced in the insulin group (3647 ± 67 g versus 3878 ± 84 g; $P < .02$ and 13% versus 45%; $P < .02$). Neonatal obesity, as reflected by skinfold measurements at three sites ($P < .005$), also was lower.

The insulin regimen used in managing women with gestational diabetes should be designed to address the patient's individual glucose profile, because some women require insulin to prevent only fasting AM hyperglycemia and others only for postprandial excursions. Typically, one to several postprandial glucose levels become consistently above target as the patient's ability to compensate for rising insulin resistance becomes inadequate with diet alone. In such cases, giving short-acting insulin such as lispro or aspart (4 to 8 units to start) before meals is helpful. If more than 10 units of short-acting insulin is needed before the noon meal, adding a 6- to 8-unit dose of NPH before breakfast helps to achieve smoother control. If the fasting glucose levels rise above 90 to 95 mg/dL, 4 to 6 units of NPH insulin should be administered between 10 to 11 PM. The doses are scaled up as necessary, twice weekly or more often, to keep glucose levels within the target range.

Use of Oral Hypoglycemic Agents

Maintaining glucose levels within the target range requires meticulous attention to diet and physical activity. For many patients, injecting insulin frequently is impossible, and there are many initiatives to augment glucose control with oral agents, particularly in patients with insulin-resistant type 2 diabetes. An ideal treatment would reduce insulin resistance, improve insulin secretion or action, and delay the uptake of glucose from the gut. Current strategies are aimed at augmentation of insulin supply (i.e., sulfonylurea and insulin therapy), amelioration of insulin resistance (i.e., exercise, weight loss, and metformin and troglitazone therapy), and limitation of postprandial hyperglycemia (i.e., acarbose therapy).

Pharmacology and Safety

Sulfonylurea compounds, commonly prescribed in the past for patients with type 2 diabetes, have been considered contraindicated during pregnancy because of the high degree of transplacental penetration of most of these agents and the clinical reports of drug concentrations in the neonate higher than maternal levels associated with prolonged and severe neonatal hypoglycemia.[253] However, rigorously designed trials have not been performed to assess these agents during pregnancy. Reports of fetal anomalies have been largely anecdotal. An increased rate of congenital malformations, particularly ear anomalies, has been reported from a small case-control study.[254] When Towner and coworkers[255] evaluated the frequency of birth defects in fetuses of patients who took oral hypoglycemics during the periconceptional period, they found that the first-trimester glycohemoglobin level and duration of diabetes were strongly associated with fetal congenital anomalies but that use of oral hypoglycemic medications was not.

Interest in glyburide, a second-generation oral sulfonylurea available in the United States since 1984, has recently been rekindled. When glyburide was compared with first-generation sulfonylureas, it was equally effective, had a lower incidence of side effects, and reduced fasting blood glucose and glycohemoglobin levels, without the inconvenience of the additional training required to administer insulin. Because of its ability to enhance target tissue insulin sensitivity, glyburide has been shown to improve glycemic control in many type 2 diabetic patients who have previously failed therapy. As adjunctive therapy, glyburide can reduce the daily dosage for those who require large amounts of insulin.[256]

Glyburide

A unique characteristic of glyburide that allows its use in pregnancy is its minimal transport across the human placenta.[257] A study by Elliott and colleagues[258] evaluated glyburide transport in 10 term human placentas with the single-cotyledon placental model and found virtually no transfer of glyburide even at concentrations 100 times the typical therapeutic levels. This surprisingly low placental transfer may result from the very high plasma-protein binding of glyburide coupled with a short elimination half-life of 4 to 8 hours.[257,259]

Based on findings consistently showing minimal transfer of glyburide across the placenta, Langer and colleagues[260] designed a randomized trial to compare this oral agent with insulin in patients with gestational diabetes. They randomized 404 women with second- and third-trimester singleton pregnancies who had gestational diabetes requiring treatment to receive glyburide or insulin in an intensified treatment protocol. At the conclusion of the trial, there was no difference between the groups in mean maternal blood glucose, percentage of infants who were LGA (12% and 13%, respectively), birth weight at or above 4000 g (7% and 4%), or neonatal complications (pulmonary, 8% and 6%; hypoglycemia, 9% and 6%; admission to neonatal intensive care unit, 6% and 7%; fetal anomalies, 2% and 2%). Only 4% of the glyburide group required insulin therapy. Glyburide was not detected in the cord serum of any infant in the glyburide group. However, only 82% of the glyburide and 88% of the insulin-treated patients achieved the target level of glycemic control, representing a glyburide "failure rate" of 18%. With regard to glyburide dosing during the trial, 31% of patients were treated with 2.5 mg, 21% with 5 mg, 19% with 10 mg, 9% with 15 mg, and 20% with 20 mg. The mean glyburide dose was 9.2 mg. Of the maternal outcome variables assessed, none was significantly different between groups except the dramatic ($P = .03$) reduction in maternal hypoglycemic episodes in the glyburide-treated group (2%) compared with the 20% rate for insulin.

Beyond this single encouraging study, further nonrandomized experience with glyburide during pregnancy is accumulating.[261,262] Chmait and coworkers,[263] describing their experience with 69 patients with gestational diabetes managed on glyburide, reported that 19% of patients required adjunctive insulin therapy to keep glucose values in the target range. The adjunctive insulin rate was higher for women diagnosed earlier in pregnancy (20 versus 27 weeks; $P < .003$) and those whose average fasting glucose in the week before starting glyburide was higher (126 versus 101 mg/dL). No cases of neonatal hypoglycemia occurred in the glyburide group.

Langer and colleagues[264] reanalyzed the previously cited randomized, controlled trial, addressing the issues of glyburide dose, GDM severity, and pregnancy outcome and grouping trial participants into low (≤10 mg) and high (>10 mg) daily glyburide dose groups and low (≤95 mg/dL) or high (>95 mg/dL) GDM severity groups based on fasting OGTT values. The rates of macrosomia were 16% versus 5%, and the rates of infants who were LGA were 22% versus 8%, ($P = .01$), respectively, in the high-dose and low-dose glyburide groups. Stratification by disease severity (using the level of fasting glucose on glucose tolerance testing) revealed equally lower rates of LGA for the glyburide- and insulin-treated subjects in the low-severity group. In the higher-severity group, the rates of macrosomia and LGA were similar in the glyburide and insulin arms. The study authors suggested that achieving an excellent level of glycemic control, rather than the mode of pharmacologic therapy, is the key to improving outcomes in cases of GDM.

There is a growing acceptance of glyburide use as a primary therapy for GDM.[265] Although no new randomized trials have been completed, several retrospective series have been published comprising 504 glyburide-treated patients, and these studies have been summarized by Moore.[266]

Jacobson and coworkers[267] performed a retrospective cohort comparison of glyburide and insulin treatment of gestational diabetes. Patients with fasting plasma glucose levels greater than 140 mg/dL on glucose tolerance testing were excluded. The insulin group ($n = 268$) consisted of those diagnosed in 1999 through 2000, and the glyburide group ($n = 236$) was diagnosed in 2001 through 2002. Glyburide dosing was begun with 2.5 mg in the morning and increased by 2.5 to 5.0 mg weekly. If the dose exceeded 10 mg daily, twice-daily dosing was considered. If glycemic goals were not met on a maximum daily dose of 20 mg, patients were changed to insulin. The study size was insufficient to detect less than a doubling of the rate of macrosomia or LGA and a 44% increase in neonatal hypoglycemia, but there were no statistically significant differences in gestational age at delivery, mode of delivery, birth weight, LGA, or percent of macrosomic infants. The rate of preeclampsia doubled in the glyburide group (12% versus 6%; $P < .02$). Women in the glyburide group also had significantly lower post-treatment fasting and postprandial blood glucose levels. The glyburide group was superior in achieving target glycemic levels (86% versus 63%; $P < .001$). The failure rate (i.e., transfer to insulin) was 12%.

Conway and associates[268] reported a retrospective cohort of 75 glyburide-treated GDM patients. Good glycemic control was achieved by 84% of the subjects with glyburide, and 16% were switched to insulin. The rate of fetal macrosomia was similar between women successfully treated with glyburide and those who converted to insulin (11.1% versus 8.3%; $P = 1.0$), and the mean birth weight was also similar. A not significantly higher proportion of infants in the glyburide group required intravenous glucose infusions because of hypoglycemia (25.0% versus 12.7%; $P = .37$).

Small cohorts reported by Kremer and colleagues[269] and Chmait and coworkers[270] demonstrated glyburide failure requiring adjunctive or substitutive insulin rates in the range of 15% to 20%. In these studies, higher GCT results (>160 to 200 mg/dL) were predictive of an approximate 50% failure rate.[271]

The recommended glyburide dosing regimen, based largely on animal studies and a few human studies of nonpregnant subjects, is to administer the agent once daily, with twice-daily doses reserved for refractory cases. Later studies of glyburide pharmacodynamics suggest that the previously recommended dosing protocols may not be optimal in pregnancy. During development of the drug in the late 1960s, single-dose studies in nondiabetic subjects demonstrated glyburide absorption within 1 hour, peak levels at about 4 hours, and low but detectable levels at 24 hours. The decrease of glyburide in the serum yielded a terminal half-life of about 10 hours, and the glucose-lowering effect could be expected to persist for 24 hours after a single morning dose.

Later data have shown that glyburide peaks earlier in the serum and has a significantly shorter half-life than previously believed. These effects reflect the fact that glyburide has two major hydroxyl metabolites, both of which are biologically active and excreted equally in the bile and urine. Although advice in the *Physician's Desk Reference* indicates that the glyburide metabolites provide no significant contribution to glyburide's hypoglycemic action ($^1/_{400}$ and $^1/_{40}$, respectively, of glyburide's potency), these data were obtained in rabbits.

Yin and associates[272] studied the glucose and insulin responses to glyburide in a group of nonpregnant, nondiabetic subjects. After a 5-mg oral dose, serum glyburide levels peaked at 2.75 hours and had sustained levels with a half-life ranging from 2 to 4 hours, considerably shorter than the quoted half-life of 10 hours.

To clarify the potential difference in drug action when given as a single dose or chronically over weeks, Jaber and colleagues[273] studied glyburide pharmacodynamics during multiple-dose administration. A significant prolongation in the half-life (week 0 = 4.0 ± 1.9 hr; week 6 = 13.7 ± 10.5 hr; and week 12 = 12.1 ± 8.2 hr) was observed during chronic dosing. These results suggest possible drug accumulation or tissue sensitization by glyburide.

Yogev and coworkers[274] examined the prevalence of undiagnosed, asymptomatic hypoglycemic events in diabetic patients using a continuous glucose monitoring system for 72 consecutive hours. Hypoglycemia was defined as more than 30 consecutive minutes of a glucose value below 50 mg/dL. Asymptomatic hypoglycemic events were recorded in 63% of insulin-treated patients but in only 28% of glyburide-treated patients. The mean number of hypoglycemic episodes per day was significantly higher in insulin-treated patients (4.2 ± 2.1) than in glyburide-treated patients (2.1 ± 1.1; $P = .03$). In insulin-treated patients, most hypoglycemic events were nocturnal (84%), whereas in glyburide-treated patients, episodes occurred equally during the day and night, suggesting a potential benefit of glyburide over insulin therapy in clinical use.

Based on these data, glyburide should be taken at least 30 minutes—and preferably 60 minutes—before meals so that the peak action (2.5 hours after dosing) covers the postprandial glucose surge. Because of its extended duration of action, glyburide taken at 10 to 11 PM is effective in lowering fasting plasma glucose levels in the morning. Significant interprandial hypoglycemia can occur with glyburide, and patients should carry glucose tablets with them at all times as a precaution. The maximum dose is 20 mg per day, and no more than 7.5 mg should be taken at a single time.

Other Agents

Metformin is frequently employed in patients with polycystic ovary syndrome and type 2 diabetes to improve insulin resistance and fertility.[275] Although it has been documented that metformin therapy improves the success of ovulation induction[276] and probably reduces first-trimester pregnancy loss in women with polycystic ovary syndrome,[181] the effects of continuing metformin during pregnancy are not clear. Coetzee and Jackson[277] treated pregestational and gestational diabetics with metformin, but the treatment failed in 54% and 29%, respectively. The perinatal mortality rate among the metformin patients was 61 per 1000, and the rate of neonatal jaundice was increased. Hellmuth and colleagues[278] reported a series of women with gestational diabetes treated with metformin or tolbutamide before 1984. Women treated with metformin had a fourfold increase in preeclampsia and a higher perinatal mortality rate compared with those who were receiving tolbutamide. However, metformin-treated women were older, more obese, and treated later in pregnancy.

A cohort study of metformin in pregnancy reported by Hughes and associates[187] in 2006 included 93 women with metformin treatment (only 32 continued until delivery) and 121 controls. There was no difference in perinatal outcomes between the groups. Glueck and coworkers[183] compared nondiabetic women with polycystic ovary syndrome (n = 28) who conceived while taking metformin and continued the agent through delivery with matched women without metformin therapy (n = 39). Gestational diabetes developed in 31% of women who did not take metformin and in 3% of those who did (OR = 0.115; CI, 0.014 to 0.938).

Because of the beneficial effect of metformin on first-trimester miscarriage, many patients with polycystic ovary syndrome enter prenatal care taking this medication. Because metformin readily crosses the placenta,[184] greater experience with this agent is necessary before it can be recommended for use throughout pregnancy.[279] A large, properly powered, randomized, controlled trial is in progress to explore these issues.[280]

The α-glucosidase inhibitors, another class of oral agents, reversibly inhibit pancreatic amylase and α-glucosidase enzymes in the small intestine, delaying cleavage of complex sugars to monosaccharides and reducing the increase of blood glucose levels after a meal. Although these agents offer particular promise in pregnant women because of limited uptake from the gut, only a few studies of the drugs in pregnancy are available. Bertini and colleagues[281] compared insulin treatment (n = 27), glyburide (n = 24), and acarbose (n = 19) in gestational diabetes. No difference was observed in maternal glucose levels or in mean birth weight, although the rates of LGA fetuses were 3.7%, 25%, and 10.5% for the groups, respectively. Neonatal hypoglycemia was observed in eight newborns, six of whom were from the glyburide group. Glucose control was not achieved in five (20.8%) of the patients using glyburide and in eight (42.1%) of the patients using acarbose. Acarbose is given before meals, initially in a dose of 25 mg taken orally three times daily up to a maximum of 100 mg taken orally three times daily.

Pregnancy Management of the Diabetic Patient and Fetus

Fetal Surveillance

The goals of third-trimester management of diabetic pregnancy are to prevent stillbirth and asphyxia while optimizing the opportunity for a safe vaginal delivery. This involves monitoring fetal growth to determine the proper timing and route of delivery and testing for fetal well-being at frequent intervals.

A regimen for fetal surveillance throughout pregnancy is provided in Table 46-19. The goals are to

- Verify fetal viability in the first trimester
- Validate fetal structural integrity in the second trimester
- Monitor fetal growth during most of the third trimester
- Ensure fetal well-being in the late third trimester

TABLE 46-19 FETAL SURVEILLANCE IN TYPES I AND II DIABETIC PREGNANCIES

Time	Test
Preconception	Maternal glycemic control
8-10 wk	Sonographic crown-rump measurement
16 wk	Maternal serum α-fetoprotein level
20-22 wk	High-resolution sonography, fetal cardiac echography in women in suboptimal diabetic control (abnormal Hb A_{1c} value) at first prenatal visit
24 wk	Baseline sonographic growth assessment of the fetus
28 wk	Daily fetal movement counting by the mother
32 wk	Repeat sonography for fetal growth
34 wk	Biophysical testing: Two times weekly nonstress test or Weekly contraction stress test or Weekly biophysical profile
36 wk	Estimation of fetal weight by sonography
37-38.5 wk	Amniocentesis and delivery for patients in poor control (persistent daily hyperglycemia)
38.5-40 wk	Delivery without amniocentesis for patients in good control who have excellent dating criteria

A variety of fetal biophysical tests are available, including fetal heart rate testing, fetal movement counting, ultrasound biophysical scoring, and fetal Doppler studies. These tests, which are described in Chapter 21, are summarized in Table 46-20.

Testing should be initiated early enough to avoid the risk of stillbirth but not so early that a high rate of false-positive results is encountered. Because the risk of fetal death is roughly proportional to the degree of hyperglycemia, testing should begin as early as 28 weeks' gestation in patients with poor glycemic control or significant hypertension. In lower-risk patients, testing should begin at 34 to 36 weeks. Fetal movement counting should be performed in all pregnancies from 28 weeks onward. A fetal movement card for monitoring fetal movement is shown in Figure 46-16.

Timing and Route of Delivery

Assessing Fetal Size

Monitoring fetal growth and predicting birth weight continue to be challenging and highly inexact processes. The purpose of such monitoring is to identify the obese fetus and, if possible, avoid birth injury. Newborns weighing more than 4000 g are responsible for 42% to 74% of shoulder dystocias and 56% to 76% of all brachial plexus injuries, even though they account for only 6% of births.[282] To identify the highest-risk fetuses, use of third-trimester ultrasound has been proposed, including serial plotting of biometric parameters, using a cutoff value for estimated fetal weight and applying a cutoff to a specific parameter (e.g., abdominal circumference).[283]

Because the risk of birth injury is proportional to birth weight,[142] much effort has been focused on sonographic estimation of fetal weight (EFW). Several polynomial formulas using combinations of head, abdomen, and limb measurements have been developed.[284,285] Unfortunately, even small errors in measurements of the head, abdomen, and femur are multiplied together in such formulas, resulting in accuracies of no better than ± 15%. In the obese fetus, the inac-

TABLE 46-20 TESTS OF FETAL WELL-BEING

Test	Frequency	Reassuring Result	Comment
Fetal movement counting	Every night from 28 wk	10 movements in <60 min	Performed in all patients
Nonstress test	Twice weekly	2 heart-rate accelerations in 20 min	Begin at 28-34 wk with insulin-dependent diabetes; start at 36 wk in diet-controlled gestational diabetes
Contraction stress test	Weekly	No heart-rate decelerations in response to ≥3 contractions in 10 min	Same as for nonstress test
Ultrasound biophysical profile	Weekly	Score of 8 in 30 min	3 movements = 2 1 flexion = 2 30-sec breathing = 2 2-cm amniotic fluid = 2

FETAL MOVEMENT RECORD

Name: ______________________

Due Date: ______________________

Start Date	Number of weeks pregnant

INSTRUCTIONS

1. Count the baby's movements **EVERY NIGHT.**
2. A movement may be a kick, swish or roll. Do not count hiccups or small flutters.
3. You can start counting any time in the evening when the baby is active. **BUT: COUNT EVERY NIGHT.**
4. Count baby's movement while lying down, preferably on your left side.
5. Mark down the **time** you feel the baby move for the first time.
6. Mark down the **time** you feel the 10th fetal movement.
7. You should feel at least 10 fetal movements within one hour. Call Labor and Delivery **immediately** if
   a) you do not feel 10 movements with 1 hour;
   b) it takes longer and longer for your baby to move 10 times;
   c) you have not felt the baby move all day

DO NOT WAIT UNTIL TOMORROW.

Date	Time First Movement Felt	Time 10th Movement Felt	Total Time
EXAMPLE 11/4/91	6:50 p.m.	7:28 p.m.	38 minutes

FIGURE 46-16 Fetal movement card. The patient is instructed to note the time at which she begins monitoring fetal movements and then note the time at which the 10th movement is felt. If she has not recorded 10 movements in 1 hour, she is to call her physician.

curacies are further magnified. Perhaps this is why no single formula has proved adequate for identifying the macrosomic fetus.[286] In the study by Combs and colleagues,[287] an EFW of 4000 g had a sensitivity of 45% and a positive predictive value of 81%. To achieve 90% sensitivity would have required using an EFW cutoff of 3535 g, which would have included 46% of the population and produced a 42% false-positive rate.

In an attempt to improve detection of macrosomia, Hackmon and coworkers[288] performed a retrospective comparison of sonographic imaging results (i.e., EFW and amniotic fluid index [AFI]) for 50 newborns with severe macrosomia (birth weight ≥ 97th percentile) and 100 infants of normal weight. The mean middle-third-trimester AFI percentile and EFW percentiles for severe macrosomic infants were significantly higher than for controls ($P < .0001$). Significant correlations were detected for birth weight and the AFI and EFW percentiles (r = 0.44 and r = 0.72, respectively; $P < .0001$). The best predictors of macrosomia were an AFI equal to the 60th percentile or higher and an EFW equal to the 71st percentile or higher, with a positive predictive value of 85%. However, even this enhanced protocol had a high-false positive rate.

Considering the inaccuracy of weight prediction from a single set of sonographic measurements, serial analysis of parameters every 1.5 to 3 weeks is commonly used. However, trended serial EFW calculations compared with a single measurement appear to be no better than a single estimate performed near term. Predictions based on the average of serial EFWs, linear extrapolation from two estimates, or extrapolation by second-order equations fitted to four estimates were no better than the prediction from the last estimate before delivery.[289]

In view of the inadequate methods used to diagnose macrosomia antenatally, the widespread practice of estimating fetal weight using ultrasound near term in diabetic pregnancy must be questioned. Parry and colleagues[290] compared the cesarean rate for neonates falsely diagnosed on ultrasound as macrosomic (i.e., false positives) with the rate for those correctly diagnosed as nonmacrosomic (i.e., true negatives). They found that the cesarean rate was significantly higher among the false-positive macrosomics than among the true negatives (42.3% versus 24.3%; RR = 1.74; $P < .05$). Even with nonmacrosomic fetuses, the availability to the clinician of a sonographic estimate of fetal weight significantly increases the risk of cesarean delivery.

Predicting Shoulder Dystocia

Because of the asymmetrical adipose deposition around the fetal chest and trunk, deliveries of macrosomic infants from women with diabetes are at high risk for shoulder dystocia and injury. However, prediction of this risk is not possible with adequate precision to avoid excessive unnecessary interventions.[291]

In a subanalysis of the ACHOIS trial, Athukorala and associates[138] identified a linear increase in the risk of shoulder dystocia and the fasting glucose level on the glucose tolerance test, with an 18-mg/dL (1-mmol) increase in the fasting oral glucose tolerance test result leading to a relative risk of 2.09 (CI, 1.03 to 4.25). As reported by others, shoulder dystocia was 10-fold more common with operative vaginal delivery of GDM infants. However, there was no clear cutoff for the glucose tolerance test fasting value that was adequately predictive of shoulder dystocia.

In an effort to minimize the incidence of shoulder dystocia and associated birth injury associated with suspected macrosomia, a number of management schemes have been proposed. Weeks and colleagues[292] assessed the management of 500 pregnancies with suspected macrosomia and found a high bias toward cesarean section and failed induction. Patients with a sonographic EFW greater than 4200 g underwent induction more often (42.5% versus 26.6%), failed to achieve active labor more frequently (49% versus 16.5%), and underwent cesarean section more frequently (52% versus 30%), regardless of actual birth weight. Despite these changes in labor management, the incidence of shoulder dystocia in the predicted and nonpredicted groups was the same (11.8% and 11.7%, respectively).

There is no clinical method of reliably identifying the fetus likely to experience shoulder dystocia and injury during birth without an unacceptably high false-positive rate. Because 8% to 20% of fetuses from diabetic pregnancy weighing 4500 g or more will have shoulder dystocia, 15% to 30% of these will have recognizable brachial plexus injury, and 5% to 15% of these injuries will result in permanent deficit, approximately 443 to 489 cesarean sections would have to be performed for suspected macrosomia to prevent one case of permanent injury from shoulder dystocia.[293]

Delivery Timing

Timing of delivery should minimize neonatal morbidity and mortality while maximizing the likelihood of vaginal delivery. Delaying delivery to as near the estimated due date as possible increases cervical ripeness and improves the chances of vaginal birth. However, the risks of fetal macrosomia, birth injury, and fetal death increase as the due date approaches. Earlier delivery may reduce the risk of shoulder dystocia, but the increase in failed labor inductions and neonatal respiratory distress is appreciable.

Rayburn and colleagues[294] reported a case-control study of outcomes of women with GDM requiring insulin who delivered at 38 weeks compared with normoglycemic controls. The study group was more likely to have an unfavorable cervix, but cesarean rates were not different between the study and control groups (12.7% versus 11.7%; $P < .8$). Mean birth weights and the frequency of birth weights greater than 4000 g were not different between the groups, suggesting that delivery at 38 to 39 weeks does not compromise maternal and infant outcomes significantly.

When all these factors are considered, the optimal time for delivery of most diabetic pregnancies is between 38.5 and 40 weeks. Indications for delivery of the diabetic pregnancy are summarized in Table 46-21. Because of the apparent delay in fetal lung maturity in diabetic pregnancies, delivery before 38.5 weeks' gestation should be performed only for compelling maternal or fetal reasons.

It may be tempting to consider early delivery in a diabetic pregnancy with evolving macrosomia identified on ultrasonography. Because fetal growth between 37 and 40 weeks' gestation in a 90th-percentile fetus is approximately 100 to 150 g per week, inducing labor 2 weeks early may reduce the risk of shoulder dystocia in some cases. Kjos and coauthors[295] compared the outcomes associated with labor induction at 38 weeks with expectant management of women with gestational diabetes. They found that expectant management increased the gestational age at delivery by 1 week, but the cesarean delivery rate was not significantly different. Macrosomia was present in 23% of the expectantly managed group versus 10% in those induced at 38 weeks.

Fetal lung maturity should be verified in all patients delivered before 38.5 weeks by the presence of greater than 3% phosphatidylglycerol or the equivalent on an amniocentesis specimen (Table 46-22). If obstetric dating is suboptimal, amniocentesis should be performed.

TABLE 46-21 INDICATIONS FOR DELIVERY IN DIABETIC PREGNANCY

Type	Indications for Delivery
Fetal	Nonreactive, positive contraction stress test
	Reactive positive contraction stress test, mature fetus
	Sonographic evidence of fetal growth arrest
	Decline in fetal growth rate with decreased amniotic fluid
	40-41 weeks' gestation
Maternal	Severe preeclampsia
	Mild preeclampsia, mature fetus
	Markedly falling renal function (creatinine clearance <40 mL/min)
Obstetric	Preterm labor with failure of tocolysis
	Mature fetus, inducible cervix

TABLE 46-22 CONFIRMATION OF FETAL MATURITY BEFORE INDUCTION OF LABOR OR PLANNED CESAREAN DELIVERY IN DIABETIC PREGNANCIES

Phosphatidylglycerol >3% in amniotic fluid collected from vaginal pool or by amniocentesis
Completion of 38.5 weeks' gestation
Normal last menstrual period
First pelvic examination before 12 wk confirms dates
Sonogram before 24 wk confirms dates
Documentation of more than 18 wk of unamplified (fetoscope) fetal heart tones

After more than 40 weeks, the benefits of continued conservative management are less than the danger of fetal compromise. Induction of labor before 42 weeks in diabetic pregnancy—regardless of the readiness of the cervix—is prudent.

Labor or Cesarean

The ACOG[296] has recommended that primary cesarean delivery be discussed with diabetic gravidas with an EFW greater than 4500 g. This may reduce the risk of shoulder dystocia to some degree for an individual patient, but the effect on the larger obstetric population is less clear.

Gonen and associates[297] retrospectively assessed the impact of a policy of elective cesarean in cases with an EFW above 4500 g. During the 4 years of the study with more than 16,000 deliveries, macrosomia was correctly predicted in only 18% of cases. Of the 115 undiagnosed macrosomic cases, 13 infants were delivered by emergency cesarean, and 99 were delivered vaginally. Three infants (3%) with macrosomia and 14 infants (0.1%) without macrosomia sustained brachial plexus injury. The policy of preemptive cesarean for an EFW greater than 4500 g prevented at most a single case of brachial palsy.

Conway and Langer[298] performed a prospective trial enrolling diabetic women among whom those with an EFW of 4250 g or more underwent elective cesarean section. Ultrasonography correctly identified the presence or absence of macrosomia in 87% of patients. The cesarean section rate increased slightly after the protocol was initiated (22% versus 25%), but overall, shoulder dystocia was less common (2.4% versus 1.1%).

Herbst[299] conducted a cost-effectiveness analysis of "prophylactic" delivery (i.e., induction or cesarean) of the fetus with an EFW greater than 4500 g using risk and benefit rates estimated from the existing medical literature.[299] For an infant of a normoglycemic pregnancy weighing 4500 g or more, routine obstetric management was the least expensive ($4014 per injury-free child) compared with elective cesarean cost of $5212 and induction cost of $5165. However, a sensitivity analysis suggested that with a shoulder dystocia risk higher than 10% (as is the case with a fetus weighing more than 4500 g in a diabetic pregnancy), primary cesarean or early induction is somewhat more financially advantageous. The current recommendation that cesarean section be considered when fetal weight is suspected to exceed 4500 g appears to confer a modest improvement in neonatal outcome.

The decision to attempt vaginal delivery or perform a cesarean delivery is inevitably based on limited data. The patient's obstetric history, the best EFW, a fetal adipose profile (i.e., abdomen larger than head), and clinical pelvimetry should all be considered. Midpelvic operative deliveries should be avoided when macrosomia is suspected, and low pelvic or even outlet operative deliveries must be approached with extreme caution if labor is protracted. With an EFW greater than 4500 g, a prolonged second stage of labor or arrest of descent in the second stage is an indication for cesarean delivery.[296] Most large series of diabetic pregnancies report a cesarean section rate of 30% to 50%. The best means by which this rate can be lowered is by early and strict glycemic control in pregnancy. Conducting long labor inductions in patients with a large fetus and a marginal pelvis may increase, rather than lower, morbidity and costs.

TABLE 46-23 INTRAPARTUM MATERNAL GLYCEMIC CONTROL

Insulin Infusion Method

1. Withhold AM insulin injection.
2. Begin and continue glucose infusion (5% dextrose in water) at 100 mL/hr throughout labor.
3. Begin infusion of regular insulin at 0.5 U/hr.
4. Begin oxytocin as needed.
5. Monitor maternal glucose levels hourly using a capillary reflectance meter at bedside or laboratory determinations, or both.
6. Adjust insulin infusion.

Plasma/Capillary Glucose (mg/dL)	Infusion Rate (U/hr)
<80	Insulin off
80-100	0.5*
101-140	1.0
141-180	1.5
181-220	2.0*
>220	2.5*

Intermittent Subcutaneous Injection Method

1. Give one half of the usual insulin dose in AM.
2. Begin and continue glucose infusion (5% dextrose in water) at 100 mL/hr throughout labor.
3. Begin oxytocin as needed.
4. Monitor maternal glucose levels hourly using a capillary reflectance meter at bedside or laboratory determinations, or both.
5. Administer regular insulin in small doses (2 to 5 U) to maintain glucose levels of 80 to 120 mg/dL.

*Intravenous bolus of 2 to 5 units when the rate increases.

Intrapartum Glycemic Management

Perinatal asphyxia and neonatal hypoglycemia correlate with maternal hyperglycemia during labor.[300] Unfortunately, strict maternal euglycemia during labor does not guarantee newborn metabolic stability in infants with macrosomia and islet cell hypertrophy. The use of a combined insulin and glucose infusion during labor maintains the maternal plasma glucose level in a narrow range (80 to 110 mg/dL) and reduces the incidence of neonatal hypoglycemia.[301] A protocol for administration of a continuous insulin infusion in labor is outlined in Table 46-23. Typical infusion rates are 5% dextrose in Ringer's lactate at 100 mL per hour and lispro or aspart insulin at 0.5 to 1 units per hour. Capillary blood glucose is monitored hourly in these patients. For patients with diet-controlled GDM or mild type 2 diabetes, avoiding dextrose in all intravenous fluids during labor usually maintains excellent glucose control.

When cesarean section is planned in a woman with diabetes, the procedure should be performed early in the day to avoid prolonged periods of fasting. On the night before surgery, patients should be instructed to take their full dose of NPH or glyburide. No morning insulin or glyburide should be taken. A glucose-containing intravenous line should be established promptly on arrival at the hospital, with insulin given as intravenous boluses on a sliding scale as needed every 1 to 4 hours to maintain maternal plasma glucose in the range of 80 to 160 mg/dL.

Postpartum Metabolic Management

In the recovery room and after delivery, insulin can be given subcutaneously to women with type 2 diabetes using a sliding scale until a regular diet is established. The insulin doses required after delivery are typically 30% to 50% of the preprandial doses required during pregnancy just before delivery. Type 1 diabetes patients require more intensive glucose monitoring after delivery, because many experience a honeymoon phase, in which insulin requirements fall dramatically. The glucose-insulin intravenous infusion should be continued in type 1 diabetes patients, especially those who have had a cesarean delivery, until the diet has normalized.

Management of the Neonate

Neonatal Transitional Management

Unmonitored and uncorrected neonatal hypoglycemia can lead to neonatal seizures, brain damage, and death. The degree of hypoglycemia correlates roughly with the degree of maternal glycemic control during the 6 weeks before birth. Pancreatic hypertrophy and chronic fetal hyperinsulinemia—holdovers from the chronically glucose-rich intrauterine environment—can lead to significant hypoglycemia after the umbilical supply of nutrients is interrupted by delivery. IDMs also appear to have disorders of catecholamine and glucagon metabolism and have diminished capability to mount normal compensatory responses to hypoglycemia. The current recommendations specify frequent blood glucose checks and early oral feeding when possible (ideally from the breast), with infusion of intravenous glucose if oral measures prove insufficient.

Ordinarily, blood glucose levels can be controlled satisfactorily with an infusion of 10% glucose. If greater amounts of glucose are required, bolus administration of 5 mL/kg of 10% glucose is recommended, with gradually increasing concentrations of glucose administered every 30 to 60 minutes, if necessary.

Breastfeeding

Considering the number of perinatal complications experienced by many women with diabetes (e.g., preeclampsia, macrosomia-induced cesarean section, neonatal hypoglycemia), achieving a high rate of breastfeeding may seem to be a superfluous goal. However, mounting evidence indicates that breastfed infants have a much lower risk of developing diabetes than do those exposed to the proteins in cow's milk.[302,303] Pettitt and associates[304] found that children who were exclusively breastfed had significantly lower rates of non–insulin-dependent diabetes mellitus than did those who were exclusively bottle-fed in all age groups. The odds ratio for non–insulin-dependent diabetes mellitus in exclusively breastfed persons, compared with exclusively bottle-fed individuals, was 0.41 (CI, 0.18 to 0.93), adjusted for age, sex, birth date, parental diabetes, and birth weight. A study by Gimeno and de Souza[305] found that a shorter duration of exclusive breastfeeding was a risk factor for childhood diabetes (OR = 2.13, CI, 1.8 to 3.55) and that the introduction to cow's milk products before age 8 days was an important risk factor for the disease. Given the increased risk of diabetes in offspring of women with diabetes, these data underscore the importance of encouraging breastfeeding in all postpartum women with diabetes.

Most neonatologists maintain strict monitoring of glucose levels in newborn IDMs for at least 4 to 6 hours (frequently 24 hours), often necessitating admission to a newborn special care unit. This early separation of mother and neonate impedes breastfeeding and infant attachment, and it may delay the onset of lactogenesis in the diabetic mother. Neubauer and colleagues[306] observed that milk of women with insulin-dependent diabetes came in later than it did in controls and had significantly lower lactose and higher total nitrogen at 2 to 3 days after delivery. The infants of these diabetic mothers had significantly less milk intake 7 to 14 days after delivery than did those of the control women. Delayed lactogenesis in the women with insulin-dependent diabetes most likely occurred in those with poor metabolic control. A study by van Beusekom and coauthors[307] analyzed concentrations of micronutrients and macronutrients in milk and capillary blood and found that tight glycemic control was associated with normal proportions of milk nutrients, compared with the multitude of milk abnormalities seen with moderate and poor control.

Evidence indicates that with proper encouragement, sustained breastfeeding is possible for a significant proportion of patients with overt diabetes. Webster and coworkers[308] longitudinally compared breastfeeding habits between women with diabetes and normal women. At discharge, 63% of mothers with insulin-dependent diabetes and 78% of mothers without diabetes were breastfeeding. At 8 weeks, the proportions of each were nearly identical (58% and 56%, respectively), and when the infants were 3 months old, 47% of mothers with insulin-dependent diabetes and 33% of women without diabetes continued to breastfeed. The study showed that IDMs were delivered atraumatically, and infants who are well oxygenated with mature lungs and who have excellent antecedent glucose control can be kept with their mothers under close glycemic monitoring for the first 1 to 2 hours of life. This permits early breastfeeding, which may reduce the need for intravenous glucose therapy.

The actual techniques of infant nursing require some modification in women with overt diabetes, especially insulinopenic patients with type 1 diabetes. Increased maternal calorie and fluid intake is necessary to maintain milk supply in all women. The calorie expenditure during nursing and for the 30 to 45 minutes thereafter (probably during post-nursing lactogenesis) may precipitate severe hypoglycemia if compensatory calories are not ingested. This is especially common during nursing late at night. Breastfeeding women with type 1 diabetes should be encouraged to take in fluids and food (100 to 300 calories per feeding episode) while nursing to avoid reactive hypoglycemia.

Fortunately, studies of breastfeeding women with diabetes indicate that lactation, even for a short duration, has a beneficial effect on overall maternal glucose and lipid metabolism. For postpartum women who have GDM during their pregnancies, breastfeeding may offer a practical, low-cost intervention that helps to reduce or delay the risk of subsequent diabetes.

References

1. Wild S, Roglic G, Green A, et al: Global prevalence of diabetes. Estimates for the year 2000 and projections for 2030. Diabetes Care 27:1047-1053, 2004.

2. National Institute of Diabetes and Digestive and Kidney Diseases (NIDDK): Prevalence of Diabetes by Race/Ethnicity Among People Aged 20 Years or Older, United States, 2005. Available at http://diabetes.niddk.nih.gov/pubs/statistics/index.htm#age (accessed January 2008).
3. Ferrara A, Kahn HS, Quesenberry CP, et al: An Increase in the Incidence of Gestational Diabetes Mellitus: Northern California, 1991-2000. Obstet Gynecol 103:526-533, 2004.
4. Harris MI, Flegal KM, Cowie CC: Prevalence of diabetes, impaired fasting glucose and impaired glucose tolerance in US adults. Diabetes Care 21:518, 1998.
5. American Diabetes Association: ADA consensus statement: Type 2 diabetes in children and adolescents. Diabetes Care 12:381-389, 2000.
6. Yang JE, Cummings EA, O'Connell C, Jangaard K: Fetal and neonatal outcomes of diabetic pregnancies. Obstet Gynecol 108(Pt 1):644-650, 2006.
7. McElvy SS, Miodovnik M, Rosenn B, et al: A focused preconceptional and early pregnancy program in women with type 1 diabetes reduces perinatal mortality and malformation rates to general population levels. J Matern Fetal Med 9:14, 2000.
8. Wylie BR, Kong J, Kozak SE, et al: Normal perinatal mortality in type 1 diabetes mellitus in a series of 300 consecutive pregnancy outcomes. Am J Perinatol 19:169, 2002.
9. Macintosh MC, Fleming KM, Bailey JA, et al: Perinatal mortality and congenital anomalies in babies of women with type 1 or type 2 diabetes in England, Wales, and Northern Ireland: Population based study. BMJ 333:177, 2006.
10. Rudge MV, Calderon IM, Ramos MD, et al: Perinatal outcome of pregnancies complicated by diabetes and by maternal daily hyperglycemia not related to diabetes: A retrospective 10-year analysis. Gynecol Obstet Invest 50:108-112, 2000.
11. Kjos SL, Schaefer-Graf U, Sardesi S, et al: A randomized controlled trial using glycemic plus fetal ultrasound parameters versus glycemic parameters to determine insulin therapy in gestational diabetes with fasting hyperglycemia. Diabetes Care 24:1904-1910, 2001.
12. Expert Committee on the Diagnosis and Classification of Diabetes Mellitus: Report of the Expert Committee on the Diagnosis and Classification of Diabetes Mellitus. Diabetes Care 20:1183-1197, 1997.
13. Expert Committee on the Diagnosis and Classification of Diabetes Mellitus: Follow up Report on the diagnosis of diabetes mellitus. Diabetes Care 26:3160-3167, 2003.
14. Hare JW, White P: Gestational diabetes and the White classification. Diabetes Care 3:394, 1980.
15. American Diabetes Association: Clinical practice recommendations—2007: Diagnosis and classification of diabetes. Diabetes Care 30(Suppl 1): S42-S47, 1997.
16. Bergman RN, Phillips LS, Cobelli C: Physiologic evaluation of factors controlling glucose disposition in man. Measurement of insulin sensitivity and B-cell sensitivity from the response to intravenous glucose. J Clin Invest 68:1456-1467, 1981.
17. Bloomgarden ZT: Development of diabetes and insulin resistance. Diabetes Care 29:161-167, 2006.
18. Flegal KM, Carroll MD, Ogden Cl, Johnson LL: Prevalence and trends in obesity among U.S. Adults, 1999-2000. JAMA 288:1728-1732, 2002.
19. American Diabetes Association: Clinical practice recommendations 2007. Standards of Medical Care—2007. Diabetes Care 30(Suppl 1):S4-S41, 2007.
20. Proceedings of the Fourth International Workshop Conference on Gestational Diabetes Mellitus. Diabetes Care 21:B161-B167, 1998.
21. Mauricio D, de Leiva A: Autoimmune gestational diabetes mellitus: A distinct clinical entity. Diabetes Metab Res Rev 17:422-428, 2001.
22. Catalano PM, Tyzbir ED, Sims EAH: Incidence and significance of islet cell antibodies in women with previous gestational diabetes mellitus. Diabetes Care 13:478-482, 1990.
23. Saker PJ, Hattersley AT, Barrow B, et al: High prevalence of a missense mutation of the glucokinase gene in gestational diabetes due to a founder-effect in a local population. Diabetalogia 39:1125-1128, 1996.
24. Zaidi FK, Wareham NJ, McCarthy MI, et al: Homozygosity for a common polymorphism in the islet specific promoter of the glucokinase gene is associated with a reduced early insulin response to oral glucose in pregnant women. Diabet Med 14:228-234, 1997.
25. Hattersley AT, Beards F, Ballantyne E, et al: Mutations in the glucokinase gene of the fetus result in reduced birth weight. Nat Genet 19:268-270, 1998.
26. Hytten FE: Weight gain in pregnancy. In Hytten F, Chamberlain G (eds): Clinical Physiology in Obstetrics. Oxford, UK: Blackwell Scientific, 1991, pp 173-203.
27. Catalano PM, Tyzbir ED, Wolfe RR, et al: Longitudinal changes in basal hepatic glucose production and suppression during insulin infusion in normal pregnant women. Am J Obstet Gynecol 167:913-919, 1992.
28. Catalano PM, Huston L, Amini SB, Kalhan SC: Longitudinal changes in glucose metabolism during pregnancy in obese women with normal glucose tolerance and gestational diabetes. Am J Obstet Gynecol 180:903-916, 1999.
29. Matthews DR, Hosker JP, Rudenski AS, et al: Homeostasis model assessment: Insulin resistance and β cell function from fasting plasma glucose and insulin concentrations in man. Diabetes 28:412-419, 1985.
30. Matsuda M, DeFronzo R: Insulin sensitivity indices obtained from oral glucose tolerance testing. Diabetes Care 22:1462-1470, 1999.
31. Pacini G, Bergman RN: MINMOD: A computer program to calculate insulin sensitivity and pancreatic responsitivity from the frequently sampled intravenous glucose tolerance test. Comput Methods Programs Biomed 23:113-122, 1986.
32. DeFronzo RA, Tobin JD, Andres R: Glucose clamp technique: A method for quantifying insulin secretion and resistance. Am J Physiol 237:E214-E223, 1979.
33. Catalano PM, Tyzbir ED, Roman NM, et al: Longitudinal changes in insulin release and insulin resistance in non-obese pregnant women. Am J Obstet Gynecol 165:1667-1672, 1991.
34. Catalano PM, Tyzbir ED, Wolfe RR, et al: Carbohydrate metabolism during pregnancy in control subjects and women with gestational diabetes. Am J Physiol 264:E60-E67, 1993.
35. Catalano PM, Bernstein IM, Wolfe RR, et al: Subclinical abnormalities of glucose metabolism in former gestational diabetics subjects. Am J Obstet Gynecol 155:1255-1262, 1986.
36. Buchanan TA: Pancreatic β-cell defects in gestational diabetes: Implications for the pathogenesis and prevention of type 2 diabetes. J Clin Endocrinol Metab 86:989-993, 2001.
37. Schmitz O, Klebe J, Moller J, et al: In vivo insulin action in type 1 (insulin-dependent) diabetic pregnant women as assessed by the insulin clamp technique. J Clin Endocrinol Metab 61:877-81, 1985.
38. Ryan EA, O'Sullivan MJ, Skyler JS: Insulin action during pregnancy. Studies with the euglycemic clamp technique. Diabetes 34:380-389, 1985.
39. Ryan EA, Enns L: Role of gestational hormones in the induction of insulin resistance. J Clin Endocrinol Metab 67:341-347, 1988.
40. Kalkoff RK, Kissebah AH, Rim H-J: Carbohydrate and lipid metabolism during normal pregnancy: Relationship to gestational hormone action. In Merkatz IR, Adam PAJ (eds): The Diabetic Pregnancy: A Perinatal Perspective. New York, Grune & Stratton, 1979, pp 3-21.
41. Barbieri RL: Endocrine disorders in pregnancy. In Yan SSC, Jaffe RB, Barbier RL (eds): Reproductive Endocrinology, 4th ed. Philadelphia, WB Saunders, 1999.
42. Kirwan JP, Hauguel-de Mouzon S, Lepercq J, et al: TNFα is a predictor of insulin resistance in human pregnancy. Diabetes 51:2207-2213, 2002.
43. Xiang AH, Peters RH, Trigo E, et al: Multiple metabolic defects during late pregnancy in women at high risk for type 2 diabetes. Diabetes 48:848-854, 1999.
44. Friedman JE, Ishizuka T, Shao J, et al: Impaired glucose transport and insulin receptor tyrosine phosphorylation in skeletal muscle from obese women with gestational diabetes. Diabetes 49:1807-1814, 1999.
45. Aguirre V, Werner ED, Giraud J, et al: Phosphorylation of Ser307 in insulin receptor substrate-1 blocks interactions with the insulin receptor and inhibits insulin action. J Biol Chem 272:1531-1537, 2002.

46. Evers IM, de Valk HW, Visser GH: Risk of complications of pregnancy in women with type 1 diabetes: Nationwide prospective study in the Netherlands. BMJ 328:915, 2004.
47. Elman KD, Welch RA, Frank RN, et al: Diabetic retinopathy in pregnancy: A review. Obstet Gynecol 75:119, 1990.
48. Bhavsar AR: Diabetic retinopathy: The latest in current management. Retina 26:S71-S79, 2006.
49. Schocket LS, Grunwald JE, Tsang AF: The effect of pregnancy on retinal hemodynamics in diabetic versus nondiabetic mothers. Am J Ophthalmol 128:477, 1999.
50. Verier-Mine O, Chaturvedi N, Webb D, Fuller JH: Is pregnancy a risk factor for microvascular complications? The EURODIAB Prospective Complications Study. Diabet Med 22:1503-1509, 2005.
51. The Kroc Collaborative Study Group: Diabetic retinopathy after two years of intensified insulin treatment. Follow-up of the Kroc Collaborative Study. JAMA 260:37-41, 1988.
52. Temple RC, Aldridge VA, Sampson MJ, et al: Impact of pregnancy on the progression of diabetic retinopathy in type 1 diabetes. Diabet Med 18:573-577, 2001.
53. American Diabetes Association. Standards of medical care in diabetes. Diabetes Care 28(Suppl 1):S4-S36, 2005.
54. U.S. Renal Data System, USRDS 2006 Annual Data Report: Atlas of End-Stage Renal Disease in the United States. Bethesda, MD, National Institutes of Health, National Institute of Diabetes and Digestive and Kidney Diseases, 2006.
55. Eknoyan G, Hostetter T, Bakris GL, et al: Proteinuria and other markers of chronic kidney disease: A position statement of the National Kidney Foundation (NKF) and the National Institute of Diabetes and Digestive and Kidney Diseases (NIDDK). Am J Kidney Dis 42:617-622, 2003.
56. Reece EA, Winn HN, Hayslett JP, et al: Does pregnancy alter the rate of progression of diabetic nephropathy? Am J Perinatol 7:193, 1990.
57. Imbasciati E, Gregorini G, Cabiddu G, et al: Pregnancy in CKD stages 3 to 5: Fetal and maternal outcomes. Am J Kidney Dis 49:753-762, 2007.
58. Rossing K, Jacobsen P, Hommel E, et al: Pregnancy and progression of diabetic nephropathy. Diabetologia 45:36, 2002.
59. Jovanovic R, Jovanovic L: Obstetric management when normoglycemia is maintained in diabetic pregnant women with vascular compromise. Am J Obstet Gynecol 149:617, 1984.
60. Reece EA, Leguizamon G, Homko C: Pregnancy performance and outcomes associated with diabetic nephropathy. Am J Perinatol 15:413, 1998.
61. Purdy LP, Hantsch CE, Molitch ME, et al: Effect of pregnancy on renal function in patients with moderate-to-severe diabetic renal insufficiency. Diabetes Care 19:1067-1074, 1996.
62. Ekbom P, Damm P, Feldt-Rasmussen B, et al: Pregnancy outcome in type 1 diabetic women with microalbuminuria. Diabetes Care 24:1739, 2001.
63. Hou S: Historical perspective of pregnancy in chronic kidney disease. Adv Chronic Kidney Dis 14:116-118, 2007.
64. Reddy SS, Holley JL: Management of the pregnant chronic dialysis patient. Adv Chronic Kidney Dis 14:146-155, 2007.
65. Romao JE Jr, Luders C, Kahhale S, et al: Pregnancy in women on chronic dialysis: A single-center experience with 17 cases. Nephron 78:416, 1998.
66. Gomez Vazquez JA, Martinez Calva IE, Mendiola Fernandez R, et al: Pregnancy in end-stage renal disease patients and treatment with peritoneal dialysis: Report of two cases. Perit Dial Int 27:353-358, 2007.
67. Davison JM: Renal transplantation in pregnancy. Am J Kidney Dis 9:374, 1987.
68. Yassaee F, Moshiri F: Pregnancy outcome in kidney transplant patients. Urol J 4:14-17, 2007.
69. Kashanizadeh N, Nemati E, Sharifi-Bonab M, et al: Impact of pregnancy on the outcome of kidney transplantation. Transplant Proc 39:1136-1138, 2007.
70. Gabbe SG, Mestman JH, Freeman RK, et al: Management and outcome of diabetes mellitus. Am J Obstet Gynecol 127:465, 1977.
71. Gabbe SG, Mestman JH, Freeman RK, et al: Management and outcome of diabetes mellitus, classes B to R: Am J Obstet Gynecol 129:723, 1977.
72. Feig DS, Razzaq A, Sykora K, et al: Trends in deliveries, prenatal care, and obstetrical complications in women with pregestational diabetes: A population-based study in Ontario, Canada, 1996-2001. Diabetes Care 29:232-235, 2006.
73. Chobanian AV, Bakris GL, Black HR, et al: The seventh report of the Joint National Committee on Prevention, Detection, Evaluation, and Treatment of High Blood Pressure: The JNC 7 report. JAMA 289:2560-2572, 2003.
74. Sibai BM: Risk factors, pregnancy complications, and prevention of hypertensive disorders in women with pregravid diabetes mellitus. J Matern Fetal Med 9:62, 2000.
75. Leguizamon G, Reece EA: Effect of medical therapy on progressive nephropathy: Influence of pregnancy, diabetes and hypertension. J Matern Fetal Med 9:70-78, 2000.
76. Peterson CM, Jovanovic-Peterson L, Mills JL, et al: Changes in cholesterol, triglycerides, body weight, and blood pressure: The National Institute of Child Health and Human Development—the Diabetes in Early Pregnancy Study. Am J Obstet Gynecol 166:513, 1992.
77. Airaksinen KEJ, Ikaheimo MJ, Salmela PI, et al: Impaired cardiac adjustment to pregnancy in type 1 diabetes. Diabetes Care 9:376, 1986.
78. Silfen SL, Wapner RL, Gabbe SG: Maternal outcome in class H diabetes mellitus. Obstet Gynecol 56:749, 1980.
79. Gordon MC, Landon MB, Boyle J, et al: Coronary artery disease in insulin-dependent diabetes mellitus of pregnancy (class H): A review of the literature. Obstet Gynecol Surv 51:437, 1996.
80. Reece EA, Egan JFX, Coustan DR, et al: Coronary artery disease in diabetic pregnancies. Am J Obstet Gynecol 154:150, 1986.
81. Carroll MA, Yeomans ER: Diabetic ketoacidosis in pregnancy. Crit Care Med 33:S347-S353, 2005.
82. Cullen MT, Reece EA, Homko CJ, et al: The changing presentations of diabetic ketoacidosis during pregnancy. Am J Perinatol 13:449, 1996.
83. American College of Obstetricians and Gynecologists (ACOG): Clinical management guidelines for obstetrician-gynecologists. ACOG practice bulletin no. 60, March 2005. Pregestational diabetes mellitus. Obstet Gynecol 105:675-685, 2005.
84. Sutherland HW, Pritchard CW: Increased incidence of spontaneous abortion in pregnancies complicated by maternal diabetes mellitus. Am J Obstet Gynecol 155:135, 1986.
85. Miodovnik M, Lavin JP, Knowles HC, et al: Spontaneous abortion among insulin-dependent diabetic women. Am J Obstet Gynecol 150:372, 1984.
86. Jovanovic L, Knopp RH, Kim H, et al: Elevated pregnancy losses at high and low extremes of maternal glucose in early normal and diabetic pregnancy: Evidence for a protective adaptation in diabetes. Diabetes Care 28:1113-1117, 2005.
87. Platt MJ, Stanisstreet M, Casson IF, et al: St Vincent's declaration 10 years on: Outcomes of diabetic pregnancies. Diabet Med 19:216, 2002.
88. Reece EA, Sivan E, Francis G, et al: Pregnancy outcomes among women with and without diabetic microvascular disease (White's classes B to FR) versus non-diabetic controls. Am J Perinatol 15:549, 1998.
89. Miller E, Hare JW, Cloherty JP, et al: Elevated maternal hemoglobin A1c in early pregnancy and major congenital anomalies in infants of diabetic mothers. N Engl J Med 304:1331, 1981.
90. Lucas MJ, Leveno KJ, Williams ML, et al: Early pregnancy glycosylated hemoglobin, severity of diabetes, and fetal malformations. Am J Obstet Gynecol 161:426, 1989.
91. Eriksson UJ, Borg LA, Cederberg J, et al: Pathogenesis of diabetes-induced congenital malformations. Ups J Med Sci 105:53, 2000.
92. Warso MA, Lands WEM: Lipid peroxidation in relation to prostacyclin and thromboxane physiology and pathophysiology. Br Med Bull 39:277, 1983.
93. Pinter E, Reece EA, Leranth CZ, et al: Arachidonic acid prevents hyperglycemia-associated yolk sac damage and embryopathy. Am J Obstet Gynecol 155:691, 1986.
94. El-Bassiouni EA, Helmy MH, Abou Rawash N, et al: Embryopathy in experimental diabetic gestation: Assessment of oxidative stress and antioxidant defence. Br J Biomed Sci 62:71-76, 2005.

95. Cederberg J, Eriksson UJ: Antioxidative treatment of pregnant diabetic rats diminishes embryonic dysmorphogenesis. Birth Defects Res A Clin Mol Teratol 73:498-505, 2005.
96. Fuhrmann K, Reiher H, Semmler K, et al: Prevention of congenital malformations in infants of insulin-dependent diabetic mothers. Diabetes Care 6:219, 1983.
97. Cederberg J, Siman CM, Eriksson UJ: Combined treatment with vitamin E and vitamin C decreases oxidative stress and improves fetal outcome in experimental diabetic pregnancy. Pediatr Res 49:755, 2001.
98. Van Assche FA, Holemans K, Aerts L: Long-term consequences for offspring of diabetes during pregnancy. Br Med Bull 60:173, 2001.
99. Padmanabhan R, Shafiullah M: Intrauterine growth retardation in experimental diabetes: Possible role of the placenta. Arch Physiol Biochem 109:260, 2001.
100. Moulton CR: Age and chemical development in mammals. J Biol Chem 57:79-97, 1923.
101. Sparks JW: Human intrauterine growth and nutrient accretion. Semin Perinatol 8:74-93, 1984.
102. Girard J, Ferre P: Metabolic and hormonal changes around birth. In Jones CT (ed): Biochemical Development of the Fetus and Neonate. New York, Elsevier Biomedical Press, 1982, p 517.
103. Ogata ES, Sabbagha R, Metzger B, et al: Serial ultrasonography to assess evolving fetal macrosomia. Studies in 23 pregnant diabetic women. JAMA 243:2405-2408, 1980.
104. Kehl RJ, Krew MA, Thomas A, Catalano PM: Fetal growth and body composition in infants of women with diabetes mellitus. J Matern Fetal Med 5:273-280, 1996.
105. Reece EA, Winn HN, Smikle C, et al: Sonographic assessment of growth of the fetal head in diabetic pregnancies compared with normal gestations Am J Perinatol 7;18-22, 1990
106. Bernstein IM, Goran MI, Amini SB, Catalano PM: Differential growth of fetal tissues during the second half of pregnancy. Am J Obstet Gynecol 176:28-32, 1997.
107. Catalano PM, Thomas A, Huston-Presley L, Amini SB: Increased fetal adiposity: A very sensitive marker of abnormal in utero development. Am J Obstet Gynecol 189:1698-1704, 2003.
108. Jovanovic-Peterson L, Peterson CM, Reed GF, et al: Maternal postprandial glucose levels and infant birth weight: The diabetes in early pregnancy study. The National Institutes of Child Health and Human Development—Diabetes in Early Pregnancy study. Am J Obstet Gynecol 164:103-111, 1991.
109. Combs CA, Gunderson E, Kitzmiller J, et al: Relationship of fetal macrosomia to maternal postprandial glucose control during pregnancy. Diabetes Care 15:1251-1257, 1992.
110. Persson B, Hason U: Fetal size at birth in relation to quality of blood glucose control in pregnancies complicated by pregestational diabetes mellitus. BJOG 103:427-433, 1996.
111. Uvena-Celebrezze J, Fung C, Thomas AJ, et al: Relationship of neonatal body composition to maternal glucose control in women with gestational diabetes mellitus. J Matern Fetal Neonatal Med 12:396-401, 2002.
112. Pedersen J: The pregnant diabetic and her newborn. In Problems and Management, 2nd ed. Baltimore, MD, Williams & Wilkins, 1977.
113. Susa JB, Boylan JM, Sehgal P, Schwartz R: Impaired insulin secretion in the neonatal monkey after chronic hyperinsulinemia in utero. Proc Soc Exp Biol Med 194:209-215, 1990.
114. Schwartz R, Grupposo PA, Petzold K, et al: Hyperinsulinemia and macrosomia in the fetus of the diabetic mother. Diabetes Care 17:640-648, 1994.
115. Salvesen DR, Brudenell JM, Proudler AJ, et al: Fetal pancreatic beta-cell function in pregnancies complicated by maternal diabetes mellitus: Relationship to fetal academia and macrosomia. Am J Obstet Gynecol 168:1363-1369, 1993.
116. Krew MA, Kehl RJ, Thomas A, Catalano PM: Relationship of amniotic fluid C-peptide levels to neonatal body composition. Obstet Gynecol 84:96-100, 1994.
117. Carpenter MW, Canick JA, Hogan JW, et al: Amniotic fluid insulin at 14-20 weeks' gestation: Association with maternal glucose intolerance and birth macrosomia. Diabetes Care 24:1259-1263, 2001.
118. Ong K, Kratzsch J, Kiess W, et al: Size at birth and cord blood levels of insulin, insulin-like growth factors I (IGF-I), IGF-II, IGF-binding protein-1 (IGFBP-1), IGFBP-3 and the soluble IGF-II/mannose-6-phosphate receptor in term human infants. The ALSPAC Study Team. Avon Longitudinal Study of Pregnancy and Childhood. J Clin Endocrinol Metab 85:4266-4269, 2000.
119. Baker J, Liu JP, Robertson EJ, Efstratiadis A: Role of insulin-like growth factors in embryonic and postnatal growth. Cell 75:73-82, 1993.
120. Liu YJ, Tsushima T, Minei S, et al: Insulin-like growth factors (IGFs) and IGF-binding proteins (IGFBP-1, -2 and -3) in diabetic pregnancy: Relationship to macrosomia. Endocr J 43:221-231, 1996.
121. Delmis J, Drazancic A, Ivanisevic M, Suchanek E: Glucose, insulin HGH and IGF-I levels in maternal serum, amniotic fluid and umbilical venous serum: A comparison between late normal pregnancy and pregnancies complicated with diabetes and fetal growth retardation. J Perinat Med 20:47-56, 1992.
122. Lauszus FF, Klebe JG, Flyvbjerg A: Macrosomia associated with maternal serum insulin-like growth factor-I and -II in diabetic pregnancy. Obstet Gynecol 97:734-741, 2001.
123. Roth S, Abernathy MP, Lee WH, et al: Insulin-like growth factors I and II peptide and messenger RNA levels in macrosomic infants of diabetic pregnancies. J Soc Gynecol Invest 3:78-84, 1996.
124. Radaelli T, Uvena-Celebrezze J, Minium J, et al: Maternal interleukin-6: Marker of fetal growth and adiposity. J Soc Gynecol Invest 13:53-57, 2006.
125. World Health Organization (WHO): Obesity: Preventing and Managing a Global Epidemic. Technical support series no. 894. Geneva, World Health Organization, 2000, pp 1-4.
126. Vohr BR, McGarvey ST, Coll CG: Effects of maternal gestational diabetes and adiposity on neonatal adiposity and blood pressure. Diabetes Care 18:467-475, 1995.
127. Catalano PM, Ehrenberg HM: The short and long term implications of maternal obesity on the mother and her offspring. BJOG 113:1126-1133, 2006.
128. Freinkel N: The Banting Lecture, 1980: Of pregnancy and progeny. Diabetes 29:1023, 1980.
129. Duggleby SL, Jackson AA: Protein, amino acid and nitrogen metabolism during pregnancy: How might the mother meet the needs of her fetus? Curr Opin Clin Nutr Metab Care 5:503-509, 2002.
130. Butte NF, Hsu HW, Thotathuchery M, et al: Protein metabolism in insulin-treated gestational diabetes. Diabetes Care 22:806-811, 1999,
131. Metzger BE, Phelps RL, Freinkel N, Navickas IA: Effects of gestational diabetes on diurnal profiles of plasma glucose, lipids and individual amino acids. Diabetes Care 3:402-409, 1980.
132. Zimmer DM, Golichowski AM, Karn CA, et al: Glucose and amino acid turnover in untreated gestational diabetes. Diabetes Care 19:591-596, 1996.
133. Kalhan SC, Denne SC, Patel DM, et al: Leucine kinetics during a brief fast in diabetes in pregnancy. Metab Clin Exp 43:378-384, 1994.
134. Knopp RH, Humphrey J, Irvin S: Biphasic metabolic control of hypertriglyceridemia in pregnancy. Clin Res 25:161A, 1977.
135. Knopp RH, Chapman M, Bergelin RO, et al: Relationship of lipoprotein lipids to mild fasting hyperglycemia and diabetes in pregnancy. Diabetes Care 3:416-420, 1980.
136. Xiang AH, Peters RK, Trigo E, et al: Multiple metabolic defects during late pregnancy in women at high risk for type 2 diabetes. Diabetes 48:848-854, 1999.
137. Knopp RH, Magee MS, Walden CE, et al: Prediction of infant birth weight by GDM screening test. Importance of plasma triglyceride. Diabetes Care 15:1605-1613, 1992.
138. Kitajima M, Satoshi O, Yasuhi I, et al: Maternal serum triglyceride at 24-32 weeks' gestation and newborn weight in nondiabetic women with positive diabetic screens. Obstet Gynecol 97:776-789, 2001.

139. Gilbert WM, Nesbitt TS, Danielsen B: Associated factors in 1611 cases of brachial plexus injury. Obstet Gynecol 93:536, 1999.
140. Athukorala C, Crowther CA, Willson K: Women with gestational diabetes mellitus in the ACHOIS trial: Risk factors for shoulder dystocia. Aust N Z J Obstet Gynaecol 47:37-41, 2007.
141. Langer O, Berkus MD, Huff RW, et al: Shoulder dystocia: Should the fetus weighing greater than or equal to 4000 grams be delivered by cesarean section? Am J Obstet Gynecol 165:831, 1991.
142. Nesbitt TS, Gilbert WM, Herrchen B: Shoulder dystocia and associated risk factors with macrosomic infants born in California. Am J Obstet Gynecol 179:476, 1998.
143. Sandmire HF, O'Halloin TJ: Shoulder dystocia: Its incidence and associated risk factors. Int J Gynaecol Obstet 26:65, 1988.
144. Widness JA, Teramo KA, Clemons GK, et al: Direct relationship of antepartum glucose control and fetal erythropoietin in human type 1 (insulin dependent) diabetic pregnancy. Diabetologia 33:378, 1990.
145. Alam M, Raza SJ, Sherali AR, Akhtar AS: Neonatal complications in infants born to diabetic mothers. J Coll Physicians Surg Pak 16:212-215, 2006.
146. Banerjee S, Ghosh US, Banerjee D: Effect of tight glycaemic control on fetal complications in diabetic pregnancies. J Assoc Physicians India 52:109-113, 2004.
147. Taylor R, Lee C, Kyne-Grzebalski D, et al: Clinical outcomes of pregnancy in women with type 1 diabetes (1). Obstet Gynecol 99:537, 2002.
148. Cordero L, Treuer SH, Landon MB, et al: Management of infants of diabetic mothers. Arch Pediatr Adolesc Med 152:249, 1998.
149. Halliday HL: Hypertrophic cardiomyopathy in infants of poorly-controlled diabetic mothers. Arch Dis Child 56:258, 1981.
150. Mace S, Hirschfeld SS, Riggs T, et al: Echocardiographic abnormalities in infants of diabetic mothers. J Pediatr 95:1013, 1979.
151. Kjos SL, Walther FJ, Montoro M, et al: Prevalence and etiology of respiratory distress in infants of diabetic mothers: Predictive value of fetal lung maturation tests. Am J Obstet Gynecol 163:898, 1990.
152. Jaeggi ET, Fouron JC, Proulx F: Fetal cardiac performance in uncomplicated and well-controlled maternal type I diabetes. Ultrasound Obstet Gynecol 17:311, 2001.
153. Hayati AR, Cheah FC, Tan AE, Tan GC: Insulin-like growth factor-1 receptor expression in the placentae of diabetic and normal pregnancies. Early Hum Dev 83:41-46, 2007.
154. Halse KG, Lindegaard ML, Goetze JP, et al: Increased plasma pro-B-type natriuretic peptide in infants of women with type 1 diabetes. Clin Chem 51:2296-2302, 2005.
155. Cooper MJ, Enderlein MA, Dyson DC, et al: Fetal echocardiography: Retrospective review of clinical experience and an evaluation of indications. Obstet Gynecol 86:577, 1995.
156. Frantz ID, Epstein MF: Fetal lung development in pregnancies complicated by diabetes. Semin Perinatol 2:347-352, 1978.
157. Robert MF, Neff RK, Hubbell JP, et al: Association between maternal diabetes and the respiratory distress syndrome. N Engl J Med 12:357, 1976.
158. Kulovich MV, Gluck L: The lung profile. II. Complicated pregnancy. Am J Obstet Gynecol 135:64, 1979.
159. Tabsh KM, Brinkman CR III, Bashore RA: Lecithin: sphingomyelin ratio in pregnancies complicated by insulin-dependent diabetes mellitus. Obstet Gynecol 59:353, 1982.
160. Ojomo EO, Coustan DR: Absence of evidence of pulmonary maturity at amniocentesis in term infants of diabetic mothers. Am J Obstet Gynecol 163:954, 1990.
161. Tyden O, Berne C, Eriksson UJ, et al: Fetal maturation in strictly controlled diabetic pregnancy. Diabetes Res 1:131, 1984.
162. Landon MB, Gabbe SG, Piana R, et al: Neonatal morbidity in pregnancy complicated by diabetes mellitus: Predictive value of maternal glycemic profiles. Am J Obstet Gynecol 156:1089, 1987.
163. Moore TR: A comparison of amniotic fluid fetal pulmonary phospholipids in normal and diabetic pregnancy. Am J Obstet Gynecol 186:641, 2002.
164. Garn SM, Clark DC: Trends in fatness and the origins of obesity. Pediatrics 57:443-456, 1976.
165. Curhan GC, Cherton GM, Willet WC, et al: Birth weight and adult hypertension and obesity in women. Circulation 94:1310-1315, 1996.
166. Curhan GC, Willett WC, Rimm EB, et al: Birth weight and adult hypertension, diabetes mellitus and obesity in U.S. men. Circulation 94:3246-3250, 1996.
167. Martorell R, Stein AD, Schroeder DG: Early nutrition and adiposity. J Nutr 131:8745-8805, 2001.
168. Mokdad AH, Ford ES, Bowman BA, et al: Diabetes trends in the U.S. 1990-1998. Diabetes Care 23:1278-1283, 2000.
169. Sinha R, Fisch G, Teague B, et al: Prevalence of impaired glucose tolerance among children and adolescents with marked obesity. N Engl J Med 346:802-810, 2002.
170. Whitaker RC: Predicting preschooler obesity at birth: The role of maternal obesity in early pregnancy. Pediatrics 114:29-36, 2004.
171. Langer O, Yogev Y, Xenakis EMJ, Brustman L: Overweight and obese in gestational diabetes: The impact on pregnancy outcome. Am J Obstet Gynecol 192:1368-1376, 2005.
172. Dabelea D, Hanson RL, Lindsay RS, et al: Intrauterine exposure to diabetes conveys risks for type 2 diabetes and obesity: A study of discordant sibships. Diabetes 49:2208-2211, 2000.
173. Boney CM, Verma A, Tucker R, Vohr BR: Metabolic syndrome in childhood: Association with birth weight, maternal obesity and gestational diabetes mellitus. Pediatrics 115:290-296, 2005.
174. Rizzo TA, Metzger BE, Burns WJ, et al: Correlations between antepartum maternal metabolism and intelligence of offspring. N Engl J Med 325:911, 1991.
175. Ornoy A, Ratzon N, Greenbaum C, et al: School-age children born to diabetic mothers and to mothers with gestational diabetes exhibit a high rate of inattention and fine and gross motor impairment. J Pediatr Endocrinol Metab 14(Suppl 1):681, 2001.
176. Varughese GI, Chowdhury SR, Warner DP, Barton DM: Preconception care of women attending adult general diabetes clinics—are we doing enough? Diabetes Res Clin Pract 76:142-145, 2007.
177. Jovanovic L, Nakai Y: Successful pregnancy in women with type 1 diabetes: From preconception through postpartum care. Endocrinol Metab Clin North Am 35:79-97, vi, 2006.
178. Dunne FP, Brydon P, Smith T, et al: Pre-conception diabetes care in insulin-dependent diabetes mellitus. QJM 92:175, 1999.
179. Rendell MS, Jovanovic L: Targeting postprandial hyperglycemia. Metabolism 55:1263-1281, 2006.
180. UK Prospective Diabetes Study Group: Tight blood pressure control and risk of macrovascular and microvascular complications in type 2 diabetes. BMJ 317:703, 1998.
181. Jakubowicz DJ, Iuorno MJ, Jakubowicz S, et al: Effects of metformin on early pregnancy loss in the polycystic ovary syndrome. J Clin Endocrinol Metab 87:524, 2002.
182. Glueck CJ, Phillips H, Cameron D, et al: Continuing metformin throughout pregnancy in women with polycystic ovary syndrome appears to safely reduce first-trimester spontaneous abortion: A pilot study. Fertil Steril 75:46, 2001.
183. Glueck CJ, Wang P, Kobayashi S, et al: Metformin therapy throughout pregnancy reduces the development of gestational diabetes in women with polycystic ovary syndrome. Fertil Steril 77:520, 2002.
184. Nanovskaya TN, Nekhayeva IA, Patrikeeva SL, et al: Transfer of metformin across the dually perfused human placental lobule. Am J Obstet Gynecol 195:1081-1085, 2006.
185. Charles B, Norris R, Xiao X, Hague W: Population pharmacokinetics of metformin in late pregnancy. Ther Drug Monit 28:67-72, 2006.
186. Gilbert C, Valois M, Koren G: Pregnancy outcome after first-trimester exposure to metformin: A meta-analysis. Fertil Steril 86:658-663, 2006.
187. Hughes RC, Rowan JA: Pregnancy in women with type 2 diabetes: Who takes metformin and what is the outcome? Diabet Med 23:318-322, 2006.
188. Glueck CJ, Wang P: Metformin before and during pregnancy and lactation in polycystic ovary syndrome. Expert Opin Drug Saf 6:191-198, 2007.

189. Arauz-Pacheco C, Parrott MA, Raskin P: The treatment of hypertension in adult patients with diabetes. Diabetes Care 25:134-147, 2002.
190. Buttar HS: An overview of the influence of ACE inhibitors on fetal-placental circulation and perinatal development. Mol Cell Biochem 176:61, 1997.
191. Briggs GG, Nageotte MP: Fatal fetal outcome with the combined use of valsartan and atenolol. Ann Pharmacother 35:859, 2001.
192. American Diabetes Association: Gestational diabetes mellitus. Diabetes Care 27(Suppl 1):S88, 2004.
193. Naylor CD, Sermer M, Chen E, et al: Selective screening for gestational diabetes mellitus. N Engl J Med 337:1591, 1997.
194. Metzger BE, Coustan DR: Summary and recommendations of the Fourth International Workshop-Conference on Gestational Diabetes Mellitus. The Organizing Committee. Diabetes Care 21(Suppl 2):B161, 1998.
195. Metzger BE, Buchanan TA, Coustan DR, et al: Summary and Recommendations of the Fifth International Workshop-Conference on Gestational Diabetes Mellitus. Diabetes Care 30:S251-S260, 2007.
196. American College of Obstetricians and Gynecologists (ACOG): Clinical management guidelines for obstetrician-gynecologists. ACOG practice bulletin no. 30, September 2001. Obstet Gynecol 98:525, 2001.
197. Mello G, Elena P, Ognibene A, et al: Lack of concordance between the 75-g and 100-g glucose load tests for the diagnosis of gestational diabetes mellitus. Clin Chem 52:1679-1684, 2006.
198. Brody SC, Harris R, Lohr K: Screening for gestational diabetes: A summary of the evidence for the U.S. Preventive Services Task Force. Obstet Gynecol 101:380-392, 2003.
199. Dooley SL, Metzger BE, Cho NH, et al: The influence of demographic and phenotypic heterogeneity on the prevalence of gestational diabetes mellitus. Int J Gynaecol Obstet 35:13, 1991.
200. Bobrowski RA, Bottoms SF, Micallef JA, Dombrowski MP: Is the 50-gram glucose screening test ever diagnostic? J Matern Fetal Med 5:317, 1996.
201. Berkus MD, Langer O: Glucose tolerance test: degree of glucose abnormality correlates with neonatal outcome. Obstet Gynecol 81:344, 1993.
202. Langer O, Brustman L, Anyaegbunam A, et al: The significance of one abnormal glucose tolerance test value on adverse outcome in pregnancy. Am J Obstet Gynecol 157:758, 1987.
203. McLaughlin GB, Cheng YW, Caughey AB: Women with one elevated 3-hour glucose tolerance test value: Are they at risk for adverse perinatal outcomes? Am J Obstet Gynecol 194:e16-e19, 2006.
204. Roberts AB, Court DJ, Henley P, et al: Fructosamine in diabetic pregnancy. Lancet 2:998, 1983.
205. Roberts AB, Baker JR: Relationship between fetal growth and maternal fructosamine in diabetic pregnancy. Obstet Gynecol 70:242, 1987
206. Page RC, Kirk BA, Fay T, et al: Is macrosomia associated with poor glycaemic control in diabetic pregnancy? Diabet Med 13:170, 1996.
207. Nasrat H, Fageeh W, Abalkhail B, et al: Determinants of pregnancy outcome in patients with gestational diabetes. Int J Gynaecol Obstet 53:117, 1996.
208. Huter O, Brezinka C, Sölder E, et al: Postpartum diabetes screening: Value of fructosamine determination [in German]. Zentralbl Gynakol 114:18, 1992.
209. Shah BD, Cohen AW, May C: Comparison of glycohemoglobin determination and the one-hour oral glucose screen in the identification of gestational diabetes. Am J Obstet Gynecol 144:774, 1982.
210. Baxi L, Barad D, Reece EA, et al: Use of glycosylated hemoglobin as a screen for macrosomia in gestational diabetes. Obstet Gynecol 64:347, 1984.
211. Artal R, Mosley GM, Dorey FJ: Glycohemoglobin as a screening test for gestational diabetes. Am J Obstet Gynecol 148:412, 1984.
212. Agarwal MM, Hughes PF, Punnose J, et al: Gestational diabetes screening of a multiethnic, high-risk population using glycated proteins. Diabetes Res Clin Pract 51:67, 2001.
213. Moses R, Griffiths RD, Davis W: Gestational diabetes: Do all women need to be tested? Aust N Z J Obstet Gynaecol 35:387, 1995.
214. American College of Obstetricians and Gynecologists (ACOG): Gestational diabetes. ACOG practice bulletin no. 30. Obstet Gynecol 98:525, 2001.
215. Coustan DR, Widness JA, Carpenter MW, et al: Should the fifty-gram, one-hour plasma glucose screening test for gestational diabetes be administered in the fasting or fed state? Am J Obstet Gynecol 154:1031, 1986.
216. Sermer M, Naylor CD, Gare D, et al: Impact of time since last meal on the gestational glucose challenge test. Am J Obstet Gynecol 171:607, 1994.
217. Major CA, Henry MJ, De Veciana M, et al: The effects of carbohydrate restriction in patients with diet-controlled gestational diabetes. Obstet Gynecol 91:600, 1998.
218. Crapo PA, Insel J, Sperling MA, et al: Comparison of serum glucose, insulin and glucagon responses to different types of complex carbohydrate in non–insulin-dependent diabetic patients. Am J Clin Nutr 34:184, 1981.
219. Churchill JA, Berrendes H, Nemore W, et al: Neuropsychological deficits in children of diabetic mothers: A report from the Collaborative Study of Cerebral Palsy. Am J Obstet Gynecol 105:257, 1969.
220. Coetzee EJ, Jackson WPU, Berman PA: Ketonuria in pregnancy—with special reference to calorie-restricted food intake in obese diabetics. Diabetes 29:177, 1980.
221. Parfitt VJ, Clark JD, Turner GM, et al: Use of fructosamine and glycated haemoglobin to verify self blood glucose monitoring data in diabetic pregnancy. Diabet Med 10:162, 1993.
222. Goldberg JD, Franklin B, Lasser D, et al: Gestational diabetes: Impact of home glucose monitoring on neonatal birth weight. Am J Obstet Gynecol 154:546, 1986.
223. Jovanovic-Peterson L: What is so bad about a prolonged pregnancy? J Am Coll Nutr 10:1, 1991.
224. de Veciana M, Trail PA, Evans AT, et al: A comparison of oral acarbose and insulin in women with gestational diabetes mellitus. Am J Obstet Gynecol 99(Suppl):S5, 2002.
225. Cousins L, Rigg L, Hollingsworth D, et al: The 24-hour excursion and diurnal rhythm of glucose, insulin and C peptide in normal pregnancy. Am J Obstet Gynecol 136:483, 1980.
226. Parretti E, Mecacci F, Papini M, et al: Third-trimester maternal glucose levels from diurnal profiles in nondiabetic pregnancies: Correlation with sonographic parameters of fetal growth. Diabetes Care 24:1317, 2001.
227. Yogev Y, Ben-Haroush A, Chen R, et al: Diurnal glycemic profile in obese and normal weight nondiabetic pregnant women. Am J Obstet Gynecol 191:949-953, 2004.
228. Lepore M, Pampanelli S, Fanelli C, et al: Pharmacokinetics and pharmacodynamics of subcutaneous injection of long-acting human insulin analog glargine, NPH insulin, and Ultralente human insulin and continuous subcutaneous infusion of insulin lispro. Diabetes 49:2142, 2000.
229. Langer O: Maternal glycemic criteria for insulin therapy in gestational diabetes mellitus. Diabetes Care 21(Suppl 2):B91, 1998.
230. Holcberg G, Tsadkin-Tamir M, Sapir O, et al: Transfer of insulin lispro across the human placenta. Eur J Obstet Gynecol Reprod Biol 115:117-118, 2004.
231. Bhattacharyya A, Brown S, Hughes S, et al: Insulin lispro and regular insulin in pregnancy. QJM 94:255, 2001.
232. Hermansen K, Vaaler S, Madsbad S, et al: Postprandial glycemic control with biphasic insulin aspart in patients with type 1 diabetes. Metabolism 51:896, 2002.
233. Bode B, Weinstein R, Bell D, et al: Comparison of insulin aspart with buffered regular insulin and insulin lispro in continuous subcutaneous insulin infusion: A randomized study in type 1 diabetes. Diabetes Care 25:439, 2002.
234. Cypryk K, Sobczak M, Pertynska-Marczewska M, et al: Pregnancy complications and perinatal outcome in diabetic women treated with Humalog (insulin lispro) or regular human insulin during pregnancy. Med Sci Monit 10:PI29-PI32, 2004.
235. Di Cianni G, Volpe L, Ghio A, et al: Maternal metabolic control and perinatal outcome in women with gestational diabetes mellitus treated with lispro or aspart insulin: Comparison with regular insulin. Diabetes Care 30:e11, 2007.
236. Mathiesen ER, Kinsley B, Amiel SA, et al: Maternal glycemic control and hypoglycemia in type 1 diabetic pregnancy: A randomized trial of insulin

aspart versus human insulin in 322 pregnant women. Diabetes Care 30:771-776, 2007.
237. Pettitt DJ, Ospina P, Kolaczynski JW, Jovanovic L: Comparison of an insulin analog, insulin aspart, and regular human insulin with no insulin in gestational diabetes mellitus. Diabetes Care 26:183, 2003.
238. Gillies PS, Figgitt DP, Lamb HM: Insulin glargine. Drugs 59:253, 2000.
239. Price N, Bartlett C, Gillmer M: Use of insulin glargine during pregnancy: A case-control pilot study. BJOG 114:453-457, 2007.
240. Wooderink JM, van Loon AJ, Storms F, et al: Use of insulin glargine during pregnancy in seven type 1 diabetic women. Diabetes Care 28:2594, 2005.
241. Hofmann T, Horstmann G, Stammberger I: Evaluation of the reproductive toxicity and embryotoxicity of insulin glargine (LANTUS) in rats and rabbits. Int J Toxicol 21:181, 2002.
242. Gabbe SG, Holing E, Temple P, et al: Benefits, risks, costs, and patient satisfaction associated with insulin pump therapy for the pregnancy complicated by type 1 diabetes mellitus. Am J Obstet Gynecol 182:1283, 2000.
243. Simmons D, Thompson CF, Conroy C, et al: Use of insulin pumps in pregnancies complicated by type 2 diabetes and gestational diabetes in a multiethnic community. Diabetes Care 24:2078, 2001.
244. Gimenez M, Conget I, Nicolau J, et al: Outcome of pregnancy in women with type 1 diabetes intensively treated with continuous subcutaneous insulin infusion or conventional therapy. A case-control study. Acta Diabetol 44:34-37, 2007.
245. Hieronimus S, Cupelli C, Bongain A, et al: Pregnancy in type 1 diabetes: Insulin pump versus intensified conventional therapy [in French]. Gynecol Obstet Fertil 33:389-394, 2005.
246. Lapolla A, Dalfra MG, Masin M, et al: Analysis of outcome of pregnancy in type 1 diabetics treated with insulin pump or conventional insulin therapy. Acta Diabetol 40:143-149, 2003.
247. Caruso A, Lanzone A, Bianchi V, et al: Continuous subcutaneous insulin infusion (CSII) in pregnant diabetic patients. Prenat Diagn 7:41, 1987.
248. McFarland MB, Langer O, Conway DL, et al: Dietary therapy for gestational diabetes: How long is long enough? Obstet Gynecol 93:978, 1999.
249. Crowther CA, Hiller JE, Moss JR, et al: Effect of treatment of gestational diabetes mellitus on pregnancy outcomes. N Engl J Med 352:2477-2486, 2005.
250. Pirc LK, Owens JA, Crowther CA, et al: Mild gestational diabetes in pregnancy and the adipoinsular axis in babies born to mothers in the ACHOIS randomised controlled trial. BMC Pediatr 7:18, 2007.
251. Jovanovic-Peterson L, Bevier W, Peterson CM: The Santa Barbara County Health Care Services Program: Birth weight change concomitant with screening for and treatment of glucose-intolerance of pregnancy: A potential cost-effective intervention? Am J Perinatol 14:221, 1997.
252. Buchanan TA, Kjos SL, Montoro MN, et al: Use of fetal ultrasound to select metabolic therapy for pregnancies complicated by mild gestational diabetes. Diabetes Care 17:275, 1994.
253. Zucker P, Simon G: Prolonged symptomatic neonatal hypoglycemia associated with maternal chlorpropamide therapy. Pediatrics 42:824, 1968.
254. Piacquadio K, Hollingsworth DR, Murphy H: Effects of in-utero exposure to oral hypoglycaemic drugs. Lancet 338:866, 1991.
255. Towner D, Kjos SL, Leung B, et al: Congenital malformations in pregnancies complicated by NIDDM. Diabetes Care 18:1446, 1995.
256. Kolterman OG: Glyburide in non-insulin-dependent diabetes: An update. Clin Ther 14:196, 1992.
257. Koren G: Glyburide and fetal safety: Transplacental pharmacokinetic considerations. Reprod Toxicol 15:227, 2001.
258. Elliott BD, Langer O, Schenker S, et al: Insignificant transfer of glyburide occurs across the human placenta. Am J Obstet Gynecol 165:807, 1991.
259. Elliott BD, Schenker S, Langer O, et al: Comparative placental transport of oral hypoglycemic agents in humans: A model of human placental drug transfer. Am J Obstet Gynecol 171:653, 1994.
260. Langer O, Conway DL, Berkus MD, et al: A comparison of glyburide and insulin in women with gestational diabetes mellitus. N Engl J Med 343:1134, 2000.
261. Langer O, Yogev Y, Xenakis EM, et al: Insulin and glyburide therapy: Dosage, severity level of gestational diabetes, and pregnancy outcome. Am J Obstet Gynecol 192:134-139, 2005.
262. Lim JM, Tayob Y, O'Brien PM, Shaw RW: A comparison between the pregnancy outcome of women with gestation diabetes treated with glibenclamide and those treated with insulin. Med J Malaysia 52:377381, 1997.
263. Chmait R, Dinise T, Moore T: Prospective observational study to establish predictors of glyburide success in women with gestational diabetes mellitus. J Perinatol 24:617-622, 2004.
264. Langer O: Oral anti-hyperglycemic agents for the management of gestational diabetes mellitus. Obstet Gynecol Clin North Am 34:255-274, 2007.
265. Coustan DR: Pharmacological management of gestational diabetes: An overview. Diabetes Care 30:S206-S208, 2007.
266. Moore TR: Glyburide for the treatment of gestational diabetes: A critical appraisal. Diabetes Care 30:S209-S213, 2007.
267. Jacobson GF, Ramos GA, Ching JY, et al: Comparison of glyburide and insulin for the management of gestational diabetes in a large managed care organization. Am J Obstet Gynecol 193:118-124, 2005.
268. Conway DL, Gonzales O, Skiver D: Use of glyburide for the treatment of gestational diabetes: The San Antonio experience. J Matern Fetal Neonatal Med 15:51-55, 2004.
269. Kremer CJ, Duff P: Glyburide for the treatment of gestational diabetes. Am J Obstet Gynecol 190:1438, 2004.
270. Chmait R, Dinise T, Moore T: Prospective observational study to establish predictors of glyburide success in women with gestational diabetes mellitus. J Perinatol 24:617-622, 2004.
271. Rochon M, Rand L, Roth L, Gaddipati S: Glyburide for the management of gestational diabetes: Risk factors predictive of failure and associated pregnancy outcomes. Am J Obstet Gynecol 195:1090-1094, 2006.
272. Yin OQ, Tomlinson B, Chow MS: CYP2C9, but not CYP2C19, polymorphisms affect the pharmacokinetics and pharmacodynamics of glyburide in Chinese subjects. Clin Pharmacol Ther 78:370-377, 2005.
273. Jaber LA, Antal EJ, Slaughter RL, Welshman IR: Comparison of pharmacokinetics and pharmacodynamics of short- and long-term glyburide therapy in NIDDM. Diabetes Care 17:1300-1306, 1994.
274. Yogev Y, Ben Haroush A, Chen R, et al: Undiagnosed asymptomatic hypoglycemia: Diet, insulin, and glyburide for gestational diabetic pregnancy. Obstet Gynecol 104:88-93, 2004.
275. Legro RS, Barnhart HX, Schlaff WD, et al: Clomiphene, metformin, or both for infertility in the polycystic ovary syndrome. N Engl J Med 356:551-566, 2007.
276. Vandermolen DT, Ratts VS, Evans WS, et al: Metformin increases the ovulatory rate and pregnancy rate from clomiphene citrate in patients with polycystic ovary syndrome who are resistant to clomiphene citrate alone. Fertil Steril 75:310-315, 2001.
277. Coetzee EJ, Jackson WP: Metformin in management of pregnant insulin-independent diabetics. Diabetologia 16:241, 1979.
278. Hellmuth E, Damm P, Molsted-Pedersen L: Oral hypoglycaemic agents in 118 diabetic pregnancies. Diabet Med 17:507, 2000.
279. Metzger BE: Diet and medical therapy in the optimal management of gestational diabetes mellitus. Nestle Nutr Workshop Ser Clin Perform Programme 11:155-165; discussion 165-169, 2006.
280. Rowan JA, on behalf of the Metformin in Gestational Diabetes Trial: A trial in progress: Gestational diabetes: Treatment with metformin compared with insulin (the Metformin in Gestational Diabetes [MiG] trial). Diabetes Care 30:S214-S219, 2007.
281. Bertini AM, Silva JC, Taborda W, et al: Perinatal outcomes and the use of oral hypoglycemic agents. J Perinat Med 33:519, 2005.
282. Sacks DA, Chen W: Estimating fetal weight in the management of macrosomia. Obstet Gynecol Surv 55:229, 2000.
283. Chauhan SP, West DJ, Scardo JA, et al: Antepartum detection of macrosomic fetus: Clinical versus sonographic, including soft-tissue measurements. Obstet Gynecol 95:639, 2000.
284. O'Reilly-Green C, Divon M: Sonographic and clinical methods in the diagnosis of macrosomia. Clin Obstet Gynecol 43:309, 2000.

285. Sokol RJ, Chik L, Dombrowski MP, et al: Correctly identifying the macrosomic fetus: Improving ultrasonography-based prediction. Am J Obstet Gynecol 182:1489, 2000.
286. Landon MB: Prenatal diagnosis of macrosomia in pregnancy complicated by diabetes mellitus. J Matern Fetal Med 9:52, 2000.
287. Combs CA, Rosenn B, Miodovnik M, et al: Sonographic EFW and macrosomia: Is there an optimum formula to predict diabetic fetal macrosomia? J Matern Fetal Med 9:55, 2000.
288. Hackmon R, Bornstein E, Ferber A, et al: Combined analysis with amniotic fluid index and estimated fetal weight for prediction of severe macrosomia at birth. Am J Obstet Gynecol 196:333.e1-e4, 2007.
289. Hedriana H, Moore TR: Comparison of single vs multiple growth sonography in predicting birthweight. Am J Obstet Gynecol 170:1600, 1994.
290. Parry S, Severs CP, Sehdev HM, et al: Ultrasonographic prediction of fetal macrosomia: Association with cesarean delivery. J Reprod Med 45:17-22, 2000.
291. Chauhan SP, Lynn NN, Sanderson M, et al: A scoring system for detection of macrosomia and prediction of shoulder dystocia: A disappointment. J Matern Fetal Neonatal Med 19:699-705, 2006.
292. Weeks JW, Pitman T, Spinnato JA. Fetal macrosomia: Does antenatal prediction affect delivery route and birth outcome? Am J Obstet Gynecol 173:1215, 1995.
293. Rouse DJ, Owen J: Prophylactic cesarean delivery for fetal macrosomia diagnosed by means of ultrasonograph—a Faustian bargain? Am J Obstet Gynecol 181:332, 1999.
294. Rayburn WF, Sokkary N, Clokey DE, et al: Consequences of routine delivery at 38 weeks for A-2 gestational diabetes. J Matern Fetal Neonatal Med 18:333-337, 2005.
295. Kjos SL, Henry OA, Montoro M, et al: Insulin-requiring diabetes in pregnancy: A randomized trial of active induction of labor and expectant management. Am J Obstet Gynecol 169:611, 1993.
296. American College of Obstetricians and Gynecologists (ACOG): Fetal macrosomia. ACOG practice bulletin no. 22, 2000.
297. Gonen R, Bader D, Ajami M: Effects of a policy of elective cesarean delivery in cases of suspected fetal macrosomia on the incidence of brachial plexus injury and the rate of cesarean delivery. Am J Obstet Gynecol 183:1296, 2000.
298. Conway DL, Langer O: Elective delivery of infants with macrosomia in diabetic women: Reduced shoulder dystocia versus increased cesarean deliveries. Am J Obstet Gynecol 178:922, 1998.
299. Herbst MA: Treatment of suspected fetal macrosomia: A cost-effectiveness analysis. Am J Obstet Gynecol 193:1035-1039, 2005.
300. Mimouni F, Tsang RC: Pregnancy outcome in insulin-dependent diabetes: Temporal relationships with metabolic control during specific pregnancy periods. Am J Perinatol 5:334-338, 1988.
301. Balsells M, Corcoy R, Adelantado JM, et al: Gestational diabetes mellitus: Metabolic control during labour. Diabetes Nutr Metab 13:257, 2000.
302. McKinney PA, Parslow R, Gurney KA, et al: Perinatal and neonatal determinants of childhood type 1 diabetes: A case-control study in Yorkshire, UK. Diabetes Care 22:928, 1999.
303. Schrezenmeir J, Jagla A: Milk and diabetes. J Am Coll Nutr 19(Suppl):176S, 2000.
304. Pettitt DJ, Forman MR, Hanson RL: Breastfeeding and incidence of non–insulin-dependent diabetes mellitus in Pima Indians. Lancet 350:166, 1997.
305. Gimeno SG, de Souza JM: IDDM and milk consumption: A case-control study in Sao Paulo, Brazil. Diabetes Care 20:1256, 1997.
306. Neubauer SH, Ferris AM, Chase CG, et al: Delayed lactogenesis in women with insulin-dependent diabetes mellitus. Am J Clin Nutr 58:54, 1993.
307. van Beusekom CM, Zeegers TA, Martini IA, et al: Milk of patients with tightly controlled insulin-dependent diabetes mellitus has normal macronutrient and fatty acid composition. Am J Clin Nutr 57:938, 1993.
308. Webster J, Moore K, McMullan A: Breastfeeding outcomes for women with insulin dependent diabetes. J Hum Lact 11:195, 1995.

Chapter 47

Thyroid Disease and Pregnancy

Shahla Nader, MD

Thyroid disorders are among the most common endocrinopathies in young women of childbearing age. In large areas of the world, iodine deficiency is the predominant cause of these disorders. In the Western Hemisphere, these disorders are most often related to altered immunity. The hormonal and immunologic perturbations of pregnancy and the postpartum period and the dependence of the fetus on maternal iodine and thyroid hormone have profound influences on maternal thyroid function and consequently on fetal well-being. Appropriate antepartum and postpartum care requires a basic knowledge of thyroid function, its alteration in pregnancy, and the more common thyroid diseases afflicting women in the setting of pregnancy, all of which are addressed in this chapter. The combination of thyroid disease and pregnancy has been the topic of several reviews,[1,2] and the Endocrine Society's guidelines for management of thyroid dysfunction during pregnancy and after delivery have recently been published.[3]

Maternal-Fetal Thyroid Physiology

Normal Thyroid Physiology

The thyroid gland is located in the anterior neck below the hyoid bone and above the sternal notch. Consisting of two lobes and connected by the isthmus, it weighs approximately 20 to 25 g. Each lobe is divided into lobules, each of which contains 20 to 40 follicles. The follicle consists of follicular cells, which surround a glycoprotein material called colloid.

The hypothalamic-pituitary axis governs the production of thyroid hormone by the follicular cells. Tonic stimulation of thyrotropin-releasing hormone (TRH) is required to maintain normal thyroid function, and hypothalamic injury or disruption of the stalk results in hypothyroidism. TRH, a tripeptide, is produced in the paraventricular nucleus of the hypothalamus, and its local production as determined by mRNA is inversely related to concentrations of circulating thyroid hormones. Traversing the pituitary stalk, TRH is delivered to the pituitary thyrotroph by the pituitary portal circulation, and it affects the production and release of thyrotropin (i.e., thyroid-stimulating hormone [TSH]). A glycoprotein, TSH is composed of α and β subunits, and the β subunit confers specificity. Control of TSH secretion occurs by negative feedback (from circulating thyroid hormone, somatostatin, dopamine) or by stimulation by TRH.

Thyroid gland production of thyroxine (T_4) and triiodothyronine (T_3) is regulated by TSH. On binding to its receptor, TSH induces thyroid growth, differentiation, and all phases of iodine metabolism from uptake of iodine to secretion of the two thyroid hormones. In the nonpregnant state, 80 to 100 μg of iodine are taken up by the gland daily. Dietary iodine is reduced to iodide, which is absorbed and cleared by the kidney (80%) and thyroid (20%). Iodide is actively trapped by the thyroid and is the rate limiting step in hormone biosynthesis. The iodide is converted back to iodine and organified by binding to tyrosyl residues, which are part of the glycoprotein thyroglobulin. This process requires the enzyme thyroid peroxidase. Iodination can give rise to monoiodotyrosine or diiodotyrosine, with the ratio depending on prevailing iodine availability. Coupling of two diiodotyrosine molecules forms T_4, and one diiodotyrosine and one monoiodotyrosine form T_3. Thyroglobulin is extruded into the colloid space at the center of the follicle, and thyroid hormone is stored as colloid.

Hormone secretion by thyroid cells, which is also under TSH control, involves digestion of thyroglobulin and extrusion of T_4 and T_3 into the capillaries. Daily secretion rates approximate 90 μg of T_4 and 30 μg of T_3. Both circulate highly bound to protein (mainly thyroxine-binding globulin [TBG]), with less than 1% in free form (0.3% of T_3 and 0.03% of T_4). Other binding proteins include thyroxine-binding prealbumin and albumin. It is the free hormone that enters cells and is active.

Whereas T_4 is completely thyroidal in origin, only approximately 20% of T_3 comes directly from the thyroid. Thyroxine is metabolized in most tissues (particularly in the liver and kidneys) to T_3 by deiodination. It is also metabolized to reverse T_3, a metabolically inactive hormone. Removal of an iodine by 5′ monodeiodination from the outer ring of T_4 results in T_3, which is metabolically active. When iodine is removed from the inner ring, reverse T_3 is produced (Fig. 47-1) Monodeiodinase type I and type II catalyze the formation of T_3, whereas reverse T_3 is catalyzed by monodeiodinase type III. Normally, approximately 35% of T_4 is converted to T_3, and 40% is converted to reverse T_3, but this balance is shifted in favor of the metabolically inert reverse T_3 in illness, starvation, or other catabolic states.[4,5] About 80% of circulating T_3 is derived from peripheral conversion. The half-life of T_4 is 1 week; 5 to 6 weeks are necessary before a change in dose of T_4 therapy is reflected in steady-state T_4 values. The half-life of T_3 is 1 day.

Free thyroid hormone enters the cell and binds to nuclear receptors and in this way signals its cellular responses.[6] The affinity of T_3 for nuclear receptors is tenfold that of T_4, which helps to explain the greater biologic activity of T_3. Thyroid hormone receptors belong to a large superfamily of nuclear-hormone receptors that include the steroid hormone, vitamin D, and retinoic acid receptors. Thyroid hormones have diverse effects on cellular growth, development, and metabolism. The major effects of thyroid hormones are genomic,

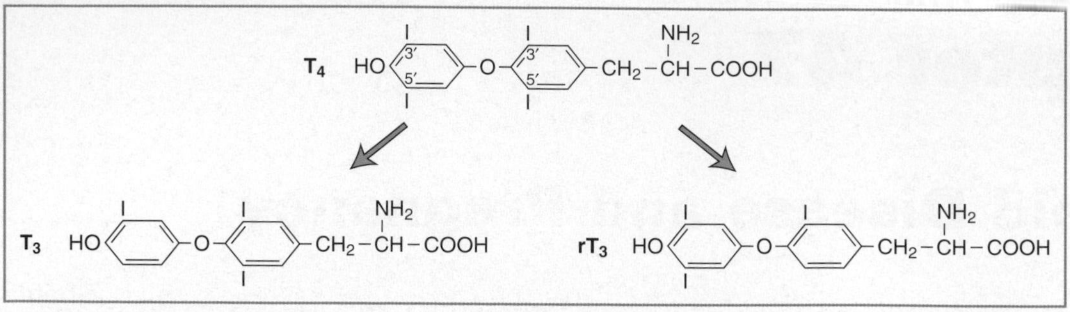

FIGURE 47-1 Iodine removal. Removal of an iodine atom by 5′-monodeiodination from the outer ring of thyroxine (T_4) results in the formation of metabolically active triiodothyronine (T_3). Removal of an iodine atom from the inner ring results in formation of the metabolically inactive reverse triiodothyronine (rT_3).

stimulating transcription and translation of new proteins in a concentration- and time-dependent manner.

Maternal Thyroid Physiology

Pregnancy alters the thyroidal economy, and the hormonal changes of pregnancy result in profound alterations in the biochemical parameters of thyroid function. This section reviews maternal thyroid physiology, the role of maternal hormones in fetal growth and development, and the development of the fetal hypothalamic-pituitary-thyroid axis. This topic was reviewed by Glinoer.[7]

Three series of events occur at different times during gestation. Starting in the first half of gestation and continuing until term, there is an increase in TBG, a direct effect of increasing circulating estrogen concentrations. Basal levels increase twofold to threefold. This increase is accompanied by a trend toward lower free hormone concentrations (T_4 and T_3), which results in stimulation of the hypothalamic-pituitary-thyroid axis. Under conditions of iodine sufficiency, the decrease in free hormone levels is marginal (10% to 15% on average). When the supply of iodine is insufficient, more pronounced effects occur, and these are addressed in later sections. There is usually a trend toward a slight increase in TSH between the first trimester and term.

The second event takes place transiently during the first trimester and is a consequence of thyroid stimulation by increasing concentrations of human chorionic gonadotropin (hCG). As hCG peaks late in the first trimester, there is partial inhibition of the pituitary and transient lowering of TSH between 8 and 14 weeks' gestation (Fig. 47-2). In about 20% of women, TSH falls below the lower limit of normal, and these women often have significantly higher hCG concentrations.[8] The stimulatory action of hCG has been broadly quantified; an increment of 10,000 IU/L is associated with a lowering of basal TSH of 0.1 mU/L. In most normal pregnancies, this is of minor consequence.[9]

In the third series of events, alterations in the peripheral metabolism of thyroid hormone occur throughout pregnancy but are more prominent in the second half. Three enzymes deiodinate thyroid hormones: deiodinase types I, II, and III. Type I is not significantly modified. Type II, which is expressed in the placenta, can maintain T_3 production locally, which can be critical when maternal T_4 concentrations are reduced. Type III is also found abundantly in the placenta, and it catalyzes the conversion of T_4 to reverse T_3 and conversion of T_3 to T_2; this abundance may explain the low T_3 and high reverse T_3 concentrations characteristic of fetal thyroid hormone metabolism.[10]

These physiologic adaptations to pregnancy, depicted in Figure 47-3, are attained without difficulty by the normal thyroid gland in a state of iodine sufficiency. This does not apply when thyroid function is compromised or iodine supply is insufficient.

Iodine Deficiency and Goiter

Increased vascularity and some glandular hyperplasia can result in mild thyroid enlargement, but frank goiter occurs because of iodine deficiency or other thyroidal disease. Although iodine deficiency is usually not a problem in the United States, Japan, and parts of Europe, 1 to 1.5 billion people in the world are at risk, with 500 million living in areas of overt iodine deficiency. The World Health Organization recommends 150 μg iodine per day for adults and 200 μg for pregnant women. There is increased renal iodine clearance during pregnancy, and in the latter part of gestation, a significant amount of iodine is diverted toward the fetoplacental unit to allow the fetal thyroid to produce its own thyroid hormones. This physiologic adaptation occurs easily with minimal hypothyroxinemia and no goiter formation in areas of iodine sufficiency. Through hypothalamic-pituitary feedback, borderline iodine intake chronically enhances thyroid stimulation. The iodine deficiency manifests as greater hypothyroxinemia, which increases TSH and thyroglobulin levels and produces thyroid hypertrophy (Fig. 47-4).

In a study of otherwise healthy pregnant women living under conditions of relative iodine restriction, thyroid volume, as assessed by ultrasonography, increased an average of 30% during pregnancy.[11] In a selected group of these women with goitrogenesis, follow-up a year after delivery did not show a return of thyroid volumes to those found in early pregnancy. Iodine intake should also be increased after delivery, especially in breastfeeding women. Ultrasonography of neonates revealed that thyroid volume was 38% larger in neonates of untreated mothers compared with neonates of mothers treated with iodine supplementation.[12]

Other than iodine deficiency, goiter in pregnancy can be related to the following:

- Graves disease
- Hashimoto thyroiditis
- Excessive iodine intake
- Lymphocytic thyroiditis
- Thyroid cancer
- Lymphoma
- Therapy with lithium or thionamides

In the United States, clinical studies of pregnant women and nonpregnant controls have not revealed an increase in goiter during preg-

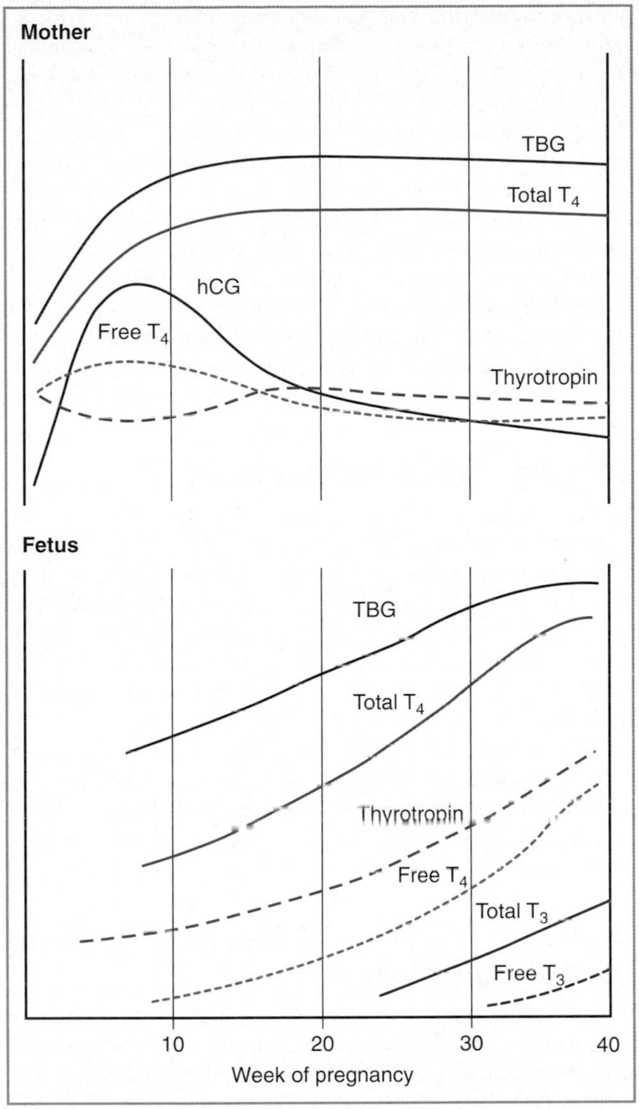

FIGURE 47-2 Relative changes in maternal and fetal thyroid function during pregnancy. The effects of pregnancy on the mother include a marked and early increase in hepatic production of thyroxine-binding globulin (TBG) and placental production of human chorionic gonadotropin (hCG). The increased level of serum TBG increases total serum thyroxine (T_4) concentrations; hCG has thyrotropin-like activity and stimulates maternal T_4 secretion. The transient hCG-induced increase in the serum level of free T_4 inhibits maternal secretion of thyrotropin. (Reprinted by permission from Burrow GN, Fisher DA, Larsen PR: Maternal and fetal thyroid function. N Engl J Med 331:1072, 1994.)

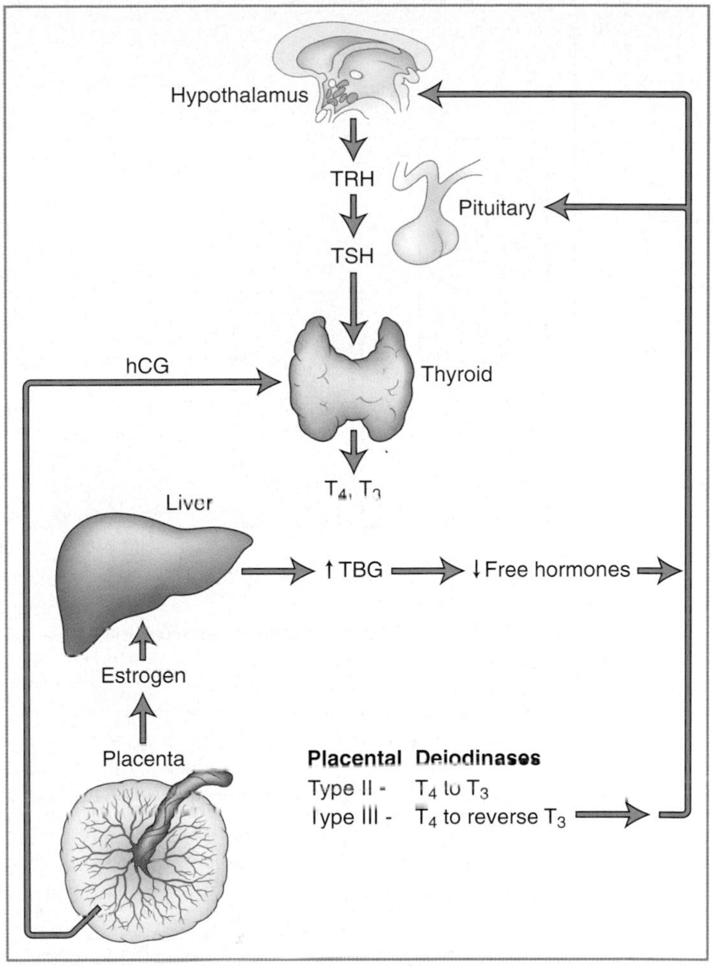

FIGURE 47-3 Physiologic adaptation to pregnancy. Schematic representation of the physiologic adaptation to pregnancy shows increased thyroxine-binding globulin (TBG) concentrations, increased levels of human chorionic gonadotropin (hCG) with its thyrotropin-like activity, and alterations in the peripheral metabolism of thyroid hormones in the placenta. TRH, thyrotropin-releasing hormone; TSH, thyroid-stimulating hormone, T4, thyroxine, T3, triiodothyronine. (Adapted from Glinoer D: What happens to the normal thyroid during pregnancy? Thyroid 9:631, 1999.)

nancy.[13] Ultrasound studies from other areas replete with iodine have confirmed these findings.[14,15]

Iodine Metabolism in Pregnancy

Although radioactive iodine is absolutely contraindicated in pregnancy, early studies using ^{132}I showed a threefold increase in thyroidal iodine clearance in pregnant women. Another set of studies enrolling 25 pregnant women also revealed increased radioactive iodine uptake during pregnancy compared with the nonpregnant or postpartum state.[16,17] The mean renal iodine clearance almost doubles because of increased renal blood flow and an increase in glomerular filtration rate of as much as 50%.[18] If iodine excretion is greater than 100 μg in a 24-hour period, the patient's iodine intake is assumed to be sufficient.[19f]

Placental-Fetal Thyroid Physiology

The thyroid gland forms as a midline outpouching of the anterior pharyngeal floor, migrates caudally, and reaches its final position by 7 weeks' gestation. Lateral contributions from the fourth and fifth pharyngeal pouches give it its bilateral shape by 8 to 9 weeks' gestation. Active trapping of iodide is detectable by week 12, and the first indication of T_4 production is detectable by week 14. Hypothalamic TRH is detectable at weeks 8 to 9, and the pituitary portal circulation is func-

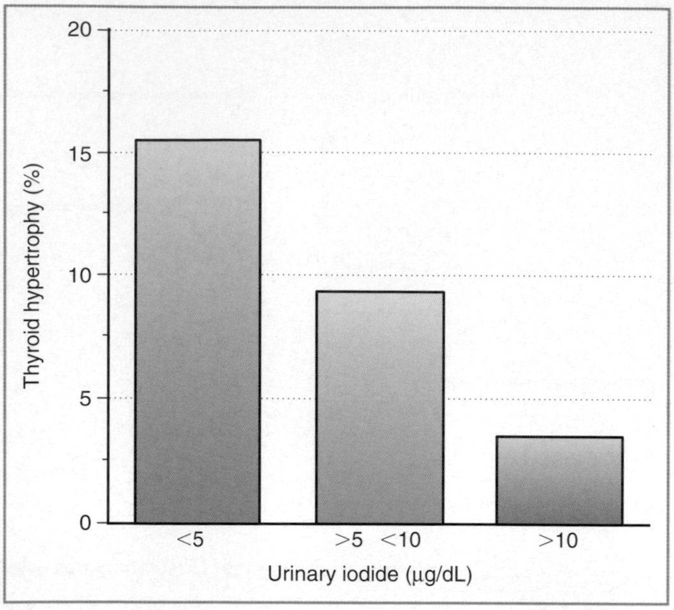

FIGURE 47-4 Iodine deficiency can manifest as thyroid hypertrophy. The percentage of maternal thyroid hypertrophy (thyroid volume > 18 mL) is plotted against the urinary iodine concentration measured during the first trimester of pregnancy. (Reprinted by permission from Caron P, Hoff M, Bassi S, et al: Urinary iodine excretion during normal pregnancy in healthy women living in the southwest of France: Correlation with maternal thyroid parameters. Thyroid 7:749, 1997.)

tional by weeks 10 to 12. Until mid-gestation, fetal TSH and T_4 concentrations remain low. At 18 to 20 weeks' gestation, the fetal thyroid gland's iodine uptake and serum T_4 concentrations begin to increase.[20] Concentrations of T_4 increase from 2 μg /dL at 20 weeks to 10 μg/dL at term, with increasing TBG concentrations contributing to this rise. Similarly, free fetal T_4 concentrations increase from 0.1 ng/dL at 12 weeks' gestation to 1.5 ng/dL near term. Increases in T_3 and free T_3 are smaller, presumably because of the availability of placental type III deiodinase, which converts T_4 rapidly to reverse T_3. Fetal serum T_3 increases from 6 ng/dL at 12 weeks' gestation to 45 ng/dL near term. Fetal serum TSH increases from 4 to 8 mU/L between weeks 12 and term.[21,22] In summary, most fetal T_4 is inactivated to reverse T_3. The T_3 (from T_4 conversion or direct fetal thyroid secretion) has limited availability. Fetal tissues that depend on T_3 for development (e.g., brain structures) are supplied by local T_4 to T_3 conversion by means of deiodinase type II.[22]

Placental Transfer of Thyroid Hormones

Although earlier studies suggested only limited T_4 and T_3 transfer through the placenta, later studies have shown that T_4 can be found in first-trimester celomic fluid by 6 weeks' gestation. Nuclear T_3 receptors can be identified in the brain of 10-week-old fetuses, and they increase tenfold by 16 weeks' gestation before the fetal thyroid becomes fully functional.[24] These studies suggest that maternal T_4 transfer occurs early in gestation and that low levels of T_4 are sustained in the fetus at this time.[25] Vulsma and colleagues[26] reported that cord serum T_4 levels in hypothyroid neonates with glandular agenesis represented as much as 30% of normal circulating values, a strong indication of maternal T_4 transfer, although this has not been a uniform finding.[27]

It appears that the first phase of maximum growth velocity of developing brain structures—neuronal multiplication and organization occurring during the second trimester—corresponds to a phase during which the supply of thyroid hormones to the fetus is almost exclusively of maternal origin.[20] In the second phase of maximum fetal brain growth velocity, occurring from the third trimester to 2 to 3 years postnatally, the supply of thyroid hormone is of fetal and neonatal origin. Low maternal thyroxine concentrations in the second trimester can result in irreversible neurologic deficit in offspring. When it occurs later, the damage to the fetal brain is less and is partially reversible. The need for T_3 by mid-gestation for development of the human cerebral cortex was also demonstrated by Kester and associates.[28] Concentrations of TSH, T_4, T_3, and reverse T_3 are measurable in the amniotic fluid and correlate with the fetal rather than maternal serum.

Neonatal Thyroid Function

Immediately after birth, there is a surge of TRH and TSH that is followed by an increase in T_3 (from increased T_4 to T_3 conversion) and a moderate increase in T_4.[10] Within a few days, the increased TSH falls to adult levels through T_4 and T_3 negative-feedback inhibition. Neonatal T_4 and T_3 concentrations return to normal adult levels within 4 to 6 weeks.[29] The transient hyperthyroxinemia can be triggered by neonatal cooling and may represent an adaptation of thermogenesis to extrauterine life.[30,31]

In premature neonates, free T_4 levels are low, TSH levels are normal (adult), and T_4 levels are related to gestational age. The clinical consequence of this transient hypothalamic hypothyroidism is unknown, but it has been associated with impaired neurologic and mental development.[32-34]

Placental Transfer of Drugs Affecting Thyroid Function

The potential influence of the placenta on fetal thyroid and neurologic development is evident by the ready transfer of several agents that affect thyroid function.[35,36] These agents include the following:

- Iodine
- Thionamides
- β-Adrenergic receptor blockers
- Somatostatin
- Exogenous TRH
- Dopamine agonists and antagonists
- Thyroid-stimulating immunoglobulins and other antibodies

TSH does not cross the placenta. TRH and corticosteroid administered antenatally before 32 weeks' gestation stimulates T_4 release and decreases the frequency of chronic lung disease among neonates.[37] Intra-amniotic administration of T_4 in the preterm setting increases fetal maturation, as reflected by an increase in the lecithin-to-sphingomyelin ratio and decrease in respiratory distress syndrome of the newborn.[38]

Pregnancy, the Immune System, and Thyroid Disease

Chapter 6 offers a detailed review of pregnancy immunology. The fetus, with its complete set of paternal antigens, survives because of adjustments in the maternal-placental-fetal immune systems. This immunologic compromise of pregnancy is orchestrated primarily by the placental tissues and passaged fetal cells that are able to modulate the local and systemic maternal immune responses.[39,40] Autoimmune responses are usually reduced in pregnancy, as evidenced by amelioration of Graves disease, rheumatoid arthritis, and multiple sclerosis.[41-43] Although there is a shift from proinflammatory T_H1 cytokines to T_H2 cytokines, driven perhaps by progesterone,[44] it is occurring against a background of reduced B-cell reactivity. The reduced B-cell responses are likely orchestrated by placental sex steroids, which are powerful negative regulators of B-cell activity. Whereas most of the immune changes in pregnancy return to normal by 12 months after delivery, there is a marked increase after most pregnancies in many different types of autoantibody secretion and an exacerbation of autoimmune disease. In most studies, total immunoglobulin G and autoantibody levels rise above pre-pregnancy levels during the first 6 months after delivery, suggesting continuing nonspecific immune stimulation.[39]

Laboratory Evaluation of Thyroid Function during Pregnancy

Thyrotropin and Thyroid Hormones

Total T_4 and total T_3 are elevated because of increased TBG production and reduced clearance induced by the hyperestrogenic state of pregnancy.[45] The normal reference range for total T_4 should be adjusted by a factor of 1.5 for pregnant patients.[2] The T_3 resin uptake (i.e., indirect laboratory measure of available TBG binding sites) is reduced in pregnancy because increased TBG binding sites take up more of the added T_3, leaving less to bind to resin. The free thyroxine index, which is a product of the total T_4 and T_3 resin uptake, usually falls to within the normal range in pregnancy. Because free T_4 can be determined, however, third-generation TSH and free T_4 assessments are the best ways to evaluate thyroid function in pregnancy. However, automated free T_4 assays are sensitive to alternations in binding proteins as occurs in pregnancy. Because these proteins change, they can falsely elevate or lower the free T_4 assay result. The free T_4, as measured by equilibrium dialysis, is not affected by these protein changes. Trimester-specific normative data for iodine-sufficient women using specific commercially available assays is not available. This topic is discussed further in the section on Subclinical Hypothyroidism and Hypothyroxinemia.

If the TSH is suppressed, suggesting overproduction of thyroid hormones, free T_3 can be determined. The third-generation TSH assays can differentiate profound from marginal suppression. Trimester-specific TSH concentrations were obtained by Dashe and colleagues,[46] who determined these concentrations at each point during gestation in singleton and twin pregnancies. They constructed nomograms for both using regression analysis and showed significantly lower TSH concentrations in the first trimester. These levels were lower in twin pregnancies, as would be expected from the known effects of hCG. Values were converted to multiples of the median for singleton pregnancies at each week of gestation, and they suggested that values expressed this way might facilitate comparison across laboratories and populations. In another study, using sensitive TSH assays, 9% of nonsymptomatic first-trimester women were found to have TSH values higher than 0.05 mU/L (i.e., lower limit of assay detection) but less than 0.4 mU/L, and another 9% had TSH values below the detection limit.[8] Free T_3 and T_4 concentrations can be in the high-normal range

TABLE 47-1 FACTORS INFLUENCING THYROXINE-BINDING GLOBULIN

Factors Increasing TBG Levels	Factors Decreasing TBG Levels
Oral contraceptives	Testosterone
Pregnancy	Nephrotic syndrome
Estrogen	Cirrhosis
Hepatitis	Glucocorticoids
Acute intermittent porphyria	Severe illness
Inherited defect	Inherited defect

TBG, thyroxine-binding globulin.

early in pregnancy because of the stimulatory effects of hCG. Free T_4 levels tend to fall through the rest of pregnancy and occasionally to levels below those of nonpregnant women.[2] Free hormone levels then fall through the rest of the pregnancy but usually not below the lower limit of normal.[47] Table 47-1 outlines factors that influence TBG and therefore total hormone concentrations.

Resistance to thyroid hormone is a rare condition encompassing a number of different defects. The pituitary and other peripheral tissues can manifest this resistance. These patients present with an increased free T_4 concentration along with an inappropriately elevated or nonsuppressed TSH, and they may have goiters. Whereas patients with thyroid hormone resistance have normal α-subunit concentrations, patients with TSH-secreting tumors (i.e., differential diagnosis of thyroid hormone resistance) often have elevated serum α-subunit levels.[48] In a case reported by Anselmo and colleagues,[49] transient thyrotoxicosis occurred during pregnancy in a woman with resistance to thyroid hormone caused by a mutation in the thyroid receptor β gene. This thyrotoxicosis manifested clinically by hypermetabolic features and paralleled the rise and peak of hCG concentrations. Symptoms ameliorated and thyroid hormone concentrations declined as pregnancy progressed and hCG concentrations fell.

Concern has been raised regarding unaffected fetuses of mothers with thyroid hormone resistance. Outcomes of pregnancies in an extended Azorean family with resistance to thyroid hormone were analyzed; miscarriages were found to be more common, and unaffected infants born to affected mothers had lower birth weights, demonstrating a direct toxic effect of thyroid hormone excess on the fetus.[30]

Thyrotropin Receptor Antibodies

Several functional types of TSH receptor antibodies are recognized. Some antibodies promote gland function (i.e., thyroid-stimulating immunoglobulins [TSIs]), some inhibit binding of TSH to its receptor (i.e., thyroid-binding inhibitory immunoglobulins [TBIIs]), and some enhance or inhibit thyroid growth. These antibodies can be measured by a variety of bioassays and receptor assays. For example, maternal production of TSIs causes maternal Graves disease, is transferred across the placenta, and can lead to neonatal Graves disease. Excess TBIIs can cause maternal and neonatal hypothyroidism.

Antithyroid Antibodies

Patients with autoimmune thyroid disease commonly develop antibodies to thyroid antigens. The two most commonly determined antibodies are those to thyroglobulin and to thyroid peroxidase (anti-TPO).[51] Among nonpregnant women, the incidence of anti-TPO

TABLE 47-2 EFFECTS OF DRUGS ON THYROID HORMONES AND FUNCTION TEST RESULTS

Inhibition of thyroid function	
	Iodine
	Lithium
Inhibition of T_4 to T_3 conversion	
	Glucocorticoid
	Ipodate
	Propranolol
	Amiodarone
	Propylthiouracil
Increased level of TSH	
	Iodine
	Lithium
	Dopamine antagonists
Decreased level of TSH	
	Glucocorticoids
	Dopamine agonists
	Somatostatin
Inhibition of T_4 and T_3 binding to binding proteins	
	Phenytoin
	Salicylates
	Sulfonylureas
Inhibition of gastrointestinal absorption of thyroid hormone	
	Ferrous sulfate
	Sucralfate
	Cholestyramine
	Aluminum hydroxide

TSH, thyroid-stimulating hormone; T_3, l-triiodothyronine; T_4, l-thyroxine.

antibodies is about 3%, with the incidence ranging from 5% to 15% among pregnant women. A substantial proportion of women with positive anti-TPO antibodies in early pregnancy develop postpartum thyroiditis.[52,53]

Drugs and Thyroid Function

Table 47-2 outlines drug effects on thyroid function and metabolism, absorption of thyroid hormones, and interpretation of thyroid function tests. Iodine and lithium inhibit thyroid function. Propranolol and ipodate block T_4 to T_3 conversion, as do glucocorticoids; however, glucocorticoids also reduce release of TSH from the pituitary, as do dopamine, dopamine agonists, and somatostatin. The antiseizure medication phenytoin reduces total T_4 levels (up to 30%) by inhibiting the binding of thyroid hormones to binding proteins and increasing T_4 clearance. Ferrous sulfate, aluminum hydroxide, and sucralfate may inhibit thyroid hormone absorption substantially—an important interaction in pregnant women who are taking both iron and thyroid hormones.

Amiodarone, an iodine-rich drug, has been used in pregnancy for maternal or fetal tachyarrhythmias. Amiodarone and the iodine are transferred across the placenta, exposing the fetus to the drug and iodine overload. This iodine overload can cause fetal or neonatal hypothyroidism and goiter, because the fetus acquires the capacity to escape from the acute Wolff-Chaikoff effect (i.e., decrease in peroxidase activity and organification that follow iodine excess) only late in gestation. Among 64 pregnancies in which amiodarone was given to the mother, 17% of progeny developed hypothyroidism (goitrous and nongoitrous). Hypothyroidism was transient, although a few of the infants were treated short term with thyroid hormones. Only two newborns had transient hyperthyroxinemia. Although breastfeeding resulted in substantial infant amiodarone ingestion, it did not cause major changes in neonatal thyroid function. The study authors concluded that amiodarone should be used only when tachyarrhythmias are unresponsive to other drugs and are life threatening and that hypothyroid neonates (and perhaps the fetus in utero) should be treated. It is prudent to monitor the infants of breastfeeding mothers who continue to use the medication.[54]

Nonthyroidal Illness and Thyroid Function

Nonthyroidal illness has been the topic of various reviews and commentaries.[4,5,55] Severely ill patients can manifest thyroid function test abnormalities that may correlate with functional inhibition of the hypothalamic-pituitary-thyroid axis, impaired T_4 to T_3 conversion (a constant accompaniment of nonthyroidal illness), and abnormalities in binding and clearance of thyroid hormone. Reverse T_3 levels are substantially elevated because of increased T_4 to reverse T_3 conversion and impaired metabolic clearance of reverse T_3. TSH concentrations can be low, normal, or elevated, although seldom higher than 20 mU/L.[55] The more severe the illness, the lower the T_4 values, and this relationship has been used as a prognostic indicator, because a high correlation has been found between a low T_4 value and a fatal outcome.[56] The best test for assessing thyroid function in severely or chronically ill patients is the free T_4 concentration. Despite the low T_3 and total T_4 state, this situation does not represent true hypothyroidism, but rather an adaptation to stress, and it should not be treated.

Thyroid Dysfunction and Reproductive Disorders

Thyroid hormones are important for normal reproductive function. Deficiency of thyroid hormone can result in delayed sexual development. As reviewed by Winters and Berga[57] and Krassas,[58] all women with infertility and menstrual disturbances should have thyroid function tests, usually T_4, T_3, and TSH. Women with type 1 diabetes, who have a relatively high incidence of hypothyroidism, should probably undergo screening before conception. This topic has been reviewed by Trokoudes and coworkers.[59]

Hyperthyroidism

Hyperthyroidism has been linked to oligomenorrhea, hypomenorrhea, amenorrhea, and infertility, although many thyrotoxic women remain ovulatory. In one survey, only 21.5% of 214 thyrotoxic patients had menstrual disturbances, compared with 50% to 60% in older series.[60] Thyroxine upregulates the production of sex hormone–binding globulin. Elevated levels of circulating testosterone and estrogen may be observed, and the clearance of testosterone is reduced. Gonadotropin concentrations can be tonically elevated.[61,62] The substantial weight loss seen in some hyperthyroid patients can affect the hypothalamic-pituitary-gonadal axis and can contribute to the infertility of severe hyperthyroidism.

Hypothyroidism

Hypothyroidism in fetal life does not affect the development of the reproductive tract, but during childhood, it leads to sexual immaturity and usually a delay in puberty, followed by anovulatory cycles. Almost 25% of women with untreated hypothyroidism have menstrual irregularities. Menorrhagia occurs frequently and can reflect interference with the endometrial maturational process and response to ovarian steroids; it usually responds to thyroxine treatment.[63] The increased miscarriage rate seen in hypothyroid patients may reflect disrupted endometrial maturation. Hypothyroidism, through increased TRH, can be associated with hyperprolactinemia, which itself can disrupt reproductive function and menstrual cyclicity,[64] leading to oligomenorrhea or amenorrhea. Galactorrhea can sometimes be seen in this setting, as can elevated levels of luteinizing hormone, possibly through diminished dopamine secretion.[65]

Women with hypothyroidism have diminished rates of metabolic clearance of androstenedione and estrone and an increase in peripheral aromatization. Whereas plasma concentrations of testosterone and estradiol are decreased because of diminished binding activity, their unbound fractions are actually increased. Several studies have suggested increased risk of miscarriage in the presence of thyroid antibodies, even in the face of a euthyroid status. Although previous studies did not demonstrate benefit in using T_4 to treat euthyroid women with recurrent spontaneous abortions,[66-68] benefit was shown by Negro and colleagues[69] in a group of 115 antibody-positive women, one half of whom received thyroxine. Treatment decreased miscarriages and prematurity by 75% and 69%, respectively. In a thoughtful accompanying editorial, Glinoer[70] stated that the statistical strength of the association between miscarriages and autoimmune thyroid disease has been largely confirmed, with a threefold increase in the overall miscarriage rate. Because there is no reason to believe that thyroxine treatment altered autoimmunity, it was thought that the subtle deficiency in thyroid hormone concentration or reduced ability of maternal thyroid function to adapt adequately in women with autoimmune thyroid disease was the main reason for the beneficial effects of thyroid hormone administration.

Radioiodine and Gonadal Function

The prevalence of infertility, premature births, miscarriage, and genetic damage in the offspring of women treated with radioactive iodine for thyrotoxicosis does not seem to be increased.[71,72] Although thyroid cancer doses of ^{131}I may be associated with subsequent menstrual irregularities, exposure to radioiodine does not appear to reduce fecundity.[73] In a study of 32 women who conceived after ^{131}I treatment for thyroid cancer (resulting in 60 term deliveries), two children conceived within a year of ^{131}I therapy had birth defects, but no anomalies were seen in the remaining 58.[74] Contraception has been recommended for 1 year after ^{131}I treatment. In a large study, Schlumberger and associates[75] obtained data on 2113 pregnancies conceived after exposure to 30 to 100 mCi of radioiodine given for thyroid cancer. The incidences of stillbirths, preterm labor, low birth weight, congenital malformations, and death during the first year of life were not significantly different between pregnancies conceived before or after radioiodine therapy. Miscarriages were more common for the women treated with ^{131}I in the year preceding conception (40%).

All women need pregnancy tests before ^{131}I treatment. Treatment late in the first trimester and in the second trimester may result in irreversible hypothyroidism in the fetus. Lactating mothers who have received diagnostic or therapeutic doses of ^{131}I should not breastfeed their infants. These topics are reviewed by Gorman[76] and Berlin.[77]

Hyperthyroidism and Pregnancy

Signs and Symptoms

The prevalence of hyperthyroidism in pregnant women ranges from 0.05% to 0.2%.[78] The signs and symptoms of mild to moderate hyperthyroidism—heat intolerance, diaphoresis, fatigue, anxiety, emotional lability, tachycardia, and a wide pulse pressure—can be mimicked by the hypermetabolic state of normal pregnancy. However, weight loss, tachycardia greater than 100 beats/min, and diffuse goiter are features that may suggest hyperthyroidism. Graves ophthalmopathy can be helpful but does not necessarily indicate active thyrotoxicosis.[79] Gastrointestinal symptoms such as severe nausea and excessive vomiting can accompany thyrotoxicosis in pregnancy, as can diarrhea, myopathy, lymphadenopathy, and congestive heart failure.

Diagnosis

Biochemical confirmation of the hyperthyroid state can be obtained through laboratory measurement of free T_4, free T_3, and TSH. Typically, elevated values of free T_4 and T_3 and greatly suppressed TSH values are found, but a normal free T_4 level can be seen in cases of T_3 toxicosis. Other laboratory features include normochromic, normocytic anemia; mild neutropenia; elevated levels of liver enzymes and alkaline phosphatase; and mild hypercalcemia. Patients may test positive for antithyroid antibodies (i.e., antithyroglobulin and antithyroid peroxidase), but they are not specific to Graves disease. TSIs are considered to be the antibodies specific to Graves disease and can be measured by bioassays or receptor assays.[80]

Differential Diagnosis

Causes of hyperthyroidism are outlined in Table 47-3. Approximately 90% to 95% of hyperthyroid pregnant women have Graves disease, and this can be diagnosed with certainty in a thyrotoxic pregnant woman who has diffuse thyromegaly with a bruit and ophthalmopathy. Whereas excess circulating thyroid hormones cause lid retraction and lid lag, proptosis and external ocular muscle palsies reflect infiltrative ophthalmopathy of Graves disease. Graves disease is an autoimmune disease mediated by antibodies (i.e., TSIs) that activate the TSH recep-

TABLE 47-3 CAUSES OF HYPERTHYROIDISM IN PREGNANCY

Graves disease
Toxic adenoma
Toxic multinodular goiter
Hyperemesis gravidarum
Gestational trophoblastic disease
TSH-producing pituitary tumor
Metastatic follicular cell carcinoma
Exogenous T_4 and T_3
De Quervain (subacute) thyroiditis
Painless lymphocytic thyroiditis
Struma ovarii

TSH, thyroid-stimulating hormone; T_3, l-triiodothyronine; T_4, l-thyroxine.

tor and stimulate the thyroid follicular cell. It affects 3% of women of reproductive age.[81]

Treatment

The outcome of treatment before pregnancy is better than that of treatment in pregnancy,[82] and hyperthyroidism is therefore best treated before conception. If untreated or treated inadequately, women may have more complications during pregnancy and delivery. Very mild cases of hyperthyroidism, with adequate weight gain and appropriate obstetric progress, may be followed carefully, but moderate or severe cases must be treated. In a retrospective study of 60 thyrotoxic pregnant women, preterm delivery, perinatal mortality, and maternal heart failure were significantly increased among women who remained thyrotoxic. Thyroid hormone status at delivery correlated directly with pregnancy outcome.[82] In another study by Momotani and Ito,[83] hyperthyroidism at conception was associated with a 25% rate of abortion and 15% rate of premature delivery, compared with 14% and 10%, respectively, for euthyroid patients. Preeclampsia has also been associated with uncontrolled hyperthyroidism.[84]

Thionamide Therapy

Thionamide therapy has been reviewed by Cooper[85] and Clark and associates.[86] The thionamides inhibit the iodination of thyroglobulin and thyroglobulin synthesis by competing with iodine for the enzyme peroxidase. Propylthiouracil (PTU) is more frequently prescribed in the United States. Carbimazole (a drug metabolized to methimazole) and methimazole itself are used often in Europe and Canada. PTU (but not methimazole) also inhibits the conversion of T_4 to T_3. The goal of therapy is to control the hyperthyroidism without causing fetal or neonatal hypothyroidism.[87] Maternal free T_4 should be maintained in the high-normal range. PTU is given every 8 hours at doses of 100 to 150 mg (300 to 450 mg total daily dosage) according to thyrotoxicosis severity. The occasional patient may require higher doses (e.g., 600 mg or more) because the risk of uncontrolled maternal hyperthyroidism is greater than that of high-dose PTU.[82] It can take 6 to 8 weeks for major clinical effects to manifest. After the patient is euthyroid (reflected by monthly free T_4 and free T_3 values), the dose of PTU should be tapered (e.g., halved), with further reduction as the pregnancy progresses. For many patients, PTU can be discontinued by 32 to 36 weeks' gestation, because remission of Graves disease during pregnancy is commonly observed, often with relapse after delivery. It has been suggested that a change from stimulatory to blocking antibody activity may contribute to this remission.[88]

Maternal side effects of PTU treatment can include rash (≈5%), pruritus, drug-related fever, hepatitis, a lupus-like syndrome, and bronchospasm. An alternative thionamide can be used, although cross-sensitivity occurs in 50% of patients. Agranulocytosis, which is the most serious side effect, develops in only 0.1%, occurring especially in older women and those receiving higher doses.[89] All patients experiencing fever or unexpected sore throat on therapy should discontinue the drug and have white blood cell count monitoring. Agranulocytosis is a contraindication to further thionamide therapy; the blood count gradually improves over days or weeks.

Methimazole is not used in the United States. Although the transplacental passage is similar,[90] methimazole may cause cutis aplasia, a scalp deformity.[91-93] Although rare, there are reports of methimazole and carbimazole embryopathy, with choanal atresia, tracheoesophageal fistula, and facial anomalies.[94-97]

The risks of untreated hyperthyroidism need to be considered in relation to the risk of antithyroid medications. They appear to relate directly to the control and severity of the hyperthyroidism. In a study of hyperthyroid pregnant women, the odds ratio for low birth weight was 2.4 for those treated during pregnancy and 9.2 for those uncontrolled during pregnancy compared with a group who was euthyroid and remained so. Similarly, prematurity was more common in the hyperthyroid group; the odds ratio was 2.8 for the controlled group and 16.5 for the uncontrolled group. Similar findings related to preeclampsia, with an odds ratio of 4.7 for the controlled group.[84] This was confirmed by a later study.[98] In other reports, higher frequencies of small-for-gestational-age births, congestive heart failure, and stillbirths have been found.[82,99] It is uncertain whether untreated Graves disease is associated with a higher frequency of congenital malformation.[87,100]

Infants of mothers receiving thionamides should be evaluated ultrasonographically for signs of hypothyroidism, such as goiter, bradycardia, and intrauterine growth restriction. If needed, cordocentesis may be performed and fetal thyroid function determined; reference ranges have been reported.[101] Doses of PTU should be adjusted to keep free T_4 level in the upper normal range and TSH level less than 0.5 mU/L during pregnancy to avoid hypothyroidism in the fetus. PTU often can be stopped in late gestation.

PTU is not significantly concentrated in breast milk (10% of serum) and does not appear to affect the infant's thyroid hormone levels in any major way. Methimazole also does not appear to affect subsequent somatic or intellectual growth in children exposed to it during lactation.[87,102,103] Antithyroid medication should be taken just after breastfeeding, allowing a 3- to 4-hour interval before the woman lactates again.

β-Blockers

β-Blockers are useful for the control of adrenergic symptoms, particularly maternal heart rate. Propranolol is commonly used in doses of 20 to 40 mg two or three times daily, and it inhibits T_4 to T_3 conversion. Alternatively, atenolol (50 to 100 mg daily) may be used, and in an emergency, esmolol, an ultra-short-acting cardioselective intravenous β-blocker, has been used successfully.[104] Prolonged therapy with β-blockers can be associated with intrauterine growth restriction, fetal bradycardia, and hypoglycemia.

Iodides

Iodides decrease circulating T_4 and T_3 levels by up to 50% within 10 days by acutely inhibiting the release of stored hormone. Their use is appropriate in combination with thionamides (which should be started before the iodide) and β-blockers in patients with severe thyrotoxicosis or thyroid storm. Potassium iodide (SSKI, 5 drops every 8 hours) is given. Sodium ipodate, a radiographic contrast agent, is an alternative and has the added benefit of inhibiting conversion of T_4 to T_3. Its safety in pregnancy has not been documented.

Because iodides cross the placenta readily, they should be used for no longer than 2 weeks, or fetal goiter can result. Inadvertent use of iodides also follows use of Betadine cleansing solutions, iodine-containing bronchodilators, and the drug amiodarone.

^{131}I thyroid ablation is contraindicated in pregnancy because the radioactive iodine is concentrated in the fetal thyroid after 10 to 12 weeks' gestation. If a woman inadvertently receives ^{131}I during pregnancy, SSKI should be given immediately, along with PTU, to block organification and reduce radiation exposure to the fetal thyroid by a factor of 100 and to the fetal whole body by a factor of 10. To be of benefit, SSKI and PTU treatment must be given within 7 to 10 days of exposure.[76]

Surgery

In select cases of thyrotoxicosis with severe complications or noncompliance, surgery can be performed in the pregnant patient. Two weeks of low-dose iodine therapy, such as one or two drops of SSKI daily, can reduce gland vascularity preoperatively. Surgery is best performed in the second trimester, although it can be done in the first or third trimester.[105] The risks are those of anesthesia, hypoparathyroidism, and recurrent laryngeal nerve paralysis.

Thyroid Storm

Thyroid storm is a life-threatening exacerbation of thyrotoxicosis. Criteria for its diagnosis have been introduced,[106] and the classic findings are various degrees of thermoregulatory dysfunction, central nervous system effects (e.g., agitation, delirium, coma), gastrointestinal dysfunction, and cardiovascular problems manifesting as tachycardia or heart failure. For example, a patient with a temperature of 102°F who is agitated and tachycardic with a pulse rate exceeding 130 beats/min would be diagnosed with thyroid storm. Although rare in pregnancy, it may be seen and can be precipitated by labor and delivery, cesarean section, infection, or preeclampsia.[107] Thyrotoxic cardiomyopathy may also lead to heart failure in pregnancy.[108] Intensive care treatment with fluid and nutritional support is necessary for thyroid storm and heart failure. A loading dose of PTU of 600 mg may be given orally or through a nasogastric tube, and 200 to 300 mg of PTU is continued every 6 hours. An hour after the initial dose of PTU, iodine is given as five drops of SSKI every 8 hours (or 500 to 1000 mg of intravenous sodium iodide every 8 hours) to inhibit thyroid hormone release. If the patient is iodine allergic, lithium (300 mg every 6 hours) is an alternative. Dexamethasone (2 mg every 6 hours) is also given to block T_4 to T_3 conversion. For tachycardia exceeding 120 beats/min, β-blockers such as propranolol, labetalol, or esmolol may be used.[1] Table 47-4 summarizes the management of thyroid storm.

Subclinical Hyperthyroidism

Subclinical hyperthyroidism, as defined by suppressed TSH and normal free T_4 and free T_3 levels, is also seen in pregnancy. In a study by Casey and associates,[109] 1.7% of women screened had subclinical hyperthyroidism, which they defined as TSH values at or below the 2.5th percentile for gestational age and a free T_4 level of 1.75 ng/dL or less. Pregnancy complications, morbidity, and mortality were not increased among these women, and it was recommended that treatment in pregnancy was unwarranted.

Fetal and Neonatal Hyperthyroidism

The topic of fetal and neonatal hyperthyroidism has been reviewed by Zimmerman.[110] Hyperthyroidism in fetuses and neonates is usually produced by transplacental passage of TSIs. Although they are a common component of active Graves disease, the antibodies can continue to be present in the maternal circulation after surgical (Fig. 47-5) or radioactive iodine ablation or even in patients with Hashimoto thyroiditis. Fetal hyperthyroidism occurs when TSIs cross the placenta and activate the fetal thyroid; this occurs in 1% of infants born to these women.

Maternal TSI levels in excess of 300% of control values are predictive of fetal hyperthyroidism[99] and should be measured at 28 to 30 weeks. The assay used should be a functional one, because TSH-receptor antibodies are heterogeneous and can stimulate or block the TSH receptor.[99,111] Neonatal syndromes have been caused by transplacental passage of stimulating and blocking antibodies.[112]

Fetal Thyrotoxicosis

Features of fetal thyrotoxicosis include a heart rate greater than 160 beats/min, growth retardation, advanced bone age, and craniosynostosis, all of which can be detected by ultrasound examination.[113] Occasionally, nonimmune fetal hydrops and fetal death occur with associated diminished subcutaneous fat and thyroid enlargement. In utero, most cases are likely treated by the PTU given to the mother. This problem can arise if the mother is euthyroid but has elevated levels of TSIs.[114] Cordocentesis can be used for diagnosis and for monitoring therapy. A combination of PTU and T_4 treats the fetal hyperthyroidism while keeping the mother euthyroid.

Neonatal Thyrotoxicosis

Features of thyrotoxicosis in the neonate include hyperkinesis, diarrhea, poor weight gain, vomiting, exophthalmos, arrhythmias, cardiac failure, hypertension (systemic and pulmonary), hepatosplenomegaly,

TABLE 47-4 TREATMENT OF THYROID STORM

Treatment	Rationale and Cautions	Dosage
General care	Intensive management achieved with intravenous fluid hydration and nutritional support	
Propylthiouracil		Initial: 600 mg orally or crushed and given by NG tube Maintenance: 200-300 mg every 6 hr given orally or by NG tube
Iodide	Initial dose to be given 1 hr after start of PTU	5 drops of supersaturated solution of potassium iodide every 8 hr *or* 500-1000 mg of intravenous sodium iodide infusion every 12 hr
Lithium carbonate	Used if patient is allergic to iodine	300 mg every 6 hr
Dexamethasone	Given to block T_4 to T_3 conversion	2 mg every 6 hr for four doses
β-Blockers	Given to control tachycardia ≥ 120 beats/min (use cautiously if patient in heart failure)	IV propranolol at 1 mg/min up to several doses until blockade is achieved and concurrent 60 mg of propranolol (PO or NG tube) every 6 hours *or* IV loading dose of 250-500 μg/kg of esmolol, followed by infusion at 50-100 μg/kg/min

IV, intravenous; NG, nasogastric; PO, orally; PTU, propylthiouracil.

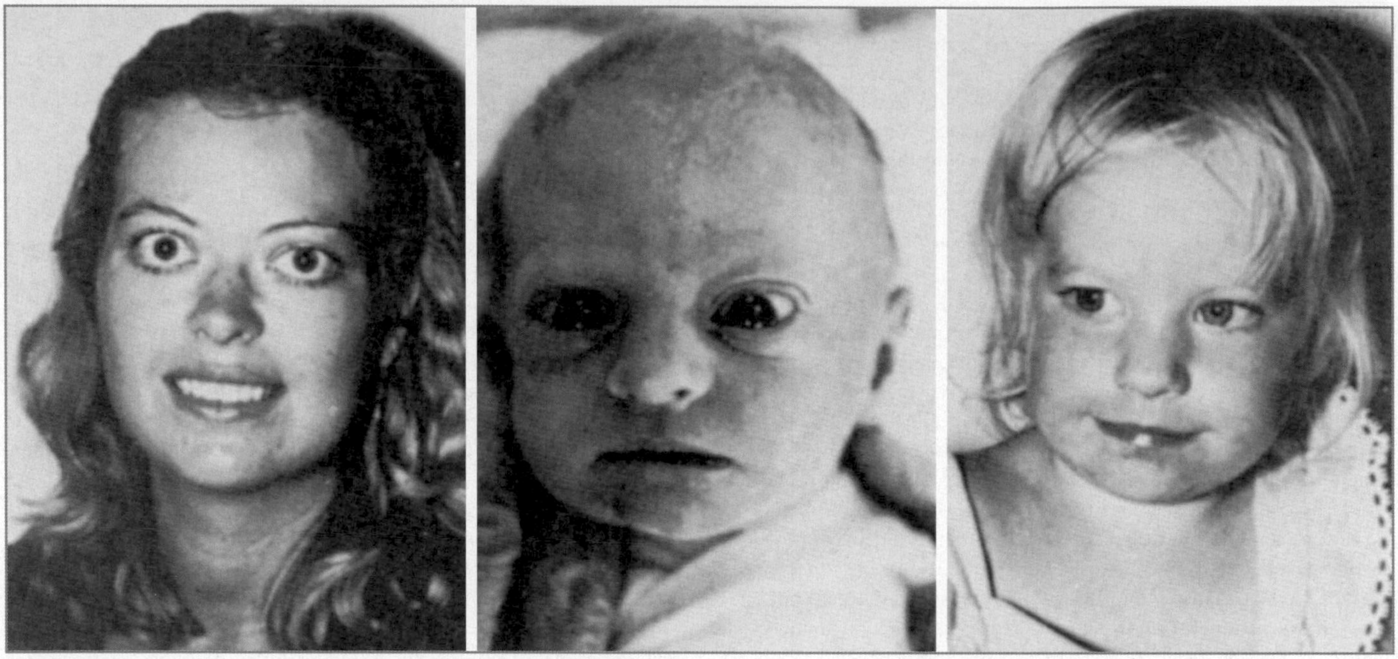

FIGURE 47-5 Graves disease. **A,** Hypothyroid 21-year-old woman who developed Graves disease at age 7 was treated by subtotal thyroidectomy. She was given maintenance therapy with thyroid hormone (0.15 mg of Synthroid) throughout pregnancy. **B,** Her daughter was born at term with severe Graves disease, goiter, and exophthalmos that persisted for 6 months. **C,** The child was normal at 20 months old.

thrombocytopenia, and craniosynostosis. The infant should be examined immediately after birth. Cord blood reflects the in utero environment, and by day 2 of life, the maternal antithyroid drug effects have receded. Affected neonates are treated with PTU, β-blockers, iodine, and glucocorticoids and digoxin, as needed. Ipodate may be preferable because it blocks T_4 to T_3 conversion. Remission by 20 weeks is common, and it usually occurs by 48 weeks; occasionally, there is persistent disease when there is a strong family history of Graves disease.

Other mechanisms of fetal and neonatal hyperthyroidism include activating mutations of the stimulatory G protein in McCune-Albright syndrome and activating mutations of the TSH receptor.[115,116]

Hyperthyroidism Related to Human Chorionic Gonadotropin

When hyperthyroidism is diagnosed during the first trimester, the physician has a challenging differential diagnosis, usually that of Graves disease versus hCG-mediated hyperthyroidism. The hCG has TSH-like stimulatory activity, which can result in overproduction of thyroid hormone when the concentrations are high or when there is a change in its molecular structure. Molecular variants of hCG with increased thyrotropic potency include basic molecules with reduced sialic acid content, truncated molecules lacking the C-terminal tail, or molecules in which the 47-48 peptide bond in the β-subunit loop is nicked.[117] This relationship is further complicated by differences in clearance rates of different hCG glycoforms.[118] In vivo thyrotropic activity is regulated by the glycoforms and the plasma half-life.

The hCG concentrations peak at 6 to 12 weeks and then decline to a plateau after 18 to 20 weeks. The stimulation of thyroid hormone production can suppress the TSH to low or suppressed values in up to 20% of normal pregnancies. Twin pregnancies can be associated with biochemical hyperthyroidism,[9] as may pregnancies complicated by trophoblastic disease. Several clinical scenarios can arise and are described in the following sections.

Gestational Transient Thyrotoxicosis

Gestational transient thyrotoxicosis (GTT) occurs in the first trimester in women without a personal or family history of autoimmune disease. It results directly from hCG stimulation of the thyroid. Glinoer and colleagues[8] found an overall prevalence of GTT in 2.4% in a prospective cohort study between 8 and 14 weeks' gestation. Symptoms compatible with thyrotoxicosis were often present, and elevated free T_4 concentrations were found. The GTT was transient, paralleled the decline in hCG, and usually did not require treatment. The thyroid gland was not enlarged. Occasionally, β-blockers were used. GTT was not associated with a less favorable outcome of pregnancy.

Hyperemesis Gravidarum

Hyperemesis gravidarum is a serious pregnancy complication associated with weight loss and severe dehydration, often necessitating hospitalization.[119] Biochemical hyperthyroidism is found in most women with this condition.[120,121] Whereas Goodwin and colleagues[120,121] found that the severity of disease varied directly with the hCG concentration, Wilson and associates[122] did not find such a correlation. As in the case of GTT, certain hCG fractions may be more important than total hCG as thyroid stimulators.[123] The duration of the hyperthyroidism varies widely from 1 to 10 weeks but is usually self-limited. Vomiting and normalization of T_4 levels occur by 20 weeks, though TSH may remain suppressed a little longer. Treatment is usually supportive, with correction of dehydration, antiemetics, and occasionally, parenteral nutrition. The vomiting may not be controlled by normalization of

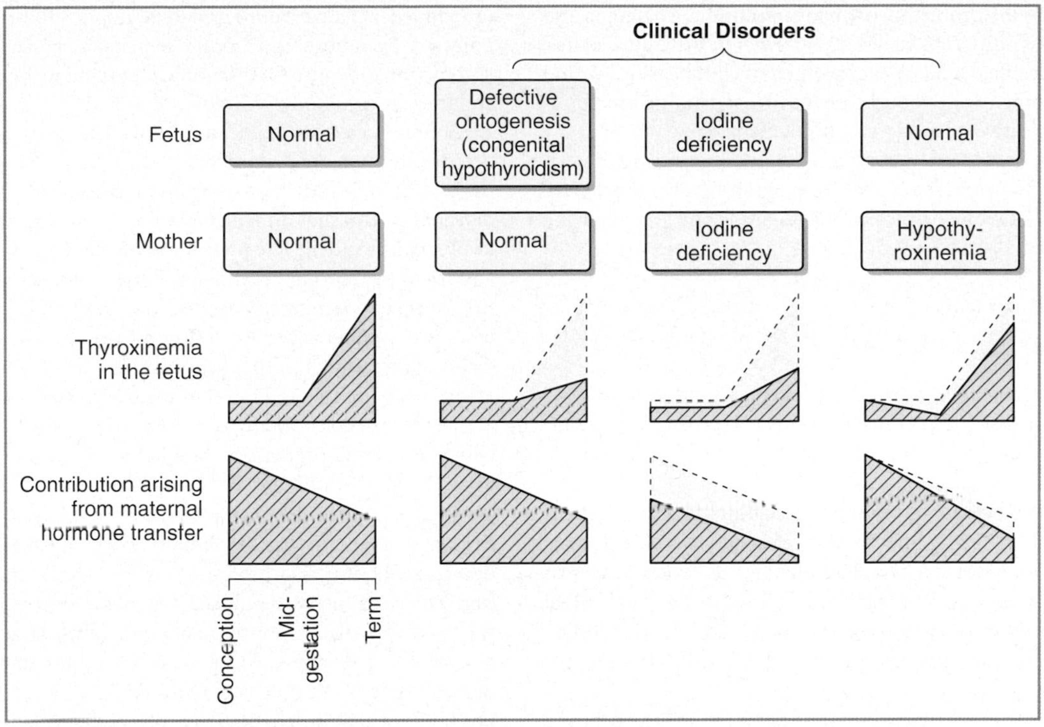

FIGURE 47-6 Thyroid function disorders. Schematic representation of the three sets of clinical conditions that can affect thyroid function in the mother alone, in the fetus alone, or in the fetomaternal unit shows the relative contributions of impaired maternal or fetal thyroid function that may eventually lead to alterations in fetal thyroxinemia. (Reprinted by permission from Glinoer D, Delange F: The potential repercussions of maternal, fetal and neonatal hypothyroxinemia on the progeny. Thyroid 10:871, 2000.)

thyroid hormones. In patients who require treatment, PTU therapy can be attempted if tolerated; methimazole suppositories can also be used.

Gestational Trophoblastic Disease

Both hydatidiform mole and choriocarcinoma can be associated with hCG levels that are greater than 1000 times normal and thus can cause hyperthyroidism (biochemically seen in approximately 50% of such women). The thyroid is usually not enlarged. Treatment of the hydatidiform mole or choriocarcinoma restores thyroid function to normal. Treatment with antithyroid drugs and β-blockers is frequently necessary, however, before surgical treatment of the mole.[124]

Recurrent Gestational Hyperthyroidism

Cases of recurrent gestational hyperthyroidism have been described.[125,126] In the case described by Rodien and colleages,[126] the hyperthyroidism was caused by a mutant TSH receptor that was hypersensitive to hCG.

Other Causes of Hyperthyroidism

Much less common causes of hyperthyroidism include thyrotoxicosis factitia (i.e., ingestion of exogenous hormone surreptitiously); in such cases, serum thyroglobulin, which is produced by the thyroid, is suppressed.[127] Women with large nodular goiters may have hyperthyroidism from autonomously functioning nodules within such goiters. Alternatively, women can have hyperthyroidism from a single toxic adenoma. If either of these entities is diagnosed during pregnancy, the correct treatment is control of hyperthyroidism with antithyroid drugs until definitive treatment (i.e., surgery or radioactive iodine) can be administered after delivery.

Even less common causes of hyperthyroidism in pregnancy are listed in Table 47-3. They include TSH-producing pituitary tumors, metastatic follicular thyroid cancer, viral (de Quervain) thyroiditis, and struma ovarii, which is an ovarian dermoid tumor in which more than 50% of the neoplasm consists of thyroid tissue.

Iodine Deficiency, Hypothyroidism, and Pregnancy

A schematic representation of the clinical conditions that can affect thyroid function in the mother, fetus, or fetomaternal unit is provided in Figure 47-6. Although iodine deficiency is rare in the United States, it is a common cause of maternal, fetal, and neonatal hypothyroidism in the world, where 1 to 1.5 billion are at risk and 500 million live in areas of overt iodine deficiency. Worldwide, it is the most common cause of mental retardation.

In the past few decades, the physiology of maternal and fetal iodine metabolism, thyroid hormone metabolism, and fetal brain development and the pathophysiology of iodine deficiency have been unraveled. These findings have revealed a fascinating aspect of pregnancy physiology. Iodine deficiency and hypothyroidism in pregnancy continue to be a worldwide problem worthy of resolution. This topic also has been a subject of numerous reviews.[128-131] Even in the United States, iodine intake has declined, and 15% of women of childbearing age and 7% of pregnant women were found to have urinary iodine excretions below 50 µg/L, indicative of moderate iodine deficiency.[132]

Pregnancy is an environmental trigger for the thyroid machinery, inducing changes in people who live in geographic areas that have iodine deficiency. Four biochemical markers are useful for following the changes induced:

1. Relative hypothyroxinemia
2. Preferential T_3 secretion as reflected by an elevated T_3/T_4 molar ratio
3. Increased TSH after the first trimester, progressing until term
4. Supranormal thyroglobulin concentrations correlating with gestational goitrogenesis

Goitrogenesis also occurs in the fetus, indicating the exquisite sensitivity of the fetal thyroid gland to the consequences of maternal iodine deficiency. This process can start during the earliest stages of fetal thyroid development. It occurs against a background of low initial maternal intrathyroidal iodine stores, the increased need for iodine after pregnancy occurs, and the insufficiency of iodine intake throughout the gestation.

It appears that maternal thyroxine, traversing the placenta during the first trimester and subsequently, is necessary for fetal brain development. Even before fetal thyroid hormone synthesis, T_3 receptors are found in fetal brain tissues, and local conversion of T_4 to T_3 can occur. Iodine deficiency perpetuates the process, because the fetus is less able to synthesize thyroid hormones even when the fetal thyroid has developed.

In severe iodine deficiency (intake of 20 to 25 µg/day), a condition known as endemic cretinism occurs, with a prevalence up to 15% in severely affected populations. These infants are characterized by severe mental retardation with a neurologic picture including deaf-mutism, squint, and pyramidal and extrapyramidal syndromes. There are few clinical signs of thyroid failure. A remarkable exception to this picture has emerged from Africa, where the cretins have less mental retardation and less in the way of neurologic deficits. The clinical picture is that of severe thyroid failure with dwarfism, delayed sexual maturation, and myxedema. Thyroid function is grossly impaired.

The consensus is that the neurologic picture of endemic cretinism results from insults to the developing brain, occurring perhaps during the first trimester (in the case of deafness) and mostly during the second trimester, with the cerebellar abnormalities resulting from postnatal insult. This is supported by the observation that the full picture can be prevented only when the iodine deficiency is corrected before the second trimester and, optimally, even before conception.[133] In Africa, iodine deficiency is complicated by selenium deficiency. The deficiency of selenium leads to accumulation of peroxide, and excess peroxide leads to destruction of thyroid cells and hypothyroidism.[134] Selenium deficiency also induces monodeiodinase I (a selenoenzyme) deficiency, resulting in reduced T_4 to T_3 conversion and increased availability of maternal T_4 for the fetal brain. This protective mechanism may prevent the development of neurologic cretinism, and the combined iodine-selenium deficiency prevalent in Africa may help explain the predominance of the myxedematous type observed there.

The neurologic abnormalities and mental retardation depend ultimately on the timing and severity of the brain insult. Endemic cretinism constitutes only the extreme expression of the spectrum of physical and intellectual abnormalities. In a meta-analysis of 18 studies in areas of iodine deficiency, it appeared to be responsible for an IQ loss of 13.5 points.[135] Even borderline iodine deficiency, as seen in Europe, can be accompanied by impaired school achievements by apparently normal children, as reviewed by Glinoer.[129]

Actions taken to eradicate iodine deficiency have prevented the occurrence of mental retardation in millions of infants throughout the world. In a study by Xue-Yi and coauthors[136] of a severely iodine-deficient area of the Xinjiang region of China, iodine was administered to pregnant women. The prevalence of moderate or severe neurologic abnormalities among 120 infants whose mothers received iodine in the first or second trimester was 2%, compared with 9% (of 952 infants) when the mothers received iodine in the third trimester (P = .008). Although treatment in the third trimester did not improve neurologic status, head growth and developmental quotients improved slightly.

The importance of thyroid hormone to fetal and neonatal well-being and development was highlighted by a remarkable case of an infant born to a mother with strongly positive TSH receptor-blocking antibodies. The mother was profoundly hypothyroid when tested after delivery. The infant was delivered by cesarean section because of bradycardia. She was also profoundly hypothyroid and required intubation. Her brain size was reduced, and her auditory brainstem response was absent at age 2 months. The audiogram at age 4 years revealed sensorineural deafness. At age 6 years, motor development was the same as at age 4 months. She required T_4 for 8 months until the antibody effect had worn off. Her physical growth was normal. The outcome of severe thyroid hormone deficiency in utero was fetal distress, permanent auditory deficit, brain atrophy, and severely impaired neuromotor development despite adequate neonatal treatment.[137]

The Institute of Medicine of the National Academy of Sciences has set the iodine requirement as 110 µg for infants 0 to 6 months, 130 µg for infants 7 to 12 months, 90 µg for children 1 to 8 years, 120 µg for those 9 to 13 years, and 150 µg for those older than 13 years. The recommended intake for pregnancy and lactation is 200 µg/day. Even higher intakes (300 to 400 µg/day) have been suggested.[138]

Hypothyroidism

Signs and Symptoms

Hypothyroidism occurs with a frequency of 1 case in 1600 to 2000 deliveries.[67] Population screening studies have revealed a higher incidence. In a study in the United States, serum TSH levels were determined in 2000 women between gestational weeks 15 to 18; 49 (2.5%) had TSH levels greater than or equal to 6 mU/L, and positive thyroid antibodies were found in 58% of these 49 women, compared with 11% of control euthyroid pregnant women.[139] In a Japanese study, only 0.29% had an elevated TSH level.[140] In another U.S. study, 1 infant in 1629 deliveries had hypothyroidism.[141]

Women with hypothyroidism have higher pregnancy complication rates. As well as miscarriages, complications include preeclampsia, placental abruption, low birth weight, prematurity, and stillbirths.[142] These outcomes can be improved with early therapy. Gestational hypertension is also more common.[141]

The symptoms of hypothyroidism are insidious and can be masked by the hypermetabolic state of pregnancy. Symptoms can include modest weight gain, decrease in exercise capacity, lethargy, and intolerance to cold. In moderately symptomatic patients, constipation, hoarseness, hair loss, brittle nails, and dry skin also can occur. Physical signs may include a goiter, a thyroidectomy scar, and delay in the relaxation phase of deep tendon reflexes.

Laboratory confirmation is obtained from an elevated TSH level, with or without suppressed free T_4. Test results for thyroid autoantibodies (antithyroglobulin and antithyroid peroxidase) may be positive. Other laboratory abnormalities can include elevated levels of creatine phosphokinase, cholesterol, and carotene and liver function abnormalities. Patients may have macrocytic or normochromic, normocytic anemia. Hypothyroidism may occur more frequently in pregnant women with type 1 diabetes, and T_4 replacement therapy can increase insulin requirements.[143]

Differential Diagnosis

Hashimoto thyroiditis, also known as chronic lymphocytic thyroiditis, an autoimmune disease, is the most common cause of hypothyroidism and can occur in 8% to 10% of women of reproductive age. It is characterized by the presence of antithyroid antibodies, and the patient may have a goiter. Titers of antithyroglobulin are elevated in 50% to 70% of patients, and almost all have antithyroid peroxidase antibodies.[53] The goiter is firm and diffusely enlarged and painless, and the gland is infiltrated by lymphocytes and plasma cells. Many patients with Hashimoto thyroiditis are actually euthyroid but can subsequently develop hypothyroidism. The thyroid gland can be atrophic and the test result for antibodies negative—so-called idiopathic hypothyroidism. Patients with other autoimmune disease also can develop Hashimoto thyroiditis.

Other important and common causes of hypothyroidism include ^{131}I therapy, ablation for Graves disease, and thyroidectomy (e.g., for thyroid cancer). Of patients who receive ^{131}I therapy, 10% to 20% are hypothyroid within the first 6 months, and 2% to 4% become hypothyroid each year thereafter.[144] Hypothyroidism can result from subacute viral thyroiditis and, much less commonly, from suppurative thyroiditis.

Drugs known to inhibit the synthesis of thyroid hormones include thionamide, iodides, and lithium. Carbamazepine, phenytoin, and rifampin can increase thyroid clearance. Aluminum hydroxide, cholestyramine, and, most important, ferrous sulfate and sucralfate can interfere with the intestinal absorption of thyroxine.

Hypothyroidism resulting from hypothalamic or pituitary disease is rare but can occur in the setting of pituitary tumors, after pituitary surgery or irradiation, and in Sheehan's syndrome and lymphocytic hypophysitis, an autoimmune disease with a predilection for women, especially in the setting of pregnancy (see Chapter 48). In secondary hypothyroidism, the TSH level may be low or normal, but the free T_4 level is low.

Treatment

Hypothyroidism must be treated promptly, and a dose of 0.1 to 0.15 mg of T_4 per day, should be initiated. The dose is adjusted every 4 weeks until the TSH concentration is in the lower end of the normal range. In women with little or no functioning thyroid tissue, a dose of 2 μg/kg/day may be required. Women who are euthyroid on T_4 need to be checked as soon as pregnancy is established; the dose should be adjusted and rechecked in 4 to 8 weeks,[145] because the requirements for thyroid hormone increase as early as the fifth week of gestation. Alternatively, the patient can be instructed to increase her dose by one extra dose per week and be checked a few weeks later. The amount of dose increase may depend on the cause. For example, women who have had total thyroidectomy may need a greater increase than women with mild hypothyroidism. Increased dosage requirements may plateau by the 20th week,[145] but the need for increased dosage may be seen as late as the third trimester in about one third of patients.[2] In a study of 12 pregnant women with hypothyroidism, 9 required a higher T_4 dose, with a mean dose increase of 45%.[146] In a review of 77 pregnancies in 65 hypothyroid women, serum TSH levels became abnormal in 70% of women with prior ^{131}I ablation therapy and in 47% of women with chronic thyroiditis. When data from other studies were pooled, overall, TSH levels increased above normal in 45% with a mean daily thyroxine dose of 146 μg.[147,148] It was estimated that the increment in dose could be predicted according to the TSH value at the first evaluation. The TSH concentration should be determined again 4 to 6 weeks after dose adjustment.

The causes of increased T_4 requirements include a real increased demand for T_4 in pregnancy[149] in patients whose thyroid reserve is compromised and, in some cases, iron therapy. Ferrous sulfate interferes with T_4 absorption and should be taken at a different time of day from thyroxine therapy.[150] Patients with thyroid cancer whose target TSH concentration is below the normal range almost uniformly require an increased dose to maintain their suppressed TSH levels, and they should be followed closely.[150] After delivery, the dose should be reduced to pre-pregnancy levels in all patients, and the TSH concentration should be measured 6 to 8 weeks later.

The topic of thyroid hormone and intellectual development has received widespread publicity and has been the subject of articles and reviews in the past few years.[128,151,152] In 1969, Man and Jones[153] studied a cohort of 1349 children and concluded that mild maternal hypothyroidism alone was associated with lower IQ levels in the offspring. In 1990, Matsuura and Konishi[154] documented that fetal brain development is affected adversely when both mother and fetus have hypothyroidism caused by chronic autoimmune thyroiditis. With the background of this information and the associations of iodine deficiency, its consequent maternal hypothyroxinemia, and abnormal fetal brain development, Haddow and associates[151] conducted a study measuring TSH levels from stored samples in more than 25,000 pregnant women. They located 62 women with high TSH levels and 124 matched women with normal values. Their 7- to 9-year-old children, none of whom had hypothyroidism as newborns, underwent 15 tests relating to intelligence, attention, language, reading ability, school performance, and visual-motor performance. The full-scale IQ in children of hypothyroid women was 4 points lower ($P = .06$); 15% had scores of 85 or less compared with 5% of controls. The IQ of the children of 48 women whose hypothyroidism was not treated averaged 7 points lower than the 124 controls ($P = .005$), and 19% had scores of 85 or lower. The researchers concluded that undiagnosed hypothyroidism can affect fetuses adversely and recommended screening for hypothyroidism in pregnancy. Fukushi and coworkers[155] reported on such screening in Japan and found hypothyroidism in 1 of 692 pregnancies.

In a study by Pop and colleagues,[156] even the presence of antithyroid peroxidase antibodies in the maternal circulation was shown to have deleterious effects on child development. In two similar studies, thyroid antibody–positive women had lower free T_4 levels, and lower scores on psychomotor tests were found in children of mothers whose free T_4 value was below the 5th and 10th percentiles as measured at 12 weeks' gestation.[157,158]

Subclinical Hypothyroidism and Hypothyroxinemia

Subclinical hypothyroidism is defined as an elevated TSH level when the free T_4 level is in the normal range. More than 90% of hypothyroidism diagnosed in pregnancy is subclinical. Its estimated prevalence in the general population is between 4% and 8.5%. The prevalence in pregnancy was 2.3% in a study of more than 17,000 women enrolled for prenatal care at 20 weeks' gestation or less.[159] In this study, pregnancies in patients with subclinical hypothyroidism were three times more likely to be complicated by placental abruption, and the rate of preterm birth (i.e., delivery at or before 34 weeks) was almost twofold higher.

Hypothyroidism has been associated with impaired neurodevelopment of the fetus.[151] However, most of the patients in this study had a TSH level of 10 mU/L or greater, and most had a low free T_4 level; that is, they had overt rather than subclinical hypothyroidism. Nonetheless, this study has prompted rigorous debate on the merits of universal screening of all pregnant women. The nuances of this debate were carefully addressed by Casey.[160] Although a panel from the American Thyroid Association, the Endocrine Society, and the American Association of Clinical Endocrinologists did not find sufficient evidence to recommend routine screening in pregnancy in 2003, leaders of the same societies later published a consensus statement, recommending screening and treatment.[161] The American College of Obstetricians and Gynecologists (ACOG) suggests it is premature to recommend universal screening for hypothyroidism, because efficacy of treatment has not been demonstrated. The ACOG and the various endocrine associations recommend TSH measurements in women with a family history of thyroid disease, prior thyroid dysfunction, symptoms of hypothyroidism, an abnormal thyroid gland, type 1 diabetes, or personal history of autoimmune disease. However, targeting high-risk cases may miss significant numbers with hypothyroidism, as was shown by Vaidya and coworkers.[162] The investigators evaluated more than 1500 consecutive pregnancies and found increased TSH levels in 40 women (2.6%). Although the prevalence of high TSH levels was higher in the high-risk group (6.8% versus 1% in low-risk patients), 30% of women with high TSH levels were in the low-risk group.

Isolated maternal hypothyroxinemia (i.e., low free T_4 and normal TSH levels) during early pregnancy has been associated with impaired neurodevelopment of the fetus.[158,163] The issue of detecting and treating isolated maternal hypothyroxinemia is an area of equal uncertainty. Unfortunately, assays of true free T_4 (e.g., equilibrium dialysis, ultrafiltration, gel filtration) are expensive and labor intensive. Clinical laboratories use a variety of tests that estimate the free hormone concentrations in the presence of protein-bound hormone, and they are binding protein dependent to some extent. This negatively affects the accuracy of free hormone assays.[164] Free T_4 assays usually result in lower values in late pregnancy.[165,166] Nonetheless, in a "Clinical Perspectives" article in the *Journal of Clinical Endocrinology and Metabolism*, Morreale de Escobar and colleagues[167] made a compelling case for screening pregnant women for hypothyroxinemia, pointing out that maternal T_4 (as opposed to T_3) is the required substrate for the ontogenetically regulated production of T_3 in the amounts needed for optimal temporal and spatial development in different brain structures. This issue is important for women with relative iodine deficiency, because T_3 is preferentially synthesized.

To address these dilemmas, the National Institute of Child Health and Human Development Maternal-Fetal Medicine Units Network initiated a randomized trial of T_4 treatment for subclinical hypothyroidism or hypothyroxinemia diagnosed during pregnancy. The primary end point is the intellectual function of the children and secondary end points include determination of the frequency of pregnancy complications, including preterm delivery, preeclampsia, abruption, and stillbirth.

What do we do in the meantime? In an editorial by Brent[67] accompanying the paper on low-risk versus high-risk case finding, it was felt that until the results of large, randomized trials become available, the extant evidence supports the benefits of T_4 therapy, at least to reduce pregnancy loss and preterm delivery.[69] This view was also held and previously stated by Larsen.[168] I recommend screening at least high-risk women (as defined by ACOG and others) for TSH and free T_4 levels. Subclinical hypothyroidism should be treated with thyroxine. Adequate iodine intake should be ensured in those with isolated hypothyroxinemia and treatment with thyroxine initiated if the hypothyroxinemia does not resolve. I also recommend screening patients who have delivered or had a miscarriage within 1 year of the index pregnancy, because postpartum or postmiscarriage thyroid disease is commonly found in the general population.

Fetal and Neonatal Hypothyroidism

The relationship between iodine deficiency and fetal development was previously discussed. Severe neurologic deficits also occur in children with congenital deficiency of thyroid hormone unrelated to iodine deficiency. Neurologic development is impaired if infants are untreated before they are 3 months old. Screening of neonates for thyroid hormone deficiency is mandatory in some states, and with early therapy, their development is reasonably normal.[29] Causes include thyroid agenesis and inborn errors of metabolism, such as peroxidase deficiency. Congenital pituitary and hypothalamic hypothyroidism also occur but are rare. Thyroid hormone deficiency can result from maternal blocking antibodies that are transferred to the fetus and that block TSH action or thyroid growth and development.[169,170]

Gruner and associates[171] reported a case of fetal goitrous hypothyroidism in which fetal TSH levels were determined on three occasions by cordocentesis to monitor weekly intra-amniotic administration of T_4. This therapy was initiated to reduce the fetal goiter and polyhydramnios (which it did) and to aid in fetal neurologic development. They also reviewed other reported cases of such therapy and concluded that the optimal dose of T_4 necessary to correct hypothyroidism could more accurately be determined by cordocentesis than by measurement of amniotic fluid hormone concentrations.

Thyroid Nodules, Malignant Tumors, and Nontoxic Goiter in Pregnancy

Thyroid tumors are the most common endocrine neoplasms. Most nodules are benign hyperplastic (or colloid) nodules, but between 5% and 20% are true neoplasms, which are benign follicular adenomas or carcinomas of follicular or parafollicular (C) cell origin. Nodular thyroid disease is common, especially in women. A prospective study found that the incidence of incipient thyroid nodules increased from 15% in the first trimester to 24% after delivery, with an increase in the growth of existing nodules.[172] There is no evidence that thyroid cancer arises more frequently in pregnancy.

When a solitary or a dominant nodule is found within the thyroid, biopsy is recommended. Cytopathologic diagnosis of fine-needle aspiration biopsy (FNAB) in women between the ages of 15 and 40 years seen at the Mayo Clinic revealed benign findings in 64% and suspicious findings in 12%; FNAB was positive for cancer in 7% and nondiagnostic in 17%.[173] The topic of nodular thyroid disease in pregnancy was also reviewed. During a 10-year period, 40 pregnant women were evaluated at the Mayo Clinic, and 39 had FNAB, 95% of which were diagnostic.[174] Most (64%) were benign. Three (8%) were positive for papillary thyroid cancer, and nine (23%) were suspicious for papillary cancer or a follicular (Hurthle cell) neoplasm. Comparable findings were reported by others.[175]

The principles of nodular thyroid disease diagnosis in pregnancy resemble those for nonpregnant women. Serum TSH and free T_4 levels should be obtained, and an FNAB should be performed on dominant nodules. Radionucleotide scanning is contraindicated, but ultrasound is often performed and can demonstrate other nodules, lymphadenopathy, or abnormal calcification. FNAB is safe in pregnancy and can be performed at any stage. If a nodule is benign, ultrasound can monitor growth of the nodule during pregnancy. If the nodule is suspicious for a follicular or Hurthle cell neoplasm, it usually represents a 10% to 15% risk of malignancy. It is generally recommended that surgery be performed after delivery, but if a malignancy is diagnosed in early pregnancy, surgery may be performed in the second trimester for the patient needing reassurance. If the FNAB result is positive or suspicious for papillary thyroid cancer, the risk is high (50% for suspicious and 100% for positive), and neck exploration should be performed at the soonest safe date. Figure 47-7 outlines the decision-making process.

The impact of pregnancy on papillary thyroid cancer was evaluated by Moosa and Mazzaferri.[176] They compared outcomes in pregnant and nonpregnant women and found no difference in the rates of recurrence, distant spread, or cause-specific mortality. Outcomes were similar when neck surgery was performed during or after pregnancy. A similar conclusion was reached in a study of thyroid cancer cases from the New Mexico Tumor Registry.[177] If medullary thyroid cancer is suspected, early surgery is advised.

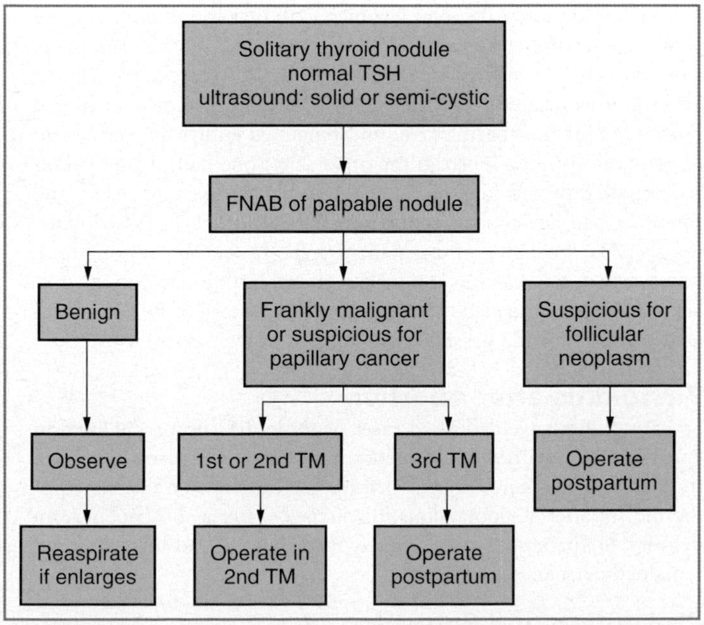

FIGURE 47-7 **Evaluation of thyroid nodules.** The decision-making process is outlined for management of a solitary thyroid nodule in pregnancy. (Adapted from Tan GH, Gharib H, Goellner JR, et al: Management of thyroid nodules in pregnancy. Arch Intern Med 156:2317, 1996. Copyright © 1996, American Medical Association. All rights reserved.)

Postpartum Thyroid Disease

Autoimmune thyroid disease, which is suppressed during pregnancy, is exacerbated in the postpartum period. New-onset autoimmune thyroid disease occurs in up to 10% of all postpartum women.[39] Up to 60% of Graves patients in the reproductive years give a history of postpartum onset.[178] Most of the immune changes of pregnancy gradually return to normal in the 12-month postpartum period. Unlike pregnancy, the major immune changes in T and B cells in the postpartum period are overall T-cell deactivation, enhanced T_H1-type T-cell function, loss of tolerance for fetal alloantigens, enhanced IgG secretion, and autoantibody secretion. Possible mechanisms explaining postpartum autoimmune exacerbation suggested by Davies[39] include a reduced number of fetal cells, leading to loss of maternal tolerance to remaining microchimeric cells, and a loss of placental major histocompatibility complex-peptide complexes, which were inducing T-cell anergy during pregnancy.

Postpartum Graves Disease

The onset of Graves disease after delivery correlates with the development of TSIs. Peak antibody production is observed 3 to 6 months after delivery. Almost all patients with persisting TSIs at the end of pregnancy have a recurrence of Graves if antithyroid drugs are withdrawn. The prevalence of postpartum Graves disease, which can be transient or persistent, is estimated at 11% of those with postpartum thyroid dysfunction.[179]

Postpartum Thyroiditis

The topic of postpartum thyroiditis (PPT) has been the focus of numerous reviews.[39,179-183] For the diagnosis of PPT, there must be a documented abnormal TSH level (suppressed or elevated) during the first postpartum year in the absence of a positive result for TSIs (excluding Graves) or a toxic nodule.

Classically, PPT manifests with a transient hyperthyroid phase of 6 weeks to 6 months after delivery. A hypothyroid phase follows and can last up to 1 year after delivery. Figure 47-8 schematically demonstrates this and the accompanying changes in serum thyroid antibody concentrations. A review of 11 studies of PPT[184] revealed that only 26% of patients presented in this classic manner. Most patients present with hyperthyroidism alone (38%) or hypothyroidism alone (36%). The incidence of PPT is 6% to 9%. It is an autoimmune disorder, and patients with type 1 diabetes have an increased incidence, which was found to be approximately 25% in two North American studies.[185,186] Women with a history of PPT in a prior pregnancy had a 69% recurrence rate in the subsequent pregnancy.

Symptoms of the hyperthyroid phase of PPT include fatigue, palpitations, heat intolerance, and nervousness. This destructive hyperthyroid phase always has a limited duration (a few weeks to a few months). Although β-blockers may reduce symptoms, antithyroid medications have no role to play.

The hypothyroid phase can be marked by fatigue, hair loss, depression, impairment of concentration, and dry skin. The hypothyroid phase frequently requires treatment, but it is reasonable to wean the patient off therapy 6 months after initiation. Some authorities recommend maintaining T_4 therapy in these patients until the childbearing years are over and then attempting to wean them off the therapy a year after the last delivery.

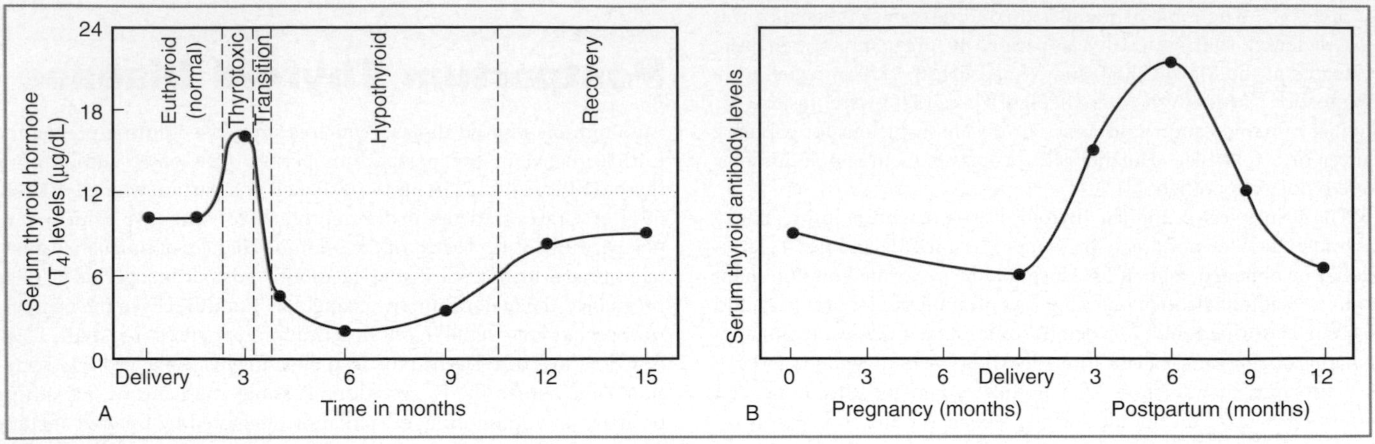

FIGURE 47-8 **Postpartum thyroiditis and changes in thyroid antibody concentrations.** **A,** Postpartum thyroiditis manifests with a transient hyperthyroid phase, during which serum levels of thyroxine (T_4) are elevated. A hypothyroid phase follows. **B,** Serum thyroid antibody levels fluctuate during and after pregnancy. (From Smallridge RC, Fein HC, Hayship CC: Postpartum thyroiditis. Bridge Newslett Thyroid Found Am 3:3, 1988.)

The thyroid gland is enlarged in PPT, and thyroid hypoechogenicity appears to be the characteristic ultrasonographic finding.[187] PPT is an autoimmune disorder, and there is an association between it and HLA-DR3, HLA-DR4, and HLA-DR5 status. The lymphocytic infiltration is similar to that seen in Hashimoto thyroiditis. Stagnaro-Green[182] reported that 33% of women who were antithyroid antibody positive in the first trimester of pregnancy had PPT, compared with 3% of women who were antibody negative.

The laboratory hallmarks of PPT, which is a destructive process, are positive test results for antithyroid antibodies (i.e., antithyroglobulin and antithyroid peroxidase), suppressed TSH levels, and high T_4 levels (released from destroyed thyroid cells) in the hyperthyroid phase, along with a profoundly suppressed radioactive iodine uptake (contraindicated in a breastfeeding woman). The absence of TSIs usually rules out Graves disease, which can also be distinguished by high radioactive iodine uptake.

Depression and Postpartum Thyroiditis

Depression and PPT are common postpartum events.[188] Four large-scale studies have been performed to evaluate their association. Harris and colleagues[189] evaluated 147 women (65 were thyroid antibody positive, and 82 were negative) at 6 to 8 weeks after delivery for thyroid status and depression. Although there was a positive correlation between PPT and postpartum depression, there was no association between antibody positivity and depression.

Pop and associates[190] evaluated 293 women during the third trimester and then every 6 weeks up to 34 weeks after delivery. They found that 38% of women with PPT experienced depression compared with 9.5% of women in a matched control group, and the difference was highly significant. Status of antibodies was not reported.

Harris and coauthors[191] investigated the association between depression and PPT in 232 women (110 were thyroid antibody positive). The women had psychiatric assessment five times during the first 28 weeks after delivery. No association was found between PPT and depression, but an association was found between depression and antibody positivity. They concluded that 4% of women experience postpartum depression that has an autoimmune origin.

Pop and colleagues[192] performed a further analysis of the same 293 women in their earlier study; antibody status was determined during the pregnancy, but only a slightly increased association between the presence of antibody and depression was found, and they concluded that antibody status during pregnancy was an important predictor of PPT but not of depression. In a subsequent study, Pop and associates[193] reported an association between thyroid antibodies and depression in postmenopausal women.

In summary, the data suggest some association for PPT, thyroid antibodies, and depression. Of the four clinical trials, two demonstrated an association between PPT and depression, whereas two demonstrated an association between thyroid antibodies and depression. The role of potential interventions such as T_4 therapy has not been evaluated systematically.

Hypothyroidism and Postpartum Thyroiditis

Recovery of thyroid function in women with PPT is not universal, and some women remain permanently hypothyroid. In a study of 44 women with PPT with a mean follow-up of 8.7 years after delivery, Tachi and associates[194] reported that 77% of the women recovered during the first postpartum year and remained euthyroid. Permanent hypothyroidism developed in the other 23%; one half of these never recovered euthyroid function after the initial postpartum insult, and the other half developed hypothyroidism during the years of follow-up. A 23% incidence of permanent hypothyroidism at long-term follow-up (mean, 3.5 years) was also reported by Othman and coworkers.[195] It is recommended that women with a history of PPT be evaluated annually for the possible development of hypothyroidism.

Thyroiditis after Abortion

Several studies have described cases of thyroiditis occurring after an abortion.[196,197] Neither the incidence nor clinical sequelae are known. In the case of Stagnaro-Green,[196] the patient developed transient hypothyroidism after a spontaneous miscarriage. After a subsequent term delivery, the patient became severely hypothyroid, and this condition remained permanent.

Prevention and Screening of Postpartum Thyroiditis

Levothyroxine (0.1 mg daily) or iodide (0.15 mg daily) was administered for 40 weeks after delivery to women who were thyroid antibody positive during pregnancy. A control group of antibody-negative women received no treatment. The incidence of PPT was similar in all three groups, and the degree of postpartum elevation of thyroid peroxidase antibodies was indistinguishable in the three groups.[198]

Whether screening for PPT is worthwhile is a contentious issue. A "Therapeutic Controversy" article in the *Journal of Clinical Endocrinology and Metabolism* addressed this topic.[179] Arguments for and against screening were presented. It was suggested that screening and treatment of symptomatic hypothyroidism would improve the quality of life of the mother, and the importance of recognizing postpartum depression was stressed. Contradicting arguments posited that the optimal screening strategy was undefined and that no cost-benefit analysis has been performed. It is agreed that women who present with symptoms should have a TSH assay performed. High-risk women (i.e., women with a history of PPT and women with type 1 diabetes) should be screened.[186,199]

References

1. Casey BM, Leveno KJ: Thyroid disease in pregnancy. Obstet Gynecol 108:1283, 2006.
2. LeBeau SO, Mandel SJ: Thyroid disorders during pregnancy. Endocrinol Metab Clin North Am 35:117, 2006.
3. Abalovich M, Amino N, Barbour LA, et al: Management of thyroid dysfunction during pregnancy and postpartum: An Endocrine Society clinical practice guideline. J Clin Endocrinol Metab 92(suppl):S1, 2007.
4. Brennan MD, Bahn RS: Thyroid hormones and illness. Endocr Pract 4:396, 1998.
5. DeGroot LJ: Dangerous dogmas in medicine: The non-thyroidal illness syndrome. J Clin Endocrinol Metab 84:151, 1999.
6. Brent GA: The molecular basis of thyroid hormone action. N Engl J Med 331:847, 1994.
7. Glinoer D: What happens to the normal thyroid during pregnancy? Thyroid 9:631, 1999.
8. Glinoer D, De Nayer P, Robyn C, et al: Serum levels of intact human chorionic gonadotropin (hCG) and its free α and β subunits, in relation to maternal thyroid stimulation during normal pregnancy. J Endocrinol Invest 16:881, 1993.
9. Grün JP, Meuris S, DeNayer P, et al: The thyrotropic role of human chorionic gonadotropin (hCG) in the early stages of twin (versus single) pregnancy. Clin Endocrinol 46:719, 1997.
10. Burrow GN, Fisher DA, Larsen PR: Maternal and fetal thyroid function. N Engl J Med 331:1072, 1994.
11. Glinoer D, De Nayer P, Delange F, et al: A randomized trial for the treatment of mild iodine deficiency during pregnancy: Maternal and neonatal effects. J Clin Endocrinol Metab 80:258, 1995.
12. Glinoer D: The regulation of thyroid function in pregnancy: Pathways of endocrine adaptation from physiology to pathology. Endocr Rev 18:404, 1997.
13. Levy RP, Newman M, Rejah LS, et al: The myth of goiter in pregnancy. Am J Obstet Gynecol 137:701, 1980.
14. Nelson M, Wickos GG, Caplan RH, et al: Thyroid gland size in pregnancy. J Reprod Med 32:888, 1987.
15. Brander A, Kivsaari L: Ultrasonography of the thyroid during pregnancy. J Clin Ultrasound 17:403, 1989.
16. Halnan KE: The radioiodine uptake of the human thyroid in pregnancy. Clin Sci 17:281, 1958.
17. Abdoul-Khair SA, Crooks J, Turnbull AC, et al: The physiological changes in thyroid function during pregnancy. Clin Sci 27:195, 1964.
18. Ferris TF: Renal disease. In Burrow GN, Ferris TF (eds): Medical Complications During Pregnancy. Philadelphia, WB Saunders, 1988, p 277.
19. Beckers C: Iodine economy in and around pregnancy. In Beckers C, Reinwein D (eds): The Thyroid and Pregnancy. New York, John Wiley and Sons, 1992.
20. Glinoer D, Delange F: The potential repercussions of maternal, fetal and neonatal hypothyroxinemia on the progeny. Thyroid 10:871, 2000.
21. Radunovic N, Domez Y, Mandelbrot L, et al: Thyroid function in fetus and mother during the second half of normal pregnancy. Biol Neonate 59:139, 1991.
22. LaFranchi S: Thyroid function in the preterm infant. Thyroid 9:71, 1999.
23. Fisher DA: Hypothyroxinemia in premature infants: Is thyroxine treatment necessary? Thyroid 9:715, 1999.
24. Bernal J, Perkonen F: Ontogenesis of the nuclear 3,5,3′-triiodothyronine receptor in the human fetal brain. Endocrinology 114:677, 1984.
25. Santini F, Chiovato L, Ghirri P, et al: Serum iodothyronine in the human fetus and the newborn: Evidence for an important role of placenta in fetal thyroid hormone homeostasis. J Clin Endocrinol Metab 84:493, 1999.
26. Vulsma T, Gons MH, de Vijlder JJ: Maternal-fetal transfer of thyroxine in congenital hypothyroidism due to a total organification defect or thyroid agenesis. N Engl J Med 321:13, 1989.
27. Delange F, de Vilder JJ, Morreale de Escobar G, et al: Significance of early diagnostic data in congenital hypothyroidism: Report of the Subcommittee on Neonatal Hypothyroidism of the European Thyroid Association. In Delange F, Fisher DA, Glinoer D (eds): Research in Congenital Hypothyroidism. New York, Plenum Press, 1989, pp 225-234.
28. Kester MHA, Martinez de Mena R, Obregon MJ, et al: Iodothyronine levels in the human developing brain: Major regulatory roles of iodothyronine deiodinases in different areas. J Clin Endocrinol Metab 9:3117, 2004.
29. Fisher DA, Polk DH: Development of the thyroid. Baillieres Clin Endocrinol Metab 3:627,1989.
30. Fisher DA, Dussault JH, Sack J, et al: Ontogenesis of hypothalamic-pituitary-thyroid function and metabolism in man, sheep and rat. Recent Prog Horm Res 3:59, 1977.
31. Polk DH: Thyroid hormone effects on neonatal thermogenesis. Semin Perinatol 12:151, 1988.
32. Reuss ML, Paneth N, Pinto-Martin JA, et al: The relation of transient hypothyroxinemia in preterm infants to neurologic development at two years of age. N Engl J Med 443:821, 1996.
33. Vulsma Y, Kok JK: Prematurity-associated neurological and development abnormalities and neonatal thyroid function. N Engl J Med 3343:857, 1996.
34. Williams FLR, Mires GJ, Barnett C, et al: Transient hypothyroxinemia in preterm infants: The role of cord sera thyroid hormone levels adjusted for prenatal and antepartum factors. J Clin Endocrinol Metab 90:4599, 2005.
35. Burrow GN, May PB, Spaulding SW, et al: TRH and dopamine interactions affecting pituitary hormone secretion. J Clin Endocrinol Metab 45:65, 1977.
36. Roti E, Gnudi A, Braverman LE: The placental transport, synthesis and metabolism of hormones and drugs, which affect thyroid function. Endocr Rev 4:131, 1983.
37. Ballard RA, Ballard PL, Creasy RK, et al: Respiratory disease in very-low-birthweight infants after prenatal thyrotropin-releasing hormone and glucocorticoid. Lancet 339:510, 1992.
38. Romaguera J, Ramirez M, Adamsons K: Intra-amniotic thyroxine to accelerate fetal maturation. Semin Perinatol 17:260, 1993.
39. Davies TF: The thyroid immunology of the postpartum period. Thyroid 9:675, 1999.
40. Weetman AP: The immunology of pregnancy. Thyroid 9:643, 1999.
41. Nelson JL, Hughes KA, Smith AG, et al: Maternal fetal disparity in HLA class II alloantigens and the pregnancy induced amelioration of rheumatoid arthritis. N Engl J Med 329:466, 1993.
42. Buyon JP, Nelson JL, Lockshine MD: The effects of pregnancy on autoimmune thyroid diseases. Clin Immunol Immunopathol 79:99, 1996.
43. Confavreuz C, Hutchinson M, Hours MH, et al: Rate of pregnancy related relapse in multiple sclerosis. New Engl J Med 339:285, 1998.
44. Piccinini MP, Giudizi MG, Biagiotti R, et al: Progesterone favors the development of human T helper cells producing Th2-type cytokines and promotes both IL-4 production and membrane CD30 expression in established Th1 cell clones. J Immunol 155:128, 1995.
45. Ain KB, Mori Y, Refetoff F: Reduced clearance rate of thyroxine-binding globulin (TBG) with increased sialylation: A mechanism for estrogen induced elevation of serum TBG concentration. J Clin Endocrinol Metab 65:689, 1987.

46. Dashe JS, Casey BM, Wells CE, et al: Thyroid stimulating hormone in singleton and twin pregnancy: Importance of gestational age-specific reference ranges. Obstet Gynecol 106:753, 2005
47. Glinoer D, Soto MF, Bouroux P, et al: Pregnancy in patients with mild thyroid abnormalities: Maternal and neonatal repercussions. J Clin Endocrinol Metab 73:421, 1991.
48. Weintraub BD: Inappropriate secretion of thyroid-stimulating hormone. Ann Intern Med 95:339, 1981.
49. Anselmo J, Kay T, Dennis K, et al: Resistance to thyroid hormone does not abrogate the transient thyrotoxicosis associated with gestation: Report of a case. J Clin Endocrinol Metab 86:4273, 2001.
50. Anselmo J, Cao D, Karrison T, et al: Fetal loss associated with excess thyroid hormone exposure. JAMA 292:691, 2004.
51. Mariotti S, Chiovato L, Vitti P, et al: Recent advances in the understanding of humoral and cellular mechanisms implicated in thyroid autoimmune disorders. Clin Immunol Immunopathol 50:573, 1989.
52. Learoyd DL, Fund HYM, McGregor AM: Postpartum thyroid dysfunction. Thyroid 2:73, 1992.
53. Weetman AP, McGregor AM: Autoimmune thyroid disease: Further developments in our understanding. Endocr Rev 15:788, 1994.
54. Bartalena L, Bogazzi F, Braverman LE, et al: Effect of amiodarone administration during pregnancy on neonatal thyroid function and subsequent neurodevelopment. J Endocrinol Invest 24:116, 2001.
55. Wartofsky L, Burman KD: Alterations in thyroid function in patients with systemic illness: The "euthyroid sick syndrome." Endocr Rev 3:164, 1982.
56. Brent GA, Hershman JM: Thyroxine therapy in patients with severe nonthyroidal illnesses and low serum thyroxine concentration. J Clin Endocrinol Metab 63:1, 1986.
57. Winters SJ, Berga SL: Gonadal dysfunction in patients with thyroid disease. Endocrinologist 7:167, 1997.
58. Krassas GE: Thyroid disease and female reproduction. Fertil Steril 74:1063, 2000.
59. Trokoudes KM, Skordis N, Picolos MK: Infertility and thyroid disorders. Curr Opin Obstet Gynecol 18:446, 2006.
60. Krassas GE, Pontikides N, Kaltsas TH, et al: Menstrual disturbances in thyroidism. Clin Endocrinol 40:641, 1994.
61. Akande EO, Hockaday TD: Plasma estrogen and luteinizing hormone concentrations in thyrotoxic menstrual disturbances. Proc R Soc Med 65:789, 1972.
62. Tanaka T, Tamin H, Kuma K, et al: Gonadotropin response to luteinizing hormone releasing hormone in hyperthyroid patients with menstrual disturbances. Metabolism 30:323, 1981.
63. Wilansky DL, Greisman B: Early hypothyroidism in patients with menorrhagia. Am J Obstet Gynecol 160:673, 1989.
64. Del Pozo E, Wyss H, Tolis G, et al: Prolactin and deficient luteal function. Obstet Gynecol 53:282, 1979.
65. Thomas R, Reid RL: Thyroid disease and reproductive dysfunction. Obstet Gynecol 70:789, 1987.
66. Wasserstrum N, Anania CA: Perinatal consequences of maternal hypothyroidism in early pregnancy and inadequate replacement. Clin Endocrinol 42:343, 1997.
67. Brent GA: Diagnosing thyroid dysfunction in pregnant women: Is case finding enough? J Clin Endocrinol Metab 92:39, 2007.
68. Montoro MN: Management of hypothyroidism during pregnancy. Clin Obstet Gynecol 40:65, 1997.
69. Negro R, Fomoso G, Manieri T, et al: Levothyroxine treatment in euthyroid pregnant women with autoimmune thyroid disease: Effects on obstetrical complications. J Clin Endocrinol Metab 91:2587, 2006.
70. Glinoer D: Miscarriage in women with positive anti-TPO antibodies: Is thyroxine the answer [editorial]? J Clin Endocrinol Metab 91:2500, 2006.
71. Greig WR: Radioactive iodine therapy for thyrotoxicosis. Br J Surg 758:765, 1973.
72. Safa AM, Schumacher OP, Rodriguez-Antunez A: Long-term follow-up results in children and adolescents treated with radioactive iodine (^{131}I) for hyperthyroidism. N Engl J Med 292:167, 1975.
73. Sioka C, Kouaklis G, Zafirakis, et al: Menstrual cycle disorders after therapy with iodine-131. Fertil Steril 86:625, 2006.
74. Smith MB, Xue H, Takahashi H, et al: Iodine ^{131}I thyroid ablation in female children and adolescents: Long term risk of infertility and birth defects. Ann Surg Oncol 1:128, 1994.
75. Schlumberger M, deVathaire F, Ceccarelli C, et al: Exposure to radioactive iodine ^{131}I for scintigraphy or therapy does not preclude pregnancy in thyroid cancer patients. J Nucl Med 37:606, 1996.
76. Gorman CA: Radio iodine and pregnancy. Thyroid 9:721, 1999.
77. Berlin L: Malpractice issues in radiology. Iodine ^{131}I and the pregnant patient. Am J Radiol 176:869, 2001.
78. Fernandez-Soto ML, Jovanovic LG, Gonzalez-Jimenez A, et al: Thyroid function during pregnancy and the postpartum period iodine metabolism and disease status. Endocr Pract 4:97, 1998.
79. Seely BL, Burrow GN: Thyrotoxicosis in pregnancy. Endocrinologist 7:409, 1991.
80. Costagliola S, Morgenthaler NG, Hoermann R, et al: Second generation assay for thyrotoxicosis receptor and bodies has superior diagnostic sensitivity for Graves disease. J Clin Endocrinol Metab 84:90, 1999.
81. Varner MW: Autoimmune disorders and pregnancy. Semin Perinatol 15:238, 1991.
82. Davis LE, Lucas MJ, Hankins GDV, et al: Thyrotoxicosis complicating pregnancy. Am J Obstet Gynecol 160:63, 1989.
83. Momotani N, Ito K: Treatment of pregnant patients with Basedow's disease. Exp Clin Endocrinol 97:268, 1991.
84. Millar LK, Wing DA, Leung AS, et al: Low birth weight and preeclampsia in pregnancies complicated by hyperthyroidism. Obstet Gynecol 84:946, 1994.
85. Cooper DS: Antithyroid drugs. N Engl J Med 352:905, 2005.
86. Clark SM, Saade GR, Sodgrass WR, et al: Pharmacokinetics and pharmacotherapy of thionamides in pregnancy. Ther Drug Monit 28:477, 2006.
87. Momotani N, Noh J, Oyanagi H, et al: Antithyroid drug therapy for Graves' disease during pregnancy. N Engl J Med 315:24, 1986.
88. Kung AWC, Jones BM: A change from stimulatory to blocking antibody activity in Graves' disease during pregnancy. J Clin Endocrinol Metab 8:514, 1998.
89. Cooper DS, Goldminz D, Levin AA, et al: Agranulocytosis associated with antithyroid drugs. Ann Intern Med 98:26, 1983.
90. Mortimer RH, Cannell GR, Addison RS, et al: Methimazole and propylthiouracil equally cover the perfused human term placental lobule. J Clin Endocrinol Metab 82:3099, 1997.
91. Milham S, Elledge W: Maternal methimazole and congenital defects in children. Teratology 5:525, 1972.
92. Van Djihe UP, Heydendael RJ, De Kleine MR: Methimazole, carbimazole and congenital skin defects. Ann Intern Med 106:60, 1987.
93. Martinez-Frias ML, Cereijo A, Rodriguez-Pinella E, et al: Methimazole in animal feed and congenital aplasia cutis. Lancet 399:742, 1992.
94. Johnsson E, Larsson G, Ljunggren M: Severe malformations in infants born to hyperthyroid women on methimazole. Lancet 350:1520, 1997.
95. Clementi M, DiGianantonio E, Pelo E, et al: Methimazole embryopathy: Delineation of the phenotype. Am J Med Genet 83:43, 1999.
96. Di Gianantonio E, Schaefer C, Mastroiacovo PP, et al: Adverse effects of prenatal methimazole exposure. Teratology 64:262, 2001.
97. Wolf D, Foulds N, Daya H: Antenatal carbimazole and choanal atresia: A new embryopathy Arch Otolaryngol Head Neck Surg 132:1009, 2006.
98. Phoojaroenchanachai M, Sriussadaporn S, Peerapatdir T, et al: Effect of maternal hyperthyroidism during late pregnancy on the risk of neonatal low birth weight. Clin Endocrinol 54:365, 2001.
99. Mitsuda N, Tamaki H, Amino N, et al: Risk factors for development disorders in infants born to women with Graves' disease. Obstet Gynecol 80:359, 1992.
100. Wing DA, Millar LK, Kooings PP, et al: A comparison of propylthiouracil versus methimazole in the treatment of hyperthyroidism in pregnancy. Am J Obstet Gynecol 170:90, 1994.
101. Thorpe-Beeston JG, Nicolaides KH, Felton CV, et al: Maturation of the secretion of thyroid hormone and thyroid-stimulating hormone in the fetus. N Engl J Med 324:532, 1991.

102. Kampmann JP, Johansen K, Hansen JM, et al: Propylthiouracil in human milk: Revision of a dogma. Lancet 1:736, 1980.
103. Azzizi F: Effect of methimazole treatment of maternal thyrotoxicosis on thyroid function in breast-feeding infants. J Pediatr 128:855, 1996.
104. Isley WL, Dahl S, Gibbs H: Use of esmolol in managing a thyrotoxic patient needing emergency surgery. Am J Med 89:122, 1990.
105. Burrow GN: The management of thyrotoxicosis in pregnancy. N Engl J Med 313:562,1985.
106. Burch HB, Wartofsky L: Life threatening thyrotoxicosis: Thyroid storm. Endocrinol Metab Clin North Am 22:263, 1993.
107. Waltman PA, Brewer JM, Lobert S: Thyroid storm during pregnancy. A medical emergency. Crit Care Nurse 24:74, 2004.
108. Sheffield JS, Cunningham FG: Thyrotoxicosis and heart failure that complicate pregnancy. Am J Obstet Gynecol 190:211, 2004.
109. Casey BM, Dashe JS, Wells CE, et al: Clinical hyperthyroidism and pregnancy outcomes. Obstet Gynecol 107:337, 2006.
110. Zimmerman D: Fetal and neonatal hyperthyroidism. Thyroid 9:727, 1999.
111. Clavel S, Madec A, Bornet H, et al: Anti TSH-receptor antibodies in pregnant patients with autoimmune thyroid disorder. BJOG 97:1003, 1990.
112. Zakarija M, McKenzie JM: Pregnancy-associated changes in thyroid-stimulating antibody of Graves' disease and the relationship to neonatal hyperthyroidism. J Clin Endocrinol Metab 57:1036, 1983.
113. Becks GP, Burrow G. Thyroid disease and pregnancy. Med Clin North Am 75:121, 1991.
114. Houck JA, Davis RE, Sharma HM: Thyroid-stimulating immunoglobulin as a cause of recurrent intrauterine fetal death. Obstet Gynecol 71:1018, 1988.
115. Yoshimoto M, Nakayama Itoi, Baba P, et al: A case of neonatal McCune-Albright syndrome with Cushing syndrome and hyperthyroidism. Acta Pediatr Scand 89:984, 1991.
116. Kopp P, Van Sande J, Parmer J, et al: Brief report: Congenital hyperthyroidism caused by a mutation in the thyrotropin receptor gene. N Engl J Med 322:150, 1995.
117. Hershman JM: Human chorionic gonadotropin and the thyroid: Hyperemesis gravidarum and trophoblastic tumors. Thyroid 9:653, 1999.
118. Talbot JA, Lambert A, Anobile LJ, et al: The nature of human chorionic gonadotropin glycoforms in gestational thyrotoxicosis. Clin Endocrinol 55:33, 2001.
119. Bashiri A, Neumann L, Maymon E, et al: Hyperemesis gravidarum: Epidemiologic features, complications and outcome. Eur J Obstet Gynecol Reprod Biol 63:135, 1995.
120. Goodwin TM, Montoro M, Mestman JH: The role of chorionic gonadotropin in transient hyperthyroidism of hyperemesis gravidarum. J Clin Endocrinol Metab 75:1333, 1992.
121. Goodwin TM, Montoro M, Mestman JH: Transient hyperthyroidism and hyperemesis gravidarum: Clinical aspects. Am J Obstet Gynecol 167:648, 1992.
122. Wilson R, McKillop JH, MacLean M, et al: Thyroid function tests are rarely abnormal in patients with severe hyperemesis gravidarum. Clin Endocrinol (Oxf) 37:331, 1992.
123. Pekary AE, Jackson IM, Goodwin TM, et al: Increased in vitro thyrotropic activity of partially sialated human chorionic gonadotropin extracted from hydatidiform moles of patients with hyperthyroidism. J Clin Endocrinol Metab 76:70, 1993.
124. Morgan LS: Hormonally active gynecologic tumors. Semin Surg Oncol 6:83, 1990.
125. Nader S, Mastrobattista J: Recurrent hyperthyroidism in consecutive pregnancies characterized by hyperemesis. Thyroid 6:465, 1996.
126. Rodien P, Bremont C, Sanson M-LR, et al: Familial gestational hyperthyroidism caused by a mutant thyrotropic receptor hypersensitive to human chorionic gonadotropin. N Engl J Med 339:1823, 1998.
127. Mariotti S, Martino E, Cupini C: Low serum thyroglobulin as a clue to the diagnosis of thyrotoxicosis factitia. N Engl J Med 307:410, 1982.
128. Lazarus JH: Thyroid hormone and intellectual development: A clinician's view. Thyroid 9:659, 1999.
129. Glinoer D: Pregnancy and iodine. Thyroid 11:471, 2001.
130. Dunn JT, Delange F: Damaged reproduction: The most important consequence of iodine deficiency. J Clin Endocrinol Metab 86:2360, 2001.
131. Delange F, de Benoist B, Pretell E, et al: Iodine deficiency in the world: Where do we stand at the turn of the century? Thyroid 11:437, 2001.
132. Hollowell JG, Staehling NW, Hannon WH, et al: Iodine nutrition in the United States. Trends from public health implications: Iodine excretion data from National Health and Nutrition Examination Surveys I and III (1971-1974 and 1988-1994). J Clin Endocrinol Metab 83:3401, 1998.
133. Pharoah PQ, Butterfield IH, Hetzel BS: Neurological damage to the fetus resulting from severe iodine deficiency during pregnancy. Lancet 1:308, 1971.
134. Vanderpas JB, Contempré B, Dvale NL, et al: Iodine and selenium deficiency associated with cretinism in Northern Zaire. Am J Clinic Nutr 52:1087, 1990.
135. Bleichrodt N, Born MP: A meta-analysis of research on iodine and its relationship to cognitive development. In Stanbury JB (ed): The Damaged Brain of Iodine Deficiency. New York, Cognizant Communication, 1994, p 195.
136. Xue-Yi C, Xin-Min J, Zhi-Hong D, et al: Time of vulnerability of the brain to iodine deficiency in endemic cretinism. N Engl J Med 331:1739, 1994.
137. Yasuda T, Ohnishi H, Wataki K, et al: Outcome of a baby born from a mother with acquired juvenile hypothyroidism having undetectable thyroid hormone concentrations. J Clin Endocrinol Metab 84:2630, 1999.
138. Utiger RD: Iodine nutrition: More is better. N Engl J Med 354:26, 2006.
139. Klein RZ, Haddow JE, Faix JD, et al: Prevalence of thyroid deficiency in pregnant women. Clin Endocrinol 35:41, 1991.
140. Kamijo K, Saito T, Saito M, et al: Transient subclinical hypothyroidism in early pregnancy. Endocrinol Jpn 37:387, 1990.
141. Leung AS, Millar LK, Koonings PP, et al: Perinatal outcome in hypothyroid patients. Obstet Gynecol 81:349, 1993.
142. Davis LE, Leveno KJ, Cunningham FG: Hypothyroidism complicating pregnancy. Obstet Gynecol 72:108, 1988.
143. Jovanovic-Peterson L, Peterson CM: De novo clinical hypothyroidism in pregnancies complicated by type I diabetes, subclinical hypothyroidism and proteinuria. Am J Obstet Gynecol 159:442, 1988.
144. Werner S: Modification of the classification of eye changes of Graves' disease: Recommendation of the Ad Hoc Committee of the American Thyroid Association. J Clin Endocrinol Metab 44:203, 1977.
145. Alexander EK, Marqusee E, Lawrence J, et al: Timing and magnitude of increases in levothyroxine requirements during pregnancy in women with hypothyroidism. N Engl J Med 351:241, 2004.
146. Mandel SJ, Larsen PR, Seely EW, et al: Increased need for thyroxine during pregnancy in women with primary hypothyroidism. N Engl J Med 323:91, 1990.
147. Kaplan MM: Monitoring thyroxine treatment during pregnancy. Thyroid 2:147, 1992.
148. Kaplan MM: Management of thyroxine therapy during pregnancy. Endocr Pract 2:281, 1996.
149. Mestman JH: Thyroid disease in pregnancy other than Graves' and post partum thyroid dysfunction. Endocrinologist 9:294, 1999.
150. Brent GA: Maternal hypothyroidism recognition and management. Thyroid 9:661, 1999.
151. Haddow JE, Palomaki GE, Alan WC, et al: Maternal thyroid deficiency during pregnancy and subsequent neuropsychological development of the child. N Engl J Med 341:549, 1999.
152. Klein RZ, Mitchell ML: Maternal hypothyroidism and child development. Horm Res 52:55, 1999.
153. Man EB, Jones WS: Thyroid function in human pregnancy. V. Incidence of maternal serum low butanol-extractable iodines and of normal gestational TBG and TBPA capacities: Retardation of 8-month old infants. Am J Obstet Gynecol 104:898, 1969.
154. Matsuura N, Konishi J: Transient hypothyroidism in infants born to mothers with chronic thyroiditis—a nationwide study of 23 cases. Endocrinol Jpn 37:767, 1990.

155. Fukushi M, Honma IC, Fujita K: Maternal thyroid deficiency during pregnancy and subsequent neuropsychological development of the child [letter]. N Engl J Med 341:556, 1999.
156. Pop VJM, deVries E, van Baar AL, et al: Maternal thyroid peroxidase antibodies during pregnancy: A marker of impaired child development? J Clin Endocrinol Metab 80:3561, 1995.
157. Lazarus JH, Aloa A, Parkes AB, et al: The effect of anti-TPO antibodies on thyroid function in early gestation: Implications for screening. Presented at the American Thyroid Association meeting, Portland, Oregon, 1998.
158. Pop VJM, Kuijpens JV, van Baar AL, et al: Low maternal FT_4 concentrations during early pregnancy associated with impaired psychomotor development in infancy. Clin Endocrinol 50:149, 1999.
159. Casey BM, Dashe JS, Wells CE, et al: Clinical hypothyroidism and pregnancy outcomes. Obstet Gynecol 105:239, 2005.
160. Casey BM: Subclinical hypothyroidism and pregnancy. Obstet Gynecol Surv 61:415, 2006.
161. Gharib H, Cobin RH, Dickey RA: Subclinical hypothyroidism during pregnancy: Position statement from the American Association of Clinical Endocrinologists. Endocr Pract 5:367, 1999.
162. Vaidya B, Anthony S, Bilous M, et al: Detection of thyroid dysfunction in early pregnancy: Universal screening or targeted high risk case finding. J Clin Endocrinol Metab 92:203, 2007.
163. Pop VJ, Brouwers EP, Vader HL, et al: Maternal hypothyroxinemia during early pregnancy and subsequent child development: A 3-year follow-up study. Clin Endocrinol 59:282, 2003.
164. Demers L, Spencer CA: Laboratory medicine practice guidelines: Laboratory support for the diagnosis and monitoring of thyroid disease. Thyroid 13:6,2003.
165. Glinoer D, De Nayer P, Bourdoux P, et al: Regulation of maternal thyroid during pregnancy. J Clin Endocrinol Metab 71:276, 1990.
166. Mandel SJ, Spencer CA, Hollowell JG: Are detection and treatment of thyroid insufficiency in pregnancy feasible? Thyroid 15:44, 2005.
167. Morreale de Escobar G, Obregon MJ, Escobar del Rey F: Is neuropsychological development related to maternal hypothyroidism or to maternal hypothyroxinemia? J Clin Endocrinol Metab 85:3975, 2000.
168. Larsen PR: Detecting and treating hypothyroidism during pregnancy. Nat Clin Pract Endocrinol Metab 2:59, 2006.
169. Dussault JH, Rousseau F: Immunologically mediated hypothyroidism. Endocrinol Metab Clin North Am 16:417, 1987.
170. Bogner U, Gruters A, Sigle B, et al: Cytotoxic antibodies in congenital hypothyroidism. J Clin Endocrinol Metab 68:671, 1989.
171. Gruner C, Kollert A, Wildt L, et al: Intrauterine treatment of fetal goitrous hypothyroidism controlled by determination of thyroid-stimulating hormone in fetal serum. A case report and review of the literature. Fetal Diagn Ther 16:47, 2001.
172. Kung A, Chau M, Lao T, et al: The effect of pregnancy on thyroid nodule formation. J Clin Endocrinol Metab 87:1010, 2002.
173. Hay ID: Nodular thyroid disease diagnosed during pregnancy: How and when to treat. Thyroid 9:667, 1999.
174. Tan GH, Gharib H, Goellner JR, et al: Management of thyroid nodules in pregnancy. Arch Intern Med 156:2317, 1996.
175. Marley EF, Oertil YC: Fine needle aspiration of thyroid lesions in 57 pregnant and postpartum women. Diagn Cytopathol 16:122, 1997.
176. Moosa M, Mazzaferri EL: Outcome of differentiated thyroid cancer diagnosed in pregnant women. J Clin Endocrinol Metab 82:2862, 1997.
177. Herzon FS, Morris DM, Segal MN, et al: Coexistent thyroid cancer and pregnancy. Arch Otolaryngol Head Neck Surg 120:1191, 1994.
178. Janssen R, Dahlberg PA, Winsa B, et al: The postpartum period constitutes an important risk for the development of clinical Graves' disease in young women. Acta Endocrinol 116:321, 1987.
179. Amino N, Tada H, Hidaka Y, et al: Therapeutic controversy. Screening for postpartum thyroiditis. J Clin Endocrinal Metab 84:1813, 1999.
180. Lazarus JH: Clinical manifestations of postpartum thyroid disease. Thyroid 9:685, 1999.
181. Lucas A, Pizarro E, Granada ML, et al: Postpartum thyroiditis: Epidemiology and clinical evolution in a non-selected population. Thyroid 10:71, 2000.
182. Stagnaro-Green AS: Recognizing, understanding and treating postpartum thyroiditis. Endocrinol Metab Clinics NA 29:417, 2000.
183. Pearce EN, Farwell AP, Braverman LE: Thyroiditis [published erratum appears in N Engl J Med 349:62, 2003]. N Engl J Med 348:2646, 2003.
184. Stagnaro-Green AS: Postpartum thyroiditis: Prevalence, etiology, and clinical implications. Thyroid Today 16:1, 1993.
185. Gerstein HC: Incidence of postpartum thyroid dysfunction in patients with type I diabetes mellitus. Ann Intern Med 188:419, 1993.
186. Alvarez-Marfany M, Roman SH, Drexler AJ, et al: Long-term prospective study of postpartum thyroid dysfunction in women with insulin dependent diabetes mellitus. J Clin Endocrinol 79:10, 1994.
187. Adams H, Jones MC, Othman S, et al: The sonographic appearances in postpartum thyroiditis. Clin Radiol l45:311, 1992.
188. Pedersen CA: Postpartum mood and anxiety disorders: A guide for the non-psychiatric clinician with an aside on thyroid associations with postpartum mood. Thyroid 9:691, 1999.
189. Harris B, Fung H, Johns S, et al: Transient postpartum thyroid dysfunction and postnatal depression. J Affect Disord 17:243, 1989.
190. Pop VJM, de Rooy HAM, Vader HL, et al: Postpartum thyroid dysfunction and depression in an unselected population. N Engl J Med 324:1815, 1991.
191. Harris B, Othman S, Davies JA, et al: Association between postpartum thyroid dysfunction and thyroid antibodies and depression. BMJ 305:152, 1992.
192. Pop VJM, de Rooy HAM, Vader VL, et al: Microsomal antibodies during gestation in relation to postpartum thyroid dysfunction and depression. Acta Endocrinol 129:26, 1993.
193. Pop VJM, Maarteens LH, Levsink G, et al: Are autoimmune thyroid dysfunction and depression related? J Clin Endocrinol Metab 83:3194, 1998.
194. Tachi J, Amino N, Tamaski H, et al: Long-term follow-up and HLA association in patients with postpartum hypothyroidism. J Clin Endocrinol Metab 66:480, 1988.
195. Othman S, Phillips DL, Parkes AB, et al: Long-term follow-up of postpartum thyroiditis. Clin Endocrinol 32:559, 1990.
196. Stagnaro-Green AS: Post-miscarriage thyroid dysfunction. Obstet Gynecol 803:490, 1992.
197. Marqusee E, Hill JA, Mandel SJ: Thyroiditis after pregnancy loss. J Clin Endocrinol Metab 82:2455, 1997.
198. Kampe O, Jansson R, Karlsson FA: Effects of L-thyroxine and iodide on the development of autoimmune postpartum thyroiditis. J Clin Endocrinol Metab 70:1014, 1990.
199. Weetman AP: Editorial: Insulin-dependent diabetes mellitus and postpartum thyroiditis: An important association. J Clin Endocrinol Metab 79:7, 1994.

Chapter 48

Other Endocrine Disorders of Pregnancy

Shahla Nader, MD

The staggering advancements made in endocrinology over the past few decades have delineated both normal physiology and pathophysiology. In tandem, technologic and pharmaceutical advances have followed that allow correction and management of prevailing problems with a precision that is lacking in many other fields of medicine. When pregnancy is superimposed on abnormal endocrine function in the mother, the consequences for the mother and the fetus can be adverse and sometimes disastrous. Awareness of this danger, combined with the knowledge that accurate diagnostic and therapeutic measures are often available, places a substantial burden on the obstetrician caring for the pregnant patient. This chapter summarizes the normal maternal endocrine adaptation to pregnancy (see also Chapters 8, 9, 46, and 47) and outlines maternal disorders, some of which are almost specific to pregnancy.

Hypothalamus and Pituitary

The sella turcica of the sphenoid bone, which is lined by dura mater, is occupied by the pituitary gland. The dura covering the roof, called the diaphragm sella, is perforated centrally by the pituitary stalk. Directly above this diaphragm and anterior to the stalk lies the optic chiasm. The gland consists of an anterior lobe (i.e., adenohypophysis) and a posterior lobe (i.e., neurohypophysis); the former accounts for more than 80% of the gland's volume. The pituitary stalk comprises the direct neural connections between the hypothalamic nuclei and the posterior lobe, and it is the vascular link between the hypothalamus and the anterior lobe, enabling hypothalamic neurohumoral secretions to influence the activity of the anterior lobe cells. Paired superior hypophyseal arteries arising from the internal carotids anastomose around the upper part of the stalk. These terminate within elongated coiled capillary loops into which the hypothalamic hormones are discharged. The capillary bed drains into portal veins that empty into sinusoids of the anterior lobe (Fig. 48-1). Paired inferior hypophyseal arteries supply the posterior lobe. The venous drainage of both lobes flows into the cavernous sinuses.

Figure 48-2 is a diagram of the interrelationships and feedback mechanisms of the higher brain centers, hypothalamus, pituitary, and target endocrine glands in normal, nonpregnant women. The adenohypophysis produces gonadotropins (e.g., luteinizing hormone [LH], follicle-stimulating hormone [FSH]), growth hormone (GH), thyrotropin or thyroid-stimulating hormone (TSH), prolactin, and adrenocorticotropin or adrenocorticotropic hormone (ACTH) and its related peptide β-lipotropin, from which melanocyte-stimulating hormone (β-MSH) is derived.

Since the 1940s, when the concept that control of the anterior pituitary is exerted through a neurohumoral mechanism was formulated, several peptides have been isolated from the hypothalamus that function in this capacity. Thyrotropin-releasing hormone (TRH) causes release of TSH (and prolactin); growth hormone–releasing hormone (GHRH) releases GH; gonadotropin-releasing hormone (GnRH) allows release of LH and FSH; and corticotropin-releasing hormone (CRH) releases ACTH. Substances with an inhibitory rather than a stimulatory influence have been identified. Somatostatin inhibits the release of GH (and many other hormones), and dopamine inhibits the release of prolactin. This inhibition of the lactotroph is clinically important; disturbances of the stalk or vascular dissociation of the hypothalamus from the anterior pituitary results in deficiency of all anterior pituitary hormones with the exception of prolactin. The lactotroph is normally under predominantly inhibitory control.

Physiologic Changes during Pregnancy

During pregnancy and in the immediate postpartum period, the anterior lobe of the pituitary can double or triple in size because of hyperplasia and hypertrophy of lactotrophs. This is evident at 1 month and continues throughout gestation. At delivery, involution of pregnancy cells occurs for a period of several months but seems to be retarded by lactation.[1] Magnetic resonance imaging (MRI) studies of normal primigravid patients have confirmed progressively increasing pituitary volumes during gestation[2]; at the end of pregnancy, there is an overall increase in pituitary gland size of 136% compared with control nulliparous subjects. Similar results have been obtained by Dinc and colleagues,[3] who found changes in pituitary gland volume of 40%, 75%, and a maximum of 120% in the second, third, and immediate postpartum periods, respectively. The major accompanying physiologic change is a progressive increase in serum prolactin concentrations,[4] with an approximately tenfold increase during gestation (Fig. 48-3).

Placental estrogens stimulate lactotroph DNA synthesis, mitotic activity, and prolactin secretion. Prolactin prepares the breasts for initiation and maintenance of lactation (see Chapter 9). Despite this dramatic increase, the lactotroph maintains its ability to respond to TRH, its releasing hormone (unlike prolactinomas, in which this response is usually blunted or absent).

Other physiologic changes during pregnancy include the following[5]:

1. Gonadotropin concentrations decline, with a progressively diminishing response to GnRH.

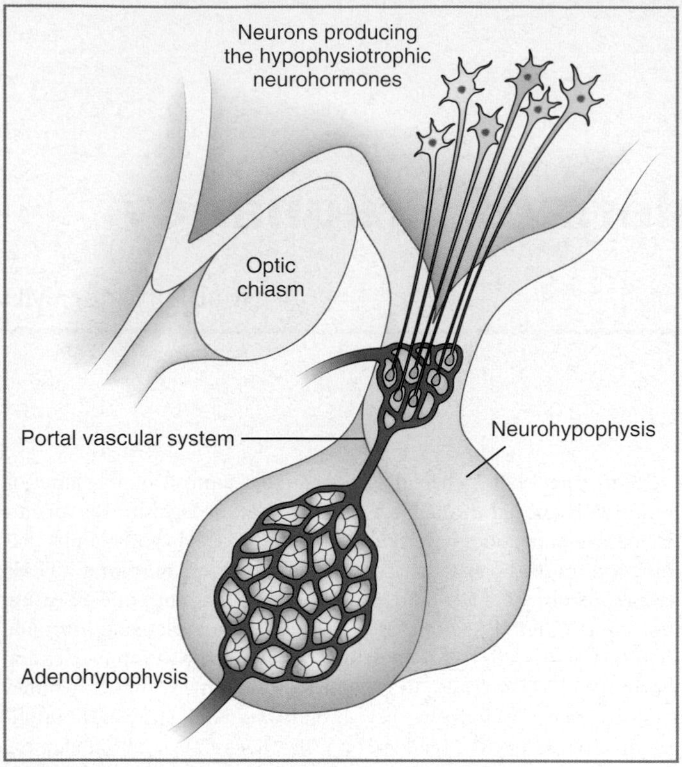

FIGURE 48-1 Neural and vascular connections of the hypothalamus and pituitary. Schematic illustration of the hypothalamus and pituitary gland indicates the neurohumoral mechanism controlling the anterior pituitary. (From Halasz B: Introduction to neuroendocrinology. In Fluckiger E, Muller EE, Thorner MO: Basic and Clinical Aspects of Neuroscience: The Dopaminergic System. Berlin, Springer-Verlag, 1985, p 1; courtesy of Sandoz, East Hanover, NJ.)

2. Pituitary GH levels decline, with an increase of a placental variant of GH. This variant has similar somatogenic but less lactogenic bioactivity than pituitary GH, with increases in insulin-like growth factor 1 (IGF-1 or somatomedin-C) commensurate with elevated levels of the GH variant. Pituitary GH is the only detectable form during the first trimester. Thereafter, the amount of placental GH increases progressively.
3. The levels of CRH of placental origin increase during the second and third trimesters.
4. A twofold to fourfold increase in ACTH concentrations occurs, despite elevations of bound and free plasma cortisol. The placenta provides an alternative source of ACTH.

The diurnal variation of cortisol, although blunted, is preserved during pregnancy (discussed in the Adrenal Glands section). Thyrotropin, decreasing slightly in the first trimester, is otherwise essentially unchanged.

The posterior pituitary is a storage terminal for the neurohypophyseal hormones oxytocin and vasopressin. Produced by the supraoptic and paraventricular hypothalamic nuclei along with their respective binding proteins or neurophysins, these hormones are transported as neurosecretory granules along the supraopticohypophysial tract to the pituitary, and from there, they find their way into the circulation. Vasopressin plays a central role in osmolarity and volume regulation. Osmoreceptors are located in the anterior hypothalamus, and vasopressin release increases when plasma osmolality rises (Fig. 48-4).

Early in pregnancy, plasma osmolality decreases to values of 5 to 10 mOsm/kg below the normal mean of 285 mOsm/kg in nonpregnant women.[6] Plasma levels of vasopressin and its response to water loading and dehydration, however, are normal in pregnancy, indicating a resetting of the threshold—that is, vasopressin is secreted at a lower plasma osmolality (see Fig. 48-4). Similarly, the plasma osmolality at which thirst is experienced is lower in the pregnant state. Along with these changes, the metabolic clearance of vasopressin increases markedly between gestational week 10 and mid-pregnancy. This is paralleled by the appearance and increase of circulating vasopressinase.[7]

Oxytocin is involved in the process of parturition[8] and in suckling. Although the role of oxytocin in the initiation of labor is unclear, there is significant preterm increase in plasma concentrations of oxytocin. During nursing, nipple stimulation initiates a neurogenic reflex that is transmitted to the hypothalamus, triggering oxytocin release from the posterior pituitary. Oxytocin then induces contraction of the myoepithelial cells and mammary duct smooth muscle, resulting in milk ejection.

Fetal Hypothalamic and Pituitary Development

The development of the structural and functional aspects of the neuroendocrine system in the fetus occurs as follows.[9] By 10 to 13 weeks' gestation, fetal pituitary and hypothalamic tissues can respond in vitro to stimulatory or inhibitory stimuli. By mid-gestation, the fetal hypothalamic-pituitary axis is a functional and autonomous unit subject to feedback control mechanisms. The posterior lobe of the fetal pituitary serves as a storage depot for neuropeptides.

Disorders of the Hypothalamus

Disorders of the hypothalamus can be congenital (e.g., Lawrence-Moon-Bardet-Biedl syndrome) or acquired inflammatory (e.g., meningitis, encephalitis), space occupying (e.g., tumors, cysts), vascular, or degenerative. For many women with these conditions, reproduction is impossible or undesirable. Among female patients with the autosomal recessive Lawrence-Moon-Bardet-Biedl syndrome of polydactyly, obesity, retinitis pigmentosa, and mental retardation, 45% to 53% are hypogonadal, but several pregnancies have been reported in such patients.[10] Craniopharyngiomas are derived from vestigial remnants of the Rathke pouch or craniopharyngeal anlage. Manifestations can include headaches, visual disturbances, and hypothalamic dysfunction, including diabetes insipidus. Seven craniopharyngiomas have been reported during pregnancy. In two, the tumor recurred, and its enlargement resulted in loss of vision in a subsequent pregnancy.[11] Two of the case reports of craniopharyngiomas, previously undiagnosed, said that patients presented with diabetes insipidus in pregnancy.[12] One of these patients also had visual field disturbances and symptoms of raised intracranial pressure. Surgery was performed 3 days after delivery at 34 weeks' gestation because of deteriorating visual acuity. Craniopharyngiomas may require surgery during pregnancy. It has even been suggested that the hormonal stimulation of pregnancy may potentiate growth of this congenital tumor. Craniopharyngioma was diagnosed in a pregnant woman who had had a normal MRI result 4 years earlier.[13]

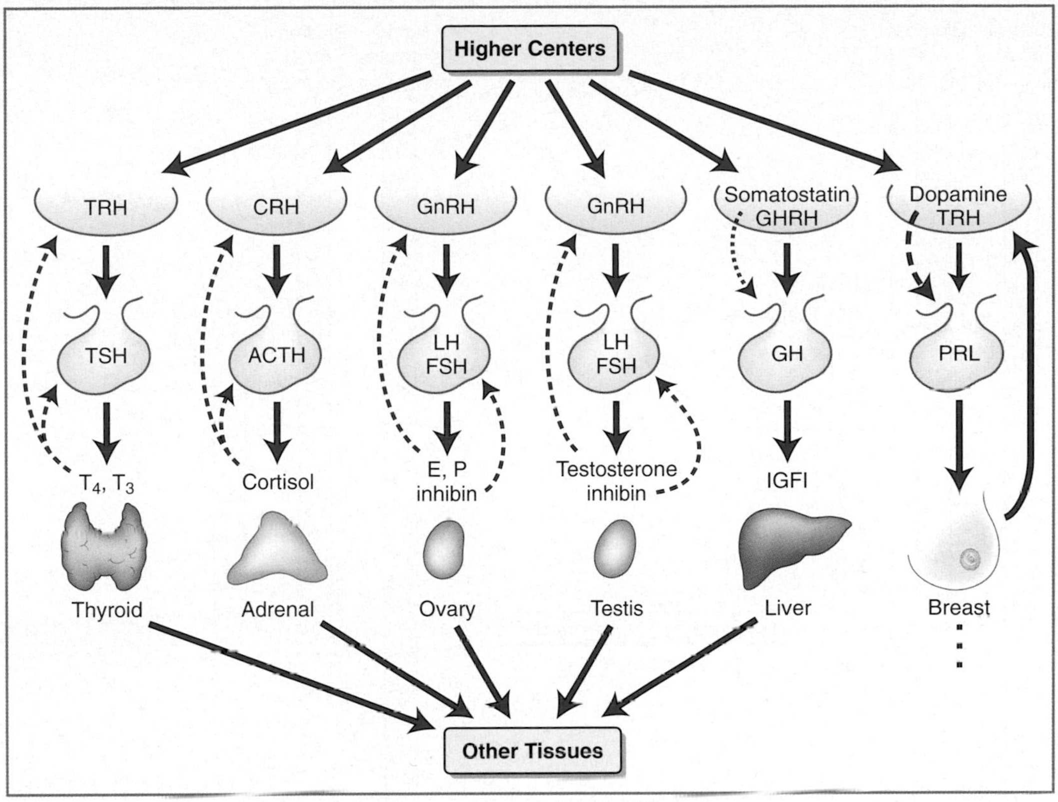

FIGURE 48-2 Relationships and feedback mechanisms of the neuroendocrine and endocrine systems. The components shown in the schematic drawing include the central nervous system, hypothalamus, anterior pituitary gland, and target glands and tissues. *Solid lines* indicate hormone secretion through stimulatory pathways; *dotted lines* indicate an inhibitory effect. ACTH, adrenocorticotropin; CRH, corticotropin-releasing hormone; E, estradiol; FSH, follicle-stimulating hormone; GH, growth hormone; GHRH, growth hormone–releasing hormone; GnRH, gonadotropin-releasing hormone; IGF-1, insulin-like growth factor 1; LH, luteinizing hormone; P, progesterone; PRL, prolactin; TRH, thyrotropin-releasing factor; TSH, thyroid-stimulating hormone; T_3, triiodothyronine; T_4, thyroxine.

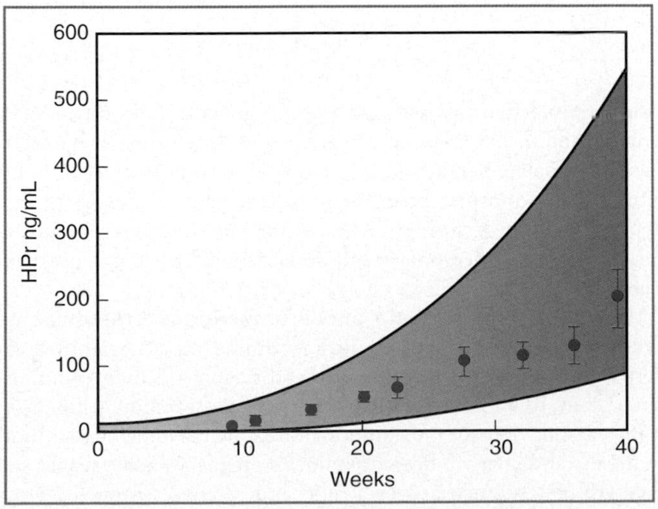

FIGURE 48-3 Prolactin levels during normal pregnancy. Basal serum prolactin (HPr) levels increase throughout a normal gestation. *Points* represent the mean ± standard error of the mean (SEM); *solid lines* represent the range of prolactin levels found during pregnancy. (From Tyson JE, Hwang P, Guyden A, et al: Studies of prolactin secretion in human pregnancy. Am J Obstet Gynecol 113:14, 1972.)

Disorders of the Pituitary

Anterior Lobe Disorders

Most commonly, tumors and, less commonly, vascular mishaps and inflammatory changes affect the anterior lobe. In their evaluation, the physician must consider anatomic derangements and the effects of excess or deficient hormones that can accompany these disorders. Because of the additional physiologic changes in pregnancy outlined previously, the combination of pregnancy and pituitary disorders poses a challenge to the obstetrician and endocrinologist in their endeavors for a safe outcome for the mother and fetus.

PITUITARY TUMORS

The topic of pituitary tumors in pregnancy has been reviewed by Molitch[5] and Gillam and colleagues.[14] Pituitary tumors can be classified as hormonally functioning or functionless lesions. Examples of the former include GH-producing tumors resulting in acromegaly, ACTH-producing tumors giving rise to Cushing disease, and prolactinomas. Prolactinoma is by far the most common pituitary tumor encountered in pregnancy. Hormonally functionless pituitary tumors are less common (although some of these produce subunits of pituitary hormones, they are clinically hormonally functionless). Because they are functionless, these pituitary tumors are relatively asymptomatic in

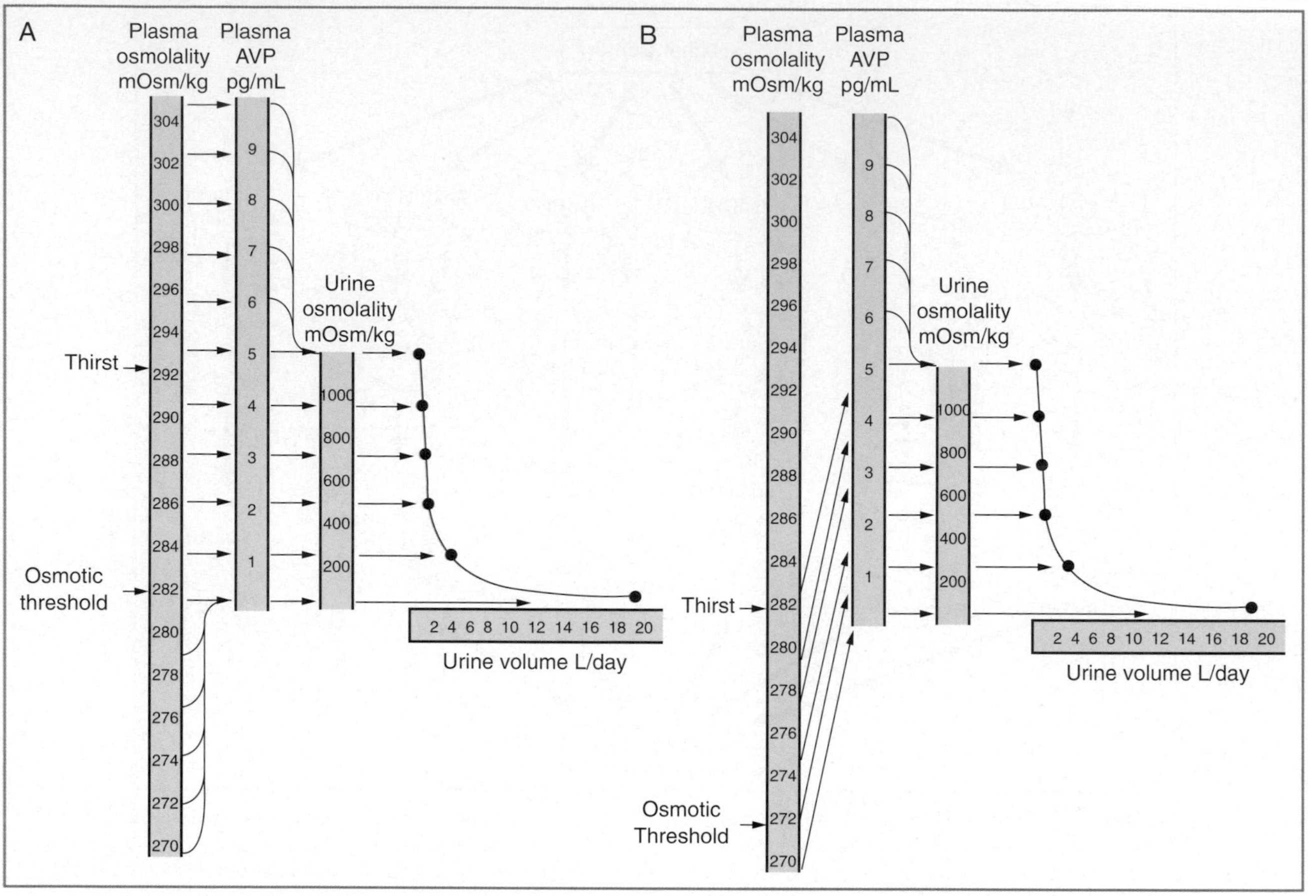

FIGURE 48-4 Osmolarity and volume regulation. **A,** Idealized schematic diagram of normal physiologic relationships shows the direct associations between plasma osmolality and plasma vasopressin and between plasma vasopressin and urine osmolality. The osmotic threshold is illustrated as a floor for plasma osmolality below which the plasma osmolality does not normally fall because of excretion of a high volume of dilute urine. Thirst is illustrated as a physiologic ceiling for plasma osmolality, because, above this level, thirst is sensed and water imbibed to avoid further elevation of plasma osmolality. **B,** Idealized schematic diagram shows the reset osmostat, as occurs in pregnancy. For the patient to function normally with a lower osmolality, thirst and the osmotic threshold must be lowered and maintain their relative relationships with one another. Urine osmolality and urine volume follow appropriately for the level of vasopressin in plasma. Subjects experience extreme thirst if the osmolality is raised into the normal range. (From Robinson AG: Disorders of antidiuretic hormone secretion. Clin Endocrinol Metab 14:55, 1985.)

their early stages and tend to be larger at the time of diagnosis. If diagnosed, the patient should undergo appropriate surgical treatment before becoming pregnant. Tumor expansion with visual field defects during pregnancy has been reported.[15,16] In the case reported by Masding and coworkers,[16] there was prompt response to bromocriptine, and this response presumably was related to shrinkage of lactotroph hyperplasia.

PROLACTINOMA

The advent of prolactin radioimmunoassay in the early 1970s permitted the correct diagnosis of prolactinomas in many patients previously thought to have functionless pituitary tumors. Because of the negative effect of excess prolactin on the hypothalamic-pituitary-gonadal axis, most of these women, who were in their childbearing years, presented with amenorrhea and, consequently, with infertility. Parallel with the development of the prolactin assay and improved radiologic techniques for diagnosing these tumors came the development and refinement of transsphenoidal microsurgical techniques and a powerful new drug, bromocriptine mesylate, which can suppress elevated prolactin concentrations to normal levels. Numerous pregnancies resulted from restoring normal gonadal function in these women, and in the 1980s, information concerning these pregnancies was consolidated. Because of the physiologic changes that occur in the pituitary in a normal pregnancy—enlargement of the gland and hyperplasia of the lactotrophs with a tenfold increase in serum prolactin—concerns about women with prolactinomas becoming pregnant were reasonable.

Effects of Prolactinoma and Bromocriptine Treatment on Pregnancy and the Fetus. Bromocriptine mesylate is an ergot derivative with potent dopamine receptor agonist activity. Administered orally, it is a potent inhibitor of prolactin secretion, with effects usually lasting only for the duration of treatment. Numerous accounts of the use and safety of bromocriptine in pregnancy are available, but they are best summarized by Krupp and Monka[17] (from the Drug Monitoring Center, Clinical Research, Sandoz, Basel, Switzerland). They collected data from 2587 pregnancies in 2437 women treated with bromocriptine during some stage of gestation. The results showed that its use was not associated with an increased risk of spontaneous abortion, multiple pregnancy, or congenital malformation in their progeny.

These investigators followed 546 children postnatally up to the age of 9 years and found no adverse effect on postnatal development. In most women treated, bromocriptine was discontinued on confirmation of pregnancy. These results are important insofar as investigations indicate that bromocriptine crosses the placental barrier and can be found in dose-related concentrations in fetal blood and in the amniotic fluid.[18] The use of bromocriptine throughout pregnancy was limited to approximately 100 patients; one infant had an undescended testicle, and another a talipes deformity.[5] The newer synthetic dopamine agonist, cabergoline, is also approved for treatment of prolactinomas. As with bromocriptine, the drug should be discontinued after pregnancy is established. Its twice-weekly administration and reduced side-effect profile makes it more palatable for some patients.[19] The experience with cabergoline use in pregnancy, albeit in fewer patients, appears to be similar to that with bromocriptine.[20,21] Given the longer safety record of bromocriptine, it is the drug of choice in patients desiring pregnancy. There have been reports of cardiac valvular defects in patients using cabergoline in large doses for Parkinson disease.[22] Although the doses used in prolactinoma patients is much smaller and the relevance of these studies to its use in such patients is unknown, caution should be exercised, and the patient should be informed.

Effects of Pregnancy on Prolactinomas. Prolactinomas are subclassified according to size as microadenomas (<10 mm in diameter) (Fig. 48-5) and macroadenomas (≥10 mm in diameter). In a review of the subject with data collected and combined from many studies, Albrecht and Betz[23] found that of 352 pregnant patients with untreated microadenomas, 8 (2.3%) experienced visual disturbances, 17 (4.8%) experienced headaches, and 2 (0.6%) had diabetes insipidus. The corresponding figures for 144 pregnant women with macroadenomas were visual disturbances in 22 (15.3%), headaches in 22 (15.3%), and diabetes insipidus in 2 (1.4%).

In the same review, the outcomes of 318 pregnancies in patients with microadenomas and macroadenomas treated (i.e., surgery, radiation therapy, or both) before pregnancy were analyzed. There were visual disturbances in 10 (3.1%), headaches in 12 (3.8%), and diabetes insipidus in 1 (0.3%). In a further compilation of series published in the world literature,[14] of 457 patients with microadenomas, 12 (2.6%) had symptomatic tumor enlargement, but none required surgery. Of 140 macroadenomas previously treated by surgery or radiation, 7 (5%) had symptomatic enlargement, and none required surgery. In contrast, of 142 macroadenomas not previously treated by surgery or radiation, 45 (31%) had symptomatic enlargement, and 12 (8.5%) had surgical treatment. Symptoms related to a pregnancy-induced increase in the size of a pituitary tumor can begin as early as the first trimester, with a mean time for the onset of visual symptoms at 14 weeks' gestation.[24] Headaches usually precede visual changes.

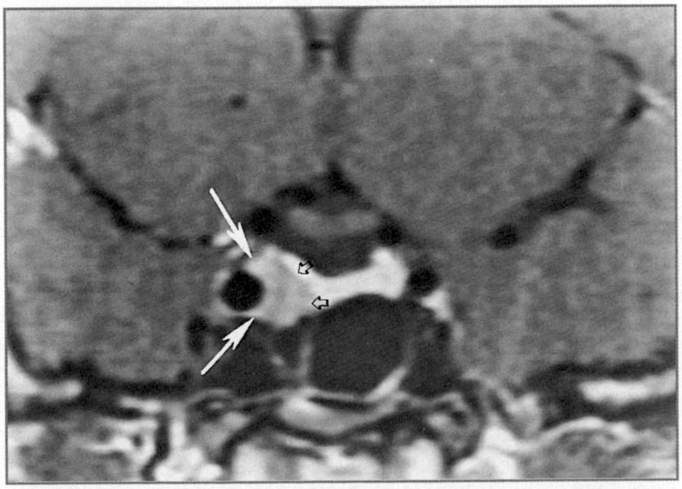

FIGURE 48-5 Prolactinoma in a 26-year-old woman. Coronal magnetic resonance imaging (SE = 600/25) after injection of gadolinium-DTPA reveals a 9 × 8 mm, solid mass *(open arrows)* of intermediate signal intensity involving the right side of the pituitary gland. The mass is abutting the dura *(solid arrows)*, which surrounds the right internal carotid artery. The gadolinium-DTPA has increased the signal intensity of normal pituitary tissue, enhancing the contrast between normal and adenomatous areas.

The data previously given can be used to counsel patients with prolactinomas who are planning pregnancy.[14,25] Patients with microadenomas can safely be given bromocriptine. Visual field testing and MRI should be performed in patients with visual changes or symptoms suggestive of tumor expansion. For patients with small intrasellar or inferiorly expanding macroadenomas, bromocriptine may also be given as primary therapy. If tumor reduction is demonstrated, pregnancy should be allowed and the drug stopped when pregnancy is diagnosed. The rate of clinically serious complications is unlikely to be high in such cases. In patients with large macroadenomas with suprasellar extension, the risk of tumor expansion is significant when using bromocriptine to establish pregnancy. Pre-pregnancy tumor debulking can significantly reduce the risk of tumor expansion in pregnancy in these patients. Alternatively, bromocriptine may be administered throughout pregnancy as discussed previously and in the Management of Prolactinoma Complications during Pregnancy section. For patients with macroadenomas treated with bromocriptine or surgically, follow-up at 1- to 3-month intervals is recommended, along with visual field testing. Repeat MRI is performed for patients with symptoms or signs of tumor expansion. Recommendations for management of patients with prolactinomas are outlined in Tables 48-1 and 48-2.

Despite prior surgical intervention, complications can occur during pregnancy.[26] Monthly measurement of serum prolactin is not necessary. Prolactin concentrations measured in a group of patients with surgically untreated microadenomas were found to be elevated early in gestation but did not increase further with advancing gestation,[27] in contrast with normal pregnant controls (Fig. 48-6). A small subset of women appears to experience decrease or normalization of prolactin levels after delivery. Tumor necrosis might have occurred in some, and use of bromocriptine has been associated with tumor fibrosis.[28]

Management of Prolactinoma Complications during Pregnancy. Bromocriptine (and cabergoline) has tumor-shrinking properties. It has been used successfully in the treatment of such complications and is the initial treatment of choice.[5] It should be administered with food and the dose adjusted according to symptoms (e.g., 2.5 to 5 mg given two or three times daily). Glucocorticoids may also be given to expedite recovery of visual defects. Surgery is recommended only if there is no response to bromocriptine.

Most patients with microadenomas have uncomplicated pregnancies, whereas a disturbing number of patients with untreated macroadenomas have symptomatic tumor enlargement. Given the tumor-shrinking properties of bromocriptine, it is not surprising that the continuous use of bromocriptine in pregnancy has been advocated and carried out in patients with macroadenomas.[29] Experience with its use throughout gestation is limited to approximately 100 patients.[5] Although the rates of abortion and perinatal mortality do not differ in women with pituitary tumors that are untreated or treated before or during pregnancy, there is a significant increase in prematurity among those treated (i.e., surgery, radiotherapy, or both) during pregnancy, compared with those not requiring such treatment or with those

TABLE 48-1 RECOMMENDATIONS FOR TREATMENT OF PATIENTS WITH PROLACTINOMAS WHO DESIRE PREGNANCY

Treatment	Microadenomas and Intrasellar Macroadenomas	Suprasellar Macroadenomas
Primary	Bromocriptine	Transsphenoidal surgery followed by bromocriptine
Alternative	Transsphenoidal surgery followed by bromocriptine (if necessary)	Radiotherapy plus bromocriptine *or* continuous bromocriptine

TABLE 48-2 MANAGEMENT OF PATIENTS HARBORING PROLACTINOMAS DURING GESTATION

Status of Patient	Microadenomas	Macroadenomas
Asymptomatic	Stop bromocriptine. Provide routine obstetric care with evaluation for symptoms of tumor expansion.	Stop bromocriptine. Perform monthly evaluation for symptoms of tumor expansion. Check visual fields every 1 to 3 months.
Symptomatic	Check visual fields. Measure the serum prolactin concentration. Obtain magnetic resonance imaging of the pituitary gland. Initiate bromocriptine with or without dexamethasone for visual complications. Perform transsphenoidal surgery if unresponsive to bromocriptine.	Check visual fields. Measure the serum prolactin concentration. Obtain magnetic resonance imaging of the pituitary gland. Initiate bromocriptine with or without dexamethasone for visual complications. Perform transsphenoidal surgery if unresponsive to bromocriptine.

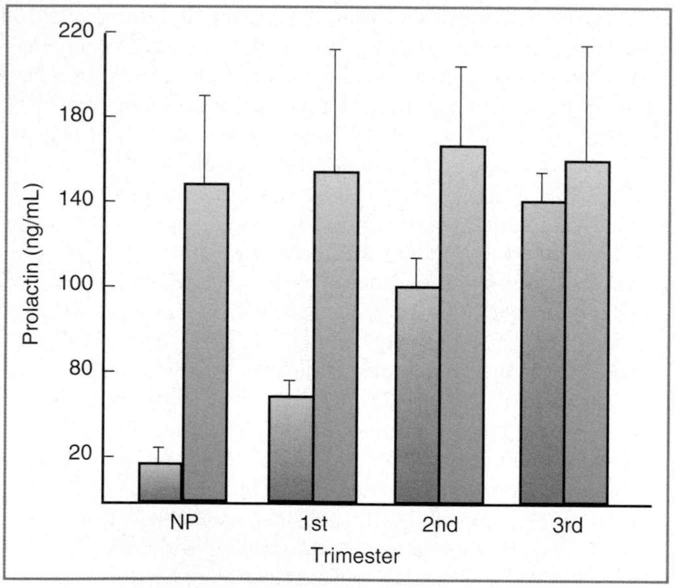

FIGURE 48-6 Prolactin concentrations. Maternal serum prolactin levels (mean ± SEM) were measured in patients with microadenomas (*blue bars*, *n* = 237) and controls (*purple bars*, *n* = 215) while nonpregnant (NP) and during each trimester of pregnancy. (From Divers WA, Yen SSC: Prolactin producing microadenomas in pregnancy. Obstet Gynecol 62:425, 1983; reprinted with permission of the American College of Obstetricians and Gynecologists.)

treated before pregnancy.[24] Pituitary apoplexy, which is a rare event, has been reported in a patient with a macroadenoma in early pregnancy.[30]

Breastfeeding and Postpartum Care. There is no reason to avoid breastfeeding when a patient with prolactinoma wishes to nurse her child. In a small study of 14 women with microadenomas who breastfed for 6 to 14 months, the level of serum prolactin was not significantly higher than it was before pregnancy.[31] In another study, the increase in prolactin associated with suckling was absent in women with pathologic hyperprolactinemia. For those wishing to inhibit lactation, bromocriptine is the treatment of choice in a dose of approximately 2.5 mg given three times daily with food.

Although occasional case reports have described seizures or strokes in women who used bromocriptine to inhibit postpartum lactation—and it should be kept in mind that suppression of lactation is no longer an approved indication for the use of this agent—a recent case-control study failed to link these events to the actual use of bromocriptine.[32] Estrogen should not be used to inhibit lactation because the tumor can expand. Ophthalmologic and radiologic evaluation and determination of serum prolactin concentrations are in order 6–8 weeks after delivery. In most instances, the sella returns to its original size and prolactin decreases to previous levels. Further pregnancies are not contraindicated in patients with prolactinomas. Decreases in prolactin and tumor size have been reported in patients with multiple bromocriptine-induced pregnancies.[33]

EXCESSIVE GROWTH HORMONE SECRETION: ACROMEGALY

Acromegaly is the result of excessive GH secretion in adults, and it is associated with acidophilic or chromophobic pituitary adenomas. About 60% of patients have macroadenomas. Women with acromegaly slowly develop coarse facial features, prognathism, and spadelike hands and feet. When clinical evidence exists, a glucose tolerance test is performed; lack of suppression of GH below 2 ng/mL during this test is in keeping with a diagnosis of acromegaly in nonpregnant patients. Because the biologic effect of GH is mediated through somatomedin-C, elevation of serum concentration of this growth factor is considered a useful confirmatory test and has been used to monitor the progression of the disease. In the context of pregnancy, however, somatomedin-C concentrations should be interpreted with caution because they can be elevated.[34] Because of the production of a placental variant of GH, special assays using antibodies that recognize specific epitopes on the two hormones are necessary to differentiate normal from placental GH.[35] The placental variant is undetectable within 24 hours after delivery. TRH testing may distinguish pituitary from placental GH; 70% of patients with acromegaly experience a GH response to TRH, whereas the placental variant does not cause a response.[36] Pituitary GH secretion is pulsatile, with 13 to 19 pulses daily, as opposed to the placental variant, which is nonpulsatile.

Menstrual irregularity or amenorrhea is an extremely common finding in acromegalic women. Nonetheless, pregnancy can occur in women with acromegaly and has been reported in 70 patients.[37] It can be accompanied by tumor expansion in approximately 10%, necessitating hypophysectomy. Despite other soft tissue changes, no major changes occur in the genital tract that would complicate delivery. Definitive treatment before conception is the treatment of choice in acromegalic women desiring children. Carbohydrate intolerance occurs in up to 50% and overt diabetes in up to 20% of acromegalic women, and the insulin resistance of pregnancy is additive. Hypertension occurs in 25% to 35% of acromegalic women, and cardiac disease is common. An additional six cases with favorable outcomes have been reported.[38]

An algorithm for the management of acromegaly in pregnancy has been presented by Herman-Bonert and colleagues.[37] Management was also reviewed by Molitch.[5] The observation that levodopa (L-dopa) causes a paradoxical decrease in GH in acromegaly led to the use of dopaminergic agonists in the treatment of acromegaly. In two reported cases, pregnancy occurred in acromegalic women during bromocriptine therapy. Continuation of treatment during pregnancy did not lead to tumor expansion.[39] Tumor expansion resulting in visual field defects, however, has been reported in one of two patients with acromegaly and macroadenomas during pregnancy.[15]

If acromegaly is diagnosed in a pregnant patient, management depends on the activity of the disease, the tumor size, and the stage of pregnancy. Active disease during pregnancy may respond to bromocriptine until fetal lung maturation is documented. If signs and symptoms related to suprasellar extension do not abate with bromocriptine, transsphenoidal surgery could be necessary.

In a case reported by Yap and associates,[40] acromegaly was diagnosed in the second trimester. Bromocriptine corrected visual field defects and suppressed prolactin secretion but did not reduce fasting GH levels. It was suggested that suppression of physiologic lactotroph hyperplasia by bromocriptine might permit noninvasive management of the pituitary adenoma in pregnancy. The somatostatin analogues octreotide and lanreotide have been used in at least 10 patients.[41,42] In three patients, the drug was continued throughout pregnancy without reported ill effects on the fetus, despite documented transplacental passage.[43] Somatostatin analogues should be discontinued in acromegalic patients contemplating pregnancy, but they may be considered an alternative to transsphenoidal surgery in pregnancy for an expanding tumor if the patient does not respond to dopaminergic agonists such as bromocriptine. The maternal-fetal transfer of GH it thought to be negligible, and apart from the effect of glucose intolerance, the fetus is not thought to be affected by acromegaly.

THYROTROPIN-SECRETING TUMORS

Three cases of TSH-secreting tumors and pregnancy have been reported. One patient was treated with octreotide before pregnancy, stopped the medication with the pregnancy diagnosis, but developed symptomatic growth at 6 months. The second, whose pregnancy was uncomplicated, received octreotide throughout gestation. The third had tumor enlargement and visual loss despite bromocriptine, necessitating transsphenoidal surgery.[44]

CUSHING SYNDROME

The hypothalamic-pituitary-adrenal axis in pregnancy was the subject of a review by Lindsay and Nieman[45] and Cushing syndrome in pregnancy the subject of a specific review by Lindsay and associates.[46] Cortisol secretion is controlled by the hypothalamic-pituitary axis. Cushing syndrome is a state of hypercortisolism that can arise from excess ACTH produced by the pituitary or an ectopic ACTH source such as a tumor, both of which can lead to bilateral adrenal hyperplasia. An adrenal lesion (i.e., adenoma or carcinoma) may be the direct source of excess cortisol.

Pregnancy is uncommon in patients with Cushing syndrome because of its association with a high incidence of menstrual disturbances and anovulation. Pituitary-dependent Cushing syndrome, also called Cushing disease, gives rise to bilateral adrenal hyperplasia and a state of hypercortisolism. Although pituitary-dependent Cushing syndrome is the most common cause in nonpregnant patients, it is relatively less commonly associated with pregnancy, because hyperfunctioning adrenal tumors are relatively more common in pregnant patients with this syndrome. A possible explanation for this discrepancy is the greater degree of ovulatory disturbance in patients with pituitary-dependent Cushing syndrome.[47]

In 136 pregnancies in 122 women,[45] the mean gestational age at diagnosis was 18 weeks. Adrenal adenomas accounted for almost one half of the cases (compared with 15% in nonpregnant women), with adrenal carcinomas occurring in 10%. Pituitary-dependant Cushing syndrome (i.e., Cushing disease) was less common, occurring in a third of the 122 women, compared with 70% in the general population. Ectopic ACTH occurred in four patients. Exacerbation of Cushing syndrome in pregnancy with amelioration or remission after pregnancy has been reported.[48,49]

Diagnosis. The diagnosis of Cushing syndrome in pregnancy can be rendered more difficult because weight gain, hypertension, striae, edema, and pigmentation may occur in normal pregnancy. More specific signs, such as thinning of the skin, spontaneous bruising, and muscle weakness, should be sought. The laboratory diagnosis is complicated by the changes in adrenal function that occur during normal pregnancy. These include an increase in bound and free serum cortisol levels, increased levels of urinary free cortisol, and a lack of adequate suppression of cortisol after low-dose dexamethasone treatment.

Urinary free cortisol excretion is less than 50 μg/24 hours in nonpregnant women with the use of mass spectroscopy assays. Excretion is increased during normal pregnancy. The mean 24 urinary free cortisol level is increased at least 180% during gestation. Levels of total and free plasma cortisol increase twofold to threefold, with a wide range of normal variation in morning cortisol ranging from 16.3 to 55 μg/dL.[45] The diurnal variation is blunted. The suppressibility of cortisol was shown to be 40% after 1 mg of dexamethasone in second- and third-trimester normal pregnancies, compared with 80% in nongravid controls; loss of suppression increased with increasing gestation. In a collected series and review of the literature with 136 cases of Cushing syndrome in pregnancy in 122 women, the following features were identified[45]:

1. There was a mean eightfold elevation in urinary free cortisol (range, 2- to 22-fold).
2. Diurnal variation of cortisol was absent.
3. Midnight cortisol level was elevated (mean, 30.9 μg/dL).
4. Using 1 mg overnight or 2-day low-dose (2 mg daily) dexamethasone suppression testing, the median suppressibility of cortisol was approximately 30% in women with Cushing disease and 10% in those with adrenal Cushing syndrome; dexamethasone suppress-

ibility was not considered a sensitive test for Cushing syndrome in pregnancy.

5. In the differential diagnosis of Cushing syndrome, 8 of 16 with the adrenal form or ACTH-independent hyperplasia had ACTH assay results below the detection limit of 10 pg/mL. Conversely, of 18 patients with Cushing disease, 2 had ACTH values below 10 pg/mL (i.e., inappropriately low).
6. Using high-dose dexamethasone (8 mg daily) and a criterion of 80% suppression as indicative of pituitary-dependant Cushing syndrome, all patients with ACTH-independent Cushing syndrome failed to suppress. However, 3 of 7 with pituitary-dependent Cushing syndrome did not have suppression.
7. MRI of the pituitary identified an adenoma in 5 of 8 subjects.
8. Adrenal imaging correctly identified the lesion in 11 of 15 by ultrasound; MRI or computed tomography were uniformly successful in identifying the lesion. Bearing these changes in mind, urinary free cortisol excretion of more than three times the upper limit of normal in the second or third trimesters may suggest Cushing syndrome.

To distinguish pituitary-dependent Cushing disease from hyperfunctioning adrenal tumors, a high-dose dexamethasone suppression test is recommended (8 mg/day for at least 2 days). Significant (≥50%) suppression of plasma cortisol is the rule in pituitary-dependent Cushing syndrome, and failure of suppression with high-dose dexamethasone, along with low or undetectable ACTH concentrations, strongly suggests an adrenal source. Because the placenta also produces ACTH, this test may not always be reliable. Ectopic ACTH syndrome also causes failure to suppress. In determining the differential diagnosis, high-dose dexamethasone suppression testing and plasma ACTH should be performed. The pituitary can be evaluated during pregnancy by means of MRI.[2,49] CRH testing in pregnancy can also aid in the differential diagnosis. Although the ACTH response to CRH is blunted in the third trimester, a substantial rise in cortisol after CRH stimulation in Cushing syndrome is consistent with pituitary-dependent disease. One microgram of ovine CRH was given per kilogram of body weight (U. S. Food and Drug Administration [FDA] pregnancy category C drug), and a rise in cortisol (44% to 130%) was seen in those with pituitary disease confirmed surgically.[45] Pituitary disease can also be distinguished from ectopic ACTH by inferior petrosal sinus sampling combined with CRH stimulation. There is one report of such testing in pregnancy.[50]

Maternal-Fetal Complications. Although congenital malformations are not more common in Cushing syndrome than in normal pregnancy,[48] maternal and fetal complications can occur. In the 136 pregnancies reported by Lindsay and Nieman,[45] maternal morbidity and mortality included hypertension (68%), diabetes or impaired glucose tolerance (25%), preeclampsia (14%), osteoporosis and fracture (5%), heart failure (3%), psychiatric disturbances (4%), wound infections (2%), and maternal deaths (2%). Fetal morbidity was also significant, with a prematurity rate of 43%, stillbirth rate of 6%, and spontaneous abortion rate of 5%, and there were two infant deaths. Intrauterine growth restriction is prevalent, occurring in approximately one half of reported cases.[47] Possible causes include hypertension and cortisol excess itself. Neonatal adrenal insufficiency has been reported and is presumably caused by suppression of the fetal hypothalamic-pituitary-adrenal axis from transplacental transport of excess maternal cortisol.

Therapy. Because of the poor fetal outcome, therapy aimed at controlling the hypercortisolism is recommended. In the 136 pregnancies discussed previously with outcomes available, when no active treatment was given, there was a 76% rate of live births, compared with 89% among women treated at a mean gestational age of 20 weeks. The following recommendations for treatment have been suggested.[46]

In the first trimester, pituitary surgery for pituitary-dependent Cushing syndrome and adrenal surgery for tumors of adrenal origin (especially to rule out carcinoma) should be performed. In the third trimester, early delivery of the fetus—preferably vaginal—may be attempted. Metyrapone therapy (to block cortisol secretion) may reduce hypercortisolism until fetal maturity is attained.[51] In the second trimester, treatment should be individualized; the alternatives are definitive surgery or medical therapy aimed at ameliorating hypercortisolism. Successful transsphenoidal surgery has been reported in the second trimester.[52] The risks of treatment with metyrapone, ketoconazole, and aminoglutethimide, all of which block cortisol secretion, are uncertain because transplacental passage occurs and fetal adrenal steroid synthesis may be affected.[53] The risk of teratogenicity, virilization of female fetuses (with aminoglutethimide) or inadequate masculinization of a male fetus (with ketoconazole) discourages the use of these two agents. Metyrapone is the drug of choice, although there is a potential for exacerbation of hypertension. Mitotane is teratogenic and should not be used.

Nelson Syndrome. When a patient with pituitary-dependent Cushing syndrome undergoes bilateral adrenalectomy as definitive treatment for hypercortisolism and the pituitary lesion is not adequately addressed, a syndrome of hyperpigmentation along with an expanding intrasellar ACTH-producing tumor can result. This is called Nelson syndrome. The association of this syndrome and pregnancy is rare. In a series involving 10 cases, 5 required postpartum treatment of their pituitary tumors, 5 were only observed, and 1 required surgical treatment during the pregnancy, with successful outcomes for the mother and child.[54] A later case documented an uncomplicated pregnancy and normal lactation.[55]

HYPOPITUITARISM

Diminished or decreased production of anterior pituitary hormones results in inadequate activity of target organs, such as the thyroid, adrenals, and gonads. The deficiency can be partial—affecting trophic hormones in various degrees—or it can be complete, resulting in panhypopituitarism. The role of the obstetrician-gynecologist in this context is twofold: to be alert to and aware of the possibility of two disease processes that can affect the pregnant patient—Sheehan syndrome and lymphocytic hypophysitis—and to recognize and treat hypopituitarism in a pregnant patient, thereby avoiding undesirable consequences.

Sheehan Syndrome. In 1937, Sheehan[56] drew attention to the relationship between postpartum hemorrhage and anterior pituitary necrosis. Because the syndrome is distinctly uncommon, with other conditions associated with shock and vascular collapse, it is assumed that the hyperplastic gland in pregnancy is more vulnerable to an inadequate blood supply. In a retrospective survey by Hall,[57] pregnant patients admitted for hemorrhagic collapse were subsequently traced and evaluated for hypopituitarism; the incidence was approximately 3.6%. There is said to be no direct correlation between the severity of the hemorrhage and the occurrence of Sheehan syndrome, but the major part of the pituitary must be destroyed before symptoms become evident.[57] In one review, small sella size was suggested as a risk.[58]

In a series of 25 cases,[59] 50% of patients had permanent amenorrhea, and the remainder had rare and scanty menses. Only one patient menstruated normally, and in most, lactation was poor or absent. There was a surprisingly long interval between the obstetric event and diagnosis (>10 years) for more than one half of the patients. In a later series of 20 cases, the mean time between diagnosis and date of last delivery was 26.8 years. Amenorrhea and absent lactation occurred in 70%. Some degree of hypogonadism, GH deficiency, and low prolactin levels occurred in all; 90% were hypothyroid, and 55% had adrenal failure.[61]

Although pregnancy in hypopituitary patients is rare, the inability to establish the diagnosis and institute proper therapy can have lethal consequences for the mother and fetus. Grimes and Brooks[61] reviewed the pregnancies of their patients with Sheehan syndrome. There was an 87% rate of live births, 13% rate of abortions, and no stillbirth or maternal death in 15 pregnancies among patients receiving hormonal therapy. In sharp contrast, in 24 pregnancies among 11 women in whom hormone replacement was not provided, there was a 58% rate of live births, 42% rate of abortions, one stillbirth, and three maternal deaths.

In nonpregnant patients thought to have Sheehan syndrome, the diagnosis and the extent of pituitary damage can be determined by tests of target organ function (e.g., thyroid function tests, cortisol concentration) and tests of pituitary reserve.[62] An ongoing pregnancy does not constitute evidence against the diagnosis of Sheehan syndrome, and it should be considered for all patients with a history of postpartum hemorrhage, especially if the patient is currently symptomatic. The finding of a low serum thyroxine level and low TSH level is in keeping with secondary hypothyroidism; low cortisol concentrations (compared with those of normal pregnant women) and failure of cortisol and ACTH to increase during times of stress are in keeping with diminished ACTH reserve. Imaging studies are likely to reveal an empty sella turcica.[63]

Treatment of pituitary insufficiency during pregnancy does not present special problems. Oral L-thyroxine (0.1 to 0.2 mg/day) and cortisol (20 mg in the morning and 10 mg in the evening) or prednisone (5 mg in the morning and 2.5 mg in the evening) are administered. There is no need for mineralocorticoids. The dose of L-thyroxine required in pregnancy is likely to be higher, and free thyroxine concentrations should be kept in the mid-normal range. TSH is not useful for monitoring treatment. As in the nonpregnant state, glucocorticoid requirements may increase during episodes of intercurrent illness. During labor, a good state of hydration should be maintained and parenteral glucocorticoids administered. This is most easily achieved by the intravenous infusion of hydrocortisone (cortisol). The dose can be adjusted as appropriate for the patient's state, ranging from 25 to 75 mg every 6 hours. After delivery, parenteral glucocorticoids should be continued in smaller doses for a few days along with intravenous fluids.

Pituitary Necrosis. Spontaneous pituitary necrosis and hypopituitarism can occur in pregnant diabetic patients, possibly related to diabetic vascular changes and the general susceptibility of the anterior pituitary to ischemia in pregnancy. It is manifested by severe, midline headaches and vomiting during the third trimester, followed by a decrease in insulin requirements. In three of eight patients reported, the condition was associated with fetal death followed by maternal death.[64] Early recognition and prompt management are essential. Pituitary apoplexy in a nondiabetic patient presenting during pregnancy with headaches and circulatory collapse has also been reported.[65]

Lymphocytic Adenohypophysitis. In 1962, Goudie and Pinkerton[66] described the case of a 22-year-old woman who died of circulatory collapse 8 hours after appendectomy. This occurred 14 months after a normal pregnancy and delivery, but she had developed secondary amenorrhea after delivery. Autopsy revealed lymphocytic infiltration of the pituitary and of the thyroid; the investigators postulated an autoimmune mechanism to explain both.

Lymphocytic adeno hypophysitis (LAH) was the subject of a review.[67] As was previously known, there is a striking temporal association of LAH with pregnancy. Of a total of 245 cases of LAH reported, 210 occurred in women, and of these women, 120 (57%) presented during pregnancy or after delivery, most in the last month of pregnancy or within the 2 months after delivery. There were no fetal complications, but one patient died in labor. Sixteen women had subsequent pregnancies. Release of pituitary antigens during pregnancy-related changes and alterations in pituitary blood supply have been suggested as links to altered immunity. Anti-pituitary antibodies have been demonstrated in a significant number of cases.[67,68] Exacerbation of the disease after delivery, even when it initially manifests in pregnancy, has been described.[69]

Table 48-3 inventories the characteristics of patients with LAH. Hypocortisolism is the most important hormone deficiency, followed by TSH, gonadotropin, and prolactin. Hyperprolactinemia may also occur, manifesting as amenorrhea or galactorrhea. Stalk compression, an inflammatory process in the lactotroph inducing release of prolactin, and antibodies stimulating prolactin synthesis are potential mechanisms leading to hyperprolactinemia.

The association of this disease with pregnancy was highlighted in an immunohistochemical study performed on pituitary material obtained at autopsy of 69 women who were pregnant or who had undergone delivery; among these were five cases of mild LAH.[1] In four of the five cases, the patients died at 38 to 41 weeks' gestation.

This is a potentially life-threatening condition, but it is a treatable disease affecting young women during or after pregnancy. The diag-

TABLE 48-3 CHARACTERISTICS OF 245 PATIENTS WITH LYMPHOCYTIC ADENOHYPOPHYSITIS

Characteristic	Quantity or Percent
Mean age of women (n = 210)	35 yr
Mean age of men (n = 35)	45 yr
History of onset in pregnant or postpartum women (120 women)	57%
Hypocortisolism	42%
Hypothyroidism	18%
Hypogonadism	12%
Inability to lactate	11%
Hyperprolactinemia	23%
Polyuria or polydipsia	1%
Headaches	53%
Visual disturbances	43%
Association with other autoimmune disease*	18%
Median duration of symptoms with diagnosis outside pregnancy	12 mo
Median duration of symptoms with diagnosis associated with pregnancy	4 mo
Required long-term hormonal treatment	56%
Deaths	8.6%
Disease resolved spontaneously	4.5%

*Includes 131 patients with infundibulo-neurohypophysitis and panhypophysitis and 245 patients with lymphocytic adenohypophysitis.

Adapted from Caturegli P, Newschaffer C, Olivi A, et al: Autoimmune hypophysitis. Endocr Rev 26:599, 2005.

nosis should be considered in women of reproductive age presenting with signs and symptoms of anterior pituitary hormone deficiencies (isolated or combined) before or after delivery, especially in the absence of significant bleeding during labor. The diagnosis should also be considered in pregnant or postpartum women with visual symptoms and changes. In the absence of a threat to vision, such patients should be treated medically with hormone replacement and their progress observed. MRI should be used to delineate and follow the anatomic defects. It typically shows a symmetrically enlarged gland and a thickened stalk, and in contrast to macroadenomas, MRI shows strong and homogeneous enhancement after gadolinium contrast.

The use of steroids has been associated with amelioration of visual symptoms,[70,71] and the sellar mass has been shown to regress spontaneously. In another reported case,[71] partial hypopituitarism resolved after delivery in a biopsy-diagnosed case of LAH. Glucocorticoids should be the first line of treatment for the pituitary mass. Other immunosuppressive drugs, such as azathioprine and methotrexate, have also been used. Decompressive surgery is indicated only for progressive visual deficit. Although considered a disease of the anterior pituitary, LAH can manifest as diabetes insipidus with thickening and prominence of the pituitary stalk.[72] LAH has recurred in a subsequent pregnancy in a case of histologically documented hypophysitis.[73] One case was associated with postpartum cardiomyopathy.[74]

Posterior Lobe Disorders

DIABETES INSIPIDUS

Vasopressin and oxytocin, produced in the supraoptic and paraventricular nuclei of the hypothalamus, are released into the posterior lobe and then into the circulation. No disease process with oxytocin deficiency or excess has been described. Lack of vasopressin results in diabetes insipidus, however, and this can occur as a primary or idiopathic disorder (≈30% of cases) or can be acquired secondary to a variety of pathologic lesions, including cranial injuries (16%), infections, sellar and suprasellar tumors (25%), and vascular lesions. The main symptoms are polyuria, polydipsia, and low urinary specific gravity. The diagnosis is confirmed by water deprivation. During this test, increasing serum osmolality in the face of low urine osmolality is diagnostic of diabetes insipidus; a return toward normal after vasopressin administration confirms vasopressin deficiency.

Effect of Diabetes Insipidus on Pregnancy. In a comprehensive review, Hendricks[75] concluded that the prior existence of diabetes insipidus in a woman did not appear to alter her fertility, the course of pregnancy, the effectiveness of labor, or lactation. Because oxytocin is also produced in the same hypothalamic nuclei, diabetes insipidus is of particular interest in managing the pregnant woman because of the possible relationship of decreased oxytocin with decreased uterine contractions during labor. Despite one report of uterine atony,[76] it appears that labor is normal in most patients with diabetes insipidus.

Effect of Pregnancy on Diabetes Insipidus. The effect of pregnancy on diabetes insipidus has been reviewed by Durr and Lindheimer.[77] Diabetes insipidus during pregnancy appears to be characterized by several distinct clinical entities: pregnancy in patients with diabetes insipidus antedating gestation; transient arginine vasopressin (AVP)–resistant but L-deamino, 8-D-arginine vasopressin (DDAVP)–responsive diabetes insipidus; transient diabetes insipidus during pregnancy in patients with acquired or hereditary latent diabetes insipidus; diabetes insipidus after a complicated delivery; and transient de novo nephrogenic diabetes insipidus, resistant to AVP and DDAVP.

For pregnancy in patients with diabetes insipidus antedating gestation, the effect of pregnancy on established diabetes insipidus varies. In a review of the subject, Hime and Richardson[78] found that 58% of patients deteriorated, 20% improved, and 15% remained the same. The metabolic clearance of vasopressin markedly increases between gestational week 10 and mid-pregnancy, and it is associated with parallel increases in circulating vasopressinase. Placental inactivation of vasopressin with the production of large quantities of vasopressinase by the placenta may contribute to this increase in clearance rate.[7] In a few patients in whom preeclampsia developed, the diabetes insipidus improved. The decreased contribution of the placenta to destruction of vasopressin is thought to explain this improvement.[79]

Transient AVP-resistant but DDAVP-responsive diabetes insipidus is attributable to excessively high quantities of circulating vasopressinase.[80] It is often associated with liver abnormalities in the mother, such as acute fatty liver or HELLP syndrome (*h*emolysis, *e*levated *l*iver enzymes, *l*ow *p*latelets). Vasopressinase isoenzymes are proteins that are cleared by the liver, and under these circumstances, excessive amounts are made available. Two cases were reported by Brewster and Hayslett[81] that were unassociated with liver disease. An accompanying commentary stated that a sodium level of 140 mEq/L should be considered hypernatremia in most pregnant women, and early recognition and treatment were advised.[82] A case of transient diabetes insipidus in pregnancy showed absence of the hyperintensity of the posterior pituitary lobe on MRI during pregnancy with restoration after delivery, presumably reflecting depletion and restoration of neurosecretory granules.[83]

Transient diabetes insipidus during pregnancy can occur in patients with acquired or hereditary latent diabetes insipidus. Patients with limited vasopressin-secreting capacity (latent-central defect) may be unable to sustain the increased production rates necessary during gestation. Clinically, transient diabetes insipidus manifests in the latter part of gestation coinciding with peak vasopressinase levels, and subsequent pregnancies may involve many recurrences. History of prior insult to the area, such as histiocytosis X or Sheehan syndrome, may be obtained. Classic hereditary nephrogenic diabetes insipidus is caused by an X-linked recessive mutation of the renal vasopressin receptor gene, and symptomatic diabetes insipidus in female carriers is rare. Some carriers, however, do have defects in renal concentrating ability, and it has been hypothesized that nonrandom X-chromosome inactivation in the kidneys could be responsible for the variable expression. Unmasking of a mild defect in vasopressin action (i.e., nephrogenic diabetes insipidus) may occur. The increased disposal of vasopressin could lead to decompensation. Lowering of the osmotic threshold for thirst, which occurs normally in pregnancy (see Fig. 48-4), causes polydipsia and unacceptable polyuria in a patient with previously compensated nephrogenic diabetes insipidus.[84]

Diabetes insipidus can occur after a complicated delivery. This is often associated with severe blood loss leading to some degree of pituitary apoplexy or Sheehan syndrome.

Transient de novo nephrogenic diabetes insipidus may be resistant to AVP and DDAVP. During pregnancy, the concentration of prostaglandin E_2 in the kidney physiologically increases. Ford and Lumpkin[85] found high prostaglandin E_2 concentrations. Reduced renal sensitivity to vasopressin has been proposed[86] to explain this.

Treatment. The treatment of choice for central diabetes insipidus is DDAVP or desmopressin acetate, a synthetic analogue of vasopressin, administered intranasally or orally. Clinical experience with DDAVP, in a study involving many infants exposed during gestation, has confirmed its safety.[87,88] Dosages range from 10 to 20 μg given once or twice daily intranasally or 0.05 to 0.1 mg administered twice daily orally, titrating up if needed. In a study by Burrow and coauthors,[89] the drug was administered and DDAVP concentrations were measured as vasopressin by radioimmunoassay in maternal serum and breast milk. Whereas maternal serum concentrations rose about sevenfold, breast milk concentrations showed little change. This suggests that, given the low levels of DDAVP in milk, these mothers may breastfeed. DDAVP has little pressor or uterotonic action, and it is not affected by vasopressinase.

PRIMARY POLYDIPSIA DURING GESTATION

Primary polydipsia has rarely been reported during gestation.[90] Pregnancy was merely incidental and had no role in the polydipsia.

Adrenal Glands

The adrenal cortex plays an important and essential metabolic role in humans. Adrenal steroidogenesis leads to the production of three types of steroids. Mineralocorticoids are produced by the zona glomerulosa, glucocorticoids produced primarily in the zona fasciculata, and sex steroids produced in the zona reticularis. Figure 48-7 depicts the biosynthetic pathways.

Control of Adrenocortical Hormones

Aldosterone is primarily under the control of the renin-angiotensin system, although ACTH and hyperkalemia also have a stimulatory role. Renin, which is secreted by the juxtaglomerular apparatus of the kidney, converts angiotensinogen (an α_2-globulin produced by the liver) to angiotensin I, which is converted to angiotensin II. Angiotensin II, in addition to its pressor action, stimulates aldosterone secretion. Although an increase in angiotensin II suppresses renin production, volume and sodium depletion stimulate its release.

Cortisol secretion is controlled by the hypothalamic-pituitary axis. CRH is secreted by the paraventricular nucleus of the hypothalamus. It is a 1-41-NH_2 polypeptide that binds to the corticotroph membrane, activating the adenyl cyclase system. ACTH is a 1-39 polypeptide derived from a much larger precursor, pro-opiomelanocortin (POMC). This precursor is processed mainly into ACTH. Cortisol secretion has a diurnal rhythm; the main secretory phase occurs during the late hours of sleep and early morning. Long- and short-loop negative feedback mechanisms are operating. In the long loop, the adrenal inhibits the anterior pituitary through the plasma cortisol by inhibiting ACTH release and by inhibition of the genome responsible for POMC synthesis. In the short loop, ACTH regulates its own secretion by inhibiting CRH release.

ACTH has a stimulatory effect on adrenal androgen synthesis, and production declines with age. The major androgens are androstenedione, dehydroepiandrosterone, and dehydroepiandrosterone sulfate. Androstenedione is converted peripherally to testosterone and to estrone and estradiol.

Physiologic Changes during Pregnancy

The plasma level of CRH increases progressively during the second and third trimesters, peaking at delivery. It has been isolated from the placenta, which is its likely source.[91,92] ACTH concentrations increase threefold from the first to third trimester, and its production by the placenta has been demonstrated.[93] The diurnal variation of cortisol and ACTH, although blunted, is maintained. Corticosteroid-binding globulin concentrations increase by three times during pregnancy, resulting in an increase in the total plasma cortisol and a decrease in its metabolic clearance. The unbound fraction also increases (free cortisol elevations of twofold to fourfold have been shown), and this is reflected by a rise in urinary free cortisol. These changes are depicted in Figure 48-8. In the third trimester, the 9 AM plasma cortisol level ranges between 25 and 46 μg/dL, and the mean urinary free cortisol excretion is elevated at east 180% during gestation. Neither placental

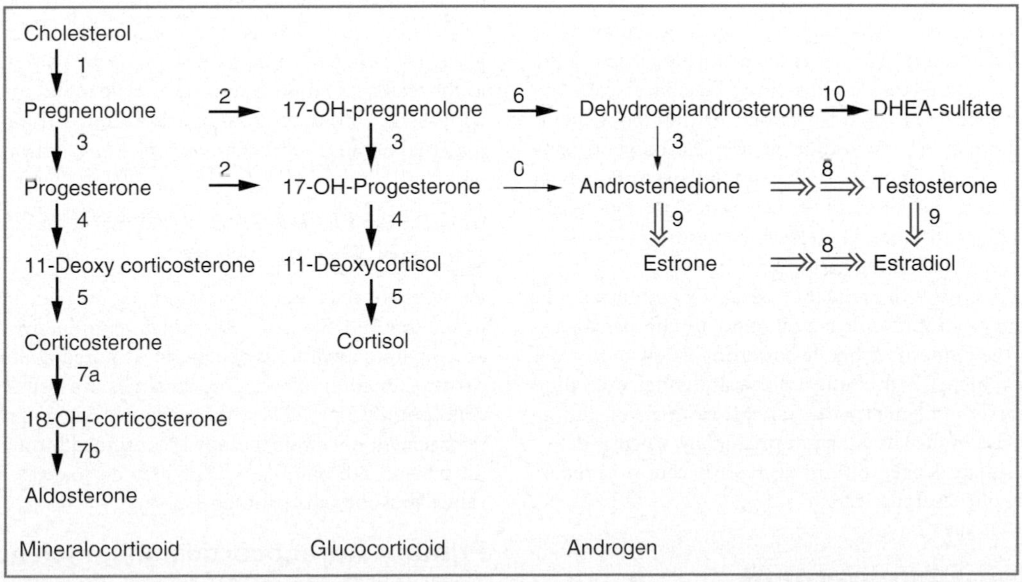

FIGURE 48-7 Adrenal steroidogenic pathways of mineralocorticoid, glucocorticoid, and androgen synthesis. Major pathways are indicated by *thick arrows* and minor ones by *thin arrows*. Extra-adrenal conversion of sex steroids is denoted by *double arrows*. Numbers indicate enzymatic steps as follows: 1,20α-hydroxylase, 22-hydroxylase, 20,22-desmolase; 2, 17α-hydroxylase; 3, 3β-hydroxysteroid dehydrogenase, Δ5-4-isomerase; 4,21-hydroxylase; 5, 11β-hydroxylase; 6, C17,20-lyase; 7a, 18-hydroxylase; 7b, 18-dehydrogenase; 8, 17β-hydroxysteroid dehydrogenase; 9, aromatase; 10, sulfatase.

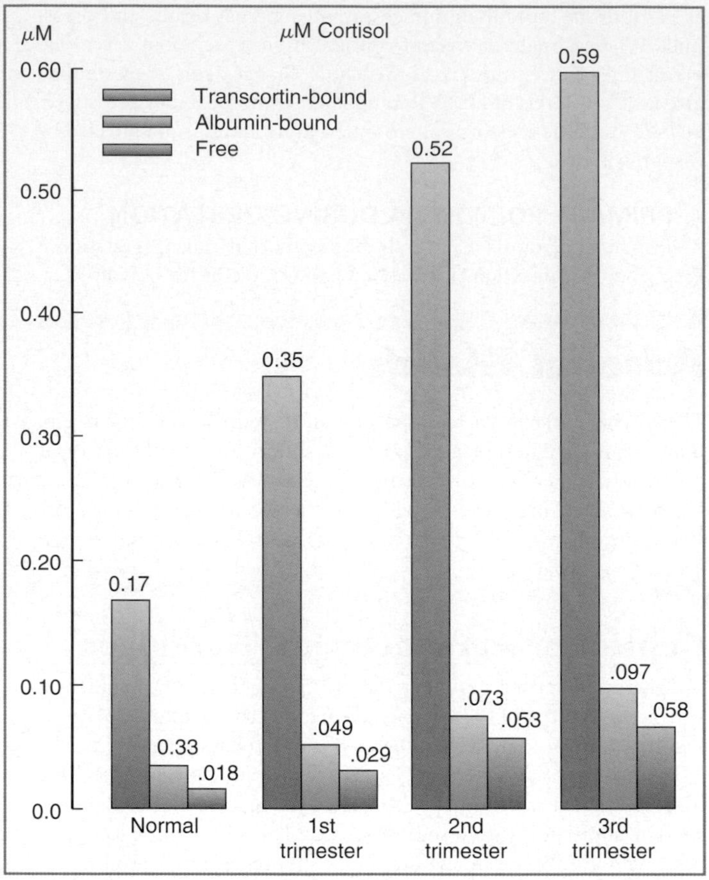

FIGURE 48-8 **Distribution of bound and free cortisol (μM/L) pregnancy plasma.** Corticosteroid-binding globulin concentrations increase during pregnancy, resulting in increased total plasma cortisol and decreased metabolic clearance. The unbound fraction also increases and is reflected by an increase in the urinary free cortisol level. (From Rosenthal HE, Slaunwhite WR, Sandberg AA: Transcortin: A corticosteroid-binding protein of plasma X. Cortisol and progesterone interplay and unbound levels of these steroids in pregnancy. J Clin Endocrinol Metab 29:352, 1969. Copyright © The Endocrine Society.)

ACTH nor CRH are suppressible in vitro with exogenous glucocorticoids. In the future, salivary assays of free cortisol may become more widely available. The normal response to ACTH has been evaluated.[94]

Renin activity increases early, peaking at 12 weeks' gestation, with a decline in the third trimester.[95] The decline is probably related to the rise in angiotensin II that occurs at this time. Plasma aldosterone concentrations reach values up to 20 times that of the nonpregnant state by the third trimester. The activation of the renin-angiotensin-aldosterone axis may result from the fall in blood pressure, which in itself results from decreased vascular responsiveness to angiotensin II and decreased vascular resistance. High levels of serum progesterone block aldosterone action, preventing kaliuresis.

Total testosterone increases in pregnancy because of an increase in sex hormone–binding globulin with a reduction in the percentage unbound; although the amount of free testosterone is low to normal in the first 28 weeks, it increases thereafter, with values often exceeding the normal range for nonpregnant women.[96] Mean levels of androstenedione also increase in the latter part of pregnancy, whereas dehydroepiandrosterone sulfate concentrations decrease because of a major increase in the metabolic clearance rate.

Fetal Adrenal Development

Fetal adrenal development has been reviewed by Keller-Wood and Wood.[97] The fetal adrenal can synthesize cortisol in vitro by 8 weeks' gestation. In vivo, placental 5-pregnenolone and 4-progesterone are used to synthesize steroids.[98] Two adrenal cortical zones can be identified in the fetus. The inner, or fetal, zone, which accounts for about 80% of the cortex in utero, involutes in the first few months of extrauterine life. The outer zone becomes the adult adrenal cortex. The fetal zone lacks 3β-hydroxysteroid dehydrogenase and is therefore unable to synthesize glucocorticoids or mineralocorticoids. The most abundant product is dehydroepiandrosterone, which forms the substrate for placental estrogen synthesis. During most of gestation, most cortisol in the fetal circulation is supplied by the mother through transplacental passage, although fetal cortisol concentrations are lower than maternal because of placental cortisol metabolism.

Disorders of the Adrenal Cortex during Pregnancy

Disorders of the adrenal cortex during pregnancy have been reviewed by Lindsay and Nieman.[99] Disrupted reproductive function commonly accompanies significant genetic or acquired abnormalities of adrenal cortical function. These abnormalities are usually diagnosed before conception. In patients with previously recognized adrenal disorders, replacement hormone therapy is continued throughout gestation, and the patient is monitored. The pregnancy-associated changes in normal values must be borne in mind.

Primary Adrenocortical Insufficiency: Addison Disease

Atrophy of the adrenals on an autoimmune basis is the most common cause of adrenal failure, accounting for 83% of cases.[100] Other causes include hemorrhage (usually associated with sepsis and burns), infections (viral, fungal, or tuberculous), and infiltrative disorders, including metastases, lymphoma, and amyloidosis. With the availability of hormone replacement, pregnancy is no longer contraindicated.

DIAGNOSIS DURING PREGNANCY

In a review of 40 cases of Addison disease in pregnancy about 5 decades ago, 18 died during pregnancy; 12 of 22 who delivered had a crisis in the puerperium, and 7 of these died.[101] The diagnosis of Addison disease in pregnancy is uncommon and may be related to the fetal contribution to maternal steroids. The symptoms include weakness, lassitude, nausea with or without vomiting, pigmentation, weight loss, anorexia, and abdominal pain. Some of these symptoms are also common in normal pregnant women. Suspicion should be heightened when a thin pregnant woman complains of prolonged nausea and vomiting, weakness, postural hypotension, and personality changes. A history of polyendocrine autoimmune disorders, type 1 diabetes, adrenogenital syndrome, tuberculosis, and acquired immunodeficiency syndrome (AIDS) places the pregnant woman at increased risk for adrenocortical insufficiency.

The signs, symptoms, and laboratory findings for primary adrenal insufficiency during pregnancy are outlined in Table 48-4. In acutely ill patients, replacement therapy must be initiated immediately and the diagnosis of primary adrenocortical insufficiency during pregnancy confirmed retrospectively by a pretreatment serum or plasma sample for measuring electrolytes, cortisol, and ACTH. In patients whose illness is less severe, a rapid ACTH stimulation test using synthetic ACTH may be performed; 250 μg is administered intravenously and blood samples are obtained at baseline, 30 minutes, and 60 minutes. Although a cortisol level exceeding 18 μg/dL and an increment exceeding 7 μg/dL are considered normal in the nonpregnant state, the mean increments have been reported as 18, 23, and 26 μg/dL in the first, second, and third trimester of pregnancy, respectively.[102] Responses to 1 μg of ACTH have shown mean peak cortisol levels of 44 μg/dL in normal pregnant women.[103] It has been suggested that adrenal insufficiency may be excluded if he basal or ACTH stimulated (250 μg) cortisol exceeds 30 μg/dL in the third trimester.

TABLE 48-4 DIAGNOSIS OF PRIMARY ADRENAL INSUFFICIENCY DURING PREGNANCY

Signs and Symptoms
Nausea with or without vomiting, anorexia
Systolic blood pressure < 100 mm Hg with postural decrease
Increased pigmentation
Abdominal pain
Personality changes
Weakness, fatigue
Muscle and joint pain
Salt craving
Laboratory Findings
Decreased sodium concentration
Increased potassium, BUN, and creatinine levels
Hypoglycemia
Plasma cortisol level below normal pregnancy level
Urinary-free cortisol: 24-hour excretion below normal pregnancy level
Increased plasma level of ACTH
Abnormal cortisol response to rapid ACTH stimulation test

ACTH, adrenocorticotropic hormone; BUN, blood urea nitrogen.

TREATMENT

Replacement regimens are similar to those used in nonpregnant women. This is usually accomplished by hydrocortisone (cortisol) at a dose of 20 mg in the morning and 10 mg in the evening, along with 0.05 to 0.1 mg of 9α-fludrocortisone administered daily. The dose of 9α-fludrocortisone is increased if postural hypotension or hyperkalemia persists and is decreased if hypertension or hypokalemia occurs. The dose of cortisol should be doubled or tripled in any situation associated with stress, including systemic illness or trauma. Breastfeeding has been discouraged because of the potential hazard of corticosteroids passing into the maternal milk, but some investigators disagree.[104] Less than 0.5% of the absorbed dose is excreted per liter of breast milk. Labor should be managed with stress doses of 300 mg of hydrocortisone over 24 hours, with subsequent tapering.

ACUTE ADRENAL INSUFFICIENCY DURING PREGNANCY, LABOR, DELIVERY, OR THE PUERPERIUM

Addisonian crisis is a rare but life-threatening event in pregnant women.[105] The onset can be confused with an abdominal surgical emergency because of the prominence of abdominal pain, nausea, vomiting, and shock. After necessary blood samples are obtained for electrolytes, cortisol, and ACTH determinations, intravenous therapy should be started immediately with 100 mg of hydrocortisone sodium succinate along with an infusion of normal saline and 5% glucose. During the first 24 hours, 300 to 400 mg of intravenous hydrocortisone sodium succinate should be given continuously, and this can conveniently be added to the replacement fluids administered.

Recovery occurs quickly, and by 24 hours, the patient may be able to return to oral feedings and replacement doses of oral hydrocortisone and 9α-fludrocortisone. If not, hydrocortisone may be continued intravenously, usually at a diminished dosage. An effort should be made to determine the cause of the adrenal crisis, and the patient should receive careful post-pregnancy supervision. Patients with mild deficiency are especially at risk during labor, delivery, and the immediate postpartum period.[104]

EFFECT OF MATERNAL ADDISON DISEASE ON THE NEWBORN

Infants born to mothers with Addison disease usually do not have any recognizable defects. Fetal growth, however, can be suboptimal, with lower-than-normal birth weights, especially if the diagnosis is confirmed late in pregnancy or during the postpartum period.[106] Fetal death has also been reported.[97] Maternal antibodies to the adrenal cortex do cross the placenta but do not significantly affect neonatal adrenal function.

Cushing Syndrome

Cushing syndrome results from an excess of glucocorticoids and is rare during pregnancy. Hypothalamic and pituitary disorders were discussed previously and have been reviewed by Buescher[107] and Lindsay and colleagues.[46]

Primary Hyperaldosteronism

Primary hyperaldosteronism has been reviewed by Lindsay and Nieman.[99] The autonomous secretion of aldosterone in primary hyperaldosteronism may result from an adrenal adenoma, bilateral hyperplasia, or, rarely, an adrenocortical carcinoma. In pregnancy, the clinical picture of hyperaldosteronism is similar to that of the nonpregnant patient with hypertension, hypokalemia, and often, kaliuresis and elevated serum bicarbonate.[108] The electrolyte disturbances and hypertension may first be apparent in the peripartum period, coinciding with the removal of the protective antialdosterone effect of progesterone. Of 31 patients reported, most have harbored adenomas.[109]

DIAGNOSIS

After standardizing the patient for dietary sodium (100 to 150 mEq daily) and posture (i.e., recumbent) and the replacement of plasma potassium, the physician measures renin activity and aldosterone concentrations. The renin activity is lower and the aldosterone concentration higher than those found in normal pregnancy.[108] Suppression of the aldosterone axis can also be attempted with salt loading (200 to 300 mEq/day for 3 to 5 days); the hallmark of primary hyperaldosteronism is a lack of suppression of serum aldosterone concentration. If surgery is contemplated, MRI may be used to localize the adenoma. The course of pregnancy is one of difficult-to-treat hypertension. Neonatal morbidity and mortality are related to placental insufficiency.

TREATMENT

Medical treatment with standard antihypertensive drugs should be provided, along with potassium supplements. Surgery in the second trimester may be required if medical treatment fails; surgery has gained wider acceptance since the advent of laparoscopic adrenalectomy. Spironolactone is contraindicated in pregnancy, especially in the first trimester, because of its possible feminizing effects. In the first case report of a pregnant patient with hyperaldosteronism associated with bilateral hyperplasia, documented by Neerhof and colleagues,[110] enalapril maleate, an angiotensin-converting enzyme inhibitor, successfully lowered blood pressures in a patient unresponsive to other medications. However, later reports of adverse effects preclude the use of angiotensin-converting enzyme inhibitors in pregnancy.[111]

Congenital Adrenal Hyperplasia

The congenital adrenal hyperplasias (CAHs) involve inherited enzymatic defects of adrenal steroidogenesis. The most severe and life-threatening disorders occur early in the biosynthetic cascade and are usually fatal or incompatible with successful reproduction. Deficiency of 21-hydroxylase is the most common defect (see Fig. 48-7), accounting for 90% to 95% of cases with an incidence of about 1 in 14,000, although in some areas, such as Alaska, it is more common.[112] The second most common form is 11-hydroxylase deficiency. CAH in pregnancy and its prenatal treatment was reviewed in 2001 by New.[113]

GENETICS

All CAHs are autosomal recessive disorders. The parents of an affected child have at least one haplotype for the defect, giving each subsequent offspring a 25% chance of having the condition and a 50% chance of being a carrier. An affected individual produces 100% carriers if her partner is not affected; if her partner is a carrier, 50% of the offspring are affected, and the other 50% are carriers. Siblings or spouses who want to know whether they are heterozygotes for 21-hydroxylase deficiency can be tested by undergoing measurements of adrenal steroids (notably 17-hydroxyprogesterone) before and after ACTH stimulation.[114]

21-HYDROXYLASE DEFICIENCY

21-Hydroxylase deficiency arises because of genetic mutations of the 21-hydroxylase gene located at a site linked to the human leukocyte antigen (HLA) histocompatibility complex on the short arm of the sixth chromosome. The variation in severity of the deficiency can be accounted for by allelic variation at the gene locus.[115] The enzyme block results in inadequate synthesis of 11-deoxycortisol and cortisol; the resulting excess ACTH stimulates adrenal precursors, notably 17-hydroxyprogesterone. Shunting of these excess precursors results in excess androgens, leading to masculinization of genitalia of the female fetus and excess masculinization of the male infant.

If the defect is severe, mineralocorticoid deficiency occurs with salt wasting. Diagnosis is confirmed by the finding of excess basal 17-hydroxyprogesterone concentrations; in milder forms, ACTH stimulation is necessary and shows an excessive increase in 17-hydroxyprogesterone. Physiologic replacement doses of glucocorticoids (usually cortisol) are used as therapy, and the dosage is based on surface area. Concentrations of 4-androstenedione, testosterone, and 17-hydroxyprogesterone are used to monitor adequacy of suppression. Fludrocortisone is indicated in salt-losing forms and in non–salt-losing forms with increased plasma renin activity. Virilized females may require surgical reconstruction of the genitalia to provide for normal appearance, intercourse, and pregnancy.

MATERNAL AND FETAL CONSIDERATIONS

Although poor control of CAH results in irregular or absent menses, patients in whom the condition is well controlled may achieve pregnancy, although less often than expected, possibly because of postnatal intervals of excess androgen exposure. Usually, the same dose of cortisol can be continued through gestation, with additional amounts given during labor, delivery, and the immediate postpartum period. Cesarean section rates may be higher because of abnormal maternal external genitalia or a small bony pelvis from premature closure of the epiphyses.[116] Most children of mothers with CAH are normal, although women receiving suboptimal doses of replacement therapy have elevated circulating androgens, which may cross the placenta and virilize the fetus.

Free testosterone levels do not change significantly during gestation and can be used as a marker for monitoring therapy. Conversely, excessive glucocorticoid therapy of the mother with CAH may result in suppression of fetal adrenals with resulting transient adrenocortical insufficiency of the neonate.

PRENATAL DIAGNOSIS AND TREATMENT

Prenatal diagnosis of 21-hydroxylase deficiency for offspring of known heterozygotes first became possible with the finding of elevated levels of 17-hydroxyprogesterone in amniotic fluid obtained by amniocentesis.[117] By the time amniocentesis is performed in the second trimester, it is too late to prevent virilization. Dexamethasone is administered in a pregnancy at risk before the end of the seventh week from conception (9 weeks' gestation). This treatment results in suppression of 17-hydroxyprogesterone and renders it unreliable for diagnosis. After HLA profiles were found to be linked to CAH, diagnoses were made with HLA linkage marker analysis using amniotic cells. To avoid errors resulting from recombination or haplotype sharing, however, direct DNA analysis of the 21-hydroxylase gene *(CYP21)* with molecular genetic techniques is recommended. Chorionic villus sampling should preferably be used to obtain fetal tissue sooner (9 to 11 weeks' gestation) for diagnosis by molecular genetic analysis.[118]

Prenatal treatment of the mother with high-dose glucocorticoids has been effective in preventing virilization of the affected female fetus; the glucocorticoid crosses the placenta and suppresses ACTH secretion from the fetal pituitary.[117] The current approach is to treat all such mothers with glucocorticoids. Dexamethasone (20 μg/kg of pre-pregnancy weight) is given orally in divided daily doses after pregnancy has been confirmed. This treatment must be given before the end of the seventh week from conception. Chorionic villus sampling is then performed. If the fetus is male, maternal treatment is discontinued; if female, the treatment is continued until the results of DNA analysis of the 21-hydroxylase gene are available. The glucocorticoids are discontinued only if the female fetus is considered unaffected.

A review of 532 pregnancies prenatally diagnosed using amniocentesis or chorionic villus sampling between 1978 and 2001 was reported by New and associates.[118] Of these 532 pregnancies, 281 were treated prenatally for congenital adrenal hyperplasia because of the risk of 21-hydroxylase deficiency. Of 116 babies affected with CAH, 61 were female, and 49 of them were treated prenatally with dexamethasone. If given in proper dosage, dexamethasone administered at or before week 9 of gestation was effective in reducing virilization. With the exception of striae, weight gain, and edema, there were no other differences in the symptoms of treated and untreated mothers. Prenatally treated newborns had weights that matched untreated and unaffected newborns, and no enduring side effects were observed. Prenatal diagnosis and treatment of 21-hydroxylase deficiency is possible and effective. An algorithm showing prenatal management of pregnancies in families at risk for a fetus affected by 21-hydroxylase deficiency is provided in Figure 48-9. An updated review has been provided by Nimkarn and New.[119] However, there are few data on long-term risks. A study based on a maternal survey showed that 174 children (48 had CAH) who received dexamethasone did not differ in cognitive or motor development from 313 unexposed children.[120] However, a later study showed impaired cognitive function in at-risk children who were treated prenatally.[121] A consensus conference recommended that only an experienced team direct this therapy, preferably under a research protocol, with consent and with prospective and long-term follow-up of the children.[122]

11-HYDROXYLASE DEFICIENCY

11-Hydroxylase deficiency, an enzyme defect that is not HLA linked, results in blocked production of cortisol and aldosterone with resulting excess precursors, 11-deoxycortisol and deoxycorticosterone.[117] A

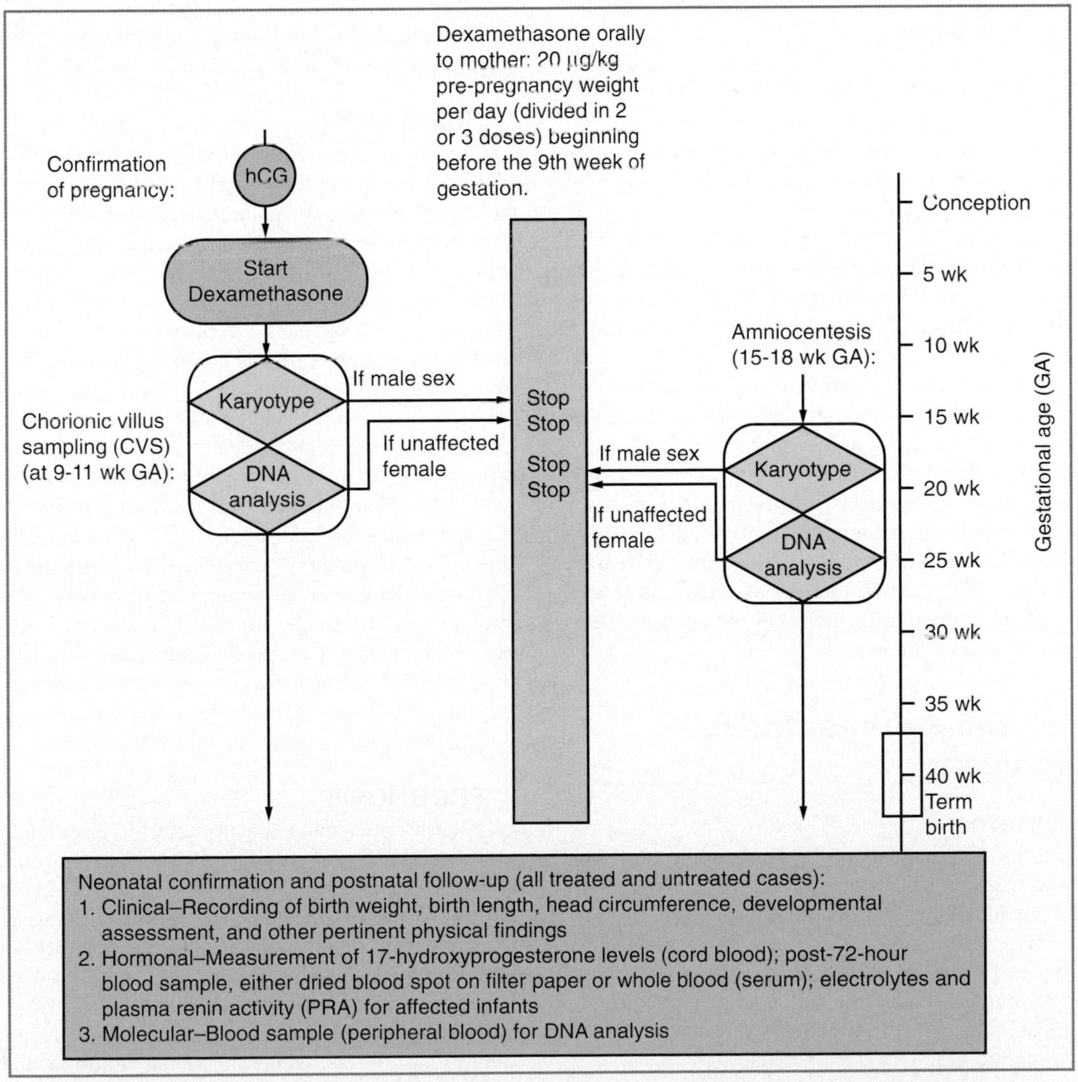

FIGURE 48-9 Algorithm for prenatal management of pregnancy in families at risk for a fetus with 21-hydroxylase deficiency. Prenatal diagnosis and treatment of 21-hydroxylase deficiency are possible and effective. (From New MI, Carlson A, Obeid J, et al: Extensive personal experience: Prenatal diagnosis for congenital adrenal hyperplasia in 532 pregnancies. J Clin Endocrinol Metab 86[12]:5651-5657, 2001. Copyright © The Endocrine Society.)

shunt toward excess androgens occurs, and the presentation is that of androgen excess and hypertension. Diagnosis is based on elevated 11-deoxycortisol and deoxycorticosterone concentrations determined basally or after ACTH stimulation. Heterozygotes have no demonstrable biochemical abnormality, even with ACTH stimulation. Treatment is with glucocorticoid replacement. Prenatal diagnosis is confirmed by measuring amniotic fluid 11-deoxycortisol concentrations.[123] Prenatal treatment of the mother with dexamethasone, as in 21-hydroxylase deficiency, has been reported, resulting in a female without virilization or ambiguous genitalia who was genetically affected.[124] Mutations in the 11-hydroxylase gene that may facilitate prenatal diagnosis have been reported.[125]

OTHER CONGENITAL ADRENAL HYPERPLASIA ENZYME DEFICIENCIES

There are a few other rare forms of CAH (see Fig. 48-7). In 17-hydroxylase deficiency, the sex steroid pathway is blocked in the adrenal cortex and gonad, resulting in a hypogonadal state and primary amenorrhea. Deficiency of 3β-hydroxysteroid dehydrogenase, if severe, manifests as lack of pubertal development. Milder forms manifest pubertally with hyperandrogenism.[126]

Long-Term Therapy with Pharmacologic Doses of Steroids

The occurrence of congenital anomalies in animal experiments—cleft palate in particular—raised concerns about pregnant women receiving glucocorticoids during pregnancy. In a review involving 260 pregnancies in which glucocorticoids had been administered to women in pharmacologic doses, only two infants had cleft palate.[127] Both mothers had received steroids in large doses early in pregnancy. Because closure of the palatal process occurs by the 12th week of gestation, it is possible that the anomaly was related to the medication. Although other, smaller studies have not supported this association,[128] a prospective cohort study and meta-analysis of epidemiologic studies concluded that prednisone increases the risk of oral clefts by an order of 3.4-fold.[129]

The hypothalamic-pituitary-adrenal axis is suppressed with long-term supraphysiologic doses of glucocorticoids, and abrupt withdrawal should be avoided because it can precipitate maternal adrenocortical insufficiency. Glucocorticoids are excreted in breast milk and have the potential to cause growth restriction in the neonate. Neonatal adrenal insufficiency, although rare, can occur in infants born to mothers being treated with exogenous glucocorticoids.[127]

Disorders of the Adrenal Medulla during Pregnancy

Pheochromocytoma

Pheochromocytomas have been reviewed by Lindsay and Nieman.[99] Pheochromocytomas are tumors of chromaffin cells. These cells cluster predominantly in the adrenal medulla, and 90% of pheochromocytomas are found in this location. Sites of extra-adrenal tumors range from the carotid body to the pelvic floor. They occur sporadically or as part of the familial multiple endocrine neoplasia type 2 syndrome. Approximately 12% are malignant, although this percentage is higher in pheochromocytomas occurring in extra-adrenal sites.

SYMPTOMS

Pheochromocytoma is a rare but potentially lethal cause of hypertension in pregnancy. Its possibility should be considered in women with intermittent, labile hypertension or paroxysmal symptoms such as anxiety, diaphoresis, headache, and palpitations. Other symptoms include chest or abdominal pain, unusual reactions to drugs affecting catecholamine release and actions, visual disturbances, convulsions, and collapse. Symptoms tend to be similar in pregnant and nonpregnant women. The occurrence of symptoms during pregnancy only, with recurrence in subsequent pregnancies, has also been described. Increased vascularity of the tumor in pregnancy and the mechanical effect of an enlarging uterus may explain this phenomenon. In many cases, severe symptoms develop in the peripartum and postpartum periods. At least 200 cases have been diagnosed in pregnancy, with an estimated prevalence of 1 in 54,000 at term.

LABORATORY DIAGNOSIS

Laboratory diagnosis involves biochemical demonstration of elevated levels of vanillylmandelic acid, catecholamines, and fractionated metanephrines in the 24-hour urine specimen. Plasma catecholamine and metanephrine levels can also be determined. Values in pregnant women are similar to those in nonpregnant subjects, but they are elevated for 24 hours after eclamptic seizures. Because methyldopa interferes with catecholamine measurements, it should be discontinued before testing. If necessary, the tumor may be localized during pregnancy by means of ultrasonography[130] or MRI.[131]

TREATMENT

Treatment of pheochromocytoma in pregnancy is somewhat controversial. Most physician agree that when the diagnosis is confirmed in the second half of pregnancy, α-adrenergic blockade with phenoxybenzamine is the treatment of choice. This drug is given orally, starting with 10 mg twice daily and gradually increasing by 10 to 20 mg daily until hypertension is controlled. When fetal maturity is achieved, cesarean section should be performed, with simultaneous or subsequent excision of the tumor[132,133] during adrenergic blockade. Phentolamine (1 to 5 mg) can be used for a hypertensive crisis.

In tumors detected before 24th weeks' gestation, surgery during pregnancy has been advocated[133] to avoid fetal wasting. Laparoscopic adrenalectomy can be performed.[134] However, a number of such cases have been managed successfully during pregnancy with α- and β-blockade with good fetal outcome.[135,136] The arguments against medical therapy are the unknown effects of α-blockade and β-blockade on the fetus in the long term, the teratogenic potential of phenoxybenzamine, and the risk of a malignant lesion. β-Blockade alone should not be used without prior α-blockade because unopposed α-adrenergic activity can lead to generalized vasoconstriction and a steep rise in blood pressure. Anesthetic management of pheochromocytoma resection during pregnancy requires special consideration.[137]

PROGNOSIS

Pheochromocytoma constitutes a life-threatening disease for the mother and the fetus, although with better management and the availability of α-adrenergic and β-adrenergic blockade, the prospects for both have improved. Table 48-5 shows the changes in maternal and fetal mortality rates over the past few decades and indicates the improved prognosis when the diagnosis is made during pregnancy.[133,138] However, a 36-year-old woman died at 27 weeks' gestation from an autopsy-diagnosed pheochromocytoma.[139] Fetal growth restriction can result from reduced uteroplacental perfusion, and fetal death may occur during acute hypertensive crises.

Four cases of malignant pheochromocytomas in pregnancy were reviewed by Ellison and associates[140] and another by Devoe and coworkers;[141] α-methyl paratyrosine, a dopamine synthesis inhibitor, was used in the latter case. Several cases of pregnancy with pheochro-

TABLE 48-5 CHANGES IN MATERNAL AND FETAL MORTALITIES IN MORE THAN 200 PREGNANCIES COMPLICATED BY PHEOCHROMOCYTOMA

	Maternal Mortality (%)			Fetal Mortality (%)		
Time of Diagnosis	Before 1969	1969-1979	1980-1987	Before 1969	1969-1979	1980-1987
During pregnancy	18	4	0	50	42	15
Postpartum period	58	50	17	56	56	35

TABLE 48-6 APPROACH TO MATERNAL HIRSUTISM AND VIRILIZATION IN PREGNANCY

Findings	Indicated Action	Possible Virilization of Female Fetus
History		
Acute onset in pregnancy	Investigate with studies as indicated below.	—
Androgenic drug exposure	Stop the drug.	—
Physical Examination or Ovarian Ultrasound		
Bilateral cystic: theca lutein cysts	Exclude high levels of human chorionic gonadotropin.	No
Bilateral solid: luteoma very likely		Yes
Unilateral solid	Perform surgery to exclude malignancy.	Yes
No ovarian mass	Investigate adrenal glands.	Yes

mocytoma as part of type 2 multiple endocrine neoplasia have been reported.[133,142,143]

Hirsutism and Virilization in Pregnancy

Hirsutism and virilization in pregnancy have been reviewed by McClamrock and Adashi.[144] Women and their female fetuses are protected from the increased concentrations of androgens by the enhanced binding to sex hormone–binding globulin, competition by progestins for binding to the androgen receptor or for disposition of androgens to more biologically potent compounds, and placental aromatization of androgens. Nevertheless, maternal hirsutism and virilization can occur in pregnancy and usually results from ovarian disease or iatrogenic insult. The female fetus can be affected by elevated circulating maternal androgens. Differentiation of the female external genitalia occurs between 7 and 12 weeks' gestation, and exposure to excess androgens can result in partial or complete labial fusion and clitoromegaly. Clitoromegaly may still occur after 12 weeks' gestation. The approach to maternal hirsutism and virilization in pregnancy is outlined in Table 48-6.

The two major causes of gestational hyperandrogenism are luteomas and hyperreactio luteinalis (i.e., gestational ovarian theca-lutein cysts). Luteomas are benign, solid tumors of the ovary; they are often multinodular and bilateral, and they are usually yellow to tan. Regardless of their virilizing effect, luteomas have been associated with elevated levels of circulating maternal androgens.

Not all luteomas cause maternal virilization (overall incidence is 35%); it depends on the amount of androgen secreted, the end-organ sensitivity, and the degree of aromatization by the placenta to nonandrogenic steroids. Approximately 80% of female infants born to mothers with virilizing luteomas are virilized and usually exhibit clitoromegaly. Although luteomas are considered intrapartum lesions that regress after delivery, this concept has been challenged and could account for recurrence of virilization in subsequent pregnancies as shown in a case of severe maternal virilization.[145] In contrast with hyperreactio luteinalis, luteomas occur more frequently in black multiparas and are not associated with toxemia, erythroblastosis, or multiple gestation.

Hyperreactio luteinalis is characterized by ovarian enlargement with many large-follicle cysts or corpora lutea, or both, with marked edema of the stroma. It usually is bilateral, affects white primigravidas, and is often associated with conditions resulting in increased human chorionic gonadotropin (hCG), such as molar pregnancies and multiple gestation. Maternal hirsutism or virilization has been documented in approximately 30% of reported cases. There are no reported cases of fetal masculinization, even if the mother is virilized. The condition may represent an excessive ovarian sensitivity to hCG. The lack of fetal virilization in this condition is intriguing and has been attributed to androgen aromatization in the placenta. As with luteomas, recurrence of hyperreactio luteinalis in consecutive pregnancies has been reported.[146] Recurrent, severe hyperandrogenism during pregnancy has also been reported without the presence of luteomas or hyperreactio luteinalis.[147]

Placental aromatase deficiency is a rare cause of maternal and fetal virilization, which may be suspected if maternal hyperandrogenism is associated with low maternal estrogen levels.[148] Only 1% enzyme activity appears necessary to prevent virilization.

Another rare cause of maternal and fetal virilization is[149] cytochrome P450 oxidoreductase (PORD) deficiency; it is an autosomal recessive disorder caused by mutations in the gene encoding an electron donor of all P450 enzymes.[149,150] This enzyme is an essential redox partner for CYP17 and CYP21 hydroxylases. Abnormal function of these enzymes can lead to maternal virilization and virilization of the female fetus together with low estriol secretion in pregnancy. Variable clinical manifestations include skeletal malformations referred to as the Antley-Bixler syndrome with insufficient glucocorticoids and increased 17-hydroxyprogesterone in both sexes.

In a few cases,[151,152] insulin-resistant polycystic ovary syndrome patients who achieve pregnancy may become extremely androgenized during pregnancy. Metformin was used in one of these cases.[151] Other ovarian lesions that can cause maternal virilization include Sertoli-Leydig cell tumors (i.e., arrhenoblastomas), Krukenberg tumors, Brenner tumors, lipoid cell tumors, dermoid cysts, and mucinous and serous cystadenocarcinomas. Most Sertoli-Leydig cell tumors coexisting with pregnancy are associated with maternal virilization, and virilization of the female fetus can occur. The malignancy rate for these tumors is high (44%), with substantial maternal (31%) and perinatal (50%) mortality rates. Krukenberg tumors, which are gastrointestinal tumors metastatic to the ovary, are often bilateral and have caused maternal and fetal virilization in all reported cases.

Adrenal tumors, including adrenocortical carcinoma, can cause maternal and fetal virilization.[153] Masculinization of the female fetus has been associated with the gestational administration of progestins and androgens and can be unaccompanied by maternal virilization.

Parathyroid Glands and Calcium Metabolism

Maternal and Fetal Physiology and Lactation

The serum calcium level is tightly regulated and maintained within normal limits by parathyroid hormone (PTH) and vitamin D. Vitamin D can be synthesized in the skin under the influence of ultraviolet irradiation or can be absorbed from dietary sources through the gastrointestinal tract. The 25(OH)D form of vitamin D (i.e., 25-hydroxycholecalciferol or vitamin D_3) is 25-hydroxylated in the liver and then 1-hydroxylated in the kidney. The physiologically active form of vitamin D is $1,25(OH)_2D$ (i.e., 1α,25-dihydroxycholecalciferol, calcitriol, or vitamin D_2), which is responsible for increasing intestinal absorption of calcium and for bone resorption. The parathyroid glands, which produce PTH, are stimulated by hypocalcemia and suppressed by high concentrations of calcium, magnesium, and $1,25(OH)_2D$ and by hypomagnesemia. PTH influences calcium metabolism by directly resorbing bone and by stimulating $1,25(OH)_2D$ formation. There are three major forms of circulating calcium: ionized, protein-bound, and chelated fractions. The ionized fraction is physiologically active and homeostatically regulated.

Calcium homeostasis in pregnancy was reviewed by Kovacs[154] and Kovacs and Fuleihan.[155] Large amounts of calcium and phosphorus are transferred against a concentration gradient from the mother to the fetus,[156] with the net accumulation of calcium being 25 to 30 g by term (mostly in the third trimester). Maternal calcium absorption doubles during pregnancy to meet these demands. Doubling of $1,25(OH)_2D$ synthesis of placental and maternal renal origin (from increased 1α-hydroxylase, itself resulting from increased prolactin, estrogen, human placental lactogen, and parathyroid related peptide) leads to the opening of voltage-gated calcium channels in the enterocyte membrane, increasing calcium absorption.[157] In the maternal circulation, there is little change in ionized calcium,[158] whereas total serum calcium concentrations fall during gestation, paralleling a decline in serum albumin.

In addition to placental calcium transfer, an expanding extracellular volume and increased urinary calcium losses place further stress on maternal calcium homeostasis. Studies of PTH using traditional radioimmunoassays have supported a concept of physiologic hyperparathyroidism in pregnancy.[158] The advent of newer immunoradiometric assays for intact PTH have shown a decline in PTH during pregnancy to 10% to 30% of pre-pregnancy values, increasing toward term.[159] This decline, however, appears to be offset by increased parathyroid-related protein (PTHrP) of fetal origin. This peptide shares considerable homology with PTH and a common receptor. It appears that PTHrP is produced by the fetal parathyroid glands and by the placenta and is the predominant regulator of active placental calcium transport. Transtrophoblastic calcium transfer also depends on an increase in calcium-binding protein, which reaches maximal concentrations in the third trimester when fetal growth is most rapid. Serum calcitonin concentrations have been variously reported as showing a rise or no consistent change during pregnancy.[160] The level of PTHrP also increases during pregnancy and is produced by fetal and maternal tissues. It likely contributes to increased $1,25(OH)_2D$ and decreased PTH concentrations, and it regulates placental calcium transport to the fetus. Urinary calcium excretion is also increased.

Fetal parathyroid tissue has been identified by 6 weeks' gestation, and skeletal mineralization is apparent by the eighth week. Total and ionized calcium concentrations are elevated in the fetus at term and decrease to normal in the newborn period. PTH levels are low in the fetus and increase after birth.[156] PTHrP is produced by fetal parathyroid glands and is the main regulator of fetal serum calcium. The calcitonin level is elevated in the fetus. These events are summarized in Table 48-7. During lactation, the average daily loss of calcium in human milk is 220 to 340 mg. There is a small drop in serum calcium accompanied by a rise in PTH and $1,25(OH)_2D$ concentrations. The ionized calcium concentration increases a little, remaining within the normal range; the serum phosphorus level increases. Intact PTH is reduced 50%, rising to normal with weaning. In contrast to the high levels in pregnancy, serum $1,25(OH)_2D$ concentrations fall to normal within days of parturition. PTHrP levels (of mammary origin) are significantly higher in lactating women, and the protein plays a key role during lactation in regulating demineralization of the skeleton, stimulating resorption of bone, and in renal tubular reabsorption of calcium and suppression of PTH. Higher PTHrP levels correlate with greater losses of bone.[155] Calcitonin levels are high in the first 6 weeks of lactation and may modulate the rate of skeletal resorption. Figure 48-10 depicts maternal calcium homeostasis during pregnancy and lactation, contrasting the mechanisms at work in these two situations.

TABLE 48-7 LEVELS OF MINERALS AND HORMONES INVOLVED IN CALCIUM HOMEOSTASIS

Mineral or Hormone	Mother	Fetus	Newborn
Total calcium*	Low	High	Decreases†
Ionized calcium*	Low normal	High	Decreases
Magnesium*	Low normal	High normal	Decreases
Phosphorus*	Low	High	Increases†
PTH	Low	Low	Increases
Calcitonin	Normal or high	High	Decreases
25(OH)D*	Variable	Variable	Variable
$1,25(OH)_2D$	High	Low	Increases
PTHrP	High‡	High	—

*Placental transfer.
†Toward nonpregnant adult values.
‡Of fetal origin.
PTH, parathyroid hormone; PTHrP, parathyroid hormone–related protein; $1,25(OH)_2D$, 1α,25-dihydroxycholecalciferol calcitriol, or vitamin D_2, the physiologically active form of vitamin D; 25(OH)D, 25-hydroxycholecalciferol, calcidiol, or vitamin D_3.

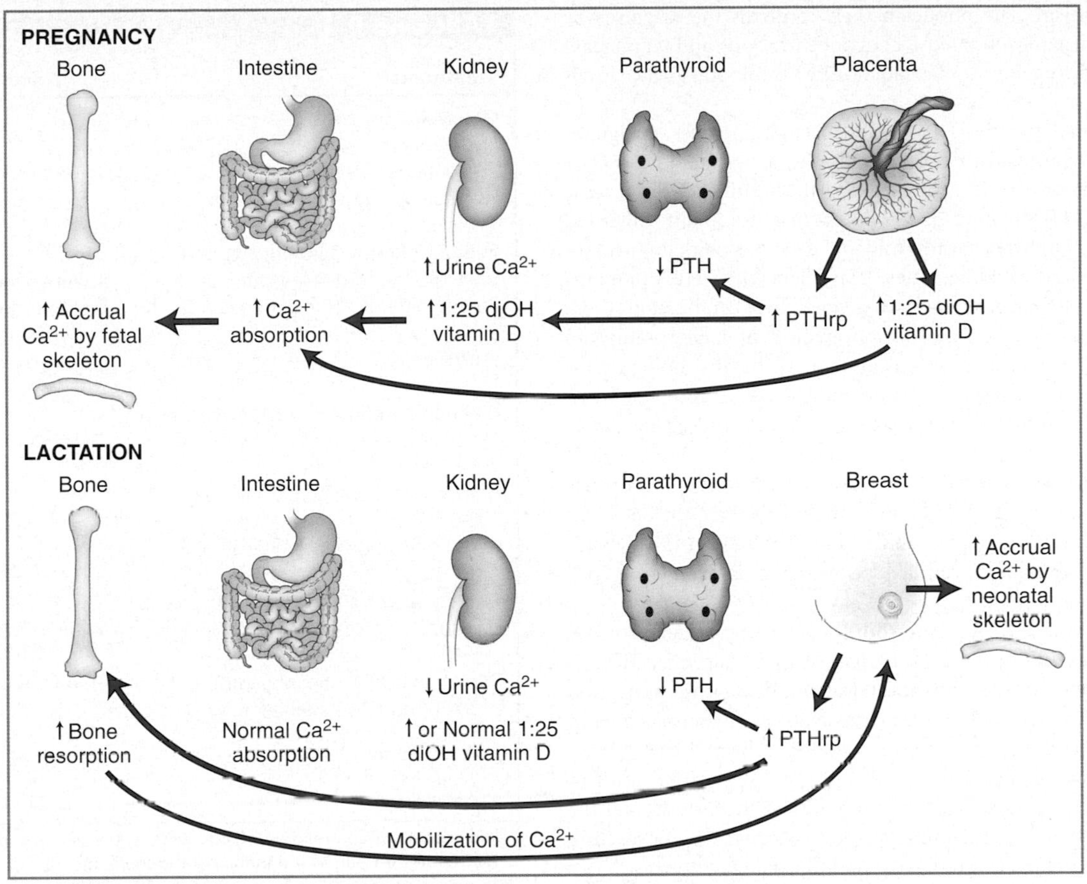

FIGURE 48-10 **Factors regulating maternal calcium metabolism during pregnancy and lactation.** Calcium (Ca^{2+}) accrual by the fetus and neonate is achieved during pregnancy and lactation, but the mechanisms are different. In pregnancy 1,25-dihydroxycholecalciferol (1:25 diOH vitamin D)–mediated increased calcium absorption plays the dominant role, whereas in lactation, parathyroid hormone–related peptide (PTHrP)–mediated bone resorption makes calcium available to the neonate. (Adapted from Kovacs CK, Fuleihan GEH: Calcium and bone disorders during pregnancy and lactation. Endocrinol Metab Clin North Am 35:21, 2006.)

Disorders of the Parathyroid Glands

Primary Hyperparathyroidism and Hypercalcemia

Hyperparathyroidism is rare in pregnancy. Of 750 cases of parathyroid surgery performed over a 21-year period,[161] only 6 occurred in pregnant women (0.8%). The topic of parathyroid disorders in pregnancy was reviewed by Mestman.[162] As in nonpregnant women, the histopathology of hyperparathyroidism involves a single adenoma in most reported cases in pregnant women, although hyperplasia and carcinoma have also been reported.[163,164] Although many patients are asymptomatic, clinical features of the associated hypercalcemia are summarized in Table 48-8.

In the 102 pregnancies (in 73 women) reported by Kristofferson and coauthors,[163] the clinical history was known in 45. Abdominal symptoms, including nausea, vomiting, pain, and renal colic, were the most common, followed by muscular weakness, mental symptoms, and polyuria; 20% were asymptomatic. The diagnosis of hyperparathyroidism during pregnancy is suggested by hypercalcemia. The decline in total serum calcium during pregnancy may mask the diagnosis or be associated with a postpartum flare-up, and ionized serum calcium should be measured in patients suspected of having primary

TABLE 48-8 MATERNAL FEATURES OF HYPERCALCEMIA

Affected System	Clinical Features
Urinary	Nephrolithiasis
	Nephrocalcinosis
	Polyuria
Neuromuscular	Weakness
Gastrointestinal	Peptic ulcer disease
	Constipation
	Anorexia
	Nausea and vomiting
Cardiovascular	Hypertension
	Arrhythmias
Skeletal	Osteitis fibrosa cystica
	Osteopenia and fractures
Neuropsychiatric	Depression
	Psychosis
	Obtundation
	Coma
Miscellaneous	Thirst
	Pruritus

hyperparathyroidism. The physician then confirms the diagnosis by finding inappropriately elevated PTH concentrations and an increase in urinary nephrogenic cyclic adenosine monophosphate levels (cAMP).

The differential diagnosis of hypercalcemia includes malignant disease, granulomatous disease, thyrotoxicosis, hypervitaminosis D or A, milk-alkali syndrome, immobilization, and familial hypocalciuric hypercalcemia (FHH), which is an autosomal dominant, inherited form of mild, benign hyperparathyroidism associated with low urinary calcium excretion. Affected neonates of mothers with FHH can manifest symptomatic hypercalcemia; if unaffected, they can develop severe neonatal hypocalcemia because of suppression of fetal parathyroid function. Severe neonatal hypercalcemia may be the homozygous variant of FHH. An altered calcium ion–sensing receptor gene, changing the set point for PTH secretion, is the underlying defect in FHH.

Hypercalcemia associated with increased production of PTHrP has been described during pregnancy and after delivery.[165] In one case, production of PTHrP by hypertrophied breast tissue led to hypercalcemia.[166] In another, hypercalcemia developed after delivery in a hypoparathyroid woman on vitamin D.[167]

During pregnancy, calcium transport across the placenta provides a degree of protection in the mother against hypercalcemia, and this protection is greatest during the third trimester. Loss of this protection with delivery can cause acute postpartum maternal hypercalcemia. In many patients, the diagnosis is confirmed after delivery by the occurrence of neonatal tetany. Ten of 15 cases of hyperparathyroidism reported by Gelister and colleagues[164] manifested in this way, and the others manifested with hyperemesis, hypertension, and a jaw fracture in a patient who turned out to have a parathyroid carcinoma.

TABLE 48-9 TREATMENT OF HYPERCALCEMIA

Treatment	Adverse Effects
General Approach	
Hydration	
Discontinue offending drugs	
Restrict calcium	
Increase Renal Calcium Excretion	
0.9% Saline, 200-500 mL/hr	Volume overload
Furosemide, 20-60 mg IV every 2-4 hr	Volume depletion, hypokalemia
Dialysis	
Calcium Chelation with Phosphates	
Oral: Neutra-phos, 500-750 mg every 6-8 hr	Extraskeletal calcification
Rectal: Phospho-soda, 5 mL every 6-8 hr	
IV: 50 mM phosphate over 8-12 hr	
Decrease Bone Resorption	
Calcitonin, 4-8 IU/kg IM or SC every 6-12 hr*	Allergic reaction, nausea
Pamidronate (bisphosphonate), 30-60 mg IV as a single infusion over 24 hr	Renal toxicity
Mithramycin, 25 μg/kg IV† every 48-72 hr	Low platelet count, renal toxicity, hepatotoxicity

*No reports of congenital defects; does not cross placenta.
†No reports on use in pregnancy; antineoplastic.
IV, intravenously; IM, intramuscularly; SC, subcutaneously.

COMPLICATIONS

Complications of hyperparathyroidism affect the mother and infant. Maternal complications include hyperemesis, renal calculi (36%), pancreatitis (13%), hypertension (10%), bone disease (19%), hypercalcemic crises (8%), and psychiatric problems. The overall maternal mortality rate remains low (1 of 73 in the collected series of Kristofferson and colleagues[162]).

Fetal morbidity and mortality rates are significant. A 30% rate of spontaneous abortion or stillbirth, 50% rate of tetany, and 25% rate of neonatal death have been reported.[168]

Although neonatal hypocalcemia with tetany is usually a transient phenomenon related to suppression of fetal parathyroid glands resulting from maternal-fetal hypercalcemia, it can be more prolonged in less mature infants or in infants with birth asphyxia. Hypercalcemic crisis also can occur during pregnancy or after delivery with high serum calcium level (>14 mg/dL), generalized weakness, vomiting, and altered mental status. Aggravation of hypercalcemia can occur because of an increase in placental production of $1,25(OH)_2D$ by the end of gestation and the removal of the placenta, with the loss of the shunt that transfers calcium from mother to fetus.

TREATMENT

For hyperparathyroidism presenting during pregnancy, standard practice favors surgical treatment. In the collected series of Kristofferson and colleagues,[163] there were 79 pregnancies among 50 women who did not undergo surgery; there were complications in 41 of the pregnancies (52%), and neonatal tetany occurred in 21 (26.6%). This contrasts with the more favorable outcome in 23 pregnancies involving 23 women who underwent surgical treatment during pregnancy; 5 (22%) had complications, and there were three cases of neonatal tetany (13%). Ideally, surgery should be performed in the second trimester, when fetal organs are developed and the uterus is less likely to undergo labor.[169] Conservative treatment of mildly affected, asymptomatic patients has also been suggested.[170]

In a case reported by Haenel and Mayfield,[171] oral phosphate and parenteral saline were used to sustain the patient during the third trimester. However, even milder forms have adverse fetal effects and risk.[172]

The treatment of life-threatening hypercalcemia can be problematic and may require hydration, furosemide, phosphates, and even hemodialysis.[173-175] Treatment is summarized in Table 48-9. Calcitonin inhibits bone resorption; its effects are generally short lived, and it does not cross the placenta. It has been used briefly in pregnancy in the third trimester in one case.[176] In life-threatening situations, Mithramycin (plicamycin) lowers calcium by inhibiting bone resorption. It is an antineoplastic agent and toxic to the fetus. In nonpregnant patients, bisphosphonates (e.g., pamidronate) given intravenously are also effective in lowering calcium levels. Transplacental passage has been shown in animal studies. For a patient with milk-alkali syndrome who presented with severe hypercalcemia related to excessive use of calcium carbonate, a single dose of the bisphosphonate etidronate was given, with prompt reduction of serum calcium and subsequent hypocalcemia.[177]

PARATHYROID CARCINOMA IN PREGNANCY

Four cases of parathyroid carcinoma during pregnancy were reviewed by Montoro and associates.[178] Severe hypercalcemia, hypertension, and a palpable neck mass were consistent features, whereas palpable masses were found in only 5% and hypertension in 10% of pregnant

TABLE 48-10 CLASSIFICATION OF HYPOPARATHYROID DISORDERS

Defect	Cause
Absence of parathyroid hormone (PTH) or insufficiency	Previous thyroid or parathyroid surgery Idiopathic hypoparathyroidism (familial or sporadic) DiGeorge syndrome Iron overload (rare) Previous irradiation with ^{131}I (rare)
Absence of and resistance to PTH	Magnesium depletion
PTH resistance	Pseudohypoparathyroidism

patients with parathyroid adenomas. Because survival depends on complete initial resection, early surgical intervention is important.

Hypoparathyroidism

Hypoparathyroidism has been reviewed by Mestman.[162] Hypoparathyroidism in pregnancy usually occurs in patients who have previously undergone neck surgery, but it can occur in less common circumstances (Table 48-10). The diagnosis is confirmed by the combination of hypocalcemia with low PTH, 1,25$(OH)_2$D, and nephrogenous cAMP concentrations. Other hypocalcemic states that need to be differentiated from hypoparathyroidism include vitamin D deficiency (with a finding of a high PTH level), excessive chelation (after blood transfusion), pancreatitis, and septic states.

Clinical features include tetany, which may be elicited in latent form by the Chvostek test (i.e., tapping of the facial nerve) and the Trousseau test (i.e., occurrence of tetany within 3 minutes of the induction of ischemia in the upper extremity). Other symptoms include paresthesia, stridor, muscle cramps, and mental changes, including frank psychosis. The electrocardiogram may reveal prolongation of the QT interval.

COMPLICATIONS

Neonatal hyperparathyroidism may result from maternal hypocalcemia. It can cause fetal bone demineralization and growth restriction.[179] Although this condition is transient, death from the complications of skeletal fractures can occur. Loughhead and colleagues[180] reviewed 16 cases of congenital hyperparathyroidism resulting from maternal hypocalcemia; bone features of hyperparathyroidism were documented in 13 cases. Six of the neonates died within the first 3 months of life. The investigators concluded that the presentation varied greatly, ranging from clinically and radiologically silent cases to neonates with severe skeletal disease and bone demineralization.

TREATMENT

The maternal serum calcium level should be maintained within normal limits. Vitamin D (50,000 to 100,000 units/day or more) and calcium salts (1.0 or 1.5 g of elemental calcium per day) may be given to maintain normocalcemia. Alternatively, calcitriol (1,25$[OH]_2$D), which has a more rapid onset of action and a shorter half-life, can be used. The usual dose is 0.5 to 1.0 μg/day.[181]

The normal replacement dose of vitamin D in a hypoparathyroid woman may need to be increased, possibly because of increased binding of vitamin D to vitamin D–binding protein. In a patient treated with calcitriol, the dose had to be doubled during pregnancy to maintain normocalcemia, similar to the physiologic twofold rise in 1,25$(OH)_2$D during pregnancy.[182] The aim should be serum calcium concentrations in the range of 8 to 9 mg/dL, with avoidance of hypercalciuria (>250 mg/24 hr), which can lead to nephrolithiasis. In late pregnancy, the dose of calcitriol may need to be reduced, and this is likely to be related to the increased PTHrP levels in late pregnancy. In limited reports of pseudohypoparathyroidism (i.e., resistance to PTH), pregnancy has normalized serum calcium, decreased PTH, and increased 1,25$(OH)_2$D levels. The presence of PTHrP cannot explain these changes, because they are resistant to PTH and PTHrP. The mechanism is unclear but may include increased placental secretion of 1,25$(OH)_2$D.[183] In the hypoparathyroid patient, a prompt decrease to pre-pregnancy doses of vitamin D is necessary after delivery so that hypercalcemia can be avoided.[184] Although lactating women usually require continuation of pregnancy doses of vitamin D, hypercalcemia has been reported,[184] and close monitoring is prudent. This finding may be related to the production of PTHrP by the breasts[167,185] or to induction of 1α-hydroxylase by prolactin.

Acute symptomatic hypocalcemia is a medical emergency. It should be treated with intravenous calcium (e.g., 10 mL of 10% calcium gluconate over 10 minutes, followed by an infusion of 0.5 to 2.0 mg/kg/hr of elemental calcium, diluted with dextrose to avoid irritation to veins).

Infants receiving breast milk from mothers consuming large doses of vitamin D should undergo periodic calcium determinations, because the breast milk will have higher-than-normal levels of vitamin D.[186] The elevated levels of vitamin D can cause hypercalcemia and impaired linear growth in the infant.

Pregnancy-Related Osteoporosis

Osteoporosis is a disorder characterized by loss of bone mass and microarchitectural deterioration, resulting in an increased risk of fracture. Normally, bone formation and resorption are coupled. Bone loss because of reduced formation or increased resorption may occur in estrogen-deficiency states, glucocorticoid-excess syndromes, thyrotoxicosis, and other circumstances.

The effect of pregnancy on bone turnover was evaluated by Black and colleagues,[187] Oliveri and coworkers,[188] and Karlsson and associates.[189] In a detailed study using biochemical markers of bone formation and resorption and dual-energy x-ray absorptiometry (DEXA) before, during (i.e., in the forearm), and after pregnancy (i.e., in the hip, spine, and forearm), Black and colleagues[187] reported increased markers of bone resorption by 14 weeks' gestation and further by 28 weeks, whereas markers of bone formation did not increase significantly until 28 weeks. Lumbar spine and hip bone mineral density decreased significantly during pregnancy. It appeared that bone remodeling became uncoupled, with an increase in resorption during the first two trimesters, and the increase in formation became evident only in the third trimester. In a study of 34 women during pregnancy, peripheral computed tomography measurements showed no change in cortical bone but tremendous variability in loss of trabecular bone. Fast losers had high serum levels of osteocalcin (a marker of bone formation), and it was suggested that this could be used as a marker of the change.[190]

In 1955, Nordin and Roper[191] described four young women with backache and vertebral compression fractures diagnosed with idiopathic osteoporosis. Their symptoms developed during or shortly after pregnancy and improved with follow-up. These investigators suggested that the association between osteoporosis and pregnancy might not have been fortuitous. Since that time, sporadic cases and small series of patients with osteoporosis in relation to pregnancy and lactation have been reported.[192,193] Smith and coworkers[194] suggested that failure of calcium accretion by the maternal skeleton, normally facilitated by increased calcium absorption in response to higher 1,25$(OH)_2$D concentrations, might explain this occurrence; these vitamin concentrations were low in several patients with osteoporosis. They suggested failure of the calcitonin response to pregnancy as another mechanism; calcitonin has anti-resorptive properties, and levels may increase during pregnancy.

In a study of 29 women with idiopathic osteoporosis associated with pregnancy,[195] it was observed that pain occurring late in the first full-term pregnancy was the most common presentation and that the natural history was improvement over time. Adult-related fractures occurring at an earlier age were more prevalent in the mothers of these women, suggesting possible genetic factors in the cause of osteoporosis. Low 1,25$(OH)_2D$ concentrations were demonstrated in a case by Khan and colleagues;[196] the abnormality reversed over time. Subsequent pregnancies are not necessarily affected.

During lactation, a substantial part of the calcium demand is mobilized from the maternal skeleton because of low estrogen and high PTHrP levels from the breasts.[197] In a study of 18 exclusively breastfeeding women, compared with 18 women in whom lactation was inhibited by bromocriptine, there was a significant decrease in lumbar spine and distal radius and in bone density, and there was biochemical evidence of increased bone turnover during breastfeeding, with an incomplete recovery 6 months after breastfeeding cessation.[198] In the bromocriptine-treated women, bone mineral density did not change. Overall, it appears that healthy young women have significant early losses of bone mineral density at the axial spine and hip during 6 months of lactation.[199] Loss, however, does not continue beyond 6 months despite continuing lactation, and bone mineral density loss usually is restored with the return of normal menses. In a study of 60 women, 47% of breastfeeders lost more than 5% of bone at the lumbar spine, and the bottle-feeders maintained bone mineral density. At 1 year after delivery, all but seven had returned to within 5% of preconception values at the spine, but recovery of the total hip loss was less complete. Several women became transiently osteoporotic.[200]

The calcium demands of late pregnancy and lactation are about 0.3 g per day. There are limited long-term data on the effects of extended and repeated lactation. Whereas some studies have shown an adverse effect,[201] parity and lactation have not been associated with low bone mineral density or osteoporotic fracture risk in epidemiologic or case-control cohort studies.[202] In a study of 11 women with pregnancy and lactation-associated osteoporosis, 10 of whom had vertebral fractures and one a nonvertebral fracture, at least one recognized risk factor (e.g., low body weight, smoking, family history, vitamin D deficiency) was present in 9 patients. Nine patients received bisphosphonates for a median of 24 months, with increase in bone mineral density of 23% after 2 years. Of five women who had subsequent pregnancies, one sustained a fracture after delivery, and two patients followed for more than 10 years sustained fractures outside pregnancy.[203] The study authors concluded that bisphosphonate therapy administered soon after presentation substantially increased spine bone density. However, because bisphosphonates can have an extremely long half-life and stay in bone for a long period, caution should be exercised if the patient wishes to conceive again, because the effects of bisphosphonates on the developing fetal skeleton has not been well studied, and the long-term safety as far as the fetus is concerned is unknown. In cases of severe osteoporosis it is reasonable to discourage lactation.

References

Hypothalamus and Pituitary

1. Scheithauer BW, Sano T, Kovacs KT, et al: The pituitary gland in pregnancy: A clinicopathologic and immunohistochemical study of 69 cases. Mayo Clin Proc 65:461, 1990.
2. Gonzalez JF, Elizondo G, Saldivar D, et al: Pituitary gland growth during normal pregnancy: An in vivo study using magnetic resonance imaging. Am J Med 85:217, 1988.
3. Dinc H, Esen F, Demirci A, et al: Pituitary dimensions and volume measurements in pregnancy and postpartum. Acta Radiol 39:64, 1998.
4. Tyson JE, Hwang P, Guyden A, et al: Studies of prolactin secretion in human pregnancy. Am J Obstet Gynecol 113:14, 1972.
5. Molitch ME: Pituitary disorders during pregnancy. Endocrinol Metab Clin North Am 35:99, 2006.
6. Davison JM, Gilmore EA, Durr JS, et al: Altered osmotic thresholds for vasopressin secretion and thirst in human pregnancy. Am J Physiol 246:105, 1983.
7. Lindheimer MD, Barron WM, Davison JM: Osmotic volume control of vasopressin release in pregnancy. Am J Kidney Dis 17:105, 1991.
8. Dawood MY, Khan-Dawood FS: The posterior pituitary pathway. In Droegemveller W, Sciarra J (eds): Gynecology and Obstetrics, vol 5. Philadelphia, JB Lippincott, 1990.
9. Decherney A, Naftolin F: Hypothalamic and pituitary development in the fetus. Clin Obstet Gynecol 23:749, 1980.
10. Green JS, Parfrey PS, Harnett JD, et al: The cardinal manifestations of Bardet-Biedl syndrome, a form of Lawrence-Moon-Biedl syndrome. N Engl J Med 321:1002, 1989.
11. Aydin Y, Can SM, Gulkilik A, et al: Rapid enlargement and recurrence of a preexisting intrasellar craniopharyngioma during the course of two pregnancies. J Neurosurg 91:322, 1999.
12. Hiett AK, Barton JR: Diabetes insipidus associated with craniopharyngioma in pregnancy. Obstet Gynecol 76:982, 1990.
13. Magge SN, Brunt M, Scott RM: Craniopharyngioma presenting during pregnancy 4 years after a normal magnetic resonance imaging scan: Case report. Neurosurgery 49:1014, 2001.
14. Gillam MP, Molitch ME, Lombardi G, et al: Advances in the treatment of prolactinomas. Endocr Rev 27:485, 2006.
15. Kupersmith MJ, Rosenberg C, Kleinberg D: Visual loss in pregnant women with pituitary adenomas. Ann Intern Med 121:473, 1994.
16. Masding MG, Lees PD, Gawne-Cain L, et al: Visual compression by a non-secreting pituitary tumor during pregnancy. J R Soc Med 96:27, 2003.
17. Krupp P, Monka C: Bromocriptine in pregnancy: Safety aspects. Klin Wochenschr 65:823, 1987.
18. del Pozo E, Krupp P: Endocrine effects of dopamine receptor stimulation on the feto-maternal unit. In Krauer B, et al (eds): Drugs and Pregnancy. London, Academic Press, 1984, p 191.
19. Colao A, Sarno AD, Sarnacchiaro F, et al: Prolactinomas resistant to standard dopamine agonists respond to chronic cabergoline treatment. J Clin Endocrinol Metab 82:876, 1997.
20. Robert E, Musatti L, Piscitelli G, et al: Pregnancy outcome after treatment with the ergot derivative cabergoline. Reprod Toxicol 10:333, 1996.
21. Ricci E, Parazzini F, Motta A, et al: Pregnancy outcome after cabergoline treatment in early weeks of gestation. Reprod Toxicol 16:791, 2002.
22. Schade R, Andersohn F, Suissa S, et al: Dopamine agonists and the risk of cardiac-valve regurgitation. N Engl J Med 356:29, 2007.
23. Albrecht BH, Betz G: Prolactin-secreting pituitary tumors and pregnancy. In Olefsy JM, Robbins RJ (eds): Contemporary Issues in Endocrinology and Metabolism: Prolactinomas, vol 2. New York, Churchill Livingstone, 1986, p 195.
24. Magyar DM, Marshall JR: Pituitary tumors and pregnancy. Am J Obstet Gynecol 132:739, 1978.
25. Casnueva FF, Molitch ME, Schleche JA, et al: Guidelines of the Pituitary Society for the Diagnosis and Management of Prolactinomas. Clin Endocrinol 65:265, 2006.
26. Belchetz PE, Carty A, Clearkin LG: Failure of prophylactic surgery to avert massive pituitary expansion in pregnancy. Clin Endocrinol 25:325, 1986.
27. Divers WA, Yen SSC: Prolactin-producing microadenomas in pregnancy. Obstet Gynecol 62:425, 1983.
28. Borges F, Horta C, Mendes P, et al: Factors of cure in hyperprolactinemic women [abstract]. Proceedings of the 11th International Congress of Endocrinology, Sydney, Australia, 2000. Endocrinologist 11:402, 2000.

29. Ruiz-Velasco V, Tolis G: Pregnancy in hyperprolactinemic women. Fertil Steril 41:793, 1984.
30. O'Donovan PA, O'Donovan PJ, Ritchie EH: Apoplexy into a prolactin secreting macroadenoma during early pregnancy with successful outcome. BJOG 93:389, 1986.
31. Zarate A, Canales ES, Alger M: The effect of pregnancy and lactation on pituitary prolactin secreting tumors. Acta Endocrinol 92:407, 1979.
32. Rothman KJ, Funch DP, Dreyer NA: Bromocriptine and puerperal seizures. Epidemiology 1:232, 1990.
33. Ahmed M, Al-Dossary E, Woodhouse NJY: Macroprolactinoma with suprasellar extension: Effect of bromocriptine withdrawal during one or more pregnancies. Fertil Steril 58:492, 1992.
34. Furlanetto RW, Underwood LE, Van Wyk JJ, et al: Serum immunoreactive somatomedin-C is elevated late in pregnancy. J Clin Endocrinol Metab 47:695, 1978.
35. Frankenne F, Closset J, Gomez F, et al: The physiology of growth hormones in pregnant women and partial characterization of the placental GH variant. J Clin Endocrinol Metab 66:1171, 1988.
36. Beckers A, Stevenaert A, Foidart JM, et al: Placental and pituitary growth hormone secretion during pregnancy in acromegalic women. J Clin Endocrinol Metab 71:725, 1990.
37. Hermann-Bonert V, Seliverstov M, Melmed S: Pregnancy in acromegaly: Successful therapeutic outcome. J Clin Endocrinol Metab 83:727, 1998.
38. Cozzi R, Attanasio R, Barausse M: Pregnancy in acromegaly: A one-center experience. Eur J Endocrinol 155:279, 2006.
39. Luboshitzky R, Dickstein G, Barzilai D: Bromocriptine induced pregnancy in an acromegalic patient. JAMA 244:584, 1980.
40. Yap AS, Clouston WM, Mortimer RH, et al: Acromegaly first diagnosed in pregnancy: The role of bromocriptine therapy. Am J Obstet Gynecol 163:477, 1990.
41. de Menis E, Billeci D, Marton E, et al: Uneventful pregnancy in an acromegalic patient treated with slow-release lanreotide: A case report. J Clin Endocrinol Metab 84:1489, 1999.
42. Neal JM: Successful pregnancy in a women with acromegaly treated with octreotide. Endocr Pract 6:148, 2000.
43. Caron P, Gerbeau C, Pradayrol L, et al: Successful pregnancy in an infertile woman with a thyrotropin-secreting macroadenoma treated with somatostatin analog (octreotide). J Clin Endocrinol Metab 81:1164, 1996.
44. Chaiamnuay S, Moster M, Katz MR, et al: Successful management of a pregnant woman with a TSH secreting pituitary adenoma with surgical and medical therapy. Pituitary 6:109, 2003.
45. Lindsay JR, Nieman LK: The hypothalamic-pituitary-adrenal axis in pregnancy: Challenges in disease detection and treatment. Endocr Rev 26:775, 2005.
46. Linday JR, Jonklaas J, Oldfield EH, et al: Cushing's syndrome during pregnancy: Personal experience and review of the literature J Clin Endocrinol Metab 90:3077, 2005.
47. Buescher MA: Cushing's syndrome in pregnancy. Endocrinologist 6:357, 1996.
48. Pickard J, Jochen AL, Sadur CN, et al: Cushing's syndrome in pregnancy. Obstet Gynecol Surv 45:87, 1990.
49. Schultz CL, Haaga JR, Fletcher BD, et al: Magnetic resonance imaging of the adrenal glands: A comparison with computed tomography. AJR Am J Roentgenol 143:1235, 1984.
50. Pinette NG, Pan YQ, Oppenheim D, et al: Bilateral inferior petrosal sinus corticotropin sampling with corticotropin releasing hormone stimulation in a pregnant patient with Cushing's syndrome. Am J Obstet Gynecol 171:563, 1994.
51. Close CF, Mann MC, Watts JF, et al: ACTH independent Cushing's syndrome in pregnancy with spontaneous resolution after delivery: Control of the hypercortisolism with metyrapone. Clin Endocrinol (Oxf) 39:375, 1993.
52. Mellor A, Harvey RD, Pobereskin LH, et al: Cushing's disease treated by trans-sphenoidal selective adenomectomy in mid-pregnancy. Br. J Anaesth 80:850, 1998.
53. Gormley MJJ, Hadden DR, Kennedy TL, et al: Cushing's syndrome in pregnancy: Treatment with metyrapone. Clin Endocrinol 16:283, 1982.
54. Surrey ES, Chang RJ: Nelson's syndrome in pregnancy. Fertil Steril 44:548, 1985.
55. Beasley EW: Pregnancy and lactation in Nelson's syndrome. Endocrinologist 9:313, 1999.
56. Sheehan HL: Post-partum necrosis of the anterior pituitary. J Pathol Bacteriol 45:189, 1937.
57. Hall MRP: Incidence of anterior pituitary deficiency following postpartum hemorrhage: Cases reviewed from the Oxfordshire and Buckinghamshire area. Proc Soc Med 55:468, 1962.
58. Kelestimur F: Sheehan's syndrome. Pituitary 6:181, 2003.
59. Drury MI, Keelan DM: Sheehan's syndrome. J Obstet Gynaecol Br Commonw 73:802, 1966.
60. Dokmetas HS, Kilicli F, Korkmaz S, et al: Characteristic features of 20 patients with Sheehan's syndrome. Gynecol Endocrinol 22:279, 2006.
61. Grimes HG, Brooks MH: Pregnancy in Sheehan's syndrome: Report of a case and review. Obstet Gynecol Surv 35:481, 1980.
62. Lufkin EG, Kao PC, O'Fallon WM, et al: Combined testing of anterior pituitary gland with insulin, thyrotropin-releasing hormone and luteinizing hormone-releasing hormone. Am J Med 75:471, 1983.
63. Scheller TJ, Nader S: Magnetic resonance imaging in Sheehan's syndrome. Case report and literature review of imaging studies. Endocr Pract 3:82, 1997.
64. Dorfman SG, Dillaplain RP, Gambrell RD: Antepartum pituitary infarction. Obstet Gynecol 53(Suppl):21S, 1979.
65. De Heide LJ, van Tol KM, Doorenbos B: Pituitary apoplexy presenting during pregnancy. Neth J Med 62:393, 2004.
66. Goudie RB, Pinkerton PH: Anterior hypophysitis and Hashimoto's disease in a young woman. J Pathol Bacteriol 83:585, 1962.
67. Caturegli P, Newschaffer C, Olivi A, et al: Autoimmune hypophysitis. Endocr Rev 26:599, 2005.
68. Nader S, Orlander P: Lymphocytic hypophysitis: A case report and review of the literature. Infertility 13:145, 1990.
69. Meichner RH, Riggio S, Manz HJ, et al: Lymphocytic adenohypophysitis causing pituitary mass. Neurology 37:158, 1987.
70. Stelmach M, O'Day J: Rapid change in visual fields associated with suprasellar lymphocytic hypophysitis. J Clin Neuroophthalmol 11:19, 1991.
71. Bitton RN, Slavin M, Decker RE, et al: The course of lymphocytic hypophysitis. Surg Neurol 36:40, 1991.
72. Ober KP, Elster A: Spontaneously resolving lymphocytic hypophysitis as a cause of postpartum diabetes insipidus. Endocrinologist 4:107, 1994.
73. Sinha D, Sinha A, Pirie AM: A case of recurrent lymphocytic hypophysitis in pregnancy. J Obstet Gynaecol 26:255, 2006.
74. Parikh A, Ezzat S: Complete anterior pituitary failure and postpartum cardiomyopathy. Endocr Pract 12:284, 2006.
75. Hendricks CH: The neurohypophysis in pregnancy. Obstet Gynecol Surv 9:323, 1954.
76. Maranon G: Diabetes insipidus and uterine atony. BMJ 2:769, 1947.
77. Durr JA, Lindheimer MD: Diagnosis and management of diabetes insipidus during pregnancy. Endocr Pract 2:353, 1996.
78. Hime MC, Richardson JA: Diabetes insipidus and pregnancy: Case report, incidence and review of literature. Obstet Gynecol Surv 33:375, 1978.
79. Campbell JW: Diabetes insipidus and complicated pregnancy. JAMA 243:1744, 1980.
80. Hamai Y, Fujii T, Nishina H, et al: Differential clinical courses of pregnancies complicated by diabetes insipidus, which does or does not predate the pregnancy. Hum Reprod 12:1816, 1997.
81. Brewster UC, Hayslett JP: Diabetes insipidus in the third trimester of pregnancy. Obstet Gynecol 105:1173, 2005.
82. Lindheimer MD: Polyuria and pregnancy: Its cause, its danger. Obstet Gynecol 105:1171, 2005.
83. Yamamoto T, Ishii T, Yamagami K, et al : Transient diabetes insipidus in pregnancy with peculiar change in signal intensity on T1-weighted magnetic resonance images. Intern Med 42:513, 2003.
84. Robinson AG, Amico JA: "No-sweet" diabetes of pregnancy. N Engl J Med 324:556, 1991.

85. Ford SM, Lumpkin HL: Transient vasopressin-resistant diabetes insipidus of pregnancy. Obstet Gynecol 68:726, 1986.
86. Nakamura Y, Takagi H, Sakurai S, et al: Transient diabetes insipidus during and after pregnancy. N Engl J Med 325:285, 1991.
87. Kallen BAJ, Carlsson SS, Bengtsson BKA: Diabetes insipidus and use of desmopressin during pregnancy. Eur J Endocrinol 132:144, 1995.
88. Ray JG: DDAVP use during pregnancy: An analysis of its safety for mother and child. Obstet Gynecol Surv 53:450, 1998.
89. Burrow GN, Wassenaar W, Robertson GL, et al: DDAVP treatment of diabetes insipidus during pregnancy and the postpartum period. Acta Endocrinol 97:23, 1981.
90. Shalev E, Goldstein D, Zuckerman H: Compulsive water drinking in pregnancy. Int J Gynaecol Obstet 18:465, 1980.

Adrenal Glands

91. Sasaki A, Liotta AS, Luckey MM, et al: Immunoreactive corticotropin-releasing factor is present in human maternal plasma during the third trimester of pregnancy. J Clin Endocrinol Metab 59:812, 1984.
92. Hillhouse EW, Grammatopoulos DK: Role of stress peptides during pregnancy and human labour. Reproduction 124:323, 2002.
93. Waddell BJ, Burton PJ: Release of bioactive ACTH by perfused human placenta at early and late gestation. J Endocrinol 136:345, 1993.
94. Suri D, Moran JU, KaszaK, et al: Assessment of adrenal reserve in pregnancy: Defining the normal response to adrenocorticotropin stimulation test. J Clin Edocrinol Metab 91:3866, 2006.
95. Wilson M, Morganti AA, Zervoudakis I, et al: Blood pressure, the renin-aldosterone system and sex steroids throughout normal pregnancy. Am J Med 68:97, 1980.
96. Kerian V, Nahoul K, LeMartelot MT, et al: Longitudinal study of maternal plasma bioavailable testosterone and androstenediol glucuronide levels during pregnancy. Clin Endocrinol (Oxf) 40:263, 1994.
97. Keller-Wood M, Wood CE: Pituitary-adrenal physiology during pregnancy. Endocrinologist 11:159, 2001.
98. Peterson RE: Cortisol. In Fuchs F, Klopper A (eds): Endocrinology of Pregnancy, 2nd ed. Hagerstown, Md, Harper & Row, 1977.
99. Lindsay JR, Nieman LK: Adrenal disorders and pregnancy. Endocrinol Metab Clin North Am 35:1, 2006.
100. Betterle C, Dal Pra C, Mantero F, et al: Autoimmune adrenal insufficiency and autoimmune polyendocrine syndromes: Autoantibodies, autoantigens, and their applicability in diagnosis and disease prediction. Endocr Rev 23:327, 2002.
101. Brent F: Addison's disease and pregnancy. Am J Surg 79:645, 1950.
102. Nolten WE, Lindheimer MD, Oparil S, et al: Deoxycorticosterone in normal pregnancy. Am J Obstet Gynecol 132:414, 1978.
103. McKenna DS, Wittber GM, Nahaaja HN, et al: The effects of repeat doses of antenatal corticosteroids on maternal adrenal function. Am J Obstet Gynecol 183:669, 2000.
104. Albert E, Dalaker K, Jorde R, et al: Addison's disease and pregnancy. Acta Obstet Gynecol Scand 68:185, 1989.
105. Seaward PGR, Guidozzi F, Sonnendecker EWW: Addisonian crisis in pregnancy: Case Report. BJOG 96:1348, 1989.
106. Drucker D, Shumak S, Angel A: Schmidt syndrome presenting with intrauterine growth retardation and postpartum addisonian crises. Am J Obstet Gynecol 149:229, 1984.
107. Buescher MA: Cushing's syndrome in pregnancy. Endocrinologist 6:357, 1996.
108. Lotgering FK, Derhx FMH, Wallenburg HCS: Primary hypoaldosteronism in pregnancy. Am J Obstet Gynecol 155:986, 1986.
109. Okawa T, Asano K, Hashimoto T, et al: Diagnosis and management of primary hyperaldosteronism in pregnancy: Case report and review of the literature. Am J Perinatol 19:31, 2002.
110. Neerhof MG, Shlossman PA, Ludomirsky A, et al: Idiopathic aldosteronism in pregnancy. Obstet Gynecol 78:489, 1991.
111. Kreft-Jais C, Plovin PF, Tchobrovtsky C, et al: Angiotensin-converting enzyme inhibitors during pregnancy: A survey of 22 patients given captopril and nine given enalapril. BJOG 95:420, 1988.
112. Pang S, Wallace MA, Hofman L, et al: Worldwide experience in newborn screening for classical congenital adrenal hyperplasia due to 21-hydroxylase deficiency. Pediatrics 81:866, 1988.
113. New MI: Prenatal treatment of congenital adrenal hyperplasia: The United States Experience. Endocrinol Metab Clin North Am 30:1, 2001.
114. White PC, New MI, Dupont BO: Congenital adrenal hyperplasia. N Engl J Med 316:1519, 1987.
115. White PC, New MI: Genetic basis of endocrine disease. 2. Congenital adrenal hyperplasia due to 21-hydroxylase deficiency. J Clin Endocrinol Metab 74:6, 1992.
116. Mori N, Miyakawa I: Congenital adrenogenital syndrome and successful pregnancy. Obstet Gynecol 35:394, 1970.
117. White PC, New MI, Dupont BO: Congenital adrenal hyperplasia. N Engl J Med 316:1580, 1987.
118. New MI, Carlson A, Obeid J, et al: Prenatal diagnosis for congenital adrenal hyperplasia in 532 pregnancies. J Clin Endocrinol Metab 86:5651, 2001.
119. Nimkarn S, New MI: Prenatal diagnosis and treatment of congenital adrenal hyperplasia. Horm Res 67:53, 2007.
120. Meyer-Bahlburg HF, Dolezal C, Baker SW, et al: Cognitive and motor development of children with and without congenital adrenal hyperplasia after early-prenatal dexamethasone. J Clin Endocrinol Metab 89:610, 2004.
121. Hirvikoski T, Nordenstrom A, Lindolm T, et al: Cognitive functions in children at risk for congenital adrenal hyperplasia treated prenatally with dexamethasone. J Clin Endocrinol Metab 92:542-548, 2007.
122. Clayton PE, Miller WL, Oberfield SE, et al: Consensus statement on 21-hydroxylase deficiency from the European Society for Paediatric Endocrinology and the Lawson Wilkins Pediatric Endocrine Society. Horm Res 58:188, 2002.
123. Rosler A, Leiberman E, Rosenmann A, et al: Prenatal diagnosis of 11 beta hydroxylase deficiency congenital adrenal hyperplasia. J Clin Endocrinol Metab 49:546, 1979.
124. Cerame BI, Newfield RS, Pascoe L, et al: Prenatal diagnosis and treatment of 11 β-hydroxylase deficiency congenital adrenal hyperplasia resulting in a normal female genitalia. J Clin Endocrinol Metab 84:3129, 1999.
125. White PC, Curnow KM, Pascoe L: Disorders of steroid 11 beta-hydroxylase isoenzymes. Endocr Rev 15:421, 1994.
126. Rosenfeld RL, Rich BL, Wolfsdorf JI, et al: Pubertal presentation of congenital 5-3β-hydroxysteroid dehydrogenase deficiency. J Clin Endocrinol Metab 51:345, 1980.
127. Bongiovanni AM, McPadden AJ: Steroids during pregnancy and possible fetal consequences. Fertil Steril 11:181, 1960.
128. Snyder RD, Snyder D: Corticosteroids for asthma during pregnancy. Ann Allergy 41:340, 1978.
129. Park-Wyllie L, Mazzotta P, Pastuszak A, et al: Birth defects after maternal exposure to corticosteroids: Prospective cohort study and meta-analysis of epidemiological studies. Teratology 62:385, 2000.
130. Griffin J, Brooks N, Patricia F, et al: Pheochromocytoma in pregnancy. Diagnosis and collaborative management. South Med J 77:1325, 1984.
131. Glazer GM, Woolsey EJ, Borrello J, et al: Adrenal tissue characterization using MR imaging. Radiology 158:73, 1986.
132. Fudge TL, McKinnon WMP, Greary WL: Current surgical management of pheochromocytoma during pregnancy. Arch Surg 115:1224, 1980.
133. Harper A, Murnaghan GA, Kennedy L, et al: Pheochromocytoma in pregnancy. Five cases and a review of the literature. BJOG 96:594, 1989.
134. Janetschek G, Neumann HP: Laparoscopic surgery for pheochromocytoma. Urol Clin North Am 28:97, 2001.
135. Lyons CW, Colmorgen GHC: Medical management of pheochromocytoma in pregnancy. Obstet Gynecol 72:450, 1988.
136. Oliver MD, Brownjohn AM, Vinali PS: Medical management of pheochromocytoma in pregnancy. Aust N Z J Obstet Gynaecol 30:268, 1990.
137. Dugas G, Fuller J, Singh S, et al: Pheochromocytoma and pregnancy: A case report and review of anesthetic management. Can J Anesth 51:134, 2004.
138. Schenker JG, Granat M: Pheochromocytomas and pregnancy—an updated appraisal. Aust N Z J Obstet Gynaecol 22:1, 1982.

139. Harrington JL, Farley DR, Van Heerden JA, et al: Adrenal tumors and pregnancy. World J Surg 23:182, 1999.
140. Ellison GT, Mansberger JA, Mansberger AR: Malignant recurrent pheochromocytoma during pregnancy. Case report and review of the literature. Surgery 103:484, 1988.
141. Devoe LD, O'Dell BE, Castillo RA, et al: Metastatic pheochromocytoma in pregnancy and fetal biophysical assessment after maternal administration of α-adrenergic, β-adrenergic, and dopamine antagonists. Obstet Gynecol 68:155, 1986.
142. van der Vaart CH, Heringa MP, Dullaart RPF, et al: Multiple endocrine neoplasia presenting as phaeochromocytoma during pregnancy. BJOG 100:1144, 1993.
143. Tewari KS, Steiger RM, Lam ML, et al: Bilateral pheochromocytoma in pregnancy, heralding multiple endocrine neoplasia syndrome IIA. J Reprod Med 46:385, 2001.

Hirsutism and Virilization in Pregnancy

144. McClamrock HD, Adashi EY: Gestational hyperandrogenism. Fertil Steril 57:257, 1992.
145. Ogilvie M, Davidson JS, Cuttance P, et al: Severe maternal virilization of benign etiology in two successive pregnancies. BJOG 112:1443, 2005.
146. Bachman R, Gennser G, Hakfelt B, et al: Steroid studies in a case of ovarian hyperluteinization with virilism in two consecutive pregnancies. Acta Endocrinol 76:747, 1974.
147. Holt HB, Medbak S, Kirk D, et al: Recurrent severe hyperandrogenism during pregnancy: A case report. J Clin Pathol 58:439, 2005.
148. Morishima A, Grumbach MM, Simpson E, et al: Aromatase deficiency in male and female siblings caused by a novel mutation and the physiologic role of estrogens. J Clin Endocrinol Metab 84:930, 1995.
149. Fukami M, Hasegawa T Horikawa R, et al: Cytochrome P450 oxidoreductase deficiency in three patients initially regarded as having 21-hydroxylase deficiency: Diagnostic value of urine steroid hormone analysis. Pediatr Res 59:276, 2006.
150. Miller WL: P450 Oxidoreductase deficiency: A new disorder of steroidogenesis with multiple clinical manifestations. Trends Endocrinol Metab 15:311, 2004.
151. Sarlis NJ, Weil SJ, Nelson LM: Administration of metformin to a diabetic woman with extreme hyperandrogenemia of non-tumoral origin: Management of infertility and prevention of inadvertent masculinization of a female fetus. J Clin Endocrinol Metab 84:1510, 1999.
152. de Butros A, Hatipoglu B: Testosterone storm during pregnancy. Endocrinologist 11:57, 2001.
153. Miyata M, Nishihara M, Tokunaka KS, et al: A maternal functioning adrenocortical adenoma causing fetal female pseudohermaphroditism. J Urol 142:806, 1989.

Parathyroid Glands and Calcium Metabolism

154. Kovacs CK: Calcium and bone metabolism during pregnancy and lactation. J Mammary Gland Biol Neoplasia 10:105, 2005.
155. Kovacs CK, Fuleihan GEH: Calcium and bone disorders during pregnancy and lactation. Endocrinol Metab Clin North Am 35:21, 2006.
156. Pitkin RM: Calcium metabolism in pregnancy and the perinatal period: A review. Am J Obstet Gynecol 151:99, 1985.
157. Steinchen JJ, Tsang RC, Grafton TL, et al: Vitamin D homeostasis in the perinatal period: 1,25-Dihydroxyvitamin D in maternal, cord and neonatal blood. N Engl J Med 302:315, 1980.
158. Pitkin RM, Reynolds WA, Williams GA, et al: Calcium metabolism in normal pregnancy: A longitudinal study. Am J Obstet Gynecol 133:781, 1979.
159. Seki K, Wada S, Nagata N, et al: Parathyroid hormone–related protein during pregnancy and the perinatal period. Gynecol Obstet Invest 37:83, 1994.
160. Kato T, Seki K, Matsui, et al: Monomeric calcitonin in pregnant women and in cord blood. Obstet Gynecol 92:241,1998.
161. Kort KC, Schiller HJ, Numann PJ: Hyperparathyroidism and pregnancy. Am J Surg 177:66, 1999.
162. Mestman JH: Parathyroid disorders of pregnancy. Semin Perinatol 22:485, 1998.
163. Kristofferson A, Dahlgren S, Lithner F, et al: Primary hyperparathyroidism and pregnancy. Surgery 97:326, 1985.
164. Gelister JSK, Sanderson JD, Chapple CR, et al: Management of hyperparathyroidism in pregnancy. Br J Surg 76:1207, 1989.
165. Lepre F, Grill V, Martin TJ: Hypercalcemia in pregnancy and lactation associated with parathyroid hormone related protein. N Engl J Med 328:666, 1993.
166. Khosla S, Van Heerden JA, Gharib H, et al: Parathyroid hormone related protein and hypercalcemia secondary to massive mammary hyperplasia. N Engl J Med 322:1157, 1990.
167. Shomali ME, Ross DS: Hypercalcemia in a woman with hypoparathyroidism associated with increased parathyroid hormone related protein during lactation. Endocr Pract 5:198, 1999.
168. Kovacs CS, Kronenberg HM: Maternal-fetal calcium and bone metabolism during pregnancy, puerperium and lactation. Endocr Rev 18:832, 1997.
169. Nudelman J, Deutsch A, Sternberg A, et al: The treatment of primary hyperparathyroidism during pregnancy. Br J Surg 71:217, 1984.
170. Lowe DK, Orwoll ES, McClung MR, et al: Hyperparathyroidism and pregnancy. Am J Surg 145:611, 1983.
171. Haenel LC, Mayfield RK: Primary hyperparathyroidism in a twin pregnancy and review of fetal-maternal calcium homeostasis. Am J Med Sci 319:191, 2000.
172. Schnatz PF: Surgical treatment of primary hyperparathyroidism during the third trimester. Obstet Gynecol 99:961, 2002.
173. Monturo MN, Collea JV, Mestman JH: Management of hyperparathyroidism in pregnancy with oral phosphate therapy. Obstet Gynecol 55:431, 1980.
174. Kleinman GE, Rodriguez H, Good MC, et al: Hypercalcemic crisis in pregnancy associated with excessive ingestion of calcium carbonate antacid: Successful treatment with hemodialysis. Obstet Gynecol 78:496, 1991.
175. Iqbal N, Aldasouqi S, Peacock M, et al: Life threatening hypercalcemia associated with primary hyperparathyroidism during pregnancy: Case report and review of literature. Endocr Pract 5:337, 1999.
176. Murray JA, Newman WA, Dacus JV: Hyperparathyroidism in pregnancy: Diagnostic dilemma. Obstet Gynecol Surv 52:202, 1997.
177. Picolos MK, Sims CR, Mastrobattista JM, et al: Milk-alkali syndrome in pregnancy. Obstet Gynecol 104:1201, 2004.
178. Montoro MN, Paler RJ, Goodwin TM, et al: Parathyroid carcinoma during pregnancy. Obstet Gynecol 95:841, 2000.
179. Fleischman AR: Fetal parathyroid gland and calcium homeostasis. Clin Obstet Gynecol 23:791, 1980.
180. Loughead JL, Mughal Z, Mimouni F, et al: Spectrum and natural history of congenital hyperparathyroidism secondary to maternal hypocalcemia. Am J Perinatol 7:350, 1990.
181. Salle BL, Berthezene F, Glorieux FH, et al: Hypoparathyroidism during pregnancy: Treatment with calcitriol. J Clin Endocrinol Metab 52:810, 1981.
182. Sadeghi-Nejad A, Wolfsdorf JI, Senior B: Hypoparathyroidism and pregnancy: Treatment with calcitriol. JAMA 243:254, 1980.
183. Breslau NA, Zerwekh JE: Relationship of estrogen and pregnancy to calcium homeostasis in pseudohypoparathyroidism. J Clin Endocrinol Metab 62:45, 1986.
184. Caplan RH, Beguin EA: Hypercalcemia in a calcitriol-treated hypoparathyroid woman during lactation. Obstet Gynecol 76:485, 1990.
185. Mather KJ, Chik CL, Corenblum B: Maintenance of serum calcium by parathyroid hormone related peptide during lactation in a hypoparathyroid patient. J Clin Endocrinol Metab 84:424, 1999.
186. Greer FR, Hollis BW, Napoli JL: High concentrations of vitamin D_2 in human milk associated with pharmacologic doses of vitamin D_2. J Pediatr 105:61, 1984.
187. Black AJ, Topping J, Durham B, et al: A detailed assessment of alterations in bone turnover, calcium homeostasis and bone density in normal pregnancy. J Bone Miner Res 15:557, 2000.

188. Oliveri B, Parisi MS, Zeni S, et al: Mineral and bone mass changes during pregnancy and lactation. Nutrition 20:235, 2004.
189. Karlsson MK, Ahlborg HG, Karlsson C: Maternity and bone mineral density. Acta Orthop 76:2, 2005.
190. Wisser J, Florio I, Neff M, et al: Changes in bone density and metabolism in pregnancy. Acta Obstet Gynecol Scand 84:349, 2005.
191. Nordin BEC, Roper A: Post-pregnancy osteoporosis. A syndrome? Lancet 1:431, 1955.
192. Di Gregorio S, Danilowicz K, Rubin Z, et al: Osteoporosis with vertebral fractures associated with pregnancy and lactation. Nutrition 16:1052, 2000.
193. Honjo S, Mizunuma H: Changes in biochemical parameters of bone turnover and bone mineral density in post-pregnancy osteoporosis. Am J Obstet Gynecol 185:246, 2001.
194. Smith R, Stevenson JC, Winearls CG, et al: Osteoporosis of pregnancy. Lancet 1:1178, 1985.
195. Dunne F, Walters B, Marshall T, et al: Pregnancy associated osteoporosis. Clin Endocrinol (Oxf) 39:487, 1993.
196. Khan AA, Ahmed MM, Pritzker KPH: Osteoporosis associated with pregnancy: Case report and review. Endocr Pract 1:236, 1995.
197. Grill V, Hillary J, Ho PM, et al: Parathyroid hormone related protein: A possible endocrine function on lactation. Clin Endocrinol (Oxf) 37:405, 1992.
198. Affinito P, Tommaselli GA, Carlo CD, et al: Changes in bone mineral density and calcium metabolism in breast feeding women. A one year follow-up study. J Clin Endocrinol Metab 81:2314, 1996.
199. Eisman J: Relevance of pregnancy and lactation to osteoporosis [commentary]. Lancet 352:504, 1998.
200. Pearson D, Kaur M, San P, et al: Recovery of pregnancy mediate bone loss during lactation. Bone 34:570, 2004.
201. Lissner L, Bengtsson C, Hansson T: Bone mineral content in relation to lactation history in pre- and postmenopausal women. Calcif Tissue Int 48:319, 1991.
202. Tuppuraineen M, Kroger H, Honkanen R, et al: Risks of perimenopausal fractures—a prospective population-based study. Acta Obstet Gynecol Scand 7:624, 1995.
203. O'Sullivan SM, Grey AB, Singh R, et al: Bisphosphonates in pregnancy and lactation-associated osteoporosis. Osteoporos Int 17:1008, 2006.

Chapter 49

Gastrointestinal Disease in Pregnancy

Thomas F. Kelly, MD, and Thomas J. Savides, MD

Pregnancy alters the anatomy and physiology of the gastrointestinal tract. These changes result in significant maternal symptoms that are experienced even in uncomplicated gestations. Difficulty arises in differentiating normal pregnancy complaints from those associated with pathology. The workup of suspected gastrointestinal disease is hampered by the potential risks of radiation or endoscopy to the fetus. Similarly, therapy for many gastrointestinal disorders must be altered because of the adverse or unknown effects of medical or surgical treatment. In this chapter, we review the common gastrointestinal disorders occurring in pregnancy and describe how pregnancy affects the presentation, diagnosis, and treatment of these disorders.

Alterations in Normal Gastrointestinal Function in Pregnancy

Esophagus

The esophagus normally maintains an alkaline pH, mainly by peristalsis of orally produced saliva and the lower esophageal sphincter preventing reflux of gastric contents.[1] Van Thiel and colleagues[2,3] found decreased tone of the gastroesophageal sphincter during pregnancy and with the use of progesterone-containing oral contraceptives. However, Fisher and associates[4] found no change in lower esophageal pressure in early pregnancy, but the sphincter's responses to hormonal and physiologic stimuli were reduced.[4] These investigators observed in opossums decreased responses of the lower esophageal sphincter circular muscle to gastrin and acetylcholine.[5] Whether arising from reduced sphincter tone or response to stimuli during pregnancy, the potential for gastrointestinal reflux appears to increase compared with nonpregnant individuals.

Stomach

The stomach receives, mixes, and propels food. It has mechanical and secretory properties. Peristaltic contractions are triggered by the gastric pacemaker located between the fundus and the corpus on the greater curvature with a normal frequency of three cycles per minute. Gastric emptying is difficult to measure in pregnancy because the typical use of radioisotopes in test meals must be avoided during human pregnancy. Measuring serial blood levels of acetaminophen, an agent that is poorly absorbed from the stomach, but quickly absorbed from the small intestine, Macfie and coworkers[6] found that gastric emptying was not delayed in pregnancy. Another study found no differences in pregnant compared with nonpregnant individuals, with the exception of delayed emptying 2 hours after delivery.[7] Using hydrogen breath testing, there were no delays in gastric emptying, but there were increases in orocecal transit time as pregnancy advanced.[8] Results of indirect studies suggest that gastric motility is not altered in pregnancy. Studies of gastric acid secretory function during pregnancy have produced conflicting results, with suggestions that acid production is decreased, unchanged, or increased.[9-11]

Small Intestine

Small intestinal transit time is prolonged during pregnancy[12] and during the luteal phase in nonpregnant women. It may be caused by elevated progesterone levels during pregnancy and their relaxing effect on smooth muscle.[13] The teleologic advantage is presumed to be increased nutrient absorption. Vitamin B_{12} absorption and transluminal transport of some amino acids in animals are increased during pregnancy.[14,15] The weight of the small intestine is increased during pregnancy in animals and is probably accounted for by the larger mucosal surface, supporting the theory of increased absorptive surface.

Colon

The functional changes of the colon in human pregnancy are inadequately studied. In pregnant animal models, colonic transit time is increased, and the smooth muscle is less responsive to stimulation.[16,17] Because progesterone is known to inhibit colonic smooth muscle activity,[18] it appears plausible that colonic motor activity is diminished during human pregnancy.

Nausea and Vomiting

Epidemiology

Up to 80% of pregnant women experience nausea and vomiting during pregnancy.[19] Annually, 4 million women in the United States and 350,000 in Canada are affected.[1] Symptoms usually occur between 4 and 10 weeks' gestation and resolve by week 20. Nausea and vomiting usually occur in the first trimester, but they occur only in the third trimester in 3% of patients. One half of pregnant women experience nausea in the morning, whereas nausea peaks in the evening in 7% of patients, and 36% experience symptoms constantly.[20]

The term *morning sickness* is somewhat misleading in that a prospective study suggested that nausea occurring only during the morning affected 2% of patients, whereas 80% of symptomatic patients had nausea or vomiting throughout the day.[21] Demographic factors associated with vomiting include first pregnancy, younger age, fewer than 12 years of education, nonsmoking status, and obesity.[22] Nausea and vomiting are more common in the Western countries and Japan and rare in Africa, Asia, and Alaska among Native Americans,[23] indicating that factors other than pregnancy contribute to the pathogenesis.

Etiology

The cause of nausea and vomiting is unknown. Genetic influences have been suggested by the concordance of frequency in monozygotic twins[24] and the fact that family members are more likely to be affected.[25,26]

Human chorionic gonadotropin has been implicated in causing nausea and vomiting. The close temporal association of peak human chorionic gonadotropin levels and nausea and vomiting symptoms and the fact that conditions associated with elevated levels, including female fetal sex, twins, and hydatidiform moles, have higher rates of hyperemesis tend to confer a causal relationship.[26-33] Fifteen prospective comparative studies have been published since 1990, and 11 have shown a significantly higher level of human chorionic gonadotropin in women with hyperemesis.[34] Estrogens also can cause nausea and vomiting. Women who experience nausea after oral contraceptive use have a higher incidence of nausea and vomiting during pregnancy.[20] In the past 29 years, there have been 17 studies of the relationship between nonthyroid hormones and nausea and vomiting, and only human chorionic gonadotropin and estrogen have shown a consistent association.[35]

Prostaglandin E_2 may contribute to this disorder, in that levels are elevated during symptomatic episodes.[36] *Helicobacter pylori* has been implicated as an etiologic agent for hyperemesis gravidarum,[37-39] although later studies have not confirmed this.[40]

Physiologic causes of nausea and vomiting of pregnancy historically have been underemphasized compared with the psychosocial factors, although these issues do have an association.[41] Some authorities have proposed that nausea and vomiting of pregnancy is an evolutionary adaptation, protecting the woman and fetus from potentially harmful foods, and is therefore a healthy adaptive response.[42]

Physiologic studies suggest that gastric dysrhythmias may have a role. Electrogastrographic recordings during pregnancy indicate that women with nausea and vomiting of pregnancy have alterations of the typical nonpregnant frequency of three cycles per minute and that these altered peristaltic contractions correlate temporally with the symptoms.[43] Altered gastric motility and gastroesophageal reflux appear to contribute to the mechanisms of nausea and vomiting in pregnancy, but the exact details are unknown.

Diagnosis of Nausea and Vomiting

Evaluation of the patient is based mainly on history. The nausea usually lasts all day. Pain is usually absent unless recurrent retching leads to painful abdominal and rib muscles. Similarly the physical exam is unremarkable unless the patient is severely dehydrated, a picture more consistent with hyperemesis gravidarum. Laboratory studies usually are not indicated or helpful. However, they are important in evaluating other potential causes that may mimic the condition, including hepatitis, pancreatitis, pyelonephritis, and uncontrolled diabetes.

TABLE 49-1 EFFECTIVENESS OF THERAPIES FOR NAUSEA AND VOMITING DURING PREGNANCY COMPARED WITH PLACEBO

Therapy	Number of Trials	Odds Ratio	95% Confidence Interval
Bendectin	3	0.23	0.007 to 0.70
Antihistamines	6	0.20	0.06 to 0.63
Phenothiazines	2	0.09	0.00 to 1.88
Vitamin B_6	2	0.64	0.18 to 2.26
Ginger	1	0.31	0.12 to 0.85
Acupuncture	2	0.35	0.12 to 1.06

Adapted from Jewell D, Young G: Interventions for nausea and vomiting in early pregnancy. Cochrane Database Syst Rev (4): CD000145, 2003.

Treatment of Nausea and Vomiting

Therapy can be instituted before the development of symptoms. Two studies have suggested that multivitamin therapy at the time of conception may reduce the incidence of nausea and vomiting.[44,45] Nonpharmacologic treatment may include ginger (500 to 1500 mg in divided doses daily).[46,47] Six randomized, controlled trials of vitamin B_6 have suggested superior or equivalent efficacy in improving symptoms over placebo, with no reports of adverse events. Acupressure or electrical stimulation on the P6 point of the wrist has shown conflicting results. The bulk of the literature suggests a benefit, but many of the studies have methodologic flaws or reveal no improvement over sham stimulation.[48-51]

Pharmacologic therapy may be effective for nausea and vomiting of pregnancy (Table 49-1). Vitamin B_6 in doses of 10 to 25 mg taken three times daily is likely the best initial treatment, and it has a low likelihood of side effects.[48,52,53] Doxylamine (10 mg) and vitamin B_6 were used until the early 1980s with apparent good effect. The compound Bendectin was removed from the market in 1983, and there was a subsequent increase in hospital admissions for nausea and vomiting.[54] For other pharmacologic treatments, including antihistamines and phenothiazines, there are no well-controlled trials.[1] Phenothiazines such as promethazine, prochlorperazine, chlorpromazine, and trimethobenzamide have shown some clinical efficacy, but their safety in pregnancy has not been proved.[1] Metoclopramide improves gastric emptying and corrects gastric dysrhythmias, and it has been safe and effective in small series.[55-57] Droperidol and ondansetron have been used for postoperative nausea and vomiting, but their use in pregnancy has been limited to case reports.[1]

Hyperemesis Gravidarum

Epidemiology

A more severe form of nausea and vomiting in pregnancy is hyperemesis gravidarum, which occurs in approximately 0.5% of live births.[34,58] It is responsible for increased hospitalization and disability, and it can result in weight loss, electrolyte imbalances, and nutritional deficiencies.[59,60] Maternal factors shown to increase the rate of hospitalization because of hyperemesis gravidarum include hyperthyroidism, psychiatric disorders, diabetes, gastrointestinal disorders, and asthma. Multiple gestations and singleton female fetuses were also associated with a higher risk.[61] Infants born to women with poor weight gain due to hyperemesis frequently have low birth weights.[60,62]

Severe rare complications of hyperemesis include Wernicke encephalopathy, a neurologic manifestation of thiamine deficiency, and pneumomediastinum and esophageal rupture.[34,63] This disorder leads to elective pregnancy termination in approximately 2% of affected pregnancies.[20] Hyperemesis gravidarum is more likely in multiple gestations, gestational trophoblastic disease, hydrops fetalis, and fetal karyotypic abnormalities, including triploidy and trisomy 21.[1] Although it typically begins in the first trimester, 10% of patients continue with symptoms throughout the pregnancy.[19]

Diagnosis

Symptoms of hyperemesis gravidarum include dry mouth, sialorrhea, hyperolfaction, and altered taste. Physical examination usually reveals dry mucous membranes, poor skin turgor, and hypotension.[1] Unlike standard nausea and vomiting of pregnancy, electrolyte abnormalities and ketonuria are identified in patients with hyperemesis gravidarum. Severely affected individuals may have elevated levels of hepatic transaminases and abnormalities in renal function.

Management

Intravenous fluid resuscitation is the initial treatment for hyperemesis gravidarum. Up to 2 L of Ringer's lactate should be infused over 3 to 5 hours, and continuing infusion subsequently is adjusted to maintain urine output above 100 mL/hr. Thiamine (100 mg) should be given intravenously before the infusion of dextrose to avoid Wernicke encephalopathy. Electrolyte levels, including magnesium and ionized calcium, should be monitored regularly.

Pharmacologic treatment includes the various antiemetics previously discussed. Pulsed steroids have been used in refractory cases. Methylprednisolone and hydrocortisone have been used in refractory cases with conflicting results. A randomized trial of oral methylprednisolone (initial doses of 16 mg three times daily followed by a 2-week taper) resulted in a reduction in readmission to the hospital when compared with oral promethazine.[64] Intravenous hydrocortisone 300 mg daily for 3 days followed by a taper over a week reduced vomiting episodes and subsequent readmission when compared with a regimen of metoclopramide.[65] Another study compared the use of intravenous methylprednisolone followed by an oral prednisone taper plus promethazine and metoclopramide with the use of only the latter drugs and found no difference in the rates of rehospitalization (35%).[66] Another randomized trial using oral prednisolone that was converted to intravenous hydrocortisone for no response was inconclusive, with a trend toward reduced vomiting, but patients had an improved sense of well-being and weight gain.[67]

The mechanism by which steroids affect nausea is not clear. The nuclei of the solitary tract, area postrema, and raphe have glucocorticoid receptors and are known to participate in the regulation of nausea and vomiting responses.[68] Corticosteroid exposure in the first trimester may be weakly associated with an increased rate of facial clefting, potentially accounting for one or two cases per 1000 treated women.[69-71] Steroids therefore should be used with caution and should be avoided if possible during the period of fetal organogenesis.[48]

Total parenteral nutrition has been used for hyperemesis gravidarum with reportedly improved outcomes.[72] Significant complications of lipid emulsions have been reported, primarily with the use of cottonseed oil, and they have included placental infarction, ketonemia, and increased uterine activity. Subsequent case reports using soybean- or soybean and safflower oil–based emulsions have not shown the same adverse events.[73] However, there is an increased risk of complications directly related to therapy, including infusion catheter sepsis (25%) and venous thrombosis (3%).[74,75] Centrally placed venous catheters have higher morbidity rates (50%) compared with peripherally inserted lines (9%).[76] One series of 52 patients receiving peripherally inserted central catheters had a complication rate of 50%.[77] The use of total parenteral nutrition should be considered as a last resort.

Adverse outcomes for women with hyperemesis and low maternal weight gain compared with those for patients without hyperemesis include higher rates of small-for-gestational-age fetuses, low birth weight, prematurity, and 5-minute Apgar scores less than 7.[60] Among women who experienced hyperemesis gravidarum in their first gestation, 15% to 19% will be affected in the second pregnancy, compared with 0.7% who had unaffected first pregnancies.[60,78]

Gastroesophageal Reflux Disease

Epidemiology

Heartburn is the most common gastrointestinal complaint in Western populations, with up to 20% of the population having heartburn symptoms on a weekly basis. During pregnancy, up to 80% of women experience heartburn at some point, and 25% have daily heartburn.[79,80] The prevalence and severity of heartburn progressively increase during pregnancy and resolve after delivery.[81,82] One large study found the prevalence of heartburn symptoms to be 22% for patients in the first trimester, 39% for those in the second trimester, and 72% for patients in the third trimester.[82] Factors associated with increased risk of heartburn symptoms were increasing gestational age, pre-pregnancy heartburn, and parity.[82]

Pathogenesis

The exact cause of gastroesophageal reflux disease (GERD) during pregnancy in unknown. The resting lower esophageal sphincter (LES) pressure is decreased during pregnancy, and progesterone seems to mediate LES relaxation in the setting of elevated estrogen levels.[83] Other possible mechanisms for gastroesophageal reflux during pregnancy include increased intra-abdominal pressure causing gastric fluid reflux, ineffective esophageal motility to clear esophageal acid reflux, and decreased gastric emptying, which can result in reflux of gastric contents.

Diagnosis

The symptoms of gastroesophageal reflux in pregnancy are the same as in the general adult population. They can include substernal burning, epigastric discomfort, dyspepsia, mild dysphagia, and regurgitation. Patients may have extraesophageal manifestations, such as hoarseness, chronic cough, chronic laryngitis, and asthma. Complications of GERD, such as gastrointestinal bleeding and esophageal strictures, are rare during pregnancy.

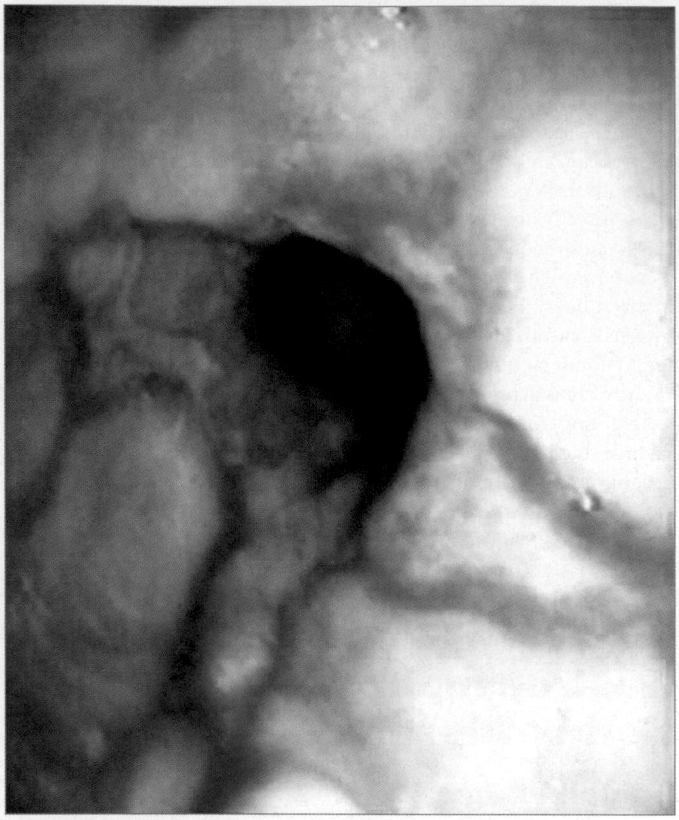

FIGURE 49-1 Endoscopic image of severe erosive esophagitis.

TABLE 49-2	FETAL SAFETY OF MEDICATIONS USED TO TREAT GASTROESOPHAGEAL REFLUX DISEASE OR PEPTIC ULCER DISEASE	
Drug	**FDA Pregnancy Category***	**Comments**
Antacids	Unrated	Generally safe
Simethicone	C	
Sucralfate	B	
Histamine$_2$ (H_2) receptor antagonists		
Cimetidine	B	
Ranitidine	B	
Famotidine	B	
Nizatidine	B	
Proton pump inhibitors		
Omeprazole	C	
Lansoprazole	B	
Rabeprazole	B	
Pantoprazole	B	
Esomeprazole	B	
Misoprostol	X	Abortifacient
Helicobacter pylori treatments		
Amoxicillin	B	
Clarithromycin	C	
Bismuth subsalicylate	C	
Tetracycline	D	
Metronidazole	B	

***U.S. Food and Drug Administration (FDA) classification of teratogenic drug risk:**

A: Well-controlled studies in pregnant women have failed to demonstrate an increased risk of fetal abnormalities.

B: Animal studies show no fetal risk, and no human data are available, *or* animal studies show a risk, but well-controlled studies in pregnant women have failed to show a risk to the fetus.

C: Risk cannot be ruled out because animal studies have shown an adverse effect, and there are no adequate, well-controlled studies in pregnant women, *or* no animal studies have been conducted, and there are no adequate, well-controlled studies in pregnant women.

D: Well-controlled or observational studies in pregnant women have demonstrated a risk to the fetus, but the benefits of therapy may outweigh potential risk.

X: Well-controlled or observational studies in animals or pregnant women have demonstrated positive evidence of fetal abnormalities, and the product is contraindicated in women who are or may become pregnant.

The diagnosis usually is made by clinical symptoms only. There is rarely reason to do invasive diagnostic tests such as barium radiographs, esophageal pH studies, or esophageal manometry studies. Upper gastrointestinal endoscopy is rarely needed, except in exceptional cases of symptoms refractory to medical management. The endoscopic appearance of GERD ranges from no mucosal breaks to severe ulceration of the distal esophagus (Fig. 49-1).

Management

For mild to moderate symptoms, lifestyle and dietary changes may help. Patients should avoid eating late at night or within a few hours of bedtime, elevate the head of the bed 6 inches, sleep on the left shoulder, and avoid things that can make GERD worse, including alcohol, cigarette smoking, caffeine, chocolate, and peppermint.

Medication is commonly used as first-line therapy for GERD in the general adult population, but in pregnancy, therapeutics are complicated by the small potential risk of teratogenicity from GERD medications. Most medications for GERD are not routinely or rigorously tested in pregnant women, and recommendations therefore come from small case series. The risks and benefits of medications for GERD, as well as the limited knowledge of the effects of these medications during pregnancy, must be discussed with the patient by the provider. Because the risk of teratogenicity is greatest in the first 10 weeks, efforts should be made to avoid all unnecessary medications during that period. Table 49-2 shows the U.S. Food and Drug Administration (FDA) classification of drug therapy for GERD and peptic ulcer disease during pregnancy. Most drugs are FDA class B.

Antacids are considered safe to use during pregnancy and can be expected to relieve symptoms in 30% to 50% of pregnant women.[84] Sucralfate is a mucosal protectant that can help relieve GERD symptoms in pregnancy. Promotility drugs such as metoclopramide can also be used to help gastric emptying and increase LES pressure, although these drugs are infrequently used because of poor tolerance to their side effects.

Histamine type 2 (H_2) receptor antagonists are apparently safe and effective in pregnancy.[85,86] Proton pump inhibitors are more effective than H_2-blockers for healing esophagitis and treating GERD, but they are less well studied in pregnancy than H_2-blockers. Omeprazole is categorized as a class C drug by the FDA because of embryotoxicity and fetotoxicity in animals and because of a few case reports

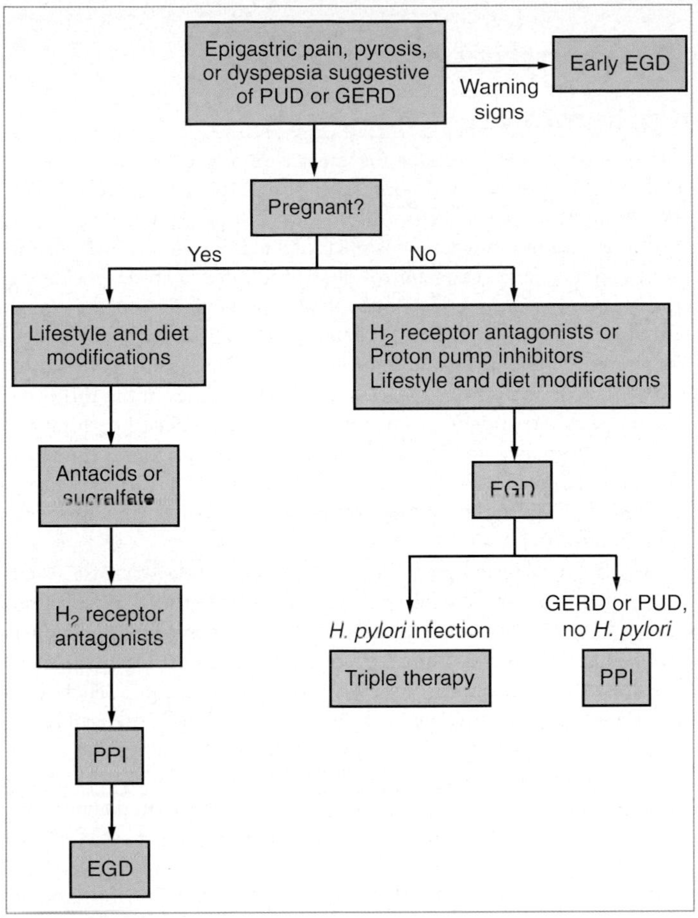

FIGURE 49-2 Stepwise management of gastroesophageal reflux disease (GERD) or peptic ulcer disease (PUD). EGD, esophagogastroduodenoscopy; PPI, proton pump inhibitor. (Modified from Cappell MS: Gastric and duodenal ulcers during pregnancy. Gastroenterol Clin North Am 32:263-308, 2003.)

of fetal birth defects in humans.[83] However, a meta-analysis of the risk of fetal malformations during the first trimester found no increase with the use of proton pump inhibitors in general and with omeprazole specifically by pregnant women.[87] A large study from Europe comparing several proton pump inhibitors, including omeprazole, also found no increase in major fetal anomalies compared with patients not exposed to proton pump inhibitors.[88]

A recommended algorithm for treating GERD in pregnancy is shown in Figure 49-2. Patients should initially be reassured and treated with lifestyle modifications. If these are unsatisfactory, use of antacids or sucralfate should be considered. Persistent symptoms, especially after the first trimester, can be treated with H_2-blockers. If symptoms persist despite H_2-blockers, consideration can be given to using proton pump inhibitors or undergoing upper endoscopy to assess the cause of GERD.

Peptic Ulcer Disease

Epidemiology

Because the incidence of peptic ulcer disease (PUD) during pregnancy is estimated from case reports and retrospective studies, it may be unreliable.[89] Epidemiologic studies suggest a decreased incidence of PUD during pregnancy, and there appears to be an improvement in patients with PUD during pregnancy. Clark[90] found that in 313 pregnancies occurring after a diagnosis of PUD, 45% had no symptoms, 44% improved, and 12% experienced no improvement. Hypotheses for this improvement include physiologic changes, including increased plasma histaminase or estrogen levels leading to reduced gastric acid; increased gastric mucosal protection induced by progesterone; immunologic tolerance allowing *H. pylori* colonization without injury; and elevated epidermal growth factor levels stimulating mucosal growth. Maternal alterations such as avoidance of alcohol, smoking, and nonsteroidal anti-inflammatory drugs; increased rest; and improved nutrition have also been postulated.[89]

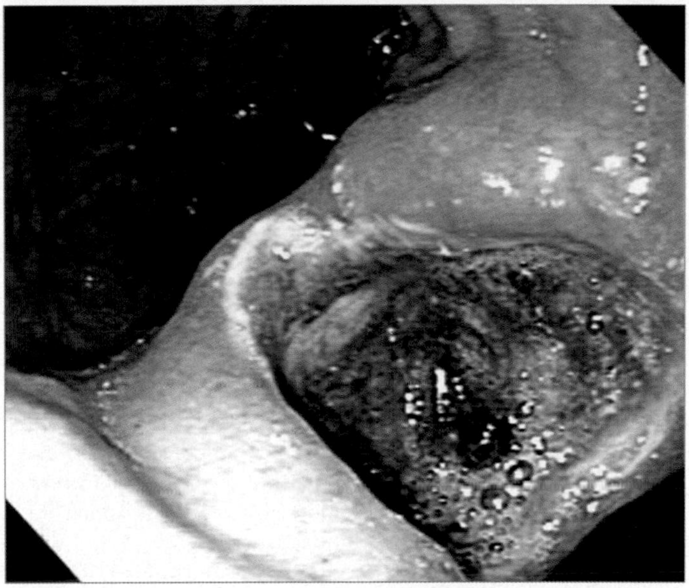

FIGURE 49-3 Endoscopic image of a deep gastric ulcer.

Diagnosis

Symptoms of PUD are similar to those in the nonpregnant population and include epigastric pain, anorexia, postprandial nausea, and vomiting. Duodenal ulcer pain can occur several hours after a meal or at nighttime, and pain usually improves with eating.[91] Gastric ulcers may not follow the classic pattern of symptoms (Fig. 49-3), and older patients who use antiulcer medication and NSAIDs may be asymptomatic.[92] Gastrointestinal reflux disease, which is more common in pregnancy, differs in that there may be a sense of substernal chest burning and fluid reflux, and it can often be worse after meals. Results of the physical examination are nonspecific, and they essentially are helpful in ruling out complicated ulcer disease or other causes of abdominal pain, including pancreatitis, cholecystitis, and appendicitis.

In the nonpregnant population, esophagogastroduodenoscopy (EGD) is preferable mainly because of its ability to accurately diagnose ulcers and to obtain histologic specimens that are tested for *H. pylori* infection.[89] EGD is relatively safe in pregnancy.[93] In the largest study, there were no maternal complications in 83 procedures, and EGD did not induce preterm delivery. Despite its presumed safety, most cases of PUD can be managed without imaging. EGD should be reserved for cases refractory to medical management.

Management

Management begins with empiric treatment (see Fig. 49-2). Because PUD and GERD therapies are similar, a stepwise scheme should be followed before considering EGD. Dietary and lifestyle alterations include avoidance of fat-laden foods, acidic drinks, caffeine, chocolate, NSAIDs, and alcohol. Smoking, stress, anxiety, and nighttime snacks should be avoided.[89]

Antacids should be used as first-line medical therapy because they have been effective in approximately 75% of duodenal ulcers.[94,95] Dosages range from 15 to 30 mL taken 1 hour after meals and at bedtime. Extra doses may be taken 3 hours after meals.[89] Aluminum- and magnesium-containing antacids have little systemic absorption and appear to be safe in pregnancy. Sucralfate, an aluminum-based polysaccharide complex, attaches to the surface of an ulcer, protecting the mucosa from further injury, and it may suppress *H. pylori* infection.[96,97] Seventy-five percent of duodenal ulcers heal with 4 weeks of sucralfate therapy.[97] Because of its minimal systemic absorption, it is a preferred drug for treating PUD in pregnancy.[98]

H_2-receptor antagonists are an effective treatment for PUD; about 80% of duodenal ulcers heal with this therapy in the general population.[99] Before the discovery of *H. pylori* and the introduction of proton pump inhibitors, H_2-blockers were the mainstay of treatment. Their safety profile in pregnancy has not been adequately demonstrated. H_2-receptor antagonists cross the placenta, but their use is justifiable if significant clinical conditions warrant.[100] Cimetidine and ranitidine have had considerable use over the past 20 years. In animal studies, cimetidine has caused a reduction in the size of fetal testes, prostate, and seminal vesicles, presumably by means of a weak antiandrogenic effect.[101] Ranitidine has no such effects in animals, and neither drug has had reports of genital malformations in humans.[84,102] More than 2000 pregnancies in database studies with exposure to cimetidine or ranitidine have been assessed, and there has not been an associated risk of congenital malformations.[84] There is less information reported for famotidine and nizatidine. Because of nizatidine's conflicting animal data, it is preferable to use more extensively studied H_2-receptor antagonists as first-line agents.[84]

Proton pump inhibitors suppress gastric acid secretion at the level of the H^+,K^+-ATPase on the parietal cell surface.[89] These agents are highly effective in the treatment of esophagitis and gastroduodenal ulcers, and they are often used in combination therapy for eradication of *H. pylori* infection. Omeprazole, the first agent in the class, produced dose-related embryonic and fetal death in animal studies. Because of these concerns and cases reported to the FDA, it has remained an FDA category C drug.[84] However, a meta-analysis comprising 593 infants suggested a nonsignificant risk for congenital malformations.[87] A multicenter, prospective, controlled study involving proton pump inhibitors in 295 pregnancies also suggested no increased teratogenic risk.[88] Although the other proton pump inhibitors are category B drugs, omeprazole is the only one available over the counter, and it is less expensive than the others.[84]

In the nonpregnant population, proton pump inhibitors are usually the initial treatment for suspected or documented reflux esophagitis and PUD. H_2-receptor antagonists, sucralfate, and antacids are used as secondary medications and for symptomatic relief.[89] During pregnancy, therapy should be modified to avoid fetal harm and because PUD usually improves during gestation. EGD is usually avoided unless the patient is failing empiric therapy with H_2-receptor antagonists. There appears to be little benefit in diagnosing *H. pylori* infection during pregnancy, because treatment involves triple drug therapy, including antibiotics, and it is usually deferred until after delivery.[89]

Appendicitis

Epidemiology

Acute appendicitis is one of the most common causes of an acute abdomen in pregnancy. It occurs in 1 in 1500 pregnancies[103] and has an approximate incidence of 0.15 to 2.10 per 1000 gestations.[104] Previous studies suggested similar incidences for nonpregnant adults, but a large case-control study indicated a lower incidence than among nonpregnant individuals, particularly in the third trimester.[105] Overall incidence rates in the first trimester range between 19% and 36%, and rates increase in the second trimester to between 27% and 60%.[105-107] The incidence decreases in the third trimester, with rates ranging from 15% to 30%. Appendiceal perforation rates in pregnancy are higher when compared with those for nonpregnant populations (55% versus 4% to 19%).[107-109] This is likely explained by confounding variables leading to the delay of diagnosis and therapy.

Fetal and maternal morbidity and mortality rates increase when appendicitis occurs during pregnancy, particularly if perforation occurs.[110,111] The fetal loss rate associated with appendectomy is higher (2.6%) than for other surgical procedures (1.2%) during pregnancy, and the rate approximates 10% if peritonitis is present.[112] There is a high rate of appendicitis-induced delivery (4.6%), and if preterm labor occurs, it is usually within 5 days of the surgery.[110,112] The advancing pregnancy appears to impair the ability of making an accurate diagnosis. Cunningham and McCubbin[111] identified delays in diagnosis of 18% and 75% in the second and third trimester, respectively, which corresponded to the higher rates of complications, including perforation and peritonitis, found in other series.[107] Hee and Viktrup[106] found the ratio of perforated appendicitis to nonperforated appendicitis to be 1.0, 2.1, and 1.6 in the first, second, and third trimesters, respectively, and they found the overall rate of appendicitis confirmed by pathologic analysis to be 50%.

Diagnosis

Right lower quadrant pain appears to be the most common symptom of appendicitis, regardless of gestational age, and it occurs in about 80% of patients.[103,106,110] Right upper quadrant pain varies, and it occurs in about 10% to 55% of patients.[103,107] Nausea and vomiting may be absent in approximately 20% of patients, and anorexia is not a reliable marker. Objective findings are similarly confusing. Fever, tachycardia, a dry tongue, and localized abdominal tenderness are common in nonpregnant individuals, but they are less reliable findings during pregnancy.[113] The Rovsing and psoas signs have not been shown to have clinical significance.[110]

Laboratory evaluation of patients with appendicitis is important, primarily for its ability to exclude alternative diagnoses (Table 49-3). Urinalysis and chest radiography should be strongly considered because urinary tract infection and right lower lobe pneumonia may manifest with lower abdominal pain. However, pyuria may occur in 40% of pregnant patients with appendicitis.[114] White blood cell (WBC) counts are not predictive, mainly because of the physiologic leukocytosis of pregnancy. Mean WBC counts in acute appendicitis are in the range of 16,000 cells/mm^3.[103]

Imaging modalities help to make the diagnosis of acute appendicitis (Table 49-4). Abdominal plain film radiography should be avoided, unless there is concern about bowel obstruction or visceral perforation. Ultrasound with a graded compression technique is usually available in most hospitals, and it avoids ionizing radiation. However, ultrasound detection of appendicitis is operator dependent. Studies assessing the accuracy of ultrasound for the diagnosis of appendicitis have been of insufficient quality or fraught by small numbers or selection bias.[115] The utility of the graded compression technique diminishes as the uterus enlarges, or the appendix is often not visualized.

Helical computed tomography (CT) in the nonpregnant population is highly sensitive and specific (approximately 98% each) for appendicitis.[116] CT scans are considered abnormal if there is an enlarged appendix (>6-mm maximal diameter) or if there are periappendiceal inflammatory changes, such as fat stranding, phlegmon, fluid collection, and extraluminal gas.[117] Radiation exposure is 300 mrad with a limited helical CT scan, which is one third of the amount of the average abdominopelvic CT scan.[118] Unfortunately, published experience with this technique in pregnancy is limited. Magnetic resonance imaging (MRI) during pregnancy has no known adverse fetal effects, and its use has been advocated in patients for whom the diagnosis has not been confirmed by other techniques.[119,120] Two reports have suggested that MRI is an excellent modality for use in the diagnosis of appendicitis in pregnancy.[121,122] A normal appendix was suggested by a diameter of less than or equal to 6 mm or if it was filled with air or oral contrast. Conversely, a fluid-filled appendix greater than 7 mm in diameter was considered abnormal.[122] However, these studies were small and retrospective.

TABLE 49-3 DIFFERENTIAL DIAGNOSIS OF ACUTE APPENDICITIS

Evaluation	Alternative Diagnosis
Surgical	Acute cholecystitis
	Pancreatitis
	Mesenteric adenitis
	Diverticulitis
	Intestinal obstruction
	Meckel's diverticulum
Medical	Gastroenteritis
	Pneumonia
	Inflammatory bowel disease
	Lupus serositis
	Diabetic ketoacidosis
	Porphyria
Gynecologic	Ruptured adnexal cyst
	Torsion
	Uterine myoma degeneration
Urologic	Ureteral colic
	Pyelonephritis
	Urinary tract infection

Treatment

Prompt surgical intervention remains the standard treatment. Appendectomy may be delayed during active labor, but it should be performed immediately after delivery or if labor is abnormally prolonged or perforation is suspected.[123] If an open procedure is chosen, a muscle-splitting incision is made over the point of maximal tenderness. If diffuse peritonitis is present, a midline incision is usually performed. A periappendiceal abscess can be treated with percutaneous drainage followed by an interval appendectomy 2 to 3 months later.[123] Perioperative antibiotics should be administered, usually a second-generation cephalosporin, expanded-spectrum penicillin, or even triple-agent therapy.

Laparoscopic appendectomy was first performed in 1980, and it spawned controversy about its use in pregnancy that continues to the present.[124] Its use in pregnancy has been documented with a good safety record,[125] and it has a complication rate similar to that for nonpregnant laparoscopy.[126] It may have advantages over open appendectomy of less abdominal wall trauma, less pain and narcotic use, and faster return to normal activity.[124,127] However, the presence of the enlarged uterus does increase the risk of inadvertent puncture with a trocar or Veress needle.[128] In the second half of pregnancy, pen laparoscopy may be preferred to avoid such complications. Unlike non pregnant laparoscopy, no instrument should be applied to the cervix. The primary trocar is inserted after determining the height of the uterus, and the secondary trocars are inserted under direct visualization. Consideration of supraumbilical, subxiphoid insertions may be necessary. Limiting intra-abdominal pressure to less than 12 mm Hg and reducing operative time can reduce concerns about maternal hypercarbia and subsequent fetal acidosis.[127,129]

Inflammatory Bowel Disease

Inflammatory bowel disease (IBD) refers to ulcerative colitis and Crohn disease. Their similarities and differences are outlined in Table 49-5. These entities are similar in that both are inflammatory conditions of the luminal gastrointestinal tract. They differ in terms of the layer of involvement of the intestinal wall, the anatomic location of involvement within the gastrointestinal tract, and the response to surgical resection. Both are treated with similar medications. The cause of ulcerative colitis and Crohn disease is unknown. There seems to be a genetic component in some patients, but there is also the possibility of an environmental trigger such as an infection. The final common

TABLE 49-4 IMAGING FOR ACUTE APPENDICITIS

Modality	Diagnostic Criteria	Evidence
Plain radiography	None	No role in the diagnosis of acute appendicitis
Ultrasound[115]	Aperistaltic and noncompressible structure with a diameter >6 mm	Sensitivity of 67-100%, specificity of 83-96%
Computed tomography[118]	Abnormal appendix identified or calcified appendicolith seen in association with periappendiceal inflammation or a diameter >6 mm	Sensitivity of 94%, specificity of 95%
Magnetic resonance imaging[122]	Appendix diameter >7 mm or 6-7 mm with periappendiceal inflammation	Sensitivity 100%, specificity 94%

TABLE 49-5 COMPARISON OF ULCERATIVE COLITIS AND CROHN DISEASE

Feature	Ulcerative Colitis	Crohn Disease
Extent of inflammation	Limited to mucosa	Involves all layers (transmural)
Intestine involved	Colon only	Throughout the gastrointestinal tract, especially the terminal ileum
Rectal involvement	Always	Sometimes
Pattern of spread	Contiguous	Skip lesions
Granulomas	No	Yes (sometimes)
Fistula	No	Yes
Strictures	No	Yes
Abscess	No	Yes
Perianal disease	No	Yes
Bloody diarrhea	Yes	Maybe
Ileal disease on computed tomography	No	Yes
Increased colon cancer risk	Yes	Maybe (if colonic involvement)
Cure with surgery	Yes	No
Percent of patients who will require surgery	20%	70%

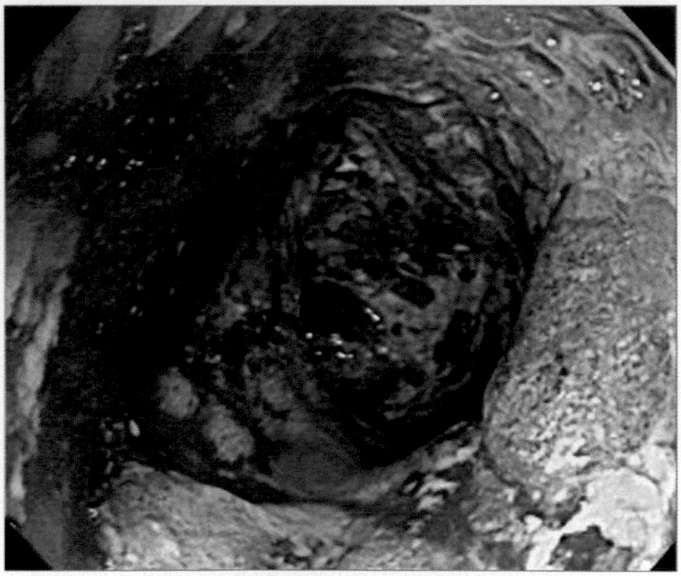

FIGURE 49-4 Endoscopic image of severe ulcerative colitis.

pathology is an increased inflammatory response against the tissues of the gastrointestinal tract.

Ulcerative colitis is characterized by inflammation limited to the mucosal surface of the colon (Fig. 49-4). It always starts at the dentate line of the rectum and extends proximally but only involves the colon. Patients usually present with bloody diarrhea. Patients usually are managed with medical therapy consisting of 5-aminosalicylates, prednisone, 6-mercaptopurine or azathioprine, and occasionally infliximab. Surgery, which is occasionally performed for refractory disease, results in complete cure of the ulcerative colitis.

Crohn disease is characterized by inflammation that can be transmural, involving all wall layers. It often involves the terminal ileum, but it can involve any part of the luminal gastrointestinal tract. Transmural inflammation may result in intestinal strictures or intestinal fistulas or abscesses. Patients are usually managed medically with 5-aminosalicylates, prednisone, 6-mercaptopurine or azathioprine, and infliximab. They also can benefit from antibiotics such as metronidazole and ciprofloxacin.

Effect of Inflammatory Bowel Disease on Pregnancy

If a woman has quiescent IBD, the pregnancy can be expected to proceed without increased complications.[130,131] Patients with ulcerative colitis and Crohn disease usually have healthy deliveries at the same rate as the general population, although some studies have suggested a greater incidence of preterm births and low-birth-weight infants.[132-138] However, it is unclear from these studies whether the degree of disease activity correlated with the differences in outcomes.

Effect of Pregnancy on Inflammatory Bowel Disease

Active ulcerative colitis or Crohn disease at the time of conception tends to remain active, and inactive disease tends to remain inactive.[136,139,140] Pregnant patients with active ulcerative colitis or Crohn disease have the same risks for complications from IBD as nonpregnant women.

Diagnostic Testing for Inflammatory Bowel Disease during Pregnancy

Patients with known IBD can be managed based on their history, physical examination findings, and blood test results. It is important to determine whether a patient with IBD who is having a flare of diarrhea during pregnancy has an intestinal infection, especially with *Clostridium difficile*, before starting any new immunosuppressive therapy (Fig. 49-5). In selected pregnant IBD patients, stool studies for infectious causes are needed. Flexible sigmoidoscopy appears to be safe during pregnancy, and it is usually the only endoscopic procedure needed in selected IBD patients. Abdominal CT or MRI may be used in carefully selected cases if the benefits outweigh potential risks.

Safety of Inflammatory Bowel Disease Medications during Pregnancy

Pregnant patients with IBD should stay on the medications that are maintaining them in remission. Stopping the medications can induce a relapse or flare of disease. Table 49-6 shows the safety of various IBD medications during pregnancy.

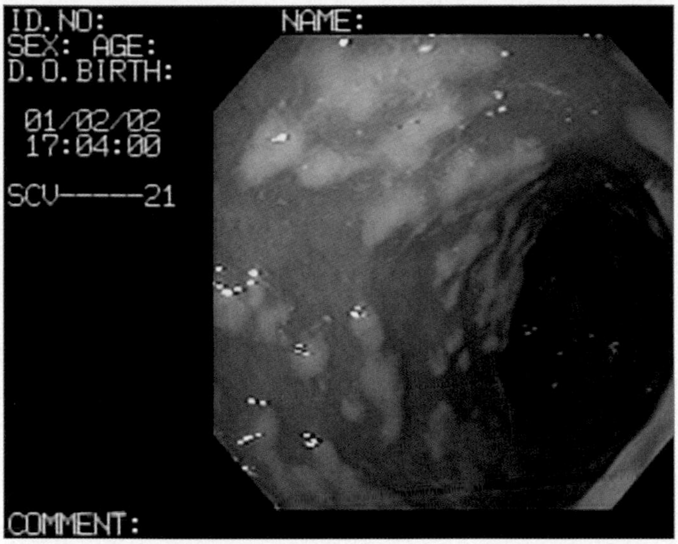

FIGURE 49-5 *Clostridium difficile* colitis.

TABLE 49-6 SAFETY OF INFLAMMATORY BOWEL DISEASE MEDICATIONS DURING PREGNANCY

Safe to Use	Probably Safe but Limited Data	Contraindicated
Sulfasalazine	Azathioprine	Methotrexate
5-Aminosalicylates	6-Mercaptopurine	Diphenoxylate
Corticosteroids	Cyclosporine	
	Metronidazole	
	Ciprofloxacin	
	Infliximab	
	Loperamide	

Antidiarrheal Medications

Loperamide (Imodium) appears to be safe during pregnancy because it has not been associated with increased rates of fetal malformations, spontaneous abortions, low birth weight, or prematurity.[141] In contrast, there have been reports of fetal malformations in patients exposed to diphenoxylate with atropine (Lomotil) during the first trimester, and it should be avoided.[142] It is probably best to avoid antidiarrheal drugs, if possible, during pregnancy and instead rely on supplemental fiber or psyllium seed.

Antibiotics

Metronidazole and ciprofloxacin are occasionally used in the management of patients with Crohn disease. Several studies have shown that short-term use of metronidazole is safe during pregnancy.[143,144] Some animal studies suggested that musculoskeletal abnormalities resulted from ciprofloxacin, but small clinical series have not reported any fetal malformations or arthropathies.[145,146]

Sulfasalazine and 5-Aminosalicylate Drugs

Sulfasalazine and 5-aminosalicylate drugs are often used for long-term maintenance of mild or moderately active IBD. These drugs appear to be safe to use in pregnancy.[88,147-150]

Corticosteroids

Oral corticosteroids such as prednisone are commonly used to manage active ulcerative colitis and Crohn disease. They are typically used for short periods to induce remission but are not used for maintenance of remission. The use of prednisone for IBD appears to be relatively safe in pregnancy, although an increased incidence of low-birth-weight neonates has been reported.[149,151]

Immunomodulators

Azathioprine and 6-mercaptopurine are increasingly used to maintain remission in patients with ulcerative colitis or Crohn disease. Azathioprine and 6-mercaptopurine cross the placenta. The largest experience with azathioprine in pregnancy comes from the renal transplant literature, which suggests it is safe to use.[152] There is less information on 6-mercaptopurine in pregnancy, but it also appears safe to use in pregnant IBD patients to keep them in remission.[153,154]

Methotrexate is occasionally used in challenging cases of IBD. Methotrexate is associated with fetal malformations and fetal demise, and it should not be used during pregnancy and ideally for at least 3 months before conception.

Biologic Agents

Infliximab (Remicade) is increasingly being used for induction and maintenance of remission of Crohn disease and occasionally for ulcerative colitis. Infliximab inhibits tumor necrosis factor. There are only small case series of infliximab being continued intentionally during pregnancy for Crohn disease, but the limited data show no obvious adverse effects.[155] Because patients who are taking maintenance infliximab usually have been refractory to other treatments, it is likely that their Crohn disease will flare during pregnancy if infliximab is stopped. The unknown risks and benefits must be discussed with the patient.

Surgery for Inflammatory Bowel Disease during Pregnancy

Surgery for IBD during pregnancy is done for emergencies such as intestinal obstruction, perforation, abscess, or fulminant colitis. In these cases, the surgery is required for the mother's health.

Irritable Bowel Syndrome

Irritable bowel syndrome (IBS) is characterized by chronic abdominal pain and altered bowel habits without obvious organic cause. It is the most commonly diagnosed gastrointestinal pathology. The estimated prevalence of IBS in the United States is between 10% and 15%.[156] IBS tends to affect younger women more than other demographic groups, which means many pregnant women also have IBS. IBS accounts for 25% to 50% of clinic referrals to gastroenterologists and approximately 10% of referrals to primary care physicians.[156]

It is unclear whether pregnancy worsens IBS symptoms, because many pregnant women develop constipation or loose stools during pregnancy. Because IBS usually poses no threat to maternal or fetal health, it can be treated symptomatically during pregnancy.

Symptoms

IBS is a heterogeneous collection of symptoms. The most common include chronic abdominal pain and altered bowel habits. Upper abdominal symptoms can also occur. The abdominal pain is often described as crampy, lower abdominal discomfort (often in left side), which can become worse with stress and better after bowel movements. Patients with IBS often complain of altered bowel movements, with constipation, diarrhea, or alternating constipation and diarrhea. When describing constipation, they often have stools resembling rabbit pellets. They often describe needing to have bowel movements several consecutive times in the morning to completely empty the rectum. They may have mucus in their stools. The diarrhea never wakes them from sleep. Upper gastrointestinal symptoms such as GERD, dyspepsia, and nausea are common, as are symptoms of gas and bloating. Extraintestinal symptoms include dyspareunia, increased urinary frequency and urgency, and fibromyalgia.[157]

Symptoms that do not suggest IBS include blood in the bowel movements, weight loss, and being awakened from sleep for abdominal pain or bowel movements. These symptoms should prompt additional evaluation.

Diagnostic Criteria

The most common diagnostic criteria for standardizing the diagnosis of IBS are the Manning criteria and the Rome III criteria (Table 49-7). The Manning criteria include abdominal pain relieved with bowel movements, looser and more frequent stools with onset of pain, passage of mucus, and sense of incomplete evacuation.[158] The Rome III diagnostic criteria for IBS are recurrent abdominal discomfort with two or more of the following: improvement with defecation, onset associated with a change in stool frequency, and onset associated with a change in stool appearance or form.[159] The Rome III criteria also describes four subtypes of IBS: IBS with constipation, IBS with diarrhea, mixed diarrhea and constipation IBS, and unsubtyped IBS.

Pathophysiology

The pathogenesis of IBS is unknown but likely multifactorial. The most common possibilities include altered motility of the gastrointestinal tract and visceral hypersensitivity. There may also be a central nervous system component because IBS patients have an increased frequency of psychiatric abnormalities such as depression, somatization disorders, and generalized anxiety disorders. There also is a subgroup of patients with postinfectious IBS.

Diagnosis

IBS should be suspected with the appropriate clinical symptoms and lack of alarming symptoms (i.e., blood in stool, weight loss, waking from sleep because of pain or bowel movements). The diagnostic evaluation is often geared to symptoms and may include blood work and endoscopic evaluations. IBS often is a diagnosis of exclusion in the correct clinical setting.

Management

There is no specific treatment for IBS because it tends to be a chronic condition. Reassurance of the patient by an understanding physician is important. Dietary changes may identify foods that worsen symptoms (e.g., dairy products, fatty foods). Supplemental fiber can help a subset of patients, although the mechanism is uncertain. Medications are needed only by a minority of IBS patients. These drugs can include antispasmodic medicines such as hyoscyamine. Low-dose antidepressants can be used to modify chronic abdominal pain. Probiotics have been reported to help symptoms. Diarrhea can be controlled with antidiarrheal medications, and constipation can be controlled by laxatives or lubiprostone. Antibiotics may help the gas and bloating symptoms of IBS in selected patients.[160]

Celiac Disease

Epidemiology and Etiology

Celiac disease is also known as celiac sprue or gluten-sensitive enteropathy.[161] Gliadin and related proteins activate the immune system, resulting in the inflammation of the small intestinal mucosa and malabsorption.[161] Celiac sprue is caused by an abnormal T-cell response against gluten in genetically predisposed people.[162]

Celiac disease is often underdiagnosed. The prevalence of this disorder ranges between 1 in 80 to 1 in 300 individuals.[163,164] The highest reported prevalence is in Western Europe and places to which Europeans immigrate.[164-166] Genetic predisposition for celiac disease is confirmed by a high rate of concordance in monozygotic twins.[167] The diagnosis may be associated with other conditions such as diabetes, lymphocytic colitis, irritable bowel syndrome, diarrhea, and unexplained anemia. Survival of these patients has improved with appropriate therapy.[168]

Diagnosis

Although celiac disease often begins in childhood, clinical symptoms of the disease may begin at any age.[169] One fourth of individuals are diagnosed after the age of 15 years.[170]

Celiac sprue may manifest in pregnancy or after delivery, and the diagnosis should be entertained when encountering severe anemia in a gravid patient.[161,171] Adults usually present with episodic diarrhea,

TABLE 49-7 DIAGNOSTIC CRITERIA FOR IRRITABLE BOWEL SYNDROME

Manning Criteria	Rome III Criteria
Pain relieved with defecation More frequent stools at the onset of pain Looser stools at the onset of pain Visible abdominal distention Mucus in stool Sense of incomplete evacuation	Recurrent abdominal discomfort at least 3 days per month in the last 3 months associated with two or more of the following: 1. Improvement with defecation 2. Onset associated with change in stool frequency 3. Onset associated with change in form of stool Supporting features: abnormal stool frequency (<3 bowel movements per week or >3 bowel movements per day), abnormal stool form, defecation straining, urgency, sense of incomplete bowel movement, mucus passage, bloating

flatulence, and weight loss. They also may have lactose intolerance and steatorrhea. Patients have abdominal discomfort, bloating, malaise, and recurrent aphthous stomatitis ulcers.[161]

Laboratory abnormalities include iron deficiency, macrocytic anemia, and vitamin D and K deficiencies. The most widely available screening test for celiac disease is the antiendomysial IgA test. The test has excellent specificity (approaching 100%), but its sensitivity as a stand-alone screen is less because of an increased prevalence of selective IgA deficiency in patients with celiac disease.[168] IgA and IgG antigliadin antibodies have moderate sensitivity but are less specific than antiendomysial antibodies; normal individuals and those with gastrointestinal inflammation from other causes test positive.[172] IgA antigliadin antibody levels are useful for monitoring dietary compliance, because they become detectable within 6 months of maintaining a gluten-free diet.[161] A rapid bedside screening test has been developed that detects IgA and IgG tissue trans-glutaminase. The sensitivity is higher than that for IgA endomysial antibodies.[173] The gold standard of diagnosis remains biopsy of the small intestine during upper gastrointestinal biopsy from the distal duodenum.[161]

Management

Management consists of eliminating gluten from the diet. Seventy percent of patients improve symptomatically within 2 weeks.[174] This includes avoidance of wheat, rye, and barley gluten. During the initial phase of treatment, oats and lactose-containing products should also be eliminated.[161] Because of problems of malabsorption, multivitamin therapy and specific replacement of vitamin D and calcium may be necessary.

The importance of recognition of celiac disease may be reflected in the studies suggesting that uncontrolled disease may be associated with adverse pregnancy outcome.[175-179] Studies of untreated and treated celiac patients revealed an increased rate of spontaneous miscarriages in the untreated cases.[175,176] The rate of intrauterine growth restriction is higher among untreated patients.[180-182] Whether these outcomes imply causation or merely association is debatable. An epidemiologic study involving 1521 women with celiac disease suggested that fertility in these patients is similar to that for the general female population.[183] Although the researchers found somewhat higher miscarriage and cesarean section rates in the affected population, there was also a trend toward delayed childbearing, which may influence the statistics. It appears the negative effects of celiac disease, including miscarriage, is reduced by treatment with a gluten-free diet.[168]

Pregnancy may unmask or reactivate celiac disease and should lead the obstetrician to evaluate signs such as anemia refractory to iron, hypokalemia, and hypocalcemia in the absence of clinical symptoms. The reason for worsening symptoms is unknown, but it is speculated to be the loss of borderline tolerance to gluten due to hormonal or endocrine mechanisms.[171]

Bariatric Surgery

Obesity has become an epidemic in the United States, with 18% of women meeting the criteria of a body mass index (BMI) of 30 kg/m^2.[184] The prevalence of morbid obesity, defined as a BMI exceeding 40 kg/m^2 or 35 kg/m^2 plus comorbidities, also is increasing. Pregnancy outcomes for these women are worse than those with a normal BMI.[185] Complications include gestational diabetes, hypertension, preeclampsia, macrosomia, and an increased cesarean section rate.

The 1991 National Institutes of Health Consensus Developmental Conference concluded that bariatric surgery is the most effective treatment for morbidly obese patients.[186] A consequence of the increased rate of obesity is the increased numbers of gastrointestinal operations performed for weight loss. The number of operations increased from 16,000 in the early 1990s to 103,000 in 2003.[187]

Two types of procedures dominate the practice of bariatric surgery. One is diversionary, which constructs a proximal gastric pouch to an outlet of a Y-shaped limb of small bowel (i.e., Roux-en-Y procedure). Variants include biliopancreatic diversion and long limb gastric bypass, which are usually reserved for heavier patients.[188] The second type involves reducing the volume of the stomach and includes gastric banding. The former procedure results in more weight loss, but it is associated with nutritional deficiencies and the dumping syndrome. Because of the lack of functional proximal small bowel, patients can have iron, vitamin B_{12}, vitamin D, and folic acid deficiencies (Table 49-8). Parenteral replacement may be necessary if oral supplementation is not successful. After bariatric surgery, patients can have acute postgastric reduction surgery (APGARS) neuropathy. Prominent features include progressive vomiting, weakness, and hyporeflexia. This disorder overlaps with other syndromes caused by deficiencies of many nutrients.[189] Gastric banding, although less successful, minimizes the risk of deficiencies due to malabsorption.

Pregnancy outcomes in patients with prior bariatric surgery appear to be relatively good. Early case reports described complications, including gastrointestinal bleeding,[190] intrauterine growth restriction,[191] and fetal anomalies.[192] However, population-based studies suggest very acceptable outcomes. Sheiner and associates[181] identified 298 deliveries complicated by an open or laparoscopic bariatric procedure. They found no differences between procedures, but compared with no prior bariatric surgery, there was a higher rate of labor inductions, fetal macrosomia, cesarean sections, and premature membrane rupture.[181] Specifically addressing gastric bypass, Dao and colleagues[193] evaluated 2423 patients who underwent a Roux-en-Y procedure. Of these, 34 became pregnant, and 21 became pregnant within a year of the surgery. There were no significant differences with respect to outcome compared with those who became pregnant more than a year after surgery.[193]

As the frequency of bariatric operations has increased, so has awareness of the complications of these procedures. Case reports of

TABLE 49-8 VITAMIN AND MINERAL DEFICIENCIES AFTER BARIATRIC SURGERY

Procedure	Iron	Folate	Vitamin B_{12}	Calcium	Vitamin D	Thiamine
Gastric banding*	↑	↑	±	±	±	±
Gastric bypass†	↑↑↑	↑↑	↑↑↑	↑↑	↑↑	±

*Vertical or adjustable gastric banding.
†Roux-en-Y or biliopancreatic diversion.
↑, mild risk of deficiency; ↑↑, moderate risk of deficiency; ↑↑↑, significant risk of deficiency; ±, negligible risk.

internal hernias causing acute surgical emergencies, including intestinal infarction, have been published in the obstetric literature.[194,195] Gastric ulcer perforation and gastrointestinal hemorrhage have also been reported.[190,196] More common problems are the nutritional deficiencies that are associated primarily with gastric bypass. They include iron, vitamin B_{12}, folate, and calcium deficiencies (see Table 49-8).

Constipation

Constipation is defined as difficult defecation and infrequent bowel movements that do not result from an underlying cause.[197] The estimated incidence during pregnancy is between 10% and 40%, as derived from studies done 2 decades ago.[198,199] The diagnosis is based on the patient's history, and the physician can use the Rome II criteria—12 weeks (not necessarily consecutive) in the prior 12 months when two of the following have occurred: straining, lumpy or hard stools, sensation of incomplete evacuation or anorectal obstruction or manual maneuvers to assist in more than 25% of defecations, and less than three bowel movements per week.[200] Problems with adherence to the Rome criteria were highlighted in a study in which 40% to 50% of patients who fulfilled the criteria did not feel constipated.[201] Constipation can arise de novo during gestation or be a chronic condition that is exacerbated by pregnancy.

Factors contributing to constipation during pregnancy include iron supplementation, decreased activity, uterine enlargement, hemorrhoids, and hormonal factors, including increased progesterone and estrogen and decreased motilin levels.[199] In animal studies, progesterone decreases smooth muscle contractility and slows gastrointestinal transit.[202] Pregnant and ovariectomized rats given estrogen and progesterone had longer colonic transit compared with nonpregnant or ovariectomy control animals.[16] Human studies of sex hormone effects have relied on orocecal transit times. In nonpregnant women, the transit time was significantly longer during the luteal phase, when progesterone levels are usually higher.[13] A study involving seven women with intractable constipation and documented slow transit times who required colectomy were compared with six women requiring colectomy for adenocarcinoma. Progesterone receptors were overexpressed in the patients with constipation. This overexpression was reproduced in normal colonic cells treated with progesterone.[203] Plasma motilin levels are depressed during pregnancy but return to normal within 1 week after delivery.[204] Although colonic transit times during pregnancy have not been studied, diaries of patients' symptoms have suggested increased problems with bowel movements in all three trimesters.[198] The causes and treatment of constipation appear to be similar to those for the general population.[199]

Education should be the first-line treatment. Patients should be instructed to increase fluid and fiber intake, exercise, and attempt defecation in the morning or after meals, when colonic activity is the highest. Dietary habits should be explored. If needed, 2 to 6 tablespoons of bran should be added to each meal, followed by a glass of water. However, the laxative effect may take 3 to 5 days.[199] Psyllium, polycarbophil, and methylcellulose act by increasing fecal water content and decreasing stool transit time. Hyperosmolar laxatives such as polyethylene glycol, sorbitol, and lactulose are poorly absorbed and increase fecal water content. Because prolonged use may lead to electrolyte imbalances, they should be used with caution. Stimulant laxatives have a fast onset of action and may be considered in patients who fail to respond to bulk or osmotic agents.[199] Their short-term use is generally safe, but long-term use is not recommended. Tolerance, although uncommon in most users, can occur in patients with severe forms of slow colonic transit.[205] A list of these agents is provided in Table 49-9.

Hemorrhoids

Hemorrhoids are common in adults.[206] One third of pregnant women are symptomatic, and approximately 10% require treatment for hemorrhoids.[207] Etiologic factors include constipation and straining at defecation, vascular engorgement from increased intra-abdominal pressure and blood volume, and the absence of valves in hemorrhoidal veins.[199] Internal hemorrhoids originate above the dentate line, and they are supplied by the superior hemorrhoidal plexus and covered with columnar epithelium. External hemorrhoids are below the dentate line, and they are supplied by the inferior hemorrhoidal plexus and covered with squamous epithelium.

TABLE 49-9 PREFERRED LAXATIVES IN PREGNANCY

Laxative	Usual Dose	Advantages	Disadvantages
Bulk forming		Long-term use in patients with uncomplicated constipation	Slow onset of action; risk of mechanical obstruction; unpleasant taste
Psyllium	7 g/day		Potential for anaphylaxis
Methylcellulose	4-6 g/day		
Hyperosmolar		Fast onset of action	Prolonged use may cause electrolyte imbalance; unsuitable for long-term use
Polyethylene glycol	8-25 g/day	Less abdominal bloating and flatulence than lactulose and sorbitol	
Lactulose	15-30 mL/day		Should be avoided in diabetics and those requiring a low-galactose diet; may exacerbate nausea
Sorbitol	15-30 mL/day	Less expensive than lactulose	
Glycerin	3-g suppository		
Stimulant		Fast onset of action.	Long-term use limited to 3 days per week
Bisacodyl	30 mg PO, 10 mg PR		More colic than with senna and cascara
Senna	17-34 mg		
Cascara	2-5 mL	Produces little or no colic	

External hemorrhoids infrequently require treatment unless complicated by thrombosis. For mild discomfort, conservative treatment includes stool softeners, sitz baths, and mild analgesics. If the pain is severe, surgical excision under local anesthesia can be performed during pregnancy.[199,207] Clot incision with removal is less efficacious, mainly because of recurrent thrombosis.[208] Internal hemorrhoids usually manifest as painless bleeding, although they can manifest with discomfort caused by prolapse or incarceration. Diagnosis may require anoscopy. Treatment usually is conservative and includes increased fiber and stool softeners. Local measures, including skin protectants and topical anesthetics, can improve symptoms. Patients with refractory symptoms may require band ligation, injection, sclerotherapy, or coagulation.[199] Rubber band ligation is effective for internal hemorrhoids that are reducibly prolapsed. Sclerotherapy using 5% phenol is safe in pregnancy, and infrared photocoagulation and laser coagulation for first- and second-degree hemorrhoids are theoretically safe.[207] Surgical hemorrhoidectomy is reserved for internal hemorrhoids that prolapse and incarcerate or that have failed conservative office measures.[199]

Gastrointestinal Endoscopy in Pregnancy

Upper Gastrointestinal Endoscopy and Colonoscopy

Upper gastrointestinal endoscopy (i.e., esophagogastroduodenoscopy [EGD]) and colonoscopy play vital roles in the diagnosis and treatment of a variety of gastrointestinal disorders. Few pregnant patients with gastrointestinal disorders need gastrointestinal endoscopy, but if they do, the main risks are related to the endoscopy itself (e.g., perforation, bleeding, infection) and complications of sedation (e.g., cardiovascular events, pulmonary aspiration, teratogenic risks of medications). Results from several small studies suggest that careful upper endoscopy and colonoscopy are safe during pregnancy.[93,209-213]

The American Society for Gastrointestinal Endoscopy (ASGE), with input from the American College of Obstetricians and Gynecologists (ACOG) Committee on Obstetric Practice, has published guidelines related to endoscopy in pregnant women.[214] They have developed general indications for endoscopy in pregnancy (Table 49-10).

Sedation for the procedure poses the greatest risk to the fetus, and consideration should be given in these cases to having anesthesiology supervision. Gastroenterologists usually perform upper endoscopy and colonoscopy on adults using moderate sedation. The drugs commonly used for gastrointestinal endoscopy sedation, and their FDA category regarding safety during pregnancy, are as follows: meperidine (B), fentanyl (C), naloxone (B), benzodiazepines (D), flumazenil (C), propofol (B), simethicone (C), glucagon (B), and polyethylene glycol (C).

Regarding patient positioning, it is recommended that the patient not lie on her back in the second and third trimesters because the pregnant uterus compresses the aorta and inferior vena cava, causing maternal hypotension and decreasing placental perfusion. Because most procedures are done with the patient in the left lateral position, this is usually not an issue.

TABLE 49-10 INDICATIONS FOR ENDOSCOPY IN PREGNANCY

Significant or ongoing gastrointestinal bleeding
Severe or refractory nausea and vomiting or abdominal pain
Dysphagia or odynophagia
Strong suspicion of a mass in the upper gastrointestinal tract or colon
Severe diarrhea with negative result for noninvasive evaluation
Choledocholithiasis or cholangitis
Biliary or pancreatic duct injury

Adapted from Qureshi WA, Rajan E, Adler DG, et al: ASGE guidelines for endoscopy in pregnant and lactating women. Gastrointest Endosc 61:357-362, 2005.

Endoscopic Ultrasound

The endoscopic ultrasound (EUS) technique uses an ultrasound probe that is incorporated into the tip of the endoscope. This allows ultrasound imaging from within the luminal gastrointestinal tract. This technique is commonly used to stage gastrointestinal malignancy and to evaluate pancreatic lesions. EUS is used during pregnancy only to look for stones in the common bile duct because it is more sensitive than MRI, CT, or ultrasound and much safer than endoscopic retrograde cholangiopancreatography because of the lack of radiation and no risk of pancreatitis.

Small Bowel Wireless Capsule Endoscopy

The small intestine had been unreachable with the standard endoscopic techniques of EGD and colonoscopy. Wireless capsule endoscopy can visualize the entire small intestine. The procedure involves swallowing a miniaturized camera that has been placed in a large pill. Images are sent back to an external recording device for a total of 8 hours of video as the pill camera moves by peristalsis through the small intestine. It would be unusual to have a pregnant woman swallow a pill camera, unless there was unexplained severe or recurrent gastrointestinal bleeding.[215] The safety and efficacy of wireless capsule endoscopy of the small bowel has not been tested in humans, and pregnancy therefore is considered a relative contraindication to capsule endoscopy.[216]

Double-Balloon Enteroscopy

A technique using a scope with a balloon on the tip and an overtube with a balloon on the distal end is used to advance a thin endoscope from the mouth into the mid-ileum. Double-balloon enteroscopy allows the endoscopist for the first time to gain access to the middle of the small intestine to obtain biopsies or to perform therapeutic maneuvers. Because this is a time-intensive procedure with a large amount of pushing and stretching in the abdomen, it would rarely be considered for use during pregnancy.

References

1. Koch KL, Frissora CL: Nausea and vomiting during pregnancy. Gastroenterol Clin North Am 32:201-234, vi, 2003.
2. Van Thiel DH, Gavaler JS, Stremple J: Lower esophageal sphincter pressure in women using sequential oral contraceptives. Gastroenterology 71:232-234, 1976.
3. Van Thiel DH, Gavaler JS, Joshi SN, et al: Heartburn of pregnancy. Gastroenterology 72:666-668, 1977.
4. Fisher RS, Roberts GS, Grabowski CJ, Cohen S: Altered lower esophageal sphincter function during early pregnancy. Gastroenterology 74:1233-1237, 1978.

5. Fisher RS, Roberts GS, Grabowski CJ, Cohen S: Inhibition of lower esophageal sphincter circular muscle by female sex hormones. Am J Physiol 234: E243-E247, 1978.
6. Macfie AG, Magides AD, Richmond MN, Reilly CS: Gastric emptying in pregnancy. Br J Anaesth 67:54-57, 1991.
7. Whitehead EM, Smith M, Dean Y, O'Sullivan G: An evaluation of gastric emptying times in pregnancy and the puerperium. Anaesthesia 48:53-57, 1993.
8. Chiloiro M, Darconza G, Piccioli E, et al: Gastric emptying and orocecal transit time in pregnancy. J Gastroenterol 36:538-543, 2001.
9. Gryboski WA, Spiro HM: The effect of pregnancy on gastric secretion. N Engl J Med 255:1131-1134, 1956.
10. Hunt JN, Murray FA: Gastric function in pregnancy. J Obstet Gynaecol Br Emp 65:78-83, 1958.
11. Waldum HL, Straume BK, Lundgren R: Serum group I pepsinogens during pregnancy. Scand J Gastroenterol 15:61-63, 1980.
12. Wald A, Van Thiel DH, Hoechstetter L, et al: Effect of pregnancy on gastrointestinal transit. Dig Dis Sci 27:1015-1018, 1982.
13. Wald A, Van Thiel DH, Hoechstetter L, et al: Gastrointestinal transit: The effect of the menstrual cycle. Gastroenterology 80:1497-500, 1981.
14. Brown J, Robertson J, Gallagher N: Humoral regulation of vitamin B_{12} absorption by pregnant mouse small intestine. Gastroenterology 72:881-888, 1977.
15. Dugas MC, Hazelwood RL, Lawrence AL: Influence of pregnancy and-or exercise on intestinal transport of amino acids in rats. Proc Soc Exp Biol Med 135:127-131, 1970.
16. Ryan JP, Bhojwani A: Colonic transit in rats: Effect of ovariectomy, sex steroid hormones, and pregnancy. Am J Physiol 251:G46-G50, 1986.
17. Scott LD, DeFlora E: Cholinergic responsiveness of intestinal muscle in the pregnant guinea pig. Life Sci 44:503-508, 1989.
18. Gill RC, Bowes KL, Kingma YJ: Effect of progesterone on canine colonic smooth muscle. Gastroenterology 88:1941-1947, 1985.
19. Gadsby R, Barnie-Adshead AM, Jagger C: A prospective study of nausea and vomiting during pregnancy. Br J Gen Pract 43:245-248, 1993.
20. Jarnfelt-Samsioe A, Samsioe G, Velinder GM: Nausea and vomiting in pregnancy—a contribution to its epidemiology. Gynecol Obstet Invest 16:221-229, 1983.
21. Lacroix R, Eason E, Melzack R: Nausea and vomiting during pregnancy: A prospective study of its frequency, intensity, and patterns of change. Am J Obstet Gynecol 182:931-937, 2000.
22. Klebanoff MA, Koslowe PA, Kaslow R, Rhoads GG: Epidemiology of vomiting in early pregnancy. Obstet Gynecol 66:612-616, 1985.
23. Semmens JP: Female sexuality and life situations. An etiologic psycho-socio-sexual profile of weight gain and nausea and vomiting in pregnancy. Obstet Gynecol 38:555-563, 1971.
24. Corey LA, Berg K, Solaas MH, Nance WE: The epidemiology of pregnancy complications and outcome in a Norwegian twin population. Obstet Gynecol 80:989-994, 1992.
25. Gadsby R, Barnie-Adshead AM, Jagger C: Pregnancy nausea related to women's obstetric and personal histories. Gynecol Obstet Invest 43:108-111, 1997, 1997.
26. Vellacott ID, Cooke EJ, James CE: Nausea and vomiting in early pregnancy. Int J Gynaecol Obstet 27:57-62, 1988.
27. Askling J, Erlandsson G, Kaijser M, et al: Sickness in pregnancy and sex of child. Lancet 354:2053, 1999.
28. Basso O, Olsen J: Sex ratio and twinning in women with hyperemesis or pre-eclampsia. Epidemiology 12:747-749, 2001.
29. del Mar Melero-Montes, Jick H: Hyperemesis gravidarum and the sex of the offspring. Epidemiology 12:123-124, 2000.
30. Furneaux EC, Langley-Evans AJ, Langley-Evans SC: Nausea and vomiting of pregnancy: Endocrine basis and contribution to pregnancy outcome. Obstet Gynecol Surv 56:775-782, 2001.
31. Goodwin TM, Hershman JM, Cole L: Increased concentration of the free beta-subunit of human chorionic gonadotropin in hyperemesis gravidarum. Acta Obstet Gynecol Scand 73:770-772, 1994.
32. James WH: The associated offspring sex ratios and cause(s) of hyperemesis gravidarum. Acta Obstet Gynecol Scand 80:378-379, 2001.
33. Steier JA, Bergsjo PB, Thorsen T, Myking OL: Human chorionic gonadotropin in maternal serum in relation to fetal gender and utero-placental blood flow. Acta Obstet Gynecol Scand 83:170-174, 2004.
34. Verberg MF, Gillott DJ, Al-Fardan N, Grudzinskas JG: Hyperemesis gravidarum: A literature review. Hum Reprod Update 11:527-539, 2005.
35. Goodwin TM: Nausea and vomiting of pregnancy: An obstetric syndrome. Am J Obstet Gynecol 186:S184-S189, 2002.
36. North RA, Whitehead R, Larkins RG: Stimulation by human chorionic gonadotropin of prostaglandin synthesis by early human placental tissue. J Clin Endocrinol Metab 73:60-70, 1991.
37. Frigo P, Lang C, Reisenberger K, et al: Hyperemesis gravidarum associated with *Helicobacter pylori* seropositivity. Obstet Gynecol 91:615-617, 1998.
38. Kazerooni T, Taallom M, Ghaderi AA: *Helicobacter pylori* seropositivity in patients with hyperemesis gravidarum. Int J Gynaecol Obstet 79:217-220, 2002.
39. Kocak I, Akcan Y, Ustun C, et al: *Helicobacter pylori* seropositivity in patients with hyperemesis gravidarum. Int J Gynaecol Obstet 66:251-254, 1999.
40. Lee RH, Pan VL, Wing DA: The prevalence of *Helicobacter pylori* in the Hispanic population affected by hyperemesis gravidarum. Am J Obstet Gynecol 193:1024-1027, 2005.
41. Atanackovic G, Wolpin J, Koren G: Determinants of the need for hospital care among women with nausea and vomiting of pregnancy. Clin Invest Med 24:90-93, 2001.
42. Sherman PW, Flaxman SM: Nausea and vomiting of pregnancy in an evolutionary perspective. Am J Obstet Gynecol 186:S190-S197, 2002.
43. Koch KL, Stern RM, Vasey M, et al: Gastric dysrhythmias and nausea of pregnancy. Dig Dis Sci 35:961-968, 1990.
44. Czeizel AE, Dudas I, Fritz G, et al: The effect of periconceptional multivitamin-mineral supplementation on vertigo, nausea and vomiting in the first trimester of pregnancy. Arch Gynecol Obstet 251:181-185, 1992.
45. Emelianova S, Mazzotta P, Einarson A, Koren G: Prevalence and severity of nausea and vomiting of pregnancy and effect of vitamin supplementation. Clin Invest Med 22:106-110, 1999.
46. Borrelli F, Capasso R, Aviello G, et al: Effectiveness and safety of ginger in the treatment of pregnancy-induced nausea and vomiting. Obstet Gynecol 105:849-856, 2005.
47. Boone SA, Shields KM: Treating pregnancy-related nausea and vomiting with ginger. Ann Pharmacother 39:1710-1713, 2005.
48. American College of Obstetrics and Gynecology (ACOG): Practice Bulletin: Nausea and vomiting of pregnancy. Obstet Gynecol 103:803-814, 2004.
49. Roscoe JA, Matteson SE: Acupressure and acustimulation bands for control of nausea: A brief review. Am J Obstet Gynecol 186:S244-S247, 2002.
50. Norheim AJ, Pedersen EJ, Fonnebo V, Berge L: Acupressure treatment of morning sickness in pregnancy. A randomised, double-blind, placebo-controlled study. Scand J Prim Health Care 19:43-47, 2001.
51. Werntoft E, Dykes AK: Effect of acupressure on nausea and vomiting during pregnancy. A randomized, placebo-controlled, pilot study. J Reprod Med 46:835-839, 2001.
52. Jewell D, Young G: Interventions for nausea and vomiting in early pregnancy. Cochrane Database Syst Rev (4):CD000145, 2003.
53. Vutyavanich T, Wongtra-ngan S, Ruangsri R: Pyridoxine for nausea and vomiting of pregnancy: A randomized, double-blind, placebo-controlled trial. Am J Obstet Gynecol 173:881-884, 1995.
54. Neutel CI, Johansen HL: Measuring drug effectiveness by default: The case of Bendectin. Can J Public Health 86:66-70, 1995.
55. Berkovitch M, Elbirt D, Addis A, et al: Fetal effects of metoclopramide therapy for nausea and vomiting of pregnancy. N Engl J Med 343:445-446, 2000.
56. Berkovitch M, Mazzota P, Greenberg R, et al: Metoclopramide for nausea and vomiting of pregnancy: A prospective multicenter international study. Am J Perinatol 19:311-316, 2002.
57. Einarson A, Koren G, Bergman U: Nausea and vomiting in pregnancy: A comparative European study. Eur J Obstet Gynecol Reprod Biol 76:1-3, 1998.

58. Kallen B: Hyperemesis during pregnancy and delivery outcome: A registry study. Eur J Obstet Gynecol Reprod Biol 26:291-302, 1987.
59. Attard CL, Kohli MA, Coleman S, et al: The burden of illness of severe nausea and vomiting of pregnancy in the United States. Am J Obstet Gynecol 186:S220-S227, 2002.
60. Dodds L, Fell DB, Joseph KS, et al: Outcomes of pregnancies complicated by hyperemesis gravidarum. Obstet Gynecol 107:285-292, 2006.
61. Fell DB, Dodds L, Joseph KS, et al: Risk factors for hyperemesis gravidarum requiring hospital admission during pregnancy. Obstet Gynecol 107:277-284, 2006.
62. Bailit JL: Hyperemesis gravidarum: Epidemiologic findings from a large cohort. Am J Obstet Gynecol 193:811-814, 2005.
63. Chiossi G, Neri I, Cavazzuti M, et al: Hyperemesis gravidarum complicated by Wernicke encephalopathy: Background, case report, and review of the literature. Obstet Gynecol Surv 61:255-268, 2006.
64. Safari HR, Fassett MJ, Souter IC, et al: The efficacy of methylprednisolone in the treatment of hyperemesis gravidarum: A randomized, double-blind, controlled study. Am J Obstet Gynecol 179:921-924, 1998
65. Bondok RS, El Sharnouby NM, Eid HE, Abd Elmaksoud AM: Pulsed steroid therapy is an effective treatment for intractable hyperemesis gravidarum. Crit Care Med 34:2781-2783, 2006.
66. Yost NP, McIntire DD, Wians FH Jr, et al: A randomized, placebo-controlled trial of corticosteroids for hyperemesis due to pregnancy. Obstet Gynecol 102:1250-1254, 2003.
67. Nelson-Piercy C, Fayers P, de Swiet M: Randomised, double-blind, placebo-controlled trial of corticosteroids for the treatment of hyperemesis gravidarum. BJOG 108:9-15, 2001.
68. Watcha MF, White PF: Postoperative nausea and vomiting. Its etiology, treatment, and prevention. Anesthesiology 77:162-184, 1992.
69. Park-Wyllie L, Mazzotta P, Pastuszak A, et al: Birth defects after maternal exposure to corticosteroids: Prospective cohort study and meta-analysis of epidemiological studies. Teratology 62:385-392, 2000.
70. Rodriguez-Pinilla E, Martinez-Frias ML: Corticosteroids during pregnancy and oral clefts: A case-control study. Teratology 58:2-5, 1998.
71. Shepard TH, Brent RL, Friedman JM, et al: Update on new developments in the study of human teratogens. Teratology 65:153-161, 2002.
72. Lee RV, Rodgers BD, Young C, et al: Total parenteral nutrition during pregnancy. Obstet Gynecol 68:563-571, 1986.
73. Amato P, Quercia RA: A historical perspective and review of the safety of lipid emulsion in pregnancy. Nutr Clin Pract 6:189-192, 1991.
74. Folk JJ, Leslie-Brown HF, Nosovitch JT, et al: Hyperemesis gravidarum: outcomes and complications with and without total parenteral nutrition. J Reprod Med 49:497-502, 2004.
75. Paranyuk Y, Levine G, Figueroa R: Candida septicemia in a pregnant woman with hyperemesis receiving parenteral nutrition. Obstet Gynecol 107:535-537, 2006.
76. Russo-Stieglitz KE, Levine AB, Wagner BA, Armenti VT: Pregnancy outcome in patients requiring parenteral nutrition. J Matern Fetal Med 8:164-167, 1999.
77. Ogura JM, Francois KE, Perlow JH, Elliott JP: Complications associated with peripherally inserted central catheter use during pregnancy. Am J Obstet Gynecol 188:1223-1225, 2003.
78. Trogstad LI, Stoltenberg C, Magnus P, et al: Recurrence risk in hyperemesis gravidarum. BJOG 112:1641-1616, 2005.
79. Bassey OO: Pregnancy heartburn in Nigerians and Caucasians with theories about aetiology based on manometric recordings from the oesophagus and stomach. BJOG 84:439-443, 1977.
80. Nebel OT, Fornes MF, Castell DO: Symptomatic gastroesophageal reflux: Incidence and precipitating factors. Am J Dig Dis 21:953-956, 1976.
81. Bainbridge ET, Temple JG, Nicholas SP, et al: Symptomatic gastro-oesophageal reflux in pregnancy. A comparative study of white Europeans and Asians in Birmingham. Br J Clin Pract 37:53-57, 1983.
82. Marrero JM, Goggin PM, de Caestecker JS, et al: Determinants of pregnancy heartburn. BJOG 99:731-734, 1992.
83. Richter JE: Gastroesophageal reflux disease during pregnancy. Gastroenterol Clin North Am 32:235-261, 2003.
84. Richter JE: Review article: The management of heartburn in pregnancy. Aliment Pharmacol Ther 22:749-757, 2005.
85. Larson JD, Patatanian E, Miner PB Jr, et al: Double-blind, placebo-controlled study of ranitidine for gastroesophageal reflux symptoms during pregnancy. Obstet Gynecol 90:83-87, 1997.
86. Ruigomez A, Garcia Rodriguez LA, Cattaruzzi C, et al: Use of cimetidine, omeprazole, and ranitidine in pregnant women and pregnancy outcomes. Am J Epidemiol 150:476-481, 1999.
87. Nikfar S, Abdollahi M, Moretti ME, et al: Use of proton pump inhibitors during pregnancy and rates of major malformations: A meta-analysis. Dig Dis Sci 47:1526-1529, 2004.
88. Av-Citrin O, Arnon J, Shechtman S, et al: The safety of proton pump inhibitors in pregnancy: A multicentre prospective controlled study. Aliment Pharmacol Ther 21:269-275, 2005.
89. Cappell MS: Gastric and duodenal ulcers during pregnancy. Gastroenterol Clin North Am 32:263-308, 2003.
90. Clark DH: Peptic ulcer in women. BMJ 1:1254-1257, 1953.
91. DeVore GR: Acute abdominal pain in the pregnant patient due to pancreatitis, acute appendicitis, cholecystitis, or peptic ulcer disease. Clin Perinatol 7:349-369, 1980.
92. Pounder R: Silent peptic ulceration: Deadly silence or golden silence? Gastroenterology 96:626-631, 1989.
93. Cappell MS, Colon VJ, Sidhom OA: A study of eight medical centers of the safety and clinical efficacy of esophagogastroduodenoscopy in 83 pregnant females with follow-up of fetal outcome with comparison control groups. Am J Gastroenterol 91:348-354, 1996.
94. Ching CK, Lam SK: Antacids. Indications and limitations. Drugs 47:305-317, 1994.
95. Peterson WL, Sturdevant RA, Frankl HD, et al: Healing of duodenal ulcer with an antacid regimen. N Engl J Med 297:341-345, 1997.
96. Banerjce S, El-Omar E, Mowat A, et al: Sucralfate suppresses *Helicobacter pylori* infection and reduces gastric acid secretion by 50% in patients with duodenal ulcer. Gastroenterology 110:717-724, 1996.
97. McCarthy DM: Sucralfate. N Engl J Med 325:1017-1025, 1991.
98. Charan M, Katz PO: Gastroesophageal reflux disease in pregnancy. Curr Treat Options Gastroenterol 4:73-81, 2001.
99. Jones DB, Howden CW, Burget DW, et al: Acid suppression in duodenal ulcer: A meta-analysis to define optimal dosing with antisecretory drugs. Gut 28:1120-1127, 1987.
100. Magee LA, Inocencion G, Kamboj L, et al: Safety of first trimester exposure to histamine H2 blockers. A prospective cohort study. Dig Dis Sci 41:1145-1149, 1996.
101. Finkelstein W, Isselbacher KJ: Drug therapy: Cimetidine. N Engl J Med 299:992-996, 1978.
102. Parker S, Schade RR, Pohl CR, et al: Prenatal and neonatal exposure of male rat pups to cimetidine but not ranitidine adversely affects subsequent adult sexual functioning. Gastroenterology 86:675-680, 1984.
103. Mourad J, Elliott JP, Erickson L, Lisboa L: Appendicitis in pregnancy: new information that contradicts long-held clinical beliefs. Am J Obstet Gynecol 182:1027-1029, 2000.
104. Guttman R, Goldman RD, Koren G: Appendicitis during pregnancy. Can Fam Physician 50:355-357, 2004.
105. Andersen B, Nielsen TF: Appendicitis in pregnancy: Diagnosis, management and complications. Acta Obstet Gynecol Scand 78:758-762, 1999.
106. Hee P, Viktrup L: The diagnosis of appendicitis during pregnancy and maternal and fetal outcome after appendectomy. Int J Gynaecol Obstet 65:129-135, 1999.
107. Tracey M, Fletcher HS: Appendicitis in pregnancy. Am Surg 66:555-559, 2000.
108. Hale DA, Molloy M, Pearl RH, et al: Appendectomy: A contemporary appraisal. Ann Surg 225:252-261, 1997.
109. Tamir IL, Bongard FS, Klein SR: Acute appendicitis in the pregnant patient. Am J Surg 160:571-575, 1990.
110. Al-Mulhim AA: Acute appendicitis in pregnancy. A review of 52 cases. Int Surg 81:295-297, 1996.
111. Cunningham FG, McCubbin JH: Appendicitis complicating pregnancy. Obstet Gynecol 45:415-420, 1975.

112. Cohen-Kerem R, Railton C, Oren D, et al: Pregnancy outcome following non-obstetric surgical intervention. Am J Surg 190:467-473, 2005.
113. Humes DJ, Simpson J: Acute appendicitis. BMJ 333:530-534, 2006.
114. Weingold AB: Appendicitis in pregnancy. Clin Obstet Gynecol 26:801-809, 1983.
115. Williams R, Shaw J: Ultrasound scanning in the diagnosis of acute appendicitis in pregnancy. Emerg Med J 24:359-360, 2007.
116. Rao PM, Rhea JT, Novelline RA, et al: Effect of computed tomography of the appendix on treatment of patients and use of hospital resources. N Engl J Med 338:141-146, 1998.
117. Rao PM, Rhea JT, Novelline RA, et al: Helical CT technique for the diagnosis of appendicitis: Prospective evaluation of a focused appendix CT examination. Radiology 202:139-144, 1997.
118. Ames CM, Shipp TD, Castro EE, et al: The use of helical computed tomography in pregnancy for the diagnosis of acute appendicitis. Am J Obstet Gynecol 184:954-957, 2001.
119. Kanal E, Borgstede JP, Barkovich AJ, et al: American College of Radiology White Paper on MR Safety: 2004 update and revisions. AJR Am J Roentgenol 182:1111-1114, 2004.
120. Shellock FG, Kanal E: Policies, guidelines, and recommendations for MR imaging safety and patient management. SMRI Safety Committee. J Magn Reson Imaging 1:97-101, 1991.
121. Cobben LP, Groot I, Haans L, et al: MRI for clinically suspected appendicitis during pregnancy. AJR Am J Roentgenol 183:671-675, 2004.
122. Pedrosa I, Levine D, Eyvazzadeh AD, et al: MR imaging evaluation of acute appendicitis in pregnancy. Radiology 238:891-899, 2006.
123. Malangoni MA: Gastrointestinal surgery and pregnancy. Gastroenterol Clin North Am 32:181-200, 2003.
124. McKinlay R, Mastrangelo MJ Jr: Current status of laparoscopic appendectomy. Curr Surg 60:506-512, 2003.
125. Affleck DG, Handrahan DL, Egger MJ, Price RR: The laparoscopic management of appendicitis and cholelithiasis during pregnancy. Am J Surg 178:523-529, 1999.
126. Fatum M, Rojansky N: Laparoscopic surgery during pregnancy. Obstet Gynecol Surv 56:50-59, 2001.
127. Al-Fozan H, Tulandi T: Safety and risks of laparoscopy in pregnancy. Curr Opin Obstet Gynecol 14:375-379, 2002.
128. Friedman JD, Ramsey PS, Ramin KD, Berry C: Pneumoamnion and pregnancy loss after second-trimester laparoscopic surgery. Obstet Gynecol 99:512-513, 2002.
129. Rollins MD, Chan KJ, Price RR: Laparoscopy for appendicitis and cholelithiasis during pregnancy: A new standard of care. Surg Endosc 18:237-241, 2004.
130. Miller JP: Inflammatory bowel disease in pregnancy: A review. J R Soc Med 79:221-225, 1986.
131. Mogadam M, Korelitz BI, Ahmed SW, et al: The course of inflammatory bowel disease during pregnancy and postpartum. Am J Gastroenterol 75:265-269, 1981.
132. Baiocco PJ, Korelitz BI: The influence of inflammatory bowel disease and its treatment on pregnancy and fetal outcome. J.Clin Gastroenterol 6:211-216, 1984.
133. Baird DD, Narendranathan M, Sandler RS: Increased risk of preterm birth for women with inflammatory bowel disease. Gastroenterology 99:987-994, 1990.
134. Elbaz G, Fich A, Levy A, et al: Inflammatory bowel disease and preterm delivery. Int J Gynaecol Obstet 90:193-197, 2005.
135. Kornfeld D, Cnattingius S, Ekbom A: Pregnancy outcomes in women with inflammatory bowel disease—a population-based cohort study. Am J Obstet Gynecol 177:942-946, 1997.
136. Nielsen OH, Andreasson B, Bondesen S, Jarnum S: Pregnancy in ulcerative colitis. Scand J Gastroenterol 18:735-742, 1983.
137. Norgard B, Fonager K, Sorensen HT, Olsen J: Birth outcomes of women with ulcerative colitis: A nationwide Danish cohort study. Am J Gastroenterol 95:3165-3170, 2000.
138. Schade RR, Van Thiel DH, Gavaler JS: Chronic idiopathic ulcerative colitis. Pregnancy and fetal outcome. Dig Dis Sci 29:614-619, 1984.
139. Hanan IM, Kirsner JB: Inflammatory bowel disease in the pregnant woman. Clin Perinatol 12:669-682, 1985.
140. Rogers RG, Katz VL: Course of Crohn's disease during pregnancy and its effect on pregnancy outcome: A retrospective review. Am J Perinatol 12:262-264, 1995.
141. Einarson A, Mastroiacovo P, Arnon J, et al: Prospective, controlled, multicentre study of loperamide in pregnancy. Can J Gastroenterol 14:185-187, 2000.
142. Lewis JH, Weingold AB: The use of gastrointestinal drugs during pregnancy and lactation. Am J Gastroenterol 80:912-923, 1985.
143. Caro-Paton T, Carvajal A, Martin DI, et al: Is metronidazole teratogenic? A meta-analysis. Br J Clin Pharmacol 44:179-182, 1997.
144. Czeizel AE, Rockenbauer M: A population based case-control teratologic study of oral metronidazole treatment during pregnancy. BJOG 105:322-327, 1998.
145. Berkovitch M, Pastuszak A, Gazarian M, et al: Safety of the new quinolones in pregnancy. Obstet Gynecol 84:535-538, 1994.
146. Loebstein R, Addis A, Ho E, et al: Pregnancy outcome following gestational exposure to fluoroquinolones: A multicenter prospective controlled study. Antimicrob Agents Chemother 42:1336-1339, 1998.
147. Bell CM, Habal FM: Safety of topical 5-aminosalicylic acid in pregnancy. Am J Gastroenterol 92:2201-2202, 1997.
148. Habal FM, Hui G, Greenberg GR: Oral 5-aminosalicylic acid for inflammatory bowel disease in pregnancy: Safety and clinical course. Gastroenterology 105:1057-1060, 1993.
149. Mogadam M, Dobbins WO III, Korelitz BI, Ahmed SW: Pregnancy in inflammatory bowel disease: Effect of sulfasalazine and corticosteroids on fetal outcome. Gastroenterology 80:72-76, 1981.
150. Trallori G, d'Albasio G, Bardazzi G, et al: 5-Aminosalicylic acid in pregnancy: Clinical report. Ital J Gastroenterol 26:75-78, 1994.
151. Warrell DW, Taylor R: Outcome for the foetus of mothers receiving prednisolone during pregnancy. Lancet 1:117-118, 1968.
152. Muirhead N, Sabharwal AR, Rieder MJ, et al: The outcome of pregnancy following renal transplantation—the experience of a single center. Transplantation 54:429-432, 1992.
153. Alstead EM, Ritchie JK, Lennard-Jones JE, et al: Safety of azathioprine in pregnancy in inflammatory bowel disease. Gastroenterology 99:443-446, 1990.
154. Francella A, Dyan A, Bodian C, et al: The safety of 6-mercaptopurine for childbearing patients with inflammatory bowel disease: A retrospective cohort study. Gastroenterology 124:9-17, 2003.
155. Mahadevan U, Kane S, Sandborn WJ, et al: Intentional infliximab use during pregnancy for induction or maintenance of remission in Crohn's disease. Aliment Pharmacol Ther 21:733-738, 2005.
156. Everhart JE, Renault PF: Irritable bowel syndrome in office-based practice in the United States. Gastroenterology 100:998-1005, 1991.
157. Whorwell PJ, McCallum M, Creed FH, Roberts CT: Non-colonic features of irritable bowel syndrome. Gut 27:37-40, 1986.
158. Manning AP, Thompson WG, Heaton KW, Morris AF: Towards positive diagnosis of the irritable bowel. BMJ 2:653-654, 1978.
159. Longstreth GF, Thompson WG, Chey WD, et al: Functional bowel disorders. Gastroenterology 130:1480-1491, 2006.
160. Pimentel M, Park S, Mirocha J, et al: The effect of a nonabsorbed oral antibiotic (rifaximin) on the symptoms of the irritable bowel syndrome: A randomized trial. Ann Intern Med 145:557-563, 2006.
161. Farrell RJ, Kelly CP: Celiac sprue. N Engl J Med 346:180-188, 2002.
162. Schuppan D: Current concepts of celiac disease pathogenesis. Gastroenterology 119:234-242, 2000.
163. Catassi C, Ratsch IM, Fabiani E, et al: Coeliac disease in the year 2000: Exploring the iceberg. Lancet 343:200-203, 1994.
164. Not T, Horvath K, Hill ID, et al: Celiac disease risk in the USA: High prevalence of antiendomysium antibodies in healthy blood donors. Scand J Gastroenterol 33:494-498, 1998.
165. Catassi C, Fabiani E, Ratsch IM, et al: The coeliac iceberg in Italy. A multicentre antigliadin antibodies screening for coeliac disease in school-age subjects. Acta Paediatr Suppl 412:29-35, 1996.

166. Johnston SD, Watson RG, McMillan SA, et al: Coeliac disease detected by screening is not silent—simply unrecognized. QJM 91:853-860, 1998.
167. Greco L, Romino R, Coto I, et al: The first large population based twin study of coeliac disease. Gut 50:624-628, 2002.
168. Moodie S, Ciclitira P: Recent developments in celiac disease. Curr Opin Gastroenterol 18:182-186, 2002.
169. Corazza GR, Gasbarrini G: Coeliac disease in adults. Baillieres Clin Gastroenterol 9:329-350, 1995.
170. Ventura A, Magazzu G, Greco L: Duration of exposure to gluten and risk for autoimmune disorders in patients with celiac disease. SIGEP Study Group for Autoimmune Disorders in Celiac Disease. Gastroenterology 117:297-303, 1999.
171. Corrado F, Magazzu G, Sferlazzas C: Diagnosis of celiac disease in pregnancy and puerperium: Think about it. Acta Obstet Gynecol Scand 81:180-181, 2002.
172. Uibo O, Uibo R, Kleimola V, et al: Serum IgA anti-gliadin antibodies in an adult population sample. High prevalence without celiac disease. Dig Dis Sci 38:2034-2037, 1993.
173. Baldas V, Tommasini A, Trevisiol C, et al: Development of a novel rapid non-invasive screening test for coeliac disease. Gut 47:628-631, 2000.
174. Fink IJ, Creamer B: Response to a gluten-free diet of patients with the coeliac syndrome. Lancet 1:300-304, 1967.
175. Ciacci C, Cirillo M, Auriemma G, et al: Celiac disease and pregnancy outcome. Am J Gastroenterol 91:718-722, 1996.
176. Ferguson R, Holmes GK, Cooke WT: Coeliac disease, fertility, and pregnancy. Scand J Gastroenterol 17:65-68, 1982.
177. Sheiner E, Peleg R, Levy A: Pregnancy outcome of patients with known celiac disease. Eur J Obstet Gynecol Reprod Biol 129:41-45, 2006.
178. Ludvigsson JF, Ludvigsson J: Coeliac disease in the father affects the newborn. Gut 49:169-175, 2001.
179. Ludvigsson JF, Montgomery SM, Ekbom A: Celiac disease and risk of adverse fetal outcome: A population-based cohort study. Gastroenterology 129:454-463, 2005.
180. Norgard B, Fonager K, Sorensen HT, Olsen J: Birth outcomes of women with celiac disease: A nationwide historical cohort study. Am J Gastroenterol 94:2435-2440, 1999.
181. Sheiner E, Levy A, Silverberg D, et al: Pregnancy after bariatric surgery is not associated with adverse perinatal outcome. Am J Obstet Gynecol 190:1335-1340, 2004.
182. Salvatore S, Finazzi S, Radaelli G, et al: Prevalence of undiagnosed celiac disease in the parents of preterm and/or small for gestational age infants. Am J Gastroenterol 102:168-173, 2007.
183. Tata LJ, Card TR, Logan RF, et al: Fertility and pregnancy-related events in women with celiac disease: A population-based cohort study. Gastroenterology 128:849-855, 2005.
184. Mokdad AH, Serdula MK, Dietz WH, et al: The spread of the obesity epidemic in the United States, 1991-1998. JAMA 282:1519-1522, 1999.
185. Cnattingius S, Bergstrom R, Lipworth L, Kramer MS: Prepregnancy weight and the risk of adverse pregnancy outcomes. N Engl J Med 338:147-152, 1998.
186. Gastrointestinal surgery for severe obesity. Proceedings of a National Institutes of Health Consensus Development Conference. March 25-27, 1991, Bethesda, MD. Am J Clin Nutr 55:487S-619S, 1992.
187. Steinbrook R: Surgery for severe obesity. N Engl J Med 350:1075-1079, 2004.
188. Kral JG: ABC of obesity. Management: Part III—surgery. BMJ 333:900-903, 2006.
189. Chang CG, Adams-Huet B, Provost DA: Acute post-gastric reduction surgery (APGARS) neuropathy. Obes Surg 14:182-189, 2004.
190. Ramirez MM, Turrentine MA: Gastrointestinal hemorrhage during pregnancy in a patient with a history of vertical-banded gastroplasty. Am J Obstet Gynecol 173:1630-1631, 1995.
191. Granstrom L, Granstrom L, Backman L: Fetal growth retardation after gastric banding. Acta Obstet Gynecol Scand 69:533-536, 1990.
192. Haddow JE, Hill LE, Kloza EM, Thanhauser D: Neural tube defects after gastric bypass. Lancet 1:1330, 1986.
193. Dao T, Kuhn J, Ehmer D, et al: Pregnancy outcomes after gastric-bypass surgery. Am J Surg 192:762-766, 2006.
194. Kakarla N, Dailey C, Marino T, et al: Pregnancy after gastric bypass surgery and internal hernia formation. Obstet Gynecol 105:1195-1198, 2005.
195. Moore KA, Ouyang DW, Whang EE: Maternal and fetal deaths after gastric bypass surgery for morbid obesity. N Engl J Med 351:721-722, 2004.
196. Erez O, Maymon E, Mazor M: Acute gastric ulcer perforation in a 35 weeks' nulliparous patient with gastric banding. Am J Obstet Gynecol 191:1721-122, 2004.
197. Tytgat GN, Heading RC, Muller-Lissner S, et al: Contemporary understanding and management of reflux and constipation in the general population and pregnancy: A consensus meeting. Aliment Pharmacol Ther 18:291-301, 2003.
198. Derbyshire EJ, Davies J, Detmar P: Changes in bowel function: Pregnancy and the puerperium. Dig Dis Sci 52:324-328, 2007.
199. Wald A: Constipation, diarrhea, and symptomatic hemorrhoids during pregnancy. Gastroenterol Clin North Am 32:309-322, vii, 2003.
200. Thompson WG, Longstreth GF, Drossman DA, et al: Functional bowel disorders and functional abdominal pain. Gut 45(Suppl 2):II43-II47, 1999.
201. Pare P, Ferrazzi S, Thompson WG, et al: An epidemiological survey of constipation in Canada: Definitions, rates, demographics, and predictors of health care seeking. Am J Gastroenterol 96:3130-3137, 2001.
202. Scott LD, Lester R, Van Thiel DH, Wald A: Pregnancy-related changes in small intestinal myoelectric activity in the rat. Gastroenterology 84:301-305, 1983.
203. Xiao ZL, Pricolo V, Biancani P, Behar J: Role of progesterone signaling in the regulation of G-protein levels in female chronic constipation. Gastroenterology 128:667-675, 2005.
204. Christofides ND, Ghatei MA, Bloom SR, et al: Decreased plasma motilin concentrations in pregnancy. BMJ (Clin Res Ed) 285:1453-1454, 1982.
205. Muller-Lissner SA, Kamm MA, Scarpignato C, Wald A: Myths and misconceptions about chronic constipation. Am J Gastroenterol 100:232-242, 2005.
206. Johanson JF, Sonnenberg A: The prevalence of hemorrhoids and chronic constipation. An epidemiologic study. Gastroenterology 98:380-386, 1990.
207. Medich DS, Fazio VW: Hemorrhoids, anal fissure, and carcinoma of the colon, rectum, and anus during pregnancy. Surg Clin North Am 75:77-88, 1995.
208. Saleeby RG Jr, Rosen L, Stasik JJ, et al: Hemorrhoidectomy during pregnancy: Risk or relief? Dis Colon Rectum 34:260-261, 1991.
209. Cappell MS, Sidhom O: Multicenter, multiyear study of safety and efficacy of flexible sigmoidoscopy during pregnancy in 24 females with follow-up of fetal outcome. Dig Dis Sci 40:472-479, 1995.
210. Cappell MS, Colon VJ, Sidhom OA: A study at 10 medical centers of the safety and efficacy of 48 flexible sigmoidoscopies and 8 colonoscopies during pregnancy with follow-up of fetal outcome and with comparison to control groups. Dig Dis Sci 41:2353-2361, 1996.
211. Cappell MS: The safety and efficacy of gastrointestinal endoscopy during pregnancy. Gastroenterol Clin North Am 27:37-71, 1998.
212. Cappell MS: The fetal safety and clinical efficacy of gastrointestinal endoscopy during pregnancy. Gastroenterol Clin North Am 32:123-179, 2003.
213. Cappell MS: Endoscopy in pregnancy: Risks versus benefits. Nat Clin Pract Gastroenterol Hepatol 2:376-377, 2005.
214. Qureshi WA, Rajan E, Adler DG, et al: ASGE guidelines for endoscopy in pregnant and lactating women. Gastrointest Endosc 61:357-362, 2005.
215. Hogan RB, Ahmad N, Hogan RB III, et al: Video capsule endoscopy detection of jejunal carcinoid in life-threatening hemorrhage, first trimester pregnancy. Gastrointest Endosc 66:205-207, 2007.
216. Storch I, Barkin JS: Contraindications to capsule endoscopy: Do any still exist? Gastrointest Endosc Clin North Am 16:329-336, 2006.

Chapter 50

Diseases of the Liver, Biliary System, and Pancreas

Catherine Williamson, MD, and Lucy Mackillop, BM BCh, MA

Liver disorders may be unique to or commonly associated with pregnancy. Liver disease may precede or develop de novo during pregnancy. Some of these disorders are so uncommon that even an experienced maternal-fetal medicine specialist may rarely encounter them. In this chapter, we review preexisting liver conditions and those that are primarily associated with pregnancy.

Liver Function in Normal Pregnancy

There is no evidence that enlargement of the liver occurs during human gestation. Hepatomegaly should be considered a potential pathologic finding, signifying the need to determine whether underlying liver disease exists. The liver is frequently elevated superiorly, especially in the third trimester as a result of the expanding uterus. There is little evidence that the liver undergoes any major histologic changes during pregnancy. Hepatic blood flow remains constant in pregnancy (i.e., 25% to 33% of cardiac output).

Major changes occur in the serum concentration of plasma proteins during gestation, and these alterations may persist for a few months after delivery. Total serum protein concentration decreases largely because of a 20% to 40% decrease in serum albumin concentration. Some of this may be explained by hemodilution secondary to the increase in total plasma volume associated with pregnancy. Maher and colleagues[1] suggested a reciprocal relationship between rising levels of α-fetoprotein and the decline in serum albumin concentration.

Fibrinogen biosynthesis and manufacture of other coagulation factors (i.e., VII, VIII, IX, and X) are increased in pregnancy and with estrogen administration. Estrogens increase hepatic rough endoplasmic reticulum and accelerate synthesis of proteins. Increased amounts of progesterone lead to proliferation of smooth endoplasmic reticulum and an increase in cytochrome P450 isoenzyme levels. The serum levels of other proteins, such as ceruloplasmin and transferrin, also increase with gestation. The concentrations of specific binding proteins, such as thyroxine-binding globulin (TBG) and corticosteroid-binding globulin (CBG), increase in normal pregnancy, which affects the concentration of the bound portion of these hormones.

This chapter is based upon a similar chapter in the 5th edition, authored by Mark B. Landon, MD.

A prospective, cross-sectional study of 430 women at a single center was carried out to determine the reference ranges for liver function test in uncomplicated pregnancies.[2] The study confirmed that there is a decrease in the upper limit of aspartate transaminase (AST), alanine transaminase (ALT), and γ-glutamyl transferase (GGT) in normal pregnancy (Table 50-1). The investigators[2] also demonstrated a decrease in bilirubin concentration, but this finding has not been demonstrated in other studies.[3]

Total serum alkaline phosphatase (ALP), largely because of placental production, increases dramatically during pregnancy. It may be two to four times baseline by the third trimester, but it returns to normal levels within a few weeks after delivery. Occasionally, the ALP concentration may increase to more than 1000 U/L, and although this is invariably of placental origin, isoenzyme testing may be requested to exclude ALP from liver or bone. Most articles concerning plasma lipids in pregnancy agree that total cholesterol and triglycerides are increased during pregnancy.

Liver function test results change significantly in the puerperium (Table 50-2) and are affected by common obstetric events, such as cesarean section.[4] This can be a confounding factor in clinical interpretation of women recovering from liver-related illnesses after delivery.

Diagnosis of Liver Disease

Hepatomegaly may signify infiltrative disease (e.g., acute fatty liver of pregnancy [AFLP]), an inflammatory condition (e.g., hepatitis), passive congestion (e.g., right-sided heart failure), Budd-Chiari syndrome, or rarely, a malignancy.

Dermatologic findings of chronic liver disease and acute liver failure, such as palmar erythema and spider nevi, are often found in normal pregnancy. Jaundice and scleral icterus are abnormal findings and warrant further evaluation. Causes of jaundice not related to pregnancy are summarized in Table 50-3, with interpretation of serum and urine bilirubin test results.

Imaging of the liver may be required during pregnancy. Ultrasound remains the primary imaging tool because of its safety record in pregnancy, but it may have limited value in assessing liver architecture. Computed tomography (CT) and endoscopic retrograde cholangiopancreatography (ERCP) can also be used during pregnancy. However, precautions should be taken to shield the fetus from radiation or to provide dosimetry estimates if significant exposure is likely. Magnetic

TABLE 50-1 LIVER FUNCTION TEST RESULTS IN NORMAL PREGNANCY

Test	Not Pregnant	First Trimester	Second Trimester	Third Trimester
AST (IU/L)	7-40	10-28	11-29	11-30
ALT (IU/L)	0-40	6-32	6-32	6-32
Bili (μmol/L)	0-17	4-16	3-13	3-14
GGT (IU/L)	11-50	5-37	5-43	5-41
Alk phos (IU/L)	30-130	32-100	43-135	130-418

Alk phos, alkaline phosphatase; ALT, alanine transaminase; AST, aspartate transaminase; Bili, bilirubin; GGT, gamma-glutamyl transferase.
Adapted from Girling JC, Dow E, Smith JH: Liver function tests in pre-eclampsia: Importance of comparison with a reference range derived for normal pregnancy. BJOG 104:246-250, 1997.

TABLE 50-2 LIVER FUNCTION TEST RESULTS AFTER DELIVERY IN NORMAL PREGNANCY

Test	Postnatal Peak (day)	Mean Increase (%)	Range of Increase (%)
AST	2-5	88	0-500
ALT	5	147	0-1140
GGT	5-10	62	0-450
Alk phos	Before delivery	—	—

Alk phos, alkaline phosphatase; ALT, alanine transaminase; AST, aspartate transaminase; GGT, gamma-glutamyl transferase.
Adapted from David AL, Kotecha M, Girling JC: Factors influencing postnatal liver function tests. BJOG 107:1421-1426, 2000.

TABLE 50-3 SERUM AND URINE FINDINGS USED TO DETERMINE THE CAUSE OF JAUNDICE

	Serum Bilirubin		Urine Bilirubin	
Cause of Jaundice	Unconjugated	Conjugated	Bilirubin	Urobilinogen
Hemolysis	↑	N	A	↑
Gilbert syndrome	↑↑	N	A	N/↓
Crigler-Najjar syndrome	↑↑↑	N	A	N/↓
Hepatocellular carcinoma	↑	↑	P	↑/↓/N
Hepatocanalicular injury	↑	↑	P	↑/↓/N
Extrahepatic disorders	N	↑	P	↓/N

A, absent; N, normal; P, present; ↑, increased; ↓, decreased.

resonance imaging (MRI) has the advantage of no radiation exposure, and it has an established safety profile in pregnancy.

Rarely, histologic diagnosis may be essential to management of a pregnant woman, such as when AFLP is being considered in the differential diagnosis and the biopsy is likely to influence the decision to proceed with delivery. The procedure remains safe in expert hands if coagulation parameters are within normal limits.

Liver Disorders Unique to Pregnancy

Intrahepatic Cholestasis of Pregnancy

Epidemiology

Intrahepatic cholestasis of pregnancy (ICP) affects 0.7% of white pregnant women,[5] approximately twice as many South Asian women,[5] and up to 5% of Chilean women.[6] The geographic variation in prevalence of the condition is likely to be explained by genetic and environmental influences, particularly because ICP is seen less frequently in Chile and Scandinavia than it was in the past.[6,7] ICP occurs more frequently in winter months.[7,8] The reasons for these epidemiologic fluctuations is not clear, but they indicate that environmental factors must play a role in the cause of ICP. There have been reports of ICP occurring more commonly in women with multiple gestation[9] and in women older than 35 years.[10] The recurrence rate of ICP varies from 60% to 90% in different populations.[6]

Pathogenesis

The cause of ICP is complex, with genetic, endocrine, and environmental factors playing roles. Evidence for a genetic origin includes the demonstration that parous sisters of affected women have a 20-fold increased risk of developing ICP.[11] This idea is further supported by pedigree studies[12,13] and the demonstration of genetic variation in biliary bile acid receptors and transporters. A few women with ICP have relatively highly penetrant heterozygous mutations in biliary transporters that result in abnormal biliary transport and accumulation of bile acids, which produces a clinical picture of cholestasis. Mutations have been reported in the *ABCB4* and *ATP8B1* genes that encode phospholipid transporters,[14-16] the *ABCB11* gene that encodes the principal bile salt transporter,[17] and the primary hepatic bile acid receptor.[18] Women who carry these mutations do not usually have symptoms when they are not pregnant, but they develop cholestasis in pregnancy.

Evidence that elevated levels of reproductive hormones cause susceptible women to develop cholestasis includes the increased prevalence of ICP in multiple pregnancy[9] and the recurrence of cholestatic symptoms when women who previously had ICP are given exogenous estrogens or the oral contraceptive (OC) pill.[13,19] Progestogens may also play a role; 34 (68%) of 50 women in a French prospective series of OC cases had been treated with oral micronized natural progesterone for risk of premature delivery.[20]

Other environmental factors may influence susceptibility to ICP. Women with hepatitis C infection develop cholestasis more commonly than other pregnant women.[21] Plasma selenium levels were significantly reduced in pregnant women on OCs compared with controls in Finnish[22] and Chilean studies,[23] and it has been proposed that selenium deficiency in women on OCs may contribute to estrogen-induced oxidation damage to hepatocytes.[23] The Chilean study demonstrated that plasma selenium levels have increased in nonpregnant individuals since the 1980s, and the investigators suggested that this may partly explain the reduction in the prevalence of ICP among women on OCs in Chile since then.[23]

The pathogenesis of the symptom of pruritus in ICP is not fully understood. Treatments that have some efficacy in treating cholestasis-related pruritus in nonpregnant patients include anion exchange resins, rifampicin, opiate antagonists, ondansetron, and phototherapy.[24]

Fetal complications that occur more commonly in ICP pregnancies include preterm labor, fetal asphyxial events, meconium staining of amniotic fluid, and intrauterine death. Three studies have demonstrated that ICP patients with higher maternal serum bile acid levels (>40 μmol/L in two studies) more commonly have pregnancies complicated by meconium-stained liquor and fetal asphyxial events,[25-27] and the largest study also demonstrated that patients with higher levels of bile acids had higher rates of spontaneous preterm labor.[27]

The likely pathogenesis of the fetal complications of ICP is related to increased levels of fetal serum bile acids, but the precise mechanisms are not understood. Most stillborn infants are of appropriate weight and have no evidence of uteroplacental insufficiency.[28,29] The evidence suggests that the intrauterine death is a sudden event. Studies have shown an abnormal fetal heart rate[26,30] or arrhythmia[31] in pregnancies complicated by ICP, and in vitro studies of neonatal heart cells indicate that they are susceptible to bile acid–induced arrhythmia.[32] The increased frequency of preterm labor may be a consequence of bile acid–induced release of prostaglandins, which may initiate labor.[33] The increased rates of meconium-stained liquor[27,28,30,34] may be related to fetal distress caused by the toxic effects of bile acids or may be a consequence of bile acids stimulating gut motility.[35]

Diagnosis

ICP should be suspected in pregnant women with pruritus but without a rash. The pruritus is commonly generalized or affects the palms and soles, but it can occur on any part of the body. There is no consensus about the most reliable biochemical test for diagnosing ICP. We recommend measuring levels of liver transaminases and serum bile acids. Because some patients have elevated transaminase levels several weeks before the levels of bile acids are increased, this is a useful screening test. However, there are also cases of ICP with elevated concentrations of serum bile acids and normal levels of liver transaminases. It is therefore advisable to test both.

Cholestasis may also occur in conjunction with other liver diseases. It is advisable to perform a liver ultrasound scan to exclude biliary obstruction. Affected women commonly have gallstones, and this is partly explained by a genetic cause, because some of the genes implicated in ICP are also mutated in pedigrees with familial gallstones.[36] However, the gallstones are unlikely to be the cause of the cholestasis unless the woman has symptoms of biliary obstruction. Other conditions that can be associated with ICP are hepatitis C, autoimmune hepatitis, and primary biliary cirrhosis. These conditions have important implications for the subsequent health of the mother, and it is therefore advisable to screen for them.

Management

MATERNAL DISEASE

Ursodeoxycholic acid (UDCA) is the only drug that has consistently been shown to improve the maternal symptoms and biochemical features of ICP. There have been several reports about the efficacy of UDCA in ICP,[37,38] but there have been few randomized, controlled trials. The largest trial showed that UDCA reduced levels of pruritus, liver transaminases, and bilirubin compared with dexamethasone or placebo and that it was particularly effective in women with serum levels of bile acids higher than 40 μmol/L.[39] UDCA is usually started at a dose of 500 mg twice daily, and the dose may be increased further.

A variety of other drugs have been proposed as treatments for ICP, including dexamethasone, *S*-adenosyl methionine, cholestyramine, and guar gum, but there is less evidence for their efficacy than there is for UDCA.[37] Aqueous cream with menthol may improve the symptoms of ICP, although it does not affect the disease process. It is advisable to give affected women vitamin K because of the theoretical risk of hemorrhage in association with ICP.

FETAL CONCERNS

No treatments have been shown to reduce fetal risks associated with ICP. However, it is likely that treatments that reduce levels of maternal bile acids also reduce fetal risk because of the data that implicate bile acids in pregnancies complicated by spontaneous preterm delivery, fetal asphyxial events, and meconium-stained amniotic fluid.[25-27] None of the UDCA trials has been powered to investigate whether the drug protects the fetus. However, it is known that UDCA treatment improves the serum bile acid levels measured in cord blood and amniotic fluid at the time of delivery.[40] In vitro studies have shown that maternal cholestasis causes impairment of placental bile acid transfer and that this is restored to normal in the placentas of women treated with UDCA.[41] Studies of neonatal rat cardiomyocytes have also shown that pre-incubation of cells in culture medium containing UDCA or dexamethasone protects networks of contracting cells from the arrhythmogenic effect of bile acids.[42]

The only forms of fetal surveillance that have been shown to predict which fetuses may be at risk are amniocentesis[28] and amnioscopy[43] for meconium. However, such an approach is likely to be considered too intrusive to be used routinely by most obstetricians. Many obstetric units review women with ICP several times per week for fetal assessment by electronic fetal monitoring and/or biophysical profile, or both. Although there is no guarantee that this approach can prevent subsequent fetal complications, there are a few reports of abnormal electronic fetal monitoring traces having been identified and emergency cesarean section performed as a consequence. Many women with ICP find this strategy reassuring.

Prevention

The recurrence rate of ICP varies from 40% to 90%.[6] It is not possible to prevent the condition in predisposed women, although it is possible to screen for biochemical abnormalities before symptoms occur. If a woman with a history of ICP requires antibiotics, it is advisable to avoid drugs that more commonly cause cholestasis in susceptible individuals, such as erythromycin, flucloxacillin, and amoxicillin with clavulanic acid. Women with a history of ICP should be advised to use hormonal contraception with care, because there is a 10% chance of developing pruritus or hepatic impairment, or both.[19]

Overlap Syndromes with Liver Dysfunction

Preeclampsia, HELLP syndrome (*h*emolysis, *e*levated *l*iver enzymes, and *l*ow *p*latelets), AFLP, and liver rupture are separate but similar conditions that usually occur during the third trimester and after delivery. They are often characterized by hypertension, elevated levels of liver enzymes, and thrombocytopenia, and resolution usually follows delivery (see Chapter 35). In some cases, however, there may be progressive disease with multisystem organ failure and possibly maternal death. HELLP syndrome is most often a variant of severe preeclampsia because hypertension and proteinuria are generally accompanying features. There is also overlap between AFLP and preeclampsia, which is present in approximately 50% of patients of AFLP.[44,45] It is essential for the clinician to differentiate the overlap syndromes from unrelated conditions, which do not improve after delivery. A multidisciplinary team approach consisting of maternal-fetal medicine and liver specialists is recommended to guide therapy.

Fatty Acid Oxidation Pathways

Disorders of fatty acid β-oxidation play a role in the cause of AFLP, the HELLP syndrome, and preeclampsia. Fatty acids are a major metabolic fuel for humans. In the presence of oxygen, fatty acids are catabolized to carbon dioxide and water, and approximately 40% of the free energy produced in this process is conserved as adenosine triphosphate (ATP). The remainder of the energy is released as heat, a process that occurs in the mitochondria by β-oxidation. This enzymatic process is particularly important for the provision of energy when glycogen stores are depleted. It consists of many transport processes and four enzymic reactions that cause two-carbon fragments to be successively removed from the carboxyl end of the fatty acid, which has been described in detail by Ibdah.[46]

An enzyme that plays a central role in this pathway is long-chain 3-hydroxyacyl-coenzyme A dehydrogenase (LCHAD). It is part of an enzyme complex, the mitochondrial trifunctional protein (MTP), which is located on the inner mitochondrial membrane. In LCHAD deficiency, there is accumulation of long-chain hydroxylacylcarnitines, free plasma hydroxyl-long-chain fatty acids, and dicarboxylic acids, which results in cell toxicity. MTP defects are autosomal recessive conditions that cause nonketotic hypoglycemia and hepatic encephalopathy in early infancy and that may progress to coma and death if untreated. They also can cause cardiomyopathy, peripheral neuropathy, myopathy, and sudden death, although the latter clinical features are not characteristically seen in isolated LCHAD deficiency. It is important to diagnose MTP disorders because the clinical complications can be avoided with dietary manipulation.

Several case series have demonstrated an increased prevalence of AFLP and, to a lesser extent, HELLP syndrome and severe preeclampsia among heterozygous mothers of children that are homozygous for LCHAD deficiency.[46-48] A subsequent study of 27 pregnancies complicated by AFLP demonstrated that 5 had fetuses with MTP mutations and that at least one copy of the common E474Q mutation was present in each case.[49] The study authors recommended that the neonates of women whose pregnancies are complicated by AFLP should be screened for MTP disorders or for the E474Q mutation. Several studies of pregnancies complicated by HELLP syndrome have not demonstrated that MTP disorders are common in the fetuses,[49-51] and therefore screening of these offspring is not recommended.

Maternal liver disease also occurs in pregnancies in which the fetus is affected by a spectrum of fatty acid oxidation disorders, including short-chain and medium-chain defects.[52] In a case-control series of 50 infants from pregnancies complicated by severe maternal liver disease, including AFLP and HELLP syndrome, long-chain defects were 50 times more common in cases than controls, and short-chain and medium-chain defects were 12 times more likely to occur.[52]

Acute Fatty Liver of Pregnancy

Epidemiology

AFLP is a rare, potentially life-threatening, pregnancy-related disease that affects 1 in 7000 to 16,000 pregnancies.[53,54] The condition occurs more commonly in primigravidas, multiple pregnancy, and pregnancies carrying a male fetus.[45,53] In two case series of 32 and 16 affected women admitted to tertiary centers, the maternal mortality rate was 12.5%.[44,45] However, there were no maternal deaths in two other series of 11 and 28 consecutive patients seen in a district hospital in Chile and the United States, respectively.[53,54] Perinatal mortality rates are reported as approximately 10% in the latest series,[44,45,54] although they were higher in another series,[52] and the investigators proposed that this was principally as a consequence of premature delivery.

Pathogenesis

The pathogenesis of AFLP is not well understood. It is clear from the studies described previously above that fatty acid oxidation disorders contribute to approximately 20% of cases.[49] In these cases, it is likely that the heterozygous mother has a reduced hepatic capacity to metabolize long-chain fatty acids. Although there is sufficient capacity in the nonpregnant state, when a heterozygous woman becomes pregnant, her liver is required to metabolize fatty acids from the fetoplacental unit in addition to her own. This increased metabolite load likely results in hepatotoxicity. This may be further compounded by the alternations in lipid metabolism that occur in normal pregnancy.

Diagnosis

AFLP typically manifests in the third trimester with symptoms of nausea, malaise, and anorexia. Later symptoms include vomiting and abdominal pain. Polydipsia and polyuria may also occur.[7,55] Liver function tests should be requested for any pregnant woman reporting these symptoms because quick diagnosis of an acute fatty liver allows stabilization of the patient and rapid delivery.

It is often difficult to differentiate AFLP from HELLP syndrome. Patients with AFLP more commonly have high levels of bilirubin, creatinine, uric acid, and neutrophils; a prolonged prothrombin time; acidosis; and hypoglycemia. Patients frequently have disseminated intravascular coagulation. Although levels of liver transaminases can be markedly increased, they can also be barely higher than normal. The level of ALT or AST should not be taken as a marker of severity of disease, because hepatocytes cannot release transaminases if they have been destroyed by severe injury. Typical biochemical features of AFLP are summarized in Table 50-4.

Imaging modalities that have been used to diagnose AFLP include liver ultrasound, MRI, and CT. A study that compared the three techniques found that CT was the best modality for demonstrating fat in the liver.[56] However, CT was successful in only 50% of cases. Liver biopsy may be used to obtain a definitive diagnosis using an oil red O stain or electron microscopy. However, this is not always practical, particularly if there is a coagulopathy and rapid delivery is required.

TABLE 50-4 BIOCHEMICAL FEATURES OF ACUTE FATTY LIVER OF PREGNANCY

Biochemical Feature*	Average at Diagnosis	Range at Diagnosis	Peak or Nadir
AST (<32 IU/L)	523	120-2317	692
ALT (<32 IU/L)	423	43-1504	493
BR (3-22 μmol/L)	99.18	15-203	180
LDH (<250 IU/L)	1483	244-3992	1709
Glucose (3.9-5.8 mmol/L)	4.5	0.6-8.7	3.1
Creatinine (μmol/L)	212.2	44-389	4950
Platelets (×10^3)	88	33-303	88

*Parenthetical values are average normal values in pregnancy.
ALT, alanine transaminase; AST, aspartate transaminase; BR, bilirubin; LDH, lactate dehydrogenase.
Modified from Fesenmeier MF, Coppage KH, Lambers DS, et al: Acute fatty liver of pregnancy in 3 tertiary care centers. Am J Obstet Gynecol 192:1416-1419, 2005.

There may be a different underlying diagnosis in some women who present with AFLP. In a series of 32 patients seen in a tertiary referral unit in London, 6 had an additional diagnosis. Two patients had malignancy, one had alcohol-induced fatty liver, another had veno-occlusive disease with antiphospholipid syndrome, and another had acute viral hepatitis A infection.[44] Poisoning with acetaminophen can cause a clinical presentation that is hard to distinguish from AFLP.

Management

Women with AFLP should be managed by a multidisciplinary team that includes obstetricians, hepatologists, anesthetists, obstetric physicians, neonatologists, and intensivists. The mother should be cared for in an intensive care setting. Blood should be taken every 6 hours to ensure that biochemical and hematologic abnormalities are diagnosed and corrected. It is essential to monitor the prothrombin time and other markers of coagulopathy, plasma glucose, platelets, creatinine, liver function test results, and arterial blood gases. Fresh-frozen plasma should be given as required. Women often require large amounts of glucose intravenously to correct hypoglycemia. If multisystem failure develops, it may be necessary to use dialysis and ventilation. *N*-Acetylcysteine is often used by liver units to treat AFLP, and we advocate its use.

Women with AFLP should be assessed regularly for encephalopathy. Mild encephalopathy manifests with confusion, fetor hepaticus (i.e., unpleasant breath), and asterixis (i.e., liver flap). A more objective assessment can be performed by asking women to draw a five-pointed star or a clock face. It is advisable to discuss patients who have AFLP with a liver unit specialist at the time of presentation for advice on the detailed management of fulminant liver failure and because assessment of suitability for orthotopic liver transplantation may be necessary.

The most important management strategy is delivery of the infant. The decision about the mode of delivery is often complex because the mother is likely to have a coagulopathy. Although vaginal delivery reduces the risk of hemorrhage, induction of labor often takes longer, and prompt delivery can improve the maternal outcome. Regional anesthesia should be avoided or used with caution and in conjunction with close monitoring. Blood tests should be performed frequently to ensure that coagulopathy is rapidly corrected in the days after delivery. In a series of 28 cases from a U.S. referral center, many of the patients who had operative delivery subsequently had wound separation, which was thought to be related to coagulopathy.[54]

Prevention

AFLP does not commonly recur in subsequent pregnancies, although there are recurrent cases reported in the literature. In women who are heterozygous for disorders of fatty acid oxidation, it may be possible to establish whether the fetus is affected, and this can indicate the magnitude of the mother's risk. If she is carrying a fetus that is homozygous for the disease, she will have a greater chance of recurrence. For heterozygous mothers who do not have affected fetuses and for others who do not have a fatty acid oxidation disorder, the recurrence risk is lower. However, the disease has potentially disastrous consequences, and women who have had one affected pregnancy should be managed in an obstetric clinic specializing in high risk pregnancies. One case series found elevated antithrombin and creatinine levels in women with AFLP several weeks before the onset of clinical symptoms.[54] It can be helpful to monitor the levels of these markers in a subsequent pregnancy of a woman who previously had AFLP.

Preeclampsia and HELLP Syndrome

Liver involvement often signifies the development of severe preeclampsia. Elevation of liver enzyme levels may also occur as an isolated laboratory abnormality or as a component of the HELLP syndrome. Although severe hypertension may be absent in women with HELLP syndrome, in most instances, there is some degree of accompanying hypertension that helps to differentiate this disorder from other diseases. Although there may be overlap between HELLP syndrome and AFLP, isolated serum transaminase elevations in severe preeclampsia rarely exceed 500 U/L. Elevated serum bilirubin levels occur in women with the HELLP syndrome, partly as a consequence of liver damage and partly in response to hemolysis, but bilirubin levels usually are higher in AFLP. Hepatic failure with encephalopathy and coagulopathy are uncommon in preeclampsia and should prompt consideration of a different diagnosis, including fatty liver and other causes of hepatic dysfunction.

Hepatic involvement occurs in approximately 10% of women with severe preeclampsia.[57] Most of these women have only liver enzyme elevations and no epigastric pain. The development of right upper quadrant pain usually signifies liver involvement, and liver function tests should be promptly obtained in this setting. Because the pain likely results from hepatic ischemia, the increased transaminase levels may occur several hours after the onset of pain in a manner similar to cardiac enzymes after a myocardial infarction. Histologic descriptions of hepatic involvement in preeclampsia include periportal hemorrhage, sinusoidal fibrin deposition, and cellular necrosis.[58] The pathophysiologic basis of these findings is likely to include ischemia, although hepatic blood flow primarily depends on the portal venous system.

Women with preeclampsia and liver involvement usually should undergo delivery, although administration of steroids first to promote fetal lung maturity can be undertaken in preterm cases when the maternal condition is otherwise stable. Laboratory abnormalities generally improve within 5 days after delivery, although they may become worse before they resolve. Because HELLP syndrome may develop during the postpartum period in 20% of cases, liver function testing and imaging should be undertaken if abdominal pain, thrombocytopenia, or other clinical features suggesting preeclampsia occur after delivery.

Liver Rupture and Infarction

Epidemiology

Rupture of the liver during pregnancy is a rare but often catastrophic event, with substantial risk for fetal and maternal death.[59] More than 95% of cases during pregnancy involve severe preeclampsia and HELLP syndrome.[44,60] However, liver rupture occurs only in a small proportion of women with preeclampsia. For example, in one series, subcapsular liver hematoma was reported in approximately 1% (4 of 442) of women with HELLP syndrome.[61] Hepatic hematoma and rupture may also occur after uncomplicated pregnancy[62,63] or in association with biliary disease, infection, aneurysm, and hepatic neoplasm.[64]

Pathogenesis

Although the pathogenesis of hepatic rupture remains unclear, subcapsular hemorrhage is a common finding at autopsy in cases of maternal preeclampsia. The right lobe of the liver is affected more commonly than the left. As major hemorrhage might have occurred by the time the patient is seen, there may be minimal or no hypertension. Subcapsular hemorrhage produces stretching of the liver capsule, and significant right upper quadrant pain can result from the distention. If stretching is expanded, rupture will occur. The resultant hemoperitoneum produces peritoneal signs and probable hypovolemic shock.

Diagnosis

Hepatic rupture most often occurs in the setting of HELLP syndrome, and the most common presenting symptoms are right upper quadrant pain, hypertension, and shock. Hypertension may not be present at the time of diagnosis because of hypovolemia, and it may become obvious only after fluid resuscitation. Symptoms that may occur include nausea, vomiting, shoulder pain, and headache.[60] Diagnostic imaging is required to establish a diagnosis.[65] Bedside ultrasonography often demonstrates hemoperitoneum. However, CT or MRI is the preferred technique for visualizing liver hematomas. Imaging is critical before consideration of liver biopsy if the diagnosis is unclear, because liver biopsy is contraindicated for patients with suspected subcapsular hemorrhage. To confirm the presence of intraperitoneal bleeding, paracentesis may occasionally be helpful.

Laboratory evaluation of women with subcapsular hematoma or rupture reveals thrombocytopenia, hypofibrinogenemia, or prolonged prothrombin and partial thromboplastin times. Anemia and hemolysis are present, and levels of bilirubin, lactate dehydrogenase, and liver transaminases are elevated. The differential diagnosis for unruptured liver hematoma includes AFLP, placental abruption with coagulopathy, thrombotic thrombocytopenic purpura, and cholangitis with sepsis.

Management

Conservative management is recommended for an intact hematoma without rupture, particularly if the patient is hemodynamically stable.[65] It is necessary to closely follow these patients in an intensive care setting, with serial imaging studies to define the extent of the subcapsular hemorrhage, its progression, and whether leaking has occurred. Sudden increases in intra-abdominal pressure from coughing or emesis should be avoided, and palpation of the liver should be kept to a minimum.

Management options for hepatic rupture include hepatic resection, hepatic artery ligation, embolization of the hepatic artery and exploration with digital compression of the hepatic artery and portal vein to temporarily arrest the hemorrhage (i.e., Pringle maneuver), and evacuation of hematoma and temporary packing with gauze swabs. When faced with a woman with hepatic rupture, it is likely that surgical exploration by a team skilled in the management of liver trauma will be used to make the diagnosis and for treatment. Fluid replacement, multiple transfusions, and correction of coagulopathy are necessary components in conjunction with an attempt to control the hepatic bleeding. In a patient who is relatively stable, angiography may be attempted while making preparations for potential laparotomy.

Maternal and fetal mortality rates may approach 50% in cases of liver rupture. In a series of seven cases, the four survivors were managed with packing and drainage.[59] The three women undergoing hepatic lobectomy did not survive. In another series of 10 patients, 9 were treated surgically with a combination of stitching of the lesion, omental patching, hepatic artery embolization, and ligation. The 10th patient was dead on arrival at the hospital. Five patients were treated with hepatic artery ligation, and all survived.[66] An analysis of all cases in the English language literature from 1960 to 1997 showed an improvement in maternal mortality over time.[60] This study compared management strategies for 141 cases.[60] However, because of the retrospective nature of the study, it was not possible to conclude which treatment modality was most effective. In many cases, the diagnosis was made at laparotomy, and this group of patients had a high survival rate that might have been related to the aggressive surgical approach. However, the group that received arterial embolization, whether it was performed with or without a laparotomy, also had a better prognosis than other groups.

Death is often caused by massive blood loss and coagulopathy. Patients who survive commonly experience respiratory insufficiency from adult respiratory distress syndrome or pulmonary edema and acute liver failure. Critical care of fluid and respiratory status monitoring (see Chapter 57) are essential, as is ongoing hepatic imaging to be certain that stabilization has occurred.

Liver Infarction

Infarction involving many areas of liver parenchyma may be a feature of severe preeclampsia or HELLP syndrome.[67] Presenting signs usually include abdominal pain and frequently fever. Thrombocytopenia is common, and transaminase levels are frequently very high. CT demonstrates clearly demarcated areas of poor vascularization involving many liver segments. Biopsy of these areas demonstrates hemorrhage and leukocyte infiltration in areas adjacent to hemorrhage. In the setting of HELLP syndrome, many adjacent areas of periportal hemorrhage most likely form these infarcted segments. Improvement after delivery can be expected, even in face of laboratory evidence of severe liver inflammation.

Maternal Disorders Coincidental to Pregnancy

Viral Hepatitis

Viral hepatitis is the most common cause of jaundice during pregnancy.[68] There are six primary subtypes of hepatitis virus: A, B, C, D, E, and G (Table 50-5). The incubation periods vary, and clinical features of acute infection may overlap. The diagnosis ultimately requires specific serologic markers for acute and chronic infection (Tables 50-6 and 50-7; see Table 50-5). The clinical implications of each virus for maternal and fetal or neonatal health vary considerably.

TABLE 50-5 COMPARISON OF VARIOUS FORMS OF VIRAL HEPATITIS

Feature	Hepatitis A	Hepatitis B	Hepatitis C	Hepatitis D	Hepatitis E
Viral type	RNA	DNA	RNA	RNA	RNA
Incubation period	14-50 days	30-180 days	30-160 days	30-180 days	14-63 days
Transmission	Fecal-oral	Parenteral	Parenteral	Parenteral	Fecal-oral
Diagnosis	IgM anti-HAV Ab	HBsAg, anti-HBs, anti-HBc, HBeAg, HBV DNA	Hepatitis C antibody	Delta Ag, IgM-specific Ab	IgM anti-HEV Ab
Carrier risk of chronic infection	0	10-15%	50-85%	Up to 80% when superinfection with Hep D occurs	0
Vertical transmission risk	No	Yes	Yes	Yes	Yes
Vaccination available	Yes	Yes	No	No	No

Ab, antibody; anti-HAV Ab, IgM-specific antibody to hepatitis A; anti-HBc, antibody to hepatitis B core antigen; anti-HBs, antibody to hepatitis B surface antigen; anti-HEV Ab, IgM-specific antibody to hepatitis E; anti-HEV, antibody to hepatitis E virus; HBeAg, hepatitis B e antigen; HBsAg, hepatitis B surface antigen.

TABLE 50-6 INTERPRETATIONS OF SEROLOGIC TESTING IN PATIENTS WITH HEPATITIS B VIRUS INFECTION

HBsAg	HBsAb	HBcAb	HBeAg	HBeAb	Possible Interpretation
–	–	–	–	–	Never infected
+	–	–	–	–	1. Early acute infection 2. Transient (up to 18 days) after vaccination
+	–	IgM	+	–	Acute HBV infection, highly infectious
+	–	IgG	+	–	Chronic HBV infection, highly infectious
+	–	IgG	–	+	Late acute or chronic HBV infection, low infectivity
–	–	IgM	±	±	Acute HBV infection
–	–	IgG	–	±	1. Low-level HBsAg carrier or remote past infection 2. Passive transfer to infant of HBsAg-positive mother
–	+	IgG	–	±	Recovery from HBV infection and immune
–	+	–	–	–	1. Immune if concentration ≥10 mIU/mL 2. Passive transfer after hepatitis B immune globulin

HBcAb, hepatitis B core antibody; HBeAb, hepatitis B e antibody; HBeAg, hepatitis B e antigen; HBsAb, hepatitis B surface antibody; HBsAg, hepatitis B surface antigen; HBV, hepatitis B virus; IgG, immunoglobulin G; IgM, immunoglobulin M; –, negative; +, positive; ±, equivocal.

The maternal management of viral hepatitis is not altered greatly by pregnancy. Supportive therapy is usually sufficient, although some cases of certain viral subtypes may lead to progressive liver failure. Hepatitis A and B remain the most common viruses responsible for acute hepatitis in pregnancy in North America and Europe. Infection during the third trimester is most common. There is evidence that infection with hepatitis E during pregnancy, which is rare in the United States, can lead to acute liver failure, and this is associated with high mortality rates.[69] The severity of infection with viruses A through D is not influenced by gestation. Prematurity and perinatal death are uncommon, but their rates are slightly increased over background rates for the general population. In contrast, miscarriage, fetal intrauterine growth restriction, and congenital malformation rates are not increased.

Hepatitis A

Hepatitis A virus (HAV) is a major cause of acute hepatitis in the United States. The virus is a ubiquitous RNA picornavirus, which is primarily transmitted from person to person through fecal-oral contamination, facilitated by poor hygiene and poor sanitation, resulting in contaminated food and water. The disease is more common among immigrants, drug users, and homosexual men.[70]

The incubation period of HAV ranges from 14 to 50 days and is followed by the nonspecific symptoms of malaise, headache, fatigue, anorexia, nausea, vomiting, and diarrhea. Cholestasis shortly follows with jaundice, acholic stools, and dark urine. Some patients, especially children, may be asymptomatic and therefore represent a key group who has a role in transmission of infection.

The diagnostic test most commonly used is an IgM-specific antibody to HAV. The presence of IgG antibody to HAV indicates postinfection status and immunity. In developing countries with poor sanitation, childhood infection is common and therefore acute HAV infection is uncommon in adult populations. In the United States, seasonal variation and an increasing frequency in adults have been observed. IgM antibody is detectable 1 month after exposure and may persist for as long as 6 months. IgG antibody to HAV appears within 35 to 40 days of exposure and signifies lifelong immunity.

Acute HAV infection rarely requires more than general supportive care. Hepatitis A is a self-limited disease without the chronic process that complicates other viral hepatitis infections, and recovery follows typically within 4 to 6 weeks. HAV infection has been associated with an increased risk for complications such as threatened preterm labor and preterm rupture of membranes.[71] Only 1 in 10,000 patients has a severe or aggressive course.[72] These individuals may require intensive care for treatment of coagulopathy and encephalopathy.

HAV is excreted in large amounts in stool before the onset of symptoms of jaundice. Affected patients should be advised of their potential

TABLE 50-7 HEPATITIS B VACCINATION RECOMMENDATIONS

Maternal HBsAg Testing
All pregnant women should be tested routinely for HBsAg.

Vaccination of Infants
At Birth
Infants born to HBsAg-positive mothers should receive hepatitis B vaccine and HBIG within ≤12 hours of birth.
Infants who are born to mothers whose HBsAg status is unknown should receive hepatitis B vaccine within ≤12 hours of birth.
Term infants ≥2000 g at birth and medically stable who are born to HBsAg-negative mothers should receive hepatitis B vaccine before hospital discharge.
Preterm infants ≤2000 g at birth who are born to HBsAg-negative mothers should receive their first dose of hepatitis B vaccine 1 month after birth.

After the Birth Vaccination
All infants should complete the hepatitis B vaccine series.
Infants born to HBsAg-positive mothers should be tested for HBsAg and HBsAb after completion of the hepatitis B vaccine series at age 9 to 18 months.

HBIG, hepatitis B immune globulin; HBsAb, hepatitis B surface antibody; HBsAg, hepatitis B surface antigen.
Adapted from Centers for Disease Control and Prevention (CDC): A comprehensive immunization strategy to eliminate transmission of hepatitis B virus infection in the United States. MMWR Morb Mortal Wkly Rep 54(RR16):1-23, 2005.

risk for transmission. For short-term protection, immune globulin (IG) is used prophylactically and after exposure. Pregnant women embarking on travel to endemic areas should be screened for immunity to HAV, and if IgG negative, they should receive vaccination because it appears safe for use in pregnancy.[72]

Perinatal transmission of HAV is rare. In such cases, fecal contamination occurs when maternal incubation coincides with delivery. Infants of mothers manifesting acute hepatitis A should receive IG to prevent horizontal transmission. Although not licensed for children younger than 2 years, vaccination appears to be efficacious in small studies of this age group.[72] Breastfeeding is not contraindicated, and the HAV vaccine is safe for lactating mothers.

Hepatitis B

Hepatitis B virus (HBV) infection is a worldwide health problem, and it is most prevalent in Asia, Southern Europe, and Latin America. Prevalence of hepatitis B surface antigen (HBsAg) carriers in the general population is 2% to 20%. HBV accounts for 40% to 45% of all cases of hepatitis in the United States.[73,74] Acute HBV infection occurs in 1 or 2 per 1000 pregnancies.[75] In the United States each year, approximately 20,000 infants are delivered of HBsAg-positive women.[76] Infection with HBV in infancy or early childhood may lead to a high rate of chronic infection. In most endemic areas, infection occurs mainly during infancy, and early childhood and mother-to-infant transmission accounts for approximately 50% of the chronic infection cases. The high risk of vertical transmission from carrier pregnant women to their offspring and its potential prevention by screening and immunization are areas of special interest to the practicing obstetrician and maternal-fetal specialist.

ACUTE HEPATITIS B

HBV is a DNA virus with three major structural antigens: HBsAg, core antigen (HBcAg), and e antigen (HBeAg) (see Table 50-6). The core antigen is present only in the hepatocytes and does not circulate in the serum. The intact virus is known as the Dane particle. Transmission occurs principally through parenteral drug use, during sexual intercourse, and vertically after perinatal exposure. The peak prevalence of disease occurs in the reproductive age group, and for females, heterosexual contact represents the most common method of infection. Population groups at increased risk include drug addicts, transfusion recipients, dialysis patients, and non-Hispanic blacks.[74]

Onset of the acute disease is usually insidious, with infants and young children typically asymptomatic. When present, clinical symptoms and signs include anorexia, malaise, nausea, vomiting, abdominal pain, and jaundice. Patients also may have rashes, arthralgias, and arthritis.

HBsAg is found in blood 2 to 8 weeks before the development of symptoms or laboratory abnormalities. Serum HBsAg usually remains detectable until the convalescent phase. HBeAg becomes detectable after HBsAg and indicates a high viral inoculum and viral replication. The diagnosis of acute hepatitis B requires the detection of surface antigen and IgM antibody to the core antigen (IgM HBcAb). Identification of IgM HBcAb is important because certain individuals with fulminant acute hepatitis B may experience a period when HBsAg is not easily detectable. Clinical recovery is accompanied by clearance of HBV DNA followed by HBeAg and HBsAg antigenemia within 1 to 3 months, along with the presence of IgG HBcAb and antibody to HBeAg (HBeAb). The presence of HBeAb indicates recovery, clearance of the virus, and immunity.

CHRONIC CARRIER STATE

Chronic infection occurs in approximately 90% of infected infants, 30% of infected children younger than 5 years, and less than 5% of infected persons older than 5 years.[77] Of these chronically infected people, 15% to 30% develop chronic acute hepatitis or cirrhosis, and a small but significant group eventually develops hepatocellular carcinoma. Chronic infection is more likely in those who remain HBeAg positive or become superinfected with hepatitis D.[73] Other factors associated with the chronic carrier state include infection early in life, symptomless infection, immunosuppression, Asian background, and Down syndrome.

Liver damage is related primarily to immunologic events. Cytotoxic T-cell destruction of infected hepatocytes manifesting core antigen results in massive liver injury over time. Exacerbations of inflammatory activity follow viral replication and mirror the load of HBV DNA detectable in serum.

PERINATAL ASPECTS OF HEPATITIS B

Pregnancy does not increase maternal morbidity or mortality from HBV or the risk of fetal complications such as fetal death or congenital abnormalities. However, spontaneous abortions in the first trimester and preterm labor in the third trimester have been increased among mothers with acute HBV infection, although the rates may be no higher than those for other febrile illnesses.[78]

Women with chronic HBV infection who become pregnant while on therapy can continue treatment, but the stage of the mother's liver disease and the potential benefit of treatment must be weighed against the small risk to the fetus. Lamivudine has been classified as a category C drug by the U.S. Food and Drug Administration (FDA), and it is not recommended in the first trimester. Lamivudine crosses the placenta freely and can be found in breast milk in equivalent concentrations to those of the mother's serum. Interferon α (IFN-α) does not cross the placenta, but it is a FDA category C drug, and its use must be carefully considered in pregnancy.

In most cases, the principal concern is potential transmission of the virus to contacts and the fetus during pregnancy and delivery. The age at which HBV infection occurs is an important factor affecting outcome. Without neonatal immunoprophylaxis, perinatal transmission occurs from 70% to 90% of individuals positive for HBsAg and HBeAg, but this high rate is reduced to less than 10% of infants born to HBsAg-positive, HbeAg-negative women.[79] This compares with 5% to 10% of individuals infected in adulthood. High viral loads and coinfection with human immunodeficiency virus (HIV) are additional risk factors for vertical transmission. The presence of HBeAg beyond the second month of life denotes likely chronic carriage. The risk of becoming a chronic carrier is independent of gestational age, birth weight, and viral subtype.

In patients with acute HBV infection, the frequency of transmission depends on gestation, with 10% of neonates becoming infected if infection occurs in the first trimester, increasing to 80% to 90% if infected in the third trimester.[77] Transmission during labor and birth likely results from the mixing of maternal and fetal blood and contact with infected cervicovaginal secretions and amniotic fluid. Transplacental transmission may occur and explains some failures of immunoprophylaxis.[80] Delivery by cesarean and avoidance of breastfeeding do not prevent infection of the newborn.

Women who present in labor with unknown HBsAg status should be considered potentially infectious until serologic testing confirms otherwise. In the absence of known natural serologic status, some institutions have used neonatal combined immunoprophylaxis as a cautionary approach.

PREVENTION AND TREATMENT

The American College of Obstetricians and Gynecologists (ACOG) and the Centers for Disease Control and Prevention (CDC)[76] continue to endorse universal prenatal screening for hepatitis B. This strategy has been deemed cost-saving in identifying 20,000 HBsAg-positive women and preventing 3000 chronically infected neonates per year in the United States. High-risk status, including admitted intravenous drug use and prostitution, may identify no more than 50% of infected women. Screening is performed at the first prenatal visit; however, testing should be repeated later in pregnancy and after delivery in seronegative mothers at high risk.[81]

A combination of passive and active immunization can effectively prevent most cases of horizontal and vertical transmission of hepatitis B. Individuals who have had household or sexual contact with infected individuals should undergo serologic testing to determine their immune status. If they are found to be seronegative, hepatitis B immune globulin (HBIG) in addition to hepatitis B vaccination may be given. HBIG is also recommended for the neonate immediately after birth; the hepatitis B vaccination series is then instituted within 12 hours of birth (see Table 50-7). This vaccine is composed of inactivated portions of the surface antigen manufactured by recombinant DNA technology. The strategy of neonatal immunoprophylaxis is between 85% and 95% effective in preventing neonatal hepatitis B infection.[82]

Despite recommendations for maternal screening and newborn immunoprophylaxis, approximately 10% of neonates of infected mothers fail to receive HBIG and vaccination after birth.[76] Each institution should provide a systematic review of maternal hepatitis B status. Postimmunization testing is important for high-risk groups likely to have carriers within a household. The CDC has recommended universal hepatitis B vaccination for all infants.[81] Testing is recommended at 12 months to ensure presence of antibodies to HBsAg. The detection of IgM anti-HBc suggests recent infection, whereas maternal IgG anti-HBc may persist beyond 12 months. Immunization failures are thought to result from a genetically predetermined response, in utero infection, immunosuppression (e.g., from intercurrent HIV infection), other diseases, or the emergence of antibody escape variants of HBV.[83]

MEDICAL PERSONNEL CONCERNS

Health care workers may acquire hepatitis B infection from patients. Approximately 380,000 American hospital-based workers sustain percutaneous injury each year.[84] Transmission of HBV, HCV, and HIV is well described, and it is estimated that percutaneous injuries account for up to 37% of HBV infections among health care workers.[85] Prevention of these infections is promoted by vaccination of health care workers, vaccination of individuals at high risk for contracting hepatitis B, and following universal precautions about sharp objects and handling of body fluids. Testing for antibodies to HBsAg (HBsAb) approximately 1 month after the third vaccine dose is advisable, because poor responders account for 20% of vaccinated individuals. Levels of HBsAb decline greatly over time; however, immunocompetence is demonstrated in most individuals by an appropriate increase in antibody to an antigen challenge (i.e., immune memory). The minimum level of protective anti-HBs is unknown. Individuals who are poor responders to vaccination should receive HBIG after an exposure.

Infected health care workers may pose a risk to patients by transmitting HBV during invasive procedures. If a patient does not have immunity to hepatitis B, an infected health care worker is obligated to inform the patient about the possibility of transmission of the virus if blood-to-blood exposure occurs. After consent is obtained, great care and caution should be used to prevent any sharp injury.

Hepatitis C

Hepatitis C virus (HCV) infection affects more than 1% of the world population and approximately 4 million individuals in the United States, where it is the leading cause of chronic liver disease. The prevalence of HCV infection among pregnant women varies from 1% to 5%, with the highest rates of infection found in urban populations.[86]

Because HCV is blood-borne, it is more common among intravenous drug users and individuals who have received many transfusions. Sexual and vertical transmission may be alternative modes of transmission. Blood transfusion donors have been routinely tested for HCV since 1990, and the risk of HCV infection is less than 1 case per million screened units of blood. The disease has a peak incidence in people between the ages of 30 and 49 years; however, a large percentage of those affected report no risk factors. Only 24% of infected pregnant women gave a history of receiving blood products, and a similar percentage (27%) denied transfusion or intravenous drug use.[87,88]

Acute HCV infection has an incubation period of 14 to 180 days. Seventy-five percent of acute cases are asymptomatic, and this means that only 25% to 30% of infected individuals are diagnosed.[89] However, the data suggest that 80% of infected patients will develop chronic liver disease with biochemical evidence of liver dysfunction, 35% will develop cirrhosis, and 5% will progress to hepatocellular carcinoma.[90,91] HCV infection follows an indolent course in most patients, and the average time is 10 years to significant hepatitis, 20 years to cirrhosis, and 30 years to hepatocellular carcinoma. This course may be altered and accelerated by coinfection with HIV.

The diagnosis of HCV infection relies on the identification of anti-hepatitis C antibody. Initial screening consists of an enzyme

TABLE 50-8 DEFINITIONS OF HEPATITIS C VIRUS INFECTIONS

Type of Infection	Status of Patient
HCV	HCV Ab positive
Chronic HCV	HCV Ab positive and HCV RNA positive for 6 months
Chronic active HCV	HCV Ab positive and HCV RNA positive for 6 months and abnormal liver function test results

Ab, antibody; HCV, hepatitis C virus.

immunoassay. Confirmation is then obtained through a recombinant immunoblot assay against four specific viral antigens. Antibody may not be present until 4 to 5 months after acute infection. The presence of antibody does not differentiate acute from chronic disease or determine the extent of viremia. Branched-chain DNA and reverse-transcriptase polymerase chain reaction assays may be used to quantify HCV RNA and viral loads (Table 50-8).

PREGNANCY CONCERNS

There is no evidence that HCV infection affects fertility. The indolent nature of the disease, with the peak incidence occurring in the childbearing-age group, makes potential HCV infection a primary concern for the obstetrician. Pregnancy does not appear to affect the clinical course of acute or chronic hepatitis C, and there appears to be no increased risk for adverse pregnancy outcomes among HCV-infected women; specifically, there is no increased risk of miscarriage, preterm delivery, or increased obstetric intervention.[92] Vertical transmission of HCV may occur, although less frequently than HBV infection. However, the diagnosis of vertical transmission is not a straightforward one. Many infants born to HCV-infected mothers are found to have passively acquired transplacental IgG antibodies for up to 18 months of life, making antibody testing of the newborn of little value. Diagnosis can be reliably established by a positive HCV RNA identification on two occasions 3 to 4 months apart after the infant is at least 2 months old and by detection of anti-HCV antibodies after the infant is 18 months old.[93]

Overall, the risk of perinatal transmission is approximately 5%.[94,95] HIV coinfection, drug abuse, and high HCV viral loads are associated with an increased risk of perinatal transmission.[96,97] In a review of 383 cases of vertical transmission,[98] weighted transmission rates were calculated to adjust for sample size and variance. For a mother who was HCV antibody positive but RNA negative, the vertical transmission rate was 1.7%, compared with 4.3% for an RNA-positive mother, and this increased to 36% in another study if titers were more than 10^6 copies/mL.[99] Vertical transmission rates were higher (19.4%) for RNA-positive mothers coinfected with HIV. There is some evidence that treatment of HIV infection with highly active antiretroviral therapy (HAART) during pregnancy reduces the risk of HCV vertical transmission.

PREGNANCY MANAGEMENT

There is no contraindication to pregnancy in HCV-infected women. The risk of perinatal infection must be discussed and the extent of maternal disease considered before making recommendations. IFN-α and pegylated interferon in combination with oral ribavirin may ameliorate disease and are being used as first-line therapy for chronically infected individuals. IFN-α does not cross the placenta, but it is a category C drug, and its use must be carefully considered in pregnancy. Ribavirin is a category X drug and should not be used in pregnant women, women attempting to become pregnant, or their male partners because of its risk of teratogenicity.

There is no association between mother-to-infant transmission and gestational age,[100] but prolonged rupture of membranes (>6 hours) may increase the risk of transmission.[93] There is conflicting evidence about whether the practice of using fetal scalp electrodes increases the risk of transmission, and this practice is discouraged.[78]

There appears to be no benefit in cesarean delivery to prevent vertical transmission in HIV-negative, HVC-positive women. Gibb and colleagues[101] reported an overall transmission rate of 6.7%, with no cases of perinatal transmission in 31 elective cesarean sections. A large study of 275 HCV-positive women[94] found no difference in vertical transmission rates (4% vaginal versus 6% cesarean). Breastfeeding is not considered a risk factor for vertical transmission.

There is no vaccine available for HCV. Whereas passive immunization with immunoglobulin is recommended after percutaneous exposure, immunoprophylaxis of the newborn has not been beneficial in clinical trials.

Hepatitis D

Hepatitis D is an RNA virus that depends on the hepatitis B virus for replication and expression. HDV infection is found only as a simultaneous (coinfection) acute infection acquired with HBV or as a superinfection in an individual who is a chronic HBV carrier. Epidemiologic features of hepatitis D are similar to those for hepatitis B.

Coinfection with HBV is generally self-limited and carries a similar risk of progression to chronic liver disease as isolated acute hepatitis B infection. However, superinfection with hepatitis D is associated with an 80% progression to chronic hepatitis. Superinfection ultimately occurs in 25% of chronic HBV carriers. Those who develop chronic hepatitis have a 75% to 80% risk of cirrhosis with potential for liver failure. HDV is transmitted by blood and blood products, and the risk factors for infection are similar to those for HBV.

The diagnosis of acute coinfection is confirmed by the presence of delta antigen or IgM-specific antibody in sera of an individual demonstrating HBsAg and core antigen IgM. Superinfection is marked by delta antigen or IgM to HDV and positive hepatitis B core antigen IgG, indicating chronic hepatitis B infection.

Women with acute hepatitis D are managed supportively as with acute hepatitis of other causes. Those with chronic infection require monitoring of liver function, including coagulation parameters. Perinatal transmission of HDV has been reported[102]; however, active measures to prevent transmission of HBV to the neonate can prevent HDV transmission.

Hepatitis E

The hepatitis E virus (HEV) is an RNA virus found most frequently in Asia, Africa, and South America. It is similar to hepatitis A in that it is transmitted by the fecal-oral route and does not progress to chronicity. The incubation period is 2 to 9 weeks, with an average of 45 days.[103] In the nonpregnant person, HEV infection is usually self-limiting and mild. However, pregnancy seems to be associated with an increased risk of contracting the virus, which leads to a particularly poor outcome. Acute liver failure has been reported for approximately 20% of pregnant women with acute HEV infection, and mortality rates in these cases are 10% to 20%.[104,105] The incidence of acute liver failure due to HEV infection increases with advancing gestation and is most common during the third trimester. HEV-associated acute liver failure is associated with significant obstetric complications such as antepartum hemorrhage, intrauterine death, poor fetal outcome, and preterm delivery.[69]

Diagnosis of hepatitis E relies on identification of IgM antibody to HEV in the sera of infected individuals. Women with HEV infection may require intensive care if liver failure develops. Although perinatal transmission is uncommon, it has been reported and may be associated with biochemical evidence of liver injury, hypoglycemia, and neonatal death.[106] Precautions should be taken when caring for infected women to minimize contact with infected feces and contaminated clothing.

Hepatitis G

Hepatitis G virus (HGV) is a single-stranded RNA flavivirus that was first described in the 1960s. Although it is found in approximately 1% of blood donors in the United States and persistent viremia is common, clinical disease and chronic hepatitis rarely occur. There are scarce data about this disease in pregnancy; however, a few case reports have documented vertical transmission.

Other Hepatic Viruses

Primary herpes simplex virus (HSV) infection is a rare cause of hepatitis in pregnancy, but it may lead to severe maternal illness and may be associated with transplacental virus transmission with consequences such as abortion, stillbirth, and congenital malformations.[107] Maternal and perinatal mortality rates of 39% have been reported for HSV hepatitis during pregnancy.[108] A high index of suspicion is warranted when disseminated maternal herpes simplex infection is present because typical mucocutaneous lesions and jaundice may be absent in affected patients. Antiviral therapy with acyclovir may be used in affected patients.[106]

Primary cytomegalovirus (CMV) infections affect 1% to 4% of seronegative women during pregnancy, and the risk of transmission to the fetus is 30% to 40%.[109] Acute CMV infection in pregnancy is usually asymptomatic. However, it may cause maternal hepatitis, and it is the most common viral cause of congenital infection that is associated with hearing loss and neurodevelopmental disability in the neonate.[110] CMV hepatitis is more common in individuals with advanced HIV infection and transplant recipients. Serious CMV infections, including hepatitis, are treated with intravenous ganciclovir. There are few data regarding the use of this medication during pregnancy, and it is unknown whether maternal treatment prevents fetal infection. Similarly, data are sparse regarding the safety of phosphonoformate (foscarnet), another drug used to treat severe CMV infections. No vaccine is available, and prevention includes hygienic measures such as hand washing after contact with saliva or urine.

Hepatitis is a well-described feature of Epstein-Barr virus infection (i.e., mononucleosis). Most cases are self-limited, although liver failure may occasionally follow infection.

Human Immunodeficiency Virus Infection

Liver disease is common in patients with advanced HIV infection and acquired immunodeficiency syndrome (AIDS) (see Chapter 38). Liver abnormalities may follow drug-induced hepatotoxicity with HIV drugs such as nevirapine and with the concomitant use of the antituberculosis drugs isoniazid and trimethoprim-sulfamethoxazole for the treatment of *Pneumocystis jiroveci* (formerly *Pneumocystis carinii*) infection. Acute and chronic hepatitis may be caused by common etiologic agents and by herpes viruses. Opportunistic and fungal infections may lead to inflammation and obstruction of the biliary tract, cholestasis, and right upper quadrant pain. Potential agents include *Cryptosporidium*, CMV, toxoplasmosis, *Cryptococcus*, histoplasmosis, and *Mycobacterium* species. Intrahepatic neoplasms most likely associated with HIV infection include non-Hodgkin lymphoma and Kaposi sarcoma.

The clinical presentation of most liver diseases in women with HIV infection is nonspecific. Fever, hepatomegaly, right upper quadrant pain, and biochemical abnormalities consistent with cholestasis are typical features. Viral loads (RNA levels) usually are high in such cases. Imaging studies are valuable in differentiating HIV-related processes from other causes of cholestatic jaundice. To avoid irradiation of the fetus, ultrasound or MRI is preferable to CT. Liver biopsy may be valuable in securing tissue for culture and diagnosis.

Chronic Liver Disease in Pregnancy

Chronic Nonviral Hepatitis

Chronic nonviral hepatitis may result from a variety of autoimmune conditions, alcoholism, and drug- or toxin-induced injury. Most cases of chronic nonviral hepatitis in reproductive-age women result from autoimmune disease. Autoantibodies to smooth muscle and liver-specific proteins are present, as are antinuclear antibodies in most cases.

Amenorrhea and infertility are common in affected women, but treatment with immunosuppressive regimens commonly stalls progression of disease and results in renewed fertility. The most commonly used immunosuppressive agents are prednisolone and azathioprine, although cyclosporin and tacrolimus may also be used.[111] If disease activity is well controlled, most women have a good prognosis for pregnancy. However, approximately 30% of cases have a flare of the disease after delivery.[111] A review of 101 pregnancies in 58 women with autoimmune hepatitis reported a perinatal mortality rate of 4%,[112] and a subsequent study of 63 pregnancies in 35 Scandinavian women reported one stillbirth and one infant who died of severe liver disease soon after delivery.[111] Rates of prematurity and fetal growth restriction are higher than in the general population, although congenital malformation rates are not. Flares in some women are related to stopping treatment. Given the reassuring data available related to the use of azathioprine[113] in pregnancy and breastfeeding,[114] women with autoimmune hepatitis should continue treatment because the risk of a flare outweighs the potential risk from treatment.

Primary Biliary Cirrhosis

Primary biliary cirrhosis is an autoimmune liver disease that is characterized by the presence of antimitochondrial antibodies. It occurs more commonly in women and classically manifests at a later age than autoimmune hepatitis. Data about the disease in pregnancy are limited.

Affected women commonly have pruritus with elevated serum levels of bile acids in addition to cholestatic hepatic impairment, and it is reasonable to anticipate that the fetal risks related to increased concentrations of bile acids will be the same as in ICP. Primary biliary cirrhosis is treated with UDCA or cholestyramine. Both drugs should be continued in pregnancy if their use is associated with an improvement in the maternal disease. However, cholestyramine binds fat-soluble vitamins, and vitamin K supplementation should be given. Fetal surveillance strategies should be the same as for ICP.

Primary Sclerosing Cholangitis

Primary sclerosing cholangitis (PSC) is a chronic cholestatic disease of unknown origin that is characterized by fibrosis and inflammation of the intrahepatic and extrahepatic bile ducts. The disorder follows a progressive course, leading to biliary cirrhosis, hepatic failure, and ultimately, death. Affected individuals are also at risk for the development of cholangiocarcinoma. PSC usually occurs in patients with ulcerative colitis and to a lesser extent in those with Crohn disease. In most cases, the onset of inflammatory bowel disease precedes the development of PSC. The cause of PSC remains obscure, but the disorder may have an immunologic basis.

The diagnosis of PSC is based on clinical, laboratory, and histology findings and includes a characteristic cholangiographic appearance of diffuse irregularity and narrowing of the hepatic bile ducts. Pruritus, jaundice, and abdominal pain are typical clinical features. Itching usually is severe enough to require UDCA or other therapies. Favorable pregnancy outcomes have been reported for women with PSC.[115,116] In one series of 13 pregnancies, including three women with onset of PSC during gestation, no significant maternal or neonatal morbidity was observed.[116] Individual case reports have detailed variable courses for PSC during pregnancy. In one report, the cholestatic process paradoxically improved with advancing gestation, followed by a decline in hepatic function after delivery.[115] Other reports have described deterioration of liver function[117] and the need for transplantation during pregnancy.[118] Severe elevations in fetal bile acid levels have been documented, indicating placental transfer.[115] Meconium passage is common, and fetal surveillance is recommended for maternal PSC in the same way as for patients with ICP.

Wilson Disease

Wilson disease is a rare disorder of copper metabolism characterized by liver failure and neurologic dysfunction. Kayser-Fleischer corneal rings are a hallmark of diagnosis; however, they may be absent in patients with liver disease. Levels of ceruloplasmin are depressed in Wilson disease but may increase to normal with advanced liver disease. The diagnosis must be considered in reproductive-age women presenting with advanced liver disease of unknown origin.

Treatment of Wilson disease consists primarily of penicillamine or trientine, both of which are well tolerated during pregnancy and should be continued. Deterioration in hepatic function may occur if these medications are abruptly discontinued.[119] Several series have reported successful pregnancies in women with treated Wilson disease.[120-122] The drug crosses the placenta and may result in copper deficiency in the fetus. Most women with Wilson disease are treated with lower doses than those used to treat cystinuria and from which the data on teratogenicity were derived.

Budd-Chiari Syndrome

Budd-Chiari syndrome is a rare disorder primarily of women that results from hepatic vein occlusion, which has been linked to pregnancy and oral contraceptive use.[123] In one series, almost 15% of cases were associated with pregnancy.[123] The disease may present acutely with obstruction of major hepatic veins or may be chronic and marked by involvement of smaller interlobular veins. The chronic variety is associated with a better prognosis. Both varieties produce congestion and necrosis of centrilobular areas of the liver.[124] Large-vein obstruction is often associated with pregnancy and preeclampsia.[125] Some have suggested that Budd-Chiari syndrome complicating pregnancy is associated with thrombophilias, including antiphospholipid antibodies and factor V Leiden mutation.[126,127]

The disorder manifests with abdominal pain, distention, and ascites. Ascitic fluid has a high protein content. Some patients have fever, nausea, vomiting, and jaundice. Laboratory evaluation shows marked elevation of the alkaline phosphatase level beyond that of normal pregnancy levels. Concentrations of liver enzymes are modestly elevated. The results of histologic examination are nonspecific, demonstrating centrilobular zonal congestion with hemorrhage and necrosis. Diagnosis can be achieved by pulsed-wave Doppler imaging demonstrating the direction and amplitude of flow. Percutaneous hepatic venous catheterization can demonstrate elevated hepatic vein pressures, venous occlusion, and collateral circulation. MRI may also aid in the diagnosis.[125]

Women who develop acute major venous obstruction often deteriorate rapidly, with portal hypertension, variceal bleeding, and fulminant hepatic failure. Pregnancy outcome depends on maternal status. Porta caval shunting may improve portal hypertension and ascites, although many pregnant women are not surgically stable enough to undergo this procedure. These procedures have been primarily accomplished in postpartum cases. There are reports of successful pregnancies after mesocaval shunting.[128] Patients developing Budd-Chiari syndrome should be evaluated for underlying thrombophilias. Even in the absence of such disorders, treatment with anticoagulation is advised, although therapy does not eliminate the risk of recurrent thrombosis.

Cirrhosis

Pregnancy in women with cirrhosis is uncommon because most of these women experience oligomenorrhea and infertility. Nonetheless, there have been considerable reports of end-stage liver disease coexisting with pregnancy. It is doubtful that any single institution or maternal-fetal specialist has managed a large number of such cases. Many of the series in the literature are 25 years or older.

Cirrhosis is associated with an increased risk for premature delivery and perinatal mortality. In a series of 95 pregnancies in 78 women with cirrhosis, 10 stillbirths were observed, and no significant change in liver function occurred in two thirds of the women.[129] Prematurity (20% risk) and need for early termination (18% risk) have also been reported.[130] Maternal complications associated with cirrhosis include anemia, preeclampsia, postpartum hemorrhage, and bleeding from esophageal varices.[130]

Bleeding from esophageal varices remains the most feared complication of cirrhosis and pregnancy. Esophageal bleeding is a cause of maternal death. Bleeding occurred in 18 of 23 women with known esophageal varices in an older series.[131] Portal decompression procedures were used successfully in several cases without adverse maternal-fetal effects. The risk for variceal bleeding is thought to increase as pregnancy advances because of increased circulating blood volume, elevation in portal pressure, and vena cava compression resulting in enhanced flow through the azygos venous system. Most bleeds occur during the second and third trimesters, with some occurring in the postpartum period. The likelihood of bleeding may be decreased in individuals who have undergone portal caval decompression procedures before pregnancy. In a study that aimed to address this topic, only one death occurred among 21 women who had undergone previous portosystemic shunting, and it was caused by hepatic coma in the postpartum period.[130] It follows that the pregnant woman with cirrhosis must be evaluated endoscopically for varices and appropriate treatment undertaken (see the Portal Hypertension section).

Because most women with cirrhosis have uncomplicated pregnancies, careful monitoring should allow progression to term. Nutritional intervention such as limiting protein intake is advised only in advanced cases and after surgical portal decompression. Maneuvers to reduce straining and thereby portal pressure are advised if varices have been documented. Vaginal delivery is the preferred route of delivery, with an attempt to shorten the second stage by forceps or vacuum extraction to limit excessive pushing and increases in intra-abdominal pressure. The pharmacokinetics and metabolism of anesthetic agents must be carefully considered. Postpartum bleeding may be increased, and vitamin K, fresh-frozen plasma, and platelets should be available.

Portal Hypertension

Although studies indicate that the pregnant woman with cirrhosis will most often have an uncomplicated pregnancy, the substantial risk of hemorrhage from bleeding varices must be emphasized to the patient and her family. The death rate for pregnant women with cirrhosis ranges from 10% to 18%, with most of these cases complicated by massive gastrointestinal bleeding.[132] Women at highest risk are those with a history of gastrointestinal bleeding antedating pregnancy.

Management of bleeding varices may be accomplished with sclerotherapy as an alternative to portacaval anastomosis. Some authorities suggest it is superior to portosystemic shunting in reducing recurrent bleeding episodes. In a study of 11 women with cirrhosis during pregnancy, 4 of 6 with documented varices experienced gastrointestinal hemorrhage requiring endoscopic sclerotherapy.[132] Five of these women also had significant coagulation disorders. In the entire series, there were six growth-restricted infants, three preterm deliveries, and one neonatal death. In addition to sclerotherapy, portal pressure may be reduced with β-blocker therapy and vasodilators. Portal decompression surgery has been accomplished during pregnancy, but it is used less often than endoscopic sclerotherapy.

Another feared complication associated with portal hypertension is the development of splenic artery aneurysm. Pulsed-wave Doppler and CT imaging may be helpful in establishing the diagnosis. Elective laparoscopic surgery with ligation should be strongly considered before pregnancy because rupture carries with it an enormous risk of maternal and fetal death.

The emerging literature describes the outcome of pregnancy in women with noncirrhotic portal hypertension, which is most commonly caused by noncirrhotic portal fibrosis, Budd-Chiari syndrome, or extrahepatic portal venous obstruction. Affected women are more likely to be of childbearing age than are women with cirrhosis. This group of women rarely has abnormal liver function, and their fertility rates are the same as controls.[133,134] There are varied reports on the fetal risks associated with noncirrhotic portal hypertension. An Indian series of 116 pregnancies in 44 patients[133] and a U.S. series of 38 cases[135] reported fetal loss rates between 7% and 8%. Two other series that included only women with extrahepatic portal venous obstruction reported fetal loss rates of 23% to 28%,[131,132] which may reflect the different causes of portal hypertension in this group.

The frequency of variceal bleeding in pregnant women with noncirrhotic portal hypertension is lower if they have had treatment for esophageal varices before pregnancy by endoscopic injection sclerotherapy or a decompression operation. In an Indian study of 50 pregnancies in 27 women, the rate of bleeding for 35 women for whom the disease was diagnosed and treated before conception was 8.6%, compared with a rate of 93% for 15 women whose disease was diagnosed during pregnancy.[134] In women with bleeding varices during pregnancy, treatment with sclerotherapy is safe.[133] For prevention of rebleeding, it is advisable to use β-blocker therapy in addition to sclerotherapy. In summary, the overall prognosis for women with noncirrhotic portal hypertension in pregnancy is better than for those with cirrhosis, particularly if the disease was diagnosed and treated before conception.

Acute Liver Failure during Pregnancy

Acute liver failure is an uncommon medical emergency during pregnancy that is associated with significant maternal and fetal morbidity and mortality. Acute liver failure is defined as the development of hepatic encephalopathy caused by severe liver dysfunction within 12 weeks of onset of symptoms in a patient with previously normal liver function.[136] It may be further categorized as hyperacute, acute, or subacute liver failure, depending on the interval between jaundice and encephalopathy of 0 to 7 days, 8 to 28 days, or 29 days to 12 weeks, respectively.

Clinical features of acute liver failure are not diagnostic. Cutaneous stigmata such as spider nevi and palmar erythema can be seen in acute liver failure, chronic liver disease, and healthy pregnancy. Other symptoms include nausea, vomiting, fatigue, and abdominal pain. Clinical signs may include hepatomegaly, splenomegaly, and ascites. Altered mental state and icterus are the clinical hallmarks of severe liver disease, and early recognition of this is essential because affected individuals should be promptly transferred to a tertiary facility where transplantation is available.

Laboratory investigations compatible with acute liver failure include abnormal liver function test results for bilirubin, AST, ALT, ALP, and GGT. Levels of transaminases higher than 2000 IU/L suggest liver ischemia, rupture, or infarction. However, low or declining levels may indicate extensive hepatocellular necrosis and lack of regenerating hepatocytes, which carries a poor prognosis. Other laboratory indices that carry a poor prognosis include low serum levels of albumin and an elevated prothrombin time, which are markers of poor hepatic synthetic function. Acidosis (pH < 7.35) and renal impairment are associated with acute liver failure, as is profound and sometimes refractory hypoglycemia. These features also indicate a poor prognosis. Hyponatremia and thrombocytopenia ($<100 \times 10^9/L$) are commonly found in acute and chronic liver disease. The causes of acute liver failure are summarized in Table 50-9.

TABLE 50-9 CAUSES OF ACUTE LIVER FAILURE

Viral hepatitis (e.g., CMV, HIV, HSV, EBV, hepatitis A, B, C, D, or E virus)
Acetaminophen overdose
Idiosyncratic drug reactions
Pregnancy-related causes (e.g., AFLP, HELLP syndrome, preeclampsia, severe hyperemesis gravidarum)
Budd-Chiari syndrome
Ischemic necrosis
Wilson disease
Autoimmune hepatitis
Toxin exposure (e.g., alcohol)
Malignancy (e.g., lymphoma, hepatocellular carcinoma)

AFLP, acute fatty liver of pregnancy; CMV, cytomegalovirus; EBV, Epstein-Barr virus; HELLP, *h*emolysis, *e*levated *l*iver enzymes, and *l*ow *p*latelets; HIV, human immunodeficiency virus; HSV, herpes simplex virus.

TABLE 50-10 KING'S COLLEGE HOSPITAL CRITERIA FOR PREDICTING POOR OUTCOMES FOR PATIENTS WITH ACUTE LIVER FAILURE

Patients Taking Acetaminophen
pH < 7.30 (regardless of encephalopathy grade)
Or
PT > 100 seconds (INR > 6.5) and serum creatinine level >300 μmol/L (>3.4 mg/dL) in patients with grade III or IV encephalopathy
Patients Not Taking Acetaminophen
PT > 100 seconds (INR > 6.5, regardless of encephalopathy grade)
Or any three of the following variables (regardless of encephalopathy grade):
Age <10 or >40 years
Cause: non-A, non-B hepatitis; halothane hepatitis; idiosyncratic drug reactions
Duration of jaundice before onset of encephalopathy >7 days
PT > 50 seconds (INR > 3.5)
Serum bilirubin >300 μmol/L (>17.5 mg/dL)

INR, international normalized ratio; PT, prothrombin time.

In the nonpregnant woman, acetaminophen overdose and viral hepatitis are the most common causes of acute liver failure in the United States.[137] There have been no epidemiologic studies of acute liver failure in pregnancy, but viral hepatitis (particularly hepatitis B and E) is probably the most common cause in the developing world, with acetaminophen overdose and pregnancy-related causes being more common in more developed nations.

Management

It is imperative to rule out pregnancy-associated diagnoses such as acute fatty liver, HELLP, or preeclampsia because delivery often leads to improvement or resolution of the maternal condition. There is no evidence that delivery affects the course of liver failure in cases of viral hepatitis. However, delivery of a viable fetus should be considered because the fetal mortality rate is high for these patients.

Patients with acute liver failure should be considered for transfer to a tertiary care center with transplantation facilities. King's College Hospital criteria (Table 50-10) are widely used in Europe and to a lesser extent in the United States, and they have been shown to accurately predict poor outcome and indicate those who should be transferred.[138]

Management comprises strenuous efforts to confirm the cause of acute liver failure coupled with intensive monitoring and supportive treatment until recovery begins or transplantation is undertaken. *N*-Acetylcysteine has been shown to improve the prognosis of women with acetaminophen overdose. Therapy should be commenced as soon as possible, and in practice, it is given to most patients until acetaminophen overdose has been ruled out.

Administration of fresh-frozen plasma without overt bleeding does not alter the outcome and obscures results of the prothrombin time test. Parenteral vitamin K_1 and folic acid should be given routinely. Fresh blood and blood products should be available to support any obstetric or surgical intervention. Gastrointestinal bleeding from gastric erosions is decreased by the prophylactic administration of a proton pump inhibitor. The stomach should be emptied hourly to prevent aspiration of gastric contents. Early enteral feeding reduces translocation of microbes from the intestinal wall into the circulation and reverses the catabolic state. Elective endotracheal intubation may be required to protect the airway (particularly before transfer and surgical procedures, including delivery) before the development of overt cerebral edema. Intubation must be performed by an experienced anesthetist.

Profound hypoglycemia remains a common cause of fetal and maternal death. Blood glucose levels should be closely monitored and immediate provisions made to administer large quantities of glucose by a central venous catheter. The patient should be maintained at 10 to 20 degrees of elevation with minimal turning and stimulation. Early manifestations of cerebral edema include peaks of systolic hypertension and tachycardia and should be treated by mannitol (0.5 to 1.0 g/kg given as a bolus) to induce a diuresis. Mannitol is potentially nephrotoxic and is ineffective in renal failure. Serum osmolalities should be maintained between 290 and 315 mOsm/L. Ultrafiltration and hemodialysis may be required to remove excess fluid. Levels of blood urea may be misleadingly low, and the renal function is best monitored by serial levels of blood creatinine and creatinine clearance. Hyperventilation to reduce the partial pressure of carbon dioxide further reduces the limited brain flow and is no longer recommended. Intracranial pressure monitoring should be considered early in the patient likely to progress to grade IV coma and in transplantation candidates. Seizures seem to be more common than previously realized and should be suspected in a deteriorating patient without specific elevations in intracranial pressure. They should be considered for assisted ventilation, especially if they require benzodiazepines and other sedative drugs. Detailed microbiologic cultures and analysis should be performed serially on all body fluids, including blood, urine, and sputum. Infections, including fungal infections, are common in patients with liver failure.

Prognosis

The overall survival rate with medical treatment is 10% to 40%. The prognosis depends on the cause. It is best for patients with acetaminophen overdose or hepatitis A and less favorable for other causes. The time to the onset of encephalopathy also affects the prognosis, with hyperacute failure having a better prognosis than subacute failure. The outcome for transplantation for acute liver failure is improving, and success rates are 75% to 90%.[139]

Liver Transplantation and Pregnancy

Several case reports,[140-143] registry data,[144,145] and two retrospective reviews[146,147] have cumulatively described pregnancy outcomes for more than 200 women with liver transplants. In contrast to the reduced fertility and menstrual dysfunction associated with end-stage liver failure, restoration of menses occurs, and fertility rates increase within months after liver transplantation. Successful outcomes for pregnancy can be expected in these women, although they are at increased risk for preeclampsia, preterm birth, and low-birth-weight and small-for-gestational-age infants.

Pregnancy should be delayed for at least 1 year after transplantation because pregnancies occurring within that period appear to have an increased incidence of prematurity, low birth weight, and acute cellular rejection compared with those occurring later than 1 year.[147] Liver transplant recipients with biopsy-proven acute rejection during pregnancy are at greater risk for poorer outcomes and recurrent rejection episodes.[148] However, pregnancy itself does not seem to impair graft function or accelerate graft rejection if the patient is adequately immunosuppressed.

Immunosuppressive therapy, such as cyclosporin and tacrolimus, that is commonly used in liver transplant recipients does not appear to be teratogenic, and breastfeeding is advocated. Careful monitoring of plasma levels is advised because of the physiologic changes in pregnancy that can alter the pharmacokinetics of immunosuppressive therapy.[149] Malabsorption due to hyperemesis gravidarum may decrease plasma levels of the drug.

Liver transplantation has been described during pregnancy for a number or pregnancy-related and coexistent conditions, including Budd-Chiari syndrome, viral hepatitis, AFLP, and HELLP syndrome with associated hepatic rupture and necrosis. In women who do survive acute liver failure and transplantation operation during pregnancy, increased risks for impaired homeostasis as a result of coagulopathy remain throughout pregnancy and delivery. Infection, renal failure, hypoglycemia, and adult respiratory distress syndrome are common complications.

Gallbladder Disease

Epidemiology

Cholelithiasis is common in the adult population. Cross-sectional studies of nonpregnant women in the United States found that 6.5% of women between 20 and 29 years old and 10.2% of women between 30 and 39 years old have gallstones or have had a cholecystectomy.[150] Pregnancy and the postpartum period appear to predispose women to gallstone formation. This is attributed to the increase in sex steroid hormone levels in pregnancy, causing biliary stasis, prolonged intestinal transit, and increased cholesterol saturation of bile. Multiparity is a risk factor; one study found that gallstones occurred in 7% of nulliparous women, with the rate rising to 19% of women with two or more pregnancies.[151] Pre-pregnancy obesity is associated with an increased risk of gallbladder disease with an odds ratio of 4.45 (95% confidence interval, 2.59 to 7.64) for a body mass index greater than 30 kg/m^2.[152] The risk of gallstones appears to increase during gestation, with sludge (i.e., precursor to stones) or stones being found in 5.1% of 3254 prospectively studied women in the second trimester, 7.9% in the third trimester, and 10.2% by 4 to 6 weeks after delivery.[152] Gallbladder disease is the most common non-obstetric cause of maternal hospitalization in the first year after delivery.[153]

Despite the high prevalence of gallstones, pregnant women are usually asymptomatic, with biliary colic reported in only 1.2% of pregnant women with known gallbladder disease.[152] However, biliary colic was a common presenting complaint of 43 (55%) of 78 symptomatic pregnant women admitted with biliary tract disease.[154] Acute cholecystitis accounted for 25% (20 of 78) of symptomatic pregnant women in the same study. However, for those who develop symptoms, the frequency of recurrence of symptoms during pregnancy is high.

Clinical Features and Diagnosis

Table 50-11 summarizes the most common gallbladder diseases. The symptoms of gallbladder disease in pregnancy are similar to those in the nonpregnant population. Biliary colic can manifest as intermittent right upper quadrant pain. More serious symptoms include anorexia, nausea, vomiting, and severe right upper quadrant or epigastric pain.

TABLE 50-11 GALLBLADDER DISEASES

Biliary colic*
Acute cholecystitis
Common bile duct obstruction
Ascending cholangitis
Gallstone ileus
Pancreatitis

***Gallbladder disease may be complicated by any combination of the disorders listed.**

Symptoms may be associated with signs of infection—classically, a mild leukocytosis and elevated temperature.

Laboratory investigations may reveal elevated serum bilirubin and ALP levels, although the level of ALP is commonly increased in normal pregnancy because of placental production. Levels of AST and ALT may also be increased. Jaundice or hyperamylasemia may be signs of complicated gallbladder disease (see Table 50-11). The differential diagnosis includes appendicitis, pancreatitis, peptic ulcer disease, pyelonephritis, AFLP, and HELLP syndrome.

Abdominal ultrasound should be performed. It has an accuracy of 97% in diagnosing cholelithiasis. If extrahepatic ductal stones are suspected but not demonstrated on ultrasound, MR cholangiography may be performed. ERCP, with its associated radiation exposure, should be limited to cases in which treatment for documented ductal stones is required.

Management

Operative management for complicated gallbladder disease is advocated as in nonpregnant women. However, the appropriate management for biliary colic and acute cholecystitis during pregnancy is controversial. Traditional conservative measures include withdrawal of oral food and fluids, administering intravenous fluids, nasogastric aspiration, and providing analgesia and antibiotics, with avoidance of surgical intervention when possible. A more aggressive approach has been advocated, leading to more surgical interventions in pregnancy. A retrospective review of 78 pregnancies in 76 patients showed that nonoperative management of symptomatic cholelithiasis (i.e., biliary colic or acute cholecystitis) led to suboptimal clinical outcomes in 38% of patients, including a 34% relapse rate and significantly higher rates of labor induction, cesarean section for treatment, and preterm delivery compared with the operative group.[154] Of the 10 patients undergoing operative management, 8 underwent surgery in the second trimester and 2 in the early third trimester. Operative management was associated with an increased risk for premature contractions, which were treated successfully with tocolytics. The laparoscopic approach appears to be feasible even in the third trimester of pregnancy.[155] Perioperative fetal monitoring and low pneumoperitoneum pressures are recommended.

Pancreatitis

Epidemiology

Acute pancreatitis is a rare and serious complication during pregnancy. The true incidence of pancreatitis complicating pregnancy is difficult to ascertain and may range from 1 case in 1000 to more than 3000 pregnancies.[156] In a series of 500 patients with acute pancreatitis, only

7 women developed the disease while pregnant.[157] Although alcohol is the most common cause in nonpregnant patients, studies have repeatedly shown that gallstones are the most common cause in pregnancy.[158] Other causes, particularly hyperlipidemia, have been described in pregnancy, as has an association between AFLP and pancreatitis, which carries a particularly poor prognosis.[159]

Clinical Features and Diagnosis

The clinical presentation of pancreatitis is not significantly altered in pregnancy. The disease may occur at any stage in gestation but is more common in the third trimester and the puerperium. Epigastric pain, which may radiate to the flanks or shoulders along with abdominal tenderness, should prompt appropriate laboratory investigations. Occasionally, a patient presents with nausea and vomiting as her only complaints. She may have mild fever and leukocytosis, and radiologic examination of the abdomen may reveal an adynamic ileus. Ultrasound imaging of the pancreas can be difficult. If significant pancreatic necrosis is suspected, CT becomes preferable. In most cases, this radiologic study is unnecessary.

In evaluating the pregnant patient with suspected pancreatitis, the differential diagnosis includes most causes of abdominal pain in young women. These are principally peptic ulcer diseases, including perforation, acute cholecystitis, biliary colic, and intestinal obstruction. Elevated amylase levels should suggest pancreatitis, although they may occur with other conditions, such as cholecystitis. Serum amylase concentrations greater than three times normal suggest pancreatitis.

Management

In most cases, acute pancreatitis resolves spontaneously within several days.[156] However, 10% of patients have a more severe course, and they are best managed in an intensive care environment. The general principles of management are the same as for nonpregnant women: bowel rest with or without nasogastric aspiration, intravenous fluids and electrolyte replacement, and parenteral analgesics. Meperidine is the drug of choice for analgesia because, unlike morphine, it does not constrict the sphincter of Oddi. Important additional measures for the pregnant patient include fetal monitoring, attention to the choice of medications, consideration of radiation to the fetus, and positioning of the mother to avoid inferior vena cava constriction. Because there is a high likelihood of associated gallstone disease, ERCP may be beneficial if common duct obstruction has occurred. Early surgical intervention is advocated for gallstone pancreatitis in all trimesters, because 70% of these patients will otherwise relapse before delivery.[160]

For women with mild disease that is responsive to conservative management, the prognosis for mother and fetus is excellent. However, for women with more severe disease, fetal morbidity and mortality rates increase. Of 43 women with acute pancreatitis, perinatal outcomes were available for 39.[156] Thirty-two newborns were delivered at term without complications, and six were delivered before term, including two stillbirths and one early neonatal demise.[156] One patient underwent therapeutic abortion. The mechanisms of demise included placental abruption and profound metabolic disturbance, including acidosis. This highlights the importance of regular fetal monitoring and consideration of delivery if the maternal disease is deteriorating.

Pancreatic Transplantation

The National Transplant Pregnancy Registry reported 56 pregnancies in 36 patients with kidney-pancreas transplants.[161] Maternal and fetal morbidity rates were high, with maternal hypertension complicating 75% of pregnancies, preeclampsia occurring in 34%, and infection occurring in 55%. The mean gestational age at birth was 34 weeks (compared with 36 weeks for kidney-only recipients), and the mean birth weight was significantly lower, with 68% being below 2500 g. Twenty-six infants had neonatal complications, including one death due to sepsis. There were six graft losses within 2 years. Adverse outcomes for the mother and fetus appear to be greater for kidney-pancreas recipients than for kidney-only recipients.

Pregnancy in transplant recipients should be planned, and multidisciplinary care is imperative. Women desiring pregnancy should be encouraged to wait until immunosuppression doses are stable. Couples should consider waiting until a minimum of 1 year after transplantation, when the risks for the mother and fetus are lower. After 1 year, it is presumed that there is a reduced risk of graft rejection and lower medication doses,[162] but there is a paucity of data to confirm this. Attention to the effects of medication on the fetoplacental unit and, if necessary, substitution of immunosuppressants should be undertaken before conception. Drug concentrations in maternal blood should be monitored throughout pregnancy because the physiologic changes associated with pregnancy can affect drug bioavailability. Increased surveillance of the mother and fetus should be undertaken to quickly detect any complications.

References

1. Maher J, Goldenberg R, Tamura T, et al: Albumin levels in pregnancy: A hypothesis—decreased levels of albumin are related to increased levels of alpha-fetoprotein. Early Hum Dev 34:209, 1993.
2. Girling JC, Dow E, Smith JH: Liver function tests in pre-eclampsia: Importance of comparison with a reference range derived for normal pregnancy. BJOG 104:246-250, 1997.
3. Bacq Y, Zarka O, Brechot JF, et al: Liver function tests in normal pregnancy: A prospective study of 103 pregnancy women and 103 matched controls. Hepatology 23:1030-1034, 1996.
4. David AL, Kotecha M, Girling JC: Factors influencing postnatal liver function tests. BJOG 107:1421-1426, 2000.
5. Abedin P, Weaver JB, Egginton E: Intrahepatic cholestasis of pregnancy: Prevalence and ethnic distribution. Ethn Health 4:35-37, 1999.
6. Germain A, Carvajal JA, Glasinovic JC, et al: Intrahepatic cholestasis of pregnancy. An intriguing pregnancy specific disorder. J Soc Gynecol Invest 9:10-14, 2002.
7. Reyes H: Intrahepatic cholestasis. A puzzling disorder of pregnancy [review]. J Gastroenterol Hepatol 12:211-216, 1997.
8. Berg B, Helm G, Petersohn I, et al: Cholestasis of pregnancy. Clinical and laboratory studies. Acta Obstet Gynecol Scand 65:107-113, 1986.
9. Gonzalez MC, Reyes H, Arrese M, et al: Intrahepatic cholestasis of pregnancy in twin pregnancies. J Hepatol 9:84-90, 1989.
10. Heinonen S, Kirkinen P: Pregnancy outcome with intrahepatic cholestasis. Obstet Gynecol 94:189-193, 1999.
11. Eloranta ML, Heinonen S, Mononen T, et al: Risk of obstetric cholestasis in sisters of index patients. Clin Genet 60:42-45, 2001.
12. Reyes H, Ribalta J, Gonzalez-Ceron M: Idiopathic cholestasis of pregnancy in a large kindred. Gut 17:709-713, 1976.
13. Holzbach RT, Sivak DA, Braun WE: Familial recurrent intrahepatic cholestasis of pregnancy: A genetic study providing evidence for transmission of a sex-limited, dominant trait. Gastroenterology 85:175-179, 1983.
14. Dixon PH, Weerasekera N, Linton KJ, et al: Heterozygous MDR3 missense mutation associated with intrahepatic cholestasis of pregnancy: Evidence for a defect in protein trafficking. Hum Mol Genet 9:1209-1217, 2000.
15. Mullenbach R, Linton KJ, Wiltshire S, et al: ABCB4 gene sequence variation in women with intrahepatic cholestasis of pregnancy. J Med Genet 40:e70, 2003.

16. Mullenbach R, Bennett A, Tetlow N, et al: ATP8B1 mutations in British cases with intrahepatic cholestasis of pregnancy. Gut 54:829-834, 2005.
17. Pauli-Magnus C, Lang T, Meier Y, et al: Sequence analysis of bile salt export pump (ABCB11) and multidrug resistance p-glycoprotein 3 (ABCB4, MDR3) in patients with intrahepatic cholestasis of pregnancy. Pharmacogenetics 14:91-102, 2004.
18. van Mil SW, Milona A, Dixon PH, et al: Functional variants of the central bile acid sensor FXR identified in intrahepatic cholestasis of pregnancy. Gastroenterology 133:507-516, 2007.
19. Williamson C, Hems LM, Goulis DG, et al: Clinical outcome in a series of cases of obstetric cholestasis identified via a patient support group. BJOG 111:676-681, 2004.
20. Bacq Y, Sapey T, Brechot MC, et al: Intrahepatic cholestasis of pregnancy: A French prospective study. Hepatology 26:358-364, 1997.
21. Locatelli A, Roncaglia N, Arreghini A, et al: Hepatitis C virus infection is associated with a higher incidence of cholestasis of pregnancy. BJOG 106:498-500, 1999.
22. Kauppila A, Korpela H, Makila UM, et al: Low serum selenium concentration and glutathione peroxidase activity in intrahepatic cholestasis of pregnancy. BMJ 294:150-152, 1987.
23. Reyes H, Baez ME, Gonzalez MC, et al: Selenium, zinc and copper plasma levels in intrahepatic cholestasis of pregnancy, in normal pregnancies and in healthy individuals in Chile. J Hepatol 32:542-549, 2000.
24. Jones EA, Bergasa NV: Evolving concepts of the pathogenesis and treatment of the pruritus of cholestasis. Can J Gastroenterol 14:33-40, 2000.
25. Laatikainen T, Ikonen E: Serum bile acids in cholestasis of pregnancy. Obstet Gynecol 50:313-318, 1977.
26. Laatikainen T, Tulenheimo A: Maternal serum bile acid levels and fetal distress in cholestasis of pregnancy. Int J Gynaecol Obstet 22:91-94, 1984.
27. Glantz A, Marschall HU, Mattsson LA: Intrahepatic cholestasis of pregnancy: Relationships between bile acid levels and fetal complication rates. Hepatology 40:467-474, 2004.
28. Fisk NM, Storey GNB: Fetal outcome in obstetric cholestasis. BJOG 95:1137-1143, 1988.
29. Davies MH, da Silva RCMA, Jones SR, et al: Fetal mortality associated with cholestasis of pregnancy and the potential benefit of therapy with ursodeoxycholic acid. Gut 37:580-584, 1995.
30. Reid R, Ivey KJ, Rencoret RH, Storey B: Fetal complications of obstetric cholestasis. BMJ 1:870-872, 1976.
31. Al Inizi S, Gupta R, Gale A: Fetal tachyarrhythmia with atrial flutter in obstetric cholestasis. Int J Gynaecol Obstet 93:53-54, 2006.
32. Gorelik J, Shevchuk A, de Swiet M, et al: Comparison of the arrhythmogenic effects of tauro- and glycoconjugates of cholic acid in an in vitro study of rat cardiomyocytes. BJOG 111:867-870, 2004.
33. Campos G, Guerra F, Israel E: Effects of cholic acid infusions in fetal lambs. Acta Obstet Gynecol Scand 65:23-26, 1986.
34. Shaw D, Frohlich J, Wittmann B, Willms M: A prospective study of 18 patients with cholestasis of pregnancy. Am J Obstet Gynecol 142:621-625, 1982.
35. Mauricio AC, Slawik M, Heitzmann D, et al: Deoxycholic acid (DOC) affects the transport properties of distal colon. Pflugers Arch 439:532-540, 2000.
36. Rosmorduc O, Hermelin B, Poupon R: *MDR3* gene defect in adults with symptomatic intrahepatic and gallbladder cholesterol cholelithiasis. Gastroenterology 120:1459-1467, 2001.
37. Williamson C: Drugs in pregnancy. Gastrointestinal disease. Best Pract Res Clin Obstet Gynaecol 15:937-952, 2001.
38. Zapata R, Sandoval L, Palma J, et al: Ursodeoxycholic acid in the treatment of intrahepatic cholestasis of pregnancy. A 12-year experience. Liver Int 25:548-554, 2005.
39. Glantz A, Marschall HU, Lammert F, et al: Intrahepatic cholestasis of pregnancy: A randomized controlled trial comparing dexamethasone and ursodeoxycholic acid. Hepatology 42:1399-1405, 2005.
40. Mazzella G, Nicola R, Francesco A, et al: Ursodeoxycholic acid administration in patients with cholestasis of pregnancy: Effects on primary bile acids in babies and mothers. Hepatology 33:504-508, 2001.
41. Serrano MA, Brites D, Larena MG, et al: Beneficial effect of ursodeoxycholic acid on alterations induced by cholestasis of pregnancy in bile acid transport across the human placenta. J Hepatol 28:829-839, 1998.
42. Gorelik J, Shevchuk A, Diakonov I, et al: Dexamethasone and ursodeoxycholic acid protect against the arrhythmogenic effect of taurocholate in an in vitro study of rat cardiomyocytes. BJOG 110:467-474, 2003.
43. Roncaglia N, Arreghini A, Locatelli A, et al: Obstetric cholestasis: outcome with active management. Int J Gynaecol Obstet 100:167-170, 2002.
44. Pereira SP, O'Donohue J, Wendon J, et al: Maternal and perinatal outcome in severe pregnancy-related liver disease. Hepatology 26:1258-1262, 1997.
45. Fesenmeier MF, Coppage KH, Lambers DS, et al: Acute fatty liver of pregnancy in 3 tertiary care centers. Am J Obstet Gynecol 192:1416-1419, 2005.
46. Ibdah JA: Acute fatty liver of pregnancy: An update on pathogenesis and clinical implications. World J Gastroenterol 12:7397-7404, 2006.
47. Ibdah JA, Bennett MJ, Rinaldo P, et al: A fetal fatty-acid oxidation disorder as a cause of liver disease in pregnant women. N Engl J Med 340:1723-1731, 1999.
48. Wilcken B, Leung KC, Hammond J, et al: Pregnancy and fetal long chain 3 hydroxyacyl coenzyme A dehydrogenase deficiency. Lancet 341:407-408, 1993.
49. Yang Z, Yamada J, Zhao Y, et al: Prospective screening for pediatric mitochondrial trifunctional protein defects in pregnancies complicated by liver disease. JAMA 288:2163-2166, 2002.
50. den Boer ME, Ijlst L, Wijburg FA, et al: Heterozygosity for the common LCHAD mutation (1528G > C) is not a major cause of HELLP syndrome and the prevalence of the mutation in the Dutch population is low. Pediatr Res 48:151-154, 2000.
51. Mutze S, Ahillen I, Rudnik-Schoeneborn S, et al: Neither maternal nor fetal mutation (E474Q) in the alpha-subunit of the trifunctional protein is frequent in pregnancies complicated by HELLP syndrome. J Perinat Med 35:76-78, 2007.
52. Browning MF, Levy HL, Wilking-Haug LE, et al: Fetal fatty acid oxidation defects and maternal liver disease in pregnancy. Obstet Gynecol 107:115-120, 2006.
53. Reyes H, Sandoval L, Wainstein A, et al: Acute fatty liver of pregnancy: A clinical study of 12 episodes in 11 patients. Gut 35:101-106, 1994.
54. Castro MA, Fasset MJ, Reynolds TB, et al: Reversible peripartum liver failure: A new perspective on the diagnosis, treatment, and cause of acute fatty liver of pregnancy based on 28 cases. Am J Obstet Gynecol 181:389-395, 2000.
55. Kennedy S, Hall PM, Seymour AE, et al: Transient diabetes insipidus and acute fatty liver of pregnancy. BJOG 101:387-391, 1994.
56. Castro MA, Ouzounian JG, Colletti PM, et al: Radiologic studies in acute fatty liver of pregnancy. A review of the literature and 19 new cases. J Reprod Med 41:839-843, 1996.
57. Weinstein L: Syndrome of hemolysis elevated liver enzymes, and low platelet count: A severe consequence of hypertension in pregnancy. Am J Obstet Gynecol 142:159, 1982.
58. Barton JR, Riely CA, Adamec TA, et al: Hepatic histopathologic condition does not correlate with laboratory abnormalities in HELLP syndrome. Am J Obstet Gynecol 167:1538, 1992.
59. Smith LG, Moise KJ Jr, Dildy GA III, et al: Spontaneous rupture of liver during pregnancy: Current therapy. Obstet Gynecol 77:171, 1999.
60. Rinehart BK, Terrone DA, Magann EF, et al: Preeclampsia-associated hepatic hemorrhage and rupture: Mode of management related to maternal and perinatal outcome. Obstet Gynecol Surv 54:196-202, 1999.
61. Sibai B, Ramadan M, Usta I, et al: Maternal morbidity and mortality in 442 pregnancies with hemolysis elevated liver enzymes with low platelets (HELLP syndrome). Am J Obstet Gynecol 169:1000, 1993.
62. Abdi S, Cameron IC, Nakielny RA, et al: Spontaneous hepatic rupture and maternal death following an uncomplicated pregnancy and delivery. BJOG 108:431-433, 2001.
63. Shaw C, Fattah N, Lynch D, et al: Spontaneous rupture of the liver following a normal pregnancy and delivery. Ir Med J 98:27-28, 2005.

64. Carlson KL, Cheryl LB: Ruptured subcapsular liver hematoma in pregnancy: A case report of non-surgical management. Am J Obstet Gynecol 190:558-560, 2004.
65. Barton JR, Sibai BM: Hepatic imaging findings in HELLP syndrome (hemolysis, elevated liver enzymes and low platelet count). Am J Obstet Gynecol 174:1820, 1996.
66. Araujo ACPF, Leao MD, Nobrega MH, et al: Characteristics and treatment of hepatic rupture caused by HELLP syndrome Am J Obstet Gynecol 195:129-133, 2006.
67. Krueger K, Hoffman B, Lee W: Hepatic infarction associated with eclampsia. Am J Gastroenterol 85:588, 1990.
68. Sookoian S: Liver disease during pregnancy: Acute viral hepatitis. Ann Hepatol 5:231-236, 2006
69. Patra S, Kumar A, Trivedi SS, et al: Maternal and fetal outcomes in pregnant women with acute hepatitis E virus infection. Ann Intern Med 147:28-33, 2007.
70. Centers for Disease Control and Prevention (CDC): Hepatitis A among homosexual men—United States, Canada, and Australia. MMWR Morb Mortal Wkly Rep 4:155, 1992.
71. Elinav E, Ben-Dov IZ, Shapira Y, et al: Acute hepatitis A infection in pregnancy is associated with high rates of gestational complications and preterm labor. Gastroenterology 130:1129-1134, 2006.
72. Centers for Disease Control and Prevention (CDC): Prevention of hepatitis A through active or passive immunization. MMWR Morb Mortal Wkly Rep 55:1-23, 2006.
73. Alter MJ, Mast EE: The epidemiology of viral hepatitis in the United States. Gastroenterol Clin North Am 23:437-55, 1994.
74. Centers for Disease Control and Prevention (CDC): Surveillance for acute viral hepatitis—United States, 2005. MMWR Morb Mortal Wkly Rep 56:1-24, 2007.
75. Dinsmoor MJ: Hepatitis in the obstetric patient. Infect Dis North Am 11:77, 1997.
76. Centers for Disease Control and Prevention (CDC): Prevention of perinatal hepatitis B by enhanced case management. MMWR Morb Mortal Wkly Rep 45:584, 1996.
77. Centers for Disease Control and Prevention (CDC): A comprehensive immunization strategy to eliminate transmission of hepatitis B virus infection in the United States. MMWR Morb Mortal Wkly Rep 54:1-23, 2005.
78. American Society of Reproductive Medicine: Hepatitis and reproduction. Fertil Steril 86(Suppl 4):S131-S141, 2006.
79. Zuckerman JN: Hepatitis B immune globulin for prevention of hepatitis B infection [review]. J Med Virol 79:919-921, 2007.
80. Tang S: Study on the HBV intrauterine infection and its rate. Zhonghua Liu Xing Bing Xue Za Zhi 11:328-330, 1990.
81. Centers for Disease Control and Prevention (CDC): Public health service interagency guidelines for screening donors of blood, plasma, organs, tissues, and semen for evidence of hepatitis B and hepatitis C. MMWR Morb Mortal Wkly Rep 40:1, 1991.
82. Lee C, Gong Y, Brok J, et al: Effect of hepatitis B immunisation in newborn infants of mothers positive for hepatitis B surface antigen: Systematic review and meta-analysis. BMJ 332:328-336, 2006.
83. Carmen WF, Zanetti AR, Karayiannis P, et al: Vaccine-induced escape mutant of hepatitis B virus. Lancet 336:325, 1990.
84. Panlilio AL, Orelien JG, Srivastava PU, et al, for the NaSH Surveillance Group and EPINet Data Sharing Network: Estimate of the annual number of percutaneous injuries among hospital-based healthcare workers in the United States, 1997-1998. Infect Control Hosp Epidemiol 25:556-562, 2004.
85. Prüss-Ustün A, Rapiti E, Hutin Y: Estimation of the global burden of disease attributable to contaminated sharps injuries among health-care workers. Am J Ind Med 48:482-490, 2005.
86. Berger A: Mother to child transmission of hepatitis C virus: Prospective study of risk factors and timing of infection in children born to women seronegative for HIV-1. Science commentary: Behavior of hepatitis C virus. BMJ 317:440, 1998.
87. Reinus JF, Leikin EL, Alter HJ, et al: Failure to detect vertical transmission of hepatitis C virus. Ann Intern Med 117:881, 1992.
88. Ward C, Tudor-Williams G, Cotzias T, et al: Prevalence of hepatitis C among pregnant women attending an inner London obstetric department: Uptake and acceptability of named antenatal testing. Gut 27:277, 2000.
89. Centers for Disease Control and Prevention (CDC): Recommendations for prevention and control of hepatitis C virus (HCV) infection and HCV-related disease. MMWR Morb Mortal Wkly Rep 15:1, 1997.
90. Schreiber GB, Busch MP, Kleinman SH, Korelitz JJ: The risk of transfusion-transmitted viral infections. The retrovirus Epidemiology Donor Study. N Engl J Med 334:1685-1690, 1996.
91. Shakil AO, Conry-Cantilena C, Alter HJ, et al: Volunteer blood donors with antibody to hepatitis C virus: Clinical, biochemical, virologic and histological features. The Hepatitis C Study Group. Ann Intern Med 123:330-337, 1995.
92. Jabeen T, Cannon B, Hogan M, et al: Pregnancy and pregnancy outcome in hepatitis type 1b. Q J Med 15:1083-1085, 2000.
93. Mast EE, Huang L, Seto DS: Risk factors for perinatal transmission of hepatitis C virus and the natural history of HCV infection acquired in infancy. J Infect Dis 192:1880-1889, 2005.
94. Resti M, Azzari C, Mannelli F, et al, for the Tuscany Study Group on Hepatitis C Virus Infection in Children: Mother to child transmission of hepatitis C virus: Prospective study of risk factors and timing of infection in children born to women seronegative for HIV-1. BMJ 317:437, 1998.
95. Conte D, Fraquelli M, Prati D, et al: Prevalence and clinical course of chronic hepatitis C virus (HVC) infection and rate of HCV vertical transmission in a cohort of 15,250 pregnant women. Hepatology 31:751, 2000.
96. Ohto H, Terazawa S, Sasaki N, et al, for the Vertical Transmission of Hepatitis C Collaborative Study Group: Transmission of hepatic C virus from mother to infants. N Engl J Med 330:744, 1994.
97. Granovsky MO, Minkoff HL, Tess BH, et al: Hepatitis C virus infection in the mothers and infants cohort study. Pediatrics 102:355, 1998.
98. Yeung LT, King SM, Roberts EA: Mother-to-infant transmission of hepatitis C virus. Hepatology 34:223-229, 2001.
99. Alter HJ: Epidemiology of hepatitis C in the west. Semin Liver Dis 15:5-14, 1995.
100. Airoldi J, Berghella V: Hepatitis C and pregnancy. Obstet Gynecol Surv 61:666-672, 2006.
101. Gibb DM, Goodall RL, Dunn DT, et al: Mother-to-child transmission of hepatitis C virus: Evidence for preventable peripartum transmission. Lancet 356:904-907, 2000.
102. Deinhardt F, Gust I: Viral hepatitis. Bull WHO 60:661, 1982.
103. Chauhan A, Jameel S, Chawla YK, et al: Common etiological agent for epidemic and sporadic non-A, non-B hepatitis. Lancet 339:1509, 1992.
104. Rab MA, Bile MK, Mubarik MM, et al: Water-borne hepatitis E virus epidemic in Islamabad, Pakistan: A common source outbreak traced to the malfunction of a modern water treatment plant. Am J Trop Med Hyg 57:151-7, 1997.
105. Aggarwal R: Hepatitis E and pregnancy. Indian J Gastroenterol 26:3-5, 2007.
106. Khuroo MS, Kamali S, Jameel S: Vertical transmission of hepatitis E virus. Lancet 345:1025-1026, 1995.
107. Sauerbrei A, Wutzler P: Herpes Simplex and varicella-zoster virus infections during pregnancy: Current concepts of prevention, diagnosis and the therapy. Part 1. Herpes simplex virus infections. Med Microbiol Immunol 196:89-94, 2007.
108. Kang AH, Graves CR: Herpes simplex hepatitis in pregnancy: A case report and review of the literature. Obstet Gynecol Surv 54:463-468, 1999.
109. Stagno S, Pass RF, Dworsky ME: Congenital cytomegalovirus infection, the relative importance of primary and recurrent maternal infection. N Engl J Med 306:945-949, 1982.
110. Malm G, Engman ML: Congenital cytomegalovirus infections. Semin Fetal Neonatal Med 12:154-159, 2007.

111. Werner M, Bjornsson E, Prytz H, et al: Autoimmune hepatitis among fertile women: Strategies during pregnancy and breastfeeding? Scand J Gastroenterol 42:986-991, 2007.
112. Candia L, Marquez J, Espinoza LR: Autoimmune hepatitis and pregnancy: A rheumatologist's dilemma. Semin Arthritis Rheum 35:49-56, 2005.
113. Ostensen M: Rheumatological disorders. Best Pract Res Clin Obstet Gynaecol 15:953-969, 2001.
114. Sau A, Clarke S, Bass J, et al: Azathioprine and breastfeeding: is it safe? BJOG 114:498-501, 2007.
115. Landon MB, Soloway RD, Freeman LJ, et al: Primary sclerosing cholangitis. Obstet Gynecol 69:457, 1987.
116. Janczewska T, Olsson R, Hultcrantz R, et al: Pregnancy in patients with primary sclerosing cholangitis. Liver 16:326, 1996.
117. Nolan DG, Martin LS, Nataragan S, et al: Fetal complications associated with extreme fetal bile acids and maternal primary sclerosing cholangitis. Obstet Gynecol 84:695, 1994.
118. Paternoster DM, Floreani A, Burra P: Liver transplantation and pregnancy. Int J Gynaecol Obstet 50:199, 1995.
119. Shimono N, Ishibashi H, Ikematsu H, et al: Fulminant hepatic failure during perinatal period in a pregnant woman with Wilson's disease. Gastroenterol Jpn 26:69, 1991.
120. Toaff R, Toaff M, Peyser M, et al: Hepatolenticular degeneration (Wilson's disease) and pregnancy. Obstet Gynecol Surv 32:497, 1977.
121. Fukuda K, Ishii A, Matsue Y, et al: Pregnancy and delivery in penicillamine treated patients with Wilson's disease. Tohoku J Exp Med 123:279, 1977.
122. Walshe JM: The management of pregnancy in Wilson's disease treated with trientine. Q J Med 58:81, 1986.
123. Khuroo M, Datta D: Budd-Chiari syndrome following pregnancy: Report of 16 cases with roentgenologic hemodynamic and histologic studies of the hepatic outflow tract. Am J Med 8:113, 1980.
124. Dilawari JB, Bambery P, Chawla Y, et al: Hepatic outflow obstruction (Budd-Chiari syndrome): Experience with 177 patients and a review of the literature. Medicine (Baltimore) 73:21, 1994.
125. Gordon S, Polson D, Shirkhoda A: Budd-Chiari syndrome complicating pre-eclampsia: Diagnosis by magnetic resonance imaging. J Clin Gastroenterol 13:460, 1991.
126. Fickert P, Ramschak H, Kenner L, et al: Acute Budd-Chiari syndrome with fulminant hepatic failure in a pregnant woman with factor V Leiden mutation. Gastroenterology 111:1670, 1996.
127. Segal S, Shenhav S, Segal O, et al: Budd-Chiari syndrome complicating severe preeclampsia in a parturient with primary antiphospholipid syndrome. Eur J Obstet Gynaecol Reprod Biol 68:227, 1996.
128. Huguet C, Deliere T, Oliver JM, et al: Budd-Chiari syndrome with thrombosis of the inferior vena cava: Long-term patency of mesocaval and cavoatrial prosthetic bypass. Surgery 95:108, 1984.
129. Huchzermeyer H: Pregnancy in patients with liver cirrhosis and chronic hepatitis. Acta Hepatosplenol (Stuttg) 18:294, 1971.
130. Schreyer P, Caspi E, El-Hindi J, et al: Cirrhosis—pregnancy and delivery: A review. Obstet Gynecol Surv 37:304, 1982.
131. Cheng YS: Pregnancy in liver cirrhosis and/or portal hypertension. Am J Obstet Gynecol 128:812, 1977.
132. Pajor A, Lehoczky D: Pregnancy in liver cirrhosis—assessment of maternal and fetal risks in eleven patients and review of management. Gynecol Obstet Invest 38:45, 1994.
133. Kocchar R, Kumar S, Goel RC, et al: Pregnancy and its outcome in patients with noncirrhotic portal hypertension. Dig Dis Sci 44:1356-1361, 1999.
134. Aggarwal N, Sawhney H, Vasishta K, et al: Non-cirrhotic portal hypertension in pregnancy. Int J Gynecol Obstet 72:1-7, 2001.
135. Britton RC: Pregnancy and esophageal varices. Am J Surg 143:421-425, 1982.
136. O'Grady JG, Schalm SW, Williams R: Acute liver failure: Redefining the syndromes. Lancet 342:273-275, 1993.
137. Ostapowicz G, Fontana RJ, Schiodt FV, et al: Ann Intern Med 137:947-954, 2002.
138. Shakil AO, Kramer D, Mazariegos GV, et al: Acute liver failure: Clinical features, outcome analysis and applicability of prognostic criteria. Liver Transpl 6:163-169, 2000.
139. O'Grady JG: Acute liver failure. Postgrad Med J 81:148-154, 2005.
140. Jankovic Z, Stamenkovic D, Duncan B, et al: Successful outcome after a technically challenging liver transplant during pregnancy. Transplant Proc 39:1704-1706, 2007.
141. Malatesta MF, Rossi M, Rocca B, et al: Pregnancy after liver transplantation: Report of 8 new cases and a review of the literature. Transpl Immunol 15:297-302, 2006.
142. Jabiry-Zieniewicz Z, Kaminski P, Pietrzak B, et al: Outcome of 4 high-risk pregnancies in female liver transplant recipients on tacrolimus immunosuppression. Transplant Proc 38:255-7, 2006.
143. Pan GD, Yan LN, Li B, et al: A successful pregnancy following liver transplantation. Hepatobiliary Pancreat Dis Int 6:98-100, 2007.
144. Kallen B, Westgren M, Aberg A, Olausson PO: Pregnancy outcome after maternal organ transplantation in Sweden. BJOG 112:904-909, 2005.
145. Armenti VT, Radomski JS, Moritz MJ, et al: Report from the National Transplantation Pregnancy Registry (NTPR): Outcomes of pregnancy after transplantation. Clin Transpl (nv):103-114, 2004.
146. Christopher V, Al-Chalabi T, Richarson PD, et al: Pregnancy outcome after liver transplantation: A single-center's experience of 71 pregnancies in 45 recipients. Liver Transpl 12:1137-1139, 2006.
147. Jabiry-Zieniewicz Z, Cyganek A, Luterek K, et al: Pregnancy and delivery after liver transplantation. Transplant Proc 35:1197-1200, 2005.
148. Armenti VT, Herrine SK, Radonski JS, Moritz MJ: Pregnancy after liver transplantation. Liver Transpl 6:671-685, 2000.
149. Deierhoi MH, Haug M 3rd: Review of selective transplant subpopulations at high risk of failure from standard immunosuppressive therapy. Clin Transplant. 14:439-448, 2000.
150. Everhart JE, Khare M, Hill M, Maurer KR: Prevalence and ethnic differences in gallbladder disease in the United States. Gastroenterology 117:632-639, 1999.
151. Gilat T, Konikoff F: Pregnancy and the biliary tract. Can J Gastroenterol 14(Suppl D):55D-59D, 2000.
152. Ko CW, Beresford SAA, Schulte SJ, et al: Incidence, natural history, and risk factors for biliary sludge and stones during pregnancy. Hepatology 41:359-365, 2005.
153. Lydon-Rochelle M, Holt VL, Martin DP, Easterling TR: Association between method of delivery and maternal rehospitalization. JAMA 283:2411-2416, 2000.
154. Lu EJ, Curet MJ, El-Sayed YY, Kirkwood KS: Medical versus surgical management of biliary tract disease in pregnancy. Am J Surg 188:755-759, 2004.
155. Peter SG, Veverka TJ: Laparoscopic cholecystectomy in pregnancy. Curr Surg 59:74-78, 2002.
156. Ramin KD, Ramin SM, Richey SD, et al: Acute pancreatitis in pregnancy. Am J Obstet Gynecol 173:187-191, 1995.
157. McKay AJ, O'Neill J, Imrie CW: Pancreatitis, pregnancy, and gallstones. BJOG 87:47, 1980.
158. Robertson KW, Stewart IS, Imrie CW: Severe acute pancreatitis and pregnancy. Pancreatology 6:309-315, 2006.
159. Moldenhauer JS, O'Brien JM, Barton JR, Sibai B: Acute fatty liver of pregnancy associated with pancreatitis: A life threatening complication. Am J Obstet Gynaecol 190:502-505, 2004.
160. Swisher SG, Hunt KK, Schmidt PJ, et al: Management of pancreatitis complicating pregnancy. Am Surg 60:759-762, 1994.
161. Armenti VT, Radomski JS, Moritz MJ, et al: Report from the National Transplantation Pregnancy Registry (NTPR): Outcomes of pregnancy after Transplantation. In Cecka JM, Terasaki PI (eds): Clinical Transplants. Los Angeles, UCLA Immunogenetics Center, 2004.
162. Larsen JL: Pancreas transplantation: Indications and consequences. Endocr Rev 25:919-946, 2004.

Chapter 51

Pregnancy and Rheumatic Diseases

Michael D. Lockshin, MD, Jane E. Salmon, MD, and Doruk Erkan, MD

Epidemiology

The systemic rheumatic illnesses commonly complicating pregnancy are systemic lupus erythematosus (SLE), antiphospholipid syndrome, rheumatoid arthritis, scleroderma, juvenile arthritis, spondyloarthropathy, and Takayasu arteritis. SLE and Takayasu arteritis affect 15- to 45-year-old women in a ratio of 9 women to 1 man. Antiphospholipid syndrome has a female-to-male ratio of 7 to 1; rheumatoid arthritis and scleroderma have a ratio of 3 to 1; juvenile arthritis is almost gender neutral; and spondyloarthropathy has a ratio of about 1 to 3. Rheumatoid arthritis and scleroderma affect middle-aged more than young women. SLE has a higher prevalence among African Americans than among whites (4 to 1). Up to 1% of all women have rheumatoid arthritis. One of 5000 to 10,000 women have SLE, and antiphospholipid syndrome may be as common as SLE, whereas the other diseases are less common.

Because of these epidemiologic patterns, the autoimmune illnesses most frequently encountered in obstetric practices are SLE and antiphospholipid syndrome. Rheumatoid arthritis is a more common illness, but it occurs most often after the childbearing years and is therefore seen less often in pregnant women.

Diagnosis of the systemic rheumatic diseases rests more on clinical than on serologic criteria (discussed with the individual diseases). Features common to all are arthralgia or arthritis; fever, myalgia, and malaise; and markers of inflammation. Current theories consider the systemic rheumatic diseases to be driven by disordered immune mechanisms, probably resulting from a genetic defect in processing exogenous infectious material, but the mechanisms and possible triggers are different among the illnesses. Systemic rheumatic illnesses are chronic and relapsing, with temporary remissions. It is more likely that a new pregnancy will be diagnosed in a woman with an established diagnosis of rheumatic illness than that a new diagnosis will be made for a previously healthy pregnant woman. Table 51-1 provides the epidemiologic, clinical, and laboratory characteristics of the rheumatic diseases most often encountered in pregnant women.

Pathogenesis

No single theory of pathogenesis explains all autoimmune diseases. Each has a clear genetic association; most prominent are the spondyloarthropathies, in which human leukocyte antigen (HLA)-B27 is present in more than 80% of patients, compared with an incidence of less than 5% in general European white populations, less in Asian and African populations, and more in some Native American populations.[1] Class II HLA and non-HLA genetic associations occur in people with SLE and rheumatoid arthritis.[2,3] Complement protein deficiencies and other immune deficits appear to predispose to SLE.[4] Smoking increases the risk of rheumatoid arthritis.[5] Deficits in T-cell regulation or uncontrolled B-cell upregulation or other abnormalities in the relevant cytokine profiles are common in autoimmune disease, although no dominant abnormality explains the pathogenesis of any rheumatic illness. Rheumatoid arthritis is successfully treated with agents that block the effect of tumor necrosis factor α (TNF-α), suggesting a critical role of that cytokine in pathogenesis.[6] Interferon upregulation characterizes SLE.[7] Details of how these abnormalities lead to the specific symptoms of arthritis, nephritis, and vasculitis are conjectural.

Serologic abnormalities potentially precede the clinical onset of illness by decades.[8] High prevalence and titer of antibodies to Epstein-Barr virus in lupus patients suggest that this virus may have an etiologic role.[9]

With regard to immunologic phenomena of pregnancy that may be relevant to autoimmune disease, in vitro data show that estrogens upregulate and androgens downregulate T-cell responses, immunoglobulin synthesis, and leukocyte production of interleukin 1 (IL-1), IL-2, IL-6, and TNF-α, though changes in these cytokines are quantitatively small and remain within physiologic ranges.[10] In pregnancy, cell-mediated immunity is depressed, as reflected by abnormal lymphocyte stimulation, decreased ratios of T cells to B cells, increased ratios of suppressor T cells to helper T cells, and decreased ratios of lymphocytes to monocytes, all of which vary with the stage of pregnancy.[11,12] The pregnancy-specific proteins α-fetoprotein, β_1-glycoprotein, and β_2-macroglobulin suppress in vitro lymphocyte function. IL-1, IL-3, TNF-α, interferon γ, and granulocyte-macrophage colony-stimulating factor are critical in sustaining pregnancy.[13] IL-3 levels are low in women with repeated pregnancy loss. In normal pregnancy, total C3, C4, and hemolytic (CH_{50}) complement levels are usually unchanged or raised relative to nonpregnant levels, but increases in classic pathway complement activation products suggest that low-grade classic pathway activation is a normal phenomenon in pregnant women. Complement activation products can alter the balance of angiogenic factor production by inflammatory cells and result in excess soluble vascular endothelial growth factor receptor type 1 (sFlt-1), which has implications for placental development and the risk for preeclampsia.[14] Inhibition of complement activation in the placenta may be essential for fetal survival,[15] and the trophoblast may be a target of autoimmunity.[16] Theoretically,

TABLE 51-1 EPIDEMIOLOGIC, CLINICAL, AND LABORATORY CHARACTERISTICS AND PREGNANCY ISSUES OF COMMON AUTOIMMUNE RHEUMATIC ILLNESSES

Disease	Epidemiology	Common Symptoms	Laboratory Results	Pregnancy Issues
Systemic lupus erythematosus	Age 15-45 yr 9:1 female to male 4:2:1 black to Asian/Hispanic to white	Arthritis, rash, fever, anemia, thrombocytopenia, nephritis, neurologic disease, alopecia	High positive ANA value Anti-DNA and/or Smith (diagnostic) Antiphospholipid, anti-SSA/Ro, SSB/La, RNP antibodies (common) Raised ESR level Anemia, thrombocytopenia Proteinuria Low complement level	Fetal loss, neonatal lupus, organ system flare
Antiphospholipid syndrome	Age 15-60 yr Female > male White > black	Blood clots, fetal loss, livedo reticularis, thrombocytopenia, cardiac valve disease	Anticardiolipin Anti-β_2-glycoprotein 1 Lupus anticoagulant test Thrombocytopenia Proteinuria	Fetal loss, HELLP syndrome
Rheumatoid arthritis	Age 35-75 yr 3:1 female to male White = black	Destructive arthritis	Anti-cyclic citrullinated peptide antibody Rheumatoid factor Raised ESR, CRP levels Bone erosions at joints	Remission in some cases during pregnancy; positioning for delivery a problem
Spondyloarthropathy	Age 15-60 yr Male > female HLA-B27	Spinal and sacroiliac arthritis	Raised ESR, CRP values HLA-B27 Radiographic sacroiliitis Spinal fusion Enthesitis	Arthritis management
Takayasu arteritis	Age 15-60 yr 9:1 female to male	Large vessel vasculitis, cardiac valve disease	Raised ESR, CRP levels Alternating narrowing and aneurysm formation in aorta and great vessels	Vascular integrity, measurement of blood pressure, cardiac failure
Scleroderma	3:1 female to male	Raynaud phenomenon, skin disease, pulmonary hypertension, hypertensive renal failure, esophageal reflux, pulmonary fibrosis	Fibrosis on skin biopsy Pulmonary fibrosis Esophageal and intestinal hypomotility Reduced pulmonary diffusion capacity Urinary protein, raised creatinine level	Complications related to esophagus, lung, heart, kidneys
Juvenile arthritis	Before age 18 yr Female > male for some types	Polyarthritis; high fever and rash (Still's type)	Raised ESR, CRP levels Raised ferritin level Erosions of joints	Complications related to joint disease

ANAs, antinuclear antibodies; CRP, C-reactive protein; ESR, erythrocyte sedimentation rate; HELLP, hemolysis, elevated liver enzymes, and low platelets; RNP, ribonucleoprotein.

these pregnancy-related changes may alter the course of specific autoimmune diseases, but clear documentation that they do is lacking.

Diagnosis

Establishing a diagnosis of a systemic rheumatic illness requires combining symptoms and physical findings with compatible serologic abnormalities, markers of inflammation, and sometimes, imaging abnormalities. Established criteria exist for diagnosis of many of these diseases.[17-19] Critical clinical and laboratory findings that can differentiate the various rheumatic diseases are displayed in Table 51-1.

Inflammatory arthritis may be indistinguishable in patients with SLE, rheumatoid arthritis, or juvenile arthritis, but in the latter two, it is more likely to be sustained than transient, and it is more likely to cause deformity. In patients with these illnesses, arthritis involves peripheral joints; in spondyloarthropathy, axial joint involvement predominates. The rashes of SLE and scleroderma are diagnostic. Livedo reticularis is common in antiphospholipid syndrome but is not specific for this diagnosis. Asymptomatic or minimally symptomatic pulselessness or vascular bruits suggest Takayasu arteritis; arterial occlusion due to antiphospholipid syndrome is usually abrupt and symptomatic.

A diagnosis of SLE in an untreated patient requires a strongly positive result for antinuclear antibody and anti-DNA or anti-Smith antibody. However, the concept of "lupus-like" is accepted, and these patients are managed as if they had unequivocal lupus. Similarly, the diagnosis of antiphospholipid syndrome requires the presence of one or more of the following: a moderate to high titer (>40 IU) of anticardiolipin antibody of the IgG or IgM isotypes, lupus anticoagulant defined by the International Society on Thrombosis and Haemostasis standards,[20] or IgG or IgM antibody to β_2-glycoprotein 1 present for at least 12 weeks. Diagnoses of rheumatoid arthritis, scleroderma, and juvenile arthritis can be made on clinical grounds alone. A diagnosis of Takayasu arteritis requires a biopsy, angiogram, or magnetic resonance or positron emission image that documents involves of the aorta or its great branches.

Management and Prevention

Knowledge of the pharmacology of drugs specific to systemic rheumatic disease is essential to the management of pregnant patients.[21-23] Because these diseases are chronic and likely to exacerbate, withdrawal of medications before or during pregnancy is usually ill advised. Planning for pregnancy must take into consideration the medications that the patient can take safely when she conceives.

Nonsteroidal anti-inflammatory drugs (NSAIDs) may cause oligohydramnios or, rarely, injure fetal kidneys or induce premature closure of the ductus arteriosus. Prednisone and methylprednisolone are largely inactivated by a placental hydroxylase and do not reach the fetus in significant concentrations. Fluorinated corticosteroids (i.e., dexamethasone and betamethasone) are not inactivated and should be used only when there is intent to treat the fetus. Whether the commonly used pulse administration of corticosteroid (1000 mg of methylprednisolone by rapid intravenous infusion, usually on 3 consecutive days) is safe in pregnancy is unknown.

Azathioprine, which is widely used in renal transplant recipients and patients with Crohn disease, is relatively safe,[24] but fetal malformations have occurred in animal models.[25] Cyclophosphamide, methotrexate, and leflunomide are contraindicated in early pregnancy because of their teratogenic and abortifacient properties, although a few infants of women given cyclophosphamide late in pregnancy have been normal.[26] The TNF-α inhibitors (i.e., etanercept, infliximab, and adalimumab) are rated relatively safe, despite the lack of long-term experience with these drugs.[21-23,27] Table 51-2 summarizes conclusions of an international review group that systematically reviewed the published data.[21]

Patients with SLE, antiphospholipid syndrome, or spondyloarthropathy have normal fertility, and those with rheumatoid arthritis and scleroderma probably have slightly lower than normal fertility. Oral contraceptives likely do not induce exacerbation of SLE; they have a small or no effect on disease incidence.[28] Ovulation induction for purposes of enhancing fertility likely does not induce flares of lupus nor induce thrombosis in patients with antiphospholipid syndrome.[29] Except for imparting genetic susceptibility, paternal rheumatic illness does not cause infertility nor affect the child.

Rheumatic Diseases

Systemic Lupus Erythematosus

Although SLE patients may have intrinsic hormonal abnormalities, they are quantitatively minor and have no discernible effect on pregnancy outcome.[30-32] Pregnancy probably does not induce serious lupus flare.[33,34] Diagnosing flare during pregnancy is difficult because pregnancy-induced thrombocytopenia, preeclamptic proteinuria, and palmar and facial erythema resemble SLE flare. Flare is most confidently diagnosed when a pregnant patient has new or increasing diagnostic rash (not erythema alone), lymphadenopathy, arthritis, fever, or anti–double-stranded DNA (anti-dsDNA) antibody.

Fetal health is threatened because approximately one third of all SLE patients have anti-Ro or anti-La antibodies, or both, as do a few patients with discoid lupus, most with subacute cutaneous lupus, and most with Sjögren syndrome. These antibodies predispose to neonatal lupus. One third to one half of SLE patients have antiphospholipid antibodies, predisposing to fetal loss (discussed later).

Maternal Complications

Maternal complications are best considered by affected organ system, because global SLE exacerbation is rare. Approximately one fourth of all SLE patients develop thrombocytopenia during pregnancy, compared with about 7% of normal women.[35] Patients with antiphospholipid antibodies often have asymptomatic, low-grade thrombocytopenia ($>50 \times 10^9$/L) that worsens slightly during pregnancy. Abrupt, severe thrombocytopenia of the immune thrombocytopenia (ITP) type and lupus-related, low-grade chronic thrombocytopenia occur independent of pregnancy. No specific test clearly differentiates types of thrombocytopenia in pregnant patients with SLE. In our experience, in pregnant patients with lupus, thrombocytopenia equally often results from antiphospholipid antibodies, active SLE, and preeclampsia.

In patients with proteinuria, clinical signs of active SLE, rising levels of anti-dsDNA antibody, very low concentrations of complement, and urinary erythrocyte casts favor a diagnosis of lupus nephritis rather than preeclampsia. Rapid worsening over days suggests preeclampsia. Hypertension, thrombocytopenia, hyperuricemia, and hypocomplementemia occur in both; normal complement levels suggest preeclampsia. Two thirds of pregnant lupus patients who entered pregnancy with renal disease develop preeclampsia, compared with less than 20% of those without prior kidney disease.[36] In women with preexisting renal disease who develop preeclampsia, renal function may not return to its pre-pregnancy baseline.

Because skin blood flow increases in pregnancy, existing rash may become more prominent as pregnancy progresses. Patients who discontinue hydroxychloroquine for pregnancy often have recurrence of rash.

Joints previously damaged by lupus arthritis may develop noninflammatory effusions when ligament loosening occurs in late pregnancy. Neurologic lupus during pregnancy is rare, but case reports document chorea and transverse myelitis induced or exacerbated by pregnancy. In patients with seizures late in pregnancy accompanied by hypertension and renal failure, it may not be possible to distinguish between cerebral SLE and eclampsia. Treatment for both is usually indicated. Pulmonary hypertension may develop or worsen during pregnancy. Concomitant care with the obstetrician and rheumatologist is advisable.

Fetal Complications

If antiphospholipid antibodies, anti-Ro and anti-La antibodies, maternal fever, severe anemia, uremia, hypertension, and preeclampsia are absent, active SLE itself does not compromise the fetus. Infants born of SLE mothers with IgG-induced thrombocytopenia usually have normal platelet counts. Rarely, Coombs antibody causes hemolysis in the fetus; anti-dsDNA antibody has no apparent pathologic effect. Thrombosis due to antiphospholipid antibodies rarely occurs in the fetus.

The *neonatal lupus syndrome* includes photosensitive rash, thrombocytopenia, hepatitis, and hemolytic anemia, all of which are transient, and congenital complete heart block, which is not.[37] The syndrome occurs exclusively in neonates of women with high-titer anti-Ro/SSA or anti-La/SSB antibodies, or both, many of whom are clinically well (a small number later develop SLE or Sjögren syndrome). With the exception of neonatal lupus syndrome, there are no congenital abnormalities associated with SLE.

Congenital heart block is first diagnosable in utero by fetal electrocardiography, ultrasound, or cardiac rate monitoring between 18 and 25 weeks' gestation (average, 23 weeks). Among SLE patients with anti-

TABLE 51-2 PREGNANCY-RELEVANT CHARACTERISTICS OF COMMONLY USED ANTIRHEUMATIC DRUGS

Drug	FDA Pregnancy Class*	FDA Lactation Class†	Safety	Comments
Aspirin‡	D§	S(?)	Variable: depends on dose and time of use	Low dose may be partially protective against fetal death in antiphospholipid syndrome; may cause maternal and fetal bleeding if administered near term; high dose of uncertain safety
Naproxen, ibuprofen, ketoprofen nabumetone, and similar drugs‡	B/D§	S(*)	Variable, depends on dose and time of use	Experience largely accumulated through treatment of headache or dysmenorrhea; no major teratogenicity; use after 34 weeks not advised
Ketorolac‡	C	S(*)	Causes dystocia and neonatal death in animals	Insufficient human experience
Celecoxib‖	C	S(?)	Few data	Insufficient human experience; not protective against thromboembolic disease
Indomethacin‡	B/D§	S(*)	Variable, depends on dose and time of use	Fetal pulmonary hypertension if used at term in third trimester; oligohydramnios
Prednisone	B	S	Generally safe	Trivial passage across placenta; safe in lactation but may suppress milk production
Methylprednisolone	B	NS	Probably safe	Similar to prednisone but fewer data available
Dexamethasone, betamethasone	C	NS	Probably safe in late pregnancy	Important transfer across placenta; used to induce fetal lung maturation
Hydroxychloroquine	C	S	Likely safe	Small published experience indicating safety
Azathioprine	D	NS	Safety uncertain	Large experience with renal transplant patients indicates no immediate danger to offspring if maternal dose is < 2 mg/kg/day; rare reports of congenital anomalies, including immunodeficiency
Cyclosporine	C	NS	Probably safe	Little experience, none suggesting high fetal risk
Cyclophosphamide	D	NS	Dangerous	Abortifacient, teratogenic
Methotrexate	X	NS	Dangerous	Abortifacient, teratogenic
Leflunomide	X	NS	Dangerous	Abortifacient, teratogenic
Etanercept	B	S(?)	Appears to be safe	No long-term studies in children
Infliximab	B	S(?)	Appears to be safe	No long-term studies in children
Adalimumab	B	S(?)	Appears to be safe	No long-term studies in children
Heparin	B	S	Appears to be safe	Anticoagulant of choice; causes osteoporosis
Low-molecular-weight heparin	B	S(?)	Similar to heparin	Similar to heparin, fewer data
Warfarin	X	S	Teratogenic and possibly fetotoxic	Fetal warfarin syndrome when given in first trimester; may cause central nervous system defects in second and third trimesters; risk of severe neonatal hemorrhage when given near term
Intravenous immunoglobulin	B	—	Appears to be safe	Administered antibodies carried to fetus

***U.S. Food and Drug Administration (FDA) pregnancy risk classification: A, controlled trials show no risk in humans; B, animal studies show no risk but no definitive studies in humans; C, animal studies show risk *or* no studies in humans *or* no information; D, positive evidence of risk but risk-benefit ratio may be acceptable in some circumstances; X, fetal risk and risk-benefit ratio always unacceptable.**

†Lactation classification: S, safe; S(*), potential for significant effects on nursing infants, give only with caution; S(?) unknown, theoretically safe, insufficient literature; NS, not safe, contraindicated, known danger.

‡All inhibitors of prostaglandin synthesis activity may inhibit labor and prolong gestation. There is also a risk of in utero closure of the ductus arteriosus, particularly when used after 34 weeks' gestation.

§Risk category D when used in the third trimester.

Adapted from Ostensen M, Khamashta M, Lockshin M, et al: Anti-inflammatory and immunosuppressive drugs and reproduction. Arthritis Res Ther 8:209, 2006.

‖Drug use restricted in patients with arterial occlusive disease.

Ro antibody, the risk that a liveborn child will have neonatal lupus rash is 25%, and congenital complete heart block is less than 3%. However, the risks of recurrent congenital heart block and neonatal lupus rash are 18% and 25%, respectively. Cardiac injury may be related to expression of the cardiac 52B Ro antigen after apoptosis of cardiomyocytes and to induction of profibrotic cytokines around the conducting system.[38,39] No specific antibody pattern predicts neonatal lupus rash. Several dizygotic twins and at least one monozygotic twin pair have been discordant for neonatal lupus, suggesting fetal contribution to illness.

Dexamethasone and plasmapheresis for the mother and early delivery have been used, with variable success, to treat fetal incomplete heart block, myocarditis, heart failure, and hydrops fetalis. Complete heart block in a newborn usually requires a permanent pacemaker. Even with a pacemaker, progressive fibrosis of the conducting system, cardiac failure, and sudden death may occur before age 5.

Preliminary data suggest that boys of SLE mothers have increased risk for learning disabilities but have normal intelligence, compared with sex- and gestational age-matched controls.[40] Children with complete congenital heart block remain at risk for cardiac death. Although case reports have described survivors of neonatal lupus who developed systemic lupus when they became adults, such events are rare. Other than the inherited tendency to develop rheumatic illness, there are no other known risks to children of other rheumatic disease mothers.

Antiphospholipid Syndrome

(See Chapter 40 for in-depth discussion of coagulation effects of antiphospholipid antibodies.)

Untreated patients with antiphospholipid syndrome and history of a fetal loss have a high frequency of mid-pregnancy intrauterine growth restriction or fetal death. Very high levels of antibody worsen the prognosis, and the simultaneous presence of several antiphospholipid antibodies increases risk, as does a prior fetal death.[41] Low level IgM and IgG anticardiolipin antibodies are not associated with poor fetal outcome, nor is an isolated false-positive test result for syphilis in the absence of other markers. Anti-β_2-glycoprotein 1 antibodies predict fetal death in the occasional patient who tests negative for anticardiolipin and lupus anticoagulant.[42] Few antiphospholipid syndrome patients suffer thromboses during pregnancy, possibly because most are prophylactically treated with heparin and low-dose aspirin. Risk of stroke and thrombophlebitis increases after delivery, especially after discontinuation of anticoagulant therapy. Ischemic cardiomyopathy and myocardial infarction may also occur after delivery. Thrombocytopenia, if a new occurrence during pregnancy, usually remits after delivery.

A pregnancy compromised by antiphospholipid antibodies is often initially uneventful, but the fetal growth rate then slows. Antepartum fetal heart rate monitoring studies show nonreactive fetal heart rate pattern, spontaneous bradycardia, diminished fetal motion, decreased amniotic fluid, reduced placental size, and, if delivery is not accomplished, fetal death. The mother may show no evidence of illness or may develop severe preeclampsia or HELLP syndrome (i.e., *h*emolysis, *e*levated *l*iver enzymes, and *l*ow *p*latelets). With treatment, fetal survival rates of more than 80% are possible, compared with less than 20% in the earliest series of untreated patients. After a patient has had a strongly positive test result for antiphospholipid antibodies during pregnancy, the fetal prognosis does not improve if lupus anticoagulant activity disappears or if anticardiolipin antibody levels decrease.

Placentas of SLE patients without antiphospholipid antibodies exhibit ischemic-hypoxic change and chronic villitis, whereas those of patients with antiphospholipid antibodies can also have decidual vasculopathy, extensive maternal floor infarction (Fig. 51-1) due to uteroplacental or spiral artery thrombosis, endothelial cell proliferation, or other fetoplacental vasculopathy.[43,44] Antiphospholipid antibody, β_2-glycoprotein 1, and placenta anticoagulant protein 1 (PAP-1) deposit together in placentas of mothers with antiphospholipid syndrome.[45] Studies[46,47] underscore the importance of inflammatory infiltrates and complement deposits in placentas from patients with antiphospholipid antibodies.

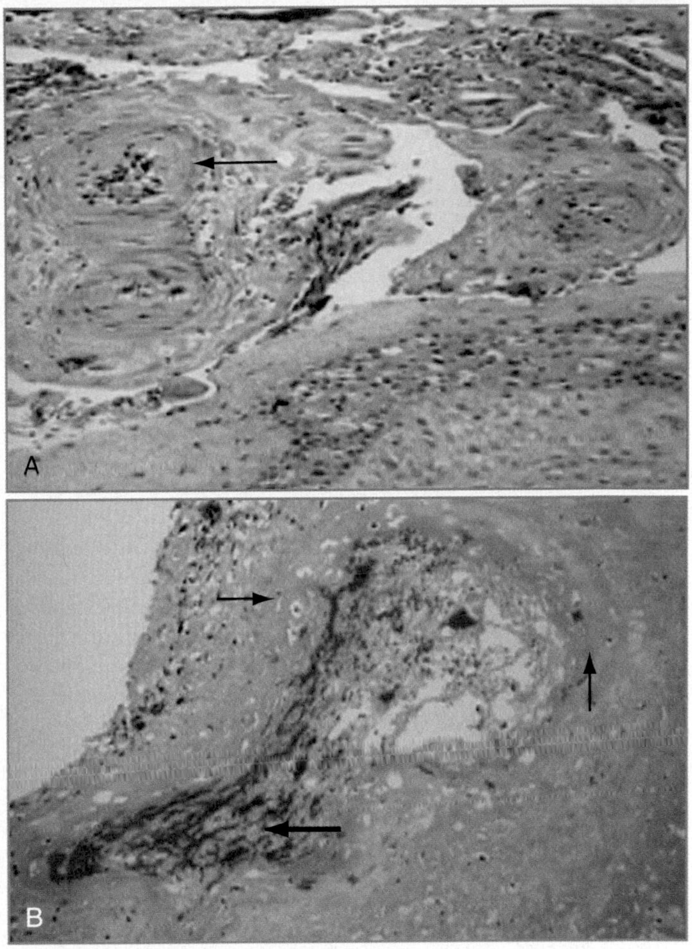

FIGURE 51-1 **Patients with antiphospholipid antibodies may have decidual vasculopathy, extensive maternal floor infarction, endothelial cell proliferation, and other fetoplacental vasculopathy.** **A,** Placental biopsy specimen demonstrates a lack of physiologic conversion, resulting in decidual vasculopathy. *Arrow* indicates spiral arterioles with smooth muscular walls and a small lumen. **B,** Placental biopsy specimen demonstrates fibrinoid necrosis in the decidual vessel wall *(small arrows)* and thrombosis in the decidual vessel *(large arrow)*. (George D, Vasanth L, Erkan D, et al: Primary antiphospholipid syndrome presenting as HELLP syndrome. Hosp Special Surg J 3:216-221, 2007).

Monitoring of antiphospholipid syndrome pregnancies consists of ultrasound evaluation of the fetal growth rate and placental volume and appearance. Weekly antepartum fetal heart rate testing may begin as early as 25 weeks. In the 25- to 32-week period, a reactive nonstress test is defined as 2 accelerations of at least 10 bpm during a 20-minute interval. Thereafter, 15 bpm is used. Nonreassuring fetal testing indicates a need to deliver. Choice of the route of delivery is determined by obstetric criteria, as well as maternal and fetal platelet counts. Newborns who test positive rarely have pathologic clotting. Short-term follow-up studies of infant survivors of lupus patients indicate that these children develop normally compared with children of equivalent prematurity, but detailed information regarding children of non-SLE patients with antiphospholipid syndrome is not available.

The relationship of autoantibodies, particularly antiphospholipid antibodies, to failure of in vitro fertilization (IVF) and embryo transfer is unproven. Murine models of antiphospholipid syndrome show abnormal blastocyst development and impairment of embryo implantation.[48] In animal models, fetal death depends on complement and adhesion molecules, and prevention of complement activation prevents fetal death. Heparin, the standard of care for pregnant patients with antiphospholipid syndrome, inhibits activation of complement and blocks leukocyte adhesion.[15,49] Further evidence that these antibodies do not appear to be associated with very early pregnancy loss is found in a meta-analysis of seven studies examining the impact of antiphospholipid antibodies on IVF outcomes. Hornstein and associates[50] reported no significant association between antiphospholipid antibodies and clinical pregnancy (OR = 0.99; 95% confidence interval [CI], 0.64 to 1.53) or live birth rates (OR = 1.07; 95% CI, 0.66 to 1.75). The investigators concluded that measurement of antiphospholipid antibodies is not warranted in patients undergoing IVF. Moreover, there is no evidence that treating patients who have antiphospholipid antibodies improves IVF success rates.[51] Other than placental insufficiency, with its risk of intrauterine growth restriction or fetal death, there are no special risks to the fetus.

Treatment recommendations for antiphospholipid syndrome pregnancy are presented in Table 51-3. Controlled treatment trials of women with two or more pregnancy losses demonstrate that low-dose aspirin (81 mg/day) plus subcutaneous unfractionated heparin (5000 to 12,000 units twice daily) begun after ultrasonographic confirmation of a viable pregnancy results in a rate of live births (not necessarily term) of more than 80%.[52,53] The lower heparin dose is as effective as higher doses, but patients who have had prior thromboses require full anticoagulant doses. Low-molecular-weight heparin has been used successfully but has not been tested in controlled trials. In a small, controlled trial, intravenous immunoglobulin did not show benefit in the primary treatment of antiphospholipid syndrome patients,[54] but it is often used in those in whom heparin has failed. Warfarin is contraindicated because it is teratogenic. Osteoporosis remains a major potential side effect of heparin treatment,[55] although it is less common with low-molecular-weight heparin.

Based on empiric data of postpartum thromboses, treated women with no prior thromboses should receive oral warfarin for 6-12 postpartum weeks. Aspirin, if used during pregnancy, should also continue for at least 3 months.

Rheumatoid Arthritis

Whether women have a high rate of pregnancy loss before developing rheumatoid arthritis is controversial. Patients with established rheumatoid arthritis frequently improve during pregnancy. Proposed reasons include the immunosuppressive effects of endogenous corticosteroid, pregnancy-associated plasma protein A, and maternal-fetal human leukocyte antigen HLA-DQ and -DR disparity. The latest data favor the latter explanation.[56] Flare of rheumatoid arthritis often follows delivery, as does new development of rheumatoid arthritis.

Pregnancy is usually uneventful in rheumatoid arthritis patients. Rheumatoid joints may become unstable in late pregnancy as physiologic joint loosening occurs and as the patient's weight distribution changes. Undiagnosed cervical spine subluxation is a particular concern. Bacteremia occurring during labor, although rare, may seed involved joints. Antiphospholipid, anti-Ro, and anti-La antibodies are uncommon, and neonatal lupus therefore occurs infrequently. High-risk pregnancy monitoring usually is not necessary. There is a slight increase in risk of fetal growth restriction and maternal hypertension, and hospitalizations are slightly longer than normal for patients with rheumatoid arthritis.[57]

Most patients need to continue their pre-pregnancy medications, including NSAIDs, corticosteroids, hydroxychloroquine, azathioprine, and TNF-α inhibitors. Low-dose prednisone is the safest option. Concomitant care with the obstetrician and rheumatologist is advisable.

Before delivery, the team managing the patient must take special care to identify the patient's disabilities to prepare for labor. Points for special emphasis are hip, knee, and neck arthritis and the potential risks of forcing joint motion beyond disease-imposed constraints,

TABLE 51-3 TREATMENT RECOMMENDATIONS FOR PREGNANT WOMEN WITH POSITIVE ANTIPHOSPHOLIPID ANTIBODY RESULTS AND NO OTHER EXPLANATION FOR PREGNANCY LOSSES

Patient Characteristic	Recommendation
High-Titer IgG or IgM aCL (>40 IU) or Positive LA Test*	
Primipara, multipara with most recent liveborn pregnancy or multipara with most recent pregnancy failure < 10 weeks (one loss)	Consider aspirin, 81 mg/day or no therapy initially; if modest (>50 × 10^9/L) and thrombocytopenia occurs, add aspirin*
Multipara, multipara with most recent pregnancy failure < 10 weeks (more than one loss), or multipara with most recent pregnancy failure ≥ 10 weeks (fetal loss)	Aspirin while trying to conceive; add heparin, 5000 units bid or low-dose LMWH at confirmation of fetal heartbeat, continue for duration of pregnancy
Multipara with prior premature birth due to preeclampsia or IUGR	Aspirin beginning after first trimester; consider heparin, depending on blood pressure control and renal function
Low-Titer IgG or IgM aCL	
Primipara, multipara with most recent liveborn pregnancy or multipara with most recent pregnancy failure < 10 weeks (one loss)	No therapy
Multipara, multipara with most recent pregnancy failure < 10 weeks (more than one loss), or multipara with most recent pregnancy failure ≥ 10 weeks (fetal loss)	Aspirin while trying to conceive; add heparin, 5000 units bid or low-dose LMWH at confirmation of fetal heartbeat, continue for duration of pregnancy
Multipara with prior premature birth due to preeclampsia or IUGR	Aspirin beginning after first trimester; consider heparin, depending on blood pressure control and renal function

*For thrombocytopenia <50 × 10^9/L, consider intravenous immunoglobulin or prednisone, or both.
aCL, anticardiolipin antibody; aPL, antiphospholipid antibody; Ig, immunoglobulin; IUGR, intrauterine growth restriction; LA, lupus anticoagulant; LMWH, low-molecular-weight heparin.

causing fracture or other injury. Elective cesarean delivery may be necessary. If intubation is planned, an anesthesiologist familiar with temporomandibular arthritis and rheumatoid cervical spine disease should be available. There are no special risks to the fetus other than those related to maternal therapy.

Sjögren Syndrome

Sjögren syndrome is characterized by generally less severe arthritis but keratoconjunctivitis sicca. Sjögren syndrome often results from another autoimmune disease, and little is known about the interaction of pregnancy with the primary syndrome. About 80% of Sjögren patients have anti-Ro/SSA and anti-La/SSB antibodies, and their children are therefore at risk for neonatal lupus.[58] Intrauterine growth restriction is uncommon. Management of patients with Sjögren syndrome is the same as that for rheumatoid arthritis, except for the monitoring necessary for neonatal lupus. Treatment of the eye and mouth manifestations of primary Sjögren syndrome is the same as in the nonpregnant patient, but the effect of pilocarpine or cevimeline (U.S. Food and Drug Administration [FDA] category C drugs) on a fetus is unknown.

Scleroderma

Scleroderma often affects women in their late reproductive years, and pregnancy during established disease is uncommon. Patients with scleroderma generally do well but may tolerate pregnancy poorly if they have limited pulmonary, cardiac, or renal function. Occasionally, scleroderma renal crisis occurs during pregnancy; it may be difficult to distinguish from preeclampsia.[59,60] Problems derive from nondistensible vascular beds and from preexisting renal, cardiac, and pulmonary insufficiency. Gastroesophageal reflux, which is common during pregnancy even in women with normal esophageal motility, can be disabling. Treatment is standard: small meals, elevating the head of the bed, histamine$_2$-blockers (FDA category B), and proton pump inhibitors (FDA category C), but not the prostaglandin E_1 analogue misoprostol (FDA category X). Maternal preeclampsia, congestive heart failure, pulmonary hypertension, pulmonary insufficiency, and renal insufficiency may occur. Renal scleroderma may be indistinguishable from preeclampsia; it may justify termination of pregnancy.[61] Angiotensin-converting enzyme inhibitors and receptor antagonists are contraindicated in the periconceptional period because of their teratogenicity (risk ratio [RR] = 2.71; 95% CI, 1.72 to 4.27) and during pregnancy because of their potential to induce renal failure and fetal deformation due to prolonged oligohydramnios, except if renal hypertensive crisis refractory to all other antihypertension medications occurs.[62] Patients with severe atonic small bowel disease can carry a pregnancy to term with the use of parenteral nutritional support. Prematurity and intrauterine growth restriction are the greatest risks to the infant. A high and persistent degree of transplacental transfer of fetal cells occurs in scleroderma patients, but the relationship of this finding to disease pathogenesis is unknown. Years after pregnancy is over, fetal cells can still be found in affected maternal skin sites.[63,64]

Spondyloarthropathy

Women with ankylosing spondylitis have normal fertility. Most patients experience no change or modest worsening of complaints during pregnancy; those who worsen return to baseline after delivery.[65] Patients with psoriatic arthritis may improve during pregnancy. Other than the specific anatomic problems of spondyloarthropathy (i.e., restricted motion of the hips and lower back that may impede vaginal delivery), patients have no unusual problems with pregnancy. Treatment for painful back is problematic because indomethacin and other NSAIDs may cause fetal harm.

Vasculitis

Patients with Takayasu disease may do well, but renovascular occlusive disease, pulmonary hypertension, and aortic insufficiency remain important potential problems. Preeclampsia is common. Management during pregnancy involves careful monitoring and treatment of hypertension (diagnosis and monitoring of which is difficult when arm arteries are occluded) and aggressive hemodynamic and pharmacologic management in the peripartum period. Sixty percent of infants have intrauterine growth restriction related to maternal aortic involvement, hypertension, and preeclampsia.

Miscellaneous Disorders

Hip disease of any kind may interfere with normal vaginal delivery, because abduction may be severely limited. Forcing a patient's joint motion beyond the point at which she feels pain or at which resistance is encountered is painful and risks fracture, dislocation, or other permanent harm. Antibiotic coverage (i.e., a cephalosporin plus gentamicin or vancomycin plus gentamicin) may be indicated in women with artificial joint replacements undergoing vaginal delivery. Pelvic and back pain may be caused by laxity of the pubic symphysis and sacroiliac joints, which is associated with increased serum levels of relaxin. Labor and delivery are occasionally complicated after delivery by infectious sacroiliitis or osteitis pubis. For diagnosis of back pain in pregnant patients, magnetic resonance imaging is preferable to computed tomography. Ultrasound, infrared therapy, and warm water therapeutic pool therapy may injure the fetus.

Pregnancy Management

Monitoring recommendations for patients with rheumatic disease are presented in Table 51-4. Unexplained elevations of maternal α-fetoprotein and human chorionic gonadotropin occur in patients with lupus and with antiphospholipid antibodies. These abnormalities correlate with preterm delivery, requirements for a higher prednisone dose, and fetal death.[66] Because intervention with dexamethasone at the earliest sign of cardiac dysfunction may reverse myocarditis and possibly congenital heart block, women with high-titer anti-Ro and anti-La antibodies and those who have previously given birth to a child with any form of neonatal lupus should undergo fetal cardiac monitoring weekly during the vulnerable period of 18 to 25 weeks' gestation. In women known to be strongly positive for lupus anticoagulant and anticardiolipin antibody, repeat testing for these antibodies during pregnancy is unnecessary, because spontaneous correction of the lupus anticoagulant level and a decrease in the anticardiolipin antibody level does not improve prognosis. In women with low antibody levels or negative test results, repetition at least once each trimester is useful because overall prognosis is that of the highest level seen during the pregnancy. The platelet count should be repeated monthly. Women significantly positive for antiphospholipid antibodies and who have had a prior fetal loss should be treated with low-dose aspirin and unfractionated or low-molecular-weight heparin.

Decisions regarding timing and route of delivery are dictated by the status of the fetus but may be influenced by maternal illness and its

TABLE 51-4 RECOMMENDED EVALUATION OF PREGNANT PATIENTS WITH AUTOIMMUNE RHEUMATIC DISEASE

Recommended Frequency	Monitoring Test
First visit	Complete blood count and urinalysis* Creatinine clearance Antiphospholipid antibodies Anti-Ro and anti-La antibodies Anti-dsDNA antibody (SLE patients) Complement (C3 and C4 or CH_{50}) (SLE patients)
Monthly	Platelet count†
Each trimester	Creatinine clearance† A 24-hour urine protein assay if screening urinalysis is abnormal† Complement† and anti-dsDNA antibody†
Weekly (last trimester, mothers with antiphospholipid antibodies)	Antenatal fetal heart rate testing (nonstress test), and/or biophysical profile‡
Between 18 and 25 weeks (mothers with anti-Ro/La antibodies)	Fetal echocardiogram, fetal electrocardiogram (?)

*The erythrocyte sedimentation rate is often abnormal in uncomplicated pregnancy.
†More frequently if abnormal.
‡Measure of fetal size, activity, and amniotic fluid volume.
CH_{50}, hemolytic complement level; dsDNA, double-stranded DNA; SLE, systemic lupus erythematosus.
Adapted from Lockshin MD: Pregnancy and rheumatic disease. In Koopman WJ, Moreland LW (eds): Arthritis and Allied Conditions, 15th ed. Philadelphia, Lippincott Williams & Wilkins, 2005, pp 1719-1728.

complications. Approximately one third of SLE patients undergo operative delivery. The usual indications for cesarean delivery are fetal distress, prior cesarean delivery, prolonged ruptured membranes, failure to progress at labor and other obstetric reasons, thrombocytopenia, and severe maternal illness.

There is little information about the use of tocolytics or stimulators of labor in pregnant women with rheumatic disease. Ritodrine, magnesium sulfate, and prostaglandin suppositories have been used without incident. At delivery, stress corticosteroid doses (usually 100 mg of hydrocortisone every 8 hours from the onset of labor until 24 hours after delivery) are administered to patients currently or recently taking corticosteroids. Asymptomatic bacteremia occurs in 3.6% of vaginal deliveries. Because of limited hip joint movement or risk of bacterial seeding, osteonecrosis of the hip may justify a decision for operative rather than vaginal delivery. The mode of delivery for patients with total hip replacements need not be surgical; patients have been delivered vaginally with appropriate attention paid to the positioning of the patient.

References

1. Khan MA, Mathieu A, Sorrentino R, et al: The pathogenetic role of HLA-B27 and its subtypes. Autoimmun Rev 6:183, 2007.
2. van der Helm-van Mil AH, Verpoort KN, le Cessie S, et al: The HLA-DRB1 shared epitope alleles differ in the interaction with smoking and predisposition to antibodies to cyclic citrullinated peptide. Arthritis Rheum 56:425, 2007.
3. Graham RR, Ortmann W, Rodine P, et al: Specific combinations of HLA-DR2 and DR3 class II haplotypes contribute graded risk for disease susceptibility and autoantibodies in human SLE. Eur J Hum Genet 15:823, 2007.
4. Boeckler P, Meyer A, Uring-Lambert B, et al: Which complement assays and typings are necessary for the diagnosis of complement deficiency in patients with lupus erythematosus? A study of 25 patients. Clin Immunol 121:198, 2006.
5. Klareskog L, Stolt P, Lundberg K, et al: A new model for an etiology of rheumatoid arthritis: Smoking may trigger HLA-DR (shared epitope)-restricted immune reactions to autoantigens modified by citrullination. Arthritis Rheum 54:38, 2006.
6. Skomsvoll JF, Wallenius M, Koksvik HS, et al: Drug insight: Anti-tumor necrosis factor therapy for inflammatory arthropathies during reproduction, pregnancy and lactation. Nat Clin Pract Rheumatol 3:156, 2007.
7. Hua J, Kirou K, Lee C, et al: Functional assay of type I interferon in systemic lupus erythematosus plasma and association with anti-RNA binding protein autoantibodies. Arthritis Rheum 54:1906, 2006.
8. Arbuckle MR, McClain MT, Rubertone MV, et al: Development of autoantibodies before the clinical onset of systemic lupus erythematosus. N Engl J Med 349:1526, 2003.
9. James JA, Harley JB, Scofield RH: Epstein-Barr virus and systemic lupus erythematosus. Curr Opin Rheumatol 18:462, 2006.
10. Cohen-Solal JF, Jeganathan V, Grimaldi CM, et al: Sex hormones and SLE: Influencing the fate of autoreactive B cells. Curr Top Microbiol Immunol 305:67, 2006.
11. Piccinni M-P: Role of immune cells in pregnancy. Autoimmunity 36:1, 2003.
12. Munoz-Valle JF, Vazquez-Del Mercado M, Garcia-Iglesias T, et al: T(H)1-T(H)2 cytokine profile, metalloprotease-9 activity and hormonal status in pregnant rheumatoid arthritis and systemic lupus erythematosus patients. Clin Exp Immunol 131:377, 2003.
13. Berman J, Girardi G, Salmon JE: TNF-alpha is a critical effector and a target for therapy in antiphospholipid antibody-induced pregnancy loss. J Immunol 174:485, 2005.
14. Girardi G, Yarilin D, Thurman JM, et al: Complement activation induces dysregulation of angiogenic factors and causes fetal rejection and growth restriction. J Exp Med 203:2165, 2006.
15. Girardi G, Redecha P, Salmon JE: Heparin prevents antiphospholipid antibody-induced fetal loss by inhibiting complement activation. Nat Med 10:1222, 2004.
16. Bulla R, Bossi F, Radillo O, et al: Placental trophoblast and endothelial cells as a target of maternal immune response. Autoimmunity 36:11, 2003.
17. Hochberg MC: Updating the American College of Rheumatology revised criteria for the classification of systemic lupus erythematosus [letter]. Arthritis Rheum 40:1725, 1997.
18. Arnett FC, Edworthy SM, Bloch DA, et al: The American Rheumatism Association 1987 revised criteria for the classification of rheumatoid arthritis. Arthritis Rheum 31:315, 1988.
19. Miyakis S, Lockshin MD, Atsumi T, et al: International consensus statement on an update of the classification criteria for definite antiphospholipid syndrome (APS). J Thromb Haemost 4:295, 2006.
20. Brandt JT, Triplett DA, Alving B, et al: Criteria for the diagnosis of lupus anticoagulants: An update. On behalf of the Subcommittee on Lupus Anticoagulant/Antiphospholipid Antibody of the Scientific and Standardisation Committee of the ISTH. Thromb Haemost 74:1185, 1995.
21. Ostensen M, Khamashta M, Lockshin M, et al: Anti-inflammatory and immunosuppressive drugs and reproduction. Arthritis Res Ther 8:209, 2006.
22. Hyrich KL, Symmons DP, Watson KD, et al, for the British Society for Rheumatology Biologics Register: Pregnancy outcome in women who were exposed to anti-tumor necrosis factor agents: results from a national population register. Arthritis Rheum 54:2701, 2006.

23. Salmon JE, Alpert D: Are we coming to terms with tumor necrosis factor inhibition in pregnancy? Arthritis Rheum 54:2353, 2006.
24. Langagergaard V, Pedersen L, Gislum M, et al: Birth outcome in women treated with azathioprine or mercaptopurine during pregnancy: A Danish nationwide cohort study. Aliment Pharmacol Ther 25:73-81, 2007.
25. Schmid BP: Monitoring of organ formation in rat embryos after in vitro exposure to azathioprine, mercaptopurine, methotrexate or cyclosporin A. Toxicology 31:9-21, 1984.
26. Ramsey-Goldman R, Mientus JM, Kutzer JE, et al: Pregnancy outcome in women with systemic lupus erythematosus treated with immunosuppressive drugs. J Rheumatol 20:1152-1157, 1993.
27. Chambers CD, Tutuncu ZN, Johnson D, et al: Human pregnancy safety for agents used to treat rheumatoid arthritis: Adequacy of available information and strategies for developing post-marketing data. Arth Res Ther 8:215, 2006.
28. Petri M, Kim MY, Kalunian KC, et al: OC-SELENA trial. Combined oral contraceptives in women with systemic lupus erythematosus. N Engl J Med 353:2550, 2005.
29. Guballa N, Sammaritano L, Schwartzman S, et al: Ovulation induction and in vitro fertilization in systemic lupus erythematosus and antiphospholipid syndrome. Arthritis Rheum 43:550, 2000.
30. McMurray RW: Steroid hormones in lupus pregnancy: In control? Arthritis Rheum 47:116, 2002.
31. Costenbader KH, Feskanich D, Stampfer MJ, et al: Reproductive and menopausal factors and risk of systemic lupus erythematosus in women. Arthritis Rheum 56:1251, 2007.
32. Lockshin MD, Buyon JP: Estrogens and lupus: Bubbling cauldron or another overrated Witches' Brew? Arthritis Rheum 56:1048, 2007.
33. Ruiz-Irastorza G, Lima F, Alves J, et al: Increased rate of lupus flare during pregnancy and the puerperium: A prospective study of 78 pregnancies. Br J Rheumatol 35:133, 1996.
34. Lockshin MD, Sammaritano LR: Lupus pregnancy. Autoimmunity 36:33, 2003.
35. Parnas M, Sheiner E, Shoham-Vardi I, et al: Moderate to severe thrombocytopenia during pregnancy. Eur J Obstet Gynecol Reprod Biol 128:163, 2006.
36. Meng C, Lockshin M: Pregnancy in lupus. Curr Opin Rheumatol 11:348, 1999.
37. Buyon JP, Clancy RM: Neonatal lupus: review of the proposed pathogenesis and clinical data from the US-based research registry for neonatal lupus. Autoimmunity 36:41, 2003.
38. Buyon JP, Tseng C-E, DiDonato F, et al: Cardiac expression of 52b, an alternative transcript of the congenital heart block–associated 52-kd SS-A/Ro autoantigen, is maximal during fetal development. Arthritis Rheum 40:655, 1997.
39. Clancy RM, Askanase AD, Kapur RP, et al: Transdifferentiation of cardiac fibroblasts, a fetal factor in anti-SSA/Ro-SSB/La antibody-mediated congenital heart block. J Immunol 169:2156, 2002.
40. Ross G, Sammaritano L, Nass R, et al: Effects of mothers' autoimmune disease during pregnancy on learning disabilities and hand preference in their children. Arch Pediatr Adolesc Med 157:397, 2003.
41. Lockshin MD, Druzin ML, Qamar T: Prednisone does not prevent recurrent fetal death in women with antiphospholipid antibody. Am J Obstet Gynecol 160:439-443, 1989.
42. Di Simone N, Raschi E, Testoni C, et al: Pathogenic role of anti-beta 2-glycoprotein I antibodies in antiphospholipid associated fetal loss: Characterisation of beta 2-glycoprotein I binding to trophoblast cells and functional effects of anti-beta 2-glycoprotein I antibodies in vitro. Ann Rheum Dis 64:462-467, 2005.
43. Magid MS, Kaplan C, Sammaritano LR, et al: Placental pathology in systemic lupus erythematosus: A prospective study. Am J Obstet Gynecol 179:226, 1998.
44. Sebire NJ, Regan L, Rai R: Biology and pathology of the placenta in relation to antiphospholipid antibody-associated pregnancy failure. Lupus 11:641, 2002.
45. La Rosa L, Meroni PL, Tincani A, et al: Beta-2-glycoprotein I and placental anticoagulant protein I in placentae from patients with antiphospholipid antibody syndrome. J Rheumatol 21:1684, 1994.
46. Shamonki JM, Salmon JE, Hyjek E, et al: Excessive complement activation is associated with placental injury in patients with antiphospholipid antibodies. Am J Obstet Gynecol 6:167, 2007.
47. Stone S, Pijnenborg R, Vercruysse L, et al: The placental bed in pregnancies complicated by primary antiphospholipid syndrome Placenta 27:457, 2006.
48. Sthoeger ZM, Mozes E, Tartakovsky B: Anti-cardiolipin antibodies induce pregnancy failure by impairing embryonic implantation. Proc Natl Acad Sci U S A 90:6464, 1993.
49. Wang L, Brown JR, Varki A, et al: Heparin's anti-inflammatory effects require glucosamine 6-O-sulfation and are mediated by blockade of L- and P-selectins. J Clin Invest 110:127, 2002.
50. Hornstein M, Davis O, Massey J, et al: Antiphospholipid antibodies and in vitro fertilization success: A meta-analysis. Fertil Steril 73:330-333, 2000.
51. Stern C, Chamley L, Norris H, et al: A randomized, double-blind, placebo-controlled trial of heparin and aspirin for women with in vitro fertilization implantation failure and antiphospholipid or antinuclear antibodies. Fertil Steril 80:376-383, 2003.
52. Kutteh WH, Ermel LD. A clinical trial for the treatment of aPL associated recurrent pregnancy loss with lower dose heparin and aspirin. Am J Reprod Immunol 35:402, 1996.
53. Rai R, Cohen H, Dave M, et al: Randomized controlled trial of aspirin and aspirin plus heparin in pregnant women with recurrent miscarriage associated with phospholipid antibodies (or antiphospholipid antibodies). BMJ 314:253, 1997.
54. Triolo G, Ferrante A, Ciccia F, et al: Randomized study of subcutaneous low molecular weight heparin plus aspirin versus intravenous immunoglobulin in the treatment of recurrent fetal loss associated with antiphospholipid antibodies. Arthritis Rheum 48:728, 2003.
55. Ruiz-Irastorza G, Khamashta MA, Hughes GRV: Heparin and osteoporosis during pregnancy: 2002 update. Lupus 11:680, 2002.
56. Nelson JL: Microchimerism in human health and disease. Autoimmunity 36:5, 2003.
57. Chakravarty EF, Nelson L, Krishnan E: Obstetric hospitalizations in the United States for women with systemic lupus erythematosus and rheumatoid arthritis. Arthritis Rheum 54: 899, 2006.
58. Julkunen H, Kaaja R, Kurki P, et al: Fetal outcome in women with primary Sjögren's syndrome: A retrospective case-control study. Clin Exp Rheum 13:65, 1995.
59. Chung L, Flyckt RL, Colon I, et al: Outcome of pregnancies complicated by systemic sclerosis and mixed connective tissue disease. Lupus 15:595-599, 2006.
60. Steen VD, Medsger TA Jr: Fertility and pregnancy outcome in women with systemic sclerosis. Arthritis Rheum 42:763-7681999.
61. Steen VD, Medsger TA Jr: Fertility and pregnancy outcome in women with systemic sclerosis. Arthritis Rheum 42:763, 1999.
62. Cooper WD, Hernandez-Diaz S, Arbogast PG, et al: Major congenital malformations after first-trimester exposure to ACE inhibitors. N Engl J Med 354:2443-2451, 2006.
63. Lambert NC, Pang JM, Yan Z, et al: Male microchimerism in women with systemic sclerosis and healthy women who have never given birth to a son. Ann Rheum Dis 64:845, 2005.
64. Artlett CM, Smith JB, Jimenez SA: Identification of fetal DNA and cells in skin lesions from women with systemic sclerosis. N Engl J Med 338:1186, 1998.
65. Gran JT, Östensen M: Spondylarthritides in females. Baillieres Clin Rheumatol 12:695, 1998.
66. Petri M, Ho AC, Patel J, et al: Elevation of maternal alpha-fetoprotein in systemic lupus erythematosus: A controlled study. J Rheum 22:1365, 1995.

Chapter 52

Neurologic Disorders

Michael J. Aminoff, MD, DSc

Women are as susceptible to neurologic disorders during gestation as at other times, and certain disorders may be aggravated or influenced by pregnancy. Investigation and management of many neurologic disorders may be complicated by the pregnancy and by concern about the safety of the developing fetus. This chapter describes some of the special problems posed by neurologic disorders during pregnancy and by pregnancy in patients with neurologic disorders.

Epilepsy

Women with epilepsy should be advised about possible interactions between anticonvulsant drugs and oral contraceptive agents. Whether oral contraceptives affect seizure frequency or blood levels of antiepileptic drugs is unclear, but certain anticonvulsants, including phenytoin, phenobarbital, primidone, carbamazepine, oxcarbazepine, and topiramate, may interfere with the effectiveness of oral contraceptives, leading to unwanted pregnancy.[1,2] The possibility of contraceptive failure must be discussed with women taking these anticonvulsants and documented in the records. Regular counseling of women with epilepsy is necessary during the reproductive years, because unplanned pregnancy may occur. Valproic acid and the newer anticonvulsants (i.e., zonisamide, vigabatrin, gabapentin, lamotrigine, levetiracetam, pregabalin, and tiagabine) have not been reported to cause contraceptive failure.[2,3] When oral contraception is desired in women taking enzyme-inducing anticonvulsants, a formulation that includes at least 50 μg of ethinyl estradiol or mestranol is preferred.

Between 0.3% and 0.6% of pregnant women have epilepsy. Pregnancy may affect the seizure disorder, and the disorder may affect the course of the pregnancy and the manner in which it is best managed. Moreover, recurrent seizures and drugs given to the mother in an attempt to control them may affect fetal development.

Effect of Pregnancy on Seizure Disorders

Pregnancy has an unpredictable and variable influence on epilepsy. When seizure frequency increases, it most commonly does so in the first trimester and usually reverts to the pregestational pattern at the conclusion of the pregnancy, although a few patients experience a permanent deterioration in seizure control. In general, control in patients with frequent seizures (i.e., more than one a month) before pregnancy is likely to deteriorate during the gestational period, whereas only about 25% of patients with infrequent attacks (i.e., less than one every 9 months) experience an exacerbation during pregnancies.

In a prospective study of 136 pregnancies in 122 epileptic women, seizure frequency increased in 50 pregnancies (37%), often in association with noncompliance with a therapeutic regimen.[4] Among several other series, seizures increased during pregnancy in 23% to 75% of instances.[5] Tanganelli and Regesta[6] found that seizures were more likely to be exacerbated during pregnancy in women with more frequent seizures before the pregnancy and in those with partial (focal) seizure disorders. Seizure control is unchanged in 53% to 67% of patients.[7]

It is usually not possible to predict the outcome in individual cases, regardless of the maternal age, the outcome of previous pregnancies, or any apparent relationship between seizures and the menstrual cycle. None of these provides a guide to the effect that pregnancy will have on the course of epilepsy. Moreover, attacks may occur during pregnancy in patients who have been free of seizures for several years.

Epilepsy may appear for the first time during or immediately after pregnancy. It is uncommon for patients in the latter group to have seizures only in relation to pregnancy and at no other time (i.e., gestational epilepsy). Some patients with true gestational epilepsy experience recurrent seizures during pregnancy, and the remainder have only a single convulsion. The occurrence of seizures in one pregnancy is no guide to the course of subsequent pregnancies.

The seizures that occur during pregnancy do not differ clinically from those occurring in other circumstances. Improved compliance with an anticonvulsant drug regimen may sometimes account for the reduction in seizure frequency that occasionally occurs during pregnancy in an epileptic woman.

The increase in seizure frequency that occurs in some epileptic patients during pregnancy may relate to the metabolic, hormonal, or hematologic changes of the gestational period or to fatigue or sleep deprivation. A rapid and excessive gain in weight sometimes occurs before an increase in seizure frequency, providing some support for the belief that fluid retention may occasionally be a factor, perhaps by a dilutional effect on anticonvulsant drug concentration. It is tempting to relate any change in seizure frequency to hormonal factors because estrogens are epileptogenic in animals and progesterone has both convulsant and anticonvulsant properties. Nausea, vomiting, reduced gastric motility, or use of antacids may also lead to reduced absorption of anticonvulsant drugs.

There is sometimes difficulty in maintaining adequate treatment with anticonvulsant drugs during pregnancy. Serum levels of the older antiepileptic drugs generally decline in pregnancy and rise in the postpartum period. For phenytoin, carbamazepine, and valproate (but not phenobarbital), the decline is less for free levels than total levels. An increase in dosage is frequently required to maintain plasma levels at pre-pregnancy values, but in this regard, it is important to appreciate that the free level, rather than the total level, of the drug correlates best with therapeutic efficacy. Several new antiepileptic drugs, such as felbamate, gabapentin, and lamotrigine, have become available, but the effect of pregnancy on their pharmacokinetics is unclear.

The reason for the changes in drug requirements is unknown. Among the various possibilities are the dilutional effect of increasing plasma volume and extracellular fluid volume. Poor compliance with the anticonvulsant drug regimen, perhaps because of nausea and vomiting or concerns about the effect of medication on the fetus, may also be an important contributory factor, as may decreased plasma protein binding and changes in the absorption and excretion of drugs. The increased metabolic capacity of the maternal liver in pregnancy and possible fetal or placental metabolism of part of the anticonvulsant dose may influence the changes in anticonvulsant drug requirements that occur in epileptic women during pregnancy.

Folic acid therapy may lower the plasma phenytoin level, sometimes to below the therapeutic range, and other drugs taken concomitantly with an anticonvulsant medication also may lead to reduced plasma levels of the anticonvulsant. Antacids and antihistamines merit particular mention, because it is not uncommon for them to be taken during pregnancy.

Status epilepticus sometimes complicates pregnancy and may occur without any preceding increase in seizure frequency, occasionally because of the injudicious discontinuation of anticonvulsant drugs. Fortunately, this is a rare occurrence, but it may lead to a fatal outcome for the mother or fetus. The absence of hypertension, proteinuria, and edema helps in distinguishing this condition from eclamptic convulsions. As in the nonpregnant patient, it is essential to obtain control of the seizures as rapidly as possible, but the former practice of terminating pregnancy is usually unnecessary.

Status epilepticus is treated with anticonvulsant drug therapy, with the pregnancy being allowed to continue to term. Intravenous diazepam (10 to 30 mg) or lorazepam (4 to 8 mg) usually provides temporary control of the seizures, but other anticonvulsant drugs are needed as well to prevent seizure recurrence. Intravenous phenytoin is usually given but is best administered in the form of fosphenytoin sodium, the dose of which is expressed in terms of phenytoin equivalents. Fosphenytoin sodium is water soluble, may be infused with dextrose or saline, is better tolerated at the infusion site than phenytoin, and may be infused three times more rapidly than intravenous phenytoin, with the same pharmacologic effects. It is converted in the body to phenytoin, which may be cardiotoxic, and cardiac monitoring is required while the fosphenytoin is given in a loading dose of 15 to 20 mg of phenytoin equivalents per kilogram, infused at a rate of up to 150 mg of phenytoin equivalents per kilogram. Other anticonvulsants may also be required, including intravenous phenobarbital or midazolam. It is essential to maintain control of the airway and of glucose and electrolyte balance.

Effect of Epilepsy on Pregnancy and Lactation

Only a few studies have attempted to document the effect of epilepsy on pregnancy. The results are often difficult to evaluate because of the limited number of cases reported; the lack of comparative data on non-epileptic women attending the same institutions; differences in the severity of the epilepsy and how it has been treated; differences in age, medical background, and socioeconomic status of the patients reported; and the lack of information concerning relevant social habits such as cigarette smoking and alcohol ingestion.

The incidence of vaginal hemorrhage and of toxemia during pregnancy among epileptic women was found to be increased in some studies but not others. Whether preterm labor occurs more commonly in epileptic women, as is sometimes reported, is unclear. There is a significantly higher rate of stillbirths among epileptic patients, but there does not seem to be an increased incidence of low-birth-weight infants, at least in some studies. Cesarean section is not indicated simply because of maternal epilepsy, except when seizures occur frequently or during labor, when they are precipitated by physical activity, or when patients cannot cooperate during labor because of their neurologic disorder or mental abnormality.[8] Fetal death can result from maternal seizures, presumably because of the accompanying hypoxia and acidosis. The effect on placental blood flow of maternal seizures is not established, but changes in fetal heart rate suggestive of hypoxia have been described[5,9]; they may relate to reduced placental blood flow or to metabolic changes in the mother.

An increased incidence of neonatal death has been reported for the offspring of epileptic mothers. The increased rate may relate to several factors, including congenital malformations, iatrogenic neonatal hemorrhage, seizures, socioeconomic issues, and preterm delivery.

Anticonvulsant drugs taken by the mother may be present in breast milk, but their concentration is usually insufficient to have any major effect on the infant. The transmission rate of antiepileptic drugs into breast milk varies with the agent and is about 2% for valproic acid; 30% to 45% for phenytoin, phenobarbital, and carbamazepine; 60% for primidone; and 90% for ethosuximide.[1] When obvious sedation develops in an infant that is likely related to antiepileptic drugs in breast milk, breastfeeding should be discontinued, and the infant should be observed for signs of drug withdrawal. Breastfeeding does not need to be discouraged for reasons related to its content of anticonvulsant medication.

Effect of Maternal Epilepsy and Anticonvulsant Drugs on the Fetus and Neonate

The epileptic woman who becomes pregnant usually is concerned that her unborn child may inherit a similar susceptibility to seizures. The risk of epilepsy in the child depends on the nature of the mother's seizure disorder; it is higher in idiopathic than acquired maternal epilepsy. Precise quantification of the risk is not possible, but it is probably about 2% to 3%. The cause of this increased risk to the offspring of epileptic mothers is unknown. It may relate to genetic factors, seizures arising during pregnancy, or the metabolic and toxic consequences of seizures or anticonvulsant drugs. In general, pregnancy in epileptic women does not need to be discouraged on these grounds, but reassurance and support are necessary.

A major problem in management of epileptic patients during pregnancy is the possibility that certain anticonvulsant drugs may induce fetal abnormalities. However, epilepsy has a relatively low prevalence rate, can occur for a multitude of reasons, can vary markedly in severity, can be treated by a variety of drugs singly or in combination, and can itself be associated with an increased risk of fetal malformations. Some patients may have a common genetic predisposition to seizures and to fetal malformation. Environmental factors may be important in the genesis of congenital abnormalities, and socioeconomic backgrounds must be matched as much as is possible when comparisons are made of the incidence of malformations in different patient populations.

All the commonly used older antiepileptic drugs are teratogenic to some extent, and malformation rates are higher for the offspring of mothers taking drug combinations. The study by Jones and associates[10] revealed a relatively high incidence of craniofacial defects, fingernail hypoplasia, and developmental delay in children exposed prenatally to carbamazepine. Its use during pregnancy, particularly in combination with other drugs, has been associated with an increased risk for spina bifida.[11] Valproic acid has an especially high (1% to 2%) rate of neural tube defects[12,13]; it may also cause cleft lip or palate, delayed development, and disorders of the cardiovascular, genitourinary, and endocrine systems.[14,15] Trimethadione seems particularly dangerous and causes fetal malformations and mental retardation in more than 50% of exposed infants. This drug, which is now rarely used, should be avoided during pregnancy when possible. Whether newer anticonvulsant drugs, such as felbamate, gabapentin, lamotrigine, tiagabine, topiramate, oxcarbazepine, and vigabatrin, are teratogenic is unknown, but some evidence suggests that lamotrigine and oxcarbazepine are teratogenic.[16]

Animal studies lend support to the belief that some anticonvulsants are teratogenic. The mechanism involved is unclear but may include folate deficiency or antagonism. Dansky and associates,[17] for example, showed that low blood folate levels before or early in pregnancy are significantly associated with spontaneous abortion and the occurrence of developmental anomalies. It has also been suggested that certain oxidative intermediary metabolites of anticonvulsants may affect cell division and migration.

Although most children born to epileptic mothers are cognitively normal, prenatal antiepileptic drug exposure may be associated with developmental delay,[18] particularly when more than one drug has been taken by the mother. The mechanisms involved are unclear, but a genetic predisposition may be important.[19] It is also unclear whether some anticonvulsant drugs pose a greater risk than others.

Maternal use of phenytoin during pregnancy has been associated with the fetal hydantoin syndrome, which is characterized by prenatal and postnatal growth deficiency, microcephaly, dysmorphic facies, and mental deficiency. Among infants exposed to phenytoin in utero, 11% have enough clinical features to be classified as having this syndrome, and almost three times as many may show lesser degrees of impairment of performance or morphogenesis. The syndrome is not unlike that ascribed to phenobarbital and carbamazepine,[10] and it resembles the fetal alcohol syndrome. A consistent facial phenotype has also been reported in children exposed to valproic acid or sodium valproate in utero.[20,21]

Maternal use of barbiturates (60 to 120 mg daily) in late pregnancy may be associated with neonatal withdrawal symptoms beginning a week after birth. They include restlessness, constant crying, irritability, tremulousness, difficulty in sleeping, and vasomotor instability but not seizures.

Clinical or subclinical coagulopathy may occur in the neonate whose mother received anticonvulsants during pregnancy. In affected infants, levels of factors II, VII, IX, and X are decreased, and levels of factors V and VIII and fibrinogen are normal. The abnormalities are similar to those produced by vitamin K deficiency. Bleeding in affected infants tends to occur within 24 hours of birth, rather than on the second or third day, as in classic hemorrhagic diseases of the newborn, and at relatively unusual sites, such as the pleural and abdominal cavities. Prevalence rates average about 10%, but the mortality rate may exceed 30%.[5] Bleeding may also occur in utero, resulting in stillbirth. No evidence of coagulopathy is found in the mothers.

Maternal ingestion of vitamin K_1 (10 mg daily) during the last month of pregnancy may prevent these hemorrhagic complications in the offspring of treated epileptic mothers,[22] but it is unclear whether routine prophylaxis in this manner is justifiable because some studies suggest that such hemorrhagic complications are rare.[23,24] Vitamin K_1 administration to the newborn infant usually reverses the bleeding tendency, but the infant may die despite such therapy. It is therefore recommended that prothrombin and partial thromboplastin times of cord blood be measured at delivery if the mother received anticonvulsant drugs. If the value is abnormally low or if there is clinical evidence of a coagulopathy during the neonatal period, treatment with infusion of fresh-frozen plasma or concentrates of factors II, VII, IX, and X may have to be considered in addition to the routine administration of vitamin K_1.

General Therapeutic Approaches

It is difficult to make more than general therapeutic recommendations about pregnancy in the epileptic woman. Epilepsy should be treated with the smallest effective dose of an anticonvulsant drug, and monotherapy is preferable to polytherapy. Drug selection is based on seizure type, clinical status, and the maternal and fetal risks.[25] Folate supplementation (4 mg daily) usually is provided.

Prenatal counseling is important. If a nonpregnant epileptic woman asks about pregnancy, it is appropriate to inform her that there is a small risk of having a malformed child because of the seizure disorder or the drugs used in its treatment. This risk is probably about double that for the non-epileptic patient, but there is still a more than 90% chance that she will have a normal child.

Data concerning the relative safety and therapeutic effectiveness of different anticonvulsant drugs in the management of pregnant epileptic patients are insufficient to guide the physician responsible for the care of these patients. It seems clear, however, that trimethadione should not be used and that valproic acid should be avoided. If valproic acid must be used, amniocentesis is advisable to detect any increase in α-fetoprotein levels (which is associated with neural tube defects) so that therapeutic abortion can be considered if necessary. Substitution of one anticonvulsant drug for another in epileptic women who are initially seen after the first trimester should be avoided, because major malformation of the fetus has probably occurred already if it is going to occur.

The principles of drug management of a seizure disorder in the pregnant woman are the same as in the nonpregnant woman. Anticonvulsant drugs are as necessary to epileptic patients during pregnancy as at other times. A detailed account of the drugs used in the treatment of epilepsy is unnecessary here, but several points are worthy of comment.

A solitary seizure, unrelated to toxemia, should not lead to a diagnosis of epilepsy because there may be no further attacks. Only time will tell whether an individual who has a single seizure is going to have further attacks, thereby justifying a diagnosis of epilepsy and necessitating prophylactic anticonvulsant drug treatment.

Although some physicians start a patient on anticonvulsant medication after one convulsion, others prefer to withhold medication until the patient has had at least two seizures, at least in the nonpregnant state. During pregnancy, many physicians initiate anticonvulsant therapy after even a single seizure and arrange for neurologic reevaluation after delivery. This approach merits emphasis because many patients with so-called gestational epilepsy have only a single convulsion, and continued treatment in such circumstances may be unnecessary. Simple medical and neurologic investigations are indicated in an adult who has an isolated seizure and is otherwise well with no neurologic signs: hematologic and biochemical screening tests, electroencephalogram, and particularly in the nonpregnant patient, magnetic resonance imaging (MRI) of the head and a chest radiograph. If the findings of such investigations are unremarkable, I discuss the controversial issue of anticonvulsant drug treatment with the patient but generally recommend that treatment be withheld unless a future attack occurs.

Pregnant women experiencing two or more seizures merit prophylactic anticonvulsant drug treatment. In those with a progressive history, abnormal neurologic signs, or a focal electroencephalographic abnormality, it is necessary to exclude an underlying structural lesion by means of MRI of the head. The management of such a lesion is described later in this chapter.

If prophylactic anticonvulsant drug treatment is necessary, it is generally continued until the patient has been seizure free for at least 2 or 3 years. Treatment is started with a small dose of one of the anticonvulsants, depending on the type of seizure experienced by the patient and the considerations outlined earlier. The dose is increased until seizures are controlled, blood concentrations reach the upper end of the optimal therapeutic range, or side effects limit further increments. If seizures continue despite optimal blood levels of the anticonvulsant drug selected, a second drug should be substituted for the first. Patients often respond preferentially to one or another of the various drugs that are available. Experience during pregnancy with certain newer antiepileptic agents (e.g., felbamate, lamotrigine, gabapentin, topiramate) is limited, however, and their effect on the developing fetus is uncertain.

Patients must take medication as prescribed, and treatment should be controlled by frequent monitoring of the plasma anticonvulsant drug concentration. Monthly follow-up visits during pregnancy usually permit satisfactory supervision of the patient. At the initial visit, trough values of total and free concentrations of each drug should be measured. Total levels should then be measured each month in patients whose seizures are well controlled; free levels should be monitored monthly in those with poor seizure control, seizures during pregnancy, or a marked (>50%) decline in total level. Poor compliance with an anticonvulsant drug regimen can often be improved by encouragement and by explanation of the importance of taking medication regularly. Simplifying the dosage schedule so that medication is taken just once or twice daily may be helpful.

As the pregnancy continues, the dose of the anticonvulsant drug may need to be increased if seizures become more common or the free level of the anticonvulsant drug declines by more than about 30%. In some instances, the required dose may reach a level that would probably cause toxic side effects in a nonpregnant patient. If the anticonvulsant dosage is increased during the pregnancy, reductions will probably be necessary in the puerperium to prevent toxicity, but this change must be based on clinical evaluation and measurement of the plasma concentration of the drug, because the period over which drug requirements decline varies considerably. Because of the poorly defined risks of increased obstetric complications among pregnant epileptic women, close supervision of these patients by the obstetrician is mandatory, and delivery in a hospital is advised.

After delivery, the infant must be inspected for congenital malformations and given an injection of vitamin K_1 (1 mg/kg intramuscularly). Clotting factors should be studied after about 4 hours, and further injections of vitamin K_1 should be given if necessary. If hemorrhage occurs, infusions of fresh-frozen plasma or of factors II, VII, IX, and X may also be necessary. Breastfeeding of a healthy infant by an epileptic mother should not be discouraged.

Headache

Headache is a common complaint and may have many causes. Among patients attending headache clinics, symptoms are most frequently attributed to migraine, tension, or depression. Tension headaches are commonly chronic, last all day, are worse in the evening, may have a tight quality to them, may be accompanied by local soreness and concern about lumps or bumps on the head, and are often accompanied by poor concentration and nonspecific symptoms such as dizziness. The pain frequently commences or is most intense in the neck and the back of the head. If treatment with mild tranquilizers (e.g., diazepam) is unsuccessful, a trial of antimigraine preparations may be worthwhile. Depression headaches are somewhat similar but are often worse in the mornings, may be accompanied by other symptoms of depression, and often respond to a limited extent to tricyclic antidepressant drugs.

Most patients presenting with headache do not have severe underlying structural disease, but it is important to consider this possibility. About one third of patients with brain tumors present with a primary complaint of headache. The headache in such patients is often an intermittent, dull, nonthrobbing ache that is exacerbated by exercise and may be associated with nausea or vomiting, but these features do not in themselves permit any reliable distinction from migraine. Similarly, the severity of the headache is unhelpful in this regard. Headaches that disturb sleep, however, suggest an underlying structural lesion, as do exertional headaches and late-onset paroxysmal headaches.

The duration and course of a headache provide a guide to the underlying cause. A long history of chronic headache without other accompaniments is unlikely to reflect serious disease unless associated with drowsiness, visual disturbances, limb symptoms, seizures, intellectual changes, or other neurologic symptoms. The sudden development of severe headache in a previously well patient is more ominous and may be caused by acute intracranial abnormality (e.g., subarachnoid hemorrhage), glaucoma, or another condition requiring specific treatment.

The evaluation of patients with headaches demands a full general and neurologic examination together with an assessment of mental status. It may be necessary to include examination of the teeth, eyes, paranasal sinuses, and urine, and various investigative procedures may be indicated, depending on the initial clinical impression. If intracranial disease is suspected on the basis of the history or presence of neurologic signs, the need for computed tomography (CT) or MRI of the head, an electroencephalogram, and examination of the cerebrospinal fluid must be decided on an individual basis. Cranial arteritis and cervical spondylosis are important causes of headache but are not expected among patients in the childbearing age group.

Post-traumatic headaches usually pose no diagnostic problem because of the relationship to previous injury, and they usually respond to simple analgesics, mild tranquilizers, or antimigraine preparations. Acute sinusitis typically produces a localized, throbbing headache accompanied by tenderness; the relationship of symptoms to a respiratory tract infection and the radiologic findings permit the diagnosis to be made with confidence, and treatment is directed at the underlying infection.

Migraine

Among women of childbearing age, migraine is an important cause of headache. In classic migraine, episodic headache is preceded by visual, sensory, or motor symptoms, but in other types, there may be no premonitory focal symptoms. Headaches may be lateralized or generalized, usually have a gradual onset, and usually last for less than a day, although they may persist for longer. They may be dull or throbbing; are commonly accompanied by nausea, vomiting, and photophobia; and are often associated with blurring of vision, lightheadedness, and scalp tenderness. Photopsia, fortification spectra, and other focal neurologic symptoms may precede or accompany the headache, and consciousness is sometimes impaired or lost (syncopal attacks or seizures).

Many women with migraine link the periodicity of some of their attacks to the menstrual cycle, with headaches occurring usually just before or during menstruation. Migrainous attacks without aura are most likely to be related to the menstrual cycle.[26] Some patients may have headaches that occur only in relation to the menstrual cycle, although this pattern is much less common. The manner in which hormonal factors provoke migraine remains unclear.[26,27]

Migraine headaches are commonly exacerbated in women using oral contraceptives, but improvement can occur in some patients. Such exacerbation usually becomes apparent within the first few months of oral contraceptive use. Preparations with a relatively high estrogen content are most likely to influence the headache pattern and are generally not as well tolerated as low-estrogen preparations. Recurrent headache provoked by the use of oral contraceptives may persist despite withdrawal of the offending medications, but whether this is anything more than fortuitous is unclear.[28] Of special concern is evidence suggesting that women with migraine exacerbated by oral contraceptives are at increased risk for cerebral infarction,[29] perhaps caused by intimal hyperplasia of arteries supplying the brain.[30]

Migraine often improves considerably after the first trimester of pregnancy, regardless of whether the attacks are related to the menstrual cycle. It occasionally worsens or occurs for the first time during pregnancy, most commonly during the first 3 months of gestation.[31] The response of migraine to pregnancy does not correlate with sex of the fetus or with differences in plasma levels of hormones.

Management of migraine consists of the avoidance of precipitating factors coupled with prophylactic or symptomatic drug treatment, if necessary. In general populations, when simple analgesics do not provide relief, treatment with extracranial vasoconstrictors (e.g., ergotamine, dihydroergotamine), β-adrenergic blockers (e.g., propranolol), serotonin agonists (e.g., sumatriptan), tricyclic antidepressants (e.g., amitriptyline), or other drugs may be necessary. Menstrual migraine may improve with standard pharmacologic therapy. Hormonal interventions are usually unsuccessful, but bromocriptine (2.5 mg three times daily) is sometimes worthwhile.[32]

During pregnancy, medication is best avoided if possible. Dietary and other precipitants of headache should be avoided. When drugs are required, simple analgesics should be used. Acetaminophen is preferred over aspirin, because aspirin may cause hemorrhagic complications and, in large doses in late pregnancy, may prolong labor and increase the incidence of stillbirth.[33,34] Tryptamine-based drugs should be avoided during pregnancy and breastfeeding, although there is no definite evidence of teratogenicity.[35] Meperidine suppositories (50 mg) may be prescribed for severe pain.[36] An effort should be made to avoid ergotamine-containing preparations because of the effect this drug may have on the gravid uterus and its potential teratogenicity. Propranolol is also best avoided during pregnancy because it may mildly impair fetal growth[37] and may theoretically lead to β-adrenergic blockade in the fetus or newborn. Inhibition of normal β-adrenergic responsiveness to asphyxia or to other stresses may theoretically increase the harmful effects of the latter.[38] Other reported potential neonatal complications include prematurity, respiratory depression, hypoglycemia, and hyperbilirubinemia.[39,40] In patients with frequent headaches, comorbidities such as depression require special consideration.

A study of the possible association of maternal migraine during pregnancy with outcome revealed that women with severe migraine have a higher prevalence of preeclampsia and severe nausea or vomiting but a lower prevalence of threatened abortion and preterm delivery.[41] This did not appear to influence delivery outcome.[41]

Postnatal Headache

About one third of women experience headaches in the week after delivery, and most of them have a personal or family history of migraine. The headaches, which are usually mild and bifrontal, respond well to simple analgesics and are self-limited.

Tumors

Any type of intracranial tumor can appear during the gestational period, and accurate diagnosis may then be delayed because symptoms are erroneously ascribed to toxemia of pregnancy. Although the relationship between the tumor and pregnancy is usually fortuitous, pituitary adenomas, meningiomas, neurofibromas, hemangioblastomas, and vascular malformations occasionally exhibit relapses in relation to pregnancy, with symptoms developing or rapidly worsening during gestation, remitting to some extent after delivery, and recurring in a subsequent pregnancy. Attention here focuses on the aspects of intracranial tumors that relate to pregnancy rather than on a more general account of intracranial neoplasms.

Visual field defects sometimes develop during pregnancy in patients with a pituitary adenoma or a craniopharyngioma, which must be excluded in such circumstances. Meningiomas in the suprasellar or parasellar region or on the medial sphenoidal wing may produce symptoms such as diplopia and unilateral scotoma or ptosis, which relapse and remit in relation to pregnancy over several years. Symptoms tend to develop in the last 4 months of gestation and often lead to a mistaken initial diagnosis of multiple sclerosis. Early surgical intervention may help to preserve vision and prevent other neurologic catastrophes.

Symptoms caused by acoustic neuroma may begin or may be aggravated in the latter stages of pregnancy.[42,43] The symptoms in different patients include hearing loss, tinnitus, headaches, vertigo, dysequilibrium, facial weakness, and diplopia. Aggravation of symptoms in one pregnancy does not necessarily indicate that exacerbation will occur in subsequent ones. Cerebellar hemangioblastomas,[44] medulloblastomas,[45] and other tumors may occur during pregnancy. Atypical psychiatric symptoms in the antenatal or postnatal period may result from an intracranial structural lesion that is unrecognized unless the patient is examined neurologically and investigated by neuroimaging studies.

How pregnancy may precipitate or exacerbate symptoms caused by intracranial tumors is unclear. The most likely explanation is that pregnancy leads to a slight increase in the size of the tumor. Tumors with symptoms consistently related to pregnancy are usually located so that only slight enlargement leads to significant involvement of important neural structures. Symptoms of spinal meningiomas may be exacerbated by pregnancy, but convexity meningiomas, which have room for expansion, are unlikely to show any particular relationship of symptoms to pregnancy.

Several possibilities have been advanced to account for the manner in which pregnancy might influence tumor size. Suggested mechanisms include accelerated growth rate, vascular engorgement, and increased fluid content, but supportive evidence for these proposals is lacking. Nevertheless, there is accumulating evidence for sex steroid–binding sites in a number of human tumors, especially meningiomas.[46] The presence of such receptors in tumors suggests that the natural

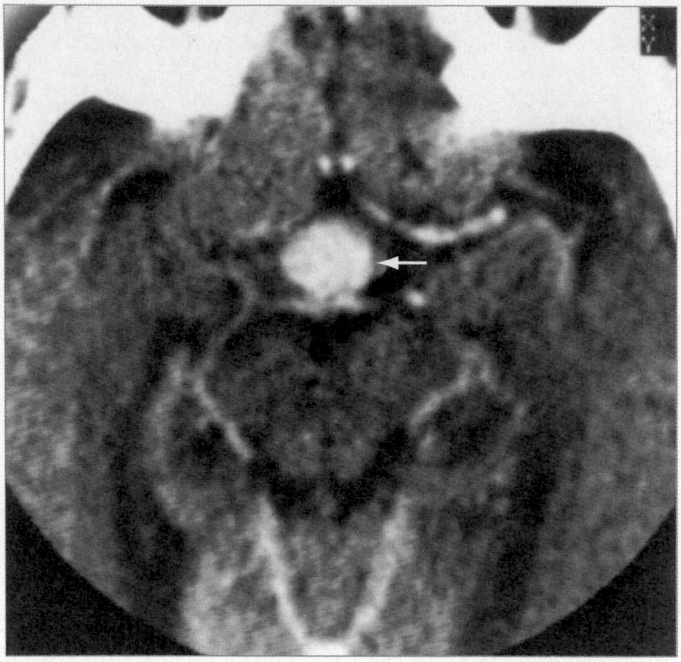

FIGURE 52-1 Computed tomography (CT) of a pituitary adenoma. CT shows an enhancing lesion *(arrow)* in the suprasellar cistern. More inferior axial scans showed this lesion arising from the sella.

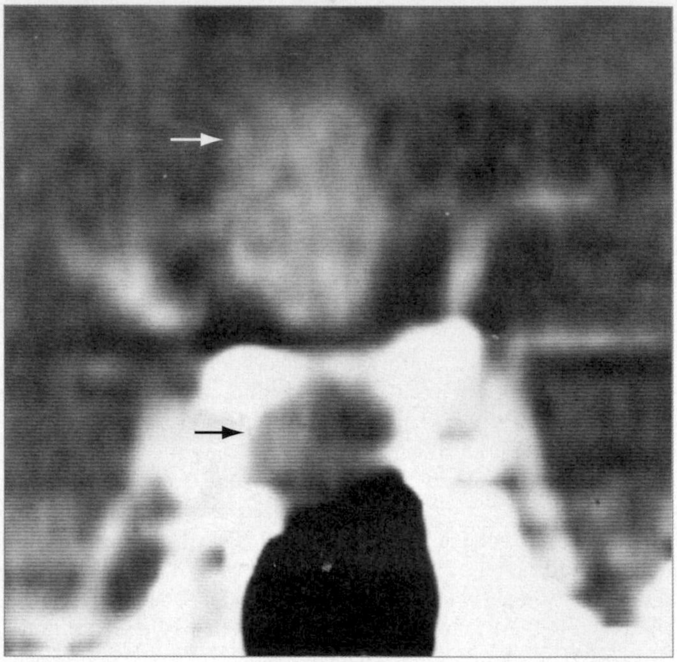

FIGURE 52-2 Coronal reformation of computed tomography (CT) of a pituitary adenoma. In the CT scan of the same patient as in Figure 52-1, the intrasellar extent *(black arrow)* and suprasellar extent *(white arrow)* of the pituitary adenoma can be seen.

history of these tumors may be modified by these hormones or their antagonists.

Patients with intracranial neoplasms may have nonspecific symptoms of cerebral dysfunction, with evidence of raised intracranial pressure or some characteristic combination of symptoms and signs that reflect the location of the lesion. The history and physical findings guide the manner in which these patients are evaluated further. MRI or CT of the head (Figs. 52-1 and 52-2) can provide an enormous amount of additional information noninvasively. MRI is more sensitive for the diagnosis of an intracranial tumor and is safe in pregnant women because it does not involve exposure to radiation. When CT or other radiologic investigations are necessary, shielding may help to protect the fetus from excessive radiation.

Each patient must be treated on an individual basis, and essential neurosurgical treatment should not be delayed because of the pregnancy. For pituitary adenomas or other benign tumors encountered in the latter half of pregnancy, operations can sometimes be delayed until a more propitious time if the patient is carefully observed. However, signs of increased intracranial pressure, visual deterioration, an increasing neurologic deficit, or the clinical features of an infratentorial lesion mandate early or immediate intervention. For patients with pituitary adenomas, pharmacologic intervention (e.g., corticosteroids, bromocriptine) may be adequate. In most instances, visual disturbances improve spontaneously after delivery, regardless of any pharmacologic measures. Cranial irradiation during the first trimester for the treatment of malignant brain tumors is associated with an increased risk of fetal loss or malformation; during later pregnancy, it is associated with an increased risk of childhood leukemia.[47] A detailed discussion of radiotherapy during pregnancy is provided by Kal and Struiksmans.[48]

In general, pregnancy can be allowed to proceed—at least until the fetus is viable and often to term—in patients with intracranial neoplasms; however, therapeutic abortion may be justifiable for some patients with malignant brain tumors and if significant symptoms, such as uncontrollable seizures, occur during pregnancy, particularly when the tumor cannot be removed completely. Obstetric management must also be determined on an individual basis. Some investigators have proposed that delivery by cesarean section is safer than spontaneous vaginal delivery in women with cerebral tumors because the vaginal delivery may enhance any increase in intracranial pressure caused by the neoplasm. However, vaginal delivery with adequate regional anesthesia and judicious shortening of the second stage of labor by use of low forceps (to prevent any increase in intracranial pressure associated with the abdominal pushing efforts of this stage) is often satisfactory.

Pregnancy may be followed by the development of choriocarcinoma, which commonly metastasizes to the brain[49] (see Chapter 43). Neurologic presentation is typically with symptoms of a space-occupying cerebral lesion or with an acute deficit resulting from hemorrhage into the lesion. Treatment of cerebral metastases may involve chemotherapy, radiation therapy, and for isolated metastases, surgery.

Pseudotumor Cerebri

Benign intracranial hypertension is associated with pregnancy and with the use of oral contraceptive preparations. When symptoms do develop during pregnancy, they usually occur in the first trimester or the month after delivery, but they may occur at any time during the gestational period. Symptoms consist of headache and visual disturbances caused by papilledema and possibly diplopia resulting from abducens weakness. The patient looks well despite the grossly abnormal appearance of the optic disks, and neither electroencephalography nor MRI reveals any evidence of a space-occupying lesion. Although lumbar puncture reveals increased pressure of the cerebrospinal fluid, the composition of the fluid is unremarkable. The possibility of intracranial venous sinus thrombosis must be considered when the patient is being evaluated.

Although benign intracranial hypertension is self-limiting, remission may not occur until well after delivery, and the disorder sometimes recurs in a subsequent pregnancy.[50] If the condition is left untreated, there is a risk of secondary optic atrophy and subsequent permanent impairment of vision. Several therapeutic approaches to lowering intracranial pressure have been reported, including use of high-dose steroids, acetazolamide, furosemide, repeated lumbar punctures, and lumboperitoneal or other shunting procedures. If the response to these measures is unsatisfactory and intracranial pressure remains high enough to endanger vision, optic nerve decompression may be required, as may early delivery of the fetus. There are no specific obstetric complications, and the patient can be expected to give birth to a normal infant.

Occlusive Cerebrovascular Disease

Cerebrovascular disease may develop during an otherwise normal pregnancy as a result of arterial or venous disease. Pregnancy increases the risk of cerebral infarction to about 13 times the rate expected outside of pregnancy.[51] The risk seems to be greatest in the few days around the time of delivery.[52]

Arterial Occlusive Disease

Arterial disease is not unusual, even in the absence of diabetes or severe hypertension, in women of childbearing age. Major arterial occlusion accounts for most cases of nonhemorrhagic hemiplegia that develop during pregnancy or the puerperium.[53] Numerous cases of occlusion of the middle cerebral artery or one of the other major intracranial arteries have been described during pregnancy, with occlusion usually occurring in the third trimester or the postpartum period. Such a stroke usually is caused by the development of a thrombus on a preexisting atheromatous plaque. Predisposing factors may be anemia, hormonal influences, hypertension, increased platelet aggregation, reduced tissue plasminogen activity, changes in blood coagulation factors (especially factors V, VII, VIII, IX, X, and XII and fibrinogen) during late pregnancy, preeclamptic toxemia with hypertension, and puerperal septicemia. Other causes of stroke in young women include protein C, protein S, and antithrombin III deficiencies; hyperhomocysteinemia; arteritis; meningovascular syphilis; sickle cell disease; antiphospholipid antibodies; polycythemia and other hematologic disorders; prosthetic cardiac valvular disease; and cardiomyopathy.

An embolus resulting from rheumatic or ischemic heart disease, subacute bacterial endocarditis, or a cardiac myxoma may occur. Rare instances of arterial occlusion by paradoxical embolization from a pelvic vein through a patent foramen ovale have also been described. Rarely, fat, air, or amniotic fluid embolism may occur in relation to childbirth and may have a fatal outcome.[54] Hypotension as a consequence of hemorrhage or related to anesthesia during labor may lead to watershed cerebral infarction.

Transient cerebral ischemic attacks may precede occlusion of one of the major intracranial arteries. The neurologic disorder and the underlying arterial disease must be investigated and treated as in nonpregnant patients. Investigations should include complete blood cell count, blood smear, erythrocyte sedimentation rate, serum cholesterol and triglyceride levels, prothrombin and partial thromboplastin times, electrocardiogram, echocardiography, and radiologic procedures. CT is an important means of excluding intracranial hemorrhage. Angiography enables the major cerebral vessels to be visualized and may permit recognition of degenerative atherosclerotic disease that can be remedied by transluminal disobliteration (Fig. 52-3). The role of thrombolytic agents such as tissue plasminogen activator for treating acute ischemic stroke in pregnant or nursing women is unclear; they may make hemorrhagic complications more likely in the first few days after delivery.

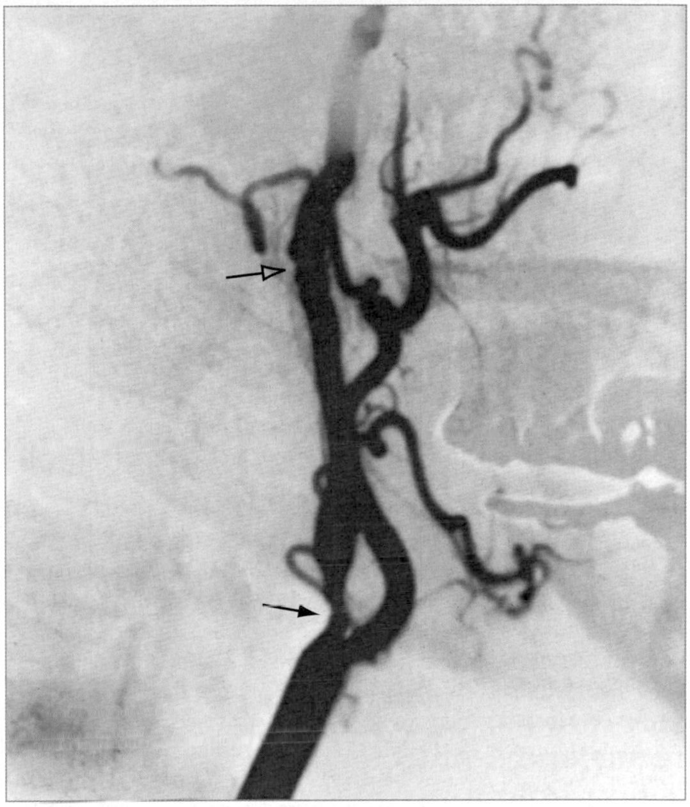

FIGURE 52-3 Common carotid angiogram. The angiogram shows atherosclerotic narrowing of the internal carotid artery *(solid arrow)* at its origin. There is some corrugation of the internal carotid artery more rostrally at the level of C1 and C2, reflecting fibromuscular dysplasia *(open arrow)*.

Surgically inaccessible disease of the intracranial arteries may serve as a source of emboli, and treatment with anticoagulants or aspirin should be considered. Warfarin is best avoided, if possible, because it crosses the placenta and increases hemorrhagic complications and because of the risks of teratogenicity and fetal wastage, especially during the first trimester.[51] Patients requiring anticoagulation during pregnancy are maintained instead on subcutaneously administered heparin, which usually is discontinued when labor begins and resumed about 12 hours after vaginal delivery or 24 hours after cesarean section. With regard to subsequent obstetric management, vaginal delivery, unless specifically contraindicated, is preferable to cesarean section. Other diseases that may be associated with arterial occlusive disease in pregnancy (e.g., eclampsia, thrombotic thrombocytopenic purpura) are discussed in Chapters 35 and 42.

Cerebral angiopathy may complicate an otherwise normal pregnancy or the postpartum period. It is sometimes associated with hypertension or the use of vasoactive drugs, and it may simulate vasculitis.[55]

The association of stroke with oral contraceptive use is widely accepted. The risk can probably be reduced by lowering other risk factors, such as hypertension. A variety of mechanisms may be involved, including a predisposition to hypercoagulability, but the precise mechanisms have not been defined.

Intracranial Venous Occlusive Disease

Intracranial venous occlusive disease is an uncommon complication of pregnancy and childbirth. When the thrombosis occurs in the first trimester, it usually follows a complication such as spontaneous abortion, therapeutic abortion, or stillbirth, but it may occur in an otherwise normal pregnancy. Intracranial venous thrombosis is more likely in the third trimester or in the puerperium and is sometimes related to preeclampsia.

Intracranial venous thrombosis is characterized clinically by headache, weakness, focal or generalized convulsions, drowsiness, and confusion. Disturbances of speech, sensation, or vision may also occur, and patients may have mild pyrexia. There may be signs of meningeal irritation resulting from subarachnoid bleeding caused by cortical infarction, and fluctuating hypertension is sometimes found. Papilledema may be present, particularly if the superior sagittal sinus is involved. The cerebrospinal fluid pressure may be increased, and the protein or cell content often is elevated; occasionally, the fluid is frankly bloodstained. The diagnosis may be confirmed by CT and magnetic resonance angiography, which are also necessary to exclude arterial pathology and vascular malformation (Figs. 52-4 and 52-5). The symptoms and signs of intracranial venous thrombosis are sometimes ascribed mistakenly to eclampsia, but the absence of previous signs of preeclampsia should help in preventing diagnostic confusion.

The prognosis is not encouraging. In about one third of cases, intracranial venous thrombosis has a fatal outcome. Moreover, if patients do survive, thrombosis may recur later in the same pregnancy, the puerperium, or subsequent pregnancies.

The etiologic basis of aseptic intracranial venous thrombosis is uncertain; coagulation abnormalities, changes in the constituents of the peripheral blood, and intimal damage to the dural sinuses have been suggested as causes. Protein C, protein S, and antithrombin III deficiencies are common inherited prothrombotic states. Protein S deficiency in particular has been associated with cerebral venous thrombosis.[56] Low levels of protein C and S have been reported during pregnancy.[57] Activated protein C resistance has been observed in a number of patients with venous thromboembolic events and in those with cerebral venous thrombosis. Deschiens and associates[58] found that 6 of 40 patients with cerebral venous thrombosis had protein C or S deficiency or activated protein C resistance, and 3 of 12 patients were similarly found by Weih and coworkers[59] to have the factor V Leiden mutation, a common cause of activated protein C resistance.

The treatment of intracranial venous thrombosis is controversial. It may include anticonvulsant drugs if seizures have occurred; antiedemic agents, such as dexamethasone and mannitol, to reduce the intracranial pressure; and anticoagulant drugs to prevent extension of thrombosis.[60] Although anticoagulants may provoke hemorrhagic intracranial complications,[61] the risk has probably been exaggerated; one study suggests that anticoagulation with dose-adjusted intravenous heparin is effective treatment.[60,62] Labor can usually be allowed to commence spontaneously, with forceps assistance of delivery, if the thrombosis occurred early in pregnancy. If thrombosis occurs shortly before or during labor, however, cesarean section may be necessary.

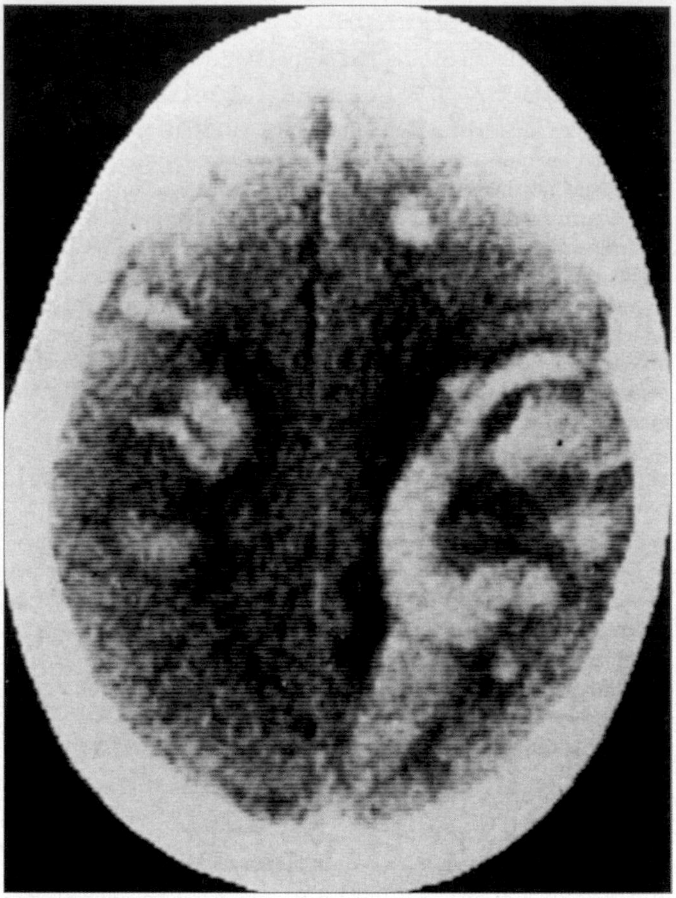

FIGURE 52-4 **Superior sagittal sinus thrombosis.** Computed tomography shows curvilinear areas of high density, which represent cortical venous thromboses and adjacent parenchymal venous infarcts.

Several reports have stressed that a strong relationship exists between factor V Leiden mutation and cerebral venous thrombosis,[63-65] particularly in women taking oral contraceptive preparations.[66] Whether all women should be tested for factor V Leiden before receiving oral contraceptive agents is unsettled. It does seem reasonable, however, to test for activated protein C resistance in patients experiencing a stroke during pregnancy, in the postpartum period, or while receiving oral contraceptives.

Pituitary Infarction

Sheehan syndrome is a well-recognized complication of the peripartum period (see Chapter 48).

Intracranial Hemorrhage

Intracranial (subarachnoid) hemorrhage is more common in women than in men. Mhurchu and colleagues[67] found that menstrual and reproductive history (other than an older age at birth of the first child) did not influence the risk of hemorrhage; the risk was not affected by use of oral contraceptive agents. Okamoto and associates[68] found an increased risk of subarachnoid hemorrhage with an earlier age of menarche and with nulligravity; they found no association with regu-

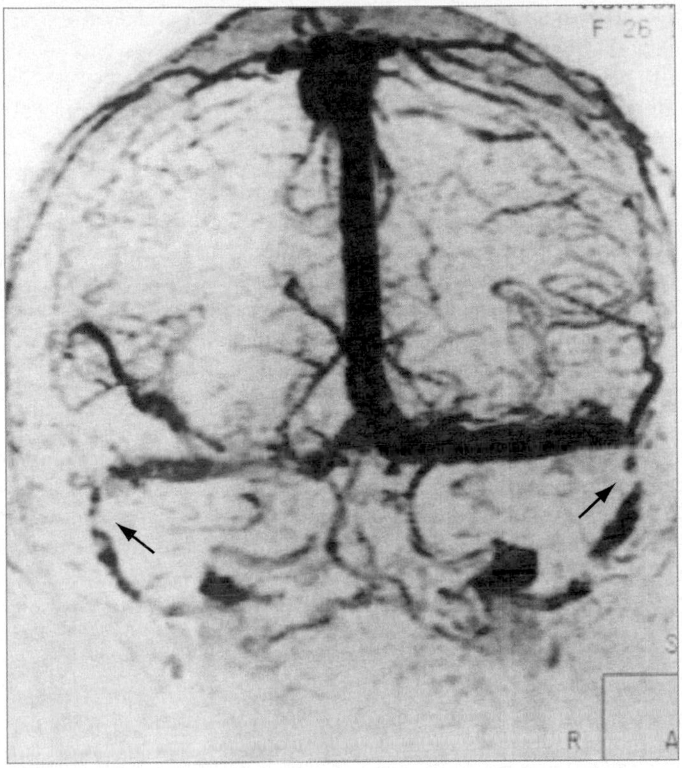

FIGURE 52-5 Intracranial venous thrombosis. A 26-year-old woman presented in the middle trimester of pregnancy with headache, and she had bilateral papilledema. The brain appeared normal in imaging studies. This coronal view of her magnetic resonance venogram (obtained using a two-dimensional time-of-flight technique) shows loss of flow-related enhancement in both transverse sinuses *(arrows)*, which is consistent with thrombus formation.

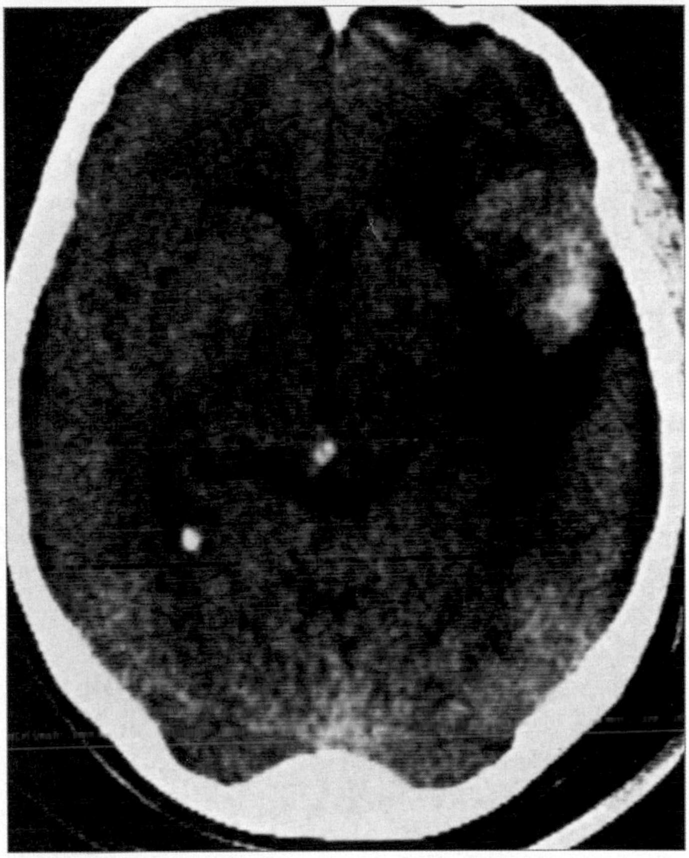

FIGURE 52-6 Evaluation of intracranial hemorrhage. Computed tomography shows hemorrhage into the sylvian fissure and adjacent parenchyma, with surrounding edema or ischemia. The findings are indicative of subarachnoid and intracerebral hemorrhage and localize the source of bleeding to the middle cerebral artery.

larity of menstrual cycle, age at pregnancy or first birth, or number of births.

When intracranial hemorrhage occurs during pregnancy, it is usually, at least in part, into the subarachnoid space. Sudden, severe headache, sometimes accompanied by nausea and vomiting, is the main symptom. Examination reveals signs of meningeal irritation that may be accompanied by depressed consciousness, cranial nerve abnormalities, and a neurologic deficit in the limbs.

In patients in whom subarachnoid hemorrhage complicates otherwise normal pregnancies, the underlying source is most commonly an aneurysm and less often an angioma or of indeterminate cause. Other less common causes of intracranial hemorrhage include mycotic aneurysms, vasculitides, various hematologic disorders, disseminated intravascular coagulation, eclampsia, and metastatic choriocarcinoma. Treatment focuses on the underlying cause. Although bleeding may occur at any time during the pregnancy, aneurysms are somewhat more likely to bleed in the latter half of the gestational period.

Cerebral angiomas, which are located supratentorially in at least 70% of patients, may appear at any age. Intracranial or subarachnoid hemorrhage is the most common manifestation, and the peak age for hemorrhage is between 15 and 20 years. The mortality rate for an initial hemorrhage is approximately 10%, but it has varied in different series; survivors are more likely to experience further hemorrhage than patients who have never had one. Other patients with intracranial angiomas may present with focal or generalized seizures, headache, focal neurologic deficits, or nonspecific neurologic symptoms. Robinson and colleagues[69] reported that pregnancy has a deleterious effect on intracranial angiomas, making them more likely to bleed, but their impression has not been substantiated by others[70] unless there is a history of earlier bleeds.[71]

Intracranial saccular aneurysms arise from a developmental arterial defect, and with increasing age, they become more common sources of hemorrhage than angiomas. They usually are located at sites of vessel branching, commonly occurring in relation to the anterior or posterior communicating arteries. Although such aneurysms sometimes cause focal symptoms that relate to compression of neighboring structures, patients usually present with hemorrhage that occurs without warning because of aneurysmal rupture. This type of hemorrhage seems to occur more commonly in the late stages of pregnancy,[72] and occurrence during labor and delivery has been reported only rarely. In addition to the signs of subarachnoid hemorrhage, focal or lateralizing neurologic signs may be present and help to localize the source of bleeding.

In the evaluation of patients presenting with symptoms of intracranial hemorrhage, the first diagnostic study performed is usually a CT of the head, which is a reliable means of detecting recent subarachnoid or intracerebral hemorrhage and may permit the source of bleeding to be localized (Fig. 52-6). In patients with angiomas, nonhomogeneous areas of mixed density with irregular calcifications are typical, and vermiform areas of enhancement are seen after infu-

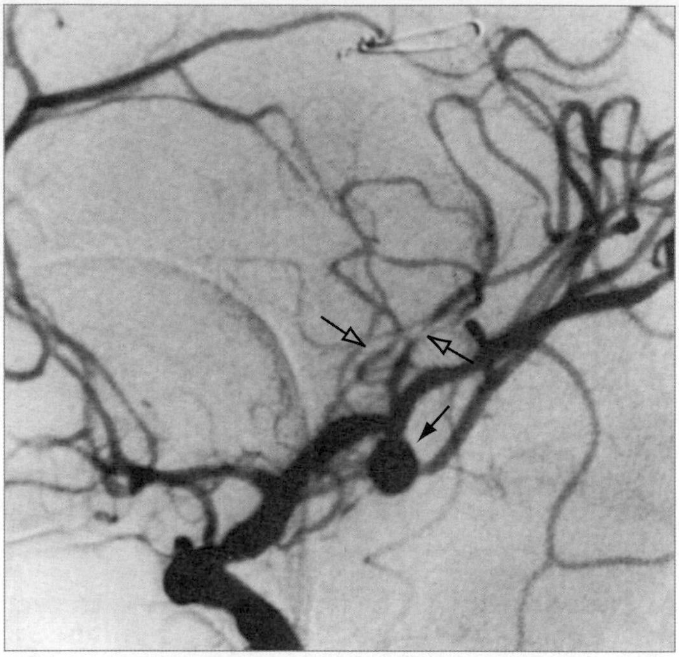

FIGURE 52-7 **Evaluation of aneurysm.** In the carotid angiogram of the same patient as in Figure 52-6, an aneurysm *(solid arrow)* is shown at the trifurcation of the middle cerebral artery. There is some spasm of vessels in the vicinity of the aneurysm *(open arrows).*

sion of contrast material. Aneurysms are seen as small, round, dense areas after infusion of contrast material and are sometimes evident even without contrast. If CT findings are normal, the cerebrospinal fluid should be examined and angiography undertaken if the fluid is bloodstained or xanthochromic.

Angiography enables the identity of the lesion to be established with certainty and provides important additional information concerning its anatomic features (Fig. 52-7). Special shielding during this and other radiologic procedures should be provided for pregnant patients. All the major intracranial vessels should be opacified; feeding vessels to angiomas sometimes arise from the contralateral side, and many aneurysms may be seen. Angiography does not always reveal the malformation in a patient with a suspected angioma, possibly because the lesion was small and destroyed itself when it bled (i.e., cryptic malformation). Nevertheless, if angiography shows neither an angioma nor an aneurysm in a patient presenting with subarachnoid hemorrhage, the study should be repeated after about 14 days because vascular spasm after a bleed may obscure an aneurysm.

The management of subarachnoid hemorrhage consists of bed rest, with sedation and analgesia as necessary and operative or endovascular treatment of the underlying lesion if feasible. Surgical treatment is aimed at preventing further hemorrhages, but induction of hypotension during the course of the intracranial operation should be avoided unless it is essential because it may be followed by premature labor or fetal death; hypothermia is well tolerated.[69]

If the anomalous vessels constituting an angioma are surgically accessible and do not involve a critical vessel or area of the brain, they can often be excised. Surgery is commonly preceded by embolization of the main vessels feeding the malformation in an attempt to reduce its size. Other obliterative techniques have been developed. The optimal time for treatment of an angioma is uncertain, but therapeutic intervention is often delayed until after childbirth.[72] In the patient with an aneurysm that has bled, the risk of further bleeding is much greater, especially in the weeks after the initial hemorrhage. Obliterative treatment, if indicated by the angiographic findings and the condition of the patient, should not be delayed because of the pregnancy.[73] An endovascular approach may be successful[74] and is favored increasingly over surgery.

In patients with aneurysms that have been successfully obliterated or that ruptured before the last trimester, pregnancy and delivery usually can proceed normally. In patients with incompletely obliterated or unoperated aneurysms that ruptured in the last 2 months of pregnancy, cesarean section is probably advisable at 38 weeks' gestation. Some authorities advocate delivery by elective cesarean section at 38 weeks in patients with arteriovenous malformations and further recommend that concomitant sterilization be considered,[69] presumably if the malformation itself is inoperable. However, the need for either procedure in this context is unclear, and arguments for them are without adequate foundation. In patients showing a steady deterioration in neurologic status and for whom a fatal outcome seems likely, preparations should be made so that the fetus, if viable, can be delivered before it dies of anoxia.

Vascular Anomalies and the Nervous System

The most important vascular anomalies that occur in relation to the nervous system are intracranial aneurysms and cerebral angiomas (discussed earlier). However, several other types of vascular anomalies may manifest during pregnancy, and they merit brief discussion.

Intracranial Dural Vascular Anomalies

Certain intracranial dural vascular anomalies may become evident for the first time during pregnancy. They consist of abnormal arteriovenous shunts involving meningeal branches of the carotid and vertebral arteries and the dural veins and sinuses. Although some represent a developmental anomaly, others are acquired in adult life, occasionally after trauma, presumably because of the close anatomic relationship of certain meningeal arteries and veins.

Shunts involving the anteroinferior group of dural sinuses (i.e., cavernous, intercavernous, sphenoparietal, superior and inferior petrosal, and basilar plexus) are characterized clinically by unilateral orbital or head pain, diplopia, a red or protruding eye, and tinnitus. The onset of symptoms sometimes follows abortion or occurs in the postpartum period, possibly because of rupture of the thin-walled dural arteries during the straining of labor or because of the circulatory changes that occur in pregnancy.

On examination, there is usually a mild proptosis, distended conjunctival veins, increased intraocular pressure, transient sixth nerve palsy, or a bruit over the eye. Angiography reveals a low-volume shunt supplied from meningeal branches of the internal or external carotid arteries, sometimes from the contralateral side. Drainage may be directly into the cavernous sinus or into a more distant dural sinus or venous structure that communicates with the cavernous sinus. The fistula may close spontaneously, but if it remains patent, embolization of the feeding vessels may help to relieve intolerable symptoms or failing vision.

Arteriovenous shunts to the superoposterior group of dural sinuses (i.e., superior and inferior sagittal, straight, transverse, sigmoid, and occipital) may occur, with a female predominance among the reported cases. Symptoms and signs may relate to the shunt itself, to subarachnoid hemorrhage, to increased intracranial pressure, or to cerebral ischemia.

Tinnitus is the most common complaint, but headache, visual deterioration, subarachnoid hemorrhage, seizures, and various neurologic deficits may also occur. A bruit is often present and may be the sole finding on examination; it is best heard over the mastoid region or behind the ear. Papilledema may be present, and other neurologic signs are sometimes encountered. The arterial supply is commonly derived from branches of the external carotid artery, tentorial branches of the internal carotid artery, and meningeal branches of the vertebral artery. Ligation or embolization of feeding vessels or a direct surgical approach to the lesion may be helpful in patients with disabling symptoms or a history of hemorrhage.

Dural and Intradural Spinal Vascular Anomalies

Spinal arteriovenous fistulas are uncommon but are important to recognize because many are readily treated by surgery. Most are dural; if intradural, they are commonly extramedullary, are posterior to the cord, and are fed by one or more arteries that fail to supply the cord or contribute only to the posterior spinal circulation.[75]

Spinal arteriovenous fistulas may lead to spinal subarachnoid hemorrhage but more commonly give rise to a gradual disturbance in the function of the cord or nerve roots, or both. Spinal subarachnoid hemorrhage is much more common in patients with a cervical malformation than a more caudal lesion, may sometimes occur from an associated (arterial) aneurysm, and is associated with an overall mortality rate of at least 15%. It may be the first symptom produced by the lesion. Approximately one half of the patients who survive the first hemorrhage have a second, and one half of the subsequent survivors have further bleeding episodes unless the underlying malformation is treated. The spinal source of the hemorrhage may not be recognized until the later development of symptoms and signs of cord dysfunction, despite the local occurrence of sudden severe pain at the onset of bleeding, accompanied by signs of meningeal irritation.

Myelopathy or radiculopathy, or both, of gradual or sudden onset is the more common manifestation. By the time of diagnosis, approximately two thirds of patients complain of leg weakness, sensory symptoms, pain, and a sphincter disturbance. In some patients, symptoms, especially pain, are precipitated or aggravated by exercise and relieved by rest, whereas symptoms in other patients may relate to specific postures, such as sitting or bending forward. Symptoms occasionally relate to pregnancy, the menstrual cycle, nonspecific infective illness, a transient increase in body temperature, or trauma. On examination, signs of an upper or lower motor neuron disturbance or a mixed motor deficit are usually found in the legs; sensory deficits are common and are usually extensive, but occasionally, they may be restricted to a radicular distribution. There may be a coexisting cutaneous angioma that occasionally relates segmentally to the spinal lesion, and a bruit may be audible over the spine on auscultation.

Numerous case reports illustrating the influence of pregnancy on these lesions have been published. In one case that I encountered, symptoms occurred during each of three pregnancies, with complete clearing after delivery. Their basis was not recognized until the patient later experienced leg weakness and urinary retention that necessitated immediate hospitalization. Myelography and spinal angiography then demonstrated an arteriovenous malformation that was treated surgically.

The relationship of symptoms to pregnancy in such cases may be based in part on enhancement of preexisting cord ischemia by hemodilution and anemia. Moreover, pressure on pelvic and abdominal veins by an enlarged uterus may aggravate symptoms of caudally situated malformations by obstructing venous return to the heart, with a consequent reduction in the intramedullary arteriovenous pressure gradient and in cord blood flow.[75]

Diagnosis depends on radiologic investigations, which must not be postponed out of concern for the developing fetus, because any delay in establishing the diagnosis may lead to increased, often irreversible, disability in the mother. Spinal MRI may fail to detect the lesion. On myelography, the characteristic abnormality consists of vermiform defects caused by vascular impressions in the column of contrast material, usually without any obstruction in the subarachnoid space. If myelography suggests a vascular malformation, spinal angiography is undertaken to determine the level and extent of the vascular abnormality; the position of the arteriovenous shunt in relation to the cord; the number, origin, and anatomic location of arteries feeding the malformation; and the main supply to the cord in the region of the malformation.

Treatment is indicated in all patients who have progressive symptoms or functional incapacity or who have had a hemorrhage. Delay in these cases may lead to irreversible disability or death. When the fistula is dural or intradural but mainly or completely extramedullary, is posterior to the cord, and is fed by vessels that do not contribute to the anterior spinal circulation, surgical treatment or embolization generally poses no specific problem. Feeding vessels are obliterated, and the fistulous portion of the lesion is removed. Fistulas located anterior to or within the cord are more difficult to treat because of their inaccessibility and because they are often supplied by the anterior spinal artery or one of its feeders. These lesions are often regarded as inoperable, and experience in their treatment remains limited.

Infections

The central nervous system may be infected by bacterial, viral, fungal, or other organisms through the blood supply, by extension from infected adjacent structures, or by direct inoculation such as may follow trauma. The neural parenchyma may be involved diffusely (e.g., encephalitis) or focally (e.g., cerebral abscess), or infection may primarily involve the meninges and parameningeal structures (e.g., meningitis, subdural empyema). Although the resulting neurologic disorder may complicate pregnancy or delivery or may necessitate antimicrobial therapy that can harm the developing fetus, the clinical features, diagnosis, and management of infections during pregnancy are essentially the same as at other times. Further discussion is limited to certain infections that pose some particular problem when they occur during pregnancy or are especially likely to develop in relation to pregnancy.

Poliomyelitis

The development of an effective vaccine has all but eradicated paralytic poliomyelitis in developed countries. Even pregnant women can be included safely in programs of mass vaccination with live oral poliovirus vaccine.[76] Nevertheless, the disorder still occurs in unprotected persons and remains common in many parts of the world. Moreover, people with residual disability from previous poliomyelitis are seen fairly regularly in most large medical centers, and obstetric management of such patients may be complicated by their neurologic deficits.

Most patients infected with poliovirus are asymptomatic or have only minor, nonspecific respiratory or gastrointestinal symptoms. Nervous system involvement occurs in only a few instances; its clinical manifestations are described in standard neurologic textbooks. Patients with neurologic involvement should be hospitalized, with care taken to provide for any circulatory or respiratory complications that may develop. Simple analgesics can be provided for relief of pain, and physical therapy may be helpful after muscle weakness has stabilized.

During pregnancy, women are more susceptible to clinical poliomyelitis, but it is unclear whether this is because they are more susceptible to the initial viral infection or to invasion of the nervous system. Pregnancy may also alter the course of the infection. The course is unaffected if poliomyelitis develops early in pregnancy, but an increase in severity or distribution of the muscle weakness may occur if childbirth takes place during the acute phase or shortly thereafter.

In early pregnancy, especially during the first trimester, spontaneous abortion may occur in association with a febrile reaction in the acute phase of poliomyelitis or in relation to apparently mild nonparalytic attacks of the disease. Abortion or fetal loss may also occur spontaneously in the second or third trimester but often with maternal illness of such severity that assisted respiration may be necessary.

Even patients with severe poliomyelitis necessitating respirator assistance can usually be managed supportively, and labor can be managed similarly to that in normal women unless there are specific obstetric indications for operative delivery or induction of labor. The uterine muscle is not paralyzed.

Fetal poliomyelitis is rare. Normal offspring can generally be anticipated, but neonatal cases of poliomyelitis are well recognized. If an infant is affected within the first 5 days of life, the disorder is assumed to result from transplacental transmission of the virus. These neonatal cases are associated with a mortality rate of at least 50%, but subclinical infection with poliovirus may also occur in newborn infants.

Tetanus

A worldwide disease, tetanus is rarely encountered in developed countries where immunizations are freely available. *Clostridium tetani* infection by means of tetanus spores may follow injury, surgical procedures, childbirth, abortion, and injections. If the spores are converted into vegetative gram-positive rods and favorable anaerobic conditions exist, tetanospasmin, a toxin that is responsible for the symptoms of tetanus, is produced.

The incubation period varies. In patients with generalized tetanus, the most common presenting symptom is trismus, and the disorder itself is characterized by frequent spasms of various muscles that can be provoked by minor external stimuli and may occur against a background of continuous tonic muscle contractions. Typically, the trunk is hyperextended, the arms are flexed, and the legs are extended; laryngospasm may lead to respiratory obstruction.

Localized tetanus is more benign and is characterized by persistent rigidity of muscles close to the site of inoculation with the organism. A splanchnic form is described after abdominal and pelvic operations or uterine trauma, with prominent involvement of the muscles of deglutition and respiration.

The morbidity and mortality rates vary. Respiratory complications are a leading cause of death, as is the autonomic hyperactivity that sometimes complicates tetanus. Treatment is directed at the following:

- Neutralizing unbound toxin with antitoxin
- Reducing further toxin production by surgical toilet and antibiotic treatment
- Controlling tetanic spasms by drugs such as diazepam, chlorpromazine, and barbiturates
- Assisting respiration mechanically if necessary
- Undertaking general supportive measures

Tetanus may develop as a complication of childbirth or abortion, especially in underdeveloped countries. It leads to abortion in many instances and has a maternal mortality rate that often exceeds 50%. In addition to the measures listed, evacuation of products retained in the uterus may be necessary, and hysterectomy is sometimes required.

Tetanus is a common cause of neonatal death in underdeveloped countries. Infection usually results from a lack of hygiene during delivery, with consequent contamination of the umbilical cord. The clinical manifestations differ from those in older children or adults, in that dysphagia and respiratory problems are often more marked, fever is usually higher, and the disease is generally more severe, often fulminating. Most affected infants are 6 to 9 days old when admitted and have a typical history of continuous crying for up to 48 hours, followed by cessation of sucking and then of crying, accompanied by convulsions and often by fever.

In regions where neonatal tetanus is common, the infant mortality rate is high. Improvement of delivery practices and obstetric services may prevent the disorder, as may the active immunization of pregnant women or of all women of childbearing potential[77] and the substitution of disinfectants for traditional cord-care practices.[78] Unfortunately, in most areas with a high incidence of tetanus neonatorum, there are no widely available maternity services, and any prophylactic approach that depends on the early identification of pregnant women is impractical.

Miscellaneous Maternal Infections

Clinical or subclinical maternal infection may involve the fetus and may affect the developing nervous system and therefore the neonate. The resulting neurologic complications merit brief comment here. Fetal infection may be inconsequential or may result in abortion, stillbirth, growth retardation, congenital disease, or developmental anomalies. Gestational age at the time of infection influences the effects (see Chapter 38).

Infection with *Listeria monocytogenes* is an important cause of habitual abortion, and it may lead to a variety of other manifestations in pregnant women. In neonates, infection may take an early-onset, predominantly septicemic form, characterized by prematurity, respiratory distress, heart failure, and increased neonatal mortality, or take a late-onset, predominantly meningitic or meningoencephalitic form. Diagnosis depends on the bacteriologic and serologic findings. Treatment consists of appropriate antibiotic therapy, usually with ampicillin.

Maternal rubella, especially when it occurs in the first 2 months of pregnancy, may cause fetal infection and a congenital syndrome characterized by ocular abnormalities, deafness, mental retardation, seizures, focal neurologic deficits, cardiac anomalies, hepatosplenomegaly, and other abnormalities in a variety of combinations. In rare patients with congenital rubella, pyramidal and extrapyramidal signs, seizures, and dementia occur as part of a progressive panencephalitic illness during the second decade of life; high antibody titers to rubella virus occur in blood and cerebrospinal fluid, and the virus may even be isolated from the brain.[79]

In congenital toxoplasmosis, seizures and pyramidal defects may result from meningoencephalitis together with chorioretinitis, obstructive hydrocephalus, and cerebral calcification. There may be respiratory and feeding difficulties. Later mental development may be retarded. For prophylactic purposes, pregnant women should be advised to avoid contact with cat feces and ingestion of raw or undercooked meat.

Fetal infections with cytomegalovirus may cause hepatosplenomegaly, jaundice, petechiae, ocular defects, cardiac defects, and other abnormalities. Involvement of the nervous system may lead to cerebral malformation, microcephaly, mental retardation, seizures, obstructive hydrocephalus, cerebral calcification, deafness, or chorioretinitis.

Herpes simplex virus infection in the neonate is characterized primarily by visceral involvement, but the brain may be affected. Seizures, irritability, motor deficits, increased intracranial pressure, and depression of consciousness may occur, sometimes in the apparent absence of more widespread disease.

Children born to women infected with the human immunodeficiency virus (HIV) are at risk of infection with the virus. The risk varies in different series for uncertain reasons. The virus may infect the fetus in utero or the neonate during birth or through breast milk. Infected children may develop acquired immunodeficiency syndrome (AIDS) after an interval ranging from several months to several years. This leads typically to developmental delay and regression as a result of progressive encephalopathy. Calcification of the basal ganglia may occur. Systemic features include failure to thrive, pneumonitis, hepatosplenomegaly, and recurrent bacterial infections. Management of pregnant women with HIV infection therefore includes minimizing the risk of transmitting the infection to offspring, recognizing neonatal infection early, reducing the risk of opportunistic infection, and managing psychosocial aspects. Antiretroviral therapy for infected women during pregnancy and zidovudine therapy for neonates for 6 weeks (or longer and with combination therapy if necessary) may be helpful. The protective effect of maternal therapy depends on the complexity and duration of treatment, and highly active antiretroviral therapy (HAART) is associated with the lowest transmission rates.[80] Compared with no antiretroviral treatment or monotherapy, combination therapy does not seem to be associated with increased risks of prematurity or other adverse outcomes of pregnancy,[81] although some antiviral agents may be teratogenic (there are limited data concerning safety during pregnancy).[82,83] The use of infant formula to prevent postnatal transmission through breast milk has helped to reduce the incidence of infection in developed countries.[84,85] Infants may require monitoring for 1 to 2 years with testing for HIV to exclude infection (see Chapter 38). Fetal infection itself may lead to teratogenicity, with nervous system malformations that are associated with vasculitic microinfarcts of the fetal brain.[82,83]

The possibility of syphilitic infection must be considered during the evaluation of all pregnant women. Effective treatment of maternal syphilis at an early stage of pregnancy usually prevents fetal involvement, and treatment in later pregnancy affects both mother and fetus. Syphilis may severely affect pregnancy, leading to increased chances of abortion and perinatal mortality and to symptomatic congenital syphilis in many of the surviving infants. Infants may also be infected at birth if they come into contact with an infective lesion. The possibility of congenital infection can be confirmed by various serologic tests. The clinical features of congenital neurosyphilis, which may become apparent after the first few weeks of life or may be delayed for several years, are essentially the same as those of neurosyphilis in adults. Infants with clinical or laboratory evidence of infection require treatment to prevent its occurrence, and penicillin is the drug of choice.

Metabolic Disorders

Several metabolic disorders are considered elsewhere in this chapter, including Wilson disease, hepatic porphyria, and the Wernicke-Korsakoff syndrome. In this section, attention is confined to two other disorders that are important to recognize for therapeutic purposes: vitamin B_{12} deficiency and phenylketonuria (PKU).

Vitamin B_{12} Deficiency

Vitamin B_{12} deficiency is a well-known cause of neurologic disease (i.e., myelopathy characterized predominantly by pyramidal and posterior column deficits, polyneuropathy, mental changes, optic neuropathy) in adults, in whom it may arise from malabsorption, dietary inadequacy, or other causes. Patients may have accompanying megaloblastic anemia, but this may be obscured if folic acid supplements have been taken. Clinical presentation during pregnancy does not differ from that in the nongestational period. Treatment with parenteral vitamin B_{12} prevents further progression and may lead to partial improvement of the neurologic disorder.

It is not widely recognized that maternal vitamin B_{12} deficiency during pregnancy and the puerperium may lead to a similar deficiency in the fetus and neonate. A reduced content of vitamin B_{12} in maternal milk may then lead to frank deficiency in breastfed infants. The resulting clinical syndrome in these infants is characterized by megaloblastic anemia, cutaneous pigmentation, apathy, developmental delay or regression, and involuntary movements. The clinical and biochemical abnormalities are rapidly corrected by vitamin supplementation.

Phenylketonuria

An autosomal recessive disorder, PKU is an important cause of mental retardation, which develops in the absence of adequate dietary treatment. Screening programs for neonates with PKU have enabled identification and treatment of affected infants to prevent intellectual deterioration, but the optimal duration of treatment remains unclear. Women with PKU have a high rate of spontaneous abortion, and their nonphenylketonuric (heterozygote) offspring have a high incidence of certain abnormalities. Among the offspring of pregnancies during which the maternal PKU is untreated, there are marked increases in the incidence of mental retardation, microcephaly, and congenital heart disease compared with the normal population, and these increases correlate with maternal blood levels of phenylalanine.

The fetal effects of maternal PKU occur because of the high maternal blood levels of phenylalanine, not because the infant has PKU. Dietary treatment before or during early pregnancy (i.e., within the first 2 months) may prevent or lessen the fetal effects.[86-90] Treatment may need to be in effect at conception for maximal benefit. Even so, a normal child cannot be ensured.

The mother with undiagnosed PKU poses different problems. Antenatal screening for maternal PKU or testing for PKU at the first antenatal visit of a woman with a family history of the disease, low intelligence of uncertain origin, or a history of microcephalic offspring is appropriate.

The newborn offspring of a mother with PKU will be homozygous or heterozygous for the disorder. The homozygotes definitely require a diet low in phenylalanine, but the proper nutritional management of heterozygotes is less clear. The mother should be advised against breastfeeding because her milk will contain a high concentration of phenylalanine. Elevation of blood phenylalanine levels is only minimal during pregnancy in mothers who are heterozygous for the disorder, and the incidence of congenital anomalies and brain damage does not appear to be increased in their offspring.

Movement Disorders

When dystonia develops during pregnancy, it usually manifests acutely as a consequence of treatment with antiemetic dopamine antagonists (e.g., metoclopramide), neuroleptic drugs, or levodopa. For patients with established dystonia, genetic counseling may be prudent if the disorder has a hereditary basis, and the need to continue on pharmacologic treatment should be evaluated before planned pregnancy. Parkinson disease shows no consistent change during pregnancy, but little information is available concerning the safety of antiparkinsonian agents when taken during the gestational period.

Chorea Gravidarum

The term *chorea* refers to involuntary rapid muscle jerks that occur unpredictably in different parts of the body. When the disorder is florid, choreic limb movements and facial grimacing are unmistakable and distort any concomitant voluntary activity. In mild cases, there may be no more than a persistent restlessness and clumsiness.

Sydenham chorea is regarded as a complication of infection with group A hemolytic streptococci, and the underlying pathology may be an arteritis. When it occurs during pregnancy, it is referred to as *chorea gravidarum*. This disease occurs most commonly in primigravidas, with symptoms tending to occur in the early part of pregnancy and remitting after delivery. A history of chorea and rheumatic fever is obtained in about two thirds of patients, and the other third have clinical signs of rheumatic heart disease. Psychological disturbance may occasionally be conspicuous. Chorea gravidarum may recur in later pregnancies. Death, primarily caused by underlying rheumatic heart disease, is rare.

Symptomatic benefit follows bed rest and sedation, and there is no indication for termination of pregnancy. The prognosis is essentially that of any cardiac complication. No specific obstetric complications are associated with chorea gravidarum, and a normal, healthy infant can generally be anticipated.

Although many cases of chorea gravidarum result from preceding streptococcal infection, in other instances, there is no clinical or laboratory evidence of such an association. Instead, clinical impression suggests that pregnancy has in some way merely exacerbated some preexisting disturbance that then becomes clinically evident. Similarly, chorea is occasionally induced by oral contraceptives in women with preexisting basal ganglia abnormalities resulting from various causes. The dyskinesia in such cases usually begins within about 3 months of the introduction of contraceptive therapy, evolves subacutely, is often asymmetrical or unilateral, and resolves with discontinuation of the offending substance. The pathophysiologic basis of hormonal contraceptive-induced chorea is uncertain, but a vascular or immunologic mechanism or a hormone-dependent alteration in central dopaminergic activity has tentatively been advanced as the underlying cause.

Chorea developing for the first time during pregnancy must not automatically be regarded as a variant of Sydenham chorea, because it may arise for other reasons. The choreic movements of Huntington disease occasionally occur for the first time during pregnancy, but the subsequent course of events and the family history will point to the correct diagnosis. Systemic lupus erythematosus may also cause chorea that sometimes commences during pregnancy, and a thorough search for evidence of this disorder should be made in all patients without clear evidence of a rheumatic basis for chorea. Finally, as in nonpregnant patients, chorea may result from polycythemia vera rubra, thyrotoxicosis, hypocalcemia, Wilson disease, and treatment with phenytoin or a major tranquilizing drug.

Restless Legs Syndrome

Between 10% and 20% of pregnant patients experience unpleasant creeping sensations deep in the legs and occasionally in the arms.[91] Symptoms generally occur when patients are relaxed, especially at night, and prompt a need to move about. These symptoms usually develop in the latter half of pregnancy, subsiding soon after delivery. Similar symptoms may also occur without any relation to pregnancy.

No abnormalities are found on neurologic examination. The cause of the disorder is unknown, but symptoms sometimes resolve after correction of any coexisting anemia or iron deficiency. Persistent or intolerable symptoms may respond to treatment with drugs such as diazepam or clonazepam. Other drugs that are sometimes helpful include levodopa, dopamine agonists, clonazepam, and opiates, but these drugs are better avoided during pregnancy if possible. Symptoms usually resolve spontaneously within a few weeks of the end of pregnancy.

Wilson Disease

An autosomal recessive disorder caused by a gene defect on the long arm of chromosome 13, Wilson disease is characterized by the accumulation of copper in the brain, liver, and other organs. Neurologic and mental symptoms such as intellectual disturbances, abnormal movements of all sorts, dysarthria, dysphagia, and rigidity are common presenting complaints. After neurologic signs are identified, careful examination of the eyes invariably shows the presence of Kayser-Fleischer rings, which are brown deposits of copper along the edge of the cornea in Descemet membrane. Clinical evidence of hepatic involvement may be present but is variable.

The diagnosis is suggested by the family history, low serum copper and ceruloplasmin concentrations, and increased 24-hour urinary excretion of copper. Treatment with a low-copper diet and with penicillamine, a chelating agent that promotes copper excretion, may lead to marked improvement of neurologic and hepatic status.

Patients with untreated Wilson disease have a high miscarriage rate. Pregnancy generally proceeds normally in patients who have received adequate chelation therapy and carries no particular hazard for the mother or fetus.[92,93] Although penicillamine therapy has been associated with mesenchymal birth defects, several reports document normal pregnancies and infants in mothers on treatment with it. An alternative approach is treatment with trientine and zinc, but experience with oral zinc salts taken during pregnancy is limited, and trientine is teratogenic in rats.[94] Labor and delivery may be complicated in patients with portal hypertension. Hemorrhage from esophageal varices may occur, especially during the second or third trimesters. Extradural analgesia helps to avoid straining during vaginal delivery; cesarean section is best reserved for obstetric indications.[95]

Multiple Sclerosis

Multiple sclerosis is a disorder in which plaques of demyelination develop at different times and in different sites throughout the central nervous system. Its cause remains uncertain; clinical onset usually occurs in early adult life. There is considerable variability in the tempo and character of neurologic symptoms and signs. The disorder is classically associated with unpredictable exacerbations during which neurologic deficits develop, followed by remissions during which symptoms and signs may partially or completely resolve. With time, patients become increasingly disabled, although perhaps not for many years after appearance of the initial symptoms. In other patients, the disorder follows a progressive course from its onset.

Several epidemiologic studies have suggested a tendency for remissions during pregnancy and an increased frequency of multiple sclerosis exacerbations in the first 3 to 6 months after childbirth.[96-98] Pregnancy itself or the number of pregnancies has no effect on subsequent neurologic disability.[99-101] The remission of multiple sclerosis during pregnancy probably relates to a gestational immunosuppressive state that has a multifactorial basis.[98] Similarly, multiple sclerosis does not influence the natural course of pregnancy or childbirth,[102] although some investigators have reported an increased incidence of small infants for age or of deliveries requiring forceps, vacuum extractor, or cesarean section.[103] When patients on interferon β therapy become pregnant, they have a higher incidence of miscarriages or stillbirths or of small babies.[104]

The possibility of a familial incidence of multiple sclerosis is widely known, but this pattern is uncommon and tends to involve siblings rather than different generations. It may merely reflect common exposure to some unrecognized etiologic agent rather than genetic predisposition to the disorder. With these points in mind, inquiries by a pregnant woman with multiple sclerosis who is worried that her child may later become affected should be met with firm reassurance. A patient with multiple sclerosis does not need to be discouraged from pregnancy unless she is already so disabled by the disorder that she will clearly be incapable of coping with the responsibilities and physical demands of parenthood. Patients with minimal incapacity who are anxious to have a child will usually do so anyway and do not need to be discouraged as long as they have some understanding of the nature of their disorder and its unpredictable course. In discussions between such patients and physicians, it seems reasonable to provide optimistic assurance that multiple sclerosis does not shorten life and that significant disability may not occur for many years, if at all.

The management of multiple sclerosis during pregnancy is supportive. The treatment of acute exacerbations consists of bed rest and prescription of a brief course of steroids, which may hasten recovery without necessarily influencing its extent. Patients with sphincter disturbances or who are paraplegic may experience increased difficulties during pregnancy. The method of delivery should depend solely on obstetric factors.

Optic Neuritis

Any type of optic neuropathy may develop fortuitously during gestation. Optic neuritis may develop during pregnancy or lactation[105] in patients with established multiple sclerosis or in patients who will later develop other manifestations of that disorder. Optic nerve involvement by tumors or vascular malformations may also appear for the first time in the gestational period, as may the optic neuropathy that sometimes complicates vitamin deficiency. Optic nerve involvement may complicate hyperemesis gravidarum, with rapid onset of marked, usually bilateral, visual loss; the entity is rare, but if vomiting is unresponsive to treatment, it may be necessary to terminate the pregnancy.

Leber optic atrophy is a hereditary disorder that usually occurs in early adult life. It commonly has a sex-linked recessive mode of inheritance, so that the male offspring of women carriers of the disorder may be affected. Other modes of inheritance have also been described. The clinical deficit commences abruptly with visual loss and leads ultimately to bilateral central scotoma with optic atrophy. No abnormalities are found in the neonate. Other forms of hereditary optic atrophy have been described in which the disorder is congenital or develops in infancy or early childhood and may have a dominant or a recessive mode of transmission. The family pedigree is important for diagnostic and counseling purposes in all such instances.

Traumatic Paraplegia

When spinal cord injury resulting in paraplegia occurs during the course of an established pregnancy, it may be followed by spontaneous abortion or stillbirth. If the pregnancy continues, the detailed radiologic investigations that are needed to determine the nature and extent of the spinal injury may be hazardous to the developing fetus, especially if it is still very immature (see Chapter 20). In such circumstances, the interests of the mother are of paramount importance.

Many patients with established paraplegia are eager to experience motherhood, and because they are capable of sexual intercourse, they inquire about the possibility and potential hazards of childbirth. Urinary tract infection, a common complication of paraplegia, can be exacerbated by pregnancy but is not a contraindication to pregnancy if there is no gross impairment of renal function. In the management of paraplegics, it is important to re-educate the paralyzed bladder so that only a minimal amount of residual urine remains after micturition. If this is achieved, difficulty with micturition can usually be postponed to the last stages of pregnancy, when catheterization is often necessary.

Pregnancy may increase the likelihood of development of pressure sores in paraplegic women. Patients and their families should be informed about the cause of these sores and the manner in which prolonged pressure can be avoided. Because anemia lowers the resistance of paraplegic patients to infection and pressure, particular care must be taken to prevent its development during pregnancy.

The uterus itself contracts normally in labor despite interruption of its nerve supply. However, patients with complete spinal cord lesions above the tenth thoracic segment cannot appreciate the onset of labor or feel any pain during it because afferent fibers from the uterus enter the cord more caudally. Medical attendants need to examine the state of the cervix to identify the onset of labor with certainty. Because labor often commences before term in such circumstances, the cervix is examined at each antenatal visit after 24 to 26 weeks' gestation; the patient should be hospitalized if the cervix is dilated.

The occurrence of symptoms such as leg spasms in association with uterine contractions may be helpful in signaling the onset of labor, as may uterine palpation by the patient's spouse. Routine hospitalization after the 32nd week should be considered. In patients with cord lesions below the 10th or 11th thoracic segment, uterine contractions produce normal pain sensations. A patient with spasticity resulting from the cord lesion may develop painful flexor spasms and ankle clonus during uterine contractions.

Pregnant women with complete cord lesions above the fifth or sixth thoracic segment (i.e., above the splanchnic outflow) may develop the syndrome of autonomic hyperreflexia with excessive activity of a viscus. This is characterized by throbbing headache, hypertension, reflex bradycardia, sweating, nasal congestion, and cutaneous vasodilatation and piloerection above the level of the lesion. During labor, these symptoms are most conspicuous with uterine contractions and become especially prominent just before delivery. Electrocardiographic monitoring may facilitate recognition of any changes in cardiac rate or rhythm that occur during uterine contractions. Symptoms are caused by the sudden release of catecholamines.

Treatment in the past has relied on reserpine (which depletes catecholamines from sympathetic nerve terminals but also can cause potentially dangerous nasal congestion in the nasal-breathing neonate), atropine, clonidine, glyceryl trinitrate, or hexamethonium (a ganglion blocker). The syndrome can be prevented or treated by spinal or epidural anesthesia extending to the level of the tenth thoracic segment, and early consultation with an anesthesiologist may therefore be helpful.

Cesarean section is not indicated by paraplegia per se, but it may be required because of bony deformity of the spine or pelvis. If the patient has a permanent suprapubic cystostomy, a vertical incision rather than a lower segment transverse incision must be used. Forceps delivery or vacuum extraction is often required because the muscles responsible for the expulsive efforts of the second stage are paralyzed and because severe hypertension sometimes necessitates shortening the second stage.

Absorbable sutures, such as catgut, are poorly absorbed in paraplegics, and sterile abscesses commonly form around buried catgut. Nonabsorbable sutures, such as nylon, are preferred for repairing an episiotomy. Paraplegic and quadriplegic patients can successfully breastfeed their infants, and they have a normal letdown (i.e., milk ejection) reflex during suckling.

Root Lesions

Prolapsed Intervertebral Disk and Pregnancy

The symptoms and signs of lumbar disk protrusion during pregnancy are similar to those occurring in nonparous women. Radicular pain and low back pain are usually conspicuous features, and there may be a segmental motor and sensory disturbance in the limbs. When the disk prolapses centrally rather than laterally, symptoms and signs in the legs may be bilateral, and sphincter disturbances occur more commonly.

Lumbar disk protrusion must be distinguished from other causes of leg weakness developing during or soon after pregnancy. Lumbosacral palsy may arise during labor from compressive injury of the plexus, but tenderness and rigidity of the lumbar spine, sciatica, and signs of root tension favor the diagnosis of protruded disk. The distribution of muscle weakness may also be helpful; depending on their location, plexus lesions cause weakness and sensory symptoms in a polyradicular or peripheral nerve distribution in the legs. Because only the anterior primary rami contribute to the plexus, a proximal radiculopathy can be distinguished from a plexus lesion by electromyographic examination of muscles supplied by the posterior primary rami (i.e., paraspinal muscles), involvement of which therefore favors a root lesion.

Management is the same as for nonpregnant women. MRI has no known effects on the fetus, but contrast agents are probably best avoided. In patients with lateral protrusion of a lumbar disk, simple analgesics provide symptomatic relief. Surgery can usually be deferred until after childbirth. However, laminectomy and excision of the protruded disk may be necessary during pregnancy, especially if symptoms are bilateral or if there is any disturbance of sphincter function.

Other Lumbosacral Root Lesions

Most disk lesions involve the L5 or S1 roots. Although a disk lesion may occasionally affect the L4 root, involvement of an upper lumbar nerve root suggests other compressive disease. In a patient presenting with an L5 or S1 radiculopathy, there may be a more rostrally situated lesion if no abnormality, such as a protruded disk, is seen in the L4-5 or L5-S1 region, because the spinal cord ends at the lower border of L1 and the roots then descend intradurally before exiting through their respective intervertebral foramina. In such circumstances, the possibility of other compressive lesions must be considered. As with nonpregnant patients, each case is best managed on an individual basis.

Plexus Lesions and Peripheral Mononeuropathies

Certain peripheral entrapment neuropathies are particularly liable to develop in pregnancy and may lead to troublesome symptoms. Recognition of the basis of such symptoms is important because, with reassurance about their benign nature, most patients can tolerate them until they give birth, when the symptoms usually subside spontaneously. Other peripheral nerve or plexus lesions may develop during labor or obstetric surgical procedures as a result of compression or stretch of nerves, especially in anesthetized patients.

Disorders of peripheral nerves may be characterized by slowing or blocking of conduction along intact axons or by axonal degeneration. The former carries a much more favorable prognosis for recovery than the latter, because after axonal degeneration has occurred, recovery can take place only by regeneration, a process that may take many months and may never be complete.

Electrophysiologic Evaluation

In the evaluation of patients with suspected nerve lesions, electrophysiologic techniques have been helpful in several ways.[106] Electromyography can aid in determining whether weakness is neurogenic; if so, the electromyographically demonstrated pattern of affected muscles may indicate the location of the lesion (i.e., whether root, plexus, or an individual peripheral nerve has been affected). The findings may also indicate whether neurogenic weakness is a consequence of impaired conduction along otherwise intact axons or of axonal degeneration, a distinction that has prognostic importance.

The motor responses to nerve stimulation provide complementary information. If axonal degeneration results from a focal lesion in a peripheral nerve, the motor responses to electrical stimulation proximal or distal to the lesion become small or absent about a week after injury, depending on the completeness of the lesion. In contrast, in patients with a conductive disturbance caused by an acute focal lesion, the motor responses to stimulation beyond (distal to) the lesion are generally normal, whereas those elicited by more proximal stimulation may be small.

Motor and sensory conduction velocity can be measured in various accessible segments of peripheral nerves, and focal slowing may provide confirmatory evidence of an underlying entrapment or focal neuropathy. In patients presenting with a mononeuropathy, nerve conduction studies can be used to exclude the real possibility of an underlying subclinical polyneuropathy.

Lumbosacral Plexus Lesion

The roots of the sciatic nerve may be compressed in the pelvis by the fetal head or obstetric forceps, and the brunt of the resulting motor deficit is then borne by muscles supplied by the common peroneal fibers because of their relationship to the bony pelvis. This type of injury to the maternal lumbosacral plexus is more likely when a short patient with a small pelvis carries a rather large infant, so that labor is complicated by minor disproportion, or when mid-forceps are used during delivery because of malpresentation. The features of the pelvis that predispose to this complication include a straight sacrum, a flat wide posterior pelvis, posterior displacement of the transverse diameter of the inlet, wide sacroiliac notches, and prominent ischial spines.

Symptoms usually are unilateral and develop immediately after delivery, but they may not be noticed until the patient is allowed out of bed. When the common peroneal fibers are involved, the main complaint is of leg weakness, which is sometimes erroneously attributed to a painful episiotomy. In more severe cases, there is footdrop. Numbness and paresthesias may occur over the dorsum of the foot and lateral aspect of the leg, and cutaneous sensation may be impaired in this distribution.

Unless the injury has been severe, the predominant pathologic change is demyelination of the affected fibers, and this is reflected in the electrophysiologic findings. With mild injuries, the prognosis for recovery is excellent; if wallerian degeneration has occurred, recovery may take many months and may never be complete. Physical therapy is all that is needed for the treatment of mild cases, but calipers and night casts may be required in more severe instances to prevent contracture.

Subsequent pregnancies can be allowed to proceed normally if an easy vaginal delivery is anticipated. Low forceps can be used with caution if necessary, but the use of mid-forceps may be hazardous. It seems sensible to advise cesarean section if the infant is very large or if premonitory symptoms suggesting nerve compression occur with attempted engagement of the fetal head in the pelvic brim during the last 4 weeks of pregnancy in a patient with a history of obstetric lumbosacral plexus palsy.

Acute Familial Brachial Neuritis

Several reports document the rare occurrence of brachial plexus neuropathy on a familial basis. Taylor[107] reported that 24 of 119 members of a family covering five generations had experienced single or multiple attacks of acute brachial neuropathy. This disorder was characterized by pain, weakness, atrophy, and sensory loss that was usually unilateral but occasionally bilateral and from which gradual recovery generally occurred. Male and female family members were affected, but among the women, there was a striking association of attacks with pregnancy or the puerperium, in contrast to the more common idiopathic disorder, which is rarely associated with pregnancy. In some instances of the familial disease, the lower cranial nerves were involved, and isolated mononeuropathies of the other extremities were present. Other cases have been described. Treatment with oral steroids may be helpful in relieving pain but does not seem to affect the rate of recovery.

Carpal Tunnel Syndrome

Compression of the median nerve may occur in the carpal tunnel at the wrist, especially when the normal size of the carpal tunnel is reduced, as by degenerative arthritis, or when the volume of its contents is increased, as in inflammatory disorders involving the tendons and connective tissues at the wrist. Carpal tunnel syndrome is common during pregnancy,[108] perhaps because of excessive fluid retention. Pain and paresthesias are early symptoms and frequently occur at night, awakening the patient from sleep. The symptoms usually involve the first three digits and the lateral border of the ring finger, but some patients report that all digits are affected. Pain may occur in the forearm and occasionally occur in the upper arm. With time, weakness of the thenar muscles may develop. On examination, it is often possible to elicit the Tinel sign (percussion of the nerve at the wrist causing paresthesias in its distal distribution), and the Phalen maneuver (flexion at the wrist for more than a minute) sometimes reproduces or enhances symptoms. There may be mild weakness and wasting of the abductor pollicis brevis and opponens pollicis muscles, impaired cutaneous sensation in a median nerve distribution in the hand, or both motor and sensory signs.

Electrophysiologic testing usually suggests or confirms the diagnosis (Fig. 52-8). In the evaluation of patients, it is important to remember that the carpal tunnel syndrome is commonly bilateral, even though it may be unilaterally symptomatic, and an entrapment neuropathy may be the first manifestation of a subclinical polyneuropathy. These possibilities can be excluded by appropriate electrophysiologic studies.

Symptoms developing or worsening during pregnancy usually respond to the nocturnal use of a wrist splint and clear within about 3 months of delivery, often settling within 1 or 2 weeks.[109] They may recur in subsequent pregnancies. The splint is placed on the dorsal surface so that the wrist can be maintained in a neutral or slightly flexed position. Some patients are helped by injection of steroids into the carpal tunnel and others by treatment with diuretics. The physician must explain to the patient that her symptoms are benign and will generally subside spontaneously after the pregnancy. With such reassurance, most patients accept their symptoms without difficulty.

Surgical division of the anterior carpal ligament may be necessary if symptoms are intolerable or do not clear in the weeks after delivery. Surgical treatment may also be necessary in a patient with clinical or electrophysiologic evidence of increasing nerve dysfunction despite conservative measures, but it can usually be avoided during the pregnancy.

Meralgia Paresthetica

The lateral femoral cutaneous nerve, a purely sensory nerve derived from the L2 and L3 roots, is particularly susceptible to compression or stretch injury during pregnancy, especially during the third trimester. Obesity and diabetes mellitus are other predisposing factors. The nerve usually runs under the outer portion of the inguinal ligament to reach the thigh, but the ligament sometimes splits to enclose the nerve. In the latter circumstance, hyperextension of the hip or an increased lumbar lordosis, such as occurs during pregnancy, leads to compression of the nerve by the posterior fascicle of the ligament. Entrapment of the nerve at any point along its course may lead to similar symptoms, and several anatomic variations may predispose the nerve to damage when it is stretched. Pain, paresthesias, and numbness may occur about the outer aspect of the thigh and are sometimes relieved by sitting. Symptoms are unilateral in approximately 80% of cases.

Little may be found on physical examination, but in severe cases cutaneous sensation is disturbed in the affected area. Symptoms, which are usually mild, subside spontaneously in the puerperium or within

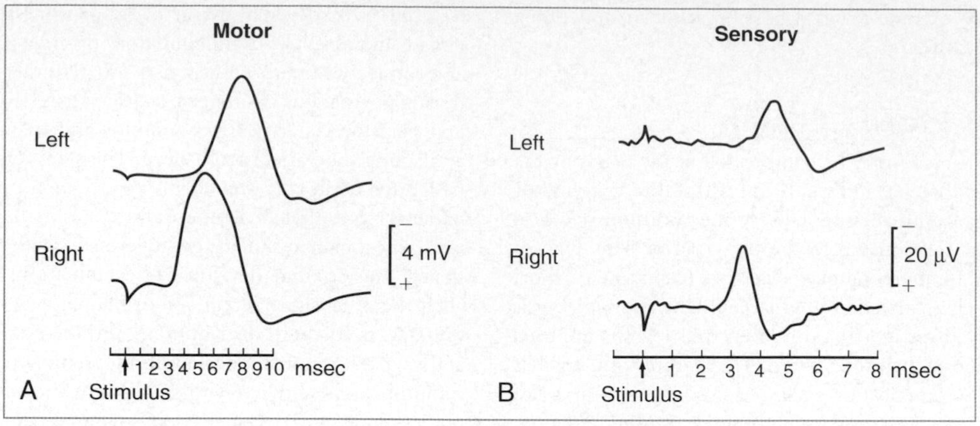

FIGURE 52-8 Nerve conduction studies in a patient with left-sided carpal tunnel syndrome. **A,** Responses are shown for the abductor pollicis brevis muscle to supramaximal electrical stimulation of the median nerves at the wrist. The latency of the response on the left is prolonged. **B,** The sensory action potentials are recorded over the median nerve at the wrist after electrical stimulation of digital sensory fibers in the index fingers. Those on the left have a smaller amplitude and more prolonged latency than those on the right. Maximal motor conduction velocity in the forearm segments of the median nerves was normal.

a few weeks of delivery. Patients should be reassured about the benign nature of the disorder. In a few instances, however, pain has been so severe that labor had to be induced early. Hydrocortisone injections in the region where the nerve lies medial to the anterior superior iliac spine may relieve persistent symptoms for a time, and low-dose tricyclic antidepressant drugs may also be helpful. Anticonvulsant agents, which are sometimes helpful for neuropathic pain, are best avoided during pregnancy. Nerve decompression by transposition may provide more lasting relief but is rarely required.

Traumatic Mononeuropathies

Certain causes and clinical features of traumatic mononeuropathies are likely to develop in relation to obstetric procedures.

The obturator nerve originates within the psoas muscle from the L2, L3, and L4 nerves; it emerges from the medial border of the psoas and enters the pelvis immediately in front of the sacroiliac joint. It sweeps around the lateral pelvic wall and then passes through the obturator foramen, dividing into branches that supply the adductor, gracilis, and external obturator muscles; the skin over part of the medial thigh; and the hip joint. The nerve may be injured during genitourinary operations involving the lithotomy position because of angulation as it leaves the obturator foramen or compression between the fetal head (or a pelvic mass) and the bony pelvic wall.[110] An obturator nerve palsy leads to impaired gait, because of weakness of the adductor muscles, and to a sensory disturbance involving particularly the medial part of the middle thigh and lower thigh. Pain may also occur and tends to radiate from the groin down the inner side of the thigh.

The femoral nerve originates within the psoas muscle from the L2, L3, and L4 nerves and passes beneath the inguinal ligament to enter the thigh. It innervates the iliacus, sartorius, pectineus, and quadriceps femoris muscles, and its cutaneous branches supply anterior and medial portions of the thigh and, through the saphenous nerve, the medial portions of the lower leg. Clinical features of a femoral nerve palsy are weakness and, in severe cases, wasting of the quadriceps muscle, sensory impairment over the anteromedial aspect of the thigh and occasionally of the leg to the medial malleolus, and depression or absence of the knee jerk. This type of palsy can occur as an isolated phenomenon in the patient with diabetes mellitus, a bleeding tendency, or retroperitoneal neoplasm, and it may sometimes arise by angulation and pressure from the inguinal ligament when the thighs are markedly flexed and abducted, as in the lithotomy position in anesthetized patients.

The saphenous nerve, the branch of the femoral nerve that supplies sensation to the medial aspect of the leg below the knee, may be damaged by pressure from leg braces when the patient is improperly suspended in the lithotomy position. The compressive injury leads to numbness and paresthesias that are usually fairly short-lived.

Sciatic or common peroneal nerve palsies are easy to confuse with a plexus palsy because their constituent fibers are susceptible to compressive injury in the sacral plexus during labor. Misplaced deep intramuscular injections are probably still the most common cause of sciatic nerve palsy. The sciatic nerve may also be injured by stretching when a patient is positioned in stirrups on the obstetric table. To avoid this injury, the knee and hip joints should be well flexed, and extreme external rotation of the hip should be avoided.

In patients with sciatic nerve palsy, the resulting weakness and sensory disturbance depend on whether the entire nerve has been affected or certain fibers are selectively involved. In general, the peroneal fibers of the sciatic nerve are much more likely to be damaged than fibers destined for the tibial nerve. The clinical features of a sciatic nerve lesion may simulate those of a peroneal neuropathy, although electromyographic evidence of involvement of the short head of the biceps femoris muscle favors the former. The common peroneal nerve is vulnerable to compression or direct trauma in the region of the head and neck of the fibula and may be injured at this site by pressure from the leg braces of the obstetric table, especially in anesthetized patients.[111] Weakness of dorsiflexion and eversion of the foot are accompanied by numbness or blunted sensation of the anterolateral aspect of the calf and the dorsum of the foot.

Bell Palsy

Sir Charles Bell first established the motor function of the seventh cranial nerve in the early 19th century. His name soon came to be associated with all forms of facial paralysis, but the designation of Bell palsy is now used for facial paresis of lower motor neuron type when no specific etiologic agent can be found. Some cases are probably caused by viral infection or an inflammatory reaction involving the facial nerve near the stylomastoid foramen or in the bony facial canal.

The incidence of Bell palsy is increased during pregnancy. The ideas of a relationship with hypertension or preeclampsia is supported by the study of Shmorgun and coworkers.[112]

The clinical features of Bell palsy are well known. The facial paresis usually is abrupt in onset, although it may worsen over the following day. Pain around the ear may precede or accompany the weakness in about half the cases but usually lasts for only a few days. The face itself feels stiff and pulled to one side. It may be difficult to close the eye on the affected side, and ipsilateral epiphora may occur. The patient may have difficulty with eating and with fine facial movements (e.g., when applying cosmetics). A disturbance of taste, caused by involvement of chorda tympani fibers, is common, and hyperacusis, caused by involvement of fibers to the stapedius, is occasionally troublesome.

Treatment is controversial. Most patients recover without treatment, and only about 10% of all patients are seriously dissatisfied with the final outcome because of permanent disfigurement or other long-term sequelae. Treatment is best reserved for patients in whom an unsatisfactory outcome can be predicted soon after onset. To be effective, treatment should commence within the first 5 or 6 days.

The best clinical guide to prognosis at an early stage is the severity of the palsy. Patients who have clinically complete palsy when they are first seen are less likely to recover fully than those with an incomplete palsy. Other clinical indicators for a poor prognosis for recovery include advancing age, hyperacusis, and severe initial pain.

The only medical treatment that may influence the outcome of Bell palsy is steroid therapy, although rigorously controlled trials have not always demonstrated benefit. Despite or because of the uncertainty about their effectiveness, many physicians routinely prescribe steroids to patients who are seen within 5 days of onset. Surgical procedures to decompress the facial nerve have not been beneficial.

Polyneuropathies

There were several early reports of the occasional occurrence of a polyneuropathy during pregnancy, but there does not appear to be any specific polyneuritis of pregnancy. Any type of polyneuropathy, such as that caused by diabetes mellitus, may develop during the gestational period. Discussion here is limited to those most likely to manifest clinically or to pose a management problem during pregnancy.

Nutritional Neuropathies

Nutritional deficiency may be the most probable cause of peripheral nerve involvement in patients who come from underdeveloped countries or have hyperemesis. Signs of peripheral nerve involvement may be found in patients with hyperemesis gravidarum who have Wernicke encephalopathy. In the limbs, numbness, paresthesias, and dysesthesias are accompanied by cutaneous sensory loss, depressed tendon reflexes, and distal weakness. Retrobulbar neuropathy may also occur, and tachycardia, postural hypotension, exertional dyspnea, and sphincter disturbances are sometimes conspicuous. The polyneuropathy is accompanied by ophthalmoplegia (e.g., horizontal and vertical nystagmus, impaired lateral gaze, conjugate gaze palsies), ataxia of gait, and a confusional state. The features of Korsakoff psychosis, which consists of impaired memory and an inability to acquire new information, sometimes accompanied by confabulation, may also be conjoined.

The diagnosis is confirmed by the finding of a marked reduction in blood transketolase activity and a marked thiamine pyrophosphate effect. Treatment consists of thiamine (50 mg), which is given once intravenously and then intramuscularly for several days until a satisfactory dietary intake is assured.

In other instances, a severe polyneuropathy may develop without an accompanying encephalopathy, presumably in relation to a nutritional deficiency, although the specific factors responsible for the peripheral nerve involvement are not known. Patients may complain about pain, paresthesias, and dysesthesias in the extremities; limb weakness; or ataxia. There may be accompanying cardiac involvement, with tachycardia, exertional dyspnea, and heart failure. Treatment consists of a balanced diet and supplements of vitamins, especially B vitamins. Vitamin B_{12} deficiency may lead to maternal polyneuropathy and other neurologic abnormalities and can affect the fetus and neonate.

Acute Idiopathic Polyneuropathy: Guillain-Barré Syndrome

An acute or subacute polyneuropathy that sometimes follows infective illnesses, inoculations, or surgical procedures but often occurs without any obvious preceding event characterizes acute idiopathic polyneuropathy. In many such instances, the neuropathy follows clinical or subclinical infection with *Campylobacter jejuni*. The disorder may have an immunologic basis, but the precise mechanism is unclear. It can pose an especially difficult management problem when it occurs during pregnancy.

The main complaint is of weakness that varies widely in severity in different patients, is often more marked proximally than distally, and is often symmetrical in distribution. It usually begins in the legs, frequently comes to involve the arms, and often affects one side or both sides of the face. Weakness may progress to total paralysis and may be life-threatening if the muscles of respiration or deglutition are involved. Sensory symptoms are common but are usually less conspicuous than motor symptoms. Autonomic dysfunction may manifest with tachycardia, cardiac irregularities, hypotension or hypertension, facial flushing, disturbances of sweating, disturbed pulmonary function, and other signs and symptoms.

Examination of the cerebrospinal fluid reveals characteristic changes; the protein content is significantly increased, but the cell content is normal. Measurement of motor and sensory conduction velocity in the peripheral nerves may reveal marked slowing, but the chronology of this reduction does not necessarily parallel that of the clinical disorder. In some patients, the conduction velocity remains normal, presumably because disease is restricted to the nerve roots or proximal segments of the nerves. Most patients eventually make a good recovery, but it may take many months, and some patients have persistent disability.

The Guillain-Barré syndrome does not occur more commonly during gestation than at other times, and the course of the disorder does not seem to be influenced by pregnancy. Improvement in neurologic status may occur before delivery and is not necessarily delayed until the infant is born.

Treatment is symptomatic, with attention directed at the prevention of complications, such as respiratory failure and vascular collapse. Plasmapheresis or treatment with intravenous immunoglobulins is helpful in patients with rapidly advancing or severe disease, but experience with such approaches is limited during pregnancy. Severely affected patients are best managed in intensive care units, where respiratory and circulatory function can be monitored and assisted respiration can be started as soon as is necessary. Ventilatory support may help to avert fetal hypoxia.[113] Ultrasonographic fetal monitoring generally reveals normal fetal movements even when the mother is severely paralyzed.[114]

Approximately 3% of patients with acute idiopathic polyneuropathy have one or more relapses, sometimes several years after the initial illness. Such relapses, which are clinically similar to the original illness, occasionally occur during pregnancy.

Porphyric Neuropathy

In the hepatic forms of porphyria, the central and peripheral nervous systems may be affected. Acute intermittent porphyria, inherited as an autosomal recessive trait, is characterized by increased production and urinary excretion of porphobilinogen and δ-aminolevulinic acid. Colicky abdominal pain is often the most conspicuous symptom, but the usual neurologic manifestation is a polyneuropathy that is predominantly motor but sometimes occurs with pronounced autonomic involvement, which may take weeks or months to regress, depending on its severity. Cerebral manifestations may also occur, often preceding the development of a severe polyneuropathy and similarly clearing after a variable time. Clinical indicators of disease activity include tachycardia, fever, and a peripheral leukocytosis. In variegate porphyria, cutaneous sensitivity to sunlight is an additional clinical feature.

Attacks may be precipitated by pharmacologic agents such as barbiturates, sulfonamides, and estrogens. Some women have found that relapses are most likely to occur premenstrually; long-term combination oral contraceptives may prevent attacks in these patients.[115] In other patients, oral contraceptives may precipitate exacerbations, and this form of contraception is probably best avoided in women with a blood relative who has a hepatic type of porphyria.[116]

Pregnancy may lead to an acute exacerbation and may even have a fatal outcome, but many patients tolerate attacks without apparent ill effect. When relapses occur, they usually do so in early pregnancy and may lead to spontaneous abortion.[116] However, exacerbations may occur at any time during pregnancy or after delivery. The implications and uncertain outcome must be explained to patients who are contemplating pregnancy, and close supervision should be provided during the gestational period. Latent cases may be exacerbated by medication used during or after labor, and particular care must be exercised in this regard. In general, if the pregnancy proceeds satisfactorily, a healthy infant can be anticipated.

Myasthenia Gravis

Variable weakness and fatigability of skeletal muscles, resulting from defective neuromuscular transmission, are the clinical hallmarks of myasthenia gravis. The disorder has an autoimmune basis. It is characterized by a reduced number of available acetylcholine receptors at the neuromuscular junctions. Myasthenia gravis is more common in females. In some patients, the external ocular muscles or levator palpebrae are especially affected; in others, the facial and bulbar muscles are selectively involved; and in other patients, the limb muscles, especially the proximal ones, are predominantly affected. Weakness may remain localized to a few muscle groups or may become generalized, and it can be a life-threatening disorder if the muscles of respiration or deglutition are involved.

Patients are particularly sensitive to even small doses of neuromuscular-blocking agents, such as tubocurarine, but improvement results from treatment with acetylcholinesterase inhibitors. Thymectomy often leads to a remission of symptoms, and myasthenia gravis may be associated with thymoma. Repetitive supramaximal electrical stimulation of motor nerves may lead to an abnormal decline in size of the evoked muscle action potentials. This finding is sometimes of diagnostic help, as is the finding of elevated levels of circulating acetylcholine receptor antibodies or antibodies to muscle-specific kinase and the clinical response to edrophonium or neostigmine. In addition to thymectomy in appropriate cases, treatment may involve the use of anticholinesterases, steroids, intravenous immunoglobulins, and plasmapheresis.

Exacerbations of myasthenia gravis sometimes occur shortly before the onset of the menstrual period and tend to improve after menstruation has begun. This association may disappear after thymectomy.

Myasthenia gravis may first appear during or shortly after pregnancy, but it is difficult to predict the influence of pregnancy on a patient with the disorder. Moreover, the effect of pregnancy may vary on different occasions, so that the outcome in individual cases cannot be predicted on this basis. Relapses can occur in early pregnancy, with partial or complete remission often occurring at a later stage. Batocchi and associates[117] found during pregnancy that myasthenia relapsed in 17% of asymptomatic patients who were not on treatment before conception; among patients on therapy, symptoms improved in 39% of pregnancies, were unchanged in 42%, and worsened in 19%. Further, myasthenic symptoms worsened after delivery in 28% of pregnancies. It may be tempting to terminate a pregnancy because of the severity of myasthenic symptoms—death has been reported in pregnancy complicated by myasthenia gravis—and because of the difficulties in their treatment, but termination does not necessarily lead to clinical benefit. Myasthenia gravis should be managed in pregnant patients as it is in nonpregnant patients.

Myasthenia gravis has little effect on the pregnancy itself. Moreover, there may be a marked contrast during labor between the strength of uterine contractions in the second stage and the skeletal muscle weakness exhibited by the patient. If the expulsive phase of labor is prolonged, instrumental assistance may help to avoid maternal exhaustion. Cesarean section should be reserved for patients in whom it is indicated on obstetric grounds. Regional analgesia is preferable to general anesthesia, and the use of muscle relaxant drugs is avoided if possible. Similarly, the use of magnesium sulfate for eclampsia should be avoided because it may precipitate myasthenic crisis. No differences were found in perinatal mortality, gestational age, or birth weight between the offspring of myasthenic and nonmyasthenic women in a population-based cohort study.[118]

Infants born to myasthenic patients should be carefully watched during the week after delivery for signs of neonatal myasthenia. Such signs include a poor cry, respiratory difficulties, weakness in sucking, a weak Moro reflex, and feeble limb movements, usually becoming apparent within the first 72 hours of birth. Symptoms are usually not evident immediately after birth, and this delay has been attributed to protection of the infant by placental transfer of maternal anticholinesterase drugs.

Neonatal myasthenia is a transient disorder that results from placental transfer of maternal antibody against acetylcholine receptors. It occurs in 10% to 15% of infants born to myasthenic mothers and does not seem to be related to the duration or severity of maternal illness, although disease in mothers of myasthenic newborns is usually generalized rather than localized. It can be treated with anticholinesterase drugs and usually subsides within 6 weeks of delivery, but it may result in death caused by aspiration or respiratory failure. Facilities should be available for the immediate resuscitation of affected infants or those at risk of being affected. Immunosuppressive therapy is sometimes required. Maternal myasthenia has also been incriminated as a rare cause of congenital arthrogryposis.[119]

The birth of a child with neonatal myasthenia does not necessarily imply that future children will also have the disorder, although they often do. The transient neonatal disorder that may occur in the offspring of a myasthenic mother must not be confused with congenital myasthenia gravis. The latter is rare, occurs in children born of healthy mothers, and is usually permanent.

Disorders of Muscle

Myotonic Dystrophy

Myotonic dystrophy type 1 is a slowly progressive, dominantly inherited disorder that usually appears in early adult life but may manifest in childhood. It has been related to an expanded trinucleotide repeat in a gene localized to 19cen-q13.2. Increasing numbers of triplet repeat expansions govern clinical expression of disease; prenatal detection of the disorder is possible.[120,121] Myotonia is accompanied by weakness of the facial, sternomastoid, and distal limb muscles. Associated features may include cataracts, frontal baldness, cardiac and endocrine disturbances, and intellectual changes. During pregnancy, the weakness and myotonia may be aggravated, and the course of the disorder is sometimes accelerated. When deterioration does occur, it often begins at about the sixth or seventh month of pregnancy.

In the antepartum period, the major reported obstetric complications of myotonic dystrophy include threatened, spontaneous, and habitual abortion. Hydramnios is well described. Ectopic pregnancy and placenta praevia may occur, and perinatal loss is increased.[122] Premature onset of labor in patients with myotonic dystrophy has been attributed in some instances to abnormalities of uterine muscle. Labor may be abnormal because of failure of the uterus to contract normally. The first stage may be prolonged, and retention of the placenta and postpartum hemorrhage may occur. Manual removal of the placenta is sometimes necessary. Skeletal muscle weakness may also lead to poor voluntary assistance in the second stage.

Type 2 myotonic dystrophy (CCTG expansion involving the *ZNF9* gene) may first manifest during pregnancy, with worsening occurring in subsequent pregnancies for uncertain reasons; improvement often follows delivery.[122] Preterm labor is more likely in women who developed initial manifestations or a deterioration of the disorder during pregnancy compared with those in whom pregnancy did not appear to influence the disease course, but obstetric risk is not increased.[122]

Myotonic dystrophy type 1 may manifest in infancy, occurring congenitally among the offspring of mothers who have the disorder, sometimes only mildly. In such cases, it is often possible to obtain a history of hydramnios or reduced fetal movements during the latter part of pregnancy. Some affected infants die within hours or a few days of birth. The clinical features in affected infants include facial diplegia, hypotonia, neonatal respiratory distress, feeding difficulties, delayed motor development, and mental retardation.[123] Myotonia, a cardinal feature of the adult disease, is absent in the congenital form. The neonatal respiratory distress may result from involvement of the respiratory muscles, pulmonary immaturity, aspiration pneumonia, and impaired neural control of respiration. Talipes is present at birth in about one half of all cases and may require surgical correction. Myotonic dystrophy type 2 has not been described in congenital form.

Familial studies have indicated that in almost every case of congenital myotonic dystrophy, transmission occurred from the mother. This type of transmission does not fit with an autosomal dominant pattern of inheritance. Genetic data suggest that the congenital form results from the combination of the gene responsible for the disorder in adults and some maternally transmitted factor, the nature of which is unclear. Others have suggested that the maternal transmission of the congenital form is associated with relative male infertility.

The management of patients requiring anesthesia for obstetric or other reasons merits comment. Depolarizing muscle relaxant drugs should be avoided because they may cause myotonic spasm, and nondepolarizing agents, such as tubocurarine, can be used but should be given in reduced dosage to patients receiving quinine for myotonia. Thiopental sodium (Pentothal) may lead to marked respiratory depression and is best avoided, as are other respiratory-depressant drugs, especially if the patient already has impaired respiratory function. Electrocardiographic monitoring permits the early recognition of any cardiac arrhythmias, to which patients with myotonic dystrophy are prone. For these reasons, regional analgesia is the preferred method of management.

Myotonia Congenita

The dominant form of myotonia congenita, Thomsen disease, is usually present from birth, although symptoms may not appear until early childhood. Patients complain of muscle stiffness (i.e., myotonia) that is enhanced by cold or inactivity and is relieved by exercise; power is full, but the muscles may be diffusely hypertrophied. Pregnancy may aggravate the myotonia, especially in the latter half of the gestational period, and improvement occurs after delivery.

Polymyositis

In polymyositis or dermatomyositis, which can occur at any age, there is weakness and wasting, especially of the proximal musculature, as a result of inflammatory infiltration of muscles and destruction of muscle fibers. The muscles are often painful and tender. There may be an association with malignancy or one of the collagen diseases. The erythrocyte sedimentation rate and serum creatine kinase levels are elevated. Histologic examination of a muscle biopsy specimen usually permits the diagnosis to be made with confidence so that treatment with steroids can be instituted. Pregnancy has a variable effect on the muscle weakness, but a high perinatal mortality rate has been reported.[124]

Psychiatric Disorders

Pregnancy may occur during the course of established psychiatric illness, and psychiatric disorders may first develop during or shortly after pregnancy, although no specific disorders are associated with this period. In the evaluation of patients with psychiatric disorders, physicians must consider that pregnancy can have a number of different psychopathologic implications, depending on the patient's social, cultural, educational, emotional, and medical background. The attitude of a patient to pregnancy, especially with regard to whether it was desired, influences her psychological response, and her capacity to cope with pregnancy depends on her acceptance of it. If the pregnancy was planned, the factors that motivated it are of some relevance because the aim might have been to overcome marital disharmony or to keep up with peers. These aspects clearly govern the response of an individual patient to pregnancy. Chapter 53 discusses psychiatric disorders.

References

1. Janz D, Beck-Mannagetta G, Andermann E, et al: Guidelines for the care of epileptic women of childbearing age. Epilepsia 30:409, 1989.
2. Zupanc ML: Antiepileptic drugs and hormonal contraceptives in adolescent women with epilepsy. Neurology 66(Suppl 3):S37, 2006.
3. Quality Standards Subcommittee, American Academy of Neurology: Practice parameter: Management issues for women with epilepsy [summary statement]. Neurology 51:944, 1998.
4. Schmidt D, Canger R, Avanzini G, et al: Change of seizure frequency in pregnant epileptic women. J Neurol Neurosurg Psychiatry 46:751, 1983.
5. Yerby MS: Pregnancy and epilepsy. Epilepsia 32(Suppl 6):S51, 1991.
6. Tanganelli P, Regesta G: Epilepsy, pregnancy, and major birth anomalies: An Italian prospective, controlled study. Neurology 42(Suppl 5):89, 1992.
7. European Registry of Antiepileptic Drugs and Pregnancy (EURAP) Study Group: Seizure control and treatment in pregnancy. Observations from the EURAP Epilepsy Pregnancy Registry. Neurology 66:354, 2006.
8. Hiilesmaa VK: Pregnancy and birth in women with epilepsy. Neurology 42(Suppl 5):8, 1992.
9. Teramo K, Hiilesmaa V, Bardy A, et al: Fetal heart rate during a maternal grand mal epileptic seizure. J Perinat Med 7:3, 1979.
10. Jones KL, Lacro RV, Johnson KA, et al: Pattern of malformations in the children of women treated with carbamazepine during pregnancy. N Engl J Med 320:1661, 1989.
11. Rosa FW: Spina bifida in infants of women treated with carbamazepine during pregnancy. N Engl J Med 324:674, 1991.
12. Bjerkedal T, Czeizel A, Goujard J, et al: Valproic acid and spina bifida. Lancet 2:1096, 1982.
13. Robert E, Guibaud P: Maternal valproic acid and congenital neural tube defects. Lancet 2:937, 1982.
14. Alsdorf R, Wyszynski DF: Teratogenicity of sodium valproate. Expert Opin Drug Saf 4:345, 2005.
15. Wyszynski DF, Nambisan M, Surve T, et al: Increased rate of major malformations in offspring exposed to valproate during pregnancy. Neurology 64:961, 2005.
16. Perucca E: Birth defects after prenatal exposure to antiepileptic drugs. Lancet Neurol 4:781, 2005.
17. Dansky LV, Rosenblatt DS, Andermann E: Mechanisms of teratogenesis: Folic acid and antiepileptic therapy. Neurology 42(Suppl 5):32, 1992.
18. Dean JC, Hailey H, Moore SJ, et al: Long term health and neurodevelopment in children exposed to antiepileptic drugs before birth. J Med Genet 39:251, 2002.
19. Meador KJ: Neurodevelopmental effects of antiepileptic drugs. Curr Neurol Neurosci Rep 2:373, 2002.
20. DiLiberti JH, Farndon PA, Dennis NR, et al: The fetal valproate syndrome. Am J Med Genet 19:473, 1984.
21. Kini U, Adab N, Vinten J, et al: Dysmorphic features: An important clue to the diagnosis and severity of fetal anticonvulsant syndromes. Arch Dis Child Fetal Neonatal Ed 91:F90, 2006.
22. Deblay MF, Vert P, Andreá M, et al: Transplacental vitamin K prevents haemorrhagic disease of infant of epileptic mother [letter]. Lancet 1:1247, 1982.
23. Hey E: Effect of maternal anticonvulsant treatment on neonatal blood coagulation. Arch Dis Child Fetal Neonatal Ed 81:F208, 1999.
24. Choulika S, Grabowski E, Holmes LB: Is antenatal vitamin K prophylaxis needed for pregnant women taking anticonvulsants? Am J Obstet Gynecol 190:882, 2004.
25. Bruno MK, Harden CL: Epilepsy in pregnant women. Curr Treat Options Neurol 4:31, 2002.
26. Silberstein SD: Headache and female hormones: What you need to know. Curr Opin Neurol 14:323, 2001.
27. Martin VT, Behbehani M: Ovarian hormones and migraine headache: Understanding mechanisms and pathogenesis: Part 2. Headache 46:365, 2006.
28. Raskin NH: Headache, 2nd ed. New York, Churchill Livingstone, 1988.
29. Collaborative Group for the Study of Stroke in Young Women: Oral contraceptives and stroke in young women: Associated risk factors. JAMA 231:718, 1975.
30. Irey NS, McAllister HA, Henry JM: Oral contraceptives and stroke in young women: A clinicopathologic correlation. Neurology 28:1216, 1978.
31. Ratinahirana H, Darbois Y, Bousser MG: Migraine and pregnancy: A prospective study in 703 women after delivery. Neurology 40(Suppl 1):437, 1990.
32. Hertzog AG: Continuous bromocriptine therapy in menstrual migraine. Neurology 48:101, 1997.
33. Niederhoff H, Zahrodnik HP: Analgesics during pregnancy. Am J Med 75(Suppl):117, 1983.
34. Sawle GV, Ramsay MM: The neurology of pregnancy. J Neurol Neurosurg Psychiatry 64:711, 1998.
35. Evans RW, Lipton RB: Topics in migraine management: A survey of headache specialists highlights some controversies. Neurol Clin 19:1, 2001.
36. Welch KMA: Migraine and pregnancy. In Devinsky O, Feldmann E, Hainline B (eds): Neurological Complications of Pregnancy. New York, Raven Press, 1994, p 77.
37. Schoenfeld N, Epstein O, Nemesh L, et al: Effects of propranolol during pregnancy and development of rats. 1. Adverse effects during pregnancy. Pediatr Res 12:747, 1978.
38. Rosen TS, Lin M, Spector S, et al: Maternal, fetal, and neonatal effects of chronic propranolol administration in the rat. J Pharmacol Exp Ther 208:118, 1979.
39. Ueland K, McAnulty JH, Ueland FR, et al: Special considerations in the use of cardiovascular drugs. Clin Obstet Gynecol 24:809, 1981.
40. Jackson CD, Fishbein L: A toxicological review of beta-adrenergic blockers. Fundam Appl Toxicol 6:395, 1986.
41. Bánhidy F, Acs N, Horváth-Púho E, et al: Pregnancy complications and delivery outcomes in pregnant women with severe migraine. Eur J Obstet Gynecol Reprod Biol 134:157, 2007.
42. Beni-Adani L, Pomeranz S, Flores I, et al: Huge acoustic neurinomas presenting in the late stage of pregnancy. Treatment options and review of literature. Acta Obstet Gynecol Scand 80:179, 2001.
43. Kachhara R, Devi CG, Nair S, et al: Acoustic neurinomas during pregnancy: Report of two cases and review of the literature. Acta Neurochir 143:587, 2001.
44. Erdogan B, Sen O, Aydin MV, et al: Cerebellar hemangioblastoma in pregnancy. A case report. J Reprod Med 47:864, 2002.
45. Razak AR, Nasser Q, Morris P, et al: Medulloblastoma in two successive pregnancies. J Neurooncol 73:89, 2005.
46. Schipper HM: Sex hormones and the nervous system. In Aminoff MJ (ed): Neurology and General Medicine, 3rd ed. New York, Churchill Livingstone, 2001, p 365.
47. DeAngelis LM: Central nervous system neoplasms in pregnancy. In Devinsky O, Feldmann E, Hainline B (eds): Neurological Complications of Pregnancy. New York, Raven Press, 1994, p 139.
48. Kal HB, Struikmans H: Radiotherapy during pregnancy: Fact and fiction. Lancet Oncol 6:328, 2005.
49. Weed JC, Hunter VJ: Diagnosis and management of brain metastasis from gestational trophoblastic disease. Oncology 5:48, 1991.
50. Gumma AD: Recurrent benign intracranial hypertension in pregnancy. Eur J Obstet Gynecol Reprod Biol 115:244, 2004.
51. Wiebers DO: Ischemic cerebrovascular complications of pregnancy. Arch Neurol 42:1106, 1985.
52. Salonen Ros H, Lichtenstein P, Bellocco R, et al: Increased risk of circulatory diseases in late pregnancy and puerperium. Epidemiology 12:456, 2001.
53. Jaigobin C, Silver FL: Stroke and pregnancy. Stroke 31:2948, 2000.
54. Tuffnell DJ: Amniotic fluid embolism. Curr Opin Obstet Gynecol 15:119, 2003.

55. Singhal AB: Cerebral vasoconstriction syndromes. Top Stroke Rehabil 11:1, 2004.
56. Confavreux C, Brunet P, Petiot P, et al: Congenital protein C deficiency and superior sagittal sinus thrombosis causing isolated intracranial hypertension. J Neurol Neurosurg Psychiatry 57:655, 1994.
57. Markus HS, Hambley H: Neurology and the blood: Haematological abnormalities in ischaemic stroke. J Neurol Neurosurg Psychiatry 64:150, 1998.
58. Deschiens MA, Conard J, Horellou MH, et al: Coagulation studies, factor V Leiden, and anticardiolipin antibodies in 40 cases of cerebral venous thrombosis. Stroke 27:1724, 1996.
59. Weih M, Vetter B, Ziemer S, et al: Increased rate of factor V Leiden mutation in patients with cerebral venous thrombosis. J Neurol 245:149, 1998.
60. Appenzeller S, Zeller CB, Annichino-Bizzachi JM, et al: Cerebral venous thrombosis: Influence of risk factors and imaging findings on prognosis. Clin Neurol Neurosurg 107:371, 2005.
61. Gettelfinger DM, Kokmen E: Superior sagittal sinus thrombosis. Arch Neurol 34:2, 1977.
62. Einhaupl KM, Villringer A, Meister W, et al: Heparin treatment in sinus venous thrombosis. Lancet 338:597, 1991.
63. Dulli DA, Luzzio CC, Williams EC, et al: Cerebral venous thrombosis and activated protein C resistance. Stroke 27:1731, 1996.
64. Martinelli I, Landi G, Merati G, et al: Factor V gene mutation is a risk factor for cerebral venous thrombosis. Thromb Haemost 75:393, 1996.
65. Pugliese D, Nicoletti G, Andreula C, et al: Combined protein C deficiency and protein C activated resistance as a cause of caval, peripheral, and cerebral venous thrombosis. Angiology 49:399, 1998.
66. Bloemenkamp KW, Rosendaal FR, Helmerhorst FM, et al: Enhancement by factor V Leiden mutation of risk of deep-vein thrombosis associated with oral contraceptives containing a third-generation progestagen. Lancet 346:1593, 1995.
67. Mhurchu CN, Anderson C, Jamrozik K, et al: Hormonal factors and risk of aneurysmal subarachnoid hemorrhage: An international population-based, case-control study. Stroke 32:606, 2001.
68. Okamoto K, Horisawa R, Kawamura T, et al: Menstrual and reproductive factors for subarachnoid hemorrhage risk in women: A case-control study in Nagoya, Japan. Stroke 32:2841, 2001.
69. Robinson JL, Hall CS, Sedzimir CB: Arteriovenous malformations, aneurysms, and pregnancy. J Neurosurg 41:63, 1974.
70. Parkinson D, Bachers G: Arteriovenous malformations: Summary of 100 consecutive supratentorial cases. J Neurosurg 53:285, 1980.
71. Horton JC, Chambers WA, Lyons SL, et al: Pregnancy and the risk of hemorrhage from cerebral arteriovenous malformations. Neurosurgery 27:867, 1990.
72. Sadasivan B, Malik GM, Lee C, et al: Vascular malformations and pregnancy. Surg Neurol 33:305, 1990.
73. Stoodley MA, Macdonald RL, Weir BK: Pregnancy and intracranial aneurysms. Neurosurg Clin North Am 9:549, 1998.
74. Piotin M, de Souza Filho CB, Kothimbakam R, et al: Endovascular treatment of acutely ruptured intracranial aneurysms in pregnancy. Am J Obstet Gynecol 185:1261, 2001.
75. Aminoff MJ: Spinal vascular disease. In Critchley EMR, Eisen A (eds): Diseases of the Spinal Cord, 2nd ed. London, Springer, 1997, p 423.
76. Harjulehto-Mervaala T, Aro T, Hiilesmaa VK, et al: Oral polio vaccination during pregnancy: Lack of impact on fetal development and perinatal outcome. Clin Infect Dis 18:414, 1994.
77. Demicheli V, Barale A, Rivetti A: Vaccines for women to prevent neonatal tetanus. Cochrane Database Syst Rev (4):CD002959, 2005.
78. Axelsson I: A Cochrane review on the umbilical cord care and prevention of infections. Lakartidningen 99:1563, 2002.
79. Frey TK: Neurological aspects of rubella virus infection. Intervirology 40:167, 1997.
80. Cooper ER, Charurat M, Mofenson L, et al: Combination antiretroviral strategies for the treatment of pregnant HIV-1-infected women and prevention of perinatal HIV-1 transmission. J Acquir Immune Defic Syndr 29:484, 2002.
81. Tuomala RE, Shapiro DE, Mofenson LM, et al: Antiretroviral therapy during pregnancy and the risk of an adverse outcome. N Engl J Med 346:1842, 2002.
82. Capparelli E, Rakhmanina N, Mirochnick M: Pharmacotherapy of perinatal HIV. Semin Fetal Neonatal Med 10:161, 2005.
83. Jacqz-Aigrain E, Koren G: Effects of drugs on the fetus. Semin Fetal Neonatal Med 10:139, 2005.
84. Fowler MG, Simonds RJ, Roongpisuthipong A: Update on perinatal HIV transmission. Pediatr Clin North Am 47:21, 2000.
85. Mofenson LM, McIntyre JA: Advances and research directions in the prevention of mother-to-child HIV-1 transmission. Lancet 355:2237, 2000.
86. Koch R, Friedman E, Azen C, et al: The International Collaborative Study of Maternal Phenylketonuria: Status report 1998. Eur J Pediatr 159(Suppl 2):S156, 2000.
87. Clarke JT: The Maternal Phenylketonuria Project: A summary of progress and challenges for the future. Pediatrics 112:1584, 2003.
88. Waisbren SE, Azen C: Cognitive and behavioral development in maternal phenylketonuria offspring. Pediatrics 112:1544, 2003.
89. Feillet F, Abadie V, Berthelot J, et al: Maternal phenylketonuria: The French survey. Eur J Pediatr 163:540, 2004.
90. Lee PJ, Ridout D, Walter JH, et al: Maternal phenylketonuria: Report from the United Kingdom Registry 1978-97. Arch Dis Child 90:143, 2005.
91. Goodman JDS, Brodie C, Ayida GA: Restless leg syndrome in pregnancy. BMJ 297:1101, 1988.
92. Pellecchia MT, Criscuolo C, Longo K, et al: Clinical presentation and treatment of Wilson's disease: A single-centre experience. Eur Neurol 50:48, 2003.
93. Sinha S, Taly AB, Prashanth LK, et al: Successful pregnancies and abortions in symptomatic and asymptomatic Wilson's disease. J Neurol Sci 217:37, 2004.
94. Hartard C, Kunze K: Pregnancy in a patient with Wilson's disease treated with D-penicillamine and zinc sulfate. Eur Neurol 34:337, 1994.
95. Furman B, Bashiri A, Wiznitzer A, et al: Wilson's disease in pregnancy: Five successful consecutive pregnancies of the same woman. Eur J Obstet Gynaecol Reprod Biol 96:232, 2001.
96. Korn-Lubetzki I, Kahana E, Cooper G, et al: Activity of multiple sclerosis during pregnancy and puerperium. Ann Neurol 16:229, 1984.
97. Birk K, Rudick R: Pregnancy and multiple sclerosis. Arch Neurol 43:719, 1986.
98. Abramsky O: Pregnancy and multiple sclerosis. Ann Neurol 36(Suppl):38, 1994.
99. Thompson DS, Nelson LM, Burns A, et al: The effects of pregnancy in multiple sclerosis: A retrospective study. Neurology 36:1097, 1986.
100. Weinshenker BG, Hader W, Carriere W, et al: The influence of pregnancy on disability from multiple sclerosis: A population-based study in Middlesex County, Ontario. Neurology 39:1438, 1989.
101. Sadovnick AD, Eisen K, Hashimoto SA, et al: Pregnancy and multiple sclerosis: A prospective study. Arch Neurol 51:1120, 1994.
102. Poser S, Poser W: Multiple sclerosis and gestation. Neurology 33:1422, 1983.
103. Dahl J, Myhr KM, Daltveit AK, et al: Pregnancy, delivery, and birth outcome in women with multiple sclerosis. Neurology 65:1961, 2005.
104. Boskovic R, Wide R, Wolpin J, et al: The reproductive effects of beta interferon therapy in pregnancy: A longitudinal cohort. Neurology 65:807, 2005.
105. Retzloff MG, Kobylarz EJ, Eaton C: Optic neuritis with transient total blindness during lactation. Obstet Gynecol 98:902, 2001.
106. Aminoff MJ: Electromyography in Clinical Practice, 3rd ed. New York, Churchill Livingstone, 1998.
107. Taylor RA: Heredofamilial mononeuritis multiplex with brachial predilection. Brain 83:113, 1960.
108. Sax TW, Rosenbaum RB: Neuromuscular disorders in pregnancy. Muscle Nerve 34:559, 2006.
109. Finsen V, Zeitlmann H: Carpal tunnel syndrome during pregnancy. Scand J Plast Reconstr Surg Hand Surg 40:41, 2006.
110. Nogajski JH, Shnier RC, Zagami AS: Postpartum obturator neuropathy. Neurology 63:2450, 2004.

111. Mabie WC: Peripheral neuropathies during pregnancy. Clin Obstet Gynecol 48:57, 2005.
112. Shmorgun D, Chan WS, Ray JG: Association between Bell's palsy in pregnancy and pre-eclampsia. QJM 95:359, 2002.
113. Gauthier PE, Hantson P, Vekemans MC, et al: Intensive care management of Guillain-Barré syndrome during pregnancy. Intensive Care Med 16:460, 1990.
114. Nelson LH, McLean WT: Management of Landry-Guillain-Barré syndrome in pregnancy. Obstet Gynecol 65(Suppl):25S, 1985.
115. Perlroth MG, Marver HS, Tschudy DP: Oral contraceptive agents and the management of acute intermittent porphyria. JAMA 194:1037, 1965.
116. Donaldson JO: Neurology of Pregnancy. Philadelphia, Saunders, 1978.
117. Batocchi AP, Majolini L, Evoli A, et al: Course and treatment of myasthenia gravis during pregnancy. Neurology 52:447, 1999.
118. Hoff JM, Daltveit AK, Gilhus NE: Myasthenia gravis: consequences for pregnancy, delivery, and the newborn. Neurology 61:1362, 2003.
119. Polizzi A, Huson SM, Vincent A: Teratogen update: Maternal myasthenia gravis as a cause of congenital arthrogryposis. Teratology 62:332, 2000.
120. Redman JB, Fenwick RG, Fu YH, et al: Relationship between parental trinucleotide CGT repeat length and severity of myotonic dystrophy in offspring. JAMA 269:1960, 1993.
121. Shelbourne P, Davies J, Buxton J, et al: Direct diagnosis of myotonic dystrophy with a disease-specific DNA marker. N Engl J Med 328:471, 1993.
122. Rudnik-Schoneborn S, Zerres K: Outcome in pregnancies complicated by myotonic dystrophy: A study of 31 patients and review of the literature. Eur J Obstet Gynecol Reprod Biol 114:44, 2004.
123. Harper PS: Myotonic Dystrophy, 2nd ed. Philadelphia, WB Saunders, 1989.
124. Tsai A, Lindheimer MD, Lamberg SI: Dermatomyositis complicating pregnancy. Obstet Gynecol 41:570, 1973.

Chapter 53

Management of Depression and Psychoses in Pregnancy and the Puerperium

Kimberly A. Yonkers, MD

Epidemiology

Approximately one in five women will experience an episode of major depressive disorder over the course of her lifetime. Chronic psychotic disorders are less common but occur in about 1% of women. The risk of developing any type of depressive disorder, bipolar disorder, or a chronic psychotic disorder such as schizoaffective disorder or schizophrenia peaks when women are in their early 20s.[1]

The risk of relapse for a woman with bipolar disorder is increased during the postpartum period compared with a nonpregnant woman,[2,3] but it is less clear whether the postpartum period confers increased risk for a woman with unipolar depression. Pregnancy does not protect against the development of an episode of depression[4,5] or mania,[2] making it likely that pregnant patients with these conditions will need behavioral and pharmacologic treatment.

The risk of developing a unipolar mood disorder, such as major or minor depressive disorder, is increased during the third trimester in some reports,[6,7] but meta-analyses did not find significant differences in risk across pregnancy.[4,8] The risk may increase in later pregnancy because some women discontinue psychopharmacologic treatment when they become pregnant, which increases the likelihood of relapse at a later point in the pregnancy.[5] Women with schizophrenia and schizoaffective disorder have chronic conditions with symptoms that are kept under control under optimal conditions because they are taking antipsychotic medication or mood-stabilizing drugs. Unipolar depression and bipolar disorder are characterized by recurrent episodes of illness that may last several weeks to several months.[9] A lack of symptoms during one trimester does not indicate that a woman with one of these illnesses will remain well throughout her pregnancy.

Whether the postpartum time, compared with pregnancy, constitutes a period of increased risk for a depressive disorder is debated. Although some reports find no increase in depressive symptoms in the puerperium compared with pregnancy,[6] others find that psychotic depression[10] and severe episodes of depression[11] increase after delivery and that women seek treatment more often after delivery than during pregnancy.[12]

Diagnostic Nomenclature for Depressive and Psychotic Disorders

Several features of the various mood and psychotic disorders overlap, but there are specific elements. They are briefly described here because they directly relate to how mood and psychotic disorders are managed clinically (Tables 53-1 and 53-2).

A depressive episode includes symptoms of low mood and diminished capacity to experience pleasure. The condition can occur in pregnant or postpartum women who suffer from a unipolar depressive disorder (e.g., major depressive disorder, minor depressive disorder, dysthymic disorder), bipolar disorder, or schizoaffective disorder. If a woman also experiences episodes of mania or hypomania (see Table 53-2), she has bipolar disorder or schizoaffective disorder, not unipolar depression. Psychotic symptoms such as auditory hallucinations or delusions can also occur in women who have unipolar depression, bipolar disorder, or schizoaffective disorder. However, if a woman is psychotic and is not having an episode of mania or depression, she has schizoaffective disorder. This diagnosis is appropriate because she has psychosis in the absence of mood symptoms. Mood symptoms can occur among women with schizophrenia, but they are not a cardinal feature of that disorder. Psychosis is chronic and central to a diagnosis of schizophrenia and schizoaffective disorder.

Identifying Psychiatric Illness during Pregnancy and the Puerperium

The typical age of onset for schizophrenia and bipolar disorder is in the late teens to early 20s. Many women with these conditions have been diagnosed previously and are usually able to provide this information and describe their lifetime treatment. The first onset of

TABLE 53-1 SYMPTOMS OF DEPRESSION, MANIA, AND PSYCHOSIS

Criteria*	Depressive Episode	Manic Episode	Psychosis
Sad, blue, depressed mood	Yes		
Persistently elevated, expansive, or irritable mood		Yes	
Decreased interest in pleasurable activities	Yes		
Increased interest in pleasurable activities likely to lead to painful consequences (e.g., shopping sprees, sexual indiscretions)		Yes	
Decreased or increased appetite or weight	Yes		
Undersleeping	Yes	Yes	
Oversleeping	Yes		
Physical or mental slowing (includes catatonia)	Yes		Yes
Agitation	Yes (fidgety, cannot relax)	Yes (increase in goal related activities)	Yes (purposeless movements)
More talkative than usual (e.g., excessive, pressured speech)		Yes	
Racing thoughts		Yes	
Decreased energy	Yes		
Increased energy		Yes	
Worthlessness, guilt	Yes		
Grandiose, inflated self-esteem		Yes	
Poor concentration, indecision, distractibility	Yes (unfocused, difficulty concentrating, difficulty making decisions))	Yes (key feature: extremely distractible by irrelevant external stimuli)	Yes (includes incoherence, disorganized speech)
Suicide ideation, intent, or plan	Yes	Yes	
Delusions			Yes
Hallucinations			Yes
Disorganized behavior			Yes
Flat affect, "no emotion"			Yes

***These items comprise criteria for the diagnosis. Patients with any of these diagnoses may have one or more of these symptoms, even if the item is not part of the diagnosis. A depressive episode requires ≧5 symptoms, including low mood or diminished pleasure, persisting for 2 weeks. Mania requires ≧3 symptoms for at least 1 week. Schizophrenia requires 2 symptoms for 4 weeks.**

bipolar disorder may occur during the puerperium, and a woman who develops symptoms listed in Table 53-1 should immediately be evaluated by a psychiatrist. Women with major and minor depressive disorders are somewhat more difficult to identify because they may or may not have had an episode before pregnancy. During pregnancy, they may remit and relapse. Depression screening scales can be helpful in identifying women who are symptomatic. However, the benefits of screening are realized only if practitioners have the skills and resources available to deliver adequate interventions or provide appropriate referrals.

Well-validated screening instruments measure general distress and dysphoria and are often less specific for depression. Appropriate tools for pregnant women include the Edinburgh Postnatal Depression Scale (EPDS),[13] Inventory of Depressive Symptomatology (IDS),[13] or Primary Care Evaluation of Mental Disorders (PRIME-MD) depression module.[14] The EPDS is designed specifically for use with perinatal women, although it is less comprehensive than the IDS and does not include all of the criteria for major depressive disorder. The EPDS has 10 items and a mood and anxiety subscale. The IDS measures severity of cognitive features of depression and anxiety and atypical depressive symptoms, such as overeating and oversleeping (rather than undersleeping and undereating); it has a self-report and clinician administered version, as well as a brief version. The PRIME-MD records diagnoses of major depressive disorder and minor depressive disorder and has been used in obstetric-gynecologic settings; it takes 5 to 20 minutes to complete.

Management

Impact of Mood and Psychotic Disorders on Pregnancy Outcomes

Developing a treatment plan for a pregnant or postpartum woman necessitates considering the risks of the underlying illness and risks associated with the various treatment options. Women with an untreated mood or psychotic disorder face a number of risks. These illnesses can lead to poor self-care, partial or total disability that can impair the care of others, and in the worst scenario, suicide or homicide because of psychotic thoughts. Compared with women without a mood or psychotic disorder, those with such conditions are more likely to smoke, use hazardous substances (i.e., alcohol or illicit drugs), and have a concurrent medical condition, and they are less likely to receive adequate prenatal care.[15-18] The review that follows addresses the risk of standard obstetric outcomes, including spontaneous abortion, preterm delivery, growth restriction, and congenital malformations, but it does not address the maternal morbidity occurring because of a psychiatric illness, for which there are few systematic data.

Schizophrenia

Information on the possible impact of schizophrenia on birth outcomes and other post-neonatal complications largely derives from linked administrative databases[19-22] that allow investigators to obtain

TABLE 53-2 DEPRESSIVE AND PSYCHOTIC DISORDERS

Psychiatric Disorder	Depressive Episodes?*	Manic Episodes?†	Psychotic Symptoms?‡	Lifetime Prevalence	Typical Treatment Needed
Major depressive disorder	Yes, central feature of the condition	No	Can have a psychotic variant	21%	Antidepressant or psychotherapy; antipsychotic needed for psychotic features
Minor depressive disorder	Yes, central feature of the condition	No	Does not typically have a psychotic variant		Psychotherapy often sufficient in pregnancy, but antidepressant may be useful after delivery
Dysthymic disorder	Yes, chronic	No	Does not typically have a psychotic variant		Psychotherapy often sufficient in pregnancy, but antidepressant may be useful after delivery
Bipolar disorder	Yes, may have depressive episodes or episodes with mixed depressive and manic symptoms	Yes, may have manic or hypomanic episodes; depressive and manic symptoms can coexist	Psychotic symptoms commonly occur but only when the patient is in episode of mania or depression	0.5-1%	Mood stabilizer and/or antipsychotic agent typically needed to maintain stability
Schizoaffective disorder	Yes, may have depressive episodes or episodes with mixed depressive and manic symptoms	Yes, may have manic or hypomanic episodes; depressive and manic symptoms can coexist	Psychotic symptoms commonly occur, even when the patient is not in episode of mania or depression	0.5-1%	Antipsychotic agent typically needed to maintain stability
Schizophrenia	Yes, but mood symptoms are neither necessary nor central feature	No	Yes, central feature of the condition	1%	Antipsychotic agent typically needed to maintain stability

***Depressive symptoms include low mood; decreased interest; alterations in sleep, energy, and appetite; guilt; poor concentration; psychomotor retardation; and suicidal ideation.**
†Manic symptoms include diminished need for sleep, decreased appetite, increased energy, racing thoughts, pressured speech, and grandiosity.
‡Psychotic symptoms include auditory hallucinations, visual hallucinations, paranoia, and other delusions.

sufficient sample sizes for relatively uncommon disorders (≈1% for psychotic disorders) and birth outcomes that are seen less frequently. When interpreting findings from these studies, it is important to observe their limitations. For example, most studies were not able to adequately control for smoking and illicit drug use, both of which are more common among schizophrenic women.[18,23] The possible role of medication treatment in poor birth outcomes has been inadequately addressed because of heterogeneity in medication use and limited cohort sizes.[24]

Given these limitations, women with schizophrenia appear to have worse birth outcomes than women without the disorder.[19-21,24,25] In a linked Danish database,[23] women with schizophrenia had a 46% higher relative risk of preterm delivery (95% confidence interval [CI], 1.19 to 1.79), 57% higher likelihood of delivering a low-birth-weight infant (95% CI, 1.36 to 1.82), and 35% higher risk for a small-for-gestational-age (SGA) infant (95% CI, 1.17 to 1.53) compared with the overall population of women. These adverse outcomes had been found earlier by other investigators.[21,25] Other complications reported for women with schizophrenia include placental abruption[21] and delivery of offspring with malformations,[20] including specific cardiac defects.[21]

Some[22,24] but not all[20] studies show an increased risk of stillbirth and neonatal death for women with psychotic disorders (including women with schizophrenia and bipolar disorder[22]) and specifically with schizophrenia.[24] There were also differences in the rates of post-neonatal deaths for infants born to women with schizophrenia compared with mortality rates for the general population.[20] Postneonatal death occurred at a rate of 0.73% among children born to women with schizophrenia, compared with 0.26% for those in the general population (relative risk [RR] = 2.76; 95% CI, 1.67 to 4.56). Most of the deaths were attributable to sudden infant death syndrome (SIDS), which occurred at a rate of 0.46% for children born to women with schizophrenia and 0.1% for the general population (RR = 5.23; 95% CI, 2.82 to 9.69).

Bipolar Disorder and Schizoaffective Disorder

There is little information regarding birth outcomes among women with bipolar disorder. The largest study is the Australian study that investigated outcomes for women with bipolar disorder (n = 1301), schizophrenia (n = 618), unipolar psychotic depression (n = 1255), and controls (n = 3129).[21] However, some studies assessed outcomes and found difficulties for all women with a psychotic disorder and did not differentiate among the types of disorders. For example, the increased risk of stillbirth (OR = 4.03; 95% CI, 1.14 to 4.25) described in one report occurred for mothers with psychotic disorders that included pregnant women with schizophrenia or bipolar illness.[22] Placenta previa and antepartum hemorrhage occur at a significantly higher rate among women with bipolar disorder than controls (4.2 versus 2.4%; OR = 1.66; 95% CI, 1.15 to 2.39). There were no differences for women with bipolar disorder compared with controls for birth weights, duration of pregnancy, or risk of malformations in one large cohort study.[21] The latter findings are curious because of the need for treatment with mood stabilizers of individuals with bipolar disorder and the association between these compounds and malformations.[26]

Unipolar Major Depressive Disorder

Some research suggests that high levels of stress are associated with spontaneous pregnancy loss in chromosomally normal offspring.[27] Because depression is a stress-related illness, similar results may be expected for depressed women. Unfortunately, studies looking specifically at depression are small, and the results are mixed, making it difficult to draw definitive conclusions.[28-30]

Most research addressing the relationship between depression and pregnancy outcomes has assessed women with depressive symptoms rather than a diagnosed depressive disorder. This is important because individuals with a number of psychiatric conditions have elevated scores on depressive screening or severity measures. With this caveat in mind, adult women with high levels of depressive symptoms as measured by the Beck Depression Inventory (>21 with a range of 0 to 63) had a 3.4-fold increased risk (95% CI, 3.3 to 3.6) for delivering preterm and a 3.9-fold increased risk (95% CI, 3.8 to 4.2) for delivering a low-birth-weight infant, compared with women with lower depression scores.[31] Similarly, pregnant, African-American women scoring in the top decile of the Center for Epidemiological Studies Depression Scale (CES-D) were almost twofold more likely (12.7% versus 8%; 95% CI, 1.04 to 3.7) to have spontaneous preterm delivery compared with the remaining women in the cohort.[32]

Of 10 prospective studies of depression and preterm birth reviewed by an Institute of Medicine panel, two reported an association. Although depression was not consistently or strongly linked to preterm birth in the general population, behaviors such as smoking, drug abuse, and alcohol use might have explained observed associations between the two.

It is possible that socioeconomic status mediates the effect of psychiatric distress on birth outcomes. In a prospective cohort of 666 pregnant women, elevated CES-D scores at 28 weeks for women with lower socioeconomic status were significantly associated with birth weight, even after controlling for smoking, social support, and other demographic and obstetric factors.

In contrast to earlier studies, a prospective cohort study from Sweden failed to find an association between maternal depressive or anxiety disorders and adverse birth outcomes among 1465 mothers. Power may be limited, however, because only 46 women had major depressive disorders and 86 had an anxiety disorders.[33] No studies were found that specifically assessed differences in risk of congenital anomalies among mothers with a depressive disorder compared with those without depression (Table 53-3).

TABLE 53-3 ANTIPSYCHOTICS AND MOOD STABILIZERS

Drug Name	Dose (mg/day)
Antipsychotics	
Aripiprazole (Abilify)	10-15
Clozapine (Clozaril)	12.5-900
Ziprasidone (Geodon)*	20-160
Risperidone (Risperdal)*	1-8
Quetiapine (Seroquel)*	150-800
Thioridazine (Mellaril)	50-800
Thiothixene (Navane)	6-60
Olanzapine (Zyprexa)*	2.5-20
Mood Stabilizers	
Valproic acid (Depakote)	750
Lamotrigine (Lamictal)	25-200
Carbamazepine (Tegretol and Tegretol-XR)	200-400

***These antipsychotic medications are also approved for the treatment of mania.**

Risks of Psychopharmacologic Treatment during Pregnancy

Antipsychotic Agents

Antipsychotic agents include the older, typical antipsychotic agents and the newer, atypical antipsychotic agents. The older, typical antipsychotic agents are further divided into the low-potency medications, such as the phenothiazines, and high-potency agents, such as the butyrophenones.

There is limited information on the risk of antipsychotic agent use in pregnancy. A comprehensive meta-analysis showed a small increase in the overall malformation rate (increase of 4 cases for every 1000 women) among women who took low-potency agents, but there was no specific pattern to the reported anomalies.[34] The lack of a pattern leaves open the possibility that factors other than the drugs contributed to this association.

There is also limited information regarding the high-potency butyrophenones and birth outcomes. The largest prospective cohort study ($n = 206$ first-trimester exposures versus 631 controls) found that elective terminations (8.8% versus 3.8%) and preterm birth (13.9% versus 6.9%) were more common for women who used this class of antipsychotic agent[35]; mothers also delivered significantly lighter infants if they were taking a butyrophenone. However, there were no differences in the rates of malformations. This small study had limited power to detect malformations unless the rates were greatly elevated.

Information regarding the risks associated with atypical antipsychotics is sparse but is increasing. Postmarketing data regarding pregnancy exposure to risperidone showed rates of malformations and spontaneous abortion that were consistent with population rates (3.8% and 16.9%, respectively).[36] However, the findings were based on prospective outcomes for 68 women. The retrospectively reported cases had much higher rates of malformations, but these data were confounded by ascertainment bias.

The atypical antipsychotic olanzapine is approved for use in treating mania. The pharmaceutical company registry of prospectively followed cases found associated rates of 13% for spontaneous abortion, 5% for stillbirth, 5% for preterm delivery, and 0% for malformations.[37] Although these are uncontrolled data, the rates are within the range expected for non-exposed populations. Limited data suggest that there may be a risk of gestational diabetes and preeclampsia[38] with the use of olanzapine. Diabetes that may be a consequence of insulin resistance and weight gain[39] has been associated with the use of this agent in nonpregnant populations.[40]

Mood Stabilizers

LITHIUM

The use of lithium during pregnancy has been comprehensively reviewed by the Institute for Evaluating Health Risks.[41] Early reports from the International Registry of Lithium Babies,[42] a voluntary physician-reporting database, described a 400-fold increased rate for cardiovascular malformations, most notably Ebstein anomaly, in offspring who were exposed in utero. It is likely that reporting bias led to overestimates because subsequent investigations identified a risk of Ebstein anomaly among lithium users at between 2 per 1000 (0.05%) and 1 per 1000 (0.1%), or 20 to 40 times higher than the rates for the general population.[43-45] A population-based study[46] found that the odds ratio for any cardiac malformation was 7.7 (95% CI, 1.9 to 7.7), although none of these anomalies was an Ebstein type. The odds ratio for any malformation was 3.3 (95% CI, 1.2 to 9.2) in this study.

Other complications found among women who used lithium in pregnancy include growth reduction,[41,44] acute lithium toxicity in neonates,[41,47] and possibly neonatal mortality.[41,48] There is little support for long-term neurodevelopmental complications from in utero exposure to lithium.[44,49]

VALPROIC ACID

Valproic acid use during pregnancy is associated with neural tube defects in about 5% to 9% of exposed offspring.[50,51] Neural tube–related teratogenicity occurs between 17 and 30 days after conception and is dose related.[52,53] Valproic acid is more commonly associated with lumbosacral than anencephalic lesions.[53]

Other complications from valproic acid use in pregnancy include growth restriction,[53] growth decelerations,[53] and withdrawal symptoms of irritability, jitteriness, feeding difficulties, abnormal tone,[51,54] and hypoglycemia.[55] Reductions in neonatal fibrinogen levels[56] have also been reported, as has possible mental retardation.[57]

CARBAMAZEPINE

Like valproic acid, carbamazepine is considered a human teratogen. Neural tube defects are prominent, occurring in 0.5% and 1% of offspring exposed in utero.[58,59] Other anomalies include craniofacial defects (11%), fingernail hypoplasia (26%), and developmental delay (20%) among liveborn offspring.[58]

The teratogenic potential of carbamazepine is frequently attributed to the toxic epoxide metabolites.[60] Oxcarbazepine, which does not produce the epoxide metabolite, may be less teratogenic, although this has not been confirmed by empiric data.

Other complications associated with carbamazepine use include reduction in birth weight (about 250 g),[61] mean head circumference (standardized for gestational age and sex),[62] and hepatic dysfunction.[63]

LAMOTRIGINE

Data regarding the possible consequences of lamotrigine use among 785 exposures with prospective follow-up data were published by the Lamotrigine Pregnancy Registry maintained by GlaxoSmithKine.[64] Rates of defects among infants exposed were similar to the base rate estimated for non-exposed populations. However, unpublished results from the North American Antiepileptic Drug Pregnancy Registry suggest a possible association between cleft palate and in utero lamotrigine exposure (personal communication with GlaxoSmithKine representative, July 2007). A follow-up study of 23 infants exposed demonstrated no alterations in development at 12 months of age.[65]

Antidepressants

Increasing numbers of women are undergoing antidepressant treatment during pregnancy.[66] According to one estimate,[66] 13% of women took an antidepressant at some point during pregnancy, and information about exposure to antidepressants and birth outcomes is therefore important.

There are several classes of antidepressants, including monoamine oxidase inhibitors (MAOIs), tricyclic antidepressants (TCAs), selective serotonin reuptake inhibitors (SSRIs), serotonin-norepinephrine reuptake inhibitors (SNRIs), and others (e.g., bupropion) (Table 53-4). SSRIs are the most frequently prescribed antidepressants during pregnancy, whereas MAOIs are rarely used.[66,67] Information about antidepressant use in pregnancy is greatest for the SSRIs and TCAs.[66]

MISCARRIAGE

A 45% higher risk (95% CI, 1.19 to 1.77) for miscarriage has been associated with the use of antidepressants in early pregnancy according

TABLE 53-4 ANTIDEPRESSANTS

Drug Class	Drug Name	Dose (mg/day)
Selective serotonin reuptake inhibitors (SSRIs)	Citalopram (Celexa)	20-40
	Escitalopram (Lexapro)	10-20
	Paroxetine (Paxil)	20-50
	Paroxetine controlled release (Paxil-CR)	25-62.5
	Fluoxetine (Prozac)	20-80 or 90 on a weekly basis
	Sertraline (Zoloft)	50-200
	Fluvoxamine (Luvox)	50-300
Monoamine oxidase inhibitors (MAOIs)	Selegiline (Emsam)	6-12 mg patch
	Tranylcypromine (Parnate)	
Tricyclic antidepressants (TCAs)	Amitriptyline (Elavil)	50-200
	Clomipramine (Anafranil)	25-250
	Desipramine (Norpramin)	100-300
	Doxepin (Sinequan)	25-150
	Imipramine (Tofranil)	75-200
	Nortriptyline (Pamelor)	25-150
	Protriptyline (Vivactil)	15-60
	Trimipramine (Surmontil)	75-200
Serotonin-norepinephrine reuptake inhibitors (SNRIs)	Duloxetine (Cymbalta)	20-60
	Venlafaxine (Effexor)	25-375
	Venlafaxine (Effexor XR)	37.5-225
Other	Bupropion (Wellbutrin)	200-450
	Bupropion sustained release (Wellbutrin S)	150-400
	Bupropion extended release (Wellbutrin XL)	150-450

to one meta-analysis.[68] The absolute risk in this analysis ($n = 3567$) was 12.4% and 8.7%, respectively, for exposed and non-exposed mothers, raising the question of ascertainment bias in some of the studies included. Information about other maternal illnesses or confounding health habits was not available in most of the studies constituting the meta-analysis.

FETAL GROWTH AND PREMATURITY

Several studies have reported that antidepressant use during pregnancy is associated with shorter gestations,[69-74] particularly for exposures occurring during the third trimester.[69,70,73] Overall, the effect on length of gestation is modest, with differences of 1 week or less between exposed and non-exposed offspring, but very large sample sizes would be necessary to see the less common, earlier preterm deliveries.[71,74-79] Of the two studies that attempted to control for a depressive illness, the effect remained in one[80] but not the other investigation.[74]

Reductions in birth weight, including low-birth-weight and SGA infants, have been associated with SSRI use during pregnancy.[74,80,81] Study findings regarding the risk of delivering an SGA infant after maternal TCA use in pregnancy are mixed.[73,81] The differences between exposed and non-exposed infants are small (e.g., increases from 7.4% to 8.5% for rates of SGA infants in one study after exposure to an SSRI[80]). Statistical attempts to control for maternal illness did not account for the possible effects of SSRIs on birth weight.[74,80]

STRUCTURAL MALFORMATIONS

Available information does not suggest that TCAs increase the risk of structural malformations.[34,74,82] Older studies did not find an association between SSRIs and structural malformations,[83,84] but later reports suggest a modestly increased risk of malformations for infants born to mothers exposed to SSRIs in early pregnancy.[85] Findings of the National Birth Defects Prevention Study[86] show an association between SSRI use during the month before and the first 3 months of pregnancy with anencephaly (OR = 2.4; 95% CI, 1.1 to 5.1), craniosynostosis (OR = 2.5; 95% CI, 1.5 to 4.0), and omphalocele (OR = 2.8; 95% CI, 1.3 to 5.7). Somewhat different findings were reported by a similar case-control study,[87] in which the overall malformation rate among SSRI users was not increased, but the rate of omphalocele and septal defects was higher among offspring specifically exposed to sertraline (OR = 5.7; 95% CI, 1.6 to 20.7 for omphalocele, and OR = 2.0; 95% CI, 1.2 to 4.0 for septal defects). Right ventricular outflow tract obstruction defects occurred at a significantly higher rate among paroxetine-exposed infants (OR = 3.3, 95% CI, 1.3 to 8.8). Other studies find an increased risk of cardiac malformations among offspring specifically exposed to paroxetine, compared with those exposed to drugs deemed nonteratogenic[88] or population-based controls.[79,89,90] Most defects were atrial or ventricular septum defects, and one report suggests an elevated risk occurred only for infants whose mothers took 25 mg per day or more of paroxetine.[91]

If these defects are associated with the class of SSRIs or individual SSRI agents as suggested, the absolute risk remains small. A twofold to fivefold increased risk is small in absolute numbers for the rates of omphalocele (background rate = 1 in 5000), craniosynostosis (background rate = 1 in 1800), and anencephaly (background rate = 1 in 1000). The most common anomalies are cardiac, for which the incidence is 1.8% to 2% for the exposed population compared with about 1% for an unexposed population. It is precisely because these events remain so rare that there are inconsistencies among studies. An editorial acknowledged a possible increased risk of malformations for infants born to mothers who used SSRIs in the first trimester but argued that these data also show that SSRIs are not major teratogens.[92] Given the sources for most reports (e.g., linked databases, surveillance database) and the lack of information about maternal illness or concurrent hazardous substance use, confounding effects remain possible.

The newer, non-SSRI antidepressants include bupropion, venlafaxine, duloxetine, reboxetine, nefazodone, and mirtazapine (see Table 53-4). These agents have far less information regarding possible teratogenic effects, and they vary in chemical structure. The largest analysis of risks associated with these agents found no statistically significant difference in the rate of congenital anomalies for offspring exposed to any one of them compared with the offspring exposed to antidepressants in aggregate[90] or to nonteratogens.[71,77-79]

OTHER PERINATAL COMPLICATIONS

Compared with unexposed infants, newborns exposed to TCAs and SSRIs in utero are more likely to experience jitteriness, irritability, and, rarely, convulsions.[70,73,93,94] The underlying mechanisms related to prenatal antidepressant exposure and short-term sequelae are not known but may be a sort of pharmacologic toxicity.[95] These symptoms are transient and usually resolve by 2 weeks of age.[96]

Persistent pulmonary hypertension has been reported in infants exposed to SSRIs after 20 weeks' gestation,[97] for whom the likelihood was sixfold higher compared with controls. This translated into an absolute risk of 6 to 12 cases per 1000 exposed, compared with 1 or 2 cases per 1000 non-exposed infants. Neither exposure to SSRI medications before 20 weeks' gestation nor exposure to non-SSRI antidepressants affects the risk of persistent pulmonary hypertension.

Clinical Approach to Treatment during Pregnancy

Clinical guidelines for managing pregnant women with unipolar depression are available from the American Psychiatric Association[98] and experts in the field.[99] There are also guidelines available from the American College of Obstetricians and Gynecologists, the American Psychiatric Association, and the American Medical Association. Guidelines for managing women with bipolar illness are available from the American Psychiatric Association.[26] There are no American Psychiatric Association guidelines for managing women with schizophrenia who are pregnant, but Trixler and colleagues[100] contributed a thorough review in 2005.

A treatment plan for a pregnant or postpartum woman with depression should begin by determining whether the patient has had recent or past symptoms of mania or psychosis, because this can help to determine the optimal treatment approach. In general, individuals with unipolar depression may need antidepressant treatment (see Table 53-2). If they have psychotic symptoms, treatment with an antipsychotic agent is also required. Because antidepressants can trigger or promote mania, antidepressant treatment must be used judiciously in women with a history of mania. Instead, mood stabilizers or antipsychotic agents with mood-stabilizing properties (e.g., atypical antipsychotics) are necessary (see Table 53-3). Women with schizophrenia or schizoaffective disorder require treatment with an antipsychotic agent and, in the latter case, a mood stabilizer.

Unipolar Depression

Factors that need to be considered to determine optimal therapy for a woman with mood disorders include her treatment preferences, her clinical history and current illness status, and her resources. An evaluation before conception allows a discussion of all treatment options and may allow a change in therapy, if so desired. Some women prefer not to take any medication, but others want to continue medication, especially if they have a history of severe, recurrent illness and relapse after medication discontinuation. A discussion about therapeutic options and the patient's preferences should be documented in the chart. If appropriate, women may be encouraged to engage in psychotherapy, which may allow them to be medication free during pregnancy or may improve the response to pharmacologic treatment. A healthy mother is the goal. Her well-being promotes the health of her fetus.

Women who do not have a history of severe recurrences after medication has been discontinued may be candidates for a behavioral therapy. Empirically validated psychotherapies include interpersonal psychotherapy[101] and cognitive-behavioral therapy.[102] Engaging in psychotherapy may allow the patient to carry her pregnancy to term without medication, with resumption of pharmacotherapy after delivery as needed. Women often have a sense of whether they can or cannot safely discontinue medication during pregnancy. They might have tried to stop pharmacotherapy in the past to prepare for pregnancy. A woman who discontinues pharmacotherapy should be monitored closely for relapse because her risk for a depressive recurrence may be as much as sixfold higher than that for a pregnant woman who continues pharmacotherapy.[5] For women whose history precludes medication discontinuation, treatment with the lowest effective dose of an agent that has been helpful to them is indicated. Because of the data regarding paroxetine use in pregnancy (discussed earlier), some clinicians and experts prefer using another medication as a first-line agent. However, because the newer data have not confirmed septal defects and other antidepressants have also been associated with low risks of malformations, this recommendation may not be necessary. If this or another agent has been the only agent to which a woman has responded, it should be the medication of choice for that patient.

Women who are already pregnant and develop a depressive disorder may be referred for psychotherapy as a first-line intervention or to augment pharmacotherapy. If the woman relapsed in the setting of discontinuing an antidepressant to which she had responded, she might need to have that medication restarted.

Bipolar Disorder

Because of the seriousness of bipolar disorder and the need for pharmacotherapy, pregnant women with bipolar disorder should be comanaged by a psychiatrist. Women who have a history of mania, whether they are in an episode of depression or not, should be treated with pharmacotherapy. Psychotherapy may be a helpful adjunct for these women, but is not likely to supplant the efficacy of pharmacotherapy. Unfortunately, many of the medications used to treatment bipolar disorder, including selected anticonvulsants such as valproate and carbamazepine, have teratogenic effects as described previously and in Chapter 20. Teratogenic effects have also been found after first-trimester exposure to lithium. As an alternative to these agents, some experts rely on the use of older antipsychotic agents, at least during the first trimester or longer.[99] Lithium may be reinstated again after the first trimester. Lamotrigine is a possible treatment during pregnancy. It needs to be titrated slowly from about 25 mg daily to about 200 mg daily, and it is therefore not an option for women who need to discontinue another mood stabilizer (e.g., valproic acid, lithium) and rapidly start another one.

Women with bipolar disorder need to be monitored carefully throughout pregnancy. Changes in renal and hepatic function and volume of distribution in pregnancy mean that dosage requirements may increase. This is particularly notable with lithium[41] and lamotrigine.[103] Not all pregnant women with bipolar disorder can remain euthymic without a mood stabilizer. The beginning signs of relapse should prompt clinicians to restart these treatments. Difficulties sleeping during pregnancy and after delivery may trigger mania or signify incipient relapse. Women who report this symptom should be prescribed adjunctive antipsychotics with soporific effects to aid in sleep and mood stabilization.

Schizophrenia and Schizoaffective Disorder

As for women with bipolar disorder, women who suffer from schizophrenia and schizoaffective disorder typically require pharmacologic treatment to control symptoms. A mood stabilizer may also be indicated, although first-trimester use of valproate, carbamazepine, and lithium should be avoided if possible. There are substantial data about the use of older, typical antipsychotic agents in pregnancy, and clinicians may elect to rely on these agents in pregnancy. Women with these conditions are at high risk for developing a mood disorder after delivery and are liable to experience worsening of their psychosis.[22]

Perinatal Complications

Women treated with lithium or lamotrigine during pregnancy require adjustment in dosage after delivery. Some experts recommend withholding lithium for about 24 hours before parturition because of the risk of maternal toxicity when the patient's volume contracts.[104]

Neonates exposed to lithium in utero are at risk for neuromuscular complications, respiratory difficulties, cardiac arrhythmias, and renal and hepatic dysfunction.[41,104] Because neonatal complication rates increase with maternal dosage, maintaining the lowest effective dose is optimal for the infant.[104] In utero exposure to antipsychotic agents may lead to complications among neonates, including hypertonicity, motor restlessness, tremor, and difficulty with feeding.[100] Similarly, in utero exposure to TCAs and SSRIs are associated with increased perinatal complications, including jitteriness, irritability, and convulsions in as many as 20% to 30% of infants.[34,70,73,105] Acute signs of anticholinergic effects of TCA, such as functional bowel obstruction and urinary retention, have also been described. These problems resolve within a few days to a week.

Studies examining the long-term developmental outcomes of children exposed to TCAs, SSRIs, and lithium in utero have failed to demonstrate that exposure to these agents affects global IQ, language development, or behavioral development, but these investigations were relatively small.[19,62,106-108]

Pharmacotherapy during Lactation

Psychotropic medications usually are alkaline and lipid soluble. They diffuse into breast milk. Infants have immature renal and hepatic systems, their blood-brain barrier is more permeable, and they may be more vulnerable to side effects. The use of psychotropic medications in lactating women has been extensively reviewed[109] (see Chapter 9).

Several factors should be considered before prescribing psychotropic medications to nursing mothers, including the benefits of breastfeeding for the infant, the severity of the mother's symptoms if left untreated, mothers' preferences, and the potential risk to the infant if psychotropic drugs are ingested through breast milk. With the exception of lithium, which equilibrates well in breast milk,[110] the amount of psychotropic drugs excreted in the mother's breast milk is modest.[109] Infants who are younger than 2 months old[109] and those exposed to medication in utero will achieve higher psychotropic drug levels and be at greater risk for side effects.[111] Fortunately, the data suggest that an infant's exposure to these drugs through breast milk does not seem to have any deleterious effects on growth or development.[109] Because of the narrow therapeutic index of lithium and the immature renal status of neonates, some experts recommend avoiding this agent during lactation,[109] although the American Academy of Pediatrics does not absolutely contraindicate breastfeeding for women receiving lithium therapy.[112]

Another drug to be avoided is the atypical antipsychotic clozapine (Clozaril), because of agranulocytosis may occur in the infant or mother. If a mother decides to breastfeed while taking antidepressant, antipsychotic, or mood-stabilizing agents, she should monitor her infant carefully for irritability, poor feeding, difficulty with arousal, muscle rigidity, tremors, fever, and difficulty gaining weight. Such symptoms should prompt reevaluation and consideration of a trial off breast milk.

Summary

Pregnancy does not protect women from developing or continuing to experience a mood or psychotic disorder. Schizophrenia and bipolar disorder have been associated with severe complications, including stillbirth, neonatal and postneonatal deaths, and low-birth-weight and preterm deliveries.[113] Women with these psychiatric illnesses should be considered to have high-risk pregnancies. Some women with recurrent major depressive disorder may be at risk for preterm delivery or delivery of a low-birth-weight infant. The psychotropic agents most frequently associated with malformations are the antiepileptic mood stabilizers, valproic acid and carbamazepine, and the standard bipolar therapy, lithium. First-trimester use of these agents should be avoided if possible. Women of reproductive potential who are taking these agents should consider taking folate prophylactically in case of unintended pregnancy. Antidepressant agents are not major teratogens, although possible perinatal complications and a low risk of malformations have been associated with the use of some of these agents. Collaboration between obstetric and psychiatric providers in managing pregnant women with mood and psychotic disorders can enhance maternal and infant health and well-being.

References

1. Kessler RC, Berglund P, Demler O, et al: Lifetime prevalence and age-of-onset distributions of DSM-IV disorders in the National Comorbidity Survey Replication [see comment] [erratum appears in Arch Gen Psychiatry 62:768, 2005]. Arch Gen Psychiatry 62:593-602, 2005.
2. Viguera A: Risk of recurrence of bipolar disorder in pregnant and nonpregnant women after discontinuing lithium maintenance. Am J Psychiatry 157:179-184, 2000.
3. Robertson E, Jones I, Haque S, et al: Risk of puerperal and non-puerperal recurrence of illness following bipolar affective puerperal (post-partum) psychosis [see comment]. Br J Psychiatry 186:258-259, 2005.
4. Gaynes B, Gavin N, Meltzer-Brody S, et al: Perinatal Depression: Prevalence, Screening Accuracy and Screening Outcomes. Evidence report/technology assessment no. 119. AHRQ publication no. 05-E006-2. Rockville, MD, Agency for Healthcare Research and Quality, 2005.
5. Cohen L, Altshuler L, Harlow B, et al: Relapse of major depressive during pregnancy in women who maintain or discontinue antidepressant treatment. JAMA 295:499-507, 2006.
6. Evans J, Heron J, Francomb H, et al: Cohort study of depressed mood during pregnancy and after childbirth. BMJ 323:257-260, 2001.
7. Hobfoll SE, Ritter C, Lavin J, et al: Depression prevalence and incidence among inner-city pregnant and postpartum women. J Consult Clin Psychol 63:445-453, 1995.
8. Bennett H, Einarson A, Taddio A, et al: Prevalence of depression during pregnancy: Systematic review [erratum in Obstet Gynecol 103:1344, 2004]. Obstet Gynecol 103:698-709, 2004.
9. Kendler K, Walters E, Kessler R: The prediction of length of major depressive episodes: Results from an epidemiological sample of female twins. Psychol Med 27:107-117, 1997.
10. Kendell RE, Chalmers JC, Platz C: Epidemiology of puerperal psychoses. Br J Psychiatry 150:662-673, 1987.
11. Cox JL, Murray D, Chapman G: A controlled study of the onset, duration and prevalence of postnatal depression. Br J Psychiatry 163:27-31, 1993.
12. Munk-Olsen T, Laursen TM, Pedersen CB, et al: New parents and mental disorders: A population-based register study. JAMA 296:2582-2589, 2006.
13. Cox J, Holden J: Perinatal Psychiatry. Use and Misuse of the Edinburgh Postnatal Depression Scale. Glasgow, The Royal College of Psychiatrists, 1994.
14. Spitzer R, Williams J, Kroenke K, et al: Validity and utility of the Patient Health Questionnaire (PHQ) in assessing 3000 obstetric gynecology patients: The Prime-MD PHQ obstetric gynecology study. Am J Obstet Gynecol 183:759-769, 2000.
15. Kitamura T, Shima S, Sugawara M, et al: Psychological and social correlates of the onset of affective disorders among pregnant women. Psychol Med 23:967-975, 1993.
16. Misra D, O'Campo P, Strobino D: Testing a sociomedical model for preterm delivery. Paediatr Perinat Epidemiol 15:110-122, 2001.
17. Pritchard CW: Depression and smoking in pregnancy in Scotland. J Epidemiol Community Health 48:377-382, 1994.
18. McKenna K, Koren G, Tetelbaum M, et al: Pregnancy outcome of women using atypical antipsychotic drugs: A prospective comparative study [see comment]. J Clin Psychiatry 66:444-449, 546, 2005.
19. Bennedsen B: Adverse pregnancy outcome in schizophrenic women: Occurrence and risk factors. Schizophr Res 33:1-26, 1998.
20. Bennedsen BE, Mortensen PB, Olesen AV, et al: Congenital malformations, stillbirths, and infant deaths among children of women with schizophrenia. Arch Gen Psychiatry 58:674-679, 2001.
21. Jablensky AV, Morgan V, Zubrick SR, et al: Pregnancy, delivery, and neonatal complications in a population cohort of women with schizophrenia and major affective disorders. Am J Psychiatry 162:79-91, 2005.
22. Howard LM, Goss C, Leese M, et al: The psychosocial outcome of pregnancy in women with psychotic disorders [see comment]. Schizophr Res 71:49-60, 2004.
23. Bennedsen BE, Mortensen PB, Olesen AV, et al: Preterm birth and intrauterine growth retardation among children of women with schizophrenia. Br J Psychiatry 175:239-245, 1999.
24. Rieder RO, Rosenthal D, Wender P, et al: The offspring of schizophrenics. Fetal and neonatal deaths. Arch Gen Psychiatry 32:200-211, 1975.
25. Sacker A, Done DJ, Crow TJ: Obstetric complications in children born to parents with schizophrenia: A meta-analysis of case-control studies. Psychol Med 26:279-287, 1996.
26. Yonkers K, Stowe Z, Cohen L, et al: Management of bipolar disorder during pregnancy and the postpartum period. Am J Psychiatry 161:608-620, 2004.
27. Boyles SH, Ness RB, Grisso JA, et al: Life event stress and the association with spontaneous abortion in gravid women at an urban emergency department. Health Psychol 19:510-514, 2000.
28. Sugiura-Ogasawara M, Furukawa T, Nakano Y, et al: Depression as a potential causal factor in subsequent miscarriage in recurrent spontaneous aborters. Hum Reprod 17:2580-2584, 2002.
29. Nakano Y, Oshima M, Sugiura-Ogasawara M, et al: Psychosocial predictors of successful delivery after unexplained recurrent spontaneous abortions: A cohort study. Acta Psychiatr Scand 109:440-446, 2004.
30. Nelson DB, McMahon K, Joffe M, et al: The effect of depressive symptoms and optimism on the risk of spontaneous abortion among inner-city women. J Womens Health 12:569-576, 2003.
31. Steer RA, Scholl TO: Self-reported depression and negative pregnancy outcomes. J Clin Epidemiol 45:1093-1099, 1992.
32. Orr S, James S, Prince CB: Maternal prenatal depressive symptoms and spontaneous preterm births among African-American women in Baltimore, MD. Am J Epidemiol 156:797-802, 2002.

33. Andersson L, Sundstrom-Poromaa I, Wulff M, et al: Neonatal outcome following maternal antenatal depression and anxiety: A population-based study. Am J Epidemiol 159:872-881, 2004.
34. Altshuler LL, Cohen L, Szuba MP, et al: Pharmacologic management of psychiatric illness during pregnancy: Dilemmas and guidelines [see comments]. Am J Psychiatry 153:592-606, 1996.
35. Diav-Citrin O, Shechtman S, Ornoy S, et al: Safety of haloperidol and penfluridol in pregnancy: A multicenter, prospective, controlled study. J Clin Psychiatry 66:317-322, 2005.
36. Coppola D, Russo LJ, Kwarta RF Jr, et al: Evaluating the postmarketing experience of risperidone use during pregnancy: Pregnancy and neonatal outcomes. Drug Saf 30:247-264, 2007.
37. Goldstein D: Olanazpine-exposed pregnancies and lactation: early experience. J Clin Psychopharmacol 20:399-403, 2000.
38. Kirchheiner J, Berghofer A, Bolk-Weischedel D: Healthy outcome under olanzapine treatment in a pregnant woman. Pharmacopsychiatry 33:78-80, 2000.
39. Dickson R: Olanzapine and pregnancy. Can J Psychiatry 43:196-197, 1998.
40. Guo JJ, Keck PE Jr, Corey-Lisle PK, et al: Risk of diabetes mellitus associated with atypical antipsychotic use among Medicaid patients with bipolar disorder: A nested case-control study. Pharmacotherapy 27:27-35, 2007.
41. Moore JA: An assessment of lithium using the IEHR evaluative process for assessing human developmental and reproductive toxicity of agents. Reprod Toxicol 9:175-210, 1995.
42. Schou M, Goldfield M, Weinstein M, et al: Lithium and pregnancy. I. Report from the register of lithium babies. BMJ 2:135-136, 1973.
43. Edmonds LD, Oakley GP: Ebstein's anomaly and maternal lithium exposure during pregnancy. Teratology 41:551-552, 1990.
44. Jacobson SJ, Jones K, Johnson K, et al: Prospective multicentre study of pregnancy outcome after lithium exposure during first trimester. Lancet 339:530-533, 1992.
45. Cohen L, Friedman J, Jefferson J, et al: The risk of in utero exposure to lithium. JAMA 271:1828-1829, 1994.
46. Kallen B, Tandberg A: Lithium and pregnancy. A cohort study on manic-depressive women. Acta Psychiatr Scand 68:134-139, 1983.
47. Ananth J: Side effects on fetus and infant of psychotropic drug use during pregnancy. Int Pharmacopsychiatry 11:256-260, 1976.
48. Stewart DE: Prophylactic lithium in postpartum affective psychosis. J Nerv Ment Dis 176:485-489, 1988.
49. Schou M: What happened later to the lithium babies? A follow-up study of children born without malformations. Acta Psychiatr Scand 54:193-197, 1976.
50. Omtzigt J: The risk of spina bifida aperta after first trimester exposure to valproate in a prenatal cohort. Neurology 42:119-125, 1992.
51. Kennedy D, Koren G: Valproic acid use in psychiatry: Issues in treating women of reproductive age. J Psychiatry Neurosci 23:223-228, 1998.
52. Omtzigt J, Nau H, Los FJ, et al: The disposition of valproate and its metabolites in the late first trimester and early second trimester of pregnancy in maternal serum, urine, and amniotic fluid: Effect of dose, co-medication, and the presence of spina bifida. Eur J Clin Pharmacol 43:381-388, 1992.
53. Jager-Roman E: Fetal growth, major malformations, and minor anomalies in infants born to women receiving valproic acid. J Pediatr 108:997-1004, 1986.
54. Felding I, Rane A: Congenital liver damage after treatment of mother with valproic acid and phenytoin. Acta Paediatr 73:565-568, 1984.
55. Thisted E, Ebbesen F: Malformations, withdrawal manifestations, and hypoglycaemia after exposure to valproate in utero. Arch Dis Child 69:288-191, 1993.
56. Majer R, Green P: Neonatal afibrinogenaemia due to sodium valproate. Lancet 2:740-741, 1987.
57. DiLiberti J, Farndon P, Dennis N, et al: The fetal valproate syndrome. Am J Med Genet 19:473-481, 1984.
58. Jones KL, Lacro RV, Johnson KA, et al: Pattern of malformations in the children of women treated with carbamazepine during pregnancy. N Engl J Med 320:1661-1666, 1989.
59. Rosa F: Spina bifida in infants of women treated with carbamazepine during pregnancy. N Engl J Med 324:674-677, 1991.
60. Lindhout D: Antiepileptic drugs and teratogenesis in two consecutive cohorts: Changes in prescription policy paralleled by changes in pattern of malformations. Neurology 42:94-110, 1992.
61. Diav-Citrin O, Shechtman S, Arnon J, et al: Is carbamazepine teratogenic? A prospective controlled study of 210 pregnancies. Neurology 57:321-324, 2001.
62. Hillesmaa V, Teramo K, Granstrom M, et al: Fetal head growth retardation associated with maternal antiepileptic drugs. Lancet 2:165-167, 1981.
63. Frey B, Braegger C, Ghelfi D: Neonatal cholestatic hepatitis from carbamazepine exposure during pregnancy and breastfeeding. Ann Pharmacother 36:644-647, 2002.
64. Cunnington M, Tennis P, for the International Lamotrigine Pregnancy Registry Scientific Advisory Committee: Lamotrigine and the risk of malformations in pregnancy [see comment]. Neurology 64:955-60, 2005.
65. Mackay F, O'Brien T, Hitchcock A: Safety of long term lamotrigine in epilepsy. Epilepsia 38:881-886, 1997.
66. Cooper WO, Willy ME, Pont SJ, et al: Increasing use of antidepressants in pregnancy. Am J Obstet Gynecol 196:544.e1, 2007.
67. Reefhuis J, Rasmussen SA, Friedman JM, et al: Selective serotonin-reuptake inhibitors and persistent pulmonary hypertension of the newborn. N Engl J Med 354:2188-2190, 2006.
68. Hemels ME, Einarson A, Koren G, et al: Antidepressant use during pregnancy and the rates of spontaneous abortions: A meta-analysis. Ann Pharmacother 39:803-809, 2005.
69. Chambers CD, Johnson KA, Dick LM, et al: Birth outcomes in pregnant women taking fluoxetine. N Engl J Med 335:1010-1015, 1996.
70. Costei A, Kozer E, Ho T, et al: Perinatal outcome following third trimester exposure to paroxetine. Arch Pediatr Adolesc Med 156:1129-1132, 2002.
71. Djulus J, Koren G, Einarson TR, et al: Exposure to mirtazapine during pregnancy: A prospective, comparative study of birth outcomes. J Clin Psychiatry 67:1280-1284, 2006.
72. Ericson A, Kallen B, Wilholm B: Delivery outcome after the use of antidepressants in early pregnancy. Eur J Clin Pharmacol 55:503-508, 1999.
73. Kallen B: Neonate characteristics after maternal use of antidepressants in late pregnancy [see comment]. Arch Pediatr Adolesc Med 158:312-316, 2004.
74. Simon G, Cunningham M, Davis R: Outcomes of prenatal antidepressant exposure. Am J Psychiatry 159:2055-2061, 2002.
75. Sivojelezova A, Shuhaiber S, Sarkissian L, et al: Citalopram use in pregnancy: Prospective comparative evaluation of pregnancy and fetal outcome. Am J Obstet Gynecol 193:2004, 2005.
76. Einarson A, Bonari L, Voyer-Lavigne S, et al: A multicentre prospective controlled study to determine the safety of trazodone and nefazodone use during pregnancy. Can J Psychiatry 48:106-110, 2003.
77. Chun-Fai-Chan B, Koren G, Fayez I, et al: Pregnancy outcome of women exposed to bupropion during pregnancy: A prospective comparative study. Am J Obstet Gynecol 192:932-936, 2005.
78. Einarson A: Pregnancy outcome following gestational exposure to venlafaxine: A multicenter prospective controlled study. Am J Psychiatry 158: 1728-1730, 2001.
79. Kallen B, Otterblad Olausson P: Antidepressant drugs during pregnancy and infant congenital heart defect. Reprod Toxicol 21:221, 2006.
80. Oberlander TF, Warburton W, Misri S, et al: Neonatal outcomes after prenatal exposure to selective serotonin reuptake inhibitor antidepressants and maternal depression using population-based linked health data. Arch Gen Psychiatry 63:898-906, 2006.
81. Kallen B: Fluoxetine use in early pregnancy [comment]. Birth Defects Res B Dev Reprod Toxicol 71:395-396, 2004.
82. Nulman I, Koren G: The safety of fluoxetine during pregnancy and lactation. Teratology 53:304-308, 1996.
83. Einarson TR, Einarson A: Newer antidepressants in pregnancy and rates of major malformations: A meta-analysis of prospective comparative studies. Pharmacoepidemiol Drug Saf 14:823-827, 2005.

84. Malm H, Klaukka T, Neuvonen PJ: Risks associated with selective serotonin reuptake inhibitors in pregnancy. Obstet Gynecol 106:1289-1296, 2005.
85. Wogelius P, Norgaard M, Gislum M, et al: Maternal use of selective serotonin reuptake inhibitors and risk of congenital malformations. Epidemiology 17:701-704, 2006.
86. Alwan S, Reefhuis J, Rasmussen SA, for the National Birth Defects Prevention Study: Use of selective serotonin-reuptake inhibitors in pregnancy and the risk of birth defects. N Engl J Med 356:2684-2692, 2007.
87. Louik C, Lin AE, Werler MM, et al: First-trimester use of selective serotonin-reuptake inhibitors and the risk of birth defects. N Engl J Med 356:2675-2683, 2007.
88. Diav-Citrin O, Shechtman S, Weinbaum D, et al: Paroxetine and fluoxetine in pregnancy: A multicenter, prospective, controlled study. Reprod Toxicol 20:459, 2005.
89. Källén BAJ, Olausson PO: Maternal use of selective serotonin re-uptake inhibitors in early pregnancy and infant congenital malformations. Birth Defects Res A Clin Mol Teratol 79:301-308, 2007.
90. GlaxoSmithKine: Updated Preliminary Report on Bupropion and Other Antidepressants including Paroxetine in pregnancy, and the Occurrence of Cardiovascular and Other Major Malformations. Available at http://us.qsk.com/does_pdf/media_news/ingenix_study.pdf (accessed June 2006).
91. Bérard A, Ramos E, Rey E, et al: First trimester exposure to paroxetine and risk of cardiac malformations in infants: The importance of dosage. Birth Defects Res B Dev Reprod Toxicol 80:18-27, 2007.
92. Greene MF: Teratogenicity of SSRIs—serious concern or much ado about little? N Engl J Med 356:2732-2733, 2007.
93. Sanz E, De-las-Cuevas C, Kiuru A, et al: Selective serotonin reuptake inhibitors in pregnant women and neonatal withdrawal syndrome: A database analysis. Lancet 365:482-487, 2005.
94. Moses-Kolko E, Bogen D, Perel J, et al: Neonatal signs after late in utero exposure to serotonin reuptake inhibitors: Literature review and implications for clinical applications. JAMA 293:2372-2383, 2005.
95. Oberlander TF, Misri S, Fitzgerald CE, et al: Pharmacologic Factors associated with transient neonatal symptoms following prenatal psychotropic medication exposure. J Clin Psychiatry 65:230-237, 2004.
96. Isbister GK, Dawson A, Whyte IM, et al: Neonatal paroxetine withdrawal syndrome or actually serotonin syndrome [comment]? Arch Dis Child Fetal Neonatal Ed 85:F147-F148, 2001.
97. Chambers C, Hernandez-Diaz H, Marter LV, et al: Selective serotonin-reuptake inhibitors and risk of persistent pulmonary hypertension of the newborn. N Engl J Med 354:579-587, 2006.
98. Wisner K, Gelenberg A, Leonard H, et al: Pharmacologic treatment of depression during pregnancy. JAMA 282:1264-1269, 1999.
99. Altshuler L, Cohen L, Moline M, et al: Treatment of depression in Women, 2001. The Expert Consensus Guideline Series. New York, McGraw-Hill, 2001.
100. Trixler M, Gati A, Fekete S, et al: Use of antipsychotics in the management of schizophrenia during pregnancy. Drugs 65:1193-1206, 2005.
101. Weissman M: Mastering Depression: A Patient's Guide to Interpersonal Psychotherapy. Albany, NY, Graywind Publications, 1995.
102. Beck AT, Rush AJ, Shaw BF, et al: Cognitive Therapy of Depression. New York, Guilford Press, 1979.
103. Tomson T, Battino D: Pharmacokinetics and therapeutic drug monitoring of newer antiepileptic drugs during pregnancy and the puerperium. Clin Pharmacokinet 46:209-219, 2007.
104. Newport DJ, Viguera AC, Beach AJ, et al: Lithium placental passage and obstetrical outcome: Implications for clinical management during late pregnancy. Am J Psychiatry 162:2162-2170, 2005.
105. Chambers C, Dick L, Felix R, et al: Pregnancy outcome in women who use sertraline. N Engl J Med 59:375-379, 1999.
106. Koren G, Nulman I, Addis A: Outcome of children exposed in utero to fluoxetine: A critical review. Depress Anxiety 8:27-31, 1998.
107. Loebstein R, Koren G: Pregnancy outcome and neurodevelopment of children exposed in utero to psychoactive drugs: The Motherisk experience. J Psychiatry Neurosci 22:192-196, 1997.
108. Oberlander TF, Reebye P, Misri S, et al: Externalizing and attentional behaviors in children of depressed mothers treated with a selective serotonin reuptake inhibitor antidepressant during pregnancy. Arch Pediatr Adolesc Med 161:22-29, 2007.
109. Eberhard-Gran M, Eskild A, Opjordsmoen S: Use of psychotropic medications in treating mood disorders during lactation: Practical recommendations. CNS Drugs 20:187-198, 2006.
110. Schou M: Lithium treatment during pregnancy, delivery, and lactation: An update. J Clin Psychiatry 51:410-413, 1990.
111. Wisner KL, Perel JM: Nortriptyline treatment of breast-feeding women. Am J Psychiatry 153:295, 1996.
112. American Academy of Pediatrics Committee on Drugs: The transfer of drugs and other chemicals into human milk. Pediatrics 108:776-789, 2001.
113. Behrman RE, Stith Butler A (eds): Preterm birth: Causes, consequences and prevention. Committee on Understanding Preterm Birth and Assuring Healthy Outcomes. Board on Health Sciences Policy. Washington, DC, Institute of Medicine, 2006.

Chapter 54

The Skin and Pregnancy

Ronald P. Rapini, MD

The physical and hormonal alterations induced by pregnancy, childbirth, and the puerperium are associated with numerous cutaneous changes. Some occur so frequently that they are not considered abnormal and vary only in degree. This chapter discusses these physiologic changes, the pathologic rashes of pregnancy, and the effects of pregnancy on preexisting dermatologic diseases.

Common Skin Changes Induced by Pregnancy

Pigmentary Changes

Hyperpigmentation occurs in at least 91% of pregnant women.[1] Much of this is presumed to result from the effects of increased levels of melanocyte-stimulating hormone (MSH)[2] or estrogen and progesterone on the melanocytes in the epidermis (see Chapter 8). Other bioactive molecules, such as placental lipids, can stimulate tyrosinase activity, which increases pigmentation. Pigmentation is typically most accentuated in the areolar and genital skin. The neck and axillae can become hyperpigmented, but if those areas become velvety or papillomatous, the physician should consider acanthosis nigricans associated with diabetes mellitus and other endocrinopathies. Hyperpigmentation of the linea alba, the longitudinal demarcation line on the midline of the abdomen, is called *linea nigra*. Pigmentary demarcation lines may also appear in other locations.[3] All of these pigmentary changes regress after delivery.

Melasma is diffuse macular hyperpigmentation of the face, usually involving the forehead, cheeks, and bridge of the nose. Although the antiquated term *chloasma* has often been used as a synonym, it was typically restricted to cases occurring during pregnancy (i.e., mask of pregnancy). Melasma occurs in about 70% of pregnant women but can occur in women who are not pregnant, especially those taking oral contraceptives and other hormones. Increased expression of α-MSH has been found in lesional skin.[4] The hyperpigmentation is usually blotchy and poorly demarcated, and it is bilaterally symmetrical. It usually resolves after delivery, although it persists for months or years in about 30% of patients.

Avoidance of exposure to sun during pregnancy helps to prevent or minimize the formation of melasma. Topical sunscreen lotions with sun protective factor (SPF) ratings of 15 or greater should be used. For troublesome hyperpigmentation that persists after delivery, topical hydroquinone bleaching creams and solutions (U.S. Food and Drug Administration [FDA] pregnancy category C), such as Lustra, Alustra, Melanex, or Solaquin, are sometimes useful.[5] In the United States, 4% hydroquinone cream is available as a generic prescription medication, and lower concentrations are available over the counter, but the FDA has been considering removing them from the market. Treatment is frequently prolonged for months. Cosmetics are useful for covering irregular pigmentation. Additional therapeutic options for melasma persisting after pregnancy include daily topical retinoic acid (tretinoin [Retin-A, Avita]), salicylic acid (SalAc cleanser), or azelaic acid (Azelex, Finacea). A combination of topical fluocinolone, hydroquinone, and tretinoin (Tri-Luma cream) is FDA approved. Chemical peels with trichloroacetic acid, phenol, glycolic acid, Jessner's solution, or kojic acid may be effective. Although the Q-switched lasers (i.e., yttrium-aluminum-garnet, ruby, or alexandrite) have been useful for many other pigmentary problems, they provide little help for melasma. Intense pulsed light (IPL) and the fractionated photolysis laser (Fraxel) have produced good results in some patients.

Pregnancy can produce new melanocytic nevi or enlarge preexisting nevi, but the incidence of changes in nevi and the formation of melanoma seems to be no greater than for nonpregnant women.[6] Most melanomas exhibit asymmetry, an irregular border, variegated colors (i.e., red or white in addition to black or blue), and a diameter greater than 6 mm. Suspicious lesions should be excised immediately.[7] Local anesthetic agents, such as lidocaine, are generally regarded as safe. The use of epinephrine in low doses along with lidocaine can expedite surgery. The subject of melanoma during pregnancy is addressed in Chapter 43.

Vascular Changes

Pregnancy induces dilation and proliferation of blood vessels. Although this is thought to result largely from estrogen, the mechanism is not completely understood. Telangiectasias (i.e., persistently dilated blood vessels) that resemble those seen with chronic sunlight or radiation exposure can occur during pregnancy. Spider angioma (i.e., nevus araneus) is characterized by a central arteriole with radiating vascular "legs" resembling those of a spider and is most prevalent in sun-exposed areas. Multiple spider angiomas also can occur in liver disease (resulting from decreased hepatic estrogen catabolism), with estrogen therapy, and in normal, nonpregnant women. These lesions can regress spontaneously. Persistent lesions are best treated with low-energy electrocoagulation or laser ablation.

Palmar erythema occurs in many normal pregnant women and can be associated with liver disease, estrogen therapy, and collagen vascular diseases. These vascular changes require no therapy and usually resolve after delivery.

Pyogenic granuloma is a misnomer for a red, nodular, often pedunculated, exuberant proliferation of blood vessels and inflammatory cells. This is granulation tissue that is not really a granuloma, which is a nodular aggregate in which macrophages predominate. The surface is often ulcerated, with yellowish purulence (i.e., pyogenic appearance). These lesions can occur anywhere on the skin, most commonly on the scalp, upper trunk, fingers, and toes. They are especially common on the gums, often resulting from gingivitis or trauma, where they have been called *epulis gravidarum*. The terms lobular capillary hemangioma, pregnancy tumor, and granuloma gravidarum are other synonyms for pyogenic granuloma.[8] Therapy consists of surgical excision or electrosurgical destruction,[9] but this can often be delayed until after delivery because some lesions regress spontaneously. Regression is associated with apoptosis of endothelial cells and a dramatic decrease in expression of vascular endothelial growth factor (VEGF),[10] mediated by a decline in estrogen and progesterone levels.[11] Immediate biopsy should be performed if there is problematic bleeding or if the clinical diagnosis is in doubt because some neoplasms, such as amelanotic melanomas, can resemble pyogenic granulomas.

Venous congestion and increased vascular permeability during pregnancy commonly cause gingivitis and edema of the skin and subcutaneous tissue, particularly of the vulva and lower legs.[12] Severe labial edema has occasionally been reported during pregnancy,[13] and a search for other causes is sometimes warranted. Varicosities are common on the legs and around the anus (i.e., hemorrhoids). They may regress after delivery but usually not completely.

Connective Tissue Changes

The mechanisms by which collagen and other connective tissue elements are influenced during pregnancy are poorly understood. Striae (i.e., stretch marks) represent linear tears in dermal connective tissue and appear as red or purple atrophic bands over the abdomen, breasts, thighs, buttocks, groin, and axillae. Sometimes, these lesions are pruritic. At least a few striae occur in 50% to 80% of pregnancies, and they are severe in about 10%, especially in teenagers.[14] Risk factors for more severe striae include maternal family history of striae, young maternal age, nonwhite race, larger baseline and delivery body mass index (weight gain >15 kg), increased abdominal and hip girths, increased newborn weight, and larger fetal height and head circumference.[15,16] Women with striae have an increased incidence of subsequent pelvic relaxation (i.e., prolapse).[17]

Despite numerous anecdotal claims of therapeutic efficacy, no topical therapy prevents or affects the course of striae, which ordinarily become less apparent as the red or purple color fades after delivery. There are numerous testimonials regarding the value of olive oil, cocoa butter, vitamin E, tretinoin, and nutritional therapy, but none of these has proved valuable in controlled studies.[18] The pulsed dye laser has been helpful, particularly in obliterating the red color of early lesions, but it is difficult to determine whether the short-term improvement is better than that after long-term observation.

Skin tags (i.e., acrochordons, soft fibromas, fibroepithelial polyps, or molluscum fibrosum gravidarum) are soft, papular or pedunculated growths of fibrous and epithelial tissue that are common in obesity and in pregnancy. They are usually skin colored to dark brown and usually appear on the neck, axillae, or groin. Skin tags often persist after delivery and can easily be electrocoagulated or snipped off with scissors.

Hair Cycle and Growth Changes

The hair growth cycle is divided into three phases: anagen, catagen, and telogen. The duration of the growing phase (i.e., anagen) of each scalp hair follicle persists 3 to 4 years, with an average daily growth rate of approximately 0.34 mm. Growth activity is followed by a relatively short transitional (i.e., catagen) phase that lasts about 2 weeks, followed by a resting phase (i.e., telogen) that lasts several weeks. When the next hair cycle starts, newly forming hair causes shedding of the older telogen hairs.

The activity of each of about 100,000 follicles on the human scalp cycles randomly and independently from the activity of neighboring follicles. At any given time, approximately 10% to 15% of hair follicles are in the telogen phase. If the average duration of growth of each follicle is approximately 1000 days (3 years), it can be calculated that about 100 hairs are shed normally each day.

In late pregnancy, hormones appear to increase the number of anagen hairs and decrease those in telogen. Estrogen receptors found in hair follicles may play a role in this. After hormone withdrawal in the postpartum period, telogen hairs can increase to 35% or more of scalp hairs, resulting in a transient hair loss peaking about 3 to 4 months after parturition. This diffuse hair loss has been called *telogen effluvium*, whether it occurs after delivery, surgery, illness, crash dieting, or some other stressful event.[19] The severity varies greatly, and it takes a total hair loss of 40% to 50% to become noticeable. Telogen effluvium usually is easy to distinguish from other causes of hair loss, and patients should be reassured that regrowth is likely to occur by 9 months after delivery without any treatment.

Hirsutism of the lower facial or sexual skin areas is uncommon, but it occasionally occurs in the second half of pregnancy and can be accompanied by acne. It is presumed to result from the effects of ovarian and placental androgens on the pilosebaceous unit. The possibility of an underlying androgen-secreting tumor of the ovary, of a luteoma, or of a lutein cyst should be considered, although polycystic ovary disease appears to be the most frequent cause. Options for hair removal include waxing, electrolysis, and laser ablation. Shaving does not increase the coarseness or growth of hair, but many women are not inclined to want to treat increased hair by this method.

Several types of nail changes have been reported during pregnancy but do not occur regularly. These changes include transverse grooving, increased brittleness, softening, or distal onycholysis.

Skin Conditions Specific to Pregnancy

Table 54-1 lists the rashes specific to pregnancy. Because of a lack of understanding of the pathogenesis of most of these conditions and the lack of specific diagnostic criteria, the terminology has been confusing.[20] Many of these diseases have been described by different investigators using different names for the same conditions.[21] In general, all tend to be pruritic and usually resolve within a few weeks after delivery. They all can recur in subsequent pregnancies, except the polymorphic eruption of pregnancy and prurigo gestationis. Three of the diseases may be associated with increased fetal mortality. Pregnant women also can experience dermatoses other than those specific to pregnancy. For example, contact dermatitis, eczema, superficial fungal infections, folliculitis,[22] erythema multiforme, urticaria, vasculitis, viral exanthems, scabies, secondary syphilis, and drug eruptions can occur, and it can

TABLE 54-1 RASHES OF PREGNANCY

Disease	Estimated Percentage of Pregnancies	Lesion Morphology	Most Common Location	Important Laboratory Features	Usual Trimester of Onset	Increased Fetal Mortality
Pruritus gravidarum	1.5-2.0%	Pruritus, no rash	Anywhere, abdomen	Sometimes increased bile salts, results of LFTs	3	Yes (?)
Pruritic urticarial papules and plaques of pregnancy (PUPPP)	0.6%	Papules, plaques, urticaria	Abdomen, thighs, especially in striae	None	3	No
Atopic eruption of pregnancy (prurigo gestationis)	0.3%	Excoriated papules	Extremities	None	2	No
Pemphigoid gestationis (herpes gestationis)	0.002%	Papules, vesicles	Anywhere, periumbilical	Direct IF biopsy	2 or 3	Yes (?)
Impetigo herpetiformis	Rare	Pustules	Intertriginous, trunk	Biopsy subcorneal pustule	1, 2, or 3	Yes
Autoimmune progesterone dermatitis	Rare	Acneiform, urticarial	Buttocks, extremities	Progesterone intradermal skin test	1	(?)

IF, immunofluorescence; LFTs, liver function tests.

be difficult to distinguish these from some of the pregnancy-specific rashes.

General Treatment

The same treatment principles apply to all of the specific dermatoses of pregnancy. Few drugs have been proved safe during pregnancy, and the risk-benefit ratio must be considered. Milder disease is treated with topical emollients, calamine lotion, cool compresses or baths, and topical corticosteroids. Topical corticosteroids (e.g., hydrocortisone and triamcinolone) are classified as FDA pregnancy risk category C drugs, but they are still widely used during pregnancy when the possible benefits outweigh the risks of minimal percutaneous absorption. Some of the very-high-potency topical corticosteroids, such as clobetasol, have potential for significant absorption on large body surface areas.

Many oral antihistamines, including the nonsedating fexofenadine (Allegra) and desloratadine (Clarinex), are labeled as FDA pregnancy risk category C drugs because available data are insufficient. Hydroxyzine (Atarax) is not recommended in the first trimester because it has been associated with a slightly increased rate (5.8%) of congenital malformations, but otherwise, it is in category C.[23] Oral antihistamines classified as category B (e.g., cetirizine [Zyrtec], chlorpheniramine, cyproheptadine [Periactin], diphenhydramine [Benadryl], loratadine [Claritin]) may be worth trying in patients with bothersome pruritus. Cetirizine and loratadine are relatively nonsedating agents. The favorite antihistamine in pregnancy appears to be diphenhydramine, even though it produces annoying drowsiness. One study associated diphenhydramine with cleft palate, but this finding has been disputed in other studies.[23] There has been an increased rate of retrolental fibroplasia reported in premature infants whose mothers took antihistamines within 2 weeks of delivery. No antihistamines are recommended during lactation by the manufacturers, but the American Academy of Pediatrics considers diphenhydramine to be safe during lactation because levels in breast milk are low.

Use of systemic corticosteroids (e.g., prednisone, prednisolone) in patients with severe disease appears to be relatively safe in humans (pregnancy class B). Although cleft palates have occurred in offspring of pregnant rabbits undergoing such therapy, this relationship has not been demonstrated in humans. Infants of mothers treated with systemic corticosteroids should be monitored for evidence of adrenal insufficiency. Ultraviolet phototherapy can be offered to pregnant women with severe pruritus if the benefits outweigh the risks of burning and excessive heat.[24]

Pruritus Gravidarum

Pruritus gravidarum is generalized itching during pregnancy without the presence of a rash, although excoriations can occur. Up to 14% of pregnant women complain of itching, but pruritus associated with cholestasis (i.e., intrahepatic cholestasis of pregnancy [see Chapter 50]) occurs in only about 1.5% to 2% of pregnant women, with onset usually in the third trimester. Some authorities seem to confuse definitions by reserving the term *pruritus gravidarum* for patients with cholestasis of pregnancy. Frank clinical jaundice occurs in only 0.02% of pregnancies. Pruritus limited to the anterior abdominal wall is common and is usually caused by skin distention and development of striae rather than cholestasis. Pruritus usually disappears shortly after delivery but recurs in approximately 50% of subsequent pregnancies.

Cholestatic itching correlates better with elevated serum bile acid levels than with other biochemical liver function tests such as alkaline phosphatase, aspartate aminotransferase (AST [SGOT]), alanine aminotransferase (ALT [SGPT]), and bilirubin. Elevated glutathione *S*-transferase α (GSTA), a specific marker of hepatocellular integrity, identifies women with intrahepatic cholestasis and distinguishes them from those with benign pruritus gravidarum.[25] Abnormal plasma lipid profiles are common in those with cholestasis. Biliary obstruction in pregnancy is discussed in more detail in Chapter 50. It has been stressed that some patients with skin lesions indicative of one of the other pregnancy rashes described in this chapter have coexisting cholestasis of pregnancy, and screening with liver function tests may be reasonable for patients with pregnancy-related rashes and for those experiencing pruritus without rash. Pruritus can precede abnormal findings of liver function tests or total serum bile acids, and follow-up testing for obstetric cholestasis may be needed for itchy pregnant patients with initially normal findings.[26]

Pruritus gravidarum is associated with twin pregnancies, fertility treatments, diabetes mellitus, and nulliparity, but it is not associated with adverse perinatal outcomes for patients without cholestasis.[27] Reported increases in rates of premature delivery and perinatal mortality appear to be restricted to those in whom frank clinical jaundice develops.

Treatment is symptomatic, and mild cases usually respond to adequate skin lubrication and topical antipruritics (discussed previously). Oral antihistamines can be of some benefit. Ultraviolet light treatment or judicious sun exposure can decrease pruritus. In more severe cases of cholestasis, phenobarbital or bile-sequestering agents such as cholestyramine (Questran), supplemented with fat-soluble vitamins, can be beneficial, although there is no agreement about efficacy.[20] A review of published studies concluded that there is insufficient evidence to recommend corticosteroids, guar gum, activated charcoal, *S*-adenosylmethionine, and ursodeoxycholic acid.[28] Other authorities are convinced that ursodeoxycholic acid reduces premature labor, fetal distress, and fetal deaths.[20] It is not clear whether early delivery by 38 weeks' gestation reduces perinatal complications for patients with cholestasis.[29]

Pruritic Urticarial Papules and Plaques of Pregnancy

Pruritic urticarial papules and plaques of pregnancy (PUPPP)[30] is a designation for a rash characterized by erythematous papules, plaques, and urticarial lesions that usually begins in the third trimester. It is the most common pregnancy rash. The rash has also been named polymorphic eruption of pregnancy (PEP) by Holmes and Black in 1982,[20] and this term is preferred in Europe. PUPPP is the most popular term in the United States. The eruption was called toxemic rash of pregnancy[31] and late-onset prurigo of pregnancy[32] in the older literature.

PUPPP is almost always pruritic, and itching is severe in 80% of patients. The lesions begin on the abdomen in 80% to 90% of patients, often sparing the umbilicus (Fig. 54-1). The striae become involved in 67% of women, suggesting that abdominal distention may contribute to the inflammation occurring with this rash (Figs. 54-2 and 54-3). In many cases, the eruption spreads to the proximal thighs, buttocks, and proximal arms. The face is usually spared. Sometimes, erythema multiforme–like target lesions are present.

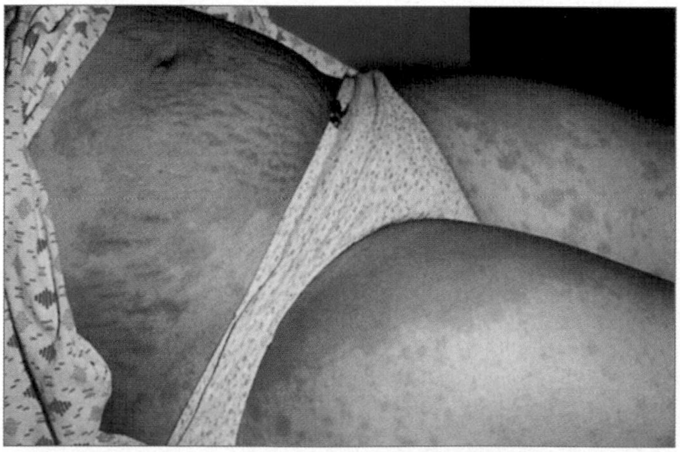

FIGURE 54-1 Pruritic urticarial papules and plaques of pregnancy. Lesions commonly begin in the abdominal striae. Confluent, erythematous, urticarial papules and plaques are seen on the thighs in this patient.

The rash usually resolves before or within several weeks after delivery, but, rarely, it may persist or even begin after delivery.[33] Some patients have had significant reductions in serum cortisol levels.[34] The disease is most prevalent among primigravidas. There is an association with increased maternal weight gain, increased twin pregnancy rate, hypertension, and induction of labor.[35] Unlike most of the other rashes of pregnancy, PUPPP does not tend to recur with subsequent pregnancies. There is no increase in the fetal morbidity or mortality rate.

Routine skin biopsies show nonspecific changes, including variable parakeratosis, spongiosus, acanthosis, dermal edema, and perivascular lymphocytes and eosinophils. Vesicles occur in a minority of cases and can cause confusion with pemphigoid gestationis, but the results of direct immunofluorescence of skin biopsy specimens are usually negative. Treatment depends on the severity of the condition. Topical corticosteroids are adequate for most patients with PUPPP.[36]

Atopic Eruption of Pregnancy

Atopic eruption of pregnancy is a newly proposed term to encompass what was formerly called prurigo gestationis and folliculitis of preg-

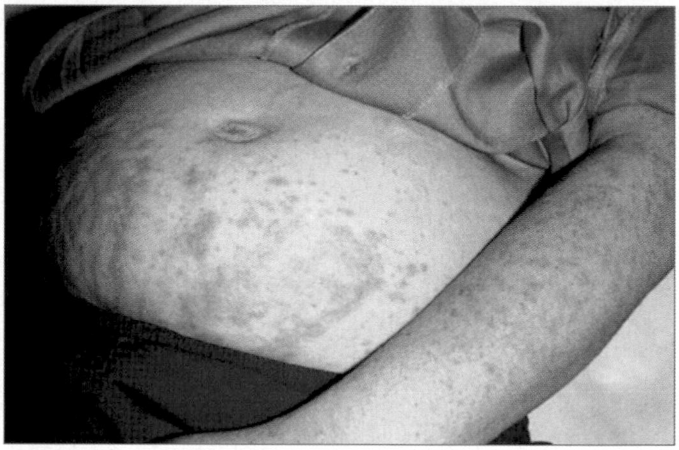

FIGURE 54-2 Pruritic urticarial papules and plaques of pregnancy. Urticarial involvement of striae occurs with papular eruption on the arms.

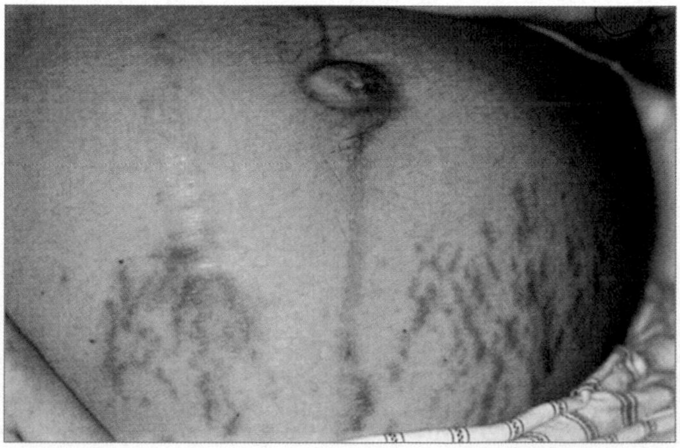

FIGURE 54-3 Pruritic urticarial papules and plaques of pregnancy. The eruption often begins in itchy, red striae. Notice the linea nigra.

nancy.[37] The general term *prurigo* designates an intensely pruritic skin eruption in which excoriation predominates, suggesting a prominent emotional component. Many of these patients have a genetic predisposition for atopic dermatitis (i.e., atopic eczema), and many examples of this disorder may instead be eczema or dermatitis.[34] Atopic dermatitis in pregnancy is considered later in this chapter.

Prurigo gestationis was first described by Besnier in 1904 and is similar to the early prurigo of pregnancy later described by Nurse in 1968.[32,34] The lesions consist of excoriated papules or nodules mostly over the extremities, usually beginning in the middle of pregnancy, whereas most of the other specific pregnancy rashes start later in pregnancy (Figs. 54-4 to 54-6). Elevated liver function test results have been reported in some cases, but this probably represents an overlap of patients with pruritus gravidarum. The eruption usually clears by 3 months after delivery, and the recurrence rate in subsequent pregnancies is low. Treatment depends on the severity of the condition.

Papular dermatitis of pregnancy was designated a distinct entity by Spangler and coauthors[38] on the basis of markedly elevated levels of 24-hour urinary human chorionic gonadotropin (hCG) levels for that stage of pregnancy and decreased levels of plasma and urinary estriol and plasma cortisol levels. The lesions were more widespread than lesions of the other pregnancy rashes. Whether these criteria are sufficient to determine a separate disease is questionable.

There have been few case reports, and some of the reported cases of papular dermatitis have been questionable because of the lack of appropriate laboratory studies to exclude the other pregnancy rashes discussed in this chapter. Vaughan Jones and coworkers[34] concluded that papular dermatitis of Spangler is not a separate entity because they were unable to identify any patients with decreased estradiol levels in a large series of patients with pregnancy rashes.

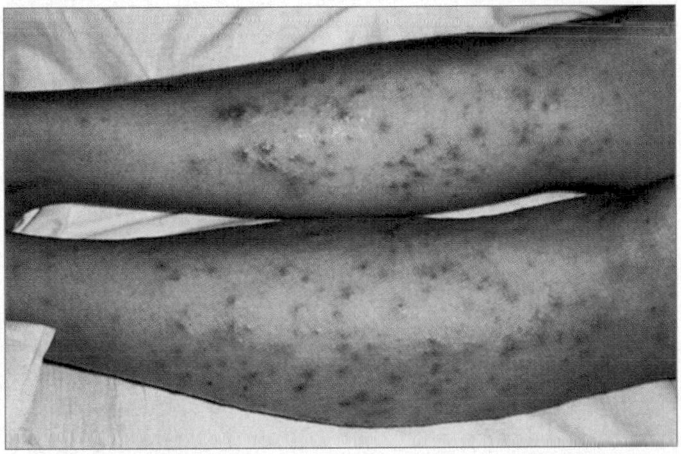

FIGURE 54-4 Prurigo gestationis. The predominant lesions are excoriated papules.

Pemphigoid Gestationis

Pemphigoid gestationis is a rare, autoimmune, blistering dermatosis of pregnancy and the immediate postpartum period.[39] It is not related to infection by herpesvirus; the unfortunately common synonym *herpes gestationis* refers to the grouped (herpetiform) nature of the blisters, which often are not herpetiform.[20] It is best to avoid the term *herpes gestationis* because of the risk of misleading patients and misinformed health care workers; not using the term avoids potentially inappropriate treatments for herpesvirus. Onset usually occurs during the second or third trimester, but cases beginning in the first trimester or the immediate postpartum period have been well documented. A high frequency of human leukocyte antigen (HLA) haplotypes B8 and DR3/DR4 has been reported.[40]

Lesions often begin around the umbilicus (Fig. 54-7). Other commonly involved areas include the trunk, buttocks, and extremities. The face and mucous membranes are usually not affected. Vesicles and bullae are the most important clinical lesions (Figs. 54-8 and 54-9). Erythematous plaques, often annular or urticaria-like, frequently are present, and they can resemble PUPPP. The extent of the disease process and the degree of accompanying pruritus can be mild to severe.

A mortality rate for infants born to affected mothers has been estimated to be as high as 30%, although this figure has been disputed.[41] Increased likelihood of prematurity has also been reported.[42] With systemic corticosteroid treatment of severe cases, fetal risk appears to be minimal. There is an increase in premature and small-for-gestational-age infants.[41] Most infants do not have skin lesions, although transient urticarial and vesicular lesions thought to be caused by transplacental antibody transfer have been observed in less than 5% of infants born of affected mothers (Figs. 54-10 and 54-11).

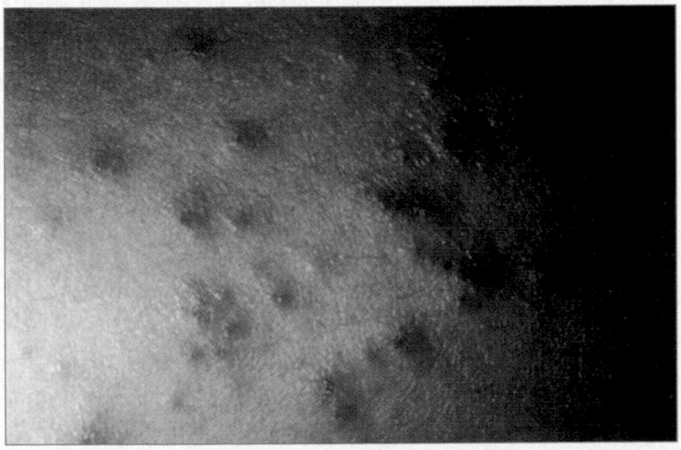

FIGURE 54-5 Prurigo gestationis. Close-up view of excoriated papules on the same patient as in Figure 54-4.

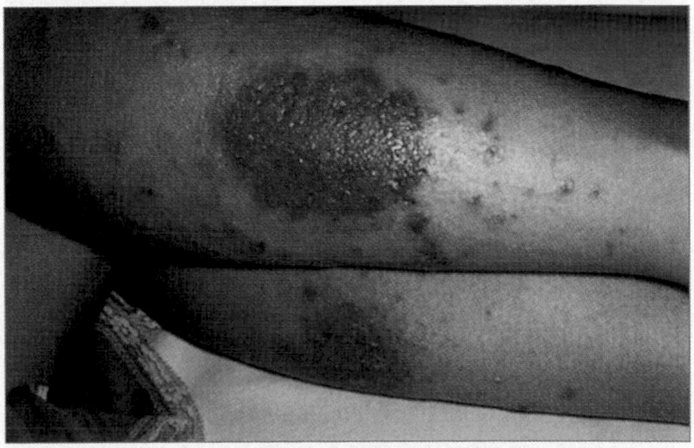

FIGURE 54-6 Prurigo gestationis. Although papules are more common, lesions occasionally coalesce into crusty plaques.

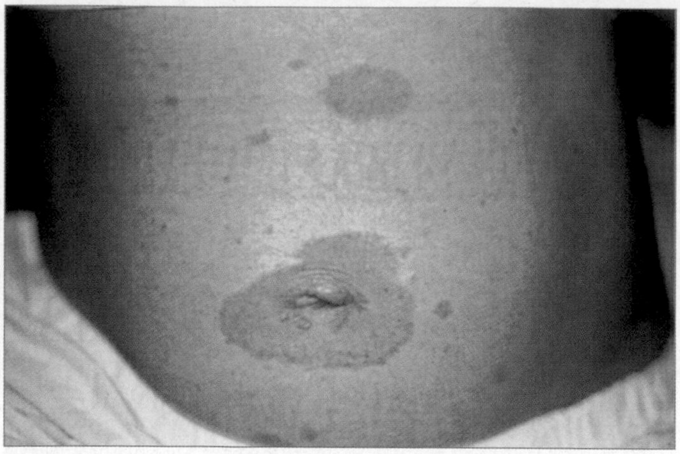

FIGURE 54-7 **Pemphigoid gestationis.** The patient has characteristic periumbilical urticarial plaque. Blisters may or may not be present.

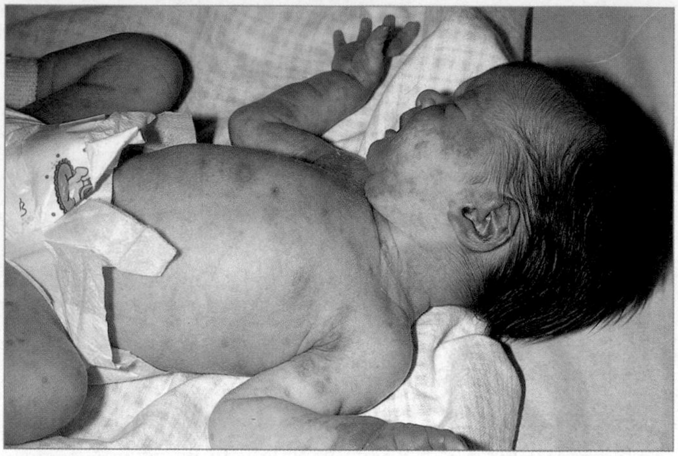

FIGURE 54-10 **Pemphigoid gestationis.** Newborn child of the mother seen in Figure 54-8 has urticarial, erythematous patches with rare blisters.

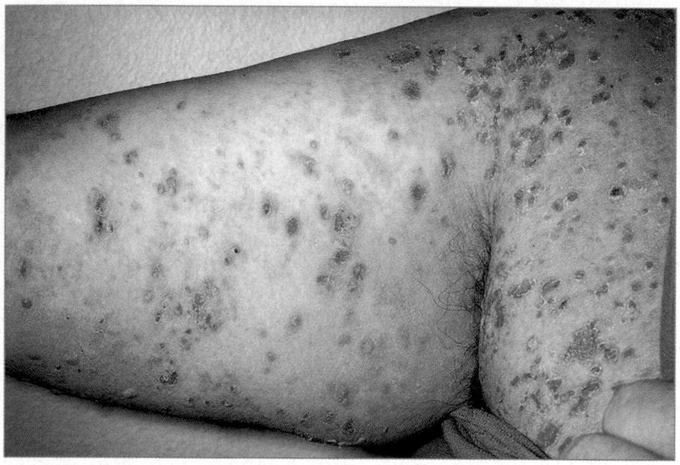

FIGURE 54-8 **Pemphigoid gestationis.** Crusts and blisters on the mother of the child seen in Figure 54-10.

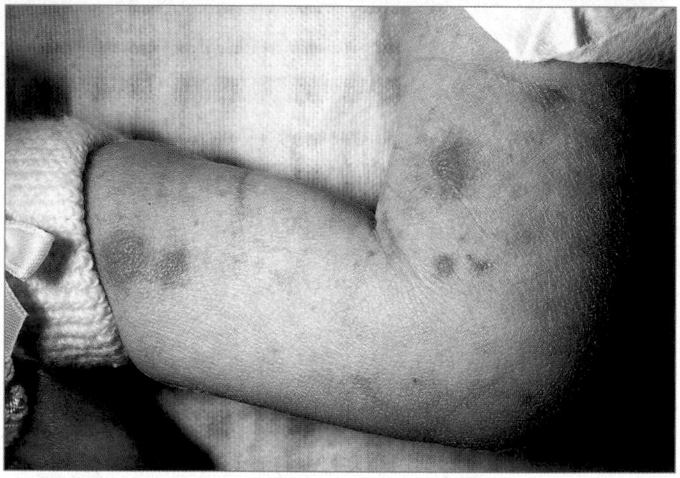

FIGURE 54-11 **Pemphigoid gestationis.** Close-up view of the erythematous patches seen in Figure 54-10.

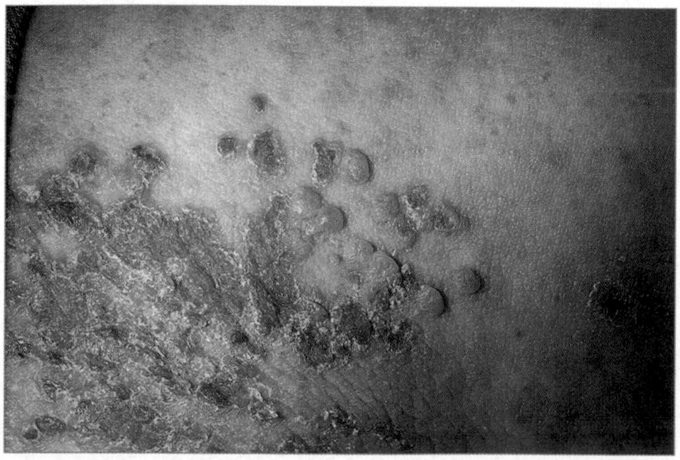

FIGURE 54-9 **Pemphigoid gestationis.** Close-up view of crusts and blisters on the mother seen in Figure 54-8.

Postpartum flares occur in 50% to 75% of patients with pemphigoid gestationis. Exacerbation typically begins within 24 to 48 hours after delivery and can last for several weeks or months. Skin lesions have been reported to persist for more than a year in women who do not breastfeed compared with those who do (average postpartum duration is 1 to 6 months).[43] Flares also can occur with subsequent pregnancies, subsequent menses, ovulation, or treatment with estrogen or progesterone. About 20% to 50% of patients who have had pemphigoid gestationis experience recurrent skin lesions when treated with oral contraceptives.

The routine histopathologic location of the blisters is usually subepidermal, but blisters sometimes are intraepidermal as a result of spongiosus. Focal necrosis of basal keratinocytes can occur. There are perivascular lymphocytes in the dermis with a significant number of eosinophils, and those nonspecific dermal changes are found if nonblistering sites are sampled for biopsies. A biopsy for direct immunofluorescence from red macules or perilesional blisters is recommended, because the routine biopsy changes are often not specific.

Immunopathologically, pemphigoid gestationis and bullous pemphigoid (an autoimmune disease most prevalent among the elderly

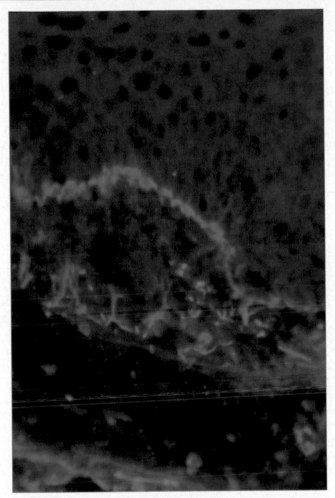

FIGURE 54-12 Pemphigoid gestationis. The skin biopsy specimen taken for direct immunofluorescence assay demonstrates a linear band of C3 at the basement membrane zone.

and with HLA-DQ3) are strikingly similar. Heavy linear deposits of C3 are present in the epidermal basement membrane zone (BMZ) of pemphigoid gestationis perilesional skin (Fig. 54-12), usually in the absence of IgG deposits when direct immunofluorescence staining methods are used. BMZ C3 deposits have also been described in some infants born to affected mothers with pemphigoid gestationis. In contrast, direct immunofluorescence of bullous pemphigoid shows both C3 and IgG.

Unlike cases of bullous pemphigoid, circulating anti-BMZ IgG autoantibodies are measurable in the serum by indirect immunofluorescence in only 10% to 20% of cases of pemphigoid gestationis. When antibodies are present, titers are usually low, in contrast to bullous pemphigoid. Circulating IgG1 autoantibodies (i.e., herpes gestationis factor, also called pemphigoid gestationis factor) avidly fix complement to the BMZ in pemphigoid gestationis. They are present in such low levels, however, that they often escape detection by routine methods. Bullous pemphigoid IgG subclasses are more heterogeneous, with IgG4 predominating over IgG1. Pemphigoid gestationis autoantibodies usually react with the NC16a domain of a 180-kDa protein associated with hemidesmosomes of basal keratinocytes,[44] whereas bullous pemphigoid autoantibodies potentially react with two protein bands, almost always with a 230-kDa protein (i.e., dystonin [DST], formerly designated BPAG1) and sometimes with the same NC16a domain of the 180-kDa protein that is the main target in pemphigoid gestationis (i.e., collagen type XVII-α1 [COL17A1], formerly designated BPAG2). Only a small number of patients with pemphigoid gestationis have autoantibodies directed against the DST protein. Studies have found that immunoblotting and enzyme-linked immunosorbent assay (ELISA) are sensitive methods for detecting the COL17A1 in the sera of patients with pemphigoid gestationis, in contrast to the often negative results obtained with indirect immunofluorescence of sera.[45] If these tests are made commercially available, they may eliminate the need for skin biopsy for direct immunofluorescence, which has been the standard test required in these patients.

There is an increased incidence of antithyroid antibodies in pemphigoid gestationis, but clinically apparent thyroid dysfunction is rare.[46] Patients are at an increased risk for Graves disease, but this usually does not occur simultaneously with pemphigoid gestationis.

Because placental antibody deposition may result in placental insufficiency, it has been suggested (based on the study of one patient) that pregnant women with pemphigoid gestationis undergo frequent umbilical artery Doppler studies to document end-diastolic velocity even without the ultrasound finding of intrauterine growth restriction.[47]

Treatment of pemphigoid gestationis should not be designed to suppress the disease process entirely, because the higher doses of therapy needed to suppress disease activity completely can have serious side effects. Instead, therapy should be directed toward suppressing the appearance of new lesions and relieving the intense pruritus. Potent topical corticosteroids can be attempted in mild to moderate cases. In moderate to severe cases, prednisone (20 to 40 mg/day) is often adequate to suppress new blister formation and relieve symptoms. After new blister formation has been suppressed, the prednisone dose can be tapered to lower doses or to just enough to maintain control and relieve symptoms. Eventually, alternate-day therapy may become more appropriate and should be attempted.

If the disease flares in the immediate postpartum period, treatment with prednisone (20 to 40 mg/day) should be reinstituted. Higher doses may be instituted at this time if necessary. Infants of mothers treated with prednisone should be monitored for evidence of adrenal insufficiency. Minocycline and nicotinamide have been used anecdotally as alternatives to prednisone in pregnancy.[48] Plasmapheresis or intravenous immunoglobulin is used for severe cases.[49] Dapsone is often used for other autoimmune blistering disorders but is contraindicated during pregnancy, because it can cause hemolytic disease of the newborn. Other treatment modalities useful for all pregnancy rashes have been discussed previously.

Impetigo Herpetiformis

First described in 1872 by von Hebra, impetigo herpetiformis is a severe, generalized pustular dermatosis associated with pregnancy.[50] The name is unfortunate because it is unrelated to bacterial infection (i.e., impetigo) or herpesvirus infection. It probably represents pustular psoriasis in pregnancy, mostly occurring in patients who have never had psoriasis before pregnancy.

Onset of the disease usually occurs in the third trimester, but well-documented cases have occurred as early as the first trimester. The disease usually subsides between pregnancies but can recur with subsequent pregnancies and usually occurs earlier in a subsequent pregnancy. Patients may have hypoparathyroidism, hypocalcemia, hypophosphatemia, decreased vitamin D levels, elevated erythrocyte sedimentation rate, and leukocytosis.[51] The cause remains unknown,

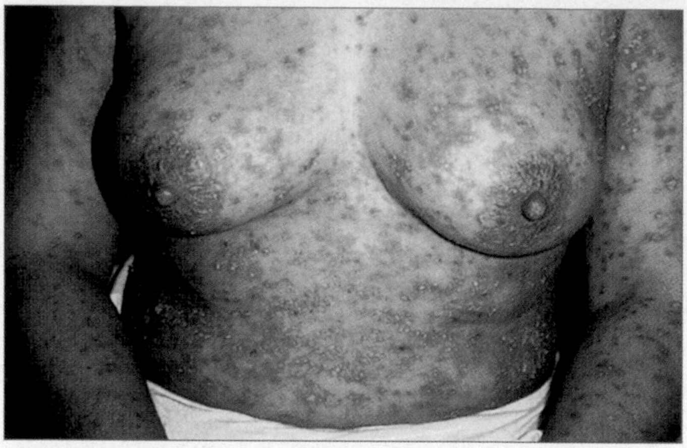

FIGURE 54-13 Impetigo herpetiformis (i.e., pustular psoriasis). The patient has extensive sterile pustules.

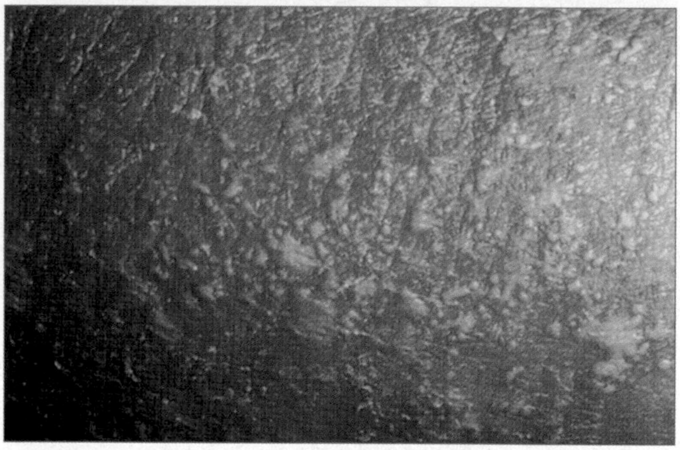

FIGURE 54-14 Impetigo herpetiformis (i.e., pustular psoriasis). Close-up view of superficial pustules occurring just beneath the stratum corneum shows the characteristic coalescence into "lakes of pus."

but it may be a reaction to drugs or occult infection in a genetically predisposed patient.

Clinically, the disease is characterized by hundreds of translucent, white, sterile pustules (Figs. 54-13 and 54-14) that arise on irregular erythematous bases or plaques. These lesions extend peripherally while central pustules rupture because of their superficial locations, leaving denuded surfaces with crusts, as occur in some forms of pemphigus. Common areas of involvement include the axillae, inframammary areas, umbilicus, groin, and gluteal crease. Pustular lesions can also occur on the hands and involve the nails with subsequent nail loss or onycholysis.

Constitutional symptoms are common and include fever, chills, nausea, vomiting, and diarrhea with severe dehydration. Delirium, tetany, and convulsions are rare complications that are usually associated with hypocalcemia. Death may occur in association with these complications and septicemia.

Impetigo herpetiformis is thought to be a form of generalized pustular psoriasis that occurs during pregnancy. The clinical presentation and histopathology of both disease entities are identical. Most pregnant patients do not have a history of psoriasis.

Histopathologically, impetigo herpetiformis is characterized by subcorneal pustules containing neutrophils and degenerated keratinocytes. Cultures of pustular lesions are usually negative disease agents unless secondarily infected.

Differential diagnosis includes acute generalized exanthematous pustulosis, which is a severe pustular drug reaction, and it is more likely to have eosinophils in the biopsy specimen. Scabies, bacterial impetigo, fungal infections, folliculitis, and acne can be pustular, but they usually look different to an experienced clinician. Cultures, potassium hydroxide preparations, and biopsies can be done when necessary.

Systemic corticosteroid therapy is the treatment of choice for impetigo herpetiformis. Usually, 20 to 40 mg of prednisone per day is sufficient to control new lesion formation. Systemic antibiotics may help when secondary infection is present. Topical measures, such as wet compresses with or without topical corticosteroid preparations, are also useful as general treatment for itchy pregnancy rashes. Intravenous fluids and electrolytes are important for patients with diarrhea, vomiting, high fever, and extensive skin pustulation. Cyclosporin has been used successfully in pregnancy for severe cases.[52] Acitretin (a synthetic vitamin A derivative given orally) and methotrexate, both used commonly for generalized pustular psoriasis, are contraindicated during pregnancy.

Autoimmune Progesterone Dermatitis

Autoimmune progesterone dermatitis is a rare, poorly defined, urticarial, papular, vesicular, or pustular eruption thought to be caused by hypersensitivity to progesterone.[53] It usually appears as a recurrent, cyclic eruption during the luteal phase of the menstrual cycle.[53] It often resembles erythema multiforme. Very few cases have involved onset or worsening of this condition with pregnancy. Two of these cases were associated with spontaneous abortion. In other cases of autoimmune progesterone dermatitis, the rash improved or cleared during pregnancy.

Estrogen dermatitis has been described in seven patients, all of whom had severe premenstrual exacerbations of a variety of skin eruptions.[54] Skin test results were positive for estrogen in all seven cases.

Autoimmune progesterone dermatitis has been documented by the use of intradermal or intramuscular test injections of progesterone.[55] Intradermal tests usually produce an immediate local urticarial reaction or a delayed reaction. Intramuscular challenges have caused exacerbations of the rash or even angioedema. Progesterone antibodies have been demonstrated in four cases by indirect immunofluorescence. An indirect basophil degranulation test has also been used, in which the patient's serum is mixed with synthetic progesterone and rabbit basophils.

Specific therapy for autoimmune progesterone dermatitis during pregnancy is unclear. Nonpregnant patients have responded to estrogens (if the allergen was progesterone), birth control pills (e.g., Loestrin, which contains ethinyl estradiol plus norethindrone), the antiestrogen tamoxifen, the anabolic androgen danazol, thalidomide, or oophorectomy.[56] Spontaneous remission can occur after successful treatment.[20] Regional anesthesia may be preferred over general anesthesia for patients with progesterone dermatitis who are also prone to angioedema and need to undergo obstetric procedures.[57]

Skin Disorders Affected by Pregnancy

The effect of pregnancy on preexisting skin diseases varies.[58] Table 54-2 lists some skin diseases that improve or become aggravated by preg-

TABLE 54-2 EFFECT OF PREGNANCY ON SKIN DISEASES

Usually Improved by Pregnancy
Fox-Fordyce disease
Hidradenitis suppurativa
Usually Aggravated by Pregnancy
Condylomata acuminata
Ehlers-Danlos syndrome
Erythema multiforme
Erythema nodosum
Herpes simplex
Lupus erythematosus
Neurofibromatosis
Pemphigus
Pityriasis rosea
Porphyrias
Pseudoxanthoma elasticum
Scleroderma (increased renal disease)
Tuberous sclerosis (increased seizures)
Unpredictable Response to Pregnancy
Acne
Acquired immunodeficiency syndrome
Atopic dermatitis
Dermatomyositis
Melanoma
Psoriasis

nancy, although the course of a disease in a given patient is not always predictable.[29,59] Most skin diseases do not affect fetal outcome.[60] Cutaneous infections are discussed in Chapter 38, and connective tissue diseases involving the skin are discussed in Chapter 51. Some infectious, autoimmune, or rheumatic diseases tend to worsen during pregnancy.

Acne

Acne is a disease of the pilosebaceous unit. It is partially influenced by androgens such as testosterone and dehydroepiandrosterone sulfate (DHEAS), which increase sebaceous gland activity. Estrogen reduces sebaceous gland size and activity, but this is probably a function of negative feedback on androgen production by the ovary. Sebaceous gland activity is increased during pregnancy. Montgomery tubercles are small sebaceous glands on the areolae of the breasts, and their papular enlargement is one of the first signs of pregnancy.

Acne consists of erythematous papules, pustules, comedones, and cysts on the face, back, and chest. Some cases reported as "pruritic folliculitis of pregnancy" of widespread locations may represent hormonally induced acne.[61] Pregnancy has a variable effect on acne, probably because many other factors are involved in its pathogenesis besides the hormonal influences discussed.

Acne can be controlled during pregnancy or lactation with topical benzoyl peroxide (category C), salicylic acid, azelaic acid (Azelex, category B), or topical antibiotics such as erythromycin (category B) or clindamycin (Cleocin T, category B).[62] Topical and oral sulfonamides should be avoided near term. Forms of topical metronidazole (MetroLotion, MetroGel, MetroCream, and Noritate cream, all category B) typically are used if other alternatives have failed. More severe disease can be treated with the apparent oral antibiotic of choice, erythromycin, starting with 1 g daily (category B), even though its efficacy has been dwindling because of the increasing resistance of bacterial flora. It appears to be safe during lactation. Erythromycin estolate has been implicated as a cause of hepatotoxicity in pregnancy after prolonged use, and it should be avoided. Tetracycline should be avoided because of its potential risk of fatty liver of pregnancy and adverse effects on fetal dentition. Vitamin A derivatives (i.e., retinoids) such as oral isotretinoin are contraindicated because of teratogenic effects. Topical retinoids such as tretinoin (Retin-A or Avita, category C) or topical adapalene (Differin, category C) are not contraindicated, but different topical drugs are probably better during pregnancy. Topical tazarotene is a category X drug, but healthy infants have been born to six women using it.

Atopic Dermatitis

Atopic dermatitis is an allergic skin disease characterized by intensely pruritic, eczematous lesions that become lichenified when patients are caught in a scratch-itch cycle.[63] There appears to be an inherited irritability of the skin (i.e., the "itch that rashes" instead of the rash that itches), and many patients have a personal or family history of eczema, asthma, hay fever, food allergies, or allergic rhinitis beginning in childhood. This disease can worsen (52%) or improve (24%) during pregnancy.[64] Exacerbation of atopic dermatitis changes in pregnancy has been called *atopic eruption of pregnancy* (previously discussed).

Some studies show that breastfeeding reduces the incidence of atopy in infants because cow's milk has been implicated as a significant aggravating factor. Soya milk is often substituted, but it also can be allergenic.[65] The mother's diet has not been shown to make a significant difference during pregnancy and breastfeeding.[66] An increased incidence of atopy in children has been associated with a wide variety of confusing factors in various studies, such as increased fetal growth and a larger head circumference,[67] increased gestational age,[68] low parity, febrile infections in pregnancy, the use of contraceptives before pregnancy,[69] and maternal smoking.[70]

Treatment with topical emollients, topical corticosteroids, and oral antihistamines is usually effective. If the skin is extremely dry and scaly, greasy ointments may be more effective than creams. Patients should be instructed to use soap sparingly and should always apply topical emollient lotions or creams after bathing. The newer immunomodulators, topical pimecrolimus (Elidel cream) and tacrolimus (Protopic ointment), are FDA pregnancy category C drugs. Exceptional patients may require systemic corticosteroids.

Erythema Nodosum

Erythema nodosum is characterized by tender nodules on the anterior lower legs, usually considered to be a reaction to a drug or an infection somewhere else, such as streptococcal pharyngitis or coccidioidomycosis.[71] Sarcoidosis and inflammatory bowel disease are also common causes.[72] Women account for 90% of patients. Erythema nodosum is known to be precipitated by pregnancy and by oral contraceptives,[73] which suggests an estrogen influence on this disease.[74]

Treatment begins with specific therapy for the underlying inciting cause. Nonsteroidal anti-inflammatory agents other than acetaminophen are usually not recommended because they can constrict the ductus arteriosus or cause prolonged labor because of prostaglandin synthesis inhibition. Systemic corticosteroids may be used in more severe noninfectious cases.

Fox-Fordyce Disease

Fox-Fordyce disease is a rare entity, often called apocrine miliaria because it can be similar to the prickly heat or heat rash involving eccrine glands. Fox-Fordyce disease occurs mainly in women, with onset occurring usually shortly after puberty.[75] Many pruritic, dome-shaped, follicular papules develop in the axillae and anogenital region, areas rich in apocrine glands.

The disease usually improves during pregnancy or with oral contraceptive therapy, probably because of an estrogen effect. Apocrine activity, unlike eccrine activity, appears to be decreased during pregnancy. Response to topical corticosteroids or pimecrolimus varies.

Genodermatoses

A long list of inherited severe cutaneous diseases involving the mother or other family members can affect fetal mortality or morbidity. Newer techniques that make it possible to study the molecular, enzymatic, and ultrastructural basis of these conditions are continually evolving. It is impossible to provide up-to-date information on this rapidly changing field in a textbook. More details of prenatal diagnosis are given in Chapter 17.

Modalities useful for detecting severe fetal skin diseases include chorionic villus sampling, amniocentesis, fetal skin biopsy,[76] and preimplantation genetic diagnosis. DNA-based tests involve screening by nucleotide sequencing, restriction enzyme digests, or linkage analysis.[77] Although ichthyosis and epidermolysis bullosa are the two most important groups of disorders, prenatal diagnosis has been successful in many other skin diseases.[78]

There are many types of ichthyosis, all of which cause extensively thickened, scaly skin resembling the scales of a fish. A variety of ichthyotic syndromes have been described that involve abnormalities other than the skin. Ichthyosiform erythroderma is subdivided into dominant and recessive forms, and generalized involvement is usually present at birth. The collodion and harlequin fetuses are severe examples of ichthyosis in which an infant with grotesque deformities, often resulting in death, is born encased in a horny sheet. Genetic defects have been discovered in many forms of ichthyosis.[79-81]

The many forms of epidermolysis bullosa are characterized by extensive blistering that can contribute to excessive fluid loss or predispose to scarring, deformities, and fatal neonatal infection. The dystrophic and letalis forms of the disease can be distinguished from the less severe simplex form by using electron microscopy or immunofluorescent staining of BMZ antigens to determine the level of blistering in the skin.[82] DNA-based prenatal diagnosis also has been used.[83]

Psoriasis

Psoriasis is a papulosquamous skin condition found in 1% to 3% of the population.[84] It is usually mild but sometimes can become severe, generalized, or associated with psoriatic arthritis. The pustular form of psoriasis was discussed earlier in the section on impetigo herpetiformis. In one study, psoriasis remained unchanged during pregnancy in 43% of patients, improved in 41%, and worsened in 14%. In the postpartum period, it remained unchanged in 37%, improved in 11%, and worsened in 49%.[85]

Psoriasis in pregnancy is commonly treated with topical corticosteroids (mostly category C agents). Low-potency hydrocortisone is used commonly on delicate skin areas such as the face and intertriginous areas, and medium-potency triamcinolone is used on most other areas. The topical vitamin D derivative calcipotriene (Dovonex, category C) has not been evaluated during pregnancy or lactation, and use of large quantities can result in hypercalcemia. The topical retinoid tazarotene is a category X agent. For severe disease, oral cyclosporin (category C) has been used without an apparent increase in problems. Ultraviolet B light therapy is safe in pregnancy. Oral psoralen combined with ultraviolet A light (PUVA) has a category C designation. The oral retinoid acitretin and the antimetabolite methotrexate are both category X drugs and should not be used during pregnancy.

References

1. Kumari R, Jaisankar TJ, Thappa DM: A clinical study of skin changes in pregnancy. Indian J Dermatol Venereol Leprol 73:141, 2007.
2. Nussbaum R, Benedetto AV: Cosmetic aspects of pregnancy. Clin Dermatol 24:133, 2006.
3. Amichai B, Grunwald MH: Pigmentary demarcation lines of pregnancy. Eur J Obstet Gynecol Reprod Biol 131:239, 2007.
4. Im S, Kim J, On WY, et al: Increased expression of alpha-melanocyte-stimulating hormone in the lesional skin of melasma. Br J Dermatol 146:165, 2002.
5. Gupta AK, Gover MD, Nouri K, et al: The treatment of melasma: A review of clinical trials. J Am Acad Dermatol 55:1048, 2006.
6. Katz VL, Farmer RM, Dotters D: Focus on primary care: from nevus to neoplasm: Myths of melanoma in pregnancy. Obstet Gynecol Surv 57:112, 2002.
7. Gormley DE: Cutaneous surgery and the pregnant patient. J Am Acad Dermatol 23:269, 1990.
8. Demir Y, Demir S, Aktepe F: Cutaneous lobular capillary hemangioma induced by pregnancy. J Cutan Pathol 31:77, 2004.
9. Sills ES, Zegarelli DJ, Hoschander MM, et al: Clinical diagnosis and management of hormonally responsive oral pregnancy tumor (pyogenic granuloma). J Reprod Med 41:467, 1996.
10. Yuan K, Lin MT: The roles of vascular endothelial growth factor and angiopoietin-2 in the regression of pregnancy pyogenic granuloma. Oral Dis 10:179, 2004.
11. Yuan K, Wing LY, Lin MT: Pathogenetic roles of angiogenic factors in pyogenic granulomas in pregnancy are modulated by female sex hormones. J Periodontol 73:701, 2002.
12. Torgerson RR, Marnach ML, Bruce AJ, et al: Oral and vulvar changes in pregnancy. Clin Dermatol 24:122, 2006.
13. Morris LF, Rapini RP, Hebert AA, et al: Massive labial edema in pregnancy. South Med J 83:846, 1990.
14. Atwal GSS, Manku LK, Griffiths CEM, et al: Striae gravidarum in primiparae. Br J Dermatol 155:965, 2006.
15. Ghasemi A, Gorouhi F, Rashighi-Firoozabadi M, et al: Striae gravidarum: Associated factors. J Eur Acad Dermatol Venereol 21:743, 2007.
16. Osman H, Rubeiz N, Tamim H, et al: Risk factors for the development of striae gravidarum. Am J Obstet Gynecol 196:62, 2007.
17. Salter SA, Batra RS, Rohrer TE, et al: Striae and pelvic relaxation: Two disorders of connective tissue with a strong association. J Invest Dermatol 126:1688, 2006.
18. Salter SA, Kimball AB: Striae gravidarum. Clin Dermatol 24:97, 2006.
19. Millikan L: Hirsutism, postpartum telogen effluvium, and male pattern alopecia. J Cosmet Dermatol 5:81, 2006.
20. Black MM, McKay M, Braude PR, et al: Obstetric and Gynecologic Dermatology, 2nd ed. London, Mosby, 2002.
21. Kroumpouzos G, Cohen LM: Specific dermatoses of pregnancy: An evidence-based systematic review. Am J Obstet Gynecol 188:1083, 2003.
22. Zoberman E, Farmer ER: Pruritic folliculitis of pregnancy. Arch Dermatol 117:20, 1981.
23. Hale EK, Pomeranz MK: Dermatologic agents during pregnancy and lactation: An update and clinical review. Int J Dermatol 41:197, 2002.
24. Weisshaar E, Diepgen TL, Luger TA, et al: Pruritus in pregnancy and childhood: Do we really consider all relevant differential diagnoses? Eur J Dermatol 15:320, 2005.

25. Dann AT, Kenyon AP, Seed PT, et al: Glutathione *S*-transferase and liver function in intrahepatic cholestasis of pregnancy and pruritus gravidarum. Hepatology 40:1406, 2004.
26. Kenyon AP, Piercy CN, Girling J, et al: Pruritus may precede abnormal liver function tests in pregnant women with obstetric cholestasis: A longitudinal analysis. BJOG 108:1190, 2001.
27. Sheiner E, Ohel I, Levy A, et al: Pregnancy outcome in women with pruritus gravidarum. J Reprod Med 51:394, 2006.
28. Burrows RF, Clavisi O, Burrows E: Interventions for treating cholestasis in pregnancy. Cochrane Database Syst Rev (4):CD000493, 2001.
29. Tunzi M, Gray GR: Common skin conditions during pregnancy. Am Fam Physician 75:211, 2007.
30. Lawley TJ, Hertz KC, Wade TR, et al: Pruritic urticarial papules and plaques of pregnancy. JAMA 241:1696, 1979.
31. Bourne G: Toxaemic rash of pregnancy. J R Soc Med 55:462, 1962.
32. Nurse DS: Prurigo of pregnancy. Australas J Dermatol 9:258, 1968.
33. Buccolo LS, Viera AJ. Pruritic urticarial papules and plaques of pregnancy presenting in the postpartum period: A case report. J Reprod Med 50:61, 2005.
34. Vaughan Jones SA, Hern S, Nelson-Piercy C, et al: A prospective study of 200 women with dermatoses of pregnancy correlating clinical findings with hormonal and immunopathological profiles. Br J Dermatol 141:71, 1999.
35. Ohel I, Levy A, Silberstein T, et al: Pregnancy outcome of patients with pruritic urticarial papules and plaques of pregnancy. J Matern Fetal Neonatal Med 19:305, 2006.
36. Rudolph CM, Al-Fares S, Vaughan-Jones SA, et al: Polymorphic eruption of pregnancy: Clinicopathology and potential trigger factors in 181 patients. Br J Dermatol 154:54, 2006.
37. Ambros-Rudolph CM, Mullegger RR, Vaughan-Jones SA, et al: The specific dermatoses of pregnancy revisited and reclassified: Results of a retrospective two-center study on 505 pregnant patients. J Am Acad Dermatol 54:395, 2006.
38. Spangler AS, Reddy W, Bardawil WA, et al: Papular dermatitis of pregnancy: A new clinical entity? JAMA 181:577, 1962.
39. Castro LA, Lundell RB, Kraus PK, et al: Clinical experience in pemphigoid gestationis: Report of 10 cases. J Am Acad Dermatol 55:823, 2006.
40. Al-Fouzan AW, Galadari I, Oumeish I, et al: Herpes gestationis (pemphigoid gestationis). Clin Dermatol 24:109, 2006.
41. Shornick JK, Black MM: Fetal risks in herpes gestationis. J Am Acad Dermatol 26:63, 1992.
42. Mascaro JM Jr, Lecha M, Mascaro JM: Fetal morbidity in herpes gestationis. Arch Dermatol 131:1209, 1995.
43. Black MM, Stephens CJ: The specific dermatoses of pregnancy: The British perspective. Adv Dermatol 7:105-126, 1992.
44. Powell AM, Sakuma-Oyama Y, Oyama N, et al: Usefulness of BP180 NC16a enzyme-linked immunosorbent assay in the serodiagnosis of pemphigoid gestationis and in differentiating between pemphigoid gestationis and pruritic urticarial papules and plaques of pregnancy. Arch Dermatol. 2005 141:705, 2005.
45. Sitaru C, Powell J, Messer G: Immunoblotting and enzyme-linked immunosorbent assay for the diagnosis of pemphigoid gestationis. Obstet Gynecol 103:757, 2004.
46. Shornick JK: Herpes gestationis. Dermatol Clin 11:527, 1993.
47. Dokart L, Harter M, Snyder M: Pemphigoid gestationis: Report of a case with umbilical artery Doppler assessment. J Reprod Med 51:591,2006.
48. Loo WJ, Dean D, Wojnarowska F: A severe persistent case of pemphigoid gestationis successfully treated with minocycline and nicotinamide. Clin Exp Dermatol 26:726, 2001.
49. Rodrigues Cdos S, Filipe P, Solana Mdel M, et al: Persistent herpes gestationis treated with high-dose intravenous immunoglobulin. Acta Derm Venereol 87:184, 2007.
50. Oumeish OY, Parish JL: Impetigo herpetiformis. Clin Dermatol 24:101, 2006.
51. Wolf Y, Groutz A, Walman I, et al: Impetigo herpetiformis during pregnancy: Case report and review of the literature. Acta Obstet Gynecol Scand 74:229, 1995.
52. Imai N, Watanabe R, Fujiwara H, et al: Successful treatment of impetigo herpetiformis with oral cyclosporine during pregnancy. Arch Dermatol 138:128, 2002.
53. Cocuroccia B, Gisondi P, Gubinelli E, et al: Autoimmune progesterone dermatitis. Gynecol Endocrinol 22:54, 2006.
54. Shelley WB, Shelley ED, Talanin NY, et al: Estrogen dermatitis. J Am Acad Dermatol 32:25, 1995.
55. Stranahan D, Rausch D, Deng A, et al: The role of intradermal skin testing and patch testing in the diagnosis of autoimmune progesterone dermatitis. Dermatitis 17:39, 2006.
56. Vasconcelos C, Xavier P, Vieira AP, et al: Autoimmune progesterone urticaria. Gynecol Endocrinol 14:245, 2000.
57. O'Rourke J, Khawaja N, Loughrey J, et al: Autoimmune progesterone dermatitis in a parturient for emergency caesarean section. Int J Obstet Anesth 13:275, 2005.
58. Oumeish OY, Al-Fouzan AW: Miscellaneous diseases affected by pregnancy. Clin Dermatol 24:113, 2006.
59. Winton GB: Skin diseases aggravated by pregnancy. J Am Acad Dermatol 20:1, 1989.
60. Seeger JD, Lanza LL, West WA, et al: Pregnancy and pregnancy outcome among women with inflammatory skin diseases. Dermatology 214:32, 2007.
61. Black MM: Prurigo of pregnancy, papular dermatitis of pregnancy, and pruritic folliculitis of pregnancy. Semin Dermatol 8:23-5, 1989.
62. Al Hammadi A, Al-Haddab M, Sasseville D: Dermatologic treatment during pregnancy: Practical overview. J Cutan Med Surg 10:183, 2006.
63. Weatherhead S, Robson SC, Reynolds NJ: Eczema in pregnancy. BMJ 335:152, 2007.
64. Kemmett D, Tidman MJ: The influence of the menstrual cycle and pregnancy on atopic dermatitis. Br J Dermatol 125:59, 1991.
65. Kramer MS: Maternal antigen avoidance during lactation for preventing atopic eczema in infants. Cochrane Database Syst Rev (2):CD000131, 2000.
66. Herrmann M-E, Dannemann A, Gruters A, et al: Prospective study on the atopy preventive effect of maternal avoidance of milk and eggs during pregnancy and lactation. Eur J Pediatr 155:770, 1996.
67. Leadbitter P, Pearce N, Cheng S, et al: Relationship between fetal growth and the development of asthma and atopy in childhood. Thorax 54:905, 1999.
68. Olesen AB, Ellingsen AR, Olesen H, et al: Atopic dermatitis and birth factors: Historical follow up by record linkage. BMJ 314:1003, 1997.
69. Xu B, Jarvelin MR, Pekkanen J: Prenatal factors and occurrence of rhinitis and eczema among offspring. Eur J Allergy Clin Immunol 54:829, 1999.
70. Schafer T, Dirschedl P, Kunz B, et al: Maternal smoking during pregnancy and lactation increases the risk for atopic eczema in the offspring. J Am Acad Dermatol 36:550, 1997.
71. Arsura EL, Kilgore WB, Ratnayake SN: Erythema nodosum in pregnant patients with coccidioidomycosis. Clin Infect Dis 27:1201, 1998.
72. Brodell RT, Mehrabi D: Underlying causes of erythema nodosum. Lesions may provide clue to systemic disease. Postgrad Med 108:147, 2000.
73. Coaccioli S, Donati L, Di Cato L, et al: Onset of erythema nodosum during pregnancy: A case report. Clin Exp Obstet Gynecol 25:50, 1998.
74. Buckshee K, Chadha S: Post-tonsillitic erythema nodosum in pregnancy. Int J Gynaecol Obstet 55:293, 1996.
75. Ghislain PD, van Der Endt JD, Delescluse J: Itchy papules of the axillae. Arch Dermatol 138:259, 2002.
76. Elias S, Emerson DS, Simpson JL, et al: Ultrasound-guided fetal skin sampling for prenatal diagnosis of genodermatoses. Obstet Gynecol 83:337, 1994.
77. Fassihi H, Eady RA, Mellerio JE, et al: Prenatal diagnosis for severe inherited skin disorders: 25 years' experience. Br J Dermatol 154:106, 2006.
78. Holbrook KA, Smith LT, Elias S: Prenatal diagnosis of genetic skin disease using fetal skin biopsy samples. Arch Dermatol 129:1437, 1993.
79. Bichakjian CK, Nair RP, Wu WW, et al: Prenatal exclusion of lamellar ichthyosis based on identification of two new mutations in the transglutaminase 1 gene. J Invest Dermatol 110:179, 1998.

80. Di Mario M, Ferrari A, Morales V, et al: Antenatal molecular diagnosis of X-linked ichthyosis by maternal serum screening for Down's syndrome. Gynecol Obstet Invest 45:277, 1998.
81. Bitoun E, Bodemer C, Amiel J, et al: Prenatal diagnosis of a lethal form of Netherton syndrome by SPINK5 mutation analysis. Prenat Diagn 22:121, 2002.
82. Shimizu H: Prenatal diagnosis of epidermolysis bullosa. Prenat Diagn 26:1260, 2006.
83. Pfendner EG, Nakano A, Pulkkinen L, et al: Prenatal diagnosis for epidermolysis bullosa: A study of 144 consecutive pregnancies at risk. Prenat Diagn 23:447, 2003.
84. Weatherhead S, Robson SC, Reynolds NJ: Management of psoriasis in pregnancy. BMJ 334:1218, 2007.
85. Dunna SF, Finlay AY: Psoriasis: Improvement during and worsening after pregnancy. Br J Dermatol 120:584, 1989.

Chapter 55

Benign Gynecologic Conditions in Pregnancy

Alessandro Ghidini, MD, and Patrizia Vergani, MD

Pathologies involving the genital organs are often detected for the first time during pregnancy because of the closer clinical and ultrasonographic surveillance that is usually instituted during gestation. Diagnosis of uterine or ovarian pathology, although benign in nature, can engender concern among the affected women and health care providers. When such pathologies are diagnosed before pregnancy, providers must carefully weigh the risks and benefits of interventions (e.g., surgical removal of myomas) before attempting conception.

Uterine Leiomyomas

Epidemiology

Leiomyomas are the most common uterine solid masses. Their prevalence ranges between 1.6% and 4%, according to series that used routine ultrasound screening in cohorts of women who presented for prenatal care.[1,2] The prevalence of leiomyomas primarily correlates to maternal age and African-American ethnicity.[3,4] Reported associations between leiomyomas and other risk factors, such as tobacco use, parity, history of diabetes mellitus, or chronic hypertension, are possibly mediated by the confounding effects of race and age.

Pathogenesis

Effect of Pregnancy on Myomas

It has been hypothesized that several changes in the myometrium associated with pregnancy can affect the size of uterine myomas, including hypertrophy, edema, stretching of the myometrium due to progressive expansion of the amniotic cavity, and degenerative changes related to ischemia. Whereas approximately 40% (range, 25% to 60%) of myomas remain stable in size during pregnancy, the remaining myomas demonstrate an increase or decrease by more than 10% of the original size. One third of myomas larger than 5 cm grow during pregnancy, in contrast to less than 10% of myomas smaller than 5 cm.[1] An increase in size occurs most commonly in the first trimester, independent of the original size of the myoma.[5-7] This may be related to the effect of the hormone human chorionic gonadotropin (hCG), receptors for which have been found in leiomyoma cells.[8] Rapid growth of the myoma does not suggest an underlying sarcoma, because most leiomyosarcomas occur in women beyond reproductive years and they originate from myometrial cells outside of myomas.[9]

Effects of Myomas on Pregnancy

Conflicting evidence has associated the presence of myomas with increased rates of infertility and obstetric complications, including spontaneous abortion, preterm delivery, placental abruption, fetal growth restriction, and malpresentation. The most reliable conclusions are derived from prospective cohort studies of women in whom myomas are detected at routine ultrasound screening in early pregnancy, allowing inclusion of asymptomatic women and of myomas of any size. Not surprisingly, the frequency of myoma-related obstetric complications is generally lower among cohorts of women identified with myomas at ultrasonographic screening than from series derived from referral radiology centers or registries of hospital admissions during pregnancy, with the inherent potential biases associated with the latter reports.

Several mechanisms have been suggested to explain the association between uterine fibroids and pregnancy complications:

- A large submucous fibroid projecting into the uterine cavity may lead to spontaneous pregnancy loss by disturbing perfusion of the endometrium at the site of blastocyst implantation, or it may interfere with normal placentation and development of the uteroplacental circulation.[10]
- Rapid fibroid growth may lead to increased uterine contractility or decreased placental oxytocinase activity,[10] both of which may disrupt placentation, or may result in a localized increase in oxytocin levels and preterm contractions
- As blood flow has been shown to be reduced within fibroids and the adjacent myometrium, it has been hypothesized that myomas may cause placental ischemia and decidual necrosis, which may lead to abruption.[11]
- Large myomas distorting the shape of the uterine cavity may cause fetal malpresentation and placenta previa.
- By decreasing the force and coordination of uterine contractions, fibroids may predispose to postpartum hemorrhage and uterine atony.[12]

INFERTILITY

There are no randomized, controlled trials testing the benefit of pre-conceptual removal of myomas on fertility. Case series have reported an improved conception rate after removal of myomas, suggesting that myomas may be associated with infertility.[13] A meta-analysis has shown that in infertile women with no identifiable infertility factors, submucous myomas are associated with lower pregnancy rates compared with infertile women without myomas (relative risk [RR] = 0.32; 95% confidence interval [CI], 0.13 to 0.70), whereas there was no effect of intramural or subserosal myomas.[14] However, subsequent retrospective and prospective observational studies have suggested that subserosal or intramural myomas without intracavitary involvement also may affect fertility.[15]

SPONTANEOUS ABORTION

Although most reviews on the effects of myomas on pregnancy quote an increased risk of miscarriage associated with myomas, the supporting evidence is scant and mostly based on case series often biased by a retrospective design, a lack of control groups, and the presence of multiple confounders. Although studies using control populations have found increased rates of threatened abortion in women with myomas compared with controls without myomas,[2] no significant differences have been reported in rates of first-trimester losses,[2,16] even in women with a history of miscarriages. The largest study found significantly increased rates of miscarriage among women with myomas compared with controls (14% versus 8%) had significantly higher rates of assisted reproductive techniques among women with myomas (15% versus 6%), an important confounder.[17] There is no conclusive evidence that number, size, or location of myomas influences rates of spontaneous abortions.

FETAL DEATH

In one small study with design limitations, the rate of second-trimester losses was significantly higher before than after myomectomy (7 of 14 versus 0 of 6; $P = .04$).[18] Another study found increased rates of second-trimester fetal losses between 18 and 23 weeks' gestation in two groups of 128 women with myomas undergoing (group 1) or not (group 2) genetic amniocentesis compared with controls without myomas (group 3) undergoing amniocentesis that were matched for maternal age, nulliparity, prior abortion or preterm birth, and gestational age at amniocentesis or sonogram (6%, 7%, and 1%, respectively; $P = .02$).[19] Although the investigators concluded that the presence of myomas increases the risk of second-trimester fetal losses, the strength of the conclusions is weakened by several biases, such as lack of information on the criteria for the choice of controls and on the indications for sonogram or amniocentesis.

PRETERM DELIVERY

Women with myomas seem to have higher rates of hospital admissions for preterm labor,[2,11,20] and the risk of preterm uterine activity has been correlated with the size of the myoma.[2,11] It is controversial, however, whether this increase in uterine contractility leads to higher rates of preterm delivery. After exclusion of series without control groups, only a few studies have dealt with the risk of preterm delivery for women with myomas (Table 55-1). The three series that observed a significant increase in risk for preterm delivery in the presence of myomas deserve special comment. Two of them[4,21] used the hospital discharge diagnosis of myoma to identify cases, a design prone to potential ascertainment biases. In the third series, logistic regression analysis demonstrated that presence of uterine myomas remained significantly associated with risk of preterm delivery after controlling for several potential confounders, including maternal age, body mass index, race, parity, insurance status, diabetes, and chronic hypertension (odds ratio [OR] = 1.4; 95% CI, 1.1 to 2.0).[3] However, the study showed no correlation between the number of myomas or myoma size and the risk of preterm delivery. In a later series of almost 25,000 women, no association was reported between presence of myomas larger than 5 cm and preterm delivery compared with women without myomas (7.6% versus 7.3%).[22]

PLACENTAL ABRUPTION

An increased rate of placental abruption has been described among women with myomas admitted to antepartum hospital care compared with those without myomas (10 [11%] of 93 versus 48 [0.7%] of 6613).[11] The study authors found that the risk of abruption was associated with myomas larger than 3 cm in diameter and with those with a retroplacental location. Similarly, Coronado and colleagues,[4] using hospital ICD9 codes and multivariate analysis to control for confounders, found that a diagnosis of abruption was significantly associated with a code for myomas compared with the absence of such a code (OR = 3.8; 95% CI, 1.6 to 9.2). Sheiner and associates,[21] using a similar design, found an odds ratio of 2.6 (95% CI, 1.6 to 4.2) for abruption in the presence of myomas. A subsequent large cohort study in which abruption was defined as placental separation at ultrasonographic examination or based on histopathologic placental examination, with or without vaginal bleeding or fetal compromise, confirmed an association between abruption and myomas (7.5% versus 0.9%) and reported that abruption was more common with large than small myomas and with submucosal myomas than myomas in other locations.[2]

TABLE 55-1 PRETERM DELIVERY IN WOMEN WITH MYOMAS

Study	Definition of PTD	Type of Study	Myomas	No Myomas	OR (95% CI)
Rice et al, 1989[11,‡]	<36 wk	Cohort	12% (11/93)	7% (440/6613)	1.9 (1.0-3.5)
Davis et al, 1990[19,*]	<37 wk	Case-control	12% (10/85)	6% (5/85)	2.1 (0.7-6.2)
Exacoustos and Rosati, 1993[2,*]	<37 wk	Cohort	9% (46/492)	9% (1099/12,216)	1.0 (0.8-1.4)
Vergani et al, 1994[22,*]	<37 wk	Cohort	10% (16/167)	10% (537/5595)	1.0 (0.6-1.7)
Coronado et al, 2000[4,†]	<38 wk	Case-control	12% (242/2065)	8% (305/4,243)	1.7 (1.4-2.0)
Sheiner et al, 2004[20,†]	<2500 g	Cohort	15% (101/690)	8% (7845/105,219)	2.1 (1.7-2.6)
Qidwai et al, 2006[3,*]	<37 wk	Cohort	19% (77/401)	13% (1867/14,703)	1.6 (1.3-2.1)

*Cases identified with ultrasonography.
†Cases identified using hospital discharge codes (ICD9) after delivery.
‡Cases identified from database of antepartum admissions.
CI, confidence interval; OR, odds ratio; PTD, preterm delivery.

At variance with these findings, two large cohort studies of myomas detected prospectively at ultrasonography[3,23] found no significant association between presence of myomas and occurrence of abruption (Vergani and colleagues[23]: 1.2% versus 0.4%; Qidwai and coworkers[3]: 2.2% versus 1.8%). Moreover, a case-control study of myomas larger than 5 cm detected prospectively at routine sonographic screening found no significant association between myomas and abruption.[22] Another case-control study found no association between abruption and retroplacental location of myomas.[20] In summary, there is conflicting evidence about a possible association between myomas and abruption.

PLACENTA PREVIA

Presence of uterine myomas may facilitate an abnormally low placental implantation. A large sonographic series of almost 15,000 women found significantly higher rates of placenta previa among patients with myomas (3.5% versus 1.8%), and a trend was identified between myoma size (≥10 cm) and risk of placenta previa.[3] In line with these findings, a cohort of almost 25,000 women undergoing sonographic screening reported significantly higher rates of placenta previa among women with myomas larger than 5 cm in diameter than among those without myomas (2.4% versus 0.6%).[22] Unlike size, the number of myomas does not seem to correlate with occurrence of placenta previa.[3]

FETAL MALPRESENTATION

A significant association (odds ratios of 1.6 to 4.0) between myomas and fetal malpresentation has been reported in large, prospective series in which multivariate analysis was used to control for confounders, including gestational age and parity.[3,4,22] Size of the myoma plays an important role. One series reported significantly higher rates of malpresentation at term in women with myomas larger than 5 cm than in controls without myomas (12% versus 5%).[22] Other investigators found a progressive increase in rates of malpresentation with myoma size: 8% in women without myomas, 10% in those with myomas smaller than 10 cm, and up to 23% in those with myomas larger than 10 cm.[3] Unlike myoma size, the number of myomas does not seem to affect the risk of fetal malpresentation.[3]

LABOR COMPLICATIONS

A large series using ICD9 codes found increased rates of labor complications (OR = 1.9; 95% CI, 1.6 to 2.2) in women with leiomyomas after controlling for maternal age, parity, and previous cesarean delivery.[4] Labor complications were mainly limited to dysfunctional labor (OR = 1.8; 95% CI, 1.3 to 2.7), because rates of prolonged labor were not significantly different between the two groups.[4] However, a large cohort of cases with myomas diagnosed prospectively at the second-trimester sonographic screening did not find an association between presence of myomas and duration of first or second stage of labor.[3] That leiomyomas do not disrupt uterine contractility is further supported by the observation that even women with large tumors (≥10 cm) have similar durations of first and second stage of labor and similar rates of cesarean delivery among labor-eligible women as women with small myomas.[3] Similar rates of cesarean delivery for dystocia (OR = 1.1; 95% CI, 0.4 to 2.3) and fetal distress (OR = 0.9; 95% CI 0.3 to 1.9) have been reported for women with myomas larger than 5 cm compared with those without myomas.[22] In summary, women with leiomyomas of any size can be reassured that if they are eligible for vaginal delivery and they initiate labor, they can expect similar rates of vaginal delivery as the general obstetric population.

CESAREAN SECTION

An increased rate of cesarean delivery is the obstetric complication most frequently observed for women with leiomyomas.[2,11,23,24] Consistent and cumulative evidence suggests that malpresentation,[3,4,21] placenta previa,[3,4,21] and location of the tumors in the lower uterine segment below the presenting fetal part[21] are the most common indications for cesarean delivery in women with leiomyomas. However, presence of leiomyomas remains significantly associated with increased risk for cesarean delivery before labor, even after correcting for these indications.[22]

POSTPARTUM HEMORRHAGE

Although one report[4] using ICD9 discharge codes found no relation between myomas and postpartum hemorrhage, more robust studies have reported an increased risk.[3,22,25] Size of myomas does not seem to play a role in the risk, because women with myomas 10 cm or larger have rates of postpartum hemorrhage similar to rates for those with smaller myomas.[3]

PERINATAL OUTCOME

Women with myomas can be reassured that adverse perinatal outcomes (i.e., neonatal death, small size for gestational age, low Apgar scores, and malformations) are not affected by the presence of uterine myomas.[2,4,11,22,23,26] The purported fetal compression syndrome, caused by the pressure effects of large myomas on fetal parts, is limited to isolated case reports, such as one in which a fetus born with severe oligohydramnios and fetal growth restriction had dolichocephaly, which the study authors ascribed to the presence of a large myoma.[27]

Diagnosis

Ultrasonographic diagnosis of leiomyoma rests on visualization of persistent, hypoechoic, spherical masses distorting the myometrial contour. When located within the myometrium, they should be differentiated from focal myometrial contractions, which tend to disappear during the examination or at follow-up scans. The hypoechoic sonographic appearance of leiomyomas may change when the masses undergo degeneration, which may lead to the appearance of cystic spaces or a coarse heterogeneous pattern consisting of hyperechogenic clusters within the myomas (Fig. 55-1). In such cases, myomas may have a worrisome appearance, and they can be mistaken for ovarian neoplasms or other intra-abdominal masses. When in doubt, magnetic resonance imaging (MRI) may help to confirm the diagnosis of a large, degenerating leiomyoma.[28] Pedunculated myomas can be differentiated from other pelvic masses by visualization of the blood supply by using color flow mapping (Fig. 55-2).

Myomas are often classified on the basis of their location in relation to the uterine cavity (i.e., submucosal if they distort the uterine cavity, intramural if they are predominantly located within the myometrial layer, and subserosal if they predominantly protrude out of the serosal surface of the uterus); in relation to the anatomic location within the uterus (i.e., fundal, corporal, isthmic, or cervical); and in relation to the placental insertion site (i.e., retroplacental or not). Such classifications are often difficult to apply in pregnancy because of uterine enlargement. Moreover, the location of a myoma can change during pregnancy because of changes in uterine size, so-called placental migration, and development of the lower uterine segment. Despite these difficulties, several series have attempted to correlate the location of myomas with the subsequent occurrence of pregnancy complications. The evidence for such associations is discussed subsequently.

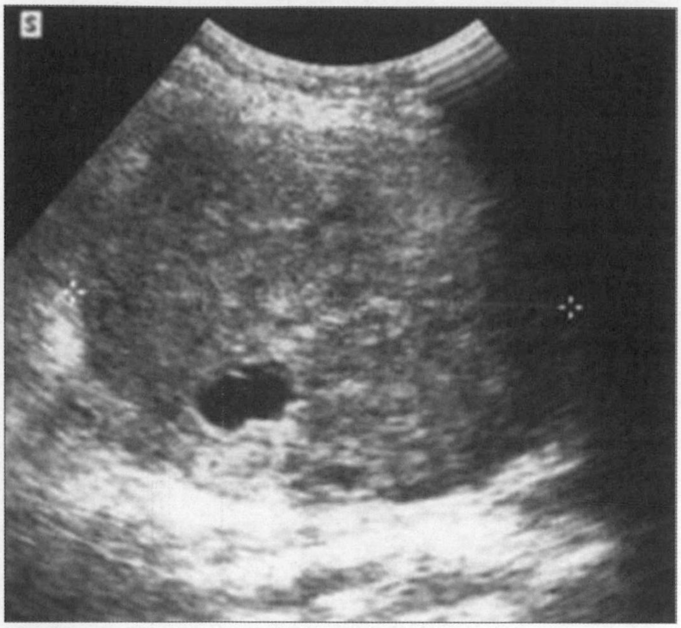

FIGURE 55-1 Degenerated myoma. Degenerated myomas have a heterogeneous echogenic pattern, with hypoechoic and hyperechogenic areas seen within the myoma.

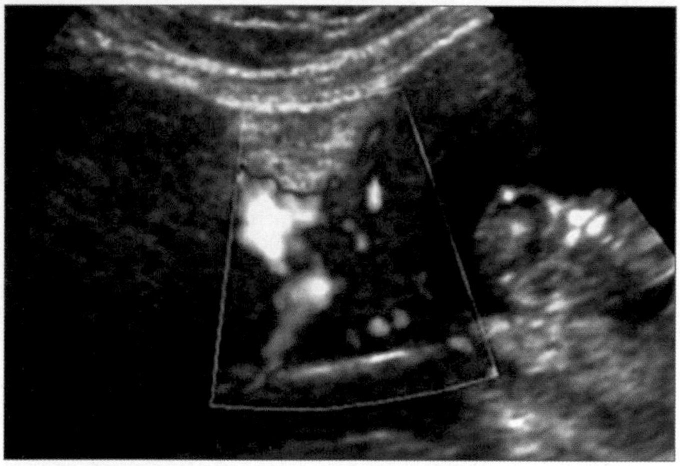

FIGURE 55-2 Pedunculated myoma. The arterial blood supply from the uterus can be demonstrated using color flow mapping.

Management

Fertility

A meta-analysis has shown that in infertile women with no identifiable infertility factors and submucous myomas, resection of the submucous myomas is followed by increased fertility rates (RR = 1.72; 95% CI, 1.13 to 2.58),[14] suggesting that resection of submucous myomas may be a treatment for infertility in selected cases.[15] Moreover, women with infertility due to submucous myomas who conceive spontaneously after myoma resection have higher pregnancy rates than those who conceive with assisted reproductive techniques.[14] Retrospective and prospective observational studies have suggested that subserosal or intramural myomas without intracavitary involvement may affect fertility and that myoma resection in such cases may improve fertility.[15] This hypothetical benefit must be weighed against the surgical risks to the woman, increased risks for future pregnancies due to the presence of the uterine scar, and risks of recurrence of myomas. Until randomized clinical trials demonstrate benefits from myoma resection in infertile women with intramural or subserosal myomas, the procedure should not be recommended.[15,29]

Miscarriages

Because of the known risks of myomectomy, the procedure should not be offered to women with myomas and history of miscarriages until prospective, observational studies with appropriate controls demonstrate an independent association between myomas and miscarriages and randomized, controlled trials document a beneficial effect of myoma resection on the risk for recurrent miscarriages.

Syndrome of Painful Myomas

The changes caused by large myomas during pregnancy may lead to the syndrome of painful myomas (i.e., red degeneration, carneous degeneration, hemorrhagic infarction, and aseptic necrobiosis) in less than 5% of patients.[1,30] The pathogenesis of the pain is unclear, although it has been attributed to ischemia and necrosis caused by rapid growth of the myoma outpacing its blood supply or acute disruption of the blood supply leading to hemorrhagic necrosis. The exquisite response of the myoma pain to cyclooxygenase inhibitors (i.e., indomethacin or ibuprofen) suggests that release of prostaglandins plays an important role in the genesis of the pain.

Clinically, the diagnosis should be considered if there is localized tenderness over the myoma; in rare cases, the syndrome may be associated with low-grade pyrexia, mild leukocytosis, nausea, and vomiting. The differential diagnosis is extensive because of the lack of specificity of the symptoms, and it includes appendicitis, ureteral stones and pyelonephritis, adnexal torsion, and preterm labor. Ultrasonography plays a critical role in establishing a correct diagnosis by demonstrating the topographic association between the site of pain and the myoma, as well as the presence of cystic areas related to myoma degeneration in 70% of cases. If the diagnosis is uncertain, MRI may be indicated.[31]

Experts' opinions and case series suggest that nonselective cyclooxygenase inhibitors are more effective in the treatment of myoma-related pain than standard analgesics or narcotics.[24,32] Use of indomethacin (25 mg every 6 hours) or ibuprofen (600 to 800 mg every 6 hours) usually leads to resolution of the symptoms within 48 hours. Intravenous therapy with ketoprofen (100 mg every 6 hours) is similarly useful, particularly in cases with gastrointestinal symptoms. An infected myoma (i.e., pyomyoma) is a rare cause of syndrome of painful myoma. It can be suspected in the presence of fever, moderate leukocytosis, and lack of response to appropriate medical therapy.[33-35] Most cases are associated with termination of pregnancy or occur in the puerperium. Intravenous antibiotics together with myomectomy[33,36] or hysterectomy[34] are the mainstays of therapy in such cases.

Myomectomy during Pregnancy

Myomas in pregnancy are best treated conservatively because of the risks of myomectomy in a pregnant uterus (chiefly bleeding and preterm delivery). Surgery should be reserved to cases of syndrome of painful myomas refractory to medical therapy. Because these cases are frequently related to torsion of pedunculated subserosal myomas, surgery is relatively safe and facilitated by clamping of the myoma pedicle.[37] A few small series have explored the effects of myomectomy in pregnancy for rapid myoma growth or recurrent myoma pain.[26,30,38] Their conclusions have been contradictory, with some finding improved pregnancy outcome with myomectomy, and others reporting higher rates of preterm delivery. The small sample size of the reports, with the associated lack of adequate statistical power, does not allow firm conclusions.

Cesarean Myomectomy

Occasionally, myomas need to be removed at the time of cesarean section to facilitate closure of the uterine incision or, rarely, to facilitate access to the fetus. With the exception of pedunculated myomas, which can be safely removed at the time of cesarean section, cesarean myomectomy carries significant risks of hemorrhagic complications. Bleeding significant enough to require transfusion, uterine artery ligation, embolization, or hysterectomy has been reported for an average of 11% of cases of myomectomy at cesarean section (range, 0% to 33%) in published series, with the number of cases ranging from 5 to 25.[2,37,39-43]

In light of the risk of severe bleeding, appropriate planning is desirable for women with large uterine myomas located in the anterior uterine wall or lower uterine segment, including careful ultrasound mapping of the myoma location in relation to placental insertion and fetal position before surgery and the availability of blood products and appropriate support personnel in case of complications. Extensive cesarean myomectomies with removal of many myomas should be seen as an elective procedure to be discouraged because of the risk of bleeding and the natural history of myomas, which tend to undergo involution after delivery.

Pregnancy after Myomectomy

The main concern for pregnancies after any type of myomectomy is the risk of uterine rupture before or during labor. The risk seems to depend on the location of the myoma and the type of surgery. After *laparotomic myomectomy*, the risk of uterine rupture is mainly limited to myomectomies with entry into the uterine cavity. After *laparoscopic myomectomy*, the risk of uterine rupture seems to be related to the location of the myoma and to inadequate suturing. Uterine rupture in pregnancies after *hysteroscopic myomectomy* is a rare event, and it has been reported only in cases of uterine perforation at the time of the procedure.

Particular risks may affect pregnancies after uterine artery embolization for myomas. A total of 144 pregnancies have been reported in women after uterine artery embolization, resulting in 83 deliveries.[44-46] The preterm delivery rate was 20% (17 of 83), and the average cesarean section rate was in excess of 50%. Rates of fetal growth restriction and birth weight were not consistently reported, but they did not seem to be significantly affected.[45] Several series reported occurrences of abnormal placentation (including accreta and previa) in pregnancies after uterine artery embolization, which contributed to increased rates of severe postpartum hemorrhage. Although these complications should be kept in the context of additional risk factors, including advanced maternal age, previous uterine surgeries, and presence of residual myomas, they raise serious concerns that uterine artery embolization may permanently alter myometrial function and induce changes in the uterine vasculature. Only one case of uterine rupture has been reported in a woman after uterine artery embolization, and it occurred at the scar of a previous cesarean section.[45]

In summary, the available evidence suggests that pregnancy and delivery can be achieved after uterine artery embolization in most cases, but the risks of complications, including prematurity and placental abnormalities, may be higher than expected for the general population. Because of the generally benign outcome associated with untreated myomas in pregnancy, uterine artery embolization should be proposed cautiously for women planning future pregnancies.

Adnexal Masses

The detection of ovarian cysts in pregnancy is not uncommon. Small cysts discovered in early pregnancy are often functional, and expectant management is recommended because most of them resolve spontaneously and do not pose a risk to the pregnancy. Larger or complex cysts pose more of a clinical dilemma. Although some clinicians often remove them in the second trimester because of the risk for complications, even large and complex masses may be followed expectantly if they appear to be benign.[47,48]

Epidemiology

The prevalence of adnexal masses depends on the gestational age. During the first 5 weeks of pregnancy, adnexal masses have been reported in 8.8% of women undergoing ultrasonographic examination; the rate decreases to 0.4% by 16 to 20 weeks.[47,49] Similarly, Condous and associates[50] identified ovarian cysts in 6.2% of pregnant women examined before 14 weeks.

Spontaneous resolution during pregnancy occurs for most adnexal masses.[47,50] In a series of 123 asymptomatic ovarian cysts detected at prenatal ultrasound examinations and followed conservatively, complete resolution was observed in 89% of cases, including 82% of the cysts larger than 6 cm in diameter.[51] Similarly, spontaneous resolution was reported for 72% (119 of 166) of ovarian cysts followed with ultrasonography[50] and for 69% (70 of 102) of simple or complex adnexal masses larger than 5 cm in diameter.[47] The high rate of resolution reflects the physiologic nature of most ovarian masses detected early in pregnancy; expectancy is a reasonable management option.[47,52]

Pathogenesis

The frequency and classification of persistent ovarian masses is limited to masses removed during or immediately after pregnancy, generating an inevitable bias because most ovarian masses with a benign appearance are not surgically removed. A review of the latest series reveals that three types of benign ovarian pathology account for most ovarian masses in pregnancy: corpus luteum cysts, mature teratomas, and cystoadenomas (Table 55-2).

TABLE 55-2 HISTOLOGIC PREVALENCE OF OVARIAN CYSTS IN PREGNANCY

Behavior	Type of Pathology	Frequency (%)
Benign	Corpus luteum	15-20
	Mature teratoma	7-42
	Luteoma or functional cyst	11-19
	Endometrioma	1-5
	Leiomyomas or adenofibromas	4-5
	Serous and mucinous cystoadenomas	9-16
Borderline	Borderline (serous, mucinous, other)	1-2
Malignant	Epithelial ovarian cancer, germ cell tumor, sex-cord stromal tumors	2-7

Data from references 52, 59, 82, 83.

Diagnosis

Most functional cysts are asymptomatic. Older series reported 10% to 30% rates of symptomatic or complicated adnexal masses during pregnancy. However, such series were prone to ascertainment bias because screening ultrasonography was not performed.[53,54] In one series of ovarian cysts detected during the course of ultrasonographic examination in the first trimester, the rates of complications were much lower (7 [4%] of 166).[50] The most common complications of adnexal masses in pregnancy are malignancy; torsion, rupture, or hemorrhage; and dystocia at delivery.

Malignancy

The potential for malignancy is the paramount concern for the managing clinicians. Among women of reproductive years, germ cell tumors are common in young women, whereas epithelial ovarian cancers occur more frequently in older patients. The rate of malignancy for adnexal masses identified during pregnancy is commonly reported as 2% to 3% of surgically removed ovarian masses. The largest series on the subject, involving 9375 patients with a hospital discharge diagnosis of an ovarian mass, found a 2.1% incidence of malignancy, including 87 (0.9%) ovarian cancers of various histologic types and 115 (1.2%) ovarian tumors of low malignant potential.[55]

Several algorithms have been proposed to differentiate benign from malignant ovarian tumors and to stratify the risk of malignancy using ultrasonographic characteristics.

Ultrasound Characteristics

Although malignant masses tend to be larger than benign ones, the size of an ovarian mass in pregnancy cannot be used to predict malignancy. In a case-control series, the average size of nonmalignant tumors was 7.6 cm and that of malignant neoplasms was 11.5 cm.[56] All masses smaller than 6 cm were benign.

Zanetta and colleagues[48] proposed a triage system to identify those who were candidates for expectant management (Table 55-3 and Fig. 55-3). The system was applied to 79 pregnant women with adnexal masses followed prospectively. Only pregnant patients with suspicious masses were triaged to surgical intervention at diagnosis, and women with masses of all the other categories were considered candidates for expectant management. There were no malignant tumors among the 23 women who underwent surgery because of persistent masses, torsion or rupture, or nonreassuring ultrasonographic findings, and all three borderline tumors were correctly suspected prenatally. Similarly, in a series of 131 tumors, ultrasonography accurately identified 95% of dermoid cysts, 80% of endometriomas, and 71% of simple cysts during pregnancy, and, more importantly, it correctly suspected the only case of malignancy.[52] In a case-control study of 40 patients (Table 55-4), 3 of whom had malignant neoplasms and 5 of whom had tumors of low malignant potential, a uniform cystic appearance of the tumors had high specificity, whereas the presence of internal papillary excrescences had high sensitivity for diagnosis of malignancy.[56]

Wheeler and Fleisher[57] prospectively investigated 34 ovarian masses with ultrasonography and color Doppler sonography, and compared their results with histologic diagnoses (Fig. 55-4). The mean pulsatility index in morphologically suspect areas within the tumor was significantly lower for malignant than for benign masses (0.7 [range, 0.4 to 1.3] versus 1.2 [range, 0.4 to 2.8]; $P = .03$), suggesting low impedance to flow in malignant masses. A pulsatility index less than 1.0 correctly identified three malignant ovarian lesions and five tumors of low malignant potential, with a sensitivity of 89%, positive predictive value of 42%, and negative predictive value of 93%. However, the overlap in blood flow patterns between benign and malignant tumors was such that the false-positive rate was almost 48%, causing incorrect assignment of malignant potential to some benign lesions and offering no advantage over the use of sonographic morphology indexing alone.

Other studies of nonpregnant women with ovarian masses have confirmed a partial role for Doppler sonography in differentiating benign from malignant ovarian tumors. However, the wide range in values makes the use of Doppler in differentiating benign from malignant perhaps most useful as an adjunct to morphologic assessment.

Serologic Markers

Serum tumor markers are primarily used for surveillance of known, treated ovarian malignancies, but they are of limited benefit in the initial assessment of ovarian masses. The level of cancer antigen 125 (CA 125) is elevated in 80% of women with epithelial ovarian malignancies, with mucinous adenocarcinomas being a notable exception. CA 125 has inadequate diagnostic accuracy in premenopausal women

TABLE 55-3 ULTRASONOGRAPHIC CLASSIFICATION OF OVARIAN MASSES IN PREGNANCY

Category	Sonographic Features
Simple cyst	Anechoic cyst without septa or vegetations
Endometriosis-like or corpus luteum–like	Hypoechoic content, homogeneous or trabecular, no papillae
Dermoid-like	Combination of hyperechogenic and hypoechogenic content, shadows
Complex benign	Septa, thick content but no papillae
Borderline-like	Smooth capsule, presence of intracystic papillae, absence of gross solid parts
Suspicious	Solid parts, irregular capsule or border, ascites, irregular vascularization

Modified from Zanetta G, Mariani E, Lissoni A, et al: A prospective study of the role of ultrasound in the management of adnexal masses in pregnancy. BJOG 110:578-583, 2003.

TABLE 55-4 RISK OF OVARIAN MALIGNANCIES BASED ON SONOGRAPHIC CRITERIA

Characteristic	Benign $n = 32$	Malignant $n = 8$
Morphology		
Complex	66% (21)	87% (7)
Solid	13% (4)	12% (1)
Cystic	22% (7)	0%
Discriminator		
Internal excrescences	0%	50%
Echogenic focus	3% (1)	0%
Septate	9% (3)	13% (1)

Reproduced with permission from Sherard GB, Hodson CA, Williams J, et al: Adnexal masses and pregnancy: A 12-year experience. Am J Obstet Gynecol 189:358-363, 2003.

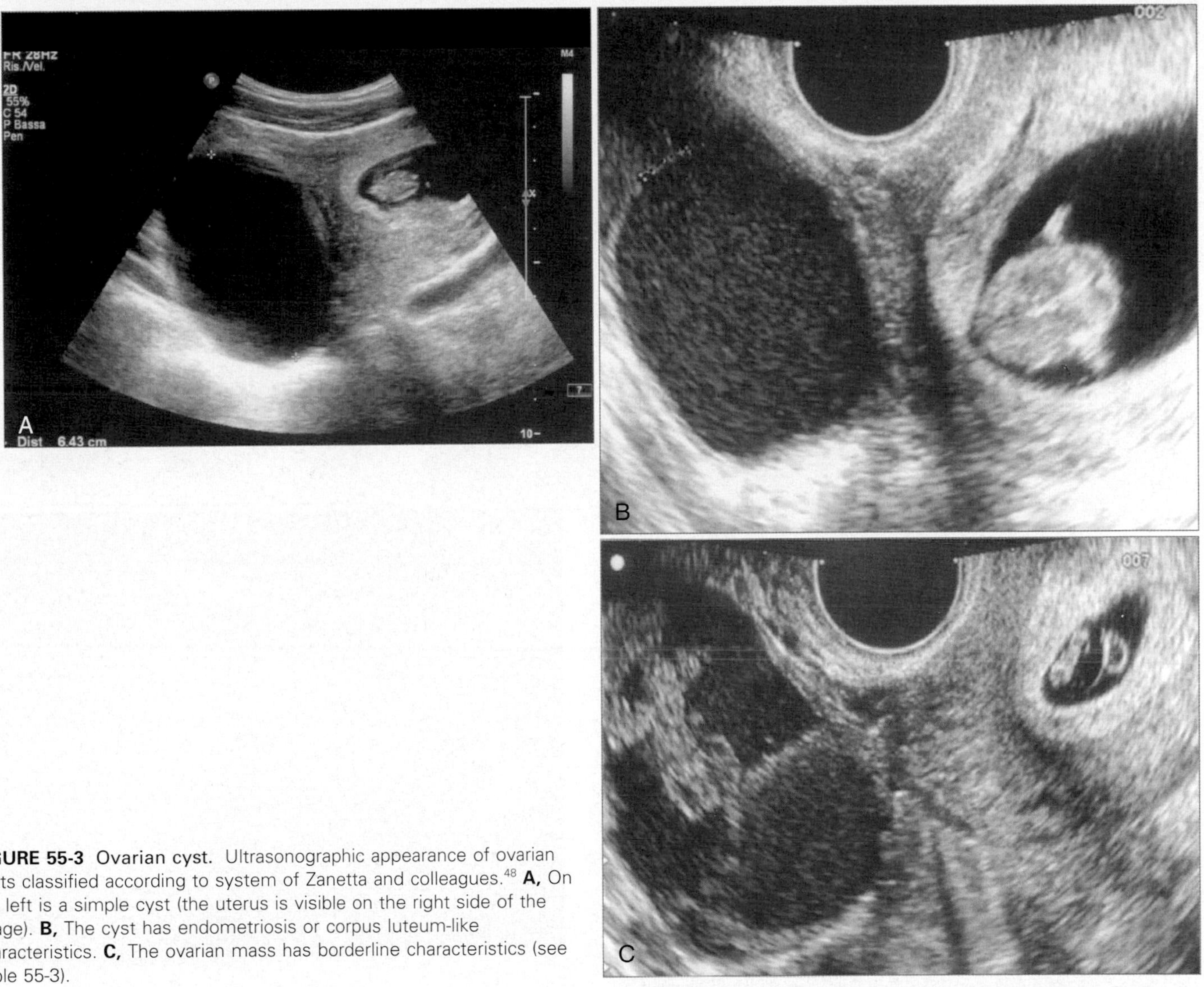

FIGURE 55-3 Ovarian cyst. Ultrasonographic appearance of ovarian cysts classified according to system of Zanetta and colleagues.[48] **A,** On the left is a simple cyst (the uterus is visible on the right side of the image). **B,** The cyst has endometriosis or corpus luteum-like characteristics. **C,** The ovarian mass has borderline characteristics (see Table 55-3).

because many benign gynecologic conditions, such as uterine fibroids, and especially pregnancy, are associated with elevated values. When elevated, the CA 125 level can provide a baseline value before treatment of ovarian cancer, but it does not help to differentiate benign from malignant masses during pregnancy.

Various other tumor markers are used to monitor germ cell tumors: α-fetoprotein (AFP) for endodermal sinus tumor, hCG for choriocarcinoma, and lactate dehydrogenase for dysgerminoma. Although germ cell tumors are among the most common ovarian malignancies seen in pregnancy, hCG and AFP have very limited use as tumor markers during pregnancy. Levels of tumor markers should be obtained before any surgical intervention when there is a suspicion of ovarian malignancy to provide a baseline value in case a malignancy is diagnosed. Any elevation in the levels of tumor markers should be considered in conjunction with the results of the imaging tests to avoid unnecessary intervention when possible.

Magnetic Resonance Imaging

MRI can be safely used during pregnancy to evaluate adnexal masses. The primary advantages of MRI are its capacity to develop three-dimensional planar images, delineate tissue planes, and characterize tissue composition. This is particularly helpful for lesions in the pelvis, where ultrasonography has a limited role in assessing the bony and muscular structures. Kier and colleagues[58] reported that MRI is a useful complement to ultrasonography for patients with adnexal masses in pregnancy. In their series of 17 patients, MRI correctly identified the cause in 17 (100%) of 17, whereas ultrasonography was accurate in 12 (71%) of 17.[58] Three patients with ultrasonographic findings of suspicious ovarian masses were found to have pedunculated uterine leiomyomas on MRI, and unnecessary surgery was avoided.

MRI can be considered as an alternate imaging strategy when the ultrasound diagnosis is uncertain, if ultrasonography raises suspicion of uterine leiomyoma or shows a solid adnexal mass, and when a radiologist experienced in interpreting MRI of adnexal masses and pregnancy is available. Both ultrasonography and MRI greatly depend on the experience of the operator.

Complications

TORSION AND RUPTURE

During pregnancy, the progressive enlargement of the uterus displaces the ovaries and fallopian tubes out of the pelvis. This phenomenon and the rapid return of these structures to their normal anatomic

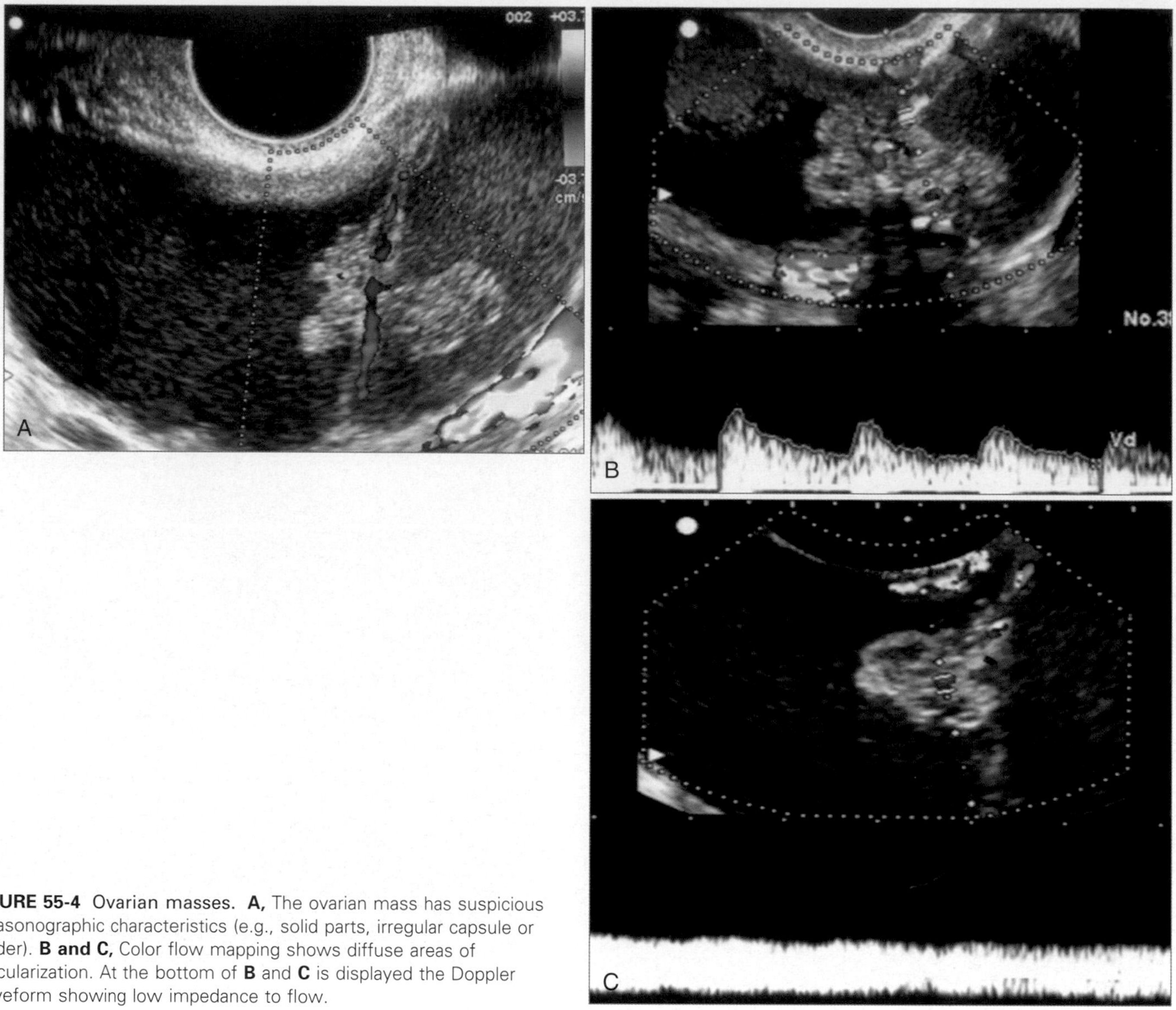

FIGURE 55-4 Ovarian masses. **A,** The ovarian mass has suspicious ultrasonographic characteristics (e.g., solid parts, irregular capsule or border). **B and C,** Color flow mapping shows diffuse areas of vascularization. At the bottom of **B** and **C** is displayed the Doppler waveform showing low impedance to flow.

location after parturition place adnexal masses at increased risk of torsion, particularly at the beginning of the second trimester and during postpartum involution. The rate of torsion in published series varies from 1% to 22%.[50,52] Rupture appears to be less common, with rates ranging from 0% to 9%.[52,59,60] Less frequent complications include bleeding and infection.

In a series of 130 women with adnexal masses, 16 required emergency laparotomy for acute abdominal pain, and 11 of 16 had documented or presumptive ovarian torsion.[59] Struyk and Treffers[60] observed a relationship between tumor size and the risk of complications; complications occurred in 35% of tumors between 5 and 6 cm in diameter and in up to 85% of larger tumors.[60] Overall, torsion occurred in 12% and rupture in 9%. A far lower rate of antepartum complications was reported by Bromley and Benacerraf[52] in a series of 131 ovarian masses among 125 pregnant women; only one patient had an ovarian torsion, and another patient underwent exploratory laparotomy. Similarly, Bernhard and coworkers[47] reported a 1% risk of torsion in their series of 102 ovarian masses; the only torsion occurred in a patient with a palpable mass.

Overall, it appears that later studies report lower risks of torsion and rupture than earlier ones. This may reflect a higher proportion of asymptomatic, ultrasound-detected ovarian masses and therefore may more accurately reflect the risk of this complication in pregnancy.

RISK OF DYSTOCIA AT DELIVERY

Obstruction of labor is a complication that can occur when large adnexal masses are lodged between the presenting fetal part and the birth canal. Obstruction of labor occurs in 2% to 17% of patients with large adnexal masses.[60,61]

Management

Optimal management of adnexal masses should be based on an accurate assessment of the risks of the complications previously outlined. Ultrasonographic criteria can successfully stratify the risk by identifying the few masses with suspicious complex features that warrant surgical management. Most masses have a benign ultrasonographic appearance, and they are suitable for conservative (expectant) management.

Surgical Management

Surgical management of adnexal masses during the first trimester should be limited to lesions with complications (i.e., torsion or rupture). Persistence of adnexal pathology during the second and third trimester may warrant intervention in if there is a strong suspicion of malignancy or large size (>6 cm) or there are symptomatic complaints. A large size may signal increased risk of torsion, rupture, or obstruction during labor. Before undergoing surgical removal, patients should be appropriately counseled about the possibility of an underlying malignancy and be prepared for possible ovarian cancer staging and related evaluation of tumor serum markers. Although the risks to mother and fetus have been substantially reduced with the improvement of anesthesia, intraoperative and postoperative care, and prenatal care, surgery during pregnancy requires a trained team of surgeons and anesthesiologists and close monitoring postoperatively.

Laparoscopy offers clear advantages to exploratory laparotomy for surgical management of adnexal masses, including less invasive surgical management and a shorter postoperative course with fewer complications.[62] Patients with an ovarian mass that is not suspected to be malignant in the first or second trimester of pregnancy potentially benefit the most by laparoscopic surgery. Sound clinical judgment is critical for patient selection, and caution is strongly advised when considering laparoscopic management of possible ovarian cancer. Although many case series proposed aspiration of simple unilocular cysts to avoid the need for major surgery, provide symptomatic relief, or allow these masses to fit into endoscopic bags, aspiration of a complex ovarian cyst runs the potential risk of malignant fluid spillage, which is associated with decreased survival.[63] Ovarian masses, especially those suspicious for cancer, should be removed intact when possible, and surgical intervention for large, complex ovarian masses should be performed by laparotomy.

Whether by laparoscopy or laparotomy, consideration can be given to ovarian cystectomy if the imaging criteria for a benign mass are met. Otherwise, oophorectomy is appropriate.

Timing of Surgery

Delaying surgery because of fear about the risks of the operation may potentially lead to increased fetal and maternal complications. Adverse fetal outcomes associated with abdominal surgery are most commonly the result of an abdominal catastrophe, such as ovarian torsion or rupture as indications for the surgery. In elective surgical cases, there seems to be no association between surgery and adverse perinatal outcome. Hess and colleagues[64] reported that patients who underwent emergency surgery because of adnexal torsion or hemorrhage had a greater incidence of abortion and preterm delivery compared with patients who underwent elective laparotomy. Elective surgical intervention is preferably timed for the second trimester, when the risk of fetal loss is minimal. Whitecar[59] found that adverse pregnancy outcomes, including preterm deliveries and fetal loss, were significantly less common if laparotomy occurred before rather than after 23 weeks' gestation (OR = 0.15; $P = .005$). Laparotomy in the third trimester was associated with a 50% risk of preterm delivery.

Other Management Considerations

If there is a risk of disrupting a corpus luteum cyst at up to 12 weeks' gestation, progesterone supplementation is indicated. The effectiveness of tocolytics for suppression of preterm delivery associated with adnexal surgery is similar to that of tocolysis administered for preterm labor. In Whitecar's series, [59] tocolytics were administered to 13 patients who had operations in the second and third trimesters; 6 of 13 had preterm deliveries, although only 2 delivered within 2 weeks of laparotomy. Given the potential for preterm delivery unresponsive to tocolysis and the negligible risks of steroids, consideration may be given to a prophylactic course of steroids for fetal maturity enhancement if the surgery is performed between 24 and 34 weeks' gestation.

Congenital Uterine Anomalies

Epidemiology

The mean overall prevalence of uterine malformations in the general population and the population of fertile women is 4.3%.[65] The mean incidence of müllerian defects in infertile patients is 3.4%, which is similar to the prevalence of 4.3% found in the general population and in fertile women. This is an indirect indication that müllerian defects have no impact on women's fertility.[65] Congenital uterine malformations complicate 1 in 594 pregnancies.[66]

Pathogenesis

Uterine malformations consist of a group of congenital anomalies of the female genital system. They are the result of disturbances in the development, formation, or fusion of the müllerian or paramesonephric ducts during fetal life. They are usually classified as six major anatomic types:

- Type I: hypoplasia or agenesis (usually with infertility)
- Type II: unicornuate uterus (i.e., normal differentiation of only one müllerian duct), often with a contralateral communicating or noncommunicating rudimentary horn
- Type III: didelphys uterus (i.e., complete failure of the müllerian ducts to fuse in the midline)
- Type IV: bicornuate uterus (i.e., two normally differentiated ducts are partially fused in the region of the fundus)
- Type V: septate uterus (i.e., failure of resorption of medial segment of the müllerian ducts)
- Type VI: arcuate uterus (i.e., minor change in the uterine cavity shape with no external dimpling)

Table 55-5 shows the prevalence of the different types of uterine anomalies.

Uterine malformations result in an abnormal uterine cavity, which is thought to impair the reproductive performance by increasing the incidence of early and late abortions, preterm deliveries, and obstetric complications. Other factors may be associated with the anatomic anomalies and may have the potential to affect pregnancy outcomes. Anomalies in uterine arterial circulation may result in uterine hypoperfusion; abnormalities in thickness of uterine walls may affect blastocyst implantation and result in poor decidualization and placentation; and associated cervical structural or functional anomalies may result in cervical incompetence. Such factors may explain why even a minor uterine anomaly, such as arcuate uterus, has been found by some investigators to result in an excess of spontaneous abortions, second-trimester losses, and preterm deliveries.[65,67] One study[68] reported significantly higher blood pressure values and higher rates of fetal growth restriction among 16 primigravidas with congenital uterine malformations compared with controls matched for parity, age and gestation, suggesting altered uteroplacental circulation in pregnancies with uterine anomalies.

Diagnosis

Diagnosis of uterine anomalies is usually made after a workup for recurrent pregnancy losses. The rates of uterine malformations in patients with recurrent pregnancy losses range from 1.8% to 37.6%,[67,69] with a mean overall rate of 12.6%.[65] Less commonly, a diagnosis of uterine anomaly is made during the course of sonographic evaluation of an ongoing pregnancy, serendipitously during the course of imaging testing, or at laparoscopy or laparotomy.

Accurate identification of the type of uterine malformation is important because each type of uterine anomaly is associated with different rates of obstetric complications.[65,67,70-72] Visualization of the uterine cavity and the fundal uterine contour is essential to differentiate uterine anomalies (e.g., between septate and bicornuate uteri). Traditionally, diagnosis rested on hysteroscopy, chromotubation, or sonohysterography for visualization of the uterine cavity and laparoscopy or laparotomy for intra-abdominal views. Three-dimensional ultrasound and saline contrast sonohysterography appear promising for reliable diagnosis and classification of congenital uterine anomalies in a noninvasive way. Although MRI is often helpful, incorrect diagnoses have been reported with the use of MRI alone, frequently mistaking a unicornuate uterus that has an associated contralateral rudimentary horn for a bicornuate or didelphic uterus. Because urinary tract anomalies occur in about 60% of congenital uterine anomalies, imaging of the urinary tract is indicated.

TABLE 55-5 UTERINE MALFORMATIONS: PREVALENCE OF THE DIFFERENT TYPES

Type of Malformation	Cases *N* (%)
Arcuate	255 (18.3)
Septate	486 (34.9)
Bicornuate	362 (26.0)
Unicornuate	134 (9.6)
Didelphys	114 (8.2)
Agenesis	40 (2.9)
Total	1392

Adapted from Grimbizis GF, Camus M, Tarlatzis BC, et al: Clinical implications of uterine malformations and hysteroscopic treatment results. Hum Reprod Update 7:161-174, 2001.

Management

Certain complications seem to be more common or unique in certain types of malformations (Table 55-6). For women with bicornuate uteri, some investigators have found poorer pregnancy outcomes when the division is partial rather than complete,[67] whereas others have been unable to confirm a difference between these two types.[72] The septate uterus has been associated with the poorest reproductive outcome, mainly because of a high rate of spontaneous abortions.[71,73-75] Didelphys, bicornuate uteri, and septate uteri are associated with rates of preterm delivery that are two to three times higher than expected in the general pregnant population.[65] Uterine rupture is a frequent complication (about 50% of cases) in pregnancies in rudimentary horns, which are frequently associated with a unicornuate uterus.[76] Although prophylactic tocolysis has been suggested for pregnancies in rudimentary horns to minimize uterine contractility and attainment of fetal viability,[76] its efficacy has not been adequately tested. A rare complication specific to uterus didelphys is hemiuterus torsion.[77]

Approaching delivery, women with uterine anomalies are at increased risk for fetal malpresentation, and fetal presentation should be verified with ultrasonography. Because major uterine anomalies (i.e., types II to IV) are associated with an increased risk for uterine rupture,[78] induction of labor should be undertaken cautiously.

Prevention

Hysteroscopic metroplasty offers the possibility of correction of the uterine cavity, mainly in cases of septate and arcuate uterus and in some cases of partial bicornuate uterus. Hysteroscopic metroplasty is associated with a significant decrease in the abortion and preterm delivery rates.[65,79,80] Transabdominal metroplasty remains the only approach in cases of bicornuate uterus.[81]

It is not known whether closer sonographic surveillance of fetal growth and mid-trimester sonographic assessment of cervical length in women with uterine anomalies may improve outcome by identification of fetal growth restriction in a timely fashion and recognition of increased risk for preterm delivery.

TABLE 55-6 PREGNANCY OUTCOMES FOR PATIENTS WITH UNTREATED UTERINE ANOMALIES

	Type of Malformation				
Feature	II Unicornuate *n* (%)	III Didelphys *n* (%)	IV Bicornuate *n* (%)	V Septate *n* (%)	VI Arcuate *n* (%)
Total patients	151	114	261	198	102
Total pregnancies	260	152	627	499	241
Ectopic pregnancies	3 (1.2)	2 (1)	2 (0.3)	3 (1)	7 (3)
Abortions	95 (37)	49 (32)	226 (36)	221 (44)	62 (26)
Preterm deliveries	42 (16)	43 (28)	144 (23)	112 (22)	18 (8)
Term deliveries	116 (45)	55 (36)	255 (41)	165 (83)	151 (63)
Live birth	141 (54)	85 (56)	346 (55)	250 (50)	159 (66)

Modified with permission from Grimbizis GF, Camus M, Tarlatzis BC, et al: Clinical implications of uterine malformations and hysteroscopic treatment results. Hum Reprod Update 7:161-174, 2001.

References

1. Strobelt N, Ghidini A, Cavallone M, et al: Natural history of uterine leiomyomas in pregnancy. J Ultrasound Med 13:399-401, 1994.
2. Exacoustos C, Rosati P: Ultrasound diagnosis of uterine myomas and complications in pregnancy. Obstet Gynecol 82:97-101, 1993.
3. Qidwai GI, Caughey AB, Jacoby AF: Obstetric outcomes in women with sonographically identified uterine leiomyomata. Obstet Gynecol 107:376, 2006.
4. Coronado GD, Marshall LM, Schwartz SM: Complication in pregnancy, labor, and delivery with uterine leiomyomas: A population-based study. Obstet Gynecol 95:764-769, 2000.
5. Lev-Toaff AS, Coleman BG, Arger PH, et al: Leiomyomas in pregnancy: Sonographic study. Radiology 164:375-377, 1987.
6. Rosati P, Exacoustos C, Mancuso S: Longitudinal evaluation of uterine myoma growth during pregnancy. J Ultrasound Med 11:511-515, 1992.
7. Aharoni A, Reiter A, Golan D, et al: Patterns of growth of uterine leiomyomas during pregnancy. A prospective longitudinal study. BJOG 95:510-513, 1988.
8. Horiuchi A, Nikaido T, Yoshizawa T, et al: HCG promotes proliferation of uterine leiomyomal cells more strongly than that of myometrial smooth muscle cells in vitro. Mol Hum Reprod 6:523-528, 2000.
9. Schwartz PE: Malignant transformation of myomas: myth or reality? Obstet Gynecol Clin North Am 33:183-198, 2006.
10. Wallach EE, Vu KK: Myomata uteri and infertility. Obstet Gynecol Clin North Am 22:791-799, 1995.
11. Rice JP, Kay HH, Mahony BS: The clinical significance of uterine leiomyomas in pregnancy. Am J Obstet Gynecol 160:1212-1216, 1989.
12. Szamatowicz J, Laudanski T, Bulkszas B, et al: Fibromyomas and uterine contraction. Acta Obstet Gynecol Scand 76:973-976, 1997.
13. Vercellini P, Maddalena S, De Giorgi O, et al: Abdominal myomectomy for infertility: A comprehensive review. Hum Reprod 13:873-879, 1998.
14. Pritts EA: Fribroids and infertility: A systematic review of the evidence. Obstet Gynecol Surv 56:483-491, 2001.
15. Klatsky PC, Tran ND, Caughey AB, et al: Fibroids and reproductive outcomes: A systematic review from conception to delivery. Am J Obstet Gynecol 198:357-366, 2008.
16. Roberts WE, Fulp KS, Morrison JC, et al: The impact of leiomyomas on pregnancy. Aust N Z Obstet Gynaecol 39:43-47, 1999.
17. Benson CB, Chow JS, Chang-Lee W, et al: Outcome of pregnancies in women with uterine leiomyomas identified by sonography in the first trimester. J Clin Ultrasound 29:261-264, 2001.
18. Li TC, Mortimer R, Cooke ID: Myomectomy: A retrospective study to examine reproductive performance before and after surgery. Hum Reprod 14:1735-1740, 1999.
19. Salvador E, Bienstock J, Blakemore KJ, et al: Leiomyomata uteri, genetic amniocentesis, and the risk of second-trimester spontaneous abortion. Am J Obstet Gynecol 186:913-915, 2002.
20. Davis JL, Ray-Mazumder S, Hobel CJ, et al: Uterine leiomyomas in pregnancy: A prospective study. Obstet Gynecol 75:41-44, 1990.
21. Sheiner E, Bashiri A, Levy A, et al: Obstetric characteristics and perinatal outcome of pregnancies with uterine leiomyomas. J Reprod Med 49:182-186, 2004.
22. Vergani P, Locatelli A, Ghidini A, et al: Large uterine leiomyomata and risk of cesarean delivery. Obstet Gynecol 109:410-414, 2007.
23. Vergani P, Ghidini A, Strobelt N, et al: Do uterine leiomyomas influence pregnancy outcome? Am J Perinatol 11:356-358, 1994.
24. Katz VL, Dotters DJ, Droegemueller W: Complications of uterine leiomyomas in pregnancy. Obstet Gynecol 73:593-596, 1989.
25. Ohkuchi A, Onagawa T, Usui R, et al: Effect of maternal age on blood loss during parturition: A retrospective multivariate analysis of 10053 cases. J Perinat Med 31:209-215, 2003.
26. Cooper NP, Okolo S: Fibroids in pregnancy—common but poorly understood. Obstet Gynecol Surv 60:132-138, 2005.
27. Chuang J, Tsai HW, Hwang JL: Fetal compression syndrome caused by myoma in pregnancy: A case report. Acta Obstet Gynecol Scand 80:472-473, 2001.
28. Chang G, Levine D: Imaging of adnexal masses of pregnancy. J Ultrasound Med 23:805-819, 2004.
29. Lefebvre G, Vilos G, Allaire C, et al, for the Clinical Practice Gynaecology Committee, Society for Obstetricians and Gynecologists of Canada: The management of uterine leiomyomas. J Obstet Gynaecol Can 25:396-418, 2003.
30. Lolis DE, Kalantaridou SN, Makrydimas G, et al: Successful myomectomy during pregnancy. Hum Reprod 18:1699-1702, 2003.
31. Birchard KR, Brown MA, Hyslop WB, et al: MRI of acute abdominal and pelvic pain in pregnant patients. AJR Am J Roentgenol 184:452-458, 2005.
32. Moyse KJ: Ultrasound diagnosis of uterine myomas and complications of pregnancy. Obstet Gynecol 82:881, 1993.
33. Grunc B, Zikulnig E, Gembruch U: Sepsis in second trimester of pregnancy due to an infected myoma. A case report and review of the literature. Fetal Diagn Ther 16:245-247, 2001.
34. Prahlow JA, Cappellari JO, Washburn SA: Uterine pyomyoma as a complication of pregnancy in an intravenous drug user. South Med J 89:892-895, 1996.
35. Tobias DH, Koeningsberg M, Kogan M, et al: Pyomyoma after uterine instrumentation. A case report. J Reprod Med 41:375-378, 1996.
36. Lee WL, Chiu LM, Wang PK, et al: Fever of unknown origin in the puerperium. A case report. J Reprod Med 43:149-152, 1998.
37. Burton CA, Grimes DA, March CM: Surgical management of leiomyomata during pregnancy. Obstet Gynecol 74:707-709, 1989.
38. Ouyang DW, Economy KE, Norwitz ER: Obstetric complications of fibroids. Obstet Gynecol Clin North Am 33:153-169, 2006.
39. Ehigiegba AE, Ande AB, Ojobo SI: Myomectomy during cesarean section. Int J Gynecol Obstet 75:21-25, 2001.
40. Buttram VC, Reiter RC: Uterine leiomyomata: Etiology, symptomatology, and management. Fertil Steril 36:433-435, 1981.
41. Hasan F, Arumugam K, Sivanesaratnam V: Uterine leiomyomata in pregnancy. Int J Obstet Gynecol 34:45-48, 1991.
42. Ortac F, Gungor M, Sommezer M: Myomectomy during cesarean section. Int J Obstet Gynecol 67:189-190, 1999.
43. Brown D, Fletcher HM, Myrie MO, et al: Caesarean myomectomy—a safe procedure. A retrospective case controlled study. J Obstet Gynaecol 19:139-141, 1999.
44. Mashburn PB, Matthews ML, Hurst BS: Uterine artery embolization as a treatment option for uterine myomas. Obstet Gynecol Clin North Am 33:125-144, 2006.
45. Walker WJ, McDowell SJ: Pregnancy after uterine artery embolization for leiomyomata: A series of 56 completed pregnancies. Am J Obstet Gynecol 195:1266-1271, 2006.
46. Kim MD, Kim NK, Kim HJ, et al: Pregnancy following uterine artery embolization with polyvinyl alcohol particles for patients with uterine fibroid or adenomyosis. Cardiovasc Intervent Radiol 28:611-615, 2005.
47. Bernhard LM, Klebba PK, Gray DL, et al: Predictors of persistence of adnexal masses in pregnancy. Obstet Gynecol 93:585-589, 1999.
48. Zanetta G, Mariani E, Lissoni A, et al: A prospective study of the role of ultrasound in the management of adnexal masses in pregnancy. BJOG 110:578-583, 2003.
49. Lavery JP, Koontz WL, Layman L, et al: Sonographic evaluation of the adnexa during early pregnancy. Surg Gynecol Obstet 163:319-323, 1986.
50. Condous G, Khalid A, Okaro E, et al: Should we be examining the ovaries in pregnancy? Prevalence and natural history of adnexal pathology detected at first-trimester sonography. Ultrasound Obstet Gynecol 24:62-66, 2004.
51. Hogston P, Lilford RJ: Ultrasound study of ovarian cysts in pregnancy: Prevalence and significance. BJOG 93:625-628, 1986.
52. Bromley B, Benacerraf B: Adnexal masses during pregnancy: Accuracy of sonographic diagnosis and outcome. J Ultrasound Med 16:447-452, 1997.
53. Buttery BW, Beischer NA, Fortune DW, et al: Ovarian tumours in pregnancy. Med J Aust 1:345-349, 1973.
54. Tawa K: Ovarian tumors in pregnancy. Am J Obstet Gynecol 90:511-516, 1964.
55. Leiserowitz GS, Xing G, Cress R, et al: Adnexal masses in pregnancy: How often are they malignant? Gynecol Oncol 101:315-321, 2006.

56. Sherard GB, Hodson CA, Williams J, et al: Adnexal masses and pregnancy: A 12-year experience. Am J Obstet Gynecol 189:358-363, 2003.
57. Wheeler TC, Fleischer AC: Complex adnexal mass in pregnancy: Predictive value of color Doppler sonography. J Ultrasound Med 16:425-428, 1997.
58. Kier R, McCarthy SM, Scoutt LM, et al: Pelvic masses in pregnancy: MR imaging. Radiology 176:709-713, 1990.
59. Whitecar P, Turner S, Highby K: Adnexal masses in pregnancy: A review of 130 cases undergoing surgical management. Am J Obstet Gynecol 181:19-24, 1999.
60. Struyk AP, Treffers PE: Ovarian tumors in pregnancy. Acta Obstet Gynecol Scand 63:421-424, 1984.
61. Ueda M, Ueki M: Ovarian tumors associated with pregnancy. Int J Gynaecol Obstet 55:59-65, 1996.
62. Al-Fozan H, Tulandi T: Safety and risks of laparoscopy in pregnancy. Curr Opin Obstet Gynecol 14:375-379, 2002.
63. Vergote I, De Brabanter J, Fyles A, et al: Prognostic importance of degree of differentiation and cyst rupture in stage I invasive epithelial ovarian carcinoma. Lancet 357:176-182, 2001.
64. Hess W, Peaceman A, O'Brien WF, et al: Adnexal mass occurring with intrauterine pregnancy: Report of fifty-four patients requiring laparotomy for definitive management. Am J Obstet Gynecol 158:1029-1034, 1988.
65. Grimbizis GF, Camus M, Tarlatzis BC, et al: Clinical implications of uterine malformations and hysteroscopic treatment results. Hum Reprod Update 7:161-174, 2001.
66. Nahum GG: Uterine anomalies: How common are they and what is their distribution among subtypes? J Reprod Med 43:877-887, 1998.
67. Acien P: Reproductive performance of women with uterine malformations. Hum Reprod 8:122-126, 1993.
68. Tranquilli AL, Giannubilo SR, Corradetti A: Congenital uterine malformations are associated to increased blood pressure in pregnancy. Hypertens Pregnancy 23:191-196, 2004.
69. Clifford K, Rai R, Watson H, Regan L: An informative protocol for the investigation of recurrent miscarriage: Preliminary experience of 500 consecutive cases. Hum Reprod 9:1328-1332, 1994.
70. Heinonen PK, Saarikoski S, Pystynen P: Reproductive performance of women with uterine anomalies. An evaluation of 182 cases. Acta Obstet Gynecol Scand 61:157-162, 1982.
71. Buttram VC Jr: Mullerian anomalies and their management. Fertil Steril 40:159-163, 1983.
72. Raga F, Bauset C, Remohi J, et al: Reproductive impact of congenital mullerian anomalies. Hum Reprod 12:2277-2281, 1997.
73. Harger JH, Archer DF, Marchese SG, et al: Etiology of recurrent pregnancy losses and outcome of subsequent pregnancies. Obstet Gynecol 62:574-581, 1983.
74. Golan A, Langer R, Bukovsky I, Caspi E: Congenital anomalies of the mullerian system. Fertil Steril 51:747-755, 1989.
75. Proctor JA, Haney AF: Recurrent first trimester pregnancy loss is associated with uterine septum but not with bicornuate uterus. Fertil Steril 80:1212-1215, 2003.
76. Nahum GG: Rudimentary uterine horn pregnancy: The 20th century worldwide experience of 588 cases. J Reprod Med 47:151-163, 2002.
77. Demaria F, Goffinet F, Jouannic JM, et al: Preterm torsion of a gravid uterus didelphys horn of a twin pregnancy. Obstet Gynecol 106:1186-1187, 2005.
78. Nahum GG: Uterine anomalies, induction of labor, and uterine rupture. Obstet Gynecol 106:1150-1152, 2005.
79. Fedele L, Arcaini L, Parazzini F, et al: Reproductive prognosis after hysteroscopic metroplasty in 102 women: Life-table analysis. Fertil Steril 59:768-772, 1993.
80. Homer HA, Li TC, Cooke ID: The septate uterus: A review of management and reproductive outcome. Fertil Steril 73:1-14, 2000.
81. Papp Z, Mezei G, Gavai M, et al: Reproductive performance after transabdominal metroplasty: A review of 157 consecutive cases. J Reprod Med 51:544-552, 2006.
82. Schmeler KM, Mayo-Smith WW, Piepert JF, et al: Adnexal masses in pregnancy: Surgery compared with observation. Obstet Gynecol 105(Pt 1):1098-1103, 2005.
83. Soriano D, Yefet Y, Seidman DS, et al: Laparoscopy versus laparotomy in the management of adnexal masses during pregnancy. Fertil Steril 71:955-960, 1999.

Chapter 56

Anesthetic Considerations for Complicated Pregnancies

Krzysztof M. Kuczkowski, MD

The physiologic changes that occur during normal pregnancy must be considered by the anesthesiologist to facilitate selecting the most appropriate and safest anesthetic drugs and techniques. When pregnancy is complicated by a significant medical disorder, the anesthetic considerations are even more challenging. This chapter reviews the special concerns posed by the more common and complex medical disorders superimposed on pregnancy and the most prudent technical solutions to the specific problems. Epidural and combined spinal-epidural analgesia and anesthesia frequently are recommended for the parturient with medical or obstetric complications because of the great flexibility and utility of these techniques for virtually any obstetric procedure.

Preeclampsia

The patient with preeclampsia has multiple organ system alterations that affect the selection of analgesia and anesthesia for labor and delivery.[1] The patient with mild preeclampsia rarely poses a major problem regarding anesthesia. Consequently, the focus here is on the patient with severe preeclampsia and eclampsia. Throughout this chapter, intensive care monitoring and the use of pulmonary artery occlusion pressure monitoring are emphasized (see Chapter 57).

Intravascular Volume Depletion

Intravascular volume depletion is a well-recognized occurrence in women with severe preeclampsia.[1,2] The anesthesiologist is concerned about inducing epidural, combined spinal-epidural, or spinal anesthesia in the patient with relative hypovolemia because the ensuing sympathetic blockade can lead to precipitous declines in blood pressure, which can seriously impair critical organ and uteroplacental blood flow. Preanesthetic volume expansion is used with caution to prevent this undesired effect. Replacement may require the use of central venous pressure or pulmonary artery pressure monitoring.[1,3] Because many patients with preeclampsia have low central filling pressures, they often require large volumes of fluid to bring the pressures into the middle of the normal range. This measure, however, can result in pulmonary edema in the postpartum period, when colloid osmotic pressure reaches its nadir.[4] More judicious fluid management with slow advancement of an epidural block, particularly for those undergoing cesarean delivery, is proving effective at maintaining maternal blood pressure while minimizing the risk of fluid overload.

The choice of fluid—crystalloid or colloid—remains controversial. Studies have demonstrated the beneficial effects of albumin administration for these patients.[5] Its use is justified in part by the fact that preeclamptic women tend to demonstrate significant reductions in plasma protein levels and colloid osmotic pressure as a result of protein loss through the kidney. Arguments against the routine use of albumin emphasize that the functional changes in membranes that allow edema to occur also allow protein to leak into the tissues, making removal of interstitial fluid more difficult. To avoid volume overload, the judicious administration of crystalloid solution (up to 2000 mL) is guided by central venous or pulmonary artery occlusion pressure monitoring. This is accomplished with simultaneous advancement of the regional block, thereby titrating the effects of one against the other. If the patient has marked edema or low colloid osmotic pressure or has not responded to crystalloid infusion, 25% salt-poor albumin is administered to maintain intravascular volume. The objective is to provide sufficient volume to allow the patient to undergo anesthesia and maintain an adequate urine flow rather than totally correct an estimated volume deficit.[1]

Vascular Reactivity

Vascular reactivity is enhanced in preeclampsia, and the increased sensitivity to vasopressor agents such as angiotensin II and catecholamines is well documented.[6,7] Systemic vascular resistance (SVR) can be increased, and uteroplacental crucial organ blood flow can be compromised. The anesthesiologist must consider the possibility that the administration of regional anesthesia and its attendant sympathetic blockade to a patient who is already experiencing volume depletion and vasoconstriction may result in sudden hypotension. The initiation of epidural blockade with maintenance of an acceptable maternal blood pressure, however, results in increases in uteroplacental blood flow.[1] An acceptable maternal blood pressure is defined as no more than a 25% reduction in systolic blood pressure.

Vasoreactivity alerts the anesthesiologist to use lower doses of vasopressors to correct maternal hypotension. An arterial catheter can be helpful in monitoring beat-to-beat blood pressure responses in patients requiring aggressive therapy. Patients who undergo general anesthesia for cesarean delivery are at risk for hypertensive crisis at the time of laryngoscopy and intubation as a result of the associated increase in sympathetic tone. This can lead to intracranial hemorrhage or pulmonary edema, and measures should be taken to block this response when general anesthesia is required.[4,8]

Coagulation

Coagulation system changes are frequently observed in patients with severe preeclampsia. The most common alteration is a decrease in platelet count. This is usually not a concern unless the level falls below 100,000/mm^3. Many anesthesiologists are reluctant to administer regional anesthesia when the platelet count is at or below this level for fear that an epidural hematoma may occur.[9,10] A possible platelet functional defect has also been identified in these patients.[11] This results in a prolonged bleeding time by the Ivy method (<5 minutes from the stab until all bleeding from the wound stops) despite a normal platelet count. The absolute limit beyond which it is thought unwise to perform regional anesthesia is arbitrary and variable, because there are no documented reports of an epidural hematoma occurring in association with epidural anesthesia in preeclamptic patients with lowered platelet counts or a prolonged Ivy bleeding time, and some have questioned the diagnostic and predictive ability of the bleeding time.[12]

There is retrospective evidence to suggest that many epidural agents have been placed in such patients without incident.[13] Nevertheless, the potential complication is so serious that the arbitrary limit generally used is as follows. If the bleeding time is less than 12 minutes or if another test of primary hemostasis indicates good platelet function, it is probably safe to use regional anesthesia even if the platelet count is below 100,000/mm^3. Other tests of whole-blood clotting (e.g., thromboelastogram, Sonoclot, Platelet Function Analyzer-100) have been evaluated in preeclamptic and healthy parturients, but their usefulness as predictors of surgical or epidural bleeding remains to be defined. Disseminated intravascular coagulation is an infrequent occurrence in preeclamptic patients, but it significantly alters other tests of coagulation.

Edema

Edema is a frequent finding in patients with preeclampsia. Limb edema can make vascular access difficult. Edema in the neck can obscure landmarks for performing internal jugular vein cannulation for central line insertion. The most worrisome edema for the anesthesiologist is that which can occur in the pharynx and larynx. Difficult or impossible intubation has been encountered, with severe maternal consequences. General anesthesia for markedly edematous preeclamptic patients should be avoided, and when absolutely necessary, preparation for alternative methods of securing the airway must be made.[1] Postextubation airway obstruction resulting from edema at the level of the glottis is a serious complication that occurs frequently in these patients.

Pulmonary edema is another complication of preeclampsia. Most of these patients have normal cardiac function with imbalances in pulmonary artery pressure and colloid osmotic pressure.[4]

The observed reduction of colloid osmotic pressure in normal pregnancy is further decreased in preeclampsia. This results from the loss of albumin, which is the major contributor to colloid osmotic pressure. Modest elevations in pulmonary artery occlusion pressure from exogenous fluid administration and mobilization of endogenous fluid alter the gradient between colloid osmotic pressure and pulmonary artery pressure so that transudation of fluid into the interstitium is likely.

Drugs

Pharmacologic agents are often required to treat patients with preeclampsia. These drugs can interact with anesthetic agents to produce an undesired effect, and the obstetrician and anesthesiologist should be aware of the pharmacology of the drugs employed, their dosages, and the time of administration.[14]

Magnesium sulfate is the most commonly administered agent in the management of preeclampsia. Adverse effects are few when it is administered appropriately, and overdosage is treated easily with intravenous calcium. Magnesium exerts several important effects at the neuromuscular junction. It inhibits the release of acetylcholine from the presynaptic nerve terminal, depresses the postjunctional membrane response, and depresses the response of the underlying myofibrils.[14] These effects are responsible for the muscle weakness and respiratory depression observed with overdosage. Neuromuscular blocking agents are used to facilitate endotracheal intubation and to maintain a relaxed surgical field when general anesthesia is provided for cesarean delivery.[15] Magnesium potentiates and prolongs the action of depolarizing agents (e.g., succinylcholine) and nondepolarizing agents (e.g., rocuronium, vecuronium, atracurium).[16] Lower doses of these drugs are necessary, and electronic monitoring of the neuromuscular junction is helpful.[17]

The patient must be evaluated carefully at the end of the procedure to ensure that she has regained sufficient muscle strength to maintain and protect her airway and to sustain adequate ventilation. Because drugs used to provide anesthesia are anticonvulsant in nature, it is prudent to discontinue magnesium sulfate therapy in the operating room when general anesthesia is used and to reinitiate use after the patient has regained full neuromuscular function.

The anesthetic options for a patient with severe preeclampsia depend on the mode of delivery. Analgesia for the first stage of labor reduces maternal catecholamine output and perhaps maintains or improves uteroplacental blood flow. Systemic analgesia with narcotics is acceptable, although continuous lumbar epidural analgesia provides the best pain relief with minimal or no sedation.[18] The use of segmental epidural analgesia avoids extensive sympathetic blockade. Opioids may be added to the local anesthetic solution to enhance the quality of pain relief without additional sympathetic or motor blockade. If sympathetic blockade must be totally avoided, intrathecal narcotics (e.g., morphine, fentanyl, sufentanil, meperidine) can be administered by single injection or continuous technique. Anesthesia for vaginal delivery may be provided by pudendal nerve block, low spinal anesthesia, or lumbar or caudal epidural anesthesia. Although the choice of anesthetic in the patient who is to undergo cesarean delivery has been controversial, the careful use of epidural anesthesia, with meticulous attention to left uterine displacement and fluid management, is associated with good maternal and fetal outcomes and is the preferred approach.[1,4]

When general anesthesia is required, measures must be taken to avoid the hypertensive response to laryngoscopy and to intubation and extubation. Labetalol administered just before induction in doses up to 1 mg/kg have proved effective in reducing this response. Alternative or adjunctive drugs, such as sodium nitroprusside and nitroglycerin, may also be used. Sodium nitroprusside, because of its short half-life, provides the advantage of allowing for minute-to-minute blood pressure control.

Inability to intubate the trachea is the leading cause of maternal death associated with general anesthesia. Alternative means of providing oxygenation and ventilation (e.g., laryngeal mask airway, the Combitube, transtracheal jet ventilation) must be readily available.[19,20]

Transtracheal jet ventilation provides adequate oxygenation and ventilation to pregnant patients.[20,21] If airway difficulty is anticipated, an awake intubation, perhaps aided by a fiberoptic bronchoscope, may be necessary.

In the past, spinal anesthesia was usually avoided for cesarean delivery of patients with severe preeclampsia because of concern about rapid onset of profound sympathetic blockade, which resulted in catastrophic hypotension difficult to treat.[22] As a result, epidural anesthesia became the preferred regional technique for cesarean section in women with severe preeclampsia because of a more gradual onset of sympathetic block.[1,23,24]

In 2003, Aya and colleagues[25] demonstrated that severely preeclamptic patients receiving spinal anesthesia for cesarean delivery were at no greater risk for profound hypotension than normotensive patients when using a standard single dose of spinal anesthesia.[25] In 2005, two more studies[26,27] supported the use of single-dose spinal anesthesia in women with severe preeclampsia.

Although the optimal anesthetic technique for cesarean section in women with severe preeclampsia still poses a dilemma for some obstetricians and obstetric anesthesiologists, it appears that spinal anesthesia in stable and noncoagulopathic parturient may be a reasonable alternative to epidural anesthesia, especially in emergency situations and particularly if it avoids the use of general anesthesia. The lower arterial blood pressure that follows induction of spinal anesthesia is far less a concern than the risk of failed ventilation, intubation, and the risk of hypertensive crisis during laryngoscopy when general anesthesia is selected for women with severe preeclapmsia.[1,24]

Neurologic Disorders

Multiple Sclerosis

Multiple sclerosis is a disease of young adults that may occur in pregnant women. The disease process is characterized by chronic inflammation, demyelination, and gliosis in the central nervous system. The cause of multiple sclerosis is not known, and there is no curative treatment. Pregnancy does not negatively affect the long-term prognosis of multiple sclerosis.[28,29]

Although there have been many attempts to associate anesthesia and surgery with relapses of symptoms, no controlled studies have directly linked any form of anesthesia to exacerbation of multiple sclerosis.[30] Nevertheless, the routine administration of anticholinergic agents is not recommended because they may induce an elevation in body temperature, known to be associated with exacerbations of multiple sclerosis. Concern has been raised that local anesthetics may be more histotoxic to neural tissue already compromised by multiple sclerosis. All local anesthetic agents are potentially neurotoxic in doses that far exceed those used clinically. Neurotoxicity from local anesthetic drugs has not been demonstrated in patients with multiple sclerosis, and epidural analgesia and anesthesia have been safely and successfully used for labor and delivery in these patients.[30,31] The lowest concentration of local anesthesia capable of producing the desired effect should be selected.[30,31] Epidural and intrathecal narcotics have also been administered without apparent adverse effect. Although peripartum and surgical stress (and general anesthesia) have been linked to exacerbation of symptoms of multiple sclerosis, published data regarding this association are limited. Diagnostic lumbar puncture is not associated with an increased rate of relapse.[32]

In summary, the review of published data does not contraindicate the use of regional anesthesia for labor, vaginal delivery, and cesarean section in patients with multiple sclerosis.[31,32] However, it is important to inform the patient that there is a high incidence of disease relapse during the postpartum period, regardless of the choice of anesthesia and mode of delivery.[32]

Paraplegia

Each year, more than 2000 women of childbearing age in the United States sustain a spinal cord injury.[33] As a result of increased survival rates for women with spinal cord injury, the number of parturients with paraplegia is increasing. The level and extent of the lesion determine the patient's response to labor. If the spinal cord lesion is below the 10th thoracic dermatome, the patient will have the sensation of labor.[33] If it is above this level, she will have minimal or no awareness of contractions. Paraplegic parturients tend to have a normal course of labor but a higher percentage of forceps-assisted deliveries because of weakness of the abdominal muscles and consequent impairment of the ability to bear down effectively in the second stage.[34] The major anesthetic issues are the management of analgesia and anesthesia for labor and delivery, the possibility of autonomic hyperreflexia, and hyperkalemia with the administration of succinylcholine.

The phenomenon of autonomic hyperreflexia occurs in patients whose spinal cord lesion is at the seventh thoracic dermatome or higher.[35,36] This condition is characterized by severe hypertension, bradycardia, headache, premature ventricular contractions, flushing, sweating, and pilomotor erection. The hypertension can be severe and, if uncontrolled, can lead to central nervous system hemorrhage, cardiac decompensation, or death. It is triggered by stimulation below the level of the spinal cord lesion.[35,36] Common initiating events include bladder or rectal distention, rubbing of the skin, genital stimulation, and contraction of any hollow viscus, including the uterus. The triggering impulse is conducted to the spinal cord, where a reflex response occurs that cannot be modulated or inhibited by higher centers because of the isolation invoked by the cord lesion. This results in an uncontrolled adrenergic discharge with norepinephrine release from the peripheral sympathetic nerve endings.[35] The release of adrenal catecholamines may also be involved.

Although a large percentage of patients at risk do exhibit this reflex, some do not. A careful history should reveal those who exhibit such a response. Because preterm labor may be unrecognized by these patients, the sudden onset of paroxysmal hypertension should prompt a search for uterine contractions before the diagnosis of pregnancy-induced hypertension is considered.

During labor, adequate blockade of the afferent impulses can be provided by regional anesthesia, even if no pain is perceived by the patient. Continuous epidural anesthesia with a local anesthetic and narcotic agents has been employed successfully to treat autonomic hyperreflexia during labor and delivery.[35,36] Spinal anesthesia in single-injection and continuous forms has been used to control blood pressure.[33-36] With regional anesthesia, it is difficult to determine whether an adequate block is present, because the usual sensory tests are useless below the level of the lesion. The anesthetic block must therefore be titrated to just above the existing sensory level. Autonomic hyperreflexia can be controlled by a variety of antihypertensive agents, such as phentolamine and sodium nitroprusside.

General anesthesia can effectively inhibit the hyperreflexia response.[35,36] If general anesthesia is required for a complex vaginal or cesarean delivery, however, the anesthesiologist must determine when the spinal cord injury initially occurred, because there is a significant release of potassium from the denervated muscle after the use of succinylcholine for endotracheal intubation if it is administered 6 months to 1 year after the injury. The elevation in serum potassium can reach life-threatening levels.[33]

Ordinarily, although a general anesthetic agent may be used safely, an epidural anesthetic agent is preferred. Regional anesthesia has the advantage of blocking afferent input, thereby avoiding autonomic hyperreflexia. If the lesion is in the upper thoracic region, the patient will have weak abdominal and thoracic musculature. The use of epidural anesthesia is preferable to spinal anesthesia because the degree of motor impairment is less and profound muscle relaxation is not required. The block can be advanced gradually, avoiding sudden hypotension from a rapid extensive sympathetic blockade.

Subarachnoid Hemorrhage

Subarachnoid hemorrhage from an intracranial vascular lesion is an uncommon but serious complication of pregnancy.[37-39] The stress induced by the increased cardiac output and blood volume, combined with the softening of vascular connective tissue by the hormonal changes of pregnancy, may predispose a patient to such an event. The diagnosis can be obscured initially because nausea and vomiting are common findings during pregnancy.

Treatment is usually surgical if the lesion is an aneurysm because this approach significantly improves maternal chances of survival. The decision to treat surgically should be influenced not by the pregnancy but by the site and type of lesion, the clinical condition of the patient, and the presence or absence of vasospasm. Medical management appears to be as effective as surgical management for arteriovenous malformations during pregnancy. After a patient has undergone surgical correction of an aneurysm, there are no special considerations for anesthetic management of labor and delivery.[39]

The anesthetic concerns regarding the patient *without* surgical correction are focused on two different clinical situations. The first relates to the patient undergoing neurosurgery for a ruptured aneurysm; the second is anesthetic management of labor and delivery for a patient who has not undergone surgical repair. Anesthesia for the patient having a neurosurgical procedure has the same primary goals as for all patients having surgery during pregnancy—maintaining uteroplacental blood flow and fetal oxygenation and preventing preterm delivery.[40-42]

The usual neurosurgical anesthetic approach to patients with these types of lesions includes the following:

- Deliberate hypotension to reduce the risk of cerebral hemorrhage
- Hypothermia to reduce cerebral metabolism
- Hyperventilation to reduce cerebral blood flow and brain size
- Diuresis to promote shrinkage of the brain

Deliberate hypotension can be produced with a volatile anesthetic, sodium nitroprusside, or nitroglycerin. Each agent carries its own potential hazards in addition to reduction in uteroplacental blood flow. A reduction in systolic blood pressure of 25% to 30% or a mean arterial blood pressure of less than 70 mm Hg leads to reductions in uteroplacental blood flow.[40] The hypotensive agents also cross the placenta and can induce hypotension in the fetus. Nitroprusside is converted to cyanide, and cyanide accumulation and toxicity in the human fetus pose at least a theoretical risk. If this agent is used, it should be for only a short time. It should be discontinued if the required infusion rate exceeds 0.5 mg/kg/hr, if maternal metabolic acidosis ensues, or if resistance to the agent is apparent.

Nitroglycerin has not been associated with adverse fetal effects. It is metabolized to nitrites, which have produced methemoglobinemia experimentally. This agent, however, is less predictable in its hypotensive effect than sodium nitroprusside. Fetal heart rate monitoring should be employed, and hypotension should be limited to the shortest period possible. Although it is preferable to avoid or limit the period of hypotension in the pregnant patient, successful neonatal outcome after induced hypotension with careful control has been observed.[42]

Hypothermia is used occasionally to decrease cerebral metabolic requirements and blood flow. The usual goal is to achieve a temperature of approximately 30° C. This measure induces similar temperature changes in the fetus, and fetal bradycardia occurs. The heart rate increases again with rewarming. Hyperventilation is commonly used during neuroanesthesia, because the decrease in P_{CO_2} reduces cerebral blood flow.[43] The goal is to reach a Pa_{CO_2} of approximately 20 to 25 mm Hg.[44,45] This degree of respiratory alkalosis should not be a problem for the healthy fetus, because a Pa_{CO_2} of 32 mm Hg is the norm for pregnant women. Fetal heart rate monitoring should alert the anesthesiologist to compromises in fetal oxygenation, and adjustments may be made accordingly.

Diuresis is often accomplished with osmotic agents or loop diuretics to shrink the brain intraoperatively and postoperatively.[44,45] These agents can cause significant negative fluid shifts for the fetus. Diuretic agents should be given only as necessary and not strictly by protocol for the pregnant patient.

The objectives in managing a patient for labor and delivery who has not undergone surgical repair are to avoid hypertension and to avoid elevations in intracranial pressure. The Valsalva maneuver should be avoided, because the sudden pressure changes at the end of the maneuver can produce a gradient that favors rupture of the lesion. Epidural analgesia and anesthesia can most effectively provide conditions to meet these goals. It may be relatively contraindicated for patients who already have marked increases in intracranial pressure, inasmuch as an unintentional dural puncture can lead to herniation of the cerebellum.[43-45] There is also a theoretical risk of further increasing intracranial pressure from the volume of fluid placed in the epidural space. This pressure increase is minimal and transient in the normal parturient when the volume administered is kept relatively small and the rate of injection slow.

Other commonly used forms of analgesia may be employed as long as maternal respiratory depression is avoided. Cesarean delivery anesthesia is best provided by the continuous epidural technique. Spinal anesthesia may be used if intracranial hypertension does not exist. If general anesthesia is required, the steps outlined previously for preventing the hypertensive response to laryngoscopy and intubation will be necessary. More information about these neurologic complications is provided in Chapter 52.

Respiratory Disorders

Significant alterations occur in the pulmonary system during pregnancy, which primarily serve to meet the increased oxygen consumption by the growing fetus. When pregnancy is complicated by a respiratory tract disorder such as asthma, cystic fibrosis, or tobacco-related respiratory complications, obstetric and anesthetic management during the peripartum period may become challenging. To understand the implications of anesthesia superimposed on a pregnant woman with respiratory disease, the physician should be well acquainted with the physiologic alterations in the respiratory tract during pregnancy. These changes and the various respiratory disorders in pregnancy are reviewed in Chapter 45.

Asthma

Asthma is the most common respiratory problem encountered in women of childbearing age. The disease is characterized by bronchial constriction, bronchial secretions, and bronchial edema. Therapy commonly includes theophylline preparations, inhaled β-adrenoceptor agonists, anticholinergic agents, corticosteroids, and occasionally, cromolyn sodium. Magnesium sulfate has also been effective in alleviating acute symptoms.[46] The effect of pregnancy on the condition of the asthmatic has been controversial, but it does appear that with proper management and prompt attention to acute episodes, most patients fare well.[46-48] Maintenance of the patient's medications and hydration are of major importance during labor and delivery.

Analgesia and anesthesia for labor and delivery of the asthmatic patient can alleviate anxiety and hyperventilation. Hyperventilation can precipitate an attack and lead to increased fluid losses and dehydration. Narcotic analgesia administered in a judicious fashion may be used, but narcotics are bronchoconstrictors and should be avoided if the patient is actively wheezing or in respiratory distress. Epidural analgesia with local anesthetics or opioids, or both, is extremely beneficial because pain can be relieved while respiratory depression is avoided.[49,50] If the patient is severely asthmatic, it is essential to avoid a high and dense level of anesthesia because accessory muscles of respiration can be impaired. A high thoracic level can completely block sympathetic pathways, and the unopposed parasympathetic tone can lead to bronchoconstriction. Low spinal anesthesia or a pudendal block is a reasonable choice for vaginal delivery if epidural analgesia is not used.

Regional anesthesia is preferred because the insertion of an endotracheal tube at the light levels of anesthesia traditionally favored for obstetrics frequently results in bronchospasm.[50,51] Even though pulmonary mechanics are reasonably well maintained under spinal, combined spinal-epidural, or epidural anesthesia to the fourth thoracic dermatome, the patient should receive an inhaled β-agonist before the procedure and bring her inhaler with her to the operating room because bronchospasm may occur.[50-52] Appropriate attention to hydration and maintenance of blood pressure are required, and supplemental oxygen is recommended.

General anesthesia for cesarean delivery in the asthmatic patient poses additional risk. Careful attention to detail is necessary to avoid life-threatening bronchospasm, and general anesthesia should be used only if regional anesthesia is contraindicated.[49,50] Preoperative preparation should include adequate hydration, intravenous aminophylline, treatment with a β_2-agonist inhaler, antacid therapy, and sufficient time for preoxygenation (≥3 minutes). A rapid-sequence induction may then be undertaken. The induction agent of choice is ketamine because it is a bronchodilator and does not release histamine.[49,51] Propofol decreases the response to airway manipulation and may prove to be a reasonable alternative. Thiopental administered in the commonly used doses for cesarean delivery produces a plane of anesthesia that is too light to prevent bronchospasm. Larger doses are an alternative to ketamine and may be employed with the small risk that the newborn will be depressed from the anesthetic in the immediate postdelivery period.

The patient with active wheezing requiring a general anesthetic for cesarean delivery may require a slower induction. Anesthesia is induced intravenously, a muscle relaxant is administered, cricoid pressure is applied and maintained, and the patient is ventilated by mask with a volatile anesthetic agent to promote bronchodilation. When a deep plane of anesthesia is reached, the patient is intubated. This technique exposes the patient to a greater risk of regurgitation and aspiration of gastric contents and should be employed only when there are no other reasonable options.[49,51]

After anesthesia is induced and the patient has been intubated successfully, maintenance includes the administration of a volatile agent in a humidified gas mixture because all gases used (e.g., isoflurane, sevoflurane, desflurane) produce direct bronchial muscle relaxation.[53] If intraoperative wheezing occurs, a β_2-agonist may be aerosolized through the endotracheal tube. Although the effect is synergistic with the halogenated agents, two potential problems must be considered. First, administration of some halogenated agents (primarily halothane, which is very infrequently used) in the presence of therapeutic or higher levels of aminophylline has been associated with serious ventricular arrhythmias and cardiac arrest.[54] Isoflurane, sevoflurane, or desflurane is a safer alternative. Second, the volatile agents tend to relax uterine musculature at concentrations that are effective as bronchodilators, and the possibility of enhanced uterine bleeding exists. This effect can usually be counteracted by the administration of oxytocin. The use of prostaglandins to control hemorrhage is not recommended because prostaglandin $F_{2\alpha}$ is a bronchoconstrictor. After the infant has been delivered, ventilation with bag and mask oxygen eliminates most of the volatile agent from the infant in a few minutes.

Muscle relaxation can be maintained with a nondepolarizing neuromuscular-blocking agent. Curare and atracurium are associated with histamine release in large doses, whereas vecuronium, rocuronium, and *cis*-atracurium are not. When a nondepolarizing agent is used, it usually must be reversed at the end of the procedure with an anticholinesterase drug such as neostigmine or edrophonium. This group of nondepolarizing drugs can produce bronchoconstriction and increased production of secretions. Consequently, a sufficient dose of an anticholinergic agent such as atropine or glycopyrrolate must be administered before use. The nonpregnant asthmatic patient is usually extubated in a deep plane of anesthesia to avoid the stimulus of the endotracheal tube, but the pregnant patient should be extubated while awake because of the risks of vomiting and aspiration. Intravenous lidocaine can prevent coughing and bronchoconstriction on emergence.[49,51]

Postoperative care includes humidified oxygen, incentive spirometry, and the required pharmacologic agents. Epidural and intrathecal narcotics provide excellent postoperative analgesia with minimal sedation.

Cystic Fibrosis

The meticulous use of pulmonary toilet and aggressive antibiotic therapy has made it possible for many women with cystic fibrosis to survive well into their childbearing years.[55] The pulmonary complications of patients with cystic fibrosis provide significant anesthetic challenges. Thick, excessive mucus production results in obstruction of the small and medium-sized airways, with subsequent bronchitis and bronchiectasis. Pneumothorax, atelectasis, progressive hypoxemia, and cor pulmonale commonly occur with the disease.

Therapy consists of postural drainage and chest percussion (often on a daily basis), antibiotics for symptoms of infection, bronchodilators for wheezing, intermittent mucolytic therapy (*N*-acetylcysteine), vitamins, and pancreatic enzyme replacement. Preoperative evaluation should include pulmonary function studies, cardiac evaluation, and measurement of arterial blood gases. Successful completion of pregnancy with careful attention to medical management is well established.[55]

Optimal analgesia during the first stage of labor is provided by continuous lumbar epidural or combined spinal-epidural anesthesia.[49,51] Intrathecal opioids should be avoided because they have occasionally been associated with severe respiratory depression, particularly if parenteral opioids have been administered.[56,57] Management concerns are similar to those of the severe asthmatic patient. The state of hydration needs to be maintained because these patients often lose excessive amounts of fluid through sweating. Narcotics should be used in very small amounts because they suppress the cough reflex and produce respiratory depression. Nitrous oxide should probably be avoided because of the frequency of pneumothorax from ruptured bullae. Anesthesia for vaginal delivery may be provided with low spinal, combined-spinal, epidural, or pudendal nerve block.

Anesthesia for cesarean delivery carries with it the same management concerns as for the patient with severe asthma, and carefully titrated continuous epidural anesthesia is recommended. Although general anesthesia can be used safely for patients with cystic fibrosis, the risk of maternal hypoxemia during induction is greater than for asthmatic patients, and the possibility of pneumothorax exists during positive-pressure ventilation.[49,51,58,59] Anticholinergics (i.e., drying agents) and narcotics are usually excluded from the regimen, and gases should be humidified. Patients with very advanced disease may require postoperative mechanical ventilation until they regain their full preoperative capabilities.

Morbid Obesity

Morbid obesity is defined as an accumulation of adipose tissue that causes the body mass index (BMI) to increase by 30% or more, as shown by the following equation:

$$\text{BMI} = \frac{\text{weight (kg)}}{[\text{height (m)}]^2}$$

In the equation, weight is in kilograms and height is in meters.

Morbid obesity is perhaps the most common nutritional disorder seen in pregnancy, and morbidly obese parturients have more pregnancy complication than normal-BMI pregnant patients.[60] Substantial change takes place over time in the respiratory system. A restrictive lung disease pattern develops, and pulmonary function testing reveals a decrease in expiratory reserve volume, vital capacity, inspiratory capacity, and total lung capacity. Compliance decreases, and the work of breathing increases. There is also a ventilation-perfusion imbalance, leading to hypoxemia, particularly in the supine or Trendelenburg position.

Pregnancy imposes changes in lung volumes similar to those resulting from obesity.[60,61] Fortunately, these effects are not additive. An important study evaluating 12 obese pregnant women revealed that the usual pulmonary changes of pregnancy occurred, but they were not accentuated by the obesity. Hypoxemia existed but was not worsened by pregnancy.[62]

Labor should be conducted in the sitting or semirecumbent position with left uterine displacement. Supplemental oxygen administration and pulse oximeter monitoring are advised. Epidural or combined spinal-epidural analgesia is recommended but may be technically difficult or impossible to perform because of obscured landmarks, difficult positioning, and excessive layers of adipose tissue.[61] Other forms of analgesia, including intrathecal narcotics, intravenous narcotics, and inhalation of nitrous oxide plus oxygen, are all suitable. The anesthetic for vaginal delivery may be any of the commonly used forms; the patient should remain in a semi-sitting position, if possible, to prevent small airway closure.

Cesarean delivery anesthesia may be provided by the spinal, epidural, or combined spinal-epidural route.[63] Technical difficulties can be encountered, and the dosage of drug needs to be reduced because spread in the subarachnoid and epidural spaces is enhanced with morbid obesity.[61,63] Care must be taken to avoid a significant motor block, which can compromise ventilation and result in hypoxemia. The Trendelenburg position should be avoided because it shifts the weight of the abdominal viscera and the panniculus toward the chest and diaphragm, further compromising respiration.

Technically, general anesthesia poses several challenges.[15,19,20] First, the airway must be secured. Endotracheal intubation can be extremely difficult as a result of excessive tissue and edema. Exceedingly large breasts can interfere with the insertion of a conventional laryngoscope. A careful assessment of the airway must be made, and if standard intubation appears to be extremely difficult, a fiberoptic intubation is recommended with the patient awake. If a rapid-sequence induction is attempted and the airway cannot be conventionally secured, an alternative means, such as a laryngeal mask airway, Combitube, or transtracheal jet ventilation, must be at hand because hypoxia and acidosis can develop at an extremely rapid rate.

After the airway is secured, mechanical ventilation is required, and the pressures generated need to be high to move the large body mass. Large tidal volumes help to prevent airway closure. Extubation should be performed only when the patient is fully awake and has regained her full strength.[15,19,20] Postoperative analgesia, preferably by the epidural route, is extremely helpful in allowing for deep breathing exercises to avoid atelectasis and pneumonia.

Cardiac Disease

The pregnant patient with heart disease represents a unique challenge for the anesthesiologist.[64,65] Determination of the appropriate analgesic and anesthetic modalities requires a thorough understanding of the parturient's pathophysiology, pharmacologic therapy, and how these factors interact with anesthetic care. Chapter 39 offers an in-depth discussion of the various cardiac disorders in pregnancy.

Over the past 25 years, greater awareness of the physiologic burden that pregnancy places on an already compromised cardiovascular system in this subset of pregnant women has led to better counseling before conception and to major advances in treatment. Formerly, rheumatic heart disease was the most common cardiac disorder in pregnancy, with mitral stenosis the single most prevalent resulting lesion. The incidence of rheumatic heart disease has decreased dramatically in the United States and Western Europe, but in many other regions of the world, it remains an important cause of maternal morbidity and mortality.[64-66] Many more women with congenital heart defects are reaching childbearing age as a consequence of surgical correction. As more women delay childbearing to later reproductive years, ischemic cardiac disease may be expected to become increasingly prevalent.[64-66]

General Considerations

Pregnancy normally results in dramatic changes in the cardiovascular system, and these changes and the cardiac disorders in pregnancy are reviewed in Chapters 7 and 39. Four principal changes that present unique problems to the patient with cardiac disease have been well delineated and have special anesthetic implications.[67]

First, there is a 50% increase in intravascular volume that usually peaks by the early-to-middle third trimester. This relative volume overload may be poorly tolerated in women whose cardiac output is limited by myocardial dysfunction from ischemic, intrinsic, or valvular lesions.

Second, there is a progressive decrease in SVR throughout pregnancy, so that mean arterial pressure is preserved at normal values despite a 30% to 40% increase in cardiac output. This can be important for patients at risk for right-to-left shunting and for patients with some types of valvular disease (e.g., aortic stenosis).

Third, the compromised cardiovascular system is further stressed by the marked fluctuations in cardiac output observed during labor. Pain and apprehension can precipitate an increase in cardiac output to as much as 45% to 50% above the levels seen in the late second stage of labor. Each uterine contraction serves as an autotransfusion to the central blood volume, resulting in an increase in cardiac output of 10% to 25%.[64,65] The Valsalva maneuver results in wide swings in venous and arterial pressures, which have been associated with acute cardiac decompensation. The increases in cardiac output reach a maximum of 80% higher than antepartum levels immediately after delivery because of relief of inferior vena cava obstruction and a final autotransfusion of approximately 500 mL from uterine contraction.

The fourth consideration is the hypercoagulability associated with pregnancy and the possible need for appropriate anticoagulation, especially in patients at increased risk for arterial thrombosis and embolization (i.e., prosthetic heart valve or chronic atrial fibrillation). Therapeutic anticoagulation affects the options for anesthetic management, as well as the placement and location of invasive monitors, and increases the risk of postpartum hemorrhage.

Optimal anesthetic management requires a thorough assessment of the anatomic and functional capacity of the diseased heart, along with an analysis of how the described major physiologic changes are likely to affect the specific limitations imposed by the intrinsic disease. To determine the most appropriate anesthetic regimen, the anesthesiologist must consider the following:

- Patient's tolerance to pain during labor or surgery
- Impact of uterine contraction-induced autotransfusion
- Postpartum changes induced by relief of vena caval obstruction
- Potential for postpartum hemorrhage
- Use of uterine oxytocic agents

The most basic principles of obstetric anesthesia management must always apply[64,65]:

- Provisions for maintenance of uteroplacental perfusion by avoidance of aortocaval compression
- Minimizing sympathetic blockade coupled with intravascular volume maintenance
- Standard-of-care monitoring of parturient and fetus
- Provision for aspiration prophylaxis

Analgesia during the first stage of labor is focused on reducing the pain-related rises in catecholamine levels and avoiding aortocaval compression. Intravenous fluid management should be carefully monitored to avoid a lack of or an excess of fluids. Arterial, central venous, and pulmonary artery monitoring may be required to manage the patient optimally. Although such lines are generally reserved for symptomatic women, patients who have critical aortic stenosis, coarctation of the aorta, aortic aneurysm, right-to-left shunts, or primary pulmonary hypertension may benefit from invasive monitoring, even if they have minimal symptoms. Chapters 39 and 57 provide more detailed information.

Appropriate analgesia should be supplied. All of the available modalities have application for some patients. Continuous lumbar epidural analgesia with local anesthetics or narcotics, or both, is frequently optimal. Limited sympathetic blockade can prove helpful for patients with mitral valve lesions because of the effects on preload and afterload. For a patient whose condition is so compromised that even the modest changes induced by segmental epidural analgesia are worrisome, the use of intrathecal narcotic analgesia by single injection or continuous catheter may be beneficial because all of the hemodynamic alterations of sympathetic blockade are avoided.[64-66]

After the patient with significant cardiac disease has entered the second stage of labor, it is prudent for her to avoid pushing. The lithotomy position may need to be avoided for patients with lesions such as mitral stenosis, inasmuch as this position results in an acute increase in central blood volume.

For second-stage management, analgesia for uterine contractions and anesthesia of the perineum are the objectives. Uterine contractions spontaneously bring the infant's head to a deliverable position, and delivery can then be assisted by the application of the vacuum extractor or forceps. A regional technique is optimal. Epidural analgesia or anesthesia may be continued. Attention must be paid to extension of the sympathetic blockade. If an epidural block is not used, a low spinal anesthetic may be appropriate. Pudendal nerve block, although it does not provide as complete an analgesia as an epidural, can be employed satisfactorily as an adjunct to regional anesthesia or can be used alone.[64-66]

It is thought that cesarean delivery should be reserved for obstetric indications only and that the presence of heart disease should not influence that decision. The overall stresses of labor and vaginal delivery, as measured by alterations in cardiac output, are approximately the same as with cesarean delivery. Some circumstances, however, may lead to the decision to perform an elective cesarean delivery. The choice of anesthesia depends on the lesion and its severity. Epidural anesthesia provides the least amount of alteration in hemodynamics during cesarean delivery, although general anesthesia can be equally as safe when the abrupt changes associated with laryngoscopy and intubation, as well as suction and extubation, are blunted by the appropriate choice of pharmacologic agents and anesthetic technique.

Anesthesia for Cardiac Surgery during Pregnancy

Cardiac surgery is avoided during pregnancy because of potential compromise to the fetus. The developing fetus may experience teratogenic effects from drugs administered during the course of anesthesia. This has been demonstrated in animals with a multitude of anesthetic adjuvants but has never been clearly documented in humans.[68-70] Teratogenic changes can be induced by hypoxia during the procedure or by decreased uteroplacental perfusion. Premature labor is often associated with surgery during pregnancy, particularly abdominal procedures. If surgery is indicated during the course of pregnancy, it is usually performed during the second trimester whenever possible. This strategy avoids the period of organogenesis, and premature labor is said to be less likely. Many centers use tocolytic therapy as part of their routine for the surgical patient who is pregnant. Although this can be useful for patients without cardiovascular disease, most of these drugs have potent cardiovascular side effects and are less desirable for the patient with heart disease.[64-66,70]

The pregnant patient with heart disease is often managed with medical therapy, which can include long periods of bed rest if necessary. If a surgical lesion is present, every attempt is made to delay the definitive procedure until after delivery of the fetus. Some patients decompensate so severely from the cardiovascular stress imposed by pregnancy that their chance of survival is very small unless surgical correction is attempted. These patients usually suffer from rheumatic valvular disease, most often mitral stenosis.

The first cardiac operations performed during pregnancy in 1952 were closed mitral commissurotomies for severe congestive heart failure caused by mitral stenosis. A review of 514 cases by Ueland revealed a maternal mortality rate of 1.75% and a fetal loss rate of 8.6%.[71] These results were quite favorable compared with a maternal mortality rate of 4.2% to 18.7% among pregnant patients with New York Heart Association (NYHA) class III and IV cardiac disease who were managed with medical therapy; the fetal loss rate for that group of patients was approximately 50%. The extremely good surgical survival figures in the cardiac surgery group probably reflect the fact that these patients are young with relatively healthy hearts that were overburdened by the circulatory changes of pregnancy and that the operations did not involve cardiopulmonary bypass. The use of cardiopulmonary bypass for open-heart procedures in the pregnant patient soon followed. The risks for the mother and fetus increase with this more complex procedure. A multi-institutional study of cardiopulmonary bypass in this subset of patients by Zitnik and colleagues[72] revealed a 5% maternal mortality rate and a fetal loss rate of 33%. Current data indicate a maternal mortality rate of 0% to 2.9% and a fetal loss rate of 20%.[73] The high rate of fetal loss has been attributed to several factors that may affect fetal oxygen delivery during cardiopulmonary bypass, including nonpulsatile perfusion, inadequate perfusion pressure, embolic events to the uteroplacental circulation, disturbance of uteroplacental blood flow by cannulas, release of catecholamines and renin, and hypothermia.[74,75] When cardiopulmonary bypass becomes mandatory, the shortest possible periods of mildly hypothermic or normothermic cardiopulmonary bypass are recommended, and a strategy of high-flow and high-pressure perfusion should be followed.[76] Some of these potential hazards can be avoided by the use of fetal monitoring during the operation.

Several reports of the benefit of fetal monitoring during cardiopulmonary bypass have appeared in the literature.[77-79] In one instance, a fetal heart rate of 60 was restored to 100 by an increase in pump flow from 3100 to 3600 mL/mi.[77] In addition to identifying potentially threatening events, all physicians have reported a sustained fetal bradycardia between 80 and 100 beats/min during hypothermic cardiopulmonary bypass, which resolves with the restoration of maternal temperature and normal circulation. One meta-analysis revealed that the fetal mortality rate was reduced to 0% when normothermic cardiopulmonary bypass was used.[73]

Based on the available knowledge of the physiologic changes of pregnancy, the pharmacology of drugs employed during cardiopulmonary bypass, the physiology of extracorporeal circulation, and experiences reported, the following recommendations for cardiopulmonary bypass during pregnancy can be made. Although it is desirable to avoid surgery until after pregnancy, no pregnant patient should be denied a definitive operation because of gestation.[64-66,70] Whenever possible, the period of organogenesis should be avoided and the second trimester favored. If cardiopulmonary bypass is required after 28 weeks' gestation, it has been suggested that cesarean delivery immediately before the cardiac surgery is a reasonable and safe procedure.[64-66,70,74] Hemostasis must be meticulous in such cases, because full anticoagulation is necessary.[80,81]

Every effort to ensure adequate fetal oxygenation and perfusion during the procedure should be exercised. Maternal inspired oxygen concentration should be maintained as high as possible, and arterial blood gases should be checked frequently. Maternal ventilation should be adjusted to avoid respiratory alkalosis, because this causes a shift in the oxyhemoglobin dissociation curve to the left, potentially decreasing oxygen transport to the fetus. Aortocaval compression must be minimized by using a wedge to provide left uterine displacement if the patient is at 20 weeks' gestation or more. Calculation of pump flows should include a 30% to 50% increase above normal to compensate for the increase in cardiac output that occurs with pregnancy. Pomini and coworkers[73] recommend maintaining flows at 2.7 L/m^2/min or greater. Perfusion pressures of 60 mm Hg or greater appear optimal for maintaining uteroplacental perfusion. Perfusion times should be kept to a minimum, and normothermic bypass should be used whenever possible. Electrolyte balance should be maintained, and the impact of vasopressors on the uteroplacental circulation should be considered before they are instituted. Electronic fetal monitoring should be used, and a member of the health care team experienced in its interpretation should be available. Monitoring of uterine activity can be desirable, because increased uterine activity has been associated with cardiopulmonary bypass.[64-66,70]

Valvular Heart Disease

Rheumatic fever continues to be the predominant cause of valvular heart disease in pregnancy. Acquired or congenital valvular heart disease in a pregnant woman poses a clinical challenge to physicians involved in her antepartum and peripartum care.[64-66,70] Complications during pregnancy include univentricular or biventricular failure, atrial dysrhythmias, systemic or pulmonary embolism, and infective endocarditis, with an overall incidence of complications estimated at 15% among all patients with valvular disease. In general, regurgitant lesions are well tolerated during pregnancy because the increased plasma volume and lowered SVR result in increased cardiac output. In contrast, stenotic valvular disease is poorly tolerated with advancing pregnancy because of the inability to increase cardiac output sufficiently to accommodate the augmented plasma volume; this situation leads to pulmonary venous congestion and possibly to frank pulmonary edema.[64]

Mitral Stenosis

Mitral stenosis can occur as an isolated lesion or in conjunction with right-sided or aortic valvular disease. It accounts for nearly 90% of rheumatic heart disease in pregnancy, with 25% of patients first experiencing symptoms during pregnancy.[64] The principal pathophysiologic derangement is a decrease in mitral valve orifice, resulting in obstruction to left ventricular filling. This hemodynamic aberration leads to a relatively fixed cardiac output. Although the left atrium initially may overcome this obstruction, with progression of disease, left atrial volume and pressure ultimately increase and lead to a progressive and chronic elevation in pulmonary capillary wedge pressure and pulmonary venous pressure; pulmonary hypertension and right ventricular hypertrophy and failure can ensue.[82,83] An anatomically moderate lesion can become functionally severe with the marked increase in cardiac output that accompanies normal pregnancy, labor, and delivery.

Anesthetic management is oriented toward the avoidance of tachycardia, because the time required for left ventricular diastolic filling is prolonged. Patients who are asymptomatic at term usually require increased vigilance but should not require invasive monitoring. Patients with marked symptoms are at significant risk in the peripartum period and should receive arterial and pulmonary artery catheter monitoring continuing through a minimum of 24 hours after delivery.[64-66,70] An increase in central circulating blood volume can occur suddenly in the immediate postpartum period, and tolerance of this intravascular load may be poor, especially for patients with a fixed cardiac output.[64-66]

Vaginal delivery is best accomplished with segmental lumbar epidural analgesia to minimize hemodynamic changes. The combined spinal-epidural analgesia is an attractive alternative to the conventional epidural block.[64,84,85] A sudden decrease in SVR may be poorly tolerated after the development of reflex tachycardia. Although other analgesic modalities may be employed, segmental epidural analgesia allows for careful titration to the desired result while minimizing undesirable changes. The addition of opioids, such as fentanyl or sufentanil, to the dilute local anesthetic mixture enhances the quality of analgesia but does not add to the sympathetic blockade. Opioids alone may be administered by the epidural or intrathecal route for the critically ill patient. Adequate segmental and perineal anesthesia reduces catecholamine-induced increases in heart rate and the urge to push, allowing fetal descent to be accomplished by uterine contractions and avoiding the deleterious effects of the Valsalva maneuver during the second stage of labor. When epidural anesthesia has not been used, a low spinal anesthetic may be administered to allow for a controlled second stage and delivery.

Caudal anesthesia is another reasonable option. Pudendal nerve block can provide adequate, although not ideal, pain relief for some patients.

Cesarean section should be reserved for obstetric indications. Anesthetic options for cesarean delivery must take into account the additional potential hazards of marked fluid shifts resulting from anesthetic technique, operative blood loss, and the mobilization of fluid in the postpartum period. Regional or general anesthesia may be used. Epidural anesthesia is preferred over spinal anesthesia because the former results in slower onset of blockade and therefore more controllable hemodynamic alterations. Prophylactic ephedrine and arbitrary intravascular volume loading are best avoided; instead, a careful titration of anesthetic level allows judicious and appropriate intravenous fluid administration, which should be guided by hemodynamic monitoring in the symptomatic patient. These patients may be prone to hypotension with epidural anesthesia because of a combination of venous pooling and prior β-adrenergic blockade and diuretic therapy.[70,86] The usual vasopressor choice of ephedrine should be avoided, because it can result in tachycardia. Instead, judicious use of metaraminol or low-dose (20 to 40 μg) phenylephrine assists in restoration of maternal blood pressure with little or no unwanted effect on uteroplacental perfusion.[64]

Some patients with mitral stenosis may require general anesthesia. General anesthesia also can provide a very stable hemodynamic course if the sympathetic stimulation associated with laryngoscopy and intubation and with suction and extubation is minimized.[87] This can be accomplished with anesthetic agents or β-adrenergic blockade, or both. Induction of general anesthesia should be accomplished carefully, without drugs that commonly produce tachycardia. Depending on the severity of the disease, the need to blunt the hemodynamic response to endotracheal intubation may necessitate the use of a high-dose, narcotic-based technique. This strategy also avoids myocardial depression and the decreases in SVR that can occur with commonly employed short-acting barbiturates. Anesthesia is maintained with narcotics, muscle relaxants, nitrous oxide, and oxygen. Emergence must be controlled carefully to ensure return of protective reflexes and avoidance of tachycardia.

Aortic Stenosis

Congenital aortic defects are the usual causes of aortic stenosis in reproductive-age women. Rheumatic disease–related aortic stenosis rarely complicates pregnancy, primarily because the natural history of this lesion resulting from rheumatic heart disease typically requires 3 to 4 decades to achieve severity adequate to produce symptoms.[88,89] Women with congenitally bicuspid aortic valves and patients with a history of bacterial endocarditis, however, can present in pregnancy with severe aortic stenosis. Unlike mitral stenosis, with aortic stenosis, symptoms of congestive heart failure, angina, and syncope develop relatively late in the course of the disease. The pathophysiology of severe aortic stenosis entails narrowing of the valve orifice to less than 1 cm^2, associated with a transvalvular gradient of 50 mm Hg, which results in significant increases in afterload to left ventricular ejection. The left ventricle appropriately and concentrically hypertrophies and becomes markedly less compliant, although contractility is usually well preserved. The transvalvular gradient increases progressively throughout pregnancy as a result of increasing blood volume and decreasing SVR.[64,65]

Anesthetic management encompasses the following goals:

- Avoiding tachycardia and bradycardia
- Maintaining adequate preload so the left ventricle may generate an adequate cardiac output across the stenotic valve
- Maintaining hemodynamic parameters within a narrow therapeutic window

Patients with transvalvular gradients greater than 50 mm Hg and patients with symptomatic aortic stenosis warrant invasive monitoring with arterial and pulmonary artery catheters in the peripartum period.[64]

Provision of labor analgesia with segmental epidural or combined spinal-epidural anesthesia remains a controversial issue because these patients may not be able to tolerate the decreases in preload and afterload due to sympathetic blockade.[88,89] Easterling and associates[90] described a series of four patients with moderate to severe aortic stenosis who were managed successfully with epidural anesthesia without untoward sequelae; adequate time was allowed to titrate the level of block carefully and initiate appropriate compensatory actions to correct hemodynamic alterations associated with the anesthetic agent. Kuczkowski and Chow[89] described a case of a parturient with severe aortic stenosis who received uneventful combined spinal-epidural analgesia with levobupivacaine and fentanyl for the first stage of labor, but in the second stage of labor, cesarean section under general anesthesia was required for fetal indications (i.e., fetal distress). The investigators concluded that anesthetic management of a parturient with aortic stenosis must be based on individual assessment of cardiac function and reserve and anticipation of the impact of selected anesthetic technique (regional or general for vaginal or abdominal delivery) on cardiac performance.[89] Subarachnoid or epidural opioids, whether alone or in combination with an epidural segmental anesthetic, are other appropriate choices. Spinal opioids have no cardiovascular effects. In particular, myocardial contractility is unaltered, preload is preserved, and, most importantly, SVR is not diminished by this technique. Local anesthetics and opioids are believed to act synergistically, allowing for a decrease in concentration of both drugs when they are used together. Effective analgesia can prevent the tachycardia associated with labor pain.

For cesarean delivery, judiciously titrated epidural anesthesia or general endotracheal anesthesia may be used. General anesthesia can be accomplished with the same caution that applies for parturients with mitral stenosis; myocardial depression associated with halogenated volatile anesthetics should be avoided.[64,65,91]

Mitral Insufficiency

Mitral valve insufficiency and regurgitation is the second most prevalent valvular lesion in pregnancy. Chronic left ventricular volume overload and work are usually well tolerated, with symptoms developing relatively late in life after childbearing age; most patients with mitral regurgitation tolerate pregnancy well.[64-66,70] Complications include an increased risk of atrial fibrillation during pregnancy, bacterial endocarditis requiring antibiotic prophylaxis, systemic embolization, and pulmonary congestion during pregnancy.[87]

Congenital mitral valve prolapse is much more common during pregnancy than mitral regurgitation, and it can be present in 10% to 17% of pregnancies. It is a well-tolerated and generally benign form of mitral regurgitation, and therapeutic interventions are rarely necessary.[64-66]

The pathophysiology of regurgitation through an incompetent mitral valve results in chronic volume overload of the left ventricle and dilatation. If left ventricular compromise is sufficiently long-standing and severe, the increase in plasma volume with pregnancy progression can result in pulmonary venous congestion. In contrast, the decreasing SVR associated with pregnancy may improve forward flow across the aortic valve at the expense of regurgitant flow. Increases in SVR, which occur with labor pain, uterine contractions, or surgical stimulation, can result in an increase in the proportion of regurgitant blood flow, perhaps leading to acute left ventricular failure.[92]

Anesthetic management of labor and delivery can be provided safely with any of the available techniques, including segmental lumbar epidural anesthesia or combined spinal-epidural anesthesia.[64,85] Adequate analgesia and anesthesia minimize the peripheral vasoconstriction, attenuating the increase in left ventricular afterload associated with labor pain and thereby augmenting the forward flow of blood. Sympathetic blockade also decreases SVR and is beneficial in this regard; the caveat is that venous capacitance will increase, and the physician must be prepared to augment preload cautiously with intravenous fluid infusion to maintain left ventricular filling volume.

Asymptomatic patients at term are unlikely to require invasive monitoring. Continuous electrocardiographic (ECG) monitoring is a reasonable addition to basic standards of peripartum monitoring. In symptomatic patients, invasive monitoring with arterial and pulmonary arterial catheter should be used.

Aortic Insufficiency

Aortic insufficiency can be congenital or acquired. If congenital, it is commonly associated with other lesions; if acquired, it may result from rheumatic heart disease or endocarditis in association with aortic root dissection. Symptoms after rheumatic fever usually develop during the fourth or fifth decade of life, and most women in whom this is the dominant lesion have uneventful pregnancies.[64-66,70]

The basic pathophysiology is chronic volume overloading of the left ventricle resulting in hypertrophy and dilation associated with increased compliance. Because of hypertrophy, myocardial oxygen requirements are higher than normal, but perfusion pressure (and oxygen supply) can be decreased by a reduction in diastolic pressure and an increased left ventricular end-diastolic pressure.[64-66]

Anesthetic considerations focus on the following goals:

- Minimizing pain and therefore catecholamine-induced increases in SVR
- Avoiding bradycardia, which increases time for regurgitant flow
- Avoiding myocardial depressants, which can exacerbate failure

Because the anesthetic concerns are similar to those for patients with mitral regurgitation, epidural anesthesia for labor and delivery is desirable to prevent increases in peripheral vasoconstriction. Epidural anesthesia is also appropriate as a surgical anesthetic agent, as is general anesthesia with judicious avoidance of direct myocardial depressants. Invasive monitoring is a requirement in any patient with symptoms of congestive heart failure.[64-66,70]

The parturient who has undergone mitral or aortic valve replacement faces several potential problems, such as thromboembolism, valvular outflow obstruction, endocarditis, and hemolysis.[93,94] These patients have received anticoagulation, usually with coumarin derivatives, to prevent the thrombotic problems mentioned. Heparin is usually substituted for coumarin anticoagulants during pregnancy to avoid potential congenital anomalies.[64] Full anticoagulation is a direct contraindication to the use of regional anesthesia because of the risk of causing epidural or spinal hematoma. The use of low-molecular-weight heparin (e.g., enoxaparin) has been associated with spinal epidural hematoma when regional anesthesia was used or attempted in Europe and in the United States,[95,96] probably because of its longer half-life than unfractionated heparin. It is therefore recommended that regional anesthesia not be administered unless the drug has been discontinued for at least 12 to 24 hours, depending on the dosage. One alternative is to continue heparinization throughout labor and delivery and use systemic analgesia for labor and general anesthesia for delivery. Another option with unfractionated heparin is to discontinue heparin therapy just before labor and delivery, normalize the coagulation results, use regional anesthesia, and restart heparin 12 hours later. This may not be practical in an obstetric setting. The choice of strategies depends on the severity of the patient's hemodynamic derangement and the optimal analgesic management.[64,65]

Congenital Heart Disease

Congenital heart disease is becoming the most common cardiac problem encountered in pregnant patients. Patients are increasingly likely to survive to childbearing age with the advent of palliative surgery or total correction of their defects. Many of these patients can be expected to have an uneventful pregnancy and delivery.[64,65]

Left-to-Right Shunts

VENTRICULAR SEPTAL DEFECT

Ventricular septal defect (VSD) occurs in 7% of adults with congenital heart disease. Patients with uncorrected lesions in the absence of pulmonary hypertension fare well during pregnancy. In the small percentage of patients with large VSDs and coexisting pulmonary hypertension, maternal mortality rates range from 7% to 40%. Severe right ventricular failure with shunt reversal (i.e., Eisenmenger syndrome) is the major ensuing complication. During pregnancy, elevation of plasma volume, cardiac output, and heart rate can increase left-to-right shunt and can further worsen the degree of pulmonary hypertension.[64,65,70]

The major goals in peripartum management include awareness that marked increases in peripheral vascular resistance and heart rate may be poorly tolerated, with ventricular failure a distinct possibility. Conversely, acute increases in pulmonary vascular resistance (PVR) and right ventricular compromise can lead to shunt reversal and hypoxia.

Optimal anesthesia for labor and vaginal delivery is achieved with segmental epidural or combined spinal-epidural anesthesia consisting of local anesthetics, opioids, or their combination to permit control of painful stimuli, minimizing changes in heart rate and SVR. Anesthesia for cesarean delivery can be accomplished with slow titration of an epidural or combined spinal-epidural anesthetic agent to allow time for correction of pressure changes or with a general anesthetic agent that combines opioid and inhalation technique to depress the adrenergic response to endotracheal intubation and minimize myocardial depression.[64,65]

ATRIAL SEPTAL DEFECT

Atrial septal defect is one of the most common congenital cardiac lesions in women of childbearing age, and pregnancy is generally well tolerated even when pulmonary blood flow is increased. However, the risk of left ventricular failure is increased during pregnancy. Increases in atrial volume result in biatrial enlargement, and supraventricular dysrhythmias are likely.

Pregnancy-associated increases in plasma volume and cardiac output accentuate the left-to-right shunt, right ventricular volume work, and pulmonary blood flow, with the possible development of pulmonary hypertension and left and right ventricular failure. Peripartum management centers on avoiding vascular resistance changes that can increase the degree of shunt. Increases in SVR or decreases in PVR may not be well tolerated.[64,65,87]

Although all of the common methods of providing labor analgesia are useful, lumbar epidural analgesia for labor, vaginal delivery, or cesarean delivery attenuates the hazards of increased SVR. General anesthesia for cesarean delivery is also well tolerated, provided that increases in SVR are avoided and sinus rhythm is maintained.

PATENT DUCTUS ARTERIOSUS

Patent ductus arteriosus (PDA) accounts for 15% of all cases of congenital heart disease, and most patients with a large PDA (>1 cm) receive early surgical intervention. Patients with a small PDA typically have normal pregnancies, but for those pregnant women with superimposed pulmonary hypertension, the maternal mortality rate can reach 5% to 6% because of ventricular failure. The progressive decrease in SVR development throughout pregnancy can be associated with shunt reversal and peripheral cyanosis.[64,87]

Anesthetic considerations include avoidance of increases in SVR and hypervolemia. Conversely, acute decreases in SVR may result in reversal of shunt in patients with preexisting pulmonary hypertension and right ventricular compromise. All modalities may be used, depending on the severity of the disease. Continuous lumbar epidural analgesia for labor and delivery diminishes the increase in SVR associated with pain. Epidural or general anesthesia is appropriate for cesarean delivery if increases in SVR associated with endotracheal intubation and surgical stimulation are addressed adequately.

Right-to-Left Shunts

Eisenmenger syndrome consists of pulmonary hypertension, a right-to-left intracardiac shunt resulting from pulmonary hypertension superimposed on a previously left-to-right shunt, and arterial hypoxemia.[97,98] Pregnancy is not well tolerated by patients with this condition. The maternal mortality rate is estimated at 30% to 50%. This entity is responsible for approximately 50% of the maternal mortality rate among parturients with congenital heart disease.[64]

Anesthetic considerations center on avoidance of any decrease in SVR and therefore on avoidance of hypotension or myocardial depression. Hypotension from any cause, including conduction block or hemorrhage, can progress to insufficient right ventricular pressures to perfuse the hypertensive pulmonary arterial bed and can result in sudden death.

Analgesia for vaginal delivery can be accomplished with systemic narcotics, intrathecal narcotics, or cautious application of a segmental epidural if SVR is maintained. During the first stage of labor, epidural or intrathecal opioid administration can be a useful adjunct, and its sole administration has been recommended as the safest approach.[64-66] If an epidural block is employed, epinephrine should be omitted from the test dose because peripheral β-adrenergic effects can decrease SVR.

For second-stage analgesia and anesthesia, a caudal epidural block may be preferable to the lumbar route because dense perineal analgesia can be provided without extensive sympathetic blockade. Cesarean delivery can be safely accomplished with the use of general anesthesia, although regional anesthesia for elective cesarean delivery has been reported.[99-102]

Regardless of the anesthetic technique employed, the postpartum period is probably the most likely time for life-threatening complications of hypoxemia, cardiac dysrhythmias, and thromboembolic events to occur; most maternal deaths occur in the first postpartum week.[64-66,102,103] Martin and colleagues[102] conducted an extensive literature search that identified 57 articles describing 103 anesthetics administered to patients with Eisenmenger syndrome.[102] The overall perioperative mortality rate was 14%; patients receiving regional anesthesia had a mortality rate of 5%, whereas those receiving general anesthesia had a mortality rate of 18%. This trend favored the use of regional anesthesia but was not statistically significant. A better predictor of outcome was the nature of the surgery and presumably the surgical disease. Patients requiring major surgery had mortality rate of 24%, whereas those requiring minor surgery had mortality rate of 5%. Patients in labor receiving regional anesthesia had a mortality rate of 24%, and most of these deaths occurred several hours after delivery.[102] The study authors concluded that most deaths probably occurred as a result of the surgical procedure and disease, not anesthesia.[102]

The use of invasive monitoring is highly recommended in the management of these patients in the peripartum period. Pulmonary artery catheters and serial arterial blood gas determinations allow early detection of changes in cardiac output, pulmonary artery pressures, and shunt fraction. Serial measurements of cardiac output and especially of SVR are useful in this regard. the technical difficulties in passage of a pulmonary artery catheter and obtaining wedge pressures are well documented, and a central venous catheter may have to suffice.[104]

TETRALOGY OF FALLOT

Tetralogy of Fallot comprises 15% of all congenital heart disease and is the most common etiologic factor in right to left shunt in women of childbearing age. Improvements in early diagnosis and treatment of patients with tetralogy of Fallot have led to an increase in the number of women who survive to reproductive age.[64-66,106] Particularly poor prognostic signs include a history of syncope, polycythemia (hematocrit <60), decreased arterial oxygen saturation (<80%), right ventricular hypertension, and congestive heart failure.[64,105] Increased right-to-left shunt can accompany pregnancy-induced decreases in SVR. The stress of labor can increase PVR and increase the degree of shunt. Most complications occur in the postpartum period when SVR is lowest, exacerbating the right-to-left shunting of blood and worsening the degree of arterial hypoxemia.[106]

Anesthetic considerations must focus on minimizing the hemodynamic changes that would exacerbate the degree of shunt. Strict avoidance of decreased SVR, decreased venous return, and myocardial depression are essential. Analgesia for labor and vaginal delivery in these patients is most safely provided by systemic medication, inhalational nitrous oxide analgesia, or pudendal block. Intrathecal opioids can prove optimal in some circumstances. Regional anesthetic techniques should be used with extreme caution because the decrease in SVR can result in increased shunt. Historically, general anesthesia has been regarded as the safer (than regional) option for abdominal delivery in pregnant women with uncorrected tetralogy of Fallot.[105] However, in many cases of tetralogy of Fallot, corrective heart surgery results in nearly complete or complete repair and nearly normal or normal cardiovascular function. If the extent of surgical repair (i.e., correction) cannot be fully established in the peripartum period, the obstetric and anesthetic management of these parturient can become challenging and complex. Anesthesia for cesarean delivery should be provided by general anesthesia in patients with uncorrected lesions. Invasive monitoring with arterial and pulmonary artery catheters to evaluate cardiac filling pressures and SVR is warranted in patients with uncorrected tetralogy or only palliative correction.

PRIMARY PULMONARY HYPERTENSION

Primary pulmonary hypertension predominantly affects women of childbearing age and is associated with a maternal mortality rate greater than 50%. Most deaths occur during labor and the puerperium.[64-66,70,87,106,107] Signs and symptoms depend on severity of the disease and are caused by a fixed low cardiac output, the degree of pulmonary hypertension, and the degree of right ventricular compromise. Pulmonary hypertension is a major component of Eisenmenger syndrome.[97,98]

Anesthetic considerations focus on the following goals:

- Evaluating the severity of the disease and its responsiveness to therapy
- Maintaining hemodynamic stability
- Administering the appropriate analgesia and anesthesia for labor and delivery

In selecting an analgesic or anesthetic regimen, the physician must consider primarily the prevention of increases in PVR from underventilation, pharmacologic agents, pulmonary hyperinflation, and stress. Decreases in right ventricular volume from intravascular volume depletion, venodilation, or aortocaval compression are poorly tolerated. Significant decreases in SVR from sympathetic blockade from regional anesthesia or volatile anesthetic agents can produce severe decompensation because the cardiovascular system may be unable to compensate for the decline in afterload.[64-66] Right ventricular contractility may be marginal, and the addition of negative inotropic anesthetic agents can lead to marked depression in cardiac function. The parturient should be monitored with an ECG, pulse oximetry, radial artery catheter, and a pulmonary artery catheter throughout labor and the postpartum period. The use of a pulmonary artery catheter allows early detection of changes in PVR or right ventricular function and serves as a guide to fluid and pharmacologic therapy.[87]

Labor and vaginal delivery can best be managed by the judicious use of systemic narcotic analgesics and pudendal nerve block. Epidural analgesia with local anesthesia may be provided only if the block is slowly titrated in a limited dermatomal fashion from T10 to L1 to avoid extensive sympathetic blockade. Intrathecal or epidural opioids also provide effective first-stage analgesia. Vaginal delivery can be managed by the addition of a caudal catheter or pudendal block.

Regional anesthesia is best avoided for cesarean delivery, and a slow induction with high-dose narcotics or an inhalation agent is recommended.[108] This practice is necessary to avoid marked increases in PVR with laryngoscopy. Cricoid pressure must be maintained throughout the induction to prevent the aspiration of gastric contents. Ventilation must be adequate, but pulmonary hyperinflation must be avoided. Uterine stimulants should be omitted because they can be associated with significant elevations in PVR.[64-66]

Coronary Artery Disease

Coronary artery disease is uncommon in women of childbearing age, with a reported incidence of 1 case in 10,000 pregnancies.[64] In one study, it was determined that only 13% of gravidas who had a myocardial infarction had a known history of coronary artery disease; the overall maternal mortality rate was 37%, increasing to 45% if the infarction occurred in the third trimester.[109]

The pathophysiology and clinical manifestations of coronary artery disease in pregnant women are identical to those in nonpregnant patients. The hemodynamic demands that pregnancy places on the myocardium stress the coronary circulation.[110] General management guidelines include efforts to reduce the cardiac workload with measures such as bed rest, nitrate therapy for preload reduction, and conduction anesthesia during delivery. Cardiac medications, such as β-blockers and nitrates, should be continued throughout the pregnancy, labor, delivery, and puerperium.[111,112] Effort must be directed toward optimizing myocardial oxygen supply; supplemental oxygen should be provided, anemia treated, and respiratory depression caused by sedation meticulously avoided.

Although reasonable pain relief can be achieved with systemic narcotic analgesia, the early institution of continuous regional anesthesia (e.g., epidural or combined spinal-epidural anesthesia) for labor and delivery is recommended to minimize the pain and stress that have the potential to precipitate ischemia and angina.[64-66] Beneficial effects associated with regional anesthesia may also include decreased preload and afterload so that myocardial work is diminished. Marked and sudden decreases in afterload must be avoided because coronary artery perfusion depends on diastolic pressure. Significant decreases in SVR can precipitate reflex tachycardia, which may increase cardiac workload sufficiently to produce ischemia. Epidural anesthesia effectively attenuates the progressive increase in central venous pressure and cardiac output that occurs during labor in the unanesthetized parturient. Multiple-lead ECG monitoring should be instituted early in labor so that ischemia can be detected and treated promptly.[87]

When establishing an epidural blockade, epinephrine should be omitted from the test dose to avoid potential tachycardia, and the block should be established by administration of slower-onset local anesthetic agents, such as bupivacaine, ropivacaine, or levobupivacaine.[113] Supplementation of a dilute local anesthetic solution with an epidural opioid has been advocated.[114,115] Fetal descent during the second stage of labor should be by force of uterine contraction, with avoidance of the Valsalva maneuver, according to the patient's baseline ejection fraction and analysis of the hemodynamic response to contractions. When epidural analgesia for first-stage labor is not employed, a low spinal anesthetic (i.e., saddle block) provides excellent conditions for an assisted delivery with minimal hemodynamic trespass.

Elective cesarean delivery can be performed safely with a slowly titrated level of epidural anesthesia, allowing judicious intravenous fluid infusion to maintain pulmonary capillary wedge pressure and blood pressure.[116] Spinal anesthesia is much less desirable, because the rapid onset of sympathetic block has great potential for hypotension and reflex tachycardia. When administering general anesthesia for cesarean delivery, the anesthesiologist considers the importance of minimizing the cardiovascular response to the stress of endotracheal intubation and surgery. In the absence of congestive heart failure, an inhalation technique is recommended.[64]

Myocardial infarction (especially in the third trimester) occurring less than 6 weeks earlier, congestive heart failure, or unstable or crescendo angina warrants invasive monitoring with arterial and pulmonary artery catheters.[117] Monitoring should be continued for a minimum of 24 hours into the postpartum period to assess increases in pulmonary capillary wedge pressure as intravascular volume increases after delivery and as anesthesia subsides.

Hypertrophic Obstructive Cardiomyopathy

Hypertrophic obstructive cardiomyopathy (HOCM), also called asymmetrical septal hypertrophy (ASH) or idiopathic hypertrophic subaortic stenosis (IHSS), is a disease without a defined cause, but at least one third of the subjects have a familial history, and it appears to be inherited as an autosomal dominant trait.[118-121] The primary features of this cardiomyopathy include marked hypertrophy of the left ventricle and interventricular septum and obstruction of the left ventricular outflow tract during systole by the hypertrophied muscle. The anterior leaflet of the mitral valve can be displaced by the hypertrophied muscle and contribute to the obstruction in some patients.

The disease commonly manifests during the second to fourth decades of life. Common symptoms include angina pectoris, dizziness, and exertional dyspnea.[64-66,118-121] Physical findings include signs of left ventricular hypertrophy, a systolic ejection murmur, and a third heart sound. The ECG pattern indicates left ventricular hypertrophy and, in many cases, evidence of Wolff-Parkinson-White syndrome and abnormal Q waves. There is wide variability in the findings and the symptoms of the disease.[118-121]

The hemodynamic limitations of HOCM are produced as the ventricle contracts. The hypertrophied walls narrow the outflow region during systole. The determinants of the degree of obstruction are the volume of the left ventricle at systole, the force of left ventricular contraction, and the degree of left ventricular distention during systolic contraction. The patient therefore requires a high preload to maintain a full left ventricle, a reduced contractile force to minimize outflow tract narrowing, and a high SVR to maintain distention of the left ventricle during systole.

Therapy primarily focuses on the administration of β-adrenergic blocking agents to reduce myocardial contractility and heart rate. Some patients also receive calcium channel blocking drugs. Patients with HOCM do not tolerate hypovolemia, decreased SVR, or increases in myocardial contractility very well.[118-121] The cardiovascular and hemodynamic changes of pregnancy have a variable effect on patients with HOCM, depending on the severity and the nature of the disorder. The increase in blood volume associated with pregnancy should yield a beneficial effect because it increases preload. The usually observed increase in heart rate and stroke volume during pregnancy can have a negative effect, and the decrease in SVR, which begins during the second trimester, may also negatively affect cardiac performance. Although the potential for left ventricular failure and cardiac arrhythmias during pregnancy exists, the outcome of patients with HOCM has been reasonably good.[64-66]

There are several therapeutic objectives during parturition:

- Minimizing pain-associated increases in catecholamine levels
- Maintaining preload by adequate intravenous fluid administration
- Avoiding a Valsalva maneuver, which decreases preload abruptly

Invasive monitoring with an arterial line and a pulmonary artery catheter can yield the information necessary to provide precise management. Recommendations for analgesia during the first stage of labor have been to employ systemic narcotics, inhaled analgesics, or paracervical block. Regional analgesia has been considered a substantial risk because of the potential for venodilation (i.e., decreased preload) and arterial dilation resulting in decreased SVR. Decreased SVR can be avoided if careful incremental titration of continuous lumbar epidural analgesia is carried out. A limited segmental level of analgesia from T10 to L2 provides adequate analgesia with minimal sympathetic blockade, preserving preload. Dilute solutions of a local anesthetic agent with the addition of a narcotic, such as fentanyl or sufentanil, provide optimal analgesia.[64-66] Intrathecal narcotics may be used, eliminating the risk of sympathetic blockade but adding the potential side effects of respiratory depression, pruritus, and nausea, all of which are easy to treat.

A combined spinal and epidural analgesic approach has been used successfully for a patient with HOCM.[122] Vaginal delivery can be accomplished with pudendal block, carefully extended epidural analgesia, and combined spinal-epidural or low spinal anesthesia (i.e., saddle block).[64-66,123] The saddle block involves the spinal segments from L2 to S5 and avoids most sympathetic nerve elements. Regional anesthesia is effective at blocking the uncontrollable urge to bear down. If hypotension necessitating a vasopressor does occur, the use of ephedrine is relatively contraindicated because it causes tachycardia and increased myocardial contractility. Metaraminol or a pure vasoconstricting drug, such as phenylephrine (20 to 40 µg), should be employed in the lowest effective doses to minimize its effect on the uterine arteries.

Anesthesia for cesarean delivery offers additional challenges. Left uterine displacement must be maintained and volume requirements carefully assessed in view of the increased blood loss. Invasive monitoring is needed. Regional anesthesia is usually avoided for the aforementioned reasons, and the level of anesthesia required is likely to produce extensive sympathetic blockade with undesirable consequences.[64,65,87] Nonetheless, a carefully titrated epidural anesthetic with ongoing compensation for the induced hemodynamic changes can prove acceptable. General anesthesia is preferred by many, although the ideal technique has not been established and experience is limited. Although the use of volatile anesthetic agents is advantageous because they reduce myocardial contractility, they also decrease uterine contractility and SVR. Modest doses should have a minimal effect on both.

As with the preeclamptic patient, the stimulating effects of laryngoscopy and intubation on patients with HOCM need to be blunted pharmacologically. Oxytocin must be administered cautiously because it tends to decrease SVR and results in tachycardia when administered rapidly. The parturient with HOCM requires careful attention by means of appropriate monitoring and immediate availability of the necessary vasopressors, β-blockers, and intravenous volume expanders.

Marfan Syndrome

Marfan syndrome is an autosomal dominant disorder characterized by connective tissue abnormalities of the cardiovascular, skeletal, and ocular systems. The principal cardiovascular involvement is weakness of the aortic media, which can result in progressive aortic dilatation or acute dissection.[91] Dilatation can begin as early as the first year of life and typically occurs first in the coronary sinuses. Profound aortic regurgitation can predate clinical evidence of aortic dissection, and dissection may not be heralded by the classic chest pain with radiation to the back that usually accompanies aortic dissection from other causes. These patients also can experience coronary artery involvement, pulmonary artery dilatation, redundant chordae tendineae, or an increased incidence of aortic coarctation.

Anesthetic management options for labor and delivery or cesarean delivery has been only rarely reported. In one case report of two patients with Marfan syndrome and evidence of aortic dissection, epidural anesthesia was provided successfully for cesarean delivery with invasive monitoring by means of a pulmonary artery catheter and an arterial line.[124] In another report, Brar[125] described a case of a Stanford type B aortic dissection (i.e., originating distal to the left subclavian artery and extending to the aortic bifurcation and proximal left iliac artery) in a primigravid woman at term who had Marfan syndrome. The dissection was managed conservatively. Cesarean section was performed under epidural anesthesia with aggressive control of hypertension. Postoperatively, there was no extension of the dissection and no aneurysm formation.[125] In the asymptomatic patient without cardiovascular manifestations and a normal echocardiographic examination, segmental epidural anesthesia for labor and vaginal delivery without invasive hemodynamic monitoring are appropriate and inherently safe if the severity of associated scoliosis does not preclude the success of this technique. Adequate analgesia provided by an epidural block is distinctly advantageous in decreasing pain and catecholamine output, diminishing the stress on the aortic wall. Anesthesia for cesarean delivery may be provided by regional or general technique.

General anesthesia for cesarean delivery in the presence of cardiovascular complications must be tailored to minimize the hemodynamic response to endotracheal intubation and surgical stimuli.[91] Prophylactic β-adrenergic blockade and inhalational agents that produce decreased myocardial contractility and slow the force of cardiac ejection have been advocated.[91] Control of blood pressure alone with vasodilators may only increase left ventricular ejection velocity and, unless combined with β-adrenergic blockade, may not prevent dissection. The potential for temporomandibular joint laxity and dislocation on endotracheal intubation also exists, although difficult intubation has not been reported.

Ehlers-Danlos Syndrome

Ehlers-Danlos syndrome is a rare, genetically transmitted connective tissue disorder that is not specific to pregnancy. Because of the multiorgan involvement and varied presentations of this disease, no uniform or routine anesthetic recommendations can be made.[126] The features of Ehlers-Danlos syndrome that have the greatest impact on the management of anesthesia include fragile, poorly healing skin; excessive bleeding; spontaneous pneumothorax; easy joint dislocation; valvular prolapse; and spontaneous dissections or ruptures of major vessels.

Some of the problems in Ehlers-Danlos syndrome may have implications for the administration of regional anesthesia.[126] Although bruising, bleeding, and hematomas are common, no coagulation disorder has been consistently associated with Ehlers-Danlos syndrome. Nevertheless, bleeding can complicate arterial, peripheral, or central line and neuraxial needle placement. If general anesthesia is selected for these parturients, the airway must be managed gently in view of the possible presence of spine involvement, periodontal disease, propensity for gingival bleeding, and oropharyngeal tissue fragility.[127,128] Cardiac function must be evaluated preoperatively, and anesthetic implications must be considered. Intraoperatively, low airway pressures are needed because of the increased risk of pneumothorax. If possible, spontaneous ventilation is recommended. Elaborate padding of pressure points is indicated.

Spinal Abnormalities

Kyphoscoliosis occurs in approximately 0.4% to 1% of the population in the United States and is associated with obstetric and anesthetic concerns during pregnancy and delivery.[91] Specific obstetric concerns relate to concomitant disease and the risk of dystocia in labor. Lesions involving the upper spine are commonly associated with disordered cardiorespiratory function. The natural history of an untreated severe curve is progression of deformity over time, resulting in early death from cardiorespiratory failure.

Anesthetic management for labor and vaginal delivery must be designed to minimize respiratory depression from systemic opioids or respiratory embarrassment from excessive intercostal muscle paralysis during high levels of regional anesthesia in patients with preexisting pulmonary dysfunction.[129] It is equally important to emphasize the need for adequate analgesia to minimize catecholamine-induced increases in cardiac output that can precipitate high-output, right-sided heart failure. A closely monitored segmental epidural analgesic technique can serve all of these purposes and avoid systemic opioid-induced respiratory depression.

Although an epidural analgesic is optimal for the aforementioned reasons, it can be difficult to achieve in the kyphoscoliotic obstetric patient. Distortion of the spinal column and of the epidural space can prevent proper placement of an epidural catheter and uniform distribution of the local anesthetic solution, resulting in an incomplete block. Subarachnoid catheter placement and segmental block have been reported for use in labor and vaginal delivery when epidural anesthesia had been unsuccessful.[91]

Continuous epidural and subarachnoid approaches have been employed to provide surgical anesthesia for cesarean delivery. Both techniques offer the distinct advantage of slow titration of anesthetic level, which allows time for assessment of adequacy of respiratory function and for compensatory hemodynamic mechanisms to become operative. Another significant factor favoring regional anesthesia is that it provides superior analgesia after cesarean delivery in the patient with scoliosis and respiratory impairment.

General anesthesia for cesarean delivery is indicated when severe scoliosis and cardiorespiratory impairment (i.e., cor pulmonale) are apparent at presentation, because respiratory embarrassment is likely to develop in these patients if a high regional anesthetic block is administered. These patients also warrant invasive monitoring of central venous pressure and serial arterial blood gas measurements.

Previous Spinal Surgery

Administration of lumbar epidural analgesia in a parturient who has had previous spinal surgery presents a unique challenge to the anesthesiologist. The difficulties include an inability to identify the epidural space, multiple attempts before catheter insertion, vascular trauma, and subdural local anesthetic injection to accidental dural puncture. In the past, previous spinal surgery was thought by some to represent a relative contraindication to regional anesthesia.[130-134] A potential problem is obliteration of the epidural space from adhesions, which can limit spread of local anesthetics and increase the risk of dural puncture. Insertion of an epidural needle in the fused area can be relatively contraindicated or impossible to perform because of the presence of bone graft material and scar tissue, degenerative changes that occur in the spine after fusion, persistent back pain, and the risk of introducing infection in the area of foreign bodies.[130] These patients may express considerable anxiety and reluctance regarding catheter insertion in their backs.

Patients who have undergone earlier spinal surgery should be seen in antepartum consultation by the anesthesiologist, and the options for analgesia and anesthesia for labor and delivery should be discussed in detail. Epidural anesthesia may be offered if the patient accepts the higher incidence of complications and failure rate. Alterations in dosage with larger-than-usual doses of local anesthesia required have been described, and, with adjustments and vigilance, this technique has been used successfully.[132]

Achondroplastic Dwarfism

Although achondroplastic dwarfism is a rare complication of pregnancy, the patient may have a number of anatomic and physiologic abnormalities that contribute to problems with the administration of anesthesia.[91] The airway in a patient with achondroplasia typically has narrowed nasal passages and pharyngeal and maxillary hypoplasia. The base of the skull is shortened (because of early fusion of constituent bones) and angulated, yielding limited extension and making endotracheal intubation potentially difficult. However, easy mask general anesthetic ventilation has been described.[135] Kyphoscoliosis is a common associated clinical finding in dwarfs, and respiratory problems caused by decreased functional residual capacity because of scoliosis and advancing enlargement of the uterus throughout pregnancy may be encountered.[91] Obstructive sleep apnea has become recognized as an insidious cause of morbidity in patients with achondroplasia, and it is more common than central apnea because of cervicomedullary cord compromise. Acquired pulmonary hypertension leading to cor pulmonale can occur in women with achondroplasia, with contributions by restrictive lung disease associated with scoliosis, chronic upper airway obstruction, and sleep apnea.

Abnormalities of the spinal cord can result from severe kyphosis and scoliosis or from odontoid hypoplasia with cervical instability, leading to spinal cord and nerve root compression.[91] The vertebral bodies are abnormally shallow, with underdeveloped vertebral arches causing narrowing of the subarachnoid and epidural space. Adults with the condition have hypoplastic intervertebral disks that can prolapse easily into a congenitally stenotic canal and produce neural compression. All of these factors can make regional anesthesia difficult or impossible to achieve, with unpredictable spread of local anesthetic solutions and increased risk of unintentional dural puncture.

Cesarean delivery is inevitable for these women because the maternal pelvis is invariably small and contracted, resulting in cephalopelvic disproportion. In this setting, the anesthesiologist must fully understand the previously described problems to facilitate the safe delivery of anesthesia and select methods of minimizing the risk of maternal aspiration and avoiding fetal depression.

Pregnancy in achondroplasia compounds many of the outlined problems and presents a unique challenge to the obstetrician and anesthesiologist. General endotracheal anesthesia has traditionally been considered the technique of choice in women with achondroplasia, even though case reports have detailed difficult endotracheal intubation.[91] In those instances, extension of the neck was difficult or impossible. These patients warrant early discussion of the probability of intubation while awake after a thorough examination of the airway and review of any available cervical radiographs.

Technically challenging problems are also associated with regional anesthesia because of the skeletal abnormalities encountered. Epidural anesthesia has been administered successfully.[136-138] A relative contraindication to regional anesthesia has been a concern that neurologic sequelae can be attributed to the anesthetic agent. Patients who have received successful epidural anesthesia have not experienced preoperative or postoperative neurologic dysfunction. Epidural anesthesia is theoretically preferable to spinal anesthesia because it lends itself to titration of the level of block. A smaller dose of anesthesia than usual may be required because of maternal short stature and kyphoscoliosis. The dangers of intraoperative hypotension and high or total spinal block are greater for spinal than for epidural anesthesia.

Substance Abuse

Substance abuse has crossed social, economic, and geographic borders, and throughout the world, it remains one of the major problems facing society. The prevalence of substance abuse in young adults (including women) has increased markedly over the past 20 years. Almost 90% of drug-abusing women are of childbearing age.[139-144] Substance abuse is "self-administration of various drugs that deviates from medically or socially accepted use, which if prolonged, can lead to the development of physical and psychological dependence."[145] Most often, abuse of an illicit substance is first suspected or diagnosed during medical management of another condition, such as hepatitis, human immunodeficiency virus (HIV) infection, or pregnancy.[139-150] Illicit substances most commonly abused in pregnancy include cocaine, amphetamines, opioids, ethanol, tobacco, marijuana, caffeine, and toluene-based solvents. Polysubstance abuse is common.[139-144,146-157] Regardless of the drugs ingested and the clinical manifestations, it is always difficult to predict the exact anesthetic implications in chemically dependent patients. Most patients with a history of drug abuse deny it when interviewed preoperatively by anesthesiologists or obstetricians.[158-160]

Anesthesiologists become involved in the care of drug-abusing patients in emergency situations, such as fetal distress, placental abruption, or uterine rupture, or in more controlled situations, such as a request for labor analgesia. Of the drugs abused, cocaine has the most profound implications for the obstetric anesthesiologist. Regional and general anesthesia in the cocaine-abusing parturient can be associated with serious complications.[139,144,148,150,152,158] When regional anesthesia is selected, combative behavior, altered pain perception, cocaine-induced thrombocytopenia, and ephedrine-resistant hypotension may be encountered. Low doses of phenylephrine titrated to the effect usually restore blood pressure to normal. Pronounced abnormalities in endorphin levels and changes in mu and kappa opioid receptor densities resulting from cocaine addiction can result in perception of pain despite adequate spinal or epidural anesthesia sensory levels.[139]

Hypertension, cardiac arrhythmias, and myocardial ischemia may be encountered under general anesthesia. Propranolol is contraindicated in cocaine-intoxicated patients because of the potential for unopposed α-adrenergic stimulation following -blockade.[161] Although esmolol may provide effective control of tachycardia and hypertension, β-blockade has also been shown to enhance cocaine-induced coronary vasoconstriction. The short elimination half-life of esmolol can offer some advantages if the drug administration is deemed necessary.

The administration of hydralazine has become a standard drug therapy for the treatment of hypertension in cocaine-addicted parturients. The action of this drug includes vasodilation and a decrease in SVR, leading to reflex tachycardia, which may not always be desirable in the patient who is already tachycardic from cocaine intake. Labetalol, a combined, nonselective β- and α-adrenergic blocker, rapidly restores blood pressure without affecting heart rate or uterine blood flow and has been recommended by many in treating cocaine toxicity. Some authorities have suggested, however, that labetalol should not be used to treat cocaine-induced hypertension because labetalol's antagonism of β-adrenergic receptors is greater than its effect on α-adrenergic receptors.[139] The use of calcium channel blockers in drug-abusing parturients remains unclear. Many other drugs, such as nitroglycerin and nitroprusside, have been recommended, although the best drug intervention remains to be established.

All potent volatile anesthetic agents can produce cardiac arrhythmias and increased SVR in cocaine-intoxicated parturients. Halothane has been found to sensitize the myocardium to the effects of catecholamines and therefore should be avoided. When ketamine is used in cocaine-abusing patients, caution is indicated, because it can stimulate the central nervous system and potentiate the cardiac effects of cocaine by further increasing catecholamine levels.[143,159] Nitroglycerin is safe and effective in the treatment of anginal chest pain resulting from acute cocaine ingestion.

References

1. Kuczkowski KM: Labor analgesia for the parturient with pregnancy-induced hypertension: What does an obstetrician need to know? Arch Gynecol Obstet 272:214, 2005.
2. Tihtonen KM, Koobi T, Uotila JT: Arterial stiffness in preeclamptic and chronic hypertensive pregnancies. Eur J Obstet Gynecol Reprod Biol 128:180, 2006.
3. Tihtonen K, Koobi T, Yli-Hankala A, et al: Maternal haemodynamics in pre-eclampsia compared with normal pregnancy during caesarean delivery. BJOG 113:657, 2006.
4. Ramanathan J, Bennett K: Pre-eclampsia: Fluids, drugs, and anesthetic management. Anesthesiol Clin North Am 21:145, 2003.
5. Ganzevoort W, Rep A, Bonsel GJ, et al: A randomised controlled trial comparing two temporising management strategies, one with and one without plasma volume expansion, for severe and early onset pre-eclampsia. BJOG 112:1358, 2005.
6. Blaauw J, Graaff R, van Pampus MG, et al: Abnormal endothelium-dependent microvascular reactivity in recently preeclamptic women. Obstet Gynecol 105:626, 2005.
7. Fischer T, Schneider MP, Schobel HP, et al: Vascular reactivity in patients with preeclampsia and HELLP (hemolysis, elevated liver enzymes, and low platelet count) syndrome. Am J Obstet Gynecol 183:1489, 2000.
8. Dyer RA, Els I, Farbas J, et al: Prospective, randomized trial comparing general with spinal anesthesia for cesarean delivery in preeclamptic patients with a nonreassuring fetal heart trace. Anesthesiology 99:561, 2003.
9. Beilin Y, Bodian CA, Haddad EM, et al: Practice patterns of anesthesiologists regarding situations in obstetric anesthesia where clinical management is controversial. Anesth Analg 83:735, 1996.
10. Moeller-Bertram T, Kuczkowski KM, Benumof JL: Uneventful epidural labor analgesia in a parturient with immune thrombocytopenic purpura and platelet count of 26,000/mm^3 which was unknown preoperatively. J Clin Anesth 16:51, 2004.
11. Nadar S, Lip GY: Platelet activation in the hypertensive disorders of pregnancy. Expert Opin Investig Drugs 13:523, 2004.
12. Channing-Rogers RP, Levin J: A critical reappraisal of the bleeding time. Semin Thromb Hemost 16:1, 1990.
13. Gambling DR: Hypertensive Disorders. In Chestnut DH (ed): Obstetric Anesthesia: Principles and Practice. Philadelphia, Elsevier Mosby, 2004, p 794.
14. Kuczkowski KM: The safety of anaesthetics in pregnant women. Expert Opin Drug Saf 5:251, 2006.
15. Kuczkowski KM, Reisner LS, Lin D: Anesthesia for cesarean section. In Chestnut DH (ed): Obstetric Anesthesia—Principles and Practice. Philadelphia, Elsevier Mosby, 2004, p 421.
16. Naguib M, Lien CA: Pharmacology of muscle relaxants and their antagonists. In Miller RD (ed): Miller's Anesthesia. Philadelphia, Elsevier Churchill Livingstone, 2005, p 481.
17. Viby-Mogensen J: Neuromuscular monitoring. Curr Opin Anaesthesiol 14:655, 2001.
18. Kuczkowski KM: Anesthetic management of labor pain: What does an obstetrician need to know? Arch Gynecol Obstet 271:97, 2005.
19. Kuczkowski KM, Reisner LS, Benumof JL: Airway problems and new solutions for the obstetric patient. J Clin Anesth 15:491, 2003.
20. Kuczkowski KM, Reisner LS, Benumof LJ: The difficult airway: Risk, prophylaxis, and management. In Chestnut DH (ed): Obstetric Anesthesia: Principles and Practice. Philadelphia, Elsevier Mosby, 2004, p 535.
21. Ezri T, Szmuk P, Warters RD, et al: Difficult airway management practice patterns among anesthesiologists practicing in the United States: Have we made any progress? J Clin Anesth 15:418, 2003.
22. Cunningham FG, Lindheimer MD: Hypertension in pregnancy. N Engl J Med 326:927, 1992.
23. Santos AC, Birnbach DJ: Spinal anesthesia in the parturient with severe preeclampsia: Time for reconsideration. Anesth Analg 97:621, 2003.
24. Santos AC, Birnbach DJ: Spinal anesthesia for cesarean delivery in severely preeclamptic women: Don't throw out the baby with the bathwater! Anesth Analg 101:859, 2005.
25. Aya AG, Mangin R, Vialles N, et al: Patients with severe preeclampsia experience less hypotension during spinal anesthesia for elective cesarean delivery than healthy parturients: A prospective cohort comparison. Anesth Analg 97:867, 2003.
26. Visalyaputra S, Rodanant O, Somboonviboon W, et al: Spinal versus epidural anesthesia for cesarean delivery in severe preeclampsia: A prospective randomized, multicenter study. Anesth Analg 101:862, 2005.
27. Aya AG, Vialles N, Tanoubi I, et al: Spinal anesthesia-induced hypotension: A risk comparison between patients with severe preeclampsia and healthy women undergoing preterm cesarean delivery. Anesth Analg 101:869, 2005.
28. Karnad DR, Guntupalli KK: Neurologic disorders in pregnancy. Crit Care Med 33:10(Suppl):S362, 2005.
29. Ferrero S, Pretta S, Ragni N: Multiple sclerosis: Management issues during pregnancy. Eur J Obstet Gynecol Reprod Biol 15:3, 2004.
30. Drake E, Drake M, Bird J, et al: Obstetric regional blocks for women with multiple sclerosis: A survey of UK experience. Int J Obstet Anesth 15:115, 2006.
31. Kuczkowski KM: Labor analgesia for the parturient with neurological disease: What does an obstetrician need to know? Arch Gynecol Obstet 274:41, 2006.
32. Bader AM: Neurologic and neuromuscular disease. In Chestnut DH (ed): Obstetric Anesthesia: Principles and Practice. Philadelphia, Elsevier Mosby, 2004, p 856.
33. Kuczkowski KM: Labor analgesia for the parturient with spinal cord injury: What does an obstetrician need to know? Arch Gynecol Obstet 274:108, 2006.
34. Pereira L: Obstetric management of the patient with spinal cord injury. Obstet Gynecol Surv 58:678, 2003
35. Osgood SL, Kuczkowski KM: Autonomic dysreflexia in a parturient with spinal cord injury. Acta Anaesthesiol Belg 57:161, 2006.
36. Kuczkowski KM: Peripartum anaesthetic management of a parturient with spinal cord injury and autonomic hyperreflexia. Anaesthesia 58:823, 2003.
37. Dias MS, Sekhar LM: Intracranial hemorrhage from aneurysms and arteriovenous malformations during pregnancy and the puerperium. Neurosurgery 25:855, 1990.
38. Horton JC, Chambers WA, Lyons SL, et al: Pregnancy and the risk of hemorrhage from cerebral arteriovenous malformations. Neurosurgery 27:867, 1990.
39. Riviello C, Ammannati F, Bordi L, et al: Pregnancy and subarachnoid hemorrhage: A case report. J Matern Fetal Neonatal Med 16:245, 2004.
40. Kuczkowski KM: Nonobstetric surgery during pregnancy: What are the risks of anesthesia? Obstet Gynecol Surv 59:52, 2004.

41. Kuczkowski KM: Nonobstetric surgery in the parturient: Anesthetic considerations. J Clin Anesth 18:5, 2006.
42. Ni Mhuireachtaigh R, O'Gorman DA: Anesthesia in pregnant patients for nonobstetric surgery. J Clin Anesth 18:60, 2006.
43. Kuczkowski KM: Trauma in pregnancy: Perioperative anesthetic considerations for the head-injured pregnant trauma victim. Anaesthetist 53:180, 2004.
44. Kuczkowski KM: Trauma in the pregnant patient. Curr Opin Anaesthesiol 17:145, 2004.
45. Kuczkowski KM: Trauma during pregnancy: A situation pregnant with danger. Acta Anaesthesiol Belg 56:13, 2005.
46. Liccardi G, Cazzola M, Canonica GW, et al: General strategy for the management of bronchial asthma in pregnancy. Respir Med 97:778, 2003.
47. Greenberger PA: Asthma during pregnancy. J Asthma 27:341, 1990.
48. Holland SM, Thomson KD: Acute severe asthma presenting in late pregnancy. Int J Obstet Anesth 15:75, 2006.
49. Kuczkowski KM: Labor analgesia for the parturient with respiratory disease: What does an obstetrician need to know? Arch Gynecol Obstet 272:160, 2005.
50. Kuczkowski KM, Moeller-Bertram T, Benumof JL: Differential diagnosis of shortness of breath and bronchospasm following eclamptic seizures: Aspiration vs. asthma? Ann Fr Anesth Reanim 23:757, 2004.
51. Lindeman KS: Respiratory disease. In Chestnut DH (ed): Obstetric Anesthesia: Principles and Practice. Philadelphia, Elsevier Mosby, 2004, p 915.
52. McGough EK, Cohen JA: Unexpected bronchospasm during spinal anesthesia. J Clin Anesth 2:35, 1990.
53. Eger EI: Inhaled anesthetics: Uptake and distribution. In Miller RD (ed): Miller's Anesthesia. Philadelphia, Elsevier Churchill Livingstone, 2005, p 131.
54. Richards W, Thompson J, Lewis G, et al: Cardiac arrest associated with halothane anesthesia in a patient receiving theophylline. Ann Allergy 61:83, 1988.
55. Wexler ID, Johannesson M, Edenborough FP, et al: Pregnancy and chronic progressive pulmonary disease. Am J Respir Crit Care Med 15:300, 2007.
56. Jaffee JB, Drease GE, Kelly T, et al: Severe respiratory depression in the obstetric patient after intrathecal meperidine or sufentanil. Int J Obstet Anesth 6:182, 1997.
57. Kuczkowski KM: Respiratory arrest in a parturient following intrathecal administration of fentanyl and bupivacaine as part of a combined spinal-epidural analgesia for labour. Anaesthesia 57:939, 2002.
58. Muammar M, Marshall P, Wyatt H, et al: Caesarean section in a patient with cystic fibrosis. Int J Obstet Anesth 14:70, 2005.
59. Cameron AJ, Skinner TA: Management of a parturient with respiratory failure secondary to cystic fibrosis. Anaesthesia 60:77, 2005.
60. Kuczkowski KM: Labor analgesia for the morbidly obese parturient: An old problem—new solution. Arch Gynecol Obstet 271:302, 2005.
61. Mhyre JM: Anesthetic management for the morbidly obese pregnant woman. Int Anesthesiol Clin 45:51, 2007.
62. Eng M, Butler J, Bonica JJ: Respiratory function in pregnant obese women. Am J Obstet Gynecol 123:241, 1975.
63. Kuczkowski KM, Benumof JL: Repeat cesarean section in a morbidly obese parturient: A new anesthetic option. Acta Anaesthesiol Scand 46:753, 2002.
64. Kuczkowski KM: Labor analgesia for the parturient with cardiac disease: What does an obstetrician need to know? Acta Obstet Gynecol Scand 83:223, 2004.
65. Gomar C, Errando CL: Neuroaxial anaesthesia in obstetrical patients with cardiac disease. Curr Opin Anaesthesiol 18:507, 2005.
66. Harnett M, Mushlin PS, Camann WR: Cardiovascular disease. In Chestnut DH (ed): Obstetric Anesthesia: Principles and Practice. Philadelphia, Elsevier Mosby, 2004, p 707.
67. Clark SL: Cardiac disease in pregnancy. Crit Care Obstet 18:237, 1991.
68. Littleford J: Effects on the fetus and newborn of maternal analgesia and anesthesia: A review. Can J Anesth 51:586, 2004.
69. Cohen-Kerem R, Railton C, Oren D, et al: Pregnancy outcome following non-obstetric surgical intervention. Am J Surg 190:467, 2005.
70. Nuevo FR: Anesthesia for nonobstetric surgery in the pregnant patient. In Birnbach DJ, Gatt SP, Datta S (eds): Textbook of Obstetric Anesthesia. New York, Churchill Livingstone, 2000, p 289.
71. Ueland K: Cardiac surgery and pregnancy. Am J Obstet Gynecol 92:148, 1975.
72. Zitnik RS, Brandenberg RO, Sheldon R, et al: Pregnancy and open heart surgery. Circulation 39(Suppl):1257, 1969.
73. Pomini F, Mercogliano D, Cavalletti C, et al: Cardiopulmonary bypass in pregnancy. Ann Thorac Surg 61:259, 1996.
74. Parry AJ, Westaby S: Cardiopulmonary bypass during pregnancy. Ann Thorac Surg 61:1865, 1996.
75. Crucean A, Murzi B, Giorgi A, et al: Cardiopulmonary bypass in ewe's fetus: Advances and setbacks in our learning curve. ASAIO J 51:649, 2005.
76. Iscan ZH, Mavioglu L, Vural KM, et al: Cardiac surgery during pregnancy. J Heart Valve Dis 15:686, 2006.
77. Koh KS, Friesen RM, Livingstone RA, et al: Fetal monitoring during maternal cardiac surgery with cardiopulmonary bypass. Can Med Assoc J 112:1102, 1975.
78. Eilen B, Kaiser IH, Becker RM, et al: Aortic valve replacement in the third trimester of pregnancy: Case report and review of the literature. Obstet Gynecol 57:119, 1981.
79. DeLaRosa J, Sharoni E, Guyton RA: Pregnancy and valvular heart disease. Heart Surg Forum 6:E7, 2002.
80. Malhotra M, Sharma JB, Tripathii R, et al: Maternal and fetal outcome in valvular heart disease. Int J Gynaecol Obstet 84:11, 2004.
81. Soeda M, Shiono M, Inoue T, et al: A successfully operated case of prosthetic valve thrombosis during planned pregnancy. Ann Thorac Cardiovasc Surg 12:66, 2006.
82. Lim ST: Rheumatic heart diseases in pregnancy. Ann Acad Med Singapore 31:340, 2002.
83. Bonow RO, Carabello BA, Kanu C, et al: for the American College of Cardiology/American Heart Association Task Force on Practice Guidelines; Society of Cardiovascular Anesthesiologists; Society for Cardiovascular Angiography and Interventions; Society of Thoracic Surgeons: ACC/AHA 2006 guidelines for the management of patients with valvular heart disease: A report of the American College of Cardiology/American Heart Association Task Force on Practice Guidelines (writing committee to revise the 1998 guidelines for the management of patients with valvular heart disease): Developed in collaboration with the Society of Cardiovascular Anesthesiologists: Endorsed by the Society for Cardiovascular Angiography and Interventions and the Society of Thoracic Surgeons. Circulation 114:84, 2006.
84. Kuczkowski KM: The combined spinal-epidural analgesia for labor pain. Rev Esp Anestesiol Reanim 8:517, 2006.
85. Kuczkowski KM: Labor pain and its management with the combined spinal-epidural analgesia: What does an obstetrician need to know? Arch Gynecol Obstet 275:183, 2007.
86. Ziskind S, Etchin A, Frenkel Y, et al: Epidural anesthesia with the Trendelenburg position for cesarean section with or without a cardiac surgical procedure in patients with severe mitral stenosis: A hemodynamic study. J Cardiothorac Anesth 3:354, 1990.
87. Mangano DT: Anesthesia for the pregnant cardiac patient. In Hughes SC, Levinson G, Rosen MA (eds): Shnider and Levinson's Anesthesia for Obstetrics. Philadelphia, Lippincott Williams & Wilkins, 2002, p 345.
88. Reimold SC, Rutherford JD: Clinical practice. Valvular heart disease in pregnancy. N Engl J Med 349:52, 2003.
89. Kuczkowski KM, Chow I: Peripartum anesthetic management of the parturient with severe aortic stenosis: Regional vs. general anesthesia? Ann Fr Anesth Reanim 23:758, 2004.
90. Easterling TR, Chadwick HS, Otto CM, et al: Aortic stenosis in pregnancy. Obstet Gynecol 72:113, 1988.
91. Kuczkowski KM: Labor analgesia for the parturient with an uncommon disorder: A common dilemma in the delivery suite. Obstet Gynecol Surv 58:800, 2003.

92. Scott H, Bateman C, Price M: The use of remifentanil in general anaesthesia for caesarean section in a patient with mitral valve disease. Anaesthesia 53:695, 1998.
93. Elkayam U, Bitar F: Valvular heart disease and pregnancy. Part II. Prosthetic valves. J Am Coll Cardiol 46:403, 2005.
94. Elkayam U, Bitar F: Valvular heart disease and pregnancy. Part I. Native valves. J Am Coll Cardiol 46:223, 2005.
95. Porterfield WR, Wu CL: Epidural hematoma in an ambulatory surgical patient. J Clin Anesth 9:74, 1997.
96. Horlocker TT, Wedel DJ, Benzon H, et al: Regional anesthesia in the anticoagulated patient: Defining the risks (the second ASRA Consensus Conference on Neuraxial Anesthesia and Anticoagulation). Reg Anesth Pain Med 28:172, 2003.
97. Kandasamy R, Koh KF, Tham SL, et al: Anaesthesia for caesarean section in a patient with Eisenmenger's syndrome. Singapore Med J 41:356, 2000.
98. Phupong V, Ultchaswadi P, Charakorn C, et al: Fatal maternal outcome of a parturient with Eisenmenger's syndrome and severe preeclampsia. Arch Gynecol Obstet 267:163, 2003.
99. Spinnato JA, Kraynack BJ, Cooper MW: Eisenmenger's syndrome in pregnancy: Epidural anesthesia for elective cesarean section. N Engl J Med 304:1215, 1981.
100. Hytens L, Alexander JP: Maternal and neonatal death associated with Eisenmenger's syndrome. Acta Anaesth Belg 37:45, 1986.
101. Cole PJ, Cross MH, Dresner M: Incremental spinal anaesthesia for elective caesarean section in a patient with Eisenmenger's syndrome. Br J Anaesth 86:723, 2001.
102. Martin JT, Tautz TJ, Antognini JF: Safety of regional anesthesia in Eisenmenger's syndrome. Reg Anesth Pain Med 27:509, 2002.
103. Gilman DH: Caesarean section in undiagnosed Eisenmenger's syndrome: Report of a patient with a fatal outcome. Anaesthesia 46:371, 1991.
104. Pollack KL, Chestnut DH, Wenstrom KD: Anesthetic management of a parturient with Eisenmenger's syndrome. Anesth Analg 70:212, 1990.
105. Fernandez CL, Kuczkowski KM: "Once a tetralogy of Fallot patient—always a tetralogy of Fallot patient (?)": Time for reconsideration? Ann Fr Anesth Reanim 23:1107, 2004.
106. Findlow D, Doyle E: Congenital heart disease in adults. Br J Anaesth 78:416, 1997.
107. Roberts NV, Keast PJ: Pulmonary hypertension and pregnancy: A lethal combination. Anaesth Intensive Care 18:366, 1990.
108. Monnery L, Nanson J, Charlton G: Primary pulmonary hypertension in pregnancy: A role for novel vasodilators. Br J Anaesth 87:295, 2001.
109. Burlew BS: Managing the pregnant patient with heart disease. Clin Cardiol 13:757, 1990.
110. Gil S, Atienzar C, Filella Y, et al: Anaesthetic management of acute myocardial infarction during labour. Int J Obstet Anesth 15:71, 2006.
111. Kulka PJ, Scheu C, Tryba M, et al: Coronary artery plaque disruption as cause of acute myocardial infarction during cesarean section with spinal anesthesia. J Clin Anesth 12:335, 2000.
112. Kuczkowski K.M: Advanced maternal age parturient: Is there reason for concern? Acta Obstet Gynecol Scand 82:681, 2003.
113. Kuczkowski KM: Levobupivacaine and ropivacaine: The new choices for labor analgesia. Int J Clin Pract 58:604, 2004.
114. Hands ME, Johnson MD, Saltzman DH, et al: The cardiac, obstetric, and anesthetic management of pregnancy complicated by acute myocardial infarction. J Clin Anesth 2:258, 1990.
115. Kuczkowski KM: Ambulatory labor analgesia: What does an obstetrician need to know? Acta Obstet Gynecol Scand 83:415, 2004.
116. Aglio LS, Johnson MD: Anesthetic management of myocardial infarction in a parturient. Br J Anaesth 65:258, 1990.
117. Frenkel Y, Etchin A, Barkai G, et al: Myocardial infarction during pregnancy: A case report. Cardiology 78:363, 1991.
118. Tessler MJ, Hudson R, Naugler-Colville M, et al: Pulmonary oedema in two parturients with hypertrophic obstructive cardiomyopathy (HOCM). Can J Anaesth 37:469, 1990.
119. Matthews T, Dickinson JE: Considerations for delivery in pregnancies complicated by maternal hypertrophic obstructive cardiomyopathy. Aust N Z J Obstet Gynaecol 45:526, 2005.
120. Ferguson EA, Paech MJ, Veltman MG: Hypertrophic cardiomyopathy and caesarean section: Intraoperative use of transthoracic echocardiography. Int J Obstet Anesth 15:311, 2006.
121. Spirito P, Autore C: Management of hypertrophic cardiomyopathy. BMJ 27:1251, 2006.
122. Ho KW, Kee WDN, Poon MCM: Combined spinal and epidural anesthesia in a parturient with idiopathic hypertrophic subaortic stenosis. Anesthesiology 87:168, 1997.
123. Kuczkowski KM: Ambulation with combined spinal-epidural labor analgesia: The technique. Acta Anaesthesiol Belg 55:29, 2004.
124. Mor-Yosef S, Younis J, Granat M, et al: Marfan's syndrome in pregnancy. Obstet Gynecol Surv 43:382, 1988.
125. Brar HB: Anaesthetic management of a caesarean section in a patient with Marfan's syndrome and aortic dissection. Anaesth Intensive Care 29:67, 2001.
126. Kuczkowski KM: Ehlers-Danlos syndrome in the parturient: An uncommon disorder—common dilemma in the delivery room. Arch Gynecol Obstet 273:60, 2005.
127. Garahan MB, Licata A: Dermatoses. In Gambling DR, Douglas MJ (eds): Obstetric Anesthesia and Uncommon Disorders. Philadelphia, WB Saunders, 1998, p 353.
128. Volkov N, Nisenblat V, Ohel G, et al: Ehlers-Danlos syndrome: Insights on obstetric aspects. Obstet Gynecol Surv 62:51, 2007.
129. Daley MD, Rolbin S, Hew E, et al: Continuous epidural anaesthesia for obstetrics after major spinal surgery. Can J Anaesth 37:S112, 1990.
130. Kuczkowski KM: Labor analgesia for the parturient with prior spinal surgery: What does an obstetrician need to know? Arch Gynecol Obstet 274:373, 2006.
131. Daley MD, Rolbin SH, Hew EM, et al: Epidural anesthesia for obstetrics after spinal surgery. Reg Anesth 15:280, 1990.
132. Crosby ET, Halpern SH: Obstetric epidural anaesthesia in patients with Harrington instrumentation. Can J Anaesth 36:693, 1989.
133. Moeller-Bertram T, Kuczkowski KM, Ahadian F: Labor analgesia in a parturient with prior Harrington rod instrumentation: Is caudal epidural an option? Ann Fr Anesth Reanim 23:925, 2004.
134. Kuczkowski KM: Labor analgesia for pregnant women with spina bifida: What does an obstetrician need to know? Arch Gynecol Obstet 275:53, 2007.
135. Mayhew JF, Katz J, Miner M, et al: Anaesthesia for the achondroplastic dwarf. Can J Anaesth 33:216, 1986.
136. Wardall GJ, Frame WT: Extradural anaesthesia for caesarean section in achondroplasia. Br J Anaesth 64:367, 1990.
137. DeRenzo JS, Vallejo MC, Ramanathan S: Failed regional anesthesia with reduced spinal bupivacaine dosage in a parturient with achondroplasia presenting for urgent cesarean section. Int J Obstet Anesth 14:175, 2005.
138. McGlothlen S: Anesthesia for cesarean section for achondroplastic dwarf: A case report. AANA J 68:305, 2000.
139. Kuczkowski KM: Labor analgesia for the drug abusing parturient: Is there cause for concern? Obstet Gynecol Surv 58:599, 2003.
140. Kuczkowski KM: Crack cocaine–induced long QT interval syndrome in a parturient with recreational cocaine use. Ann Fr Anesth Reanim 24:697, 2005.
141. Kuczkowski KM: Anesthetic implications of drug abuse in pregnancy. J Clin Anesth 15:382, 2003.
142. Birnbach DJ: Anesthetic management of the drug-abusing parturient: Are you ready? J Clin Anesth 15:325, 2003.
143. Kuczkowski KM: The cocaine abusing parturient: A review of anesthetic considerations. Can J Anaesth 51:145, 2004.
144. Kuczkowski KM, Benumof JL: Cesarean section in the parturient with HIV and recent cocaine and alcohol intake: Anesthetic implications. Int J Obstet Anesth 11:135, 2002.
145. Stoelting RK, Dierdorf SF: Psychiatric illness and substance abuse. In Stoelting RK, Dierdorf SF (eds): Anesthesia and Co-Existing Disease. New York, Churchill Livingstone, 1993, p 517.
146. Kuczkowski KM: Social drug use in the parturient: Implications for the management of obstetrical anaesthesia. Med J Malaysia 58:144, 2003.

147. Kuczkowski KM: Human immunodeficiency virus in the parturient. J Clin Anesth 15:224, 2003.
148. Kuczkowski KM, Benumof JL: Amphetamine abuse in pregnancy: Anesthetic implications. Acta Anaesthesiol Belg 54:161, 2003.
149. Kuczkowski KM: Solvents in pregnancy: An emerging problem in obstetrics and obstetric anaesthesia. Anaesthesia 58:1036, 2003.
150. Kuczkowski KM: Caesarean section in a cocaine-intoxicated parturient: Regional vs. general anaesthesia? Anaesthesia 58:1042, 2003.
151. Cassidy B, Cyna AM: Challenges that opioid-dependent women present to the obstetric anaesthetist. Anaesth Intensive Care 32:494, 2004.
152. Kuczkowski KM: Inhalation induction of anesthesia with sevoflurane for emergency Cesarean section in an amphetamine-intoxicated parturient without an intravenous access. Acta Anaesthesiol Scand 47:1181, 2003.
153. Kuczkowski KM, Le K: Substance use and misuse in pregnancy: Peripartum anesthetic management of a parturient with recent methanol, toluene and isopropanol intake. Acta Anaesthesiol Belg 55:53, 2004.
154. Kuczkowski KM: Crack cocaine as a cause of acute postoperative pulmonary edema in a pregnant drug addict. Ann Fr Anesth Reanim 24:437, 2005.
155. Kuczkowski KM: Marijuana in pregnancy. Ann Acad Med Singapore 33:336, 2004.
156. Kuczkowski K.M: Labor analgesia for the tobacco and ethanol abusing parturient: A routine management? Arch Gynecol Obstet 271:6, 2005
157. Kuczkowski KM: Liquid ecstasy during pregnancy. Anaesthesia 59:926, 2004.
158. Kuczkowski KM: Cardiovascular complications of recreational cocaine use in pregnancy: Myth or reality? Acta Obstet Gynecol Scand 84:100, 2005.
159. Kuczkowski KM: Peripartum care of the cocaine abusing parturient: Are we ready? Acta Obstet Gynecol Scand 84:108, 2005.
160. Kuczkowski KM: Herbal ecstasy: Cardiovascular complication of khat chewing in pregnancy. Acta Anaesthesiol Belg 56:19, 2005.
161. Lange RA, Hillis LD: Cardiovascular complications of cocaine use. N Engl J Med 345:351, 2001.

Chapter 57

Intensive Care Monitoring of the Critically Ill Pregnant Patient

Stephanie Rae Martin, DO, and Michael Raymond Foley, MD

Less than 1% of pregnant women will become critically ill and require admission to an intensive care unit (ICU).[1-8] Between 47% and 93% of ICU admissions result from an obstetric complication, primarily hemorrhage and hypertensive disorders. Other common causes include respiratory failure and sepsis. Common non-obstetric indications for ICU admission include maternal cardiac disease, trauma, anesthetic complications, cerebrovascular accidents, and drug overdosage. In many series, most obstetric ICU admissions occur in the immediate postpartum period and are most likely caused by complications of acute hemorrhage.[1,4-6,9]

An intimate understanding of the physiologic changes of pregnancy is essential in managing critically ill patients. This chapter addresses basic critical care monitoring in obstetrics and discusses conditions in which more intensive management of the pregnant patient may be indicated.

Maternal Mortality

Epidemiology

Maternal mortality is defined as the number of maternal deaths (direct and indirect) per 100,000 live births. Direct obstetric deaths result primarily from thromboembolic events, hemorrhage, hypertensive disorders of pregnancy, and infectious complications. Indirect obstetric deaths arise from preexisting medical conditions, including diabetes, systemic lupus erythematosus, pulmonary disease, and cardiac disease aggravated by the physiologic changes of pregnancy. Figure 57-1 shows specific causes of pregnancy-related mortality for three time periods as reported by the Centers for Disease Control and Prevention.[10-12]

Maternal mortality rates are periodically surveyed by various local, state, and national agencies. Because these data are primarily collected from death certificates, some have suggested that the numbers underestimate the mortality rate by as much as 20% to 50%.[13] Variations in the definition of maternal death, medicolegal concerns, and physicians untrained in the proper completion of death certificates further confuse these investigations. To address these concerns, the Division of Reproductive Health at the Centers for Disease Control and Prevention, in collaboration with the American College of Obstetricians and Gynecologists (ACOG) and state health departments, began in 1987 to systematically collect these data in the Pregnancy-Related Mortality Surveillance System.

Mortality rates have declined precipitously in the United States over the past century, but a slight increase has been observed in more recent years, as shown in Figure 57-2.[11] Some of this increase has been attributed to better ascertainment of data collected prospectively and to the use of multiple source documents. Although this trend is exhibited for all races, wide discrepancies still exist between white and non-white populations, even when controlling for age and use of prenatal care (Fig. 57-3).[12] The reasons for this discrepancy remain unclear. Geographic differences in maternal mortality rates are also apparent and are likely influenced by racial disparities. States with higher percentages of births to African-American women are also those with the highest maternal mortality rates. The data on pregnancy-related mortality in the United States between 1990 and 1997 indicate a rate of 11.8 deaths per 100,000 pregnant women (8.1 deaths per 100,000 whites, 30.0 deaths per 100,000 African Americans).[12] Advancing maternal age and lack of education are also associated with an increased risk for death in pregancy.[12] Potential explanations for this increased risk include a higher incidence of underlying or undiagnosed chronic disease.

Prediction of Maternal Mortality

Predicting the risk of mortality for pregnant patients remains a challenge. The overall maternal mortality rate for critically ill gravidas admitted to an ICU ranges from 0% to 20%, with most series reporting maternal mortality rates of less than 5% for all obstetric ICU admissions.[1,3-5,8] Several scoring systems are routinely employed in critical care settings in an attempt to objectively describe the severity of the critical illness and accurately predict mortality risks. The Acute Physiologic and Chronic Health Evaluation (APACHE) scoring system,[14,15] Simplified Acute Physiologic Score (SAPS),[16] and Mortality Prediction Model (MPM)[17] are three widely used methods that track a variety of variables in nonpregnant patients.

Several authors have evaluated the applicability of the scoring systems in critically ill pregnant patients.[18-20] In a study of obstetric ICU patients, the APACHE III score did not accurately predict maternal mortality.[18] In the largest series, 93 gravidas were compared with 96 nonpregnant women. The overall mortality rate in the obstetric population was 10.8%. The APACHE II, SAPS II, and MPM II scoring systems each performed well in predicting mortality (14.7%, 7.8%, and 9.1%, respectively).[19] The predicted mortality rate was significantly higher among obstetric patients compared with non-obstetric

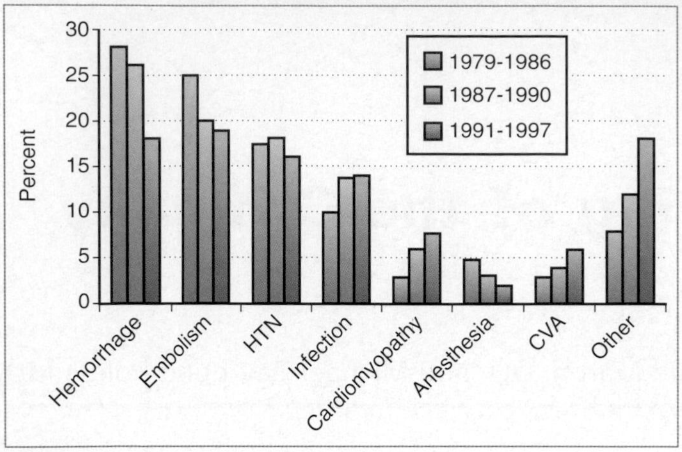

FIGURE 57-1 **Causes of maternal mortality for three time periods.** Obstetric deaths are caused by thromboembolic events, hemorrhage, hypertension, infections, and preexisting medical conditions, such as diabetes, systemic lupus erythematosus, pulmonary disease, and cardiac disease aggravated by the physiologic changes of pregnancy. CVA, cerebrovascular accident; HTN, hypertension. (From Berg CJ, Chang J, Callaghan WM, et al: Pregnancy-related mortality in the United States, 1991-1997. Obstet Gynecol 101:289-296, 2003.)

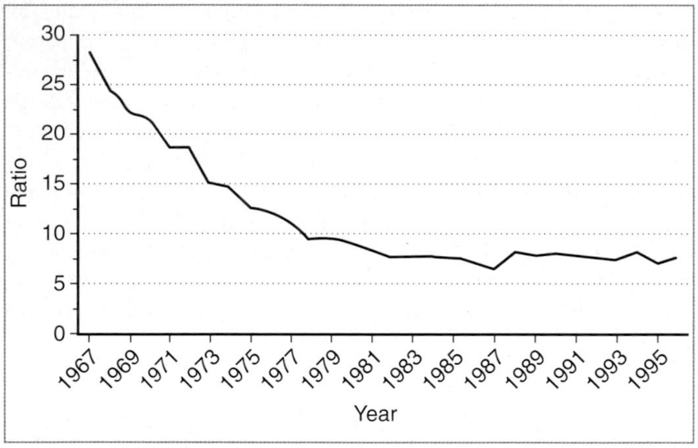

FIGURE 57-2 **Maternal mortality ratios in the United States by year for 1967 to 1996.** Ratios are the number of maternal deaths per 100,000 live births. The term *ratio* is used instead of rate because the numerator includes some maternal deaths that were not related to live births and therefore were not included in the denominator. (From Centers for Disease Control and Prevention: Maternal Mortality—United States, 1982-1996. MMWR Morb Mortal Wkly Rep 47:705-707, 1998.)

patients for each of the three scoring tools, despite no difference in actual mortality between the two groups (10.8 versus 10.4%).

None of the scoring systems includes adjustments for normal obstetric physiologic changes such as decreased blood pressure and increased respiratory rate. Laboratory abnormalities such as elevated liver function test results and low platelet counts, which are common in obstetric disorders such as HELLP syndrome (*h*emolysis, *e*levated *l*iver enzymes, and *l*ow *p*latelets), are not included in the assessments and may limit their potential applicability. In summary, although the available critical care mortality scoring systems can possibly be applied

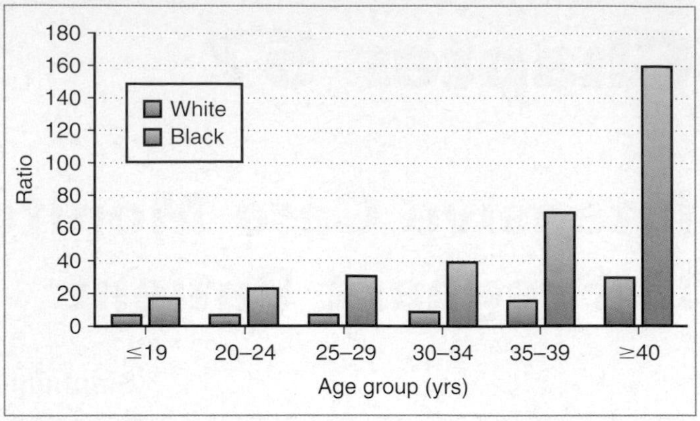

FIGURE 57-3 Pregnancy-related mortality ratios by age and race in the United States for 1991 to 1999. The mortality ratios are the number of deaths per 100,00 live births.

to the obstetric population, they have the potential to overestimate the mortality risk for critically ill gravidas.

Invasive Central Hemodynamic Monitoring

Background and Insertion Technique

Placement of a central venous catheter may be indicated to provide central venous access for fluid replacement, medication administration, or hemodynamic measurements. Since its introduction in the early 1970s,[21] invasive hemodynamic monitoring with a pulmonary artery catheter (PAC) has become quite common in critically ill patients. The most commonly available Swan-Ganz catheters are multilumen devices that enable direct monitoring of central venous pressure (CVP, right ventricular preload), pulmonary capillary wedge pressure (PCWP, left ventricular preload), cardiac output (CO), systemic vascular resistance (SVR, left ventricular afterload), pulmonary artery pressures, and mixed venous oxygen saturation. CO and mixed venous oxygen saturation can be measured in the conventional manner by thermodilution and direct distal port aspiration, respectively, or by newer fiberoptic technology that allows continuous monitoring of CO and mixed venous oxygen saturation.

PACs (i.e., Swan-Ganz catheters) are typically inserted percutaneously through an introducer sheath and in a sterile manner through the left subclavian or right internal jugular veins and advanced into the right heart. The right internal jugular vein is usually preferred because it offers the shortest and most direct entry into the right heart. Access through the femoral vein offers the advantage of compressibility in a patient with a coagulopathy, but it is most distant from the right heart and may require fluoroscopic guidance. As the catheter is advanced, characteristic oscilloscopic pressure waveforms are used to establish the catheter's location within the heart. A 1.5-mL balloon is positioned close to the tip of the catheter. Inflation of the balloon allows the catheter to be carried through the heart by flowing blood.

After the inflated balloon reaches the pulmonary artery, it travels distally until it wedges in a smaller-caliber artery and occludes blood flow. This results in a nonpulsatile waveform from which the PCWP is measured. When the balloon is deflated, return of an identifiable pulmonary artery systolic and diastolic pressure tracing should occur. A portable chest radiograph is indicated after placement of a PAC to verify appropriate catheter positioning and exclude pneumothorax.

Indications for Pulmonary Artery Catheterization

The most common indications for PAC placement in the obstetric population include the following[22]:

- Hypovolemic shock unresponsive to initial volume resuscitation attempts
- Septic shock with refractory hypotension or oliguria
- Severe preeclampsia with refractory oliguria or pulmonary edema
- Ineffective intravenous antihypertensive therapy
- Adult respiratory distress syndrome (ARDS)
- Intraoperative or intrapartum cardiac failure
- Severe mitral or aortic valvular stenosis
- New York Heart Association (NYHA) class III or IV heart disease in labor
- Anaphylactoid syndrome of pregnancy (i.e., amniotic fluid embolism)

Although use of the PAC in nonpregnant critically ill patients is widespread, until recently, randomized trials demonstrating a clear benefit of PAC directed care were lacking. Several small studies suggested a decrease in mortality when PACs are used to direct therapies,[23-25] while others reported an increase in mortality associated with the use of PACs[26-29] or no benefit.[30-32] The large Canadian Critical Care Clinical Trials Group study prospectively randomized 1994 high-risk surgical patients to receive a PAC to direct therapy or standard therapy and reported no survival benefit when therapy was directed by a PAC (7.8% versus 7.7% for controls).[33] A British trial randomized more than 1000 critically ill patients to management with or without a PAC and failed to demonstrate a survival benefit (68.4% versus 65.7% for controls).[34] The Evaluation Study of Congestive Heart Failure and Pulmonary Artery Catheterization Effectiveness (ESCAPE trial) also demonstrated no difference in mortality or length of stay for 433 patients with congestive heart failure randomized to PAC or no catheter.[35]

A meta-analysis of 13 trials published since 1985 included 5051 patients randomized to a PAC or to no PAC to guide management. No difference was identified in mortality or length of hospital stay. Conversely, the use of a PAC was significantly associated with more frequent use of inotropes and vasodilators.[36] In summary, although placement of PACs remain widespread, the available data do not support the routine use of PACs for all critically ill patients. Data addressing the role of PACs in pregnant critically ill patients are lacking.

Complications of Central Venous Catheters

Common complications associated with initial venous access, advancement, and maintenance of a PAC are listed in Table 57-1.[37] Some complications, such as pulmonary infarction and pulmonary artery rupture, are specific to placement of a PAC and do not occur with central venous access alone. Minimal available data address specific complication rates associated with PAC use in pregnant women. Initial complication rates decline as operator experience increases, and only properly trained personnel should insert catheters for invasive hemodynamic monitoring.[38] Several studies have also demonstrated that ultrasound-guided placement results in fewer failed attempts at placement, fewer complications such as hematoma or arterial puncture, and less time for placement.[39]

TABLE 57-1 POTENTIAL PULMONARY ARTERY CATHETER COMPLICATIONS

At Insertion	After Placement
Pneumothorax	Pulmonary infarction
Thrombosis	Pulmonary artery rupture
Arterial puncture	Infection
Air embolization	Balloon rupture
Catheter knotting	Endocardial or valvular damage
Cardiac arrhythmias (transient, sustained)	

Complications encountered at initial insertion include arterial puncture, pneumothorax, and air embolism. Pneumothorax risks are highest with a subclavian approach. Transient cardiac arrhythmias are commonly encountered during placement and advancement of the PAC. The majority consist of premature ventricular contractions or nonsustained ventricular tachycardia, and they resolve with withdrawal or advancement of the catheter. The overall incidence of transient minor arrhythmias during advancement of a PAC exceeds 20% in most studies.[37] Significant arrhythmias such as sustained ventricular tachycardia or fibrillation are less common, occurring in less than 4% of patients in most series, and they are more likely to be encountered in patients with cardiac ischemia.[37]

Infections related to central venous catheters are common and may involve a superficial skin infection, colonization, or a more serious bacteremia. Skin flora, particularly *Staphylococcus* species, are most commonly involved. Positive cultures from the tip of a PAC are common and are considered evidence of colonization. However, for bacteremia or sepsis to be diagnosed, the patient must also have positive blood cultures with the same organism and clinical evidence of systemic infection, such as fever or hypotension.[40] The risk of bacteremia is approximately 0.5% per catheter day, and the risk increases with each day the catheter remains indwelling. Bacteremia resulting from central venous catheters accounts for 87% of bloodstream infections in critically ill patients.[41] Infectious complications can be minimized by adherence to strict sterile technique, placement in the subclavian site, use of antimicrobial-coated catheters, avoiding antibiotic ointments that can increase fungal colonization, avoiding empiric catheter changes, and removing the catheter as soon as possible.[42]

Venous thrombosis risk can be minimized by placement at the subclavian site and by limiting the duration of catheter placement. Pulmonary infarction may occur as a result of direct occlusion of a pulmonary artery branch caused by drifting of the catheter or thromboembolic events. Catheter knotting can be avoided during placement if the operator remains aware of the centimeter markings on the advancing catheter. The right ventricle usually is reached when the catheter has been inserted 25 to 30 cm from the jugular vein site. Few patients require more than 50 cm of catheter to reach the pulmonary artery. Inflated catheter balloons should be checked before insertion to reduce the risk of air leakage and balloon rupture. Overinflation of the balloon with air (>1.5 mL) should be avoided. A pressure-release balloon has been described that limits overinflation and thereby minimizes pulmonary

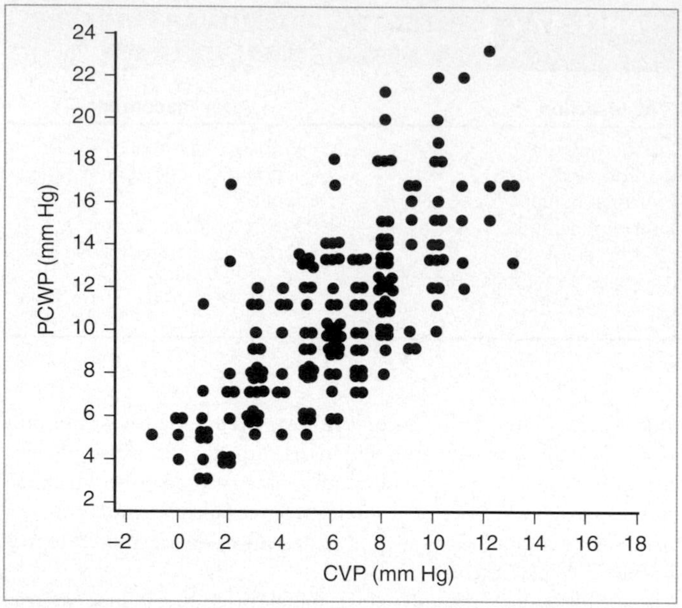

FIGURE 57-4 Relationship of central venous pressure (CVP) to pulmonary capillary wedge pressure (PCWP) in severe pregnancy-induced hypertension. If an accurate assessment of left ventricular preload is deemed important in the management of the patient's cardiovascular complications, insertion of a pulmonary artery catheter may be indicated. (From Cotton DB, Gonik B, Dorman K, et al: Cardiovascular alterations in severe pregnancy-induced hypertension: Relationship of central venous pressure to pulmonary capillary wedge pressure. Am J Obstet Gynecol 151:762, 1985.)

TABLE 57-2 FORMULAS FOR CALCULATING HEMODYNAMIC VARIABLES

$SVR = [(MAP - RAP)]/CO \times 80$
$PVR = (PAP - PCWP/CO) \times 80$
$CO = VO_2/(CaO_2 - CvO_2)$
$DO_2 = CO \times CaO_2 \times 10$
$VO_2 = (CaO_2 - CvO_2) \times CO \times 10$
$CaO_2 = (1.34 \times Hb \times SaO_2) + (0.003 \times PaO_2)$
$CvO_2 + (1.34 \times Hb \times SvO_2) + (0.003 \times PvO_2)$
O_2 extraction $= VO_2/ DO_2$
$Qs/Qt = CcO_2 - CaO_2/CcO_2 - CvO_2$

CaO_2, arterial oxygen concentration; CcO_2, end capillary O_2 content; CO, cardiac output; CvO_2, venous oxygen concentration; DO_2, oxygen delivery; Hb, hemoglobin; MAP, mean arterial pressure; O_2, oxygen; PaO_2, arterial partial pressure of oxygen; PAP, pulmonary artery pressure; PCWP, pulmonary capillary wedge pressure; PvO_2, venous partial pressure of oxygen; PVR, pulmonary vascular resistance; Qs/Qt, shunt fraction; RAP, right atrial pressure; SaO_2, arterial oxygen saturation; SvO_2, venous oxygen saturation; SVR, systemic vascular resistance; VO_2, oxygen consumption.

vessel injury. Pulmonary artery rupture is a rare but often fatal complication that occurs more commonly in patients with pulmonary artery hypertension or who are anticoagulated. Valvular damage can occur from chronic catheter irritation or during insertion when the catheter balloon is not deflated before retrograde movement.

CVP monitoring alone should not be considered equivalent to PAC monitoring. Preeclampsia and its complications, such as oliguria and pulmonary edema, may prompt central venous access. However, several investigators have described poor correlation between the central venous catheter and PCWP in gravidas with pregnancy-induced hypertension (Fig. 57-4).[43,44] If an accurate assessment of left ventricular preload is deemed important in the management of the patient's cardiovascular complications, insertion of a PAC may be indicated. Whether this holds true for pregnant women with critically ill disease states other than pregnancy-induced hypertension remains unknown.

Hemodynamic Considerations

With a PAC, the following hemodynamic variables can be directly measured in the patient:

- Heart rate (beats/min)
- CVP (mm Hg)
- Pulmonary artery systolic and pulmonary artery diastolic pressures (mm Hg)
- PCWP (mm Hg)
- CO (L/min)
- Mixed venous oxygen saturation (%)

By use of a sphygmomanometer or by peripheral artery catheterization, direct measurements of systemic arterial pressures can also be obtained. Table 57-2 lists formulas for calculating selected hemodynamic variables.

Hemodynamic variables often are expressed in an "indexed" fashion (i.e., cardiac index). To do this, the original nonindexed CO value must be divided by body surface area. Because standard body surface area calculations have never been established specifically for pregnancy, this traditional way of expressing hemodynamic data is somewhat controversial in obstetrics. Those who argue for its use point out that indexing allows direct comparison of hemodynamic parameters for pregnant women of different sizes, a critical issue when interpreting these values.

Mean hemodynamic measurements for pregnant and nonpregnant patients are presented in Table 57-3. They are paired data from 10 healthy subjects, taken between 36 and 38 weeks' gestation and between 11 and 13 weeks after delivery.[45] Using the noninvasive technique of M-mode echocardiography, other investigators have demonstrated that many of these physiologic alterations in hemodynamics begin in the early phases of pregnancy.[46] Position changes late in pregnancy significantly influenced central hemodynamic stability. The standing position increased pulse by 50%, left ventricular stroke work index by 21%, and pulmonary vascular resistance by 54%.[47] Compared with the nonpregnant state, the pregnant state seemed to result in a buffering of orthostatic-related hemodynamic changes. The investigators speculated that the increased intravascular volume during pregnancy accounted for this stabilizing effect.

Hemodynamics of Specific Conditions during Pregnancy

Mitral Valve Stenosis

Mitral stenosis is the most common rheumatic valvular lesion encountered in pregnancy (see Chapter 39). When the valve area falls below 1.5 cm^2, filling of the left ventricle during diastole is severely limited, resulting in a fixed CO. Prevention of tachycardia and maintenance of adequate left ventricular preload is essential in these patients. As the heart rate increases, less time is allowed for the left atrium to adequately empty and fill the left ventricle during diastole. The left atrium may become overdistended, resulting in dysrhythmias (primarily atrial

TABLE 57-3 NORMAL CENTRAL HEMODYNAMIC PARAMETERS IN HEALTHY NONPREGNANT AND PREGNANT PATIENTS

Hemodynamic Parameter	Nonpregnant Values	Pregnant Values
Cardiac output (L/min)	4.3 ± 0.9	6.2 ± 1.0
Heart rate (beats/min)	71 ± 10	83 ± 10
Systemic vascular resistance (dyne × cm × sec^{-5})	1530 ± 520	1210 ± 266
Pulmonary vascular resistance (dyne × cm × sec^{-5})	119 ± 47	78 ± 22
Colloid oncotic pressure (mm Hg)	20.8 ± 1.0	18.0 ± 1.5
Colloid oncotic pressure – pulmonary capillary wedge pressure (mm Hg)	14.5 ± 2.5	10.5 ± 2.7
Mean arterial pressure (mm Hg)	86.4 ± 7.5	90.3 ± 5.8
Pulmonary capillary wedge pressure (mm Hg)	6.3 ± 2.1	7.5 ± 1.8
Central venous pressure (mm Hg)	3.7 ± 2.6	3.6 ± 2.5
Left ventricular stroke work index (g × m × m^{-2})	41 ± 8	48 ± 6

From Clark SL, Cotton DB, Lee W, et al: Central hemodynamic assessment of normal term pregnancy. Am J Obstet Gynecol 161:1439, 1989.

fibrillation, which increases the risk of thromboembolic complications) or pulmonary edema. Adequate preload, however, is essential to maintain left ventricular filling pressure. Alternatively, if preload is excessive, pulmonary edema and atrial dysrhythmias may result. Medical management of these patients involves activity restriction, treatment of dysrhythmias, β-blockers to control heart rate, and careful diuretic use. The goal of diuretic therapy is to treat pulmonary edema, with care not to overly reduce left ventricular preload. Adequate analgesia and anesthesia during labor and delivery also reduce excessive cardiac demands associated with pain and anxiety.

The other important hemodynamic consideration for patients with mitral valve stenosis relates to the potential for misinterpretation of the invasive monitoring data. Because of the stenotic mitral valve, PCWP readings do not accurately reflect left ventricular diastolic pressure. In some instances, very high PCWP values are recorded (and are needed to maintain an adequate CO). Overt pulmonary edema is usually not associated with these high readings. During attempts at maintaining a relatively constricted intravascular volume, the CO should be concomitantly monitored and maintained. For each individual patient, optimal PCWP and CO values (i.e., values that maintain blood pressure and tissue perfusion) should be determined.

Aortic Stenosis

The major problem encountered with aortic stenosis is the patient's potential inability to maintain CO because of severe obstruction or in the setting of decreasing left ventricular preload (see Chapter 39). Unlike mitral valve stenosis, aortic valve stenosis requires that attempts be made to maintain the patient in a relatively hypervolemic state, although the fixed CO may lead to pulmonary edema. The time surrounding labor and delivery is particularly risky for these patients. To maintain an adequate CO, adequate venous return to the heart is crucial. Decreased venous return can result from excess blood loss, hypotension, and ganglionic blockade from a regional anesthetic or even vena caval occlusion in the supine position. Pulmonary artery catheterization may be indicated in patients with significant aortic stenosis to accurately estimate intravascular volume and guide fluid replacement.

Pulmonary Hypertension

Pulmonary artery hypertension may arise as a primary lesion or result from an underlying cardiac abnormality (see Chapter 39). Primary pulmonary hypertension is characterized by an unexplained elevation in pulmonary artery pressures (>25 to 30 mm Hg). Prognosis is grim for patients with primary pulmonary hypertension; mean survival is 2.8 years from the diagnosis. Maternal mortality rates for patients with pulmonary hypertension have been as high as 50%.[48-50] These patients are at increased risk for complications from placement of a PAC. Pulmonary hypertension may also result from unrepaired congenital intracardiac shunts such as a ventricular septal defect, atrial septal defect, or patent ductus arteriosus, which lead to chronic overperfusion of the pulmonary vasculature. Over time, pulmonary arterial pressures may become significant enough to reverse the direction of flow across the shunt. This reversal of shunt flow to a right-to-left pattern defines Eisenmenger syndrome. The estimated maternal mortality rate for Eisenmenger syndrome is between 30% and 40%.[50,51] In a review of 73 patients with Eisenmenger syndrome, the overall mortality rate was 36%, which has been essentially unchanged during the past 2 decades.[50]

The underlying problem in patients with this condition is obstruction to right ventricular outflow caused by a fixed and elevated pulmonary vascular resistance. This can ultimately lead to right-to-left shunting of deoxygenated blood with resultant hypoxemia. Reductions in blood return to the heart can decrease right ventricular preload so that the pulmonary vasculature is further hypoperfused. The resultant hypoxemia has been associated with sudden death. Intrapartum management requires maintenance of a relatively hypervolemic state, and any interventions that may lead to significant reduction in preload or decrease in SVR should be avoided. Placement of a PAC may be quite challenging in these patients, and many experts believe the risks of placement may outweigh any potential benefit.

Anaphylactoid Syndrome of Pregnancy

Anaphylactoid syndrome of pregnancy (i.e., amniotic fluid embolus) is a rare but devastating complication of pregnancy characterized by acute onset of hypoxia, hypotension or cardiac arrest, and coagulopathy occurring during labor, during delivery, or within 30 minutes after delivery.[52,53] This same constellation of findings may have other causes, such as hemorrhage, uterine rupture, or sepsis, and each should be excluded before assigning a diagnosis of amniotic fluid embolism. The combination of sudden cardiovascular and respiratory collapse with a coagulopathy is similar to that observed in patients with anaphylactic or septic shock. In each of these settings, a foreign substance (e.g., endotoxin) is introduced into the circulation. This initiates a cascade of events resulting in activation and release of mediators such as histamines, thromboxane, and prostaglandins, which lead to disseminated intravascular coagulation (DIC), hypotension, and hypoxia. The inciting factor is presumed to be present in amniotic fluid that is introduced into the maternal circulation, but the precise factor that initiates the sequence have not been identified. It is a commonly held misconception that the presence of fetal debris in the pulmonary circulation is diagnostic of an amniotic fluid embolus. Fetal debris can be found in the pulmonary circulation in most normal laboring patients, and it is identified only in 78% of patients who meet the criteria for the diagnosis of amniotic fluid embolism.[52,53]

Management of amniotic fluid embolism is entirely supportive. Replacement of blood and clotting factors, adequate hydration and blood pressure support, ventilatory support, and invasive cardiac monitoring in addition to resuscitation efforts usually are required for these patients. The data suggest mortality rates approach 61% or higher. Most patients do not survive the initial course and die within 5 days. For those who survive, neurologic impairment is common.[52]

Hypertensive Disorders of Pregnancy

Most clinical hemodynamic monitoring studies in obstetrics have enrolled patients with hypertensive disorders of pregnancy (see Chapter 35). From a purely clinical perspective, clear indications for this invasive technology have not been established. Arguments for its use center on reports demonstrating a broad spectrum of hemodynamic findings in this group of patients. For patients identified to be relatively hypovolemic, optimizing intravascular volume status should improve uteroplacental perfusion, reduce SVR, and blunt hypotensive complications associated with conduction anesthesia and antihypertensive therapy. Oliguria (particularly if unresponsive to fluid therapy) and refractory pulmonary edema, both recognized complications of severe preeclampsia, may also be better defined and managed with invasive monitoring.

Vasospasm is a central feature of preeclampsia. In one series of 51 untreated preeclamptic patients, an elevated SVR value was identified with invasive monitoring.[54] Preeclampsia likely represents an overall vasoconstrictive condition that is frequently influenced by underlying disease processes such as chronic hypertension, duration and severity of illness, and various therapeutic modalities.

Using ventricular function curves that correlate PCWP (i.e., left ventricular preload) with left ventricular stroke work index (i.e., myocardial contractility), investigators found that most preeclamptic and eclamptic patients fall into a relatively hyperdynamic range.[55] The values shown in Figure 57-5 are superimposed on ventricular function graphs derived from nonpregnant subjects. The preeclamptic patient probably has at least a normal and probably a somewhat hyperdynamic functioning heart during pregnancy. As expected, this cardiac function, as estimated by CO, appears to be inversely related to SVR.

Some investigators have recommended that patients with pregnancy-induced hypertension be classified by different hemodynamic subsets so that management protocols can be tailored to individual needs. Clark and associates[56] first reported the use of this approach for dealing with the oliguric preeclamptic patient. They found that these patients had low PCWP values (i.e., hypovolemic) and elevated SVR (i.e., severe vasoconstriction) or were volume replete with normal to elevated vascular resistances. A third group had markedly elevated PCWP and SVR readings with depressed cardiac function.[56] Management of these groups of oliguric patients varies. In the first subset, patients respond favorably to volume expansion therapy. The next two groups of patients are best managed with vasodilators and aggressive afterload reduction therapy.

Another important issue in the management of oliguric patients with preeclampsia is the use of standard urinary diagnostic indices, such as urine-to-plasma ratios of osmolality, urea nitrogen, and creatinine or fractional excretion of sodium. Although these urinary parameters are routinely used in non-obstetric patients to differentiate prerenal and renal causes of oliguria, they have proved to be unreliable in patients with preeclampsia. In preeclampsia complicated by oliguria, urinary diagnostic indices may suggest a prerenal cause despite normal intravascular volume, demonstrated by invasive pressure measurement determinations. From a physiologic standpoint, it is postulated that the kidney misinterprets local renal artery vasospasm to indicate a volume-depleted state.

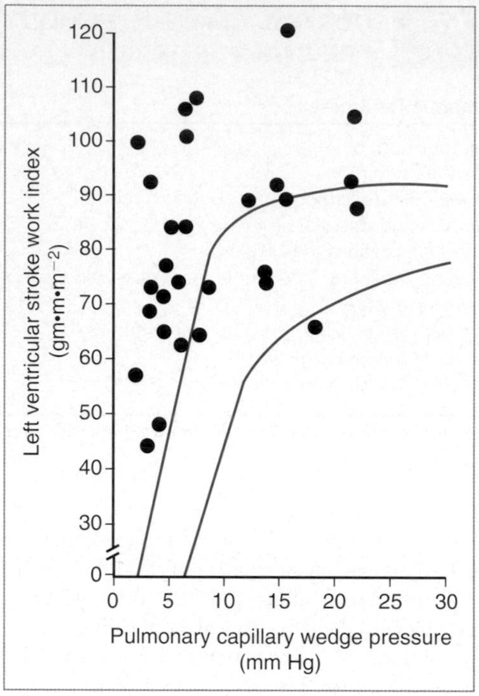

FIGURE 57-5 Ventricular function in pregnancy-induced hypertensive patients. On plots of ventricular function curves that correlate pulmonary capillary wedge pressure with left ventricular stroke work index, most preeclamptic and eclamptic patients fall into a relatively hyperdynamic range. (Combined data from Benedetti TK, Cotton DB, Read JC, et al: Hemodynamic observations in severe pre-eclampsia with a flow-directed pulmonary artery catheter. Am J Obstet Gynecol 136:465, 1980; Hankins GDV, Wendel GP, Cunningham FG, et al: Longitudinal evaluation of hemodynamic changes in eclampsia. Am J Obstet Gynecol 15:506, 1984; Phelan JP, Yurth DA: Severe preeclampsia. I. Peripartum hemodynamic observations. Am J Obstet Gynecol 144:17, 1982; and Rafferty TD, Berkowitz RL: Hemodynamics in patients with severe toxemia during labor and delivery. Am J Obstet Gynecol 138:263, 1980.)

Septic Shock

Septic shock refers to the systemic inflammatory response syndrome associated with infection, persistent hypotension, and major organ dysfunction despite initial fluid resuscitation.[57] Although the hemodynamic effects of septic shock have been well described in the non-obstetric literature, limited information is available for obstetric patients. One study described the hemodynamic profiles of 10 obstetric patients at various gestational ages, who were identified to have septic shock and required invasive monitoring. In this small series, SVR and myocardial function were depressed but improved with therapy.[58] Mabie and coworkers[59] described similar findings in a more recent series of 18 obstetric patients with septic shock. The main hemodynamic characteristics of those who succumbed to septic shock included lower blood pressure, stroke volume, and left ventricular stroke work index than survivors.[59] Sepsis and septic shock are addressed in more detail later in this chapter.

Noninvasive Hemodynamic Assessment

The PAC is the gold standard for measurement of hemodynamic status in the critically ill patient. However, according to available data, use of the PAC to guide therapy does not favorably affect survival and carries substantial risks.

Transesophageal echocardiography (TEE) has emerged as a noninvasive tool for the bedside assessment of the hemodynamic status of nonpregnant, critically ill adults. In an anesthetized patient, a small transducer is introduced into the esophagus and real-time data collected. TEE can accurately measure left ventricular preload, left ventricular filling pressure, CO, left ventricular ejection fraction, and severe right ventricular dysfunction.[60-62] TEE is often used in hypotensive patients to determine the cause of the hypotension, such as inadequate filling or depressed contractility (Table 57-4). TEE can detect other abnormalities, including left ventricular obstruction, structural abnormalities, proximal pulmonary emboli, and valvular disease. It is also useful in evaluating the left atrium and mitral valve because of the proximity of these structures to the transducer, and it appears to be superior in evaluating congenital cardiac defects.

Only a few small series have compared data derived from a PAC with two-dimensional transthoracic and Doppler echocardiography in obstetric patients. In one report of 12 patients requiring PAC for preeclampsia management, CO measured by Doppler echocardiography correlated well with CO assessed by thermodilution using a PAC.[63] Another study of 16 obstetric patients found good correlation between thermodilution assessment of CO and Doppler echocardiography.[64] In a study of 11 critically ill obstetric patients, Belfort and colleagues[65] demonstrated no difference between Doppler echocardiographic and PAC-derived estimation of stroke volume, CO, cardiac index, left ventricular filling pressure, pulmonary artery systolic pressure, and right atrial pressure.[65] The data from these reports are encouraging, but echocardiographic estimation of pulmonary artery pressure was significantly overestimated in 32% of obstetric patients with suspected pulmonary artery hypertension.[66] The technique appears to be well-tolerated, but further study is warranted.

Respiratory Failure

Substantial anatomic and physiologic changes occur over the course of pregnancy that impact respiratory function (see Chapter 7). Minute ventilation increases in a normal pregnancy and is determined by respiratory rate and tidal volume. The 40% increase in tidal volume (i.e., amount of air exchanged during a cycle of inspiration and expiration) primarily drives the increase in minute ventilation. As a result, the levels of CO_2 decline, creating an alkalotic state. To accommodate for the decrease in CO_2, the kidneys excrete bicarbonate (HCO_3^-). An arterial blood gas determination in a normal pregnant woman therefore reflects a slightly increased pH, decreased PCO_2, and decreased serum HCO_3– (i.e., respiratory alkalosis with compensatory metabolic acidosis), as outlined in Table 57-5. As the pregnancy progresses, increasing abdominal girth leads to an upward displacement of the diaphragm, widening of the subcostal angle by 50%, and increased chest circumference. The end result is a decrease in the functional residual capacity by 20%. The functional residual capacity reflects the amount of air remaining in the alveoli at the completion of expiration. As the functional residual capacity decreases, the alveoli collapse, and gas exchange decreases.[67]

Common causes for respiratory failure in pregnancy include pulmonary edema, asthma, infection, and pulmonary embolus.[68,69] In a series of 43 gravidas requiring mechanical ventilation while undelivered, 86% delivered during the admission, and of these, 65% underwent cesarean section, with an associated mortality rate of 36% for those delivered by cesarean section. Overall maternal and perinatal mortality rates were high (14% and 11%, respectively).[68]

Debate continues about whether delivery improves respiratory status in these patients. Tomlinson and coworkers[70] described their experience with 10 patients who delivered while mechanically ventilated. In all but one patient, the cause of respiratory failure was pneumonia.[70] The only demonstrable benefit after delivery was a 28% reduction in FIO_2 in the ensuing 24 hours. The investigators concluded that routine delivery of these patients was not recommended. This is the only study published that was designed specifically to address this question. However, data from other series support the conclusion that delivery does not uniformly result in significant maternal improvement. Mortality rates after delivery while requiring ventilatory support range from 14% to 58%, and cesarean section may further increase this risk.[68,69,71]

TABLE 57-4 ORIGIN OF HYPOTENSION

End-Diastolic Cross-Sectional Area	Ejection Fraction	Cause
Decreased	>0.8	Hypovolemia
Increased	<0.2	Left ventricular failure
Normal	>0.5	Low SVR or severe MR, AR, or VSD

AR, aortic regurgitation; MR, mitral regurgitation; SVR, systemic vascular resistance; VSD, ventricular septal defect.
From Cahalan MK: Intraoperative Transesophageal Echocardiography: An Interactive Text and Atlas. New York, Churchill Livingstone, 1996.

TABLE 57-5 CHANGES IN ARTERIAL BLOOD GAS MEASUREMENTS IN PREGNANCY

Measurements	Pregnant Values	Nonpregnant Values
pH	7.4-7.46	7.38-7.42
PCO_2 (mm Hg)	26-32	38-45
PO_2 (mm Hg)	75-106	70-100
HCO_3^- (mEq/L)	18-21	24-31
O_2 saturation (%)	95-100	95-100

Modified from Dildy G, Clark SL, Phelan JP, et al: Maternal-fetal blood gas physiology. In Critical Care Obstetrics, 4th ed. New York, Blackwell, 2004.

Acute Respiratory Distress Syndrome

Acute respiratory distress syndrome (ARDS) is characterized by rapid onset of progressive respiratory distress. Evaluation reveals bilateral pulmonary infiltrates without evidence of cardiac failure or increased hydrostatic pressure (i.e., PCWP < 18 mm Hg). These patients require high concentrations of oxygen and frequently need intubation. ARDS is also defined by a diminished ratio of the partial pressure of oxygen to the fraction of inspired oxygen ($PaO_2/FIO_2 \leqq 200$). If the ratio falls between 200 and 300, acute lung injury is present that is not severe enough to be called ARDS.

In pregnant women, infections with varicella or herpes simplex virus, severe preeclampsia, eclampsia, and hemorrhage most commonly precipitate respiratory failure.[68,72] Septic patients are at particular risk for developing acute pulmonary injury and ARDS as a consequence of pulmonary vascular damage that facilitates the leakage of intravascular fluid into the pulmonary interstitial spaces. Mortality rates are quite high, and patients who survive often have pulmonary function compromised by fibrosis and scarring of pulmonary tissue.

The treatment of ARDS focuses on identifying and treating underlying causes such as infection and then providing respiratory, hemodynamic, and nutritional support to facilitate lung healing. Respiratory support may precipitate additional lung injury, and efforts to maintain adequate oxygen delivery should also minimize lung trauma in an effort to facilitate healing of the lungs.

Management of respiratory failure in nonpregnant, critically ill patients has historically used a goal of maintaining a tidal volume of 10 to 15 mL/kg. In ARDS, high tidal volumes may lead to alveolar overdistention or repeated recruitment and collapse of alveoli, predisposing to alveolar damage and release of inflammatory mediators that worsen pulmonary damage. In 2000, the ARDSNet published results of 861 patients with ARDS randomized to traditional tidal volumes (12 mL/kg) or to a low tidal volume of 6 mL/kg.[73] The traditional tidal volume group also maintained a goal of 50 cm of H_2O or less, compared with lower peak pressures of 30 cm of H_2O in the low tidal volume group. Low tidal volumes and lower peak pressures were associated with lower mortality rates (31% versus 40%) and shorter periods of intubation compared with conventional tidal volumes and peak pressure goals. Increased tidal volume and other normal changes in pulmonary physiology may affect the utility of this approach in pregnant women.

Prone Ventilation

Mechanical ventilation in the prone position has improved oxygenation in up to 80% of patients with ARDS and acute lung injury. Approximately 50% of patients maintain improved oxygenation after they return to the supine position.[74] Mechanical ventilation in the prone position is believed to achieve several beneficial physiologic changes: improved aeration of well-perfused dorsal atelectatic lung areas, improved alveolar recruitment, relief of cardiac compression on the lung posteriorly, and improved mobilization of secretions.

Several randomized trials have compared supine with prone positioning in nonpregnant patients with ARDS and acute lung injury. In one randomized trial of 304 patients, prone positioning maintained for an average of 7 hours daily was not associated with a decrease in mortality, but significant improvement in oxygenation was observed in 70% of patients, with most of the benefit occurring in the first hour of prone positioning.[75] Another multicenter, randomized trial of 791 patients with hypoxemic respiratory failure with multiple causes, including ARDS, found similar results. In addition to improved oxygenation with prone positioning at least 6 hours daily, a decrease in ventilator-associated pneumonia was observed. However, no difference in mortality was demonstrated by prone positioning.[76] Only one study has shown a mortality benefit with early and prolonged prone positioning of ARDS patients. The major difference in this study was the length of time patients were maintained prone—on average 17 hours daily for a mean of 10 days. The 136 patients were randomized within 48 hours of intubation.[77]

Prone positioning can be accomplished manually or with a special bed designed to rotate the patient. Complications related to prone positioning include pressure sores, endotracheal tube displacement or obstruction, loss of venous access, vomiting, and edema. Data on prone ventilation in the pregnant patient are lacking. Anticipated problems include the gravid abdomen and difficulties in accomplishing fetal monitoring while prone.

Pulmonary Edema

Pregnant women are predisposed to developing pulmonary edema for various reasons, including increased plasma volume and CO in conjunction with decreased colloid oncotic pressure (COP), which occurs normally over the course of pregnancy. Alterations in the balance of hydrostatic and oncotic pressure between the pulmonary vessels and the interstitial spaces can lead to an egress of fluid from the vascular space into the interstitium and manifest clinically as pulmonary edema. Approximately 1 in 1000 pregnancies is complicated by pulmonary edema. In a review of almost 63,000 pregnancies, Sciscione and coworkers[78] reported pulmonary edema occurring most often during the antepartum period (47%), with 39% occurring in the postpartum period and the remaining 14% in the intrapartum period.[78] In this series, the two most common attributable causes of pulmonary edema were cardiac disease and tocolytic use (25.5% each). The remaining cases of pulmonary edema were caused by fluid overload (21.5%) and preeclampsia (18%). The management of patients with pulmonary edema is focused on establishing the diagnosis, determining the cause, and improving oxygenation.

Colloid Oncotic Pressure Abnormalities

Four forces affect fluid balance between vascular and interstitial spaces. The COP is the force exerted primarily by albumin and other proteins within the capillary, which holds fluid within the vascular space. The oncotic pressure within the interstitial space also works to hold fluid in the interstitium. Hydrostatic forces within the vessel and the interstitium exert the opposite effect.

COP decreases over the course of pregnancy, and by term, it approximates 22 mm Hg.[79] This is approximately 3 mm Hg lower than pre-pregnancy values as a result of the dilutional effect from plasma expansion. An isolated decrease in oncotic pressure, as may occur in pregnancy or in patients with nephrotic syndrome, is usually well compensated and does not lead to pulmonary edema unless complicated by additional factors such as increased intravascular pressure or pulmonary injury resulting in vascular permeability.[80] Excessive intravenous fluids, blood loss, decreasing COP after delivery, and the postpartum autotransfusion effect can place patients at further increased risk for pulmonary edema.

Hydrostatic or Cardiogenic Pulmonary Edema

Pulmonary edema due to primary cardiac issues with or without alterations in COP is referred to as *hydrostatic* or *cardiogenic pulmonary edema*. CO is controlled through continuous adjustments in heart rate and stroke volume. At some point, the heart is no longer able to increase the CO in response to increasing preload because of intrinsic cardiac abnormalities or excessive fluid administration, resulting in overload. If left ventricular outflow is restricted, blood intended to empty into the left atrium remains in the pulmonary vasculature, which is reflected by the increased PCWP, left ventricular end-diastolic pressure, and pulmonary artery pressure. The net result is an increase in the pulmonary intravascular hydrostatic pressure. When this pressure exceeds the interstitial pressures, fluid is forced out of the pulmonary vasculature into the interstitial spaces, resulting in pulmonary edema.

A transthoracic or transesophageal echocardiogram can distinguish whether pulmonary edema is cardiogenic in origin. Evidence of poor ventricular systolic function is identified by a decreased ejection fraction, as seen in patients with a cardiomyopathy. Echocardiography may also identify valvular abnormalities that may lead to compromised cardiac function and predispose patients to pulmonary edema, such as aortic or mitral stenosis.

Pulmonary Edema in the Setting of Preeclampsia

Pulmonary edema develops in approximately 2.5% of patients with preeclampsia, most commonly in the postpartum period.[43,81,82] The cause is not completely understood, but it likely results from a combination of problems. Impaired left ventricular function may be a result of chronic hypertension, particularly if it develops in the antepartum period. Substantially increased SVR may also impair left ventricular function and lead to pulmonary edema, especially in the setting of iatrogenic fluid overload. Preeclamptic patients often lose significant amounts of albumin through the urine and exhibit decreased albumin production, both of which can lower the COP. In preeclamptic patients, the COP can decrease to 18 mm Hg by term and drop further after delivery to 14 mm Hg.[43] Endothelial damage also leads to increased capillary permeability. Preeclamptic patients with pulmonary edema that fails to respond to oxygen, diuresis, and fluid restriction, especially when combined with oliguria, may require pulmonary artery catheterization to guide further therapy. In a series of 10 patients with severe preeclampsia who underwent placement of a PAC, the findings varied. Five patients demonstrated a decreased gradient between the COP and PCWP, but two patients had a cardiac explanation for the pulmonary edema, and three patients had increased pulmonary vascular permeability.[83]

Tocolytic-Induced Pulmonary Edema

In the past, the use of parenteral β-agonists such as terbutaline and ritodrine was more common and became associated with the development of pulmonary edema.[78,84] However, as the use of intravenous β-agonists for tocolysis has decreased, the incidence of pulmonary edema related to tocolytic use appears to have diminished. Magnesium does not appear to independently increase the risk of pulmonary edema.[85]

Shock

Shock is the physiologic response to impaired tissue oxygenation. Oxygen deficiency at the cellular level may result from inadequate delivery of oxygen, such as in hypovolemic states, cardiac failure, and hemorrhage or from improper uptake or use of oxygen, as in septic states and neurogenic shock. In obstetric patients, shock most commonly results from hemorrhage and sepsis. Regardless of the cause, therapy is directed at restoring tissue oxygenation by eliminating the originating cause, providing adequate volume replacement, and improving cardiac function and circulation. Difficulty in reversing this phenomenon explains the high mortality rates for patients with shock.

Sepsis and Septic Shock

Incidence and Mortality

Sepsis accounts for 9.3% of deaths occurring in the United States and complicates approximately 1 in 8000 deliveries.[86] Fortunately, only a small percentage of these deaths can be attributed to gynecologic or obstetric problems. Bacteremia is not uncommon in obstetric patients, but these patients appear to be less likely to progress to septic shock.[59,87,88] An epidemiologic review of sepsis in the United States gathered discharge data on more than 10 million cases of sepsis over a 22-year period ending in 2000.[89] According to this study, the incidence of sepsis in the population is increasing at a rate of 8.7% annually. However, the percentage of pregnant women diagnosed with sepsis in that period decreased by 50%, from 0.6% to 0.3%. African Americans and men appear to be at higher risk for developing sepsis, but mortality rates did not appear to differ from those of whites and women, respectively.

Mortality rates overall have declined significantly to approximately 17%, but the marked increase in sepsis diagnosis in the population accounts for tripling of the rate of hospital death from sepsis. Between 1987 and 1997, infectious causes accounted for 13% of maternal deaths.[10,11] Mortality rates associated with septic shock in pregnancy are uncertain and are derived primarily from older, small series of cases, but they generally appear to be much lower than for the nonpregnant population. Estimates range from 12% to 28% for obstetric septic patients[58,59,87,90] to 40% to 80% for the nongravid population.[91] Improved outcomes for pregnant patients have been attributed to a younger patient population, type of organisms, sites of infection more easily accessed and treated, and lower rates of coexistent diseases.

Definitions

The American College of Chest Physicians and the Society of Critical Care Medicine published consensus guidelines in 1991 that were designed to create consistency in the definitions used to describe septic conditions. Updated guidelines were published in 2003.[57] These definitions represent the understanding that these conditions exist along a continuum of increasing severity while sharing a common pathophysiology. This continuum begins after the body develops a systemic response to an infection and may progress to multiorgan dysfunction with hemodynamic instability and even death.

The later classification system questions the utility of the diagnosis of systemic inflammatory response syndrome (SIRS), suggesting that the criteria previously set forth are too sensitive and nonspecific. SIRS was defined as the clinical response to infection manifested by two or more of the following: temperature of 38° C or higher or 36° C or lower; pulse of 90 beats/min or higher; respiration rate of 20 breaths/min or higher or a $PaCO_2$ less than 32 mm/Hg; or a white blood cell count of 12,000 or more or 4000 or less or more than 10% immature neutrophils. When SIRS criteria are met and infection is confirmed or suspected, the patient is then considered to be septic. The latest guidelines expanded on this concept in the definitions (Table 57-6). These definitions do not take into account the physiologic changes of pregnancy and therefore may overdiagnose sepsis.

TABLE 57-6 DIAGNOSTIC CRITERIA OF SEPSIS SYNDROMES

Condition	Definition
Infection	Pathologic process caused by the invasion of normally sterile tissue or fluid or body cavity by pathogenic or potentially pathogenic microorganisms
Bacteremia	Presence of bacteria in the bloodstream
Sepsis	Systemic inflammation accompanied by infection
Severe sepsis	Sepsis complicated by major organ dysfunction
Septic shock	Persistent unexplained arterial hypotension in the setting of severe sepsis

Data from Levy MM, Fink MP, Marshall JC, et al: 2001 SCCM/ESICM/ACCP/ATS/SIS International Sepsis Definitions Conference. Crit Care Med 31:1250-1256, 2003.

Gram-positive organisms have surpassed gram-negative organisms as the most common cause of sepsis in the general population, unlike the situation for pregnant patients. Common organisms isolated from pregnant patients in septic shock include *Escherichia coli*, groups A and B streptococci, *Klebsiella* species, and *Staphylococcus aureus*.[59] The source of infection in pregnant women is typically the genitourinary tract and includes lower urinary tract infections, pyelonephritis, chorioamnionitis, endometritis, and rarely, septic abortion, necrotizing fasciitis, and toxic shock syndrome.[58,59,87,88,92]

Pathophysiology of Sepsis

Sepsis is a complex phenomenon that originates with invasion of the host by an offending organism. After infection, macrophages are recruited, bind to the organism, and initiate a collection of responses resulting in the activation of the inflammatory and coagulation cascades. Initially, the sepsis response was postulated to be the result of an exaggerated inflammatory response. Initial pharmacologic approaches therefore targeted suppression of the inflammation process, including corticosteroids and agents to block cytokines such as tumor necrosis factor α (TNF-α) and interleukin 1β (IL-1β).[93] These approaches have been largely unsuccessful, a testament to the complexity of the sepsis syndromes. The roles of anti-inflammatory mediators and genetics in the sepsis cascade has been increasingly appreciated.[94] Activation of the inflammatory cascade after infection causes release of interleukins, tumor necrosis factors, interferons, prostaglandins, platelet-activation factor, oxygen free radicals, nitric oxide, complement, and fibrinolysins.[95]

Hemostatic mechanisms are also affected in severe sepsis. Initiation of the clotting cascade results from macrophages and monocytes involved in production of inflammatory mediators. Endothelial damage also contributes to the procoagulant effect, causing platelet activation and suppression of protein C activity. These derangements in the hemostatic balance lead to clotting factor consumption, fibrin deposition, thrombin generation, and decreased platelet levels.[96] The resultant microthrombi are thought to negatively affect end-organ damage and contribute to the clinical features of severe sepsis and septic shock, such as oliguria, ARDS, and hepatic dysfunction. In severe cases, consumption of clotting factors is substantial enough to cause hemorrhagic complications from DIC. Figure 57-6 outlines the sepsis cascade.

Clinical Manifestations

Septic shock has been classified as three progressive clinical stages: warm shock, cold shock, and irreversible (secondary) shock, which are summarized in Table 57-7. The initial phase is characterized by vasodilation, increased capillary permeability, and endothelial damage. Clinically, the patient may have evidence of infection or fever and may have positive blood cultures. Peripheral vasodilation causes flushing and warm extremities. It also leads to a decrease in blood pressure with diminished cardiac preload, which leads to a tachycardic response in an effort to maintain or increase the CO. Initial laboratory findings vary. An elevated white blood cell count may be followed by neutropenia. Hyperglycemia is typical as a result of altered adrenal responsiveness, insulin resistance, and increased levels of catecholamines and cortisol.

If uninterrupted, sepsis progresses and is characterized by intense vasoconstriction. This leads to poor perfusion, which is manifested by cool extremities and altered organ function as a result of inadequate oxygenation (i.e., cold shock). Oliguria is typical, as are respiratory failure and ARDS. The CO decreases as a result of inadequate venous return and increasing peripheral resistance. In the advanced stages of septic shock (i.e., secondary or irreversible shock), symptoms progress and reflect the global effects of inadequate tissue perfusion and oxygenation: hypotension, respiratory failure, renal failure, DIC, myocardial depression, electrolyte disturbances, obtundation, and metabolic acidosis.

Management

If the patient is at a viable gestational age and is undelivered with evidence of sepsis or septic shock, the fetal status should be monitored closely with continuous fetal heart rate monitoring and ultrasound evaluation to estimate fetal weight, assess amniotic fluid volume, and confirm gestational age. Uterine perfusion and oxygenation are adversely affected as the sepsis progresses. Contractions are often encountered, possibly as a result of decreased uterine perfusion and decreased oxygen delivery to the myometrium. Tocolysis should be undertaken with caution because the side effects of the medications (e.g., tachycardia, vasodilation) may impair physiologic adaptations to sepsis. If maternal status can be corrected and fetal status remains reassuring, delivery can be avoided. The decision about whether to proceed with delivery may be challenging, particularly if maternal status is deteriorating. The fetus may not tolerate labor because of poor uterine perfusion and maternal hypoxemia; conversely, the mother may be too unstable to safely undergo a surgical procedure. If the source of infection is the uterus, as in septic abortion or chorioamnionitis, evacuation of the uterus is necessary.

Sepsis management has several goals:

- Identification of the source of infection
- Institution of empiric antibiotic therapy
- Early, aggressive improvement in circulating volume
- Optimization of hemodynamic performance
- Maintenance of oxygenation
- Volume resuscitation

Aggressive fluid replacement to improve circulating intravascular volume is a mainstay of sepsis management and has improved CO, oxygen delivery, and survival. Studies have demonstrated a survival benefit for patients with septic shock managed with protocol-driven, early, aggressive volume resuscitation. Early goal-directed therapy (EGDT) involves tailoring treatments and resuscitative efforts to achieve specified endpoints, which include normal mixed venous oxygen saturation, arterial lactate concentration, base deficit, and pH in an effort to reduce end-organ dysfunction and ultimately reduce mortality.

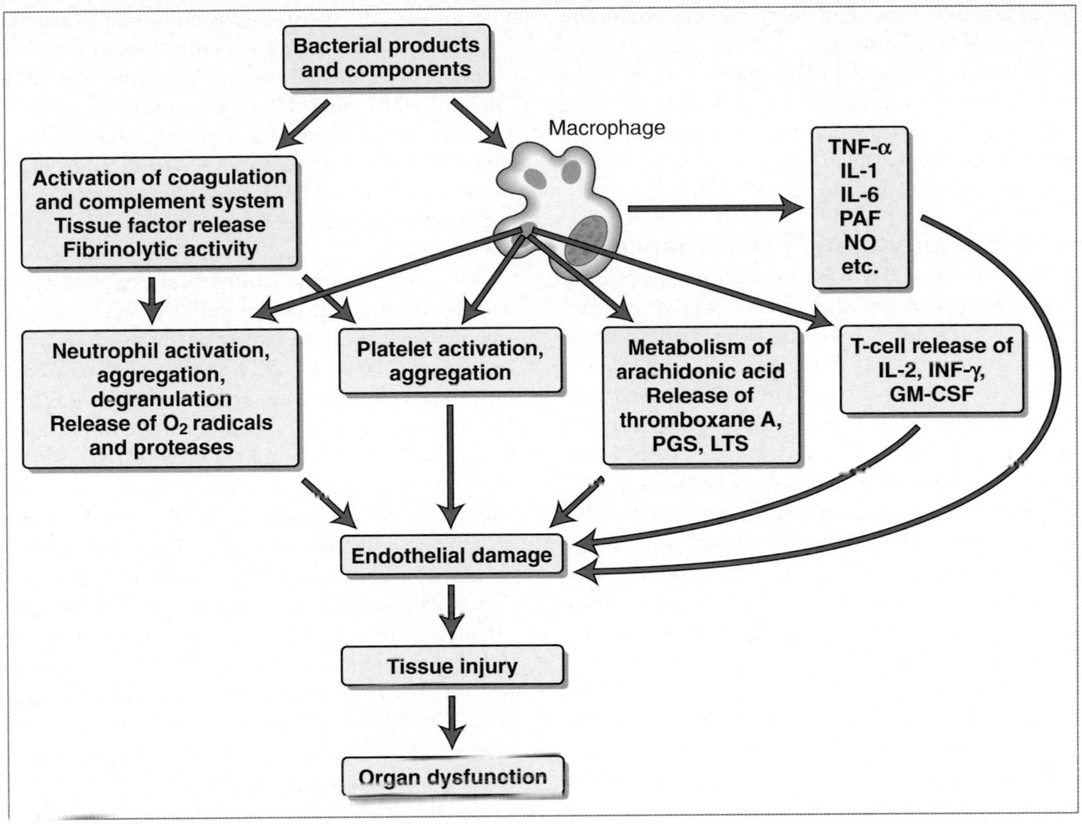

FIGURE 57-6 The sepsis cascade. Hemostatic mechanisms are affected in patients with severe sepsis, and derangements in the hemostatic balance lead to clotting factor consumption, fibrin deposition, thrombin generation, decreased platelets, tissue injury, and organ dysfunction. GM-CSF, granulocyte-macrophage colony-stimulating factor; IL, interleukin; LTS, leukotrienes; NO, nitric oxide; PAF, platelet-activating factor; PGS, prostaglandin synthesis; TNF-α, tumor necrosis factor α. (Modified from Bone RC: The pathogenesis of sepsis. Ann Intern Med 115:457-469, 1991.)

TABLE 57-7 STAGES OF SHOCK

Warm (Early) Shock	Cold (Late) Shock	Secondary (Irreversible) Shock
Flushing	Cyanosis	Renal failure
Warm extremities	Cool extremities	Disseminated intravascular coagulopathy
Rapid capillary refill	Delayed capillary refill	Myocardial failure
Decreased mental status	Increased vascular resistance	Refractory hypotension
Hypotension	Decreased cardiac output	Obtundation
Increased cardiac output	Respiratory failure or adult respiratory distress syndrome	
Tachycardia	Oliguria	
Tachypnea		

In 2001, Rivers and colleagues[97] published the results of a prospective, randomized trial of EGDT compared with standard therapy for patients in septic shock in a single institution. Therapy for patients in the EGDT group was initiated in the emergency room setting before transfer to the intensive care unit and included placement of central venous catheters with the ability to measure continuous venous oxygen saturation ($ScvO_2$). An elevated $ScvO_2$ value reflects inadequate perfusion and uptake of oxygen in the tissues. Red blood cell transfusions were administered to maintain the hematocrit at 30% or higher, and inotropic agents were added if the $ScvO_2$ level was inadequately corrected (<70%). The protocol called for a 500-mL crystalloid bolus every 30 minutes until the CVP reached 8 to 12 mm Hg. The volume of fluid administered to both groups of patients was similar in the first 72 hours (>13 L), but the EGDT group received more volume in the initial 6 hours of therapy (5 versus 3.5 L). This aggressive approach decreased the mortality rate by 16% (30.5% versus 46.5%).

Clinicians have questioned whether modification of this protocol, particularly elimination of continuous venous oxygen saturation ($ScvO_2$), could produce similar results. In 2006, Lin and coworkers[98] randomized patients to EGDT without measurement of $ScvO_2$ and confirmed survival benefit. Patients randomized to receive modified EGDT were significantly less likely to die (71.6% versus 53.7%), spent fewer days in the hospital, were intubated for a shorter time, and were at less risk for developing sepsis-associated central nervous system and renal dysfunction compared with controls.

Because of the encouraging survival and morbidity data, EGDT is being widely adopted in the management of severe sepsis, but it remains to be confirmed whether this approach will produce similarly improved outcomes in a pregnant population. The precise goals to appropriately guide therapy in a pregnant population also must be defined.

Optimization of Hemodynamic Performance

In addition to replacing intravascular volume to improve perfusion and cardiac preload, early pharmacologic interventions to improve vascular tone, cardiac contractility, and cardiac preload confer a considerable survival advantage.[97,98] If the patient fails to respond appropriately to aggressive fluid resuscitation efforts, vasopressors are indicated to improve vascular tone, resulting in improved cardiac return and CO, peripheral perfusion, and oxygen delivery. In the initial publication on EGDT, the requirement for vasopressors was significantly diminished by early, aggressive fluid resuscitation (37% versus 51%), but there was no difference in the requirement for inotropic agents between the two groups (9% versus 15%).[97] In this study, vasopressors were initiated to maintain mean arterial pressure above 65 mm Hg. Use of a similar protocol minimized the delay in initiation of vasopressors and reduce mortality.[98]

Dopamine hydrochloride is the most commonly employed first-line vasopressor in the intensive care setting. Dopamine's α- and β-adrenergic effects are dose dependent. Low doses (<10 µg/kg/min) improve myocardial contractility, CO, and renal perfusion without negatively affecting myocardial oxygen consumption. As the dose increases (>20 mg/kg/min), α-adrenergic effects predominate, resulting in increasing SVR in addition to increased CO. In a viable gestation requiring vasopressor support, fetal monitoring is essential because dopamine has decreased uterine perfusion in an animal model.[99] Dobutamine is similar to dopamine, but it has primarily β1-adrenergic effects. Dobutamine therefore improves CO with minimal impact on heart rate or vascular resistance. In the EGDT protocol, dobutamine was used to improve oxygen consumption in patients who failed to respond to fluid resuscitation, dopamine infusion to improve mean arterial pressure, and red cell transfusion to correct anemia.[97] Table 57-8 lists other commonly used vasopressor agents for the management of severe sepsis and septic shock.

Source Control and Antimicrobial Therapy

Prompt identification of the probable source of infection is essential to initiate appropriate antimicrobial therapy and improve outcomes for septic patients. In an obstetric population, common sources of infection are the uterus and genitourinary tract, and gram-negative bacteria constitute the primary organisms. In the non-obstetric population, gram-positive organisms represent most of the organisms isolated in septic patients, followed closely by gram-negative bacteria.[89] Cultures should be collected from blood and any suspected site, including the uterus if necessary, for identification of the organism and determination of antibiotic sensitivities. Empiric antimicrobial therapy targeted at the suspected organism should not be delayed pending culture results.[100-103]

TABLE 57-8 INOTROPIC DRUGS FOR MANAGEMENT OF SHOCK

Agent	Dose	Hemodynamic Effect
Dopamine		
Low dose	<10 µg/kg/min	↑ CO, vasodilation of renal arteries
High dose	10-20 µg/kg/min	↑ CO, ↑ SVR
Dobutamine	2.5-15 µg/kg/min	↑ CO, ↓ SVR or ↑ SVR
Phenylephrine	40-180 µg/min	↑ SVR
Norepinephrine	2-12 µg/min	↑ CO, ↑ SVR
Isoproterenol	0.5-5 µg/min	↓ CO, ↑ SVR

CO, cardiac output; SVR, systemic vascular resistance; ↑, increase; ↓, decrease.

In an obstetric and postpartum population, antibiotic coverage usually consists of β-lactam antibiotics (i.e., penicillins, cephalosporins, carbapenems, and monobactams) with or without an aminoglycoside (see Chapter 38). Monotherapy with a carbapenem or third- or fourth-generation cephalosporin is as effective as a β-lactam antibiotic in combination with an aminoglycoside in non-neutropenic patients with severe sepsis.[104] In undelivered patients, tetracycline derivatives and quinolones should be avoided. When culture results become available, antibiotic therapy can be adjusted if necessary.

After appropriate antibiotic therapy has been initiated and the process of stabilization of the patient has begun, attention should be directed to source control. This entails removal of indwelling lines and catheters, with replacement if necessary. Indications for more aggressive surgical approaches are less clearly defined. Generally, more invasive surgical approaches are not emergent and can be accomplished after the condition of the patient has stabilized.[105] Exceptions are infections involving clostridia and group A streptococci, such as necrotizing fasciitis. In this scenario, delay in excision of affected tissues can have a dramatic negative effect on the patient's condition.[106] Evaluation of the abdomen by ultrasound or computed tomography (CT) can assist in identification of an intra-abdominal abscess. When drainage of an intra-abdominal abscess is necessary, the percutaneous approach is preferable. In obstetric conditions, evacuation of the uterus by suction curettage in septic abortion or delivery of the neonate in viable gestations should occur after initiation of antibiotics and stabilization of the patient. Postpartum hysterectomy may be necessary if the patient fails to respond to antibiotics and the uterus is the suspected source.

Adjunctive Therapies in Sepsis Management

INSULIN THERAPY

In the critically ill population, hyperglycemia is a common phenomenon attributable to insulin resistance and escalations in glucagon, cortisol, and catecholamine levels, which promote glycogenolysis and gluconeogenesis.[107] In 2001, Van den Berghe and colleagues[108] published a large, prospective, randomized trial that demonstrated that tight glycemic control (blood glucose level of 80 to 110 mg/dL) in critically ill patients decreased overall mortality by 34%. Septic patients exhibited an even more impressive 76% reduction in mortality as a result of aggressive euglycemia with insulin therapy.[108] Other significant benefits of tight glycemic control included fewer ventilator days, less time in the ICU, decrease risk for developing septicemia, and a reduced need for dialysis.

Pregnant women demonstrate insulin resistance and to have higher circulating insulin levels than their nonpregnant counterparts. They are also predisposed to developing fasting hypoglycemia because of higher levels of insulin and continuous delivery of glucose to the fetus. However, the impact of aggressive euglycemia in the critically ill pregnant patient remains to be studied.

CORTICOSTEROIDS

Empiric administration of corticosteroids in high doses does not improve survival of unselected septic patients and may worsen outcomes because of secondary infection.[109,110] However, as the pathophysiology of sepsis has become more clearly understood, the contribution of relative adrenal insufficiency in critically ill patients and the potential benefit of lower-dose, selective corticosteroid replacement have reemerged.

Stresses such as pain, fever, hypovolemia, or severe illness normally stimulate marked increases in cortisol levels. In the patient with septic shock, the adrenal gland may not respond to adrenocorticotropic hormone (ACTH) stimulus appropriately and fail to mount adequate corticosteroid production. In the setting of septic shock, however, the levels of cortisol may be increased overall, but the magnitude of increase after ACTH administration may be blunted. This phenomenon is described as relative adrenal insufficiency.[111,112] This group of patients is being evaluated for potential benefit from lower doses of corticosteroids. A randomized trial conducted by Annane and colleagues[113] demonstrated a survival benefit (mortality rate of 37% versus 47% for controls) for patients with septic shock treated with low-dose hydrocortisone and fludrocortisone. Patients who had documented blunted adrenal responsiveness also benefited from a reduced need for vasopressor support. All of these patients had elevated baseline cortisol levels. A 2004 meta analysis of 16 trials that included more than 2000 patients suggested similar benefit from lower-dose steroid replacement in patients with severe sepsis and septic shock.[114] Steroids did not appear to confer a mortality benefit when all data were included. However, inclusion of only studies utilizing low-dose (300 mg of hydrocortisone or an equivalent), longer-duration (5 to 11 days) therapy did demonstrate a decrease in overall mortality rates. The investigators recommended initiation of low-dose glucocorticoid replacement in septic patients with blunted adrenal responsiveness confirmed by an ACTH stimulation test.

The degree of adrenal suppression in pregnant or postpartum septic shock patients and the effect of low-dose steroids on outcomes in this population are unknown. If the patient remains undelivered, care should be taken in the choice of corticosteroids. Betamethasone and dexamethasone cross the placenta and have improved neonatal outcomes for premature infants. However, both can negatively impact neonatal outcomes when administered in large doses.[115]

ACTIVATED PROTEIN C THERAPY FOR SEVERE SEPSIS

One of the pathophysiologic mechanisms thought to contribute to morbidity and mortality in sepsis patients is inappropriate activation of the coagulation system. As a result, many trials have been performed involving various antithrombotic agents, including antithrombin III and tissue factor-pathway inhibitor, without successfully identifying a treatment to reduce mortality among septic shock patients.[116] In contrast, activated protein C (APC, drotrecogin alfa) has been approved by the U.S. Food and Drug Administration (FDA) for use in severely septic patients at high risk for death as evidenced by an APACHE II score greater than 25.

Patients with severe sepsis have an acquired deficiency of protein C and are limited in their ability to convert protein C to its active form. These low protein C levels have been associated with poorer outcomes for severe sepsis patients.[117,118] APC is believed to mediate the effects of severe sepsis in several ways. APC stimulates fibrinolysis and inactivates factors Va and VIIIa, resulting in inhibition of thrombin formation.[94,119] Decreased thrombin formation then leads to decreased inflammation by inhibiting platelet activation, neutrophil recruitment, and mast cell degranulation. Two trials have evaluated APC's effect on mortality in patients with severe sepsis. In the Recombinant Human Activated Protein C Worldwide Evaluation in Severe Sepsis (PROWESS) trial, a multicenter, randomized trial, APC administration to patients in septic shock decreased the 28-day mortality rate from 30.8% in the placebo group to 24.7% ($P = .005$) in the study group. This represents a 6.1% absolute reduction in overall mortality due to septic shock and a 13% reduction in the groups with the highest predicted mortality based on APACHE II scores.[120] A subsequent single-arm trial (Extended Evaluation of Recombinant Human Activated Protein C [ENHANCE] trial) using APC in severe sepsis patients demonstrated a mortality rate (25.3%) similar to that seen in the PROWESS trial (24.7%). Patients who received the therapy in the first 24 hours after diagnosis of major organ dysfunction had the lowest mortality rate (22.9%).[121]

The most significant complication resulting from the use of APC is hemorrhage. In the PROWESS trial, 3.5% of patients receiving APC suffered a significant hemorrhagic event such as intracranial hemorrhage or need for transfusion, compared with a 2% incidence in the control group. The risk of bleeding appears to be greatest during the infusion period, because APC has a very short half-life. Because of this risk, APC is not indicated for all patients with septic shock, and its use should be limited to patients with greatest risk of mortality (i.e., APACHE II scores ≧25 and one major organ dysfunction). APC is contraindicated if the risk of bleeding is increased (i.e., active internal bleeding, hemorrhagic stroke in the preceding 3 months, intracranial or intraspinal surgery, severe head trauma in the preceding 2 months, trauma, or epidural catheter). The role of APC in managing obstetric patients has not been established. Significant changes in the coagulation cascade occur, including elevated factor VIII levels. The impact of these changes on the responsiveness to APC is unknown; however, pregnancy is not a contraindication to its use.

Hemorrhagic Shock

Incidence and Etiology

Obstetric hemorrhage is the leading cause of maternal death after an intrauterine gestation. The overall incidence of maternal death from hemorrhage is 1.4 per 100,000 live births. When ectopic gestations are excluded, placental abruption is the most common cause of death (18.5%).[122] The cause of hemorrhage varies by pregnancy outcome; maternal deaths after a live birth are most likely associated with postpartum hemorrhage. Stillbirths are most likely to be associated with death from placental abruption, and undelivered pregnancies occur most often with lacerations or uterine ruptures.[122] A significant increase in risk of death from hemorrhage is seen in nonwhite women and with advancing age. In an analysis of maternal morbidity and mortality, hemorrhage accounted for 39% of near-miss morbidities. The investigators estimated that 46% of these near-miss events were preventable and were related to communication issues, policies and procedures, failure to identify high-risk status, failure to transfer to a higher level of care, or inappropriate care. The presence of a significant disease state, such as preeclampsia, was also a contributor.[123]

Causes of obstetric hemorrhage associated with an intrauterine gestation include placental abruption or previa, uterine rupture, surgical lacerations, invasive placentation, uterine inversion, and postpartum hemorrhage, usually caused by atony or retained products of conception. The source of hemorrhage can usually be determined by assessment of the patient. Concealed hemorrhage (e.g., abruption, liver capsule rupture in HELLP syndrome) is also possible and should be considered in a patient with evidence of shock and no obvious source of hemorrhage.

Obstetric hemorrhage has been arbitrarily defined as an estimated blood loss of more than 500 mL in a vaginal delivery and greater than

TABLE 57-9 CLINICAL STAGING OF HEMORRHAGIC SHOCK BY VOLUME OF BLOOD LOSS

Severity of Shock	Findings	Blood Loss (%)	Volume (mL)*
None	None	Up to 20	Up to 900
Mild	Tachycardia (<100 beats/min) Mild hypotension Peripheral vasoconstriction	20-25	1200-1500
Moderate	Tachycardia (100-120 beats/min) Hypotension (80-100 mm Hg) Restlessness Oliguria	30-35	1800-2100
Severe	Tachycardia (>120 beats/min) Hypotension (<60 mm Hg) Altered consciousness Anuria	>35	>2400

*Based on an average blood volume of 6000 mL at 30 weeks' gestation.

1000 mL for cesarean section.[124] Other definitions describe a decrease in the hematocrit by 10% or the need for transfusion.[125] However, estimates of blood loss are inaccurate and can vary widely. The true incidence of obstetric hemorrhagic shock is unknown.

Clinical Staging of Hemorrhage

Because of the normal blood volume expansion in pregnancy, clinical evidence of hypovolemia becomes evident much later than expected. Relatively minor symptoms such as orthostatic hypotension and tachycardia typically do not appear until at least 20% to 25% of the blood volume is lost. Table 57-9 outlines the clinical staging of hemorrhagic shock, depending on severity.

Management

The goal of management of hemorrhagic shock is to identify and control the bleeding source while restoring circulating blood volume and clotting factors. Baseline laboratory evaluation is recommended on recognition of the hemorrhage and should include a complete blood cell count, blood type and crossmatch, fibrinogen level, prothrombin time (international normalized ratio), and activated partial thromboplastin time. A basic metabolic panel is potentially useful to assess renal function and electrolyte disturbances. These laboratory tests should be repeated at regular intervals until the situation is resolved. The Lee-White whole-blood clotting time test can be used as a crude method to assess for the presence of DIC. Whole blood is collected in an unheparinized tube and observed. A stable clot should form between 5 and 15 minutes.

VOLUME REPLACEMENT THERAPY

Adequate and timely replacement of circulating volume is essential in the management of hemorrhagic shock. This is accomplished by administering crystalloid solutions such as normal saline or colloids such as albumin or blood products. Controversy exists about the most appropriate combination of fluids to replace circulating volume. Crystalloid solutions appear to be as effective as colloid solutions in most settings.[126] The Advanced Trauma Life Support (ATLS) course has proposed widely accepted standards for management of the trauma patient. For the patient in hemorrhagic shock, initial resuscitation with 2 L of crystalloid solution is followed by packed red cell transfusions.[127] The degree of volume resuscitation is also a matter of debate. Historically, aggressive, early fluid resuscitation was thought to result in improved outcomes. However, later data suggest that excessive fluid resuscitation may destabilize clot formation and stability, worsen hypothermia, and contribute to hemodilution without providing the expected benefit in survival. Some physicians recommend resuscitation to allow for *permissive hypotension* (i.e., systolic blood pressure >80 mm Hg).[127]

TABLE 57-10 COLLOID INFUSIONS

Colloid	Dose (mL)	Crystalloid Volume Expansion Equivalent	Estimated Duration of Effect (hr)
Albumin			
5% solution	500-700	Similar to crystalloid	24
25% solution	100-200	3.5 times crystalloid	24
Hetastarch	500-1000	Similar to crystalloid	24-36
Dextran (70)	500	1050 mL over 2 hours	24

COLLOID SOLUTIONS

Colloid solutions are intravenous fluids containing particles larger than 10,000 daltons. Packed red cells are considered a colloid, but this discussion focuses on additional colloid products. The major advantage provided by a colloid solution is the significant increase in plasma volume compared with a crystalloid solution. Colloid solutions increase intravascular COP and draw fluid into the intravascular space. In achieving this effect, extravascular volume can become depleted, and fluid resuscitation should include adequate administration of crystalloids. The degree of plasma expansion depends on the availability of extravascular fluid. In certain clinical settings such as sepsis, surgical trauma, or preeclampsia, vascular permeability is altered, and colloid solutions can escape into extravascular spaces, particularly the lungs, and lead to pulmonary edema. Available colloid solutions include albumin, dextran, and hetastarch. Table 57-10 compares the effects of these agents.

Albumin solutions are available in concentrations of 5% or 25%. A 25-g infusion of albumin temporarily increases intravascular volume by roughly 450 mL over 60 minutes as a result of its considerable oncotic activity. Albumin is cleared rapidly from the circulation, particularly in patients with shock or sepsis.

Dextran solution contains large glucose polymers with mean molecular weights of 40,000 daltons (dextran 40) or 70,000 daltons (dextran 70). Dextran 40 is rarely used for the purposes of volume expansion. A 500-mL infusion of 6% dextran 70 should rapidly expand intravascular volume by more than 1000 mL. Adverse effects of dextran administration include increased bleeding risk and allergic reaction. Anaphylactic reactions affect 1 in 3300 patients receiving dextran. In higher doses (>20 mL/kg/24 hr), dextran may negatively affect platelet function and clotting factor activation, and it may interfere with fibrin function. It also may interfere with laboratory cross-matching of blood. Dextran should be used cautiously in patients with hypovolemia due to hemorrhage who may already have a coagulopathy and require further cross-matching of blood.

Hydroxymethyl starch (i.e., hetastarch) is a synthetic molecule available in a 6% solution in normal saline (Hespan) or lactated electrolyte solution (Hextend). Like the other available colloid solutions of albumin and dextran, hetastarch also induces intravascular volume expansion by increasing oncotic pressure. The effects of hetastarch can persist for 24 to 36 hours. As with dextran, hetastarch may negatively affect the clotting system. Hetastarch can prolong prothrombin and partial thromboplastin times, decrease platelet counts, and reduce clot tensile strength, and it should be used with caution in patients who may have a coagulopathy. Hextend is a newer hetastarch formulation with smaller-molecular-weight particles in addition to electrolytes and lactate similar to plasma levels. It may have less effect on the coagulation profile compared with other colloids and therefore offer a theoretical advantage in the setting of hemorrhage.[128]

BLOOD COMPONENT THERAPY

Blood product replacement is the cornerstone of successful management of hemorrhagic shock. The variety of blood product components available for transfusion is summarized in Table 57-11, along with anticipated effects. Whole blood has not been separated into the various components and therefore offers a theoretical advantage because it contains clotting factors and platelets in addition to red blood cells. The major limitation to the use of whole blood is the inability to store the product beyond 24 hours. After 24 hours of extravascular storage, platelets and granulocytes are completely lost and 2,3-diphosphoglycerate is depleted, significantly compromising the oxygen carrying capacity of the red blood cells. Prolonged storage results in depletion of clotting factors and increasing levels of potassium and ammonia. For these reasons, whole blood is typically separated into its individual components and stored for later use; it is essentially unavailable in the United States. Individual components can then be administered to address specific derangements according to clinical indications. The routine administration of clotting factors after every 4 to 6 units of packed red blood cells has not been demonstrated to improve outcomes.[129]

A single unit of packed red cells has a hematocrit of approximately 80% and can increase the hemoglobin level by 1 g/dL in a 70-kg individual. Removal of white blood cells from the unit of blood (i.e., leukocyte-poor blood) decreases the risk of febrile transfusion reactions. Patients with evidence of acute hemorrhage (>30% blood volume loss), hemoglobin level between 6 and 10 g/dL with evidence of tachycardia and hypotension, or hemoglobin concentration less than 6 g/dL should be considered candidates for transfusion.[130,131]

Dilutional thrombocytopenia can occur as a result of massive transfusion in a hemorrhaging patient. After replacement of one blood volume, 35% to 40% of a patient's platelets usually remain, and platelet replacement is recommended in the setting of bleeding and significant thrombocytopenia. Platelet counts equilibrate within 10 minutes and can be assessed immediately after completion of the transfusion.

Fresh-frozen plasma (FFP) is plasma that is extracted from whole blood within 6 hours of collection and frozen. A single unit of FFP contains 700 mg of fibrinogen in addition to factors II, V, VII, IX, X, and XI. It is indicated for the replacement of multiple clotting factors in patients with acute hemorrhage and evidence of DIC. The goal is to correct clotting factor deficiencies and to achieve a post-transfusion serum fibrinogen level of approximately 100 mg/dL.

Cryoprecipitate is obtained from FFP and contains factor VIII (80 to 120 units), fibrinogen (200 mg), von Willebrand factor, and factor XIII. One unit of cryoprecipitate and one unit of FFP have similar effects on the fibrinogen level (increase of 10 to 15 mg/dL). However, because of its smaller volume, cryoprecipitate more efficiently raises the fibrinogen level compared with FFP.

COMPLICATIONS OF TRANSFUSION

Complications resulting from blood component transfusion vary from infections to immunologic responses. Table 57-12 outlines the frequency of various transfusion-related complications.

Minor transfusion reactions are relatively common occurrences and are not caused by hemolysis. Common clinical findings include low-grade fever, urticaria, or hives, and they result from exposure to incompatible platelet or white blood cell antigens. The use of leukocyte-poor packed red cells minimizes these types of reactions. Nonhemolytic reactions do not require discontinuation of the transfusion. Symptoms can be managed with antipyretic agents and antihistamines, as needed.

TABLE 57-11 BLOOD COMPONENTS

Component	Contents	Indications	Volume	Shelf Life	Expected Effect
Packed RBCs	Red cells, some plasma, few WBCs	Correct anemia	300 mL	21 days	Increase HCT 3%/unit, Hgb 1 g/unit
Leukocyte-poor blood	RBCs, some plasma, few WBCs	Correct anemia, reduce febrile reactions	250 mL	21-24 days	Increase HCT 3%/unit, Hgb 1 g/unit
Platelets	Platelets, some plasma, RBCs, few WBCs	Bleeding due to thrombocytopenia	50 mL	Up to 5 days	Increase total platelet count 7500 μL/unit
Fresh-frozen plasma	Plasma, clotting factors V, XI, XII	Treatment of coagulation disorders	250 mL	2 hours thawed, 12 months frozen	Increase total fibrinogen 10-15%/unit
Cryoprecipitate	Fibrinogen, factors V, VIII, XIII, von Willebrand factor	Hemophilia A, von Willebrand disease, fibrinogen deficiency	40 mL	4-6 hours thawed	Increase total fibrinogen 10-15 mg/dL per unit

HCT, hematocrit; Hgb, hemoglobin; RBCs, red blood cells; WBCs, white blood cells.

TABLE 57-12 TRANSFUSION-RELATED RISKS

Disease or Disorder	Risk
Hepatitis B	1/137,000
Hepatitis C	<1/1,000,000
Human immunodeficiency virus type 1 (HIV-1)	<1/1,900,000
Bacterial contamination	1/38,565
Acute hemolytic reaction	1/250,000-1/1,000,000
Delayed hemolytic reaction	1/1,000
Transfusion-related acute lung injury	1/5,000

Adapted from Goodnough LT, Brecher ME, Kanter MH, et al: Transfusion medicine. Part 1. Blood transfusion. N Engl J Med 340:438-447, 1999; and the American Association of Blood Banks 2002. Available at www.aabb.org.

Severe reactions after transfusion are usually the result of a hemolytic reaction to the administration of an incompatible unit of blood. Historically, administration of ABO-incompatible blood was thought to occur at a rate of 1 in 600,000 units, but a later report suggests it occurs with much greater frequency (1 in 25,000 units). Administrative error is the culprit in most of these events, underscoring the need for accurate accounting of transfused units, particularly in an emergent situation.[132] Cardiovascular decompensation with DIC, fever, and renal failure usually develop rapidly after initiation of an incompatible transfusion. Treatment entails immediate discontinuation of the transfusion and supportive care.

ADDITIONAL SUPPORTIVE MEASURES

Red Blood Cell–Saving Devices. In patients anticipated to be at risk for excessive intraoperative blood loss, such as suspected placenta accreta, use of an autologous transfusion device (Cell Saver) should be considered.[124,133] Theoretical risks of inducing amniotic fluid embolism have caused some concern regarding the use of intraoperative cell salvage during cesarean section. However, several reports have validated its safety in this arena.[134-137] After delivery of the fetus and clearing the operating field of amniotic fluid, the suction device is changed, and blood is collected into the Cell Saver. In approximately 3 minutes, a unit of blood with a hematocrit of 50% is generated. In one study comparing patients who received blood salvage and autotransfusion during cesarean section with those receiving allogeneic blood transfusions, no differences in the rates of infection, coagulation abnormalities, or respiratory problems could be identified.[135] This technology may be particularly valuable for patients who have the potential for severe blood loss or who have religious preferences mandating the avoidance of transfused blood products.

Acute Normovolemic Hemodilution. Acute normovolemic hemodilution offers an additional option for patients at significant risk for intraoperative hemorrhage. The principle behind this approach is to dilute the patient's circulating volume so that when bleeding occurs, it has a lower hematocrit. This is accomplished by collecting blood from the patient preoperatively and placing it into special storage bags that can be obtained from the blood bank. Simultaneously, the patient is given crystalloid solution in a 3:1 ratio, resulting in a dilutional effect and a decrease in the maternal hematocrit. Intraoperatively, after achieving control of the blood loss, or at the discretion of the surgeon, the patient's blood is then reinfused, resulting in an increase in the hematocrit.

Potential advantages include preservation of clotting factors, a decreased likelihood of allogeneic transfusion, and therefore a decreased risk of infectious morbidity, alloimmunization, and immunologic complications. Adverse fetal effects have not been described during this process.[138,139] Acute normovolemic hemodilution is a time-consuming process and is not appropriate for an acutely hemorrhaging patient. Suggested criteria for acute normovolemic hemodilution include an increased likelihood of transfusion; preoperative hemoglobin level of 12 g/dL or higher; absence of clinically significant coronary, pulmonary, renal, or liver disease; absence of severe hypertension; and absence of infection and risk of bacteremia.[140]

Other Measures. Supplemental oxygenation and elevation of the lower extremities are recommended for patients with hemorrhage. The use of antishock (MAST) trousers has fallen out of favor after publication of a randomized trial that failed to demonstrate survival benefit.[141]

Massive transfusion and blood loss place the patient at significant risk for concomitant abnormalities that can compromise successful resuscitation. Maintenance of the airway and ventilation cannot be ignored. Management of the hemorrhaging patient should include regular assessment for coagulation abnormalities and recurrent bleeding, correction of electrolyte abnormalities, particularly calcium and potassium, and maintenance of temperature above 35° C. After control of bleeding is achieved, resuscitation is considered complete if the following goals are met[142]:

- Normal or hyperdynamic vital signs
- Hematocrit higher than 20% (transfusion threshold determined by the patient's age)
- Normal serum electrolyte levels
- Normal coagulation function, with a platelet count of at least 50,000
- Restoration of adequate microvascular perfusion, as indicated by a pH of 7.40 with a normal base deficit, normalized serum lactate level, normal mixed venous oxygenation, normal or high CO, and normal urine output.

DEFINITIVE THERAPY FOR HEMOSTASIS

Control of obstetric hemorrhage must take into consideration the apparent cause of the hemorrhage. For example, the most likely cause of postpartum hemorrhage is uterine atony, which would be expected to respond to uterine massage and uterotonic agents as first-line therapy. Hemorrhage due to placenta accreta or previa requires surgical intervention. Recombinant factor VIIa (rFVIIa, NovoSeven) is approved for the management of bleeding in hemophiliacs, but its role is emerging as an off-label adjunctive therapy for the control of catastrophic, coagulopathic bleeding. Recombinant factor VIIa functions by activating factor X, thereby enhancing thrombin production and formation of a stable clot. It is not intended as first-line therapy for control of hemorrhage, and most physicians recommend use of rFVIIa only after other attempts to control hemorrhage have failed. This includes any necessary surgical approach, appropriate replacement of blood products, and correction of severe acidosis, hypothermia, and hypocalcemia.[143,144] rFVIIa has been employed for the control of obstetric hemorrhage.[145-148] Table 57-13 outlines pharmacologic agents useful in controlling hemorrhage from an atonic uterus.

Hemorrhage after a vaginal delivery should prompt a thorough evaluation for and repair of cervical or vaginal lacerations, particularly if an instrumented delivery was performed. If uterine atony fails to respond to uterine massage and uterotonic agents, evaluation for potential retained placental fragments should be performed. Ultrasound may be of assistance in this assessment process, particularly if uterine curettage is necessary. Intrauterine pressure packs to control

TABLE 57-13 PHARMACOLOGIC AGENTS USEFUL FOR CONTROLLING UTERINE ATONY

Agent	Dose	Considerations/Side Effects
Oxytocin (Pitocin)	10-40 units/L IV 10 units IM	IV bolus may cause PVCs and hypotension
Methylergonovine (Methergine)	0.2 mg IM every 2-4 hours, maximum of 5 doses	Increased SVR, increased MAP, increased CVP Side effects include pulmonary edema, seizures, intracranial hemorrhage, retinal detachment, and coronary vasospasm. Avoid in patients with hypertension
Prostaglandin 15-methyl $F_{2\alpha}$ (Hemabate)	0.25 mg IM every 15-90 minutes, maximum dose of 2 mg	Diarrhea Bronchoconstriction Increased CO, increased heart rate, and increased right heart pressure Increased PVR Decreased SVR Decreased coronary artery perfusion Avoid in patients with asthma
Dinoprostone (prostaglandin E_2)	20 mg per rectum or vagina every 2 hours	Diarrhea, nausea, vomiting Tachypnea, pyrexia, tachycardia Decreased SVR Decreased MAP Increased CO
Misoprostol (Cytotec, prostaglandin E_1)	800-1000 μg per rectum	Diarrhea, vomiting Abdominal pain Headache
Recombinant factor VIIa (NovoSeven)	200 μg/kg initial dose; may repeat with 100 μg/kg at 1 and 3 hours after the first dose	Indicated with persistent bleeding despite adequate first-line therapies May increase risk for thromboembolic events

CVP, central venous pressure; CO, cardiac output; IM, intramuscular; IV, intravenous; MAP, mean arterial pressure; PVC, premature ventricular contraction; PVR, pulmonary vascular resistance; SVR, systemic vascular resistance.

life-threatening postpartum hemorrhage have been successful according to some reports.[149,150] However, the technique used to place the packing is integral to its success and can be challenging. Other physicians have attempted to provide packing by modifying various inflatable devices such as Foley catheters or Sengstaken-Blakemore tubes.[151,152] The SOS Bakri tamponade balloon has been introduced specifically to provide intrauterine compression in the management of postpartum hemorrhage.[153] The SOS Bakri tamponade balloon has been placed vaginally and at cesarean section.

Surgery to Control Obstetric Hemorrhage. If uterine hemorrhage after vaginal delivery fails to respond to the previously described measures, exploratory laparotomy should be performed. If the bleeding is encountered at cesarean section, the same techniques for control of hemorrhage may be applied. The B-Lynch uterine body compression suture has been performed successfully to control hemorrhage due to unresponsive uterine atony, and it is demonstrated in Figure 57-7.[154,155] The B-Lynch suture has been performed in conjunction with placement of an SOS Bakri balloon to achieve hemostasis.[156]

Suture ligation of the ascending uterine arteries (i.e., O'Leary suture) is another option and is technically straightforward to perform in most scenarios. O'Leary and O'Leary[157,158] reported the successful use of this technique (Fig. 57-8) in controlling postpartum and postcesarean bleeding. The uterine artery can be visualized and accessed anteriorly or posteriorly. The uterine arteries are readily accessible with uterine manipulation, and minimal or no vessel dissection is necessary for uterine artery ligation. Hypogastric artery ligation is more technically challenging, requiring dissection of the retroperitoneal space through the broad ligament. Bilateral ligation usually is necessary to achieve adequate reduction in pulse pressure. The surgeon must be familiar with pelvic vascular anatomy to avoid ureteral injury or inadvertent ligation of the common or exterior iliac artery, which will obstruct blood flow to the lower extremity. If possible, ligation of the vessel should occur below the branch of the superior gluteal artery, as demonstrated in Figure 57-9. Because of the technical challenges and questionable efficacy of the procedure (hemorrhage controlled in approximately 40% of cases), hypogastric artery ligation is not commonly performed.[159]

The incidence of emergent peripartum hysterectomy for obstetric hemorrhage is less than 0.8%.[160-164] Cesarean delivery, prior cesarean delivery, and multiple gestation are significant risk factors.[164,165] Other indications for peripartum hysterectomy include uterine rupture, extension of the uterine incision, infection, and myomas. A study reported peripartum hysterectomy data from a national database between 1998 and 2003 and included more than 18,000 hysterectomies. Although some case series have suggested that invasive placentation appears to be supplanting uterine atony as the leading indication for peripartum hysterectomy, other data suggest they may be equally common.[160,161,164,166] Complications from emergency peripartum hysterectomy include excessive blood loss and the need for blood product replacement, fever, wound infection, ureteral injury, thromboembolic events, cardiac arrest, and death.[160,162,163,166] Supracervical and total hysterectomy have been described for the management of obstetric hemorrhage, although data are lacking to determine whether one approach is superior to the other.

Pelvic Artery Embolization. Interventional radiologists have become proficient in arteriography for a variety of diagnostic and therapeutic approaches. It is no surprise then that selective pelvic artery embolization for the management of obstetric hemorrhage is gaining in experience. Many case series have described its effectiveness in this scenario, with success rates exceeding 90%.[167-170] In addition to avoiding the added morbidity of surgical exploration, it preserves future fertility.[170,171]

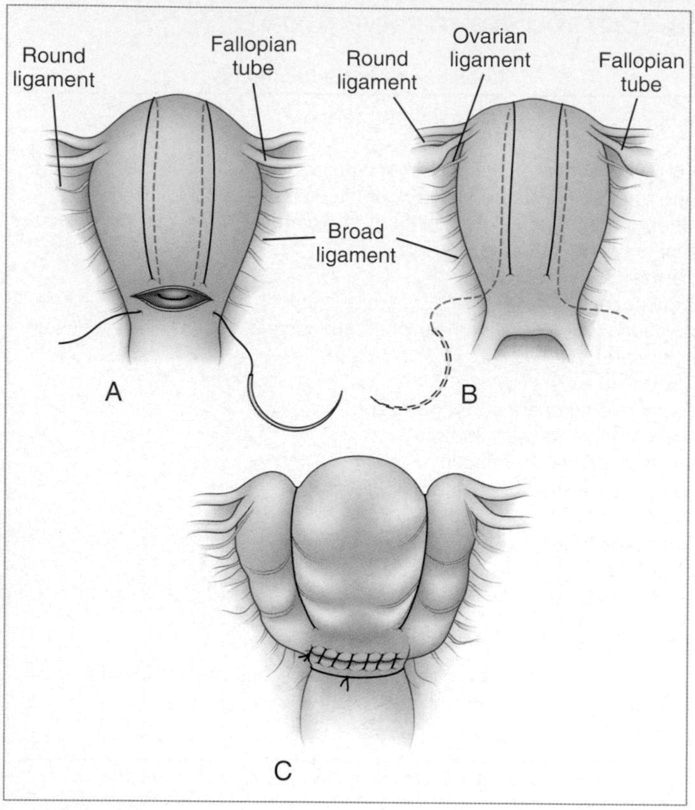

FIGURE 57-7 B-Lynch surgical technique. **A,** Anterior view of the B-Lynch stitch placement. **B,** Posterior view of the B-Lynch stitch placement. **C,** Anterior view of the completed procedure. (From B-Lynch C, Coker A, Lawal AH, et al: The B-Lynch surgical technique for the control of massive postpartum haemorrhage: An alternative to hysterectomy? Five cases reported. BJOG 104:372, 1997. Reprinted with permission.)

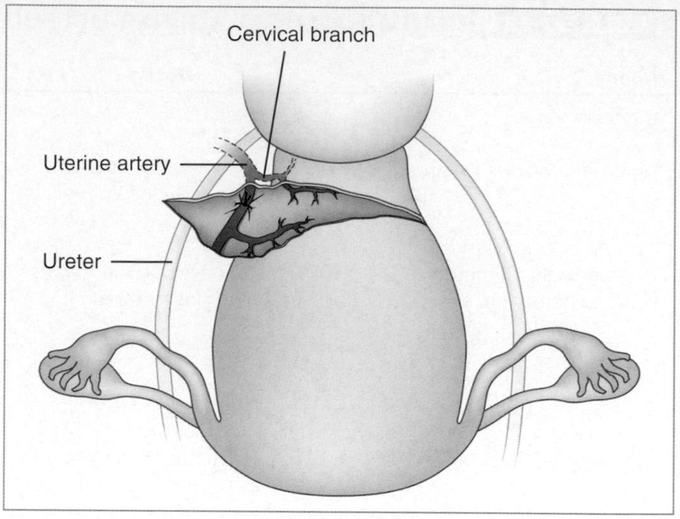

FIGURE 57-8 Anterior approach to the uterine artery ligation technique for postpartum obstetric hemorrhage.

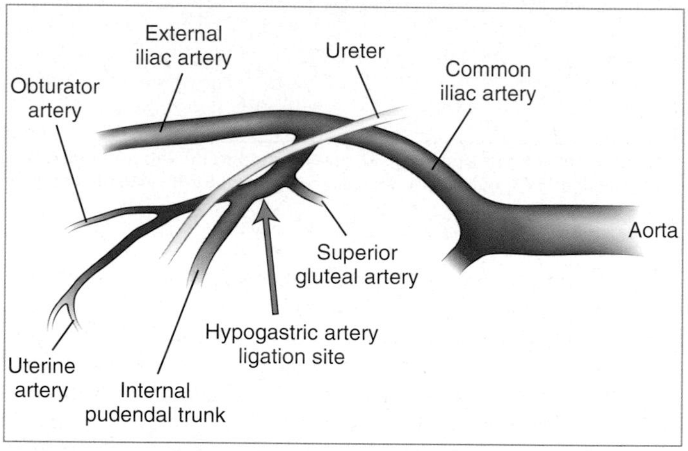

FIGURE 57-9 Localization of the hypogastric artery along the right pelvic side wall.

The procedure is performed in the interventional radiology suite. The femoral artery is accessed and diagnostic arteriography performed with fluoroscopic imaging to localize the target arteries for embolization. A variety of options are available for arterial occlusion, including an absorbable gelatin sponge (Gelfoam) or another type of particulate material.

Potential adverse results from the procedure include ischemia or tissue necrosis, infection, nephrotoxicity due to contrast medium, and bleeding at the access site or failure of the embolization. Failure of this approach does not preclude a subsequent surgical attempt at hemorrhage control. Conversely, after hypogastric artery ligation is performed, successful arteriographic embolization is much more difficult to achieve.

Trauma in Pregnancy

Trauma is a leading cause of non-obstetric deaths in the United States, and it is estimated to complicate 6% to 7% of all pregnancies.[172] About 4000 fetuses are lost annually due to complications from trauma in pregnancy.[173] Most incidents are considered minor, and less than 0.4% of patients require hospitalization. Of those requiring admission, 24% proceed to delivery during the hospitalization.[174,175] Motor vehicle accidents and falls account for most traumatic events affecting pregnant women, followed by domestic violence, assault, and suicide attempts.[172,176-178] Domestic violence escalates during pregnancy and is estimated to affect as many as 20% of pregnant patients.[179] A high index of suspicion for domestic violence is warranted for any pregnant woman presenting for evaluation after a traumatic event.

Blunt Abdominal Trauma

The gravid uterus is particularly vulnerable to blunt trauma from motor vehicle accidents, assaults, and falls. When a pregnant woman is injured severely, it most likely involved a motor vehicle accident. Three-point restraint seatbelts are safe for use by pregnant women, they significantly decrease the risk of serious maternal injury and fetal loss, and they are recommended by ACOG.[180-183] Proper use of seatbelts appears to be a significant predictor of maternal and fetal outcomes.[181,184] Approximately one third of pregnant women do not wear seat belts because of discomfort, inconvenience, or fears about hurting the fetus. Prenatal education regarding seat belt use significantly improves proper seat belt use.[173] The addition of airbags does not appear to be problematic for pregnant patients and may further reduce risk of injury.[182]

Placental abruption is a particularly serious complication after blunt trauma and motor vehicle accidents, because it may lead to premature labor and delivery, concealed hemorrhage, consumptive coagulopathy, fetomaternal hemorrhage, fetal distress, and death. Detection of an abruption in the patient without vaginal bleeding presents a challenge. Abruption occurs in approximately 7% of patients after trauma, but the severity of the injury does not appear to correlate with the presence of an abruption or to predict outcome. Most placental abruptions occur in patients after relatively minor trauma without evidence of serious injury.[172,178,185-187] Unfortunately, a negative ultrasound result does not reliably exclude the possibility of a placental abruption. At best, the sensitivity of ultrasound to detect abruption is 25%.[188] However, the sonographic identification of an abruption correlates with a higher likelihood of adverse outcome.[188,189]

The Injury Severity Score (ISS) is often used to quantify the risk of adverse outcomes for nonpregnant patients.[190] Unfortunately, the ISS does not translate well to the pregnant population and has not been shown to reliably predict outcomes in this group. El-Kady and colleagues[174] published a large, population-based study of more than 10,000 trauma evaluations in pregnant women.[174] Patients were divided into those delivering during the admission for trauma and those discharged to deliver at a later date. Falls were most common among women requiring delivery, followed by motor vehicle accidents. The likelihood of abruption, uterine rupture, maternal death, and adverse neonatal outcomes, including fetal and neonatal death, was significantly higher for the group that delivered during the trauma admission. Those women discharged undelivered after trauma had improved maternal outcomes compared with the delivered patients, but they remained at increased risk for preterm delivery, abruption, and the need for blood products compared with uninjured controls. These risks could not accurately be predicted by the ISS. Adverse fetal and neonatal outcomes were not increased after discharge. In contrast, for the group of patients who delivered during the trauma admission, a high ISS (>10) was associated with the highest risk for adverse outcomes. However, a lower ISS score (<10) was still associated with a significant increase in serious adverse events, including abruption, uterine rupture, and maternal or fetal death. The Revised Trauma Score (RTS), which includes the Glasgow Coma Scale, also appears to be limited in its ability to accurately predict pregnancy outcome after trauma.[191]

External monitoring of the fetal heart rate and contraction monitoring are recommended after blunt trauma in a viable gestation. Pearlman and associates[178] performed a prospective study monitoring patients for a minimum of 4 hours after blunt trauma. Eighty-eight percent of the patients had no visible trauma; 2.4% were critically injured. Most patients had contractions, and 70% required admission beyond the initial 4-hour observation period. Of these, 19% went on to deliver, with one fetal death. The abruption incidence in this subgroup was 9.4%. No adverse events occurred in the group of patients for whom contractions did not occur more frequently than every 15 minutes. However, all women suffering an adverse perinatal outcome had contractions every 2 to 5 minutes at some point during the initial 4-hour observation period. The severity of injury did not predict abruption or adverse outcomes.[178] Other investigators have since validated the concept that less than one contraction every 15 minutes is not associated with adverse outcomes after blunt trauma in pregnant patients.[172,185,192] A minimum of 4 hours of fetal heart rate and contraction monitoring is recommended after blunt trauma in pregnant women, regardless of injury severity. Beyond the initial observation period, the recommended duration for monitoring is not clear, particularly for patients with evidence of contractions. Most physicians recommend at least 24 hours because most serious complications occur shortly after the traumatic event.

$$\text{Fetal red blood cells} = \frac{\text{MBV} \times \text{maternal Hct} \times \%\ \text{fetal cells (KB)}}{\text{Newborn Hct}}$$

If KB result is 0.9% : 0.9% of maternal blood volume (MBV) is fetal origin.
MBV is assumed to be 5000 mL for an average-size woman at term.
Maternal hematocrit (Hct) should be measured; assume approximately 35%.
Normal Hct for term newborn infant can be assumed to be 50%, if the patient is undelivered.

$$\text{Fetal red blood cells} = \frac{5000 \times 0.35 \times 0.009}{0.5} = 31.5\ \text{mL}$$

Therefore, the fetus has hemorrhaged 31.5 mL of red cells into the maternal circulation. At term, the neonatal blood volume is 125 mL/kg. If the Hct is assumed to be approximately 50% at term, the actual amount of blood lost is 63 mL. In a term infant assumed to weigh 3500 g, the blood volume is approximately 438 mL, and the fetus has lost 7% of its blood volume.

FIGURE 57-10 Calculation of the volume of fetomaternal hemorrhage using the Kleihauer-Betke results.

Fetomaternal hemorrhage is another potential concern after blunt trauma in pregnancy. A Kleihauer-Betke test can provide an estimate of the amount of fetal blood within the maternal circulation, which is particularly important in determining if additional doses of RhoGAM are necessary in Rh-negative women. The test is based on the detection of fetal hemoglobin. If the presence of fetal hemoglobin within maternal red cells, such as in a hemoglobinopathy, is detected, the result will be falsely elevated. Figure 57-10 describes how to interpret a Kleihauer-Betke result and calculate volume of fetomaternal hemorrhage. Spontaneous fetomaternal hemorrhage can occur throughout pregnancy in the absence of any identified precipitating event, but the volumes appear to be low.[193] Fetomaternal hemorrhage is thought to occur with greater frequency after blunt trauma, and Kleihauer-Betke testing is often recommended. However, the available data suggest that a positive Kleihauer-Betke result does not alter management. In four studies of 730 pregnant women who had Kleihauer-Betke testing performed after blunt trauma, 95 (13%) had evidence of fetomaternal hemorrhage.[172,178,192,194] Of these, in only two cases (0.02%) did the result potentially alter management; one patient had significant hemorrhage requiring delivery as a result of fetal distress, and one underwent umbilical cord blood sampling but did not require transfusion or delivery. For the remainder, the result did not appear to affect management. In another study, no difference was found in the frequency of positive Kleihauer-Betke tests between normal controls and pregnant women being evaluated for trauma.[194]

Because of the gravid uterus, patterns of traumatic injury are somewhat different in pregnant patients after blunt abdominal trauma, particularly motor vehicle accidents. Upper abdominal injury to the spleen and liver are more common, whereas bowel injuries occur less frequently.[192,195] Traumatic uterine rupture has been reported, but it is rare with minor trauma.[174,196] The risk increases with increasing severity of trauma and the size of the uterus. Most ruptures occur in the fundal or posterior regions. With traumatic rupture of the uterus, fetal mortality approaches 100%.

Pelvic fractures are typically related to trauma as a result of a motor vehicle accident. The presence of a pelvic fracture should raise concern about significant bleeding risk and coexistent intra-abdominal trauma, such as splenic or hepatic laceration or urinary tract injury. Pelvic fracture is not a contraindication to vaginal delivery. The decision should be based on the stability of the fracture and presence of pelvic deformities. Fetal head injuries are also more common if a pelvic fracture is sutained.[197]

Penetrating Abdominal Trauma

Gunshot and stab wounds are the most common penetrating injuries in pregnant women, usually as a result of assault or suicide attempt. The enlarged uterus increases the likelihood that the uterus and fetus will sustain injury, and the prognosis is generally less favorable for the fetus. Penetrating trauma to the lower abdomen carries a lower likelihood of maternal bowel injury. The impact of gunshot wounds is less predictable and varies according to the entry site and angle, size of uterus and distance from the gun. Visceral injuries occur in 19% of pregnant patients, compared with 82% in nonpregnant patients. Mortality rates are correspondingly lower in pregnant victims (3.9% versus 12.5%).[198] Stab wounds are more likely to involve the upper abdomen during pregnancy, and in these cases, bowel injury should be considered.[198,199]

Evaluation of the patient after penetrating abdominal trauma should include an assessment of the likelihood of intra-abdominal bleeding. Ultrasound and CT are useful in this regard, and exploratory laparotomy is recommended if there is suspicion of bowel perforation or active hemorrhage. Diagnostic peritoneal lavage can help determine if bleeding is likely in hemodynamically stable patients with equivocal findings on abdominal ultrasound or CT. Lavage is performed by entering the abdomen through a small incision and infusing a saline wash. The presence of blood in the recovered lavage fluid supports the presence of intra-abdominal bleeding and warrants exploration. Tetanus toxoid prophylaxis should be used for the same indications as in the nonpregnant patient.

Trauma Management Issues

On initial presentation, the pregnant trauma patient should be evaluated similar to the nonpregnant patient. Assessment and stabilization of the airway, breathing, and circulation are the primary steps, followed by systematic evaluation for evidence of traumatic injuries. If the patient is pregnant, rapid confirmation of gestational age and assessment of fetal well-being are necessary. This evaluation can be performed simultaneous to any required maternal stabilization efforts.

Care should be taken to provide displacement of the gravid uterus off the aorta and vena cava. Compression of the great vessels occurs after the uterus reaches a size consistent with 20 weeks' gestation, and it decreases the CO. Displacement can be accomplished manually, by moving the patient to a lateral position, or by placing a wedge under the hip.

Evaluation of a pregnant trauma patient must take into consideration the physiologic changes of pregnancy that affect the clinical presentation. Pregnant women near term have expanded their circulating blood volume by 40% to 50%. As a result, significant intra-abdominal or intrauterine blood loss can occur with minimal change in maternal vital signs. Prognosis is worse if the patient develops hypotension and tachycardia.[187] In a viable gestation, a reassuring fetal heart rate tracing demonstrates adequate uterine perfusion and acts as a barometer of maternal status. As maternal cardiovascular status deteriorates, uterine perfusion suffers and manifests as contractions and fetal heart rate abnormalities. Fibrinogen levels decrease in the setting of hemorrhage as a result of consumption. In pregnancy, fibrinogen levels are substantially elevated, and low and even normal-range fibrinogen should raise concern about the pregnant patient.

TABLE 57-14 ESTIMATES OF FETAL RADIATION EXPOSURE FROM COMMON RADIOLOGIC PROCEDURES IN A TRAUMA PATIENT

Radiologic Examination	Fetal Radiation Exposure (cGy)
Chest (posteroanterior, lateral)	<<0.1
Abdomen	0.15-0.26
Pelvis	0.2-0.35
Hip	0.13-0.2
Computed tomography of head	<<0.1
Computed tomography of abdomen	0.04
Computed tomography of pelvis	2.5

Delivery timing and route are dictated by maternal and fetal status and need to be individualized. If laparotomy is necessary, hysterotomy is not automatically indicated. If there is evidence of uterine injury, delivery may be necessary. Pregnancy should not preclude the use of diagnostic testing thought to be otherwise indicated for a pregnant trauma patient. No single diagnostic radiologic imaging study exists that can provide enough radiation exposure to adversely affect a developing fetus. Radiation exposure of less than 5 rads has not been associated with fetal abnormalities or pregnancy loss, and the radiation associated with abdominal and pelvic CT scans falls substantially below this threshold.[200] Magnetic resonance imaging (MRI) does not produce ionizing radiation, and no adverse fetal effects have been reported from in utero exposure. However, because of theoretical concerns, ACOG states that the "National Radiological Protection Board arbitrarily advises against its use in the first trimester."[200] Table 57-14 lists anticipated dose of radiation exposure to the fetus from examinations commonly required for a trauma patient.

Burns in Pregnancy

Background

According to the American Burn Association, 40,000 people require hospitalization because of burns each year. Of these, 60% are admitted to one of the 125 specialized burn centers in the United States. These centers admit 200 patients per year on average, compared with the average of three burn admissions to nonspecialized burn centers.[201,202] Although current U.S. statistics are not available, burn injuries appear to be more common in developing countries, as evidenced by fewer case reports from the United States In two larger series of burns in pregnancy collected in India and Iran, approximately 7% of burn victims were pregnant patients. Burns resulting from flames or scalds account for 78% of cases; the remainder resulted from hot object contact (8%) or electrical (4%), chemical (3%), or other (6%) causes.[203]

Classification

Burns are characterized by the depth and size of the involved area. Partial-thickness burns (formerly classified as first-degree and second-degree burns) involve superficial skin layers and are capable of re-

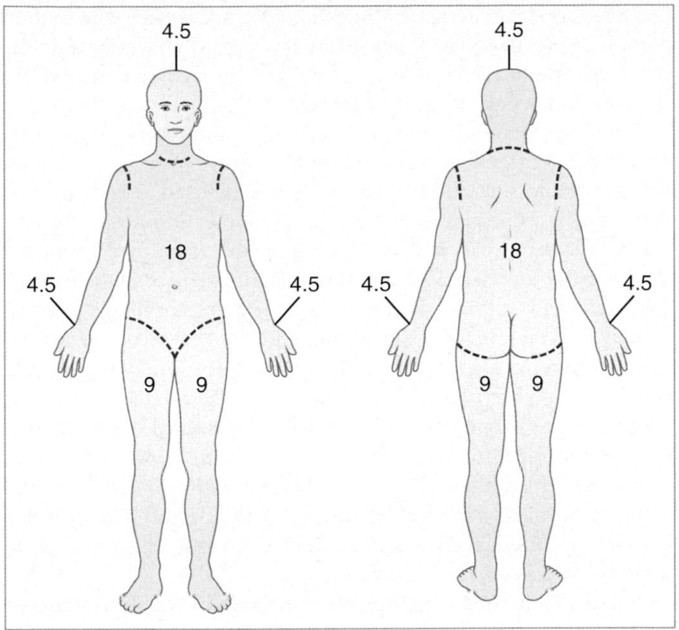

FIGURE 57-11 Body surface area diagram depicts the relative percentage of the total body surface area of defined anatomic areas in nonpregnant adults. (From Wolf SE, Hernon DN: Burns. In Townsend CM, Beauchamp RD, Evers BM, et al [eds]: Sabiston's Textbook of Surgery, 17th ed. Philadelphia, Elsevier Saunders, 2004.)

TABLE 57-15 CLASSIFICATION OF BURN SEVERITY

Classification	Defined Body Surface Areas
Minor	<15% partial thickness <2% full thickness
Moderate	15-25% 2-10% full thickness
Major	>25% >10% full thickness Any burn involving the face, eyes, ears, feet, or perineum Inhalation injury or electrical injury

epithelialization. These burns are painful, blistering injuries that can be red, white, or pink. These wounds are usually managed with topical agents and dressings. If healing does not occur within 3 weeks, management converts to that for more serious burns. Full-thickness burns (formerly called third-degree burns) are the most severe, and epithelium does not regenerate. These burns are not blistering and are painless. They can be gray, white, or brown.

Early surgical excision of the eschar is the standard of management in the United States. Full-thickness wounds hold the greatest potential for scarring, contractures, and infection and should be referred to a burn center.[204,205] The prognosis for pregnant and nonpregnant patients is directly related to the percentage of body surface area involved. Figure 57-11 shows one method of estimating the percentage of total body surface burned in nonpregnant adults. A modification for the pregnant patient has not been created, but the gravid abdomen should be taken into account when estimating body surface area involvement. The severity of the burn increases in proportion to the degree of involvement, as outlined in Table 57-15.

Outcomes

Severe burns are morbid events with significant short-term and long-term consequences. The pregnancy does not appear to negatively affect the outcome after a burn, but the burn has the potential to significantly affect the pregnancy outcome. Maternal and fetal survival depends most on the severity of the burn itself.[201,202,206] In one of the largest series of burns in pregnancy, Maghsoudi and colleagues[202] prospectively collected data on 51 pregnant burn victims admitted to a referral burn center in Iran over a 9-year period. The overall maternal mortality rate was 39%, and the fetal mortality rate was 45%. The most significant predictor of maternal and fetal mortality was total body surface area involvement exceeding 40% and the presence of inhalation injury. These patients suffered severe burns; the mean burn surface area was 38%. In nonsurvivors, the mean burn surface area was 69%. Other studies have found similar results.[201]

Management

Management of the pregnant burn patient is similar to that of a nonpregnant patient. Acute management of the burn victim should address aggressive fluid resuscitation, evaluation for inhalation injury and airway maintenance, assessment of carbon monoxide poisoning, anemia, prevention of infection, and wound management.

The initial priority is recognition of smoke inhalation injury, carbon monoxide poisoning, and airway management. Carbon monoxide crosses the placenta easily, and fetal hemoglobin has a higher affinity for carbon monoxide than adult hemoglobin. Hyperbaric oxygen may play a role in treating carbon monoxide poisoning.[207] Early intubation should be considered to maximize oxygen delivery in a patient with inhalation injury and to protect against aspiration.

Fluid losses after a serious burn are substantial as a result of third spacing due to edema and evaporative loss from damaged skin. The fluid deficit is easily underestimated in a pregnant patient. The normal physiologic adaptations of pregnancy, including up to 40% increase in blood volume, 40% increase in CO, and 20% decrease in SVR, are not reflected in the fluid replacement strategies recommended for nonpregnant burn patients. One commonly used formula, the Parkland formula, recommends replacement with Ringer's lactate at a rate of 4 mL/kg of body weight per percent of body surface area burned. Fifty percent of the calculated replacement volume is administered over the initial 8 hours and the remainder over the subsequent 16 hours. In one report,[208] the Parkland formula underestimated fluid requirement in a pregnant burn patient by almost 10 L. Given the lack of guidelines for pregnant patients, fluid resuscitation should be individualized to achieve hemodynamic stability, adequate urine output, and uterine perfusion. Electrolyte disturbances should also be anticipated and addressed.

Burns are associated with a significant hypermetabolic state and markedly increased nutritional requirements. Hypermetabolism can be minimized by providing adequate pain relief; supplying aggressive wound management with excision, grafting, and occlusive dressings; and managing temperature and adequate fluid replacement. Attention to adequate nutrition is essential and usually requires enteral and parenteral feeds.[209]

Wound infection and sepsis are significant risks after burn injury. Bacteremia results from colonization of the burn area. The most common organisms encountered are *S. aureus*, *Pseudomonas aeruginosa*, and *Candida albicans*.[210] Aggressive management of the wound with excision of the eschar, grafting, and occlusive dressings, in addition to topical and systemic antibiotics, helps to prevent infectious complications. The patient may be at increased risk for venous thromboembolic events.

Assessment of fetal well-being in a viable gestation should not be overlooked. Intravascular depletion, hypoxemia, hypermetabolism, and infection can adversely affect the fetus. Continuous monitoring is recommended in a viable gestation, particularly during the early stages of management. If the abdomen is involved with burn, direct auscultation may be limited and continuous fetal heart rate monitoring not feasible. Sterile coverings are available for the heart rate monitor and ultrasound probes to minimize infection risk. Vaginal ultrasound assessment may also be considered in some settings.

Contractions and preterm labor are to be expected, particularly in a severely burned pregnant patient, although the frequency is unknown. Few data are available to guide the use of tocolytic medications. Tocolysis should therefore be undertaken cautiously and judiciously, with an appreciation of the hemodynamic effects and other side effects of the drug. Hypovolemic patients may not tolerate β-agonists such as terbutaline, because they may already be in a high output state. Given the high fetal mortality rates with severe burns, delivery may be the most judicious alternative in a viable gestation. Most physicians recommend cesarean section for the usual obstetric indications. Delivery by cesarean section through a burned abdomen and vaginal delivery through a burned perineum have been reported.[208,211-213]

Cardiopulmonary Resuscitation and Perimortem Cesarean Section

Cardiac arrest in a pregnant patient is a rare event. According to the most recent available data on United States maternal mortality, the most likely neonatal outcome in the setting of a maternal death is a live birth.[12] The data do not reflect the frequency of arrest occurring before delivery. In a review of 38 patients delivered perimortem by cesarean section, the causes included trauma, cardiac abnormalities, embolism, magnesium overdose, sepsis, intracranial hemorrhage, anesthetic complications, eclampsia, and uterine rupture.[214] The causes of cardiac arrest in pregnant women are more likely to be acute and therefore may be more amenable to aggressive interventions. Several physiologic changes of pregnancy negatively affect attempts at cardiopulmonary resuscitation (CPR):

- Increased CO and requirement for uterine perfusion
- Aortocaval compression by the gravid uterus in the supine position
- Reduced functional residual capacity and increased oxygen consumption
- Reduced chest wall compliance
- Delayed stomach emptying and decreased esophageal sphincter tone, which increase the aspiration risk

Aortocaval obstruction should be relieved by placing the patient in a more lateral recumbent position or by manually displacing the uterus. CPR can provide only 30% of the CO when the patient is supine.[215] The effectiveness of compressions increases dramatically when the patient is tilted in the lateral position.[214] Early intubation is recommended to minimize aspiration risk. The use of sodium bicarbonate to correct maternal acidosis should be undertaken with caution because of the potential for worsening fetal acidosis. Electrocardioversion can be performed in a pregnant patient; the recommendations are the same as for nonpregnant patients.[216]

Rapid restoration of maternal circulation and reversal of hypoxia are the most effective ways to minimize negative effects on the fetus. If this is not possible, attention must then be directed to evacuation of the uterus by cesarean section. Cesarean section in the setting of maternal cardiac arrest can improve the likelihood of an intact neonatal outcome and simultaneously improve maternal resuscitative efforts. In 1986, Katz and colleagues[217] initially advocated performing a cesarean section at 4 minutes after instituting CPR.[217] This recommendation was based on the theory that emptying the uterus would improve CO generated by chest compressions after the obstructing uterus was emptied. Maternal neurologic injury could be avoided if cerebral perfusion improved by 6 minutes, the time at which cerebral injury occurs after cessation of blood flow. They then reviewed the literature and reported neonatal outcomes at various time intervals after delivery. From these data, delivery within 5 minutes of arrest was most likely to result in good neonatal outcomes.[52,217]

Subsequently, Katz and coworkers[214] reviewed 34 published cases of perimortem cesarean section performed between 1985 and 2004 to assess whether the "4-minute rule" was valid. In this series, 79% delivered live infants (30 of 38; 3 sets of twins and 1 set of triplets). Data were available regarding the arrest-to-delivery interval for 25 infants and are presented in Table 57-16. Similar to data presented in earlier series, prolonging the arrest-to-delivery interval decreased the likelihood of intact survival, although apparently normal neonates were delivered even after more than 15 minutes.

Data were also provided about perimortem cesarean section potentially negatively impacting maternal survival. Twenty (59%) of 34 cases provided information regarding maternal hemodynamic status and indicated a beneficial effect on maternal resuscitation efforts after perimortem cesarean. None of the cases had worsening maternal

TABLE 57-16 PERIMORTEM CESAREAN DELIVERIES WITH SURVIVING INFANTS WITH REPORTS OF TIME FROM MATERNAL CARDIAC ARREST TO DELIVERY OF THE INFANT, 1985-2004

Time (min)	Gestational Age (wk)	Number of Patients
0-5	25-42	8 (normal infant) 1 (retinopathy of prematurity and hearing loss) 3 (condition not reported)
6-10	28-37	1 (normal infant) 2 (neurologic sequelae) 1 (condition not reported)
11-15	38-39	1 (normal infant) 1 (neurologic sequelae)
>15	30-38	4 (normal infants) 2 (neurologic sequelae) 1 (respiratory sequelae)
Total		25

From Katz V, Balderston K, DeFreest M: Perimortem cesarean delivery: Were our assumptions correct? Am J Obstet Gynecol 192:1916-1920, 2005.

status as a result of perimortem cesarean section; 12 women had "sudden" and "profound" improvement at the time of emptying the uterus.[214]

The following guidelines are being suggested for the management of maternal cardiac arrest with a viable gestation:

1. Begin maternal CPR immediately.
2. Establish an airway.
3. Establish intravenous access simultaneously.
4. Institute cesarean delivery if there is no evidence of a maternal pulse by 4 minutes.
5. Sterile technique is not necessary, and the patient need not be moved to an operating room.
6. Continue CPR efforts during and after delivery.
7. Continuous fetal monitoring is not possible because of interference from resuscitative efforts. The maternal condition dictates whether perimortem cesarean section is necessary.

Cesarean section is not recommended in an unstable patient because of anticipated cardiac arrest. This may inadvertently precipitate a worse maternal outcome. If CPR is effective at restoring circulation, perimortem cesarean section is not recommended.

Brain Death and Somatic Support during Pregnancy

Brain death is defined as the complete absence of brain function, which is determined clinically by lack of consciousness, movement, respiratory effort, and most reflexes. It is confirmed by the lack of activity on electroencephalogram. It is considered distinct from coma and persistent vegetative state (Table 57-17).[218]

Maternal brain death has been rarely reported in the obstetric and critical care literature. Two reviews on the topic identified only 12 reported cases since 1982.[218,219] Two additional cases were identified.[220,221] The most common reason for brain death was subarachnoid hemorrhage, followed by trauma and infection.

After brain death occurs, the options include immediate delivery, withdrawal of maternal support, or prolongation of maternal life to

TABLE 57-17 FEATURES OF COMA, PERSISTENT VEGETATIVE STATE, AND BRAIN DEATH

Feature	PVS	Coma	Brain Death
Self-awareness	Absent	Absent	Absent
Suffering	No	No	No
Motor function	No purposeful movement	No purposeful movement	None or only reflex spinal movements
Sleep-wake cycles	Intact	Absent	Absent
Respiratory function	Normal	Depressed, variable	Absent
Electroencephalographic activity	Polymorphic delta or theta, sometimes slow alpha	Polymorphic delta or theta	Electrocerebral silence
Cerebral metabolism	Reduced by 50% or more	Reduced by 50% or more, variable	Absent
Life expectancy	Usually 2-5 yr	Varies	Death within 2-4 wk (Harvard criteria)
Neurologic recovery	Nontraumatic: rare after 3 mo Traumatic: rare after 12 mo	Usually recovery, PVS, or death in 2-4 wk	No recovery

PVS, persistent vegetative state.

Adapted from Ashwal S, Cranford R: Medical aspects of the persistent vegetative state—first of two parts. The Multi-Society Task Force on PVS. N Engl J Med 330:1499-1508, 1994.

TABLE 57-18 INTENSIVE CARE MANAGEMENT OF PREGNANT PATIENTS WITH SEVERE NEUROLOGIC INJURY

Condition	Therapy	Physiologic Goal
Respiratory failure	Controlled hyperventilation, PEEP	Physiologic hypercarbia, decrease intracranial pressure, avoid neurogenic pulmonary edema
Fluid-resistant hypotension	Left lateral position, vasopressors	Maintain uteroplacental circulation
Hypothermia	Warming blankets	Prevent fetal bradycardia and IUGR
Hyperthermia	Cooling blankets	Prevent fetal death
Nutritional support	Enteral or parenteral insulin	Maintain positive nitrogen balance (energy intake of 126-147 kJ/kg of ideal body weight), avoid hyperglycemia
Panhypopituitarism	DDAVP, thyroxine, cortisol	Adjust for central diabetes insipidus and adrenocortical insufficiency
Infection prevention	Frequent cultures, catheter line changes	Prevent sepsis
Deep venous thrombosis prophylaxis	Heparin	Prevent pulmonary embolism
Preterm labor	Betamethasone or dexamethasone, consider tocolysis	Prolong gestation
General condition	Expert nursing care	

DDAVP, L-deamino-8-D-arginine vasopressin; IUGR, intrauterine growth restriction; PEEP, positive end-expiratory pressure.

improve the neonatal prognosis by advancing gestational age. The challenges in providing life support to the brain-dead gravida cannot be underestimated and include hemodynamic instability, panhypopituitarism, ventilatory support, temperature regulation, nutrition, infectious complications, hypercoagulability, and premature contractions (Table 57-18).[215] Given these challenges, it is surprising that two patients experienced a latency exceeding 100 days, with a mean latency of longer than 50 days from the diagnosis of brain death.[218-220,222,223] Delivery timing is based on assessment of fetal well-being or maturity unless there is evidence of maternal deterioration. Preparation for immediate bedside cesarean section should be made. Discussion of the ethical and legal considerations that surround these cases is beyond the scope of this chapter.

References

1. Baskett TF, Sternadel J: Maternal intensive care and near-miss mortality in obstetrics. BJOG 105:981-984, 1998.
2. Graham SG, Luxton MC: The requirement for intensive care support for the pregnant population. Anaesthesia 44:581-584, 1989.
3. Heinonen S, Tyrvainen E, Saarikoski S, et al: Need for maternal critical care in obstetrics: A population-based analysis. Int J Obstet Anesth 11:260-264, 2002.
4. Kilpatrick SJ, Matthay MA: Obstetric patients requiring critical care. A five-year review. Chest 101:1407-1412, 1992.
5. Lapinsky SE, Kruczynski K, Seaward GR, et al: Critical care management of the obstetric patient. Can J Anaesth 44:325-329, 1997.
6. Loverro G, Pansini V, Greco P, et al: Indications and outcome for intensive care unit admission during puerperium. Arch Gynecol Obstet 265:195-198, 2001.
7. Mabie WC, Sibai BM: Treatment in an obstetric intensive care unit. Am J Obstet Gynecol 162:1-4, 1990.
8. Mahutte NG, Murphy-Kaulbeck L, Le Q, et al: Obstetric admissions to the intensive care unit. Obstet Gynecol 94:263-266, 1999.
9. Zeeman GG, Wendel GD Jr, Cunningham FG: A blueprint for obstetric critical care. Am J Obstet Gynecol 188:532-536, 2003.
10. Berg CJ, Atrash HK, Koonin LM, Tucker M: Pregnancy-related mortality in the United States, 1987-1990. Obstet Gynecol 88:161-167, 1996.
11. Berg CJ, Chang J, Callaghan WM, et al: Pregnancy-related mortality in the United States, 1991-1997. Obstet Gynecol 101:289-296, 2003.
12. Chang J, Elam-Evans LD, Berg CJ, et al: Pregnancy-related mortality surveillance—United States, 1991-1999. MMWR Surveill Summ 52:1-8, 2003.
13. Atrash HK, Alexander S, Berg CJ: Maternal mortality in developed countries: Not just a concern of the past. Obstet Gynecol 86(Pt 2):700-705, 1995.
14. Knaus WA, Draper EA, Wagner DP, et al: APACHE II: A severity of disease classification system. Crit Care Med 13:818-829, 1985.
15. Knaus WA, Wagner DP, Draper EA, et al: The APACHE III prognostic system. Risk prediction of hospital mortality for critically ill hospitalized adults. Chest 100:1619-1636, 1991.
16. Stevens TA, Carroll MA, Promecene PA, et al: Utility of Acute Physiology, Age, and Chronic Health Evaluation (APACHE III) score in maternal admissions to the intensive care unit. Am J Obstet Gynecol 194:e13-e15, 2006.
17. Le G Jr, Lemeshow S, Saulnier F: A new Simplified Acute Physiology Score (SAPS II) based on a European/North American multicenter study. JAMA 270:2957-2963, 1993.
18. Lemeshow S, Teres D, Klar J, et al: Mortality Probability Models (MPM II) based on an international cohort of intensive care unit patients. JAMA 270:2478-2486, 1993.
19. El-Solh AA, Grant BJ: A comparison of severity of illness scoring systems for critically ill obstetric patients. Chest 110:1299-1304, 1996.
20. Lewinsohn G, Herman A, Leonov Y, et al: Critically ill obstetrical patients: Outcome and predictability. Crit Care Med 1412-1414, 1994.
21. Swan HJ, Ganz W, Forrester J: Catheterization of the heart in man with use of a flow-directed balloon- tipped catheter. N Engl J Med 283:447-451, 1970.
22. American College of Obstetricians and Gynecologists (ACOG): Invasive hemodynamic monitoring in obstetrics and gynecology. ACOG technical bulletin no. 175, December 1992. Int J Gynaecol Obstet 42:199-205, 1993.
23. Boyd O, Grounds RM, Bennett ED: A randomized clinical trial of the effect of deliberate perioperative increase of oxygen delivery on mortality in high-risk surgical patients. JAMA 270:2699-2707, 1993.
24. Del Guercio LR, Cohn JD: Monitoring operative risk in the elderly. JAMA 243:1350-1355, 1980.
25. Older P, Smith R: Experience with the preoperative invasive measurement of haemodynamic, respiratory and renal function in 100 elderly patients scheduled for major abdominal surgery. Anaesth Intensive Care 389-395, 1988.
26. Gore JM, Goldberg RJ, Spodick DH, et al: A community-wide assessment of the use of pulmonary artery catheters in patients with acute myocardial infarction. Chest 92:721-727, 1987.
27. Zion MM, Balkin J, Rosenmann D, et al: Use of pulmonary artery catheters in patients with acute myocardial infarction. Analysis of experience in 5,841 patients in the SPRINT Registry. SPRINT Study Group. Chest 98:1331-1335, 1990.
28. Connors AF Jr, Speroff T, Dawson NV, et al: The effectiveness of right heart catheterization in the initial care of critically ill patients. SUPPORT Investigators. JAMA 276:889-897, 1996.
29. Hayes MA, Timmins AC, Yau EH, et al: Elevation of systemic oxygen delivery in the treatment of critically ill patients. N Engl J Med 330:1717-1722, 1994.
30. Polanczyk CA, Rohde LE, Goldman L, et al: Right heart catheterization and cardiac complications in patients undergoing noncardiac surgery: An observational study. JAMA 286:309-314, 2001.
31. Heyland DK, Cook DJ, King D, et al: Maximizing oxygen delivery in critically ill patients: A methodologic appraisal of the evidence. Crit Care Med 24:517-524, 1996.
32. Ivanov RI, Allen J, Sandham JD, et al: Pulmonary artery catheterization: A narrative and systematic critique of randomized controlled trials and recommendations for the future. New Horiz 5:268-276, 1997.
33. Sandham JD, Hull RD, Brant RF, et al: A randomized, controlled trial of the use of pulmonary-artery catheters in high-risk surgical patients. N Engl J Med 2;348:5-14, 2003.
34. Harvey S, Stevens K, Harrison D, et al: An evaluation of the clinical and cost-effectiveness of pulmonary artery catheters in patient management in intensive care: A systematic review and a randomised controlled trial. Health Technol Assess 10:iii-xi, 1, 2006.
35. Binanay C, Califf RM, Hasselblad V, et al: Evaluation study of congestive heart failure and pulmonary artery catheterization effectiveness: The ESCAPE trial. JAMA 294:1625-1633, 2005.
36. Shah MR, Hasselblad V, Stevenson LW, et al: Impact of the pulmonary artery catheter in critically ill patients: Meta-analysis of randomized clinical trials. JAMA 294:1664-1670, 2005.
37. Practice guidelines for pulmonary artery catheterization: An updated report by the American Society of Anesthesiologists Task Force on Pulmonary Artery Catheterization. Anesthesiology 99:988-1014, 2003.
38. Nolan TE, Wakefield ML, Devoe LD: Invasive hemodynamic monitoring in obstetrics. A critical review of its indications, benefits, complications, and alternatives. Chest 101:1429-1433, 1992.
39. Randolph AG, Cook DJ, Gonzales CA, et al: Ultrasound guidance for placement of central venous catheters: A meta-analysis of the literature. Crit Care Med 24:2053-2058, 1996.
40. John F McConville, Kress JP: Intravascular devices. In: Jesse B, Hall M, Gregory A, Schmidt M, et al (eds): Principles of Critical Care, 3rd ed. New York, McGraw-Hill, 2007.
41. Richards MJ, Edwards JR, Culver DH, et al: Nosocomial infections in combined medical-surgical intensive care units in the United States. Infect Control Hosp Epidemiol 21:510-515, 2000.

42. McGee DC, Gould MK: Preventing complications of central venous catheterization. N Engl J Med 20;348:1123-1133, 2003.
43. Benedetti TJ, Cotton DB, Read JC, et al: Hemodynamic observations in severe pre-eclampsia with a flow-directed pulmonary artery catheter. Am J Obstet Gynecol 136:465-470, 1980.
44. Bolte AC, Dekker GA, van Eyck J, et al: Lack of agreement between central venous pressure and pulmonary capillary wedge pressure in preeclampsia. Hypertens Pregnancy 19:261-271, 2000.
45. Clark SL, Cotton DB, Lee W, et al: Central hemodynamic assessment of normal term pregnancy. Am J Obstet Gynecol 161(Pt 1):1439-1442, 1989.
46. Capeless EL, Clapp JF: Cardiovascular changes in early phase of pregnancy. Am J Obstet Gynecol 161(Pt 1):1449-1453, 1989.
47. Clark SL, Cotton DB, Pivarnik JM, et al: Position change and central hemodynamic profile during normal third-trimester pregnancy and post partum. Am J Obstet Gynecol 164:883-887, 1991.
48. Bonnin M, Mercier FJ, Sitbon O, et al: Severe pulmonary hypertension during pregnancy: Mode of delivery and anesthetic management of 15 consecutive cases. Anesthesiology 102:1133-1137, 2005.
49. Smedstad KG, Cramb R, Morison DH: Pulmonary hypertension and pregnancy: A series of eight cases. Can J Anaesth 41:502-512, 1994.
50. Weiss BM, Zemp L, Seifert B, et al: Outcome of pulmonary vascular disease in pregnancy: A systematic overview from 1978 through 1996. J Am Coll Cardiol 31:1650-1657, 1998.
51. Yentis SM, Steer PJ, Plaat F: Eisenmenger's syndrome in pregnancy: Maternal and fetal mortality in the 1990s. BJOG 105:921-922, 1998.
52. Clark SL, Hankins GD, Dudley DA, et al: Amniotic fluid embolism: Analysis of the national registry. Am J Obstet Gynecol 172(Pt 1):1158-1167, 1995.
53. Davies S: Amniotic fluid embolus: A review of the literature. Can J Anaesth 48:88-98, 2001.
54. Visser W, Wallenburg HC: Central hemodynamic observations in untreated preeclamptic patients. Hypertension 17(Pt 2):1072-1077, 1991.
55. Easterling TR, Benedetti TJ, Schmucker BC, et al: Maternal hemodynamics in normal and preeclamptic pregnancies: A longitudinal study. Obstet Gynecol 76:1061-1069, 1990.
56. Clark SL, Greenspoon JS, Aldahl D, et al: Severe preeclampsia with persistent oliguria: Management of hemodynamic subsets. Am J Obstet Gynecol 154:490-494, 1986.
57. Levy MM, Fink MP, Marshall JC, et al: 2001 SCCM/ESICM/ACCP/ATS/SIS International Sepsis Definitions Conference. Crit Care Med 31:1250-1256, 2003.
58. Lee W, Clark SL, Cotton DB, et al: Septic shock during pregnancy. Am J Obstet Gynecol 159:410-416, 1988.
59. Mabie WC, Barton JR, Sibai B: Septic shock in pregnancy. Obstet Gynecol 90(Pt 1):553-561, 1997.
60. Vignon P: Hemodynamic assessment of critically ill patients using echocardiography Doppler. Curr Opin Crit Care 11:227-234, 2005.
61. Laupland KB, Bands CJ: Utility of esophageal Doppler as a minimally invasive hemodynamic monitor: A review. Can J Anaesth 49:393-401, 2002.
62. Vezina DP, Cahalan MK: Transesophageal echocardiogram. In Ronald D.Miller MD (ed): Miller's Anesthesia, 5th ed. Philadelphia, Elsevier, 2005.
63. Easterling TR, Watts DH, Schmucker BC, et al: Measurement of cardiac output during pregnancy: Validation of Doppler technique and clinical observations in preeclampsia. Obstet Gynecol 69:845-850, 1987.
64. Lee W, Rokey R, Cotton DB: Noninvasive maternal stroke volume and cardiac output determinations by pulsed Doppler echocardiography. Am J Obstet Gynecol 158(Pt 1):505-510, 1988.
65. Belfort MA, Rokey R, Saade GR, et al: Rapid echocardiographic assessment of left and right heart hemodynamics in critically ill obstetric patients. Am J Obstet Gynecol 171:884-892, 1994.
66. Penning S, Robinson KD, Major CA, et al: A comparison of echocardiography and pulmonary artery catheterization for evaluation of pulmonary artery pressures in pregnant patients with suspected pulmonary hypertension. Am J Obstet Gynecol 184:1568-1570, 2001.
67. Crapo RO: Normal cardiopulmonary physiology during pregnancy. Clin Obstet Gynecol 39:3-16, 1996.
68. Jenkins TM, Troiano NH, Graves CR, et al: Mechanical ventilation in an obstetric population: Characteristics and delivery rates. Am J Obstet Gynecol 188:549-552, 2003.
69. Mabie WC, Barton JR, Sibai BM: Ault respiratory distress syndrome in pregnancy. Am J Obstet Gynecol 167:950-957, 1992.
70. Tomlinson MW, Caruthers TJ, Whitty JE, et al: Does delivery improve maternal condition in the respiratory-compromised gravida? Obstet Gynecol 91:108-111, 1998.
71. Collop NA, Sahn SA: Critical illness in pregnancy. An analysis of 20 patients admitted to a medical intensive care unit. Chest 103:1548-1552, 1993.
72. Karetzky M, Ramirez M: Acute respiratory failure in pregnancy. An analysis of 19 cases. Medicine (Baltimore) 77:41-49, 1998.
73. Ventilation with lower tidal volumes as compared with traditional tidal volumes for acute lung injury and the acute respiratory distress syndrome. The Acute Respiratory Distress Syndrome Network. N Engl J Med 342:1301-1308, 2000.
74. Pelosi P, Brazzi L, Gattinoni L: Prone position in acute respiratory distress syndrome. Eur Respir J 20:1017-1028, 2002.
75. Gattinoni L, Tognoni G, Pesenti A, et al: Effect of prone positioning on the survival of patients with acute respiratory failure. N Engl J Med 345:568-573, 2001.
76. Guerin C, Gaillard S, Lemasson S, et al: Effects of systematic prone positioning in hypoxemic acute respiratory failure: A randomized controlled trial. JAMA 292:2379-2387, 2004.
77. Mancebo J, Fernandez R, Blanch L, et al: A multicenter trial of prolonged prone ventilation in severe acute respiratory distress syndrome. Am J Respir Crit Care Med 173:1233-1239, 2006.
78. Sciscione AC, Ivester T, Largoza M, et al: Acute pulmonary edema in pregnancy. Obstet Gynecol 101:511-515, 2003.
79. Wu PY, Udani V, Chan L, et al: Colloid osmotic pressure: Variations in normal pregnancy. J Perinat Med 11:193-199, 1983.
80. Ronald H, Ingram J, Braunwald E: Dyspnea and Pulmonary edema. In Kasper DL, Fauci AS, Longo DL, et al (eds): Harrison's Principles of Internal Medicine, 16th ed. New York, McGraw-Hill, 2005.
81. Zhang J, Meikle S, Trumble A: Severe maternal morbidity associated with hypertensive disorders in pregnancy in the United States. Hypertens Pregnancy 22:203-212, 2003.
82. Sibai BM, Mabie BC, Harvey CJ, et al: Pulmonary edema in severe preeclampsia-eclampsia: Analysis of thirty-seven consecutive cases. Am J Obstet Gynecol 156:1174-1179, 1987.
83. Benedetti TJ, Kates R, Williams V: Hemodynamic observations in severe preeclampsia complicated by pulmonary edema. Am J Obstet Gynecol 152:330-334, 1985.
84. Benedetti TJ: Life-threatening complications of betamimetic therapy for preterm labor inhibition. Clin Perinatol 13:843-852, 1986.
85. Yeast JD, Halberstadt C, Meyer BA, et al: The risk of pulmonary edema and colloid osmotic pressure changes during magnesium sulfate infusion. Am J Obstet Gynecol 169:1566-1571.
86. Angus DC, Wax RS: Epidemiology of sepsis: An update. Crit Care Med 29(Suppl):S109-S116, 2001.
87. Blanco JD, Gibbs RS, Castaneda YS: Bacteremia in obstetrics: Clinical course. Obstet Gynecol 58:621-625, 1981.
88. Bryan CS, Reynolds KL, Moore EE: Bacteremia in obstetrics and gynecology. Obstet Gynecol 64:155-158, 1984.
89. Martin GS, Mannino DM, Eaton S, et al: The epidemiology of sepsis in the United States from 1979 through 2000. N Engl J Med 348:1546-1554, 2003.
90. Sheffield JS: Sepsis and septic shock in pregnancy. Crit Care Clin 20:651-660, 2004.
91. Friedman G, Silva E, Vincent JL: Has the mortality of septic shock changed with time. Crit Care Med 26:2078-2086, 1998.
92. Ledger WJ, Norman M, Gee C, Lewis W: Bacteremia on an obstetric-gynecologic service. Am J Obstet Gynecol 121:205-212, 1975.

93. Zeni F, Freeman B, Natanson C: Anti-inflammatory therapies to treat sepsis and septic shock: A reassessment. Crit Care Med 25:1095-1100, 1997.
94. Hotchkiss RS, Karl IE: The pathophysiology and treatment of sepsis. N Engl J Med 348:138-150, 2003.
95. Shapairo N, Zimmer G, Barkin A: Sepsis syndromes. In Marx JA (ed): Rosen's Emergency Medicine: Concepts and Clinical Practice, 6th ed. Philadelphia, Mosby Elsevier, 2006.
96. Aird WC: Sepsis and coagulation. Crit Care Clin 21:417-431, 2005.
97. Rivers E, Nguyen B, Havstad S, et al: Early goal-directed therapy in the treatment of severe sepsis and septic shock. N Engl J Med 345:1368-1377, 2001.
98. Lin SM, Huang CD, Lin HC, et al: A modified goal-directed protocol improves clinical outcomes in intensive care unit patients with septic shock: A randomized controlled trial. Shock 26:551-557, 2006.
99. Rolbin SH, Levinson G, Shnider SM, et al: Dopamine treatment of spinal hypotension decreases uterine blood flow in the pregnant ewe. Anesthesiology 51:37-40, 1979.
100. Kollef MH, Sherman G, Ward S, et al: Inadequate antimicrobial treatment of infections: A risk factor for hospital mortality among critically ill patients. Chest 115:462-474, 1999.
101. Kreger BE, Craven DE, McCabe WR: Gram-negative bacteremia. IV. Re-evaluation of clinical features and treatment in 612 patients. Am J Med 68:344-355, 1980.
102. Leibovici L, Paul M, Poznanski O, et al: Monotherapy versus beta-lactam-aminoglycoside combination treatment for gram-negative bacteremia: A prospective, observational study. Antimicrob Agents Chemother 41:1127-1133, 1997.
103. Ibrahim EH, Sherman G, Ward S, et al: The influence of inadequate antimicrobial treatment of bloodstream infections on patient outcomes in the ICU setting. Chest 118:146-155, 2000.
104. Bochud PY, Glauser MP, Calandra T: Antibiotics in sepsis. Intensive Care Med 27(Suppl 1):S33-S48, 2001.
105. Jimenez MF, Marshall JC: Source control in the management of sepsis. Intensive Care Med 27(Suppl 1):S49-S62, 2001.
106. Bilton BD, Zibari GB, McMillan RW, et al: Aggressive surgical management of necrotizing fasciitis serves to decrease mortality: A retrospective study. Am Surg 64:397-400, 1998.
107. Brierre S, Kumari R, Deboisblanc BP: The endocrine system during sepsis. Am J Med Sci 328:238-247, 2004.
108. Van den Berghe G, Wouters P, Weekers F, et al: Intensive insulin therapy in the critically ill patients. N Engl J Med 345:1359-1367, 2001.
109. Cronin L, Cook DJ, Carlet J, et al: Corticosteroid treatment for sepsis: A critical appraisal and meta-analysis of the literature. Crit Care Med 23:1430-1439, 1995.
110. Lefering R, Neugebauer EA: Steroid controversy in sepsis and septic shock: A meta-analysis. Crit Care Med 23:1294-1303, 1995.
111. Shenker Y, Skatrud JB: Adrenal insufficiency in critically ill patients. Am J Respir Crit Care Med 163:1520-1523, 2001.
112. Annane D: Corticosteroids for septic shock. Crit Care Med 29(Suppl): S117-S120, 2001.
113. Annane D, Sebille V, Charpentier C, et al: Effect of treatment with low doses of hydrocortisone and fludrocortisone on mortality in patients with septic shock. JAMA 288:862-871, 2002.
114. Annane D, Bellissant E, Bollaert PE, et al: Corticosteroids for severe sepsis and septic shock: A systematic review and meta-analysis. BMJ 329:480, 2004.
115. NIH Consensus Development Conference on Antenatal Corticosteroids Revisited: Repeat Courses. Bethesda, National Institutes of Health, 2000.
116. Warren HS, Suffredini AF, Eichacker PQ, et al: Risks and benefits of activated protein C treatment for severe sepsis. N Engl J Med 347:1027-1030, 2002.
117. Fisher CJ Jr, Yan SB: Protein C levels as a prognostic indicator of outcome in sepsis and related diseases. Crit Care Med 28(Suppl):S49-S56, 2000.
118. Yan SB, Helterbrand JD, Hartman DL, et al: Low levels of protein C are associated with poor outcome in severe sepsis. Chest 120:915-922, 2001.
119. Matthay MA: Severe sepsis—a new treatment with both anticoagulant and antiinflammatory properties. N Engl J Med 344:759-762, 2001.
120. Bernard GR, Vincent JL, Laterre PF, et al: Efficacy and safety of recombinant human activated protein C for severe sepsis. N Engl J Med 344:699-709, 2001.
121. Vincent JL, Bernard GR, Beale R, et al: Drotrecogin alfa (activated) treatment in severe sepsis from the global open-label trial ENHANCE: further evidence for survival and safety and implications for early treatment. Crit Care Med 33:2266-2277, 2005.
122. Chichakli LO, Atrash HK, Mackay AP, et al: Pregnancy-related mortality in the United States due to hemorrhage: 1979-1992. Obstet Gynecol 94(Pt 1):721-725, 1999.
123. Geller SE, Rosenberg D, Cox SM, et al: The continuum of maternal morbidity and mortality: factors associated with severity. Am J Obstet Gynecol 191:939-944, 2004.
124. American College of Obstetricians and Gynecologists (ACOG): Clinical management guidelines for obstetrician-gynecologists: Postpartum hemorrhage. ACOG practice bulletin no. 76, October 2006: Obstet Gynecol 108:1039-1047, 2006.
125. Combs CA, Murphy EL, Laros RK Jr: Factors associated with postpartum hemorrhage with vaginal birth. Obstet Gynecol 77:69-76, 1991.
126. Velanovich V: Crystalloid versus colloid fluid resuscitation: A meta-analysis of mortality. Surgery 105:65-71, 1989.
127. Alam HB, Rhee P: New developments in fluid resuscitation. Surg Clin North Am 87:55-72, vi, 2007.
128. Martin G, Nett-Guerrero E, Wakeling H, et al: A prospective, randomized comparison of thromboelastographic coagulation profile in patients receiving lactated Ringer's solution, 6% hetastarch in a balanced-saline vehicle, or 6% hetastarch in saline during major surgery. J Cardiothorac Vasc Anesth 16:441-446, 2002.
129. American College of Obstetricians and Gynecologists (ACOG): Blood component therapy. ACOG technical bulletin no. 199, November 1994. Committee on Technical Bulletins of the American College of Obstetricians and Gynecologists. Int J Gynaecol Obstet 48:233-238, 1995.
130. Simon TL, Alverson DC, AuBuchon J, et al: Practice parameter for the use of red blood cell transfusions: Developed by the Red Blood Cell Administration Practice Guideline Development Task Force of the College of American Pathologists. Arch Pathol Lab Med 122:130-138, 1998.
131. Practice guidelines for perioperative blood transfusion and adjuvant therapies: An updated report by the American Society of Anesthesiologists Task Force on Perioperative Blood Transfusion and Adjuvant Therapies. Anesthesiology 105:198-208, 2006.
132. Stainsby D: ABO incompatible transfusions—experience from the UK Serious Hazards of Transfusion (SHOT) scheme Transfusions ABO incompatible. Transfus Clin Biol 12:385-388, 2005.
133. American Academy of Obstetricians and Gynecologists (ACOG): Placenta accreta. ACOG Committee opinion no. 266, January 2002. Obstet Gynecol 99:169-170, 2002.
134. Potter PS, Waters JH, Burger GA, Mraovic B: Application of cell-salvage during cesarean section. Anesthesiology 90:619-621, 1999.
135. Rebarber A, Lonser R, Jackson S, et al: The safety of intraoperative autologous blood collection and autotransfusion during cesarean section. Am J Obstet Gynecol 179(Pt 1):715-720, 1998.
136. Waters JH, Biscotti C, Potter PS, et al: Amniotic fluid removal during cell salvage in the cesarean section patient. Anesthesiology 92:1531-1536, 2000.
137. Weiskopf RB: Erythrocyte salvage during cesarean section. Anesthesiology 92:1519-1522, 2000.
138. Estella NM, Berry DL, Baker BW, et al: Normovolemic hemodilution before cesarean hysterectomy for placenta percreta. Obstet Gynecol 90(Pt 2):669-670, 1997.
139. Grange CS, Douglas MJ, Adams TJ, et al: The use of acute hemodilution in parturients undergoing cesarean section. Am J Obstet Gynecol 178(Pt 1):156-160, 1998.
140. Monk TG: Acute normovolemic hemodilution. Anesthesiol Clin North Am 23:271-281, vi, 2005.

141. Mattox KL, Bickell W, Pepe PE, et al: Prospective MAST study in 911 patients. J Trauma 29:1104-1111, 1989.
142. Dutton RP: Current concepts in hemorrhagic shock. Anesthesiol Clin 25:23-34, 2007.
143. Spahn DR, Cerny V, Coats TJ, et al: Management of bleeding following major trauma: A European guideline. Crit Care 11:R17, 2007.
144. Levi M, Peters M, Buller HR: Efficacy and safety of recombinant factor VIIa for treatment of severe bleeding: A systematic review. Crit Care Med 33:883-890, 2005.
145. Boehlen F, Morales MA, Fontana P, et al: Prolonged treatment of massive postpartum haemorrhage with recombinant factor VIIa: Case report and review of the literature. BJOG 111:284-287, 2004.
146. Bouwmeester FW, Jonkhoff AR, Verheijen RH, et al: Successful treatment of life-threatening postpartum hemorrhage with recombinant activated factor VII. Obstet Gynecol 101:1174-1176, 2003.
147. Segal S, Shemesh IY, Blumental R, et al: The use of recombinant factor VIIa in severe postpartum hemorrhage. Acta Obstet Gynecol Scand 83:771-772, 2004.
148. Tanchev S, Platikanov V, Karadimov D: Administration of recombinant factor VIIa for the management of massive bleeding due to uterine atonia in the post-placental period. Acta Obstet Gynecol Scand 84:402-403, 2005.
149. Hallak M, Dildy GA III, Hurley TJ, et al: Transvaginal pressure pack for life-threatening pelvic hemorrhage secondary to placenta accreta. Obstet Gynecol 78(Pt 2):938-940, 1991.
150. Maier RC: Control of postpartum hemorrhage with uterine packing. Am J Obstet Gynecol 169(Pt 1):317-321, 1993.
151. Condous GS, Arulkumaran S, Symonds I, et al: The "tamponade test" in the management of massive postpartum hemorrhage. Obstet Gynecol 101:767-772, 2003.
152. De Loor JA, van Dam PA: Foley catheters for uncontrollable obstetric or gynecologic hemorrhage. Obstet Gynecol 88(Pt 2):737, 1996.
153. Bakri YN, Amri A, Abdul JF: Tamponade-balloon for obstetrical bleeding. Int J Gynaecol Obstet 74:139-142, 2001.
154. Lynch C, Coker A, Lawal AH, et al: The B Lynch surgical technique for the control of massive postpartum haemorrhage: An alternative to hysterectomy? Five cases reported. BJOG 104:372-375, 1997.
155. Allam MS, Lynch C: The B-Lynch and other uterine compression suture techniques. Int J Gynaecol Obstet 89:236-241, 2005.
156. Nelson WL, O'Brien JM: The uterine sandwich for persistent uterine atony: Combining the B-Lynch compression suture and an intrauterine Bakri balloon. Am J Obstet Gynecol 196:e9-e10, 2007.
157. O'Leary JA, O'Leary JL: Uterine artery ligation for control of postcesarean hemorrhage. Surg Forum 19:409-410, 1968.
158. O'Leary JL, O'Leary JA: Uterine artery ligation in the control of intractable postpartum hemorrhage. Am J Obstet Gynecol 94:920-924, 1966.
159. Clark SL, Phelan JP, Yeh SY, et al: Hypogastric artery ligation for obstetric hemorrhage. Obstet Gynecol 66:353-356, 1985.
160. Zelop CM, Harlow BL, Frigoletto FD Jr, et al: Emergency peripartum hysterectomy. Am J Obstet Gynecol 168:1443-1448, 1993.
161. Stanco LM, Schrimmer DB, Paul RH, et al: Emergency peripartum hysterectomy and associated risk factors. Am J Obstet Gynecol 168(Pt 1):879-883, 1993.
162. Clark SL, Yeh SY, Phelan JP, et al: Emergency hysterectomy for obstetric hemorrhage. Obstet Gynecol 64:376-380, 1984.
163. Forna F, Miles AM, Jamieson DJ: Emergency peripartum hysterectomy: A comparison of cesarean and postpartum hysterectomy. Am J Obstet Gynecol 190:1440-1444, 200.
164. Whiteman MK, Kuklina E, Hillis SD, et al: Incidence and determinants of peripartum hysterectomy. Obstet Gynecol 108:1486-1492, 2006.
165. Francois K, Ortiz J, Harris C, et al: Is peripartum hysterectomy more common in multiple gestations? Obstet Gynecol 105:1369-1372, 2005.
166. Kastner ES, Figueroa R, Garry D, et al: Emergency peripartum hysterectomy: Experience at a community teaching hospital. Obstet Gynecol 99:971-975, 2002.
167. Pelage JP, Le DO, Jacob D, et al: Selective arterial embolization of the uterine arteries in the management of intractable post-partum hemorrhage. Acta Obstet Gynecol Scand 78:698-703, 1999.
168. Tourne G, Collet F, Seffert P, et al: Place of embolization of the uterine arteries in the management of post-partum haemorrhage: A study of 12 cases. Eur J Obstet Gynecol Reprod Biol 110:29-34, 2003.
169. Gilbert WM, Moore TR, Resnik R, et al: Angiographic embolization in the management of hemorrhagic complications of pregnancy. Am J Obstet Gynecol 166:493-497, 1992.
170. Ornan D, White R, Pollak J, et al: Pelvic embolization for intractable postpartum hemorrhage: Long-term follow-up and implications for fertility. Obstet Gynecol 102(Pt 1):904-910, 2003.
171. Descargues G, Mauger TF, Douvrin F, et al: Menses, fertility and pregnancy after arterial embolization for the control of postpartum haemorrhage. Hum Reprod 19:339-343, 2004.
172. Connolly AM, Katz VL, Bash KL, et al: Trauma and pregnancy. Am J Perinatol 14:331-336, 1997.
173. Pearlman MD, Phillips ME: Safety belt use during pregnancy. Obstet Gynecol 88:1026-1029, 1996.
174. El-Kady D, Gilbert WM, Anderson J, et al: Trauma during pregnancy: An analysis of maternal and fetal outcomes in a large population. Am J Obstet Gynecol 190:1661-1668, 2004.
175. Williams JK, McClain L, Rosemurgy AS, et al: Evaluation of blunt abdominal trauma in the third trimester of pregnancy: Maternal and fetal considerations. Obstet Gynecol 75:33-37, 1990.
176. Weiss HB, Songer TJ, Fabio A: Fetal deaths related to maternal injury. JAMA 286:1863-1868, 2001.
177. Crosby WM: Traumatic injuries during pregnancy. Clin Obstet Gynecol 26:902-912, 1983.
178. Pearlman MD, Tintinallli JE, Lorenz RP: A prospective controlled study of outcome after trauma during pregnancy. Am J Obstet Gynecol 162: 1502-1507, 1990.
179. Gazmararian JA, Lazorick S, Spitz AM, et al: Prevalence of violence against pregnant women. JAMA 275:1915-1920, 1996.
180. American College of Obstetricians and Gynecologists (ACOG): Automobile passenger restraints for children and pregnant women. ACOG technical bulletin no. 151, January 1991. Int J Gynaecol Obstet 37:305-308, 1992.
181. Pearlman MD, Viano D: Automobile crash simulation with the first pregnant crash test dummy. Am J Obstet Gynecol 175(Pt 1):977-981, 1996.
182. Moorcroft DM, Stitzel JD, Duma GG, et al: Computational model of the pregnant occupant: Predicting the risk of injury in automobile crashes. Am J Obstet Gynecol 189:540-544, 2003.
183. Hyde LK, Cook LJ, Olson LM, et al: Effect of motor vehicle crashes on adverse fetal outcomes. Obstet Gynecol 102:279-286, 2003.
184. Pearlman MD, Klinich KD, Schneider LW, et al: A comprehensive program to improve safety for pregnant women and fetuses in motor vehicle crashes: A preliminary report. Am J Obstet Gynecol 182:1554-1564, 2000.
185. Dahmus MA, Sibai BM: Blunt abdominal trauma: Are there any predictive factors for abruptio placentae or maternal-fetal distress? Am J Obstet Gynecol 169:1054-1059, 1993.
186. Schiff MA, Holt VL: The injury severity score in pregnant trauma patients: Predicting placental abruption and fetal death. J Trauma 53:946-949, 2002.
187. Baerga-Varela Y, Zietlow SP, Bannon MP, et al: Trauma in pregnancy. Mayo Clin Proc 75:1243-1248, 2000.
188. Glantz C, Purnell L: Clinical utility of sonography in the diagnosis and treatment of placental abruption. J Ultrasound Med 21:837-840, 2002.
189. Nyberg DA, Mack LA, Benedetti TJ, et al: Placental abruption and placental hemorrhage: Correlation of sonographic findings with fetal outcome. Radiology 164:357-361, 1987.
190. Baker SP, O'Neill B, Haddon W Jr, et al: The injury severity score: A method for describing patients with multiple injuries and evaluating emergency care. J Trauma 14:187-196, 1974.

191. Biester EM, Tomich PG, Esposito TJ, et al: Trauma in pregnancy: Normal Revised Trauma Score in relation to other markers of maternofetal status—a preliminary study. Am J Obstet Gynecol 176:1206-1210, 1997.
192. Goodwin TM, Breen MT: Pregnancy outcome and fetomaternal hemorrhage after noncatastrophic trauma. Am J Obstet Gynecol 162:665-671, 1990.
193. Choavaratana R, Uer-Areewong S, Makanantakosol S: Feto-maternal transfusion in normal pregnancy and during delivery. J Med Assoc Thai 80:96-100, 1997.
194. Dhanraj D, Lambers D: The incidences of positive Kleihauer-Betke test in low-risk pregnancies and maternal trauma patients. Am J Obstet Gynecol 190:1461-1463, 2004.
195. Kuhlmann RS, Cruikshank DP: Maternal trauma during pregnancy. Clin Obstet Gynecol 37:274-293, 1994.
196. Maull KI: Maternal-fetal trauma. Semin Pediatr Surg 10:32-34, 2001.
197. Palmer JD, Sparrow OC: Extradural haematoma following intrauterine trauma. Injury 25:671-673, 1994.
198. Lavery JP, Staten-McCormick M: Management of moderate to severe trauma in pregnancy. Obstet Gynecol Clin North Am 22:69-90, 1995.
199. Esposito TJ: Trauma during pregnancy. Emerg Med Clin North Am 12:167-199, 1994.
200. American College of Obstetricians and Gynecologists (ACOG): Guidelines for diagnostic imaging during pregnancy. ACOG committee opinion no. 158, 1995.
201. Akhtar MA, Mulawkar PM, Kulkarni HR: Burns in pregnancy: Effect on maternal and fetal outcomes. Burns 20:351-355, 1994.
202. Maghsoudi H, Samnia R, Garadaghi A, et al: Burns in pregnancy. Burns 32:246-250, 2006.
203. Sidney F Miller C: National Burn Repository 2005 report, version 2.0. 2006. Available at www.ameriburn.org.
204. Pham TN, Gibran NS: Thermal and electrical injuries. Surg Clin North Am 87:185, viii, 2007.
205. Alsbjorn B, Gilbert P, Hartmann B, et al: Guidelines for the management of partial-thickness burns in a general hospital or community setting—recommendations of a European working party. Burns 33:155-160, 2007.
206. Rayburn W, Smith B, Feller I, et al: Major burns during pregnancy: Effects on fetal well-being. Obstet Gynecol 63:392-395, 1984.
207. Shah AJ, Kilcline BA: Trauma in pregnancy. Emerg Med Clin North Am 21:615-629, 2003.
208. Pacheco LD, Gei AF, VanHook JW, et al: Burns in pregnancy. Obstet Gynecol 106(Pt 2):1210-1212, 2005.
209. Prelack K, Dylewski M, Sheridan RL: Practical guidelines for nutritional management of burn injury and recovery. Burns 33:14-24, 2007.
210. Demling R, Gates J: Medical aspects of trauma and burn care. In Goldman L, Ausiello D (eds): Cecil Textbook of Medicine, 22nd ed. Philadelphia, WB Saunders, 2004.
211. Guo SS, Greenspoon JS, Kahn AM: Management of burn injuries during pregnancy. Burns 27:394-397, 2001.
212. Jain ML, Garg AK: Burns with pregnancy—a review of 25 cases. Burns 19:166-167, 1993.
213. Polko LE, McMahon MJ: Burns in pregnancy. Obstet Gynecol Surv 53:50-56, 1998.
214. Katz V, Balderston K, DeFreest M: Perimortem cesarean delivery: Were our assumptions correct? Am J Obstet Gynecol 192:1916-2190, 2005.
215. Mallampalli A, Powner DJ, Gardner MO: Cardiopulmonary resuscitation and somatic support of the pregnant patient. Crit Care Clin 20:747-761, x, 2004.
216. Nanson J, Elcock D, Williams M, et al: Do physiological changes in pregnancy change defibrillation energy requirements? Br J Anaesth 87:237-239, 2001.
217. Katz VL, Dotters DJ, Droegemueller W: Perimortem cesarean delivery. Obstet Gynecol 68:571-576, 1986.
218. Bush MC, Nagy S, Berkowitz RL, et al: Pregnancy in a persistent vegetative state: Case report, comparison to brain death, and review of the literature. Obstet Gynecol Surv 58:738-748, 2003.
219. Powner DJ, Bernstein IM: Extended somatic support for pregnant women after brain death. Crit Care Med 31:1241-1249, 2003.
220. Feldman DM, Borgida AF, Rodis JF, et al: Irreversible maternal brain injury during pregnancy: A case report and review of the literature. Obstet Gynecol Surv 55:708-714, 2000.
221. Hussein IY, Govenden V, Grant JM, et al: Prolongation of pregnancy in a woman who sustained brain death at 26 weeks of gestation. BJOG 113:120-122, 2006.
222. Nettina M, Santos E, Ascioti KJ, et al: Sheila's death created many rings of life. Nursing 23:44-48, 1993.
223. Wuermeling HB: Brain-death and pregnancy. Forensic Sci Int 69:243-245, 1994.

Part V

THE NEONATE

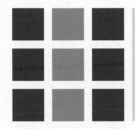

Chapter 58

Neonatal Morbidities of Prenatal and Perinatal Origin

James M. Greenberg, MD, Vivek Narendran, MD, Kurt R. Schibler, MD, Barbara B. Warner, MD, Beth Haberman, MD, and Edward F. Donovan, MD

Obstetric and Postnatal Management Decisions

The nature of obstetric clinical practice requires consideration of two patients: mother and fetus. The intrinsic biologic interdependence of one with the other creates challenges not typically encountered in other realms of medical practice. Often, there is a paucity of objective data to support the evaluation of risks and benefits associated with a given clinical situation, forcing obstetricians to rely on their clinical acumen and experience. Family perspectives must be integrated in clinical decision making, along with the advice and counsel of other clinical providers. In this chapter, we review how to best use neonatologic expertise in the obstetric decision-making process.

Optimal perinatal care often derives from collaboration between the obstetrician and neonatologist during pregnancy and especially around the time of labor to eliminate ambiguity and confusion in the delivery room and to ensure that patients and families understand the rationale for obstetric and postnatal management decisions. The neonatologist can provide information regarding risks to the fetus associated with delaying or initiating preterm delivery and can identify the optimal location for delivery to ensure that skilled personnel are present to support the newborn infant.

In addition to contributing information about gestational age–specific outcomes, the neonatologist can anticipate neonatal complications related to maternal disorders such as diabetes mellitus, hypertension, and multiple gestations or to prenatally detected fetal conditions such as congenital infections, alloimmunization, or developmental anomalies. When a lethal condition or high risk of death in the delivery room is anticipated, the neonatologist can assist with the formulation of a birth plan and develop parameters for delivery room intervention.

Preparing parents by describing delivery room management and resuscitation of a high-risk infant can demystify the process and reduce some of the fear anticipated by the expectant family. Premature infants are susceptible to thermal instability and are moved rapidly after birth to a warming bed to prevent hypothermia while assessing the infant's cardiorespiratory status and vigor. The need for resuscitation is determined by careful evaluation of cardiorespiratory parameters and appropriate response according to published Neonatal Resuscitation Program guidelines.[1]

Common Morbidities of Pregnancy and Neonatal Outcomes

Complications of pregnancy that affect infant well-being may be immediately evident after birth, such as hypotension related to maternal hemorrhage, or may manifest hours later, such as hypoglycemia related to maternal diabetes or thrombocytopenia related to maternal preeclampsia. Anemia and thyroid disorders related to transplacental passage of maternal IgG antibodies to platelets or thyroid, respectively, may manifest days after delivery.

Diabetes during pregnancy serves as an example. Infants born to women with diabetes are often macrosomic, increasing the risk of shoulder dystocia and birth injury. After delivery, these infants may have significant hypoglycemia, polycythemia, and electrolyte disturbances, which require close surveillance and treatment. Lung maturation is delayed in the infants born to women with diabetes, increasing the incidence of respiratory distress syndrome (RDS) at a given gestational age. Infants of diabetic mothers may also have delayed neurologic maturation, with decreased tone typically leading to delayed feeding competence. Less common complications include an increased incidence of congenital heart disease and skeletal malformations. These neonatal complications are typically managed without long-term sequelae, but they are not without consequences, such as prolonged hospital stay. Neonatal complications for the infant of a woman with diabetes are a function of maternal glycemic control. Careful antenatal attention to optimal control of blood glucose can reduce neonatal morbidity due to maternal diabetes.

Table 58-1 summarizes other morbidities of pregnancy and their effects on neonatal outcome. The list is not exhaustive and does not take into account how multiple morbidities may interact to create additional complications. All of these problems may contribute to increased length of hospital stay after delivery and to long-term morbidity.

Chorioamnionitis has diverse effects on the fetus and neonatal outcome. It is associated with premature rupture of membranes and preterm delivery. Elevated levels of proinflammatory cytokines may predispose neonates to cerebral injury.[2] Although suspected or proven neonatal sepsis is more common in the setting of chorioamnio-

TABLE 58-1 MANAGEMENT CONSIDERATIONS ASSOCIATED WITH NEONATAL MANAGEMENT OF CONGENITAL MALFORMATIONS

Malformation	Management Considerations
Clefts	Alternative feeding devices (e.g., Haberman feeder), genetics evaluation, occupational or physical therapy
Congenital diaphragmatic hernia	Skilled airway management, pediatric surgery, immediate availability of mechanical ventilation, nitric oxide, ECMO
Upper airway obstruction or micrognathia	Skilled airway management, otolaryngologic evaluation, genetics evaluation and management, immediate availability of mechanical ventilation
Hydrothorax	Skilled airway management, nitric oxide, ECMO, chest tube placement, immediate availability of mechanical ventilation
Ambiguous genitalia	Endocrinology, urologic consultation, genetic profile available for immediate evaluation
Neural tube defects	Dressings to cover defect, IV fluids, neurosurgery, urologic evaluation, orthopedics evaluation and management
Abdominal wall defects	Saline-filled sterile bag to contain exposed abdominal contents, IV fluids, pediatric surgery, genetics evaluation and management
Cyanotic congenital heart disease	IV access, prostaglandin E_1, immediate availability of mechanical ventilation

ECMO, extracorporeal membrane oxygenation; IV, intravenous.

nitis, many neonates born to mothers with histologically proven chorioamnionitis are asymptomatic and appear uninfected. Animal models and associated epidemiologic data suggest that chorioamnionitis can accelerate fetal lung maturation, as measured by surfactant production and function. However, preterm infants born to mothers with chorioamnionitis are more likely to develop bronchopulmonary dysplasia (BPD).[3-5] The neonatal consequences of chorioamnionitis are likely related to the timing, severity, and extent of the infection and the associated inflammatory response.

The effects of preeclampsia on the neonate include intrauterine growth retardation, hypoglycemia, neutropenia, thrombocytopenia, polycythemia, and electrolyte abnormalities such as hypocalcemia. Most of these problems appear related to placental insufficiency, with diminished oxygen and nutrient delivery to the fetus. With delivery and supportive care, most of these problems will resolve with time, although some patients will require treatment with intravenous calcium or glucose, or both, in the early neonatal period. Similarly, severe thrombocytopenia may require platelet transfusion therapy. Preeclampsia may protect against intraventricular hemorrhage (IVH) in preterm infants, perhaps because of maternal treatment or other unknown factors.[6] Unlike intrauterine inflammation, preeclampsia does not appear to accelerate lung maturation.[7]

Maternal autoimmune disease may affect the neonate through transplacental transfer of autoantibodies. Symptoms are a function of the extent of antibody transfer. Treatment is supportive and based on the affected neonatal organ systems. For example, maternal Graves disease may cause neonatal thyrotoxicosis requiring treatment with propylthiouracil or β-blockers. Maternal lupus or connective tissue disease is linked to congenital heart block that may require long-term pacing after delivery. Myasthenia gravis during pregnancy occasionally results in a transient form of the disease in the neonate. Supportive therapy during the early neonatal period addresses most issues associated with maternal autoimmune disorders. Passively transferred autoantibodies gradually clear from the neonatal circulation with a half-life of 2 to 3 weeks.

Neonatal outcome associated with maternal nutritional status during pregnancy is of growing interest. The Dutch famine of 1944 to 1945 created a unique circumstance for studying the consequences of severe undernutrition during pregnancy (i.e., caloric intake <1000 kcal/day). Mothers experienced significant third-trimester weight loss, and offspring were underweight.[8] There is growing evidence that infants undernourished during fetal life are at higher risk for "adult" diseases such as atherosclerosis and hypertension. Poor maternal nutrition during intrauterine life may signal the fetus to modify metabolic pathways and blood pressure regulatory systems, with health consequences lasting into late childhood and beyond.[9] Conversely, maternal overnutrition (i.e., excessive caloric intake) predisposes mothers to insulin resistance and large-for-gestational-age infants.[10,11]

Neonatal anemia may be a consequence of perinatal events such as placental abruption, ruptured vasa previa, or fetal-maternal transfusion. At delivery, the neonate may be asymptomatic or display profound effects of blood loss, including high-output heart failure or hypovolemic shock. The duration and extent of blood loss along with any fetal compensation typically determine neonatal clinical status at delivery and subsequent management. In the delivery room, prompt recognition of acute blood loss and transfusion with type O, Rh-negative blood can be a lifesaving intervention.

Neonates from a multifetal gestation are, on average, smaller at a given gestational age than their singleton counterparts. They are also more likely to deliver before term and therefore are more likely to experience the complications associated with low birth weight and prematurity described in this chapter. Monochorionic twins may experience twin-twin transfusion syndrome. The associated discordant growth and additional problems of anemia, polycythemia, congestive heart failure, and hydrops may further complicate the clinical course after delivery, even after amnioreduction or fetoscopic laser occlusion. Cerebral lesions such as periventricular white matter injury and ventricular enlargement may occur more frequently in the setting of twin-twin transfusion syndrome.[12] Additional epidemiologic studies and long-term follow-up are needed to further address this issue.

Congenital malformations present significant challenges for caregivers and families, and prenatal diagnosis is an opportunity to provide anticipatory guidance. The neonatologist can facilitate delivery coverage and ensure availability of appropriate equipment, medications, and personnel. Table 58-1 summarizes some of the important considerations associated with management of congenital malformations and reflects the importance of multidisciplinary input. Typically, these patients are best delivered in a setting where experienced delivery room attendance is available. If the needed consultative services and equipment are not readily available, arrangement should be made for prompt transfer to a tertiary center. Successful transports depend on clear communication between centers, for example, regarding delivery of an infant with gastroschisis, so that the delivering hospital provides adequate intravenous hydration and protection of exposed abdominal organs, and the referral center can mobilize pediatric surgical intervention immediately on arrival of the infant.

In settings of premature, preterm, or prolonged rupture of membranes and premature labor, mothers are frequently treated with antibiotics and tocolytic agents. Maternal medications administered during pregnancy for non-obstetric diseases can have a significant impact on the neonate. A common challenge in many centers is the treatment of opiate-addicted mothers on methadone. The symptoms of neonatal abstinence syndrome vary as a function of the degree of prenatal opiate exposure and age after delivery. Many infants appear neurologically normal at delivery, only to exhibit symptoms later on the first or second day or extrauterine life. Infants with neonatal abstinence syndrome typically demonstrate irritability, poor feeding, loose and frequent stools, and in severe cases, seizures. Treatment options include nonpharmacologic intervention (e.g., swaddling, minimal stimulation), methadone, or non-narcotic drugs such as phenobarbital. These infants often require hospitalization for many days or weeks until their irritability is under sufficient control to allow for care in a home setting. There is clinical evidence that neonates may also exhibit similar symptoms after withdrawal from antenatal nicotine exposure.[13,14] The consequences of other illicit drug use during pregnancy have been widely studied but are difficult to assess because of difficulties with diagnosis and confounding variables. Maternal cocaine abuse has been associated with obstetric complications such as placental abruption. Vascular compromise may predispose neonates to cerebral infarcts and bowel injury. Developmental delay and behavioral problems are observed, although associated factors such as poverty, lack of prenatal care, and low socioeconomic status also contribute.

Alloimmune hemolytic disorders such as Rh hemolytic disease and ABO incompatibility can cause neonatal morbidity ranging from uncomplicated hyperbilirubinemia to severe anemia, hydrops, and high-output congestive heart failure. Although it is uncommon, Rh hemolytic disease must be considered as a cause of unexplained hydrops, anemia, or heart failure in infants born to Rh-negative mothers, especially if there is a possibility of maternal sensitization. ABO incompatibility is common, with up to 20% of all pregnancies potentially at risk. The responsible isohemagglutinins have weak affinity for blood group antigens, and the degree of hemolysis and subsequent jaundice varies among patients. Indirect immunoglobulin (Coombs) testing has limited value in predicting clinically significant jaundice. Neonatal morbidity is typically restricted to hyperbilirubinemia requiring treatment with phototherapy.

Prematurity

The mean duration of a spontaneous singleton pregnancy is 280 days or 40 menstrual weeks, 38 weeks after conception. An infant delivered before completion of 37 weeks' gestation is considered to be preterm according to the World Health Organization (WHO) definition. Infant morbidity and mortality increase with decreasing gestational age at birth. The risk of poor outcome, defined as death or lifelong handicap, increases dramatically as gestational age decreases, especially for very low birth weight (VLBW) infants (Fig. 58-1).

Complications of Prematurity

Besides increased mortality risk, prematurity is associated with an increased risk for morbidity in almost every major organ system. BPD, retinopathy of prematurity, necrotizing enterocolitis, and IVH are particularly linked to preterm births. Intrauterine growth restriction and increased susceptibility to infection are not restricted to the preterm infant but are complicated in the immature infant. Table 58-2 summarizes common complications of prematurity by organ system.

The rate of preterm birth increased by 30% between 1983 and 2004, from 9.6% to 12.5%. Three major causes have been identified to explain the rise (see Chapter 29): improved gestational dating associated with increased use of early ultrasound,[16] the substantial rise in multifetal gestation associated with assisted reproductive technology, and an increase in "indicated" preterm births.[17] The latter category is important because decisions affecting the timing and management of preterm delivery can have a profound effect on neonatal outcome. The risk of death before birth hospital discharge doubles when the gestational age decreases from 27.5 weeks (10%) to 26 weeks (20%). Delaying delivery even for a few days may substantially improve outcome, especially before 32 weeks, assuming that the intrauterine environment is safe to support the fetus. However, in some clinical situations with a high potential for preterm delivery, it is difficult to assess the quality of the intrauterine environment. Three common examples are preterm, premature rupture of membranes (see Chapter 31), placental abruption (see Chapter 37), and preeclampsia (see Chapter 35). In each case, prolonging gestation to allow continued fetal growth and maturation in utero is accompanied by an uncertain risk of rapid change in maternal status with a corresponding increased risk of fetal compromise. Tests of fetal well-being are discussed in Chapter 21, and clinical decision making in obstetrics is addressed in Chapters 28 and 29.

Obstetric decisions about the timing of delivery in the setting of uncertain in utero risk are a significant contributing factor to the increase in late preterm births, after 32 to 34 weeks. The contribution of elective delivery must also be considered. Although perinatal mor-

TABLE 58-2 COMMON COMPLICATIONS OF PREMATURITY BY ORGAN SYSTEM

Organ System	Morbidity
Pulmonary	Respiratory distress syndrome Bronchopulmonary dysplasia Pulmonary hypoplasia Apnea of prematurity
Cardiovascular	Patent ductus arteriosus Apnea and bradycardia Hypotension
Gastrointestinal, hepatic	Necrotizing enterocolitis Dysmotility or reflux Feeding difficulties Hypoglycemia
Central nervous system	Intraventricular hemorrhage Periventricular leukomalacia
Visual	Retinopathy of prematurity
Skin	Excess insensible water loss Hypothermia
Immunologic, hematologic	Increased incidence of sepsis and meningitis Anemia of prematurity

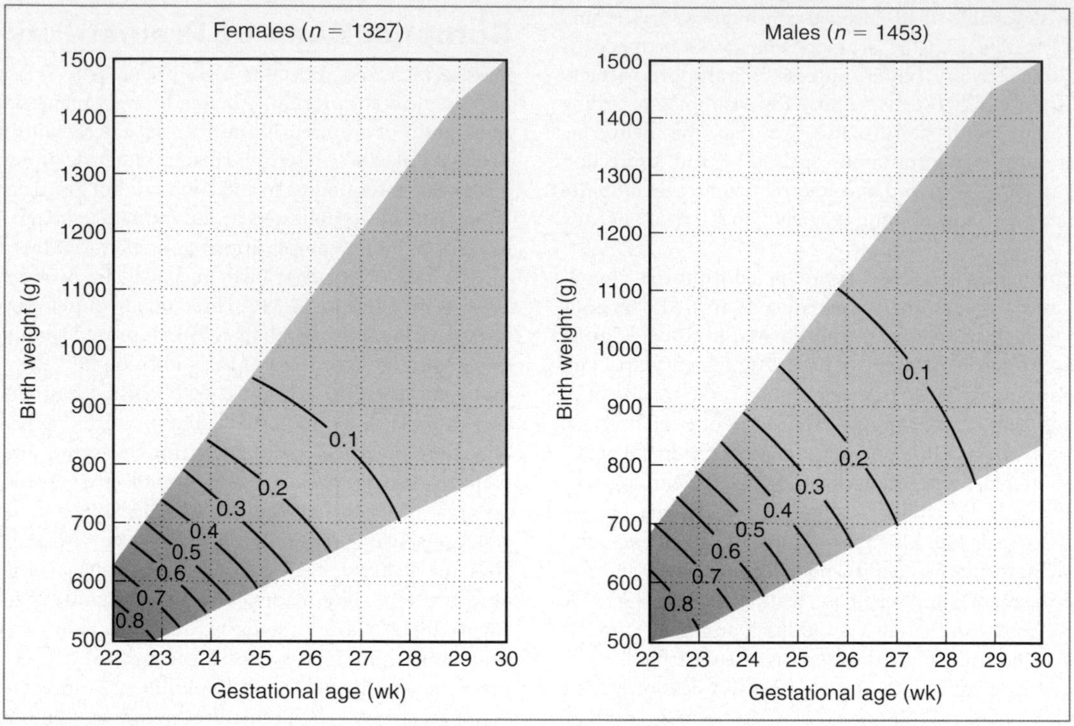

FIGURE 58-1 Estimated mortality risk by birth weight and gestational age based on singleton infants born in National Institute of Child Health and Human Development (NICHD) Neonatal Research Network centers between January 1, 1995, and December 31, 1996. Numeric values represent age- and weight-specific mortality rates per 100 births. (From Lemons JA, Bauer CR, Oh W, et al: Very low birth weight outcomes of the National Institute of Child Health and Human Development Neonatal Research Network, January 1995 through December 1996. NICHD Neonatal Research Network. Pediatrics 107:E1, 2001. Used with permission of the American Academy of Pediatrics.)

tality continues to decrease, in part due to a decline in stillbirths,[17] interest in understanding the extent of morbidity associated with late preterm deliveries has intensified because of the large number of these late preterm infants and the potential to avoid morbidities, such as temperature instability, feeding problems, hyperbilirubinemia requiring treatment, suspected sepsis, and respiratory distress. Infants born at 35 weeks' gestation are nine times more likely to require mechanical ventilation than those born at term.[18]

Most complications of late preterm delivery are easily treated, but their economic and social effects are substantial, and long-term sequelae are not well understood. For example, brain growth and development proceed rapidly during the third trimester and continue for the first several years of life. An infant born at 35 weeks' gestation has approximately one-half the brain volume of a term infant. Although IVH is unusual after 32 weeks' gestation, regions including the periventricular white matter continue to undergo rapid myelination during this period. Studies by Stein and colleagues[19] and Kirkegaard and coworkers[20] demonstrate an association between late preterm delivery and long-term neurodevelopmental problems, including learning disabilities and attention deficit disorders. Careful neurologic and epidemiologic studies will be required to define any mechanistic connection between late preterm delivery and these long-term outcomes.

Our growing recognition of the morbidity and mortality risks associated with preterm delivery clearly deserve close scrutiny and further study. Table 58-3 compares estimates of complication rates between preterm and late preterm infants.

Classic preterm infants, typically defined as those born before 32 weeks' gestation or weighing less than 1500 g, or both, comprise only 1.5% of all deliveries, whereas the late preterm population accounts for 8% to 9% of all births. Even uncommon complications in the later preterm population may represent a significant health care burden. As the number of late preterm infants continues to increase, clinicians and policymakers will likely focus additional attention on the causes and prevention of such deliveries (Fig. 58-2).

Decisions at the Threshold of Viability

Decisions regarding treatment of infants at the "limit of viability" are often the most difficult for families and health care professionals. The difficulty stems in part from the lack of clarity in defining what that limit is, which has fallen by approximately 1 week every decade over the past 40 years. Among developed countries, most identify the limit of viability at 22 to 25 weeks' gestation.[29-31] Making decisions at this early gestation requires accurate information about mortality and morbidity for this population. At 22 weeks (22 0/7days to 22 6/7 days), survival is rare and typically not included in studies of survival or long-term outcome. Rates of survival to hospital discharge for infants born at 23 weeks' gestation (23 0/7 to 23 6/7 days) range from 15% to 30%. Survival increases to between 30 and 55% for infants born at 24 weeks' gestation.[15,23,30,32-35] The Vermont-Oxford Network reported weight-based survival for more than 4000 infants born between 401 and 500 g (mean gestational age of 23.3 ± 2.1 weeks) from 1996 to 2000. Survival to hospital discharge was 17%.[36] Although mortality

TABLE 58-3 ESTIMATED COMPLICATION RATES FOR PRETERM AND LATE PRETERM INFANTS

Complication of Prematurity	Incidence for Preterm Infants*	Incidence for Late Preterm Infants†
Respiratory distress syndrome	65% surf Rx < 1500 g 80% < 27 wk[21]	5%
Bronchopulmonary dysplasia	23% < 1500 g[15]	Uncommon
Retinopathy of prematurity	Approx 40% < 1500 g[22-24]	
Intraventricular hemorrhage with ventricular dilation or parenchymal involvement	11% < 1500 g[15]	Rare
Necrotizing enterocolitis	5-7% < 1500 g[15]	Uncommon
Patent ductus arteriosus	30% < 1500 g[15]	Uncommon
Feeding difficulty	>90%	10-15%[25]
Hypoglycemia	NA	10-15%[25]

***Defined as <32 weeks and/or <1500 g.**
†Defined as 32-37 weeks and/or 1500-2500 g.
NA, not available; surf Rx, surfactant treatment.

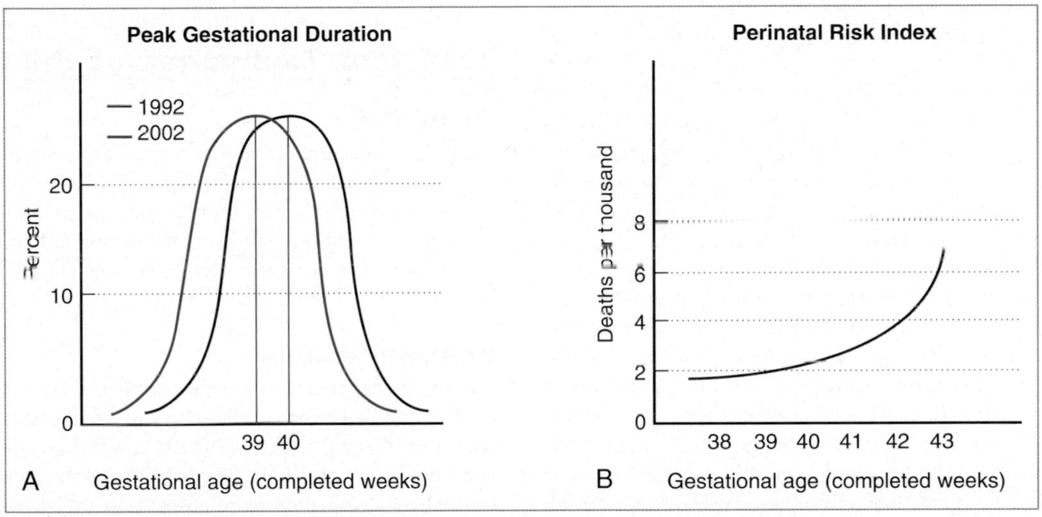

FIGURE 58-2 Peak gestational age duration and risk of intrauterine fetal demise. **A,** Change in peak gestational duration between 1992 and 2002. The duration of gestation decreased by a full week during that decade, from 40 weeks to 39 weeks. **B,** The risk of intrauterine fetal demise increases with increasing gestational age, especially beyond 40 weeks. The risk of intrauterine fetal demise likely influences obstetric decision making regarding the timing of delivery in pregnancies approaching 40 weeks' gestation. (Data from Davidoff MJ, Dias T, Damus K, et al: Changes in the gestational age distribution among U.S. singleton births: Impact on rates of late preterm birth, 1992 to 2002. Semin Perinatol 30:8-15, 2006; Yudkin PL, Wood L, Redman CW: Risk of unexplained stillbirth at different gestational ages. Lancet 1:1192-1194, 1987; and Smith GC: Life-table analysis of the risk of perinatal death at term and post term in singleton pregnancies. Am J Obstet Gynecol 184:489-496, 2001.)

rates decline for each 1-week increase in gestational age at delivery, long-term neurodevelopmental outcomes do not improve proportionately. Of infants born at less than 25 weeks' gestation, 30% to 50% will have moderate to severe disability, including blindness, deafness, developmental delays and cerebral palsy.[23,30,32] The National Institute of Child Health and Human Development reported neurodevelopmental outcomes for more than 5000 infants born between 22 and 26 weeks' gestation from 1993 to 1998. Bayley mental development index (MDI) and nonverbal development index (NDI) scores improved and blindness was reduced, but rates of severe cerebral palsy, hearing loss, shunted hydrocephalus, and seizures were unchanged.[37]

Birth weight and gender also affect survival rates. Higher weights within gestational age categories and female sex consistently show a survival advantage and better neurodevelopmental outcomes.[15,37] Survival and long-term outcomes of very preterm infants are improved with delivery at a tertiary center, rather than neonatal transfer from an outlying facility.[38-40] When families desire resuscitation or dating is uncertain, every attempt should be made to transfer to a tertiary center for delivery. Maternal transfer to a tertiary center and administration of corticosteroids (see Chapter 23) are the only antenatal interventions that have been significantly and consistently related to improved neonatal neurodevelopmental outcomes.[37] Other attempted strategies are discussed in Chapter 29.

Planning for Delivery at the Limits of Viability

Ideally, discussion between physicians and parents should begin before birth in a nonemergent situation, and include both obstetric and neonatal care providers. Even during active labor, communication with the family should be initiated as a foundation for postnatal discussions. The family should understand that plans made before delivery are influenced by maternal and fetal considerations and are based on limited information. It should be emphasized that information available only after delivery, such as birth weight and neonatal physical findings, may change the infant's prognosis.[30]

Neonatal Resuscitation at the Limits of Viability

If time allows before delivery of an infant whose gestational age is near the threshold of viability, a thoughtful birth plan developed by the parents in consultation with maternal-fetal medicine specialists and the neonatologist should be established. The neonatologist can assist families in making decisions regarding a birth plan for their infant by providing general information about the prognosis, the hospital course, potential complications, survival information, and general health and well-being of infants delivered at the similar gestational age. When time does not permit such discussions, careful evaluation of gestational age and response to resuscitation are instrumental in assisting families in making decisions regarding viability or nonviability of an extremely premature infant. The presence of an experienced pediatrician at delivery is recommended to assess weight, gestational age and fetal status, and to provide medical leadership in decisions to be made jointly with families.[29,31] In cases of precipitous deliveries when communication with families has not occurred, physicians should use their best judgment on behalf of the infant to initiate resuscitation until families can be brought into the discussion, erring on the side of resuscitation if the appropriate course is uncertain.[29,41]

Under ideal circumstances, the health care team and the infant's family should make shared management decisions regarding these infants. The American Medical Association and American Academy of Pediatrics endorse the concept that "the primary consideration for decisions regarding life-sustaining treatment for seriously ill newborns should be what is best for the newborn," and they recognize parents as having the primary role in determining the goals of care for their infant.[1,29,42] Discussions with the family should include local and national information on mortality as well as long-term outcomes. Parental participation should be encouraged with open communication regarding their personal values and goals.

Decisions about resuscitation should be individualized to the case and the family but should begin with parameters for care that are based on global reviews of the medical and ethical literature and expertise. The Nuffield Council on Bioethics in the United Kingdom has proposed parameters for treating extremely premature infants that parallel guidance from the American Academy of Pediatrics.[1,29] When gestation or birth weight are associated with almost certain early death and anticipated morbidity is unacceptably high, resuscitation is not indicated. Exceptions to comply with parental requests may be appropriate in specific cases, such as for infants born at less than 23 weeks' gestation or with a birth weight of 400 g. When the prognosis is more uncertain, survival is borderline with a high rate of morbidity, such as at 23 to 24 weeks' gestation, parental views should be supported.

Decisions regarding care of extremely preterm infants is always difficult for all involved. Parental involvement, active listening, and accurate information are critical to an optimal outcome for infants and their families. Although parents are considered the best surrogate for their infant, health care professionals have a legal and ethical obligation to provide appropriate care for the infant based on medical information. If agreement with the family cannot be reached, it may be appropriate to consult the hospital ethics committee or legal council. If the situation is emergent and the responsible physician concludes the parents wishes are not in the best interest of the infant, it is appropriate to resuscitate against parental objection.[35]

Respiratory Problems in the Neonatal Period

No aspect of the transition from fetal to neonatal life is more dramatic than the process of pulmonary adaptation. In a normal term infant, the lungs expand with air, pulmonary vascular resistance rapidly decreases, and vigorous, consistent respiratory effort ensues within a minute of separation from the placenta. The process depends on crucial physiologic mechanisms, including production of functional surfactant, dilation of resistance pulmonary arterioles, bulk transfer of fluid from air spaces, and physiologic closure of the ductus arteriosus, foramen ovale. Complications such as prematurity, infection, neuromuscular disorders, developmental defects, or complications of labor may interfere with neonatal respiratory function. Common respiratory problems of neonates are reviewed in the following sections.

Transient Tachypnea of the Newborn

Definition

Transient tachypnea of the newborn (TTN), commonly known as *wet lungs*, is a mild condition affecting term and late preterm infants. This is the most common respiratory cause of admission to the special care nursery. Transient tachypnea is self-limiting, with no risk of recurrence or residual pulmonary dysfunction. It rarely causes hypoxic respiratory failure.[43]

Pathophysiology

During the last trimester, a series of physiologic events led to changes in the hormonal milieu of the fetus and its mother to facilitate neonatal transition.[44] Rapid clearance of fetal lung fluid is essential for successful transition to air breathing. The bulk of this fluid clearance is mediated by transepithelial sodium re-absorption through amiloride sensitive sodium channels in the respiratory epithelial cells.[45] The mechanisms for such an effective "self-resuscitation" soon after birth are not completely understood. Traditional explanations based on Starling forces and vaginal squeeze for fluid clearance account only for a fraction of the fluid absorbed.

Risk Factors

Transient tachypnea is classically seen in infants delivered near term, especially after cesarean birth before the onset of spontaneous labor.[46,47] Absence of labor is accompanied by impaired surge of endogenous steroids and catecholamines necessary for a successful transition.[48] Additional risk factors such as multiple gestations, excessive maternal sedation, prolonged labor, and complications resulting from excessive maternal fluid administration have been less consistently observed.

Clinical Presentation

The clinical features of TTN include a combination of grunting, tachypnea, nasal flaring, and mild intercostal and subcostal retractions along with mild central cyanosis. The grunting can be fairly significant and sometimes misdiagnosed as RDS resulting from surfactant deficiency. The chest radiograph usually shows prominent perihilar streaks that represent engorged pulmonary lymphatics and blood vessels. The radiographic appearance and clinical symptoms rapidly improve within the first 24 to 48 hours. The presence of fluid in the fissures is a common nonspecific finding. TTN is a diagnosis of exclusion and it is important that other potential causes of respiratory distress in the newborn are excluded. The differential diagnosis of TTN includes pneumonia or sepsis, air leaks, surfactant deficiency, and congenital heart disease. Other rare diagnoses are pulmonary hypertension, meconium aspiration, and polycythemia.

Diagnosis

TTN is primarily a clinical diagnosis. Chest radiographs typically demonstrate mild pulmonary congestion with hazy lung fields. The pulmonary vasculature may be prominent. Small accumulations of extrapleural fluid, especially in the minor fissure on the right side, may be seen.

Management

Management is mainly supportive. Supplemental oxygen is provided to keep the oxygen saturation level greater than 90%. Infants are usually given intravenous fluids and not fed orally until their tachypnea resolves. Rarely, infants may need continuous positive airway pressure to relieve symptoms. Diuretic therapy has been shown to be ineffective.[49]

Neonatal Implications

TTN can lead to significant morbidity related to delayed initiation of oral feeding, which may interfere with parental bonding and establishment of successful breastfeeding. The hospital stay is prolonged for mother and infant. The existing perinatal guidelines[50] recommend scheduling elective cesarean births only after 39 completed weeks' gestation to reduce the incidence of TTN (Fig. 58-3).

Pulmonary Hypoplasia

Lung development begins during the first trimester when the ventral foregut endoderm projects into adjacent splanchnic mesoderm (see Chapter 15). Branching morphogenesis, epithelial differentiation, and acquisition of a functional interface for gas exchange ensue through the remainder of gestation and are not completed until the second or third year of postnatal life. Clinical conditions associated with pulmonary hypoplasia and approaches to prevention and treatment are discussed here.

Perturbation of lung development at anytime during gestation may lead to clinically significant pulmonary hypoplasia. Two general pathophysiologic mechanisms contribute to pulmonary hypoplasia: extrinsic compression and neuromuscular dysfunction. Infants with aneuploidy such as trisomy 21 and those with multiple congenital anomalies or hydrops fetalis have a high incidence of pulmonary hypoplasia.

Oligohydramnios, whether caused by premature rupture of membranes or diminished fetal urine production, can lead to pulmonary hypoplasia. The reduction in branching morphogenesis and surface area for gas exchange may be lethal or clinically imperceptible. Clinical studies link the degree of pulmonary hypoplasia to the duration and severity of the oligohydramnios. Similarly, pulmonary hypoplasia is a hallmark of congenital diaphragmatic hernia (CDH), caused by extrinsic compression of the developing fetal lung by the herniated abdominal contents. The degree of pulmonary hypoplasia in CDH is directly related to the extent of herniation. Large hernias occur earlier in gestation. In most cases, the contralateral lung is also hypoplastic.

Lindner and associates[51] report a significant mortality risk for infants born to women with premature rupture of membranes and oligohydramnios before 20 weeks' gestation. Their retrospective analysis demonstrated 69% short-term mortality risk. However, the remaining infants fared well and were discharged with apparently normal pulmonary function. Prediction of clinical outcome is difficult for these infants.

Prenatal diagnosis and treatment of pulmonary hypoplasia are discussed in Chapters 18 and 24. Postnatal treatment for pulmonary hypoplasia is largely supportive. A subset of infants with profound hypoplasia have insufficient surface area for effective gas exchange. These patients typically display profound hypoxemia, respiratory acidosis, pneumothorax, and pulmonary interstitial emphysema. At the other end of the spectrum, some infants have no clinical evidence of pulmonary insufficiency at birth but have diminished reserves

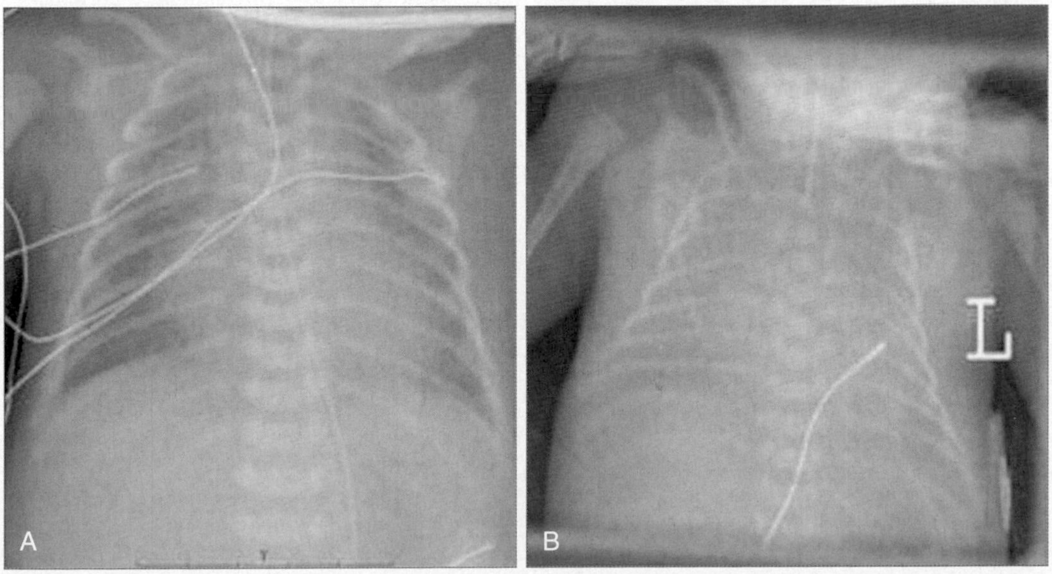

FIGURE 58-3 Radiographic appearance of transient tachypnea of the newborn (TTN) (**A**) and respiratory distress syndrome RDS (**B**). The radiographic characteristics of TTN include perihilar densities with fairly good aeration, bordering on hyperinflation. In contrast, neonates with RDS have diminished lung volumes on chest radiographs reflecting atelectasis associated with surfactant deficiency. Diffuse "ground-glass" infiltrates along with air bronchograms make the cardiothymic silhouette indistinct.

when stressed. In between is a cohort of patients with respiratory insufficiency responsive to mechanical ventilation and pharmacologic support. Typically, these patients have adequate oxygenation and ventilation, suggesting adequate gas exchange capacity. However, many develop pulmonary hypertension. The pathophysiologic sequence begins with limited cross-sectional area of resistance arterioles, followed by smooth muscle hyperplasia in these same vessels. Early use of pulmonary vasodilators such as nitric oxide is the mainstay of management for increased pulmonary vasoreactivity. Optimizing pulmonary blood flow reduces the potential for hypoxemia thought to stimulate pathologic medial hyperplasia. If oxygenation, ventilation, and acid-base balance are maintained, nutritional support and time can allow sufficient lung growth to support the infant's metabolic demands. In many cases, the process is lengthy, requiring mechanical ventilation and treatment with pulmonary vasodilators such as sildenafil, bosentan, or prostacyclin for weeks to months. Just as prenatal prognosis is difficult to assess, predicting outcome for patients with pulmonary hypoplasia managed in the neonatal intensive care unit is hampered by limited data.

Respiratory Distress Syndrome

RDS is a significant cause of early neonatal mortality and long-term morbidity. However, in the past 3 decades, significant advances have been made in the management of RDS, with consequent decreases in associated morbidity and mortality.

Perinatal Risk Factors

The classic risk factors for RDS are prematurity and low birth weight. Factors that negatively affect surfactant synthesis include maternal diabetes, perinatal asphyxia, cesarean delivery without labor, and genetic factors (i.e., white race, history of RDS in siblings, male sex, and surfactant protein B deficiency).[52] Congenital malformations that lead to lung hypoplasia such as diaphragmatic hernia are also associated with significant surfactant deficiency. Prenatal assessment of fetal lung maturity and treatment to induce fetal lung maturity are discussed in detail in Chapter 23.

Clinical Presentation

Symptoms are typically evident in the delivery room, including tachypnea, nasal flaring, subcostal and intercostal retractions, cyanosis, and expiratory grunting. The characteristic expiratory grunt results from expiration through a partially closed glottis, providing continuous distending airway pressure to maintain functional residual capacity and thereby prevent alveolar collapse. These signs of respiratory difficulty are not specific to RDS and have a variety of pulmonary and nonpulmonary causes, such as transient tachypnea, air leaks, congenital malformations, hypothermia, hypoglycemia, anemia, polycythemia, and metabolic acidosis. Progressive worsening of symptoms in the first 2 to 3 days, followed by recovery, characterizes the typical clinical course. This timeline (curve) is modified by administration of exogenous surfactant with a more rapid recovery. Classic radiographic findings include low-volume lungs with a diffuse reticulogranular pattern and air bronchograms. The diagnosis can be established chemically by measuring surfactant activity in tracheal or gastric aspirates, but this is not routinely done.[53]

Management

Infants are managed in an incubator or under a radiant warmer in a neutral thermal environment to minimize oxygen requirement and consumption. Arterial oxygen tension (PaO_2) is maintained between 50 and 80 mm Hg, with saturations between 88% and 96%. Hypercarbia and hyperoxia are avoided. Heart rate, blood pressure, respiratory rate, and peripheral perfusion are monitored closely. Because sepsis cannot be excluded, screening blood culture and complete blood cell counts with differential counts are performed, and infants are started on broad-spectrum antibiotics for at least 48 hours.

SURFACTANT THERAPY

Surfactant replacement is one of the safest and most effective interventions in neonatology. The first successful clinical trial of surfactant use was reported in 1980 using surfactant prepared from an organic solvent extract of bovine lung to treat 10 infants with RDS.[54] By the early 1990s, widespread use of surfactant leads to a progressive decrease in RDS-associated mortality. Two strategies for treatment are commonly used: prophylactic surfactant, in which surfactant is administered before the first breath to all infants at risk for developing RDS, and rescue therapy, in which surfactant is given after the onset of respiratory signs. The advantages of prophylactic administration include a better distribution of surfactant when instilled into a partially fluid filled lung along with the potential to decrease trauma related to resuscitation. Avoiding treatment of unaffected infants and related cost savings are the advantages of rescue therapy. Biologically active surfactant can be prepared from bovine, porcine, human, or synthetic sources. When administered to patients with surfactant deficiency and RDS, all these preparations show improvement in oxygenation and a decreased need for ventilatory support, along with decreased air leaks and death.[55] The combined use of antenatal corticosteroids and postnatal surfactant improves neonatal outcome more than postnatal surfactant therapy alone.

CONTINUOUS POSITIVE AIRWAY PRESSURE

In infants with acute RDS, continuous positive airway pressure (CPAP) appears to prevent atelectasis, minimize lung injury, and preserve surfactant function, allowing infants to be managed without endotracheal intubation and mechanical ventilation. Early delivery room CPAP therapy decreases the need for mechanical ventilation and the incidence of long-term pulmonary morbidity.[56,57] Increasing use of CPAP has led to decreased use of surfactant and decreased incidence of BPD.[58] Common complications of CPAP include pneumothorax and pneumomediastinum. Rarely, the increased transthoracic pressure leads to progressive decrease in venous return and decreased cardiac output. Brief intubation and administration of surfactant followed by extubation to CPAP is an additional RDS treatment strategy increasingly used in Europe and Australia.[59] Prospective, randomized trials enrolling extremely low birth weight (ELBW) infants and comparing early delivery room CPAP with early prophylactic surfactant therapy are being conducted in the National Institute of Child Health and Human Development (NICHD) Neonatal Network (i.e., SUPPORT trial).

MECHANICAL VENTILATION

The goal of mechanical ventilation is to limit volutrauma and barotrauma without causing progressive atelectasis while maintaining adequate gas exchange. Complications associated with mechanical ventilation include pulmonary air leaks, endotracheal tube displacement or dislodgement, obstruction, infection, and long-term complications such as BPD and subglottic stenosis.

Complications

Acute complications include air leaks such as pneumothorax, pneumomediastinum, pneumopericardium, and pulmonary interstitial emphysema. The incidence of these complications has decreased significantly with surfactant treatment. Infection, intracranial hemorrhage, and patent ductus arteriosus occur more frequently in VLBW infants with RDS. Long-term complications and comorbidities include BPD, poor neurodevelopmental outcomes, and retinopathy of prematurity. Incidence of these complications is inversely related to decreasing birth weight and gestation.

Promising new therapies for the treatment of RDS include early inhaled nitric oxide and supplementary inositol for prevention of long-term pulmonary morbidity (e.g., BPD).[60-62] Noninvasive respiratory support techniques such as synchronized nasal intermittent positive ventilation (SNIPPV) and high-flow nasal cannulas are being studied to decrease ventilator associated lung injury.[63,64]

Bronchopulmonary Dysplasia

The classic form of BPD was first described[65] in a group of preterm infants who were mechanically ventilated at birth and who later developed chronic respiratory failure with characteristic radiological findings. These infants were larger, late preterm infants with lung changes attributed to mechanical trauma and oxygen toxicity. Smaller, extremely preterm infants with lung immaturity who have received antenatal glucocorticoids have developed a milder form, called *new BPD*.[66] This disease primarily occurs in infants weighing less than 1000 g who have very mild or no initial respiratory distress. The clinical diagnosis is based on the need for supplemental oxygen at 36 weeks' corrected gestational age.[67] A physiologic definition of BPD based on the need for oxygen at the time of diagnosis has been developed.[68]

Clinically, the transition from RDS to BPD is subtle and gradual. Radiologically, classic BPD is marked by areas of shifting focal atelectasis and hyperinflation with or without parenchymal cyst formation. Chest radiographs of infants with the new BPD show bilateral haziness, reflecting diffuse microatelectasis without multiple cystic changes. These changes lead to ventilation-perfusion mismatching and increased work of breathing. Preterm infants with BPD gradually wean off respiratory support and oxygen or continue to worsen with progressively severe respiratory failure, pulmonary hypertension, and a high mortality risk.

Pathophysiology

Risk factors predisposing preterm infants to BPD include extreme prematurity, oxygen toxicity, mechanical ventilation, and inflammation.[69] The pathologic findings characterized by severe airway injury and fibrosis in the old BPD have been replaced in the new BPD with large, simplified alveolar structures, impaired capillary configuration, and various degrees of interstitial cellularity or fibroproliferation.[70] Airway and vascular lesions tend to be associated with more severe disease.

Oxygen-induced lung injury is an important contributing factor. Exposure to oxygen in the first 2 weeks of life and as chronic therapy has been associated in clinical studies with the severity of BPD.[71,72] In animal models, hyperoxia has been shown to mimic many of the pathologic findings of BPD. Two large, randomized trials in preterm infants suggested that the use of supplemental oxygen to maintain higher saturations resulted in worsening pulmonary outcomes.[73,74] Barotrauma and volutrauma associated with mechanical ventilation have been identified as major factors causing lung injury in preterm infants.[75,76] Surfactant replacement therapy is beneficial in decreasing symptoms of RDS and improving survival. The efficacy of surfactant to decrease the incidence of subsequent BPD is less well established. Chronic inflammation and edema associated with positive-pressure ventilation cause surfactant protein inactivation.

Because intrauterine inflammation is increasingly recognized as a cause of preterm parturition, antenatal inflammation is gaining more attention in the pathogenesis of BPD and other morbidities of prematurity.[77] Chorioamnionitis has been strongly associated with impaired pulmonary and vascular growth, a typical finding in the new BPD.

Most deliveries before 30 weeks' gestation are associated with histologic chorioamnionitis, which except for preterm initiation of labor is otherwise clinically silent. The more preterm the delivery, the more often histologic chorioamnionitis is detected. Increased levels of proinflammatory mediators in amniotic fluid, placental tissues, tracheal aspirates, lung, and serum of ELBW preterm infants support an important role for both intrauterine and extrauterine inflammation in the development and severity of BPD. The proposed interaction between the proinflammatory and anti-inflammatory influences on the developing fetal and preterm lung is detailed in Figure 58-4. Several animal models and preterm studies demonstrate that mediators of inflammation, including endotoxins, tumor necrosis factor, IL-1, IL-6, IL-8, and transforming growth factor α can enhance lung maturation but concurrently impede alveolar septation and vasculogenesis, contributing to the development of BPD.[78-81] Chorioamnionitis alone is associated with BPD, but the probability is increased when these infants receive a second insult such as mechanical ventilation or postnatal infection.[82-84]

Maternal genital mycoplasmal infection, particularly with *Mycoplasma hominis* and *Ureaplasma urealyticum*, is associated with preterm delivery.[85] Numerous studies have isolated these organisms from amniotic fluid and placentas in women with spontaneous preterm birth (i.e., preterm birth due to preterm labor or preterm rupture of membranes). After birth, these organisms are known to colonize and elicit a proinflammatory response in the respiratory tract, leading to BPD.

The unpredictable variation in the incidence of BPD, despite adjusting for low birth weight and prematurity, suggests a genetic predisposition to the occurrence and the severity of BPD. Expression of genes critical to surfactant synthesis, vascular development, and inflammatory regulation are likely to play a role in the pathogenesis of BPD. Twin studies have shown that the BPD status of one twin, even after correcting for contributing factors, is a highly significant predictor of BPD in the second twin. In this particular cohort, after controlling for covariates, genetic factors accounted for 53% of the variance in the liability for BPD.[86] Genetic polymorphisms in the inflammatory response are increasingly recognized as important in the pathogenesis of preterm parturition (see Chapter 28), and may be similarly important in the genesis of inflammatory morbidities in the preterm neonate as well.

Long-Term Complications

Infants with BPD have significant pulmonary sequelae during childhood and adolescence. Reactive airway disease occurs more frequently, with increased risk of bronchiolitis and pneumonia. Up to 50% of infants with BPD require readmission to hospital for lower respiratory tract illness in the first year of life.[87]

BPD is an independent predictor of adverse neurologic outcomes. Infants with BPD exhibit lower average IQs, academic difficulties, delayed speech and language development, impaired visual-motor integration, and behavior problems.[88] Sparse data also suggest an increased risk for attention deficit disorders, memory and learning deficits. Delayed growth occurs in 30% to 60% of infants with BPD at 2 years. The degree of long-term growth delay is inversely proportional to birth weight and directly proportional to the severity of BPD.

Prevention Strategies

Several strategies to decrease the incidence of BPD have been tried, including administration of surfactant in the delivery room, antioxidant superoxide dismutase and vitamin A supplementation, optimizing fluid and parenteral nutrition, aggressive treatment of patent ductus arteriosus, minimizing mechanical ventilation, limiting exposure to high levels of oxygen, and infection prevention. Table 58-4 enumerates current strategies and their relative effectiveness in preventing BPD.[89] Large, controlled clinical trials and meta-analysis have not demonstrated a significant impact of these pharmacologic and nutritional interventions.[90] The multifactorial nature of BPD suggests that targeting individual pathways is unlikely to have a significant effect on outcome. Strategies to address several pathways simultaneously are more promising (Fig. 58-4).

Meconium-Stained Amniotic Fluid and Meconium Aspiration Syndrome

The significance and management of meconium-stained amniotic fluid has evolved with time. Meconium is present in the fetal intestine by the second trimester. Maturation of intestinal smooth muscle and the myenteric plexus progresses through the third trimester. Intrauterine passage of meconium is unusual before 36 weeks and does not typically occur for several days after preterm delivery. The potential for intrauterine meconium passage increases with each week of gestation thereafter.[91] The physiologic stimuli for passage of meconium are still incompletely understood. Clinical experience and epidemiologic data suggest that a stressed fetus may pass meconium before birth. Infants born through meconium-stained amniotic fluid have a lower pH and are likely to have nonreassuring fetal heart tracings.[92] Meconium-stained amniotic fluid at delivery occurs in 12% to 15% of all deliveries and occurs more frequently in post-term gestation and in African Americans.[93]

In contrast to meconium-stained amniotic fluid, meconium aspiration syndrome is unusual. Meconium aspiration syndrome is a clinical diagnosis that includes delivery through meconium-stained amniotic fluid along with respiratory distress and a characteristic appearance on chest radiographs. Approximately 2% of deliveries with meconium-stained amniotic fluid are complicated by meconium aspiration syndrome, but the reported incidence varies widely.[94,95] The severity of the syndrome varies. The hallmarks of severe disease are the need for positive-pressure ventilation and the presence of pulmonary hypertension. Severe meconium aspiration is associated with significant mortality and morbidity risk, including air leak, chronic lung disease, and developmental delay.

A relationship between meconium-stained amniotic fluid and meconium aspiration syndrome has been presumed since the 1960s, when the strategy of tracheal suctioning in the delivery room to prevent meconium aspiration was proposed.[96] By the 1970s, this practice was clinically established and affirmed by retrospective reviews. Oropharyngeal suctioning on the perineum before delivery of the chest to complement tracheal suctioning was also recommended. However, additional studies did not verify the benefit of tracheal suctioning. Tracheal suctioning did not affect the incidence of meconium aspiration syndrome in vigorous infants in large, prospective, randomized trial.[97] Another prospective, randomized, controlled study in 2514 infants to determine the efficacy of oropharyngeal suctioning before delivery of the fetal shoulders in infants born through meconium-stained amniotic fluid also found no reduction in meconium aspiration syndrome.[98] Amnioinfusion during labor to dilute the concentration of meconium has also been studied to prevent meconium aspiration, but a randomized trial found no reduction in the incidence or severity of meconium aspiration.[99] These well-designed clinical trials support the notion that meconium-stained amniotic fluid may

TABLE 58-4 BRONCHOPULMONARY DYSPLASIA PREVENTION STRATEGIES

Intervention	Relative Effectiveness	Evidence or Quality of Data
Antenatal steroids	+	Strong
Early surfactant	++	Strong
Postnatal systemic steroid	++	Moderate
Vitamin A	+	High
Antioxidants	–	Moderate
Permissive hypercapnia	+++	Minimal
Fluid restriction	++	Moderate
High-frequency ventilation	±	Moderate
Delivery room management	++++	Animal data
Inhaled nitric oxide	+	Minimal
Continuous positive airway pressure used early	+++	Moderate

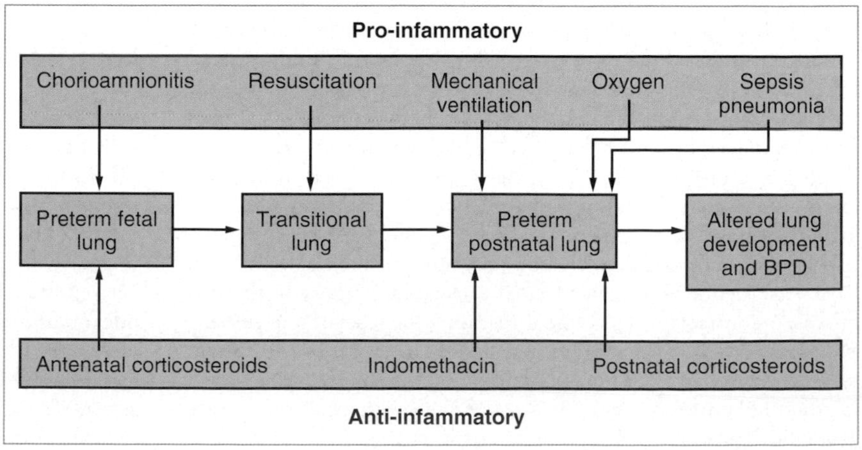

FIGURE 58-4 Role of inflammation in the pathogenesis of bronchopulmonary dysplasia (BPD).

not have a true mechanistic, pathophysiologic connection with meconium aspiration syndrome.

In 2001, Ghidini and Spong[100] questioned the connection between meconium-stained amniotic fluid and meconium aspiration syndrome. Reports describe infants born through clear amniotic fluid with respiratory distress with pulmonary hypertension and other clinical characteristics of meconium aspiration syndrome.[101] Experimental data suggest that factors promoting fetal acidosis and hypoxemia promote remodeling of resistance pulmonary arteries. These same factors can promote intrauterine meconium passage. However, the remodeling, perhaps exacerbated by inflammation from infection or by meconium, produces a clinical syndrome called *meconium aspiration syndrome.*[102,103] The incidence of meconium aspiration syndrome has decreased in several centers over the past several years, perhaps a consequence of improvements in obstetric assessment and management,[104,105] including a reduction in the incidence of post-term deliveries. Our center has experienced a decline in meconium aspiration syndrome while concurrently pursuing a policy of no routine tracheal suctioning for infants born through meconium-stained amniotic fluid.

Treatment of severe meconium aspiration syndrome has dramatically improved in recent years, leading to decreases in morbidity and mortality. Significant advances have come from treatment of pulmonary hypertension with selective pulmonary vasodilators, including inhaled nitric oxide, sildenafil, and bosentan. These improve oxygenation and enable less injurious ventilator strategies with reduced subsequent morbidity from air leak and chronic lung disease. Exogenous surfactant administration may be another useful treatment modality. Although the mechanism is unclear, this intervention reduces ventilation-perfusion mismatch and probably reduces the risk of ventilator-associated lung injury.[106]

The current state of knowledge regarding meconium-stained amniotic fluid and meconium aspiration syndrome presents challenges for obstetricians and neonatologists. The incidence of meconium aspiration syndrome has decreased, but the reasons for the decline are not readily apparent. The Neonatal Resuscitation Program[35] protocol for delivery room management no longer recommends tracheal suctioning for vigorous infants, implying that airway management leading to establishment of ventilation should take precedence. Meconium or other material obstructing the airway should be cleared, but suctioning an unobstructed airway at the expense of delaying initiation of effective ventilation may be deleterious. A collaborative approach between obstetrician and neonatologist is paramount. Personnel skilled in establishment of ventilation and airway patency should attend any infant expected to be depressed at delivery.

Pulmonary Hypertension

At delivery the normal transition from fetal to neonatal pulmonary circulation is mediated by a rapid, dramatic decrease in pulmonary vascular resistance. Endothelial cell shape change, relaxation of pulmonary arteriolar smooth muscle, and alveolar gaseous distention all contribute to this process. Several pathologic processes, including congenital malformations, sepsis, and pneumonia, can alter this sequence to produce neonatal pulmonary hypertension. It typically accompanies pulmonary hypoplasia when diminished surface area for gas exchange and inadequate pulmonary blood flow lead to hypoxia and remodeling of the resistance pulmonary arterioles. These vessels are more prone to constriction under conditions of acidosis and hypoxemia, resulting in the right to left shunting of deoxygenated blood characteristic of neonatal persistent pulmonary hypertension. In neonates, pulmonary hypertension tends to mimic prenatal physiology when pulmonary vascular resistance is necessarily high.

First principles of management include optimal oxygenation and ventilation through elimination of ventilation-perfusion mismatch. When positive-pressure ventilation is employed, overdistention must be avoided to minimize the risk of lung injury and BPD. Treatment of pulmonary hypertension has been revolutionized by pharmacologic interventions that specifically reduce pulmonary vascular resistance. Of these, nitric oxide is the best studied, with clear evidence of efficacy for treatment of pulmonary hypertension in the setting of meconium aspiration syndrome or sepsis.[107] Clinical experience with other pulmonary vasodilators, including sildenafil, bosentan, and prostacyclin, is increasing and has proved useful in certain clinical situations.[108]

Excessive proliferation of medial smooth muscle or its presence in vessels ordinarily devoid of smooth muscle complicates the treatment of pulmonary hypertension. This pathologic remodeling can occur in utero or during postnatal life. The stimuli for this process are not understood, but typically include hypoxic stress of extended duration and volutrauma associated with mechanical ventilation. Pulmonary vasodilators become less effective as remodeling progresses, prompting clinicians to pursue "gentle" ventilation strategies.[109] By focusing on preductal rather than postductal oxygen saturations, lower ventilator settings can be achieved, reducing the risk of remodeling.

Gastrointestinal Problems in Neonatal Period

Necrotizing enterocolitis (NEC) is a devastating complication of prematurity and the most common gastrointestinal emergency in the neonatal period. It affects 1% to 5% of infants admitted to neonatal intensive care units.[110] The reported incidence is 4% to 13%[111] in VLBW infants (<1500 g). NEC is characterized by an inflammation of the intestines, which can progress to transmural necrosis and perforation. The onset typically occurs within the first 2 to 3 weeks of life, but it can occur well beyond the first month. The mortality rate related to NEC ranges from 10% to 30% for all cases and up to 50% for infants requiring surgery.[111-114] As more preterm and low-birth-weight infants survive the initial days of life, the number of infants at risk for NEC has increased. From 1982 to 1992, although overall U.S. neonatal mortality rates declined, the mortality rates for NEC increased.[26]

A variety of antenatal and postnatal exposures have been suggested as risk factors for the development of NEC.[112,113,115] Gestational age and birth weight are consistently related to NEC. Among prenatal factors, indomethacin tocolysis has been most often reported. Some studies report reduced incidence of NEC in infants treated with antenatal steroids.[116-118]

Initial trials on use of indomethacin as a tocolytic showed no adverse neonatal affects although sample sizes were small.[119,120] Although some subsequent case reports and retrospective reviews suggested indomethacin might be associated with adverse neonatal outcomes, including NEC,[121,122] others found no association[123,124] of indomethacin tocolysis with NEC when used as a single agent but did find an increased risk when used as part of double-agent tocolytic therapy, even after controlling for neonatal sepsis. A meta-analysis of randomized, controlled trials and observational studies from 1966 though 2004 found no significant association between indomethacin tocolysis and NEC in either study type, although the pooled sample size of the published randomized, controlled trials limited statistical power.[125] There is insufficient evidence to alter use of antenatal indomethacin in relationship to NEC (see Chapter 29).

Postnatal interventions to prevent the development of NEC include alterations in feeding type and advancements, oral antibiotics, immune globulin use and vitamin supplementation. Decreased incidence of NEC has been demonstrated only for human milk. A meta-analysis of randomized, controlled trials evaluating use of human milk and NEC found a fourfold decrease (relative risk [RR] = 0.25; 95% confidence interval [CI], 0.06 to 0.98) with the use of human milk.[126] Mothers of infants at risk, particularly those less than 32 weeks' gestation, should be encouraged to supply breast milk for their infant. Providing early prenatal and postnatal counseling on use of human milk increases the initiation of lactation and neonatal intake of mother's milk without increasing maternal stress or anxiety.[127] Newer preventive interventions being explored include the use of probiotics and growth factors aimed at protecting the gut epithelium.[128]

NEC may present slowly or as a sudden catastrophic event. Abdominal distention occurs early, with bloody stools present in 25% of cases.[110] The radiographic hallmark is the presence of pneumatosis intestinalis or portal venous gas (see Fig. 58-2). Progression may be rapid, resulting in bowel perforation with evidence of free air on the radiograph. Early management consists of bowel decompression, intravenous antibiotics, and respiratory and cardiovascular support as indicated. The single absolute indication for surgical intervention is pneumoperitoneum (Fig. 58-5).

For infants who survive NEC, morbidity is high, including high rates of growth failure, chronic lung disease, and nosocomial infections.[129-131] Lengths of stay and hospital costs are significantly lengthened, particularly in surgical NEC.[131] Long-term neurologic outcomes are adversely affected. NEC is an independent risk factor for development of cerebral palsy and developmental delay.[129,130,132] For infants with surgical NEC, depending on the amount of bowel lost, there is risk of short gut syndrome requiring parenteral nutrition and, ultimately, small bowel or liver transplantation. NEC is the single most common cause of the short gut syndrome in children.[27-29]

Hyperbilirubinemia

Hyperbilirubinemia is common; 60% of term infants and 80% of preterm infants develop jaundice in the first week of life.[133] Bilirubin levels are elevated in neonates due to increased production coupled with decreased excretion. Increased production is related to higher rates of red cell turnover and shorter red cell life span.[134] Rates of excretion are lower because of diminished activity of glucoronosyltransferase, limiting bilirubin conjugation, and increased enterohepatic circulation. In most cases, jaundice has no clinical significance because bilirubin levels remain low, and it is transient. Less than 3% develop levels greater than 15 mg/dL.[133] Risk factors for development of severe jaundice are outlined in Table 58-5.

Several important risk factors have their origin in the prenatal and perinatal environment. Hyperbilirubinemia is seen more frequently in infants of mothers who are diabetic (IDM). The pathogenesis of increased bilirubin in IDM infants is uncertain but has been attributed to polycythemia as well as increased red cell turnover.[136,137] Prenatally, maternal blood group immunization may result from blood transfusion or fetal maternal hemorrhage. Although the prevalence of Rh(D) immunization has significantly decreased with the advent of prevention programs, including use of Rh immune globulin, antibodies to other blood group antigens may still occur. ABO hemolytic disease, a common cause of severe jaundice in the newborn, rarely causes hemo-

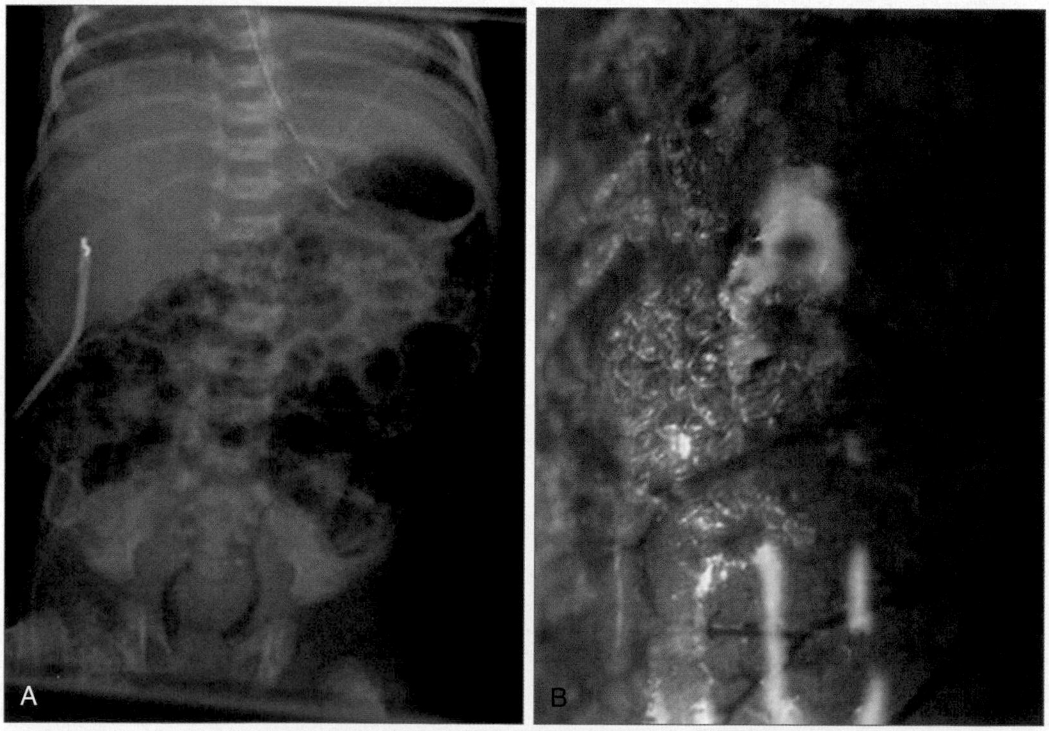

FIGURE 58-5 Diagnosis and pathology of necrotizing enterocolitis. **A,** Typical radiographic appearance of necrotizing enterocolitis, demonstrating pneumatosis and intramural gas. **B,** Intraoperative photograph of the small bowel, which contains intramural gas.

TABLE 58-5 COMMON CLINICAL RISK FACTORS FOR SEVERE HYPERBILIRUBINEMIA

Jaundice in the first 24 hours
Visible jaundice before discharge
Previous jaundiced sibling
Exclusive breastfeeding
Bruising, cephalohematoma
East Asian, Mediterranean, or Native American origin or ethnicity
Maternal age >25 years
Male sex
Unrecognized hemolysis (i.e., ABO, Rh, c, C, E, Kell, and other minor blood group antigens)
Glucose-6-phosphate dehydrogenase deficiency
Infant of a diabetic mother

Adapted from Centers for Disease Control and Prevention: Kernicterus in full-term infants; United States, 1994-1998. Report No.: 50(23), 2001.

lytic disease in the fetus. Other antibodies associated with hemolytic disease in the fetus and newborn are discussed in Chapter 26. A fetus who is apparently unaffected in utero may have continued hemolysis postnatally; physicians caring for the newborn should be notified of any maternal sensitization.

Other perinatal factors associated with severe hyperbilirubinemia include delivery before 38 weeks. Infants born at 36 to 37 weeks' gestation have an almost sixfold increase of significant hyperbilirubinemia[138] and require close surveillance and monitoring, especially if breastfed.[139] Feeding difficulties, also common for the near term infant, increase this risk still further and may result in delayed hospital discharge or readmission for the infant. The presence of bruising or a cephalohematoma, more common after instrumented or difficult deliveries, will also increase risk. Polymorphisms of genes coding for enzymes mediating bilirubin catabolism may also contribute to the development of severe hyperbilirubinemia.[140]

The primary consequence of severe hyperbilirubinemia is potential neurotoxicity. Kernicterus is a neurologic syndrome resulting from deposition of unconjugated bilirubin in the basal ganglia and brainstem nuclei, and neuronal necrosis.[141] Clinical features may be acute or chronic, resulting in tone and movement disorders such as choreoathetosis and spastic quadriplegia, mental retardation, and sensorineural hearing loss.[142] A number of factors influence the neurotoxic effects of bilirubin, making prediction of outcome difficult. Bilirubin more easily enters the brain if it is not bound to albumin, is unconjugated, or there is increased permeability of the blood brain barrier.[142] Conditions such as prematurity that alter albumin levels or that alter the blood brain barrier such as infection, acidosis, and prematurity affect bilirubin entry into the brain. As a result, there is no serum level of bilirubin that predicts outcome. In early studies of infants with Rh hemolytic disease, kernicterus developed in 8% of infants with serum bilirubin concentrations of 19 to 24 mg/dL, 33% with levels of 25 to 29 mg/dL, and 73% of infants with levels of 30 to 40 mg/dL.[141]

Levels of indirect bilirubin below 25 mg/dL in otherwise term healthy infants without hemolytic disease are unlikely to result in kernicterus without other risk factors, as indicated in a study of 140 term and near-term infants with levels above 25 mg/dL, in which no cases of kernicterus occurred.[143] Kernicterus has however been reported in otherwise healthy breastfed term newborns at levels above 30 mg/dL.[144] One of the most important of these risk factors is prematurity. The less mature the infant the greater the susceptibility of the neonatal brain.[141] At what level more subtle neurologic abnormalities appear remains unclear.[139]

Management of hyperbilirubinemia is aimed at the prevention of bilirubin encephalopathy while minimizing interference with breastfeeding and unnecessary parental anxiety. Key elements in prevention include systematic evaluation of newborns before discharge for the presence of jaundice and its risk factors, promotion and support of successful breastfeeding, interpretation of jaundice levels based on the hour of life, parental education, and appropriate neonatal follow-up based on time of discharge.[139] Treatment of severe hyperbilirubinemia should be initiated promptly when identified. Guidelines for treatment with phototherapy and exchange transfusion vary with gestational age, the presence or absence of risk factors, and the hour of life. Nomograms to guide patient management are available from the American Academy of Pediatrics.[139] Kernicterus is largely preventable. It requires close collaboration between prenatal and postnatal caretakers for accurate dissemination of information regarding risk factors for parents and caregivers.

Feeding Problems

Feeding problems related to complications of prematurity, congenital anomalies, or gastrointestinal disorders contribute significantly to length of stay for hospitalized newborns. In a study of children referred to an interdisciplinary feeding team, 38% were born preterm.[145] Premature infants with a history of neonatal chronic lung disease or neurologic injury such as IVH or periventricular leukomalacia (PVL) and those with a history of NEC are at the highest risk for long-term feeding problems. These medically complex infants often have other comorbidities, such as tracheomalacia, chronic aspiration, and gastroesophageal reflux (GER), that interfere with normal maturational patterns of feeding. Premature infants with complex medical problems often require prolonged intubation and mechanical ventilation with delayed initiation of enteral feeding, all of which have been associated with subsequent feeding difficulties. These infants often have difficulty integrating sensory input because of medical interventions and neurologic immaturity. All of these factors combine to increase the risk of developing oral aversion.

Infants with congenital anomalies are also at high risk for feeding disorders. Infants with tracheoesophageal fistula with esophageal atresia often have difficulty feeding due to tracheomalacia, recurrent esophageal stricture, and GER, which are known associates of this disorder. Infants with CDH have an extremely high incidence of oral aversion and growth problems in addition to the pulmonary complications. Surviving infants and children with CDH have a 60% to 80% incidence of associated GER which has been shown to persist into adulthood.[146-151] Often, GER is severe, refractory to medical therapy, and requires a surgical antireflux procedure. Infants with CDH often have inadequate caloric intake due to fatigue or oral aversion and increased energy requirements leading to poor growth. Often these infants require supplemental tube feedings by nasogastric, nasojejunal, or gastrostomy feeding tube. These feeding difficulties may last several years and are often accompanied by a behavioral-based feeding component.

Infants with congenital or acquired gastrointestinal abnormalities often have associated feeding difficulties. Infants with conditions such as gastroschisis with or without associated intestinal atresias often require prolonged hospitalization because of a slow tolerance of enteral feedings and a higher risk for NEC after gastroschisis repair.[152,153] They often have dysmotility and severe GER with oral aversion.[154] A small percentage of patients have long-term intolerance of enteral feedings and require prolonged total parenteral nutrition (TPN). Patients requiring long-term TPN may develop liver injury or cholestasis and ultimately may require liver or small bowel transplantation. Infants who develop short bowel syndrome resulting from NEC also have difficulties tolerating enteral feeds, depending on the length and function of the remaining bowel. Like patients with gastroschisis, infants with severe short bowel syndrome may require prolonged TPN and go on to develop liver or intestinal failure requiring transplantation.

In summary, premature infants and infants with congenital anomalies or acquired gastrointestinal abnormalities are at high risk for long-term feeding problems. It is important to counsel families regarding this risk. Minimizing iatrogenic oral aversion is crucial. Involving a feeding specialist early in a medically complex infant's course may help reduce these problems.

Neurologic Problems in the Neonatal Period

Hypoxic-Ischemic Encephalopathy

Injury to the brain sustained during the perinatal period was once thought to be one of the most common causes of death or severe, long-term neurologic deficits in children.[155] However, data show that only 10% of brain injury is related to perinatal or intrapartum events.[156,157] There is increasing recognition that events occurring well before labor contribute significantly to the cause of brain injury. Despite improvements in perinatal practice, the incidence of hypoxic-ischemic encephalopathy has remained stable at 1 or 2 cases per 1000 term births.[158,159] Strategies for prevention of brain injury have been mainly supportive because prevention has been difficult because of the lack of clinically reliable indicators and the occurrence of the initiating event well before the onset of labor. However, because brain injury initiated by a hypoxic-ischemic event is also affected by a "reperfusion phase" of injury, strategies targeting this process of ongoing injury are being developed for neuroprotection.[160,161]

Definition of Asphyxia

The brain injury referred to as hypoxic-ischemic encephalopathy occurs due to impaired cerebral blood flow likely as a consequence of interrupted placental blood flow leading to impaired gas exchange.[162] If gas exchange is persistently impaired, hypoxemia and hypercapnia develop with resultant fetal acidosis or what has been referred to as *asphyxia*. Severe fetal acidemia, defined as an umbilical arterial pH of less than 7.00, is associated with an increased risk of adverse neurologic outcome.[163,164] However, even with this degree of acidemia, only a small portion of infants develop significant encephalopathy and subsequent sustained neurologic injury.[165-167] Fetal scalp blood sampling and umbilical cord gas data do not have great sensitivity to predict long-term neurologic impairment.

Clinical Markers

Other clinical measures to identify fetal stress (such as fetal heart rate abnormalities, meconium-stained amniotic fluid, low Apgar scores, and need for cardiopulmonary resuscitation CPR) in the delivery room do not reliably identify infants at high risk for brain injury when used in isolation. Despite the widespread use of electronic fetal heart rate monitoring (EFM) which detects changes in fetal heart rate related to fetal oxygenation, there has been no reduction in the incidence of cerebral palsy.[163] In 2005, an American College of Obstetricians and Gynecologists (ACOG) practice bulletin called "Clinical Management Guidelines for Obstetrician-Gynecologists"[164] concluded that EFM has a high false-positive rate to predict adverse outcomes and is associated with an increase in operative deliveries without any reduction in cerebral palsy. Meconium-stained amniotic fluid is commonly seen during labor, but no data exist to associate it with adverse neurologic outcome. Apgar scores were originally introduced to identify infants in need of resuscitation, not to predict neurologic outcome. Apgar scores are not specific to an infant's acid-base status but can reflect drug use, metabolic disorder, trauma, hypovolemia, infection, neuromuscular disorder, and congenital anomalies. However, a persistently low Apgar score after 5 minutes despite intensive CPR has been associated with increased morbidity and mortality.[162,168-170] The combination of a low 5-minute Apgar score with other markers such as fetal acidemia and the need for CPR in the delivery room, predicts a significantly increased risk of brain injury.[171,172] Perlman and Risser[172] found a 340-fold increased risk of seizures and associated moderate to severe encephalopathy in association with a 5-minute Apgar score of 5, delivery room intubation or CPR, and an umbilical arterial cord pH less than 7.00.

Neonatal Encephalopathy

Neonatal encephalopathy is clinically characterized by depressed level of consciousness, abnormal muscle tone and reflexes, abnormal respiratory pattern, and seizures.[155] These findings may result from a hypoxic-ischemic event but can also be due to other conditions such as metabolic disorders, neuromuscular disorders, toxin exposure, and chromosomal abnormalities or syndromes. Not all infants with neonatal encephalopathy go on to develop permanent neurologic impairment. The Sarnat staging system is frequently used to classify the degree of encephalopathy and predict neurologic outcome.[166] Infants with mild encephalopathy (Sarnat stage 1) generally have a favorable outcome. Infants with moderate encephalopathy (Sarnat stage 2) develop long-term neurologic compromise in 20% to 25% of cases, and infants with severe encephalopathy (Sarnat stage 3) have a greater than 80% risk of death or long-term neurologic sequelae.[155]

Multiorgan Injury

In addition to neurologic compromise, the interruption of placental blood flow can result in systemic organ injury. Animal models and clinical studies have demonstrated that the kidney is exquisitely sensitive to reductions in renal blood flow.[173,174] The result of decreased renal perfusion is acute tubular necrosis with varying degrees of oliguria and azotemia. Other organ systems are also sensitive to reduced blood flow. Decreased blood flow to the gastrointestinal tract can lead to luminal ischemia and increased risk for NEC. Decreased pulmonary blood flow can result in persistent pulmonary hypertension of the newborn. Lack of blood flow to the liver can result in hepatocellular injury and impaired synthetic function, leading to hypoglycemia and disseminated intravascular coagulation. Fluid retention and hyponatremia can develop due to the combination of impaired renal function and the release of antidiuretic hormone. Suppression of parathyroid hormone release can lead to hypocalcemia and hypomagnesemia. These electrolyte abnormalities can further affect myocardial function. Muscle can be affected by electrolyte abnormalities and direct cellular injury, leading to rhabdomyolysis.[162]

Neuropathology

The reduction in cerebral blood flow associated with a hypoxic-ischemic event sets off a complex cascade of regional circulatory factors and biochemical changes at the cellular level. Hypoxia induces a switch from normal oxidative phosphorylation to anaerobic metabolism, leading to depletion of high-energy phosphate reserves, accumulation of lactic acid, and inability to maintain cellular functions.[161,175] The end result is cellular energy failure, metabolic acidosis, release of glutamate and intracellular calcium, lipid peroxidation, build-up of nitric oxide, and eventual cell death.[155,161,176] It is this process of cellular injury that is being targeted for neuroprotection strategies.

Neuroimaging

Diffusion-weighted magnetic resonance imaging (MRI) has become the gold standard to define the extent and potentially the timing of the brain injury. Diffusion-weighted techniques can detect signal changes due to reduced brain water diffusivity within the first 24 to 48 hours of the insult.[162,177-179] Magnetic resonance spectroscopy can also detect alterations in metabolites such as lactate, *N*-acetyl aspartate, choline, and creatinine in specific regions of the brain indicating injury.[177,180] However, MRI is difficult to perform in an unstable patient, and computed tomography (CT) may be preferable as the initial study for term infants and ultrasound for preterm infants.

Neuroprotection Strategies

Brain cooling by selective cooling of the head or systemic hypothermia has been studied as a potential therapy for neonates with hypoxic-ischemic encephalopathy. The Cool Cap Study Group found no significant improvement in survival or severe neurodevelopmental disability in 234 term infants with moderate to severe neonatal encephalopathy and abnormal amplitude integrated electroencephalography (aEEG) in a multicenter, randomized trial of selective head cooling.[165] However, there was improvement in infants with less severe aEEG changes in a subgroup analysis.[165] A large, multicenter, randomized trial of brain cooling using whole-body hypothermia for infants of 36 weeks' gestation with moderate or severe encephalopathy found that systemic hypothermia resulted in an 18% reduction of death or moderate or severe disability at 18 to 22 months of age.[181] Proposed reasons for the greater benefit in the latter study from the NICHD Neonatal Research Network are earlier initiation of cooling and possible differences in the severity of brain injury (Cool Cap study required the additional evidence of an abnormal aEEG).[165] There are insufficient data to suggest that one method of brain cooling is superior to the other. Until more data are available, treatment with brain cooling is best considered an experimental technique.[167]

Because the therapeutic window for effective treatment may be limited to within 6 hours of delivery, future efforts are being focused on early identification of infants at the greatest risk for hypoxic-ischemic injury. Infants at highest risk are those with evidence of a sentinel event during labor, pronounced respiratory and neuromuscular depression at delivery with persistently low Apgar scores, the need for delivery room resuscitation, severe fetal acidemia (umbilical artery pH less than7.00 or base deficit of 16 mEq/L), and evidence of an early abnormal neurologic examination, seizures, or an abnormal aEEG.[161,172,182-184]

Summary of Hypoxic-Ischemic Brain Injury

Hypoxic-ischemic brain injury due to intrapartum asphyxia is a rare but serious cause of long-term neurodevelopmental disability. It is often difficult to define a specific intrapartum event because the initiating event may occur before the onset of labor. Early identification of at-risk newborns by neuroimaging techniques, aEEG findings, history, and clinical examination may provide an opportunity to ameliorate the effects of ongoing brain injury using neuroprotective strategies. The goal of these therapeutic interventions is the reduction of long-term neurodevelopmental disabilities, including cerebral palsy.

Intraventricular Hemorrhage

IVH (i.e., germinal matrix hemorrhage) occurs most commonly in preterm infants and is a major cause of mortality and long-term disability. Bleeding originates in the subependymal germinal matrix but may rupture through the ependyma into the ventricular system. IVH is graded into four categories:

Grade I: Bleeding is localized to the germinal matrix
Grade II: Bleeding into the ventricle but the clot does not distend the ventricle
Grade III: Bleeding into the ventricle with ventricular dilation
Grade IV: Intraparenchymal extension

Incidence

Diagnosis is made most commonly by cranial ultrasound, with most hemorrhages occurring within 6 hours of birth and 90% within the first 5 days of life.[185] The incidence of IVH has decreased significantly with improvements in perinatal care such as maternal transfer and antenatal steroids. From 1990 to 1999, the incidence of IVH reported for infants with birth weights of less than 1000 g was 43%, and 13% were grade III or grade IV. In 2000 and 2002, the overall incidence of IVH decreased to 22%; only 3% were severe despite improvements in survival.[186] Lower gestational age is associated with an increased risk of severe IVH.[168]

Pathogenesis

Anatomic and physiologic factors have been implicated in the pathogenesis of IVH. The germinal matrix is composed of thin-walled blood vessels that lack supportive tissue. These fragile vessels have a tendency to rupture spontaneously or in response to stress, such as hypoxia-ischemia, changes in blood pressure or cerebral perfusion, and pneumothoraces. In addition to these structural factors, premature infants have an immature cerebrovascular autoregulation system (so-called pressure-passive circulation) in response to systemic hypotension, which makes them more susceptible to hemorrhage.[174,185,187] Immaturities in the coagulation system and increased fibrinolytic activity of premature infants may also play a role.[169,188-190]

Outcomes

Although it has been generally thought that infants with grade I or II IVH have similar outcomes to those without cranial ultrasound abnormalities, extremely-low-birth-weight infants with grade I or II IVH had worse neurodevelopmental outcomes at 20 months corrected age compared with those with normal cranial ultrasound scans in a 2006 report.[191] About 35% of infants with grade III IVH have adverse neurologic outcomes. In those who develop post-hemorrhagic hydrocephalus requiring surgical intervention, the disability rate increases to about 60%.[169] Grade IV IVH is associated with the highest mortality rates, and 80% to 90% are associated with poor neurologic outcomes.[170]

Antenatal Prevention

The only therapies shown to decrease the incidence of IVH in premature infants are antenatal corticosteroid administration and maternal transfer to a tertiary care center for delivery. Multiple studies have shown that the administration of corticosteroids before preterm delivery to induce lung maturity has significantly reduced the incidence of RDS, mortality, and severe IVH. According to a meta-analysis of four trials that included 596 infants of 24 to 33 weeks' gestation, prenatal corticosteroid therapy was associated with a relative risk reduction for

IVH of 0.57 (95% CI, 0.41 to 0.78).[171] Maternal transfer to a tertiary care center for gestational age less than 32 weeks decreased the incidence of death or major morbidity, including IVH.[39] Antenatal phenobarbital, vitamin K, and magnesium sulfate have failed to demonstrate a consistent decrease in overall IVH, severe IVH, or death.[192-194]

Postnatal Prevention

The goal of postnatal prevention has been blood pressure stabilization to prevent fluctuations in cerebral perfusion, correction of coagulation disturbances, and stabilization of germinal matrix vasculature.[185] Postnatal administration of phenobarbital and muscle paralysis have been shown to stabilize blood pressure, but neither has been found to decrease the incidence of IVH or neurologic impairment.[195,196] Fresh-frozen plasma and ethamsylate to promote platelet adhesiveness and correct coagulation disorders also do not reduce the incidence of IVH.[194,197-199] Indomethacin remains the most promising preventive therapy for IVH because of its ability to constrict the cerebral vasculature, inhibit prostaglandin and free radical production, and mature the germinal matrix vasculature.[197,200-202] Prophylactic indomethacin decreases the incidence of severe IVH. Follow-up studies have shown slight improvement in cognitive function in infants who received prophylactic indomethacin but no difference in the incidence of cerebral palsy.[203-205] Prophylactic indomethacin is reserved for preterm infants at high risk for IVH until further studies clarify the appropriate candidates for prophylaxis.

Post-hemorrhagic Hydrocephalus

The most serious complication of IVH is post-hemorrhagic hydrocephalus due to obstruction of cerebrospinal fluid (CSF) flow. This occurs when multiple blood clots obstruct CSF reabsorption channels, leading to transforming growth factor β1 (TGF-β1)–stimulated production of extracellular matrix proteins such as fibronectin and laminin, which ultimately lead to scar formation.[206] Progressive ventricular dilatation can worsen brain injury because of damage to periventricular white matter resulting from increased intracranial pressure and edema.[172] Therapies such as serial lumbar punctures, diuretics, and intraventricular fibrinolytic therapy are ineffective and may even be harmful.[207] Although surgical shunt placement carries significant risk of shunt complications and infection, it remains the definitive therapy for progressive post-hemorrhagic hydrocephalus.

Summary of Intraventricular Hemorrhage

IVH due to a fragile germinal matrix and an unstable cerebrovascular autoregulatory system remains a significant cause of neurologic morbidity in preterm infants. Infants with cardiorespiratory complications are at highest risk. Antenatal corticosteroids are the most effective preventive therapy available. Despite significant reduction in the incidence of severe IVH, new prevention and treatment therapies for hydrocephalus are needed.

Periventricular Leukomalacia

PVL refers to injury to the deep cerebral white matter in two characteristic patterns, described as *focal periventricular necrosis* and *diffuse cerebral white matter injury*. This type of brain injury typically affects premature infants and is a common cause of cerebral palsy. Preterm infants who have suffered an IVH or have cardiopulmonary instability are at the highest risk. Other intrauterine factors, such as infection, premature prolonged rupture of membranes, first-trimester hemorrhage, placental abruption, and prolonged tocolysis, have been associated with increased risk of PVL.[174,208-211] The reported incidence of PVL detected by ultrasound examination in VLBW infants is 5% to 15%.[212] However, ultrasound often fails to identify the more subtle evidence of diffuse white matter injury. The incidence of PVL diagnosed at autopsy is much higher, indicating that the true incidence of PVL is likely underestimated.

Neuropathology

Focal necrosis most commonly occurs in the cerebral white matter at the level of the trigone of the lateral ventricles and around the foramen of Monro.[212] These sites make up the border zones of the long penetrating arteries. Classically, these lesions undergo a coagulative necrosis that results in cyst formation or focal glial scars.[174] The more diffuse type of injury may also occur in conjunction with focal necrosis but is more frequently recognized as an independent entity. Diffuse white matter injury seems to affect premyelinating oligodendrocytes and leads to global loss of these cells and an increase in hypertrophic astrocytes in response to the diffuse injury.[174,212-214] This loss of oligodendrocytes leads to white matter volume loss and ventriculomegaly.

Pathogenesis

The pathogenesis of PVL primarily occurs by hypoxia-ischemia leading to neuronal injury due to free radical exposure, cytokine toxicity, and exposure to excessive excitatory neurotransmitters such as glutamate.[174] Vascular anatomic factors also seem to play a role. PVL tends to occur in arterial end zones or so-called border zones.[215] The arterial supply is composed of long penetrating arteries that terminate deep in the periventricular white matter, basal penetrating arteries, which supply the immediate periventricular area, and short penetrating arteries, which supply the subcortical white matter. Focal necrosis occurs most commonly in the anterior and posterior periventricular border zones because in premature infants these vessels are immature. Diffuse white matter injury may also occur due to vascular immaturity. At early gestations (24 to 28 weeks), there are few anastomoses between the long and short penetrators. Arterial border zones may occur in the subcortical and remote periventricular areas, resulting in a more diffuse type of injury.[212]

The preterm brain is vulnerable to ischemia because of impaired cerebrovascular regulation. Preterm infants exhibit a pressure-passive circulation; a decrease in systemic blood pressure is associated with a decrease in cerebral perfusion, leading to ischemia.[212,216,217] Immature oligodendrocytes seem to be more sensitive to free radical injury, cytokine effects, and the presence of glutamate.

Clinical Outcomes

The most common long-term sequela of PVL is spastic diplegia, a form of cerebral palsy in which the lower extremities are more affected than the upper extremities. The descending fibers of the motor cortex, which regulate function of the lower extremities, traverse the periventricular area and are most likely to be injured. More severe injury with lateral extension may be associated with spastic quadriplegia or other manifestations such as cognitive, visual, or auditory impairments.

Summary of Periventricular Leukomalacia

PVL is a major cause of neurologic morbidity in premature infants, especially those who weigh less than 1000 g at birth. Prevention is the only strategy to treat PVL. Avoidance of fluctuations in blood pressure and cerebral vasoconstrictors, such as extreme hypocarbia, is important because of the known immaturity in cerebrovascular autoregulation of preterm infants. Investigational strategies targeting the cascade of oligodendroglial death may be promising.

Perinatal Stroke

Arterial ischemic stroke (AIS) in neonates is defined as a cerebrovascular event around the time of birth with resultant clinical or radiographic evidence of focal cerebral arterial infarction. Most occur in the distribution of the middle cerebral artery.[176,218-220] AIS accounts for most perinatal ischemic strokes. When the diagnosis is based on symptoms in the neonatal period, the reported incidence is 1 case in 4000 live births.[176,221,222] The incidence of perinatal ischemic strokes that were asymptomatic in the neonatal period and diagnosed at a later time is unknown.

Clinical Presentation

Neonatal seizures are the most common clinical presentation and usually are focal in origin without other signs of neonatal encephalopathy.[176,223] However, some infants are systemically ill, and the diagnosis is made with neuroimaging to rule out evidence of hypoxic-ischemic injury or bleeding. Neonates with focal neurologic signs account for less than 25% of cases.[218,222,224,225]

Perinatal stroke may also be identified retrospectively in initially well-appearing infants who present in later months with signs of hemiparesis, developmental delay, or seizures.[176,226] In these cases, neuroimaging reveals a remote injury, often occurring in the middle cerebral artery territory.

Pathophysiology and Risk Factors

The mechanisms of perinatal stroke are thought to be multifactorial. Regional ischemia with subsequent hypoxia and infarction plays a role. A relative hypercoagulable state in newborns due to the presence of fetal hemoglobin, polycythemia, and activation of coagulation factors in the fetus and mother around the time of birth seems to increase the risk of a thromboembolic event leading to stoke.[176,227] Risk factors for perinatal stroke include maternal and placental disorders, neonatal hypoxic-ischemic injury, hematologic disorders, infection, cardiac disorders, trauma, and drugs. Often, a combination of risk factors is identified.

Neuroimaging and Electroencephalographic Assessment

Although cranial ultrasound is the easiest to perform, it is not a sensitive indicator of perinatal stroke.[175] Little information exists on prenatal cranial ultrasound, but prenatal ultrasound scans may show areas of unilateral echolucencies, which may represent areas later identified as prenatal stroke. CT imaging can usually be performed readily in neonates and usually does not require sedation. CT evidence of perinatal ischemic stroke includes focal hypodensity with or without intraparenchymal hemorrhage, abnormal gray-white differentiation, and evidence of volume loss or porencephaly if the injury is remote from the time of delivery[176] (Fig. 58-6).

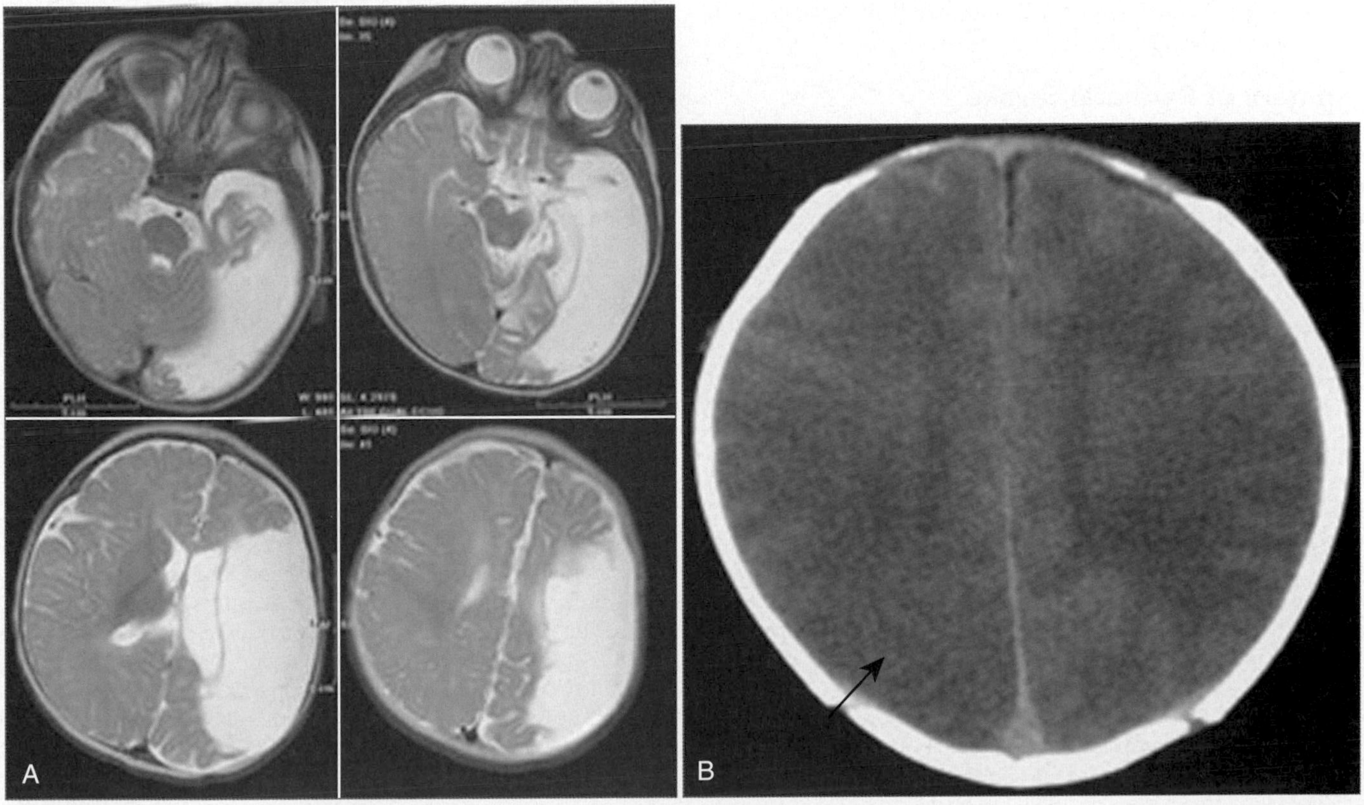

FIGURE 58-6 Diagnostic imaging studies of neonatal stroke. **A,** Magnetic resonance imaging study of a 6-month-old infant demonstrates a large region of encephalomalacia involving most of the left temporal lobe and large regions of the left frontal and parietal lobes. The distribution is consistent with a remote infarction of the left middle cerebral artery. The infant had a history of sepsis and disseminated intravascular coagulation during the early neonatal period. An ultrasound scan when the infant was 1 day old was unremarkable. **B,** Computed tomography of a 1-day-old term infant who presented with a focal seizure. The perinatal history was unremarkable. There is loss of gray-white matter differentiation involving the right parietal and occipital regions *(arrow)*. There is a smaller area of involvement in the right frontal region. A cranial ultrasound examination was normal.

MRI with diffusion-weighted imaging is the most sensitive, especially in the setting of early infarction. MRI may be able to demonstrate restricted diffusion within a vascular distribution for acute stroke as well as chronic changes such as encephalomalacia, gliosis, and ventriculomegaly for remote events (see Fig. 58-6). MR angiography may be useful in some cases to confirm arterial occlusion although it is not commonly used unless a vascular malformation is suspected. Functional MRI may be valuable in the future to understand how the brain reorganizes after perinatal stroke.[218,228,229] EEG may be useful to detect subclinical seizures that may cause secondary brain injury.[218]

Further diagnostic studies focused on risk factors for perinatal ischemic stroke should include blood tests for coagulation disturbances and genetic predispositions, urine toxicology for metabolic disorders and toxins such as cocaine, echocardiography, infectious workup including lumbar puncture, maternal testing for acquired coagulation disorders such as antiphospholipid antibodies, and an assessment of the placenta.[176]

Outcomes

Perinatal ischemic stroke is the most common cause of hemiplegic cerebral palsy (CP).[176] Although not all survivors of perinatal stroke suffer long-term disabilities, 50% to 75% of infants who suffered a perinatal stroke will have a neurologic deficit or seizures.[215,218,230-232] Lee and colleagues[215] reported a population-based study of neonatal AIS showing that 32% of infants with AIS who presented with symptoms in the neonatal period went on to develop CP, whereas 82% of infants diagnosed retrospectively developed CP. Because patients identified retrospectively presented because of hemiparesis, they were more likely to be classified as having CP.

Summary of Perinatal Stroke

Perinatal ischemic stroke is a major cause of long-term neurologic disability. Treatment is purely supportive, and management is rehabilitation focusing on muscle strengthening and prevention of contractures. Neuroprotective strategies and approaches to prevention are needed. Advanced neuroimaging techniques to better understand how the brain reorganizes after this type of injury are being used as research tools.

Cerebral Palsy

Cerebral palsy (CP) is a clinical diagnosis that refers to a group of nonprogressive motor impairments. As early as 1862, William John Little described the relationship between children with motor abnormalities and pregnancy complications such as difficult labor, neonatal asphyxia, and premature birth.[177] In 2005, the International Committee on Cerebral Palsy Classification defined CP as "a group of developmental disorders of movement and posture, which cause activity limitations that are attributed to nonprogressive disturbances that occurred in the developing fetal or infant brain. The motor disorders of cerebral palsy are often accompanied by disturbances of sensation, cognition, communication, perception, and behavior and by a seizure disorder."[178] Despite improvements in perinatal care, the prevalence of CP has remained relatively unchanged over the past 50 years, with an incidence of 1.5 to 2.5 cases per 1000 live births.[155,233,234]

Classification

Traditionally, CP has been classified by topography based on the affected limb involvement (i.e., monoplegia, hemiplegia, diplegia, triplegia, and quadriplegia) and a description of the predominant type of tone or movement abnormality (i.e., spastic, dyskinetic, ataxic, hypotonic, or mixed). The International Committee on Cerebral Palsy Classification proposed a new classification system that takes into account the presence or absence of associated impairments, other anatomic involvement besides limbs, radiologic findings, and causation (Table 58-6).

TABLE 58-6 COMPONENTS OF CEREBRAL PALSY CLASSIFICATION

1. Motor abnormalities
   - A. Nature and typology of the motor disorder: the observed tonal abnormalities assessed on examination (e.g., hypertonia, hypotonia) and the diagnosed movement disorders, such as spasticity, ataxia, dystonia, or athetosis
   - B. Functional motor abilities: the extent to which the individual is limited in his or her motor function in all body areas, including oromotor and speech function
2. Associated impairments
   - A. Presence of absence of associated nonmotor neurodevelopmental or sensory problems, such as seizures, hearing or vision impairments, and attentional, behavioral, communicative, or cognitive deficits
   - B. Extent to which impairments interact in individuals with cerebral palsy
3. Anatomic and radiologic findings
   - A. Anatomic distribution: parts of the body (e.g., limbs, trunk, bulbar region) affected by motor impairments or limitations
   - B. Radiologic findings: neuroanatomic findings on computed tomography or magnetic resonance imaging, such as ventricular enlargement, white matter loss, or brain anomaly
4. Causation and timing
   - A. Whether there is a clearly identified cause, as is usually the case with postnatal cerebral palsy (e.g., meningitis, head injury), or when brain malformations are present
   - B. Presumed time frame during which the injury occurred, if known

Adapted from Bax M, Goldstein M, Rosenbaum P, et al: Proposed definition and classification of cerebral palsy, April 2005. Dev Med Child Neurol 47:571-576, 2005.

Etiology

Cerebral palsy is a result of injury to the developing brain that occurs prenatally, perinatally, or postnatally. Between 75% and 80% of cases of CP have been attributed to events during pregnancy. Ten percent are attributable to intrapartum events such as birth asphyxia,[156,235,236] and 10% follow postnatal causes such as head injury or central nervous system infection.[179,180] Risk factors for cerebral palsy include prematurity, multiple gestation, growth restriction, intracranial hemorrhage, PVL, infections, placental pathology, genetic syndromes, structural brain abnormalities, birth asphyxia or trauma, and kernicterus. The origins of CP tend to be multifactorial, but in some cases, no cause is identified. Some of the more common risk factors will be discussed in detail. The roles of intracranial hemorrhage, PVL, and birth asphyxia contributing to CP have been discussed in a previous section of this chapter.

Prematurity

Prematurity and low birth weight seem to be the most important risk factors for CP, with an increased prevalence of CP associated with decreasing gestational age and decreasing birth weight as compared with term infants. It is important first to consider the rates of CP and neurosensory impairments in term infants. Msall and coworkers[237] reported rates of disability in term infants as follows: 0.2% for CP, 2% to 3% for cognitive impairment, 0.1% to 0.3% for hearing loss, and 0.1% for visual impairment.[237] With improvements in survival for ELBW infants, defined as less than 1000 g, there are concerns that disability rates will increase as well. Several investigators have reported neurodevelopmental disability rates among ELBW infants born in the 1990s. Reported rates range from 8% to 19% with CP, 19% to 49% with developmental disability, 1% to 4% with hearing impairment, and 1% to 4% with visual impairment.[23,32,132,238-240] When extreme prematurity is considered, Shankaran and associates[181] showed that surviving infants born at the threshold of viability (i.e., birth weight <750 g, gestational age <24 weeks, and a 1-minute Apgar of 3), had neurodisability rates of 60%, with almost one third of infants having CP. The increase in disability rates may be related to heavy use of postnatal steroids to treat neonatal chronic lung disease and high rates of sepsis during this period. Poor neurodevelopmental outcomes have been associated with widespread use of postnatal steroids in the 1990s, and routine use of this therapy to treat chronic lung disease is now discouraged.[31,241-243] The association between sepsis and cerebral palsy has also been identified in many studies and is discussed in a later section.

Because further reduction in mortality of ELBW infants is unlikely, strategies to reduce neonatal morbidity are increasingly important. Decreased rates of CP have been reported in ELBW infants born between 2000 and 2002, a period associated with increased use of antenatal steroids, decreased use of postnatal steroids, and decreased incidence of nosocomial sepsis.[186] Chronic lung disease is an independent risk factor for neurodevelopmental disability for which improved strategies are needed. Inhaled nitric oxide for preterm infants with respiratory failure has been studied, and improved cognitive outcome in infants treated with inhaled nitric oxide has been reported,[244,245] but this effect has not been consistently observed in ELBW infants.[246,247]

Multiple Births

The risk of developing CP is significantly higher in multiple gestations compared with singleton births. Data from CP registries show that the risk for developing CP in twins is four or five times greater than singletons. For triplets the risk is 12 to 13 times greater.[183,248-250] Although twins comprise only 1.6% of the population, they have a 5% to 10% incidence of CP.[251] The higher rate of CP in multiple births may relate to preterm birth and to other complications associated with multiple gestation such as placental and cord abnormalities, intra-placental shunting, structural anomalies, and difficulties at delivery.

The incidence of CP increases as birth weight decreases. Only 0.9% of singletons weigh less than 1500 g at birth, compared with 9.4% of twins, 32.2% of triplets, and 73.3% of quadruplets.[183,252] Population-based registries have also broken down the risks of CP related to birth weight groups as follows: 66.5 per 1000 surviving infants born weighing less than 1000 g, 57.4 per 1000 surviving infants with birth weights between 1000 and 1499 g, and 8.9 per 1000 surviving infants with birth weights between 1500 and 2499 g.[182] However, twins with birth weight above 2500 g still have a threefold to fourfold increased risk of developing CP compared with singletons.[183] It is unclear why this risk remains increased near term, but it may be linked to an increased risk of asphyxia or fetal growth restriction, which occurs more commonly in multiples.

The risk of CP is increased with the fetal death of a co-twin and is higher for same-sex twins than for different-sex twins.[253-256] When both twins are born alive and one twin dies in infancy, the risk is even greater than if one twin died in utero, with same-sex twins having a greater risk than different-sex twins.[183] These data suggest that monochorionic placentation has a significant role in the pathogenesis of CP, likely because of placental vascular anastomoses.

Multiple gestations have significantly increased because of assisted reproductive technology (ART). The increased risk of CP associated with ART is likely because of the higher rate of preterm births because ART is typically not associated with monochorionicity unless monozygotic division occurs. However, the increased risk of CP associated with ART requires further study. A Danish study suggests that IVF pregnancies may carry an increased risk of CP not attributable to birth weight or gestation[184] (see Chapter 29).

Growth Restriction

There is much debate in the literature about whether infants with fetal growth restriction have an increased incidence of CP. Many investigators have reported an increased risk of CP for infants who are small for gestational age (SGA).[257-262] However, fetal growth restriction is a separate entity from SGA (see Chapter 34). *Fetal growth restriction* refers to failure of a fetus to grow at an optimal predicted rate, using fetal growth standards derived from ultrasound measurements of healthy fetuses in utero at each gestational age. Fetal growth curves can account for variables, including fetal sex, ethnicity, parity, and maternal height and weight.[263-265] SGA refers to infants who weigh less than a given percentile (usually the 10th) for gestational age and does not take into account potential etiologies of SGA such as constitutional small stature, chromosomal anomalies, congenital infections, or structural malformations. Studies of risk of cerebral palsy often use birth weight alone to define their population of interest, which may explain the observed increased risk of CP associated with low birth weight. This increased risk of CP may result from the effects of intrauterine growth restriction, because these cohort studies include more mature SGA term infants and preterm infants with equivalent birth weights.[266,267] The terminology used affects how the data may be interpreted.

Many studies have demonstrated that SGA term or preterm infants beyond 33 weeks' gestation have the highest risk of developing CP.[259-261] The Surveillance of Cerebral Palsy in Europe (SCPE) Collaborative Group reported that infants born between 32 and 42 weeks' gestation with a birth weight below the 10th percentile were four to six times more likely to develop CP than infants with a birth weight between the 25th and 75th percentile.[267,268] For infants born before 33 weeks' gestation with fetal growth restriction, the association is less clear, because this population has the highest risk of adverse neurodevelopmental outcome. It is therefore difficult to separate the risk purely due to growth restriction from the effect of prematurity in general. Other factors that increase the risk of CP are the severity of SGA, male sex, and perinatal asphyxia.[269]

Growth-restricted infants may be more susceptible to intrapartum hypoxia, which leads to adverse neurologic outcome. Data from the Collaborative Perinatal Project showed that infants with intrauterine growth restriction (IUGR) had similar incidences of CP compared with non-IUGR infants when examined at 7 years of age in the absence of intrapartum hypoxia. However, when intrapartum hypoxia was identified, children with IUGR had an increased incidence of neurodevelopmental disability compared with those without IUGR.[197] The relative risk of CP due to intrapartum hypoxia was actually lower in a study of infants who were SGA compared with appropriate for gestational age (AGA) infants.[262] Based on conflicting results it seems clear that other factors may be involved.

Perinatal Infections

Maternal, intrauterine, and neonatal infections have all been associated with cerebral palsy. Congenital viral infections such as toxoplasmosis, rubella, cytomegalovirus (CMV), herpes simplex virus, and syphilis may account for 5% to 10% of CP cases.[270] Maternal infection and inflammation has been associated with an increased incidence of preterm birth and are risk factors for the development of CP. Intra-amniotic infection, also referred to as clinical chorioamnionitis, has been associated with preterm labor, preterm premature rupture of the fetal membranes, and subsequent preterm birth.[271,272] Chorioamnionitis also has been associated with an increased risk for developing CP through several likely mechanisms. An increased risk of IVH and PVL has been associated with maternal chorioamnionitis and premature rupture of membranes in numerous studies.[210,211,273-275] Histologic chorioamnionitis without clinical signs of intra-amniotic infection has also been linked to increased risk of IVH, PVL, and CP.[276-280]

Laboratory and clinical evidence has emerged that supports the hypothesis that intrauterine infection and inflammation leads to the production of proinflammatory cytokines, which are responsible for white matter brain injury and ultimately for CP. These cytokines are potentially toxic to developing oligodendrocytes in fetal white matter and cause reduced myelination and subsequent white matter injury.[270,273,281,282] Various cytokines may have a direct toxic effect on cerebral white matter by increasing the production of nitric oxide synthase, cyclooxygenase, other associated free radicals, and excitatory amino acids.[270,282-285] This relationship between elevated cytokine levels and the development of white matter injury has been seen in both preterm and term infants. A fourfold to sixfold increased risk for white matter injury has been associated with elevated levels of interleukin (IL) 1β from amniotic fluid and from umbilical cord blood in preterm infants.[2,286] In a study of term infants who went on to develop CP, stored blood samples had significantly increased levels of the cytokines IL-1, IL-8, IL-9, tumor necrosis factor β, and RANTES.[287] The combination of intrauterine infection and intrapartum hypoxia has been correlated with a dramatic increase in the incidence of CP.[288]

Neonatal infection has been associated with the development of CP due to direct central nervous system damage, e.g., in meningitis, or to a systemic inflammatory response syndrome (SIRS) that leads to sepsis, shock, and multiorgan system failure.[270] Preterm infants who develop infection seem to be at higher risk.[289,290] A study of 6093 ELBW survivors born between 1993 and 2001 found an 8% incidence of CP among infants who did not develop a postnatal infection and a 20% incidence of CP in infants whose hospital course was complicated by sepsis, NEC, or meningitis.[240] The infected infants also had an extremely high risk of cognitive impairment, defined as a Bayley MDI score less than 70 at 18 months compared with noninfected infants (33% to 42% versus 22%).[240] Another study of ELBW survivors found that NEC requiring surgical intervention was associated with a significant increase in both the incidence of CP and developmental disabilities compared with those without NEC.[129]

Placental Abnormalities

Because the placenta supplies nutrients to the developing fetus and serves as a barrier that protects the fetus from influences such as infectious organisms, toxins, trauma, and immune mediators, placental abnormalities can predispose fetuses to adverse outcomes. Placental abnormalities associated with CP can fall into three categories. The first encompasses events that occur during or before labor, also known as *sentinel lesions*, that can cause fetal hypoxia. These lesions include uteroplacental separation, fetal hemorrhage, and umbilical cord occlusion.[291] The next category is made up of thromboinflammatory processes that affect fetal circulation and include fetal thrombotic vasculopathy, chronic villitis, meconium-associated fetal vascular necrosis, and fetal vasculitis related to chorioamnionitis.[291,292] The third category includes processes that cause decreased placental reserve, such as chronic placental insufficiency, chronic villitis, chronic abruption, chronic vascular obstruction, and perivillous fibrin deposition.[293] Evaluation of the placenta in the cause of neonatal encephalopathy may provide some insight into the fetal intrauterine environment and its contribution to the neurologic impairment.

Coexisting Impairments

Historically, CP has been defined strictly by the location and degree of motor impairment. However, associated coimpairments such as disturbances in sensation, cognition, communication, perception, and behavior are common, as are seizures. A new definition that includes coimpairments has been proposed.[178,234] A Dutch population study of children with CP reported that 40% had seizures, 65% had cognitive deficits (IQ < 85), and 34% had visual impairments.[294] Hearing impairments and feeding difficulties are also common.

Strategies to Reduce Cerebral Palsy

Strategies to reduce CP have focused on asphyxia and premature birth because these factors seem to be the most amenable to intervention to prevent CP. Strategies commonly used to reduce intrapartum hypoxia such as fetal heart monitoring, maternal oxygen administration, repositioning, and strict guidelines for oxytocin use have not affected the rate of CP. Fetal heart rate monitoring increases the rate of operative interventions without reducing the rate of CP[164] and may theoretically increase the prevalence of CP by increasing the risk of chorioamnionitis.[295,296] Reduction of perinatal intracranial injuries associated with the decreased use of forceps and vacuum extraction in the past 20 years is a positive trend that may contribute to a reduction in the incidence of CP.[155,297]

Preterm birth accounts for approximately 35% of cerebral palsy cases.[298] Strategies to reduce the incidence of preterm birth have been sought to reduce the incidence of CP, provided the risk of an in utero insult is not increased by prolonging pregnancy. Prevention of preterm birth has proved elusive, making strategies to reduce morbidity more immediately promising. Antenatal steroids decrease the incidence of several morbidities strongly associated with cerebral palsy, including IVH, PVL,[171,299] RDS, and chronic lung disease. Postnatal steroids used to treat neonatal chronic lung disease, however, are associated with a significantly increased risk of CP.[241,300-302]

Another strategy under study to reduce CP in preterm infants is the administration of magnesium sulfate before delivery. The proposed beneficial mechanism is the ability of magnesium sulfate to stabilize vascular tone, reduce reperfusion injury, and reduce cytokine mediated injury.[303,304] Several observational studies have found an association between maternal administration of magnesium sulfate (given for preeclampsia or preterm labor) and a reduced risk of CP.[305-308] However, other investigators have reported no protective effect of magnesium.[309-314] The Australasian Collaborative Trial of Magnesium Sulphate examined the efficacy of magnesium sulfate given to women at risk for preterm birth less than 30 weeks' gestation solely for neuroprotection. This study was a much larger, randomized, controlled trial ($N = 1062$), and the investigators reported a lower incidence of CP, although the difference was not statistically significant (6.8% versus 8.2%), and no serious harmful effects to women or their children.[194] Although the use of prenatal magnesium sulfate cannot be recommended based on this study alone, this intervention is being further investigated (see Chapter 29). A large, 10-year NIH trial of intrapartum administration of magnesium sulfate as neuroprotective agent found a reduced rate of moderate to severe cerebral palsy among survivors at 2 years of age who received antenatal magnesium.[315]

Summary of Cerebral Palsy

Cerebral palsy is a significant adverse event with origins in pregnancy. Many risk factors have been identified, although sometimes no etiologic factor is found. Strategies to reduce asphyxia and prevent preterm birth have not shown a significant decrease in rates of CP. Because most CP is related to extremely preterm birth and the survival rates of these ELBW infants is improving, strategies to reduce neonatal brain injury, such as the use of antenatal steroids, are the most promising. Future trials of antenatal neuroprotection for preterm infants may prove beneficial to combat inflammation- or cytokine-mediated brain injury.

Infectious Disease Problems in the Neonatal Period

Neonatal infection is a significant cause of neonatal morbidity and mortality in preterm and term infants. The risk of infection is inversely related to gestational age. The clinical manifestations of neonatal infection vary by pathogen and age of acquisition. The spectrum of pathogens causing neonatal infection is broad and has changed over the decades.[316] However, the cornerstones of management remain prevention when possible, early detection, and focused treatment.

Compared with older children and adults, neonatal host defense is blunted by incomplete development and experience with self versus non-self discrimination.[317] All components of the immune system are deficient. Nonspecific immunity is defective at several levels. Skin and mucosal barriers are immature, especially in preterm infants. Levels of nonspecific antibacterial proteins such as lysozyme and lactoferrin are low. Neutrophil numbers are low, with limited storage pools available to clear bacteria. Key neutrophil functions, including chemotaxis, phagocytosis, and intracellular killing, are limited. The neonate is poorly equipped to clear transient bacteremia and localize bacterial infection. Specific humoral and cell-mediated immune functions are also limited. Circulating immunoglobulin levels are very low compared with adult levels. The neonate acquires virtually all of its circulating IgG from the mother through transplacental transport. The bulk of this antibody is transferred during the third trimester, making the preterm infant profoundly deficient. B-cell function is immature as well. The primary antibody response to infection mediated by the infant is production of IgM. Although T lymphocytes are present at birth, their function is almost undetectable by standard functional assays.

The nature of neonatal immune function accounts for the clinical manifestations of most early-onset infections. Nonspecific signs such as lethargy, poor feeding, temperature instability, decreased tone, apnea, and altered perfusion may or may not be present. Fever is uncommon, as are localized processes such as cellulitis, abscesses, or osteomyelitis. When present, they are usually accompanied by bacteremia. Similarly, bacteremia must always be suspected in neonates with meningitis or urinary tract infections.

Chorioamnionitis

The relationship between chorioamnionitis and neonatal infection is complex and remains incompletely understood. Some studies demonstrate a direct correlation between chorioamnionitis and neonatal infection. Other poor neonatal outcomes, including RDS and BPD, are associated with chorioamnionitis.[84,318] However, other clinical series and studies using animal model systems reach essentially the opposite conclusion—that chorioamnionitis protects against these same outcomes.[319,320] Some of the confusion is grounded in definitions of chorioamnionitis. Clinical chorioamnionitis, as characterized by maternal fever and uterine tenderness, is probably a very different disease from clinically silent histologic chorioamnionitis commonly seen in preterm deliveries. Whether these represent different disease entities or different manifestations of the same disease spectrum is not evident. The fetal response to infection has important consequences for neonatal outcome. Studies using proteomic analysis of amniotic fluid show promise for relating the diagnosis of chorioamnionitis to the neonatal clinical course.[321,322]

Group B β-Hemolytic Streptococci

Infection with group B β-hemolytic streptococci (GBS) was first recognized as a cause of early-onset neonatal sepsis in the 1970s. By the 1990s, GBS was a leading cause of serious neonatal infections. The organism is a common colonizing constituent of the vagina and rectum in 10% to 30% of pregnant women. GBS colonization is more common in African-American women and those with a previous history of a neonate with GBS disease or a history of a GBS urinary tract infection. Epidemiologic studies demonstrate that most invasive, early-onset neonatal GBS disease involves vertical transmission from the mother to the fetus during labor. This observation led to studies of intrapartum antibiotic prophylaxis with penicillin G or ampicillin. The success of this strategy prompted the publication of guidelines for intrapartum antibiotic prophylaxis by the Centers for Disease Control and Prevention.[323] A follow-up study completed in 2005 confirmed the success of this strategy.[324] Most infants with invasive, serious GBS now seen are born to mothers with negative GBS screening cultures who have presumably converted to GBS-positive carrier status in the interval between screening and delivery.[325] In the future, rapid GBS screening technology may allow for identification of these women when they present in labor.[326] There is some concern that intrapartum antibiotic prophylaxis may be associated with a higher incidence of serious bacterial infections later in infancy. This was most pronounced when broad-spectrum antibiotics were used for intrapartum prophylaxis rather than penicillin G.[327] The advantages of intrapartum antibiotic prophylaxis to reduce the risk of invasive neonatal GBS disease clearly outweigh any risks, especially if penicillin is employed.

Viral Infections

Cytomegalovirus

Human cytomegalovirus (CMV) is transmitted horizontally (i.e., direct person-to-person contact with virus-containing secretions) and vertically (i.e., from mother to infant before, during, or after birth) and through transfusion of blood products or organ transplantation from previously infected donors. Vertical transmission of CMV to infants occurs by one of the following routes of transmission: in utero by transplacental passage of maternal blood borne virus, through an infected maternal genital tract, and postnatally by ingestion of CMV-positive human milk.[328,329]

Approximately 1% of all liveborn infants are infected in utero and excrete CMV at birth. Risk to the fetus is greatest in the first half of gestation. Although fetal infection can occur after maternal primary infection or after reactivation of infection during pregnancy, sequelae are far more common in infants exposed to maternal primary infection, with 10% to 20% of infants manifesting neurodevelopmental impairment or sensorineural hearing loss in childhood.[330]

Congenital CMV infection is usually clinically silent. Some infected infants who appear healthy at birth are subsequently found to develop hearing loss or learning disabilities. Approximately 10% of infants with congenital CMV infection exhibit evidence of profound involvement at birth, including intrauterine growth restriction, jaundice, purpura, hepatosplenomegaly, microcephaly, intracerebral calcifications, and retinitis.[331] Although ganciclovir has been used to treat some infants with congenital CMV infection, it is not recommended routinely because of insufficient efficacy data. One study of ganciclovir treatment provided to infants with congenital CMV with central nervous system involvement suggested that treatment decreased progression of hearing impairment.[332] Because of the potential toxicity of long-term ganciclovir therapy, additional investigation is required before a recommendation can be made.

Infection acquired during pregnancy from maternal cervical secretions or after delivery from human milk usually is not associated with clinical illness. Infections resulting from transfusion of blood products with CMV-seropositive donors and from human milk to preterm infants have been associated with serious systemic infections, including lower respiratory tract infection. Transmission of CMV by transfusion to newborn infants has been reduced by using CMV-antibody negative donors, by freezing erythrocytes in glycerol, or by removal of leukocytes by filtration before administration.[333] CMV transmission by human milk can be decreased by pasteurization.[334] However, freeze-thawing is probably not effective.[335] If fresh donor milk is needed for infants born to CMV-antibody negative mothers, provision of these infants with milk from only CMV-antibody negative women should be considered.

Hepatitis B

HBV is a DNA virus whose important components include an outer lipoprotein envelope containing antibody to hepatitis B surface antigen (HBsAg) and an inner nucleocapsid containing the hepatitis B core antigen. Only antibody to HBsAg (anti-HBs) provides protection from HBV infection. Perinatal transmission of HBV is highly efficient and usually occurs from blood exposure during labor and delivery. In utero transmission of HBV is rare, accounting for less than 2% of perinatal infections in most studies. The risk of an infant acquiring HBV from an infected mother as a result of perinatal exposure is 70% to 90% for infants born to mothers who are HBsAg and HBeAg positive. The risk is 5% to 20% for infants born to mothers who are HBeAg negative. Age at the time of acute infection is the primary determinant of risk of progression to chronic HBV infection. More than 90% of infants with perinatal infection will develop chronic HBV infection. Between 25% and 50% of children infected between 1 to 5 years of age become chronically infected, whereas only 2% to 6% of older children or adults develop chronic HBV infection.[336]

The goals of HBV prevention programs are to prevent the acute HBV infection and to decrease the rates of chronic HBV infection and HBV-related chronic liver disease. Over the past 2 decades a strategy has been progressively implemented in the United States to prevent HBV transmission. This includes the following components: universal immunization of infants beginning at birth, prevention of perinatal HBV infection by routine screening of all pregnant women and appropriate immunoprophylaxis of infants born to HBsAg-positive women and infants born to women with unknown HBsAg status, routine immunization of children and adolescents who have previously not been immunized, and immunization of previously nonimmunized adults at increased risk of infection.

Two types of products are available for hepatitis B immunoprophylaxis. Hepatitis B immune globulin (HBIG) provides short-term protection (3 to 6 months) and is indicated only in postexposure circumstances. Hepatitis B vaccine is used for pre-exposure and post-exposure protection and provides long-term protection. Pre-exposure immunization with hepatitis B vaccine is the most effective means to prevent HBV transmission. To decrease the HBV transmission rate universal immunization is necessary. Postexposure prophylaxis with hepatitis B vaccine and HBIG or hepatitis B vaccine alone effectively prevents infection after exposure to HBV. The effectiveness of postexposure immunoprophylaxis is related to the time elapsed between exposure and administration. Immunoprophylaxis is most effective if given within 12 to 24 hours of exposure. Serologic testing of all pregnant women for HBsAg is essential for identifying women whose infants will require postexposure prophylaxis beginning at birth.

Hepatitis B vaccines are highly effective and safe. These vaccines are 90% to 95% efficacious for preventing HBV infection. Studies in preterm infants and low-birth-weight infants (<2000 g) have demonstrated decreased seroconversion rates after administration of hepatitis B vaccination. However, by 1 month chronological age medically stable preterm infants should be immunized, regardless of initial birth weight or gestational age. Routine postimmunization testing for anti-HBs is not necessary for most infants. However, postimmunization testing for HBsAg and anti-HBs at 9 to 18 months is recommended for infants born to HBsAg-positive mothers.

Immunization of pregnant women with hepatitis B vaccine has not been associated with adverse effects on the developing fetus. Because HBV infection may result in severe disease in the mother and chronic infection in the newborn infant, pregnancy is not considered a contraindication to immunization. Lactation is also not a contraindication to immunization.

Herpes Simplex Virus

Neonatal herpes simplex virus infections range from localized skin lesions to overwhelming disseminated disease. The latter has a case-fatality rate in excess of 50%, even with prompt initiation of antiviral therapy. Vertical transmission is the likely mode of transmission for most cases. Mothers with a history of previous disease appear to convey at least some type-specific immunity to the neonate. Most mothers of severely infected infants have no recognized history of HSV and no evidence of active disease on physical examination. No screening protocols for HSV are available, and there is no vaccine.[337,338]

Human Immunodeficiency Virus

Landmark studies[339,340] in the 1990s demonstrated the value of intrapartum antiretroviral therapy to reduce the risk of maternal to fetal transmission of human immunodeficiency virus (HIV). Improvements in the quality and availability of rapid HIV testing holds promise for timely and accurate identification of infected women and their newborn infants. The risk of congenital HIV is reduced to approximately 1% when HIV-positive mothers receive antiretroviral therapy during labor and treatment is continued for the neonate within 12 hours of delivery, Breastfeeding is contraindicated, unless there is no access to clean water and infant formula.

Laboratory diagnosis of HIV infection during infancy depends on detection of virus or viral nucleic acid. Cord blood should not be used for this early test because of possible contamination by maternal blood. A positive result identifies infants who have been infected in utero. Approximately 93% of infected infants have detectable HIV DNA at 2 weeks, and almost all HIV-infected infants have positive HIV DNA PCR assay results by 1 month of age. A test within the first 14 days of age can facilitate decisions regarding initiation of antiretroviral therapy. Transplacental passage of antibodies complicates use of antibody-based assays for diagnosis of infection in infants because all infants born to HIV-seropositive mothers have passively acquired maternal antibodies.

Antiretroviral therapy is indicated for most HIV-infected children. Initiation of therapy depends on virologic, immunologic, and clinical criteria. Because HIV infection is a rapidly changing area, consultation with an expert in pediatric HIV is recommended.

Rubella

Humans are the only source of infection. Peak incidence of infection is in late winter and early spring. Before widespread use of rubella vaccine, rubella was an epidemic disease with most cases occurring in children. The incidence of rubella has decreased 99% from the prevaccine era. Although the number of susceptible people has decreased since introduction and widespread use of rubella vaccine, serologic surveys indicate that approximately 10% of the U.S. population older than 5 years is susceptible. The percentage of susceptible people who are foreign born or from areas with poor vaccine coverage is higher. The risk of congenital rubella syndrome is highest among infants of women born outside the United States. Epidemiologic data suggests that rubella is no longer endemic in the United States.[341]

Congenital rubella syndrome is characterized by a constellation of anomalies, which may include ophthalmologic (i.e., cataracts, microphthalmos, pigmentary retinopathy, and congenital glaucoma), cardiac (i.e., patent ductus arteriosus and peripheral pulmonary artery stenosis), auditory (i.e., sensorineural hearing impairment), and neurologic (i.e., meningoencephalitis, behavioral abnormalities, and mental retardation) abnormalities. Neonatal manifestations of congenital rubella syndrome include growth retardation, interstitial pneumonia, radiolucent bone disease, hepatosplenomegaly, thrombocytopenia, and dermal erythropoiesis, also called blueberry muffin lesions. The occurrence of congenital defects varies with timing of the maternal infection.

Detection of rubella-specific IgM antibody usually indicates recent postnatal infection or congenital infection in a newborn infant, but false-positive and false-negative results occur. Congenital infection can be confirmed by stable or increasing rubella-specific IgG over several months. Rubella virus can be isolated most consistently from throat or nasal swabs by inoculation of appropriate cell culture. Blood, urine, CSF, and pharyngeal swab specimens can also yield virus in congenitally infected infants.

Infants with congenital rubella should be considered contagious until at least 1 year old, unless nasopharyngeal and urine cultures are repeatedly negative for rubella virus. Infectious precautions should be considered for children up to 3 years old who are hospitalized for congenital cataract extraction. Caregivers of these infants and children should be made aware of the potential hazard to susceptible pregnant contacts.

Sexually Transmitted Infections

Chlamydia

In the newborn period, *Chlamydia trachomatis* is associated with conjunctivitis and pneumonia. Acquisition of *C. trachomatis* occurs in approximately 50% of infants born vaginally to infected mothers and in some infants delivered by cesarean section with intact membranes.[342] Neonatal chlamydial conjunctivitis is characterized by ocular congestion, edema, and discharge developing a few days to several weeks after birth and usually lasting 1 to 2 weeks. Pneumonia in infants is usually an insidious afebrile illness occurring between 2 and 20 weeks after birth. It is characterized by a staccato cough, tachypnea, and rales on physical examination. Pulmonary hyperinflation and infiltrates are demonstrated on the chest radiograph.

Topical prophylaxis with silver nitrate, erythromycin, or tetracycline for all newborn infants to avert gonococcal ophthalmia does not prevent chlamydial conjunctivitis or extraocular infections.[343] Infants with chlamydial conjunctivitis are treated with oral erythromycin base or ethylsuccinate (50 mg/kg per day in four divided doses) for 14 days. Alternatively, oral sulfonamides may be used after the immediate neonatal period for infants who do not tolerate erythromycin. Because the efficacy of treatment is about 80%, follow-up of infants is recommended. In some instances, a second course of therapy may be required.

Chlamydial pneumonia is treated with oral azithromycin (20 mg/kg/day) for 3 days or erythromycin base or ethylsuccinate (50 mg/kg per day in four divided doses) for 14 days. Detection and treatment of *C. trachomatis* infections before delivery is the most effective way to reduce the risk of neonatal conjunctivitis and pneumonia.

Gonococcal Infections

Infection with *Neisseria gonorrhoeae* in the newborn infant usually involves the eyes. Other types of gonococcal infections include arthritis, disseminated disease with bacteremia, meningitis, scalp abscess, or vaginitis.

Microscopic examination of Gram-stained smears of exudates from the eyes, skin lesions, synovial fluid, and, when clinically warranted, CSF may be useful in the initial evaluation. Identification of gram-negative intracellular diplococci in these smears can be helpful, in particular if the organism is not recovered in culture. *N. gonorrhoeae* can be cultured from normally sterile sites such as blood, CSF, and synovial fluid.

For routine ophthalmia neonatorum prophylaxis of infants immediately after birth, a 1% silver nitrate solution, 1% tetracycline, or 0.5% erythromycin ophthalmic ointment is instilled into each eye. Prophylaxis may be delayed for as long as 1 hour after birth to facilitate parent-infant bonding. Topical antimicrobial agents cause less chemical irritation than silver nitrate. None of the topical agents is effective against *C. trachomatis*.[343]

When prophylaxis is administered, infants born to mothers with known gonococcal infection rarely develop gonococcal ophthalmia. However, because gonococcal ophthalmia or disseminated disease occasionally can occur in this situation, infants born to mothers known to have gonorrhea should receive a single dose of ceftriaxone (125 mg) given intravenously or intramuscularly. Preterm and low-birth-weight infants are given 25 to 50 mg/kg of ceftriaxone to a maximum dose of 125 mg.

Infants with clinical evidence of ophthalmia neonatorum, scalp abscess, or disseminated disease should be hospitalized. Cultures of the blood, eye discharge, or other sites of infection such as CSF should be performed to confirm the diagnosis and determine antimicrobial susceptibility. Tests for concomitant infection with *C. trachomatis*, syphilis, and HIV infection should be performed. Recommended treatment, including for ophthalmia neonatorum, is ceftriaxone (25 to 50 mg/kg, given intravenously or intramuscularly, not to exceed 125 mg) given once. Infants with gonococcal ophthalmia should receive eye irrigations with saline solution immediately and at frequent intervals until the discharge is eliminated. Topical antimicrobial treatment alone is inadequate and is unnecessary when recommended systemic antimicrobial treatment is provided. Infants with gonococcal ophthalmia should be hospitalized and evaluated for disseminated infection. Recommended therapy for arthritis and septicemia is ceftriaxone or cefotaxime for 7 days. If meningitis is documented, treatment should continue for a total of 10 to 14 days.

Syphilis

Congenital syphilis is contracted from an infected mother through transplacental transmission of *Treponema pallidum* at any time during the pregnancy or birth. Intrauterine syphilis can result in stillbirth, hydrops fetalis, or preterm birth. The infant can present with edema, hepatosplenomegaly, lymphadenopathy, mucocutaneous lesions, osteochondritis, pseudoparalysis, rash, or snuffles at birth or within the first 2 months of life. Hemolytic anemia or thrombocytopenia may be identified on laboratory evaluation. Untreated infants, regardless of whether they have manifestations in infancy, may develop late manifestations, usually after 2 years of age and involving the bones, central nervous system, eyes, joints, and teeth. Some consequences of intrauterine infection may not become apparent until many years after birth.

Definitive diagnosis is established by identification of spirochetes by microscopic dark field examination or by direct fluorescent antibody tests of lesion exudates or tissue such as the placenta or umbilical cord. Presumptive diagnosis is possible using nontreponemal and treponemal tests. The use of only one type of test is insufficient for diagnosis, because false-positive nontreponemal test results occur with various medical conditions and false-positive treponemal test results can occur with other spirochetal diseases.

No newborn infant should be discharged from the hospital without determination of the mother's serologic status for syphilis.[344] All infants born to seropositive mothers require a careful examination and a quantitative nontreponemal syphilis test. The test performed in the infant should be the same as that performed on the mother so that comparison of titer results is facilitated. An infant should be evaluated for congenital syphilis if the maternal titer has increased fourfold, if the infant titer is fourfold greater than the mother's titer, or if the infant has clinical manifestations of syphilis. The infant should be evaluated if born to a mother with positive nontreponemal and treponemal test results if the mother has any of the following conditions. First, the syphilis has not been treated or treatment has not been documented. Second, syphilis during pregnancy was treated with a nonpenicillin regimen. Third, syphilis was treated less than 1 month before delivery because treatment failures occur and efficacy cannot be assumed. Fourth, syphilis was treated before pregnancy but with insufficient follow-up to assess the response to treatment and current infection status.

Evaluation for syphilis in an infant should include a physical examination, quantitative nontreponemal syphilis test of serum from the infant, VDRL test of the CSF and analysis of the CSF for cells and protein concentration, long bone radiographs, and a complete blood cell and platelet counts. Other clinically indicated tests may include a chest radiograph, liver function tests, ultrasonography, ophthalmologic examination, and an auditory brainstem response test. Pathologic examination of the placenta or umbilical cord using specific antitreponemal antibody staining is also recommended.

Infants should be treated for congenital syphilis if they have proven or probable disease demonstrated by one or more of the following: physical, laboratory, or radiographic evidence of active disease; positive placenta or umbilical cord test results for treponemes using direct fluorescent antibody *T. pallidum* staining or dark-field test; a reactive result on VDRL on testing of CSF; or 4a serum quantitative nontreponemal titer is at least fourfold higher than the mother's titer using the same test and preferably the same laboratory. If the infant's titer is less than four times that of the mother, congenital syphilis still can be present. When circumstances warrant evaluation of an infant for syphilis, the infant should be treated if test results cannot exclude infection, if the infant cannot be adequately evaluated, or if adequate follow-up cannot be ensured.

Infants with proven congenital syphilis should be treated with aqueous crystalline penicillin G. The dosage should be based on chronologic age, not gestational age. The dose of penicillin G is 100,000 to 150,000 U/kg per day, administered as 50,000 U/kg per dose intravenously every 12 hours during the first 7 days of life and then every 8 hours thereafter for a total of 10 days. Alternatively, penicillin G procaine (50, 000 U/kg/day) given intramuscularly for 10 days may be considered, but adequate CSF concentrations may not be achieved with this regimen.

References

1. American Academy of Pediatrics, American Heart Association: Ethics and care at the end of life. In Textbook of Neonatal Resuscitation Textbook, 5th ed. Elk Grove Village, IL, American Academy of Pediatrics and American Heart Association, 2006, pp 9-1 to 9-16.
2. Yoon BH, Jun JK, Romero R, et al: Amniotic fluid inflammatory cytokines (interleukin-6, interleukin-1beta, and tumor necrosis factor-alpha), neonatal brain white matter lesions, and cerebral palsy. Am J Obstet Gynecol 177:19-26, 1997.
3. Watterberg KL, Demers LM, Scott SM, et al: Chorioamnionitis and early lung inflammation in infants in whom bronchopulmonary dysplasia develops. Pediatrics 97:210-215, 1996.
4. Moss TJ, Nitsos I, Ikegami M, et al: Experimental intrauterine *Ureaplasma* infection in sheep. Am J Obstet Gynecol 192:1179-1186, 2005.
5. Richardson BS, Wakim E, daSilva O, et al: Preterm histologic chorioamnionitis: Impact on cord gas and pH values and neonatal outcome. Am J Obstet Gynecol 195:1357-1365, 2006.
6. Perlman JM: Intrapartum hypoxic-ischemic cerebral injury and subsequent cerebral palsy: Medicolegal issues. Pediatrics 99:851-859, 1997.
7. Schiff E, Friedman SA, Mercer BM, et al: Fetal lung maturity is not accelerated in preeclamptic pregnancies. Am J Obstet Gynecol 169:1096-1101, 1993.
8. Lumey LH, Ravelli AC, Wiessing LG, et al: The Dutch famine birth cohort study: Design, validation of exposure, and selected characteristics of subjects after 43 years follow-up. Paediatr Perinat Epidemiol 7:354-367, 1993.
9. Barker DJ: Fetal origins of coronary heart disease. BMJ 311:171-174, 1995.
10. Ehrenberg HM, Mercer BM, Catalano PM: The influence of obesity and diabetes on the prevalence of macrosomia. Am J Obstet Gynecol 191:964-968, 2004.
11. Callaway LK, Prins JB, Chang AM, et al: The prevalence and impact of overweight and obesity in an Australian obstetric population. Med J Aust 184:56-59, 2006.
12. Lopriore E, Sueters M, Middeldorp JM, et al: Neonatal outcome in twin-to-twin transfusion syndrome treated with fetoscopic laser occlusion of vascular anastomoses. J Pediatr 147:597-602, 2005.
13. Godding V, Bonnier C, Fiasse L, et al: Does in utero exposure to heavy maternal smoking induce nicotine withdrawal symptoms in neonates? Pediatr Res 55:645-651, 2004.
14. Law KL, Stroud LR, LaGasse LL, et al: Smoking during pregnancy and newborn neurobehavior. Pediatrics 111(Pt 1):1318-1323, 2003.
15. Lemons JA, Bauer CR, Oh W, et al: Very low birth weight outcomes of the National Institute of Child Health and Human Development Neonatal Research Network, January 1995 through December 1996. NICHD Neonatal Research Network. Pediatrics 107:E1, 2001.
16. Kramer MS, Demissie K, Yang H, et al: The contribution of mild and moderate preterm birth to infant mortality. Fetal and Infant Health Study Group of the Canadian Perinatal Surveillance System. JAMA 284:843-849, 2000.

17. Smulian JC, Shen-Schwarz S, Vintzileos AM, et al: Clinical chorioamnionitis and histologic placental inflammation. Obstet Gynecol 94:1000-1005, 1999.
18. Escobar GJ, Clark RH, Greene JD: Short-term outcomes of infants born at 35 and 36 weeks' gestation: We need to ask more questions. Semin Perinatol 30:28-33, 2006.
19. Stein RE, Siegel MJ, Bauman LJ: Are children of moderately low birth weight at increased risk for poor health? A new look at an old question. Pediatrics 118:217-223, 2006.
20. Kirkegaard I, Obel C, Hedegaard M, et al: Gestational age and birth weight in relation to school performance of 10-year-old children: A follow-up study of children born after 32 completed weeks. Pediatrics 118:1600-1606, 2006.
21. Hulsey TC, Alexander GR, Robillard PY, et al: Hyaline membrane disease: The role of ethnicity and maternal risk characteristics. Am J Obstet Gynecol 168:572-576, 1993.
22. Mikkola K, Ritari N, Tommiska V, et al: Neurodevelopmental outcome at 5 years of age of a national cohort of extremely low birth weight infants who were born in 1996-1997. Pediatrics 116:1391-1400, 2005.
23. Hintz SR, Kendrick DE, Vohr BR, et al: Changes in neurodevelopmental outcomes at 18 to 22 months' corrected age among infants of less than 25 weeks' gestational age born in 1993-1999. Pediatrics 115:1645-1651, 2005.
24. Ho S, Saigal S: Current survival and early outcomes of infants of borderline viability. Neoreviews 6:e123-e132, 2005.
25. Wang ML, Dorer DJ, Fleming MP, et al: Clinical outcomes of near-term infants. Pediatrics 114:372-376, 2004.
26. Davidoff MJ, Dias T, Damus K, et al: Changes in the gestational age distribution among U.S. singleton births: Impact on rates of late preterm birth, 1992 to 2002. Semin Perinatol 30:8-15, 2006.
27. Yudkin PL, Wood L, Redman CW: Risk of unexplained stillbirth at different gestational ages. Lancet 1:1192-1194, 1987.
28. Smith GC: Life-table analysis of the risk of perinatal death at term and post term in singleton pregnancies. Am J Obstet Gynecol 184:489-496, 2001.
29. Nuffield Council on Bioethics: Critical Care Decisions in Fetal and Neonatal Medicine: Ethical Issues. London, Nuffield Council on Bioethics, 2006.
30. MacDonald H: Perinatal care at the threshold of viability. Pediatrics 110:1024-1027, 2002.
31. Committee on the Fetus and Newborn: Postnatal corticosteroids to treat or prevent chronic lung disease in preterm infants. Pediatrics 109:330-338, 2002.
32. Wood NS, Marlow N, Costeloe K, et al: Neurologic and developmental disability after extremely preterm birth. EPICure Study Group. N Engl J Med 343:378-384, 2000.
33. Costeloe K, Hennessy E, Gibson AT, et al: The EPICure study: Outcomes to discharge from hospital for infants born at the threshold of viability. Pediatrics 106:659-671, 2000.
34. Vanhaesebrouck P, Allegaert K, Bottu J, et al: The EPIBEL study: Outcomes to discharge from hospital for extremely preterm infants in Belgium. Pediatrics 114:663-675, 2004.
35. American Academy of Pediatrics, American Heart Association: Ethics and care at the end of life. In Textbook of Neonatal Resuscitation Textbook, 5th ed. Elk Grove Village, IL, American Academy of Pediatrics and American Heart Association, 2006, pp 9-5 to 9-6.
36. Lucey JF, Rowan CA, Shiono P, et al: Fetal infants: The fate of 4172 infants with birth weights of 401 to 500 grams—the Vermont Oxford Network experience (1996-2000). Pediatrics 113:1559-1566, 2004.
37. Vohr BR, Wright LL, Poole WK, et al: Neurodevelopmental outcomes of extremely low birth weight infants <32 weeks' gestation between 1993 and 1998. Pediatrics 116:635-643, 2005.
38. Cifuentes J, Bronstein J, Phibbs CS, et al: Mortality in low birth weight infants according to level of neonatal care at hospital of birth. Pediatrics 109:745-751, 2002.
39. Warner B, Musial MJ, Chenier T, et al: The effect of birth hospital type on the outcome of very low birth weight infants. Pediatrics 113(Pt 1):35-41, 2004.
40. Haberland CA, Phibbs CS, Baker LC: Effect of opening midlevel neonatal intensive care units on the location of low birth weight births in California. Pediatrics 118:e1667-e1679, 2006.
41. Bell EF: Noninitiation or withdrawal of intensive care for high-risk newborns. Pediatrics 119:401-403, 2007.
42. Committee on Bioethics: Ethics and care of critically ill infants and children. Pediatrics 98:149-152, 2006.
43. Dudell GG, Jain L: Hypoxic respiratory failure in the late preterm infant [abstract]. Clin Perinatol 33:803-830; viii-ix, 2006.
44. Jain L, Dudell GG: Respiratory transition in infants delivered by cesarean section. Semin Perinatol 30:296-304, 2006.
45. Jain L, Eaton DC: Physiology of fetal lung fluid clearance and the effect of labor. Semin Perinatol 30:34-43, 2006.
46. Riskin A, Abend-Weinger M, Riskin-Mashiah S, et al: Cesarean section, gestational age, and transient tachypnea of the newborn: Timing is the key. Am J Perinatol 22:377-382, 2005.
47. Kolas T, Saugstad OD, Daltveit AK, et al: Planned cesarean versus planned vaginal delivery at term: Comparison of newborn infant outcomes. Am J Obstet Gynecol 195:1538-1543, 2006.
48. Ronca AE, Abel RA, Ronan PJ, et al: Effects of labor contractions on catecholamine release and breathing frequency in newborn rats. Behav Neurosci 120:1308-1314, 2006.
49. Lewis V, Whitelaw A: Furosemide for transient tachypnea of the newborn. Cochrane Database Syst Rev (1):CD003064, 2002.
50. ACOG Committee on Obstetric Practice and AAP Committee on Fetur and Newborn: Intrapartum and postpartum care of the mother. In Lockwood CJ, Lemmons JA (eds): Guidelines for Perinatal Care, 6th ed. Elk Grove Village, IL, American Academy of Pediatrics and American College of Obstetricians and Gynecologists, 2007, pp 139-174.
51. Lindner W, Pohlandt F, Grab D, et al: Acute respiratory failure and short-term outcome after premature rupture of the membranes and oligohydramnios before 20 weeks of gestation. J Pediatr 140:177-182, 2002.
52. Gerten KA, Coonrod DV, Bay RC, et al: Cesarean delivery and respiratory distress syndrome: Does labor make a difference? Am J Obstet Gynecol 193(Pt 2):1061-1064, 2005.
53. Eckert Seitz E, Fiori HH, Luz JH, et al: Stable microbubble test on tracheal aspirate for the diagnosis of respiratory distress syndrome. Biol Neonate 87:140-144, 2005.
54. Kallapur S, Ikegami M: The surfactants. Am J Perinatol 17:335-343, 2000.
55. Halliday HL: Recent clinical trials of surfactant treatment for neonates. Biol Neonate 89:323-329, 2006.
56. Ammari A, Suri M, Milisavljevic V, et al: Variables associated with the early failure of nasal CPAP in very low birth weight infants. J Pediatr 147:341-347, 2005.
57. Ho JJ, Henderson-Smart DJ, Davis PG: Early versus delayed initiation of continuous distending pressure for respiratory distress syndrome in preterm infants. Cochrane Database Syst Rev (2):CD002975, 2002.
58. Stevens T, Harrington E, Blennow M, et al: Early surfactant administration with brief ventilation vs. selective surfactant and continued mechanical ventilation for preterm infants with or at risk for respiratory distress syndrome. Cochrane Database Syst Rev (4):CD003063, 2007.
59. Stevens TP, Blennow M, Soll RF: Early surfactant administration with brief ventilation vs. selective surfactant and continued mechanical ventilation for preterm infants with or at risk for respiratory distress syndrome. Cochrane Database Syst Rev (3):CD003063, 2004.
60. Howlett A, Ohlsson A: Inositol for respiratory distress syndrome in preterm infants. Cochrane Database Syst Rev (4):CD000366, 2003.
61. Kinsella JP, Cutter GR, Walsh WF, et al: Early inhaled nitric oxide therapy in premature newborns with respiratory failure. N Engl J Med 355:354-364, 2006.
62. Ballard RA, Truog WE, Cnaan A, et al: Inhaled nitric oxide in preterm infants undergoing mechanical ventilation. N Engl J Med 355:343-353, 2006.
63. Aghai ZH, Saslow JG, Nakhla T, et al: Synchronized nasal intermittent positive pressure ventilation (SNIPPV) decreases work of breathing (WOB) in premature infants with respiratory distress syndrome (RDS)

compared to nasal continuous positive airway pressure (NCPAP). Pediatr Pulmonol 41:875-881, 2006.
64. Kulkarni A, Ehrenkranz RA, Bhandari V: Effect of introduction of synchronized nasal intermittent positive-pressure ventilation in a neonatal intensive care unit on bronchopulmonary dysplasia and growth in preterm infants. Am J Perinatol 23:233-240, 2006.
65. Northway WH Jr, Rosan RC, Porter DY: Pulmonary disease following respirator therapy of hyaline-membrane disease. Bronchopulmonary dysplasia. N Engl J Med 276:357-368, 1967.
66. Jobe AH: Severe BPD is decreasing. J Pediatr 146:A2, 2005.
67. Bancalari E, Claure N: Definitions and diagnostic criteria for bronchopulmonary dysplasia. Semin Perinatol 30:164-170, 2006.
68. Walsh MC, Yao Q, Gettner P, et al: Impact of a physiologic definition on bronchopulmonary dysplasia rates. Pediatrics 114:1305-1311, 2004.
69. Chess PR, D'Angio CT, Pryhuber GS, et al: Pathogenesis of bronchopulmonary dysplasia. Semin Perinatol 30:171-178, 2006.
70. Coalson JJ: Pathology of bronchopulmonary dysplasia. Semin Perinatol 30:179-184, 2006.
71. Tin W, Gupta S: Optimum oxygen therapy in preterm babies. Arch Dis Child Fetal Neonatal Ed 92:F143-F147, 2007.
72. Tin W, Milligan DW, Pennefather P, et al: Pulse oximetry, severe retinopathy, and outcome at one year in babies of less than 28 weeks' gestation. Arch Dis Child Fetal Neonatal Ed 84:F106-F110, 2001.
73. Askie LM, Henderson-Smart DJ, Irwig L, et al: Oxygen-saturation targets and outcomes in extremely preterm infants. N Engl J Med 349:959-967, 2003.
74. Supplemental Therapeutic Oxygen for Prethreshold Retinopathy of Prematurity (STOP-ROP), a randomized, controlled trial. I. Primary outcomes. Pediatrics 105:295-310, 2000.
75. Donn SM, Sinha SK: Minimising ventilator induced lung injury in preterm infants. Arch Dis Child Fetal Neonatal Ed 91:F226-F230, 2006.
76. Woodgate PG, Davies MW: Permissive hypercapnia for the prevention of morbidity and mortality in mechanically ventilated newborn infants. Cochrane Database Syst Rev (2):CD002061, 2001.
77. Yoon BH, Romero R, Kim KS, et al: A systemic fetal inflammatory response and the development of bronchopulmonary dysplasia. Am J Obstet Gynecol 181:773-779, 1999.
78. Kallapur SG, Jobe AH: Contribution of inflammation to lung injury and development. Arch Dis Child Fetal Neonatal Ed 91:F132-F135, 2006.
79. Kallapur SG, Bachurski CJ, Le Cras TD, et al: Vascular changes after intra-amniotic endotoxin in preterm lamb lungs. Am J Physiol Lung Cell Mol Physiol 287:L1178-L1185, 2004.
80. Kallapur SG, Moss TJ, Ikegami M, et al: Recruited inflammatory cells mediate endotoxin-induced lung maturation in preterm fetal lambs. Am J Respir Crit Care Med 172:1315-1321, 2005.
81. Le Cras TD, Hardie WD, Deutsch GH, et al: Transient induction of TGF-alpha disrupts lung morphogenesis, causing pulmonary disease in adulthood. Am J Physiol Lung Cell Mol Physiol 287:L718-L729, 2004.
82. Jobe AH: Antenatal associations with lung maturation and infection. J Perinatol 25(Suppl 2):S31-S35, 2005.
83. Van Marter LJ: Progress in discovery and evaluation of treatments to prevent bronchopulmonary dysplasia. Biol Neonate 89:303-312, 2006.
84. Van Marter LJ, Dammann O, Allred EN, et al: Chorioamnionitis, mechanical ventilation, and postnatal sepsis as modulators of chronic lung disease in preterm infants. J Pediatr 140:171-176, 2002.
85. Witt A, Berger A, Gruber CJ, et al: Increased intrauterine frequency of *Ureaplasma urealyticum* in women with preterm labor and preterm premature rupture of the membranes and subsequent cesarean delivery. Am J Obstet Gynecol 193:1663-1669, 2005.
86. Bhandari V, Gruen JR: The genetics of bronchopulmonary dysplasia. Semin Perinatol 30:185-191, 2006.
87. Bhandari A, Panitch HB: Pulmonary outcomes in bronchopulmonary dysplasia. Semin Perinatol 30:219-226, 2006.
88. Anderson PJ, Doyle LW: Neurodevelopmental outcome of bronchopulmonary dysplasia. Semin Perinatol 30:227-232, 2006.
89. Jobe AH, Bancalari E: Bronchopulmonary dysplasia. Am J Respir Crit Care Med 163:1723-1729, 2001.
90. Baveja R, Christou H: Pharmacological strategies in the prevention and management of bronchopulmonary dysplasia. Semin Perinatol 30:209-218, 2006.
91. Ramon y Cajal CL, Martinez RO: Defecation in utero: A physiologic fetal function. Am J Obstet Gynecol 188:153-156, 2003.
92. Manning FA, Harman CR, Morrison I, et al: Fetal assessment based on fetal biophysical profile scoring. IV. An analysis of perinatal morbidity and mortality. Am J Obstet Gynecol 162:703-709, 1990.
93. Sriram S, Wall SN, Khoshnood B, et al: Racial disparity in meconium-stained amniotic fluid and meconium aspiration syndrome in the United States, 1989-2000. Obstet Gynecol 102:1262-1268, 2003.
94. Rossi EM, Philipson EH, Williams TG, et al: Meconium aspiration syndrome: Intrapartum and neonatal attributes. Am J Obstet Gynecol 61:1106-1110, 1989.
95. Cleary GM, Wiswell TE: Meconium-stained amniotic fluid and the meconium aspiration syndrome: An update. Pediatr Clin North Am 45:511-529, 1998.
96. Keenan WJ: Recommendations for management of the child born through meconium-stained amniotic fluid. Pediatrics 113(Pt 1):133-134, 2004.
97. Wiswell TE, Gannon CM, Jacob J, et al: Delivery room management of the apparently vigorous meconium-stained neonate: Results of the multicenter, international collaborative trial. Pediatrics 105(Pt 1):1-7, 2000.
98. Vain NE, Szyld EG, Prudent LM, et al: Oropharyngeal and nasopharyngeal suctioning of meconium-stained neonates before delivery of their shoulders: Multicentre, randomised controlled trial. Lancet 364:597-602, 2004.
99. Fraser WD, Hofmeyr J, Lede R, et al: Amnioinfusion for the prevention of the meconium aspiration syndrome. N Engl J Med 353:909-917, 2005.
100. Ghidini A, Spong CY: Severe meconium aspiration syndrome is not caused by aspiration of meconium. Am J Obstet Gynecol 185:931-938, 2001.
101. Kinsella JP, Truog WE, Walsh WF, et al: Randomized, multicenter trial of inhaled nitric oxide and high-frequency oscillatory ventilation in severe, persistent pulmonary hypertension of the newborn. J Pediatr 131(Pt 1):55-62, 1997.
102. Hall SM, Hislop AA, Wu Z, et al: Remodelling of the pulmonary arteries during recovery from pulmonary hypertension induced by neonatal hypoxia. J Pathol 203:575-583, 2004.
103. Thureen PJ, Hall DM, Hoffenberg A, et al: Fatal meconium aspiration in spite of appropriate perinatal airway management: Pulmonary and placental evidence of prenatal disease. Am J Obstet Gynecol 176:967-975, 1997.
104. Dargaville PA, Copnell B: The epidemiology of meconium aspiration syndrome: Incidence, risk factors, therapies, and outcome. Pediatrics 117:1712-1721, 2006.
105. Yoder BA, Kirsch EA, Barth WH, et al: Changing obstetric practices associated with decreasing incidence of meconium aspiration syndrome. Obstet Gynecol 99(Pt 1):731-739, 2002.
106. Soll RF, Dargaville P: Surfactant for meconium aspiration syndrome in full term infants. Cochrane Database Syst Rev (2):CD002054, 2002.
107. Inhaled nitric oxide in full-term and nearly full-term infants with hypoxic respiratory failure. The Neonatal Inhaled Nitric Oxide Study Group. N Engl J Med 336:597-604, 1997.
108. Ostrea EM, Villanueva-Uy ET, Natarajan G, et al: Persistent pulmonary hypertension of the newborn: Pathogenesis, etiology, and management. Paediatr Drugs 8:179-188, 2006.
109. Boloker J, Bateman DA, Wung JT, et al: Congenital diaphragmatic hernia in 120 infants treated consecutively with permissive hypercapnea/spontaneous respiration/elective repair. J Pediatr Surg 37:357-366, 2002.
110. Piazza AJ, Stoll BJ: Digestive system disorders. In Kliegman RM, Behrman RE, Jenson HB, et al (eds): Nelson Textbook of Pediatrics, 18th ed: Philadelphia, WB Saunders, 2007.

111. Jesse Na, Neu J: Necrotizing enterocolitis: Relationship to innate immunity. Clinical features, and strategies for prevention. Neoreviews 7:e143-e148, 2006.
112. Uauy RD, Fanaroff AA, Korones SB, et al:. Necrotizing enterocolitis in very low birth weight infants: Biodemographic and clinical correlates. J Pediatr 119:630-638, 1991.
113. Stoll BJ: Epidemiology of necrotizing enterocolitis. Clin Perinatol 21:205-218, 1994.
114. Moss RL, Dimmitt RA, Barnhart DC, et al: Laparotomy versus peritoneal drainage for necrotizing enterocolitis and perforation. N Engl J Med 354:2225-2234, 2006.
115. Llanos AR, Moss ME, Pinzon MC, et al: Epidemiology of neonatal necrotising enterocolitis: A population-based study. Paediatr Perinat Epidemiol 16:342-349, 2002.
116. Bauer CR, Morrison JC, Poole WK, et al: A decreased incidence of necrotizing enterocolitis after prenatal glucocorticoid therapy. Pediatrics 73:682-688, 1984.
117. Halac E, Halac J, Begue EF, et al: Prenatal and postnatal corticosteroid therapy to prevent neonatal necrotizing enterocolitis: A controlled trial. J Pediatr 117(Pt 1):132-138, 1990.
118. Roberts D, Dalziel S: Antenatal corticosteroids for accelerating fetal lung maturation for women at risk of preterm birth. Cochrane Database Syst Rev (3):CD004454, 2006.
119. Niebyl JR, Blake DA, White RD, et al: The inhibition of premature labor with indomethacin. Am J Obstet Gynecol 136:1014-1019, 1980.
120. Zuckerman H, Shalev E, Gilad G, et al: Further study of the inhibition of premature labor by indomethacin. Part II. Double-blind study. J Perinat Med 12:25-29, 1984.
121. Norton ME, Merrill J, Cooper BA, et al. Neonatal complications after the administration of indomethacin for preterm labor. N Engl J Med 329:1602-1607, 1993.
122. Major CA, Lewis DF, Harding JA, et al: Tocolysis with indomethacin increases the incidence of necrotizing enterocolitis in the low-birth-weight neonate. Am J Obstet Gynecol 170(Pt 1):102-106, 1994.
123. Vermillion ST, Newman RB: Recent indomethacin tocolysis is not associated with neonatal complications in preterm infants. Am J Obstet Gynecol 181(Pt 1):1083-1086, 1999.
124. Parilla BV, Grobman WA, Holtzman RB, et al: Indomethacin tocolysis and risk of necrotizing enterocolitis. Obstet Gynecol 96:120-123, 2000.
125. Loe SM, Sanchez-Ramos L, Kaunitz AM: Assessing the neonatal safety of indomethacin tocolysis; A systematic review with meta-analysis. Obstet Gynecol 106:173-179, 2005.
126. McGuire W, Anthony MY: Donor human milk versus formula for preventing necrotising enterocolitis in preterm infants: Systematic review. Arch Dis Child Fetal Neonatal Ed 88:F11-F14, 2003.
127. Sisk PM, Lovelady CA, Dillard RG, et al: Lactation counseling for mothers of very low birth weight infants: Effect on maternal anxiety and infant intake of human milk. Pediatrics 117:e67-e75, 2006.
128. Lin HC, Su BH, Chen AC, et al: Oral probiotics reduce the incidence and severity of necrotizing enterocolitis in very low birth weight infants. Pediatrics 115:1-4, 2005.
129. Hintz SR, Kendrick DE, Stoll BJ, et al: Neurodevelopmental and growth outcomes of extremely low birth weight infants after necrotizing enterocolitis. Pediatrics 115:696-703, 2005.
130. Salhab WA, Perlman JM, Silver L, et al: Necrotizing enterocolitis and neurodevelopmental outcome in extremely low birth weight infants <1000 g. J Perinatol 24:534-540, 2004.
131. Bisquera JA, Cooper TR, Berseth CL: Impact of necrotizing enterocolitis on length of stay and hospital charges in very low birth weight infants. Pediatrics 109:423-428, 2002.
132. Vohr BR, Wright LL, Dusick AM, et al: Neurodevelopmental and functional outcomes of extremely low birth weight infants in the National Institute of Child Health and Human Development Neonatal Research Network, 1993-1994. Pediatrics 105:1216-1226, 2000.
133. Nelson KB, Ellenberg JH: Apgar scores as predictors of chronic neurologic disability. Pediatrics 68:36-44, 1981.
134. Avery GB, Fletcher M, MacDonald MG (eds): Neonatology: Pathophysiology and Management of the Newborn, 4th ed. Philadelphia, JB Lippincott, 1994.
135. Centers for Disease Control and Prevention (CDC): Kernicterus in full-term infants; United States, 1994-1998. MMWR Morb Mortal Wkly Rep 50:23, 2001.
136. Peevy KJ, Landaw SA, Gross SJ: Hyperbilirubinemia in infants of diabetic mothers. Pediatrics 66:417-419, 1980.
137. Cowett RM: Neonatal Care of the Infant of the Diabetic Mother. Neoreviews 13:e190-e5, 2002.
138. Newman TB, Xiong B, Gonzales VM, Escobar GJ: Prediction and prevention of extreme neonatal hyperbilirubinemia in a mature health maintenance organization. Arch Pediatr Adolesc Med 154:1140-1147, 2000.
139. American Academy of Pediatrics: Guidelines for clinical practice: Management of hyperbilirubinemia in the newborn infant 35 or more weeks of gestation. Pediatrics 114:297-316, 2004.
140. Huang MJ, Kua KE, Teng HC, et al. Risk factors for severe hyperbilirubinemia in neonates. Pediatr Res 56:682-689, 2004.
141. Volpe JJ: Bilirubin and brain injury. Neurology of the Newborn, 3rd. ed. Philadelphia, WB Saunders, 1995, pp 490-515.
142. Dennery PA, Seidman DS, Stevenson DK: Neonatal hyperbilirubinemia. N Engl J Med 344:581-590, 2001.
143. Newman TB, Liljestrand P, Jeremy RJ, et al: Outcomes among newborns with total serum bilirubin levels of 25 mg per deciliter or more. N Engl J Med 4;354:1889-1900, 2006.
144. Maisels MJ, Newman TB: Kernicterus in otherwise healthy, breast-fed term newborns. Pediatrics 96(Pt 1):730-733, 1995.
145. Burklow KA, Phelps AN, Schultz JR, et al: Classifying complex pediatric feeding disorders. J Pediatr Gastroenterol Nutr 27:143-147, 1998.
146. Stolar CJ, Levy JP, Dillon PW, et al: Anatomic and functional abnormalities of the esophagus in infants surviving congenital diaphragmatic hernia. Am J Surg 159:204-207, 1990.
147. Van Meurs KP, Robbins ST, Reed VL, et al: Congenital diaphragmatic hernia: Long-term outcome in neonates treated with extracorporeal membrane oxygenation. J Pediatr 122:893-899, 1993.
148. Kieffer J, Sapin E, Berg A, et al: Gastroesophageal reflux after repair of congenital diaphragmatic hernia. J Pediatr Surg 30:1330-1333, 1995.
149. D'Agostino JA, Bernbaum JC, Gerdes M, et al: Outcome for infants with congenital diaphragmatic hernia requiring extracorporeal membrane oxygenation: The first year. J Pediatr Surg 30:10-15, 1995.
150. Vanamo K, Rintala RJ, Lindahl H, et al: Long-term gastrointestinal morbidity in patients with congenital diaphragmatic defects. J Pediatr Surg 31:551-554, 1996.
151. Muratore CS, Utter S, Jaksic T, et al: Nutritional morbidity in survivors of congenital diaphragmatic hernia. J Pediatr Surg 36:1171-1176, 2001.
152. Ledbetter DJ: Gastroschisis and omphalocele. Surg Clin North Am 86:249-260, vii, 2006.
153. Molik KA, Gingalewski CA, West KW, et al: Gastroschisis: A plea for risk categorization. J Pediatr Surg 36:51-55, 2001.
154. Beaudoin S, Kieffer G, Sapin E, et al: Gastroesophageal reflux in neonates with congenital abdominal wall defect. Eur J Pediatr Surg 5:323-326, 1995.
155. Volpe JJ (ed): Neurology of the Newborn. Philadelphia, WB Saunders, 2001.
156. Nelson KB, Ellenberg JH: Antecedents of cerebral palsy. Multivariate analysis of risk. N Engl J Med 315:81-86, 1986.
157. Gaffney G, Sellers S, Flavell V, et al: Case-control study of intrapartum care, cerebral palsy, and perinatal death. BMJ 308:743-750, 1994.
158. Gunn AJ: Cerebral hypothermia for prevention of brain injury following perinatal asphyxia. Curr Opin Pediatr 12:111-115, 2000.
159. Dixon G, Badawi N, Kurinczuk JJ, et al: Early developmental outcomes after newborn encephalopathy. Pediatrics 109:26-33, 2002.
160. Vannucci RC, Perlman JM: Interventions for perinatal hypoxic-ischemic encephalopathy. Pediatrics 100:1004-10014.
161. Perlman JM: Intervention strategies for neonatal hypoxic-ischemic cerebral injury. Clin Ther 28:1353-1365, 2006.

162. Perlman JM: Intrapartum asphyxia and cerebral palsy: Is there a link? Clin Perinatol 33:335-353, 2006.
163. Thacker SB, Stroup D, Chang M: Continuous electronic heart rate monitoring for fetal assessment during labor. Cochrane Database Syst Rev (2): CD000063, 2001.
164. American College of Obstetricians and Gynecologists (ACOG): Clinical management guidelines for obstetrician-gynecologists: Intrapartum fetal heart rate monitoring. ACOG practice bulletin no. 70, December 2005. Obstet Gynecol 106:1453-1460, 2005.
165. Gluckman PD, Wyatt JS, Azzopardi D, et al: Selective head cooling with mild systemic hypothermia after neonatal encephalopathy: Multicentre randomised trial. Lancet 365:663-670, 2005.
166. Sarnat HB, Sarnat MS: Neonatal encephalopathy following fetal distress. A clinical and electroencephalographic study. Arch Neurol 33:696-705, 1976.
167. Papile LA: Systemic hypothermia—a "cool" therapy for neonatal hypoxic-ischemic encephalopathy. N Engl J Med 353:1619-1620, 2005.
168. Batton DG, Holtrop P, DeWitte D, et al: Current gestational age-related incidence of major intraventricular hemorrhage. J Pediatr 125:623-625, 1994.
169. Whitelaw A: Intraventricular haemorrhage and posthaemorrhagic hydrocephalus: Pathogenesis, prevention and future interventions. Semin Neonatol 6:135-146, 2001.
170. Volpe JJ (ed): Neurology of the Newborn. 3rd ed. Philadelphia, WB Saunders, 1995.
171. Crowley P: Prophylactic corticosteroids for preterm birth. Cochrane Database Syst Rev (2):CD000065, 2000.
172. Kaiser AM, Whitelaw AG: Cerebrospinal fluid pressure during post haemorrhagic ventricular dilatation in newborn infants. Arch Dis Child 60:920-924, 1985.
173. Dauber IM, Krauss AN, Symchych PS, et al: Renal failure following perinatal anoxia. J Pediatr 88:851-855, 1976.
174. Folkerth RD: Periventricular leukomalacia: Overview and recent findings. Pediatr Dev Pathol 9:3-13, 2006.
175. Golomb MR, Dick PT, MacGregor DL, et al: Cranial ultrasonography has a low sensitivity for detecting arterial ischemic stroke in term neonates. J Child Neurol 18:98-103, 2003.
176. Nelson KB, Lynch JK: Stroke in newborn infants. Lancet Neurol 3:150-158, 2004.
177. Little WJ: On the influence of abnormal parturition, difficult labours, premature birth, and asphyxia neonatorum, on the mental and physical condition of the child, especially in relation to deformities. Clinical orthopaedics and related research 46:7-22, 1996.
178. Bax M, Goldstein M, Rosenbaum P, et al: Proposed definition and classification of cerebral palsy, April 2005. Dev Med Child Neurol 47:571-576, 2005.
179. Paneth N, Kiely J: The frequency of cerebral palsy: A review of population studies in industrialized nations since 1950. Clin Dev Med 87:46-56, 1984.
180. Stanley F, Blair E: Postnatal risk factors in the cerebral palsies. Clin Dev Med 87:135-149, 1984.
181. Shankaran S, Johnson Y, Langer JC, et al: Outcome of extremely-low-birth-weight infants at highest risk: gestational age < or =24 weeks, birth weight < or = 750 g, and 1-minute Apgar < or = 3. Am J Obstet Gynecol 191:1084-1091, 2004.
182. Pharoah PO, Cooke T, Johnson MA, et al: Epidemiology of cerebral palsy in England and Scotland, 1984-1989. Arch Dis Child 79:F21-F25, 1998.
183. Pharoah PO: Risk of cerebral palsy in multiple pregnancies. Clin Perinatol 33:301-313, 2006.
184. Lidegaard O, Pinborg A, Andersen AN: Imprinting diseases and IVF: Danish National IVF cohort study. Hum Reprod 20:950-954, 2005.
185. Hill A: Intraventricular hemorrhage: Emphasis on prevention. Semin Pediatr Neurol 5:152-160, 1998.
186. Wilson-Costello D, Friedman H, Minich N, et al: Improved neurodevelopmental outcomes for extremely low birth weight infants in 2000-2002. Pediatrics 119:37-45, 2007.
187. Tsuji M, Saul JP, du Plessis A, et al: Cerebral intravascular oxygenation correlates with mean arterial pressure in critically ill premature infants. Pediatrics 106:625-632, 2000.
188. Andrew M, Castle V, Saigal S, et al: Clinical impact of neonatal thrombocytopenia. J Pediatr 110:457-464, 1987.
189. Whitelaw A, Haines ME, Bolsover W, et al: Factor V deficiency and antenatal intraventricular haemorrhage. Arch Dis Child 59:997-999, 1984.
190. Gilles FH, Price RA, Kevy SV, et al: Fibrinolytic activity in the ganglionic eminence of the premature human brain. Biol Neonate 18:426-432, 1971.
191. Patra K, Wilson-Costello D, Taylor HG, et al: Grades I-II intraventricular hemorrhage in extremely low birth weight infants: Effects on neurodevelopment. J Pediatr 149:169-173, 2006.
192. Crowther CA, Henderson-Smart DJ: Phenobarbital prior to preterm birth for preventing neonatal periventricular haemorrhage. Cochrane Database Syst Rev (3):CD000164, 2003.
193. Crowther CA, Henderson-Smart DJ: Vitamin K prior to preterm birth for preventing neonatal periventricular haemorrhage. Cochrane Database Syst Rev (1):CD000229, 2001.
194. Crowther CA, Hiller JE, Doyle LW, et al: Effect of magnesium sulfate given for neuroprotection before preterm birth: A randomized controlled trial. JAMA 290:2669-2676, 2003.
195. Whitelaw A: Postnatal phenobarbitone for the prevention of intraventricular hemorrhage in preterm infants. Cochrane Database Syst Rev (2): CD001691, 2000.
196. Cools F, Offringa M: Neuromuscular paralysis for newborn infants receiving mechanical ventilation. Cochrane Database Syst Rev (4):CD002773, 2000.
197. Berg AT: Indices of fetal growth-retardation, perinatal hypoxia-related factors and childhood neurological morbidity. Early Hum Dev 19:271-283, 1989.
198. Benson JW, Drayton MR, Hayward C, et al: Multicentre trial of ethamsylate for prevention of periventricular haemorrhage in very low birthweight infants. Lancet 2:1297-1300, 1986.
199. The EC randomised controlled trial of prophylactic ethamsylate for very preterm neonates: Early mortality and morbidity. The EC Ethamsylate Trial Group. Arch Dis Child Fetal Neonatal Ed 70:F201-F205, 1994.
200. Pryds O, Greisen G, Johansen KH: Indomethacin and cerebral blood flow in premature infants treated for patent ductus arteriosus. Eur J Pediatr 147:315-316, 1988.
201. Pourcyrous M, Leffler CW, Bada HS, et al: Brain superoxide anion generation in asphyxiated piglets and the effect of indomethacin at therapeutic dose. Pediatr Res 34:366-369, 1993.
202. Ment LR, Stewart WB, Ardito TA, et al: Indomethacin promotes germinal matrix microvessel maturation in the newborn beagle pup. Stroke 23:1132-1137, 1992.
203. Fowlie PW: Intravenous indomethacin for preventing mortality and morbidity in very low birth weight infants. Cochrane Database Syst Rev (2): CD000174, 2000.
204. Ment LR, Vohr B, Allan W, et al: Outcome of children in the indomethacin intraventricular hemorrhage prevention trial. Pediatrics 105(Pt 1):485-491, 2000.
205. Vohr BR, Allan WC, Westerveld M, et al: School-age outcomes of very low birth weight infants in the indomethacin intraventricular hemorrhage prevention trial. Pediatrics 111(Pt 1):e340-e346, 2003.
206. Whitelaw A, Christie S, Pople I: Transforming growth factor-beta1: A possible signal molecule for posthemorrhagic hydrocephalus? Pediatr Res 46:576-580, 1999.
207. Whitelaw A: Repeated lumbar or ventricular punctures for preventing disability or shunt dependence in newborn infants with intraventricular hemorrhage. Cochrane Database Syst Rev (2):CD000216, 2000.
208. Spinillo A, Capuzzo E, Stronati M, et al: Obstetric risk factors for periventricular leukomalacia among preterm infants. BJOG 105:865-871, 1998.
209. Resch B, Vollaard E, Maurer U, et al: Risk factors and determinants of neurodevelopmental outcome in cystic periventricular leucomalacia. Eur J Pediatr159:663-670, 2000.

210. Perlman JM, Risser R, Broyles RS: Bilateral cystic periventricular leukomalacia in the premature infant: Associated risk factors. Pediatrics 97(Pt 1):822-827, 1996.
211. Zupan V, Gonzalez P, Lacaze-Masmonteil T, et al: Periventricular leukomalacia: Risk factors revisited. Dev Med Child Neurol 38:1061-1067, 1996.
212. Volpe JJ: Brain injury in the premature infant: Overview of clinical aspects, neuropathology, and pathogenesis. Semin Pediatr Neurol 5:135-151, 1998.
213. Golden JA, Gilles FH, Rudelli R, et al: Frequency of neuropathological abnormalities in very low birth weight infants. J Neuropathol Exp Neurol 56:472-478, 1997.
214. Gilles FH, Leviton A, Dooling EC: The Developing Human Brain: Growth and Epidemiologic Neuropathology. Boston, John Wright 1983.
215. Lee J, Croen LA, Lindan C, et al: Predictors of outcome in perinatal arterial stroke: A population-based study. Ann Neurol 58:303-308, 2005.
216. Lou HC, Lassen NA, Tweed WA, et al: Pressure passive cerebral blood flow and breakdown of the blood-brain barrier in experimental fetal asphyxia. Acta Paediatr Scand 68:57-63, 1979.
217. Pryds O, Greisen G, Lou H, et al: Heterogeneity of cerebral vasoreactivity in preterm infants supported by mechanical ventilation. J Pediatr 115:638-645, 1989.
218. Kirton A, deVeber G: Cerebral palsy secondary to perinatal ischemic stroke. Clin Perinatol 33:367-386, 2006.
219. Schulzke S, Weber P, Luetschg J, et al: Incidence and diagnosis of unilateral arterial cerebral infarction in newborn infants. J Perinat Med 33:170-175, 2005.
220. de Vries LS, Groenendaal F, Eken P, et al: Infarcts in the vascular distribution of the middle cerebral artery in preterm and fullterm infants. Neuropediatrics 28:88-96, 1997.
221. Lynch JK, Nelson KB: Epidemiology of perinatal stroke. Current opinion in pediatrics 13:499-505, 2001.
222. deVeber G, Roach ES, Riela AR, et al: Stroke in children: Recognition, treatment, and future directions. Semin Pediatr Neurol 7:309-317, 2000.
223. Lee J, Croen LA, Backstrand KH, et al: Maternal and infant characteristics associated with perinatal arterial stroke in the infant. JAMA 293:723-729, 2005.
224. Miller V: Neonatal cerebral infarction. Semin Pediatr Neurol 7:278-288, 2000.
225. Mercuri E, Cowan F: Cerebral infarction in the newborn infant: Review of the literature and personal experience. Eur J Paediatr Neurol 3:255-263, 1999.
226. Golomb MR, MacGregor DL, Domi T, et al: Presumed pre- or perinatal arterial ischemic stroke: Risk factors and outcomes. Ann Neurol 50:163-168, 2001.
227. Suarez CR, Walenga J, Mangogna LC, et al: Neonatal and maternal fibrinolysis: Activation at time of birth. Am J Hematol 19:365-372, 1985.
228. Heller SL, Heier LA, Watts R, et al: Evidence of cerebral reorganization following perinatal stroke demonstrated with fMRI and DTI tractography. Clin Imaging 29:283-287, 2005.
229. Staudt M, Grodd W, Gerloff C, et al: Two types of ipsilateral reorganization in congenital hemiparesis: A TMS and fMRI study. Brain 125(Pt 10):2222-2237, 2002.
230. deVeber GA, MacGregor D, Curtis R, et al: Neurologic outcome in survivors of childhood arterial ischemic stroke and sinovenous thrombosis. J Child Neurol 15:316-324, 2000.
231. Mercuri E, Barnett A, Rutherford M, et al: Neonatal cerebral infarction and neuromotor outcome at school age. Pediatrics 113(Pt 1):95-100, 2004.
232. Sreenan C, Bhargava R, Robertson CM: Cerebral infarction in the term newborn: Clinical presentation and long-term outcome. J Pediatr 137:351-355, 2000.
233. Kuban KC, Leviton A: Cerebral palsy. N Engl J Med 330:188-195, 1994.
234. Wood E: The child with cerebral palsy: Diagnosis and beyond. Semin Pediatr Neurol 13:286-296, 2006.
235. MacLennan A: A template for defining a causal relation between acute intrapartum events and cerebral palsy: International consensus statement. BMJ 319:1054-1059, 1999.
236. Blair E, Stanley FJ: Intrapartum asphyxia: A rare cause of cerebral palsy. J Pediatr 112:515-519, 1988.
237. Msall ME: The panorama of cerebral palsy after very and extremely preterm birth: Evidence and challenges. Clin Perinatol 33:269-284.
238. Vohr BR, Msall ME, Wilson D, et al: Spectrum of gross motor function in extremely low birth weight children with cerebral palsy at 18 months of age. Pediatrics 116:123-129, 2005.
239. Wilson-Costello D, Friedman H, Minich N, et al: Improved survival rates with increased neurodevelopmental disability for extremely low birth weight infants in the 1990s. Pediatrics 115:997-1003, 2005.
240. Stoll BJ, Hansen NI, Adams-Chapman I, et al: Neurodevelopmental and growth impairment among extremely low-birth-weight infants with neonatal infection. JAMA 292:2357-2365, 2004.
241. Stark AR, Carlo WA, Tyson JE, et al: Adverse effects of early dexamethasone in extremely-low-birth-weight infants. National Institute of Child Health and Human Development Neonatal Research Network. N Engl J Med 344:95-101, 2001.
242. Yeh TF, Lin YJ, Lin HC, et al: Outcomes at school age after postnatal dexamethasone therapy for lung disease of prematurity. N Engl J Med 350:1304-1313, 2004.
243. Wood NS, Costeloe K, Gibson AT, et al: The EPICure study: Associations and antecedents of neurological and developmental disability at 30 months of age following extremely preterm birth. Arch Dis Child Fetal Neonatal Ed 90:F134-F140, 2005.
244. Schreiber MD, Gin-Mestan K, Marks JD, et al: Inhaled nitric oxide in premature infants with the respiratory distress syndrome. N Engl J Med 349:2099-2107, 2003.
245. Mestan KK, Marks JD, Hecox K, et al: Neurodevelopmental outcomes of premature infants treated with inhaled nitric oxide. N Engl J Med 353:23-32, 2005.
246. Field D, Elbourne D, Truesdale A, et al: Neonatal ventilation with inhaled nitric oxide versus ventilatory support without inhaled nitric oxide for preterm infants with severe respiratory failure: The INNOVO multicentre randomised controlled trial (ISRCTN 17821339). Pediatrics 115:926-936, 2005.
247. Van Meurs KP, Wright LL, Ehrenkranz RA, et al: Inhaled nitric oxide for premature infants with severe respiratory failure. N Engl J Med 353:13-22, 2005.
248. Pharoah PO, Cooke T: Cerebral palsy and multiple births. Arch Dis Child Fetal Neonatal Ed 75:F174-F177, 1996.
249. Watson L, Stanley F: Report of the Western Australian Cerebral Palsy Register. Perth, Telethon Institute for Child Health Research, 1999.
250. Scher AI, Petterson B, Blair E, et al: The risk of mortality or cerebral palsy in twins: A collaborative population-based study. Pediatr Res 52:671-681, 2002.
251. Javier LF, Root L, Tassanawipas A: Cerebral palsy in twins. Dev Med Child Neurol 34:1053-1063, 1992.
252. Garite TJ, Clark RH, Elliott JP, et al: Twin and triplets: The effect of plurality and growth on neonatal outcome compared with singleton infants. Am J Obstet Gynecol 191:700-707, 2004.
253. Pharoah PO, Adi Y: Consequences of in-utero death in a twin pregnancy. Lancet 355:1597-1602, 2000.
254. Pharoah PO: Cerebral palsy in the surviving twin associated with infant death of the co-twin. Arch Dis Child Fetal Neonatal Ed 84:F111-F116, 2001.
255. Pharoah PO, Price TS, Plomin R: Cerebral palsy in twins: A national study. Arch Dis Child Fetal Neonatal Ed 87:F122-F124, 2002.
256. Glinianaia SV, Pharoah PO, Wright C, et al: Fetal or infant death in twin pregnancy: Neurodevelopmental consequence for the survivor. Arch Dis Child Fetal Neonatal Ed 86:F9-F15, 2002.
257. Jarvis S, Glinianaia SV, Torrioli MG, et al: Cerebral palsy and intrauterine growth in single births: European collaborative study. Lancet 362:1106-1111, 2003.

258. Liu J, Li Z, Lin Q, et al: Cerebral palsy and multiple births in China. International journal of epidemiology 29:292-299, 2000.
259. Ellenberg JH, Nelson KB: Birth weight and gestational age in children with cerebral palsy or seizure disorders. Am J Dis Child 133:1044-1048, 1979.
260. Blair E, Stanley F: Intrauterine growth and spastic cerebral palsy. I. Association with birth weight for gestational age. Am J Obstet Gynecol 162:229-237, 1990.
261. Topp M, Langhoff-Roos J, Uldall P, et al: Intrauterine growth and gestational age in preterm infants with cerebral palsy. Early Hum Dev 44:27-36, 1996.
262. Uvebrant P, Hagberg G: Intrauterine growth in children with cerebral palsy. Acta Paediatr 81:407-412, 1992.
263. Hadlock FP, Harrist RB, Martinez-Poyer J: In utero analysis of fetal growth: A sonographic weight standard. Radiology 181:129-133, 1991.
264. Marsal K, Persson PH, Larsen T, et al: Intrauterine growth curves based on ultrasonically estimated foetal weights. Acta Paediatr 85:843-848, 1996.
265. Mongelli M, Gardosi J: Longitudinal study of fetal growth in subgroups of a low-risk population. Ultrasound Obstet Gynecol 6:340-344, 1995.
266. Jarvis S, Glinianaia SV, Blair E: Cerebral palsy and intrauterine growth. Clin Perinatol 33:285-300, 2006.
267. Yanney M, Marlow N: Paediatric consequences of fetal growth restriction. Semin Fetal Neonatal Med 9:411-418, 2004.
268. Surveillance of cerebral palsy in Europe: A collaboration of cerebral palsy surveys and registers. Surveillance of Cerebral Palsy in Europe (SCPE). Dev Med Child Neurol 42:816-824, 2000.
269. Jarvis S, Glinianaia SV, Arnaud C, et al: Case gender and severity in cerebral palsy varies with intrauterine growth. Archives of disease in childhood 90:474-479, 2005.
270. Hermansen MC, Hermansen MG: Perinatal infections and cerebral palsy. Clin Perinatol 33:315-333, 2006.
271. Goldenberg RL, Hauth JC, Andrews WW: Intrauterine infection and preterm delivery. N Engl J Med 342:1500-1507, 2000.
272. Goldenberg RL, Culhane JF, Johnson DC: Maternal infection and adverse fetal and neonatal outcomes. Clin Perinatol 32:523-559, 2005.
273. Dammann O, Leviton A: Maternal intrauterine infection, cytokines, and brain damage in the preterm newborn. Pediatr Res 42:1-8, 1997.
274. Dammann O, Leviton A: The role of perinatal brain damage in developmental disabilities: An epidemiologic perspective. Ment Retard Dev Disabil Res Rev 3:13-21, 1997.
275. Alexander JM, Gilstrap LC, Cox SM, et al: Clinical chorioamnionitis and the prognosis for very low birth weight infants. Obstet Gynecol 91(Pt 1):725-729, 1998.
276. Wu YW, Colford JM Jr: Chorioamnionitis as a risk factor for cerebral palsy: A meta-analysis. JAMA 284:1417-1424, 2000.
277. Grafe MR: The correlation of prenatal brain damage with placental pathology. J Neuropathol Exp Neurol 53:407-415, 1994.
278. Salafia CM, Minior VK, Rosenkrantz TS, et al: Maternal, placental, and neonatal associations with early germinal matrix/intraventricular hemorrhage in infants born before 32 weeks' gestation. Am J Perinatol 12:429-436, 1995.
279. De Felice C, Toti P, Parrini S, et al: Histologic chorioamnionitis and severity of illness in very low birth weight newborns. Pediatr Crit Care Med 6:298-302, 2005.
280. Kraus FT: Cerebral palsy and thrombi in placental vessels of the fetus: Insights from litigation. Hum Pathol 28:246-248, 1997.
281. Leviton A: Preterm birth and cerebral palsy: Is tumor necrosis factor the missing link? Dev Med Child Neurol 35:553-558, 1993.
282. Adinolfi M: Infectious diseases in pregnancy, cytokines and neurological impairment: An hypothesis. Dev Med Child Neurol 35:549-558, 1993.
283. Dammann O, Leviton A: Brain damage in preterm newborns: Might enhancement of developmentally regulated endogenous protection open a door for prevention? Pediatrics 104(Pt 1):541-550, 1999.
284. Chao CC, Hu S, Ehrlich L, et al: Interleukin-1 and tumor necrosis factor-alpha synergistically mediate neurotoxicity: Involvement of nitric oxide and of *N*-methyl-D-aspartate receptors. Brain Behav Immun 9:355-365, 1995.
285. Okusawa S, Gelfand JA, Ikejima T, et al: Interleukin 1 induces a shock-like state in rabbits. Synergism with tumor necrosis factor and the effect of cyclooxygenase inhibition. J Clin Invest 81:1162-1172, 1988.
286. Yoon BH, Romero R, Yang SH, et al: Interleukin-6 concentrations in umbilical cord plasma are elevated in neonates with white matter lesions associated with periventricular leukomalacia. Am J Obstet Gynecol 174:1433-1440, 1996.
287. Nelson KB, Grether JK: Potentially asphyxiating conditions and spastic cerebral palsy in infants of normal birth weight. Am J Obstet Gynecol 179:507-513, 1998.
288. Nelson KB, Dambrosia JM, Grether JK, Phillips TM: Neonatal cytokines and coagulation factors in children with cerebral palsy. Ann Neurol 44:665-675, 1998.
289. Wheater M, Rennie JM: Perinatal infection is an important risk factor for cerebral palsy in very-low-birthweight infants. Dev Med Child Neurol 42:364-367, 2000.
290. Murphy DJ, Hope PL, Johnson A: Neonatal risk factors for cerebral palsy in very preterm babies: Case-control study. BMJ 314:404-408, 1997.
291. Redline RW: Placental pathology and cerebral palsy. Clin Perinatol 33:503-516, 2006.
292. Redline RW: Severe fetal placental vascular lesions in term infants with neurologic impairment. Am J Obstet Gynecol 192:452-457, 2005.
293. Redline RW, Patterson P: Patterns of placental injury. Correlations with gestational age, placental weight, and clinical diagnoses. Arch Pathol Lab Med118:698-701, 1994.
294. Wichers MJ, Odding E, Stam HJ, et al: Clinical presentation, associated disorders and aetiological moments in cerebral palsy: A Dutch population-based study. Disabil Rehabil 27:583-589, 2005.
295. Shy KK, Luthy DA, Bennett FC, et al: Effects of electronic fetal-heart-rate monitoring, as compared with periodic auscultation, on the neurologic development of premature infants. N Engl J Med 322:588-593, 1990.
296. Nelson KB, Dambrosia JM, Ting TY, Grether JK: Uncertain value of electronic fetal monitoring in predicting cerebral palsy. N Engl J Med 334:613-618, 1996.
297. Martin JA, Hamilton BE, Sutton PD, et al: Births: Final data for 2003. Natl Vital Stat Rep 54:1-116, 2005.
298. Thorngren-Jerneck K, Herbst A: Perinatal factors associated with cerebral palsy in children born in Sweden. Obstet Gynecol 108:1499-1505, 2006.
299. Crowley PA: Antenatal corticosteroid therapy: A meta-analysis of the randomized trials, 1972 to 1994. Am J Obstet Gynecol 173:322-335, 1995.
300. Yeh TF, Lin YJ, Huang CC, et al: Early dexamethasone therapy in preterm infants: A follow-up study. Pediatrics 101:E7, 1998.
301. O'Shea TM, Kothadia JM, Klinepeter KL, et al: Randomized placebo-controlled trial of a 42-day tapering course of dexamethasone to reduce the duration of ventilator dependency in very low birth weight infants: Outcome of study participants at 1-year adjusted age. Pediatrics 104(Pt 1):15-21, 1999.
302. Shinwell ES, Karplus M, Reich D, et al: Early postnatal dexamethasone treatment and increased incidence of cerebral palsy. Arch Dis Child Fetal Neonatal Ed 83:F177-F181, 2000.
303. McDonald JW, Silverstein FS, Johnston MV: Magnesium reduces *N*-methyl-D-aspartate (NMDA)–mediated brain injury in perinatal rats. Neurosci Lett 109:234-238, 1990.
304. Weglicki WB, Phillips TM, Freedman AM, et al: Magnesium-deficiency elevates circulating levels of inflammatory cytokines and endothelin. Molecular and cellular biochemistry 110:169-173, 1992.
305. Wiswell TE, Graziani LJ, Caddell JL, et al: Maternally administered magnesium sulphate protects against early brain injury and long-term adverse neurodevelopmental outcomes in preterm infants: A prospective study. Pediatr Res 39:253A, 1996.
306. Nelson KB, Grether JK: Can magnesium sulfate reduce the risk of cerebral palsy in very low birthweight infants? Pediatrics 95:263-269, 1995.
307. Hauth JC, Goldenberg RL, Nelson KB, et al: Reduction of cerebral palsy with maternal $MgSO_4$ treatment in newborns weighing 500-1000 g [abstract]. Am J Obstet Gynecol 172(Pt 2):419, 1995.
308. Schendel DE, Berg CJ, Yeargin-Allsopp M, et al: Prenatal magnesium sulfate exposure and the risk for cerebral palsy or mental retardation

among very low-birth-weight children aged 3 to 5 years. JAMA 276:1805-1810, 1996.
309. Paneth N, Jetton J, Pinto-Martin J, Susser M: Magnesium sulfate in labor and risk of neonatal brain lesions and cerebral palsy in low birth weight infants. The Neonatal Brain Hemorrhage Study Analysis Group. Pediatrics 99:E1, 1997.
310. O'Shea TM, Klinepeter KL, Dillard RG: Prenatal events and the risk of cerebral palsy in very low birth weight infants. Am J Epidemiol 147:362-369, 1998.
311. Boyle CA, Yeargin-Allsopp M, Schendel DE, et al: Tocolytic magnesium sulfate exposure and risk of cerebral palsy among children with birth weights less than 1,750 grams. American journal of epidemiology 152:120-124, 2000.
312. Grether JK, Hoogstrate J, Walsh-Greene E, et al: Magnesium sulfate for tocolysis and risk of spastic cerebral palsy in premature children born to women without preeclampsia. Am J Obstet Gynecol 183:717-725, 2000.
313. Mittendorf R, Covert R, Boman J, et al: Is tocolytic magnesium sulphate associated with increased total paediatric mortality? Lancet 350:1517-1518, 1997.
314. Mittendorf R, Dambrosia J, Pryde PG, et al: Association between the use of antenatal magnesium sulfate in preterm labor and adverse health outcomes in infants. Am J Obstet Gynecol 186:1111-1118, 2002.
315. Rouse D for the NICHD MFMU Network. A randomized controlled trial of magnesium sulfate for the prevention of cerebral palsy. Abstract 1 at the 2008 meeting of the Society for Maternal Fetal Medicine. Am J Obstet Gynecol 197:S2, 2008.
316. Bizzarro MJ, Raskind C, Baltimore RS, et al: Seventy-five years of neonatal sepsis at Yale: 1928-2003. Pediatrics 116:595-602, 2005.
317. Schelonka RL, Infante AJ: Neonatal immunology. Semin Perinatol 22:2-14, 1998.
318. Andrews WW, Goldenberg RL, Faye-Petersen O, et al: The Alabama Preterm Birth study: Polymorphonuclear and mononuclear cell placental infiltrations, other markers of inflammation, and outcomes in 23- to 32-week preterm newborn infants. Am J Obstet Gynecol 195:803-808, 2006.
319. Willet KE, Kramer BW, Kallapur SG, et al: Intra-amniotic injection of IL-1 induces inflammation and maturation in fetal sheep lung. Am J Physiol Lung Cell Mol Physiol 282:L411-L4120, 2002.
320. Nogueira-Silva C, Santos M, Baptista MJ, et al: IL-6 is constitutively expressed during lung morphogenesis and enhances fetal lung explant branching. Pediatr Res 60:530-536, 2006.
321. Gravett MG, Novy MJ, Rosenfeld RG, et al: Diagnosis of intra-amniotic infection by proteomic profiling and identification of novel biomarkers. JAMA 292:462-469, 2004
322. Buhimschi CS, Buhimschi IA, Abdel-Razeq S, et al: Proteomic biomarkers of intra-amniotic inflammation: Relationship with funisitis and early-onset sepsis in the premature neonate. Pediatr Res 61:318-324, 2007.
323. Schrag S, Gorwitz R, Fultz-Butts K, et al: Prevention of perinatal group B streptococcal disease. Revised guidelines from CDC. MMWR Recomm Rep 51:1-22, 2002.
324. Centers for Disease Control and Prevention (CDC): Perinatal group B streptococcal disease after universal screening recommendations—United States, 2003-2005. MMWR Morb Mortal Wkly Rep 56:701-705, 2007.
325. Puopolo KM, Madoff LC, Eichenwald EC: Early-onset group B streptococcal disease in the era of maternal screening. Pediatrics 115:1240-1246, 2005.
326. Honest H, Sharma S, Khan KS: Rapid tests for group B *Streptococcus* colonization in laboring women: A systematic review. Pediatrics 117:1055-1066, 2006.
327. Glasgow TS, Young PC, Wallin J, et al: Association of intrapartum antibiotic exposure and late-onset serious bacterial infections in infants. Pediatrics 116:696-702, 2005.
328. Dworsky M, Yow M, Stagno S, et al: Cytomegalovirus infection of breast milk and transmission in infancy. Pediatrics 72:295-299, 1983.
329. Hamprecht K, Maschmann J, Vochem M, et al: Epidemiology of transmission of cytomegalovirus from mother to preterm infant by breastfeeding. Lancet 357:513-518, 2001.
330. Fowler KB, Stagno S, Pass RF, et al: The outcome of congenital cytomegalovirus infection in relation to maternal antibody status. N Engl J Med 326:663-667, 1992.
331. Noyola DE, Demmler GJ, Nelson CT, et al: Early predictors of neurodevelopmental outcome in symptomatic congenital cytomegalovirus infection. J Pediatr 138:325-231, 2001.
332. Kimberlin DW, Lin CY, Sanchez PJ, et al. Effect of ganciclovir therapy on hearing in symptomatic congenital cytomegalovirus disease involving the central nervous system: A randomized, controlled trial. J Pediatr 143:16-25, 2003.
333. Gilbert GL, Hayes K, Hudson IL, et al: Prevention of transfusion-acquired cytomegalovirus infection in infants by blood filtration to remove leucocytes. Neonatal Cytomegalovirus Infection Study Group. Lancet 1:1228-1231, 1989.
334. Hamprecht K, Maschmann J, Muller D, et al: Cytomegalovirus (CMV) inactivation in breast milk: Reassessment of pasteurization and freeze-thawing. Pediatr Res 56:529-535, 2004.
335. Maschmann J, Hamprecht K, Weissbrich B, et al: Freeze-thawing of breast milk does not prevent cytomegalovirus transmission to a preterm infant. Arch Dis Child Fetal Neonatal Ed 91:F288-F290, 2006.
336. Shepard CW, Finelli L, Fiore AE, et al: Epidemiology of hepatitis B and hepatitis B virus infection in United States children. Pediatr Infect Dis J24:755-760, 2005.
337. Kropp RY, Wong T, Cormier L, et al: Neonatal herpes simplex virus infections in Canada: Results of a 3-year national prospective study. Pediatrics 117:1955-1962, 2006.
338. O'Riordan DP, Golden WC, Aucott SW: Herpes simplex virus infections in preterm infants. Pediatrics 118:e1612-e1620, 2006.
339. Connor EM, Sperling RS, Gelber R, et al: Reduction of maternal-infant transmission of human immunodeficiency virus type 1 with zidovudine treatment. Pediatric AIDS Clinical Trials Group Protocol 076 Study Group. N Engl J Med 331:1173-1180, 1994.
340. Volmink J, Siegfried NL, van der Merwe L, et al: Antiretrovirals for reducing the risk of mother-to-child transmission of HIV infection. Cochrane Database Syst Rev (1):CD003510, 2007.
341. Reef SE, Redd SB, Abernathy E, et al: The epidemiological profile of rubella and congenital rubella syndrome in the United States, 1998-2004: The evidence for absence of endemic transmission. Clin Infect Dis 43(Suppl 3):S126-S132, 2006.
342. Schachter J, Grossman M, Sweet RL, et al: Prospective study of perinatal transmission of *Chlamydia trachomatis*. JAMA 255:3374-3377, 1986.
343. Hammerschlag MR, Cummings C, Roblin PM, et al: Efficacy of neonatal ocular prophylaxis for the prevention of chlamydial and gonococcal conjunctivitis. N Engl J Med 320:769-772, 1989.
344. Kumar P: Physician documentation of neonatal risk assessment for perinatal infections. J Pediatr 149:265-267, 2006.

INDEX

Note: Page numbers followed by f indicate figures; those followed by t indicate tables.

A

Abacavir (Ziagen), for HIV infection, 772t
ABCB4 gene, 1060
ABCB11 gene, 1060
Abdominal circumference, fetal
  in intrauterine growth restriction, 642, 643f
  maternal diabetes and, 964
Abdominal situs, fetal echocardiography of, 307, 310–311, 311f
Abdominal trauma
  blunt, 1184–1186, 1185f
  penetrating, 1186
Abdominal wall defects, 293–294, 294f
  neonatal management of, 1198t
Abdominal wound infection, 761–762
Abilify (aripiprazole), dosage of, 1116t
ABO hemolytic disease, hyperbilirubinemia in, 1208–1209
ABO incompatibility, neonatal outcomes with, 1199
Abortion(s)
  of conjoined twins, 468
  and preterm birth, 557
  selective
    of acardiac twin, 434t, 468
    of anomalous fetus, 469–470
    for TRAP sequence, 439–440
    for twin-to-twin transfusion syndrome, 437, 439
  spontaneous
    chromosomal abnormalities in, 21, 21t, 22, 22t
    and first-semester screening, 231–232
    with uterine anomalies, 1144t
    uterine myomas and, 1136, 1138
  thyroiditis after, 1010
Abortuses, chromosome abnormalities in, 21, 21t, 22, 22t
Abruptio placentae, 731–734
  defined, 731
  diagnosis of, 732
  epidemiology of, 731
  factor V Leiden mutation and, 832
  fetal loss due to, 624
  hyperhomocysteinemia and, 834
  management of, 732–733, 733t
  pathogenesis of, 731–732, 731f
  preterm labor due to, 529, 529f
  prevention of, 734
  prothrombin gene mutation and, 833
  risk factors and associations for, 731–732
  due to trauma, 1185
  uterine myomas and, 1136–1137
Abscess
  pelvic, 762
  periappendiceal, 1047
Absent end-diastolic velocities (AEDV)
  in middle cerebral artery, 375
  in umbilical artery, 372–373, 373f, 374t
Absent pulmonary valve (APV), tetralogy of Fallot with, 332–333, 333f
ACA(s) (anticardiolipin antibodies)
  fetal loss due to, 625
  thrombophilia due to, 829, 830t
Acarbose, for diabetes, 982
Acardiac twinning, 64–65, 65f, 66f, 467–468
  invasive fetal therapy for, 434t, 468
Accelerations, in fetal heart rate, 406
Accessory mammary glands, 128
Accessory nipples, 128
Accolate (zafirlukast), for asthma, 940t, 942
ACE (angiotensin-converting enzyme) inhibitors (ACEIs)
  for chronic hypertension, 678
  during pregnancy, 801t
  as teratogens, 349, 351t, 353, 800
Acetaminophen, for influenza, 785
Acetylcholinesterase (AChE), prenatal screening for, 234–235, 234t
  in twins, 459
ACHOIS (Australian Carbohydrate Intolerance Study in Pregnant Women) trial, 979–980, 984
Achondroplastic dwarfism, anesthesia with, 1161
Acid-base balance, fetal. *See* Fetal acid-base balance.
Acidemia
  defined, 401, 401t
  fetal responses to, 399–400
  metabolic, 401, 401t
  mixed, 401, 401t
  pathologic fetal, 402–403, 403t
  respiratory, 401, 401t
Acidosis
  defined, 401, 401t
  metabolic, 401–402
  respiratory, 401
Acitretin, as teratogen, 353–354
Acne, 1131
Acoustic neuroma, 1093
Acquired immunodeficiency syndrome (AIDS). *See* Human immunodeficiency virus (HIV).
Acrocentric chromosomes, 17
Acrochordons, 1124
Acromegaly, 1020–1021
ACTH. *See* Adrenocorticotropic hormone (ACTH).
Actin, in myometrial contraction, 78f
Action potentials, in myometrial contractility, 76
Activated protein C (aPC)
  in anticoagulant system, 828, 828f
  for septic shock, 763, 1179
Activated protein C (aPC) resistance, and fetal loss, 625, 626t
Active phase, of labor, 691, 692, 692t
Activin, during pregnancy, 120
Acupressure, for nausea and vomiting, 1042, 1042t
Acute familial brachial neuritis, 1105
Acute fatty liver of pregnancy (AFLP), 1062–1063, 1063t
  acute renal failure due to, 909
Acute idiopathic polyneuropathy, 1107–1108
Acute liver failure, 1071–1072, 1071t, 1072t
Acute lymphoid leukemia (ALL), in pregnancy, 899
Acute myeloid leukemia (AML), in pregnancy, 899
Acute neurologic injury, umbilical cord acid-base balance and, 403–404
Acute normovolemic hemodilution, 1182
Acute Physiologic and Chronic Health Evaluation (APACHE) scoring system, 1167
Acute promyelocytic leukemia (APL), in pregnancy, 899
Acute renal cortical necrosis (ARCN), 908–909
Acute renal failure, 907–909, 907t
Acute respiratory distress syndrome (ARDS), 1174
  with acute pyelonephritis, 755
Acyclovir, for herpes simplex, 770
ADA (American Diabetes Association), classification and diagnostic criteria of, 953
Adalimumab, for rheumatic disease, 1081, 1082t
ADAM 12, prenatal screening for, 230
ADAMTS13, 842, 843, 843t, 908
Adaptive immunity, 87–88
ADCC (antibody-dependent cell-mediated cytotoxicity) assay, for RhD antibody, 481
Addison disease, 1026–1027, 1027t
Addisonian crisis, 1027
Adducts, 6
Adenohypophysis. *See* Anterior pituitary lobe.
Adenohypophysitis, lymphocytic, 1023–1024, 1023t
Adenomas
  pituitary, 1017–1022, 1093, 1094f
  thyroid, 1008
Adenosine, during pregnancy, 801t
Adenoviruses, breastfeeding with, 137t
Adnexal masses, 1139–1143
  complications of, 1141–1142
  diagnosis of, 1140–1142, 1140t, 1141f, 1142f
    MRI for, 1141
    serologic markers for, 1140–1141
    ultrasonic characteristics in, 1140, 1140t, 1141f, 1142f
  epidemiology of, 1139
  malignant, 885–886, 886t, 1140, 1140t
  management of, 1142–1143
  pathogenesis of, 1139, 1139t
ADO (allele dropout), 260
ADPKD (autosomal dominant polycystic kidney disease)
  pregnancy with, 913, 916t
  prenatal diagnosis of, 248t, 295–296
Adrenal cortex
  disorder(s) of, 1026–1030
    Addison disease as, 1026–1027, 1027t
    congenital adrenal hyperplasia as, 1028–1030, 1029f
    Cushing syndrome as, 1027
    primary hyperaldosteronism as, 1027–1028, 1028f
  fetal development of, 1026
Adrenal corticosteroids. *See* Corticosteroid(s).

Adrenal glands
  control of adrenocortical hormones by, 1025
  fetal development of, 1026
  physiology of, 1025, 1025f
  during pregnancy, 1025–1026, 1026f
Adrenal hyperplasia, congenital
  pregnancy with, 1028–1030, 1029f
  prenatal diagnosis of, 248t, 262
Adrenal insufficiency, relative, in septic shock, 1179
Adrenal medulla
  disorder(s) of, 1030–1031, 1031t
  in fetal cardiovascular regulation, 165
  in fetal heart rate, 398
Adrenal neuroblastomas, hydrops fetalis due to, 509
Adrenal steroidogenesis, 1025, 1025f
Adrenergic control, of fetal cardiovascular system, 164–165
β-Adrenergic receptor agonists
  after premature rupture of the membranes, 606
  as uterine relaxants, 81
β_2-Adrenergic receptor agonists, for asthma, 940, 940t, 941
α-Adrenergic receptor blocking agents, for pheochromocytoma, 1030
β-Adrenergic receptor blocking agents
  for chronic hypertension, 677–678
  for hyperthyroidism, 1002
  for pheochromocytoma, 1030
  during pregnancy, 800, 801t
  for thyroid storm, 1003, 1003t
Adrenocortical hormones, control of, 1025, 1025f
Adrenocortical insufficiency, primary, 1026–1027, 1027t
Adrenocorticotropic hormone (ACTH)
  control of, 1025
  in Cushing syndrome, 1022
  ectopic, 1022
  during pregnancy, 1016, 1025
  in preterm labor, 529, 530f
Adrenocorticotropic hormone (ACTH) stimulation test, 1027
Adrenomedullin
  in fetal cardiovascular regulation, 166–167
  as uterine relaxant, 80
Adult polycystic kidney disease, 295–296
  prenatal diagnosis of, 248t
Adult respiratory distress syndrome (ARDS), 1174
  with acute pyelonephritis, 755
Advair (fluticasone and salmeterol), for asthma, 940t
Adverse case reports, on safety of exposures, 349
Adynamic ileus, postcesarean, 709
AEDV (absent end-diastolic velocities)
  in middle cerebral artery, 375
  in umbilical artery, 372–373, 373f, 374t
AF. *See* Amniotic fluid (AF).
AFI (amniotic fluid index), 366
  with post-term pregnancy, 615
Afibrinogenemia, 844t, 845t, 848
AFLP (acute fatty liver of pregnancy), 1062–1063, 1063t
  acute renal failure due to, 909
AFP. *See* α-Fetoprotein (AFP).
African-Americans
  fetal loss in, 622
  fetal pulmonary maturity in, 421
  preeclampsia and eclampsia in, 654
  preterm birth in, 551, 552f, 554, 554t, 555f, 557
Afterload, fetal, 162, 163
AGCs (atypical glandular cells), 887
Age
  gestational. *See* Gestational age.
  maternal
    and fetal loss, 619–620, 623
    and preeclampsia and eclampsia, 654
    and prenatal screening, 222, 222t, 232–233, 233t
Agenerase (amprenavir), for HIV infection, 772t
AIDS. *See* Human immunodeficiency virus (HIV).
AIF (anti-intrinsic factor antibody), 870t
Airway branching, in fetal lung development, 194–195, 195f
AIS (arterial ischemic stroke), perinatal, 1213–1214, 1213f
Alanine, during pregnancy, 120t
Alanine transaminase (ALT), in pregnancy, 1059, 1060t
Albumin, for hydrops fetalis, 512
Albumin solutions, for hemorrhagic shock, 1180, 1180t
Albuterol, for asthma, 940, 940t, 941
  with acute exacerbations, 943, 943t, 944t
Alcohol, as teratogen, 348–349, 351t, 354–355, 354f
Alcohol consumption
  intrauterine growth restriction due to, 640
  and preterm birth, 555
Alcohol-related birth defects (ARBD), 354
Alcohol-related neurodevelopmental abnormalities (ARND), 354
Aldosterone
  control of, 1025, 1025f
  during pregnancy, 1026
ALIFE (Anticoagulants for Living Fetuses) study, 628
Alkaline phosphatase (ALP), in pregnancy, 1059, 1060t
Alkalosis, respiratory, 401
  during pregnancy, 104, 927
ALL (acute lymphoid leukemia), in pregnancy, 899
Allele(s), 6
Allele dropout (ADO), 260
Allelic heterogeneity, 25
Allergic phenomena, preterm labor due to, 531
Allergic rhinitis, asthma exacerbated by, 942
Allograft, pregnancy as, 87
Allograft function, with renal transplantation, 919
Allograft rejection, with renal transplantation, 919
Alloimmune hemolytic disorders, neonatal outcomes with, 1199
Alloimmune thrombocytopenia, neonatal, 840–842, 840t
Alloimmunization
  due to non-Rh antibodies, 495–499, 495t, 497t
  due to Rh antibodies. *See* Rhesus (Rh) alloimmunization.
ALP (alkaline phosphatase), in pregnancy, 1059, 1060t
Alpha error, 213, 214
ALSPAC (Avon Longitudinal Study of Parents and Children), 153
ALT (alanine transaminase), in pregnancy, 1059, 1060t
Alveolar buds, 128
Alveolar collapse, in respiratory distress syndrome, 419
Alveolar stage, of fetal lung development, 194f, 194t, 195–196, 195t, 196f
Alveolarization, 194f, 194t, 195–196, 195t, 196f
Alveoli, development of, 127f, 128
Alzheimer's disease, 34
Amastia, 128
Ambiguous genitalia, 1198t
Ambulation, for arrest of labor, 696
Amenorrhea, due to acromegaly, 1021
American Diabetes Association (ADA), classification and diagnostic criteria of, 953
Amino acid(s), during pregnancy, 107, 120t
Amino acid turnover, and fetal obesity, 965–966
Aminoglycosides
  for acute pyelonephritis, 756
  nephrotoxicity of, 909
Aminopterin, as teratogen, 351t, 352
5-Aminosalicylates, for inflammatory bowel disease, 1049
Amiodarone
  during pregnancy, 801t
  and thyroid function, 1000
Amitriptyline (Elavil), dosage of, 1117t
AML (acute myeloid leukemia), in pregnancy, 899
Amniocentesis, 247–251
  chorionic villus sampling *vs.*, 258–259
  complications of, 250
  early, 251
  fluorescence in situ hybridization in, 249–250
  historical perspective on, 247
  laboratory considerations for, 249–250
  to monitor Rh-immunized pregnancies, 483–484, 484f
  mosaic results of, 249
  with multiple gestation, 257–258, 258t, 459
  pregnancy loss after, 250–251, 250t
  serial reduction, for twin-to-twin transfusion syndrome, 465–466
  technique of, 247–249, 248f
Amniochorion, permeability of, 50
Amnion, 39–40, 39f, 40f, 599
Amnion nodosum, in twin-to-twin transfusion syndrome, 62, 64
Amnionitis. *See* Chorioamnionitis.
Amnioreduction, for twin-to-twin transfusion syndrome, 437, 438–439, 439t
Amniostat-FLM PG, impact of contaminants on, 422t
Amniotic bands, invasive fetal therapy for, 434t
Amniotic cavity, 47, 599
  preterm labor due to microbial invasion of, 525
Amniotic fluid (AF), 47–52
  composition of, 47, 48–49
  ΔOD_{450} of, 483, 484f
  functions of, 47
  homeostasis of, 50–51
  intramembranous flow of, 50–51
  meconium-stained, 1206–1207
  membrane water flow of, 50–51
  production of, 47–49, 48f
  resorption of, 49
  subjectively reduced, 365
  volume of, 47, 48–49, 48f
Amniotic fluid density, 420
Amniotic fluid embolus, hemodynamics of, 1171–1172
Amniotic fluid evaluation, for fetal pulmonary maturity, 419–420
Amniotic fluid index (AFI), 366
  with post-term pregnancy, 615
Amniotic fluid infection. *See* Chorioamnionitis.
Amniotic fluid measurement, in biophysical profile score, 365–366, 365t, 366f
Amniotic fluid turbidity, 420

Amniotic fluid volume, 365
with intrauterine growth restriction, 644
with post-term pregnancy, 615
Amniotic infection syndrome, 744
Amniotic sac, 38–39, 39f, 599
Amniotic septostomy, for twin-to-twin transfusion syndrome, 437, 465
Amniotomy, for induction of labor, 701
Amorphic allele, 6
Amoxicillin
for acute pyelonephritis, 756t
for asymptomatic bacteriuria and acute cystitis, 752t, 906
for *Chlamydia trachomatis,* 748, 748t
for preterm premature rupture of the membranes, 606
Amoxicillin-clavulanate
for acute pyelonephritis, 756t
for preterm premature rupture of the membranes, 606
for puerperal endometritis, 761
Ampicillin
for acute pyelonephritis, 756, 756t
for asymptomatic bacteriuria and acute cystitis, 752t
for group B *Streptococcus* infection, 768
for listeriosis, 773
for pelvic abscess, 762
for preterm premature rupture of the membranes, 606
for puerperal endometritis, 760
for septic shock, 763
Ampicillin-sulbactam
for acute pyelonephritis, 756t
for septic shock, 763
Amplicor *Mycobacterium tuberculosis* (MTB) Test, 935
Amprenavir (Agenerase), for HIV infection, 772t
Anafranil (clomipramine), dosage of, 1117t
Anagen, 1124
Anal incontinence, cesarean delivery to prevent, 708, 711
Analgesia
for labor and delivery, 715–717
while breastfeeding, 139t
Anaphase
meiotic, 8f
mitotic, 7f, 8
Anaphase lag, 15
Anaphylactoid syndrome of pregnancy, hemodynamics of, 1171–1172
Anastomotic vessels, laser ablation of, for twin-to-twin transfusion syndrome, 437–439, 438f, 439t, 465–466
Ancillary test(s), for fetal health assessment, 380–383
contraction stress test and oxytocin challenge test as, 381–382, 381f
fetal movement counting as, 383, 383t
vibroacoustic stimulation as, 382–383
β-Adrenergic agonists
after premature rupture of the membranes, 606
as uterine relaxants, 81
β_2-Adrenergic agonists, for asthma, 940, 940t, 941
β-Adrenergic blocking agents
for chronic hypertension, 677–678
for hyperthyroidism, 1002
for pheochromocytoma, 1030
during pregnancy, 800, 801t
for thyroid storm, 1003, 1003t
Androgen(s), as teratogens, 351t
Androgen synthesis, pathways of, 1025, 1025f
Android pelvis, labor with, 693
Androstenedione, during pregnancy, 1026
Anemia(s), 869–882
aplastic and hypoplastic, 875–876
associated with systemic disease, 881–882
autoimmune hemolytic, 874–875
classification of
morphologic, 869, 872
by pathophysiologic mechanisms, 869, 870t
clinical presentation of, 869
Cooley, 877
defined, 869
evaluation of, 869–870, 870t
due to glucose-6-phosphate dehydrogenase deficiency, 875
due to hemoglobinopathies, 877–881
structural, 878–881, 878t, 880t, 881t
thalassemia syndromes as, 877–878, 877f, 878t, 879f
hereditary spherocytosis and elliptocytosis as, 874
hydrops fetalis due to, 510
iron deficiency, 870, 872, 873–874
macrocytic, 869, 872
megaloblastic, 874
microcytic, 869, 872
with multiple gestation, 461
neonatal, 1198
normocytic, 869, 872
paroxysmal nocturnal hemoglobinuria as, 876–877
and perinatal morbidity and mortality, 872–873
due to renal insufficiency, 917
sickle cell, 878t, 879–880, 880t
Anencephaly, 281, 282f
Anesthesia, 1147–1162
with asthma, 945
for breech presentation, 704
with cardiac disease, 1152–1160
congenital, 1156–1158
coronary artery, 1158–1159
general considerations with, 1152–1153
hypertrophic obstructive cardiomyopathy as, 1159
due to Marfan syndrome, 1159–1160
valvular, 1154–1156
for cardiac surgery, 1153–1154
for cesarean delivery, 712–713
with Ehlers-Danlos syndrome, 1160
for labor and delivery, 715–717
with neurologic disorders, 1149–1150
for placenta previa, 727–728
with preeclampsia, 1147–1149
with respiratory disorders, 1150–1152
with spinal abnormalities, 1160–1161
with substance abuse, 1161–1162
Aneuploidy, 14–15, 15f, 18f
in abortuses and stillbirths, 21, 21t, 22t
fetal loss due to, 619–620, 623, 626
and intrauterine growth restriction, 227t, 638
in multiple gestation, 256, 256t, 458–459, 458t
noninvasive diagnosis of, 262–263
prenatal screening for, 227–229, 227t, 228f, 228t, 229f
X-chromosomal, 19–20, 20t
Aneurysm(s)
aortic, due to Marfan syndrome, 818, 818f, 819f
intracranial saccular, 1097–1098, 1098f
ANF (atrial natriuretic factor), in preeclampsia, 665
Angelman syndrome, 30
Angina, unstable, 816–817
Angina pectoris, stable, 816
Angiography
of intracranial hemorrhage, 1098, 1098f
of occlusive cerebrovascular disease, 1095, 1095f
Angiomas, cerebral, 1097–1098
Angiotensin I, 1025
Angiotensin II, 1025
in fetal cardiovascular regulation, 165
Angiotensin II receptor antagonists, as teratogens, 353
Angiotensin sensitivity, in preeclampsia, 662, 662f
Angiotensin-converting enzyme (ACE) inhibitors (ACEIs)
for chronic hypertension, 678
during pregnancy, 801t
as teratogens, 349, 351t, 353, 800
Angiotensinogen, 1025
Animal models
of developmental origins of health and disease, 154
of fetal behavioral state activity, 171–172, 172f
Anion gap, 401–402
Ankylosing spondylitis, 1085
Anogenital gonorrhea, 744
ANP (atrial natriuretic peptide), in fetal cardiovascular regulation, 165–166
Antacids
for GERD, 1044, 1044t, 1045f
for peptic ulcer disease, 1046
Antenatal screening. *See* Prenatal screening.
Antepartum hemorrhage, 725–734
due to abruptio placentae, 730f, 731–734, 733t
epidemiology of, 725
due to placenta accreta, 728–729, 728f
due to placenta previa, 725–729, 726f, 726t, 727t, 728f
due to vasa previa, 729–730, 730f
Anterior abdominal wall, anomalies of, 293–294, 294f
Anterior pituitary lobe
anatomy and physiology of, 1015, 1016f, 1017f
during pregnancy, 1015
Anterior pituitary lobe disorder(s), 1017–1024
acromegaly as, 1020–1021
Cushing syndrome as, 1021–1022
hypopituitarism as, 1022–1024, 1023t
pituitary tumors as, 1017–1022
prolactinoma as, 1018–1020, 1019f, 1020f, 1020t
thyrotropin-secreting tumors as, 1021
Anthropoid pelvis, labor with, 693
Antiarrhythmic medications, for fetal arrhythmias, 336t
Antibiotic(s)
while breastfeeding, 139t
with cesarean delivery, 709
for inflammatory bowel disease, 1049
for preterm labor, 561, 570
for preterm premature rupture of the membranes, 209, 209f, 210f, 604, 605–606
for septic shock, 1178
Antibiotic-resistant *Neisseria gonorrhoeae,* 745
Antibody titer, maternal, 481
Antibody-dependent cell-mediated cytotoxicity (ADCC) assay, for RhD antibody, 481
Anti-c antibody, 496
Anticardiolipin antibodies (ACAs)
fetal loss due to, 625
thrombophilia due to, 829, 830t
Anticipation, 29

Anticoagulant(s)
with prosthetic heart valves, 819–820, 820t, 864
as teratogens, 348, 351–352, 351t, 800
for venous thromboembolism, 862–864
Anticoagulant system, 826–828, 828f
Anticoagulants for Living Fetuses (ALIFE) study, 628
Anticonvulsants
effect on fetus and neonate of, 1090–1091
for epilepsy, 1089–1092
and oral contraceptives, 1089
for preeclampsia, 671–673, 672t
as teratogens, 348, 351t, 352, 1090–1092
Antidepressants
clinical approach to, 1118–1119
dosage of, 1117t
during lactation, 1119–1120
perinatal complications of, 1119
as teratogens, 351t, 353, 1117–1118
Antidiarrheal medications, for inflammatory bowel disease, 1049
Antiendomysial IgA test, 1051
Antiepileptic drugs. *See* Anticonvulsants.
Antigen(s), 87
Antigen recognition, and preeclampsia, 666
Antihistamines
for nausea and vomiting, 1042, 1042t
for skin conditions, 1125
Antihypertensive medications
for chronic hypertension, 676–678, 678t
with diabetes, 970
for preeclampsia, 673, 673t
as teratogens, 351t, 353
while breastfeeding, 139t
Anti-inflammatory agent, progesterone as, 73
Anti-inflammatory cytokines, in preterm labor, 527
Anti-inflammatory state, pregnancy as, 88–89, 89f
Anti-intrinsic factor antibody (AIF), 870t
Anti-k antibody, 497, 497t
Anti-K1 antibody, 478, 478f, 479, 496–497, 497t
Anti-K2 antibody, 497, 497t
Anti-M antibody, 497–498
Antimorphic allele, 6
Anti-N antibody, 498
Antioxidant therapy, for prevention of preeclampsia, 675–676
Antiparallel strands, 4, 4f
Antiphospholipid syndrome (APS), 829–831, 1083–1084
diagnosis of, 829, 1080, 1080t
diagnostic criteria for, 829, 830t
epidemiology of, 1079
fertility with, 1081
fetal loss due to, 625, 1083
and infertility, 830
and in vitro fertilization, 1083–1084
obstetric complications of, 829–830
placenta in, 1083, 1083f
treatment for, 830–831, 1084, 1084t
and venous thromboembolism, 829, 830, 855
Antiplatelet treatment, for prevention of preeclampsia, 675
Antipsychotic agents
clinical approach to, 1119
dosage of, 1116t
during lactation, 1119–1120
perinatal complications of, 1119
risks of, 1116
Anti-RhC antibody, 496
Anti-Rhc antibody, 496
Anti-Rh(D) immune globulin, 478, 479–481
for idiopathic thrombocytopenic purpura, 839
Anti-RhE antibody, 496
Anti-Rhe antibody, 496
Antirheumatic drugs, 1081, 1082t
Anti-RhG antibody, 496
Anti-S antibody, 498
Anti-s antibody, 498
Antiseizure medications. *See* Anticonvulsants.
Antisense strand, 5
Antithrombin (AT), in anticoagulant system, 828, 828f
Antithrombin (AT) deficiency, 831t, 834
and fetal loss, 625t, 626t, 834
and venous thromboembolism, 856t, 863
Anti-thyroglobulin, 999
Antithyroid antibodies
fetal loss due to, 620
in postpartum thyroiditis, 1009, 1010, 1010f
during pregnancy, 999–1000
Antithyroid peroxidase (anti-TPO) antibodies, 999–1000, 1007
α_1-Antitrypsin deficiency, prenatal diagnosis of, 248t
Anti-U antibody, 498
Aorta, coarctation of, 330–331, 331f
maternal, 808–809
Aortic aneurysm, due to Marfan syndrome, 818, 818f, 819f
Aortic arch
fetal echocardiography of, 314–315, 314f–316f
in hypoplastic left heart syndrome, 329, 329f
Aortic atresia, hypoplastic left heart syndrome with, 329
Aortic insufficiency, anesthesia with, 1156
Aortic regurgitation, 813–814
Aortic root, fetal echocardiography of, 309, 314–315
Aortic stenosis
fetal, 330, 330f
invasive fetal therapy for, 277t, 445, 446t
maternal, 805–806, 806f, 813, 813f
anesthesia with, 1155
hemodynamics of, 1171
Aortic valve, fetal echocardiography of, 309, 314
Aortic valvuloplasty, fetal, 277t, 445, 446t
APACHE (Acute Physiologic and Chronic Health Evaluation) scoring system, 1167
aPC (activated protein C)
in anticoagulant system, 828, 828f
for septic shock, 763, 1179
aPC (activated protein C) resistance, and fetal loss, 625, 626t
Apgar score, with intrauterine growth restriction, 646
APL (acute promyelocytic leukemia), in pregnancy, 899
Aplastic anemia, 875–876
Apocrine miliaria, 1132
Apolipoprotein E gene *(APOE)*, 34
Appendectomy, 1047
Appendicitis, 1046–1047, 1047t
APS. *See* Antiphospholipid syndrome (APS).
Aptivus (tipranavir), for HIV infection, 772t
APV (absent pulmonary valve), tetralogy of Fallot with, 332–333, 333f
Aquaporins (AQPs), 51
Aqueductal stenosis, 280, 280f
Arachidonic acid cascade, 74–75, 75f
Arachidonic acid metabolites, in fetal cardiovascular regulation, 166
ARBD (alcohol-related birth defects), 354
Arborized crystals, due to premature rupture of the membranes, 602, 602f
ARCN (acute renal cortical necrosis), 908–909
Arcuate uterus, 1143, 1144t
ARDS (acute/adult respiratory distress syndrome), 1174
with acute pyelonephritis, 755
Areolae
anatomy of, 129–130, 129f
development of, 127f, 128
L-Arginine, as uterine relaxant, 80
Arginine vasopressin (AVP)
for diabetes insipidus, 1024
in fetal cardiovascular regulation, 165
Aripiprazole (Abilify), dosage of, 1116t
Armenti, Vincent T., 920
ARND (alcohol-related neurodevelopmental abnormalities), 354
Aromatase deficiency, 117
Arrest disorders, 695–696
Arrhythmias
fetal, 336–340, 337f–340f
hydrops fetalis due to, 507–508
medications for, 336, 336t
"respiratory," 368f
maternal, 818
ART (assisted reproductive technologies)
and cerebral palsy, 1215
perinatal risks of, 260–261
and preterm birth, 558
Arterial blood gases
fetal, 162, 162t, 386, 386t
in pregnancy, 1173, 1173t
for pulmonary embolus, 859
umbilical cord, 402–405, 403t–405t
Arterial blood pressure, during pregnancy, 102
Arterial circulation, fetal, with intrauterine growth restriction, 644
Arterial ischemic stroke (AIS), perinatal, 1213–1214, 1213f
Arterial occlusive disease, intracranial, 1095–1096, 1095f
Arterial oxygen content (CaO_2), 928
Arteriolar narrowing, in preeclampsia, 661
Arteriovenous fistulas, spinal, 1099
Arteriovenous shunts, intracranial, 1098–1099
Arteritis, Takayasu, 1085
diagnosis of, 1080–1081, 1080t
epidemiology of, 1079
Arthritis
juvenile, 1079, 1080, 1080t
psoriatic, 1085
rheumatoid, 1084–1085
diagnosis of, 1080, 1080t
epidemiology of, 1079
fertility with, 1081
labor and delivery with, 1084–1085
pathogenesis of, 1079
pregnancy loss with, 1084
Artificial heart valves, pregnancy with, 819–820, 820t, 864
ASB (asymptomatic bacteriuria), 750–753, 752t, 905–906
and preterm labor and birth, 568, 751
Ascending aorta, fetal echocardiography of, 309, 314–315
Ascites, fetal, 307, 307f
due to nonimmune hydrops, 506, 506f
ASCs (atypical squamous cells), 887
ASD (atrial septal defect)
fetal, 321, 322
maternal, 800–802, 802f
anesthesia with, 1157
ASH (asymmetrical septal hypertrophy), anesthesia with, 1159
Asherman syndrome, and pregnancy loss, 622
Ashkenazi Jewish population, carrier screening in, 238t, 240–243, 241t, 242t

Aspartate transaminase (AST), in pregnancy, 1059, 1060t
Aspartoacylase deficiency, carrier screening for, 238t, 242
Asphyxia, 1210
 and cerebral palsy, 1216
 defined, 401t
 fetal heart rate with, 410f, 411t
Aspiration pneumonia, 930
Aspirin
 for antiphospholipid antibody syndrome, 830–831, 1084, 1084t
 for intrauterine growth restriction, 645
 for pregnancy loss, 628t
 for prevention of preeclampsia, 675
 for rheumatic disease, 1082t
Assisted reproductive technologies (ART)
 and cerebral palsy, 1215
 perinatal risks of, 260–261
 and preterm birth, 558
AST (aspartate transaminase), in pregnancy, 1059, 1060t
Asthma, 937–945
 anesthesia with, 1151
 breastfeeding with, 945
 classification of, 938, 938t
 diagnosis of, 938
 effects of pregnancy on, 938
 effects on pregnancy of, 938–939, 939t
 epidemiology of, 937
 management of, 939–945
  for acute exacerbations, 943, 943t, 944t
  antenatal, 942–945, 943t, 944t
  assessment and monitoring in, 939–940
  avoiding or controlling asthma triggers in, 940
  exacerbated by allergic rhinitis, 942
  during labor and delivery, 943–945
  patient education in, 940
  pharmacologic therapy in, 940–942, 940t, 941t
 overview during pregnancy of, 945
Asthma triggers, 940
Asymmetrical septal hypertrophy (ASH), anesthesia with, 1159
Asymptomatic bacteriuria (ASB), 750–753, 752t, 905–906
 and preterm labor and birth, 568, 751
Asynchronous delivery, 463
AT. *See* Antithrombin (AT)
Atazanavir (Reyataz), for HIV infection, 772t
Atherosclerotic disease, intracranial, 1095, 1095f
Atherosclerotic heart disease, and diabetes, 961–962
Atherosis, in preeclampsia, 660, 660f, 661
Atopic dermatitis, 1131
Atopic eruption of pregnancy, 1125t, 1126–1127, 1127f, 1131
Atopy, breastfeeding and, 1131
Atosiban, for preterm labor, 564
ATP8B1 gene, 1060
Atrial bigeminy, blocked, in fetus, 338
Atrial bradycardia, in fetus, 338
Atrial contractions, premature, 336–337, 337f
Atrial flutter, in fetus, 338, 340
Atrial natriuretic factor (ANF), in preeclampsia, 665
Atrial natriuretic peptide (ANP), in fetal cardiovascular regulation, 165–166
Atrial septal defect (ASD)
 fetal, 321, 322
 maternal, 800–802, 802f
  anesthesia with, 1157
Atrial septostomy, fetal, 446t
Atrial septum, fetal echocardiography of, 312, 313f
Atrioventricular block, maternal, 810
Atrioventricular canal (AVC) defect, 324–326, 325f, 326f
Atrioventricular valves, fetal echocardiography of, 308f, 312–313
Atripla (efavirenz + emtricitabine + tenofovir), for HIV infection, 772t
Attention deficit hyperactivity disorder, biophysical profile score and, 389t
Atypical glandular cells (AGCs), 887
Atypical squamous cells (ASCs), 887
Augmentation mammoplasty, breastfeeding after, 132
Auscultation, electronic fetal monitoring *vs.*, 413
Australian Carbohydrate Intolerance Study in Pregnant Women (ACHOIS) trial, 979–980, 984
Autoimmune disease, maternal, neonatal outcomes with, 1198
Autoimmune hemolytic anemia, 874–875
Autoimmune hepatitis, 1069
Autoimmune progesterone dermatitis, 1125t, 1130
Autoimmune thrombocytopenic purpura, 837–840
Autoimmune thyroid disease
 miscarriage due to, 620, 1001
 postpartum, 1009–1011, 1010f
Autoimmunity, in rheumatic diseases, 1079–1080
Autologous transfusion device (Cell Saver), 1182
Automated Lumadex-FSI, 420
Autonomic hyperreflexia, 1103–1104
 anesthesia with, 1149–1150
Autonomic nervous system, in fetal cardiovascular regulation, 163–165
Autosomal deletions, 15, 16t
Autosomal dominant inheritance, 23–24, 24f
Autosomal dominant myotonic dystrophy, 30
Autosomal dominant polycystic kidney disease (ADPKD)
 pregnancy with, 913, 916t
 prenatal diagnosis of, 248t, 295–296
Autosomal duplications, 15
Autosomal recessive inheritance, 24, 24f
Autosomal recessive polycystic kidney disease, 295, 296f
Autosomes, 7
AVC (atrioventricular canal) defect, 324–326, 325f, 326f
Avon Longitudinal Study of Parents and Children (ALSPAC), 153
AVP (arginine vasopressin)
 for diabetes insipidus, 1024
 in fetal cardiovascular regulation, 165
Axillary dissection, 893
Axillary staging, of breast cancer, 892
Azathioprine
 for inflammatory bowel disease, 1049
 for renal transplantation, 918, 919, 920
 for rheumatic disease, 1081, 1082t
Azithromycin
 for *Chlamydia trachomatis,* 748, 748t
 for HIV infection, 771
AZT (zidovudine), for HIV infection, 771, 772t, 773
Aztreonam
 for acute pyelonephritis, 756t
 for pelvic abscess, 762

B

Bacillus Calmette-Guérin (BCG) vaccine, 935
Bacteremia
 due to burns, 1187–1188
 defined, 1176t
Bacterial pneumonia, 930–932, 931f
Bacterial vaginosis (BV), 741–742, 742f, 742t, 743t
 and premature rupture of the membranes, 599
 and preterm birth, 556, 568, 570, 741, 742, 742t
Bacteriuria
 asymptomatic, 750–753, 752t, 905–906
  and preterm labor and birth, 568, 751
 postcesarean, 709
Balanced complete atrioventricular canal defect, 325, 325f
"Banana sign," in neural tube defects, 281, 283f
Banding patterns, 12, 12f
Barbiturates, effect on fetus and neonate of, 1091
Bariatric surgery, 1051–1052, 1051t
Baroreceptors, in fetal heart rate, 398
Baroreflex regulation, of fetal cardiovascular system, 164
Base deficit, fetal, 400, 401t
Base excess, fetal, 400, 401t
 during labor, 402t
Baseline features, of fetal heart rate patterns, 405–406
Baseline fetal heart rate, 405, 406–407, 407f
BCG (bacillus Calmette-Guérin) vaccine, 935
Beating four-chamber view, in fetal echocardiography, 307–308, 308f, 311–314, 312f–314f
Becker muscular dystrophy, prenatal diagnosis of, 248t
Beclomethasone, for asthma, 941, 941t
Bed rest, for prevention of preterm labor and birth, 569
 with multiple gestation, 460
Behavior(s), fetal
 absent, 363–364, 364f
 basic functions of, 361
 coupled, 362, 362f
 individual, 361
 normal, 361–362
 patterned, 361–362
 and transition to neonatal behavior, 362
Behavioral state(s), fetal, 362
Behavioral state activity, fetal, 171–174
 animal studies of, 171–172, 172f
 developmental changes in, 173–174, 173t
 effect of hypoxia and intrauterine growth restriction on, 174, 174f
 human studies of, 172–173, 173f
Bell, Charles, 1106
Bell palsy, 1106–1107
Bendectin (doxylamine succinate and pyridoxine hydrochloride with or without dicyclomine hydrochloride)
 for nausea and vomiting, 1042, 1042t
 as teratogen, 347
Benign intracranial hypertension, 1094–1095
Benzathine penicillin G, for syphilis, 781, 781t
Bernard-Soulier syndrome, 844t–846t, 845–846
Beta error, 213–214
Betamethasone
 developmental effects of, 153–154
 fetal biophysical effects of, 425–426
 and fetal lung development, 196f
 for hemolytic disease of the fetus and newborn, 494

Betamethasone (Continued)
for induction of fetal pulmonary maturity
dosage of, 423, 423t
experimental results of, 203, 203f
maternal consequences of, 426
neonatal outcomes of, 424–425, 424f, 425f
repeated courses of, 427
after preterm premature rupture of the membranes, 605
for rheumatic disease, 1081, 1082t
Bias, 211
Bicarbonate (HCO_3^-)
for diabetic ketoacidosis, 962t
in fetal acid-base balance, 400
during labor, 402t
during pregnancy, 1173, 1173t
Bicornuate uterus, 1143, 1144, 1144t
and pregnancy loss, 622t
Biliary cirrhosis, primary, 1069
Biliary colic, 1073
Biliopancreatic diversion, 1051, 1051t
Bilirubin
in anemia, 869–870, 870t
in jaundice, 1060t, 1209
in pregnancy, 1059, 1060t
Binding proteins, in placental tissues, 117t
Biologic agents, for inflammatory bowel disease, 1049
Biophysical profile score (BPS), 175, 364–369
in diabetic pregnancy, 983t
with Doppler ultrasound abnormalities, 371, 372t
factors that influence, 369, 369t
and fetal pH on cordocentesis, 383–384, 384f
with intrauterine growth restriction, 644
and neurologic outcome, 389, 389f, 389t
outcome prediction using, 364, 365f
and perinatal mortality, 369, 369f, 387–388, 388t
scoring technique for, 366–369, 368t, 387–388, 388t
systematic application of, 366, 368t
variable(s) in, 364, 365–366
amniotic fluid measurement as, 365–366, 365t, 366f
cardiotocogram as, 365t, 366, 367f, 368f
fetal breathing movements as, 365t, 366
fetal movement and tone as, 365t, 366
Biopsy(ies)
breast, 892
cervical, 887, 888
cervical insufficiency due to, 586–587
for prenatal diagnosis, 259
renal, 912
thyroid, 1008–1009, 1009f
Biparietal diameter
and fetal pulmonary maturity, 420
in intrauterine growth restriction, 642
Bipolar disorder
diagnostic criteria for, 1113, 1114t, 1115t
epidemiology of, 1113
identification of, 1113–1114
impact on pregnancy outcomes of, 1114, 1115
treatment of
clinical approach to, 1119
dosage for, 1116t
during lactation, 1119–1120
perinatal complications of, 1119
risks of, 1116–1117
Birth. *See* Labor and delivery.
preterm. *See* Preterm labor and birth.
Birth defects, with in vitro fertilization, 260–261
Birth injury, diabetes and, 966–967, 966f
Birth weight
and adult disease, 151–154, 152f
extremely low. *See* Extremely low birth weight (ELBW).
and gestational age, 636, 636t
low. *See* Low birth weight (LBW).
maternal obesity and, 144
with multiple gestation, 454
and survival and morbidity with preterm birth, 550–551, 550f, 551f
very low. *See* Very low birth weight (VLBW).
Bisacodyl, for constipation, 1052t
Bishop score, for post-term pregnancy, 616
Bisphosphonates, for hypercalcemia, 1034, 1034t
Bladder exstrophy, 294
Blastocyst, 37, 38f
Blastocyst adhesion, 619
Blastocyst apposition, 619
Bleeding. *See also* Hemorrhage.
after chorionic villus sampling, 255
in late pregnancy, 725–734
due to abruptio placentae, 730f, 731–734, 733t
epidemiology of, 725
due to placenta accreta, 728–729, 728f
due to placenta previa, 725–729, 726f, 726t, 727t, 728f
due to vasa previa, 729–730, 730f
and preterm labor and birth, 527–529, 529f, 558
Bleeding disorders, 844t–846t, 847–848
Bleeding time, in abruptio placentae, 733t
Blindness, cortical, biophysical profile score and, 389t
Blocked atrial bigeminy, in fetus, 338
β-Blockers. *See* β-Adrenergic blocking agents.
Blood component therapy, for hemorrhagic shock, 1181–1182, 1181t, 1182t
Blood flow patterns, fetal, 159–162, 160f–162f, 162t
Blood gases
fetal, 162, 162t, 386, 386t
in pregnancy, 1173, 1173t
for pulmonary embolus, 859
umbilical cord, 402–405, 403t–405t
Blood glucose
during pregnancy, 975–976, 975f, 976f, 976t
self-monitoring of, 974–976, 975t
Blood loss, during delivery, 104
Blood pH, fetal, 162, 162t, 386, 386t
determination of, 400–401
in labor, 402t
Blood pressure
during labor, 104
in preeclampsia, 656–657
during pregnancy, 102–103, 102f, 652, 653f
Blood pressure monitoring, during pregnancy, 103
Blood product replacement
for abruptio placentae, 733, 733t
for hemorrhagic shock, 1181–1182, 1181t, 1182t
Blood transfusions, for hemorrhagic shock, 1181–1182, 1181t, 1182t
Blood typing, fetal, 262
Blood volume
control of fetal, 398
during pregnancy, 101, 799, 870–871, 871f
Bloom syndrome, carrier screening for, 242t
Blunt abdominal trauma, 1184–1186, 1185f
B-Lynch uterine body compression suture, for obstetric hemorrhage, 1183, 1184f
BNP (B-type natriuretic peptide), in fetal cardiovascular regulation, 165–166
Body composition, in developmental origins of health and disease, 154–155
Body mass index (BMI), 143–144
and preterm birth, 555–556, 555f
Body movements, fetal, 172, 173f, 175, 177, 361
in biophysical profile score, 365t, 366
counting of, 383, 383t
Body stalk, 39f, 41
Body stalk anomaly, 294
Body surface area, of burns, 1187, 1187f
Bohr effect, 186
Bone marrow transplantation, for aplastic and hypoplastic anemia, 876
Bone resorption, pregnancy effect on, 1035
Bone turnover, pregnancy effect on, 1035
Borrelia burgdorferi
breastfeeding with, 136t
fetal loss due to, 623
BPD. *See* Bronchopulmonary dysplasia (BPD).
BPS. *See* Biophysical profile score (BPS).
BPS (bronchopulmonary sequestration), 286, 286f
Brachial neuritis, acute familial, 1105
Brachial plexus injury, due to shoulder dystocia, 697
Bradycardia, fetal, 338, 338f
baseline, 405, 406, 407f
due to complete heart block, 408f
after cordocentesis, 385–386
in utero treatment of, 411f, 411t
Brain cooling, for hypoxic-ischemic encephalopathy, 1211
Brain death, 1189–1190, 1189t
Brain growth and development, fetal, 175–176, 176t
Brain tumors, 1093–1094, 1094f
headaches due to, 1092
Breast(s), 127–130
abnormalities of, 128–129, 128t, 129t
accessory, 128
candidiasis of, 135, 137t, 138–139
development of, 127–128, 127f, 128f, 130t
examination of, 126
during lactation, 130
mature, 127f, 128, 129f
nipple and areola of, 129–130, 129f
in pregnancy, 130
Breast augmentation, breastfeeding after, 132
Breast biopsy, 892
Breast cancer
clinical presentation and diagnosis of, 891–892, 892t
epidemiology of, 891
follow-up of, 894
monitoring of, 894
pathology of, 892–893
in pregnancy, 891–894, 892t, 893f
pregnancy after, 894–895
prognosis for, 894
staging of, 892
treatment of, 893–894, 893f
Breast engorgement, 134, 138t
Breast hyperplasia, 128–129, 129t
Breast hypoplasia, 128, 129t
Breast mass, differential diagnosis of, 892, 892t
Breast milk
components of, 125
drugs in, 139–141, 139t, 140f, 140t
production of, 127f, 130–131, 130t, 131f
Breast reduction, breastfeeding after, 126, 132
Breast stimulation, for cervical ripening, 702t
Breast-conservation surgery, 893

Breastfeeding, 125–141. *See also* Lactation.
with Addison disease, 1027
adequacy of, 133, 134
with asthma, 945
and atopy, 1131
benefits of, 125–126
after breast augmentation, 132
after breast reduction, 126, 132
complications of, 138–139, 138f, 138t
and contraception, 134–135
contraindications to, 125–126
and developmental origins of health and disease, 153, 155
with diabetes, 986
with epilepsy, 1090
hypercalcemia due to, 1035
initiation of, 131–133, 133f
let-down (ejection) reflex in, 131, 132f, 133, 133f
maternal infections during, 135–138, 136t–137t
medications while, 126, 139–141, 139t, 140f, 140t
milk production in, 127f, 130–131, 130t, 131f
and necrotizing enterocolitis, 1208
with nipple piercing, 126
and osteoporosis, 1036
with phenylketonuria, 1101–1102
postpartum issues in, 134
after premature or multiple births, 134
with prolactinoma, 1020
promotion of, 126–127
psychotropic medications during, 1119–1120
recommendations on, 134
with renal transplantation, 920
timing of, 133
with vitamin B_{12} deficiency, 1101
Breathing movements, fetal, 172f–174f, 175, 176–177, 361, 362, 362f
in biophysical profile score, 365t, 366
Breech delivery
umbilical cord acid-base balance with, 405
vaginal, 704–705, 705t
Breech presentation, 703–706, 705t
Breech-breech twins, 462–463
Breech-vertex twins, 462–463
Bromocriptine
for acromegaly, 1021
to inhibit lactation, 1020
for migraines, 1093
for prolactinoma, 1018–1019
Bronchogenic cyst, 285, 286f
Bronchopulmonary dysplasia (BPD), 1205–1206
long-term complications of, 1205
pathophysiology of, 1205, 1206f
prematurity and, 1201t
prevention of, 1206, 1206t
risk factors for, 1205
Bronchopulmonary sequestration (BPS), 286, 286f
Brow presentation, 706–707
B-type natriuretic peptide (BNP), in fetal cardiovascular regulation, 165–166
Budd-Chiari syndrome, 1070
Budesonide, for asthma, 941, 941t
Buffers, in fetal acid-base balance, 400
Bulk-forming laxatives, for constipation, 1052, 1052t
Bupropion (Wellbutrin), dosage of, 1117t
Burkholderia cepacia, with cystic fibrosis, 947
Burkitt lymphoma, 898, 899
Burns, 1186–1188, 1187f, 1187t
Butoconazole, for vulvovaginal candidiasis, 740t
BV (bacterial vaginosis), 741–742, 742f, 742t, 743t
and premature rupture of the membranes, 599
and preterm birth, 556, 568, 570, 741, 742, 742t

C

C bands, 12
CA 125 (cancer antigen 125), 1140–1141
Cabergoline, for prolactinoma, 1019
CAD (coronary artery disease), maternal, 816–817
anesthesia with, 1158–1159
CAH (congenital adrenal hyperplasia)
pregnancy with, 1028–1030, 1029f
prenatal diagnosis of, 248t, 262
Calcitonin
in fetus, 1032
for hypercalcemia, 1034, 1034t
in lactation, 1032
Calcitonin gene–related peptide (CGRP)
in fetal cardiovascular regulation, 166–167
as uterine relaxant, 80
Calcitriol, for hypoparathyroidism, 1035
Calcitriol (1α,25-dihydroxycholecalciferol), 1032
Calcium
elemental, for hypocalcemia, 1035
in myometrial contraction, 78, 78f
Calcium channel blockers
for preterm labor, 562–563
as uterine relaxants, 81
Calcium chelation, for hypercalcemia, 1034, 1034t
Calcium excretion, during pregnancy, 106
Calcium gluconate, for hypocalcemia, 1035
Calcium metabolism, parathyroid glands and, 1032, 1032f, 1033f
Calcium salts, for hypoparathyroidism, 1035
Calcium supplementation
during pregnancy, 146, 146t
for prevention of preeclampsia, 675
Caldesmon, in myometrial contraction, 78
Caliceal dilation, during pregnancy, 105
Calmodulin (CaM), in myometrial contraction, 78
Caloric intake, with multiple gestation, 455
Calorie restriction, for diabetes, 974
Calponin, in myometrial contraction, 78
Camptomelic dysplasia, 298
Campylobacter jejuni, Guillain-Barré syndrome due to, 1107
Canadian Critical Care Clinical Trials Group study, 1170
Canalicular stage, of fetal lung development, 194, 194f, 194t
Canavan disease, carrier screening for, 238t, 242, 242t
Cancer, 885–899
breast, 891–895, 892t, 893f
cervical, 886–889, 886t
colon, 895–896
epidemiology of, 885
gestational trophoblastic neoplasia as, 891
hematologic, 896–899, 897t
malignant melanoma as, 895
ovarian, 885–886, 886t
treatment of, 889–891, 889t
Cancer antigen 125 (CA 125), 1140–1141
Candidiasis, 739–741, 740t
breastfeeding with, 135, 136t, 137t, 138–139
with HIV infection, 771
CaO_2 (arterial oxygen content), 928
CAOS (chronic abruption-oligohydramnios sequence), 732
CAP(s) (contraction-associated proteins), 79
CAPD (continuous ambulatory peritoneal dialysis), 917–918
Capillary fluid shift, in fetal blood volume control, 398
Capillary glucose levels, target, 975–976, 975f, 976f, 976t
Capillary glucose monitoring, timing of, 974–975, 975t
Capreomycin, for tuberculosis, 937t
Carbamazepine (Tegretol)
dosage of, 1116t
as teratogen, 348, 351t, 352, 1117
Carbohydrate(s), in diet, 147
Carbohydrate counting, 978
Carbohydrate restriction, for diabetes, 974
Carbon dioxide arterial partial pressure ($PaCO_2$), during pregnancy, 927
Carbon dioxide partial pressure (PCO_2)
fetal, in labor, 402t
during pregnancy, 104, 1173
Carbon dioxide transfer, placental, 190–191
Carbon monoxide poisoning, 1187
Carbonic acid (H_2CO_3), in fetal acid-base balance, 400
Carbonic anhydrase, during pregnancy, 927
Carboprost tromethamine, for postpartum hemorrhage, 698–699
Cardiac anomalies, 278–279, 278t
Cardiac arrest, 1188–1189
Cardiac arrhythmias. *See* Arrhythmias.
Cardiac disease. *See* Heart disease.
Cardiac looping, 279
Cardiac output (CO)
with aortic stenosis, 1171
fetal, 161–162, 161f, 162f, 162t
and fetal oxygenation, 188–189, 189f
during labor, 104, 1153
with mitral stenosis, 1170, 1171
noninvasive assessment of, 1173
nonpregnant, 1171t
postpartum, 104
in preeclampsia, 661
during pregnancy, 101–102, 102f, 103t, 799, 1171t
Cardiac performance, during pregnancy, 799
Cardiac rhabdomyoma, 335, 335f
Cardiac surgery, during pregnancy, 820–821
anesthesia for, 1153–1154
Cardiac transplantation, pregnancy after, 817
Cardiac tumors, 335–336, 336f, 337f
Cardioactive drugs, during pregnancy, 801t
Cardiogenic pulmonary edema, 1174–1175
Cardiomyopathy
in infants of diabetic mothers, 967
maternal, 814–816, 815f
anesthesia with, 1159
Cardiopulmonary bypass, during pregnancy, 1154
Cardiopulmonary resuscitation (CPR), 1188–1189
Cardiotachometer, 399
Cardiotocogram (CTG)
of abruptio placentae, 732
in biophysical profile score, 365t, 366, 367f, 368f
computerized, 370–371, 371f
Cardiovascular adaptations
to multiple gestation, 455
to pregnancy, 799, 1152–1153
Cardiovascular anomalies. *See* Congenital heart disease (CHD).

Cardiovascular causes, of hydrops fetalis, 507–509, 508t
Cardiovascular changes, in preeclampsia, 661–662, 662f
Cardiovascular complications
of diabetes, 961–962, 961f
of prematurity, 1199t
Cardiovascular disease
low birth weight and, 152, 152f
preeclampsia and subsequent, 655–656, 656f
Cardiovascular drugs
during pregnancy, 800, 801t
while breastfeeding, 139t
Cardiovascular system
fetal, 159–167
blood flow patterns and oxygen delivery in, 159–162, 160f–162f, 162t
cardiac output and its distribution in, 161–162, 161f, 162f, 162t
control of, 164–167
ductus arteriosus in, 160f, 167
intracardiac and vascular pressures in, 162, 163f
myocardial function in, 162–164
venous return to heart in, 159–160, 160f, 161f
during pregnancy, 101–104, 102f, 103t
Carotid angiogram, of intracranial aneurysm, 1098f
Carpal tunnel syndrome, 1105, 1106f
Carrier screening, 238–246
for cystic fibrosis, 238–240, 238t–240t, 242t
for fragile X syndrome, 245–246, 246t
for hemoglobinopathies, 238t, 243–245, 244t
informed consent for, 238
in Jewish population, 238t, 240–243, 241t, 242t
recommendations on, 238, 238t
Cartilage oligomeric matrix protein (COMP), in skeletal growth, 297
Cascara, for constipation, 1052t
Case reports, 207–208
Case series, 207–208
Case-control studies, 208, 208t
on safety of exposures, 350
Castor oil, for cervical ripening, 702t
Catagen, 1124
Catecholamines, in pheochromocytoma, 1030
Catecholestrogens, in pregnancy, 115–116
CBC (complete blood count), in anemia, 869
CCAM (congenital cystic adenomatoid malformation), 286–287, 287f
hydrops fetalis due to, 444, 509
invasive fetal therapy for, 277t, 444
CCAM volume ratio (CVR), 444
CCTG (computerized cardiotography), 370–371, 371f
CDH. *See* Congenital diaphragmatic hernia (CDH).
Cefazolin
for acute pyelonephritis, 756t
for group B *Streptococcus* infection, 768
for mastitis, 764
for puerperal endometritis, 761
Cefepime, for acute pyelonephritis, 756t
Cefixime, for gonorrhea, 745, 746
Cefotaxime
for acute pyelonephritis, 756t
for gonorrhea, 745, 745t
Cefotetan
for acute pyelonephritis, 756t
for puerperal endometritis, 760
Cefoxitin, for gonorrhea, 745
Ceftizoxime, for gonorrhea, 745, 745t
Ceftriaxone
for acute pyelonephritis, 756, 756t
for gonorrhea, 745, 745t, 746
for ophthalmia neonatorum, 1219
Cefuroxime, for acute pyelonephritis, 906
Celecoxib, for rheumatic disease, 1082t
Celexa (citalopram), dosage of, 1117t
Celiac disease, 28, 1050–1051
Celiac sprue, 28, 1050–1051
Cell cycle, 7, 7f
meiotic, 8–10, 8f–11f
Cell division
meiotic, 8–10, 8f–11f
mitotic, 7–8, 7f
Cell Saver (autologous transfusion device), 1182
Cellular immunity, 87
Central nervous system (CNS)
embryologic development of, 279
in fetal heart rate, 398
infections of, 1099–1101
Central nervous system (CNS) anomalies, 279–282, 279f–283f
Central nervous system (CNS) complications, of prematurity, 1199t
Central venous catheter, 1168
complications of, 1169–1170
Central venous pressure (CVP)
nonpregnant, 1171t
during pregnancy, 103t, 1171t
and pulmonary capillary wedge pressure, 1170, 1170f
Centric fusion, 18f
Centromere, 7, 7f
Centrosomes, 7
Cephalexin
for acute pyelonephritis, 906
for asymptomatic bacteriuria and acute cystitis, 752t, 906
for mastitis, 764
Cephalopelvic disproportion (CPD)
arrest disorders due to, 695
brow presentation due to, 707
Cerebral angiomas, 1097–1098
Cerebral angiopathy, 1095–1096
Cerebral edema
in acute liver failure, 1072
in preeclampsia, 658
Cerebral infarction, 1095–1096, 1095f–1097f
Cerebral oxygen consumption, fetal, 176, 176t
Cerebral palsy (CP), 1214–1217
biophysical profile score and, 389, 389f, 389t
chorioamnionitis and, 758–759, 758t
classification of, 1214, 1214t
coexisting impairments with, 1216
defined, 1214
etiology of, 1214
hemiplegic, due to perinatal stroke, 1214
intrauterine growth restriction and, 646
after intrauterine transfusion, 492
multiple gestation and, 1215
perinatal infections and, 1215–1216
placental abnormalities and, 1216
preterm birth and, 552, 1214–1215, 1216–1217
prevalence of, 1214
risk factors for, 1214
strategies to reduce, 1216
Cerebrovascular disease, occlusive, 1095–1096, 1095f–1097f
Cervical biopsy, 887, 888
cervical insufficiency due to, 586–587
Cervical cancer, 886–889, 886t
Cervical carcinoma, 887–889
Cervical cerclage, 589–594
complications after, 594, 594f
efficacy of, 591–592
emergency, 594
indications for, 592–593, 592f
McDonald, 590, 593
with multiple gestation, 460
perioperative and intraoperative care for, 593–594, 593f
placement of second, 594
pre-conceptional, 589
during pregnancy, 589–591, 590f
for preterm birth prevention, 568–569, 571–572, 591–592
preterm premature rupture of the membranes with, 594, 606–607
removal of, 594
Shirodkar, 590, 590f, 593
transabdominal, 590–591, 591f
transvaginal, 590, 590f
Wurm, 593
Cervical coefficient, 691
Cervical competence, defined, 583
Cervical dilation, 70, 523, 583, 584f
cervical cerclage for, 593
in preterm labor, 560
rate of, 692, 692f, 692t, 695
Cervical disorders, preterm labor due to, 531
Cervical effacement, 69, 584, 585f, 702
in preterm labor, 560, 568
Cervical examination, for preterm labor, 568–569
Cervical inflammation, cervical insufficiency due to, 587, 587f
Cervical injury, cervical insufficiency due to, 586–587
Cervical insufficiency, 583–595
causes of, 585–587
acquired, 586–587, 587f
congenital, 585–586, 586f
defined, 583
diagnosis of, 587–589, 588f
preterm labor and birth due to, 531, 559–560, 568–569, 571–572
treatment of, 589–594
cervical cerclage for, 589–594
complications after, 594, 594f
efficacy of, 591–592
indications for, 592–593, 592f
perioperative and intraoperative care for, 593–594, 593f
pre-conceptional, 589
during pregnancy, 589–591, 590f
transabdominal, 590–591, 591f
transvaginal, 590, 590f
nonsurgical, 589
Cervical intraepithelial neoplasia (CIN), 887
and preterm birth, 557–558
Cervical length
cervical insufficiency due to, 586, 586f, 588–589
cervical cerclage for, 593
in multiple gestation, 457, 460
and premature rupture of the membranes, 600
and preterm birth, 558–560, 559f, 560f
Cervical polyp, cervical insufficiency due to, 587, 587f
Cervical remodeling
during labor and delivery, 523
during pregnancy, 583–584, 584f, 585f
Cervical repair, 583, 584f
Cervical ripening, 523, 583, 584f, 702
cervical insufficiency due to, 587
methods of, 702–703, 702t, 703t

Cervical ripening *(Continued)*
for post-term pregnancy, 615, 616
and premature labor, 530, 568
Cervical softening, 523, 583, 584f, 702
cervical insufficiency due to, 587
Cervical surgery
cervical cerclage after, 592–593
and preterm birth, 557–558
Cervidil Rx (dinoprostone)
for cervical ripening, 702t, 703t
for post-term pregnancy, 615, 616
for uterine atony, 1183t
Cervix
anatomy of, 583
in pregnancy, 69, 583–584, 584f, 585f
Cesarean delivery, 707–713
anesthesia for, 712–713
for breech presentation, 703–704
with cervical cancer, 889
with cervical cerclage, 594
complications of, 708–710
in diabetic pregnancy, 985–986
elective, 707–708
electronic fetal monitoring and, 413
excessive weight gain and, 145
and fetal lung fluid, 197
history of, 707–708
incision for, 713
indications for, 707, 708, 710–711
induction of labor and, 700
maternal obesity and, 144
of monoamniotic twins, 467
myomectomy during, 1039
for neonatal alloimmune thrombocytopenia, 842
perimortem, 1188–1189, 1188t
for placenta previa, 727–728
to prevent pelvic floor dysfunction, 708, 711
rates of, 707, 708
reducing morbidity of, 712–713
with renal transplantation, 920
repeat, 710
trial of labor after, 710, 711–712
uterine myomas and, 1137
uterine rupture after, 710, 712
vaginal birth after, 708, 711–712
wound infection after, 761–762
Cesarean hysterectomy, 713
CF. *See* Cystic fibrosis (CF).
CGRP (calcitonin gene–related peptide)
in fetal cardiovascular regulation, 166–167
as uterine relaxant, 80
Chain termination method, 32
Chancre, 778, 779
CHB (complete heart block), in fetus, 338, 338f
bradycardia due to, 408f
CHD. *See* Congenital heart disease (CHD).
Chediak-Higashi syndrome, 846, 846t
Chemical cleavage method, 32
Chemical pneumonitis, 930
Chemoreceptors, in fetal heart rate, 397–398
Chemoreflex regulation, of fetal cardiovascular system, 164
Chemotherapy
for breast cancer, 894
for hemolytic disease of the fetus and newborn, 494–495
for Hodgkin lymphoma, 898
for leukemia, 899
for non-Hodgkin lymphoma, 898–899
during pregnancy, 890
teratogenicity of, 351t, 352
Chest radiography, of pulmonary embolus, 859, 861f, 862
CHF (congestive heart failure), fetal, 315–316, 316t
Chiasmata, 9, 9f
Chickenpox, 783–784
Childhood growth, and developmental origins of health and disease, 153
Childhood neurologic abnormalities, diabetes and, 968–969
Chimeras, 66
Chi-square test, 213
Chlamydia, in newborn period, 1219
Chlamydia pneumoniae, pneumonia due to, 931
Chlamydia trachomatis, 746–748
breastfeeding with, 136t
diagnosis of, 747
epidemiology of, 746
with gonorrhea, 745, 746
life cycle of, 93f
pathogenesis of, 746–747
and postpartum endometritis, 747
and pregnancy outcome, 93–96, 93f–95f, 747
and preterm birth, 556
prevention of, 748
treatment of, 747–748, 748t
Chloasma, 1124
Cholangitis, primary sclerosing, 1070
Choledochal cyst, fetal, 293
Cholelithiasis, 1073
Cholestasis, intrahepatic, of pregnancy, 1060–1061, 1125
Cholesterol, during pregnancy, 120t
Chondrodysplasias, hydrops fetalis due to, 508t, 511–512
Chondroectodermal dysplasia, 298
Chorea gravidarum, 1102
Chorioallantoic vessels, 40
Chorioamnion, permeability of, 50
Chorioamnionitis, 757–759, 758t
and bronchopulmonary dysplasia, 1205
and cerebral palsy, 1216
due to cervical cerclage, 594
clinical, 757
neonatal outcomes with, 1197–1198, 1217
after premature rupture of the membranes, 600, 604, 605, 606
umbilical cord acid-base balance with, 404, 404t
Chorioangioma
hydrops fetalis due to, 509
invasive fetal therapy for, 434t
Choriocarcinoma, 1094, 1141
Chorion, 38, 39f, 599
Chorion laeve, 38, 39f
Chorionic 15-hydroxy-prostaglandin dehydrogenase (PGDH), in control of labor, 72
Chorionic fusion, irregular, 58
Chorionic villus sampling (CVS), 251–256
accuracy of, 253–255
amniocentesis *vs.*, 258–259
complications of, 255–256
confined placental mosaicism in, 254–255
history of, 251–252
laboratory aspects of, 253
maternal cell contamination in, 253–254
with multiple gestation, 258, 258t, 459
pregnancy loss after, 255
risk of fetal abnormality after, 256
transabdominal, 252–253, 253f
transcervical, 252, 252f, 253
Chorionicity, 57, 57f–60f, 58, 454–456, 455f
Choroid plexus cysts, 284, 284f
and aneuploidy, 227, 227t
Chromatids, sister, 7
Chromatin, 7
Chromosomal arms, 7, 12, 12f
Chromosomal mosaicism, in amniocentesis, 249
Chromosomally mediated *Neisseria gonorrhoeae,* 745
Chromosome(s), 6–22
acrocentric, 17
in cell cycle, 7, 7f
iso-, 18
in meiosis, 8–10, 8f–11f
in mitosis, 7–8, 7f
number of, 6–7
abnormalities in, 14–15, 15f
ring, 15, 16f
segregation of, 10
sex, 7, 19
abnormalities of, 19–20, 20t
structure of, 7
Chromosome abnormalities, 14–18
in abortuses and stillbirths, 21, 21t, 22t
fetal loss due to, 619–620, 623, 626
hydrops fetalis due to, 508t, 509
and intrauterine growth restriction, 227t, 638
in multiple gestation, 256, 256t, 458–459, 458t
selective termination for, 469–470
in number, 14–15, 15f
prevalence of, 20–21, 21t
sex, 19–20, 20t
in structure, 15–18, 16f–19f, 16t
Chromosome analysis, 10–14, 12f–14f
indications for, 21–22
Chromosome paint probe, 12–13
Chronic abruption-oligohydramnios sequence (CAOS), 732
Chronic kidney disease (CKD), 910–912
antenatal strategy and decision making with, 911–912
impact of pregnancy on, 910–911, 911t
and perinatal outcome, 911
postpartum care with, 912
preconception counseling with, 910–911
due to preeclampsia, 907
stages of, 910, 910t
Chronic lymphocytic thyroiditis, 1007
Chronic renal disease, in preeclampsia, 653t
Chylothorax, in fetus, 289, 289f
Cigarette smoking
and abruptio placentae, 731
and biophysical profile score, 369t
intrauterine growth restriction due to, 640
neonatal outcomes of, 1199
and preterm birth, 554, 568, 572
teratogenicity of, 348, 351t, 355–356, 355f, 356f
Cimetidine, for peptic ulcer disease, 1046
CIN (cervical intraepithelial neoplasia), 887
and preterm birth, 557–558
Ciprofloxacin
for asymptomatic bacteriuria, 753
for gonorrhea, 745
for inflammatory bowel disease, 1049
Circulation
fetal, 159–160, 160f
maternal
fetal cell-free RNA in, 263
prenatal diagnosis using fetal cells in, 261–262
Cirrhosis, 1070–1071
primary biliary, 1069
Citalopram (Celexa), dosage of, 1117t
CKD. *See* Chronic kidney disease (CKD).
Cleft lip and palate, 27, 27t, 284–285
neonatal management of, 1198t

Clindamycin
for bacterial vaginosis, 741, 742t
for group B *Streptococcus* infection, 768
for mastitis, 764
for pelvic abscess, 762
for puerperal endometritis, 760, 761
for septic shock, 763
Clinical research, 207–217
importance of, 207
on screening and diagnosis in, 214–217, 215t, 216f
sources of error in, 210–214, 212t, 213t
types of studies in, 207–210, 208t, 209f, 210f
Clinical trial, randomized, 208–209
Clomiphene, and preterm birth, 558
Clomipramine (Anafranil), dosage of, 1117t
Clonidine, for chronic hypertension, 678t
Clostridium difficile colitis, 1048, 1049f
Clostridium tetani, 1100
Clotrimazole, for vulvovaginal candidiasis, 740t
Clotting cascade, 826, 827f
Clozapine (Clozaril)
dosage of, 1116t
during lactation, 1120
Clubfoot, early amniocentesis and, 251
CMV. *See* Cytomegalovirus (CMV).
CNS. *See* Central nervous system (CNS).
CNVs (copy number variations), 3, 14, 31, 32
CO. *See* Cardiac output (CO).
CO_2. *See* Carbon dioxide *entries.*
Coagulation, disseminated intravascular
due to abruptio placentae, 624
in preeclampsia, 662–663, 674
Coagulation cascade, 826, 827f
Coagulation disorder(s), 825–848
after abruptio placentae, 733, 733t
bleeding disorders as, 844t–846t, 847–848
neonatal, due to maternal use of anticonvulsants, 1091
platelet disorder(s) as, 837–847
acquired, 837–843
Bernard-Soulier syndrome as, 844t–846t, 845–846
congenital, 843–847
drug-induced thrombocytopenia and functional platelet defects as, 843
idiopathic thrombocytopenic purpura as, 837–840
neonatal alloimmune thrombocytopenia as, 840–842, 840t
of platelet secretion, 844t, 846–847
thrombotic thrombocytopenic purpura and hemolytic uremic syndrome as, 842–843, 843t
von Willebrand disease as, 843–845, 844t–846t
in preeclampsia, 662–663, 674, 1148
thrombophilia(s) as, 829–837
acquired, 829–831, 830t
inherited, 831–835
due to antithrombin deficiency, 831t, 834
due to factor V Leiden mutation, 831–833, 831t
hyperhomocysteinemia as, 833–834
due to mutations in fibrinolytic pathway genes, 835
due to other factor V mutations, 833
due to protein C deficiency, 831t, 834
due to protein S deficiency, 831t, 834–835
due to protein Z-dependent protease inhibitor and protein Z deficiency, 835
Coagulation disorder(s) *(Continued)*
due to prothrombin gene mutation, 831t, 833
screening for, 835–837
Coagulation factors, in preeclampsia, 658, 662–663
Coarctation of the aorta, 330–331, 331f
maternal, 808–809
Cocaine, as teratogen, 356
Cocaine abuse, neonatal outcomes with, 1199
Cochrane Database of Systemic Reviews, 209–210, 209f, 210f
Cochrane Review, on tocolytic agents, 562–566
Coding strand, 5
Codominant trait, 23
Codons, 5
Cohort studies, 208, 208t
Coitus, and preterm birth, 555, 569
Colic, biliary, 1073
Colitis
Clostridium difficile, 1048, 1049f
ulcerative, 1047–1049
clinical characteristics of, 1047–1048, 1048f, 1048t
diagnostic testing for, 1048, 1048f, 1049f
effect of pregnancy on, 1048
effect on pregnancy of, 1048
treatment of, 1048–1049, 1049t
Collaborative Group on Antenatal Steroid Therapy, 427
Collagen, in platelet plug formation, 825
Collagen disorders, cervical insufficiency due to, 585–586
Collagen gene loci, in skeletal growth, 297
Collodion fetus, 1132
Colloid osmotic pressure (COP)
abnormalities of, 1174
nonpregnant, 1171t
during pregnancy, 103t, 1171t, 1174
Colloid solutions, for hemorrhagic shock, 1180–1181, 1180t
Colon, in pregnancy, 1041
Colon cancer, 895–896
Colonoscopy, 895, 1053
Colorectal cancer, 895–896
Colposcopy, 887
Colton antigen, 495t
Coma, 1189–1190, 1189t
Combivir (zidovudine and lamivudine), for HIV infection, 771–772, 772t
Common carotid arteriogram, 1095f
Common pathway of parturition, 521–524, 522f, 524f
COMP (cartilage oligomeric matrix protein), in skeletal growth, 297
Complete atrioventricular canal defect, 325–326, 325f, 326f
Complete blood count (CBC), in anemia, 869
Complete heart block (CHB), in fetus, 338, 338f
bradycardia due to, 408f
Complex inheritance, 26–27, 27t
Compound presentation, 707
Computed tomography (CT)
of appendicitis, 1047, 1047t
of perinatal stroke, 1213, 1213f
Computed tomography pulmonary angiography (CTPA), for pulmonary embolus, 859, 860, 861, 861f, 862
Computerized cardiotography (CCTG), 370–371, 371f
Condyloma acuminatum, 748
Cone biopsy, 887, 888
Confidence intervals, 212
Confined placental mosaicism, 254–255
Confounding, 210–211
Congenital adrenal hyperplasia (CAH)
pregnancy with, 1028–1030, 1029f
prenatal diagnosis of, 248t, 262
Congenital anomalies
antenatal recognition of, 275–276, 276f
of anterior abdominal wall, 293–294, 294f
antidepressants and, 1118
cardiovascular. *See* Congenital heart disease (CHD).
central nervous system, 279–282, 279f–283f
craniofacial, 284–285, 285f
defined, 275
diabetes and, 963–964, 963t
feeding problems due to, 1209
fetal heart rate with, 413
of gastrointestinal tract, 290–293, 290f–293f
of genitourinary tract, 294–297, 295f–297f
incidence and recurrence of, 278t
intracranial cystic lesions as, 282–284, 283f, 284f
and intrauterine growth restriction, 638
of lungs, 285–289, 286f–289f
major, 275
management of, 277–278, 277t, 278t
in multiple gestation, 456, 457–459, 458t
selective termination for, 469–470
of neck and chest, 285–290, 286f–289f
neonatal outcomes with, 1198–1199, 1198t
population frequency of, 275
prognosis for, 277
progression of, 277–278
skeletal, 297–299, 298t
Congenital cystic adenomatoid malformation (CCAM), 286–287, 287f
hydrops fetalis due to, 444, 509
invasive fetal therapy for, 277t, 444
Congenital deafness, carrier screening for, 242t
Congenital diaphragmatic hernia (CDH), 287–289
and aneuploidy, 227t
feeding problems due to, 1209
incidence of, 440
invasive fetal therapy for, 277t, 288, 434t, 442–444
lung area to head circumference ratio in, 288, 441, 442t, 443f
postnatal management of, 442, 1198t
prenatal diagnosis of, 287, 288f, 440, 441f
prognosis for, 287–289, 441, 442t, 443f
pulmonary arterial hypotension due to, 441–442
pulmonary hypoplasia due to, 196–197, 1203
types of, 440
Congenital heart disease (CHD)
anesthesia with, 1156–1158
and aneuploidy, 227t
aortic stenosis as
fetal, 330, 330f
maternal, 805–806, 806f
anesthesia with, 1155
atrial septal defect as
fetal, 321, 322
maternal, 800–802, 802f
anesthesia with, 1157
atrioventricular block as, maternal, 810
atrioventricular canal defect as, fetal, 324–326, 325f, 326f
cardiac tumors as, fetal, 335–336, 335f, 336f
coarctation of the aorta as
fetal, 330–331, 331f
maternal, 808–809

Congenital heart disease (CHD) *(Continued)*
cyanotic, neonatal management of, 1198t
double-outlet right ventricle as, fetal, 333
Ebstein anomaly as
fetal, 326–327, 326f, 327f
maternal, 810, 810f
Eisenmenger syndrome as, maternal, 804–805, 804f
anesthesia with, 1157
epidemiology of, 28–29, 28t
fetal, 305–340
aortic stenosis as, 330, 330f
arrhythmia(s) as, 336–340, 336t
antiarrhythmic medications for, 336, 336t
premature atrial contractions as, 336–337, 337f
sustained bradycardia as, 338, 338f
sustained tachycardia as, 338–340, 339f, 340f
atrial septal defect as, 321, 322
atrioventricular canal defect as, 324–326, 325f, 326f
cardiac tumors as, 335–336, 335f, 336f
classification of, 320t
coarctation of the aorta as, 330–331, 331f
double-outlet right ventricle as, 333
Ebstein anomaly as, 326–327, 326f, 327f
echocardiography of, 310–317
atrial septum in, 312, 313f
atrioventricular valves in, 312–313
beating four-chamber view in, 307–308, 308f, 311–314, 312f–314f
congestive heart failure in, 315–316, 316f
general imaging in, 310
great arteries and ductal and aortic arches in, 309, 309f, 314–315, 314f–316f
during heart beating, 308
heart size in, 307–308
heart structure in, 308
heart symmetry in, 308
hydrops in, 310
indications for, 306
outflow tracts in, 309, 309f, 314–315, 314f–316f
screening, 307–309, 308f, 309f
semilunar valves in, 309, 314
sensitivity of, 310
three-dimensional, 307, 309–310, 316–317, 317f–319f
umbilical cord in, 310, 310f
venous drainage in, 311–312, 312f
ventricles in, 313, 313f
ventricular septum in, 309, 313–314, 314f
visceroatrial situs in, 307, 310–311, 311f
embryologic development of, 279
etiology of, 28, 29, 279, 306t
hypoplastic left heart syndrome as, 328–330, 329f
invasive fetal therapy for, 277t, 434t, 445, 446t
pulmonary atresia with intact ventricular septum as, 328, 328f
risk factors for, 305–306, 306t
screening for, 306–310
background of, 306–307
technique of, 307–309, 307f–309f
with three-dimensional imaging, 307, 309–310
tetralogy of Fallot as, 324, 324f, 331–333, 332f, 333f
transposition of the great arteries as, 333–334, 333f, 334f

Congenital heart disease (CHD) *(Continued)*
tricuspid atresia as, 327–328, 327f
tricuspid valve dysplasia as, 326–327, 326f, 327f
truncus arteriosus as, 334–335, 335f
venous anomalies as
pulmonary, 321–322, 321f
systemic, 318–320, 319f–321f
ventricular septal defect as, 313–314, 322–324, 323f, 324f
hydrops fetalis due to, 507
hypoplastic left heart syndrome as, fetal, 328–330, 329f
incidence of, 28, 278, 305
and intrauterine growth restriction, 638
left-to-right shunt as, maternal, 800–804, 802f–804f
anesthesia with, 1156–1157
maternal, 800–810
aortic stenosis as, 805–806, 806f
anesthesia with, 1155
atrial septal defects as, 800–802, 802f
anesthesia with, 1157
atrioventricular block as, 810
coarctation of the aorta as, 808–809
Ebstein anomaly as, 810, 810f
Eisenmenger syndrome as, 804–805, 804f
anesthesia with, 1157
left-to-right shunt as, 800–804, 802f–804f
mitral stenosis as, 805
anesthesia with, 1154–1155
obstructive, 805–809, 806f–809f
patent ductus arteriosus as, 803–804, 804f
anesthesia with, 1157
primary pulmonary hypertension as, 805
pulmonic stenosis as, 806–807, 806f, 807f
tetralogy of Fallot as, 807–808, 807f–809f
anesthesia with, 1157–1158
ventricular septal defect as, 802–803, 803f
anesthesia with, 1156–1157
mitral stenosis as, maternal, 805, 811–812, 811f
anesthesia with, 1154–1155
nuchal translucency and, 237, 237t
obstructive, maternal, 805–809, 806f–809f
patent ductus arteriosus as, maternal, 803–804, 804f
anesthesia with, 1157
primary pulmonary hypertension as, maternal, 805
pulmonary atresia with intact ventricular septum as, fetal, 328, 328f
pulmonic stenosis as, maternal, 806–807, 806f, 807f
recurrence risk of, 28–29, 28t, 278–279, 278t
right-to-left shunts as, anesthesia with, 1157–1158
risk factors for, 305–306, 306t
tetralogy of Fallot as
fetal, 324, 324f, 331–333, 332f, 333f
maternal, 807–808, 807f–809f
anesthesia with, 1157–1158
transposition of the great arteries as, fetal, 333–334, 333f, 334f
tricuspid atresia as, fetal, 327–328, 327f
tricuspid valve dysplasia as, fetal, 326–327, 326f, 327f
truncus arteriosus as, fetal, 334–335, 335f
venous anomalies as
pulmonary, 321–322, 321f
systemic, 318–320, 319f–321f
ventricular septal defect as
fetal, 313–314, 322–324, 323f, 324f
maternal, 802–803, 803f
anesthesia with, 1156–1157

Congenital Minimata disease, 354
Congenital nephrosis, 235
Congenital rubella syndrome (CRS), 775–776.1219
Congenital uterine anomalies. *See* Uterine anomalies.
Congenital varicella syndrome, 933
Congestive cardiomyopathy, in infants of diabetic mothers, 967
Congestive heart failure (CHF), fetal, 315–316, 316t
Conization, cervical cerclage after, 592–593
Conjoined twins, 57, 60, 468–469, 468f
Connective tissue changes, in pregnancy, 1124
Connective tissue disease, neonatal outcomes with, 1198
Consanguinity, 24, 24f
Consensus Development Statement of Cesarean Childbirth, 711
Consent, informed, for carrier screening, 238
CONSORT statement, 208
Constipation, 1052, 1052t
Continuous ambulatory peritoneal dialysis (CAPD), 917–918
Continuous positive airway pressure (CPAP), for respiratory distress syndrome, 1204
Continuous subcutaneous insulin infusion (CSII), 977f, 979, 979t
Contraception
breastfeeding and, 134–135
with renal transplantation, 921
Contractile phase, of myometrial remodeling, 522
Contractility, fetal, 162
Contraction(s), 76–82
defined, 522
in diagnosis, 70
effectiveness of, 522
fetal heart rate with, 410f, 411t
hormonal regulation of, 79–81, 79f, 80t
during labor, 522–523
measurement of, 399
mechanics of, 76–79, 78f
in pregnancy, 691
and preterm birth, 558, 560
regulation of electrical activity in, 76, 77f
Contraction monitoring, after trauma, 1185
Contraction stress test (CST), 381–382, 381f
in diabetic pregnancy, 983t
Contraction-associated proteins (CAPs), 79
Contractures, 522
Contrast venography, of deep venous thrombosis, 857
Cool Cap Study Group, 1211
Cooley anemia, 877
Coombs test, direct, in anemia, 870, 870t, 872
COP (colloid osmotic pressure)
abnormalities of, 1174
nonpregnant, 1171t
during pregnancy, 103t, 1171t, 1174
Copper supplementation, during pregnancy, 146t
Copy number variations (CNVs), 3, 14, 31, 32
Cordocentesis, 383–386
biophysical profile score and, 383–384, 384f
complications of, 385–386, 385t, 386f
fetal respiratory status by, 386, 386t
for idiopathic thrombocytopenic purpura, 839
indications for, 383–384, 384t
to monitor Rh-immunized pregnancies, 484
monitoring after, 385
for neonatal alloimmune thrombocytopenia, 841
procedure for, 384–385, 384f, 385f
technique of, 259

Coronary artery disease (CAD), maternal, 816–817
anesthesia with, 1158–1159
Coronary heart disease, and diabetes, 961–962
Coronary sinus, fetal echocardiography of, 311, 312f, 313f
Corpus luteum cyst, 1143
Corpus mammae, 129
Cortical blindness, biophysical profile score and, 389t
Corticosteroid(s)
for asthma
with acute exacerbations, 944t
inhaled, 940–941, 940t, 941t
during labor and delivery, 943
oral, 940t, 942
in breastfeeding, 131
for cervical ripening, 702t
developmental effects of, 153–154
for hemolytic disease of the fetus and newborn, 494
for idiopathic thrombocytopenic purpura, 838
for induction of fetal pulmonary maturity, 423–428
dosage of, 423, 423t
experimental models of, 203, 203f
maternal consequences of, 426
mechanism of action of, 423
neonatal outcomes of, 424–425, 424f–426f
NIH Consensus Panel guidelines for, 427t, 428
other fetal and neonatal effects of, 425–426
repeated courses of, 426–428
for inflammatory bowel disease, 1049
long-term therapy with, 1030
for neonatal alloimmune thrombocytopenia, 841–842
for preterm labor, 561
for preterm premature rupture of the membranes, 604, 605
for rheumatic disease, 1081, 1082t
for septic shock, 1178–1179
for skin conditions, 1125
as teratogens, 351t, 352
Corticosteroid-binding globulin, during pregnancy, 1025, 1026f
Corticotropin-releasing hormone (CRH)
in control of labor, 72
and fetal lung development, 203
in neurohormonal control, 1015
during pregnancy, 120, 1016, 1025
in preterm labor, 529, 530f
secretion of, 1025
Corticotropin-releasing hormone (CRH) testing, for Cushing syndrome, 1022
Corticotropin-releasing hormone–binding protein (CRH-BP)
in control of labor, 72
during pregnancy, 120
Cortisol
for Addison disease, 1027
control of, 1025, 1025f
in control of labor, 72
excessive secretion of, 1021–1022
and fetal lung development, 203
for hypopituitarism, 1023
during pregnancy, 120, 1016, 1025, 1026f
and progesterone, 73–74
Cortisone, for induction of fetal pulmonary maturity, 423t
Coumadin. *See* Warfarin (Coumadin).
Coupled behaviors, fetal, 362, 362f
COX (cyclooxygenase) inhibitors, for preterm labor, 563–564
COX-2 (cyclooxygenase-2), in control of labor, 74
CP. *See* Cerebral palsy (CP).
CPAP (continuous positive airway pressure), for respiratory distress syndrome, 1204
CPD (cephalopelvic disproportion)
arrest disorders due to, 695
brow presentation due to, 707
CPR (cardiopulmonary resuscitation), 1188–1189
Craniofacial anomalies, 284–285, 285f
Craniopagus, 468
Craniopharyngiomas, 1016, 1093
Craniosynostosis, 284, 299
Creatinine, serum, during pregnancy, 910
Creatinine clearance, in preeclampsia, 657
Creatinine concentration, in preeclampsia, 657
Cretinism, endemic, 1006
CRH. *See* Corticotropin-releasing hormone (CRH).
Crigler-Najjar syndrome, jaundice due to, 1060t
Crista dividens, fetal, 160
Crista interveniens, fetal, 160
Critical oxygen delivery, 929, 929f
Crixivan (indinavir), for HIV infection, 772t
Crohn disease, 1047–1049
clinical characteristics of, 1047–1048, 1048f, 1048t
diagnostic testing for, 1048, 1049f
effect of pregnancy on, 1048
effect on pregnancy of, 1048
genetics of, 28
treatment of, 1048–1049, 1049t
Cromolyn, for asthma, 940t, 941t, 942
Crossing over, 8f, 9, 9f
CRS (congenital rubella syndrome), 775–776.1219
Cryoprecipitate
for abruptio placentae, 733t
for hemorrhagic shock, 1181, 1181t
Crystalloid solutions, for hemorrhagic shock, 1180
CSII (continuous subcutaneous insulin infusion), 977f, 979, 979t
CST (contraction stress test), 381–382, 381f
in diabetic pregnancy, 983t
CT (computed tomography)
of appendicitis, 1047, 1047t
of perinatal stroke, 1213, 1213f
CTG (cardiotocogram)
of abruptio placentae, 732
in biophysical profile score, 365t, 366, 367f, 368f
computerized, 370–371, 371f
CTPA (computed tomography pulmonary angiography), for pulmonary embolus, 859, 860, 861, 861f, 862
Cushing disease, 1021
Cushing syndrome
adrenal, 1027
pituitary, 1021–1022
Cutoff values, 221, 222t
CVP (central venous pressure)
nonpregnant, 1171t
during pregnancy, 103t, 1171t
and pulmonary capillary wedge pressure, 1170, 1170f
CVR (CCAM volume ratio), 444
CVS. *See* Chorionic villus sampling (CVS).
Cyanotic congenital heart disease, neonatal management of, 1198t
Cyclooxygenase (COX) inhibitors, for preterm labor, 563–564
Cyclooxygenase-2 (COX-2), in control of labor, 74
Cyclophosphamide
for rheumatic disease, 1081, 1082t
as teratogen, 352
Cyclopia, 285
Cycloserine, for tuberculosis, 937t
Cyclosporine
for renal transplantation, 918, 919
for rheumatic disease, 1082t
Cymbalta (duloxetine), dosage of, 1117t
Cyst(s)
bronchogenic, 285, 286f
choledochal, 293
choroid plexus, 284, 284f
and aneuploidy, 227, 227t
corpus luteum, 1143
Dandy-Walker, 280–281, 281f
milk-retention, 138
ovarian, 1139–1143
complications of, 1141–1142
diagnosis of, 1140–1142, 1140t, 1141f, 1142f
MRI for, 1141
serologic markers for, 1140–1141
ultrasonic characteristics in, 1140, 1140t, 1141f, 1142f
epidemiology of, 886, 1139
management of, 886, 1142–1143
pathogenesis of, 1139, 1139t
posterior fossa, and aneuploidy, 227t
Cystic adenomatoid malformation, congenital, 286–287, 287f
hydrops fetalis due to, 444, 509
invasive fetal therapy for, 277t, 444
Cystic fibrosis (CF), 31f, 946–948
anesthesia with, 1151–1152
carrier screening for, 238–240, 238t–240t, 242t
effect of pregnancy on, 946–947
epidemiology of, 946
fetal risks with, 948
labor and delivery with, 948
management of, 948
preconception counseling on, 947
pregnancy outcome with, 947
prenatal diagnosis of, 248t
Cystic hygroma, 289–290, 289f
and aneuploidy, 227t
hydrops fetalis due to, 509
Cystic lymphangioma, 289–290, 289f
Cystitis, 753–754, 906
Cytochrome P450 oxidoreductase (PORD) deficiency, 1031
Cytogenetic abnormalities, fetal loss due to, 619–620
Cytogenetics, molecular, 12–14, 13f, 14f
Cytokines
and immune response, 88
in placental tissues, 117t
in pregnancy, 88–89, 89f
in preterm labor and birth, 526–527, 526f, 556
Cytokinesis, 8
Cytomegalovirus (CMV), 764–766
breastfeeding with, 136t
clinical manifestations of, 765
congenital
clinical manifestations of, 765, 1217–1218
diagnosis of, 765
pathogenesis of, 765
treatment of, 765–766, 1218
diagnosis of, 765
epidemiology and pathogenesis of, 764–765
fetal infection with, 1101
fetal loss due to, 624
hepatitis due to, 1069

Cytomegalovirus (CMV) *(Continued)*
  hydrops fetalis due to, 510–511
  intrauterine growth restriction due to, 638
  intrauterine transfusion with, 492
  in newborn period, 1217–1218
  prevention of, 766
  risk factors for, 765
  treatment of, 765–766
Cytosine, deamination of, 6, 6f
Cytotec. *See* Misoprostol (Cytotec).
Cytotoxic drugs, while breastfeeding, 139t, 140
Cytotrophoblast, 41, 42, 42f, 43f

D

d4T (stavudine), for HIV infection, 772t
Dairy products, in diet, 147
Dalteparin, for venous thromboembolism, 863
  prevention of, 836
Damage-associated molecular patterns (DAMPs), 92
Dandy-Walker malformation, 280–281, 281f
Dapsone, for *Pneumocystis jiroveci* pneumonia, 934
Darunavir (Prezista), for HIV infection, 772t
Database cohorts, on safety of exposures, 349–350
Daughter cells, 7
DDAVP (L-deamino,8-D-arginine vasopressin)
  for diabetes insipidus, 1024–1025
  for von Willebrand disease, 843–844, 845t
ddC (zalcitabine), for HIV infection, 772t
DDi (didanosine), for HIV infection, 772t
D-dimer assays
  for deep venous thrombosis, 857–858, 858f
  for pulmonary embolus, 861, 861f, 862
Deafness, congenital, carrier screening for, 242t
Deamination, of cytosine, 6, 6f
L-Deamino,8-D-arginine vasopressin (DDAVP, desmopressin acetate)
  for diabetes insipidus, 1024–1025
  for von Willebrand disease, 843–844, 845t
Decelerations, in fetal heart rate
  early, 406, 411t
  late, 406, 408–409.409f, 410f, 411t
  prolonged, 406
  variable, 406, 409–410, 410f, 411t
Decidua, 37
  basalis, 37
  capsularis, 37, 38
  vera, 37, 38
Decidual hemorrhage, preterm labor due to, 527–529, 529f
Decidual/membrane activation, in labor and delivery, 523
Decision analysis, 210
Deep venous thrombosis (DVT)
  clinical presentation of, 856, 856t
  diagnosis and evaluation of, 856–858, 856t, 858f, 861
  epidemiology of, 855
  postcesarean, 709
  prevention of, 835–837, 864–865
  risk factors for, 855–856, 856t
  treatment of, 862–864, 862t
Deflection abnormalities, 706–707
Dehydroepiandrosterone sulfate (DHEAS)
  in control of labor, 70, 72
  in pregnancy, 115
Deiodinases, during pregnancy, 996
Deiodination
  in normal thyroid physiology, 995, 996f
  during pregnancy, 996
Delavirdine (Rescriptor), for HIV infection, 772t
Delayed interval delivery, 463
Deletions, 15, 16f, 16t
  in linkage analysis, 33
Delivery. *See* Labor and delivery.
Delta base, 400, 401t
Delta infection (hepatitis D virus), 786, 787t, 1065t, 1068
Delta storage pool disease, 846–847
Delta virus infection, 786
ΔOD_{450}, of amniotic fluid, 483, 484f
Dengue virus, breastfeeding with, 135
Deoxyribonucleic acid. *See* DNA (deoxyribonucleic acid).
Depakote (valproic acid)
  dosage of, 1116t
  as teratogen, 348, 351t, 352, 1117
Dependent edema, 104
Depression
  diagnostic criteria for, 1113, 1114t, 1115t
  epidemiology of, 1113
  identification of, 1114
  impact on pregnancy outcomes of, 1114, 1116
  postpartum, and thyroiditis, 1010
  and preterm birth, 555
  symptoms of, 1113, 1114t, 1115t
  treatment of
    clinical approach to, 1118–1119
    dosage for, 1117t
    during lactation, 1119–1120
    perinatal complications of, 1119
    risks of, 1117–1118
Depression headaches, 1092
Depression screening scales, 1114
Depressive episode, 1113, 1114t, 1115t
Dermatitis
  atopic, 1131
  autoimmune progesterone, 1125
  estrogen, 1130
  papular, of pregnancy, 1127
Dermatomyositis, 1109
Dermatosis(es), 1124–1130, 1125t
  atopic eruption of pregnancy (prurigo gestationis) as, 1125t, 1126–1127, 1127f
  autoimmune progesterone dermatitis as, 1125t, 1130
  general treatment of, 1125
  impetigo herpetiformis as, 1125t, 1129–1130, 1130f
  pemphigoid gestationis (herpes gestationis) as, 1125t, 1127–1129, 1128f, 1129f
  pruritic urticarial papules and plaques of pregnancy as, 1125t, 1126, 1126f
  pruritus gravidarum as, 1125–1126, 1125t
DES (diethylstilbestrol), as teratogen, 351t
Descent, during labor, 691–692, 692t, 693
  abnormalities of, 696–697, 696f, 696t
Descriptive studies, 207–208
Desensitization, for penicillin allergy, 780, 781t
Desipramine (Norpramin), dosage of, 1117t
Desmopressin acetate (L-deamino,8-D-arginine vasopressin)
  for diabetes insipidus, 1024–1025
  for von Willebrand disease, 843–844, 845t
Development, 37–44
  fetal, 175–177, 176t
    in diabetic pregnancy, 982–984, 985
    in multiple gestation, 456–457, 461
    with post-term pregnancy, 614
    rate of, 636, 636f, 636t, 637f
  macroscopic, 37–41, 38f–40f
  microscopic, 41–44, 42f–44f
  postfertilization, 37, 38f, 39f
  with post-term pregnancy, 616–617
Developmental delay, after intrauterine transfusion, 492
Developmental effects, of post-term pregnancy, 616–617
Developmental origins, of health and disease, 151–156
  animal models of, 154
  antenatal glucocorticoids in, 153–154
  breastfeeding in, 153
  childhood growth in, 153
  for diabetes, 152–156
  interventions based on, 154–155
  low birth weight in, 151–152, 152f
  and maternal body composition, 154–155
  maternal weight in, 152–154, 155
  mechanistic insights into, 154
  and neonatal feeding regimens, 155
  and nutrient supplementation, 154
  thrifty phenotype hypothesis in, 155
Dexamethasone
  developmental effects of, 153
  fetal biophysical effects of, 425–426
  for hemolytic disease of the fetus and newborn, 494
  for 21-hydroxylase deficiency, 1028–1029, 1029f
  for induction of fetal pulmonary maturity
    dosage of, 423, 423t
    neonatal outcomes of, 424–425, 424f, 425f
  for neonatal alloimmune thrombocytopenia, 841
  after preterm premature rupture of the membranes, 605
  for rheumatic disease, 1001, 1002t
  for thyroid storm, 1003, 1003t
Dexamethasone suppression test, for Cushing syndrome, 1021–1022
Dextran solution, for hemorrhagic shock, 1180–1181, 1180t
Dextrose, for diabetic ketoacidosis, 962t
Dextro-transposition of the great arteries (D-TGA), 333–334, 333f
DGI (disseminated gonococcal infection), 744, 746
DHEAS (dehydroepiandrosterone sulfate)
  in control of labor, 70, 72
  in pregnancy, 115
Diabetes, 953–986
  antenatal corticosteroids with, 426
  antihypertensive medications for, 973–982
  breastfeeding with, 986
  childhood neurologic abnormalities with, 968–969
  classification and pathobiology of, 953–955, 954t
  diagnosis of, 970–973, 971t–973t
  diagnostic criteria for, 955, 955t
  epidemiology of, 953, 954f
  fetal loss due to, 624–625
  fetal lung development with, 421
  fetal morbidity and mortality with, 963–967
    birth injury as, 966–967, 966f
    congenital anomalies as, 963–964, 963t
    fetal obesity as, 964–966, 965t, 966t
    miscarriage as, 963
    perinatal mortality as, 963, 963t
  and fetal pulmonary maturity, 421
  fetal surveillance with, 982, 982t, 983f, 983t
  genetic and other causes of, 955
  gestational, 955
    defined, 955
    developmental effect of, 152–153
    diagnosis of, 971–973, 971t–973t
    epidemiology of, 955
    glyburide for, 981
    insulin for, 979–980

Diabetes *(Continued)*
maternal-fetal metabolism in, 956–958, 957f
pathophysiology of, 955
risk factor screening for, 971, 971t, 973, 973t
hydrops fetalis due to, 512
intrapartum glycemic management with, 985–986, 985t
intrauterine growth restriction due to, 641
maternal morbidity with, 958–963
due to cardiovascular complications, 961–962, 961f
due to diabetic ketoacidosis, 962–963, 962t
nephropathy as, 959–961, 959f, 959t, 960f
retinopathy as, 958
maternal obesity and, 144
maternal-fetal metabolism in, 956–958, 957f
maturity-onset, of young, 955
metabolic management of, 973–982
avoiding ketosis in, 974
avoiding nocturnal hypoglycemia in, 974
dietary therapy in, 973–974
glucose monitoring in, 974–976
pregestational, 970
target levels in, 975–976, 975f, 976f, 976t
timing of, 974–975, 975t
insulin therapy in, 976–980, 977f, 977t, 979t
low glycemic foods in, 974
oral hypoglycemic agents in, 970, 980–982
postpartum, 986
preconceptional, 970
principles of, 973–974
neonatal morbidity and mortality with, 967–968, 968f, 986, 1197
neonatal transitional management with, 986
obesity and, 955
overt, 970–971
preconceptional management of, 969–970, 969t
and preeclampsia, 654
pregestational, 973–982
antihypertensive medications for, 973–982
dietary therapy for, 973–974
glucose monitoring for, 970, 974–976, 975f, 975t, 976f, 976t
insulin therapy for, 976–980, 977f, 977t, 979t
oral hypoglycemic agents for, 970, 980–982
preconceptional management of, 969–970, 969t
with renal transplantation, 920
timing and route of delivery with, 982–985, 984t, 985t
type 1, 954, 970–971
type 2, 954–955, 971
Diabetes in Early Pregnancy (DIEP) study, 961, 964, 974
Diabetes insipidus, 1024–1025
Diabetic ketoacidosis (DKA), 962–963, 962t
Diabetic mothers, infants of
hyperbilirubinemia in, 1208
morbidity and mortality in, 967–968, 968f, 986
Diabetic nephropathy, 913–914, 959–961
categories of, 959, 959t
course during pregnancy of, 916t, 959–960, 960f
effect of pregnancy on progression of, 959, 959f
epidemiology of, 959
pathophysiology of, 959
renal dialysis for, 960
renal transplantation for, 960–961
Diabetic retinopathy, 958
Diagnosis, prenatal. *See* Prenatal diagnosis.
Diagnostic tests
assessing research on, 214–217, 215t, 216f
prenatal. *See* Prenatal diagnosis.
Diakinesis, 8f, 9
Dialysis
for diabetic nephropathy, 960
hemo-, 915–917, 916t
peritoneal, 917–918
Diamniotic twins, 57, 57f, 58
acardiac, 65f
dichorionic, 57–58, 58f, 59f
monochorionic, 58, 58f, 60–61, 61f, 62f
twin-to-twin transfusion syndrome with, 63f
Diaphragm
during pregnancy, 927–928
sella, 1015
Diaphragmatic hernia, congenital. *See* Congenital diaphragmatic hernia (CDH).
Diastolic blood pressure
defined, 651
during pregnancy, 102, 102f, 103
Diastrophic dysplasia, 298
Diastrophic dysplasia sulfate transporter (DTDST), in skeletal growth, 297
Diazepam, for status epilepticus, 1090
Diazoxide, for preeclampsia, 675
DIC (disseminated intravascular coagulation)
due to abruptio placentae, 624
in preeclampsia, 662–663, 674
Dichorionic twins, 57, 57f–59f, 58
diagnosis of, 455–456, 456f
selective termination with, 470
Didanosine (DDi, Videx), for HIV infection, 772t
Didelphys uterus, 1143, 1144, 1144t
Diego antigen, 495t
DIEP (Diabetes in Early Pregnancy) study, 961, 964, 974
Diet. *See also* Nutrition.
for celiac disease, 1050
for constipation, 1052
for cystic fibrosis, 946
for diabetes, 973–974
for GERD, 1044, 1045f
for irritable bowel syndrome, 1050
vegetarian, 146t, 147–148
Dietary guidelines, 147–148, 147t
Diethylstilbestrol (DES)
cervical insufficiency due to, 586, 592–593
as teratogen, 351t
Diffuse, large B-cell lymphoma, 898–899
Diffuse cerebral white matter injury, 1212
Diffusion, simple, 50
Digoxin
during pregnancy, 801t
for supraventricular tachycardia, 339
1α,25-Dihydroxycholecalciferol (1,25(OH)$_2$D, calcitriol, vitamin D$_2$), 1032
Diiodotyrosine, in normal thyroid physiology, 995
Dilated cardiomyopathy, maternal, 814
Dilation and curettage, cervical insufficiency due to, 586
Diltiazem, during pregnancy, 801t
Dinoprostone (Prepidil, Cervidil Rx)
for cervical ripening, 702t, 703t
for post-term pregnancy, 615, 616
for uterine atony, 1183t
Diphenylhydantoin, as teratogen, 351t, 352
Diphtheria, breastfeeding with, 135
Diploid number, 8
Diplonema, 9
Diplotene, 8f
Direct assays, 30
Direct obstetric deaths, 1167
Disease, developmental origins of, 151–156
animal models of, 154
antenatal glucocorticoids in, 153–154
breastfeeding in, 153
childhood growth in, 153
for diabetes, 152–156
interventions based on, 154–155
low birth weight in, 151–152, 152f
and maternal body composition, 154–155
maternal weight in, 152–154, 155
mechanistic insights into, 154
and neonatal feeding regimens, 155
and nutrient supplementation, 154
thrifty phenotype hypothesis in, 155
Disk lesions, 1104
Disk prolapse, 1104
Disomy, uniparental, 247, 254
Disopyramide, during pregnancy, 801t
Disposition index, 957
Disseminated gonococcal infection (DGI), 744, 746
Disseminated intravascular coagulation (DIC)
due to abruptio placentae, 624
in preeclampsia, 662–663, 674
Diuretics
for chronic hypertension, 677, 679
for preeclampsia, 675
during pregnancy, 800, 801t
for subarachnoid hemorrhage, 1150
Dizygotic (DZ) twins, 55
causes of, 56
frequency of, 56
identification of, 66–67
placentation of, 57–58, 58f, 59f
DKA (diabetic ketoacidosis), 962–963, 962t
DNA (deoxyribonucleic acid)
free fetal, prenatal diagnosis using, 261–262
structure of, 3–5, 4f
synthesis of, 4–5, 4f
transcription of, 5, 5f
DNA diagnostics, 30–34, 30f–32f
DNA polymorphisms, 33
DNA probes, 12, 13f, 30f, 32
DNA sequencing, 32
DO$_2$. *See* Oxygen delivery (DO$_2$).
Dobutamine, for septic shock, 763, 1178, 1178t
Dombrock antigen, 495t
Dominant trait, 22–23
Dopamine
for acute renal failure due to preeclampsia, 908
in neurohormonal control, 1015
for septic shock, 763, 1178, 1178t
Dopaminergic agonists, for acromegaly, 1021
Doppler ultrasound
application of, 378–379, 379f
fetal, 371–377
and frequency of biophysical profile scoring, 371, 372t
with intrauterine growth restriction, 644–645
of middle cerebral artery, 374–375, 375f
in Rh-immunized pregnancy, 485–488, 485f, 486f, 490
of umbilical artery, 175, 372–374, 373f, 374f, 374t
venous studies in, 375–377, 376f, 377f
maternal, 377–378, 378f, 379f
patterns of deterioration in, 378–379, 379f, 380f
Doppler ultrasound transducer, for fetal heart rate monitoring, 399
Dose response, to teratogens, 348

Double-balloon enteroscopy, 1053
"Double-bubble" sign, 291, 291f
Double-outlet right ventricle (DORV), 333
Douching, and preterm birth, 555
Down syndrome
  prenatal screening for, 222–233
    ADAM 12 in, 230
    combined first- and second-trimester, 232
    cutoff values in, 222t
    ductus venosus wave form in, 231
    first-trimester
      impact of spontaneous miscarriages on, 231–232
      serum markers in, 229–230, 230t
      ultrasound markers in, 227–229, 230–231, 230t, 231f
    human chorionic gonadotropin in, 229–230
    integrated aneuploidy screening as, 232
    likelihood ratios in, 221–222, 222t, 225, 226, 226t
    maternal age in, 222, 222t, 232–233, 233t
    with multiple gestation, 458–459
    nasal bone in, 225, 230–231, 231f, 232
    nuchal translucency in, 228, 230
    PAPP-A in, 229
      in twins, 257, 459
    receiver operating curve in, 222f
    second-trimester
      serum markers in, 222–225, 224t, 226
      ultrasound markers in, 225–226, 225t, 226t
    sequential testing as, 232
    serum markers in
      first-trimester, 229–230, 230t
      second-trimester, 222–225, 224t, 226
    tricuspid regurgitation in, 231
    ultrasound markers in
      first-trimester, 227–229, 230–231, 230t, 231f
      second-trimester, 225–226, 225t, 226t
  recurrence risk for, 246–247
  due to robertsonian translocation, 247, 247t
  in twins, 256, 256t, 257, 257t, 458–459, 458t
  due to uniparental disomy, 247
Doxepin (Sinequan), dosage of, 1117t
Doxylamine, for nausea and vomiting, 1042
Doxylamine succinate and pyridoxine hydrochloride with or without dicyclomine hydrochloride (Bendectin)
  for nausea and vomiting, 1042, 1042t
  as teratogen, 347
Drug(s)
  and biophysical profile score, 369t
  and breastfeeding, 126, 139–141, 139t, 140f, 140t
  hydrops fetalis due to, 512
  and neonatal outcomes, 1199
  and thyroid function, 1000, 1000t
Drug abuse. *See* Substance abuse.
Drug-induced hypothyroidism, 1007
Drug-induced thrombocytopenia, 843
Drug-induced valvular heart disease, 814
DTDST (diastrophic dysplasia sulfate transporter), in skeletal growth, 297
D-TGA (dextro-transposition of the great arteries), 333–334, 333f
Duchenne muscular dystrophy, prenatal diagnosis of, 248t
Ductal arches, fetal echocardiography of, 314–315, 314f
Ductus arteriosus
  fetal, 160f, 167
    echocardiography of, 314f, 315
    patent, prematurity and, 1201t
    premature closure or narrowing of, hydrops fetalis due to, 509
  maternal, patent, 803–804, 804f
    anesthesia with, 1157
Ductus venosus, fetal, 159–160, 160f
  Doppler studies of, 376–377, 376f
Ductus venosus wave form, prenatal screening for, 231
Duffy antigen, 478f, 495t, 497t, 498–499
Duloxetine (Cymbalta), dosage of, 1117t
Dumping syndrome, 1051
Duodenal atresia, 291–292, 291f
  and aneuploidy, 227t
Duplications, 15
Dural vascular anomalies
  intracranial, 1098–1099
  spinal, 1099
DVT. *See* Deep venous thrombosis (DVT).
Dwarfism, achondroplastic, anesthesia with, 1161
Dynamic mutations, 29–30
Dynamic ultrasound, of fetal anomalies, 275–276, 276f
Dysautonomia, familial, carrier screening for, 242t
Dysgerminoma, ovarian, 886, 1141
Dyslipidemia, in preeclampsia, 658
Dysmature offspring, 616–617
Dyspnea, during pregnancy, 103
Dysrhythmias. *See* Arrhythmias.
Dysthymic disorder, diagnostic criteria for, 1113, 1115t
Dystocia
  due to adnexal masses, 1142
  cesarean delivery for, 711
  shoulder, 697–698
    diabetes and, 966–967, 966f, 984
    umbilical cord acid-base balance with, 405
Dystonia, 1102
Dystrophy, myotonic, 1109
DZ twins. *See* Dizygotic (DZ) twins.

E

E_1 (estrone), in pregnancy, 114f, 116f
E_2 (estradiol)
  in implantation, 111
  in pregnancy, 114f, 116f
Early decelerations, in fetal heart rate, 406, 411t
Early goal-directed therapy (EGDT), for septic shock, 1176–1178
EB(s) (elementary bodies), of *Chlamydia*, 93f, 95f, 747
Ebola virus, breastfeeding with, 135
Ebstein anomaly
  fetal, 326–327, 327f
  maternal, 810, 810f
ECG (electrocardiography)
  fetal, ST analysis of, 415
  for pulmonary embolus, 859
ECG (electrocardiographic) changes, during pregnancy, 799
Echocardiography
  fetal. *See* Fetal echocardiography.
  for pulmonary embolus, 859
  transesophageal, 1173
Echogenic bowel, 292–293, 292f
Eclampsia
  defined, 651
  postpartum, 674
  risk factors for, 654
Eclampsia *(Continued)*
  seizure prophylaxis and treatment in, 671–673, 671t, 672t
  symptoms preceding, 671, 671t
ECoG (electrocorticogram), fetal, 171, 172f, 173, 174, 174f
Economic status, and preterm birth, 554
Ectoderm, 39f
Ectopic ACTH syndrome, 1022
Ectopic pregnancy
  after cesarean delivery, 710
  with renal transplantation, 918
  with uterine anomalies, 1144t
Edema
  cerebral
    in acute liver failure, 1072
    in preeclampsia, 658
  dependent, 104
  labial, 1124
  due to preeclampsia, 651, 652f
    anesthetic considerations with, 1148
    cerebral, 658
    pulmonary, 674, 1175
      anesthetic considerations with, 1148
  pulmonary, 1174–1175
    colloid osmotic pressure abnormalities and, 1174
    hydrostatic or cardiogenic, 1174–1175
    in preeclampsia, 674, 1175
      anesthetic considerations with, 1148
    tocolytic-induced, 1175
  skin, due to nonimmune hydrops, 507, 507t
Edinburgh Postnatal Depression Scale (EPDS), 1114
EDNO (endothelium-derived nitric oxide), in fetal cardiovascular regulation, 166
Educational status, and preterm birth, 554, 554t
Efavirenz (Sustiva), for HIV infection, 772t
Efavirenz + emtricitabine + tenofovir (Atripla), for HIV infection, 772t
Effexor (venlafaxine), dosage of, 1117t
EFM. *See* Electronic fetal monitoring (EFM).
EFW (estimation of fetal weight), in diabetic pregnancy, 982–984, 985
EGD (esophagogastroduodenoscopy), 1045, 1045f, 1046, 1053
EGDT (early goal-directed therapy), for septic shock, 1176–1178
EGF (epidermal growth factor)
  in implantation, 113, 113t
  in pregnancy, 118
  as uterine stimulant, 80
Ehlers-Danlos syndrome, anesthesia with, 1160
Eicosanoid cascade, 74–75, 75f
Eisenmenger syndrome
  hemodynamics of, 1171
  maternal, 804–805, 804f
    anesthesia with, 1157
Ejection reflex, 131, 132f, 133, 133f
Elavil (amitriptyline), dosage of, 1117t
ELBW (extremely low birth weight)
  and cerebral palsy, 1125
  defined, 545
  and survival and morbidity with preterm birth, 550–551, 551f
Electrocardiographic (ECG) changes, during pregnancy, 799
Electrocardiography (ECG)
  fetal, ST analysis of, 415
  for pulmonary embolus, 859
Electrocorticogram (ECoG), fetal, 171, 172f, 173, 174, 174f
Electromechanical coupling, 76
Electromyography, 1104

Electronic fetal monitor (EFM), 399
  adjuncts to, 414–415
  vs. auscultation, 413
  with multiple gestation, 462
Electro-oculogram (EOG), fetal, 171, 172f
Electrophysiologic evaluation, of nerve lesions, 1104–1105, 1106f
Elementary bodies (EBs), of *Chlamydia*, 93f, 95f, 747
Elliptocytosis, hereditary, 874
Ellis–van Creveld syndrome, 298
Embolus
  amniotic fluid, hemodynamics of, 1171–1172
  pulmonary. *See* Pulmonary embolus (PE).
Embryonic demise
  due to endocrine disorders, 620–621
  due to genetic abnormalities, 619–620
  management of, 627–629, 627t, 628t
  peri-implantation, 619
  recurrent
    immunologic causes of, 621–622
    management of, 628–629, 628t
    due to uterine abnormalities, 622, 622t
Embryonic development, 37–44
  of breast, 127–128, 127f, 128f
  macroscopic, 37–41, 38f–40f
  microscopic, 41–44, 42f–44f
  postfertilization, 37, 38f, 39f
Embryonic stage, of fetal lung development, 193, 194f, 194t
Employment, and preterm birth, 555
Emsam (selegiline), dosage of, 1117t
Emtricitabine (Emtriva), for HIV infection, 772t
Enalapril, for chronic hypertension, 678, 678t
Encephalitis, measles, 776–777
Encephalocele, 281, 282f
Encephalopathy
  hepatic, 1071
  neonatal, 1210
    hypoxic-ischemic, 1210–1211
  Wernicke, 1107
End-diastolic velocities
  in middle cerebral artery
    absent, 375
    reverse, 375
  in umbilical artery
    absent, 372–373, 373f, 374t
    reverse, 372, 373–374, 374f
Endemic cretinism, 1006
Endocarditis, infective, prophylaxis against, 798, 821
Endocervical curettage, 887
Endocrine changes, in pregnancy, 119–122
Endocrine disorders, fetal loss due to, 620–621
Endocrine organ, fetoplacental unit as, 115–119
  estrogens in, 115–117, 116f
  growth factors as, 117–119, 117t, 118f, 119f
  progesterone in, 115
Endocrine system, relationships and feedback mechanisms of, 1015, 1017f
Endocrinology
  of fetoplacental unit, 115–119
  of implantation, 111–114, 112f, 113t
  of pregnancy, 111–122
    corticotropin-releasing hormone and corticotropin-releasing hormone–binding protein system in, 120
    early, 114
    estrogens in, 115–117, 116f
    growth factors in, 117–119, 118t, 119f, 120f
    human chorionic gonadotropin in, 113–114, 114f
    inhibin-related proteins in, 120
    insulin as, 118–120, 118f–120f, 120t
Endocrinology *(Continued)*
    luteal-phase shift in, 114–115, 115f
    metabolic changes in, 119–122
    oxytocin in, 121
    progesterone in, 115
    prolactin in, 121–122, 121f
    prostaglandins in, 122
    relaxin in, 118f, 121
Endoderm, 38
Endodermal sinus tumors, 886, 1141
Endogenous pressors, sensitivity to, in preeclampsia, 661–662, 662f
Endometritis, puerperal, 760–761
  breastfeeding with, 136t
  Chlamydia trachomatis and, 747
Endomyometritis, postcesarean, 709
Endoscopic fetal surgery, 433
Endoscopic ultrasound (EUS), 1053
Endoscopy, gastrointestinal, 1053, 1053t
Endothelial cell dysfunction, in preeclampsia, 663
Endothelial-derived factors, in fetal cardiovascular regulation, 166–167
Endothelin (ET)
  in fetal cardiovascular regulation, 166–167
  and patent ductus arteriosus, 167
  as uterine stimulant, 80
Endothelin-1, in preeclampsia, 661
Endothelium-derived nitric oxide (EDNO), in fetal cardiovascular regulation, 166
Endotoxin, and fetal lung development, 196f, 203, 203f
End-stage renal disease (ESRD), diabetic nephropathy and, 959, 959t, 960
Enfuvirtide (Fuzeon), for HIV infection, 772t
Engagement, during labor, 693
Engorgement, 134, 138t
ENHANCE (Extended Evaluation of Recombinant Human Activated Protein C) trial, 1179
Enhancer sequences, 5
Enigmatic fever, 764
Enoxaparin
  with mechanical heart valves, 864
  for venous thromboembolism, 863
    prevention of, 836
Enterobacteriaceae, breastfeeding with, 137t
Enterocolitis, necrotizing, 1207–1208, 1208f
  feeding problems due to, 1210
  prematurity and, 1201t
Enteroscopy, double-balloon, 1053
Environmental agents, as teratogens, 354. *See also* Teratogen(s).
Environmental toxins, intrauterine growth restriction due to, 640
EOG (electro-oculogram), fetal, 171, 172f
EPCOT (European Prospective Cohort on Thrombophilia) study, 625
EPDS (Edinburgh Postnatal Depression Scale), 1114
Epidermal growth factor (EGF)
  in implantation, 113, 113t
  in pregnancy, 118
  as uterine stimulant, 80
Epidermolysis bullosa, 1132
Epidural analgesia and anesthesia
  for cesarean delivery, 712
  for labor and delivery, 716–717
Epigenetic changes, in developmental origins of health and disease, 154
Epilepsy, maternal, 1089–1092
  effect of pregnancy on, 1089–1090
  effect on fetus and neonate of, 1090–1091
  effect on pregnancy and lactation of, 1090
  epidemiology of, 1089
Epilepsy, maternal *(Continued)*
  general therapeutic approaches to, 1091–1092
  gestational, 1089, 1091
Epinephrine, sensitivity to, in preeclampsia, 662
Episiotomy infection, 759–760, 759f
Episodic changes, in fetal heart rate patterns, 405
Epivir (lamivudine)
  for hepatitis B virus, 1066–1067
  for HIV infection, 772t
Epstein-Barr virus, hepatitis due to, 1069
Epulis gravidarum, 1124
ER(s) (estrogen receptors), 74
Erb palsy, due to shoulder dystocia, 697
Ergonovine maleate, for postpartum hemorrhage, 698
Erosive esophagitis, 1044f
Error(s)
  random, 210, 211–213, 212t, 213t
  sources of, in clinical research, 210–214, 212t, 213t
  systematic, 210–211
  type I and type II, 213–214
Ertapenem
  for pelvic abscess, 762
  for puerperal endometritis, 760
  for septic shock, 763
Erythema
  infectiosum, 774
  nodosum, 1131
  palmar, 1123–1124
Erythroblastosis fetalis. *See* Hemolytic disease of the fetus and newborn (HDFN).
Erythrocyte membrane therapy, for hemolytic disease of the fetus and newborn, 494
Erythroderma, ichthyosiform, 1132
Erythromycin
  for *Chlamydia trachomatis,* 748, 748t
  for preterm premature rupture of the membranes, 606
Erythropoietin
  for iron deficiency anemia, 874
  recombinant human, 917
ESCAPE (Evaluation Study of Congestive Heart Failure and Pulmonary Artery Catheterization Effectiveness) trial, 1170
Escitalopram (Lexapro), dosage of, 1117t
Esmolol, for thyroid storm, 1003, 1003t
Esophageal atresia, 290–291, 290f
Esophageal varices, 1070, 1071
Esophagitis, erosive, 1044f
Esophagogastroduodenoscopy (EGD), 1045, 1045f, 1046, 1053
Esophagus, in pregnancy, 1041
ESRD (end-stage renal disease), diabetic nephropathy and, 959, 959t, 960
Essential thrombocytopenia, 838
Estetrol, in pregnancy, 115, 116f
Estimation of fetal weight (EFW), in diabetic pregnancy, 982–984, 985
Estradiol (E_2)
  in implantation, 111
  in pregnancy, 114f, 116f
Estriol
  in pregnancy, 115, 116–117, 116f
  prenatal screening for, 223, 224–225
    in twins, 257, 257t, 458
Estrogen(s)
  for cervical ripening, 702t
  in control of labor, 74
  and fetoplacental unit, 115–117, 116f
  in implantation, 111
  in pregnancy, 114f, 115–117, 116f
Estrogen dermatitis, 1130
Estrogen receptors (ERs), 74

Estrone (E_1), in pregnancy, 114f, 116f
ET. *See* Endothelin (ET).
Etanercept, for rheumatic disease, 1081, 1082t
Ethambutol, for tuberculosis, 936–937, 937t
Ethionamide, for tuberculosis, 937t
Ethnic differences
in fetal loss, 622
in fetal pulmonary maturity, 421
in preeclampsia and eclampsia, 654
in preterm birth, 551, 552f, 554, 554t, 555f, 557
Etretinate, as teratogen, 353–354
Euglobulin clot lysis time, in abruptio placentae, 733t
Euploidy, 14
Eurofetus trial, 438, 439t
European Prospective Cohort on Thrombophilia (EPCOT) study, 625
EUS (endoscopic ultrasound), 1053
Evaluation Study of Congestive Heart Failure and Pulmonary Artery Catheterization Effectiveness (ESCAPE) trial, 1170
Evidence-based practice, 207–217
assessing research on screening and diagnosis in, 214–217, 215t, 216f
defined, 207
importance of, 207
sources of error in clinical research in, 210–214, 212t, 213t
types of clinical research studies in, 207–210, 208t, 209f, 210f
Ex utero intrapartum treatment (EXIT) procedure, 435
Exercise, intrauterine growth restriction due to, 641
Exocoelom, 37
Exocoelomic cavity, 47
Exocoelomic fluid, 47
Exons, 5
Expanded polyglutamine repeats, 29
Expectant management, of preeclampsia, 669–671
Expiratory reserve volume, during pregnancy, 105t
Extended Evaluation of Recombinant Human Activated Protein C (ENHANCE) trial, 1179
External cephalic version, of twin, 462
External version
for breech presentation, 705–706
for transverse lie, 706
Extra-amniotic prostaglandin, for cervical ripening, 702t
Extravillous trophoblast, 41, 43, 43f
Extremely low birth weight (ELBW)
and cerebral palsy, 1125
defined, 545
and survival and morbidity with preterm birth, 550–551, 551f
Eye movements, fetal, 171, 172f, 173

F

Face presentation, 706–707
Facial anomalies, 284–285, 285f
Facial cleft, 284–285, 285f
and aneuploidy, 227t
Factor V Leiden (FVL) mutation, 831–833, 831t
and fetal loss, 625, 625t, 626t, 832
and IUGR, 832–833
and placental abruption, 832
and preeclampsia, 832
and venous thromboembolism, 855, 856t
Factor V mutations, 833
Factor VII, in fibrin plug formation, 826, 827f
Factor VII deficiency, 844t–846t, 847
Factor VIII deficiency, 24, 844t–846t, 847
prenatal diagnosis of, 248t
Factor VIII inhibitors, 847
Factor IX deficiency, 844t–846t, 847
Factor X deficiency, 844t–846t, 847
Factor Xa, in fibrin plug formation, 826, 827f
Factor XI deficiency, 844t, 845t, 847–848
Factor XII deficiency, 844t, 845t, 848
Factor XIII deficiency, 844t, 845t, 847, 848
Famciclovir (Famvir), for genital herpes, 770
Familial brachial neuritis, acute, 1105
Familial dysautonomia, carrier screening for, 242t
Familial hypocalciuric hypercalcemia (FHH), 1034
Familial risk, of preterm birth, 553
Fanconi anemia, carrier screening for, 242t
FAS (fetal alcohol syndrome), 348–349, 354–355, 354f
Fas ligand (FasL), expression of, 90, 90f
FASD (fetal alcohol spectrum disorders), 354–355
Fasting, during pregnancy, 119–120
Fasting glucose
in diabetes, 955, 955t, 975
impaired, 955, 971
in pregnancy, 955, 955t
Fats, in diet, 147
Fatty acid oxidation pathways, 1062
Fatty liver of pregnancy, acute, 1062–1063, 1063t
acute renal failure due to, 909
FBMs (fetal breathing movements), 172f–174f, 175, 176–177, 361, 362, 362f
in biophysical profile score, 365t, 366
FBS (fetal blood sampling). *See* Cordocentesis.
FDA (Food and Drug Administration), teratogenic risk assessments of, 350, 350t, 351
FDPs (fibrin degradation products)
in abruptio placentae, 733t
in fibrinolysis, 828, 828f
Fecal incontinence, cesarean delivery to prevent, 708, 711
Feeding problems
in neonatal period, 1209–1210
prematurity and, 1201t
Femoral nerve palsy, 1106
Femur length
in Down syndrome, 225
in intrauterine growth restriction, 642, 643f
FEP (free erythrocyte protoporphyrin), 870, 872
Fern test, for premature rupture of the membranes, 602, 602f
Ferritin, serum, 870, 870t
Ferrous sulfate, for iron deficiency anemia, 873
Fertilization, 10, 11f
development after, 37, 38f, 39f
Fetal abdominal circumference
in intrauterine growth restriction, 642, 643f
maternal diabetes and, 964
Fetal acid-base balance, 400–405, 401t–405t
with acute chorioamnionitis, 404, 404t
and acute neurological injury, 403–404
with breech delivery, 405
buffers in, 400
carbonic acid in, 400
determination of, 400–401
factors affecting, 401–402, 402t
with fetal heart rate abnormalities, 404, 404t
with meconium, 404
noncarbonic acids in, 400
normal values for, 402, 403t
with nuchal cords, 404
with operative vaginal delivery, 405, 405t
with oxytocin, 405
pathologic acidemia in, 402–403, 403t
physiology of, 400–401
Fetal acid-base balance *(Continued)*
in prolonged pregnancy, 404
with shoulder dystocia, 405
terminology of, 401, 401t
umbilical cord analysis of, 402–405
Fetal alcohol spectrum disorders (FASD), 354–355
Fetal alcohol syndrome (FAS), 348–349, 354–355, 354f
Fetal allograft analogy, 87
Fetal anomalies
antenatal recognition of, 275–276, 276f
of anterior abdominal wall, 293–294, 294f
cardiovascular. *See* Congenital heart disease (CHD).
central nervous system, 279–282, 279f–283f
craniofacial, 284–285, 285f
defined, 275
of gastrointestinal tract, 290–293, 290f–293f
of genitourinary tract, 294–297, 295f–297f
incidence and recurrence of, 278t
intracranial cystic lesions as, 282–284, 283f, 284f
of lungs, 285–289, 286f–289f
management of, 277–278, 277t, 278t
in multiple gestation, 456, 457–459, 458t
selective termination for, 469–470
of neck and chest, 285–290, 286f–289f
population frequency of, 275
prognosis for, 277
progression of, 277–278
skeletal, 297–300, 298t
Fetal arrhythmias, 336–340, 336t, 337f–340f
"respiratory," 368f
Fetal autopsy, after pregnancy loss, 626
Fetal behavior(s)
absent, 363–364, 364f
basic functions of, 361
coupled, 362, 362f
individual, 361
normal, 361–362
patterned, 361–362
and transition to neonatal behavior, 362
Fetal behavioral state(s), 362
Fetal behavioral state activity, 171–174
animal studies of, 171–172, 172f
developmental changes in, 173–174, 173t
effect of hypoxia and intrauterine growth restriction on, 174, 174f
human studies of, 172–173, 173f
Fetal blood gases, 162, 162t, 386, 386t
Fetal blood pH, 162, 162t, 386, 386t
determination of, 400–401
in labor, 402t
Fetal blood sampling (FBS). *See* Cordocentesis.
Fetal blood typing, for RhD, 481–483, 482f–484f, 482t
Fetal body measurements, in intrauterine growth restriction, 642, 643f
Fetal body movements, 172, 173f, 175, 177, 361
Fetal breathing movements (FBMs), 172f–174f, 175, 176–177, 361, 362, 362f
in biophysical profile score, 365t, 366
Fetal cardiovascular system, 159–167
blood flow patterns and oxygen delivery in, 159–162, 160f–162f, 162t
cardiac output and its distribution in, 161–162, 161f, 162f, 162t
control of, 164–167
ductus arteriosus in, 160f, 167
intracardiac and vascular pressures in, 162, 163f
myocardial function in, 162–164
venous return to heart in, 159–160, 160f, 161f

Fetal cell(s), in maternal circulation, prenatal diagnosis using, 261–262
Fetal cell-free RNA, in maternal circulation, 263
Fetal circulation, 159, 160f
Fetal compensatory responses, to hypoxemia, 362–363, 363f
Fetal compromise, 363
Fetal demise, 619–629
due to antiphospholipid syndrome, 625
after chorionic villus sampling, 255
after cordocentesis, 385, 385t
defined, 622
diagnostic considerations for, 626–627, 627t
early, 622
due to endocrine disorders, 620–621
epidemiology of, 622–623
due to fetomaternal hemorrhage, 624
due to genetic abnormalities, 619–620, 623
gestational age and, 1201f
due to infection, 623–624
due to inherited thrombophilia, 625–626, 625t, 626t, 628, 831–835, 836–837
intermediate, 622
late, 622
management of, 627–629, 627t, 628t
maternal obesity and, 144–145
medical conditions causing, 624–625
after mid-trimester amniocentesis, 250–251, 250t
in multiple gestation, 469, 625
due to placental abruption, 624
recurrent, 626
cervical cerclage for, 592, 592f
immunologic causes of, 621–622
management of, 627, 627t, 628–629, 628t
due to uterine abnormalities, 622, 622t
uterine myomas and, 62, 1136, 1138
due to vasa previa, 729
Fetal development, 37–44
macroscopic, 37–41, 38f–40f
microscopic, 41–44, 42f–44f
postfertilization, 37, 38f, 39f
Fetal distress, cesarean delivery for, 711, 713
Fetal Doppler velocimetry, 371–377
and frequency of biophysical profile scoring, 371, 372t
of middle cerebral artery, 374–375, 375f
of umbilical artery, 175, 372–374, 373f, 374f, 374t
venous studies in, 375–377, 376f, 377f
Fetal echocardiography, 310–317
of atrial septum, 312, 313f
of atrioventricular valves, 308f, 312–313
beating four-chamber view in, 307–308, 308f, 311–314, 312f–314f
of congestive heart failure, 315–316, 316t
general imaging in, 310
of great arteries and ductal and aortic arches, 309, 309f, 314–315, 314f–316f
during heart beating, 308
of heart size, 307–308
of heart structure, 308
of heart symmetry, 308
of hydrops, 310
indications for, 306
of outflow tracts, 309, 309f, 314–315, 314f–316f
screening, 307–309, 308f, 309f
of semilunar valves, 309, 314
sensitivity of, 310
three-dimensional, 307, 309–310, 316–317, 317f–319f
of umbilical cord, 310, 310f
of venous drainage, 311–312, 312f
Fetal echocardiography *(Continued)*
of ventricles, 313, 313f
of ventricular septum, 309, 313–314, 314f
of visceroatrial situs, 307, 310–311, 311f
Fetal electrode, 399
Fetal endoscopic tracheal occlusion (FETO), for congenital diaphragmatic hernia, 443–444
Fetal growth and development, 175–177, 176t
in diabetic pregnancy, 982–984, 985
in multiple gestation, 456–457, 461
with post-term pregnancy, 614
rate of, 636, 636f, 636t, 637f
Fetal head circumference, in intrauterine growth restriction, 643f
Fetal health assessment, 175, 361–389
ancillary test(s) for, 380–383
contraction stress test and oxytocin challenge test as, 381–382, 381f
fetal movement counting as, 383, 383t
vibroacoustic stimulation as, 382–383
biophysical profile score for, 364–369
with Doppler ultrasound abnormalities, 371, 372t
factors that influence, 369, 369t
and fetal pH on cordocentesis, 383–384, 384f
and neurologic outcome, 389, 389f, 389t
outcome prediction using, 364, 365f
and perinatal mortality, 369, 369f, 387–388, 388t
scoring technique for, 366–369, 368t
systematic application of, 366, 368t
variable(s) in, 364, 365–366
amniotic fluid measurement as, 365–366, 365t, 366f
cardiotocogram as, 365t, 366, 367f, 368f
fetal breathing movements as, 365t, 366
fetal movement and tone as, 365t, 366
cordocentesis for, 383–386
biophysical profile score and, 383–384, 384f
complications of, 385–386, 385t, 386f
fetal respiratory status by, 386, 386t
indications for, 383–384, 384t
monitoring after, 385
procedure for, 384–385, 384f, 385f
in diabetic pregnancy, 982, 982t, 983f, 983t
Doppler ultrasound for
application of, 378–379, 379f
fetal, 371–377
and frequency of biophysical profile scoring, 371, 372t
of middle cerebral artery, 374–375, 375f
of umbilical artery, 372–374, 373f, 374f, 374t
venous studies in, 375–377, 376f, 377f
maternal, 377–378, 378f, 379f
patterns of deterioration in, 378–379, 379f, 380f
evaluation of testing for, 388–389, 388t, 389f, 389t
fetal heart rate monitoring for, 369–371, 370t, 371f
Growth Restriction Intervention Trial on, 379, 388, 388t
indications for, 387–388, 387t
integrated testing for, 379–380, 380f, 380t
for intrauterine growth restriction, 644–645
invasive testing for, 383–386
in multiple gestation, 457, 461
normal behavior in, 361–362, 362f
objectives of, 364
and perinatal mortality, 387–388, 388t
Fetal health assessment *(Continued)*
with post-term pregnancy, 615
with preeclampsia, 669, 671
after pregnancy loss, 628–629
principles of monitoring in, 364
recommendations for, 387, 387t
responses to hypoxemia in, 362–364, 363f, 364f
Fetal heart rate (FHR), 172, 173f, 175, 361
accelerations in, 406
average, 397
baseline, 405, 406–407, 407f
cardiotocogram of, 365t, 366, 367f, 368f
decelerations in
early, 406, 411t
late, 406, 408–409, 409f, 410f, 411t
prolonged, 406
variable, 406, 409–410, 410f, 411t
factors controlling, 397–399
"minimal variable," 366, 367f
normal pattern of, 406, 407f
normal variations in, 397
saltatory, 413, 413f
sinusoidal, 410–413, 412f
variability in, 406–408, 408f, 411t
Fetal heart rate (FHR) abnormalities, umbilical cord acid-base balance with, 404, 404t
Fetal heart rate (FHR) monitoring, 369–371, 370t, 371f, 399
with multiple gestation, 462
after trauma, 1185
Fetal heart rate (FHR) patterns, 405–413
accelerations in, 406
baseline features of, 405–406
baseline rate in, 405, 406–407, 407f
bradycardia in, 405, 406, 407f, 411f, 411t
with congenital anomalies, 413
early decelerations in, 406, 411t
episodic changes in, 405
in utero treatment of, 410, 411f, 411t
late decelerations in, 406, 408–409, 409f, 410f, 411t
normal, 406, 407f
periodic patterns in, 405, 407, 408–410, 409f–411f
prolonged decelerations in, 406
quantification in, 406
saltatory, 413, 413f
sinusoidal, 410–413, 412f
tachycardia in, 405, 406–407, 411f
variability in, 406–408, 408f, 411t
variable decelerations in, 406, 409–410, 410f, 411t
Fetal hydantoin syndrome, 352, 1091
Fetal hydrops. *See* Hydrops fetalis.
Fetal inflammatory response syndrome (FIRS), 527, 528f
Fetal karyotyping, after pregnancy loss, 626
Fetal loss. *See* Fetal demise.
Fetal lung development, 193–204, 194t
alveolar stage of, 194f, 194t, 195–196, 195t, 196f
canalicular stage of, 194, 194f, 194t
diabetes and, 967–968, 968f
embryonic stage of, 193, 194f, 194t
fetal breathing movements and, 176–177
fetal lung fluid in, 197
induced maturation in, 202–204, 203f, 203t
pseudoglandular stage of, 193, 194f, 194t
and pulmonary hypoplasia, 196–197, 196t
saccular stage of, 194–195, 194f, 194t, 195f
surfactant in, 197–202
composition of, 197–198, 197f

Fetal lung development (Continued)
metabolism of, 198–200, 199f, 201f
physiologic effects of, 200–202, 201f
for respiratory distress syndrome, 202, 202f
Fetal lung fluid, 197
Fetal lung maturity. *See* Fetal pulmonary maturity.
Fetal lung profile, 419
Fetal malpresentation, 703–707
breech as, 703–706, 705t
compound, 707
deflection abnormalities as, 706–707
transverse lie as, 706
uterine anomalies and, 1144
uterine myomas and, 1137
Fetal methylmercury syndrome, 354
Fetal monitoring, 717. *See also* Fetal health assessment.
for breech presentation, 704–705
electronic, 399
adjuncts to, 414–415
vs. auscultation, 413
with multiple gestation, 462
Fetal movement(s), 172, 173f, 175, 177, 361
in biophysical profile score, 365t, 366
Fetal movement counting (FMC), 383, 383t
in diabetic pregnancy, 983f, 983t
"Fetal origins of disease" hypothesis, 646
Fetal oxygenation, 187–189, 187t, 188f, 189f
oxygen therapy and, 189–190, 189f, 189t, 190f
Fetal pain, during fetoscopy, 435
Fetal posture, in biophysical profile score, 365t, 366
Fetal pulmonary maturity, 419–428
assessment of, 419–423
in diabetic pregnancy, 421, 984–985, 985t
by direct evaluation of amniotic fluid, 419–420
impact of contaminants on, 422, 422t
impact of gestational age on, 420–421, 421f
with multiple gestation, 421, 461
noninvasive, 420
racial and gender differences in, 421
from vaginal fluid specimens, 423
induction of, 202–204
corticosteroids for, 423–428
dosage of, 423, 423t
experimental models of, 203, 203f
maternal consequences of, 426
neonatal outcomes of, 424–425, 424f–426f
NIH Consensus Panel guidelines for, 427t, 428
other fetal and neonatal effects of, 425–426
repeated courses of, 426–428
experimental models of, 203, 203f, 203t
thyrotropin-releasing hormone for, 203–204
thyroxine for, 423–424
with preterm premature rupture of the membranes, 423, 601
Fetal pulse oximetry, 414–415
Fetal respiratory status, by cordocentesis, 386, 386t
Fetal scalp sampling, for idiopathic thrombocytopenic purpura, 839
Fetal size, in diabetic pregnancy, 982–984, 985
Fetal stress, preterm labor due to, 529, 530f
Fetal surveillance
antepartum. *See* Fetal health assessment.
with chronic kidney disease, 912
in diabetic pregnancy, 982, 982t, 983f, 983t
with dialysis, 917
Fetal surveillance (Continued)
intrapartum. *See* Intrapartum fetal surveillance.
with renal transplantation, 920
Fetal swallowing, 49
Fetal therapy, invasive. *See* Invasive fetal therapy.
Fetal tissue, oxygen transport to, 187–189, 187t, 188f, 189f
Fetal tone, in biophysical profile score, 365t, 366
Fetal valvuloplasty, 445, 446t
Fetal warfarin syndrome, 351, 864
Fetal weight
estimation of, in diabetic pregnancy, 982–984, 985
and gestational age, 636, 636f
in intrauterine growth restriction, 642, 643f
Fetal-pelvic index, 695
Fetal-placental cotyledons, 40–41, 44, 44f
Fetal-to-placental ratio, 41
Feticide, selective. *See* Selective termination.
FETO (fetal endoscopic tracheal occlusion), for congenital diaphragmatic hernia, 443–444
Fetomaternal hemorrhage (FMH), 478, 480–481
fetal loss due to, 624
hydrops fetalis due to, 510
due to trauma, 1185, 1185f
Fetoplacental unit, as endocrine organ, 115–119
estrogens in, 115–117, 116f
growth factors as, 117–119, 117t, 118f, 119f
progesterone in, 115
α-Fetoprotein (AFP)
and abruptio placentae, 732
after chorionic villus sampling, 255–256
and endodermal sinus tumor, 1141
prenatal screening for, 223, 224, 224t
for neural tube defects, 233–235, 234t
in twins, 257, 257t, 458, 459
Fetoscopic laser coagulation, for twin-to-twin transfusion syndrome, 437–439, 438f, 439t, 465–466
Fetoscopic tracheal occlusion, for congenital diaphragmatic hernia, 289
Fetoscopy, 435
fetal pain relief during, 435
instrumentation for, 435
risk for pPROM after, 435, 435t
Fetus, oxygen uptake by, 181–187, 182f
Fetus compressus, 64, 64f, 65f
Fetus papyraceus, 64, 64f, 65f
FEV_1 (forced expiratory volume in 1 second)
in asthma, 938, 939–940
in cystic fibrosis, 947
Fever
enigmatic, 764
puerperal, 760–761
FFP (fresh-frozen plasma)
for abruptio placentae, 733t
for hemorrhagic shock, 1181, 1181t
FGFRs (fibroblastic growth factor receptors), in skeletal growth, 297
FGS (focal glomerular sclerosis), 916t
FHH (familial hypocalciuric hypercalcemia), 1034
FHR. *See* Fetal heart rate (FHR).
Fibrin degradation products (FDPs)
in abruptio placentae, 733t
in fibrinolysis, 828, 828f
Fibrin plug formation, 826, 827f
Fibrinogen
in abruptio placentae, 733t
in platelet plug formation, 825
pregnancy effect on, 829
Fibrinoid, of placenta, 43
Fibrinolysis, 828–829, 828f
Fibrinolytic pathway genes, mutations in, 835
Fibroblastic growth factor receptors (FGFRs), in skeletal growth, 297
Fibroepithelial polyps, 1124
Fibroids. *See* Uterine leiomyomas.
Fibromas, soft, 1124
Fibronectin(s)
in decidual/membrane activation, 523
and preterm labor, 560–561, 568
Fick principle, 181, 182f
Fifth disease, 774
FIGO (International Federation of Gynecology and Obstetrics), 888
Filtration capacity, during pregnancy, 106
Filtration coefficient, 50
Filtration fraction, during pregnancy, 106
Fine-needle aspiration biopsy (FNAB), of thyroid nodule, 1008–1009, 1009f
FIRS (fetal inflammatory response syndrome), 527, 528f
First- and Second-Trimester Evaluation of Risk (RASTER) study, 567
FISH (fluorescence in situ hybridization), 12, 13f
in amniocentesis, 249–250
Fish consumption, 147, 147t
Fish oil supplements, 147
for preterm birth prevention, 569, 570t
Fisher's exact test, 213
Flecainide, during pregnancy, 801t
Flow cytometry, 12–13
Fluconazole
for HIV infection, 771
for vulvovaginal candidiasis, 740–741, 740t
Fludrocortisone
for Addison disease, 1027
for septic shock, 1179
Fluid accumulation, fetal, due to nonimmune hydrops, 506–507, 506f, 507f
Fluid deficit, due to burns, 1187
Fluid pocket, in amniotic fluid measurement, 365, 366f
Fluid replacement
for acute renal failure due to preeclampsia, 908
for septic shock, 1176
Fluid resuscitation
for acute pyelonephritis, 755
for diabetic ketoacidosis, 962–963, 962t
for hyperemesis gravidarum, 1043
for septic shock, 763
Flunisolide, for asthma, 941t
Fluorescence in situ hybridization (FISH), 12, 13f
in amniocentesis, 249–250
Fluorescent treponemal antibody absorption (FTA-ABS) test, 779
Fluoxetine (Prozac), dosage of, 1117t
Fluticasone, for asthma, 941t
Fluticasone and salmeterol (Advair), for asthma, 940t
Fluvoxamine (Luvox), dosage of, 1117t
FMC (fetal movement counting), 383, 383t
in diabetic pregnancy, 983f, 983t
FMH. *See* Fetomaternal hemorrhage (FMH).
FMR1 gene, 30
FMR-1 (fragile X mental retardation 1) protein, 245–246
FNAB (fine-needle aspiration biopsy), of thyroid nodule, 1008–1009, 1009f
Foam Stability Index (FSI), 420
Focal glomerular sclerosis (FGS), 916t
Focal periventricular necrosis, 1212

Folate
 in anemia, 870, 870t
 in pregnancy, 871–872
Folate deficiency
 and fetal loss, 620
 megaloblastic anemia due to, 874
Folate supplementation, 143, 146t, 871–872
 with multiple gestation, 461
Foley catheter, for cervical ripening, 703t
Follicle-stimulating hormone (FSH), in pregnancy, 114f
Folliculitis of pregnancy, 1125t, 1126–1127, 1127f
Follistatin, during pregnancy, 120
Fondaparinux, for type 2 heparin-induced thrombocytopenia, 863–864
Food and Drug Administration (FDA), teratogenic risk assessments of, 350, 350t, 351
Food-borne infections, 147
Foramen ovale, 160
 premature closure of, hydrops fetalis due to, 508–509
 restricted, in hypoplastic left heart syndrome, 329, 329f
Forced expiratory volume in 1 second (FEV_1)
 in asthma, 938, 939–940
 in cystic fibrosis, 947
Forceps delivery, 713–714
 for breech presentation, 705
Formoterol, for asthma, 941
Formula feeding, and developmental origins of health and disease, 153, 155
Fortovase (saquinavir), for HIV infection, 772t
Fosphenytoin sodium, for status epilepticus, 1090
Fox-Fordyce disease, 1132
Fractures, pelvic, 1185–1186
Fragile X mental retardation 1 (FMR-1) protein, 245–246
Fragile X syndrome, 5, 30
 carrier screening for, 245–246, 246t
 prenatal diagnosis of, 248t
Fragile X–associated tremor/ataxia syndrome (FXTAS), 245
Fragmin in Pregnant Women with a History of Uteroplacental Insufficiency and Thrombophilia (FRUIT) study, 628
Frank-Starling mechanism, 398–399
FRDA (frataxin) gene, 29
Free erythrocyte protoporphyrin (FEP), 870, 872
Free fatty acids, during pregnancy, 120t
Free fetal DNA, prenatal diagnosis using, 261–262
Free thyroxine index, 999
Fresh whole blood, for abruptio placentae, 733t
Fresh-frozen plasma (FFP)
 for abruptio placentae, 733t
 for hemorrhagic shock, 1181, 1181t
Friedreich ataxia, 29–30
Fructosamine screening, for gestational diabetes mellitus, 972
Fruit(s), in diet, 147
FRUIT (Fragmin in Pregnant Women with a History of Uteroplacental Insufficiency and Thrombophilia) study, 628
FSH (follicle-stimulating hormone), in pregnancy, 114f
FSI (Foam Stability Index), 420
FTA-ABS (fluorescent treponemal antibody absorption) test, 779
Functional residual capacity, during pregnancy, 104, 105t, 1173
Fundal implantation, of placenta, 699
Funipuncture. *See* Cordocentesis.
Furosemide
 for acute renal failure due to preeclampsia, 908
 for hypercalcemia, 1034, 1034t
Fusion inhibitor, for HIV infection, 772t
Fuzeon (enfuvirtide), for HIV infection, 772t
FVL mutation. *See* Factor V Leiden (FVL) mutation.
FXTAS (fragile X–associated tremor/ataxia syndrome), 245

G

G bands, 12, 12f, 13f
G_1 phase, 7, 7f
G_2 phase, 7, 7f
G6PD (glucose-6-phosphate dehydrogenase) deficiency, 875
 hydrops fetalis due to, 510
Galactocele, 138
Gallbladder disease, 1073, 1073t
Gallstones, 1073
Gap junctions
 between myometrial cells, 79f
 in myometrial contractions, 522
Gardnerella vaginalis vaginitis. *See* Bacterial vaginosis (BV).
Gastric banding, 1051, 1051t
Gastric bypass, 1051, 1051t
Gastric emptying, in pregnancy, 1041
Gastroesophageal reflux disease (GERD), 1043–1045
 asthma exacerbated by, 942
 diagnosis of, 1043–1044, 1044f
 epidemiology of, 1043
 management of, 1044–1045, 1044t, 1045t
 in newborn period, 1209
 pathogenesis of, 1043
Gastrointestinal causes, of hydrops fetalis, 508t, 512
Gastrointestinal complications, of prematurity, 1199t
Gastrointestinal disease, 1041–1053
 appendicitis as, 1046–1047, 1047t
 celiac disease as, 1050–1051
 constipation as, 1052, 1052t
 gastroesophageal reflux disease as, 1043–1045, 1044f, 1044t, 1045f
 hemorrhoids as, 1052–1053
 hyperemesis gravidarum as, 1042–1043
 inflammatory bowel disease as, 1047–1049, 1048f, 1048t, 1049f, 1049t
 irritable bowel syndrome as, 1049–1050, 1050t
 nausea and vomiting as, 1041–1042, 1042t
 peptic ulcer disease as, 1045–1046, 1045f
Gastrointestinal endoscopy, 1053, 1053t
Gastrointestinal function, in pregnancy, 1041
Gastrointestinal manifestations, of cystic fibrosis, 946
Gastrointestinal problem(s) in neonatal period, 1207–1210
 feeding problems as, 1209–1210
 hyperbilirubinemia as, 1208–1209, 1209t
 necrotizing enterocolitis as, 1207–1208, 1208f
Gastrointestinal tract anomalies, 290–293, 290f–293f
Gastroschisis, 293–294, 294f
 feeding problems due to, 1209–1210
Gaucher disease
 carrier screening for, 242, 242t
 hydrops fetalis due to, 511
GBS infection. *See* Group B *Streptococcus* (GBS) infection.
GCT (glucose challenge test), 971–972, 972t
GDM. *See* Gestational diabetes mellitus (GDM).
Gel electrophoresis, 32
Gender detection, prenatal, 262
Gender differences
 in fetal pulmonary maturity, 421
 in meiosis, 9–10, 10f, 11f
Gene(s), 3–6, 4f–6f, 6t
 chemical nature of, 3–5, 4f
 defined, 3
 in information transfer, 5, 5f
 mutations of, 5–6, 6f, 6t
Gene expression, quality control in, 5, 5f
Gene function, biochemistry of, 5, 5f
Gene-environment interaction, in preterm labor and birth, 527, 553
General anesthesia, for cesarean delivery, 712–713
Genetic abnormalities, fetal loss due to, 619–620, 623
Genetic association, 33–34
Genetic code, 5, 5f
Genetic evaluation, of stillbirth, 263
Genetic factors, in intrauterine growth restriction, 637–638
Genetic influences, on timing of labor, 70
Genetic predisposition, to preterm birth, 553
Genetic screening, preimplantation, 259–261
Genetic susceptibility, to teratogens, 348
Genetic testing, 30–34, 30f–32f
Genetics, 3–34
 chromosomes in, 6–22
  abnormalities of, 14–18
   in abortuses and stillbirths, 21, 21t, 22t
   in number, 14–15, 15f
   prevalence of, 20–21, 21t
   with sex chromosomes, 19–20, 20t
   in structure, 15–18, 16f–19f, 16t
  analysis of, 10–14, 12f–14f
   indications for, 21–22
  in cell cycle, 7, 7f
  in meiosis, 8–10, 8f–11f
  in mitosis, 7–8, 7f
  sex, 7, 19
   abnormalities of, 19–20, 20t
 dynamic mutations and trinucleotide repeats in, 29–30
 genes in, 3–6, 4f–6f, 6t
 genetic testing and DNA diagnostics in, 30–34, 30f–32f
 Human Genome Project and genomics in, 34
 impact on medicine of, 3
 imprinting in, 30
 online resources for, 6t
 patterns of inheritance in, 22–29
  autosomal dominant, 23–24, 24f
  autosomal recessive, 24, 24f
  Mendel's laws for, 22–23, 23f
  mitochondrial, 29
  multifactorial, 25–29, 27t, 28t
  sex-linked, 24–25, 25f
  symbols for, 23, 23f
 of preeclampsia, 667
Genital herpes, 769–770
Genital tract infections
 and premature rupture of the membranes, 599
 and preterm labor and birth, 556, 568
Genital warts, 748, 749, 750
Genitalia, ambiguous, 1198t
Genitourinary tract anomalies, 294–297, 295f–297f
Genodermatoses, 1132
Genome-wide association studies (GWAS), 26
Genomic imprinting, 30
Genotypes, 9

Gentamicin
  for acute pyelonephritis, 756, 756t, 906
  for listeriosis, 773
  for pelvic abscess, 762
  for puerperal endometritis, 760, 761
  for septic shock, 763
Geodon (ziprasidone), dosage of, 1116t
Gerbich antigen, 495t
GERD. *See* Gastroesophageal reflux disease (GERD).
Germ cell cancers, 885, 1141
German measles. *See* Rubella.
Gestational age
  birth weight and, 636, 636t
  blood pressure and, 652, 653f
  determination of, 546
  and fetal demise, 1201f
  and fetal pulmonary maturity, 420–421, 421f
  fetal weight and, 636, 636f
  last menstrual period (LMP) and, 613
  and survival and morbidity with preterm birth, 549, 550f
Gestational diabetes mellitus (GDM), 955
  defined, 955
  developmental effect of, 152–153
  diagnosis of, 971–973, 971t–973t
  epidemiology of, 955
  glyburide for, 981
  insulin for, 979–980
  maternal-fetal metabolism in, 956–958, 957f
  pathophysiology of, 955
  risk factor screening for, 971, 971t, 973, 973t
Gestational hypertension, 652
  excessive weight gain and, 145
  maternal obesity and, 144
Gestational thrombocytopenia, 838
Gestational timing, of teratogenic exposure, 348
Gestational transient thyrotoxicosis (GTT), 1004
Gestational trophoblastic disease, hyperthyroidism due to, 1005
Gestational trophoblastic neoplasia (GTN), 891
GFBMs (gross fetal body movements), 172, 173f, 175, 177
GFR (glomerular filtration rate)
  in preeclampsia, 663–664
  during pregnancy, 105–106, 910
GGT (γ-glutamyl transferase), in pregnancy, 1059, 1060t
GH (growth hormone)
  excessive secretion of, 1020–1021
  placental, 1020–1021
  during pregnancy, 1016
GHRH (growth hormone–releasing hormone), in neurohormonal control, 1015
Giemsa banding, 12, 12f, 13f
Gigantomastia, 128–129
Gilbert syndrome, jaundice due to, 1060t
Ginger, for nausea and vomiting, 1042, 1042t
Gingivitis, 1124
GISP (Gonococcal Isolate Surveillance Project), 745
Glanzmann thrombasthenia, 825, 844t–846t, 847
Gliadin, in celiac disease, 1050
Glomerular capillary endotheliosis, in preeclampsia, 659, 659f
Glomerular filtration rate (GFR)
  in preeclampsia, 663–664
  during pregnancy, 105–106, 910
Glomerular functional changes, in preeclampsia, 663–664
Glomerular pathology, in preeclampsia, 659, 659f
Glomeruloendotheliosis, in preeclampsia, 653t
Glomerulonephritis
  acute and chronic, 912
  in preeclampsia, 653t
Glucagon, during pregnancy, 120t
Glucocorticoids
  developmental effects of, 153–154
  and fetal lung development, 196, 196f, 203, 203f
  for hemolytic disease of the fetus and newborn, 494
  for 21-hydroxylase deficiency, 1028–1029, 1029f
  for idiopathic thrombocytopenic purpura, 838
  for induction of fetal pulmonary maturity, 423–428
    dosage of, 423, 423t
    experimental models of, 203, 203f
    maternal consequences of, 426
    mechanism of action of, 423
    neonatal outcomes of, 424–425, 424f–426f
    NIH Consensus Panel guidelines for, 427t, 428
    other fetal and neonatal effects of, 425–426
    repeated courses of, 426–428
  long term therapy with, 1030
  for neonatal alloimmune thrombocytopenia, 841–842
  pathways of synthesis of, 1025, 1025f
  for preterm labor, 561
Glucokinase mutation, 955
Glucose
  blood
    during pregnancy, 975–976, 975f, 976f, 976t
    self-monitoring of, 974–976, 975t
  for diabetic ketoacidosis, 962t
  fasting
    in diabetes, 955, 955t, 975
    impaired, 955, 971
    in pregnancy, 975, 975t, 976t
  and intrauterine growth restriction, 639
  maternal concentrations of, and fetal obesity, 964
  plasma, in diabetes, 955t
  during pregnancy, 120t
Glucose challenge test (GCT), 971–972, 972t
Glucose excretion, during pregnancy, 106
Glucose homeostasis, in pregnancy, 956, 956f, 957f
Glucose metabolism, in normal and diabetic pregnancy, 955–958, 956f, 957f
Glucose monitoring, 974–976
  pregestational, 970
  target levels in, 975–976, 975f, 976f, 976t
  timing of, 974–975, 975t
Glucose production, in normal and diabetic pregnancy, 956, 956f
Glucose tolerance
  impaired, 955, 971
  in pregnancy, 956, 956f, 957f
Glucose tolerance test
  for acromegaly, 1020
  oral, 955, 955t, 971, 971t, 972, 972t
Glucose-6-phosphate dehydrogenase (G6PD) deficiency, 875
  hydrops fetalis due to, 510
α-Glucosidase inhibitors, for diabetes, 982
γ-Glutamyl transferase (GGT), in pregnancy, 1059, 1060t
Gluten-sensitive enteropathy, 28, 1050–1051
Glyburide, for diabetes, 980–981, 982
Glycemic control, for septic shock, 1178
Glycemic index, 974
Glycemic management, intrapartum, 985–986, 985t
Glycerin, for constipation, 1052t
Glyceryl trinitrate (GTN), for preterm labor, 564–565
Glycogen storage disease type IA, carrier screening for, 242t
Glycohemoglobin, 974
Glycosylated hemoglobin, 974
GnRH (gonadotropin-releasing hormone), in neurohormonal control, 1015
Goiter
  fetal, 1006, 1008
  maternal, 996–997, 1005, 1006
    due to Hashimoto thyroiditis, 1007
  neonatal, 1004f
Gonadal function, radioiodine and, 1001
Gonadotropin(s), during pregnancy, 1015
Gonadotropin-releasing hormone (GnRH), in neurohormonal control, 1015
Gonococcal infections
  disseminated, 744, 746
  in newborn period, 1219–1220
Gonococcal Isolate Surveillance Project (GISP), 745
Gonococcal ophthalmia, neonatal, 744, 1219
Gonocytes, 9
Gonorrhea, 742–746
  anogenital, 744
  breastfeeding with, 136t
  chlamydial infection with, 745, 746
  clinical manifestations of, 744
  diagnosis of, 744–745
  epidemiology of, 742–743, 743f
  pathogenesis of, 743–744
  pharyngeal, 744
  prevention of, 746
  treatment of, 745–746, 745t
Graduated elastic compression stockings, for prevention of venous thromboembolism, 864
Granulocyte(s), during pregnancy, 90
Granulocyte colony-stimulating factor, for septic shock, 763
Granuloma, pyogenic, 1124
Granulomatosis, Wegener, renal dysfunction in, 914
Granulosa cell tumors, 886
Graves disease
  maternal
    neonatal outcomes with, 1198
    postpartum, 1009
    in pregnancy, 1001–1002, 1003, 1004f
  neonatal, 1004f
Gray platelet syndrome, 846, 846t
Great arteries
  fetal echocardiography of, 309, 309f, 314–315, 314f–316f
  transposition of, 333–334, 333f, 334f
    tricuspid atresia with, 327
Great vessel defects, nuchal translucency and, 237, 237t
Gregg, Norman, 347
GRIT (Growth Restriction Intervention Trial), 379, 388, 388t, 645
Gross fetal body movements (GFBMs), 172, 173f, 175, 177
Group A β-hemolytic *Streptococcus,* 766
Group A *Streptococcus* infection, breastfeeding with, 135, 137t
Group B *Streptococcus* (GBS) infection, 766–769
  breastfeeding with, 135, 136t
  clinical manifestations of
    in mother, 767
    in neonate, 766–767, 766t
  diagnosis of, 767

Group B *Streptococcus* (GBS) infection *(Continued)*
epidemiology of, 766
in neonatal period, 1217
clinical manifestations of, 766–767, 766t
and premature rupture of the membranes, 599, 606
and preterm labor, 561
prevention of, 767–769, 768f
treatment of, 767
Growth and development
fetal, 175–177, 176t
in diabetic pregnancy, 982–984, 985
in multiple gestation, 456–457, 461
with post-term pregnancy, 614
rate of, 636, 636f, 636t, 637f
with post-term pregnancy, 616–617
Growth factors
and fetal obesity, 965
in implantation, 113, 113t
placenta and, 117–119, 117t, 118f, 119f
Growth hormone (GH)
excessive secretion of, 1020–1021
placental, 1020–1021
during pregnancy, 1016
Growth hormone–releasing hormone (GHRH), in neurohormonal control, 1015
Growth Restriction Intervention Trial (GRIT), 379, 388, 388t, 645
GTN (gestational trophoblastic neoplasia), 891
GTN (glyceryl trinitrate), for preterm labor, 564–565
GTT (gestational transient thyrotoxicosis), 1004
Guillain-Barré syndrome, 1107–1108
Gummas, 778
Gunshot wounds, 1186
GWAS (genome-wide association studies), 26
Gynecoid pelvis, labor with, 693
Gynecologic cancers, 885–889, 886t

H

H_2 (histamine type 2) receptor antagonists
for GERD, 1044, 1044t, 1045f
for peptic ulcer disease, 1046
H_2CO_3 (carbonic acid), in fetal acid-base balance, 400
HAART (highly active antiretroviral therapy), for HIV infection, 771–772
Haemophilus influenzae, pneumonia due to, 930
Haemophilus vaginalis vaginitis. *See* Bacterial vaginosis (BV).
Hair changes, in pregnancy, 1124
Hair growth cycle, 1124
Hamartoma, lymphatic, 289–290, 289f
Hantavirus, breastfeeding with, 135
Haploid number, 8, 9
Haploinsufficiency, 25
Haptoglobin, serum, 869, 870t
Harlequin fetus, 1132
Hartman sign, 37
Hashimoto thyroiditis, 1007
HAV (hepatitis A virus), 785, 787t, 1065–1066, 1065t
breastfeeding with, 135, 136t
Havrix (hepatitis A vaccine), 785
Hb. *See* Hemoglobin (Hb) *entries.*
HBIG (hepatitis B immune globulin), 786, 1066t, 1067, 1218
HBsAg (hepatitis B surface antigen), in newborn period, 1218
HBV. *See* Hepatitis B virus (HBV).
hCG. *See* Human chorionic gonadotropin (hCG).
hCGH (high-resolution comparative genomic hybridization), 14
HCO_3^-. *See* Bicarbonate (HCO_3^-).
hCS (human chorionic somatomammotropin), in pregnancy, 118–119, 118f, 120f
Hct (hematocrit)
in anemia, 871, 871f
during pregnancy, 101
HCV. *See* Hepatitis C virus (HCV).
HDFN. *See* Hemolytic disease of the fetus and newborn (HDFN).
HDN (hemolytic disease of the newborn). *See* Hemolytic disease of the fetus and newborn (HDFN).
HDV (hepatitis D virus), 786, 787t, 1065t, 1068
Head circumference, fetal, in intrauterine growth restriction, 642, 643f
Head compression, fetal heart rate with, 411t
Headache, 1092–1093
Health and disease, developmental origins of, 151–156
animal models of, 154
antenatal glucocorticoids in, 153–154
breastfeeding in, 153
childhood growth in, 153
for diabetes, 152–156
interventions based on, 154–155
low birth weight in, 151–152, 152f
and maternal body composition, 154–155
maternal weight in, 152–154, 155
mechanistic insights into, 154
and neonatal feeding regimens, 155
and nutrient supplementation, 154
thrifty phenotype hypothesis in, 155
Hearing loss, after intrauterine transfusion, 493
Heart
anatomic changes in
postpartum, 104
during pregnancy, 101
development of, 279
Heart block, complete, 338, 338f
bradycardia due to, 408f
Heart defects, congenital. *See* Congenital heart disease (CHD).
Heart disease
congenital. *See* Congenital heart disease (CHD).
maternal, 797–821
anesthesia with, 1152–1160
aortic regurgitation as, 813–814
aortic stenosis as, 805–806, 806f, 813, 813f
anesthesia with, 1155
arrhythmia as, 818
cardiomyopathy as, 814–816, 815f
congenital, 800–810
aortic stenosis as, 805–806, 806f
atrial septal defects as, 800–802, 802f
atrioventricular block as, 810
coarctation of the aorta as, 808–809
Ebstein anomaly as, 810, 810f
Eisenmenger syndrome as, 804–805, 804f
left-to-right shunt as, 800–804, 802f–804f
mitral stenosis as, 805
obstructive, 805–809, 806f–809f
patent ductus arteriosus as, 803–804, 804f
primary pulmonary hypertension as, 805
pulmonic stenosis as, 806–807, 806f, 807f
tetralogy of Fallot as, 807–808, 807f–809f
ventricular septal defect as, 802–803, 803f
coronary artery disease as, 816–817
anesthesia with, 1158–1159
diagnosis of, 797
Heart disease *(Continued)*
drug-induced valvular, 814
general guidelines for management of, 799–800, 800t, 801t
heart failure as, 817
in Marfan syndrome, 818, 818f, 819f
mitral regurgitation as, 812, 812f, 813
anesthesia with, 1155–1156
mitral stenosis as, 805, 811–812, 811f
anesthesia with, 1154–1155
mitral valve prolapse as, 812, 812f
anesthesia with, 1156
pre-conception counseling for, 797–799, 798t
prophylactic antibiotics with, 821
rheumatic, 810–812, 811f
Heart failure, maternal, 817
Heart murmurs, during pregnancy, 104
Heart rate
fetal, 172, 173f, 175
nonpregnant, 1171t
during pregnancy, 102, 102f, 103t, 1171t
with multiple gestation, 455
Heart sounds, during pregnancy, 104
Heart surgery, during pregnancy, 820–821
Heart transplantation, pregnancy after, 817
Heart valves, artificial, pregnancy with, 819–820, 820t, 864
Heartburn, 1043
Helicobacter pylori, 1044t, 1045, 1045f, 1046
HELLP syndrome, 653
anemia in, 872
diabetes in, 961
differential diagnosis of, 843, 843t
liver disease in, 1062, 1063
Hemabate (prostaglandin 15-methyl $F_{2\alpha}$), for uterine atony, 1183t
Hematocrit (Hct)
in anemia, 871, 871f
during pregnancy, 101
Hematologic causes, of hydrops fetalis, 508t, 510
Hematologic complications, of prematurity, 1199t
Hematologic events, in pregnancy, 799, 870–872, 871f, 871t
Hematologic malignancies, during pregnancy, 896–899, 897t
Hematoma(s)
after cordocentesis, 386, 386f
postcesarean wound, 709
Hemodialysis, 915–917, 916t
for diabetic nephropathy, 960
Hemodilution, acute normovolemic, 1182
Hemodynamic assessment, noninvasive, 1173, 1173t
Hemodynamic monitoring, invasive central, 1168–1173
for anaphylactoid syndrome of pregnancy, 1171–1172
for aortic stenosis, 1171
background and insertion technique for, 1168–1169
complications of, 1169–1170, 1169t
hemodynamic considerations in, 1170, 1170t, 1171t
for hypertensive disorders of pregnancy, 1172, 1172f
indications for, 1169
for mitral valve stenosis, 1170–1171
and pulmonary capillary wedge pressure, 1170, 1170f
for pulmonary hypertension, 1171
for septic shock, 1172–1173
Hemodynamic parameters, 1170, 1171t
Hemodynamic variables, 1170, 1170t

Hemodynamics
of anaphylactoid syndrome of pregnancy, 1171–1172
antepartum, 103, 103t
of aortic stenosis, 1171
of hypertensive disorders of pregnancy, 1172, 1172f
intrapartum, 104
of mitral valve stenosis, 1170–1171
postpartum, 104
of pulmonary hypertension, 1171
of septic shock, 1172–1173
Hemoglobin (Hb), glycosylated, 974
Hemoglobin A_{1c} (Hb A_{1c}), with diabetes, 970, 971, 972, 974
Hemoglobin C (Hb C), carrier screening for, 243
Hemoglobin C (Hb C) disease, 878t, 881
Hemoglobin C (Hb C) trait, 878t, 881
Hemoglobin (Hb) concentration, and stillbirth, 623
Hemoglobin D (Hb D), carrier screening for, 243
Hemoglobin E (Hb E), carrier screening for, 243
Hemoglobin E (Hb E) disease, 881, 881t
Hemoglobin (Hb) electrophoresis, 243, 870t
Hemoglobin H (Hb H) disease, 245, 877, 877f, 878t
Hemoglobin (Hb) level
in anemia, 869, 870t
normal, 869
Hemoglobin (Hb) oxygen saturation, fetal, 160, 161, 161f
Hemoglobin S (Hb S), carrier screening for, 243
Hemoglobin S (Hb S)–β thalassemia, 878t, 881
Hemoglobin S (Hb S)–high F, 878t
Hemoglobin sickle C (Hb SC) disease, 878t, 880–881
Hemoglobinopathies, 877–881
carrier screening for, 238t, 243–245, 244t
prenatal diagnosis of, 248t
structural, 878–881, 878t, 880t, 881t
thalassemia syndromes as, 877–878, 877f, 878t, 879f
Hemoglobinuria, paroxysmal nocturnal, 876–877
Hemolysis, jaundice due to, 1060t
Hemolytic anemia, autoimmune, 874–875
Hemolytic disease of the fetus and newborn (HDFN), 477–499
clinical management of, 486–495
chemotherapeutic agents for, 494–495
in first affected pregnancy, 486–488, 487f
intrauterine transfusion for, 488–493
access site for, 488
adjunctive measures with, 491
amount of, 490, 490t
method of, 488–490, 490f
outcome of, 492–493
with severely anemic early-second-trimester fetus, 491
source of red blood cells in, 491–492
timing of, 492
intravenous immune globulin for, 493–494
nasal tolerance for, 495
oral tolerance for, 494
plasmapheresis for, 493, 494
with previously affected fetus or infant, 488, 489f
sensitization to paternal leukocyte antigens for, 495
diagnosis of, 481–483
fetal blood typing through genetics for, 481–483, 482f–484f, 482t
in vitro tests for, 481
maternal antibody determination for, 481
Hemolytic disease of the fetus and newborn (HDFN) *(Continued)*
genetics of, 479, 479f
historical perspectives on, 477
incidence of, 478, 478f
monitoring of, 483–486
amniocentesis for, 483–484, 484f
fetal blood sampling for, 484
ultrasound for, 484–486, 484f, 485f
due to non-RhD antibodies, 495–499, 495t, 497t
pathophysiology of, 478–479
prevention of, 479–481
terminology for, 477
Hemolytic disease of the newborn (HDN). *See* Hemolytic disease of the fetus and newborn (HDFN).
Hemolytic uremic syndrome (HUS), 842–843, 843t
acute renal failure due to, 908
Hemophilia A, 24, 844t–846t, 847
prenatal diagnosis of, 248t
Hemophilia B, 844t–846t, 847
Hemorrhage. *See also* Bleeding.
antepartum, 725–734
due to abruptio placentae, 730f, 731–734, 733t
epidemiology of, 725
due to placenta accreta, 728–728, 728f
due to placenta previa, 725–729, 726f, 726t, 727t, 728f
due to vasa previa, 729–730, 730f
fetomaternal, 478, 480–481
fetal loss due to, 624
hydrops fetalis due to, 510
due to trauma, 1185, 1185f
intracranial (subarachnoid)
fetal
due to idiopathic thrombocytopenic purpura, 839
due to neonatal alloimmune thrombocytopenia, 840, 841–842
maternal, 1096–1098, 1097f, 1098f
anesthesia with, 1150
intraventricular, 1211–1212
prematurity and, 1201t
obstetric, 1179–1184
clinical staging of, 1180, 1180t
defined, 1179–1180
incidence and etiology of, 1179–1180
management of, 1180–1184
additional supportive measures in, 1182
hemostasis in, 1182–1184, 1183t, 1184f
volume replacement in, 1180–1182, 1180t–1182t
protocol for, 727, 727t
postpartum, 698–699
uterine myomas and, 1137
Hemorrhagic fevers, breastfeeding with, 135
Hemorrhagic shock, 1179–1184
clinical staging of, 1180, 1180t
incidence and etiology of, 1179–1180
management of, 1180–1184
additional supportive measures in, 1182
hemostasis in, 1182–1184, 1183t, 1184f
volume replacement in, 1180–1182, 1180t–1182t
Hemorrhoids, 1052–1053
Hemostasis, for hemorrhagic shock, 1182–1184, 1183t, 1184f
Hemostatic system, 825–829
anticoagulant system in, 826–828, 828f
disorders of. *See* Coagulation disorder(s).
effect of pregnancy on, 829
fibrin plug formation in, 826, 827f
fibrinolysis in, 828–829, 828f
platelet plug formation in, 825–826, 826f
Heparin
for antiphospholipid antibody syndrome, 830–831, 1084, 1084t
for preeclampsia, 674
during pregnancy, 801t
with prosthetic heart valves, 819, 820, 820t
for recurrent pregnancy loss due to inherited thrombophilia, 628
for rheumatic disease, 1082t
for septic pelvic vein thrombophlebitis, 764
for venous thromboembolism, 862–863, 862t
prevention of, 836
Heparin-induced thrombocytopenia (HIT), 863–864
Hepatic complications, of prematurity, 1199t
Hepatic encephalopathy, 1071
Hepatic length, in Rh-immunized pregnancy, 485
Hepatic lesions, in preeclampsia, 658, 658f
Hepatic masses, fetal, 293, 293f
Hepatic rupture, 1064
Hepatic venous return, fetal, 159–160, 159f
Hepatitis, 785–786, 787t
autoimmune, 1069
breastfeeding with, 135–137, 136t
chronic nonviral, 1069
viral, 1064–1069, 1065t, 1066t, 1068t
Hepatitis A vaccine (Vaqta, Havrix), 785
Hepatitis A virus (HAV), 785, 787t, 1065–1066, 1065t
breastfeeding with, 135, 136t
Hepatitis B immune globulin (HBIG), 786, 1066t, 1067, 1218
Hepatitis B surface antigen (HBsAg), in newborn period, 1218
Hepatitis B vaccination, 1066t, 1067, 1218
Hepatitis B virus (HBV), 786, 787t, 1065t, 1066–1067
acute, 1066
breastfeeding with, 135, 136t
chronic carrier state of, 1066
coinfection with hepatitis D virus, 1068
diagnosis of, 1065t, 1066
epidemiology of, 1066
medical personnel concerns with, 1067
in newborn period, 1218
perinatal aspects of, 1066–1067
prevention and treatment of, 1067
transfusion-related, 1182t
Hepatitis C virus (HCV), 786, 787t, 1065t, 1067–1068
breastfeeding with, 135–137, 136t
chronic, 1068t
active, 1068t
diagnosis of, 1067–1068, 1068t
epidemiology of, 1067
and intrahepatic cholestasis of pregnancy, 1061
pregnancy concerns with, 1068
pregnancy management with, 1068
transfusion-related, 1182t
transmission of, 1067
Hepatitis D virus (HDV, delta infection), 786, 787t, 1065t, 1068
Hepatitis E virus (HEV), 786, 787t, 1065t, 1068–1069
Hepatitis G virus (HGV), 786, 787t, 1069
Hepatocanalicular injury, jaundice due to, 1060t
Hepatocellular carcinoma, jaundice due to, 1060t

Hepatomegaly
fetal, 293
maternal, 1059
Hereditary elliptocytosis, 874
Hereditary nephritis, 912
Hereditary spherocytosis, 874
Heritability, 25, 26
Hermansky-Pudiak syndrome, 846, 846t, 847
Hernia, congenital diaphragmatic. *See* Congenital diaphragmatic hernia (CDH).
Herpes gestationis, 1125t, 1127–1129, 1128f, 1129f
Herpes simplex virus (HSV), 769–770
breastfeeding with, 136t
hepatitis due to, 1069
in neonate, 1101, 1218
after premature rupture of the membranes, 607
Herpes zoster, 783–784
Hespan (hydroxymethyl starch), for hemorrhagic shock, 1180t, 1181
Hetastarch (hydroxymethyl starch), for hemorrhagic shock, 1180t, 1181
Heteroplasmy, 29
Heteroploidy, 14
HEV (hepatitis E virus), 786, 787t, 1065t, 1068–1069
Hexosaminidase A deficiency, carrier screening for, 238t, 240–241, 241t
Hextend (hydroxymethyl starch), for hemorrhagic shock, 1180t, 1181
HGV (hepatitis G virus), 786, 787t, 1069
Hiccups, fetal, 361, 366
HIFs (hypoxia-inducing factors), in preeclampsia, 665
HIG (hyperimmune globulin), for cytomegalovirus, 624, 765
Highly active antiretroviral therapy (HAART), for HIV infection, 771–772
High-resolution comparative genomic hybridization (hCGH), 14
Hirschsprung disease, 28
Hirsutism, 1031–1032, 1031t, 1124
Histamine type 2 (H_2) receptor antagonists
for GERD, 1044, 1044t, 1045f
for peptic ulcer disease, 1046
Histones, 7
HIT (heparin-induced thrombocytopenia), 863–864
HIV. *See* Human immunodeficiency virus (HIV).
Hivid (zalcitabine), for HIV infection, 772t
HLA. *See* Human leukocyte antigen (HLA).
HLHS (hypoplastic left heart syndrome), 328–330, 329f
invasive fetal therapy for, 445
HOCM (hypertrophic obstructive cardiomyopathy), anesthesia with, 1159
Hodgkin lymphoma (HL), in pregnancy, 896–898, 897t
Hofbauer cells, 41, 43
Holoprosencephaly, 282–283, 283f
and aneuploidy, 227t
Homan sign, 856
Homeobox *(HOX)* genes, in skeletal growth, 297
Homoplasmy, 29
Hormonal adaptations, to multiple gestation, 455
Hormonal contraceptives, with breastfeeding, 134–135
Hormonal control
of labor, 70–76
cascade of events in, 70–72, 71f
estrogens in, 74
fetal hypothalamic-pituitary-adrenal axis in, 72–73
Hormonal control *(Continued)*
oxytocin in, 75–76
progesterone in, 73–74
prostaglandins in, 74–75, 75f
of myometrial contractions, 79–81, 79f, 80t
Hormonal disorders, preterm labor due to, 531–532
Hormonal regulation, of fetal heart rate, 398
Hormones, maternal and fetal, and intrauterine growth restriction, 641
HOX (homeobox) genes, in skeletal growth, 297
HPA(s) (human platelet antigens), in neonatal alloimmune thrombocytopenia, 840, 840t
HPA (hypothalamic-pituitary-adrenal) axis, of fetus, in control of labor, 72–73
HPV (human papillomavirus), 748–750, 749f
and cervical intraepithelial neoplasia, 887
11β-HSD (11β-hydroxysteroid dehydrogenase), in control of labor, 72–73
3β-HSD (3β-hydroxysteroid dehydrogenase) deficiency, 1030
HSV. *See* Herpes simplex virus (HSV).
HTLV-I (human T-cell leukemia virus type I), breastfeeding with, 136t, 138
Humalog (insulin lispro), 977f, 977t, 978, 979
Human chorionic gonadotropin (hCG)
and abruptio placentae, 732
and choriocarcinoma, 1141
and gestational trophoblastic neoplasia, 891
hyperthyroidism related to, 1004–1005
and maternal thyroid physiology, 996, 997f
and nausea and vomiting, 1042
in pregnancy, 113–114, 114f
prenatal screening for, 223, 224, 229–230
in twins, 257, 257t, 458, 459
Human chorionic somatomammotropin (hCS), in pregnancy, 118–119, 118f, 120f
Human Genome Project, 3, 34
Human immunodeficiency virus (HIV), 770–773
acute phase of, 771
breastfeeding with, 136t, 137–138
diagnosis of, 771
epidemiology of, 770–771
fetal blood sampling with, 386
latent phase of, 771
liver disease with, 1069
myocarditis or cardiomyopathy with, 816
in newborn period, 1218–1219
pathogenesis of, 771
perinatal transmission of, 771, 1101
pneumonia with, 771, 929–930, 933–934, 934f
symptomatic phase of, 771
transfusion-related, 1182t
treatment of, 771–773, 772t, 1101
Human immunodeficiency virus (HIV)-associated nephropathy, 915
Human leukocyte antigen (HLA)
lack of expression of, 89–90
sensitization to paternal, for hemolytic disease of the fetus and newborn, 495
Human leukocyte antigen C (HLA-C), in preeclampsia, 661
Human leukocyte antigen G (HLA-G), and early pregnancy loss, 619
Human papillomavirus (HPV), 748–750, 749f
and cervical intraepithelial neoplasia, 887
Human placental growth hormone, in pregnancy, 119
Human platelet antigens (HPAs), in neonatal alloimmune thrombocytopenia, 840, 840t
Human T-cell leukemia virus type I (HTLV-I), breastfeeding with, 136t, 138
Humerus, in Down syndrome, 225–226
Humoral immunity, 87
Huntington disease, prenatal diagnosis of, 248t
HUS (hemolytic uremic syndrome), 842–843, 843t
acute renal failure due to, 908
Hyaluronidase, for cervical ripening, 702t
Hybridization-based methods, 31–32, 31f
Hydatidiform mole, 42, 891
hyperthyroidism due to, 1005
and preeclampsia, 654
Hydralazine
for chronic hypertension, 678, 678t
for preeclampsia, 673, 673t
during pregnancy, 801t
Hydramnios
due to nonimmune hydrops, 507
in twin-to-twin transfusion syndrome, 62
Hydrencephaly, 283–284
Hydrocephalus, 279–280
and aneuploidy, 227t
diagnosis of, 279–280, 279f, 280f
invasive fetal therapy for, 277t, 280
post-hemorrhagic, 1212
prognosis for, 280
Hydrocortisone
for Addison disease, 1027
for asthma, 943
for hyperemesis gravidarum, 1043
for hypopituitarism, 1023
for induction of fetal pulmonary maturity, 423t
for septic shock, 763, 1179
Hydronephrosis
and aneuploidy, 227t
during pregnancy, 105
Hydrops fetalis, 505–513
defined, 478, 505
delivery considerations with, 513
diagnostic approach to, 512–513
echocardiography of, 310
epidemiology of, 505
etiology of, 507–512, 508t
cardiovascular, 507–509, 508t
chondrodysplasia as, 508t, 511–512
chromosomal, 508t, 509
congenital cystic adenomatoid malformation as, 444, 509
diabetes in, 512
gastrointestinal, 508t, 512
hematologic, 508t, 510
hemolytic disease of the fetus and newborn as, 478–479
infectious, 508t, 510–511
malformation sequence in, 508t
medications in, 512
metabolic, 508t, 511
parvovirus as, 511, 774
thoracic, 508t, 509–510
twin pregnancy in, 508t, 510
urinary, 508t, 512
experimental management of idiopathic, 512
fetal fluid accumulation in, 444, 506–507, 506f, 507f
homozygous, 877f
management of, 513
mirror syndrome due to, 505–506
presenting signs and symptoms of, 505–506
recurrence risks for, 513
scoring system for, 506
ultrasonography of, 506, 506f, 507f
Hydroquinone cream, for melasma, 1124
Hydrostatic pulmonary edema, 1174–1175
Hydrothorax
hydrops fetalis due to, 509–510
invasive fetal therapy for, 444
neonatal management of, 1198t

Hydroureter, during pregnancy, 105
Hydroxychloroquine, for rheumatic disease, 1082t
25-Hydroxycholecalciferol [25(OH)D, vitamin D_3], 1032
2-Hydroxyestradiol, in pregnancy, 115
2-Hydroxyestriol, in pregnancy, 115
2-Hydroxyestrone, in pregnancy, 115–116
11-Hydroxylase deficiency, 1029–1030
17-Hydroxylase deficiency, 1030
21-Hydroxylase deficiency, 1028–1029, 1029f
Hydroxymethyl starch (hetastarch, Hespan, Hextend), for hemorrhagic shock, 1180t, 1181
17α-Hydroxyprogesterone (17-OHP), in pregnancy, 114f, 115
17α-Hydroxyprogesterone caproate (17P), for preterm labor, 532, 570–571, 570t, 571f
3β-Hydroxysteroid dehydrogenase (3β-HSD) deficiency, 1030
11β-Hydroxysteroid dehydrogenase (11β-HSD), in control of labor, 72–73
Hygroma, cystic, 289–290, 289f
  and aneuploidy, 227t
  hydrops fetalis due to, 509
Hyperaldosteronism, primary, 1027–1028, 1028f
Hyperandrogenism, gestational, 1031–1032, 1031t
Hyperbilirubinemia
  in infants of diabetic mothers, 967
  after intrauterine transfusion, 493
  in neonatal period, 1208–1209, 1209t
Hypercalcemia, 1033–1035, 1033t, 1034t
  familial hypocalciuric, 1034
Hypercoagulability, in pregnancy, 1153
Hypercortisolism, 1021–1022
Hyperechoic bowel, and aneuploidy, 226, 227t
Hyperemesis gravidarum, 1004–1005, 1042–1043
Hyperglycemia
  and biophysical profile score, 369t
  transient maternal, due to antenatal corticosteroids, 426
Hyperhomocysteinemia, 833–834
  and fetal loss, 625t, 834
Hyperimmune globulin (HIG), for cytomegalovirus, 624, 765
Hyperinsulinemic-euglycemic clamp, 956, 956f
Hyperlipidemia, in preeclampsia, 658
Hypermastia, 128
Hypermetabolism, due to burns, 1187
Hypermorphic allele, 6
Hyperosmolar laxatives, for constipation, 1052, 1052t
Hyperoxia, maternal, for intrauterine growth restriction, 645
Hyperparathyroidism, primary, 1033–1035, 1033t, 1034t
Hyperpigmentation, in pregnancy, 1124
Hyperreactio luteinalis, 1031
Hyperreflexia, in preeclampsia, 657
HyperRHO, 479–480
Hypertension
  benign intracranial, 1094–1095
  chronic, 676–679
    defined, 651
    with diabetes, 961
    diagnosis of, 652–653, 676
    effects on fetus of, 676
    effects on mother of, 676
    epidemiology of, 676
    obstetric management of, 679
    pathogenesis of, 676
    pharmacologic management of, 676–679, 678t
    preeclampsia superimposed on, 651–652
Hypertension *(Continued)*
  with chronic kidney disease, 912
  classification of, 651–653, 652f, 653f, 653t
  with diabetes, 970
  in diabetic nephropathy, 913–914
  with dialysis, 917
  in eclampsia, 651
  fetal loss due to, 624
  gestational, 652
    excessive weight gain and, 145
    maternal obesity and, 144
  in HELLP syndrome, 652
  hemodynamics of, 1172, 1172f
  portal, 1071
  in preeclampsia. *See* Preeclampsia.
  pulmonary
    fetal, congenital diaphragmatic hernia and, 441–442
    maternal, 805
      anesthesia with, 1158
      hemodynamics of, 1171
    in neonatal period, 1207
  with renal transplantation, 919
Hypertensive emergencies, in preeclampsia, 673, 673t
Hyperthyroidism
  diagnosis of, 1001
  differential diagnosis of, 1001–1002
  fetal and neonatal, 1003–1004, 1004f
  in pregnancy, 1001–1003, 1001t, 1003t
  recurrent gestational, 1005
  related to human chorionic gonadotropin, 1004–1005
  signs and symptoms of, 1001
  subclinical, 1003
  thyroid storm due to, 1003, 1003t
  treatment of, 1002–1003
  in women, 1000
Hypertrophic cardiomyopathy
  idiopathic, 815–816, 815f
  in infants of diabetic mothers, 967
Hypertrophic obstructive cardiomyopathy (HOCM), anesthesia with, 1159
Hyperventilation
  during pregnancy, 104, 927
  for subarachnoid hemorrhage, 1150
Hyperviscosity, in infants of diabetic mothers, 967
Hypocalcemia
  in infants of diabetic mothers, 967
  maternal, 1035
Hypofibrinogenemia, 844t, 845t, 848
Hypogastric artery ligation, for obstetric hemorrhage, 1183, 1184f
Hypoglycemia
  in acute liver failure, 1072
  avoidance of nocturnal, for diabetes, 974
  and biophysical profile score, 369t
  in infants of diabetic mothers, 967
  prematurity and, 1201t
Hypoglycemic agents, oral, 970, 980–982
Hypomorphic allele, 6
Hypoparathyroidism, 1035, 1035t
Hypophyseal arteries, 1015
Hypophysis-pituitary-adrenal-placental axis, fetal, in preterm labor, 529, 530f
Hypopituitarism, 1022–1024, 1023t
Hypoplastic anemia, 875–876
Hypoplastic left heart syndrome (HLHS), 328–330, 329f
  invasive fetal therapy for, 445
Hypotension
  fetal heart rate with, 409f, 411t
  maternal, due to cesarean delivery, 710
Hypotension *(Continued)*
  noninvasive assessment of, 1173, 1173f
  for subarachnoid hemorrhage, 1150
Hypothalamic-pituitary-adrenal (HPA) axis, of fetus, in control of labor, 72–73
Hypothalamus
  anatomy and physiology of, 1015, 1016f, 1017f
  disorders of, 1016
  fetal development of, 1016
  during pregnancy, 1015–1016, 1016f, 1017f
Hypothermia
  for hypoxic-ischemic encephalopathy, 1211
  for subarachnoid hemorrhage, 1150
Hypothesis generation, 208
Hypothesis testing, 208, 211–212, 212t
Hypothyroidism
  differential diagnosis of, 1007
  drug-induced, 1007
  fetal and neonatal, 1008
  idiopathic, 1007
  iodine deficiency and, 1005–1006, 1005f
  mental retardation due to, 1007
  and postpartum thyroiditis, 1010
  in pregnancy, 1005–1008
  screening for, 1008
  signs and symptoms of, 1006–1007
  subclinical, 1007–1008
  treatment of, 1007
  in women, 1000–1001
Hypothyroxinemia, 1005f
  subclinical, 1008
Hypotonic fluids, for preeclampsia, 674
Hypoventilation, maternal, and fetal respiratory acidosis, 401
Hypoxemia
  defined, 401, 401t
  fetal responses to, 362–364, 363f, 364f
Hypoxia
  and cerebral palsy, 1216
  defined, 401, 401t
  fetal, and behavioral state activity, 174, 174f
  fetal responses to, 399–400
  maternal, and fetal respiratory acidosis, 401
  physiologic, 188
  saltatory fetal heart rate due to, 413, 413f
Hypoxia-inducing factors (HIFs), in preeclampsia, 665
Hypoxic-ischemic encephalopathy, in neonatal period, 1210–1211
Hyrtl anastomosis, 40
Hysterectomy
  for cervical cancer, 888, 889
  cesarean, 713
  for obstetric hemorrhage, 1183
  for placenta accreta, 729
Hysteroscopic myomectomy, 1039

I

IAP (intrapartum antibiotic prophylaxis), for group B *Streptococcus* infection, 766, 767–768, 768f
IBD. *See* Inflammatory bowel disease (IBD).
IBS (irritable bowel syndrome), 1049–1050, 1050t
Ibuprofen, for rheumatic disease, 1082t
ICH. *See* Intracranial hemorrhage (ICH).
Ichthyosiform erythroderma, 1132
Ichthyosis, 1132
ICP (intrahepatic cholestasis of pregnancy), 1060–1061, 1125
ICSI (intracytoplasmic sperm injection), perinatal risks of, 260–261
Ideogram, 12, 12f
Idiopathic hypertrophic cardiomyopathy, 815–816, 815f

Idiopathic hypertrophic subaortic stenosis (IHSS), anesthesia with, 1159
Idiopathic thrombocytopenic purpura (ITP), 837–840
IDMs (infants of diabetic mothers)
  hyperbilirubinemia in, 1208
  morbidity and mortality in, 967–968, 968f, 986
IDO (indolamine 2,3-dioxygenase), 90, 94, 95f
IDS (Inventory of Depressive Symptomatology), 1114
IE (infective endocarditis), prophylaxis against, 798, 821
IFG (impaired fasting glucose), 955, 971
IFN-α (interferon-α), for hepatitis C virus, 1068
IgA nephropathy, 916t
IGFs. *See* Insulin-like growth factors (IGFs).
IGT (impaired glucose tolerance), 955, 971
IL. *See* Interleukin (IL) *entries.*
Ileus, adynamic, postcesarean, 709
Illicit drugs, as teratogens, 356
IM (intramembranous) pathway, 49, 50–51
Imipenem-cilastin
  for pelvic abscess, 762
  for puerperal endometritis, 760
  for septic shock, 763
Imipramine (Tofranil), dosage of, 1117t
Immune globulin
  hepatitis A, 785
  hepatitis B, 786, 1066t, 1067, 1218
  intravenous. *See* Intravenous immune globulin (IVIG).
  rhesus, 478, 479–481
    for idiopathic thrombocytopenic purpura, 839
  varicella zoster, 783
Immune privileged site, pregnant uterus as, 88–90, 89f, 90f
Immune response(s)
  cytokines and, 88
  to trophoblast, 88–90, 89f–91f, 91–92
  types of, 87–88
Immune suppression
  local, 90, 90f
  systemic, 88
Immunity
  adaptive, 87–88
  cellular, 87
  humoral, 87
  natural or innate, 87
    in pregnancy, 90–92, 91f
Immunologic causes, of pregnancy loss, 621–622, 628
Immunologic changes, in preeclampsia, 666, 667
Immunologic complications, of prematurity, 1199t
Immunology
  general concept of, 87–88
  of pregnancy, 87–96
    defining, 87
    infection in, 92–96, 93f–95f
    innate immune system in, 90–92, 91f
    maternal immune response to trophoblast in, 88–90, 89f, 90f
    and rheumatic diseases, 1079–1080
    and thyroid system, 998–999
Immunomodulators, for inflammatory bowel disease, 1049
Immunosuppressive agents
  for renal transplantation, 918, 919, 920, 921
  as teratogens, 351t, 352
Imodium (loperamide), for inflammatory bowel disease, 1049
Impaired fasting glucose (IFG), 955, 971
Impaired glucose tolerance (IGT), 955, 971
Impetigo herpetiformis, 1125t, 1129–1130, 1130f
Implantation, 37, 38f, 40
  endocrinology of, 111–114, 112f, 113t
  site of, 112
  steps in, 111, 112f, 619
  timing of, 619
  window for, 111
Imprinting, 30
In vitro fertilization (IVF)
  antiphospholipid antibodies and, 1083–1084
  implantation with, 111
  perinatal risks of, 260–261
  and preterm birth, 558
Incidental thrombocytopenia of pregnancy, 838
Incontinence, cesarean delivery to prevent, 708, 711
Independent assortment, 22, 23f
Indinavir (Crixivan), for HIV infection, 772t
Indirect assays, 30
Indirect obstetric deaths, 1167
Indolamine 2,3-dioxygenase (IDO), 90, 94, 95f
Indomethacin
  for cervical insufficiency, 589
  and necrotizing enterocolitis, 1207–1208
  for preterm labor, 563–564
  for rheumatic disease, 1082t
Induction of labor, 700–703
  for breech presentation, 705
  and cesarean delivery, 700
  contraindications for, 701
  in diabetic pregnancy, 985
  elective, 700–701, 700t
  for fetal demise, 627–628
  incidence of, 700, 700f
  indicated, 701–703, 702t, 703t
  for post-term pregnancy, 615–616
  after premature rupture of the membranes, 604
Infant mortality rate
  defined, 548
  with preterm birth, 548–551, 549f–552f, 553t
Infantile polycystic kidney, 295, 296f
Infants of diabetic mothers (IDMs)
  hyperbilirubinemia in, 1208
  morbidity and mortality in, 967–968, 968f, 986
Infection(s), 739–787
  with bacterial vaginosis, 741–742, 742f, 742t, 743t
    and premature rupture of the membranes, 599
    and preterm birth, 556, 568, 570, 741, 742, 742t
  during breastfeeding, 135–138, 136t–137t
  with candidiasis, 739–741, 740t
    breastfeeding with, 135, 136t, 137t, 138–139
  due to central venous catheters, 1170
  and cerebral palsy, 1215–1216
  with *Chlamydia trachomatis,* 746–748
    breastfeeding with, 136t
    diagnosis of, 747
    epidemiology of, 746
    and gonorrhea, 745, 746
    life cycle of, 93f
    pathogenesis of, 746–747
    and postpartum endometritis, 747
    and pregnancy outcome, 93–96, 93f–95f, 747
    and preterm birth, 556
    prevention of, 748
    treatment of, 747–748, 748t
  chorioamnionitis as, 757–759, 758t
    and bronchopulmonary dysplasia, 1205
    and cerebral palsy, 1216
    due to cervical cerclage, 594
Infection(s) *(Continued)*
    clinical, 757
    in neonatal period, 1197–1198, 1217
    after premature rupture of the membranes, 600, 604, 605, 606
    umbilical cord acid-base balance with, 404, 404t
  after chorionic villus sampling, 255
  of CNS, 1099–1101
  cytomegalovirus, 764–766
    breastfeeding with, 136t
    clinical manifestations of, 765
    congenital
      clinical manifestations of, 765
      diagnosis of, 765
      pathogenesis of, 765
      treatment of, 765–766
    diagnosis of, 765
    epidemiology and pathogenesis of, 764–765
    fetal loss due to, 624
    hydrops fetalis due to, 510–511
    intrauterine growth restriction due to, 638
    intrauterine transfusion with, 492
    in neonatal period, 1217–1218
    prevention of, 766
    risk factors for, 765
    treatment of, 765–766
  defined, 1176t
  disseminated gonococcal, 744, 746
  episiotomy, 759–760, 759f
  fetal loss due to, 623–624
  food-borne, 147
  with gonorrhea, 742–746
    anogenital, 744
    breastfeeding with, 136t
    and chlamydia, 745, 746
    clinical manifestations of, 744
    diagnosis of, 744–745
    epidemiology of, 742–743, 743f
    pathogenesis of, 743–744
    pharyngeal, 744
    prevention of, 746
    treatment of, 745–746, 745t
  group A *Streptococcus,* breastfeeding with, 135, 137t
  group B *Streptococcus,* 766–769
    breastfeeding with, 135, 136t
    clinical manifestations of
      in mother, 767
      in neonate, 766–767, 766t
    diagnosis of, 767
    epidemiology of, 766
    in neonatal period, 1217
      clinical manifestations of, 766–767, 766t
    and premature rupture of the membranes, 599, 606
    and preterm labor, 561
    prevention of, 767–769, 768f
    treatment of, 767
  with hepatitis, 785–786, 787t
    autoimmune, 1069
    breastfeeding with, 135–137, 136t
    chronic nonviral, 1069
    viral, 1064–1069, 1065t, 1066t, 1068t
  with herpes simplex virus, 769–770
    breastfeeding with, 136t
    hepatitis due to, 1069
    after premature rupture of the membranes, 607
  with human immunodeficiency virus, 770–773
    acute phase of, 771
    breastfeeding with, 136t, 137–138
    diagnosis of, 771
    epidemiology of, 770–771

Infection(s) *(Continued)*
fetal blood sampling with, 386
latent phase of, 771
liver disease with, 1069
myocarditis or cardiomyopathy with, 816
in newborn period, 1218–1219
pathogenesis of, 771
perinatal transmission of, 771
pneumonia with, 771, 929–930, 933–934, 934f
symptomatic phase of, 771
transfusion-related, 1182t
treatment of, 771–773, 772t
with human papillomavirus, 748–750, 749f
and cervical intraepithelial neoplasia, 887
hydrops fetalis due to, 508t, 510–511
with influenza, 784–785
pneumonia due to, 930, 932
intrauterine growth restriction due to, 638–639
with listeriosis, 773
fetal loss due to, 623
mastitis as, 138, 138f, 138t, 764
breastfeeding with, 135, 137t
with mumps, 773–774
in neonatal period, 1217–1220
chorioamnionitis as, 1217
with group B β-hemolytic streptococci, 1217
sexually transmitted, 1219–1220
viral, 1217–1219
and cerebral palsy, 1216
with parvovirus, 774–775, 774t
fetal loss due to, 623
hydrops fetalis due to, 511
pelvic abscess as, 762
postcesarean, 709
and pregnancy, 92–96, 93f–95f
preterm labor and birth due to, 524–527, 525f, 526f, 528f, 556, 568
with puerperal endometritis, 760–761
breastfeeding with, 136t
with renal transplantation, 919–920
with rubella, 775–776
intrauterine growth restriction due to, 638
in newborn period, 1219
as teratogen, 347, 799
with rubeola, 776–777
septic pelvic vein thrombophlebitis as, 763–764
septic shock as, 762–763, 1175–1179
clinical manifestations of, 1176, 1177t
cold (late), 1176, 1177t
definitions for, 1175–1176, 1176t
epidemiology of, 1175
hemodynamics of, 1172–1173
hemostatic mechanisms in, 1176, 1177f
management of, 1176–1179, 1178t
pathophysiology of, 1176, 1177f
secondary (irreversible), 1176, 1177t
warm (early), 1176, 1177t
with syphilis, 777–782
congenital
case definition for, 780, 780t
clinical manifestations of, 778–779
diagnosis of, 780
epidemiology of, 777–778, 778f, 779
pregnancy outcome with, 779
transmission of, 779
treatment of, 782
diagnosis of, 779–780, 780t
epidemiology of, 777–778, 778f
fetal loss due to, 623
hydrops fetalis due to, 510
Jarisch-Herxheimer reaction in, 781–782

Infection(s) *(Continued)*
latent, 778, 782
neuro-, 779–780, 781
pathogenesis of, 778
prevention of, 782
primary, 778, 782
secondary, 778, 782
tertiary, 778
treatment of, 780–782, 781t
with toxoplasmosis, 782–783
with *Trichomonas vaginalis*, 741
breastfeeding with, 137t
and preterm birth, 556
urinary tract, 750–756, 905–907
acute pyelonephritis as, 754–756, 755t, 756t, 906–907
asymptomatic bacteriuria as, 750–753, 752t, 905–906
classification of, 750, 750t
cystitis as, 753–754
diagnosis of, 905
epidemiology of, 750
treatment of, 906
with varicella-zoster virus, 783–784
wound, 761–762
due to burns, 1187–1188
Infective endocarditis (IE), prophylaxis against, 798, 821
Inferior vena cava (IVC), fetal, 159–160, 160f
Doppler studies of, 377
interrupted, 320, 320f, 321f
Inferior vena cava (IVC) filters, 865
Infertility
antiphospholipid antibodies and, 830
after cesarean delivery, 710
and chromosomal defects, 22
myomas and, 1135–1136, 1138
Inflammation
anemia and, 881
and bronchopulmonary dysplasia, 1205, 1206f
cervical insufficiency due to, 587, 587f
and pregnancy, 88–89, 89f
preterm labor and birth due to, 524–527, 525f, 526f, 528f, 556
Inflammatory bowel disease (IBD), 1047–1049
clinical characteristics of, 1047–1048, 1048f, 1048t
diagnostic testing for, 1048, 1048f, 1049f
effect of pregnancy on, 1048
effect on pregnancy of, 1048
genetics of, 28
treatment of, 1048–1049, 1049t
Inflammatory responses, in preeclampsia, 666
Infliximab (Remicade)
for inflammatory bowel disease, 1049
for rheumatic disease, 1081, 1082t
Influenza
pneumonia due to, 930, 932
viral, 784–785
Influenza vaccine, 785
Information bias, 211
Informed consent, for carrier screening, 238
INH (isoniazid)
for HIV infection, 771
for tuberculosis, 936, 937, 937t
Inheritance patterns, 22–29
autosomal dominant, 23–24, 24f
autosomal recessive, 24, 24f
Mendel's laws for, 22–23, 23f
mitochondrial, 29
multifactorial, 25–29, 27t, 28t
sex-linked, 24–25, 25f
symbols for, 23, 23f
Inhibin, during pregnancy, 120

Inhibin A, prenatal screening for, 223
Inhibin-related proteins, during pregnancy, 120
Injury Severity Score (ISS), 1185
Innate immunity, 87
in pregnancy, 90–92, 91f
Insertions, 15, 17f
in linkage analysis, 33
Inspiratory capacity, during pregnancy, 105t
Inspiratory reserve volume, during pregnancy, 105t
Insulin
in breastfeeding, 131
continuous subcutaneous infusion of, 977f, 979, 979t
for diabetes, 976–980, 977f, 977t, 979t
for diabetic ketoacidosis, 962t, 963
fetal concentrations of, and fetal obesity, 964–965
intermediate-acting, 976, 977f, 977t, 978
intrapartum, 985–986, 985t
long-acting, 976, 977f, 977t
NPH, 977f, 977t, 978, 980
postpartum, 986
during pregnancy, 118–120, 118f–120f, 120t
regular, 977t, 978
for septic shock, 1178
short-acting, 976, 977t, 978
types of, 976, 977f, 977t
typical regimens for, 976–978, 977f
ultralente, 977f
Insulin aspart (Novolog), 977t, 978
Insulin glargine (Lantus), 977f, 977t, 978
Insulin lispro (Humalog), 977f, 977t, 978, 979
Insulin pump, 977f, 979, 979t
Insulin receptor substrate-1 (IRS-1), 958
Insulin resistance
birth weight and, 152
in normal and diabetic pregnancy, 119, 119f, 956, 956f, 958
peripheral, 956
and preeclampsia, 654, 656, 658
Insulin response
in normal and diabetic pregnancy, 956–957, 957f
in type 2 diabetes, 954–955
Insulin secretion, in normal and diabetic pregnancy, 956–957, 957f
Insulin sensitivity
in normal and diabetic pregnancy, 956–957, 957f, 958
in type 2 diabetes, 954–955
Insulin-like growth factor(s) (IGFs)
and fetal obesity, 965
in pregnancy, 118, 118f
Insulin-like growth factor 1 (IGF-1)
and fetal loss, 621
during pregnancy, 1016
Insulin-like growth factor–binding proteins (IGFBPs), and fetal obesity, 965
Insulin-resistant polycystic ovary syndrome, 1031–1032
Integrated aneuploidy screening, for Down syndrome, 232
Integrated fetal testing, 379–380, 380f, 380t
Integrins, in implantation, 112–113, 113t
Interferon-α (IFN-α), for hepatitis C virus, 1068
Interleukin-1 (IL-1), in preterm labor, 526, 526f
Interleukin-1α (IL-1α)
for fetal lung maturation, 203, 203f
in preterm labor, 526, 526f
Interleukin-1β (IL-1β)
in implantation, 113, 113t
in preterm labor, 526, 526f

Interleukin-6 (IL-6), in preterm labor and birth, 527, 528f, 553
Interleukin-8 (IL-8)
  in cervical insufficiency, 587
  in preterm labor, 529
Interleukin-10 (IL-10)
  in implantation, 113t
  in preterm labor, 527
Interleukin-11 (IL-11), in preterm labor, 529
Intermittent pneumatic compression devices, for prevention of venous thromboembolism, 864–865
International Federation of Gynecology and Obstetrics (FIGO), 888
Interphase, 7, 7f
Interrupted inferior vena cava, 320, 320f, 321f
Interstitial deletion, 15, 16f
Interstitial translocations, 17f
Interventional studies, 208–209
Intervertebral disk, prolapsed, 1104
Intestinal atresia, 292, 292f
Intra-abdominal version, for transverse lie, 706
Intra-amniotic catheter, 399
Intra-amniotic endotoxin, and fetal lung development, 196f, 203, 203f
Intra-amniotic infection. *See* Chorioamnionitis.
Intracardiac pressures, fetal, 162, 163f
Intracervical inflammation, cervical insufficiency due to, 587, 587f
Intracranial arterial occlusive disease, 1095–1096, 1095f
Intracranial cystic lesions, fetal, 282–284, 283f, 284f
Intracranial dural vascular anomalies, 1098–1099
Intracranial hemorrhage (ICH)
  fetal
    due to idiopathic thrombocytopenic purpura, 839
    due to neonatal alloimmune thrombocytopenia, 840, 841–842
  maternal, 1096–1098, 1097f, 1098f
    anesthesia with, 1150
Intracranial hypertension, benign, 1094–1095
Intracranial saccular aneurysms, 1097–1098, 1098f
Intracranial tumors
  fetal, 284
  maternal, 1093–1094, 1094f
    headaches due to, 1092
Intracranial venous occlusive disease, 1096, 1096f, 1097f
Intracranial venous thrombosis, 1096, 1096f, 1097f
Intracytoplasmic sperm injection (ICSI), perinatal risks of, 260–261
Intradural vascular anomalies, spinal, 1099
Intrahepatic cholestasis of pregnancy (ICP), 1060–1061, 1125
Intramembranous (IM) pathway, 49, 50–51
Intrapartum antibiotic prophylaxis (IAP), for group B *Streptococcus* infection, 766, 767–768, 768f
Intrapartum fetal surveillance, 397–415
  electronic monitoring *vs.* auscultation for, 413–415
  of fetal acid-base balance, 400–405, 401t–405t
  fetal heart rate monitor for, 399
  of fetal heart rate patterns, 405–413
    accelerations in, 406
    baseline rate in, 405, 406–407, 407f
    bradycardia in, 406, 407f, 411f, 411t
    with congenital anomalies, 413
    early decelerations in, 406, 411t
    in utero treatment of, 410, 411f, 411t
Intrapartum fetal surveillance *(Continued)*
    late decelerations in, 406, 408–409.409f, 410f, 411t
    normal, 406, 407f
    periodic patterns in, 407, 408–410, 409f–411f
    prolonged decelerations in, 406
    quantification in, 406
    saltatory, 413, 413f
    sinusoidal, 410–413, 412f
    tachycardia in, 406–407, 411f
    variability in, 406–408, 408f, 411t
    variable decelerations in, 406, 409–410, 410f, 411t
  of fetal responses to hypoxia/acidemia, 399–400
  of uterine activity, 399
Intrapartum infection. *See* Chorioamnionitis.
Intrapericardial teratoma, 335–336, 336f
Intraperitoneal fetal transfusion (IPT), 477, 488, 490
Intraplacental pressures, in fetal blood volume control, 398
Intrauterine fetal demise. *See* Fetal demise.
Intrauterine fetal invasive treatment. *See* Invasive fetal therapy.
Intrauterine growth restriction (IUGR), 635–646
  antenatal fetal testing for, 379–380, 380t, 644–645
  asymmetric, 642
  and behavioral state activity, 174
  and cerebral palsy, 1215
  definitions for, 635–636
  diabetes and, 964
  diagnosis of, 641–642, 642t, 643f
  etiology of, 637–641
    aneuploidy in, 227t, 638
    congenital anomalies in, 638
    environmental toxins in, 640
    genetic factors in, 637–638
    inadequate maternal nutrition in, 639–640
    infection in, 638–639
    maternal and fetal hormones in, 641
    maternal obesity in, 144
    maternal vascular disease in, 640–641
    multiple gestation in, 639
    placental factors in, 640
  factor V Leiden mutation and, 832–833
  incidence of, 636
  labor and delivery with, 645–646
  management of, 644–646, 645t
  neonatal complications and long-term sequelae of, 646
  and perinatal mortality and morbidity, 637, 637f
  and placental respiratory gas exchange, 185–186, 186f
  preeclampsia and, 654–655, 670
  prothrombin gene mutation and, 833
  rate of fetal growth and, 636, 636f, 636t, 637f
  symmetric, 642
Intrauterine infection, preterm labor and birth due to, 524–527, 525f, 526f, 556
Intrauterine pressure catheters, 695–696
Intrauterine transfusion (IUT), for Rh alloimmunization, 488–493
  access site for, 488
  adjunctive measures with, 491
  amount of, 490, 490t
  method of, 488–490, 490f
  outcome of, 492–493
  with severely anemic early-second-trimester fetus, 491
  source of red blood cells in, 491–492
  timing of, 492
Intravascular fetal transfusion (IVT), 477, 488–490, 490f, 491, 492
Intravascular volume, in pregnancy, 1152
Intravascular volume depletion, in preeclampsia, 1147
Intravenous immune globulin (IVIG)
  for antiphospholipid antibody syndrome, 831
  for hemolytic disease of the fetus and newborn, 493–494
  for idiopathic thrombocytopenic purpura, 838
  for neonatal alloimmune thrombocytopenia, 841–842
  for pregnancy loss, 628t
  for rheumatic disease, 1082t
Intraventricular hemorrhage (IVH), 1211–1212
  prematurity and, 1201t
Introns, 5
Invasive central hemodynamic monitoring, 1168–1173
  for anaphylactoid syndrome of pregnancy, 1171–1172
  for aortic stenosis, 1171
  background and insertion technique for, 1168–1169
  complications of, 1169–1170, 1169t
  hemodynamic considerations in, 1170, 1170t, 1171t
  for hypertensive disorders of pregnancy, 1172, 1172f
  indications for, 1169
  for mitral valve stenosis, 1170–1171
  and pulmonary capillary wedge pressure, 1170, 1170f
  for pulmonary hypertension, 1171
  for septic shock, 1172–1173
Invasive fetal testing. *See* Cordocentesis.
Invasive fetal therapy, 277–278, 433–447
  for amniotic bands, 434t
  for chorioangioma, 434t
  for congenital cystic adenomatoid malformation, 277t, 444
  for congenital diaphragmatic hernia, 277t, 434t, 440–444, 441f, 442t, 443f
  for congenital heart defects, 277t, 434t, 445, 446t
  criteria for, 433, 434t
  endoscopic, 433
  EXIT procedure for, 435
  fetoscopy for, 435, 435t
  for fetus acardiacus and discordant anomalies, 434t, 468
  history of, 433
  for hydrocephalus, 277t
  for hydrothorax, 444
  indications for, 277t, 433, 434t
  for lower urinary tract obstruction, 277t, 434t, 444–445, 445t
  for neural tube defects, 277t, 434t, 445–447, 447t
  open, 433–435
  for pleural effusion, 277t, 444
  for sacrococcygeal teratoma, 434t
  for thoracic space-occupying lesions, 434t
  for TRAP sequence, 439–440
  for twin-to-twin transfusion syndrome, 434t, 436–439, 436t, 438f, 439t
  for umbilical cord occlusion, 440
Inventory of Depressive Symptomatology (IDS), 1114
Inversion(s)
  chromosomal, 15–16, 17f, 18f
  of uterus, 699–700
Invirase (saquinavir), for HIV infection, 772t

Iodide
for hyperthyroidism, 1002
in normal thyroid physiology, 995
for prevention of postpartum thyroiditis, 1010–1011
for thyroid storm, 1003, 1003t
Iodination, in normal thyroid physiology, 995
Iodine, in normal thyroid physiology, 995
Iodine deficiency, 996–997, 998f, 1005–1006, 1005f
Iodine metabolism, in pregnancy, 997
Ionizing radiation, as teratogen, 354
Ipratropium bromide, for asthma, 940t, 944t
IPT (intraperitoneal fetal transfusion), 477, 488, 490
Iron, plasma, 870, 870t
Iron deficiency anemia, 870, 872, 873–874
Iron dextran, for iron deficiency anemia, 873–874
Iron kinetics, during pregnancy, 871, 871t
Iron requirements, for pregnancy, 871, 871f
Iron sucrose, for iron deficiency anemia, 873, 874
Iron supplementation, during pregnancy, 146, 146t
with multiple gestation, 461
Irregular chorionic fusion, 58
Irritable bowel syndrome (IBS), 1049–1050, 1050t
IRS-1 (insulin receptor substrate-1), 958
Ischiopagus, 468
Isochromosomes, 18
Isoniazid (INH)
for HIV infection, 771
for tuberculosis, 936, 937, 937t
Isoproterenol, for septic shock, 1178t
Isotretinoin, as teratogen, 348, 351t, 353–354
ISS (Injury Severity Score), 1185
ITP (idiopathic thrombocytopenic purpura), 837–840
IUGR. *See* Intrauterine growth restriction (IUGR).
IUT. *See* Intrauterine transfusion (IUT).
IVC. *See* Inferior vena cava (IVC).
IVF. *See* In vitro fertilization (IVF).
IVH (intraventricular hemorrhage), 1211–1212
prematurity and, 1201t
IVIG. *See* Intravenous immune globulin (IVIG).
IVT (intravascular fetal transfusion), 477, 488–490, 490f, 491, 492

J
Jackson, Edith, 132
Jarisch-Herxheimer reaction, 781–782
Jaundice, 1059, 1060t
in neonatal period, 1208–1209, 1209t
Jewish population, carrier screening in, 238t, 240–243, 241t, 242t
Juvenile arthritis, 1079, 1080, 1080t

K
k antigen, 497, 497t
K1 antigen, 478, 478f, 479, 496–497, 497t
K2 antigen, 497, 497t
Kaletra (lopinavir/ritonavir), for HIV infection, 772, 772t
Kanamycin, for tuberculosis, 937t
Karyogram, 12, 13f
Karyotype analysis, preimplantation genetic screening for, 260
Karyotyping, spectral, 13–14, 14f
KCl (potassium chloride), for diabetic ketoacidosis, 962t
Kefauver-Harris Amendment, 347
Kell antigen, 478, 478f, 479, 495t, 496–497, 497t
Kernicterus, 1209
Ketoacidosis, diabetic, 962–963, 962t
Ketonuria, avoidance of, for diabetes, 974
Ketoprofen, for rheumatic disease, 1082t
Ketorolac, for rheumatic disease, 1082t
Ketosis, avoidance of, for diabetes, 974
Kidd antigen, 478f, 495t, 497t, 499
Kidney(s)
fetal
anomalies of, 295–296, 295f, 296f
development of, 294–295
multicystic dysplastic, 295, 295f
polycystic, 295–296, 296f
during pregnancy, 105–107, 106f
ectopic, 915
solitary, 909, 915, 916t
Kidney biopsy, fetal, 259
Kidney development, small birth weight and, 154
Kidney disease. *See* Renal disorder(s).
Kidney stones, 913, 916t
Kidney transplantation, 918–921, 918t
for diabetic nephropathy, 960–961
Killer immunoglobulin receptors (KIRs), in preeclampsia, 661
Klebsiella pneumoniae, pneumonia due to, 930
Kleihauer-Betke test, 1185, 1185f
Klinefelter syndrome, 20
Koplik spots, 776
Korsakoff psychosis, 1107
Krukenberg tumors, 1032
Kyphoscoliosis, anesthesia with, 1160

L
Labetalol
for chronic hypertension, 678, 678t, 679
for preeclampsia, 673, 673t
Labial edema, 1124
Labor and delivery, 69–81
abnormal presentation(s) in, 703–707
breech as, 703–706, 705t
compound, 707
deflection abnormalities as, 706–707
transverse lie as, 706
uterine anomalies and, 1144
uterine myomas and, 1137
abnormality(ies) of, 693–700
arrest disorders as, 695–696
of first stage, 693–696, 694t
inversion of uterus as, 699–700
of placental separation and control of uterine bleeding, 698
postpartum hemorrhage as, 698–699
prolonged latent phase as, 694–695
protraction disorders as, 695
retained placenta as, 698
of rotation and descent, 696–697, 696f, 696t
of second stage, 696–698, 696f, 696t
shoulder dystocia as, 697–698
of third stage, 698–700
uterine myomas and, 1137
achieving successful, 81
active phase of, 691, 692, 692t
analgesia and anesthesia for, 715–717
asynchronous, 463
blood loss during, 104
cervical dilation in, 692, 692f, 692t, 695
cervical remodeling in, 523
cesarean. *See* Cesarean delivery.
with chronic kidney disease, 912
common pathway of, 521–524, 522f, 524f
with cystic fibrosis, 948
decidual/membrane activation in, 523
defined, 69
delayed interval, 463
descent during, 691–692, 692t, 693
abnormalities of, 696–697, 696f, 696t
Labor and delivery *(Continued)*
with diabetes, 982–986, 984t, 985t
diagnosis of, 70
with dialysis, 917
fetal heart rate during, 410f, 411f
fetal scalp blood values in, 402, 402t
forceps, 713–714
for breech presentation, 705
hemodynamics during, 104
hormonal control of, 70–76, 71f
cascade of events in, 70–72, 71f
estrogens in, 74
fetal hypothalamic-pituitary-adrenal axis in, 72–73
oxytocin in, 75–76
progesterone in, 73–74
prostaglandins in, 74–75, 75f
with hydrops fetalis, 513
induction of, 700–703
for breech presentation, 705
and cesarean delivery, 700
contraindications for, 701
in diabetic pregnancy, 985
elective, 700–701, 700t
for fetal demise, 627–628
incidence of, 700, 700f
indicated, 701–703, 702t, 703t
for post-term pregnancy, 615–616
after premature rupture of the membranes, 604
with intrauterine growth restriction, 645–646, 645t
latent phase of, 691, 692, 692t
prolonged, 694–695
at limits of viability, 1201–1202
mechanisms of, 521–524
monitoring of, 717
with monoamniotic twins, 467
with morbid obesity, 1152
with multiple gestation, 461–463
myometrial contractility in, 522–523
normal, 691–692, 692f, 692t
onset of, 691, 694
pelvis in, 692–693
with preeclampsia, 668, 669–670
preterm. *See* Preterm labor and birth.
progression of, 691–692, 692f, 692t
documentation of, 693
prostaglandins in, 523–524, 524f
with renal transplantation, 920
rotation during, 693
abnormalities of, 696–697
stages of, 691–692, 692f, 692t
stations of, 696t
timing of, 70
in diabetic pregnancy, 984–985, 984t, 985t
with intrauterine growth restriction, 645
vacuum extraction for, 714–715
"Labor genes," 79
Lactate dehydrogenase, and dysgerminoma, 1094, 1141
Lactation. *See also* Breastfeeding.
calcium metabolism during, 1032, 1033f
and contraception, 134–135
with epilepsy, 1090
inhibition of, 1020
initiation of, 131–133
and osteoporosis, 1036
parathyroid glands in, 1032, 1032f, 1033f
physiology of, 130–133
psychotropic medications during, 1119–1120
Lactation specialists, 132

Lactiferous ducts
anatomy of, 129
development of, 127–128, 127f, 128f
plugged, 138, 138t
Lactogenesis, 127f, 130–131, 130t, 131f
Lactotrophs
neurohormonal control of, 1015
during pregnancy, 1015
Lactulose, for constipation, 1052, 1052t
LAH (lymphocytic adenohypophysitis), 1023–1024, 1023t
Lambda sign, 456
Lamellar body count (LBC), 420
in diabetic pregnancy, 421
impact of contaminants on, 422, 422t
from vaginal fluid specimens, 423
Laminaria, for cervical ripening, 703t
Lamivudine (3TC, Epivir)
for hepatitis B virus, 1066–1067
for HIV infection, 772t
Lamotrigine (Lamictal)
dosage of, 1116t
risks of, 1117, 1119
Lanreotide, for acromegaly, 1021
Lantus (insulin glargine), 977f, 977t, 978
Laparoscopic appendectomy, 1047
Laparoscopic myomectomy, 1039
Laparoscopic surgery, during pregnancy, 890–891
Laparoscopy, of adnexal masses, 1143
Laparotomic myomectomy, 1039
Laparotomy, for postpartum hemorrhage, 699
Large bowel obstruction, 293
Large-for-gestation-age (LGA) infants
health and disease in, 153
maternal diabetes and, 964–966, 965t, 966t
maternal obesity and, 144
Laryngeal papilloma, 748–749
Laser ablation, of anastomotic vessels, for twin-to-twin transfusion syndrome, 437–439, 438f, 439t, 465–466
Lassa fever, breastfeeding with, 135
Last menstrual period (LMP), and gestational age, 613
Late decelerations, in fetal heart rate, 406, 408–409.409f, 410f, 411t
Latent phase, of labor, 691, 692, 692t
prolonged, 694–695
Lateral femoral cutaneous nerve compression, 1105–1106
Lawrence-Moon-Bardet-Biedl syndrome, 1016
Laxatives, 1052, 1052t
LBC. *See* Lamellar body count (LBC).
LBW. *See* Low birth weight (LBW).
LCHAD (long-chain 3-hydroxyacyl-coenzyme A dehydrogenase) deficiency, 1062
LDA (low-dose aspirin), for antiphospholipid antibody syndrome, 830–831
Lead, as teratogen, 354
Leber optic atrophy, 1103
Lecithin/sphingomyelin (L/S) ratio, 419
in diabetic pregnancy, 421
impact of contaminants on, 422, 422t
from vaginal fluid specimens, 423
LEEP. *See* Loop electrosurgical excision procedure (LEEP).
Leflunomide, for rheumatic disease, 1081, 1082t
Left ventricle, fetal echocardiography of, 313, 313f
Left ventricular dysfunction, asymptomatic, 817
Left ventricular stroke work index, 1171t
Left-sided vena cava (LSVC), persistent, 318–320, 319f, 320f
Left-to-right shunt, maternal, 800–804, 802f–804f
anesthesia with, 1156–1157
Legionella pneumophila, pneumonia due to, 931, 932
Leiomyomas. *See* Uterine leiomyomas.
"Lemon sign," in spina bifida, 281, 283f
Leptin, and intrauterine growth restriction, 641
Leptonema, 8f, 9
Leptotene, 8f
LES (lower esophageal sphincter), in pregnancy, 1041, 1043
Let-down reflex, 131, 132f, 133, 133f
Leukemia
congenital, hydrops fetalis due to, 510
in pregnancy, 898, 899
Leukemia inhibitory factor, in implantation, 113t
Leukocyte-poor blood, for hemorrhagic shock, 1181t
Leukomalacia, periventricular, 1212
chorioamnionitis and, 758–759, 758t
Leukotriene mediators, for asthma, 940t, 941t, 942
Levofloxacin, for pelvic abscess, 762
Levothyroxine (L-thyroxine)
for hypopituitarism, 1023
for prevention of postpartum thyroiditis, 1010–1011
Levo-transposition of the great arteries (L-TGA), 334, 334f
Lexapro (escitalopram), dosage of, 1117t
LGA (large-for-gestation-age) infants
health and disease in, 153
maternal diabetes and, 964–966, 965t, 966t
maternal obesity and, 144
LH (luteinizing hormone), in pregnancy, 114f
LHR (lung area to head circumference ratio), in congenital diaphragmatic hernia, 288, 441, 442t, 443f
Lidocaine, during pregnancy, 801t
Lifestyle modifications, for GERD, 1044, 1045, 1045f
Likelihood ratios, 215–216
in Down syndrome, 221–222, 222t, 225, 226, 226t
Liley, William, 477
Limb reduction defects (LRD), after chorionic villus sampling, 256
Limits of viability, 1200–1202
Linea nigra, 1124
Linezolid, for mastitis, 764
Linkage analysis, 30–31, 30f, 33–34
Linkage disequilibrium, 34
Lipid(s)
in surfactant, 197, 197f
total plasma, during pregnancy, 119
Lipoproteins, during pregnancy, 119
Listeriosis, 773, 1100
fetal loss due to, 623
Lithium
during lactation, 1119–1120
perinatal complications of, 1119
as teratogen, 351t, 353, 1116–1117
for thyroid storm, 1003, 1003t
Little, William John, 1214
Livedo reticularis, 1080
Liver
acute fatty, 1062–1063, 1063t
acute renal failure due to, 909
imaging of, 1059–1060
Liver disease, 1059–1073
acute fatty liver of pregnancy as, 1062–1063, 1063t
acute liver failure as, 1071–1072, 1071t, 1072t
Budd-Chiari syndrome as, 1070
chronic, 1069–1071
Liver disease *(Continued)*
cirrhosis as, 1070–1071
primary biliary, 1069
coincidental to pregnancy, 1064–1069, 1065t, 1066t, 1068t
diagnosis of, 1059–1060, 1059t
in HELLP syndrome, 1063
hepatitis as
nonviral, 1069
viral, 1064–1069, 1065t, 1066t, 1068t
due to herpes simplex virus, 1069
due to HIV infection, 1069
intrahepatic cholestasis of pregnancy as, 1060–1061
liver infarction as, 1064
liver rupture as, 1064
liver transplantation for, 1072–1073
overlap syndromes with, 1062–1064, 1063t
portal hypertension as, 1071
in preeclampsia, 1063
primary sclerosing cholangitis as, 1070
unique to pregnancy, 1060–1064, 1063t
Wilson disease as, 1070
Liver failure, acute, 1071–1072, 1071t, 1072t
Liver function, in pregnancy, 1059, 1060t
Liver function tests
in acute fatty liver of pregnancy, 1062, 1063t
in acute liver failure, 1071
in preeclampsia, 658
in pregnancy, 1059, 1060t
Liver infarction, 1064
Liver rupture, 1064
Liver transplantation, 1072–1073
Liver tumors, fetal, 293
LMP (last menstrual period), and gestational age, 613
LMWH. *See* Low molecular weight heparin (LMWH).
Local immune suppression, 90, 90f
Locus heterogeneity, 25
Long arm, 12, 12f
Long limb gastric bypass, 1051, 1051t
Long-chain 3-hydroxyacyl-coenzyme A dehydrogenase (LCHAD) deficiency, 1062
Loop electrosurgical excision procedure (LEEP), 887, 888
cervical cerclage after, 592–593
cervical insufficiency due to, 586–587
and preterm birth, 557–558
Loperamide (Imodium), for inflammatory bowel disease, 1049
Lopinavir/ritonavir (Kaletra), for HIV infection, 772, 772t
Lorazepam, for status epilepticus, 1090
Low birth weight (LBW)
and adult disease, 151–152, 152f, 153
antidepressants and, 1118
defined, 545
extremely. *See* Extremely low birth weight (ELBW).
incidence of, 545–546, 546f
and preterm labor and birth, 545–546
prevention of, 154
very. *See* Very low birth weight (VLBW).
Low molecular weight heparin (LMWH)
for antiphospholipid antibody syndrome, 830–831, 1084, 1084t
with prosthetic heart valves, 819, 820t, 864
for recurrent pregnancy loss due to inherited thrombophilia, 628
for rheumatic disease, 1082t
for venous thromboembolism, 863
prevention of, 836, 865

Low spinal anesthesia, for labor and delivery, 716
Low-dose aspirin (LDA), for antiphospholipid antibody syndrome, 830–831
Lower esophageal sphincter (LES), in pregnancy, 1041, 1043
Lower urinary tract obstruction (LUTO)
invasive fetal therapy for, 277t, 434t, 444–445, 445t
pathophysiology of, 444
Low-glycemic foods, for diabetes, 974
Low-lying placenta, 725, 726f
LRD (limb reduction defects), after chorionic villus sampling, 256
L/S ratio. *See* Lecithin/sphingomyelin (L/S) ratio.
LSVC (left-sided vena cava), persistent, 318–320, 319f, 320f
L-TGA (levo-transposition of the great arteries), 334, 334f
L-thyroxine (levothyroxine)
for hypopituitarism, 1023
for prevention of postpartum thyroiditis, 1010–1011
Lumbar disk protrusion, 1104
Lumbosacral plexus lesion, 1105
Lumbosacral root lesions, 1104
Lung(s), wet, 1202–1203, 1203f
Lung anomalies, 285–289, 286f–289f
Lung area to head circumference ratio (LHR), in congenital diaphragmatic hernia, 288, 441, 442t, 443f
Lung bud, 193, 194f
Lung development, fetal, 193–204, 194t
alveolar stage of, 194f, 194t, 195–196, 195t, 196f
canalicular stage of, 194, 194f, 194t
embryonic stage of, 193, 194f, 194t
fetal breathing movements and, 176–177
fetal lung fluid in, 197
induced maturation in, 202–204, 203f, 203t
pseudoglandular stage of, 193, 194f, 194t
and pulmonary hypoplasia, 196–197, 196t
saccular stage of, 194–195, 194f, 194t, 195f
surfactant in, 197–202
composition of, 197–198, 197f
metabolism of, 198–200, 199f, 201f
physiologic effects of, 200–202, 201f
for respiratory distress syndrome, 202, 202f
Lung fluid, fetal, 49, 197
Lung maturation, induced. *See* Fetal pulmonary maturity, induction of.
Lung profile, fetal, 419
Lupus erythematosus, systemic. *See* Systemic lupus erythematosus (SLE).
Lupus flare, 914, 1081
Lupus nephritis, 914, 916t
Luteal phase defect, fetal loss due to, 620
Luteal-placental shift, timing of, 114–115, 115f
Luteinizing hormone (LH), in pregnancy, 114f
Luteomas, 1031
Lutheran antigen, 478f
LUTO (lower urinary tract obstruction)
invasive fetal therapy for, 277t, 434t, 444–445, 445t
pathophysiology of, 444
Luvox (fluvoxamine), dosage of, 1117t
Lyme disease, breastfeeding with, 136t
Lymphadenectomy, for cervical cancer, 888, 889
Lymphangioma, cystic, 289–290, 289f
Lymphatic hamartoma, 289–290, 289f
Lymphocytic adenohypophysitis (LAH), 1023–1024, 1023t
Lymphocytic thyroiditis, chronic, 1007
Lymphoma
Burkitt, 899
diffuse, large B-cell, 898–899
Hodgkin, 896–898, 897t
non-Hodgkin, 897t, 898–899
Lysosomal storage diseases, hydrops fetalis due to, 511

M

M antigen, 497–498
MacLayne, Eufame, 715
Macroadenoma, 1019, 1020t
Macrobid (nitrofurantoin monohydrate macrocrystals), for asymptomatic bacteriuria and acute cystitis, 752t, 906
Macrocytic anemia, 869, 872
Macronutrient intake, 147
Macrophages, during pregnancy, 90
Macrosomia
excessive weight gain and, 145
maternal diabetes and, 964–966, 965t, 966t, 982–984
maternal obesity and, 144
with post-term pregnancy, 614
Magma reticulare, 38
Magnesium
for preterm labor, 561
as uterine relaxant, 80–81
Magnesium sulfate ($MgSO_4$)
anesthesia with, 1148
for preeclampsia, 671–672, 672t
for preterm labor, 565–566
and cerebral palsy, 1216
Magnetic resonance arteriography (MRA), for pulmonary embolus, 860, 861f, 862
Magnetic resonance imaging (MRI)
of adnexal masses, 1141
of appendicitis, 1047, 1047t
of breast cancer, 892
of hypoxic-ischemic encephalopathy, 1211
of perinatal stroke, 1213f, 1214
Magnetic resonance (MR) venography, of deep venous thrombosis, 857
Major depressive disorder
diagnostic criteria for, 1113, 1115t
epidemiology of, 1113
identification of, 1114
impact on pregnancy outcomes of, 1116
treatment of
clinical approach to, 1118–1119
dosage for, 1117t
during lactation, 1119–1120
perinatal complications of, 1119
risks of, 1117–1118
Malalignment ventricular septal defects, 324, 324f
Malformation sequence, hydrops fetalis due to, 508t
Malignancy(ies), 885–899
breast cancer as, 891–895, 892t, 893f
cervical, 886–889, 886t
colon cancer as, 895–896
epidemiology of, 885
gestational trophoblastic neoplasia as, 891
hematologic, 896–899, 897t
malignant melanoma as, 895, 1123
ovarian, 885–886, 886t
treatment of, 889–891, 889t
Malignant melanoma, 895, 1123
Malnutrition
intrauterine growth restriction due to, 639–640
neonatal outcomes with, 1198
Malpresentation, 703–707
breech as, 703–706, 705t
compound, 707
deflection abnormalities as, 706–707
transverse lie as, 706
uterine anomalies and, 1144
uterine myomas and, 1137
Mammary fat pad, 129, 129f
Mammary gland(s)
accessory, 128
development of, 127–128, 127f, 128f, 130t
during lactation, 130
in pregnancy, 130
Mammary lobulus, 129f
Mammary lobus, 129f
Mammary pit, 127
Mammogenesis, 127–128, 127f, 128f, 130t
Mammography, 892
Mammoplasty
augmentation, breastfeeding after, 132
reduction, breastfeeding after, 126, 132
Management of Myelomeningocele study (MOMS), 446
Mania. *See also* Bipolar disorder.
symptoms of, 1113, 1114t, 1115t
Manic episode, 1113, 1114t, 1115t
Mannitol, for cerebral edema, in acute liver failure, 1072
MAOIs (monoamine oxidase inhibitors), dosage of, 1117t
Maple syrup urine disease, carrier screening for, 242t
Marburg virus, breastfeeding with, 135
Marfan syndrome
maternal, 818, 818f, 819f
anesthesia with, 1159–1160
prenatal diagnosis of, 248t
Markers, defined, 225
Mastectomy, 893
Mastitis, 138, 138f, 138t, 764
breastfeeding with, 135, 137t
Matched study design, 213
Maternal age
and fetal loss, 619–620, 623
and preeclampsia and eclampsia, 654
and prenatal screening, 222, 222t, 232–233, 233t
Maternal antibody titer, 481
Maternal blood donation, for intrauterine transfusion, 491–492
Maternal circulation
fetal cell-free RNA in, 263
prenatal diagnosis using fetal cells in, 261–262
Maternal monitoring, with preeclampsia, 668–669
Maternal mortality and morbidity
due to cesarean delivery, 708–710
due to chronic hypertension, 676
defined, 1167
due to diabetes, 958–963
epidemiology of, 1167, 1168f
with multiple gestation, 454–455
prediction of, 1167–1168
due to preeclampsia, 655
Maternal serum α-fetoprotein (MSAFP)
and abruptio placentae, 732
after chorionic villus sampling, 255–256
prenatal screening for, 223, 224, 224t, 233–235, 234t
in twins, 257, 257t, 458, 459
Maternal stress, preterm labor and birth due to, 529, 530f, 555
Maternal-fetal metabolism, in normal and diabetic pregnancy, 955–958, 956f, 957f

Maternal-fetal tolerance, 87
Maternal-placental tolerance, 87
Matrilineal inheritance, 29
Matrix metalloproteinases (MMPs)
in implantation, 113t
in membrane rupture, 599
in preterm labor, 523, 528
Maturity-onset diabetes of the young (MODY), 955
MCA. *See* Middle cerebral artery (MCA).
McDonald cerclage, 590, 593
MCP-1 (monocyte chemoattractant protein-1), 73
McRoberts maneuver, for shoulder dystocia, 697
MDK (multicystic dysplastic kidney), 295, 295f
Mean, regression to the, 26
Mean arterial pressure, 1171t
Mean corpuscular hemoglobin concentration (MCHC), in anemia, 870t
Mean corpuscular volume (MCV), in anemia, 870t
Measles, 776–777
atypical, 777
German (3-day). *See* Rubella.
Measles encephalitis, 776–777
Measles vaccine, 777
Mechanical heart valves, pregnancy with, 819–820, 820t, 864
Mechanical ventilation, for respiratory distress syndrome, 1174, 1204
Meconium, umbilical cord acid-base balance with, 404
Meconium aspiration syndrome, 1206–1207
with intrauterine growth restriction, 646
with post-term pregnancy, 614–615
Meconium staining, 1206–1207
with post-term pregnancy, 614–615
Medawar, Peter, 87
Median nerve compression, 1105, 1106f
Medications. *See* Drug(s).
Megacystis, 296–297, 297f
obstructive, 296–297, 297f
Megacystis-microcolon-intestinal hypoperistalsis syndrome (MMIHS), 296
Megaloblastic anemia, 874
Megaureter, 296
Meiosis, 8–10, 8f–11f
clinical significance of, 10
sex differences in, 9–10, 10f, 11f
stages of, 8–9, 8f, 9f
Meiotic cell division, 8–10, 8f–11f
Meiotic division I, 8–9, 8f
Meiotic division II, 8f, 9
Meiotic nondisjunction, 10, 14–15, 15f
Melanocytic nevi, 1124
Melanoma, malignant, 895, 1123
Melasma, 1124
Mellaril (thioridazine), dosage of, 1116t
Membrane(s), 599
stripping (sweeping) of, for cervical ripening, 702t
Membrane activation, in labor and delivery, 523
Membrane permeability, 50
Membrane rupture. *See also* Abruptio placentae.
physiology of, 599–600
premature. *See* Premature rupture of the membranes (PROM).
spontaneous, 599
Membrane transfer, 50
Membrane water flow, 50–51
Membranous twin, 64, 64f, 65f
Membranous ventricular septal defects, 323–324, 323f
Memory T cells, and pregnancy loss, 621
Mendel, Gregor, 22
Mendelian disorders, 22
Mendelson syndrome, 930
Meningiomas, 1093
Menstrual disturbances
due to acromegaly, 1021
due to hyperthyroidism, 1000
due to hypothyroidism, 1000–1001
due to radioiodine, 1001
Mental retardation
biophysical profile score and, 389t
due to hypothyroidism, 1007
due to iodine deficiency, 1006
Meperidine
for labor and delivery, 715
for migraines, 1093
Meralgia paresthetica, 1105–1106
6-Mercaptopurine, for inflammatory bowel disease, 1049
Mercury, in fish, 147, 147t
Meropenem, for pelvic abscess, 762
Mesoderm, 38, 39f, 40
Mesomelic dysplasia, 298
Messenger RNA (mRNA), 5, 5f
Meta-analysis, 209–210, 209f, 210f
Metabolic acidemia, 401, 401t
Metabolic acidosis, 401–402
Metabolic changes
in preeclampsia, 658
in pregnancy, 119–122
Metabolic disorders
hydrops fetalis due to, 508t, 511
neurologic manifestations of, 1101–1102
Metabolic factors, affecting fetal acid-base balance, 401–402
Metabolic homeostasis, in pregnancy, 120f
Metabolic management, of diabetes, 973–982
avoiding ketosis in, 974
avoiding nocturnal hypoglycemia in, 974
dietary therapy in, 973–974
glucose monitoring for, 974–976
pregestational, 970
target levels in, 975–976, 975f, 976f, 976t
timing of, 974–975, 975t
insulin therapy in, 976–980, 977f, 977t, 979t
low glycemic foods in, 974
oral hypoglycemic agents in, 970, 980–982
preconceptional, 970
principles of, 973–974
Metabolic syndrome
in childhood and adolescence, 152–153
maternal diabetes and, 968
preeclampsia and, 656
Metanephrine, in pheochromocytoma, 1030
Metaphase
meiotic, 8f, 9
mitotic, 7f, 8
Metaphase chromosomes, preparation of, 11–12, 12f, 13f
Metastasis, of breast cancer, 892
Metformin, for diabetes, 970, 981–982
Methadone, neonatal outcomes with, 1199
Methotrexate
for inflammatory bowel disease, 1049
for rheumatic disease, 1081, 1082t
as teratogen, 351t, 352, 894
α-Methyl paratyrosine, for pheochromocytoma, 1030
Methylcellulose, for constipation, 1052, 1052t
Methyldopa
for chronic hypertension, 678, 678t, 679
for preeclampsia, 673
Methylene tetrahydrofolate reductase (MTHFR) gene mutations, 833–834
Methylergonovine (Methergine)
for postpartum hemorrhage, 698
for uterine atony, 1183t
Methylmercury, as teratogen, 354
Methylprednisolone
for asthma, 942
for hyperemesis gravidarum, 1043
for induction of fetal pulmonary maturity, 423t
for rheumatic disease, 1081, 1082t
Metoclopramide
for GERD, 1044
for hyperemesis gravidarum, 1043
for nausea and vomiting, 1042
Metronidazole
for bacterial vaginosis, 741, 742, 742t
for inflammatory bowel disease, 1049
for pelvic abscess, 762
for puerperal endometritis, 760
for septic shock, 763
for trichomoniasis, 741
Metyrapone, for Cushing syndrome, 1022
MFPR (multifetal pregnancy reduction), 470–471, 471t
$MgSO_4$. *See* Magnesium sulfate ($MgSO_4$).
MI (myocardial infarction), 817
Miconazole, for vulvovaginal candidiasis, 740t
Microadenoma, 1019, 1020f, 1020t
Microalbuminuria, 959, 959t, 960, 960f
Microbial invasion of the amniotic cavity (MIAC), preterm labor due to, 525
Microcephaly, 284
Microcytic anemia, 869, 872
Microdeletion syndrome, 15, 16t
Microduplication syndromes, 15
Micrognathia, 285, 1198t
Microsatellites, 31, 33
Middle cerebral artery (MCA)
Doppler studies of
fetal, 374–375, 375f
with intrauterine growth restriction, 644
in Rh-immunized pregnancy, 485–488, 485f, 486f, 490
maternal, 377–378, 379f
occlusion of, 1095
Mid-forceps delivery, 713, 714
Mifepristone (RU-486), 73
for cervical ripening, 702t
Migraine headaches, 1092–1093
Milk ducts
anatomy of, 129
development of, 127–128, 127f, 128f
plugged, 138, 138t
Milk ejection reflex, 131, 132f, 133, 133f
Milk line, 127
Milk production, 127f, 130–131, 130t, 131f
Milk rejection sign, 891
Milk ridge, 127
Milk streak, 127
Milk supply, faltering, 134
Milk-alkali syndrome, 1034
Milk-retention cysts, 138
Milk-to-plasma ratio, 140–141
β-Mimetic drugs, for preterm labor, 566
Mineral deficiencies, after bariatric surgery, 1051, 1051t
Mineral supplementation, during pregnancy, 146, 146t
Mineralocorticoids, pathways of synthesis of, 1025, 1025f
Minimata disease, congenital, 354
Mini-sequencing, 32

Minor depressive disorder
diagnostic criteria for, 1113, 1115t
epidemiology of, 1113
identification of, 1114
Minute ventilation, during pregnancy, 927, 1173
Mirror syndrome, 654
due to nonimmune hydrops, 505–506
Miscarriage(s). *See also* Pregnancy loss; Spontaneous abortion.
antidepressants and, 1117–1118
uterine myomas and, 1136, 1138
Misoprostol (Cytotec)
for cervical ripening, 702–703
for fetal demise, 627–628
for postpartum hemorrhage, 699
for post-term pregnancy, 616
for uterine atony, 1183t
Mithramycin, for hypercalcemia, 1034, 1034t
Mitochondrial DNA (mtDNA), in developmental origins of health and disease, 154
Mitochondrial inheritance, 29
Mitochondrial trifunctional protein (MTP), 1062
Mitosis, 7–8, 7f
clinical significance of, 10
Mitotic cell division, 7–8, 7f
Mitotic nondisjunction, 10
Mitral atresia, hypoplastic left heart syndrome with, 329, 329f
Mitral insufficiency, anesthesia with, 1155–1156
Mitral regurgitation, maternal, 812, 812f, 813
anesthesia with, 1155–1156
Mitral stenosis, maternal, 805, 811–812, 811f
anesthesia with, 1154–1155
hemodynamics of, 1170–1171
Mitral valve, fetal echocardiography of, 313
Mitral valve prolapse (MVP), maternal, 812, 812f
anesthesia with, 1156
Mixed acidemia, 401, 401t
Mixed venous oxygen saturation (SVO_2), 929
Mixed venous oxygen tension, 929
Mixed venous oxygenation, 929
MLCK (myosin light-chain kinase)
in myometrial contraction, 78
in tocolysis, 562
MMC (myelomeningocele), invasive fetal therapy for, 277t, 445–447, 447t
MMIHS (megacystis-microcolon-intestinal hypoperistalsis syndrome), 296
M-mode analysis, of fetal arrhythmias, 337, 337f
MMPs (matrix metalloproteinases)
in implantation, 113t
in membrane rupture, 599
in preterm labor, 523, 528
MNS antigens, 478f, 495t, 497–498, 497t
MODY (maturity-onset diabetes of the young), 955
Molar pregnancy, 42, 891
hyperthyroidism due to, 1005
and preeclampsia, 654
Molecular cytogenetics, 12–14, 13f, 14f
Molluscum fibrosum gravidarum, 1124
Mometasone, for asthma, 941t
MOMS (Management of Myelomeningocele study), 446
Monilial vaginitis, 739–741, 740t
Monoamine oxidase, in fetal heart, 163
Monoamine oxidase inhibitors (MAOIs), dosage of, 1117t
Monoamniotic twins, 57, 58, 59f, 60, 61, 466–467, 466f
Monochorionic twins, 57, 57f, 58, 60
acardiac, 65f
antenatal diagnosis of, 455–456, 456t
diamniotic, 58, 58f, 60–61, 61f, 62f
Monochorionic twins *(Continued)*
intrauterine demise of one fetus with, 469
invasive fetal therapy with, 436–440, 436t, 438f, 439t
monoamniotic, 60
selective termination with, 470
twin-to-twin transfusion syndrome with, 62f, 63f
Monocyte(s), during pregnancy, 90
Monocyte chemiluminescence test, for RhD antibody, 481
Monocyte chemoattractant protein-1 (MCP-1), 73
Monocyte monolayer assay, for RhD antibody, 481
5′-Monodeiodination, in normal thyroid physiology, 995, 996f
Monogenetic disorders, preimplantation genetic screening for, 160
Monoiodotyrosine, in normal thyroid physiology, 995
Mononeuropathies
peripheral, 1104–1107, 1106f
traumatic, 1106
Monosomy, 15, 17, 18f
Monozygotic (MZ) twins, 55
causes of, 56, 57f
frequency of, 55–56
heterokaryotic, 66
identification of, 66–67
placentation of, 57, 58, 58f
Montelukast (Singulair), for asthma, 940t, 942
Montgomery glands, 129, 129f
Mood disorders, 1113–1120
diagnostic criteria for, 1113, 1114t, 1115t
epidemiology of, 1113
identification of, 1113–1114
impact on pregnancy outcomes of, 1114, 1115–1116
symptoms of, 1114t
treatment of, 1116–1120
clinical approach to, 1118–1119
dosage for, 1116t, 1117t
during lactation, 1119–1120
perinatal complications of, 1119
risks of, 1116–1118
Mood stabilizers
clinical approach to, 1119
dosage of, 1116t
during lactation, 1119–1120
perinatal complications of, 1119
risks of, 1116–1117
Morning sickness, 1042
Morphine sulfate, for prolonged latent phase, 694
Mortality Prediction Model (MPM), 1167
Morula, 37, 38f
Mosaic results
of amniocentesis, 249
of chorionic villus sampling, 254–255
Mosaicism
in amniocentesis, 249
confined placental, 254–255
Motor vehicle accidents, 1184–1186, 1185f
Movement(s), fetal, 172, 173f, 175, 177, 361
in biophysical profile score, 365t, 366
counting of, 383, 383t
Movement disorders, 1102
MPM (Mortality Prediction Model), 1167
MR (magnetic resonance) venography, of deep venous thrombosis, 857
MRA (magnetic resonance arteriography), for pulmonary embolus, 860, 861f, 862
MRI. *See* Magnetic resonance imaging (MRI).
mRNA (messenger RNA), 5, 5f
MSAFP. *See* Maternal serum α-fetoprotein (MSAFP).
MTD (*Mycobacterium tuberculosis* Direct) Test, 935
mtDNA (mitochondrial DNA), in developmental origins of health and disease, 154
MTHFR (methylene tetrahydrofolate reductase) gene mutations, 833–834
MTP (mitochondrial trifunctional protein), 1062
Mucolipidosis type IV, carrier screening for, 242t
Mueller-Hillis maneuver, 697
Müllerian duct fusion anomalies
cervical insufficiency due to, 586
pregnancy loss due to, 622, 622t
and preterm birth, 557
Multicolor karyotyping, 13–14, 14f
Multicystic dysplastic kidney (MDK), 295, 295f
Multifactorial inheritance, 25–29, 27t, 28t
Multifetal gestation. *See* Multiple gestation.
Multifetal pregnancy reduction (MFPR), 470–471, 471t
Multiorgan injury, due to hypoxic-ischemic encephalopathy, 1210
Multiple gestation, 55–67, 453–471
abnormalities of, 64–66, 64f–66f
acardiac twin in, 64–65, 65f, 66f, 467–468
invasive fetal therapy for, 434t, 468
amniocentesis in, 257–258, 258t, 459
aneuploidy in, 256, 256t, 458–459, 458t
antepartum management of, 459–461
birth weight with, 454
breastfeeding after, 134
causes of, 56, 57f
and cerebral palsy, 1215
cervical length in, 457, 460
chimeras in, 66
chorionic villus sampling with, 258, 258t, 459
chorionicity of, 57, 57f–60f, 58, 455f, 454–456
conjoined, 57, 60, 468–469, 468f
diagnosis of, 455
diamniotic, 57, 57f, 58
acardiac, 65f
dichorionic, 57–58, 58f, 59f
monochorionic, 58, 58f, 60–61, 61f, 62f
twin-to-twin transfusion syndrome with, 63f
dichorionic, 57, 57f–59f, 58
diagnosis of, 455–456, 456f
selective termination with, 470
disappearance of twin in, 66
dizygotic, 55
causes of, 56
frequency of, 56
identification of, 66–67
placentation of, 57–58, 58f, 59f
Down syndrome in, 256, 256t, 257, 257t, 458–459, 458t
fetal anomalies in, 456, 457–459, 458t
fetal growth in, 456–457
fetal loss with, 625
fetal pulmonary maturity in, 421, 461
fetal surveillance in, 457, 461
fetal well-being in, 457
fraternal, 55
higher-order
labor and delivery with, 463
pregnancy reduction with, 470–471, 471t
identical, 55
incidence of, 55, 453, 454t
intrapartum management of, 461–463
intrauterine demise of one fetus in, 469
intrauterine growth restriction due to, 639
maternal adaptations to, 454–455
maternal complications of, 461
maternal mortality and morbidity with, 454

Multiple gestation *(Continued)*
membranous, 64, 64f, 65f
monoamniotic, 57, 58, 59f, 60, 61, 466–467, 466f
monochorionic, 57, 57f, 58, 60f
acardiac, 65f
antenatal diagnosis of, 455–456, 456t
diamniotic, 58, 58f, 60–61, 61f, 62f
intrauterine demise of one fetus with, 469
invasive fetal therapy with, 436–440, 436t, 438f, 439t
monoamniotic, 60
selective termination with, 470
twin-to-twin transfusion syndrome with, 62f, 63f
monozygotic, 55
causes of, 56, 57f
frequency of, 55–56
heterokaryotic, 66
identification of, 66–67
placentation of, 57, 58, 58f
neonatal outcomes with, 1198
neural tube defects with, 459
nutrition with, 148
perinatal mortality and morbidity with, 453–454, 454f, 461
placentation in, 57–61, 57f–60f
preeclampsia with, 460–461, 654
pregnancy reduction with, 470–471, 471t
prenatal diagnosis with, 256–258, 256t–258t
preterm labor and birth with
interventions for, 460
pathogenesis of, 529–531, 531f, 558
rates of, 460, 546, 547f, 558, 559f, 559t
selective termination of anomalous fetus in, 469–470
twin reversed arterial perfusion sequence in, 64–65, 65f, 66f, 467–468
twin-to-twin transfusion syndrome in, 61–64, 61f–63f, 463–466, 463f
types of, 55–56
ultrasonography of, 455–457, 456f, 456t
velamentous insertion of umbilical cord and vasa praevia in, 59, 60f
zygosity in, 66–67, 67f
Multiple sclerosis, 1102–1103
anesthesia with, 1149
Multivariable analysis, 213
Multivitamins
for nausea and vomiting, 1042
during pregnancy, 146, 146t
Mumps, 773–774
Mumps vaccine, 774
Muscle biopsy, fetal, 259
Muscle disorders, 1109
Muscular dystrophy, prenatal diagnosis of, 248t
Muscular ventricular septal defects, 323, 323f
Musculoskeletal development, fetal, 177
Mutation(s), 5–6, 6f, 6t
dynamic, 29–30
new, 24
silent, 5f
MVP (mitral valve prolapse), maternal, 812, 812f
anesthesia with, 1156
Myasthenia gravis, 1108–1109
neonatal outcomes with, 1198
Mycobacterium avium-intracellulare, with HIV infection, 771
Mycobacterium tuberculosis. See Tuberculosis.
Mycobacterium tuberculosis Direct (MTD) Test, 935
Mycoplasma hominis
breastfeeding with, 136t
and bronchopulmonary dysplasia, 1205
Mycoplasma pneumoniae, pneumonia due to, 931
Myelomeningocele (MMC), invasive fetal therapy for, 277t, 445–447, 447t
Myocardial function, fetal, 162–164
Myocardial infarction (MI), 817
Myocardial ischemia, 816–817
Myocarditis
with HIV infection, 816
hydrops fetalis due to, 509
Myocardium, fetal, 163
Myomas. *See* Uterine leiomyomas.
Myomectomy
cesarean, 1039
hysteroscopic, 1039
laparoscopic, 1039
laparotomic, 1039
during pregnancy, 1138–1139
pregnancy after, 1039
Myometrial contractions, 76–82
defined, 522
in diagnosis, 70
effectiveness of, 522
fetal heart rate with, 410f, 411t
hormonal regulation of, 79–81, 79f, 80t
during labor, 522–523
measurement of, 399
mechanics of, 76–79, 78f
in pregnancy, 691
and preterm birth, 558, 560
regulation of electrical activity in, 76, 77f
Myometrial differentiation, 79
Myometrial hyperplasia, 69
Myometrial remodeling, in pregnancy, 522
Myometrial stretch, preterm labor due to, 529–531, 531f
Myometrium, regulation of electrical activity within, 76, 77f
Myonecrosis, at episiotomy incision site, 760
Myosin, in myometrial contraction, 76
Myosin head, in myometrial contraction, 76–78, 78f
Myosin light-chain kinase (MLCK)
in myometrial contraction, 78
in tocolysis, 562
Myosin-actin crossbridge, in myometrial contraction, 78f
Myotonia congenita, 1109
Myotonic dystrophy, 1109
autosomal dominant, 30
prenatal diagnosis of, 248t
MZ twins. *See* Monozygotic (MZ) twins.

N

N antigen, 498
NAATs (nucleic acid amplification tests)
for *Chlamydia trachomatis,* 747
for gonorrhea, 744, 745
Nabumetone, for rheumatic disease, 1082t
NAEPP (National Asthma Education and Prevention Program), 938, 941, 942, 943
Nafcillin
for mastitis, 764
for wound infection, 761
Nail changes, in pregnancy, 1124
NAIT (neonatal alloimmune thrombocytopenia), 840–842, 840t
Naproxen, for rheumatic disease, 1082t
Narcosis, therapeutic, for prolonged latent phase, 694
Narcotic analgesics, for labor and delivery, 715
Nasal anomalies, 285
Nasal bone (NB), in Down syndrome, 225, 230–231, 231f, 232
Nasal bone (NB) contingency screening, for Down syndrome, 232
Nasal tolerance, to RhD antigen, 495
National Asthma Education and Prevention Program (NAEPP), 938, 941, 942, 943
National Institute of Child Health and Human Development Maternal-Fetal Medicine Units (NICHD-MFMU) Network study, 427
National Institutes of Health (NIH) Consensus Panel on Antenatal Steroids, 427t, 428
National Transplantation Pregnancy Registry (NTPR), 920
Natriuretic peptides, in fetal cardiovascular regulation, 165–166
Natural immunity, 87
in pregnancy, 90–92, 91f
Natural killer (NK) cells
during pregnancy, 90
and pregnancy loss, 621
Nausea and vomiting, 1041–1042, 1042t
nutrition with, 148
Navane (thiothixene), dosage of, 1116t
NB (nasal bone), in Down syndrome, 225, 230–231, 231f, 232
NB (nasal bone) contingency screening, for Down syndrome, 232
Necrotizing enterocolitis (NEC), 1207–1208, 1208f
feeding problems due to, 1210
prematurity and, 1201t
Necrotizing fasciitis
due to abdominal wound infection, 761–762
at episiotomy incision site, 760
Negative predictive value (NPV), 214–215, 215t, 221
Neisseria gonorrhoeae. See Gonorrhea.
Nelfinavir (Viracept), for HIV infection, 772t
Nelson syndrome, 1022
Neomorphic allele, 6
Neonatal abstinence syndrome, 1199
Neonatal alloimmune thrombocytopenia (NAIT), 840–842, 840t
Neonatal behavior, transition from fetal to, 362
Neonatal complications
of cesarean delivery, 710
of diabetes, 967–968, 968f, 986
of intrauterine growth restriction, 646
of placenta previa, 729
after premature rupture of the membranes, 601
of renal transplantation, 920
Neonatal encephalopathy, 1210
Neonatal gonococcal ophthalmia, 744
Neonatal lupus syndrome, 1081
Neonatal management decisions, 1197
Neonatal morbidity and mortality
with alloimmune hemolytic disorders, 1199
with chorioamnionitis, 1197–1198
with congenital malformations, 1198–1199
with diabetes, 967–968, 968f, 986, 1197
excessive weight gain and, 145
with maternal autoimmune disease, 1198
with maternal malnutrition, 1198
with maternal medications, 1199
with multifetal gestation, 1198
with preeclampsia, 1198
with substance abuse, 1199
Neonatal outcomes, common morbidities of pregnancy and, 1197–1199, 1198t
Neonatal period
gastrointestinal problem(s) in, 1207–1210
feeding problems as, 1209–1210
hyperbilirubinemia as, 1208–1209, 1209t
necrotizing enterocolitis as, 1207–1208, 1208f

Neonatal period *(Continued)*
infectious disease(s) in, 1217–1220
chorioamnionitis as, 1217
with group B β-hemolytic streptococci, 1217
sexually transmitted, 1219–1220
viral, 1217–1219
neurologic problem(s) in, 1210–1217
cerebral palsy as, 1214–1217, 1214t
hypoxic-ischemic encephalopathy as, 1210–1211
intraventricular hemorrhage as, 1211–1212
perinatal stroke as, 1213–1214, 1213f
periventricular leukomalacia as, 1212
respiratory problem(s) in, 1202–1207
bronchopulmonary dysplasia as, 1205–1206, 1206f, 1206t
meconium aspiration syndrome as, 1206–1207
pulmonary hypertension as, 1207
pulmonary hypoplasia as, 1203–1204
respiratory distress syndrome as, 1203f, 1204–1205
transient tachypnea of the newborn as, 1202–1203, 1203f
Neonatal resuscitation, at limits of viability, 1202
Nephritis
hereditary, 912
lupus, 914, 916t
Nephropathy
diabetic, 913–914, 959–961
categories of, 959, 959t
course during pregnancy of, 916t, 959–960, 960f
effect of pregnancy on progression of, 959, 959f
epidemiology of, 959
pathophysiology of, 959
renal dialysis for, 960
renal transplantation for, 960–961
HIV-associated, 915
IgA, 916t
reflux, 913, 916t
Nephrosclerosis, in preeclampsia, 653t
Nephrosis, congenital, 235
Nephrotic syndrome, 915
Nephrotoxic drugs, 909
Nerve conduction studies, 1104–1105, 1106f
Neural tube defect(s) (NTDs), 281–282
anencephaly as, 281, 282f
diagnosis of, 281, 282f
encephalocele as, 281, 282f
folic acid deficiency and, 143
genetics of, 27–28, 27t
invasive fetal therapy for, 277t, 434t, 445–447, 447t
neonatal management of, 1198t
prenatal screening for, 233–235, 234t, 236f
in twins, 257, 459
spina bifida as, 281–282, 283f
Neuritis
acute familial brachial, 1105
optic, 1103
Neuroblastomas, adrenal, hydrops fetalis due to, 509
Neurodevelopmental abnormalities, childhood, diabetes and, 968–969
Neuroendocrine system, relationships and feedback mechanisms of, 1015, 1017f
Neurofibromatosis type 1, prenatal diagnosis of, 248t
Neurohormones, in placental tissues, 117t
Neurohypophysis. *See* Posterior pituitary lobe.
Neurologic disorder(s), 1089–1110
anesthesia with, 1149–1150
childhood, diabetes and, 968–969
epilepsy as, 1089–1092
headache as, 1092–1093
due to infections, 1099–1101
intracranial hemorrhage as, 1096–1098, 1097f, 1098f
due to metabolic disorders, 1101–1102
of movement, 1102
multiple sclerosis as, 1102–1103
of muscle, 1109
myasthenia gravis as, 1108–1109
occlusive cerebrovascular disease as, 1095–1096, 1095f–1097f
optic neuritis as, 1103
plexus lesions and peripheral mononeuropathies as, 1104–1107, 1106f
polyneuropathies as, 1107–1108
pseudotumor cerebri as, 1094–1095
psychiatric, 1109–1110
root lesions as, 1104
traumatic paraplegia as, 1103–1104
tumors as, 1093–1094, 1094f
due to vascular anomalies, 1098–1099
Neurologic injury
acute, umbilical cord acid-base balance and, 403–404
severe, 1189–1190, 1189t
Neurologic morbidity
due to intrauterine demise of one fetus in multiple gestation, 469
after intrauterine transfusion, 492
preterm birth and, 552
Neurologic outcome, with biophysical profile score management, 389, 389f, 389t
Neurologic problem(s), in neonatal period, 1210–1217
cerebral palsy as, 1214–1217, 1214t
hypoxic-ischemic encephalopathy as, 1210–1211
intraventricular hemorrhage as, 1211–1212
perinatal stroke as, 1213–1214, 1213f
periventricular leukomalacia as, 1212
Neuroma, acoustic, 1093
Neuropathy(ies)
nutritional, 1107
porphyric, 1108
retrobulbar, 1107
Neuropeptides, in placental tissues, 117t
Neuroprotectants, for preterm labor, 561
Neurosyphilis, 779–780, 781
Neutra-Phos, for hypercalcemia, 1034t
Nevirapine (Viramune), for HIV infection, 772t
Nevus(i)
araneus, 1123
melanocytic, 1124
NF-κB (nuclear factor kappa B), 92
NHL (non-Hodgkin lymphoma), in pregnancy, 897t, 898–899
NICHD-MFMU (National Institute of Child Health and Human Development Maternal-Fetal Medicine Units) Network study, 427
Nicotine. *See* Cigarette smoking.
Niemann-Pick disease type A, carrier screening for, 242t
Nifedipine
for chronic hypertension, 678t, 679
for preeclampsia, 673, 673t
during pregnancy, 801t
for preterm labor, 562–563
NIH. *See* Nonimmune hydrops (NIH).
NIH (National Institutes of Health) Consensus Panel on Antenatal Steroids, 427t, 428
Nipple(s)
accessory, 128
anatomy of, 129–130, 129f
candidiasis of, 135, 137t, 138–139
development of, 127, 127f
sore, 134
Nipple piercing, breastfeeding with, 126
Nipple tenderness, 134
Nitrates, during pregnancy, 801t
Nitrazine test, for premature rupture of the membranes, 602
Nitric oxide (NO)
in fetal cardiovascular regulation, 166
and patent ductus arteriosus, 167
in preeclampsia, 663
as uterine relaxant, 80
Nitric oxide (NO) donors, for preterm labor, 564–565
Nitrofurantoin, for acute pyelonephritis, 756
Nitrofurantoin monohydrate macrocrystals (Macrobid), for asymptomatic bacteriuria and acute cystitis, 752t, 906
Nitroglycerin, for retained placenta, 698
NK (natural killer) cells
during pregnancy, 90
and pregnancy loss, 621
NO. *See* Nitric oxide (NO).
Nocturnal hypoglycemia, avoidance of, for diabetes, 974
NOD (nucleotide-binding oligomerization domain) proteins, 92, 94–96, 94f, 95t
Noncarbonic acids, in fetal acid-base balance, 400
Nondisjunction, 14–15, 15f
meiotic, 10, 14–15, 15f
mitotic, 10
Nonhistone proteins, 7
Non-Hodgkin lymphoma (NHL), in pregnancy, 897t, 898–899
Nonimmune hydrops (NIH), 505–513
defined, 478, 505
delivery considerations with, 513
diagnostic approach to, 512–513
echocardiography of, 310
epidemiology of, 505
etiology of, 507–512, 508t
cardiovascular, 507–509, 508t
chondrodysplasia as, 508t, 511–512
chromosomal, 508t, 509
congenital cystic adenomatoid malformation as, 444, 509
diabetes in, 512
gastrointestinal, 508t, 512
hematologic, 508t, 510
hemolytic disease of the fetus and newborn as, 478–479
infectious, 508t, 510–511
malformation sequence as, 508t
medications in, 512
metabolic, 508t, 511
thoracic, 508t, 509–510
twin pregnancy as, 508t, 510
urinary, 508t, 512
experimental management of idiopathic, 512
fetal fluid accumulation in, 444, 506–507, 506f, 507f
management of, 513
mirror syndrome due to, 505–506
presenting signs and symptoms of, 505–506
recurrence risks for, 513
scoring system for, 506
ultrasonography of, 506, 506f, 507f
Non-nucleoside reverse transcriptase inhibitors, for HIV infection, 772t

Non–rapid eye movement (NREM) sleep, fetal, 171, 173–174, 176, 176t
Nonreflex late decelerations, in fetal heart rate, 409, 410f
Nonsense codons, 5f
Nonspecific vaginitis. *See* Bacterial vaginosis (BV).
Nonsteroidal anti-inflammatory drugs (NSAIDs)
  nephrotoxicity of, 909
  for preterm labor, 563
  for rheumatic disease, 1081, 1082t
Nonstress test (NST), 370
  in diabetic pregnancy, 983t
  nonreactive, 363–364, 364f, 370, 370t
  problems with using, 370, 370t
  reactive, 367f, 370, 370t
Nonvertex first twin, 462–463
Norepinephrine
  in fetal heart, 163
  sensitivity to, in preeclampsia, 662, 662f
  for septic shock, 1178t
Normocytic anemia, 869, 872
Norpramin (desipramine), dosage of, 1117t
Norprogesterones, as teratogens, 351t
Nortriptyline (Pamelor), dosage of, 1117t
Norvir (ritonavir), for HIV infection, 772, 772t
Novolog (insulin aspart), 977t, 978
NovoSeven (recombinant factor VIIa), for obstetric hemorrhage, 1182, 1183t
NPH insulin, 977f, 977t, 978, 980
NPV (negative predictive value), 214–215, 215t, 221
NREM (non–rapid eye movement) sleep, fetal, 171, 173–174, 176, 176t
NSAIDs (nonsteroidal anti-inflammatory drugs)
  nephrotoxicity of, 909
  for preterm labor, 563
  for rheumatic disease, 1081, 1082t
NST. *See* Nonstress test (NST).
NT (nuchal translucency), 227–229, 228f, 228t, 229f, 230
  with normal karyotype, 237, 237t
  in twins, 257, 459
NTDs. *See* Neural tube defect(s) (NTDs).
NTPR (National Transplantation Pregnancy Registry), 920
NTQR (Nuchal Translucency Quality Review), 229
Nuchal cords, umbilical cord acid-base balance with, 404
Nuchal muscle activity, fetal, 171, 172f
Nuchal skin fold
  in Down syndrome, 225, 227t
  in various aneuploidies, 227t
Nuchal translucency (NT), 227–229, 228f, 228t, 229f, 230
  with normal karyotype, 237, 237t
  in twins, 257, 459
Nuchal Translucency Quality Review (NTQR), 229
Nuclear factor kappa B (NF-κB), 92
Nucleic acid(s), fetal, in other body fluids, 262–263
Nucleic acid amplification tests (NAATs)
  for *Chlamydia trachomatis,* 747
  for gonorrhea, 744, 745
Nucleic acid hybridization, 31–32, 31f
Nucleoside analogues, for HIV infection, 772t
Nucleosomes, 7
Nucleotide analogue, for HIV infection, 772t
Nucleotide bases, 3–4, 4f, 5, 5f
Nucleotide-binding oligomerization domain (NOD) proteins, 92, 94–96, 94f, 95f
Null allele, 6
Nutrition, 143–148. *See also* Diet.
  with burns, 1187
  with cystic fibrosis, 946
  in developmental origins of health and disease, 154–155
  with dialysis, 917
  fish in, 147, 147t
  fish oil supplements in, 147
  folic acid in, 143
  and food-borne infections, 147
  guidelines for, 147–148, 147t
  inadequate maternal, intrauterine growth restriction due to, 639–640
  macronutrient intake in, 147
  with multiple gestation, 148, 455
  with nausea and vomiting, 148
  and obesity, 143–145
  pre-conception, 143–144
  underweight in, 143–144
  vegetarian diet in, 146t, 147–148
  vitamin and mineral supplementation in, 146, 146t
  and weight gain, 143, 145–146, 145t, 146t
Nutritional neuropathies, 1107
Nutritional status, and preterm birth, 555–556, 555f
Nutritional supplements
  for intrauterine growth restriction, 645
  for preterm birth prevention, 567–568, 569, 570t, 572
Nystatin, for vulvovaginal candidiasis, 740t

O

O_2. *See* Oxygen *entries.*
Obesity, 143–145
  bariatric surgery for, 1051–1052, 1051t
  in developmental origins of health and disease, 152–154, 155
  diabetes and, 955
    fetal, 964–966, 965t, 966t
    maternal, 955, 965, 966t, 968
  fetal, maternal diabetes and, 964–966, 965t, 966t, 984–986
  and fetal loss, 625
  maternal
    and adolescent metabolic syndrome, 968
    and diabetes, 955, 965, 966t, 968
    and fetal obesity, 965, 966t
  morbid
    anesthesia with, 1152
    defined, 1152
    labor and delivery with, 1152
  and preeclampsia, 654, 656
  prevalence of, 1051
Observational cohort studies, on safety of exposures, 349
Observational studies, 208, 208t
Obstetric deaths, direct *vs.* indirect, 1167
Obstetric forceps delivery, 713–714
  for breech presentation, 705
Obstetric hemorrhage, 1179–1184
  clinical staging of, 1180, 1180t
  defined, 1179–1180
  incidence and etiology of, 1179–1180
  management of, 1180–1184
    additional supportive measures in, 1182
    hemostasis in, 1182–1184, 1183t, 1184f
    volume replacement in, 1180–1182, 1180t–1182t
  protocol for, 727, 727t
Obstetric injury, cervical insufficiency due to, 586
Obstructive heart disease, maternal, 805–809, 806f–809f
Obturator nerve palsy, 1106
OC(s). *See* Oral contraceptives (OCs).
Occlusive cerebrovascular disease, 1095–1096, 1095f–1097f
Octreotide, for acromegaly, 1021
Odds ratio, 212, 213
Office of Women's Health, 351
Ofloxacin, for pelvic abscess, 762
Ogilvie syndrome, postcesarean, 709
OGTT (oral glucose tolerance test), 955, 955t, 971, 971t, 972, 972t
25(OH)D (25-hydroxycholecalciferol), 1032
1,25OH$_2$D (1α,25-dihydroxycholecalciferol), 1032
17-OHP (17α-hydroxyprogesterone), in pregnancy, 114f, 115
Olanzapine (Zyprexa)
  dosage of, 1116t
  risks of, 1116
Oligohydramnios, 47, 49, 50
  in biophysical profile score, 365–366, 367
  fetal breathing movements with, 177
  with post-term pregnancy, 615
  and pulmonary hypoplasia, 1203
Oliguria, in preeclampsia, 673–674, 1172
Omega-3 fatty acids
  in fish, 147
  for preterm birth prevention, 569, 570t
Omeprazole
  for GERD, 1044–1045
  for peptic ulcer disease, 1046
Omphalocele, 293, 294f
  and aneuploidy, 227t
Omphalomesenteric vessels, 40
Omphalopagus, 468
Oocytes, 9, 11f
Oogonia, 9
Open fetal surgery, 433–435
Operative vaginal delivery, umbilical cord acid-base balance with, 405, 405t
Ophthalmia
  gonococcal, neonatal, 744, 1219
  neonatorum, 1219
Opiate(s), for labor and delivery, 715
Opiate addiction, neonatal outcomes with, 1199
Opioids, for labor and delivery, 715
Opportunistic diseases, with HIV infection, 771
Optic neuritis, 1103
Oral contraceptives (OCs)
  anticonvulsants and, 1089
  and intrahepatic cholestasis of pregnancy, 1060, 1061
  and migraine headaches, 1093
  and stroke, 1096
Oral desensitization, for penicillin allergy, 780, 781t
Oral erythrocyte membrane therapy, for hemolytic disease of the fetus and newborn, 494
Oral glucose tolerance test (OGTT), 955, 955t, 971, 971t, 972, 972t
Oral hypoglycemic agents, 970, 980–982
Oral tolerance, to RhD antigen, 494
Orbits, fused, 285
Organ blood flow, fetal, 162, 162t
Organization of Teratology Information Specialists (OTIS), 350–351
Oseltamivir, for influenza, 785
Osmolarity, during pregnancy, 1016, 1018f
Osmotic threshold, during pregnancy, 1018f
Osteogenesis imperfecta, 298
Osteoporosis, pregnancy-related, 1035–1036
Ostium primum atrial septal defects
  fetal, 322
  maternal, 802f

Ostium secundum atrial septal defect, maternal, 802f
OTIS (Organization of Teratology Information Specialists), 350–351
Outflow tracts, fetal echocardiography of, 309, 309f, 314–315, 314f–316f
Ovarian cancer, 885–886, 886t, 1140, 1140t
Ovarian cysts, 1139–1143
 complications of, 1141–1142
 diagnosis of, 1140–1142, 1140t, 1141f, 1142f
  MRI for, 1141
  serologic markers for, 1140–1141
  ultrasonic characteristics in, 1140, 1140t, 1141f, 1142f
 epidemiology of, 886, 1139
 management of, 886, 1142–1143
 pathogenesis of, 1139, 1139t
Ovarian dysgerminoma, 886, 1141
Ovarian masses, 1139–1143
 complications of, 1141–1142
 diagnosis of, 1140–1142, 1140t, 1141f, 1142f
  MRI for, 1141
  serologic markers for, 1140–1141
  ultrasonic characteristics in, 1140, 1140t, 1141f, 1142f
 epidemiology of, 1139
 malignant, 885–886, 886t, 1140, 1140t
 management of, 1142–1143
 pathogenesis of, 1139, 1139t
Ovarian rupture, 1141–1142, 1143
Ovarian torsion, 886, 1141–1142, 1143
Ovarian vein syndrome, 763
Ovary, fetal, 115
Overdistention syndrome, 909
Overweight, 143–145
Ovulation stimulation, and preterm birth, 558
β-Oxidation, 1062
Oxidative stress, in preeclampsia, 666–667, 675–676
Oxygen capacity, of fetus, 187
Oxygen consumption (VO_2), 929, 929f
 placental, 185
 during pregnancy, 105, 929
 reduction of, by fetus, 363
Oxygen content
 arterial, 928
 fetal, 188
Oxygen delivery (DO_2), 928–929, 928f, 929f
 critical, 929, 929f
 fetal, 159–162, 160f–162f, 162t
 during pregnancy, 929
Oxygen diffusing capacity, placental, 184
Oxygen distribution, control of, by fetus, 363
Oxygen extraction ratio, 929
Oxygen partial pressure (PO_2)
 fetal, 362
  and intrauterine growth restriction, 640
  in labor, 402t
 during pregnancy, 1173t
 in uterine and umbilical circulations, 182–185, 182t, 183f, 184f, 186f
Oxygen saturation
 fetal, 160, 161, 161f, 414–415
  and behavioral state activity, 174, 174f
 and intrauterine growth restriction, 640
 mixed venous, 929
 during pregnancy, 1173t
 of uterine venous blood, 186–187
Oxygen supplementation, for septic shock, 763
Oxygen supply, increase in, by fetus, 362–363
Oxygen therapy, and fetal oxygenation, 189–190, 189f, 189t, 190f
Oxygen transport
 to fetal tissue, 187–189, 187t, 188f, 189f
 transplacental, 183–186, 183f, 184f, 186f
 to uterus, 181, 182f, 182t
Oxygen uptake, by uterus and fetus, 181–187, 182f
Oxygenation
 fetal, 187–189, 187t, 188f, 189f
  oxygen therapy and, 189–190, 189f, 189t, 190f
 mixed venous, 929
Oxygen-binding curve, 928, 928f
Oxygen-induced lung injury, and bronchopulmonary dysplasia, 1205
Oxyhemoglobin dissociation curve, 928, 928f
 maternal *vs.* fetal, 188, 188f
Oxytocin (Pitocin)
 in breastfeeding, 131, 132f, 133, 133f
 for cervical ripening, 702t
 in control of labor, 75–76
 fetal bradycardia due to, 407f
 with multiple gestation, 461
 for postpartum hemorrhage, 698
 during pregnancy, 121, 1016
 umbilical cord acid-base balance with, 405
 for uterine atony, 1183t
 as uterine stimulant, 80
Oxytocin augmentation
 for arrest disorders, 695
 for breech presentation, 705
 for prolonged latent phase, 694
 for protraction disorders, 695
Oxytocin challenge test, 381–382, 381f
Oxytocin induction
 for breech presentation, 705
 after premature rupture of the membranes, 604
Oxytocin receptor antagonists
 for preterm labor, 564
 as uterine relaxants, 81

P

17P (17α-hydroxyprogesterone caproate), for preterm labor, 532, 570–571, 570t, 571f
p region, 12, 12f
PAC. *See* Pulmonary artery catheter (PAC).
PAC(s) (premature atrial contractions), 336–337, 337f
Pachynema, 9
Packed red blood cells
 for abruptio placentae, 733t
 for hemorrhagic shock, 1181, 1181t
$PaCO_2$ (carbon dioxide arterial partial pressure), during pregnancy, 927
PAF (platelet activating factor), in preterm labor, 526f
PAI. *See* Plasminogen activator inhibitor (PAI) *entries.*
Pain, fetal, during fetoscopy, 435
Palmar erythema, 1123–1124
Pamelor (nortriptyline), dosage of, 1117t
Pamidronate, for hypercalcemia, 1034, 1034t
p-amino-salicylic acid, for tuberculosis, 937t
PAMPs (pathogen-associated molecular patterns), 92
Pancreatic transplantation, 1074
Pancreatitis, 1073–1074
Panhypopituitarism, 1022
Pap smear results, atypical, 887
Papilloma, laryngeal, 748–749
Papillomatosis, respiratory, 748–749
PAPP-A (pregnancy-associated plasma protein A), 229
 in twins, 257, 459
Papular dermatitis of pregnancy, 1127
PAPVR (partial anomalous pulmonary venous return), 321–322
PAR-1 (protease-activated receptor type 1), in preterm labor, 528
Paracentric inversion, 15
Paracervical block, for labor and delivery, 716
Paraplegia
 anesthesia with, 1149–1150
 traumatic, 1103–1104
Parasympathetic innervation, of fetal heart, 163–164
Parasympathetic nervous system, in fetal heart rate, 397
Parathyroid carcinoma, 1034–1035
Parathyroid glands
 disorders of, 1033–1036, 1033t–1035t
 fetal development of, 1032
 in lactation, 1032, 1032f, 1033f
 maternal and fetal physiology of, 1032, 1032f, 1033f
Parathyroid hormone (PTH), in calcium metabolism, 1032
Parathyroid hormone–related protein (PTHrP), 1032, 1032f, 1033f
 hypercalcemia due to increased production of, 1034
 as uterine relaxant, 80
Parathyroid hormone–related protein receptor (PTHrPR), in skeletal growth, 297
PARIS (Perinatal Antiplatelet Review of International Studies) Collaborative Group, 675
Parkland formula, for burns, 1187
Parnate (tranylcypromine), dosage of, 1117t
Paroxetine (Paxil), dosage of, 1117t
Paroxetine controlled release (Paxil-CR), dosage of, 1117t
Paroxysmal nocturnal hemoglobinuria (PNH), 876–877
Parran, Thomas, 777
Partial anomalous pulmonary venous return (PAPVR), 321–322
Partial atrioventricular canal defect, 325
Partial thromboplastin time, in abruptio placentae, 733t
Partogram, 693
Parturition. *See also* Labor and delivery.
 biology of, 69–81
 cervical ripening in, 523, 583–587
 membrane rupture in, 523
 myometrial activation in, 522–523
 parturition cascade, pathologic, 521–532
Parturition cascade, 70–72, 71f
Parvovirus, 774–775, 774t
 fetal loss due to, 623
 hydrops fetalis due to, 511, 774
Patent ductus arteriosus (PDA)
 maternal, 803–804, 804f
  anesthesia with, 1157
 prematurity and, 1201t
Paternal leukocyte immunization
 for hemolytic disease of the fetus and newborn, 495
 for pregnancy loss, 628t
Paternal zygosity testing, for RhD, 481–483, 482f–484f, 482t
Pathogen-associated molecular patterns (PAMPs), 92
Patient education
 for asthma, 940
 for constipation, 1052
Pattern recognition receptors (PRRs), 87, 91, 92
 in preterm labor, 526

Patterned behavior, fetal, 361–362
Paxil (paroxetine), dosage of, 1117t
Paxil-CR (paroxetine controlled release), dosage of, 1117t
PC. *See* Protein C (PC).
PCO_2 (carbon dioxide partial pressure)
  fetal, in labor, 402t
  during pregnancy, 104, 1173
PCOS (polycystic ovarian syndrome)
  fetal loss due to, 620–621
  insulin-resistant, 1031–1032
PCP (*Pneumocystis carinii* pneumonia). *See* *Pneumocystis jiroveci* pneumonia (PJP).
PCR (polymerase chain reaction), 30, 31f, 32, 32f
PCWP. *See* Pulmonary capillary wedge pressure (PCWP).
PDA (patent ductus arteriosus)
  maternal, 803–804, 804f
    anesthesia with, 1157
  prematurity and, 1201t
PE. *See* Pulmonary embolus (PE).
Peak expiratory flow rate (PEFR), in asthma, 938, 940
Peak systolic velocity (PSV), in fetal middle cerebral artery, 374–375, 374f
Pedigree, 23, 23f
Pegylated interferon, for hepatitis C virus, 1068
Pelvic abscess, 762
Pelvic artery embolization, for obstetric hemorrhage, 1183–1184
Pelvic floor dysfunction, cesarean delivery to prevent, 708, 711
Pelvic fractures, 1185–1186
Pelvic inflammatory disease, breastfeeding with, 136t
Pelvic vein thrombophlebitis, septic, 763–764
Pelvis, in labor, 692–693
Pemphigoid gestationis, 1125t, 1127–1129, 1128f, 1129f
Penetrance, 23–24, 26
Penetrating abdominal trauma, 1186
Penicillamine, as teratogen, 351t
Penicillin
  for pelvic abscess, 762
  for puerperal endometritis, 760
  for septic shock, 763
Penicillin allergy, oral desensitization for, 780, 781t
Penicillin G
  for group B *Streptococcus* infection, 767, 768, 768f
  for listeriosis, 773
  for syphilis, 780–781, 781t
Penicillinase-producing *Neisseria gonorrhoeae,* 745
Pentamidine, for *Pneumocystis jiroveci* pneumonia, 934
PEP (polymorphic eruption of pregnancy), 1125t, 1126, 1126f
Peptic ulcer disease (PUD), 1045–1046, 1045f
Peptide hormones, in placental tissues, 117t
Percutaneous umbilical blood sampling (PUBS). *See* Cordocentesis.
Periappendiceal abscess, 1047
Periarteritis nodosa, renal dysfunction in, 914, 916t
Pericardial effusions, due to nonimmune hydrops, 506, 507f
Pericentric inversion, 15–16, 17f
Peri-implantation loss, 619
Perinatal Antiplatelet Review of International Studies (PARIS) Collaborative Group, 675
Perinatal infections, and cerebral palsy, 1215–1216
Perinatal mortality and morbidity
  anemia and, 872–873
  antidepressants and, 1117–1118, 1119
  biophysical profile score and, 369, 369f, 387–388, 388t
  due to chronic hypertension, 676
  with chronic kidney disease, 911
  defined, 548
  with diabetes, 963–967, 963t
  with Doppler velicometry, 388, 388t
  electronic fetal monitoring and, 413
  with intrauterine growth restriction, 637, 637f
  lithium and, 1119
  with monoamniotic twins, 466–467
  with multiple gestation, 453–454, 454f, 461
  with post-term pregnancy, 614, 614f
  due to preeclampsia, 654–655
  with premature rupture of the membranes, 601
  with preterm birth, 548–551, 549f–552f, 553t, 1199, 1200f
  uterine myomas and, 1137
Perinatal stroke, 1213–1214, 1213f
Periodic fetal heart rate patterns, 405, 407, 408–410, 409f–411f
Periodontal disease, and preterm birth, 556, 568
Peripartum cardiomyopathy, 814–815
Peripheral entrapment neuropathies, 1104–1107, 1106f
Peripheral mononeuropathies, 1104–1107, 1106f
Peritoneal dialysis, 917–918
Periventricular leukomalacia (PVL), 1212
  chorioamnionitis and, 758–759, 758t
Peroneal nerve palsy, 1105, 1106
Persistent left-sided superior vena cava, 318–320, 319f, 320f
Persistent umbilical vein, 318, 319f
Persistent vegetative state, 1189–1190, 1189t
Pessaries, for cervical insufficiency, 589
PET (positron emission tomography), of Hodgkin lymphoma, 897
PG. *See* Phosphatidylglycerol (PG).
PGD_2 (prostaglandin D_2), in control of labor, 74
PGDH (prostaglandin dehydrogenase), in control of labor, 72
PGE_1. *See* Prostaglandin E_1 (PGE_1).
PGE_2. *See* Prostaglandin E_2 (PGE_2).
$PGF_{2\alpha}$ (prostaglandin $F_{2\alpha}$)
  in control of labor, 74
  for postpartum hemorrhage, 698–699
PGH (placental growth hormone), in pregnancy, 120f
PGH_2 (prostaglandin H_2), in control of labor, 74
PGHS (prostaglandin H synthase), in control of labor, 72
PGHS (prostaglandin H_2 synthase), in control of labor, 74–75
PGI_2 (prostaglandin I_2)
  in control of labor, 74
  in fetal cardiovascular regulation, 166
PGM (prothrombin gene mutation), 831t, 833
  and venous thromboembolism, 856t
PGS (preimplantation genetic screening), 259–261
pH
  defined, 401t
  fetal blood, 162, 162t, 386, 386t
    determination of, 400–401
    in labor, 402t
  during pregnancy, 1173, 1173t
  umbilical cord, 402–403, 403t
Phagocytic cells, in immune response, 87
Phalen maneuver, 1105
Pharyngeal gonorrhea, 744
Phenobarbital
  for hemolytic disease of the fetus and newborn, 494–495
  for preterm labor, 561
Phenocopy, 25
Phenolsulfonphthalein, excretion of, in preeclampsia, 664
Phenothiazines, for nausea and vomiting, 1042, 1042t
Phenotype, 22
Phenoxybenzamine, for pheochromocytoma, 1030
Phentolamine, for pheochromocytoma, 1030
Phenylephrine, for septic shock, 1178t
Phenylketonuria (PKU), 1101–1102
  prenatal diagnosis of, 248t
Phenytoin
  for preeclampsia, 672
  as teratogen, 348, 351t, 352, 1091
Pheochromocytoma, 679, 1030–1031, 1031t
Phosphates, for hypercalcemia, 1034, 1034t
Phosphatidylcholine, in surfactant, 197, 197f
  metabolism of, 199f, 200
Phosphatidylglycerol (PG)
  in amniotic fluid, 419
    in diabetic pregnancy, 421, 967, 968f
    impact of contaminants on, 422, 422t
  in surfactant, 197, 197f
    metabolism of, 199f, 200
  in vaginal fluid specimens, 423
Phosphatidylinositol (PI)
  in amniotic fluid, 419
    in diabetic pregnancy, 421
  in vaginal fluid specimens, 423
Phosphatidylinositol glycan class A *(PIGA)* gene, 876
Phospholipase A_2 (PLA_2), in control of labor, 74
Phospholipids
  in amniotic fluid, 419
  in surfactant, 197, 197f
    metabolism of, 199–200, 199f
Phospho-soda, for hypercalcemia, 1034t
Physical activity, and preterm birth, 555, 569
Phytohemagglutinin, 11
PI (phosphatidylinositol)
  in amniotic fluid, 419
    in diabetic pregnancy, 421
  in vaginal fluid specimens, 423
Pica, due to iron deficiency anemia, 873
Pierre Robin syndrome, 285
PIGA (phosphatidylinositol glycan class A) gene, 876
Pigmentary changes, in pregnancy, 1123
Pinopodes, 619
PIOPED (Prospective Investigation of Pulmonary Embolism Diagnosis), 860
Piperacillin-tazobactam
  for acute pyelonephritis, 756t
  for puerperal endometritis, 760
  for septic shock, 763
Pitocin. *See* Oxytocin (Pitocin).
Pituitary adenomas, 1017–1022, 1093, 1094f
Pituitary apoplexy, 1020
Pituitary disorder(s), 1017–1025
  of anterior lobe, 1017–1024
    acromegaly as, 1020–1021
    Cushing syndrome as, 1021–1022
    hypopituitarism as, 1022–1024, 1023t
    pituitary tumors as, 1017–1022
    prolactinoma as, 1018–1020, 1019f, 1020f, 1020t
    thyrotropin-secreting tumors as, 1021
  of posterior lobe, 1024–1025
    diabetes insipidus as, 1024–1025
    primary polydipsia as, 1025

Pituitary gland
anatomy and physiology of, 1015, 1016f, 1017f
fetal development of, 1016
during pregnancy, 1015–1016, 1016f, 1017f
Pituitary infarction, 1096
Pituitary insufficiency, 1022–1024, 1023t
Pituitary necrosis, 1022, 1023
Pituitary stalk, 1015
Pituitary tumors, 1017–1022
PJP. *See Pneumocystis jiroveci* pneumonia (PJP).
PKD1, 913
PKD2, 913
PKU (phenylketonuria), 1101–1102
prenatal diagnosis of, 248t
PLA_2 (phospholipase A_2), in control of labor, 74
Placenta(s)
accreta, 698, 728–729, 728f
development of, 37–38, 38f, 39f
examination of, after pregnancy loss, 626
expulsion of, 698
fibrinoid of, 43
fundal implantation of, 699
fused, 59f, 60, 67f
and growth factors, 117–119, 117t, 118f, 119f
increta, 728
low-lying, 725, 726f
as mechanical barrier, 88
normal term, 41
oxygen consumption by, 185
oxygen transport across, 183–186, 183f, 184f, 186f
percreta, 728
previa, 37, 725–729
complete, 725
complications of, 728–729, 728f
defined, 725
diagnosis of, 726–727, 726f
epidemiology of, 725
management of, 727–728, 727t
marginal, 725
pathogenesis of, 725–726
risk factors for, 725, 726t
uterine myomas and, 1137
retained, 698
surface vessels of, 40
in twinning, 57–61, 57f–60f
Placental abnormalities, and cerebral palsy, 1216
Placental abruption. *See* Abruptio placentae.
Placental aromatase deficiency, 1031
Placental carbon dioxide transfer, 190–191
Placental clock, 72
Placental factors, intrauterine growth restriction due to, 640
Placental growth hormone (PGH), in pregnancy, 120f
Placental migration, 725–726
Placental mosaicism, 254–255
Placental pathology, in preeclampsia, 661
Placental respiratory gas exchange, 181–187
Placental separation, 698
Placental site giant cells, 43, 43f
Placental size, intrauterine growth restriction due to, 640
Placental steroid sulfatase deficiency, 225
Placental thickening, due to nonimmune hydrops, 507
Placental tumors, hydrops fetalis due to, 509
Placental villi, 41–44, 42f, 44f
Placental-fetal thyroid physiology, 997–998
Placental-site vessels, in preeclampsia, 660–661, 660f
Plasma osmolality, during pregnancy, 1016, 1018f
Plasma volume, during pregnancy, 101, 107, 870, 871f
Plasmapheresis, for hemolytic disease of the fetus and newborn, 493, 494
Plasmin, in fibrinolysis, 828, 828f
Plasminogen activator inhibitor 1 (PAI-1)
and fetal loss, 620–621
in fibrinolysis, 828, 828f
mutations in, 835
pregnancy effect on, 829
Plasminogen activator inhibitor 1 (PAI-1) deficiency, 848
Plasminogen activator inhibitor 2 (PAI-2)
in fibrinolysis, 828, 828f
pregnancy effect on, 829
Platelet(s), for hemorrhagic shock, 1181t
Platelet activating factor (PAF), in preterm labor, 526f
Platelet activation, 825, 826f
Platelet adhesion, 825, 826f
Platelet aggregation, 825, 826f
Platelet concentrate, for abruptio placentae, 733t
Platelet count
in abruptio placentae, 733t
in preeclampsia, 1148
Platelet disorder(s), 837–847
acquired, 837–843
Bernard-Soulier syndrome as, 844t–846t, 845–846
congenital, 843–847
drug-induced thrombocytopenia and functional platelet defects as, 843
idiopathic thrombocytopenic purpura as, 837–840
neonatal alloimmune thrombocytopenia as, 840–842, 840t
of platelet secretion, 844t, 846–847
thrombotic thrombocytopenic purpura and hemolytic uremic syndrome as, 842–843, 843t
von Willebrand disease as, 843–845, 844t–846t
Platelet plug formation, 825–826, 826f
Platelet secretion, 825, 826f
Platelet secretion defects, 844t, 846–847
Platelet storage pool deficiencies, 844t, 845t
Platelet transfusions, for idiopathic thrombocytopenic purpura, 838
Pleural effusions, in fetus, 289, 289f
in hydrops fetalis, 444, 506, 506f
invasive fetal therapy for, 277t, 444
Plexus lesions, 1104–1107, 1106f
Plicamycin, for hypercalcemia, 1034, 1034t
Plugged ducts, 138, 138t
Pneumococcal pneumonia, 930, 931–932, 931f
Pneumococcal polysaccharide vaccination, 932
Pneumocystis carinii pneumonia (PCP). *See Pneumocystis jiroveci* pneumonia (PJP).
Pneumocystis jiroveci pneumonia (PJP)
diagnosis of, 931, 933, 934f
with HIV infection, 771, 933–934
therapy for, 933–934
Pneumonia, 929–934
aspiration, 930
atypical, 931
bacterial, 930–932, 931f
bacteriology of, 930
epidemiology of, 929–930
with HIV infection, 771, 929–930, 933–934, 934f
maternal and fetal outcome with, 930
viral, 932–933, 933f
Pneumonitis, chemical, 930
PNH (paroxysmal nocturnal hemoglobinuria), 876–877
PO_2. *See* Oxygen partial pressure (PO_2).
POF (premature ovarian failure), fragile X syndrome and, 245, 246
Polar bodies, 9, 11f, 37
Poliomyelitis, 1099–1100
Polycystic kidney disease
autosomal dominant (adult)
pregnancy with, 913, 916t
prenatal diagnosis of, 248t, 295–296
autosomal recessive (infantile), 295, 296f
Polycystic ovarian syndrome (PCOS)
fetal loss due to, 620–621
insulin-resistant, 1031–1032
Polycythemia, in infants of diabetic mothers, 967
Polydipsia, primary, 1025
Polyethylene glycol, for constipation, 1052, 1052t
Polygenic inheritance, 26
Polyglutamine repeats, expanded, 29
Polyhydramnios, 47, 50
Polymerase chain reaction (PCR), 30, 31f, 32, 32f
Polymorphic eruption of pregnancy (PEP), 1125t, 1126, 1126f
Polymorphisms, 6
Polymyositis, 1109
Polyneuropathy(ies), 1107–1108
acute idiopathic, 1107–1108
Polyp(s)
cervical, cervical insufficiency due to, 587, 587f
fibroepithelial, 1124
Polyploidization, 14
Polyploidy, 15
Polypyrimidine tract binding protein–associated splicing factor (PSF), 73
Polythelia, 128
Polyunsaturated fatty acids (PUFA), for preterm birth prevention, 569, 570t
POMC (pro-opiomelanocortin), 1025
Ponderal index, 635
PORD (cytochrome P450 oxidoreductase) deficiency, 1031
Porencephaly, 283–284
Porphyric neuropathy, 1108
Portal hypertension, 1071
Portal venous return, fetal, 159, 160f
Positive predictive value (PPV), 214, 215, 215t, 221
Positron emission tomography (PET), of Hodgkin lymphoma, 897
Posterior fossa cyst, and aneuploidy, 227t
Posterior pituitary lobe
anatomy and physiology of, 1015, 1016f, 1017f
during pregnancy, 1016
Posterior pituitary lobe disorder(s), 1024–1025
diabetes insipidus as, 1024–1025
primary polydipsia as, 1025
Posterior urethral valves, 296, 297, 297f
Post-hemorrhagic hydrocephalus, 1212
Postnatal growth, and developmental origins of health and disease, 153
Postnatal headache, 1093
Postnatal management decisions, 1197
Postpartum hemorrhage, 698–699
uterine myomas and, 1137
Postpartum thyroiditis (PPT), 1009–1011, 1010f
Postprandial glucose levels, 974–975, 975t
Post-term pregnancy, 613–617
defined, 613
developmental effects of, 616–617
fetal evaluation and management of, 615–616
incidence of, 613
labor induction for, 615–616
pathogenesis of, 613
perinatal risks of, 614–615, 614f
risk factors for, 613–614
umbilical cord acid-base balance with, 404
Post-test odds, 215–216
Potassium chloride (KCl), for diabetic ketoacidosis, 962t

Potassium excretion, during pregnancy, 106
Power, statistical, 214
Power stroke, in myometrial contraction, 78f
PPD (purified protein derivative), 935, 936, 936f
pPROM. *See* Preterm premature rupture of the membranes (pPROM).
PPT (postpartum thyroiditis), 1009–1011, 1010f
PPV (positive predictive value), 214, 215, 215t, 221
PR. *See* Progesterone receptor (PR) *entries.*
Prader-Willi syndrome, 30
Prazosin, for chronic hypertension, 678t
Preconception counseling
  with chronic kidney disease, 910, 910t
  with maternal heart disease, 797–799, 798t
Pre-conceptional care, for preterm birth prevention, 572–573
Predictive adaptive response hypothesis, 155
Predictive values, 214–215, 215t, 221
Prednisolone, for induction of fetal pulmonary maturity, 423t
Prednisone
  for asthma, 940t
  for hyperemesis gravidarum, 1043
  for hypopituitarism, 1023
  for idiopathic thrombocytopenic purpura, 838
  for impetigo herpetiformis, 1130
  for induction of fetal pulmonary maturity, 423t
  for inflammatory bowel disease, 1049
  for neonatal alloimmune thrombocytopenia, 841–842
  for pemphigoid gestationis, 1129
  for renal transplantation, 918
  for rheumatic disease, 1081, 1082t
Preeclampsia, 653–676
  acute renal failure due to, 907–908
  anesthesia with, 1147–1149
  and cardiovascular disease in later life, 655–656, 656f
  clinical presentation of, 656–661, 656t
  coagulation system changes with, 1148
  diabetes and, 961, 961f
  diagnostic criteria for, 651
  edema in, 651, 652f, 1148
  epidemiology of, 653–656
  excessive weight gain and, 145
  factor V Leiden mutation and, 832
  fetal heart rate with
    late decelerations in, 409f
    no variability of, 408f, 410f
  fetal loss due to, 624
  genetics of, 666
  hemodynamics of, 1172
  intravascular volume depletion due to, 1147
  laboratory findings in, 657–658, 657t
  liver disease in, 1062, 1063
  management of, 666–675
    antepartum, 668–671
    antihypertensive therapy in, 673, 673t
    delivery in, 668, 669–670
    for disseminated intravascular coagulation, 674
    expectant, 669–671
    fetal observation in, 669, 671
    follow-up assessment in, 675
    initial, 669
    intrapartum, 671–674, 671t–673t
    maternal monitoring in, 668–669
    for oliguria, 673–674
    philosophy of, 666–667
    postpartum, 674–675
    for pulmonary edema, 674
Preeclampsia *(Continued)*
    seizure prophylaxis and treatment in, 671–673, 671t, 672t
    therapies no longer recommended for, 675
  and maternal mortality, 655
  maternal obesity and, 144
  with multiple gestation, 460–461, 654
  neonatal outcomes with, 1198
  oliguria in, 673–674, 1172
  pathologic changes in, 658–661
    in brain, 658
    in kidney, 653, 653t, 658–660, 659f
    in liver, 658, 658f
    placental, 661
    vascular, 660–661, 660f
  pathophysiologic change(s) in, 661–667
    cardiovascular, 661–662, 662f
    in coagulation, 662–663
    endothelial cell dysfunction as, 663
    immunologic and inflammatory, 666, 667
    oxidative stress as, 666–667, 675–676
    in renal function, 663–666, 664f, 665t
  and perinatal mortality, 654–655
  prevention of, 675–676
  prothrombin gene mutation and, 833
  pulmonary edema in, 674, 1175
    anesthetic considerations with, 1148
  recurrence of, 655, 655t
  with renal transplantation, 919
  risk factors for, 653–654
  short-term prognosis for, 654–655
  signs and symptoms of, 656–657, 656t
  spectrum of, 653
  superimposed on chronic hypertension, 651–652
  vs. thrombotic thrombocytopenic purpura and hemolytic uremic syndrome, 843, 843t, 908
  vascular reactivity due to, 1147–1148
  vasospasm in, 1172
Pregnancy
  as allograft, 87
  duration of, 70
  ectopic
    after cesarean delivery, 710
    with renal transplantation, 918
    with uterine anomalies, 1144t
  maintenance of early, 114
  as prothrombotic state, 855
  symptoms and signs of, 103–104
Pregnancy loss, 619–629
  with diabetes, 963, 963t
  embryonic
    due to endocrine disorders, 620–621
    due to genetic abnormalities, 619–620
    management of, 627–629, 627t, 628t
    peri-implantation, 619
    recurrent
      immunologic causes of, 621–622
      management of, 627, 627t, 628–629, 628t
      due to uterine abnormalities, 622, 622t
  fetal
    due to antiphospholipid syndrome, 625
    after chorionic villus sampling, 255
    after cordocentesis, 385, 385t
    diagnostic considerations for, 626–627, 627t
    due to endocrine disorders, 620–621
    epidemiology of, 622–623
    due to fetomaternal hemorrhage, 624
    due to genetic abnormalities, 619–620, 623
    due to infection, 623–624
    due to inherited thrombophilia, 625–626, 625t, 626t, 628, 831–835, 836–837
    management of, 627–629, 627t, 628t
Pregnancy loss *(Continued)*
    medical conditions causing, 624–625
    after mid-trimester amniocentesis, 250–251, 250t
    in multiple gestation, 625
    due to placental abruption, 624
    recurrent, 626
      cervical cerclage for, 592, 592f
      immunologic causes of, 621–622
      management of, 627, 627t, 628–629, 628t
      due to uterine abnormalities, 622, 622t
    uterine myomas and, 62, 1136, 1138
  due to hypothyroidism, 1001
  due to vasa previa, 729
Pregnancy reduction, multifetal, 470–471, 471t
Pregnancy registries, on safety of exposures, 349
Pregnancy termination
  with conjoined twins, 468
  and preterm birth, 557
  selective
    of acardiac twin, 434t, 468
    of anomalous fetus, 469–470
    for TRAP sequence, 439–440
    for twin-to-twin transfusion syndrome, 437, 439
Pregnancy-associated plasma protein A (PAPP-A), 229
  in twins, 257, 459
Pregnancy-induced hypertension. *See* Hypertension; Preeclampsia.
Pregnancy-Related Mortality Surveillance System, 1167
Preimplantation genetic screening (PGS), 259–261
Preload, fetal, 162
Premature atrial contractions (PACs), 336–337, 337f
Premature infants
  arterial blood gas values for, 403t
  breastfeeding of, 134
Premature ovarian failure (POF), fragile X syndrome and, 245, 246
Premature rupture of the membranes (PROM), 599–608
  clinical course of, 600
  complications after, 600–601
  defined, 599
  diagnosis of, 601–602, 602f
  epidemiology of, 600
  initial evaluation of, 602
  management of, 602–607, 603f
  oxytocin induction after, 604
  pathophysiology of, 599–600
  prediction and prevention of, 600
  preterm. *See* Preterm premature rupture of the membranes (pPROM).
  risk factors for, 599–600
  due to trichomoniasis, 741
Prematurity, 1199–1202. *See also* Preterm labor and birth.
  defined, 1199
  at limit of viability, 1200–1202
Premutation alleles, 29
Prenatal diagnosis, 246–259
  amniocentesis for, 247–251
    chorionic villus sampling *vs.*, 258–259
    complications of, 250
    early, 251
    historical perspective on, 247
    laboratory considerations for, 249–250
    with multiple gestation, 257–258, 258t, 459
    pregnancy lost after, 250–251, 250t
    technique of, 247–249, 248f
  biopsies for, 259
  chorionic villus sampling for, 251–256

Prenatal diagnosis *(Continued)*
accuracy of, 253–255
amniocentesis *vs.*, 258–259
complications of, 255–256
history of, 251–252
laboratory aspects of, 253
with multiple gestation, 258, 258t
pregnancy loss after, 255
risk of fetal abnormality after, 256
transabdominal, 252–253, 253f
transcervical, 252, 252f, 253
of fragile X syndrome, 246
indication(s) for, 246–247, 247t, 248t
maternal age as, 232–233, 233t
with multiple gestation, 256–258, 256t–258t
of neural tube defects, 235, 236f
noninvasive, 261–263
percutaneous umbilical blood sampling for, 259
for Tay Sachs disease, 241
for β-thalassemia, 244–245
Prenatal screening, 221–246
for acetylcholinesterase, 234–235, 234t
cutoff values in, 221, 222t
for Down syndrome, 222–233
ADAM 12 in, 230
combined first- and second-trimester, 232
cutoff values in, 222t
ductus venosus wave form in, 231
first-trimester
impact of spontaneous miscarriages on, 231–232
serum markers in, 229–230, 230t
ultrasound markers in, 227–229, 230–231, 230t, 231f
human chorionic gonadotropin in, 229–230
likelihood ratios in, 221–222, 222t, 225, 226, 226t
maternal age in, 222, 222t, 232–233, 233t
nasal bone in, 225, 230–231, 231f, 232
nuchal translucency in, 228, 230
PAPP-A in, 229
in twins, 257, 459
receiver operating curve in, 222f
second-trimester
serum markers in, 222–225, 224t, 226
ultrasound markers in, 225–226, 225t, 226t
serum markers in
first-trimester, 229–230, 230t
second-trimester, 222–225, 224t, 226
tricuspid regurgitation in, 231
ultrasound markers in
first-trimester, 227–229, 230–231, 230t, 231f
second-trimester, 225–226, 225t, 226t
first-trimester
impact of spontaneous miscarriages on, 231–232
serum markers in, 229–230, 230t
with twins, 257, 459
ultrasound markers in, 227–229, 228f, 228t, 229f, 230–231, 231f
for gene mutations, 238–246
in cystic fibrosis, 238–240, 238t–240t, 242t
in fragile X syndrome, 245–246, 246t
in hemoglobinopathies, 238t, 243–245, 244t
informed consent for, 238
in Jewish population, 238t, 240–243, 241t, 242t
recommendations on, 238, 238t
goal of, 238
for human chorionic gonadotropin, 223, 224, 229–230
in twins, 257, 257t, 458, 459
Prenatal screening *(Continued)*
ideal test for, 221
likelihood ratios in, 221–222, 222t, 225, 226, 226t
maternal age as indication for, 222, 222t, 232–233, 233t
for maternal serum α-fetoprotein, 223, 224, 224t, 233–235, 234t
in twins, 257, 257t, 458, 459
with multiple gestation, 256–257, 256t, 257t, 458, 459
for neural tube defects, 233–235, 234t, 236f
in twins, 257, 459
for pregnancy-associated plasma protein A, 229
receiver operating curve in, 221, 222f
second-trimester
serum markers in, 223–224, 224t, 226
with twins, 256–257, 257t, 458–459
ultrasound markers in, 225–227, 225t–228t
value of, 236–237, 237t
sensitivity and specificity of, 221
serum markers in
first-trimester, 229–230, 230t
with twins, 257, 459
second-trimester, 223–224, 224t, 226
with twins, 256–257, 257t, 458
for twins, 256–257, 256t, 257t, 458–459
ultrasound markers in
first-trimester, 227–229, 228f, 228t, 229f, 230–231, 231f
second-trimester, 225–227, 225t–228t
value of, 236–237, 237t
Prepidil (dinoprostone)
for cervical ripening, 702t, 703t
for post-term pregnancy, 615, 616
for uterine atony, 1183t
Preprandial glucose levels, 975t, 978–979
Presentation(s), abnormal, 703–707
breech as, 703–706, 705t
compound, 707
deflection abnormalities as, 706–707
transverse lie as, 706
uterine anomalies and, 1144
uterine myomas and, 1137
Preterm and growth-restricted neonates, defined, 635
Preterm labor and birth, 545–573. *See also* Prematurity.
antidepressants and, 1118
body mass index and, 144
and cerebral palsy, 552, 1214–1215, 1216–1217
cigarette smoking and, 356, 356f
clinical presentations of, 547–548
in common pathway of parturition, 521–524, 522f, 524f
complications of, 1199–1200, 1199t, 1201f, 1201t
consequence(s) of, 548–552, 549f–554f, 553t
long-term, 551–552, 553f, 554f
perinatal and infant mortality as, 548–551, 549f–552f, 1199, 1200f
perinatal morbidity as, 551, 552f, 553t
defined, 521, 545
diagnosis of, 560–561
incidence of, 521, 545–546, 546f, 547f
indicated, 521, 545, 548, 548f, 569
infant morbidity and mortality with, 1199, 1200f
interventional strategy(ies) for, 560–567
after acute treatment, 567
antenatal corticosteroids as, 561
antibiotics as, 561
neuroprotectants as, 561
Preterm labor and birth *(Continued)*
primary, 560
to reduce morbidity and mortality, 561
regionalization of care as, 561
secondary, 560
tertiary, 560
tocolytic therapy as, 561–567
calcium channel blockers for, 562–563
choice of agent for, 562
clinical uses of, 566–567
contraindications to, 561
cyclooxygenase inhibitors for, 563–564
goals of, 561–562
magnesium sulfate for, 565–566
nitric oxide donors for, 564–565
oxytocin antagonists for, 564
β-sympathomimetic drugs as, 566
and low birth weight, 545–546
with multiple gestation
interventions for, 460
pathogenesis of, 529–531, 531f, 558
rates of, 460, 546, 547f, 558, 559f, 559t
pathogenesis of, 521–532
allergic phenomena in, 531
cervical disorders in, 531
genetic factors in, 70
hormonal disorders in, 531–532
infection and inflammation in, 524–527, 525f, 526f, 528f
maternal and fetal stress in, 529, 530f
mechanisms of, 521–524, 522f, 524f
uterine overdistention in, 529–531, 531f
uteroplacental vascular disease and decidual hemorrhage in, 527–529, 529f
prevention of, 567–573
antibiotics for, 570
cervical cerclage for, 568–569, 571–572
cervical examination for, 568–569
with clinical risk factors, 569–573, 570t, 571f
modification of maternal activity for, 569
nutritional supplements for, 567–568, 569, 570t, 572
periodontal care for, 568
before pregnancy, 572–573
progestational agents for, 570–571, 570t, 571f
in routine prenatal care, 567–569
screening for, 568–569
smoking cessation for, 568, 572
recurrence of, 556–557, 557t, 572
risk factor(s) for, 552–560
assisted reproductive technologies as, 558
asymptomatic bacteriuria as, 568, 751
bleeding as, 558
cervical length as, 558–560, 559f, 560f
cervical surgery as, 557–558
current pregnancy characteristics as, 558–560, 559f, 559t, 560f
educational and economic status as, 554, 554t
familial, 553
infections as, 556
maternal behaviors and environment as, 554–555
maternal characteristics as, 553–556, 554t, 555f
multiple gestation as, 558, 559f, 559t
nutritional status as, 555–556, 555f
physical activity as, 555, 569
pregnancy termination as, 557
prior preterm birth as, 556–557, 557t
psychological, 555
race and ethnic background as, 551, 552f, 554, 554t, 555f, 557

Preterm labor and birth *(Continued)*
reproductive history as, 556–558, 557t
scoring of, 568
uterine anomalies as, 557
uterine contractions as, 558
uterine volume as, 558
spontaneous, 521, 545, 548, 548f
prevention of, 569–572, 570t, 571f
as syndrome, 524, 525f
with uterine anomalies, 1144t
uterine myomas and, 1136, 1136t
and viability, 521
Preterm lung, physiologic effects of surfactant on, 200–202, 201f
Preterm neonates, defined, 635
Preterm premature rupture of the membranes (pPROM)
with cervical cerclage, 594, 606–607
early, 601, 603f, 604–607
epidemiology of, 600
due to fetal inflammatory response syndrome, 527, 528f
and fetal pulmonary maturity, 423, 601
after fetoscopic procedures, 435, 435t
late, 603f, 604
management of, 602–607, 603f
antibiotics for, 209, 209f, 210f, 604, 605–606
corticosteroids for, 604, 605
initial evaluation in, 602
tocolysis for, 606
due to maternal herpes infection, 607
due to microbial invasion of the amniotic cavity, 525
prediction and prevention of, 600
previable, 601, 603f, 607
risk factors for, 599–600
due to uteroplacental vascular disease or decidual hemorrhage, 527–529, 529f
Pretest odds, 215
Previable premature rupture of the membranes, 601, 603f, 607
Prezista (darunavir), for HIV infection, 772t
Primary biliary cirrhosis, 1069
Primary Care Evaluation of Mental Disorders (PRIME-MD), 1114
Primary immune thrombocytopenic purpura, 837–840
Primary pulmonary hypertension, maternal, 805
anesthesia with, 1158
Primary sclerosing cholangitis (PSC), 1070
Probability value, 212
Probenecid, for gonorrhea, 745
Procainamide, during pregnancy, 801t
Procaine penicillin, for syphilis, 781t
Professional policies, for preterm birth prevention, 572
Progestational agents, for preterm birth prevention, 570–571, 570t, 571f
Progesterone
as anti-inflammatory agent, 73
in cervical remodeling, 523
constipation due to, 1052
in control of labor, 73–74
and cortisol, 73–74
and fetal loss, 620–621, 628, 628t
and fetoplacental unit, 115
and hyperventilation of pregnancy, 927
in implantation, 111
in pregnancy, 114–115, 114f, 115f, 117
for prevention of preterm labor and birth, 570–571, 570t, 571f
with multiple gestation, 460
suspension of action of, preterm labor due to, 531–532
Progesterone blockage, 73
Progesterone dermatitis, autoimmune, 1125
Progesterone receptor A (PR-A), 73
Progesterone receptor (PR) antagonist, 73
Progesterone receptor B (PR-B), 73
Progesterone receptor (PR) cofactors, 73
Progestins
during pregnancy, 117
for preterm labor, 532
Proinflammatory cytokines, in preterm labor and birth, 526–527, 526f, 556
Prolactin
in breastfeeding, 131, 132f
and fetal loss, 621
neurohormonal control of, 1015
during pregnancy, 121–122, 121f, 1015, 1017f
Prolactinoma, 1018–1020, 1019f, 1020f, 1020t
Prolapsed intervertebral disk, 1104
Proliferative phase, of myometrial remodeling, 522
Prolonged deceleration, in fetal heart rate, 406
Prolonged latent phase, 694–695
Prolonged pregnancy. *See* Post-term pregnancy.
PROM. *See* Premature rupture of the membranes (PROM).
Promethazine
for hemolytic disease of the fetus and newborn, 494
for hyperemesis gravidarum, 1043
Promoter sequences, 5
Promotility drugs, for GERD, 1044, 1045f
Prone ventilation, for acute respiratory distress syndrome, 1174
Pronucleus, 11f
Pro-opiomelanocortin (POMC), 1025
Propafenone, during pregnancy, 801t
Prophase, 7–8, 7f
Propranolol
for chronic hypertension, 678t
for thyroid storm, 1003, 1003t
Propylthiouracil (PTU), for thyroid storm, 1003, 1003t
Prospective cohort study, 208
Prospective Investigation of Pulmonary Embolism Diagnosis (PIOPED), 860
Prostacyclin, in preeclampsia, 663
Prostaglandin(s)
for cervical ripening, 702t
in control of labor, 74–75, 75f
in fetal cardiovascular regulation, 166
in fetal heart rate, 398
for induction, with multiple gestation, 461
in labor and delivery, 523–524, 524f
and patent ductus arteriosus, 167
during pregnancy, 122
in preterm labor and birth, 526f, 556
as uterine stimulants, 80
Prostaglandin 15-methyl $F_{2\alpha}$ (Hemabate), for uterine atony, 1183t
Prostaglandin D_2 (PGD_2), in control of labor, 74
Prostaglandin dehydrogenase (PGDH), in control of labor, 72
Prostaglandin E_1 (PGE_1)
for cervical ripening, 702–703, 702t, 703t
for fetal demise, 627–628
for postpartum hemorrhage, 699
for post-term pregnancy, 616
for uterine atony, 1183t
Prostaglandin E_2 (PGE_2)
for cervical ripening, 702t, 703t
in control of labor, 74
in fetal cardiovascular regulation, 166
and nausea and vomiting, 1042
Prostaglandin E_2 (PGE_2) *(Continued)*
and patent ductus arteriosus, 167
for post-term pregnancy, 615, 616
for uterine atony, 1183t
Prostaglandin $F_{2\alpha}$ ($PGF_{2\alpha}$)
in control of labor, 74
for postpartum hemorrhage, 698–699
Prostaglandin H synthase (PGHS), in control of labor, 72
Prostaglandin H_2 (PGH_2), in control of labor, 74
Prostaglandin H_2 synthase (PGHS), in control of labor, 74–75
Prostaglandin I_2 (PGI_2)
in control of labor, 74
in fetal cardiovascular regulation, 166
Prostaglandin induction, after premature rupture of the membranes, 604
Prostaglandin inhibitors, for cervical insufficiency, 589
Prostaglandin synthesis inhibitors
for preterm labor, 563–564
as uterine relaxants, 81
Prosthetic heart valve, pregnancy with, 819–820, 820t, 864
Protease inhibitors, for HIV infection, 772t
Protease-activated receptor type 1 (PAR-1), in preterm labor, 528
Protein(s)
in diet, 147
serum, 1059
in surfactant, 198
Protein C (PC)
activated
in anticoagulant system, 828, 828f
for septic shock, 763, 1179
in anticoagulant system, 828, 828f
Protein C (PC) deficiency, 831t, 834
and fetal loss, 625, 625t, 626t, 834
and venous thromboembolism, 856t
Protein hormones, in placental tissues, 117t
Protein S (PS) deficiency, 831t, 834–835
and fetal loss, 625, 625t, 626t, 834–835
and venous thromboembolism, 856t
Protein synthesis, 5, 5f
Protein Z (PZ), in anticoagulant system, 828, 828f
Protein Z (PZ) antigen, and fetal loss, 625t
Protein Z (PZ) deficiency, 835
Protein Z–dependent protease inhibitor (ZPI), in anticoagulant system, 828, 828f
Protein Z-dependent protease inhibitor (ZPI) deficiency, 835
Proteinuria
defined, 651
in preeclampsia, 657, 664, 670
Prothrombin G20201A, 833
and fetal loss, 625, 625t, 626t, 833
Prothrombin gene mutation (PGM), 831t, 833
and venous thromboembolism, 856t
Prothrombin time, in abruptio placentae, 733t
Prothrombotic state, pregnancy as, 855
Proton pump inhibitors
for GERD, 1044–1045, 1044t, 1045f
for peptic ulcer disease, 1046
Protraction disorders, 695
Protriptyline (Vivactil), dosage of, 1117t
PROWESS (Recombinant Human Activated Protein C Worldwide Evaluation in Severe Sepsis) trial, 1179
Prozac (fluoxetine), dosage of, 1117t
PRRs (pattern recognition receptors), 87, 91, 92
in preterm labor, 526
Prurigo gestationis, 1125t, 1126–1127, 1127f
Prurigo of pregnancy, 1125t, 1126–1127, 1127f

Pruritic urticarial papules and plaques of pregnancy (PUPPP), 1125t, 1126, 1126f
Pruritus
gravidarum, 1125–1126, 1125t
due to intrahepatic cholestasis of pregnancy, 1061, 1125
PS (protein S) deficiency, 831t, 834–835
and fetal loss, 625, 625t, 626t, 834–835
and venous thromboembolism, 856t
PSC (primary sclerosing cholangitis), 1070
Pseudoglandular stage, of fetal lung development, 193, 194f, 194t
Pseudohypoparathyroidism, 1035
Pseudomosaicism, 249
Pseudotumor cerebri, 1094–1095
Pseudo–von Willebrand disease (pseudo-vWD), 843–845, 844t, 845t
PSF (polypyrimidine tract binding protein–associated splicing factor), 73
Psoriasis, 1132
pustular, 1125t, 1129–1130, 1130f
Psoriatic arthritis, 1085
PSV (peak systolic velocity), in fetal middle cerebral artery, 374–375, 374f
Psychiatric disorder(s), 1109–1110, 1113–1120
diagnostic criteria for, 1113, 1114t, 1115t
epidemiology of, 1113
identification of, 1113–1114
impact on pregnancy outcome of, 1114–1116
treatment of, 1114–1120
clinical approach to, 1118–1119
dosage for, 1116t, 1117t
during lactation, 1119–1120
perinatal complications of, 1119
risks of, 1116–1118
Psychological factors, and preterm birth, 555
Psychopharmacologic treatment
clinical approach to, 1118–1119
dosages for, 1116t, 1117t
during lactation, 1119–1120
perinatal complications of, 1119
risks of, 1116–1118
teratogenicity of, 351t, 353
Psychosis
diagnostic criteria for, 1113, 1114t, 1115t
epidemiology of, 1113
identification of, 1113–1114
impact on pregnancy outcomes of, 1114–1115
Korsakoff, 1107
treatment of
clinical approach to, 1118, 1119
dosages for, 1116t
during lactation, 1119–1120
perinatal complications of, 1119
risks of, 1116
Psychotherapeutic medications
clinical approach to, 1118–1119
dosages for, 1116t, 1117t
during lactation, 1119–1120
perinatal complications of, 1119
risks of, 1116–1118
as teratogens, 351t, 353
Psychotic symptoms, 1113, 1114t, 1115t
Psychotropic medications
clinical approach to, 1118–1119
dosages for, 1116t, 1117t
during lactation, 1119–1120
perinatal complications of, 1119
risks of, 1116–1118
as teratogens, 351t, 353
Psyllium, for constipation, 1052, 1052t
PTH (parathyroid hormone), in calcium metabolism, 1032
PTHrP (parathyroid hormone–related protein), 1032, 1032f, 1033f
hypercalcemia due to increased production of, 1034
as uterine relaxant, 80
PTHrPR (parathyroid hormone–related protein receptor), in skeletal growth, 297
PTU (propylthiouracil), for thyroid storm, 1003, 1003t
Pubertal development, of breast, 127f, 128
Public educational interventions, for preterm birth prevention, 572
Public policies, for preterm birth prevention, 572
PUBS (percutaneous umbilical blood sampling). *See* Cordocentesis.
PUD (peptic ulcer disease), 1045–1046, 1045f
Pudendal block, for labor and delivery, 716
Puerperal endometritis, 760–761
breastfeeding with, 136t
Chlamydia trachomatis and, 747
Puerperal fever, 760–761
PUFA (polyunsaturated fatty acids), for preterm birth prevention, 569, 570t
Pulmonary arterial hypertension
congenital diaphragmatic hernia and, 441–442
hemodynamics of, 1171
Pulmonary arteriography, for pulmonary embolus, 860–861, 862
Pulmonary artery, fetal echocardiography of, 309, 309f, 314–315, 314f
Pulmonary artery catheter (PAC), 1168
complications of, 1169–1170, 1169t
hemodynamic variables measured by, 1170, 1170t, 1171t
indications for, 1169
insertion of, 1168–1169
Pulmonary atresia
with intact ventricular septum, 328, 328f
tetralogy of Fallot with, 332, 332f
Pulmonary capillary wedge pressure (PCWP)
central venous pressure and, 1170, 1170f
with hypertension, 1172
with mitral stenosis, 1171
nonpregnant, 1171t
during pregnancy, 103t, 1168, 1171t
Pulmonary complications, of prematurity, 1199t
Pulmonary edema, 1174–1175
colloid osmotic pressure abnormalities and, 1174
hydrostatic or cardiogenic, 1174–1175
in preeclampsia, 674, 1175
anesthetic considerations with, 1148
tocolytic-induced, 1175
Pulmonary embolus (PE)
clinical findings with, 858–859
diagnosis and evaluation of, 858–862, 859t, 861f
epidemiology of, 855
prevention of, 835–837, 864–865
risk factors for, 855–856, 856t
risk score for, 859, 859t
treatment of, 862–864, 862t
Pulmonary hypertension
fetal, congenital diaphragmatic hernia and, 441–442
maternal, 805
anesthesia with, 1158
hemodynamics of, 1171
in neonatal period, 1207
Pulmonary hypoplasia, 196–197, 196t, 1203–1204
with preterm premature rupture of the membranes, 601
Pulmonary stenosis
fetal
invasive fetal therapy for, 277t, 445, 446t
tetralogy of Fallot with, 324f, 331–332, 332f
maternal, 806–807, 806f, 807f
Pulmonary valve
absent, tetralogy of Fallot with, 332–333, 333f
fetal echocardiography of, 309, 314
Pulmonary valvuloplasty, fetal, 277t, 445, 446t
Pulmonary vascular resistance (PVR)
nonpregnant, 1171t
during pregnancy, 103t, 1171t
Pulmonary veins, fetal echocardiography of, 308f, 311, 312f
Pulmonary venous anomalies, 321–322, 321f
Pulmonary venous return
partial anomalous, 321–322
total anomalous, 321f, 322
Pulse oximetry, fetal, 414–415
Pump twin, 467
PUPPP (pruritic urticarial papules and plaques of pregnancy), 1125t, 1126, 1126f
Purified protein derivative (PPD), 935, 936, 936f
Purpura, thrombocytopenic
idiopathic (primary immune, autoimmune), 837–840
thrombotic, 842–843, 843t
acute renal failure due to, 908
Pustular psoriasis, 1125t, 1129–1130, 1130f
PVL (periventricular leukomalacia), 1212
chorioamnionitis and, 758–759, 758t
PVR (pulmonary vascular resistance)
nonpregnant, 1171t
during pregnancy, 103t, 1171t
Pyelectasis, in Down syndrome, 225
Pyelonephritis
acute, 754–756, 906–907
asymptomatic bacteriuria and, 751
diagnosis of, 754–755, 906
epidemiology of, 754
fetal risks from, 906
pathogenesis of, 754
prevention of, 756, 907
signs and symptoms of, 906
treatment of, 755–756, 755t, 756t, 906–907
chronic, 913
Pygopagus, 468
Pyloric stenosis, 27, 27t, 28
Pyogenic granuloma, 1124
Pyomyoma, 1138
Pyrazinamide, for tuberculosis, 937t
Pyridoxine
for HIV infection, 771
for tuberculosis, 936
Pyrimethamine, for toxoplasmosis, 783
Pyuria, 905
PZ. *See* Protein Z (PZ).

Q

Q bands, 12
q region, 12, 12f
QRNG (quinolone-resistant *Neisseria gonorrhoeae*), 745
Quad screen, for Down syndrome, 223
Quadrivalent, 17, 18f
Qualitative traits, 26
Quantitative traits, 26
Queenan curve, to monitor Rh-immunized pregnancies, 483–484, 484f
Quetiapine (Seroquel), dosage of, 1116t
Quinidine, during pregnancy, 801t
Quinolone-resistant *Neisseria gonorrhoeae* (QRNG), 745

Quintero staging system, for twin-to-twin transfusion syndrome, 436, 436t
Quinupristin/dalfopristin, for mastitis, 764
QUOROM statement, 210

R

R bands, 12
RAAS (renin-angiotensin-aldosterone system), in preeclampsia, 664–665, 664f
Racial differences
  in fetal loss, 622
  in fetal pulmonary maturity, 421
  in preeclampsia and eclampsia, 654
  in preterm birth, 551, 552f, 554, 554t, 555f, 557
Radial aplasia, 299
Radiation exposure
  teratogenicity of, 354
  for trauma patients, 1186, 1186t
Radiation therapy
  for breast cancer, 893–894
  for cervical cancer, 888, 889, 890
  for Hodgkin lymphoma, 898–899
  for non-Hodgkin lymphoma, 898–899
  during pregnancy, 890
Radical trachelectomy, for cervical cancer, 889
Radioactive compounds, while breastfeeding, 139t, 140
Radiographic imaging, during pregnancy, 889–890, 890t
Radioiodine
  goiter due to, 1007
  and gonadal function, 1001
RADIUS (Routine Antenatal Diagnostic Imaging with Ultrasound) study, 236, 615
Random error, 210, 211–213, 212t, 213t
Randomized clinical trial, 208–209
Ranitidine, for peptic ulcer disease, 1046
Rapid eye movement (REM) sleep, fetal, 171, 173–174, 176, 176t
Rapid plasma reagin (RPR) test, 779
Rapid postnatal growth hypothesis, and developmental origins of health and disease, 153
RAS. *See* Renin-angiotensin system (RAS).
Rash(es), 1124–1130, 1125t
  atopic eruption of pregnancy (prurigo gestationis) as, 1125t, 1126–1127, 1127f
  autoimmune progesterone dermatitis as, 1125t, 1130
  general treatment of, 1125
  impetigo herpetiformis as, 1125t, 1129–1130, 1130f
  pemphigoid gestationis (herpes gestationis) as, 1125t, 1127–1129, 1128f, 1129f
  pruritic urticarial papules and plaques of pregnancy as, 1125t, 1126, 1126f
  pruritus gravidarum as, 1125–1126, 1125t
RASTER (First- and Second-Trimester Evaluation of Risk) study, 567
RB(s) (reticulate bodies), of *Chlamydia,* 93f, 95f, 747
RBCs. *See* Red blood cell(s) (RBCs).
RdD pseudogene, 479
RDS. *See* Respiratory distress syndrome (RDS).
Recall bias, 211
Receiver operating characteristic (ROC) curves, 216–217, 216f, 221, 222f
Recessive trait, 22
Reciprocal translocation, 16–17, 18f
Recombinant factor VIIa (rFVIIa, NovoSeven), for obstetric hemorrhage, 1182, 1183t
Recombinant Human Activated Protein C Worldwide Evaluation in Severe Sepsis (PROWESS) trial, 1179
Recombinant human erythropoietin (rHuEPO), 917
Recurrence risk, 25–26, 27, 27t
Red blood cell(s) (RBCs)
  in anemia, 869
  for intrauterine transfusion, 491–492
  packed
    for abruptio placentae, 733t
    for hemorrhagic shock, 1181, 1181t
Red blood cell (RBC) count, in anemia, 870t
Red blood cell genotype determination, fetal, 262
Red blood cell mass, during pregnancy, 101
Red blood cell morphology, in abruptio placentae, 733t
Red blood cell (RBC)-saving devices, 1182
Red blood cell (RBC) volume, in anemia, 870–871, 871f
Red cell alloimmunization, 477–479. *See also* Hemolytic disease of the fetus and newborn (HDFN).
Red cell isoimmunization, 477
Reduction mammoplasty, breastfeeding after, 126, 132
REDV (reverse end-diastolic velocities)
  in middle cerebral artery, 375
  in umbilical artery, 372, 373–374, 374f
Reflex late decelerations, in fetal heart rate, 408–409, 409f
Reflux nephropathy, 913, 916t
Regional anesthesia
  for cesarean delivery, 712–713
  for placenta previa, 727–728
Regression to the mean, 26
Reinversion, of uterus, 699
Relative risk, 212
Relaxin
  for cervical ripening, 702t
  in pregnancy, 118f, 121
  as uterine relaxant, 80
REM (rapid eye movement) sleep, fetal, 171, 173–174, 176, 176t
Remicade (infliximab)
  for inflammatory bowel disease, 1049
  for rheumatic disease, 1081, 1082t
Renal agenesis, 295, 295f
Renal anomalies, and aneuploidy, 227t
Renal biopsy, 912
Renal blood flow, during pregnancy, 102, 105
Renal calculi, 913, 916t
Renal cortical necrosis, acute, 908–909
Renal dialysis
  for diabetic nephropathy, 960
  hemo-, 915–917, 916t
  peritoneal, 917–918
Renal disorder(s), 905–921
  acute fatty liver of pregnancy as, 909
  acute renal cortical necrosis as, 908–909
  acute renal failure as, 907–909, 907t
  acute renal obstruction as, 909
  autosomal dominant polycystic kidney disease as, 913, 916t
  chronic kidney disease as, 910–912, 910t, 911t
  diabetic nephropathy as, 913–914, 916t
  effect of pregnancy on, 915, 916t
  factors affecting prognosis for, 915, 916t
  focal glomerular sclerosis as, 916t
  glomerulonephritis as, 912, 916t
  hemodialysis for, 915–917, 916t
  in hemolytic uremic syndrome and thrombotic thrombocytopenic purpura, 908
  HIV-associated nephropathy as, 915
Renal disorder(s) *(Continued)*
  IgA nephropathy as, 916t
  nephrotic syndrome as, 915
  due to nephrotoxic drugs, 909
  in periarteritis nodosa, 914, 916t
  peritoneal dialysis for, 917–918
  in preeclampsia, 907–908
  due to previous urinary tract surgery, 914–915, 916t
  pyelonephritis as
    acute, 906–907
    chronic, 913, 916t
  reflux nephropathy as, 913, 916t
  renal transplantation for, 918–921, 918t
  solitary kidney as, 909, 915, 916t
  in systemic lupus erythematosus, 914, 916t
  in systemic sclerosis (scleroderma), 914, 916t
  tubulointerstitial disease as, 913, 916t
  urinary tract infection as, 905–907
  urolithiasis as, 913, 916t
  in Wegener granulomatosis, 914
Renal failure
  acute, 907–909, 907t
  anemia in, 881–882
Renal function
  in preeclampsia, 657, 657t, 663–666, 664f, 665t
  during pregnancy, 105–106, 910
Renal insufficiency, anemia due to, 917
Renal obstruction, acute, 909
Renal pathology, in preeclampsia, 653, 653t, 658–660, 659f
Renal plasma flow, during pregnancy, 102, 105
Renal transplantation, 918–921, 918t
  for diabetic nephropathy, 960–961
Renal tubular function
  in preeclampsia, 664–666, 664f, 665t
  during pregnancy, 106–107, 106f
Renin
  physiology of, 1025
  during pregnancy, 1026
Renin-angiotensin system (RAS), 1025
  in fetal cardiovascular regulation, 165–167
  in fetal heart rate, 398
  in preeclampsia, 664–665, 664f
Renin-angiotensin-aldosterone system (RAAS), in preeclampsia, 664–665, 664f
Replication, 5, 5f
  errors in, 5–6, 6f
Replicative segregation, 29
Reproductive history, and preterm birth, 556–558, 557t
Reproductive tract, during pregnancy, 69
REPROTOX, 350
Rescriptor (delavirdine), for HIV infection, 772t
Research, clinical, 207–217
  importance of, 207
  on screening and diagnosis in, 214–217, 215t, 216f
  sources of error in, 210–214, 212t, 213t
  types of studies in, 207–210, 208t, 209f, 210f
Reserpine, for chronic hypertension, 678t
Residual volume, during pregnancy, 105t, 927
Respiratory acidemia, 401, 401t
Respiratory acidosis, 401
Respiratory alkalosis, 401
  during pregnancy, 104, 927
"Respiratory arrhythmia," 368f
Respiratory disease(s), 927–948
  anesthesia with, 1150–1152
  asthma as, 937–945
    breastfeeding with, 945
    classification of, 938, 938t
    diagnosis of, 938
    effects of pregnancy on, 938

Respiratory disease(s) *(Continued)*
effects on pregnancy of, 938–939, 939t
management of, 939–945
antenatal, 942–945, 943t, 944t
assessment and monitoring in, 939–940
avoiding or controlling asthma triggers in, 940
exacerbated by allergic rhinitis, 942
during labor and delivery, 943–945
patient education in, 940
pharmacologic therapy in, 940–942, 940t, 941t
overview during pregnancy of, 945
cystic fibrosis as, 946–948
pneumonia as, 929–934
aspiration, 930
bacterial, 930–932, 931f
bacteriology of, 930
epidemiology of, 929–930
with HIV infection, 933–934, 934f
viral, 932–933, 933f
restrictive, 945–946
sarcoidosis as, 945–946
tuberculosis as, 934–937
diagnosis of, 935–936, 935f, 935t
epidemiology of, 934
multidrug-resistant, 934–935
prevention of, 936, 936f
treatment of, 936–937, 937t
Respiratory distress syndrome (RDS), 419
adult (acute), 1174
with acute pyelonephritis, 755
chorioamnionitis and, 758, 759
clinical presentation of, 1204
complications of, 1204–1205
continuous positive airway pressure for, 1204
in infants of diabetic mothers, 967–968, 968f
management of, 1204, 1205
mechanical ventilation for, 1204
in neonatal period, 1203f, 1204–1205
perinatal risk factors for, 1204
prematurity and, 1201t
after preterm premature rupture of the membranes, 605
surfactant for, 202, 202f, 1204
surfactant in, 200, 201f
Respiratory factors, affecting fetal acid-base balance, 401
Respiratory failure, 1173–1175, 1173t
Respiratory gas exchange, placental, 181–187
Respiratory papillomatosis, 748–749
Respiratory problem(s), in neonatal period, 1202–1207
bronchopulmonary dysplasia as, 1205–1206, 1206f, 1206t
after cesarean delivery, 710
meconium aspiration syndrome as, 1206–1207
pulmonary hypertension as, 1207
pulmonary hypoplasia as, 1203–1204
respiratory distress syndrome as, 1204–1205
transient tachypnea of the newborn as, 1202–1203, 1203f
Respiratory rate, during pregnancy, 104
Respiratory system, during pregnancy, 104–105, 105t, 927–928
Restless legs syndrome, 1102
Restriction enzymes, 31–32, 31f
Restriction fragment length polymorphisms (RFLPs), 30, 30f, 33
Restrictive lung disease, 945–946
Retained placenta, 698
Reticulate bodies (RBs), of *Chlamydia,* 93f, 95f, 747
Reticulocyte count, in anemia, 869, 870t
Retinal changes, in preeclampsia, 657
Retinoids, as teratogens, 348, 351t, 353–354
Retinol, as teratogen, 353
Retinopathy
diabetic, 958
of prematurity, 1201t
Retrobulbar neuropathy, 1107
Retrospective cohort study, 208
Retrospective secondary analysis of prospectively collected data, 208
Retrovir (zidovudine), for HIV infection, 771, 772t, 773
Reverse dot-blot analysis, 31, 31f
Reverse end-diastolic velocities (REDV)
in middle cerebral artery, 375
in umbilical artery, 372, 373–374, 374f
Reverse transcriptase inhibitors, for HIV infection, 772t
Reverse transcription, 5
Reverse triiodothyronine (reverse T_3), 995, 996f
Reyataz (atazanavir), for HIV infection, 772t
RFLPs (restriction fragment length polymorphisms), 30, 30f, 33
rFVIIa (recombinant factor VIIa), for obstetric hemorrhage, 1182, 1183t
Rh alloimmunization. *See* Rhesus (Rh) alloimmunization.
Rh (rhesus) blood group, prenatal determination of, 262
Rh gene locus, 479, 479f
Rhabdomyoma, cardiac, 335, 335f
RhC antigen, 496
Rhc antigen, 496
RHCE gene, 479, 479f
RhD (rhesus D) antibody, 477, 478
maternal titer of, 481
RhD gene, 479, 479f
RhE antigen, 496
Rhe antigen, 496
Rhesus (Rh) alloimmunization, 477–495
due to amniocentesis, 250
clinical management of, 486–495
chemotherapeutic agents for, 494–495
in first affected pregnancy, 486–488, 487f
intrauterine transfusion for, 488–493
access site for, 488
adjunctive measures with, 491
amount of, 490, 490t
method of, 488–490, 490f
outcome of, 492–493
with severely anemic early-second-trimester fetus, 491
source of red blood cells in, 491–492
timing of, 492
intravenous immune globulin for, 493–494
nasal tolerance for, 495
oral tolerance for, 494
plasmapheresis for, 493, 494
with previously affected fetus or infant, 488, 489f
sensitization to paternal leukocyte antigens for, 495
due to cordocentesis, 386
diagnosis of, 481–483
fetal blood typing through genetics for, 481–483, 482f–484f, 482t
in vitro tests for, 481
maternal antibody determination for, 481
genetics of, 479, 479f
historical perspectives on, 477
incidence of, 478, 478f
neonatal outcomes with, 1199
due to non-RhD antibodies, 496, 497t
pathophysiology of, 478–479
Rhesus (Rh) alloimmunization *(Continued)*
prevention of, 479–481
sinusoidal fetal heart rate due to, 410–413, 412f
terminology for, 477
Rhesus (Rh) blood group, prenatal determination of, 262
Rhesus D (RhD) antibody, 477, 478
maternal titer of, 481
Rhesus immune globulin (RhIG), 478, 479–481
for idiopathic thrombocytopenic purpura, 839
Rheumatic disease(s), 1079–1086
antiphospholipid syndrome as, 1080t, 1083–1084, 1083f, 1084t
diagnosis of, 1080 1081, 1080t
epidemiology of, 1079
juvenile arthritis as, 1080t
management and prevention of, 1081, 1082t
pathogenesis of, 1079–1080
pregnancy management with, 1085–1086, 1086t
rheumatoid arthritis as, 1080t, 1084–1085
scleroderma as, 1080t, 1085
Sjögren syndrome as, 1085
spondyloarthropathy as, 1080t, 1085
systemic lupus erythematosus as, 1080t, 1081–1083
Takayasu arteritis as, 1080t, 1085
Rheumatic fever, maternal, 810
Rheumatic heart disease, maternal, 810–812, 811f
Rheumatoid arthritis, 1084–1085
diagnosis of, 1080, 1080t
epidemiology of, 1079
fertility with, 1081
labor and delivery with, 1084–1085
pathogenesis of, 1079
pregnancy loss with, 1084
RhG antigen, 496
RhIG (rhesus immune globulin), 478, 479–481
for idiopathic thrombocytopenic purpura, 839
Rhinitis, asthma exacerbated by, 942
RhoGAM, 479–480
Rhophylac, 480
rHuEPO (recombinant human erythropoietin), 917
Ribavirin, for hepatitis C virus, 1068
Ribonucleic acid (RNA), 3
messenger, 5, 5f
translation of, 5, 5f
Rifampin, for tuberculosis, 937, 937t
Right ventricle
double-outlet, 333
fetal echocardiography of, 313, 313f
Right ventricular outflow tract (RVOT), fetal echocardiography of, 309
Right-to-left shunt
anesthesia with, 1157–1158
without pulmonary hypertension, 807–808, 807f, 808f
Ring chromosome, 15, 16f
Ringer's lactate, for burns, 1187
Risk assessments, teratogenic, 350–351, 350t
Risk difference, 212
Risperidone (Risperdal), dosage of, 1116t
Ritodrine, for preterm labor, 566
Ritonavir (Norvir), for HIV infection, 772, 772t
RNA (ribonucleic acid), 3
messenger, 5, 5f
translation of, 5, 5f
Robertson, W. R. B., 17
Robertsonian translocation, 17–18, 18f, 19f
Down syndrome due to, 247, 247t
ROC (receiver operating characteristic) curves, 216–217, 216f, 221, 222f

Root lesions, 1104
Rotation, during labor and delivery, 693
  abnormalities of, 696–697
Route of administration, of teratogens, 348
Routine Antenatal Diagnostic Imaging with Ultrasound (RADIUS) study, 236, 615
Roux-en-Y procedure, 1051, 1051t
RPR (rapid plasma reagin) test, 779
RU-486 (mifepristone), 73
  for cervical ripening, 702t
Rubella, 775–776, 1100
  intrauterine growth restriction due to, 638
  in newborn period, 1219
  as teratogen, 347, 799
Rubella vaccine, 776
Rubeola, 776–777
Rupture of the membranes. *See also* Abruptio placentae.
  physiology of, 599–600
  premature. *See* Premature rupture of the membranes (PROM).
  spontaneous, 599
RVOT (right ventricular outflow tract), fetal echocardiography of, 309

S

S antigen, 498
s antigen, 498
S phase, 7, 7f
S/A ratio. *See* Surfactant/albumin (S/A) ratio.
Saccular aneurysms, intracranial, 1097–1098, 1098f
Saccular stage, of fetal lung development, 194–195, 194f, 194t, 195f
Sacrococcygeal teratoma
  hydrops fetalis due to, 509
  invasive fetal therapy for, 434t
Saddle block, for labor and delivery, 716
Salmeterol, for asthma, 940t, 941
Saltatory fetal heart rate, 413, 413f
Sample size, 213–214
Saphenous nerve palsy, 1106
SAPS (Simplified Acute Physiologic Score), 1167
Saquinavir (Invirase, Fortovase), for HIV infection, 772t
Sarcoidosis, 945–946
Sarcopenia, 177
SCA (sickle cell anemia), 878t, 879–880, 880t
Schilling test, 872
Schizoaffective disorder
  diagnostic criteria for, 1113, 1115t
  epidemiology of, 1113
  impact on pregnancy outcomes of, 1115
  treatment of
    clinical approach to, 1118, 1119
    dosage for, 1116t
    during lactation, 1119–1120
    perinatal complications of, 1119
    risks of, 1116
Schizophrenia
  diagnostic criteria for, 1113, 1114t, 1115t
  epidemiology of, 1113
  identification of, 1113
  impact on pregnancy outcomes of, 1114–1115
  treatment of
    clinical approach to, 1118, 1119
    dosage for, 1116t
    during lactation, 1119–1120
    perinatal complications of, 1119
    risks of, 1116
Schlusskoagulum, 37
Scianna antigen, 495t
Sciatic nerve palsy, 1105, 1106
Scleroderma, 1085
  diagnosis of, 1080, 1080t
  epidemiology of, 1079
  fertility with, 1081
  renal, 914, 916t, 1085
Sclerosing cholangitis, primary, 1070
Sclerotherapy, for hemorrhoids, 1053
Scottish Pregnancy Intervention (SPIN) study, 628
SCPE (Surveillance of Cerebral Palsy in Europe) Collaborative Group, 1215
Screening
  carrier, 238–246
    for cystic fibrosis, 238–240, 238t–240t, 242t
    for fragile X syndrome, 245–246, 246t
    for hemoglobinopathies, 238t, 243–245, 244t
    informed consent for, 238
    in Jewish population, 238t, 240–243, 241t, 242t
    recommendations on, 238, 238t
  for congenital heart disease, 306–310
    background of, 306–307
    technique of, 307–309, 307f–309f
    with three-dimensional imaging, 307, 309–310
  defined, 214
  preimplantation genetic, 259–261
  prenatal. *See* Prenatal screening.
  successful program for, 214
Screening tests
  assessing research on, 214–217, 215t, 216f
  defined, 214
Secundum atrial septal defect, 322
Sedatives, for labor and delivery, 715
Segregation, 22, 23f
Seizure(s)
  due to perinatal stroke, 1213, 1213f
  in preeclampsia, 671–673, 671t, 672t, 674
Seizure disorders, maternal, 1089–1092
  effect of pregnancy on, 1089–1090
  effect on fetus and neonate of, 1090–1091
  effect on pregnancy and lactation of, 1090
  epidemiology of, 1089
  general therapeutic approaches to, 1091–1092
L-selectin, in implantation, 113t
Selection bias, 211
Selective serotonin reuptake inhibitors (SSRIs)
  dosage of, 1117t
  perinatal complications of, 1119
  as teratogens, 351t, 353, 1118
Selective termination
  of acardiac twin, 434t, 468
  of anomalous fetus, 469–470
  for TRAP sequence, 439–440
  for twin-to-twin transfusion syndrome, 437, 439
Selegiline (Emsam), dosage of, 1117t
Sella turcica, 1015
Semilunar valves, fetal echocardiography of, 309, 314
Senna, for constipation, 1052t
Sense strand, 5
Sensitivity, 214, 221
Sentinel lesions, in cerebral palsy, 1216
Sentinel lymph node biopsy, for breast cancer, 892
Sepsis, 1175–1179
  due to burns, 1187–1188
  clinical manifestations of, 1176, 1177t
  definitions for, 1175–1176, 1176t
  epidemiology of, 1175
  management of, 1176–1179, 1178t
  pathophysiology of, 1176, 1177f
  severe, 1176t
Septal defects, 313–314, 322–324, 323f, 324f
Septal hypertrophy, in infants of diabetic mothers, 967
Septate uterus, 1143, 1144, 1144t
  and pregnancy loss, 622t
Septic pelvic vein thrombophlebitis, 763–764
Septic shock, 762–763, 1175–1179
  clinical manifestations of, 1176, 1177t
  cold (late), 1176, 1177t
  definitions for, 1175–1176, 1176t
  epidemiology of, 1175
  hemodynamics of, 1172–1173
  hemostatic mechanisms in, 1176, 1177f
  management of, 1176–1179, 1178t
  pathophysiology of, 1176, 1177f
  secondary (irreversible), 1176, 1177t
  warm (early), 1176, 1177t
Septostomy, for twin-to-twin transfusion syndrome, 437, 465
Sequential testing, for Down syndrome, 232
Serial reduction amniocentesis, for twin-to-twin transfusion syndrome, 465–466
Seroquel (quetiapine), dosage of, 1116t
Serotonin-norepinephrine reuptake inhibitors (SNRIs), dosage of, 1117t
Sertoli-Leydig cell tumors, 886, 1032
Sertraline (Zoloft), dosage of, 1117t
Serum screening
  for adnexal masses, 1140–1141
  first-trimester, 229–230, 230t
    with twins, 257, 459
  second-trimester, 223–224, 224t, 226
    with twins, 256–257, 257t, 458–459
"7-3" rule, for fluid resuscitation, 763
Sex chromosomes, 7, 19
  abnormalities of, 19–20, 20t
Sex cord–stromal tumors, 886
Sex determination, prenatal, 262
Sex differences
  in fetal pulmonary maturity, 421
  in meiosis, 9–10, 10f, 11f
Sex-linked inheritance, 24–25, 25f
Sexual intercourse, for cervical ripening, 702t
Sexually transmitted infections
  in neonatal period, 1219–1220
  and preterm birth, 556
SGA infant. *See* Small-for-gestational-age (SGA) infant.
Shake test, 420
Sheehan syndrome, 1022–1023, 1096
Shingles, 783–784
Shirodkar cerclage, 590, 590f, 593
Shock, 1175–1184
  hemorrhagic, 1179–1184
    clinical staging of, 1180, 1180t
    incidence and etiology of, 1179–1180
    management of, 1180–1184
      additional supportive measures in, 1182
      hemostasis in, 1182–1184, 1183t, 1184f
      volume replacement in, 1180–1182, 1180t–1182t
  septic, 762–763, 1175–1179
    clinical manifestations of, 1176, 1177t
    cold (late), 1176, 1177t
    definitions for, 1175–1176, 1176t
    epidemiology of, 1175
    hemodynamics of, 1172–1173
    hemostatic mechanisms in, 1176, 1177f
    management of, 1176–1179, 1178t
    pathophysiology of, 1176, 1177f
    secondary (irreversible), 1176, 1177t
    warm (early), 1176, 1177t
Short arm, 12, 12f
Short tandem repeats, 33

Shoulder dystocia, 697–698
diabetes and, 966–967, 966f, 984
umbilical cord acid-base balance with, 405
Shoulder presentation, 706
Sickle cell anemia (SCA), 878t, 879–880, 880t
Sickle cell disease, carrier screening for, 238t, 243
Sickle cell trait, 878–879, 878t
Sickle cell–hemoglobin C disease, 878t, 880–881
Sickle thalassemias, carrier screening for, 243
"Significance," 212
Silent mutations, 5f
Silent substitutions, 6
Simethicone, for GERD, 1044t
Simple diffusion, 50
Simple sequence repeat length polymorphisms (SSLPs), 31, 32, 33
Simple sequence repeats, 33
Simplified Acute Physiologic Score (SAPS), 1167
Simpson, James, 715
Sinequan (doxepin), dosage of, 1117t
Single gene disorders, noninvasive diagnosis of, 262
Single nucleotide polymorphisms (SNPs), 3, 31, 32, 33
Single-gene traits, 22
Singulair (montelukast), for asthma, 940t, 942
Sinus bradycardia, in fetus, 338
Sinus rhythm, fetal, 336, 337f
Sinus venosus atrial septal defects, 321, 322
Sinusitis, asthma exacerbated by, 942
Sinusoidal fetal heart rate, 410–413, 412f
Sirenomelia, 60
SIRS (systemic inflammatory response syndrome), 1175
Sister chromatids, 7, 7f
Sjögren syndrome, 1085
Skeletal anomalies, 297–299, 298t
Skeletal dysplasia, 297–299, 298t
Skeletal growth, 297
Skin biopsy, fetal, 259
Skin changes, induced by pregnancy, 1123–1124
Skin disorder(s), 1124–1132
affected by pregnancy, 1130–1132, 1131t
acne as, 1131
atopic dermatitis as, 1131
erythema nodosum as, 1131
Fox-Fordyce disease as, 1132
genodermatoses as, 1132
psoriasis as, 1132
with prematurity, 1199t
specific to pregnancy, 1124–1130, 1125t
atopic eruption of pregnancy (prurigo gestationis) as, 1125t, 1126–1127, 1127f
autoimmune progesterone dermatitis as, 1125t, 1130
general treatment of, 1125
impetigo herpetiformis as, 1125t, 1129–1130, 1130f
pemphigoid gestationis (herpes gestationis) as, 1125t, 1127–1129, 1128f, 1129f
pruritic urticarial papules and plaques of pregnancy as, 1125t, 1126, 1126f
pruritus gravidarum as, 1125–1126, 1125t
Skin edema, due to nonimmune hydrops, 507, 507f
Skin tags, 1124
SLE. *See* Systemic lupus erythematosus (SLE).
Sleep state activity, fetal, 171–174
animal studies of, 171–172, 172f
and brain development, 176, 176t
developmental changes in, 173–174, 173t
effect of hypoxia and intrauterine growth restriction on, 174, 174f
human studies of, 172–173, 173f
Sleep-wake cycle, in fetus, 364–364, 364f
Small bowel obstruction, 292, 292f
Small bowel wireless capsule endoscopy, 1053
Small intestine, in pregnancy, 1041
Small-for-gestational-age (SGA) infant
antidepressants and, 1118
and cerebral palsy, 1215
defined, 635
inadequate weight gain and, 145
maternal obesity and, 144
with post-term pregnancy, 614
Smellie, William, 713
Smith-Lemli-Opitz syndrome, 224
Smoke inhalation injury, 1187
Smoking. *See* Cigarette smoking.
Smoking cessation, for preterm labor prevention, 568, 572
SNPs (single nucleotide polymorphisms), 3, 31, 32, 33
SNRIs (serotonin-norepinephrine reuptake inhibitors), dosage of, 1117t
Social and illicit drugs, as teratogens, 351t, 354–356, 354f–356f
Socioeconomic status
and preeclampsia and eclampsia, 654
and preterm birth, 554
Sodium dicloxacillin, for mastitis, 764
Sodium excretion, during pregnancy, 106
Sodium ferric gluconate, for iron deficiency anemia, 873, 874
Sodium nitroprusside
for preeclampsia, 673t, 675
during pregnancy, 801t
Sodium restriction, for preeclampsia, 675
Sodium retention, in preeclampsia, 665–666, 665t
Soft fibromas, 1124
Solenoids, 7
Somatic support, 1189–1190, 1189t
Somatomedin-C
in acromegaly, 1020
during pregnancy, 1016
Somatostatin, in neurohormonal control, 1015
Somatostatin analogues, for acromegaly, 1021
Sorbitol, for constipation, 1052, 1052t
Sore nipples, 134
Sotalol, during pregnancy, 801t
Source control, for septic shock, 1170
Southampton Women's Survey, 153
Southern blotting, 30, 31–32, 31f
SP-A (surfactant protein A), 198, 199f
Spastic diplegia, 1212
SP-B (surfactant protein B), 198, 199f
SP-C (surfactant protein C), 198, 199f
SP-D (surfactant protein D), 198, 199f
Species specificity, of teratogens, 348
Specificity, 214, 221
Spectinomycin, for gonorrhea, 745, 745t
Spectral Doppler evaluation, of fetal arrhythmias, 336, 337f
Spectral karyotyping, 13–14, 14f
Spectrum of outcomes, of teratogenic exposure, 348–349
Spermatid, 10f
Spermatocytes, 9, 10f
Spermatogenesis, 9, 10f
Spermatogonia, 9, 10f
Spermatozoa, 10f
Spherocytosis, hereditary, 874
Spider angioma, 1123
SPIN (Scottish Pregnancy Intervention) study, 628
Spina bifida, 281–282, 283f
Spinal abnormalities, anesthesia with, 1160–1161
Spinal anesthesia
for cesarean delivery, 712
for labor and delivery, 716
Spinal arteriovenous fistulas, 1099
Spinal cord injury, 1103–1104
anesthesia with, 1149–1150
Spinal muscular atrophy, 5
prenatal diagnosis of, 248t
Spinal root lesions, 1104
Spinal surgery, anesthesia with previous, 1160–1161
Spinal vascular anomalies, 1099
Spiral arteries, in preeclampsia, 660, 660f, 661
Spiral artery vasculopathy, preterm labor due to, 527, 529f
Splenectomy, for idiopathic thrombocytopenic purpura, 838–839
Splenic artery aneurysm, 1071
Splenic perimeter, in Rh-immunized pregnancy, 485
Splicing, 5, 5f
Spondylitis, ankylosing, 1085
Spondyloarthropathy, 1085
diagnosis of, 1080, 1080t
epidemiology of, 1079
fertility with, 1081
pathogenesis of, 1079
Spontaneous abortion
chromosomal abnormalities in, 21, 21t, 22, 22t
and first-semester screening, 231–232
with uterine anomalies, 1144t
uterine myomas and, 1136, 1138
Spontaneous rupture of the membranes (SROM), 599
SSLPs (simple sequence repeat length polymorphisms), 31, 32, 33
SSRIs (selective serotonin reuptake inhibitors)
dosage of, 1117t
perinatal complications of, 1119
as teratogens, 351t, 353, 1118
ST analysis (STAN), of fetal electrocardiography, 415
Stab wounds, 1186
Staphylococcus aureus
breastfeeding with, 137t
pneumonia due to, 930
Staphylococcus infection, breastfeeding with, 135
Stations, of labor and delivery, 696t
Status epilepticus, 1090
Stavudine (d4T, Zerit), for HIV infection, 772t
Steroids. *See* Corticosteroid(s).
Stillbirth. *See also* Pregnancy loss.
chromosome abnormalities in, 21
epidemiology of, 622–623
genetic evaluation of, 263
maternal obesity and, 144–145
with multiple gestation, 453, 454f, 461
preeclampsia and, 654
recurrent, 626
Stimulant laxatives, for constipation, 1052, 1052t
Stomach, in pregnancy, 1041
STOX1, in preeclampsia, 667
Stratified analysis, 213, 213t
Streptococcal pneumonia, 930, 931–932, 931f
Streptococcus infection, breastfeeding with, 135, 136t, 137t
Streptococcus pneumoniae, pneumonia due to, 930, 931–932, 931f
Streptococcus pyogenes. See Group B *Streptococcus* (GBS) infection.
Streptomycin
as teratogen, 351t
for tuberculosis, 937t

Stress, maternal and fetal, preterm labor and birth due to, 529, 530f, 555
Stretch, myometrial, preterm labor due to, 529–531, 531f
Stretch marks, 1124
Striae, 1124
Stripping of membranes, for cervical ripening, 702t
Stroke
  maternal, 1095–1096, 1095f–1097f
  perinatal, 1213–1214, 1213f
Stroke volume
  with multiple gestation, 455
  during pregnancy, 102, 102f
Stromelysin-3, 43
Student *t* test, 213
Study design, 207–210, 208t, 209f, 210f
Subarachnoid hemorrhage
  fetal
    due to idiopathic thrombocytopenic purpura, 839
    due to neonatal alloimmune thrombocytopenia, 840, 841–842
  maternal, 1096–1098, 1097f, 1098f
    anesthesia with, 1150
Subarterial ventricular septal defects, 324
Subcostal angle, during pregnancy, 927
Subpubic arch, in labor, 693
Substance abuse
  anesthesia with, 1161–1162
  neonatal outcomes with, 1199
  and pregnancy loss, 626–627
  and preterm birth, 554–555
  while breastfeeding, 139t, 140
Sucralfate
  for GERD, 1044t, 1045f
  for peptic ulcer disease, 1046
Sulfadiazine, for toxoplasmosis, 783
Sulfatase deficiency, 117
Sulfisoxazole, for asymptomatic bacteriuria and acute cystitis, 752t
Sulfsasalazine, for inflammatory bowel disease, 1049
Summary estimate, 209, 209f, 210f
Sun exposure, avoidance of, 1124
Superfecundation, 56
Superior sagittal sinus thrombosis, 1096f
Superior vena cava (SVC), persistent left-sided, 318–320, 319f, 320f
Supine hypotensive syndrome, 102
Supraventricular tachycardia (SVT), in fetus, 339, 339f, 407
Surfactant, 197–202
  composition of, 197–198, 197f
  metabolism of, 198–200, 199f, 201f
  physiologic effects of, 200–202, 201f
  for respiratory distress syndrome, 202, 202f, 1204
Surfactant deficiency, primary, 202
Surfactant protein A (SP-A), 198, 199f
Surfactant protein B (SP-B), 198, 199f
Surfactant protein C (SP-C), 198, 199f
Surfactant protein D (SP-D), 198, 199f
Surfactant/albumin (S/A) ratio, 420, 421f
  in diabetic pregnancy, 421
  impact of contaminants on, 422t
  from vaginal fluid specimens, 423
Surmontil (trimipramine), dosage of, 1117t
Surveillance of Cerebral Palsy in Europe (SCPE) Collaborative Group, 1215
Sustiva (efavirenz), for HIV infection, 772t
SVC (superior vena cava), persistent left-sided, 318–320, 319f, 320f
SVO_2 (mixed venous oxygen saturation), 929
SVR. *See* Systemic vascular resistance (SVR).
SVT (supraventricular tachycardia), in fetus, 339, 339f, 407
Swallowing, fetal, 49
Sweeping of membranes, for cervical ripening, 702t
Sydenham chorea, 1102
Sympathetic innervation, of fetal heart, 163–164
Sympathetic nervous system, in fetal heart rate, 397
β-Sympathomimetic drugs, for preterm labor, 566
Synaptonemal complex, 9
Syncytiotrophoblast, 41, 42f, 44
  in preeclampsia, 661
Syncytium, 42
Syndrome of painful myomas, 1138
Synthetic phase, of myometrial remodeling, 522
Syphilis, 777–782
  congenital
    case definition for, 780, 780t
    clinical manifestations of, 778–779, 1101
    diagnosis of, 780
    epidemiology of, 777–778, 778f, 779
    pregnancy outcome with, 779, 1101
    transmission of, 779, 1101, 1220
    treatment of, 782
  diagnosis of, 779–780, 780t
  epidemiology of, 777–778, 778f
  fetal loss due to, 623
  hydrops fetalis due to, 510
  Jarisch-Herxheimer reaction in, 781–782
  latent, 778, 782
  neuro-, 779–780, 781
  in newborn period, 1220
  pathogenesis of, 778
  prevention of, 782
  primary, 778, 782
  secondary, 778, 782
  tertiary, 778
  treatment of, 780–782, 781t, 1101
Systematic error, 210–211
Systematic reviews, 209–210, 209f, 210f
Systemic diseases, anemia associated with, 881–882
Systemic immune suppression, 88
Systemic inflammatory response syndrome (SIRS), 1175
Systemic lupus erythematosus (SLE), 1081–1083
  antiphospholipid antibodies and, 829, 830t
  diagnosis of, 1080, 1080t
  epidemiology of, 1079
  fertility with, 1081
  fetal complications of, 1081–1082
  flare in, 914, 1081
  maternal complications of, 1081
  neonatal outcomes with, 1198
  pathogenesis of, 1079
  renal dysfunction in, 914, 916t
Systemic sclerosis, renal dysfunction in, 914, 916t
Systemic vascular resistance (SVR)
  with hypertension, 1172
  nonpregnant, 1171t
  in preeclampsia, 1147
  during pregnancy, 103, 103t, 1153, 1171t
Systemic venous anomalies, 318–320, 319f–321f
Systolic blood pressure, during pregnancy, 102, 102f
Systolic murmurs, during pregnancy, 104

T

T bands, 12
T helper lymphocytes (T_H cells), 88, 89f
T regulatory cells (Tregs), 90
t test, 213
T_3. *See* Triiodothyronine (T_3).
T_4. *See* Thyroxine (T_4).
Tachycardia, fetal, 338–340, 339f, 340f
  baseline, 405, 406–407
  in utero treatment of, 411f
Tachypnea of the newborn, transient, 1202–1203, 1203f
Tacrolimus, for renal transplantation, 918
TAFI (thrombin-activated fibrinolytic inhibitor), in fibrinolysis, 828–829, 828f
Takayasu arteritis, 1085
  diagnosis of, 1080–1081, 1080t
  epidemiology of, 1079
Talipes, and aneuploidy, 227t
Talipes equinovarus, early amniocentesis and, 251
Tap test, 420
TAPVR (total anomalous pulmonary venous return), 321f, 322
TAR (thrombocytopenia with absent radii), 846, 847
TAT (thrombin/antithrombin) complexes, in preterm labor, 528
Tay-Sachs disease
  carrier screening for, 238t, 240–241, 241t, 242t
  prenatal diagnosis of, 248t
TBG (thyroxine-binding globulin)
  in normal thyroid physiology, 995
  during pregnancy, 996, 997f, 999, 999t
TBIIs (thyroid-binding inhibitory immunoglobulins), during pregnancy, 999
3TC (lamivudine)
  for hepatitis B virus, 1066–1067
  for HIV infection, 772t
TCAs (tricyclic antidepressants)
  dosage of, 1117t
  risks of, 1118, 1119
TDx FLM assay, 420, 421f
  impact of contaminants on, 422, 422t
  from vaginal fluid specimens, 423
TE (tracheoesophageal) fistula, 290–291, 290f
  feeding problems due to, 1209
TEE (transesophageal echocardiography), 1173
Tegretol (carbamazepine)
  dosage of, 1116t
  as teratogen, 348, 351t, 352, 1117
Telangiectasias, 1123
Telogen, 1124
Telogen effluvium, 1124
Telomere, 7, 7f
Telophase
  meiotic, 8f
  mitotic, 7f, 8
Tenofovir (Viread), for HIV infection, 772t
Tension headaches, 1092
Teratogen(s), 347–356, 351t
  androgens and norprogesterones as, 351t
  antiepileptic drugs as, 351t, 352
  antihypertensive medications as, 351t, 353
  cervical insufficiency due to, 586
  chemotherapeutic and immunosuppressive agents as, 351t, 352
  congenital cardiac defects due to, 279
  corticosteroids as, 351t, 352
  defined, 347
  diethylstilbestrol as, 351t
  dose response to, 348
  environmental agents as, 354
  genetic susceptibility to, 348
  historical perspective on, 347–348
  ionizing radiation as, 354
  penicillamine as, 351t
  psychotherapeutic medications as, 351t, 353
  retinoids as, 351t, 353–354
  risk assessments and sources of information on, 350–351, 350t

Teratogen(s) *(Continued)*
route of administration of, 348
social and illicit drugs as, 351t, 354–356, 354f–356f
species specificity of, 348
streptomycin as, 351t
tetracycline as, 351t
trimethadione as, 351t
vitamin K antagonists as, 351–352, 351t
Teratogenic exposure
defined, 347
gestational timing of, 348
sources of safety data on, 349–350
specific mechanisms leading to pathogenesis with, 349
spectrum of outcomes of, 348–349
Teratology, principles of, 348–349
Teratoma
intrapericardial, 335–336, 336f
sacrococcygeal
hydrops fetalis due to, 509
invasive fetal therapy for, 434t
Terbutaline
for asthma, 941, 943
for external version, 705
for preterm labor, 566
Terconazole, for vulvovaginal candidiasis, 740t
TERIS, 350
Term growth-restricted neonates, defined, 635
Terminal deletion, 15, 16f
Termination of pregnancy
with conjoined twins, 468
and preterm birth, 557
selective
of acardiac twin, 434t, 468
of anomalous fetus, 469–470
for TRAP sequence, 439–440
for twin-to-twin transfusion syndrome, 437, 439
thyroiditis after, 1010
Testes, fetal, 115
Testosterone, during pregnancy, 1026
Tetanus, 1100
Tetracycline, as teratogen, 351t
Tetracycline-resistant *Neisseria gonorrhoeae,* 745
Tetralogy of Fallot (TOF)
fetal, 324, 331–333
with absent pulmonary valve, 332–333, 333f
with pulmonary atresia, 332, 332f
with pulmonary stenosis, 324f, 331–332, 332f
maternal, 807–808, 807f–809f
anesthesia with, 1157–1158
TF (tissue factor)
in fibrin plug formation, 826, 827f
pregnancy effect on, 829
TFPI (tissue factor pathway inhibitor), in anticoagulant system, 828, 828f
TGA (transposition of the great arteries), 333–334, 333f, 334f
tricuspid atresia with, 327
T_H cells (T helper lymphocytes), 88, 89f
α-Thalassemia, 877
carrier screening for, 238t, 245, 878, 879f
genotypes of, 877, 877f
hematologic and clinical aspects of, 878t
hydrops fetalis due to, 510
prenatal diagnosis of, 248t
silent carrier for, 878t
β-Thalassemia, 877–878
carrier screening for, 238t, 243–245, 244t, 878, 879f
hematologic and clinical aspects of, 878t
major, 877
β-Thalassemia *(Continued)*
minor, 877–878
prenatal diagnosis of, 248t
Thalassemia syndromes, 877–878, 877f, 878t, 879f
α-Thalassemia trait, 878t
β-Thalassemia trait, 877–878
Thalidomide, as teratogen, 347
Theophylline, for asthma, 940t, 941t, 942
Therapeutic narcosis, for prolonged latent phase, 694
Thiamine
for hyperemesis gravidarum, 1043
for Korsakoff psychosis, 1107
Thiazide, for chronic hypertension, 678t
Thiazide diuretics, during pregnancy, 800
Thick filament, in myometrial contraction, 78f
Thin filament, in myometrial contraction, 78f
Thionamide, for hyperthyroidism, 1002
Thioridazine (Mellaril), dosage of, 1116t
Thiothixene (Navane), dosage of, 1116t
Third circulation, 62
Third-trimester bleeding, 725–734
due to abruptio placentae, 730f, 731–734, 733t
epidemiology of, 725
due to placenta accreta, 728–729, 728f
due to placenta previa, 725–729, 726f, 726t, 727t, 728f
due to vasa previa, 729–730, 730f
Thoms, Herbert, 132
Thomsen disease, 1109
Thoracic abnormalities, hydrops fetalis due to, 508t, 509–510
Thoracic compression syndromes, pulmonary hypoplasia due to, 196, 196t
Thoracic space-occupying lesions, invasive fetal therapy for, 434t
Thoracopagus, 468, 468f
Three-dimensional fetal cardiac imaging, 307, 309–310, 316–317, 317f–319f
Threshold traits, 26
Thrifty phenotype hypothesis, 155
Thrombasthenia, Glanzmann, 825, 844t–846t, 847
Thrombin
in anticoagulant system, 828, 828f
in preterm labor, 528, 529, 529f
Thrombin time, in abruptio placentae, 733t
Thrombin-activated fibrinolytic inhibitor (TAFI), in fibrinolysis, 828–829, 828f
Thrombin/antithrombin (TAT) complexes, in preterm labor, 528
Thrombin-thrombomodulin complex, in fibrinolysis, 828f, 829
Thrombocytopenia
drug-induced, 843
heparin-induced, 863–864
incidental (essential, gestational), 838
neonatal alloimmune, 840–842, 840t
Thrombocytopenia with absent radii (TAR), 846, 847
Thrombocytopenic purpura
idiopathic (primary immune, autoimmune), 837–840
thrombotic, 842–843, 843t
acute renal failure due to, 908
Thromboembolism, venous. *See* Venous thromboembolism (VTE).
Thrombolytic therapy, 864
Thrombophilia(s), 829–837
acquired, 829–831, 830t
inherited, 831–835
due to antithrombin deficiency, 831t, 834
due to factor V Leiden mutation, 831–833, 831t
Thrombophilia(s) *(Continued)*
fetal loss due to, 625–626, 625t, 626t, 628
hyperhomocysteinemia as, 833–834
due to mutations in fibrinolytic pathway genes, 835
due to other factor V mutations, 833
due to protein C deficiency, 831t, 834
due to protein S deficiency, 831t, 834–835
due to protein Z-dependent protease inhibitor and protein Z deficiency, 835
due to prothombin gene mutation, 831t, 833
and venous thromboembolism, 855–856, 856t
screening for, 835–837
Thrombophilia in Pregnancy Prophylaxis Study (TIPPS), 628
Thrombophlebitis, septic pelvic vein, 763–764
Thromboprophylaxis, with mechanical heart valves, 819–820, 820t, 864
Thrombosis, prevention of, 826–828, 828f
Thrombotic thrombocytopenic purpura (TTP), 842–843, 843t
acute renal failure due to, 908
Thyroarytenoid muscle, phasic activity of fetal, 172f
Thyroglobulin, in normal thyroid physiology, 995
Thyroid adenomas, 1008
Thyroid biopsy, 1008 1009, 1009f
Thyroid cancer, 1008–1009, 1009f
radioiodine for, 1001
Thyroid disease, 995–1011
autoimmune
miscarriage due to, 620, 1001
postpartum, 1009–1011, 1010f
fetal loss due to, 620, 1001
hyperthyroidism as, 1000
diagnosis of, 1001
differential diagnosis of, 1001–1002
fetal and neonatal, 1003–1004, 1004f
in pregnancy, 1001–1003, 1001t, 1003t
related to human chorionic gonadotropin, 1004–1005
signs and symptoms of, 1001
subclinical, 1003
thyroid storm due to, 1003, 1003t
treatment of, 1002–1003
hypothyroidism as, 1000–1001
differential diagnosis of, 1007
fetal and neonatal, 1008
iodine deficiency and, 1005–1006, 1005f
in pregnancy, 1005–1008
signs and symptoms of, 1006–1007
subclinical, 1007–1008
treatment of, 1007
intrauterine growth restriction due to, 641
iodine deficiency and goiter as, 996–997, 998f
postpartum, 1009–1011
Graves disease as, 1009
thyroiditis as, 1009–1011, 1010f
pregnancy immunology and, 998–999
thyroid nodules, malignant tumors, and nontoxic goiter as, 1008–1009, 1009f
Thyroid function
drug effects on, 1000, 1000t
laboratory evaluation of, 999–1000, 999t, 1000t
neonatal, 998
nonthyroidal illness and, 1000
placental transfer of drugs affecting, 998
Thyroid gland
anatomy of, 995
development of, 997–998

Thyroid hormone(s)
fetal, 998
in normal thyroid physiology, 995–996, 996f
placental transfer of, 998
during pregnancy, 996, 997f, 999
resistance to, 999
Thyroid hormone receptors, 995
Thyroid hypertrophy, due to iodine deficiency, 996, 998f
Thyroid nodules, 1008–1009, 1009f
Thyroid peroxidase, in normal thyroid physiology, 995
Thyroid physiology
maternal-fetal, 996–997, 997f, 998f
normal, 995–996, 996f
placental-fetal, 997–998
Thyroid storm, 1003, 1003t
Thyroid tumors, 1008–1009, 1009f
Thyroid-binding inhibitory immunoglobulins (TBIIs), during pregnancy, 999
Thyroiditis
after abortion, 1010
Hashimoto (chronic lymphocytic), 1007
postpartum, 1009–1011, 1010f
Thyroid-stimulating hormone (TSH, thyrotropin)
fetal, 998
neonatal, 998
in normal thyroid physiology, 995
during pregnancy, 999, 1016
Thyroid-stimulating immunoglobulins (TSIs), during pregnancy, 999
fetal and neonatal hyperthyroidism due to, 1003
Thyrotoxicosis
factitia, 1005
fetal, 1003
gestational transient, 1004
neonatal, 1003–1004
Thyrotropin. *See* Thyroid-stimulating hormone (TSH, thyrotropin).
Thyrotropin receptor antibodies, during pregnancy, 999
Thyrotropin-releasing hormone (TRH)
fetal, 997
for fetal lung maturation, 203–204
neonatal, 998
in neurohormonal control, 1015
in normal thyroid physiology, 995
Thyrotropin-secreting tumors, 1021
Thyroxine (T_4)
fetal, 997, 998
free
fetal, 998
neonatal, 998
in normal thyroid physiology, 995
during pregnancy, 999
for hypothyroidism, 1007, 1008
for induction of fetal pulmonary maturity, 423–424
neonatal, 998
in normal thyroid physiology, 995, 996f
placental transfer of, 998
during pregnancy, 996, 997f, 999
Thyroxine-binding globulin (TBG)
in normal thyroid physiology, 995
during pregnancy, 996, 997f, 999, 999t
Thyroxinemia, in fetus, 1005f
TIBC (total iron-binding capacity), 870, 870t, 872
Ticarcillin-clavulanic acid
for puerperal endometritis, 760
for septic shock, 763
Tidal volume
in acute respiratory distress syndrome, 1174
during pregnancy, 104, 105t, 927, 1173
TIMPs (tissue inhibitors of matrix metalloproteinases), in membrane rupture, 599
Tinel sign, 1105
Tinidazole, for trichomoniasis, 741
Tinzaparin, for venous thromboembolism, 863
Tioconazole, for vulvovaginal candidiasis, 740t
TIPPS (Thrombophilia in Pregnancy Prophylaxis Study), 628
Tipranavir (Aptivus), for HIV infection, 772t
Tissue factor (TF)
in fibrin plug formation, 826, 827f
pregnancy effect on, 829
Tissue factor pathway inhibitor (TFPI), in anticoagulant system, 828, 828f
Tissue inhibitors of matrix metalloproteinases (TIMPs), in membrane rupture, 599
Tissue-type plasminogen activator (tPA), in fibrinolysis, 828, 828f
TLRs (toll-like receptors), 91f, 92–93
in preterm labor, 526
TMP-SMX. *See* Trimethoprim-sulfamethoxazole (TMP-SMX).
TNF-α (tumor necrosis factor-α)
and insulin sensitivity, 958
in preterm labor, 526, 526f, 527
Tobacco. *See* Cigarette smoking.
Tocodynamometer, 399
Tocolytic therapy, 561–567
calcium channel blockers for, 562–563
choice of agent for, 562
clinical uses of, 566–567
contraindications to, 561
cyclooxygenase inhibitors in, 563–564
goals of, 561–562
magnesium sulfate in, 565–566
with multiple gestation, 460
nitric oxide donors in, 564–565
oxytocin antagonists in, 564
for preterm premature rupture of the membranes, 606
pulmonary edema due to, 1175
β-sympathomimetic drugs in, 566
TOF. *See* Tetralogy of Fallot (TOF).
Tofranil (imipramine), dosage of, 1117t
Tolerance
maternal-fetal, 87
maternal-placental, 87
Toll-like receptors (TLRs), 91f, 92–93
in preterm labor, 526
Total anomalous pulmonary venous return (TAPVR), 321f, 322
Total iron-binding capacity (TIBC), 870, 870t, 872
Total lung capacity, during pregnancy, 105t
Total parenteral nutrition, for hyperemesis gravidarum, 1043
Total-body irradiation, for aplastic and hypoplastic anemia, 876
Toxemia, 661. *See also* Preeclampsia.
Toxins, intrauterine growth restriction due to, 640
Toxoplasmosis, 782–783, 1100–1101
tPA (tissue-type plasminogen activator), in fibrinolysis, 828, 828f
TP-PA (*Treponema pallidum* particle agglutination) test, 779
Tracheal occlusion, in utero, for congenital diaphragmatic hernia, 288–289, 442–444
Trachelectomy, radical, for cervical cancer, 889
Tracheoesophageal (TE) fistula, 290–291, 290f
feeding problems due to, 1209
Transabdominal cervicoisthmic cerclage, 590–591, 591f
Transabdominal chorionic villus sampling, 252–253, 253f
Transabdominal ultrasound, of placenta previa, 726, 726f
Transcervical chorionic villus sampling, 252, 252f, 253
Transcription, 5, 5f
Transesophageal echocardiography (TEE), 1173
Transferrin saturation, 870t
Transforming growth factor α, in pregnancy, 118
Transforming growth factor β, in implantation, 113, 113t
Transfusion(s)
for hemorrhagic shock, 1181–1182, 1181t, 1182t
intrauterine, for Rh alloimmunization, 488–493
access site for, 488
adjunctive measures with, 491
amount of, 490, 490t
method of, 488–490, 490f
outcome of, 492–493
with severely anemic early-second-trimester fetus, 491
source of red blood cells in, 491–492
timing of, 492
Transfusion reactions, 1181–1182
Transient cerebral ischemic attacks, 1095
Transient tachypnea of the newborn (TTN), 1202–1203, 1203f
Transitional atrioventricular canal defect, 326
Translation, 5, 5f
Translocation(s), 16–18
interstitial, 17f
reciprocal, 16–17, 18f
robertsonian, 17–18, 18f, 19f
Down syndrome due to, 247, 247t
Transplacental exchange, venous equilibration model of, 183–184, 183f
Transplantation
heart, pregnancy after, 817
liver, 1072–1073
pancreatic, 1074
renal, 918–921, 918t
for diabetic nephropathy, 960–961
Transposition of the great arteries (TGA), 333–334, 333f, 334f
tricuspid atresia with, 327
Transvaginal cerclage, 590, 590f
Transvaginal ultrasound (TVUS)
of placenta previa, 726, 726f
of preterm labor, 560
Transverse lie, 706
Transverse sinus thrombosis, 1097f
Tranylcypromine (Parnate), dosage of, 1117t
TRAP (twin reversed arterial perfusion) sequence, 64–65, 65f, 66f, 467–468
invasive fetal therapy for, 439–440
Trastuzumab, for breast cancer, 894
Trauma
cervical insufficiency due to, 586–587
in pregnancy, 1184–1186, 1185f, 1186t
Traumatic mononeuropathies, 1106
Traumatic paraplegia, 1103–1104
Tregs (T regulatory cells), 90
Treponema pallidum. *See* Syphilis.
Treponema pallidum particle agglutination (TP-PA) test, 779
TRH. *See* Thyrotropin-releasing hormone (TRH).
Trial of labor, after cesarean section, 710, 711–712

Triamcinolone
for asthma, 941t
for induction of fetal pulmonary maturity, 423t
Trichomonas vaginalis, 741
breastfeeding with, 137t
and preterm birth, 556
Tricuspid atresia, 327–328, 327f
Tricuspid regurgitation
fetal echocardiography of, 313
prenatal screening for, 231
Tricuspid valve
Ebstein anomaly of, 326–327, 327f
maternal, 810, 810f
fetal echocardiography of, 308f, 313
Tricuspid valve dysplasia, 326–327, 326f, 327f
Tricyclic antidepressants (TCAs)
dosage of, 1117t
risks of, 1118, 1119
Triggers, for asthma, 940
Triglyceride(s), during pregnancy, 119
Triglyceride concentrations, and fetal obesity, 966
Triiodothyronine (T_3)
fetal, 998
free
fetal, 998
in normal thyroid physiology, 995
during pregnancy, 999
neonatal, 998
in normal thyroid physiology, 995, 996f
placental transfer of, 998
during pregnancy, 996, 997f, 999
reverse, 995, 996f
Triiodothyronine (T_3) resin uptake, during pregnancy, 999
Trimethadione, as teratogen, 351t
Trimethoprim, for urinary tract infections, 906
Trimethoprim-sulfamethoxazole (TMP-SMX)
for acute pyelonephritis, 756, 756t
for asymptomatic bacteriuria and acute cystitis, 752t, 753
for HIV infection, 771
for *Pneumocystis jiroveci* pneumonia, 933–934
Trimipramine (Surmontil), dosage of, 1117t
Trinucleotide repeats, 29–30
Triple screen, for Down syndrome, 223
Triplets, breastfeeding of, 134
Triploidy, 15
Trisomy, 15, 17, 18f
Trisomy 18, prenatal screening for, 227, 227t, 228t
Trisomy 21. *See* Down syndrome.
Trizivir (zidovudine + lamivudine + abacavir), for HIV infection, 772t
Trophoblast, 37, 41
maternal immune response to, 88–90, 89f–91f, 91–92
response to infection by, 92–93
chlamydial, 94–96, 95f
Trophoblast invasion, 619
Trophoblastic shell, 41, 42f
Trophotropism, 725–726
Tropomyosin, in myometrial contraction, 78, 78f
Troponin complex, in myometrial contraction, 78f
Truncus arteriosus, 334–335, 335f
TSH. *See* Thyroid-stimulating hormone (TSH, thyrotropin).
TSIs (thyroid-stimulating immunoglobulins), during pregnancy, 999
fetal and neonatal hyperthyroidism due to, 1003
TTN (transient tachypnea of the newborn), 1202–1203, 1203f
TTP (thrombotic thrombocytopenic purpura), 842–843, 843t
acute renal failure due to, 908
TTTS. *See* Twin-to-twin transfusion syndrome (TTTS).
Tuberculosis, 934–937
breastfeeding with, 125, 135, 137t, 937
diagnosis of, 935–936, 935f
epidemiology of, 934
extrapulmonary, 935–936
multidrug-resistant, 934–935, 937
prevention of, 936, 936f
risk factors for, 935, 935t
treatment of, 936–937, 937t
Tubulin, 7–8
Tubulointerstitial disease, 913, 916t
Tumor necrosis factor-α (TNF-α)
and insulin sensitivity, 958
in preterm labor, 526, 526f, 527
Turner syndrome, 19–20, 20t
TVUS (transvaginal ultrasound)
of placenta previa, 726, 726f
of preterm labor, 560
TWAR agent, pneumonia due to, 931
Twin(s), 55–67, 453–471
abnormalities of, 64–66, 64f–66f
acardiac, 64–65, 65f, 66f, 467–468
invasive fetal therapy for, 434t, 468
amniocentesis with, 257–258, 258t, 459
aneuploidy in, 256, 256t, 458–459, 458t
antepartum management of, 459–461
birth weight of, 454
breastfeeding of, 134
causes of, 56, 57f
cerebral palsy in, 1215
cervical length with, 457, 460
chimeras with, 66
chorionic villus sampling with, 258, 258t, 459
conjoined, 57, 60, 468–469, 468f
diagnosis of, 455
diamniotic, 57, 57f, 58
acardiac, 65f
dichorionic, 57–58, 58f, 59f
monochorionic, 58, 58f, 60–61, 61f, 62f
twin-to-twin transfusion syndrome with, 63f
dichorionic, 57, 57f–59f, 58
diagnosis of, 455–456, 456f
selective termination with, 470
disappearance of, 66
dizygotic, 55
causes of, 56
frequency of, 56
identification of, 66–67
placentation of, 57–58, 58f, 59f
Down syndrome in, 256, 256t, 257, 257t, 458–459, 458t
fetal loss with, 625
fetal pulmonary maturity in, 421, 461
fetal surveillance in, 457, 461
fetal well-being of, 457
fraternal, 55
hydrops fetalis in, 508t, 510
identical, 55
identification of zygosity in, 66–67, 67f
incidence of, 55, 453, 454t
intrapartum management of, 461–463
intrauterine demise of one, 469
intrauterine growth restriction in, 639
maternal adaptations to, 454–455
maternal complications of, 461
maternal mortality and morbidity with, 454
membranous, 64, 64f, 65f
Twin(s) *(Continued)*
monoamniotic, 57, 58, 59f, 60, 61, 466–467, 466f
monochorionic, 57, 57f, 58, 60f
acardiac, 65f
antenatal diagnosis of, 455–456, 456t
diamniotic, 58, 58f, 60–61, 61f, 62f
intrauterine demise of one fetus with, 469
invasive fetal therapy with, 436–440, 436t, 438f, 439t
monoamniotic, 60
selective termination with, 470
twin-to-twin transfusion syndrome with, 62f, 63f
monozygotic, 55
causes of, 56, 57f
frequency of, 55–56
heterokaryotic, 66
identification of, 66–67
placentation of, 57, 58, 58f
neural tube defects with, 459
nonvertex first, 462–463
perinatal mortality and morbidity with, 453–454, 454f, 461
placentation in, 57–61, 57f–60f
preeclampsia with, 460–461, 654
prenatal diagnosis with, 256–258, 256t–258t
preterm labor and birth with
interventions for, 460
pathogenesis of, 529–531, 531f, 558
rates of, 460, 546, 547f, 558, 559f, 559t
pump, 467
selective termination of anomalous fetus with, 469–470
third, 56
twin reversed arterial perfusion sequence in, 64–65, 65f, 66f, 467–468
twin-to-twin transfusion syndrome in, 61–64, 61f–63f, 463–466, 463f
types of, 55–56
ultrasonography of, 455–457, 456f, 456t
vanishing, 469
velamentous insertion of umbilical cord and vasa praevia in, 59, 60f
vertex-nonvertex, 462
vertex-vertex, 462
Twin reversed arterial perfusion (TRAP) sequence, 64–65, 65f, 66f, 467–468
invasive fetal therapy for, 439–440
Twin studies, 26
Twinning impetus, 56
Twin-peak sign, 456
Twin-to-twin transfusion syndrome (TTTS), 61–64, 463–466
background of, 463
clinical and sonographic features of, 61f–63f, 463f, 464
diagnosis of, 436, 464
etiology and pathogenesis of, 61–64, 62f, 436, 463–464
fetal loss due to, 625
hydrops fetalis due to, 510
incidence of, 436, 463
invasive fetal therapy for, 434t, 436–439, 438f, 439t
management of, 464–466
staging of, 436, 436t
Type I error, 213, 214
Type II error, 213–214

U
U antigen, 498
UDCA (ursodeoxycholic acid), for intrahepatic cholestasis of pregnancy, 1061

Ulcer(s), peptic, 1045–1046, 1045f
Ulcerative colitis, 1047–1049
clinical characteristics of, 1047–1048, 1048f, 1048t
diagnostic testing for, 1048, 1048f, 1049f
effect of pregnancy on, 1048
effect on pregnancy of, 1048
treatment of, 1048–1049, 1049t
Ultralente insulin, 977f
Ultrasound
of abruptio placentae, 732
of adnexal masses, 1140, 1140t, 1141f, 1142f
of appendicitis, 1046–1047, 1047t
of breast cancer, 892
of cervical insufficiency, 588–589, 588f
of cervix, 583–584, 584f, 585f
of deep venous thrombosis, 856–858, 858f
Doppler
application of, 378–379, 379f
fetal, 371–377
and frequency of biophysical profile scoring, 371, 372t
with intrauterine growth restriction, 644–645
of middle cerebral artery, 374–375, 375f
in Rh-immunized pregnancy, 485–488, 485f, 486f, 490
of umbilical artery, 175, 372–374, 373f, 374f, 374t
venous studies in, 375–377, 376f, 377f
maternal, 377–378, 378f, 379f
patterns of deterioration in, 378–379, 379f, 380f
dynamic, of fetal anomalies, 275–276, 276f
endoscopic, 1053
of intrauterine growth restriction, 642, 643f
to monitor Rh-immunized pregnancies, 484–486, 485f, 486f
of multiple gestation, 455–457, 456f, 456t
of neural tube defects, 235, 236f
of nonimmune hydrops, 506, 506f, 507f
of placenta accreta, 728–729, 728f
of placenta previa, 726, 726f
of preterm labor, 560
of uterine myomas, 1137, 1138f
of vasa previa, 729, 730f
Ultrasound Doppler velocimetry
application of, 378–379, 379f
fetal, 371–377
and frequency of biophysical profile scoring, 371, 372t
of middle cerebral artery, 374–375, 375f
of umbilical artery, 175, 372–374, 373f, 374f, 374t
venous studies in, 375–377, 376f, 377f
maternal, 377–378, 378f, 379f
patterns of deterioration in, 378–379, 379f, 380f
Ultrasound screening
first-trimester, 227–229, 228f, 228t, 229f, 230–231, 231f
second-trimester, 225–227, 225t–228t
value of, 236–237, 237t
Umbilical artery(ies), 40
anatomy and physiology of, 372
Doppler ultrasound velocimetry of, 175, 372–374, 373f, 374f, 374t
with intrauterine growth restriction, 644
single, and intrauterine growth restriction, 638
Umbilical artery resistance, 372, 373f, 374f
Umbilical blood flow, 188, 399
nicotine and, 355, 355f
Umbilical blood sampling, percutaneous, 259
Umbilical circulation. *See* Umbilical venous PO_2.
Umbilical cord(s)
development of, 40
fetal echocardiography of, 310, 310f
fusion of, 60
knots in, 40, 60
velamentous insertion of, 59, 60f
Umbilical cord blood, acid-base analysis of, 402–405, 403t–405t
Umbilical cord compression, fetal heart rate with, 411t
Umbilical cord occlusion, invasive fetal therapy for, 440
Umbilical vascular resistance, nicotine and, 355, 355f
Umbilical vein, 40
fetal Doppler studies of, 377, 377f
persistent, 318, 319f
Umbilical venous oxygen saturation, of fetus, 187
Umbilical venous PO_2, 182–186
developmental changes in, 185–186, 186f
with intrauterine growth restriction, 185–186, 186f
levels of, 182, 182t
uterine and, 182–185, 183f, 184f
Umbilical venous return, 159, 160f
Undernutrition
intrauterine growth restriction due to, 639–640
neonatal outcomes with, 1198
Underweight, 143–144
Unicornuate uterus, 1143, 1144t
intrauterine growth restriction due to, 641
and pregnancy loss, 622t
Uniparental disomy (UPD), 247, 254
Univariate data analysis, 213
uPA (urokinase-type plasminogen activator), in fibrinolysis, 828, 828f
UPJ (uteropelvic junction) obstruction, 296, 296f
Upper airway obstruction, neonatal, 1198t
Upper gastrointestinal endoscopy, 1053
Urate clearance, in preeclampsia, 657, 657t, 664
Urea nitrogen, during pregnancy, 910
Ureaplasma urealyticum
breastfeeding with, 136t
and bronchopulmonary dysplasia, 1205
Ureteral dilation, during pregnancy, 105
Ureteric calculi, 913, 916t
Urethral valves, posterior, 296, 297, 297f
Uric acid clearance, in preeclampsia, 657, 657t, 664
Uric acid concentration, in preeclampsia, 657
Uric acid levels, during pregnancy, 106–107
Urinary concentrating capacity, in preeclampsia, 664
Urinary disorders, hydrops fetalis due to, 508t, 512
Urinary diversion, 914
Urinary incontinence, cesarean delivery to prevent, 708, 711
Urinary tract, during pregnancy, 105–107, 106f
Urinary tract infection(s) (UTIs), 750–756, 905–907
acute pyelonephritis as, 754–756, 755t, 756t, 906–907
asymptomatic bacteriuria as, 750–753, 752t, 905–906
classification of, 750, 750t
cystitis as, 753–754
diagnosis of, 905
epidemiology of, 750
treatment of, 906
Urinary tract obstruction, lower
invasive fetal therapy for, 277t, 434t, 444–445, 445t
pathophysiology of, 444
Urinary tract reconstruction, 914–915
Urinary tract surgery, previous, 914–915, 916t
Urine, fetal output of, 47, 48–49
and intramembranous flow, 50, 51
Urine osmolality, during pregnancy, 1016, 1018f
Urokinase-type plasminogen activator (uPA), in fibrinolysis, 828, 828f
Urolithiasis, 913, 916t
Ursodeoxycholic acid (UDCA), for intrahepatic cholestasis of pregnancy, 1061
Uterine activity
detection of, 399
excessive, fetal heart rate with, 407f, 411t
Uterine activity monitoring, for prevention of preterm labor and birth, with multiple gestation, 460
Uterine agenesis, 1143, 1144t
Uterine anomalies, 1143–1144
cervical insufficiency due to, 586, 592–593
diagnosis of, 1144
epidemiology of, 1143
intrauterine growth restriction due to, 641
management of, 1144, 1144t
pathogenesis of, 1143–1144, 1144t
pregnancy loss due to, 622, 622t
and preterm birth, 557
prevention of, 1144
Uterine artery(ies)
Doppler studies of, 377, 378f
in preeclampsia, 660, 660f
Uterine artery ligation, for obstetric hemorrhage, 1183, 1184f
Uterine atony, 698, 699, 1182–1184, 1183t, 1184f
Uterine bleeding, from placental separation, 698
Uterine blood flow, during pregnancy, 69, 102
Uterine circulation, oxygen pressures in. *See* Uterine venous PO_2.
Uterine contractions, 76–82
defined, 522
in diagnosis, 70
effectiveness of, 522
fetal heart rate with, 410f, 411t
hormonal regulation of, 79–81, 79f, 80t
during labor, 522–523
measurement of, 399
mechanics of, 76–79, 78f
in pregnancy, 691
and preterm birth, 558, 560
regulation of electrical activity in, 76, 77f
Uterine factors, and preterm birth, 558–560, 559f, 560f
Uterine fibroids. *See* Uterine leiomyomas.
Uterine hypoplasia, 1143
Uterine inversion, 699–700
Uterine leiomyomas, 1135–1139
and cesarean section, 1137
classification of, 1137
degenerated, 1137, 1138f
diagnosis of, 1137, 1138f
effect of pregnancy on, 1135
effects on pregnancy of, 1135–1137, 1136t
epidemiology of, 1135
and fetal malpresentation, 1137
infected, 1138
and infertility, 1135–1136, 1138
and labor complications, 1137
management of, 1138–1139
pathogenesis of, 1135–1137, 1136t
pedunculated, 1137, 1138f
and perinatal outcome, 1137
and placenta previa, 1137
and placental abruption, 1136–1137
and postpartum hemorrhage, 1137

Uterine leiomyomas *(Continued)*
and pregnancy loss, 622, 1136, 1138
and preterm delivery, 1136, 1136t
syndrome of painful, 1138
Uterine myomas. *See* Uterine leiomyomas.
Uterine overdistention, preterm labor due to, 529–531, 531f
Uterine relaxants, 80–81, 80t
Uterine rupture
in trial of labor after cesarean delivery, 710, 712
uterine anomalies and, 1144
Uterine stimulants, 80, 80t
Uterine synechiae, and pregnancy loss, 622
Uterine venous blood, oxygen saturation of, 186–187
Uterine venous PO_2, 182–187
factors that determine, 186–187, 186f, 187f
with intrauterine growth restriction, 186–187, 186f
levels of, 182, 182t
umbilical *vs.*, 182–185, 183f, 184f
Uterine volume
with multiple gestation, 454
and preterm birth, 558
Uteropelvic junction (UPJ) obstruction, 296, 296f
Uteroplacental blood flow, intrauterine growth restriction due to deficits in, 640–641
Uteroplacental vascular disease, preterm labor due to, 527–529, 529f
Uterus
as immune privileged site, 88–90, 89f, 90f
inversion of, 699–700
oxygen transport to, 181, 182f, 182t
oxygen uptake by, 181–187, 182f
during pregnancy, 69
regulation of electrical activity within, 76, 77f
Uterus didelphys, and pregnancy loss, 622t
UTIs. *See* Urinary tract infection(s) (UTIs).

V

VACTERL association, 291
Vacuum extraction, 714–715
Vaginal birth after cesarean (VBAC), 708, 711–712
with multiple gestation, 461, 463
Vaginal bleeding. *See* Bleeding.
Vaginal fluid specimens, assessment of fetal pulmonary maturity from, 423
Vaginitis
Gardnerella vaginalis. See Bacterial vaginosis (BV).
Haemophilus vaginalis. See Bacterial vaginosis (BV).
monilial, 739–741, 740t
nonspecific. *See* Bacterial vaginosis (BV).
Vaginosis, bacterial, 741–742, 742f, 742t, 743t
and premature rupture of the membranes, 599
and preterm birth, 556, 568, 570, 741, 742, 742t
Vagus nerve, in fetal heart rate, 397
Valacyclovir (Valtrex), for genital herpes, 770
Valproic acid (Depakote)
dosage of, 1116t
as teratogen, 348, 351t, 352, 1117
Valve replacement, pregnancy after, 819–820, 820t, 864
Valvular aortic stenosis, 330, 330f
maternal, 805–806, 806f, 813, 813f
anesthesia with, 1155
Valvular heart disease
fetal
aortic stenosis as, 330, 330f
invasive fetal therapy for, 277t, 445, 446t
pulmonary stenosis as
invasive fetal therapy for, 277t, 445, 446t
tetralogy of Fallot with, 324f, 331–332, 332f
maternal, 797, 798t
anesthesia in, 1154–1156
aortic regurgitation as, 813–814
aortic stenosis as, 805–806, 806f, 813, 813f
anesthesia with, 1155
artificial valves for, 819–820, 820t, 864
drug-induced, 814
mitral regurgitation as, 812, 812f, 813
anesthesia with, 1155–1156
mitral stenosis as, 805, 811–812, 811f
anesthesia with, 1154–1155
mitral valve prolapse as, 812, 812f
anesthesia with, 1156
pulmonic stenosis as, 806–807, 806f, 807f
Valvuloplasty, fetal, 445, 446t
Vancomycin
for group B *Streptococcus* infection, 768
for mastitis, 764
for pelvic abscess, 762
Vanillylmandelic acid, in pheochromocytoma, 1030
Vanishing twin, 469
Vaqta (hepatitis A vaccine), 785
Variable decelerations, in fetal heart rate, 406, 409–410, 410f, 411t
Variable expressivity, 23
Variable number tandem repeats, 33
Varicella, 783–784
Varicella pneumonia, 930, 932–933, 933f
Varicella vaccine (Varivax), 784, 933
Varicella zoster immune globulin (VZIG), 783
Varicella-zoster virus (VZV), 783–784
Varices, esophageal, 1070, 1071
VAS (vibroacoustic stimulation), 382–383
Vasa previa, 59, 60f, 729–730, 730f
Vascular anomalies, and nervous system, 1098–1099
Vascular changes
in placental site, in preeclampsia, 660–661, 660f
in pregnancy, 1123–1124
Vascular disease, maternal, intrauterine growth restriction due to, 640–641
Vascular endothelial growth factor (VEGF)
in implantation, 113t
and intramembranous flow, 51
Vascular pressures, fetal, 162, 163f
Vascular reactivity, in preeclampsia, 1147–1148
Vasculitis, 1085
Vasomotor centers, in fetal heart rate, 398
Vasopressin
deficiency in, 1024–1025
in fetal cardiovascular regulation, 165
during pregnancy, 1016, 1018f
Vasoreactivity, in preeclampsia, 1147–1148
Vasospasm, in preeclampsia, 662, 662f, 1172
VBAC (vaginal birth after cesarean), 708, 711–712
with multiple gestation, 461, 463
VDRL (Venereal Disease Research Laboratory) test, 779
Vecuronium, for intrauterine transfusion, 491
Vegetables, in diet, 147
Vegetarian diet, 146t, 147–148
VEGF (vascular endothelial growth factor)
in implantation, 113t
and intramembranous flow, 51
Velamentous insertion, 40
Venereal Disease Research Laboratory (VDRL) test, 779
Venlafaxine (Effexor), dosage of, 1117t
Venous anomalies
pulmonary, 321–322, 321f
systemic, 318–320, 319f–321f
Venous circulation, fetal, with intrauterine growth restriction, 644–645
Venous compliance, during pregnancy, 103
Venous Doppler studies, fetal, 375–377, 376f, 377f
Venous drainage, fetal echocardiography of, 311–312, 312f
Venous equilibration model, of transplacental exchange, 183–184, 183f
Venous occlusive disease, intracranial, 1096, 1096f, 1097f
Venous return, fetal, 159–160, 160f, 161f
Venous thromboembolism (VTE), 855–865
diagnosis and evaluation of, 856–862
for acute pulmonary embolus, 858–862, 859t, 861f
for deep venous thrombosis, 856–858, 856t, 858f
epidemiology of, 855
pregnancy and risk of, 829
prevention of, 835–837, 864–865
risk factors for, 855–856, 856t
due to thrombophilia. *See* Thrombophilia(s).
treatment of, 862–864, 862t
Venous thrombosis
due to central venous catheters, 1170
deep. *See* Deep venous thrombosis (DVT).
intracranial, 1096, 1096f, 1097f
Venous ultrasonography (VUS)
of deep venous thrombosis, 856–858, 858f
for pulmonary embolus, 861–862, 861f
Venous vascular bed, during pregnancy, 103
Ventilation-perfusion (V/Q) scanning, for pulmonary embolus, 859–860, 861f, 862
Ventricles, fetal echocardiography of, 313, 313f
Ventricular function, in pregnancy-induced hypertension, 1172, 1172f
Ventricular septal defect (VSD)
fetal, 313–314, 322–324, 323f, 324f
epidemiology of, 278
maternal, 802–803, 803f
anesthesia with, 1156–1157
Ventricular septum, fetal echocardiography of, 309, 313–314, 314f
Ventricular tachycardia, in fetus, 340, 340f
Ventriculomegaly, 279–280
and aneuploidy, 227t
diagnosis of, 279–280, 279f, 280f
invasive fetal therapy for, 277t, 280
prognosis for, 280
Verapamil, during pregnancy, 801t
Vernix caseosa, in amniotic fluid, 420
Vertex-breech twins, 462
Vertex-nonvertex twins, 462
Vertex-transverse twins, 462
Vertex-vertex twins, 462
Very low birth weight (VLBW)
defined, 545
incidence of, 546
and survival and morbidity with preterm birth, 550–551, 551f, 553t
Viability, 521, 1200–1202
Vibroacoustic stimulation (VAS), 382–383
Videx (didanosine), for HIV infection, 772t
Villous capillaries, 41–42
Viracept (nelfinavir), for HIV infection, 772t

Viral hepatitis, 785–786, 787t
  breastfeeding with, 135–137, 136t
Viral infections, in neonatal period, 1217–1219
Viral influenza, 784–785
Viral pneumonias, 932–933
Viramune (nevirapine), for HIV infection, 772t
Viread (tenofovir), for HIV infection, 772t
Virilization, in pregnancy, 1031–1032, 1031t
Visceroatrial situs, fetal echocardiography of, 307, 310–311, 311f
Visual complications, of prematurity, 1199t
Vital capacity, during pregnancy, 105t
Vitamin A, as teratogen, 353
Vitamin B_6
  for nausea and vomiting, 1042, 1042t
  for tuberculosis, 936
Vitamin B_{12}
  in anemia, 870, 870t
  in pregnancy, 872
Vitamin B_{12} deficiency, 1101
  megaloblastic anemia due to, 874
Vitamin C, for prevention of preeclampsia, 675
Vitamin D
  in calcium metabolism, 1032
  for hypoparathyroidism, 1035
Vitamin D_2 (1α,25-dihydroxycholecalciferol), 1032
Vitamin D_3 (25-hydroxycholecalciferol), 1032
Vitamin deficiencies, after bariatric surgery, 1051, 1051t
Vitamin E, for prevention of preeclampsia, 675
Vitamin K antagonists, as teratogens, 348, 351–352, 351t
Vitamin K_1, with anticonvulsants, 1091
Vitamin supplementation, during pregnancy, 146, 146t
Vitelline vessels, 40
Vivactil (protriptyline), dosage of, 1117t
VLBW (very low birth weight)
  defined, 545
  incidence of, 546
  and survival and morbidity with preterm birth, 550–551, 551f, 553t
VO_2. *See* Oxygen consumption (VO_2).
Volume depletion, intravascular, in preeclampsia, 1147
Volume expansion, during pregnancy, 101, 107
Volume homeostasis, during pregnancy, 107
Volume regulation, during pregnancy, 1016, 1018f
Volume replacement, for hemorrhagic shock, 1180–1182, 1180t–1182t
Volume resuscitation, for septic shock, 1176
Vomiting, 1041–1042, 1042t
  nutrition with, 148
von Willebrand disease (vWD), 843–845, 844t–846t
von Willebrand factor (vWF)
  deficiency in, 843
  in platelet plug formation, 825
V/Q (ventilation-perfusion) scanning, for pulmonary embolus, 859–860, 861f, 862
VSD (ventricular septal defect)
  fetal, 313–314, 322–324, 323f, 324f
    epidemiology of, 278
  maternal, 802–803, 803f
    anesthesia with, 1156–1157
VTE. *See* Venous thromboembolism (VTE).
Vulvovaginal candidiasis (VVC), 739–741, 740t
VUS (venous ultrasonography)
  of deep venous thrombosis, 856–858, 858f
  for pulmonary embolus, 861–862, 861f
vWD (von Willebrand disease), 843–845, 844t–846t
vWF (von Willebrand factor)
  deficiency in, 843
  in platelet plug formation, 825
VZIG (varicella zoster immune globulin), 783
VZV (varicella-zoster virus), 783–784

W

Wakefulness, fetal, 171–174
  animal studies of, 171–172, 172f
  developmental changes in, 173–174, 173t
  effect of hypoxia and intrauterine growth restriction on, 174, 174f
  human studies of, 172–173, 173f
Warfarin (Coumadin)
  during pregnancy, 801t
  with prosthetic heart valves, 819–820, 820t, 864
  for rheumatic disease, 1082t
  as teratogen, 351–352, 351t
Warfarin embryopathy syndrome, 800
Warts, genital, 748, 749, 750
Water channels, 51
Wegener granulomatosis, renal dysfunction in, 914
Weight gain, during pregnancy, 143, 145–146, 145t, 146t
  inadequate, intrauterine growth restriction due to, 639
  with multiple gestation, 455
Wellbutrin (bupropion), dosage of, 1117t
Wernicke encephalopathy, 1107
West Nile virus (WNV), breastfeeding with, 135
Wet lungs, 1202–1203, 1203f
WGAS (whole-genome association studies), 26
White classification, of diabetes in pregnancy, 954, 954t
White, Priscilla, 953
Whole blood, for hemorrhagic shock, 1181
Whole blood clotting time, in abruptio placentae, 733t
Whole-genome association studies (WGAS), 26
Williams syndrome, 13f
Wilson disease, 1070, 1102
Window of receptivity, 37
WinRHO-SDF, 480
Wireless capsule endoscopy, 1053
Wiskott-Aldrich syndrome, 846, 846t
WNV (West Nile virus), breastfeeding with, 135
Woods maneuver, for shoulder dystocia, 697
Work, and preterm birth, 555
Wound hematomas, postcesarean, 709
Wound infection, 761–762
  due to burns, 1187–1188
Wurm cerclage, 593

X

X cells, 43, 43f
X chromosome, 7, 19
  aneuploidies of, 19–20, 20t
X inactivation, 19, 24
Xiphopagus, 468
XIST gene, 19
X-linked dominant inheritance, 25, 25f
X-linked inheritance, 24–25, 25f
X-linked recessive inheritance, 24–25, 25f
X-rays, during pregnancy, 889–890, 890t

Y

Y chromosome, 7, 19
Yolk sac, 38–39, 39f
Yolk sac tumors, 886

Z

Zafirlukast (Accolate), for asthma, 940t, 942
Zalcitabine (ddC, Hivid), for HIV infection, 772t
ZAM (zone of altered morphology), in decidual/membrane activation, 523
Zanamivir, for influenza, 785
Zavanelli maneuver, for shoulder dystocia, 697
Zerit (stavudine), for HIV infection, 772t
Ziagen (abacavir), for HIV infection, 772t
Zidovudine (AZT, Retrovir), for HIV infection, 771, 772t, 773
Zidovudine + lamivudine + abacavir (Trizivir), for HIV infection, 772t
Zidovudine and lamivudine (Combivir), for HIV infection, 771–772, 772t
Zinc, and intrauterine growth restriction, 639
Zinc supplementation, during pregnancy, 146t
Ziprasidone (Geodon), dosage of, 1116t
Zoloft (sertraline), dosage of, 1117t
Zona pellucida, 37
Zone of altered morphology (ZAM), in decidual/membrane activation, 523
ZPI (protein Z–dependent protease inhibitor), in anticoagulant system, 828, 828f
ZPI (protein Z-dependent protease inhibitor) deficiency, 835
Zygonema, 8f, 9
Zygosity, identification of, 66–67, 67f
Zygotene, 8f
Zyprexa (olanzapine)
  dosage of, 1116t
  risks of, 1116